PEDIATRIC GASTROINTESTINAL DISEASE

Pathophysiology, Diagnosis, Management

PEDIATRIC GASTROINTESTINAL DISEASE

Pathophysiology, Diagnosis, Management

Robert Wyllie, M.D.
Head, Section of Pediatric Gastroenterology and Nutrition
Cleveland Clinic Foundation
Cleveland, Ohio

Jeffrey S. Hyams, M.D.
Division of Pediatric Gastroenterology
Hartford Hospital
Hartford, Connecticut

W.B. SAUNDERS COMPANY
Harcourt Brace Jovanovich, Inc.
Philadelphia London Toronto Montreal Sydney Tokyo

W.B. SAUNDERS COMPANY
Harcourt Brace Jovanovich, Inc.

The Curtis Center
Independence Square West
Philadelphia, Pennsylvania 19106

Library of Congress Cataloging-in-Publication Data

Pediatric gastrointestinal disease: pathophysiology, diagnosis, management / [edited by] Robert Wyllie, Jeffrey S. Hyams.

p. cm

ISBN 0-7216-3128-2

1. Pediatric gastroenterology. I. Wyllie, R. (Robert) II. Hyams, Jeffrey S.

[DNLM: 1. Gastrointestinal Diseases—in infancy & childhood. WS 310 P37145]

RJ446.P44 1993

618.92′33—dc20

DNLM/DLC 92-11720

Pediatric Gastrointestinal Disease:
Pathophysiology, Diagnosis, Management ISBN 0-7216-3128-2

Printed in Mexico

Last digit is the print number: 9 8 7 6 5 4 3 2 1

To ***Elaine***

To ***Susan*** *and* ***Eli, Shirley*** *and* ***Ben***

Contributors

ANA ABAD-SINDEN, M.S., R.D.
Nutritionist, Pediatric Nutrition Support Service, University of Virginia Medical Center, Charlottesville, Virginia
The Practical Use of Infant Formulas

THOMAS E. ADRIAN, PH.D., M.R.C.PATH.
Professor and Head of Physiology, Creighton University School of Medicine, Omaha, Nebraska
Gastrointestinal Hormones

FREDERICK ALEXANDER, M.D., F.A.C.S.
Director, Surgical Residency Program; Staff Surgeon and Director, Section of Pediatric Surgery, Cleveland Clinic Foundation, Cleveland, Ohio
Inguinal Hernia and Hydrocele; Anterior Abdominal Wall Defects

STEVEN M. ALTSCHULER, M.D.
Assistant Professor of Pediatrics, University of Pennsylvania School of Medicine; Chief, Division of Gastroenterology and Nutrition, Children's Hospital of Philadelphia, Philadelphia, Pennsylvania
Neurology of the Gut

MARVIN E. AMENT, M.D.
Professor of Pediatrics, University of California, Los Angeles, School of Medicine; Chief, Division of Pediatric Gastroenterology and Nutrition, UCLA Medical Center, Los Angeles, California
Parenteral Nutrition in Infants and Children

JOEL M. ANDRES, M.D.
Professor and Chief, Pediatric Gastroenterology, University of Florida College of Medicine; Chief, Pediatric Gastroenterology, Shands Hospital, Gainesville, Florida
Polyps and Polyposis Syndromes

DEAN L. ANTONSON, M.D.
Associate Professor of Pediatrics, University of Nebraska School of Medicine and Creighton University Medical Center; Attending Staff, University of Nebraska Medical Center and Creighton University Medical Center; Active Staff, Children's Memorial Hospital; Consulting Staff, Methodist Hospital, St. Elizabeth's Hospital-Lincoln, Omaha Veterans Administration Hospital, Omaha, Nebraska
Anatomy and Physiology of the Small and Large Intestine

ERIC A. ARGAO, M.D.
William Cooper Procter Research Scholar, Division of Basic Science Research; Fellow, Division of Pediatric Gastroenterology and Nutrition, Children's Hospital Medical Center, Cincinnati, Ohio
Bile Acid Physiology and Alterations in the Enterohepatic Circulation

SALVATORE AURICCHIO, M.D., PH.D.
Full Professor, Department of Pediatrics; Head, First Division of Pediatrics, Second Faculty of Medicine, University of Naples, Italy
Celiac Disease

BARBARA BAETZ-GREENWALT, M.D.
Section Head, Pediatric Infectious Disease, Cleveland Clinic Foundation, Cleveland, Ohio
Intra-abdominal Infection

WILLIAM F. BALISTRERI, M.D.
Dorothy M. M. Kersten Professor of Pediatrics, University of Cincinnati College of Medicine; Director, Division of Pediatric Gastroenterology and Nutrition, Children's Hospital Medical Center, Cincinnati, Ohio
Bile Acid Physiology and Alterations in the Enterohepatic Circulation

KEITH J. BENKOV, M.D.
Assistant Professor, Mt. Sinai School of Medicine; Clinical Director, Division of Pediatric Gastroenterology, Mt. Sinai Hospital, New York, New York
Gastrointestinal Aspects of Acquired Immunodeficiency Syndrome in Children

STEVEN K. BERGSTROM, M.D.
Assistant Professor of Pediatrics, Division of Hematology/Oncology, University of Connecticut Health Center, Farmington, Connecticut
Neoplasms of the Gastrointestinal Tract

SCOTT J. BOLEY, M.D.
Professor of Surgery and Pediatrics, Albert Einstein College of Medicine; Chief of Pediatric Surgical Services, Montefiore Medical Center, Bronx, New York
Hirschsprung's Disease; Imperforate Anus

ATHOS BOUSVAROS, M.D.
Instructor of Pediatrics, Harvard Medical School; Assistant Staff, Children's Hospital Combined Program in Pediatric Gastroenterology and Nutrition, Children's Hospital, Boston, Massachusetts
Immunology and Gastrointestinal Disease

JOHN T. BOYLE, M.D.
Associate Professor of Pediatrics, Case Western Reserve University School of Medicine; Chief, Division of Gastroenterology and Nutrition, Rainbow Babies and Children's Hospital, Cleveland, Ohio
Protracted Diarrhea

CHRISTOPHER W. BROWN, M.D.
Assistant Professor of Pediatrics, Medical College of Wisconsin; Medical Director of the Feeding Team, Children's Hospital of Wisconsin, Milwaukee, Wisconsin
Gastrointestinal Motility

KENNETH H. BROWN, M.D.
Professor, Department of Nutrition; Director, Program in International Nutrition, University of California-Davis, Davis, California
Management of Acute Diarrhea

PATRICE BURKE, R.N.
Nutrition Support Nurse Clinician, Mt. Sinai Medical Center, New York, New York
Enteral Nutrition

A. WESLEY BURKS, M.D.
Associate Professor of Pediatrics, University of Arkansas for Medical Sciences; Staff, Arkansas Children's Hospital, Little Rock, Arkansas
Allergic Gastroenteropathy

WILLIAM J. BYRNE, M.D.
Associate Clinical Professor of Pediatrics, University of California, San Francisco; Director, Division of Gastroenterology/Nutrition, Children's Hospital Oakland, Oakland, California
Foreign Bodies and Bezoars

MAUREEN E. CAULFIELD, M.D.
Staff, Department of Pediatric and Adolescent Medicine, Section of Pediatric Gastroenterology and Nutrition, Cleveland Clinic Foundation, Cleveland, Ohio
Ulcerative Colitis

PETER J. CERA, Jr., M.D.
Associate, Laboratory Medicine, Geisinger Medical Center, Danville, Pennsylvania
Intestinal Biopsy

CEWIN CHAO, M.S., R.D.
Pediatric Nutrition Support Dietician, Mt. Sinai Medical Center, New York, New York
Enteral Nutrition

ANUPAMA CHAWLA, M.D.
Instructor of Pediatrics, Cornell University Medical College; Attending Physician, Division of Pediatric Gastroenterology and Nutrition, Department of Pediatrics, North Shore University Hospital, Manhasset, New York
Defects in Fat Transport

JOSEPH H. CLARK, M.D.
Associate Professor of Pediatrics, Medical College of Georgia; Director, Pediatric Gastroenterology and Nutrition, Medical College of Georgia Hospital and Clinics, Augusta, Georgia
Anatomy and Physiology of the Esophagus

MITCHELL B. COHEN, M.D.
Associate Professor of Pediatrics and Medicine, University of Cincinnati; Attending Physician, Children's Hospital Medical Center, Cincinnati, Ohio
Infectious Diarrhea

STEVEN J. CZINN, M.D.
Associate Professor, Department of Pediatrics, Case Western Reserve University School of Medicine; Attending Physician, Division of Pediatric Gastroenterology and Nutrition, Rainbow Babies and Children's Hospital, Cleveland, Ohio
Helicobacter Pylori *Gastroduodenal Disease in Infants and Children*

BEVERLY BARRETT DAHMS, M.D.
Associate Professor of Pathology and Pediatrics, Case Western Reserve University

School of Medicine; Director, Pediatric Pathology, University Hospitals of Cleveland, Cleveland, Ohio
Gastrointestinal Mucosal Biopsy

FREDRIC DAUM, M.D.
Professor of Pediatrics, Cornell University Medical College; Chief, Division of Pediatric Gastroenterology and Nutrition, North Shore University Hospital, Manhasset, New York
Defects in Fat Transport

RICHARD J. DECKELBAUM, M.D., C.M., F.R.C.P.(C)
Professor of Pediatrics, Columbia University College of Physicians and Surgeons; Director, Division of Gastroenterology and Nutrition, Babies Hospital, Columbia Presbyterian Medical Center, New York, New York
Enteric Parasites

CARLO DiLORENZO, M.D.
Visiting Assistant Professor of Pediatrics, University of California, Los Angeles School of Medicine; Assistant Professor of Pediatrics, Charles R. Drew University of Medicine and Science, Los Angeles; Staff, Division of Pediatric Gastroenterology, Harbor-UCLA Medical Center, Torrance, California
Gastrointestinal Motility; Chronic Intestinal Pseudo-obstruction

CHRISTOPHER DUGGAN, M.D.
Fellow, Combined Program in Pediatric Gastroenterology and Nutrition, Harvard Medical School; Staff, Children's Hospital and Massachusetts General Hospital, Boston, Massachusetts
Management of Acute Diarrhea

SIGMUND H. EIN, M.D., C.M., F.R.C.S.(C), F.A.C.S., F.A.A.P.
Associate Professor, Department of Surgery, University of Toronto Faculty of Medicine; Staff Surgeon, Division of General Surgery, Hospital for Sick Children; Consultant Staff, Division of Pediatrics, Women's College Hospital; Associate Staff, Department of Surgery, Mount Sinai Hospital, Toronto, Ontario, Canada
Esophageal Atresia and Tracheoesophageal Fistula

STEVEN H. ERDMAN, M.D.
Assistant Professor of Pediatrics, Steele Memorial Children's Research Center, University of Arizona College of Medicine; Staff, Pediatric Gastroenterology, University of Arizona Health Sciences Center, Tucson, Arizona
Maldigestion and Malabsorption

ARTHUR R. EULER, M.D.
Director, Zantac Clinical Development, Glaxo Pharmaceuticals, a Division of Glaxo, Inc., Research Triangle Park, North Carolina
Gastritis

JONATHAN S. EVANS, M.D.
Staff, Pediatric Gastroenterology and Nutrition, Nemours Children's Clinic, Jacksonville, Florida
Abnormalities of the Bile Ducts

MICHAEL K. FARRELL, M.D.
Associate Professor of Pediatrics, University of Cincinnati College of Medicine; Director, Nutrition Support Team, Attending Gastroenterologist, Children's Hospital Medical Center, Cincinnati, Ohio
Failure to Thrive

GEORGE D. FERRY, M.D.
Associate Professor of Clinical Pediatrics, Baylor College of Medicine; Chief, Gastroenterology Ambulatory Service, and Head, Hepatology Unit, Texas Children's Hospital, Houston, Texas
Caustic Indigestion

HUGH V. FIROR, M.D.
Professor and Chairman, Department of Surgery, University of Illinois College of Medicine-Peoria; Vice Chairman, Department of Surgery, St. Francis Medical Center; Active Staff, Children's Hospital of Illinois at St. Francis Medical Center, Peoria, Illinois
Congenital Anomalies of the Midgut

JOSEPH F. FITZGERALD, M.D.
Professor of Pediatrics, Indiana University School of Medicine; Director, Gastrointestinal/Liver Disease Section, James Whitcomb Riley Hospital for Children, Indianapolis, Indiana
Ascites

JUDAH FOLKMAN, M.D.
Julia Dyckman Andrus Professor of Pediatric Surgery, Professor of Anatomy and Cellular Biology, Harvard Medical School; Senior Associate in Surgery and Director, Surgical Research Laboratory, Children's Hospital, Boston, Massachusetts
Appendicitis

E. A. FRANKEN, Jr., M.D.
Professor and Head, Department of Radiology, University of Iowa College of Medicine; Director, Department of Radiology, University of Iowa Hospitals and Clinics, Iowa City, Iowa
Gastrointestinal Imaging

SOUHEIL GEBARA, M.D.
Head, Section of Pediatric Gastroenterology, Department of Pediatrics, Henry Ford Hospital, Detroit, Michigan
Congenital Anomalies of the Midgut

MARK A. GILGER, M.D.
Assistant Professor of Pediatrics, Baylor College of Medicine; Director, GI Procedures Suite; Attending Physician, Gastroenterology and Nutrition, Texas Children's Hospital, Houston, Texas
Cholelithiasis and Cholecystitis

WALLACE A. GLEASON, Jr., M.D.
Associate Professor of Pediatrics and Chief, Division of Gastroenterology and Nutrition, University of Texas Medical School at Houston; Director of Gastroenterology and Nutrition, Hermann Children's Hospital; Associate Pediatrician, University of Texas M. D. Anderson Cancer Center, Houston, Texas
Protein-Losing Enteropathy

REGINO P. GONZALEZ-PERALTA, M.D.
Fellow, Pediatric Gastroenterology, University of Florida College of Medicine; Staff, Pediatric Gastroenterology, Shands Hospital, Gainesville, Florida
Polyps and Polyposis Syndromes

SHERWOOD L. GORBACH, M.D.
Professor of Community Health and Medicine, Tufts University School of Medicine; Attending Physician, New England Medical Center Hospital and St. Elizabeth's Hospital, Boston, Massachusetts
Indigenous Flora

MARILYN J. GOSKE, M.D.
Section Head, Pediatric Radiology, Cleveland Clinic Children's Hospital, Cleveland Clinic Foundation, Cleveland, Ohio
Intra-abdominal Infection

GLENN R. GOURLEY, M.D.
Associate Professor, Department of Pediatrics, University of Wisconsin School of Medicine and Waisman Center on Mental Retardation and Human Development; Staff, University of Wisconsin Hospital and Clinics, Madison, Wisconsin
Jaundice

WILLIAM B. GREENOUGH III, M.D.
Professor of Medicine, School of Medicine; Professor of International Health, School of Hygiene and Public Health, The Johns Hopkins University; Attending Physician, Francis Scott Key Medical Center and The Johns Hopkins Hospital, Baltimore, Maryland
Management of Acute Diarrhea

JEFFREY K. GRIFFITHS, M.D., M.P.H., T.M.
Assistant Professor of Medicine, Tufts University School of Medicine; Director of Clinical Microbiology, St. Elizabeth's Hospital; Division of Infectious Diseases, St. Elizabeth's Hospital, and Division of Geographic Medicine and Infectious Diseases, Tufts-New England Medical Center, Boston, Massachusetts
Indigenous Flora

JAY L. GROSFELD, M.D.
Chairman and Lafayette F. Page Professor, Department of Surgery, Indiana University School of Medicine; Surgeon-in-Chief, James Whitcomb Riley Hospital for Children; Staff Surgeon, Indiana University Hospital; Staff Surgeon, Wishard Memorial Hospital, Indianapolis, Indiana
Intussusception

JOYCE D. GRYBOSKI, M.D.
Professor of Pediatrics, Yale University School of Medicine; Staff, Yale-New Haven Hospital, New Haven, Connecticut
Peptic Ulcer in Children

MOISES GUELRUD, M.D.
Professor, University of Venezuela Medical School; Chief, Division of Gastroenterology, Hospital General del Oeste, MSAS, Caracas, Venezuela
Endoscopic Retrograde Cholangiopancreatography

WILLIAM J. GUSS, Ph.D.
Clinical Pharmacy Specialist, Department of Pharmaceutical Services, UCLA Medical Center, Los Angeles, California
Parenteral Nutrition in Infants and Children

ERIC HASSALL, M.B.Ch.B., F.R.C.P.(C)
Assistant Professor, Department of Pediatrics, University of British Columbia Faculty of Medicine; Head, Division of Gastroenterology, British Columbia Children's Hospital, Vancouver, British Columbia, Canada
Portal Hypertension

EDWIN I. HATCH, Jr., M.D.
Clinical Associate Professor of Surgery, University of Washington School of Medicine; Attending Surgeon, Children's Hospital and Medical Center, Seattle, Washington
The Acute Abdomen

PATRICK J. HEALEY, M.D.
Senior Surgical Resident, Hartford Hospital, Hartford, Connecticut
Abdominal Masses

LEO A. HEITLINGER, M.D.
Assistant Professor of Pediatrics, Ohio State University School of Medicine; Staff, Section of Gastroenterology, Children's Hospital, Columbus, Ohio
Anatomy and Physiology of the Pancreas

JOHN J. HERBST, M.D.
Professor and Chief, Pediatric Gastroenterology, Lousiana State University School of Medicine-Shreveport; Staff, Lousiana State University Medical Center-Shreveport, Shreveport, Louisiana
Achalasia and Other Motor Disorders

DONALD W. HIGHT, M.D.
Director, Section of Pediatric Surgery; Clinical Associate Professor of Surgery, University of Connecticut School of Medicine, Farmington; Senior Attending Surgeon, Newington Children's Hospital, Newington, Connecticut
Abdominal Masses

A. CRAIG HILLEMEIER, M.D.
Associate Professor of Pediatrics, University of Michigan Medical School; Director, Division of Pediatric Gastroenterology, C. S. Mott Children's Hospital, Ann Arbor, Michigan
Gastrointestinal Hemorrhage

JEFFREY S. HYAMS, M.D.
Professor of Pediatrics, University of Connecticut Health Center; Director, Division of Pediatric Gastroenterology and Nutrition, Hartford Hospital, Hartford, Connecticut
Crohn's Disease

PAUL E. HYMAN, M.D.
Associate Professor of Pediatrics, University of California, Los Angeles; Chief, Division of Pediatric Gastroenterology, Harbor-UCLA Medical Center, Torrance, California
Gastrointestinal Motility; Chronic Intestinal Pseudo-obstruction

DAVID ISRAEL, M.D., F.R.C.P.(C)
Clinical Assistant Professor, University of British Columbia Faculty of Medicine; Staff Gastroenterologist, Division of Gastroenterology, British Columbia Children's Hospital, Vancouver, British Columbia, Canada
Portal Hypertension

MAUREEN M. JONAS, M.D.
Assistant Professor of Pediatrics, Harvard Medical School; Associate in Gastroenterology, Children's Hospital, Boston, Massachusetts
Bacterial Overgrowth in the Small Bowel

SIMON C. S. KAO, M.D.
Associate Professor, Department of Radiology, University of Iowa College of Medicine; Staff, Pediatric Radiology, University of Iowa Hospitals and Clinics; Iowa City, Iowa
Gastrointestinal Imaging

MARSHA H. KAY, M.D.
Staff, Section of Pediatric Gastroenterology and Nutrition, Cleveland Clinic Foundation, Cleveland, Ohio
Esophagogastroduodenoscopy, Colonoscopy, and Related Techniques

BENNY KERZNER, M.D.
Professor, Department of Pediatrics, the George Washington University School of Medicine and Health Sciences; Chairman, Department of Gastroenterology and Nutrition, Children's National Medical Center, Washington, D.C.
Breath Testing

SYLVAIN KLEINHAUS, M.D.
Professor of Surgery and Pediatrics, Albert Einstein College of Medicine; Director, Pediatric Surgery, Montefiore Medical Center (Moses Division), North Central Bronx Hospital, Bronx, New York
Hirschsprung's Disease; Imperforate Anus

RONALD E. KLEINMAN, M.D.
Associate Professor of Pediatrics, Harvard Medical School; Chief, Pediatric Gastroenterology and Nutrition, Massachusetts General Hospital, Boston, Massachusetts
Immunology and Gastrointestinal Disease

ROBERT M. KLIEGMAN, M.D.
Professor of Pediatrics, Case Western Reserve University School of Medicine; Vice Chairman and Associate Director of Pediatrics, Rainbow Babies and Children's Hospital, Cleveland, Ohio
Neonatal Necrotizing Enterocolitis

WILLIAM J. KLISH, M.D.
Professor of Pediatrics, Baylor College of Medicine; Chief, Nutrition and Gastroenterology, Texas Children's Hospital, Houston, Texas
Nutritional Assessment

SAMUEL A. KOCOSHIS, M.D.
Associate Professor of Pediatrics, University of Pittsburgh School of Medicine; Director of Gastroenterology, Children's Hospital of Pittsburgh, Pittsburgh, Pennsylvania
Other Diseases of the Small Intestine and Colon

HINDA R. KOPELMAN, M.D., F.R.C.P.(C)
Assistant Professor of Pediatrics, McGill University; Director, Division of Gastroenterology and Nutrition, Montreal Children's Hospital, Montreal, Quebec, Canada
Pancreatic Function Testing; Cystic Fibrosis

STANLEY H. KORMAN, M.B.B.S., F.R.A.C.P.
Lecturer in Pediatrics, Hebrew University–Hadassah Medical School; Staff Pediatric Gastroenterologist, Hadassah University Hospital, Mt. Scopus, Jerusalem, Israel
Enteric Parasites

ALAN M. LAKE, M.D.
Associate Professor of Pediatrics, The Johns Hopkins University School of Medicine; Staff, Division of Pediatric Gastroenterology and Nutrition, Johns Hopkins Hospital, Baltimore, Maryland
Anatomy and Physiology of the Stomach

D. WAYNE LANEY, JR., M.D.
Research Scholar, Division of Pediatric Gastroenterology and Nutrition, Children's Hospital Medical Center, Cincinnati, Ohio
Infectious Diarrhea

NEAL S. LeLEIKO, M.D., PH.D.
Associate Professor of Pediatrics, Mt. Sinai School of Medicine; Chief, Division of Pediatric Gastroenterology, Liver Diseases, and Clinical Nutrition, Mt. Sinai Medical Center, New York, New York
Enteral Nutrition

STEVEN N. LICHTMAN, M.D.
Associate Professor of Pediatrics, University of North Carolina at Chapel Hill School of Medicine; Staff, Department of Pediatric Gastroenterology, University of North Carolina Hospitals, Chapel Hill, North Carolina
Basic Aspects of Digestion and Absorption

DENNIS P. LUND, M.D.
Instructor, Department of Surgery, Harvard Medical School; Assistant in Surgery and Director of Trauma, Department of Surgery, Children's Hospital, Boston, Massachusetts
Appendicitis

MARTIN MAKSIMAK, M.D.
Clinical Assistant Professor, Jefferson Medical College of Thomas Jefferson University, Philadelphia; Director of Pediatric Gastroenterology, Geisinger Clinic, Danville, Pennsylvania
Intestinal Biopsy

JAMES F. MARKOWITZ, M.D.
Associate Professor of Pediatrics, Cornell University Medical College; Associate Director, Division of Pediatric Gastroenterology, North Shore University Hospital, Manhasset, New York
Intestinal Obstruction and Ileus

H. JUHLING McCLUNG, M.D.
Associate Professor of Pediatrics, Ohio State University College of Medicine; Staff, Section of Gastroenterology, Children's Hospital, Columbus, Ohio
Anatomy and Physiology of the Pancreas

CATHERINE F. MEWS, M.B.B.S., F.C.A.C.P.
Fellow, Gastroenterology and Nutrition, Children's Hospital of Los Angeles, Los Angeles, California
Abdominal Pain

ADAM G. MEZOFF, M.D.
Assistant Professor of Pediatrics, Wright State University School of Medicine; Staff, Children's Medical Center, Dayton, Ohio
Irritable Bowel Syndrome

WILLIAM M. MICHENER, M.D., M.S.(PED)
Senior Physician, Pediatric and Adolescent Gastroenterology, Cleveland Clinic Foundation, Cleveland, Ohio
Ulcerative Colitis

ANN MILANESE, M.D.
Assistant Professor of Pediatrics, University of Connecticut School of Medicine, Farmington; Assistant Medical Director

and Associate Director of Pediatrics, Newington Children's Hospital, Newington, Connecticut
Eating Disorders and Obesity

J. ROBERTO MORAN, M.D.
Director, Pediatric Nutrition, Gastroenterology, and Allergy, Mead Johnson Research Center, Evansville, Indiana
Vitamins and Trace Elements

KATHLEEN J. MOTIL, M.D., PH.D.
Assistant Professor of Pediatrics, Children's Nutrition Research Center, Baylor College of Medicine; Active Staff, Texas Children's Hospital and Harris County Hospital District, Houston, Texas
Development of the Gastrointestinal Tract

MARY SUSAN MOYER, M.D.
Associate Professor of Pediatrics, Yale University School of Medicine; Staff, Yale–New Haven Hospital, New Haven, Connecticut
Peptic Ulcer in Children

HILLEL NAON, M.D.
Fellow, Pediatric Gastroenterology and Nutrition, Children's Hospital of Los Angeles, Los Angeles, California
Secretory Neoplasms of the Pancreas

ALLAN D. OLSON, M.D.
Assistant Professor of Pediatrics, Division of Pediatric Gastroenterology, University of Michigan School of Medicine; Staff, C. S. Mott Children's Hospital, Ann Arbor, Michigan
Gastrointestinal Hemorrhage

SUSAN R. ORENSTEIN, M.D.
Associate Professor of Pediatrics, University of Pittsburgh School of Medicine; Staff, Pediatric Gastroenterology Division, Children's Hospital of Pittsburgh, Pittsburgh, Pennsylvania
Dysphagia and Vomiting; Gastroesophageal Reflux

DAVID PICCOLI, M.D.
Assistant Professor of Pediatrics, University of Pennsylvania School of Medicine; Director, Clinical Services, Division of Gastroenterology and Nutrition, Children's Hospital of Pennsylvania, Philadelphia, Pennsylvania
Chronic Pancreatitis

ROY PROUJANSKY, M.D.
Assistant Professor of Pediatrics, Jefferson Medical College of Thomas Jefferson University, Philadelphia, Pennsylvania; Chief, Division of Gastroenterology and Nutrition, Alfred I. duPont Institute, Wilmington, Delaware
Eosinophilic Gastroenteritis

LAURIE REYEN, R.N., M.N., C.N.S.N.
Assistant Clinical Professor, University of California, Los Angeles School of Nursing; Clinical Nurse Specialist, Nutrition Support, UCLA Medical Center, Los Angeles, California
Parenteral Nutrition in Infants and Children

ALLAN J. ROSENBERG, M.D.
Professor of Pediatrics, East Carolina University School of Medicine; Staff, Pitt County Memorial Hospital, Greenville, North Carolina
Constipation and Encopresis

THOMAS M. ROSSI, M.D.
Associate Professor of Pediatrics, Department of Pediatrics, State University of New York at Buffalo; Division Chief, Gastroenterology and Nutrition, Children's Hospital of Buffalo, Buffalo, New York
Pseudomembranous Colitis

MATHURAM SANTOSHAM, M.D., M.P.H., F.A.A.P.
Professor, Department of International Health, School of Hygiene and Public Health, and Department of Pediatrics, The Johns Hopkins University; Staff, Johns Hopkins Hospital, Baltimore, Maryland
Management of Acute Diarrhea

ROBERT SAWIN, M.D.
Assistant Professor of Surgery, University of Washington School of Medicine; Attending Surgeon, Children's Hospital and Medical Center, Seattle, Washington
The Acute Abdomen

RICHARD A. SCHREIBER, M.D., F.R.C.P.(C)
Assistant Professor, Department of Pediatrics, McGill University Faculty of Medicine; Staff, Division of Gastroenterology and Nutrition, Montreal Children's Hospital, Montreal, Quebec, Canada
Congenital Diseases of the Exocrine Pancreas

MARSHALL Z. SCHWARTZ, M.D.
Professor of Surgery and Pediatrics, George Washington University School of Medicine; Surgeon-in-Chief and Chair-

man, Department of Surgery, Children's National Medical Center, Washington, D.C.
Meckel's Diverticulum and Other Omphalomesenteric Duct Remnants

FRANK R. SINATRA, M.D.
Professor of Pediatrics, University of Southern California School of Medicine; Head, Division of Gastroenterology and Nutrition, Children's Hospital of Los Angeles and Los Angeles County/USC Medical Center, Los Angeles, California
Abdominal Pain

MICHAEL V. SIVAK, JR., M.D.
Chairman, Department of Gastroenterology, Cleveland Clinic Foundation, Cleveland, Ohio
Endoscopic Retrograde Cholangiopancreatography

IVA SMOLENS, M.D.
Resident, Department of Surgery, University of California, Davis, Medical Center, Sacramento, California
Meckel's Diverticulum and Other Omphalomesenteric Duct Remnants

RITA STEFFEN, M.D.
Staff, Section of Pediatric Gastroenterology and Nutrition, Department of Pediatric and Adolescent Medicine, Cleveland Clinic Foundation, Cleveland, Ohio
Endoscopic Retrograde Cholangiopancreatography

JAMES L. SUTPHEN, M.D., PH.D.
Associate Professor of Pediatrics, University of Virginia School of Medicine; Chief, Pediatric Gastroenterology, University of Virginia Medical Center, Charlottesville, Virginia
The Practical Use of Infant Formulas

DANIEL W. THOMAS, M.D.
Associate Professor of Pediatrics, University of Southern California School of Medicine; Attending Staff Gastroenterologist, Children's Hospital of Los Angeles and Los Angeles County/USC Medical Center, Los Angeles, California
Secretory Neoplasms of the Pancreas

WILLIAM R. TREEM, M.D.
Associate Professor of Pediatrics, University of Connecticut School of Medicine, Farmington; Associate Director, Division of Pediatric Gastroenterology and Nutrition, Hartford Hospital, Hartford, Connecticut
Short Bowel Syndrome

RICCARDO TRONCONE, M.D.
Assistant Professor, Department of Pediatrics, Second Faculty of Medicine, University of Naples, Italy
Celiac Disease

JOHN N. UDALL, JR., M.D., PH.D.
Professor of Pediatrics, Louisiana State University Medical School; Chief, Division of Pediatric Gastroenterology and Nutrition, Children's Hospital, New Orleans, Louisiana
Maldigestion and Malabsorption

MARTIN H. ULSHEN, M.D.
Associate Professor of Pediatrics, University of North Carolina at Chapel Hill School of Medicine; Chief of Pediatric Gastroenterology, University of North Carolina Hospitals, Chapel Hill, North Carolina
Basic Aspects of Digestion and Absorption

JON A. VANDERHOOF, M.D.
Professor and Chairman, Department of Pediatrics, Creighton University School of Medicine; Chief, Department of Pediatrics, Saint Joseph Hospital, Omaha, Nebraska
Diarrhea

STEVEN J. WEISMAN, M.D.
Associate Professor of Pediatrics, Division of Hematology/Oncology, University of Connecticut School of Medicine, Farmington, Connecticut
Neoplasms of the Gastrointestinal Tract

ZVI WEIZMAN, M.D.
Associate Professor of Pediatrics, Ben-Gurion University Faculty of Health Sciences; Head, Pediatric Gastroenterology and Nutrition Unit, Department of Pediatrics, Soroka Medical Center, Beer-Sheva, Israel
Acute Pancreatitis

STEVEN L. WERLIN, M.D.
Professor of Pediatrics, Medical College of Wisconsin; Director of Gastroenterology, Children's Hospital of Wisconsin, Milwaukee, Wisconsin
Gastrointestinal Motility

KAREN W. WEST, M.D.
Associate Professor, Department of Surgery, Indiana University School of Medicine; Staff Surgeon, James Whitcomb Riley Hospital for Children, Indiana University Hospital, Wishard Memorial Hospital, Indianapolis, Indiana
Intussusception

ROBERT WYLLIE, M.D.
Head, Section of Pediatric Gastroenterology and Nutrition, Cleveland Clinic Foundation, Cleveland, Ohio
Esophagogastroduodenoscopy, Colonoscopy, and Related Techniques

Preface

Pediatric gastroenterology has undergone a dramatic evolution in the past three decades, from the initial training of a few pediatricians within adult gastroenterology programs to the establishment of dedicated pediatric gastroenterology programs, national and international meetings, and subspecialty board certification. Basic and clinical research in pediatric gastroenterology have increased our scientific understanding of gastrointestinal disease processes in infants and children and have provided data to facilitate the diagnosis and treatment of a growing list of disorders. Technologic advances allow us to image the gastrointestinal and hepatobiliary systems in even the smallest infants. These developments have firmly established the identity of pediatric gastroenterology as an important discipline, and pediatric gastroenterology clinicians are available at most major medical facilities.

Although pediatric gastroenterologists are often called on to diagnose and manage complex and uncommon disorders, more often they are consulted on more common childhood complaints such as diarrhea, constipation, vomiting, and abdominal pain. These tasks put them in contact with other caretakers of children, including those in primary care roles, other pediatric subspecialists, and adult physicians called on to see children. The purpose of this book is to comprehensively review the field of clinical pediatric gastroenterology. We hope it is a useful reference for all those health care professionals faced with evaluating and treating children with gastrointestinal complaints. To accomplish this task, we have enlisted the aid of a distinguished group of pediatric subspecialists, including gastroenterologists, surgeons, radiologists, allergists, pathologists, and nutritionists. We have asked them to present a scientific basis for clinical observations to facilitate our understanding of disease pathogenesis and treatment.

The book is organized into several distinct sections that sequentially review the basic aspects of gastrointestinal function, common gastrointestinal problems, and organ-specific disorders of the esophagus, the stomach, the small and large bowel, and the pancreas. It then proceeds with a comprehensive review of diagnostic modalities, including endoscopy and biopsy, motility, breath testing, radiologic imaging, and interpretation of biopsy material. The text concludes with several chapters concerning important aspects of pediatric nutrition and nutritional support.

Although this text includes several excellent chapters on pediatric hepatobiliary disease, we have not attempted an encyclopedic review of the topic, and readers are encouraged to consult several currently available fine textbooks in hepatology. Likewise, those readers who desire a more detailed discussion of pediatric nutrition should consult any of several textbooks devoted to this subject.

Even though the production of this textbook has occasionally been associated with H_2 receptor–resistant dyspepsia, we are pleased with the product and hope that it will serve an important role in facilitating the care of children with gastrointestinal disease.

We would like to thank our chapter authors for their contributions to this text, the staff at W. B. Saunders for their help and encouragement (especially Judith Fletcher, Sue Reilly, and Bill Preston), and, most importantly, our families, who extended their support and patience as we went through the many steps involved in the book's production. We look forward to hearing the comments and suggestions of our readers.

ROBERT WYLLIE, M.D.
JEFFREY S. HYAMS, M.D.

Contents

Section One

BIOLOGIC ASPECTS OF GASTROINTESTINAL FUNCTION

Chapter 1

Development of the Gastrointestinal Tract

KATHLEEN J. MOTIL

OVERVIEW OF THE ONTOGENY OF THE GASTROINTESTINAL TRACT

The ontogeny of the gastrointestinal tract, the hepatobiliary system, and the pancreas is divided classically into six stages according to the major anatomic and physiologic events that occur from conception through maturation. These stages include (1) gametogenesis, or the formation of the egg and sperm; (2) fertilization of the gametocytes; (3) cleavage, or cellular multiplication of the organism without substantial change in size; (4) gastrulation, or the formation of the three germinal layers, the ectoderm, mesoderm, and endoderm, from which subsequent body tissues are derived; (5) organogenesis, or the formation of the basic organ structures of the body; and (6) growth and differentiation of the organism such that essential physiologic functions may be accomplished and promote survival. These last two stages of ontogeny dominate the process of development in the human infant.

The gastrointestinal tract is formed during the fourth week of gestation and appears as a small, 4-mm, hollow tube (Fig. 1–1). The epithelial tissues of the gut are derived from the endodermal layer, whereas the muscles and connective tissues are derived from the mesodermal layer of the embryo during invagination of the embryonic disc. The *foregut* comprises the esophagus, stomach, duodenum, liver, gallbladder, and pancreas; the *midgut* is composed of the jejunum, ileum, and the ascending and transverse colon; and the *hindgut* comprises the descending and rectosigmoid colon. These organs constitute the major anatomic structures of the human gastrointestinal tract.

Several major events occur during the first two trimesters of pregnancy. During the third and seventh weeks of gestation, respectively, the buccopharyngeal and cloacal membranes of the primitive gut rupture, thereby establishing continuity between the amniotic fluid and the intraluminal contents of the gut. Herniation and rotation of the gut, as well as descent of the cecum, are complete by the end of the fourth month of gestation. Elongation of the gut, the formation of identifiable organ structures, and tissue differentiation proceed until 20 to 24 weeks of gestation. By the end of the second trimester of pregnancy, the esophagus, stomach, liver, gallbladder, pancreas, small intestine, and colon are well formed and display the rudimentary structures consistent with early physiologic function. The third trimester is the period of maximal intrauterine growth and differentiation of the gastrointestinal tract.

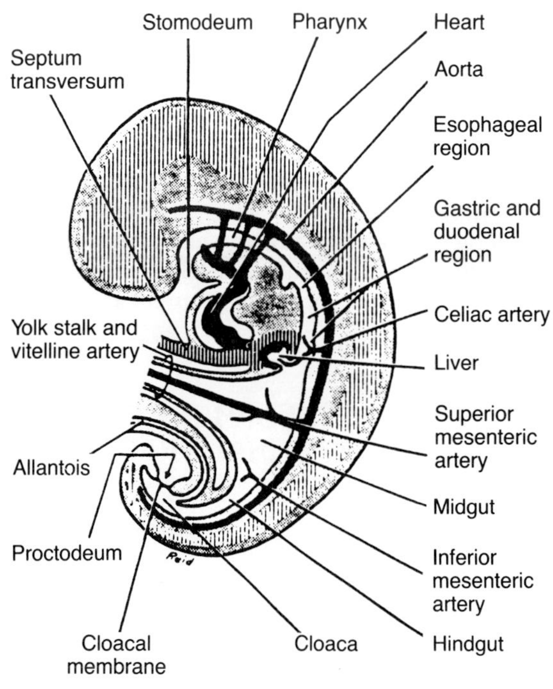

Figure 1–1. Midsagittal section of a 4-week embryo showing the early digestive system and its blood supply. (From Moore KL: The Developing Human. 4th ed. Philadelphia, WB Saunders, 1988, p 218; with permission.)

This work is a publication of the USDA/ARS Children's Nutritional Research Center, Department of Pediatrics, Baylor College of Medicine, and Texas Children's Hospital, Houston, Texas. This project has been funded in part with federal funds from the U.S. Department of Agriculture, Agricultural Research Service, under Cooperative Agreement number 58-6250-1-003. The contents of this publication do not necessarily reflect the views or policies of the U.S. Department of Agriculture, nor does mention of trade names, commercial products, or organizations imply endorsement by the U.S. government.

Many regulatory factors are involved in the ontogeny of the gastrointestinal tract.[1,2] These factors include the genetic endowment of the individual, a biologic clock that directs developmental chronology, and endogenous substances such as hormones and neurotransmitters. The development of the gastrointestinal tract can be altered by environmental factors, particularly those related to feeding. Although differences in feeding practices may appear inconsequential, it is noteworthy that the type of nourishment may influence the functional development of the gastrointestinal tract in the infant.

The three major physiologic functions of the gastrointestinal tract are (1) motility, (2) absorption and secretion, and (3) immunologic protection. The development of these functions is sustained by two primary nutrient sources: (1) amniotic fluid, during gestation, and (2) colostrum and human milk or commercially prepared formulas, after birth. Enteral nutrition is initiated at 3 weeks of gestation, when amniotic fluid circulates through the gastrointestinal tract. However, the limited volume and type of nutrients in amniotic fluid to which the gut is exposed minimize the extent of its function. The transition from amniotic fluid, in conjunction with placental blood flow, to milk as a source of nutritional support requires a coordinated functional response by the gastrointestinal tract in terms of (1) effective sucking, swallowing, gastric emptying, intestinal peristalsis, and defecation; (2) regulated salivary, gastric, pancreatic, and hepatobiliary secretions; (3) availability of intestinal brush border enzymes and transport systems; and (4) appropriate antigenic responses to foreign material within the gut. The most important feature of the human gastrointestinal tract is its ability to adapt at birth to a variety of nutrients and to use these nutrients effectively for further growth and functional development. The second most important feature of the ontogeny of the gastrointestinal tract in humans is that some aspects of these physiologic functions of the gut may not be fully developed until preschool age.

Although several good reviews of gut ontogeny are available,[3,4] information is limited about developmental gastroenterology in humans. This chapter focuses on what is known about the functional aspects of human gastrointestinal development and, when information is available, the influence of feeding on gut development and adaptation.

FUNCTIONAL DEVELOPMENT OF THE GASTROINTESTINAL TRACT IN THE INFANT

Oropharynx

Amniotic fluid circulates passively through the gastrointestinal tract at the beginning of the third week of gestation. The fetus actively swallows amniotic fluid as early as 12 weeks of gestation. The volume of fluid swallowed increases from 5 ml per day at 12 weeks to 15 ml per day at 20 weeks and 400 ml per day at term. The ingestion of amniotic fluid by the fetus is thought to regulate the volume or composition of the amniotic fluid or to exert a trophic effect on the developing gut.

Non-nutritive sucking begins at approximately 20 weeks of gestation, whereas nutritive sucking develops at approximately 34 weeks of gestation.[5,6] Both types of movements are reflex behaviors, and their development is dependent on gestational age. After birth, other factors, such as the length of time the infant has to acquire feeding experience, the flow rate, and the taste of the feeding, may influence the effectiveness of sucking and swallowing.[6]

Non-nutritive sucking is characterized by mouthing movements that occur twice as fast as those of nutritive sucking. Swallows may precede or follow these nonspecific movements and generally inhibit respiration. Premature infants may have non-nutritive sucking movements that persist throughout the first week of life.[7] Non-nutritive sucking is thought to enhance the rate of gastric emptying and weight gain in preterm infants, presumably as a result of hormonal mechanisms associated with enhanced gastrin secretion and inhibited somatostatin release.[8] Thus, the early occurrence of non-nutritive sucking in premature infants may enable earlier tolerance of oral feeding.

Nutritive sucking requires a mature sucking and swallowing pattern, particularly during periods of feeding.[9] The mature pattern is characterized by prolonged bursts of sucking; individual sucking movements occur at a rate of two per second and contain one to four swallows during each burst. This pattern is nutritionally efficient, because large volumes of milk are consumed during each sucking movement. In term infants, the mature pattern of sucking and swallowing develops within a few days of birth and indicates adequate relaxation and contraction of the upper and lower esophageal sphincters and the unidirectional propagation of esophageal contractions.[7,10]

An immature nutritive sucking and swallowing pattern may persist in premature infants longer than in term infants.[10] This immature pattern is inefficient and is characterized by shorter bursts of sucking (individual sucking movements occurring at a rate of one per second) and by the ingestion of smaller volumes of milk during each sucking movement. Regardless of an efficient or inefficient nutritive pattern, sucking, swallowing, and breathing occur in a coordinated fashion during feeding. Sucking may decrease respiratory rate, but respiratory arrests do not occur.

Nutritive sucking may be influenced by the type of feeding or the concentration of specific nutrients provided. Milk feedings appear to elicit higher sucking frequencies than do water or dextrose feedings, although sweet-tasting solutions, such as sucrose, appear to elicit a higher sucking frequency than does water alone or salty-tasting solutions.[11] The frequency of sucking also increases with increasing concentrations of carbohydrates in solution. These differences in feeding preferences presumably are related to the sensation of taste. Little information is available, however, on the ontogeny of taste in infants.

Esophagus

The esophagus can be identified at 4 weeks of gestation. The primary function of the esophagus is to propel amniotic fluid or milk feedings from the mouth to the stomach during swallowing. After birth, the esophageal sphincters prevent the reflux of gastric secretions and feedings into the esophagus, mouth, or lungs. From a functional point of view, esophageal motility requires an organized progression of peristaltic movement through the body of the esophagus and coordination of relaxation and contraction of the upper and lower esophageal sphincter.

The upper esophageal sphincter (UES) is composed of the cricopharyngeal muscle and the inferior pharyngeal constrictors. The UES is present by 32 weeks of gestation and is functional in the early newborn period.[7] In term infants the UES pressure averages 29 ± 10 cm H_2O and is 1 to 7 mm Hg higher than that of the esophageal body.[7, 12] UES pressure generally increases with the presence of acid and fluid in the esophagus and with esophageal distention. UES pressure does not increase in response to acid stimulation, however, in infants younger than 10 weeks of postnatal age.[12] The developmental significance of the UES is in the role it plays in the pathogenesis of acid reflux associated with respiratory complications, such as reactive airway disease and apnea.[12]

The developmental features that permit motility throughout the body of the esophagus include the appearance of neuroblasts and the inner circular muscle by 5 weeks of gestation, and the outer longitudinal muscle by 8 weeks of gestation. The functional activity of the esophageal body includes primary, secondary, and tertiary peristalsis. Primary peristalsis occurs with swallowing, whereas secondary peristalsis is initiated by esophageal distention unrelated to swallowing. Tertiary peristalsis refers to simultaneous or reverse contractions of the esophageal body. Tertiary waves are nonperistaltic and are considered to be pathologic. The regulation of esophageal peristalsis is mediated by the brain, the vagus nerve, and the sympathetic fibers of the submucosal and myenteric plexuses.

Esophageal peristalsis is present in the premature infant, although in the early newborn period (<12 hours of life) and in very low birth weight infants, tertiary peristaltic waves appear in response to poorly coordinated swallows.[7] Esophageal peristalsis becomes more coordinated, the rate of peristalsis slows, and tertiary contractions decrease in frequency with increasing postnatal age. Esophageal peristalsis may be influenced by the temperature of the feeding and by intra-abdominal pressure. Cold solutions inhibit and warm solutions enhance peristaltic contractions, whereas increased intra-abdominal pressure reduces the speed of peristalsis. Thus, the manner of feeding may influence the efficiency of esophageal function in the newborn infant.

The lower esophageal sphincter (LES) is the most studied component of esophageal ontogeny and comprises the longitudinal and circular muscles in continuity with those of the esophageal body. LES function is mediated by the vagus nerve and sympathetic fibers of the myenteric and submucosal plexuses. The length of the LES increases from an average of 0.6 cm at 27 weeks of gestation to 1 cm at term[13] and presumably displays asymmetry comparable to that of the adult. The basal pressure of the LES fluctuates in response to respiration, because of its intra-abdominal and intraesophageal location. Although earlier studies suggested that LES pressures are low at birth and increase with increasing postnatal age,[7] recent studies using continuously perfused catheters suggest that the LES is well developed in the early postnatal period.[13, 14] In term infants younger than 4 days of age, LES pressures average 42 ± 11 mm Hg.[14, 15] Additional studies document LES pressures of 43 ± 8 mm Hg in term infants 2 to 6 weeks of age[13] and 24 ± 2 mm Hg in term infants younger than 6 months of age. These values suggest that LES pressure falls with increasing postnatal age.

In premature infants with an average weight of 1,500 gm, LES pressures are low (5 ± 1 mm Hg) at 27 weeks of gestation and increase with increasing gestational, but not postnatal, age (23 ± 2 mm Hg at 37 weeks).[16] Despite low values, LES pressures are always higher than gastric fundal pressures by 4 ± 1 mm Hg to 18 ± 1 mm Hg at 27 weeks and 37 weeks of gestation, respectively. The functional aspects of the LES in premature infants are developmentally less mature than those in term infants.

LES pressure is regulated by neurogenic, myogenic, and hormonal factors. Tonic closure of the LES is thought to be intrinsic to its smooth muscle. Gastrin also has been suggested as a mediator of basal LES tone, particularly in newborn infants, because of their elevated serum gastrin levels at birth.[15] No correlation is apparent, however, between serum gastrin levels and basal LES pressures. There does not appear to be an adrenergic influence on tonic LES pressure even though alpha- and beta-blockers alter LES pressures. The vagus nerve mediates the LES response to stimulation through cholinergic innervation but does not alter basal tone. In children, cholinergic agonists, such as bethanecol, increase basal LES pressure by 32 ± 6 mm Hg for approximately a half hour.[13] Other substances increase basal LES pressures, including metoclopramide, cisapride, and protein meals, whereas anticholinergics, dopamine, caffeine, theophylline, morphine, diazepam, fatty meals, vasoactive intestinal polypeptide (VIP), gastrointestinal inhibitory polypeptide (GIP), and cholecystokinin (CCK) decrease basal LES pressures. From a functional viewpoint, dietary factors that influence LES pressure may be important to consider when high-calorie feedings are administered to the infant, particularly when gastroesophageal reflux or apnea is present.

Stomach

The stomach can be identified as a dilatation of the gut by 4 weeks of gestation. As the stomach matures, the dorsal border, which becomes the greater curvature, grows faster than the ventral border, or lesser curvature.

Between 5 and 7 weeks of gestation, the stomach rotates 90 degrees in a clockwise direction around its longitudinal axis (Fig. 1–2). The primary functions of the stomach are related to motility and secretion. The features that make gastric motility and secretion possible include the sequential appearance during gestation of the circular and longitudinal muscles by 9 weeks, the development of the pylorus by 14 weeks, the presence of parietal and endocrine cells by 10 weeks, and the appearance of mucous neck and chief cells by 12 weeks. By the end of the first trimester, hydrochloric acid and intrinsic factor are produced by the parietal cells, pepsin by the chief cells, and gastrin and renin by the endocrine cells in the stomach, whereas mucous secretion from mucous neck cells is delayed until 16 weeks of gestation.

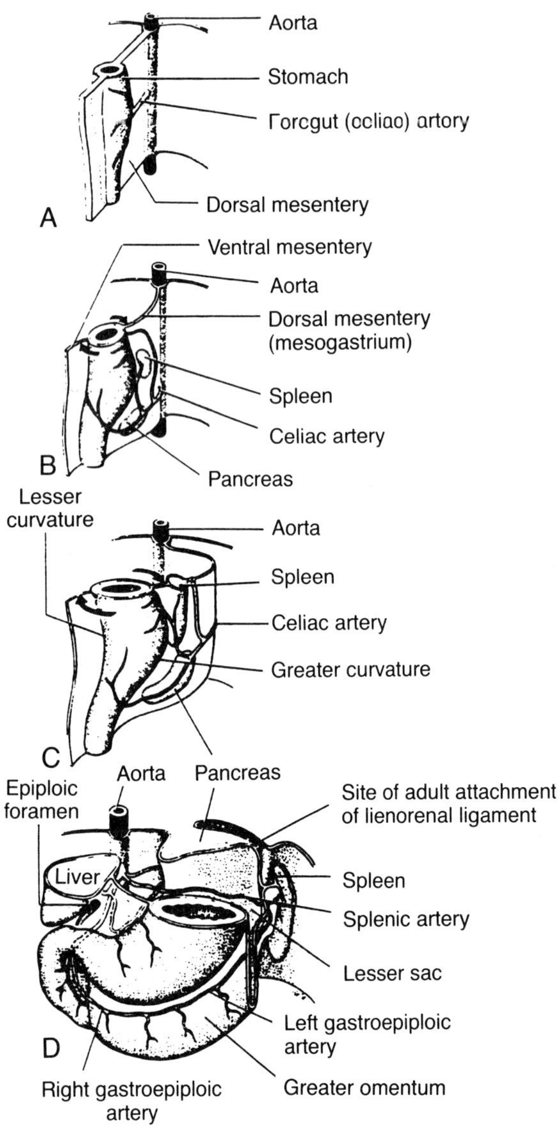

Figure 1–2. Development and rotation of the stomach and formation of the greater omentum. *A,* ~ 4 weeks; *B,* ~ 5 weeks; *C,* ~ 6 weeks; *D,* ~ 7 weeks. (From Moore KL: The Developing Human. 4th ed. Philadelphia, WB Saunders, 1988, p 219; with permission.)

The regulation of the maturation of the stomach has not been well defined but is thought to include neuroendocrine factors, such as gastrin, VIP, thyroxine, cortisol, and epidermal growth factor.[17, 18]

Acid secretion begins shortly after birth. In term infants, basal acid output is low throughout the first 5 hours of life.[19] Further acid secretion in response to pentagastrin stimulation does not occur during this early period.[20] Acid production subsequently increases throughout the first 10 days of life, decreases between 10 and 30 days of life, and then approaches adult levels of 0.02 mEq per kg per hour by 3 months of age.[21] Basal acid output in premature infants is lower than that in term infants but increases with increasing postnatal age.[22] Acid secretion in premature infants increases in response to pentagastrin stimulation, but this response depends on both postnatal and gestational age. Maximal acid production in premature infants, however, remains less than that in term infants.

The mechanisms that control acid secretion in infants are not well defined. Maximal acid output is generally proportional to parietal cell mass, although the density of parietal cells in the newborn infant has not been determined. Gastrin levels at birth are higher than those at subsequent postnatal ages,[23] presumably because acid is not secreted or the amount secreted is low. Nutrients such as calcium and protein are thought to influence the maturation processes of acid production in the infant.[24]

Pepsinogen has been identified in fetal stomachs by 8 weeks of gestation. There are a variety of pepsinogens that demonstrate differential development.[25] Pepsin activity appears at 16 weeks of gestation and increases thereafter in proportion to gestational age. The mechanisms that regulate chief cell function and pepsin activity in the human are not well studied.

Intrinsic factor (IF) has been identified in the human at 11 weeks of gestation. Parietal cells in newborn infants are thought to have a greater capacity to produce IF than acid.[26] Similar amounts of IF are produced by the parietal cells of term and preterm infants. Adult production rates occur by 3 months of age. IF production is independent of enteral feeds.[26]

Gastric motility and emptying involve complex interactions between neurogenic, myogenic, and hormonal activities. During the first few days of life in term infants, gastric motility is characterized by a continuance of esophageal peristaltic waves rather than independent, rhythmic, propagated contractions.[7] After feeding, the stomach contracts in a repetitive, but nonmigrating, pattern.[27] Gastric emptying occurs through a combination of increased gastric tone, fundal contraction, and hydrostatic pressure. Similar gastric contractions have been reported in premature infants throughout the end of the first week of life.[28] Although information about the development of the functional aspects of the stomach is limited, additional studies indicate that the type of feeding affects gastrointestinal motility. Thus, infants fed human milk have more rapid gastric emptying[29] and return more rapidly to the fasting pattern of gut motility, that is, the reappearance of the migrating motor complex,[30] compared with formula-fed infants.

Pancreas

The dorsal and ventral buds of the pancreas can be identified at 4 weeks of gestation. The major function of the pancreas is in the digestion and utilization of dietary nutrients. The developmental features that make the secretory functions of the pancreas possible have not been well characterized in the infant.

Rotation and fusion of the dorsal and ventral buds and their ducts are complete by 7 weeks of gestation (Fig. 1–3). Primitive pancreatic acini appear at 12 weeks, and rough endoplasmic reticulum and zymogen granules within the acini can be detected at 14 weeks of gestation. Trypsin, chymotrypsin, phospholipase A, and lipase are present in low concentrations in the pancreas at this time. Amylase is present by 16 weeks of gestation. Maturation of the acini is complete by 20 weeks of gestation. The exocrine pancreas, however, triples in size during the first year of life.

Islet cells can be detected at 12 weeks of gestation. Endocrine cells, primarily of the alpha type, can be identified by 13 weeks of gestation and predominate until late gestation, when the numbers of beta and delta cells increase. However, immunoreactive insulin can be detected as early as 12 weeks of gestation. At birth, three types of endocrine cells are concentrated in islets: 75% are beta cells (insulin), 20% are alpha cells (glucagon), and 5% are delta cells (gastrin, somatostatin, and pancreatic polypeptide).

Pancreatic enzymes, including trypsin, chymotrypsin, amylase, and lipase, are secreted continuously and in response to vagal stimulation or food ingestion. The major mediator of vagal stimulation is acetylcholine, whereas cholecystokinin is released in response to a fat or protein meal. These mediators interact with a second messenger cascade, leading to the fusion of zymogen granules, their extrusion into the pancreatic ducts, and the secretion of their contents from the pancreas into the gut. Secretin is the mediator of fluid and electrolyte secretions from the pancreas. Secretin also interacts with a second messenger cascade, resulting in the efflux of water, bicarbonate, chloride, sodium, and potassium from the pancreas.

Trypsin, lipase, and amylase are found in the duodenum of premature infants at 32 weeks of gestation.[31] The concentrations of these enzymes, however, are lower than those in term infants. In addition, the levels of individual enzymes are influenced by the type of carbohydrate present in the feeding. For example, duodenal amylase levels are high in infants who are fed starch-containing formulas, whereas duodenal trypsin and lipase levels are high in infants fed glucose-containing formulas. In premature and term infants, pancreatic enzymes do not develop in parallel with each other; trypsin appears in greatest quantity first, followed by chymotrypsin, carboxypeptidase, lipase, and then amylase.[32] Secretory responses to secretin and cholecystokinin are poor during the first postnatal month of life and do not differ in response to either protein or carbohydrate milk sources, for example, cow's milk versus soy formula. The pancreatic secretory response

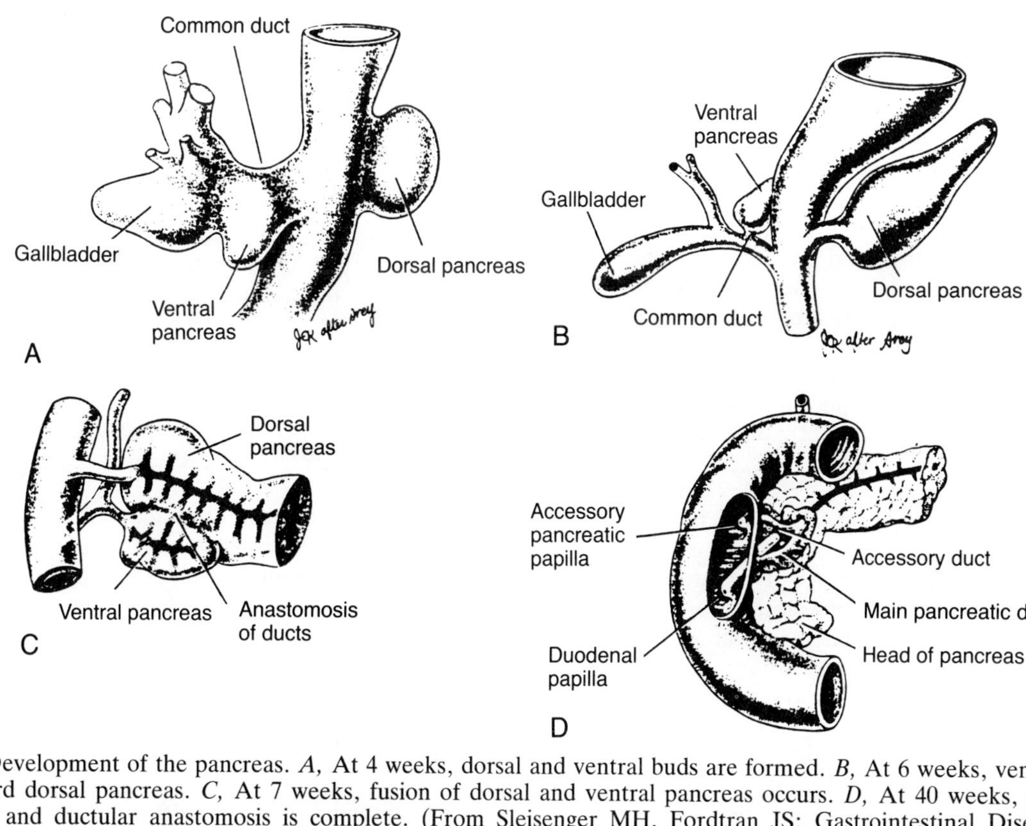

Figure 1–3. Development of the pancreas. *A,* At 4 weeks, dorsal and ventral buds are formed. *B,* At 6 weeks, ventral pancreas extends toward dorsal pancreas. *C,* At 7 weeks, fusion of dorsal and ventral pancreas occurs. *D,* At 40 weeks, pancreas is a single organ, and ductular anastomosis is complete. (From Sleisenger MH, Fordtran JS: Gastrointestinal Disease. 4th ed. Philadelphia, WB Saunders, 1989, p 1772; with permission.)

to human milk, however, varies.[33] Salivary amylase is present, whereas pancreatic amylase cannot be found. Although the amounts of enzymes vary, the ratios between enzymes, such as trypsin and chymotrypsin, are relatively constant.

Although pancreatic secretory function appears immature, fat malabsorption does not pose a major problem in premature and term infants, presumably because lingual and gastric lipases are present. In contrast with fat, however, the digestion of complex carbohydrates and starches varies.[34] In term infants, blood glucose levels fail to rise in response to starch ingestion, and the duodenal hydrolysis of amylopectin is low.[35] Nevertheless, formulas containing glucose polymers and corn syrup solids are generally well tolerated and support growth in infants, presumably because of digestion by salivary amylase.[36] Moreover, negligible amounts of carbohydrate are found in the stools of infants, presumably as a result of colonic salvage via bacterial fermentation.[37]

Secretory function of both acini (pancreatic enzymes) and ducts (water, bicarbonate) increases with increasing postnatal age.[31, 37] As postnatal age advances, pancreatic secretory function can be modulated by dietary factors. A high-protein diet, for example, increases trypsin and lipase secretion, whereas a high-fat diet does not alter lipase secretion. Similarly, a high-starch diet increases amylase secretion.[31] Soy protein formula enhances trypsin and lipase secretion relative to cow's milk protein formula.[38]

Liver

The liver appears during the fourth week of gestation as a diverticulum arising from the duodenum. The cranial portion differentiates into hepatic parenchymal tissue and bile ducts. The caudal portion forms the gallbladder and cystic duct. Hepatic lobes are present by 6 weeks of gestation. The liver reaches its peak size by 10 weeks of gestation and constitutes 10% of fetal weight. Throughout gestation, hepatocytes increase in size, number, and glycogen content.

Bile canaliculi are well developed by 6 weeks of gestation. The formation of intrahepatic bile ducts from cell plates derived from the hepatic duct is complete by 12 weeks of gestation. The gallbladder and cystic duct canalize by 8 weeks of gestation.

The fetal liver synthesizes bile acids from cholesterol as early as 14 weeks of gestation. Bile acid metabolism, however, is immature in newborn premature and term infants relative to that in adults. The rate of bile acid synthesis increases throughout gestation and with increasing postnatal age.[39, 40] There are qualitative differences, however, in the type of primary bile acids synthesized and secreted. Chenodeoxycholate is the predominate bile acid early in gestation, whereas increasing concentrations of cholic acid are found in late gestation. Various atypical bile acids are found in the fetus, but their significance has not been determined.[41] The bile acid pool size in both premature and term infants is one sixth and one half, respectively, that of adults.[39] However, the pool size increases with increasing postnatal age. The process of bile acid detoxification also changes quantitatively throughout development. Taurine conjugation is the primary excretory pathway for bile acids throughout gestation and in the early postnatal period. Glycine conjugation increases with increasing postnatal age and gradually replaces taurine conjugation. In addition, bile acids are also sulfated in the fetus to enhance their solubility,[42] and sulfation increases postnatally. Secondary bile acids (deoxycholic and lithocholic) are not found in the stools of infants during the first week of life, because bacterial colonization of the colon is limited. When bile acids appear in the duodenum of premature infants, their concentration is less than that found in term infants and adults. In addition, a critical micellar concentration, sufficient to maintain adequate dispersion of the products of fat digestion, may not be achieved.[39]

The enterohepatic pathway of bile salt absorption is also immature in the human infant. Taurine-conjugated bile acids are passively absorbed by the fetal gut[43]; active ileal transport begins after birth.[44] Intestinal motility also contributes to the regulation of the enterohepatic circulation of bile salts. Presumably bile salt absorption is inefficient in premature infants younger than 34 weeks of gestation, because coordinating migrating motor complexes and peristaltic activity have not developed.[45] Thus, it is likely that the immaturity of bile acid synthesis, secretion, metabolism, and enterohepatic circulation contribute to the presence of steatorrhea in premature infants.

Although the factors that regulate the development of bile acid metabolism and the enterohepatic pathway in the human are not known, likely candidates are hormones, such as glucocorticoids and thyroxine, and growth and dietary factors.[46] Corticosteroids increase bile acid pool sizes, synthesis rates, and intraduodenal concentrations by a factor of three in premature infants.[39] Epidermal growth factor, a polypeptide found in human milk, enhances postnatal growth and differentiation of the liver, including bile salt secretion and pool size in the animal model. Malnutrition, on the other hand, is associated with a reduction in liver growth, bile flow, and bile salt–independent flow.

Small Intestine

At 4 weeks of gestational age, the duodenum can be distinguished from the stomach and the cecal bulge. The small bowel epitomizes the functional development of the gastrointestinal tract in that it specializes in all aspects of gut function: motility, digestion, absorption, and immunoprotection.

The gut lengthens rapidly between 6 and 12 weeks of gestation. Because of its rapid increase in size, the small intestine transiently herniates into the umbilical cord between 6 and 12 weeks of gestation. On re-entry into the abdominal cavity, the intestine rotates counterclockwise by 270 degrees around an axis formed by the superior mesenteric artery (Fig. 1–4). At this time, continuity is lost with the embryonic yolk sac via the vitelline duct. Further positioning of the small bowel continues until 20 weeks of gestation, when the gastrointestinal tract achieves its final anatomic position. The small bowel continues to lengthen throughout gestation such that its overall size increases by a factor of nearly 1,000 and measures approximately 270 cm at term. The small bowel does not achieve its adult length of 4 to 5 m until approximately 4 years of age.[47]

The circular muscles of the small intestine appear at 6 weeks of gestation, and the longitudinal muscles at 8 weeks. The muscularis mucosa, however, is not present until 17 weeks of gestation. Neuroblasts appear at 7 weeks, and differentiation into the myenteric and submucosal plexuses occurs at 9 and 13 weeks, respectively. Peristalsis occurs shortly thereafter. However, jejunal contractions remain disorganized in the premature infant before 30 weeks of gestation.[48] With the appearance of migrating myoelectric complexes at 34 weeks, duodenal and jejunal contractions become coordinated, resulting in the propagation of peristaltic waves in an organized manner.

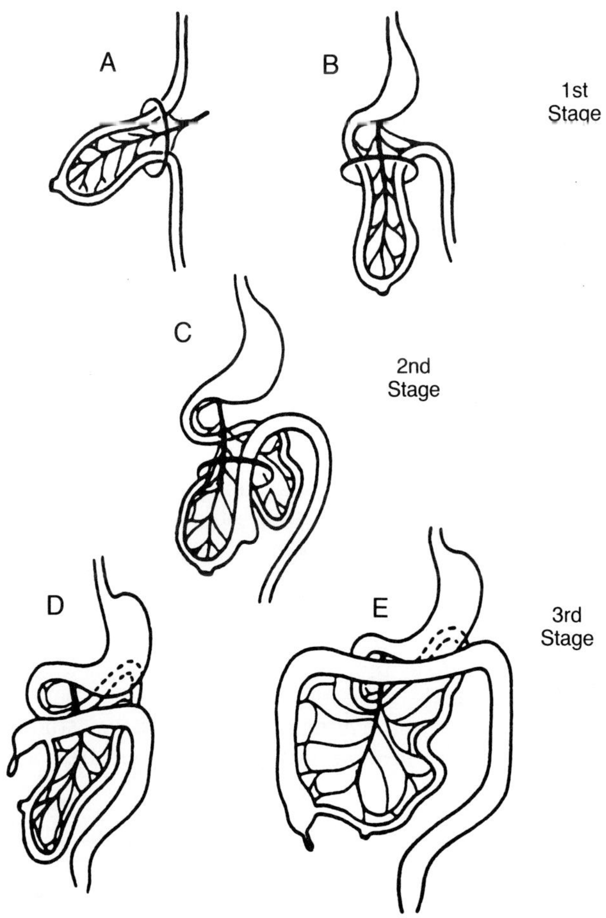

Figure 1–4. Rotation of the intestine. *A,* At 6 weeks, duodenojejunal loop rotates 270° counterclockwise around superior mesenteric artery. *B,* At 8 weeks, incomplete rotation. *C,* At 9 weeks, incomplete rotation. *D,* At 11 weeks, incomplete rotation. *E,* At 12 weeks, descent of cecum. (Modified from Snyder WH Jr, Chaffin L: Embryology of the intestinal tract. Ann Surg 1954; 140:368–380; with permission.)

Villi appear in the duodenum at 8 weeks of gestation and reach the terminal ileum by 11 weeks. Because of the rapid proliferation of epithelial tissue, the duodenum becomes obstructed temporarily, then reopens by 9 weeks of gestation. However, obstruction of the small bowel distal to the duodenum does not occur, despite proliferation of villi throughout the gut. The villi acquire their tall, slender, fingerlike shape in the proximal intestine by 14 weeks of gestation. The villi are shorter, wider, and fewer in number in the duodenum and shorter and more pointed in the ileum. Villi of maximum density, 40 per m^2, are found in the jejunum. The net result is that the surface area of the duodenum and jejunum is fourfold greater than that of the ileum. Microvilli also appear at 8 weeks of gestation, and, by 12 weeks, have a partially developed glycocalyx, glycogen deposits, mitochondria, Golgi bodies, and a junctional complex. By 14 weeks of gestation, enterocytes are morphologically mature and display a well-organized brush border. The enterocyte also has a tubular system that disappears after 22 weeks of gestation. This structure is thought to be involved in the uptake of macromolecules.

The crypts of Lieberkühn appear in the duodenum at 10 weeks of gestation and in the ileum and colon by 11 weeks. The crypts are approximately one third the size and three times the number of the villi. Paneth's cells appear in the crypts at 12 weeks of gestation. The crypts are the site of enterocyte proliferation. As migration occurs along the crypt and villus, enterocytes differentiate and mature by the time they reach the upper third of the villus. The typical adult appearance of the enterocyte is seen by 14 weeks of gestation. Further subcellular maturation is complete by the end of the second trimester of pregnancy. However, the process of enterocyte migration and maturation in the newborn infant is slower than that in adults and requires at least 6 days for epithelial renewal.

Endocrine cells appear in the gut by 9 weeks of gestation. Between approximately 9 and 12 weeks, mature secretory granules containing gastrin, secretin, cholecystokinin, motilin, serotonin, somatostatin, GIP, and substance P subsequently appear in the endocrine cells of the crypts. Enteroglucagon appears in the ileum at the same time, whereas VIP is found in the epithelial cells after 18 weeks of gestation. The concentrations of these peptide hormones and neurotransmitters increase throughout gestation and reach adult levels by term.[49] Other specialized cells, such as mucus-secreting goblet cells, appear at the same time as the endocrine cells, whereas Brunner's glands are detected in the duodenum after 14 weeks of gestation.

Despite the mature appearance of the intestinal epithelium by the end of the second trimester, its brush border membrane is functionally immature. Fetal hydrolytic enzymes, including sucrase-isomaltase[50] and several peptidases,[51] differ from those of adults. These functional differences are probably related to developmental differences in glycosylation and result in altered receptor responsiveness. Although information in the human is lacking, similar changes presumably occur in the composition of mucus and the lipid portion of the epithelial membrane. These developmental differences in membrane structure may influence the functional aspects of enterocyte transport and uptake of antigens in the infant.

DIGESTION AND TRANSPORT OF NUTRIENTS

Carbohydrates

Lactase and sucrase-isomaltase activities are detected in the brush border membrane of mature enterocytes at 8 weeks of gestation and develop in a cephalocaudad direction. Lactase activity is highest in the proximal jejunum and decreases distally. Lactase activity increases at 14 weeks of gestation but remains at 30% of the newborn level of activity until birth.[52, 53] Despite an apparent lactase deficiency, term and preterm infants tolerate lactase-containing formulas owing to the process of carbohydrate salvage by colonic bacteria. Peak lactase activity is found during early postnatal life. Within the first few years of life, lactase activity decreases to the adult level (one tenth that at birth). In contrast, sucrase-isomaltase activity rises steadily, but at variable rates; 70% of adult levels is achieved at 34 weeks of gestation, and adult levels are achieved at birth.[53] Sucrase-isomaltase activity remains highest in the proximal and mid-jejunum. However, the structural form of sucrase-isomaltase in the fetus differs from that in adults. Glucoamylase (maltase) and trehalase activities have been detected at 13 weeks of gestation. Glucoamylase activity remains low, although significant activity is present in premature infants.[53] In contrast, trehalose activity rises steadily and reaches adult levels by 23 weeks of gestation. Recent studies suggest that, in the absence of pancreatic amylase, premature infants can digest alpha-glucosidases, such as glucose polymers, more readily than lactose because of the presence of disaccharidase and glucoamylase. Salivary amylase also is present early in gestation and contributes to the digestion of glucose polymers.

The rate of glucose transport in the jejunum is low at 11 weeks of gestation and increases by a factor of four at 16 weeks as the number of transport sites increases. The development of sodium-coupled glucose transport progresses in a cephalocaudad direction and reaches a similar transport capacity in the terminal ileum at 21 weeks of gestation. The maximal glucose transport rate in the jejunum of infants is 20 to 25% that of adults and apparently increases throughout the first year of life.[54] The maximal rate of galactose transport is similar to that of glucose and is lower in infants than in adults. The development of fructose transport in humans, however, has not been studied.

Proteins and Peptides

Hydrochloric acid and pepsin initiate protein digestion in the stomach. Although acid and pepsinogen levels are lower than those in adults, they are capable of initiating limited protein digestion in the stomach of both term and preterm infants.

Most protein hydrolysis occurs in the proximal gut and is dependent on the presence of enterokinase, pancreatic proteases, and brush border and cytosolic peptidases. Enterokinase initiates the process of protein digestion by the activation of trypsinogen. Enterokinase is detected in the duodenum at 24 weeks of gestation and increases by a factor of three at birth.[52] The appearance of enterokinase also progresses in a cephalocaudad direction but remains highest in the duodenum. Activity levels of enterokinase at birth are 25% of those at 1 year of age and 10% of those in adulthood and increase thereafter until adult levels are achieved at approximately 4 years of age. The relative deficiency of enterokinase activity, however, is not rate limiting for protein digestion. Trypsin, chymotrypsin and carboxypeptidase B are present in the gut lumen and respond to secretin, pancreozymin, and a protein meal in term and preterm infants. Although levels of these enzymes are lower than those in older children, they are sufficient to permit efficient digestion of protein to peptides.

Peptides may be hydrolyzed first by brush border enzymes in the lumen of the small bowel and absorbed as amino acids. Most of the activities of the brush border peptidases (oligoaminopeptidase, carboxypeptidase, aminopeptidase, dipeptidylpeptidase IV, gamma-glutamyl transpeptidase) are present at 8 weeks of gestation. By the end of the first trimester, activities of dipeptidylpeptidase IV, carboxypeptidase, and oligoaminopeptidase in the fetus are similar to those in adults, whereas gamma-glutamyl transpeptidase is higher and aminopeptidase is lower. Although the developmental aspects of the remaining brush border peptidases have not been well-studied in humans, the structure of fetal peptidases is known to differ from those in adults, presumably owing to differences in glycosylation.[51] Cytoplasmic peptidases, also not well studied in humans, are present in intestinal mucosa at 11 weeks of gestation. Cytoplasmic peptidase activities increase at birth; activities in the jejunum are higher than those in the ileum.

Amino acid transport across gut mucosa is detected at 12 weeks of gestation. Throughout the second trimester, sodium-coupled amino acid transport increases as the number of transport sites increases. The capacity differs, however, in the transport of neutral, acid, and basic amino acids. The development of the peptide transport systems in the human has not been well studied but appears to be present early in the second trimester of pregnancy.

Fat

The digestion and absorption of fat occur in two phases: (1) the luminal and (2) the mucosal. The luminal phase, which is dependent on the presence of bile acids and pancreatic enzymes, involves the emulsification and hydrolysis of triglycerides to free fatty acids and beta-monoglycerides. These products of fat digestion subsequently enter into bile acid aggregates to form mixed micelles. The mucosal phase involves the movement of mixed micelles through the unstirred water layer at the mucosal cell surface and subsequent release and diffusion of free fatty acids and monoglycerides into the cell. Within the cell, the free fatty acids and monoglycerides are re-esterified to triglycerides. The latter are assimilated into chylomicrons and released into the lymphatic vessels.

The efficiency of long-chain triglyceride absorption ranges from 70 to 95% in term infants and from 40 to 90% in premature infants. Medium-chain triglycerides are digested and absorbed more efficiently than are long-chain triglycerides because they do not require bile salts for esterification or solubilization. Medium-chain triglycerides also are neither re-esterified nor incorporated into mixed micelles but rather are taken up directly by the portal vein.

The developmental immaturity of the biliary and pancreatic aspects of fat digestion in the infant has been described earlier. In premature infants, rates of bile acid synthesis are lower and pool size is smaller than those in term infants and adults, thereby leading to intraluminal bile salt concentrations that are decreased to levels below the critical micellar concentrations essential for solubilizing fat into micelles. In conjunction with limited pancreatic lipase activity, fat malabsorption is the expected result. Alternative mechanisms for facilitating fat digestion, however, are present in the infant. Lingual lipase, secreted by serous glands located on the tongue, is detected by 26 weeks of gestation and approaches levels similar to those found in term infants by 34 weeks of gestation. Gastric lipase, secreted by glands in the stomach, also facilitates fat digestion in the infant. A third lipase, bile salt–stimulated lipase, is found in human milk after 26 weeks of gestation and may contribute to the lower degree of fat malabsorption noted in breast-fed infants. Thus, the combined action of lingual, gastric, and bile salt–stimulated lipases in human milk effectively substitutes for pancreatic lipase and minimizes the consequences of fat maldigestion in infants.

In contrast with fat digestion, the details of fat absorption in the human have not been well characterized. Most knowledge of these processes at the level of the enterocyte has been derived from animal studies. However, the presence of circulating chylomicrons after a fat-containing feeding in infants suggests that enzymes such as apolipoproteins develop prenatally, although they may be structurally immature.[55] Apolipoprotein B_{100} is the only form of this transport protein found in fetuses younger than 20 weeks of gestation, whereas apolipoprotein B_{48} is found in adults.

Water and Electrolytes

Absorption of electrolytes occurs in the villous cells, and secretion occurs from the crypt cells. Because crypt cells differentiate into villous cells, electrolyte balance depends on the ratio of villous cells to crypt cells and their rate of turnover. Water movement across the intestinal mucosa follows the movement of electrolytes. Transport across the intestinal epithelium is regulated by extracellular factors, such as glucose and amino acids, that facilitate sodium entry into the cell and by fatty acids that modulate second-messenger cascades involved in transport processes. Intracellular factors, such as cyclic AMP, ionized calcium, and transmembrane potentials, also regulate electrolyte transport. Most of the processes involved in the transport of fluid and electrolytes, however, have not been studied in infants; instead, they have been inferred from studies in animals.

Vitamins and Minerals

Information regarding the development of vitamin digestion and absorption in infants is limited. Folate absorption in infants is lower than that in adults. Similarly, the decreased secretion of IF in term and preterm infants may influence the absorption of vitamin B_{12}.

Calcium absorption occurs primarily in the duodenum by an active transport process and is dependent on gestational age and the source of the milk feeding. Phosphorus absorption occurs primarily in the jejunum by an active, vitamin D–dependent process and by simple diffusion. Phosphorus absorption is influenced by dietary calcium and phosphorus intake. Magnesium absorption occurs throughout the gut and is independent of gestational and postnatal age. Copper and iron are absorbed from the duodenum, whereas zinc is absorbed from the duodenum and proximal jejunum. The efficiency of absorption of the trace minerals is dependent on the milk source, that is, 50 to 70% for infants fed human milk versus 5 to 50% for infants fed cow milk–based formulas.

IMMUNE FUNCTION OF THE GUT

The gastrointestinal-associated lymphoid tissues comprise the lymphocytes scattered throughout the lamina propria as well as organized aggregates of lymphocytes in Peyer's patches. Lymphocytes are detected in the gut mucosa at 8 weeks of gestation and may proliferate in response to mitogens by 12 weeks. Peyer's patches appear in the small bowel between 16 and 18 weeks of gestation. M cells overlying the Peyer's patches appear in the terminal ileum at 17 weeks of gestation. M cells are the specialized surface cells of Peyer's patches that permit uptake of macromolecules by the gut and antigenic processing within enteric lymphoid tissues. However, lymphoid tissues within Peyer's patches require sufficient antigenic stimulation for activation, and such stimulation does not develop until several weeks after birth.

Absorption of macromolecules by pinocytosis and transport to intercellular spaces is found in the human gut between 10 and 12 weeks of gestation. Although gut closure occurs with the disappearance of the amino tubular system during the third trimester, permeability of the gut to undigested macromolecules is greater in the human infant than in the adult.[56] These macromolecules include proteins, e.g., milk, as well as disaccharides, e.g., lactose. Gut closure may be enhanced by oral feedings; the rate of maturation is more rapid when human milk, rather than commercially prepared formulas, is consumed.[57] The clinical correlates of altered gut permeability in infancy are cow's milk and soy protein sensitivities.

Altered permeability of the infant gut may be a consequence of immature immunologic and nonimmunologic host defense factors. Immaturity of the enteric immune system is reflected in a deficiency of immunoglobulin (Ig)-containing cells and secretory IgA in the intestine of infants throughout the first 12 days of life.[58] In addition, when premature infants younger than 35 weeks of gestation are fed exogenous protein, they are unable to form antibodies to foreign antigens.[59] The process of immune maturation may be enhanced not only by increasing gestational age and antigenic exposure but also by factors found in human milk, such as lymphocytes, macrophages, and immunoglobulins. Nutritional deficiencies have an adverse affect on the secretory and cellular responsiveness of the enteric and systemic immune systems.[60] The consequences of nutrient deficiencies in infants include increased macromolecular uptake by the gut and may lead to the development of allergy in children.

Colon

The cecal bulge appears at 4 weeks of gestation and undergoes a series of longitudinal foldings at 8 weeks. Haustra and teniae appear between 8 and 12 weeks. After the rotation of the midgut is complete by 12 weeks, the cecum descends into the right iliac fossa. The rectum forms from the cloaca and fuses with the colon by 8 weeks. The circular muscles appear at 8 weeks of gestation, and the longitudinal muscles appear at 10 weeks, whereas the muscularis mucosa is detected at 15 weeks. Neuroblasts begin to migrate at 5 weeks, and Meissner's and Auerbach's plexuses are detected at 8 and 12 weeks, respectively. The migration of the ganglion cells is complete at 24 weeks of gestation.

Villi and crypts appear in the colon at 13 weeks of gestation and develop in a caudocephalad direction in contrast with that of the small bowel. The villi persist until 22 weeks of gestation, then regress, and disappear at birth. The development of colonic villi parallels that of small intestinal villi. Commensurate with villus formation is the presence of disaccharidase activities, although activity levels are much lower than those in the small intestine. Brush border and cytosolic peptidase activities also are present in fetal colonic mucosa. However, unlike the case with the appearance and disappearance of their activities in the small bowel, colonic oligoaminopeptidase levels persist throughout infancy and into adulthood.[53, 61] Endocrine and goblet cells appear in the colon at 5 and 12 weeks, respectively, as they do in the small bowel. Enterochromaffin cells, which secrete serotonin and motilin, as well as other peptide-secreting (somatostatin, pancreatic polypeptide) endocrine cells, are found throughout the colon during the second trimester. The development of absorptive and transport activities in colonic mucosa has not been studied in humans except for those of chloride and bicarbonate. The coupled transport system for chloride absorption and bicarbonate secretion is poorly developed in the preterm infant.

Gut Flora

The gut is a sterile organ before the birth of the infant. Colonization of the gut by intestinal bacteria begins at birth and progresses rapidly in the immediate postnatal period. The pattern of microbial growth in the gut is influenced by the type of maternal and environmental organisms to which the infant is exposed, the type and composition of infant feedings, and the level of immaturity of gut structure and function, including the enteric immune system.

The endogenous rectovaginal flora of the mother is thought to contribute to the colonization of the infant gut, although not all studies support this theory. Gestational age and route of delivery also affect the pattern of microbial colonization of the gut. Premature infants have lower colony counts than do term infants. Similarly, infants born by cesarean section have lower colony counts than do infants born by the vaginal route. Stability of the colonic flora occurs during the first 2 weeks of postnatal life. In healthy infants, aerobic organisms (primarily species of *Enterobacter*) are the first to appear in the gut, after which anaerobic organisms appear (primarily *Bifidobacterium,* and to a lesser extent, *Clostridium* and *Bacteroides*).[62]

Different patterns of colonization are found in the gut of human milk– and formula-fed infants.[63] The stools of breast-fed infants have a predominance of *Bifidobacterium,* whereas those of formula-fed infants have a predominance of *Bacteroides* and *Clostridium. Bifidobacterium* produces acetate as the major volatile fatty acid in stools of breast-fed infants; colonization of the gut by facultative anaerobes is inhibited, therefore, because of the acid pH of the stool. In contrast, the stool pH of formula-fed infants is high because of the presence of butyric and propionic acid; therefore, the stool has a more heterogeneous population of potentially pathogenic enteric flora. Human milk also contains factors such as *N*-acetyl-D-glucosamine and lactose, which promote the growth of lactobacilli, whereas other nutrients found in higher concentrations in formulas, such as glucose and casein, inhibit the growth of this bacterium. Similarly, the low level of iron in human milk promotes the growth of *Bifidobacterium* in contrast with the higher iron content of infant formulas.[64] Nonspecific factors in human milk, such as lysozyme and lactoferrin, also may influence enteric colonization by suppressing the growth of coliforms. Human milk presumably mediates bacterial colonization of the gut by secretory IgA antibodies specific for a wide variety of *Escherichia coli* antigens. With the introduction of solid foods, bacterial colonization of the gut shifts toward an adult pattern.

Host defense mechanisms that mediate enteric colonization include gastric acidity, immaturity of the microvilli, and intestinal motility. The decrease in acid production at birth may permit the more viable passage of ingested bacteria into the gut. Similarly, the immaturity of the microvilli may permit enhanced bacterial adherence or attachment as a result of alterations in receptor binding sites. The absence of the migrating myoelectric complexes before 34 weeks of gestation predisposes the infant to small bowel bacterial overgrowth. Coupled with sepsis or other illness, altered gastrointestinal motility leads to clinical features consistent with the blind loop syndrome. Malnutrition places the infant at risk for the consequence of diarrhea and the propensity for altered bacterial flora in conjunction with gut mucosal injury.

ENDOCRINE SYSTEM OF THE GASTROINTESTINAL TRACT

The endocrine system of the gastrointestinal tract presumably facilitates the postnatal process of adaptation to extrauterine nutrition. During this time, major changes occur in the structure, motility, digestion, absorption, and immunologic function of the gastrointestinal tract. The adaptive responses of the gastrointestinal tract to postnatal nutrition depend on the presence of regulatory peptide hormones released from the endocrine cells of the gut in conjunction with hormones from the pancreas, pituitary, thyroid, and adrenal glands.

Regulatory peptides in the gut appear between 6 and 16 weeks of gestation. Some peptides persist, whereas others disappear during development.[65] These changes in peptide hormones may facilitate the regulation of growth and functional development of the fetal gut. Several peptide hormones, including enteroglucagon, neurotensin, gastrin, GIP, pancreatic polypeptide, and motilin, have been measured in the fetal circulation between 16 and 20 weeks of gestation. These peptide hormones, as well as glucagon and secretin, are found in the term infant at birth. Fasting hormone concentrations in the term infant generally are similar to those in fasting adults, although fasting gastrin and VIP levels are significantly higher. These same peptides are different from those in the term infant. The functional significance of many of these hormones in infants remains to be elucidated. For example, the surge in pancreatic glucagon immediately after birth is important for the initiation of glycogenolysis and gluconeogenesis before enteral feeding. Similarly, after fetal distress, the levels of several of these gut hormones, particularly motilin, rise,[66] and they are associated with the intrauterine passage of meconium.

Before birth, the enteral assimilation of amniotic fluid, which is composed primarily of protein and minerals, has a minor role in the nutrition of the fetus. After birth, the gut is exposed to other nutrients, such as carbohydrate and fat. The exposure to these intraluminal nutrients may enhance or alter the digestive and absorptive capabilities of the gut. For example, the first feed of human milk in term infants is followed by a significant rise in insulin, growth hormone, gastrin, and enteroglucagon, but not in GIP or pancreatic glucagon.[67] In contrast, these peptide hormones show no change in response to the first feed in premature infants.[68] During the first 2 postnatal weeks in term and premature infants, basal peptide hormone levels rise three- to tenfold. The hormonal surges in response to feedings also increase with increasing postnatal age in both groups of infants.[69] The mode of delivery and the composition of the feed also have important influences on the development of the neonatal gastrointestinal tract.[70–72] In term infants, a feeding of milk, but not glucose, leads to a surge in enteroglucagon. In premature infants, bolus, but not continuous, feedings lead to surges in multiple peptide hormones. Human milk feedings result in concentrations of pancreatic polypeptide that are higher and GIP concentrations that are lower than those measured after formula feedings. Breast-fed premature infants also show postnatal preprandial hormonal surges, but these responses are smaller than those seen in term infants. These changes in the secretion of gut hormones do not occur in infants who have never been fed.[73] However, hormonal surges follow rapidly when feedings are instituted. Gut development is delayed when enteral feedings are withheld in animal studies. Thus, the timing, type, and mode of enteral feeding may have a beneficial effect on gut development in the human infant.

CLINICAL IMPLICATIONS OF GASTROINTESTINAL ONTOGENY

The clinical implications of the ontogeny of the gastrointestinal tract in the human infant lead to obvious questions regarding enteral feedings and the gastrointestinal problems encountered with early feedings, particularly in the premature infant. The timing of the initial feeding, the source of milk, and the method of providing milk feedings to the premature infant require further investigations to optimize the use of dietary nutrients and to enhance further development of the immature gut. Not infrequently, the functional immaturity of the neonatal gut, in conjunction with enteral feedings, leads to transient clinical problems. The developmental mechanisms that account for these clinical abnormalities often are unknown.

Feeding

Controversy persists as to the time to initiate enteral feedings in the premature infant. For the very low birth weight infant whose course is complicated by ventilator-dependent lung disease, the correct time to institute enteral feedings is unclear. The delay of hypocaloric feedings in sick premature infants does not increase the risk of necrotizing enterocolitis. Early feedings also are associated with earlier full enteral feedings, fewer days of parenteral nutrition, and a reduced incidence of cholestasis.[74] Until further studies are completed, it is recommended that enteral feedings be withheld for the first 1 to 2 weeks of postnatal life until symptoms associated with shock, hypotension, and ileus are resolved and the infant is no longer ventilator and umbilical-line dependent. In contrast, for the larger, healthy premature infant whose birth weight is greater than 1,500 gm, small amounts of enteral feedings at frequent intervals, for example, 3 to 5 ml per kg every 2 to 3 hours, may be initiated within the first postnatal day.

The choice of feeding sources for the premature infant is limited to human milk or specialized, commercially prepared formulas. Human milk has a unique role in the feeding of the premature infant because of its composition, and it has substances that are functionally significant in the development of the gastrointestinal tract. These substances include digestive enzymes such as bile salt–dependent lipase; hormones, such as cortisol and thyroxine; growth factors, such as epidermal growth factor and nucleotides; and nonspecific and cellular immunoprotective factors, such as lactoferrin, lysozyme, complement, immunoglobulins, lymphocytes, and macrophages. Despite these unique components, human milk is nutritionally insufficient in protein, sodium, calcium, and phosphorus and requires fortification to meet the nutritional needs of the rapidly growing premature infant.[75] Banked, pooled human milk is not suitable for premature infants. Its composition differs from that produced by mothers who deliver premature infants, and if it is frozen or pasteurized, it loses its immunoprotective capabilities from white blood cells and other nonspecific factors.

Commercially prepared formulas for premature infants also have been modified to meet the nutritional needs of the rapidly growing premature infant. These modifications are based on current concepts consistent with the developmental capabilities of the gut. These formulas contain higher protein concentrations, with a predominance of the whey component; higher calcium, phosphorus, sodium, zinc, and copper contents; and a broader distribution of carbohydrate and fat sources that includes lower lactose and long-chain triglyceride concentrations balanced with higher glucose polymer and medium-chain triglyceride concentrations, respectively. Premature infants may be fed with unfortified human milk or standard cow milk–based formulas fortified with iron after they have attained a weight of 2,000 gm. Soy formulas are not recommended for routine use in premature infants because of the reduced bioavailability of phosphorus and increased risk of osteopenia or rickets of prematurity.

The method by which the infant is fed depends on the level of maturity and state of health of the infant. Nipple feeding, whether by breast or bottle, is the preferred method for feeding the infant. However, immaturity of the suck-swallow reflex before 34 weeks of gestation may prevent effective feeding by this route. Premature infants also may have cardiopulmonary disease, neurologic disorders, or gastrointestinal anomalies that preclude effective nipple feedings. Under these circumstances, nasogastric, gastrostomy, or transpyloric tube feedings are necessary to maintain adequate nutritional intake. Bolus tube feedings rely on adequate gastric emptying and may aggravate esophageal dysfunction or respiratory disease in premature infants. In contrast, continuous tube feedings offer better bioavailability of nutrients to premature infants with short gut syndrome and diarrhea,[76] enhance weight gain in very low birth weight infants, and benefit those with delayed gastric emptying and gastroesophageal reflux who are at risk for complications of these entities. Nonetheless, continuous tube feedings do not challenge the enteric hormonal response, the consequence of which may adversely affect further gut development.

Early Gastrointestinal Problems

Symptoms associated with gastrointestinal dysfunction are common features of the early postnatal period. Anorexia, vomiting, constipation, diarrhea, or bleeding may occur. The precise cause of these symptoms in any particular case usually becomes obvious with careful observation, examination, and testing when appropriate.

Newborn infants may eat poorly at first because of an apparent lack of the sensation of hunger. However, the possibility of neurologic disorders should be ruled out. Choanal atresia also leads to poor feeding because of the infant's inability to breathe while feeding.

Regurgitation or vomiting may be functional or suggest partial or complete obstruction at some point along the gastrointestinal tract. Incoordination of swallowing and esophageal dysmotility are present in premature and term infants younger than 12 hours of age and may contribute to functional symptoms such as regurgitation. Similarly, gastric emptying in premature infants may be delayed, particularly in conjunction with cow's milk–based formulas. Such formulas have a high-caloric density that contains a greater proportion of nonprotein energy from monosaccharides and disaccharides than from glucose polymers or from long-chain rather than medium-chain triglycerides. Small bowel motility also is ineffective until 32 weeks of gestation, at which time the migrating motor complex appears. Despite the greater frequency of the migrating motor complex in premature infants, transit time through the small bowel may be as long as 9 hours, or twice as long as that in term infants, because of the twofold shorter propagation rate of the migrating motor complex.

If vomiting is present, the nature of the vomitus may provide clues to the site of obstruction. Mucus or saliva alone suggests obstruction proximal to the stomach, for example, esophageal atresia, whereas coagulated milk suggests gastroesophageal reflux or obstruction at the level of the pylorus. Bile-stained material suggests obstruction distal to the ampulla of Vater, whereas fecal-stained vomitus indicates obstruction low in the gastrointestinal tract. Hematemesis may result from the ingestion of maternal blood or the presence of esophagitis, stress ulcers, or clotting abnormalities. Metabolic and neurologic disorders should be considered in the differential diagnosis of vomiting.

The first meconium stool is passed by 81% of term infants within 12 hours, by 96% within 24 hours, and by nearly all infants at 48 hours.[77] Failure to pass stool within this time may suggest sepsis or obstruction, particularly Hirschsprung's disease. However, delayed passage of stool may be found in 20% of premature infants[78] and is related to gestational age, the time of the first feed, and the presence of ileus. Subsequent stool patterns in healthy infants are extremely variable and range from as few as one every 3 days to as many as ten daily. Although breast-fed infants have more frequent episodes of liquid stools than do formula-fed infants, it is neither uncommon nor abnormal for breast-fed infants to have as few as one bowel movement every 7 to 10 days. This latter pattern does not constitute a problem of constipation unless the stools are hard and dry. In contrast, the premature infant may pass hard, dry stools at infrequent intervals, leading to symptoms of anorexia, abdominal distention, and vomiting. The reason for this bowel pattern is unknown, but the problem may be treated successfully with glycerin suppositories.

Many healthy infants, particularly those who are breast fed, pass eight to ten loose or watery stools daily, usually in conjunction with feedings, but continue to thrive. This pattern of bowel movements does not constitute a problem of diarrhea unless the infant appears ill. Diarrhea may be associated with the presence of sepsis, an enteric infection, intolerance to milk protein, or, rarely, a deficiency of monosaccharide absorption, disaccharidase deficiency, or fat malabsorption. The presence of blood in the stool frequently leads to diarrhea and may be associated with intolerance to milk protein, an ulcerated Meckel's diverticulum, intussusception, duplication, or hemangioma of the bowel.

SUMMARY

The development of the gastrointestinal tract in the human infant is complete by the end of the second trimester of pregnancy. However, functional immaturity is present during early postnatal life and may persist in some areas throughout the preschool age. The uniqueness of the human gut is seen in its ability to adapt to a variety of nutrient sources and to utilize these nutrients for further growth and development. Human milk has a unique place in the development of the infant's gastrointestinal tract because of its special properties that stimulate growth and differentiation and provide immunoprotection to the gut. Nevertheless, many issues related to the developmental aspects of the gut and feeding of the premature infant are unresolved and require further investigation.

ACKNOWLEDGEMENT

The author appreciates the preparative and editorial assistance of Angela Cavese and E. Roseland Klein.

REFERENCES

1. Lebenthal E, Lee PC: Interactions of determinants in the ontogeny of the gastrointestinal tract: A unified concept. Pediatr Res 1983; 17:19–24.
2. Lebenthal E: Gastrointestinal ontogeny and its impact on infant feeding. Monogr Paediatr 1982; 16:17–38.
3. Walker WA, Durie PR, Hamilton JR, et al: Pediatric Gastrointestinal Disease. Philadelphia, BC Decker, 1991.
4. Grand RJ, Watkins JB, Torti FM: Development of the human gastrointestinal tract. Gastroenterology 1976; 70:790–810.
5. Herbst JJ: Development of suck and swallow. J Pediatr Gastroenterol Nutr 1983; 2:S131–S135.
6. Casaer P, Daniels H, Devlieger H, et al: Feeding behavior in preterm neonates. Early Hum Dev 1982; 7:331–346.
7. Gryboski JD: The swallowing mechanisms of the neonate: I. Esophageal and gastric motility. Pediatrics 1965; 35:445–452.
8. Widstrom AM, Marchini G, Matthiesen AS, et al: Nonnutritive sucking in tube-fed preterm infants: Effects on gastric motility and gastric contents of somatostatin. J Pediatr Gastroenterol Nutr 1988; 7:517–523.
9. Cortial C, Lezine I: Comparative study of nutritive sucking in the newborn (premature and full term). Early Child Dev Care 1974; 3:211–228.
10. Daniels H, Casaer P, Devlieger H, et al: Mechanisms of feeding efficiency in preterm infants. J Pediatr Gastroenterol Nutr 1986; 5:593–596.
11. Ashmead DH, Reilly BM, Lipsitt LP: Neonates' heart-rate, sucking rhythm, and sucking amplitude as a function of sweet taste. J Exp Child Psychol 1980; 29:264–281.
12. Sondheimer JM: Upper esophageal sphincter and pharyngoesophageal motor function in infants with and without gastroesophageal reflux. Gastroenterology 1983; 85:301–305.
13. Moroz S, Espinoza J, Cumming W, et al: Lower esophageal sphincter function in children with and without gastroesophageal reflux. Gastroenterology 1976; 71:236–241.
14. Vanderhoof JA, Rapoport PJ, Paxson CL Jr: Manometric diagnosis of lower esophageal sphincter incompetence in infants: Use of small, single-lumen perfused catheter. Pediatrics 1978; 62:805–808.
15. Moroz SP, Beiko P: Relationship between lower esophageal sphincter pressure and serum gastrin concentration in the newborn infant. J Pediatr 1981; 99:725–728.
16. Newell SJ, Sarkar PK, Durbin GM, et al: Maturation of the lower esophageal sphincter in the preterm baby. Gut 1988; 29:167–172.
17. O'Loughlin EV, Chung M, Hollenger M, et al: Effect of epidermal growth factor on ontogeny of the gastrointestinal tract. Am J Physiol 1985; 249:G674–G678.
18. Woll PJU, Rozengurt E: Neuropeptides as growth regulators. Br Med Bull 1989; 45:492–505.
19. Euler AR, Byrne WJ, Cousins LM, et al: Increased serum gastrin concentrations and gastric acid hyposecretion in the immediate newborn period. Gastroenterology 1977; 72:1271–1273.
20. Euler AR, Byrne WJ, Meis PJ, et al: Basal and pentagastrin-stimulated acid secretion in newborn human infants. Pediatr Res 1979; 13:36–37.
21. Christie DL: Development of gastric function during the first month of life. *In* Lebenthal E, ed: Textbook of Gastroenterology and Nutrition in Infancy. New York, Raven Press, 1981, p. 109
22. Human PE, Clarke DD, Everett SL, et al: Gastric acid secretory function in preterm infants. J Pediatr 1985; 106:467–471.
23. Euler AR, Ament ME, Walsh JH: Human newborn hypergastrinemia: An investigation of prenatal and perinatal factors and their effects on gastrin. Pediatr Res 1978; 12:652–654.
24. Hyman PE, Feldman EJ, Ament ME, et al: Effect of enteral feeding on the maintenance of gastric acid secretory function. Gastroenterology 1983; 84:341–345.
25. Adamson I, Esangbedo A, Okolo AA, et al: Pepsin and its multiple forms in early life. Biol Neonate 1988; 53:267–273.
26. Marino LR, Bacon BR, Hines JD, et al: Parietal cell function of full-term and premature infants: Unstimulated gastric acid and intrinsic factor secretion. J Pediatr Gastroenterol Nutr 1984; 3:23–27.
27. Tomomasa T, Itoh Z, Koizumi T, et al: Nonmigrating rhythmic activity in the stomach and duodenum of neonates. Biol Neonate 1985; 48:1–9.
28. Hancock PJ, Bancalari E: Gastric motility in premature infants fed two different formulas. J Pediatr Gastroenterol Nutr 1984; 3:696–699.
29. Cavell B: Gastric emptying in infants fed human milk or infant formula. Acta Paediatr Scand 1981; 70:639–641.

30. Tomomasa T, Hyman PE, Itoh K, et al: Gastroduodenal motility in neonates: Response to human milk compared with cow's milk formula. Pediatrics 1987; 80:434–438.
31. Zoppi G, Andreotti G, Pajno-Ferrara F, et al: Exocrine pancreas function in premature and full-term infants. Pediatr Res 1972; 6:880–886.
32. Lebenthal E, Lee PC: Development of functional responses in human exocrine pancreas. Pediatrics 1980; 66:556–560.
33. Norman A, Strandvik B, Ojamae O: Bile acids and pancreatic enzymes during absorption in the newborn. Acta Paediatr Scand 1972; 61:571–576.
34. De Vizia B, Ciccimarra F, De Cicco N, et al: Digestibility of starches in infants and children. J Pediatr 1975; 86:50–55.
35. Auricchio S, Della-Pietra D, Vegnente A: Studies on intestinal digestion of starch in man: II. Intestinal hydrolysis of amylopectin in infants and children. Pediatrics 1967; 39:853–862.
36. Cicco R, Holzman IR, Brown DR, et al: Glucose polymer tolerance in premature infants. Pediatrics 1981; 67:498–501.
37. Shulman RJ, Wong WW, Irving CS, et al: Utilization of dietary cereal by young infants. J Pediatr 1983; 103:23–28.
38. Lebenthal E, Choi TS, Lee PC: The development of pancreatic function in premature infants after milk-based and soy-based formulas. Pediatr Res 1981; 15:1240–1244.
39. Watkins JB, Szczepanik P, Gould JB, et al: Bile salt metabolism in the human premature infant. Gastroenterology 1975; 69:706–713.
40. Heubi JE, Balistreri WF, Suchy FJ: Bile salt metabolism in the first year of life. J Lab Clin Med 1982; 100:127–136.
41. Lester R, St Pyrek J, Little JM, et al: Diversity of bile acids in the fetus and newborn infant. J Pediatr Gastroenterol Nutr 1983; 2:355–364.
42. Watkins JB: Placental transport: Bile acid conjugation and sulfation in the fetus. J Pediatr Gastroenterol Nutr 1983; 2:365–373.
43. Lester R, Smallwood RA, Little JM, et al: Fetal bile salt metabolism: The intestinal absorption of bile salt. J Clin Invest 1977; 59:1009–1016.
44. de Belle RC, Vaupshas V, Vitullo BB, et al: Intestinal absorption of bile salts: Immature development in the neonate. J Pediatr 1979; 94:472–476.
45. Bisset WM, Watt JB, Rivers RPA, et al: Ontogeny of fasting small intestinal motor activity in the human infant. Gut 1988; 29:483–488.
46. Henning SJ: Postnatal development: Coordination of feeding, digestion, and metabolism. Am J Physiol 1981; 241:G199–G214.
47. Siebert JR: Small-intestine length in infants and children. Am J Dis Child 1980; 134:593–595.
48. Morriss FH Jr, Moore M, Weisbrodt NW, et al: Ontogenic development of gastrointestinal motility: IV. Duodenal contractions in preterm infants. Pediatrics 1986; 78:1106–1113.
49. Bryant MG, Buchan AM, Gregor M, et al: Development of intestinal regulatory peptides in the human fetus. Gastroenterology 1982; 83:47–54.
50. Triadou N, Zweibaum A: Maturation of sucrase-isomaltase complex in human fetal small and large intestine during gestation. Pediatr Res 1985; 19:136–138.
51. Caporale C, Fontana P, Fontanella A, et al: Isolation and characterization of two particle-bound oligoaminopeptidases from human meconium that are different from oligoaminopeptidase of adult small intestine. J Pediatr Gastroenterol Nutr 1985; 4:908–916.
52. Antonowicz I, Lebenethal E: Developmental pattern of small intestinal enterokinase and disaccharidase activities in the human fetus. Gastroenterology 1977; 72:1299–1303.
53. Raul F, Lacroix B, Aprahamian M: Longitudinal distribution of brush border hydrolases and morphological maturation in the intestine of the preterm infant. Early Hum Dev 1986; 13:225–234.
54. Younoszai MK: Jejunal absorption of hexose in infants and adults. J Pediatr 1974; 85:446–448.
55. Glickman RM, Rogers M, Glickman JN: Apolipoprotein B synthesis by human liver and intestine in vitro. Proc Natl Acad Sci U S A 1986; 83:5296–5300.
56. Udall JN, Walker WA: The physiologic and pathologic basis for the transport of macromolecules across the intestinal tract. J Pediatr Gastroenterol Nutr 1982; 1:295–301.
57. Weaver LT, Laker MF, Nelson R, et al: Milk feeding and changes in intestinal permeability and morphology in the newborn. J Pediatr Gastroenterol Nutr 1987; 6:351–358.
58. Burgio GR, Lanzavecchia A, Plebani A, et al: Ontogeny of secretory immunity: Levels of secretory IgA and natural antibodies in saliva. Pediatr Res 1980; 14:1111–1114.
59. Rieger CHL, Rothberg RM: Development of the capacity to produce specific antibody to an ingested food antigen in the premature infant. J Pediatr 1975; 87:515–518.
60. Watson RR, McMurray DN, Martin P, et al: Effect of age, malnutrition and renutrition on free secretory component and IgA in secretions. Am J Clin Nutr 1985; 42:281–289.
61. Lacroix B, Kedinger M, Simon-Assmann P, et al: Developmental pattern of brush border enzymes in the human fetal colon: Correlation with some morphogenetic events. Early Hum Dev 1984; 9:95–103.
62. Cooperstock MS, Zedd AJ: Intestinal flora of infants. *In* Hentges D, ed: Human Intestinal Microflora in Health and Disease. New York, Academic Press, 1983, p 79.
63. Simhon A, Douglas JR, Drasar BS, et al: Effect of feeding on infant's fecal flora. Arch Dis Child 1982; 57:54–58.
64. Mevissen-Verhage EA, Marcelis JH, Harmsen-Van Amerongen WC, et al: Effect of iron on neonatal gut flora during the first week of life. Eur J Clin Microbiol 1985; 4:14–18.
65. Bloom SR: Development of regulatory peptides in the human fetal intestine. *In* Bloom SR, Polak JM, eds: Gut Hormones. Edinburgh, Churchill Livingstone, 1981, p 119.
66. Lucas A, Christofides ND, Adrian TE, et al: Fetal distress, meconium, and motilin. Lancet 1979; 1:718.
67. Aynsley-Green A, Bloom SR, Williamson DH, et al: Endocrine and metabolic responses in human newborn to first feed of breast milk. Arch Dis Child 1977; 52:291–295.
68. Lucas A, Bloom SR, Aynsley-Green A: Metabolic and endocrine events at the time of the first feed of human milk in preterm and term infants. Arch Dis Child 1978; 53:731–736.
69. Lucas A, Bloom SR, Aynsley-Green A: Postnatal surges in gut hormones in term and preterm infants. Biol Neonate 1982; 41:63–67.
70. Aynsley-Green A, Lucas A, Bloom SR: The effect of feeds of different composition on entero-insular hormone secretion in the first hours of life in human neonates. Acta Paediatr Scand 1979; 68:265–270.
71. Aynsley-Green A, Adrian TE, Bloom SR: Feeding and the development of enteroinsular hormone secretion in the preterm infant: Effects of continuous gastric infusions of human milk compared with intermittent boluses. Acta Paediatr Scand 1982; 71:379–383.
72. Calvert SA, Soltesz G, Jenkins PA, et al: Feeding premature infants with human milk or preterm milk formula: Effects of postnatal growth, intermediary metabolism and regulatory peptides. Biol Neonate 1985; 47:189–198.
73. Lucas A, Bloom SR, Aynsley-Green A: Metabolic and endocrine consequences of depriving preterm infants of enteral nutrition. Acta Paediatr Scand 1983; 72:245–249.
74. Dunn L, Hulman S, Weiner J, et al: Beneficial effects of early hypocaloric enteral feeding on neonatal gastrointestinal function: Preliminary report of a randomized trial. J Pediatr 1988; 112:622–629.
75. Modanlou HD, Lim MO, Hansen JW, et al: Growth, biochemical status, and mineral metabolism in very-low-birth-weight infants receiving fortified preterm human milk. J Pediatr Gastroenterol Nutr 1986; 5:762–767.
76. Parker R, Stroop S, Greene H: A controlled comparison of continuous versus intermittent feeding in the treatment of infants with intestinal disease. J Pediatr 1981; 99:360–364.
77. Ogala WN, Amiebenomo CS: The time of passage of the first urine and stool by Nigerian neonates. Trop Geogr Med 1987; 38:415–417.
78. Jhaveri MK, Kumar SP: Passage of the first stool in very low birth weight infants. Pediatrics 1987; 79:1005–1007.

Chapter 2

Basic Aspects of Digestion and Absorption

MARTIN H. ULSHEN and STEVEN N. LICHTMAN

The gastrointestinal tract and accessory organs of digestion constitute a highly specialized system for the assimilation of ingested nutrients. Ultimately, nutrients must enter the intestinal mucosa to be transported or utilized; the luminal surface of the mucosa is lined by a continuous sheet of differentiated epithelium with digestive and absorptive capacities. In the small bowel, epithelial cells proliferate in the crypts and migrate up the fingerlike villi while simultaneously undergoing maturation. The presence of villi increases the luminal surface area of the bowel; the absorptive surface is further increased by the occurrence of microvilli (i.e., the brush border) on the epithelial cell surface. Mature epithelial cells are lost at the villus tip; in humans, the continuous renewal of proximal small bowel epithelium occurs over a 5- to 7-day period. The gastrointestinal tract is metabolically active, consuming a significant fraction of the total body oxygen need. The surface epithelium utilizes the majority of this oxygen requirement, largely to provide adenosine triphosphate (ATP) for Na^+,K^+–ATPase-dependent Na^+ transport, which is the ultimate driving force for many nutrient transporters. Glutamine is the major energy source for the small bowel mucosa, utilized primarily by the surface epithelium and taken up from products of intraluminal protein digestion and from the plasma.[1] Collectively, ketone bodies are the next major source of energy for the small bowel.

DIGESTION AND ABSORPTION OF CARBOHYDRATES

Monosaccharides are the only carbohydrates that are able to cross the mucosal membrane of the small intestine in large amounts in an unaltered state. Starches and oligosaccharides are the major form of carbohydrate in the human diet but must undergo digestion to monosaccharides before they can be assimilated (Fig. 2–1). A small amount of dietary disaccharide (a few percentage points) and as much as 10 to 20% of starch ingested by normal persons are not absorbed in the small bowel but pass into the colon to be converted to short-chain fatty acids (SCFAs) by colonic bacteria.[2–4] The SCFAs are absorbed in the colon, and this process is known as *colonic conservation of carbohydrate* (see discussion on absorption of SCFAs in the section on digestion and absorption of fat). In addition to conserving calorie intake, this process prevents the diarrhea that might result from physiologic carbohydrate malabsorption. The process may also be protective in limiting the symptoms of pathologic carbohydrate malabsorption (e.g., in association with short bowel or adult-onset lactose intolerance), as illustrated in Fig. 2–2.

Digestion of Starch

Dietary starch occurs principally as straight chains of glucose with alpha-1,4 bonds (amylose) or as similar straight chains with intermittent alpha-1,6 branches, accounting for about 5% of the total linkages (amylopectin). Dietary starch exists primarily in the latter form. The most important enzyme in the digestion of starch is alpha-amylase, which acts only on the interior alpha-1,4 bonds of starch (Table 2–1). The hydrolytic products of the action of this enzyme on amylopectin are maltose (2 glucose units), maltotriose (3 glucose units), and the alpha-limit dextrins. Oligosaccharides in the alpha-limit dextrin group consist of as many as 6 glucose units with one or more alpha-1,6 branches. The amount of glucose release by alpha-amylase is negligible; in addition, this enzyme does not act at alpha-1,6 bonds or at the beta-1,4 links of cellulose.

The first step in carbohydrate digestion is the oral exposure of starch to salivary alpha-amylase. This enzyme is thought to make a minor contribution to overall starch digestion, except perhaps in neonates, because it is inactivated at gastric pH. Human milk, in contrast with bovine milk, is rich in alpha-amylase activity.[5, 6] Although pancreatic secretion of alpha-amylase is quite low in the first months of life, in the adult, secretion is in excess of normal requirements for starch hydrolysis. Therefore, digestion of starch is completed before intes-

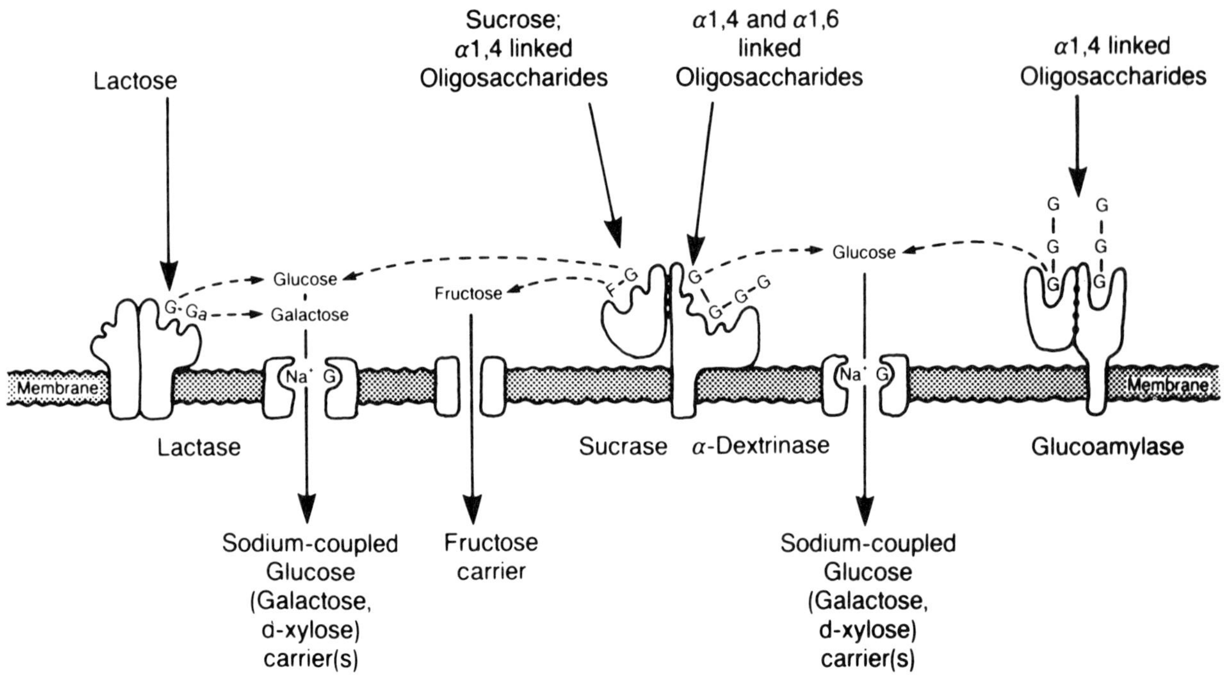

Figure 2–1. Overview of brush border digestion and absorption of carbohydrate in the small bowel. The alpha-1,4–linked and alpha-1,6–linked oligosaccharides are products of intraluminal alpha-amylase digestion of starch. Passive diffusion of monosaccharides across the brush border membrane is not shown but occurs as well. Sucrase alpha-dextrinase and sucrase-isomaltase represent the same enzyme complex. G, glucose; Ga, galactose; F, fructose. (Modified from Van Dyke RW: Mechanisms of digestion and absorption of food. *In* Sleisenger MH, Fordtran JS, eds: Gastrointestinal Disease: Pathophysiology, Diagnosis, Management. 4th ed. Philadelphia, WB Saunders, 1989, p 1066; with permission.)

tinal contents reach the distal duodenum.[7] The form in which starch is taken in the diet influences the degree to which it is digested.[4, 8] For example, the starch from low-gluten wheat or rice bread is nearly completely digested in the small bowel, whereas about 10 to 20% of the carbohydrate from wheat flour bread may pass into the colon. Wheat flour consists of granules of starch surrounded by a protein shell, and this layering effect may be the cause of the resistance to digestion. For similar reasons, digestibility of starch has been shown to vary among different cereals.[9]

Regulation of pancreatic enzyme secretion is the result of a complex and incompletely understood interaction of the cholinergic nervous system and gut hormone activity.[10, 11] Exposure of the duodenum to nutrient (i.e., the intestinal phase of pancreatic secretion) is the major stimulus for pancreatic enzyme secretion. Fats have the greatest effect, amino acids have an intermediate effect, and carbohydrate has the lowest effect on enzyme secretion. The hormone cholecystokinin (CCK) is secreted by the intestine on exposure to fat, protein, and amino acid. Administration of a CCK receptor antagonist eliminates the response to CCK and reduces meal-stimulated pancreatic enzyme secretion by 60%. However, atropine causes nearly complete suppression of pancreatic enzyme secretion in response to intraduodenal fat administration. Therefore, the cholinergic system appears to have a greater effect than does CCK on enzyme output during the intestinal phase of pancreatic secretion. Secretin promotes alpha-amylase secretion but has less effect on lipase and little effect on pancreatic protease release. CCK, secretin, and the cholinergic system appear to work in concert to regulate stimulation of pancreatic enzyme secretion. Secretin is the major stimulant of pancreatic bicarbonate and fluid secretion. Other gut peptides, such as vasoactive intestinal peptide (VIP) and pancreatic polypeptide, may contribute to stimulation of pancreatic secretion as well. A number of neuropeptides, including VIP, have been identified in the pancreas and appear to be important mediators of the cholinergic effects on the pancreas.

Table 2–1. ENZYMES OF CARBOHYDRATE DIGESTION

Enzyme	Main Substrates
Amylase (from human milk, saliva, pancreas)	Alpha-1,4 interior bonds of amylose and amylopectin
Oligosaccharidases (from small bowel mucosa)	
Sucrase-isomaltase (alpha-dextrinase)	Sucrose and alpha-limit dextrins (alpha-1,4 and alpha-1,6 bonds)
Lactase-phlorizin hydrolase	Lactose
Maltase-glucoamylase	Alpha-limit dextrins (alpha-1,4 bonds) Glucose oligomers
Trehalase	Trehalose (found principally in mushrooms)

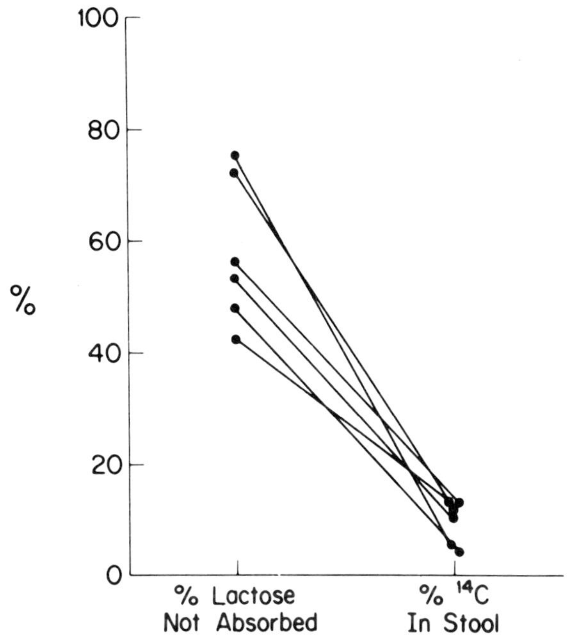

Figure 2–2. Colonic conservation of carbohydrate is illustrated by studies in a group of six people with lactase deficiency, each ingesting 12.5 gm of radiolabeled lactose. The percentage of administered lactose malabsorbed in the small bowel was determined by ileal aspiration. By comparison, the much lower percentage of ^{14}C derived from lactose and found in the stool demonstrates that most of this disaccharide passing through the small bowel was assimilated in the colon. (From Bond JH, Levitt MD: Quantitative measurement of lactose absorption. Gastroenterology 1976; 70:1061; with permission.)

Digestion of Oligosaccharides

Oligosaccharides from the diet include the disaccharides (especially sucrose and lactose) and the hydrolytic products of starch digestion, described earlier. These oligosaccharides cannot be absorbed intact but must first be split to monosaccharides in the small bowel or metabolized by bacteria to SCFAs in the colon (absorption of SCFAs is described later). In the small intestine, these carbohydrates are hydrolyzed at the luminal surface of the brush border in the presence of a group of enzymes known as the *oligosaccharidases* or *disaccharidases* (see Table 2–1). These enzymes are membrane glycoproteins; each includes a hydrophobic region serving as a membrane anchor and an intraluminal hydrophilic region containing the active site.[12] Oligosaccharidase activity is found associated with the mature villous enterocyte; levels of activity are maximal in the proximal jejunum.[13] The genes for sucrase-isomaltase and lactase have been located on chromosomes 3 and 2, respectively. Regulation of lactase activity in adult-onset lactase deficiency appears to be most commonly related to gene expression.[13a, 13b]

The oligosaccharidases are classified, according to the bonds on which they act, as alpha-glucosidases, including sucrase-isomaltase and maltase-glucoamylase, or the beta-galactosidase lactase (also known as *lactase-phlorizin*). Alpha-glucosidase activity appears to be stimulated by the presence of substrate, but this does not appear to be true for lactase.[14, 15] Because the half-life of these enzymes is a matter of hours but migration of the villous enterocyte to the villous tip takes several days, these enzymes must be continuously synthesized and degraded. Pancreatic enzymes and possibly bile acids and lysolecithin play a major role in the degradation of these enzymes.[16, 17]

With the exception of lactase, the oligosaccharidases have the capacity to hydrolyze substrate at a rate more rapid than the rate of absorption of the resultant monosaccharides.[18, 19] Thus, monosaccharide absorption is usually the rate-limiting step in assimilation of oligosaccharides. In contrast with the other oligosaccharidases, lactase is the rate-limiting step in the digestion and absorption of lactose.

The alpha-limit dextrins that result from amylopectin hydrolysis are digested by the complementary action of three brush border oligosaccharidases: sucrase, isomaltase, and glucoamylase.[20] Glucose monomers are removed in sequence from the nonreducing end of the oligosaccharide. Isomaltase is most active in promoting cleavage of alpha-1,4 bonds when four or more glucose residues remain; when fewer glucose residues remain, sucrase is most active. The alpha-1,6 branches can be hydrolyzed by isomaltase alone. This may be the most important role of isomaltase in digestion, and therefore it is also known as *alpha-dextrinase.* Glucoamylase is especially active for straight-chain glucose polymers with about 6 glucose units.[21] Studies in normal volunteers demonstrate that starch and oligosaccharides ingested in test meals are essentially completely absorbed before the intestinal contents have reached the distal jejunum.[7, 22, 23]

Absorption of Monosaccharides

Dietary starch and oligosaccharides are the major source of absorbed monosaccharides. During meals, glucose is absorbed down a concentration gradient, but absorption continues as this gradient is reversed. Glucose and galactose are transported by the same active, Na^+-coupled, carrier-mediated process.[24] The Na^+,K^+-ATPase pump at the basolateral membrane of the enterocyte maintains a low intracellular Na^+ concentration; movement of Na^+ down an electrochemical gradient is the driving force for coupled glucose-galactose transport. The intestinal Na^+-glucose cotransporter has been isolated recently and appears to be a 75-kd polypeptide.[25] On addition of Na^+ to this transport protein, it undergoes a conformational change that results in an increase in affinity for glucose. Immunohistochemical studies have localized this polypeptide to the microvillus membrane (present from crypt to villus tip); the concentration is greatest in the jejunum.[26] This cotransporter appears to be homologous, but not identical, to a renal glucose transport protein. An Na^+-independent glucose transporter has been identified in the basolateral membrane and is immunochemically distinct from the brush border glucose cotransporter. Studies of transport func-

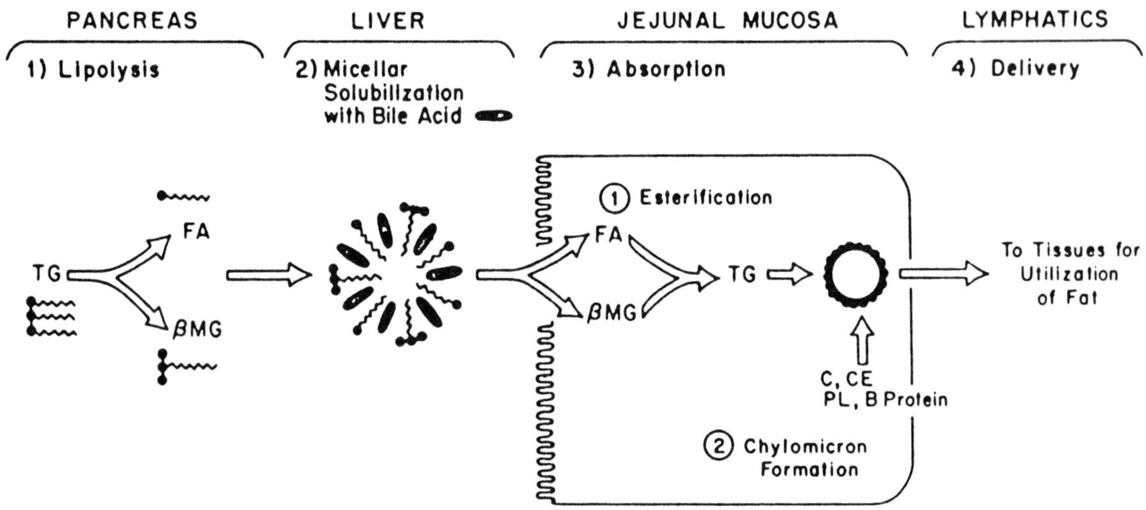

Figure 2–3. Overview of the major steps of lipid digestion and absorption. The steps include (1) lipolysis of triglyceride (TG) to fatty acids (FA) and beta monoglycerides (βMG); (2) micellar solubilization by bile salts; (3) absorption of fatty acids and beta monoglycerides into the enterocyte; and (4) delivery to tissues for utilization, re-esterification and formation of chylomicrons. C, cholesterol; CE, cholesterol ester; PL, phospholipid; B protein, apoprotein. (From Wilson FA, Dietschy JM: Differential diagnostic approach to clinical problems of malabsorption. Gastroenterology 1971; 61:912; with permission.)

tion suggest that activity is greatest at the villus tips. Activation of the Na^+-coupled cotransporter by glucose has been associated with loosening of tight junctions and, thereby, an increase in paracellular transport of small molecules. This may be the major route for assimilation of glucose and other nutrients, such as oligopeptides, following a meal.[27, 28] Fructose transport across the intestinal mucosa occurs by facilitated transport (i.e., a carrier-mediated process, not requiring energy).[29] The capacity to absorb fructose is limited in humans and can be suppressed in some people during ingestion of a diet rich in fructose.[30]

DIGESTION AND ABSORPTION OF FAT

Fat constitutes 30 to 60% of the caloric intake in the Western diet. Dietary fat is composed of triglyceride (90%); essential fatty acids (linoleic and linolenic acid); phospholipids; vitamins A, D, and E; and cholesterol. Triglycerides consist of three fatty acids on a glycerol backbone; the outer sites are known as the alpha and alpha-1 positions, and the center fatty acid is at the beta position. Each fatty acid on the glycerol moiety is usually different; the most common long-chain fatty acids are C16 (oleate) and C18 (palmitate). Certain fatty acids are found preferentially on specific sites on the glycerol molecule. For example, among the many fatty acids available, the palmitic and stearic acids often occupy the alpha and alpha–1 position in animal fats, whereas linoleic acid often occupies the beta position in vegetable oils. This explains why saturated fatty acids are usually located at the alpha position of phosphoglyceride and unsaturated fatty acids are located at the beta position.

By themselves, triglycerides are insoluble in water and form an unstable emulsion, but when they interact with phospholipids in the dietary proportions of approximately 30:1, respectively, a stable emulsion is formed. The phospholipid functions as an emulsifier enveloping the triglyceride. Phospholipids, especially lecithin (phosphatidylcholine), are derived from plant and animal cell membranes in the adult diet (4–8 gm per day), as well as from cells shed from the intestinal tract and bile (7–22 gm per day). In water, lecithin disperses to form concentric lamellar structures called *liposomes*.

Polyunsaturated fatty acids are needed for synthesis of prostaglandins. Phospholipase A_2 cleaves the desired polyunsaturated fatty acid from the beta position of a phospholipid. Linoleic (18:2ω6) and linolenic (18:3ω3) acid are essential polyunsaturated fatty acids because they cannot be synthesized by animals. Although other polyunsaturated fatty acids are also important for prostaglandin synthesis (e.g., arachidonic [20:4ω6], eicosapentanoic [20:5ω3], and docosahexaenoic [22:6ω3]), these can be synthesized by chain elongation from linoleic and linolenic acids.

Once ingested, dietary fat requires several well-defined stages for digestion, absorption, and transport to the lamina propria from the enterocyte (Fig. 2–3). Despite the complexity of the process, absorption from the lumen into the enterocyte and then to the lamina propria requires only 12 minutes. In the normal state, more than 95% of intraluminal fat is absorbed.

Emulsification and Solubilization of Fat

As triglycerides are released from food, shearing forces and mixing within the stomach and small intestine produce emulsified particles smaller than 0.5 μm in diameter. These particles form an oily phase separate from the water phase; digestion occurs at the oil-water interphase. Triglyceride emulsions are stabilized by several components, including phospholipids, bile salts, polysaccharides, monoglycerides, and diglycerides, many of which arise simultaneously from initial fat digestion. Bile salts are important in solubilization and in the promotion of pancreatic lipase activity, but 75% of dietary triglyceride can be absorbed without bile salts. Cholesterol and sterol vitamin absorption are affected more severely by bile acid deficiency than is triglyceride absorption.

Hydrolysis and Dispersion of Fat

Lipid digestion consists mainly of hydrolysis of ester bonds within triglyceride and phospholipids (Table 2–2). There are six lipases, if one considers gastric lipase as distinct from lingual lipase. It appears that lingual lipase is the most prevalent preduodenal lipase in some laboratory animals, whereas gastric lipase is most prevalent in others.[31, 32] It is likely that the predominant preduodenal lipase in humans is gastric lipase.[33, 34]

Lingual and gastric lipases are active at a low pH (2.0–7.5). Lingual lipase originates from Ebner's gland, which is located beneath the circumvallate papillae. Gastric lipase has been identified in biopsies from the body of the stomach but not the antrum or duodenum.[35] Lingual and gastric lipases are immunologically distinct from other lipases that originate from the pancreas and from each other. These enzymes initiate hydrolysis in the stomach and may account for 10 to 40% of total fat hydrolysis in neonates, because pancreatic sources of lipases are not fully developed at this time. Because these enzymes are also active at a higher pH, they may continue to function in the duodenum and be important in people who have pancreatic insufficiency, such as those with cystic fibrosis.[36] Gastric lipase hydrolyzes medium-chain triglycerides five to eight times faster than long-chain triglycerides. The products of hydrolysis are fatty acids and diacylglycerol. In neonates, medium-chain triglycerides disappear more rapidly than long-chain triglycerides from stomach contents following a meal because neonates appear to absorb medium-chain triglycerides directly from the stomach; in addition, gastric lipase hydrolyzes medium-chain triglycerides at a higher rate than long-chain triglycerides.[37]

Table 2–2. ENZYMES OF LIPID ABSORPTION

Enzyme	Source	Site of Action	Product
Human milk lipase	Mammary gland	Small intestine	FA, glycerol, MG, free sterol
Lingual lipase	Ebner's glands (circumvallate papillae)	Stomach	FA, DG
Gastric lipase	Body of stomach	Stomach	FA, DG
Pancreatic lipase	Pancreas	Small intestine	FA, 2-MG
Colipase	Pancreas	Small intestine	
Phospholipase A_2	Pancreas	Small intestine	FA, lysophospholipids
Pancreatic nonspecific lipase	Pancreas	Small intestine	Hydrolysates of sterol, vitamin esters, and cholesterol esters

MG, monoglyceride; DG, diglyceride; FA, fatty acids.

The role of lingual and gastric lipases has been controversial; some data indicate that these lipases are responsible for only 10% of fat digestion in newborns. Bile salts inhibit lingual lipase activity, so function in the duodenum is probably limited. Free fatty acids also inhibit this activity. Recent studies suggest that digestion of human milk triglyceride depends on three lipases (gastric, human milk, and pancreatic), each with a unique but overlapping function.[38]

Intestinal lipolysis is the result of four enzymes, including human milk lipase (in nursing infants), pancreatic lipase, phospholipase A_2, and nonspecific lipase. Human milk lipase is important in the newborn because fat intake accounts for 50 to 60% of total calories but pancreatic lipase secretion is not fully developed. This enzyme is resistant to acid and is activated by bile salts in the duodenum. Pancreatic lipase, in conjunction with its cofactor colipase, is responsible for the major proportion of triglyceride hydrolysis (see section on digestion of starch for discussion of pancreatic secretion). Colipase is a small molecule of molecular weight 10 kd. In the presence of bile salts and phospholipid, colipase binds lipase to the triglyceride emulsion for hydrolysis of triglyceride at the alpha and alpha-1 positions. The products are monoglyceride, diglycerides, and free fatty acids. Colipase is initially synthesized as procolipase, which is activated by trypsin. Paradoxically, pancreatic lipase is inhibited by a high critical micellar concentration of bile acids. However, this obstacle is overcome by the presence of colipase, which attaches to the ester bond of the triglyceride and brings the lipase close to the triglyceride, thereby eliminating the inhibitory effect of bile acids. In persons with steatorrhea secondary to pancreatic insufficiency, fecal fat output correlates better with colipase secretion than with lipase secretion (Fig. 2–4).[39] As little as 2% of normal lipase secretion can be compatible with normal fat digestion if colipase secretion is adequate.

The luminal concentration of lipase decreases as it travels distally in the small intestine due to digestion by pancreatic proteases.[40] Diversion of pancreatic juice or inhibition of protease activity causes increased pancreatic protease production owing to interruption of a negative feedback loop.[41] Less work has been done with regard to feedback inhibition of pancreatic lipase. Perfusion of camostat, a protease inhibitor, causes increased lipase production,[41] but in other studies, instillation of amylase or purified lipase in the intestine did not affect pancreatic lipase synthesis and secretion.[42]

Phospholipase A_2 is a calcium-dependent bile salt–activated lipase secreted by the pancreas. It is the major enzyme in the digestion of intestinal phospholipids; it cleaves both dietary and biliary phospholipids. The

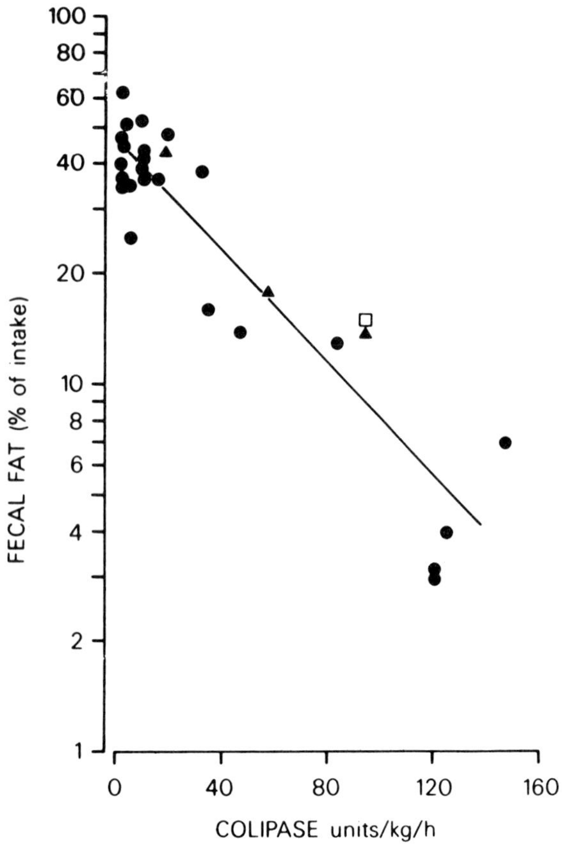

Figure 2–4. Correlation of fecal fat output (percentage of intake) with colipase secretion in persons with cystic fibrosis *(closed circles),* Shwachman's syndrome *(closed triangles),* and pancreatic hypoplasia *(open squares).* $r = -0.92$; $P < 0.001$. (From Gaskin KJ, Durie PR, Lee L, et al: Colipase and lipase secretion in childhood-onset pancreatic insufficiency: Delineation of patients with steatorrhea secondary to relative colipase deficiency. Gastroenterology 1984; 86:5; with permission.)

pancreas also produces a nonspecific lipase, called *cholesterol esterase,* which is important in hydrolysis of ester bonds in cholesterol and sterol vitamins (A, D, and E). It forms free sterols that are readily absorbed.

The pH of chyme coming from the stomach is in the range of 2 to 3, but changes to approximately 6.5 in the duodenum because of bicarbonate secretion from the pancreas. It is important that the pH stay above 5 because (1) pancreatic lipase, trypsin, and amylase all have diminished function when pH is below 5; (2) bile acids conjugated to glycine will precipitate spontaneously at pH below 5; and (3) partitioning of fatty acids into the aqueous phase is diminished below pH of 6 in vitro.

The Unstirred Water Layer

As a solute passes from the bulk phase within the lumen toward the enterocyte, it first passes through the unstirred water layer (UWL) adjacent to the microvillus membrane (Fig. 2–5). To understand how the UWL may function as a rate-limiting step, the dimensions of the villus structure must be considered. A villus is about 200 to 500 μm in length, projecting into the lumen of the intestine. Each human jejunal enterocyte has approximately 700 microvilli.[43] Microvilli are approximately 1 μm long and 0.1 μm wide. The space between two microvilli is about 0.02 to 0.05 μm. The UWL thickness is approximately 115 to 330 μm,[44] which is greater than the length of many villi. The glycocalyx is only 0.1 to 0.5 μm deep but may be responsible for protecting the acid microenvironment at the epithelial cell surface. In addition to the glycocalyx, mucus lies over the microvillus membrane, but neither causes significant resistance to absorption of solutes.[45] It is the UWL that provides resistance to passive absorption of solutes. Rather than an anatomic barrier, it is a diffusion barrier between the enterocyte cell surface and the bulk emulsion phase in the lumen. Once lipids reach the cell membrane, diffusion into the enterocytes is rapid.

The UWL consists of a series of water lamellae extending out from the enterocyte cell membrane, each becoming progressively more stirred, until they blend with the bulk water phase. Movement by solute flux *(J)* is determined by the equation

$$J = [(C1 - C2) \times S_w \times D]/d$$

where C1 is the concentration of the luminal solute, C2 is the concentration of the solute just at the epithelial cell membrane, S_w is the surface area of the UWL, D is

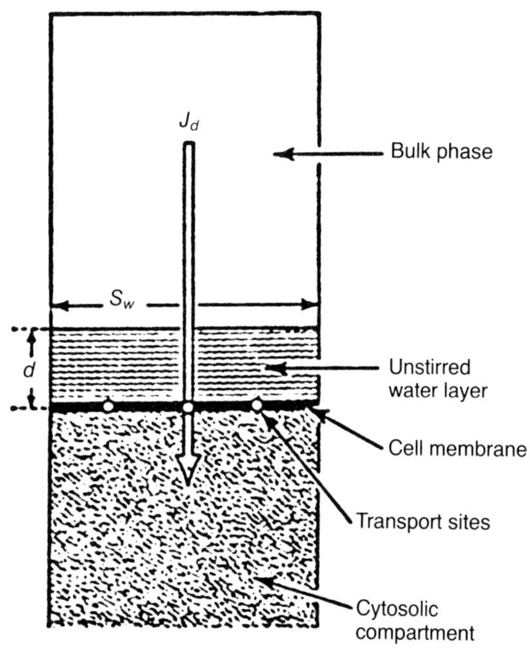

Figure 2–5. The unstirred water layer (UWL). The two major barriers to uptake of solute molecules from the bulk phase (lumen) into the cytosolic compartment of the cell are the UWL and luminal cell membrane. Resistance due to the UWL is d/S_w. J_d, rate of uptake of solute molecules (solute flux); S_w, surface area of UWL; d, thickness of UWL. (From Thomson ABR, Dietschy JM: Derivation of the equations that describe the effects of unstirred water layers on the kinetic parameters of active transport processes in the intestine. J Theor Biol 1977; 64:280; with permission.)

the aqueous diffusion constant of the solute, and *d* is the thickness of the UWL.[45] Recently, the previously described magnitude of the UWL has been questioned as physiologically impossible; an alternative proposal is that the width of the UWL is only 40 mm and that mixing is achieved by contraction of villi.[45a]

Absorption of Lipid

Lipids are released into the stomach from ingested food by the actions of lingual and gastric lipases. Emulsification is assisted by gastric and pyloric contractions and by addition of by-products of early hydrolysis and bile salts in the duodenum. Lipolysis continues in the small intestine with the help of pancreatic lipase, phospholipase A_2, and nonspecific lipase. Gradually, the triglyceride-oil phase of large droplets (0.5 μm) shrinks by release of fatty acids and monoglycerides into the oil-water viscous phase. This is followed by creation of smaller mixed micelles, liposomes, and unilamellar vesicles. The products of fat digestion are free fatty acids, monoglycerides, phosphatidylcholine, free cholesterol, and free sterols, which are solubilized in bile acid micelles. Most absorption of digested fat occurs in the proximal small bowel at the villous tips and is complete by the midjejunum.[46] Lipids traverse two barriers: the UWL and the brush border membrane.

The bile acid micelle further dissociates owing to the low pH of the microenvironment just outside the enterocyte.[47] SCFAs and medium-chain fatty acids are absorbed as monomers and are rate-limited by the brush border membrane, whereas the absorption of long-chain fatty acids and cholesterol is rate-limited by the UWL.[48] Once the products of lipolysis reach the cell membrane, they rapidly diffuse by passive transport into the enterocyte. The rate of fatty acid transfer is directly related to the length of the fatty acid and inversely related to polarity. An Na^+-dependent transporter for fatty acids has been described.[49, 50] Phosphatidylcholine is passively absorbed as lysophospholipid.

Using microelectrodes and dye indicators, the acid microenvironment around the enterocyte has been shown to be approximately 400 to 700 μm in rats.[51] The mucous coat protects the microenvironment, and there is no evidence for a hydrogen ion secretion mechanism. A change in luminal pH may affect the pH of the microenvironment and, therefore, may affect lipid absorption. It is important that the pH of the microenvironment remains acidic because this pH promotes dissociation of micelles into products that are the necessary form for absorption into the enterocyte.

Long-chain fatty acids, such as oleic acid, linoleic acid, and arachidonic acids, are absorbed in a fashion that demonstrates saturation kinetics. The reasons for saturation kinetics are unknown but may include the effect of the UWL, limited solubility of long-chain fatty acids in the aqueous phase, or saturation of the fatty acid–binding protein in the cytosol of the enterocyte.

Processing of Fat Within the Enterocyte

Once within the enterocyte, the products of lipolysis are bound to fatty acid–binding protein (molecular weight 15 kd) and transported to specific organelles for further processing. Triglyceride is resynthesized from fatty acids and glycerol in the smooth endoplasmic reticulum (SER) via a monoacylglycerol pathway. Phosphatidylcholine is resynthesized from lysophospholipid, glycerol, and fatty acids using the acyltransferase or alpha-glycerophosphate pathway in the SER. Cholesterol is re-esterified in the SER by acyl CoA:cholesterol acyltransferase.

To transport fat (especially cholesterol, which is essential for all cell membrane synthesis) from the enterocyte, chylomicrons are assembled in the tubular SER and Golgi bodies. After ingestion of fat, chylomicrons are the major lipoprotein found in blood. Phospholipid and apoprotein make up the surface coat, which allows the inner fatty substances to be transported in the aqueous blood medium. Several apoproteins (apo A_1, apo A_4, and apo B) are synthesized by the enterocyte, but Apo B is essential for chylomicron production and may exist as a stored pool in the enterocyte. The usual phospholipid source is dietary and biliary, but if the source is limited, then the enterocyte can synthesize phospholipids de novo within the SER. Therefore, the absence of phospholipid is not a rate-limiting step for chylomicron formation. In their final form, chylomicrons consist of an apoprotein and phosphatidylcholine coat, a triglyceride core, cholesterol esters, and free cholesterol.

Chylomicrons are released into the intercellular space as vesicles by exocytosis across the basolateral membrane of the enterocyte. They enter lacteals within the lamina propria and subsequently reach the lymphatic vessels. After transport to the lymph from the enterocyte, chylomicrons acquire additional apoproteins, including apo C and apo E.

Absorption of Short-Chain Fatty Acids

SCFAs, composed of six carbons or fewer, are the end products of anaerobic bacterial fermentation of undigested carbohydrate residue, especially cellulose and pectin. They are important products of the colonic salvage pathway for carbohydrate (see section on digestion and absorption of carbohydrates). Absorption of SCFAs may account for up to 550 kcal in an adult.[52] Three SCFAs (acetate, propionate, and butyrate) are quantitatively the most abundant anions in feces in a ratio of approximately 60:25:15, respectively.

Colonic bacteria produce 300 to 600 mmol of SCFAs per day, but only 10 mmol are lost in stool daily, indicating an efficient and complete mechanism of absorption within the colon. SCFAs are weak acids, so at the colonic pH of 7.0, they are in the ionized form, which makes simple passive absorption unlikely. In rabbits, absorption is linked to electroneutral Na^+ absorption through an Na^+-H^+ exchanger.[53] In the distal rat colon, SCFAs stimulate active sodium and chloride absorption, a result of uptake of nonionized butyrate and coupled Na^+-H^+ and chloride-butyrate exchange.[54]

Although the majority of SCFAs are produced in the colon (60–150 mmol per L), small amounts (less than 1.5 mmol per L) are detectable in the jejunum[55, 56] and distal ileum (7–15 mmol per L).[57] The mechanism of absorption and importance of the small intestinal SCFAs are unknown.

SCFAs appear to have an important role in colonic homeostasis. It is likely that SCFAs serve as the major energy source for colonocytes. They may stimulate epithelial cell division and function as a trophic factor in the gut.[55] SCFAs have a role in the regulation of sodium, bicarbonate, and pH of fecal water. Recently, SCFAs have been shown to play an important role in the treatment of diversion colitis.[58]

Bile Acid Absorption

The primary bile acids, cholic and chenodeoxycholic acid, are synthesized in the liver. Secondary bile acids are metabolic products of bacteria within the intestinal lumen. Bile salts are conjugated to taurine or glycine. The bile salt concentration of hepatic bile is approximately 35 mmol per L, which is further diluted to 10 to 20 mmol per L in the proximal intestine and is only 2 to 3 mmol per L at the terminal ileum in rats. Bile acids are absorbed by active transport in the terminal ileum as well as by passive diffusion in the jejunum. Below the critical micellar concentration, bile acids exist as monomers, but above the critical micellar concentration, they aggregate to form micelles. Dissociation must occur in the low pH microenvironment of the UWL near the enterocyte cell surface because bile acids are absorbed only as monomers.

Jejunal hyperacidity, which occurs in pancreatic insufficiency, does not affect bile acid secretion but does cause precipitation of bile acids. This process may worsen steatorrhea in patients with pancreatic insufficiency.[59]

Cholesterol Absorption

Cholesterol is absorbed as a monomer. Bile salts affect both the luminal and the mucosal stages of cholesterol absorption. A surface mucosal protein binds cholesterol prior to absorption into the enterocyte.[60] Surface mucin may bind cholesterol and diminish its absorption. Unsaturated fatty acids and phosphatidylcholine inhibit cholesterol absorption because these lipids enhance solubility of the micellar fraction and allow less monomer to dissociate from the micelle. Only 40 to 50% of dietary cholesterol is absorbed by enterocytes in normal persons.[61]

Medium-Chain Triglyceride Absorption

Medium-chain triglycerides (i.e., triglycerides composed of fatty acids with 8 to 12 carbons) are absorbed intact by passive diffusion into the enterocyte. This probably accounts for about 30% of medium-chain triglyceride absorption. Medium-chain triglycerides are easily hydrolyzed by pancreatic lipase to free fatty acids and glycerol, both of which are also rapidly absorbed. Medium-chain triglyceride is not re-esterified within the enterocyte or packaged into chylomicrons.

DIGESTION AND ABSORPTION OF PROTEINS

Assimilation of dietary protein involves a complex series of complementary steps (Fig. 2–6). This process begins in the stomach, where gastric acid denatures dietary protein and promotes the peptic digestion of protein to large polypeptides. Pancreatic proteases secreted into the small bowel are endopeptidases and

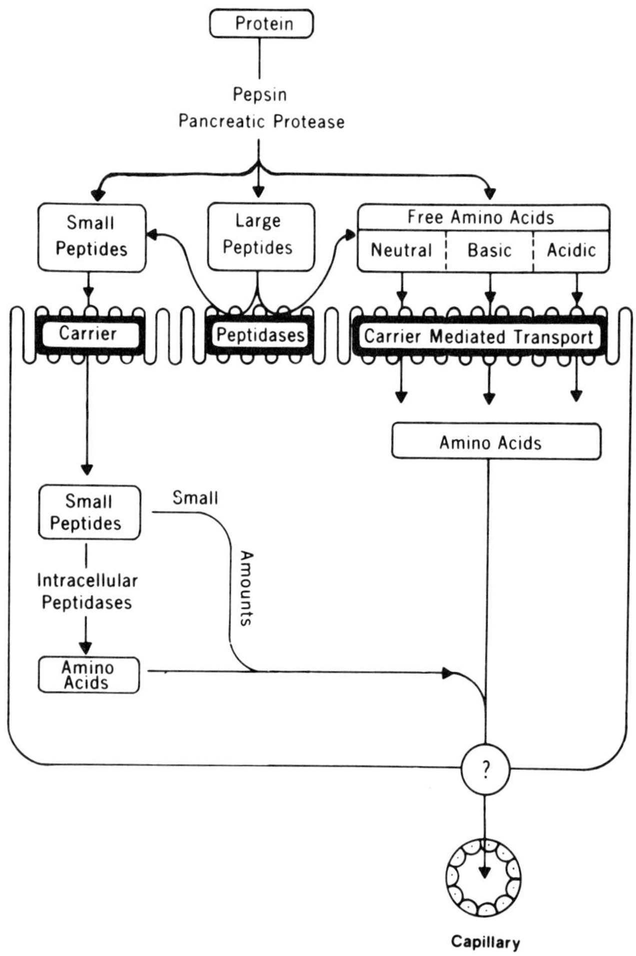

Figure 2–6. Overview of digestion and absorption of protein in the small bowel. (From Castro GA: Digestion and absorption. *In* Johnson LR, ed: Gastrointestinal Physiology. 4th ed. St Louis, Mosby Year Book, 1991, p 120; with permission.)

Table 2–3. PANCREATIC PROTEASES

Endopeptidases—act at internal peptide bonds to yield peptides with the carboxy-terminal amino acids shown below:

Enzyme	Carboxy-terminal Amino Acid of Product
Trypsin	Basic amino acids
Chymotrypsin	Aromatic amino acids, leucine, glutamine, methionine
Elastase	Nonpolar amino acids

Exopeptidases—act at the carboxy-terminal amino acids shown below:

Enzyme	Carboxy-terminal Amino Acids
Carboxypeptidase A	Aromatic or Nonpolar amino acids
Carboxypeptidase B	Basic amino acids

exopeptidases, which act in a sequential fashion to split large polypeptides and proteins, mainly to oligopeptides of six or fewer amino acid residues. Bile and bicarbonate secreted into the small bowel lumen provide a stable environment promoting pancreatic proteolysis. Recently identified neutral endopeptidases on the brush border of the small intestine digest larger polypeptides as well.

Peptide hydrolases of the small bowel are enzymes that hydrolyze oligopeptides and are present on the brush border surface and within the cytosol of the surface epithelial cells. These enzymes split oligopeptides of six or fewer amino acid residues. Dipeptides and tripeptides may be hydrolyzed at the enterocyte surface or transported into the cell intact and split in the presence of cytosol peptide hydrolases. In contrast with the brush border enzymes, cytosol peptide hydrolases do not cleave oligopeptides more than three amino acids in length. Therefore, the surface enzymes seem most important in the digestion of oligopeptides more than three amino acids in length. At the luminal surface of the small bowel, there are carriers for amino acids, dipeptides, and tripeptides. Digested protein enters the portal vein almost exclusively as free amino acid.

The average adult excretes only 6 to 12 gm of fecal protein despite ingesting 60 to 100 gm of protein and adding another 60 gm of endogenous protein to the intestinal contents each day.[62, 63] Therefore, a large proportion of the endogenous protein from secretions and intestinal desquamation must be reabsorbed. Studies in persons offered a protein-free diet have demonstrated that the small intestine participates in the digestion of endogenous protein.[62] After a balanced meal, about 60% of the protein content is removed before reaching the proximal jejunum.[63] The majority of the remaining nonprotein, alpha-amino nitrogen, is in the form of oligopeptides two to six amino acids in length; free amino acids are present to a lesser extent. Although dietary protein can be identified in the proximal ileal contents, nearly complete digestion and absorption occur by the time that the intestinal contents arrive at the terminal ileum. Less than 1 gm of protein, oligopeptides, and free amino acids passes into the colon.

Gastric Phase of Protein Digestion

Initial digestion of protein in the stomach in the presence of acid and pepsin does not seem essential, as people with total gastrectomy or pernicious anemia with achlorhydria are able to assimilate protein normally.[64] A number of pepsinogens are secreted by the chief cells of the stomach and Brunner's glands of the duodenum and are converted to pepsin at pH less than 5. Pepsins are labile at pH greater than 6. The pepsins are proteases that release large polypeptides and are most active at peptide bonds that include phenylalanine, tyrosine, leucine, and glutamic acid. Hydrochloric acid (HCl) is probably active in protein digestion, because protein absorption from isolated loops of small bowel in animals can be improved by preincubating the protein with either pepsin and HCl or HCl alone.[65]

Small Intestine: Intraluminal Phase of Digestion

Digestion of proteins and large polypeptides in the small intestine is the result of the combined action of pancreatic proteases and mucosal enzymes. Pancreatic proteases are secreted by the pancreas in inactive form, known as *zymogens* (see section on digestion of starch for discussion of pancreatic secretion). Conversion of inactive trypsinogen to active trypsin requires the removal of an N terminal peptide and is catalyzed initially by a mucosal enzyme, enterokinase. In humans, this enzyme appears to be localized to the proximal small bowel. Trypsin activates the other zymogens and trypsinogen itself. Therefore, in persons with enterokinase deficiency, none of the zymogens are activated.[66]

Each pancreatic protease has a unique hydrolytic action at an internal peptide bond (endopeptidase) or terminal peptide bond (exopeptidase) that is complementary to the other enzymes (Table 2–3).[67] Chymotrypsin and elastase expose carboxy-terminal aromatic and nonpolar amino acid residues to the action of carboxypeptidase A. Basic amino acid residues exposed by trypsin at the carboxy-terminal can be split by carboxypeptidase B. The products of pancreatic digestion are oligopeptides of as many as six amino acid residues and, to a small extent, free amino acids. These oligopeptides are resistant to the action of the pancreatic proteases.

In humans, trypsin activity in the proximal bowel is maximal at about 30 minutes after a meal and remains elevated for at least 4 hours.[63] The quantity of trypsin in luminal contents decreases in an aboral gradient. However, as the volume of contents decreases in this direction as well, the concentration of trypsin remains uniform throughout the small bowel and, in the ileum, is still adequate for protein digestion. Fecal nitrogen content does not become abnormal until the pancreatic output of trypsin is less than 10% of normal (Fig. 2–7).[68] This is the same level of pancreatic function at which steatorrhea begins to appear. Bile salts appear to maintain the stability of pancreatic enzymes by increasing the solubility of calcium salts.[69]

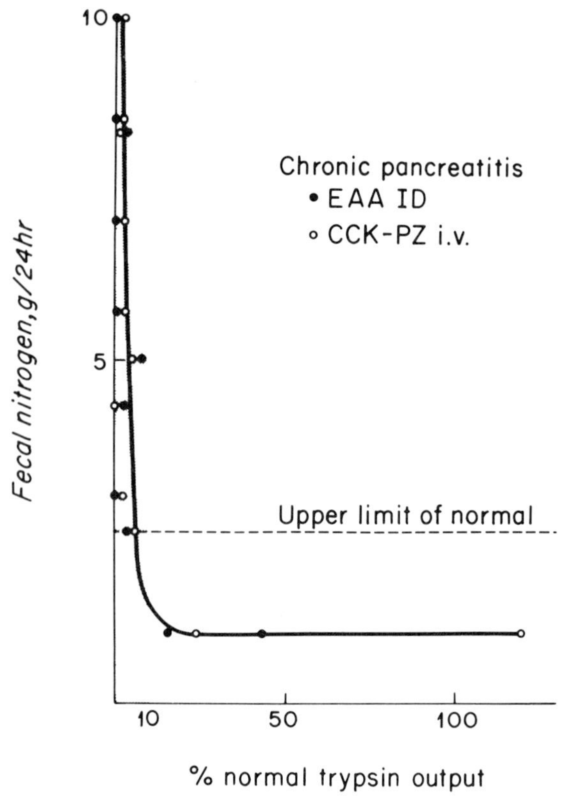

Figure 2–7. Relationship of daily fecal nitrogen excretion to pancreatic trypsin output in adults with chronic pancreatitis. The open and closed circles represent the manner in which pancreatic trypsin secretion was stimulated (intravenous cholecystokinin and intraduodenal essential amino acids, respectively). Nitrogen content of stool does not increase above normal until trypsin output is less than 10% of normal. (Reprinted with permission from DiMagno EP, Go VLW, Summerskill WHJ: Relations between pancreatic enzyme outputs and malabsorption in severe pancreatic insufficiency. *The New England Journal of Medicine,* vol. 288, p. 814, 1973.)

Small Intestine: Mucosal Phase of Digestion

Brush Border Endopeptidase

Persons with severe pancreatic insufficiency nevertheless absorb a portion of ingested protein. The mucosa of the small intestine appears capable of digestion of proteins; animals with nearly total pancreatic insufficiency (secondary to ligation of the pancreatic duct) are able to absorb nearly 40% of a protein meal.[65] Furthermore, when a protein meal is placed in an isolated loop of bowel, 30% of the protein is absorbed over 4 hours. Absorption in this loop is improved by pretreatment of the meal with pepsin and HCl or HCl alone. A group of brush border membrane endopeptidases, distinct from the pancreatic proteases, has been identified and characterized in animals.[70] Initially, three enzymes have been identified. These enzymes have optimum activity at neutral pH, and activity is maximally expressed in the mature region of the villus. The products of action of these enzymes on polypeptides are then further hydrolyzed by aminopeptidase N, suggesting that this group of enzymes acts in concert with this oligopeptidase. Neutral endopeptidases have subsequently been identified in small bowel samples from humans.[71]

Mucosal Peptide Hydrolases

Venous blood from the small intestine contains absorbed protein almost exclusively as free amino acids. Therefore, the small intestine must split oligopeptides that result from pancreatic protease digestion prior to movement into the blood. The mucosal enterocytes of the small intestine contain a group of enzymes that split these oligopeptides, which are known as *peptide hydrolases.*[72–76] Distinctly different enzymes are found at the brush border and in the cytosol of the enterocyte. The brush border enzymes are located on the villous epithelium and act at the mucosal surface in the intestinal lumen. The cytosol peptide hydrolases, which differ from the brush border group in physicochemical and immunochemical properties, act within the surface epithelial cells and are not in contact with the luminal contents. Brush border peptide hydrolases are unique to the small bowel, whereas the cytosol enzymes have been demonstrated in a number of tissues.

About 90% of the total mucosal peptide hydrolase activity for dipeptides and 40% of the activity for tripeptides are found in the cytosol fraction. However, oligopeptides with a chain length of more than three amino acids are not split by the cytosol enzymes. These oligopeptides of four to six amino acid residues are cleaved to shorter peptides and free amino acids by the brush border enzymes. Many dipeptides and tripeptides are potential substrates for either group of hydrolases. Some dipeptides—for example, those with proline—cannot be split by brush border enzymes.

In nature, a huge number of unique dipeptides (400) and tripeptides (8,000) are possible. Therefore, no comprehensive study of digestion and absorption of all the possible oligopeptides has been performed. Most brush border and cytosol peptide hydrolases are aminopeptidases, releasing amino acids singly from the amino-terminal end of the peptide. Carboxypeptidase splits the carboxy-terminal amino acid from those oligopeptides in which proline is the penultimate carboxy-terminal residue.[77] Dipeptidyl aminopeptidase IV splits dipeptides from the amino-terminal when arginine or lysine is the amino-terminal amino acid or proline or alanine is the penultimate amino-terminal residue. Substrate specificity overlaps widely among the peptide hydrolases. Free hydrophobic amino acids (e.g., leucine) inhibit peptide hydrolase activity.[78] Peptide hydrolase activity is responsive to diet, as animals offered a high-protein diet have greater brush peptide hydrolase activity than do animals offered a low-protein diet.[79, 80]

Peptide Absorption

Dipeptides and tripeptides, in contrast with oligosaccharides, can cross the surface epithelium of the small bowel intact. Furthermore, amino acids from a number of oligopeptides have been shown to be assimilated more rapidly than their constituent amino acids from an equimolar solution (Fig. 2–8).[81, 82] The rate of absorption of amino acid from a complex protein hydrolysate is greater than from an amino acid mixture that is based on the composition of the original protein.[81, 83] This observation appears to be the result of a carrier-mediated, active transport process specific for oligopeptides. After a meal, more than half of the nonprotein amino acid in the intestinal contents is in the form of oligopeptides.[62, 63] It is likely that the intact absorption of oligopeptides with two or three amino acid residues is a quantitatively important route for protein assimilation.

A number of lines of evidence have led to the conclusion that dipeptides and tripeptides can be absorbed intact. Persons with congenital defects in transport of specific amino acids by the enterocyte are able, nevertheless, to absorb these amino acids when bound in dipeptides. When the dipeptide GlyGly has been infused into the small intestines of volunteers, low levels of this dipeptide have been found intact in the plasma.[81] Dipeptides that are poorly hydrolyzed at the brush border can be assimilated, although uptake can be decreased by metabolic inhibitors.[84, 85] Some tripeptides are absorbed intact, whereas others may first be split to dipeptides and free amino acids or free amino acids alone. Evaluation of tetrapeptides has been limited, but intact peptide transport has not yet been demonstrated.[86, 87]

Demonstration in humans that dipeptide transport can be saturated and that peptides can competitively inhibit the transport of one another during perfusion studies has confirmed that dipeptide transport is carrier mediated.[81, 88] Free amino acids do not compete with dipeptides for this carrier, and therefore it is distinct from the amino acid carriers. In vitro, transport has been demonstrated to be active, as it occurs against an electrochemical gradient and can be inhibited by anoxia or metabolic inhibitors.[85, 86] An electrochemical gradient for H^+ appears to be the driving force and suggests that H^+ is cotransported with oligopeptides. It appears that there is only one peptide carrier.[89] Affinity to the carrier is influenced by characteristics of both the carboxy- and the amino-terminal amino acids of a peptide.[88–90] Tripeptides have lower affinity than dipeptides.[91] The rate of disappearance of dipeptides during intestinal perfusion in humans is only slightly greater in jejunum than in ileum.[81] A recent study demonstrating paracellular movement of oligopeptide suggests that diffusion of peptides (or solvent drag, or both) may be quantitatively important in protein assimilation.[28]

In human subjects, the amino acid in a tryptic digest of casein is absorbed more rapidly than the amino acid in a comparable mixture of free amino acids.[92] In addition, absorption of the individual amino acids from the casein digest is more uniform than from the amino acid mixture. However, no difference in amino acid absorption was noted when human subjects ingested a fish protein hydrolysate or a comparable mixture of amino acids.[93] The rate of absorption of amino acids from a defined mixture of 12 dipeptides was greater than that from an equimolar mixture of the constituent amino acids in human subjects.[94] This difference is most notable for amino acids with slow rates of absorption. The rates of absorption of amino acids were also more uniform from the dipeptide mixture. This observation is consistent with in vitro studies of hamster jejunum demonstrating more uniform affinity for transport and maximal

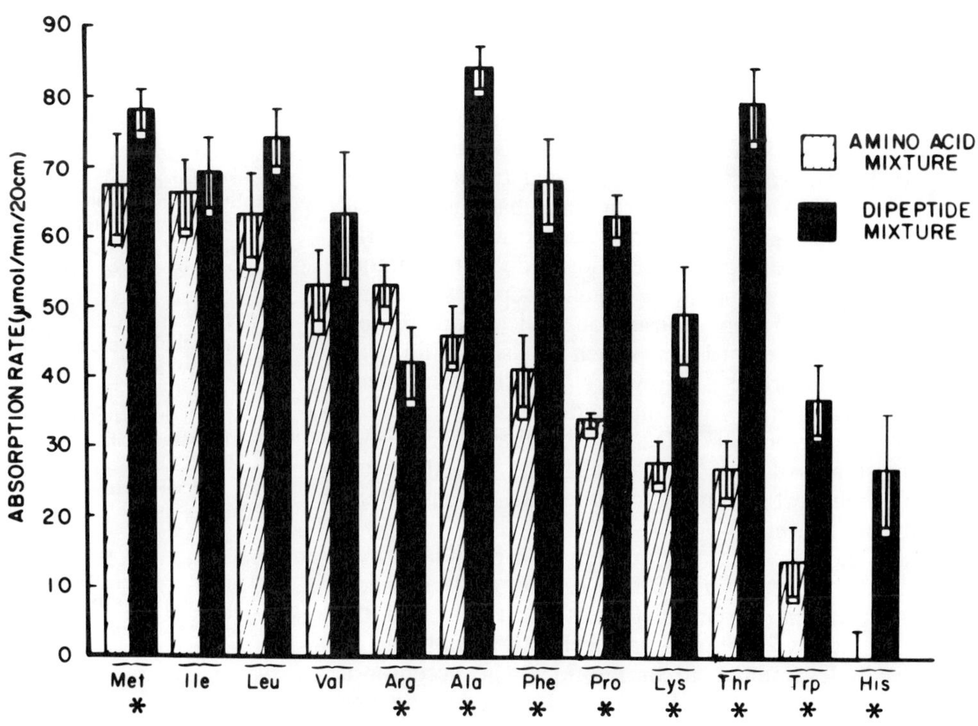

Figure 2–8. Rate of absorption of amino acids from a mixture of 12 glycyl-dipeptides and from a similar mixture of free amino acids. Concentration of each dipeptide and free amino acid was 6 mmol per L. The asterisk signifies a statistically significant difference. Overall, the rate of absorption of individual amino acids is greater from the dipeptide than from the free amino acid mixture. In addition, the rates of assimilation of amino acids from the dipeptide mixture tend to be more uniform. (From Steinhardt HJ, Adibi SA: Kinetics and characteristics of absorption from an equimolar mixture of 12 glycyl-dipeptides in human jejunum. Gastroenterology 1986; 90:579; with permission.)

rate of transport among a group of peptides as compared with the group of free amino acids from which the peptides were composed.[95] In persons with gluten-sensitive enteropathy, the rate of absorption of dipeptides is less severely affected than absorption of amino acids in the jejunum.

Amino Acid Absorption

Absorption of free amino acids in the small intestine can occur by active, Na^+-coupled transport, facilitated transport, or simple diffusion.[96] During active transport, amino acid and Na^+ couple to a carrier molecule at the luminal surface of the microvillus membrane and are then transported across the membrane to be released within the enterocyte. The basolateral Na^+ pump maintains a low intracellular Na^+ concentration, providing the electrochemical gradient that drives Na^+–amino acid transport. In contrast with the single carrier for peptide absorption, it appears that there are multiple amino acid transporters with overlapping specificity. Therefore, some amino acids are carried by more than one system; for example, there are at least four different Na^+-dependent transport systems for neutral amino acids. Oligopeptides and amino acids do not compete for absorption, indicating that the carriers differ. Furthermore, free amino acids are absorbed more rapidly in proximal than in distal small bowel, whereas peptides are absorbed uniformly throughout the small intestine.[81, 97, 98] The relative role of carrier-mediated transport versus diffusion is dependent on the intraluminal concentration of amino acid.[99] At high concentrations, diffusion becomes quantitatively more important. As described for glucose assimilation, activation of the Na^+ cotransporters (including amino acid) is associated with a loosening of tight junctions and an increase in paracellular transport. Facilitated transport appears to have a minor role in amino acid transport.

The existence of hereditary disorders of amino acid transport has been the best evidence that more than one route of absorption of amino acids occurs in humans. Each of these rare autosomal recessive disorders is associated with a defect in amino acid absorption occurring in both enterocytes and proximal tubular cells of the kidney.[100] Defects in neutral and dibasic amino acid absorption occur in Hartnup's disease and cystinuria, respectively. The capacity to absorb adequate amounts of the affected amino acids in oligopeptides prevents more serious nutritional consequences. Lysinuric protein intolerance is a disorder in which dibasic amino acids are poorly absorbed.[101] However, dibasic amino acids are not assimilated from dipeptides as well, and this disorder represents a defect in basolateral transport. The existence of this disorder suggests that there are specific transport systems associated with the basolateral membrane as well.

Brush border gamma-glutamyl transpeptidase may participate in transport of free amino acids or short peptides.[102] This enzyme catalyzes the transfer of the gamma-glutamyl group of intracellular glutathione to the acceptor amino acid or peptide. The acceptor is translocated across the brush border membrane and then released in the presence of gamma-glutamyl cyclotransferase. Activity of gamma-glutamyl transpeptidase is greatest in the proximal small intestine and greatest at the villus tip. Thus, a number of characteristics of this enzyme are consistent with a potential role in amino acid absorption; however, this role is not established.

In healthy volunteers, the rate of absorption of different amino acids at equal concentrations varies.[97, 103, 104] Methionine and the branched-chain amino acids are taken up at the greatest rate, and aspartic and glutamic acid at the lowest rate, from an equimolar mixture of the 18 common dietary amino acids.[103] Similar observations have been made when equimolar mixtures of the eight essential amino acids have been studied.[104] Overall, essential amino acids are somewhat better absorbed than nonessential amino acids. In mixtures, some amino acids competitively inhibit absorption of other amino acids. Among the neutral amino acids, the longer the side chain the greater the affinity for the carrier (e.g., leucine > valine > glycine).[97] Neutral amino acids are absorbed more rapidly than charged amino acids. The L-form of an amino acid is better absorbed than the D-form. Separation of the carboxyl group from the alpha-carbon or substitution of the alpha-amino group slows the rate of absorption of an amino acid.

Intact Protein Absorption

The gastrointestinal tract is the major route of transfer of maternal immunoglobulin for neonates of some species (e.g., rodents and piglets). However, humans absorb intact protein in only trace amounts, and immunoglobulin transfer is transplacental. This process of absorption of minor quantities of macromolecules has relevance for the development of dietary protein hypersensitivity but has little consequence for overall assimilation of protein from diet.

REFERENCES

1. Windmueller HG: Glutamine utilization by the small intestine. Adv Enzymol 1982; 53:201–237.
2. Bond JH, Levitt MD: Quantitative measurement of lactose absorption. Gastroenterology 1976; 70:1058–1062.
3. Bond JH, Currier BE, Buchwald H, et al: Colonic conservation of malabsorbed carbohydrate. Gastroenterology 1980; 78:444–447.
4. Anderson IH, Levin AS, Levitt MD: Incomplete absorption of the carbohydrate in all-purpose wheat flour. N Engl J Med 1981; 304:891–892.
5. Jones JB, Mehta NR, Hamosh M: Alpha-amylase in preterm human milk. J Pediatr Gastroenterol Nutr 1982; 1:43–48.
6. Lindberg T, Skude G: Amylase in human milk. Pediatrics 1982; 70:235–238.
7. Fogel MR, Gray GM: Starch hydrolysis in man: An intraluminal process not requiring membrane digestion. J Appl Physiol 1973; 35:263–267.
8. Stephen AM, Haddad AC, Phillips SF: Passage of carbohydrate into the colon: Direct measurements in humans. Gastroenterology 1983; 85:589–595.
9. Snow P, O'Dea K: Factors affecting the rate of hydrolysis of starch in food. Am J Clin Nutr 1981; 34:2721–2727.
10. Adler G, Beglinder C: Hormones as regulators of pancreatic secretion in man. Eur J Clin Invest 1990; 20:S27–S32.

11. Holst JJ: Neuronal control of pancreatic exocrine secretion. Eur J Clin Invest 1990; 20:S33–S39.
12. Brunner J, Hauser H, Braun H, et al: The mode of association of the enzyme complex sucrase-isomaltase with the intestinal brush border membrane. J Biol Chem 1979; 254:1821–1828.
13. Newcomer AD, McGill DB: Distribution of disaccharidase activity in the small bowel of normal and lactase-deficient subjects. Gastroenterology 1966; 51:481–488.
14. Deren JJ, Broitman SA, Zamcheck N: Effect of diet upon intestinal disaccharidases and disaccharide absorption. J Clin Invest 1967; 46:186–195.
15. Rosensweig NS, Herman RH: Time response of jejunal sucrase and maltase activity to a high-sucrose diet in normal man. Gastroenterology 1969; 56:500–505.
16. Alpers DH, Tedesco FJ: The possible role of pancreatic proteases in the turnover of intestinal brush border protein. Biochim Biophys Acta 1975; 401:28–40.
17. Cook RM, Powell PM, Moog F: Influence of biliary stasis on the activity and distribution of maltase, sucrase, alkaline phosphatase, and leucylnaphthylamidase in the small intestine of the mouse. Gastroenterology 1973; 64:411–420.
18. Gray GM, Santiago NA: Disaccharide absorption in normal and diseased human intestine. Gastroenterology 1966; 51:489–498.
19. McMichael HB, Webb J, Dawson AM: The absorption of maltose and lactose in man. Clin Sci 1967; 33:135–145.
20. Gray GM, Lally GB, Conklin KA: Action of intestinal sucrase-isomaltase and its free monomers on an α-limit dextrin. J Biol Chem 1979; 254:6038–6043.
21. Kelly JJ, Alpers DH: Properties of human intestinal glucoamylase. Biochim Biophys Acta 1973; 315:113–122.
22. Borgstrom B, Dahlqvist A, Lundh G, et al: Studies of intestinal digestion and absorption in the human. J Clin Invest 1957; 36:1521–1536.
23. Dahlqvist A, Borgstrom B: Digestion and absorption of disaccharides in man. Biochem J 1961; 81:411–418.
24. Crane RK: Na^+-dependent transport in the intestine and other animal tissues. Fed Proc 1965; 24:1000–1006.
25. Peerce BE, Clarke RD: Isolation and reconstitution of the intestinal Na^+/glucose cotransporter. J Biol Chem 1990; 265:1731–1736.
26. Haase W, Heitmann K, Friese W, et al: Characterization and histochemical localization of the rat intestinal Na^+–D-glucose cotransporter by monoclonal antibodies. Eur J Cell Biol 1990; 52:297–309.
27. Madara JL: Loosening tight junctions: Lessons from the intestine. J Clin Invest 1989; 83:1089–1094.
28. Atisook K, Madara JL: An oligopeptide permeates intestinal tight junctions at glucose-elicited dilatations. Gastroenterology 1991; 100:719–724.
29. Guy MJ, Deren JJ: Selective permeability of the small intestine for fructose. Am J Physiol 1971; 221:1051–1056.
30. Ravich WJ, Bayless TM, Thomas M: Fructose: Incomplete intestinal absorption in humans. Gastroenterology 1983; 84:26–29.
31. DeNigris SJ, Homash M, Kasbekar DK, et al: Lingual and gastric lipases: Species differences in the origin of prepancreatic digestive lipases and in the localization of gastric lipase. Biochim Biophys Acta 1988; 959:38–45.
32. Moreau H, Gargouri Y, Lecat D, et al: Screening of preduodenal lipases in several mammals. Biochim Biophys Acta 1988; 959:247–252.
33. Tiruppathi C, Balasubramanian KA: Purification and properties of an acid lipase from human gastric juice. Biochim Biophys Acta 1982; 712:692–697.
34. Moreau H, Langier R, Gargouri Y, et al: Human preduodenal lipase is entirely of gastric fundic origin. Gastroenterology 1988; 95:1221–1226.
35. DiPalma J, Kirk CL, Hamosh M, et al: Lipase and pepsin activity in the gastric mucosa of infants, children, and adults. Gastroenterology 1991; 101:116–121.
36. Abrams CK, Hamosh M, Dutta SK, et al: Role of nonpancreatic lipolytic activity in exocrine pancreatic insufficiency. Gastroenterology 1987; 92:125–129.
37. Hamosh M, Bitman J, Liao TH, et al: Gastric lipolysis and fat absorption in preterm infants: Effect of medium-chain triglyceride- or long-chain triglyceride–containing formulas. Pediatrics 1989; 83:86–92.
38. Bernback S, Blackberg L, Hernell O: The complete digestion of human milk triacylglycerol in vitro requries gastric lipase, pancreatic colipase–dependent lipase and bile salt–stimulated lipase. J Clin Invest 1990; 85:1221–1226.
39. Gaskin KJ, Durie PR, Lee L, et al: Colipase and lipase secretion in childhood-onset pancreatic insufficiency: Delineation of patients with steatorrhea secondary to relative colipase deficiency. Gastroenterology 1984;86:1–7.
40. Layer P, Go VLW, DiMagno EP: Fate of pancreatic enzymes during aboral small intestinal transit in humans. Am J Physiol 1986; 251:G475–G480.
41. Layer P, Jansen JB, Cherian L, et al: Feedback regulation of human pancreatic secretion. Gastroenterology 1990; 98:1311–1319.
42. Slaff J, Jacobson D, Tillman CR, et al: Protease-specific suppression of pancreatic exocrine secretion. Gastroenterology 1984; 87:44–52.
43. Brown AL: Microvilli of the human jejunal epithelial cell. J Cell Biol 1962; 12:623–627.
44. Westergaard H, Kietschy JM: Delineation of the dimensions and permeability characteristics of the two major diffusion barriers to passive mucosal uptake in the rabbit intestine. J Clin Invest 1974; 54:718–732.
45. Thomson ABR, Dietschy JM: The role of the unstirred water layer in intestinal permeation. *In* Csaky TZ, ed: Pharmacology of Intestinal Permeation. Vol 2. Berlin, Springer-Verlag, 1984, pp 166–269.
45a. Strocchi A, Levitt MD: A reappraisal of the magnitude and implications of the intestinal unstirred layer. Gastroenterology 1991; 101:843–847.
46. Simmonds WJ, Hofmann AF, Theodur E: Absorption of cholesterol from a micellar solution: Intestinal perfusion studies in man. J Clin Invest 1967; 46:874–890.
47. Shiau Y-F, Levine GM: pH dependence of micellar diffusion and dissociation. Am J Physiol 1980; 239:G177–G182.
48. Proulx P, Aubry H, Brglez I, et al: Studies on the uptake of fatty acids by brush border membranes of the rabbit intestine. Can J Biochem Cell Biol 1984; 63:249–256.
49. Stremmel W, Lotz G, Strohmeyer G, et al: Identification, isolation, and partial characterization of a fatty acid binding protein from rat jejunal microvillus membranes. J Clin Invest 1985; 75:1068–1076.
50. Stremmel W, Strohmeyer G, Berk PD: Hepatocellular uptake of oleate is energy dependent, sodium linked, and inhibited by an antibody to a hepatocyte plasma membrane fatty acid binding protein. Proc Natl Acad Sci U S A 1986; 83:3584–3588.
51. Daniel H, Neugebauer R, Kratz A, et al: Localization of acid microclimate along the intestinal villi of rat jejunum. Am J Physiol 1985; 248:G293–G298.
52. Ruppin H, Bar-Meir S, Soergel KH, et al: Absorption of short-chain fatty acids by the colon. Gastroenterology 1980; 78:1500–1507.
53. Sellin JH, DeSoignie R: Short-chain fatty acid absorption in rabbit colon in vitro. Gastroenterology 1990; 99:676–683.
54. Binder HJ, Mehta P: Short-chain fatty acids stimulate active sodium and chloride absorption in vitro in the rat distal colon. Gastroenterology 1989; 96:989–996.
55. Hoverstad T: Studies of short chain fatty acid absorption (review). Scand J Gastroenterol 1986; 21:257–260.
56. Schmitt MG, Soergel KH, Wood CM, et al: Absorption of short-chain fatty acids from the human ileum. Am J Dig Dis 1977; 22:340–347.
57. Florent C, Flourie B, Leblond A, et al: Influence of chronic lactulose ingestion on the colonic metabolism of lactulose in man (an in vivo study). J Clin Invest 1985; 75:608–613.
58. Harig JM, Soergel KH, Komorowski RA, et al: Treatment of diversion colitis with short-chain fatty acid irrigation. N Engl J Med 1989; 320:23–28.
59. Einarsson K, Angelin B, Johansson C: Biliary lipid metabolism in chronic pancreatitis: Influence of steatorrhea. Gut 1987; 28:1495–1499.
60. Mayer RM, Treadwell CR, Gallo LL, et al: Intestinal mucins and cholesterol uptake in vitro. Biochim Biophys Acta 1985; 833:34–43.
61. Ponz de Leon M, Iori R, Barbolini G, et al: Influence of small bowel transit time on dietary cholesterol absorption in human beings. N Engl J Med 1982; 307:102–103.

62. Adibi SA, Mercer DW: Protein digestion in human intestine as reflected in luminal, mucosal, and plasma amino acid concentrations after meals. J Clin Invest 1973; 52:1586–1594.
63. Chung YC, Kim YS, Shadchehr A, et al: Protein digestion and absorption in human small intestine. Gastroenterology 1979; 76:1415–1421.
64. Taylor WH: Biochemistry of pepsins. *In* Code CF, ed: Handbook of Physiology. Vol 6, Alimentary Canal. Washington, DC, American Physiological Society, 1968, pp 2567–2587.
65. Curtis KJ, Gaines HD, Kim YS: Protein digestion and absorption in rats with pancreatic duct occlusion. Gastroenterology 1978; 74:1271–1276.
66. Hadorn B, Sumida C, Tarlow MJ, et al: The activation of human pancreatic proteinases: Studies on human pancreatic juice and duodenal juice of four children with intestinal enterokinase deficiency. Acta Paediatr Scand 1971; 60:369.
67. Keller PJ: Pancreatic proteolytic enzymes. *In* Code CF, ed: Handbook of Physiology. Vol 6, Alimentary Canal. Washington, DC, American Physiological Society, 1968, pp 2605–2628.
68. DiMagno EP, Go VLW, Summerskill WHJ: Relations between pancreatic enzyme outputs and malabsorption in severe pancreatic insufficiency. N Engl J Med 1973; 288:813–815.
69. Green GM, Nasset ES: Importance of bile in regulation of intraluminal proteolytic enzyme activities in the rat. Gastroenterology 1980; 79:695–702.
70. Song IS, Yoshioka M, Erickson RH, et al: Identification and characterization of brush-border membrane-bound neutral metalloendopeptidases from rat small intestine. Gastroenterology 1986; 91:1234–1242.
71. Guan D, Yoshioka M, Erickson RH, et al: Protein digestion in human and rat small intestine: Role of new neutral endopeptidases. Am J Physiol 1988; 255:G212–G220.
72. Kim YS, Birthwhistle W, Kim YW: Peptide hydrolases in the brush border and soluble fractions of small intestinal mucosa of rat and man. J Clin Invest 1972; 51:1419–1430.
73. Kim YS, Kim YW, Sleisenger MH: Studies on the properties of peptide hydrolases in the brush border and soluble fractions of small intestinal mucosa of rat and man. Biochim Biophys Acta 1974; 370:283–296.
74. Noren O, Dabelsteen W, Sjostrom H, et al: Histological localization of two dipeptidases in the pig small intestine and liver, using immunofluorescence. Gastroenterology 1977; 72:87–92.
75. Tobey N, Heizer W, Yeh R, et al: Human intestinal brush border peptidases. Gastroenterology 1985; 88:913–926.
76. Tobey NA, Lyn-Cook LE, Ulshen MH, et al: Intestinal brush border peptidases: Activities in normal and abnormal peroral intestinal biopsy specimens. J Lab Clin Med 1986; 107:221–227.
77. Aurricchio S, Greco L, Vizia B, et al: Dipeptidyl aminopeptidase and carboxypeptidase activities of the brush border of rabbit small intestine. Gastroenterology 1978; 75:1073–1079.
78. Kim YS, Brophy EJ: Effect of amino acids on purified rat intestinal brush-border membrane aminoologopeptidase. Gastroenterology 1979; 76:82–87.
79. Nicholson JA, McCarthy DM, Kim YS: The responses of rat intestinal brush border and cytosol peptide hydrolase activities to variation in dietary protein content: Dietary regulation of intestinal peptide hydrolases. J Clin Invest 1974; 54:890–898.
80. Reisenauer AM, Gray GM: Abrupt induction of a membrane digestive enzyme by its intraintestinal substrate. Science 1985; 227:70–72.
81. Adibi SA: Intestinal transport of dipeptides in man: Relative importance of hydrolysis and intact absorption. J Clin Invest 1971; 50:2266–2275.
82. Silk DBA, Perrett D, Clark ML: Intestinal transport of two dipeptides containing the same two neutral amino acids in man. Clin Sci Mol Med 1973; 45:291–299.
83. Silk DBA, Nicholson JA, Kim YS: Hydrolysis of peptides within lumen of small intestine. Am J Physiol 1976; 231:1322–1329.
84. Fogel MR, Adibi SA: Assessment of the role of brush border peptide hydrolases in luminal disappearance of dipeptides in man. J Lab Clin Med 1974; 84:327–333.
85. Matthews DM, Addison JM, Burston D: Evidence for active transport of the dipeptide carnosine (β-alanyl-L-histidine) by hamster jejunum in vitro. Clin Sci Mol Med 1974; 46:693–705.
86. Addison JM, Burston D, Payne JW, et al: Evidence for active transport of tripeptides by hamster jejunum in vitro. Clin Sci Mol Med 1975; 49:305–312.
87. Adibi SA, Morse EL: The number of glycine residues which limits intact absorption of glycine oligopeptides in human jejunum. J Clin Invest 1977; 60:1008–1016.
88. Adibi SA, Soleimanpour MR: Functional characterization of dipeptide transport system in human jejunum. J Clin Invest 1974; 53:1368–1374.
89. Das MN, Radhakrishnan AN: Studies on a wide-spectrum intestinal dipeptide uptake system in the monkey and in the human. Biochem J 1975; 146:133–139.
90. Addison JM, Burston D, Dalrymple JA, et al: A common mechanism for transport of di- and tripeptides by hamster jejunum in vitro. Clin Sci Mol Med 1975; 49:313–322.
91. Sleisenger MH, Burston D, Dalrymple JA, et al: Evidence for a single common carrier for uptake of a dipeptide and a tripeptide by hamster jejunum in vitro. Gastroenterology 1976; 71:76–81.
92. Silk DBA, Marrs TC, Addison JM, et al: Absorption of amino acids from an amino acid mixture simulating casein and a tryptic hydrolysate of casein in man. Clin Sci Mol Med 1973; 45:715–719.
93. Silk DBA, Chung YC, Berger KL, et al: Comparison of oral feeding of peptide and amino acid meals to normal human subjects. Gut 1979; 20:291–299.
94. Steinhardt HJ, Adibi SA: Kinetics and characteristics of absorption from an eqimolar mixture of 12 glycyl-dipeptides in human jejunum. Gastroenterology 1986; 90:577–582.
95. Burston D, Matthews DM: Kinetics of influx of peptides and amino acids into hamster jejunum in vitro: Physiological and theoretical implications. Clin Sci 1990; 79:267–272.
96. Hopfer U: Membrane transport mechanisms for hexoses and amino acids in the small intestine. *In* Johnson LR, ed: Physiology of the Gastrointestinal Tract. 2nd ed. New York, Raven Press, 1987, pp 1499–1526.
97 Adibi SA: The influence of molecular structure of neutral amino acids on their absorption kinetics in the jejunum and ileum of human intestine in vivo. Gastroenterology 1969; 56:903–911.
98. Silk DBA, Webb JPW, Lane AE, et al: Functional differentiation of human jejunum and ileum: A comparison of the handling of glucose, peptides, and amino acids. Gut 1974; 15:444–449.
99. Webb KE: Intestinal absorption of protein hydrolysis products: A review. J Anim Sci 1990; 68:3011–3022.
100. Silk DBA: Disorders of nitrogen absorption. Clin Gastroenterol 1982; 11:47–72.
101. Desjeux JF, Rajantie J, Simell O, et al: Lysine fluxes across the jejunal epithelium in lysinuric protein intolerance. J Clin Invest 1982; 65:1382–1387.
102. Garvey TQ, Hyman PE, Isselbacher KJ: γ-Glutamyl transpeptidase of rat intestine: Localization and possible role in amino acid transport. Gastroenterology 1976; 71:778–785.
103. Adibi SA, Gray SJ, Menden E: The kinetics of amino acid absorption and alteration of plasma composition of free amino acids after intestinal perfusion of amino acid mixtures. Am J Clin Nutr 1967; 20:24–33.
104. Adibi SA, Gray SJ: Intestinal absorption of essential amino acids in man. Gastroenterology 1967; 52:837–845.

Chapter 3

Bile Acid Physiology and Alterations in the Enterohepatic Circulation

ERIC A. ARGAO and WILLIAM F. BALISTRERI

Adequate elimination of cholesterol from the body and proper digestion and absorption of dietary lipids require bile acids. The enterohepatic circulation is a critical conservation mechanism; interruption of the enterohepatic circulation allows for fecal loss of bile acids, causing a contracted pool size that may lead to malabsorption and cholesterol gallstone formation. In the immature members of many species, there is an altered bile acid physiology and underdevelopment of the enterohepatic circulation, thereby predisposing to physiologic cholestasis and steatorrhea. This chapter reviews both normal bile acid physiology and the developmental changes seen in immature states. The recent advances that have led to a greater understanding of bile acid physiology and the characterization of defects in bile acid biosynthesis and metabolism and their clinical consequences likewise are presented.

CHEMISTRY

Bile acids are acidic steroid compounds. Their structure consists of a cyclopentanoperhydrophenanthrene nucleus (ABCD rings) that is connected at position 17 to a side chain of variable length with a terminal carboxyl group. In mammals, the side chain is branched and is five carbons (C_{20}–C_{24}) long. The orientation of the hydrogen atom at the C_5 position determines the stereochemistry of the A/B ring junction. The common human bile acids are 5-β (A/B *cis*). The bile acid structure, in the absence of hydroxyl substituents, is referred to as *cholanoic acid* (Fig. 3–1); hence, the term *5-β cholanoic acid* is used to refer to the major bile acids in humans. Bile acids are classified as amphipathic molecules because they contain dissymmetric polar and nonpolar regions, thereby possessing characteristic physicochemical properties in water under appropriate conditions.[1] The polarity (or hydrophilicity) is determined by the pattern (number and orientation) of hydroxyl substituents in the nuclear rings. The addition of a single hydroxyl group can significantly enhance the aqueous solubility of bile acids.[2]

SYNTHESIS

Hepatic catabolism of cholesterol to highly polar bile acids is the major pathway by which cholesterol is eliminated from the body.[3] In humans, about one half of the daily net cholesterol removal is achieved via conversion to bile acids, with the remainder being transported across the canaliculus for elimination from the body in the form of biliary free cholesterol.[4] Conversion of cholesterol to bile acid involves multiple specific reactions, which include hydroxylation, oxidation, and reduction processes; the end product is an unconjugated primary bile acid, either cholic acid or chenodeoxycholic acid (Fig. 3–2).[5, 6]

SECRETION AND BIOTRANSFORMATION

Cholic acid is a *trihydroxy* bile acid (3α,7α,12α-trihydroxy-5β cholanoic acid), whereas chenodeoxycholic

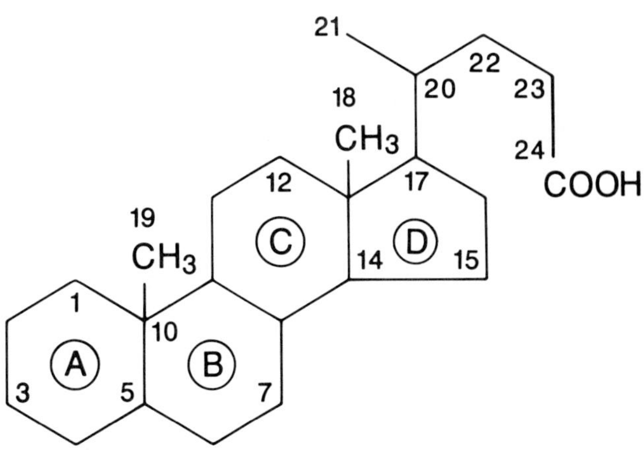

Figure 3–1. Bile acid structure in the absence of hydroxyl substituents is referred to as *cholanoic acid,* consisting of a steroid moiety (ABCD rings) and a side chain terminating in a carboxyl group (C_{24}).

CHOLESTEROL

↓ (1) 7α-hydroxylase*

7α-hydroxycholesterol

↓ (2) 3β-hydroxy steroid dehydrogenase (HSD)/isomerase*

7α-hydroxy-5-cholesten-3-one

↓ (3) 3β-HSD/isomerase*

7α-hydroxy-4-cholesten-3-one

↓ (4) 12α-hydroxylase*

7α,12α-dihydroxy-4-cholesten-3-one

↓ (5) Δ^4-3-oxosteroid-5β-reductase**

7α,12α-dihydroxy-5β-cholestan-3-one

↓ (6) 3α-HSD**

5β-cholestane-3α,7α,12α-triol

↓ (7) C_{26}-hydroxylase***

5β-cholestane-3α,7α,12α26-tetrol

↓ (8) alcohol/aldehyde dehydrogenase**

3α,7α,12α-trihydroxy-5β-cholestan-26-oic acid

↓ (9) peroxisomal oxidation

3α,7α,12α-trihydroxy-5β-cholanoic acid
(CHOLIC ACID)

Figure 3–2. Pathway for biosynthesis of one of the primary bile acids (cholic acid) from cholesterol. Asterisks denote cellular localization of each step: * microsome; ** cytosol; *** mitochondria; note peroxisomal metabolism at step 9. (Modified from Setchell KDR: Disorders of bile acid synthesis. *In* Walker WA, Durie PR, et al, eds: Pediatric Gastrointestinal Disease: Pathophysiology, Diagnosis, Management. Philadelphia, BC Decker, 1991, pp 992–1013; with permission.)

acid is a *dihydroxy* bile acid (3α,7α-dihydroxy-5β cholanoic acid) (Fig. 3–3). Following biosynthesis from cholesterol, unconjugated bile acids must undergo selective side chain amidation at the carboxyl site with glycine or taurine before secretion into bile.[7, 8] The first step in this conjugation process is the formation of a coenzyme A (CoA) derivative (Fig. 3–4).[9] The human liver preferentially conjugates bile acids with taurine.[10] However, because of the relative abundance of glycine compared with taurine in the mature human, bile acid conjugation with glycine normally predominates; typically the glycine to taurine ratio is 3:1.[11–13] Glycine and taurine conjugates are fully resistant to pancreatic digestion with carboxypeptidases,[14] and their passive absorption from the biliary tract is minimal,[15] thereby allowing efficient delivery to the small bowel of all molecules secreted by the liver.[7]

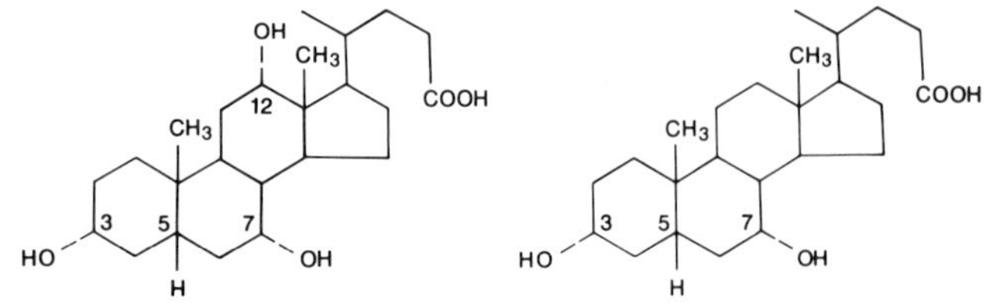

CHOLIC ACID CHENODEOXYCHOLIC ACID

Figure 3–3. Structure of the two primary bile acids found in adult humans: cholic acid (3α,7α,12α-trihydroxy-5β-cholanoic acid) and chenodeoxycholic acid (3α,7α-dihydroxy-5β-cholanoic acid).

The canalicular transport of bile acids is an uphill, saturable, carrier-mediated process that presumably requires an electrical gradient.[16, 17] Bile acid secretion into bile has been shown to stimulate bile flow.[18] The rate of hepatic bile acid secretion in adult humans is approximately 20 to 30 gm per day. Conjugated bile acids are temporarily concentrated in the gallbladder and are released when the gallbladder contracts in response to meal stimulation. Once they reach the intestinal lumen, the small percentage of primary bile acids that escape reabsorption are further metabolized to yield secondary bile acids.

Bile is a mixture of both primary and secondary bile acids. Analysis of normal adult human bile shows that 60 to 80% of the total bile acids are primary bile acids (cholic acid and chenodeoxycholic acid), 25 to 30% deoxycholic acid, and the remainder (about 1%) lithocholic acid, which makes up only a small proportion of the total bile acid pool.[6, 8] Similar to other species, therefore, human bile contains predominantly primary bile acids, whereas feces has mostly secondary bile acids, deoxycholic acid and lithocholic acid.[8, 19–21]

Intestinal bacterial flora release hydrolase enzymes that catalyze the deconjugation process, restoring the

CHOLIC ACID

↓ ATP | coenzyme A

cholyl CoA

↓ glycine ↓ taurine

GLYCOCHOLATE TAUROCHOLATE

Figure 3–4. Bile acid conjugation. The first step in bile acid conjugation is an ATP-driven reaction resulting in formation of a coenzyme A derivative (cholyl CoA). The subsequent step, linkage with either glycine or taurine, is catalyzed by the enzymes, *N*-acyl transferase and ligase; the end product is a glycine- or taurine-conjugated bile acid. In health, the usual glycine to taurine ratio is approximately 3–5:1 owing to the relative abundance of glycine compared with taurine. Conjugation with other compounds, such as glucuronic acid and sulfuric acid, may also occur.

free (unconjugated) cholic acid and chenodeoxycholic acid structure. A subsequent reaction involves 7α-dehydroxylation of cholic acid and chenodeoxycholic acid to form deoxycholic acid (3α, 12α-dihydroxy-5β cholanoic acid) and lithocholic acid (3α-hydroxy-5β cholanoic acid), respectively, the so-called secondary bile acids (Fig. 3–5). Ursodeoxycholic acid is a minor bile acid in human bile but is found in abundance in the bile of various bear species. Ursodeoxycholic acid can either be synthesized directly by the liver (primary bile acid) or produced by hydrogenation and epimerization of 7-keto lithocholic acid (making it a tertiary bile acid). It is quite similar to chenodeoxycholic acid in structure, differing only in spatial orientation of the C_7-hydroxyl group, which is equatorial (beta) in the ursodeoxycholic acid molecule and axial (alpha) in chenodeoxycholic acid.

Quantitatively, 7α-dehydroxylation is the most important bacterial transformation of bile acids.[22] In vitro studies have shown that before the hydroxyl group can be cleaved by bacteria from the C_7 position, deconjugation must first occur in the ileum, impeding ileal bile acid absorption and promoting delivery into the large bowel.[8, 23] Dehydroxylation of the free bile acids is believed to take place mainly in the colon.[8, 24] Numerous anaerobic intestinal bacteria possess deconjugating capacity[25–28]; the dehydroxylating enzymes are far less ubiquitous.[23] In addition to dehydroxylation, bacteria can oxidize the hydroxyl groups to form keto groups.

ENTEROHEPATIC CIRCULATION

The enterohepatic circulation of bile acids is represented in Figure 3–6. The major component of bile acid conservation from the intestinal lumen is reabsorption of conjugated bile acids by active transport. This process accounts for about 80% of the total bile acid reabsorbed. *Active* bile salt transport is localized exclusively to the ileum.[29–37] The efficiency of this transport system for different bile acids is variable.[34] Trihydroxy bile acids are more efficiently absorbed than dihydroxy bile acids, and bile acids conjugated with taurine are more efficiently transported than glycine conjugates. Evidence suggests that ileal bile acid transport requires energy derived from oxidative processes,[30] which allows the mucosal cells to accumulate bile acids against a concentration gradient. Unconjugated bile acids (dihydroxy > trihydroxy) undergo *passive* diffusion throughout the small intestine and the colon.[38–47] Glycine conjugates, especially of the dihydroxy bile acids, chenodeoxycholic and deoxycholic acid, are also typically absorbed passively as a result of their high pKa. Per unit length, the jejunum is thought to be two to three times more effective than the colon in passive bile acid absorption.[48] Although the role of passive absorption at extraileal sites may be of minor importance in the normal enterohepatic circulation, it becomes significant at times when the enterohepatic circulation is interrupted, for example, following ileal resection.[6]

Approximately 0.2 to 0.6 gm,[21, 49, 50] or 5 mg per kg per day,[51] of bile acid appears in feces as bile acid excretory products. This fecal loss is compensated for by synthesis of new primary bile acids in the liver. Fecal excretion accounts for the majority of bile acid loss from the enterohepatic circulation[6]; a small amount (about 2%) is lost through urinary and skin excretion.[49]

After intestinal absorption, bile acids are transported

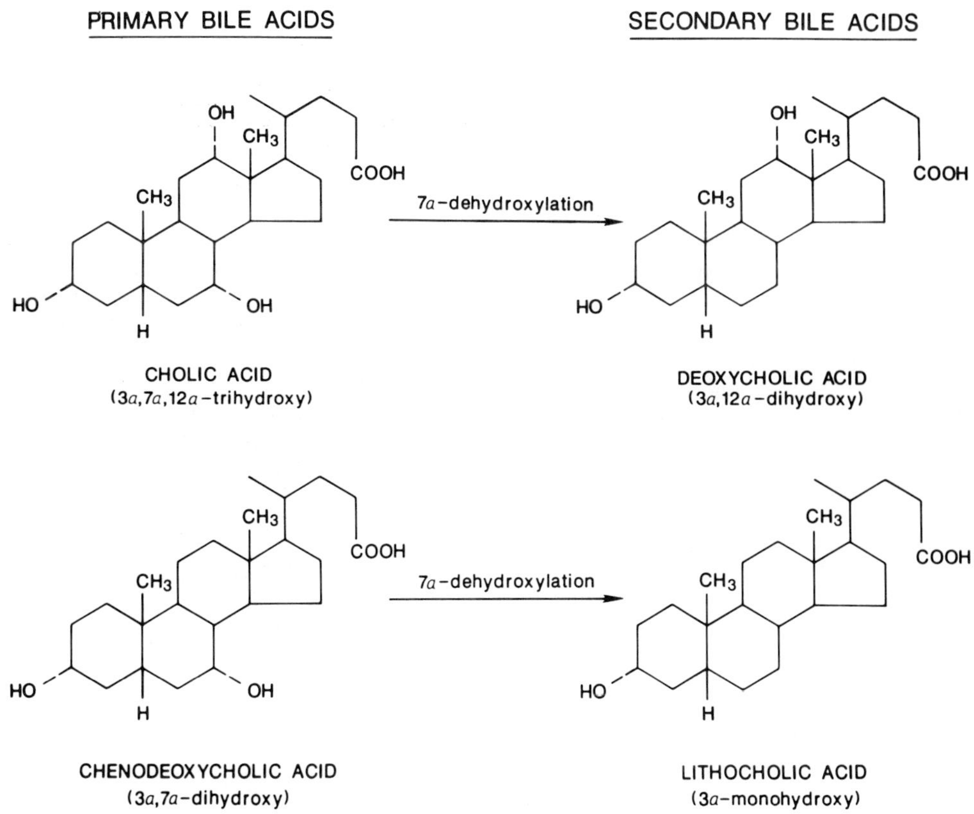

Figure 3–5. Conversion of primary bile acids (cholic acid and chenodeoxycholic acid) to secondary bile acids (deoxycholic acid and lithocholic acid) by intestinal bacterial 7α-dehydroxylation.

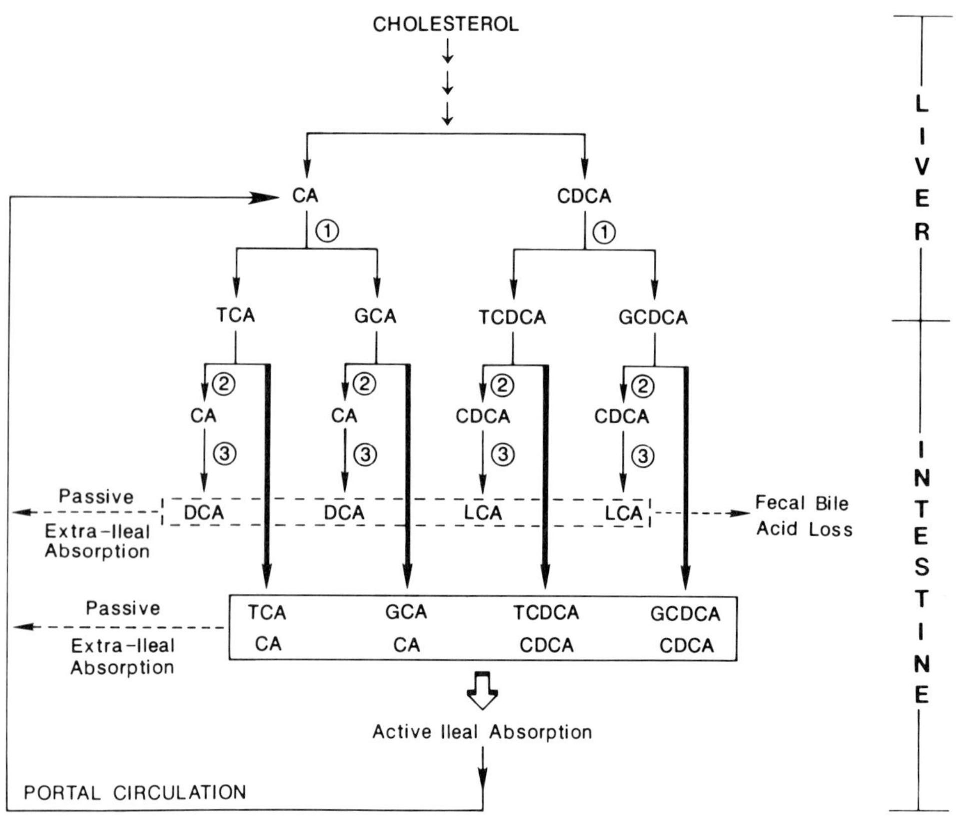

Figure 3–6. The enterohepatic circulation of bile acids. (1) In the liver—conjugation of primary bile acids, cholic acid (CA) and chenodeoxycholic acid (CDCA), with taurine or glycine to form taurocholic acid (TCA), glycocholic acid (GCA), taurochenodeoxycholic acid (TCDCA), and glycochenodeoxycholic acid (GCDCA) prior to secretion. (2) In the intestinal lumen—deconjugation by intestinal bacteria restores primary bile acid structure; followed by (3) bacterial 7α-dehydroxylation to yield the secondary bile acids, deoxycholic acid (DCA) and lithocholic acid (LCA). The primary bile acids are conserved through the enterohepatic circulation; their absorption may occur via passive absorption throughout the small intestine and colon or via active transport in the ileum. Secondary bile acids may be either passively absorbed or lost in feces. After intestinal absorption, bile acids enter the portal circulation and are transported back to the liver, thereby reinitiating the cycle.

back to the liver via the portal vein,[52, 53] bound predominantly to albumin and a smaller proportion to other proteins.[54] The phenomenon of bile acid "spillover" from portal venous blood to the systemic circulation is seen in cases of impaired liver uptake. This results in elevated 2-hour postprandial levels of serum bile acid. On reaching the liver, the bile acids are filtered through endothelial cells and move across the space of Disse to reach the hepatocyte basolateral (or sinusoidal) membrane. Passive diffusion may allow the more hydrophobic bile acids (i.e., unconjugated monohydroxy and dihydroxy forms) to traverse the sinusoidal membrane.[55, 56] In humans, however, most of the bile acids to be cleared from portal blood by the hepatocyte are amidates of cholic acid, chenodeoxycholic acid, and deoxycholic acid[9]; these require an active transport system that utilizes the Na^+ gradient across the basolateral membrane as a driving force.[57] What was formerly believed to be an Na^+-independent transport mechanism[58] is now suggested to be a nonionic diffusion process.[59]

Once inside the liver, unconjugated primary and secondary bile acids are again conjugated with glycine or taurine, together with newly synthesized bile acids, before secretion into bile. For this reason, there are normally *no* unconjugated bile acids in bile.[6] In addition, 7-rehydroxylation does not occur in humans; therefore, the reabsorbed secondary bile acids, lithocholic acid and deoxycholic acid, remain intact throughout the enterohepatic circulation.[60]

Lithocholic acid is considered to be a hepatotoxic bile acid[61]; it is known to induce cholestasis in experimental animals,[62, 63] and, together with deoxycholic acid, may promote intestinal carcinogenesis.[64] Lithocholic acid undergoes sulfation in the liver at the 3α-hydroxyl group prior to its excretion into bile[65]; despite being only about 60% complete in healthy subjects,[66] this process is believed to be vital for detoxification.[62, 65–68] Sulfation may be responsible for the limited passive absorption of lithocholic acid in the jejunum and active absorption in the ileum, resulting in a small pool size for this bile acid.[67] In primary rat hepatocyte studies, sulfation of lithocholate and its conjugates was shown to be a slow process, unlike amidation of the free (unconjugated) form, which was rapid and nearly complete.[69] Sulfated glycolithocholic acid (SGLC) is the major metabolite of lithocholic acid in normal human bile[66, 68, 70] and is the form of lithocholic acid that has been shown to be highly cholestatic in rat; the taurine conjugate is less cholestatic.[71] SGLC has a strong binding activity to free calcium ions and may coprecipitate when a critical solubility concentration is achieved inside the hepatocyte or in the canaliculus.[72] Taurine conjugation prevents biliary calcium–dependent precipitation.[73] If calcium precipitation does not occur prior to bile acid release from the liver and biliary tract, sulfated lithocholic acid conjugates may bind to insoluble calcium phosphate in the intestine and potentially prevent accumulation of lithocholic acid in the enterohepatic circulation.[74] Bile acid sulfation is increasingly recognized as a significant biotransformation process in disease states. Primary bile acid conjugates may be sulfated and excreted in the urine in cholestasis.[66]

INTERRUPTION OF THE ENTEROHEPATIC CIRCULATION

The enterohepatic circulation of bile acids may be disrupted in various ways. Pharmacologic agents such as cholestyramine and colestipol (i.e., bile acid–binding resins), external diversion of bile flow as in a biliary fistula, and ileal resection all interrupt the normal recycling of bile acids. Bile acid malabsorption resulting from the use of cholestyramine or as a consequence of ileal disease (or resection) alters the bile acid pool in both size and composition. Malabsorbed conjugated bile acids enter the colon, where they may be deamidated and, to some extent, reabsorbed as free bile acids.[74] This results in increased levels of unconjugated bile acids in the portal circulation. In healthy subjects, approximately 30 to 40% of total serum bile acids is accounted for by unconjugated cholic acid, whereas in patients with ileal resection, this proportion may exceed 50%. The loss of malabsorbed bile acids into the colon and stool is compensated for by hepatic biosynthesis of bile acids. When the loss far exceeds the rate of synthesis, however, contraction of the bile acid pool size occurs. The overall bile acid deficit seen in these conditions has numerous consequences. Intraluminal bile salt deficiency is known to impair the formation of micelles, thereby causing malabsorption of fat and fat soluble vitamins. Biliary bile acid depletion may jeopardize cholesterol solubility in bile, which predisposes to cholesterol gallstone formation.[6]

When the primary bile acids are prevented from contact with intestinal bacteria (as in biliary diversion or malabsorption), 7α-dehydroxylation and formation of secondary bile acids does not occur, and deoxycholic acid rapidly disappears from the circulation. A dramatic rise in the glycine:taurine bile salt ratio from a normal level of 2 to 3:1 to 12 to 20:1[13, 75, 76] is thought to occur because of taurine depletion.[6] A clinical consequence of the increased glycine:taurine bile salt ratio is the development of hyperoxaluria and formation of renal calculi.[76, 77] When the bile acids conjugated with glycine are not absorbed from the small bowel, colonic bacteria are able to mediate deconjugation, liberating increased quantities of glycine. Glycine can then be further metabolized by bacterial enzymes to glyoxalate that, when absorbed, undergoes hepatic oxidation to oxalic acid, finally to appear as oxalate crystals in the kidney and urine during excretion.[6] This problem is further complicated by changes in colonic mucosal permeability caused by chenodeoxycholic acid and deoxycholic acid, which may result in increased absorption of dietary oxalate.[78] Taurine administration to patients who have undergone ileal resection has been shown to correct and treat the hyperoxaluric state.[76, 77]

Another major consequence of interruption of the enterohepatic circulation is a marked change in bile acid synthesis rate, owing to a lack of feedback inhibition; this will be discussed in greater detail in the following section.

REGULATION OF BILE ACID SYNTHESIS

Much effort has been expended in an attempt to define the mechanisms and modulating factors that regulate bile acid synthesis. Growth hormone, thyroid hormone, insulin, and adrenal cortical hormones all have been considered to be important factors in the regulation of bile acid synthesis. Studies using a rat model have suggested that growth hormone can modulate bile acid synthesis.[79] In growth hormone–deficient children, increased micellar bile acid concentrations were detected in jejunal aspirates following growth hormone treatment,[80] suggesting that growth hormone causes an increase in secretion of bile acids or in bile acid synthesis. Another study has demonstrated increased hepatic bile acid synthesis and bile acid pool size after 6 months of hormonal replacement therapy in growth hormone–deficient patients, with no change in total cholesterol synthesis, suggesting an effect mediated via the enzyme cholesterol 7α-hydroxylase.[81] Cholesterol 7α-hydroxylase activity is believed to exhibit a circadian rhythm that may be hormonally regulated, as evidenced by inhibition following adrenalectomy or hypophysectomy, or both.[82] In the rat, the level of cholesterol 7α-hydroxylase activity parallels the diurnal fluctuation in plasma corticotropin and corticosterone concentration.[83] Glucocorticoids, especially dexamethasone, have been shown to stimulate the synthesis of bile acids by inducing cholesterol 7α-hydroxylase activity in hybrid cells of rat hepatocytes and hepatoma cells[84] and in primary monolayer rat hepatocyte cultures.[83] Metabolism of 7α-hydroxycholesterol to bile acids, an intermediate step in the bile acid pathway, was unaffected. Conversely, the activity of cholesterol 7α-hydroxylase may be inhibited by ethinyl estradiol, thereby blocking bile acid synthesis.[85, 86] Cholesterol 7α-hydroxylase is a microsomal enzyme that is not barbiturate inducible,[87] although small doses of phenobarbital may enhance bile acid synthesis in primates.[88]

The concept of bile acid "negative biofeedback regulation" was developed to account for the stimulation of bile acid synthesis that occurs in conditions in which the enterohepatic circulation is interrupted.[89] In 1957, Eriksson[90] first reported a marked increase (10- to 20-fold) in hepatic bile acid synthesis in bile fistula rats. This finding was subsequently confirmed in other animal and human experiments in which bile acid depletion was induced, using either cholestyramine feeding or bile duct diversion, to enhance the synthesis of bile acids through increased 7α-hydroxylase activity.[90–101]

Unlike the stimulatory effect seen with bile acid depletion, the effect of bile acid feeding or infusion on bile acid synthesis has remained controversial. Attempts to reconstruct the enterohepatic circulation in bile fistula rats by bile acid infusion have yielded discordant findings with regard to the suppressive effect on the synthesis of bile acids. When Bergstrom and Danielsson[91] reinfused bile acids into the terminal portion of the common bile duct in biliary-diverted rats, the expected rebound (compensatory increase) in bile acid synthesis was suppressed. Subsequent animal and human experiments have shown that reinfusion of bile acids inhibited the synthesis of bile acids and the activity of cholesterol 7α-hydroxylase.[102–109] The dihydroxy bile acids, chenodeoxycholic acid and deoxycholic acid, have been noted to be potent inhibitors of bile acid synthesis in vivo in humans as well as in rats[110–114] and also in cultured hepatocytes of young weaned pigs.[115] Although this inhibition of bile acid synthesis is believed to be mediated at the level of cholesterol 7α-hydroxylase, direct suppression of enzyme activity does not seem to be a key factor.[116–119] Regulation is thought to be achieved by modulation of enzyme turnover rate, that is, increased synthesis or decreased degradation.[119–121] A recent study has suggested that bile acids regulate 7α-hydroxylase at the transcriptional level.[122] Bile acids are also known to inhibit the activity of 3-hydroxy-3-methylglutaryl-coenzyme A (HMG-CoA) reductase, which is the rate-limiting enzyme in cholesterol synthesis. Intravenous infusion of mevinolin, a potent inhibitor of HMG-CoA reductase, has been shown to inhibit cholesterol and bile acid secretion in rat studies both in vivo[89] and in vitro.[118, 123–125] Cholesterol availability may therefore be significant in regulating bile acid synthesis. Taurocholic acid is believed to inhibit cholesterol synthesis or enhance biliary cholesterol secretion, or both, resulting in depletion of a critical cholesterol pool in the liver. This effect, in turn, may suppress bile acid synthesis because of decreased cholesterol substrate availability.[126] Another mechanism of feedback inhibition was proposed by Stange and associates in 1988.[114] In a study comparing intact and colectomized rats, they noted that dietary cholic acid or taurocholic acid suppressed bile acid formation indirectly via colonic formation and absorption of the secondary bile acid deoxycholic acid.

The concept of feedback regulation of synthesis of bile acids has been challenged. No inhibition of synthesis was seen when bile acids, at concentrations exceeding those measured in portal blood, were added to freshly suspended or monolayer cultured hepatocytes of rat and rabbit.[118, 123, 124, 127] Similar absence of inhibition of bile acid synthesis has been reported in in vivo infusion studies in humans and bile-diverted rats using taurocholic acid or ursodeoxycholic acid.[89, 110, 112, 113, 126, 128] Varying the infusion rate of taurocholate into either the jugular vein or the duodenum of bile-diverted rats was shown to enhance biliary cholesterol secretion and bile flow but not to suppress bile acid synthesis.[89] The conflicting observations obtained from different laboratories may be related to the difficulty in achieving normal physiologic bile acid hepatic flux rates in the laboratory without causing injury or death to the animal.[129] The use or nonuse of bicarbonate supplementation in bile fistula rat studies,[129] the structure (hydrophobicity) of the bile acids utilized, the hydrophobic-hydrophilic balance of the bile salt pool,[121] and the level of differentiation of cultured cells used can also affect the outcome of experiments on bile acid regulation. Recent work by Lillienau and colleagues[130] suggested that negative feedback regulation of the enterohepatic circulation may also occur at the active ileal bile acid transport level.

PHYSIOLOGIC FUNCTIONS OF BILE ACIDS

In addition to being involved in feedback regulation of bile acid synthesis, bile acids are known to play a major role in other multiple physiologic hepatobiliary and intestinal processes (Table 3–1).

Hepatobiliary

In the absence of bile acid secretion, the liver is able to secrete a watery bile, commonly referred to as *bile acid–independent bile flow*.[132, 133] Active bile acid transport in the liver and secretion into bile, however, accounts for the predominant regulatory mechanism of bile formation and secretion.[134] This portion is known as *bile acid–dependent flow*, associated with simultaneous biliary lipid, phospholipid, and cholesterol secretion. Unconjugated bile acids, in general, have been shown to induce a greater rate of bile flow compared with their conjugated forms.[135]

Bile acids may modulate the synthesis of cholesterol via effects on the HMG-CoA reductase enzyme. In vitro studies using human liver slices have shown that bile acids regulate phospholipid synthesis.[136] Gurantz and Hofmann[135] demonstrated that the nuclear (hydroxyl substituents) and side chain structure of bile acids are major determinants of their capacity to induce lipid and cholesterol secretion. Using a bile fistula hamster model, they infused pure bile acids at physiologic rates into the proximal small bowel and showed that, regardless of the conjugation state, most of the bile acids induced secretion of cholesterol and phospholipid in a dose-related manner. The ursocholic acid conjugate had negligible secretory effects. The induction ability of the various bile acids, in order of potency from the highest to the lowest, was as follows: chenodeoxycholic acid > urso-

Table 3–1. PHYSIOLOGIC FUNCTIONS OF BILE ACIDS

Liver and Biliary Tract
Induce choleresis (bile acid–dependent flow)
Regulate phospholipid and cholesterol synthesis and transport across the canaliculus
Induce phospholipid and cholesterol secretion
Solubilize and transport biliary cholesterol
Desaturate bile (decrease cholesterol concentration)
Precipitate calcium
Intestine
Micelle formation
Aid in fat digestion
Allow absorption of fat and fat-soluble compounds
Regulate colonic absorption of water and electrolytes
Regulate gastrointestinal motility
Cathartic effect
Effect on neurotransmitters
Increase intracellular Ca^{2+} concentration
Modulate secretin release

Modified from Balistreri WF, Setchell KDR: Clinical implications of bile acid metabolism. *In* Silverberg M, Daum F, eds: Textbook of Pediatric Gastroenterology. Chicago, Year Book Medical Publishers, 1987, pp 72–89; with permission.

deoxycholic acid > cholic acid > ursocholic acid. The same pattern was observed for the conjugated derivatives. Others have confirmed that bile acid–dependent biliary cholesterol and phospholipid secretion increases as a function of bile acid hydrophobicity.[137]

Among several pure bile acids studied, chenodeoxycholic acid has been proved to produce unsaturated bile.[138, 139] This property has been the basis for the use of chenodeoxycholic acid for dissolution of cholesterol gallstones.

Bile acid anions are important potential buffers for intraluminal calcium.[140] This may prevent calcium from precipitating with other anions (e.g., bilirubinate to form pigment gallstones) and may likewise affect calcium interaction in the intestinal lumen.

Intestinal

After secretion into the hepatobiliary tract or release from the gallbladder, or both, bile acids enter the duodenum as mixed micelles. Micelles consist of an external surface that is hydrophobic and an internal hydrophilic core.[141] A minimal concentration of bile acids (critical micellar concentration [CMC]) must be present in the proximal small intestine to carry out designated functions vital for the process of fat absorption, which include (1) modulation of fat hydrolysis by lipase; (2) solubilization of products of lipolysis; and (3) delivery of free fatty acids and monoglycerides to the enterocyte absorptive surface.[142–144] In addition to dietary fatty acids, monoglycerides, phospholipids, and cholesterol, fat-soluble vitamins may be solubilized in micellar form to facilitate absorption. The CMC of an individual bile acid is significantly influenced by nuclear and side chain structure. Hydroxyl substitution of the steroid nucleus results in loss of micelle-forming ability; trihydroxy conjugates have a higher CMC than do dihydroxy conjugates.[143] Likewise, shortening of the side chain length results in a higher CMC.[145]

Bile acids are known to have a striking effect on colonic absorptive activity. In vivo studies of the human colon have demonstrated that dihydroxy bile acid solutions induced continuous secretion or inhibition of absorption of sodium, potassium, and water.[146] This may explain the cathartic action of excessive quantities of bile acids in the colon. Furthermore, bile acids in the colon have also been shown to accelerate motility in both animal and human models.[147–149] Studies on the effect of various bile acids on colonic myoelectrical activity in dogs suggested that deoxycholic acid may enhance motility through effects on the action of neurotransmitters of colonic smooth muscle or by increasing intracellular calcium ion concentrations by enhancing its absorption.[150]

Bile acids have also been demonstrated to have a potential role in regulating gastrointestinal hormone output. Based on in vivo studies involving bile salt infusion into the duodenum of human subjects, it was concluded that bile acids, in concentration and composition similar to that in the gallbladder, have the ability to induce the release of immunoreactive secretin from human intestine.[151] The mechanism remains to be studied.

PHYSIOLOGIC IMMATURITY OF BILE ACID METABOLISM AND THE ENTEROHEPATIC CIRCULATION

Developmental maturation must occur in the liver and gastrointestinal tract to allow a successful transition from the intrauterine to the extrauterine environment.[152] Immaturity of bile acid metabolism and the enterohepatic circulation is seen in the immature members of many species, including preterm and term human infants (Table 3–2).[153–158] Human fetal bile acid synthesis has been demonstrated beginning at the 12th to the 16th week of gestation.[160, 161] Hepatic α-hydroxylation is thought to be underdeveloped in the fetus, resulting in a decreased cholic acid:deoxycholic acid ratio compared with adults.[162] In a study of normal newborn infants, Watkins and coworkers[153] showed that the mean infant cholate pool size was significantly less than that found in adults (290 versus 605 mg per m^2), with a similar decrease in bile acid synthetic rate (110 for infants versus 194 mg per m^2 per day for adults). Further evidence indicating immaturity of bile acid synthesis is the qualitative difference of the bile acid pool, that is, the presence of "atypical" bile acids formed via fetal biosynthetic pathways.[163] Many of the bile acids identified in meconium and amniotic fluid are also found in human fetal bile.[162–166] These include compounds hydroxylated at the C_1, C_4, and C_6 positions of the steroid moiety and coplanar bile acid molecules such as allo-bile acids and the 3β-hydroxy-Δ-5 compounds. These compounds are typically not detected in significant amounts in healthy adults; in fact, at term, the monohydroxy bile acids, lithocholic and 3β-hydroxy-5-cholenoic acids, account for only a small percentage of the total bile acids.[167] It is unlikely that these atypical bile acids are of maternal origin; rather, their presence may reflect a primary fetal

Table 3–2. EXPERIMENTAL DATA THAT DELINEATE THE PERIOD OF *IMMATURITY* OF BILE ACID SYNTHESIS AND METABOLISM IN EARLY LIFE

Elevated serum bile acid levels (physiologic cholestasis)
Contracted bile acid pool size
Altered (qualitative and quantitative) bile acid synthesis
Decreased synthesis rate
Presence of "atypical" bile acids
Impaired bile acid biotransformation (amidation, sulfation)
Altered distribution of bile acid pool (predominantly enterohepatic)
Low rate of hepatic bile acid excretion and bile flow
Decreased concentration of intraluminal bile acids
Inefficient active ileal bile acid transport (decreased functional bile acid carriers?)
Impaired hepatic bile acid uptake from portal venous blood
Absence of portal to centrilobular gradient for bile acid uptake

Modified from Balistreri WF, Schubert WK: Liver disease in infancy and childhood. *In* Schiff L, Schiff ER, eds: Diseases of the Liver. 6th ed. Philadelphia, JB Lippincott, 1986, pp 1337–1426; with permission.

hepatic biosynthetic pattern. Atypical bile acids may be unable to mediate bile flow and thus play a role in the low rates of hepatic excretion. In addition, monohydroxy bile acids are thought to be cholestatic, thereby impairing bile acid excretion and bile flow.[168] It has been suggested that measurement of the monohydroxy bile acids in amniotic fluid may provide an indication of fetal immaturity.[165] Moreover, it appears that a resurgence of the fetal bile acid synthetic pathway occurs during conditions of cholestasis.[163] Another type of atypical bile acid, nonsulfated tetrahydroxylated bile acid, is seen in the urine of healthy newborns[169] as well as in cholestatic children and adults.[163] Polyhydroxylation renders bile acids more soluble and may therefore allow elimination by an alternate route.

Bile acid conjugation and sulfation are not fully developed in fetal and suckling rats.[170–172] The rate of bile acid conjugation in the late fetal and newborn liver is approximately 5 to 10% of that noted in adult rats. A rapid maturation of conjugation is observed at weaning and is fully developed by the age of 2 months. During human gestation, primary bile acids are predominantly conjugated with taurine.[173] Taurine conjugates remain as the major bile acid form until well into the first year of life, after which the glycine:taurine ratio approaches the adult level of 3:1.[160, 174, 175] A similar pattern of predominance of taurine conjugation in early life is seen in fetal and newborn rabbits and rats.[176, 177]

The ability to excrete bile acids seems to vary from species to species. Mature hepatic excretory function has been reported in near-term fetal dogs (excretory rate of 80% of administered cholic acid in 6–10 hours),[178] whereas monkeys of comparable gestational age were found to have a lower capacity for bile salt turnover and excretion (excretion of 33% of infused dose).[179] A similar reduced rate of bile acid secretion has been shown in fetal and newborn sheep.[180]

Studies using the guinea pig model have demonstrated that passive diffusion of taurocholate is the only route for intestinal transport and absorption during the fetal and neonatal stages and is the single mode of jejunal transport throughout life.[181] It has been suggested previously that in many animal species, including humans, ileal active transport is either absent or inefficiently developed at birth and that the maturation process may proceed at a rate that varies from species to species.[155, 181–184] In the guinea pig, for example, active ileal transport appears on postnatal day 5 and persists into adulthood[181]; maturation takes place in dogs between 2 and 5 weeks of age.[183] Rat ileal uptake is exclusively passive on postnatal days 14 to 16; this changes to a combined active and passive process by day 18.[185] The postnatal appearance of ileal active taurocholate transport occurs during the third postnatal week in rats[182, 184, 186, 187]; kinetic analysis suggests that this may be the result of an increase in functional bile acid carriers within the ileal brush border membrane.[184] Other rat studies have shown that although the absence of thyroxine or glucocorticoids may alter the active transport system expression,[188, 189] these hormones do not seem essential for the appearance of the transport system.[185, 189] In vitro human experiments using everted jejunal and ileal rings have also shown that the active ileal transport mechanism is absent in the fetus and neonate.[155] Kinetic studies using isotopes of cholate and chenodeoxycholate, however, failed to show results consistent with interruption of enterohepatic circulation in newborn infants, suggesting immaturity, and not complete absence, of active ileal bile salt transport.[190] Uphill active transport was demonstrated in ileal specimens beginning only at 8 months of life. Aside from developmental changes seen in bile acid transport and absorptive capacity of ileal brush border membrane, another intraluminal event that undergoes changes with age is the distribution of taurocholate pool size, as shown by Little and associates[191] in the rat model. On day 19 of the 21-day gestation in rats, the gut contains only 1/17th as much taurocholate as the liver; by day 21, there is an equal proportion in gut and liver. On postnatal day 5, the amount of taurocholate found in the intestine is six times that in the liver, which in the adult is 20 times higher. This developmental change in taurocholate pool distribution may indicate maturation of hepatic enzyme systems or secretory mechanism, or both.

Utilizing hepatocyte basolateral membrane vesicles isolated from 14-day-old rats, Suchy and colleagues[192] demonstrated marked impairment in hepatic uptake of taurocholate. A progressive increase in uptake is seen with maturation.[193] Studies carried out in the suckling rat, using labeled bile acid analogue (^{125}I-cholylglycyltyrosine) injected into the portal vein, showed a homogeneous pattern of distribution throughout the acinus, suggesting absence of a lobular gradient for bile acid uptake.[194] This is in contrast with the portal to centrilobular gradient for uptake observed in the adult rat.[195]

Impaired hepatic uptake, transport, or secretion of bile acids in the immature species may be reflected in elevated serum bile acid concentrations in early life.[196] This becomes even more impressive in the context of a contracted bile acid pool size and an undeveloped (or underdeveloped) ileal active transport mechanism. Human infants demonstrate high levels of serum bile acids from birth up to about 6 to 8 weeks, followed by a gradual decline to adult concentrations during the first 4 to 6 months of life.[197] An exaggerated rise in serum bile acid levels in response to meals is also seen in infants but not older children, suggesting defective uptake by the liver.

Hormones may modulate the development of the enterohepatic circulation and changes in bile acid metabolism. Administration of glucocorticoids to pregnant rats and human subjects is known to result in expansion of the bile salt pool in the offspring,[154, 177, 191] presumably mediated by enhanced hepatic bile acid synthesis or transport, or both. Bile salt synthesis and secretion were likewise stimulated (50-fold) by cortisol in in vitro studies using fetal hepatocyte culture.[198] Dexamethasone has been shown to cause redistribution of the taurocholate pool to the intestine,[191] suggesting enhanced bile flow. Thyroid hormone does not appear to be directly involved in changes in the enterohepatic circulation and bile acid metabolism, including cholate turnover rate and bile acid pool size.[199, 200]

Immaturity at multiple sites of the enterohepatic circulation of bile acids predisposes an infant to cholestasis during times of stress or injury. These include sepsis, drugs, toxins, viral insults, or chemical agents (organic and inorganic), such as in total parenteral nutrition solutions. The newborn likewise undergoes a state of "physiologic steatorrhea," during which fat is poorly digested and is therefore malabsorbed. This may arise secondary to the contracted bile salt pool size, impaired bile flow, decreased hepatic bile acid secretion, low concentration of intraluminal bile acids, and impaired bile acid transport and absorption from the intestine because of a poorly developed ileal active transport system.

INBORN ERRORS OF BILE ACID SYNTHESIS AND METABOLISM

Inborn errors of bile acid synthesis and metabolism may be classified as *primary*, related to a specific enzyme deficiency, or *secondary*, arising from organellar (such as peroxisomal) or organ dysfunction (Table 3–3).[201]

Primary Defect

Cerebrotendinous xanthomatosis is a disorder involving a defect in cholesterol side chain degradation.[202] Two other known enzyme deficiencies affecting bile acid synthesis include 3β-hydroxy-Δ^5-C_{27} steroid dehydrogenase/isomerase deficiency[203, 204] and Δ^4-3-oxosteroid-5β-reductase deficiency,[205] both of which result in defective transformation of the steroid moiety. In 3β-hydroxy-Δ^5-C_{27} steroid dehydrogenase deficiency (see Fig. 3–2, step 2), cholic acid and chenodeoxycholic acid are not synthesized. A marked elevation in 7-hydroxy-cholesterol level, the substrate for the deficient enzyme, is found in serum. Oral bile acid replacement (chenodeoxycholic acid) has been used successfully in one case.[206] Δ^4-3-Oxosteroid-5β-reductase, the enzyme required for the conversion of Δ^4-3-oxo-C_{27}-intermediates to 3α-hydroxy-5β(H) compounds in the bile acid biosynthetic pathway, has been shown to be deficient in identical twin infants with severe intrahepatic cholestasis and giant cell hepatitis (see Fig. 3–2, step 5). The rate of bile acid synthesis was markedly diminished in this disorder; bile contained trace quantities of bile acids, whereas urinary bile acid consisted mainly of Δ^4-3-oxo-bile acids. Evidence of hepatocellular damage and cholestasis was seen in both biochemical testing of serum and histopathologic examination of liver tissue.[205, 207] Combination bile acid therapy with cholic acid and ursodeoxycholic acid normalized hepatic biochemical abnormalities and bile canalicular morphology associated with decreased Δ^4-3-oxo- and allo-bile acids.[201, 202, 208]

Table 3–3. INBORN ERRORS OF BILE ACID SYNTHESIS AND METABOLISM

Primary Defect
Defect in cholesterol side chain degradation
Cerebrotendinous xanthomatosis
Defect in steroid nucleus transformation
3β-hydroxy steroid dehydrogenase/isomerase deficiency
Δ^4-3-oxosteroid–5β reductase deficiency
Secondary Defect (Due to Peroxisomal Dysfunction)
Defect with loss of all peroxisomal functions (peroxisomes absent)
Zellweger's (cerebrohepatorenal) syndrome
Neonatal adrenoleukodystrophy
Infantile Refsum's disease
Hyperpipecolic acidemia
Leber's congenital amaurosis
Defect with loss of several peroxisomal functions
Zellweger-like syndrome
Rhizomelic chondrodysplasia punctata
Defect with loss of a single peroxisomal function
Adrenoleukodystrophy
Pseudo-Zellweger (thiolase deficiency) syndrome
Bifunctional protein deficiency
Acatalasemia
Hyperoxaluria type I
Acyl-CoA oxidase deficiency (pseudoneonatal adrenoleukodystrophy)

Modified from Balistreri WF: Fetal and neonatal bile acid synthesis and metabolism: Clinical implications. J Inher Metab Dis 1991; 14:459–477; with permission.

Secondary Defect

Peroxisomes play an important role in β-oxidation of bile acids; they contain catalases and oxidases. In Zellweger's (cerebrohepatorenal) syndrome, there is complete absence of hepatic peroxisomes. The primary defect is thought to be impaired delivery of matrix protein into peroxisomes.[209] The disorder is characterized by severe global developmental delay, characteristic facies, renal cortical cysts, hypotonia, and intrahepatic cholestasis with hepatomegaly and icterus.[210, 211] Markedly high concentrations of dihydroxycoprostanic and trihydroxycoprostanic acid and varanic acid are seen in the urine; these are bile acid precursors formed prior to complete oxidation of the side chain.[212] Other abnormalities include impaired phytanic acid oxidation, increased levels of pipecolic acid (product of lysine degeneration), and increased very long chain fatty acids in the absence of peroxisomal oxidation.[213–215] Zellweger's syndrome is a fatal disorder in most instances. A "Zellweger-like" syndrome has been reported in infants with phenotypic features similar to Zellweger's syndrome; in these patients, peroxisomes are demonstrable in the liver, but peroxisomal enzymes may be deficient. The primary defect is believed to be in the transport of matrix enzymes.

The recognition of other forms of inborn errors of bile acid metabolism and synthesis will allow for a clearer understanding of bile acid physiology and identification of other causes of neonatal cholestasis. These may be potentially treatable disorders when diagnosed early (even prenatally). With advances in bile acid technology, especially the use of gas chromatography–mass spectrometry and fast atom bombardment–mass spectrometry,[202, 203, 205] and applications of techniques of molecular biology, these disorders may be better defined. Management of these cholestatic diseases with oral bile acid therapy is promising.

BILE ACID–INDUCED DIARRHEA (Cholerrheic Enteropathy)

Bile acids are thought to play a significant role in initiating or perpetuating a cycle of intestinal dysfunction, diarrhea, malabsorption, and, potentially, malnutrition.[216] Bile acids, in varying concentrations, exert an effect on colonic motility; electrolyte and water absorption or secretion, or both; mucosal permeability; and cyclic AMP via adenylate cyclase. Any or all of these mechanisms may contribute to bile acid–induced diarrhea. The induction of diarrhea (net secretion) by bile acids will occur when certain physiologic derangements occur.[217] To induce diarrhea, bile acids in the colon must be (1) dihydroxylated (chenodeoxycholic acid or deoxycholic acid); (2) present in concentrations greater than or equal to 1.5 mmol per L; (3) present in aqueous phase; and (4) in an alkaline media with an appropriate pH of 7.5 to 8.0.

Bile acid malabsorption may be primary or secondary. *Primary bile acid malabsorption* is characterized by an absent or inefficient bile acid active transport system in the ileum. This may manifest itself as a form of protracted infantile diarrhea syndrome or as idiopathic bile acid catharsis in adults.[218] Affected persons have high concentrations of fecal bile acid, low levels of intraluminal bile acid, and contracted bile acid pool size with increased fractional turnover rate.[219–221] Fasting serum bile acid levels are below normal, and there is no rise in serum concentration after a meal.

Secondary bile acid malabsorption arises in patients with ileal disease or dysfunction as seen following a bout of infectious enteritis. These children may develop a clinical picture characterized by poor weight gain despite a seemingly optimal nutrient intake. Transient ileal dysfunction in these patients results in excessive fecal bile acid excretion, intraluminal bile acid deficiency, impaired lipid digestion and absorption, and steatorrhea.[222] Other forms of ileal dysfunction where secondary bile acid malabsorption is expected include ileal resection or bypass and Crohn's disease.

Diagnosis

To rule out bile acid–induced diarrhea, stool pH and duodenal intubation will provide useful clinical data. Fecal bile acid excretion may be measured in 24- to 72-hour stool collection. With oral administration of isotope-labeled bile acid and tracer studies, the course of the bile acid in the enterohepatic circulation can be followed. The use of the bile acid meal study provides a simple screening test based on the principle of postprandial bile acid spillover from portal venous blood (following active ileal absorption) into the peripheral circulation.[223, 224]

Therapy

Administration of a bile acid–binding resin (e.g., cholestyramine) or aluminum-containing antacid (with bile acid–binding properties) may improve the diarrhea.[225, 226] Codeine, atropine, and loperamide have been tried in an attempt to retard intestinal motility and enhance net colonic fluid and electrolyte uptake.[227–229] Propranolol is thought to abolish deoxycholic acid–induced diarrhea by its action as an adenylate cyclase inhibitor.[230]

UTILITY OF SERUM BILE ACID CONCENTRATION DETERMINATION

Measurement of serum bile acid levels plays an important role in the evaluation of hepatobiliary and some intestinal diseases (Table 3–4).

Elevated *fasting* levels of serum bile acids suggest reduced hepatic uptake, impaired secretion by the liver, or the existence of a portosystemic shunt. When used to further evaluate patients with abnormalities on routine liver function testing, high serum bile acid concentrations may help strengthen a diagnosis of hepatobiliary disease. Serial determination of fasting levels may be a reliable indicator of the degree of cholestasis in patients with resolving cholestasis after serum conjugated bilirubin levels normalize. This may be beneficial in deciding when to discontinue fat-soluble vitamin supplementation.

Two-hour postprandial serum bile acid levels may be a sensitive indication of hepatocyte uptake function ("clearance" test). Impaired uptake by the liver results in spillover of bile acids from the portal venous circulation to systemic venous blood. Ileal disease or dysfunction causes malabsorption of conjugated primary bile acids. This results in a contracted pool size and decreased fasting serum levels of primary bile acids. The expected postprandial rise in serum bile acid concentration is absent or markedly diminished. In cases of small

Table 3–4. SERUM PRIMARY BILE ACID LEVELS IN DISEASE STATES

Increased
Cholestasis
Intrahepatic
Extrahepatic
Hepatocellular damage (decreased bile acid uptake and altered synthesis)
Portacaval shunt
Decreased
Ileal disease or dysfunction (bile acid malabsorption)
Ileal resection
Crohn's disease
Radiation
Celiac disease (decreased gallbladder emptying and altered transit time)
Postcholecystectomy
Normal
Gilbert's disease
Newborn (physiologic jaundice)

Modified from Balistreri WF, Setchell KDR: Clinical implications of bile acid metabolism. *In* Silverberg M, Daum F, eds: Textbook of Pediatric Gastroenterology. Chicago, Year Book Medical Publishers, 1987, pp 72–89; with permission.

bowel bacterial overgrowth, bile acids may be more rapidly deconjugated in the proximal small bowel resulting in an increased load of free bile acids in the intestinal lumen. Passive absorption of these deamidated bile acids results in elevated serum concentration of unconjugated bile acids.[231-234] When this loss exceeds the ability of the liver to compensate (by increasing bile acid synthesis), bile acid pool size decreases, and fasting serum primary bile acid levels decline.

REFERENCES

1. Hofmann AF: The function of bile salts in fat absorption. Biochem J 1963; 89:57–68.
2. Hofmann AF, Small DM: Detergent properties of bile salts: Correlation with physiological function. Annu Rev Med 1967; 18:333–376.
3. Siperstein MD, Jayko ME, Chaikoff IL, et al: Nature of the metabolic products of C^{14}-cholesterol excreted in bile and feces. Proc Soc Exp Biol Med 1952; 81:720–724.
4. Schwartz CC, Berman M, Vlahcevic ZR, et al: Multicompartmental analysis of cholesterol metabolism in man: I. Characterization of the hepatic bile acid and biliary cholesterol precursor sites. J Clin Invest 1978; 61:408–423.
5. Setchell KDR: Disorders of bile acid synthesis. *In* Walker WA, Durie PR, Hamilton JR, et al, eds: Pediatric Gastrointestinal Disease: Pathophysiology, Diagnosis, Management. Philadelphia, BC Decker, 1991, pp 992–1013.
6. Dowling RH: The enterohepatic circulation. Gastroenterology 1972; 62:122–140.
7. Hofmann AF, Strandvik B. Defective bile acid amidation: Predicted features of a new inborn error of metabolism. Lancet 1988; 2:311–313.
8. Farkkila M, Miettinen TA: Lipid metabolism in bile acid malabsorption. Ann Med 1990; 22:5–13.
9. Hofmann AF: Bile acid secretion, bile flow and biliary lipid secretion in humans. Hepatology 1990; 12:17S–25S.
10. Bengmark S, Ekdahl PH, Olsson R: Effect of taurine and glycine treatment on the conjugation of bile acids in partialy hepatectomised rats. Acta Chir Scand 1964; 128:180–185.
11. Sjovall J: Dietary glycine and taurine on bile acid conjugation in man. Proc Soc Exp Biol Med 1959; 100:676–678.
12. Encrantz JC, Sjovall J: On the bile acids in duodenal contents of infants and children. Clin Chim Acta 1959; 4:793–799.
13. McLeod GM, Wiggins HS: Bile salts in small intestinal contents after ileal resection and in other malabsorption syndromes. Lancet 1968; 1:873–876.
14. Huijghebaert SM, Hofmann AF: Pancreatic carboxypeptidase hydrolysis of bile acid–amino acid conjugates: selective resistance of glycine and taurine amidates. Gastroenterology 1986; 90:306–315.
15. Hofmann AF, Mysels KJ: Bile salts as biological surfactants. Colloids Surfaces 1988; 30:145–173.
16. Yanagisawa J, Ho M, Ishibaki M, et al: Microanalysis of bile acid in human liver by selected ion monitoring. Anal Biochem 1980; 104:75–86.
17. Weinman SA, Graf J, Boyer JL: Voltage-driven, taurocholate-dependent secretion in isolated hepatocyte couplets. Am J Physiol 1989; 256:G826–G832.
18. Schersten T, Nilsson S, Cahlin E, et al: Relationship between the biliary excretion of bile acids and the excretion of water, lecithin, and cholesterol in man. Eur J Clin Invest 1971; 1:242–247.
19. Hofmann AF: Chemistry and enterohepatic circulation of bile acids. Hepatology 1984; 4:4S–14S.
20. Danielsson H: Present status of research on catabolism and excretion of cholesterol. Adv Lipid Res 1963; 1:335–385.
21. Eneroth P, Gordon B, Sjovall J: Characterization of trisubstituted cholanoic acids in human feces. J Lipid Res 1966; 7:524–530.
22. Batta AK, Salen G, Arora R, et al: Side chain conjugation prevents bacterial 7-dehydroxylation of bile acids. J Biol Chem 1990; 265:10925–10928.
23. Norman A: Metabolism of glycocholic acid in man. Scand J Gastroenterol 1970; 5:231–236.
24. Norman A, Shorb MS: In vitro formation of deoxycholic and lithocholic acid by human intestinal microorganisms. Proc Soc Exp Biol Med 1962; 110:552–555.
25. Nair PP, Gordon M, Reback J: The enzymatic cleavage of the carbon-nitrogen bond in 3α, 7α, 12α-trihydroxy-5β-cholan-24-oylglycine. J Biol Chem 1967; 242:7–11.
26. Midtvedt T, Norman A: Bile acid transformations by microbial strains belonging to genera found in intestinal contents. Acta Pathol Microbiol Scand 1967; 71:629–638.
27. Hill MJ, Drasar BS: Degradation of bile salts by human intestinal bacteria. Gut 1968; 9:22–27.
28. Shimada K, Bricknell KS, Finegold SM: Deconjugation of bile acids by intestinal bacteria: Review of literature and additional studies. J Infect Dis 1969; 119:273–281.
29. Baker RD, Searle GW: Bile salt absorption at various levels of rat small intestine. Proc Soc Exp Biol Med 1960; 105:521–523.
30. Lack L, Weiner IM: In vitro absorption of bile salts by small intestine of rats and guinea pigs. Am J Physiol 1961; 200:313–317.
31. Holt PR: Intestinal absorption of bile salts in the rat. Am J Physiol 1964; 207:1–7.
32. Playoust MR, Isselbacher KJ: Studies on the transport and metabolism of conjugated bile salts by intestinal mucosa. J Clin Invest 1964; 43:467–476.
33. Glassner JE, Weiner IM, Lack L: Comparative physiology of intestinal taurocholate transport. Am J Physiol 1965; 208:359–362.
34. Lack L, Weiner IM: Intestinal bile salt transport: structure-activity relationships and other properties. Am J Physiol 1966; 210:1142–1152.
35. Lack L, Weiner IM: The role of the intestine during the enterohepatic circulation of bile salts. Gastroenterology 1967; 52:282–287.
36. Buchwald H, Gebhard RL: Localization of bile salt absorption in vivo in the rabbit. Ann Surg 1968; 167:191–198.
37. Dietschy JM: Mechanisms for the intestinal absorption of bile acids. J Lipid Res 1968; 9:297–309.
38. Samuel P, Saypol GM, Meilman E, et al: Absorption of bile acids from the large bowel in man. J Clin Invest 1968; 47:2070–2078.
39. Gustafsson BE, Norman A: Bile acid absorption from the caecal contents of germ-free rats. Scand J Gastroenterol 1969; 4:585–590.
40. Sullivan MF: Bile salt absorption in the irradiated rat. Am J Physiol 1965; 209:158–164.
41. Norman A, Sjovall J: On the transformation and enterohepatic circulation of cholic acid in the rat: Bile acids and steroids 68. J Biol Chem 1958; 233:872–885.
42. Portman OW: Further studies of the intestinal degradation products of cholic acid–24-C^{14} in rats: Formation of deoxycholic acid. Arch Biochem Biophys 1958; 78:125–137.
43. Tidball CS: Intestinal and hepatic transport of cholate and organic dyes. Am J Physiol 1964; 206:239–242.
44. Dietschy JM, Salomon HS, Siperstein MD: Bile acid metabolism: I. Studies on the mechanisms of intestinal transport. J Clin Invest 1966; 45:832–846.
45. Davenport HW: Absorption of taurocholate–24–^{14}C through the canine gastric mucosa. Proc Soc Exp Biol Med 1967; 125:670–673.
46. Hislop IG, Hofmann AF, Schoenfield LJ: Determinants of the rate and site of bile acid absorption in man (abstract). J Clin Invest 1967; 46:1070.
47. Small NC, Dietschy JM: Characterization of the monomer and micelle components of the passive diffusion process of bile acids across the small intestine of the rat (abstract). Gastroenterology 1968; 54:1272.
48. Dowling RH, White J, Perry PM: Conservation of intestinal bile acid concentration after ileal resection. Helv Med Acta 1973; 37:103–111.
49. Grundy SM, Ahrens EH, Miettinen TA: Quantitative isolation and gas-liquid chromatographic analysis of total fecal bile acids. J Lipid Res 1965; 6:397–410.

50. Evrard E, Janssen G: Gas-liquid chromatographic determination of human fecal bile acids. J Lipid Res 1968; 9:226–236.
51. Miettinen TA, Kesaniemi YA: Cholesterol balance and lipoprotein metabolism in man. *In* Grundy SM, ed: Bile Acids and Atherosclerosis. New York, Raven Press, 1986, pp 113–155.
52. Josephson B, Rydin A: The resorption of the bile acids from the intestines. Biochem J 1936; 30:2224–2228.
53. Olivecrona T, Sjovall J: Bile acids in rat portal blood. Acta Physiol Scand 1959; 46:284–290.
54. Rudman D, Kendall FE: Bile acid content of human serum: II. The binding of cholanic acids by human plasma proteins. J Clin Invest 1957; 36:538–542.
55. van Dyke RW, Stephens JE, Scharschmidt BF: Bile acid transport in cultured rat hepatocytes. Am J Physiol 1982; 243:G484–G492.
56. Cabral DJ, Small DM, Lilly HS, et al: Transbilayer movement of bile acids in model membranes. Biochemistry 1987; 26:1801–1804.
57. Zimmerli B, Valantinas J, Meier PJ: Multispecificity of Na^+-dependent taurocholate uptake in basolateral (sinusoidal) rat liver plasma membrane vesicles. J Pharm Exp Ther 1989; 250:301–308.
58. Blitzer BL, Terzakis C, Scott KA: Hydroxyl/bile acid exchange: A new mechanism for the uphill transport of cholate by basolateral liver plasma membrane vesicles. J Biol Chem 1986; 261:12042–12046.
59. Meier PJ: Transport polarity of hepatocytes. Semin Liver Dis 1988; 8:293–307.
60. Hofmann AF: Bile acids. *In* Arias IM, Jakoby WB, Popper H, et al, eds: The Liver: Biology and Pathobiology. New York, Raven Press, 1988, pp 553–572.
61. Bagheri SA, Bolt MG, Boyers JL, et al: Stimulation of thymidine incorporation in mouse liver and biliary tract epithelium by lithocholate and deoxycholate. Gastroenterology 1978; 74:188–192.
62. Palmer RH: Bile acids, liver injury, and liver disease. Arch Intern Med 1972; 130:606–617.
63. Kakis G, Yousef IM: Pathogenesis of lithocholate- and taurolithocholate-induced intrahepatic cholestasis in rats. Gastroenterology 1978; 75:595–607.
64. Crowther JS, Drasar BS, Goddard P, et al: The effect of a chemically defined diet on the faecal flora and faecal steroid concentration. Gut 1973; 14:790–793.
65. Palmer RH: The formation of bile acid sulfates: A new pathway of bile acid metabolism in humans. Proc Natl Acad Sci U S A 1967; 58:1047–1050.
66. Cowen AE, Korman MG, Hofmann AF, et al: Metabolism of lithocholate in healthy man: I. Biotransformation and biliary excretion of intravenously administered lithocholate, lithocholylglycine, and their sulfates. Gastroenterology 1975; 69:59–66.
67. Cowen AE, Korman MG, Hofmann AF, et al: Metabolism of lithocholate in healthy man: II. Enterohepatic circulation. Gastroenterology 1975; 69:67–76.
68. Palmer RH, Bolt MG: Bile acid sulfates: I. Synthesis of lithocholic acid sulfates and their identification in human bile. J Lipid Res 1971; 12:671–679.
69. Galle PR, Theilmann L, Raedsch R, et al: Taurine and glycine conjugation and sulfation of lithocholate in primary hepatocyte cultures. Biochim Biophys Acta 1989; 1003:250–253.
70. Stiehl A, Becker M, Czygan P, et al: Bile acids and their sulphated and glucuronidated derivatives in bile, plasma, and urine of children with intrahepatic cholestasis: Effects of phenobarbital treatment. Eur J Clin Invest 1980; 10:307–316.
71. Yousef IM, Tuchweber B, Vonk RJ, et al: Lithocholate cholestasis—sulfated glycolithocholate-induced intrahepatic cholestasis in rats. Gastroenterology 1981; 80:233–241.
72. Bellentani S, Armocida C, Pecorari M, et al: The role of calcium precipitation in the sulfoglycolithocholate-induced cholestasis of the bile fistula hamster. J Hepatol 1990; 10:356–363.
73. van der Meer R, Vonk RJ, Kuipers F: Cholestasis and the interactions of sulfated glyco- and taurolithocholate with calcium. Am J Physiol 1988; 254:G644–G649.
74. Einarsson K, Reihner E, Ewerth S, et al: Serum concentrations of unconjugated and conjugated cholic acid in portal venous and systemic venous blood of fasting man. Scand J Clin Lab Invest 1989; 49:83–91.
75. Van Deest BW, Fordtran JS, Morawski SG, et al: Bile salt and micellar fat concentration in proximal small bowel contents of ileectomy patients. J Clin Invest 1968; 47:1314–1324.
76. Dowling RH, Rose GA, Sutor DJ: Hyperoxaluria and renal calculi in ileal disease. Lancet 1971; 1:1103–1106.
77. Admirand WH, Earnest D, Williams H: Hyperoxaluria and bowel disease. Clin Res 1971; 19:562.
78. Chadwick VS, Elias E, Bell GD, et al: The role of bile acids in the increased intestinal absorption of oxalate after ileal resection. *In* Matern S, Hackenschmidt J, Back P, et al, eds: Advances in Bile Acid Research. Stuttgart, Schattauer-Verlag, 1974, pp 435–440.
79. Beher WT, Beher ME, Semenuk G: The effect of pituitary and thyroid hormones on bile acid metabolism in the rat. Metabolism 1966; 15:181–188.
80. Poley JR, Smith JD, Thompson JB, et al: Improved micellar dispersal of dietary lipid by bile acids during replacement therapy in growth hormone–deficient children. Pediatr Res 1977; 11:1186–1191.
81. Heubi JE, Burstein S, Sperling MA, et al: The role of human growth hormone in the regulation of cholesterol and bile acid metabolism. J Clin Endocrinol Metab 1983; 57:885–891.
82. Myant NB: Hormonal control of cholesterol metabolism. *In* Bittar EE, Bittar N, eds: The Biological Basis of Medicine. Vol 2. New York, Academic Press, 1968, pp 193–220.
83. Princen HMG, Meijer P, Hofstee B: Dexamethasone regulates bile acid synthesis in monolayer cultures of rat hepatocytes by induction of cholesterol 7α-hydroxylase. Biochem J 1989; 262:341–348.
84. Everson GT: Bile acid synthesis by liver cell hybrids (rat): Studies of the regulation of bile acid synthesis by dexamethasone. *In* Paumgartner G, Stiehl A, Gerok W, eds: Falk Symposium 45: Bile Acids and the Liver with an Update on Gallstone Disease. Lancaster, MTP Press, 1987, pp 61–63.
85. Bonorris GC, Coyne MJ, Chung A, et al: Mechanism of estrogen-induced saturated bile in the hamster. J Lab Clin Med 1977; 90:963–970.
86. Davis RA, Elliott TS, Lattier GR: Regulation of bile acid synthesis via direct effects on the microsomal membrane. Biochemistry 1986; 25:1632–1636.
87. Boyd GS, Scholan NA, Mitton JR: Factors influencing cholesterol 7α-hydroxylase activity in the rat liver. *In* Holmes WL, Carlson LA, Paoletti R, eds: Drugs Affecting Lipid Metabolism (Adv Exp Med Biol, vol 4). New York, Plenum Press, 1969, pp 443–456.
88. Redinger RN, Small DM: Primate biliary physiology: VIII. The effect of phenobarbital upon bile salt synthesis and pool size, biliary lipid secretion, and bile composition. J Clin Invest 1973; 52:161–172.
89. Davis RA, Musso CA, Malone-McNeal M, et al: Examination of bile acid negative feedback regulation in rats. J Lipid Res 1988; 29:202–211.
90. Eriksson S: Biliary excretion of bile acids and cholesterol in bile fistula rats: Bile acids and steroids. Proc Soc Exp Biol Med 1957; 94:578–582.
91. Bergstrom S, Danielsson H: On the regulation of bile acid formation in the rat liver. Acta Physiol Scand 1958; 43:1–7.
92. Tennent DM, Siegel H, Zanetti ME, et al: Plasma cholesterol lowering action of bile acid binding polymers in experimental animals. J Lipid Res 1960; 1:469–473.
93. Myant NB, Eder HA: The effect of biliary drainage upon the synthesis of cholesterol in the liver. J Lipid Res 1961; 2:363–368.
94. Beher WT, Beher ME, Rao B: Bile acid and cholesterol metabolism in the mouse as affected by cholestyramine. Proc Soc Exp Biol Med 1966; 122:881–884.
95. Danielsson H, Einarsson K, Johansson G: Effects of biliary drainage on individual reactions in the conversion of cholesterol to taurocholic acid. Eur J Biochem 1967; 2:44–49.
96. Shefer S, Hauser S, Mosbach EH: 7α-Hydroxylation of cholesterol by rat liver microsomes. J Lipid Res 1968; 9:328–333.
97. Shefer S, Hauser S, Bekersky I, et al: Feedback regulation of bile acid biosynthesis in the rat. J Lipid Res 1969; 10:646–655.
98. Shefer S, Hauser S, Bekersky I, et al: Biochemical site of regulation of bile acid biosynthesis in the rat. J Lipid Res 1970; 11:404–411.
99. Moutafis CD, Myant NB: The metabolism of cholesterol in two

hypercholesterolemic patients treated with cholestyramine. Clin Sci 1969; 37:443–454.
100. Dowling RH, Mack E, Small DM: Effects of controlled interruption of the enterohepatic circulation of bile salts by biliary diversion and by ileal resection on bile salt secretion, synthesis, and pool size in the rhesus monkey. J Clin Invest 1970; 49:232–242.
101. Kempen HJM, Vos-Van Holstein MPM, de Lange J: Bile acids and lipids in isolated rat hepatocytes: Content, synthesis, and release, as affected by cholestyramine treatment of donor rats. J Lipid Res 1982; 23:823–830.
102. Mosbach EH, Rothschild MA, Bekersky I, et al: Bile acid synthesis in the isolated, perfused rabbit liver. J Clin Invest 1971; 50:1720–1730.
103. Shefer S, Hauser S, Lapar V, et al: Regulatory effects of sterols and bile acids on hepatic 3-hydroxy-3-methylglutaryl CoA reductase and cholesterol 7α-hydroxylase in the rat. J Lipid Res 1973; 14:573–580.
104. Danzinger RG, Hofmann AF, Thistle JL, et al: Effect of oral chenodeoxycholic acid on bile acid kinetics and biliary lipid composition in women with cholelithiasis. J Clin Invest 1973; 52:2809–2821.
105. Einarsson K, Hellstrom K, Kallner M: Feedback regulation of bile acid formation in man. Metabolism 1973; 22:1477–1483.
106. Schoenfield LJ, Bonorris GG, Ganz P: Induced alterations in the rate-limiting enzymes of hepatic cholesterol and bile acid synthesis in the hamster. J Lab Clin Med 1973; 82:858–868.
107. LaRusso NF, Hoffman NE, Hofmann AF, et al: Effect of primary bile acid ingestion on bile acid metabolism and biliary lipid secretion in gallstone patients. Gastroenterology 1975; 69:1301–1314.
108. Key PH, Bonorris GG, Marks JW, et al: Biliary lipid synthesis and secretion in gallstone patients before and during treatment with chenodeoxycholic acid. J Lab Clin Med 1980; 95:816–826.
109. Pries JM, Gustafson A, Wiegand D, et al: Taurocholate is more potent than cholate in suppression of bile salt synthesis in the rat. J Lipid Res 1983; 24:141–146.
110. Nilsell K, Angelin B, Leyd B, et al: Comparative effects of ursodeoxycholic acid and chenodeoxycholic acid on bile acid kinetics and biliary lipid secretion in humans. Gastroenterology 1983; 85:1248–1256.
111. Bertolotti M, Carulli N, Menozzi D, et al: In vivo evaluation of cholesterol 7α-hydroxylation in humans: Effect of disease and drug treatment. J Lipid Res 1986; 27:1278–1286.
112. Pooler PA, Duane WC: Effects of bile acid administration on bile acid synthesis and its circadian rhythm in man. Hepatology 1988; 8:1140–1146.
113. Heuman DM, Vlahcevic ZR, Bailey ML, et al: Regulation of bile acid synthesis. II. Effect of bile acid feeding on enzymes regulating hepatic cholesterol and bile acid synthesis. Hepatology 1988; 8:892–897.
114. Stange EF, Scheibner J, Lutz C, et al: Feedback regulation of bile acid synthesis in the rat by dietary vs. intravenous cholate or taurocholate. Hepatology 1988; 8:879–886.
115. Kwekkeboom J, Van Voorthuizen EM, Princen HMG, et al: Feedback inhibition of bile acid synthesis in cultured pig hepatocytes. Biochem Biophys Res Commun 1988; 155:850–856.
116. Van Cantfort J, Gielen J: Cholesterol 7α-hydroxylase: II. Biochemical properties and participation of endogenous cholesterol in the assay in vitro. Eur J Biochem 1975; 55:33–40.
117. Schwartz MA, Margolis S: Effects of drugs and sterols on cholesterol 7α-hydroxylase activity in rat liver microsomes. J Lipid Res 1983; 24:28–33.
118. Kubaska WM, Gurley EC, Hylemon PB, et al: Absence of negative feedback control of bile acid biosynthesis in cultured rat hepatocytes. J Biol Chem 1985; 260:13459–13463.
119. Kwekkeboom J, Princen HMG, Van Voorthuizen EM, et al: Bile acids exert negative feedback control on bile acid synthesis in cultured pig hepatocytes by suppression of cholesterol 7α-hydroxylase activity. Hepatology 1990; 12:1209–1215.
120. Einarsson K, Johansson G: Effect of actinomycin D and puromycin on the conversion of cholesterol into bile acids in bile fistula rats. FEBS Lett 1968; 1:219–222.
121. Heuman DM, Hylemon PB, Vlahcevic ZR: Regulation of bile acid synthesis: III. Correlation between biliary bile salt hydrophobicity index and the activities of enzymes regulating cholesterol and bile acid synthesis in the rat. J Lipid Res 1989; 30:1161–1171.
122. Pandak WM, Li YC, Chiang JYL, et al: Regulation of cholesterol 7α-hydroxylase mRNA and transcriptional activity by taurocholate and cholesterol in the chronic biliary diverted rat. J Biol Chem 1991; 266:3416–3421.
123. Botham KM, Lawson ME, Beckett GJ, et al: The effect of portal blood bile acid concentrations on bile salt synthesis in rat liver: Studies with isolated hepatocytes. Biochim Biophys Acta 1981; 666:238–245.
124. Davis RA, Highsmith WE, Malone-McNeal M, et al: Bile acid synthesis by cultured hepatocytes: Inhibition by mevinolin, but not by bile acids. J Biol Chem 1983; 258:4079–4082.
125. Davis RA, Hyde PM, Kuan JCW, et al: Bile acid synthesis by cultured rat hepatocytes: Regulation by cholesterol availability. J Biol Chem 1983; 258:3661–3667.
126. Heuman DM, Hernandez CR, Hylemon PB, et al: Regulation of bile acid synthesis. I. Effects of conjugated ursodeoxycholate and cholate on bile acid synthesis in chronic bile fistula rat. Hepatology 1988; 8:358–365.
127. Whiting MJ, Wishart RA, Growing MR, et al: Bile acid synthesis and secretion by rabbit hepatocytes in primary monolayer culture: Comparison with rat hepatocytes. Biochim Biophys Acta 1989; 1001:176–184.
128. Davis RA, Musso CA, Lattier GR: Regulation of bile acid synthesis by microsomal cholesterol. *In* Paumgartner G, Stiehl A, Gerok W, eds: Falk Symposium 42: Enterohepatic Circulation of Bile Acids and Sterol Metabolism. Lancaster, MTP Press, 1985, pp 37–45.
129. Duane WC, McHale AP, Hamilton JN: Studies of feedback suppression of bile salt synthesis in the bile-fistula rat. J Lipid Res 1988; 29:212–214.
130. Lillienau J, Munoz J, Longmire-Cook SJ: Negative feedback regulation of the ileal bile acid transport system: The second site of regulation of the enterohepatic circulation. *In* Paumgartner G, Stiehl A, Gerok W, eds: Falk Symposium 58: Bile Acids as Therapeutic Agents—from Basic Science to Clinical Practice. Lancaster, Kluwer, 1991, pp 163–165.
131. Balistreri WF, Setchell KDR. Clinical implications of bile acid metabolism. *In* Silverberg M, Daum F, eds: Textbook of Pediatric Gastroenterology. Chicago, Year Book Medical Publishers, 1987, pp 72–89.
132. Blitzer BL, Boyer JL: Cellular mechanisms of bile formation. Gastroenterology 1982; 83:346–357.
133. Javitt NB: Hepatic bile formation. N Engl J Med 1976; 295:1511–1516.
134. Boyer JL: New concepts of mechanisms of hepatocyte bile formation. Physiol Rev 1980; 60:303–326.
135. Gurantz D, Hofmann AF: Influence of bile acid structure on bile flow and biliary lipid secretion in the hamster. Am J Physiol 1984; 247:G736–G748.
136. Nilsson S, Schersten T: Synthesis of phospholipids and triglycerides in human liver slices. Scand J Clin Lab Invest 1969; 24:237–249.
137. Carulli N, Loria P, Bertolotti M, et al: Effects of acute changes of bile acid pool composition on biliary lipid secretion. J Clin Invest 1984; 74:614–624.
138. Thistle JL, Hofmann AF: Efficacy and specificity of chenodeoxycholic acid therapy for dissolving gallstones. N Engl J Med 1973; 289:655–659.
139. Thistle JL, Schoenfield LJ: Induced alterations in composition of bile of persons having cholelithiasis. Gastroenterology 1971; 61:488–496.
140. Moore EW, Celic L, Ostrow JD: Interactions between ionized calcium and sodium taurocholate: Bile salts are important buffers for prevention of calcium-containing gallstones. Gastroenterology 1982; 83:1079–1089.
141. Sherlock S: Gall-stones and inflammatory gallbladder disease. *In* Sherlock S, ed: Diseases of the Liver and Biliary System. 7th ed. Oxford, Blackwell Scientific Publications, Alden Press, 1985, pp 506–530.
142. Hofmann AF: Trends in bile acid research: The past and the future. *In* Paumgartner G, Stiehl A, Gerok W, eds: Falk Symposium 52: Trends in Bile Acid Research. Dordrecht, Kluwer, 1988, pp 19–49.
143. Hofmann AF: The function of bile salts in fat absorption: The

solvent properties of dilute micellar solutions of conjugated bile salts. Biochem J 1963; 89:57–68.
144. Hofmann AF, Borgstrom B: The intraluminal phase of fat digestion in man: The lipid content of the micellar and oil phases of intestinal content obtained during fat digestion and absorption. J Clin Invest 1964; 43:247–257.
145. Hofmann AF, Roda A: Physicochemical properties of bile acids and their relationship to biological properties: An overview of the problem. J Lipid Res 1984; 25:1477–1489.
146. Mekhjian HS, Phillips SF, Hofmann AF: Colonic secretion of water and electrolytes induced by bile acids: Perfusion studies in man. J Clin Invest 1971; 50:1569–1577.
147. Galapeaux EA, Templeton RD, Borkon EL: The influence of bile on the motility of the dog's colon. Am J Physiol 1938; 121:130–136.
148. Meyer AE, McEwan JP: Bile acids and their choline salts applied to the inner surface of isolated colon and ileum of guinea pig. Am J Physiol 1948; 153:386–392.
149. Bergmann M: Uber die peristaltische Wirksamkeit der Gallensauren und ihre klinische anwendung. Wien Klin Wochenschr 1952; 64:704–707.
150. Flynn M, Darby C, Hyland J, et al: The effect of bile acids on colonic myoelectrical activity. Br J Surg 1979; 66:776–779.
151. Hanssen LE: Pure synthetic bile salts release immunoreactive secretin in man. Scand J Gastroenterol 1980; 15:461–463.
152. Balistreri WF, Heubi JE, Suchy FJ: Immaturity of the enterohepatic circulation in early life: Factors predisposing to "physiologic" maldigestion and cholestasis. J Pediatr Gastroenterol Nutr 1983; 2:346–354.
153. Watkins JB, Ingall D, Szczepanik P, et al: Bile salt metabolism in the newborn: Measurement of pool size and synthesis by stable isotope technique. N Engl J Med 1973; 288:431–434.
154. Watkins JB, Szczepanik P, Gould JB, et al: Bile salt metabolism in the human premature infant. Gastroenterology 1975; 69:706–713.
155. de Belle RC, Vaupshas V, Vitullo BB, et al: Intestinal absorption of bile salts: Immature development in the neonate. J Pediatr 1979; 94:472–476.
156. Heubi JE, Balistreri WF: Bile salt metabolism in infants and children after protracted infantile diarrhea. Pediatr Res 1980; 14:943–946.
157. Heubi JE, Balistreri WF, Suchy FJ: Bile salt metabolism in the first year of life. J Lab Clin Med 1982; 100:127–136.
158. Watkins JB, Jarvenpaa AL, Szczepanik-Van Leeuwen P, et al: Feeding the low birth weight infant: V. Effects of taurine, cholesterol and human milk on bile acid kinetics. Gastroenterology 1983; 85:793–800.
159. Balistreri WF, Schubert WK: Liver disease in infancy and childhood. *In* Schiff L, Schiff ER, eds: Diseases of the Liver. 6th ed. Philadelphia, JB Lippincott, 1986, pp 1337–1426.
160. Poley JR, Dower JC, Owen CA, et al: Bile acids in infants and children. J Lab Clin Med 1964; 63:838–846.
161. Sharp HL, Peller J, Carey JB, et al: Primary and secondary bile acids in meconium. Pediatr Res 1971; 5:274–279.
162. Colombo C, Zuliani G, Ronchi M, et al: Biliary bile acid composition of the human fetus in early gestation. Pediatr Res 1987; 21:197–200.
163. Back P, Walter K: Developmental pattern of bile acid metabolism as revealed by bile acid analysis of meconium. Gastroenterology 1980; 78:671–676.
164. Setchell KDR, Dumaswala R, Colombo C, et al: Hepatic bile acid metabolism during early development revealed from the analysis of human fetal gallbladder bile. J Biol Chem 1988; 263:16637–16644.
165. Deleze G, Paumgartner G, Karlaganis G, et al: Bile acid pattern in human amniotic fluid. Eur J Clin Invest 1978; 8:41–45.
166. St Pyrek J, Sterzycki R, Lester R, et al: Constituents of human meconium. II. Identification of steroidal acids with 21 and 22 carbon atoms. Lipids 1982; 17:241–249.
167. Nakagawa M, Setchell KDR: Bile acid metabolism in early life: Studies of amniotic fluid. J Lipid Res 1990; 31:1089–1098.
168. Balistreri WF, Belknap WM, Suchy FJ, et al: Immaturity of the enterohepatic circulation of bile acids in early life: Factors responsible for increased peripheral serum bile acid concentrations. *In* Paumgartner G, Stiehl A, Gerok W, eds: Falk Symposium 42: Enterohepatic Circulation of Bile Acids and Sterol Metabolism. Lancaster, MTP Press, 1985, pp 87–93.
169. Strandvik B, Wikstrom SA: Tetrahydroxylated bile acids in healthy human newborns. Eur J Clin Invest 1982; 12:301–305.
170. Suchy FJ, Courchene SM, Balistreri WF: Ontogeny of hepatic bile acid conjugation in the rat. Pediatr Res 1985; 19:97–101.
171. Balistreri WF, Zimmer L, Suchy FJ, et al: Bile salt sulfotransferase: Alterations during maturation and non-inducibility during substrate ingestion. J Lipid Res 1984; 25:228–235.
172. Balistreri WF, Suchy FJ, Heubi JE, et al: Physiological immaturity of the enterohepatic circulation of bile acids. *In* Barbara L, Dowling RH, Hofmann AF, et al, eds: Bile Acids in Gastroenterology. Lancaster, MTP Press, 1982, pp 192–199.
173. Haber LR, Vaupshas V, Vitullo BB, et al: Bile acid conjugation in organ culture of human fetal liver. Gastroenterology 1978; 74:1214–1223.
174. Encrantz JC, Sjovall J: On the bile acids in duodenal contents of infants and children. Clin Chim Acta 1959; 4:793–799.
175. Challacombe DN, Edkins S, Brown GA: Duodenal bile acids in infancy. Arch Dis Child 1975; 50:837–843.
176. Subbiah MTR, Marai L, Dinh DM, et al: Sterol and bile acid metabolism during development: I. Studies on the gallbladder and intestinal bile acids of newborn and fetal rabbit. Steroids 1977; 29:83–92.
177. Graham TO, Van Thiel DH, Little JM, et al: Synthesis of taurocholate by rat fetal liver in organ culture: Effects of cortisol in vitro. Am J Physiol 1979; 237:E177–E184.
178. Jackson BT, Smallwood RA, Piasecki GJ, et al: Fetal bile salt metabolism: I. The metabolism of sodium cholate-^{14}C in the fetal dog. J Clin Invest 1971; 50:1286–1294.
179. Little JM, Smallwood RA, Lester R, et al: Bile-salt metabolism in the primate fetus. Gastroenterology 1975; 69:1315–1320.
180. Hardy KJ, Hoffman NE, Mihaly G, et al: Bile acid metabolism in fetal sheep: Perinatal changes in the bile acid pool. J Physiol (Lond) 1980; 309:1–11.
181. Heubi JE, Fondacaro JD: Postnatal development of intestinal bile salt transport in the guinea pig. Am J Physiol 1982; 243:G189–G194.
182. Little JM, Lester R: Ontogenesis of intestinal bile salt absorption in the neonatal rat. Am J Physiol 1980; 239:G319–G323.
183. Lester R, Smallwood RA, Little JM, et al: Fetal bile salt metabolism. The intestinal absorption of bile salt. J Clin Invest 1977; 59:1009–1016.
184. Moyer MS, Heubi JE, Goodrich AL, et al: Ontogeny of bile acid transport in brush border membrane vesicles from rat ileum. Gastroenterology 1986; 90:1188–1196.
185. Heubi JE, Gunn TD: The role of glucocorticoids in the postnatal development of ileal active bile salt transport. Pediatr Res 1985; 19:1147–1151.
186. Heubi JE, Fellows JL: Postnatal development of intestinal bile salt transport: Relationship to membrane physico-chemical changes. J Lipid Res 1985; 26:797–805.
187. Barnard JA, Ghishan FK, Wilson FA: Ontogenesis of taurocholate transport by rat ileal brush border membrane vesicles. J Clin Invest 1985; 75:869–873.
188. Barnard JA, Ghishan FK: Methylprednisolone accelerates the ontogeny of sodium-taurocholate cotransport in rat ileal brush border membranes. J Lab Clin Med 1986; 108:549–555.
189. Heubi JE: Role of thyroxine on postnatal development of ileal active bile salt transport. Am J Physiol 1986; 251:G237–G242.
190. Heubi JE, Fondacaro JD, Balistreri WF: Bile salt absorption in neonates. J Pediatr 1979; 95:1085–1086.
191. Little JM, Richey JE, Van Thiel DH, et al: Taurocholate pool size and distribution in the fetal rat. J Clin Invest 1979; 63:1042–1049.
192. Suchy FJ, Courchene SM, Blitzer BL: Taurocholate transport by basolateral plasma membrane vesicles isolated from developing rat liver. Am J Physiol 1985; 248:G648–G654.
193. Suchy FJ, Balistreri WF: Uptake of taurocholate by hepatocytes isolated from developing rats. Pediatr Res 1982; 16:282–285.
194. Suchy FJ, Balistreri WF, Breslin JS, et al: Absence of an acinar gradient for bile acid uptake in developing rat liver. Pediatr Res 1987; 21:417–421.
195. Suchy FJ, Balistreri WF, Hung J, et al: Intracellular bile acid transport in rat liver as visualized by electron microscope autoradiography using a bile acid analogue. Am J Physiol 1983; 245:G681–G689.
196. Belknap WM, Balistreri WF, Suchy FJ, et al: Physiologic cho-

lestasis II. Serum bile acid levels reflect the development of the enterohepatic circulation in rats. Hepatology 1981; 1:613–616.
197. Suchy FJ, Balistreri WF, Heubi JE, et al: Physiologic cholestasis: Elevation of the primary serum bile acid concentrations in normal infants. Gastroenterology 1981; 80:1037–1041.
198. Graham TO, Van Thiel DH, Lester R, et al: Synthesis of taurocholate by rat fetal liver in organ culture: Effects of cortisol in vitro. Am J Physiol 1979; 237:E177–E184.
199. Middleton WRJ: Thyroid hormones and the gut. Gut 1971; 12:172–177.
200. Hellstrom K, Lindstedt S: Cholic acid turnover and biliary bile acid composition in humans with abnormal thyroid function: Bile acids and steroids 139. J Lab Clin Med 1964; 63:666–679.
201. Balistreri WF: Fetal and neonatal bile acid synthesis and metabolism: Clinical implications. J Inher Metab Dis 1991; 14:459–477.
202. Setchell KDR, Street JM: Inborn errors of bile acid synthesis. Semin Liver Dis 1989; 7:85–99.
203. Clayton PT, Leonard JV, Lawson AM, et al: Familial giant cell hepatitis associated with synthesis of 3β,7α-dihydroxy- and 3β,7α,12α-trihydroxy-5-cholenoic acids. J Clin Invest 1987; 79:1031–1038.
204. Buchmann MS, Kvittingen EA, Nazer H, et al: Lack of 3β-hydroxy-Δ^5-C_{27}-steroid dehydrogenase/isomerase in fibroblasts from a child with urinary excretion of 3β-hydroxy-Δ^5-bile acids: A new inborn error of metabolism. J Clin Invest 1990; 86:2034–2037.
205. Setchell KDR, Suchy FJ, Welsh MB, et al: Δ^4-3-Oxosteroid 5β-reductase deficiency described in identical twins with neonatal hepatitis: A new inborn error in bile acid synthesis. J Clin Invest 1988; 82:2148–2157.
206. Ichimiya H, Nazer H, Gunasekaran T, et al: Treatment of chronic liver disease caused by 3β-hydroxy-Δ^5-C_{27}-steroid dehydrogenase deficiency with chenodeoxycholic acid. Arch Dis Child 1990; 65:1121–1124.
207. Daugherty CC, Setchell KDR, Balistreri WF: Bile canalicular abnormalities in an inborn error of bile acid (BA) metabolism (Δ^4-3-oxosteroid 5β-reductase deficiency) (abstract). Lab Invest 1991; 64:3P.
208. Balistreri WF, Hofmann AF, A-Kader HH, et al: Successful bile acid therapy in 3 siblings with neonatal hepatitis due to an inborn error of bile acid biosynthesis (abstract). Pediatr Res 1991; 29:99A.
209. Santos MJ, Imanaka T, Shio H, et al: Peroxisomal membrane ghosts in Zellweger syndrome: Aberrant organelle assembly. Science 1988; 239:1536–1538.
210. Passarge E, McAdams AJ: Cerebro-hepato-renal syndrome. J Pediatr 1967; 71:691–702.
211. Smith DW, Opitz JM, Inhorn SL: A syndrome of multiple developmental defects including polycystic kidneys and intrahepatic biliary dysgenesis in 2 siblings. J Pediatr 1965; 67:617–624.
212. Hanson RF, Isenberg JN, Williams GC, et al: The metabolism of 3α,7α,12α-trihydroxy-5β-cholestan-26-oic acid in two siblings with cholestasis due to intrahepatic bile duct anomalies. J Clin Invest 1975; 56:577–587.
213. Govaerts LCP, van den Berg GA, Theeuwes A, et al: Urinary polyamine and metabolite excretion by children with Zellweger's syndrome. Clin Chim Acta 1990; 192:61–68.
214. Schrakamp G, Roosenboom CFP, Schutgens RBH, et al: Alkyl dihydroxyacetone phosphate synthase in human fibroblasts and its deficiency in Zellweger syndrome. J Lipid Res 1985; 26:867–873.
215. Schrakamp G, Schutgens RB, Wanders RJ, et al: The cerebro-hepato-renal (Zellweger) syndrome: Impaired de novo biosynthesis of plasmalogens in cultured skin fibroblasts. Biochim Biophys Acta 1985; 833:170–174.
216. Balistreri WF: Bile acid–induced intestinal dysfunction: Implications to protracted infantile diarrhea and malnutrition. *In* Lebenthal E, ed: Chronic Diarrhea in Children. New York, Nestle, Vevey/Raven Press, 1984, pp 347–364.
217. McJunkin B, Fromm H, Sarva RP, et al: Factors in the mechanism of diarrhea in bile acid malabsorption: Fecal pH—a key determinant. Gastroenterology 1981; 80:1454–1464.
218. Hess-Thaysen E, Pedersen L: Idiopathic bile acid catharsis. Gut 1978; 17:569–570.
219. Balistreri WF, Partin JC, Schubert WK: Bile acid malabsorption—a consequence of terminal ileal dysfunction in protracted diarrhea of infancy. J Pediatr 1977; 90:21–28.
220. Heubi JE, Balistreri WF, Partin JC, et al: Refractory infantile diarrhea due to primary bile acid malabsorption. J Pediatr 1979; 94:546–551.
221. Heubi JE, Balistreri WF, Partin JC, et al: Enterohepatic circulation of bile acids in infants and children with ileal resection. J Lab Clin Med 1980; 95:231–240.
222. Jonas A, Arigao S, Diver-Haber A, et al: Disturbed fat absorption following infectious gastroenteritis in children. J Pediatr 1979; 95:366–372.
223. Balistreri WF, Suchy FJ, Heubi JE: Serum bile acid response to a test meal stimulus: A sensitive test of ileal function. J Pediatr 1980; 96:582–594.
224. Suchy FJ, Balistreri WF: Ileal dysfunction in Crohn's disease assessed by postprandial serum bile acid response. Gut 1981; 22:948–952.
225. Sali A, Murray WR, Mackay C: Aluminum hydroxide in bile salt diarrhoea. Lancet 1977; 2:1051–1054.
226. Clain JE, Malagelada JR, Chadwick VS, et al: Binding properties in vitro of antacids for conjugated bile acids. Gastroenterology 1977; 73:556–559.
227. Mainguet P, Fiasse R: Double-blind placebo-controlled study of loperamide (Imodium) in chronic diarrhoea caused by ileocolic disease or resection. Gut 1977; 18:575–579.
228. Schiller LR, Davis GR, Santa Ana CA, et al: Studies of the mechanism of the antidiarrheal effect of codeine. J Clin Invest 1982; 70:999–1008.
229. Takagi T, Takeda M: Chenodeoxycholic acid–induced diarrhea in rats: Effects of atropine and codeine. Arch Int Pharmacodyn 1979; 240:328–339.
230. Coyne MJ, Bonorris GG, Chung A, et al: Propranolol inhibits bile acid and fatty acid stimulation of cyclic AMP in human colon. Gastroenterology 1977; 73:971–974.
231. Lewis B, Panveliwalla AD, Tabaqchali S, et al: Serum bile acids in the stagnant-loop syndrome. Lancet 1969; 1:219–220.
232. Setchell KDR, Harrison DL, Gilbert JM, et al: Serum unconjugated bile acids: Qualitative and quantitative profiles in ileal resection and bacterial overgrowth. Clin Chim Acta 1985; 152:297–306.
233. Stellaard F, Sauerbruch T, Luderschmidt C, et al: Intestinal involvement in progressive systemic sclerosis detected by increased unconjugated serum bile acids. Gut 1987; 28:446–450.
234. Masclee A, Tangerman A, Van Schaik A, et al: Unconjugated serum bile acids as a marker of small intestinal bacterial overgrowth. Eur J Clin Invest 1989; 19:384–389.

Chapter 4

Indigenous Flora

JEFFREY K. GRIFFITHS and SHERWOOD L. GORBACH

The gut of the infant is colonized soon after birth with a plethora of microorganisms, predominantly anaerobic bacteria. Diet strongly influences the microbial composition, with bottle-fed infants having a more complex flora than that of breast-fed babies. After weaning, the flora approximates that seen in older children and adults. At each stage, the flora forms a complex ecosystem that is resistant to change, but it can be perturbed by dietary alteration or antimicrobial drugs. In an important and incompletely understood way, the indigenous flora of the gut plays a major role in the development of the mucosal immune system, the maturation of the gut itself, and the overall nutrition of the child. In this chapter, we discuss the relationship between the flora and its host in health and disease. We emphasize the complex role that the entire flora plays, rather than focus on a list of the bacteria found at different times or places.

NORMAL FLORA OF THE PEDIATRIC GUT: AGE- AND DIET-RELATED CHANGES

At birth, the sterile gut is rapidly colonized by facultative organisms such as *Escherichia coli* and streptococci, presumably acquired from the vaginal flora of the mother during birth.[1] Soon thereafter, strict anaerobes are found, and a heterogeneous, complex flora begins to develop[2–4] (Table 4–1). In infants delivered by cesarean section, Enterobacteriaceae other than *E. coli* are more frequently found, and the appearance of anaerobes is somewhat delayed.[4, 5] Rather than resembling the mother's flora, the flora of the infant delivered by cesarean section reflects the environment to which it is first exposed, for example, a hospital birthing room. Thus, both the route of delivery and the microbiologic milieu to which the infant is exposed play a role in the development of the flora.

It has been suggested that the slower colonization by anaerobes in infants born prematurely or by cesarean section increases the risk of the infant's acquiring a nosocomial pathogen.[6] Certainly, breast-fed babies are less frequently colonized by highly resistant hospital bacteria.

The initial bacterial flora of a breast-fed baby is rapidly replaced by lactobacilli and bifidobacteria, with some *Clostridium* and *Bacteroides* species also detectable. At 1 week of age, normal breast-fed infants are found to have 100 to 1,000 times more *Bifidobacterium* than members of Enterobacteriaceae in their stools.[7–9] In formula-fed infants, however, members of Enterobacteriaceae usually predominate in the fecal flora. In some urban hospitals in developed countries, *Lactobacillus* may be more common than *Bifidobacterium* in the gut flora of breast-fed infants.[10, 11]

Iron in infant formulas may favor the development of a complex flora composed of members of Enterobacteriaceae, *Bacteroides*, and *Clostridium* species.[12] Because breast milk and unsupplemented cow's milk are relatively low in iron, a less complicated flora of *Lactobacillus* or *Bifidobacterium* usually prevails.

With weaning come changes in the flora of the gut; these changes relate in part to the relative mixture of milk and other foods, but little is known about this process. Increases in the number of *E. coli, Streptococcus*, and *Clostridium* are observed, with a concomitant increase in the isolation of *Bacteroides* and anaerobic gram-positive cocci.[13]

After weaning, the "adult" pattern of flora is seen:

Table 4–1. FECAL FLORAL DEVELOPMENT IN NEONATES DURING FIRST FOUR DAYS OF LIFE*

Bacterial Group	Day 1 (% of neonates)	Day 2 (% of neonates)	Day 3 (% of neonates)	Day 4 (% of neonates)
Enterobacteria	0	52	70	83
Enterococci	4	91	100	100
Pseudomonads	0	0	0	4
Streptococci	9	17	17	35
Staphylococci	26	74	74	48
Anaerobic gram-positive cocci	0	9	26	35
Bacteroides	0	30	61	78
Bifidobacteria	0	74	91	100
Clostridia	0	26	70	78
Eubacteria	0	13	35	35
Fusobacteria	0	0	0	0
Lactobacilli	0	22	27	39
Veillonellae	0	4	9	52

*Percentage of neonates colonized by various bacteria.

Adapted from Rotimi VO, Duerden B: The development of the bacterial flora in normal neonates. J Med Microbiol 1981; 14:51–62; with permission.

Bacteroides and other anaerobic gram-positive organisms tend to equal the numbers of *Bifidobacterium* and *Streptococcus; Clostridium* and *E. coli* are isolated at lower concentrations than before weaning. This stable, or "mature," stage of the fecal flora has been termed an *ecologic climax stage*, or the *C flora*.[14] During the climax stage, the flora is remarkably resistant to invasion by new organisms.[15]

The discussion so far has related to the colonic flora. The stomach, under the influence of stomach acid, has few isolatable organisms, which, if present, reflect the oral and nasopharyngeal floras[16] (Table 4–2). The duodenum and the upper jejunum harbor a sparse flora, generally fewer than 10^4 organisms per ml, which also reflects the oral and nasopharyngeal floras.[17, 18] Further down the small bowel, the number of bacteria increases, and the flora changes to resemble the colonic flora, although facultative bacteria still predominate over anaerobic bacteria. Distal to the ileocecal sphincter, a sharp increase in the number of bacteria is encountered, especially among strict anaerobic forms, which now outnumber aerobic-facultative types by 1,000 to 1.[19–21] The importance of the ileocecal sphincter is illustrated by the observation that cecectomy causes colonization of the upper small bowel in humans and reduction in colonization resistance in the mouse.[22]

Control of the flora is mediated at the portal of entry by gastric acid, which suppresses intrusion by environmental organisms. Normal peristalsis of the intestine is another important control mechanism in the small bowel because it helps clear the upper gut of bacteria. Stasis, such as seen in blind loop syndrome, leads to profoundly higher numbers of bacteria in the upper small bowel.[23–25]

A number of changes occur in the intestinal tract during early development and growth. Developmentally regulated molecules, such as receptors in the microvillus membrane, may account for age-related changes in susceptibility to microbial pathogens or their toxins.

Table 4–2. MATURE HUMAN GASTROINTESTINAL FLORA

	Microbial Concentrations*			
Bacteria	***Stomach***	***Upper Small Bowel***	***Lower Small Bowel***	***Feces***
Aerobic or facultative microorganisms	$0–10^3$	$0–10^5$	$10^3–10^7$	$10^7–10^{12}$
Enterobacteria	$0–10^2$	$0–10^3$	$10^2–10^6$	$10^4–10^{10}$
Streptococci	$0–10^3$	$0–10^4$	$10^2–10^6$	$10^5–10^{10}$
Staphylococci	$0–10^2$	$0–10^3$	$10^2–10^5$	$10^4–10^7$
Lactobacilli	$0–10^3$	$0–10^4$	$10^2–10^5$	$10^6–10^{10}$
Anaerobic bacteria				
Bacteroides	Rare	$0–10^2$	$10^3–10^7$	$10^{10}–10^{12}$
Bifidobacteria	Rare	$0–10^3$	$10^3–10^5$	$10^8–10^{12}$
Streptococci†	Rare	$0–10^3$	$10^2–10^4$	$10^8–10^{11}$
Clostridia	Rare	Rare	$10^2–10^4$	$10^6–10^{11}$
Eubacteria	Rare	Rare	Rare	$10^9–10^{12}$

*Numbers of microorganisms per milliliter or gram of intestinal contents.
†Includes *Peptostreptococcus* and *Peptococcus*.
Adapted from Simon GL, Gorbach SL: Intestinal flora and gastrointestinal function. *In* Johnson R, ed: Physiology of the Gastrointestinal Tract. 2nd ed. New York, Raven Press, 1987, pp 1729–1747; with permission.

Although data from humans are scanty, some information is available from other mammalian systems. Immature rats are more susceptible to *E. coli* heat-stable enterotoxin than are mature rats,[26] and jejunal tissue of the immature rat has more receptors for this molecule than does the jejunal tissue of mature animals.[27] Further, the gut of the preweanling rat is markedly more susceptible to cholera toxin than is that of the postweanling rat.[28] As discussed later, the gut of the human infant appears to be resistant to the effects of *Clostridium difficile* toxins, which are associated with diarrhea and pseudomembranous enterocolitis. In human neonates, jejunal contractions are irregular before 30 weeks of age, and this probably interferes with the normal flux of nutrients and bacteria; stasis may occur in some neonates on a developmental basis.[29]

SMALL BOWEL OVERGROWTH AND TROPICAL SPRUE: CONTRASTS IN FLORA

Gustave Dammin, working in Guatemala in 1945, noted that the intestine of children dying of malnutrition harbored increased numbers of bacteria. Now termed the *small bowel overgrowth syndrome*, this condition is characterized by chronic diarrhea; intestinal malabsorption; and large numbers of bacteria, often anaerobes, in the upper intestine.[30] Steatorrhea, vitamin deficiencies, and carbohydrate malabsorption are frequently present.

Small bowel bacterial overgrowth can be secondary to localized anatomic disorders, such as surgical blind loops, Meckel's or small bowel diverticula, and small bowel strictures caused by surgery or tuberculosis. Overgrowth is also associated with motility derangements, such as seen in chronic malnutrition, diabetes, scleroderma, or abdominal radiation. Another cause of small bowel bacterial overgrowth is the short-gut syndrome, caused by extensive resection of the gut for congenital malformations or necrotizing enterocolitis.

Diagnosis of the overgrowth syndrome is difficult because no simple diagnostic tests are available. The breath hydrogen test may be unreliable,[31] as some bacteria do not produce hydrogen in vitro.[32] Quantitative cultures of jejunal-aspirated fluid remain the gold standard.

Clinical disease is associated with colonization by anaerobic bacteria in the overgrowth syndrome. Merely suppressing the aerobic-facultative bacteria does not reverse the malabsorption of nutrients and the diarrhea. On the other hand, antimicrobial therapy directed against anaerobes is often successful.[21] The processes that cause malabsorption may not be those that lead to diarrhea. Small bowel colonization with *E. coli* alone can cause fluid secretion and diarrhea in rabbit gut loops but does not produce malabsorption.[33] It has been suggested that bile salt deconjugation by enteric bacteria leads to impaired micelle formation in the gut and subsequent fat malabsorption. Although anaerobes such as *Bacteroides, Bifidobacterium, Veillonella, Clostrid-*

ium, and *Enterococcus* perform this deconjugation, coliforms lack the necessary enzymatic systems to do so.[34]

Vitamin B_{12} malabsorption is often seen in the small bowel overgrowth syndrome, and it may cause vitamin B_{12} deficiency and megaloblastic anemia. Again, anaerobes play a major role in vitamin B_{12} malabsorption; metronidazole, but not penicillin or kanamycin, corrects vitamin B_{12} malabsorption in surgically created blind loops in rats.[35] Increased carbohydrate fermentation occurs in the altered milieu of small intestinal overgrowth. D-Xylose absorption is decreased as a result of utilization of the D-xylose by bacteria within the gut lumen.[36] The end products of gut carbohydrate fermentation can be detected in the urine of neonates by gas chromatography; the explanation of this finding is increased intestinal permeability, unabsorbed lactose in the colon, and colonization with nosocomial organisms such as *Klebsiella, Serratia*, and *Enterobacter*.[37]

Because a key part of the overgrowth syndrome is excessive bacterial colonization, Gracey[38] has proposed that it be called the *contaminated small bowel syndrome*. There is merit to this appellation, because antimicrobial therapy directed at reduction of the bacterial flora or surgical correction of an anatomic defect usually cures the disease.

The metabolic activities of colonic bacteria are diverse, and, if colonization is present in abnormal locations such as the upper small bowel, the normal homeostasis between the gut microflora and the host can be altered. For example, tropical sprue, which is associated with malabsorption and vitamin deficiency, is also related to small bowel colonization with aerobic-facultative flora. Obligate anaerobes, which are the hallmark of the overgrowth syndrome, are present only in low numbers in the jejunum of patients with tropical sprue.[39–41] In contrast with the normal or near-normal mucosal architecture in bacterial overgrowth syndromes, the bowel mucosa in patients with tropical sprue demonstrates marked alterations of the mucosal architecture, with blunting of villi and inflammatory infiltration of the lamina propria. Suppression of the small bowel flora by broad-spectrum antibiotics, such as tetracyclines, ameliorates the diarrhea symptoms and malabsorption derangements of tropical sprue. Some researchers have suggested that the coliform flora in tropical sprue contains enterotoxin-producing strains,[42] but this view has not been confirmed. At present, it appears that the primary process in tropical sprue is damage to the mucosa, leading to the secondary effects of bacterial colonization and subsequent malabsorption. Whether the primary cause is a previous viral infection or a toxin disease remains a conundrum.

CHANGES IN THE INTESTINAL FLORA ASSOCIATED WITH ANTIMICROBIAL THERAPY AND DIET

In certain diarrheal diseases, the gut flora is substantially replaced by a pathogen, and antimicrobial therapy is directed to eliminating the pathogen. Cholera is the classic example. Normal gut bacteria decline in number while cholera vibrios colonize the entire gut from the mouth to the anus; only with suppression of the vibrios does the normal flora return to normal levels.[43–45]

Antimicrobials affect all susceptible bacteria, regardless of their pathogenic potential, and treatment of one infection may allow another illness associated with a change of the flora to occur. An example is *C. difficile*–associated diarrhea and colitis. Treatment with various types of antimicrobial drugs has been implicated as a principal precipitant of the disease. The antimicrobial drugs suppress the normal flora and allow *C. difficile* to overgrow in this "microbial vacuum." Diarrhea and colitis are caused by the toxins of *C. difficile*, which cause fluid secretion and cell damage. Interestingly, the large bowel of the neonate is relatively resistant to the toxins. Thus, rates of colonization with *C. difficile* and the presence of its toxin are high (as much as 70% in newborn nurseries), yet clinical disease is rare. Gryboski and coworkers[46] have commented on the frequency of immune defects in infants and children who have symptomatic *C. difficile* infection, thus accounting for the presence of disease in the naturally resistant gut at this age.

Other examples of the adverse effects of suppressing the flora are found in the child who is admitted to the intensive care unit and treated with potent broad-spectrum antimicrobials, and the child who is administered immunosuppressive treatment and concurrent antimicrobial prophylaxis. Stool cultures yield highly resistant gram-negative bacilli and yeasts. In this setting, the normal flora has been replaced by the hospital flora, and the gut then serves as a reservoir for resistant organisms that cause systemic infections in the vulnerable patient.[47]

Dietary intake can also influence the bacterial composition of the intestinal flora. Changes in bacterial populations are associated with altered metabolic reactions in the gut. In general, adults eating low-fat, high–complex-carbohydrate diets have higher fecal counts of aerobic bacteria and lower numbers of anaerobic bacteria.[48] This observation is the functional equivalent of the differences seen in breast- versus bottle-fed infants. These shifts in the flora are not dramatic and are of uncertain clinical importance. These differences may be more important in the long term, however, as some components of the bacterial flora have the ability to convert dietary compounds into carcinogens, as discussed later.

METABOLIC EFFECTS OF THE GUT FLORA

The normal flora of the gut contains more than 400 species of bacteria.[49] Because of this diversity, it is difficult to show changes associated with any specific bacterium in the setting of a disease or an altered diet. However, the metabolic activity of the gut microflora *as a whole* can be assessed in response to various factors.

To the patient and to the clinician, these changes in metabolic activity of the microflora are more important than the specific names of the multitudinous bacteria.

A classic example of the metabolic activity of the microflora is the ability of the gut flora to inactivate certain antibiotics. The microflora, capable of esterifying primary amino groups, can inactivate sulfonamides and aminoglycosides. De-esterification also occurs with chloramphenicol, with release of the dichloracetyl group and loss of activity of the drug.

Compounds that undergo enterohepatic circulation are strongly affected by the metabolic alterations of the microflora. Estrogens, vitamins (folic acid, vitamin B_{12}, and derivatives of vitamin D), cholesterol, protoporphyrin, and bile acids are naturally occurring compounds that undergo circulation through the liver, biliary excretion, reabsorption from the intestine, and deliverance via the portal vein to the liver. Drugs that undergo this circulation include morphine, digoxin, rifampin, promethazine, and colchicine. The gut flora removes polar molecules, such as glucuronic acid or sulfate, which are conjugated to compounds in the liver for solubilization and excretion in the biliary system. The deconjugated, or "free," molecule can then be reabsorbed by the bowel and returned to the liver. The liver once again attaches a polar group to the compound and then excretes the conjugated compound via the bile.[50] The gut flora may remove the polar group, and the cycle may occur once again or the molecule may be excreted in the feces.

Diet can alter the balance of deconjugation and reabsorption versus excretion. Vegetarian women, for example, excrete more estrogen in their stool and have lower serum levels of estrogen than do omnivore women.[51] The mechanism that contributes to these findings is related to reduced deconjugating enzyme activity in the microflora of vegetarian women. Conjugated estrogen excreted in bile is reabsorbed to a lower extent in vegetarian women, leading to higher fecal levels and lower serum levels.

In a related manner, in the 1970s, oral contraceptive failures were reported in some women taking a variety of antimicrobial drugs, including rifampin, ampicillin, chloramphenicol, and nitrofurantoin. In a small group of women who were taking oral contraceptives and who were studied while taking ampicillin and tetracycline, urinary excretion of ethinyl estradiol, the synthetic estrogen in oral contraceptives, was decreased, as was the fecal level of bacterial beta-glucuronidase. The metabolism of exogenous estrogen contraceptives can be altered by antimicrobial therapy, which probably suppresses the bacteria that deconjugate estrogens.[52] More ethinyl estradiol is lost in the feces, with lower serum levels, which could permit ovulation and unexpected pregnancy.

The microflora also synthesizes helpful compounds, such as vitamin K and its homologues, biotin, thiamine, and folic acid. For vitamin K, sufficient amounts are made by the microflora so that no dietary supplementation is usually necessary to meet the human host's needs; antibiotic therapy, however, can suppress vitamin K endogenous production. Germ-free or antibiotic-treated animals require biotin in their feed, but normal animals do not need this supplementation.[53]

Any substance entering the gut is a potential foodstuff for the microflora as well as the host. For example, the dietary disaccharides sucrose, lactose, and maltose are normally hydrolyzed by the mucosal brush border enzymes of gut enterocytes in the upper small bowel. In persons with a genetic or acquired disaccharidase deficiency, these sugars remain intact and are not absorbed in the small intestine. They are delivered to the ileum and large bowel where bacterial lactases, maltases, and sucrases hydrolyze the disaccharides. These simple sugars are then fermented to short-chain fatty acids (SCFAs). The end result is diarrhea with an acidic fecal effluent.

Other carbohydrates in foods are also metabolized by the microflora. The normal small bowel is unable to absorb 5 to 20% of dietary starch, as measured by breath hydrogen excretion.[54] Unabsorbed carbohydrates include not only dietary starch but also other plant fibers and sugars, such as arabinose, xylose, mannose, and rhamnose[55]; these compounds are carried into the metabolic cauldron of the colon, where they are fermented by the colonic bacteria to SCFAs and other products. SCFAs are a major source of energy for the colonic mucosa and the host, and their rate of absorption is faster than that of sodium.[56] It has been estimated that this metabolic activity of the colonic flora contributes 5 to 10% of the total daily energy requirements, and in marginally nourished children, this amount may be significant.

When added to total parenteral nutrition, butyrate, a major SCFA, ameliorates the atrophy of the colonic mucosa usually seen with this form of therapy.[57] Indeed, butyrate appears to be a major source of energy for colonic enterocytes, even in the presence of glucose,[58] and it may be a required nutrient for the healthy colon.[59] A chronic lack of SCFAs can lead to nutritional colitis and diarrhea, known to clinicians as *diversion* or *starvation colitis*. Excluding SCFAs from the colon results in the conversion of the colonic mucosa from an absorptive to a secretory epithelium.[60] It has been suggested that ulcerative colitis could be classified as a nutritional colitis, because ulcerative colitis colonic epithelial cells are unable to utilize SCFAs, despite abundant quantities in the lumen.[61]

Other products of microflora carbohydrate fermentation, such as D-lactic acid and pyruvate, have been reported to cause a clinical illness similar to alcohol intoxication.[62] This is seen most commonly in short bowel overgrowth syndromes.

Bacterial metabolism of proteins and amino acids, whether from dietary sources or sloughed enterocytes and mucin, results in the formation of amines and short-chain organic acids. Unabsorbed dietary fatty acids in patients with steatorrhea are carried to the ileum and colon, where they can be converted to hydroxylated acids, such as stearic acid, which can stimulate fluid secretion in the colon and produce diarrhea.[50]

Dietary patterns established in childhood can have important consequences for diseases of adults. As mentioned earlier, the bacterial flora can metabolize certain exogenous and endogenous compounds to active carcinogens. Epidemiologic studies have demonstrated a strong correlation between a "Western" diet (high in animal fat and low in fiber) and the incidence of colon cancer.[63] Specific enzyme activities that are thought to promote carcinogen production are found at higher levels in the microflora of people consuming a Western diet. For example, nitroreductase and azoreductase are enzymes that reduce nitro compounds and azo compounds, respectively, to known carcinogens. These enzymes are mostly confined to the colonic flora. Common intestinal bacteria, such as *Enterococcus, Clostridium, Bacteroides*, and *Bifidobacterium*, are capable of adding a nitroso group to secondary amines, via *N*-nitrosation. Azo dyes, commonly used in the food dye, textile, and printing industries, are degraded by intestinal bacteria. Many azo compounds have been proscribed as food dyes, as evidence has accumulated of their carcinogenic potential. Vegetarians in the United States have lower levels of fecal bacterial nitroreductase and azoreductase than do Americans who ingest a Western diet.[64] Just as hypertension in children has become a concern because of adverse outcomes in adults, so should dietary patterns in childhood be considered in the development of colon cancer in adults.

PROBIOTICS: MANIPULATION OF THE GUT FLORA

Manipulation of the gut flora by administering "helpful" exogenous bacteria, known as *probiotics*, is an old idea. Many claims have been made for the beneficial effects of yogurt and other fermented dairy products. Fermentation of food with lactobacilli increases the availability, digestibility, and assimilation of nutrients. Moreover, people who are lactase-deficient are able to ingest yogurt even when they are intolerant of other milk products[65]; the yogurt organisms *Lactobacillus bulgaricus* and *Streptococcus thermophilus* provide the necessary lactase absent in the host.

There is some evidence that altering the flora with yogurt, other fermented dairy products, or lyophilized lactic acid bacteria can ameliorate diarrhea of various causes. Zychowicz and coworkers[66, 67] found that milk fermented with *Lactobacillus acidophilus* decreased the fecal shedding rate in children with chronic *Salmonella* and *Shigella* infections, and continued administration eliminated diarrhea. Gotz and colleagues[68] demonstrated that lactobacilli decreased the incidence of ampicillin-associated diarrhea from 14 to 0% in a group of children. Alm[69] reported that the duration of *Salmonella* carriage was decreased in persons given *L. acidophilus*. Gorbach and associates[70] reported that relapsing *C. difficile* colitis was successfully treated with a newly discovered human *Lactobacillus casei* strain known as *Lactobacillus* GG. It is likely that the common mechanism of action in these two reports is colonization of the gut flora. In the case of *Lactobacillus* GG, and probably other lactic acid bacteria, the organism produces an antimicrobial substance that suppresses various bacterial pathogens.[71]

Diarrhea and malnutrition in children remain major public health issues for the world.[72, 73] Recent evidence suggests that bloody diarrhea with dysentery and persistent diarrhea are the two major killers rather than acute watery diarrhea. It appears that yogurt, with its supply of lactase and increased availability of nutrients compared with whole milk or soy milk, may become an important adjunct in the treatment of these diarrheas. In 1963, Niv and coworkers[74] reported that yogurt decreased the duration of illness in infants hospitalized with acute diarrhea. More recently, Ghazalia and associates[75] demonstrated that yogurt, when compared with milk, decreased the duration of illness in infants with persistent diarrhea. In Pakistan, Bhutta and coworkers[76] have compared the effect of yogurt and kitchri (a vegetable, rice, and lentil mixture) with soya-based, lactose-free formula in the dietary management of diarrhea persisting for 14 days or longer; the yogurt-based regimen was clearly superior to the soya regimen, as measured by weight gain, stool frequency, and stool volumes. In a recent report from Finland, children hospitalized with acute diarrhea, mostly caused by rotavirus, recovered more rapidly when given either fermented milk with *Lactobacillus* GG or lyophilized *Lactobacillus* GG, compared with placebo-treated control subjects.[77] Studies currently in progress will help define the role, if any, of fermented dairy products in the treatment of diarrhea in children.

INTESTINAL MICROFLORA AND THE IMMUNE SYSTEM

Seventy percent of the daily production of immunoglobulin (Ig) is secreted into the gut.[78] One fourth of the gut mass is lymphoid tissue, composed of Peyer's patches, other lymphoid tissues, and intraepithelial lymphocytes. The normal gut has been characterized as existing in a state of "physiologic inflammation" induced by the microflora.[79] The presence of the flora not only induces but also maintains mucosal immunity, a system characterized by committed antibody-producing B cells; T helper and suppressor cells; and accessory cells, such as macrophages and mast cells. Secretory IgA is released at the mucosal surface by enterocytes. Many of the morphologic abnormalities seen in germ-free animals, such as longer intestinal villi, shorter crypts, and a sparsely populated lamina propria,[80] are the reflection of a sparsely developed immune system with few immunologically active cells in the lamina propria. Epithelial cell regulation by locally produced cytokines and precursors, like those produced by immunologically competent cells, is far different in the germ-free gut compared with the normal colonized gut.[81] Because enterocytes are capable of elaborating a number of cytokines, they may assist in the regulation of underlying lymphoid cells. It is uncertain whether the differences in the microbial composition of the intestinal flora affect the overall immunologic competency of the mucosal immune system in the normal child. Nonetheless, it is clear that the state of readiness of the mucosal immune system is maintained by the flora, and intestinal immunity may work synergistically with the microflora to resist colonization by new, potentially pathogenic microorganisms.

REFERENCES

1. Tannock GW, Fuller R, Smith SL, et al: Plasmid profiling of members of the family Enterobacteriaceae, lactobacilli, and the bifidobacteria to study the transmission of bacteria from mother to infant. J Clin Microbiol 1990; 28:1225–1228.
2. Gareau FE, Mackel DC, Boring JR III, et al: The acquisition of fecal flora by infants from their mothers during birth. J Pediatr 1959; 54:313–318.
3. Long SS, Swenson RM: Development of anaerobic fecal flora in healthy newborn infants. J Pediatr 1977; 91:298–301.
4. Rotimi VO, Duerden B: The development of the bacterial flora in normal neonates. J Med Microbiol 1981; 14:51–62.
5. Neut C, Bezirtzoglou E, Romand C, et al: Bacterial colonization of the large intestine in newborns delivered by cesarean section. Zentralbl Bakteriol Hyg 1987; A266:330–337.
6. Bhutta ZA, Naqvi SH, Muzaffar T, et al: Neonatal sepsis in Pakistan: Presentation and pathogens. Acta Paediatr Scand 1991; 80:596–601.
7. Cooperstock MS, Zedd AJ: Intestinal flora of infants. *In* Hentges D, ed: Human Intestinal Microflora in Health and Disease. New York, Academic Press, 1983, pp 79–99.
8. Benno Y, Sawada K, Mitsuoka T: The intestinal microflora of infants: composition of fecal flora in breast-fed and bottle-fed infants. Microbiol Immunol 1984; 28:975–986.
9. Tomkins AM, Bradley AK, Oswald S, et al: Diet and the faecal microflora of infants, children and adults in rural Nigeria and urban UK. J Hyg (Lond):1981; 86:285–293.
10. Lundequist B, Nord CE, Winberg J: The composition of the faecal microflora in breast-fed and bottle-fed infants from birth to eight weeks. Acta Paediatr Scand 1985; 74:45–51.
11. Hall MA, Cole CB, Smith SL, et al: Factors influencing the presence of faecal lactobacilli in early infancy. Arch Dis Child 1990; 65:185–189.
12. Mevissen-Verhage EA, Marcelis JH, de Vos MN, et al: *Bifidobacterium, Bacteroides* and *Clostridium* spp. in fecal samples from breast-fed and bottle-fed infants with and without iron supplement. J Clin Microbiol 1987; 25:285–289.
13. Mata LV, Urrutia JJ: Intestinal colonization of breast-fed children in a rural area of low socio-economic level. Ann NY Acad Sci 1971; 176:93–109.
14. Wilson KH, Patel M, Permoad P et al: Ecological succession: Use in development of synthetic microfloras. Microecol Ther 1986; 16:181–189.
15. Gorbach SL, Barza M, Guiliano M, et al: Colonization resistance of the human intestinal microflora: Testing the hypothesis in normal volunteers. Eur J Clin Microbiol Infect Dis 1988; 7:98–102.
16. Drasar BS, Shiner M, McLeod GM: Studies on the intestinal flora: I. The bacterial flora of the gastrointestinal tract in healthy and achlorhydric persons. Gastroenterology 1969; 56:71–79.
17. Justesen T, Nielsen DH, Hjelt K, et al: Normal cultivable microflora in upper jejunal fluid in children without gastrointestinal disorders. J Pediatr Gastroenterol Nutr 1984; 3:683–686.
18. Justesen T, Nielsen OH, Jacobson IE, et al: The normal cultivable microflora in upper jejunal fluid in healthy adults. Scand J Gastroenterol 1984; 19:279–282.
19. Gorbach SL, Plaut AF, Nahas L, et al: Studies of intestinal microflora: II. Microorganisms of the small intestine and their relations to oral and fecal flora. Gastroenterology 1967; 53:856–867.
20. Savage DC: Microbial ecology of the gastrointestinal tract. Annu Rev Microbiol 1977; 31:107.
21. Simon GL, Gorbach SL: The human intestinal microflora. Dig Dis Sci 1986; 1:147S–162S.
22. Voravuthikunchai SP, Lee A: Cecectomy causes long-term reduction of colonization resistance in the mouse gastrointestinal tract. Infect Immunol 1987; 55:995–999.
23. Dixon JMS: The fate of bacteria in the small intestine. J Pathol Bacteriol 1960; 79:131–140.
24. Broido PW, Gorbach SL, Nyhus LM: Microflora of the gastrointestinal tract and the surgical malabsorption syndromes. Surg Gynecol Obstet 1972; 135:449–460.
25. Drude RB Jr, Hines C Jr: The pathophysiology of intestinal bacterial overgrowth syndromes. Arch Intern Med 1980; 140:1349–1352.
26. Cohen MB, Moyer MS, Luttrell M, et al: The immature rat small intestine exhibits an increased sensitivity and response to *Escherichia coli* heat-stable enterotoxin. Pediatr Res 1986; 20:555–560.
27. Chu SH, Ely IG, Walker WA: Age and cortisone alter host responsiveness to cholera toxin in the developing gut. Am J Physiol 1989; 256:G220–G225.
28. Seo JK, Chu SW, Walker WA: Development of intestinal host defense: An increased sensitivity in the adenylate cyclase response to cholera toxin in suckling rats. Pediatr Res 1980; 25:225–227.
29. Morriss FV, Moore M, Weisbrodt NW, et al: Ontogenic development of gastrointestinal motility: IV. Duodenal contractions in preterm infants. Pediatrics 1986; 78:1106–1113.
30. King CE, Toskes PP: Small intestine bacterial overgrowth. Gastroenterology 1979; 76:1035–1055.
31. Corazza GR, Menozzi MG, Strocchi A, et al: The diagnosis of small bowel bacterial overgrowth: Reliability of jejunal culture and inadequacy of breath hydrogen testing. Gastroenterology 1990; 98:302–309.
32. Khin-Maung-U, Tin-Aye, Ku-Tin-Myint, et al: In vitro hydrogen production by enteric bacteria cultured from children with small bowel bacterial overgrowth. J Pediatr Gastroenterol Nutr 1992; 14:192–197.
33. Wanke CA, Guerrant RL: Small bowel colonization alone is a cause of diarrhea. Infect Immunol 1987; 55:1924–1926.
34. Lewis R, Gorbach S: Modification of bile acids by intestinal bacteria. Arch Intern Med 1972; 130:545–548.
35. Welkos S, Toskes P, Baer H: Importance of anaerobic bacteria in the cobalamin malabsorption of the experimental rat blind loop syndrome. Gastroenterology 1981; 80:313–320.
36. Goldstein F, Karacadag S, Wirts CW, et al: Intraluminal small intestinal utilization of D-xylose by bacteria: A limitation of the D-xylose absorption test. Gastroenterology 1970; 59:380–386.
37. Walker V, Mills GA, Hall MA, et al: Carbohydrate fermentation by gut microflora in preterm neonates. Arch Dis Child 1989; 64:1367–1373.
38. Gracey M: The contaminated small bowel syndrome: Pathogenesis, diagnosis and treatment. Am J Clin Nutr 1979; 32:234–243.
39. Bhat P, Shantakumari S, Rajan D, et al: Bacterial flora of the gastrointestinal tract in Southern Indian control subjects and patients with tropical sprue. Gastroenterology 1972; 62:11–21.
40. Gorbach SL, Mitra R, Jacobs B, et al: Bacterial contamination of the upper small bowel in tropical sprue. Lancet 1969; 1:59–61.
41. Cook GC: Etiology and pathogenesis of postinfective tropical malabsorption (tropical sprue). Lancet 1984; 1:721–723.
42. Klipstein FA, Holdeman LV, Corcino JJ, et al: Enterotoxigenic intestinal bacteria in tropical sprue. Ann Intern Med 1973; 79:632–641.
43. Gorbach SL, Banwell JG, Chatterjee BD, et al: Acute undifferentiated human diarrhea in the tropics: I. Alterations in intestinal microflora. J Clin Invest 1971; 50:881–889.
44. Gorbach SL, Banwell JG, Jacobs B: Intestinal microflora in Asiatic cholera: I. "Rice-water" stool. J Infect Dis 1970; 121:32–37.
45. Gorbach SL, Banwell JG, Jacobs B, et al: Intestinal microflora in Asiatic cholera: II. The small bowel. J Infect Dis 1970; 121:38–45.
46. Gryboski JD, Pellerano R, Young N, et al: Positive role of *Clostridium difficile* infection in diarrhea in infants and children. Am J Gastroenterol 1991; 86:685–689.
47. Bonatti H, Guggenbichler JP, Hager J: Treatment of nosocomial infections in children undergoing antimicrobial chemotherapy. Infection 1990; 18:302–306.
48. Gorbach SL: Function of the normal human microflora: The Bengt E. Gustafsson Memorial Lecture. Scand J Infect Dis 1986; 49(Suppl):17–30.
49. Finegold SM, Attebury HR, Sutter VL: Effect of diet on human fecal flora: Comparison of Japanese and American diets. Am J Clin Nutr 1974; 27:1456–1469.

50. Goldin BR, Lichtenstein AH, Gorbach SL: The role of intestinal flora. *In* Shils ME, Young V, eds: Modern Nutrition in Health and Disease. 7th ed. Philadelphia, Lea and Febiger, 1988, pp 500–515.
51. Goldin BR, Adlercreutz H, Gorbach SL, et al: Estrogen excretion patterns and plasma levels in vegetarian and omnivorous women. N Engl J Med 1982; 307:1542–1547.
52. Swenson L, Goldin BR, Gorbach SL: Effects of antibiotics of fecal/urinary excretion of ethinyl estradiol, and oral contraceptive. Gastroenterology 1980; 78:1332.
53. Coates ME, Fuller R: The gnotobiotic animal and the study of gut microbiology. *In* Clarke RTJ, Bauchop T, eds: Microbial Ecology of the Gut Flora. New York, Academic Press, 1977, pp 311–346.
54. Anderson IH, Levine AS, Levitt MD: Incomplete absorption of the carbohydrate in all-purpose wheat flour. N Engl J Med 1981; 304:891–892.
55. Vercellotti JR, Salyers AA, Ballard WS, et al: Breakdown of mucin and plant polysaccharides in the human colon. Can J Biochem 1977; 55:1190–1196.
56. McNeil NI, Cummings JH, James WPT: Short chain fatty acid absorption by the human large intestine. Gut 1978; 19:819–822.
57. Goldstein RM, Hebiguchi T, Luk GD: The effects of total parenteral nutrition on gastrointestinal growth and development. J Pediatr Surg 1985; 67:975–982.
58. Roediger WEW: Role of anaerobic bacteria in the metabolic welfare of the colonic mucosa in man. Gut 1980; 21:793–798.
59. Royall D, Wolever TMS, Jeejeebhoy KN: Clinical review: Clinical significance of colonic fermentation. Am J Gastroenterol 1990; 85:1307–1312.
60. Roediger WE, Rae DA: Trophic effect of short chain fatty acids on mucosal handling of ions by the defunctioned colon. Br J Surg 1982; 69:23–25.
61. Roediger WEW: The starved colon: Diminished mucosal nutrition, diminished absorption, and colitis. Dis Colon Rectum 1990; 33:858–862.
62. The colon, the rumen, and D-lactic acidosis (editorial). Lancet 1990; 336:559–560.
63. Goldin BR, Sullivan CE, Gorbach SL: Etiologic factors in the development of colonic cancer: Bacteria, beef and animal fat. *In* Kurtz RC, ed: Nutrition in Gastrointestinal Diseases. New York, Churchill Livingstone, 1981.
64. Goldin BR, Swenson L, Dwyer J, et al: Effect of diet and *Lactobacillus* acidophilus supplements on human fecal bacterial enzymes. J Natl Cancer Inst 1980; 64:255–261.
65. Gorbach SL: Lactic acid bacteria and human health. Ann Med 1990; 22:37–41.
66. Zychowicz C, Surazymska A, Sierwierska B, et al: Effect of *Lactobacillus acidophilus* cultures (acidophilus milk) on the carrier state of *Shigella* and *Salmonella* organisms in children. Pediatr Pol 1974; 49:997–1003.
67. Zychowicz C, Kowalczyk C, Cieplinska T: Results of administration of *Lactobacillus acidophilus* cultures (acidophilus milk) in an endemic focus of dysentery. Pediatr Pol 1975; 50:429–435.
68. Gotz V, Romankiewicz JA, Moss J, et al: Prophylaxis against ampicillin-associated diarrhea with a *Lactobacillus* preparation. Am J Hosp Pharm 1979; 36:754.
69. Alm L: The effect of *Lactobacillus acidophilus* administration upon the survival of *Salmonella* in randomly selected human carriers. Prog Food Nutr Sci 1983; 7:13–17.
70. Gorbach SL, Chang TW, Goldin BR: Successful treatment of relapsing *Clostridium difficile* colitis with *Lactobacillus* GG. Lancet 1987; 2:1519.
71. Silva M, Jacobus NV, Deneke C, et al: An antimicrobial substance from a human *Lactobacillus* strain. Antimicrob Agents Chemother 1987; 1:1231–1233.
72. Briend A: Is diarrhoea a major cause of malnutrition among the under-fives in developing countries? A review of available evidence. Eur J Clin Nutr 1990; 44:611–628.
73. Mata L: Infection, malnutrition and growth. J Gastroenterol Hepatol 1990; 1(Suppl):32–43.
74. Niv M, Levy W, Greenstein NM: Yogurt in the treatment of infantile diarrhea. Clin Pediatr 1963; 2:407–411.
75. Boudraa G, Touhami M, Pochart P, et al: Effect of feeding yogurt versus milk in children with persistent diarrhoea. J Pediatr Gastroenterol Nutr 1990; 11:509–512.
76. Bhutta ZA, Molla AM, Issani Z, et al: Dietary management of persistent diarrhea: Comparison of a traditional rice-lentil based diet with soy formula. Pediatrics 1991; 88:1010–1018.
77. Isolauri E, Juntunen M, Rautanen T, et al: A human *Lactobacillus* strain *(Lactobacillus casei* spp strain GG) promotes recovery from acute diarrhea in children. Pediatrics 1991; 88:90–97.
78. Keren DF: Gastrointestinal immune system and its disorders. Monog Pathol 1990; 31:247–285.
79. Simon GL, Gorbach SL: Intestinal flora and gastrointestinal function. *In* Johnson LR, ed: Physiology of the Gastrointestinal Tract. 2nd ed. New York, Raven Press, 1987, pp 1729–1747.
80. Abrams GD, Bauer H, Sprinz H: Influence of the normal flora on mucosal morphology and cellular renewal in the ileum: A comparison of germ-free and conventional mice. Lab Invest 1962; 12:355–364.
81. Castro GA: Immunological regulation of epithelial function. Am J Physiol 1982; 243:G321–G329.

Chapter 5

Gastrointestinal Motility

PAUL E. HYMAN and CARLO DiLORENZO

ANATOMY[1]

Visceral myocytes are spindle shaped, measuring 200 to 300 μm in length and 10 to 20 μm in diameter at rest. They may shorten to 25% of their resting length in maximal isotonic contraction. Myocytes in neonates are about half the length of myocytes in adults. The cell membrane is characterized by several distinctive features, including (1) caveolae, which are flask-shaped invaginations of unknown function that cover one third of the cell surface, increasing the total amount of the cell membrane by 50 to 70%; and (2) dense bands, which are electron-dense materials that are the attachment sites for thin (actin) filaments and intermediate filaments.

Within the myocytes are numerous microtubules, centrioles, Golgi apparatus, lysosomes, sarcoplasmic reticula, mitochondria, and three kinds of filaments. Actin, or thin filaments, are about 12 times more numerous than myosin, the thick filaments. The actin and myosin filaments interdigitate. Intermediate filaments are composed of desmin, which is a fibrous protein that forms a cytoskeletal network. Eighty to 90% of the volume of a smooth muscle cell is composed of filamentous contractile proteins and dense bodies.

Cell-to-cell communications occur through several kinds of junctions. *Intermediate junctions* occur when dense bands from adjacent cells form a symmetric junction. These intermediate junctions may provide direct mechanical links between myocytes. *Gap junctions* are oval areas of cell membrane closely opposed to an identical region of an adjacent cell. Gap junctions probably facilitate the movement of certain ions.

Myocytes are densely packed into the muscularis mucosae and muscularis externa. Cells lie parallel to each other and often form sheets. The inner layer of circular muscle and the external layer of longitudinal muscle run at right angles (orthogonal) to each other in both muscularis mucosae, which averages 38 μm in thickness, and the muscularis externa. In the colon, the muscularis externa does not surround the entire circular layer, as in the small intestine, but is arranged into three thick longitudinal bands called the taenia coli.

The relatively scant extracellular matrix within the muscle tissue contains abundant collagen fibrils, which probably transmit tension between groups of muscle. Other cells within smooth muscle tissue include interstitial Cajal cells, macrophages, mast cells, and myoblast-like cells.

The innervation of the intestinal tract consists of intrinsic and extrinsic fibers. Extrinsic nerves include the preganglionic fibers of the vagus and the postganglionic fibers of the sympathetic nerves from the celiac, superior, and inferior mesenteric ganglia. The vagal parasympathetic nerves increase contractions, whereas the sympathetic nerves decrease contractions. Nerves enter the intestinal wall through the mesentery, along branches of the large blood vessels. Most nerve fibers within the gut are entirely intrinsic. Intrinsic neurons are found in the myenteric plexus (Auerbach's plexus), situated between the circular and the longitudinal layers of the muscularis externa, and the submucous plexus (Meissner's plexus), situated between muscle layers of the submucosa. The neuroanatomy of the intestine is discussed in detail in Chapter 7.

STIMULUS-CONTRACTION COUPLING

Stimulus-contraction coupling refers to the mechanisms by which a substance interacts with a myocyte to increase cellular calcium (iCa^{2+}) and induce contraction[2] (Fig. 5–1). Muscle contraction is the biologically rele-

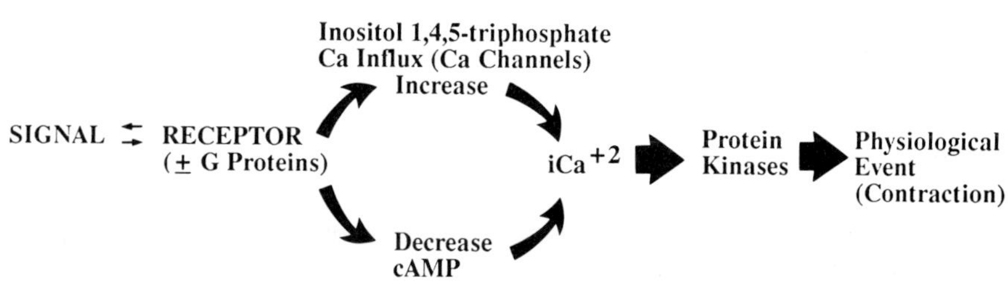

Figure 5–1. Stimulus-contraction coupling.

vant final response to cellular functions that begin with the binding of an agonist, such as acetylcholine or substance P, to a receptor on the myocyte plasma membrane. Agonist-receptor binding initiates a series of intracellular events, often beginning with activation of a G protein, one of a class of membrane proteins binding guanine nucleotides, which act as signal transducers of the intracellular response. Receptor-operated calcium channels may open, leading to an influx of extracellular calcium down a steep concentration gradient. Calcium influx causes depolarization of membrane potential; this mechanism is called *electromechanical coupling*. Influx of extracellular calcium is necessary for optimal contraction of tissues with brief, forceful phasic contractions, such as the gastric antrum and the small intestine. There may be activation of phospholipase C, which generates the second-messenger inositol 1,4,5-triphosphate (IP_3) and diacylglycerol. IP_3 mobilizes intracellular calcium stores from the sarcoplasmic reticulum and raises the concentration of free intracellular calcium. Intracellular stores of calcium are used for contraction of tonically contracting tissues, such as the gastric fundus and lower esophageal sphincter.[3] This is accomplished without changes in membrane potential and is called *pharmacomechanical coupling*. Increases in iCa^{2+} result in calcium binding to the regulatory protein calmodulin. Calmodulin then binds to another regulatory protein, caldesmon. In the relaxed state, caldesmon binds to the myosin-binding domain of actin. When the calcium-activated calmodulin complex binds to caldesmon, it causes a conformational change that allows the actin-myosin interaction. Ca^{2+}-bound calmodulin activates myosin light-chain kinase. This enzyme phosphorylates myosin light chains, the regulatory subunits of the myosin complex. Phosphorylation of the two 20-kd light chains of myosin activates the adenosine triphosphate (ATP) hydrolysis site (Mg^{+2}–ATPase) on the head region of the myosin heavy chain, resulting in actin-myosin cross-bridge formation (Fig. 5–2).

Cross-bridges appear to be the most important mechanism for tension development and shortening of the smooth muscle cell. When the iCa^{2+} decreases within the cytoplasm, myosin light chain phosphatase cleaves the phosphate from the light chains, terminating the cross-bridge. The isometric tension reflects the number of cross-bridges and so may be related to the quantity of actin and myosin in the tissue. In contrast, the maximal velocity of shortening of the tissue is related to the cross-bridge cycling rate.

Relaxation of the myocyte is mediated by membrane receptors for substances such as vasoactive intestinal peptide (VIP), which act by closing calcium channels, decreasing IP_3 production, and increasing intracellular concentrations of cyclic adenosine monophosphate. Each of these effects results in decreasing the iCa^{2+}.

SMALL INTESTINE

The small intestine measures about 270 cm in newborns and grows to about 4 to 5 m in the adult. Ingested fluid or solid will not propagate caudally by gravity but requires coordinated contractions of the bowel wall. The rate of propulsion and the vigor of mixing are linked to the effective digestion and absorption of the luminal contents. In addition to the mixing and propulsion of food, intestinal motor activity functions during fasting to sweep the small bowel clear of undigestible food particles, bacteria, and desquamated cells. In the special circumstance of vomiting, bowel contents move rapidly in the orad direction.[4]

All motor functions are executed by the coordinated contraction and relaxation of the muscle layers in the small intestinal wall. Contractions and relaxations are regulated by the intrinsic activity of the smooth muscle tissue together with the modulating actions of the autonomic nervous system and gastrointestinal hormones. The human enteric nervous system (ENS), consisting of cell bodies and processes of the neural plexi within the gut wall, contains more than 10^8 neurons, which is roughly equivalent to the number of neurons in the spinal cord. Neural networks integrate central nervous system (CNS) and the sensory information that modulates motor responses. This "decision making" is highly complex, so that the myenteric, neural, and hormonal control of the gut together are known as the "gut brain,"[5] or the "little brain" of the gut.[6]

Peristaltic Reflex

There is an intestinal peristaltic reflex consisting of coordinated contraction above, and relaxation below, the site of stimulation. The stimulant is most often food, as it contacts or distends the mucosa. The coordination of the peristaltic reflex is abolished by nicotinic antagonists, suggesting the involvement of cholinergic interneurons within the myenteric plexus. Cholinergic and tachykinin motor neurons are responsible for contraction, and VIP motor neurons regulate descending relaxation.[7] Myenteric plexus interneurons influence peristalsis through interactions with motor neurons, without directly stimulating smooth muscle cells. Somatostatin neurons release somatostatin during descending relaxation, enhancing VIP release. Opioid neurons exert a continuous inhibitory effect on VIP neurons.[8]

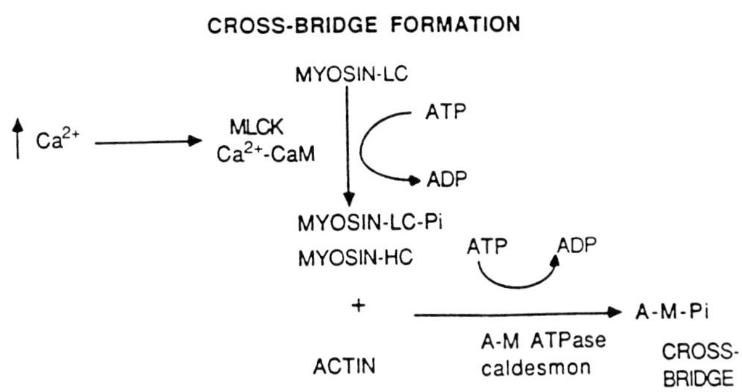

Figure 5–2. Intracellular events mediating cross-bridge formation. LC, light chain; HC, heavy chain; MLCK, myosin light-chain kinase; Pi, phosphate. (Courtesy of R. Willenbucher, MD)

Fasting Motility

During fasting, small bowel motility is organized into a recurrent pattern of three different phases that together constitute the migrating motor complex (MMC). These phases consist of a period of quiescence (phase 1), which is followed by a period of random, intermittent contractions (phase 2), similar to the normal postprandial pattern. Phase 2 is succeeded by 3 to 7 minutes of high-amplitude contractions occurring at the maximal possible frequency for each intestinal site (phase 3; Fig. 5–3). Phase 3 can start anywhere from the lower esophageal sphincter to the distal jejunum, and it propagates at a rate of 5 to 15 cm per minute toward the ileum, often stopping before reaching the ileocecal junction. As one complex reaches the terminal ileum, another complex starts in the proximal bowel. Phase 3 migrates approximately at the same speed in children and in adults. The complete MMC occurs every 90 to 300 minutes in adults and every 40 to 100 minutes in infants. The age-related changes in MMC duration have important practical implications: similar information is accrued from a shorter antroduodenal manometry in infants compared with adults. The length of phase 2 varies inversely with the length of phase 1 and appears to be associated with the level of arousal, with phase 1 dominating during sleep. Intestinal transit time is fastest during phase 3. On the other hand, intestinal absorption is reduced during phase 3, and it is best during the slow transit of phase 1.

The MMC has been called the "intestinal housekeeper," because it is thought to clear the small intestine of bacteria and undigestible food residue. Repeating high-amplitude contractions during phase 3 may dislodge small particles trapped among the villi. Phase 3 is associated with an increase in intestinal secretions.[9] Thus, the "housekeeper" may wash as well as sweep the small intestine clean.[10] Absence of the MMC is associated with bacterial overgrowth.[11]

Postprandial Motility

Ingestion of a nutrient meal disrupts the MMC in humans, leading to a prolonged period of apparently irregular activity (Fig. 5–4), similar to phase 2 during fasting. The fed pattern has fewer propagating contractions than phase 2.[12] Thus, it seems that fed activity is more likely to result in mixing than propulsion; the reverse is true for fasted activity.

The minimum amount of nutrient needed to initiate a fed pattern is unknown. Nonabsorbable iso-osmolar or hyperosmolar material does not disrupt the MMC. Mechanical distention plays only a minor role, because ingestion of saline solution disrupts MMCs for a much shorter period than does ingestion of the same volume of milk. A direct linear relationship exists between the quantity of food ingested into the stomach or infused into the duodenum and the time of phase 3 reappearance. The duration of the fed pattern correlates with gastric emptying and is influenced by the characteristics of the meal. Equal calories of fat inhibit the MMC longer than does sucrose, and sucrose inhibits the MMC longer than does protein. The effect of fat may be a consequence of fat emptying from the stomach more slowly than protein and carbohydrate and, consequently, prolonging the exposure of the upper intestine to nu-

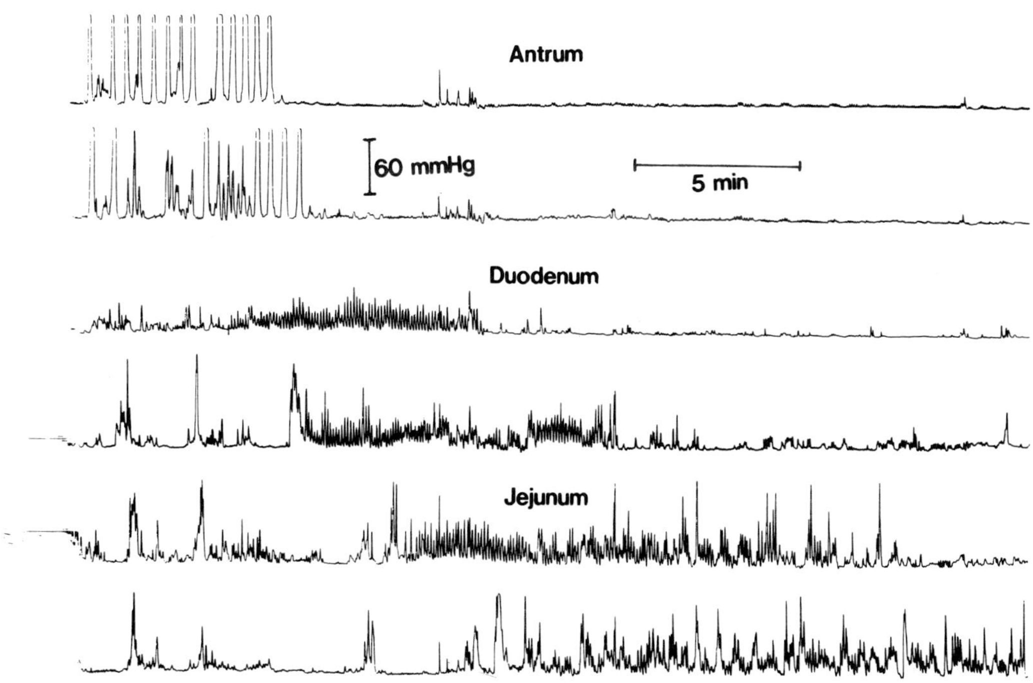

Figure 5–3. Normal phase 3 of the MMC followed by phase 1. Phase 3 starts in the antrum and migrates to the jejunum.

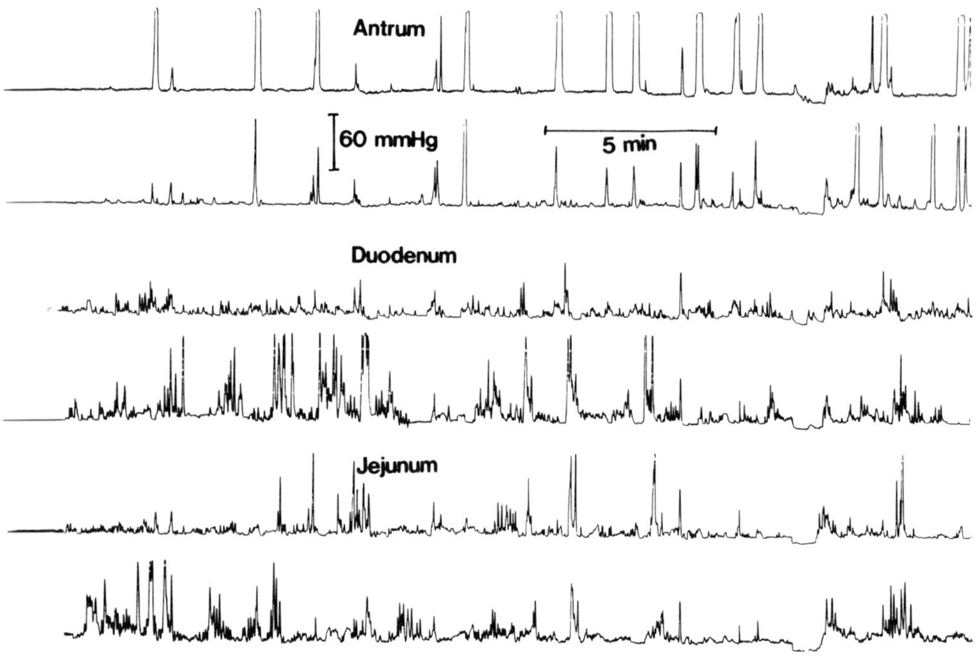

Figure 5–4. Normal postprandial motility.

trient material.[13] In adults, a mixed 450 kcal meal suppresses the MMC for an average of 3.5 hours.

Both neural and hormonal influences play a role in suppressing MMCs and initiating the fed pattern. Intravenous infusion of secretin, insulin, cholecystokinin, gastrin, or pancreatic polypeptide disrupts MMCs and induces a fed pattern.[14] Direct mucosal contact with nutrient is not essential for the inhibition of MMC. The MMC is disrupted in the distal small intestine 10 to 20 minutes after a meal, at a time when nutrients are not likely to have reached that segment. Total parenteral nutrition does not interfere with the MMC, indicating that the presence of nutrients in the blood does not activate the mechanisms that inhibit the MMC. Vagotomy inhibits the fed pattern, suggesting that vagal activity has a role in suppressing the fasting pattern.[15, 16] There is also evidence that intrinsic nerves may mediate disruption of the MMC. Local perfusion of neostigmine and of bethanechol each immediately disrupted the MMC cycle in progress up to 80 to 100 cm orad or aborad to the perfusion site,[4] suggesting that short neural reflexes are present.

Ontogeny of Intestinal Motility

When radiographic contrast material is injected into the gastrointestinal tract of a fetus in utero, before 30 weeks of gestation, there is little movement of the marker out of the stomach. With increasing gestational age, the contrast material moves into the small intestine, and by 34 weeks, it moves into the colon.[17] In the neonate, increasing gestational age results in acceleration of the luminal transit rate. Manometric studies in preterm and term infants[18–21] characterized the maturation of fasting and postprandial patterns of contractions during fasting and after a meal. Prior to 30 weeks' postconception, motor activity is poorly developed, with only low-pressure, nonpropagated contractions. After 30 week's postconception, newborns generate increased luminal pressures and develop short clusters of rhythmic contractions that become longer in duration and propagate more frequently with increased postnatal age.[22] By 38 weeks' postconception, the MMC is present.

Feedings increase the number of duodenal contractions in infants as young as 25 weeks' postconceptual age. For a given age and formula volume, the postprandial motor response is greater in previously fed infants compared with unfed infants.[23] In very preterm infants, there is often coexistence of an active fed pattern but an immature fasting pattern with no MMC.[24] Perhaps because fasting motor activity contributes considerably to the aborad movement of intestinal contents,[25] the ability to digest and absorb nutrients correlates with the maturity of the fasting motor activity.

Administration of corticosteroids accelerates maturation of the neonatal duodenal motility. Ischemia and CNS diseases slow maturation.[19]

Myogenic Control

The control of contraction within an individual muscle cell depends on the electrical activity generated by potential differences across the cell membrane.

The maximum frequency and propagation speed of small intestinal contractions are determined by the regular oscillation in the myocyte membrane potential. Two major types of activity can be detected; an omnipresent electrical control activity (ECA) and an electrical response activity (ERA).[26] ECA is also known as *slow-wave* or *pacesetter potential* and consists of rhythmic oscillations of membrane potential. ERA is also known as *spike potential* and occurs when neural or chemical

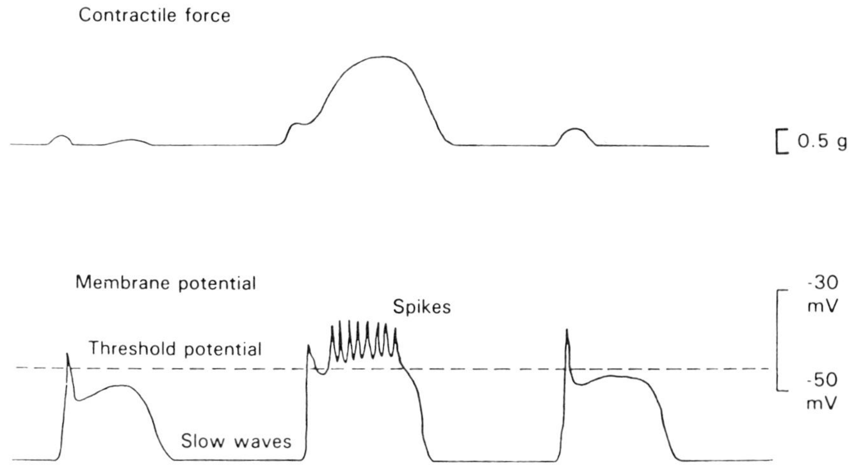

Figure 5–5. Diagram of the electrical and mechanical activity of smooth muscle showing the relationship between fluctuations in membrane potential and contractile force. (From Reed NW: Small intestinal motility physiology. *In* Physiology, Diagnosis and Therapy in GI Motility Disorders [Medicine Publishing Foundation Symposium Series, 22]. Toronto, MES Medical Education Services, 1988, pp 23–26; with permission.)

stimuli mediate a depolarization sufficient to exceed an excitation threshold (Fig. 5–5). ERA is associated with muscle cell contraction. The strength and duration of contraction are related to the amplitude and frequency of spike potentials in an ERA burst.[27] The smooth muscle cell contracts only once during one ECA, during the depolarized phase when the ERA is superimposed on the ECA. It follows that the maximum frequency of contraction in any part of the gut will be identical to the frequency of the ECA. If the required neurochemical stimulus is not present, the frequency of contraction will be less than the maximal frequency of ECA. This process is referred to as the *temporal control of contractions* because it determines the frequency and timing of contraction at each site of the intestine.[28]

The spatial coordination of contractions depends on the spatial coordination of ECA. Through interactions at cell junctions, the intestinal smooth muscle acts as a syncytium. Therefore, ECA generated in each cell interacts with ECA in adjoining cells. The frequency of ECA cycles decreases in a proximal-distal gradient. In humans, the frequency of the slow waves decreases from the duodenum (12 per minute) to the ileum (8 per minute). Orderly time lag in the distal direction ensures that a contraction will begin at a proximal site and will propagate in a distal direction.

Intrinsic Neurogenic Control

The nerves with their cell bodies in the gut wall and their interactions are referred to as the enteric nervous system (ENS). The human ENS contains more than 10^8 neurons, divided into two major plexuses; the myenteric plexus (Auerbach's plexus), situated between the longitudinal and the circular muscle layer, and the submucosal plexus (Meissner's plexus), located in the submucosa. The two plexuses contain structured networks of neurons and communicate through connecting nerve axons. Each ganglion contains numerous cell bodies that may send or receive processes, or both, from other cells in the same plexus, ganglia in other plexuses, and extrinsic nerve.

The ENS is not simply a relay station for autonomic input to the gastrointestinal tract but an integrative system with structural and functional properties analogous to the CNS (Fig. 5–6). The circuitry of the ENS is able to generate stereotypic ("hardwired") patterns of electrical activity that regulate motility, secretion, and blood flow. These intrinsic patterns are modulated by a variety of external inputs that reach the ENS by way of either extrinsic nerves or hormones.

The importance of the control of gut motility by the ENS is corroborated by the findings that a completely

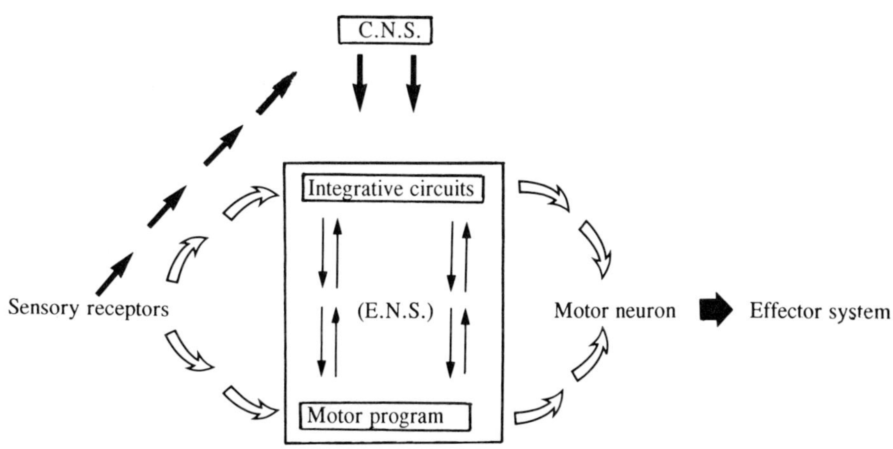

Figure 5–6. Schematic representation of the interactions between intrinsic and extrinsic neurogenic control of intestinal motility.

extrinsically denervated segment can still mix and propel its contents and that an autotransplanted segment of small bowel does not cause obstruction.[4] In a Thiry-Vella loop, the MMCs cycle independently of the MMCs in the remainder of the small intestine.[30, 31] When the small intestine is divided into small segments by multiple transections and reanastomoses, each segment generates its own MMC, which cycles independently from other segments.[4] Thus, each segment of intestine has its own mechanism for initiation of the MMCs.[32, 33] In the intact small intestine, the ENS has local neuronal circuitry coupled with each other so that a proximal circuit drives the distal circuit with a time lag.

Stimulation with the motilin receptor agonist erythromycin fails to induce MMCs in preterm infants who lack pre-existing MMCs, providing further evidence that a mature ENS is essential for normal intestinal cyclic motor activity.[34]

Extrinsic Neurogenic Control

The small intestine is supplied by parasympathetic nerves from the vagus and by sympathetic nerves from the thoracolumbar outflow. About 90% of the nerve fibers in the abdominal vagus are afferent, with cell bodies in the nodose ganglia.[35]

After recovery from truncal or selective vagotomy, MMC activity usually persists or reappears quickly. Vagotomy, freezing the cervical vagus, and atropine reduce the duration of phase 2,[36] whereas splanchnicectomy and adrenergic antagonists increase it.[37] Furthermore, initiating premature MMCs in the stomach with injections of motilin requires an intact vagus.[38] Thus, vagal integrity seems to be important in the regulation of the MMC, especially in the gastric region.

Extrinsic sympathetic nerves provide important inhibitory efferents to the gut. Sympathetic nerves mediate ileus associated with laparotomy and peritoneal irritation. In these situations, ablation of the sympathetic nerves results in return of the MMC.[39, 40]

Chemical Control

A plethora of peptides, amines, kinins, purines, eicosanoids, and nitric oxide are endogenous substances capable of modulating intestinal smooth muscle function. Specific physiologic roles are difficult to define for most of the substances, because responses vary among tissues and species. Histochemical studies have shown that the substances present in human small bowel enteric neurons include norepinephrine, enkephalin, somatostatin, neuropeptide Y, substance P, VIP, and serotonin. Regulatory substances are not all neurocrine. Other substances may be autocrine, with secreted substances mediating functions in the same cell; paracrine, with secretions mediating effects on local tissues; or endocrine, with blood-borne substances mediating effects on target tissues.

Contraction is stimulated by acetylcholine. Atropine and hexamethonium block all spontaneous contractions in the small intestine in the fasted or fed state; administration of cholinomimetics or anticholinesterases increases small bowel contractions. Other putative neurocrine excitatory substances include the tachykinins, neurokinin A and substance P. Although the excitatory effects of acetylcholine and the tachykinins seem certain, the postsynaptic inhibition is nonadrenergic and noncholinergic but its precise chemical identity is not known. Likely candidates include VIP, calcitonin gene–related peptide, nitric oxide, somatostatin, purines, and beta-endorphin.

Norepinephrine is released by postganglionic sympathetic neurons from the prevertebral ganglia. Adrenergic agonists decrease and antagonists stimulate intestinal contractions, suggesting that norepinephrine mediates smooth muscle relaxation.[41] It seems that the action of this sympathetic transmitter is an indirect—the inhibition of excitatory ganglionic transmission—rather than a direct relaxant effect on smooth muscle. The relaxation induced by sympathetic nerve stimulation is thus due to removal of an excitatory cholinergic stimulus.[42, 43]

The peptide hormone motilin may initiate MMCs originating in the stomach. MMCs that originate below the pylorus are not related to plasma motilin variation. The macrolide erythromycin is a motilin receptor agonist,[44] and erythromycin initiates MMCs at doses much lower than those required for its antibacterial properties.[45] Because it has been demonstrated that a meal produces an increase in the serum concentration of motilin in humans, motilin could also play a role in the regulation of human postprandial motility.[46]

Somatostatin can induce or suppress MMCs, depending on the dosages used and the conditions of the experiments. Somatostatin may facilitate the orderly progression of phase 3 of the MMC from the stomach into the small intestine.[47] MMCs are also stimulated by infusions of morphine, substance P, pancreatic polypeptide, histamine, and metoclopramide.

Infusion of cholecystokinin, gastrin, glucagon, insulin, and secretin all interrupt the MMC.

COLON

The colon serves two functions: absorption of water and electrolytes and storage and elimination of waste. Although a meal takes only seconds to traverse the 20- to 30-cm–long esophagus, a few minutes to pass through the stomach (15–30 cm), and 2 to 4 hours to reach the ileocolonic junction (200–500 cm), it may be 12 to 30 hours before its residua pass out from the colon (100–130 cm).[48]

Colon motility has been studied with the use of radiopaque markers[49] and barium[50] to assess colonic transit time. Newer techniques including manometry,[51] electromyography,[52] and scintiscanning[53] have been used in adults and children[54–56] for the investigation of colon motility.

Types of Contractions

The cyclic motor activity observed during the fasting condition in adults and children from the lower esoph-

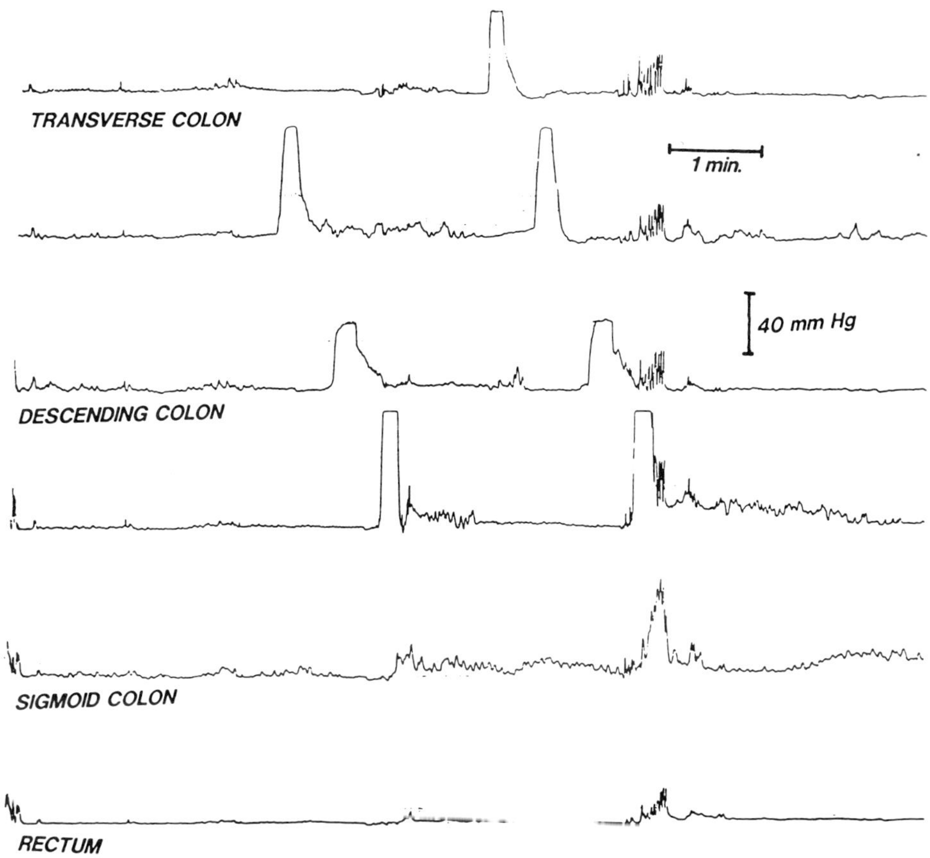

Figure 5–7. Two high-amplitude propagated contractions (HAPCs) observed after a meal in a child without constipation.

agus to the terminal ileum is not found in the human colon.[57] Only recently, a rectal motor complex (RMC), which is not synchronous with or related to the MMC, has been reported.[58] The RMC is a repetitive series of contractions that occurs in normal adults every 90 minutes at night and every 300 minutes during the day. Within each complex, contractions have a mean frequency of 4 to 7 per minute and a mean duration of 10 minutes. RMCs and the intestinal MMCs differ in that the RMCs are not abolished by feeding. The physiologic role of the RMCs is not known, but speculation is that the complexes may keep the rectum empty, thereby avoiding the sensation of rectal fullness and the desire to defecate between bowel movements.[58]

Normal features of colon motility include long periods of quiescence, as well as nonpropagating and propagating contractions at irregular intervals. Contractions can be phasic, tonic, or phasic superimposed on tonic. Flow of luminal contents through the colon is not steady or progressive; rather, nonpropulsive, segmental movements of the colon move fecal material equally in a retrograde and antegrade fashion away from the area of high pressure.[59] Mixing of colonic contents is extensive, and particles ingested on different days are frequently found in the same stool. Segmental contractions prevent the rapid forward flow of colonic contents by producing a back-and-forth movement. The transverse colon, especially, may serve as a storage area for colonic contents, because feces empty rapidly from the cecum and ascending colon but are retained in the transverse colon.[60]

Contractions are relatively infrequent before meals and during sleep, and they increase after meals and on awakening.[50] Eating is an important stimulus for colonic motility.[50] There is an increase in colon motility 20 to 40 minutes after beginning a meal that is known as the *gastrocolonic reflex*.[61] Although this reflex is clearly demonstrable in the distal colon, it is less prominent in the cecum and ascending colon.[62] The term *gastrocolonic reflex* is probably a misnomer—the phenomenon is not a reflex (because it takes 20 minutes to occur) and it does not require the presence of the stomach (because it also occurs in gastrectomized patients).[63] A more appropriate phrase would be *colonic response to food*.[64] The magnitude of the colonic response to food increases in proportion to the number of calories and the fat content of the meal.[65] The absence of the gastrocolonic response may be a marker for disease as well as a contributing factor in the pathogenesis of constipation.[55] It is absent in children and adults with chronic intestinal pseudo-obstruction.[56, 66] Other factors that can increase colonic motility in normal persons are short-term physical[67] or mental stress,[68] emotional response,[69] and caffeinated and decaffeinated coffee.[70]

Another feature of normal colon motility is the presence of high-amplitude propagated contractions (HAPCs). During colon manometries, HAPCs are identified by their high amplitude (>100 mm Hg) and propagation over at least 30 cm (Fig. 5–7). Arising from the proximal colon, HAPCs propagate to the distal sigmoid colon. One HAPC is often followed by others at 3- to 4-minute intervals during the postprandial period, and their frequency increases after a meal.[71] HAPCs are associated with caudad movement of the colonic contents and passage of stools or gas.[72, 73] There are more frequent HAPCs in children than in adults, a feature that may partially explain the increased number of bowel movements observed in infants and children.[74] Because fecal material in the colon becomes progressively harder and thicker as water is absorbed, colonic contractions, such as HAPCs, are probably required to move contents in the caudad direction.[75] It is not clear what initiates HAPCs. There is some evidence that HAPCs can be induced by distention of the lumen[76] or by luminal irritants, such as olive oil and bisacodyl.[77]

Ontogeny of Colon Motility

Colonic motor function seems to be very poor in utero, and defecation is abnormal before delivery. Meconium is usually passed within the first 24 hours of life. Exceptions are found in severely distressed infants, who pass meconium prior to delivery, and in children with Hirschsprung's disease or other forms of anatomic or physiologic obstruction, who have delayed passage of meconium. After birth, colonic motility seems rapidly to acquire characteristics similar to colon motility in adults.

Myogenic Control

Colonic myocytes exhibit regular, spontaneous changes in ionic conductance leading to ECA (slow waves). When the cell membrane potential depolarizes beyond a certain threshold, ERA (spikes) occur, and, coupled with this electrical activity, the cell contracts. ECA and ERA have been recorded from both circular and longitudinal muscle.[78, 79] In contrast with the relatively constant frequency of slow waves in the small bowel, there is a wide variation in frequency in the colon, fluctuating from 4 to 30 cycles per minute.[80] The amplitude and frequency of slow waves are sensitive to stimulatory and inhibitory neurotransmitters. ERA increases when the muscle is stretched, so distention of the colon by intraluminal contents may control the motor activity of the intact organ.[80] This is the reason that stool volume and consistency may be important factors in the overall control of colon motility.

When electrical oscillations are slower than 12 per minute, each slow wave may generate a phasic contraction characterized by a sharp rise and fall in pressure. When the electrical oscillation of either muscle layer exceeds a frequency of 12 to 14 per minute, individual contractions may fuse, because relaxation between these frequent oscillations of membrane potential is incomplete.[64] This phenomenon is known as *long spike burst*, and it is associated with prolonged, tonic contractions.[81, 82] There is great variability in ECA frequency from the colon. Thus, there are periods in the colon when the usual relationship between an electrical event and contraction is no longer present.

Intrinsic Neurogenic Control

The myenteric and submucosal enteric plexuses of the colon contain a highly organized and complex network of neurons that control motor, sensory, secretory, and absorptive functions. Thus, the gut brain continues into the colon. It is not clear whether the neurons from the submucosal plexus innervate the smooth muscle cells directly; it seems that they make synaptic connections in the myenteric plexus before reaching the smooth muscle cells.[83]

In addition to excitatory cholinergic and inhibitory adrenergic nerves, there are noncholinergic, nonadrenergic nerves that have stimulatory and inhibitory inputs. Peptidergic nerves in the colon may contain VIP, somatostatin, galanin, substance P, calcitonin gene–related peptide, neuropeptide Y, peptide YY, peptide histidine isoleucine, methionine-enkephalin, and gastrin-releasing peptide.[75]

Extrinsic Neurogenic Control

The vagus innervates the proximal colon, and the sacral pelvic nerves supply the distal colon and rectum. These predominantly cholinergic nerves stimulate the colon, but they also carry inhibitory and sensory afferent fibers.

The adrenergic innervation to the proximal colon is carried by the splanchnic nerves originating in the superior mesenteric ganglion. The adrenergic innervation to the distal colon is carried by lumbar colonic nerves originating in the inferior mesenteric ganglion. The adrenergic nerves inhibit colonic motility. The prevertebral ganglia appear to play an important role in modulating the sympathetic inhibition of colonic motility. They act as sites of relay and coordination: afferent signals from mechanoreceptors in the colon proceed to the prevertebral ganglia and are processed there,[84, 85] exerting negative feedback on other regions of the colon.

Studies in patients with spinal cord transection have suggested that the spinal cord provides a chronic neural inhibition to the colon and that supraspinal centers have a stimulatory influence. In fact, patients with lumbar spinal cord lesions have increased colonic motility, and those with high cord transection have decreased colonic motility.[86]

Chemical Control

Acetylcholine is the primary agonist for colonic smooth muscle contraction. Atropine blocks all spontaneous contractions in vivo,[87] and bethanechol[88] and neostigmine[89] enhance colonic contractions in vivo and in vitro.

Norepinephrine inhibits colonic motor activity mainly by modulating the release of acetylcholine at the synaptic junctions in the enteric ganglia. Both alpha- and beta-receptor agonists inhibit colonic contractions; the inhibition is greater in the left colon than in the right colon.[90]

Substance P has been proposed as the main noncholinergic excitatory neurotransmitter in the gastrointestinal tract. It has an excitatory effect on the colon, which is partially atropine resistant.[91] Substance P also acts directly on the smooth muscle cell, stimulating contraction of the colonic circular smooth muscle by decreasing the potassium conductance of the cell membrane.[92]

VIP has been proposed as the neurotransmitter of the nonadrenergic enteric inhibitory neurons. VIP neurons appear to originate in the submucosal plexus and spread to the myenteric plexus.[93]

Neurotensin and cholecystokinin seem to be involved in the postprandial response to food. Their serum concentration increases after the ingestion of a meal, and fat is the most potent stimulant for their release.[94, 95] Neurotensin acts at presynaptic sites to stimulate colon motor activity. The increase in motility produced by neurotensin is greater in the proximal colon than in the distal colon.[96] The stimulatory effect of cholecystokinin is most evident in the distal colon.[97, 98]

Secretin, glucagon, and progesterone inhibit colon motility.[97, 99, 100]

REFERENCES

1. Gabella G: Structure of muscles and nerves in the gastrointestinal tract. *In* Johnson LR, ed: Physiology of the Gastrointestinal Tract, 2nd ed. 1987, pp 335–351.
2. Kamm KE, Stull JT: Regulation of smooth muscle contractile elements by second messengers. Annu Rev Physiol 1989; 51:299–313.
3. Biancani P, Hillemeier K, Bitar KN, et al: Contraction mediated by Ca^{2+} reflux in esophageal muscle and by Ca^{2+} release in the LES. Am J Physiol 1987; 253:G760–G766.
4. Sarna SK, Otterson MF: Small intestinal physiology and pathophysiology. Gastroenterol Clin North Am 1989; 18:375–405.
5. Sarna SK, Condon RE, Cowles V: The enteric mechanisms of initiation of migrating myoelectric complexes (MMC's) in dogs. Gastroenterology 1983; 84:814–822.
6. Wood JD: Intrinsic neural control of intestinal motility. Annu Rev Physiol 1981; 43:33–51.
7. Grider JR: Identification of neurotransmitters regulating intestinal peristaltic reflex in humans. Gastroenterology 1989; 97:1414–1419.
8. Grider JR, Makhlouf GM: Role of opioid neurons in the regulation of intestinal peristalsis. Am J Physiol 1987; 253:G226–G231.
9. Vantrappen GR, Peeters TL, Janssens J: The secretory component of the interdigestive migrating motor complex in man. Scand J Gastroenterol 1979; 14:663–667.
10. Read NW: Small intestinal motility physiology. *In* Physiology, Diagnosis and Therapy in GI Motility Disorders (MEDICINE Publishing Foundation Symposium Series, 22). Toronto, MES Medical Education Services, 1988, pp 23–36.
11. Vantrappen G, Janssens J, Ghoos Y: The interdigestive motor complex of normal subjects and patients with bacterial overgrowth of the small intestine. J Clin Invest 1977; 59:1158–1166.
12. Sarna SK, Soergel KH, Harig JM, et al: Spatial and temporal patterns of human jejunal contractions. Am J Physiol 1989; 257:G423–G432.
13. DeWever I, Eeckhout C, Vantrappen G, et al: Disruptive effect of test meals on interdigestive motor complex in dogs. Am J Physiol 1978; 235:E661–E665.
14. Vantrappen G, Janssens J, Peeters TL: The migrating motor complex. Med Clin North Am 1981; 65:1311–1329.
15. Thompson DG, Ritchie HD, Wingate DL: Patterns of small intestinal motility in duodenal ulcer patients before and after vagotomy. Gut 1982; 23:517–523.
16. Weisbrodt NW: Motility of the small intestine. *In* Johnson LH eds: Physiology of the Gastrointestinal Tract. New York, Raven Press, 1987, pp 631–663.
17. McLain CR: Amniography studies of the gastrointestinal motility in human fetus. Am J Obstet Gynecol 1963; 86:1079–1087.
18. Tomomasa T, Itoh Z, Koizumi T, et al: Nonmigrating rhythmic activity in the stomach and duodenum of neonates. Biol Neonate 1985; 48:1–9.
19. Morriss FH, Moore M, Weisbrodt NW, et al: Ontogenic development of gastrointestinal motility: IV. Duodenal contractions in preterm infants. Pediatrics 1986; 78:1106–1113.
20. Bisset WM, Watt JB, Rivers RPA, et al: Ontogeny of fasting small intestinal motor activity in the human infant. Gut 1988; 29:453–488.
21. Berseth CL: Gestational evolution of small intestinal motility in preterm and term infants. J Pediatr 1989; 115:646–651.
22. Bisset WM: Intestinal motor activity in the preterm infant. *In* Milla PJ, Welburn P, eds: Disorders of Gastrointestinal Motility in Childhood. Chichester, John Wiley & Sons, 1988, pp 29–38.
23. Bisset WM, Watt JB, Rivers RPA, et al: The motor response of the small intestine to milk feeds in preterm infants (abstract). Dig Dis Sci 1987; 32:903.
24. Berseth CL: Neonatal small intestinal motility: Motor responses to feeding in term and preterm infants. J Pediatr 1990; 117:777–782.
25. Kerlin P, Zinsmeister A, Phillips S: Relationship of motility to flow of contents in the human small intestine. Gastroenterology 1982; 82:701–706.
26. Sarna SK: Gastrointestinal electrical activity: Terminology. Gastroenterology 1975; 68:1631–1635.
27. McCoy EJ, Bass P: Chronic electrical activity of gastroduodenal area: Effects of food and certain catecholamines. Am J Physiol 1963; 205:439–445.
28. Sarna SK: In vivo myoelectric activity: Methods, analysis and interpretation. *In* Wood JD, ed: Handbook of Physiology, Gastrointestinal Motility and Circulation. Bethesda, MD, American Physiology Society, 1989.
29. Meyer EA, Raybould H: Role of neural control in gastrointestinal motility and visceral pain. *In* Snape WJ Jr, ed: Pathogenesis of Functional Bowel Disease. New York, Plenum Publishing, 1989, pp 13–35.
30. Carlson GM, Bedi BS, Code CF: Mechanism of propagation of intestinal interdigestive myoelectric complex. Am J Physiol 1972; 222:1027–1030.
31. Aeberhard PF, Magnenat LD, Zimmerman WA: Nervous control of migratory myoelectric complex of the small bowel. Am J Physiol 1980; 238:G102–G108.
32. Itoh Z, Nakaya M, Suzuki T: Neurohormonal control of gastrointestinal motor activity in conscious dogs. Peptides 1981; 2:223–228.
33. Ormsbee HS III, Telford LG, Suter GM, et al: Mechanism of propagation of canine migrating motor complex: A reappraisal. Am J Physiol 1981; 240:G141–G146.
34. Tomomasa T, Miyazki M, Igarashi T, et al: The effect of erythromycin on the gastroduodenal motility in human premature infants. J Gastrointest Motil 1991; 3:205.
35. Evans DHL, Murray JC: Histological and functional studies on the fiber composition of the vagus nerve of the rabbit. J Anat 1954; 88:3320–3337.
36. Ruckebush Y, Bueno L: Migrating myoelectrical complex of the small intestine. Gastroenterology 1977; 73:1309–1314.
37. Marlett JA, Code CF: Effect of celiac and superior mesenteric ganglionectomy on interdigestive myoelectric complex in dogs. Am J Physiol 1979; 237:E432–E436.
38. Hall KE, Greenberg GR, El-Sharkawy TY, et al: Relationship between porcine motilin–induced migrating motor complex–like activity, vagal integrity, and endogenous motilin release in dogs. Gastroenterology 1984; 87:78–85.
39. Bueno L, Fioramonti J, Ruckebusch Y: Postoperative intestinal motility in dogs and sheep. Dig Dis Sci 1978; 23:682–689.
40. Bueno L, Ferre J-P, Ruckebusch Y: Effects of anesthesia and surgical procedures on intestinal myoelectric activity in rats. Dig Dis Sci 1978; 23:690–695.
41. Carlson GM, Ruddon RW, Hug CC Jr, et al: Effects of nicotine on gastric antral and duodenal contractile activity in the dog. J Pharmacol Exp Ther 1970; 172:367–376.

42. Norberg KA, Sjoqvist F: New possibilities for adrenergic modulation of ganglionic transmission. Pharmacol Rev 1966; 18:743–751.
43. Cowie LA, Kosterlitz HW, Waterfield AA: Factors influencing the release of acetylcholine from the myenteric plexus of the ileum of the guinea-pig and rabbit. Br J Pharmacol 1978; 64:565–580.
44. Peeters T, Matthyjs G, Depoortere I,·et al: Erythromycin is a motilin receptor agonist. Am J Physiol 1989; 257:G470–G474.
45. Tomomasa T, Kouroume T, Arai H, et al: Erythromycin induces migrating motor complex in human gastrointestinal tract. Dig Dis Sci 1986; 31:157–161.
46. Boivin M, Raymond MC, RiBerdy M, et al: Plasma motilin variation during the interdigestive end digestive states in man. J Gastrointest Motil 1990; 2:240–246.
47. Peeters TL, Janssens J, Vantrappen GR: Somatostatin and the interdigestive migrating motor complex in man. Regul Pept 1983; 5:209–217.
48. Metcalf AM, Phillips SF, Zinsmeister AR, et al: A simplified assessment of segmental colonic transit. Gastroenterology 1987; 92:40–47.
49. Hinton J, Lennard-Jones J, Young A: A new method of studying gut transit times using radio-opaque markers. Gut 1969; 10:842-847.
50. Ritchie JA: Mass peristalsis in the human colon after contact with oxyphenisatin. Gut 1972; 13:211–219.
51. Narducci F, Bassotti G, Gaburri M, et al: Twenty-four-hour manometric recording of colonic motor activity in humans. Gut 1987; 28:17–25.
52. Bueno L, Fioramonti J, Ruckebusch Y, et al: Evaluation of colon myoelectrical activity in health and functional disorders. Gut 1980; 41:480–485.
53. Krevsky B, Malmud LS, D'Ercole F, et al: Colonic transit scintigraphy: A physiologic approach to the quantitative measurement of colonic transit in humans. Gastroenterology 1986; 91:1102–1112.
54. Davidson M, Bauer CH: Studies of colonic motility in children. Pediatrics 1958; 21:746–751.
55. Di Lorenzo C, Flores AF, Reddy SN, et al: Colon motility in symptomatic children after surgery for Hirschsprung's disease: Abnormalities in "healthy" colon (abstract). Gastroenterology 1991; 100:437.
56. Di Lorenzo C, Flores A, Reddy SN, et al: Colonic manometry differentiates causes of intractable constipation in children. J Pediatr 1992; 120:690–695.
57. Kellow JE, Borody TJ, Phillips SF, et al: Human interdigestive motility: Variation in patterns from the esophagus to colon. Gastroenterology 1986; 91:386–395.
58. Orkin BA, Hanson RB, Kelly KA: The rectal motor complex. J Gastrointest Motil 1989; 1:5–8.
59. Ritchie JA: Colonic motor activity and bowel function: I. Normal movement of contents. Gut 1968; 9:442–456.
60. Krevsky B, Malmud LS, D'ercole F, et al: Colonic transit scintigraphy. Gastroenterology 1986; 91:1102–1112.
61. Wright SH, Snape WJ Jr, Battle W, et al: Effect of dietary components on gastrocolonic response. Am J Physiol 1980; 238: G228–G232.
62. Kerlin P, Zinsmeister AR, Phillips SF: Motor responses to food of the ileum, proximal colon and distal colon of healthy humans. Gastroenterology 1983; 84:762–770.
63. Duthie HL: Colonic response to eating. Gastroenterology 1978; 75:527–529.
64. Philips SF: Physiology of colon motility. *In* Physiology, Diagnosis and Therapy in GI Motility Disorders (MEDICINE Publishing Foundation Symposium Series, 22). Toronto, MES Medical Education Services, 1988, pp 37–47.
65. Wright SH, Snape WJ Jr, Battle WM, et al: Effect of dietary components on the gastrocolonic response. Am J Physiol 1980; 238:G228–G232.
66. Snape WJ, Sullivan MA, Cohen S: Abnormal gastrocolic response in patients with intestinal pseudo-obstruction. Arch Intern Med 1980; 140:386–387.
67. Bingham SA, Cummings JH: Effect of exercise and physical fitness on large intestine function. Gastroenterology 1989; 97:1389–1399.
68. Narducci F, Snape WJ Jr, Battle WM, et al: Increased colon motility during exposure to a stressful situation. Dig Dis Sci 1985; 30:40–44.
69. Welgen P, Meshkinpour H, Beeler M: Effect of anger on colon motor and myoelectric activity in irritable bowel syndrome. Gastroenterology 1988; 94:1150–1156.
70. Brown SR, Cann PA, Read NW: Effect of coffee on distal colon function. Gut 1990; 31:450–453.
71. Bassotti G, Gaburri M: Manometric investigation of high amplitude propagated contractile activity of the human colon. Am J Physiol 1988; 255:G660–G664.
72. Torsoli A, Ramorino ML, Ammaturo MV, et al: Mass movements and intracolonic pressures. Am J Dig Dis 1971; 16:693–696.
73. Hardcastle JD, Mann CV: Physical factors in the stimulation of colon peristalsis. Gut 1970; 11:41–46.
74. Weaver LT: Bowel habit from birth to old age. J Pediatr Gastroenterol Nutr 1988; 7:637–640.
75. Sarna SK: Physiology and pathophysiology of colonic motor activity: I. Dig Dis Sci 1991; 36:827–862.
76. Narducci F, Bassotti G, Gaburri M, et al: Distension stimulated motor activity of the human transverse, descending and sigmoid colon (abstract). Gastroenterology 1985; 88:1515.
77. Spiller RC, Brown ML, Phillips SF: Decreased fluid tolerance, accelerated transit and abnormal motility of the human colon induced by oleic acid. Gastroenterology 1986; 91:100–107.
78. Huizinga JD, Stern H, Diamant NE, et al: The relationship between slow electrical oscillatory activity, spikes, and contractions in human colonic circular muscle (abstract). Gastroenterology 1984; 86:1119.
79. Huizinga JD, Chow E, Stern H, et al: Alterations in electrical activity of human colon smooth muscle by adrenergic and cholinergic stimulation, in vitro (abstract). Gastroenterology 1984; 86:1119.
80. Huizinga JD, Stern H, Chow E, et al: Electrophysiological control of motility in the human colon. Gastroenterology 1985; 88:500–511.
81. Sarna SK, Waterfall WE, Bardakjian BL, et al: Types of human colonic electrical activity recorded postoperatively. Gastroenterology 1981; 81:61–70.
82. Schang JC, Devroede G: Fasting and postprandial myoelectric spiking activity in the human sigmoid. Gastroenterology 1983; 85:1048–1053.
83. Sanders KM, Smith TK: Motoneurones of the submucous plexus regulate electrical activity of the circular muscle of canine proximal colon. J Physiol 1986; 380:293–310.
84. Croweroft PH, Holman ME, Szurszewski JH: Excitatory input from the distal colon to the inferior mesenteric ganglion in the guinea pig. J Physiol (Lond) 1971; 219:443–461.
85. Weems WA, Szurszewski JH: Modulation of colonic motility by peripheral neural inputs to neurons of the inferior mesenteric ganglia. Gastroenterology 1977; 73:273–278.
86. Connell AM, Frankel H, Suttmann L: The motility of the pelvic colon following the complete lesions of the spinal cord. Paraplegia 1963; 1:98–105.
87. Wienbeck M: The electrical activity of the cat colon in vivo: II. The effects of bethanechol and morphine. Res Exp Med 1972; 158:280–287.
88. Snape WJ Jr, Cohen S: Effect of bethanechol, gastrin I, or cholecystokinin on myoelectrical activity. Am J Physiol 1979; 236:E458–E463.
89. Karaus M, Sarna SK: Giant migrating contractions during defecation in the dog colon. Gastroenterology 1987; 92:925–933.
90. Esser MJ, Mahoney JL, Robinson JC, et al: Effects of adrenergic agents on colonic motility. Surgery 1987; 102:416–423.
91. Koelbel CBM, Mayer EA, Reeve JRJ, et al: Involvement of substance P noncholinergic excitation of rabbit colonic muscle. Am J Physiol 1989; 256:G246–G253.
92. Sims SM, Walsh JV, Singer JJ: Substance P and acetylcholine both suppress the same K^+ current in dissociated smooth muscle cells. Am J Physiol 1986; 251:C580–C587.
93. Cohen S, Snape WJ: Movement of the small and large intestine. *In* Sleisenger M, Fordtran JS, eds: Gastrointestinal Disease: Pathophysiology, Diagnosis, Management. Philadelphia, WB Saunders, 1989, pp 1088–1105.
94. Mashford ML, Nilsson G, Rokaeus A, et al: The effect of food ingestion on circulating neurotensin-like immunoreactivity (NTLI) in the human. Acta Physiol Scand 1978; 104:244–246.

95. Walsh JH, Lamers CB, Valenzuela JE: Cholecystokinin-octapeptide immunoreactivity in human plasma. Gastroenterology 1982; 82:438–444.
96. Thor K, Rosell S: Neurotensin increases colonic motility. Gastroenterology 1986; 90:27–31.
97. Dinoso VP Jr, Meshkinpour H, Lorber SH, et al: Motor responses of the sigmoid colon and rectum to exogenous cholecystokinin and secretin. Gastroenterology 1973; 65:438–444.
98. Harvey RJ, Read AE: Effect of cholecystokinin on colonic motility and symptoms in patients with the irritable bowel syndrome. Lancet 1973; 1:7793–7795.
99. Taylor I, Duthie HL, Cumberland DC, et al: Glucagon and the colon. Gut 1975; 16:973–978.
100. Gill RC, Bowes KL, Kingma YJ: Effect of progesterone on canine colonic smooth muscle. Gastroenterology 1985; 88:1941–1947.

Chapter 6

Immunology and Gastrointestinal Disease

ATHOS BOUSVAROS and RONALD E. KLEINMAN

The human gastrointestinal tract is constantly exposed to dietary antigens and microorganisms. The mucosal immune system has the complex task of generating selective immune responses to potential pathogens while avoiding pathologic immune responses to normal intestinal flora or food antigens. This chapter first reviews the anatomic, functional, and developmental aspects of the human intestinal mucosal immune system and then discusses specific illnesses in which alterations in immune function are important in disease pathophysiology.

CELLULAR COMPONENTS OF THE IMMUNE RESPONSE

Lymphocytes, macrophages, dendritic cells, neutrophils, eosinophils, and mast cells compose the vast majority of immune cells in the human gastrointestinal tract. Lymphocytes are classified as either B (bone marrow–derived) cells or T (thymus-derived) cells. The B cells respond to an antigen by proliferating and differentiating into immunoglobulin (Ig)-producing plasma cells and are also involved in antigen presentation to T cells. Ig produced by plasma cells enhances effector cell phagocytosis by opsonizing target cells. Ig also can promote cytotoxicity by activating the complement pathway.[1, 2]

T cells perform either cytotoxic functions or regulatory functions. Cytotoxic T cells that possess the CD8 phenotype are antigen specific; these T cells recognize and lyse cells bearing antigens in association with class I molecules of the major histocompatibility complex (MHC).[3] In contrast, cytotoxic T cells that possess the CD16 phenotype are termed *natural killer cells;* they can lyse cells without MHC-associated antigen recognition.[4] A subset of cytotoxic T cells require stimulation by interleukins (ILs) to manifest cytotoxic properties; these particular T cells are termed *lymphokine-activated killer cells.*[5]

Regulatory T cells either enhance or inhibit the immune response by secretion of multifunctional molecules termed *cytokines* (ILs). Helper T cells, most of which belong to the CD4 phenotype, produce cytokines (e.g., IL-2, IL-4, and IL-5) that promote T cell proliferation, B cell differentiation, and Ig production.[6, 7] T cells with suppressor function may express either the CD4 or the CD8 phenotype, and they decrease Ig production either directly or via cytokine release.[8, 9]

Macrophages and dendritic cells phagocytose pathogens and antigens and then present antigenic fragments in association with proteins of the MHC to T cells, resulting in T cell activation and the initiation of the inflammatory cascade. Macrophages also release soluble cytokines (e.g., IL-1-beta, IL-6, and tumor necrosis factor alpha), which are important in the promotion of growth and differentiation of B and T lymphocytes.[10–12]

The effector cells of the immune system include neutrophils, eosinophils, and mast cells in addition to T cells. Neutrophils are primarily phagocytic cells that kill bacteria through phagocytosis and oxidation. Eosinophils possess granules that contain cytotoxic compounds, such as major basic protein and eosinophilic cationic protein; crosslinking of receptors on the eosinophil surface by IgE causes the release of these factors.[13, 14] Neutrophils as well as eosinophils are capable of metabolizing arachidonic acid via the cyclooxygenase and lipoxygenase pathways to produce prostaglandins and leukotrienes, compounds that promote chemotaxis and smooth muscle contractions. Mast cells also release pharmacologically active mediators, such as prostaglandins and histamine, when stimulated by IgE; also, they may be an important source of cytokines that regulate lymphocyte function.[15, 16]

FUNCTIONAL ANATOMY

Nonimmune host defenses reduce the amount of antigen that reaches the intestinal mucosal immune system. Gastric and pancreatic proteases digest proteins to smaller, less antigenic peptides. Intestinal peristalsis limits the exposure to potentially harmful materials by propelling them through the gastrointestinal tract. Intestinal mucin coats the mucosal surface, forming a physical barrier to antigenic penetration. Mucin contains glycoproteins that can mimic receptors on epithelial cell surfaces, thus competitively inhibiting the binding by toxins or pathogens to the gut surface. The mucous coat also acts as a framework to which secreted Igs can attach and more effectively bind luminal antigens.[17–19]

In the adult human, the epithelial cells at the mucosal surface are joined by means of a network of tight junctions that forms a physical barrier to the passage of macromolecules. Proteins that manage to enter epithelial cells intact generally undergo lysosomal degradation; therefore, only minimal amounts of antigen can penetrate the epithelial barrier. Small molecules, such as disaccharides, can pass between tight junctions (the paracellular pathway), but large peptides or proteins cannot (Fig. 6–1).[20, 21]

In the adult, antigen passage from the intestinal lumen to underlying immunocompetent cells is limited to specialized regions of the epithelial surface, which are called *follicle-associated epithelium (dome epithelium).* The dome epithelium overlies the organized aggregates of lymphoid tissue (Peyer's patches) found predominantly in the ileum and is characterized by decreased numbers of mucin-producing goblet cells and by the presence of specialized epithelial cells that are termed *M cells.*[22] M cells are flattened cells with shortened microvilli and a paucity of lysosomes. Ultrastructural studies of animal intestinal epithelium demonstrate that M cells endocytose macromolecules (e.g., horseradish peroxidase and cationized ferritin) and organisms (e.g., *Escherichia coli* RDEC-1 and reovirus) and transport these intact antigens to underlying lymphoid tissues. Thus, the M cell represents a portal of entry to the lymphoid elements of the Peyer's patch, where the initial steps in antigen processing occur (Fig. 6–2).[23, 24]

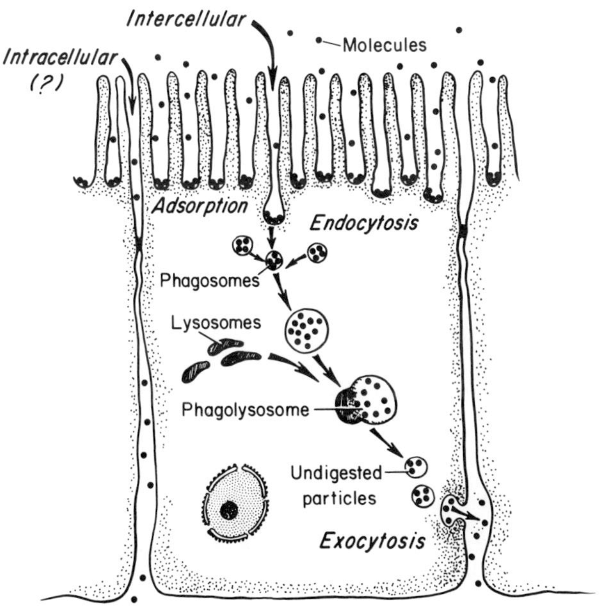

Figure 6–1. Antigen passage across the epithelial cell surface barrier. Macromolecules undigested by pepsin or pancreatic enzymes may undergo receptor-mediated or nonselective endocytosis by the enterocyte. Within the enterocyte, lysosomal degradation of protein occurs, but small peptides may still enter the systemic circulation. Small molecules, such as disaccharides, may enter the paracellular space across tight junctions. (From Walker WA, Isselbacher KJ: Uptake and transport of macromolecules by the intestine: Possible role in clinical disorders. Gastroenterology 1974; 67:531; with permission.)

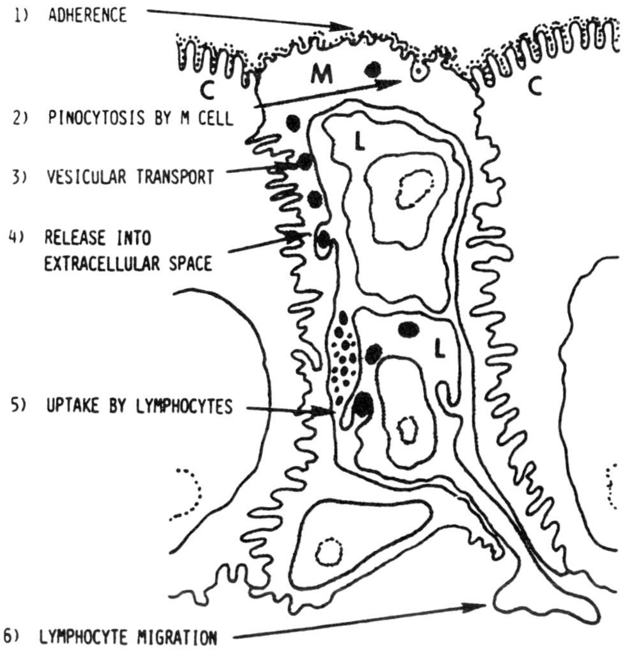

Figure 6–2. Dome epithelium. M cells overlying Peyer's patches, or lymphoid aggregates, preferentially endocytose antigens or viruses. These particles are then transported in largely unmodified form to antigen-presenting cells within the Peyer's patch. (From Owen RL: Sequential uptake of horseradish peroxidase by lymphoid follicle epithelium of Peyer's patches in the normal unobstructed mouse intestine: An ultrastructural study. Gastroenterology 1977; 72:440; with permission.)

For an antibody response to antigen within the Peyer's patch to occur, naive B cells must differentiate and proliferate into plasma cells. The initial step in B cell activation occurs when intact antigen binds to Igs on the cell surface. Further signals for B cell differentiation are provided by soluble cytokines secreted by helper T cells.[7] In contrast with B cells, T cells do not recognize antigen directly, but they do recognize antigenic fragments on the surface of antigen-presenting cells (APCs). APCs have the capability to phagocytose antigen, degrade it in lysosomes, and transfer the degraded antigenic peptides to the APC surface, where the peptides associate with molecules of the MHC. Helper T cells recognize antigenic peptide in association with MHC class II molecules by the T cell surface molecules CD4 and T cell receptor.[25] Macrophages, dendritic cells, and B cells all express surface MHC class II molecules and are thought to function as APCs within the Peyer's patch. Enterocytes also can express MHC class II molecules and can present antigen to T cells in vitro, but the in vivo significance of this finding has not been determined (Fig. 6–3).[26]

A stimulated Peyer's patch B cell undergoes migration through the lymphatics to the mesenteric lymph nodes and thoracic duct and into the systemic circulation. Once in the systemic circulation, the B cell may lodge in

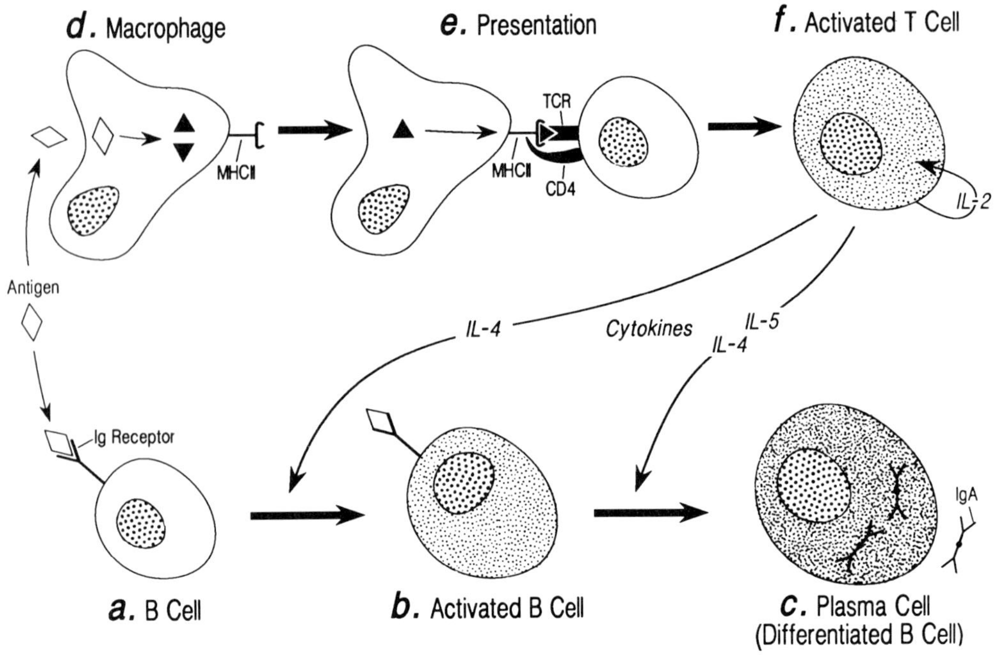

Figure 6–3. Antigen processing in Peyer's patch. Antigen may bind directly to immunoglobulin on the surface of a B cell, or it may be endocytosed by an APC and presented to a helper T cell. The helper T cell then secretes cytokines that promote B cell differentiation. (From Bousvaros A, Walker WA: *In* Bouchier I, et al, eds: Gastroenterology: Clinical Science and Practice. Bailliere-Tindall, in press; with permission.)

lymphoid organs (e.g., spleen and tonsils) or mucosal sites (e.g., urinary or respiratory tract). However, intestinal B cells preferentially return to gut lamina propria, where they may either lie dormant as "memory" B cells or mature into Ig-producing plasma cells. The process of the migration of gut B cells through the systemic circulation and the return of the cells to mucosal surfaces is termed the *IgA cell cycle* (Fig. 6–4).[27, 28]

The principal Ig produced by mucosal plasma cells, IgA, has two major subclasses: IgA1 and IgA2. Two IgA molecules of either subclass combine with a single J-chain molecule within the plasma cell to form dimeric IgA. The IgA dimer is then transported out of the plasma cell to the basal lamina of the enterocyte, where it combines with a protein synthesized by the enterocyte, termed the *secretory component.* The completed secretory IgA molecule is transported through the cytoplasm of the enterocyte into the intestinal lumen, where it then may complex with antigen. Secretory IgA can also be produced by plasma cells in conjunction with epithelial cells in bronchi, salivary glands, and breast tissue. In this way, antigens in the maternal intestine can

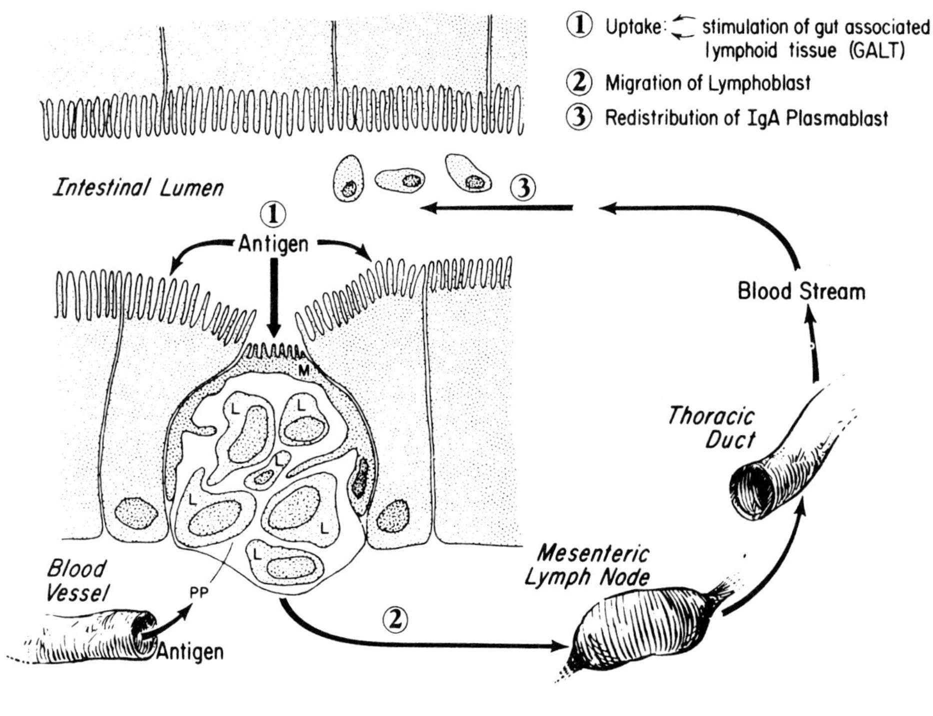

Figure 6–4. B lymphocytes activated by antigen leave the Peyer's patch and enter the mesenteric lymph nodes, thoracic duct, and systemic circulation. The B cells may then enter other mucosal sites (bronchi) or lymphoid organs (spleen, tonsils) but preferentially return to the intestinal mucosa, where they mature into IgA-producing plasma cells. (Reprinted with permission from *The New England Journal of Medicine*, vol. 297, p. 768, 1977.)

generate a specific IgA response that is transferred to the suckling infant through maternal breast milk.[29–31]

In summary, the mucosal immune response in humans begins with antigenic stimulation of B and T cells within the Peyer's patch. B cell maturation, migration, and return to the lamina propria are thought to be controlled by regulatory cytokines secreted principally by T cells. Within the lamina propria, effector cells (including plasma cells, neutrophils, and eosinophils) mediate the inflammatory response against pathogenic organisms.

SYSTEMIC TOLERANCE

Whereas orally ingested food antigens can generate a mucosal immune response (e.g., secretory IgA production), the primary systemic response to oral antigen is one of immunologic hyporesponsiveness, or tolerance. Tolerance is defined as an antigen-specific inactivation of lymphocytes resulting in the absence of an immune response. An animal exposed to a tolerance-inducing antigen (tolerogen) will not respond to a more immunogenic form of the antigen subsequently. Three major theories of tolerance development have been proposed: clonal deletion, clonal anergy, and suppressor cell activation. With clonal deletion and clonal anergy, the interaction of the tolerogen with a B lymphocyte or helper T lymphocyte results in cellular death or cellular unresponsiveness, respectively. The end result is an absence of Ig-producing cells directed against that specific antigen. In contrast, the interaction of tolerogen with a suppressor T cell clone generates a large number of suppressor T cells that, subsequently, can inhibit B cell antibody production.[32]

In murine models, orally administered ovalbumin can generate tolerance to ovalbumin administered intravenously as early as 1 hour after the oral immunization. This tolerance to ovalbumin can be passed among syngeneic mice by transferring serum from the orally immunized mouse into an unimmunized mouse. In addition, the tolerance response can be abolished by the removal of suppressor T cells with cytotoxic drugs. The degree of tolerance induction also depends on the MHC haplotype of the rodent, with BALB/B mice developing much less tolerance to orally administered ovalbumin than BALB/c mice.[33] A current hypothesis based on the these data is that intestinal antigen-processing cells (e.g., macrophages) modify an immunogenic protein (e.g., ovalbumin) into a "tolerogenic protein" that preferentially activates T suppressor cells in the systemic immune system.[34] Although tolerance in humans is poorly understood, defective tolerance is potentially important in the pathogenesis of intestinal diseases, such as milk allergy and celiac disease.

INTERLEUKINS

When stimulated by antigens or mitogens, cells of the immune system produce a host of soluble proteins that regulate growth and differentiation of lymphocytes and hematopoietic cells. An abbreviated list of these products (termed *ILs* or *cytokines*) is shown in Table 6–1. IL-1 and IL-2 are thought to be essential in the pro-

Table 6–1. PRINCIPAL ACTIONS OF SOME CYTOKINES

Compound	Chief Sources	Stimulated Process
Interleukin-1	Macrophages Lymphocytes Endothelial cells	Growth and differentiation of lymphocytes Tissue catabolism Prostaglandin E_2 synthesis Fever (endogenous pyrogen)
Interleukin-2	Activated T cells	Growth and differentiation of lymphocytes Cytotoxic activity
Interleukin-3	Activated T cells	Growth of bone marrow progenitors
Interleukin-4	T cells	Growth and differentiation of B cells Immunoglobulin production
Interleukin-5	Activated T cells	B cell differentiation
Interleukin-6	T cells Macrophages	B cell differentiation, T cell activation Hepatocyte production of acute-phase reactants
Interleukin-7	Bone marrow stromal cells, fibroblasts	B and T lymphocyte differentiation Lymphokine-activated killer cells
Interleukin-8	Macrophages	Neutrophil chemotaxis
Interleukin-9	CD4 T cells	T cell activation
Interleukin-10	T cells (murine)	Inhibition of murine T cell cytokine release
Tumor necrosis factor alpha	Macrophages	Fever (pyrogenic) Cachexia Bone resorption
Tumor necrosis factor beta	Lymphocytes	Same as tumor necrosis factor alpha
Interferon gamma	T cells, natural killer cells	Activation of macrophages, cytotoxic cells, and B cells Immunoglobulin production
Transforming growth factor beta	Platelets Macrophages	Inhibition of T cell proliferation Promotion of wound healing

From Bousvaros A, Walker WA: Basic gastrointestinal immunology. *In* Hodgson HJF, ed: Gastroenterology: Clinical Science and Practice. Bailliere-Tindall, in press; with permission.

motion of T cell growth, whereas IL-4 and IL-5 are important in the regulation of B cell differentiation. In addition, many of these compounds have important systemic effects. For example, IL-1 is a potent endogenous pyrogen and stimulator of the cyclooxygenase pathway of prostaglandin production, whereas IL-6 stimulates hepatocytes to produce acute-phase reactants. For a more detailed discussion of the compounds, the reader is referred to several review articles.[35–38]

DEVELOPMENTAL IMMUNOLOGY

In the term newborn human infant, the nonimmune mucosal defenses are relatively mature. The neonate achieves a gastric pH of 2 by the first 24 hours of life, and pancreatic protease activity is similar to that of older infants.[39, 40] However, premature infants younger than 29 weeks of age may have diminished peristaltic contractions and, therefore, decreased antigen clearance.[41]

Immunoperoxidase staining of human fetal intestine demonstrates that by 20 weeks of gestation, the cellular components of the immune system (B cells, T cells, and macrophages) all are present in the intestinal mucosa. In addition, secretory component is present in enterocytes by 22 weeks of gestation. However, the newborn human infant's intestinal mucosa possesses almost no IgA-producing plasma cells, and functionally significant IgA production does not begin until after 1 month of age.[42] Animal and human studies suggest that antigenic stimulation by feeding is important in the promotion of intestinal IgA system maturation and that the withholding of feeds may result in reduced numbers of mucosal IgA-producing plasma cells.[43, 44]

CLINICAL ASPECTS OF DISORDERED IMMUNITY

Alterations in mucosal immunity are prominent in the pathogenesis of many gastrointestinal diseases. In the primary and secondary immunodeficiencies, defective humoral or cellular immunity may predispose to infection by opportunistic pathogens or to idiopathic villous atrophy. In allergic illnesses of the gastrointestinal tract, a foreign antigen induces either IgE or cell-mediated hypersensitivity reactions, resulting in either anaphylaxis or local tissue damage. Activation of the immune system is also thought to mediate mucosal damage in celiac disease, inflammatory bowel disease, and autoimmune enteropathy.

Gastrointestinal Disease in Immunodeficiency

Table 6–2 contains a partial list of primary and secondary immunodeficiencies; for a complete list, the reader is referred to the World Health Organization immunodeficiency classification.[45] Only those diseases with prominent gastrointestinal manifestations will be discussed in the following sections.

Table 6–2. REPRESENTATIVE IMMUNODEFICIENCY DISORDERS

Primary Immunodeficiencies
Humoral Immunodeficiencies
X-linked agammaglobulinemia
Autosomal recessive agammaglobulinemia
Hyper-IgM syndrome
Selective IgA deficiency
Transient hypogammaglobulinemia of infancy
Combined Cellular and Humoral Immunodeficiencies
Common variable immunodeficiency
Severe combined immunodeficiency
Immunodeficiency with Other Systemic Disease
Ataxia telangiectasia
Wiskott-Aldrich syndrome
DiGeorge syndrome
Chronic mucocutaneous candidiasis
Defects of Phagocytic Function
Chronic granulomatous disease
Chédiak-Higashi syndrome
Myeloperoxidase deficiency
Complement Deficiencies
Secondary Immunodeficiencies
Malnutrition
Malignancy
Drug-induced
Acquired immunodeficiency syndrome

Adapted from Rosen FS, Wedgwood RJ, Eibl M, et al: Primary immunodeficiency diseases: Report of a World Health Organization scientific group on immunodeficiency. Clin Immunol Immunopathol 1986; 40:166–196; and Gurbindo C, Seidman EG: Gastrointestinal manifestations of immunodeficiency states. *In* Walker WA, Durie PR, Hamilton JR, et al, eds: Pediatric Gastrointestinal Disease: Pathophysiology, Diagnosis, Management. Philadelphia, BC Decker, 1991; pp 503–526; with permission.

Humoral Immunodeficiencies

Selective IgA deficiency, the most common primary immunodeficiency, has a prevalence of 1 in 900.[46] The decreased IgA production is thought to arise from either an arrest in B cell maturation or an inability to synthesize secretory component.[47, 48] Persons with this disorder have extremely low levels (<5 mg per dl) of serum and mucosal IgA; in addition, 15 to 20% of patients with selective IgA deficiency also have low levels of IgG subclasses IgG2 and IgG4. However, a compensatory increase in biologically active secretory IgM frequently protects against infection.[49, 50]

Most people with selective IgA deficiency are asymptomatic. However, selective IgA-deficient patients have an increased risk of developing infections and autoimmune disease (Table 6–3). Recurrent giardiasis that is refractory to antibiotic therapy may result in partial villous atrophy and secondary malabsorption. In addition, there is an increased incidence of celiac disease, food allergy, pernicious anemia, and idiopathic villous atrophy found in IgA-deficient patients.[51, 52] Therefore, the patient with IgA deficiency and chronic diarrhea should be evaluated extensively for the presence of enteric pathogens and undergo small bowel biopsy if no infectious cause is discovered. Antibiotic therapy with metronidazole, furazolidone, or quinacrine should be administered to the selected IgA-deficient patient with giardiasis.[53] If diarrhea persists and a biopsy demonstrates villous atrophy, a gluten-free diet may be thera-

Table 6–3. COMPLICATIONS OF SELECTIVE IgA DEFICIENCY

Upper respiratory infections	Primary biliary cirrhosis
Sinusitis	Henoch-Schönlein purpura
Bronchiectasis	Cholelithiasis
Giardiasis	Allergic disorders
Malabsorption	Inflammatory bowel disease
Celiac disease	Gastrointestinal lymphoma
Achlorhydria	

Adapted from Cunningham-Rundles C: Selective IgA deficiency and the gastrointestinal tract. Immunol Allergy Clin North Am 1988; 8:435–439; with permission.

peutic. Intravenous Ig should be avoided in patients with selective IgA deficiency, as it does not cross mucosal surfaces and may result in systemic anaphylaxis.[54]

X-linked (Bruton's) agammaglobulinemia presents with recurrent infections after 9 months of age. Affected males have a paucity of peripheral lymphoid tissue and low serum levels of all classes of Igs. Recurrent sinusitis, otitis media, pneumonia, and chronic echovirus infection are the most common reported illnesses. However, 10% of patients will develop chronic diarrhea, with rotavirus the most frequent identifiable pathogen. Other reported causes of chronic enteritis include *Giardia, Salmonella, Campylobacter, Cryptosporidium,* coxsackievirus, and poliovirus. Associations with sclerosing cholangitis and a sprue-like illness have also been noted, but it is unclear whether the incidence of autoimmune disease is actually increased in these patients.[55–57]

Transient hypogammaglobulinemia of infancy has been detected in as many as 10% of toddlers with chronic diarrhea. This disorder primarily affects children between 1 and 3 years of age and is characterized by low levels of serum IgG; IgA or IgM levels also may be decreased. Although the Ig deficiency generally resolves in later childhood, a subset of children will have persistent hypogammaglobulinemia. Lactose intolerance, *Giardia lamblia* infestation, and *Clostridium difficile* infection are found in as many as one third of children with low serum Igs and chronic diarrhea. Small bowel histology may show enteritis or villous atrophy in as many as 50% of patients. Antibiotic therapy or a lactose-free diet will benefit those patients with identifiable causes of the diarrhea, but otherwise no specific therapy is usually necessary.[58, 59]

Combined Cellular and Humoral Immunodeficiencies

Common variable immunodeficiency has an onset in late childhood or adulthood, with recurrent bronchitis and bronchiectasis the most common presentations. Afflicted patients have low levels of antibody production owing to a defect either in B cell differentiation or in T cell helper function. Gastrointestinal disease occurs in as many as 70% of patients and accounts for much of the morbidity (Table 6–4). *Giardia* is the most common infection detected, but *Salmonella, Campylobacter, Cryptosporidium,* or rotavirus also may be present.[60] Nodular lymphoid hyperplasia, defined as multiple, discrete lymphoid aggregates of the stomach and small bowel, is detected radiographically or endoscopically in as many as 20% of patients and may predispose to either malabsorption or gastrointestinal bleeding.[61, 62] Idiopathic sprue with subtotal villous atrophy is frequently present in those patients with no infections and is generally unresponsive to a gluten-free diet.[63, 64] Accompanying abnormalities include aphthous stomatitis, pernicious anemia, cholelithiasis, malacoplakia, and inflammatory bowel disease. Rarely, severe malabsorption may result in hyperoxaluria, vitamin B_{12} deficiency, and caloric deprivation and may require parenteral nutrition.[60]

Patients with *severe combined immunodeficiency* present in the first months of life with chronic diarrhea, failure to thrive, and persistent viral or fungal infections. A number of enzymatic and immunologic abnormalities (including adenosine deaminase deficiency, purine nucleoside phosphorylase deficiency, or abnormalities in T lymphocyte maturation) can give rise to the depressed cellular and humoral immunity seen in these patients. Gastrointestinal illness occurs in 90% of patients. Prolonged rotavirus infection is the most frequent intestinal infection and may give rise to intractable diarrhea. Other noted causes of enteropathy include *Salmonella, Shigella,* adenovirus, picornavirus, and *Cryptosporidium* infections. Although candidiasis rarely involves the intestine, candidal esophagitis should be suspected in infants with severe combined immunodeficiency and decreased oral intake.[55, 65]

Other Immunodeficiency Disorders

Chronic mucocutaneous candidiasis is characterized by a diminished T cell response to candidal antigens. Infants with this disorder present with persistent thrush or candidal dermatitis, failure to thrive, and dystrophic nails. Candidal esophagitis may result in refusal of foods. A polyglandular endocrinopathy syndrome characterized by hypoparathyroidism, hypothyroidism, adrenal insufficiency, and pernicious anemia develops in as many as 70% of older children. Malabsorption secondary to pancreatic insufficiency contributes to the poor weight gain in 10% of patients. Therapy includes eradication of *Candida* with topical antibiotics plus ketoconazole or fluconazole, as well as hormone or pancreatic enzyme replacement, when appropriate.[66, 67]

Chronic granulomatous disease is caused by the inability of an affected patient's neutrophils to generate superoxide, leading to infections with catalase-positive

Table 6–4. GASTROINTESTINAL COMPLICATIONS OF COMMON VARIABLE IMMUNODEFICIENCY

Inflammatory bowel disease	Idiopathic sprue
Giardiasis	Sprue-like disorder
Ménétrier's disease	Pernicious anemia
Nodular lymphoid hyperplasia	Gastrointestinal lymphoma

Adapted from Sperber KE, Mayer L: Gastrointestinal manifestations of common variable immunodeficiency. Immunol Allergy Clin North Am 1988; 8:423–434; with permission.

organisms, including *Staphylococcus aureus, Serratia, Aspergillus,* and *Nocardia.* Small bowel involvement may mimic Crohn's disease, with multifocal abscesses, fistulas, and granulomatous colitis. The presence of lipid-containing histiocytes in the mucosa and submucosa of colonic biopsies strongly suggests chronic granulomatous colitis. Such colitis may respond to therapy with sulfasalazine or interferon gamma, but surgical resection may be necessary for intractable colitis or acute obstruction.[68–71]

Secondary Immunodeficiencies

Human immunodeficiency virus (HIV) (see Chapter 56) was projected to infect between 1,500 and 1,800 infants each year, based on anonymous newborn screening studies, by 1992. The HIV preferentially enters and kills CD4 lymphocytes via binding of viral gp120 glycoprotein to the CD4 protein, which results in decreased helper-inducer T cell function.[72] Macrophages also can internalize HIV, but they do not kill the virus and may serve as a reservoir of infection. Systemic immune abnormalities noted in HIV-infected patients include hypergammaglobulinemia, functionally ineffective antibody, and severely impaired cell-mediated immunity.[73]

Failure to thrive and poor growth are present in at least 25% of HIV-infected children.[74] Almost every enteric or opportunistic pathogen has been identified in the gastrointestinal tract of children with acquired immunodeficiency syndrome (AIDS) (Table 6–5). Chronic parasitic infestation with *Giardia, Cryptosporidium, Isospora belli,* or *Enterocytozoon bieneusi* (a Microsporida) frequently causes watery or malabsorptive diarrhea. Small bowel histology may demonstrate the pathogen, or it may show a nonspecific plasmacytic infiltrate with villous atrophy; electron microscopy is usually necessary to identify any members of Microsporida. *Mycobacterium avium-intracellulare* and *Mycobacterium tuberculosis* infections are common in AIDS patients and are characterized by extensive macrophage infiltration of the lamina propria. Cytomegalovirus and herpes simplex virus may cause oral ulcerations, esophagitis, or proctocolitis.[75–80] The HIV genome has been identified in enterocytes by in situ hybridization, and HIV may cause mucosal damage by a direct cytopathic effect.[81]

Table 6–5. OPPORTUNISTIC GASTROINTESTINAL INFECTIONS IN PATIENTS WITH HIV

Intestine	Liver
Candida	*Mycobacterium*
Cryptosporidium	*Histoplasma*
Isospora belli	*Coccidioides immitis*
Microsporida	*Cryptococcus*
Mycobacterium avium-intracellulare	Cytomegalovirus
Giardia lamblia	
Cytomegalovirus	
Herpes simplex virus	
Adenovirus	
HIV enteropathy	

Table 6–6. SUGGESTED EVALUATION FOR A CHILD WITH IMMUNODEFICIENCY AND CHRONIC DIARRHEA

Stool Studies
- Enteric pathogens (including *Escherichia coli* 0157:H7)
- Ova and parasites
- *Clostridium difficile* toxin
- Rotavirus
- Acid-fast stain (for *Cryptosporidium*)

Tests of Mucosal Function
- D-Xylose
- Lactose breath hydrogen test
- 72-hour fecal fat

Endoscopic Evaluation
- Upper endoscopy, biopsy, histology with periodic acid–Schiff or acid-fast stain
  - Disaccharidases
  - Duodenal fluid for *Giardia,* bacterial colony count
  - Bacterial, viral, fungal cultures
  - Mycobacterial culture
  - Electron microscopy
- Flexible sigmoidoscopy

Evaluation of the HIV-infected child with failure to thrive should include an examination for identifiable infectious pathogens, a noninvasive appraisal of mucosal integrity, and an assessment of mucosal architecture (Table 6–6). An abnormal D-xylose level correlates positively with enteric infections in HIV-infected children. In contrast, lactose malabsorption occurs at an earlier age in HIV-infected children but is not associated with infections.[74] Endoscopic evaluation should include bacterial, viral, fungal, and mycobacterial cultures, as well as acid-fast stain (for *Cryptosporidium*) and electron microscopy (for viruses and Microsporida). In addition, a duodenal fluid culture may demonstrate bacterial overgrowth.[77, 78]

The causes of malnutrition in the child with HIV infection include malabsorption, increased caloric needs because of illness, and, possibly, increased levels of cachexia-inducing cytokines (e.g., tumor necrosis factor). Anorexia commonly accompanies HIV infection; therefore, in the malnourished child with HIV, aggressive enteral or parenteral nutritional therapy is necessary to improve growth and achieve a positive nitrogen balance.[82, 83]

Allergic Disease of the Gastrointestinal Tract

Food allergies in childhood (see Chapter 42) have two primary clinical presentations: immediate onset (e.g., urticaria, wheezing, or anaphylaxis) or delayed onset (e.g., milk-induced colitis or eosinophilic gastroenteritis). In the former condition, antigen stimulates B cells to secrete IgE, which causes activation of mast cells and eosinophils and release of vasoactive substances. The pathogenesis of delayed-onset symptoms is not well understood but may involve helper T cell release of cytokines with activation of eosinophils and macrophages.[84]

A wide variety of clinical symptoms may occur when the offending food is given to a child with hypersensitivity (Table 6–7). The most commonly cited allergens in infancy and childhood include cow's milk, soy, egg, wheat, and peanuts. However, many other foods as well as food additives and dyes can result in adverse immune-mediated reactions. It is desirable to determine which food protein is responsible for the adverse reaction, because excessive empiric restriction of foods can result in caloric deprivation and poor growth.[85–87] An unblinded milk or food challenge with a period of observation of several hours in the physician's office and continued observation at home for 48 hours is a simple way of screening for food allergy in infants.[88] Skin prick tests and serum immunoassay tests (radioallergosorbent test and enzyme-linked immunosorbent assay) are also helpful ancillary evaluations in confirming IgE-mediated food allergies. Although negative skin and radioallergosorbent tests correlate well with the absence of IgE-mediated food allergies, false-positive results frequently occur. Therefore, a food should not be eliminated from a child's diet on the basis of skin or immunoassay testing alone.[84, 89] The "gold standard" for diagnosis of food intolerance is the double-blinded food challenge. In one study, 28% of children followed from birth to 3 years of age had histories suggestive of food intolerance, but fewer than one third of the patients with positive histories had findings present on double-blinded food challenges.[90]

Allergic colitis, protein-induced enteropathy, and eosinophilic gastroenteritis all have been reproducibly associated with immune-mediated reactions to dietary proteins. Allergic colitis usually presents in otherwise healthy infants younger than 1 month of age with colicky behavior and frequent seedy stools that contain blood or mucus. The stool may contain fecal leukocytes or eosinophils; no infectious pathogens are identified. In the young infant, necrotizing enterocolitis and Hirschsprung's enterocolitis must be considered in the differential diagnosis. Flexible sigmoidoscopy and biopsy of the rectum demonstrate a focal colitis with eosinophilic infiltration of the colonic crypts.[91–94] Because cow's milk and soy proteins in formula are the most common causes of infantile allergic colitis, treatment requires feeding the infant with a protein hydrolysate formula for the first 6 months to 1 year of life. Some infants may develop allergic colitis while being breast fed; a subset of these infants resolve their symptoms after milk products are restricted from the maternal diet.[95] Stools generally normalize within 72 hours after withdrawal of the dietary antigen, and more than 90% of infants tolerate a rechallenge with milk or soy after 1 year of age.

Table 6–7. CLINICAL MANIFESTATIONS OF FOOD ALLERGY

Anaphylaxis	Rhinorrhea
Vomiting	Conjunctivitis
Diarrhea or malabsorption	Urticaria or angioedema
Lactose intolerance	Atopic dermatitis
Abdominal pain	Colic or irritability
Colitis	Migraine
Wheezing	

Cow's milk protein enteropathy presents in the first year of life with persistent diarrhea, poor weight gain, anemia, and hypoalbuminemia. The symptoms frequently occur following a bacterial or viral enteritis. Small bowel biopsy demonstrates partial villous atrophy and a mononuclear infiltrate and can occasionally mimic celiac disease, although the villous lesion is usually "patchy." Secondary lactose intolerance also may occur. Infants with this condition improve when placed on a lactose-free protein hydrolysate formula, and most of them tolerate milk products when they are rechallenged at 1 year of age.[95–98]

Eosinophilic gastroenteritis (see Chapter 43) occurs in older toddlers and school-aged children with and without a prior allergic history. Three principal forms of this disorder have been reported: (1) a mucosal form that affects the intestine and presents with malabsorption and protein-losing enteropathy; (2) a submucosal form that affects the gastric antrum and presents with outlet obstruction; and (3) a serosal form that presents with edema and ascites. An elevated peripheral blood eosinophil count and IgE level suggest the diagnosis. A biopsy may demonstrate eosinophils in the duodenum or antrum; however, submucosal infiltrates in the stomach may not be seen on a superficial biopsy. Therapy consists of elimination of suspected food allergens. If no response occurs, treatment with corticosteroids or oral cromolyn may provide relief.[99–101]

Graft Versus Host Disease

Allogeneic bone marrow transplant recipients are at risk for acute or chronic graft versus host disease (GVHD). Acute GVHD generally occurs 3 to 6 weeks following marrow transplantation and is characterized primarily by skin rash, transaminase elevation, abdominal cramping, and watery or greenish diarrhea. In severe cases, hematochezia, protein-losing enteropathy, and electrolyte imbalance secondary to high stool output may occur. Upper or lower endoscopy may demonstrate edema, friability, hemorrhage, or ulceration of intestinal or colonic mucosa but cannot distinguish GVHD from infectious causes. Histologically, a sparse inflammatory infiltrate with apoptosis of intestinal, colonic, or gastric crypt cells suggests the diagnosis.

Liver involvement in acute GVHD may present with cholestasis, hepatocellular necrosis, or a combination of the two, with histology that generally demonstrates varying degrees of bile duct necrosis. In contrast, chronic GVHD that occurs more than 120 days post-transplant presents in a manner similar to that of autoimmune or connective tissue disease, with skin, eye, oral, esophageal, joint, and liver involvement. Dysphagia and odynophagia frequently occur; esophageal desquamation is less common. Liver disease occurs more frequently in the chronic form of GVHD than in the acute form and can be difficult to distinguish from viral hepatitis, especially hepatitis C. Liver biopsy may be helpful, in that GVHD more commonly manifests with bile duct necrosis, whereas the inflammation seen in hepatitis C or other non-A, non-B hepatitis is more commonly parenchymal.[102–104]

SUMMARY

Major advances have occurred in our understanding of mucosal immune function during the past three decades. Immaturity of the mucosal immune system and aberrant immune responses to benign exogenous or self-antigens are responsible for the development of the significant intestinal and liver disorders of infancy and childhood. Congenital defects of immune response may produce serious, debilitating dysfunction of the gut and liver as well. As our understanding of the determinants of the intestinal immune response improves, new agents can be developed that selectively modulate mucosal immunity.

REFERENCES

1. Cooper MD: B lymphocytes: Normal development and function. N Engl J Med 1987; 317:1452–1456.
2. Davies DR, Metzger H: Structural basis of antibody function. Annu Rev Immunol 1983; 1:87–117.
3. Grey HM, Sette A, Buus S: How T cells see antigen. Sci Am 1989; 261:56–64.
4. Trinchieri G: Biology of natural killer cells. Adv Immunol 1989; 47:187–190.
5. Kanof ME, Strober W: Lymphokine-activated killer cell cytotoxicity in the immune system. Gastroenterology 1989; 97:222–224.
6. James SP, Zeitz M, Kanof ME, et al: Intestinal lymphocyte subpopulations and mechanisms of cell-mediated immunity. Immunol Allergy Clin North Am 1988; 8:369–391.
7. Abbas AK: A reassessment of the mechanisms of T cell–dependent B cell activation. Immunol Today 1988; 9:89–94.
8. Morimoto C, Letvin NL, Distaso JA, et al: The isolation and characterization of the human suppressor inducer T cell subset. J Immunol 1985; 134:1508.
9. Asherson GI, Colizzi V, Zembala M: An overview of T suppressor cell circuits. Ann Rev Immunol 1986; 4:37–68.
10. Young JW, Steinman RM: Accessory cell requirements for the mixed-leukocyte reaction and polyclonal mitogens, as studied with a new technique for enriching blood dendritic cells. Cell Immunol 1988; 111:167–182.
11. Unanue ER, Allen PM: The basis for the immunoregulatory role of macrophages and other accessory cells. Science 1987; 236:551–557.
12. Akira S, Hirano T, Taga T, et al: Biology of multifunctional cytokines: IL-6 and related molecules (IL-1 and TNF). FASEB J 1990; 4:2860–2867.
13. Weller PF: The immunobiology of eosinophils. N Engl J Med 1991; 324:1110–1118.
14. Gleich GJ, Adolphson CR: The eosinophilic leukocyte: Structure and function. Adv Immunol 1986; 39:177–253.
15. Atkins FM: Intestinal mucosal mast cells. Ann Allergy 1987; 53:44–53.
16. Gordon JR, Burd PR, Galli SJ: Mast cells as a source of multifunctional cytokines. Immunol Today 1990; 11:458–464.
17. Bousvaros A, Walker WA: Development and function of the intestinal mucosal barrier. *In* McDonald TT, ed: Ontogeny of the Immune System of the Gut. Boca Raton, CRC Press, 1990, pp 1–21.
18. Israel EJ, Walker WA: Host defense development in gut and related disorders. Pediatr Clin North Am 1988; 35:1–18.
19. Snyder JD, Walker WA: Structure and function of intestinal mucin: Developmental aspects. Int Arch Allergy Appl Immunol 1987; 82:351–356.
20. Weiner ML: Intestinal transport of macromolecules. Food Chem Toxicol 1988; 10:867–880.
21. Udall JN, Walker WA: The physiologic and pathologic basis for the transport of macromolecules across the intestinal tract. J Pediatr Gastroenterol Nutr 1982; 1:295–301.
22. Pabst E: The anatomical basis for the immune function of the gut. Anat Embryol 1987; 176:135–143.
23. Wolf JL, Bye WA: The membranous (M) cell and the mucosal immune system. Annu Rev Med 1984; 35:95–112.
24. Sneller MC, Strober W: M cells and host defense. J Infect Dis 1986; 154:737–739.
25. Abbas AK, Lichtman AH, Pober JS: Antigen presentation and T cell antigen recognition. *In* Cellular and Molecular Immunology. Philadelphia, WB Saunders, 1991, pp 115–138.
26. Bland P: MHC class II expression by the gut epithelium. Immunol Today 1988; 9:174–176.
27. Ogra PL: Ontogeny of the local immune system. Pediatrics 1979; 64(Suppl):765–773.
28. Isselbacher KJ, Walker WA: Intestinal antibodies. N Engl J Med 1977; 297:768–775.
29. Mestecky J, McGhee JR, Elson CO: Intestinal IgA system. Immunol Allergy Clin North Am 1988; 8:469–483.
30. Ahnen DJ, Brown WR, Kloppel TM: Secretory component: The polymeric immunoglobulin receptor. Gastroenterology 1985; 89:667–682.
31. Slade HB, Schwartz SA: Mucosal immunity: The immunology of breast milk. J Allergy Clin Immunol 1987; 80:346–356.
32. Abbas AK, Lichtman AH, Pober JS: Immunologic tolerance and regulation of immune responses. *In* Cellular and Molecular Immunology. Philadelphia, WB Saunders, 1991, pp 204–223.
33. Mowat AM, Lamont AG, Bruce MG: A genetically determined lack of oral tolerance to ovalbumin is due to failure of the immune system to respond to intestinally derived tolerogen. Eur J Immunol 1987; 17:1673–1676.
34. Peng HJ, Turner MW, Strobel S: The generation of a tolerogen after the ingestion of ovalbumin. Clin Exp Immunol 1990; 81:510–515.
35. Mizel SB: The interleukins. FASEB J 1989; 3:2379–2388.
36. Strober W, James SP: The interleukins. Pediatr Res 1988; 24:549–557.
37. Platanias LC, Vogelzang NJ: Interleukin-1. Am J Med 1990; 89:621–629.
38. Van Snick J: Interleukin-6: An overview. Annu Rev Immunol 1990; 8:253–278.
39. Ebers DW, Smith DI, Gibbs GE: Gastric acidity on the first day of life. Pediatrics 1956; 18:800–804.
40. Lebenthal E, Lee PC: Development of functional response in human exocrine pancreas. Pediatrics 1980; 66:556.
41. Morriss FH, Moore M, Weisbrodt NW, et al: Ontogenic development of gastrointestinal motility: IV. Duodenal contractions in preterm infants. Pediatrics 1986; 78:1106–1112.
42. Spencer J, McDonald TT: Ontogeny of human mucosal immunity. *In* McDonald TT, ed: Ontogeny of the Immune System of the Gut. Boca Raton, CRC Press, 1990, pp 23–51.
43. Rothman D, Udall JW, Pang KY, et al: The effect of short-term starvation on mucosal barrier function in the newborn rabbit. Pediatr Res 1985; 19:727–731.
44. Knox WF: Restricted feeding and human intestinal plasma cell development. Arch Dis Child 1986; 61:744–749.
45. Rosen FS, Wedgwood RJ, Eibl M, et al: Primary immunodeficiency diseases: Report of a World Health Organization scientific group on immunodeficiency. Clin Immunol Immunopathol 1986; 40:166–196.
46. Cunningham-Rundles C: Selective IgA deficiency and the gastrointestinal tract. Immunol Allergy Clin North Am 1988; 8:435–449.
47. Conley ME, Cooper MD: Immature IgA B cells in IgA-deficient patients. N Engl J Med 1981; 305:475–479.
48. Strober W, Krakauer R, Klaeveman HC, et al: Secretory component deficiency: A disorder of the IgA immune system. N Engl J Med 1976; 294:351–356.

49. Morgan G, Levinsky RJ: Clinical significance of IgA deficiency. Arch Dis Child 1988; 63:579–581.
50. Oxelius VA, Laurell AB, Lindquist B, et al: IgG subclasses in selective IgA deficiency: Common occurrence of IgG2-IgA deficiency. N Engl J Med 1981; 304:1476–1477.
51. Zinneman HH, Kaplan AP: The association of giardiasis with reduced secretory immunoglobulin A. Dig Dis 1975; 125:207.
52. Crabbe PA, Heremans JF: Selective IgA deficiency with steatorrhea: A new syndrome. Am J Med 1967; 42:319–326.
53. Shepherd RW, Boreham PF: Recent advances in the diagnosis and management of giardiasis. Scand J Gastroenterol 1989; 24(Suppl 169):60–64.
54. Burks AW, Sampson HA, Buckley RM: Anaphylactic reactions following gammaglobulin administration in patients with hypogammaglobulinemia: Detection of IgE antibodies to IgA. N Engl J Med 1986; 314:560–564.
55. Stiehm ER, Chin TW, Haas A, et al: Infectious complications of the primary immunodeficiencies. Clin Immunol Immunopathol 1986; 40:69–86.
56. Lederman HM: X-linked agammaglobulinemia: An analysis of 96 patients. Medicine 1985; 64:145–156.
57. Arbo A, Santos JI: Diarrheal diseases in the immunocompromised host. Pediatr Infect Dis J 1987; 6:894–906.
58. Perlmutter DH, Leichtner AM, Goldman H, et al: Chronic diarrhea associated with hypogammaglobulinemia and enteropathy in infants and children. Dig Dis Sci 1985; 30:1149–1155.
59. McGeady SJ: Transient hypogammaglobulinemia of infancy: Need to reconsider name and definition. J Pediatr 1987; 110:47–50.
60. Sperber KE, Mayer L: Gastrointestinal manifestations of common variable immunodeficiency. Immunol Allergy Clin North Am 1988; 8:423–434.
61. Bastlein C, Burlefinger R, Holzberg E, et al: Common variable immunodeficiency syndrome and nodular lymphoid hyperplasia in the small intestine. Endoscopy 1988; 20:272–275.
62. Bennett WG, Watson RA, Heard JK, et al: Home hyperalimentation for common variable hypogammaglobulinemia with malabsorption secondary to intestinal nodular lymphoid hyperplasia. Am J Gastroenterol 1987; 82:1091–1095.
63. Catassi C, Mirakian R, Natalini G, et al: Unresponsive enteropathy associated with circulating enterocyte autoantibodies in a boy with common variable hypogammaglobulinemia and type 1 diabetes. J Pediatr Gastroenterol Nutr 1988; 7:608–613.
64. Conley ME, Park CL, Douglas SD: Childhood common variable immunodeficiency with autoimmune disease. J Pediatr 1986; 108:915–922.
65. Jarvis WR, Middleton PJ, Gelfand EW: Significance of viral infections in severe combined immunodeficiency disease. Pediatr Infect Dis 1983; 2:187–192.
66. Kirkpatrick CH: Chronic mucocutaneous candidiasis. Eur J Clin Microbiol Infect Dis 1989; 8:448–456.
67. Herrod HG: Chronic mucocutaneous candidiasis in childhood and complications of non-*Candida* infection. J Pediatr 1990; 116:377–382.
68. Werlin SL, Chusid MJ, Caya J, et al: Colitis in chronic granulomatous disease. Gastroenterology 1982; 82:328–331.
69. Isaacs D, Wright VM, Shaw DG, et al: Chronic granulomatous disease mimicking Crohn's disease. J Pediatr Gastroenterol Nutr 1985; 4:498–501.
70. Lindahl JA, Williams FH, Newman SL: Small bowel obstruction in chronic granulomatous disease. J Pediatr Gastroenterol Nutr 1984; 3:637–640.
71. Newberger PE, Ezekowitz RAB: Cellular and molecular effects of recombinant interferon gamma in chronic granulomatous disease. Hematol Oncol Clin North Am 1988; 2:267–275.
72. Rosenberg ZF, Fauci AS: Immunopathogenetic mechanisms of HIV infection. Immunol Today 1990; 11:176–180.
73. Pinching AJ: Antibody responses in HIV infection. Clin Exp Immunol 1991; 84:181–184.
74. Miller TL, Orav J, Martin S, et al: Malnutrition and carbohydrate malabsorption in children with vertically transmitted human immunodeficiency virus 1 infection. Gastroenterology 1991; 100:1296–1302.
75. Kotler DP: Intestinal and hepatic manifestations of AIDS. Adv Intern Med 1989; 34:43–72.
76. Kotler DP, Francisco A, Clayton F, et al: Small intestinal injury and parasitic diseases in AIDS. Ann Intern Med 1990; 113:444–449.
77. Rodgers VD, Kagnoff MF: Gastrointestinal manifestations of the acquired immunodeficiency syndrome. West J Med 1987; 146:57–67.
78. Antony MA, Brandt LJ, Klein RS, et al: Infectious diarrhea in patients with AIDS. Dig Dis Sci 1988; 33:1141–1146.
79. McLoughlin LC, Nord KS, Joshi VV, et al: Severe gastrointestinal involvement in children with the acquired immunodeficiency syndrome. J Pediatr Gastroenterol Nutr 1987; 6:517–524.
80. Connolly GM, Shanson D, Hawkins DA, et al: Non-cryptosporidial diarrhea in human immunodeficiency virus–infected patients. Gut 1989; 30:195–200.
81. Ullrich R, Zeitz M, Heise W, et al: Small intestinal structure and function in patients infected with human immunodeficiency virus (HIV): Evidence for HIV-induced enteropathy. Ann Intern Med 1989; 111:15–21.
82. Bentler M, Stanish M: Nutrition support of the pediatric patient with AIDS. J Am Diet Assoc 1987; 87:488–491.
83. Winick M, Andrassy RJ, Bryan MA, et al: Guidelines for nutrition support in AIDS. Nutrition 1989; 5:39–46.
84. Wershil BK, Walker WA: Food allergy in children. Immunol Allergy Clin North Am 1988; 8:485–504.
85. Sampson HA: Differential diagnosis in adverse reactions to foods. J Allergy Clin Immunol 1986; 78:212–215.
86. Sampson HA, McCaskill CC: Food hypersensitivity and atopic dermatitis: Evaluation of 113 patients. J Pediatr 1985; 107:669–673.
87. Bishop JM, Hill DJ, Hosking S: Natural history of cow milk allergy: Clinical outcome. J Pediatr 1990; 116:862–867.
88. Goldman AS, Anderson DW, Sellar WA, et al: Oral challenges with milk and isolated milk proteins in allergic children. Pediatrics 1983; 32:425–443.
89. Sampson HA, Albergo R: Comparison of prick skin tests, RAST, and double-blind placebo-controlled food allergens in children with atopic dermatitis. J Allergy Clin Immunol 1984; 74:26–30.
90. Bock SA, Lee WY, Remigo LK, et al: Studies of hypersensitivity reactions to foods in infants and children. J Allergy Clin Immunol 1978; 62:327–332.
91. Gryboski JD, Burkle F, Hillman R: Milk-induced colitis in an infant. Pediatrics 1966; 38:299–302.
92. Goldman H, Proujansky R: Allergic proctitis and gastroenteritis in children: Clinical and mucosal biopsy features in 53 cases. Am J Surg Pathol 1986; 10:75–86.
93. Jenkins HR, Pincott JR, Soothill HF, et al: Food allergy: The major cause of infantile colitis. Arch Dis Child 1984; 59:326–329.
94. Odze RD, Bines JE, Leichtner AM, et al: Prospective biopsy evaluation of allergic proctocolitis in infants. Gastroenterology 1991; 1100:A236.
95. Harrison M, Kilby A, Walker-Smith JA, et al: Cow's milk protein intolerance: A possible association with gastroenteritis, lactose intolerance, and IgA deficiency. Br Med J 1976; 1:1501–1504.
96. Iyngkaran N, Robinson MJ, Sumithran E, et al: Cow's milk protein–sensitive enteropathy. Arch Dis Child 1978; 53:150–153.
97. Freier S, Faber J: Epidemiology, clinical manifestations and management of cow's milk protein hypersensitivity. Front Gastrointest Res 1986; 13:95–112.
98. Walker-Smith JA: Food-sensitive enteropathies. Clin Gastroenterol 1986; 15:55–69.
99. Katz A, Twarog FJ, Zelger RS, et al: Milk-sensitive and eosinophilic gastroenteropathy: Similar clinical features with contrasting mechanisms and clinical course. J Allergy Clin Immunol 1984; 74:72–78.
100. Whittington PF, Whittington GL: Eosinophilic gastroenteropathy in childhood. J Pediatr Gastroenterol Nutr 1988; 7:379–385.
101. Trounce JQ, Tanner MS: Eosinophilic gastroenteritis. Arch Dis Child 1985; 60:1186–1188.
102. McDonald GB: Graft-versus-host disease of the intestine and liver. Immunol Allergy Clin North Am 1988; 8:543–557.
103. Tutschka PJ: Early complications of bone marrow transplantation in children and adults. Bone Marrow Transplant 1989; 4(Suppl):22–26.
104. Sullivan KM, Shulman HM, Storb R: Chronic graft-vs.-host disease in 52 patients. Blood 1981; 52:267–276.

Chapter 7

Neurology of the Gut

STEVEN M. ALTSCHULER

INTRODUCTION

The control of gastrointestinal function is dependent mostly on complex neural circuits that are located within the gut wall (enteric nervous system [ENS] and the central nervous system [CNS]). These neural circuits have been subjected to intensive study using a variety of anatomic, histochemical, immunocytochemical, and neurophysiologic techniques. As a result, considerable information exists concerning the morphology, connectivity, transmitter specificity, and physiologic function of the neuronal elements that provide innervation to the gastrointestinal tract. This chapter provides a summary of our current knowledge of gut neurobiology.

NEURON STRUCTURE AND ANATOMY

Cellular Anatomy[1, 2]

The basic anatomic and functional unit of the ENS and the CNS is the neuron. Neurons are linked into complex circuits by specialized cellular processes that facilitate the transmission of information to other neurons and to muscle and glandular cells. Although many morphologic variations exist, the typical neuron consists of a cell body (soma) and a number of cellular processes that extend away from the cell body (Fig. 7–1). As with all mammalian cell types, the cell body of the neuron houses the nucleus and other intracellular organelles necessary for its functional integrity. Cellular processes extending from the cell body are classified into two types: axons and dendrites. Functionally, the axonal process of a neuron is responsible for conveying information to other cells or neurons, whereas dendritic processes along with the cell body proper act as a receptive field for receiving information from other neurons.

Anatomic and functional interactions between neurons and between neurons and other cells occur at specialized structures termed *synapses*. Interactions between neurons occur at synaptic sites formed by axons and dendrites (axodendritic), axons and cell bodies (axosomatic), and, occasionally, two axons (axoaxonal). At the ultrastructural level (electron microscopic level), synapses are characterized by a presynaptic area that is formed by the terminal process of an axon (see Fig. 7–1). Clustered within the axon's terminal are numerous vesicles that contain the neurotransmitters used in synaptic transmission. During chemical synaptic transmission, the vesicles fuse with the presynaptic membrane, and the transmitter is released into the synaptic space by an exocytotic process. Free transmitters attach to receptors on the postsynaptic membrane, thereby activating the neuron or cell. The postsynaptic area of the neuron is located on the dendritic processes, which are termed *spines*, and on the cell body (Fig. 7–2*A*). Synaptic junctions formed by dendritic spines tend to be

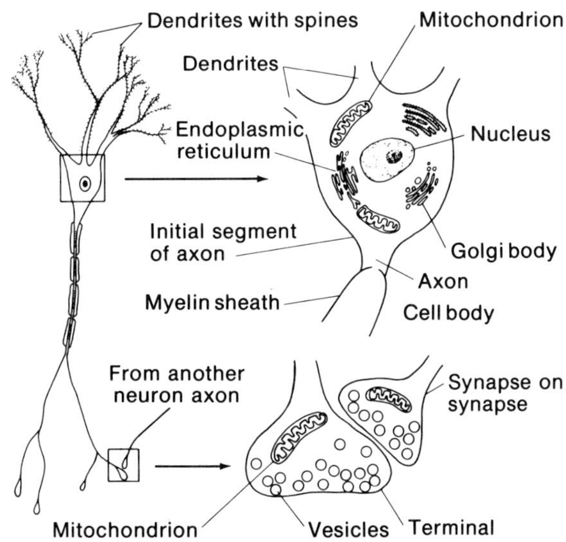

Figure 7–1. Schematic representation of a typical neuron. The neuron consists of the cell body, axon, and dendrites. The surface of the dendritic process and the cell body constitute the receptive synaptic surface of the neuron. The axonal process is usually longer than the dendritic processes, and its terminal end consists of a specialized process called the *synaptic terminal.* The synaptic terminal contains vesicles that are presumably the storage site for neurotransmitters synthesized within the cell or within the synaptic terminal. (From The Brain: An Introduction to Neuroscience. By Richard F. Thompson. Copyright © 1985 by W.H. Freeman and Company. Reprinted with permission.)

The writing of this chapter was supported by NIH grant DK-01747.

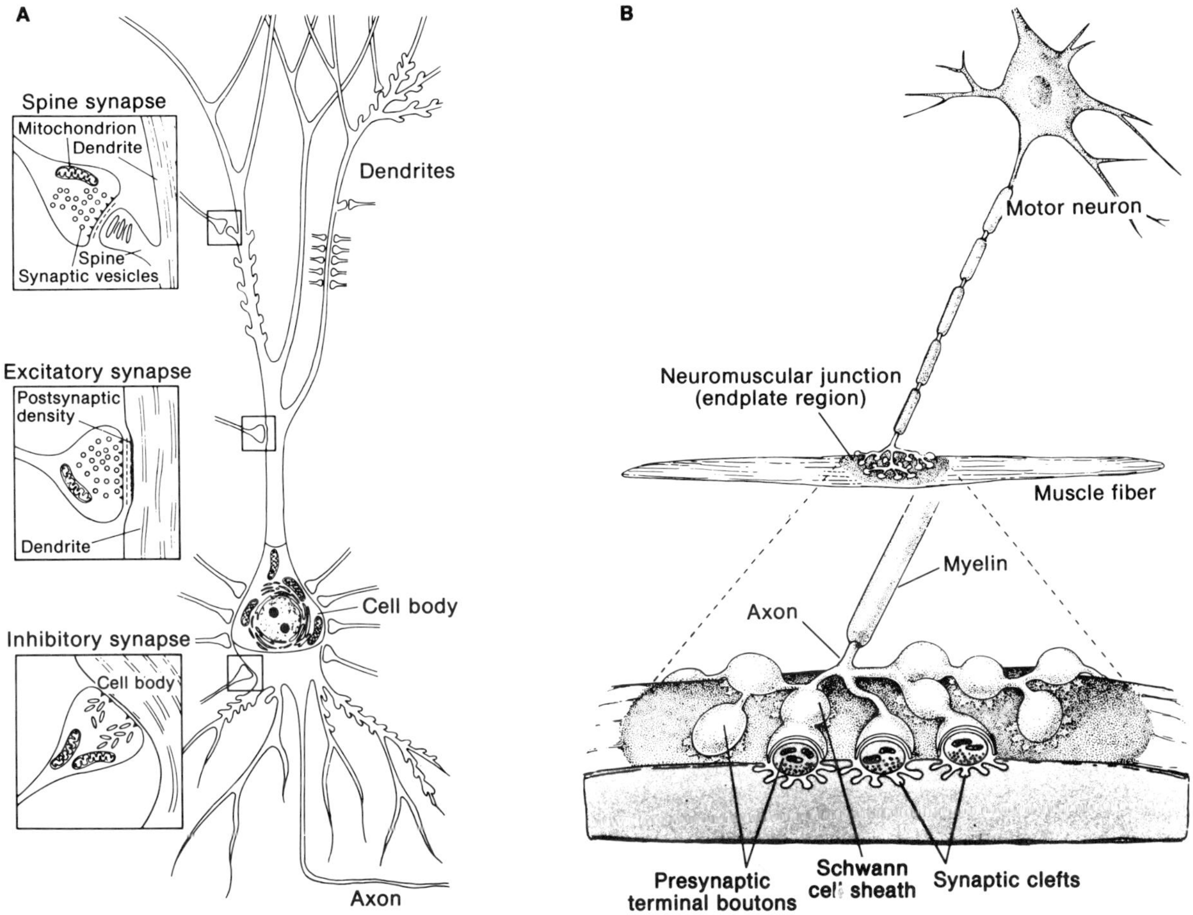

Figure 7–2. *A* and *B* are schematic representations of different types of neural synapses and nerve-muscle synapses. See text for further details. (*A*, From The Brain: An Introduction to Neuroscience. By Richard F. Thompson. Copyright © 1985 by W.H. Freeman and Company. Reprinted with permission; and *B*, From Kandel ER, Siegelbaum S: Principles underlying electrical and chemical synaptic transmission. *In* Kandel ER, Schwartz JH, eds: Principles of Neural Science. 2nd ed. New York, Elsevier, 1985, p. 94; with permission.)

excitatory, whereas those on the cell body tend to be inhibitory to the postsynaptic neuron.

The synaptic junctions formed by motoneuron axons and muscle fibers differ morphologically from the classic neuronal synapse (Fig. 7–2*B*). The terminal portion of the motoneuron axon consists of a series of varicosities called *synaptic boutons*. Mitochondria and vesicles containing the neurotransmitter acetylcholine (Ach) are located within the synaptic boutons. The postsynaptic membrane or motor endplate (see Fig. 7–2*B*) contains a high density of Ach receptors, which allows for interaction between nerve and muscle.

Cellular Function and Synaptic Transmission[2–7]

The primary functions of the neuron are the conductance and transmission of information to other cells. The efficient transmission of information depends on special properties of the neuronal cell membrane that allow for the generation and propagation of an electrical action potential as well as on the ability of the neuron to synthesize, package, and transport neurotransmitters for their use in synaptic transmission.

The ability of a neuron to generate and then propagate an action potential down the axon to a synaptic junction is dependent on its electrical properties. Typically, the neuron's resting membrane potential is about −70 mV (inside the neuron compared with outside the neuron) as result of (1) the extracellular movement of K^+ through open membrane channels; (2) the intracellular presence of many large negatively charged protein molecules that are unable to pass through the cell membrane; and (3) an active Na^+, K^+ pump that exchanges three intracellular Na^+ molecules for two extracellular K^+ molecules. Additionally, membrane channels exist for Na^+, Cl^-, and Ca^{2+}. In contrast with the K^+ channel, the channels for Na^+ and Ca^{2+} are gated in the resting state and do not allow movements of a large number of ions through the membrane.

The ability of a neuron to respond to electrical or chemical stimulation (synaptic or direct) results from a change in membrane potential. The change in membrane potential reflects an alteration in the relative permeability of stimulus-dependent ion channels (primarily Na^+, Ca^{2+}, and, to a lesser extent, K^+). Two possible membrane events can occur in response to stimulation of the cell: (1) excitation, or membrane depolarization (decreased negativity owing to an intracellular movement of Na^+ and Ca^{2+} as a result of increased membrane permeability; and (2) inhibition, or hyperpolarization (increased negativity as a result of the extracellular movement of K^+ secondary to a receptor-mediated increase in membrane permeability for this ion). The neurotransmitter Ach, by either nicotinic or muscarinic action, is commonly involved in excitatory synaptic events, and norepinephrine is commonly involved in inhibitory synaptic events.

An action potential represents a transient depolarization or excitation of the cell membrane and occurs primarily as a result of the intracellular flux of Na^+ (Fig. 7–3). The site of origin of the action potential is typically the initial segment of the axon, the area with the highest density of voltage-dependent Na^+ channels. These channels transiently open at a threshold voltage slightly higher than the resting membrane potential (initial period of membrane depolarization), which accounts for the massive influx of Na^+. An action potential, once initiated, travels peripherally in all directions from its site of origin. The action potential is propagated down the axon as the result of a spreading wave of depolarization that sequentially opens voltage-controlled (gated) Na^+ channels. Following the point of maximum depolarization, the cell membrane undergoes a rapid repolarization to a point of greater negativity (termed *after-hyperpolarization*) as a consequence of the opening of closed K^+ channels (see Fig. 7–3). The opening of these channels allows for an extracellular flux of K^+ down its concentration gradient. The conduction velocity of an action potential is dependent on two factors: (1) diameter of the conducting fiber (conduction velocity increases with increasing fiber diameter; and (2) the presence or absence of a myelin sheath. The presence of a myelin sheath on an axon, with its typical interruptions (nodes) every millimeter, provides an anatomic substrate for discontinuous conductance of an action potential down an axon. This form of conductance is faster than that observed with unmyelinated axons.

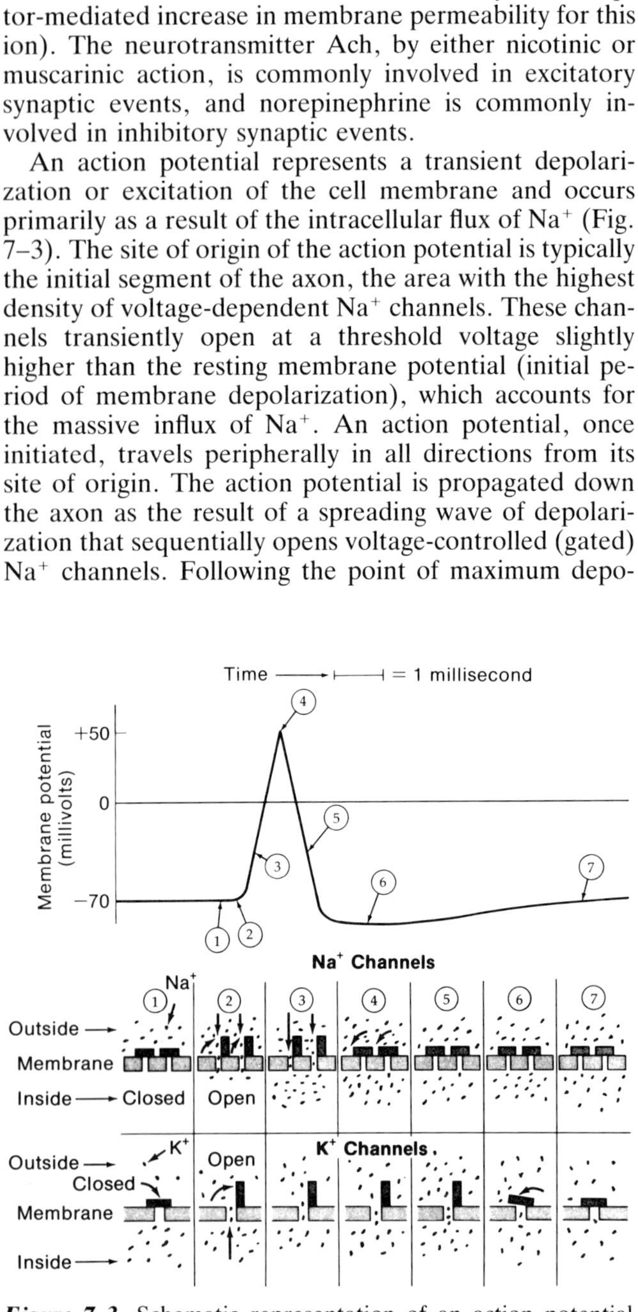

Figure 7–3. Schematic representation of an action potential and the ion fluxes that result in depolarization and hyperpolarization of the cell membrane. Membrane depolarization is due primarily to intracellular influx of sodium ions (Na^+) through voltage-gated channels. The opening of voltage-gated K^+ channels results in the repolarization of the membrane that occurs at the end of the action potential. (From The Brain: An Introduction to Neuroscience. By Richard F. Thompson. Copyright © 1985 by W.H. Freeman and Company. Reprinted with permission.)

Synaptic transmission is dependent on the action potential reaching the terminal process of an axon. Neurotransmitter release from the presynaptic terminal occurs as a result of membrane depolarization and intracellular flux of Ca^{2+} in this area. The presynaptic terminal membrane area is characterized by a high density of voltage-gated Ca^{2+} channels that open during membrane depolarization. The release of a neurotransmitter from the presynaptic terminal through an exocytotic process allows for its diffusion through the presynaptic space and its binding to receptors on the postsynaptic membrane. Alteration in postsynaptic membrane potentials occurs from an opening or closing of receptor-mediated ion channels. The postsynaptic membrane can undergo either a depolarization or a hyperpolarization, depending on the direction of ion flux and the charge of the ions. Neurotransmitters may also increase the level of a second messenger, such as cyclic adenosine monophosphate (AMP), cyclic guanosine monophosphate (GMP), and inositol triphosphate, within the postsynaptic cell. These second messengers, in turn may alter the permeability of membrane ion channels and the level of intracellular Ca^{2+}. It appears that intracellular Ca^{2+} is involved as a final mediator of many cellular processes.

NEURAL INNERVATION OF THE GASTROINTESTINAL TRACT

General Organization

Neural structures innervating the gastrointestinal tract are located in the ENS and the CNS and are conceptually divided into three levels (Fig. 7–4): (1) an afferent, or sensory, level that conveys information from the gut's sensory receptor; (2) an efferent, or motor, level that consists of motoneurons that have direct contact with effector cells (e.g., striated or smooth muscle cells, secretory cells, and absorptive cells) within the gut; (3) an organizing, or integrative, level located within both the ENS and the CNS, that consists of networks of interneurons in contact with both afferent and efferent levels. Neurons of the organizing level integrate sensory input and program the output of motoneurons.

Sensory, motor, and inter- (integrative) neurons are

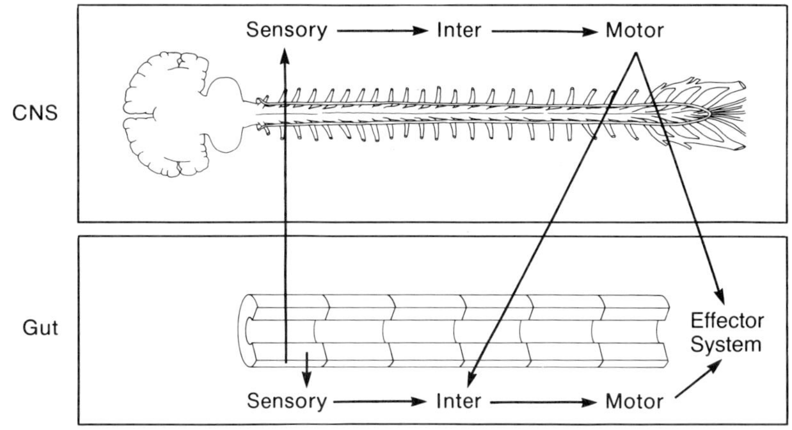

Figure 7–4. Schematic representation of the levels of innervation of the gastrointestinal tract by the CNS and ENS. Note the multiple areas of integration between the CNS and ENS. The ENS represents the final common pathway to effector cells within the gaastrointestinal tract. (Modified from Wood JD, Wingate DL: Gastrointestinal Neurobiology [The Little Brain in the Gut]. American Gastroenterological Association Teaching Project. Timonium, MD, Milner-Fenwick, 1988; with permission.)

found in both the ENS and the CNS, providing for multiple levels of neural control of gastrointestinal function. The ENS and CNS function as an integrative network, with the ENS providing the final common pathway for output to gut effectors (see Fig. 7–4). Although there are constant and direct interactions between the ENS and the CNS, the ENS is capable of mediating reflex activity within the alimentary tract independently of CNS and spinal control. Bayliss and Starling, in 1899, were the first investigators to recognize the existence of a local nervous system within the gut wall that is capable of mediating reflex activity within the intestine independently of extrinsic neural influences. Their observations, termed the *law of the intestine,* provided physiologic evidence for the existence of the ENS.

Enteric Nervous System

Definition[8]

The ENS is a system of neurons, nerve fibers, and supporting cells located within the walls of the gastrointestinal tract. A neuron is classified as an enteric neuron if its cell body is located within the ENS. Neurons whose terminal processes are located within the gut wall but whose cell bodies are found outside the ENS are termed *extrinsic neurons*. Groups of neurons located within the ENS are termed *enteric ganglia.* The number of neurons located within the ENS has been estimated to be in the range of several million.

Development of Enteric Neurons

Enteric neurons are derived from neuroblasts that originate within the vagal region of the neural crest.[9–11] These cells migrate to the gastrointestinal tract along the same pathways as do the descending fibers of the vagus nerve (Fig. 7–5).[9, 12] During their migration to the gut wall, these enteric neuron precursors continue to proliferate and transiently express cathecholamines (cells are immunoreactive for tyrosine hydroxylase, dopamine beta-hydroxylase, and aromatic L-amino acid decarboxylase) and other neural characteristics, including neurofilament immunoreactivity, peripherin, and growth and microtubule-associated proteins.[11–13] Enteric

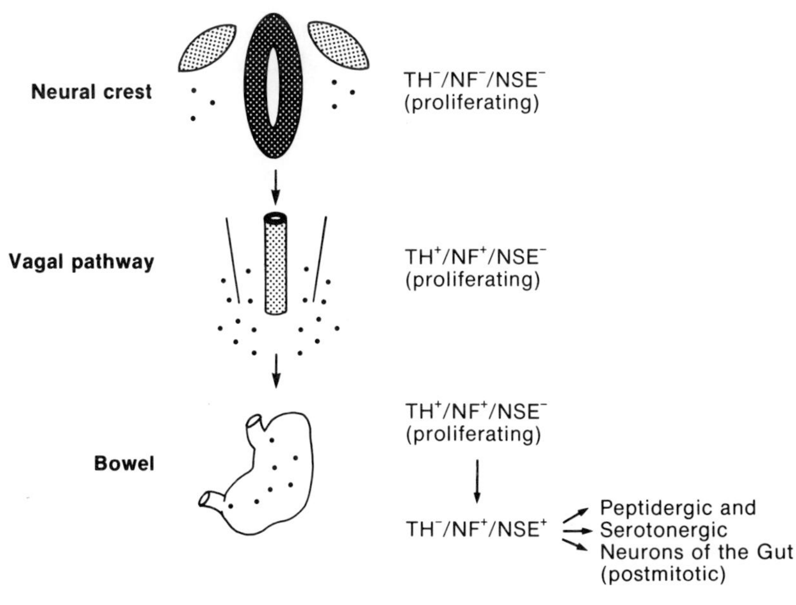

Figure 7–5. Schematic representation of the migration and development of enteric neurons. Enteric neurons are derived from neural crest cells that migrate along the vagal pathway to the bowel. During their migration and proliferation, these cell transiently express proteins (TH, tyrosine hydroxylase; NF, neurofilament) that are absent in the mature and nonproliferating enteric neuron. Mature enteric neurons are immunoreactive for neuron-specific enolase (NSE). (From Baetge G, Schneider KA, Gershon MD: Development and persistence of catecholaminergic neurons in cultured explants of fetal murine vagus nerves and bowel. Development 1990; 110:689–701; with permission of the Company of Biologists Ltd.)

precursors continue to proliferate within the gut wall before terminally differentiating into mature enteric neurons. Mature enteric neurons colonize the bowel late in fetal life and are known to influence effector cells by this stage of development.[14, 15] Phenotypically, mature enteric neurons no longer express catecholamines; however, they are immunoreactive for neuron-specific enolase.[12]

Characteristics of Enteric Neurons

A number of different criteria have been used since the turn of the century to classify enteric neurons.[16] Dogiel's work at the light microscopic level published in 1899 was the first attempt at classification of enteric neurons by objective criteria. Dogiel used the size and shape of the neuronal cell body and the axonal and dendritic morphology to classify enteric neurons into three types (I–III). Type I neurons were described as being stellate shaped, with many short stubby dendrites and one long axon. Type II and III neurons, in contrast, were identified as having a smoother cell body with fewer but longer dendritic processes. The dendritic processes of these neurons were found to extend over multiple adjacent ganglia. An example of each type of cell is presented in Figure 7–6 and illustrates the differences in the earlier mentioned characteristics.

In the myenteric plexus of the guinea pig's small intestine, eight different types of enteric neurons have been described based on ultrastructural criteria such as maximal cell diameter, location within the ganglia, location of synaptic input, and organization of intracellular organelles.[17] Some of these neurons appear (with analysis at the light microscopic level) to correspond to Dogiel type I neurons. In contrast, enteric neurons of the submucous plexus are morphologically similar at the ultrastructural level and appear similar to Dogiel type III neurons.

The morphologic difference that Dogiel observed in enteric neurons has now been correlated with differences in electrophysiologic properties.[18–20] On the basis of intracellular recording, Dogiel type I neurons have been classified primarily as S-type neurons, and Dogiel type II neurons, as AH-type neurons.[20] Although S- and AH-type neurons differ in a number of electrical properties (Table 7–1), the most obvious distinction in these cell types is the characteristics of their stimulus-evoked action potentials.[6, 21, 22]

Table 7–1. ELECTROPHYSIOLOGIC PROPERTIES OF ENTERIC NEURONS

Properties	Classification of Neuron	
	S	*AH*
Resting membrane potential	Low	High
Membrane resistance	High	Low
Repetitive action potential in response to stimulus	Yes	No
Tetrodotoxin-sensitive action potential	Yes	No
Afterhyperpolarization	No	Yes
Cholinergic input	Yes	Rare

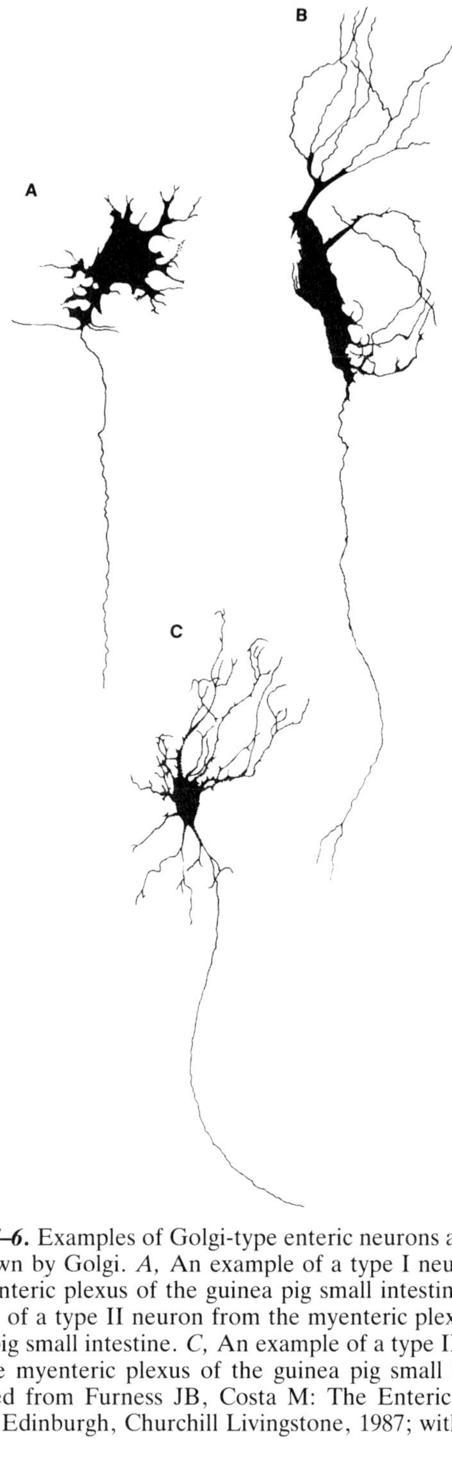

Figure 7–6. Examples of Golgi-type enteric neurons as defined and drawn by Golgi. *A,* An example of a type I neuron from the myenteric plexus of the guinea pig small intestine. *B,* An example of a type II neuron from the myenteric plexus of the guinea pig small intestine. *C,* An example of a type III neuron from the myenteric plexus of the guinea pig small intestine. (Modified from Furness JB, Costa M: The Enteric Nervous System. Edinburgh, Churchill Livingstone, 1987; with permission.)

The action potentials of S neurons are tetrodotoxin sensitive, and those of AH neurons are tetrodotoxin resistant. Because tetrodotoxins specifically block the opening of Na^+ channels, it appears that the generation of action potentials in S neurons is totally dependent on the inward movement of Na^+. The generation of action potentials in AH neurons, in contrast, occurs as a result of the inward movement of both Na^+ and Ca^{2+}, accounting for the partial resistance of these neurons to tetrodotoxin (Fig. 7–7). It also appears that the membrane

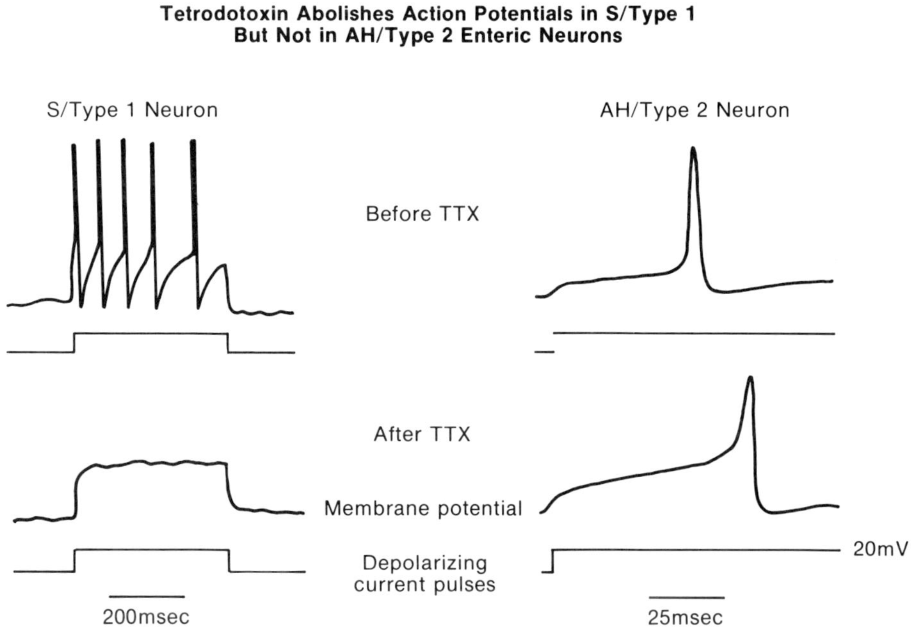

Figure 7–7. Effect of tetrodotoxin on the stimulus-induced action potentials of S- and AH-type enteric neurons. Note that tetrodotoxin has a more profound effect on the generation of an action potential in an S-type than in an AH-type enteric neuron. (Modified from Wood JD, Wingate DL: Gastrointestinal Neurobiology [The Little Brain in the Gut]. American Gastroenterological Association Teaching Project. Timonium, MD, Milner-Fenwick, 1988; with permission.)

excitability of S neurons is higher than that of AH neurons resulting in the generation of multiple action potentials in S neurons and a single action potential in AH neurons in response to a stimulus of long duration (see Fig. 7–7). In this regard, the duration of after-hyperpolarization time is much shorter in S neurons than in AH neurons (see Fig. 7–7).

Enteric Neurotransmitters

The most extensive and precise classification of enteric neurons is based on their neurochemical content. Immunocytochemical and histochemical techniques have been used with great success to localize a great variety of neuropeptides and biologically active amines within enteric neurons and their processes. Approximately 20 different established or potential neurotransmitters have been localized in enteric neurons (Table 7–2). Many of the same transmitters and neuropeptides initially described in the CNS have now been demonstrated within the ENS. It appears that an enteric neuron's neurochemical content correlates with its histologic and functional characteristics.[16] For example, Dogiel type I neurons that are immunoreactive for vasoactive intestinal peptide (VIP) demonstrate the electrophysiologic properties of an S enteric neuron. Additionally, enkephalin appears to colocalize with a number of other peptides in Dogiel type I neurons, whereas neuropeptide Y colocalizes with other peptides in Dogiel type III neurons.

The ability to localize peptide immunoreactive neurons and their projection with a high degree of anatomic resolution in conjunction with pharmacologic studies has provided a wealth of information concerning the functional role of the many described neurotransmitters within the ENS. Neurotransmitters involved in synaptic transmission at the neuromuscular junction (circular muscle of the gut wall) include Ach, bombesin, substance P, calcitonin gene-related peptide, adenosine triphosphate (ATP), galanin, and VIP. Peptide immunoreactive neurons for these transmitters are located primarily in the myenteric plexus (Table 7–3). A number of neurotransmitters, including, Ach, substance P, VIP, neuropeptide Y, and somatostatin, appear to have profound effects on the secretory properties of enterocytes. Nerve fibers immunoreactive for these transmitters have been found in the mucosal plexus (see Table 7–3) of the intestine. The neurons of origin of these fibers are located within the myenteric and submucous plexuses (see Table 7–3) and the sympathetic ganglia.

Structure of Enteric Ganglia

At the ultrastructural level, enteric ganglia closely resemble the CNS as opposed to other autonomic gan-

Table 7–2. ENS NEUROTRANSMITTERS

Established
Acetylcholine (ACH)
Adenosine triphosphate (ATP)
Bombesin or gastrin-releasing peptide (GRP)
Calcitonin gene-related peptide (CGRP)
Cholecystokinin (CCK)
Dynorphin (DYN)
Enkephalin (ENK)
Galanin (GAL)
Gamma-aminobutyric acid (GABA)
5-Hydroxytryptamine (5-HT)
Neuropeptide Y (NPY)
Norepinephrine (NA)
Somatostatin (SOM)
Substance P (SP)
Vasoactive intestinal peptide (VIP)
Potential
Adenosine
Glutamate
Glycine
Neurotensin
Peptide histidine isoleucine (HI)

Table 7–3. COMPONENT PLEXUSES OF THE GASTROINTESTINAL TRACT

Plexus	Identifying Characteristics	Ganglia Present
Subserosal	Fine nerve bundles that form connections between extrinsic nerves and nerves of the deeper layers of the gut wall	Stomach Intestine Rectum
Longitudinal muscle	Fine nerve bundles that run parallel to the muscle cell	None
Myenteric (Auerbach's)	Network of nerve fibers and small ganglia that is located in the plane between the external longitudinal and circular muscle coats of the gut wall Ganglia are found at the junction of nerve fibers	Entire gastrointestinal tract
Circular muscle	Small nerve bundles that run parallel to the long axis of muscle fibers Nerves connect with myenteric and deep muscular plexuses	None
Deep muscular	Aggregate of nerve bundles located in the inner part of the circular muscle layer Nerve bundles form continual meshwork around circumference of the gut	None
Submucous (Meissner's)	Network of small ganglia and connecting nerve fibers Continuous around circumference of the gut	Primarily in intestine
Muscularis mucosae	Fine nerve bundles that run parallel to long axis of the muscle cell Nerve fibers accompany bundles of smooth muscles that project into intestinal villi and between gastric glands	None
Mucosal	Dense network of interconnecting nerves and ganglia located within the lamina propria	Stomach Small and large intestine

glia. Neuronal cell bodies, their cell processes, and enteric glial cells form compact structures, with little intercellular space, within the connective tissue between muscle layers or in the submucosa.[23, 24] Enteric ganglia lack blood vessels, connective tissue cells, collagen, and a capsule, in contrast with other autonomic ganglia, resulting in an appearance that is similar to the CNS. The close proximity of multiple neuronal elements (cell body, axons, and dendrites) provides the anatomic substrate for the efficient transfer of information within the ENS. Synaptic transmission occurs at axoaxonal, axodendritic, and axosomatic contacts.

Most cellular elements within the enteric ganglia are either supportive or glial cells. At the ultrastructural level and by immunocytochemical criteria, enteric glial cells more closely resemble CNS astrocytes than the Schwann cells of other peripheral ganglia or nerves.[24–26] These cells are positioned around cell bodies and axons within the ganglia and form intricate structures that divide the neuronal projections into large bundles within individual nerve fibers.[24]

Anatomy of the Enteric Plexus

The ENS consists of a number of interconnected plexuses of nerve cell bodies (ganglia) and fibers that form the circuits underlying enteric reflexes (Fig. 7–8). According to Furness and Costa,[27, 28] eight different plexuses, each occupying a different layer of the gut wall, compose the ENS (see Fig. 7–8 and Table 7–3). The prominence and development of each of these plexuses vary according to anatomic location within the gastrointestinal tract and by animal species.[29–32] The myenteric (Auerbach's) plexus, located between longitudinal and circular muscle layers, and submucous (Meissner's) plexus, located between the muscularis mucosa and the circular muscle layer, constitute the two most prominent plexuses in most animal species. Most of the enteric ganglia are located within these two plexuses.

Extensive investigations of the rodent's small intestine have suggested that the myenteric plexus consists of a uniform matrix of nerve fibers (termed *internodal strands*) that intersect with large enteric ganglia at regular intervals (Fig. 7–9).[27] Together the ganglia and internodal strands provide the primary framework for the myenteric plexus and are termed the *primary plexus* (see Fig. 7–9). Two additional components of the myenteric plexus, termed the *secondary plexus* and the *tertiary plexus*, consisting primarily of smaller-diameter nerve fibers, have also been described (see Fig. 7–9). Recent investigations of the myenteric plexus in other areas of the gastrointestinal tract in a variety of animal species have demonstrated far less uniformity in matrix organization, density of enteric ganglia and neurons, and nerve bundle diameter.[27, 29, 30]

In the esophagus, for example, the matrix arrangement is quite irregular, with many internodal strand intersections lacking ganglia.[29] Many of the ganglia are located outside the major internodal strand (parafascicular ganglia). Parafascicular ganglia have also been described in the rectum and in the cardia of the stomach. The myenteric plexus of the proximal stomach and the distal colon are also characterized by the presence of thick nerve bundles, termed *shunt fascicles*, that generally do not intersect with enteric ganglia and may represent the terminal processes of extrinsic nerves.[27, 29] The structural diversity of the myenteric plexus in different regions of the gastrointestinal tract may provide an anatomic substrate for regional differences in function. The submucous plexus, like the myenteric plexus, generally consists of a regular meshwork of intercon-

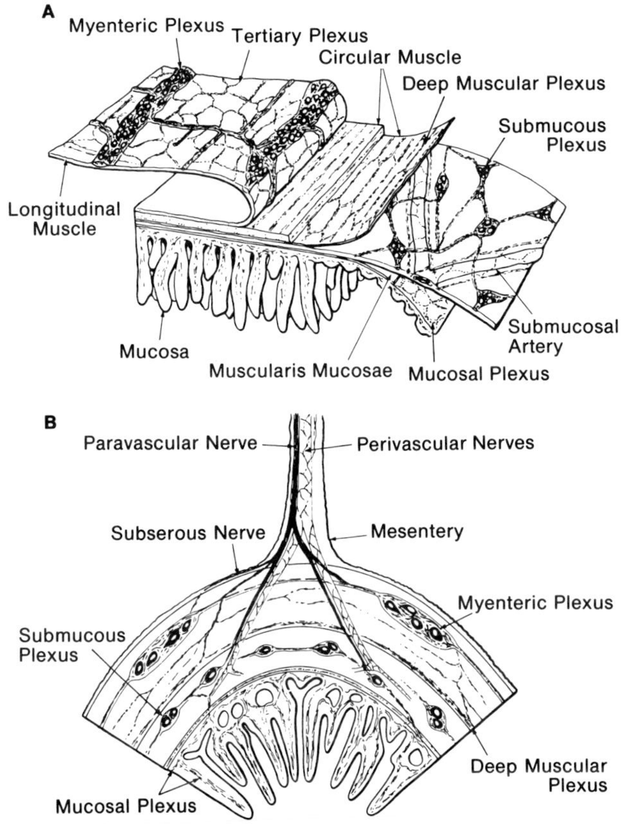

Figure 7–8. Schematic representation of the enteric plexuses of guinea pig small intestine as seen from a whole mount (*A*) and transverse (*B*) section. Although eight different plexuses are diagrammed, two plexuses (the myenteric and the submucous) are, by far, the most prominent. (From Furness JB, Costa M: The Enteric Nervous System. Edinburgh, Churchill Livingstone, 1987; with permission.)

nected nerve fibers and ganglia. However, the ganglia tend to be smaller, with a lower density of enteric neurons and nerve fibers of a smaller diameter than comparable structures in the myenteric plexus.[27] Within the small bowel, this plexus is most prominent and occupies the entire circumference and length of the intestine. The submucous plexus is far less prominent in the stomach and colon and is essentially nonexistent in the esophagus.

The enteric ganglia of the myenteric and submucous plexuses are the site of origin of intramural neural connections between the multiple layers of the bowel wall. The projections of a single enteric neuron within the ENS have been mapped using a combination of immunohistochemical and lesion techniques.[33–39] These extensive studies, which are summarized schematically in Figure 7–10, demonstrate that a number of different neurotransmitters characterize the projections. Enteric motor neurons within the myenteric plexus provide innervation to the circular muscle and the mucosal layers of the gut wall. Additionally, projections of myenteric interneurons penetrate the adjacent and distant ganglia of the myenteric plexus and the ganglia of the submucous plexus.

Enteric neurons of the submucous plexus appear to be either sensory or motor neurons. Projections of these neurons penetrate the mucosal layer of the bowel and provide the potential for local reflex activity within the mucosa. Myenteric ganglia, however, do not appear to receive projections of submucous enteric neurons.

Enteric Control of Gastrointestinal Function

The ENS, like the CNS, contains three functional classes of neurons whose interactions provide the circuitry that underlies all aspects of gastrointestinal function. Sensory or afferent innervation of the alimentary tract is provided by *specialized sensory neurons* that sense changes in mechanical or chemical stimuli and transform the information into electrical signals (action potential). The terminal endings of a sensory neuron's peripheral process generally act as the receptor that

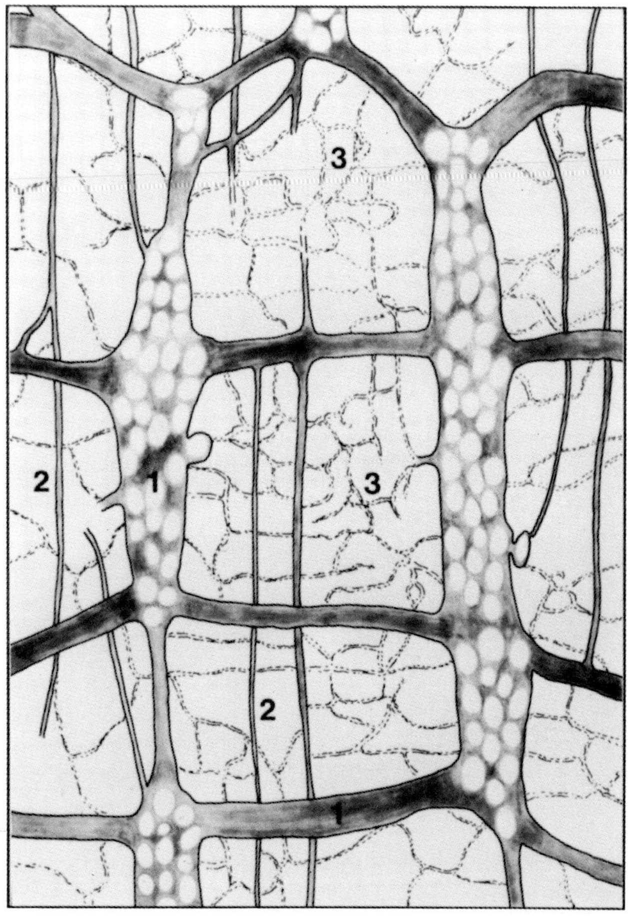

Figure 7–9. Schematic representation of the fine structure of the guinea pig's myenteric plexus. The myenteric plexus is composed of three components: (1) primary plexus—ganglia and internodal strands; (2) secondary plexus—nerve bundles running parallel to the circular muscle; and (3) tertiary plexus—fine network of nerve fibers located at the interface of the longitudinal and circular muscle layers. (From Furness JB, Costa M: The Enteric Nervous System. Edinburgh, Churchill Livingstone, 1987; with permission.)

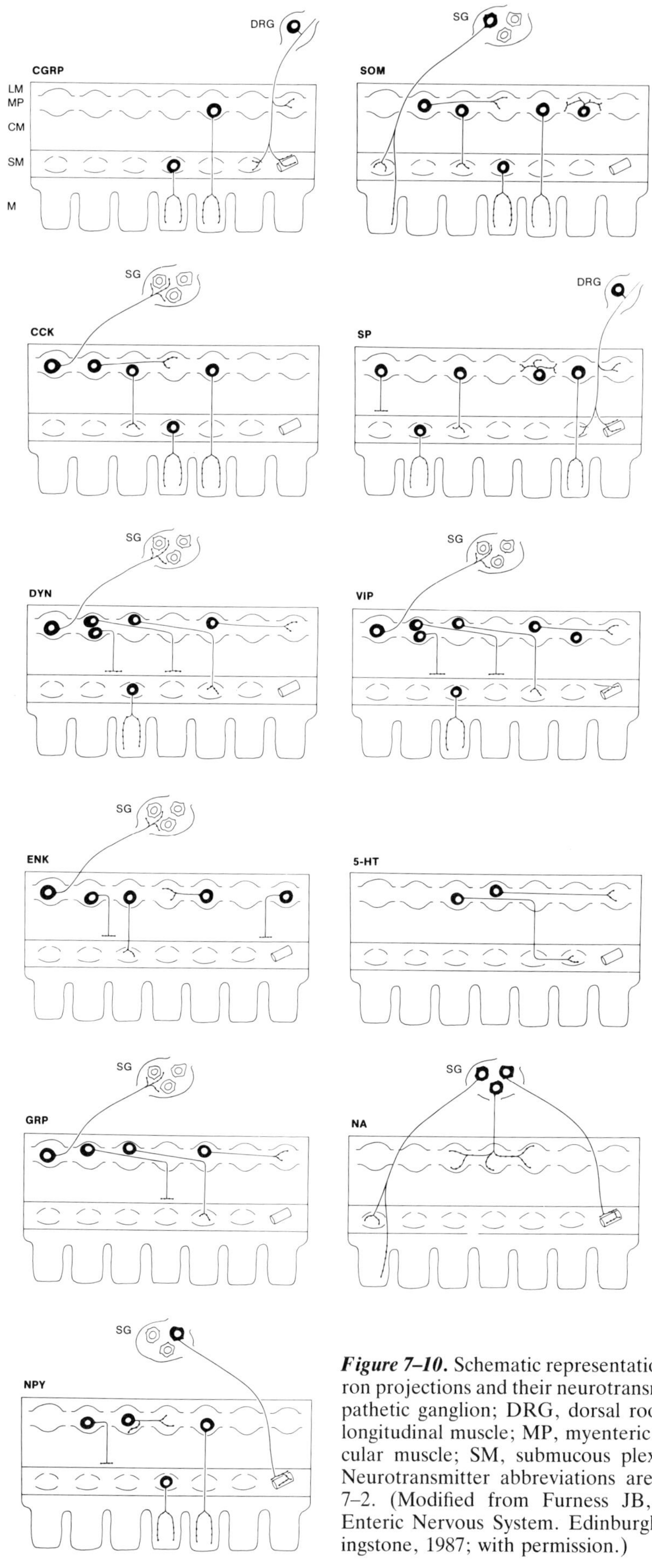

Figure 7–10. Schematic representation of enteric neuron projections and their neurotransmitters. SG, sympathetic ganglion; DRG, dorsal root ganglion; LM, longitudinal muscle; MP, myenteric plexus; CM, circular muscle; SM, submucous plexus; M, mucosa. Neurotransmitter abbreviations are found in Table 7–2. (Modified from Furness JB, Costa M: The Enteric Nervous System. Edinburgh, Churchill Livingstone, 1987; with permission.)

senses changes in mechanical or chemical stimuli. In most instances, sensory receptors are free nerve endings with no morphologic specialization. The different classes of sensory receptors include mechanoreceptors (tension and mucosal rub), chemoreceptors (glucose, fat, pH, and osmoreceptor), and thermoreceptors.

The second functional class of enteric neurons is composed of the *interneurons*. These neurons are linked synaptically with other interneurons and with sensory and motor neurons. Functionally, these neurons integrate sensory information in the form of action potentials and form pattern-generating circuits (motor programs) that drive motor neurons. The formation of pattern-generating circuits by these neurons provides the anatomic basis for the stereotyped, repetitive behaviors (e.g., peristalsis) or functions that characterize the gastrointestinal tract. Their synaptic connections with sensory neurons provide a mechanism for the constant reflex or feedback modulation and fine-tuning of their output.

Motor neurons constitute the third functional class of enteric neurons. These enteric neurons are synaptically linked with interneurons and effector structures of the gastrointestinal tract. They are either excitatory or inhibitory to the effector structures they innervate and are responsible for initiating, maintaining, or inhibiting the behavior of the effector structure.

The importance of the ENS to gastrointestinal function is evident from both animal and clinical studies. Chemical ablation of the small bowel's myenteric neurons in the rat is associated with profound longitudinal and circular muscle hypertrophy and alterations in recorded myoelectric activity.[40] Similar alterations in muscle histology and myoelectric activity have been found in the piebald mouse model for Hirschsprung's disease.[40–44]

In humans, an absence or alteration of enteric neurons is seen in a number of disorders, including achalasia, Chagas' disease, chronic intestinal pseudo-obstruction, and Hirschsprung's disease.[45–49] Each of these disorders is associated with severe derangements in gut motility and often leads to symptoms of obstruction without a fixed anatomic lesion.

Central Nervous System

General Organization

The CNS provides both afferent (sensory) and efferent (motor) innervation to the gastrointestinal tract. Sensory innervation is provided by vagal and splanchnic primary afferent fibers. These afferent fibers travel in close association with parasympathetic preganglionic fibers in the vagus nerve and sympathetic postganglionic fibers in the splanchnic nerves, respectively. Their neuronal cell bodies are located in the nodose and dorsal root ganglia, respectively.

Vagal afferents terminate as sensory receptors in the mucosal and muscular layers of the gastrointestinal tract, from the level of the soft palate through the descending colon, and in the liver, pancreas, and gallbladder.[50–59] Extracellular recordings of a single neuron's activity from the nodose ganglion or brain stem of experimental animals have revealed the existence of vagal mechanoreceptors, chemoreceptors, and thermoreceptors.[50–52, 55, 57, 60] Splanchnic afferents innervate the serosal surface and the mesentery of the bowel as well as its mucosal and muscular layers.[61] These afferents convey pain sensation from the gastrointestinal tract to the spinal cord as well as function as mechanoreceptors, chemoreceptors, and thermoreceptors.

Motor innervation is provided by the sympathetic and parasympathetic divisions of the autonomic nervous system (Fig. 7–11). The ganglia (location of the postganglionic neurons) of the sympathetic division are located along either side of the spinal cord or in a prevertebral position, whereas the ganglia of the parasympathetic division are positioned within the gastrointestinal tract. Preganglionic sympathetic and parasympathetic neurons are located in the intermediolateral cell column of spinal cord segments T2 through L2 (sympathetic) and the medulla and sacral spinal cord (parasympathetic).

The sympathetic innervation of the gastrointestinal tract is organized in a rostrocaudal topographic distribution. The esophagus, stomach, and proximal small bowel receive postganglionics from the most rostral prevertebral and trunk ganglia (celiac, superior and middle cervical, and stellate; see Fig. 7–11). The most distal parts of the gastrointestinal tract are innervated by the caudal prevertebral and trunk ganglia. Sympathetic postganglionic fibers provide rich innervation to the gut vasculature, the myenteric and submucous plexuses, and the muscular layers of the sphincteric areas. More limited innervation is evident in the circular and longitudinal muscle layers of the nonsphincteric area and the mucosal layer of the bowel.[62] Stimulation of the sympathetic efferents generally causes contraction of the sphincteric areas and the blood vessels and inhibits motility and secretion.[62]

The vagus and sacral nerves are the source of parasympathetic innervation to the gastrointestinal tract. Most of the gastrointestinal tract is innervated by the vagus nerve, with the sacral nerves generally innervating only the distal colon and rectum (see Fig. 7–11). Recent studies have demonstrated that the vagal efferents terminate primarily within the myenteric plexus of the gut.[63, 64] Because a major source of CNS innervation to the gut is provided by the vagus nerve, considerable study has been devoted to determining the brain stem organization of vagal projections from the alimentary tract.

Vagal Innervation and Brain Stem Organization

The use of axoplasmic tracing techniques in experimental animals has demonstrated a particularly strong visceral representation within the vagal motor nuclei (nucleus ambiguus [NA] and dorsal motor nucleus [DMN] of the vagus nerve) and the vagal sensory

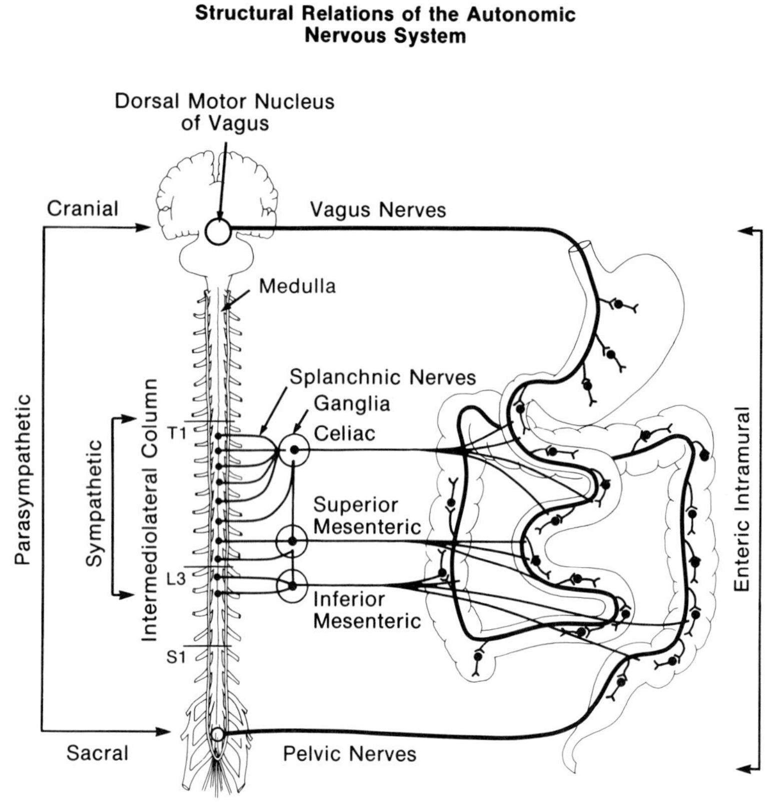

Figure 7–11. Schematic representation of the topographic organization of CNS motor projections (sympathetic and parasympathetic) to the gastrointestinal tract. (Modified from Wood JD, Wingate DL: Gastrointestinal Neurobiology [The Little Brain in the Gut]. American Gastroenterological Association Teaching Project. Timonium, MD, Milner-Fenwick, Inc. 1988; with permission.)

nucleus (nucleus tractus solitarii [NTS].[65–73] Extensive studies in the rat have demonstrated that a precise viscerotopic organization for afferent and efferent projections from the gastrointestinal tract exists within the dorsal (DMN-NTS) and ventral (NA) vagal complexes.[58, 59, 66–68, 74–85] The formulation and acceptance of viscerotopic maps for vagal innervated structures have depended heavily on the development of new neuroanatomic tracers and injection strategies to control leakage and spread of the tracers.

Ventral Vagal Complex

Nucleus Ambiguus

The NA, located in the ventrolateral medulla, comprises a continuum of rostrocaudally aligned subdivisions that begin rostrally at the level of the facial nucleus and extend caudally to the spinal medullary junction.[82] These subdivisions, which are readily discernible by their different cellular densities when the medulla is sectioned in the sagittal plane, have been designated as the *compact, semicompact, loose,* and *external formations* by Bieger and Hopkins.[82] The dorsal division of the NA comprises the compact, semicompact, and loose formations and is the source of special visceral efferents that innervate the striated muscle of the upper gastrointestinal and respiratory tracts (branchiomeric musculature). The external formation, which composes the ventral division of the NA, lies ventral and lateral to the dorsal division and is the source of the general visceral efferents that innervate the thoracic viscera. The dorsal division of the NA is no longer considered to be a source—DMN is only source—of general visceral efferent innervation to abdominal viscera.[81, 82, 86]

The viscerotopic organization of the NA discussed in this section is derived from studies conducted primarily in the rat, where direct intramuscular injections of the tracer into different parts of the upper gastrointestinal tract were performed.[82, 84] Tracer injections into the soft palate, pharynx, and cricothyroid muscle result in retrograde neuronal labeling limited to the semicompact formation, whereas, in contrast, injections of all levels of the esophagus result in neuronal labeling limited to the compact formation (Figs. 7–12 and 7–13). Injections of tracer into the intrinsic laryngeal muscles result in retrograde neuronal labeling limited to the loose formation.

Although the entire esophagus of the rat (and striated portions in other mammals[75, 87–90]) derives its vagal motor innervation from the compact formation, the population of motoneurons projecting to different levels of the esophagus is not entirely homogenous. Using fluorescent dyes as a tracer, Bieger and Hopkins[82] have demonstrated that separate populations of neurons innervate the different levels of the esophagus. The cervical esophagus has the most restricted representation; its motoneurons are limited to the most rostral and dorsal aspects of the compact formation[82, 84] (see Fig. 7–13). Motoneurons projecting to the thoracic and subdiaphragmatic esophagus, in contrast, are located throughout the entire rostrocaudal and mediolateral extent of the compact formation. Although the rostrocaudal distribution of

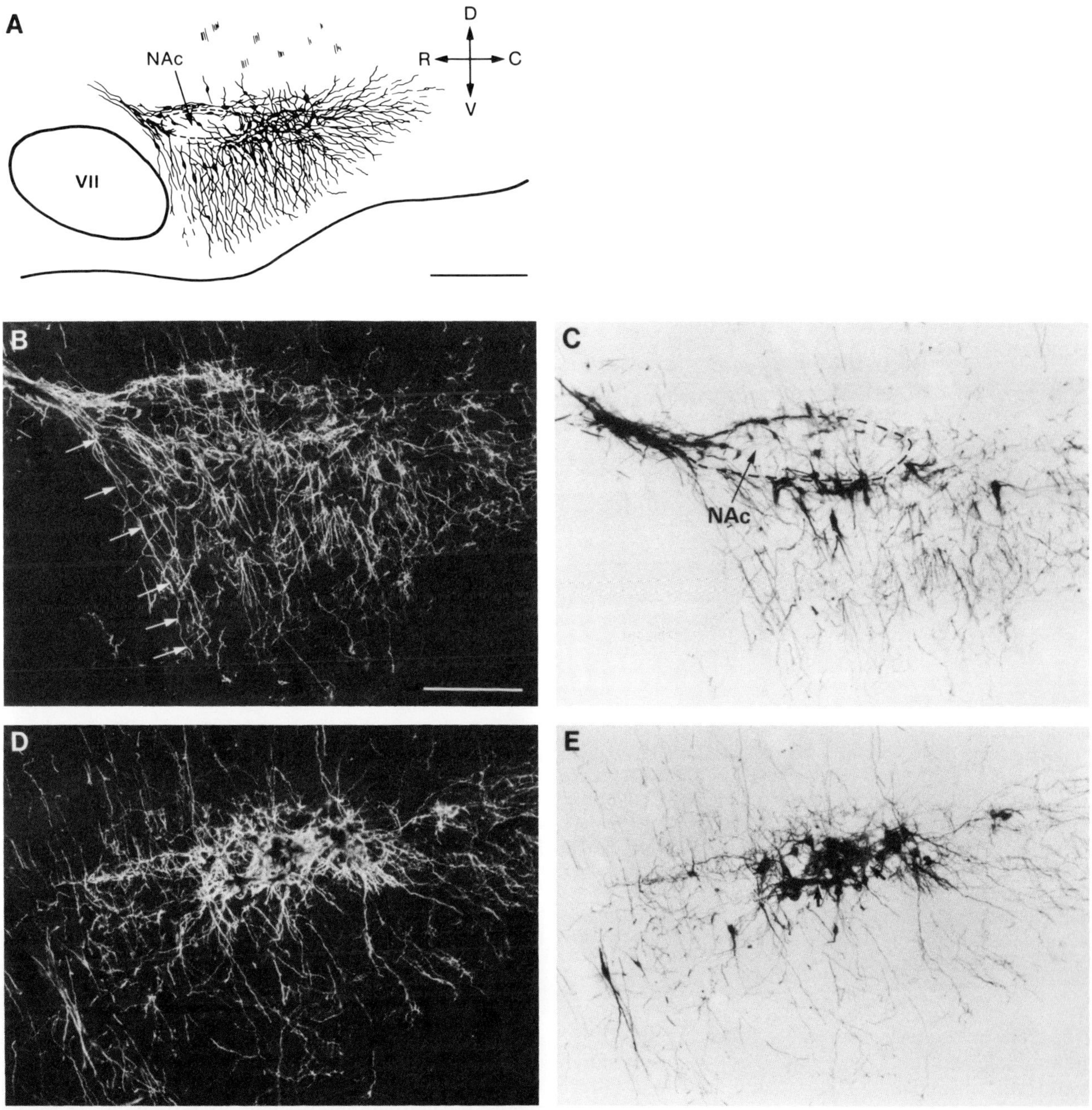

Figure 7–12. *A,* Schematic camera lucida reconstruction in the sagittal plane of six serial sections through the NA following injection of CT-HRP into the pharynx of a rat. *B* and *C,* and *D* and *E* are two sets of dark-field and bright-field photomicrographs of sagittal sections through the NA following injection of tracer into the pharynx. In *B,* the *arrows* indicate the path of one dendrite that extends 600 μm from the nucleus. The *arrows* in *E* indicate dendritic bundles within the confines of the nucleus. Calibration bar in *A* = 500 μm, and in *B* = 250 μm. Photomicrographs *B–E* are at the same magnification. R, rostral; C, caudal; D, dorsal; V, ventral. (From Altschuler SM, Bao X, Miselis RR: Dendritic architecture of nucleus ambiguus motoneurons projecting to the upper alimentary tract in the rat. J Comp Neurol 1991; 309:402–414. Copyright 1991 by Wiley-Liss; with permission.)

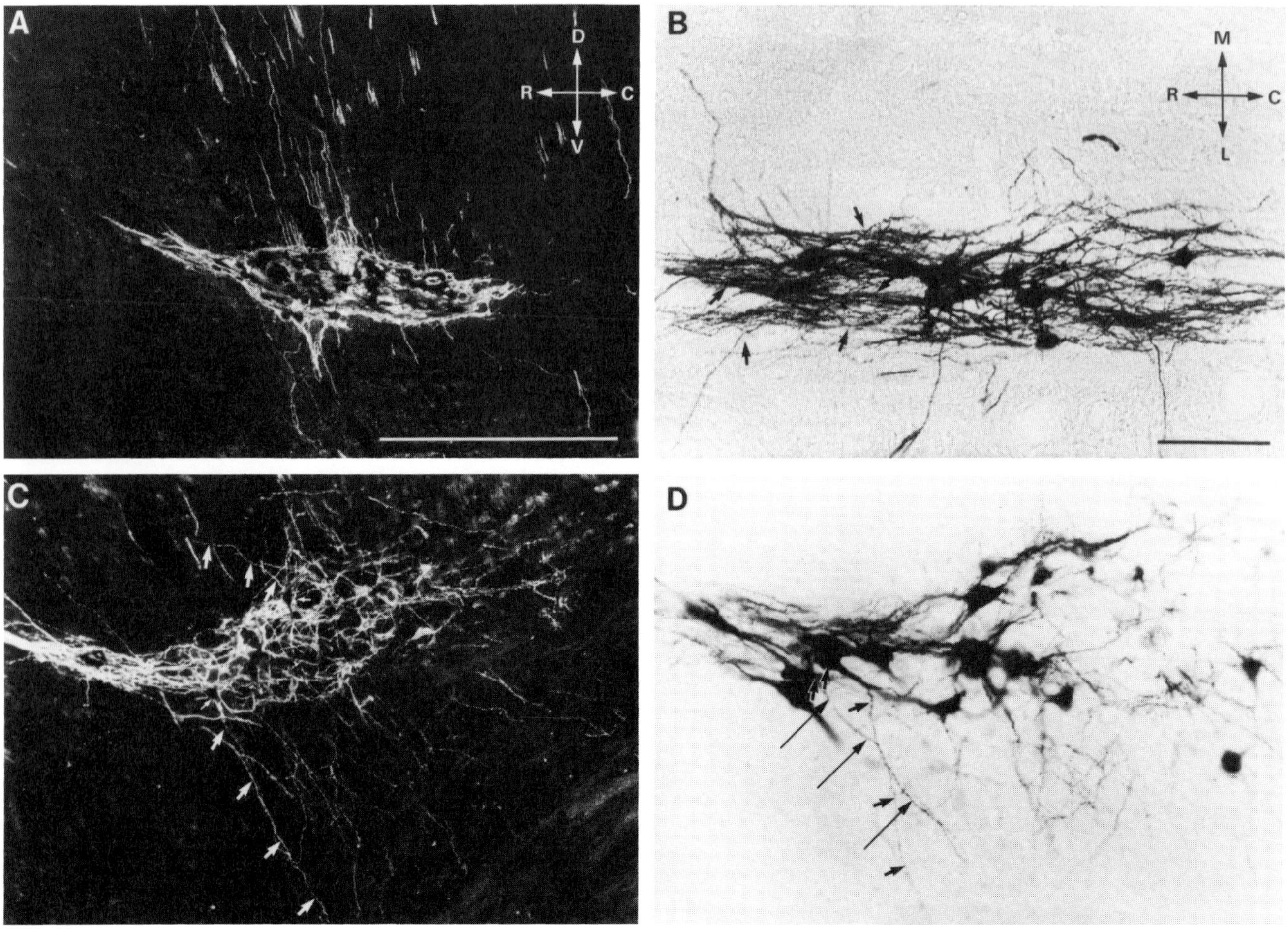

Figure 7–13. *A,* Dark-field photomicrograph of a sagittal section through the NA following injection of CT-HRP into the subdiaphragmatic esophagus of a rat. *B,* Bright-field photomicrograph of a horizontal section following injection of CT-HRP into the thoracic esophagus. Note that the dendrites form bundles (*arrows*) that run primarily in a rostrocaudal direction and are confined to the boundaries of the compact formation of the NA. *C,* Dark-field photomicrograph of a sagittal section following injection of CT-HRP into the cervical esophagus. Note that the cell bodies are located primarily in the rostral and dorsal portions of the compaction formation. *D,* Bright-field photomicrograph at higher magnification of a sagittal section 80 μm medial to the section in *C.* The sets of *arrows* in *C* and *D* indicate dendrites whose origin could be traced to cell bodies located in the NAc. Calibration bar in *A* = 500 μm, and in *B* = 125 μm. *A* and *C,* and *B* and *D* are at the same magnification. *R,* rostral; *C,* caudal; *D,* dorsal; *V,* ventral; *M,* medial; *L,* lateral. (From Altschuler SM, Bao X, Miselis RR: Dendritic architecture of nucleus ambiguus motoneurons projecting to the upper alimentary tract in the rat. J Comp Neurol 1991; 309:402–414. Copyright 1991 by Wiley-Liss; with permission.)

labeled cells overlaps considerably following injection of the thoracic and subdiaphragmatic esophagus, a more rostral level of maximal cell labeling is found after injection of the thoracic esophagus.[84] These findings suggest that a crude rostrocaudal organotropism exists within the compact formation that corresponds to rostrocaudal positioning along the esophagus.

A prominent characteristic of both the compact and the semicompact formations is the extensive bundling of motoneuronal dendrites within the confines of the nucleus.[82, 84] (see Figs. 7–12 and 7–13). These dendritic bundles are oriented primarily in the rostrocaudal direction and are evident following sectioning of the medulla in either the horizontal or the sagittal plane.[84] The semicompact formation is also the site of origin of ventrolaterally and dorsomedially oriented dendritic bundles. These bundles differ from longitudinal dendritic bundles in a number of ways. Motoneuron dendrites that contribute to these bundles are limited to the same rostrocaudal plane and do not extend rostrocaudally throughout the nucleus. Additionally, these bundles are not confined entirely to the semicompact formation but actually penetrate the adjacent reticular formation.

Dendritic bundles have been postulated to serve as networks for the generation of complex motor events where a synchronization of motoneuronal activity is required.[91–97] The extensive longitudinal bundling of dendrites found in the NA, one of the major motor nuclei involved in swallowing,[98, 99] suggests a role for these structures in maintaining a precise sequence of muscle activation through the rostrocaudal integration of motoneuronal activity during the swallowing motor sequence. In contrast, transverse dendritic bundles may provide a mechanism for the localized modification of motor output without affecting the sequence of muscle activation. Thus, it appears likely that dendritic bundles subserve a function similar to that of enteric ganglia.

Motoneurons located within the NA have been shown to have extensive extranuclear dendritic projections. The extranuclear dendritic fields for the musculature represented in the semicompact formation are more extensive than those for musculature represented in the compact formation.[84] Based on the size of the dendritic fields, the potential for modulation by multiple central afferents would appear to be greater for musculature that is represented within the semicompact formation. The potential dendritic-afferent contacts may provide an anatomic substrate for the musculature represented in the semicompact formation to participate in a variety of motor functions (swallowing, respiration, and phonation[98, 100, 101]). Because the esophagus is essentially limited to one primary motor function—peristalsis—it is not unexpected that motoneurons projecting to this structure have more limited extranuclear dendritic projections. Esophageal motoneurons are known to receive afferent projections from a limited area of the brain stem, the subnucleus centralis of the NTS.[102–106]

Dorsal Vagal Complex

Dorsal Motor Nucleus

The DMN is the sole source of the general visceral efferent fibers that make synaptic contact with postganglionic neurons located in the myenteric plexus of the bowel wall.[63, 64, 107] The smooth muscle of the gastrointestinal tract, in turn, receives its motor innervation from neurons located within the myenteric plexus, indicating that no direct contacts exist between vagal fibers that originate in the DMN and the smooth muscle of the gastrointestinal tract. In the rat, in which the entire esophagus consists of striated muscle, motoneurons of the DMN begin their innervation of the alimentary canal at the level of the stomach and continue to innervate the gastrointestinal tract as far caudad as the descending colon. Innervation of the esophagus by DMN motoneurons occurs in those mammals in which a portion of the esophagus consists of smooth muscle (e.g., the cat).

The right and left DMN contribute efferent axons, respectively, to the right and left cervical vagal nerves. These nerves cross above the diaphragm and then enter the abdominal cavity, where they have been designated as the *left* and *right subdiaphragmatic vagus nerves*, respectively. The left subdiaphragmatic vagus further divides into the celiac and left gastric nerves, whereas the right subdiaphragmatic vagus divides into the hepatic, accessory celiac, and right gastric nerves.

The ability to apply neuroanatomic tracers easily to either vagal nerve branches or the different abdominal viscera directly has led to the development of organizational maps of the DMN based on both injection strategies. Although these two injection strategies have often provided conflicting results regarding DMN organization, more recent studies in which adequate measures to control tracer spread have been employed have yielded results that permit the correlation of vagal branch-organization topology with viscerotopic representation within the DMN.[59, 81, 83, 108, 109]

The studies of Fox and Powley[108] and Norgren and Smith,[109] in which tracers have been applied directly to the branches of the subdiaphragmatic vagus in the rat, have provided conclusive evidence that the DMN is organized mediolaterally with respect to these branches. Motoneurons located within large medial columns of the right and left DMN contribute efferent axons to the left and right gastric nerves, respectively. The celiac and accessory celiac nerves are composed of axons of motoneurons located in smaller lateral columns of the right and left DMN. The representation of the hepatic branch consists of a few scattered neurons located within the left medial DMN.

Anatomic studies that use direct intramuscular injections of tracer have suggested that motoneurons innervating specific abdominal viscera are localized within either the medial or the lateral bilaterally symmetric columns. This concept has been supported by our recent experiments in the rat, in which the representation of the small and large intestine within the DMN has been investigated. These studies demonstrated a significant representation for cecum that was localized to the two lateral columns of the DMN in a rostrocaudal distribution, which conforms to the pattern of DMN labeling seen after the application of tracer to the celiac and accessory celiac branches of the vagus nerve.[59, 108, 109] Although the representations of the stomach and the cecum dominate the medial and lateral column, respectively (Fig. 7–14), other areas of the bowel have a sparse representation localized to either the medial or the lateral columns.

Motoneurons that innervate the duodenum are limited to the medial columns, whereas the jejunum, ileum, and ascending colon receive motor innervation from the lateral columns. In recent investigations, we have demonstrated that motoneurons located in the lateral columns of the DMN, through the celiac and accessory celiac branches of the vagus, provide innervation to the ascending, transverse, and descending portions of the colon (unpublished observation). DMN innervation to the level of the descending colon has been confirmed by the presence of labeled vagal fibers in this area of the bowel following the injection of either ^{3}H-leucine or the fluorescent carbocyanine dye DiI into the DMN.[64, 107]

These anatomic studies support a mediolateral organization within the DMN that corresponds to rostrocaudal positioning along the alimentary canal, with the stomach and duodenum represented in medial columns and the more distal areas of the small bowel, cecum, and colon represented in the lateral columns. Additionally, evidence is emerging that a more precise viscerotopic organization for the stomach exists within the medial column of the DMN. Recent studies in the cat and the rat have demonstrated that the antrum-pylorus is represented most medially, the fundus most laterally, and the body of the stomach diffusely throughout the mediolateral extent of this column.[81, 85, 110]

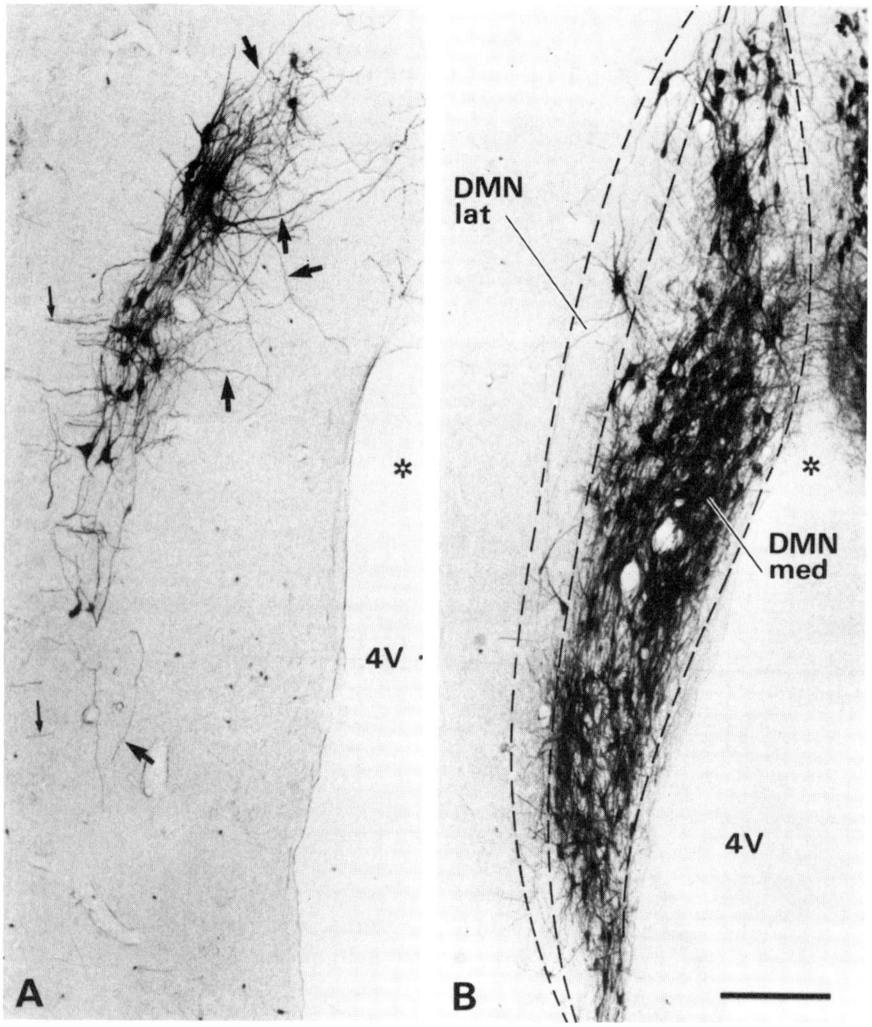

Figure 7–14. *A,* Light-field photomicrograph of a horizontal section through the DMN following injection of CT-HRP into the cecum of a rat. *B,* Light-field photomicrograph of a horizontal section through the DMN following injection of CT-HRP into the stomach of a rat. Dendrites (*filled arrows*) project medially and rostrocaudally within the DMN. Axons are marked by *thin arrows*. The *asterisk* marks the level of the obex which appears more rostrad in *A* owing to a small difference in depth of the section. Note that there is a distinct topography of the labeling of motoneurons in the DMN. The stomach is innervated by neurons of the medial column, and the cecum by neurons of the lateral column. Calibration bar = 250 μm. (From Altschuler SM, Ferenci DA, Lynn RB, et al: Representation of the cecum in lateral dorsal motor nucleus of the vagus nerve and commissural subnucleus of the nucleus tractus solitarii in rat. J Comp Neurol 1990; 304:261–274. Copyright © 1990 by Wiley-Liss. Reprinted by permission of Wiley-Liss, a division of John Wiley and Sons, Inc.)

The use of cholera toxin–horseradish peroxidase (CT-HRP) as a neural tracer has provided the first demonstration that DMN motoneurons have both extensive intranuclear and extranuclear dendritic arborizations.[59, 81, 83, 111] Within the confines of DMN, motoneurons located in both the medial and the lateral columns exhibit similar dendritic architectonics. Most of the dendrites of gastric and cecal motoneurons project primarily in a rostrocaudal direction within the confines of the medial and lateral columns, respectively[59, 81] (see Fig. 7–14). Additionally, at all rostrocaudal levels, a portion of each column's motoneuron dendritic arbors penetrates the adjacent column. The dendritic architecture of DMN motoneurons appears to provide for the coordination of efferent activity both throughout the rostrocaudal extent of the cell column and between columns.

The NTS is the major extranuclear site of termination of DMN motoneuron dendrites. The course of penetration and sites of termination within the NTS of these dendritic projections vary according to their column of origin. Dendrites of gastric and cecal motoneurons exit the DMN in trajectories that are essentially perpendicular to each other and terminate in areas of the NTS that overlap the central terminal field of their respective primary sensory neurons.[59] This anatomic arrangement of DMN motoneuron dendrites and sensory afferent terminals within the NTS would support and actually favor the organ-specific monosynaptic interactions between these anatomic structures. The existence of synaptic contacts between labeled sensory afferent terminals and motoneuron dendrites has been demonstrated at the ultrastructural level in the subnucleus gelatinosus (gastric afferent terminal field) of the NTS following injection of CT-HRP into the stomach or its application to the cervical vagus in the rat.[111] It is conceivable that most of the peripheral sensory afferent–dendritic contacts in the NTS occur on an organ-specific basis, as it has been demonstrated that the extranuclear dendrites of gastric and cecal motoneurons encircle or avoid the afferent terminal field of the other respective organ.[59] Additionally, gastric motoneuron dendrites also avoid and encircle the esophageal afferent terminal field in the subnucleus centralis of the NTS.[58]

Dorsal Vagal Complex

Nucleus Tractus Solitarii

The NTS is the first synaptic site for afferent projections from the peripheral structures conveyed through cranial nerves V, VII, IX, and X. The organization of afferent terminal fields within the NTS is broadly based on the sensory modality they subserve. The most obvious and first organizational scheme formulated for the NTS was its division into a rostral-lateral gustatory half and caudal-medial visceral half.[112] This scheme, which was based on the incubation of whole nerve branches with free HRP, has been fine-tuned by studies that have provided information on organ-specific representation within the NTS. The topographic representation of the alimentary tract within the NTS has been studied extensively by organ-specific injections of neuroanatomic tracers and is the focus of the discussion in this section.

Afferent information from the alimentary tract is conveyed to the NTS primarily through cranial nerves IX and X. The cell bodies of vagal and glossopharyngeal afferent nerve fibers are located within a fused ganglionic mass that is composed of the multiple ganglia of these nerves.[58] Within this fused ganglionic mass, sensory neurons that project to the soft palate and pharynx are located superiorly, and those that project to the esophagus, stomach, and small and large bowel are located inferiorly (Fig. 7–15), indicating the existence of a crude viscerotopic organization corresponding to rostrocaudal positioning along the alimentary tract.[58, 59]

In the rat, direct intramuscular injections of HRP conjugates into different areas of the alimentary tract result in afferent terminal labeling generally confined to the NTS.[58] The NTS is a complex nucleus made up of multiple subnuclei that have different cell morphology, packing density, intensity of Nissl's staining, neuropeptide content, and connectivity. Afferents from the gastrointestinal tract project primarily to the medial division of the NTS (area medial to the tractus solitarius) and terminate with a viscerotopic organization in distinct subnuclei. The NTS subnuclei associated with the ali-

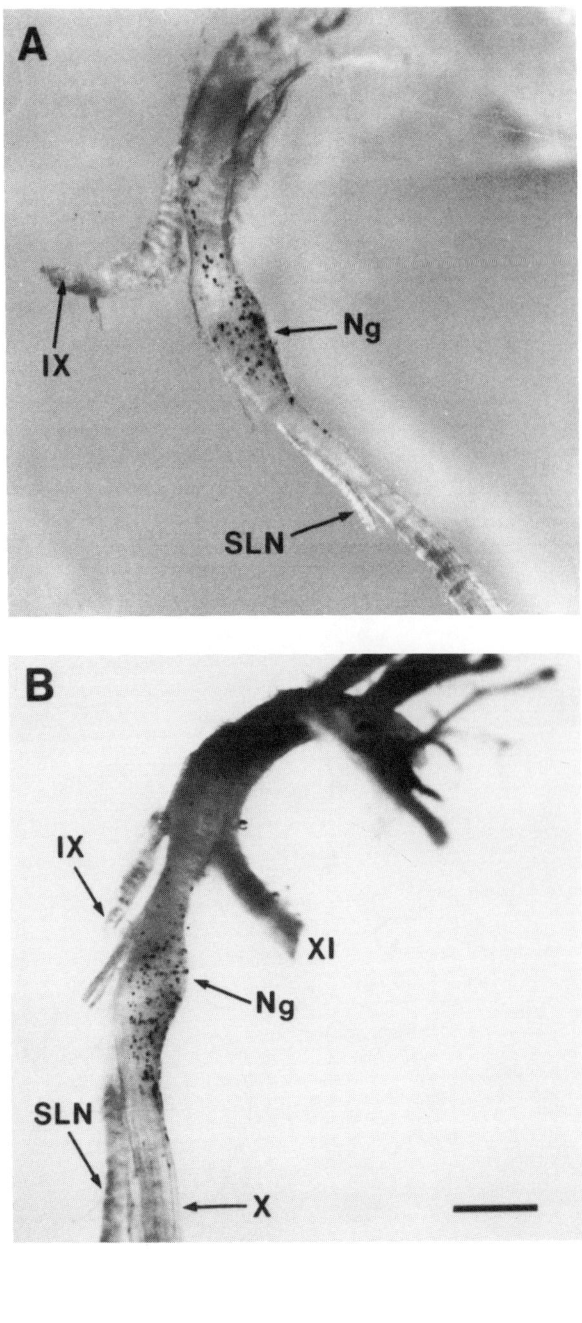

Figure 7–15. *A* and *B* are photomicrographs of neuronal labeling and nodose ganglion labeling following injection of tracer into the cecum and stomach of the rat, respectively. Calibration bar = 1 mm. Ng, Nodose ganglion; SLN, superior laryngeal nerve; IX, glossopharyngeal nerve; X, vagus nerve; XI, accessory nerve. (From Altschuler SM, Ferenci DA, Lynn RB, et al: Representation of the cecum in lateral dorsal motor nucleus of the vagus nerve and commissural subnucleus of the nucleus tractus solitarii in rat. J Comp Neurol 1990; 304:261–274. Copyright © 1990 by Wiley-Liss. Reprinted by permission of Wiley-Liss, a division of John Wiley and Sons, Inc.)

mentary tract (in the rat) include the gelatinosus, centralis, commissuralis, medialis, interstitialis, and intermedialis[58, 59] (Fig. 7–16).

When the distributions of alimentary tract afferents are reconstructed in the horizontal plane through the brain stem, the major organizational feature apparent is a rostrocaudal segregation of terminal fields that corresponds to rostrocaudal positioning along the alimentary tract.[58, 59, 81, 83] The soft palate is represented most rostrally in the NTS. Prominent labeling is present in the interstitial subnucleus, with less dense labeling extending medially into the intermediate and rostral medial subnuclei. A portion of palatal afferents terminate rostrally in the lateral division of the NTS (area lateral to the tractus solitarius), supporting the presence of gustatory receptors in this structure. The interstitial and intermediate subnuclei represent sites within the NTS where the terminal fields of the soft palate, pharynx, and larynx overlap. Within the interstitial and intermediate subnuclei, however, soft palate afferents are represented most rostrally, laryngeal afferents most caudally, and pharyngeal afferents intermediately to those of the soft palate and larynx. Afferents from the esophagus, stomach, and intestine terminate caudally and medially to palatal and pharyngeal afferents. The distribution of afferents from these structures demonstrates little overlap, in comparison with palatal and pharyngeal afferents. Esophageal afferents terminate entirely within the subnucleus centralis (Fig. 7–17), distributing throughout the entire rostrocaudal extent of this subnucleus. The terminal fields of the cervical, thoracic, and subdiaphragmatic esophagus show considerable overlap in their rostrocaudal distribution within the subnucleus. However, a crude topographic organization does appear to exist because injection of the cervical, thoracic, and subdiaphragmatic esophagus results, respectively, in the heaviest labeling within the rostral, middle, and caudal portions of the subnucleus centralis.

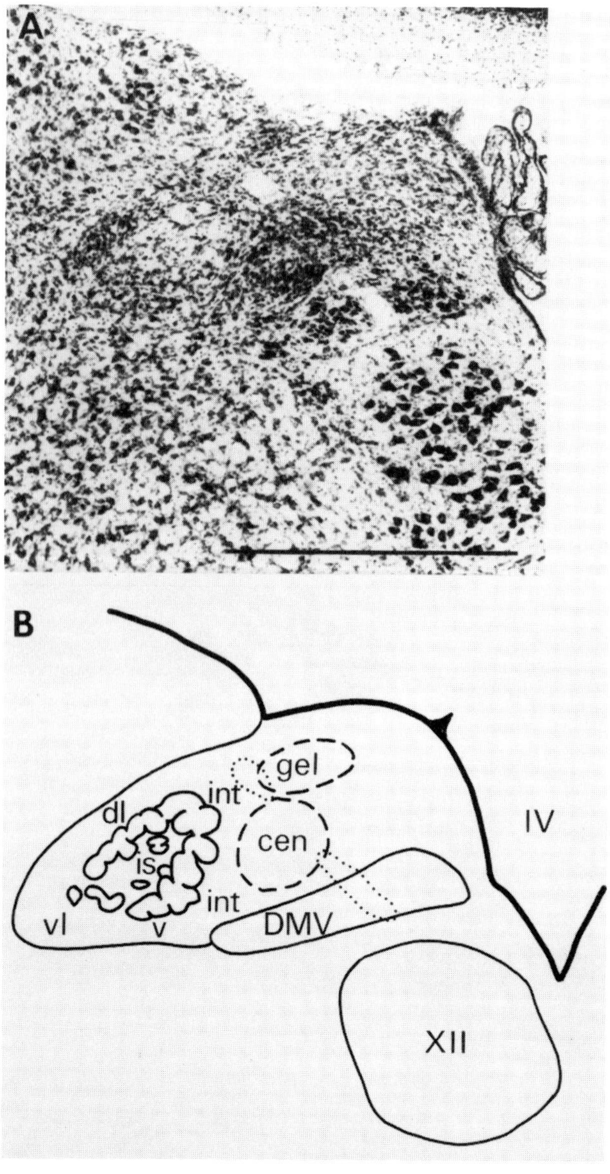

Figure 7–16. Subnuclei of the NTS in the rat that receive primary vagal afferents from the gastrointestinal tract. *A,* Photomicrograph of a transverse Nissl-stained section through the dorsal vagal complex of the rat at the level of the fourth ventricle. *B,* Schematic representation of the subnuclei of the NTS present in photomicrograph *A*. Calibration bar in *A* = 500 μm. Cen, subnucleus centralis; gel, subnucleus gelatinosus; is, subnucleus interstitialis; int, subnucleus intermedialis; dl, subnucleus dorsolateralis; vl, subnucleus ventralateralis; v, subnucleus ventralis; TS, tractus solitarius; DMV, dorsal motor nucleus of the vagus nerve; XII, hypoglossal nucleus; IV, fourth ventricle. (From Altschuler SM, Bao X, Bieger D, et al: Viscerotopic representation of the upper alimentary tract in the rat: Sensory ganglia and nuclei of the solitary and spinal trigeminal tracts. J Comp Neurol 1989; 283:248–268. Copyright © 1989 by Wiley-Liss. Reprinted by permission of Wiley-Liss, a division of John Wiley and Sons, Inc.)

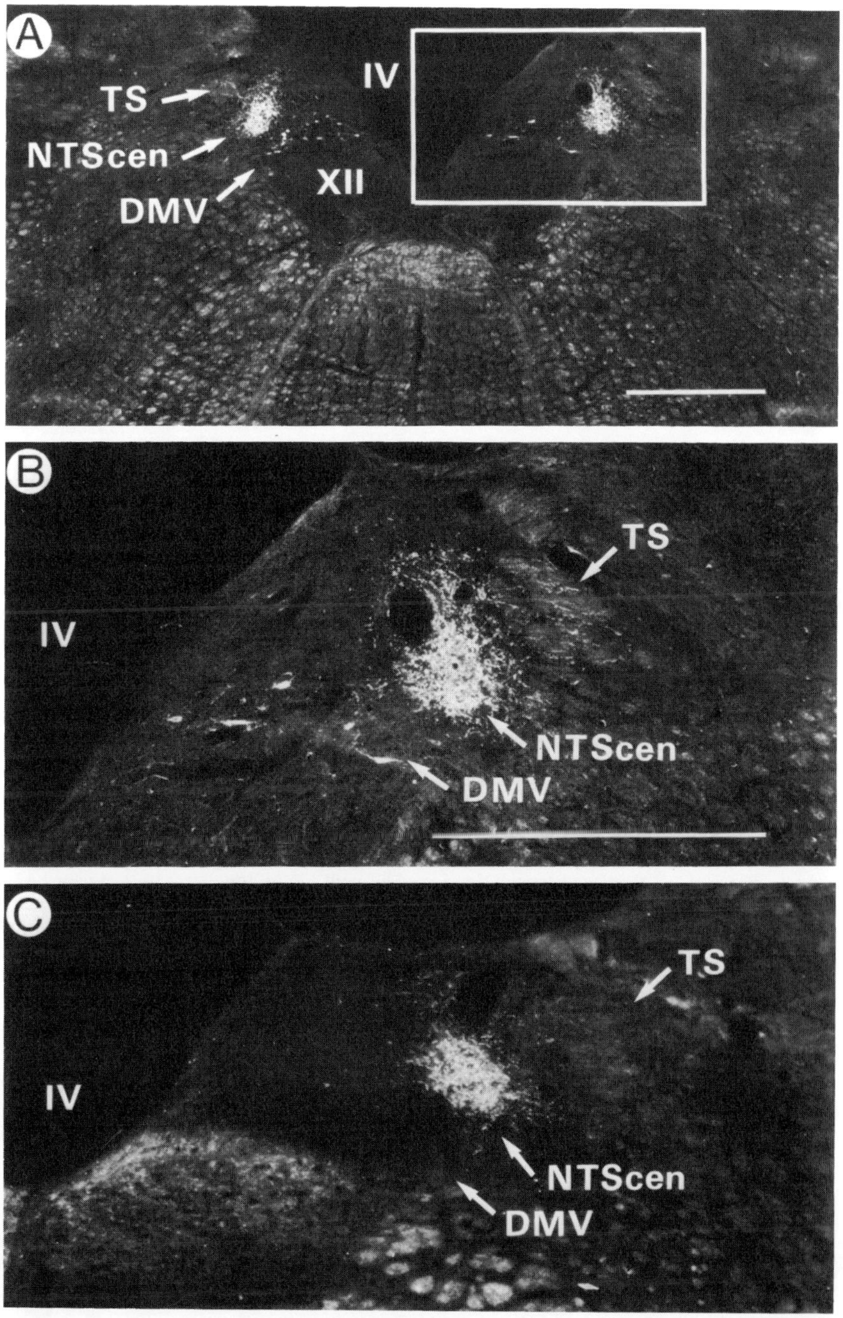

Figure 7–17. Dark-field photomicrographs of coronal sections through the dorsal vagal complex at low (*A*) and high power (*B* and *C*) following injection of tracer into esophagus of a rat. Vagal afferent terminal labeling is limited to the subnucleus centralis of the NTS (NTScen). Other subnuclei of the NTS and the DMV lack labeling (see Figure 7–16 for key to abbreviations). (From Altschuler SM, Bao X, Bieger D, et al: Viscerotopic representation of the upper alimentary tract in the rat: Sensory ganglia and nuclei of the solitary and spinal trigeminal tracts. J Comp Neurol 1989; 283:248–268. Copyright © 1989 by Wiley-Liss. Reprinted by permission of Wiley-Liss, a division of John Wiley and Sons, Inc.)

The densest concentration of gastric afferents within the NTS is found within the subnucleus gelatinosus, which is located dorsomedially to the subnucleus centralis. Gastric afferents also penetrate sites within the medial and commissural subnuclei, resulting in a more caudal distribution than that of esophageal afferents. Intestinal afferents project most prominently to the dorsolateral portion of the commissural subnucleus, with less prominent extensions rostrally into the periventricular portions of the NTS (an area dorsal and medial to the subnucleus gelatinosus) and caudally into the medial subnucleus and ventromedial portion of the commissural subnucleus.

SUMMARY

The highly organized viscerotopic representation of the gastrointestinal tract within the dorsal and ventral vagal complexes and the documented connections of these areas with higher levels of the CNS support the concept of a visceral neuraxis. The integration of different motor behaviors (e.g., swallowing or vomiting), extragastrointestinal reflexes, and visceral pain perception with gastrointestinal function may occur as a result of the precise circuitry inherent within a visceral neuraxis. Disruptions in this precise circuitry or its neurochemical regulatory mechanism may be etiologic to the development of disorders such as irritable bowel syndrome, bulimia, and recurrent abdominal pain of childhood.

ACKNOWLEDGMENTS

The author thanks Carolyn Trojan and Julie Giordano for assistance in the preparation of the manuscript.

REFERENCES

1. Thompson RF: Neuron. *In* The Brain: An Introduction to Neuroscience. New York, WH Freeman, 1985, pp 29–48.
2. Kandel ER, Schwartz JH, eds: Principles of Neural Science. 2nd ed. New York, Elsevier, 1985, pp 49–175.
3. Thompson RF: Membranes and potentials. *In* The Brain: An Introduction to Neuroscience. New York, WH Freeman, 1985, pp 49–76.
4. Thompson RF: Synaptic transmission. *In* The Brain: An Introduction to Neuroscience. New York, WH Freeman, 1985, pp 77–102.
5. Shepherd GM: Neurobiology. 2nd ed. New York, Oxford University Press, 1988, pp 65–176.
6. Wood JD: Physiology of the enteric nervous system. *In* Johnson LR, ed: Physiology of the Gastrointestinal Tract. 2nd ed. New York, Raven Press, 1987, pp 67–109.
7. North RA: Electrophysiology of enteric ganglia. Neuroscience 1982; 7:315–325.
8. Furness JB, Costa M: An overview of the enteric nervous system. *In* The Enteric Nervous System. London, Churchill Livingstone, 1987, pp 1–5.
9. Andrew A: The origin of intramural ganglia: IV. The origin of enteric ganglia: A critical review and discussion of the present state of the problem. J Anat 1971; 108:169–184.
10. Yntema CL, Hammond WS: The origin of intrinsic ganglia of trunk viscera from vagal neural crest in the chick embryo. J Comp Neurol 1954; 101:515–541.
11. Baetge G, Gershon MD: Transient catecholaminergic (TC) cells in the vagus nerves and bowels of fetal mice: Relationship to the development of enteric neurons. Dev Biol 1989; 132:189–211.
12. Baetge G, Schneider KA, Gershon MD: Development and persistence of catecholaminergic neurons in cultured explants of fetal murine vagus nerves and bowel. Development 1990; 110:689–701.
13. Baetge G, Pintar JE, Gershon MD: Transiently catecholaminergic (TC) cells in the bowel of fetal rats and mice: Precursors of non-catecholaminergic enteric neurons. Dev Biol 1990; 141:353–380.
14. Gershon MD, Thompson EB: The maturation of neuromuscular function in a multiple innervated structure: Development of the longitudinal muscle of the fetal mammalian gut and its cholinergic excitatory, adrenergic inhibitory and non-adrenergic inhibitory innervation. J Physiol (Lond) 1973; 234:257–277.
15. Rothman TP, Nilaver G, Gershon MD: Colonization of the developing murine enteric nervous system and subsequent phenotypic expression by the precursors of the peptidergic neurons. J Comp Neurol 1984; 225:13–23.
16. Furness JB, Costa M: Cytoarchitectonics of the enteric nervous system. *In* The Enteric Nervous System. London, Churchill Livingstone, 1987, pp 26–54.
17. Cook RD, Burnstock G: The ultrastructure of Auerbach's plexus in the guinea-pig: I. Neuronal elements. J Neurocytol 1976; 5:195–206.
18. Hodgkiss JP, Lees GM: Correlated electrophysiological and morphological characteristics of myenteric plexus neurons. J Physiol (Lond) 1978; 285:19P–20P.
19. Hodgkiss JP, Lees GM: Morphological studies of electrophysiologically identified myenteric plexus neurons of the guinea-pig ileum. Neuroscience 1983; 8:593–608.
20. Bornstein JC, Costa M, Furness JB, et al: Electrophysiology and enkephalin immunoreactivity of identified myenteric plexus neurons in the guinea-pig small intestine. J Physiol (Lond) 1984; 351:313–325.
21. Nishi S, North RA: Intracellular recording from the myenteric plexus of the guinea-pig ileum. J Physiol (Lond) 1973; 231:471–491.
22. Hirst GDS, Holman ME, Spence I: Two types of neurons in the myenteric plexus of duodenum in the guinea-pig. J Physiol (Lond) 1974; 236:303–326.
23. Wilson AJ, Furness JB, Costa M: The fine structure of the submucous plexus of the guinea-pig ileum: I. The ganglia, neurons, Schwann cells and neuropil. J Neurocytol 1981; 10:759–784.
24. Komuro T, Baluk P, Burnstock G: An ultrastructural study of neurons and non-neuronal cells in the myenteric plexus of the rabbit colon. Neuroscience 1982; 7:1797–1806.
25. Gabella G: Fine structure of the myenteric plexus in the guinea-pig ileum. J Anat 1972; 111:69–97.
26. Gabella G: Ultrastructure of the nerve plexuses of the mammalian intestine: The enteric glial cells. Neuroscience 1981; 6:425–436.
27. Furness JB, Costa M: Arrangement of the enteric plexuses. *In* The Enteric Nervous System. Edinburgh, Churchill Livingstone, 1987, pp 6–25.
28. Furness JB, Costa M: Types of nerves in the enteric nervous system. Neuroscience 1980; 5:1–20.
29. Christensen J, Rick JA, Robinson BA, et al: Arrangement of the myenteric plexus throughout the gastrointestinal tract of the opossum. Gastroenterology 1983; 85:890–899.
30. Christensen J, Rick GA: Nerve cell density in submucous plexus throughout the gut of cat and opossum. Gastroenterology 1985; 89:1064–1069.
31. Christensen J, Stiles MJ, Rick GA, et al: Comparative anatomy of the myenteric plexus of the distal colon in eight mammals. Gastroenterology 1984; 86:706–713.
32. Wilson AJ, Furness JB, Costa M: The fine structure of the submucous plexus of the guinea-pig ileum: II. Description and analysis of vesiculated nerve profiles. J Neurocytol 1981; 10:785–804.
33. Keast JR, Furness JB, Costa M: The origins of peptide and norepinephrine nerves in the mucosa of the guinea-pig small intestines. Gastroenterology 1984; 86:637–644.
34. Furness JB, Costa M: Projections of intestinal neurons showing immunoreactivity for vasoactive intestinal polypeptide are consistent with these neurons being enteric inhibitory neurons. Neurosci Lett 1979; 15:199–204.
35. Furness JB, Costa M: Neurons with 5-hydroxytryptamine–like immunoreactivity in the enteric nervous system: Their projections in the guinea-pig small intestines. Neuroscience 1982; 7:341–349.
36. Furness JB, Costa M, Gibbins IL, et al: Neurochemically similar myenteric and submucous neurons directly traced to the mucosa of small intestines. Cell Tissue Res 1985; 241:155–163.
37. Furness JB, Costa M, Miller RJ: Distribution and projections of nerves with enkephalin-like immunoreactivity in the guinea-pig small intestine. Neuroscience 1983; 8:653–664.
38. Ekblad E, Ekman R, Hakason R, et al: GRP neurones in the rat small intestine issue long anal projections. Regul Pept 1984; 9:279–287.
39. Ekblad E, Hankanson R, Sundler F: VIP and PHI coexist with an NPY-like peptide in intramural neurons of the small intestine. Regul Pept 1984; 10:47–55.
40. Holle GE, Forth W: Myoelectric activity of small intestine after chemical ablation of myenteric neurons. Am J Physiol 1990; 258:G519–G526.
41. Nagahama M, Ozaki T, Hama K: A study of myenteric plexus of the congenital aganglionosis rat (spotting lethal). J Anat Embryol 1985; 171:285–296.
42. Wood JD: Electrical activity of the intestines of mice with hereditary megacolon and absence of enteric ganglion cells. Dig Dis Sci 1973; 18:477–488.
43. Wood JD, Brann LR: Pharmacological analysis of rebound excitation in large intestine of piebald mouse for Hirschsprung's disease. Dig Dis Sci 1986; 31:744–752.
44. Wood JD, Brann LR, Vermillion DL: Electrical and contractile

behavior of large intestinal musculature of piebald mouse model for Hirschsprung's disease. Dig Dis Sci 1986; 31:638–650.
45. Cohen S: Motor disorders of the esophagus. N Engl J Med 1979; 301:184–192.
46. Schuffler MD, Jonah A: Chronic idiopathic intestinal pseudo-obstruction caused by degenerative disorder of the myenteric plexus: The use of Smith's method to define neuropathology. Gastroenterology 1982; 82:476–486.
47. Schuffler MD, Lowe MC, Bill A: Studies of idiopathic intestinal pseudo-obstruction: hereditary hollow visceral myopathy—clinical and pathological studies. Gastroenterology: 1977; 73:327–338.
48. Schuffler MD: Chronic intestinal pseudo-obstruction syndromes. Med Clin North Am 1981; 65:1331–1375.
49. Rohrman CA, Ricci MT, Krishnamurthy S, et al: Radiological and histological differentiation of neuromuscular disorders of the gastrointestinal tract: Visceral myopathies, visceral neuropathies, and progressive systemic sclerosis. Am J Roentgenol 1984; 143:933–941.
50. Mei N: Vagal glucoreceptors in the small intestine of the cat. J Physiol 1978; 282:485–506.
51. Ewart WE, Wingate DL: Central representation and opioid modulation of gastric mechanoreceptor activity in the rat. Am J Physiol 1983; 244:G27–G32.
52. Appia F, Ewart WR, Pittam BS, et al: Convergence of sensory information from abdominal viscera in the rat brain stem. Am J Physiol 1986; 251:G169–G175.
53. Andrews PLR, Grundy D, Scrathcherd T: Vagal afferent discharge from mechanoreceptors in different regions of the ferret stomach. J Physiol 1980; 298:513–524.
54. Davison JS: Response of single vagal afferent fibers to mechanical and chemical stimulation of the gastric and duodenal mucosa in cats. J Exp Physiol (Lond) 1972; 57:405–416.
55. El Ouazzani T, Mei N: Electrophysiologic properties and role of the vagal thermoreceptors of lower esophagus and stomach of cat. Gastroenterology 1982; 83:995–1001.
56. Christensen J: Origin of sensation in the esophagus. Am J Physiol 1984; 246:G221–G225.
57. Clerc N, Mei N: Vagal mechanoreceptors located in the lower oesophageal sphincter of the cat. J Physiol 1983; 336:487–498.
58. Altschuler SM, Bao X, Bieger D, et al: Viscerotopic representation of the upper alimentary tract in the rat: Sensory ganglia and nuclei of the solitary and spinal trigeminal tracts. J Comp Neurol 1989; 283:248–268.
59. Altschuler SM, Ferenci DA, Lynn RB, et al: Representation of the cecum in lateral dorsal motor nucleus of the vagus nerve and commissural subnucleus of the nucleus tractus solitarii in rat. J Comp Neurol 1990; 304:261–274.
60. Barber WD, Burks TF: Brain stem response to phasic gastric distension. Am J Physiol 1983; 245:G242–G248.
61. Leek BF: Abdominal and pelvic visceral receptors. Br Med Bull 1977; 2:163–168.
62. Furness JB, Costa M: Sympathetic influences on gastrointestinal function. *In* The Enteric Nervous System. Edinburgh, Churchill Livingstone, 1987, pp 207–238.
63. Kirshgessner AL, Gershon MD: Identification of vagal efferent fibers and putative target neurons in the enteric nervous system of the rat. J Comp Neurol 1989; 285:38–53.
64. Berthoud H-R, Jedrzejewska A, Powley TL: Simultaneous labeling of vagal innervation of the gut and afferent projection from the visceral forebrain with DiI injected into the dorsal vagal complex in the rat. J Comp Neurol 1990; 301:65–69.
65. Beckstead RM, Norgren R: An autoradiographic examination of the central distribution of the trigeminal, facial, glossopharyngeal, and vagal nerves in the monkey. J Comp Neurol 1979; 184:455–472.
66. Kalia M, Mesulam M-M: Brain stem projections of sensory and motor components of the vagus complex in the cat: The cervical vagus and nodose ganglion. J Comp Neurol 1980; 193:435–465.
67. Kalia M, Mesulam M-M: Brain stem projections of sensory and motor components of the vagus complex in the cat: II. Laryngeal, tracheobronchial, pulmonary, cardiac, and gastrointestinal branches. J Comp Neurol 1980; 193:467–508.
68. Kalia M: Brain stem localization of vagal preganglionic neurons. J Auton Nerv Syst 1981; 3:451–481.
69. Dennison SJ, Merritt VE, Aprison MH, et al: Redefinition of the location of the dorsal (motor) nucleus of the vagus in the rat. Brain Res Bull 1981; 6:77–81.
70. Dennison SJ, O'Connor BL, Aprison MH, et al: Viscerotopic localization of preganglionic parasympathetic cell bodies of origin of the anterior and posterior subdiaphragmatic vagus nerves. J Comp Neurol 1981; 197:259–269.
71. Kalia M, Sullivan JM: Brain stem projections of sensory and motor components of the vagus nerve in the rat. J Comp Neurol 1982; 211:248–264.
72. Contreras RJ, Beckstead RM, Norgren R: The central projections of the trigeminal, facial, glossopharyngeal and vagus nerves: An autoradiographic study in the rat. J Auton Nerv Syst 1982; 6:303–322.
73. Scharoun SL, Barone FC, Wayner MJ, et al: Vagal and gastric connections to the central nervous system determined by the transport of horseradish peroxidase. Brain Res Bull 1984; 13:573–583.
74. Hinrichsen CFL, Ryan AT: Localization of laryngeal motoneurons in the rat: Morphological evidence for dual innervation. Exp Neurol 1981; 74:341–355.
75. Yoshida Y, Miyazaki T, Hirano M, et al: Localization of efferent neurons innervating the pharyngeal constrictor muscles and the cervical esophagus muscle in the cat by means of the horseradish peroxidase method. Neurosci Lett 1981; 22:91–95.
76. Rogers RC, Hermann GE: Central connections of the hepatic branch of the vagus nerve: A horseradish peroxidase histochemical study. J Auton Nerv Syst 1983; 7:165–174.
77. Holstege G, Graveland G, Bijker-Biemond C, et al: Location of motoneurons innervating soft palate, pharynx and upper esophagus: Anatomical evidence for a possible swallowing center in the pontine reticular formation. Brain Behav Evol 1983; 23:47–62.
78. Fryscak R, Zenker W, Kantner D: Afferent and efferent innervation of the rat esophagus: A tracing study with horseradish peroxidase and nuclear yellow. Anat Embryol 1984; 170:63–70.
79. Gwyn DG, Leslie RA, Hopkins DA: Gastric afferents to the nucleus of the solitary tract in the cat. Neurosci Lett 1979; 14:13–17.
80. Katz DM, Karten HJ: Visceral representation within the nucleus of the tractus solitarius in the pigeon, *Columba livia*. J Comp Neurol 1983; 218:42–73.
81. Shapiro RE, Miselis RR: The central organization of the vagus nerve innervating the stomach of the rat. J Comp Neurol 1985; 238:473–488.
82. Bieger D, Hopkins DA: Viscerotopic representation of the upper alimentary tract in the medulla oblongata in the rat: The nucleus ambiguus. J Comp Neurol 1987; 262:546–562.
83. Rinaman L, Miselis RR: The organization of vagal innervation of rat pancreas using cholera toxin–horseradish peroxidase conjugate. J Auton Nerv Syst 1987; 21:109–125.
84. Altschuler SM, Bao X, Miselis RR: Dendritic architecture of nucleus ambiguus motoneurons projecting to the upper alimentary tract in the rat. J Comp Neurol 1991; 309:402–414.
85. Okumura T, Namiki M: Vagal motor neurons innervating the stomach are site-specifically organized in the dorsal motor nucleus of the vagus nerve in rats. J Auton Nerv Syst 1990; 29:157–162.
86. Cruz Orive L-M: On the estimation of particle number. J Microsc 1980; 120:15–27.
87. Lawn AM: The localization, in the nucleus ambiguus of the rabbit, of the cells of origin of motor fibers in the glossopharyngeal nerve and various branches of the vagus nerve by means of retrograde degeneration. J Comp Neurol 1966; 127:293–306.
88. Lawn AM: The nucleus ambiguus of the rabbit. J Comp Neurol 1966; 127:307–320.
89. Nomura S, Mizuno N: Central distribution of efferent and afferent components of the cervical branches of the vagus nerve. Anat Embryol 1983; 166:1–18.
90. Hudson LC, Cummings JF: The origins of innervation of the esophagus of the dog. Brain Res 1985; 326:125–136.
91. Kriebel ME, Bennett MV, Waxman SG, et al: Oculomotor neurons in fish: Electrotonic coupling and multiple sites of impulse initiation. Science 1969; 166:520–524.

92. Scheibel ME, Scheibel AB: Organization of spinal motoneuron dendrites in bundles. Exp Neurol 1970; 28:106–112.
93. Scheibel ME, Scheibel AB: Developmental relationship between spinal motoneuron dendrite bundles and patterned activity in the hind limb of cats. Exp Neurol 1970; 29:328–335.
94. Scheibel ME, Scheibel AB: Developmental relationship between spinal motoneuron dendrite bundles and patterned activity in the forelimb of cats. Exp Neurol 1971; 30:367–373.
95. Scheibel ME, Scheibel AB: Dendrite bundles as sites for central programs: An hypothesis. Int J Neurosci 1973; 6:195–202.
96. Roney KJ, Scheibel AB, Shaw GL: Dendritic bundles: survey of anatomical experiments and physiological theories. Brain Res Rev 1979; 1:225–271.
97. Schoenen J: Dendritic organization of the human spinal cord: The motoneurons. J Comp Neurol 1982; 211:226–247.
98. Miller AJ: Deglutition. Physiol Rev 1982; 62:129–184.
99. Miller AJ: Neurophysiological basis of swallowing. Dysphagia 1986; 1:91–100.
100. Arnold GE: Physiology and pathology of the cricothyroid muscle. Laryngoscope 1961; 71:687–752.
101. Bosma JF, Fletcher S: The upper pharynx: A review: II. Physiology. Ann Otol Rhinol Laryngol 1962; 71:134–157.
102. Bieger D: Muscarinic activation of rhombencephalic neurones controlling oesophageal peristalsis in the rat. Neuropharmacology 1984; 23:1451–1464.
103. Stuesse SL, Fish SE: Projections to the cardioinhibitory region of the nucleus ambiguus of rat. J Comp Neurol 1984; 229:271–278.
104. Ross CA, Ruggiero DA, Reis DJ: Projections from the nucleus tractus solitarii to the rostral ventrolateral medulla. J Comp Neurol 1985; 242:511–534.
105. Cunningham ET, Sawchenko PE: A circumscribed projection from the nucleus of the solitary tract to the nucleus ambiguus in the rat: Anatomical evidence for somatostatin-28–immunoreactive interneurons subserving reflex control of esophageal motility. J Neurosci 1989; 9:1668–1682.
106. Cunningham ET, Sawchenko PE: Central neural control of esophageal motility: A review. Dysphagia 1990; 5:35–51.
107. Connors NA, Sullivan JM, Kubb KS: An autoradiographic study of the distribution of fibers from the dorsal motor nucleus of the vagus to the digestive tube of the rat. Acta Anat 1983; 115:266–271.
108. Fox EA, Powley TL: Longitudinal columnar organization within the dorsal motor nucleus represents separate branches of the abdominal vagus. Brain Res 1985; 341:269–282.
109. Norgren R, Smith GP: Central distribution of subdiaphragmatic vagal branches in the rat. J Comp Neurol 1988; 273:207–223.
110. Pagani FD, Norman WP, Gillis RA: Medullary parasympathetic projections innervate specific sites in the feline stomach. Gastroenterology 1988; 95:277–288.
111. Rinaman L, Card JP, Schwaber JS, et al: Ultrastructural demonstration of a gastric monosynaptic vagal circuit in the nucleus of the solitary tract in rat. J Neurosci 1989; 9:1985–1996.
112. Hamilton RB, Norgren R: Central projections of gustatory nerves in the rat. J Comp Neurol 1984; 222:560–577.

Chapter 8

Gastrointestinal Hormones

THOMAS E. ADRIAN

REGULATORY PEPTIDES OF THE GUT

Enteric hormonal peptides play a key role in the control of gastrointestinal functions. The alimentary tract also has an extensive intrinsic nervous system in which several regulatory peptides, such as vasoactive intestinal polypeptide (VIP), substance P, bombesin, and enkephalins, function as neurotransmitters or neuromodulators. Together with central connections via the vagus and splanchnic nerves, this integrated neuronal and hormonal system controls the functions of digestion and absorption of ingested nutrients and also influences subsequent metabolism. In addition, some of the gastrointestinal hormones together with other peptides, such as epidermal growth factor and spasmolytic polypeptide, appear to play a role in maintaining the growth and integrity of the gastrointestinal mucosa. These growth factors appear to be involved in the repair of tissue damage as well as in normal growth. Although we have some insight into the role played by hormones and growth factors in the structural and functional development of the alimentary tract, our understanding of the developmental role played by the enteric nervous system is limited.

Chemistry of the Gut Regulatory Peptide Families

The gastrointestinal hormones and several neuropeptides appear to have evolved from common ancestors by the process of gene duplication. This evolutionary process is still continuing today, as is evidenced by the cosecretion of similar peptides derived from the same gene. Examples of this are glucagon and the glucagon-related peptides I and II,[1] substance P with the related tachykinin called *neurokinin A*,[2] neurotensin with neuromedin N,[3] VIP with the related peptide histidine methionine (PHM),[4] and several peptides with opiate-like activity from the enkephalin precursor.[5]

Most of the gastrointestinal hormones fit into three major families, whereas other links are more tenuous. The three families are (1) the gastrin/cholecystokinin (CCK) family; (2) the secretin/glucose-dependent insulinotrophic peptide (GIP)/glucagon/enteroglucagon family, which also has neural (VIP and PHM) and pituitary (growth hormone-releasing hormone) relatives; and (3) the pancreatic polypeptide (PP)/peptide YY (PYY) family, which has neuropeptide Y (NPY) as its neural cousin.[6] Other relationships appear more distant; for example, there is some sequence homology between motilin and gastrin, somatostatin and secretin, and also neurotensin and PYY. The metabolic hormone insulin is structurally and functionally related to the insulin-like growth factors I and II.[7] The other beta-cell–derived peptide, known as *islet amyloid polypeptide* or *amylin*, closely resembles another neuropeptide called *calcitonin gene-related peptide* (CGRP).[8, 9] Several of the gastrointestinal hormones exist in multiple molecular forms, with differences either in length or in side-chain modification, such as sulfation. Most have a C-terminal amide group which renders them resistant to carboxypeptidase activity. The structures of the individual peptides will be considered in turn.

Gastrin exists in several molecular forms, but most important are a 17–amino acid and a 34–amino acid peptide, the smaller peptide being identical in sequence to the carboxy-terminal end of the latter peptide.[10, 11] The small peptide, little gastrin, is the predominant form secreted after a meal, whereas big gastrin predominates in the basal state. Little gastrin has a potency similar to big gastrin, but its half-life in the circulation is shorter.[12] The gastrins all have a single tyrosine located six residues from the C-terminus that is sulfated in about half of the gastrin molecules in each individual person.[13] Tyrosine sulfation has no effect on the biologic activity of gastrin, however. Indeed, biologic activity resides in the C-terminal end, the minimal fragment for full activity being the tetrapeptide. Pentagastrin, used extensively for acid secretory studies, is a stabilized analogue of this active portion of the gastrin molecule.[14]

CCK, like gastrin, exists in several molecular forms. In the case of CCK, however, all forms are sulfated, and this modification is necessary for biologic activity.[15] The first forms to be isolated were a 33– and a 39–amino acid peptide, but it is now apparent that larger forms, with 83 and 58 amino acids, predominate in the circulation.[16–18] The biologic activity of all forms resides in the common, amidated, C-terminal end of the molecule.[15] The C-terminal octapeptide (CCK–8), which is the minimal fragment with full biologic activity, occurs abundantly in the central and peripheral nerves.[19] The last five amino acids in this C-terminal end of CCK are shared with the gastrins. This property, which leads to pharmacologic overlap in the actions of these peptides, created a substantial hurdle in obtaining specific antibodies for radioimmunoassay, although this problem has recently been circumvented.

Secretin is a 27–amino acid peptide with a C-terminal amide group, and only this single molecular form has been reported.[20] In contrast to gastrin or CCK, the entire secretin molecule appears to be important for biologic activity.[21] Secretin shares considerable sequence homology with the hormones glucagon and GIP, as well as with several neuropeptides, as mentioned earlier.

GIP is a 42–amino acid member of the secretin family.[22, 23] Several authors have noted the presence of a larger molecular form of GIP in the small intestine and the plasma, but the relative biologic activity of big GIP to the 42–amino acid form has not been reported.[24, 25] Small amounts of a truncated form of the peptide (GIP 3-42) have been purified from the small intestine, but this form has a greatly reduced biologic activity, suggesting that the N-terminal portion of GIP is important in this regard.[23]

Motilin is a straight, 22–amino acid peptide that has minor sequence homology with gastrin but no similarity to other peptides.[26] A large molecular form of motilin is also found in the circulation in humans.[27] Unlike the case with most other gut hormones, the N-terminal region of motilin is important for biologic activity.

Neurotensin is a 13–amino acid, straight-chain peptide that has minor sequence homology with PYY.[28] Circulating levels of whole neurotensin are low, but the N-terminal fragments neurotensin 1–8 and neurotensin 1–11, which are not biologically active, are found in higher concentrations.[29, 30] This may lead to problems in determining physiologic levels of intact neurotensin if N-terminally directed antisera are used to measure the peptide.

Enteroglucagon is a term used to describe glucagon-like immunoreactivity of gut origin. It has been known for many years that glucagon-like peptides are produced by the gut, but that the material differs in its chemical structure as well as in its biologic activity and mechanism of release.[31, 32] Now that the sequence of preproglucagon has been derived from the gene sequence, it is clear that the same gene is transcribed in both the gut and the pancreas. The post-translational processing of the glucagon precursor differs in these sites, however, giving rise to quite separate products.[33, 34] The glucagon gene encodes for three similar sequences, glucagon and the glucagon-like peptides I and II (GLP I and II). The glucagon molecule itself is flanked by both C-terminal and N-terminal peptides. In the pancreas, the glucagon sequence is cleaved from these flanking peptides, whereas GLP I and II are secreted uncleaved as a single peptide.[33] In contrast, two peptides containing the glucagon sequence are produced in the gut: the major one (glicentin) is extended by both flanking peptides, and the minor one (oxyntomodulin) is extended only in the C-terminal end.[34] The GLPs are cleaved and secreted separately in the gut (GLP I 7-36 amide and GLP II). The antibodies that are used to measure "enteroglucagon" are really N-terminally directed glucagon antibodies that cross-react with enteroglucagon (glicentin and oxyntomodulin). Glucagon levels, measured using specific C-terminally directed antisera, are subtracted from those measured using the nonspecific antibody, leaving a derived enteroglucagon concentration.

Both PYY and PP are 36–amino acid, tyrosine-rich, straight-chain polypeptides that are amidated at the C-terminal end.[35, 36] It has become clear that at least two receptor subtypes exist for PYY and NPY.[37] Structure-activity studies suggest that both ends of these peptides are involved in binding and activity at one receptor subtype, whereas C-terminal fragments are sufficient to bind to the other.

Somatostatin (derived from somatotropin release-inhibiting factor, or SRIF) exists in two molecular forms: a 14–amino acid cyclic peptide (SRIF-14) and a 28–amino acid peptide that has the SRIF-14 sequence at its C-terminus.[38, 39] Biologic activity resides within the ring, and a potent, long-acting analogue is available for clinical use.[40]

A new islet hormone was recently purified from the amyloid that is found in the pancreas of some adult-onset diabetic patients.[8, 9] This peptide, which has been named *islet amyloid polypeptide*, or *amylin*, shares considerable sequence homology with CGRP.[8]

LOCALIZATION OF GASTROINTESTINAL HORMONES

There are 10 enteric peptides that act on the alimentary tract via the circulation. These are listed in Table 8–1, together with their site of secretion and major actions. The endocrine cells that synthesize these peptides, with the exception of those that produce somatostatin, are of the open type, with luminal processes that presumably respond to nutrients and other factors such as pH within the lumen to stimulate their secretion. Gastrin is produced mainly in the gastric antrum, but some is also secreted from the duodenum.[41] Somatostatin is found in endocrine cells of the gastric fundus and antrum, in the islets of Langerhans of the pancreas, and throughout the intestinal tract.[42] Although evidence suggests that somatostatin has some actions through the blood stream, the cells that produce this peptide have processes to other endocrine and exocrine cells, which suggests a paracrine action.[42] Somatostatin is also an abundant neuropeptide of the central and peripheral nervous system and is well represented throughout the enteric nerves of the myenteric and submucous plexuses.[42] The upper small intestine contains the endocrine cells that secrete CCK, secretin, GIP, and motilin.[41] Neurotensin cells are confined to the distal ileum.[43] Enteroglucagon and PYY are colocalized and are pro-

Table 8–1. CIRCULATING GASTROINTESTINAL HORMONES

Hormone	Localization	Major Physiologic Actions
Gastrin	Gastric antrum	Stimulates gastric acid secretion
Cholecystokinin	Duodenum	Stimulates pancreatic enzymes, contracts gallbladder
Secretin	Duodenum	Stimulates pancreatic bicarbonate and hepatic bile
Pancreatic polypeptide	Pancreas	Inhibits exocrine pancreas, relaxes gallbladder
Glucose-dependent insulinotropic peptide	Upper small intestine	Potentiates glucose-stimulated release of insulin from pancreas
Motilin	Upper small intestine	Triggers migrating motor complexes, speeds gastric emptying
Neurotensin	Distal ileum	Stimulates pancreatic secretion, inhibits gastric function
Enteroglucagon	Ileum and colon	Stimulates mucosal growth, inhibits gastric function
Peptide YY	Ileum and colon	Inhibits gastric acid, slows gastric emptying and intestinal transit
Somatostatin*	Stomach, pancreas, small and large bowel	Inhibits release of all of the above hormones, inhibits secretions and motor effects

*May act locally (i.e., paracrine peptide); also is found in nerves.

duced by the same cell type, albeit from different genes.[44] Enteroglucagon concentrations are highest in the distal ileum and decrease aborally through the colon. In contrast, although PYY is found in the ileum, it is more abundant in the colon.[45] Concentrations increase distally, and the highest levels are found in the sigmoid colon and rectum.[45] PP acts as a gut hormone, although it is localized along with the metabolic hormones insulin, glucagon, and amylin in the pancreatic islets.[8, 46]

PHYSIOLOGIC FUNCTIONS OF GASTROINTESTINAL HORMONES

Gastrin

Gastrin is a hormone that, together with acetylcholine from cholinergic fibers of the vagus nerves and local histamine, stimulates gastric acid secretion.[47] Gastrin is released from the gastric antrum and proximal duodenum into the blood stream by the presence of food in the stomach, partly by distention, and also by the presence of partially digested protein.[48] Gastrin secretion is inhibited by a low pH in the gastric antrum.[48] This inhibition functions as a negative feedback mechanism that prevents overstimulation of the acid-secreting parietal cells in the gastric fundus. Thus, hypergastrinemia invariably accompanies conditions associated with achlorhydria. In addition to being an acid secretagogue, gastrin also exhibits a potent trophic effect on the gastric mucosa, an action that is probably of profound importance in the newborn infant.[49] The trophic effects of gastrin appear initially to involve hyperplasia of an endocrine cell type called the *enterochromaffin-like* (ECL) *cells*, which produce histamine in the fundic mucosa.[50] The ECL cells are then involved in mediating the fundic growth response. Drugs that cause a profound inhibition of gastric acid secretion, such as omeprazole or irreversible histamine H_2 blockers, inhibit the negative feedback elicited by low pH and cause hypergastrinemia.[50] The resulting high concentrations of gastrin stimulate ECL cell hyperplasia, which, in experimental animals, can lead to the development of gastric carcinoid tumors.[50] Tumors are not seen following short-term use of such drugs. It is tempting to speculate that the sequence of events that occurs with these drugs mirrors the situation in the early neonate, in whom inhibition of acid secretion allows the high concentration of gastrin in the circulation to exert its trophic effect.

Secretin

Secretin is a hormonal peptide, localized to the duodenal mucosa, that stimulates pancreatic and hepatic bicarbonate secretion.[21] Secretin is released when acid chyme passes through the pylorus into the duodenal bulb.[51] The ensuing bicarbonate secretion rapidly neutralizes the pH of the duodenum. This affords protection to the duodenal mucosa and provides a neutral environment for the activity of pancreatic enzymes.[51]

Cholecystokinin

CCK is responsible for postprandial pancreatic enzyme secretion and gallbladder contraction.[52, 53] Localized to the duodenum and upper jejunum, CCK is released by the presence of fat and protein in the small bowel.[53] In addition to its secretory effects, CCK stimulates hyperplasia and hypertrophy of the pancreas.[54]

Motilin

Motilin has powerful motor actions on the gastrointestinal tract. In particular, motilin stimulates formation of the interdigestive myoelectric complexes, or so-called housekeeping waves of motor activity, that move down the intestine in the interprandial period and sweep it clear of debris and undigested foodstuff.[55] Motilin also accelerates gastric emptying and increases colonic motility.[56] The physiologic importance of these motor effects induced by motilin remains uncertain, however. Macrolides, such as erythromycin, are agonists for the motilin receptor.[57] This explains the motor effects of these drugs, which have recently been used clinically in a variety of motility disorders.

Glucose-Dependent Insulinotropic Peptide

GIP is a peptide hormone that was originally called *gastric inhibitory peptide*; however, it soon became apparent that gastric inhibition was a pharmacologic rather than a physiologic action of this peptide.[22, 23] It is known that GIP releases insulin from the pancreas, although to accomplish this it requires a small elevation of blood glucose concentrations (approximately 1 mmol/L), such as that seen after the ingestion of food.[58, 59] Hence, the peptide was renamed *glucose-dependent insulinotropic peptide,* but the acronym GIP was retained. It has been known for many years that glucose ingestion causes a far greater release of insulin than does the same amount of glucose administered intravenously. Clearly, a signal from the gut (known as the *enteroinsular axis*) potentiates the effect of glucose on the beta-cell, and the name *incretin* was coined for this indirect signal. Although the enteroinsular axis appears to be complex, involving both neural and humoral factors, GIP is perhaps the most likely candidate to fulfill the role of the hormonal component. Recent studies, however, suggest that the C-terminal portion of the GLP I (GLP I 7-37 amide), which is released along with enteroglucagon in the gut, may also play an important role in this incretin effect.[60]

Pancreatic Polypeptide

Although PP is localized to the islets of Langerhans of the pancreas, along with the metabolic hormones insulin and glucagon, this peptide acts as a gastrointestinal hormone.[46] Its actions include inhibition of pancreatic enzyme secretion and relaxation of the gallbladder in the postprandial period.[61] Circulating PP levels remain high for many hours postprandially.[46] Because the PP concentration remains high long after concentrations of other hormones, such as CCK, have returned to the basal level, it has been suggested that PP may play a role in conserving bile and pancreatic enzymes in readiness for ingestion of the next meal.

Neurotensin

The endocrine cells that secrete neurotensin are localized to the terminal ileum, and the release of neurotensin is effected whenever nutrients reach the distal portion of the small bowel.[62] Thus, in normal humans, excursions of neurotensin from the basal level after food ingestion are small.[62] Neurotensin release is greater whenever unabsorbed nutrients pass through the distal small intestine. High neurotensin concentrations are seen in malabsorption states, such as celiac disease, and in patients with postgastrectomy symptoms of dumping. The actions of neurotensin include the inhibition of gastric acid secretion and the slowing of the rate of gastric emptying.[63] Neurotensin also potentiates the effect of secretin in stimulating pancreatic bicarbonate secretion.[64]

Enteroglucagon

Enteroglucagon is released by carbohydrate and fat in the intestine, whereas these nutrients inhibit the release of glucagon from the pancreas.[65] Although enteroglucagon has not been purified in sufficient quantities to undertake full physiologic studies, a mass of circumstantial evidence points to a trophic role for this peptide.[66] Enteroglucagon levels are increased, like those of neurotensin, in any situation associated with malabsorption, such as celiac disease or after small bowel resection. Enteroglucagon concentrations correlate remarkably with crypt cell hyperplasia in these conditions. A patient with an endocrine tumor that produced enteroglucagon had marked villus hypertrophy in the small bowel.[67] In addition, partially purified enteroglucagon stimulates deoxyribonucleic acid (DNA) synthesis in vitro. Enteroglucagon could therefore be considered to be the growth hormone of the intestinal mucosa. It should be emphasized, however, that the evidence linking enteroglucagon with mucosal growth is rather circumstantial.

Peptide YY

PYY is a recently discovered hormone that is localized to the distal ileum and colon in humans.[45] Concentrations of PYY increase following the ingestion of food, and the magnitude of the response reflects the size of the meal ingested.[45] PYY infusions in humans, at doses that are within the physiologic range, have revealed potent inhibitory effects on gastric secretion and emptying and also a marked delay in small bowel transit.[68, 69] These effects appear to be mediated by the inhibition of presynaptic cholinergic transmission. PYY enhances net fluid absorption in the small intestine by the inhibition of crypt cell cyclic adenosine monophosphate–mediated chloride secretion.[70] At higher concentrations, PYY infusion in animals inhibits pancreatic secretion, but this effect is not seen at physiologic levels in humans.[68]

Islet Amyloid Polypetide (Amylin)

Amylin is produced in the beta-islet cells of the pancreas and is cosecreted with insulin.[8, 9] The physiologic role for this hormone is not yet established, but it has been implicated as being involved in the development of diabetes. Amylin inhibits the secretion of insulin and thus impairs glucose tolerance. Amylin also impairs the uptake of glucose and glycogen synthesis, and it can cause profound insulin resistance in peripheral tissues.[8, 9] These effects are of considerable interest; however, they do not seem to be produced in humans at the levels of amylin found in the circulation. Evidence is thus accumulating against a major role for amylin in the pathophysiology of diabetes.[8, 9]

FETAL DEVELOPMENT OF GASTROINTESTINAL HORMONES

Appearance of Gastrointestinal Hormones

Cells that secrete gastrin, somatostatin, motilin, and GIP are detectable at 8 weeks of gestation, gastrin and somatostatin cells being most numerous.[71] In tissue extracts, these hormones and neuropeptides such as VIP are readily detectable by radioimmunoassay at this time.[72] By 14 weeks of gestation, all of the endocrine cell types are present in the intestinal mucosa, although the anatomic distribution is somewhat different from that seen in the adult.[71] For example, gastrin cells are found in the ileum, neurotensin cells in the duodenum, PP cells in the colon, and PYY cells in the pancreas early in the second trimester.[71, 73] By the end of the second trimester, however, the cellular distribution resembles that of the adult. Peptidergic nerves are first demonstrable in the myenteric plexus at about 12 weeks of gestation, correlating with the known developmental pattern of enteric nerve plexuses.[71] After 3 months, the enteric nerves migrate through to the submucous plexus. By the third trimester, all of the regulatory peptide systems appear well developed, although the tissue content of some, notably gastrin, rises dramatically just prior to birth.[72] In early fetal life, large molecular forms of peptides such as GIP and motilin predominate, suggesting that the post-translational enzymic processing pathways may be immature. At birth, the molecular forms of the gastrointestinal regulatory peptides and their distribution in the gut are similar to those of the adult.[72]

Secretion of Gastrointestinal Hormones

Several alimentary hormones can be detected in umbilical blood collected at fetoscopy in the second trimester (Fig. 8–1).[74] It is also evident that some endocrine cell types are functional, because several hormones, such as enteroglucagon, PYY, and GIP, are found in higher concentrations in blood from the umbilical artery and vein than in the maternal circulation at 18 to 21 weeks of gestation.[74] Other peptides, such as gastrin, glucagon, and PP, are also found in the fetal circulation but at concentrations below those in the maternal blood. Even with these hormones, there is evidence for activity during fetal life, as they are found in substantial quantities in amniotic fluid, which is swallowed by the fetus, and are likely to play a role in gut development.[74, 75] It is tempting to speculate that trophic peptides, such as gastrin, in amniotic fluid may play an important role in gastrointestinal development even before luminal nutrition begins at birth.

GASTROINTESTINAL HORMONES IN NEONATES

In utero, the fetus receives continuous intravenous nutrition that is controlled by the maternal metabolism.

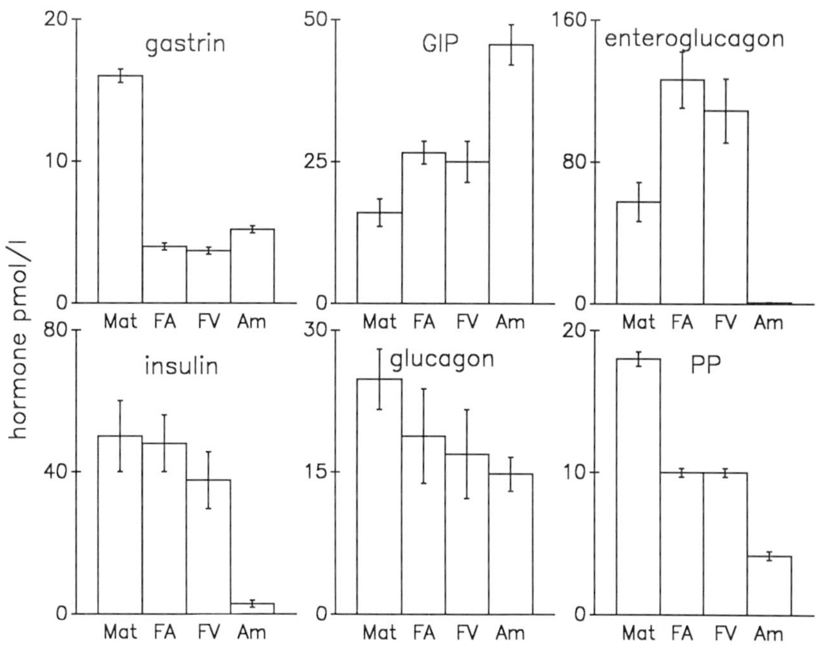

Figure 8–1. Maternal (Mat), fetal artery (FA), fetal vein (FV), and amniotic fluid (Am) concentrations of gastrointestinal and pancreatic hormones (mean ± SEM) in samples collected at fetoscopy at 16 to 20 weeks of gestation. (Modified from Aynsley-Green A: The adaptation of the human neonate to extrauterine nutrition: A pre-requisite for postnatal growth. *In* Cochburn F, ed: Fetal and Neonatal Growth. New York, John Wiley, 1988, pp 165–166. Copyright 1988. Reprinted by permission of John Wiley & Sons, Ltd.)

At birth, nutrition via the placenta ceases, and the infant has to adapt to enteral feeding with milk. In early neonatal life, there are marked changes in the functions of the alimentary tract as well as substantial growth. Gastrointestinal hormones, which are known to have trophic, secretory, and motor functions, play an important role in the control of alimentary function in the adult. These gut regulatory peptides appear to be involved in the characteristic changes in intestinal growth and function that are triggered by enteral feeding.[76]

Several interesting changes in gastrointestinal hormone secretion during the early neonatal period have been documented recently. Each of these changes will be considered in turn. However, the major changes seen in early infant life are summarized in Table 8–2.

Table 8–2. MAJOR CHANGES IN CIRCULATING GUT HORMONE LEVELS IN THE NEWBORN

Hormone	Observed Changes in Neonates
Gastrin	Hypersecretion at birth; level remains elevated without increased acid secretion
Cholecystokinin	Marked postnatal surge, levels higher than in adult
Secretin	Higher levels in first week of life compared with adult even without enteral feeding
Pancreatic polypeptide	Small postnatal surge of basal levels; postfeed response smaller than in adult
Glucose-dependent insulinotropic peptide	Low levels in first days of life, then adult pattern develops
Motilin	Massive postnatal surge of prefeed levels; postfeed decrease in levels more marked than in adult
Neurotensin	Large postnatal surge and development of massive postprandial responses compared with adult
Enteroglucagon	Massive postnatal surge and development of marked postfeed response
Peptide YY	High levels at birth; massive postnatal surge

Gastrin

At birth, cord blood levels of gastrin are already four or five times higher than those in the adult, and prefeed basal levels remain elevated for several weeks (Figs. 8–2 and 8–3).[77–79] Several groups have demonstrated postprandial gastrin responses to the first milk feed.[79, 80] After 3 or 4 weeks of life, basal gastrin levels begin to decline, and when this occurs, postprandial responses become more marked (Fig. 8–4).[77, 81] Gastric acid is detectable in the stomach at birth and reaches a peak in the first day or two.[78, 82, 83] Thereafter, acid output decreases for a period of about 1 month in spite of the hypergastrinemia and rapid growth of the stomach. It has been suggested that the lack of responsiveness could result from a lack of receptors in the oxyntic gland mucosa. This is supported by the failure of exogenous pentagastrin to stimulate gastric acid in early neonatal life.[84] However, a more likely explanation is that secretion is suppressed by some inhibitor, such as PYY or neurotensin, thus enabling gastrin to stimulate growth of the gastric mucosa without hyperstimulating acid secretion.[68, 85]

Secretin

In adults, secretin release is both transient and intermittent. It is of considerable interest, therefore, that plasma secretin levels are higher in neonates at birth than in adults. In addition, during the first 3 weeks of life, a postprandial response develops that is much more

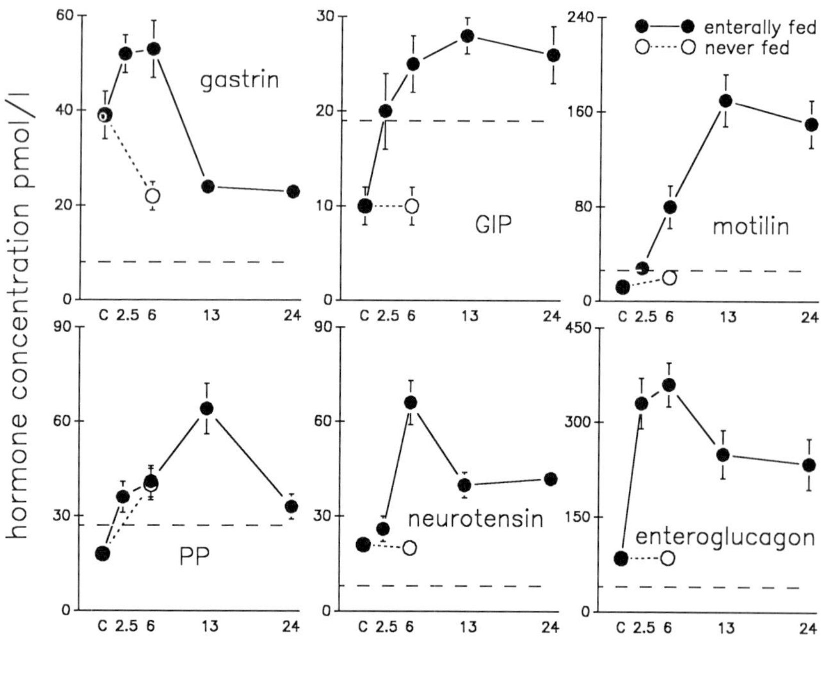

Figure 8–2. Postnatal changes in plasma concentrations of gastrointestinal hormones (mean ± SEM) in preterm infants at birth (C, cord blood) and preprandially at 2.5, 6, 13, and 24 days. *Solid circles* show samples drawn from infants fed from birth with regular boluses of human milk; *open circles* show samples taken from a group of infants who had never received any enteral feeding. *Dotted line* shows the mean adult fasting value for each hormone. (Modified from Lucas A, Bloom SR, Aynsley-Green A: Postnatal surges in plasma gut hormones in term and preterm infants. Biol Neonate 1982; 41:64; with permission of S. Karger AG, Basel.)

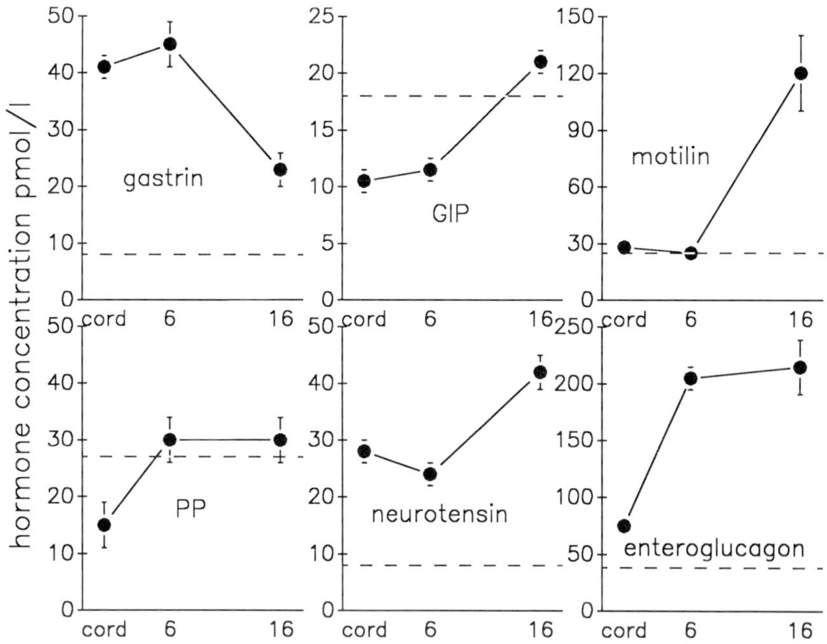

Figure 8–3. Postnatal changes in plasma concentrations of gastrointestinal hormones (mean ± SEM) in term infants at birth (C, cord blood) and preprandially at 6 and 16 days. *Dotted line* shows the mean adult fasting value for each hormone. (Modified from Lucas A, Bloom SR, Aynsley-Green A: Postnatal surges in plasma gut hormones in term and preterm infants. Biol Neonate 1982; 41:64; with permission of S. Karger AG, Basel.)

marked than that seen in adults (see Fig. 8–4).[86] Because secretin is considered to be a major factor in triggering the neutralization of acid chyme entering the duodenum, the increase in circulating secretin levels may be of considerable importance in mucosal protection during this period. It is notable that the postnatal surge of secretin, unlike that of the other alimentary hormones, occurs even in the absence of feeding, indicating the importance of this mucosal cytoprotective function.[81]

Cholecystokinin

CCK has marked trophic effects on the adult pancreas and appears responsible for regeneration following resection or acute pancreatitis.[49] It has been suggested that the observed postnatal surge of plasma CCK concentrations, therefore, may be of importance in stimulating growth of this organ (Fig. 8–5).[87] Studies in the guinea pig, using continuous peripheral CCK receptor blockade either in utero or in early neonatal life, have failed to show an effect on pancreatic development.[88] Exogenous administration of CCK also has no effect in the neonatal rat, an observation blamed on receptor immaturity.[89] This is clearly not the case in the guinea pig, however, in that secretory responses to CCK are present at birth, and the developmental responses are relatively unchanged by CCK receptor blockade.[88] Other factors are clearly involved in neonatal pancreatic development, and epidermal growth factor (or transforming growth factor-alpha, which acts on the same receptor) and secretin are likely candidates.[89, 90]

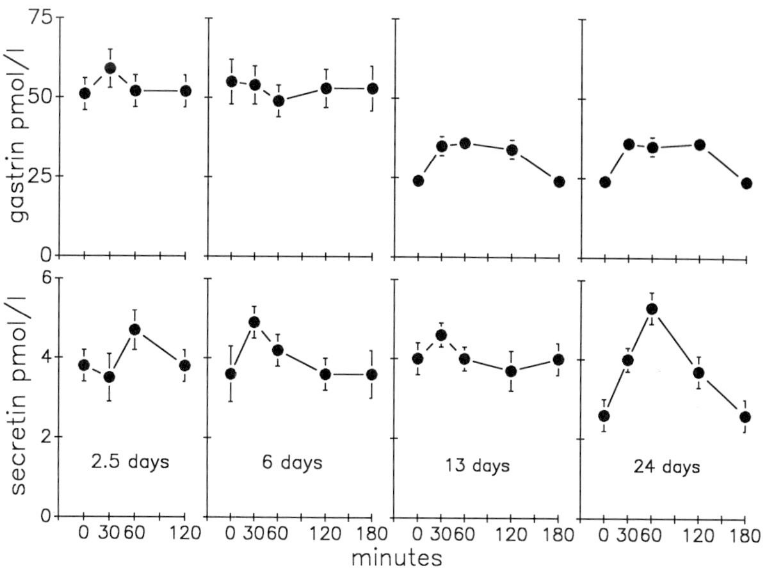

Figure 8–4. Postnatal development of the effect of milk feeding on concentrations of gastrin and secretin in healthy preterm infants. Between 8 and 13 single observations contributed to each point (mean ± SEM). (Modified from Lucas A, Bloom SR, Aynsley-Green A: Development of gut hormone responses to feeding in neonates. Arch Dis Child 1980; 55:679; with permission.)

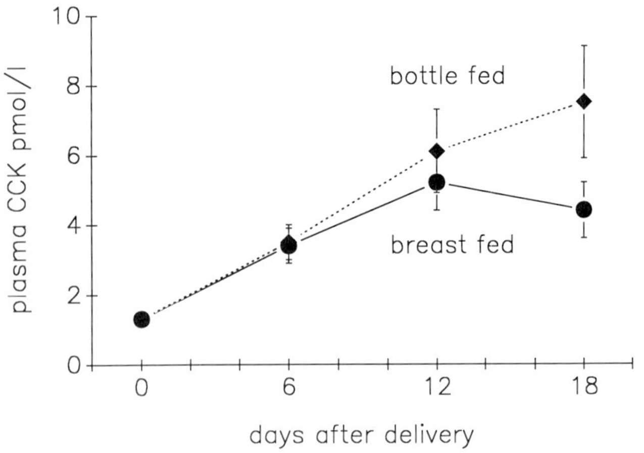

Figure 8–5. Plasma cholecystokinin (CCK) concentrations in breast- and formula-fed preterm infants at birth and preprandially at 6, 12, and 18 days after delivery (mean ± SEM). (Modified from Calvert SA, Soltesz G, Jenkins PA, et al: Feeding premature infants with human milk or preterm milk formula: Effects on postnatal growth, intermediary metabolism and regulatory peptides. Biol Neonate 1985; 47:189–198; with permission of S. Karger AG, Basel.)

Motilin

Motilin concentrations are low in cord blood, but preprandial basal concentrations show a massive 10-fold postnatal surge that is particularly evident in preterm neonates (see Figs. 8–2 and 8–3). The peak occurs at about 2 weeks of postnatal life.[81] As basal levels increase, a fall in motilin levels following milk feeding becomes evident, which is more like the pattern seen in the normal adult after a mixed meal (Fig. 8–6).[77] It is likely that this increase in circulating motilin concentrations stimulates the known increase in motor activity of the gut that occurs during the neonatal period. Interdigestive motor complexes appear normal at birth in the term infant but interdigestive cycles are incomplete in preterm neonates.[91] Premature infants exhibit abnormal motor activity with periods of motor quiescence and nonpropagating contractions. Thus, motor activity is more immature in preterm infants than in term infants.[91] The relationship between maturation of the migrating motor complexes and the late postnatal surge of motilin in the preterm neonate is not clear.

Glucose-Dependent Insulinotropic Peptide

Marked changes in insulin and glucagon release from the islets of Langerhans are seen after birth. Cutting the umbilical cord, of course, disrupts the intravenous supply of metabolites, particularly glucose. Insulin secretion is suppressed, and a glucagon surge is seen, together with increases in the counter-regulatory hormones such as cortisol and catecholamines.[92] This process initiates hepatic glycogenolysis and gluconeogenesis and leads to stabilization of blood glucose levels. These early endocrine and metabolic changes can maintain metabolic homeostasis for only a few hours, however, and the supply and utilization of exogenous nutrients then become increasingly important. GIP concentrations are low at birth, as would be expected from the low insulin levels (see Figs. 8–2 and 8–3).[81] GIP levels increase gradually throughout the first month of life together with the development of a marked postfeeding GIP response, similar to that seen in the adult after ingestion of a mixed meal (see Fig. 8–6).[93] The development of the GIP response to feeding in neonates is mirrored by the postprandial insulin response, which increases through the first month of life to maintain glucose homeostasis (Fig. 8–7).[93]

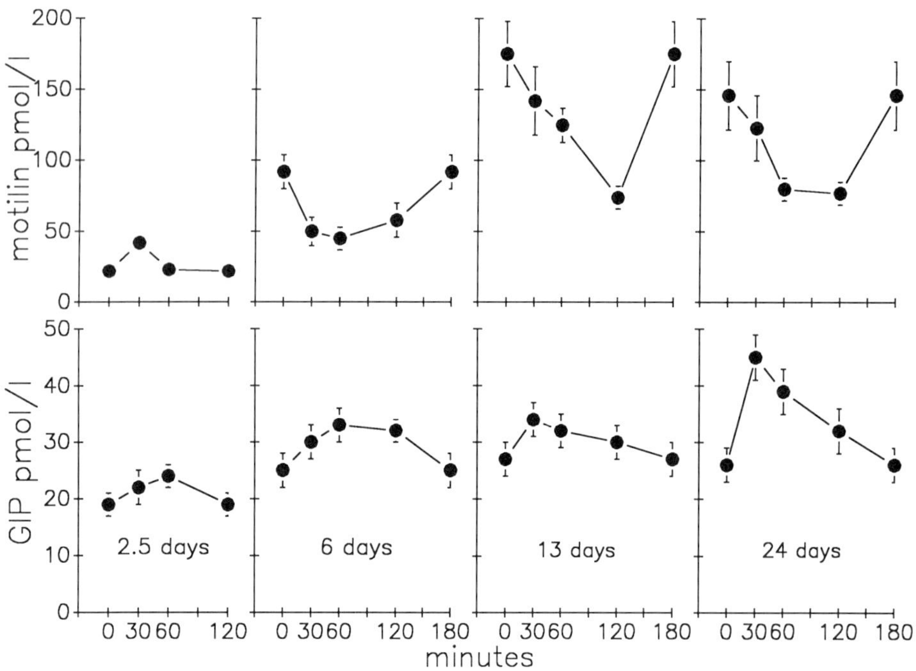

Figure 8–6. Postnatal development of the effect of milk feeding on concentrations of motilin and glucose-dependent insulinotropic peptide (GIP) in healthy preterm infants. Between 8 and 13 single observations contributed to each point (mean ± SEM). (Modified from Lucas A, Bloom SR, Aynsley-Green A: Development of gut hormone responses to feeding in neonates. Arch Dis Child 1980; 55:679; with permission.)

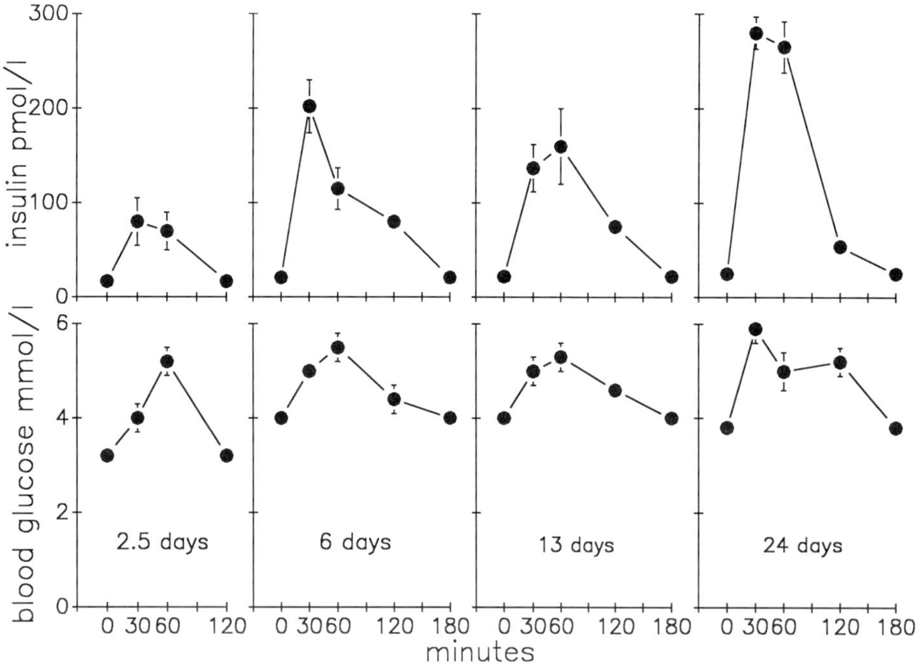

Figure 8–7. Postnatal development of the effect of milk feeding on concentrations of insulin and blood glucose in healthy preterm infants. Between 8 and 13 single observations contributed to each point (mean ± SEM). (Modified from Lucas A, Bloom SR, Aynsley-Green A: Development of gut hormone responses to feeding in neonates. Arch Dis Child 1980; 55:680; with permission.)

Pancreatic Polypeptide

Basal PP concentrations, which at birth are lower than those of the adult, show a small postnatal surge that is particularly evident in preterm infants (see Figs. 8–2 and 8–3).[81] During the first weeks of life, postprandial PP responses develop, but these are smaller in magnitude than those seen in the adult.[94] Overall, there is little evidence of a major developmental role for this peptide.

Neurotensin

Plasma neurotensin concentrations are higher in the neonate, and an enhanced postprandial response develops in the first month of life (see Figs. 8–2, 8–3, and 8–8).[95] Both the reduction of gastric secretion and the slowing of the rate of gastric emptying will decrease the rate at which acid chyme enters the duodenum and, therefore, will result in a more steady absorption of nutrients from the gut. Thus, neurotensin may be im-

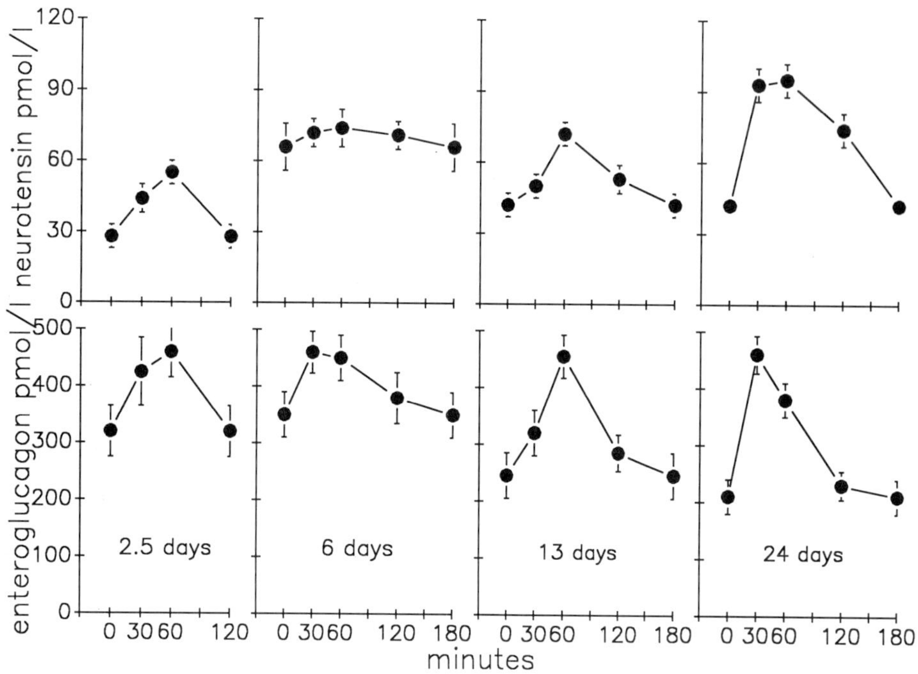

Figure 8–8. Postnatal development of the effect of milk feeding on concentrations of neurotensin and enteroglucagon in healthy preterm infants. Between 8 and 13 single observations contributed to each point (mean ± SEM). (Modified from Lucas A, Bloom SR, Aynsley-Green A: Development of gut hormone responses to feeding in neonates. Arch Dis Child 1980; 55:680; with permission.)

portant in the adaptation of the neonate to enteral nutrition.

Enteroglucagon

Plasma enteroglucagon concentrations show a marked postnatal surge that peaks within the first week and is associated with the development of a marked postprandial response (see Figs. 8–2, 8–3, and 8–8).[77, 81] Because an increased rate of small intestinal mucosal growth is known to occur during this period, one may speculate that the increase of this trophic hormone is important in neonatal alimentary maturation. The resulting mucosal growth increases the absorptive area for the uptake of nutrients from the gut.

Peptide YY

Concentrations of PYY are elevated in cord blood and rise postnatally to a peak within the first 2 weeks postpartum (Fig. 8–9).[85] At their peak, the plasma PYY concentrations are about 50 times higher than fasting levels in normal adults and 10 times higher even than the postprandial response seen after a massive 5,000-cal meal in young adults.[85] Furthermore, these neonatal plasma PYY levels are considerably higher even than levels seen in adult patients with malabsorption due to sprue or chronic pancreatitis, or after bowel resection.[85] There is evidence to suggest that gastric emptying and intestinal transit are rapid during the first week of life, in both term and preterm infants. The triggering mechanism for the changes that then take place is unknown, but it is likely that factors such as PYY play a role.[69] In addition, the potent inhibitory effect of PYY on gastric secretion may account for the prevention of acid hypersecretion during the early neonatal period, in spite of the marked hypergastrinemia.[68]

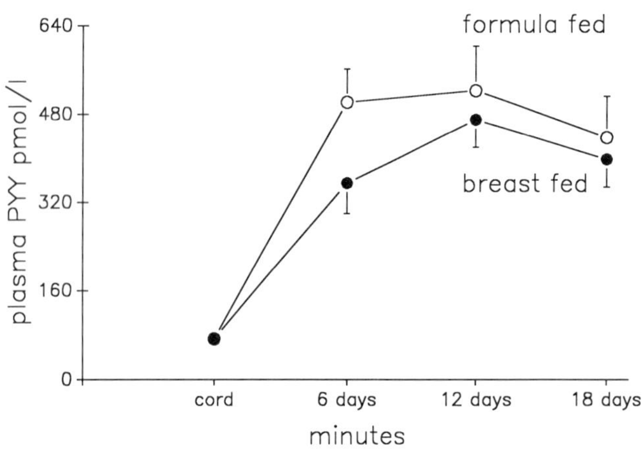

Figure 8–9. Plasma concentrations of peptide YY (PYY) at birth (cord blood), and preprandially in preterm infants receiving either human milk or formula at 6, 12, and 18 days of postnatal life (mean ± SEM). Mean fasting levels in healthy adults were 10 ± 2 pmol per L for comparison. (Modified from Adrian TE, Smith HA, Calvert SA, et al: Elevated plasma peptide YY in human neonates and infants. Pediatr Res 1986; 20:1226; with permission.)

Amylin

To date, there have been no reports on the developmental changes of amylin production or secretion.

FEEDING AND THE DEVELOPMENT OF GASTROINTESTINAL HORMONE RESPONSES

It is clear that marked changes in gastrointestinal physiology accompany the introduction of enteral feeding in the infant. Therefore, it is of considerable interest that the postnatal surges of gut hormones are not seen in infants who have never received enteral feeding (see Fig. 8–2).[81] Concentrations of all of these hormones, with the exception of secretin, remain low in infants who receive only parenteral nutrition, for example, infants with hyaline membrane disease.[96]

The composition of food and the mode of administration are also important in the development of gastrointestinal hormone responses. This can be demonstrated as early as the first feed in infants, when dextrose elicits a different response than does milk.[97] There are also differences in hormone responses between breast- and bottle-fed infants.[98]

Dietary Influences on Enteric Hormones

There is considerable evidence to suggest that endocrine peptides from the gastrointestinal tract play an important role in the growth and functional development of the gastrointestinal tract, in addition to the general regulation of alimentary functions. There are precise mechanisms of control for each of the gut hormones in adults, and, indeed, the amount of a particular hormone liberated by a meal is adequate to stimulate the appropriate digestive responses for that particular meal.[99] For example, a meal rich in long-chain triglycerides will evoke a large CCK response that is not seen with medium-chain fats.[100] The high circulating levels of CCK, in turn, stimulate the pancreatic enzyme secretion and release the bile salts (by gallbladder contraction) necessary for digestion of the long-chain fat.[100] Medium-chain triglycerides, on the other hand, are rapidly hydrolyzed by lingual and gastric lipases; they are water soluble, do not require micelle formation for digestion, and are rapidly absorbed. Thus, bile salts and pancreatic enzymes are not required for digestion of medium-chain triglycerides, and a large CCK response is not seen when they are ingested.[101] The gut endocrine system, with its sparse distribution of overlapping cell types, is designed to produce an integrated digestive response to the discontinuous stimulation of ingested food. As the type of food presented can influence the integrated hormonal response, it is apparent that differences in nutrition in early neonatal life may result in changes in the growth and functional development of the neonatal alimentary tract.

Changes in Nutrition in Fetal and Neonatal Life

The fetus makes little demand on its gastrointestinal tract because the nutritional needs are provided intravenously by the placenta. The situation changes dramatically at birth, however, when demand for nutrients necessitates the rapid maturation of the alimentary tract. This development of the gastrointestinal tract is characterized by the integrated maturation of its many functions. However, the observation that premature infants make a satisfactory transition from intravenous nutrition via the placenta to extrauterine enteral feeding suggests that external influences can exert a substantial influence. The massive postnatal surge in circulating levels of hormones that have trophic as well as secretory and motor functions is compelling circumstantial evidence of a profound gut endocrine influence on alimentary development.[81] This is further supported by the observation that these hormonal surges are not seen in sick infants who are on parenteral nutrition and have not been fed orally.[96] It is likely that the failure of trophic gut hormone secretion is responsible for the hypoplastic gut and pancreas that accompany parenteral nutrition. Appropriate enteral stimuli or hormone replacement may eventually alleviate this problem.

A further factor of potential importance in gut development is the ingestion of colostrum from early suckling. There are marked differences between the nutritional content of colostrum and midlactation milk, which may influence postnatal gut development.[102] In human milk, protein content is 10-fold lower than in colostrum, whereas lactose levels are three times higher and fat content is relatively unchanged.[102] The colostrum supplies the newborn infant with large amounts of protective immunoglobulins, but dietary protein content is also increased compared with mature milk.[102] Any advantage that the intake of colostrum confers with regard to hormone release and alimentary development will be lost in formula-fed babies.

Influence of Different Feed Types on Gastrointestinal Hormones in Neonates

The first feed of human milk given 4 to 6 hours after full-term birth is associated with a marked rise in circulating concentrations of glucose, insulin, growth hormone, gastrin, and enteroglucagon, whereas glucagon and GIP levels are unaffected.[80] The composition of the feed is important, however, as a first feed of glucose has no effect on enteroglucagon even though the increment of glucose, insulin, and gastrin is similar to the milk feed.[80]

Substantial differences in gastrointestinal hormone responses are seen between infants fed human breast milk and those fed a formula.[98] By day 6, preprandial levels of the small intestinal hormones motilin, GIP, and neurotensin were much higher in bottle-fed infants (Fig. 8–10), who also had greater postprandial changes

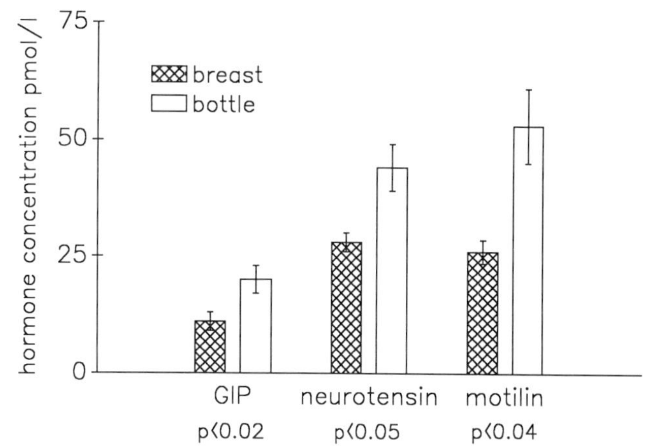

Figure 8–10. Basal levels of glucose-dependent insulinotropic peptide (GIP), neurotensin, and motilin in breast-fed and bottle-fed healthy term infants (mean ± SEM). (Modified from Lucas A, Adrian TE, Sarson DL, et al: Breast vs bottle: Endocrine responses are different with formula feeding. Lancet 1980; 1:1268; with permission.)

in levels of insulin, motilin, neurotensin, enteroglucagon, and PP.[98] The possible explanations for these alterations include (1) the differences between the composition of human milk and cow's milk formula (despite attempts to humanize it) and (2) the reduced milk intake of breast-fed infants during the first days of life, as lactation is developing. It should be noted, however, that by the sixth day of life, milk intake was similar in both groups. The differences in composition include the greater absorbability of fat in human milk and the higher total fat and branched chain amino acid content of formula.[98] Other factors may include the presence of active lipase and other enzymes as well as hormones in human breast milk. The presence of growth factors, such as epidermal growth factor, in human milk may also be of profound importance in neonatal gut development.[103, 104] Several other regulatory peptides have been reported in human milk, including gastrin, neurotensin, PYY, VIP, PHM, and bombesin.[105] Of these peptides, bombesin, which has trophic effects in a number of tissues, was present in higher concentrations in breast milk than in plasma.[105]

The differences in hormone responses between breast- and bottle-fed infants may be of considerable practical importance. The enhanced insulin response in bottle-fed infants despite a similar degree of glycemia may result from increased circulating levels of branched chain amino acids or GIP, both of which enhance glucose-stimulated insulin secretion. Because insulin enhances cellular glucose uptake and inhibits lipolysis, the greater insulin release may explain the increased deposition of subcutaneous fat seen in bottle-fed infants. Differences in motilin levels may account for the well-known differences in stool frequency between bottle- and breast-fed infants. As enteroglucagon is likely to exert a major trophic effect on the small bowel mucosa, changes in the levels of this hormone may influence postnatal gut development.[66, 106]

When soy-based and other milk substitute formulas are considered, the changes in normal gut hormone responses are likely to be even more marked. The response of some hormones varies according to the degree of fat saturation. For example, polyunsaturated fat is a more potent releaser of CCK, a hormone that has trophic effects on the gallbladder and pancreas as well as a stimulatory effect on pancreatic enzyme and bile secretion into the duodenum.[100]

Comparison of Effects of Continuous Infusion Feeding with Intermittent Boluses on Gut Hormone Release

Preterm infants receive gastric milk feedings either as continuous feeds or intermittent boluses; however, the information on the influence of these feeding modes on gastrointestinal hormones and gut development is scant. Both groups show similar increases in plasma motilin, neurotensin, enteroglucagon, and PP levels.[107] By 13 days of age, infusion-fed infants have higher levels of insulin, gastrin, and GIP.[107] Although both methods of feeding result in progressive changes in circulating enteroinsular hormone levels, the development of postprandial increases in response to bolus feeding is absent in infusion-fed infants.[107] The absence of meal-stimulated gut hormone responses possibly has effects on the developing alimentary tract but does not appear to influence body weight gain, which is similar between the two groups.[107]

Effect of Long-Term Breast Feeding on Gut Hormone Responses

There is little information on the development of gut hormone responses after the first month of life, but one study compared pancreatic and gut regulatory peptides in a group of 9-month-old infants who had been breast-fed exclusively from birth with control subjects weaned during the first 3 months of life. There were no significant differences in basal hormone levels between these two groups, but postprandial rises in insulin, PP, and CCK concentrations were significantly obtunded in the breast-fed group.[108] The insulin/glucagon ratio was also lower in the breast-fed infants despite similar degrees of glycemia. No significant differences in postprandial gastrin, GIP, secretin, motilin, neurotensin, or enteroglucagon levels were seen between the two groups.[108] Overall, the levels of these regulatory peptides were lower than those seen in the first postnatal weeks and thus were tending toward the responses seen in the adult.[108]

Effect of Minimal Enteral Feeding on Gastrointestinal Hormones

To study the relationship between the quantity of milk ingested and the development of postnatal surges of gut hormones, infants who were recovering from hyaline membrane disease were investigated. Six-day-old infants who had been exclusively fed parenterally showed no postnatal elevation of gastrin, motilin, GIP, neurotensin, or enteroglucagon. In contrast, infants who had received restricted enteral feeding over this period had hormone surges similar to those seen in healthy infants on full enteral feeds (Fig. 8–11).[109] Substantial elevations in gastrin, GIP, and enteroglucagon levels were seen after a cumulative enteral feed volume since birth of only 24 ml (12 ml per kg body weight) had been consumed (Fig. 8–12). By the time the infants had received a cumulative intake of 96 ml (50 ml per kg), the hormone surges had reached maximal levels that were identical to those of enterally fed healthy infants (see Fig. 8–12). Greater feed volumes were required to induce the normal surge of motilin and neurotensin, but even these were considerably lower than those required for full enteral feeding. These observations suggest that minimal enteral feeding may have an important therapeutic role in the maintenance of functional gastrointestinal integrity in infants who undergo prolonged parenteral nutrition.[109, 110]

Practical Significance of Alimentary Hormone Changes with Nutrition

At birth, the gastrointestinal tract is required to initiate and sustain rapid body growth. Survival of the infant is dependent on its ability to adapt successfully to enteral nutrition. The available evidence suggests that the enormous postnatal changes in levels of several circulating regulatory peptides are profoundly important in triggering the adaptive alimentary responses during this critical period. With the vast improvement in the care of preterm infants with respiratory disease, nutrition has become the critical factor for survival, and this is dependent on the state of development of the gastrointestinal tract. Clearly, preservation of the hormonal responses that trigger gut development is important; however, the mechanisms by which amniotic fluid, colostrum, and, ultimately, milk act to prime the gut endocrine system to stimulate alimentary growth and development have still not been unraveled. One group of infants likely to benefit directly from such studies are those who require total parenteral nutrition because of necrotizing enterocolitis, short bowel syndrome, hyaline membrane disease, or neonatal nesidioblastosis. In this group, preservation of the developmental triggers for the alimentary tract, either by minimal enteral nutrition or by hormone replacement therapy, may prevent the atrophic responses and gallbladder stasis that make management and subsequent enteral feeding difficult.[109] Preliminary studies suggest that tiny amounts of milk (15 ml) are sufficient to stimulate the release of trophic hormones, such as enteroglucagon, in the preterm neonate.[109, 110] Further study is needed to reveal the nutritional conditions that are optimal for normal gut growth and functional development.

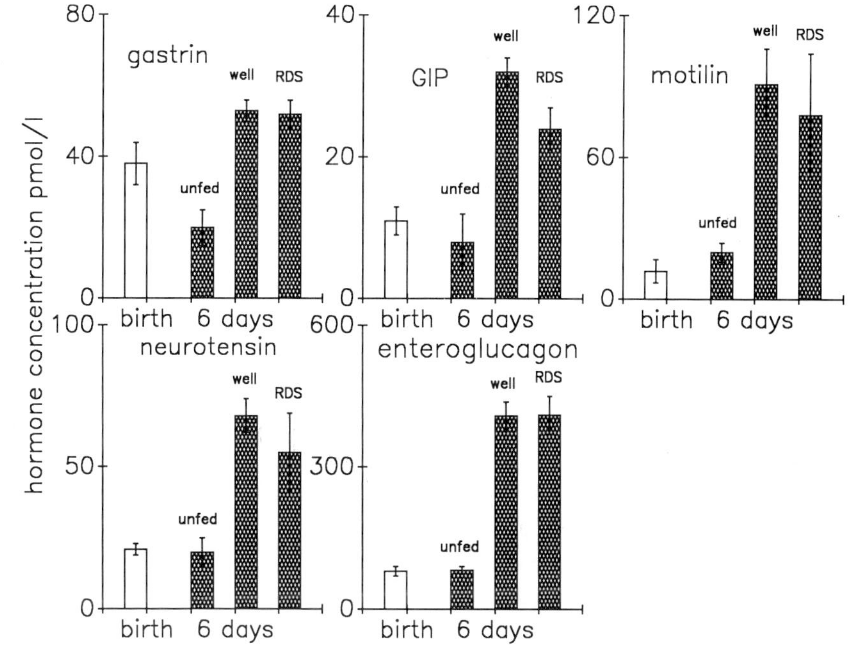

Figure 8–11. Plasma concentrations of gastrointestinal hormones at birth (cord blood) and at 6 days in infants who had received no enteral feeds since birth (unfed), in healthy enterally fed infants (well), and in infants with respiratory disease (RDS) on restricted enteral intake (mean ± SEM). (Modified from Lucas A, Bloom SR, Aynsley-Green A: Gut hormones and "minimal enteral feeding." Acta Paediatr Scand 1986; 75:720; with permission.)

PATHOPHYSIOLOGY OF GASTROINTESTINAL HORMONES

There are two ways in which secretion of gastrointestinal hormones can be changed in alimentary diseases: (1) there can be abnormal release of a peptide localized to the site of the abnormality; and (2) there can be secondary adaptive changes in other parts of the alimentary tract that tend to compensate for the abnormality. The advent of radioimmunoassay provided, for the first time, a technique with the requisite sensitivity and specificity to measure the low levels of gut hormones in the circulation. This technologic advance has enabled investigation of the role of gut hormones in several gastrointestinal diseases. Although most studies have concentrated on adult disorders, there is already a considerable volume of knowledge that is of interest to the pediatric gastroenterologist. The alimentary regulatory peptide abnormalities that accompany several childhood disorders are discussed in the following segments.

Celiac Sprue

Gluten enteropathy is characterized by villous atrophy of the upper small intestine. Therefore, it is perhaps not surprising that there is a reduced secretion of the hormonal peptides localized to the mucosa of this region.

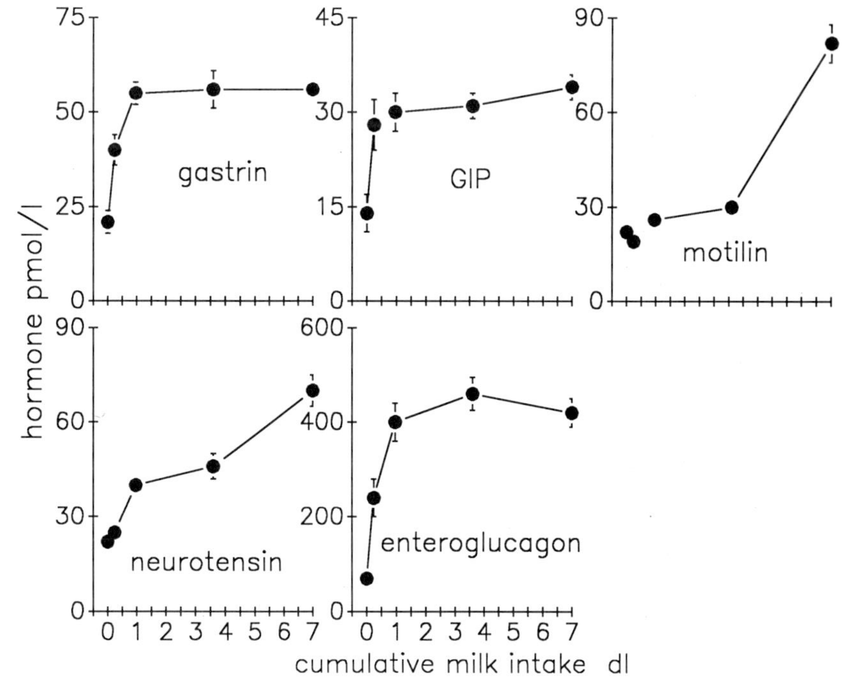

Figure 8–12. Plasma concentrations of gastrointestinal hormones according to the total cumulative enteral intake of human milk since birth in preterm infants (mean ± SEM). (Modified from Lucas A, Bloom SR, Aynsley-Green A: Gut hormones and "minimal enteral feeding." Acta Paediatr Scand 1986; 75:721; with permission.)

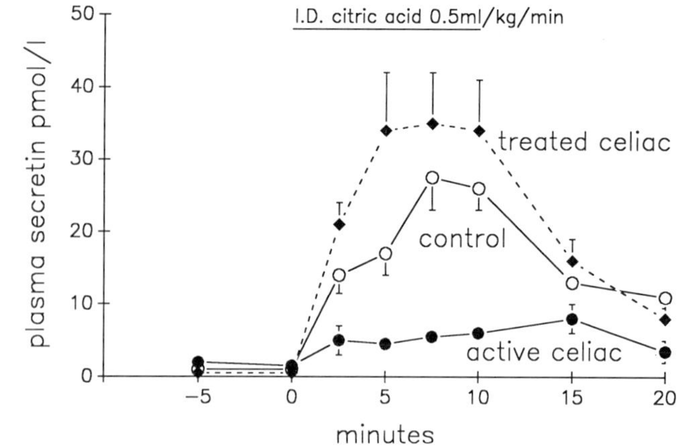

Figure 8–13. Plasma secretin response to intraduodenal citric acid (0.5 ml per kg body weight) in children with active celiac sprue, in patients treated with a gluten-free diet, and in healthy age-matched control subjects (mean ± SEM). (Modified from Besterman HS, Bloom SR, Sarson DL, et al: Gut-hormone profile in coeliac disease. Lancet 1978; 1:786; with permission.)

Responses of CCK, secretin, and GIP to normal stimuli are absent in this disease (Fig. 8–13).[111–113] The reduction in circulating levels of CCK and secretin explains the reduced pancreatic exocrine secretion that exacerbates the malabsorption of celiac disease.[111, 112] In patients with sprue, the pancreas responds normally to exogenous stimulation using intravenous CCK and secretin. In contrast with the reduced secretion of peptides from the upper small intestine, there is an increased release of those localized in the distal bowel, such as enteroglucagon, neurotensin, and PYY (Fig. 8–14).[111, 114] Enteroglucagon appears trophic to the small intestine, and crypt cell turnover is increased in celiac disease. The enhanced release of enteroglucagon may represent an adaptive response whereby unabsorbed nutrients reaching the distal ileum will stimulate the release of a hormone that stimulates growth of the intestinal mucosa in an attempt to increase the surface area available for absorption.[111] Both PYY and neurotensin have motor inhibitory effects on the foregut that tend to delay gastric emptying and intestinal transit.[63, 69] Enhanced release of these inhibitory hormones constitutes another adaptive response. Hormones that are localized to other parts of the alimentary tract, such as gastrin in the stomach and PP in the pancreas, are normal in celiac sprue.[111] When celiac patients were successfully treated with a gluten-free diet, the hormonal abnormalities disappeared.[111, 114] Thus, the gut hormone profile in celiac disease reflects the anatomic distribution of the disease process and helps explain the pathophysiology.

Cystic Fibrosis

In a series of children with cystic fibrosis with severe pancreatic insufficiency, the release of the pancreatic hormone PP was almost totally abolished (Fig. 8–15).[115] Not only were fasting levels of the peptide low, but the normal PP release in response to a milk drink was absent.[115] Plasma insulin and GIP responses were significantly reduced in patients with cystic fibrosis compared with control subjects, even though the early glucose rise was greater in the former group.[115] The reduced GIP secretion may exacerbate the glucose intolerance that accompanies pancreatic destruction. Fasting enteroglucagon concentrations were grossly elevated in the cystic fibrosis patients and remained elevated throughout the test (Fig. 8–16).[115] Once again, the increased release of enteroglucagon could be considered to be an appropriate adaptive response in this disorder. Plasma concentrations of gastrin, secretin, motilin, and glucagon all were normal in the patients with cystic fibrosis.[115]

A separate study of adult cystic fibrosis reflected the hormonal abnormalities seen in children with the disease.[116]

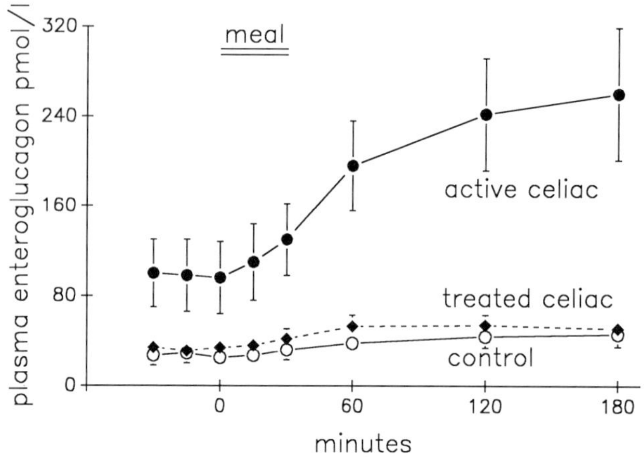

Figure 8–14. Plasma enteroglucagon response to a test breakfast in patients with active celiac sprue, in patients treated with a gluten-free diet, and in healthy age-matched control subjects (mean ± SEM). (Modified from Besterman HS, Bloom SR, Sarson DL, et al: Gut-hormone profile in coeliac disease. Lancet 1978; 1:787; with permission.)

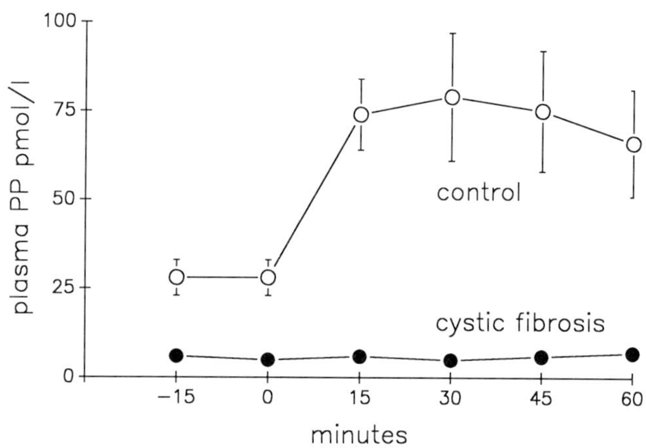

Figure 8–15. Plasma concentrations of PP in response to a milk drink (10 ml per kg) in children with pancreatic insufficiency due to cystic fibrosis (mean ± SEM). (Modified from Adrian TE, McKiernan J, Johnstone DI, et al: Hormonal abnormalities of the pancreas and gut in cystic fibrosis. Gastroenterology 1980; 79:463; with permission.)

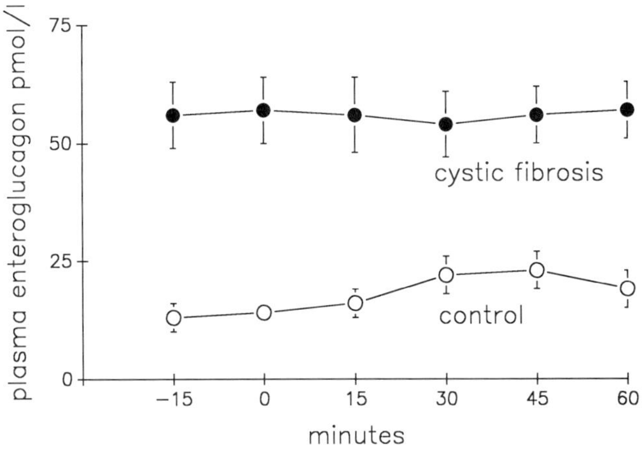

Figure 8–16. Plasma enteroglucagon concentrations in response to a milk drink (10 ml per kg) in children with pancreatic insufficiency due to cystic fibrosis (mean ± SEM). (Modified from Adrian TE, McKiernan J, Johnstone DI, et al: Hormonal abnormalities of the pancreas and gut in cystic fibrosis. Gastroenterology 1980; 79:463; with permission.)

Infective Diarrhea

Patients with acute infective diarrhea were found to have a moderate increase in enteroglucagon, PYY, and PP levels, together with a massive increase in motilin concentrations (Fig. 8–17).[114, 117] Once again, these abnormalities normalized once the patients were fully recovered. In patients with diarrhea, the plasma concentrations of motilin greatly exceeded those previously found to accelerate gastric emptying and to increase intestinal motility in healthy volunteers during exogenous infusion of motilin.[117] Motilin may therefore play a role in the motor abnormalities that are seen in this condition. Rapid transit, triggered hormonally, may be a defensive mechanism to rid the alimentary tract of pathogens and their secreted toxins.

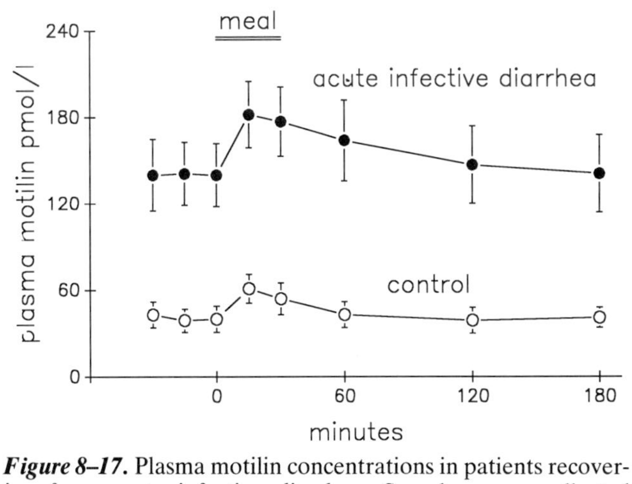

Figure 8–17. Plasma motilin concentrations in patients recovering from acute infective diarrhea. Samples were collected during fasting and during the first meal taken after recovery (mean ± SEM). (Modified from Besterman HS, Christofides ND, Welsby PD, et al: Gut hormones in acute diarrhea. Gut 1983; 24:667; with permission.)

A recent study described hormone changes in infants with acute gastroenteritis. The patients were previously well but required hospital admission for oral rehydration therapy.[118] At presentation there was a massive elevation of circulating enteroglucagon, with concentrations about 15 times higher than those in adults with acute diarrhea. Enteroglucagon levels continued to rise through the acute stage of the illness and before introduction of milk feeds, at which time no postprandial elevation was seen. The enteroglucagon levels had returned to normal 3 months later, when the infants were well again. Concentrations of PYY were similarly increased in these infants. Motilin concentrations were also elevated in these infants with gastroenteritis, but to levels similar to those seen in adults with diarrhea. However, motilin levels in these children were still elevated 3 months after an apparent complete recovery. Neurotensin, VIP, and PP concentrations in the infants with gastroenteritis were similar to those of healthy, age-matched control subjects. The evidence from this study suggested that the enteroglucagon response to infantile diarrhea may be related to the extent of mucosal damage and its repair.[118] Furthermore, the findings show that (1) the gut endocrine system in infants responds to diarrhea in a manner different from that in adults; and (2) measurement of the peptide hormones may give information on the degree of damage or recovery or of ongoing pathologic change.

Necrotizing Enterocolitis

Changes in circulating enteric hormones in six infants with necrotizing colitis were recently reported.[119] The mean gestational period for these infants was 30 weeks, and symptoms and signs of enterocolitis developed at a mean time after birth of 23 days. The concentrations of GIP, neurotensin, and enteroglucagon all were lower than the mean values for fed infants of comparable age, whereas the levels of gastrin, motilin, and PP were not significantly different.[119] These scant data are difficult to interpret given the spectrum of ages at which the disease developed, the timing at which samples were drawn, and the fact that some infants had been enterally fed for as long as 4 weeks prior to the illness, whereas others had received no nutrition via the oral route.[119]

Short Bowel Syndrome

The major changes seen after ileal resection include a massive rise in PYY levels and marked increases in concentrations of motilin, PP, and enteroglucagon (Fig. 8–18).[120, 121] Increases in levels of enteroglucagon, which is a trophic hormone, and PYY, which inhibits gastric secretion and profoundly reduces intestinal transit, are appropriate responses in this condition. Preservation or even enhancement of the PYY response would probably be of value in diminishing the rapid transit and diarrhea associated with this condition. Studies in experimental animals have revealed that improvement in transit and

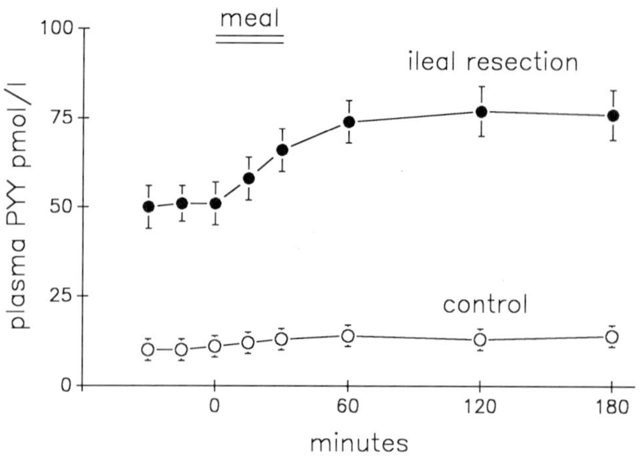

Figure 8–18. Plasma concentrations of peptide YY (PYY) following a test breakfast in patients who have undergone small bowel resection and in healthy age-matched control subjects (mean ± SEM). (Modified from Adrian TE, Savage AP, Fuessl HS, et al: Release of peptide YY (PYY) after resection of small bowel, colon or pancreas in man. Surgery 1987; 101:717; with permission.)

fluid absorption are temporally related to the development of the increased PYY response.[122]

Inflammatory Bowel Disease

Crohn's disease is accompanied by marked increases in PYY and motilin concentrations, together with smaller increments of PP and enteroglucagon.[114, 123] The reason for the increase in PYY is not apparent in the absence of malabsorption, but it may merely reflect the inflammatory response.

Fetal Distress Syndrome

Fetal distress in term infants results in a marked elevation in plasma levels of glucagon, PP, motilin, and VIP.[124] It has been suggested that the high motilin levels may be the cause of the intrauterine passage of meconium that is characteristic of this condition.[124] Glucagon, VIP, and PP all are released in other conditions associated with extreme stress.

Infantile Colic

Two studies have reported high circulating motilin concentrations in infants with colic.[125, 126] In a prospective study, motilin levels were elevated at birth as well as at 6 and 12 weeks of age in infants with colic.[126] The observation of this hormonal abnormality before the onset of feeding, on the first day of postnatal life, suggests that a change in gut motor function may be a primary event in this condition.[126]

Pseudo-obstructive Ileus

Plasma motilin concentrations measured in patients with pseudo-obstructive ileus have been found to be extremely low.[12] This finding led to attempts to initiate motor activity with intravenous motilin infusions. Results have been encouraging, with motor complexes beginning after 1 or 2 hours of motilin administration.

Obesity

Obesity in some groups of children may result from hormonal abnormalities. It is interesting, therefore, that alterations in somatostatin tissue content and plasma levels have been observed in obesity.[127] These findings suggest that somatostatin deficiency may be a causative factor in the development of obesity.[127] The alterations in somatostatin may be secondary to changes in other functions, although hyposomatostatinemia might facilitate nutrient assimilation. Other gastrointestinal hormones appear to play a role in the control of food intake. CCK has profound effects on the reduction of food intake via inhibition of gastric emptying and, independently, through effects on the central nervous system.[128] PYY stimulates appetite and also inhibits lipogenolysis. Studies on these hormones in patients with morbid obesity might provide valuable information.

FUTURE DIRECTIONS

Considerable advances have been made in our understanding of the pathophysiology of the regulatory peptides of the gut. Study of the release of these hormones in patients with gastrointestinal diseases has given us insight into the normal physiologic function of these peptides. In addition, the measurement of a profile of gut hormones has considerable diagnostic promise in being relatively easy and noninvasive. Indeed, detection of alimentary disorders by the measurement of hormones in a serum sample has particular value in a pediatric population, which is difficult to investigate by more conventional methods. Although we have a fair picture of the gut endocrine responses in celiac sprue and cystic fibrosis, there are other disorders in which abnormal gut hormone function may play a role or have diagnostic value. These include cow's milk intolerance, toddler diarrhea, and necrotizing enterocolitis in infants. Study of gut hormone secretion in these disorders is awaited with interest.

REFERENCES

1. Bell G, Sanchez-Pescador R, Laybourn P, et al: Exon duplication and divergence in the human preproglucagon gene. Nature 1983; 304:368–371.
2. Nawa H, Kotani H, Nakanishi S: Tissue-specific generation of two preprotachykinin mRNA's from one gene by alternative RNA splicing. Nature 1984; 312:729–734.

3. Minamino N, Kangawa K, Matsuo H, et al: A novel neurotensin-like peptide identified in porcine spinal cord. Biochem Biophys Res Commun 1984; 122:542–549.
4. Itoh N, Obata K, Yanaihara N, et al: Human preprovasoactive intestinal polypeptide contains a novel PHI-27 like peptide, PHM-27. Nature 1983; 304:547–549.
5. Comb M, Seeburg PH, Adelman J, et al: Primary structure of the human Met- and Leu-enkephalin precursor and its mRNA. Nature 1982; 295:663–666.
6. Walsh JH: Gastrointestinal hormones. *In* Johnson LR, ed: Physiology of the Gastrointestinal Tract. New York, Raven Press, 1991, pp 181–254.
7. Daughaday WH, Rotwein P: Insulin-like growth factors I and II: Peptide, messenger ribonucleic acid and gene structures, serum, and tissue concentrations. Endocrinol Rev 1989; 10:68–91.
8. Westermark P, Wernstedt C, Wilannder E, et al: Amyloid fibrils in human insulinoma and islets of Langerhans of the diabetic cat are derived from a neuropeptide-like protein also present in normal cells. Proc Natl Acad Sci U S A 1987; 84:3881–3885.
9. Cooper GJ, Willis AC, Clark A, et al: Purification and characterization of a peptide from amyloid-rich pancreases of type-2 diabetic patients. Proc Natl Acad Sci U S A 1987; 84:8628–8632.
10. Gregory RA, Tracy HJ: The constitution and properties of two gastrins extracted from hog antral mucosa. Gut 1964; 5:103–117.
11. Gregory RA, Tracy HJ: The chemistry of the gastrins: Some recent advances. *In* Thompson JC, ed: Gastrointestinal Hormones. Austin, University of Texas Press, 1975, pp 13–24.
12. Eysselein V, Maxwell V, Reedy T, et al: Similar acid stimulatory potencies of synthetic human big and little gastrins in man. J Clin Invest 1984; 73:1284–1290.
13. Gregory H, Hardy PM, Jones DS, et al: Structure of gastrin. Nature 1964; 204:931–933.
14. Tracy HJ, Gregory RA: Physiological properties of a series of synthetic peptides structurally related to gastrin I. Nature 1964; 204:935–938.
15. Llanos O, Konturek S, Rayford P, et al: Pancreatic bicarbonate, serum gastrin, and secretin responses to meals varying in pH. Am J Physiol 1977; 233:E41–E46.
16. Mutt V, Jorpes J: Structure of porcine cholecystokinin-pancreozymin. Eur J Biochem 1968; 6:156–162.
17. Eysselein V, Reeve J Jr, Shively J, et al: Partial structure of a large canine cholecystokinin (CCK58): Amino acid sequence. Peptides 1982; 3:687–691.
18. Eberlein GA, Eysselein VE, Goebell H: Cholecystokinin-58 is the major molecular form in man, dog and cat but not in pig, beef and rat intestine. Peptides 1988; 9:993–998.
19. Villanueva M, Collins S, Jensen R, et al: Structural requirements for action of cholecystokinin on enzyme secretion from pancreatic acini. Am J Physiol 1982; 242:G416–G422.
20. Mutt V, Jorpes J, Magnusson S: Structure of porcine secretin: The amino acid sequence. Eur J Biochem 1970; 15:513.
21. Makhlouf G, Bodanszky M, Fink M, et al: Pancreatic secretory activity of secretin 5-27 and substituted analogues. Gastroenterology 1978; 75:244–248.
22. Brown JC, Dryburgh JR: A gastric inhibitory polypeptide: The complete amino acid sequence. Can J Biochem 1971; 49:867–872.
23. Jornvall H, Carlquist M, Kwauk S, et al: Amino acid heterogeneity of gastric inhibitory polypeptide (GIP). FEBS Lett 1981; 123: 205–209.
24. Sarson DL, Bryant MG, Bloom SR: A radioimmunoassay for gastric inhibitory polypeptide in human plasma. J Endocrinol 1980; 85:487–496.
25. Brown JC, Dryburgh JR, Ross S, et al: Identification and actions of gastric inhibitory polypeptide. Recent Prog Horm Res 1975; 31:487–532.
26. Brown JC, Cook MA, Dryburgh JR: Motilin, a gastric motor activity stimulating polypeptide: The complete amino acid sequence. Can J Biochem 1973; 51:533–537.
27. Christofides ND, Bryant MG, Ghatei MA, et al: Molecular forms of motilin in the mammalian and human gut and human plasma. Gastroenterology 1981; 80:292–300.
28. Carraway R, Leeman SE: The isolation of a new hypotensive peptide, neurotensin, from bovine hypothalami. J Biol Chem 1973; 248:6854–6861.
29. Theodorsson-Norheim E, Rosell S: Characterization of human plasma neurotensin-like immunoreactivity after fat ingestion. Regul Pept 1983; 6:207–218.
30. Lee YC, Allen JM, Uttenthal LO, et al: Quantitation and characterization of human plasma neurotensin-like immunoreactivity in response to a meal. Dig Dis Sci 1985; 30:129–133.
31. Unger RH, Ketterer H, Eisentraut AM: Distribution of immunoassayable glucagon in gastrointestinal tissues. Metabolism 1966; 15:865–867.
32. Ghatei MA, Bloom SR: Enteroglucagon in man. *In* Bloom SR, Polak JM, eds: Gut Hormones. Vol 2. Edinburgh, Churchill Livingstone, 1981, pp 332–338.
33. Patzelt C, Chiltz E: Conversion of proglucagon in pancreatic alpha cells: The major endproducts are glucagon and a single peptide, the major proglucagon fragment, that contains two glucagonlike sequences. Proc Natl Acad Sci U S A 1984; 81:5007–5011.
34. Holst J: Molecular heterogeneity of glucagon in normal subjects and in patients with glucagon-producing tumours. Diabetologia 1983; 24:359–365.
35. Floyd J, Fajans S, Pek S, et al: A newly recognized pancreatic polypeptide. Plasma levels in health and disease. Recent Prog Horm Res 1977; 33:519–570.
36. Tatemoto K, Mutt V: Isolation of two novel candidate hormones using a chemical method for finding naturally occurring polypeptides. Nature 1980; 285:417–418.
37. Servin AL, Rouyer Fessars C, Laburthe M, et al: PYY and NPY inhibit VIP-stimulated cAMP production in rat small intestine: Structural requirements of peptides for interacting with PYY-preferring receptors. Endocrinology 1989; 124:692–700.
38. Brazeau P, Guillemin R: Somatostatin: Newcomer from the hypothalamus. N Engl J Med 1974; 290:963–964.
39. Pradayrol L, Jornvall H, Mutt V, et al: N-terminally extended somatostatin: The primary structure of somatostatin-28. FEBS Lett 1980; 109:55–58.
40. O'Donnell LJD, Farthing MJG: Therapeutic potential of a long-acting somatostatin analogue in gastrointestinal disease. Gut 1989; 30:1165–1172.
41. Bryant MG, Bloom SR: Distribution of the gut hormones in the primate intestinal tract. Gut 1979; 20:653–659.
42. Yamada T: Local regulatory actions of gastrointestinal peptides. *In* Johnson LR, ed: Physiology of the Gastrointestinal Tract. New York, Raven Press, 1986, pp 131–142.
43. Polak JM, Sullivan SN, Bloom SR, et al: Specific localisation of neurotensin to the N cell in human intestine by radioimmunoassay and immunocytochemistry. Nature 1977; 270:183–184.
44. Bottcher G, Sjolund K, Ekblad E, et al: Coexistence of peptide YY and glicentin immunoreactivity in endocrine cells of the gut. Regul Pept 1984; 8:261–266.
45. Adrian TE, Ferri GL, Bacarese-Hamilton AJ, et al: Human distribution and release of a putative new gut hormone, peptide YY. Gastroenterology 1985; 89:1070–1077.
46. Adrian TE, Bloom SR, Bryant MG, et al: Distribution and release of human pancreatic polypeptide. Gut 1976; 17: 940–944.
47. McGuigan J, Isaza J, Landor J: Relationships of gastrin dose, serum gastrin, and acid secretion. Gastroenterology 1971; 61:659–666.
48. Walsh JH, Grossman MI: Medical progress: Gastrin. N Engl J Med 1975; 292:1324–1332.
49. Johnson LR: Regulation of gastrointestinal growth. *In* Johnson LR, ed: Physiology of the Gastrointestinal Tract. 2nd ed. New York, Raven Press, 1987, pp 301–333.
50. Green DM, Bishop AE, Rindi G, et al: Enterochromaffin-like cell populations in human fundic mucosa: Quantitative studies of their variations with age, sex, and plasma gastrin levels. J Pathol 1989; 157:235–241.
51. Schaffalitzky De Muckadell O, Fahrenkrug J: Secretion pattern of secretin in man: Regulation by gastric acid. Gut 1978; 19:812–818.
52. O'Rourke MF, Reidelberger RD, Solomon TE: Effect of CCK antagonist L 364,718 on meal-induced pancreatic secretion in rats. Am J Physiol 1990; 258:G179–G184.
53. Liddle R, Goldfine I, Rosen M, et al: Cholecystokinin bioactivity in human plasma: Molecular forms, responses to feeding, and relationship to gallbladder contraction. J Clin Invest 1985; 75:1144–1152.

54. Peterson H, Solomon T, Grossman M: Effect of chronic pentagastrin, cholecystokinin, and secretin on pancreas of rats. Am J Physiol 1978; 234:E286–E293.
55. Vantrappen G, Janssens J, Peeters TL, et al: Motilin and the interdigestive migrating motor complex in man. Dig Dis Sci 1979; 24:497–500.
56. Christofides ND, Modlin IM, Fitzpatrick ML, et al: Effect of motilin on the rate of gastric emptying and gut hormone release during breakfast. Gastroenterology 1979; 76:903–907.
57. Depoortere I, Peeters TL, Vantrappen G: The erythromycin derivative EM-523 is a potent motilin agonist in man and in rabbit. Peptides 1990; 11:515–519.
58. Dupré J, Ross SA, Watson D, et al: Stimulation of insulin secretion by gastric inhibitory peptide in man. J Clin Endocrinol 1973; 37:826–827.
59. Sarson DL, Wood SM, Holder D, et al: The effect of glucose-dependent insulinotropic polypeptide infused at physiological concentrations on the release of insulin in man. Diabetologia 1982; 22:33–36.
60. Kreyman B, Ghatei MA, Williams G, et al: Glucagon-like peptide-I 7-36: A physiological incretin in man. Lancet 1987; 2:1300–1304.
61. Greenberg GR, McCloy RF, Adrian TE, et al: Inhibition of pancreas and gallbladder by pancreatic polypeptide. Lancet 1978; 2:1280–1282.
62. Mashford ML, Nilsson G, Rokaeus A, et al: The effect of food ingestion on circulating neurotensin-like immunoreactivity in the human. Acta Physiol Scand 1976; 104: 244–246.
63. Blackburn AM, Fletcher DR, Bloom SR, et al: Effect of neurotensin on gastrin function. Lancet 1980; 1:987–989.
64. Fletcher DR, Blackburn AM, Adrian TE, et al: Effect of neurotensin on pancreatic function in man. Life Sci 1981; 29:2157–2161.
65. Conlon JM: Proglucagon-derived peptides: Nomenclature, biosynthetic relationships, and physiological roles. Diabetologia 1988; 31:563–566.
66. Sagor GR, Al Mukhtarr MYJ, Ghatei MA, et al: The effect of altered luminal nutrition on cellular proliferation and plasma concentrations of enteroglucagon and gastrin after small bowel resection in the rat. Br J Surg 1982; 69:14–18.
67. Bloom SR: An enteroglucagon tumour. Gut 1972; 13:520–523.
68. Adrian TE, Savage AJ, Sagor GR, et al: Effect of peptide YY on gastric, pancreatic and biliary function in humans. Gastroenterology 1985; 89:494–499.
69. Savage AP, Adrian TE, Carolan G, et al: Effects of peptide YY (PYY) on mouth to cecum transit time and on the rate of gastric emptying in healthy volunteers. Gut 1987; 70:166–170.
70. Playford RJ, Domin J, Beacham J, et al: Preliminary report: Role of peptide YY in defence against diarrhoea. Lancet 1990; 335:1555–1557.
71. Buchan AMJ, Bryant MG, Polak JM, et al: Development of regulatory peptides in the human fetal intestine. *In* Bloom SR, Polak JM, eds: Gut Hormones. New York, Churchill Livingstone 1981, pp 119–124.
72. Bryant MG, Buchan AMJ, Gregor M, et al: Development of intestinal regulatory peptides in the human fetus. Gastroenterology 1982; 83:47–51.
73. Ah-Rachedi A, Vamdell I, Adrian TE, et al: Peptide YY (PYY) immunoreactivity is costored with glucagon-related immunoreactants in endocrine cells of the gut and pancreas. Histochemistry 1984; 80:487–491.
74. Aynsley-Green A: The adaptation of the human neonate to extrauterine nutrition: A pre-requisite for postnatal growth. *In* Cochburn F, ed: Fetal and Neonatal Growth. New York, John Wiley & Sons, 1988, pp 153–193.
75. Mulvihill SJ, Stone MM, Fonkalsrud EW, et al: Trophic effect of amniotic fluid on fetal gastrointestinal development. J Surg Res 1986; 40:291–296.
76. Lucas A, Bloom SR, Aynsley-Green A: Development of gut hormone responses to feeding in neonates. Arch Dis Child 1980; 55:678–682.
77. Lucas A, Adrian TE, Christofides ND, et al: Plasma motilin, gastrin and enteroglucagon and feeding in the human newborn. Arch Dis Child 1980; 55:673–677.
78. Euler AP, Byrne WJ, Cousins LM, et al: Increased serum gastrin concentrations and gastric hyposecretion in the immediate newborn period. Gastroenterology 1977; 72:1271–1273.
79. Rogers IM, Davidson DC, Lawrence J, et al: Neonatal secretion of gastrin and glucagon. Arch Dis Child 1974; 49:796–806.
80. Aynsley-Green A, Lucas A, Bloom SR: The effects of feeds of differing composition on entero-insular hormone secretion in the first hours of life in human neonates. Acta Pediatr Scand 1979; 68:265–270.
81. Lucas A, Bloom SR, Aynsley-Green A: Postnatal surges in plasma gut hormones in term and preterm infants. Biol Neonate 1982; 41:63–67.
82. Miller BA: Observations on the gastric acidity during the first month of life. Arch Dis Child 1941; 16:22–30.
83. Ahn CI, Kim KJ: Acidity and volume of gastric contents in the first week of life. J Korean Med Assoc 1963; 6:948–950.
84. Malloy MH, Morris FH, Denson SE, et al: Neonatal gastric motility in dogs: Maturation and response to pentagastrin. Am J Physiol 1979; 236:E562–E566.
85. Adrian TE, Smith HA, Calvert SA, et al: Elevated plasma peptide YY in human neonates and infants. Pediatr Res 1986; 20:1225–1227.
86. Lucas A, Adrian TE, Bloom SR, et al: Plasma secretin in neonates. Acta Pediatr Scand 1980; 69:205–210.
87. Calvert SA, Soltesz G, Jenkins PA, et al: Feeding premature infants with human milk or preterm milk formula: Effects on postnatal growth, intermediary metabolism and regulatory peptides. Biol Neonate 1985; 47:189–198.
88. Joekel CS, Herrington MK, Vanderhoof JA, et al: Are surges of plasma CCK and secretin responsible for pancreatic development in neonatal guinea pigs? Physiologist 1990; 33:117A.
89. Pollack PF, Wood JG, Solomon TE: Effect of secretin on growth of stomach, small intestine, and pancreas of developing rats. Dig Dis Sci 1990; 35:749–758.
90. Herrington MK, Joekel CS, Mohamadpour H, et al: Effect of epidermal growth factor on neonatal pancreatic growth. Gastroenterology 1991; 100:A645.
91. Berseth CL: Gestational evolution of small intestine motility in preterm and term infants. J Pediatr 1989; 115: 646–651.
92. Sperling N: Integration of fuel homeostatis by insulin and glucagon in the newborn. Monogr Pediatr 1982; 16:39–58.
93. Lucas A, Sarson DL, Bloom SR, et al: Developmental aspects of gastric inhibitory polypeptide (GIP) and its possible role in the enteroinsular axis in neonates. Acta Paediatr Scand 1980; 69:321–325.
94. Lucas A, Adrian TE, Bloom SR, et al: Plasma pancreatic polypeptide in the human neonate. Acta Paediatr Scand 1980; 69:211–214.
95. Lucas A, Aynsley-Green A, Blackburn AN, et al: Plasma neurotensin in term and preterm neonates. Acta Paediatr Scand 1981; 17:201–206.
96. Lucas A, Bloom SR, Aynsley-Green A: Metabolic and endocrine consequences of depriving preterm infants of enteral nutrition. Acta Pediatr Scand 1983; 72:245–249.
97. Aynsley-Green A, Lucas A, Bloom SR: The effects of feeds of differing composition on entero-insular hormone secretion in the first hours of life in human neonates. Acta Paediatr Scand 1979; 68:265–270.
98. Lucas A, Adrian TE, Sarson DL, et al: Breast vs bottle: Endocrine responses are different with formula feeding. Lancet 1980; 1:1267–1269.
99. Adrian TE, Bloom SR: Effect of food on the hormones of the gastrointestinal tract. *In* Hunter JO, Jones V, eds: Food and the Gut. Philadelphia, Bailliere-Tindall, 1985, pp 13–29.
100. Beardshall K, Frost G, Morarji Y, et al: Saturation of fat and cholecystokinin release: Implications for pancreatic carcinogenesis. Lancet 1989; 2:1008–1010.
101. Isaacs PET, Ladas S, Forgacs IC, et al: A comparison of the effects of ingested medium- and long-chain triglyceride on gallbladder volume and the release of cholecystokinin and other gut peptides. Dig Dis Sci 1987; 32:481–486.
102. Widdowson EM: Development of the digestive system: Comparative animal studies. Am J Clin Nutr 1985; 41:384–390.
103. Gale SM, Read LC, George-Nascimento C, et al: Is dietary epidermal growth factor absorbed by premature human infants? Biol Neonate 1989; 55:104–110.

104. Koldovsky O: Is breast-milk epidermal growth factor biologically active in the suckling? Nutrition 1989; 5:223–225.
105. Berseth CL, Michener SR, Nordyke CK, et al: Postpartum changes in pattern of gastrointestinal regulatory peptides in human milk. Am J Clin Nutr 1990; 51:985–990.
106. Gornacz GE, Ghatei MA, Al-Mukhtar MYT, et al: Plasma enteroglucagon and CCK levels and cell proliferation in defunctioned small bowel in the rat. Dig Dis Sci 1984; 29:1041–1049.
107. Aynsley-Green A, Adrian TE, Bloom SR: Feeding and the development of enteroinsular hormone secretion in the preterm infant: Effects of continuous gastric infusions of human milk compared with intermittent boluses. Acta Paediatr Scand 1982; 71:379–383.
108. Salmenpera L, Perheentupa J, Siimes MA, et al: Effects of feeding regimen on blood glucose levels and plasma concentrations of pancreatic hormones and gut regulatory peptides at nine months of age: Comparison between infants fed with milk formula and infants exclusively breast-fed from birth. J Pediatr Gastroenterol Nutr 1988; 7:651–656.
109. Lucas A, Bloom SR, Aynsley-Green A: Gut hormones and "minimal enteral feeding." Acta Paediatr Scand 1986; 75:719–723.
110. Gounaris A, Antolitou F, Costalos C, et al: Minimal enteral feeding, nasojejunal feeding and gastrin levels in premature infants. Acta Paediatr Scand 1990; 79:226–227.
111. Besterman HS, Bloom SR, Sarson DL, et al: Gut-hormone profile in coeliac disease. Lancet 1978; 1:785–788.
112. Calam J, Ellis A, Dockray G: Identification and measurement of molecular variants of cholecystokinin in duodenal mucosa and plasma. J Clin Invest 1982; 69:218–225.
113. Domschke S, Bloom SR, Adrian TE, et al: Coeliac sprue: Abnormalities of the hormone profile of gastroduodenal mucosa. Scand J Gastroenterol 1989; 24(Suppl 167): 86–88.
114. Adrian TE, Savage AP, Bacarese-Hamilton AJ, et al: Peptide YY abnormalities in gastrointestinal disease. Gastroenterology 1986; 90:379–384.
115. Adrian TE, McKiernan J, Johnstone DI, et al: Hormonal abnormalities of the pancreas and gut in cystic fibrosis. Gastroenterology 1980; 79:460–465.
116. Allen JM, Penketh ARL, Adrian TE, et al: Adult cystic fibrosis: Postprandial response of gut regulatory peptides. Gastroenterology 1983; 85:1379–1383.
117. Besterman HS, Christofides ND, Welsby PD, et al: Gut hormones in acute diarrhea. Gut 1983; 24:665–671.
118. Lawson GR, Nelson R, Laker MF, et al: Gut regulatory peptides and intestinal permeability in acute infantile gastroenteritis. Arch Dis Child 1992; 67:272–276.
119. Aynsley-Green A, Lucas A, Lawson GR, et al: Gut hormones and regulatory peptides in relation to enteral feeding, gastroenteritis, and necrotizing enterocolitis in infancy. Arch Dis Child 1990; 117:S24–S32.
120. Adrian TE, Savage AP, Fuessl HS, et al: Release of peptide YY (PYY) after resection of small bowel, colon or pancreas in man. Surgery 1987; 101:715–719.
121. Besterman HS, Adrian TE, Mallinson CN, et al: Gut hormone release after intestinal resection. Gut 1982; 23:854–861.
122. Armstrong DN, Ballantyne GH, Adrian TE, et al: Adaptive increase in peptide YY and enteroglucagon after proctocolectomy and pelvic ileal reservoir reconstruction. Dis Colon Rectum 1991; 34:119–125.
123. Besterman HS, Mallinson CN, Modigliani R, et al: Gut hormones in inflammatory bowel disease. Scand J Gastroenterol 1983; 18:845–852.
124. Lucas A, Cristofides ND, Adrian TE, et al: Fetal distress, meconium, and motilin. Lancet 1979; 1:718–719.
125. Lothe L, Ivarsson SA, Lindberg T: Motilin, vasoactive intestinal polypeptide, and gastrin in infantile colic. Acta Paediatr Scand 1987; 76:316–320.
126. Lothe L, Ivarsson SA, Ekman R, et al: Motilin and infantile colic: A prospective study. Acta Paediatr Scand 1990; 79:410–416.
127. Leung YK, Lebenthal E: Gastrointestinal peptides: Physiology, ontogeny, and clinical significance. *In* Lebenthal E, ed: Human Gastrointestinal Development. New York, Raven Press, 1989, pp 41–98.
128. Morley JE: Appetite regulation: The role of peptides and hormones. J Endocrinol Invest 1989; 12:135–147.

Section Two

CLINICAL SIGNS AND SYMPTOMS

Chapter 9

Eating Disorders and Obesity

ANN MILANESE

EATING DISORDERS

Definitions

Eating disorders represent an important health challenge to those clinicians caring for adolescents. Partially responsible for this challenge are impossible standards for achievement presented by society and the media to an uncertain, vulnerable population. The consequences are dire and include short-term catastrophes, such as sudden death, suicide, and severe psychological maladjustment. The long-term impact of chronic food deprivation, medication and exercise abuse, and enormous weight fluctuation includes poorly regulated metabolism and an increased risk of osteoporosis. Impaired interpersonal relationships also result from the chronic disruption of social and developmental adjustment. Early recognition and aggressive, balanced treatment can alleviate some of the misery brought about by extended self-abuse.

The term *eating disorders* includes anorexia nervosa and bulimia nervosa, which occur in adolescence, and pica and rumination disorder of infancy. As is done in this chapter, obesity is often considered with eating disorders. However, simple obesity is more accurately viewed as a physical condition rather than primarily as a psychological disturbance. No specific psychiatric diagnosis or psychodynamic description is uniquely associated with childhood obesity. Family members and health professionals may unwittingly reinforce eating-disordered behavior and the resulting weight loss in the sedentary, slightly overweight adolescent.

The American Psychiatric Association[1] publishes specific diagnostic criteria for anorexia nervosa and bulimia nervosa (Tables 9–1 and 9–2).

Anorexia nervosa is characterized by certain essential features, which include (1) a refusal to maintain body weight over a minimal normal weight for age and height, with 15% weight loss or weight below expected; (2) intense fear of gaining weight or becoming fat; (3) disturbance in the experience of one's body weight, size, or shape (distortion of body image); and (4) in females, amenorrhea for at least three consecutive cycles. (Note that amenorrhea is the correct label even if menstrual periods do occur but only after hormone administration.)

Although the primary mechanism for weight loss in anorexia nervosa is usually caloric restriction, starvation may be compounded by hyperactivity and intensive exercising. The physical symptoms and signs as well as behavioral characteristics, such as preoccupation with food preparation, closely mimic those found in patients subjected to starvation.[2] People with anorexia nervosa tend to deny or minimize the severity of their malnutrition. Delays in psychosexual behavioral development and compulsive behaviors, such as hand washing, may coexist with anorexia nervosa.

The diagnostic criteria for bulimia nervosa are (1) recurrent episodes of binge eating (a binge is defined as rapid consumption of a large amount of food in a discrete time period); (2) a perceived lack of control over eating during binges; (3) regular purging through self-induced vomiting, laxatives, or diuretics, strict dieting or fasting, or vigorous exercise to prevent weight gain; (4) a minimum average of two binge-eating episodes a week for at least 3 months; and (5) persistent overconcern with body shape and weight.

People with bulimia nervosa often report feeling that their life is dominated by guilt, shame, and conflictual feelings about eating.[3] There is no typical weight profile; bulimic patients may be underweight, normal, or overweight, and they may experience great fluctuations in their weight during the course of their illness. People with bulimia are prone to other disinhibited behaviors, including substance abuse, sexual promiscuity, and self-mutilation. Some authors note a history of childhood

Table 9–1. DIAGNOSTIC CRITERIA FOR ANOREXIA NERVOSA

Refusal to maintain minimal normal body weight (15% below expected)
Intense fear of obesity
Body image disturbance
Amenorrhea for three consecutive cycles

Adapted from American Psychiatric Association: Diagnostic and Statistical Manual of Mental Disorders, Third Edition, Revised. Washington, DC, American Psychiatric Association, 1987, pp 65–69; with permission.

Table 9–2. DIAGNOSTIC CRITERIA FOR BULIMIA NERVOSA

Recurrent episodes of binge eating
Perceived lack of control during binges
Purgative behaviors
Two binges per week for at least 3 months
Preoccupation with body shape and weight

Adapted from American Psychiatric Association: Diagnostic and Statistical Manual of Mental Disorders, Third Edition, Revised. Washington, DC, American Psychiatric Association, 1987, pp 65–69; with permission.

sexual or physical abuse in as many as 66% of bulimic patients. This supports the conceptualization of bulimia as a symptom of loss of control.[4]

Although anorexia nervosa and bulimia nervosa are defined as two distinct entities, approximately 47% of food-restricting anorectic patients experience bulimic symptoms at some point.[5] Behavioral differences among the patients are noted, such that fasting patients tend to be introverted, denying physical or psychological distress and bulimic patients, a slightly older group, are more extroverted and claim somatic distress as well as guilt, depression, and anxiety.

Prevalence and Predisposition

Historical accounts of eating disorders date back at least to 895 A.D.[6] What previously may have been a medical curiosity has assumed the proportions of an epidemic over the past 25 years. Prevalence studies for anorexia nervosa[7] indicate that it occurs in as many as 5 to 10% of females within the peak ages of 12 to 18 years. Because the age at onset of bulimia nervosa is slightly older, studies of this disorder focus on college students and indicate prevalence figures of 4.5[8] to 18%[9] for females. One to five percent of people with eating disorders are males. Many authors describe characteristics of presentation and family history and dynamics that are *not* gender specific.[10] However, Yager and associates[11] report a higher prevalence of certain eating-disordered behaviors, including binges, intense fear of fat, and diuretic abuse, in homosexual male students compared with heterosexual male students.

Fifty to seventy percent of high school girls describe themselves as "being on a diet,"[12, 13] whereas only about 15% are actually overweight. On a self-report measure of binging tendencies, 79% of female undergraduates reported episodes of eating that seem out of control.[14] Schwartz and associates[15] found that 10% of females at a private coeducational college used self-induced vomiting as a means of weight control.

Given the intense pressure for and high value of thinness in our society, the demarcation between "normal" weight preoccupation and dieting and symptomatic eating disorders is not distinct. Garner and associates[16] reported on this phenomenon in 1984 and cautioned for extreme perspicacity in the evaluation of persons suspected of having eating disorders. He concluded that certain hallmarks of ego or personality function must be present for the diagnosis of anorexia nervosa to be established. These were differentiated on the Eating Disorders Inventory[17] on the subscales involving "ineffectiveness," "interpersonal distrust," and "lack of interoceptive awareness." The remaining five subscales on the inventory are "drive for thinness," "bulimia," "body dissatisfaction," "perfectionism," and "maturity fears." With the exception of bulimia, the remaining four characteristics occur sufficiently often in the adolescent population to be viewed as statistically normal.

Differentiating normal from pathologic behaviors has been a source of great controversy and may account for the usage of additional designations such as "combined," "atypical," and "subclinical" eating disorders. Variations in type are complicated by differences in the definition of a "binge," which can vary from an unplanned apple for an anorectic to a bulimic's 4,000-cal extravaganza. These variations influence the results of prevalence studies.

Anorexia nervosa is common among sisters and mothers of anorectic patients. There is an increased frequency (53%) of major affective (mood) disorders, such as bipolar and manic-depressive illness and depression, among first-degree biologic relatives in both anorexia nervosa and bulimia nervosa.[18] Strober and associates[19] reported that 18% of first- and second-degree relatives of their eating-disordered patients had histories of alcoholism, and 13% had problems with substance abuse.

A combination of biologic, psychological, and social factors contributes to the evolution of an eating disorder.[20] Lucas[21] proposed using the biopsychosocial model to conceptualize the unique interplay of determinants for each patient. Predisposing factors include biologic, developmental, psychological, and social vulnerabilities, with no single area responsible for the "cause."

Pathogenetic Considerations

Self-starvation has fascinated the medical profession for many decades. In a landmark work, Keys and associates[2] described healthy, nonobese male volunteers who were placed on starvation regimens for several months and then refed. Detailed accounts of the subjects' behaviors during starvation depict relentless preoccupation with food, sexual apathy, and worsening selfishness. The observations provide an excellent resource for those people seeking human studies on both starvation and dietary-induced obesity.

Biologic Factors. Although a unifying physiologic mechanism that supports the genesis of eating disorders would be satisfying, it would be an oversimplification of what should be viewed as a multidetermined disorder. Most endocrinologic abnormalities documented in anorectic patients are distinguished not by the diagnosis of anorexia nervosa but by the presence of starvation. These abnormalities include elevated plasma cortisol and aldosterone, decreased insulin release, decreased gonadotropins and circulating norepinephrine, reduced levels of thyroxine and triiodothyronine, and inappropriate responses of growth hormone to stimulation by glucose, insulin, L-dopa, and the dopamine agonists apomorphine and bromocriptine. These have been postulated to result from diminished pituitary output secondary to some disruption in hypothalamic function.[22] Thus far, this disruption cannot be distinguished from that which occurs in simple starvation in concert with psychological stress. The irregularity in hypothalamic function and the low levels of circulating norepinephrine are believed to cause a decrease in appetite stimulation.

The majority of endocrine alterations documented in underweight eating-disordered patients revert to normal in the face of nutritional repletion.[23] Amenorrhea represents a possible exception, occurring prior to weight loss in 33 to 50% of patients with anorexia nervosa.[24] It occurs as a result of low (prepubertal) levels of luteinizing hormone, follicle-stimulating hormone, and gonadotropin-releasing hormone, apparently resulting from hypothalamic dysfunction. Frequently, weight gain alone does not ensure reinstatement of normal hypothalamic-pituitary-ovarian axis function.[23]

Males with anorexia nervosa may demonstrate a hypogonadotropic profile. They also manifest a predictable pattern of sexual apathy and impotence.[25]

Developmental Factors. Some aspects of adolescent body dissatisfaction and belief in the efficacy of dieting are normative and typical of the developmental stage. The prevalence of dieting in high school girls is 50 to 70%,[26] but especially among high school girls in grade 9 or above, the presence of low self-esteem in body image and social relations may differentiate normal from pathologic dieting.[27] Other individual psychological indicators of risk include deficient ego (self) identity and autonomy and lack of distinction in defining self and body.

Eating disorders interrupt the developmental process. The longer they actively persist, the more difficult it becomes for the patients to re-enter their peer group. They have missed transitional social experiences and must re-enter a peer group that may be more advanced, experimenting with sex or drugs and alcohol. In a survey of college students, 27% of those with bulimia nervosa cite "abuse" of alcohol or drugs compared with 36% of control subjects.[8] Unprepared for age-appropriate social and emotional challenges, patients may cling to eating-disordered behaviors that have come to constitute the core of their identity.

Familial Factors. Certain characteristics of family functioning are noted in families with eating disorders. It remains unclear whether these characteristics are primary or secondary. In anorexia nervosa, family patterns resemble patterns noted in families stressed by psychosomatic problems and other chronic illnesses. Minuchin and colleagues' description of the psychosomatic family[28] included elements of enmeshment, overprotectiveness, rigidity, and poor conflict resolution. Enmeshment applies in either direction, that is, the parent's overinvolvement in the child's world or the "adultification" of a child in the parent's world. These are the children who are treated as peers by their parent. Enmeshment with one parent may often coexist with physical or emotional distance from the other parent. Inadequate conflict resolution becomes particularly problematic when the family is required to incorporate the changing identity of an adolescent child.

Bulimic patients may have a different family experience than do anorectic patients. Typically, they experience a lack of nurturance and structure and a greater degree of overt conflict and disorganization. In keeping with the biopsychosocial model, the family cannot be implicated as the sole "cause" of an eating disorder. It can possibly be viewed as a source of significant stress and also as remiss in engendering in a child the skills necessary to cope with the challenges of maturity. This environment may accentuate the three personality features noted by Johnson and Connors[29] to be consistently present in bulimic patients: (1) behavioral self-regulatory problems; (2) social discomfort and fear of rejection; and (3) a high desire for achievement, expressed through pursuit of thinness.

Sociocultural Factors. The work of Garfinkel and Garner[30] documents the idealization of thinness that has dominated our culture and the media over the past two decades. Unrealistic standards that are incompatible with a healthy lifestyle have been set. In pursuit of perfection, anything short of these standards is defined as inadequacy. Obsession with thinness symbolizes both the feminine physical ideal and the moral virtue of self-control. This is evident in all the advertising media, but its promotion on television is of the most concern because the average American youngster views 22 to 25 hours per week.[31] This annually exceeds the time spent in the classroom! By the time this child graduates from high school, he or she will have spent 15,000 hours in front of the television and will have seen approximately 350,000 commercial messages.[32] The models in television commercials are thinner than the general population,[33] in spite of the fact that most of the foods they advertise are high–caloric density products, including non-nutritive snacks, fast foods, and sweetened cereals.[34] Popular magazines typically juxtapose articles on diet and exercise with calorically dense recipes.

Comerci[35] describes a group of adolescents and young adolescents who engage in "body-focused" activities, such as modeling, dancing, track athletics, gymnastics, and wrestling. These are examples of pursuits that focus on optimal body type and extremes of self-discipline and that may be associated with the development of eating-disorders. The tendency for these behaviors may also be encouraged or perpetuated by coaches, teachers, and other authority figures. A well-known example is George Ballanchine, the ballet master whose standards virtually demanded eating-disordered behavior of his dancers.

Medical Aspects of Diagnosis

Unlike other malnourished patients, such as those with cancer or inflammatory bowel disease, the eating-disordered population has no underlying digestive or absorptive pathology.

It is useful to divide the objective medical assessment

Table 9–3. GOALS OF OBJECTIVE ASSESSMENT

Assess current health and nutritional status
Assess effects of starvation or malnutrition
Assess effects of self-destructive behaviors
Consider differential diagnosis (see Table 9–4)

into four areas (Table 9–3). Questions and observations may overlap, but organizing thought processes around target areas helps minimize the chances of overlooking important information.

The goals of objective assessment include identifying current health and nutritional status and evaluating and documenting the effects of short-term starvation and more chronic malnutrition. Self-destructive behaviors present in eating disorders are myriad and can impact virtually every organ system. Careful consideration must also be given to the differential diagnosis (Table 9–4), because overlooking organic pathology might have catastrophic results.

In addition to documenting a patient's condition, the goal of objective medical assessment is to bridge denial and to help patients and their families realize the extent of physical impairment experienced as a result of the eating disorder. The clinical mandate is for an exhaustively thorough evaluation without wasting time, energy, and money on unnecessary diagnostic maneuvers.

Evaluation of the current nutritional status provides a sense of protein stores (condition of skin, hair, and nails) and energy stores as well as body weight compared with the usual and the ideal. These young women often appear well turned out and fashionably dressed. This may contradict or mask a state of malnutrition, particularly if extensive denial clouds the history. Therefore, one must look beyond the material trappings of fashion and prosperity to seek objective physical evidence of protein-calorie malnutrition. Acute starvation in an obese or formerly obese patient may not present as cachexia. However, serious physiologic consequences of starvation, including weakness, decreased initiative, apathy, and depression, may be present and may complicate making an accurate psychiatric diagnosis.

Self-destructive behaviors include vomiting and abuse of drugs, such as laxatives, diuretics, stimulants, hormones, and steroids. Daily laxative abuse has been reported in 3 to 25% of bulimic patients and less frequently than daily in 12 to 30%; therefore, it occurs in as many as 55% of patients with bulimia nervosa.[36] Other self-destructive behaviors include compulsive exercising and more obvious self-inflicted injuries, such as cutting, burning, or scratching.

Table 9–4. DIFFERENTIAL DIAGNOSES

Cancer
Pregnancy
Inflammatory bowel disease
Thyroid disease
Central nervous system disorders
Drug abuse

Careful differential diagnostic consideration is critical because the failure to identify other organic disorders may have dire consequences. Szmukler and Russell[37] have reported on diabetic patients who withheld insulin to prevent glucose metabolism. We have encountered one patient with cystic fibrosis who avoids pancreatic enzymes to induce fat malabsorption.

History Taking

The medical history should be taken in a supportive and nonjudgmental fashion. Adolescents and young adults are more likely to cooperate with history taking if they are given an explanation of why a particular question is being asked. The medical history should address areas specifically related to eating disorder symptoms. It should define the current symptoms in detail and elicit a description of any complications or conditions that may occur in association with the eating disorder. The patient should be questioned directly concerning dietary intake, binging, purging, exercise, and body image. Sample questions are found in Table 9–5.

Besides obtaining information about the onset, duration, and frequency of symptoms, the review of systems should include specific questions regarding changes in hair, skin, nails, teeth, and gums. Patients should also be asked about headaches, visual problems, and changes

Table 9–5. SPECIFIC QUESTIONING

Dietary Intake
What do you eat for breakfast?
What do you eat for lunch? dinner?
Do you eat meals, or do you "graze"?
What do you drink? How much?
What foods don't you eat? Why not?
Binging
Do you ever eat large amounts at one time?
What is the most you remember eating at one time?
Describe a typical "binge."
Have you ever started eating and felt unable to stop?
How often do binges occur?
Purging
Have you ever made yourself throw up?
How do you do it?
Have you ever used ipecac?
Have you ever thrown up blood or coffee ground–like material?
Have you ever taken laxatives or enemas, diuretics, hormones, or stimulants to lose weight?
Exercise
Do you get any regular form of exercise?
Do you belong to a health club?
Do you walk? jog? run?
Do you do calisthenics? aerobics?
Do you exercise in the late afternoon or early morning?
Have you ever taken steroids or manipulated your diet to develop your muscles?
What would you do if you broke your hip and could not exercise?
Body Image
Do you feel your current weight is too high, too low, or just right?
Would you like to gain or lose weight?
How much weight would you like to lose?
What clothing size would you like to be?
What part of your body is too heavy?

Table 9–6. SPECIFIC AREAS OF MEDICAL HISTORY

Textural changes in hair, skin, and nails
Hair loss
Teeth or gum problems
Headaches
Light-headedness, dizziness, fainting, blackouts
Heart palpitations, skipped beats, pulse racing
Vomiting of blood or coffee ground material
Abdominal pain
Change in stool character; constipation or diarrhea
Irregular or absent menses
Cold intolerance
Cold, blue, mottled extremities
Edema, bruisability

in alertness or cardiovascular function. Because of the risks inherent in vomiting, evidence should be sought for gastrointestinal bleeding and changes in stool pattern. The menstrual history should focus on irregular or absent menses and abnormalities in sexual function, such as loss of libido or dyspareunia. The musculoskeletal review should note complaints of cold extremities or changes in color, edema, and bruisability (Table 9–6).

Physical Examination and Nutritional Assessment

Nutritional status is best documented by a combination of objective measurements and the examiner's clinical impression. Anthropometrics, including height, weight, skin fold thickness, and arm muscle circumference measurements, allow documentation at a point in time. These measurements can be compared with established norms or with any previous values obtained on the patient. Patients may resort to spurious means of increasing weight, such as water and salt loading (consuming enormous quantities of water and shakers full of salt), inserting weighted objects into pockets or body orifices, and readjusting scales. More subjective indicators of nutritional status include the condition of the subcutaneous tissue and skin and hair quality. The rate of hair growth can be estimated by looking at the unprocessed roots in patients who color or "perm" their hair, noting a "normal" rate of about 1/2 inch per month.

Indicators of malnutrition include pallid skin; dry, brittle hair and nails; and the presence of superficial infections. Measurements of temperature, pulse, and blood pressure should be obtained. Look for evidence of bradycardia, orthostatic change, or hypothermia. Careful scrutiny should be given to the heart rate and rhythm. The abdominal examination should focus on the presence of fecal masses, an indicator of constipation. Examination of the extremities includes checking for edema and poor perfusion. The spine examination includes a careful inspection for the presence of scoliosis.

Self-destructive behaviors include vomiting, abuse of drugs, compulsive exercising, and self-inflicted injury. Oral mucosal lesions, dental enamel erosion, subconjunctival hemorrhage, or parotid swelling signal excessive vomiting. Calluses may be seen on the dorsal surface of the hand from traumatic contact with incisors when inducing vomiting. Mental status may be affected by drug abuse. Excessive exercise can manifest as joint swelling or the sacral decubiti that occur when thin persons perform extraordinary numbers of sit-ups. Examples of self-inflicted injury are slashes, scratches, or burns.

Consider differential diagnostic possibilities by looking for evidence of increased intracranial pressure and checking for breast or abdominal masses, lymphadenopathy, thyromegaly, or focal neuropathy.

Diagnostic Studies

Laboratory evaluations should be selected based on the index of suspicion generated from the history and physical examination of the individual patient. If purging behaviors are present, electrolytes, blood urea nitrogen, creatinine, and urine specific gravity are helpful, as the results might reflect hypokalemia, chronic metabolic alkalosis or acidosis, and dehydration. Dilutional hyponatremia or hypernatremia may occur from water or salt loading, respectively. If drug abuse is suspected, a toxicology screen should be obtained. Frequent vomiting or excessive use of laxatives (particularly those of the stimulant or irritant type) should prompt examination of the stool for occult blood.

Overall nutritional status can be evaluated by measuring total protein, albumin, and transferrin and calcium, phosphorus, and magnesium. Because of shorter half-lives, serum prealbumin and retinol-binding protein indicate a more immediate protein nutrition status.[38]

The complete blood count can document the effects of starvation or malnutrition. The hemoglobin level and hematocrit as well as absolute leukocyte and lymphocyte count may be decreased. Serum iron level and total iron-binding capacity reflect iron status with or without anemia.

In malnourished patients, skin testing frequently demonstrates anergy, or impaired cell-mediated immunity.[39] In amenorrheic patients, the hypothalamic-pituitary-ovarian axis can be assessed by luteinizing hormone, follicle-stimulating hormone, and estradiol. Amenorrheic exercise abusers with prepubertal levels of gonadatropins and estradiol are at risk for stress fractures. Bone densitometry may be helpful in defining the potential risks associated with high-impact exercise.[40]

Severely malnourished patients should have an electrocardiogram (ECG) with a rhythm strip. Cardiac changes can be structural, functional, and electrical. Structural cardiac changes include left ventricular wall thinning evidenced by low voltage in the chest leads. (This impression can be confirmed on echocardiogram.) On ECG, low voltage may be interpreted as "ischemic" change but is more accurately viewed as evidence of myocardial wasting. Ventricular thinning can lead to "ventriculovalvular distortion" or mitral valve prolapse and regurgitation, a risk factor for cardiac arrhythmia. Functional cardiac changes include decreased exercise tolerance and endurance and a prolonged recovery phase after exercise. Bradycardia is often seen in patients with severe eating disorders. Because of the high frequency of exercise abuse in eating disorders, it is necessary to differentiate between pathologic and physiologic bradycardia (patients generally seek the latter interpretation). Electrical changes that may be noted on ECG are prolongation of the PR interval, leading to heart block, and QT prolongation. A corrected QT interval of greater than 0.46 seconds is considered an "ECG harbinger," a window for ectopic conduction patterns. In a person with a prolonged QT interval, the potential for arrhythmia is accentuated by primary antiarrhythmic drugs, such as quinidine and procainamide, and sympathomimetic drugs, such as caffeine, nicotine, pseudoephedrine, phenylpropanolamine, and amphetamine, which may be abused for their anorexic potential.

Laboratory studies that may be useful in completing the differential diagnosis are erythrocyte sedimentation rate, urinanalysis, thyroid function studies, serum uric acid, examination of stool for occult blood, serum prolactin, pregnancy test, and possibly a chest radiograph.

Complications

The complications or morbidity associated with eating disorders reach far and wide. "Far" refers to long-term and short-term complications, and "wide" refers to the number of organ systems affected by starvation and pathologic behaviors.

Dental problems result primarily from excessive vomiting and include dental enamel erosion (on the lingual aspects of the teeth), stomatitis, pharyngitis, and parotitis. Vomiting further affects the gastrointestinal system, with esophageal erosion or tears (Mallory-Weiss syndrome) and gastroesophageal reflux. Lower gastrointestinal bleeding and deterioration of the ganglia of Auerbach's plexus, leading to severe constipation, have been noted to result from chronic abuse of stimulant laxatives.

Electrolyte, glucose, and acid-base derangements may occur as a result of vomiting (metabolic alkalosis) or laxative abuse (metabolic acidosis). Hypokalemia is the most common effect of excessive loss of gastric hydrochloric acid and may predispose to cardiac arrhythmias or paralytic ileus. Hypophosphatemia may complicate refeeding. Phosphorus levels reach their nadir at roughly 6 days into the refeeding regimen and, coupled with the QT interval prolongation that occurs in bradycardic states, may allow for the genesis of arrhythmias.

Bradycardia is the most common cardiovascular finding, reported in as many as 87% of patients with eating disorders. Orthostatic hypotension has been noted and, if present, places the patient at risk for fainting. Abuse of syrup of ipecac, used to induce vomiting, has led to reports of reversible cardiomyopathy[41] and of heart failure and death.[42]

Lanugo hair is thought to be a heat-conserving adaptation in the face of starvation and malnutrition. Decubitus ulcers over the lumbosacral spine have been noted secondary to excessive exercising (sit-ups) in fat-depleted patients.

Thermoregulatory problems are common in patients with eating disorders. One speculation is that this is related to the hypothalamic disruption that they experience. However, this view has been challenged by Davies and associates,[43] who studied temperature regulation in anorexia nervosa patients during exercise. Their findings suggest that at least in fat-depleted persons, the loss of the insulating capacity of body fat plays a more primary role in temperature instability.

Maximal bone accretion of calcium occurs normally in adolescence and young adulthood.[40] The long-term effect of the prolonged calcium deprivation associated with low estrogen levels is not entirely known. It has been suggested that low weight, deficient calcium intake, and chronically decreased estrogen levels affect bone mineralization and may predispose to postmenopausal osteoporosis.[44] The short-term effect of excessive high-impact exercise, which for behavioral and psychiatric reasons may not be limited by fatigue or discomfort, is a higher rate of stress fractures. This has been illustrated by ballerinas and distance runners.[45] Bone densitometry of the axial skeleton may assist in identifying those patients at highest risk for vertebral compression and stress fractures and for later osteoporosis.

The psychiatric complications of eating disorders include alcohol and substance abuse and suicide. Considered altogether, these complications account for most of the deaths that occur as a result of eating disorders. Forty to eighty percent of patients with eating disorders meet the criteria for a lifelong, major depression.[46]

The Physician's Role on the Treatment Team

Cultural reinforcement of external attributes that resemble eating-disordered characteristics bolsters the patient and family's denial of the diagnosis and worsens the prognosis by allowing the symptoms to become more deeply entrenched in the developing identity of the patient. The physician must assist the patient and the family in bridging the denial of the severity of an eating disorder, which often negates treatment efforts. This includes presenting them with evidence from the initial medical evaluation and differential diagnosis as well as offering ongoing medical consultation and routine follow-up appointments. Initially, the severe medical consequences may be a "ticket" to therapy for the patient and family. There is, however, a danger of overmedicalizing eating disorders such that when weight gain occurs and bradycardia resolves, there is a loss of impetus for continued psychotherapy. Collins and associates[47] described four goals of inpatient multidisciplinary treatment of anorexia nervosa. Minor modification renders them useful for either inpatient or outpatient treatment. The goals include (1) improvement in eating behavior; (2) enhancement of socialization; (3) achievement of a stable, healthy, and appropriate weight; and (4) engagement of the patient *and* the family in a psychotherapeutic relationship.

The complexity of the pathology and the multiplicity of therapeutic needs mandate some type of team approach to the optimal treatment of patients with eating disorders. This team may be a center-based multidisciplinary team or an ad hoc community-based group of treating professionals with shared goals. Both therapeutic scenarios require cross-disciplinary professional respect, frequent communication, and clear documentation of impressions and plans. Physicians may find themselves in the role of the team "bad guy," setting minimum goals for heart rate, temperature, and weight and defining guidelines for team and camp participation, exercise, and diet.

If the medical role on the team is being filled by a nonprimary care or subspecialty provider, communication with the primary care provider is crucial, because each may mistakenly neglect or undermine important aspects of care. An example of a split that might occur would be for a primary care provider to complete a physical examination form for gymnastics camp for a patient who is under activity restriction because of her eating disorder. Parents should not bear the responsibility for communication between professionals.

Medical Treatment

Acute Stabilization

The highest priority in the acute care of patients with eating disorders is to stabilize potentially life-threatening abnormalities, such as dehydration, electrolyte derangements, and hypoglycemia.

Correcting Specific Abnormalities

Iron deficiency has been called the most common nutritional deficiency in the United States. Adolescent girls are at particular risk, and runners have been cited as a subgroup at greatest risk.[48] Squire[49] described three stages of iron deficiency: iron depletion, iron deficiency without anemia, and iron deficiency anemia. Iron depletion represents the consumption of iron stores from the liver, spleen, and bone marrow. The laboratory abnormality that signals iron depletion is decreased serum ferritin. Iron depletion is thought to diminish the muscular capacity for aerobic metabolism. Iron deficiency without anemia may be reflected in decreased serum iron and increased total iron-binding capacity. Impaired athletic performance has been described in this intermediate stage of iron deficiency. Frank iron deficiency anemia is the most advanced manifestation of iron deficiency. All of the iron deficiency states may be worsened by inadequate dietary intake of iron and by intensive exercise, which may increase iron losses through the gastrointestinal tract, as well as by myoglobin breakdown that occurs during high-impact exercise.

Calcium plays many important physiologic roles, including the enhancement of bone density and muscle contraction. Adolescents with eating disorders are at particular risk for calcium deficiency because of their tendency to restrict dairy products to reduce calories and their propensity for amenorrhea because of a prepubertal regression in the hypothalamic-pituitary-ovarian axis. Carbonated beverages may be consumed in great quantities in an effort to abate hunger. These contain phosphorus, which can increase renal calcium excretion. The recommended daily allowance for calcium is 1,200 mg. This amount should be increased to 1,500 mg if the patient has amenorrhea. Dietary calcium requirements can be met by consuming dairy products, grains, and green leafy vegetables, or commercially available calcium supplements. Biologic availability is probably best when calcium is combined with vitamin D, as it is in dairy products. There is some evidence that calcium absorption is impaired by consuming the high-fiber grain foods that are high in phytates.[50]

Oral supplementation, whether potassium, iron, or calcium, is useless if the patient persists in vomiting.

Dietary Management

Specific dietary recommendations must be made to achieve a balanced caloric intake. The diet should provide enough calories for tissue maintenance and replenishment, plus an additional increment for activity. This goal usually cannot be achieved immediately in patients who are accustomed to extremes of starvation or purging. Initially, a minimal caloric level of 1,000 to 1,200 cal should be set. Subsequently, calories may be increased by 500 to 750 per week until the desired level is reached. Most patients will voluntarily consume their calories through food if the mealtime milieu is structured and supportive. An occasional patient might need additional nutrients administered through artificial means, that is, nasogastric tube or intravenous feedings (Table 9–7). A decision must be made as to whether calories should be supplied through food or through balanced nutritional supplements (e.g., Ensure Plus). Although most patients state their desire to consume calories as food, to do so is sometimes extremely anxiety producing because of the great number of choices that must be made. A trial of solid food may help illustrate to patients their inability to make such choices. If food is offered, patients tend to select those that are lowest in fat in the name of cardiovascular health. Fat is necessary for lean tissue replenishment. A fat-restricted diet is *not* in the best interest of a recuperating, malnourished patient. In addition, a diet adequate in calories and low in fat has greater bulk because of the high fiber and water content

Table 9–7. CONTRAINDICATIONS FOR NONORAL NUTRITIONAL INTERVENTION

Nasogastric Tube Feeding
Mucosal erosion or ulceration
Upper respiratory infection or aspiration
Gastrointestinal perforation
Contribution to oral aversive patterns
Intravenous Feeding
Infection from intravenous catheter
Embolic complications

of typical low-fat foods. This proves difficult to consume comfortably and reinforces restrictive tendencies.

Bowel Program

The medical care provider may be called on to devise a bowel program for patients with eating disorders. Malnutrition itself predisposes to constipation; this is worsened if a patient's access to the bathroom after meals has been restricted because of a history of purging. With nutritional rehabilitation, an underweight patient may experience an increase in abdominal girth. This may be a sign of normal replenishment, which is intensified by delays in gastric emptying time. The impact of increasing girth (and snug clothing) on body image can be quite upsetting and can negatively reinforce a patient around dietary compliance. Many bulimic patients abuse laxatives chronically and are dependent on stimulant-type laxatives for normal bowel movements; the withdrawal of these laxatives must be tapered. A balanced bowel program should include adequate intake of fluids and fiber, access to the bathroom (supervised, if necessary) when the gastric-colic reflex is likely to occur, use of stool softeners and lubricants, and, when necessary, judicious use of stimulant laxatives to promote effective bowel function. The principles of treating encopresis[51] can be quite applicable.

Exercise Program

A final area of medical treatment is the interruption and subsequent reintroduction of exercise. Many patients with eating disorders may have deeply entrenched, obsessive, or self-destructive patterns of exercise. Energy must be conserved, especially if a patient is not taking adequate calories. This precludes the possibility of exercise during the initial stages of medical treatment.

The distinction between exercise as a health-promoting behavior in healthy persons and as a self-destructive behavior in malnourished compromised persons must be made repeatedly. For example, judgment may be impaired regarding temperature ranges that are unsafe for exercising outdoors. Avoiding outdoor exertion in hot weather is particularly important for patients taking drugs such as lithium, which can promote electrolyte loss through excessive sweating. Caution patients about preventing heat stress as well and about the importance of replacing lost fluid after exercise. A loss of insulation brought about by depleted fat increases vulnerability to hypothermia, making it imperative to avoid exposure in extremely cold weather. Generally, temperatures between 40° and 80°F are optimal for light outdoor activities.

Psychopharmacologic Interventions

Psychopharmacologic interventions in patients with eating disorders have primarily addressed themselves to relief of depression and specific bulimic symptomatology. For interfering with bulimic symptoms, two drugs, amphetamine and fenfluramine, have been investigated for their appetite-suppressing characteristics.

Ong and coworkers[52] observed the effect of methylamphetamine on eight bulimic patients who had fasted overnight prior to the study. They noted that the subjective sensation of hunger was delayed for about 2 hours and that the number of calories consumed during a subsequent binge was diminished by 75%. Further, the tendency for postbinge purging was eliminated. Unfortunately, along with these benefits, amphetamine carries an increasing tolerance and a serious risk of addiction. This is highly undesirable, particularly given the dependent tendencies of many bulimic patients that make them particularly susceptible to addiction.

A typical binge is carbohydrate laden. Carbohydrate consumption is thought to be a principal mechanism for inducing the release of the neurotransmitter serotonin.[53] When a carbohydrate-rich, protein-poor meal is consumed, brain uptake of tryptophan is facilitated, leading to increased serotonin synthesis and the accompanying feelings of contentment generally associated with satiation. This has provided a rationale for specific pharmacologic intervention in obese carbohydrate-cravers. The drug D-fenfluramine, a serotonergic drug, has been noted to suppress selectively carbohydrate snacking in obese subjects.[54] Its use is at least theoretically justified in that subgroup of bulimic patients.

Positive family histories for major affective disorders have supported therapeutic trials of antidepressant medications. They have been used adjunctively in the treatment of eating disorders to combat the symptoms of depression observed in many patients, particularly those with bulimia. Most studies document improvement in patients' depressive symptoms.[55] Imipramine, a tricyclic antidepressant, and its related compounds, amitriptyline and desipramine, have been the principal agents used to treat patients with depression. The side effects of dry mouth, urinary retention, constipation, and palpitations are unpleasant and interfere with patient adherence. The side effects of hypotension, blurred vision, and a potential for cardiac arrhythmias mandate careful monitoring of patients taking these drugs. Acute overdosage of tricyclic antidepresents may be complicated by cardiac arrhythmias, seizures, and coma; therefore, extreme caution should be exercised in giving large prescriptions to potentially suicidal patients.

Monoamine oxidase inhibitors have not been widely used or studied because of the necessity for patients' taking them to maintain themselves on a tyramine-free diet. In a double-blind, placebo-controlled study, Walsh and associates[56] reported a reduction in binges in 76% of patients. However, a corresponding improvement was not demonstrated on the Harrison Depression Scale. Overall, the usefulness of monoamine oxidase inhibitors has been diminished by requisite dietary modifications and by a variety of side effects. The most serious adverse reaction is hypertensive crisis, occasionally reported to be fatal.

Fluoxetine (Prozac) is an antidepressant medication that has some advantage over tricyclic antidepressants in the treatment of eating disorders. It is at least comparably effective in reducing bulimic behavior (binging and purging), has fewer anticholinergic side effects, and offers the advantage of not increasing body weight, which is a high priority in this population.[57]

Outcomes

Outcomes in eating disorders may be defined in a number of ways. Easier to mark are the short-term, somewhat dramatic ones, including improvements in physical and physiologic appearance and the absence of specific anorectic or bulimic behaviors, or of life-threatening events such as cardiac arrhythmias, drug overdoses, catastrophic accidents, or suicide.[58] More elusive is the documentation of developmental or psychological "recovery," freedom from psychiatric illness, relief from body image preoccupation, and improved quality of interpersonal relationships.

Vomiting as a symptom carries a worse prognosis than food restriction. Keller and associates[59] describe a 43% rate of continuation after 18 months of outpatient therapy and a 65% rate of relapse within 1 year of recovery from bulimia. Two obstacles to short-term abatement of symptoms are the patients' inability to control binges and their unwillingness to tolerate the almost inevitable weight gain that accompanies normalization of dietary intake.

Long-term studies of anorexia nervosa are not optimistic for the establishment of normal eating and freedom from excessive weight preoccupation by 5 years from diagnosis. Hsu[60] and Swift[61] describe about 35% recovery in terms of these characteristics. Approximately 75% of patients with anorexia nervosa find employment and experience improvement in weight and menstrual function. Indicators of social or marital adjustment vary from 40 to 50%.[62, 63]

Patients with eating disorders require aggressive, vigilant medical care. However, in isolation this will not ensure recovery. An exclusive relationship with a medical provider may actually prolong an eating disorder by keeping the patient sick. Equally meticulous psychological care must be concurrent with medical care. Psychological factors may impede patient adherence, even in instances of severe medical compromise. Therefore, physicians should maintain close communication with mental health providers. They should question whether unresolved psychological issues are interfering with recovery, especially when a patient's clinical status deviates from the expected. Most eating disorders should be viewed as chronic, waxing and waning with a patient's life stresses and tasks.

OBESITY

Definitions

Contrary to popular belief, the two purposes of fat are not to make a portion of the population unhappy and to make diet promoters rich. An estimated $32 billion per year is spent in the diet control industry and yet data from the 1976–1980 Health and Nutrition Examination Survey (HANES II) indicate that obese persons still account for 25 to 45% of the U.S. adult population.[64]

The primary purpose of fat is to insulate the body and preserve core temperature. Fat is relatively lightweight and stores approximately 9 kcal of energy per gm. The carbon skeletons of dietary fat, carbohydrate, and amino acids all can be converted to adipose tissue triglycerides, which are the adipocyte storage forms of energy and nutrients. An average-sized adult stores energy equivalent to around 70 days' worth of intake.[65]

The term *obesity* applies to excess adiposity, or body fat, and has long been linked with excessive food intake. The word obese comes from the Latin word *obedere*, meaning "to eat away."[66] Obesity has been quantitated in many ways, ranging from cosmetic obesity, which is greater than 120% of ideal body weight (Table 9–8), to morbid obesity, which is defined as being 45 kg (100 lb) or 100% greater than ideal body weight. Some degree of obesity has been estimated to affect 15 to 20% of children and adolescents, most of whom become obese adults.[67]

Defining obesity in terms of weight alone is imprecise because it discounts variations in body composition, that is, variations in the skeletal and muscular contributions to body weight. For example, it is possible for a child to be of normal weight and have excess fat, as in a child with inadequate muscle development owing to hypotonia or primary neuromuscular disease,[68] or for a child to be abnormally heavy by virtue of increased lean body mass without excess fat, as in a muscular high school football player.

Obesity may be defined as a statistical expression of weight-for-age or weight-for-height measures. In practice, one may use the National Center for Health Statistics Percentiles for Physical Growth.[69] These charts are based on data from a large group of children of the same age according to variance from a mean weight or a mean ratio of weight to height. In a normal or gaussian distribution, the mean is the center of a bell-shaped curve. Approximately 68% of a population lies within plus or minus one standard deviation of the mean and 95% within plus or minus two standard deviations. This leaves 5%, 2.5% at each tail, with those on the plus side being defined as excessively heavy compared with the mean. The charts make no suppositions about causes or associated morbidity. They merely relate a child's weight or ratio of weight to height to a large number of same-aged U.S. children. Data from the Ten-State Nutritional Survey (TSNS)[70] indicate that far more than

Table 9–8. CALCULATION OF % IBW

1. Find "ideal" weight (use either a. or b.):
   a. The weight that corresponds to the height percentile.
   b. The weight that is at the 50th percentile for height on the weight-for-stature growth chart.
2. Calculate % IBW:

$$\% \text{ IBW} = \frac{\text{actual weight}}{\text{ideal weight}} \times 100$$

% IBW, percent ideal body weight.

2.5% of U.S. children are greater than two standard deviations above the mean, suggesting that the growth charts used today are statistically inaccurate. In fact, the TSNS data suggest that 17% of boys and 12% of girls are obese by age 13. Approximately 80% of these will become obese adults.[71]

Anthropometric measurements provide an estimate of the contribution of fat to a person's total body mass. The most widely used method is to measure height, weight, and midarm circumference and then to measure skin thickness (reflecting subcutaneous fat) at various body sites, including the triceps and subscapular skin folds. Skin fold measurements are used to estimate fatness because of a correlation with body fatness.[72] The standards were published by Frisancho[73] based on data obtained in a TSNS [70] from more than 40,000 infants, children, and adults. Obesity has been defined as a triceps skin fold greater than the 85th percentile.[74] Garn[75] designates greater than the 95th percentile as "super-obese." The implication of this negative-sounding designation is a minimal likelihood of spontaneous remission. To ensure precise, consistent measurements, a careful and experienced examiner should measure skin folds using well-calibrated calipers. Measurements are inaccurately reproduced when skin folds are greater than 30 mm,[76] because of shifts that occur in interstitial fluid when skin is compressed.

Other indirect estimates of body composition can be made, but these are best used as research techniques. Percentage of body fat can be estimated by the use of potassium-40 counting, or it can be derived from measures of total body water. Hydrostatic (underwater) weighing is another technique that derives fatness from comparison of the weight submerged in water with the weight in air.

Specific Causative Factors

Obesity should be viewed as a condition rather than a specific disease or disorder with a single specific cause. Attempts have been made to classify obesity by a pathophysiologic mechanism. One such classification includes hyperphagia and hypometabolism. Hyperphagia, or excessive food intake, might be the result of poor feeding practices, inadequate interpretation of satiety, or overeating (binging) for psychological reasons, such as anxiety or depression. Hypometabolism relates to the body's need for and storage of energy. Metabolism is influenced by many factors, including genetics, activity level, body composition, prior food intake, and drugs. Hypometabolism suggests that because of one or a number of these factors, a person's caloric needs are reduced.

Organic causes of obesity (Table 9–9) account for 1% or fewer cases of obesity. Taitz[77] has divided the organic causes into three broad categories: somatic dysmorphic syndromes, central nervous system disorders, and endocrinopathies. Patients with somatic dysmorphic syndromes have various deformities and malfunctions of the musculoskeletal and central nervous systems as well as mental retardation and growth failure. When obesity is secondary to a central nervous system disorder, excessive adiposity may result either from excessive food intake because of damage to the hypothalamic satiety center or, more rarely, from "pathologic gorging," which occurs because of abnormal cortical activity. Endocrinopathies, which constitute the third category of organic causes, affect energy utilization by decreasing metabolism. In the clinical setting, extensive laboratory investigation is generally unnecessary in seeking these diagnoses because the presence of a primary disorder can be ruled out by ascertaining normal linear growth and growth velocity, normal intellectual development, normal genitalia, and no history of central nervous system insult.

Table 9–9. ORGANIC CAUSES OF OBESITY

Somatic Dysmorphic Syndromes
Prader-Willi syndrome
Vasquez syndrome (males with X-linked short stature, mental retardation, hypogonadism, gynecomastia)
Laurence-Moon-Biedl syndrome
Cohen's syndrome (hypotonia, hyperextensible joints, unusual facies, mental retardation)
Alström's syndrome (deafness, diabetes mellitus, retinitis pigmentosa, short stature, hypogonadism)
X chromosome disorders
Pseudohypoparathyroidism
Central Nervous System Damage
Trauma
Tumor
Postinfection
Endocrinopathies
Hypothyroidism
Insulinoma
Cushing's syndrome
Exogenous corticosteroids
Mauriac's syndrome (diabetes with excessive insulin administration characterized by short stature and hepatomegaly)
Stein-Leventhal syndrome

Adapted from Merritt RJ: Obesity. Curr Prob Pediatr 1982; 12:6; with permission.

A single specific cause will not be identified for most obese patients. Therefore, efforts are better directed at determining the interacting factors that influence the development of obesity.

Factors Influencing the Development of Obesity

Garn and coworkers[78] stated, "The obese tend to replicate themselves in obesity." Families at high risk for producing obese children are those in whom one or both parents are obese. This observation does not necessarily imply genetic causes, as parent-sibling concordance may be related to lifestyle rather than genetics. Spouses tend to have similar degrees of fatness, with skin fold correlations between the parents almost as high as between siblings.[79]

The same study[79] reports on the patterns of parent-offspring obesity, demonstrating that children with two lean parents are leaner than those with one lean parent, who are leaner than those with two fat parents. Children with two obese parents are three times more likely to be obese at 17 years of age (30% risk) than those with two lean parents (10% risk). Another study by Garn and associates[80] reveals good correlation between adopted and natural siblings; the correlation becomes stronger with earlier age of adoption. The Garn hypothesis for nongenetic familial obesity is that fatness is the result of shared nutritional standards within families.

On the other hand, a Danish study[81] suggests that obesity has a strong genetic basis. A group of 540 adoptees was selected and divided into four weight classes. No relationship was established between fatness in adoptive parents and adoptee children, and a strong relationship across the whole range of adiposity was demonstrated between biologic parents and adoptee children.

Some workers have suggested a lower morbidity in genetic obesity than in the acquired type. The Pima Indians represent a well-studied example of human genetic obesity. The lowest mortality in this population occurs at a body mass index between 35 and 40 kg per m^2 body surface area, which is 50 to 90% above the actuarial standard for weight. This occurrence supports the rationale for more intense prevention and intervention in environmentally mediated obesity[82] than in genetic obesity.

Maternal obesity,[83] excessive weight gain during pregnancy,[84] and diabetes mellitus have been demonstrated to produce increased fatness in infants. In a study of 265 term newborn infants, Whitelaw[83] determined that the 61 infants born to obese mothers had greater skin fold thicknesses than babies born to mothers matched for blood pressures, smoking history, and parity who were not obese. Udall and coworkers[84] correlated both pre-pregnancy weight-for-height measures and weight gain during pregnancy with increased newborn fat. The pre-pregnancy weight-for-height measure was found to relate only to newborn fat, whereas excess weight gain during pregnancy (greater than 18 kg) influenced both newborn fatness and length. In this study, only one half of the large-for-gestational-age infants could be considered fat while the other half were proportionately large.

Agras and coworkers[85] studied variations in infant feeding style, seeking evidence for an "obese eating style." They measured factors such as sucking and volumetric flow, duration of feeding, and suck frequency. More vigorous infant feeding style was associated with increased caloric intake and greater adiposity. This work can be related to earlier work by Kessen.[86] He suggests that infants who are more distractible, stimulable, and intense on an infant temperament assessment have a greater risk of obesity.

Children whose weight places them at or above the 90th percentile in the first year of life are at relative risk for the development of obesity. In a retrospective study, Charney and associates[87] determined that 36% of infants who exceeded the 90th percentile for weight were overweight as adults compared with 14% of average and lightweight infants. The influences of birth weight and weight attained during the first 6 months of life were analyzed separately, and the latter was found to be of even greater influence than the former. Weight gain during the first 6 months may be influenced by genetic factors and by dietary practices.

A focus of ongoing investigation and controversy has been the determination of whether the type of milk given to infants influences the development of obesity. The studies have been contaminated by a tendency for earlier introduction of solid foods in bottle-fed babies and by the influence of ethnicity on feeding practices and adiposity. A recent study by Baranowski and colleagues[88] carefully considered many of the problems encumbering the infant feeding literature. Their conclusions did not support concerns about higher risk for the development of obesity in bottle-fed babies.

Excessive television viewing has been correlated with childhood obesity.[89] Data from four cycles of the HANES[64] indicate a 54% increase in the frequency of obesity in 6- to 11-year-old children and a 39% increase in 12- to 17-year-old adolescents over a period of 15 years. A strong, significant relationship is noted between obesity and television viewing such that the association with television viewing is surpassed only by that of prior obesity.

Results of studies correlating socioeconomic status with obesity indicate a direct relationship between obesity and income for most groups. The striking exception is the reverse correlation between fatness and income in older female children noted in U.S. studies by Stunkard.[90] This may be the result of variations in genetics, dietary intake related to income and culture, lifestyle, or other social factors, such as fashion.

Determination of the factors that influence the development of obesity remains a high priority if prevention is to be undertaken. Some of these factors, such as genetic predisposition, are immutable and not necessarily pathogenetic, while other lifestyle factors may lend themselves to systematic and vigorous efforts toward change. The literature demonstrates striking disagreement as to whether genetics or environment is primarily responsible for obesity. The best reconciliation of this dispute is probably that obesity is a heterogeneous condition that is influenced by genetics and environment and is perpetuated by vicious cycles of exercise avoidance and maladaptive coping through nonsocial means, such as escapism (e.g., television viewing) and overeating. If prevention measures are undertaken, they should be focused at a high risk population rather than applied indiscriminately to all people.

Energy Regulation in the Obese

The "set point" theory suggests that the human organism has an intrinsic mechanism for the maintenance of some individual-specific optimal weight. Remarkable weight constancy has been noted in most people over time.[91] This suggests that the body maintains the status quo by up- or down-regulation of metabolism and energy utilization. The work of Keys and associates in the 1950s[2] demonstrated this tendency in 36 adult men. Much earlier, Neumann[92] speculated about a mechanism called *luxus consumption* (diet-induced thermogenesis). This is the body's tendency to adjust to periods of increased caloric intake by initial weight gain followed by a plateau phase. This plateau was thought to represent acclimation, with expenditure of the extra calories through the production of heat in "futile" metabolic cycles, which in animals has been localized in brown adipose tissue.[93] It has also been demonstrated that people who take inadequate calories experience decreases in metabolism that are similar to hibernation.[2,94] Although many researchers have challenged this concept of metabolic regulation, clinical experience suggests that some type of individually determined metabolic control of weight accounts for the extremely refractory and stable nature of obesity.

Complications

Diabetes mellitus and cardiovascular disease are often cited as complications of obesity.[95] Although these complications are virtually exclusive to adults, hypertension[96] and abnormalities in glucose metabolism[97–99] have been documented in obese children and adolescents. These data provide some justification for interventive energy directed at the pediatric population.

Taitz[100] categorized three classes of physical complications of obesity: (1) potentially lethal; (2) handicapping effects of bulk; and (3) nuisance. The risk of life-threatening illness actually occurring in childhood secondary to obesity is extremely low. The exceptions are those rare cases of *pickwickian syndrome*, a name coined in the 1950s[101] that refers to a combination of extreme obesity and obstructive apnea or hypoventilation. Death from heart failure associated with cardiomyopathy is another rarely reported catastrophe.[102] A third potentially lethal complication, pancreatitis, is also rare. Handicapping effects of bulk, the second category of complications, pose the most significant obstacle to health and physical activity. They can bring about major orthopedic disorders, such as genu valgum, Blount disease (tibia vara),[103] coxa vara, and Legg-Calvé-Perthes disease, and serious respiratory disorders, such as chest wall restriction and upper airway obstruction. Included in the third class of complications are "nuisance" problems, such as intertriginous friction irritation and superficial infections.

In addition to physical risks, there are psychosocial consequences of being overweight.[104] These include peer problems and social isolation for those who are obese as children,[105] and low self-esteem and feelings of inadequacy and impotence for those whose obesity has its onset in adolescence.[106] Unfortunately, obese children and adults suffer from discrimination on many fronts. They suffer at school from the taunts of peers who also project negative attributes on obese silhouettes,[107] and from school personnel. They also suffer in the work place because of discriminatory hiring and promotion practices.[108, 109]

Obese children enter puberty slightly earlier than do their peers. This results in increased linear growth prior to puberty, easily tracking at greater than or equal to the 75th percentile using the NCHS Percentiles for Physical Growth.[69] Bone age advancement and skeletal maturation, and therefore growth cessation, occur at a younger age, and eventual height may be slightly less than that of peers. Obese children achieve earlier sexual maturation[110] and thus tend to look maturer than their peers, accentuating the differences in appearance.

Our culture epitomizes the Duchess of Windsor's remark, "You can't be too rich or too thin." Medical professionals must be careful not to perpetuate the latter prejudice in the name of "good health." This concept is called *looksism* or *weightism* and has been explored as a psychological[111] as well as a political issue. Fitzgerald[112] proposes that the well-described associated morbidity is not caused by obesity but rather by the stress of being obese in our weight-obsessed society. During the 1980s, the feminist movement noted size discrimination as a civil rights issue that affects primarily women. They challenged the assumption that people who are fat are by definition unhealthy and emphasized the morbidity and mortality associated with largely ineffective weight loss measures. The National Association to Advance Fat Acceptance was established to promote size acceptance as an individual as well as a legal right.

If medical practitioners are interested primarily in preventing serious complications, we must seek an operational definition, clarifying the degree of obesity that places patients at serious risk. Knapp[113] has proposed shifting the focus from "ideal" to "dangerous" weights. This is a more useful conceptualization than 120% ideal body weight, an amount that seems to be based on the popular definition of ideal body weight rather than on the actual level of overweight at which children's health is compromised.

Dietz[114] suggests intervention for those degrees of childhood obesity that are not likely to remit spontaneously and therefore are likely to be associated with cardiovascular sequelae in adulthood. Seven-year-old boys at 138 to 139% ideal body weight show a spontaneous obesity remission rate at age 14 years of 53%. This decreases to 30.3 percent at 149 to 156% ideal body weight and decreases to zero at greater than 165% ideal body weight. Abraham and associates[115, 116] suggest the notion of relative risk for obesity in adulthood. In obese 10- to 13-year-old children, the relative risk of becoming an obese adult is 18:1 for girls and 5 to 6:1 for boys.

Although strict criteria are not assigned, practitioners should integrate available data on risk for ongoing obesity to judge those children for whom intervention is justified and advisable. Beware of strong societal and commercial pressures that promote excess thinness, and confine recommendations for intervention to those patients whose health and well-being appear potentially or truly jeopardized.

Prevention

Sound practices for healthful habits should be initiated in infancy. Some examples of these practices are listed in Table 9–10. Good general advice is to feed children enough when they are hungry, give attention and cuddling when they need comfort, and encourage exercise

Table 9–10. FEEDING TIPS

Breast feeding is encouraged. Breast milk contains a balance of calories per volume, and the mother is not able to count the number of ounces per feeding.
Pay attention to the differentiation of the infant's cues around hunger, physical distress, and desire for attention.
Avoid feeding "empty calories," or non-nutritive foods. Avoid making formulas with less water or adding cereals or sweeteners to formula or milk.
Don't put solid foods into the bottle. They overconcentrate the formula and deny the child opportunities for learning to associate specific tastes with textures, and for enhancing oral-motor skills for chewing.
Postpone the introduction of solid foods until the child is neurodevelopmentally ready, i.e., able to maintain seated posture and adequate in oral-motor competence.
Examine family style and habits. Consider use of nonfood vs. food rewards and perceptions about "good food" vs. "junk food."

when they are restless. Whether or not obesity can be prevented remains controversial, so assumptions or blame should not be made simply because a child is fat. Many lifestyle factors associated with obesity prevention are health promoting and would be desirable for both obese and nonobese families.

Pisacano and coworkers[117] devised and studied a specific strategy for preventive intervention in infancy. They adapted the "Prudent Diet,"[118] which supplies 12% of calories as protein, 30% as fat, and 58% as carbohydrate. The diet was started at age 3 months in a study group of 80 infants who by age 3 years showed a 1.28% incidence of being overweight, compared with 25.5% in control subjects (overweight was defined as weight percentile exceeding height percentile by one standard deviation). Their findings cross ethnic and racial lines and provide a powerful stimulus for preventive dietary modification in infancy.

Management

Obesity is a complex condition with many contributors and perpetuators. If intervention is undertaken, the goal is to identify and simultaneously address as many of these as possible. The common goal of specific treatments is to induce a negative energy balance.

Dietary Manipulation

For the person whose caloric intake is excessive, a negative energy balance can be accomplished if there is a willingness and an ability to decrease food intake. Weight reduction diets span the range of possibilities from moderate restriction (balanced deficit diet, cutting 250–500 calories a day) to fasting. Usual dietary intake should be assessed by calorie counts so that realistic modifications can be made. These modifications should also be tailored according to the age and needs of the child so that specific nutrient deficiencies are avoided.

The Stop Light Diet for Children[119] is an 8-week program for children and parents. It has enjoyed widespread use in dietary intervention programs because of its flexibility and ease of application. This diet employs a color-coded exchange system of foods—which are designated green, yellow, and red according to caloric content—and incorporates behavior change concepts.

Severely restrictive diets have little use in pediatrics because (1) they *may* interfere with at least short-term linear growth[120, 121]; (2) they are philosophically not in keeping with the notions of teaching long-term healthful principles and modifying lifestyle; and (3) they suggest that there is a straightforward medical answer to a problem that is far more complicated, placing an expectation that the medical profession should provide a cure when none may be available.

The protein-sparing modified fast (semistarvation ketogenic diet) is occasionally useful in initiating weight loss in severely obese, medically compromised patients. This diet is more desirable than simple fasts in that it spares protein for growth by supplying 1.5 gm of protein per kg ideal body weight. Dietz[114] suggests basing the protein calculation on 120% ideal body weight in order to account for the potentially greater lean body mass that may occur in obese adolescents. Undesirable symptoms associated with this diet include orthostasis, decreased energy level, nausea, headaches, and constipation. Children on protein-sparing modified fasts must be closely monitored for metabolic complications, such as hypokalemia, hypocalcemia, and hyperuricemia. The diet must be monitored to ensure adequate intake of vitamins, minerals, and potassium. Dietary adherence can be monitored by ensuring the daily presence of ketonuria.

Fillers and bulking agents, such as methylcellulose and psyllium, are occasionally used to enhance a feeling of fullness after meals. These are generally taken with water, and although they promote gastric fullness from distention, the feeling of satisfaction generally associated with satiety is lacking.

Treatment is more difficult in those whose obesity is sustained by low metabolism and who therefore need fewer calories for maintenance of body weight. Further decreases in food intake undermines patients from getting adequate amounts of necessary macronutrients and micronutrients.

Exercise

Regular, sustained exercise is advisable for healthy weight loss. It exerts a stimulating effect on metabolism,[122] consumes calories (Table 9–11), conditions the cardiovascular system, and provides a sense of well-being and positive experience that children can, hopefully, incorporate into their lifestyle. Exercise may also provide a healthy means of coping with frustration and stress. Combined with dietary restriction, exercise spares lean tissue in favor of the loss of fat.[123]

When obtaining information, a detailed activity history is as important as a dietary history. Consider preferred type, frequency, intensity, and duration of physical activities. Exercise prescription should be individualized, specific, and realistic.

Table 9–11. ENERGY COST (CAL/15 MIN) OF SELECTED PHYSICAL ACTIVITIES

Activity	Weight Kg (lb) 50 (110)	59 (130)	68 (150)	77 (170)	86 (190)	95 (209)
Bicycling, leisure, 5.5 mph	48	57	66	74	82	91
Circuit training	140	164	189	213	238	264
Dance						
Aerobic	126	148	171	194	216	240
Active	78	92	105	118	134	147
Gymnastics	50	58	68	76	86	95
Hiking	62	72	84	95	106	117
Running						
5.2 mph	102	120	138	158	176	194
7.5 mph	162	188	213	240	266	291
Swimming						
Fast crawl	117	138	159	180	201	222
Slow crawl	96	114	130	148	165	183
Walking	60	71	81	93	104	114

Adapted from McArdle WD, Katch FI, Katch VL: Exercise physiology. Philadelphia, Lea & Febiger, 1981, pp 486–493.

Maximum benefit is achieved from sustained aerobic activities such as walking, running, biking, skating, and dancing. A minimum of three aerobic sessions per week will bring about a cardiovascular training response; increasing the sessions to four to six times a week will consume calories and will effect more dramatic changes in body composition.

For a sedentary child, the first thing that should be exercised is restraint! Avoid recommendation of an overly ambitious exercise program that may set the stage for an early failure because of injury, discomfort, or discouragement about not achieving goals. Set goals for frequency, intensity, and duration that the child can achieve fairly easily. Most obese people do not enjoy exercise.[124] The aim is to make physical activity become reinforcing because of the good feelings it can promote.

In planning an exercise program, account for the child's preferences and skills as well as the availability of equipment and facilities. Neurodevelopmental considerations are important in individualizing the program. Adapt the program for the child's attention span, task persistence, motor planning skills, balance, and coordination to avoid the embarrassment of spotlighting weaknesses in these areas. Children who are weak in balance and coordination fare better in repetitive activities, such as biking, walking, or swimming, because they do not involve quick, unanticipated shifts in position.

Certain activities pose mechanical and respiratory obstacles for the obese. High-impact exercises, such as jogging or high-impact aerobics, place obese children at risk for sprains or overuse injuries because of a tendency for genu valgum and foot overpronation. An early injury is a serious threat to future exercise adherence. People who are obese also have a tendency for abnormalities in resting pulmonary mechanics. These abnormalities are compounded by increased ventilatory demands during exercise. At rest, obese subjects have been described as having shallow respirations with limited diaphragmatic excursion, leading to ventilation-perfusion abnormalities. During exercise, a suboptimal increase in tidal volume, coupled with oxygen requirements and carbon dioxide production increasing in direct proportion to body fat content, compromises work capacity.[125]

For children who find it burdensome to sustain one activity because of a short attention span or low task persistence, a modified circuit routine is an enjoyable way of extending exercise time. A circuit consists of any number of stations, each with a different activity, such as an exercise bike, jump rope, distance walk or run, and exercise mat (for predefined calisthenics). The child spends a set amount of time (usually 1–2 minutes) at each station. The circuit may be repeated any number of times given the number of stations and the time spent at each one. Circuit training is beneficial because interest level is maintained during a combination of activities that may be individually difficult to sustain. In addition, a circuit is a good way of setting small, short-term, achievable goals as part of a "bigger picture." It also illustrates the most important characteristic of a successful exercise program, that is, that exercise should be *fun*.

Swimming is often recommended because it minimizes the risk of injury to joints. But it is skill dependent, and there may be limited access to pools. Many children perceive swimming as an outdoor, summer activity, whereas their physicians envision swimming laps in an indoor pool. Use of machines to row, bike, or stair-climb overcomes the threats of bad weather, but these activities depend on the availability of equipment and a child's ability to do one exercise repetitively for an extended time. In addition, most machines are scaled to adult sizes, which makes them too large for smaller children to use safely. Some parents report adapting machines with wooden blocks to compensate for size differences. Use of machines provides the advantage of more precise regulation of intensity without requiring children to monitor their own pulse. Music helps dispel the monotony, and some type of radio or tape player might be used as a reinforcer for early behavioral compliance.

Eliciting the cooperation of parent and child and accounting for individual preferences and capabilities are key factors in planning a successful exercise program. Short-term goals should be structured for success; their achievement may enhance commitment and adherence. Overall, exercise is a behavior that may correlate with successful long-term maintenance of weight loss.[126]

Behavior and Habit Alteration

Diet and exercise are intrinsic to weight loss, but this dyad alone does not represent a mechanism for successful weight reduction. The reason for this may be bad habits, with complex roots. A habit is defined as "a constant, often unconscious inclination to perform an act, acquired through its frequent repetition."[127] Examples include eating while reading, watching television, or talking on the phone. Although hunger might be the initial stimulus for eating, the distraction provided by the concurrent activity interferes with awareness of total intake or attention to satiation when that feeling occurs.

Behavioral treatment of obesity is based on recognizing patterns that perpetuate obesity, that is, overeating and sedentary lifestyle, and replacing them with health-promoting behaviors. There is a need for a structured consistent approach that is positively engineered. Prohibitions may be inappropriately seized because of a child's developmentally driven needs for independence and self-determination. In supporting a child in the adoption and maintence of new behaviors, it is helpful to categorize the behaviors as being healthy or unhealthy rather than good or bad. (Table 9–12 provides examples of reframing prohibitions as healthful behaviors.) With the child's assistance, non-health-promoting behaviors can be identified and quantitated. The child should participate in devising specific positive alternatives.

Most behaviorally based programs include the elements of contracting, stimulus control and self-monitoring, and social reinforcement and modeling.[128]

Outcomes

Although the combination of diet, exercise, and behavior modification techniques sounds promising for treatment of obesity, the long-term statistics are dismal. Brownell[124] states, "If 'cure' from obesity is defined as reduction to ideal weight and maintenance of that weight for 5 years, a person is more likely to recover from most forms of cancer than from obesity." Estimates of maintenance of weight loss range from roughly 3 or 4%[129, 130] to 25%, and thus we cannot say that there is an intervention that is permanently effective for most patients.[131]

Studies that demonstrate the best outcomes are those that incorporate behavior therapy into a program of diet and exercise modification.[132, 133] Epstein and colleagues[134] describe 10-year follow-up in a behavioral family-based program for obese children. The age at initiation of treatment was 6 to 12 years. Parental weight losses during participation in the intervention part of the study were not permanent, supporting the notion that children may have a behavioral and metabolic advantage in pursuit of long-term weight loss. This study gives the first evidence of significant improvement of obesity with intervention.

Childhood obesity represents a dilemma that is thus far insoluble. Most medical and psychological evidence suggests that reversal of obesity would benefit overall health and emotional development. However, the intervention strategies that are effective for even marginal weight loss in a small percentage of obese children are not without morbidity. Unsuccessful treatment attempts may extract a serious toll in terms of metabolic status, self-esteem, and family dynamics. Therefore, it may be that aggressive intervention should be limited to those children for whom success can be predicted based on preliminary diagnostic and treatment efforts. For the remaining children, therapeutic energy should be spent on facilitating adjustment and self-acceptance. Gains in these areas might possibly constitute the foundation for later lifestyle and behavioral changes.

Table 9–12. REFRAMING PROHIBITIONS

Negative Statement	Positive Reframe
Don't eat in front of the TV. Don't eat while talking on the phone. Don't eat while reading.	Designate one place to eat that is free of distractions. Pay attention to feelings of hunger and fullness during a meal.
Don't be sedentary.	Establish a regular exercise schedule and make time for it. Choose activities that you like.
Don't eat when you're bored, angry, or frustrated.	Eat when you truly feel hungry. Stop when you feel satisfied.
Don't eat snacks directly out of serving dishes.	Plan your snacks. Serve them to yourself on a small plate.
Don't skip meals.	Plan and eat meals and snacks to fit in with your tastes and schedule.

Remember: Everyone makes mistakes now and then. Try to understand why you slipped, and then give yourself another chance to succeed.

REFERENCES

1. American Psychiatric Association: Diagnostic and Statistical Manual of Mental Disorders. 3rd ed, rev. Washington, DC, American Psychiatric Association, 1987, pp 65–69.
2. Keys A, Brozek J, Hanschel A, et al: The Biology of Human Starvation. Minneapolis, University of Minnesota Press, 1950, pp 783–818.
3. Abraham SF, Beumont PJ: How patients describe bulimia or binge eating. Psychol Med 1982; 12:625–635.
4. Root MPP, Fallon P, Friedrich WN: Bulimia: A Systemic Approach to Treatment. 1st ed. New York, Norton, 1986.
5. Casper RC, Eckert ED, Halmi KA, et al: Bulimia: Its incidence and clinical importance in patients with anorexia nervosa. Arch Gen Psychiatry 1980; 37:1030–1035.
6. Habermas T: Friderada: A case of miraculous fasting. Int J Eat Disord 1986; 5:555–562.
7. Pope HG, Hudson JI, Yurgelun-Todd D, et al: Prevalence of anorexia nervosa and bulimia in three student populations. Int J Eat Disord 1984; 3:45–51.
8. Pyle RL, Mitchell JE, Eckert ED, et al: The incidence of bulimia in freshman college students. Int J Eat Disord 1983; 2:75–85.
9. Halmi KA, Falk JR, Schwartz E: Binge-eating and vomiting: A survey of a college population. Psychol Med 1981; 11:697–706.
10. Oyebode F, Boodhoo JA, Schapira K: Anorexia nervosa in males. Int J Eat Disord 1988; 7:121–124.
11. Yager J, Kurtzman F, Landsverk J, et al: Behaviors and attitudes related to eating disorders in homosexual male college students. Am J Psychiatry 1988; 145:495–497.
12. Kelley JT, Patten SE: Adolescent behaviors and attitudes toward weight and eating. *In* Mitchell JE, ed: Anorexia Nervosa and Bulimia: Diagnosis and treatment. Minneapolis: University of Minnesota Press, 1985, pp 191–204.
13. Rosen JC, Tacy B, Howell D: Life stress, psychological symptoms and weight reducing behavior in adolescent girls. Int J Eat Disord 1990; 9:17–26.
14. Hawkins RC, Clement PF: Development and construct validation of a self-report measure of binge eating tendencies. Addict Behav 1980; 5:219–226.
15. Schwartz DM, Thompson MG, Johnson CL: Anorexia nervosa and bulimia: The socio-cultural context. Int J Eat Disord 1982; 1:20–36.
16. Garner DM, Olmsted MP, Polivy J, et al: Comparison between weight-preoccupied women and anorexia nervosa. Psychosom Med 1984; 46:255–266.

17. Garner DM, Olmsted MP, Polivy J: Development and validation of a multidimensional eating disorder inventory for anorexia nervosa and bulimia. Int J Eat Disord 1983; 2:15–34.
18. Hudson JI, Pope HG Jr, Jonas JM, et al: Family history study of anorexia nervosa and bulimia. Br J Psychiatry 1983; 142:133–138.
19. Strober M, Salkin B, Burroughs J, et al: Validity of the bulimia-restricter distinction in anorexia nervosa: Parental personality characteristics and family psychiatric morbidity. J Nerv Ment Dis 1982; 170:345–351.
20. Yates A: Current perspectives on the Eating Disorders: I. History, psychological and biological aspects. J Am Acad Child Adolesc Psychiatry 1989; 28:813–828.
21. Lucas AR: Toward the understanding of anorexia nervosa as a disease entity. Mayo Clin Proc 1981; 56:254–264.
22. Vigersky RA, Loriaux DL: Anorexia nervosa as a model of hypothalamic dysfunction. In Vigersky RA, ed: Anorexia Nervosa. New York, Raven Press, 1977, pp 109–121.
23. Wakeling A, de Souza VFA, Gore MBR, et al: Amenorrhoea, body weight and serum hormone concentrations, with particular reference to prolactin and thyroid hormones in anorexia nervosa. Psychol Med 1979; 9:265–272.
24. Halmi KA: Anorexia nervosa: Demographic and clinical features in 94 cases. Psychosom Med 1974; 36:18–26.
25. Garfinkel PE, Garner DM, Rodin G: Eating disorders. In Kinney JM, Jeejeebhoy KN, Hill GL, et al, eds: Nutrition and Metabolism in Patient Care. Philadelphia, WB Saunders, 1988, pp 205–224.
26. Rosen JC, Tacy B, Howell D: Life stress, psychological symptoms and weight reducing behavior in adolescent girls: A prospective analysis. Int J Eat Disord 1990; 9:17–26.
27. Gralen SJ, Levine MP, Smolak L, et al: Dieting and disordered eating during early and middle adolescence: Do the influences remain the same? Int J Eat Disord 1990; 9:501–512.
28. Minuchin S, Rosman DL, Baker L: Psychosomatic Families: Anorexia Nervosa in Context. Cambridge, MA, Harvard University Press, 1978.
29. Johnson C, Connors ME: The Etiology and Treatment of Bulimia Nervosa: A Biopsychosocial Perspective. New York, Basic Books, 1987.
30. Garfinkel PE, Garner DM: Anorexia Nervosa: A Multidimensional Perspective. New York, Brunner/Mazel, 1982, p 515.
31. AC Nielsen Company: Nielsen Report on Television, 1989. Northbrook, IL, Nielsen Media Research, 1989.
32. Strasburger VC: When parents ask about the influence of TV on their kids. Contemp Pediatr 1985; May: 18–30.
33. Kaufman LL: Prime-time nutrition. J Commun 1980; 30:37–46.
34. Barcus E, McLaughlin L: Food Advertising on Childrens Television: An Analysis of Appeals and Nutritional Content. Newtonville, MA, Action for Children's Television, 1978.
35. Comerci GD: Eating disorders in adolescents. Pediatr Rev 1988; 10(2):37–47.
36. Mitchell JE, Pyle RL, Eckert ED: Bulimia. *In* Hales RE, Frances AJ, eds. Psychiatry Update: The American Psychiatric Association Annual Review. Vol 4, section 4. Washington, DC, APA Press, 1985, pp 464–480.
37. Szmukler GI, Russell GFM: Diabetes mellitus, anorexia nervosa and bulimia. Br J Psychiatry 1983; 142:305–308.
38. Katz MD, Lor E, McGhan WF: Comparison of serum prealbumin and transferring for nutritional assessment of TPN patients: A preliminary study. Nut Support Serv 1986; 6:22–24.
39. Kaminski MV Jr, Pinchcofsky-Devin GD, McCormick DC: DCH testing as a nutritional assessment tool. Nutr Support Serv 1985; 5:21–23.
40. Rigotti NA, Nussbaum SR, Herzog DB, et al: Osteoporosis in women with anorexia nervosa. N Engl J Med 1984; 311:1601–1606.
41. Palmer EP, Guay AT: Reversible myopathy secondary to abuse of ipecac in patients with major eating disorders. New Engl J Med 1985; 313:1457–1459.
42. Schiff RJ, Wurzel CL, Brunson SC, et al: Death due to chronic syrup of ipecac use in a patient with bulimia. Pediatrics 1986; 78:412–416.
43. Davies CT, Fohlin L, Thorn C: Temperature regulation in anorexia nervosa patients during prolonged exercise. Acta Med Scand 1979; 205:257–262.
44. Davies KM, Pearson PH, Huseman CA, et al: Reduced bone mineral in patients with eating disorders. Bone 1990; 11:143–147.
45. Frisch RE, Wyshak G, Vincent L: Delayed menarche and amenorrhea in ballet dancers. N Engl J Med 1980; 303:17–19.
46. Strober M, Katz JL: Do eating disorders and affective disorders share a common etiology? A dissenting opinion. Int J Eat Disord 1987; 6:171–180.
47. Collins M, Hodas GR, Liebman R: Interdisciplinary model for the inpatient treatment of adolescents with anorexia nervosa. J Adolesc Health Care 1983; 4:3–8.
48. Brown RT, McIntosh SM, Seabolt VR, et al: Iron status of adolescent female athletes. J Adolesc Health Care 1985; 6:349–352.
49. Squire DL: Female athletes. Pediatr Rev 1987; 9:183–190.
50. Heaton KW, Pomare EW: Effect of bran on blood lipids and calcium. Lancet 1974; 1:49–50.
51. Levine MD: Encopresis. *In* Carey WB, Crocker AC, Gross RT, eds: Developmental Behavioral Pediatrics. Philadelphia, WB Saunders, 1983, pp 586–595.
52. Ong YL, Checkley SA, Russell GFM: Suppression of bulimic symptoms with methylamphetamine. Br J Psychiatry 1983; 143:288–293.
53. Fernstrom JD, Wurtman RJ: Brain serotonin content: Increases following ingestion of carbohydrate diet. Science 1971; 174:1023–1025.
54. Wurtman J, Wurtman R, Mark S, et al: D-Flenfluramine selectively suppresses carbohydrate snacking by obese subjects. Int J Eat Disord 1985; 4:89–99.
55. Agras WS, Dorian B, Kirkley BG, et al: Imipramine in the treatment of bulimia: A double-blind controlled study. Int J Eat Disord 1987; 6:29–38.
56. Walsh BT, Stewart JW, Roose SP, et al: Treatment of bulimia with phenelzine. Arch Gen Psychiatry 1984; 41:1105–1109.
57. Solyom L, Solyom C, Ledwidge B: The fluoxetine treatment of low-weight chronic bulimia nervosa. J Clin Psychopharmacol 1990; 10:421–425.
58. Crisp AH: Anorexia nervosa at normal body weight: The abnormal normal weight control syndrome. Int J Psychiatr Med 1982; 11:203–233.
59. Keller MB, Lavori PW, McDonald-Scott P, et al: Reliability of lifetime diagnoses and symptoms in patients with a current psychiatric disorder. J Psychiatr Res 1981; 16:229–240.
60. Hsu LKG: Outcome in anorexia nervosa. Arch Gen Psychiatry 1980; 37:1041–1048.
61. Swift WJ: The long-term outcome of early onset anorexia nervosa: Critical review. J Am Acad Child Psychiatry 1982; 21:38–46.
62. Schwartz DM, Thompson M: Do anorectics get well? Current research and future needs. Am J Psychiatry 1981; 138:319–323.
63. Cantwell DP, Sturzenberger S, Burroughs J, et al: Anorexia nervosa: An affective disorder? Arch Gen Psychiatry 1977; 34:1087–1093.
64. Van Itallie TB: Health implications of overweight and obesity in the United States. Ann Intern Med 1985; 103:983–988.
65. Garrow JS: Luxuskonsumption, brown fat, and human obesity. Br Med J 1983; 286:1684–1686.
66. The American Heritage Dictionary. Revised edition of The American Heritage Dictionary of the English Language. New college ed. Boston, Houghton Mifflin, 1985.
67. Rolland-Cachera MF, Deheeger M, Guilloud-Bataille M, et al: Tracking the development of adiposity from one month of age to adulthood. Ann Hum Biol 1987; 14:219–229.
68. Bandini LG, Schoeller DA, Fukagawa NK, et al: Body composition and energy expenditure in adolescents with cerebral palsy or myelodysplasia. Pediatr Res 1991; 29:70–77.
69. Hamill PV, Drizd TA, Johnson CL, et al: Physical growth: National Center for Health Statistics percentiles. Am J Clin Nutr 1979; 32:607–629.
70. US Department of Health, Education, and Welfare: Ten-State Nutritional Survey: US Department of Health, Education, and Welfare Publication no. (HSM 73–8704). Washington, DC. US Government Printing Office, 1972.

71. Lloyd JK, Wolff OH, Whelan WS: Childhood obesity. Br Med J 1971; 2:145.
72. Roche AF, Sievogel RM, Chumlea WC, et al: Grading body fatness from limited anthropometric data. Am J Clin Nutr 1981; 34:2831–2838.
73. Frisancho A: New norms of upper limb fat and muscle areas for assessment of nutritional status. Am J Clin Nutr 1981; 34:2540.
74. Selzer CC, Mayer J: Simple criterion of obesity. Postgrad Med 1965; 38A:101–107.
75. Garn SM: Continuities and changes in fatness from infancy through adulthood. Curr Prob Pediatr 1985; 15:1–47.
76. Merritt RJ: Obesity. Curr Prob Pediatr 1982; 12:6.
77. Taitz LS: Classification of obesity. *In* The Obese Child. Oxford, Blackwell Scientific Publications, 1983, pp 142–156.
78. Garn SM, Bailey SM, Solomon MA, et al: Effect of remaining family members on fatness prediction. Am J Clin Nutr 1981; 34:148–153.
79. Garn SM, Clark DC: Trends in fatness and the origins of obesity: Ad hoc committee to review the Ten State Nutritional Survey. Pediatrics 1976; 57:443–456.
80. Garn SM, Bailey SM, Cole PE: Similarities between parents and their adopted children. Am J Phys Anthropol 1976; 45:539–543.
81. Stunkard AJ, Sorensen TIA, Hanis C, et al: An adoption study of human obesity. N Engl J Med 1986; 314:193–198.
82. Pettitt DJ, Lisse JR, Knowler WC, et al: Mortality as a function of obesity and diabetes mellitus. Am J Epidemiol 1982; 115:359–366.
83. Whitelaw AGL: Influence of maternal obesity on subcutaneous fat in the newborn. Br Med J 1976; 1:985–986.
84. Udall JN, Harrison GG, Vaucher Y, et al: Interaction of maternal and neonatal obesity. Pediatrics 1978; 62:17–21.
85. Agras WS, Kraemer HC, Berkowitz RI, et al: Does a vigorous feeding style influence early development of adiposity? J Pediatr 1987; 110:799–804.
86. Kessen W: Signs of risk of obesity in newborn babies. Int J Obesity 1980; 4:341–347.
87. Charney E, Goodman HC, McBride M, et al: Childhood antecedents of adult obesity. Do chubby infants become obese adults? N Engl J Med 1976; 295:6–9.
88. Baranowski T, Bryan GT, Rassin DK, et al: Ethnicity, infant feeding practices, and childhood adiposity. J Dev Behav Pediatr 1990; 11:234–239.
89. Dietz WH Jr, Gortmaker SL: Do we fatten our children at the TV set? Obesity and television viewing in children and adolescents. Pediatrics 1985; 75:807–812.
90. Stunkard AJ: Obesity and the social environment: Current status, future prospects. Ann NY Acad Sci 1977; 300:298–320.
91. Keesey RE: A set point analysis of the regulation of body weight. *In* Stunkard AJ, ed: Obesity. Philadelphia, WB Saunders, 1980, pp 144–165.
92. Neumann RO: Experimentelle Beiträge zur Lehre von dem tälichen Nahrungsbedard des Menschen unter besonderer Berücksichtigung der notwendigen Eiweissmenge. Arch Hyg (Berl) 1902; 45:1–87.
93. Rothwell NJ, Stock MJ: A role for brown adipose tissue in diet-induced thermogenesis. Nature 1979; 281:31–35.
94. Bray GA:. Effect of caloric restriction on energy expenditure in obese patients. Lancet 1969; 2:397–398.
95. Van Itallie TB: Obesity: Adverse effects on health and longevity. Am J Clin Nutr 1979; 32:2723–2733.
96. Rames LK, Clark WR, Connor WE, et al: Normal blood pressures and the evaluation of sustained blood pressure elevations in childhood: The muscatine study. Pediatrics 1978; 61:245–251.
97. Paulsen EP, Richenderfer L, Ginsberg-Fellner F: Plasma glucose, free fatty acids, and immunoreactive insulin in 66 obese children: Studies in reference to a family history of diabetes mellitus. Diabetes 1968; 17:261–269.
98. Martin MM, Martin ALA: Obesity, hyperinsulinism, and diabetes mellitus in childhood. J Pediatr 1973; 82:192–201.
99. Kida K, Watanabe N, Fujisawa Y, et al: The relation between glucose tolerance and insulin binding to circulating monocytes in obese children. Pediatrics 1982; 70:633–637.
100. Taitz LS: The Obese Child. Oxford, Blackwell Scientific Publications, 1983, p 164.
101. Finkelstein JW, Avery ME: The pickwickian syndrome: Studies on ventilation and carbohydrate metabolism: Case report of a child who recovered. Am J Dis Child 1963; 106:251–257.
102. Weekly Clinicopathologic Conferences, Barnes and Wohl Hospitals, Washington University School of Medicine: Massive obesity and cardiac failure. Am J Med 1978; 64:827–833.
103. Dietz WH, Gross WL, Kirkpatrick JA: Blount's disease (tibia vara): Another skeletal disorder associated with childhood obesity. J Pediatr 1982; 101:735–737.
104. Wadden TA, Stunkard AJ: Social and psychological consequences of obesity. Ann Intern Med 1985; 103:1062–1067.
105. Staffieri JR: A study of social stereotype of body image in children. J Pers Soc Psychol 1967; 7:101–104.
106. Stunkard AJ, Mendelson M: Obesity and the body image: I. Characteristics of disturbances in the body image of some obese persons. Am J Psychiatry 1967; 123:1296–1300.
107. Allon N: Latent social services in group dieting. Soc Prob 1975; 32:59–69.
108. Roe DA, Eickwort KR: Relationships between obesity and associated health factors with unemployment among low-income females. J Am Med Wom Assoc 1976; 31:193–194, 198–199, 203–204.
109. Wooley OW, Wooley SC, Dyrenforth SR: Obesity and women. II. A neglected feminist topic. Wom Stud Int Q 1979; 2:81–92.
110. Garn SM, Rohmann CG: Interaction of nutrition and genetics and the timing of growth and development. Pediatr Clin North Am 1966; 13:353–379.
111. Wooley SC, Wooley OW: Should obesity be treated at all? *In* Stunkard AJ, Stellar E, eds: Eating and Its Disorders. New York, Raven Press, 1984, pp 185–192.
112. Fitzgerald FT: The problem of obesity. Annu Rev Med 1981; 32:221–231.
113. Knapp TR: A methodological critique of the "ideal weight" concept. JAMA 1983; 250:506–510.
114. Dietz WH Jr: Nutrition and obesity. *In* Grand RJ, Sutphen JL, Dietz WH Jr, eds: Pediatric Nutrition. Boston, Butterworths, 1987, pp 525–538.
115. Abraham S, Collins G, Nordsieck M: Relationship of childhood weight status to morbidity in adults. HSMHA Health Rep 1971; 86:273–284.
116. Abraham S, Nordsieck M: Relationship of excess weight in childhood. Public Health Rep 1960; 75:263–273.
117. Pisacano JC, Lichter H, Ritter J, et al: An attempt at prevention of obesity in infancy. Pediatrics 1978; 61:360–364.
118. Bureau of Nutrition: The Prudent Diet. New York, Bureau of Nutrition, Department of Health, 1972.
119. Epstein LH, Squires S: The Stop Light Diet for Children: An 8-Week Program for Children and Parents. Boston, Little, Brown, 1988.
120. Brook CG, Lloyd JK, Wolff OH: Rapid weight loss in children. Br Med J 1974; 3:44–45.
121. Rayner PH, Court JM: Effect of dietary restriction and anorectic drugs on linear growth in childhood obesity. Arch Dis Child 1974; 49:822–823.
122. Thompson JK, Jarvie GJ, Lahey BB, et al: Exercise and obesity: Etiology, physiology, and intervention. Psychol Bull 1982; 91:55–79.
123. Bray GA: The Obese Patient. Philadelphia, WB Saunders, 1976, pp 94–128.
124. Brownell KD: Obesity: Understanding and treating a serious, prevalent, and refractory disorder. J Consult Clin Psychol 1982; 50:820–840.
125. Dupont DC, Freedman AP: Obesity. *In* Bove A, Lowenthal D, eds: Exercise Medicine. New York, Academic Press, 1983, pp 270–271.
126. Miller PM, Sims KL: Evaluation and component analysis of a comprehensive weight control program. Int J Obesity 1981; 5:57–66.
127. The American Heritage Dictionary. Revised edition of The American Heritage Dictionary of the English Language. New college ed. Boston, Houghton Mifflin, 1985.
128. Chapman SL, Jeffry DB: Situational management, standard setting, and self-reward in a behavior modification weight loss program. J Consult Clin Psychol 1978; 46:1588–1589.
129. Wing RR, Jeffery RW: Outpatient treatments of obesity: A

comparison of methodology and clinical results. Int J Obesity 1979; 3:261–279.
130. Kramer FM, Jeffery RW, Forster JL, et al: Long-term follow-up of behavioral treatment for obesity: Patterns of weight regain among men and women. Int J Obesity 1989; 13:123–136.
131. Stunkard AJ, Penick SB: Behavior modification in the treatment of obesity. The problem of maintaining weight loss. Arch Gen Psychiatry 1979; 36:801–806.
132. Epstein LH, Wing RR, Sternachak L, et al: Comparison of family-based behavior modification and nutrition education for childhood obesity. J Pediatr Psychol 1980; 5:25–36.
133. Graves T, Myers AW, Clark L: An evaluation of problem-solving training in the behavioral treatment of childhood obesity. J Consult Clin Psychol 1988; 56:246–250.
134. Epstein LH, Valoski A, Wing RR, et al: Ten-year follow-up of behavioral, family-based program for obese children. JAMA 1990; 264:2519–2523.

Chapter 10

Dysphagia and Vomiting

SUSAN R. ORENSTEIN

The gastrointestinal tract propels ingested material in a rostral-caudal direction through its lumen. Both dysphagia and vomiting are symptoms suggesting impairment of this process. This chapter focuses on the differential diagnosis and diagnostic evaluation of these symptoms, and briefly reviews the therapeutic options. Excellent sources for detailed information concerning the physiologic bases for these events are also available.[1, 2]

DYSPHAGIA

Normal Swallowing

Swallowing is a complex, usually automatic function of the oropharynx and esophagus that is required before the other nutrient-processing functions of the gastrointestinal system occur. Swallowing is divided into three phases: oral, pharyngeal, and esophageal. The mouth prepares food for swallowing by mastication, lubrication, and formation of a bolus, which is then presented to the pharynx by the tongue. This automatic preparation is of variable duration and under voluntary control. The pharyngeal phase is rapid (<1 sec) and reflexive. Protective mechanisms to keep food out of the airway during pharyngeal transit include elevation of the soft palate against the nasopharyngeal wall, lowering of the epiglottis over the larynx, closure of the glottis, temporary arrest of respiration, and relaxation and opening of the upper esophageal sphincter (UES). The opening of the UES directs the food into the esophagus, where the esophageal phase of deglutition begins. Esophageal peristalsis is coordinated with the pharyngeal contraction and the aftercontraction of the UES to continue the propulsion of the food toward the stomach. The lower esophageal sphincter (LES) relaxes nearly simultaneously with the UES to allow rapidly moving liquids to enter the stomach without resistance well before the peristaltic wave (traveling at about 3 cm per sec) reaches the LES.

Dysphagia and Related Symptoms

Dysphagia is generally defined as difficulty swallowing, a symptom that may be described by an older child or adolescent. An infant or young child, on the other hand, must demonstrate the difficulty swallowing, sometimes quite dramatically (Table 10–1). An infant or child may choke, cough, gag, or become cyanotic during feedings. When these symptoms occur during deglutition, the location of the disorder is usually oropharyngeal; coughing immediately following deglutition suggests a pharyngoesophageal disorder. Symptoms following a meal suggest gastroesophageal reflux or retention of material in a diverticulum or in an enlarged esophagus. If these symptoms are not attended to, a young child may begin to refuse to drink or eat, appearing hungry but turning away from offered nutrition. Weight loss or lack of normal weight gain may ensue. Recurrent aspiration pneumonias, initially seeming to be the result of a primary infection, may occur as more subtle symptoms of dysfunctional swallowing. Oral regurgitation during a meal may result from dysfunctional swallowing in some patients; nasal regurgitation during drinking may accompany severe disability of upper esophageal function; drooling because of an inability to handle even secretions may befall some children with a severe obstruction. Dysphagia may be accompanied by changes in voice quality owing to chronic laryngeal soiling and irritation by incompletely swallowed material. Finally, unusual behavior during eating may be the only manifestation of dysphagia.

Dysphagia is usually perceived as discomfort rather

Table 10–1. OTHER SYMPTOMS SOMETIMES ASSOCIATED WITH DYSPHAGIA

Aspiration
Cough, choke, gag
Recurrent pneumonia
Nasopharyngeal Regurgitation (sneezing)
Oral Regurgitation (drooling, if severe—unable to handle own secretions)
Abnormalities of Voice
"Wet" voice—due to laryngeal soiling from dysfunctional swallowing
Hoarse voice—due to laryngeal inflammation
"Nasal" voice—due to velopharyngeal insufficiency and nasopharyngeal air escape
Swallowing Behavior
Posturing of head and neck during swallowing
Rapid or slow intake; multiple swallows; pocketing of food in cheeks

than pain and may be localized substernally or in the suprasternal notch. The discomfort is commonly perceived to be proximal to the actual site of obstruction; it is rarely referred distally. Older children may be able to distinguish dysphagia from other similar symptoms, such as odynophagia (painful swallowing) or heartburn, but these symptoms are often poorly distinguished, even by adults. A recent review of 1,035 adults evaluated for dysphagia found that only 36% of them could be documented to have esophageal dysmotility, but 62% had increased esophageal acid exposure. Of the entire group with dysphagia, 74% of them also complained of heartburn.[3] Two particular forms of dysphagia have been identified: transfer dysphagia and globus. The former denotes dysphagia during the oropharyngeal phase of swallowing, and the latter refers to the sensation that something is stuck in the upper esophagus. Although originally considered to represent a psychogenic etiology, globus (originally globus hystericus) actually may have an organic basis.[4]

Table 10–2. DIFFERENTIAL DIAGNOSIS OF DYSPHAGIA

Structural Causes (fixed narrowing)
- Intrinsic: stenosis, web, stricture (see Table 10–3); tumor, polyp
- Extrinsic: vascular ring, thyromegaly, exostosis, paraesophageal hernia, esophageal diverticula

Functional Causes (dysmotility)
- Systemic neuromuscular disease
  - Corticobulbar dysfunction
    - Newborn transient pharyngeal weakness—congenital flaccid bulbar palsy
    - Congenital malformations: Arnold-Chiari, syringobulbia
    - Acquired disease: stroke (cortical, bulbar), tumor, trauma, bulbar polio
    - Cerebral palsy, pseudobulbar palsy, bulbar palsy
  - Neuropathy
    - Metabolic: diabetic neuropathy
    - Toxin: tetanus, lead poisoning, rabies
    - Drug: nitrazepam
  - Motor end plate: myasthenia gravis, botulism
  - Myopathy
    - Dystrophy: myotonic, oculopharyngeal
    - Inflammatory
      - Striated muscle: polymyositis, dermatomyositis
      - Smooth muscle: systemic lupus erythematosus
    - Metabolic: hyperthyroid, hypothyroid
- Isolated esophageal dysmotility
  - Diffuse esophageal spasm
  - Nutcracker esophagus
  - Achalasia
  - Hypertensive LES
  - Nonspecific esophageal motility disorder

Miscellaneous Causes
- Inflammatory
  - Pharyngeal: pharyngitis, pharyngeal abscess
  - Esophageal: esophagitis (reflux associated, infectious, pill induced)
- Cicatricial: tracheostomy, other neck surgery
- Foreign body
- Psychogenic: globus
- Familial dysautonomia

Adapted from Enterline H, Thompson J: Congenital defects, rings, and webs. *In* Enterline H, Thompson J, eds: Pathology of the Esophagus. New York, Springer-Verlag, 1984, pp 23–41; with permission.

Table 10–3. DIFFERENTIAL DIAGNOSIS OF ESOPHAGEAL STENOSES

Upper Esophagus
- Inflammatory: caustic ingestion, epidermolysis bullosa, other
- Congenital

Midesophagus
- Inflammatory: "peptic," due to reflux (including Barrett's stricture)
- Congenital
  - Isolated
  - Esophageal atresia associated (tracheal remnants or cartilage in some)

Lower Esophagus
- Inflammatory: "peptic" due to reflux
- Muscular ring (A ring—proximal)
- Mucosal rings, webs
  - Above squamocolumnar junction
  - At squamocolumnar junction (Schatzki's; B ring—distal)

Miscellaneous
- Postoperative, other than esophageal atresia repair
- Inflammatory, other than peptic or caustic
  - Nasogastric tubes, radiation therapy, chemotherapy
  - Drugs, infections

Adapted from Enterline H, Thompson J: Congenital defects, rings, and webs. *In* Enterline H, Thompson J, eds: Pathology of the Esophagus. New York, Springer-Verlag, 1984, pp 23–41; with permission.

Differential Diagnosis

When dysphagia for liquids is less than that for solids, a structural cause, such as a fixed esophageal narrowing, is likely; when dysphagia for liquids is the same as, or greater than, that for solids, dysmotility is suggested. A structural cause is also indicated by the need to regurgitate a bolus to gain relief, whereas dysmotility is indicated when movements of the neck or repeated swallowing permits material to pass into the stomach. This differentiation between the structural and functional aspects of dysphagia is a basic step in categorizing the causes for the condition (Table 10–2).

Structural Disorders. Structural, fixed obstruction to the propagated movement of a swallowed bolus may result from an intrinsic narrowing of the esophagus by congenital stenoses (Fig. 10–1) or webs, or by acquired strictures (Fig. 10–2) or tumors. These intrinsic obstructions of the esophagus are further categorized in Table 10–3. The age and previous history of the child, as well as the radiographic localization of the narrowing, suggest the etiology. Further diagnostic refinement is achieved endoscopically and histologically. Extrinsic compression of the esophagus also may present as dysphagia; the radiographic appearance aids in the diagnosis of entities such as vascular rings causing dysphagia lusoria (Fig. 10–3).

Functional Disorders. Most nonstructural causes of dysphagia are due to dysmotility of the oropharynx and esophagus (see Table 10–2). A host of systemic neuromuscular diseases may affect the neuromuscular foundations of normal swallowing. Cortical or brain stem disease may impair voluntary transfer of the bolus to the pharynx (i.e., the oral phase of swallowing); dysfunction of the brain stem or any of the six cranial nerves that participate in normal swallowing may affect

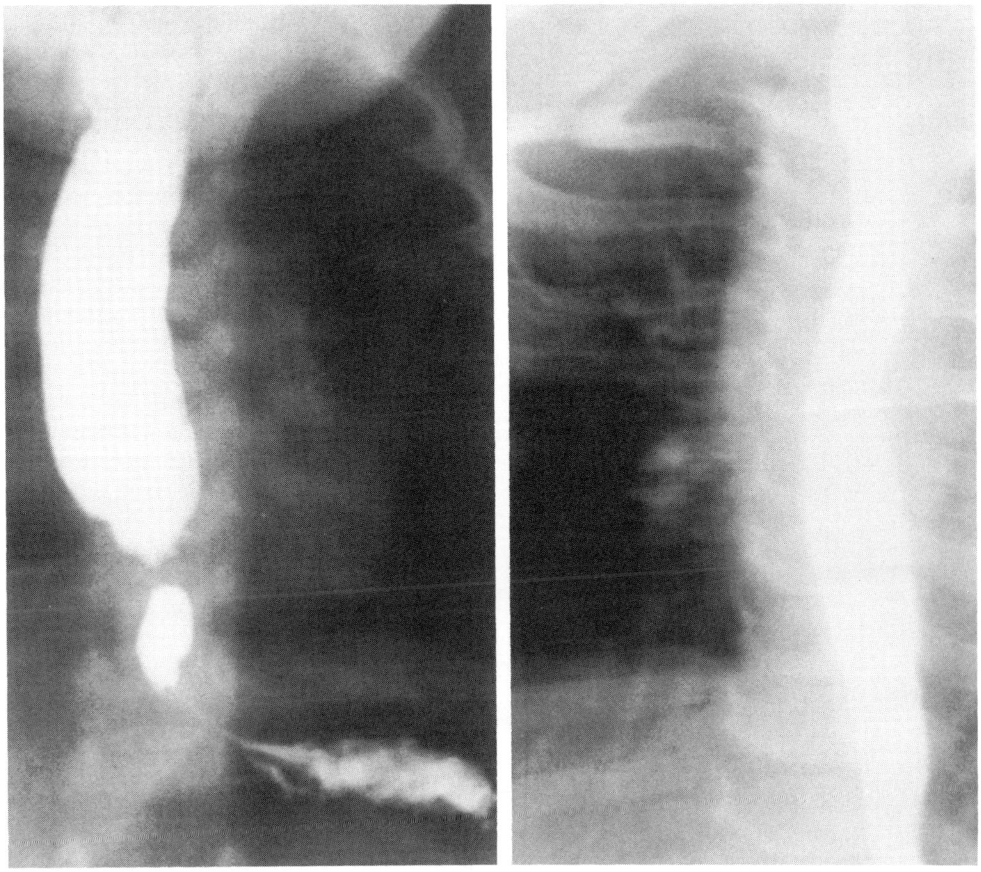

Figure 10–1. Radiograph of a congenital esophageal stenosis, before and after treatment with dilatations. This boy presented at 1 month of age with a 3-week history of coughing, gagging, and forceful emesis at each feeding; the barium esophagram (*left*) showed a very narrow stenosis with proximal dilation of the esophagus. After a series of eight endoscopic balloon dilations during the next 7 months, he remained asymptomatic, and barium esophagram at 1 year of age demonstrated resolution of the stenosis (*right*). (From Garau P, Orenstein SR: Congenital muscular esophageal stenosis treated by balloon dilation. J Pediatr Gastroenterol Nutr 1993; 16:98–101; with permission.)

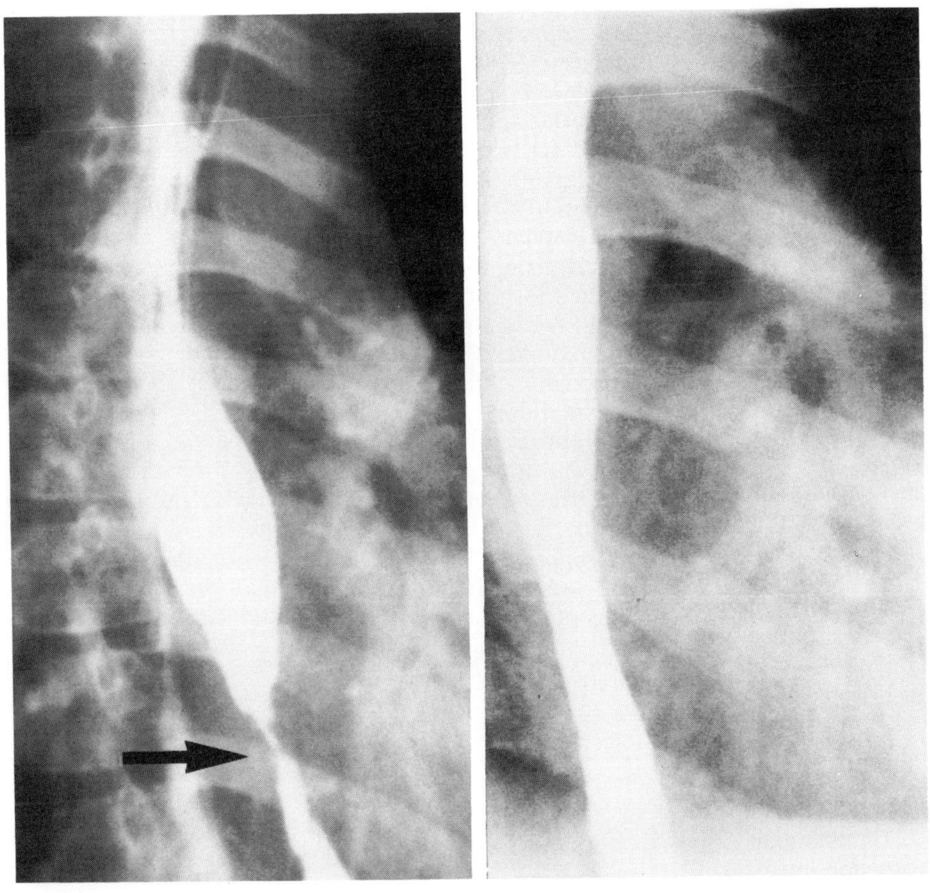

Figure 10–2. Radiograph of a peptic esophageal stricture, before and after treatment with dilatations. This 10-year-old boy had a 6-month history of dysphagia before his stricture (*arrow*) was demonstrated by barium esophagram (*left*). Weight had dropped to the 10th percentile, but height was at the 50th percentile. The stricture was improved symptomatically and radiographically (*right*) by a series of bougienage dilations, and subsequent fundoplication allowed the underlying peptic esophagitis to heal.

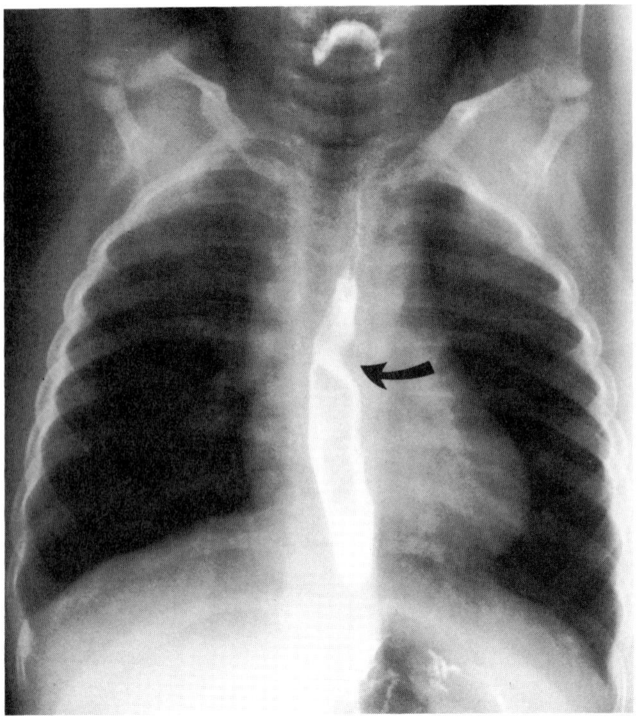

Figure 10–3. Vascular malformation producing dysphagia. Barium esophagram demonstrates a right subclavian artery in this 2-year-old girl with dysphagia for solid foods and postprandial coughing and choking. The anterior-posterior projection shows the impression on the barium column (*arrow*) made by the anomalous artery as it courses upward from left to right behind the esophagus after its origin from the aortic arch. (From Orenstein SR: Manometric demonstration of aberrant right subclavian artery associated with dysphagia. J Pediatr Gastroenterol Nutr 1984; 3:635; with permission.)

initiation of the automatic, semireflexive portion of the swallow in the pharynx; and myopathies, brain stem abnormalities, or disorders of intrinsic esophageal neurons may hinder the function of both the smooth muscle of the lower esophagus and the striated muscle of the oropharynx and upper esophagus.[5, 6]

In addition to being caused by systemic disease, dysmotility may result from isolated (primary) esophageal motility disorders. These are largely classified descriptively and are discussed in more detail in Chapter 28.

Miscellaneous Disorders. Esophageal complaints, including dysphagia, also may be due to several common disorders that do not fit clearly into the structural-functional classification discussed previously. Inflammatory disease of the pharynx and esophagus (such as that due to gastroesophageal reflux) may produce nonspecific dysmotility or may result in odynophagia, which is difficult for the patient to distinguish from dysphagia. Similarly, a pharyngeal or esophageal foreign body may temporarily disturb motor function or may cause a partial obstruction or discomfort that is difficult to distinguish from dysphagia. Scarring due to surgery in the neck, particularly tracheostomy, often impairs the laryngeal elevation, which is necessary for normal cricopharyngeal opening, and thus may cause dysphagia. Anomalies such as H-type tracheoesophageal fistula, laryngeal cleft, or unilateral vocal cord paralysis also may present as swallowing difficulties. The interactions of emotional state and esophageal function have been noted repeatedly and may underlie some of the reported associations between dysphagia and psychiatric illness.[7–11]

Cricopharyngeal Dysphagia. Cricopharyngeal dysphagia is a particularly interesting category of motor dysfunction causing dysphagia. Normal functioning of the UES (largely the cricopharyngeal muscle) demands exquisitely coordinated timing between pharyngeal contraction and UES relaxation. The pharyngeal contraction should not begin prior to UES relaxation and should end before the UES resumes its normal tone. The UES must relax completely and must be actively pulled open by the upward and forward movement of the larynx.

Abnormalities of several types have been identified in the function of this intricate unit (Table 10–4). The pharyngeal contractions may be hypotensive. The UES may fail to relax or may relax incompletely (cricopharyngeal achalasia). It may relax late or resume its tone early. Finally, it may fail to open completely owing to inadequate elevation of the larynx. These findings are demonstrable manometrically and may be suggested radiographically.

A posterior cricopharyngeal bar is sometimes seen radiographically in these instances and was formerly assumed to represent spasm of the cricopharyngeal muscle. Recently, however, such bars have been shown to be associated with normal cricopharyngeal pressure and relaxation and normal flow across the UES. The bar seems actually to represent a reduced maximal dimension of the UES owing to reduced muscle compliance; the normal rate of flow is produced by increased intrabolus pressure "upstream" from the bar.[12]

Although many cases of cricopharyngeal dysphagia in childhood remain idiopathic, discrete treatable causes of cricopharyngeal dysphagia continue to be identified. Recent examples include drooling and aspiration associated with nitrazepam (Fig. 10–4) and dysphagia associated with unsuspected Arnold-Chiari malformations (Fig. 10–5).[13, 14] Thus, it is important to investigate thoroughly children who have dysphagia before characterizing their symptoms as idiopathic.

Oropharyngeal Dysphagia. Neurologic causes for oropharyngeal dysphagia make bolus formation challenging, causing particular difficulty with thin liquids and grainy foods (such as rice or crackers).

Esophageal Diverticulum. Diverticula of the esophagus are intriguing lesions that may present with symptoms of dysphagia. Epiphrenic and Zenker's diverticula

Table 10–4. CLASSIFICATION OF CRICOPHARYNGEAL DYSPHAGIA

Pharyngeal motor weakness
Cricopharyngeal achalasia
Cricopharyngeal incoordination
Defective laryngeal elevation and cricopharyngeal opening

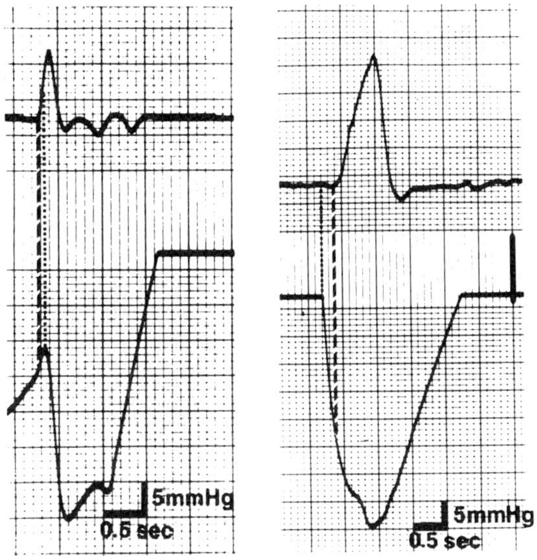

Figure 10–4. Cricopharyngeal incoordination due to nitrazepam. Manometric tracings from an 18-month-old boy with drooling and aspiration show pharyngeal (*upper tracings*) and cricopharyngeal (*lower tracings*) pressures with swallowing both before (*left panel*) and after (*right panel*) reduction of his nitrazepam dosage. Before reduction of the dosage, the peak of pharyngeal contraction occurs prior to the onset of cricopharyngeal relaxation, and 0.2 seconds prior to the nadir of relaxation; these findings, as well as his symptoms, normalized following reduction of the dosage. (Adapted from Wyllie E, Wyllie R, Cruse RP, et al. Reprinted with permission from *The New England Journal of Medicine,* vol. 314, pp 36–37, 1986.)

occur above sphincters, and are believed to be caused by high-pressure or poorly relaxing sphincters (pulsion diverticula), in contrast with the midesophageal diverticula caused by traction. This difference has implications for therapy, in that myotomy of the related sphincter is believed by many clinicians to be a necessary part of the surgical therapy of pulsion diverticula.[15] A diverticulum may also independently cause dysphagia by external compression of the nearby esophagus.

Diagnostic Evaluation

Radiology. Diagnostic evaluation of children presenting with dysphagia (Table 10–5) generally begins with radiographic evaluation.[16] Structural abnormalities can be readily identified, dysmotility of the oropharynx and esophagus can be seen, and sequelae such as laryngeal aspiration or nasopharyngeal regurgitation can be documented. Barium fluoroscopy provides a particularly vivid demonstration of intrinsic (see Figs. 10–1 and 10–2) and extrinsic (see Fig. 10–3) obstructive lesions of the esophagus, and it documents characteristic findings in functional disorders, such as the achalasia beak (Fig. 10–6) or the cricopharyngeal bar (Fig. 10–7). As with most diagnostic procedures, the yield of radiography depends on the interest and expertise of the person performing the study.

Several useful techniques for radiologic examination have been described: full column, mucosal relief, double contrast, and recording of motion.[17] The full column is optimal for demonstrating structural lesions and can be supplemented by using barium-coated solid boluses, such as marshmallows or cookies, in addition to various consistencies of liquid barium. Dense barium is used for demonstrating the mucosal surface detail, both in the collapsed esophagus (mucosal relief technique) and in the esophagus distended with gas (double-contrast technique [Fig. 10–8]). As a supplement to routine "spot films," recording of motion permits the identification of functional disorders of swallowing. Such recording is performed during fluoroscopic observation, using methods such as videotaping or cine recording. These methods allow repeated review of the motility at reduced speed and are particularly necessary in the oropharynx and at the UES, because of the rapidity and complexity of this part of the normal swallow.

Manometry. Unless a clear structural lesion is demonstrated radiographically, most patients with dysphagia will benefit from manometric evaluation. Esophageal manometry examines the motility of the esophagus, including the LES, the UES, and the pharynx. It should generally be performed with the patient unsedated, with

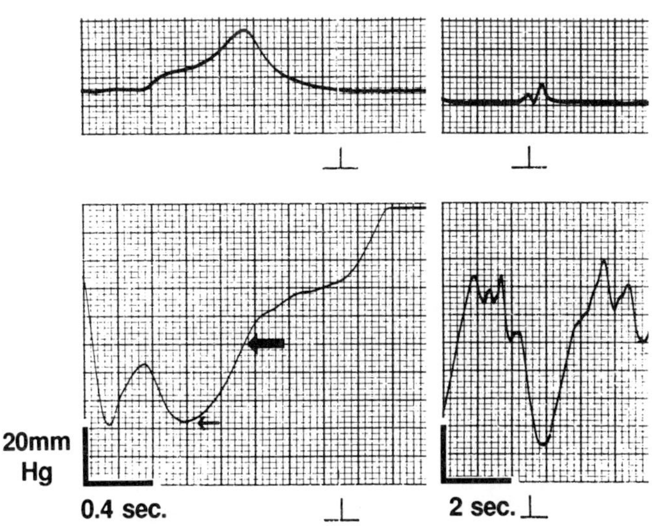

Figure 10–5. Cricopharyngeal incoordination due to Arnold-Chiari malformation. This boy presented at birth with a cervical myelomeningocele, hydrocephalus (treated with ventriculoperitoneal shunt), and a cervical syrinx. At 2 years of age, dysphagia led to manometric evaluation, which demonstrated cricopharyngeal incoordination (*left panel*). The pharyngeal wave (*upper tracing*) is not coordinated with UES relaxation (*lower tracing*) in this preoperative study; the nadir of sphincter relaxation (*small arrow*) occurs 0.3 seconds before the pharyngeal peak, and the sphincter pressure exceeds the pharyngeal pressure at the time of the pharyngeal peak (*large arrow*). Seven months later, following craniocervical decompression, resolution of dysphagia and the manometric incoordination were demonstrated (*right panel*), although duplex pharyngeal waves persisted. (Reproduced with permission from Putnam PE, Orenstein SR, Pang D, et al: Cricopharyngeal dysfunction associated with Chiari malformations. Pediatrics 1992; 89:871–876. Copyright 1992 Pediatrics.)

Table 10–5. DIAGNOSTIC EVALUATION OF DYSPHAGIA

Barium Fluoroscopy
Structural and obstructing defects
Dysmotility: tongue, palate, oropharynx, cricopharyngeus, esophagus
Aspiration: laryngeal, nasopharyngeal
Manometry—Functional Neuromuscular Defects
Abnormalities of pressure
Low- or high-amplitude waves
High-pressure or nonrelaxing sphincters
Abnormalities of duration or configuration of waves
Abnormalities of timing
Slow, rapid, simultaneous, retrograde, incomplete, or uncoordinated peristalsis
Uncoordinated relaxation of sphincters
Provocative testing
Endoscopy (± biopsy)
Structural defects
Mucosal detail
Histologic evaluation
Therapeutic intervention

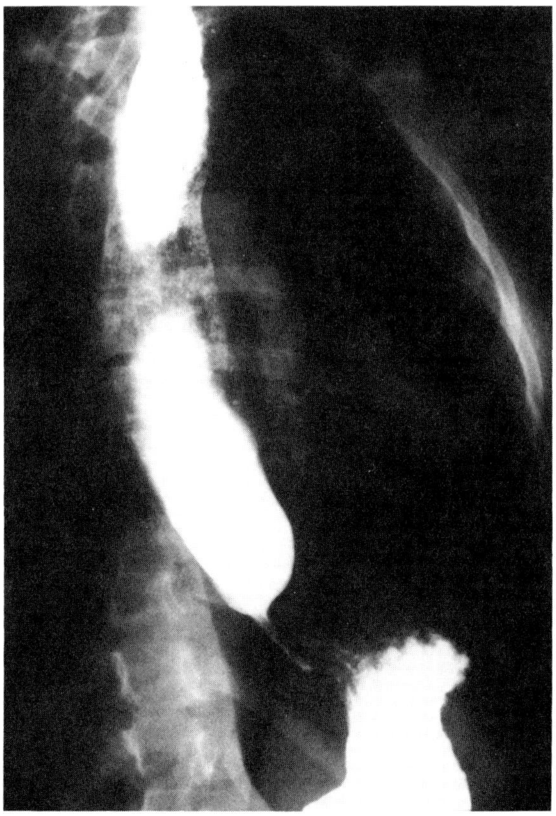

Figure 10–6. Radiographic demonstration of achalasia producing dysphagia. This 14-year-old girl had had the sensation of food getting stuck in her esophagus for 2 years and regurgitated food every 1 to 15 days, nonetheless maintaining excellent nutrition—her weight was at the 60th percentile and her height, 15th percentile. Barium esophagram showed the typical "beak" at the gastroesophageal junction, and food mixed with the barium despite fasting overnight. Esophageal manometry confirmed the diagnosis of achalasia, showing complete failure of LES relaxation and simultaneous low-pressure, repetitive waves in the esophageal body, which also had an elevated baseline pressure. She reported responding symptomatically to nifedipine but will probably eventually require dilation or myotomy.

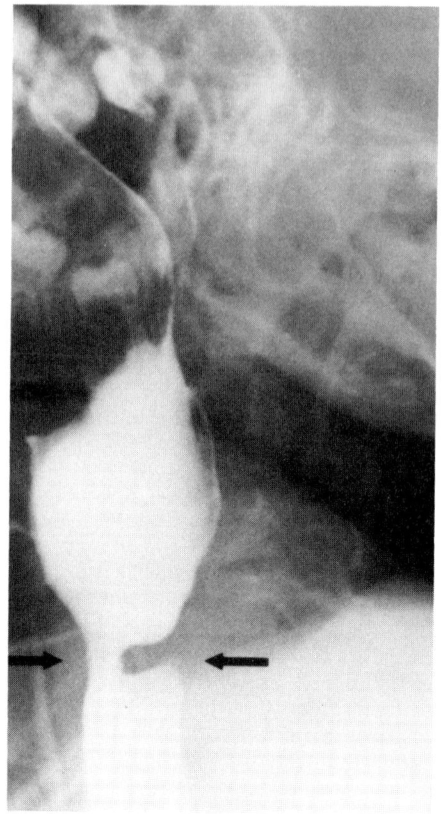

Figure 10–7. A cricopharyngeal bar. This boy presented at birth with an L4 myelomeningocele and also had hydrocephalus (treated with ventriculoperitoneal shunt) and type II Arnold-Chiari malformation. At 3 years of age, his dysphagia, gurgling voice, and nasal speech led to evaluation, which demonstrated cricopharyngeal incoordination. Although craniocervical decompression relieved the dysphagia and manometric abnormalities, it did not relieve the dysphonia or radiographic cricopharyngeal bar, shown here as a posterior impression on the barium column at the level of the upper esophageal sphincter (*arrows*) 4 years after decompression. However, the delay in bolus transit that was associated with the bar preoperatively was relieved by the decompressive surgery. (Reproduced with permission from Putnam PE, Orenstein SR, Pang D, et al. Pediatrics 1992; 89:871–876. Copyright 1992 Pediatrics.)

examination of each area during wet and dry swallows. (The latter may be achieved in infants or neurologically abnormal children using a primitive reflex: a puff of air blown on the face produces a swallow.[18]) Amplitude, duration, and speed of pressure waves are quantified. Resting tone of the UES and the LES is measured, although the marked lability of the former must be kept in mind.[19] Completeness and coordination of the relaxations of these sphincters are also noted. Occasionally, provocative maneuvers such as acid infusion, balloon distention, food ingestion, or administration of edrophonium, bethanechol, or pentagastrin are useful.[20–22] An example of a form for recording these results is shown in Figure 10–9; it is organized from the distal to the proximal areas because that is the order of examination as the motility catheter is withdrawn. Table 10–6 lists some of the disorders that are associated with various manometric abnormalities.

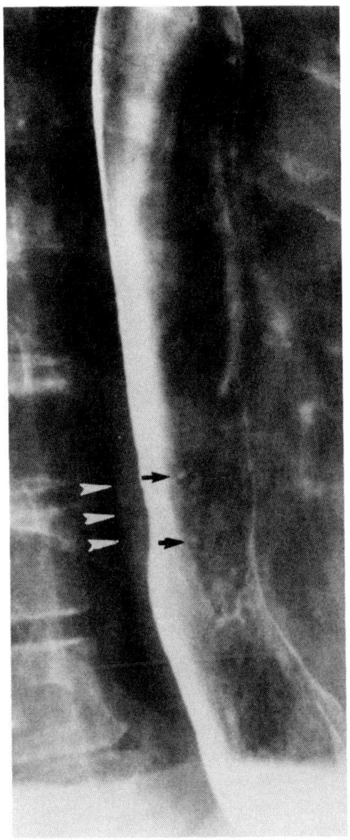

Figure 10–8. Radiographic demonstration of esophagitis. Double-contrast film in a patient with severe endoscopic esophagitis shows surface irregularity, erosions (*arrows*), and mild narrowing with wall thickening (*arrowheads*). (From Ott DJ: Barium esophagram. *In* Castell D, Wu W, Ott E, eds: Gastro-Esophageal Reflux Disease: Pathogenesis, Diagnosis, Therapy. Mount Kisco, NY, Futura, 1985, p 119; with permission.)

Endoscopy, Biopsy, and Dilatation. Endoscopy is the optimal study for examination of mucosal detail, and it permits histologic sampling and performance of some therapeutic procedures at the same time. For dysphagia that has been shown radiographically to result from intrinsic structural lesions, endoscopy provides information about whether a stenotic area (Fig. 10–10) is associated with peptic esophagitis, Barrett's esophagus (Fig. 10–11), or muscle hypertrophy (Fig. 10–12), for example, and identifies the nature of inflammatory or neoplastic causes for dysphagia. Therapeutic endoscopic procedures, such as dilatations, may be carried out at the same time, both for intrinsic structural lesions (congenital as well as acquired [see Figs. 10–1 and 10–2]) and for functional lesions such as achalasia of the LES and the UES.[23–25]

Therapy

Therapy for dysphagia is tailored to its cause (Table 10–7). Definitive therapy is available for some disorders, whereas supportive care must suffice for others. Cricopharyngeal achalasia, for example, may be treated with neurosurgical decompression if it is caused by Arnold-Chiari malformation[14]; with dilatation if it is idiopathic, persistent,[26] and associated with normal oropharyngeal function[23]; or with myotomy if dilatation is unavailable or unsuccessful.[27, 28] Pharmacologic therapy is available for some primary disorders of esophageal motility.[29–33] For disorders without any known definitive therapy, techniques that maintain nutrition while they protect the airway from aspiration are crucial. Whether oral feeding can be maintained depends on the severity of the disorder and the compensatory mechanisms available. Specialists in oral rehabilitation are found in several disciplines, including speech therapy and occupational therapy, and their expertise can be valuable in feeding a child with dysphagia.[34, 35] Oral nutrition of patients with dysphagia can often be improved by changes in food (consistency and temperature), feeding tools (straw and spoon), positioning (of the body, head, and neck), and behaviors facilitating safe swallowing. These behaviors include the Mendelsohn maneuver, which prolongs laryngeal elevation and therefore cricopharyngeal opening, and the supraglottic swallow, which uses valved expiration following the swallow to decrease aspiration. When oral feeding is not possible, other means for assuring nutrition must be used. When dysphagia is so severe that even oral secretions are hazardous, extreme measures may be required to prevent chronic aspiration.[36]

VOMITING

Vomiting and Related Symptoms

Vomiting is defined as the forceful expulsion of the contents of the stomach through the mouth. It may be seen as a protective reflex: removing toxic material from the body or relieving pressure in hollow organs distended by distal obstruction. It is often preceded by nausea and retching.

Nausea is an unpleasant, vaguely epigastric or abdominal sensation, which is difficult to define or describe. It has been quantified by subjective scales[37] and is accompanied by a variety of autonomic changes: decreased gastric tone, contractions, secretion, and mucosal blood flow; increased salivation, sweating, pupil diameter, and heart rate; and changed respiratory rhythm.[1] Duodenogastric reflux may occur during nausea, accompanied by retrograde peristalsis from the small intestine to the antrum or by generalized, simultaneous contractions of the antrum and the duodenum.[38, 39] *Retching* is defined as strong, involuntary efforts to vomit; they may be seen as preparatory maneuvers to vomiting. These efforts consist of spasmodic contractions of the somatic muscles of the diaphragm (both costal and crural) and the abdominal wall at the same time as the LES relaxes. The LES is also pulled cephalad by contraction of the striated longitudinal muscles of the upper esophagus and may herniate through the crural hiatus, preventing the increased intra-abdominal pressure from being transmitted to the LES.[40] During retching, gastric material is

CHILDREN'S HOSPITAL OF PITTSBURGH

DIGESTIVE DISORDERS

ANORECTAL / ESOPHAGEAL MOTILITY REPORT

FORM NO. 528-494 (10-84)

DATE	AGE	SEX	☐ INPATIENT ☐ OUTPATIENT IF OUTPATIENT, HANDWRITE REQUESTED PATIENT I.D. INFORMATION IN BOX AT RIGHT.

PATIENT NAME

UNIT NO.

BIRTH DATE

↑ ADDRESSOGRAPH PLATE AREA ↑

REFERRING PHYSICIAN	FILE NUMBER

CLINICAL DATA

MANOMETRIC DATA

☐ ANORECTAL

TECHNIQUE	TUBE DIAMETER	DISTENDING VOLUME

RECTUM

RECTAL RESTING PRESSURE

SPONTANEOUS RECTAL ACTIVITY

FREQUENCY	AMPLITUDE

RECTAL RESPONSE TO DISTENDING BALLOON

AMPLITUDE OF CONTRACTION	THRESHOLD OF SENSITIVITY

INTERNAL ANAL SPHINCTER

LOCATION	RESTING PRESSURE

SPONTANEOUS ANAL ACTIVITY

FREQUENCY	AMPLITUDE

INTERNAL ANAL RESPONSE TO DISTENDING BALLOON

THRESHOLD OF SENSITIVITY	CONTRACTION OR RELAXATION?	AMPLITUDE

EXTERNAL ANAL SPHINCTER

LOCATION	RESTING PRESSURE

EXTERNAL ANAL RESPONSE TO DISTENDING BALLOON

CONTRACTION?	AMPLITUDE

ANAL WINK

CONTRACTION?	AMPLITUDE

MAXIMAL VOLUNTARY SQUEEZE

AMPLITUDE OF CONTRACTION

VOLUNTARY DEFECATORY EFFORT

SPHINCTER RELAXATION?	TO BASELINE?

☐ ESOPHAGEAL

TECHNIQUE	TUBE DIAMETER

INTRAGASTRIC PRESSURE

LOWER ESOPHAGEAL SPHINCTER

LOCATION	PRESSURE INVERSION POINT

LES-GASTRIC PRESSURE GRADIENT (END EXPIRATORY)

RESPONSE TO SWALLOW

BODY OF ESOPHAGUS

END EXPIRATORY RESTING PRESSURE

RESPONSE TO SWALLOW

DROPPED SWALLOWS	PERISTALTIC WAVES
%	%
SIMULTANEOUS WAVES	AMPLITUDE OF WAVES
%	
DURATION OF WAVES	RATE OF PROPAGATION

UPPER ESOPHAGEAL SPHINCTER

LOCATION	PRESSURE
RELAXATION?	TO BASELINE?

PHARYNX

AMPLITUDE	DURATION	COORDINATION?

ADDITIONAL OBSERVATIONS

INTERPRETATION

PHYSICIAN'S SIGNATURE M.D.	DATE

Figure 10–9. Form used at the Children's Hospital of Pittsburgh for documenting manometric findings. The right side of the form is used to record the details of esophageal manometry.

Table 10–6. MANOMETRIC CLUES TO DIAGNOSIS OF DYSPHAGIA

Manometric Measure	Finding	Disorder*
LES		
Resting pressure	↑	***Hypertensive LES,*** **achalasia,** DES
	↓	***Hypotensive LES (GER),*** **scleroderma**
Relax with swallow	Incomplete	***Achalasia,*** DES, scleroderma
Body		
Resting pressure	↑	**Achalasia**
	↓	?
Waves		
Absent (or dropped)		**Achalasia,** NEMD
Pressure	↑	***Nutcracker,*** **DES**
	↓	**Myotonic dystrophy,** achalasia, NEMD
Duration	↑	**Nutcracker, DES**
	↓	?
Propagation	Slow	?
	Rapid	?
	Simultaneous	***DES,*** **vigorous achalasia,** NEMD
	Retrograde	?
	Incomplete	
	Dropped	**Achalasia, scleroderma,** NEMD
	Secondary (or decreased proximal pressure)	**DES,** NEMD, **dermatomyositis** or **polymyositis,** botulism
Configuration	Abnormal (multiple peaks)	***DES,*** **vigorous achalasia,** NEMD, **diabetes**
UES		
Resting pressure†	↑	**Globus,** GER, Plummer-Vinson syndrome
	↓	**Laryngectomy,** dystrophy,‡ myasthenia gravis
Relax with swallow	Incomplete (achalasia)	**Neuropathy,**§ botulism
	Uncoordinated (dyskinesia)	**Neuropathy**§
	Late relaxation	**Familial dysautonomia**
	Early closure	**Zenker's diverticulum**
Pharynx: Waves		
Pressure	↑	**Rabies, tetanus,** chorea,‖ **globus**
	↓	**Myopathy,**¶ **misc. pharyngeal palsy****
Duration	↑	**Myotonic dystrophy, rabies, tetanus, chorea**‖
	↓	?
Configuration	Abnormal	Chorea‖

Italic bold type* indicates "Required for Diagnosis"; plain **bold type indicates "Common Disorder"; plain type indicates "Occasional."

†UES pressure lability in normal subjects makes these associations questionable.

‡Dystrophy: oculopharyngeal or myotonic muscular dystrophy.

§Neuropathy: especially of brain stem or cranial nerves, e.g., bulbar polio, syringobulbia, Arnold-Chiari malformation, brain stem tumor, cerebrovascular accident of vertebrobasilar or posterior inferior cerebellar arteries.

‖Chorea: Sydenham chorea.

¶Myopathy: of striated or smooth muscle or motor end plate involved in swallowing, e.g., dystrophy, myasthenia gravis, myositis, systemic lupus erythematosus, thyrotoxicosis.

**Misc. pharyngeal palsy: e.g., cerebrovascular accident, bulbar polio, faucialform diphtheria, vagal or pharyngeal nerve involvement by botulism, lead, or ethanol neuropathy.

DES, diffuse esophageal spasm; NEMD, nonspecific esophageal motility disorders; GER, gastroesophageal reflux.

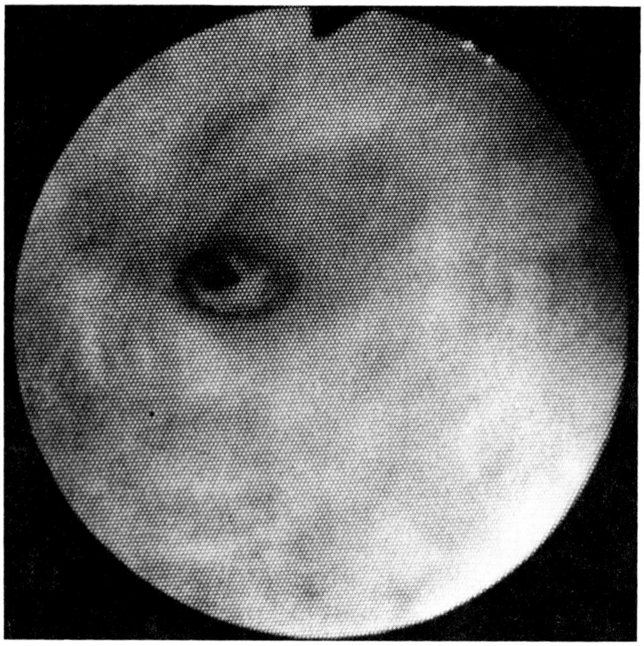

Figure 10–10. Endoscopic view of a peptic esophageal stricture. This 15-year-old boy, who had had frequent regurgitation and episodes of bronchitis during his first few years of life, had a 10-year history of dysphagia before he presented with vomiting and chest pain signaling food impaction and perforation above a stricture associated with Barrett's epithelium. Shown here is the stricture as seen endoscopically just prior to an interval repeat dilation.

Table 10–7. THERAPY FOR DYSPHAGIA

Treat Primary Disease if Possible
- Esophageal structural abnormalities: dilatation or surgery
- Systemic neuromuscular disorders
  - Neurosurgery (for brain tumor, Arnold-Chiari malformation, etc.)
  - Pharmacologic treatment (for tetanus, polymyositis, hyperthyroidism, etc.)
- Esophageal dysmotility
  - Dilatation or myotomy for hypertensive or nonrelaxing sphincters
  - Pharmacologic treatment
    - Calcium channel blocker: nifedipine, diltiazem
    - Nitrates: isosorbide dinitrate
    - Anticholinergic: propantheline bromide, valethamate bromide, L-hyoscyamine
    - Adrenoceptor antagonists?
    - Psychotropic medications (trazodone, etc.)?

Assure Nutrition and Airway Protection
- Oral feeding: slow, careful; avoid distractions
  - Nutrient characteristics
    - Bolus volume and viscosity change timing of swallow components
    - Semisolids and thick liquids generally easiest
  - Head positions
    - Neck flexion protects airway; neck extension speeds oral transit
    - Head rotation directs bolus down opposite side; head tilt, down same side
  - Maneuvers: supraglottic swallow, Mendelsohn maneuver
- Nonoral nutrition
  - Nasogastric (beware reflux) or nasoduodenal feeds
  - Gastrostomy (beware reflux) or intestinal feeds via gastrostomy
  - Jejunostomy feeds
  - Parenteral nutrition
- Laryngeal stents, etc., for patients unable to handle their secretions

moved into the esophagus by the combination of increased positive intra-abdominal pressure and increased negative intrathoracic pressure, but this material may be returned to the stomach by secondary peristalsis. Vomiting (emesis) differs from retching in that material is expelled from the mouth. This expulsion of material delivered to the esophagus by retching is fostered by relaxation of the diaphragmatic crura and reversal of intrathoracic pressure from negative to positive. The UES also relaxes, perhaps in response to the increase of intraluminal pressure in the esophagus.

Regurgitation, in contrast to vomiting, is an effortless return of gastric contents to the mouth. No nausea or retching occurs, and no contraction of the diaphragm or the abdominal muscles is evident. Regurgitation is considered to represent one form of gastroesophageal re-

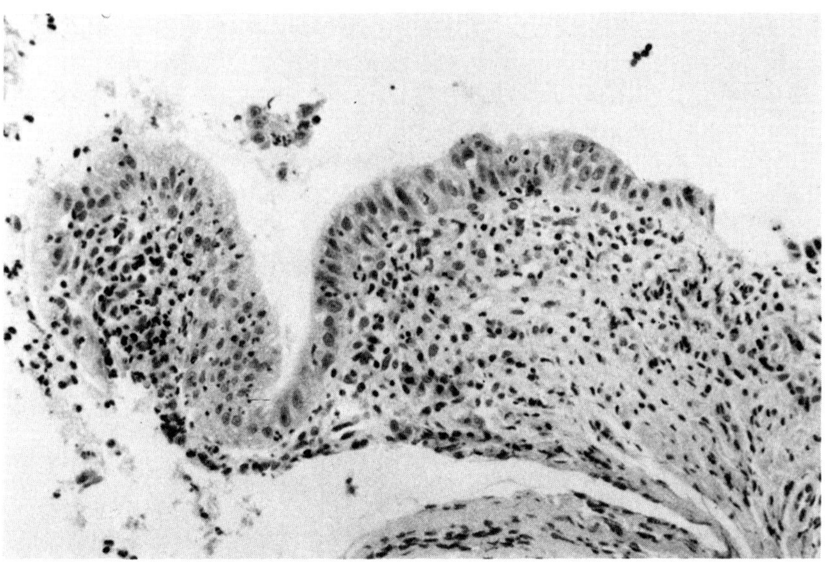

Figure 10–11. Histology of esophageal mucosa just below the esophageal stricture shown endoscopically in Figure 10–10. The epithelium is gastric type; it and the lamina propria are markedly infiltrated with inflammatory cells. That this gastric epithelium represented Barrett's metaplasia of the esophagus was supported by the finding of intestinal metaplasia with goblet cells elsewhere in the specimen.

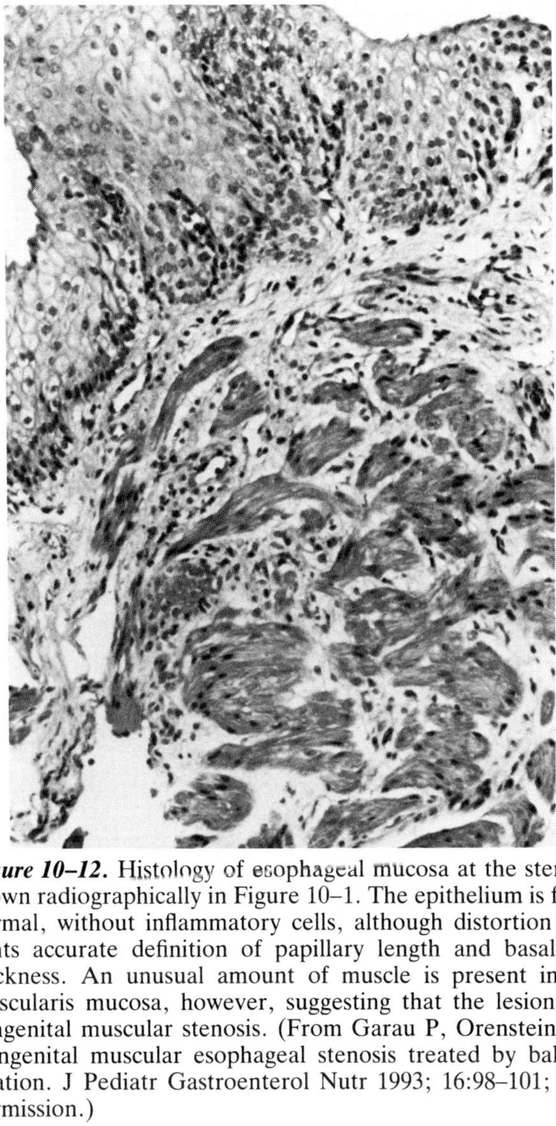

Figure 10–12. Histology of esophageal mucosa at the stenosis shown radiographically in Figure 10–1. The epithelium is fairly normal, without inflammatory cells, although distortion prevents accurate definition of papillary length and basal cell thickness. An unusual amount of muscle is present in the muscularis mucosa, however, suggesting that the lesion is a congenital muscular stenosis. (From Garau P, Orenstein SR: Congenital muscular esophageal stenosis treated by balloon dilation. J Pediatr Gastroenterol Nutr 1993; 16:98–101; with permission.)

flux; the other form is nonregurgitant or "occult" reflux, in which the refluxed material does not escape the esophagus. Whether the physiology of regurgitation is actually qualitatively different from that of vomiting is unknown, but recent work suggests that motor correlates similar to some of those associated with vomiting underlie what is termed regurgitation.[1, 41]

Neuroanatomy

The stereotypic response of vomiting is mediated by neural efferents in the vagal, phrenic, and spinal nerves (Fig. 10–13). Input to these nerves arrives from the brain stem "vomiting center." There is probably no single anatomic structure identifiable as the vomiting center, but the final common pathway for this centrally programmed complex reflex is through medullary interneurons in the solitary tract nucleus and a variety of sites in the nearby reticular formation. These interneurons probably receive cortical, vagal, vestibular, and other input, especially from the area postrema. The area postrema, the "chemoceptive trigger zone," is located on the floor of the fourth ventricle, outside the blood-brain barrier, and has been identified as a crucial source for neural input causing vomiting, particularly as a response to circulating drugs and toxins.[2, 42]

Differential Diagnosis of Vomiting

The causes of vomiting are extremely varied. Classification of the causes of vomiting may be based on (1) the anatomic locus of the proximate source of the afferent stimulation of vomiting; (2) the age of the patient; and (3) the presence of suggestive associated symptoms or signs.

Anatomic Locus of Stimulus. Table 10–8 shows a classification of causes of vomiting based on the anatomic site of origin of the stimulus. Stimuli for the vomiting center arising from the cortex, the vestibular nuclei or cerebellum, the brain stem chemoceptive trigger zone, or peripheral organs all may cause the stereotypic response of vomiting. It is thus important to keep in mind that this gastrointestinal symptom may be caused by many nongastrointestinal diseases.[43]

Age. Physicians treating children are assisted in the differential diagnosis of vomiting by the age at which the patient presents (Table 10–9). Clearly, severe congenital obstructive or metabolic diseases present in the newborn period. Developmental abnormalities and less severe congenital diseases often become symptomatic later in infancy. Feeding intolerances of various sorts also appear during infancy, as the offending food is introduced; some of these intolerances occur because the immature (or temporarily damaged) intestine is more permeable to intact antigens than is the intestine of older persons. Infants also manifest nonpathogenic regurgitant reflux (see Chapter 26). During childhood or adolescence, a wide variety of acquired disorders become symptomatic, and some subtle congenital malformations may also first become evident at these older ages. In adolescents, it is additionally important to keep in mind the disorders that may be a byproduct of this stressful period of development: vomiting due to pregnancy, drug ingestion, and eating disorders (anorexia nervosa or bulimia) are added to the diagnoses that must be considered.

Associated Symptoms or Signs. Associated symptoms or signs accompanying vomiting also help focus the evaluation for the cause of the vomiting. Such suggestive symptoms and signs are categorized in Table 10–10.

Vomiting Syndromes. Several specific syndromes featuring vomiting, which are often difficult to diagnose and manage, have been described.

Cyclic vomiting, in which episodes of severe vomiting are interspersed between intervals of normal health, is a syndrome of unknown cause, diagnosed by exclusion, managed symptomatically, and of unknown prognosis. It is probably a "wastebasket" description, perhaps

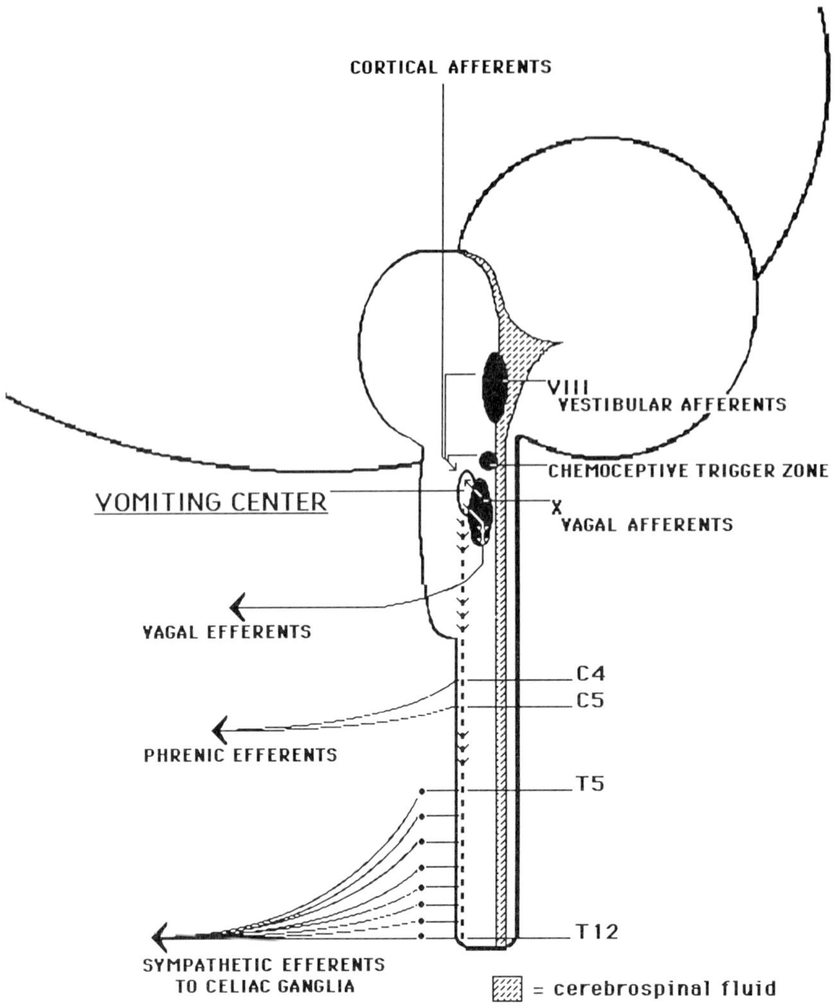

Figure 10–13. Neuroanatomy of vomiting. The diagram shows a midsagittal view of a portion of the cerebral cortex, the cerebellum, the pons, the medulla, and the spinal cord. The vomiting center receives input from the cortex, from the vestibular system (via the vestibular nucleus—VIII), from the blood (via the chemoceptive trigger zone—the area postrema), and from the gastrointestinal periphery (via the vagal nuclei—X). Output from the vomiting center through vagal, phrenic, and sympathetic nerves produces the complex stereotypic behavior associated with emesis.

including children with migrainous, epileptogenic, and psychogenic vomiting; the only advantage of considering it as a diagnosis is the mollification provided by diagnostic labeling. Such labeling should not deter the physician from being certain that treatable organic disease is not present. Reported cases of organic disease mislabeled cyclic vomiting have included intermittent intussusception or volvulus due to enteric duplication, diverticulum, or malrotation; increased intracranial pressure in shunted patients with slit ventricles; and toxic or metabolic disease.[44–47]

Psychogenic vomiting has no organic cause; this syndrome emphasizes the prominent influence that cortical and psychological inputs may have in stimulating nausea and vomiting. Characteristic features include chronicity, association with stress and with meals, suppressibility, la belle indifférence regarding the symptom itself, and relief by hospitalization. There may be no nausea or anorexia, and the vomiting may be self-induced.

Existence of the *superior mesenteric artery syndrome* is debated, but proponents of the syndrome describe extrinsic compression of the duodenum, which is trapped between the superior mesenteric artery anteriorly and the aorta posteriorly as the superior mesenteric artery crosses over the duodenum in the root of the mesentery.[48] The compression is usually just to the right of midline, where it produces a cutoff of the duodenum radiographically, often with proximal dilation. Synonyms include Wilkie's syndrome, arteriomesenteric duodenal compression, and cast syndrome. Superior mesenteric artery syndrome may be suspected when bilious emesis and epigastric discomfort relieved by vomiting occur in the context of weight loss, lordosis, body casts, lengthy bed rest, or prior abdominal surgery, particularly when crampy pain is relieved by prone or knee-chest positions. Adolescents and young adults are most often affected.

Rumination is the apparently voluntary and pleasurable regurgitation of food that is then mouthed or chewed and reswallowed. Adults and older children may regurgitate by contracting abdominal muscles[49]; infants may put their fingers or fists deep in their mouths in an apparent attempt to stimulate regurgitation. Although such apparent self-stimulation probably has a psychogenic basis in many instances, the observation of an infant whose rumination behavior ceased with treatment of her esophagitis (Orenstein SR, unpublished observation, 1986) suggests that in some instances what ap-

Table 10–8. DIFFERENTIAL DIAGNOSIS OF VOMITING BY ANATOMIC LOCUS OF STIMULUS

Stimulation of Supramedullary Receptors
- Psychogenic vomiting
- Increased intracerebral pressure (subdural effusion or hematoma, cerebral edema or tumor, hydrocephalus, meningoencephalitis, Reye's syndrome)
- Vascular (migraine, severe hypertension)
- Seizures
- Vestibular disease, "motion sickness"

Stimulation of Chemoceptive Trigger Zone
- Drugs: opiates, ipecac, digoxin, anticonvulsants
- Toxins
- Metabolic products
  - Acidemia, ketonemia (diabetic ketoacidosis, lactic acidosis, phenylketonuria, renal tubular acidosis)
  - Aminoacidemia (tyrosinemia, hypervalinemia, hyperglycinemia, lysinuria, maple syrup urine)
  - Organic acidemia (methylmalonic acidemia, proprionic acidemia, isovaleric acidemia)
  - Hyperammonemia (Reye's syndrome, urea cycle defects)
  - Uremia (renal failure)
  - Other (hereditary fructose intolerance, galactosemia, fatty acid oxidation disorders, diabetes insipidus, adrenal insufficiency, hypercalcemia, hypervitaminosis A); see also ref. 43

Stimulation of Peripheral Receptors or Obstruction of the Gastrointestinal Tract, or Both
- Pharyngeal: gag reflex (sinusitis secretions, self-induced, rumination)
- Esophageal
  - Functional: reflux, achalasia, other esophageal dysmotility
  - Structural: stricture, ring, atresia, etc.
- Gastric
  - Peptic ulcer disease (including Zollinger-Ellison syndrome), infection, dysmotility/gastroparesis
  - Obstruction (e.g., bezoar, pyloric stenosis, web, chronic granulomatous disease)
- Intestinal
  - Infection, enteritis, enterotoxin, appendicitis
  - Dysmotility (e.g., metabolic or diabetic neuropathy, intestinal pseudo-obstruction)
  - Nutrient intolerance (e.g., cow's milk, soy, gluten, eosinophilic enteropathy)
  - Obstruction (e.g., atresia, web, stenosis, adhesions, bands, volvulus, intussusception, superior mesenteric artery syndrome, duplication, meconium plug, meconium ileus, Hirschsprung's disease, distal intestinal obstruction syndrome in cystic fibrosis)
- Hepatobiliary, pancreatic: hepatitis, cholecystitis, pancreatitis
- Cardiac: intestinal ischemia
- Renal: pyelonephritis, hydronephrosis, renal calculi, glomerulonephritis
- Respiratory: pneumonia, otitis, pharyngitis, sinusitis, common cold
- Miscellaneous: peritonitis, sepsis, pregnancy; improper feeding techniques

Adapted from Orenstein SR: Gastroesophageal reflux. Curr Prob Pediatr 1991; 21:193–242; with permission.

pears to be an attempt to stimulate the gag reflex may actually be a response to pain in the throat. Other investigators have also identified rumination as a presenting symptom for gastroesophageal reflux.[50] Thus, diagnosis of, and treatment for, both psychogenic causes and esophagitis should be considered. Two types of rumination, psychogenic and self-stimulating, have been described.[51] The former tends to occur in normal infants with a disturbed parent-child relationship; the latter occurs in mentally retarded persons of any age and without regard to nurturing. Both positive and negative reinforcement have been used in behavioral therapy.[52]

Hyperemesis gravidarum is generally a problem of adults, but occasionally a pregnant pediatric patient may suffer from it. It has been suggested that esophagitis plays a role in prolonging vomiting during pregnancy.[53]

Abdominal migraine is a periodic syndrome of abdominal symptoms. Epigastric or periumbilical pain may accompany nausea and vomiting; diarrhea, fever, chills, vertigo, irritability, and polyuria have also been reported. When these abdominal symptoms coexist with head pain, which occurs in 30 to 40% of patients with migrainous headaches, the diagnosis is simpler than when they occur in isolation, which happens in about 3% of patients who later develop typical migrainous headaches. Usually, isolated abdominal migrainous attacks occur suddenly, last an hour to days, and are consistent in character within the same person. There is usually a family history of migraine, and patients are asymptomatic between attacks. Recent work has suggested criteria for diagnosis of abdominal migraine based on the visual evoked response.[54] Symptoms respond to prophylactic propranolol; ergotamine may abort an episode. These symptoms are likely to be due to vascular constriction causing ischemia of the gastrointestinal tract or of central nervous system areas innervating the gastrointestinal tract.

Anorexia nervosa and bulimia are considered to be eating disorders primarily of psychogenic origin and are treated in detail in Chapter 9. It must be kept in mind that symptoms of upper gastrointestinal dysmotility, including esophageal dysmotility, may be similar to the symptoms of these eating disorders; also, patients with primary anorexia nervosa often manifest delayed gastric emptying, which may benefit from therapy with prokinetic agents.[11]

Diagnostic Evaluation of Vomiting

The diagnostic evaluation of vomiting depends on the limited differential diagnosis arrived at by consideration

Table 10–9. DIFFERENTIAL DIAGNOSIS OF VOMITING BY AGE

Newborn
- Congenital obstructive gastrointestinal malformations
  - Atresias or webs of esophagus or intestine
  - Meconium ileus or plug; Hirschsprung's disease
- Inborn errors of metabolism

Infant
- Acquired or milder obstructive lesions: pyloric stenosis, malrotation and volvulus, intussusception
- Metabolic diseases, milder inborn errors of metabolism
- Nutrient intolerances
- Functional disorders: gastroesophageal reflux
- Psychosocial disorders: rumination, injury due to child abuse

Child—most causes from Table 10–8

Adolescent—most childhood causes, plus pregnancy, drugs (of abuse, suicide), eating disorders

Table 10–10. DIFFERENTIAL DIAGNOSIS OF VOMITING BY ASSOCIATED SYMPTOMS AND SIGNS

Contents of Vomitus
- Undigested: achalasia
- Blood or "coffee grounds": gastritis, ulcers, esophagitis, varices
- Initially without, then with, blood: Mallory-Weiss tear
- Bile: postampullary obstruction
- Clear, large volume: Zollinger-Ellison syndrome
- Malodorous, feculent: stasis with bacterial overgrowth, gastrocolic fistula, ischemic injury to gut

Force of Vomiting
- Projectile: pyloric stenosis and other gastric obstruction, gastroesophageal reflux (occasionally), metabolic disease
- Forceless regurgitation: gastroesophageal reflux

Relationship of Vomiting to Time of Day or Mealtime
- Early morning: high intracranial pressure, pregnancy, gag due to sinusitis
- Mealtime: peptic ulcer disease, psychogenic

Relationship of Vomiting to Particular Foods
- Cow, soy, gluten: protein intolerances
- Other or multiple: allergic enteropathies, eosinophilic gastroenteropathy, metabolic disease (e.g., hereditary fructose intolerance)

Periodicity of Vomiting
- Paroxysmal, cyclic: carcinoid, pheochromocytoma, porphyria, diencephalic syndrome, epilepsy, familial dysautonomia

Other Gastrointestinal Symptoms and Signs
- Nausea: lack of nausea suggests raised intracranial pressure, gut obstruction
- Esophageal pain: esophagitis (may be secondary to chronic vomiting)
- Dysphagia: esophageal disease
- Diarrhea: infectious enteritis, partial luminal obstruction, toxin
- Constipation or distension: luminal obstruction, hypercalcemia
- Delayed vomiting, succussion splash: gastric outlet obstruction or stasis
- Visible peristalsis: luminal obstruction, especially pyloric
- Bowel sounds: obstruction vs. atony
- Abdominal pain or tenderness: may localize diseased organ, define severity
- Abdominal mass
  - Lesions produced by luminal or vascular obstruction
  - Inflamed or neoplastic lesions
  - Congenital malformations, pyloric "tumor"
- Abdominal scars: postoperative adhesions or stenoses; surgical vagotomy
- Jaundice
  - Hepatitis, hepatobiliary malformation
  - Urinary tract infection or pyloric stenosis in neonate

Neurologic Symptoms and Signs: metabolic, toxic, central nervous system disease
- Headache, vertigo, visual changes (photophobia, scotomata, field cuts)
- Abnormal tone, seizures
- Fundoscopic or fontanelle evidence of increased intracranial pressure

Other Organ System Symptoms and Signs
- Cardiac (hypotension or hypertension: intestinal ischemia, paroxysmal diseases (see below)
- Urinary: pyelonephritis, hydronephrosis, renal calculi, hypertension
- Respiratory: pneumonia, otitis, aspiration due to vomiting

Degree of Well-Being
- Well
  - Gastroesophageal reflux
  - Stimulation of gag reflex
  - Rumination, psychosocial, psychogenic, malingering
- Acutely ill—often with dehydration, electrolyte abnormalities
  - Surgical emergencies (luminal or vascular obstruction)
  - Gastroenteritis, hepatitis, pancreatitis, sepsis, meningitis
  - Ingestions
  - Pain: may help localize diseased organ
  - Fever: inflammatory lesions (e.g., appendicitis, peritonitis, pyelonephritis)
- Chronically ill: often with malnutrition ("failure to thrive")
  - Metabolic disease (especially if abnormalities of tone and development)
  - Partial or intermittent obstructions

Epidemiologic Information
- Epidemics: gastrointestinal infections, toxic exposures
- Family history: migraine, peptic ulcer disease, etc.

of the differential diagnoses discussed previously. Details of the evaluation appropriate for the various disorders are discussed individually in subsequent chapters.

Complications of Vomiting

The complications of vomiting include the metabolic complications of acute vomiting (dehydration and electrolyte abnormalities), the nutritional complications of chronic vomiting, and Mallory-Weiss tears[55] from forceful vomiting.

Metabolic Complications. Metabolic sequelae of vomiting are dehydration, alkalosis, and sodium and potassium depletion.

Dehydration results from the loss of secretions in the emesis, and also from the inability to ingest fluid effectively, either because of anorexia and nausea or because ingested fluid is promptly vomited.

Alkalosis is due to the loss of gastric hydrochloric acid in the vomitus. It is exacerbated by a shift of hydrogen ions into the cells because of potassium deficiency and by a contraction of the extracellular fluid because of sodium deficiency.

Potassium is lost in the vomitus and is also wasted by the kidneys. Potassium accompanies the renal excretion of bicarbonate due to the alkalosis. This potassium wasting is increased in the setting of sodium depletion. Sodium is lost in the vomitus and in the urine.

In states of marked alkalosis, urine pH is 7 or 8, and urinary sodium and potassium levels are high despite sodium and potassium depletion. Urine chloride, however, remains low, reflecting the nonrenal losses of NaCl and KCl.

Nutritional Complications. The weight loss, or "failure to thrive," that may result from chronic vomiting is self-evident. It is crucial to attend to this complication of vomiting when devising plans of therapy.

Mallory-Weiss Tear. Mallory-Weiss tear, a linear mucosal laceration in the juxtaesophageal gastric mucosa, was first described in 1929.[56] It usually follows prolonged forceful retching or vomiting, but it occasionally produces blood in the initial vomitus.[57] Invisible radiographically, it is diagnosed endoscopically and is often best seen at withdrawal of the instrument or during retroflexion. The tear is initially seen as a red rent oriented parallel to the esophageal length; a day later, while healing, it may appear as a white streak with surrounding erythema. It usually requires no treatment but occasionally requires transfusion. Intractable cases may be treated with vasopressin infusion, balloon tamponade, angiographic embolization, or surgery.

Peptic Esophagitis. Esophagitis similar to that resulting from gastroesophageal reflux may be caused by chronic vomiting. Whether endoscopically or histologically diagnosed (see Chapter 26), it should be treated when found. Usually, histamine receptor blockade and use of a prokinetic agent are helpful. The use of antacids should be tempered by knowledge of the acid-base status of the patient.

Therapy for Vomiting

Therapy for vomiting is directed at the specific cause when one is identified. In addition, care must be taken to identify and treat any metabolic and nutritional complications that may be present. Frequent small feedings may minimize the stimulation to vomit. Esophagitis should be treated when present. Treatment of the psychobehavioral aspects of vomiting may also be important, because of the cortical influences on emesis.[58]

Antiemetic drugs are useful in situations of persistent vomiting to reduce the metabolic and nutritional consequences and perhaps to interrupt vicious cycles in which psychogenic factors may also participate. Situations that have received particular attention recently are vomiting associated with chemotherapy[59–61] and vomiting following ophthalmic surgery (the oculoemetic reflex).

Antiemetic drugs include the prokinetic agents metoclopramide, domperidone, cisapride, and bethanechol. Metoclopramide is perhaps the best general antiemetic agent currently available in the United States, but experience with cisapride abroad is encouraging. Other agents are discussed later and treated in detail elsewhere.[62] Optimal therapy for vomiting due to chemotherapy, for example, may eventually be found to include several agents to provide blockade of the multiple receptor types in the chemoceptor trigger zone.[60]

Antihistamines. Dimenhydrinate (Dramamine) is useful especially for vomiting due to motion sickness or vestibular disorders.

Anticholinergics. Scopolamine has also been useful in the treatment of vomiting due to vestibular disorders or stimulation. Transdermal administration using dermal patches is available.

Phenothiazines and Butyrophenones. Prochlorperazine (Compazine), chlorpromazine (Thorazine), and the butyrophenone haloperidol (Haldol) are recommended in adults for vomiting due to drugs, radiation, or surgery, but they have significant side effects, including irreversible extrapyramidal reactions and blood dyscrasias.

Cannabinoids. Tetrahydrocannabinol, the active component of marihuana, and nabilone, a synthetic cannabinoid derivative, have been effective for treatment of chemotherapy-induced vomiting in some series.[63] An alternative in this setting is high-dose metoclopramide, with concurrent diphenhydramine as prophylaxis against extrapyramidal side effects.[64]

Anxiolytics, Sedatives, and Tricyclic Antidepressants. Diazepam (Valium) and related drugs have shown some antiemetic properties in studies of adults and children, particularly in settings in which a psychogenic component is suspected, such as vomiting prior to chemotherapy, which may occur in 20% of children receiving chemotherapy.[65] Suggestive studies have also shown some efficacy of tricyclic antidepressants in combination antiemetic therapy.

Steroids. Steroids have been found to have some antiemetic properties. Although this group of drugs is not generally used as primary therapy for vomiting, it may have the beneficial side effect of reducing vomiting in patients who require steroid therapy for other reasons.[66]

Beta-Adrenergic Antagonists. Propranolol is useful for prevention of vomiting due to migraine.

SUMMARY

Dysphagia and vomiting are important symptoms of gastrointestinal and multisystem disease. Careful evaluation of children with these symptoms allows accurate diagnosis and appropriate treatment.

REFERENCES

1. Lang IM, Sarna SK: Motor and myoelectric activity associated with vomiting, regurgitation, and nausea. *In* Wood J, ed: Motility and Circulation. Vol 1. Schultz SG, ed: Gastrointestinal System, Section 6 of Handbook of Physiology. New York, Oxford University Press, 1989; pp 1179–1198.
2. Carpenter DO: Central nervous system mechanisms in deglutition and emesis. *In* Wood J, ed: Motility and Circulation. Vol 1. Schultz SG, ed: The Gastrointestinal System, Section 6 of Handbook of Physiology. New York, Oxford University Press, 1989; pp 685–714.
3. Decktor DL, Allen ML, Robinson M: Esophageal motility, heartburn, and gastroesophageal reflux: Variations in clinical presentation of esophageal dysphagia. Dysphagia 1990; 5:211–215.
4. Wilson JA, Pryde A, Pirir J, et al: Pharyngoesophageal dysmotility in globus sensation. Arch Otolaryngol Head Neck Surg 1989; 115:1086–1090.
5. Buchholz D: Neurologic causes of dysphagia. Dysphagia 1987; 1:152–156.
6. Bass NH: Neurogenic dysphagia: Diagnostic assessment and rehabilitation of feeding disorders in the neurologically impaired. *In* Eisenberg M, Grzesiak R, eds: Advances in Clinical Rehabilitation. New York, Springer, 1987; pp 186–228.
7. Clouse RE, Lustman PJ: Psychiatric illness and contraction abnormalities of the esophagus. N Engl J Med 1983; 309:1337–1342.
8. Clouse RE, Lustman PJ, Reidel WL: Correlation of esophageal motility abnormalities with neuropsychiatric status in diabetics. Gastroenterology 1986; 90:1146–1154.
9. Ouyang A: Esophageal motility disorders mimicking anorexia nervosa? Gastroenterology 1987; 92:2038–2039.
10. Schuster MM: Esophageal spasm and psychiatric disorder. N Engl J Med 1983; 309(22):1382–1383.
11. Stacher G, Kiss A, Wiesnagrotzki S, et al: Oesophageal and gastric motility disorders in patients categorized as having primary anorexia nervosa. Gut 1986; 27:1120–1126.
12. Dantas RO, Cook IJ, Dodds WJ, et al: Biomechanics of cricopharyngeal bars. Gastroenterology 1990; 99:1269–1274.
13. Wyllie E, Wyllie R, Cruse RP, et al: The mechanism of nitrazepam-induced drooling and aspiration. N Engl J Med 1986; 314:35–38.
14. Putnam PE, Orenstein SR, Pang D, et al: Cricopharyngeal dysfunction associated with Chiari malformations. Pediatrics 1992; 89:871–876.
15. Waters PF, DeMeester TR: Foregut motor disorders and their surgical management. Med Clin North Am 1981; 65:1235–1268.
16. Jones B, Donner MW: Examination of the patient with dysphagia. Radiology 1988; 167:319–326.
17. Ott DJ, Gelfand DW, Wu WC, et al: Radiological evaluation of dysphagia. JAMA 1986; 256:2718–2721.
18. Orenstein SR, Giarrusso VS, Proujansky R, et al: The Santmyer swallow: A new useful infant reflex. Lancet 1988; 1:345–346.
19. Davidson GP, Dent J, Willing J: Monitoring of upper oesophageal sphincter pressure in children. Gut 1991; 32:607–611.
20. Benjamin SB, Richter JE, Cordova CM, et al: Prospective manometric evaluation with pharmacologic provocation of patients with suspected esophageal motility dysfunction. Gastroenterology 1983; 84:893–901.
21. Deschner WK, Maher KA, Cattau EL Jr, et al: Manometric responses to balloon distention in patients with nonobstructive dysphagia. Gastroenterology 1989; 97:1181–1185.
22. Mellow MH: Esophageal motility during food ingestion. A physiologic test of esophageal motor function. Gastroenterology 1983; 85:570–577.
23. Dinari G, Danziger Y, Mimouni M, et al: Cricopharyngeal dysfunction in childhood. Treatment by dilatations. J Pediatr Gastroenterol Nutr 1987; 6:212–216.

24. Lindor KD, Ott BJ, Hughes RW Jr: Balloon dilatation of upper digestive tract strictures. Gastroenterology 1985; 89:545–548.
25. Bourgeois N, Coffernils M, Buset M, et al: Management of dysphagia in suspected esophageal motor disorders. Dig Dis Sci 1991; 36:268–273.
26. Frank MM, Gatewood OMB: Transient pharyngeal incoordination in the newborn. Am J Dis Child 1966; 111:178–181.
27. Bluestone CD, Stool SE, Sieber WK, et al: Congenital cricopharyngeal achalasia. Ann Otol 1977; 86:603–610.
28. Berg HM, Jacobs JB, Persky MS, et al: Cricopharyngeal myotomy: A review of surgical results in patients with cricopharyngeal achalasia of neurogenic origin. Laryngoscope 1985; 95:1337–1340.
29. Hongo M, Traube M, McAllister RG Jr, et al: Effects of nifedipine on esophageal motor function in humans: Correlation with plasma nifedipine concentration. Gastroenterology 1984; 86:8–12.
30. Hongo M, Traube M, McCallum RW: Comparison of effects of nifedipine, propantheline bromide, and the combination on esophageal motor function in normal volunteers. Dig Dis Sci 1984; 29:300–304.
31. Snyder SH, Reynolds IJ: Calcium-antagonist drugs: Receptor interactions that clarify therapeutic effects. N Engl J Med 1985; 313:995–1002
32. Traube M, McCallum RW: Primary oesophageal motility disorders: Current therapeutic concepts. Drugs 1985; 30:66–77.
33. Clouse RE, Lustman PJ, Eckert TC, et al: Low-dose trazodone for symptomatic patients with esophageal contraction abnormalities. Gastroenterology 1987; 92:1027–1036.
34. Helfrich-Miller KR, Rector KL, Straka JA: Dysphagia: Its treatment in the profoundly retarded patient with cerebral palsy. Arch Phys Med Rehabil 1986; 67:520–525.
35. Linden P: Videofluoroscopy in the rehabilitation of swallowing dysfunction. Dysphagia 1989; 3:189–191.
36. Weisberger EC: Treatment of intractable aspiration using a laryngeal stent or obturator. Ann Otol Rhinol Laryngol 1991; 100:101–107.
37. Melzack R, Rosberger Z, Hollingsworth ML, et al: New approaches to measuring nausea. Can Med Assoc J 1985; 133:755–761.
38. Ingelfinger FJ, Moss RE: The activity of the descending duodenum during nausea. Am J Physiol 1942; 136:561–566.
39. Thompson BG, Malagelada JR: Vomiting and the small intestine. Dig Dis Sci 1982; 27:1121–1125.
40. Johnson HD, Laws JW: The cardia in swallowing, eructation, and vomiting. Lancet 1966; 2:1268–1273.
41. Orenstein SR, Deneault LG, Lutz JW, et al: Regurgitant reflux, in contrast to nonregurgitant reflux, is associated with rectus abdominus contraction in infants. Gastroenterology 1991; 100:A135.
42. Malegelada JR, Camilleri M: Unexplained vomiting: A diagnostic challenge. Ann Intern Med 1984; 101:211–218.
43. Burton BK: Inborn errors of metabolism: The clinical diagnosis in early infancy. Pediatrics 1987; 79:359–369.
44. Meyers FA, Dempsey D, Caroline D, et al: Duodenal diverticulum as cause of cyclic vomiting. Dig Dis Sci 1989; 34:1148–1149.
45. Johnston JM, Harnsberger JK: Episodic vomiting due to intermittent duodenal intussusception. J Pediatr Gastroenterol Nutr 1990; 10:405–408.
46. Coker SB: Cyclic vomiting and the slit ventricle syndrome. Pediatr Neurol 1987; 3:297–299.
47. Embry CK. Toxic cyclic vomiting in an 11-year-old girl. J Am Acad Child Adolesc Psychiatry 1987; 26:447–448.
48. Fromm S, Cash JM: Superior mesenteric artery syndrome: An approach to the diagnosis and management of upper gastrointestinal obstruction of unknown etiology. South Dakota J Med 1990; 43:5–10.
49. Amarnath RP, Abell TL, Malagelada JR: The rumination syndrome in adults. Ann Intern Med 1986; 105:513–518.
50. Shepherd RW, Wren J, Evans S, et al: Gastroesophageal reflux in children. Clin Pediatr 1987; 26:55–60.
51. Mayes SD, Humphrey FJ II, Handford HA, et al: Rumination disorder: Differential diagnosis. J Am Acad Child Adolesc Psychiatry 1988; 27:300–302.
52. Winton ASW, Singh NN: Rumination in pediatric populations. A behavioral analysis. J Am Acad Child Psychiatry 1983; 22:269–275.
53. Mogadam M:. The role of esophagitis in the pathogenesis of hyperemesis gravidarum. Am J Gastroenterol 1984; 79:827.
54. Mortimer MJ, Good PA: The VER as a diagnostic marker for childhood abdominal migraine. Headache 1990; 30:642–645.
55. Graham DY, Schwartz JT: The spectrum of the Mallory-Weiss tear. Medicine 1977; 57:307–318.
56. Mallory GK, Weiss S: Hemorrhages from lacerations of the cardiac orifice of the stomach due to vomiting. Am J Med Sci 1929; 178:506.
57. Knauer CM: Mallory-Weiss syndrome. Gastroenterology 1976; 71:5.
58. Latimer PR, Malmud LS, Fisher RS: Gastric stasis and vomiting: Behavioral treatment. Gastroenterology 1982; 83:684–688.
59. Kobrinsky NS: Regulation of nausea and vomiting in cancer chemotherapy. Am J Pediatr Hematol Oncol 1988; 10:209–213.
60. Marshall G, Kerr S, Vowels M, et al: Antiemetic therapy for chemotherapy-induced vomiting: Metoclopramide, benztropine, dexamethasone, and lorazepam regimen compared with chlorpromazine alone. J Pediatr 1989; 115:156–160.
61. Vomiting and chemotherapy (editorial). Lancet 1990; 335:265–266.
62. Barnes JH: The physiology and pharmacology of emesis. Mol Aspects Med 1984; 7:397–508.
63. Chan HSL, Correia JA, MacLeod SM: Nabilone versus prochlorperazine for control of cancer chemotherapy-induced emesis in children: A double-blind crossover trial. Pediatrics 1987; 79:946–952.
64. Stoudemire A, Cotanch P, Laslo J: Recent advances in the pharmacologic and behavioral management of chemotherapy-induced emesis. Arch Intern Med 1984; 144:1029–1033.
65. Dolgin MJ, Katz ER, McGinty K, et al: Anticipatory nausea and vomiting in pediatric cancer patients. Pediatrics 1985; 75:547–552.
66. Mehta P, Gross S, Graham-Pole J, et al: Methylprednisolone for chemotherapy-induced emesis: A double-blind randomized trial in children. J Pediatr 1986; 108:774–776.

Chapter 11

Ascites

JOSEPH F. FITZGERALD

HISTORICAL NOTES

The term *ascites* finds its origin in the Greek word *askites,* which means bladder or bag. Ascites is defined as an effusion and accumulation of serous fluid in the abdominal cavity.[1] Dawson,[2] in his historical treatise on ascites published in 1960, indicated that Hippocrates had suggested in 5 B.C. that ascites resulted from the leakage of hepatic fluid into the peritoneal cavity, and that Erasistratus of Alexandria had postulated two centuries later that obstruction of hepatic blood flow was the major factor in peritoneal fluid accumulation. Ascites was produced in dogs in the seventeenth century by the ligation of the inferior vena cava, and Sydenham suggested a relationship between alcohol consumption and ascites in the same century. The association of hepatic disease with renal dysfunction was described in the second half of the nineteenth century.

Abdominal paracentesis was commonly performed during the time of Erasistratus, though he disagreed with the practice. Celsus (ca 20 B.C.) described the techniques of paracentesis, and Paul of Aegina (A.D. 625–690) wrote a detailed description of the technique of paracentesis and included the warning: "Avoid by all means a sudden evacuation, for some ignorant persons having evacuated the vital spirit with the fluid have immediately killed the patient."[2]

PATHOGENESIS OF ASCITES FORMATION

Peritoneal fluid formation is a dynamic process. The net volume of peritoneal fluid is the result of an equilibrium maintained between production and absorption. Osmotic and hydrostatic forces, as described by the Starling equilibrium, control the net flux of fluid (and proteins) between the peritoneal capillary bed and the peritoneal cavity. Movement of materials between the compartments is modified by the integrity of the peritoneal membrane and is influenced by the functioning of the lymphatic drainage system. A dynamic equilibrium is maintained between the plasma and the peritoneal cavity, even when ascites is present and there is a net increase in abdominal fluid accumulation. Every hour, 40 to 80% of intraperitoneal fluid is exchanged with the plasma.[3]

Intraperitoneal fluid accumulates when there is inflammation of either the visceral or parietal peritoneum; portal venous or lymphatic obstruction, or both; decreased plasma colloid oncotic pressure; or rupture of an intra-abdominal viscus. Inflammation of the peritoneum promotes capillary permeability and the leakage of high-protein fluid into the peritoneal cavity. This increases the colloid osmotic pressure of the intraperitoneal fluid, which in turn retards absorption of the fluid. Acute or chronic increases in portal venous pressure may result in intraperitoneal fluid accumulation. Cirrhosis is the most common cause of portal vein obstruction. Prehepatic, presinusoidal portal hypertension results from congenital anomalies of the portal vein, such as portal vein atresia with cavernous transformation, which manifests as splenomegaly in the first year of life and bleeding from esophageal varices thereafter. This condition is rarely associated with ascites. Ascites seems to develop only after multiple episodes of variceal hemorrhage lead to a sudden decrease in plasma oncotic pressure.

Congenital defects in the lymphatic system, mesenteric adenitis, intra-abdominal tuberculosis, and neoplastic disease of the abdomen, retroperitoneum, thorax, and mediastinum are characterized by the development of chylous ascites. The pathophysiologic mechanism would appear to be increased pressure in the thin-walled lymphatic channels, which leads to their rupture.

Hepatic, gastrointestinal, and renal diseases may be associated with hypoalbuminemia and a resultant decreased plasma colloid osmotic pressure. Fluid may accumulate in the peritoneal cavity as well as in other tissue spaces. Peripheral edema always accompanies the ascites due solely to hypoalbuminemia. A perforated abdominal viscus or cyst may cause fluid or blood to accumulate in the abdomen. Blunt trauma associated with rupture of the liver or spleen is not uncommon. Severe pancreatic inflammation or a disruption of the pancreatic ductal system may be associated with ascites. Neonatal ascites is often associated with urinary tract abnormalities involving a direct communication between the renal collecting system and the abdominal cavity.[4] Lysosomal storage diseases may present with congenital ascites. The ascites may be detected in utero by ultrasonography. The list of lysosomal storage diseases that have presented with neonatal ascites includes infantile sialidosis, Salla's disease, GM_1 gangliosidosis, Gaucher's disease,[5] and Niemann-Pick disease type C.[6]

CIRRHOTIC ASCITES

Traditionally, it has been proposed that ascites develops in the cirrhotic patient when the balance between the Starling forces in the hepatic sinusoids and splanchnic capillaries is altered, resulting in the formation of excessive lymph, which the thoracic duct is incapable of returning to the general circulation. The excess protein-containing lymph accumulates in the peritoneal cavity, reducing the effective plasma volume, that is, that part of the total plasma volume that effectively stimulates plasma volume receptors. The traditional concept is that the factors that lead to intraperitoneal fluid accumulation and the consequent reduction in the effective plasma volume result in decreased renal perfusion. This decrease, in turn, results in activation of the renin-angiotensin-aldosterone system, leading to renal sodium conservation and increased production and release of vasopressin. The result is (1) the conservation of free water and activation of the sympathetic nervous system, which can effect a redistribution of blood flow within the kidney and (2) alterations in poorly defined local and systemic humoral factors, such as prostaglandin E_2, humoral and atrial natriuretic factors, and the kallikrein-kinin system (Fig. 11–1). Support for the concept of a diminished effective intravascular volume as a major factor in the increased tubular reabsorption of sodium and water in cirrhotic patients comes from studies performed by Epstein and coworkers.[7, 8] Based on head-out water immersion studies on patients with decompensated cirrhosis, they observed that water immersion normalizes renal sodium handling in this patient population. Marked natriuresis and kaliuresis were noted in most patients. Water immersion results in prompt redistribution of plasma volume, which is associated with a sustained increase in central blood volume. Hence, Epstein and coworkers reversed the marked sodium retention that accompanies decompensated cirrhosis by a manipulation that altered the distribution of the total plasma volume without increasing the total plasma volume.

An alternative "overflow" theory for the development of ascites in patients with hepatic cirrhosis was promulgated by Lieberman and associates 20 years ago.[9, 10] This theory proposes that renal retention of sodium and water, leading to expansion of the total plasma volume, is the primary initiating event in the development of ascites (Fig. 11–2). Expansion of the total plasma volume in the setting of portal hypertension and a reduced plasma colloid osmotic pressure results in sequestration of fluid in the peritoneal space. Support for this concept comes from studies performed by Levy and colleagues using a dog model of cirrhosis.[11–14] Their progressive studies suggested that increases in hepatic sinusoidal pressure result in renal sodium retention prior to the appearance of ascites, and that the stimulus for sodium retention originates in the hepatic sinusoids (i.e., a baroreceptor). A humoral factor may be involved.[14] This theory seems unlikely since volume expansion appears to improve rather than impair urinary sodium and water clearance in cirrhotic patients with ascites[15]; yet it may be that a primary defect in renal sodium handling is important in the early stages of cirrhosis,[15a] and a reduced effective plasma volume is the major determinant of sodium retention once decompensation is well established.[8]

It could be that milder increases in sinusoidal pressure are associated with a concomitant retention of filtered renal sodium.[15a] This overall expansion in extracellular volume might cause a more rapid increase in sinusoidal pressure, leading to increased lymph formation and the sequestration of protein-rich hepatic lymph in the peritoneal cavity. This would then lead to a shift of fluid to the peritoneal cavity, resulting in a decreased effective circulating volume, which would activate the interrelationships described in Figure 11–1.

CLINICAL FEATURES

Ascites may develop suddenly or insidiously. Sudden development of ascites occurs more commonly with the nonhepatic etiologies, but may accompany a sudden reduction in hepatocellular function in a patient with marginally compensated cirrhosis. The latter may be caused by massive hemorrhage, septic shock, superim-

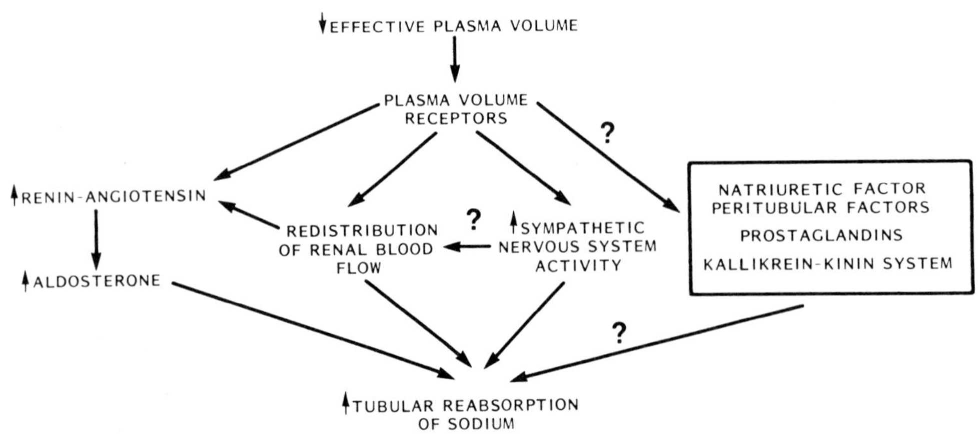

Figure 11–1. Schematic representation of the classical "underflow" theory of ascites formation. (From Wyllie R, Arasu TS, Fitzerald JF: Ascites: Pathophysiology and management. J Pediatr 1980; 97:167–176; with permission.)

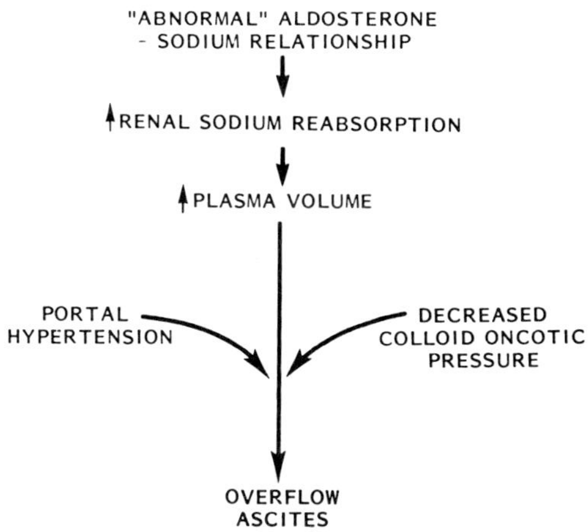

Figure 11–2. Interrelationships that contribute to ascites formation according to the "overflow" theory promulgated by Lieberman and Reynolds. (From Wyllie R, Arasu TS, Fitzgerald JF: Ascites: Pathophysiology and management. J Pediatr 1980; 97:167–176; with permission.)

posed infection, or the ingestion of hepatic toxins. Occlusion of the portal vein results in the precipitous formation of ascites in a patient with hypoalbuminemia. An insidious onset of ascites reflects a subcritical functioning hepatic mass that will be corrected, in the long term, only by transplantation.

Careful physical examination provides important diagnostic clues to the etiology of the ascites (Table 11–1). The classic decompensated cirrhotic patient appears sallow and dehydrated, with profound muscle wasting. The abdomen is distended because of dilated intestinal loops as well as the presence of intra-abdominal fluid. Fullness in the flanks is a constant finding. The umbilicus may be everted, and the distance between the symphysis pubis and the umbilicus appears to be diminished.[15] Persistently increased intra-abdominal pressure in association with decreased total body muscle mass predisposes the patient to the development of hernias (umbilical, incisional, inguinal, or femoral) and scrotal edema. Prominent anterior wall veins radiating from the umbilicus that persist after successful management of the ascites represent portosystemic collateral channels. Increased intra-abdominal pressure may result in obstruction to cephalad flow in the inferior vena cava. This is manifested by the appearance of vessels that run from the groin to the lower costal margins. These vessels disappear with satisfactory management of the ascites.

Table 11–1. HELPFUL CLUES TO ETIOLOGY OF ASCITES

Splenomegaly—portal hypertension
Prominent abdominal vasculature—portal hypertension/obstructed inferior vena cava
Cor pulmonale—congestive heart failure
Pericardial friction rub—constrictive pericarditis
Abdominal pain (diffuse)—peritonitis
Abdominal pain (radiating to back)—pancreatitis
Abdominal pain (pelvis)—uterine/ovarian disease
Lymphedema—lymphatic obstruction

Table 11–2. DETECTION OF FREE INTRA-ABDOMINAL FLUID

Fluid wave (observed on palpating one flank while tapping the opposite side of the abdomen)
Shifting dullness (when patient turns from supine to lateral decubitus position)
Ballottement (sensation of fluid displacement when palpating liver or spleen with quick, pushing motion)
Puddle sign (decreased auscultation of high-frequency vibrations in central abdomen when flicking side of abdomen with patient on hands and knees)

Various techniques have been taught to medical students to detect the presence of ascites. The first three techniques listed in Table 11–2 have been known for more than 100 years and allow detection of fluid volumes in excess of 1 L.[16] The last, the puddle sign, was described by Lawson and Weissbein in 1959.[17] The patient lies prone for 5 minutes and then rises to hands and knees for examination. The examiner flicks the flanks lightly while moving a stethoscope from the most dependent part of the abdomen to the flanks. A positive sign consists of a change in the intensity and character of the percussion note. This technique reportedly allows the detection of as little as 120 ml of free intra-abdominal fluid.

Various imaging techniques complement the assessment of a patient with ascites. Radiographic signs of ascites that are seldom seen with other intra-abdominal conditions include medial displacement of the lateral liver border, separation of the properitoneal flank strip from the colon, and "dog ears" in the pelvis, that is, densities superior and lateral to the bladder secondary to intra-abdominal fluid in the peritoneal recesses.[16] Nonspecific signs include diffuse abdominal haziness; medial displacement of the bowel; separation of gas-filled small bowel loops; bulging of the flanks; and indistinct psoas, splenic, and hepatic margins (Fig. 11–3).

Ultrasonography is quite sensitive for the detection of free or loculated fluid within the peritoneal cavity.[18] This noninvasive technology can readily distinguish fluid from solid masses and free fluid from loculated fluid. The presence of shifting echo-free zones to dependent locations, as the patient is rotated from supine to lateral positions, corroborates the presence of free intra-abdominal fluid (Fig. 11–4). Localized, nonshifting echo-free zones suggest confined collections of fluid. Differentiation of loculated fluid from other structures, for example, an ovarian cyst, a dilated urinary collecting system, or an enlarged urinary bladder, is usually possible by analysis of shape and position.

Computed tomography (CT) may be employed to evaluate the peritoneal cavity when the data generated by the sonogram are equivocal. Ascitic fluid is readily identified, since its density is invariably less than that of the abdominal viscera and greater than that of fat (Fig. 11–5). The smallest volume of fluid that may be detected is similar to that identified by ultrasound. By comparison, ultrasound images in multiple planes can more readily distinguish free from loculated collections of

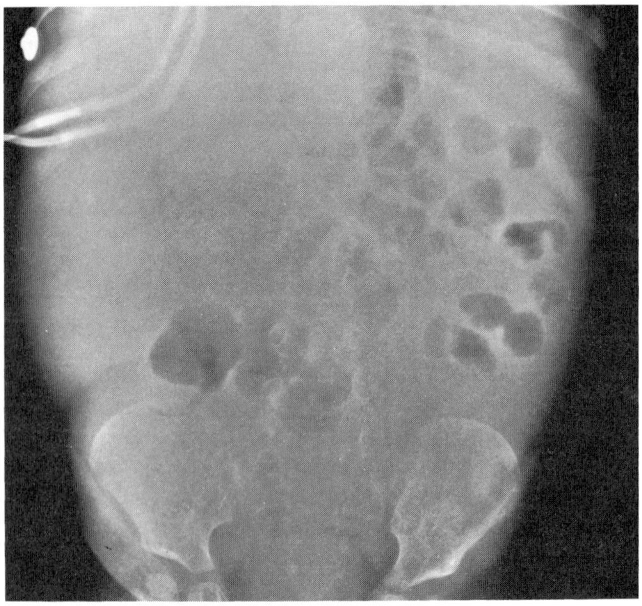

Figure 11–3. Typical abdominal radiograph from a patient with significant ascites, with abdominal haziness, separation of gas-filled small bowel loops, bulging of the flanks, and indistinct psoas, splenic, and hepatic margins.

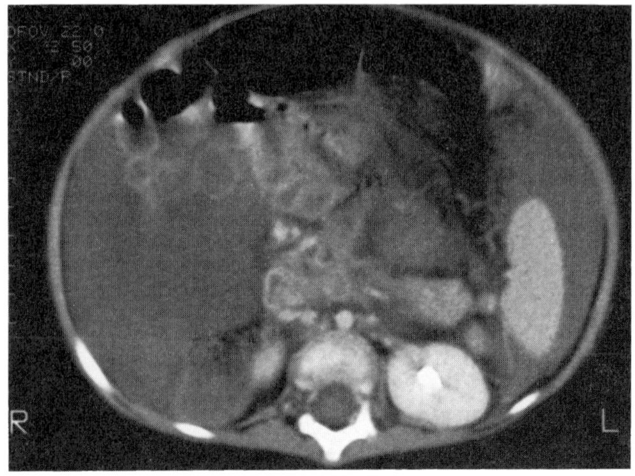

Figure 11–5. Computed tomogram revealing abundant intraperitoneal fluid surrounding intra-abdominal viscera.

fluid. Other advantages of ultrasonography over CT scanning in the evaluation of ascites include shorter scanning time, lower cost, and no ionizing radiation. Magnetic resonance (MR) imaging is sensitive for the detection of ascites, but rarely needed. The fluid has very low intensity on T_1 images and very high intensity on T_2 images[19] (Fig. 11–6).

ASCITIC FLUID EXAMINATION

Physicians have both extolled and denied the efficacy and safety of abdominal paracentesis as a diagnostic procedure since its initial proposal. In 1920, Denzer[20] established the usefulness of paracentesis in children for the diagnosis of peritonitis (prior to necropsy). Putative complications of diagnostic paracentesis in patients with cirrhosis include bowel perforation and hemorrhage.[21] These are extremely rare. The effects of entering the intestinal lumen, which occurs more frequently than is usually appreciated, are of little or no clinical significance.[22] The intestinal wall has the ability to seal a needle puncture wound quickly so that contamination of the peritoneal cavity is minimal. An occasional complication is sudden labial or scrotal edema due to dissection of fluid between the Camper and the Scarpa fascial planes,[23] which almost never occurs when small-bore needles are used. The procedure is performed under sterile conditions using a narrow-bore angiocatheter. The anterior abdominal wall is punctured through the avascular linea alba, 2 cm below the umbilicus, using a *Z* technique. The amount of fluid withdrawn for routine diagnostic studies need not exceed 10 to 20 ml. The intraperitoneal fluid obtained from a patient with parenchymal liver disease is typically straw-colored. Chylous fluid is white or yellow-white, and a creamy supernatant will develop after the fluid settles for a period. Abdominal trauma is suggested by the aspiration of blood, bile-stained fluid, air, or intestinal contents. Deeply bile-stained fluid may indicate a direct communication between the biliary tract and the peritoneal cavity. This may be seen in infants and children who develop sudden ascites following hepatic replacement therapy.

The laboratory studies that should be performed on the fluid are listed in Table 11–3. The protein content of intraperitoneal fluid obtained from cirrhotic patients tends to be low (<2.5 gm per dl). Hoefs[24] was the first researcher to suggest that the difference in albumin concentrations between serum and ascitic fluid may more reliably differentiate between exudative and transudative ascites, since albumin is the principal oncotically active protein in the serum, and since oncotic forces are important in the formation of cirrhotic ascites.

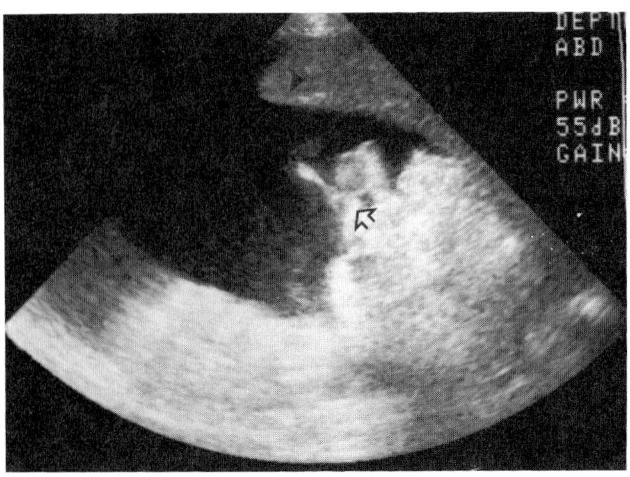

Figure 11–4. Abdominal ultrasound study revealing ascites with loop of bowel and mesenteric stalk "floating" in ascitic fluid (*open arrow*). Liver edge can be noted in the upper aspect of the photograph (*arrowhead*).

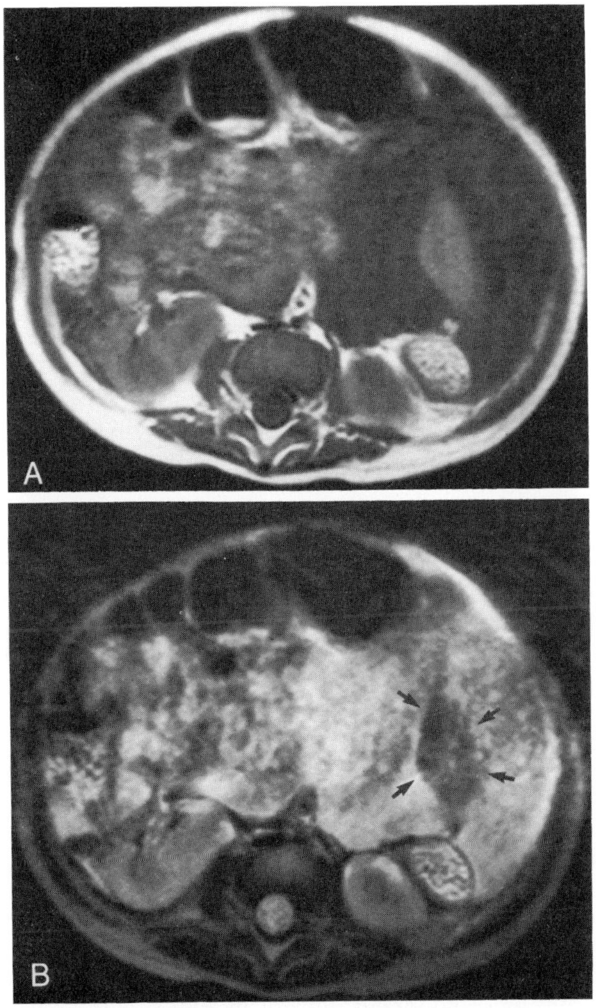

Figure 11–6. Magnetic resonance imaging from a patient with ascites. The ascitic fluid has low intensity on T_1-weighted image (*A*) and high intensity on T_2-weighted image (*B*). Fluid is surrounding a visceral structure (*arrows*).

The difference in albumin concentrations between serum and ascitic fluid should be greater than 1.0 gm per dl in patients with cirrhosis, based on studies of the albumin content of thoracic duct lymph in this patient population.[25] Patients with exudative ascites should have normal portal venous pressures, and the albumin concentration in the ascitic fluid should more closely resemble the serum concentration. Subsequent studies have supported and extended Hoefs's original observation.[26, 27]

An elevated ascitic fluid amylase level, which is usually accompanied by an increase in ascitic fluid white blood cells, protein concentration, and lactate dehydrogenase activity, allows the diagnosis of pancreatic ascites.[28] Ascitic fluid lactate dehydrogenase activity is usually elevated in patients with malignant or tuberculous ascites. Confirmation of malignant disease by paracentesis is difficult, since atypical mesothelial cells are normally found in the peritoneal fluid. The triglyceride level in chylous ascites exceeds that of the serum and is usually greater than 400 mg per dl. The total fat content is usually twice that of plasma.

The total ascitic fluid white blood cell count and differential aid in the consideration of intraperitoneal infection. Antibiotic therapy should be initiated in all patients with greater than 500 polymorphonuclear leukocytes per μl of peritoneal fluid, as well as in any patient with signs of peritonitis and greater than 250 polymorphonuclear leukocytes per μl.[29] Spontaneous bacterial peritonitis arises most commonly in decompensated cirrhotic patients with hypoalbuminemia and preexisting, large-volume ascites. Analysis of the clinical and bacteriologic features of 12 episodes of spontaneous bacterial peritonitis arising in 11 children with chronic liver disease strongly suggested that complement deficiency, most likely related to persistent hepatic dysfunction, may be important in the pathogenesis of spontaneous bacterial peritonitis.[30]

The presence of gram-positive bacteria in peritoneal fluid strongly suggests spontaneous (primary) peritonitis. The identification of both gram-positive and -negative bacteria in ascitic fluid should generate concern that intestinal perforation has occurred and that laparotomy may be necessary. A Gram stain revealing only gram-negative bacteria could be consistent with either primary or secondary peritonitis and dictates close observation during the administration of appropriate antibiotic therapy. Paracentesis should be performed again after 48 hours of therapy. The infection is usually blood borne, and it is monomicrobial in 90% of cases.[15]

MANAGEMENT

The successful management of ascites relates to the underlying cause. Hepatogenous ascites is a sign of severe hepatic dysfunction. The catastrophic complications of cirrhosis, including esophageal variceal hemorrhage, hepatorenal syndrome, and spontaneous bacterial peritonitis, occur almost exclusively in cirrhotic patients with ascites. Gastroesophageal reflux, inferior vena cava obstruction, disturbances in cardiac and renal circulation, and a predisposition to pulmonary atelectasis and hernias, as mentioned previously, result from the increased abdominal pressure associated with ascites formation. Ascites is not the root of all evil if left unat-

Table 11–3. EXAMINATION OF ASCITIC FLUID

Cell count with differential: normal finding is <250 white blood cells per μl with lymphocytic predominance; a finding of >75 neutrophils per μl suggests inflammation
Total protein/albumin
Glucose: tuberculous peritonitis is suggested by a peritoneal fluid glucose <30 mg/dl
Amylase
Cholesterol and triglyceride: chylous ascites is accompanied by a triglyceride value >400 mg/dl
Lactic dehydrogenase and leucine aminopeptidase: elevations suggest an intra-abdominal malignant process
Bilirubin and creatinine, if biliary or urinary tract leakage suspected (neonates)
Gram stain, acid-fast bacteria, and fungal smears
Bacterial (aerobic and anaerobic), mycobacterial, and fungal cultures
Cytology, when a malignant process must be considered

tended, but it is not without risk. A decision to manage ascites aggressively must be tempered by the knowledge that treatment neither alters the underlying hepatopathy nor necessarily prolongs life. Vigorous treatment of ascites is associated with severe risks, including acid-base and electrolyte imbalance, hepatic encephalopathy, hypovolemia, and renal insufficiency.

Sodium Restriction

The cornerstone of medical management of ascites is dietary sodium restriction. The rate of ascitic fluid accumulation relates directly to the amount of sodium retained (intake minus excretion). Most patients with cirrhotic ascites excrete less than 10 mEq of sodium daily. Hence, even a modest intake of sodium such as 1 g (43 mEq) results in positive sodium balance and progressive accumulation of intraperitoneal fluid. Limitation of sodium to 1 to 2 mEq per kg per day often affects a diuresis without rendering the diet totally unpalatable. Serum and urine electrolytes must be monitored in order to assure negative sodium balance. A negative balance of 120 mEq of sodium will be accompanied by the loss of approximately 1 L of water. A small percentage of patients respond to sodium restriction alone, usually within 5 days. Patients with serum sodium levels greater than 135 mEq per L who excrete greater than 15 mEq of sodium per 24 hours are likely to experience a diuresis with dietary sodium restriction alone; those with normal serum sodium levels who excrete less than 15 mEq of sodium per 24 hours usually require diuretic assistance.

Water Restriction

Impaired water excretion frequently accompanies cirrhotic ascites. This abnormality leads to the development of hyponatremia (serum sodium less than 130 mEq per L). The impaired clearance of free water is due primarily to nonosmotic release of antidiuretic hormone.[31] Hyponatremia is associated with neurologic symptoms and signs that are difficult to distinguish from those of hepatic encephalopathy. Marked hyponatremia (serum sodium less than 120 mEq per L) may result in permanent neurologic damage and even death.[32] Hyponatremia is more commonly a complication of diuretic therapy, and termination of diuretics and restriction of fluid intake to 50 to 75 percent of the calculated maintenance will usually raise the serum sodium concentration above 130 mEq per L.

Diuretic Therapy

The fundamental principle of any diuretic strategy is to use diuretics in increasing potency and in the smallest amount necessary to maintain a satisfactory diuresis. The goal of diuretic therapy is to promote negative sodium and water balance. This can be documented readily by monitoring urinary sodium excretion. Spironolactone should be prescribed initially in a dosage of 2 to 3 mg per kg per day in two to three divided doses. This synthetic steroid, which is relatively free of side effects, selectively antagonizes the effect of aldosterone on the distal renal tubule and collecting system (Fig. 11–7). There is a 3- to 4-day lag between initiation of spironolactone and optimal effect. The dosage can be increased to 5 mg per kg per day when no positive effect is noted by the fourth day; however, spironolactone may cause hyperkalemia and a hyperchloremic acidosis at this dosage.

A lack of fluid mobilization with salt restriction and a distal-acting diuretic dictates that a more proximal-acting diuretic be added to the treatment strategy. Approximately 20 to 50% of the filtered sodium load is reabsorbed in the ascending limb of Henle. Furosemide and other loop diuretics inhibit sodium transport in the thick ascending limb of the loop of Henle. The natriuretic response of furosemide relates to the concentration of drug within the renal tubular fluid rather than in the blood.[33] Loop diuretics purportedly activate renal prostaglandin synthesis, which leads to renal arteriolar dilation and increased renal blood flow.[34] Furosemide should be initially prescribed in a dosage of 0.5 mg per kg twice daily. Again, the natriuretic response must be monitored. A good response would lead to reduction of the furosemide dosage to 0.5 mg per kg daily; a suboptimal response should be followed by an increase in dosage to 1 mg per kg twice daily. Longer-acting diuretics, such as thiazides and ethacrynic acid, may continue to promote natriuresis and kaliuresis in patients with severe liver disease after electrolyte disturbances have developed.

Absorption of ascitic fluid averages 300 to 500 ml per day during spontaneous diuresis in adults, with maximal absorption of 700 to 900 ml per day with diuretic therapy.[35] A diuresis that exceeds this rate of ascitic fluid absorption in a patient without peripheral edema will lead to contraction of the effective plasma volume, which will, in turn, lead to decreased renal blood flow, azotemia, and, eventually, hyponatremia.[16] This may result in irreversible functional renal failure (hepatorenal syndrome). Rapid expansion of the circulating volume of plasma in patients with hypoalbuminemia may be accomplished by albumin infusion. A brisk diuresis may then be initiated by intravenous furosemide administration. We infuse 1 g per kg of albumin (up to 25 g) over 2 to 3 hours and then administer 0.5 to 1 mg per kg of furosemide intravenously.[16] We have found this therapy to have only short-term effectiveness, however.

Therapeutic Abdominal Paracentesis

Large-volume paracentesis was the only therapy available for the management of patients with chronic hepatogenous ascites before the introduction of effective diuretic therapy. Repeated removal of large volumes of intraperitoneal fluid was generally considered ineffec-

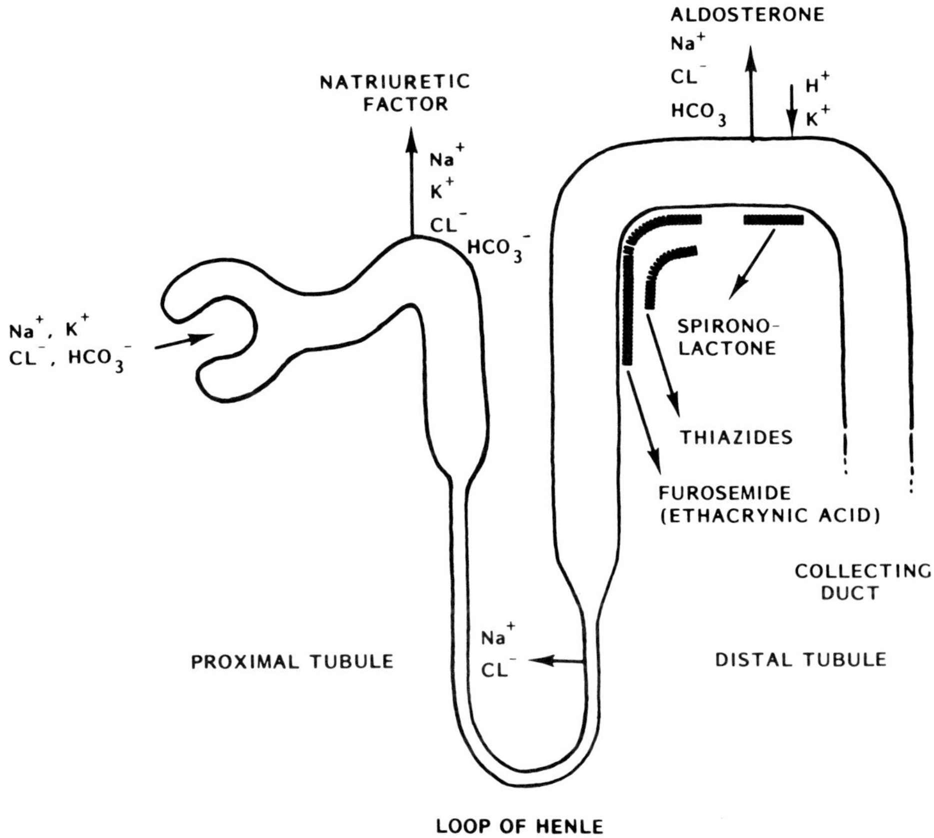

Figure 11–7. Diuretic interference with normal nephron function. (From Wyllie R, Arasu TS, Fitzgerald JF: Ascites: Pathophysiology and management. J Pediatr 1980; 97:167–176; with permission.)

tive, and it was frequently associated with complications, including hypovolemia, hyponatremia, renal insufficiency, decreased cardiac output, and hepatic encephalopathy.[35] Further, repeated paracenteses were accompanied by the loss of a significant amount of nitrogen which further compromised the marginal nutritional status of these patients. Carey and associates[36] noted in 1983 that the removal of large volumes of intraperitoneal fluid during the performance of laparoscopy in patients with decompensated cirrhosis appeared to be well tolerated. These authors suggested that the frequency of the complications just discussed may have been overestimated. Kao and colleagues[37] measured plasma volumes before and after large-volume paracentesis (5 L) in 18 cirrhotic adults. They found a 2.7% decrease in plasma volume at 24 hours postparacentesis and 2.8% by 48 hours postparacentesis. These values did not reach significance. No complications were encountered, but the serum creatinine increased at 48 hours postparacentesis. A subsequent study examining the effect of large-volume paracentesis in a similar patient population revealed an increase in cardiac output and a progressive decrease in central venous pressure, pulmonary capillary wedge pressure, and creatinine clearance in the first 24 hours following paracentesis,[38] all of which suggested that these patients became hypovolemic as the ascitic fluid reaccumulated. The hypovolemia was accompanied by elevations of plasma renin activity and the plasma aldosterone level and a decrease in the level of atrial natriuretic peptide. No serious complications were observed despite the apparent reduction in plasma volume, and it was concluded that large-volume paracenteses were satisfactorily tolerated. These observations led to the application of repeated large-volume paracenteses accompanied by intravenous administration of salt-poor albumin to prevent fluid shifts and maintain normal renal function.[39–41] Finally, the investigators who had pioneered these paracentesis studies reported their experience with total paracentesis in 38 patients with cirrhotic ascites.[42] A mean of 10 L of fluid was removed over 1 hour. The patients were administered 6 to 8 gm of albumin per L of fluid removed, with a sodium content of 30 mEq per L, at a rate of 2 ml per minute. Fifty percent of the calculated albumin was given immediately after paracentesis and the remainder 6 hours later. Their experience with total single paracentesis compared favorably with their previous results with repeated large volume paracenteses. Further, they found that subsequent administration of diuretic therapy to this patient population, previously classified as refractory, avoided reaccumulation of intraperitoneal fluid in approximately 50%. A recent study has demonstrated that albumin can be replaced with dextran 70, 100 ml for each liter of ascites removed, allowing a 30-fold reduction in cost.[42a] All of these findings suggest that abdominal paracentesis may be complementary to diuretic therapy in the management of patients with tense ascites who do not respond to sodium restriction and diuretic therapy alone.

Peritoneovenous Shunting

LeVeen and coworkers[43] developed a pressure-activated one-way valve for peritoneovenous shunting in 1974. One limb of the shunt lies free in the peritoneal cavity, and the efferent limb is within the superior vena cava near its entrance to the right atrium. Flow is maintained when there is a 3- to 5-cm H_2O pressure gradient between the valve and its venous end. When the pressure is below 3 cm H_2O the one-way valve closes, preventing blood from flowing into the tubing and, eventually, into the peritoneal cavity. Two additional shunts, modified after the LeVeen shunt, have been introduced.[44, 45] These modifications have a pumping mechanism that allows for greater shunting and improved ability to clear a partially occluded shunt. The LeVeen shunt is used most commonly. There are no data to indicate the frequency of insertion of these shunts in pediatric patients. Our limited experience with patients younger than the age of 10 years has been associated with a high incidence of shunt failures, quite possibly related to the size of the tubing in the pediatric modification. Peritoneovenous shunting is associated with numerous complications, including diffuse intravascular coagulation, central venous thrombosis, infection, and variceal hemorrhage.[45–47]

Ascites Ultrafiltration and Reinfusion

Ascitic fluid may be drained from the abdomen, concentrated by ultrafiltration, and then reinfused into a peripheral vein. Molecules greater than 50 kd are trapped by the membrane filter.[48] This technique allows the reinfusion of the patient's own proteins, rather than exogenous albumin, to maintain a normal plasma oncotic pressure. It has been successfully employed in a 6-year-old boy with intractable ascites resulting from chronic liver disease and a congestive cardiomyopathy.[49] This methodology bears the same complications as peritoneovenous shunting. It is also expensive and time consuming, and probably does not have any advantage over simple paracentesis with albumin or dextran 70 infusion.

Portosystemic Shunting

Selective types of shunts (e.g., distal splenorenal) decompress only a portion of the splanchnic circulation and are not effective in relieving ascites. The end-to-side portacaval shunt decompresses the splanchnic bed but not the hepatic sinusoids, and ascites may persist or reform after this operation. The side-to-side portacaval shunt, or its equivalent, is the only operation that decompresses both the splanchnic and hepatic vascular beds. Unfortunately, 33% of patients die following the shunt, and long-term survival is poor.[50] There may be a place for transjugular intrahepatic shunts in the management of patients with marked sinusoidal portal hypertension and intractable ascites in the future.[51]

Management of Spontaneous Bacterial Peritonitis

Therapy of spontaneous bacterial peritonitis should be directed toward (1) treatment of the vascular perfusion abnormalities that result from the rapid shifts of fluid and electrolytes; (2) reduction of the accompanying paralytic ileus; (3) correction of the effects of bacterial toxins (e.g., coagulation defects, increased vascular permeability, and shock); and (4) eradication of extra-abdominal sites of infection.[29] Antimicrobial therapy should be initiated promptly when examination of the intraperitoneal fluid suggests spontaneous bacterial peritonitis. Antibiotic therapy should be designed with three goals in mind: (1) broad-spectrum coverage of common organisms that are found in spontaneous bacterial peritonitis; (2) obtaining adequate ascitic fluid concentrations; and (3) a low incidence of nephrotoxicity and superinfection.[52] Ampicillin (200 to 300 mg per kg per 24 hours, administered intravenously in six doses) and gentamicin (7.5 mg per kg per 24 hours, administered intravenously every 8 hours) have traditionally been prescribed when spontaneous bacterial peritonitis is suspected and bacteria are *not* identified with Gram staining of the fluid.[29] There has, however, been a recent trend toward the use of a third-generation cephalosporin (e.g., cefotaxime, 150 mg per kg per 24 hours, administered intravenously in four divided doses). There is the suggestion that a third-generation cephalosporin is more effective and less toxic than ampicillin and an aminoglycoside.[52] Patients with cirrhotic ascites are purportedly more susceptible to aminoglycoside-induced nephrotoxicity,[53] and this risk is reduced when a third-generation cephalosporin is prescribed. One should be aware of the variable activity of third-generation cephalosporins against anaerobes and their apparent inactivity against *Pseudomonas* species.[54] A randomized, controlled study of 100 patients with liver disease and spontaneous bacterial peritonitis compared 5 days of therapy with intravenous cefotaxime to 10 days of therapy with the same agent.[55] Infection-related mortality, hospitalization mortality, bacteriologic cure, and recurrence were not significantly different between the two treatment groups. The authors concluded that short-course treatment of spontaneous bacterial peritonitis was as effective as long-course therapy and was significantly less expensive. Another recent study has demonstrated that selective intestinal decontamination may prevent the development of spontaneous bacterial peritonitis in hospitalized patients with low ascitic fluid protein levels (<1.5 gm per dl).[56] Norfloxacin, the antibiotic administered, produces a selective intestinal decontamination because it inhibits aerobic gram-negative intestinal flora while preserving the anaerobic flora. The study group of adult patients received 400 mg of norfloxacin per day throughout the hospitalization. Unfortunately, this antimicrobial agent is not approved for use in children and young adolescents. Diuresis of cirrhotic ascites increases the concentrations of ascitic fluid complement components and increases the opsonic activity of ascitic fluid, which may retard bacterial infection of the fluid.[57]

SUMMARY

Ascites formation is the result of a disequilibrium between intraperitoneal fluid production and absorption. The two most important factors contributing to ascites formation are impaired hepatic synthetic function, manifested by hypoalbuminemia and a reduced serum oncotic pressure, and portal hypertension. Thoughtful consideration of the principles of evaluation should precede the conceptualization of an initial treatment strategy, or, to be blunt, a loop diuretic should not be immediately prescribed in "knee-jerk" fashion. Valuable information is obtained from the measurement of urine electrolytes and examination of the intra-abdominal fluid. A rational progression of management options flows from careful assessment and monitoring.

REFERENCES

1. Dorland's Illustrated Medical Dictionary. 27th ed. Philadelphia, WB Saunders, 1988.
2. Dawson D: Historical notes on ascites. Gastroenterology 1960; 39:790–791.
3. Dykes PW, Jones JH: Albumin exchange between plasma and ascitic fluid. Clin Sci 1968; 34:185–197.
4. Garrett RA, Franken EA: Neonatal ascites: perirenal urinary extravasation with bladder outlet obstruction. J Urol 1969; 102:627–632.
5. Gillan JE, Lowden JA, Gaskin K, et al: Congenital ascites as a presenting sign of lysosomal storage disease. J Pediatr 1984; 104:225–231.
6. Maconochie IK, Chong S, Mieli-Vergani G, et al: Fetal ascites: an unusual presentation of Niemann-Pick disease. Arch Dis Child 1989; 64:1391–1393.
7. Epstein M, ed: The Kidney in Liver Disease. 3rd ed. Baltimore, Williams & Wilkins, 1988.
8. Epstein M: Functional renal abnormalities in cirrhosis: Pathophysiology and management. *In* Zakin D, Boyer TD, eds: Hepatology: A Textbook of Liver Disease. 2nd ed. Philadelphia, WB Saunders, 1990, p 493.
9. Lieberman FL, Denison EK, Reynolds TB: The relationship of plasma volume, portal hypertension, ascites and renal sodium retention in cirrhosis: The overflow theory of ascites formation. Ann NY Acad Sci 1970; 170:202–212.
10. Lieberman FL, Ito S, Reynolds TB: Effective plasma volume in cirrhosis with ascites: Evidence that a decreased value does not account for renal sodium retention, a spontaneous reduction in glomerular filtration rate (GFR) and a fall in GER during drug-induced diuresis. J Clin Invest 1969; 48:975–981.
11. Levy M: Sodium retention and ascites formation in dogs with experimental portal cirrhosis. Am J Physiol 1977; 233:F572–F585.
12. Levy M, Wexler MJ: Renal sodium retention and ascites formation in dogs with experimental cirrhosis but without portal hypertension or increased splanchnic vascular capacity. J Lab Clin Med 1978; 91:520–536.
13. Levy M, Wexler MJ, McCaffrey C: Sodium retention in dogs with experimental cirrhosis following removal of ascites by continuous peritoneovenous shunting. J Lab Clin Med 1979; 94:933–946.
14. Unikowsky B, Wexler MJ, Levy M: Dogs with experimental cirrhosis of the liver but without intrahepatic hypertension do not retain sodium or form ascites. J Clin Invest 1983; 72:1594–1604.
15. Sherlock S: Diseases of the Liver and Biliary System, 8th ed. London, Blackwell Scientific Publications, 1989, pp 129–150.
15a. Wensing G, Sabra R, Branch RA: Renal and systemic hemodynamics in experimental cirrhosis in rats: Relation to hepatic function. Hepatology 1990; 12:13–19.
16. Wyllie R, Arasu TS, Fitzgerald JF: Ascites: pathophysiology and management. J Pediatr 1980; 97:167–176.
17. Lawson JO, Weissbein AS: The puddle sign—an aid in the diagnosis of minimal ascites. N Engl J Med 1959; 260:652–654.
18. Dinkel E, Lehnart R, Troger J, et al: Sonographic evidence of intraperitoneal fluid: An experimental study and its clinical implications. Pediatr Radiol 1984; 14:299–303.
19. Cohen MD: MRI of the gastrointestinal and musculoskeletal systems in children. Appl Radiol 1987; 16:50–54.
20. Denzer BS: A new method of diagnosis of peritonitis in infancy and childhood. Am J Dis Child 1920; 20:113–114.
21. Mallory A, Schaeffer JW: Complications of diagnostic paracentesis in patients with liver disease. JAMA 1978; 239:628–630.
22. Giacobine JW, Siler VE: Evaluation of diagnostic abdominal paracentesis with experimental and clinical studies. Surg Gynecol Obstet 1960; 110:676–686.
23. Conn HO: Sudden scrotal edema in cirrhosis: A paracentesis syndrome. Ann Intern Med 1971; 74:943–945.
24. Hoefs JC: Serum protein concentration and portal pressure determine the ascitic fluid protein concentration in patients with chronic liver disease. J Lab Clin Med 1983; 102:260–273.
25. Witte MH, Witte CL, Dumont AF: Estimated net transcapillary water and protein flux in the liver and intestines of patients with portal hypertension from hepatic cirrhosis. Gastroenterology 1980; 80:265–272.
26. Pare P, Talbot J, Hoefs JC: Serum-ascites albumin concentration gradient: A physiologic approach to the differential diagnosis of ascites. Gastroenterology 1983; 85:240–244.
27. Rector WG Jr, Reynolds TB: Superiority of the serum-ascites albumin difference over the ascites total protein concentration in separation of "transudative" and "exudative" ascites. Am J Med 1984; 77:83–85.
28. Cameron JL: Chronic pancreatic ascites and pancreatic pleural effusions. Gastroenterology 1978; 74:134–140.
29. Clark JH, Fitzgerald JF, Kleiman MB: Spontaneous bacterial peritonitis. J Pediatr 1984; 104:495–500.
30. Larcher VF, Manolaki N, Vegmente A, et al: Spontaneous bacterial peritonitis in children with chronic liver disease: Clinical features and etiologic factors. J Pediatr 1985; 106:907–912.
31. Bichet D, Szatalowicz V, Chaimovitz C, et al: Role of vasopressin in abnormal excretion in cirrhotic patients. Ann Intern Med 1982; 96:413–417.
32. Arieff AI: Hyponatremia associated with permanent brain damage. Adv Intern Med 1987; 32:325–344.
33. Odlind B: Relationship between tubular secretion of furosemide and its saluretic effect. J Pharmacol Exp Ther 1979; 208:515–521.
34. Planas R, Arroyo V, Rimola A, et al: Acetylsalicylic acid suppresses the renal hemodynamic effect and reduces the diuretic action of furosemide in cirrhosis with ascites. Gastroenterology 1983; 84:247–252.
35. Liebowitz HR: Hazards of abdominal paracentesis in the cirrhotic patient. III. NY State J Med 1962; 62:2223–2229.
36. Carey WD, Kohne JC, Leatherman J, et al: Ascitic fluid removal: Does it cause renal or hemodynamic decompensation. Cleve Clin Q 1983; 50:397–400.
37. Kao HW, Rakov NE, Savage E, et al: The effect of large volume paracentesis on plasma volume—a cause of hypovolemia? Hepatology 1985; 5:403–407.
38. Simon DM, McCain JR, Bonkovsky HL, et al: Effects of therapeutic paracentesis on systemic and hepatic hemodynamics and on renal and hormonal function. Hepatology 1987; 7:423–429.
39. Quintero E, Gines P, Arroyo V, et al: Paracentesis versus diuretics in the treatment of cirrhotics with tense ascites. Lancet 1985; 1:611–612.
40. Gines P, Arroyo V, Quintero E, et al: Comparison between paracentesis and diuretics in the treatment of cirrhotics with tense ascites. Gastroenterology 1987; 93:234–241.
41. Salerno F, Badalamenti S, Incerti P, et al: Repeated paracentesis and IV albumin infusion to treat "tense" ascites in cirrhotic patients: A safe alternative therapy. J Hepatol 1987; 5:102–108.
42. Tito L, Gines P, Arroyo V, et al: Total paracentesis associated with intravenous albumin management of patients with cirrhosis and ascites. Gastroenterology 1990; 98:146–151.
42a. Terg R, Berreta J, Abecasis R, et al: Dextran administration

avoids hemodynamic changes following paracentesis in cirrhotic patients: A safe and inexpensive option. Dig Dis Sci 1992; 37:79–83.

43. LeVeen HH, Christoudias G, Ip M, et al: Peritoneovenous shunting for ascites. Ann Surg 1974; 180:580–591.
44. Lund RH, Newkirk JB: Peritoneovenous shunting system for surgical management of ascites. Contemp Surg 1979; 14:31–45.
45. Epstein M: Peritoneovenous shunt in the management of ascites and the hepatorenal syndrome. Gastroenterology 1982; 82:790–799.
46. Greig PD, Langer B, Blendis LM, et al: Complications after peritoneovenous shunting for ascites. Am J Surg 1980; 139:125–131.
47. Fulenwider JT, Smith RB, Redd SC, et al: Peritoneovenous shunts: Lessons learned from an eight-year experience with 70 patients. Arch Surg 1984; 119:1133–1137.
48. Lai KN, Leung JWC, Vallance-Owen J: Dialytic ultrafiltration by hemofilter in treatment of patients with refractory ascites and renal insufficiency. Am J Gastroenterol 1987; 82:665–668.
49. Assadi FK, Gordon D, Kecskes SA, et al: Treatment of refractory ascites by ultrafiltration-reinfusion of ascitic fluid peritoneally. J Pediatr 1985; 106:943–946.
50. Welch HF, Welch CS, Carter JH: Prognosis after surgical treatment of ascites: Results of side-to-side shunt in 40 patients. Surgery 1964; 56:75–82.
51. Wright TL, Boyer TD: Diagnosis and management of cirrhotic ascites. *In* Zakim D, Boyer TD (eds): Hepatology: A Textbook of Liver Disease. 2nd ed. Philadelphia, WB Saunders, 1990, p. 623.
52. Felisart J, Rimola A, Arroyo V, et al: Cefotaxime is more effective than is ampicillin-tobramycin in cirrhotics with severe infections. Hepatology 1985; 5:457–462.
53. Cabrera J, Arroyo V, Ballesta AM, et al: Aminoglycoside nephrotoxicity in cirrhosis. Gastroenterology 1982; 82:97–105.
54. Siegel JD: Intra-abdominal sepsis. *In* Nelson JD, ed: Current Therapy in Pediatric Infectious Disease. 2nd ed. Philadelphia, 1988, BC Decker, p 72.
55. Runyon BA, McHutchison JG, Antillon MR, et al: Short-course versus long-course antibiotic treatment of spontaneous bacterial peritonitis. Gastroenterology 1991; 100:1737–1742.
56. Soriano G, Guarner C, Teixido M, et al: Selective intestinal decontamination prevents spontaneous bacterial peritonitis. Gastroenterology 1991; 100:477–481.
57. Runyon BA, Epps DE: Diuresis of cirrhotic ascites increases its opsonic activity and may help prevent spontaneous bacterial peritonitis. Hepatology 1986; 6:396–399.

Chapter 12

Caustic Ingestion

GEORGE D. FERRY

PATHOGENESIS

The accidental ingestion of caustic agents is a significant problem for young children. The Association of Poison Control Centers National Data Collection System, serving a population of 191.7 million people, reported 1,713,462 human poison exposures in 1990.[1] The majority of these reported poisonings—1,032,959 (60.3%)—were in children 6 years of age or younger and were accidental. Caustic exposures reported in this same age group included 11,516 incidents due to alkaline agents and 4,748 due to acids. Household bleaches were also a common cause of accidental poisonings in young children, with 18,376 reported exposures. The products most often involved included automatic dishwasher agents, laundry detergents, swimming pool products, and toilet bowl and oven cleaners[1] (Table 12–1). Accidental caustic ingestion occurs most commonly between 1 and 3 years of age[2] (Fig. 12–1), with boys accounting for 50 to 62% of cases.[3, 4]

Injury to the lips, oropharynx, and upper airway may occur with many caustic agents, but esophageal burns account for most of the serious injuries and acute and chronic complications. Esophageal burns are reported in 18 to 46% of caustic ingestions occurring in children,[2, 5–7] with Liquid Drano, lye, and ammonia being the agents most likely to produce significant injury[2] (Table 12–2). Children living on farms are at an even higher risk for serious burns, since industrial-strength agents are in common use in that setting.[8] Household bleaches are among the most commonly ingested products, but their relatively neutral pH makes them less irritating than alkalis and acids.[9] It is rare to see esophageal burns with these agents, and, when present, they tend to be mild.[10–12] Solid caustic materials, which tend to adhere to the mucosa, may produce deep burns of the oral cavity and esophagus,[10] but they are less likely to reach the stomach.[13] Whether or not solid caustic agents tend to cause more serious burns than liquid agents is controversial,[2, 5] but the immediate and severe pain produced by these products may limit the amount ingested and thus lessen the extent of injury.[13] Powdered detergents tend to injure the upper airway, resulting in stridor and epiglottitis, and esophageal injury is less common.[14]

The mechanisms by which caustic agents produce tissue injury differ for alkalis and acids, as do the sites of injury. Alkalis, with a pH greater than 7, cause liquefaction necrosis with early disintegration of the mucosa, allowing deep penetration and even perforation.[9, 15] Those agents with a pH of 11 or higher frequently cause severe burns, even with ingestion of small amounts.[14] Agents with pHs ranging from 9 to 11, including many household detergents and phosphates, rarely cause serious injuries unless taken in large amounts.[16] The course of injury and repair in experimentally induced esophageal burns due to alkali has been well demonstrated in animal models.[15] Penetration into the esophageal wall by alkaline agents varies with the concentration and the length of time the agent remains in contact with the mucosa. Experimentally, a 10% solution of sodium hydroxide may require as long

Table 12–1. CAUSTIC EXPOSURE IN CHILDREN YOUNGER THAN 6 YEARS OF AGE

Agent	Number
Chemicals	
Acids	1,220
Alkali	2,772
Bleaches (household)	18,376
Drain cleaners	
Acids	87
Alkali	619
Automatic dishwasher agents	2,999
Industrial cleaners	
Acids	167
Alkali	366
Laundry detergents	9,446
Miscellaneous cleaners	
Acids	252
Alkali	3,306
Oven cleaners	
Acid	2
Alkali	1,086
Swimming pool/aquarium products	2,738
Tile cleaners	
Acid	1,611
Alkali	3,149
Toilet bowl cleaners	
Acid	1,409
Alkali	218
Unknown	1,768
TOTAL	51,591

Data from Litovitz TL, Bailey KM, Schmitz BF, et al: 1990 Annual Report of the American Association of Poison Control Centers National Data Collection System. Am J Emerg Med 1991; 9:461–509.

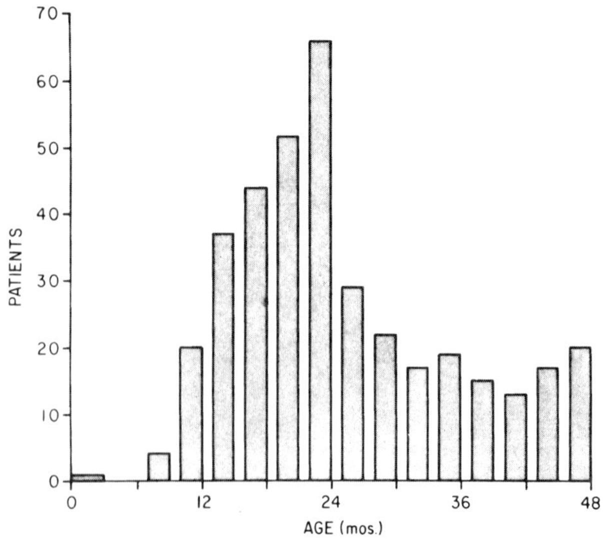

Figure 12–1. Caustic ingestion in pediatric patients by age. (From Adam JS, Birck HG: Pediatric caustic ingestion. Ann Otol Rhinol Laryngol 1982; 91:656–658; with permission.)

as 1 minute of contact to produce a deep burn, whereas as little as 1 ml of 30% sodium hydroxide can cause transmural necrosis of the esophagus within 1 second of contact.[17] Following the initial necrosis, additional destruction takes place over the first week owing to inflammation and vascular thrombosis. By 10 days there is formation of granulation tissue and weakening of the esophageal wall. It is during this early period that the esophagus is increasingly vulnerable to perforation.[18] By 3 weeks, fibrogenesis and stricture formation are well under way, and perforation is less likely.

Acids, or corrosives, with a pH less than 7, cause coagulation necrosis, and the coagulum that forms on the mucosal surface limits deeper penetration.[9] The alkaline pH and squamous epithelium of the esophagus are additional factors that may help limit the severity of esophageal injury from acids. These factors may also explain why ingested acids tend to reach the stomach in greater amounts, resulting in more serious gastric injury, including gastric perforation.[9] Since there is a tendency for pooling of contents in the antrum and some degree of antral spasm, acids tend to produce the most severe burns in the prepyloric area.[11, 19] Although perforation of the esophagus is less common with ingestion of acids, the esophagus is not spared from significant injury, as 6 to 20% of these ingestions will result in esophageal burns.[20] Upper airway injuries are also common with ingestion of acids, perhaps related to their bad taste, which tends to stimulate gagging, choking, and attempts to spit out the ingested material.[9]

Small button batteries from hearing aids, calculators, and watches have the potential to cause significant burns in the esophagus and, occasionally, in the stomach.[21] Most of these batteries measure 7.9 to 11.6 mm in diameter and pass through the esophagus and gastrointestinal tract spontaneously without producing symptoms. Larger batteries, especially those 15.6 mm or greater in size, are more likely to lodge in the esophagus, where leakage of their caustic contents can produce significant esophageal burns. The caustic material in small batteries is primarily silver or mercuric oxide, but some contain manganese dioxide, zinc, or lithium. Tracheoesophageal fistula and scarring have been reported in one case in which the retained battery was not detected promptly.[21]

Ingestion in young children and in older children who are mentally retarded is generally accidental, and the volume ingested is small. Ingestion in adults is more often deliberate and related to attempted suicide.[22] These cases are often associated with large quantities of caustic agents, and the injury to the esophagus and stomach is often severe.[23] At least one case of alkali ingestion due to child abuse has been reported, with lye being placed in a milk bottle.[24]

Table 12–2. ESOPHAGEAL BURNS WITH CAUSTIC AGENTS INGESTED BY 402 PEDIATRIC PATIENTS

Agent	+ Esoph.	− Esoph.	Total
Drano			
Liquid	21	86	107
Solid	7	41	48
Lye	14	40	51
Toilet bowl cleaner (Vanish, Saniflush, Vansol)	7	45	52
Ammonia cleanser	7	29	36
Ammonia ampules	0	18	18
Plunge	3	15	18
Clinitest tablets	0	10	10
HTH (pool cleaner)	0	10	10
Oven cleaner	0	8	8
Dry cleaning fluid	0	2	2
Unknown, miscellaneous	13	26	39

+ Esophageal burns; − No esophageal burns.
From Adam JS, Birck HG: Pediatric caustic ingestion. Ann Otol Rhinol Laryngol 1982; 91:656–658; with permission.

CLINICAL PRESENTATION

Drooling, dysphagia, retrosternal or abdominal pain, stridor, hoarseness, nasal flaring, and retractions suggest upper airway injury or complicating esophageal burns, or both. Epiglottitis may occasionally be severe, especially in children younger than 2 years of age, and prompt intubation may be required.[14, 25] Vomiting and hematemesis may also be seen with upper airway injury without esophageal involvement.[26] Although symptoms of upper airway injury usually begin rapidly after contact with caustic agents, there may be a 1- to 2-hour delay with ingestion of powdered agents.[14]

Any or all of these symptoms may also be associated with esophageal injury; however, the presence or absence of symptoms does not predict ingestion or the presence or severity of esophageal or gastric burns. In a single series of 378 caustic ingestions in children, 12% had no symptoms but had severe esophageal burns, whereas 82% who were symptomatic at presentation had minimal or no esophageal involvement (Table 12–3).[3] The presence or absence of oral lesions is also a poor predictor of esophageal injury. In a review of multiple case series totaling 489 children, 45% without oral burns had esophageal burns, and 54% with oral burns had accompanying esophageal burns.[12] Deep esophageal burns can be complicated by esophageal perforation with mediastinitis and tracheoesophageal fistula.[9]

Dysphagia is the most common symptom following caustic ingestion and results from alterations in peristalsis secondary to esophageal irritation. Dysphagia may occur without severe esophageal injury, as shown in the series of Gaudreault and associates in which 75% of 106 children who presented with dysphagia had minimal to no obvious esophageal injury.[3] Esophageal studies during the acute phase of injury have shown loss of motility with delayed transit,[27] similar to what is seen in peptic esophagitis.[28, 29] Prolonged esophageal transit time as measured by radionuclide testing may persist for several weeks following severe esophageal burns. Dysphagia persisting after the acute injury results from segmental rigidity due to fibrosis of deeper muscle layers, with or without strictures.[27] Fibrosis produces a decreased amplitude of esophageal contractions and elevated basal pressure.

There is little written about the incidence and severity of gastric lesions in caustic ingestion, partly because this type of injury is less common, and partly because of the use of rigid endoscopes that are often not advanced beyond the first visible esophageal burn.[12] In a more recent review in which flexible pediatric endoscopes were used to evaluate 156 children with caustic ingestion, 17 (11%) had esophageal and gastric burns and 14 (9%) had gastric burns only.[7] In patients taking relatively large amounts of alkali (200–300 ml), gastric injury has been reported in 86% of cases and may be more severe.[23] Large ingestions have resulted in both gastric perforation and hemorrhage and death from erosion into bronchial vessels.[10] Gastric injury is often most severe with acids, such as sulfuric acid, resulting in pyloric obstruction.[10] Duodenal erosions are reported in occasional cases.[23]

Table 12–3. SEVERITY OF ESOPHAGEAL LESION IN PATIENTS WITH OR WITHOUT SIGNS AND/OR SYMPTOMS*

	Signs and/or Symptoms			
	Present (N = 298)		Absent (N = 80)	
Esophageal Lesion	*No.*	%	*No.*	%
Grade 0 or 1**	243	82	70	88
Grade 2	55	18	10	12
Grade 3	0	0	0	0
Stricture	5	2	1	1

*P values were not significant.

**Grade 0 or 1, erythema, edema; grade 2, ulceration; grade 3, perforation.

From Gaudreault P, Parent M, McGuigan MA, et al: Predictability of esophageal injury from signs and symptoms: A study of caustic ingestion in 378 children. Pediatrics 1983; 71:767–770. Reproduced by permission of Pediatrics, vol 71; Copyright 1983.

DIAGNOSTIC EVALUATION

It is essential to document the presence or absence of esophageal or gastric injury following caustic ingestion. Radiologic examination is valuable and essential for followup to detect the presence of strictures, but barium studies are not reliable in detecting acute injury or in predicting stricture formation.[22, 26] Upper endoscopy is the most reliable method to detect injury[5, 7] and is generally performed within the first 24 to 48 hours. During this period, mucosal injury may not yet have penetrated through the entire esophageal wall, and perforation is less likely.[2, 5, 7] The objectives of early endoscopy are to establish the presence or absence of esophageal or gastric lesions, or both, and to determine the severity of involvement. Once the extent of injury is known, appropriate therapy can be initiated. Endoscopy within the first 12 hours after ingestion may be too early to appreciate the full extent of the injury,[9] but the information gained is generally adequate for proper management. Flexible fiberoptic and video endoscopes have made upper endoscopy safer, and in all but the most severe cases these endoscopes can be passed through the esophagus and into the stomach, even if esophageal burns are noted.[5, 7, 23] Rigid endoscopes are still in common use, but the risk of perforation remains a major consideration, and these endoscopes are generally not advanced beyond the first significant esophageal burn.[7] Flexible endoscopes also allow the use of conscious (intravenous) sedation in an outpatient setting.[11] In patients with severe burns and with upper airway signs or symptoms, endoscopy should be performed using general anesthesia with protection of the airway.[11] Under these controlled circumstances, endoscopy can be performed with much greater safety.

Since the history regarding ingestion is often vague, and symptoms in young children may be unreliable, some authors suggest endoscopy in all pediatric patients with any hint of caustic ingestion.[5, 7] However, in patients with a questionable history of ingestion, no evidence of oral lesions, and no dysphagia, vomiting, or other symptoms, it is generally safe to observe fluid intake and overall status over several hours. If the patient remains asymptomatic with normal swallowing, endoscopy may be unnecessary.[12] A flow chart outlining the initial indications for endoscopy and appropriate follow-up is shown in Figure 12–2. Patients who have ingested household bleaches rarely have significant tissue injury and rarely require endoscopy. Patients with a definite history or strong suggestion of ingestion, even if asymptomatic, and patients with symptoms or oral burns should be evaluated with upper endoscopy.[2, 30]

A grading system for esophageal burns has been useful in planning appropriate medical therapy, documenting the need for a nasogastric tube, and predicting later stricture formation. First-degree burns are those with injury limited to edema and erythema; second-degree burns are characterized by linear ulceration and necrotic tissue with whitish plaques; and third-degree burns include circumferential injury with sloughing of the mucosa.[5, 13] Other authors use third-degree burns to

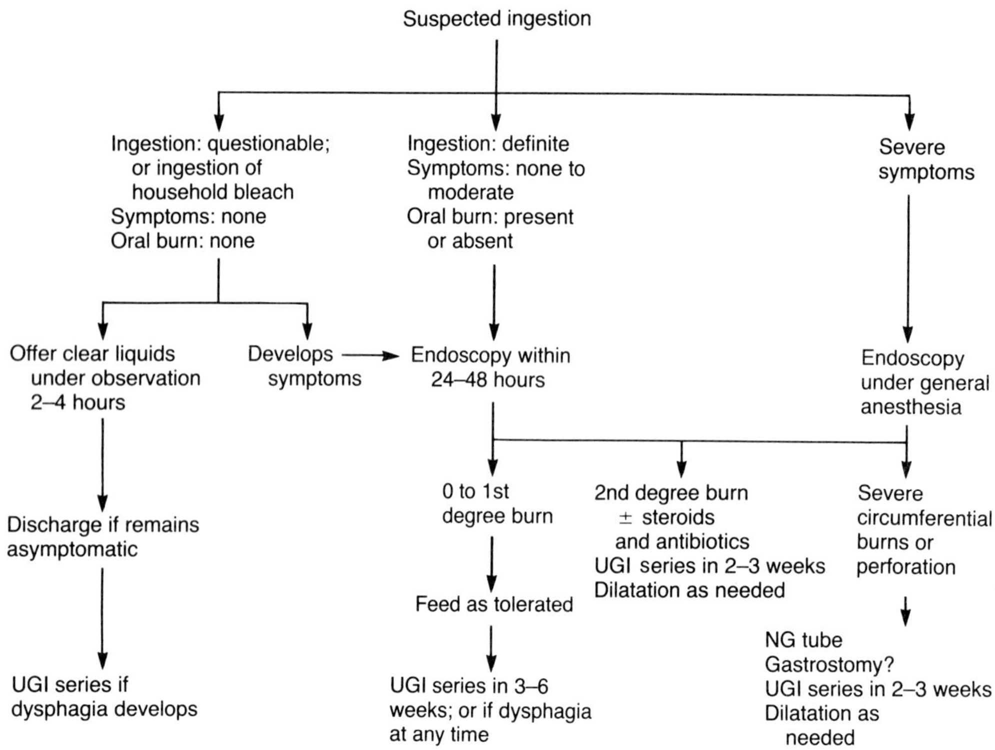

Figure 12–2. Evaluation of ingestion of caustic substances.

define patients with perforation.[3] Linear burns rarely lead to stenosis, whereas circumferential burns frequently heal with stricture formation.[31]

TREATMENT

The initial treatment of caustic ingestion is primarily observation, with an emphasis on preventing vomiting, choking, and aspiration. The induction of vomiting with ipecac or other substances is contraindicated, as this may lead to additional esophageal injury if gastric contents come in contact with the esophageal mucosa.[12] The use of neutralizing agents has been suggested, but there is concern about additional damage from heat injury during the neutralization process. Although experimental studies with neutralizing agents suggest that they are safe, this type of therapy is not generally accepted.[32] The use of diluting agents, such as milk or water, has been recommended by some authors.[12] If a large volume is taken, however, vomiting is more likely, and this may lead to further complications. In the presence of acute airway swelling and obstruction, dilution is clearly contraindicated.[12] In addition, the amount of milk or other fluids that would be necessary to dilute the caustic agent significantly is too great and cannot be used; therefore, no attempts at either dilution or neutralization can be recommended. The use of a nasogastric tube to wash out the stomach is also contraindicated, since perforation or additional injury may occur while passing the tube. With upper airway symptoms, corticosteroids may be indicated, and intubation or even tracheostomy is occasionally required.[25]

In the presence of severe esophageal injury, when there are extensive circumferential burns or a strong possibility of perforation, or both, a nasogastric tube should be placed under direct visualization at the time of upper endoscopy. This will provide a route for nutritional support during the healing phase, and it will help maintain a lumen during stricture formation. A nasogastric tube can also serve as a guide for esophageal dilatation once a stricture has formed.[33] Keeping a small channel open throughout the length of the esophagus will also allow later passage of a string for retrograde dilatation. Varying sizes of silicone nasogastric tubes, from 5 to 10 mm in diameter, have also been used as stents in circular, deeply ulcerated caustic injuries, and they may prevent the development of serious strictures.[34, 35]

The use of corticosteroids to prevent esophageal stricture formation has been a controversial issue since early animal studies demonstrated that steroids prevent esophageal scarring.[15, 36–38] Numerous small case series have suggested beneficial effects of early steroids in first- or second-degree esophageal burns, with 0 to 25% of burns resulting in strictures in treated groups versus 25 to 88% in untreated patients.[2, 10, 22, 39, 40] When corticosteroids are used, they are started as soon as an esophageal burn is documented by endoscopy. The dose used is equivalent to prednisone 1 to 2 mg per kg per day (maximum 60 mg per day) for 3 to 4 weeks.[9] Some authors have suggested that corticosteroids should be used with all ingestions, even before endoscopy, with the rationale that the earlier the use, the more effective the treatment. If endoscopy shows no evidence of burns, the corticosteroids can then be stopped.[18] Antibiotics

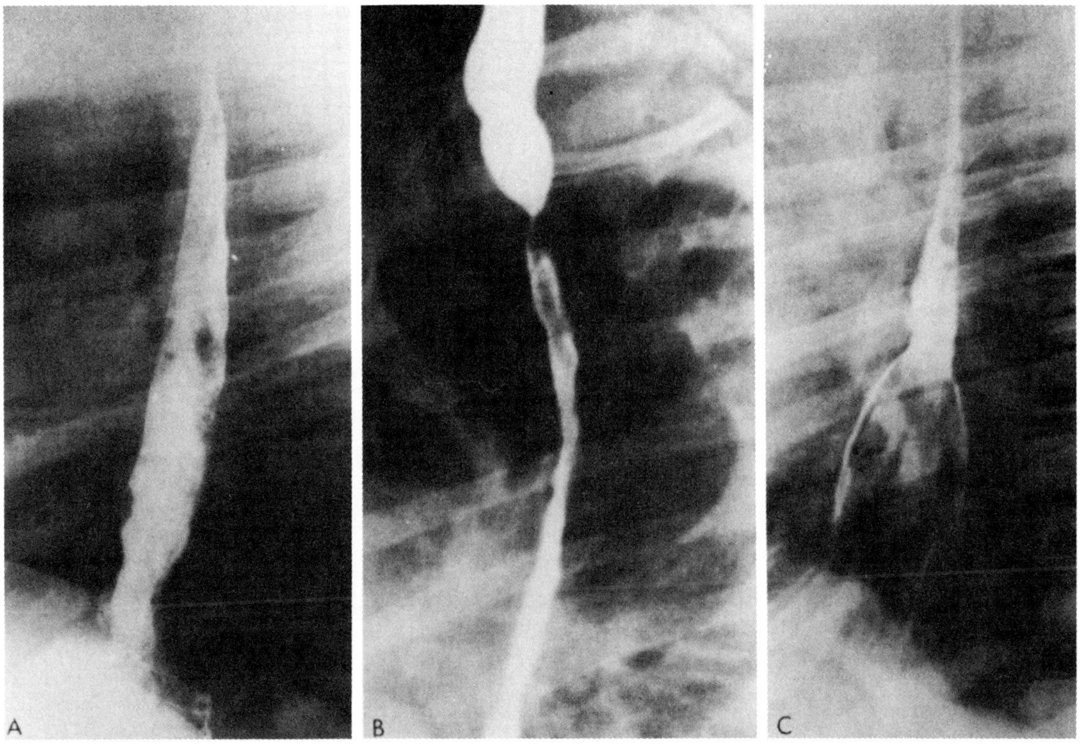

Figure 12–3. Ingestion of Drano in 2-year-old child. *A,* Initial esophagram made several hours after ingestion of the caustic agent shows ill-defined mucosa probably resulting from edema and mucus. *B,* Repeat esophagram 3 weeks later shows constriction of the thoracic portion of the esophagus with more severe stricture in the proximal portion and dilatation of the cervical esophagus. *C,* Repeat esophagram 3 months later shows esophageal stricture with retraction of the gastric cardia into the chest. (From Singleton EB, Wagner ML, Dutton RV, eds: Radiology of the Alimentary Tract in Infants and Children. Philadelphia, WB Saunders, 1977, p 86; with permission.)

are generally used whenever steroids are used because of the increased risk of infection, especially bacterial spread to the mediastinum.[37]

Other studies have failed to show any benefit from corticosteroids, reporting strictures in 20 to 38% of documented esophageal burns, regardless of treatment.[5, 13, 26] In a controlled, prospective trial in which 60 children were randomized to receive a placebo or prednisolone (2 mg per kg per day intravenously) followed by 3 weeks of oral prednisone, there was no clear-cut benefit to corticosteroids. Stricture formation appeared to be related only to the severity of the caustic injury.[5] In addition, corticosteroids are clearly contraindicated in certain settings. In third-degree burns, stricture formation is inevitable, perforation is common, and steroids may mask the onset of mediastinitis and infection. Corticosteroids are not indicated for acid burns; since strictures of the esophagus are less common, the steroids may mask any symptoms of gastric necrosis and perforation, and they do not appear to be effective.[10]

Early dilatation to prevent stricture formation has been tried with some success, but the increased incidence of perforation has limited its use.[39] In severe burns with highly caustic materials, such as industrial-strength lye, extensive esophageal injury is common, and a gastrostomy is useful in allowing placement of a string for later retrograde dilatation. All patients with significant burns and the potential for stricture formation should be evaluated with barium contrast studies 1 to 3 weeks postingestion.

Ingestion of small button batteries should be evaluated by chest and abdominal radiographs. If the battery is noted to be in the esophagus, prompt removal is indicated.[21] If the battery has reached the stomach or intestine, follow-up after 3 to 4 days is indicated to ascertain passage (see Chapter 13).

LATE COMPLICATIONS

Stricture formation is the primary complication of caustic injury and is reported in 2 to 38% of ingestions and in 3 to 57% of ingestions with documented esophageal burns.[2–5] Most third-degree (circumferential) burns lead to esophageal strictures, regardless of treatment,[5] whereas second-degree burns are less likely to result in strictures.[26] Although there are rare reports of patients developing strictures following a normal endoscopy,[2] it is likely that a burn was present but was missed using a rigid endoscope. Approximately 80% of patients with a developing stricture will have obstructive symptoms within 2 months, and in the most severe burns, there may be complete obstruction within 3 weeks.[41] The typical radiologic progression from initial injury to stricture formation is demonstrated in Figure 12–3.[42] At 3 weeks, the esophagram shows a long constriction with a more severe stricture proximally, and at 3 months there is a significant stricture with shortening of the esophagus.

Once a stricture is confirmed radiologically, esophageal dilatation is usually necessary to maintain or re-establish normal swallowing. A variety of dilators can be used, including mercury-filled bougies, Maloney antegrade dilators or Tucker dilators used in retrograde dilatation, and dilators passed over a string or guide wire. Caustic strictures appear to perforate easily; retrograde dilatation has been considered the safest method, although this does require a gastrostomy and a string for guidance.[33] Balloon dilators under endoscopic control have recently been used successfully in children.[43] Perforation should be less likely with these instruments because only radially directed force is exerted, and the longitudinal shearing force with antegrade and retrograde dilators is avoided. Balloon dilatation is not totally free from complications, as even this technique has resulted in esophageal perforation.[44]

Although esophageal dilatation may be beneficial initially, repeated dilatations are usually needed. Only 33 to 48% of patients with caustic strictures have long-term success with repeated dilatations. The remaining patients, who often have long strictures, have increasing difficulty in swallowing owing to progressive obstruction. Within 2 years following caustic ingestion, many of these patients will need colon interposition.[4, 5] Colon interposition is reserved for more extensive strictures and is generally successful; however, this bypass surgery is not without problems. Motility may be abnormal, and many patients have some persistent difficulty in swallowing. In addition, anastomotic strictures may need periodic dilatation, and reflux of gastric contents can produce gastrocolic ulceration.[45, 45a]

Pyloric stenosis has occurred with both acids and alkalis and is often associated with esophageal injury and strictures.[10] With severe injury to the stomach, gastric outlet obstruction may occur, developing over 3 to 10 weeks.[19, 46] Surgical bypass may be necessary, but endoscopic balloon dilatation has also been used successfully in one child with pyloric obstruction due to liquid alkali.[47]

Caustic injury appears to lead to an increased risk of esophageal carcinoma,[13] with an incidence following corrosive strictures of 2 to 8%.[13, 48] The time interval between ingestion and the detection of tumor has been from 16 to 42 years,[48] and there is some speculation that the true incidence of carcinoma could reach 30% or more if patients were followed for 30 years.[49] Although removing the esophagus is a difficult procedure, some authors now recommend resection at the time of bypass with colon interposition.[13, 48] Any patient with a history of caustic ingestion and the late onset or worsening of dysphagia should be promptly evaluated, and carcinoma should be suspected until proved otherwise.

REFERENCES

1. Litovitz TL, Bailey KM, Schmitz BF, et al: 1990 annual report of the American Association of Poison Control Centers National Data Collection System. Am J Emerg Med 1991; 9:461–509.
2. Adam JS, Birck HG: Pediatric caustic ingestion. Ann Otol Rhinol Laryngol 1982; 91:656–658.
3. Gaudreault P, Parent M, McGuigan MA, et al: Predictability of esophageal injury from signs and symptoms: A study of caustic ingestion in 378 children. Pediatrics 1983; 71:767–770.
4. Moazam F, Talbert JL, Miller D, et al: Caustic ingestion and its sequelae in children. South Med J 1987; 80:187–190.
5. Anderson KD, Rouse TM, Randolph JG: A controlled trial of corticosteroids in children with corrosive injury of the esophagus. N Engl J Med 1990; 323:637–640.
6. Haller JA, Andrews HG, White JJ, et al: Pathophysiology and management of acute corrosive burns of the esophagus: Results of treatment in 285 children. J Pediatr Surg 1971; 6:578–583.
7. Previtera C, Giusti F, Guglielmi M: Predictive value of visible lesions (cheeks, lips, oropharynx) in suspected caustic ingestion: May endoscopy reasonably be omitted in completely negative pediatric patients? Pediatr Emerg Care 1990; 6:176–178.
8. Edmonson MB: Caustic alkali ingestions by farm children. Pediatrics 1987; 79:413–416.
9. Friedman EM: Caustic ingestions and foreign bodies in the aerodigestive tract of children. Pediatr Clin North Am 1989; 36:1403–1410.
10. Hawkins DB, Demeter MJ, Barnett TE: Caustic ingestion: Controversies in management: A review of 214 cases. Laryngoscope 1980; 90:98–109.
11. Moore WR: Caustic ingestions: Pathophysiology, diagnosis, and treatment. Clin Pediatr 1986; 25:192–196.
12. Wason S: The emergency management of caustic ingestions. J Emerg Med 1985; 2:175–182.
13. Kirsh MM, Ritter F: Caustic ingestion and subsequent damage to the oropharyngeal and digestive passages. Ann Thorac Surg 1976; 21:74–82.
14. Einhorn A, Horton L, Altieri M, et al: Serious respiratory consequences of detergent ingestions in children. Pediatrics 1989; 84:472–474.
15. Haller JA Jr, Bachman K: The comparative effect of current therapy on experimental caustic burns of the esophagus. Pediatrics 1964; 34:236–245.
16. Muhlendahl KEV, Oberdisse U, Krienke EG: Local injuries by accidental ingestion of corrosive substances by children. Arch Toxicol 1978; 39:299–314.
17. Leape LL, Ashcraft KW, Scarpelli DG, et al: Hazard to health—liquid lye. N Engl J Med 1971; 284:578–581.
18. Tewfik TL, Schloss MD: Ingestion of lye and other corrosive agents: A study of 86 infant and child cases. J Otolaryngol 1980; 9:72–77.
19. Hodgson JH: Corrosive stricture of the stomach: Case report and review of literature. Br J Surg 1959; 46:358–361.
20. Maull KI, Scher LA, Greenfield LJ: Surgical implications of acid ingestion. Surg Gynecol Obstet 1979; 148:895–898.
21. Litovitz TL: Battery ingestions: Product accessibility and clinical course. Pediatrics 1985; 75:469–476.
22. Borja AR, Ransdell HT Jr, Thomas TV, et al: Lye injuries of the esophagus: Analysis of ninety cases of lye ingestion. J Thorac Cardiovasc Surg 1969; 57:533–538.
23. Cello JP, Fogel RP, Boland CR: Liquid caustic ingestion. Arch Intern Med 1980; 140:501–504.
24. Friedman EM: Caustic ingestions and foreign body aspirations: An overlooked form of child abuse. Ann Otol Rhinol Laryngol 1987; 96:709–712.
25. Moulin D, Bertrand JM, Buts JP, et al: Upper airway lesions in children after accidental ingestion of caustic substances. J Pediatr 1985; 106:408–410.
26. Ferguson MK, Migliore M, Staszak VM, et al: Early evaluation and therapy for caustic esophageal injury. Am J Surg 1989; 157:116–120.
27. Cadranel S, Di Lorenzo C, Piepsz A, et al: Caustic ingestion and esophageal function. J Pediatr Gastroenterol Nutr 1990; 10:164–168.
28. Cucchiara S, Staiano A, Di Lorenzo C, et al: Esophageal motor abnormalities in children with gastroesophageal reflux and peptic esophagitis. J Pediatr 1986; 108:907–911.
29. Hillemeier AC, Grill BB, McCallum R, et al: Esophageal and gastric motor abnormalities in children with gastroesophageal motor abnormalities in gastroesophageal reflux during infancy. Gastroenterology 1983; 84:741–746.

30. Viscomi GJ, Beckhuis GJ, Whitten CF: An evaluation of early esophagoscopy and corticosteroid therapy in the management of corrosive injury of the esophagus. J Pediatr 1961; 59:356–360.
31. Kleager LE, Yarington CT Jr: Emergency management of esophageal burns: A review for the primary health care physician. Nebr Med J 1974; 59:64–68.
32. Maull KI, Osmand AP, Maull CD: Liquid caustic ingestions: An in vitro study of the effects of buffer, neutralization, and dilution. Ann Emerg Med 1985; 14:1160–1162.
33. Hawkins DB: Dilation of esophageal strictures: Comparative morbidity of antegrade and retrograde methods. Ann Otol Rhinol Laryngol 1988; 97:460–465.
34. Wijburg FA, Heymans HS, Urbanus NA: Caustic esophageal lesions in childhood: Prevention of stricture formation. J Pediatr Surg 1989; 24:171–173.
35. Reyes HM, Hill JL: Modification of the experimental stent technique for esophageal burns. J Surg Res 1976; 20:65–70.
36. Spain DM, Molomut N, Haber A: The effect of cortisone on the formation of granulation tissue in mice. Am J Pathol 1950; 26:710–711.
37. Rosenberg N, Kunderman PJ, Vroman L, et al: Prevention of experimental esophageal stricture by cortisone. Arch Surg 1953; 66:593–598.
38. Weisskopf A: Effects of cortisone on experimental lye burn of the esophagus. Ann Otol Rhin Laryngol 1952; 61:681–691.
39. Cleveland WW, Thornton N, Chesney JG, et al: The effect of prednisone in the prevention of esophageal stricture following the ingestion of lye. South Med J 1958; 51:861–864.
40. Middelkamp JN, Cone AJ, Ogura JH, et al: Endoscopic diagnosis and steroid and antibiotic therapy of acute lye burns of the esophagus. Laryngoscope 1961; 71:1354–1362.
41. Webb WR, Koutras P, Ecker RR, et al: An evaluation of steroids and antibiotics in caustic burns of the esophagus. Ann Thorac Surg 1970; 9:95–102.
42. Singleton EB, Wagner ML, Dutton RV: *In* Radiology of the alimentary tract in infants and children. 2nd ed. Philadelphia, WB Saunders, 1977, p 86.
43. Sato Y, Frey EE, Smith WL, et al: Balloon dilatation of esophageal stenosis in children. Am J Roentgenol 1988; 150:639–642.
44. Ball WS, Strife JL, Rosenkrantz J, et al: Esophageal strictures in children: Treatment by balloon dilatation. Radiology 1984; 150:263–264.
45. West KW, Vane DW, Grosfeld JL: Esophageal replacement in children: Experience with thirty-one cases. Surgery 1986; 100:751–757.
45a. Han M-T: Illeocolic replacement of esophagus in children with esophageal stricture. J Pediatr Surg 1991; 26:755–757.
46. Herrington JL: Stenosis of the gastric antrum and proximal duodenum resulting from the ingestion of a corrosive agent. Am J Surg 1964; 107:580–585.
47. Treem WR, Long WR, Friedman D, et al: Successful management of an acquired gastric outlet obstruction with endoscopy-guided balloon dilation. J Pediatr Gastroenterol Nutr 1987; 6:992–996.
48. Ti TK: Esophageal carcinoma associated with corrosive injury prevention and treatment by esophageal resection. Br J Surg 1983; 70:223–225.
49. Kiviranta UK: Corrosion carcinoma of the oesophagus. Acta Otolaryngol 1952; 42:89–95.

Chapter 13

Foreign Bodies and Bezoars

WILLIAM J. BYRNE

Toddlers and young children frequently evaluate their surroundings by tasting and swallowing new and unusual objects. Indeed, the peak incidence of foreign body ingestion occurs between 6 months and 3 years of age.[1] Older children and adolescents with mental retardation or psychiatric disturbances may swallow virtually anything. These patients present the clinician with the unique challenge of deciding on the appropriate application of expectant management, endoscopy, or surgery.

Since the management of foreign bodies is based on collected experience, not on controlled studies, each case must be approached on an individual basis. The type of foreign object, its location in the gastrointestinal tract, and whether the patient is symptomatic are all important variables in the application of treatment guidelines. Table 13–1 lists the more commonly swallowed objects. Of all foreign bodies that reach the stomach, 80 to 90% will pass spontaneously, 10 to 20% will require endoscopic removal, and 1% will require surgery.[2] Objects that may not pass include those with a diameter of more than 20 mm or those that are more than 5 cm in length (Fig. 13–1).[3, 4] Because of the risk of perforation, sharp objects, such as chicken or fish bones, long pins, and toothpicks, should be removed endoscopically rather than allowed to pass spontaneously.[5]

Infants and children most often ingest coins, buttons, batteries, and toys, whereas adults experience more problems with bones and meat. The possibility of a second foreign body should always be considered when one is known to have been ingested. Recurrent ingestion is not uncommon, particularly among the mentally retarded or adolescents with psychiatric disorders. Over time, a total of 2,533 objects was retrieved from the stomach of one patient![6]

Table 13–1. FOREIGN BODIES COMMONLY INGESTED BY INFANTS, CHILDREN, AND ADOLESCENTS

Coins	Glass fragments
Disk (button) batteries	Pop tabs
Straight pins	Broken dental retainers
Hat pins	Ballpoint pen tops
Chicken or fish bones	Keys
Toothpicks	Marbles
Screws	Crayons
Nails	Silverware
Thumbtacks	Erasers
Safety pins	Bottle caps
Razor blades	Seashells
Meat	

SPECIFIC TYPES OF FOREIGN BODIES

Coins

Coins are the most frequently swallowed foreign objects and account for the majority of esophageal foreign bodies in children. More than 2,800 cases were reported by the American Association of Poison Control Centers Database in 1987.[7] Half of the patients were younger than 2 years of age, and 29% were younger than 1 year of age.[8] Coins lodged in the esophagus may not produce symptoms. Hodge and associates[9] reviewed radiographs from 80 children with a history of having swallowed a coin. In 25 (31%) the coin was stuck in the esophagus. Eleven of the patients (44%) were asymptomatic. Schunk and colleagues reported a similar experience in 52 patients.[10] In this series the coin was found in the esophagus in 30 (58%), 9 of which (30%) were asymptomatic. The authors of both studies concluded that all children who swallow coins should undergo prompt roentgenographic evaluation. Although this recommendation seems prudent, it is not without controversy.[11, 12] In the esophagus the flat surface of the coin will be seen on an anteroposterior view and the edge will be seen in a lateral view (Fig. 13–2). The opposite is true for coins in the trachea: The anteroposterior view reveals the edge, and the lateral view the flat surface.

Esophageal foreign bodies, whether symptomatic or not, should be removed. In the symptomatic patient this needs to be done as soon as possible. In the asymptomatic patient a temporizing approach should be taken. Experience dictates that the foreign body will usually pass into the stomach within 24 hours, either spontaneously or following the ingestion of liquids.[9–12] When

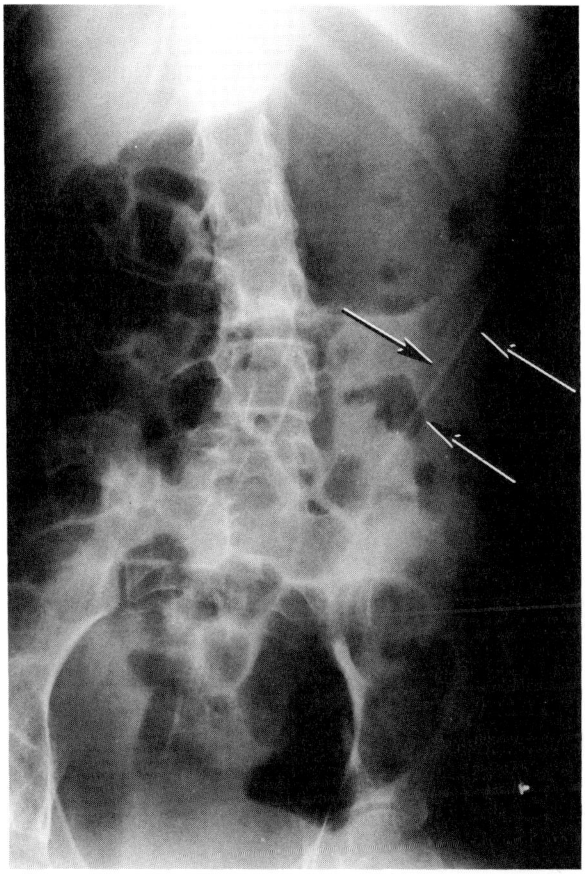

Figure 13–1. This 13-year-old girl was being followed for scoliosis. An abdominal film showed a long thin foreign body in the descending colon (*arrows*). The patient admitted to having swallowed a pencil several weeks before.

passage does not occur, the child is at risk for complications such as esophageal perforation,[13] tracheoesophageal fistula,[14] and esophagoaortic fistula.[15] These severe complications occurred after 4 months,[13] 8 years,[14] and 1 week,[15] respectively. Chaikhouni and coworkers,[16] in a review of 88 patients with esophageal foreign bodies, found that the only consistent risk factor for a major complication was the presence of the coin in the esophagus for more than 24 hours. From Schunk and associates' series,[10] two asymptomatic patients had coins removed after impactions of five days. Mucosal erosion was present in one case, and in the other the coin was embedded in the mucosa. The type of coin may be important. The new zinc penny (97.6% zinc, 2.4% copper), which replaced the copper penny (95% copper, 5% zinc) in 1982, is more corrosive in the esophagus. Although 24 hours appears to be a safe waiting period, if the coin has not passed into the stomach by then, it should be removed. A number of techniques may be employed. There are advocates for the use of rigid endoscopy,[17] flexible endoscopy,[18, 19] Foley catheters,[9, 10, 20] and bougie dilator advancement.[21] Which technique is best is controversial.

As a general rule, coins 20 mm or less in diameter in the stomach may be expected to pass spontaneously through the gastrointestinal tract. The diameters of U.S. coins are pennies, 18 mm; nickels, 21 mm; dimes, 17 mm; quarters, 24 mm; half-dollars, 30 mm; and dollars, 26 and 38 mm. Once it has been determined that the coin is in the stomach, the parents should be instructed to examine the stools for passage of the coin. Unless symptoms of gastric outlet obstruction occur (i.e., abdominal pain or vomiting, or both), endoscopic removal should be delayed. If the parents do not report passage of the coin, an abdominal film should be taken 1 week after ingestion. Subsequent films taken every 7 to 10 days may be used to monitor passage of the coin. If after 4 weeks the coin remains in the stomach, it should be removed endoscopically.

Disk (Button) Batteries

Over the last decade, disk batteries used in hearing aids, watches, calculators, cameras, and toys have become an important cause of caustic esophageal injury in infants and children.[24–28] Extrapolations from data reported to the National Poison Center Network for 1980 indicate that between 510 and 850 disk battery ingestions occur every year in the United States.[29] However, prior to 1982, only six cases had been reported in the medical literature. Two of the children died,[30, 31] and two suffered serious morbidity.[32, 33] Because of the magnitude and potential serious consequences of the problem, the National Button Battery Ingestion Study was started in 1982 to review characteristics of ingestions and provide guidelines for therapy (24-hour emergency hotline: 202-625-3333). Litovitz initially reported 119 button battery ingestions occurring over an 11-month period.[28] Seventy-

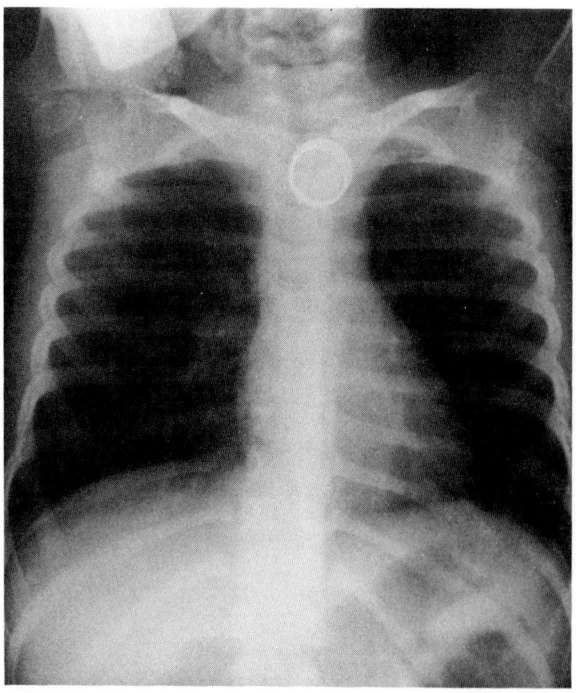

Figure 13–2. Anteroposterior (AP) view of the chest showing a bottle cap lodged in the cervical esophagus. The flat surface, as with coins, is present on the AP view.

one percent of the patients were younger than 5 years of age. Forty-eight percent of the ingested batteries were either loose or had been discarded, 34.4% were in the product, and 3.4% were in the manufacturer's packaging. The prevalence of ingested batteries that had been left out underscores the need for parental and public education regarding the prompt disposal or safe storage of these items out of the sight and reach of children. Hearing-aid batteries were the most common type swallowed (33.9%). Of interest was the fact that of the 18 swallowed hearing-aid batteries, 14 were swallowed by hearing-impaired children who had removed the batteries from their own hearing aids. A recent update of the registry analyzing 2,382 cases of cylindrical and button battery ingestion reported similar trends.[28a]

Disk batteries are composed of four systems: (1) the mercuric oxide system with mercuric oxide cathode and zinc anode; (2) the silver oxide system with a silver oxide cathode and zinc anode; (3) a manganese oxide system with a manganese dioxide cathode and zinc anode; and (4) a lithium system. All four systems contain a 20 to 45% solution of either potassium or sodium hydroxide. Batteries cause tissue injury by any one or a combination of the following mechanisms: pressure necrosis, low-voltage burns, or corrosive injury due to liquefaction necrosis induced by leakage of the alkaline solution. Mercury toxicity is more of a theoretical concern. In contrast to mercuric oxide, elemental mercury is readily absorbed. Elemental mercury is produced when mercuric oxide is reduced in the presence of gastric acid and iron from the corroding steel casing of the battery. To date, only one case of mild mercury poisoning has been documented.[34] Ninety percent of all disk batteries will pass spontaneously through the gastrointestinal tract.[28] Eighty-five percent of these will do so within 72 hours.

Management of a disk battery ingestion depends on its location. The child should be given nothing by mouth. Emetics have not been helpful and are not indicated.[24, 28] Urgent roentgenographic examination visualizing the gut from mouth to anus must be performed. When the object is lodged in the esophagus, the radiologist should be able to distinguish between a disk battery and a coin.[35] In the anteroposterior projection, disk batteries demonstrate a double-density shadow due to the bilaminar structure of the battery. On lateral view, the edges of most disk batteries are round and present a step-off at the junction of the anode and cathode. Disk batteries lodged in the esophagus demand urgent removal. Contact time of as little as 1 hour may result in mucosal injury, and within 4 hours all layers of the esophagus may be involved. Endoscopic retrieval under general anesthesia using a polyp snare, a Dormer basket, or a through-the-endoscope balloon is the procedure of choice. Advantages over the Foley catheter technique include the ability to access directly the esophageal mucosa and the avoidance of aspiration into the respiratory tree during withdrawal. The presence of significant tissue damage warrants a follow-up barium study in 10 to 14 days to rule out stricture formation or a fistula.

Once the battery is in the stomach, a more conservative course may be taken. All but the largest batteries (i.e., those greater than 20 mm in diameter) should pass. Cathartics, such as magnesium sulfate or magnesium citrate, or a prokinetic agent, such as metoclopramide, may be given to hasten transit time. Although of no proven efficacy, antacids or histamine H_2 blockers may be given to reduce acid secretion and thereby theoretically reduce the risk of mercury poisoning. Antiemetics should be avoided, since regurgitation of the battery from the stomach into the esophagus necessitating emergent endoscopy for removal has been reported.[28a] The child may be followed as an outpatient, and the parents should be instructed to strain the stools. If after 48 hours the battery has not passed, a repeat abdominal film should be taken. Continued presence of the battery in the stomach or the presence of abdominal symptoms necessitates endoscopic removal. Although the battery may temporarily "hang up" in the ileum, cecum, or ascending colon, there has been only one reported complication involving the intestine. In this patient the disk battery lodged in a Meckel's diverticulum and resulted in a fatal perforation.[33] Abdominal films should be repeated until the battery's elimination can be documented. Surgical removal becomes necessary when the battery fails to move over a period of 5 days or the patient develops symptoms of abdominal pain or peritoneal irritation.

Sharp or Elongated Foreign Bodies

Sharp or pointed foreign bodies, as well as elongated foreign bodies, can sometimes be difficult to manage (Fig. 13–3). As a group, sharp or pointed objects carry a higher risk for significant morbidity.[36–39] Fifteen to 35% of perforations from foreign body ingestion are due to sharp or pointed objects. Perforations are particularly likely to occur in the C loop of the duodenum, at the ligament of Trietz, in the terminal ileum or ileocecal region, and in the sigmoid colon. Certain objects such as bones, long straight pins, and toothpicks carry a significantly higher risk.[40, 41] As a general guideline, in adolescents or older children, an object longer than 5 cm or wider than 2 cm is not likely to pass. For infants and young children, the limit is 3 cm in length. High-risk objects or those exceeding these dimensions require urgent endoscopic removal from the stomach or proximal duodenum. Small nails, screws, pins, and thumbtacks may be managed conservatively.

Animal studies have shown that the bowel dilates locally in response to mucosal contact with a sharp object.[42] This reflex relaxation of the muscle wall, combined with axial flow in the lumen, tends to turn sharp objects around, preventing perforation. When possible, a high-roughage diet should be started. Serial abdominal films should be obtained at 4- to 5-day intervals. If a pin or other sharp object stays in place for 5 days or more or the patient develops abdominal symptoms, it is quite likely that the object has penetrated the bowel wall or is lodged in a Meckel's diverticulum or the appendix.[43] Surgical intervention is then necessary.

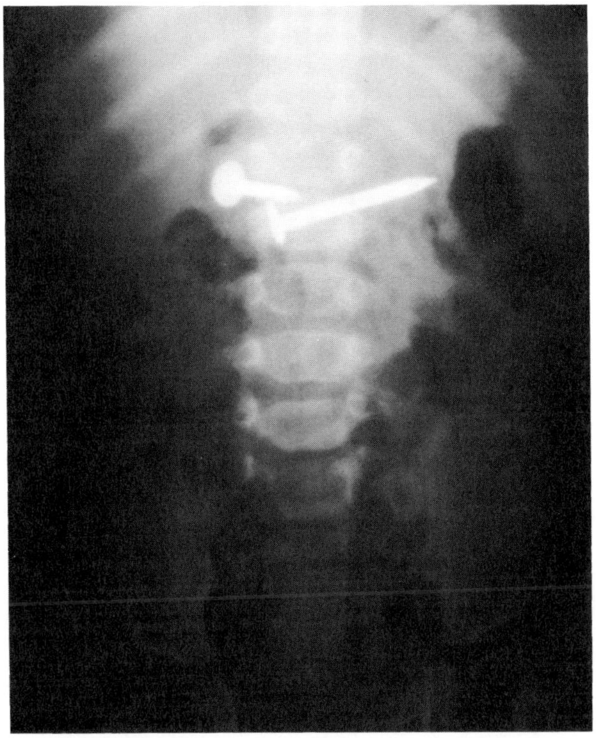

Figure 13–3. Plain radiograph of the abdomen shows two nails in the stomach of a 15-month-old infant. These were removed endoscopically.

Open safety pins present a major problem. If lodged in the esophagus with the open end proximal and the spring distal, the patient should undergo endoscopy; the pin should be carefully pushed into the stomach and then retrieved using an overtube. When the orientation is reversed, the pin should be grasped, pulled into an overtube, and withdrawn. Closed safety pins, once in the stomach, will pass and require only careful follow-up.

Razor blades in the esophagus may be removed either through the rigid esophagoscope or with a large endoscope using an overtube. Although once in the stomach, razor blades may pass, they should be removed endoscopically.

Meat

Meat impaction in the esophagus is uncommon in children. When this occurs it is usually secondary to an esophageal abnormality such as a stricture or motility disorder.[44] Hot dogs and meat are the most common offenders and usually lodge in the distal esophagus.[45] Management depends on the symptoms. If the child is having difficulty handling secretions, an urgent endoscopy for removal should be done. Because of the high risk of stricture, the object should not be pushed into the stomach unless it is known that there is no distal pathology. If there are no problems with handling secretions, endoscopy may be delayed for 12 hours. Unless the object passes, further postponement is unwise because of the increasing risk of complications.[16] Sedation or glucagon, or both, may be helpful in facilitating passage.[46–48]

Glucagon is particularly effective with objects in the distal one third of the esophagus because of its ability to decrease lower esophageal sphincter pressure.[48] Disruption of a meat impaction with papain (Adolph's Meat Tenderizer) is thought to be effective, but its use cannot be recommended.[49, 50] It is debatable whether enzymatic digestion of the meat actually occurs, and injury to the esophageal wall is a potential risk. Two deaths from perforation have been attributed to the administration of this agent.[51] Once the meat passes, an esophagram or an upper endoscopy should be done to exclude esophageal pathology.

Radiolucent Foreign Bodies

Glass, plastic, wood, and aluminum can pop tabs may be difficult to see on routine radiographs, particularly if the object is lodged in the hypopharynx or cervical esophagus. Thin barium may be used to try to outline the object (Fig. 13–4). If it is identified in the esophagus, it should be removed endoscopically. Endoscopy is also indicated if the patient is symptomatic. Failure to identify the object in an asymptomatic patient or the presence of the object in the stomach warrants only careful follow-up by the parents for its passage in the stool.

TECHNICAL ASPECTS OF FOREIGN BODY MANAGEMENT

The technique used to remove a foreign body depends on its type, its location in the gastrointestinal tract, and the age of the patient. Objects may hang up anywhere, increasing the risk of perforation. Common sites are areas of angulation or narrowing of the lumen (Fig. 13–5). Before any foreign body is extracted, the object should be duplicated, the procedure carefully preplanned, and a dry run carried out. A number of devices are available to grasp the object (Fig. 13–6). Which device to use is an individual preference. Coins are best retrieved with a basket, polyp snare, or rat-tooth jaw if the rim is present. Screws, pins, nails, and other long objects may be grasped with the alligator jaws or rubber-tipped jaws. The rat-tooth jaws are useful for removing food from the esophagus. Large objects or those with no edges, such as marbles or seeds, are best trapped in the basket. Remember Jackson's axiom when removing sharp or pointed objects: "Advancing points puncture, trailing do not."[52] Regardless of whether the procedure is done under conscious sedation or general anesthesia, a Kelly or McGill forceps and laryngoscope must be available in case the object is lost in the hypopharynx. The need for surgical removal of a foreign body is sometimes necessary and should not cloud good clinical judgment or be considered a personal defeat.

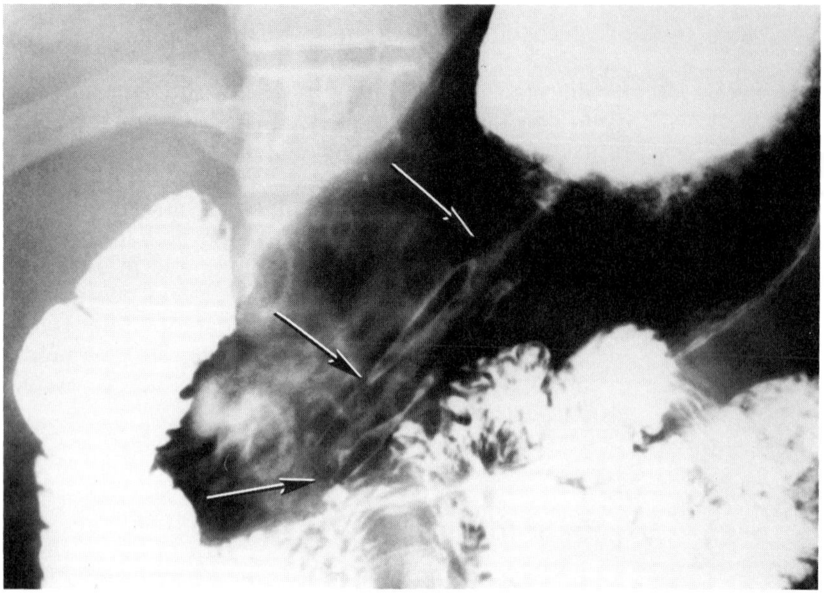

Figure 13–4. Contrast study outlining the handle (*arrows*) of a plastic fork in the stomach.

Esophagus

Most esophageal foreign bodies lodge at one of three primary sites: the level of the cricopharyngeal muscle, the level of the aortic arch, or the gastroesophageal junction. It also must be kept in mind that pathologic narrowing may be responsible for an object's failure to progress. Coins lodged in the esophagus may be given up to 24 hours to pass, but disk button batteries require urgent removal. Sharp objects may cause penetrating esophageal injury and should be removed immediately.

Clinical Manifestations. Although most patients present with symptoms of chest pain and salivation, some are asymptomatic. Therefore, the history of an ingestion must be taken seriously. Patients may initially choke or cough, which is followed by gagging in an effort to

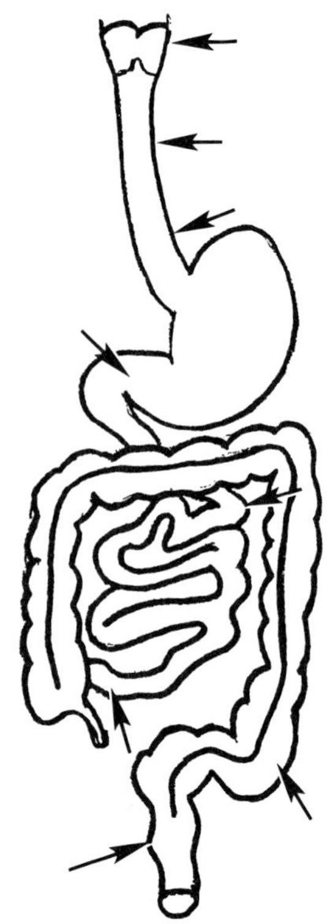

Figure 13–5. Sites (*arrows*) in the gastrointestinal tract where foreign bodies may arrest after ingestion.

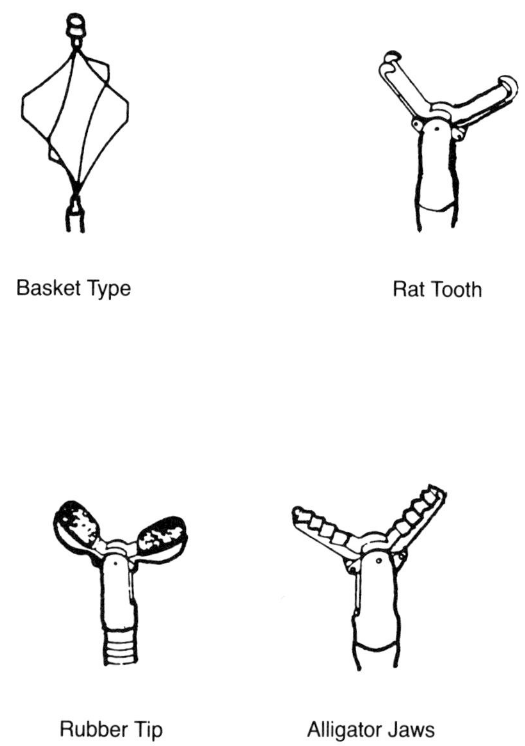

Figure 13–6. Devices available for the removal of foreign bodies. *A,* Basket for trapping coins, marbles, and other rounded objects. *B,* Rat-tooth jaws for grasping food and other soft materials. *C,* Alligator jaws and rubber-tipped jaws for grasping screws, nails, and pins.

regurgitate the object. Pain may be perceived at the level of the obstruction or referred to the sternal notch. It may be quite severe, and the patient may be in considerable distress.

Diagnosis. The history of a foreign body ingestion warrants radiographic examination from the mouth to the anus. Plain anteroposterior views of the neck, chest, and abdomen, as well as lateral views of the neck and chest, should be done. Failure to visualize the object does not preclude its presence. Objects such as plastic, wood, aluminum, glass, and bones are radiolucent and will be difficult to detect. In the symptomatic patient, failure to visualize the object warrants urgent endoscopy. Contrast radiography may be useful in the asymptomatic patient (see Fig. 13–4). Barium-coated cotton pledgets should not be used because they add another foreign body and may make subsequent endoscopic examination and retrieval more difficult.

Management. With the exception of coins, all esophageal foreign bodies should be removed under direct vision. This allows evaluation of the mucosa for underlying pathology prior to the object's extraction. Coins may be removed using a Foley catheter.[20] The procedure is relatively simple, but should be attempted only by experienced personnel. It is done under fluoroscopy after the patient has been immobilized on a papoose board or wrapped securely in a sheet. A Foley catheter is passed orally. Once the tip of the catheter passes beyond the foreign body, the balloon is inflated with contrast material. The patient is then placed into a prone oblique position, and the fluoroscopic table is turned into a head-down position. Then, applying a steady traction, the Foley catheter is withdrawn, its balloon pulling the foreign body ahead of it. Once out of the esophagus, aided by gravity, the object should fall out of the mouth. However, a laryngoscope and forceps must be available. If the object cannot be dislodged with steady traction, intravenous glucagon, 0.05 mg per kg, may be given in an effort to induce sufficient esophageal relaxation to permit successful extraction. Failure after glucagon warrants endoscopic intervention. The Foley catheter technique should not be used to remove disk button batteries.

Endoscopic retrieval of any foreign object requires careful preplanning and adequate sedation. Consideration should be given to using general anesthesia. If the object is in the cervical esophagus, or its exact location is unknown, insertion of the endoscope should be done under direct vision. Prior to removal of the object, the esophageal mucosa should be carefully inspected for signs of injury. Foreign bodies should never be extracted forcibly. Adequate insufflation of air to distend the esophagus, parenteral glucagon to induce relaxation, and orientation of the object into the frontal plane will facilitate successful removal. Trauma to the esophagus from sharp objects may be avoided by using an overtube (Fig. 13–7). The overtube is placed over the endoscope prior to beginning the procedure. Once the endoscope is in the esophagus, the overtube is introduced using the endoscope as a guide. After the object has been securely grasped, it is pulled back into the overtube, and the entire assembly is removed together. Open safety pins,

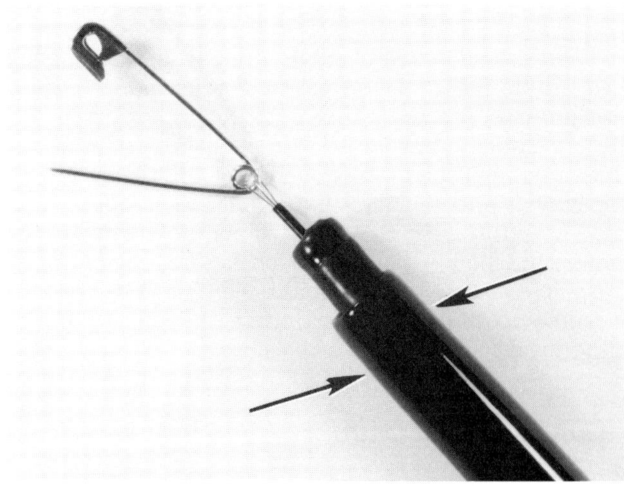

Figure 13–7. Sharp objects should be securely grasped and pulled into the overtube *(arrows),* which has been passed over the endoscope. The entire apparatus is then withdrawn.

with the spring end oriented distally, should be carefully pushed into the stomach, turned, grasped securely with the spring end oriented proximally, and removed using the overtube. An overtube is also useful to avoid repetitive intubations during the piecemeal removal of a food bolus. Severe mucosal disruption and bleeding, or the presence of chest pain following the procedure, suggests esophageal perforation. A contrast study of the esophagus should be done.

Stomach and Duodenum

Objects may fail to pass through the pylorus, or become lodged there or in the duodenal sweep. For coins, disk batteries, and other blunt objects, observation is appropriate, since those less than 20 mm in diameter will likely pass through the pylorus and subsequently through the entire digestive tract. Failure of a disk battery to pass within 48 hours warrants removal of the object. Four weeks may be allowed for coins. Sharp objects greater than 5 cm in length should be removed endoscopically because of the risk of perforation.

Clinical Manifestations. Most patients will be asymptomatic. Vomiting and pain suggest pyloric obstruction; if coupled with fever and peritoneal signs, they suggest perforation. Duodenal perforation from a sharp object such as a pin or toothpick may produce only minimal symptoms. The diagnosis requires a high index of suspicion.

Diagnosis. Metal objects will be seen on plain films of the abdomen. However, radiopaque materials, such as plastic, wood, or aluminum, may require a contrast study to document their location and whether or not perforation has occurred.

Management. Most objects that pass through the pylorus will pass safely through the intestine. Exceptions include chicken or fish bones; pins, needles, or other long thin objects longer than 5 cm; and razor blades.

These objects carry a higher risk for intestinal perforation and should be removed promptly from the stomach. Endoscopic retrieval of a gastric foreign body requires planning and practice with the correct accessory before the procedure is begun. Just prior to the procedure, an abdominal film should be done to be sure the object has not moved into the intestine. Retrieval is often facilitated by positioning the object along the greater curvature in the body of the stomach before attempting to grasp it. Sharp objects should be removed using an overtube to prevent trauma to the esophagus during withdrawal.

Colon and Rectum

Children will occasionally place objects in the rectum. Small blunt objects will pass spontaneously. Large or sharp objects require retrieval. This can be done through a sigmoidoscope or by using a vaginal speculum and Kocher clamp. Adequate sedation with local or general anesthesia is essential to relax the anal sphincter. A long foreign object should be oriented in the vertical plane before attempting to remove it. If the object is beyond the reach of the sigmoidoscope, observation for 12 to 24 hours will allow the object to descend. The other alternative is to use an upper endoscope, a retrieval forceps, and an overtube. After removal of the object, the sigmoidoscopy should be repeated to look for mucosal injury.[53]

BEZOARS

Bezoars are a rare and unique form of gastrointestinal foreign body that have held a certain mystic fascination through the ages.[54] The term *bezoar* is derived from the Arabic *badzehr* or the Persian *padzahr*, both of which mean antidote to poison. From antiquity until the late eighteenth century, a bezoar from an animal's stomach was highly revered because of its magical powers. Taken internally, it neutralized poisons, destroyed venoms, and counteracted attacks of epilepsy, dysentery, plague, and leprosy. Worn as a charm, it provided protection from evil spirits. Today the term *bezoar* refers to the accumulation of exogenous matter in the stomach and small intestine.

In an early extensive review of bezoars, DeBakey and Ochsner noted that 90% of all patients were female, and that the peak age group was between 10 and 19 years.[54] Bezoars are classified on the basis of their composition. Trichobezoars are composed primarily of the patient's own hair. Trichotillomania with trichophagia may result in bezoar formation and is indicative of a personality disorder. McGehee and Buchanan,[55] reporting on two children with trichobezoars and iron deficiency, suggested that trichophagia was a form of pica. Other sources of the fibers for bezoar formation include carpets, blankets, animal hair, or doll's hair. Trichobezoars may become quite large and can form a cast of the stomach if they have been present for many years A "tail" may extend from the gastric portion of the bezoar into the small intestine, resulting in obstructive jaundice[56] and pancreatitis.[57] Protein-losing gastroenteropathy and steatorrhea have been reported in association with trichobezoars.[58, 59] In one report,[59] the microscopic appearance of the gastric mucosa showed hyperplasia similar to that seen with chronic hypertrophic gastritis, which was suggested as the etiology of the protein loss.

Phytobezoars are composed of a heterogeneity of plant and vegetable material. Among adults this is the most common form of bezoar. In DeBakey and Ochsner's review of bezoars,[54] 92 of 126 (73%) phytobezoars were due to the ingestion of persimmons. Persimmon bezoar (diospyrobezoar) occurs following the ingestion of large amounts of the unripe fruit. The pulp, which contains phlobatannin, coagulates in the stomach on contact with acid.[60] Fortunately, persimmons are not a favorite of children because of their tart taste. Other substances that may form phytobezoars when ingested in excessive amounts include celery, pumpkin, grape skins, prunes, raisins, leeks, wild beets, and grass. Hypochlorhydria, decreased antral motility, and poor chewing of food are predisposing factors in phytobezoar formation. They have been described in patients with muscular dystrophy,[61] diabetic gastroparesis,[62] and H_2 receptor antagonist use.[63]

Although initially described in full-term infants, most lactobezoars are found in premature low-birth-weight infants.[64, 65] Early reports hypothesized that lactobezoars were due to improperly prepared hypertonic formulas or to dehydration. In the early 1980s there was an apparent increase in the incidence of lactobezoars in low-birth-weight infants, which now seems to have waned. This rise in the number of cases was attributed to specialized premature formulas and, in particular, to their high casein content. Schreiner and coworkers[66] found no lactobezoars during a 14-month period in 223 infants weighing less than 2,000 gm who were fed whey-predominant formulas, whereas they found a 6.6% incidence in a similar group fed casein-predominant formulas. However, Ross Laboratories, a major manufacturer of casein-predominant formulas, used its market share and Schreiner and coworkers' 6.6% incidence figure and concluded that 1,300 cases should occur yearly if casein is solely responsible.[67] This expected number of cases far exceeded the actual number of reported cases. Further, lactobezoars have been reported in exclusively breast-fed infants.[68] Although the firmer curds formed by casein are important contributors, other factors are involved in lactobezoar formation, including (1) a trend to earlier and more rapid advancement of feedings in very small or very ill premature infants; (2) the use of high-caloric-density formulas; (3) the higher calcium and protein content of special premature formulas; (4) continuous drip feedings; and (5) the unique physiology of gastric secretion and gastric emptying in low-birth-weight infants.

Concretions of dehydrated antacid—antacid bezoars—may form in patients with poor gastric motility. Premature infants or patients in the intensive care unit on high-dose antacid therapy for acid peptic disease or for prophylaxis against stress-related bleeding are especially at risk.[69]

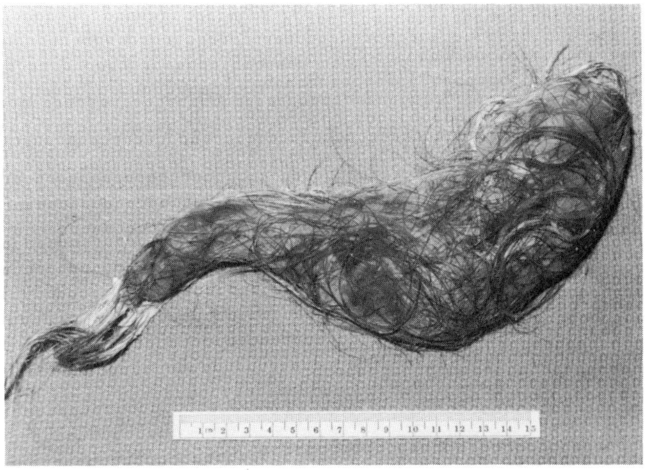

Figure 13–8. Trichobezoar removed surgically from the stomach of a 2½-year-old boy who presented with vomiting and failure to thrive.

Clinical Manifestations. Trichobezoars present with symptoms suggesting gastric outlet or intestinal obstruction, or both, including anorexia, vomiting, and weight loss. In 70% of cases there are complaints of abdominal pain, and abdominal distention is frequently noted.[54] Patchy baldness from hair pulling may be a useful clue.[55] Abdominal palpation usually reveals a firm mass in the left upper quadrant. Abdominal crepitus may also be noted. Frequently, severe halitosis is present owing to the putrefying material in the stomach. Laboratory evaluation may show iron-deficiency anemia, hypoproteinemia, or steatorrhea.

Phytobezoars present in a similar manner, although in only half of cases is a mass palpable. Peptic ulceration is also more common owing to phytobezoars' more abrasive nature.

Symptoms suggestive of the presence of a lactobezoar in a premature infant include abdominal distention, vomiting, and increasing gastric residual volumes. A mass may be palpable in the left upper quadrant. Some cases may be clinically silent, with the lactobezoar having been found incidentally on a radiographic study. Gastric perforation as a presenting manifestation has been described.[64, 70]

Diagnosis. Plain abdominal films frequently suggest the presence of a bezoar. An upper gastrointestinal series will show a movable mass within the barium field, and on a postevacuation film the mass is often outlined by a thin barium shell. Ultrasound has also been used to diagnose a bezoar. Endoscopy not only provides definitive evidence of the bezoar's presence as well as its type, but also may be a means of therapeutic dissolution.

Management. The treatment of trichobezoars is surgical—there is no way to dissolve the matted hair, and their large size makes endoscopic disruption or removal impossible (Fig. 13–8). Some phytobezoars may be physically disrupted or dissolved. Therefore, a trial of medical therapy is warranted before gastrotomy is performed. Techniques include a clear liquid lavage plus metoclopramide[71] and endoscopic fragmentation with a biopsy forceps or polyp snare.[72] Madsen and associates[73] reported the successful use of a Teledyne Water Pik (Fort Collins, CO) in five patients. Dissolving phytobezoars with papain[74] or acetylcysteine[75] has been reported, but using the enzyme cellulase has met with the most success.[76, 77] Lactobezoars are treated by withholding feedings for 48 hours and maintaining hydration with intravenous fluids. Resolution is usually prompt, and endoscopic disruption is rarely necessary.

REFERENCES

1. Alexander W, Kadish JA, Dunbar JS: Ingested foreign bodies in children. *In* Kaufmann HJ, eds: Progress in Pediatric Radiology. 2nd ed. Chicago, Year Book Medical Publishers, 1969, pp 256–285.
2. Schwartz GF, Polsky HS: Ingested foreign bodies of the gastrointestinal tract. Am Surg 1985; 51:173–179.
3. Waye JD: Removal of foreign bodies from the upper intestinal tract with fiberoptic instruments. Am J Gastroenterol 1976; 65:557–560.
4. Koch H: Operative endoscopy. Gastrointest Endosc 1977; 24:65–68.
5. Maliki M, Evans WE: Foreign body perforation of the intestinal tract. Arch Surg 1970; 101:475–482.
6. Chalk SG, Faucer H: Foreign bodies in the stomach. Arch Surg 1928; 16:494–500.
7. Litovitz TL, Schmitz BF, Matyumas N, et al: 1987 annual report of the American Association of Poison Control Centers National Data Collection System. Am J Emerg Med 1988; 6:479–515.
8. Jackson RM, Hawkins DB: Coins in the esophagus. What is the best management? Int J Pediatr Otorhinolaryngol 1986; 12:127–135.
9. Hodge D, Tecklenburg F, Fleisher G: Coin ingestion: Does every child need a radiograph? Ann Emerg Med 1985; 14:443–446.
10. Schunk JE, Cornele H, Bolte R: Pediatric coin ingestions. Am J Dis Child 1989; 143:546–548.
11. Caravati EM, Bennett DL, McElwee NE: Pediatric coin ingestion. Am J Dis Child 1989; 143:549–551.
12. Fulginiti VA: Is standard practice in pediatrics "standard"? A potential lesson for experts and practitioners. Am J Dis Child 1989; 143:529–530.
13. Nahmah BJ, Mueller C: Asymptomatic esophageal perforation by a coin in a child. Ann Emerg Med 1984; 13:627–629.
14. Obiako MN: Tracheoesophageal fistula: A complication of foreign body. Ann Otol Rhinol Laryngol 1982; 91:325–327.
15. Vella EE, Booth PJ: Foreign body in the esophagus. Br Med J 1965; 2:1042.
16. Chaikhouni A, Kratz JM, Crawford FA: Foreign bodies of the esophagus. Ann Surg 1985; 51:173–179.
17. Gracia C, Frey CF, Balaz IB: Diagnosis and management of ingested foreign bodies: A ten-year experience. Ann Emerg Med 1984; 13:30–34.
18. Christie DL, Ament ME: Removal of foreign bodies from esophagus and stomach with flexible fiberoptic panendoscopes. Pediatrics 1976; 57:931–936.
19. Bendig DW: Removal of blunt esophageal foreign bodies by flexible endoscopy without general anesthesia. Am J Dis Child 1986; 140:789–790.
20. Campbell JB, Quattromani FL, Foley LC: Foley catheter removal of blunt esophageal foreign bodies: Experience with 100 consecutive children. Pediatr Radiol 1983; 13:116–119.
21. Bonadio WA, Jona JZ, Glicklich M, et al: Esophageal bougienage technique for coin ingestion in children. J Pediatr Surg 1988; 23:917–918.
22. Euler AR: How long should a foreign body stay in the stomach? Pediatrics 1978; 61:671.
23. Ghazi A, Tan S, Wolff WI: Pediatric fiberoptic instruments—application in removal of foreign body in children's stomachs. NY State J Med 1979; 79:384–386.

24. Litovitz TL: Button battery ingestions: A review of 56 cases. JAMA 1983; 249:2495–2500.
25. Temple DM, McNeese MC: Hazards of battery ingestion. Pediatrics 1983; 71:100–103.
26. Vottler TP, Nash JC, Rudledge JC: The hazard of ingested alkaline disk batteries in children. JAMA 1983; 249:2504–2506.
27. Maves MD, Carithers JS, Birck KG: Esophageal burns secondary to disk battery ingestion. Ann Otol Rhinol Laryngol 1984; 93:364–369.
28. Litovitz TL: Battery ingestions: Product accessibility and clinical course. Pediatrics 1985; 75:469–476.
28a. Litovitz TL, Schmitz BF: Ingestion of cylindrical and button batteries: An analysis of 2382 cases. Pediatrics 1992; 89:747–757.
29. National Poison Center Network Computer System for Documenting Data in Poison Exposures. Pittsburgh, 1981.
30. Blatnik BS, Toohill RJ, Lehman RH: Fatal complications from an alkaline battery foreign body in the esophagus. Ann Otol 1977; 86:611–615.
31. Shabino CL, Feinberg AN: Esophageal perforation secondary to alkaline battery ingestion. JACEP 1979; 8:360–362.
32. Votteler TP: Warning: Ingested disk batteries. Tex Med J 1981; 77:7.
33. Willis GA, Ho WC: Perforation of Meckel's diverticulum by an alkaline hearing aid battery. Can Med Assoc J 1982; 126:497–498.
34. Kulig K, Rumack CM, Rumack BH, et al: Disk battery ingestion: Elevated urine mercury levels and enema removal of battery fragments. JAMA 1983; 249: 2502–2504.
35. Maves MD, Lloyd TV, Carithers JS: Radiographic identification of ingested disk batteries. Pediatr Radiol 1986; 16:154–156.
36. Abel RM, Fischer JE, Henderson HH: Penetration of the alimentary tract by a foreign body with migration to the liver. Arch Surg 1971; 102:227–229.
37. Grosfeld JL, Eng K: Right iliac artery–duodenal fistula in infancy due to a "whisk-broom" bristle perforation. Ann Surg 1972; 176:761–762.
38. Rosch W, Classen M: Fiberendoscopic foreign body removal from the upper gastrointestinal tract. Endoscopy 1972; 4:193–197.
39. Esposito G: Left empyema and pneumothorax after perforation of the stomach, diaphragm, and pleura by an intragastric foreign body. Ann Chir Infant 1973; 14:413–416.
40. Maleki M, Evan WE: Foreign body perforation of the intestinal tract. Arch Surg 1970; 101:475–477.
41. Schwartz JT, Graham DY: Toothpick perforation of the intestines. Ann Surg 1977; 185:64–66.
42. Carp L: Foreign bodies in the intestine. Ann Surg 1927; 85:575–585.
43. Kassner EG, Mutchler RW, Klotz DH, et al: Uncomplicated foreign bodies of appendix in children: Radiologic observations. J Pediatr Surg 1974; 9:207–209.
44. Buchin PJ: Foreign bodies of the esophagus. NY State J Med 1981; 81:1057–1059.
45. Vizcarrondo FJ, Brady PG, Nord H: Foreign bodies of the upper gastrointestinal tract. Gastrointest Endosc 1983; 29:208–210.
46. Ferrucci JR, Long JA: Radiologic treatment of esophageal food impaction using intravenous glucagon. Radiology 1977; 127:25–28.
47. Trenkner SW, Maglinte DT, Lehman G, et al: Esophageal food impaction: Treatment with glucagon. Radiology 1983; 149:401–403.
48. Friedland GW: The treatment of acute esophageal food impaction. Radiology 1983; 149:601–602.
49. Andersen HA, Bernatz PE, Grindlay JH: Perforation of the esophagus after use of a digestive agent: Report of a case and experimental study. Ann Otol Rhinol Laryngol 1959; 68:890–896.
50. Holsinger JW, Frison RL, Sealy WC: Esophageal perforation following meat impaction and papain ingestion. JAMA 1968; 204:188–189.
51. Goldmer F, Danley D: Enzymatic digestion of esophageal meat impaction. Dig Dis Sci 1985; 30:546–550.
52. Jackson C, Jackson CL: Disease of the air and food passages of foreign body origin. Philadelphia, WB Saunders, 1937.
53. Barone JE, Sohn M, Nealon TF: Perforations and foreign bodies of the rectum: Report of 28 cases. Ann Surg 1976; 184:601–606.
54. DeBakey M, Ochsner A: Bezoars and concretions: Comprehensive review of the literature with an analysis of 303 collected cases and a presentation of 8 additional cases. Surgery 1938; 4:934–963; Surgery 1939; 5:132–160.
55. McGehee FT Jr, Buchanan GR: Trichophagia and trichobezoar: Etiologic role of iron deficiency. J Pediatr 1980; 97:946–948.
56. Schreiber H, Filston HC: Obstructive jaundice due to gastric trichobezoar. J Pediatr Surg 1976; 11:103–104.
57. Shawis RN, Doig CM: Gastric trichobezoar associated with transient pancreatitis. Arch Dis Child 1984; 59:994–995.
58. Hossenbocus A, Colin-Jones DG: Trichobezoar, gastric polyposis, protein-losing gastroenteropathy and steatorrhea. Gut 1973; 14:730–732.
59. Valberg LS, McCorriston JR, Partington MW: Bezoar: An unusual cause of protein-losing gastroenteropathy. Can Med Assoc J 1966; 94:388–391.
60. Izumi S, Isida K, Iwamoto M: Mechanism of formation of phytobezoars with special reference to persimmon ball. Jpn J Med Sci Trans II Biochem 1933; 2:21–33.
61. Kuiper D: Gastric bezoar in a patient with myotonic dystrophy. Am J Dis Child 1971; 16:529–531.
62. Brady P: Gastric phytobezoars consequent to delayed gastric emptying. Gastrointest Endosc 1978; 24:159–161.
63. Nichols T: Phytobezoar formation: A new complication of cimetidine therapy. Ann Intern Med 1981; 95:70–72.
64. Erenberg A, Shaw RD, Yousefzadeh D: Lactobezoar in the low-birth-weight infant. Pediatrics 1979; 63:642–646.
65. Schreiner RL, Brady MS, Franken EA: Increased incidence of lactobezoars in low birth weight infants. Am J Dis Child 1979; 133:936–940.
66. Schreiner RL, Brady MS, Ernst JA, et al: Lack of lactobezoars in infants given predominantly whey protein formulas. Am J Dis Child 1982; 136:437–439.
67. Kashyap S: Lactobezoar risk. Pediatrics 1988; 81:177–178.
68. Yoss BS: Human milk lactobezoars. J Pediatr 1984; 105:819–822.
69. Portugeuz-Malavasi A, Aranda JV: Antacid bezoars in a newborn. Pediatrics 1979; 63:679–680.
70. Levkoff AH, Gadsden RH, Hennigar GR: Lactobezoar and gastric perforation in a neonate. J Pediatr 1970; 77:875–877.
71. Delpre G, Glanz I, Neeman A: New therapeutic approach in postoperative phytobezoars. J Clin Gastroenterol 1984; 6:231–233.
72. Diettrich N, Gaw F: Postgastrectomy phytobezoars endoscopic diagnosis and treatment. Arch Surg 1985; 120:432–437.
73. Madsen R, Skibba R, Galvan A: Gastric bezoars. A technique of endoscopic removal. Dig Dis Sci 1978; 23:717–720.
74. Sparberg M, Nielsen A, Andruczak R: Bezoar following gastrostomy. Am J Dig Dis 1968; 13:579–581.
75. Schlang H: Acetylcysteine in removal of bezoar. JAMA 1970; 214: 1329.
76. Deal D, Vitale P, Raffin S: Dissolution of a postgastrectomy bezoar by cellulase. Gastroenterology 1973; 64:467–469.
77. Stanten A, Peters H: Enzymatic dissolution of phytobezoars. Am J Surg 1975; 130:259–261.

Chapter 14

Abdominal Pain

CATHERINE F. MEWS and FRANK R. SINATRA

INTRODUCTION

Abdominal pain is a common symptom in childhood and adolescence. Chronic abdominal pain is defined as the presence of at least three discrete episodes of pain occurring over a period of 3 or more months.[1] Chronic abdominal pain that interferes with normal daily activity or performance has a reported prevalence of 10 to 15% in school-aged children between the ages of 5 and 14 years, with a slightly increased prevalence in girls.[2–6] A recent epidemiologic study of abdominal pain in 6-year-old children conducted by Faull and associates[7] suggests that at least as many children suffer from chronic abdominal pain that does not affect daily activity and are thus rarely seen by physicians. In 90 to 95% of children with chronic abdominal pain, no organic cause for the pain is identified, and the children are considered to have a functional disorder affecting the gastrointestinal tract.[1, 8, 9]

Functional gastrointestinal disorders are a poorly understood group of conditions in which there is a physiologic variation from the normal in the absence of organic (structural, infectious, inflammatory, or biochemical) disease. Throughout the pediatric literature functional chronic abdominal pain is most frequently referred to by the term *recurrent abdominal pain* (RAP) of childhood.[1, 2, 4, 7, 9] Although often discussed as a homogeneous group of patients, children with functional chronic abdominal pain probably represent a heterogeneous group of disorders. The wide variety of descriptive terms applied to these patients' symptoms—*irritable bowel syndrome of childhood*,[10] *spastic colon of childhood*,[11] *nonorganic recurrent abdominal pain*,[12] *periodic syndrome*,[13] or *psychogenic recurrent abdominal pain*[14]—reflects both the heterogeneity of the group and our lack of understanding of the pathogenesis of the symptoms. It has been suggested that a disturbance in the regulation of gastrointestinal motility provoked by physical or psychological stress may be a major contributing factor in the development of functional RAP. Functional disorders of the gastrointestinal tract seen by the pediatrician may include such common problems as colic in the infant, chronic nonspecific diarrhea in the toddler, recurrent abdominal pain in the school-aged child, and classic adult-type irritable bowel syndrome in the adolescent (see Chapter 57).

PATHOPHYSIOLOGY

The etiology and pathogenesis of functional RAP are poorly understood; however, there is general agreement that *functional* is not synonymous with *imaginary* and that the child experiences pain that is abdominal in location. The origin of the pain is presumed to be from the nerve endings in the submucosa, musculature, and serosa of the abdominal organs.[15] It has been postulated that gastrointestinal tract distention or spasm leading to increased muscle tension may result in pain.[16] Studies using distensible balloons within the gastrointestinal tract have shown that the change in muscle tension rather than the specific amount of tension developed appears to be the stimulus for pain.[17] These studies have also helped us identify the site from which specific abdominal pain is elicited.[18] Periumbilical pain, for example, is thought to originate from the small bowel distal to the duodenojejunal angle and ascending, transverse, and descending colon. Distention of the esophagus, ileocecal area, hepatic flexure, and sigmoid colon may result in specific quadrant pain. Whether the pain in functional RAP is secondary to the same pathways as the pain produced by distention of balloons within the gastrointestinal tract has yet to be proven.

It was once thought that functional RAP was associated with a lowered threshold for pain[19]; however, recent direct testing[20] has not supported any abnormality in the response of these children to painful stimuli. A genetic vulnerability or environmental influence appears evident, as there is a high frequency of pain complaints in the family members of children suffering from functional RAP.[1, 21] Various psychological and physiologic factors that have been implicated as being mediators or moderators in functional RAP are listed in Table 14–1.[11, 22–28]

A number of studies have examined the relationship between stress and functional RAP. McGrath and coworkers,[29] in a study of children with functional RAP and pain-free control subjects, found no difference in life stress experienced by each group. In contrast, Greene and associates[23] were able to identify significantly higher stress in adolescents with nonorganic abdominal pain than in those being seen for routine health care. Similarly, Hodges and associates[30] found significant differences in stress-associated life events in children with functional RAP compared with children without

Table 14–1. POSSIBLE MEDIATORS AND MODERATORS OF FUNCTIONAL RECURRENT ABDOMINAL PAIN

Psychological	Physiologic
Stress factors	Autonomic instability
Operant conditioning	Lactose intolerance
Role modeling	Gut dysmotility
Depression	Constipation
Family enmeshment	Endogenous opiates
Somatization	

RAP. There appears to be an inconsistent correlation between functional RAP and life stress in children. It seems likely that perception of life stresses rather than the severity or frequency of stress may be different in children with functional RAP. Life stresses appear to assume greater significance in a child with functional RAP than in a healthy child.

Recently, it has been hypothesized that the pain in functional RAP may be mediated by an increase in endorphinergic activity in response to stressful stimuli.[28] Endogenous opiate peptides have been identified throughout the human digestive system,[31] and their spectrum of biologic action resembles that of the exogenous opiates that affect gastrointestinal motility, gastric emptying, intestinal transit, biliary pressure, and defecation.[32] Stanghellini and colleagues[33] found elevations in plasma levels of beta-endorphin and norepinephrine in association with gastroduodenal motor disturbances in subjects submitted to cold pain and or labyrinthine stimulation. Varni and colleagues,[34] after reviewing the literature on endorphins and stress, concluded that a primary trigger for the synthesis and secretion of endorphins is the physiologic and cognitive perception of stress.

Various studies designed to investigate the prevalence of psychological problems in children with functional RAP and abdominal pain of organic origin have been undertaken.[1, 10, 35] Raymer and coworkers[35] concluded that significant psychological distress frequently accompanies both organic and nonorganic abdominal pain; whether this is secondary to the underlying chronic pain, primary in nature, or a combination of the two is not readily apparent. Several authors have commented on the strong association of functional RAP with emotional problems and certain personality types. Stone and Barbero,[10] in a study of 102 children with RAP, found many of their patients to be insecure and sensitive. Apley[1] found a higher prevalence of anxious, timid, and apprehensive children among a group of 100 children with RAP when compared with a control group. Liebman,[36] studying a group of 119 children with RAP, described 30% of them as being perfectionistic. Such behavioral profiles may be primary, reflecting a genetic vulnerability; alternatively, they may represent a psychological adaptation to both organic and nonorganic pain. Other studies of children,[29, 35] however, support the body of adult literature, which has found it impossible to identify specific personality types associated with functional gastrointestinal complaints. No definitive study confirming the psychological etiology of functional RAP has yet been conducted. The psychological aspects of functional RAP deserve further study in well-designed prospective trials, which will allow personality characteristics and psychological factors before and after the development of functional RAP to be evaluated accurately. It seems clear, however, that psychological factors and family dynamics, whether primary or secondary to the pain, may influence how the pain is perceived and managed by the child and his or her family.

Various conceptual models have been developed to help the physician understand the pathogenesis of functional RAP. The best model appears to be one that depicts a complex interplay of genetic and environmental influences and physical and psychological stress that results in an alteration or imbalance in gastrointestinal motor activity causing abdominal pain. Examples of physical stress include recent viral infections, aerophagia, chronic constipation, and recent intake of medications. Psychological stresses include school phobia, separation anxiety, marital discord, poverty, death or illness of a family member, and geographic relocation.

Several studies have described altered intestinal motor activity in children with increased amplitude and duration of rectosigmoid pressure waves in response to the parasympathetic agonist neostigmine methylsulfate (Prostigmin) in 73.4% of patients with functional RAP versus 49.5% of control subjects.[37] The heightened rectosigmoid response to stimulation with neostigmine in the children with functional RAP suggests either an increased sensitivity of the colon to parasympathetic stimulation or a more generalized autonomic imbalance.[38] Kopel and colleagues' study,[37] however, lacked direct evidence linking the patients' abdominal pain to the alteration in gastrointestinal motility described. Dimson[11] described constipation and delayed intestinal transit of carmine (a red coloring matter) in children with functional RAP triggered by emotional factors. His data suggest that delayed transit is more likely in patients with tenderness over the left colon and in those children having rectal constipation. This study, however, lacked a control population. More recently, Pineiro-Carrero and associates described altered gastroduodenal motility patterns in adolescents with functional RAP.[39] The adolescents with functional RAP had more frequent migrating motor complexes (MMC), but they were shorter in duration and had slower propagation velocities. Pain coincided with episodes of high-pressure duodenal contractions. These contractions were not observed in the normal population. In this study there was no direct evidence connecting physical or psychological stress with disturbance in motor activity. In a more heterogeneous group of patients with functional gastrointestinal symptoms, Hyman and coworkers[40] found antroduodenal manometric abnormalities in 87% of the patients studied. Further adding to the evidence that functional gastrointestinal disorders are associated with disorders in intestinal motility, Fenton and colleagues demonstrated failure of disruption of the MMC by an intraduodenal bolus of 5% dextrose in children with toddler's diarrhea but not in the control group.[41] These studies suggest that functional disorders of the gastrointestinal tract may be associated with disturbances in gastrointestinal motility and that the clinical manifestations are related to the particular pattern of disturbance of intestinal motor activity.

Many patients with functional abdominal pain have associated "autonomic" symptoms, such as pallor, headache, dizziness, and nausea. Because the autonomic nervous system, particularly the parasympathetic component, modulates the sensory and motor responses of the intestine to internal and external stimuli, it has been speculated that in patients with functional RAP, dysfunction of the autonomic nervous system may result in alteration of intestinal motility and thereby produce pain.[37] Utilizing pupillometry as a method of studying autonomic function, Rubin and coworkers[42] described an abnormal pupillary response to cold stress characterized by a slower decrement in pupillary dilatation following the stress in patients with nonorganic abdominal pain compared with a control group.[42] Apley and coworkers could not duplicate this observation; however, they did report modification of normal pupillary reactions in children with nonorganic abdominal pain.[25] In a later study, Feuerstein and associates exposed children with nonorganic RAP and control subjects to a cold pressor stimulus and were unable to demonstrate a differential autonomic, somatic, subjective, or behavioral response between the groups.[20] These studies used a physical stimulus outside the gastrointestinal tract and used extraintestinal organs for the study of the autonomic nervous system's response to stress. Such studies cannot rule out the possibility of a differential gastrointestinal response to stress.

Malabsorption of carbohydrates, especially lactose, has been reported in the setting of functional RAP. Barr and colleagues[26] documented malabsorption on the basis of elevated end expiratory breath hydrogen levels in 40% of 80 children with RAP. They reported a qualitative improvement in pain symptoms in 70% of the lactose-malabsorber group when a lactose-free diet was provided and concluded that lactose intolerance was the cause of the pain in these patients. A subsequent study[43] reported similar prevalances of lactose malabsorption in a group of patients with RAP and in a group of age-matched patients with diarrhea but without pain. It would thus appear that malabsorption of lactose does not directly cause the pain but may result in an alteration in gastrointestinal function and subsequent abdominal pain in a susceptible group of patients. Differences in the symptoms among the group of lactose malabsorbers may be related to differences in the transit time through the small intestine, the amount of lactose unabsorbed, the rate of bacterial metabolism, the quantities of gas produced, and the absorption and catabolism of bacterial metabolites.[44–46]

The use of fiberoptic endoscopic examination of the gastrointestinal tract has become more widespread in the pediatric age group in the past 10 years. As is the practice in adults, pediatric endoscopists have commenced performing routine biopsies despite a normal macroscopic appearance. Pathologists often describe nonspecific inflammation in the biopsy samples. The significance of these inflammatory changes is uncertain, and whether the inflammation bears any relationship to the pathogenesis of recurrent abdominal pain in children needs to be determined. Nonspecific inflammation is often present in biopsy samples from patients with nonulcer dyspepsia. Controversy surrounds the role that this inflammation plays in the pathogenesis of this condition, since inflammatory changes also are commonly found in biopsies of asymptomatic adult patients.[47] Controlled trials using therapy with antacids and histamine H_2 antagonists in adults with nonulcer dyspepsia and nonspecific inflammation have shown these agents to be no more effective than placebos in the relief of symptoms.[48, 49] As suggested by Boyle,[50] it will be extremely interesting over the next few years to see whether microscopic gastritis, duodenitis, and colitis studies affect our concept of recurrent abdominal pain in children.

CLINICAL MANIFESTATIONS

Functional abdominal pain tends to occur in children between the ages of 4 and 14 years, with the mean age of onset between 5 and 10 years.[1, 10] There is an increased prevalence in girls, especially between the ages of 9 and 12 years, with the female to male ratio approaching 1.5: 1 during these years. The characteristics of functional abdominal pain are listed in Table 14–2. In most patients the pain is brief in duration, episodic, and interspersed with periods of well-being.[51] The pain-free intervals are of variable length, ranging from a few days to many weeks. Most episodes of pain last less than 1 hour and rarely persist for more than 3 hours.[1, 10] Continuous pain with episodic exacerbations is described in less than 10% of patients.[1, 10] The pain is often vaguely described by the child, and most often is described as cramping or colicky. Some children complain of a dull, constant pain.[10, 51] In the vast majority of patients, the pain is periumbilical or midepigastric in location, and the child will localize the site by placing his or her entire hand over the area. If asked to localize the pain with one finger, the child often draws a circle circumscribing the umbilicus. Radiation of the pain is rare. "Apley's rule"—that the further the localization of the pain from the umbilicus, the greater the likelihood of an underlying organic disorder—has proved useful in evaluating children with recurrent abdominal pain; however, it must be appreciated that it is common for organic disease to be located in the umbilical and midepigastric regions.[1, 52]

Table 14–2. CHARACTERISTICS OF FUNCTIONAL ABDOMINAL PAIN

Age range (4–14 years)
Chronic (three or more episodes in 3 months)
Episodes of pain alternating with pain-free periods
Periumbilical or epigastric location, no radiation
Variable severity (mild to severe)
Nature of pain (cramping, dull, burning)
Inconsistent relationship to meals, bowel movements, or general activity
Disturbance of normal activity

Mild to extreme pain may be experienced by children with functional RAP, and it has been our experience that the pain can be as severe as that which accompanies organic disease. During a severe episode of pain, the child may be tearful or crying, doubled over, sitting with knees drawn to chest, or exerting pressure on the abdominal wall. A consistent relationship to meals, bowel movements, general activity, or time of day is generally not demonstrated, although some children tend to experience the pain at the onset of the evening meal. The pain may persist during the evening, making it difficult for the child to fall asleep, but once the child is asleep, the pain seldom causes him or her to awake. It is not unusual for the pain to be present during periods of relaxation or play.

Symptoms that commonly occur in association with functional RAP include headache, pallor, nausea, anorexia, dizziness, and constipation.[1, 10, 36, 53] Headache and pallor are noted to occur during the episode of abdominal pain in at least 50% of patients.[36] Other commonly reported symptoms include limb pains and lethargy.[2, 10, 36] A slight elevation in temperature is often reported by parents, but invariably the temperatures recorded are less than 38°C. Abdominal distention, vomiting, and diarrhea are uncommon. Constitutional symptoms such as growth failure, weight loss, high fevers, rashes, arthritis, anemia, and rectal bleeding are not symptoms of functional abdominal pain and, when present, should alert the physician to the presence of an organic illness.

Further information that may support the physician in the diagnosis of functional RAP may be obtained from the past medical, family, and social histories. Several reviews have suggested that prenatal (morning sickness, headaches, difficult labors) and postnatal (poor eating habits, colic) problems are likely to be present in the histories of children with functional RAP.[10, 36] None of these studies, however, included control groups. The family history is likely to be positive for functional gastrointestinal problems and migraine headaches.[1, 36] Gastrointestinal symptoms may be slightly more common in the mother (50%) than in the father (47%).[10] The environment of children with functional RAP is often reported as stressful, with marital discord, separation, or divorce having occurred in 39% of Liebman's families within the year of onset of functional RAP.[36] Some children find school a very stressful situation, and functional RAP can be a manifestation of school stress.[54, 55] Liebman[36] found that only 9% of children with functional RAP attended school regularly, with 28% missing more than 10% of school days. Geographic and school changes, financial problems, and physical illness in a parent or sibling are relatively common experiences of children with functional RAP. It is surprising, however, how infrequently the child and family relate the pain to an environmental stress. The onset of pain often evokes a response from the parents, physician, and school that serves to reinforce the pain behavior. The receipt of special privileges and parental attention or the avoidance of stressful events, such as school examinations or sports activities, directly reinforces the expression of pain. Such learned illness behavior has been clearly demonstrated in the adult irritable bowel syndrome population.[56] Despite the fact that the pain usually lasts less than an hour, the child stays away from school the entire day. Resumption of normal home activities after resolution of the pain is the norm. Further reinforcement of the pain occurs when the school sends the child home when he or she complains of pain. The prescription of multiple medications by the physician in an attempt to alleviate the pain also serves to reinforce the pain behavior.

DIAGNOSTIC APPROACH

The history and physical examination of the patient with recurrent abdominal pain is clearly the most important aspect of the diagnostic evaluation.[12, 51, 57] It is imperative that adequate time be allocated to obtain a thorough clinical history and perform a physical examination. Time to establish rapport with the patient and his or her family is also essential. We find that at least 1 hour must be allocated when initially assessing patients with this problem. About 50% of the children with RAP referred to a gastroenterologist for assessment will have been symptomatic for less than 12 months at the time of consultation. Others will have had pain complaints for 1 to 5 years.[58] At the time of referral, many patients will have already been evaluated by one or more physicians, and multiple diagnostic tests designed to rule out organic disease may have been performed. Instead of reassuring the patient and family that there is no serious underlying organic disease, this battery of negative diagnostic tests often reinforces the pain behavior and increases the family's anxiety and frustration.

The most common age of children presenting with functional RAP is between 4 and 14 years. Onset of chronic abdominal pain in a child less than 4 years of age requires a more extensive diagnostic work-up, especially for structural abnormalities. Similarly, the onset of RAP after 14 years of age is uncommon, and symptoms of the classic irritable bowel syndrome of adulthood are more likely to be observed. A history of sexual activity should be obtained from the adolescent, and gynecologic disorders should be considered.

It is not possible to distinguish patients with functional pain from those with organic pain on the basis of sex, personality traits, or intelligence. Most of the patients are of average or higher-than-average intelligence. Early reports of patients with functional pain described them as being perfectionists, constant worriers, and overachievers.[1, 10, 36] Subsequent studies have failed to confirm these traits.[29, 35]

The physical examination should be thorough and meticulous and should, if possible, be performed between and during attacks of pain. We find it beneficial, when age appropriate, to carry out the examination in the presence of the parents so that they are aware of the completeness of the examination. Height and weight should be plotted on appropriate percentile charts along with any previous recordings available. Growth and development are not altered in functional RAP despite the duration of symptoms. Signs of heightened anxiety, such as tachycardia, mild systolic hypertension, sweaty palms, cold extremities, and dilated pupils, may be present.[1, 10] The abdominal examination is generally nonspecific. There may be abdominal tenderness, but it is often vague and diffuse. Deep palpation is not associated with guarding or rebound tenderness. Generally, most discomfort is elicited over the lower abdomen, especially in the area of the descending colon and sigmoid. Rectal examination may reveal the presence of pelletlike stools in the ampulla. Notably absent from the physical examination are signs of chronic disease such as pallor, clubbing, arthritis, hepatosplenomegaly, abdominal masses, perianal disease, or stools positive for occult blood.

In most patients, a few simple screening tests are indicated (Table 14–3). These tests include complete blood count, erythrocyte sedimentation rate, urinalysis, urine culture, and studies of the stool for ova and parasites and for occult blood. According to Bain,[8] these tests can exclude 95% of organic disorders producing recurrent abdominal pain. The addition of the lactose hydrogen breath test allows that subgroup of patients with lactose intolerance to be detected.[26] In addition, we have found the measurent of random fecal alpha$_1$-antitrypsin to be a sensitive, noninvasive screen for inflammatory bowel disease.[59, 60] These basic tests are aimed at excluding inflammatory bowel disease, urinary tract infection, parasitic infection, and lactose intolerance. Once these screening tests have been performed, management of the patient can generally be initiated without further investigation, provided that routine follow-up is assured. If symptoms are somewhat atypical, further investigation may be necessary.

DIFFERENTIAL DIAGNOSIS

There are a vast number of organic diseases that may cause recurrent abdominal pain in children. Few of these are likely to elude diagnosis if the history taking and physical examination have been thorough. Abdominal pain of organic origin tends to be more consistent and is often localized. Organic pain is more likely to radiate through to the back and cause interrupted sleep and is less likely to be associated with extraintestinal autonomic manifestations than functional RAP. Table 14–4 lists certain features or "red flags" that suggest a higher risk of organic disease in children with recurrent abdominal pain. The presence of these features signals the need for a more extensive evaluation for organic disease. Most studies have found that when an organic disease is responsible for recurrent abdominal pain, the pathology is most likely to be located within the genitourinary or intestinal tract.[3, 16] Brief descriptions of some of the more common causes of organic abdominal pain (Table 14–5) that require differentiation from functional RAP are presented in the following sections.

Table 14–3. SCREENING TESTS FOR FUNCTIONAL ABDOMINAL PAIN

Complete blood count
Erythrocyte sedimentation rate
Urinalysis
Urine culture
Stool examination for ova and parasites
Stool examination for occult blood
Lactose breath hydrogen test
Random fecal alpha$_1$-antitrypsin level

Table 14–4. FINDINGS SUGGESTING ORGANIC DISEASE IN CHILDREN WITH RECURRENT ABDOMINAL PAIN

Recurrent fevers (>38°C)
Weight loss or poor weight gain
Growth failure
Pain localized away from the midline
Perianal disease
Hematemesis
Bilious emesis
Stools with gross or occult blood
Anemia
Elevated erythrocyte sedimentation rate
Elevated fecal alpha$_1$-antitrypsin

Peptic Ulcer Disease

Abdominal pain is the most prominent presenting symptom in 90% of children with peptic ulcer disease (see Chapter 33).[61, 62] The typical ulcer pain of adults that worsens with fasting and is relieved by meals is not common in children and adolescents.[62, 63] Silverman and Roy[63] suggest that the diagnosis of peptic ulceration should be considered in the following circumstances:

1. Chronic abdominal pain present at night or in the early morning hours
2. Recurrent vomiting related to meals
3. Anemia if occult blood is present in the stools
4. Vague gastrointestinal complaints in a patient with a positive family history of duodenal ulcer

Esophagitis

Peptic esophagitis (see Chapter 26) frequently presents with substernal or epigastric pain and is often more severe on lying down and during vigorous exercise. The regurgitation of fluid into the mouth is an unequivocal symptom of esophageal reflux. The pain may be associated with vomiting and may be resistant to relief by antacids.

Table 14–5. MOST FREQUENT ORGANIC CAUSES OF RECURRENT ABDOMINAL PAIN

Peptic ulcer disease	Biliary colic
Esophagitis	Carbohydrate intolerance
Inflammatory bowel disease	Parasitic infestations
Recurrent intestinal obstruction	Urinary tract disease
Constipation	Musculoskeletal pain
Pancreatitis	

Inflammatory Bowel Disease

The clinical findings in Crohn's disease and ulcerative colitis (see Chapters 59 and 60) depend on the location and extent of the inflammatory process. In small bowel Crohn's disease, the abdominal pain is frequently postprandial, cramping in nature, and periumbilical in location. Pain is due primarily to narrowing (stricturing) of the small bowel. Right lower quadrant tenderness in association with a fullness or mass, weight loss, elevated erythrocyte sedimentation rate, fever, joint pains, or rash should alert the physician to the possibility of Crohn's disease. Colitis tends to be associated with lower abdominal pain that is worse before and during defecation and is relieved by the passage of stool. Weight loss, diarrhea, urgency to defecate, and occult or overt rectal bleeding are additional features suggestive of colitis.

Recurrent Intestinal Obstruction

Intestinal obstruction (see Chapter 19) is characterized by intermittent cramping, central abdominal pain, bilious emesis, and abdominal distention. Causes of recurrent small bowel obstruction include intussusception, malrotation with midgut volvulus, and adhesions. Plain abdominal radiographs in the supine and erect positions may reveal dilated bowel with multiple air-fluid levels in cases of complete obstruction. Contrast studies of the small intestine and colon may be necessary in cases of incomplete obstruction.

Constipation

Chronic constipation (see Chapter 16) can cause lower abdominal pain and cramping, abdominal distention, diarrhea from overflow incontinence, and rectal bleeding. It may be classified as being idiopathic or secondary to gastrointestinal or systemic disease. Careful history and physical examination will allow the gastroenterologist to distinguish between idiopathic and secondary causes in most instances. Occasionally, children present with RAP and unrecognized chronic stool retention. A plain abdominal radiograph may be useful in detecting clinically significant stool retention in some patients.[27] Constipation secondary to organic disease states should be treated by appropriate medical or surgical means. Mineral oil, bulk laxatives, and a high-fiber diet along with regular toileting are the mainstays of therapy for idiopathic constipation.

Pancreatitis

The occurrence of discrete episodes of pain in the epigastric or periumbilical region associated with nausea and vomiting should lead to the consideration of pancreatitis (see Chapters 68 and 69). Pain is often initiated by meals, and resolution of symptoms generally occurs over a period of 4 to 8 days. Early in the course of chronic pancreatitis, an elevation in serum amylase is expected, but as the disease progresses serum enzymes are often normal.[64] Ultrasonography and computed tomography imaging may be helpful in the diagnosis. An enlarged, edematous pancreas is seen early in the course of the disease, but as it progresses the pancreas becomes shrunken and fibrotic. Metabolic conditions such as hypercalcemia[65] and hyperlipemia types I and IV may also result in chronic pancreatitis and recurrent pain.[66]

Biliary Colic

Although variable, the pain of biliary colic (see Chapter 72) is characteristically located in the epigastrium and right upper quadrant. The pain is acute in onset and rises to maximum intensity over 10 to 20 minutes. Biliary pain often remains constant for several hours and gradually subsides to a dull, vague discomfort. Radiation of the pain to the back and shoulder is common, especially in older children. Pain often follows meals but can occur at any time of the day or night. Nausea and vomiting may accompany a severe attack of pain. Laboratory studies are seldom useful in the diagnosis unless the serum bilirubin is elevated. Ultrasonography is the preferred method of detecting cholelithiasis or choledochal cyst.

Carbohydrate Intolerance

In children presenting with chronic abdominal pain, diarrhea, bloating, and increased flatulence, the diagnosis of carbohydrate intolerance should be considered (see Chapters 2 and 38). Dietary lactose, fructose, and sorbitol are the most frequently implicated sugars in such patients.[67–69] A comprehensive dietary history usually provides insight into the problem. A breath hydrogen test following a lactose or fructose load as indicated will generally reveal increased hydrogen production, indicating excess fermentation of these carbohydrates within the colon. Complete elimination of the offending sugar often produces a clinical response, and subsequent reintroduction of the carbohydrate up to the level tolerated should be undertaken.

Parasitic Infestations

Infestation of the gastrointestinal tract by parasites has become relatively common in industrialized parts of the world (see Chapter 49). *Giardia lamblia, Cryptosporidium, Dientamoeba fragilis,* and *Blastocystis hominis* are the parasitic infestations most frequently encountered and should be considered as possible etiologic agents in cases of abdominal pain that is accompanied by anorexia, abdominal distention, and diarrhea. Fresh stool samples should be examined for ova and parasites. In cases of suspected giardiasis, stool studies are frequently negative, and diagnosis may require obtaining duodenal fluid by either intubation or string test.

Chronic parasitic infestations may occur in children with immunodeficiency syndromes, and an investigation of immune function may be indicated in select patients.

Urinary Tract Disease

Obstructive uropathy with hydronephrosis and pyelonephritis may present with recurrent abdominal pain and must be ruled out while it is still reversible. Ureteropelvic junction obstruction may present with recurrent, cramping periumbilical pain and vomiting without clinical or laboratory findings to suggest a urologic etiology.[70, 71] If one suspects organic disease or if the abdominal pain is referred to the flank or groin, prompt investigation of the urinary tract is warranted and should include urinalysis and urine culture as well as ultrasound of the urinary tract.

Musculoskeletal Pain

Musculoskeletal trauma is an infrequently described and probably underdiagnosed organic cause of chronic abdominal pain. Muscle pain is usually well localized and sharp in nature and may be exacerbated by movement. Brown[72] reported that 79 of 100 consecutive adolescents with upper abdominal and chest pain had costochondritis. A history of antecedent trauma or strain and exacerbation by movement signal the possibility of a musculoskeletal disorder. Diagnosis of musculoskeletal pain relies on physical findings such as unilateral rectus abdominus spasm and tenderness, especially along its costal insertion. Radiologic examination of the ribs to exclude fracture or tumor may be necessary. Nonsteroidal anti-inflammatory agents may be effective in pain relief; however, in cases of intractable pain, local injection of a steroid anesthetic mixture for relief of rib pain or costochondritis may be required.[73]

TREATMENT

Management of this heterogeneous group of patients must be individualized to be effective. The goal of therapy is to treat the whole child and family and not simply the symptoms. The primary objective in the management of children with functional abdominal pain should be to normalize life and allow any abdominal discomfort to have minimal impact on daily activities. The diagnosis of functional RAP must be presented to the parents and child as a positive diagnosis based on the history, physical examination, and, if necessary, laboratory investigations. It is important to emphasize the fact that the diagnosis is not made simply by the exclusion of organic disease. It is imperative to reassure the patient and family that the pain is indeed real and abdominal in location, but that no serious organic disease is present. The physician needs to explain the nature of the symptom complex and then offer an explanation of the presumed pathophysiology of the condition. We explain that various stimuli of physical or psychological origin are thought to trigger an alteration in gastrointestinal motor activity. This alteration in motor activity causes tension to develop within the intestinal wall, resulting in pain. We explain that not all children experiencing the same stress will develop pain and that individual children may perceive stress differently. We suggest that in some instances, there may be a genetic predisposition in families with a history of functional intestinal complaints. To help convey a psychophysiologic framework, we explain that most people experience some stress-induced pain. A typical example might be tension headaches in adults. Results of any laboratory or radiologic studies the patients may have had prior to referral are reviewed and discussed with the family. Organic diseases ruled out by these studies are mentioned. We ask the parents if there is any specific disease they are particularly concerned that their child may have and then discuss this condition with them, explaining why we feel that their child does not have this disease. We find it useful to let the patient and family know that functional abdominal pain is a very common condition, with 10 to 15% of school-aged children affected.

The therapy for functional abdominal pain is directed at reassuring and educating the family. Reassurance is achieved by scheduling follow-up appointments that enable sustained contact with the child and family. Education begins at the first interview with an explanation of the pathophysiology of the condition, as outlined previously. At subsequent appointments the physician is often able to identify other environmental stresses that may be precipitating or modifying the abdominal pain. In some instances the physician may be able to suggest some approaches that will help in eliminating or minimizing these factors. Secondary gains the child receives when abdominal pain is experienced serve to reinforce the pain behavior and must be eliminated if the child is to recover. The parents should be encouraged to support the child but not the symptom of pain.[74] Regular daily activities must be undertaken despite the presence of pain. A return to full-time school activities within 1 to 2 days of the initial consultation is essential. It is often useful for the physician to communicate directly with the child's teacher or the school nurse to explain the nature of the problem. Strict criteria for allowing the child to remain home from school need to be developed; we include a temperature of greater than 38.5°C or significant diarrhea or vomiting, but not pain alone. If the child does not attend school, he or she should be seen by the pediatrician early on the day of absence and return to school if deemed fit to do so by the pediatrician. Similarly, if the child experiences pain at school, he or she may be allowed to go to the school nurse but should not return home unless one of these criteria is met. Most of the morbidity associated with functional RAP is related to the prolonged absence from school.

The use of high-fiber diets is well established in the management of adult irritable bowel syndrome. The data on the use of these diets in children with functional abdominal pain, however, are still preliminary.[75] A double-blind crossover study performed by Feldman and colleagues[76] demonstrated a 50% improvement in attacks of pain in patients whose diet was supplemented with 10 gm of corn fiber per day as compared with placebo. Few side effects of the fiber-enriched diet were reported. We generally recommend a high-fiber diet in our patients with functional abdominal pain and suggest a gradual increase in dietary fiber over at least 1-month period. If there is no response to this program, the diet is discontinued. We have found the addition of fiber to be most helpful in those patients who have constipation in association with abdominal pain.

Pharmacologic therapy has not been found to be of benefit in children with functional RAP. Various classes of drugs have been tried, including antispasmodics, anticholinergics, anticonvulsants, and antidepressants. Apley,[1] in a double-blind crossover study of 36 children with nonorganic abdominal pain, assessed the effect of phenobarbitone versus a placebo and found no consistent improvement with phenobarbitone. There are no clinical data to suggest that any of these medications are more effective at relieving symptoms than placebo, and their use is potentially harmful. Many of these drugs have a low therapeutic-toxicity ratio and may in fact aggravate symptoms. The use of medications, as mentioned previously, may be one of the major reinforcers of pain behavior.

In rare instances the symptoms of functional RAP are so persistent and severe that outpatient management does not succeed in modifying the pain behavior. These children continue to be unable to attend school or function normally. In such instances limited hospitalization may become necessary. Once these patients are hospitalized, the severe pain commonly diminishes or disappears. Stone and Barbero[10] demonstrated the disappearance of intestinal symptoms in 53% of their patients and a diminution in symptoms in another 38% during hospitalization. Observation in the hospital allows the physician to examine familial interactions in greater depth and assess the family's coping mechanisms. It also allows the physician to obtain information about the child from other hospital staff such as the primary nurse and hospital schoolteacher. It is imperative that during the hospitalization the physician continue to educate the child and family and offer firm reassurance that no organic disease is present. Unfortunately, the current insurance and government payment systems often make such potentially beneficial hospitalization impossible.

In some patients little change in abdominal pain occurs during hospitalization, and the episodes of pain continue unabated. It is not uncommon to find evidence of major stresses and significantly disturbed family dynamics in these children. Symptoms of depression may be evident in both the child and the family. The gastroenterologist's attempt to educate the child and family and to modify environmental stresses is rarely successful in this situation, and referral to a child psychiatrist is indicated. Often prolonged psychological intervention is required to return these children to normal activity and to enable them to cope with daily stress. While the child is receiving psychological therapy, it is important for the gastroenterologist to continue to see the child and family regularly to offer support and reassurance that organic disease is not present and to emphasize the importance of complying with the psychotherapy.

PROGNOSIS

A number of retrospective studies have been performed in an attempt to determine the long-term outcome of functional RAP of childhood.[21, 68, 77, 78] Reassuringly, it has been found that a diagnosis of functional abdominal pain rarely obscures that of an organic disease. Stickler and Murphy,[77] in a long-term follow-up of 161 patients with abdominal pain, found that organic disorders were missed in only three instances. In two of these patients the diagnosis of inflammatory bowel disease had been suspected on the basis of a history of weight loss and the finding of anemia but was not confirmed at the time by roentgenographic examination.[77] In 30 to 50% of patients, once a positive diagnosis of functional abdominal pain has been made, there is rapid (within 2–6 weeks) resolution of symptoms,[21, 78, 79] suggesting that the child and family accept the physician's diagnosis and reassurance that the pain is not organic in origin. However, despite the good prognosis in these patients, it has been found that regardless of treatment a sizable percentage of patients continue to have abdominal pain or other chronic pain symptoms into adulthood. In Apley and Hale's[79] series of 30 patients treated with explanation and reassurance, complete resolution of symptoms was found in nine patients. Eleven patients continued to have abdominal pain, but in only two cases did the pain restrict work or other activities. Ten patients had resolution of abdominal pain but developed other symptoms such as headache, backache, and menstrual irregularities.[79] In Apley's earlier series[1] of 30 untreated patients with recurrent abdominal pain, three fourths of those with continuing abdominal pain were not well adjusted, and their work and other activities suffered. Apley and Hale,[79] from their small series of patients, described several factors that appeared to influence prognosis in children with functional RAP. Associated with a bad prognosis were (1) coming from a "painful family," (2) male sex, (3) onset of pain prior to 6 years of age, and (4) duration of pain for greater than 6 months prior to treatment.

Treatment with explanation and reassurance does not always cure the abdominal pain, but it does seem to affect the prognosis and increase the patient's ability to live a normal life. Until further advances are made into the etiology and pathogenesis of functional abdominal complaints, explanation and reassurance will continue as the mainstays of therapy.

REFERENCES

1. Apley J: The child with abdominal pains. London, Blackwell Scientific Publications, 1975.
2. Oster J: Recurrent abdominal pain, headache and limb pain in children and adolescents. Pediatrics 1972; 50:429–436.

3. Apley J, Naish N: Recurrent abdominal pains: A field survey of 1,000 school children. Arch Dis Child 1958; 33:165–170.
4. Pringle MLK, Butler NR, Davie R: 11,000 Seven Year Olds: The National Child Development Study (1958 cohort). London, Longmans, 1966.
5. Parcel GS, Nader PR, Meyer MP: Adolescent health concerns, problems and patterns of utilization in a triethnic urban population. Pediatrics 1977; 60:157–164.
6. Dodge JA: Recurrent abdominal pain in children. Br Med J 1976; 1:385–387.
7. Faull C, Nicol AR: Abdominal pain in six year olds: An epidemiological study in a new town. J Child Psychol Psychiatry 1986; 27:251–260.
8. Bain HW: Chronic vague abdominal pain in children. Pediatr Clin North Am 1974; 21:991–1000.
9. Bury RG: A study of 111 children with recurrent abdominal pain. Aust Paediatr J 1987; 23:117–119.
10. Stone RT, Barbero GT: Recurrent abdominal pain in childhood. Pediatrics 1970; 45:732–738.
11. Dimson SB: Transit time related to clinical findings in children with recurrent abdominal pain. Pediatrics 1971; 47:666–674.
12. Maddison TG: Recurrent abdominal pain in children. Med J Aust 1977; 1:708–710.
13. Papatheophilou R, Jeavons PM, Disney ME: Recurrent abdominal pain: a clinical and electroencephalographic study. Develop Med Child Neurol 1972; 14:31–44.
14. Nicol AR: Psychogenic abdominal pain in childhood. Br J Hosp Med 1982; 27:351–353.
15. Leek BF: Abdominal and pelvic visceral receptors. Br Med Bull 1977; 33:163–168.
16. Rappaport L: Recurrent abdominal pain: Theories and pragmatics. Pediatrician 1989; 16:78–84.
17. Lipkin M, Sleisenger MH: Studies of visceral pain: Measurement of stimulus intensity and duration associated with the onset of pain in esophagus, ileum and colon. J Clin Invest 1958; 37:28–34.
18. Swarbick ET, Bat L, Hegarty JE, et al: Site of pain from the irritable bowel. Lancet 1980; 2:443–446.
19. Galler JR, Neustein S, Walker WA: Clinical aspects of recurrent abdominal pain in children. Adv Pediatr 1980; 27:31–53.
20. Feuerstein M, Barr RG, Francoeur TE, et al: Potential biobehavioral mechanisms of recurrent abdominal pain in children. Pain 1982; 13:287–298.
21. Christensen MF, Mortensen O: Long-term prognosis in children with recurrent abdominal pain. Arch Dis Child 1975; 50:110–114.
22. McGrath PJ, Feldman W: Clinical approach to recurrent abdominal pain in children. J Dev Behav Pediatr 1986; 7:56–61.
23. Greene JW, Walker LS, Hickson G, Thompson J: Stressful life events and somatic complaints in adolescents. Pediatrics 1985; 75:19–22.
24. Astrada CA, Licamele WL, Walsh TL, et al: Recurrent abdominal pain in children and associated *DSM-III* diagnoses. Am J Psychiatry 1981; 138:687–688.
25. Apley J, Haslam DR, Tulloh CG: Pupillary reaction in children with recurrent abdominal pain. Arch Dis Child 1971; 46:337–340.
26. Barr RG, Levine MD, Watkins JB: Recurrent abdominal pain of childhood due to lactose intolerance. N Engl J Med 1979; 300:1449–1452.
27. Barr RG, Levine MD, Wilkinson RH, et al: Chronic and occult stool retention. Clin Pediatr 1979; 18:674–686.
28. Gaffney A, Gaffney PR: Recurrent abdominal pain in children and the endogenous opiates: A brief hypothesis. Pain 1987; 30:217–219.
29. McGrath PJ, Goodman JT, Firestone P, et al: Recurrent abdominal pain: A psychogenic disorder? Arch Dis Child 1983; 58:888–890.
30. Hodges K, Kline JJ, Barbero G, et al: Life events occurring in families of children with recurrent abdominal pain. J Psychosom Res 1984; 28:185–188.
31. Polak JM, Bloom SR, Sullivan SN, et al: Enkephalin-like immunoreactivity in the human gastrointestinal tract. Lancet 1977; 1:972–974.
32. Konturek SJ: Opiates and the gastrointestinal tract. Am J Gastroenterol 1980; 74:285–291.
33. Stanghellini V, Malagelada JR, Zinsmeister AR, et al: Stress-induced gastroduodenal motor disturbances in humans: Possible humoral mechanism. Gastroenterology 1983; 85:83–91.
34. Varni JW, Katz ER, Dash J: Behavioural and neurochemical aspects of pediatric pain. *In* Russo DC, Varni JW, eds: Behavioural Pediatrics Research and Practice. 1st ed. New York, Plenum Press, 1982, pp 177–224.
35. Raymer D, Weininger O, Hamilton JR: Psychological problems in children with abdominal pain. Lancet 1984; 1:439–440.
36. Liebman WM: Recurrent abdominal pain in children. Clin Pediatr 1978; 17:149–153.
37. Kopel FB, Kim IC, Barbero GJ: Comparison of rectosigmoid motility in normal children, children with recurrent abdominal pain and children with ulcerative colitis. Pediatrics 1967; 39:539–545.
38. Chaudhary NA, Phil D, Truelove SC: Human colonic motility: A comparative study of normal subjects, patients with ulcerative colitis and patients with the irritable bowel syndrome. Gastroenterology 1961; 40:18–26.
39. Pineiro-Carrero VM, Andres JM, Davis RH, et al: Abnormal gastroduodenal motility in children and adolescents with recurrent functional abdominal pain. J Pediatr 1988; 113:820–825.
40. Hyman PE, Napolitano JA, Diego A, et al: Antroduodenal manometry in the evaluation of chronic functional gastrointestinal symptoms. Pediatrics 1990; 86:39–44.
41. Fenton TR, Harries JT, Milla PJ: Disordered small intestinal motility: A rational basis for toddlers' diarrhoea. Gut 1983; 24:897–903.
42. Rubin LS, Barbero GJ, Sibinga MS: Pupillary reactivity in children with recurrent abdominal pain. Psychosom Med 1967; 29:111–120.
43. Lebenthal E, Rossi TM, Nord KS, et al: Recurrent abdominal pain and lactose absorption in children. Pediatrics 1981; 67:828–832.
44. Christopher NL, Bayless TM: Role of the small bowel and colon in lactose-induced diarrhea. Gastroenterology 1971; 60:845–852.
45. Bond JH, Levitt MD: Quantitative measurement of lactose absorption. Gastroenterology 1976; 70:1058–1062.
46. Levitt MD: Production and excretion of hydrogen gas in man. N Engl J Med 1969; 281:122–127.
47. Talley NJ, Phillips SF: Non-ulcer dyspepsia: Potential causes and pathophysiology. Ann Intern Med 1988; 108:865–879.
48. Lance P, Wastell C, Schiller KFR: A controlled trial of cimetidine for the treatment of nonulcer dyspepsia. J Clin Gastroenterol 1986; 8:414–418.
49. Nyren O, Adami HO, Bates S, et al: Absence of therapeutic benefit from antacids or cimetidine in non-ulcer dyspepsia. N Engl J Med 1986; 314:339–343.
50. Boyle JT: Chronic abdominal pain. *In* Walker WA, Durie PR, Hamilton JR, et al, eds: Pediatric Gastrointestinal Disease. 1st ed. Philadelphia, BC Decker, 1991, pp 45–54.
51. Silverman A, Roy CC: Psychophysiologic recurrent abdominal pain. *In* Silverman A, Roy CC, eds: Pediatric Clinical Gastroenterology. 3rd ed. St Louis, CV Mosby, 1983, pp 342–349.
52. Gadiyar BN, Taneja PN, Ghai OP: Recurrent pain in abdomen in children. Ind J Child Health 1963; 12:289–295.
53. Varsano I, Zeidel A, Matoth Y: Recurrent abdominal pain in children. Pediatrician 1977; 6:90–99.
54. Rosenberg AJ: Recurrent abdominal pain in children. Drug Ther 1982; 12:161–176.
55. Schmitt BD: School phobia—the great imitator: A pediatrician's viewpoint. Pediatrics 1971; 48:433–441.
56. Whitehead WE, Winget C, Fedoravicius AS, et al: Learned illness behaviour in patients with irritable bowel syndrome and peptic ulcer. Dig Dis Sci 1982; 27:202–208.
57. Marshall DG: Diagnosis and treatment: Recurrent abdominal pain in children—a surgeon's viewpoint. Pediatrics 1967; 40:1024–1026.
58. Green M: Diagnosis and treatment: Psychogenic, recurrent, abdominal pain. Pediatrics 1967; 40:84–89.
59. Thomas DW, Sinatra FR, Merritt RJ: Fecal alpha-1-antitrypsin excretion in young people with Crohn's disease. J Pediatric Gastroenterol Nutr 1983; 2:491–496.
60. Thomas DW, Sinatra FR, Merritt RJ: Random fecal alpha-1-antitrypsin concentration in children with gastrointestinal disease. Gastroenterology 1981; 80:776–782.
61. Motil KJ: Peptic ulcer disease. *In* Oski FA, DeAngelis CD, Feigin RD, et al, eds: Principles and Practice of Pediatrics. 1st ed. Philadelphia, JB Lippincott, 1990, pp 1689–1694.

62. Drumm B, Rhoads JM, Stringer DA, et al: Peptic ulcer disease in children: Etiology, clinical findings, and clinical course. Pediatrics 1988; 82:410–414.
63. Silverman A, Roy CC: Disorders of stomach and duodenum. *In* Silverman A, Roy CC, eds: Pediatric Clinical Gastroenterology. 3rd ed. St Louis, CV Mosby, 1983, pp 162–189.
64. Rothstein FC, Wyllie R, Gauderer MWL: Hereditary pancreatitis and recurrent abdominal pain of childhood. J Pediatr Surg 1985; 20:535–537.
65. Grendell JH, Cello JP: Chronic pancreatitis. *In* Sleisenger MH, Fordtran JS, eds: Gastrointestinal Disease: Pathophysiology, Diagnosis, Management. 3rd ed. Philadelphia, WB Saunders, 1983, pp 1485–1514.
66. Cameron JL, Capuzzi DM, Zuidema GD, et al: Acute pancreatitis with hyperlipemia: Evidence of a persistent defect in lipid metabolism. Am J Med 1974; 56:482–489.
67. Liebman WM: Recurrent abdominal pain in children: Lactose and sucrose intolerance: A prospective study. Pediatrics 1979; 64:43–45.
68. Kneepkens CMF, Vonk RJ, Fernandes J: Incomplete intestinal absorption of fructose. Arch Dis Child 1984; 59:735–738.
69. Hyams JS: Chronic abdominal pain caused by sorbitol malabsorption. J Pediatr 1982; 100:772–773.
70. Johnston JH, Evans JP, Glassberg KI, et al: Pelvic hydronephrosis in children: A review of 219 personal cases. J Urol 1977; 117:97–101.
71. Byrne WJ, Arnold WC, Stannard MW, et al: Ureteropelvic junction obstruction presenting with recurrent abdominal pain: Diagnosis by ultrasound. Pediatrics 1985; 76:934–937.
72. Brown RT: Costochondritis in adolescents. J Adolesc Health Care 1981; 1:189–201.
73. Li BUK: Recurrent abdominal pain in childhood: An approach to common disorders. Compr Ther 1987; 13:46–53.
74. Berger HG, Honig PJ, Liebman R: Recurrent abdominal pain, gaining control of the symptom. Am J Dis Child 1977; 131:1340–1344.
75. Manning AP, Heaton KW, Harvey RF, et al: Wheat fibre and irritable bowel syndrome, a controlled trial. Lancet 1977; 2:417–418.
76. Feldman W, McGrath P, Hodgson C, et al: The use of dietary fiber in the management of simple, childhood, idiopathic, recurrent, abdominal pain. Am J Dis Child 1985; 139:1216–1218.
77. Stickler GB, Murphy DB: Recurrent abdominal pain. Am J Dis Child 1979; 133:486–489.
78. Magni G, Pierri M, Donzelli F: Recurrent abdominal pain in children: A long term followup. Eur J Pediatr 1987; 146:72–74.
79. Apley J, Hale B: Children with recurrent abdominal pain: How do they grow up? Br Med J 1973; 3:7–9.

Chapter 15

Diarrhea

JON A. VANDERHOOF, M.D.

Diarrhea is a common complaint in pediatrics. Evaluation of an infant or child with diarrhea requires an understanding of the pathophysiology of diarrhea as well as a basic understanding of fluid absorption. Following a discussion of these topics, this chapter presents an approach to the differential diagnosis of both acute and chronic diarrhea in infants and children of various ages, with most specific entities discussed in greater detail elsewhere in this book.

Diarrhea is most commonly defined as either an increase in the frequency or decrease in the consistency of stool. As there is considerable variation in stool number, volume, and consistency among individuals, or in the same individual, the definition is somewhat imprecise. In adults, the stool volume averages around 100 gm per day, the primary stool constituent being water.[1, 2] Increased fiber intake markedly increases daily stool volume.[3] Normal infants pass 5 to 10 gm per kg per day, and stool volume in excess of 10 gm per kg per day in infants is often considered diarrhea.[4] By age 3 years, stool volume reaches adult levels. Stool loss greater than 200 gm per day defines diarrhea in both children and adults. The division of diarrhea into acute and chronic is arbitrary, but most physicians accept a minimum duration of 3 weeks before labeling symptoms as chronic.

FLUID ABSORPTION

Stool consistency is determined by many factors, including such dietary factors as fiber intake. In addition, fluid and electrolyte transport plays a major role in determining stool consistency and volume. Fluid and electrolyte transport is a complex process, involving both transmembrane transport and transport through the paracellular pathway, the space between the epithelial cells.[5–7] A very high percentage of fluid and electrolytes is transported through the paracellular pathway in the proximal small intestine, because the "pores" or tight junctions between cells are large, allowing rapid osmotic flow both into and out of the upper gastrointestinal tract. It is this mechanism that rapidly renders the contents of the small intestine isotonic regardless of the osmolality upon entering the small bowel. Distally in the small intestine and in the colon, there is less back diffusion of sodium and water, as the paracellular pathway is much less permeable and water and electrolytes are conserved to a much greater extent.

Sodium is absorbed either coupled with chloride or, in the case of the ileum and colon, by a sodium-hydrogen exchange process colinked with the chloride-bicarbonate exchange process.[8, 9] Water is absorbed totally by passive diffusion, following an osmotic gradient created primarily by sodium. The sodium pump, Na^+, K^+ ATPase, is located on the basolateral membrane of the enterocyte. It is this mechanism that is responsible for maintaining a low intracellular sodium content and creating a sodium gradient across the cell membrane. Sodium, therefore, enters the enterocyte through the brush border membrane and exits through the basolateral membrane. Sodium can enter through a number of mechanisms, including passive diffusion, specific sodium channels, and protein carriers linked with chloride. Glucocorticoids and mineralocorticoids may influence sodium transport through alterations in the sodium channel mechanism.[10] The relative importance of these different entry mechanisms may vary from the proximal to the distal small intestine and colon. Sodium also enters the cell through a coupled mechanism with monosaccharides and amino acids.[11, 12] These mechanisms serve as driving forces for glucose and amino acid absorption as well as electrolyte and fluid absorption.

All water movement in the intestine is determined by osmotic gradients created by solute transport.[13] When sodium is transported into the intracellular space adjacent to the epithelial cell, the high osmotic gradient in this compartment draws fluid through the intercellular space at the tight junctional end. Water and sodium then diffuse inward through the basement membrane into the interstitium and enter lymphatics and capillaries. A perijunctional actin-myosin complex appears to regulate the permeability of the paracellular pathway, permitting opening of the tight junctions and allowing absorption of additional nutrients and electrolytes from lumen to blood through the paracellular route.[14]

In addition to sodium, other electrolytes play a significant, albeit lesser, role in fluid absorption. In some instances, chloride may be actively secreted into the small intestine, acting as a major stimulant of fluid secretion.[15] Chloride conduction channels appear to be present in the apical membrane of the crypt cell, acting as a major mechanism for chloride secretion in response to a positive intracellular chloride gradient or changes in a number of intracellular messengers. In the small intestine, potassium is absorbed primarily through the paracellular pathway in response to fluid fluxes, i.e., solvent drag and osmotic gradients. Active absorption of potassium through energy-dependent potassium-hydrogen exchange in the apical membrane may be important in the more distal small intestine and colon, where the paracellular pathway is less permeable and transcellular absorption becomes the predominant force.[16] Bicarbonate absorption is accomplished through hydrogen secretion, with resultant formation of carbon dioxide and water that subsequently diffuse back into the blood. Active secretion of bicarbonate in the ileum occurs as part of the chloride absorption process through the chloride-bicarbonate exchange mechanism.[17]

Regulation of fluid and electrolyte transport in the small intestine is a complex process. It appears to be under the control of a variety of different regulatory mechanisms, including endocrine factors and the enteric nervous system.[17–19] Gut flora, changes in the immune system, and dietary factors are also important. Gastrointestinal peptides and neurotransmitters, as well as exogenous agents such as bacterial endotoxins, all alter cyclic adenosine monophosphate (AMP) in the intestinal epithelial cell, which markedly influences electrolyte transport.[20–23]

In addition to changes in fluid and electrolyte secretion, gut motility may also influence stool volume and consistency.[24, 25] Several factors influence motility, but it is primarily under the control of the enteric nervous system, an intrinsic nervous system modulated to some degree through the autonomic nervous system. In addition, a variety of gastrointestinal hormones and neuropeptides may alter gut motility in response to numerous stimuli, including various dietary factors. This complex interrelationship is important in several pathophysiologic states that commonly affect infants and children.

Through the processes of absorption, secretion, and motility, a volume of fluid several times that of fluid consumption and stool output is commonly handled by the small intestine and colon. Approximately 9 L of fluid each day in the older child or adult will traverse the ligament of Treitz.[25, 26] This fluid includes not only ingested food but also secretions from the stomach, liver, pancreas, and duodenum, all of which must be reabsorbed along with the nutrients in the remainder of the gastrointestinal tract. This 9 L of fluid will be reduced to 1 L by the time it reaches the ileocecal valve and enters the colon.[27] The adult colon, with a normal absorptive capacity of 3 to 4 L per day, is quite capable of absorbing this volume of fluid in the nonpathologic state. However, once this capacity is exceeded, diarrhea results.[27]

PATHOPHYSIOLOGY

Diarrhea is often subdivided based on pathophysiology. Osmotic diarrhea, motility disorders, and inflammation exudation, or both, are common categories, although overlap exists. In many disease states, more than one mechanism may be responsible for the diarrhea.

Osmotic Diarrhea

Osmotic diarrhea is a term applied when malabsorption of an absorbable solute creates an osmotic load in the distal small intestine and colon resulting in increased fluid losses.[28] This commonly occurs when carbohydrates, relatively small osmotically active particles, are malabsorbed.[29] If an ingested material is hypertonic, rapid flux of fluid across the duodenal epithelium results in isotonicity by the time the solution reaches the ligament of Treitz. In this process, significant amounts of fluid are secreted into the small intestine and must be reabsorbed more distally. The proximal small bowel is highly permeable to water and ions, and sodium and chloride are continually secreted in the upper small intestine across a concentration gradient. In the more distal small intestine and colon, permeability tightens, and the osmotic pressure created by the malabsorbed carbohydrate resists the reabsorption of water normally driven by active transport of sodium and chloride. Active reabsorption of these ions in the distal small bowel in the absence of reabsorption of the malabsorbed carbohydrate results in enteric sodium concentrations much lower than that of plasma. Further metabolism of malabsorbed carbohydrate to short-chain fatty acids such as propionate and butyrate as well as hydrogen, CO_2, and methane may occur.[30] Although some of these short-chain fatty acids are reabsorbed in the colon, they exert an additional osmotic load, further exacerbating osmotic diarrhea. A major characteristic of osmotic diarrhea is that it stops when feeding is discontinued. Second, it is characterized by a sizable gap in osmolality (usually greater than 50). The "osmotic gap" is calculated by the equation:

$$(Na^+ \text{ in mEq/L}) + (K^+ \text{ in mEq/L}) \times 2 = \text{Measured fecal osmolality in mOsm/kg}$$

In the absence of osmotically active malabsorbed substances, two times the sum of the sodium and potassium concentrations should equal about 290. The lower electrolyte concentrations in osmotic diarrhea suggest that some other osmotic substance is contributing to the isotonic osmotic load in the fluid expelled from the colon. In infants, bacterial metabolism of the malabsorbed carbohydrate commonly results in a stool pH of less than 5.5, another characteristic feature of many types of osmotic diarrhea.

Malabsorption of carbohydrates in infants is usually caused by diffuse mucosal injury.[31, 32] There are some conditions in which carbohydrates are selectively malabsorbed, such as congenital sucrase isomaltase deficiency or, in the older child or adult, primary acquired lactase deficiency. In addition, laxative preparations such as lactulose or milk of magnesia may produce osmotic diarrhea. Excess carbohydrate malabsorption may occur in combination with hypermotility disorders such as irritable colon of infancy, where large volumes of hypertonic juices rapidly traverse the small intestine, further exacerbating motility-induced diarrhea. In other instances, high-carbohydrate feedings may exacerbate diarrhea in children recovering from acute viral enteritis whose absorptive process may be impaired. Juices containing large quantities of carbohydrates, such as apple juice, are a common culprit, and rapid cessation of diarrhea results upon withdrawal of the offending substance.[33]

Secretory Diarrhea

Intestinal absorption of water and electrolytes is the net difference between the fluid and electrolytes secreted and fluid and electrolytes absorbed.[34] Total net absorption may be much smaller than either of the two unidirectional processes. Therefore, a change in the balance between these two unidirectional processes can markedly alter total intestinal fluid absorption and may result in secretory diarrhea.

Some investigators believe that all enterocytes are involved in both absorption and secretion, whereas others consider crypt cells the primary anatomic site of secretion. Certainly, disorders that result in villus destruction are associated with diarrhea, a component of which is often secretory. However, many secretory diarrheas occur in morphologically normal intestines.

Secretory diarrhea in the classical sense is not related to food in the gastrointestinal tract and, as a consequence, persists even if the patient has fasted for an extended period of time.[25] In patients with pure secretory diarrhea, eating does not increase stool volume significantly. Pure secretory diarrheas typically do not exhibit evidence of inflammation, in that occult blood and white blood cells are absent from the stool. Because the diarrhea is not related to dietary constituents, the osmolality of the stool can be accounted for by normal ionic constituents. Therefore, doubling the sum of sodium and potassium concentrations should equal the fecal osmolality.

There is a pitfall in applying these definitive terms to secretory diarrhea. In the majority of patients with gastrointestinal disease who exhibit features of secretory diarrhea, other mechanistic processes may be involved.[35] Although certain inflammatory diarrheas have a secretory component, they may also have an exudative component as well as an osmotic component during feeding.

Secretory diarrhea occurs under a number of conditions. Classically, secretory diarrheas are mediated by gastrointestinal peptides such as vasoactive intestinal polypeptide (VIP) and are associated with tumors such as ganglioneuroblastoma or Zollinger-Ellison syndrome.[36–38] However, other substances may induce fluid secretion, including bile acids, fatty acids, and laxatives.[39–41] Congenital disorders of fluid transport such as congenital chloridorrhea may also produce secretory diarrhea.[17]

Motility Disorders

Although motility is not often a major cause of malabsorption, changes in motility can definitely influence absorption. Slowing intestinal transit pharmacologically or nutritionally through increased ileal fat increases absorption.[24, 25] Severe impairment of intestinal motility results in intestinal stasis with subsequent inflammation, bile acid deconjugation, and malabsorption. Hypermotility is an uncommon cause of malabsorption. However, watery diarrhea may result from rapid transit in irritable colon of infancy. Malabsorption is not significant, and growth is normal. Deranged motility may be a component of diarrhea from other causes, including thyrotoxicosis, bile acid malabsorption, and a variety of other disorders.[42, 43] Documentation of hypermotility as a cause of diarrhea is difficult, however, and pharmacologic therapy is often unrewarding.

Inflammatory Diarrhea

Inflammation in the small intestine or colon may cause diarrhea in a number of conditions.[44–50] Exudation of mucus, protein, and blood into the gastrointestinal lumen may contribute to fecal water, electrolyte, and protein loss, but this usually occurs in association with other types of diarrhea, such as osmotic or secretory. Examples include inflammatory bowel disease, infectious disorders in the distal small bowel and colon, and celiac disease in the upper small intestine.

DIFFERENTIAL DIAGNOSIS OF DIARRHEA

Acute Diarrhea

In formulating a differential diagnosis in a child with diarrhea, one must first differentiate acute and chronic diarrhea. The duration of acute diarrhea is short, usually less than two weeks. It is most often caused by an enteric infection. Differential diagnosis varies somewhat with age, but not to the extent of chronic diarrhea.

In general, viral pathogens produce injury to the proximal small intestine, and bacterial pathogens usually involve colonic inflammation. As a consequence, viral pathogens typically produce watery diarrhea and vomiting, bacterial pathogens bloody stools, mucus, and crampy abdominal pain. Many bacterial infections, however, have a toxin-producing component causing watery diarrhea. This may be the sole presentation of a bacterial infection.

Because infectious diarrhea typically presents with either vomiting and watery stools or bloody, mucousy diarrhea, it is often valuable to consider the differential diagnosis of these two clinical presentations separately. As mentioned above, vomiting and watery stools are often caused by viral organisms. Rotavirus is the most common and is frequently seen in infants and small children, especially during the winter.[51, 52] Other viral pathogens, including the Norwalk agent and enterovirus, may produce a similar clinical syndrome. The disease is often abrupt in onset, with 24 to 48 hours of vomiting followed by 3 to 5 days of diarrhea. Dehydration is a relatively common complication. Although the standard therapy has been intravenous fluid replacement to correct the dehydration, recent evidence suggests that judicious use of oral rehydration therapy will correct most cases of mild to moderate dehydration without difficulty.

Protozoal pathogens may cause proximal small bowel mucosal injury as well. Giardiasis, discussed later as a chronic pathogen (see Chapter 49), may produce an acute diarrheal syndrome. *Cryptosporidium* is a newly recognized protozoal pathogen that causes severe chronic diarrhea and malnutrition in immunocompromised patients and an acute self-limited diarrheal disorder in immunocompetent patients.[53–55] This disorder may be spread through person-to-person contact, although it is highly associated with exposure to farm animals. Patients develop nausea, vomiting, abdominal cramps, low-grade fever, and profuse watery diarrhea. The disorder is self-limited, usually lasting about two weeks, and no specific antimicrobial therapy exists. The organism may occasionally be found in the stool but is frequently diagnosed only on intestinal biopsy.

Certain bacterial pathogens may produce a watery diarrhea. In most instances, this is caused by the production of toxins, which induce fluid secretion in the small intestine.[56] Cholera is a classic example. Certain species of *Aeromonas hydrophila* and *Plesiomonas shigelloides* may produce secretory watery diarrhea.[57–60] Both, however, have also been demonstrated to produce a colitis picture with crampy abdominal pain, mucus, and blood.

Acute self-limited bloody diarrhea is usually caused by a bacterial pathogen. *Shigella* and *Salmonella* are typical examples. Enteroinvasive *Escherichia coli* may also produce such a clinical picture. Enterohemorrhagic *E. coli,* type 0157H7, is recognized as one of the more common causes of bloody diarrhea in children and frequently produces hemolytic uremic syndrome and thrombotic thrombocytopenic purpura.[61] Hemolytic uremic syndrome appears to follow approximately 10% of such infections. *Clostridium difficile* may grow in large quantities following antibiotic administration and produce a colitis syndrome.[61–64] This disorder should be considered whenever a patient develops bloody diarrhea following antibiotic therapy, especially if pseudomembranes are visualized at sigmoidoscopy.

In most instances, the sigmoidoscopic appearance of bacterial diarrheas is nonspecific. Histologic changes are likewise fairly nonspecific. Through the sigmoidoscope, one visualizes the presence of spontaneous and induced friability, granularity, and loss of ramifying vessels. These findings are quite similar to those observed in ulcerative colitis. More proximal colon disease with distal spearing should suggest the possibility of other organisms such as *Yersinia enterocolitica* or the protozoal pathogen *Entamoeba histolytica*. If symptoms of cramping and bloody diarrhea and sigmoidoscopic evidence of colitis exist beyond 2 weeks in the face of negative cultures, inflammatory bowel disease should be considered a strong possibility.

Chronic Diarrhea

Differential diagnosis of chronic diarrhea changes markedly with age, much more so than acute diarrhea. In the small infant, perhaps the most common cause of chronic diarrhea is a disorder commonly known as intractable diarrhea of infancy (Table 15–1). This term is usually utilized to describe infants with diarrhea associated with diffuse mucosal injury beginning prior to 6 months of age, lasting longer than 2 weeks, and associated with malabsorption and malnutrition.[65–67] More recently, the term *protracted diarrhea of infancy* has been utilized, sinces the prognosis for this disorder has been markedly improved through the use of parenteral nutrition and newer elemental diets.[68]

The term *intractable diarrhea of infancy* implies that a distinct disease entity exists. However, there are several different disease processes that may produce histologically similar mucosal lesions resulting in a common symptom complex and similar consequences. Postinfectious diarrheal syndromes, intestinal protein intolerance syndromes, and a few other disorders may all produce similar findings.

Perhaps the major cause of intractable diarrhea of infancy in most areas of the United States is cow's milk and soy protein intolerance.[69, 70] These infants commonly develop enterocolitis, with inflammation in both the small bowel and the colon, a few days to a few weeks after initially ingesting cow's milk protein. Although inflammation may occur in any part of the gastrointestinal tract, it may also be limited to the colon. These children present during the first 3 months of life with a constellation of vomiting, irritability, poor feeding, diarrhea, and bloody stools. Stools commonly test positive for reducing substances, suggesting small bowel mucosal injury with carbohydrate malabsorption. Stool pH is usually below 5.5 for the same reason, and stool leukocytes are often present, suggestive of colitis. When cow's milk is withdrawn, symptoms resolve in a majority of milk-intolerant infants. Many relapse after a short withdrawal of cow's milk if placed on a soy formula, because a high percentage of milk-intolerant infants are also soy intolerant. Utilization of a casein hydrolysate formula is often more effective in ameliorating symptoms. When rechallenged with cow's milk or soy protein, children may relapse abruptly, the majority of reactions occurring within 24 to 48 hours. However, occasionally the reaction is delayed for several days. Life-threatening anaphylaxis may occur in a small minority of infants.

A small percentage of patients do not respond to withdrawal of cow's milk and soy protein from the diet and continue to have diarrhea and malabsorption while on a casein hydrolysate formula. It is these infants who are often classified as having intractable diarrhea or

Table 15–1. MAJOR CAUSES OF CHRONIC DIARRHEA IN SMALL INFANTS

Intractable diarrhea of infancy
Milk and soy protein intolerance
Protracted infectious enteritis
Microvillus inclusion disease
Autoimmune enteropathy
Hirschsprung's disease
Munchausen's syndrome by proxy
Congenital transport defects
Nutrient malabsorption

protracted diarrhea of infancy.[71] A variety of histologic abnormalities may be seen in the small intestine, including blunting and flattening of the villi, increased mononuclear cells with occasional polymorphonuclear infiltrates, cuboidalization of the surface epithelium, and a mild to moderate increase in mitotic activity in the crypts. These histological lesions vary substantially and are poorly predictive of the need for long-term parenteral nutrition.[68] It is quite likely that they are patchy in their distribution, and this may well account for their unpredictability. A significant percentage of patients with intractable diarrhea of infancy start out with infectious injury. A variety of enteropathogenic microorganisms may produce small bowel mucosal injury, including adherent *Escherichia coli*, rotavirus, *Giardia*, and others. Alteration of permeability of the mucosal membrane is often thought to produce secondary cow's milk or soy protein sensitivity, which may further aggravate mucosal injury and exacerbate the intractable diarrhea state. This phenomenon may actually represent the unmasking of pre-existing subclinical milk protein intolerance. Breast-feeding may offer some protection against the development of intractable diarrhea due to the anti-infectious factors present in human milk. Histologically, intractable diarrhea produced by cow's milk protein intolerance and protracted infectious enteritis appear similar.

Chronic postenteritis diarrhea following infection may also occur in older infants. Zoppi and colleagues reviewed 48 such patients, 18 less than 12 months of age and 30 between the ages of 12 and 30 months of age.[72] All had mild malabsorption and impairment of growth and chronic low-grade inflammation on intestinal biopsy. Diets were hypocaloric and high in carbohydrates, possibly a contributing factor in malabsorption and poor growth. Iyngkaran and coworkers described several infants younger than 2 months of age who were challenged with cow's milk protein 6 weeks after recovery from infectious enteritis, all of whom had previously been exposed to cow's milk.[73] Biopsies before and after milk challenge demonstrated significant mucosal injury following milk challenge, and milk challenge was significantly associated with diarrhea, vomiting, and weight loss.

Other less common causes of chronic diarrhea and mucosal injury occur in infancy. Congenital microvillus atrophy, otherwise known as microvillus inclusion disease, presents with severe diarrhea shortly after birth and is characterized by hypoplastic atrophy of the villi.[74–77] Electron microscopy reveals ultrastructural abnormalities of the microvillus membrane consisting of shortening and depletion of the microvilli and inclusions and involutions of the brush border membrane containing microvilli. This particular lesion is considered the hallmark of congenital microvillus atrophy, and microvillus inclusions may also be seen in the colon. The disorder becomes clinically apparent a few days after birth and results in intractable diarrhea. Although long-term survival with home total parenteral nutrition is possible, the disorder is usually fatal and does not respond to corticosteroids.

Autoimmune enteropathy is another rare disorder characterized by severe proximal intestinal mucosal injury.[78, 79] Autoantibodies against gut epithelium are typically found, and the histological lesion in the small intestine is usually quite severe, with marked polymorphonuclear infiltration and total flattening of the mucosa, resembling celiac disease. This disorder usually begins somewhat later in life than either intractable diarrhea or congenital microvillus atrophy, typically around 6 months of age. Although some patients respond to an elemental diet, immunosuppressive drugs are usually more helpful. Most respond, at least partially, to corticosteroids. Addition of mercaptopurine or azathioprine may also be helpful, and recent reports have documented response to cyclosporine in a limited number of cases. Evidence of multiorgan autoimmune disease such as diabetes and renal involvement is not uncommon.

Treatment of intractable diarrhea, regardless of the cause, is heavily based on supplemental parenteral nutrition and continuous enteral infusion of an elemental diet. Recent evidence suggests that enteral feedings hasten the recovery from mucosal injury, and that parenteral nutrition can often be avoided through aggressive use of continuous enteral infusion of an elemental diet.

Hirschsprung's disease is a possible diagnosis for any infant who presents with intractable diarrhea. This diagnosis should be suggested if the child has had delayed passage of meconium during the first 24 hours of life, or if constipation preceded the diarrhea. Predisposing factors for Hirschsprung's disease such as a strong family history or the presence of Down's syndrome likewise should caution the clinician to consider this possibility. Although only a small percentage, around 10%, of infants with Hirschsprung's disease develop enterocolitis, the disorder carries a very high mortality rate, up to 50%. Prompt decompression of the colon proximal to the aganglionic segment either through the use of a tube or by surgical placement of an ostomy is indicated. The diagnosis of Hirschsprung's disease may be established through the use of rectal suction biopsy, provided the clinician and pathologist are skilled in obtaining and processing the specimen.

Another cause of chronic diarrhea in infants is Munchausen's syndrome by proxy. A small number of cases have been reported in which administration of laxatives to small infants has produced an intractable diarrhea-like syndrome.[80, 81] The histologic changes typically seen in small intestine biopsies in intractable diarrhea of infancy are not present, however, and separation of the child from the caretaker results in abrupt cessation of symptoms. Parents of these infants are often overly concerned about the infant and are in constant attendance. Like Hirschsprung's disease, Munchausen's syndrome by proxy needs to be considered in the differential diagnosis of intractable diarrhea.

Congenital transport defects may result in chronic diarrhea from birth. One classic cause of congenital secretory diarrhea is congenital chloridorrhea.[82, 83] In this disorder, the chloride-bicarbonate exchange mechanism in the ileum and colon is reversed and chloride is actively secreted. Excess bicarbonate absorption results in alkalosis, and chloride malabsorption results in secretory diarrhea because of the osmotic load of the secreted chloride in the colon. Marked hypokalemia occurs. Patients present in infancy with severe diarrhea and extremely watery stools containing no blood, no white blood cells, and no reducing substances. Biopsies of the small intestine and colon are normal. Because of the tremendous active chloride secretion, stool chloride content exceeds that of the sum of the sodium and potassium, and the diagnosis can be strongly suspected following stool electrolyte measurement in correlation with clinical presentation.

Nutrient malabsorption may cause chronic diarrhea. Congenital glucose-galactose malabsorption is a defect in monosaccharide transport in which the active transport carrier protein for glucose and galactose is absent. Upon ingestion of any formula containing glucose or galactose, which includes all complete infant formulas, chronic severe watery diarrhea ensues, resulting in failure to thrive and stools that test positive for reducing substances. As in congenital chloridorrhea, biopsies of the small intestine and colon are normal. Fructose can be transported in these patients and may be utilized as a therapeutic source of carbohydrates. It should be noted that this condition is extremely rare.

An equally rare disorder is congenital lactase deficiency, a congenital absence of lactase. This should be differentiated from primary acquired lactase deficiency, in which lactase levels drop throughout late childhood. In congenital lactase deficiency, severe watery diarrhea is present from birth, but resolves upon treatment with a lactosc-free formula. Biopsies of the small intestine are normal, and stools are positive for reducing substances but negative for occult blood and white blood cells. Again, this condition is extremely rare and must be differentiated from the much more common milk protein enterocolitis, in which diarrhea may also resolve following milk withdrawal, but in which intestinal or colonic biopsies are abnormal, and stools frequently contain occult blood or white blood cells. Congenital sucrase isomaltase deficiency is a more common congenital disaccharidase deficiency state, but it is still quite rare. As sucrose is not a common dietary carbohydrate during the first 6 months of life, these children do not develop watery stools until sucrose is administered. Again, watery diarrhea and low fecal pH are common and suggestive of carbohydrate malabsorption, but because sucrose is a nonreducing sugar, stool tests for reducing substances may be either normal or only slightly positive.

Chronic Diarrhea in the Toddler

The differential diagnosis of chronic diarrhea changes rather markedly during the latter part of the first year and into the second year of life (Table 15–2). The most common cause of chronic diarrhea in this age group is irritable colon of infancy, also known as chronic nonspecific diarrhea.[84, 85] This disorder is often thought to be a variant of irritable bowel syndrome, and it is not uncommon to find a family history of irritable bowel syndrome, especially in parents or siblings. Infants with

Table 15–2. MAJOR CAUSES OF CHRONIC DIARRHEA IN TODDLERS

Irritable colon of infancy (chronic nonspecific diarrhea)
Protracted viral enteritis
Giardiasis
Sucrase isomaltase deficiency
Tumors (secretory diarrhea)
Ulcerative colitis
Celiac disease

this disorder typically have intermittent loose watery stools. Stools vary from two to three mushy stools on some days to six to ten watery stools on others. They are frequently forcefully expelled and are quite foul smelling. The odor, however, is not at all characteristic of steatorrhea, but rather is more typical of fluid from the ileum, which is not surprising, since the disorder is one of rapid transit and stools frequently spend very little time in the colon.

There are several characteristics of the clinical presentation of this disorder that help differentiate it from other causes of chronic diarrhea simply by obtaining a careful history and performing a physical examination. The first is the intermittent nature of the diarrhea. These children often oscillate between normal and watery stools, even between diarrhea and constipation. Stools are usually not expelled at night, although it is not uncommon for children to have a very watery stool immediately after waking in the morning. Children with chronic nonspecific diarrhea typically manifest normal growth. The exception is the child who is placed on a hypocaloric diet in an attempt to control the diarrhea.

Because of the intermittent nature of the diarrhea, such children are often misdiagnosed as having food allergies or recurrent episodes of viral enteritis. The assumption of food allergy is strengthened in the minds of the parents by the common presence of vegetable or other food particles in the stool, which are simply the manifestation of rapid transit. The intermittent nature of the diarrhea also suggests recurrent bouts of viral enteritis. This frequently results in institution of hypocaloric diets, which, in turn, impair the child's growth and weight gain.

The mechanism for the diarrhea in this disorder appears to be altered gastrointestinal motility. Despite relatively rapid transit, absorption is reasonably intact and the child will grow well if fed adequately. Institution of a high-fat, low-carbohydrate diet is often helpful both because of reduced dietary osmolality and because of the effects of ileal fat on retarding gastrointestinal motility.[86–88] When fat reaches the ileum, secretion of gastrointestinal hormones from that region slows gastric emptying and small bowel transit, thereby providing some improvement in the child's diarrhea. Occasional bouts of watery stools will still occur, but significant improvement is to be anticipated.

Another disorder seen in toddlers that closely mimics chronic nonspecific diarrhea is referred to as protracted viral enteritis.[85, 89–92] This disorder starts with a viral infection such as rotavirus. The institution of high-carbohydrate, low-fat feedings results in chronic hypocaloric hyperosmotic feedings, which may further exacerbate diarrhea. Low-grade mucosal injury persists, and the primarily osmotic diarrhea continues. Mild weight loss may occur due to the hypocaloric feedings and perhaps the low-grade malabsorption. Frequently, children with this disorder consume large quantities of apple juice or other high-carbohydrate beverages. These patients respond quite dramatically to the institution of a high-fat, low-carbohydrate diet. A small percentage, mostly those less than a year of age, may be milk protein intolerant and will relapse when milk feedings are restored. Lactase deficiency is usually not evident this late in the course of the illness. Milk protein intolerance is usually a transient condition in this setting and resolves in 2 to 4 months.

One other disorder that closely mimics chronic nonspecific diarrhea is giardiasis. *Giardia* is a proximal small intestinal protozoal pathogen that causes mucosal injury resulting in malabsorption and watery diarrhea.[93] Although it is commonly thought of as a pathogen contracted from contaminated food or water, in pediatrics it is more commonly passed from individual to individual, especially in day-care centers or other crowded situations. The diarrhea in giardiasis tends to be much less intermittent than in chronic nonspecific diarrhea, and because of the proximal small bowel mucosal injury, malabsorption and weight loss are more common. Diagnosis is often difficult, because pathogens are not always recovered in the stool. In fact, stool examinations may be normal in up to 50% of patients with giardiasis. Tests recently developed to detect *Giardia* antigen in the stool appear to be somewhat more sensitive.[94, 95] Small intestinal biopsy with careful examination for the presence of the *Giardia* organisms, or aspiration of duodenal or jejunal contents, is a more sensitive means of diagnosis.

Two less common causes of watery diarrhea that can present like chronic nonspecific diarrhea are congenital sucrase isomaltase deficiency and secretory diarrhea from tumors. Sucrase isomaltase deficiency is a defect in carbohydrate digestion in which the enzyme required for hydrolysis of sucrose and alpha limit dextrins is not present in the small intestine. As a consequence, these children have watery stools from osmotic diarrhea when sucrose is introduced into the diet. This usually corresponds with the time that infants with toddler diarrhea or chronic nonspecific diarrhea develop symptoms, and, as a consequence, it must be considered in the differential diagnosis even though it is quite rare. It should be suspected when screening studies indicate a chronically low stool pH of less than 5.5. Bacterial breakdown of the malabsorbed carbohydrates in the stool to organic acids decreases the stool pH and serves as a reasonably good screening test for this disorder. Stools are often negative for reducing substances because sucrose is a nonreducing sugar. However, hydrolyzing the stool with hydrochloric acid prior to measuring reducing substances will result in a positive test. In performing these assays, it is important to obtain measurements while the child is ingesting sucrose.

There are a few tumors that cause secretory diarrhea in children. Although an uncommon cause of chronic diarrhea in toddlers, these tumors do occasionally occur and must be considered in the differential diagnosis. Neuroblastomas, ganglioneuroblastomas, and pancreatic tumors that secrete VIP are the primary ones to exclude. Twenty-four-hour urine vanillylmandelic acid determinations as well as serum VIP determinations will adequately screen for most of them. They should be considered primarily in children who have continual rather than intermittent diarrhea and in whose diarrhea continues even when feeding is stopped.

There are some other causes of chronic diarrhea that occur in toddlers but vary substantially from the clinical presentation of chronic nonspecific diarrhea. These include early presentations of inflammatory bowel disease and primary malabsorptive disorders such as celiac sprue and cystic fibrosis. Crohn's disease is very rare under the age of 5 years and, as a consequence, most inflammatory bowel disease seen in toddlers is ulcerative colitis. These disorders are discussed elsewhere (see Chapters 59 and 60)

Celiac sprue, otherwise known as celiac disease or gluten enteropathy, is a relatively uncommon disorder in North America but is much more common in Europe. This disorder results in chronic proximal small intestinal inflammation following ingestion of gluten, a protein constituent in wheat, oats, barley, and rye. The alpha gliadin fraction of gluten appears to induce a hypersensitivity reaction in the small intestine, resulting in complete flattening of the villi, deepening of the crypts, and a marked increase in mitotic activity. Patients present with failure to thrive, abdominal distention, chronic diarrhea, and weight loss. Because of the mucosal injury, they are often poor eaters. Diarrhea usually develops as a later manifestation of the disease after significant failure to thrive and anorexia have already appeared. In this way, this disorder is different from chronic nonspecific diarrhea. Although new screening studies are now available to help determine the need for intestinal biopsies, biopsy diagnosis is still required in all cases. Clinical response to withdrawing gluten is usually slow and inconsistent, and for this reason, symptomatic response to gluten withdrawal and challenge is not adequate for establishing the presence or absence of celiac disease.

Over the years, many have advocated three biopsies to diagnose celiac disease: one at the time of diagnosis, one several months to years following gluten withdrawal, and a third to demonstrate recurrence of injury following gluten challenge. However, in patients with classic clinical presentations who present later than the first year of life, when other common causes of mucosal injury occur less frequently, one biopsy at the time of diagnosis is probably adequate, provided the histologic features are totally consistent with celiac disease. The antibody screening tests, antigliadin immunoglobulin A (IgA) and IgG, antireticulin, and antiendomysium, have made it much easier to screen for the presence of this disease.[96–98] These are typically useful in children with growth failure in whom celiac disease is regarded as a minor consideration in the differential diagnosis. Studies vary, but about 95% sensitivity can be anticipated. However, all these tests can be abnormal in children with nonspecific mucosal injury.

Children with chronic diarrhea should be evaluated for celiac disease if they manifest the clinical characteristics of failure to thrive, abdominal distention, muscle wasting, and anorexia in association with their diarrhea and if screening studies suggest malabsorption such as low serum carotene or the presence of large quantities of fat in the stool or if they do not respond to conservative therapy for the other more common causes of chronic diarrhea. In no instance should a child be placed on a therapeutic trial of a gluten-free diet without adequate evaluation. Children with chronic nonspecific diarrhea will occasionally improve on this diet because it is typically lower in carbohydrate, and this response can make the whole picture terribly confusing.

Cystic fibrosis is often considered in the differential diagnosis of chronic diarrhea. However, these children have fat malabsorption from pancreatic insufficiency, and their carbohydrate and protein absorption is usually quite adequate. As a consequence, the stools are primarily steatorrhea and not diarrhea. Large, frequently passed, foul-smelling stools that are not watery in consistency occur in the presence of failure to thrive, often with a history of recurrent respiratory infections. Ten percent may present at birth with bowel obstruction secondary to meconium ileus. Because watery diarrhea is not a symptom of cystic fibrosis, sweat chloride determination to exclude cystic fibrosis is not part of the routine evaluation of a child with chronic watery diarrhea. However, in the context of malabsorption and failure to thrive with large quantities of fat in the stool and a low serum carotene, sweat chloride determination should be obtained to exclude cystic fibrosis.

Chronic Diarrhea in School-Aged Children

The differential diagnosis again changes as the child progresses into school age (Table 15–3). Inflammatory bowel disease becomes more common, disorders such as chronic nonspecific diarrhea and protracted viral enteritis disappear, and other possibilities enter the differential diagnosis.

In the school-aged child with chronic diarrhea, inflammatory bowel disease plays a major role in the differential diagnosis. After age 5 years, both Crohn's disease and ulcerative colitis are relatively common, and Crohn's disease appears to be increasing in frequency. These children typically present with blood and mucus in the stool and often with abdominal pain and cramping. In Crohn's disease, growth failure is common, and physical examination often reveals perianal abnormalities and some right lower quadrant tenderness, since ileal and proximal colonic involvement is most common. In such patients, colonoscopic evaluation of the colon is much more definitive in making the diagnosis than radiographic studies; it permits histological sampling, which improves diagnostic capabilities. These disorders are discussed extensively elsewhere in the text (see Chapters 59 and 60).

Table 15–3. ADDITIONAL CAUSES OF CHRONIC DIARRHEA IN SCHOOL-AGED CHILDREN

Inflammatory bowel disease
Appendiceal abscess
Primary acquired lactase deficiency
Constipation with encopresis

Appendicitis may cause chronic diarrhea in infants and children. Unlike appendicitis in adults, childhood appendicitis frequently results in perforation. Localized inflammation in the region of the cecum results in chronic diarrhea, often associated with chronic low-grade fever and some abdominal tenderness, which may or may not be impressive on physical examination.

Primary acquired lactase deficiency begins to present in school-aged children. Lactase levels begin to drop between ages 3 to 5 years in such children. A gradual decrease in lactase levels results in subtle chronic increases in lactose malabsorption following ingestion of milk. The child gradually develops flatulence, abdominal pain, and loose stools following milk ingestion. In the older child, flatulence and abdominal pain may be more prominent than diarrhea. The diagnosis is easily made through the use of breath hydrogen testing, in which an oral lactose load is given and the breath is sampled for hydrogen content at frequent intervals thereafter. It should be pointed out that a small number of cases of milk protein intolerance have been observed in older children, and even in adults, in which ingestion of milk protein is followed by a sudden onset of diarrhea, abdominal pain, and occasionally vomiting. In these patients, the lactose breath hydrogen test is normal, and histologic injury of the bowel following milk protein ingestion can often be demonstrated.

Finally, a number of patients with constipation may be brought to the physician by their parents for evaluation of chronic diarrhea. In this instance, the children develop a fecal impaction with overflow incontinence known as encopresis. Chronic soiling of the pants, often with loose stool, leads the parents to believe that the child has diarrhea. This disorder is quickly differentiated from diarrhea in most instances by demonstration of impaction on rectal examination. Most school-aged children, even when they have diarrhea, can usually make it to the toilet to pass their stools unless the diarrhea is extremely bad. In children with encopresis, chronic soiling occurs so frequently that it is fairly easy to differentiate the two by history alone.

Diagnostic Studies in Diarrhea

Evaluation of the patient with diarrhea should start with certain screening studies. Many of these are appropriate in children with both acute and chronic diarrhea (see Table 15–4). Stools positive for occult blood generally indicate inflammation. This test is most commonly positive in patients with colitis. In the case of acute diarrhea, this usually suggests a bacterial infection; in the case of chronic diarrhea, inflammatory bowel disease such as ulcerative colitis or Crohn's disease is more likely. The same is true for patients with stools positive for white blood cells. Stools positive for reducing sub-

Table 15–4. SCREENING TESTS IN DIARRHEA

Test	Interpretation if Abnormal
Stool for occult blood	Inflammation, usually colonic
Stool Clinitest:	Carbohydrate malabsorption—usually proximal small bowel injury
Stool pH <5.5	Carbohydrate malabsorption—usually proximal small bowel injury
1-Hour blood xylose	Diffuse small bowel injury
Sudan stain for fat	Gross steatorrhea—small bowel, pancreatic, or biliary
Stool for white blood cell count	Inflammation, usually colonic

stances or stools with a pH of less than 5.5 usually indicate carbohydrate malabsorption. The carbohydrates are fermented by colonic bacteria that produce lactic acid, and this reduces the stool pH. Although these studies are abnormal in patients with congenital defects of carbohydrate malabsorption, they usually indicate small bowel injury. In the case of acute diarrhea, viral enteritis is the most common cause. In chronic diarrhea, infants with intractable diarrhea of infancy or any other chronic enteropathy will commonly have stools positive for clinitest and/or low pH. One must remember, however, that these tests are valid only when the child is being fed adequate quantities of formula containing carbohydrates. Sucrose is a nonreducing sugar, and the presence of sucrose in the stool will not result in a stool positive for reducing substances unless bacterial action upon the carbohydrate has split the disaccharide, producing some reducing sugar. Fortunately, enough bacterial action is usually present to produce some indication of increased reducing sugars in these patients. Stools positive for Sudan stain for fat indicate gross steatorrhea, which may be of small bowel, pancreatic, or biliary origin. Because the test is not sensitive, it is not done frequently. Many have advocated the use of the one-hour blood xylose determination as an indicator of small bowel mucosal injury, especially in patients with chronic diarrhea or suspected malabsorption syndromes. This test is neither specific nor sensitive and is currently done less frequently, given the recent introduction of antibody screening tests for celiac disease and the increased use of endoscopic biopsies of the small intestine.

Screening studies help the clinician decide what further studies are indicated. In the case of acute diarrhea, stool studies positive for occult blood or white blood cells suggest the need for stool cultures. Stool cultures are often quite expensive, and utilizing the screening studies to help dictate their use is often cost-effective. In acute diarrhea, low pH stools positive for reducing substances suggest a viral pathogen and may suggest the need for viral antigen studies for common viruses such as rotavirus. Most commonly, viral diarrheas in children are self-limited, and such tests are usually not helpful in the management of the patient.

In the case of chronic diarrhea, studies indicating small bowel mucosal injury may suggest the need to look for *Giardia* in the stool or do further screening studies for celiac disease, such as antigliadin, antireticulin, and antiendomysial antibodies. In addition, the screening studies may dictate the appropriate use of endoscopic procedures. Patients with hematest positive stools containing white blood cells may benefit from colonoscopic examination and colon biopsies.

Traditionally, biopsies of the small intestine have been of great usefulness in diagnosing the cause of chronic diarrhea. Certain diseases, such as intestinal lymphangiectasia, giardiasis, cryptosporidium, and abetalipoproteinemia, can be diagnosed from biopsies because of characteristic histologic features. The presence of severe inflammation raises the question of autoimmune enteropathy. Electron microscopic examination of the biopsies can be useful in detecting microvillus inclusion disease. Disorders such as intractable diarrhea of infancy, protracted viral enteritis, milk or soy protein intolerance, malnutrition, certain immunodeficiency disorders, and even celiac disease have a fairly nonspecific inflammatory process, and it may be difficult to differentiate one from another. However, the small bowel biopsy will help to assess the exact nature of the disease and document the mucosal injury.

There is some controversy about how biopsies of the small intestine should be performed. Traditionally, biopsies have been obtained with a suction biopsy tube. The Rubin tube, the Crosby and Carey capsules, the Watson capsule, and more recently the MediTech directable biopsy apparatus have all been used with great success in obtaining histologic specimens from infants and children. The procedure is low risk but requires substantial expertise. Because of the time involved in obtaining samples and the skill necessary in placing the biopsy capsule, endoscopic biopsies of the small intestine have become more common. The procedure is easy, requires little time, and allows sampling from multiple sites. However, with this technique it is more difficult to biopsy more distally into the small intestine. Endoscopic biopsy samples are also smaller in size and susceptible to crush artifact. Mounting endoscopic biopsies on small slices of cucumber fixed in alcohol, which can be subsequently embedded, sectioned, and stained along with the biopsy sample, allows improved orientation and improved interpretation of endoscopic biopsies. We have found this technique extremely helpful when using endoscopic biopsies for the detection of small bowel mucosal disease.

SUMMARY

Diarrhea in the pediatric age group may arise through a variety of different mechanisms and from many different causes. Different etiological factors may produce diarrheal stools through one or more different mechanisms. As in most of pediatrics, the differential diagnosis of diarrhea varies markedly with age, especially in the case of chronic diarrhea. The clinician must correlate the age of the patient, the nature of the stools, the chronicity of the problem, and other relevant historic factors in order to formulate an adequate differential diagnosis upon which to base an evaluation.

REFERENCES

1. Schiller LR, Hogan RB, Morawski SG, et al: The incidence and significance of bile acid malabsorption in patients with chronic idiopathic diarrhea. Gastroenterology 1987; 92:151.
2. Goy JAE, Eastwood MA, Mitchell WD, et al: Fecal characteristics contrasted in the irritable bowel syndrome and diverticular disease. Am J Clin Nutr 1976; 29:1480.
3. Tucker DM, Sandstead HH, Logan GM, et al: Dietary fiber and personality factors as determinants of stool output. Gastroenterology 1981; 81:879.
4. Weaver LT: Bowel habit from birth to old age. J Pediatr Gastroenterol Nutr 1988; 7:637–640.
5. Powell DW: Ion and water transport in the intestine. *In* Andreoli TE, Hoffman JF, Fanestil DD, et al, eds: Physiology of Membrane Disorders. New York, Plenum, 1986, p 559.
6. Shepherd RW, Hamilton JR, Gall DG: The postnatal development of sodium transport in the proximal small intestine of the rabbit. Pediatr Res 1980; 14:250–253.
7. Phillips SF: Diarrhea: A current view of the pathophysiology. Gastroenterology 1972; 63:495–518.
8. Turnberg LA, Fordtran JS, Carter NW, et al: Mechanism of bicarbonate absorption and its relationship to sodium transport in the human jejunum. J Clin Invest 1970; 49:548.
9. Turnberg LA, Bieberdorf FA, Morawski SG, et al: Interrelationship of chloride, bicarbonate, sodium, and hydrogen transport in the human ileum. J Clin Invest 1970; 49:557.
10. Powell DW: Barrier function of epithelia. Am J Physiol 1981; 241:G275–G278.
11. Ghishan FK, Wilson FA: Developmental maturation of D-glucose transport by rat jejunum brush-border membrane vesicles. Am J Physiol 1985; 248:G87–G92.
12. Fordtran J: Stimulation of active and passive sodium absorption by sugars in the human jejunum. J Clin Invest 1975; 55:728–737.
13. Diamond JM: Solute-linked water transport in epithelia. *In* Hoffman FJ, ed: Membrane Transport Processes. New York, Raven Press, 1978, p 257.
14. Pappenheimer JR: Physiological regulation of transepithelial impedance in the intestinal mucosa of rats and hamsters. J Membrane Biol 1987; 100:137–148.
15. Field M: Intracellular mediators of secretion in the small intestine. *In* Binder HJ, ed: Mechanisms of Intestinal Secretion. New York, Alan R. Liss, 1979, p 83.
16. Smith P, McCabe R: Mechanism and regulation of small intestinal electrolyte transport. *In* Johnson LR, ed: Physiology of the Gastrointestinal Tract. 2nd ed. New York, Raven Press, 1987, p 1307.
17. Bieberdorf FA, Gorden P, Fordtran JS: Pathogenesis of congenital alkalosis with diarrhea. Implications for the physiology of normal ileal electrolyte absorption and secretion. J Clin Invest, 1972; 51:1958–1968.
18. Cooke HJ: Neural and humoral regulation of small intestinal electrolyte transport. *In* Johnson LR, ed: Physiology of the Gastrointestinal Tract. 2nd ed. New York, Raven Press, 1987, p 1307.
19. Castro GA: Immunological regulation of epithelial function. Am J Physiol 1983; 243:G321–G329.
20. Bern MJ, Sturbaum CW, Karayalcin SS, et al: Immune system control of rat and rabbit colonic electrolyte transport: Role of prostaglandins and enteric nervous system. J Clin Invest 1989; 83:1810–1820.
21. Shlatz LJ, Kimberg DV, Cattieu KA: Phosphorylation of specific rat intestinal microvillus and basal-lateral membrane proteins by cyclic nucleotides. Gastroenterology 1979; 76:293–299.
22. Field M, Graf LH, Laird WJ, et al: Heat-stable enterotoxin of *Escherichia coli:* In vitro effects on guanylate cyclase activity, cyclic GMP concentration, and ion transport in small intestine. Proc Natl Acad Sci USA 1978; 75:2800–2804.
23. Hughes JM, Murad F, Chang B, Guerrant RL: Role of cyclic GMP in the action of heat-stable enterotoxin of *Escherichia coli.* Nature 1978; 271:755–756.
24. Schiller LR, Davis GR, Santa Ana CA, et al: Studies of the mechanism of the antidiarrhea effect of codeine. J Clin Invest 1982; 70:999.
25. Fordtran JS: Speculations on the pathogenesis of diarrhea. Fed Proc 1967; 26:1405.
26. Fordtran JS, Locklear TW: Ionic constituents and osmolality of gastric and small intestinal fluids after eating. Am J Dig Dis 1966; 11:503.
27. Phillips SF, Giller J: The contribution of the colon to electrolyte and water conservation in man. J Lab Clin Med 1973; 81:733.
28. Fordtran JS, Rector FC, Ewton MF, et al: Permeability characteristics of the human small intestine. J Clin Invest 1965; 44:1935.
29. Christopher NL, Bayless TM: Role of the small bowel and colon in lactose-induced diarrhea. Gastroenterology 1971; 60:845.
30. Bond JH, Currier BE, Buchwald H, et al: Colonic conservation of malabsorbed carbohydrate. Gastroenterology 1980; 78:444.
31. Butler DG, Gall DG, Kelly MN, et al: Transmissible gastroenteritis. Mechanisms responsible for diarrhea in an acute viral enteritis in piglets. J Clin Invest 1974; 53:1335–1342.
32. Keljo DJ, MacLeod RJ, Purdue MH, et al: D-Glucose transport in piglet jejunal brush-border membranes: Insights from a disease model. Am J Physiol 1985; 249:G751–G760.
33. Hyams JS, Etienne NL, Leichtner AM, et al: Carbohydrate malabsorption following fruit juice ingestion in young children. Pediatrics 1988; 82:64–68.
34. Powell DW: Intestinal water and electrolyte transport. *In* Johnson LR, ed: Physiology of the Gastrointestinal Tract. 2nd ed. New York, Raven Press, 1987, p 1267.
35. Fordtran JS, Santa Ana CA, Morawski SG, et al: Pathophysiology of chronic diarrhoea: Insights derived from intestinal perfusion studies in 31 patients. Clin Gastroenterol 1986; 15:529.
36. Krejs GJ: VIPoma syndrome. Am J Med 1987; 82:37–47.
37. Levine MM, Edelman R: Enteropathogenic *Escherichia coli* of classic serotypes associated with infant diarrhea: Epidemiology and pathogenesis. Epidemiol Rev 1987; 6:31–50.
38. Scheibel E, Rechnitzer C, Fahrenkrug J, et al: Vasoactive intestinal polypeptide (VIP) in children with neural crest tumours. Acta Pediatr Scand 1982; 71.721–725.
39. Balistreri WF, Partin JC, Schubert WK: Bile acid malabsorption—a consequence of terminal ileal dysfunction in protracted diarrhea of infancy. J Pediatr 1977; 89:21.
40. Thaysen EH: Idiopathic bile acid diarrhoea reconsidered. Scand J Gastroenterol 1985; 20:452.
41. Cummings JH, Sladen GE, James OFW, et al: Laxative-induced diarrhoea: A continuing clinical problem. Br Med J 1974; 1:537.
42. Cassuto J, Jodal M, Tuttle R, et al: On the role of intramural nerves in the pathogenesis of cholera toxin–induced intestinal secretion. Scand J Gastroenterol 1981; 16:377–384.
43. Eklund S, Jodal M, Lundgren O: The enteric nervous system participates in the secretory response to the heat stable enterotoxins of *Escherichia coli* in rats and cats. Neuroscience 1985; 14:673–681.
44. Kerzner B, Kelly MH, Gall DG, et al: Transmissible gastroenteritis: Mechanisms responsible for diarrhea in an acute viral enteritis in piglets. Gastroenterology 1979; 76:20–24.
45. Shepherd RW, Gall DG, Butler DG, et al: Transmissible gastroenteritis: Sodium transport and the intestinal epithelium during the course of viral enteritis. Gastroenterology 1977; 72:457–561.
46. Granger DN, Hernandez LA, Grisham MB: Reactive oxygen metabolites: Mediators of cell injury in the digestive system. Viewpoints Dig Dis 1986; 18:13–16.
47. Purdue MH, Gall DG: Intestinal anaphylaxis in the rat: Jejunal response to in vitro antigen exposure. Am J Physiol 186; 250: G427–G431.
48. Rothbaum R, McAdams AJ, Giannella R, et al: A clinicopathologic study of enterocyte-adherent *Escherichia coli*: A cause of protracted diarrhea in infants. Gastroenterology 1982; 83:441–454.
49. Harris J, Shields R: Absorption and secretion of water and electrolytes by the intact human colon in diffuse untreated proctocolitis. Gut 1970; 11:27.
50. Gooptu D, Truelove SC, Warner GT: Absorption of electrolytes from the colon in cases of ulcerative colitis and in control subjects. Gut 1969; 10:555.

51. DuPont HL: Rotaviral gastroenteritis—some recent developments. J Infect Dis 1984; 149:663–666.
52. Sack DA, Rhoads M, Molla A, et al: Carbohydrate malabsorption in infants with rotavirus diarrhea. Am J Clin Nutr 1982; 36:1112–1118.
53. Sallon S, Deckelbaum RJ, Schmid II, et al: *Cryptosporidium*, malnutrition, and chronic diarrhea in children. Am J Dis Child 1988; 142:312–315.
54. Kocoshis SA, Cibull ML, Davis TE, et al: Intestinal and pulmonary cryptosporidiosis in an infant with severe combined immune deficiency. J Pediatr Gastroenterol Nutr 1984; 3:149–157.
55. Soave R, Johnson WD: *Cryptosporidium* and *Isopora belli* infections. J Infect Dis 1988; 157:225–229.
56. Moriarty KJ, Turnberg LA: Bacterial toxins and diarrhoea. Clin Gastroenterol 1986; 15:529.
57. Gracey M, Burke V, Robinson J: Aeromonas-associated gastroenteritis. Lancet 1982; 2:1304–1306.
58. Burke V, Gracey M, Robinson J, et al: The microbiology of childhood gastroenteritis: *Aeromonas* species and other infective agents. J Infect Dis 1983; 148:68–74.
59. Nime FA, Burek JK, Page DL, et al: Acute enterocolitis in a human being infected with the protozoan *Cryptosporidium*. Gastroenterology 1976; 70:592–598.
60. Stephen S, Rao KNA, Kumar MS, et al: Human infection with *Aeromonas* species: Varied clinical manifestations. Ann Intern Med 1975; 83:368–369.
61. Whitington PF, Friedman AL, Chesney RW: Gastrointestinal disease in the hemolytic-uremic syndrome. Gastroenterology 1979; 76:728–733.
62. Gransden WR, Damm MA, Anderson JD, et al: Further evidence associating hemolytic-uremic syndrome with infection by verotoxin producing *Escherichia coli* O157:H7. J Infect Dis 1986; 154:522–523.
63. Richardson SE, Karmali MA, Becker LE, et al: The histopathology of hemolytic-uremic syndrome associated with verocytotoxin-producing *Escherichia coli* infections. Hum Pathol 1988; 19:1102–1108.
64. Pai CH, Gordon R, Sims HV, et al: Sporadic cases of hemorrhagic colitis associated with *Escherichia coli* O157:H7: Clinical, epidemiologic, and bacteriologic features. Ann Intern Med 1984; 101:738–742.
65. Avery GB, Villavicencio O, Lilly JR, et al: Intractable diarrhea in early infancy. Pediatrics 1968; 41:712.
66. Larcher VF, Shepherd R, Francis DEM, et al: Protracted diarrhea of infancy. Arch Dis Child 1977; 52:597.
67. Lo CW, Walker WA: Chronic protracted diarrhea of infancy: A nutritional disease. Pediatrics 1983; 72:786.
68. Goldgar CM, Vanderhoof JA: Lack of correlation of small bowel biopsy and clinical course of patients with intractable diarrhea of infancy. Gastroenterology 1986; 90:527–532.
69. Hill DJ, Davidson FP, Cameron DJS, et al: The spectrum of cow's milk allergy in childhood. Acta Paediatr Scand 1979; 68:847.
70. Iyngkaran N, Robinson MH, Prathap K, et al: Cow's milk protein-sensitive enteropathy: Combined clinical and histological criteria for diagnosis. Arch Dis Child 1978; 53:20.
71. Mirakian R, Richardson A, Milla PJ, et al: Protracted diarrhoea of infancy: Evidence in support of an autoimmune variant. Br Med J 1986; 193:113–116.
72. Zoppi G, Deganello A, Gaburro D: Persistent post-enteritis diarrhoea. Eur J Pediatr 1977; 126:225.
73. Iyngkaran N, Robinson MH, Sumithran E, et al: Cow's milk protein-sensitive enteropathy: An important factor in prolonging diarrhoea of acute infective enteritis in early infancy. Arch Dis Child 1978; 53:150.
74. Davidson GP, Cutz E, Hamilton JR, et al: Familiar enteropathy: A syndrome of protracted diarrhea from birth, failure to thrive, and hypoplastic villous atrophy. Gastroenterology 1978; 75:783.
75. Goutet JM, Boccon-Gibod L, Chatelet F, et al: Familiar protracted diarrhoea with hypoplastic villous atrophy: Report of two cases. Pediatr Res 1982; 16:1045.
76. Phillips AD, Jenkins P, Raafat F, et al: Congenital microvillous atrophy: specific diagnostic features. Arch Dis Child 1985; 60:730.
77. Schmitz J, Ginies JL, Arnaud-Battandier F, et al: Congenital microvillous atrophy, a rare cause of neonatal intractable diarrhoea. Pediatr Res 1982; 16:1014.
78. Mirakian R, Richardson A, Milla PJ, et al: Protracted diarrhoea of infancy: Evidence in support of an autoimmune variant. Br Med J 1986; 293:1132.
79. Unsworth J, Hutchins P, Mitchell J, et al: Flat small intestinal mucosa and autoantibodies against the gut epithelium. J Pediatr Gastroenterol Nutr 1982; 1:503.
80. Ackerman NB, Strobel CT: Polle syndrome: Chronic diarrhea in Munchausen's child. Gastroenterology 1981; 81:1140.
81. Pickering LK, Kohl S: Munchausen syndrome by proxy. Am J Dis Child 1981; 135:288.
82. Holmberg C: Congenital chloride diarrhoea. Clin Gastroenterol 1986; 15:583.
83. Clark EB, Vanderhoof JA: Effects of acetazolamide on electrolyte balance in congenital chloridorrhea. J Pediatr 1977; 91:148–149.
84. Davidson M, Wasserman R: The irritable colon of childhood (chronic nonspecific diarrhea syndrome). J Pediatr 1966; 69:1027–1038.
85. Davidson M: Functional problems associated with colonic dysfunction: The irritable bowel syndrome. Pediatr Ann 1987; 16:776–795.
86. Greene HL, Ghishan FK: Excessive fluid intake as a cause of chronic diarrhea in young children. J Pediatr 1982; 102:836–840.
87. Cohen SA, Hendrics KM, Mathis RK, et al: Chronic nonspecific diarrhea: Dietary relationships. Pediatrics 1979; 64:402–407.
88. Lloyd-Still JD: Chronic diarrhea of childhood and the misuse of elimination diets. J Pediatr 1979; 95:10–13.
89. Groothuis JR, Berman S, Chapman J: Effect of carbohydrate ingested on outcome in infants with mild gastroenteritis. J Pediatr 1986; 25:85–88.
90. Klish WJ, Udall JN, Rodriguez JT, et al: Intestinal surface area in infants with acquired monosaccharide intolerance. J Pediatr 1978; 92:566–571.
91. Trounce JQ, Walker-Smith JA: Sugar intolerance complicating acute gastroenteritis. Arch Dis Child 1985; 60:986–990.
92. Phillips AD, Walker-Smith JA: Delayed recovery in childhood. *In* Walker-Smith JA, McNeish AS, eds: Diarrhoea and Malnutrition in Childhood. London, Butterworths, 1986, pp 107–112.
93. Farthing MJG, Mata LJ, Urutia JJ, et al: Natural history of *Giardia* infection of infants and children in rural Guatemala and its impact on physical growth. Am J Clin Nutr 1986; 43:393–403.
94. Goka AKJ, Rolston DDK, Mathan VI, et al: Diagnosis of giardiasis by specific IgM antibody enzyme-linked immunosorbent assay. Lancet 1986; 2:184–186.
95. Ungar BLP, Yolken RH, Nash TE, et al: Enzyme-linked immunosorbent assay for detection of *Giardia lamblia* in fecal specimens. J Infect Dis 1984; 149:90–97.
96. Maki M, Hallstrom O, Vesikari T, et al: Evaluation of serum IgA-class reticulin antibody test for the detection of childhood celiac disease. J Pediatr 1984; 105:901–905.
97. Eade DE, Lloyd RS, Lang C, et al: IgA and IgG reticulin antibodies in celiac and non-celiac patients. Gut 1977; 18:991–993.
98. Burgin-Wolff A, Bertele RM, Berger R, et al: A reliable screening test for childhood celiac disease: Fluorescent immunosorbent test for gliadin antibodies. J Pediatr 1963; 102:655–660.

Chapter 16

Constipation and Encopresis

ALLAN J. ROSENBERG

INTRODUCTION

Constipation and encopresis are common in infants and children. It is estimated that 10 to 25% of children referred to pediatric gastroenterology practices are seen for disorders of defecation.[1, 2] The pediatrician and pediatric gastroenterologist must understand and treat these disorders from infancy through adolescence. Chronic constipation in adults has been defined as a gastrointestinal disorder consisting of hard stools, fewer than three bowel movements per week, or the inability to expel stool, whether hard or soft, that lasts longer than 6 weeks.[3] No clear definition exists in pediatrics. Confusion frequently arises from a failure to appreciate the wide variation in bowel habits in normal children.

Constipation should be considered a symptom, not a diagnosis, and may be a manifestation of a wide variety of disorders and secondary to various medications (Tables 16–1 and 16–2).

Constipation is the result of impaired colonic propulsion of luminal contents (fecal retention) or an increased outlet resistance due to pelvic or anorectal dysfunction (difficulty in defecation).

In pediatrics, unresolved constipation may lead to fecal retention and impaction, with overflow incontinence causing soiling or encopresis. The term *encopresis* was originally coined by Weissenberg in 1926, building on the term *enuresis,* to describe children with true psychogenic soiling, or the voluntary passage of whole bowel movements in the underwear or another unusual place.[4]

Kanner[5] defined encopresis as "the act of involuntary defecation which is not directly due to organic illness." Subsequently, the term has been used synonymously with the broader concept of fecal incontinence or soiling and can be defined as the regular deposition by a child of formed or semiformed stools in the underwear (or other unorthodox locations) after the age of 4 years.

Confusion exists in the medical literature regarding the diagnosis and management of encopresis, which seems to stem from the failure to recognize that fecal incontinence may occur with or without constipation. The physiologic and psychological mechanisms associated with incontinence in the constipated child represent a specific entity, distinct from incontinence in the child who does not have constipation. Easson[6] has subdivided the encopretic syndrome into (1) primary infantile encopresis (never toilet trained, not constipated); (2) primary reactive encopresis (never toilet trained, constipated with overflow); (3) secondary infantile encopresis (toilet trained, regression to incontinence without constipation); and (4) secondary reactive encopresis (toilet trained, incontinence with constipation). This chapter attempts to provide an understanding of and treatment approach for the major defecation problems in children: chronic constipation and encopresis.

Although population studies are limited, soiling has been noted in 1.3% of those children older than 4 years of age[7] and in 1 to 2% of 7-year-old children.[8] In elementary school–aged children, the incidence varies from 1.5 to 7.5% of children.[9] A similar or even higher frequency of intermittent soiling in those children of school age is suspected. Bellman[10] found encopresis in 1.5% of second grade youngsters. Levine[11] studied a large general pediatric clinic population over an 18-month period and found 102 cases of encopresis, which included approximately 3% of the population older than 4 years of age.

The ratio of boys to girls varies from study to study but is approximately 6:1.[11] The disorder shows little or no preference for social class. There is no evidence that it is related to family size, ordinal position of the child in the family, or age of the parents.[12] One study has reported that concordance for constipation was fourfold higher in monozygotic than in dizygotic twins.[13] Soiling in childhood often accompanies or follows constipation. In most of the children, no organic cause can be detected, and the accumulation of feces in the rectal ampulla is the only documented abnormality.[12–14] This fecal impaction may result from either a decreased urge to defecate or difficulty in stool expulsion. Reduced feeling secondary to rectal distention[10] could explain the decreased urge to defecate. Robinson and Gibbons[15] demonstrated that active anal contraction during defecation obstructs the anal outlet, causing fecal retention in soiling children. Soiling then occurs as a consequence of a chronically filled rectum with overflow of stool. Treatment is multimodal, using lubricants and bowel

Table 16–1. CONSTIPATING CONDITIONS

Dysfunctional State
Developmental
Cognitive handicaps
Attention deficit
Situational
Excessive parental interventions
Coercive toilet training
Toilet phobia
School bathroom avoidance
Psychogenic
Depression
Anorexia nervosa
Constitutional
Genetic predisposition
Colonic inertia
Reduced volume and drying
Low-fiber diet
Dehydration
Malnutrition, underfeeding
Faulty diet—excessive milk
Altered Anatomy and Physiology
Structural
Anal stenosis
Imperforate anus
Anterior displaced anus
Acquired inflammatory stricture
Necrotizing enterocolitis
Inflammatory bowel disease
Malrotation, congenital intestinal bands
Abdominal pelvic masses
Anterior sacral meningomyelocele
Sacral teratoma
Aganglionosis and abnormal myenteric plexus
Hirschsprung's disease, congenital
Chagas' disease, acquired
Intestinal pseudo-obstruction
Abnormal abdominal musculature
Prune belly
Gastroschisis
Abnormal innervation
Meningomyelocele
Spinal cord tumor
Hypotonia
Cerebral palsy
Amyotonia congenita
Familial visceral myopathy
Connective tissue disorder
Scleroderma
Amyloidosis
Mixed connective tissue disease
Lupus erythematosus
Metabolic or Endocrine Dysfunction
Hypothyroidism
Hypercalcemia
Lead ingestion
Diabetes mellitus
Panhypopituitarism
Drugs
See Table 16–2

habit training to relieve constipation and a biofeedback training to enhance anal function and prevent soiling.

CLINICAL PRESENTATION

The diagnosis of chronic constipation and encopresis is based on an appropriate history and physical examination demonstrating a dilated rectum containing excessive stool, usually opposing the anal verge. Occasionally, other studies are indicated (Table 16–3).

The history obtained in a manner that avoids arousing defensive reactions from the parents usually proves the most rewarding investigative procedure. Call and associates[16] found three characteristic difficulties in the parent-child relationships of children with fecal retention. The first problem was the lack of a sense of comfort and security that allows the child to communicate with the parents and the parent to sense the communication, understand it, and respond in a helpful way. A second type of disturbance in the parent-child relationship that contributes to fecal withholding is the parent who is excessively preoccupied with the child's anal and bowel functions. The third characteristic difficulty is psychologically traumatic experiences with toileting. The cardinal feature of encopresis is withholding, or "hoarding," of stool. Parents frequently fail to recognize this phenomenon. To the parent, successful toilet training is a milestone in the process of normal social development. For the child, cooperation with the training process may be a rewarding experience, or the process may become a focus of the child's determination to exert his or her own will.

Levine[11] suggests three development periods that appear critical in the generation of encopresis: period I (Early Experience and Predisposition) covers the first 2

Table 16–2. AGENTS ASSOCIATED WITH CONSTIPATION IN CHILDREN AND ADULTS

Minerals
Aluminum containing (antacids and sucralfate)
Calcium supplements
Barium sulfate
Bismuth
Opiates and Antimotility Agents
Codeine
Diphenoxylate (Lomotil)
Lopramide (Imodium)
Antihypertensive and Antiarrhythmic Agents
Calcium channel blockers
Clonidine (Catapres)
Disopyramide (Norpace)
Anticholinergic and Antispasmodic Agents
Phenothiazines
Neuroleptics
Antihistamines
Dicyclomine (Bentyl)
Hyoscyamine (Levsin, Donnatol)
Tricyclic Antidepressants
Methylphenidate (Ritalin)
Antiparkinsonism Drugs
Sympathomimetic Agents
Ephedrine
Isoproterenol
Phenylephrine
Phenylpropanolamine
Pseudoephedrine
Terbutaline
Nonsteroidal Anti-inflammatory Drugs
Diuretics
Heavy Metal Ingestion
Arsenic
Lead
Mercury

Table 16–3. EVALUATION OF CHRONIC CONSTIPATION AND ENCOPRESIS

History
Bowel movements in toilet
Frequency
Consistency
Size
Encopresis—"accidents"
Age at onset
Duration
Size
Frequency
Patterns (time of day)
Past history
Birth history
Patterns of stooling in infancy
Toileting history
Dietary history—milk and fiber intake
Associated symptoms
Straining
Pain
Urgency
Diarrhea
Urinary incontinence
Physical Examination
Abdominal examination
Presence of palpable fecal material
Anorectal examination
Location of anus
Prolapse, perianal inflammation, and fissures
Tone of anal canal, "wink" reflex
Presence of fecal impaction
Initial Investigation Prior to Treatment
Stool log for daily toileting and accidents
Time
Consistency
Quantity
Diet log
Additional Studies
Plain radiograph of abdomen
Barium enema
Rectal motility and electromyography of pelvic floor and external anal sphincter
Gut transit studies
Defacography
Rectal biopsy

years of life; period II (Training and Autonomy) includes a span from ages 2 to 5 years; and period III (Extramural Function) encompasses the early school years. As children pass through these periods, constitutional predispositions, circumstances of environment, and critical life events become cumulative and potentiate the functional bowel disorder. The absence of symptoms in the first 6 months of life is important in excluding Hirschsprung's disease. The age at onset in chronic constipation and encopresis may be less than 1 year (25%) but is usually between 2 and 4 years. Of 119 children with constipation described by Davidson and coworkers,[17] when the constipation began in infancy, 76 of the 119 children were encopretic. Irrespective of when the symptoms lead to referral, many children with severe chronic idiopathic constipation experience an early onset of their problem. The incidence of both constipation and encopresis increases markedly at a time when the processes of development are allowing the toddler to gain control over defecation. Whatever the underlying cause, constipation was found by Levine[18] to have begun before the training period in nearly half of the patients.

Children whose past history suggests significant bowel dysfunction during infancy or as a toddler may be revealing a constitutional or congenital predisposition to encopresis. "Early colonic inertia" has been described as an endogenous tendency toward immature or generally inefficient bowel function.[19] Further potentiation of encopresis in this age group may be induced by parental overreaction, as extremes of joy or anger surrounding defecation may engender excessive bowel preoccupation on the part of the developing child. Aggressive management can lead to dysfunction; for example, excessive use of suppositories and enemas, digital manipulation, and other coercive offenses may create a so-called "anal stamp."[12] Anthony[12] observed: "The battle of the bowel seemingly won in the nursery is destined to be lost on the playing field at school." Infants or toddlers themselves may potentiate impaired function by voluntary withholding. As defecation starts to be perceived as a negative experience, the child "strains" during the urge to defecate. The parents observe the child standing with the legs hyperextended or in a crouched position, grunting and "squeezing," flushed, and obviously uncomfortable; and they assume this behavior represents an effort on the child's part to defecate, especially when there is a history of previous constipation. In reality, however, this is an effort to retain rather than to expel the bowel movement. During such an episode, a small portion of fecal material often escapes and is accepted as support of the parents' misinterpretation. Fissures and other forms of perianal irritation may result from constipation and potentiate chronic bowel difficulty by encouraging further withholding.

A report of voluntary stool withholding prior to the customary age of experimentation with the sphincter strongly suggests an anal fissure or other organic cause as the initiating mechanism for the child's desire to avoid defecation. A history of coercive toilet training is obtainable with many encopretic children. By the time parents seek medical attention for their child's encopresis, they often have become defensive about their toilet-training practices, and the history obtained may not be reliable. Attempts to accomplish toilet training at an inappropriately early age, that is, before the child possesses the ability to control evacuation, must be looked on as coercion. In general, encopresis is not recognized until the age at which the child is expected to be toilet trained is exceeded. Professional and lay opinions vary widely as to this age limit. The age at which toilet training begins varies substantially both in and between populations. Accepted values for a given cultural group include 2 years of age in North America and England, 3 years in France and Scandinavia, and elsewhere up to 6 years of age.[20] During the preschool years, children explore new frontiers of independence. To the developing child, bowel training and the newly acquired control it offers represent a major step forward. To some vulnerable youngsters, toileting is marred by fear, power struggles, and fantasy. During this stage, children who have demonstrated bowel vulnerability earlier are likely to continue to accumulate potentiating factors. Apprehension of the toilet may represent an initial potentiator of dysfunction in a child who has no previous history of bowel problems. It has been reported that inappropriate training techniques, such as extremes of coercion or permissiveness, can induce toilet aversion. At this age the presenting complaint may not be constipation, because the parents are inclined to attribute the child's soiling to poor sphincter control. Stool withholding and constipation bear a confused cause-effect relationship with each other. The voluntary retention of feces over a prolonged period leads to the accumulation of a large bolus from which increasing amounts of water are removed through the normal process of absorption. In turn, the presence of such a bolus may be responsible for the child's efforts to avoid any evacuation that he or she knows will be painful.

This soiling is usually the expression of so-called "paradoxical" diarrhea, in which fluid intestinal contents flow around a large bolus of hard fecal material in the rectum. It is understandable that parents, and even physicians, may misinterpret the nature of the incontinence. Of 76 such children described by Davidson and colleagues,[17] 10% had, at one time or other, been given the diagnosis of diarrhea. A distended rectum can result in diminished bladder capacity and some urinary "dribbling" during the day. Urinary problems (enuresis and urinary tract infection) are not uncommon with constipation; rectal prolapse is unusual. Treatment of the stool retention usually improves urologic symptoms. Encopresis at night is rare as compared with enuresis. Abrahamian and Lloyd-Still[21] noted that definable events, such as diet changes, rectal fissures, intercurrent illness, moving to a new home, changing schools, birth of a sibling, travel, and family problems, are present at onset in some instances. Other signs or symptoms occurring frequently in those who also soil can include abdominal pain, fecal impaction, poor appetite, and poor weight gain. Those suffering from recurrent abdominal pain tend to be children with relatively recent onset of stool retention and incontinence. Those with long-standing encopresis generally have acquired a tolerance to colonic distention and seldom complain of pain.

The typically encopretic preschool child has stools infrequently, usually once every 4 or 5 days, and, in some instances, only once every 10 to 14 days. After a week or two of retention, the child develops abdominal discomfort, is reluctant to eat, becomes irritable, and avoids play. As the urge to defecate becomes more frequent, overflow soilage and retentive posturing recur more often. Several days of increasing discomfort culminate in the very distressful passage of a stool in an amount often large enough to plug the toilet. After passing the stool, the child is dramatically relieved of discomfort. His or her mood, playfulness, and appetite immediately return to normal. Retentive posturing and overflow soiling often stop for a few days.

Regardless of its origins, stool withholding usually leads to aggressive intervention by parents to alleviate the child's apparent constipation. These efforts generally include enemas as well as a host of laxative substances. Many of these children display their aversion to enemas by struggling or crying, and those who do not are just as likely to resent the process. In one study,[22] encopretic children undergoing psychotherapy indicated by the pictures they drew that they regarded enemas as a punitive measure. Even if one ignores the element of discomfort that may attend an enema, it is not surprising that the encopretic child reacts negatively to a procedure that is contrary to the original goal, that is, withholding of stool.

Parents may fail to recognize that the olfactory sensory apparatus accommodates to odors that are constantly present, that people have limited awareness of their own body smells, and, therefore, that children with chronic incontinence are insensitive to the offensive odor of their own products.[23] During the early school years, children with other potentiating factors may be predisposed to encopresis. Children who usually defecate each morning at home may, on entering school, determine to withhold defecation until they are back in the private safety of their own home.[11] The resulting chronic rectal distention may lead to loss of rectal sensitivity and the normal defecation urge.[17, 18, 24–26] After several months, the child may develop overflow incontinence. During the early school years, children with regular bowel habits can begin to have encopresis following illnesses such as gastroenteritis. Normal bowel rhythms can be interrupted, and the child cannot compensate. When encopresis is potentiated during the school years, a number of factors may be responsible. The loss of rectal and anal sensation is a complicating factor, as is the diminution in colonic muscle tone with chronic bowel distention.

The physical examination is particularly important in assessing the abdominal contents, anal tone and placement, sacral appearance and size, and contents of the rectal ampulla. Fecal masses are often palpable above the pubic symphysis and in the left lower quadrant. Particular attention should be paid to the presence or absence of fecal material within the rectum, any evidence of lesions near the anus that might produce discomfort, and the presence of a normal anal reflex, that is, a visible contraction of the external anal sphincter in response to stroking of the perianal skin. Anterior ectopic anus has been reported by several authors as a common cause of intractable constipation in childhood.[27, 28] The onset of constipation has characteristically been in early infancy. In some children overflow incontinence may occur.[29] Studies have suggested that the internal sphincter may frequently function normally and that the difficulties in defecation may arise directly from the abnormal oblique direction of the anal canal.[30] In some children the anal orifice is located well forward of its normal location, but in others the anterior displacement may be subtle.[27] Reisner and associates[31] studied the location of the anal orifice in normal infants and children. Hendren[29] and Leape and Ramenofsky[28] each found that some patients with idiopathic constipation have an anterior anus. Bar-maor and Eitan[32] established an objective, numeric index for the proper location of the normal anus and the distances between the vagina or scrotum, anus, and coccyx. Anterior displacement was defined as a ratio of less than 0.34 in females and less than 0.46 in males. A plain abdominal radiograph may be helpful in assessing the amount of fecal retention. A barium enema to rule out Hirschsprung's disease may be indicated in the constipated infant but is rarely helpful in the older child. A physiologic definition of constipation can be obtained using rectal manometry and electromyography.[33]

PHYSIOLOGY

To understand the abnormal functioning of altered bowel habits resulting in constipation and encopresis, it is necessary to appreciate what is normal in the pediatric population. The greatest amount of objective data has been gathered on the frequency of the passage of stool.[34] Frequency of stooling is related to gastrointestinal transit time. Mean total intestinal transit times increase with age, being approximately 8.5 hours at 1 to 3 months of age,[35] 16 hours from 4 to 24 months of age,[36] and 26 hours from 3 to 13 years of age.[37] A mean transit time of 26 hours in 65 normal and 80 hours in 65 constipated English children was found by Burkitt and associates.[38] Values range from 30 to 48 hours in young adults. Stool weight appears to vary substantially across ethnic and population boundaries, largely related to diet and fiber intake. An inverse relationship between stool weight and transit time was demonstrated by Burkitt. Fecal consistency is important; the left colon and rectum are not capable of storing liquids whose transit time, from transverse colon to anus, is rapid.[39] Increased fiber intake produces larger stools, whereas diminished fiber leads to decreased stool size. Children pass soft stools weighing approximately 25 gm each. The upper limit of normal adult stool weight for the person consuming a North American diet is 200 gm.

There is a decline in the frequency of defecation with age. Studies[40, 41] from western societies have indicated that 94 to 99% of adults have a bowel action between three times daily and three times weekly. In infants the average number of daily stools rises from 1.4 on the day of birth to approximately 4 per day at 1 week of age. Ninety-seven percent of a group of 800 infants were reported by Nyhan[42] to have between one and nine bowel movements daily during the first week of life. Weaver and associates[43] reported that among 240 infants between the ages of 2 and 20 weeks, half of whom were fed breast milk and half cow's milk formula, 93% had between one and seven bowel movements each day. He found that 85% of 1- to 4-year-old children passed stool once or twice each day.

Anorectal physiology is the study of the mechanisms that ensure fecal continence and the integrity of the pelvic floor when the person is in the erect posture. Fecal continence is achieved by the control of bowel contents that approach the end of their intestinal passage, that is, the unconscious or conscious retention and voluntary release of fecal material in the act of defecation. The three major factors that contribute to fecal continence are a suitable storage organ, an appropriate consistency of stool, and a functional sphincter apparatus. If any of these fails, incontinence may result.

The colon acts as a storage organ that concentrates fecal material by withdrawing water. Motility within the colon mixes the fecal material rather than immediately propelling the contents in a caudad direction. Anal continence is a function of stool consistency, anatomic integrity of the bowel, and the coordinated action of the smooth and striated muscles. Specialized anatomy and physiology of the anorectal region determine the combination of physical factors and reflexes that control defecation.

The rectum serves as a storage compartment, whereas the pelvic floor muscles and two anal sphincters (internal and external) regulate fecal contents (air, solids, or liquid) as well as the impending desire to defecate or pass gas.[44] Colon compliance, the flap valve functions of the flexures and rectal valves, and a reverse motility gradient in the rectosigmoid area help maintain continence.

The most important structures in the process of defecation are the internal and external anal sphincters and the anorectal angle produced by the muscles of the pelvic floor.[45] It has been reported that the external sphincter can remain maximally contracted for only about 40 seconds, after which it becomes fatigued.[46, 47] The angle at the rectosigmoid junction provides an obstacle to propulsion of viscous fluids such as stools. The axis of the rectum forms approximately a right angle with the axis of the anal canal and is created by the continuous tonic contraction of the striated puborectal muscle. This angle is present except when the hips are flexed more than 90 degrees or during defecation. The lumen of the rectum ends at the pelvic floor, where it passes through the levator ani muscles and continues as the anal canal. This canal is surrounded by the internal and external anal sphincters, which overlap each other. Both the internal and the external anal sphincters have a resting tone that creates a high-pressure zone in the anal canal. This zone represents a barrier to rectal pressure and is thought to be a mechanism for continence.

The external anal sphincter contributes only 10 to 15% of the resting anal pressure but serves an important function in maintaining continence by reflex contraction in response to the transient rise in intra-abdominal pressure. The external anal sphincter contracts under voluntary control. This voluntary contraction of the external anal sphincter and puborectal muscles can extend the period of continence and presumably allow the rectum to accommodate the increased volume with a disappearance of the sense of urgency.

Continence of solid stool is not related to the external anal sphincter, because this can be divided without resulting in incontinence. Continence for flatus and liquid is a function of the closed anal canal maintained by the internal anal sphincter. The external anal sphincter functions to preserve voluntary continence when loose stool overcomes the primary mechanisms of continence.

At intervals, often during the postprandial period, the colon delivers stool to the rectal ampulla. A sensation of fullness or the urge to defecate results from activation of stretch receptors in the rectal and pelvic muscular walls when they are distended by air or stool. Distention of the rectum by a bolus of stool from the proximal bowel results in a characteristic reflex relaxation (the rectosphincteric relaxation reflex) of the internal anal sphincter. The internal anal sphincter is inhibited, reducing its tonic partial resting pressure[45, 48] and allowing defecation in response to rectal distention. Mucosal receptors detect the presence of these contents and can distinguish between solid and fluid matter; the person is thus made aware of the "call to stool."[45]

During defecation, the person adopts a sitting or squatting position and performs a Valsalva maneuver, thus increasing intra-abdominal pressure. These voluntary acts are accompanied by contraction of the levator ani and coccygeal muscles, which oppose downward descent of the pelvic floor. In the flexed squatting position, the angle formed by the puborectalis is such that its contraction cannot occlude the lumen of the distal rectum. Both increased intra-abdominal pressure and hip flexion tend to straighten the anorectal angle. Increased intra-abdominal pressure promotes the forward movement of feces from both the distal colon and the rectum. Simultaneously, the external anal sphincter relaxes, permitting the passage of feces through the anal canal. The ability to voluntarily withhold stool develops at varying ages estimated at between 6 and 18 months.

PATHOPHYSIOLOGY AND ETIOLOGY

The pattern of hoarding may begin if the child becomes motivated to avoid having a stool after having already learned how voluntarily to resist evacuation. This motivation may already be present should defecation be associated with discomfort, for example, in the presence of an anal fissure, a fistula in ano, or a tendency toward constipation on a dietary basis. Occasionally, an associated reduction in fluid intake produces transitory constipation. The accompanying discomfort from defecation may lead to withholding of stool. Such fecal withholding is ordinarily temporary but may become prolonged if the child's anxieties are increased by overly aggressive therapy leading to chronic constipation and encopresis.

New techniques are available to investigate the pathophysiology of disorders involving the anal sphincters, rectum, and pelvic floor, for example, anorectal manometry, electromyography, radiographic defecography (dynamic radiographs of defecation), intestinal transit studies, and rectal compliance.

In the absence of secondary causes of constipation, patterns of colonic dysmotility can be characterized and quantified by anorectal manometry and measurement of colonic transit time. Anorectal manometry, a technique used frequently in pediatrics, should be considered in children with severe constipation to determine the resistance to rectal distention, the anal resting tone, the strength of voluntary anal contractions, and the patient's ability to sense rectal distention (rectal sensation) and to evaluate the rectosphincteric reflex. It is important that anal manometry be performed by experienced, well-trained personnel to avoid factors that may lead to the misinterpretation of the test. This includes chronic, uncorrected rectal distention by fecal impaction. Studies of anorectal and distal colonic motility in children with chronic constipation have demonstrated functional abnormalities in nearly all cases.

Anorectal manometry measures pressure and is a means of quantifying the function of the internal and external anal sphincters. The fact that there is no accepted standardized method of performing anal sphincter manometry may account for inconsistencies that occur from study to study. Pressure measurements in the rectum and anal canal are recorded using either microtipped intraluminal pressure transducers,[49] water perfusion catheters, or stationary intra-anal balloons connected to external pressure transducers. Pressures in the anorectal canal are usually measured at 1-cm intervals using a stationary pull-through technique or a continuous pull-out method. The anal canal is defined as the region with resting tone at least 5 mm Hg higher than that in the rectum, showing a motor activity pattern (minor and major waves) different from that in the rectum and reflex relaxation of tone during rectal distention. The highest anal resting tone is located 1 to 1.5 cm from the anal verge. This region is used to study the motor activity of the internal anal sphincter as well as the reflex relaxation of that sphincter during rectal distention. The mean length of the anal canal was found by Holschneider[50] and Arhan and associates[51] to be 3 cm (range 2–5 cm) in children 4 to 12 years of age. There is wide variation in reported resting anal pressure in healthy children. Using perfused catheters, the recorded mean anal pressure was approximately 15 mm Hg. Using a balloon system, mean anal resting pressure was found to be 29 mm Hg by Varma and Stephens,[52] and 38 mm Hg by Arhan and colleagues.[51] Schuster,[53] using a similar system, reported that anal resting pressure was 50 to 90 mm Hg in infants, which is higher than those values found in other studies.

Loening-Baucke[26] found an average anal resting pressure of 53 mm Hg in normal children and 62 mm Hg in constipated children. Meunier and coworkers[54] reported an anal resting pressure at age 1 to 15 years of 52 ± 10 mm Hg. Using a solid-state intraluminal transducer probe, the author found that anal resting tone in constipated children had a range of 30 to 60 mm Hg.

An inflatable rectal balloon is attached to a catheter to study the effects of rectal distention. The rectal balloon is inflated to elicit the presence of the rectosphincteric reflex, that is, relaxation of the internal anal sphincter and contraction of the external anal sphincter. Threshold volume is the amount of air required to initiate reflex internal anal sphincter relaxation and is critical in normal defecation, particularly as it relates to the volume required to initiate internal anal sphincter relaxation. The threshold volume has been shown to be increased in constipation. The smallest volume injected into the rectal balloon that induces an amplitude of at least 5 mm Hg determines the rectosphincteric reflex threshold, which ranges from 10 to 25 ml in control patients and from 5 to 30 ml in constipated children. The mean rectosphincteric reflex threshold has not been found to be significantly different in control subjects and constipated children. However, there are a few studies[53, 55–57] that demonstrated an increased rectosphincteric reflex. The volume of constant relaxation, or threshold volume required to induce a long-lasting relaxation of the internal anal sphincter, has also been reported to be increased in children with chronic constipation.[26] The depth of reflex internal anal sphincter relaxation may be decreased in severe constipation. The volume of rectal distention required to produce conscious awareness is the rectal sensory threshold volume. Rectosphincteric reflex and rectal sensory threshold volume increase in parallel in constipation without encopresis[57]; internal anal sphincter relaxation often occurs before conscious awareness is elicited, thus increasing the risk of inadvertent soiling. This relates to a history of not sensing the urge to defecate before soiling occurs.

In normal subjects the rectosphincteric reflex is close to the threshold for conscious rectal sensation. Soiling may occur because the volume of stool required to initiate conscious rectal sensation is increased relative to the volume of stool required to initiate internal sphincter relaxation.[2, 24] Indeed, children with chronic idiopathic constipation have been found to have a decreased rectal sensitivity as demonstrated by a raised conscious threshold. The volume threshold of transient sensation has been reported to be increased in children with chronic constipation in most,[2, 58–60] but not all,[26, 61] studies. The rectum may fail to empty if its elastic properties are decreased, leading to a greater distensibility and higher threshold to trigger a rectoanal inhibitory reflex.[62]

Some children have evidence of anal outlet obstruction. They have difficulties with the expulsion of simulated stools from the rectum, and they fail to relax or actively may contract the external anal sphincter during attempted defecation. Relaxation induced by large volumes of distention may be diminished or of normal amplitude. A decreased depth of internal sphincter relaxation during defecation could result in anal outlet obstruction owing to a persistently high pressure in the distal anal canal. Increased anal pressure in chronic constipation has been reported in several studies using varied measurement techniques.[55, 56, 58] Inadequate relaxation of the puborectal muscle can also cause outlet obstruction.[63] Children who are chronically constipated may contract both the puborectal muscle and the external anal sphincter instead of relaxing them.[64, 65]

Arhan and colleagues[55] found that the anus is hypertonic in chronically constipated children and that the threshold for a rectoanal inhibitory reflex is raised. Ogorek and Reynolds[66] performed anorectal manometry on 12 normal children and 18 patients suffering from constipation and soiling. In both groups the results of the rectoanal inhibitory reflex and the squeezing anal pressure were similar. The pressure recording in all the normal children showed that the anal canal relaxed during defecation. Fourteen constipated children (78%) closed the anal canal while straining by contracting the anal sphincter. This supports the notion that paradoxical contraction appears to be the cause of chronic constipation.

However, Loening-Baucke[26] found that the resting anal tone was reduced when recorded with a pressure transducer located statically in the anal canal. Reynolds[67] and Martelli and associates[68] in separate studies demonstrated anorectal outlet obstruction in about one third of chronically constipated patients. Meunier[64] found 36% of the children with encopresis exhibited an inappropriate increase in pressure at the level of the external sphincter during simulated defecation, compared with 10% of the control children. Anal achalasia, defined as failure of anal relaxation during the Valsalva maneuver, was present initially in 60% of the author's patients and 77% of Meunier's patients.[64] Karen and coworkers[65] demonstrated an increase in anal pressure during attempted defecation in 78% of children with chronic constipation and encopresis. In control subjects there was a decrease in anal pressure during attempted defecation, and the paradoxical closure of the canal seen in the patient group differed from that seen during voluntary anal squeeze in that there was an associated rise in rectal pressure. In studying the ability to expel water-filled balloons of various volumes, constipated children exerted pressures on the water-filled rectal balloons similar to those of control children, but their ability to expel the balloon was significantly decreased. Read and Timms[69] found that adult incontinent patients were abnormal with regard to their ability to retain a solid sphere in the rectum as weights were applied and were unable to retain saline infused into the rectum. However, constipated patients were no different from control subjects in their ability to detect the presence of fluid infused into the rectum. Fourteen encopretics (45%) exhibited external sphincter contraction during expulsion, compared with only one control subject. It appears that the ability or inability to defecate balloons was independent of rectal sensation or rectal size. This finding adds to the considerable evidence that some chronically constipated children may have an abnormality of defecation dynamics characterized by a failure of external anal sphincter relaxation.

Gastrointestinal transit velocity can be measured for the entire intestinal tract or for the colon and its segments. Constipation may be defined by the delay in gastrointestinal transit that is usually in the colon.[42, 70] In adults, three patterns emerge: (1) transit is slow in all segments of the colon, with definite dysfunction of the right colon, known as *colonic inertia;* (2) delay may occur in the left colon and rectosigmoid areas, described as *hindgut dysfunction;* and (3) there may be isolated prolongation of rectosigmoid passage, termed *outlet obstruction*.

The whole-gut transit time as studied by the passage of radiopaque markers has been reported to be significantly prolonged in children with constipation.[37, 71] Markers were found to occupy various segments of the colon and the rectum for prolonged periods in 61% of those with constipation. Clearance was reported to be delayed in the distal colon or rectum, or both, in 42% and in the proximal colon and distal colon and rectum in 19%. When constipation is due to colonic inertia, the passage of markers is delayed, and they may remain distributed throughout the left and right colon for more than 5 days.[67]

A study by Vajro and associates[72] employed the breath hydrogen method to estimate anorectal transit time in children suffering from constipation. The transit rate of a lactulose test solution was unaltered, but that of a semisolid nutrient meal was significantly prolonged.

Electromyography of the pelvic floor and external sphincter is a useful method of evaluating chronically constipated patients. In normal subjects there is continuous tonic activity of the striated muscle of the pelvic floor at rest, and in most of the subjects, inhibition of this activity can be demonstrated during straining. Using external cutaneous electrodes, a decrease in activity in the external sphincter during defecation was detected in all the control children but in only 42% of those with abdominal pain and constipation. Lennard-Jones[73] reported the results of electromyography in 15 constipated patients. There was a normal response to coughing, but a marked and sustained rise in anal canal pressure occurred on straining associated with increased activity of the external sphincter. In the constipated patients no inhibition of electrical activity was seen in either the puborectal or the external sphincter muscles, but rather there was increased activity in one or both of these muscles associated with the rise in anal canal pressure. Dynamic studies of defecation to assess the anorectal angle and the ability to retain fluid infused in the rectum are now used in evaluating adult patients.

Increased anal pressure and an inability to sufficiently relax the anal canal to allow defecation may lead to retention and encopresis. Therapy aimed at normalizing anal relaxation can restore continence.[74]

MANAGEMENT

The pediatrician or family physician can help prevent chronic constipation by providing anticipatory guidance to parents concerning normal bowel function and the early detection of problems. Advice regarding toilet training should be an integral part of health supervision. The physician must remember that many parents are reluctant to ask questions and turn instead to uninformed sources. Brief discussions with the family about toilet training during routine visits for the child from 6 months to 3 years of age can help prevent toileting problems.

The goals of therapy for chronic constipation and encopresis are to terminate soiling, establish regular bowel habits, restore the urge to defecate, and prevent reimpaction. The cumulative published data suggest that treatment with multiple modalities is usually more successful than that with a single therapy.[75] Most children are successfully treated; however, children with "voluntary" fecal incontinence without megarectum or impaction are resistant to therapy.[76]

Children with evidence of initial or persisting psychosocial or emotional problems should be referred for appropriate consultation and therapy. Patients with an atypical history should prompt the physician to review the differential diagnosis of this condition, searching for other causes. Anorectal manometry effectively excludes Hirschsprung's disease and provides information about defecatory dynamics that enhances biobehavioral treatment. A few causes of constipation require surgical intervention, including Hirschsprung's disease, Chagas' disease, East African megacolon, and pseudo-obstruction in some patients.

Management of the infant begins with education of the parents concerning normal bowel habits and frequency and the occurrence of withholding behaviors. Critical features in infancy include an understanding of the variable patterns of normal stooling, correct interpretation of normal defecatory straining, and limited use of physical interventions. Overly vigorous treatment may reaffirm in the parent's or child's mind the potential for serious pathology.

Judicious use of glycerin suppositories in the infant with constipation may be helpful.[64] Local agents (enemas and suppositories) distend or irritate the colon and rectum and initiate reflex evacuation.[3] Repeated finger dilations, enemas, digital disimpactions, and frequent suppositories should be avoided. The attitudes toward enemas displayed by children in Pinkerton's study[22] indicate the potential aggravating hazards of the use of enemas for diagnostic or therapeutic purposes in encopretic children. The risk of water intoxication from large tap water enemas is as great with functional megacolon as with Hirschsprung's disease. Later in the first year, an increasingly varied solid food intake containing fiber may be helpful. Excessive milk intake leading to a low-residue, high-protein, and high-calcium diet should be avoided. Hard, pellet-like stools may respond to oral supplementation with luminally active agents, such as dark Karo syrup (up to 1 tsp per oz per feeding) and lactulose.

In the toddler and preschool child who presents with active stool-withholding behavior of short duration, therapy consisting of one to two cleansing enemas, followed by increasing dietary fiber and assisted daily evacuation for several weeks with mineral oil therapy, is usually enough to restore a normal defecation pattern and reduce soiling. Maintaining the rectum empty of retained stool over time results in a decrease in rectal size and an increase in rectal sensitivity to distention.[17]

The classic approach proposed by Davidson and associates[17] for chronic constipation in the preschool- and school-aged child still forms the basis of treatment. He divided management into three phases: the initial phase (evaluation), the second phase (regulation and motivation), and the third phase (continuation). The program described by Levine[11] for the school-aged child incorporates the traditional elements of bowel cleansing, maintenance therapy to prevent stool retention, modification of diet, habit training,[77] and behavioral modification. Rappaport and colleagues[78] noted a good outcome in children with better compliance and an internal locus of control. Locus of control reflects the child's belief that he or she can control life events. These variables were independent of each other and were not associated with perceived self-confidence or predicted by socioeconomic status, age, duration of symptoms, gender, or severity. Risk for a poor outcome has been related to poor compliance and significant coexisting psychiatric problems. Levine and Bakow[79] noted risk features, included learning disabilities, disobedience, fearlessness, difficult toilet training, school-time soiling, lack of associated constipation, and teenage occurrence. Mental deficiency associated with severe motor impairment often causes resistant constipation.

A complete history and physical examination will confirm the diagnosis in most children. The treatment program must be effectively communicated to the parents and to the child. By interview and take-home pamphlet we explain normal anatomy and bowel function, the process of stooling, the definition of medical terms, a model for understanding the abnormality in bowel function, the purpose of each intervention, the problems to be encountered, and the need for persistence. A caring relationship is established, and the need for careful, long-term follow-up emphasized.

A clean bowel is imperative to ensure early success and to avoid the complication of overflow incontinence resulting from the maintenance medication. To achieve initial catharsis the author uses one or two adult hypertonic phosphate enemas 30 to 60 minutes apart, followed by daily oral laxatives (bisacodyl 5–10 mg) for 3 to 5 days. Alternatively, an oral lavage solution can be used. Ingebo and Heyman[80] described the successful use of a balanced polyethylene glycol–electrolyte solution by oral or nasogastric administration to be safe, prompt (6–18 hours), and effective in cleansing the bowel. This approach may be effective in the patient who is unable to cooperate fully as well as in obtaining rapid cleansing in the inpatient or office setting. An abdominal radiograph and examination of the abdomen and rectum will confirm a clean bowel.

Maintenance therapy is aimed at preventing the reaccumulation of retained feces and at overcoming stool holding. Once an empty rectum is achieved, overflow soiling (encopresis) ceases. The author follows Davidson and associates' approach[17] using a high-dose mineral oil therapy (5 ml per kg twice daily) to induce two to four "pudding-like" bowel movements daily. The goal of this therapy is to maintain adequate stool frequency, avoid continued passage of large stools, and prevent withholding or stool retention. During this phase a discharge of stained oil suggests a recurrence of impacted stool, whereas clear drainage may suggest too large a dose of oil. Oil leakage from the anus is a sign that too large a dose of oil is being ingested or that there is a persistent impaction around which the oil is leaking. Physical examination of the child usually reveals whether the lubricant dose should be increased or reduced.

Only those patients exerting control by withholding will demonstrate oil and stool leakage. If the child responds to the urge to defecate with prompt passage of stool, soiling from involuntary expulsion of material does not occur. Instead of lowering the dose of oil for this symptom, increasing the dosage to overcome voluntary withholding is indicated. Alternative medications include milk of magnesia, and lactulose. The dosage of milk of magnesia is similar to that of oil. Lactulose is a semisynthetic disaccharide that is not absorbed from the gastrointestinal tract and that increases the water content of the stool. It produces osmotic diarrhea of low fecal pH. It is titrated to obtain the desired response. Cisapride, a prokinetic agent, has been studied in paraplegic subjects and others with chronic constipation, with evidence of significant improvement of symptoms. Murray and colleagues[81] showed that cisapride improved stool consistency, eliminated soiling, and promoted a diminished reliance on multiple anticonstipation therapies in most of the encopretic children evaluated. The oral liquid form was well accepted, with a minimum of side effects. Few studies have systematically compared medications. Sondheimer and Gervaise[82] compared a lubricant (mineral oil) with a laxative (Senokot), showing a lower rate of recurrence and an increased ability to discontinue treatment at 6 months in those treated with mineral oil. All medications have been used for long periods without evidence of complication. Hsiung and coworkers[83] demonstrated that absorption is interfered with to a negligible extent when an adequate interval exists between administration of the oil and ingestion of fatty material. Clark and associates[84] reported normal vitamin A and E status in children taking mineral oil for 6 months. Critical elements of this phase, in addition to mineral oil, include diet modification by increasing dietary fiber to at least 20 gm per day and retraining with toileting and biofeedback.

Biobehavioral training in combination with lubricant treatment is aimed at establishing regular bowel movements through the development of a conditioned response. Conditioning to more frequent elimination ensures softer stools and is effective in children old enough to cooperate, for example, 3 to 4 years of age. The child sits on the commode for 5 to 15 minutes after breakfast and dinner, with proper foot support for leverage. Patients refractory to treatment are evaluated by anorectal manometry and electromyography. The finding of rectoanal dyssynergy is an indication for biofeedback therapy.[85–88]

Paradoxical anal closure may be the result of a self-conditioning process. Patients may learn to contract the external anal sphincter in response to the urge and the act of defecation. Recent manometric studies in children with chronic constipation and encopresis demonstrate the frequent occurrence of paradoxical external anal sphincter contraction during defecation.[50, 61] Robinson and Gibbons[15] used rectal biofeedback to teach subjects to inhibit this contraction, with rapid disappearance of soiling. Wald and colleagues[85] compared biofeedback with mineral oil as part of a program that included disimpaction and habit training. Biofeedback was clearly superior to the use of mineral oil in children with paradoxical contraction, whereas it was inferior to mineral oil in those patients with normal expulsion.

Karen and associates[65] treated 12 children with constipation and encopresis associated with paradoxical external anal sphincter contraction using a biofeedback method designed to condition these patients to relax the external anal sphincter during defecation. They recorded a gradual transition to a normal manometric pattern, and, in general, there was an improvement in clinical symptoms that usually paralleled the normalization of the anal sphincter response. We treated 30 children with chronic constipation and encopresis who demonstrated

Table 16–4. TREATMENT OF CHRONIC CONSTIPATION AND ENCOPRESIS

Initial Consultation
- History
- Physical examination
- "Demystification" and education
- Anorectal manometry

Catharsis
- Enema—hypertonic phosphate (120 ml), 1 or 2, if necessary, twice daily for 2 days
- Laxative—bisacodyl 5–10 mg for 3–5 days or polyethylene glycol–electrolyte solution

Maintenance
- Mineral oil 5 ml/kg per day in two divided doses titrated to 2–4 loose stools per day
- Multiple vitamins 1/day
- Toileting 5–10 minutes after breakfast and dinner
- Anal sphincter biofeedback training if needed
- Fiber-rich diet, 20 g/day minimum

Continuance
- Follow-up visits every 1–3 months as necessary for support
- Biofeedback as necessary
- Restart lubricant for recurrences
- Reinforce dietary fiber

electromyographically an inability to relax the anal sphincter with biofeedback. Twenty-two of the 24 children[74] who learned to relax the anal sphincter were having fewer than one accident per month after 8 weeks of training.

For children older than 5 years of age who can cooperate, paradoxical contraction of the external anal sphincter can be eliminated with biofeedback. The procedure is painless and appears to produce sustained improvement. The final phase of treatment includes the gradual withdrawal of mineral oil over a 1- to 12-month period and reliance on dietary fiber and timed toileting. For those with more severe encopresis and megarectum, continuing on low-dose mineral oil therapy (30–60 ml at bedtime) may be recommended for longer periods to continue the bowel training. In those patients who require and respond to biofeedback training, brief retraining may be needed when symptoms recur.

Excellent responses to treatment have been reported in 45 to 100% of children followed for periods ranging from 2 months to 3 years.[26] Moderate improvement is reported in 20 to 30%, whereas failure is reported in 25 to 35%.[65, 79, 89] In Rosenberg and Whitehead's series, approximately 70% of the incontinent patients improved with a multimodal treatment program.[74]

Few long-term studies have been reported, and it is difficult to track "cures" for long intervals or to understand the long-term outcome of treatment failures.

REFERENCES

1. Fleisher DR: Diagnosis and treatment of disorders of defecation in children. Pediatr Ann 1976; 5:71–101.
2. Molnar D, Taitz LS, Urwin OM, et al: Anorectal manometry results in defecation disorders. Arch Dis Child 1983; 58:257–261.
3. Castle SC: Constipation—endemic in the elderly? Gerontopathophysiology, evaluation and management. Med Clin North Am 1989; 73:1497–1509.
4. Weissenberg S: Encopresis. Z Kinderbeilk 1926; 40:674–677.
5. Kanner L: Child Psychiatry. Springfield, IL, Charles C. Thomas, 1935, p 224.
6. Easson WM: Encopresis–psychogenic soiling. Can Med Assoc J 1960; 82:624.
7. From Birth to Seven: Report from National Child Development Survey. London, 1972, p 399.
8. Loening-Baucke VA, Younoszai MK: Effect of treatment on rectal and sigmoid motility in chronically constipated children. Pediatrics 1984; 73:199–205.
9. Doleys DM: Enuresis and encopresis. *In* Ollendick TH, Hersen M, eds: Handbook of Child Psychopathology. New York, Plenum Press, 1983, pp 201–226.
10. Bellman M: Studies on encopresis. Acta Pediatr Scand (Suppl) 1966; 1:170.
11. Levine MD: Encopresis: Its potentiation, evaluation and alleviation. Pediatr Clin North Am 1982; 29:315–330.
12. Anthony EJ: An experimental approach to the psychopathology of childhood: Encopresis. Br J Med Psychol 1957; 30:146.
13. Bakwin H, Davidson M: Constipation in twins. Am J Dis Child 1971; 121:179–181.
14. Barr RG, Levine MD, Wilkinson RH: Occult stool retention: A clinical tool for this evaluation in school-aged children. Clin Pediatr 1979; 18:674.
15. Robinson BA, Gibbons ISE: Paradoxical external anal sphincter function in fecal retention with soiling and its control by operant conditioning. Gastroenterology 1976; 70:930A.
16. Call JD, Christianson M, Penrose FR, et al: Psychogenic megacolon in three preschool boys. Am J Orthopsychiatry 1963; 33:923–928.
17. Davidson M, Kugler MM, Bauer CH: Diagnosis and management in children with severe and protracted constipation and obstipation. J Pediatr 1963; 62:261–275.
18. Levine MD: Children with encopresis: A descriptive analysis. Pediatrics 1975; 56:412–416.
19. Coekin M, Gairner D: Fecal incontinence in children: The physical factor. Br Med J 1960; 2:1175.
20. Whiting J, Child IL: Child Training and Personality. New Haven, Yale University Press, 1953.
21. Abrahamian FP, Lloyd-Still JD: Chronic constipation in childhood: A longitudinal study of 186 patients. J Pediatr Gastroenterol Nutr 1984; 3:460–467.
22. Pinkerton P: Psychogenic megacolon in children: The implications of bowel negativism. Arch Dis Child 1958; 33:371.
23. Murphy MS: Constipation. *In* Walker WA, Durie PR, et al, eds: Pediatric Gastrointestinal Diseases. Vol 1. Philadelphia, BC Decker, 1991, pp 90–110.
24. Meunier P, Mollard P, Marechal JM: Physiology of megarectum: The association of megarectum with encopresis. Gut 1976; 17:224–227.
25. Nixon HH: Megarectum in the older child. Proc R Soc Med 1967; 60:801–803.
26. Loening-Baucke VA: Sensitivity of the sigmoid colon and rectum in children treated for chronic constipation. J Pediatr Gastroenterol Nutr 1984; 3:454–459.
27. Bill AH, Johnson RJ, Foster RA: Anteriorly placed rectal opening in the perineum, "ectopic anus": A report of 30 cases. Ann Surg 1958; 147:173–179.
28. Leape LL, Ramenofsky ML: Anterior ectopic anus: A common cause of constipation in children. J Pediatr Surg 1978; 13:627–629.
29. Hendren WH: Constipation caused by anterior location of the anus and its surgical correction. J Pediatr Surg 1978; 13:505–512.
30. Kerremans PH, Penninck MA, Beckers PV: Functional evaluation of ectopic anus and its surgical consequences. Am J Dis Child 1974; 128:811–814.
31. Reisner SH, Sivan Y, Nitzan M, et al: Determination of anterior displacement of the anus in newborn infants and children. Pediatrics 1984; 73:216–217.
32. Bar-Maor JA, Eitan A: Determination of the normal position of the anus. J Pediatr Gastroenterol Nutr 1987; 6:559–601.
33. Devroede G, Arhan P, Schang JC, et al: Orderly and disorderly fecal continence. *In* Kodner IJ, Fry RD, Roe UP, eds: Colon, Rectal and Anal Surgery: Current Techniques and Controversies. St. Louis, CV Mosby, 1985, pp 40–62.

34. Weaver LT, Steiner H: The bowel habit of young children. Arch Dis Child 1984; 59:649–652.
35. Lesne E, Binet L, Paulin A: La traversee digestive chez le nourrisson variation biologiques et pathologiques. Arch Med Infants 1920; 23:449–456.
36. Triboulet H: Duree de la traverse chez l'enfant modale epreuve du carmin. Bull Soc Pediatr Paris 1909; 11:512–529.
37. Dimson SB: Carmine as an index of transit times in children with simple constipation. Arch Dis Child 1970; 45:232–235.
38. Burkitt D, Morley D, Walker A: Dietary fibre in under- and overnutrition in childhood. Arch Dis Child 1980; 55:803–807.
39. Christensen J: Motility of the colon. *In* Johnson LR, ed: Physiology of the Gastrointestinal Tract. 2nd ed. New York, Raven Press, 1987, p 665.
40. Connell AM, Hilton C, Irvine G, et al: Variation in bowel habit in two population samples. Br Med J 1965; 2:1095–1099.
41. Drossman KDA, Sandler RS, McKee DC, et al: AJ. Bowel patterns among subjects not seeking health care. Gastroenterology 1982; 83:529–534.
42. Nyhan WL: Stool frequency of normal infants in the first weeks of life. Pediatrics 1952; 10:414–425.
43. Weaver LT, Ewing G, Taylor LC: The bowel habit of milk-fed infants. J Pediatr Gastroenterol Nutr 1988; 7:568–571.
44. Wald A: Disorders of defecation and fecal continence. Cleve Clin J Med 1989; 56:491–501.
45. Lubowski DZ, Swash M, Henry MM: Neural mechanisms in disorders of defecation. Baillieres Clin Gastroenterol 1988; 2:201–223.
46. Porter NH: A physiological study of the pelvic floor in rectal prolapse. Ann R Coll Surg Engl 1962; 31:379–404.
47. Gaston EA: The physiology of fecal continence. Surg Gynecol Obstet 1948; 87:280–290.
48. Bennett DL, Duthie HL: The functional importance of the internal anal sphincter. Br J Surg 1964; 51:355–357.
49. Rosenberg AJ, Vela AD: A new simplified technique for pediatric manometry. Pediatrics 1983; 71:240–245.
50. Holschneider A: Elecktromanometrie des enddarmes: Diagnostik und therapie der Inkontinenz und der Chronischen Obstipation. 2nd ed. Munich, Urban und Schwarzenberg, 1983, pp 110–126.
51. Arhan P, Faverdin C, Thouvenot J: Ano-rectal motility in sick children. Scand J Gastroenterol 1972; 7:309.
52. Varma KK, Stephens D: Neuromuscular reflexes of rectal continence. Aust NZ J Surg 1972; 41:263.
53. Schuster MM: Diagnostic value of anal sphincter pressure measurements. Hosp Pract 1973; 8:115–122.
54. Meunier P, Marechal JM, de Beaujeu MJ: Rectoanal pressures and rectal sensitivity studies in chronic childhood constipation. Gastroenterology 1979; 77:330.
55. Arhan P, Devroede G, Jenannin B, et al: Idiopathic disorders of fecal continence in children. Pediatrics 1983; 71:774–779.
56. Suzuki H, Amano S, Honzumi M, et al: Rectoanal pressures and rectal compliance in constipated infants and children. Z Kinderchir Grenzgeb 1980; 29:330–336.
57. Sondheimer JM: Helping the child with chronic constipation. Contemp Pediatr 1985; 12:28.
58. Meunier P, Louis D, Jaubert M, et al: Physiologic investigation of primary chronic constipation in children: Comparison with the barium enema study. Gastroenterology 1984; 87:1351–1357.
59. Porter NH: Megacolon: A physiological study. Proc R Soc Med 1961; 54:1043–1047.
60. Lawson JON: The soiling child. Practitioner 1975; 214:807–808.
61. Wald A, Chandra R, Chiponis D, et al: Anorectal function and continence mechanisms in childhood encopresis. J Pediatr Gastroenterol Nutr 1986; 5:346–351.
62. Chowdhury AR, Dinoso VP, Lorber SH: Characterization of a hyperactive segment at the rectosigmoid junction. Gastroenterology 1976; 71:584–588.
63. Preston DM, Lennard-Jones JE, Thomas GM: Towards a radiological definition of idiopathic megacolon. Gastrointest Radiol 1984; 10:167–169.
64. Meunier P: Rectoanal dyssynergia in constipated children. Dig Dis Sci 1985; 30:784A.
65. Karen S, Wagner Y, Heldenberg KD, et al: Studies of manometric abnormalities of the rectoanal region during defecation in constipated and soiling children: Modification through biofeedback therapy. Am Gastroenterol 1988; 83:827–831.
66. Ogorek CP, Reynolds, JC: Chronic constipation: Diagnosis and treatment. Endosc Rev 1987; Nov/Dec:1–7.
67. Reynolds JC: Chronic severe constipation. Comtemp Iss Gastroenterol 1987; 6:95.
68. Martelli H, Devroede G, Arhan P, et al: Mechanisms of idiopathic constipation: Outlet obstruction. Gastoenterology 1978; 75:623–631.
69. Read NW, Timms JM: Defecation and the pathophysiology of constipation. Clin Gastroenterol 1986; 15:937–965.
70. Misiewicz JJ, Connell AM, Pontes FA: Comparison of the effects of meals and prostigmine on the proximal and distal colon in patients with and without diarrhea. Gut 1966; 7:468–473.
71. Corazziari E, Cocchiara S, Staiano A, et al: Gastrointestinal transit time, frequency of defecation and anorectal manometry in healthy and constipated children. J Pediatr 1985; 106:379–382.
72. Vajro P, Silano G, Longo D, et al: Orocaecal transit time in healthy and constipated children. Acta Paediatr Scand 1988; 77:583–586.
73. Lennard-Jones JE: Coloproctology and the Pelvic Floor: Constipation. Butterworths, London, 1985, pp 350–377.
74. Rosenberg AJ, Whitehead T: Achieving anal relaxation: The key to continence for encopretic children. Gastoenterology 1990; 99:1229.
75. Hatch TF: Encopresis and constipation in children. Pediatr Clin North Am 1988; 35:2.
76. Fitzgerald JF: Encopresis, soiling, constipation: What's to be done? Pediatrics 1975; 56:348–349.
77. Lowery SP, Srour JW, Whitehead WE, et al: Habit training as treatment of encopresis secondary to chronic constipation. J Pediatr Gastroenter Nutr 1985; 4:397–401.
78. Rappaport L, Landman G, Fenton T, et al: Locus of control as predictor of compliance and outcome in treatment of encopresis. J Pediatr 1986; 109:106–164.
79. Levine MD, Bakow H: Children with encopresis: A study of treatment outcome. Pediatrics 1976; 58:845.
80. Ingebo KB, Heyman MB: Polyethylene glycol–electrolyte solution for intestinal clearance in children with refractory encopresis. Am J Dis Child 1988; 142:340–342.
81. Murray RD, Li BUK, McClung HJ, et al: Cisapride for intractable constipation in children: Observations from an open trial. J Pediatr Gastroenterol Nutr 1990; 11:503–508.
82. Sondheimer JM, Gervaise EP: Lubricant versus laxative in the treatment of chronic functional constipation of children: A comparative study. J Pediatr Gastroenterol Nutr 1982; 1:223–226.
83. Hsiung JC, Riley GM, Nesbitt RM: The influence of mineral oil on the absorption of diethylstilbestrol from the gastrointestinal tract. J Urol 1948; 60:297.
84. Clark JH, Russel GJ, Fitzgerald JF: Serum beta-carotene, retinal and alpha-tocopherol levels during mineral oil therapy for constipation. Am J Dis Child 1987; 141:1210–1212.
85. Wald A, Chandra R, Gabel S, et al: Evaluation of biofeedback in childhood encopresis. J Pediatr Gastroenterol Nutr 1987; 6:554–558.
86. Riboli EB, Frascio M, Pitto G, et al: Biofeedback conditioning for fecal incontinence. Arch Phys Med Rehabil 1988; 69:29–31.
87. Dietrich S, Okamoto G: Bowel training for children with neurogenic dysfunction: A follow-up. Arch Phys Med Rehabil 1982; 63:166–170.
88. MacLeod JH: Biofeedback in the management of partial anal incontinence. Dis Colon Rectum 1983; 26:244–246.
89. Loening-Baucke V, Younoszai MK: Effect of treatment on rectal and sigmoid motility in chronically constipated children. Pediatrics 1984; 73:199–205.

Chapter 17

The Acute Abdomen

EDWIN I. HATCH, JR., and ROBERT SAWIN

One of the most challenging tasks facing the pediatric health care provider is to differentiate between abdominal pain that requires prompt surgical intervention and that which does not. Although in the broadest sense all children with stomachaches may be said to have "acute abdomens," the emphasis of this chapter is on the neonate, infant, child, or adolescent with acute abdominal pain who needs evaluation to determine whether surgical intervention is indicated.

PATHOPHYSIOLOGY OF ABDOMINAL PAIN

Pain sensed in the abdomen can arise from six different sources: visceral distention, ischemia, intra-abdominal inflammation, abdominal wall pathology, metabolic abnormalities, and neurologic abnormalities. Understanding the anatomy and physiology of each can help prevent unnecessary laparotomy or delayed laparotomy when operative intervention is essential.

Visceral pain results from noxious stimulation of the visceral pain receptors, which are similar to the somatic pain receptors. Visceral pain receptors, however, lack proprioception, touch, and temperature sensing organs and are less densely distributed. This relative paucity of receptors accounts for the poorly localized character of visceral pain in contrast to somatic pain.

The painful stimuli reach the central nervous system (CNS) via afferent sympathetic and parasympathetic fibers. In the CNS, these noxious visceral sensations travel along the spinothalamic tracts to the cerebral cortex, just as with somatic pain.

Referred Pain

When pain resulting from intra-abdominal pathology is sensed as originating in another part of the body, the pain is termed *referred pain*. Common clinical examples include the periumbilical pain experienced with appendicitis or the inguinal pain associated with a ureteral stone.

There are several theories offered to explain the neuroanatomy and neurophysiology of referred pain.[1] The two most commonly accepted hypotheses are more than 30 years old and have been corroborated in recent years with experimental evidence. The first theory is called the *visceral-somatic convergence theory,* which is based on the observation that there are both somatic and visceral afferent fibers that converge on the same neurons in the spinothalamic tracts.[2] Thus, in the example of the appendix, the visceral afferents and the somatic afferent fibers from the skin around the umbilicus interface with the spinothalamic tract at the same point. This signal transmitted to the cerebral cortex by the spinothalamic tracts is preferentially interpreted as having originated in the skin, since pain receptors are more numerous in the skin and the patient's prior pain experience has most likely been caused by the more common noxious stimuli to the skin rather than to the deep viscera. Confirmatory data for this theory have been reported in humans and experimental animals.[3]

The second commonly endorsed theory of referred pain is the *peripheral nerve branching theory,* which proposes that the axons of the dorsal root ganglion cells are bifurcated, with one branch going to the skin and the other going to the viscera.[4] This anatomic finding has been confirmed and may therefore explain, in part, the referred pain phenomenon.

Etiologies of Abdominal Pain

Distention is a potent stimulus of visceral pain. This has been demonstrated in humans by inflating balloons in the gastrointestinal tract. This pain can be eliminated or lateralized to one side by sympathetectomy.[1] The early pain associated with appendicitis and cholelithiasis, as well as the pain caused by intestinal obstruction, are examples of visceral pain caused by distention.[5]

Inflammation stimulates visceral pain as well. The inflammatory response may vary depending on the inciting agent and on the cell populations involved, but one of the products of the inflammatory cascade is frequently bradykinin. This chemical is a potent stimulus for both somatic and visceral pain. Anti-inflammatory drugs such as aspirin or ibuprofen block the experimental effects of bradykinin on autonomic nervous signals, and administration of prostaglandin E_1 or prostaglandin I_2 restores the noxious effects. An example of an inflammatory cause of abdominal pain is peritonitis from a perforated viscus.

Ischemia is a variable noxious stimulus. Patients with

ischemia of the myocardium may not experience pain, and the same is true of some patients with ischemia of an abdominal organ; more typically, however, ischemia will result in severe pain that is out of proportion to the objective findings on physical exam. The reason for this is unknown. Ischemia is followed by an intense inflammatory response, which may be a further stimulus for pain, but this inflammation is often preceded by several hours of abdominal pain.[6]

Abdominal wall pathology, such as a hematoma of the rectus abdominis sheath following trauma, can cause pain that appears to arise from within the abdomen. In this instance the somatic pain may be incorrectly interpreted as referred visceral pain.

Extra-abdominal pathology can present as abdominal pain because of the dermatomal pattern. Examples include testicular torsion or pneumonia.

Metabolic abnormalities cause abdominal pain by unknown mechanisms. Some of the abnormalities actually cause intra-abdominal pathology, such as hyperlipidemia leading to pancreatitis; others, such as lead poisoning, have no obvious explanation for the apparent localization to the abdomen.

Neurologic abnormalities, such as radiculopathy from discitis or shingles infection (varicella-zoster virus), can masquerade as an intra-abdominal process, again because of the dermatomal referral pattern.

Developmental Factors

The issue of whether newborns or infants feel pain has been controversial. Some have suggested that incomplete myelination and an incompletely developed cerebral cortex means that noxious stimuli are not transmitted to the CNS adequately, are not interpreted by the cerebral cortex as pain, or are not remembered as having been painful. However, recent studies measuring the neuroendocrine response to surgery and to painful stimuli *have* shown that neonates and infants have a hormonal and catecholamine response that is similar to that seen in adults.[7–9] It is clear that abdominal wall muscle spasm and tenderness associated with peritonitis are appreciable in neonates.

PHYSIOLOGY OF THE PERITONEUM

The peritoneum is a semipermeable membrane that lines the abdominal cavity. On the abdominal side of the diaphragm, lymphatic vessels run deep to the peritoneum. During exhalation, the diaphragm stretches, allowing the intraperitoneal fluid to flow through the peritoneal membrane into the lymphatics. With inhalation, the contraction of the diaphragmatic muscles and the decreased intrathoracic pressure facilitates the egress of fluid into the thoracic lymph vessels.[10] Also contributing to the cephalad movement of peritoneal fluid is the downward gravitational displacement of the liver, which creates a potential space over the liver, resulting in a siphonlike effect. This, plus the tendency of the peristalsing intestine to move the fluid to the lateral gutters, results in a well-established intraperitoneal circulation of fluid.[10]

In addition to fluid, particulate matter such as bacteria can be rapidly removed from the peritoneum via these diaphragmatic lymphatics. This facilitates clearance of bacterial infections, but does so at the expense of potentially producing septicemia.[10]

Other local factors protect the peritoneum from invasive infections. The inflammatory response initiated by bacteria results in the release of cytokines such as tumor necrosis factor (TNF),[11] interleukins, and activated complement.[12] Polymorphonuclear leukocytes, macrophages, and opsonins are exuded into the peritoneum from the plasma in response to inflammation. In addition, fibrin release is enhanced, and fibrinolysis is impaired, resulting in increased ability to form fibrinous adhesions. These adhesions facilitate isolation of the bacterial infection by forming loculations. Migration of the omentum to the source of inflammation enhances the loculation process. The paralytic ileus and abdominal muscle wall rigidity that result from the local inflammation further retard the movement of infectious material out of the peritoneal cavity.

The immune system of the neonate is incompletely developed. When compared with those of adult animals, neonatal neutrophils have impaired ability to function properly.[13] Nonetheless, neonatal mononuclear cells are capable of producing TNF[14, 15] and other cytokines necessary for peritonitis to occur. Little is known about intraperitoneal circulation in neonates and how it may differ from that of adults. The infant omentum appears to have the ability to migrate to a focus of inflammation but is a less substantial organ. This may explain why infants with perforated appendicitis seldom have a well-localized abscess in contrast with that seen in older children.[16]

AGE-RELATED DIFFERENTIAL DIAGNOSIS

One of the unique aspects of assessing abdominal pain in a pediatric patient is the importance of the child's age. Although many of the causes of abdominal pain can be seen in any age group, the differential diagnosis for a given age group is heavily skewed (Fig. 17–1). For instance, intussusception can be seen in adolescent patients (with distal intestinal neoplasms), but it is far less common than in 2-year-olds, where it is one of the most common causes of the "surgical abdomen." The following sections focus on several causes of the acute abdomen in the age groups in which they are most commonly seen. The reader must keep in mind, however, that most of these lesions can occur at any age.

Neonate

The ultimate challenge for the neonatologist is to diagnose the neonate with an acute abdomen at an early stage. The previously well, full-term neonate who de-

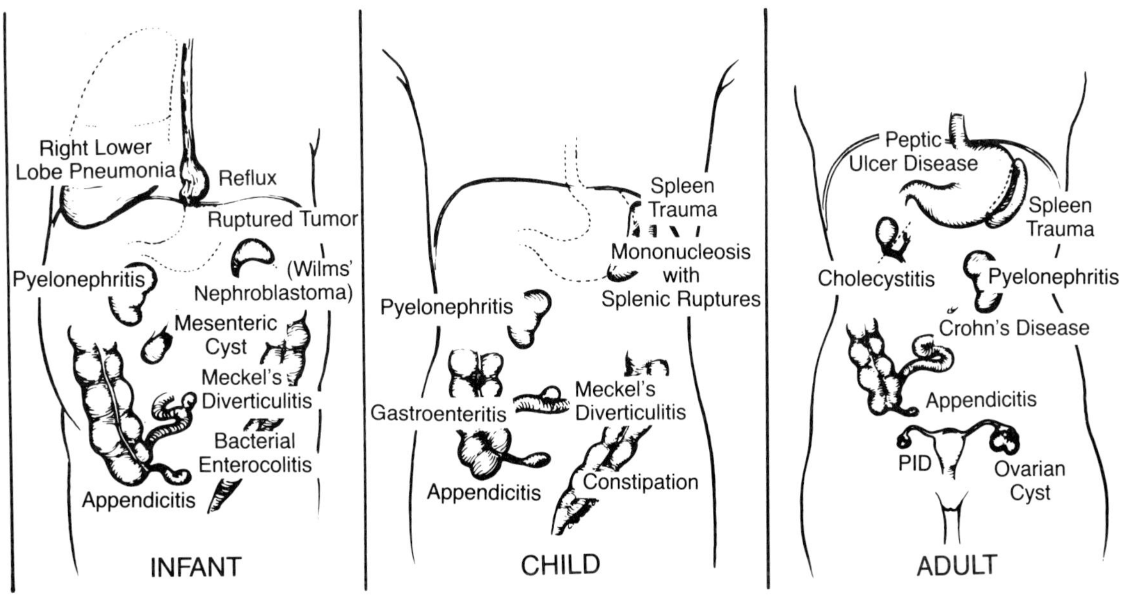

Figure 17–1. Sites of pathologic processes resulting in abdominal pain.

velops necrotizing enterocolitis, intestinal volvulus, or even a perforated viscus may not demonstrate or communicate the impending threat caused by the intra-abdominal pathology until systemic signs of sepsis are evident.[17] In contrast, the premature, critically ill neonate, who has less physiologic reserve, may make the abdominal process more obvious by showing such systemic signs as metabolic acidosis, thrombocytopenia, worsening respiratory status, or bradycardia before an intra-abdominal catastrophe occurs.[17] The differential diagnosis of the acute abdomen in the neonate is listed in Table 17–1.

In general, the neonate may exhibit nonspecific signs or symptoms, making an exact preoperative diagnosis difficult (Table 17–2). Although the laboratory and radiologic evaluation of the neonate is helpful, the most important diagnostic parameters are obtained by a complete history and thorough physical examination. Serial examination by the same skilled clinician is frequently the most reliable factor in the early diagnosis of the acute abdomen.[18]

Although the exact etiology of the acute abdomen in the neonate is often determined only at the time of operation, there are three highly morbid entities that mandate early diagnosis: malrotation with midgut volvulus, Hirschsprung's enterocolitis, and necrotizing enterocolitis. Although these diseases may be seen in infants and children, they most often affect neonates and warrant special consideration.

Malrotation with Midgut Volvulus

The neonate who feeds normally for a few days and then develops bilious vomiting must be considered an acute emergency. Midgut volvulus (see Chapter 35) must be ruled out as soon as possible. These babies are usually healthy otherwise, and 4 hours can make the difference between the presence and absence of intestinal ischemia.[19] An emergent upper gastrointestinal contrast study to verify the position of the ligament of Treitz should be followed by an exploratory laparotomy.[20] (Fig. 17–2).

Malrotation with midgut volvulus represents a spectrum of lesions ranging from an intermittent volvulus with no intestinal ischemia to that which can result in total loss of the midgut.[21] The tightness of the base of the volvulus with resulting lymphatic, venous, and finally arterial obstruction may take from hours to days to become symptomatic. At one end of the spectrum, the neonate might present with failure to thrive or signs of lymphatic congestion such as chylous ascites or mesenteric cysts. At the other end, the neonate might present with bilious vomiting associated with an acute abdomen

Table 17–1. ETIOLOGIES OF ACUTE ABDOMEN IN THE NEONATE

Malrotation with midgut volvulus	Pyelonephritis
Meconium peritonitis	Birth trauma
Perforated viscus	Ovarian torsion
Necrotizing enterocolitis	Intussusception
Appendicitis	Internal hernia
Meconium ileus	Incarcerated hernia

Table 17–2. FACTORS SUGGESTING ACUTE ABDOMEN IN THE NEONATE

Bilious vomiting	Brawny edema abdominal wall
Abdominal tenderness	Crying—pulling up legs
Abdominal distension	Irritability
Abdominal mass	Lethargy
Obstipation	Bloody stools
Feeding intolerance	Inguinal hernia at birth
Omphalitis	Fever or hypothermia

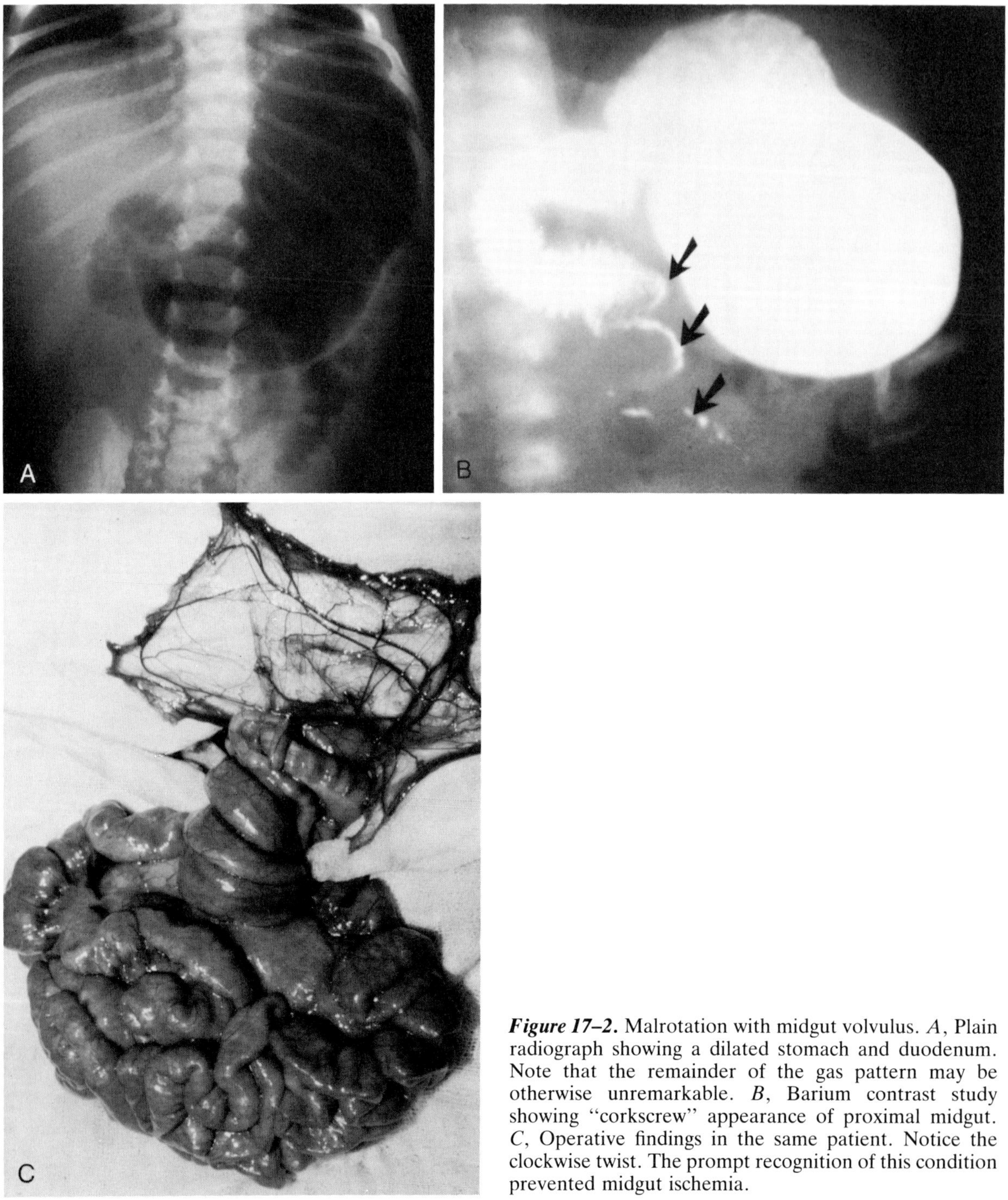

Figure 17–2. Malrotation with midgut volvulus. *A*, Plain radiograph showing a dilated stomach and duodenum. Note that the remainder of the gas pattern may be otherwise unremarkable. *B*, Barium contrast study showing "corkscrew" appearance of proximal midgut. *C*, Operative findings in the same patient. Notice the clockwise twist. The prompt recognition of this condition prevented midgut ischemia.

secondary to bowel ischemia.[22] At operation it is necessary to untwist the volvulus, divide the duodenal bands, broaden the base of the mesentery, and remove the appendix (Ladd procedure).[23] Ischemic portions of intestine should be resected, attempting to save as much small intestine as possible. If the entire midgut is ischemic, then untwisting the volvulus, deferring extensive resection, and repeating the laparotomy in 12 to 24 hours may be appropriate.[24] When the diagnosis is confirmed by an early upper gastrointestinal series and surgery is performed early, the outcome should be excellent.[6]

Hirschsprung's Enterocolitis

The neonate who fails to spontaneously pass meconium in the first 24 hours of life should be evaluated to rule out Hirschsprung's disease (see Chapter 54). If this neonate develops abdominal distention associated with tenderness and sepsis, then enterocolitis must be considered.[25] The intestinal mucosa of the neonate with Hirschsprung's disease is abnormal, perhaps explaining the predisposition for bacterial invasion and enterocolitis.[26–28] A limited barium enema by a pediatric radiologist may help with the diagnosis, but the false-negative rate is high in the neonatal period.[29, 30] Following the barium enema, careful rectal irrigations to decompress the colon may be indicated. Fluid resuscitation, antibiotics, and careful serial examinations determine whether emergency colostomy is necessary. Ideally, a suction rectal biopsy for acetyl cholinesterase stains as well as a routine histology is performed to establish the diagnosis of Hirschsprung's disease.

Necrotizing Enterocolitis

Necrotizing enterocolitis (NEC) (see Chapter 61) is a disease seen principally in preterm neonates, although 10% of cases involve full-term neonates.[17] Multiple etiologies have been proposed, including infection, ischemia, and early initiation of enteral feedings.[31–33] Although some or all of these factors may be involved, the common final pathway seems to include ischemia and ultimately leads to a picture of coagulation necrosis, inflammation, hemorrhage, and bacterial overgrowth.[34] Gas may accumulate in the bowel wall, creating the radiologic finding of pneumatosis cystoides intestinalis.

The process may involve the small intestine, colon, or both. Although the findings at laparotomy are often patchy with apparently spared regions of bowel, the entire small intestine and colon may suffer a partial thickness mucosal insult, resulting in long-term intestinal dysfunction. If full-thickness bowel wall injury occurs, perforation may result.

Systemic manifestations of NEC may include thrombocytopenia and neutropenia, which are thought to be consequences of endotoxin-induced platelet activating factor (PAF) release from the intestine, as well as TNF release from activated macrophages.[35] In addition, metabolic acidosis, disseminated intravascular coagulation, decreased left ventricular function, and hypotension may all be seen.

Gastrointestinal symptoms include paralytic ileus, bloody or bilious gastric aspirates, hematochezia, and abdominal distention. Erythema and edema of the abdominal wall may be signs of underlying peritonitis owing to the thinness of the abdominal wall musculature. This is especially true around the umbilicus, the linea alba, and the linea semilunaris. Muscular spasm and tenderness of the abdominal wall can be appreciated by careful examination and are further signs of peritonitis.

Operative management is often avoided by prompt recognition of NEC and volume resuscitation, correction of the metabolic abnormalities, and initiation of broad-spectrum antibiotic therapy. The indications for surgical treatment include evidence of perforation, failure to resolve the systemic abnormalities, or signs of gangrenous segments of bowel such as localized abdominal wall erythema or edema, palpable mass, or a persistent air-filled loop of bowel on serial x-rays.[36–38] Strictures can occur after NEC, more commonly after nonoperative management.[39, 40] The goal of any operation for NEC should be conservation of as much bowel as is safely possible. Enterostomies are indicated when gross contamination or hemodynamic instability is present. Some authors have reported fewer strictures and lower morbidity with primary anastomoses.[41]

Infant

The infant, defined as a child older than 1 month but younger than 2 years, requires many of the same considerations as the neonate. Congenital problems, however, become less common, and acquired lesions such as intussusception are more frequently seen. Although the infant is better able to communicate abdominal pain than the neonate, the early diagnosis of an acute abdomen remains a major challenge to the clinician. Serial examination is the key to the diagnosis of the acute abdomen.

The history becomes more relevant as the infant's skill in communication matures. Parents are the most accurate source of information. Common parental concerns include poor feeding, lethargy, increased crying and fussiness, vomiting, decreased playfulness, or perhaps just the vague realization that something is wrong. These subtle clues may provoke them to seek medical evaluation.

Which of the infants with these subtle complaints requires emergent evaluation? The infant who has bilious vomiting, severe pain, or bloody stools should be seen immediately. In addition, any child whose symptoms persist or worsen warrants expeditious assessment.

It is worth the extra time and effort to gain the confidence of the patient by distracting the infant with toys or sounds before getting close to the abdomen. Warm hands and patience are most helpful. Watching the infant feed helps differentiate between hunger and true discomfort. Inspect the abdomen for distention or a scaphoid appearance. Listen to the abdomen for hyperactive or hypoactive bowel sounds. The chest should also be auscultated to rule out pneumonia. Begin palpation of the abdomen only after the infant is relaxed. Gentleness is essential. Rock the infant's feet and legs up with the left hand while the right hand examines for masses, organomegaly, or tenderness. Palpation should begin away from the suspected tender area, saving the unpleasant examination for last. Peritonitis is very difficult to establish in this age group and requires serial examination by the same clinician. It is very challenging to differentiate between peritonitis and tender distended loops of bowel, especially in a fussy infant.

The rectal examination should be saved for last; its utility is operator dependent and debatable. It is helpful in detecting pelvic masses, constipation, and "currant jelly" stools, as well as the forceful stooling that follows the withdrawal of the finger in the infant with Hirschsprung's disease. Sometimes efforts to protect the infant from a painful examination are detrimental because of a delay in diagnosis. Again, the importance of the serial examination by the same clinician cannot be overemphasized.

Intussusception

Intussusception, covered in detail in Chapter 47, is the most common cause of the surgical acute abdomen in the infant age group. The triad of colicky abdominal pain, a palpable abdominal mass, and currant jelly stools is present in only 20% of patients.[42, 43] History may be more important than physical examination. Laboratory tests and plain radiographs may be unremarkable. The contrast enema is diagnostic and often therapeutic.[44–46]

The infant with suspected intussusception should be carefully evaluated by a surgeon and have intravenous fluids and antibiotics started prior to the contrast enema. The success of the contrast enema in reducing an intussusception varies from 50 to 94% in recent series utilizing air as a substitute for barium.[45, 47, 48] If reduction is unsuccessful, the infant is taken promptly to the operating room for surgical reduction, possible bowel resection, and appendectomy. The overall results should be excellent, with morbidity related to delays in diagnosis. Infants younger than 6 months of age have a higher morbidity because of risk of perforation during contrast enema.[47, 49]

Intestinal Obstruction

Although pyloric stenosis is the most common cause of bowel obstruction, it does not belong in a discussion of the acute abdomen. Incarcerated hernia is the most common cause of intestinal obstruction between the third and sixth months of life. Intussusception and malrotation with midgut volvulus, as well as Hirschsprung's disease, have already been discussed, which leaves us with a rare but difficult and important group to discuss. The infant who has an internal hernia, or a volvulus around an omphalomesenteric band, is very difficult to diagnose. Such an infant is inconsolable, but rarely has bilious vomiting or bloody stools until late. Barium enema may or may not be helpful, because the point of obstruction may be difficult to visualize in a retrograde manner. Oral contrast studies from above may be helpful. Again, the physical examination is the most important factor in making an early decision to operate on these difficult-to-diagnose infants.

The Battered Infant

The abused infant may present with an acute abdomen. Often medical help is sought late because of fear or denial. The most common injury that results in an acute abdomen is a perforation of the jejunum just distal to the ligament of Treitz.[50–52] Although the etiology is difficult to establish, it is usually secondary to a sharp blow in the midabdomen by either a fist or the heel of a foot. Other signs of child abuse may be a clue. Often a vague history, such as "he slipped in the tub," leads to an abdominal radiograph showing free air from the jejunal injury. Unfortunately, these victims often present moribund or dead in the emergency room.[52]

The physician should suspect child abuse in any infant who has an unexplained acute abdomen associated with a hollow viscus injury. Following head injuries, abdominal injuries are the leading cause of death in these innocent victims. Child abuse accounts for 11% of blunt abdominal trauma in children under 13 years of age, as reported by a major trauma center.[52] The abused child's average age was 2½ years. Often the presenting history is incompatible with the seriousness of the injuries. A high index of suspicion may be life saving in this tragic situation.

Child

Although a child can communicate better than an infant, certain factors make the differentiation between real and functional complaints more difficult. The history and physical examination far outweigh any radiologic or laboratory studies in establishing the presence of an acute abdomen in this age group. Appendicitis is by far the most common etiology of the acute abdomen in this age group and often the most difficult to diagnose before perforation occurs.[18]

Appendicitis

Although appendicitis is discussed in more detail in Chapter 53, a brief inclusion here is essential for completeness. The greatest challenge to the pediatric health care provider is to sort out from the hundreds of children with stomachaches those children with appendicitis. Promptness in making the diagnosis of appendicitis is important, since perforation occurs in the majority of cases just 20 to 36 hours from the onset.

The classic story is a child who develops periumbilical or midepigastric pain, some nausea or vomiting, anorexia, and later a low-grade fever followed by a worsening of symptoms, with pain localizing to the right lower quadrant of the abdomen. The child does not sleep well, stops playing, and gets progressively worse. On examination, he or she appears ill, does not move, and has exquisite tenderness localized in the area of McBurney's point. Unfortunately, this classic story and picture are not always present. The differential diagnosis of the child with acute abdominal pain is listed in Table 17–3.

Adolescents

Gynecologic

In the adolescent patient, the differential diagnosis of abdominal pain expands considerably, especially in the

Table 17–3. DIFFERENTIAL DIAGNOSIS OF ACUTE ABDOMEN IN THE CHILD

More Common	Less Common
Appendicitis	Cholecystitis
Viral gastroenteritis	Crohn's disease
Bacterial gastroenteritis	Nephrolithiasis
Constipation	Meckel's diverticulitis
Urinary tract infection	Mesenteric cyst
Mesenteric adenitis	Ureteropelvic junction obstruction
Pancreatitis	Diabetic ketoacidosis
Testicular torsion	Hemolytic-uremic syndrome
Ovarian cyst	Lymphoma
Pneumonia	Pneumococcal peritonitis
Trauma	Sickle-cell disease
Hepatitis	Typhlitis
Infectious mononucleosis	Gallbladder hydrops
	Henoch-Schönlein purpura
	Intussusception

female. Although appendicitis remains the most common cause of abdominal pain requiring surgical treatment, the onset of puberty introduces a variety of gynecologic diseases to be considered by the surgeon contemplating a laparotomy. Consequently, the percentage of normal appendices found at the time of appendectomy is highest in this group, ranging from 35 to 50%.

The most common of these gynecologic processes that can masquerade as appendicitis is pelvic inflammatory disease (PID). The spectrum of PID ranges from acute salpingitis, which is best managed nonoperatively, to tubo-ovarian abscess, which may require surgery. PID can be a unilateral problem, but it is generally a more diffuse pelvic process. Patients with PID have abdominal pain (90%), fever higher than 100°F (60%), and leukocytosis (70%). The history of a recent menstrual period is suggestive for PID, but when studied critically in a prospective fashion, it has failed to discriminate between appendicitis and PID.[53] The erythrocyte sedimentation rate (ESR) has also been purported to be of value in differentiating PID from appendicitis, but it is neither sensitive nor specific.[54]

PID is typically a polymicrobial inflammatory process, with anaerobes and enteric organisms frequently involved. Thus, broad-spectrum antibiotic therapy, such as ampicillin, gentamicin, and clindamycin or metronidazole, is necessary. The nonoperative management of PID is usually successful, unless the tubo-ovarian abscess has ruptured, in which case urgent operation is indicated.

Bleeding ovarian cysts may also present with abdominal pain and tenderness. The pain may be accompanied by low-grade fever or even leukocytosis. A menstrual history is important, as many of these events occur immediately following ovulation. The onset of pain is often sudden. An ectopic pregnancy must be included in the differential diagnosis, therefore mandating a pregnancy test. Ultrasound may be helpful in making the diagnosis, since free fluid may be seen in the pelvis and the cyst may be identified. The presence of an intrauterine pregnancy may also be confirmed on ultrasound.

Another pelvic source of abdominal pain is adnexal torsion. This pain is often associated with low-grade fever, unilateral tenderness, and a palpable mass. Ultrasound is helpful in making the diagnosis. The etiology of adnexal torsion in the adolescent is an enlarged ovary resulting from a functional cyst or a neoplasm.

Laparoscopy can be helpful in evaluating adolescent females with abdominal pain, especially when the history and physical exam are in any way atypical for appendicitis. In some series, laparoscopy has reduced the negative appendectomy rate in this difficult age group; in other reports, the inability to visualize the appendix well has resulted in no appreciable difference.[55]

Pancreatic and Biliary

Adolescents can develop gallstones that are symptomatic as biliary colic, cholecystitis, or gallstone pancreatitis. The risk factors for cholecystitis include hemolytic diseases such as sickle-cell anemia or hereditary spherocytosis, the use of exogenous estrogens such as oral contraceptives, cystic fibrosis, and ileal diseases such as Crohn's disease (see Chapter 72).

As in the case for adults, once the source of the right upper quadrant pain is established as cholelithiasis, it is essential to rule out concomitant cholecystitis. The presence of fever, leukocytosis, or a nonvisualizing gallbladder on radionuclide hepatobiliary scintigraphy requires antibiotic therapy followed by surgical therapy. Acalculous cholecystitis can also occur, notably in intensive-care-unit patients.

Pancreatitis in adolescents is usually idiopathic or post-traumatic. Fortunately, the other causes such as gallstones, alcohol abuse, hyperlipidemia, hypercalcemia, and medications are rare. The diagnosis is best made by elevated serum amylase and lipase levels or by pancreatic swelling on ultrasound or computerized tomography (CT) scanning of the abdomen (see Chapter 68).

Inflammatory Bowel Disease

Abdominal pain is a frequent symptom of both Crohn's disease and ulcerative colitis, although other gastrointestinal complaints are usually present as well. Pain may be the initial presenting symptom, particularly in Crohn's disease. It can also be severe enough to warrant emergency laparotomy in the patient with ulcerative colitis and toxic megacolon (see Chapters 59 and 60).

Peptic Ulcer Disease

Although uncommon in children of any age, peptic ulcer disease can present with abdominal pain with or without gastrointestinal bleeding. Fortunately, both the bleeding and pain can almost always be managed in a nonoperative manner using histamine blockers, antacids, or, more recently, the H^+ pump inactivator omeprazole. Peptic ulcers rarely perforate in children (see Chapter 33).

Urinary Tract Infections

Infections of the urinary tract may result in abdominal pain, fever, leukocytosis, and signs of peritoneal irritation at any age. The swelling of the kidney that results from pyelonephritis may even cause a paralytic ileus with nausea and vomiting. Avoidance of a laparotomy can best be assured by doing a urinalysis. Although some mild pyuria (<10 white blood cells [WBCs] per high-powered field) may be seen with appendicitis, anything more pronounced (such as urinary leukocyte esterase or bacteria) should be evaluated with a renal ultrasound or a CT scan. In severe, localized pyelonephritis, the CT scan may show lobar nephronia (Fig. 17–3).[56] If severe pyuria or bacteria are present, or if radiologic imaging shows any abnormalities of the urinary tract, then initiation of intravenous antibiotic therapy is indicated. Failure of the abdominal pain or tenderness to resolve within the next 24 to 48 hours should raise the question of concomitant intra-abdomi-

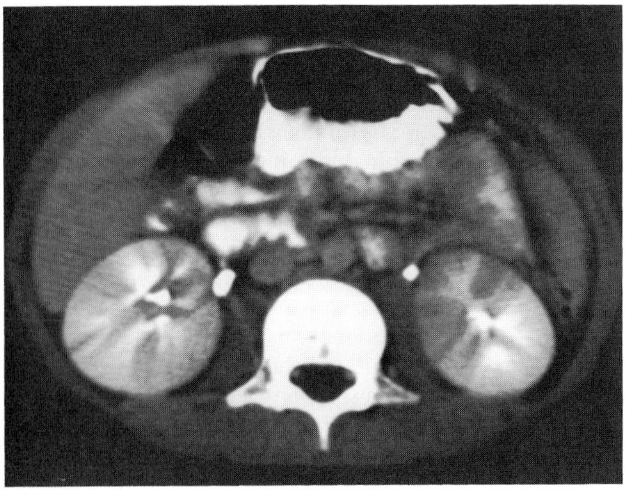

Figure 17–3. Lobar nephronia or focal pyelonephritis as seen on CT scan. Despite the appearance of a localized collection of infection, this entity can be managed nonoperatively.

nal pathology that would require laparotomy. The fever associated with pyelonephritis may take several days to resolve, especially in lobar nephronia.

MEDICAL CONDITIONS OBSCURING THE ACUTE ABDOMEN

Children with certain medical conditions, especially those involving the hematologic and reticuloendothelial cell systems, can develop problems that present as an acute abdomen. In some instances the medical condition predisposes the child to intra-abdominal pathology that may require surgical treatment; in others the underlying medical problem may masquerade as a surgical emergency. Understanding the role of the medical problem is important in expediting prompt surgical treatment or avoiding an unnecessary operation.

Henoch-Schönlein Purpura

Henoch-Schönlein purpura (HSP) is a systemic vasculitis manifesting as a purpuric rash, arthritis, nephritis, and abdominal pain and can be difficult to distinguish from intra-abdominal pathology requiring surgical therapy. Although 50 to 70% of children with HSP present with abdominal pain, only 2 to 6% have surgical lesions.[57, 58] Intussusception, often ileal-ileal, is the most common operative lesion. Because of its location in the small bowel only, this type of intussusception can often be diagnosed by barium enema, but it is not likely to be reduced nonoperatively. Other less common surgical lesions include intestinal perforation, segmental intestinal ischemia, and gastrointestinal hemorrhage. Although many patients with HSP develop gastrointestinal bleeding, few require operative therapy (see Chapter 63).

Hemolytic Uremic Syndrome

Hemolytic uremic syndrome (HUS) is a triad of hemolytic anemia, thrombocytopenia, and renal insufficiency. Many of the affected children present with severe abdominal pain and tenderness, as well as diarrhea, which appears to be caused by intestinal infections, the most common being verotoxic strains of *Escherichia coli.*[59] The toxins produced by these *E. coli* have been shown to damage endothelial cells and to produce a colonic necrosis when injected intravenously in rabbits. This experimental model mimics the human disease state in which pancreatitis, colonic necrosis, and colonic stenosis have been described. Those conditions that require surgical treatment are rare[60] (see Chapter 63).

Neutropenia

The neutropenic patient may lack the ability to localize any abdominal pathology, making diagnosis extremely difficult. Such children are prone to neutropenic enterocolitis or typhlitis, a condition characterized by mucosal ulceration of the intestine (usually ileum and cecum) resulting in bacterial invasion of the bowel wall, which can lead to a full-thickness inflammation and occasionally perforation[61] (Fig. 17– 4). Typhlitis can occur in any neutropenic patient, but it appears to be most common in leukemia patients, especially those with acute myelogenous leukemia. The chemotherapeutic drug cytarabine has been implicated as a contributing factor to the development of neutropenic enterocolitis.[62]

Since these children can also have appendicitis, pancreatitis, acalculous cholecystitis, and other diseases requiring surgical treatment, serial physical exams are essential. Nasogastric decompression and antimicrobial therapy with broad-spectrum antibiotics, including anaerobic coverage, should be initiated for all neutropenic

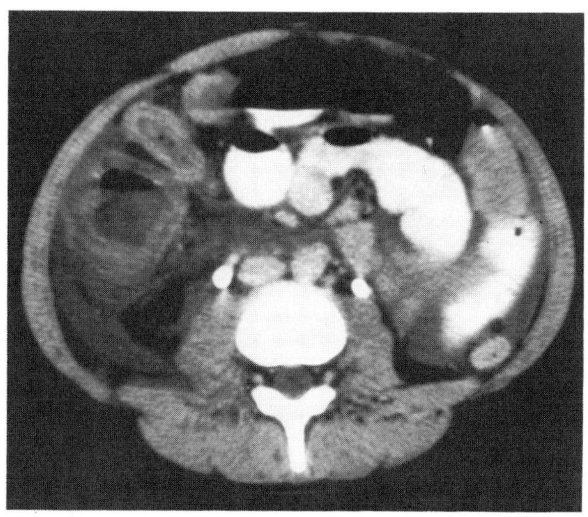

Figure 17–4. Neutropenic enterocolitis or typhlitis. Note the thickened wall of the ascending colon and neighboring bowel. Appendicitis can also be seen in neutropenic patients and may have a similar appearance on CT scan.

patients with abdominal pain and fever. The diagnosis of neutropenic enterocolitis can best be made by CT scan or ultrasonography. Unfortunately, these imaging techniques are neither 100% sensitive nor specific for typhlitis.[63]

If the pain is localized to the right upper quadrant, radionuclide hepatobiliary scanning should be done to exclude cholecystitis. If the pain and tenderness are localized anywhere else, surgical treatment may be necessary. Continued deterioration or medical instability may obviate the need for localization of the abdominal symptoms and warrant an exploratory laparotomy.

The laparotomy finding of neutropenic enterocolitis should be managed by limited resection of the involved bowel with enterostomy and mucous fistula creation. Survival from surgical therapy in neutropenic abdominal conditions is largely dependent on the patient's ability to resolve the neutropenia. A particularly poor outcome can be anticipated in patients with *Clostridium septicum* enterocolitis.[64]

Nephrotic Syndrome

Patients with ascites, regardless of the etiology, are at risk for the development of spontaneous bacterial peritonitis (SBP).[65] This is particularly true of children with nephrotic syndrome, whose renal disease results in hypoproteinemia and ascites. The ascites fluid appears to be prone to colonization by pathogenic bacteria, arising from either transient bacteremia or translocation of organisms through the intestinal wall. The most common organisms are *Streptococcus pneumoniae*, *Haemophilus influenzae*, and *E. coli*.[65]

Such patients present with diffuse abdominal pain, fever, leukocytosis, and generalized abdominal tenderness. The fact that most of these children are treated with corticosteroids for their renal disease makes the clinical assessment much more difficult. Fortunately, these patients should not require laparotomy, since appendicitis is unusual in nephrotic syndrome. Paracentesis usually yields polymorphonuclear cells and one single type of organism.

DIAGNOSTIC TESTS

Many of the diagnostic tests employed in evaluating the acute abdomen are of limited value. One must view them as only contributing pieces of evidence, to be considered in conjunction with the history and physical examination, which are usually more important. A few of the more common tests deserve some discussion.

Blood Tests

White Blood Count. This is perhaps the most frequently utilized blood test in evaluation of the acute abdomen. It is easily and rapidly obtained. Although it is generally true that leukocytosis and/or an increased percentage of immature granulocytes are seen with peritonitis or acute intra-abdominal inflammation, several significant exceptions exist. The normal leukocyte count for neonates is so variable that the WBC is seldom helpful in this age group, except when neutropenia is discovered; this suggests a bone marrow that is overwhelmed by sepsis and is a poor prognostic finding that may warrant a granulocyte transfusion. Patients who are receiving immunosuppressive medications may not manifest a leukocytosis in response to intra-abdominal inflammation. Even in the normal child, serious intra-abdominal pathology may be present without noteworthy leukocytosis. The converse is also true; an elevated WBC does not always indicate a surgical disease of the abdomen. Viral gastroenteritis may be associated with an elevated WBC as well, although it is often due to a high proportion of lymphocytes.

Serum Amylase. Pancreatitis is classically associated with hyperamylasemia and hyperlipasemia. Amylase is also secreted by the salivary glands, small intestine, kidney, and fallopian tubes. Consequently, an elevated amylase level is not specific to diseases of the pancreas. Conversely, pancreatitis may be present in the absence of hyperamylasemia. High levels of serum amylase are more typical of pancreatitis than of pathology in the other organs mentioned, however.

Blood Gas. The finding of metabolic acidosis in the patient with abdominal symptoms suggests either some intra-abdominal ischemia or a systemic insult severe enough to result in tissue hypoperfusion. This is especially true of the premature neonate. Intestinal ischemia, however, does not always result in a metabolic acidosis, even in midgut volvulus. It is likely that the occlusion of the twisted mesenteric veins prevents entry into the systemic circulation of the oxygen radicals and inflammatory mediators released by the ischemic tissue.

Radiologic Tests

Plain Abdominal Radiographs. This frequently overused examination is unnecessary when the patient has a history and physical exam that indicate peritonitis. In less obvious situations, it may be of some help. The presence of a fecalith in a patient with abdominal pain warrants an appendectomy. Pneumatosis intestinalis in the premature infant is almost diagnostic of NEC, but it can be seen with other diseases, some of which do not require surgery. Portal venous air is seen in pylephlebitis, which may result from appendicitis, neutropenic enterocolitis, and NEC. Although it is a poor prognostic finding, some authors have argued that laparotomy is not mandated by the finding of portal venous air. Free air or pneumoperitoneum is virtually always an indication for laparotomy in children, rare reports of benign pneumoperitoneum notwithstanding. Free air persisting more than 24 hours after a laparotomy in an infant is also markedly abnormal.[66]

Ultrasonography. This test has become increasingly popular for assessing abdominal pain, especially in the female adolescent population. The ability to visualize free fluid in the pelvis, adnexal masses, intrauterine pregnancy, ectopic pregnancy, and often an inflamed appendix makes this test helpful in avoiding unnecessary laparotomies. Ultrasonography can also be used to identify intussusceptions, segments of intestine with inflammatory bowel disease, neutropenic enterocolitis, midgut volvulus, biliary tract pathology, pancreatitis, and urinary tract pathology that might present with abdominal pain. Its usefulness is somewhat limited in patients with paralytic ileus, as the gas-filled loops of bowel often obscure the view.

REFERENCES

1. Bonica JJ: General considerations of acute pain. *In* Bonica JJ, ed: The Management of Pain. 2nd ed. Philadelphia, Lea and Febiger, 1990, pp 137–182.
2. Pomeranz B, Wall PD, Weber WV: Cord cells responding to fine myelinated afferents from viscera, muscle and skin. Physiol J (Lond.) 1968; 199:511–516.
3. Foreman RD, Hancock MB, Willis WD: Responses of spinothalamic tract cells in the thoracic spinal cord of the monkey to cutaneous and visceral inputs. Pain 1981; 11:149–154.
4. Kruger L, Manty HPW: Changing concepts in the anatomy of pain. Semin Anesth 1985; 4:209–213.
5. Cope Z: Cope's early diagnosis of the abdomen. 16th ed. Revised by William Silen. New York, Oxford University Press, 1983.
6. Howell CG, Vozza F, Shaw S, et al: Malrotation, malnutrition, and ischemic bowel disease. J Pediatr Surg 1982; 17:469–473.
7. Anand KJS, Brown MJ, Causon RC, et al: Can the human neonate mount an endocrine and metabolic response to surgery. J Pediatr Surg 1985; 20:41–48.
8. Ward Platt MP, Tarbit MJ, Aynsley-Green A: The effect of anesthesia and surgery on metabolic homeostasis in infancy and childhood. J Pediatr Surg 1990; 25:472–478.
9. Boix-Ochoa J, Martinez Ibanez V, Potau N, et al: Cortisol response to surgical stress in neonates. Pediatr Surg Int 1987; 2:267–270.
10. Simmons RL, Ahrenholz DH: Therapeutic principles in peritonitis. *In* Simmons RL, ed: Topics in Intraabdominal Surgical Infection. Norwalk, CT, Appleton-Century-Crofts, 1982.
11. Echternacher B, Falk W, Maennel DN, et al: Requirement of endogenous tumor necrosis factor/cachectin for recovery for experimental peritonitis. J Immunol 1990; 145:3762–3766.
12. Christou NV: Systemic and peritoneal host defenses in peritonitis. World J Surg 1990; 14:184–190.
13. Cairo MS: Neonatal neutrophil host defense. Am J Dis Child 1989; 143:40–46.
14. Silen ML, Hesse DG, Felsen D, et al: Cachectin/tumor necrosis factor production by fetal and newborn rat hepatic macrophages. J Pediatr Surg 1989; 24:34–38.
15. Imura K, Fukui Y, Yagi M, et al: Perioperative change of plasma endotoxin levels in early infants. J Pediatr Surg 1989; 24:1232–1235.
16. Graham JM, Polorny WJ, Harberg FJ: Acute appendicitis in preschool age children. Am J Surg 1980; 139:247.
17. Andrews DA, Sawin RS, Ledbetter DJ, et al: Necrotizing enterocolitis in term neonates. Am J Surg 1990; 159:507–509.
18. Hatch EI: The acute abdomen in children. Pediatr Clin North Am 1985; 32:1151–1164.
19. Howell CG, Vozza F, Shaw S, et al: Malrotation, malnutrition, and ischemic bowel disease. J Pediatr Surg 1982; 17:469–473.
20. Rasmussen L, Anderson OP, Pedersen SA: Intestinal malrotation and volvulus in infancy. Pediatr Surg Int 1990; 5:27–29.
21. Powell DM, Othersen HB, Smith CD: Malrotation of the intestines in children. The effect of age on presentation and therapy. J Pediatr Surg 1989; 24:777–780.
22. Rasmussen L, Andersen OP, Pedersen SA: Intestinal malrotation and volvulus in infancy. Pediatr Surg Int 1990; 5:27–29.
23. Ladd WE: Discussion of Penberthy GC, Benson CD, Weller CN. Trans Am Surg Assoc 1942; 50:945.
24. Moore TC: Management of midgut volvulus with extensive necrosis by "patch, drain, and wait" in early infancy and childhood. Pediatr Surg Int 1991; 6:313–317.
25. Thomas DFM, Fernie DS, Bayston R, et al: Enterocolitis in Hirschsprung's disease: A controlled study of the etiologic role of clostridium difficile. J Pediatr Surg 1986; 21:22–25.
26. Wilson-Storey D, Scobie WG: Impaired gastrointestinal mucosal defense in Hirschsprung's disease. A clue to the pathogenesis of enterocolitis. J Pediatr Surg 1989; 24:462–464.
27. Fujimoto T, Puri P: Persistence of enterocolitis following diversion of faecal stream in Hirschsprung's disease. A study of mucosal defense mechanisms. Pediatr Surg Int 1988; 3:141–146.
28. Teitelbaum DH, Caniano DA, Qualman SJ: The pathophysiology of Hirschsprung's-associated enterocolitis. Importance of histologic correlates. J Pediatr Surg 1989; 24:1271–1277.
29. Klein MD, Coran AG, Wesley JR, Drongowski RA: Hirschsprung's disease in the newborn. J Pediatr Surg 1984; 19:370–374.
30. Smith GHH, Cass D: Infantile Hirschsprung's disease—is a barium enema helpful? Pediatr Surg Int 1991; 6:318–321.
31. Czyrko C, Del Pin CA, O'Neill JA, et al: Maternal cocaine abuse and necrotizing enterocolitis: Outcome and survival. J Pediatr Surg 1991; 26:414–421.
32. Kliegman RM: Models of the pathogenesis of necrotizing enterocolitis. J Pediatrics 1990; 117(1):S2–S5.
33. Czyrko C, Del Pin CA, O'Neill JA, et al: Maternal cocaine abuse and necrotizing enterocolitis: Outcome and survival. J Pediatr Surg 1991; 26:414–421.
34. Ballance WA, Dahms BB, Shenker N, et al: Pathology of necrotizing enterocolitis. A ten-year experience. J Pediatrics 1990; 117:S6–S13.
35. Caplan MS, Hsueh W: Necrotizing enterocolitis: Role of platelet activating factor, endotoxin, and tumor necrosis factor. J Pediatrics 1990; 117:S47–S51.
36. Kosloske AM, Papile L, Burstein J: Indications for operation in acute necrotizing enterocolitis of the neonate. Surgery 1980; 87:502–505.
37. Ross MN, Wayne ER, Janik JS, et al: A standard of comparison for acute surgical necrotizing enterocolitis. J Pediatr Surg 1989; 24:998–1002.
38. Spigland N, Yazbeck S, Desjardins JG: Surgical outcome of necrotizing enterocolitis. Pediatr Surg Int 1990; 5:355–358.
39. Schwartz MZ, Hayden CK, Richarson CJ, et al: A prospective evaluation of intestinal stenosis following necrotizing enterocolitis. J Pediatr Surg 1982; 17:764–768.
40. Hartman GE, Drugas GT, Shochat SJ: Post-necrotizing enterocolitis strictures with sepsis or perforation: Risk of clinical observation. J Pediatr Surg 1988; 23:562–566.
41. Harberg FJ, McGill CW, Saleem MM, et al: Resection with primary anastomosis for necrotizing enterocolitis. J Pediatr Surg 1983; 18:743–747.
42. Bruce J, Huh YS, Cooney DR, et al: Intussusception:. Evolution of current management. J Pediatr Gastroenterol Nutr 1987; 6:663–674.
43. Beasley SW, Auldist AW, Stokes KB: The diagnostically difficult intussusception: Its characteristics and consequences. Pediatr Surg Int 1988; 3:135–138.
44. Zamir O, Mogle P, Lernau OZ, et al: The efficiency and limitations of barium enema in the treatment of intussusception in infancy and childhood. Pediatr Surg Int 1987; 2:105–107.
45. Palder SB, Ein SH, Stringer DA, et al: Intussusception: Barium or air? J Pediatr Surg 1991; 26:271–275.
46. Ravitch MM, McCune RM: Intussusception in infants and children. J Pediatr Surg 1991; 37:153–173.
47. Ein SH, Mercer S, Humphry A, MacDonald P: Colon perforation during attempted barium enema reduction of intussusception. J Pediatr Surg 1981; 16:313–315.
48. Guo J, Ma X, Zhou Q: Results of air pressure enema reduction of intussusception: 6,396 cases in 13 years. J Pediatr Surg 1986; 21:1201–1203.
49. Mitra SK, Rao PLNG, Bhattacharyya NC, et al: Rupture of intussuscipiens. J Pediatr Surg 1982; 17:300–301.
50. Gornall P, Ahmed S, Jolleys A, et al: Intra-abdominal injuries in the battered baby syndrome. Arch Dis Child 1972; 47:211–214.
51. McCort J, Vaudagna J: Visceral injuries in battered children. Radiology 1964; 82:424–428.
52. Kempe CH, Silverman FN, Steele BF, et al: The battered child syndrome. JAMA 1962; 181:17–24.

53. Robinson JA, Burch BH: An assessment of the value of the menstrual history differentiating acute appendicitis from pelvic inflammatory disease. Surg Gynecol Obstet 1984; 159:149–152.
54. Bongard F, Landers DV, Lewis F: Differential diagnosis of appendicitis and pelvic inflammatory disease: A prospective analysis. Am J Surgery 1985; 150:90–96.
55. Whitworth CM, Whitworth PW, Sanfillipo J, et al: Value of diagnostic laparoscopy in young women with possible appendicitis. Surg Gynecol Obstet 1988; 167:187–190.
56. Ratmore MH, Barton LL, Luisiri A: Acute lobar nephronia: A review. Pediatrics 1991; 87:728–734.
57. Cull DL, Rosario V, Lally KP, et al: Surgical implications of Henoch Schönlein purpura. J Pediatr Surg 1990; 25:741–743.
58. Martinez-Frontanilla LA, Silverman L, Meagher DP: Intussusception in Henoch-Schönlein purpura: Diagnosis with ultrasound. J Pediatr Surg 1988; 23:375–376.
59. Moake JL: Recent observations on the pathophysiology of thrombotic thrombocytopenic purpura and the hemolytic uremic syndrome. Hematol Pathol 1990; 4:197–201.
60. Brandt ML, Oregan S, Rousseau E, et al: Surgical complications of the hemolytic uremic syndrome. J Pediatr Surg 1990; 25:1109–1112.
61. Katz JA, Wagner ML, Gresik MV, et al: Typhilitis: An 18-year experience and postmortem review. Cancer 1990; 65:1041–1047.
62. Shambergor RC, Weinstein HJ, Delorey MJ, et al: The medical and surgical management of typhlitis in children with acute myelogenous leukemia. Cancer 1986; 57:603–609.
63. Wade DS, Douglass H, Nava HR, et al: Abdominal pain in neutropenic patients. Arch Surg 1990; 125:1119–1127.
64. Tanabe KK, Jones WG, Barie PS: Clostridial sepsis and malignant disease. Surg Gynecol Obstet 1989; 169:423–428.
65. Gorensek MJ, Lebel MH, Nelson JD: Peritonitis in children with nephrotic syndrome. Pediatrics 1988; 81:849–856.
66. Ein SH, Stephens CA, Reilly BJ: The disappearance of free air after pediatric laparotomy. J Pediatr Surg 1985; 20:422–424.

Chapter 18

Intra-abdominal Infection

BARBARA BAETZ-GREENWALT and
MARILYN GOSKE

INTRODUCTION

Prior to the development of operative therapy for intra-abdominal sepsis, more than 90% of patients died of such infections. When surgical management became available during the latter part of the nineteenth century and early part of the twentieth century, mortality rates decreased to about 50%.[1] Despite the introduction of penicillin and, subsequently, many other antibiotics, mortality from this form of sepsis remained basically unchanged from 1930 to 1970, fluctuating between 43 and 46%. In the decade of the 1980s, survival improved, probably as a result of new operative techniques and more potent antibiotics, as well as intense supportive care. In addition, new radiographic techniques for diagnosing and treating abscesses were developed.

Intra-abdominal sepsis is less common in children than it is in adults, but it is not a rare condition. Most pediatric cases of intra-abdominal sepsis are secondary in nature, with appendicitis the most common underlying cause of secondary peritonitis. Necrotizing enterocolitis, biliary tract disease, trauma, and infection related to indwelling foreign bodies make up the other most common causes of secondary peritonitis in children.

Intra-abdominal infections may occur intraperitoneally as peritonitis, or they may be localized to several different spaces or to just the retroperitoneal space. Infections may also localize between loops of bowel, or they may be contained within the intra-abdominal organs themselves (liver, spleen, pancreas, or ovaries). Retroperitoneal infections may occur in the kidney itself as an intrarenal abscess, or infection may escape the confines of the organ and involve the perinephric space as a perirenal abscess. The psoas muscle may also be involved with abscess formation, and, likewise, the retroperitoneal space as a whole may be a site for abscess formation.

Critical to understanding the pathogenesis, clinical manifestations, and treatment of intra-abdominal infection is an appreciation of intra-abdominal anatomy. The abdominal cavity is divided into spaces by the organs that are contained within it and their mesenteric attachments and peritoneal reflections (Fig. 18–1). These compartments within the abdominal cavity determine the route of spread of infected fluid. Several physical factors at work in the intra-abdominal environment normally move fluid into the dependent areas, such as the pericolic gutters and pelvis, and cephalad into the subphrenic spaces. Peristalsis normally pushes fluid laterally and downward into the lateral colic gutters. Both the right and the left pericolic gutters are in continuity with the pelvic recess. This is the most dependent part of the peritoneal cavity. In females, the space between the rectum and the body of the uterus that projects into the pelvic recess is called the *pouch of Douglas.* This lies above the posterior fornix of the vagina. In males, a pouch of peritoneal cavity between the rectum and bladder is the most dependent recess of the peritoneal cavity. Infection in the form of abscess commonly occurs in both the right and the left pericolic spaces. Because the bowel occupies the medial portion of the abdomen, infection in the gutters does not usually extend to include the medial aspect of the abdominal cavity. However, the right pericolic gutter extends in a cephalad direction and is continuous with the right subphrenic and subhepatic spaces. The cephalad limit of the left pericolic gutter is formed by the phrenocolic ligament. Therefore, an abscess located in the left pericolic gutter does not usually communicate with the left subdiaphragmatic space.

Infection tends to migrate caudad or inferiorly into the pelvis and may also be moved upward into the subphrenic area. This cephalad movement occurs because of the motion of the diaphragm during respiration and is enhanced by absorption of fluid through the diaphragmatic lymphatics. Both create a cephalad flow of peritoneal fluid. With the liver being displaced inferiorly, gravity creates the subdiaphragmatic space.

When infected fluid reaches the right subdiaphragmatic space, an abscess may form in either the subphrenic space or the subhepatic space. The right triangular and coronary ligaments form the horizontal and posterior boundaries of these two spaces. Vertical reflection of the falciform ligament further divides the right perihepatic space into right subphrenic and right

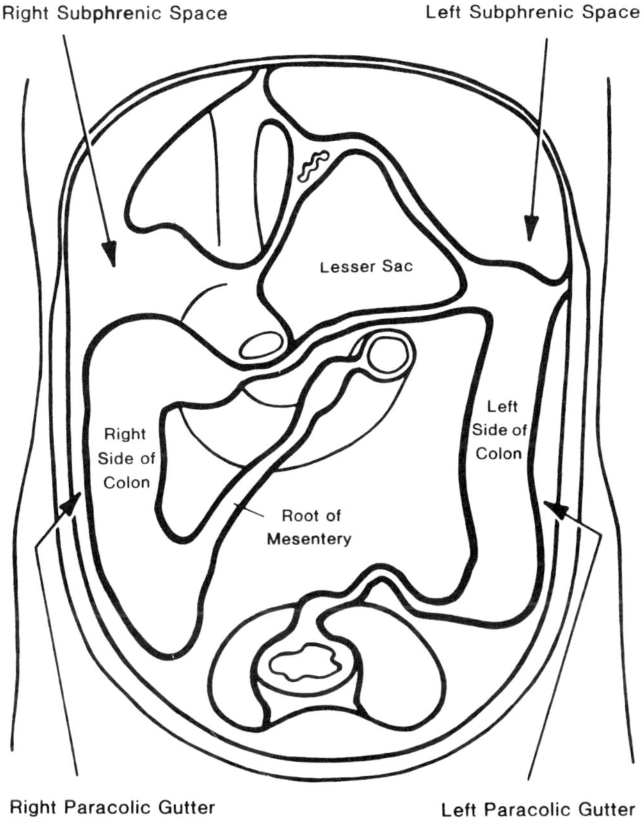

Figure 18–1. Potential spaces in which pus can collect. These spaces are determined largely by the bowel mesentery. (From Ferrucci JT, vanSonnenberg E: Intra-abdominal abscess: Radiological diagnosis and treatment. JAMA 1981; 246:2728–2733; with permission. Copyright 1981, American Medical Association.)

subhepatic spaces. The right and left subphrenic spaces are separated by the falciform ligament. This prevents the spread of pus from one subphrenic space to the other and probably explains why only 5 to 15% of subphrenic abscesses are bilateral.[2] The right perihepatic space will have abscesses in a distribution in accordance with the membranes that divide it into the subphrenic space, in which these abscesses will lie either anteriorly or posteriorly, and the subhepatic space, in which they will lie superiorly or inferiorly. The left subhepatic space is divided into the left subphrenic space and the lesser sac. The lesser sac is in continuity with the main peritoneal cavity through an opening called the *foramen of Winslow.* The boundaries of the lesser sac are made up of the pancreas and kidneys posteriorly, the stomach anteriorly, and the liver and the folds of the duodenal mesentery laterally.

In summary, fluid introduced into the peritoneal cavity first descends into the dependent pelvic recesses and then ascends via the right pericolic gutter under the influence of hydrostatic forces and intestinal movement into the right perihepatic space. Abscesses in these areas are usually due to diffuse peritoneal contamination (e.g., perforation of a viscus). Abscesses spread in this way are often multiple. Although there is some limited continuity with the peritoneal cavity through the foramen of Winslow, abscesses in the lesser sac are usually a result of disease in one of the organs that form the lesser sac boundaries.

The retroperitoneal space extends from the diaphragm to the pelvic brim, with the posterior peritoneal membrane and the transversalis fascia forming its anterior and posterior boundaries. The ascending and descending colon, duodenum, and pancreas traverse the anterior retroperitoneal space, which is defined as that area between the peritoneum and the anterior renal fascia. The kidneys and the ureters lie within the posterior retroperitoneal space. This is also known as the *perinephric space* and is bounded by the anterior and posterior renal fascia. Inferiorly, the renal fascia is open, which allows spread of any pelvic infection into the perirenal space.

The normal peritoneal cavity is lined by a thin, serous membrane with a surface area (in the adult) of 1.7 m. It is made up of a monolayer of flat polygonal cells over a basement membrane. The peritoneal membrane behaves as a semipermeable barrier and has been used for many years as a dialysis membrane, since it is highly permeable, allowing transfer of substances in both directions. Substances such as fluids, electrolytes, antibiotics, and even blood can be placed within the peritoneal cavity and transferred across the peritoneal membrane. The rate of movement across the membrane is dependent on serum oncotic pressure and hydrostatic forces in the lymphatic vessels and the portal veins. Concentration gradients also help determine the rate of water and solute movement across this membrane. The lymphatics underlie this membrane and remove particulate matter, such as bacteria, from the peritoneal cavity. Valves within the thoracic lymphatics prevent backward spread from the lymphatics into the peritoneal cavity. Diaphragmatic movements and pressure changes in the thoracic cavity enable the lymphatic fluid to flow up into the thoracic duct.

The peritoneal space contains fluid, usually in small amounts (50–75 ml of clear fluid), that ordinarily has less than 3 gm of protein per dl. Some leukocytes, usually fewer than 300 cells per mm^3 consisting of lymphocytes and macrophages, are normally found in peritoneal fluid. Inflammation within the peritoneal cavity, however, may increase the amount of intravascular fluid secreted into the peritoneal space at the rate of 300 to 500 ml per hour. This fluid shift can cause severe hypovolemia and shock.

PERITONITIS

Peritonitis is defined as a chemical or infectious inflammation of the peritoneal lining of the abdominal cavity. Chemical peritonitis will not be discussed in this chapter. Infectious peritonitis may be either primary or secondary. *Primary peritonitis,* also called *spontaneous* or *idiopathic peritonitis,* is defined as infection of the peritoneal cavity in which the source of infection arises outside the abdominal cavity and reaches the peritoneal cavity by either hematogenous or lymphatic spread. *Secondary peritonitis,* on the other hand, is infection that arises from within the abdominal cavity itself, secondary to a primary intra-abdominal catastrophe, such as appendiceal rupture or rupture of a solid organ or an abscess within an organ. Intra-abdominal infection that is manifested by peritonitis is rather common; most cases are secondary peritonitis. Occasionally, peritonitis may be secondary to bacteria introduced into the peritoneal cavity following trauma or by a foreign body, such as a ventriculoperitoneal (VP) shunt or a peritoneal dialysis catheter. In women, the genitourinary tract can also serve as a source for intra-abdominal sepsis via retrograde spread through the open fallopian tubes.

Most cases of primary peritonitis occur in children with nephrotic syndrome or cirrhosis. The incidence of primary peritonitis in children with nephrotic syndrome varies from 2[3, 4] to 17.3%.[5] Rarely, primary peritonitis may occur in otherwise normal children. The presence of ascites is a common predisposing condition associated with primary peritonitis in children.

The microbial etiology of primary peritonitis in children includes predominantly *Streptococcus pneumoniae,* group A streptococci, and gram-negative enteric bacilli. In a review of 214 children with nephrotic syndrome with 62 episodes of peritonitis, a definite microbiologic diagnosis was possible in 50% of the episodes, and 38% (24 cases) had pneumococcal disease.[5] Three episodes were caused by alpha-hemolytic streptococcus, and one was caused by enterococcus. Altogether, 45% of the total cases were caused by gram-positive organisms. There were two episodes of gram-negative peritonitis identified, one caused by *Escherichia coli* and the other by *Klebsiella,* making up 3.2% of the cases of primary peritonitis. In a retrospective study of 280 admissions of nephrotic patients from 1963 to 1967 in Boston, it was reported that gram-negative bacteria accounted for most of the cultured organisms in cases of primary peritonitis. The literature, therefore, supports a significant role for both gram-negative and gram-positive organisms in primary peritonitis in children with nephrotic syndrome.[4, 6, 7]

Spontaneous peritonitis in children who have cirrhotic ascites is caused most often by gram-negative enteric organisms, with *E. coli* and *Klebsiella pneumoniae* the most common. *S. pneumoniae,* other streptococcal species, including enterococcus, and occasionally *Staphylococcus aureus* may also cause primary peritonitis under these circumstances. The liver plays a crucial role in removing enteric organisms that have reached the circulation by intestinal transmural migration; when portal systemic shunting occurs through the liver, hepatic clearance of bacteria is reduced. This allows both persistence of bacterial contamination in the blood stream and delayed clearance from lymphatics that drain the peritoneal cavity. Bacteria can persist in the ascitic fluid as well as in the systemic circulation as a result of failure of the liver to clear these organisms. Enteric bacteria may also persist in hypertonic ascitic fluid, such as peritoneal dialysis fluid. Hypertonicity of the peritoneal fluid appears to enhance the migration of bacteria across the colonic wall, increasing the risk of peritonitis in the dialysis patient. Primary peritonitis may occasionally complicate systemic tuberculosis infection.

Clinical Presentation

The child with primary peritonitis presents with an acute febrile illness accompanied by abdominal pain, nausea, vomiting, and, occasionally, diarrhea. Diffuse abdominal tenderness reflects the inflammatory process present within the peritoneal cavity. Often, there is rebound tenderness and hypoactive or absent bowel sounds. If corticosteroids are being used, some of the clinical manifestations may be suppressed. Fever, however, is a common presenting sign and occurs in 50 to 80% of children with primary peritonitis.

Paracentesis in primary peritonitis generally reveals a peritoneal leukocyte count of more than 300 cells per mm^3 and often more than 1000 cells per mm^3 in 85% of cases, with predominance of granulocytes. In a review of ascitic fluid from uninfected patients and those with bacterial peritonitis, there were significant differences in granulocyte counts noted.[8] Uninfected fluid averaged 122 cells per mm^3, versus 2,686 cells per mm^3 for infected fluid. A fluid pH of 7.45 has been noted in uninfected patients, compared with 7.24 in those with infection, giving an arterial–ascitic fluid pH gradient of 0.02 in uninfected patients, versus 0.22 in infected patients. Ascitic lactate has been noted to be about 12 mg per dl in those who did not have infection compared with 25 mg per dl in those who did. Ascitic lactate was 15 mg per dl in noninfected fluid, compared with 45 mg per dl in infected fluid. The most reliable cutoff points for diagnosis were determined to be a polymorphonuclear leukocyte count of more than 500 cells per mm^3, an ascitic fluid pH less than 7.35, an arterial–ascitic fluid pH gradient greater than 0.1, and an ascitic fluid lactate level greater than 25 mg per dl.[8] Gram stain of the ascitic fluid is positive in only about 40% of cases; however, a positive Gram stain is diagnostic. If children with presumed primary peritonitis are found to have mixed bacterial flora in the ascites, then exploratory laparotomy may be considered in order to rule out other possible intra-abdominal sources of the peritonitis. Occasionally, bacteria may appear in the peritoneal fluid in the absence of peritonitis, for example, in primary pneumococcal pneumonia. In the setting of nephrotic syndrome or ascites, gram-positive diplococci on a Gram stain and a positive culture for *S. pneumoniae* usually reflect primary peritonitis, not peritonitis secondary to another focus.

Management

If the Gram stain is positive for gram-positive diplococci, penicillin therapy alone may be sufficient in a child with nephrotic syndrome. However, in most instances, the Gram stain is negative, and while awaiting identification of cultures of blood and peritoneal fluid, empiric therapy should include coverage for both gram-positive and gram-negative organisms. Antibiotic therapy can be tailored to specific etiologies when results become available. Primary bacterial peritonitis due to

S. pneumoniae and group A streptococci is best treated with penicillin G. For empiric broad-spectrum coverage for both gram-negative and gram-positive organisms in primary peritonitis, a variety of choices are available. Ampicillin combined with an aminoglycoside, such as gentamicin, offers broad-spectrum coverage, but there is some risk of nephrotoxicity, especially in the patient with underlying renal disease. Other alternatives, such as a beta-lactam antibiotic with a beta-lactamase inhibitor—ticarcillin/clavulanic acid (Timentin)—or a third-generation cephalosporin, such as cefotaxime and ceftriaxone, may be appropriate choices. Clinical improvement in response to antibiotic therapy should be evident within 24 to 48 hours of therapy if the diagnosis is correct. Antimicrobial therapy for *S. pneumoniae* and group A streptococci should continue for a minimum of 10 days. For gram-negative organisms, the duration of therapy should be 14 days.

SECONDARY PERITONITIS

Secondary peritonitis has multiple causes. Contamination of the peritoneal cavity can occur following rupture of an intra-abdominal visceral abscess, such as amebic or pyogenic liver abscess, splenic abscess, renal or perirenal abscess, tubo-ovarian abscess, and, rarely, pancreatic abscess. It can follow perforation of the appendix or another part of the bowel. Vascular accidents of the bowel with necrosis and perforation following intussusception or vasculitis may give rise to peritonitis. Direct trauma to the abdomen with penetrating injury to the bowel, stomach, bladder, or uterus may cause peritonitis as well. Much more rarely in children, suppurative cholecystitis or ascending cholangitis may lead to intra-abdominal infection. Peritonitis may also follow the use of catheters that are placed in the peritoneal cavity either to shunt ventricular fluid from the ventricular system in the brain or for use in peritoneal dialysis. Occasionally, in postpubertal female children, the vaginal flora (which contain *Neisseria gonorrhoeae, S. aureus,* or *S. pneumoniae*) and infections acquired from the female genital tract attain access to the peritoneal cavity via the fallopian tubes, giving rise to secondary peritonitis. There have been extremely rare cases reported in prepubertal female children of *N. gonorrhoeae* peritonitis secondary to sexual abuse, with transmission of gonococci and ascension of the infection from the prepubertal pelvic organs.[9, 10] The most common cause of peritonitis in children, however, is appendicitis and complicated appendicitis (rupture and gangrene) (see Chapter 53). The peritoneal response to contamination from the gastrointestinal tract or from trauma may be generalized in the form of peritonitis or may also occasionally give rise to attempts to localize the infection in the form of abscesses. Free intraperitoneal abscesses will be covered in this section.

Microbiology and Epidemiology

The microbiology of peritonitis secondary to disruption of the gastrointestinal tract or spillage of a visceral abscess is determined by the source of the rupture. The microbiology of the gastrointestinal tract varies, depending on which level is involved (Table 18–1).[10a, 10b]

Table 18–1. ENTERIC MICROORGANISMS

Site	Predominant Organism	Concentration (per gm contents)
Stomach	*Streptococcus viridans*	$<10^3$
	Lactobacilli	
	Occasional yeast	
Small bowel		
Proximal	Streptococci (aerobic)	$<10^5$
Distal	Coliforms (aerobic)	$<10^6$–10^7
	Bacteroides spp	
	Bifidobacilli	
Colon	Anaerobes: 99–99.9%	
	Bifidobacteria	10^9–10^{11}
	Clostridia	$<10^3$
	Bacteroides spp	10^9–10^{10}
	Anaerobic cocci	
	Aerobes: 0.1–1%	
	E. coli	
	Enterococci	
	Streptococcus viridans	

From references 10a, 10b, and 20.

Anaerobes make up the vast bulk of the bacterial population of the large intestine, accounting for more than 99% of the bacterial species present. With modern bacteriologic techniques, it has been possible to document the presence of these anaerobic bacteria in cultures of peritoneal fluid and abscesses more accurately. Brook[11] recently studied aerobic and anaerobic bacteria in intra-abdominal infections from 339 peritoneal cavity specimens (83 from abdominal abscesses and 89 from postsurgical wounds) and found that anaerobic bacteria alone were present in 43 (13%) of the peritoneal specimens, aerobic bacteria alone in 38 (11%), and mixed anaerobic and aerobic flora in 258 (76%). He found the predominant aerobes and facultative anaerobes in abdominal infections to be *E. coli* and streptococcal species and the predominant anaerobes to be *Bacteroides, Peptostreptococcus,* and *Clostridium* species. He recovered 334 isolates of *Bacteroides fragilis,* which accounted for 75% of the isolates from abscesses. In a subsequent study of intra-abdominal abscesses in children, Brook[12] studied 23 children who had undergone drainage of intra-abdominal abscesses. The etiologic factors predisposing to abscess formation were ruptured appendix in 12 patients, trauma in 5, Crohn's disease in 3, intestinal surgery in 2, and rupture of a hollow viscus in 1. Bacteria were present in all specimens, and anaerobic bacteria alone were present in 4 specimens (17%), aerobes alone were present in only 1 specimen (4%), and mixed flora were present in 18 specimens (78%). The predominant organisms in this pediatric study were *B. fragilis* group (23 isolates), *Peptostreptococcus* species (20 isolates), and *E. coli* (15 isolates). Of these isolates, 29 beta-lactamase–producing organisms were recovered from 83% of these patients. Although these organisms make up the vast majority of the isolates described in peritonitis in children, Aronoff and associates[13] reported that *Pseudomonas aeruginosa* has recently been isolated more frequently in "community-acquired" cases of peritonitis. It is known that patients who develop intra-abdominal infection while in the hospital after having received broad-spectrum antibiotics have a higher rate of recovery of highly resistant strains, such as *Serratia* and *Acinetobacter,* than do patients who have not been hospitalized.

The bacteriology of the genital tract becomes important in females who develop intra-abdominal sepsis. In addition to sexually transmitted organisms, such as *N. gonorrhoeae* and *Chlamydia trachomatis,* anaerobic flora are the predominant species in tubo-ovarian abscesses and may lead to intra-abdominal sepsis. In addition to pelvic sepsis, organisms of genitourinary origin may sometimes ascend and cause a perihepatitis syndrome, or Fitz-Hugh–Curtis syndrome. This type of infection is usually caused by *N. gonorrhoeae* or *Chlamydia.*[14] Prepubertal children can develop tubo-ovarian abscesses.[15] To date, however, direct isolation of *Chlamydia* from the liver itself has not been reported.

Peritonitis following trauma to the abdomen may involve organisms such as *S. aureus* in addition to gastrointestinal tract organisms. Penetrating injuries to the abdominal viscera, such as the liver and spleen, usually do not lead to infection, since these organs are generally sterile. Finally, peritonitis may follow rupture of an amebic hepatic abscess or an abscess arising in one of the other intra-abdominal organs, such as the spleen, pancreas, and kidney.

Pathogenesis

The bacteria involved in intra-abdominal sepsis and abscess formation cause damage through several different mechanisms. Certain bacteria produce endotoxins, which are a heterogenous group of high-molecular-weight compounds composed of polysaccharides, lipids, and proteins. These compounds are part of the cell wall of many gram-negative bacteria. The lipid component of the lipopolysaccharide appears to be associated with the majority of the toxic effects through (1) activation of many mediators of inflammation, such as tumor necrosis factor (TNF) and interleukin 1 (IL–1); (2) activation of both the classic and alternative complement pathways; and (3) activation of arachidonic acid metabolism leading to the release of prostaglandins and leukotrienes. The macrophage appears to be a central cell for effecting the release of TNF, prostaglandins, and IL–1, which cause an acute-phase response and stimulate a broad spectrum of lymphokine and collagenase production, activating many other phagocytic and endothelial cells. Increased vascular permeability, secondary to vasodilation due to these mediators, can result in hypotension and even death. Coagulation abnormalities are caused by intravascular activation of the coagulation cascade. The bone marrow is stimulated by endotoxin as well, increasing proliferation, differentiation of bone marrow cells into functional cells, and phagocytic activity.[16] TNF and IL–1 are the common mediators of endotoxin-mediated shock that occurs in gram-negative and gram-positive sepsis.[17]

Although most species of anaerobic bacteria do not possess endotoxin (only *Fusobacterium* spp. are known to possess endotoxin), they possess several other properties that increase their virulence and pathogenicity. Both *Bacteroides* species and *Fusobacterium* species are capable of adhering to epithelial cells. In addition, they produce important exoenzymes, a variety of sulfatases, hyaluronidase, heparinase, and other proteases. The exact function of these enzymes in the development of the signs and symptoms of peritonitis is not well understood. These enzymes certainly cause inflammation, necrosis, and suppuration, however.

An important virulence factor of anaerobes is the presence of a capsule. The ability of different strains of anaerobic bacteria to produce abscesses is directly related to the composition of the polysaccharide capsule.[16] It appears that immunoregulatory T cells determine whether an abscess can be contained and also regulate antibody response to *B. fragilis*–induced intra-abdominal abscesses. CD4 and CD8 lymphocytes, which are generated following immunization with the polysaccharide capsule or components of *B. fragilis,* can provide protection against the development of intra-abdominal abscesses in an animal model of experimental peritonitis. Cellular immunity appears to be important in the disease process of intra-abdominal abscesses in humans as well.[18] The anaerobic cocci, clostridia, and fusobacteria also depend on a capsule to enhance invasiveness. Both aerobic and anaerobic bacteria are protected against opsonization by the presence of a capsule. Encapsulated bacteria are better able to withstand the body's abilities to eliminate them and are therefore more infectious than nonencapsulated bacteria.

Probably the most important aspect of the mixed flora that is encountered in intra-abdominal sepsis and abscess is the synergism that occurs between anaerobic and aerobic bacteria.[19] Bacterial virulence also appears to be enhanced when certain microorganisms are combined intraperitoneally with chemical irritants such as hemoglobin, enzymes, and bile. This adjuvant effect greatly enhances the pathogenicity of the invading bacteria. Establishment of this mixed infection involving predominantly obligate and facultative anaerobes requires that certain environmental conditions exist. The oxygen tension and the oxygen reduction potential must be low, and the proper nutrients must be available to support fermentative metabolism. If these conditions are met, anaerobic organisms can rapidly reproduce and may produce gas, interrupt blood supply, and decrease the viability of surrounding tissue.[20] Anaerobes, such as *Bacteroides,* may also be able to protect aerobic bacteria from being phagocytized and from effective antibiotic therapy because of the production of beta-lactamase. *Bacteroides fragilis* strains can also produce other penicillinases and enzymes that inactivate cephalosporins and imipenem. Penicillinases are produced by many of the other anaerobic bacteria occasionally encountered in these abscesses.[21] The classic experiments of Onderdonk and associates,[22, 23] tracing the evolution of intra-abdominal infection following implantation of fecal contents intraperitoneally in rats, showed that *E. coli* initially predominated in the peritoneal exudate. Bacteremia accompanying this phase of the infection was uniformly present and was often fatal. In surviving rats, indolent late-onset intra-abdominal abscesses developed in which anaerobes such as *B. fragilis* predominated. Onderdonk and associates[22, 23] reported that elimination of *E. coli* reduced early mortality but did not prevent late-onset abscess formation, and elimination of the anaerobic component of the infection did not prevent the early mortality due to the aerobic gram-negative organisms. An understanding of the synergistic activity in intraperitoneal infections secondary to ruptured bowel or contamination of the peritoneal cavity with gastrointestinal tract flora provides a basis for empiric therapy in these infections. It is understood, however, that the environment of an abscess inhibits the activity of some antibiotics. Certain drugs, such as aminoglycosides, do not function well in the reduced-oxygen environment with low pH that exists in an abscess cavity, and beta-lactam antibiotics are often inactivated by enzymes such as beta-lactamases. Therefore, drainage remains an important component of therapy for these infections.

In addition to the local inflammatory response, there is a tremendous exudation of fluid into the peritoneal cavity through the peritoneal membrane in peritonitis. A fibrinous exudate glues together peritoneal surfaces, bowel mesentery, and omentum in an attempt to isolate and localize areas of infected tissue. A final step in the pathway to controlling the infection within the peritoneal cavity results in the formation of abscesses. If the body is unable to contain the peritoneal infection locally or by abscess formation, infection may escape the confines of the peritoneal cavity and spread throughout the abdominal contents; in addition, systemic invasion may occur, with resultant bacteremia and distant organ involvement. Large fluid shifts can affect the circulating blood volume, aggravated by fluid and electrolyte loss from vomiting and diarrhea, and the cardiovascular system may be progressively compromised. Vasodilatory effects secondary to circulating endotoxin, TNF, and IL–1 may also produce the capillary leak syndrome and further decrease cardiac output. This, in turn, may progress to lactic acidosis, oliguria, hypotension, and death.

Effects on the respiratory system from intraperitoneal sepsis can also be seen. The diaphragms are unable to function against the distended and painful abdominal contents. Basilar atelectasis and intrapulmonary shunting of blood occur, and in some patients respiratory failure can ensue. Adult respiratory distress syndrome following intra-abdominal sepsis is associated with an extremely high mortality rate.[24]

Appendicitis

Appendicitis (see Chapter 53) is the most common cause of peritonitis in infants and children. One of every 15 people will develop appendicitis at some time during life, and the peak incidence of this disease is 12 years of age.[25] Neonatal appendicitis is exceedingly rare and extremely difficult to diagnose. Perforation and generalized peritonitis are the rule, occurring in more than 95% of newborn infants with this problem, and the mortality rate has been exceedingly high, ranging from 60 to 95% in nonperforated and perforated cases, respectively. Complicated appendicitis, which is defined as appendicitis with gangrene and perforation, occurs in approximately 30 to 45% of children with appendicitis (Fig. 18–2*A* and 2*B*). The added complication of an abdominal mass occurs in another 2 to 7% of patients.

When appendicitis has progressed to a periappendiceal inflammatory mass, computed tomography (CT) has been found to be helpful. Jeffrey[26] divided adult patients into three categories with treatment based on their CT appearance. It was noted that patients with periappendiceal phlegmon and small abscesses could be treated with antibiotic therapy alone, which would result in complete resolution of the inflammatory process in 88% of patients. A second category of patients included those with a well-defined periappendiceal abscess that was larger than 3 cm and contained fluid or air. These patients were treated with CT- or ultrasound-guided percutaneous catheter drainage and broad-spectrum antibiotics. The third category included patients with extensive and poorly defined periappendiceal abscess. These patients were treated with immediate surgical exploration. CT can also demonstrate findings of acute appendicitis with pericecal inflammation (68%), abscess (55%), and a calcified appendicolith (23%). In the series of Balthazar,[27] CT's sensitivity was similar to barium enema, but the findings at surgery correlated better with the CT examination. The author notes that a normal CT scan does not exclude appendicitis, since "mild forms without periappendiceal disease may escape detection."[27]

Perforated appendicitis with massive intra-abdominal abscesses are not uncommon, particularly in the younger patient[28, 29] (Fig. 18–3*A*–*C*). Magnetic resonance (MR) imaging is sensitive in the detection of abscess, but the findings can be nonspecific and similar to those seen in neoplasm. However, typically neoplasm will have evidence of invasion and nodularity that is not seen in abscess formation.[29]

Rarely, children may develop liver abscess or inflammation of the portal vein from appendicitis that may result in portal vein thrombosis and hypertension. This was a prevalent finding in the preantibiotic era but is rarely seen today.[30]

If the patient has obvious ascites and signs of peritonitis, paracentesis can be diagnostic, as discussed in the section on primary peritonitis. The performance of paracentesis in the patient with previous abdominal surgery requires great care. One must be aware that bowel may be adherent to the underside of abdominal scars, and these areas should be avoided. Use of ultrasound or CT scan to guide the paracentesis is often helpful.

Management

The treatment of peritonitis and intra-abdominal abscess related to appendicitis requires the use of both

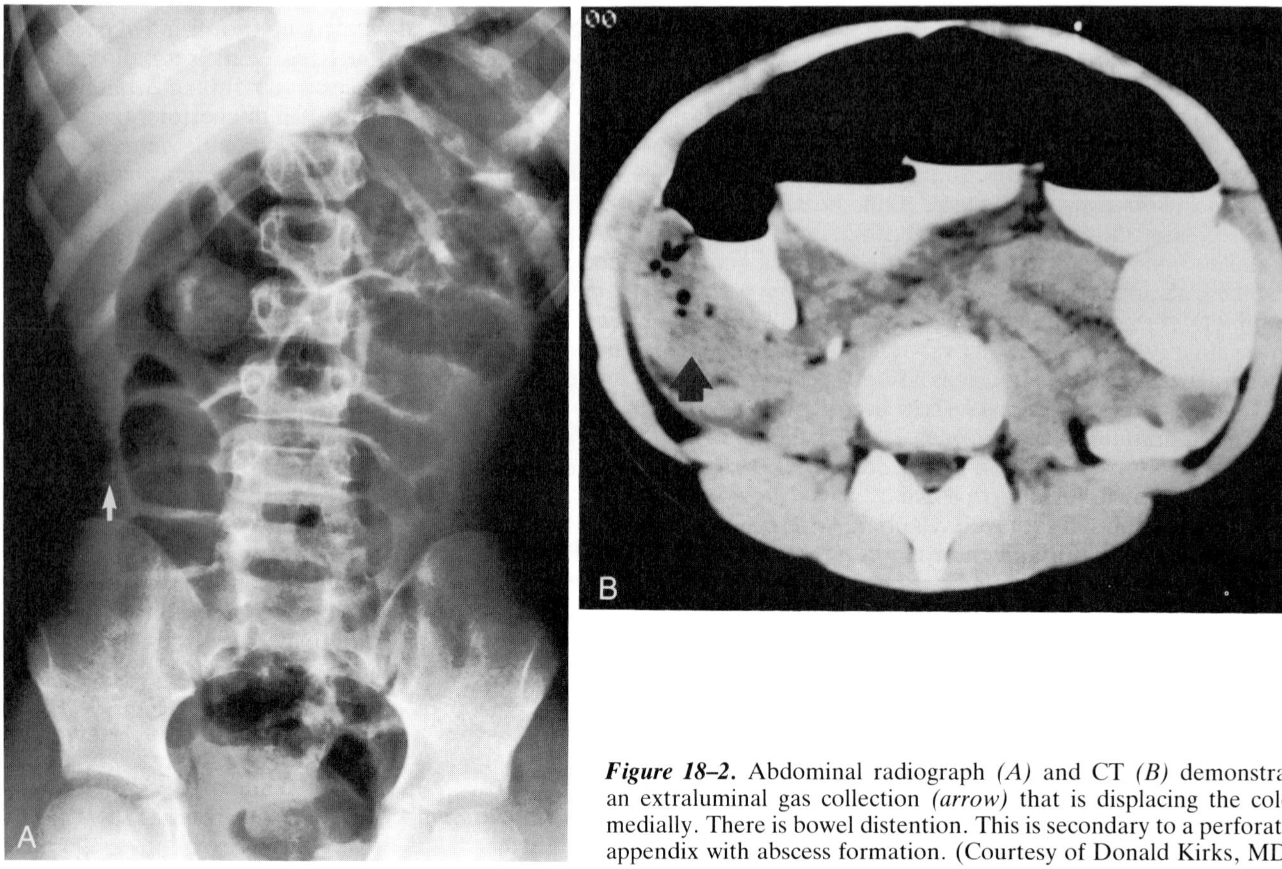

Figure 18–2. Abdominal radiograph *(A)* and CT *(B)* demonstrate an extraluminal gas collection *(arrow)* that is displacing the colon medially. There is bowel distention. This is secondary to a perforated appendix with abscess formation. (Courtesy of Donald Kirks, MD.)

antibiotics and surgical drainage. Of utmost importance is the stabilization of the patient prior to surgical intervention. This requires rehydration and correction of electrolyte abnormalities, control of fever, and administration of appropriate antibiotics. Antibiotics must cover the most common organisms usually encountered in gangrenous and perforated appendicitis. These pathogens are representative of those in the lower gastrointestinal tract, typically facultative aerobic microorganisms such as *E. coli* (most common), *Klebsiella,* and occasionally, enterococci. Anaerobic isolates include *Bacteroides,* most often *B. fragilis*. In addition, other anaerobes, such as *Peptostreptococcus, Fusobacterium,* and *Clostridium,* may occasionally be encountered. Much less commonly, organisms such as *P. aeruginosa* and *S. aureus* may be found. Antimicrobial agents must be started preoperatively and continued postoperatively to reduce the high frequency of wound infection that follows intra-abdominal sepsis from perforated appendix. Initially, empiric therapy should include coverage of all of the previously mentioned organisms. After the culture reports have been completed, one may tailor antibiotic therapy appropriately. Combinations of two or three drugs have traditionally been used, and the "gold standard" has been ampicillin, gentamicin, and clindamycin.[31–33] Because of recent reports of *Bacteroides* species and other anaerobes that are resistant to clindamycin, some have recommended the use of metronidazole in place of clindamycin for anaerobic coverage. Because metronidazole is active only against strict anaerobes, however, it cannot be relied on for coverage of the aerobic gram-negative organisms always encountered in ruptured appendicitis and abscess. An alternative to the ampicillin-gentamicin-clindamycin or ampicillin-gentamicin-metronidazole therapy for ruptured appendicitis with or without abscess may be ticarcillin–clavulanic acid and an aminoglycoside, such as tobramycin. The ticarcillin–clavulanic acid combination inhibits the beta-lactamase produced by *Bacteroides* species and therefore covers most of the anaerobic bacteria that might be active in such an infection. In addition, ticarcillin in combination with an aminoglycoside, such as tobramycin, provides broad-spectrum coverage of Enterobacteriaceae as well as *P. aeruginosa* that may be present. Another alternative is imipenem, a carbapenem antibiotic that has an extremely broad antimicrobial spectrum. It should be used in combination with an aminoglycoside for treating a serious *Pseudomonas* infection. Aztreonam, a monobactam antibiotic, has a spectrum of activity that is limited strictly to gram-negative aerobic organisms. It would not be a feasible choice unless used in combination with metronidazole to cover anaerobic organisms and possibly might require the addition of ampicillin if enterococci were isolated from the intra-abdominal cultures.[34]

Appendiceal rupture complicated by abdominal mass and abscess requires great judgment on the part of the surgeon as to whether surgery should be done immediately with drainage of the abscess or whether an interval appendectomy should be done following 4 to 6 weeks

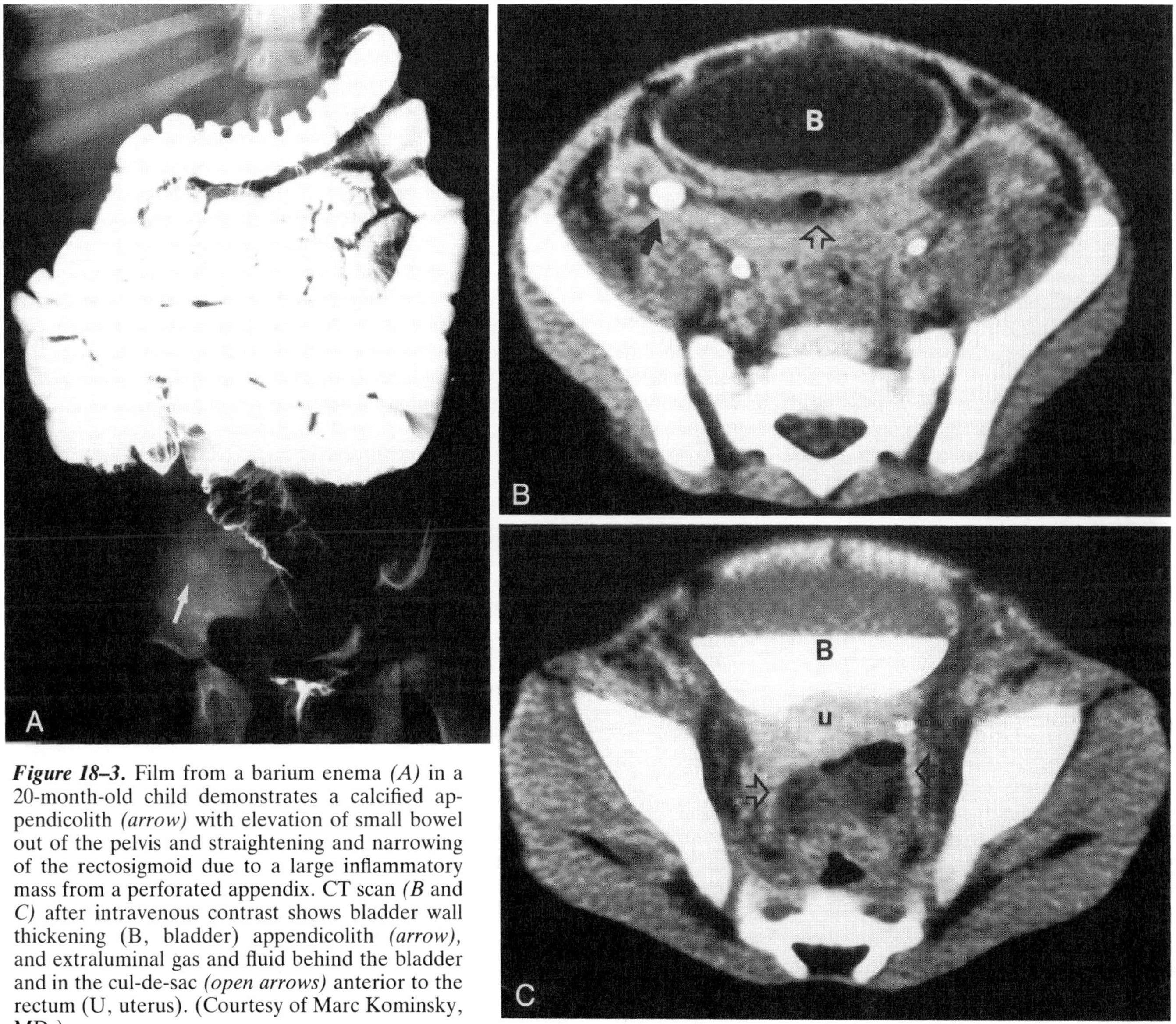

Figure 18–3. Film from a barium enema *(A)* in a 20-month-old child demonstrates a calcified appendicolith *(arrow)* with elevation of small bowel out of the pelvis and straightening and narrowing of the rectosigmoid due to a large inflammatory mass from a perforated appendix. CT scan *(B* and *C)* after intravenous contrast shows bladder wall thickening (B, bladder) appendicolith *(arrow),* and extraluminal gas and fluid behind the bladder and in the cul-de-sac *(open arrows)* anterior to the rectum (U, uterus). (Courtesy of Marc Kominsky, MD.)

of intensive antibiotic therapy. Immediate surgery for appendicitis with abdominal mass may reveal an approximately 4 to 6% frequency of phlegmon.[34] There will be little pus found in this situation, and it is known that with conservative therapy with broad-spectrum antibiotics, a large number of patients with such a phlegmon would probably resolve such a mass. However, even after conservative therapy, interval appendectomy is usually necessary because of the risk of recurrent appendicitis in as many as 20% of patients.

The duration of therapy following the demonstration of an intra-abdominal abscess varies. In the patient in whom *Candida albicans* is found along with other pathogens in the peritoneal fluid or the abscess cavity, amphotericin B should be added to the antimicrobial regimen. Amphotericin B is usually given for a 10 to 14 day course, for a total of 7.5 mg per kg for a child. Other adjunctive techniques in the management of intra-abdominal sepsis with abscess following appendicitis include drainage and various irrigation techniques.

Other Conditions

Rarely, organs other than the appendix may perforate and lead to peritonitis and intra-abdominal abscess. The most common cause of gastrointestinal perforation, other than appendicitis, is necrotizing enterocolitis (see Chapter 61). Following this, ulcers of the duodenum, stomach, and jejunum occasionally will perforate. Overall, the most likely site of perforation in infants and children is the ileum, followed by rectosigmoid, stomach, and duodenum.[35] Because the stomach has a much lower population of bacteria and especially a lower number of anaerobes, empiric antibiotic therapy may be somewhat modified following gastric or duodenal perforation in a young infant.[30, 36]

Peritonitis that occurs in relation to peritoneal dialysis usually involves *S. aureus* (coagulase-positive staphylococci), coagulase-negative staphylococci, or other skin flora; occasionally, enteric bacteria may gain access to the peritoneal cavity, stimulated in the transmural migration by the hypertonic peritoneal dialysis fluid. A polymicrobial peritoneal culture found in a child undergoing peritoneal dialysis should prompt an immediate evaluation for an underlying ruptured viscus, such as the appendix. According to several reviews of peritonitis in children on chronic ambulatory peritoneal dialysis (CAPD),[37–41] during the first year of dialysis, peritonitis occurs in about 60% of patients undergoing CAPD. Recurrent peritonitis occurs in about 20 to 30% of patients and often leads to an inability to perform CAPD because of interruption of therapy and the need to remove the catheter to treat recurrent infection. In the pediatric population, the frequency ranges from one episode of peritonitis in every 4 months to approximately one in every 14 patient months. The microbiology of these infections is remarkably similar from center to center, although some centers show more difficulty with fungi complicating peritoneal dialysis than others. A large variety of fungi have been recovered from CAPD patients. *Candida* species predominate in most areas. Unlike peritonitis related to skin contaminants such as *Staphylococcus epidermis* or *S. aureus,* peritonitis caused by fungi usually requires the removal of the catheter to eradicate the infection. Rarely, mycobacterial infections may cause peritonitis in patients undergoing CAPD. These often require removal of the catheter.

Clinical manifestations of peritonitis in CAPD patients are similar to those in patients not undergoing dialysis. Abdominal pain and tenderness are found in the majority of CAPD patients; however, fever is usually much less common. The effluent from the dialysis is cloudy in 98% of patients. Abdominal pain occurs in about 78% of patients and is accompanied by fever in 35%. Tenderness is present in 76%. Cultures of the peritoneal fluid usually grow bacteria in 80 to 90% of cases. Sterile cultures may be due to fastidious organisms or, occasionally, to a chemical peritonitis.

Treatment of peritonitis in these patients is often managed on an outpatient basis. Most transplant centers use intraperitoneal administration of antibiotics in the peritoneal dialysis solution. This may be accompanied by intravenous antibiotics; most antibiotics given intravenously reach therapeutic concentrations within the peritoneal cavity. The half-life of the drug(s) in the peritoneal cavity, of course, is dependent on the frequency of dialysis and whether the antibiotic used is transported effectively across the peritoneal membrane. Likewise, intraperitoneal administration of antibiotics also results in therapeutic systemic levels for many antibiotics.

Empiric therapy for gram-positive peritonitis in CAPD patients usually uses vancomycin or a first-generation cephalosporin. Occasionally, an aminoglycoside may be added. Vancomycin is usually administered intraperitoneally as an initial dose of 2 gm in a 2-L bag, followed by 0.1 to 0.5 gm per 24 hours. Cefazolin is administered as 1 gm per 2-L bag initially, followed by 0.25 gm per 6 hours. Gentamicin is given as 120 mg in the first 2-L bag followed by 65 mg per 48 hours. The duration of therapy is quite variable. Most centers treat gram-positive peritonitis for 7 to 10 days. Gram-negative peritonitis, on the other hand, may require 2 or more weeks of therapy, depending on clinical response. There have been no prospective, randomized clinical trials looking at the relative efficacy of various regimens for the therapy of CAPD peritonitis, so the ideal regimen has not yet been described. Mycobacterial and fungal peritonitis as well as *P. aeruginosa* peritonitis usually require catheter removal in addition to intraperitoneal and intravenous antibiotic therapy. Other indications for catheter removal may include (1) three or more episodes of peritonitis caused by the same organism; (2) three or more episodes of peritonitis occurring within 12 months of the start of CAPD; or (3) obvious catheter tunnel infection caused by *S. aureus*. Occasionally, rifampin may be used in combination with vancomycin for synergism to eradicate coagulase-negative staphylococcal peritonitis infections. Rifampin is concentrated intracellularly and is particularly effective synergistically with vancomycin in eradicating intracellular sequestration of these gram-positive organisms.[42]

Finally, secondary peritonitis may occur in association with infection of VP shunting systems. Occasionally, a pseudocyst may form in the abdomen in association with these shunting systems. Cerebrospinal fluid usually fills the pseudocyst, and occasionally this fluid may be infected. The most common organisms causing VP shunt infections are *S. aureus,* coagulase-negative staphylococci, and diphtheroids. Other complications of VP shunts may include perforation of an intra-abdominal viscus, such as the intestine, liver, and spleen, by the distal end of the shunting system. Perforation of the bowel may give rise to peritonitis due to the usual bowel organisms. In addition, these children may have an ascending infection and meningitis as a result of infection at the distal end of the VP shunt.[43, 44] Many of these children present with abdominal pain or rapidly enlarging abdominal girth. Some present with shunt malfunction in association with cerebrospinal fluid ascites or a pseudocyst in the abdomen. Although these pseudocysts may lack signs of systemic infection, most authors believe that many of these pseudocysts are actually reactions to low-grade chronic infection of the VP shunt. Management of these complications of VP shunts usually includes either revision or removal of the shunt in combination with appropriate antibiotic therapy.

LOCALIZED INTRA-ABDOMINAL ABSCESSES

Localized intra-abdominal abscesses occur within visceral intra-abdominal organs (liver, spleen, pancreas, and tubo-ovarian system) as well as in the perivisceral spaces, that is, the interintestinal loops and the periappendiceal, subdiaphragmatic, and subhepatic spaces.

Hepatic Abscess

Hepatic abscesses, pyogenic or amebic, are rare in children. There have been two autopsy reviews of liver abscesses in pediatric patients,[45, 46] as well as Pineiro-Carrero and coworkers' review of pediatric cases from 1975 to 1986.[47] Additional review of the pediatric literature reveals a total of 310 cases of pyogenic liver abscess occurring in children younger than 11 years of age.[47–65]

Although amebic liver abscesses do occur in the United States, they are exceedingly rare and usually are found in children who live in areas bordering Mexico or who have traveled to other endemic areas. Haffar and colleagues[66] described five children with amebic liver abscess and reviewed 119 other children from the world literature; they estimate that liver abscess as a complication of amebiasis occurs in fewer than 1% of children infected with ameba.

The incidence of pyogenic liver abscess in children varies from 3 to 25 per 100,000 hospital admissions.[42, 43] In the neonatal autopsy series reported by Ayra and colleagues,[51] the incidence was reported as 12 per 100,000. The incidence of liver abscesses in adults varies between 7 and 16 per 100,000, depending on which series is reviewed.[67, 68] Whether this apparent increase in the incidence of hepatic abscess in children represents a true increase in the disease or an increase in the sensitivity of the diagnostic methods is not clear. When age and sex can be ascertained in the cases reported in the literature, it appears that liver abscesses in children are predominantly a disease of children in the first year of life. In 61 of 130 cases in which age was noted, 47% occurred in children younger than 1 year of age. Twenty-one percent of cases occurred in children between ages 1 and 5 years, 19% in ages 5 through 10 years, and 13% in children from 10 to 20 years. Of 198 cases in which the sex of the child has been identified, 122 (61.6%) of the cases occurred in boys versus 76 (38.3%) of the cases in girls.

In both adults and children, certain underlying diseases predispose patients to the development of liver abscess. Travel or residence in an endemic area where ameba are prevalent predisposes to the development of amebic hepatic abscesses. In addition, close association with someone shedding ameba may also lead to the development of amebic abscess in a patient residing outside an endemic area. Certain underlying diseases, such as chronic granulomatous disease (CGD), leukemia, and other immunocompromised states, predispose both adults and children to the development of abscess formation. Bilfinger and associates[50] report hepatic abscesses in nonimmunocompromised children as a separate group. In their retrospective review covering the years 1963 to 1984, they reported 10 children, with an additional 15 from the literature, who had developed 11 bacterial and 11 amebic abscesses of the liver. Only one child was found to have CGD, and three children had appendicitis as a predisposing condition. In these immunocompetent children, the age range tended to be somewhat older (range 1–10 years in 7 of 10), with an average age of 6.3 years. In Chusid's series,[48] 26 of 61 cases of hepatic abscess occurred in children with CGD; in the remaining 40 children, leukemia was present in seven, two had recurrent infection, and one each had sickle cell anemia with immunosuppressive therapy or aplastic anemia. Approximately half of the patients reported by Chusid[48] did not have an underlying chronic disease predisposing them to the development of hepatic abscess.

The pathophysiology of pyogenic hepatic abscesses may involve access of bacteria to the liver via a number of routes. The ascending biliary pathway may be implicated in children with biliary tract disease, especially when obstruction is present. The portovenous route is important for bacterial seeding of the hepatic parenchyma in children who have appendicitis or necrotizing mesenteric adenitis. In addition, neonates who have umbilical catheters are also at risk for ascension of bacteria via the portovenous system. Trauma, either blunt or sharp, may also occasionally lead to subsequent infection. In a review of unruptured intrahepatic hematomas by Geis and coworkers,[63] 4 of 16 patients who had intrahepatic hematomas following severe blunt torso trauma developed hepatic abscess with sepsis requiring emergent surgical intervention. The hepatic arterial route can play a role in seeding the liver in cases of bacterial endocarditis or in cases in which the hepatic artery has been catheterized. The remaining category of cryptogenic pyogenic hepatic abscesses is reserved for those patients in whom no apparent source or predisposing condition can be identified.

Excluding amebic liver abscess, pyogenic liver abscesses are caused predominantly by *S. aureus* in patients with underlying immunosuppression and CGD as well as those who do not have an underlying predisposing condition. Gram-negative bacteria make up a significant minority of liver abscesses. Fungal liver abscesses are found predominantly in children with CGD or in those with underlying leukemia, especially in children who have been profoundly neutropenic for extended periods and have been exposed to broad-spectrum antibiotics (Fig. 18–4). Cat-scratch disease occasionally results in multiple liver abscesses that are characterized on biopsy

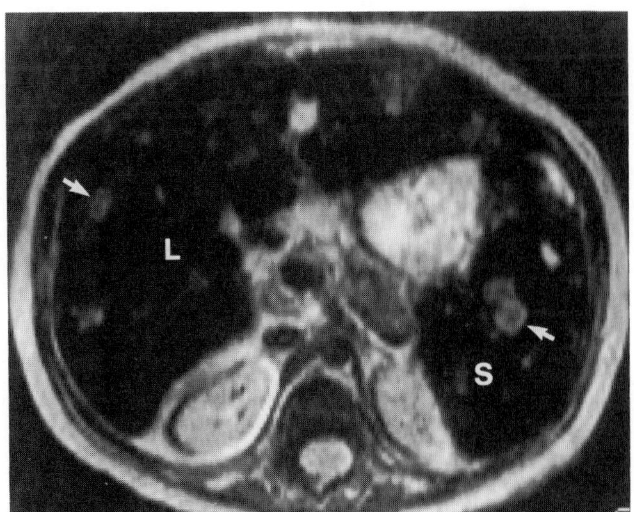

Figure 18–4. MR imaging scan in a child with leukemia receiving chemotherapy. Multiple circular "target lesions" *(arrows)* compatible with fungal abscesses are noted in the liver (L) and spleen (S).

as classic stellate abscess. When properly cultured, anaerobes are present in approximately 25 to 30% of liver abscesses, either as a single agent or as one of several bacterial species. Sterile culture results are quite rare when cultures are obtained and processed appropriately. Liver abscesses are often multiple and found predominantly within the right lobe of the liver. It is quite unusual to have both lobes of the liver involved with abscesses.

The clinical signs and symptoms of hepatic abscess are frustratingly nonspecific. In neonates especially, the diagnosis is rarely made prior to death. Most consistently, abdominal pain, fever, and hepatomegaly are present in most patients subsequently proven to have hepatic abscess. The only consistently abnormal laboratory value is an elevated erythrocyte sedimentation rate. The duration of symptoms can be as brief as 1 day or as long as 90 days. It is important to consider that a child with fever, hepatomegaly, and abdominal pain may have an amebic hepatic abscess because the management of amebic liver abscesses is different from that of pyogenic liver abscesses. The diagnosis of hepatic abscess has become much more sensitive and precise with the evolution of modern ultrasonography supplemented by scanning procedures and CT scan.

Ultrasound is probably the most common initial imaging method and is highly accurate.[69] Several authors have attempted to diagnose the causative organism (amebic versus suppurative) on the basis of the ultrasound pattern. Although overall there is overlap, certain patterns emerge.

Invasive amebiasis spreads from the intestinal tract to the liver, causing peripheral necrosis. Ultrasound studies will demonstrate indistinct lesions with internal echoes prior to liquefaction. Eventually, many of the lesions will go on to form hypoechoic, thin-walled abscesses sometimes containing air. Compared with pyogenic abscesses, amebic abscesses are better defined with a peripheral halo and are multiple in a contiguous fashion.[70] The CT appearance of amebiasis is also nonspecific; usually, low-density, well-circumscribed lesions are seen. Amebiasis can be diagnosed with some certainty only when there is direct extension through the diaphragm into the pleural or pericardial space.[71]

Immunocompromised children with pyogenic liver abscess demonstrate similar findings on CT and ultrasound. The ultrasound will demonstrate hypoechoic or mixed-echo patterns. Pyogenic abscesses are more likely to have ill-defined margins and a "honeycomb" internal pattern.[71] Again, fluid may be seen within the liquified abscess cavity. Air may be detected on ultrasound, but it is more difficult to see than on CT scanning. Dynamic CT scanning may demonstrate a "double-target sign."[72] Also, as CT spatial resolution has improved, tiny abscesses less than 2 cm in diameter may be visualized in a "cluster." This is also suggestive of early pyogenic hepatic abscess.[73]

Percutaneous aspiration for diagnosis or drainage for treatment may be done with either CT[74] or ultrasound.[75] In children with amebic abscess, diagnosis is usually made with indirect hemagglutination or immunodiffusion tests, or both, and rarely are radiologic interventional techniques necessary. However, particularly in the immunocompromised host, percutaneous drainage techniques play an important role in diagnosis and treatment.

Overall, it appears that ultrasonography, in addition to being the least invasive method, is also the most sensitive for diagnosing space-occupying lesions within the liver and defining abscess characteristics. It also provides the opportunity to guide aspiration of the abscess, thereby providing immediate information about the etiology of the infection. In addition to radiologic investigation, children, especially neonates, should have a blood culture performed, since often in children the etiologic agent can be obtained from the blood as well as from the liver itself. In addition to the usual laboratory tests, such as a complete blood count and erythrocyte sedimentation rate, antibody titers to ameba and a stool examination for ameba should be performed. When the abscess fluid is aspirated, routine bacteriologic cultures, including appropriately handled anaerobic cultures, should be performed. The aspirate should be evaluated for cytology, since it can be difficult to differentiate between a necrotic tumor and a pyogenic abscess on radiologic evaluation. A search for other underlying conditions, especially endocarditis, must be undertaken if there are multiple lesions, and a remote intra-abdominal focus, such as an occult appendiceal abscess, should be sought.

Once the diagnosis of liver abscess has been made, the number and location of abscess(es) determines which drainage procedure should be done. Drainage is essential in the management of these patients, and children who have both drainage and appropriate antibiotic therapy tend to do well in resolving this serious infection. Empiric antibiotic therapy pending results of cultures should include coverage for *S. aureus* as well as gram-negative bacteria; a penicillinase-stable penicillin combined with an aminoglycoside would be an appropriate initial choice, with the addition of anaerobic and amebic antibiotic (metronidazole) coverage initially until laboratory information becomes available. Once the underlying etiology of the abscess has been identified, antibiotic therapy should be appropriately tailored. The duration of therapy should be 4 to 6 weeks for intravenous antibiotic therapy, with oral antibiotic therapy for an additional 4 to 8 weeks, depending on clinical response. Amebic liver abscess should be treated initially with intravenous metronidazole; if there is no response after several days of intravenous therapy, then drainage should be carried out. Metronidazole therapy should be continued for at least 10 days, assuming an adequate response to therapy.

Mortality in children with liver abscesses has improved with the increased accuracy of diagnosis of this disease. Untreated liver abscess is uniformly fatal. Failure to consider the diagnosis of amebic liver abscess is particularly devastating because this disease, when appropriately diagnosed, usually has an excellent prognosis. Pyogenic liver abscess mortality rates vary with age. In neonates, liver abscess is nearly always fatal because it is so difficult to diagnose. In older children, draining the abscess appears to have a positive outcome in terms of mortality. In the series by Pineiro-Carrero and associates,[47] percutaneous drainage resulted in a zero mortality rate, and open drainage an 11% mortality rate, whereas there was 47% mortality in patients who received no drainage. In smaller series, mortality rates vary from 10 to 25%. The overall mortality rates in children appear to be lower than those in adults, for whom rates from 30 to 80% are routinely reported.

Splenic Abscess

Splenic abscesses are uncommon in children and adults. Autopsy series encompassing both adults and children in the preantibiotic years reported an incidence of splenic abscess varying from 0.14 to 0.7%. Several adult reviews[76, 77] and a pediatric review[78] note a change in the clinical spectrum of splenic abscess from preantibiotic years to the recent decades. In children, splenic abscesses occur from infancy throughout childhood without any apparent peak age of incidence. Fever occurred in the vast majority of patients (91%), often with abdominal pain (42.9%) that localized to the left upper quadrant (21%). Left-sided chest pain occurred in 19.6% of patients. Splenomegaly was noted in 46.4% of patients, with accompanying hepatomegaly in 18%; 8.5% of patients had pleural effusion, accompanied by left lower lobe rales in 12.5%. The classic symptoms of splenic abscess (left shoulder pain, left upper quadrant pain, and left chest pain) occurred in only 50% of patients. As in adults, predisposing factors frequently occur in pediatric patients who develop splenic abscess. Only 12.5% of patients appeared to have no underlying condition predisposing them to the development of splenic infection. There are several distinct categories of predisposing conditions in children who develop splenic abscess: (1) metastatic infection—endocarditis,[79] cat-scratch disease,[56] appendicitis, and metastatic tuberculosis[80, 81]; (2) an underlying hematologic abnormality, especially leukemia (patients with aplastic anemia and leukemia most frequently had associated profound neutropenia preceding the development of splenic abscesses); (3) hemoglobinopathy, including sickle cell disease, hemoglobin C sickle cell disease, and sickle cell thalassemia, which make up, together with oncologic abnormalities, 46.4% of pediatric patients with splenic abscess; and (4) an underlying anatomic abnormality, most often injury produced by external trauma or, rarely, secondary to internal trauma such as splenic torsion. Approximately 10% of patients with splenic abscess have an associated anatomic abnormality.

Splenic abscesses may be solitary or multiple. Children with infections at other sites have a slight predominance of solitary abscess formation, although endocarditis predisposes to multiple lesions. Following trauma or torsion, solitary lesions occurred in five out of six pediatric patients with splenic abscess. In patients who have multiple splenic abscesses, other organ sites are quite likely to be involved. The most commonly involved accompanying site is the liver, followed by subcutaneous sites, and, rarely, the kidney, bones, heart, or lungs.

The microbiologic etiology of splenic abscess has become much more clearly defined since 1978 with the advent of improved culturing systems for both anaerobes and fungal organisms. The two leading organisms causing splenic abscess in 38 children who had either positive blood or splenic cultures were *Candida* species and *S. aureus*.[77] Streptococci (*Streptococcus pyogenes, Streptococcus faecalis,* and *S. pneumoniae*) caused a smaller proportion of abscesses. Of gram-negative bacteria, *Salmonella* species was the leading cause, with isolated cases due to other enteric gram-negative bacteria, both anaerobic and aerobic. Blood cultures were positive in 42% of children with solitary splenic abscesses and in 31% of children who had multiple lesions. When splenic tissue was available for culture and histology, the etiologic agent was isolated in 77% of children with solitary abscesses and 89% of children with multiple abscesses. Whereas *Candida* species is the most common cause of multiple abscesses in children, staphylococci and salmonellae are the most frequent cause of solitary abscesses in children, especially in the setting of hemoglobinopathy.

Chest radiography in a child with suspected splenic abscess may reveal abnormalities in 74 to 82% of patients, regardless of predisposing clinical condition or underlying extent of involvement of the spleen. Most often, left-sided pleural effusion (33%), elevated left hemidiaphragm (59%), or both, sometimes accompanied by left lower lobe infiltrate, may be seen. In 90% of the pediatric patients reported by Keidl and Chusid,[78] a radiologic abnormality was described in the abdominal radiograph, most often splenic enlargement with displacement of the stomach. Scanning procedures, such as technetium or gallium liver-spleen scans, sometimes show decreased focal uptake in areas of abscess in the instance of technetium scans, or increased uptake in the instance of gallium scans. Gallium scans tend to be positive more often in instances in which there are multiple or large abscesses. Both ultrasound and CT readily demonstrate abscess.

On ultrasound, there is typically a poorly defined, hypoechoic, round lesion. It may develop into a complex mass containing septation and debris.[82]

CT will show an area of decreased CT density with an air-fluid or fluid-fluid level. In general, CT will more easily demonstrate small amounts of gas, allowing for a more specific diagnosis.[82]

MR imaging is quite sensitive in demonstrating inflammatory change in general; however, the appearance of abscess is variable on MR images. If an air-fluid level is present within the abscess, the diagnosis can be strongly suggested; however, the accuracy of MRI has not been determined (see Fig. 18–4).

Management of splenic abscesses includes drainage combined with antibiotic therapy. Whereas splenectomy used to be the procedure of choice in splenic abscess, percutaneous drainage with splenic salvage has been shown to be effective in selected patients.[83]

Patients who have solitary lesions documented by aspiration of purulent nonloculated fluid may undergo CT- or ultrasound-guided aspiration of the abscess, which has good results when combined with intensive antibiotic therapy. Multiloculated or complex splenic abscesses, however, most often need to be approached surgically. Splenectomy should be accompanied by appropriate immunization with pneumococcal[23] and *Haemophilus influenzae* type B vaccine to help protect against the subsequent immunologic deficit. Antibiotic therapy alone may be appropriate for patients in whom multiple small abscesses are found. These small lesions are not amenable to percutaneous drainage but may respond to prolonged antibiotic therapy. This is especially true in the instance of multifocal *C. albicans* lesions, which seem to respond best to prolonged therapy with amphotericin B, provided that the child's neutrophil count returns to normal.

Although splenic abscess is quite rare in children, it is increasing in frequency as increasing numbers of immunosuppressed children survive for extended periods. Since splenic abscesses are uniformly fatal if unrecognized and untreated, a high index of suspicion is necessary in children who have persistent fever, bacteremia, or fungemia with abdominal pain in the absence of other more specific findings.

Pancreatic Abscess

Infection of the pancreas is exceedingly rare in children. There are no prospective studies or large series of children with pancreatitis who develop abscess, infected pancreatic necrosis, or infected pseudocysts. Isolated case reports exist documenting the occurrence of pancreatic abscess in infancy,[84] as well as isolated children included in larger series of adult patients reported with pancreatic infection.[85, 86] As in adults, pancreatic abscesses follow acute pancreatitis or chronic pancreatitis in children. However, in contrast with adults with acute pancreatitis in whom the predisposing conditions are most often biliary tract disease and ethanol abuse, childhood onset of acute pancreatitis is more commonly associated with trauma, metabolic abnormalities, viral infection, anatomic abnormalities, and medications (see Chapter 68).[87, 88] Secondary pancreatic infection may manifest itself as pancreatic abscess, infected pancreatic necrosis, or infected pseudocyst. Differentiating among these infectious entities can be difficult. *Infected necrosis* is diffuse bacterial inflammation of necrotic pancreatic tissue without significant pus collections.[89] *Pancreatic abscess,* in contrast, is a localized collection of pus surrounded by a capsule. *Pancreatic pseudocyst* is a well-walled-off cystic structure, usually with sterile fluid that occasionally can become contaminated. Secondary pancreatic infections occur at rates varying from 1 to 10% of cases of acute pancreatitis. However, these infections are quite significant in that they account for approximately 80% of deaths in patients with acute pancreatitis. In the past decade, infectious complications of endoscopic retrograde cholangiopancreatography (ERCP) constitute about 8% of cases of pancreatic infection in adults. To date, there are no comparable data published on pediatric populations.

The clinical presentation in patients who develop pancreatic infection includes the usual clinical findings of acute pancreatitis with superimposed signs and symptoms of sepsis. An abdominal mass in addition to the pancreatic pain and distention accompanying the pancreatitis occasionally arouses suspicion concerning a secondary pancreatic infection. There are no specific signs or symptoms, however, that can differentiate severe pancreatitis from a complication such as an infection or pancreatic pseudocyst with or without infection. The usual time course of infection may vary from several days, for example, following an ERCP examination in which a pseudocyst might be infected, to 14 to 22 days after an episode of acute pancreatitis.

Diagnosis of secondary pancreatic infection relies on the use of CT scanning to identify the presence of a pseudocyst or intraparenchymal abscess. Ultrasound can also be useful in identifying a pseudocyst or phlegmon. However, CT scanning offers more definitive information on the anatomy of the fluid collection and its relationship to nearby structures (Fig. 18–5). Routine roentgenograms of the chest will show nonspecific abnormalities in approximately one third to one half of patients, such as basilar atelectasis, pleural effusion, and acute respiratory distress syndrome. A roentgenogram of the abdomen may show displacement of the gastric air bubble or the classic soap bubble sign of retrogastric air. However, retrogastric air is not pathognomonic for pancreatic infection. Distinguishing between pseudocysts that are sterile and those that are infected can be difficult on radiologic examination; however, the clinical situation may help define which patients are more likely to be suffering from pancreatic infection.

On CT scan, the pancreas again may appear enlarged, and the peripancreatic fat has a hazy appearance due to surrounding inflammation. Children with pancreatitis may proceed to develop a pseudocyst. The pseudocyst will demonstrate single or multiple cystic spaces. On CT, fluid-filled cysts adjacent to or remote from the

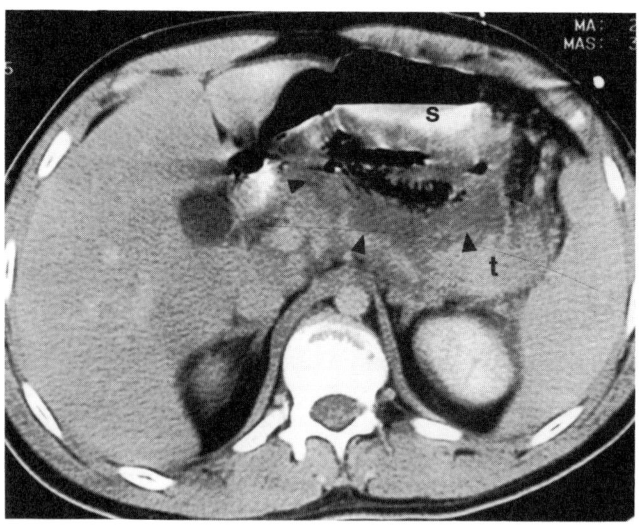

Figure 18–5. CT scan after oral and intravenous contrast demonstrates a large pancreatic abscess *(arrows)* posterior to the stomach (s). The tail (t) of the pancreas is seen at this level.

pancreas, as well as surrounding fluid, are seen. Although infected and noninfected pseudocysts have been compared by ultrasound, the most reliable indicator of infection is diagnostic needle aspiration. This greatly improves the early diagnosis of pancreatic abscess.[90] Percutaneous CT-guided aspiration of the fluid collection is the most reliable method of differentiating secondary pancreatic infection from pancreatic inflammation. Gram stain and culture results from material aspirated from such a fluid collection will help guide empiric therapy as well as formulate plans for further invention. The microbiology of secondary pancreatic infection may involve organisms from the gastrointestinal tract or, occasionally, from contrast material injected during ERCP. The organisms most frequently isolated from secondary pancreatic infections are *E. coli, K. pneumoniae, Pseudomonas,* and *Proteus*. Gram-positive species include *Staphylococcus,* enterococci, *Enterobacter,* and aerobic and anaerobic streptococci, as well as *Bacteroides* species. Occasionally, a pure culture of *Candida* may be found in a pancreatic abscess.

Surgical intervention is absolutely necessary in that patients with secondary pancreatic infection who are managed medically uniformly die. Surgical drainage of the abscess or pseudocyst, as well as removal of necrotic pancreatic and peripancreatic tissue combined with continuous drainage, provides the best outcome in combination with high-dose antibiotic therapy. The most common complications following surgery for secondary pancreatic infection involve respiratory failure, gastrointestinal tract hemorrhage, gastric outlet obstruction, transient glucose intolerance, and fistula formation. Surgical mortality is 39.3% in recent reports.[91]

Several authors have reported on percutaneous drainage of infected pseudocysts and pancreatic abscess.[92, 93] Following CT-guided percutaneous aspiration for diagnosis by Gram stain and culture to distinguish a sterile from an infected pancreatic process, percutaneous catheter drainage can be effective therapy in certain patients. Infected pancreatic necrosis would not lend itself to percutaneous catheter drainage because of the semisolid nature of the necrotic tissue; however, catheter drainage combined with antibiotics may be adequate for draining acute infected pseudocysts as well as extrapancreatic fluid collections and pancreatic abscess. There has been little experience with this approach, and there are no published cases in children as yet.

Empiric antibiotic therapy should be broad spectrum and given in high doses and should provide coverage for aerobic gram-negative, as well as anaerobic, classic colonic flora. If the infection is thought to be an infected pseudocyst following ERCP, coverage for *S. aureus* should be included as well. Choices for empiric antibiotic therapy pending culture results might include a third-generation cephalosporin, such as cefotaxime combined with metronidazole, for anaerobic coverage. Alternatively, ticarcillin–clavulanate acid, with or without an aminoglycoside, would also provide broad-spectrum aerobic and anaerobic coverage. The duration of therapy depends on the clinical response and associated septic complications, but a minimum of 14 days of coverage directed at the pathogens recovered and including anaerobic coverage is appropriate therapy.

Tubo-ovarian Abscess

Tubo-ovarian abscesses are rare in children but are an increasingly important problem in sexually active adolescents. Acute pelvic inflammatory disease (PID) is a major health problem for women of reproductive age and is the most serious complication of sexually transmitted diseases in young women. Inflammatory complications occur in approximately 15 to 25% of cases. Tubo-ovarian abscess is the major early complication associated with acute PID and occurs in 5 to 10% of patients hospitalized for treatment.[94] These infections may also present as an intra-abdominal abscess.

The criteria for the diagnosis of PID have been standardized.[95] Patients with PID have lower abdominal pain and tenderness, cervical motion tenderness, and adnexal tenderness, plus evidence of inflammatory process with fever or leukocytosis, or a positive culdocentesis with bacteria and white blood cells in peritoneal fluid. In addition, they may have an inflammatory mass, elevated erythrocyte sedimentation rate, evidence of infection with *N. gonorrhoeae* or *C. trachomatis,* or the presence of purulence in the endocervical discharge.

It is difficult to distinguish between complicated PID and a tubo-ovarian abscess. Identification of an inflammatory adnexal mass is essential and can sometimes be found on pelvic examination. However, sometimes the classic symptoms of acute PID are shared with those of urinary, gastrointestinal, or other gynecologic diseases. Ultrasound is most helpful in sorting out the etiology of the patient's pain. Through a well-distended urinary bladder, the uterus, ovaries, and surrounding pelvis are easily imaged. Early in PID, no abnormalities may be present. However, once PID has progressed to pyosalpinx and tubo-ovarian abscesses, the ultrasound becomes positive. Typically with pyosalpinx, the fallopian tube elongates and becomes redundant. A somewhat characteristic tubular fluid-filled structure is seen. The dilated tube may contain echoes within it owing to layering of purulent debris.[96] The abscess is often a complex mass with areas of solid tissue and fluid. The margins may appear irregular, or "shaggy." Abscesses tend to have a thick wall, although portions of the wall may be thin. Air or fluid levels may be seen. Free fluid within the pouch of Douglas can be associated with peritonitis. Sometimes, the free fluid may loculate and form an abscess.

In addition to ultrasound demonstrating the location and size of pelvic abscess, both endovaginal and transabdominal ultrasound have been used for guidance in draining pelvic fluid collections. Particularly in patients in whom the abscess is in the cul-de-sac, transvaginal drainage guided by an endovaginal probe may be useful and avoid surgery.[97]

Although ultrasound is the imaging study of choice for PID, occasionally a patient with pelvic pain may have had a CT scan when the diagnosis of PID was not suspected clinically. CT scan shows a thick-walled, fluid-dense mass in an adnexal location. There may be septations within the mass, and the borders between the uterus or adjacent bowel loops may be indistinct. There

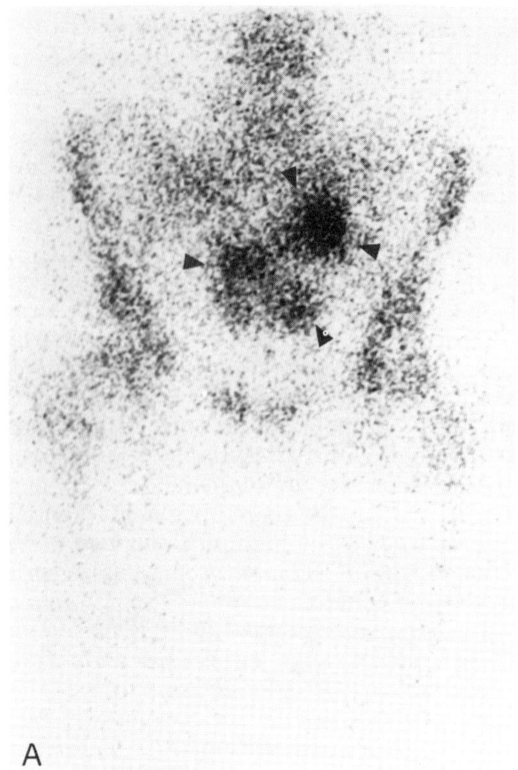

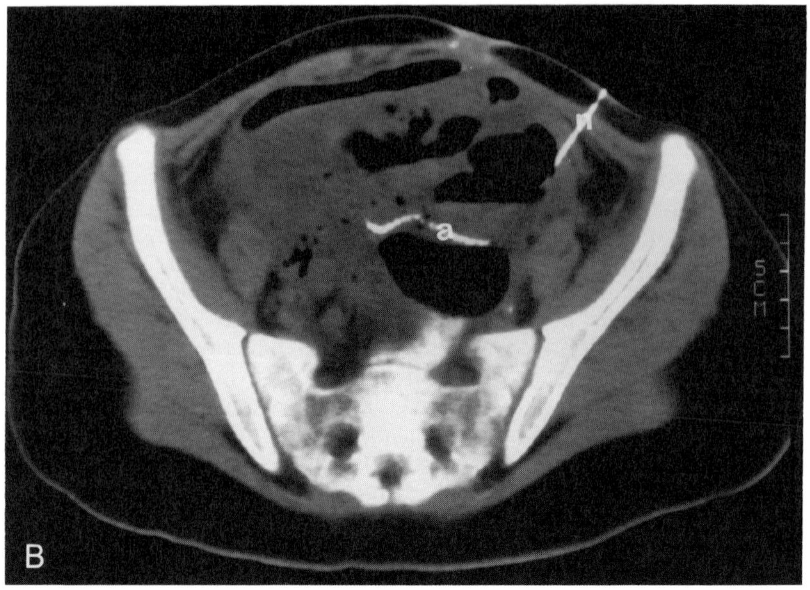

Figure 18–6. Indium-labeled white blood cell scan *(A)* and later CT scan *(B)* during drainage of a large pelvic abscess. This 11-year-old girl has had familial polyposis with two past episodes of spontaneous bowel perforation and abscess. She had undergone a total proctocolectomy and J-pouch several years ago. She presented with fever and was relatively asymptomatic. Indium scan demonstrated another abscess *(arrows)*. Owing to multiple past surgeries, percutaneous aspiration and catheter drainage were performed in this patient (a, surgical clips; n, needle).

may be unilateral or bilateral hydronephrosis due to displacement of the ureter. Gas bubbles may be present. Thickening of the uterosacral ligaments and increased density of the presacral fat are also helpful in suggesting acute inflammation in this region. Occasionally, periaortic adenopathy is seen.[98]

In contrast with the general assumption that surgical drainage is required for abscess formation, experience in the management of tubo-ovarian abscess has established primary medical management as the initial approach to these intra-abdominal infections. This conservative medical approach has been successful when broad-spectrum antibiotics were used, as summarized by Sweet.[94] In 1,075 cases of tubo-ovarian abscess treated, 67% responded to conservative medical therapy (range 16 to 95%). Keeping in mind that these abscesses not only contain *N. gonorrhoeae* and *Chlamydia* but also include gram-negative anaerobes, such as *B. fragilis* and streptococci, adequate anaerobic therapy must be included for optimal treatment. Antimicrobial regimens that included clindamycin resulted in reduction of tubo-ovarian abscess size in 86% of patients, compared with only 46.4% of patients who did not receive clindamycin. Inpatient treatment regimens for tubo-ovarian abscess traditionally have included clindamycin plus an aminoglycoside or cefoxitin alone. Alternative regimens include a third-generation cephalosporin (cefotaxime) plus metronidazole or extended-spectrum penicillins. Data using these latter regimens are not extensive.

If patients fail to respond to appropriate antibiotics after approximately 72 hours of therapy, surgical intervention should be considered. One must remember that a tubo-ovarian abscess may rupture at any time, presenting a surgical emergency that requires immediate intervention.

Once a tubo-ovarian abscess has ruptured and pelvic peritonitis develops, right subphrenic or subhepatic abscesses may occur. These can be delineated on ultrasound. Rarely, patients may present with right upper quadrant pain and fever due to Fitz-Hugh–Curtis syndrome. Large adnexal masses or bilateral adnexal involvement are also conditions that predict antibiotic failure and the need for subsequent surgical intervention. Both percutaneous and laparoscopy-directed percutaneous drainage of tubo-ovarian abscess appear to be promising approaches to drainage. No control studies comparing percutaneous or laparoscopic drainage with medical treatment have yet been published.

Perivisceral Infection

In addition to localized abscesses that occur within the intra-abdominal organs, localized abscesses can form between loops of bowel (e.g., in children with inflammatory bowel disease), and they may also collect in localized spaces under the diaphragm and under the liver (Figs. 18–6*A* and *B* and 18–7*A* and *B*). In patients with inflammatory bowel disease, intra-abdominal abscesses occur in the setting of the development of sinus tracts and fistulas as a result of chronic transmural inflammation. In a recent review of adolescents with Crohn's disease by Biller and coworkers,[99] the mean time from diagnosis of disease until the development of

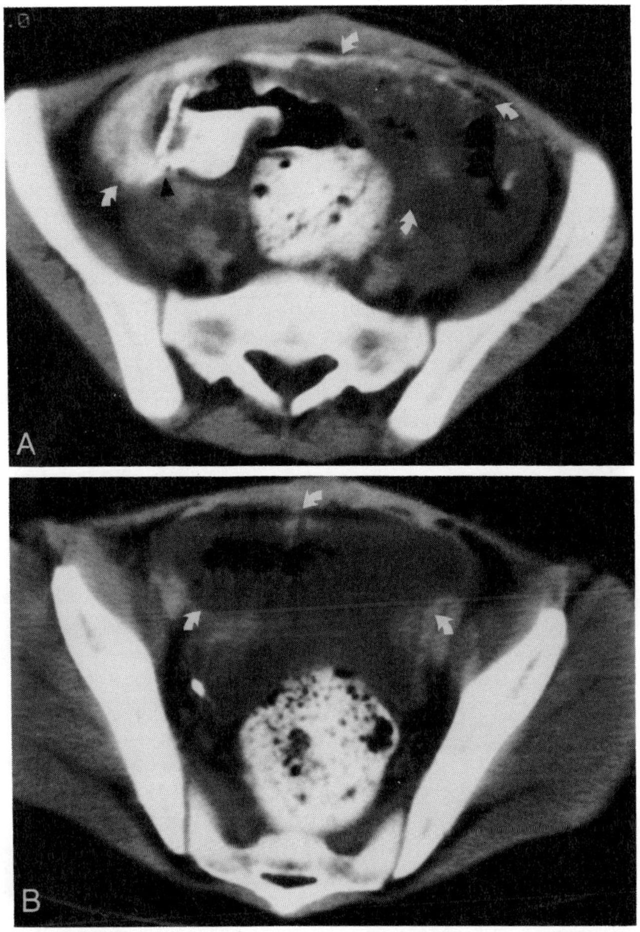

Figure 18–7. Two sequential CT images in a 16-year-old teenager who has undergone a subtotal colectomy and ileorectal anastomosis for ulcerative colitis. She was receiving steroids and was afebrile but tired. CT scan after intravenous and water-soluble rectal contrast shows a dehiscence at the ileorectal anastomosis *(arrow)*, with spillage of contrast into a large pelvic abscess *(white arrows)*.

an abdominal abscess was 1.7 years. All patients had involvement of both the terminal ileum and the right colon. This is in contrast with the development of abdominal abscesses in adults with Crohn's disease in whom the average interval from diagnosis of Crohn's disease to abscess development varied from 8 to 10 years.[99–101]

In pediatric patients with known Crohn's disease who have a changing pattern of clinical symptoms and in whom abscess is suspected, CT has been shown to be the initial study of choice. CT can demonstrate bowel wall thickening and dilatation, mesenteric abnormalities, fistulas, and perianal disease as well as abscesses and phlegmon.[102]

Abscess drainage in patients with Crohn's disease requires close cooperation between the pediatric radiologist and surgeons. The percutaneous approach may often completely resolve the abscess and the patient's clinical symptoms. Percutaneous drainage may reduce the number or extent of subsequent surgery[103]; however, this procedure has not been as successful in curing abscesses resulting from fistula.

Barium examinations are less helpful in complications of Crohn's disease, in part because they may interfere with subsequent CT and nuclear medicine examinations and cannot demonstrate extraluminal disease. However, they remain the study of choice for evaluation of mucosal disease, enteroenteric fistulas, strictures, and postsurgical anatomy.

Ultrasound may be helpful when it demonstrates round or oval hypoechoic fluid collections. However, ultrasound may have difficulty finding an abscess within the midabdomen or pelvis owing to overlying bowel that reflects the ultrasound beam. In addition, dilated loops of bowel from an ileus or obstruction that are not in peristalsis may be confused with an abscess.[104]

Indium 111–labeled leukocytes and gallium scan may be helpful in those patients who have had multiple surgeries, making CT interpretation more difficult, or in whom the CT scan has been negative.[105]

Once intra-abdominal abscess or intraloop abscess is diagnosed in the setting of Crohn's disease, and drainage has been accomplished, antibiotic management should include the usual broad-spectrum coverage for aerobic gram-negative enteric bacilli as well as anaerobic bacteria (see the section on peritonitis).

Subphrenic Abscess

Subphrenic abscess in children was reviewed by Mackenzie and associates,[106] who analyzed 19 consecutive cases over a 10-year period. All of these patients had subphrenic abscess as a complication of intra-abdominal sepsis or surgery. The most common cause of intra-abdominal infection was either appendicitis or primary peritonitis. Subphrenic abscess occurred with an incidence of 0.45%. Four patients (21%) died, and the length of hospitalization varied from 30 to 122 days. Diagnosis of a subphrenic abscess is best accomplished by CT scan to localize the fluid collection. Subphrenic gas collections, basal atelectasis, elevation of the diaphragm, and pleural effusion may also be present on the chest radiograph. Four of the 19 children had bilateral subphrenic abscess. All these were suprahepatic, in contrast with the primarily intraperitoneal location of subphrenic abscesses in the other 15 patients. Therapy of subphrenic abscess involves surgical drainage, via either CT-guided needle aspiration with catheter placement or an open drainage procedure. Antibiotic coverage must include the usual enteric flora; in addition, if primary peritonitis was the preceding event, gram-positive coverage for *S. aureus* must be included. Prompt diagnosis of appendicitis with adequate drainage of complicated appendicitis remains the primary method of preventing the development of subphrenic abscess in children.

Retroperitoneal Abscess

Intra-abdominal infection, in addition to occurring in the intraperitoneal space as either a generalized or a localized collection, may also occur in the retroperitoneal space, involving the kidney, or in the perinephric area. Occasionally, an abscess may be localized to muscles in the retroperitoneal area, such as the psoas muscle. Renal and perirenal abscesses have been reviewed.[107] Classification of intrarenal abscess has been expanded to include acute focal bacterial nephritis and acute multifocal bacterial nephritis, as well as previously recognized renocortical abscess, renocortical medullary abscess, and xanthogranulomatous pyelonephritis. These five entities exist in adults as well as in children, although in the postantibiotic era, the incidence of infections such as these is decreasing dramatically. A recent review of renal abscess in childhood[108] reiterated the inherent difference between a renocortical abscess and a corticomedullary abscess. In addition, acute focal bacterial nephritis and acute lobar nephronia have recently been reviewed in children.[109] Acute focal bacterial nephritis is an acute, nonsuppurative renal infection that represents progression of acute pyelonephritis on a spectrum toward intrarenal abscess formation. Extension of acute focal bacterial nephritis produces acute multifocal bacterial nephritis; these two entities can be distinguished radiographically and pathogenically rather than by their clinical presentations. Acute focal bacterial nephritis is limited to a single lobe of the kidney, whereas multifocal bacterial nephritis produces a heavy polymorphonuclear infiltrate throughout the kidney with some abscess formation. Xanthogranulomatous pyelonephritis is an exceedingly rare but severe chronic intrarenal infection that has been described in children.[110, 111] The etiology of xanthogranulomatous pyelonephritis is unclear. In adults, it is associated with stones and lymphatic obstruction and is characterized pathologically by macrophage endocytosis of cholesterol and other lipids. It appears to be the result of chronic urinary tract infection with obstruction.

Progression from intrarenal focal nephritis to renocortical medullary abscess can occur, especially in children whose infections are associated with vesicoureteral reflux. Parenchymal infection develops when reflux persists after bacterial inoculation of the renal medulla has taken place. This explains why corticomedullary abscess is frequently caused by typical urinary tract pathogens in contrast with renocortical abscess. The gram-negative bacillary corticomedullary infection may be somewhat more likely to perforate the renal capsule and form a perinephric abscess.

Renocortical abscess, in contrast, is a result of hematogenous spread of bacteria from a distant focus to the renal cortex. Common extrarenal foci include skin lesions, especially cutaneous carbuncles, osteomyelitis, and endovascular infections. Patients receiving hemodialysis or abusing intravenous drugs or those with diabetes mellitus are particularly predisposed to the development of staphylococcal bacteremia, with the resultant risk of renocortical infection. The interval between the original staphylococcal infection and the development of renocortical abscess varies from days to months, with the average interval of approximately 7 weeks. *Staphylococcus aureus* is the causative agent in 90% of renocortical abscesses in adults as well as in children. Unlike corticomedullary abscess, ascending infection is an infrequent cause of renocortical abscess. The cortical abscess can rupture through the renal capsule and form a perinephric abscess. However, this is an unusual complication that is seen in fewer than 10% of renocortical abscesses. The clinical features of the child with a renocortical abscess include fever and localized flank pain. Most of the patients do not have urinary tract symptoms because the circumscribed cortical process does not usually communicate with the caliceal collecting system. Infants with renal abscesses may have bulging of the flank. In addition, infants as well as older children may have abdominal pain and tenderness to palpation in the abdomen as well as along the costovertebral angle. Pulmonary examination may be abnormal, with decreased expiratory effort, dullness, diminished breath sounds, or rales on the affected side. The erythrocyte sedimentation rate is uniformly elevated, as is the peripheral white blood cell count. Blood cultures are usually sterile.

The presentation of a child with a renocortical medullary abscess, or ascending infection, differs from that of a child with renocortex abscess in that because the corticomedullary abscess drains into the urinary collecting system more commonly, urinalysis is often abnormal with bacteriuria, pyuria, and proteinuria with or without hematuria. Occasionally, urinalysis may be normal. These children often have fever, chills, and flank or abdominal pain. Nausea and vomiting are common and, especially in combination with the abdominal pain, may confuse the presentation of an intrarenal abscess by mimicking an intraperitoneal process. A flank mass and, rarely, a draining flank sinus may be present. A previous history of recurrent urinary tract infection is common, especially in association with vesicoureteral reflux or obstruction. In contrast with renocortical abscess in which *S. aureus* is the most common bacterial etiology, the pathogens recovered from corticomedullary abscesses include *E. coli, Klebsiella,* and *Proteus*.

Since the clinical presentations of these four intrarenal infections are so similar, differentiation among them depends on the use of CT scanning and ultrasound. In addition, the differential diagnosis must include renal cyst and renal tumor. Urosepsis, which is more common with corticomedullary abscess, usually does not occur in patients with cysts and tumors. Additionally, an abnormal urinalysis, found in most patients with corticomedullary abscess, is unusual in a patient with a renocortical abscess. Both ultrasonography and CT scanning have been used in the past decade to differentiate among these processes. Ultrasound is more sensitive in the diagnosis of acute focal and acute multifocal bacterial nephritis than CT scan. Ultrasound shows a poorly marginated sonolucent mass disrupting the corticomedullary junction in one or multiple renal lobes. On CT scan, a postcontrast study may show a poorly defined, wedge-shaped, hypodense area. In a more well-developed medullary cortical or renal cortex abscess, ultrasound may show an anechoic or septated mass. CT scans confirm ultrasonic findings, showing well-defined areas with low attenuation. A rim of peripheral enhancement after infusion of intravenous contrast may be present. These intrarenal abscesses may be drained with either ultrasound or CT guidance for definitive diagnosis.

Treatment of intrarenal abscess in the past has required open drainage of organized collections of pus. However, with the development of sensitive radiologic techniques for following response to therapy and with the ability percutaneously to drain collections, many authors now recommend a staged management consisting of an initial trial of intensive antibiotic therapy followed by percutaneous drainage of abscess and, finally, open surgery.[112] Fluid aspirated from intrarenal abscesses should be sent for aerobic and anaerobic culture, including for *Mycobacterium* and fungi. In addition, fluid should be sent for cytology, because necrotic tumors occasionally will appear that are indistinguishable from intrarenal abscesses.

Empiric antibiotic therapy initially should include a semisynthetic penicillin with an aminoglycoside until culture results are known. Alternatively, a first-generation cephalosporin or vancomycin may be used to cover *S. aureus*. Since positive urine cultures do not always correlate with the bacteria recovered from the abscess drainage, antibiotic therapy should not be limited to pathogens recovered in the urine in the case of corticomedullary abscess. Once culture results are known, antibiotic therapy may be modified, and parenteral antibiotics should be continued for 10 to 14 days, followed in the case of staphylococcal abscess by oral antistaphylococcal therapy for an additional 2 to 4 weeks. If response to therapy does not occur within 48 hours following the institution of intravenous therapy, percutaneous aspiration should be attempted. If fever and clinical symptoms persist for 5 to 6 days, and flank pain does not disappear after 24 hours following percutaneous drainage, open drainage should be undertaken.

Management of the infected renal cyst in patients with polycystic kidney disease who may have one or more cysts that have become infected is problematic. Most often the etiologic agents are gram-negative uropathogens, and the presentation is similar to that in patients with normal kidneys with intrarenal infection. In the patient in whom a solitary renal cyst becomes infected, management is the same as it is for a patient with an uncomplicated intrarenal abscess. Patients with polycystic kidney disease, however, are best managed with a conservative approach using prolonged (6 to 8 weeks) antibiotics because surgical intervention is extremely difficult.

Perinephric Abscess

A perinephric abscess is a collection of pus in the tissue surrounding the kidney but contained within Gerota's fascia. This uncommon disorder is a serious complication of both urinary tract and systemic infections. Despite advances in diagnostic and surgical techniques and antibiotic therapy, the overall mortality from perinephric abscess in adults has ranged from zero to 56%, with a review citing an overall mortality rate of 13%.[113] In a review of perinephric abscess in pediatric patients,[114] six cases of perinephric abscess in patients younger than 18 years of age were reviewed. Only 10 patients were reported from 1956 to 1988, compared with approximately 240 cases in children reported during the preantibiotic era. This infection in children was seen predominantly as a complication of abdominal or urologic surgery in the last 3 decades compared with children in the preantibiotic era, in whom perinephric abscess was a complication of a ruptured intrarenal abscess. In contrast with adults, perinephric abscess complicating previous urinary tract infection with stones or obstruction or diabetes mellitus was rarely reported in children. Urologic and other congenital anomalies occurred in 60% of patients reported. An important subgroup of perinephric abscess patients are those patients who have recently received kidney transplants, in whom the incidence was 0.3% in 12 years.[115] In these immunosuppressed patients, signs and symptoms of perinephric abscess were evident despite the use of prednisone. Perinephric abscesses occurred 2 weeks to 52 months after transplantation and were associated with lymphoceles in some patients.

The clinical presentation of a child with perinephric abscess can be insidious. Fever is present in all patients; flank and back pain and abdominal complaints are common as well in 30 to 50%. Unlike the case with adults, the duration of symptoms prior to presentation tends to be brief in children, ranging from 1 to 8 days. Physical examination reveals abdominal tenderness with or without a mass in 83%. Flank mass or tenderness is less frequent. Blood cultures in adults are frequently positive (40% of patients), whereas blood cultures in children are uniformly negative. Perinephric abscess should be considered in the child with fever of unknown origin, especially if that child has recently undergone urologic or gastrointestinal tract surgery. Radiologic investigation, as for other renal abscesses, depends on the use of ultrasonography and CT scanning. The presence of gas in the renal parenchyma and the perirenal space suggests a perinephric abscess. CT scan reveals the precise anatomic relationship of the retroperitoneal infection and, in particular, defines extension to the flank or psoas muscle or, superiorly, to the subphrenic area. These anatomic details are important in planning surgical drainage.

Percutaneous or open drainage of perinephric abscess seems imperative in the management of this disease. Antibiotic therapy alone is not adequate, in contrast with the therapy for intrarenal abscess. Percutaneous catheter drainage can be used in some children in conjunction with antistaphylococcal penicillins and an aminoglycoside or third-generation cephalosporin. Occasionally, complete nephrectomy must be carried out.

Psoas Abscess

The psoas muscle and the iliacus muscle, which reside in the retroperitoneal space, can occasionally become involved by an extension of infection from either a retroperitoneal appendicitis or an intrarenal or perirenal abscess. In addition, the psoas muscle can be infected secondary to other operative complications or to osteomyelitis. Rarely, a primary staphylococcal abscess can occur in the psoas muscle, presumably following hematogenous dissemination of the bacteria. Tuberculosis of the spine can occasionally involve the psoas muscle, and in the preantibiotic era, psoas abscess was presumed to be equivalent to tuberculosis of the spine or sacroiliac joints.

Psoas abscess in children is uncommon, but it enters the differential diagnosis of a child who presents with a painful limp and fever.[116, 117] Psoas abscess may also follow trauma with bacterial seeding of a hematoma, even by common respiratory pathogens such as *H. influenzae* type B.[118] Differentiating a psoas or an iliac muscle infection from an infected hip can be difficult. On close examination, however, the hip is found not to be tender, and there is full passive range of motion. Aspiration of the hip joint, if the diagnosis is in doubt, will be negative. At this point, CT scan will be helpful in identifying the abscess in the muscle and possible osteomyelitis in adjacent bones. Nuclear bone scan can also be used to assess for the coexistence of osteomyelitis. Drainage of the abscess through a percutaneous retroperitoneal approach avoids contamination of the peritoneal cavity with the abscess. Initial antibiotic coverage should take into account any underlying focus, such as gastrointestinal disease. In this instance, antibiotics should be the same as for a ruptured appendix. In the absence of underlying gastrointestinal pathology, the organism most frequently cultured is *S. aureus*. In the young child with a previous respiratory focus, *H. influenzae* coverage should be included. An antistaphylococcal penicillin with a third-generation cephalosporin or, alternatively, ticarcillin–clavulanic acid would be good initial coverage. Duration of therapy depends on clinical response and pathogens recovered, but a minimum of 10 days of therapy for *S. aureus* seems appropriate. In the setting of Crohn's disease, especially if bowel resection is carried out at the same time as abscess drainage, the incidence of recurrent abscess is relatively high (38%).[117]

REFERENCES

1. Witmann DH: Intra-abdominal infections: Introduction. World J Surg 1990; 14:145–147.
2. Sanders RC, James AE Jr, Fischer K: Correlation of liver scans and images with abdominal radiographs in perihepatic sepsis. Am J Surg 1972; 124:346–352.
3. Nohr CW, Marshall BG: Primary peritonitis in children. Can J Surg 1984; 27:179–181.
4. Speck WT, Dresdale SS, McMillan RW: Primary peritonitis and the nephrotic syndrome. Am J Surg 1974; 127:267–279.
5. Gorensek MJ, Lebel MH, Nelson JD: Peritonitis in children with nephrotic syndrome. Pediatrics 1988; 81:849–856.
6. Wilfert CM, Katz SL: Sepsis and nephrosis. Pediatrics 1968; 42:840–843.
7. McDougal WS, Izant RJ, Zollinger RM: Primary peritonitis in infancy and childhood. Ann Surg 1975; 181:310–313.
8. Garcia-Tsao G, Conn HO, Werner E: The diagnosis of bacterial peritonitis: Comparison of pH lactate concentration and leukocyte count. Hepatology 1985; 5:91–96.
9. Burry VF: Gonococcal vulvovaginitis and possible peritonitis in prepubertal girls. Am J Dis Child 1971; 121:536–537.
10. Fuld GL: Gonococcal peritonitis in a prepubertal child. Am J Dis Child 1968; 115:621–622.

10a. Cooperstock M: Indigenous flora and pathogenesis: *In* Feigin RD, Cherry JD, eds: Pediatric Infectious Diseases. 2nd ed. Philadelphia, WB Saunders, 1987, pp 106–109.

10b. Finegold SM: Peritonitis. *In* Hoeprich PD, Jordan MC, eds: Infectious Diseases. 4th ed. Philadelphia, JB Lippincott, 1989, pp 854–857.

11. Brook I: A 12-year study of aerobic and anaerobic bacteria in intra-abdominal and postsurgical-abdominal wound infections. Surg Gynecol Obstet 1989; 169:387–392.
12. Brook I: Aerobic and anaerobic microbiology of intra-abdominal abscesses in children. South Med J 1989; 82:1479–1482.
13. Aronoff SC, Olson MM, Audierer MWL, et al: *Pseudomonas aeruginosa* as a primary pathogen in children with bacterial peritonitis. J Pediatr Surg 1987; 22:861–864.
14. Echenbach D: Fitz-Hugh–Curtis syndrome. *In* Holmes KK, Mardh PA, Sparling PF, et al, eds: Sexually Transmitted Diseases. New York, McGraw-Hill, 1984, pp 633–638.
15. Mahboubi S, Caro BA: Computed tomography in the evaluation of tubo-ovarian abscesses in children. J Comp Tomogr 1986; 10:67–70.
16. Hau T: Bacteria toxins in the peritoneum. World J Surg 1990; 14:167–175.
17. Dinarello CA: The pro-inflammatory cytokines interleukin-1 and tumor necrosis factor and treatment of the septic shock syndrome. J Infect Dis 1991; 163:1177–1184.
18. Crabb JH, Finberg R, Onderdonk AB, et al: T-cell regulation of *Bacteroides fragilis* induced intra-abdominal abscess. Rev Infect Dis 1990; 12:S178–S184.
19. Bjornson HS: Bacterial synergy virulence factors and host defense mechanisms in the pathogenesis of intra-abdominal infections. *In* Simmons RL, ed: Topics in Intra-Abdominal Surgical Infection. Norwalk, CT, Appleton-Century-Crofts, 1982, pp 65–78.
20. Levison ME, Bush LM: Peritonitis and other intra-abdominal infections. *In* Mandel GL, Douglas RG, Bennett JE, eds: Principles and Practice of Infectious Diseases. 3rd ed. New York, Churchill Livingstone, 1990, pp 636–670.
21. Nord CE, Hedberg M: Resistance to beta-lactam antibiotics and anaerobic bacteria. Rev Infect Dis 1990; 12:S231–S234.
22. Weinstein WM, Onderdonk AB, Bartlett JG, et al: Antimicrobial therapy of experimental intra-abdominal sepsis. J Infect Dis 1975; 132:282–286.
23. Onderdonk AB, Bartlett JG, Louie T, et al: Microbial synergy in experimental intra-abdominal abscess. Infect Immunol 1976; 13:22–26.
24. Runcie C, Ramsay G: Intra-abdominal infection: Pulmonary failure. World J Surg 1990; 14:196–203.
25. Stevenson RJ: Abdominal pain unrelated to trauma. Surg Clin North Am 1985; 65:1181–1215.
26. Jeffrey RB Jr: Periappendiceal inflammatory masses: CT directed management and clinical outcome in 70 patients. Radiology 1988; 167:13.
27. Balthazar EJ, Megibow AJ, Hulnick D, et al: CT of appendicitis. AJR 1986; 147:705–710.
28. Singleton EB: Moderator film panel cases: Society of Pediatric Radiology. Pediatr Radiol 1990; 201:212–217.
29. Burton EM, Boulden TF, Magill HL, et al: Case of the day: Appendicitis with appendiceal rupture and pelvic abscess. Radiographics 1990; 10:372–374.
30. Slovis TL, Haller JO, Cohen HL, et al: Complicated appendiceal inflammatory disease in children: Pylephlebitis and liver abscess. Radiology 1989; 171:823.
31. Dougherty SH: Role of enterococcus in intraabdominal sepsis. Am J Surg 1984; 148:308–312.
32. Dougherty SH, Flohr AB, Simmons RL: "Breakthrough" enterococcal septicemia in surgical patients. Arch Surg 1983; 118:232–238.
33. Barrall DT, Kenney PR, Slotman GJ, et al: Enterococcal bacteremia in surgical patients. Arch Surg 1985; 120:57–63.
34. Saini S, Kellum JM, O'Leary MP, et al: Improved localization and survival in patients with intraabdominal abscesses. Am J Surg 1983; 145:136–142.
35. Emanuel B, Zlotnik P, Raffensperger JJ: Perforation of the gastrointestinal tract in infancy and childhood. Surg Gynecol Obstet 1978; 146:926–928.
36. Bell MJ, Keating JP, Turnberg JL, et al: Perforated stress ulcers in infants. J Pediatr Surg 1981; 16:998–1002.

37. Mocan H, Murphy AV, Beattie TJ, et al: Peritonitis in children on continuous ambulatory peritoneal dialysis. J Infect 1988; 16:243–251.
38. Peterson PK, Matzke G, Keane WF: Current concepts in the management of peritonitis of patients undergoing continuous ambulatory peritoneal dialysis. Rev Infect Dis 1987; 9:604–612.
39. Smith JL, Flanigan MJ: Peritoneal dialysis catheter sepsis: A medical and surgical dilemma. Am J Surg 1987; 154:602–607.
40. Golper TA, Hartstein AI: Analysis of the causative pathogens in uncomplicated CAPD-associated peritonitis: Duration of therapy, relapses and prognosis. Am J Kidney Dis 1986; 7:141–145.
41. Stone MM, Fonkalsrud EW, Salusky IV, et al: Surgical management of peritoneal dialysis catheters in children: Five-year experience with 1,800 patient month follow-up. J Pediatr Surg 1986; 21:1177–1181.
42. Buggy BP, Schaberg DR, Swartz RD: Intraleukocytic sequestration as a cause of persistent *Staphylococcus aureus* peritonitis in continuous ambulatory peritoneal dialysis. Am J Med 1984; 76:1035–1040.
43. Norfray JF, Henry HM, Givens JD, et al: Abdominal complications from peritoneal shunts. Gastroenterology 1979; 340:337–340.
44. Yount RA, Glazier MC, Mealey J, et al: Cerebrospinal fluid ascites complicating ventral peritoneal shunting. J Neurosurg 1984; 61:180–183.
45. Dehner LP, Kissane JM: Pyogenic hepatic abscesses in infancy and childhood. J Pediatr 1969; 74:763–773.
46. Moss TM, Pysher TJ: Hepatic abscesses in neonates. Am J Dis Child 1981; 135:726–728.
47. Pineiro-Carrero VM, Andrew JM: Morbidity and mortality in children with pyogenic liver abscess. Am J Dis Child 1989; 143:1424–1427.
48. Chusid MJ: Pyogenic hepatic abscess in infancy and childhood. Pediatrics 1978; 62:554–559.
49. Goldenring JM, Flores M: Primary liver abscesses in children and adolescents. Clin Pediatr 1986; 25:153–158.
50. Bilfinger TV, Hayden CK, Oldham KT, et al: Pyogenic liver abscesses in nonimmunocompromised children. South Med J 1986; 79:39–40.
51. Ayra LS, Ghani R, Abdali S, et al: Pyogenic liver abscesses in children. Clin Pediatr 1982; 21:89–93.
52. Tariq AA, Rudolph N, Levin EJ: Solitary hepatic abscess in a newborn infant. Clin Pediatr 1977; 16:577–578.
53. Paone RE, Mercer LC: Hepatic abscess caused by a ventriculoperitoneal shunt. Pediatr Infect Dis J 1991; 10:338–339.
54. Reddy SC: Subcapsular hepatic abscess: A rare complication of ventriculoperitoneal shunt. South Med J 1987; 80:1309–1311.
55. Maxwell AJ, Mantor H: Fungal liver abscesses and acute leukemia. Clin Radiol 1988; 39:197–201.
56. Delbeke D, Sandler MP, Shaff MI, et al: Cat-scratch disease: Report of a case with liver lesions and no lymphadenopathy. J Nucl Med 1988; 29:1454–1456.
57. Rizkallah MF, Meyer L, Ayoub EM: Hepatic and splenic abscesses in cat-scratch disease. Pediatr Infect Dis J 1988; 7:191–195.
58. Garty B, Conley ME, Douglas SD, et al: Recurrent infections and staphylococcal liver abscess in a child with C1r deficiency. J Allergy Clin Immunol 1987; 80:631–635.
59. Weinreb BD, Winklestein JA, Haller JA, et al: Indium 111–labeled white blood cell scintigraphy for the diagnosis of upper abdominal abscesses in a child with Wiskott-Aldrich syndrome. J Pediatr Surg 1987; 22:1041–1044.
60. Kumar A, Kapoor R, Chopra K, et al: Typhoid fever: Unusual hepatic manifestations. Clin Pediatr 1989; 28:99–100.
61. Black CT, Kupferschmid JP, West KW, et al: *Haemophilus parainfluenzae* infections in children with the report of a unique case. Rev Infect Dis 1988; 10:342–346.
62. Slovis TL, Haller JO, Cohen HL, et al: Complicated appendiceal inflammatory disease in children: Pylephlebitis and liver abscess. Radiology 1989; 171:823–825.
63. Geis WP, Schulz KA, Giaccino JL, et al: The fate of unruptured intrahepatic hematomas. Surg 1981; 90:689–697.
64. George DL, Arnow PM, Fox AS, et al: Bacterial infection as a complication of liver transplantation: Epidemiology and risk factors. Rev Infect Dis 1991;13:387–396.
65. McCorkell SJ, Niles NL: Pyogenic liver abscesses: Another look at medical management. Lancet 1985; 1:803–806.
66. Haffar A, Boland FJ, Edwards MS: Amebic liver abscess in children. Pediatr Infect Dis J 1982; 1:322–326.
67. McDonald DMI, Corey GR, Gallus HA, et al: Single and multiple pyogenic liver abscesses. Medicine 1984; 63:291–302.
68. Rubin RH, Schwartz MN, Malt R: Hepatic abscess: Changes in clinical, bacteriologic and therapeutic aspects. Am J Med 1974; 57:601–610.
69. Laurin S, Kaude JV: Diagnosis of liver-spleen abscesses in children with emphasis on ultrasound for initial and follow-up examination. Pediatr Radiol 1984; 14:198–204.
70. Oleszczuk-Raske K: Ultrasonic features of pyogenic and amoebic hepatic abscesses. Pediatric Radiol 1989; 19:203.
71. Radin DR, Ralls PW, Colletti PM, et al: CT of amebic abscess. AJR 1988; 150:1297–1301.
72. Mathieu D, Vasile M, Fagniez PL, et al: Dynamic CT features of hepatic abscesses. Radiology 1985; 154:749–752.
73. Jeffrey RB, Tolentino CS, Chang FC, et al: CT of small pyogenic hepatic abscesses: The cluster sign. AJR 1988; 151:487–489.
74. Bowers ED, Robison DJ, Doberneck RC: Pyogenic liver abscess. World J Surg 1990; 14:128–132.
75. Vachon L, Diament MJ, Stanley P: Percutaneous drainage of hepatic abscesses in children. J Pediatr Surg 1986; 21:366.
76. Chun CH, Raff MJ, Contreras L, et al: Splenic abscess. Medicine 1980; 59:50–65.
77. Malken N, Ignatius J, Skinner M, et al: Changing clinical spectrum of splenic abscess: A multicenter study and review of the literature. J Surg 1987; 154:27–34.
78. Keidl CM, Chusid MJ: Splenic abscesses in childhood. Pediatr Infect Dis J 1989; 8:368–373.
79. Johnson JD, Raff MJ, Barnwell PA, et al: Splenic abscess complicating infectious endocarditis. Arch Intern Med 1983; 143:906–912.
80. Wolff MJ, Bitran J, Northland RG, et al: Splenic abscess due to *Mycobacterium tuberculosis* in patients with AIDS. Rev Infect Dis 1991; 13:373–375.
81. Wou CC, Chow KS, Lu TN, et al: Tuberculous splenic abscess: Sonographic detection and follow-up. J Clin Ultrasound 1990; 18:205–209.
82. Van der Lann RT, Verbeeten B Jr, Smits NJ, et al: Computed tomography in the diagnosis and treatment of solitary splenic abscesses. J Comput Assist Tomogr 1989; 13:71.
83. Gleich S, Wollin DA, Herbsman H: A review of percutaneous drainage in splenic abscess. Surg Gynecol Obstet 1988; 167:211–216.
84. Katz S, Rivkind A, Cohen O, et al: Pancreatic abscess: An unusual complication of pancreatitis in infancy. J Pediatr Surg 1983; 18:306–307.
85. Hurley JE, Vargan T: Early diagnosis and outcome of pancreatic abscess and pancreatitis. Am Surg 1987; 53:29–33.
86. Ranson JHC, Balthazar E, Caccavale R, et al: Computed tomography in the prediction of pancreatic abscess in acute pancreatitis. Ann Surg 1985; 201:656–665.
87. Durie PR: Pancreatitis. *In* Walker WA, ed: Pediatric Gastrointestinal Disease. Philadelphia, BC Decker, 1991, pp 1209–1236.
88. Weizman Z, Durie PR: Acute pancreatitis in childhood. J Pediatr 1988; 113:24–29.
89. Bittner R, Block S, Bruchler M, et al: Pancreatic abscess and infected pancreatic necrosis: Different local septic complications in acute pancreatitis. Dig Dis Sci 1987; 32:1082–1087.
90. Jeffrey RB Jr, Grendell JH, Federle MP, et al: Improved survival with early CT diagnosis of pancreatic abscess. Gastrointest Radiol 1987; 12:26.
91. Lumsden A, Bradley EL III: Secondary pancreatic infections. Surg Gynecol Obstet 1990; 170:459–467.
92. Banks PA, Gerzof SG: Pancreatic pseudocyst in abscess: Is percutaneous drainage a reasonable option? *In* Barkin JS, Rogers AI, eds: Difficult Decisions in Digestive Diseases. Chicago, Yearbook Medical Publishers, 1989, pp 181–191.
93. Lang EK, Paolini RM, Pottmieyer A: The efficacy of palliative and definitive percutaneous versus surgical drainage of pancreatic abscesses and pseudocysts: A prospective study of 85 patients. South Med J 1991; 84:55–65.
94. Sweet RL: Treatment of pelvic inflammatory disease. Contemp Iss Infect Dis 1992; 9:27–46.
95. Hager WD, Eschenbach DA, Spence MR, et al: Criteria for diagnosis and grading of salpingitis. Obstet Gynecol 1983; 61:113–114.

96. Callen PW: Ultrasonography in Obstetrics and Gynecology. Philadelphia, WB Saunders, 1983.
97. Abbitt PL, Goldwag S, Urbanski S: Endovaginal sonography for guidance in draining pelvic fluid collections. Am J Roentgenol 1990; 154:849–850.
98. Wilbur A: CT of tubo-ovarian abscess. Comp Assist Tomogr 1990; 14:625.
99. Biller JA, Grand RJ, Harris BH: Abdominal abscesses in adolescents with Crohn's disease. J Pediatr Surg 1987; 22:873–876.
100. Keighley M, Eastwood D, Ambrose N, et al: Incidence in microbiology of abdominal pelvic abscess in Crohn's disease. Gastroenterology 1982; 83:1271–1275.
101. Nagler S, Poticha S: Intra-abdominal abscess in regional enteritis. Am J Surg 1979; 137:350–354.
102. Jabra A, Fishman EK, Taylor GA: Crohn's disease in the pediatric patient: CT evaluation. Radiology 1991; 179:495–498.
103. Doemeny JM, Burke DR, Meranze SG: Percutaneous drainage of abscesses in patients with Crohn's disease. Gastrointest Radiol 1988; 13:237.
104. Haaga JR: Imaging intraabdominal abscesses and nonoperative drainage procedures. World J Surg 1990; 14:204–209.
105. Gerzof SG, Oates ME: Imaging techniques for infections in the surgical patient. Surg Clin North Am 1988; 68:147–165.
106. Mackenzie M, Fordyce J, Young DG: Subphrenic abscess in children. Br J Surg 1975; 62:305–308.
107. Patterson JE, Andriole VT: Renal and perirenal abscesses. Infect Dis Clin North Am 1987; 1:907–926.
108. Wippermann CF, Schofer O, Beetz R, et al: Renal abscess in childhood: Diagnostic and therapeutic progress. Pediatr Infect Dis J 1991; 10:446–450.
109. Rathore MH, Barton LL, Luisiri A: Acute lobar nephronia: A review. Pediatrics 1991; 87:728–734.
110. Braun G, Moussali L, Balanzar JL: Xanthogranulomatous pyelonephritis in children. J Urol 1985; 133:236–239.
111. Kierce F, Carroll R, Guiney EJ: Xanthogranulomatous pyelonephritis in childhood. Br J Urol 1985; 57:261–264.
112. Wipperman CF, Schofer O, Beetz R, et al: Renal abscess in childhood: Diagnostic and therapeutic progress. Pediatric Infect Dis J 1991; 10:446–450.
113. Edelstein H, McCabe RE: Perinephric abscess: Modern diagnosis and treatment in 47 cases. Medicine 1988; 67:118–131.
114. Edelstein H, McCabe RE: Perinephric abscess in pediatric patients: Report of six cases in review of the literature. Pediatr Infect Dis J 1989; 81:167–170.
115. Edelstein H, McCabe RE, Lieberman E: Perinephric abscess in renal transplant recipients: Report of seven cases in review. Rev Infect Dis 1989; 11:569–577.
116. Schwaitzberg SD, Pokorny WJ, Thurston RS, et al: Psoas abscess in children. J Pediatr Surg 1985; 20:339–342.
117. Hoffer FA, Shamberger RC, Teele RL: Ilio-psoas abscess: Diagnosis and management. Pediatr Radiol 1987; 17:23–27.
118. Davies D, King SM, Parekh RS, et al: Psoas abscess caused by *Haemophilus influenzae* type B. Pediatr Infect Dis J 1991; 10:411–412.

Chapter 19

Intestinal Obstruction and Ileus

JAMES F. MARKOWITZ

Obstruction of the gastrointestinal tract is a clinical problem commonly encountered by physicians caring for children of any age. Obstructions can be mechanical (either simple or strangulating) or paralytic and are found at all levels of the gastrointestinal tract. Characteristically, certain entities result in obstruction during different stages of childhood. This chapter attempts to summarize the pathophysiologic events common to many causes of obstruction, particularly as they pertain to the management of children and adolescents with these conditions. The chapter also discusses the differential diagnosis of obstruction during childhood and attempts to delineate the differences between ileus and obstruction. A more detailed discussion of intestinal pseudo-obstruction can be found in Chapter 48.

MECHANICAL OBSTRUCTION

Congenital as well as acquired conditions result in mechanical obstruction of the gastrointestinal tract. Obstruction may arise from abnormalities of the wall of the gut, from lesions arising extrinsic to the gut, and from intraluminal contents. Various conditions associated with obstruction occurring in the pediatric patient are summarized in Table 19–1. Although congenital lesions commonly present within the first hours or days of life, numerous examples of congenital lesions (e.g., intraluminal webs, malrotation with obstructing bands, or Meckel's diverticulum) can present at any age.[1]

Mechanical obstruction is generally classified as simple or strangulating. In simple obstruction, the aboral flow of luminal contents is prevented, resulting in characteristic pathophysiologic events. In strangulating obstruction, blood flow to the affected segment of gut is impaired. The resulting ischemic changes can lead to more significant morbidity and mortality than that associated with simple obstruction.

Pathophysiology

Simple Obstruction

A number of different pathophysiologic events associated with the onset of simple obstruction have been described. As the aboral flow of intestinal contents is prevented, the gut proximal to the site of obstruction distends with ingested liquids and solids, swallowed air, and gastrointestinal secretions. During the first 12 hours of obstruction, fluids accumulate owing to decreased intestinal absorption of electrolytes and water. At this stage there is little change in the amount of intestinal secretion. As distention becomes more marked, continuing intraluminal accumulation of fluid and electrolytes occurs as a result of further decreases in the rate of absorption and a simultaneous increase in the rate of intestinal secretion.[2] The mechanisms underlying distention-induced intestinal secretion are not clear but may result partially from local neural rather than humoral factors.[3] In addition, distention-induced secretion may result from stimulation of local prostaglandin production.[4] Whatever the mechanism, these fluid and electrolyte shifts commonly result in isotonic intravascular depletion, often associated with hypokalemia. When obstruction occurs at the gastric outlet, hypochloremic alkalosis characteristically occurs secondary to protracted loss of hydrochloric acid.

Mechanical obstruction also results in poorly understood changes in motility. Acutely, the gut proximal to an obstruction demonstrates periods of sustained, markedly increased myoelectric spike bursts and contractile activity that then subside into a period of quiescence.[5, 6] This cycle of motor activity appears to correlate with the patient's subjective symptoms of colic. As obstruction progresses and the proximal gut dilates, contractile activity decreases until little, if any, activity is present. In addition, as fluid accumulates and distention occurs, nausea and reflex vomiting develop.

Distinct blood flow changes have been demonstrated in models of simple obstruction. In general, blood flow appears to be inversely proportional to intraluminal pressure. As intraluminal pressure increases, blood flow is shifted away from the mucosa.[7] Decreased mucosal blood flow might logically be expected to result in decreased mucosal viability and function. Although these changes appear to be especially important in closed-loop obstructions (e.g., volvulus) because of the relatively high intraluminal pressures generated, similar changes have been documented in simple, open-loop obstructions.[8]

Table 19–1. CAUSES OF MECHANICAL OBSTRUCTION IN THE PEDIATRIC PATIENT

Esophageal Obstruction
- Congenital
  - Atresia (with or without tracheoesophageal fistula)
  - Intraluminal web
  - Cartilaginous ring
- Acquired
  - Peptic stricture
  - Foreign body

Gastroduodenal Obstruction
- Congenital
  - Atresia
  - Antral web
  - Duodenal web ("windsock" obstruction)
  - Annular pancreas
  - Malrotation with extrinsic bands
- Acquired
  - Peptic ulcer disease
  - Foreign body
  - Bezoar
  - Chronic granulomatous disease
  - Crohn's disease
  - Superior mesenteric artery syndrome
  - Eosinophilic gastroenteritis
  - Gastric volvulus

Small Bowel Obstruction
- Congenital
  - Atresias (ileal more common than jejunal)
  - Meckel's diverticulum
  - Enteric duplications
  - Meconium ileus
- Acquired
  - Intussusception
  - Volvulus
  - Adhesions (postoperative or postinflammatory)
  - Hernia (external or internal)
  - Stricture secondary to:
    - Necrotizing enterocolitis
    - Crohn's disease
    - Trauma
    - Surgical anastomosis
  - Appendicitis
  - Submucosal hematoma
  - Parasites (ascariasis, tapeworm)
  - Tumor
  - Peritoneal "cocoon" encapsulation
  - Meconium ileus equivalent
  - Henoch-Schönlein purpura (intussusception or postinflammatory stricture)
  - Extrinsic compression (mesenteric cyst, ventriculoperitoneal shunt, tumor)

Colonic Obstruction
- Congenital
  - Imperforate anus
  - Atresia
  - Hirschsprung's disease
  - Neuronal intestinal dysplasia
  - Meconium plug
  - Microcolon
- Acquired
  - Fecal impaction
  - Intussusception
  - Stricture
  - Tumor
  - Sigmoid volvulus

Obstruction also results in dramatic changes in the bacteriology of the intestine. With the onset of obstruction, intraluminal bacteria rapidly proliferate in the usually sparsely colonized proximal intestine. Coliforms and anaerobes, such as *Clostridium* and *Bacteroides* species, predominate and can be found in concentrations (10^9–10^{10} per ml) comparable with that usually found in stool.[9, 10] As mucosal barriers break down, the presence of these intraluminal organisms enhances the risks of bacterial translocation and portal sepsis or endotoxemia.

Strangulating Obstruction

Mechanical obstruction associated with vascular compromise results in strangulating obstruction. If the obstruction is rapidly reversed, no irreversible injury may result. However, when the strangulation is not relieved, the resulting ischemia can lead to intestinal infarction. Vascular supply can be compromised by extrinsic compression of a mesenteric arcade resulting from a hernial ring or adhesion or from a volvulus that interrupts blood flow by mechanically twisting the mesentery. Less commonly, local pressure necrosis from progressive distention within a closed-loop obstruction can result in local areas of ischemia and resultant infarction.

The pathophysiologic events associated with simple mechanical obstruction are also important in strangulating obstruction. However, as vascular impairment results, local venous engorgement and edema develop, followed by reflex arterial vasospasm. Local hypoxia impairs tissue viability, and hemorrhage or thrombosis can develop. The increasing luminal distention and pressure cannot be vented because of the closed-loop nature of most strangulating obstructions, and significant third spacing of fluid and electrolytes occurs. Unless the obstruction is relieved, transmural infarction with associated perforation, local or generalized peritonitis, and septicemia will result.[11]

Clinical Presentation

The signs and symptoms of obstruction of the gastrointestinal tract vary to some degree with the site, cause, and chronicity of the obstruction. Although a number of studies in adult patients have attempted to identify the clinical characteristics that might differentiate simple from strangulating obstruction, no combination of symptoms or signs has proved to discriminate between the two entities with a high degree of sensitivity and specificity.[12–14] Comparable studies in pediatric patients have not been reported.

Symptoms

Classically, the cardinal symptoms of obstruction include nausea and vomiting, colicky abdominal pain, abdominal distention, and progressive obstipation.

Nausea and Vomiting. Effortful vomiting is common following most obstructions; however, in infants, distinguishing between effortful vomiting and the effortless regurgitation usually associated with gastroesophageal reflux is not always possible. Vomitus initially includes recently ingested food but becomes bilious, assuming that the level of obstruction is below the ampulla of Vater. As obstruction continues, stasis and bacterial overgrowth result in vomitus that is increasingly feculent. When obstruction is in the distal small bowel or colon, vomiting may not occur, and the patient may complain only of severe nausea. By contrast, with gastric or high small bowel obstructions, nausea and vomiting may be the sole manifestations. Recurrent episodes of vomiting that remit spontaneously can result from intermittent, spontaneously resolving high-grade partial or complete obstruction.[15] Children with a diverse etiology of lesions, such as duodenal intussusception secondary to a duodenal duplication, small bowel stricture due to necrotizing enterocolitis or Crohn's disease, and mesenteric cyst impinging extrinsically on a loop of bowel, have been described (Fig. 19–1*A* and *B*).

Pain is generally episodic and often is poorly localized to the epigastrium. Distinct episodes of colic, however, tend to occur more frequently in proximal compared with distal obstructions. These episodes are generally interspersed by periods in which the crampy pain disappears completely. This poorly localized, colicky pain is thought to be visceral in origin. Better localization of pain occurs if peritonitis develops. When apparent, this parietal pain is generally associated with more continuously persistent symptoms, marked tenderness, and abdominal rigidity.

Distention. Proximal to an obstruction, the bowel begins to fill with ingested material, gastrointestinal secretions, and gas. Abdominal distention then gradually becomes apparent. However, when obstruction occurs high in the gastrointestinal tract, distention may not be present. It may also be absent if recurrent vomiting is able to empty adequately the obstructed segments of bowel.

Obstipation. Progressive inability to defecate or pass flatus is often a late manifestation of obstruction. Early in the process, the bowel distal to an obstruction is able to empty both flatus and stool. Once the distal bowel empties, obstipation becomes evident; however, not all patients with obstruction completely stop passing material per rectum. Patients with intussusception or volvulus frequently pass bloody stool or mucus. By contrast, patients with high-grade partial obstructions may pass gas intermittently or have explosive bouts of diarrhea that tend to relieve their pain acutely.

Physical Examination

The examination of the child with obstruction is always important and often reveals the cause or site of obstruction, or both. Signs of dehydration are common, and vital signs as well as physical findings must be assessed carefully. During periods of colic, patients appear acutely ill. Infants characteristically cry incon-

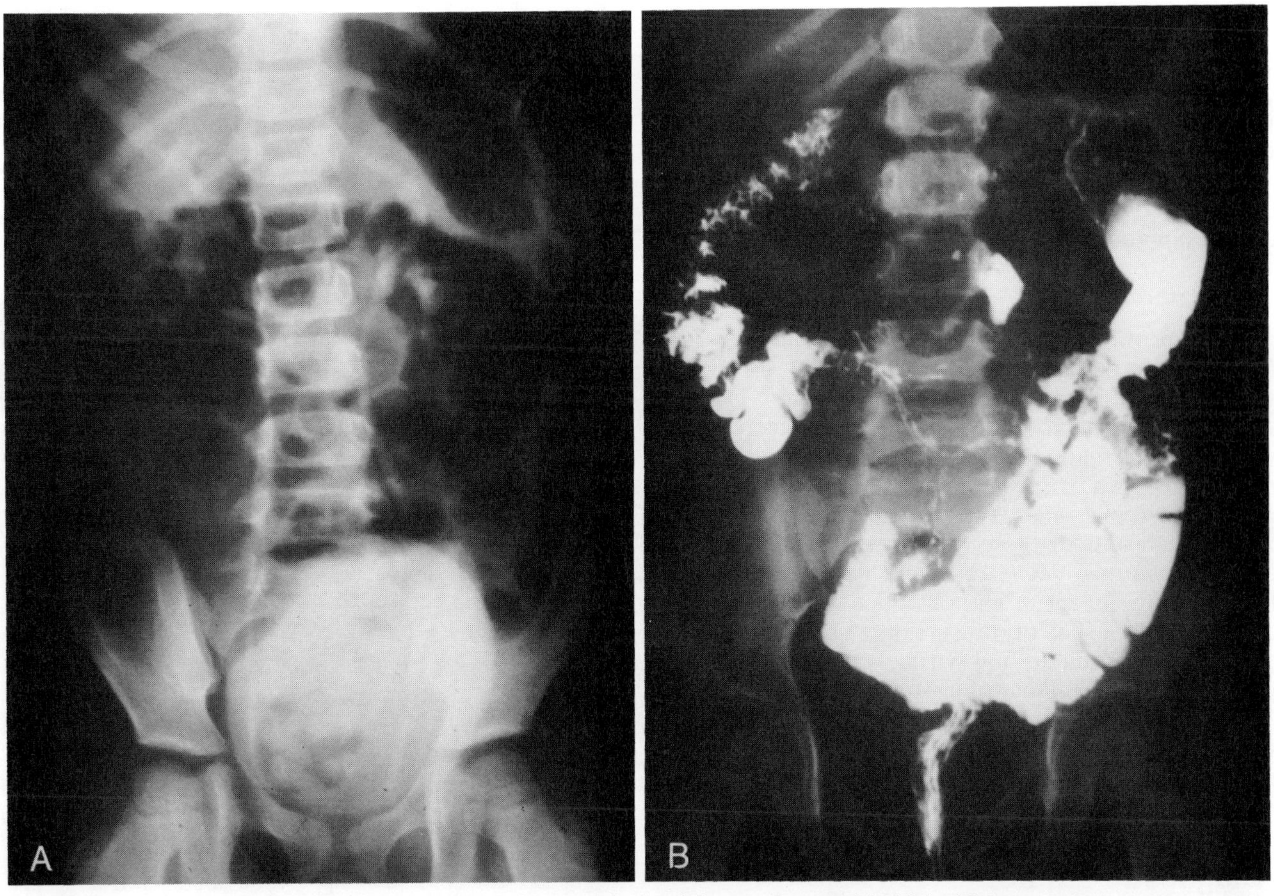

Figure 19–1. *A,* Single film from an intravenous pyelogram obtained from a 7-year-old child with recurrent vomiting. A filling defect caused by a mesenteric cyst extrinsically compresses the bladder. Note the nonspecific bowel gas pattern. *B,* Barium contrast study from the same patient, demonstrating lack of contrast-filled bowel loops in the right lower quadrant.

solably at these times and often pull up their legs and appear to be unable to find a comfortable position. Between painful attacks, however, patients can be quite comfortable, and infants often are able to fall asleep, only to be awakened again shortly thereafter with the onset of another wave of pain.

Inspection of the abdomen can reveal important clues to diagnosis. Abdominal distention is often present but can be absent in children with high intestinal obstruction or with copious vomiting. Incisional scars can suggest the possibility of postoperative adhesions. Erythema of the abdominal wall is a particularly ominous sign, as it frequently is associated with underlying peritonitis and, potentially, ischemic or necrotic bowel.

Auscultation remains important in the diagnosis of obstruction. Bowel sounds are often hypoactive, characterized by tinkles and splashes that are interspersed by loud "rushes" that commonly accompany the onset of crampy pain. A gastric succussion splash can suggest gastric outlet obstruction. In the later stages of a well-established obstruction, however, bowel sounds can be absent once significant luminal dilatation and loss of muscular contractility occur.

Palpation can reveal the presence of a hernia, a finding that should be diligently searched for in every patient with apparent obstruction. Dilated loops of bowel or masses can also be palpated. In the infant, the pyloric "olive" of pyloric stenosis, or the sausage-shaped mass of an intussusception are often sufficiently typical to allow accurate diagnosis during the physical examination. In addition, the sense of an "empty" quadrant of abdomen on palpation can also raise the suspicion of an intussusception. Although generalized tenderness may be evident in simple obstruction, the presence of distinct, localized tenderness or abdominal rigidity should be considered evidence of peritonitis and possible strangulating obstruction.

Laboratory Findings

There are no specific biochemical abnormalities that are diagnostic of obstruction or are capable of differentiating simple from strangulating obstruction. Despite this lack of specificity, serum electrolyte, blood urea nitrogen, and creatinine levels should be measured in any patient with suspected obstruction as guides to appropriate replacement of fluid and electrolytes. Although the results of these tests are not specific, characteristic abnormalities (e.g., hypochloremic metabolic alkalosis in the event of gastric outlet obstruction) can suggest potential sites of obstruction. A complete blood count is also indicated, and particular attention should be given to the possibility of a strangulating obstruction if marked leukocytosis or leukopenia is present. Other biochemical studies are indicated in particular instances to rule out possible differential diagnoses (e.g., amylase to exclude pancreatitis).

Diagnostic Studies

Obstruction of the gastrointestinal tract can almost always be suspected after the history and physical examination have been completed. However, diagnostic imaging is often necessary to confirm the clinical impression of obstruction, to localize the level of obstruction, and to rule out other conditions that must be considered in the differential diagnosis.

Plain supine and erect abdominal radiographs are the most useful studies for confirming the presence of obstruction and suggesting the level of the gastrointestinal tract affected. In the neonate, a gasless abdomen is suggestive of esophageal atresia, whereas in the older child the same finding suggests a marked degree of third-spaced fluid compatible with gastroenteritis. Distal small bowel or colonic obstruction is suggested by the finding of multiple dilated loops of bowel containing differential air-fluid levels and the lack of air in the distal colon and rectum. Care must be taken in interpreting the level of obstruction from the flat plate in the neonate, however, as it is often difficult to determine whether a given bowel loop is small bowel or colon (Fig. 19–2). A "double-bubble" sign suggests duodenal atresia in the obstructed neonate or high duodenal obstruction (often secondary to extrinsic bands) in the older child (Fig. 19–3). However, in the latter situation or, occasionally, in the child with more distal obstruction who has had copious vomiting, the radiographs can appear normal. In the child

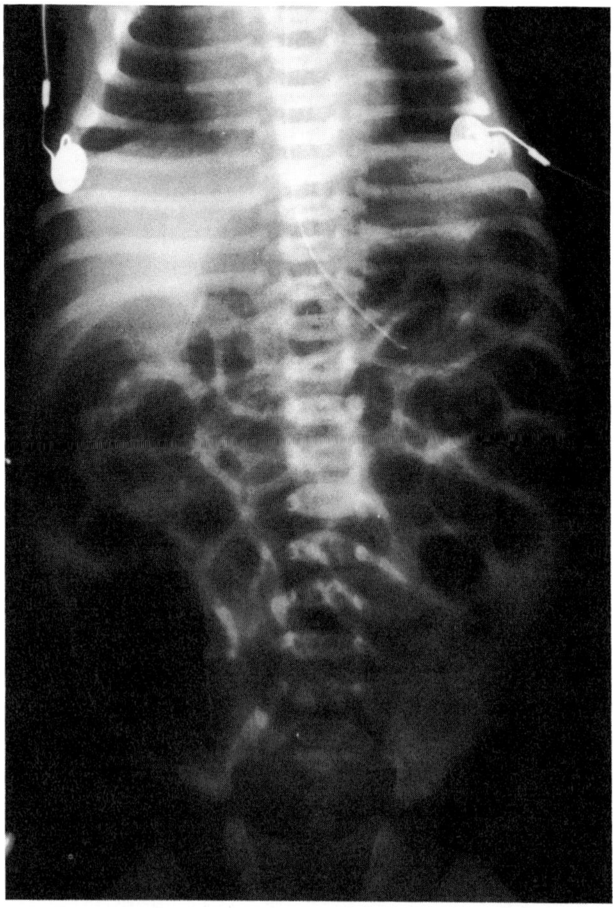

Figure 19–2. Plain radiograph of the abdomen from a 3-day-old neonate with Hirschsprung's disease. Distinguishing small from large bowel loops is often not possible in infants of this age.

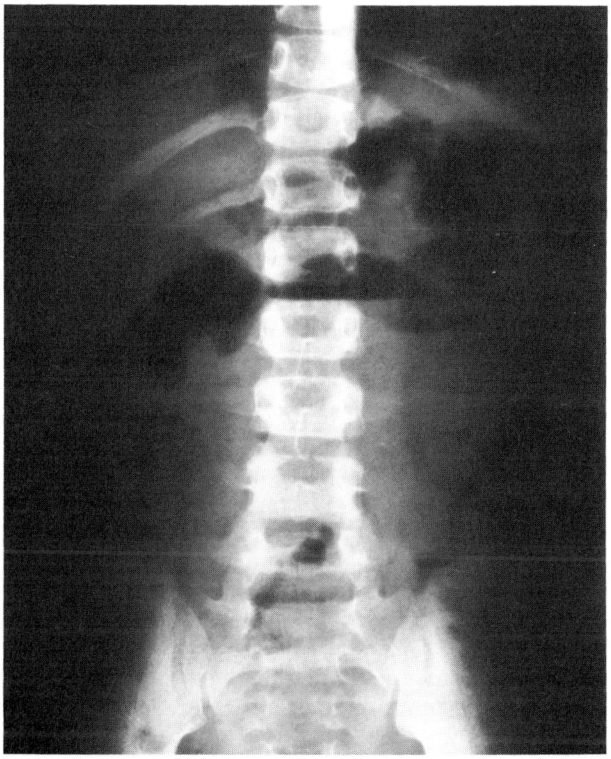

Figure 19–3. Plain radiograph of the abdomen of an 8-year-old boy with recurrent vomiting due to superior mesenteric artery syndrome. The dilated proximal duodenum and an air-fluid level in the distal stomach are readily apparent.

with ileus rather than obstruction, dilated loops of bowel throughout the gastrointestinal tract, at times associated with small air-fluid levels, will be seen (Fig. 19–4). Occasionally, the plain abdominal radiograph can also reveal the etiology of obstruction, as in the case of inguinal hernias (Fig. 19–5), meconium ileus, fecal impaction (Fig. 19–6), or volvulus.

Ultrasonography plays an important role in the diagnosis of obstruction in the child. It is particularly good at noninvasively demonstrating the hypertrophic pyloric muscle (>4 mm thick) and elongated, narrowed pyloric channel (>2 cm long) typical of pyloric stenosis.[16] Ultrasonography is therefore recommended as the imaging study of choice in the infant with a history suggestive of pyloric stenosis but in whom the typical pyloric mass cannot be palpated. Sonography can be expected to be about 90% accurate in demonstrating the lesion, and there are virtually no false-positive results. Although sonography has also been advocated for diagnosing other causes of bowel obstruction (especially small bowel intussusception[17] and midgut volvulus[18]), the multiple gas-filled, dilated loops of bowel present often obscure the area of interest. Despite these limitations, sonography can be a useful adjunctive method for identifying lesions such as duplications or tumors, which can present with obstruction.

Contrast studies of the bowel are indicated when the evaluation fails to identify the cause of obstruction. To avoid the risk of barium contamination of the peritoneum, retrograde contrast enemas using a water-soluble contrast, such as Gastrografin, are generally used for studies in infants or when there is a significant risk of perforation. These studies are useful for identifying malrotation, meconium ileus, and intussusception and, in the last two conditions, can be therapeutic as well as diagnostic. Barium enemas are preferable for delineating mucosal contours and for identifying the transition zone of Hirschsprung's disease (Fig. 19–7). Antegrade barium contrast studies can be used to delineate causes of gastric outlet or high bowel obstructions or to visualize high-grade partial obstructions of the more distal bowel, as is often seen in Crohn's disease (Fig. 19–8). Water-soluble agents are once again used when there is a risk of perforation. Because it is not diluted in the gut, metrizamide, an isotonic water-soluble agent, has been reported to be superior to the other water-soluble agents for delineating mucosal detail.[19] However, its cost makes its use prohibitive in all but the smallest infants.

Differentiation Between Simple and Strangulating Obstruction

Differentiating a simple obstruction from a strangulating obstruction becomes crucially important in determining appropriate treatment. Although studies directed

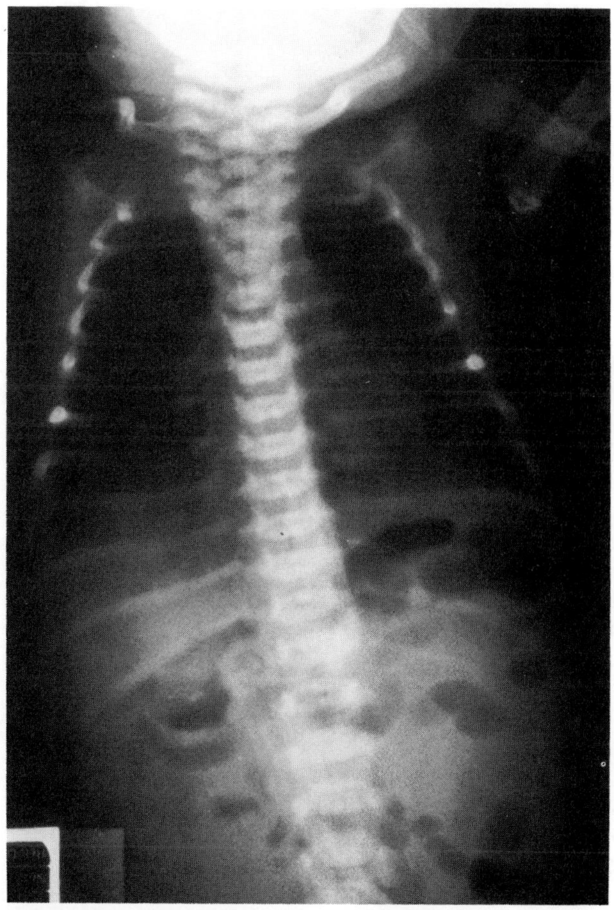

Figure 19–4. Plain radiograph of the abdomen reveals a nonspecific gas pattern in a 3-week-old child with distention secondary to ileus.

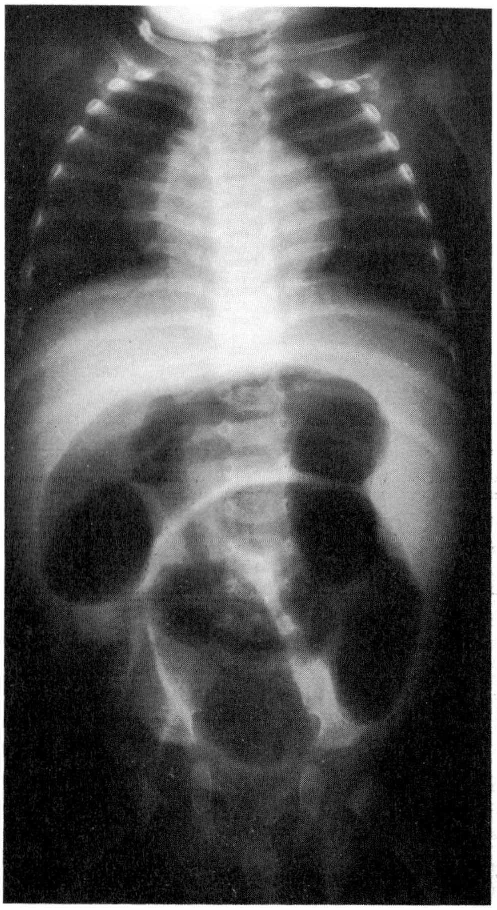

Figure 19–5. Plain radiograph of the abdomen reveals massive intestinal dilatation in a 4-month-old child with abdominal distention and vomiting secondary to intestinal obstruction from inguinal hernias. Note the presence of gas within the scrotum.

at this diagnostic challenge have been reported in adult patients, no comparable data exist for the pediatric or adolescent patient. In the worst instance, children with strangulating obstruction manifest signs of shock, acidosis, and peritonitis, and the abdominal wall often is doughy and erythematous. A patient with these signs presents little diagnostic dilemma. However, the goal of all clinicians must be to recognize early, reversible strangulation before these advanced signs develop. In adults a number of different studies have suggested that different combinations of signs, symptoms, and laboratory tests (e.g., fever, feculent vomiting, absent bowel sounds, localized abdominal tenderness, and leukocytosis) might predict strangulation.[20, 21] However, more recent prospective as well as retrospective studies[13, 14, 22, 23] refute these contentions. There appears to be no combination of symptoms, signs, or laboratory studies that reliably distinguishes simple obstruction from strangulating obstruction. When studied prospectively, even the experienced clinical judgment of a senior attending surgeon was found to have only a sensitivity of 48% and specificity of 83% in identifying strangulation.[13] This inability to accurately differentiate simple obstruction from strangulating obstruction must always be kept in mind when nonoperative therapies are instituted.

Treatment

Patients with obstruction of the gastrointestinal tract suffer not only from impeded transit of material through the gut but also from the dehydrating effects of enhanced intestinal secretion and vomiting. Patients with strangulating obstructions may also manifest signs of shock, sepsis, or hemorrhage. Treatment must first be directed at resuscitating and stabilizing the patient before further definitive therapy can safely be attempted. However, little time can be lost if strangulation has occurred, as ischemia can quickly result in frank necrosis and gangrene of the bowel if not rapidly reversed. Systemic treatment demands that appropriate intravenous access be ensured. Central venous pressure or pulmonary artery pressure monitoring can guide vigorous fluid resuscitation. Although weighted intestinal tubes have often been advocated for decompression of distal intestinal obstructions, clinical experience suggests that most children are adequately treated with a nasogastric tube attached to an intermittent suction device. Such treat-

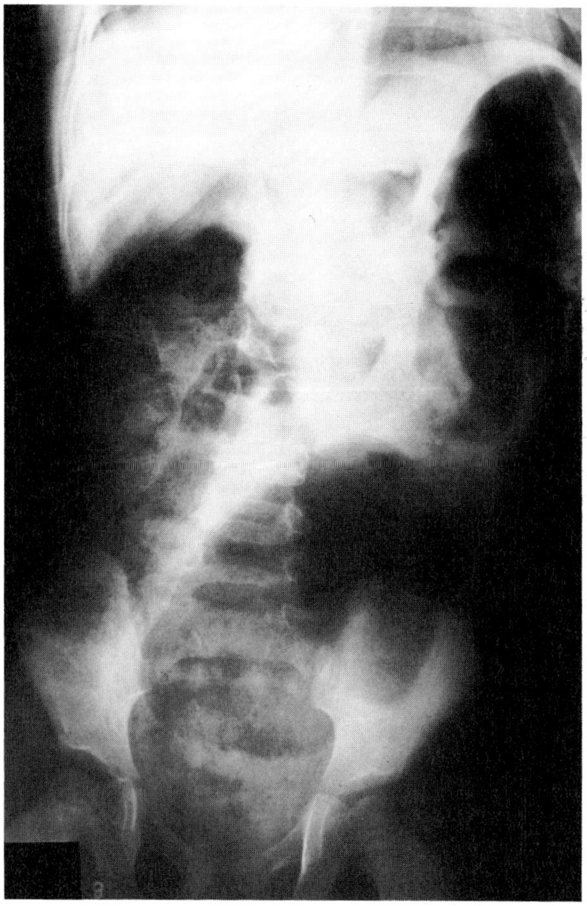

Figure 19–6. Three-year-old girl with abdominal distention and vomiting associated with fecal impaction. Shadows of stool fill the pelvis and can be seen outlining the left and right colon in this plain abdominal radiograph.

ment not only relieves pain and vomiting by decompressing the distended stomach and more distal loops of bowel but also decreases the risks of both perforation and aspiration. Blood cultures and antibiotic coverage should be instituted in the appropriate clinical circumstance (especially in the neonate, or in any child with suspected strangulating obstruction). Preparations for potentially imminent surgery, including obtaining blood for type and cross-match, should also be given high priority.

The role of nonoperative versus operative management as primary therapy in intestinal obstruction remains poorly studied in children. *Nonoperative treatment can be considered only when there is little likelihood of a strangulating obstruction.* Partial or complete obstruction due to adhesions or strictures (from Crohn's disease or as a late complication of necrotizing enterocolitis) often resolve with nasogastric decompression alone. In a recent retrospective analysis of the experience with partial adhesive obstructions, 74% of 149 episodes not requiring immediate surgery (no sign of fever, leukocytosis, localized abdominal tenderness, or complete obstruction) resolved with nonoperative management.[24] Recurrence rates were reported to be 18.75% after surgery and 36.47% after conservative management. However, complete obstructions should only rarely be treated conservatively for longer than 6 to 12 hours if obvious signs of clinical improvement are not manifest. In partial obstructions, clinical experience as well as studies in adult patients[25] suggest that almost all symptomatic responses will be found in the first 48 to 72 hours of decompression. In the study of partial adhesive obstruction in children cited previously[24] 65% of the successful nonoperative clinical trials were evident within 72 hours and 90% within 96 hours. Extended nonoperative therapy (>96 hours) offers little increased chance of success. However, more prolonged conservative management (10–14 days) can be successful in obstruction secondary to duodenal or small bowel hematoma.[26]

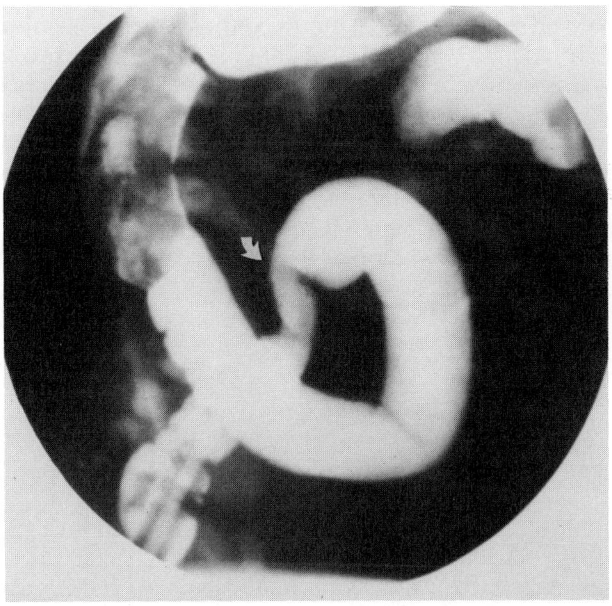

Figure 19–7. Spot film of the rectosigmoid obtained at barium enema from a 3-day-old infant with Hirschsprung's disease (same patient as in Figure 19–2). A transition zone *(arrow)* is clearly defined.

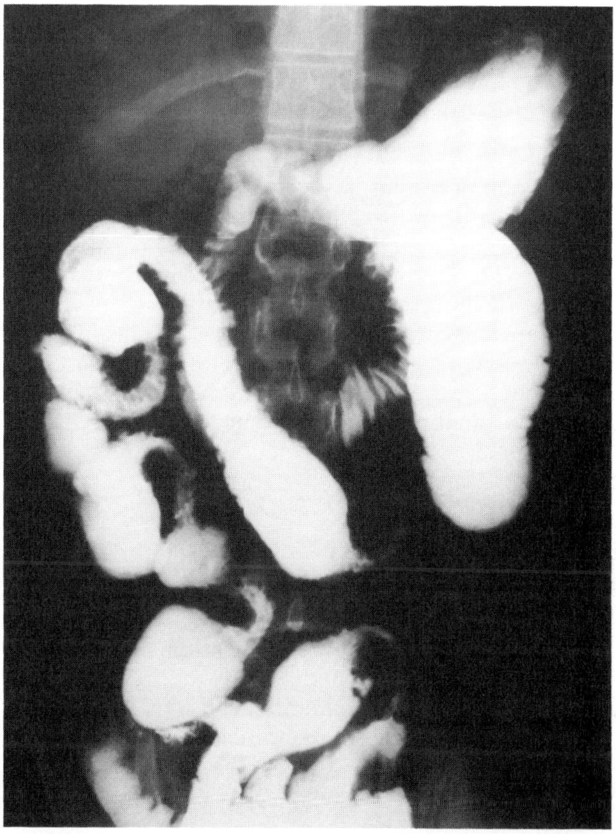

Figure 19–8. Barium contrast radiograph obtained as part of a small bowel follow-through in a 15-year-old girl with Crohn's disease and recurrent partial obstruction. Multiple stenotic lesions of the jejunum and ileum are present.

A number of different conditions resulting in obstruction are recognized as highly amenable to nonoperative management. Intussusception and meconium ileus can often be successfully treated by the radiologist. Ileocolic intussusception can be completely reduced by an air or a retrograde contrast enema.[27–29] Similarly, hypertonic water-soluble contrast enemas, at times mixed with acetylcysteine,[30] often eliminate the obstruction secondary to meconium ileus and meconium ileus equivalent.

Medical management also plays an important role preoperatively, as surgical outcome is often directly correlated with the adequacy of preoperative resuscitation. Gastric decompression and appropriate fluid and electrolyte management are critically important in the prompt return of gastric function following a pyloromyotomy for pyloric stenosis. A similar case can be made for the infant with Hirschsprung's disease. Even in the event of enterocolitis, colonic irrigations coupled with antibiotics and fluid, electrolyte, and nutritional management can stabilize a potentially critically ill neonate. This period of medical management obviates the need for emergency decompressive surgery and ultimately allows definitive repair as a single-stage surgical intervention.[31]

ILEUS

Any condition that results in abnormally slow or absent aboral transit of intestinal contents without demonstrable mechanical obstruction can be considered as an ileus. The term *ileus,* therefore, encompasses a spectrum of different clinical and pathophysiologic entities. Ileus can involve the entire gastrointestinal tract or only segments of it. In the latter situation, isolated involvement of the stomach (gastric atony) or colon or an isolated small bowel loop are most common.

Pathophysiology

The normal control of gastrointestinal motility requires a complex interaction between myogenic and neurogenic factors. Smooth muscles supply propulsive force, but the pattern and coordination of these muscular contractions are modified by both enteric and central nervous system influences and by a multitude of polypeptides acting by both endocrine and paracrine pathways.[32, 33] Imbalances among these competing influences can result in marked disruption of normal motor function and ileus.

The pediatrician most commonly sees ileus associated with either infection or surgery. Varying degrees of ileus can be seen in children with gastroenteritis, especially among those treated with antimotility drugs such as loperamide or opiates.[34] More significant ileus is often associated with sepsis. Following abdominal surgery, ileus is universal. In this circumstance, the return of gastrointestinal motor function follows a characteristic temporal sequence. The small intestine commonly resumes myoelectric and contractile activity within a few hours of surgery. The stomach generally does not resume adequate function for 24 to 48 hours postoperatively, whereas the colon often takes as long as 3 to 5 days to resume normal function.[35] The pathophysiologic mechanisms underlying ileus in these clinical circumstances have not been fully elucidated. Increased sympathetic activity is commonly found postoperatively, and the resulting imbalance between sympathetic and parasympathetic tone is believed by many clinicians to result in ileus.[36] The contribution of endogenous endorphins and exogenous opiates to ongoing motor dysfunction in these circumstances also remains unclear. A variety of other abnormalities of humoral and paracrine factors may also be important.[37]

Ileus is also seen in a number of other clinical settings. Metabolic abnormalities, including hypokalemia and uremia, can cause ileus. Lead poisoning has also been implicated.[38] Drugs can also interfere with gastrointestinal motor function. Anticholinergics (including antihistamines with anticholinergic effects), autonomic blockers, and opiates can directly interfere with normal enteric or central nervous system control, or both, of gastrointestinal smooth muscle function.[39] Phenothiazines and antidepressants also have anticholinergic or antiserotonergic effects, or both, that interfere with gut motor function.[40] Vincristine has direct toxic effects on enteric nerves and can result in prolonged motor dysfunction. Children have also been described as developing prolonged but reversible ileus secondary to an overdose of loperamide and as a consequence of the surreptitious use of ipecac.

These conditions need to be differentiated from the conditions collectively considered under the term *intestinal pseudo-obstruction.* The pseudo-obstruction syndromes represent a group of chronic disorders presenting with chronic or recurrent, self-limited episodes of nonmechanical obstruction. These conditions represent true motility disorders characterized by functionally and often histopathologically abnormal smooth muscle or enteric neurons. A complete review of these conditions can be found in Chapter 48.

Clinical Presentation

Children and adolescents with ileus generally present with increasing abdominal distention. Pain is usually minimal, and nausea and vomiting are frequently absent. Despite increasing girth, flatus and loose stools are commonly present. Physical findings are often confined to abdominal distention; there is little, if any, evidence of tenderness. In contrast with mechanical obstruction, however, bowel sounds are characteristically diminished to absent.

Diagnostic Studies

The plain abdominal radiograph demonstrates multiple, small air-fluid levels throughout the abdomen, colon, and rectum (Fig. 19–9). In contrast with mechanical obstruction in which serial abdominal radiographs reveal progressive bowel distention and the disappearance of gas from the distal bowel, serial radiographs in the child with an ileus show either no significant worsening or a gradual improvement of the bowel gas pattern. If contrast radiographs are obtained, there is usually slow transit of contrast material through dilated but mechanically patent bowel loops.

Treatment

Treatment is generally supportive, as ileus is usually a self-limited process. Patients cannot tolerate oral feedings and require intravenous fluids to maintain appropriate hydration. In children with discomfort from abdominal distention or recurrent vomiting, nasogastric decompression is useful. When possible, specific therapies directed at the associated cause of ileus (e.g., antibiotics for sepsis, correction of metabolic derangements, and discontinuation of responsible pharmacologic agents) offer the best hope of rapid resolution of the symptoms.

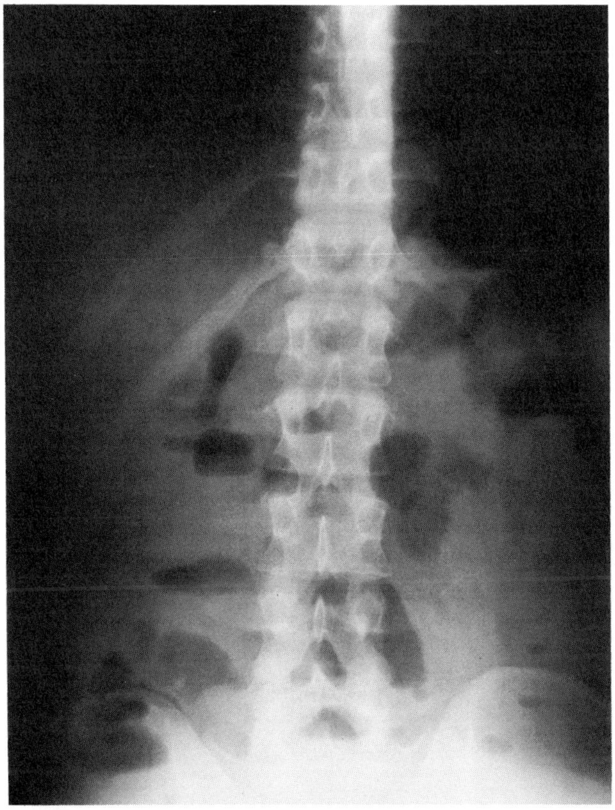

Figure 19–9. Plain abdominal radiograph shows a nonspecific bowel gas pattern in a 16-year-old boy with vomiting due to gastroenteritis.

Based on clinical and experimental data derived from experience in adults, many surgeons are increasingly enthusiastic about the early use of prokinetic agents, such as metoclopramide, in the child or adolescent with postoperative ileus. By stimulating the early return of gastric function postoperatively, the need for nasogastric decompression is often eliminated. Earlier resumption of feeding has generally not been possible, however, probably because metoclopramide lacks significant prokinetic effects in the distal bowel. Newer panintestinal prokinetic agents such as cisapride, motilin agonists such as erythromycin, serotonin antagonists, or combinations of agents designed to correct the apparent imbalance in sympathetic and parasympathetic tone may offer improved therapy in the future. The use of similar pharmacologic regimens also offers a therapeutic alternative to the unusual child with prolonged, unremitting ileus. However, no data on the use of such regimens in children have been reported apart from the experience with cisapride in the pseudo-obstruction syndromes[41, 42] and in cystic fibrosis complicated by recurrent distal intestinal obstructions.[43]

REFERENCES

1. Sheridan R: Nonrotation of the midgut presenting in the adolescent and adult. Am J Gastroenterol 1989; 84:670–673.
2. Shields R: The absorption and secretion of fluid and electrolytes by the obstructed bowel. Br J Surg 1965; 52:774–779.
3. Caren JF, Meyer JH, Grossman MI: Canine intestinal secretion during and after rapid distension of the small bowel. Am J Physiol 1974; 227:183–188.
4. MacGregor IL, Lavigne ME: Inhibition by indomethacin of intestinal distension induced secretion in the rat. J Surg Res 1979; 26:167–170.
5. Summers RW, Yanda R, Prihoda M, et al: Acute intestinal obstruction: An electromyographic study in dogs. Gastroenterology 1983; 85:1301–1306.
6. Malagelada JR, Camillari M, Stanghellini V: Manometric Diagnosis of Gastrointestinal Disorders. New York; Thieme, 1986; p 82.
7. Shikata J, Shida T, Amino K, Ishioka K, et al: Experimental studies on the hemodynamics of the small intestine following increased intraluminal pressure. Surg Gynecol Obstet 1983; 156:155–160.
8. Ruf W, Suehiro GT, Suehiro A, et al: Intestinal blood flow at various intraluminal pressures in the piglet with closed abdomen. Ann Surg 1980; 191:157–163.
9. Sykes PA, Boulter KH, Schofield PF: The microflora of the obstructed bowel. Br J Surg 1976; 63:721–725.
10. Gupta S, Reddy KRRM, Sanyal SC: Bacterial flora in acute small bowel obstruction. Chemotherapy 1980; 26:446–451.
11. Laufman H, Nora PF: Physiological problems underlying intestinal strangulation obstruction. Surg Clin North Am 1962; 42:219–229.
12. Leffal LD, Syphax B: Clinical aids in strangulation intestinal obstruction. Am J Surg 1970; 120:756–759.
13. Sarr MG, Bulkley GB, Zuidema GD: Preoperative recognition of intestinal strangulation obstruction: Prospective evaluation of diagnostic capability. Am J Surg 1983; 145:176–182.
14. Snyder EN Jr, McCranie D: Closed loop obstruction of the small bowel. Am J Surg 1966; 111:398–402.
15. Johnston JM, Harnsbarger JK: Episodic vomiting due to intermittent duodenal intussusception. J Pediatr Gastroenterol Nutr 1990; 10:405–408.
16. Blumhagen JD, Noble HGS: Muscle thickness in hypertrophic pyloric stenosis: Sonographic determination. AJR 1983; 140:221–223.
17. Bowerman RA, Silver TM, Jaffe MH: Real-time ultrasound diagnosis of intussusception in children. Radiology 1982; 143:527–529.
18. Leonidas JC, Magid N, Soberman N, et al: Midgut volvulus in infants: Diagnosis with US. Radiology 1991; 179:491–493.
19. Cohen MD, Schreiner R, Grosfeld J, et al. A new look at the neonatal bowel: Contrast studies with metrizamide (Amipaque). J Pediatr Surg 1983; 18:442–448.
20. Bizer LS, Liebling RW, Dleany HM, et al: Small bowel obstruction: The role of nonoperative treatment in simple intestinal obstruction and predictive criteria for strangulation obstruction. Surgery 1981; 89:407–413.
21. Stewardson RH, Bombeck CT, Nyhus LM: Critical operative management of small bowel obstruction. Ann Surg 1978; 187:189–193.
22. Zollinger RM, Kinsey DL: Diagnosis and management of intestinal obstruction. Am Surg 1964; 30:1–5.
23. Shatila AH, Chamberlain BE, Webb WR: Current status of diagnosis and management of strangulation obstruction of the small bowel. Am J Surg 1976; 132:299–303.
24. Akgur FM, Tanyel FC, Buyukpamukcu N, et al: Adhesive small bowel obstruction in children: The place and predictors of success for conservative treatment. J Pediatr Surg 1991; 26:37–41.
25. Peetz DJ, Gamelli RL, Pilcher DB: Intestinal intubation in acute, mechanical small-bowel obstruction. Arch Surg 1982; 117:334–336.
26. Czyrko C, Weltz CR, Markowitz R, et al: Blunt abdominal trauma resulting in intestinal obstruction: When to operate? J Trauma 1990; 30:1567–1571.
27. Kuta AJ, Benator RM: Intussusception: Hydrostatic pressure equivalents for barium and meglumine sodium diatrizoate. Radiology 1990; 175:125–126.
28. Shiels WE II, Bisset GS III, Kirks DR: Simple device for air reduction of intussusception. Pediatr Radiol 1990; 20:472–474.
29. Stringer DA, Ein SH: Pneumatic reduction: Advantages, risks and indications. Pediatr Radiol 1990; 20:475–477.

30. Wagget H, Bishop H, Koop E: Experience with Gastrogafin enema in the treatment of meconium ileus. J Pediatr Surg 1970; 5:649–654.
31. So HB, Schwartz DL, Becker JM, et al: Endorectal "pull-through" without preliminary colostomy in neonates with Hirschsprung's disease. J Pediatr Surg 1980; 15:470–471.
32. Bueno L, Fioramonti J: CNS peptidergic regulation of gut motility. *In* Tache Y, Wingate D, eds: Brain-Gut Interactions. Boca Raton, CRC Press, 1991; pp 231–244.
33. Fox JAET: Control of gastrointestinal motility by peptides: Old peptides, new tricks—new peptides, old tricks. Gastroenterol Clin North Am 1989; 18:163–178.
34. Murtaza A, Khan SR, Butt KS, et al: Paralytic ileus, a serious complication in acute diarrhoeal disease among infants in developing countries. Acta Paediatr Scand 1989; 78:701–705.
35. Woods JH, Erickson LW, Condon RE, et al: Postoperative ileus: A colonic problem? Surgery 1978; 84:527–533.
36. Smith J, Kelly KA, Weinshilboum RM: Pathophysiology of postoperative ileus. Arch Surg 1977; 113:203–209.
37. Livingston EH, Passaro EP Jr: Postoperative ileus. Dig Dis Sci 1990; 35:121–132.
38. Zweiner RJ, Owensby JE, Belknap WM: Lead poisoning presenting as intestinal ileus in a child (letter). Am J Dis Child 1990; 144:524–526.
39. George CF: Drugs causing intestinal obstruction: A review. J R Soc Med 1980; 73:200–204.
40. Sriram K, Schumer W, Ehrenpreis S, et al: Phenothiazine effect on gastrointestinal tract function. Am J Surg 1979; 137:87–91.
41. Cohen NP, Booth IW, Parashar K, et al: Successful management of idiopathic intestinal pseudo-obstruction with cisapride. J Pediatr Surg 1988; 23:229–230.
42. Hyman PE, McDiarmid SV, Napolitano JA, et al: Cisapride in children with pseudo-obstruction (abstract). Gastroenterology 1988; 94:A198.
43. Koletzko S, Corey M, Ellis L, et al: Effects of cisapride in patients with cystic fibrosis and distal intestinal obstruction syndrome. J Pediatr 1990; 117:815–822.

Chapter 20

Gastrointestinal Hemorrhage

ALLAN D. OLSON and
A. CRAIG HILLEMEIER

The clinical presentation of a child with gastrointestinal hemorrhage can vary from acute life-threatening shock to a clinically asymptomatic child with stools that are positive for occult blood. Gastrointestinal bleeding in infants and children can be a major challenge, despite our enhanced diagnostic capabilities and the recent advances in our understanding of the pathophysiology of hypovolemic shock.

In this chapter on gastrointestinal bleeding we define terms that describe its quality and location; review the pathophysiology of hypovolemic shock, concentrating on the emergency treatment of acute gastrointestinal bleeding; review the process used to localize bleeding; and discuss its differential diagnosis and therapeutic approaches.

DEFINITIONS AND CLINICAL PRESENTATIONS

Because gastrointestinal hemorrhage can present in several distinct ways, a clear understanding of the terms describing the different forms of gastrointestinal bleeding is essential. *Hematemesis* is used to describe vomiting of either bright red or coffee-ground–like material and suggests that the source of bleeding is located above the ligament of Treitz (Table 20–1). *Hematochezia*, the passage of bright red or maroon blood from the rectum, is most commonly associated with a colonic source of bleeding, but it has been estimated that in upper gastrointestinal hemorrhage slightly more than 10% of patients will present with hematochezia due to the rapid transit of blood through the intestine. When this occurs, the bleed is usually hemodynamically significant and reflected in orthostatic changes. *Melena*, the passing of dark black stools, occurs in patients bleeding from a site located above the ileocecal valve. The jet black color of melanotic stools results from the action of bacteria on hemoglobin that has been converted to hematin or other hemochromes.[1] Melena can also occur, however, in patients bleeding from the right side of the colon who have severe constipation. *Borborygmi* describes the deep rumbling abdominal sounds caused by the rapid transit of blood through the bowel, which is seen in patients with acute upper gastrointestinal bleeding and is a result of the cathartic effect of blood in the gastrointestinal tract.

EVALUATION AND STABILIZATION

Pathophysiology

Patients with gastrointestinal hemorrhage must be evaluated for shock. Recognizing the early phases of

Table 20–1. SIGNS AND SYMPTOMS IN GASTROINTESTINAL HEMORRHAGE

Sign	Indication	Site of Bleeding
Splenomegaly Caput medusa Jaundice	Portal hypertension	Esophageal varices Portal gastropathy
Hemangioma Telangiectasia	Multiple hemangioma syndrome	Vascular malformation of GI tract
Hematemesis	Bleeding from above the ligament of Treitz	Upper GI tract
Melena	Bleeding from above the ileocecal valve	Upper GI tract or small intestine
Hematochezia	Colonic bleeding, massive UGI bleeding	GI tract
Nasogastric aspirate: gross blood	Bleeding from above the ligament of Treitz	Upper GI tract
Palpable purpura	Henoch-Schönlein purpura	GI tract

shock requires a clear and complete understanding of the compensatory changes in body physiology that follow the rapid reduction in intravascular volume caused by gastrointestinal hemorrhage. More complete reviews of the pathophysiologic changes of shock are available elsewhere.[2–7]

In animal models in which hemorrhage has lowered the blood pressure to 50% of normal, there is a compensatory vasoconstriction that returns the blood pressure to near normal within 30 to 60 minutes.[2] Following this initial increase, there is a progressive drop in blood pressure due to vasodilation, resulting in irreversible hypotension and death.[2] It is therefore critical to replace intravascular volume deficits to reverse shock early and rapidly.

The major elements responsible for the initial compensation following gastrointestinal hemorrhage are outlined in Figure 20–1. Reduction in mean arterial pressure results in reflex selective vasoconstriction of skeletal, splanchnic, and cutaneous vascular beds, resulting in a redistribution of the reduced cardiac output to the heart and brain. Circulation to the renal vascular bed maintained early in hypovolemic shock due to renal vascular autoregulation is decreased in continued severe shock, resulting in renal-cortical necrosis or acute tubular necrosis. Release of antidiuretic hormone (vasopressin) and stimulation of the renin-angiotensin-aldosterone system increase retention of water and sodium, and alterations in Starling forces lead to "auto-transfusion" from the interstitial fluids to the intravascular fluids. Despite these initial compensatory responses, ongoing uncorrected shock leads to tissue ischemia. Hypotension, mental dysfunction, anuria, and respiratory and cardiac failure occur.

Assessing Clinical Status

The most important determination in evaluating a patient with gastrointestinal hemorrhage is whether hypovolemic shock is present or likely to occur.[7a] Several aspects of the physical exam are crucial in this evalua-

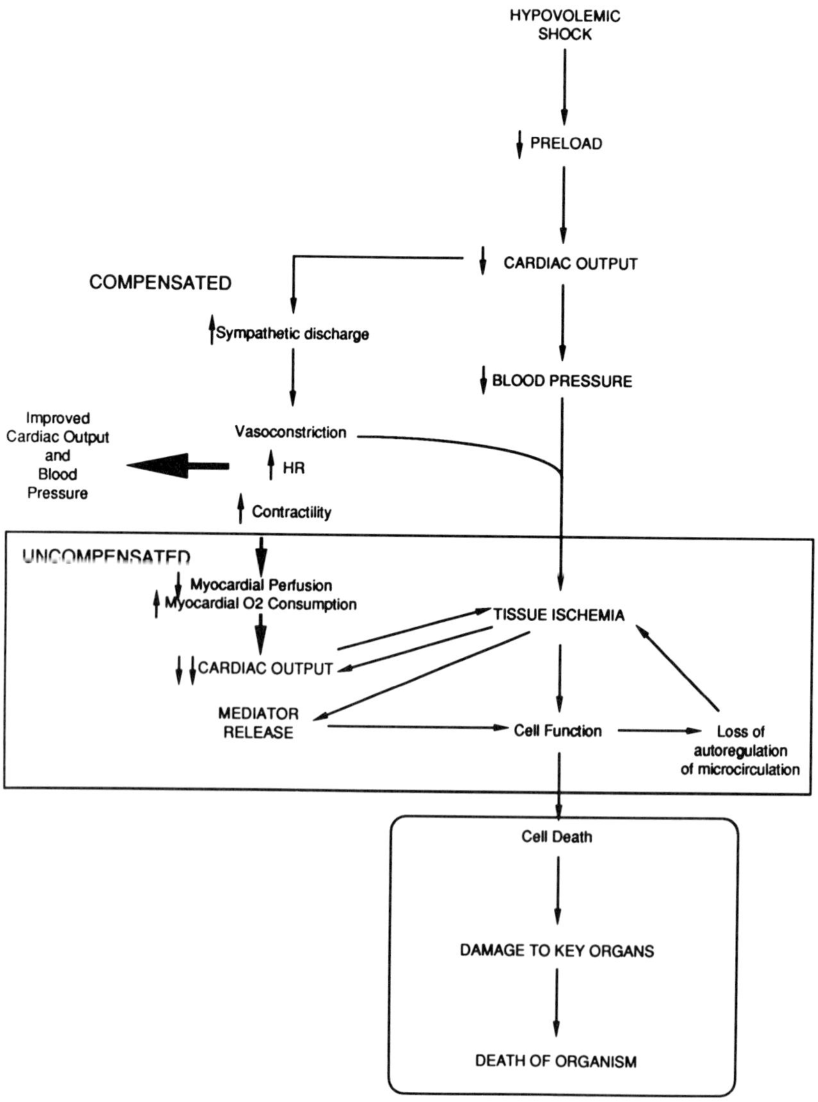

Figure 20–1. Major physiologic events following significant gastrointestinal hemorrhage.

tion. Vital signs, an essential part of this evaluation, should include the pulse rate and the blood pressure lying, sitting, and, if possible, standing. An increase in the pulse rate of more than 20 beats per minute when going from a lying to a sitting position, or a decrease in diastolic blood pressure of more than 10 mm Hg when going from a lying to a sitting position, indicates a greater than 20% loss of intravascular volume. Tachycardia, when present, suggests a significant decrease in intravascular volume. Adult patients with a 10 to 15% loss of intravascular volume have a 10 to 20% elevation in pulse rate. As blood loss increases to 20 to 25%, the pulse rate increases to more than 150 beats per minute. When the intravascular volume deficit exceeds 25%, the capillary refill is prolonged as blood is shunted from the skin to the brain and kidneys. Capillary refill can be examined by applying firm pressure over soft tissues or nail beds for five seconds and then quickly releasing the pressure. If the blanched area takes more than five seconds to regain its color, there is poor peripheral perfusion.

Progressive shock may further restrict blood flow, eventually resulting in a decrease in body surface temperature. Blood stasis secondary to peripheral vasoconstriction leads to cyanosis. As the volume deficit increases, hypovolemic shock worsens, and as the intravascular deficit exceeds 30%, the body continues to compensate by decreasing urine output. Urine output and fluid intake must be carefully monitored throughout fluid resuscitation of patients in shock. Urine output in children is normally 2 to 3 ml per kg per hour, and urine output less than 1 ml per kg per hour is indicative of renal hypoperfusion. As blood loss exceeds 40%, compensation fails, pulses are lost, cerebral perfusion decreases, and the patient passes from lethargy to coma. The respiratory rate should also be carefully monitored. Hyperventilation is an early sign of a developing acidosis induced by a decrease in central nervous system (CNS) pH. Volume overload and congestive heart failure must also be considered in a patient with hyperventilation following fluid resuscitation. An arterial blood gas can be used to confirm acidosis in a tachypneic child, which reflects decreased tissue perfusion.[8] Persistent acidosis in the face of a normal pulse or blood pressure may indicate the need to restore tissue perfusion by expanding the intravascular volume. Ultimately, as shock worsens, CNS hypoperfusion results in progressive deterioration in mentation, a late and grave prognostic sign.

An estimate of the quantity of blood lost should be attempted in all patients, but since historical estimates of blood loss can be very unreliable, the physical signs and symptoms listed above should be given priority. A hematocrit and hemoglobin should be obtained on all patients initially and repeatedly during active bleeding. However, an initial normal result should not be falsely reassuring, since in a rapid gastrointestinal hemorrhage, the patient's hematocrit and hemoglobin can remain normal for several hours following the gastrointestinal hemorrhage, until the intravascular volume deficit is replenished by equilibration with other body fluids.

Physical examination by an experienced observer to evaluate capillary perfusion, skin color for the presence of cyanosis, pulse, blood pressure, respiratory pattern, and level of consciousness should continue on an ongoing basis throughout the hemorrhage to enable rapid recognition of recurring shock. To enhance the ability to anticipate shock, it is helpful if the rate of bleeding is assessed periodically. In upper gastrointestinal bleeding this is best accomplished through lavage of the stomach by means of a nasogastric tube placed in the stomach. The amount of blood lost in the stool should also be monitored, estimated, and recorded, and any change in color from melena to bright red blood should be noted as a possible sign of increased blood loss and hypovolemic shock. It is prudent that all patients with significant gastrointestinal bleeding be monitored in a pediatric intensive care unit for changes in vital signs and urine output until they are stable and bleeding has ceased.

Table 20–2. TREATMENT GOALS IN PATIENTS WITH GASTROINTESTINAL BLEEDING AND SHOCK

Establish and maintain the intravascular volume.
Re-establish a normal oxygen-carrying capacity by transfusion with packed red blood cells.
Determine source and site of blood loss.
Stop gastrointestinal bleeding.

Treating Hypovolemic Shock from Gastrointestinal Hemorrhage

Treatment goals for the management of hypovolemic shock following gastrointestinal hemorrhage are listed in Table 20–2. The primary deficit, a decrease in intravascular volume, must be replenished as rapidly as possible (Table 20–3). A large-bore intravenous (IV) catheter should be placed immediately upon recognition of an intravascular deficit to provide adequate vascular access. Delay will make the placement of an IV catheter more difficult, because as the patient progresses further

Table 20–3. TREATMENT OF PATIENTS WITH HYPOVOLEMIC SHOCK SECONDARY TO GASTROINTESTINAL HEMORRHAGE

Establish adequate intravenous access by placing intravenous catheters: for mild shock, one intravenous catheter; for moderate or severe shock, two intravenous catheters. Recommended catheter size: Infant: 20 gauge Child: 18 gauge Adolescent: 16 gauge
Rapidly infuse saline, lactated Ringer's, or Plasmanate (10 ml/kg/10 min until vital signs normalized).
Carefully monitor pulse, blood pressure, central venous pressure, CVP to avoid fluid overload.
Monitor urine output and skin perfusion and orthostatic changes in pulse and blood pressure for early recognition of shock.
Transfuse with packed red blood cells to return oxygen-carrying capacity to normal.
Carefully record all fluids transfused and estimate and record all recognized fluids lost.

into shock, venous distension decreases. Patients with severe hypovolemic shock (a deficit of greater than 20% of the intravascular volume) should have two IVs placed. The catheter size recommended for each age is outlined in Table 20–3. Flow through the IV catheter is inversely proportional to the *fourth* power of the diameter, and it has been shown that the flow through a single 16-gauge catheter is equivalent to the combined flow through four 20-gauge catheters.[9] In patients with severe hypovolemic shock, placement of a central venous line may be a life-saving maneuver. The central venous line not only provides immediate, secure intravenous access via a large-diameter catheter but also is helpful in monitoring the changes in intravascular volume during resuscitation. Central venous pressure should range from 4 to 10 in adults and from 3 to 8 in children.[10] When IV access is not possible, an intraosseous line may be required to rapidly expand intravascular volume.

After IV access has been established, an initial bolus of 10 to 20 ml per kg of normal saline or lactated Ringer's saline should be infused rapidly over 10 minutes. The fluid bolus should be repeated as required until (1) a normal renal output is established, (2) orthostatic changes in pulse and blood pressure are abolished, and (3) cutaneous perfusion is normalized.

The choice between crystalloid or colloid solutions to replace the intravascular deficit in patients with hypovolemic shock may be difficult (Table 20–4). The advantage of crystalloid solutions such as normal saline and lactated Ringer's is that they are readily available; colloids such as Albumisol or Plasmanate are less readily available, but because of the increased oncotic pressure produced by the albumin component, they may be more effective in replacing and expanding the intravascular volume deficit.[11] Since overexpansion of the vascular space during fluid resuscitation is common, a record of all fluids administered and a sequential record of pulse, blood pressure, and orthostatic changes should be reviewed carefully throughout the resuscitation.

The second goal in patients with hypovolemic shock is to increase the oxygen-carrying capacity of the intravascular fluid. This requires transfusion of either packed red blood cells or whole blood. The decision to transfuse varies with the age of the patient, the presence of cardiovascular disease, and the presence of continued bleeding. In general, the hematocrit should be maintained above 30% in patients with cardiac disease and above 25% in healthy children until active bleeding has ceased. Blood should be warmed whenever massive transfusions are required.[12] Calcium supplementation may also be required following massive transfusions to counter the effect of calcium-binding agents.

Table 20–4. INTRAVENOUS FLUIDS FOR VOLUME RESUSCITATION

Crystalloids
0.9% sodium chloride
Lactated Ringer's solution
Colloids
5% human serum albumin in 0.9% sodium chloride
25% human serum albumin in 0.9% sodium chloride
Blood Products
Whole blood
Packed red blood cells
Fresh frozen plasma

Modified from Blumer JL: A Practical Guide to Pediatric Intensive Care. 3rd ed. St. Louis, Mosby Year Book, 1990, p 73; with permission.

Table 20–5. EVALUATION OF PATIENTS WITH GASTROINTESTINAL BLEEDING

History
History of past bleeding
Quality and quantity of blood loss
Physical Examination
Pulse, blood pressure lying and sitting
Examine for ascites
Examine for hepatosplenomegaly
Examine for caput medusa
Laboratory
Type and cross match
CBC, platelet count, and reticulocyte count
PT and PTT
ALT, AST, BUN
Guaiac or hematest suspected blood

CBC, complete blood count; PT, prothrombin time; PTT, partial thromboplastin time; ALT, alanine aminotransferase; AST, aspartate aminotransferase; BUN, blood urea nitrogen.

Calculating Transfusion Requirements

The amount of blood required to raise the hemoglobin a desired amount can be calculated by estimating the blood volume at 70 ml per kg. This quantity of packed red blood cells (ml) can be simplified as follows:

[(70 ml/kg × weight in kg) (desired hemoglobin − present hemoglobin)]/23 gm hemoglobin per 100 dl of packed red blood cells

This formula fails, however, to account for any decrease in the blood volume itself and will therefore underestimate blood requirements in a patient who has bled rapidly and has not had time to re-expand intravascular volume. A rough guideline applicable in most infants and children is that administration of 5 ml of packed red blood cells per kg will raise the hematocrit three points and the hemoglobin 1 gm per dl; the 5:3:1 ratio makes the rule easy to remember.

DIAGNOSING THE SITE OF GASTROINTESTINAL BLEEDING

Identifying the source of the gastrointestinal bleeding must wait until the patient has had cardiovascular stabilization. Hypovolemic shock should be reversed and oxygen-carrying capacity replaced as outlined above before addressing this question. The initial history obtained during resuscitation should include a family history for cardiovascular abnormalities and a history of ingesting any drugs (particularly salicylates or steroids), caustic materials, or foreign bodies (Table 20–5).[13] The character and quantity of bleeding should be evaluated, and the presence of abdominal pain or intestinal obstruction should be examined. The presence of diarrhea or a past history of abdominal pain in the patient or other family members should also be examined. In addition to evaluating orthostatic changes, the initial physical examination should determine the presence of hepatosplenomegaly, ascites, and abdominal masses. A rectal examination can evaluate polyps and anorectal lesions, determine stool color, and provide a stool sample to test for the presence of blood. The skin should be carefully examined for vascular abnormalities or the presence of a caput medusa over the abdomen.

Verifying Gastrointestinal Bleeding

Patients with epistaxis or oropharyngeal bleeding often report vomiting bright red blood. It is therefore essential that bleeding from a nasal or oropharyngeal site be considered and eliminated as a potential source of vomited blood. Red food coloring from candy, drinks, or medications frequently mimics gastrointestinal bleeding (Table 20–6). All blood or bloodlike material vomited or passed from the rectum should be tested for occult blood with either a hematest or a guaiac card to distinguish blood from cherry or strawberry candies, medications, juices, or Popsicles. The use of definitive testing for blood will avoid unnecessary concern and unnecessary and inappropriate diagnostic examinations. When occult testing of gastric aspirate is required it is important not to rely on standard stool tests, since they may be falsely negative in acidic solutions.[14] Melena can also be mimicked by several compounds, including iron medications and bismuth-containing compounds (Pepto-Bismol).

Testing for Blood

Many tests are commercially available to detect blood in the stool, but all can be grouped into four basic techniques. The most widely used test is based on the conversion of leukodyes, such as guaiac, from a colorless to a colored compound by the peroxidative effect of hemoglobin. The tests based on guaiac or other leukodyes include Hemoccult, HemoFec, Coloscreen, Colo-Rect, Hema-Check, Quick-Cult, Haemo-screen, Early Detection, and Seracult. The threshold for a positive test can vary greatly with test conditions (1 to 80 mg hemoglobin per gm stool).[15–19] Recent ingestion of red meat, plant peroxidases, or large quantities of iron preparations can lead to false-positive tests. Ascorbic acid in large quantities can create false negatives, so patients should not take vitamin C tablets prior to being screened for blood in the stool using any of these tests. The gastroccult, also based on the leukodye reaction but more reliable in an acid environment, should be used in preference to the hemoccult[20] when examining gastric contents for blood.

The second test, HemoQuant, is a recently introduced quantitative, noninvasive test that is specific for heme.[21] HemoQuant is a fluorometric assay utilizing antibodies specific for heme and heme-derived porphyrin. Since both heme and its primary breakdown product are detected,[22] the HemoQuant is less affected by degradations during storage or during passage through the gastrointestinal tract.[23] Although HemoQuant may be affected by red meat, it is not affected by dietary peroxidases and medications.

The third test uses antihemoglobin antibodies (e.g., Heme/detect and FECA-EIA). Though this test is highly specific and requires no dietary restrictions, digestion of globin during intestinal transit and storage decreases its sensitivity, especially to upper gastrointestinal blood loss.

The last approach to detecting gastrointestinal blood loss uses the injection of ^{51}Cr-labeled erythrocytes while monitoring the stool for ^{51}Cr. This approach is rarely used because it requires 3 days to perform, is expensive, and is not readily available.

Table 20–6. MIMICKERS OF GASTROINTESTINAL BLEEDING

Bleeding from the nose and oropharynx
Bright red blood may be mimicked by red colored candies, juices, and foods
Black colored stools may be caused by:
Bismuth (Pepto-Bismol)
Iron preparations
Spinach
Blueberries
Licorice

Distinguishing Between Upper and Lower Gastrointestinal Bleeding

Hematemesis is highly suggestive of upper gastrointestinal bleeding. Upper gastrointestinal bleeding is most commonly associated with melena, but when rapid upper gastrointestinal bleeding occurs, a patient can present with bright red blood from the rectum. The presence of borborygmi in these patients may help suggest an upper gastrointestinal source for the bleeding. Hematochezia suggests bleeding from a colonic lesion. As stated earlier, in rare patients, melena can occur with a bleeding site in the right side of the colon when the colonic transit time is prolonged, as in severe constipation. Elevation of the blood urea nitrogen (BUN) out of proportion to creatinine suggests that the bleeding site is in the upper gastrointestinal tract.[24, 25, 25a]

Nasogastric Tube Placement

Placement of a nasogastric tube can be helpful in distinguishing between upper and lower gastrointestinal bleeding in patients presenting with melena or hematochezia. Aspiration of visible blood from the stomach strongly suggests that the bleeding site is located proximal to the ligament of Treitz.[1, 26] Hematest, or hemoccult-positive material from a nasogastric tube aspirate, may be seen following placement of the tube. Presence of small amounts of bright red blood-tinged material immediately following tube placement may be difficult to interpret, but if bleeding clears rapidly and does not recur, it is likely due to trauma from tube placement. Absence of blood on gastric aspiration or lavage indicates that no active hemorrhage is occurring from the esophagus or stomach at the time of aspiration. Active bleeding from a duodenal lesion, though usually associated with reflux of blood into the stomach and a positive gastric aspirate, need not result in blood on aspiration of gastric contents.

In one study, the use of a nasogastric tube aspirate to distinguish between upper and lower gastrointestinal bleeding in adults presenting with gastrointestinal hemorrhage resulted in the correct identification of upper gastrointestinal bleeding more than 90% of the time. The absence of blood on gastric aspirate correlated with an identifiable lower gastrointestinal bleeding source in 50% of the patients and no identified source of bleeding in the remaining 50%.[26] The presence of esophageal varices is not a contraindication to placement of a nasogastric tube.

If the nasogastric tube aspirate shows no sign of upper gastrointestinal bleeding, the tube is generally removed. If there is evidence of gastrointestinal bleeding, the tube may be left in place to monitor ongoing bleeding.

IDENTIFYING THE SOURCE OF GASTROINTESTINAL HEMORRHAGE

Diagnostic Maneuvers

Esophagogastroduodenoscopy

Over the past 20 years, advances in fiber-optic technology and the increased number of pediatric gastroenterologists and pediatric surgeons trained in endoscopic techniques have greatly improved our ability to identify both the location and cause of gastrointestinal bleeding[27, 28, 28a] (see Chapter 74). Before the introduction of fiber-optic endoscopy, diagnostic interventions for upper gastrointestinal bleeding were limited to radiographic findings on upper GI series, and the cause of the bleeding was identified in less than 50% of patients. Since the introduction of esophagogastroduodenoscopy, both the location and the cause of upper gastrointestinal bleeding can be identified in 85 to 90% of patients.[27, 28]

Before an esophagogastroduodenoscopy is performed, the stomach should be cleared of blood and blood clots via nasogastric lavage with iced saline through a nasogastric tube.[28a] A large-bore nasogastric tube should be used with multiple ports, such as a Salem sump tube, to enhance the clearing of clots from the stomach. Care must be taken to prevent hypothermia in infants and small children.

Endoscopy may also provide important prognostic information regarding the likelihood of continued bleeding.[29] Identification of a visible vessel in the base of a bleeding ulcer (as illustrated in Figure 20–2*E*), or of an esophageal tear, has been reported to have a high association with persistent bleeding or rebleeding episodes, indicating a greater chance that the patient will require surgical intervention.[30–32] Approximately one half of patients with proven esophageal varices can be shown endoscopically to be bleeding from another source—most commonly erosive gastritis, duodenal ulcer, or gastric ulcer.[12] Endoscopy is therefore indicated in all patients with significant upper gastrointestinal bleeding. The diagnostic accuracy of esophagogastroduodenoscopy remains high for the first 12 to 24 hours after a bleeding episode.[9, 28, 33, 34] Endoscopy also provides access to the bleeding site for direct intervention.[35] Although upper gastrointestinal bleeding stops spontaneously in more than 90% of patients, establishing a definitive diagnosis will direct appropriate therapy.

The complication rate reported for emergency endoscopy is fourfold greater than that during elective endoscopy.[36] In most instances, endoscopy can and should be delayed until the patient's clinical status has stabilized. Patients undergoing endoscopy should have a normal intravascular volume and a hematocrit greater than 20 to 25% if possible. Fluid and blood infusions should be completed to correct deficits.

Ingestion of barium for an upper gastrointestinal series will preclude endoscopy for 12 to 24 hours, but endoscopy does not prevent a follow-up upper gastrointestinal series. We advocate that patients presenting with upper gastrointestinal bleeding undergo esophagogastroduodenoscopy as the primary diagnostic maneuver.[37, 38]

Colonoscopy

In colonic or lower gastrointestinal bleeding, a colonoscopy can identify the source of bleeding with more accuracy and specificity than a barium enema.[39, 40–44] In chronic colonic bleeding, the cause of the bleeding can be identified by colonoscopy in approximately 40% of patients.[45, 46] Common bleeding sources include juvenile polyps and inflammatory bowel disease.[46] Colonoscopy is more effective in identifying the presence and number of polyps in the colon than a barium enema and provides direct access for polypectomy. Colonoscopy also allows access for direct coagulation of bleeding lesions using electrocoagulation, thermocoagulation, or laser therapy. The ability to directly visualize the mucosal surface, directly remove or treat bleeding lesions, and obtain biopsies to confirm the presence of inflammation has established colonoscopy as the primary diagnostic procedure in lower gastrointestinal bleeding. During active colonic bleeding, the presence of blood throughout the colon may obscure the site of bleeding. If possible, the colon should be emptied of blood by the use of polyethylene glycol via mouth or nasogastric tube prior to colonoscopy[47] (see Chapter 74).

Meckel's Scan

Because technetium (Tc) 99m pertechnetate is actively accumulated by cells in gastric mucosa, it can be used to identify the presence of ectopic gastric mucosa in a

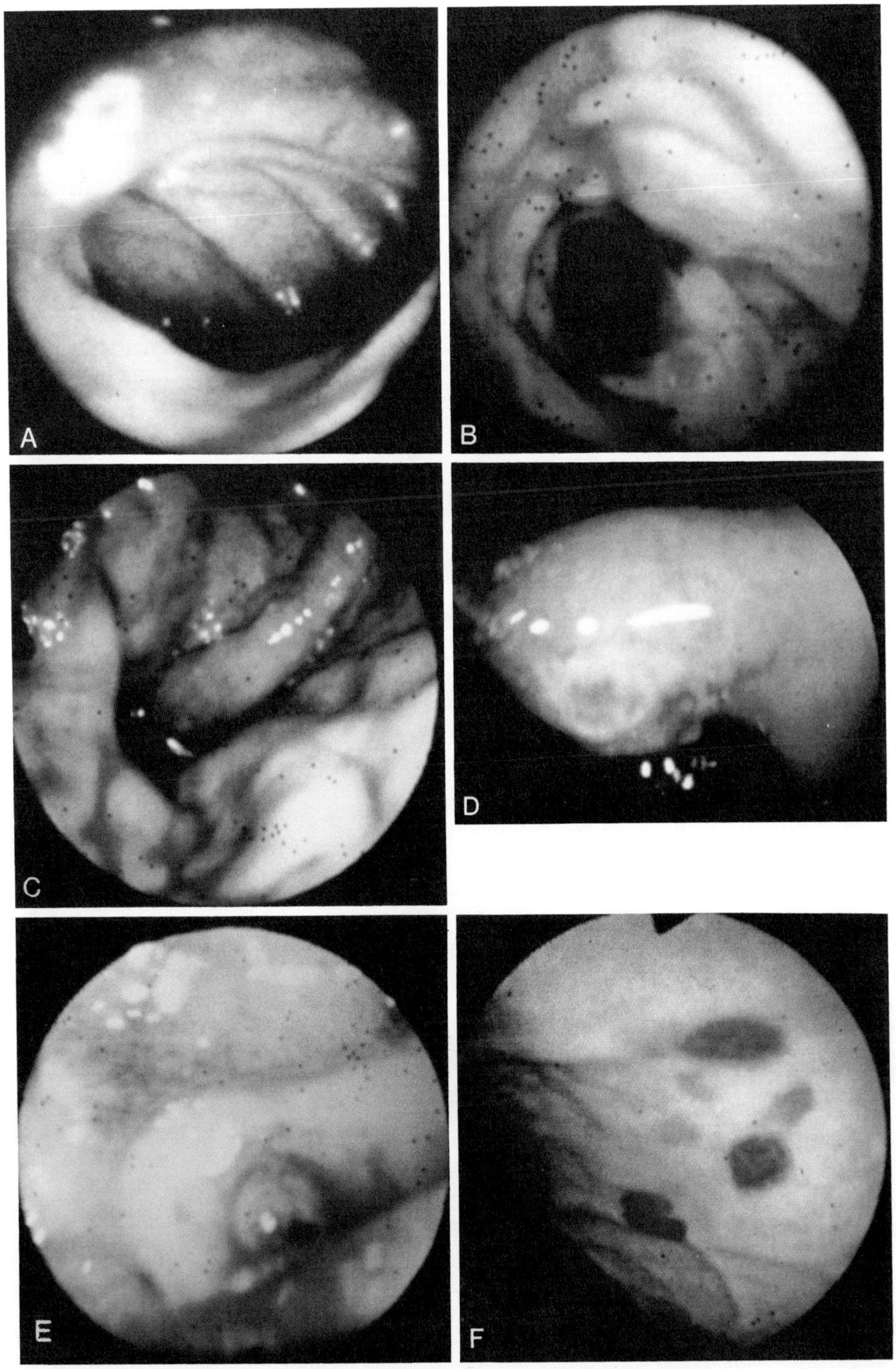

Figure 20–2. Common causes of upper gastrointestinal bleeding. *A,* duodenal ulcer. The margin of the base is sharp with an erythematous rim confined to a 1-cm zone around the ulcer base. *B,* severe acid reflux esophagitis. Lower portion of esophagus proximal to gastroesophageal junction covered with whitish exudate and hemorrhagic mucosa. *C,* bleeding esophageal varices. Note the multiple interconnecting raised undulating mucosal columns. *D,* gastric ulcer overlying a gastric leiomyoma. Note the erosive gastric ulcer where the gastric mucosa passes over the smooth submucosal mass. Leiomyoma confirmed at surgery for recurrent gastric ulcers. *E,* duodenal ulcer with a visible vessel. Note the distinct margin of the duodenal ulcer with the prominent red point indicating the visible vessel. *F,* hereditary hemangioma. Multiple prominent red lesions indicate the multiple hereditary hemangiomas. (Fig. 20–2 *A, C, E,* and *F* courtesy of Dr. Tim Nostrand, University of Michigan.)

Meckel's diverticulum or intestinal duplications.[48–52] Though the Meckel's diverticulum is the most frequent congenital anomaly of the intestinal tract, with an incidence of 0.3 to 3.0%,[53] the majority of Meckel's diverticula do not contain gastric mucosa. However, more than 90% of *bleeding* Meckel's diverticula do contain gastric mucosa. The sensitivity of a Meckel's scan can be enhanced by administration of pentagastrin.[54] Cimetidine can improve the diagnostic accuracy of the Meckel's scan by preventing secretion of the pertechnetate dye.[51] A Meckel's scan requires only 1 hour for completion, and the short half-life of this isotope allows a tagged red blood cell scan to be done within 24 to 48 hours of its completion. A Meckel's scan should be considered whenever significant lower gastrointestinal bleeding has occurred (see Chapter 50).

Bleeding Scans

Nuclear medicine studies involving a peripheral intravenous injection of technetium sulfur colloid can detect the site of bleeding when the rate of bleeding is as low as 0.1 ml per minute.[55–60] The study is noninvasive and has a low radiation exposure. The short half-life of this isotope combined with the rapid elimination of the sulfur colloid by uptake into the reticuloendothelial system limits the reliability of this imaging technique during acute bleeding. The half-time for clearance of the technetium sulfur colloid from the blood is about 2 minutes.

Although ^{99m}Tc-pertechnetate–labeled red blood cell scan requires more preparation than the sulfur colloid scan, it provides a sensitive and accurate localization of the site of active gastrointestinal bleeding.[61–63] The longer half-life of the labeled red blood cells enables the imaging of the gastrointestinal system to continue for up to 24 hours. These scans have been estimated to be slightly less sensitive than those using ^{99m}Tc-sulfur colloid, with the ability to visualize the site of bleeding when the bleeding rate is 0.5 ml per minute or higher.[64, 65] This is comparable to the bleeding rate of 0.5 ml per minute required for detecting the site of bleeding by angiography. Catheter placement, injection of contrast media, and exposure to ionizing radiation required for radiographic angiography are all avoided. Radiation exposure with ^{99m}Tc-pertechnetate–labeled red blood cells is 0.2 rad (less than that of an upper gastrointestinal series).

The ^{99m}Tc-pertechnetate–labeled blood cell scan requires that a sample of the patient's own red cells be drawn, labeled with ^{99m}Tc-pertechnetate, and reinjected into the blood stream. The ^{99m}Tc-pertechnetate–labeled blood cell scan should be considered when a small intestinal source of bleeding is suspected or when no source can be detected by endoscopy.[59, 66] Arteriovenous malformations can be detected using this technique.[67, 68] In most institutions, the ^{99m}Tc-pertechnetate–labeled red blood cell scan is used to direct subsequent localized angiography. The nuclear scan can be readily repeated in patients with intermittent bleeding.

Angiography

The usefulness of angiography as a diagnostic test is usually limited to patients with *active* gastrointestinal bleeding. It has been estimated that in order for angiography to detect the source of bleeding, the rate of bleeding must be at least 0.5 ml per minute.[69] The introduction of bleeding scans using pertechnetate, with its greater sensitivity and lower risk, has decreased angiography's role as a primary test in gastrointestinal bleeding.[57] Sedation or anesthesia is required for angiography. A catheter is introduced via the femoral artery and located in the arteries feeding the mesenteric system. Injection of contrast material can identify extravasation of the dye into the gastrointestinal tract or a characteristic blush that indicates early filling of a vascular lesion or an arteriovenous malformation.[70] When used in the appropriate situation, angiography has an accuracy of 50 to 75% but is associated with a significant complication rate of approximately 2%.[71]

Angiography's advantage is that the catheter can be left in position for therapeutic maneuvers, including infusion of vasopressin or direct embolization of vascular malformations.[72–75] Angiography is effective in identifying the source of bleeding in 40 to 86% of patients with lower gastrointestinal bleeding.[76–78] Though many patients will rebleed following cessation of vasopressin infusion, the control of bleeding enables patient stabilization and the conversion of emergency surgery to elective surgery, with a decrease in mortality from 40 to 10%.[79]

Upper Gastrointestinal Radiography

Contrast studies of the upper gastrointestinal tract have taken a secondary role in the evaluation of patients since the introduction of endoscopy.[33, 80, 81] Radiographic studies are particularly useful in defining anatomic deficits such as esophageal strictures, malrotation of the bowel, or deep ulcerations. Upper gastrointestinal radiography can outline the entire upper gastrointestinal tract from the esophagus down to the ileocecal valve. Mucosal detail can be enhanced by enteroclysis and the use of air contrast. Radiography gives important information concerning gastrointestinal tract function and can detect gastroesophageal reflux and gastrointestinal motility disorders (see Chapter 78).

Barium Enema

Barium enema is effective in identifying the anatomic location of the large bowel and is particularly important in neonates and infants presenting with signs of obstruction associated with gastrointestinal bleeding. In these patients, malrotation with secondary intestinal volvulus must be rapidly identified. Intussusception, a common problem in infants particularly between the ages of 6 months and 24 months, can be diagnosed and, in many cases, treated by barium enema. The barium enema is also effective in identifying the presence of polyps[81, 81a] (see Chapter 78).

DIFFERENTIAL DIAGNOSIS OF GASTROINTESTINAL BLEEDING

Upper Gastrointestinal Bleeding

The common causes of upper gastrointestinal bleeding in neonates, infants, toddlers, children, and adolescents are indicated in Table 20–7. Peptic ulcer disease is the most common cause of upper gastrointestinal bleeding in patients ranging in age from newborns to adolescents.[82] In newborns, hemorrhagic gastritis is the most common cause of peptic ulcer disease, with gastric lesions predominant over duodenal lesions. Esophagitis secondary to gastroesophageal reflux becomes an important cause of upper gastrointestinal bleeding in older infants. Severe erosive esophagitis (as illustrated in Fig. 20–2*B*) is a common cause of bleeding in patients with severe developmental delay and mental retardation. In adolescents, a duodenal ulcer (as illustrated in Fig. 20–2*A*) becomes the most common manifestation of peptic ulcer disease. The incidence of variceal bleeding peaks between the ages of 3 and 5 years, as children with neonatal liver disease (e.g., biliary atresia) or children with portal vein thrombosis commonly become symptomatic at this time.

Lower Gastrointestinal Bleeding

The causes of lower gastrointestinal bleeding as a function of age are listed in Table 20–8. Bright red blood from the rectum limited to the outside of stools suggests a rectal or anal site of bleeding, such as a rectal fissure.[82] This is the most common cause of rectal bleeding in infants. Hemorrhoidal bleeding is rarely seen in adolescents. Bright red blood mixed through the stool suggests a colonic source for the bleeding located higher than the rectum. Colitis in infants is most commonly due to infections or to an allergic reaction to milk and soy protein.[83–86] It has been reported that milk protein can be transferred in adequate quantities in the milk of breast-feeding mothers to induce colitis. Significant gastrointestinal bleeding suggests the presence of a Meckel's diverticulum (as illustrated in Fig. 20–3*A*).[87]

Polyps are uncommon in infants less than 1 year of age, but the incidence of polyps climbs rapidly in toddlers and children and peaks between 5 and 7 years of age (as illustrated in Fig. 20–3*D*). There is a progressive decrease in the incidence of polyps in older children and teenagers and an increasing incidence of inflammatory bowel disease in teenagers and young adults. Inflammatory bowel disease replaces polyps as the most common cause of lower gastrointestinal bleeding in teenagers.

Table 20–7. UPPER GASTROINTESTINAL BLEEDING

Age Group	Common	Less Common
Neonates (0–30 days)	Swallowed maternal blood Gastritis Duodenitis	Coagulopathy Vascular malformations Gastric/esophageal duplication Leiomyoma
Infants (30 days–1 year)	Gastritis and gastric ulcer Esophagitis Duodenitis	Esophageal varices Foreign body Aortoesophageal fistula
Children (1–12 years)	Esophagitis Esophageal varices Gastritis and gastric ulcer Duodenal ulcer Mallory-Weiss tear Nasopharyngeal bleeding	Leiomyoma Salicylates Vascular malformation Hematobilia
Adolescents (12 years–adult)	Duodenal ulcer Esophagitis Esophageal varices Gastritis Mallory-Weiss tear	Thrombocytopenia Dieulafoy's ulcer Hematobilia

Table 20–8. LOWER GASTROINTESTINAL BLEEDING

Age Group	Common	Less Common
Neonates (0–30 days)	Anorectal lesions Swallowed maternal blood Milk allergy Necrotizing enterocolitis Midgut volvulus	Vascular malformations Hirschsprung's enterocolitis Intestinal duplication Coagulopathy
Infants (30 days–1 year)	Anorectal lesions Midgut volvulus Intussusception (<3 yrs) Meckel's diverticulum Infectious diarrhea Milk allergy (<4 yrs)	Vascular malformations Intestinal duplication Acquired thrombocytopenia
Children (1–12 years)	Juvenile polyps Meckel's diverticulum Intussusception (<3 yrs) Infectious diarrhea Anal fissure Nodular lymphoid hyperplasia	Henoch-Schönlein purpura Hemolytic-uremic syndrome Vasculitis (SLE) Inflammatory bowel disease
Adolescents (12 years–adult)	Inflammatory bowel disease Polyps Hemorrhoids Anal fissure Infectious diarrhea	Arteriovascular malformation Adenocarcinomas Henoch-Schönlein purpura Pseudomembranous colitis

Gastrointestinal Bleeding in Newborns

Hematemesis during the first few days of life may result from the fetus swallowing maternal blood during

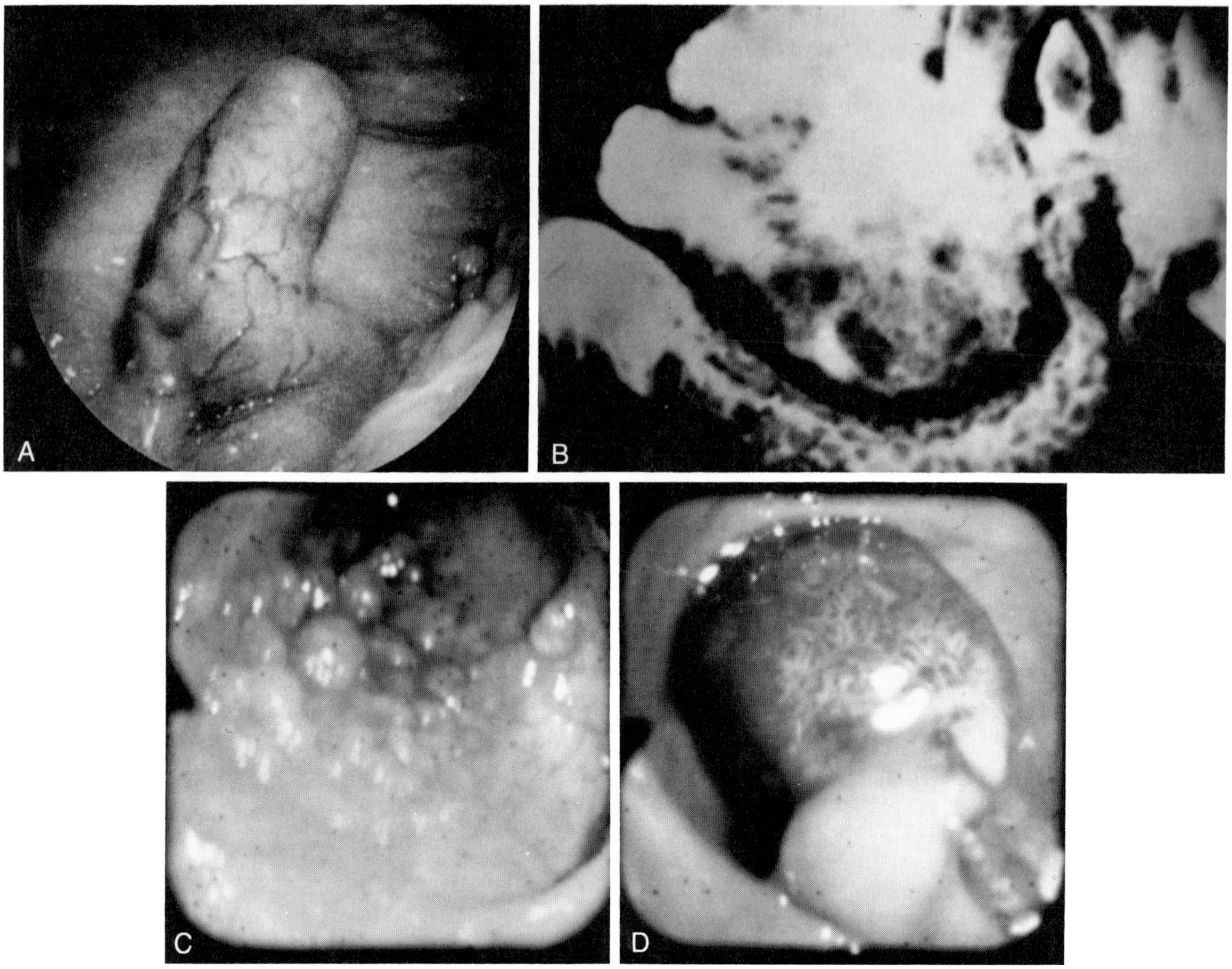

Figure 20–3. Common causes of lower gastrointestinal bleeding. *A,* Meckel's diverticulum at surgery. Prominent outpouching from the ileum prior to surgical removal of the Meckel's diverticulum. *B,* lymphonodular hyperplasia. Barium enema shows multiple small filling defects of the terminal ileum. *C,* lymphonodular hyperplasia on colonoscopy. Direct visualization shows multiple small polypoid lesions secondary to lymphocytic infiltration of mucosal surface. *D,* juvenile polyp, colonoscopy appearance. A 20-cm diameter polypoid mass with a nodular surface and a prominent stalk, consistent with juvenile polyp. (Fig. 20–3*B, C,* and *D* courtesy of Dr. Tim Nostrand, University of Michigan.)

delivery [88, 89] This possibility can be excluded rapidly by the performance of the Apt test,[90] in which blood from the stomach is placed on filter paper and mixed with 1% sodium hydroxide. Maternal adult hemoglobin will be reduced from a rusty brown to a yellow color. Fetal hemoglobin is resistant to reduction and will retain a pink or bright red color. Absence of fetal hemoglobin should eliminate concern about acute gastrointestinal hemorrhage. This test should be limited to bright red blood and cannot be applied to denatured blood found in melena or coffee-ground material. In breast-fed neonates or young infants, a cracked nipple may be the cause of blood in the vomitus or guaiac-positive stools. An Apt test can be used on fresh blood to confirm this suspicion, and a careful examination of the mother's breasts may reveal the bleeding site.

Twenty percent of neonates presenting with hematemesis have an underlying bleeding disorder.[91] The administration of parenteral vitamin K at birth has virtually eliminated hemorrhagic disease of the newborn. However, a history of nonhospital delivery should raise the possibility of this disorder and calls for prompt administration of vitamin K. Recent reports compiled following the introduction of endoscopy in infants have shown a significant incidence of gastritis, gastric erosions, and peptic ulcers in newborns.[92]

Anal fissure is the most common cause for rectal bleeding and can most commonly be identified on external examination. The presence of excoriation of the perineum and buttocks can lead to guaiac-positive stools.

Necrotizing enterocolitis (NEC) can present as hematest-positive stools but is commonly associated with both abdominal distention and bilious vomiting.[93, 94] Though most commonly found in premature patients (90%), full-term babies may also develop this disorder. Though rarely presenting as gross hemorrhage, NEC must be considered in all newborns with guaiac-positive stools. Since NEC in full-term infants is commonly associated with congenital heart disease, gastrointestinal bleeding in patients with heart disease should raise this possibility[95] (see Chapter 61).

Malrotation with intestinal volvulus is a surgical emergency that may present in the newborn period,[94, 94a] with bleeding from ischemic bowel. The presence of obstruction, suggested by vomiting and abdominal distention, should alert the observer to this diagnostic possibility.

Gastrointestinal Bleeding in Infants

Upper gastrointestinal bleeding in infants is most commonly due to gastritis, esophagitis, or peptic ulcer disease.[96] On rare occasions patients with rapidly developing portal hypertension can present during the first 2 months of life.

Lower gastrointestinal bleeding in infants is most commonly caused by anorectal fissures. Intussusception must be considered, particularly when the infant has signs of intestinal obstruction. Intussusception is most common between 6 and 24 months of life and must be considered in any patient having bright red blood from the rectum and vomiting.[94] Mucus in the stool gives it the classic "currant jelly" appearance (see Chapter 47).

A congenital malformation may present as a bleeding episode at any age, but it most commonly occurs in infants and toddlers. Meckel's diverticulum, vascular lesions, or an intestinal duplication fall under this category.[87, 97, 97a] A Meckel's diverticulum must always be considered, particularly when the bleeding is rapid and massive with a drop in hematocrit of greater than 10 points (see Chapter 50).

Infants commonly develop infectious colitis. *Salmonella, Shigella, Campylobacter, Escherichia coli,*[98–101] *Yersinia,* and *Clostridium difficile* may all cause hematochezia.

Milk or soy intolerance may present with chronic gastrointestinal tract blood loss arising from any portion of the gastrointestinal tract, including the stomach, duodenum, lower gut, and colon.[83–86]

Gastrointestinal Bleeding in Children

Upper gastrointestinal bleeding in children is most commonly due to peptic disorders including esophagitis (as illustrated in Fig. 20–2*B*), gastritis, gastric ulcer, duodenitis, and duodenal ulcer. Patients with a history of liver disease, particularly biliary atresia,[102] or umbilical venous catheterization have an increased risk of portal hypertension and of variceal bleeding. Rare causes of severe upper gastrointestinal hemorrhage include aortoesophageal fistula[103] secondary to foreign body erosions and Dieulafoy's ulcer.[104]

Lower gastrointestinal bleeding in children is most commonly due to anorectal disease and juvenile polyps.[46] Uncommon during the first year of life, colonic polyps in children usually occur between 3 and 7 years of age.[46] Bleeding from polyps is rarely massive, generally painless, often episodic, and not associated with diarrhea or vomiting. Although juvenile polyps can be found throughout the colon, many can be identified by a digital rectal exam. Polyps can also be identified by colonoscopy or air-contrast barium enema. Colonoscopy is preferred, since polypectomy can be performed during the procedure. Determination of the histology of excised polyps is important to distinguish adenomatous polyps from inflammatory or juvenile polyps[105] (see Chapter 58). Henoch-Schönlein purpura (HSP)[106] and hemolytic uremic syndrome (HUS) vasculitis can present as acute gastrointestinal bleeding. HSP, usually associated with a palpable purpuric rash and hematuria, can present initially as only acute gastrointestinal bleeding. Lymphonodular hyperplasia (illustrated in Fig. 20–3*B* and 20–3*C*) can also present with active lower gastrointestinal bleeding.[106a] Less common causes of lower gastrointestinal bleeding in children include leiomyoma (as illustrated in Fig. 20–2*D*),[107] arteriovenous malformations,[108–110] and intestinal ulcers.[111–113]

Gastrointestinal Bleeding in Adolescents

Upper gastrointestinal bleeding in older children and adolescents is most commonly due to primary peptic ulcer disease, as it is in the adult population. In adolescents the relative incidence of duodenal ulcers compared to gastric ulcers is 2:1. Acute gastrointestinal bleeding following severe vomiting episodes suggests the presence of a Mallory-Weiss tear of the esophagus.[114] Gastric masses such as leiomyoma (as illustrated in Fig. 20–2*D*) predispose to gastric ulcers and can present as acute gastrointestinal bleeding.

The increasing incidence of inflammatory bowel disease as children move from childhood into adolescence leads to displacement of colonic polyps as the most common cause of lower gastrointestinal bleeding.[42, 115] It should be noted, however, that polyps remain a significant cause of gastrointestinal bleeding throughout the adolescent period.[45, 46]

Prognostic Indicators of Upper Gastrointestinal Bleeding

Patients with variceal hemorrhage have both a higher risk of rebleeding and a higher mortality rate than those with other diagnoses.[116] The mortality rate in adults with varices is 30% during the initial hospitalization and 50% during rebleeding episodes.[116] In adult patients with ulcer disease, the presence of a visible vessel (as illustrated in Fig. 20–2*E*) or fresh or old clot observed during endoscopy has been correlated with an up to 50% higher risk of rebleeding[32] and a greater association with surgical intervention.[31, 117, 118] The ulcer location has also been associated with the risk of rebleeding. Ulcers high on the lesser curvature of the stomach or on the posterior inferior wall of the duodenum bulb are more likely to rebleed.[119]

Gastrointestinal Hemorrhage in the Immune Compromised Host

Patients with a compromised immune system require careful consideration of an expanded differential diagnosis when they present with gastrointestinal hemorrhage[120] (see Chapter 56). In B cell disorders such as agammaglobulinemia or hypogammaglobulinemia, there is an increased risk of developing both bacterial and viral illnesses.[121–123] Colitis is common with a variety of pathogens (e.g., *Salmonella*, *Shigella*, *Campylobacter*).[124, 125]

In severe combined immune deficiency disease,[126] candida esophagitis has been commonly noted. In patients with cyclic neutropenia and neutrophil defects such as chronic granulomatous disease, salmonella enteritis is common, and bacteremia is a serious complication.[124]

Infections associated with gastrointestinal hemorrhage in AIDS patients include herpes simplex virus, cytomegalovirus (CMV), or candida.[127b] CMV and herpes simplex viruses can both induce rapidly progressing colitis with severe bleeding. The other causes of colitis in AIDS patients include *Salmonella*, *Shigella*, *Campylobacter,* and *Clostridium difficile*.[128]

Acquired immune deficiency secondary to medications used to prevent rejection of kidney,[129] liver,[130] or bone marrow transplants[131–133] is also associated with opportunistic gastrointestinal infections that may result in bleeding. Esophagitis caused by herpes simplex virus or CMV infection is common.[130] Both CMV and *Clostridium difficile* colitis have been reported in immunosuppressed patients who have undergone kidney and liver transplants.[131] Hemorrhage in patients with leukemia is associated with neutropenia and colitis.[134] Bleeding and hematoma formation are more extensive in patients with platelet counts below 50,000 mm^3.[135]

The presence of immunosuppressive agents and multiple antibiotics sets the stage for fungal and invasive candida infection that may present as severe bleeding from esophagitis. Fungal and CMV infection can cause bleeding and perforation in patients with lymphomas.[136, 137]

Occult Gastrointestinal Bleeding

Pediatric gastroenterologists are commonly faced with the problem of locating occult gastrointestinal bleeding in patients presenting with iron-deficiency anemia.[138] A low hematocrit combined with a low mean corpuscular volume suggest chronic blood loss with iron deficiency. Iron deficiency can be confirmed by measurement of a serum ferritin or serum iron and serum iron binding capacity. Initial steps must be taken to ensure that the blood loss is occurring from the gastrointestinal tract. Stool guaiac tests should be done on three to five occasions before the gastrointestinal tract is excluded as a source of bleeding. Large amounts of blood may be lost into the gastrointestinal lumen and remain occult. Ingestion of 200 ml of blood is required consistently to produce melena in volunteers.[139] As in acute gastrointestinal bleeding, a careful evaluation of the patient's medical, family, and travel history may suggest clues to the cause and site of the bleeding. Presence of localized epigastric pain suggests peptic ulcer disease, with esophagitis, gastritis, or duodenal ulcer being quite probable. A history of increased stool frequency, poor weight gain, fever, or arthritis should raise the possibility of inflammatory bowel disease. Presence of white blood cells on a stool evaluation can suggest colitis, which in an infant or toddler is most commonly associated with milk-soy intolerance.[140, 141] The presence of vascular lesions on the skin suggests vascular malformation of the gastrointestinal tract as a bleeding site. Intestinal helminth infestation is a common cause of occult bleeding in tropical and subtropical countries.[142] Erosions of the esophagus, stomach, and duodenum are the most common gastrointestinal lesions associated with occult bleeding and account for 30 to 70% of adult cases.[143–146] Additional considerations are upper gastrointestinal blood loss associated with nonsteroidal analgesics[147, 148] and lower gastrointestinal blood loss associated with nodular lymphoid hyperplasia[149] (see Table 20–9).

When no clinical clues are forthcoming from the history or the physical examination, upper and lower endoscopies are often performed. Although a Meckel's diverticulum most commonly presents with a rapid drop in hematocrit associated with bright red blood from the rectum, a Meckel's scan should be done in all patients in whom esophagogastroduodenoscopy and colonoscopy have failed to identify a source of bleeding. A tagged red blood cell study can be useful in patients with intermittent blood loss that is moderately rapid; how-

Table 20–9. CAUSES OF OCCULT GASTROINTESTINAL BLEEDING

Inflammatory Causes	**Tumors and Neoplastic Causes**
Peptic esophagitis	Polyps
Crohn's disease	Lymphoma
Chronic ulcerative colitis	Leiomyoma
Mild enterocolitis	Lipoma
Celiac disease	Carcinoma
Eosinophilic gastroenteritis	**Drugs**
Meckel's diverticulum	Nonsteroidal anti-inflammatory drugs
Solitary colon ulcer	**Extragastrointestinal Causes**
Infectious Causes	Hemoptysis
Hookworm	Epistaxis
Strongyloidiasis	Oropharyngeal bleeding
Ascariasis	**Artifactual Causes**
Tuberculous enterocolitis	Hematuria
Amebiasis	Menstrual bleeding
Vascular Causes	Nonspecific test positivity
Angiodysplasia and vascular ectasias	**Miscellaneous Causes**
Gastroesophageal varices	Long-distance running
Congestive gastropathy	Coagulopathies
Hemangiomas	Factitial

Modified from Ahlquist DA: Approach to the patient with occult gastrointestinal bleeding. *In* Yamada T, ed: Textbook of Gastroenterology. Philadelphia, JB Lippincott, 1991, p 620; with permission.

ever, this study is limited by its ability to detect bleeding only when blood is lost at a rate greater than 0.5 ml per minute. Tagged red blood cell scans can also be useful in identifying vascular malformations during the initial blood study. The recent introduction of enteroscopy promises to improve our ability to identify bleeding lesions in the small intestine, although its clinical role has yet to be established.[150]

Hemorrhagic Diathesis

Patients presenting with gastrointestinal hemorrhage should have a protime and partial thromboplastin time drawn early in the clinical course to identify a hemorrhagic diathesis—whether congenital (hemophilia A and B) or acquired—vitamin K deficiency, chronic liver disease, or idiopathic thrombocytopenic purpura. The presence of anticoagulant must also be considered in patients with systemic lupus erythematosus. The use of anticoagulants such as coumadin or platelet inhibitors such as salicylates should be determined. Interestingly, in patients with hemophilia, peptic ulcer disease is still the most common cause of gastrointestinal bleeding.[151]

Medications Associated with Gastrointestinal Hemorrhage

Salicylate ingestion (specifically aspirin) has been shown to be associated with an increased incidence of gastric ulcer and is frequently the cause of hemorrhagic gastric erosions and gastritis.[152–154] It is presumed that salicylates increase the incidence of ulcers by interruption of the gastric mucosal barrier, allowing back diffusion of hydrogen ions and erosive gastritis. The ability of salicylates to inhibit prostaglandin synthesis may also decrease the cytoprotective properties of the gastric mucosa, resulting in damage. The most common finding, diffuse gastritis, responds rapidly to the removal of aspirin and inhibition of gastric acid production by H_2 antagonists.[155, 156] Gastric mucosal injury has been observed in patients treated with nonsteroidal anti-inflammatory agents, [147, 148, 153, 157, 157a] including indomethacin, ibuprofen, naproxen, tolmetin, and sulindac. These agents inhibit local production of prostaglandin in the upper gastrointestinal tract and have been associated with gastritis, gastric ulcers, and duodenal ulcers. Prophylactic treatment with prostaglandins and capsaicin is effective in preventing acute gastritis due to nonsteroidal anti-inflammatory agents.[158] Histamine H_2 antagonists and sucralfate appear effective in preventing duodenal ulcerations.[159]

The relationship of corticosteroid therapy to peptic ulcer disease is unclear.[159a] One retrospective study using meta-analysis to examine 71 clinical studies suggested that corticosteroids increase the risk of peptic ulcers and gastrointestinal hemorrhage.[160] However, such studies are complicated by the increased incidence of peptic ulcer disease in patients with the underlying illnesses for which corticosteroids are being used. Clinical experience suggests that this is a rare association in children.

Some medications have been associated with ulceration of the gastrointestinal tract, including tetracyclines and iron preparations. Chemotherapeutic agents including cytoxan and methotrexate have been implicated in the development of mucosal and gastrointestinal ulcers. Adriamycin and radiation therapy can induce esophagitis and gastrointestinal bleeding.[161]

Stress-Induced Gastritis

Stress-induced gastritis (see Chapter 32) is a common finding in patients admitted to the intensive-care unit (ICU) with hypotension, thermal burns, renal failure, or neurologic trauma.[162, 163, 163a] Clinically significant bleeding occurs in 2 to 10% of adult ICU patients, and mucosal erosions are found in up to 75%.[164] The routine use of high-dose antacids,[165] H_2 blockers, or sucralfate[166] in susceptible patients has been shown to decrease the bleeding risk. Superior results were obtained when antacids were used to maintain the pH at greater than 4.0, suggesting that this may be critically important.[167] At present, the use of a continuous infusion of H_2 blockers has not been studied in a controlled fashion.[168] In adult patients, sucralfate has been shown to be as effective as antacids in prophylaxis[169] and to have a lower rate of nosocomial pneumonia in patients on respirators.[170]

Gastrointestinal Bleeding Associated with Portal Hypertension

Up to 50% of bleeding episodes in patients with portal hypertension (see Chapter 27) and esophageal varices results from a nonvariceal source.[171] Endoscopy is therefore important to determine the source of bleeding so that appropriate therapy can be offered.

The incidence of rebleeding following an initial esophageal bleed is high in patients bleeding from esophageal varices, with one third of adult patients reported to rebleed within 6 weeks.[172] Sclerotherapy (discussed below), surgical shunts, and propranolol have all been advocated to prevent rebleeding.[173, 174, 174a] Propranolol is effective in preventing the first gastrointestinal bleed[174, 175] and decreasing mortality[174] in patients with cirrhosis. Its role in pediatric patients, however, is not defined.

Angiodysplasia

Visualization of a small bright red mucosal vascular lesion may be the first indication of angiodysplasia. Accounting for 5 to 7% of upper gastrointestinal bleeding episodes in adults, angiodysplasia in children is less common and is usually associated with hereditary hemorrhagic telangiectasia or Osler-Weber-Rendu syndrome.[176–178a] Although endoscopic coagulation of these lesions has reportedly been successful,[178a, 179] rebleeding rates are high.[180]

SPECIFIC THERAPEUTIC MODALITIES FOR GASTROINTESTINAL HEMORRHAGE

Gastric Lavage

Historically, gastric lavage with iced saline was used until gastrointestinal bleeding stopped.[181, 182] However, both clinical and experimental data have questioned the utility of this practice.[183–185] Controlled trials have not shown any therapeutic benefit from cold lavage solutions.[184] Gastric lavage with levarterenol has been proposed as treatment for gastrointestinal bleeding,[186] but it has not been shown to be more effective than simple lavage. The extensive commitment of personnel required for continuous gastric lavage, and their risk of exposure to blood products have led us to recommend that gastric lavage be used solely as a diagnostic maneuver or in preparation for endoscopy.

Decreasing Gastric Acidity with H_2 Antagonists

Gastric pH of less than 4 is believed to be important in the pathogenesis of peptic ulceration in intensive-care patients. Antacids, H_2 antagonists, and sucralfate have been shown to have a protective role in preventing bleeding, although the effect may not be dramatic.[163a, 166, 187, 188] If used, H_2 antagonists or antacids should be given in sufficient doses to maintain gastric pH at greater than 4.

Vasoactive Agents

Vasopressin and its analogue terlipressin have been used to decrease blood flow through the celiac and mesenteric vessels to decrease variceal bleeding.[189–193] Vasopressin infusion has been effective in controlling bleeding from stress ulcers, focal or diffuse gastritis, and Mallory-Weiss tears.[194] Vasopressin is reported to be effective both as a systematically delivered intravenous infusion into a peripheral vein[195] and as a direct infusion via arterial catheter into the celiac axis to treat bleeding from esophageal varices. Infusion rates of 0.2 to 0.4 U per 1.73 m² per minute have been advocated. Reported complications include abdominal pain, diarrhea, decreased urine output, and hyponatremia.

Somatostatin has been advocated as an agent to decrease variceal hemorrhage.[196, 197] It has the dual effect of decreasing gastric and gastrointestinal blood flow and inhibiting acid secretion by inhibiting both gastrin synthesis and gastric acid production. In addition, somatostatin reportedly has a lower complication rate than vasopressin. If this is confirmed, somatostatin may replace vasopressin as the agent of choice to decrease hemorrhage in patients with variceal bleeding.[198–200]

Balloon Tamponade of Esophageal Varices

The Sengstaken-Blakemore tube has been used successfully in the treatment of persistent variceal hemorrhage since its introduction in 1950[201] and may have a role in the patient whose variceal hemorrhage does not respond to other therapy. The Sengstaken-Blakemore tube consists of a triple-lumen catheter, with one lumen draining from the tip of the catheter and the other lumens available to fill a round gastric balloon located near the tip and a cylindrical esophageal balloon located more proximally. During acute hemorrhage from gastroesophageal varices, the Sengstaken-Blakemore tube is passed through the nose into the stomach, and the gastric contents are aspirated. Air is then injected to confirm the tube's location in the stomach. The gastric balloon is inflated to an appropriate size for the patient (gastric size ranges from 120 to 240 ml). Following inflation of the gastric balloon, the tube is gradually withdrawn until resistance is felt. The tube is located snug against the lower portion of the esophagus and is maintained in this position by taping the tube firmly to the nose or to a fixed external support such as a football helmet. After confirmation of the proper location of the gastric balloon, the presence of bleeding from esophageal varices should be monitored by placement of a small catheter to a point just above the esophageal balloon. If esophageal bleeding is present, the esophageal balloon should be inflated using a carefully calibrated manometric system to accurately establish and maintain the pressure within the esophageal balloon. The pressures used for tamponade range from 30 to 40 mm of mercury. Although a Sengstaken-Blakemore tube can be life saving in patients with esophageal variceal bleeding, it must be used cautiously, since even in experienced hands it can cause serious complications in up to 20% of patients.[202–206] Underinflation of the gastric balloon can lead to migration of the esophageal balloon into the hypopharynx and upper airway obstruction, and overinflation of the esophageal balloon can lead to esophageal ulcer and perforation. Periodic decompression of the esophageal balloon should occur every 12 to 24 hours to check for esophageal bleeding. If bleeding is noted when the balloon is deflated, the balloon should be reinflated. Since the risk of mucosal ulceration increases with the duration of use, it is best to limit use of this tube to less than 24 hours whenever possible. The larger gastric capacity of the Linton-Nachlas tube makes it appropriate for the treatment of gastric varices by direct tamponade.[206]

Sclerotherapy

Sclerotherapy, first described using rigid endoscopy by Crafoord and Frenckner in 1939,[207, 208] has been adapted to the use of flexible endoscopy. Although multiple techniques have been reported using different sclerosing solutions and equipment, all involve the injection of a sclerosing solution directly into or alongside esophageal varices. Choice of solution varies: 1 to 5% sodium morrhuate, 0.5 to 1% tetradecylsulfate, hypertonic glucose, ethanol, or combinations of the above have all been tried.[209] Sclerotherapy is effective in treating acute bleeding from esophageal varices.[210–213b] Repeated weekly or monthly injections lead to total obliteration of the vessels. Complication rates are substantial[214–216a] and include esophageal ulceration in approximately 2% of patients, esophageal stricture in 2%, left pleural effusion in 1.5%, mucosal sloughing in 0.5%, and esophageal perforation in 0.7%. Rare reported complications include esophageal motility disorders and a single report of thoracic spinal paralysis in a 4-year-old girl.[217] Some believe sclerotherapy to be superior to medical therapy for the prevention of rebleeding of esophageal varices[212, 213, 218, 219] and that it is as effective in the long-term prevention of rebleeding as surgical shunt[220, 221] (see Chapters 27 and 74).

Sclerosing solutions have been utilized in a limited number of adults to obliterate vascular malformations and visible vessels in bleeding peptic ulcers.[168, 222–225] Injection of epinephrine has been reported in a controlled study to produce hemostasis and decrease both infusion requirements and emergency surgery.[28a, 222]

Ligation of Esophageal Varices

Ligation of esophageal varices with endoscopically placed elastic bands in adults has proved successful with fewer complications than with sclerotherapy in several studies.[222a–222d] Currently, there is limited experience with this technique in children.

Thermal Coagulation

The heater probe consists of a heating coil within a Teflon-coated hollow aluminum cylinder. The Teflon coating on the cylinder allows the probe to make direct contact with the tissue, and precision regulation of the heating coil and probe temperature allows for a uniform depth of tissue damage.[226] After applying pressure via the probe to the point of bleeding, coagulation is produced by passing current through the heating coil.[35, 227, 228] The low complication rate of this technique, its relative lack of expense, its ease of operation, and its ready portability make it an excellent tool in treating localized bleeding lesions, including visible vessels in the base of a peptic ulcer, esophageal tears, or arteriovenous malformations.[28a, 224, 229, 229a]

Electrocoagulation

Electrocoagulation was initially introduced using a monopolar probe. Problems with the monopolar probe included a deep spread of tissue coagulation, adherence of tissue to the probe, and dispersion of coagulation energy by pooled secretions. The monopolar probe has now been largely replaced by the bipolar probe. The bipolar circumactive probe (BICAP) combines two electrodes in the same probe separated by 1 to 2 mm. By combining two electrodes, the depth of current flow into the tissue is kept constant.[230–232] A multipolar probe with six electrode plates is also available,[233] which further reduces the depth of current flow into the tissue, decreasing tissue damage and producing a more uniform superficial electrocoagulation. Both the BICAP[28a, 234, 234a] and the multipolar probe[225] have been used successfully for treatment of localized bleeding lesions, such as a visible vessel or arteriovenous malformation.

Laser Photocoagulation

The use of laser therapy has recently been limited by the introduction of the cheaper alternatives of BICAP electrocoagulation[232, 235] and thermocoagulation with the heater probe.[236]

Laser photocoagulation utilizes a quartz fiber that transmits the monochromatic light energy to the tissue via the biopsy channel of the endoscope.[230] The light is converted into heat within the tissue and coagulates tissue proteins. The two commonly available lasers are the Argon laser and the ND:YAG laser. The Argon laser has a wave length that is absorbed by hemoglobin and produces a superficial coagulation. The ND:YAG laser produces a wave length that penetrates the tissue to a greater depth and is not absorbed by hemoglobin. The ND:YAG laser has been used successfully to control active gastrointestinal bleeding.[237, 238] Hemoglobin does not interfere with its function.[235] Unfortunately, the laser's greater tissue penetration increases the risk of perforation, and it is both expensive and not readily portable. The laser is most readily applicable for lesions such as vascular malformations, where direct tissue contact may not be desirable and treatment can be elective.[239]

Surgery

Specific entities such as a Meckel's diverticulum, duplication of the small bowel, and Hirschsprung's disease may require surgical intervention as the definitive treatment. Patients requiring multiple transfusions (e.g., greater than 1½ times their blood volume) should be considered candidates for surgical exploration.[80]

REFERENCES

1. Elta G: Approach to the patient with gross gastrointestinal bleeding. *In* Yamada T, ed: Textbook of Gastroenterology. Philadelphia, JB Lippincott, 1991, pp 591–615.
2. Wetzel R: Shock. *In* Rogers MC, ed: Textbook of Pediatric Intensive Care. Baltimore, Williams & Wilkins, 1987, p 483.
3. Blumer J: Shock. *In* Blumer J, ed: A Practical Guide to Pediatric Intensive Care. St. Louis, Mosby Year Book, 1990, pp 71–81.
4. Shoemaker W: Pathophysiology and therapy of shock syndromes. *In* Shoemaker W, Thompson WL, Holbrook PR, eds: Textbook of Critical Care. Philadelphia, WB Saunders, 1984, pp 52–72.
5. Perkin R, Levin D: Shock. *In* Levin D, Morriss FC, eds:

Essentials of Pediatric Intensive Care. St. Louis, Quality Medical Publishing, 1990, pp 78–97.
6. Tuggle D: Gastrointestinal bleeding. *In* Blumer J, ed: A Practical Guide to Pediatric Intensive Care. St. Louis, Mosby Year Book, 1990, pp 567–569.
7. Rackow E, Falk J: Colloid and crystalloid fluid resuscitation. *In* Shoemaker W, Thompson WL, Holbrook DR, eds: Textbook of Critical Care. Philadelphia, WB Saunders, 1984, pp 733–745.
7a. Gostout CJ: Medical therapy of bleeding ulcers. Semin Gastrointest Dis 1992; 3:53–64.
8. Vladeck B, Bassin R, Kark A, et al: Rapid and slow hemorrhage in man: II. Sequential acid-base and oxygen transport responses. Ann Surg 1971; 173:331–336.
9. Cox K, Ament M: Upper gastrointestinal bleeding in children and adolescents. Pediatrics 1979; 63:408–413.
10. Hochman H, Grodin M, Crone R: Dehydration, diabetic ketoacidosis, and shock in the pediatric patient. Pediatr Clin North Am 1979; 26:803–826.
11. Shoemaker W: Evaluation of colloids, crystalloids, whole blood and red cell therapy in the critically ill patient. Clin Lab Med 1982; 2:35–63.
12. Boyan C: Cold or warmed blood for massive transfusions. Am Surg 1964; 160:282.
13. Hyams J, Leichtner A, Schwartz A: Recent advances in diagnosis and treatment of gastrointestinal hemorrhage in infants and children. J Pediatr 1985; 106:1–9.
14. Layne E, Mellow M, Lipman T: Insensitivity of guaiac slide tests for detection of blood in gastric juice. Ann Intern Med 1981; 94:774–776.
15. Ahlquist D, McGill D, Schwartz S, et al: HemoQuant, a new quantitative assay for fecal hemoglobin: Comparison with Hemoccult. Ann Intern Med 1984; 101:297–302.
16. Doran J, Hardcastle J: Bleeding patterns in colorectal cancer: The effect of aspirin and the implications for faecal occult blood testing. Br J Surg 1982; 69:711–713.
17. Heinrich H: Occult blood tests (letter). Lancet 1980; 1:822.
18. Ostrow J, Mulvaney C, Hansell J, et al: Sensitivity and reproducibility of chemical tests for fecal occult blood with an emphasis on false-positive reactions. Am J Dig Dis 1973; 18:930–940.
19. Stroehlein J, Fairbanks V, McGill D, et al: Hemoccult detection of fecal occult blood quantitated by radioassay. Am J Dig Dis 1976; 21:841–844.
20. Rosenthal P, Thompson J, Singh M: Detection of occult blood in gastric juice. J Clin Gastoenterol 1984; 6:119–121.
21. Schwartz S, Dahl J, Ellefson M, et al: The "Hemo Quant" test; a specific and quantitative determination of heme (hemoglobin) in feces and other materials. Clin Chem 1983; 29:2061–2067.
22. Ahlquist D, McGill D, Schwartz S, et al: Fecal blood levels in health and disease. A study using HemoQuant. N Engl J Med 1985; 312:1422–1428.
23. Goldschmiedt M, Alquist D, Wieand H, et al: Measurement of degraded fecal hemoglobin-heme to estimate gastrointestinal site of occult bleeding. Appraisal of its clinical utility. Dig Dis Sci 1988; 33:605–608.
24. Pumphrey C, Beck E: Raised blood urea concentration indicates considerable blood loss in acute upper gastrointestinal haemorrhage. Br Med J 1980; 1:527.
25. Snook J, Holdstock G, Bamforth J: Value of a simple biochemical ration in distinguishing upper and lower sites of gastrointestinal haemorrhage. Lancet 1986; 2:1064.
25a. Urashima M, Toyoda S, Nakano T, et al: BUN/Cr ratio as an index of gastrointestinal bleeding mass in children. J Pediatr Gastroenterol Nutr 1992; 15:89–92.
26. Luk G, Bynum T, Hendrix T: Gastric aspiration in localization of gastrointestinal hemorrhage. JAMA 1979; 241:576–578.
27. Cadranel S, Rodesch P, Peters J, et al: Fiberendoscopy of the gastrointestinal tract in children. A series of 100 examinations. Am J Dis Child 1977; 131:41–45.
28. Prolla J, Diehl AS, Benvenuti GA, et al: Upper gastrointestinal fiberoptic endoscopy in pediatric patients. Gastrointest Endosc 1983; 29:279–281.
28a. Freeman ML: Endoscopic control of ulcer bleeding. Semin Gastrointest Dis 1992; 3:65–74.
29. Sutton F: Upper gastrointestinal bleeding in patients with esophagael varices. What is the most common source? Am J Med 1987; 83:273–275.
30. Johnston J: The sentinel clot/visible vessel revisited. Gastrointest Endosc 1986; 32:238–239.
31. Swain C, Storey D, Bown S, et al: Nature of the bleeding vessel in recurrently bleeding gastric ulcers. Gastroenterology 1986; 90:595–608.
32. Storey D, Bown S, Swain C, et al: Endoscopic prediction of recurrent bleeding in peptic ulcers. N Engl J Med 1981; 305:915–916.
33. Gryboski JD: The value of upper gastrointestinal endoscopy in children. Dig Dis Sci 1981; 26:17S–21S.
34. Leincke J, Schaffer R, Hogan W: Emergency endoscopy in acute upper GI bleeding (UGB): Does timing affect the significance of diagnostic yield? Gastrointest Endosc 1976; 22:32–38
35. Johnston J: Endoscopic hemostasis for bleeding peptic ulcer. Gastrointest Endosc 1987; 33:260–262.
36. Katon R: Complications of upper gastrointestinal endoscopy in the gastrointestinal bleeder. Dig Dis Sci 1981; 26:47S–54S.
37. Dronfield M, Langman M, Atkinson M, et al: Outcome of endoscopy and barium radiography for acute upper gastrointestinal bleeding: Controlled trial in 1,037 patients. Br Med J 1982; 284:545–548.
38. Morris D, Levine G, Soloway R, et al: Prospective, randomized study of diagnosis and outcome in acute upper-gastrointestinal bleeding: Endoscopy versus conventional radiography. Am J Dig Dis 1975; 20:1103–1109.
39. Aldridge M, Sim A: Colonoscopy findings in symptomatic patients without x-ray evidence of colonic neoplasms. Lancet 1986; 2:833–834.
40. Tedesco F, Waye J, Raskin J, et al: Colonoscopic evaluation of rectal bleeding: A study of 304 patients. Ann Intern Med 1978; 89:907–909.
41. Cucchiara S, Guandalini S, Stainano A, et al: Sigmoidoscopy, colonoscopy and radiology in the evaluation of children with rectal bleeding. J Pediatr Gastroenterol Nutr 1983; 2:667–671.
42. Hassall E, Barclay G, Ament M: Colonoscopy in childhood. Pediatrics 1984; 73:594–599.
43. Steffen R, Wyllie R, Sivak M, et al: Colonoscopy in the pediatric patient. J Pediatr 1989; 115:507–514.
44. Rex D, Weddle R, Lehman G, et al: Flexible sigmoidoscopy plus air contrast barium enema versus colonoscopy for suspected lower gastrointestinal bleeding. Gastroenterology 1990; 98:855–861.
45. Williams C, Laage N, Campbell C, et al: Total colonoscopy in children. Arch Dis Child 1982; 57: 49–53.
46. Euler A, Seibert J: The role of sigmoidoscopy, radiographs, and colonoscopy in the diagnostic evaluation of pediatric age patients with suspected juvenile polyps. J Pediatr Surg 1981; 16:500–502.
47. Caos A, Benner K, Manier J, et al: Colonoscopy after Golytely preparation in acute rectal bleeding. J Clin Gastroenterol 1986; 8:46–49.
48. Sfakianakis G, Hasse G: Abdominal scintigraphy for ectopic gastric mucosa: A retrospective analysis of 143 studies. AJR 1982; 138:7–12.
49. Seitz W, Keim HJ, Hahn K: Abdominal scintigraphy for diagnosis of intestinal bleeding. World J Surg 1978; 2:613–619.
50. Cooney DR, Suszynski DO, Camboa E, et al: The abdominal technetium scan (a decade of experience). J Pediatr Surg 1982; 17: 611–619.
51. Baum S: Pertechnetate imaging following cimetidine administration in Meckel's diverticulum of the ileum. Am J Gastroenterol 1981; 76:464–465.
52. Zwas S, Czerniak A, Wolfstein I: Unusual scintigraphic presentation of a shifting Meckel's diverticulum. Clin Nucl Med 1985; 10:252–255.
53. Williams R: Management of Meckel's diverticulum. Br J Surg 1981; 68:477–480.
54. Treves S, Grand RJ, Eraklis A: Pentagastrin stimulation of technetium-99m uptake by ectopic gastric mucosa in a Meckel's diverticulum. Radiology 1978; 128:711–712.
55. Datz F, Thorne D, Remley K, et al: Bleeding rates necessary for imaging acute gastrointestinal bleeding with Tc99m–labeled red blood cells in an experimental model. J Nucl Med 1987; 28:514–520.
56. Alavi A, Ring E: Localization of gastrointestinal bleeding: Superiority of 99mTc sulfur colloid compared with angiography. Am J Roentgenol. 1981; 137:741–748.

57. Alavi A: Detection of gastrointestinal bleeding with 99mTc-sulfur colloid. Semin Nucl Med 1982; 12:126–138.
58. Miskowiak J, Nielsen S, Munck O, et al: Acute gastrointestinal bleeding detected with abdominal scintigraphy using technetium-99m–labeled albumin. Scand J Gastroenterol 1979; 14:389–394.
59. Driscoll D: The role of radionuclide imaging in the diagnosis of gastrointestinal bleeding in children. Radiography 1986; 52:237–239.
60. Majd M: Radionuclide imaging in pediatrics. Pediatr Clin North Am 1985; 32: 1573–1579.
61. Riff E, Hayden P, Stevenson J: The detection of acute gastrointestinal bleeding using in vivo technetium 99m pertechnetate-labeled erythrocytes. J Pediatr 1980; 97:956–958.
62. Siddiqui A, Schauwecker D, Wellman H, et al: Comparison of technetium-99m sulfur colloid and in vitro labeled technetium-99m RBCs in the detection of gastrointestinal bleeding. Clin Nucl Med 1985; 10:546–549.
63. Landry A, Hartshorne M, Bunker S, et al: Optimal technetium-99m RBC labeling for gastrointestinal hemorrhage study. Clin Nucl Med 1985; 10:491–493.
64. Steer M, Silen W: Diagnostic procedures in gastrointestinal hemorrhage. N Engl J Med 1983; 309:646–650.
65. Smith R, Copely D, Bolen F: 99mTC RBC scintigraphy: Correlation of gastrointestinal bleeding rates with scintigraphic findings. Am J Roentgenol 1987; 148:869–874.
66. Winzelberg G, Froelich J, McKusick K, et al: Radionuclide localization of lower gastrointestinal hemorrhage. Radiology 1981; 139:465–469.
67. Wesselhoeft C, DeLuca F, Luke M: Positive 99mTc-pertechnetate scan in a child with intestinal arteriovenous malformation. J Pediatr Surg 1986; 21:71–72.
68. Bunker S, Lull RJ, Tanasescu DE, et al: The superiority of 99mTc RBC over 99mTc-sulfur colloid in the detection and localization of gastrointestinal hemorrhage. AJR 1984; 143:543–548.
69. Afshani E, Berger P: Gastrointestinal tract angiography in infants and children. J Pediatr Gastroenterol Nutr 1986; 5:173–186.
70. Meyerovitz M, Fellows K: Angiography in gastrointestinal bleeding in children. Am J Roentgenol 1984; 143:837–840.
71. Keller F, Rosch J: Value of angiography in diagnosis and therapy of acute upper gastrointestinal hemorrhage. Dig Dis Sci 1981; 26:78S–89S.
72. Sheedy P, Fulton R, Atwell D: Angiographic evaluation of patients with chronic gastrointestinal bleeding. Am J Roentgenol Radium Ther Nucl Med 1975; 123:338–347.
73. Goldman M, Freeny P, Tallman J, et al: Transcatheter vascular occlusion therapy with isobutyl 2-cyanoacrylate (bucrylate) for control of massive upper gastrointestinal bleeding. Radiology 1978; 129:41–49.
74. Gomes A, Lois J, McCoy R: Angiographic treatment of gastrointestinal hemorrhage: Comparison of vasopressin infusion and embolization. AJR 1986; 146:1031–1037.
75. Clark R, Colley D, Eggers F: Acute arterial gastrointestinal hemorrhage: Efficacy of transcatheter control. AJR 1981; 136:1185–1189.
76. Leitman I, Paull D, Shires G: Evaluation and management of massive lower gastrointestinal hemorrhage. Ann Surg 1989; 209:175–180.
77. Rossle M, Richter G, Noldge G, et al: New non-operative treatment for variceal haemorrhage. Lancet 1989; 2:153.
78. Britt L, Warren L, Moore O: Selective management of lower gastrointestinal bleeding. Am Surg 1983; 49:121–125.
79. Browder W, Cerise E, Litwin M: Impact of emergency angiography in massive lower gastrointestinal bleeding. Ann Surg 1986; 204:530–536).
80. Ament M: Diagnosis and management of upper gastrointestinal tract bleeding in the pediatric patient. Pediatr Rev 1990; 12:107–116.
81. O'Connor J: Colonoscopy in children. Am J Surg 1981; 141:344–345.
81a. Jaramillo E, Slezak P: Comparison between double-contrast barium enema and colonoscopy to investigate lower gastrointestinal bleeding. Gastrointest Radiol 1992; 17:81–83.
82. Hillemeier C, Gryboski J: Gastrointestinal bleeding in the pediatric patient. Yale J Biol Med 1984; 57:135–147.
83. Coello-Ramirez P, Larrosa-Harro A: Gastrointestinal occult hemorrhage and gastroduodenitis in cow's milk protein intolerance. J Pediatr Gastroenterol Nutr 1984; 3:215–218.
84. Halpin T, Byrne W, Ament M: Colitis, persistent diarrhea and soy protein intolerance. J Pediatr 1977; 91:404–407.
85. Powell G: Milk- and soy-induced enterocolitis of infancy. J Pediatr 1978; 93:533–560.
86. Wilson N, Self T, Hamburger R: Severe cow's milk induced colitis in an exclusively breast-fed neonate. Case report and clinical review of cow's milk allergy. Clin Pediatr 1990; 29:77–80.
87. Brown C, Olshaker J: Meckel's diverticulum. Am J Emerg Med 1988; 6:157–164.
88. Glader B: Bleeding disorders in the newborn infant. *In* Avery ME, Taeusch HW, eds: Schaffer's Diseases of the Newborn. Philadelphia, WB Saunders, 1984, p 560.
89. Parikh N, Sebring E, Polesky H: Evaluation of bloody gastric fluid from newborn infants. J Pediatr 1979; 94:967–969.
90. Apt L, Downey W: Melena neonatorum; the swallowed blood syndrome, a simple test for the differentiation of adult and fetal hemoglobin in bloody stools. J Pediatr 1955; 47:6–12.
91. Sherman N, Clatworthy H: Gastrointestinal bleeding in neonates; a study of 94 cases. Surgery 1967; 62:614–619.
92. Liebman W, Thaler M, Bujanover Y: Endoscopic evaluation of upper gastrointestinal bleeding in the newborn. Am J Gastoenterol 1978; 69:607–608.
93. Kliegman R, Fanaroff A: Necrotizing enterocolitis. N Engl J Med 1984; 310:1093–1103.
94. Silber G: Lower gastrointestinal bleeding. Pediatr Rev 1990; 12:85–93.
94a. Bonadio WA, Clarkson T, Naus J: The clinical features of children with malrotation of the intestine. Pediatr Emerg Care 1991; 7:349–349.
95. Moss T, Alder R: Necrotizing enterocolitis in older infants, children and adolescents. J Pediatr 1982; 100:764–766.
96. Nord K, Rossi T, Lebenthal E: Peptic ulcer in children. The predominance of gastric ulcers. Am J Gastroentrol 1981; 75:153–157.
97. Boley S, Brandt L, Mitsudo S: Vascular lesions of the colon. Adv Intern Med 1984; 29:301–326.
97a. St Vil D, Brandt ML, Panic S, et al: Meckel's diverticulum in children: A 20-year review. J Pediatr Surg 1991; 26:1289–1292.
98. Griffin P, Ostroff S, Tauxe R, et al: Illnesses associated with *Escherichia coli* 0157:H7 infections. A broad clinical spectrum. Ann Intern Med 1988; 109:705–712.
99. Levine M: *Escherichia coli* that cause diarrhea: Enterotoxigenic, enteropathogenic, enteroinvasive, enterohemorrhagic, and enteroadherent. J Infect Dis 1987; 155:377–389.
100. Gryan B: Enterohaemorrhagic *Escherichia coli.* Scan J Infect Dis 1990; 22:1–4.
101. Griffin P, Olmstead L, Petras R: *Escherichia coli* 0157:H7-associated colitis. A clinical and histological study of 11 cases. Gastroenterology 1990; 99:142–149.
102. Lilly J, Stellin G: Variceal hemorrhage in biliary atresia. J Pediatr Surg 1984; 19:476–479.
103. Grey T, Mittleman R, Wetli C, et al: Aortoesophageal fistula and sudden death. A report of two cases and review of the literature. Am J Forensic Med Pathol 1988; 9:19–22.
104. Sarles H, Schenkein J, Hecht R, et al: Dielafoy's ulcer: A rare cause of massive gastric hemorrhage in an 11-year-old girl: Case report and literature review. Am J Gastroenterol 1984; 79:930–932.
105. Mougenot J, Baldassarre M, Mashako L, et al: Recto-colic polyps in the child. Analysis of 183 cases. Arch Fr Pediatr 1989; 46:245–248.
106. Byrn J, Fitzgerald J, Northway J, et al: Unusual manifestations of Henoch-Schönlein syndrome. Am J Dis Child 1976; 130:1335–1337.
106a. Colon AR, DiPalma JS, Leftridge CA: Intestinal lymphonodular hyperplasia of childhood: Patterns of presentation. J Clin Gastroenterol 1991; 13:163–166.
107. Nader P, Margolin F: Hemangioma causing gastrointestinal bleeding. Case report and review of the literature. Am J Dis Child 1966; 111:215–222.
108. Meyer C, Troncale F, Galloway S, et al: Arteriovenous malformations of the bowel: An analysis of 22 cases and a review of the literature. Medicine 1981; 60:36–48.

109. Sarin S: Sclerotherapy for variceal bleeding in children. Indian Pediatr 1988; 25:231–235.
110. Oldham K, Lobe T: Gastrointestinal hemorrhage in children. A pragmatic update. Pediatr Clin North Amer 1985; 32:1247–1263.
111. Sunaryo F, Boyle J, Ziegler M, et al: Primary nonspecific ileal ulceration as a cause of massive rectal bleeding. Pediatrics 1981; 68:247–250.
112. Murray F, Lombard M, Dervan P, et al: Bleeding from multifocal heterotopic gastric mucosa in the colon controlled by an H_2 antagonist. Gut 1988; 29:848–851.
113. Testart J, Maupas J, Metayer J, et al: Rectal peptic ulceration—a rare cause of rectal bleeding. Report of a case. Dis Colon Rectum 1988; 31:803–805.
114. Ballesteros J, Company J, Gaya J, et al: Mallory-Weiss syndrome. Review of 25 cases. Rev Clin Esp 1985; 176:72–73.
115. Homan W, Tang C, Thorbjarnarson B: Acute massive hemorrhage from intestinal Crohn's disease. Report of seven cases and review of the literature. Arch Surg 1976; 111:901–905.
116. Graham D, Smith J: The course of patients after variceal hemorrhage. Gastroenterology 1981; 80:800.
117. Wara P: Endoscopic prediction of major rebleeding—a prospective study of stigmata of hemorrhage in bleeding ulcer. Gastroenterology 1985; 88:1209–1214.
118. Griffiths W, Neumann D, Welsh J: The visible vessel as an indicator of uncontrolled or recurrent gastrointestinal hemorrhage. N Engl J Med 1979; 300:1411–1413.
119. Swain C, Salmon P, Northfield P: Does ulcer position influence presentation or prognosis of acute gastrointestinal bleeding? Gut 1986; 27:A632.
120. Ament M: Immunodeficiency syndromes and the gut. Scand J Gastroenterol 1985; 114(Suppl):127–135.
121. Feigin R, Shearer W: Opportunistic infection in children. II. In the compromised host. J Pediatr 1975; 87:677–694.
122. Mulholland M, Delaney J, Folker J, et al: Gastrointestinal complications of congenital immunodeficiency states. The surgeon's role. Ann Surg 1983; 198:673–680.
123. Oleske J, Minnefor A, Cooper RJ, et al: Immune deficiency syndrome in children. JAMA 1983; 249:2345–2349.
124. Arbo A, Santos J: Diarrheal diseases in the immunocompromised host. Pediatr Infect Dis 1987; 6:894–906.
125. Bodey G, Fainstein V: Infections of the gastrointestinal tract in the immunocompromised patient. Annu Rev Med 1986; 37:271–281.
126. Lauzon D, Delage G, Brochu P, et al: Pathogens in children with severe combined immune deficiency disease or AIDS. Can Med Assoc J 1986; 135:33–38.
127. Chachoua A, Dieterich D, Krasinski K, et al: 9-(1,3-dihydroxy-2 propoxymethyl) quanine (Ganciclovir) in the treatment of cytomegalovirus gastrointestinal disease with the acquired immunodeficiency syndrome. Ann Intern Med 1987; 107:133–137.
127a. Kawimbe B, Bem C, Patil PS, et al: Cytomegalovirus ileitis presenting as massive rectal bleeding in infancy. Arch Dis Child 1991; 66:883–884.
128. Berstein L, Krieger B, Novick B, et al: Bacterial infection in the acquired immunodeficiency syndrome of children. Pediatr Infect Dis 1985; 4:472–475.
129. So S, Najarian J, Nevins T, et al: Low-dose cyclosporine therapy combined with standard immunosuppression in pediatric renal transplantation. J Pediatr 1987; 111:1017–1021.
130. Breing M, Zitelli B, Starzl T, et al: Epstein-Barr virus, cytomegalovirus and other viral infections in children after liver transplantation. J Infect Dis 1987; 156:273–279.
131. Rubin R: Infection in the renal and liver transplant patient. *In* Rubin R, Young LS, eds: Clinical Approach to Infection in the Compromised Host. New York, Plenum, 1988, p 557.
132. McDonald G, Shulman H, Sullivan K, et al: Intestinal and hepatic complications of human bone marrow transplantation. Part II. Gastroenterology 1987; 90:770–784.
133. Engelhard D, Marks M, Good R: Infections in bone marrow transplant recipients. J Pediatr 1986; 108:335–346.
134. Moir D, Bale P: Necropsy findings in childhood leukemia, emphasizing neutropenic enterocolitis and cerebral calcification. Pathology 1976; 8:247–258.
135. Strober W, Brown WR: The mucosal immune system. *In* Samter M, Talmage DW, Frank M, et al, eds: Immunological Diseases. Boston, Little, Brown, 1988, p 79.
136. Eras P, Goldstein M, Sherlock P: Candida infection of the gastrointestinal tract. Medicine 1972; 51:367–379.
137. Hirsch M: Herpes group virus infections in the compromised host. *In* Rubin RH, Young LS, eds: Clinical Approach to Infection in the Compromised Host. New York, Plenum, 1988, p 347.
138. Reeves J, Vichinsky E, Addiego J, et al: Iron deficiency in health and disease. Adv Pediatr 1983; 30:281–320.
139. Schliff L, Steven R, Shapiro N, et al: Observations on the oral administration of citrate blood in man. Am J Med Sci 1942; 203:409.
140. Woodruff C: Iron deficiency in infancy and childhood. Pediatr Clin North Am 1977; 24:85–94.
141. Savilahti E, Verkasalo M: Intestinal cow's milk allergy: Pathogenesis and clinical presentation. Clin Rev Allergy 1984; 2:7–23.
142. Roche M, Layrisse M: The nature and causes of "hookworm anemia." Am J Trop Med Hyg 1966; 15:1029–1102.
143. Kerlin P, Reiner R, Davies M: Iron deficiency anemia—A prospective study. Aust NA J Med 1979; 9:402.
144. Cook I, Pavli P, Riley J, et al: Gastrointestinal investigation of iron deficiency anaemia. Br Med J 1986; 292:1380–1382.
145. Calvey H, Castleden C: Gastrointestinal investigations for anaemia in the elderly: A prospective study. Age Ageing 1987; 16:399–404.
146. Hershko C, Vitells A, Braverman D: Causes of iron deficiency anemia in an adult inpatient population. Effect of diagnostic workup on etiologic distribution. Blut 1984; 49:347–352.
147. Kaplan B, Benson J, Rothstein F, et al: Lymphonodular hyperplasia of the colon as a pathologic finding in children with lower gastrointestinal bleeding. J Pediatr Gastroenterol Nutr 1984; 3:704–708.
148. Graham D, Smith S: Gastroduodenal complications of chronic NSAID therapy. Am J Gastroenterol 1988; 83:1081.
149. Ivey K: Gastrointestinal intolerance and bleeding with nonnarcotic analgesics. Drugs 1986; 32:71–89.
150. Lewis B, Waye J: Chronic gastrointestinal bleeding of obscure origin: Role of small bowel enteroscopy. Gastroenterology 1988; 94:1117–1120.
151. Mittal R, Spero J, Lewis J, et al: Patterns of gastrointestinal hemorrhage in hemophilia. Gastroenterology 1985; 88:515–522.
152. Levy M, Miller D, Kaufman D, et al: Major upper gastrointestinal tract bleeding. Relation to the use of aspirin and other nonnarcotic analgesics. Arch Intern Med 1988; 148:281–285.
153. Silvoso G, Ivey K, Butt J, et al: Incidence of gastric lesions in patients with rheumatic disease on chronic aspirin therapy. Ann Intern Med 1979; 91:517–520.
154. Domschke S, Domschke W: Gastroduodenal damage due to drugs, alcohol and smoking. Clin Gastroenterol 1984; 13:405–436.
155. Fromm D: Salicylate and gastric mucosal damage. Pediatrics 1978; 62:938–942.
156. Graham D, Smith J: Aspirin and the stomach. Ann Intern Med 1986; 104:390–398.
157. Holzer P, Pabst M, Lippe I: Intragastric capsaicin protects against aspirin-induced lesion formation and bleeding in the rat gastric mucosa. Gastroenterology 1989; 96:1425–1433.
157a. Holvoet J, Terriere L, Van Hee W, et al: Relation of upper gastrointestinal bleeding to non-steroidal anti inflammatory drugs and aspirin: A case-control study. Gut 1991; 32:730–734.
158. Cohen M, McCready D, Clark L, et al: Protection against aspirin-induced antral and duodenal damage with enporstil. A double-blind endoscopic study. Gastroenterology 1985; 88:382–386.
159. Lanza F, Aspinall R, Swabb E, et al: Double-blind, placebo-controlled endoscopic comparison of the mucosal protective effects of misoprotol versus cimetidine on tolmetin-induced mucosal injury to the stomach and duodenum. Gastroenterology 1988; 95:289–294.
159a. Carson JL, Strom BL, Schinnar R, et al: The low risk of upper gastrointestinal bleeding in patients dispensed corticosteroids. Am J Med 1991; 91:223–228.
160. Conn H, Butzer B: Nonassociation of adrenocorticoid therapy and peptic ulcer. N Engl J Med 1976; 294:473–479.
161. Newburger P, Cassady J, Jaffe N: Esophagitis due to adriamycin and radiation therapy for childhood malignancy. Cancer 1978; 42:417–423.
162. Skillman J, Silen W: Acute gastroduodenal "stress" ulceration:

Barrier disruption of varied pathogenesis? Gastroenterology 1970; 59:478–482.

163. Skillman J, Bushnell L, Goldman H, et al: Respiratory failure, hypotension, sepsis, and jaundice. A clinical syndrome associated with lethal hemorrhage from acute stress ulceration of the stomach. Am J Surg 1969; 117:523–530.

163a. Morrissette CT, Smith JL: Stress gastritis: An intensive care unit view. Semin Gastrointest Dis 1992; 3:99–104.

164. Kamada T, Fusamoto H, Kawano S, et al: Acute gastroduodenal lesions in head injury. An endoscopic study. Am J Gastroenterol 1977; 68:249–253.

165. Hastings P, Skillman J, Bushnell L, et al: Antacid titration in the prevention of acute gastrointestinal bleeding: A controlled, randomized trial in 100 critically ill patients. N Engl J Med 1978; 298:1041–1045.

166. Lopez-Herce J, Dorao P, Elola P, et al: Frequency and prophylaxis of upper gastrointestinal hemorrhage in critically ill children. Crit Care Med 1992; 20:1082–1089.

167. Priebe H, Skillman J, Bushnell L, et al: Antacid versus cimetidine in preventing acute gastrointestinal bleeding. A randomized trial in 75 critically ill patients. N Engl J Med 1980; 302:426–430.

168. Ostro MJ, Russell JA, Soldin SJ, et al: Control of gastric pH with cimetidine boluses versus primed infusions. Gastroenterology 1985; 89:532.

169. Tryba M, Zevounou F, Torok M, et al: Prevention of acute stress bleeding with sucralfate, antacids, or cimetidine. A controlled study with pirenzepine as a basic medication. Am J Med 1985; 79:55–61.

170. Driks M, Craven D, Celli B, et al: Nosocomial pneumonia in intubated patients given sucralfate as compared with antacids or histamine type 2 blockers. The role of gastric colonization. N Engl J Med 1987; 317:1376–1382.

171. Dagradi A, Mehler R, Tan D, et al: Sources of upper gastrointestinal bleeding in patients with liver cirrhosis and large esophagogastric varices. Am J Gastroenterol 1970; 54:458–463.

172. Kleber G, Sauerbruch T, Ansari H, et al: Prediction of variceal hemorrhage in cirrhosis: A prospective follow-up study. Gastroenterology 1991; 100:1332–1337.

173. Smith J, Graham D: Variceal hemorrhage: A critical evaluation of survival analysis. Gastroenterology 1982; 82:968–973.

174. Poynard T, Cales P, Pasta L, et al: Beta-adrenergic-antagonist drugs in the prevention of gastrointestinal bleeding in patients with cirrhosis and esophageal varices. An analysis of data and prognostic factors in 589 patients from four randomized clinical trials. N Engl J Med 1991; 324:1532–1538.

174a. Carey WD: Pharmacological management of portal hypertensive upper intestinal hemorrhage. Semin Gastrointest Dis 1992; 3:75–82.

175. Garden O, Millis P, Birnie G, et al:. Propranolol in the prevention of recurrent variceal hemorrhage in cirrhotic patients. A controlled trial. Gastroenterology 1990; 98:185–190.

176. Smith C, Bartholomew L, Cain J: Hereditary hemorrhagic telangiectasia and gastrointestinal hemorrhage. Gastroenterology 1963; 44:1.

177. Vase P, Grove O: Gastrointestinal lesions in hereditary hemorrhagic telangiectasia. Gastroenterology 1986; 91:1079–1083.

178. Krane S: Case records of the Massachusetts General Hospital. N Engl J Med 1979; 300:129.

178a. Lewis BS: Vascular anomalies of the gastrointestinal tract. Semin Gastrointest Dis 1992; 3:105–112.

179. Marwick T, Kerlin P: Angiodysplasia of the upper gastrointestinal tract. Clinical spectrum in 41 cases. J Clin Gastroenterol 1986; 8:404–407.

180. Rutgeerts P, VanGompel F, Geboes K, et al: Long term results of treatment of vascular malformations of the gastrointestinal tract by neodymium YAG laser photocoagulation. Gut 1985; 26:586–593.

181. Andrus C, Ponsky J: The effects of irrigant temperature in upper gastrointestinal hemorrhage: A requiem for iced saline lavage. Am J Gastroenterol 1987; 82:1062–1064.

182. Nicoloff D, Griffen W, Salmon P, et al: Local gastric hypothermia in the management of massive gastrointestinal hemorrhage. Surg Gynecol Obstet 1962; 114:495–503.

183. Cichowicz E, Alvarez-Ruiz J: Acute upper gastrointestinal bleeding in children. Bol Assoc Med PR 1983; 75:214–220.

184. Ponsky J, Hoffman M, Swayngum D: Saline irrigation in gastric hemorrhage: The effect of temperature. J Surg Res 1980; 28:204–205.

185. Bryant L, Mobin-Uddin K, Dillon M: Comparison of ice water with iced saline solution for gastric lavage in gastroduodenal hemorrhage. Am J Surg 1972; 124:570.

186. Kiselow M, Wagner M: Intragastric instillation of levarterenol. A method for control of upper gastrointestinal tract hemorrhage. Arch Surg 1973; 107:387–389.

187. Lacroix J, Infante-Rivard C, Gauthier M, et al: Upper gastrointestinal tract bleeding acquired in a pediatric intensive care unit: Prophylaxis trial with cimetidine. J Pediatr 1986; 108:1015–1018.

188. Collins R, Langman M: Treatment with histamine H_2 antagonists in acute upper gastrointestinal hemorrhage. Implications of randomized trials. N Engl J Med 1985; 313:660–666.

189. Hussey K: Vasopressin therapy for upper gastrointestinal tract hemorrhage. Has its efficacy been proven? Arch Intern Med 1985; 145:1263–1267.

190. Freeman J, Cobden I, Lishman A, Record C: Controlled trial of terlipressin ("Glypressin") versus vasopressin in the early treatment of oesophageal varices. Lancet 1982; 2:66–68.

191. Johnson W, Widrich W, Ansell J, et al: Control of bleeding varices by vasopressin: A prospective randomized study. Ann Surg 1977; 186:369–376.

192. Resnick R: Intraarterial vasopressin: A continuing challenge. Gastroenterology 1975; 68:411–412.

193. Ready J, Robertson A, Rector W: Effects of vasopressin on portal pressure during hemorrhage from esophageal varices. Gastroenterology 1991; 100:1411–1416.

194. Goldman M: Interventional radiology. *In* Yamada I, ed: Textbook of Gastroenterology. Philadelphia, JB Lippincott, 1991, pp 2443–2455.

195. Chojkier M, Groszmann R, Atterbury C, et al: A controlled comparison of continuous intra-arterial and intravenous infusions of vasopressin in hemorrhage from esophageal varices. Gastroenterology 1979; 77:540–546.

196. Magnusson I, Ihre T, Johansson C, et al: Randomized double blind trial of somatostatin in the treatment of massive upper gastrointestinal haemorrhage. Gut 1985; 26:221–226.

197. Burroughs A, McCormick P, Hughes M, et al: Randomized, double-blind, placebo-controlled trial of somatostatin for variceal bleeding. Emergency control and prevention of early variceal rebleeding. Gastroenterology 1990; 99:1388–1395.

198. Basso N, Bagarani M, Bracci F, et al: Ranitidine and somatostatin. Their effects on bleeding from the upper gastrointestinal tract. Arch Surg 1986; 121:833–835.

199. Kravetz D, Bosch J, Teres J, et al: Comparison of intravenous somatostatin and vasopressin infusions in treatment of acute variceal hemorrhage. Hepatology 1984; 4:442–446.

200. Reichlin S: Somatostatin. N Engl J Med 1983; 309:1556–1563.

201. Sengstaken R, Blakemore A: Balloon tamponade for the control of hemorrhage from esophageal varices. Ann Surg 1950; 131:781–789.

202. Chojkier M, Conn H: Esophageal tamponade in the treatment of bleeding varices. Dig Dis Sci 1980; 25:267–272.

203. Conn H: To scope or not to scope. N Engl J Med 1981; 304:967–969.

204. Kline J: Modification of the adult Blakemore tube for use in children with bleeding esophageal varices. J Pediatr Gastroenterol Nutr 1986; 5:153–154.

205. Pitcher J: Safety and effectiveness of the modified Sengstaken-Blakemore tube: A prospective study. Gastroenterology 1971; 61:291–298.

206. Teres J, Cecilia A, Bordas J, et al: Esophageal tamponade for bleeding varices. Controlled trial between the Sengstaken-Blakemore tube and the Linton-Nachlas tube. Gastroenterology 1978; 75:566–569.

207. Crafoord C, Frenckner P: New surgical treatment of varicose veins of the esophagus. Acta Otolaryngol 1939; 27:422–429.

208. Howard E, Stamatakis J, Mowat A: Management of esophageal varices in children by injection sclerotherapy. J Pediatr Surg 1984; 19:2–5.

209. Randall G, Jensen D, Hirabayashi K, et al: Controlled study of different sclerosing agents for coagulation of canine gut arteries. Gastroenterology 1989; 96:1274–1281.

210. Pinkus J: CR—a new irritant agent. N Engl J Med 1978; 299:901–902.

211. Terabayashi H, Ohnishi K, Tsunoda T, et al: Prospective controlled trial of elective endoscopic sclerotherapy in comparison with percutaneous transhepatic obliteration of esophageal varices in patients with nonalcoholic cirrhosis. Gastroenterology 1987; 93:1205–1209.
212. O'Connor K, Lehman G, Yune H, et al: Comparison of three nonsurgical treatments for bleeding esophageal varices. Gastroenterology 1989; 96:899–906.
213. Infante-Rivard C, Esnaola S, Villeneuve J: Role of endoscopic variceal sclerotherapy in the long-term management of variceal bleeding: A meta-analysis. Gastroenterology 1989; 96:1087–1092.
213a. Hill ID, Bowie MD: Endoscopic sclerotherapy for control of bleeding varices in children. Am J Gastroenterol 1991; 86:472–476.
213b. Maksoud JG, Goncalves ME, Porta G, et al: The endoscopic and surgical management of portal hypertension in children: Analysis of 123 cases. J Pediatr Surg 1991; 26:178–181.
214. Donovan T, Ward M, Shepherd R: Evaluation of endoscopic sclerotherapy of esophageal varices in children. J Pediatr Gastroenterol Nutr 1986; 5:696–700.
215. Vane D, Boles E, Clatworthy H: Esophageal sclerotherapy: An effective modality in children. J Pediatr Surg 1985; 20:703–707.
216. Monroe P, Morrow C, Millen J, et al: Acute respiratory failure after sodium morrhuate esophageal sclerotherapy. Gastroenterology 1983; 85:693–699.
216a. Kochhar R, Goenka MD, Mehta SK: Esophageal strictures following endoscopic variceal sclerotherapy: Antecedents, clinical profile, and management. Dig Dis Sci 1992; 37:347–352.
217. Seidman E, Weber A, Morin C, et al: Spinal cord paralysis following sclerotherapy for esophageal varices. Hepatology 1984; 4:950–954.
218. Terblanche J, Northover J, Bornman P, et al: A prospective controlled trial of sclerotherapy in the long term management of patients after esophageal variceal bleeding. Surg Gynecol Obstet 1979; 148:323–333.
219. Planas R, Boix J, Broggi M, et al: Portacaval shunt versus endoscopic sclerotherapy in the elective treatment of variceal hemorrhage. Gastroenterology 1991; 100:1078–1086.
220. Cello J, Grendell J, Crass R, et al: Endoscopic sclerotherapy versus portacaval shunt in patients with severe cirrhosis and variceal hemorrhage. N Engl J Med 1984; 311:1589–1594.
221. Korula J, Balart L, Radvan G, et al: A prospective, randomized controlled trial of chronic esophageal variceal sclerotherapy. Hepatology 1985; 5:584–589.
222. Panes J, Viver J, Forne M, et al: Controlled trial of endoscopic sclerosis in bleeding peptic ulcers. Lancet 1987; 2:1292–1294.
222a. Saeed ZA, Ramirez FC: Endoscopic therapy of bleeding from portal hypertension. Semin Gastrointest Dis 1992; 2:83–98.
222b. Saeed ZA, Michaletz PA, Winchester CB: Endoscopic variceal ligation in patients who have failed endoscopic sclerotherapy. Gastrointest Endosc 1990; 36:572–574.
222c. Stiegmann GV, Goff JS, Sun JH, et al: Endoscopic elastic band ligation for active variceal hemorrhage. Am Surg 1989; 55:124–128.
222d. Stiegmann G, Goff J, Michaletz P, et al: Endoscopic variceal ligation vs. sclerotherapy for bleeding esophageal varices: Early results of a prospective randomized trial. Gastrointest Endosc 1989; 35:431–434.
223. Chen P, Wu C, Liaw Y: Hemostatic effect of endoscopic local injection with hypertonic saline-epinephrine solution and pure ethanol for digestive tract bleeding. Gastrointest Endosc 1986; 32:319–323.
224. Chung S, Leung J, Sung J, et al: Injection or heat probe for bleeding ulcer. Gastroenterology 1991; 100:33–37.
225. Laine L: Multipolar electrocoagulation versus injection therapy in the treatment of bleeding peptic ulcers. A prospective, randomized trial. Gastroenterology 1990; 99:1303–1306.
226. Protell R, Rubin C, Auth D, et al: The heater probe: A new endoscopic method for stopping massive gastrointestinal bleeding. Gastroenterology 1978; 74:257–262.
227. Johnston J: Endoscopic thermal treatment of upper gastrointestinal bleeding. Endosc Rev 1985; 2:12–26.
228. Michaletz P, Judge D: Microwave energy compared with heater probe and BICAP in canine models of peptic ulcer hemorrhage. Gastroenterology 1989; 97:676–684.
229. Fleischer D: Endoscopic therapy of upper gastrointestinal bleeding in humans. Gastroenterology 1986; 90:217–234.
229a. Tanabe S, Koizumi W, Kida M, et al: Experimental and clinical studies on heater probe hemostasis for upper gastrointestinal bleeding with special reference to comparison with ethanol injection. Gastroenterol Jpn 1991; 26:75–77.
230. Silverstein F, Gilbert D, Auth D: Endoscopic hemostasis using laser photocoagulation and electrocoagulation. Dig Dis Sci 1981; 26:31s–40s.
231. Protell R, Gilbert D, Silverstein F, et al: Computer-assisted electrocoagulation: Bipolar vs. monopolar in the treatment of experimental canine gastric ulcer bleeding. Gastroenterology 1981; 80:451–455.
232. Rutgeerts P, Vantrappen G, VanHootegem P, et al: Neodymium-YAG laser photocoagulation versus multipolar electrocoagulation for the treatment of severely bleeding ulcers: A randomized comparison. Gastrointest Endosc 1987; 33:199–202.
233. Laine L: Multipolar electrocoagulation in the treatment of active upper gastrointestinal tract hemorrhage. A prospective controlled trial. N Engl J Med 1987; 316:1613–1617.
234. O'Brien J, Day S, Burnham W: Controlled trial of small bipolar probe in bleeding peptic ulcers. Lancet 1986; 1:464–467.
234a. Ishii M, Yamada S, Shiomi M, et al: Endoscopic bipolar electrocoagulation in upper gastrointestinal bleeding. Gastroenterol Jpn 1991; 26:71–74.
235. Goff J: Bipolar electrocoagulation versus Nd-YAG laser photocoagulation for upper gastrointestinal bleeding lesions. Dig Dis Sci 1986; 31:906–910.
236. Johnston J, Sones J, Long B, et al: Comparison of heater probe and YAG laser in endoscopic treatment of major bleeding from peptic ulcers. Gastrointest Endosc 1985; 31:175–180.
237. Rutgeerts P, Vantrappen G, Broeckaert L, et al: Controlled trial of YAG laser treatment of upper digestive hemorrhage. Gastroenterology 1982; 83:410–416.
238. Fleischer D: The current status of gastrointestinal laser activity in the United States. Gastrointest Endosc 1982; 28:157–161.
239. Gostout C, Ahlquist D, Radford C, et al: Endoscopic laser therapy for watermelon stomach. Gastroenterology 1989; 96:1462–1465.

Chapter 21

Failure to Thrive

MICHAEL K. FARRELL

INTRODUCTION

An infant's most important task is to grow and develop into a mature, functioning adult. Nutrition is one of the critical factors responsible for growth, and inadequate nutrition results in suboptimal growth. Undernutrition also affects an infant psychologically, resulting in apathy, depression, developmental delay, and withdrawal from the environment. If inadequate nutrition persists, there may be long-term effects on a child's physical, emotional, and psychological development.[1] Nutrition is not the sole factor responsible for normal growth and development: Genetic endowment; environmental issues such as the availability of appropriate foods provided in a caring, nurturing milieu; and the capacity to digest, absorb, and efficiently utilize ingested food are also important.[2] This complex interaction between environmental, social, and nutritional factors results in normal growth and development; disruptions have an adverse effect.

Failure to thrive in the broadest sense is a term used to describe infants and children whose growth deviates from that expected for their sex and age. It is a symptom, not a diagnosis. It is an initial impression that requires further evaluation. It is a diagnostic challenge; the differential diagnosis encompasses all of pediatrics, since dysfunction of any organ system may result in malnutrition and impaired growth (Table 21–1 gives a partial listing of potential causes). Delayed growth is a common disorder; it may account for 3 to 5% of hospital admissions and may affect 10 to 20% of outpatients, particularly those in poor socioeconomic settings.[3, 4]

Traditionally, failure to thrive has been categorized as either organic or nonorganic.[5] Nonorganic failure to thrive is growth failure without a diagnosable medical etiology; it has been attributed to maternal deprivation or an insufficiently nurturing environment. Organic failure to thrive is growth failure due to an underlying medical disorder. This arbitrary classification has recently been challenged. Homer and Ludwig have suggested a third category, "mixed," based on the fact that the effects of medical disorders are often compounded by psychosocial problems.[6] Eighty-two children hospitalized in a tertiary referral center were retrospectively classified: 28% had organic causes, 46% had nonorganic causes, and 26% had elements of both and were thus classified as mixed in etiology. A common example of a mixed cause is a child with a chronic disorder, such as recurrent ear infections, who develops behavioral problems that result in altered eating patterns and subsequent slowed growth.

There is a long history associating environmental neglect and poor child development.[7] Throughout early recorded history, unwanted or unfit children were abandoned by their families and society. In the thirteenth century, Frederick II performed a bizarre experiment. He was interested in the "primary language of man," the language spoken "naturally" if there were no outside influences. He ordered a group of newborn infants isolated on an island with a wet nurse who was absolutely forbidden to speak to the infants. All the infants died; this is perhaps the first documented example of nonorganic failure to thrive. During the Industrial Revolution, many "foundlings" were placed in public institutions; the mortality rate among these infants was 70%. As early as 1915, Chapin urged early discharge of infants under one year of age from New York's hospitals because of the dreadful mortality.[8] Thirty years later, Bakwin described the emotional deprivation seen in hospitalized infants who were isolated because of infection: "the outstanding features are listlessness, emaciation and pallor, relative immobility . . . facial expression is unhappy, muscle tone is poor . . . the infants show no interest in the environment, lying quietly in bed, rarely crying and moving very little."[9] Following World War II, Spitz and Wolff[10] described "anaclitic depression" in orphanages where the children received minimal stimulation. Widdowson[11] found that adequate caloric intake in the face of an unfavorable psychological environment resulted in poor physical growth. Two orphanages were studied, one of which had a stern supervisor who disciplined the children at mealtimes. Although the food intake was similar, the children in the "stern" orphanage had one third the weight gain of those in the other group. In 1947 Talbot[12] linked the home environment and nonorganic failure to thrive; he described poor caloric intake due to generalized neglect. Coleman and Provence[13] again confirmed failure to thrive in the nonhospital environment and related the observed developmental delay to the mother's state of depression. Powell and associates[14] described a group of children with psychosocial dwarfism who were short, had pathological home situations, and had bizarre diet histories, such as eating from a dog dish and drinking from the

Table 21–1. DIFFERENTIAL DIAGNOSIS FOR FAILURE TO GAIN WEIGHT

Psychosocial Deprivation
Maternal depression
Emotional deprivation
Maternal deprivation
Reactive attachment disorder of infancy
Pschosocial dwarfism
Feeding Disorders
Occult neurological disorders
"Difficult" breast feeder
Improper formula mixing/administration
Oropharyngeal disorders
"Fear" syndromes
Central Nervous Systems Abnormalities
Cerebral palsy
Diencephalic syndrome
Increased intracranial pressure (tumor, chronic subdural hematomas, intoxications)
Neuromuscular disorders
Cardiac Disease (especially lesions leading to congestive failure)
Pulmonary Disease
Bronchopulmonary dysplasia
Cystic fibrosis
Gastrointestinal Diseases
Rumination
Gastroesophageal reflux
Pyloric stenosis
Malrotation
Postnecrotizing enterocolitis stricture
Hirschsprung's disease
Chronic diarrhea
Intractable diarrhea of infancy
Postenteritis enteropathy
Giardiasis
Sucrase-isomaltase deficiency
Celiac disease
Autoimmune enteropathy
Inflammatory bowel disease
Chronic cholestasis
Renal Disorders
Renal dysplasia
Renal tubular acidosis
Immunodeficiency (including HIV infection)
Perinatal Factors
Intrauterine growth retardation
Intrauterine infections
Fetal alcohol syndrome
Genetic, "Dwarfing" Syndromes
Connective Tissue Disorders
Juvenile rheumatoid arthritis
Endocrine
Growth hormone deficiency
Hypothyroidism
Hypopituitarism
Diabetes mellitus
Chronic Infections
Tuberculosis
Congenital syphilis
Cytomegalic inclusion virus
Metabolic Disorders
Altered calcium, phosphorus metabolism (rickets)
Mucopolysaccharidosis
Mucolipidosis
Sphingolipidosis
Glycogen storage disease
Organic acidosis
Aminoacidurias
Malignancies

toilet. These children also had a high incidence of behavioral problems and retarded motor and intellectual development; their endocrine studies suggested hypopituitarism. All the children improved when they were removed from the abusive environment. Initially it was thought that the growth failure was caused primarily by maternal deprivation via neuroendocrine changes. Whitten and colleagues[15] subsequently demonstrated that infants with poor weight gain improved when hospitalized even though they remained in the same deprived emotional state; infants treated with increased nurturing but not increased food did not gain weight.

Recently there have been two changes in our traditional thinking regarding poor growth. First, it is now recognized that the common biologic insult in all children with failure to thrive, regardless of cause, is malnutrition.[16] The laws of thermodynamics, particularly the law of energy conservation, still apply. When energy intake is greater than energy expenditure, weight gain and growth occur. Both sides of the equation must be considered equally. The therapeutic and diagnostic focus must be on the assessment and treatment of malnutrition and its complications rather than the detection of rare occult diseases.

Second, the transactional model of infant development has superseded the previously simplistic notion of maternal deprivation.[17] The transactional model suggests that the quality of parental care reflects both the child's and the family's individual psychodynamics as well as a spectrum of biologic and social risk factors that interact and modify one another over time (Fig. 21–1). These include economic forces, social networks, and family health beliefs. Not all children in a family are treated equally; some may be nurtured better than others, depending on the parents' own history and current stresses. This model also emphasizes that parenting quality reflects the child's as well as the caretaker's personality and characteristics. Not all children are equally easy to nurture; influencing factors may include temperament, negativity, lack of affect, ahedonism, disorganized behavioral responses due to previous medical illnesses, or underlying conditions that make the child burdensome to the caretaker[17, 18] (Table 21–2). In addition, the secondary behavioral changes of malnutrition can make a child more difficult to nurture, thus creating a vicious cycle.

A more recent phenomenon is poor growth secondary to inadequate caloric intake because of the parents' fear of obesity, cholesterol, or "junk foods" or because of personal or family religious or cultural beliefs.[19, 20] The result is growth failure and the sequelae of malnutrition, such as delayed pubarche. Pugliese and associates evaluated 14 children (9 boys and 5 girls, aged 9 to 17 years) with growth failure.[19] All had decreased growth velocity; the caloric intake ranged from 32 to 91% of the recommended dietary allowance (RDA). No underlying physical or psychiatric disorders were detected. Accelerated growth occurred after nutritional counseling and increased caloric intake.

Growth failure (malnutrition) is the sine qua non of failure to thrive. Therefore, the term *failure to thrive,* although it has long been used in pediatrics, is an

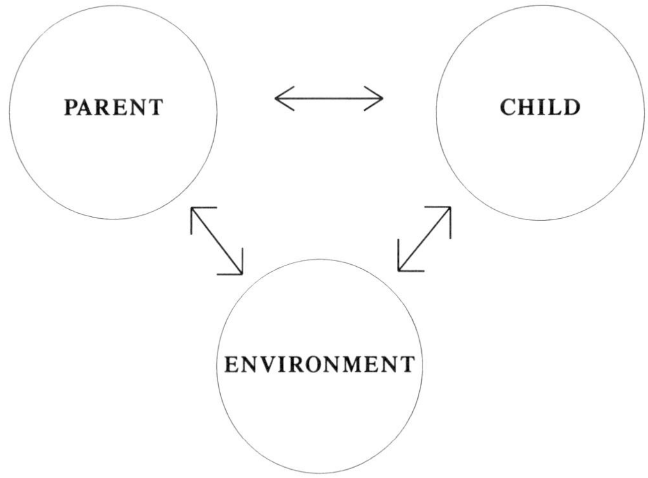

Figure 21–1. Potential interactions affecting a child's feeding behavior.

unfortunate choice of words. The concept of "thrive" is judgmental; it can evoke feelings of guilt and shame in parents and may undermine the patient-physician relationship.[21] Since inadequate nutrition and malnutrition are the major features, the author prefers the term *failure to gain weight/grow appropriately*.

The diagnosis should be applied to an infant or child who is two standard deviations below the mean weight for his or her age and sex (i.e., less than the third percentile) or has persistent deviation from his or her own previously established growth curves, usually crossing two major percentiles.[6, 15] Both parts of the definition are equally important: A child does not have to fall below the third percentile before there is concern; conversely, all children below the third percentile are not necessarily abnormal, since 3% of normal children are below the third percentile. For example, children with constitutional short stature will be below the third percentile but will have normal growth velocity and follow their own curves. Both children depicted in Figure 21–2 are having difficulty gaining weight appropriately and require further evaluation.

Table 21–2. SOCIAL AND ENVIRONMENTAL FACTORS

Organic Factors
Prenatal complications
Minor congenital anomalies
Drug, alcohol, other toxin exposure
Intrauterine growth retardation
Prematurity
Continuing medical illness (may be major or minor)
Nonorganic Factors
Individual temperament—child and parents
Inadequate support network
Help-rejecting style of coping
Overwhelmed mother
Absent father (physically or emotionally)
Feeding difficulties
Poor nonfeeding interactions resulting in neglect
Social stress
Poverty
Marital stress
Recent death in family
Other family losses
Chronic illness
Disorganized life style
Unplanned pregnancy

Infants and children normally gain weight; therefore, failure to gain weight or any loss of weight is potentially serious. However, children's weight is not constant; it fluctuates day to day, and minor illnesses may interfere with appetite. A single point on a growth curve is difficult to interpret; serial data obtained over time are much better. Suggested time intervals to prompt concern are poor weight gain over 10 to 50 days in children less than 5 months of age and 90 days for children over 5 months.[22, 23] Some weight loss, up to 10%, is normal immediately after birth, but the infant should be back to birth weight by 10 to 14 days. In general, the younger the child, the sooner the clinician should become concerned about poor growth.

Poor weight gain is usually the first finding; decreased linear growth and head circumference occur later and are signs of chronic malnutrition. The best indicator is the rate of weight gain and linear growth. Table 21–3 depicts growth rates for children in the first two years of life.[24]

EVALUATION

The evaluation of a child with poor growth must include nutritional, medical, social, family, and developmental factors.[6] This is often best done with a multidisciplinary approach.[21] The evaluation begins with a careful and thorough history and physical examination. Nowhere else in pediatrics is the old truism so applicable: The history reveals 75% of the diagnosis, the physical examination the remainder. Laboratory studies should be used only to confirm the clinical impression. Sills reviewed 118 patients hospitalized with failure to thrive; 18 had proven organic etiologies. Only 1.4% of all the laboratory studies performed were useful in making the diagnosis. The only positive studies were those that confirmed a specific indication from the history and physical examination.[5]

The initial evaluation must be planned and orderly.

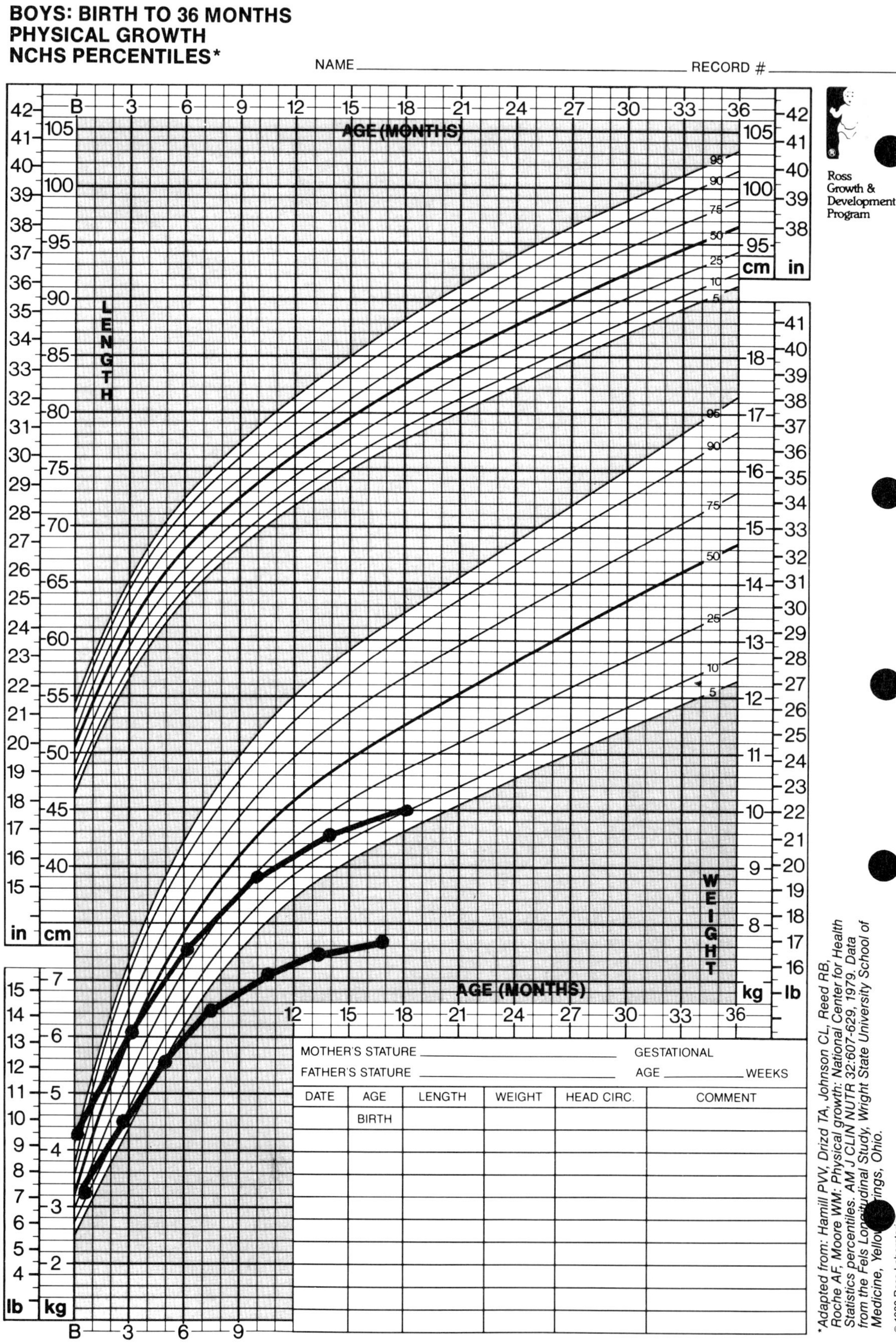

Figure 21–2. Two common forms of growth failure. Both require evaluation because the children are deviating from their established growth patterns. (© Am. J. Clin. Nutr. American Society for Clinical Nutrition.)

Table 21–3. EXPECTED DAILY CHANGES IN WEIGHT AND LENGTH

Age (months)	Weight Gain (gm/day)	Length Gain (mm/day)
0–3	25–30	0.9
3–6	20	0.7
6–9	15	0.5
9–12	10	0.4
12–18	8	0.4
18–24	6	0.3

From Karlberg PK, Engstrom I, Lichtenstein H, Svennberg I: The development of children in a Swedish urban community: A prospective longitudinal study. III. Physical growth during the first three years of life. Acta Paediatr Scand 1968; 187(Suppl):48–66; with permission.

Parents may initiate the evaluation by expressing concern about the child's growth; more commonly, careful examination of data plotted on standard growth curves alerts the clinician to potential problems. Thus it is crucial that height/length, weight, and head circumference be accurately measured and recorded at each scheduled visit to the physician's office. Growth data should be corrected for gestational age so that the truly premature infant is not misclassified. Once a problem is uncovered, potentially devastating illnesses should be excluded and common causes sought.

History

The evaluation begins with a careful history. If possible, both parents and any other caretakers should be present. The physician must make the parents comfortable and encourage them to be partners in the investigation. Spoken and unspoken accusations must be avoided. The physician must recognize that the term *failure to thrive* can be perceived as judgmental and may anger the parents. The focus should not be on thriving but rather on the reasons that the expected growth has not been achieved.

The perinatal history must be reviewed in detail. Maternal illnesses, drug and alcohol use, and smoking during pregnancy may result in low-birth-weight infants. Infants with failure to thrive are much more likely to have been small for their gestational age than controls; 10 to 40% percent of infants with failure to thrive have birth weights below 2,500 gm as compared to 7% of the general population.[4, 25, 26] Intrauterine growth retardation places the child at risk for subsequent growth problems. Placental insufficiency early in pregnancy produces infants that are symmetrically small (decreased length, weight, head circumference); these children tend to remain below the third percentile but grow along their own growth curves. Late placental insufficiency results in decreased weight with little or no effect on length or head circumference; these infants usually show "catch-up" growth by six months of age. High-risk perinatal conditions such as birth asphyxia or sepsis must be identified, since they may be the cause of unrecognized neurologic damage resulting in poor feeding. The neurologically injured child often has poor infant-parent interaction that is aggravated by the frustrations of poor feeding.[27]

The feeding history must be reviewed in detail, focusing on the type and amounts of feedings and any changes that have been made. Both the quantity and quality of the feedings should be investigated. Precise questions should be asked about the methods of formula preparation, since errors are frequent; in one study, up to 11% of infants' formula was improperly prepared.[28] The age at which solid foods were introduced should be noted; the onset of weight loss or poor gain after the introduction of cereals suggests celiac disease. Family eating patterns should be discussed, many families do not have regular mealtimes, and the child may be sipping low-calorie beverages or snacking all day.[29] Often, modifications in the infant's diet result in hypocaloric intake. Examples include dilute formula or clear liquids for gastrointestinal disorders and family health concerns about cholesterol, obesity, or other nutritional factors.[19, 20]

Both the child and the parents should be observed during a feeding. The length and vigor of the feeding are important; inability to suck or easy tiring are significant clues that may not be spontaneously volunteered. The interaction between the parents and the infant should be noted. Are the parents comfortable with feeding? What is the infant's response to feeding?

The medical history should focus on previous illnesses and hospitalizations. Any history of frequent infection must be clarified. The number and nature of the stools should be determined. Large foul-smelling stools are suggestive of fat malabsorption but may not be perceived as diarrhea by the parents. Excessive sweating or easy fatigue suggest cardiac disease. Recurring pulmonary symptoms may be the initial presentation of cystic fibrosis. Excessive urine output or a poor urinary stream in a male suggests renal disease. The infant's sleeping patterns should be examined; specifically, noisy breathing or snoring should be sought. Obstructive sleep apnea is an under-recognized cause of poor growth, perhaps because it interferes with nocturnal growth hormone secretion.[30] Factors that affect the metabolic rate should be investigated. Are there unexplained fevers? Is the child excessively active? Infants with spastic or athetoid cerebral palsy may have increased energy needs.[31]

The breast-fed infant poses a particular challenge. Two different syndromes have been reported: the infant who is underfed and responds by restless behavior and excessive crying, and the infant who fails to gain weight but offers no complaint.[32, 33] Maternal factors such as poor milk production due to inadequate diet, illness, or fatigue may cause poor weight gain. There may be interference with the normal "let-down" reflex, resulting in inadequate milk supply; smoking and excessive alcohol use may be the cause, but the most common reason is psychological inhibition due to maternal concerns, anxiety, or fear of disapproval.[34] In a group of 51 healthy Swedish women, half perceived a transient lactation crisis during which they produced insufficient milk.[35] The most common reasons were the maternal factors described earlier. However, when the crisis and noncrisis groups were compared, the mothers in the crisis group were found to have had more emotional discomfort with breast-feeding, breast-fed for the infant rather than for themselves, and weaned earlier. The infants in the crisis group had less breast-milk intake and gained weight more slowly than the infants in the noncrisis group.

Occasionally there is no obvious cause for the breast-fed infant's failure to gain weight; severe dehydration and hypernatremia have been reported.[36] For these reasons, the breast-feeding dyad should be seen at age 10 to 14 days. If there is concern about the amount of milk produced, the infant can be weighed before and after the feeding. Some perfectly normal breast-fed babies just gain weight slowly the first several weeks; they can be easily distinguished from infants with problems. The former infant gains steadily and is content, and the mother's breasts feel full. The breast-fed infant who fails to thrive is restless and cries excessively. The object after evaluation is to instill confidence in the mother; simple achievable goals should be prescribed. The mother, infant, and environment must interact harmoniously to ensure a successful breast-feeding experience.

The physical and psychological factors surrounding feeding must be examined. At the end of the interview the clinician should have a sense of the parents' comfort with feeding as well as the infant's feeding behavior and the infant-parent interaction.

The social history should be carefully reviewed. In the busy clinical setting, there is a tendency to minimize social factors. Yet a child's poor growth may be caused by social concerns and problems, the best correlation with failure to gain weight is poverty. The parents' past history should be reviewed; frequently there are "ghosts in the nursery."[37] Parents, when given the opportunity, often describe their own parental deprivation. The loss or death of a previous child may be the source of unresolved grief. The circumstances of the conception may be important: Was the child wanted? What financial burdens does this child place on the family? What supports are available? Is the father physically and emotionally involved? Parents may express feelings of being overwhelmed by the responsibilities associated with the infant; there may be feelings of loneliness, inadequate support, and depression.[38–41] During the interview, the physician must obtain an idea of the parents' level of functioning; one of the common causes of failure to thrive is a mother previously unrecognized as mildly retarded who has inadequate family support.[42]

The developmental history must be reviewed; 50 to 70% of infants with failure to thrive suffer some developmental delay, including lowered IQ and speech and reading delays.[3] The initial assessment should evaluate the severity and types of delay, since they are typically uneven. Gross motor function and speech tend to be the most affected; fine motor and visual areas are relatively spared. Cognitive function is decreased, but it is difficult to evaluate due to the depression that accompanies malnutrition. There may also be abnormalities of posture and muscle tone. Developmental catch-up may be noted after nutritional therapy; follow-up evaluations are helpful.

The timing of the onset of inadequate weight gain must be clarified. Many parents express concern about a child's decreased weight gain during the second year of life. This is usually due to the child's negativism and natural decrease in appetite at this age, and parental reassurance is usually all that is needed. However, any delay in reaching developmental milestones raises the possibility of central nervous system disease. The loss of previously acquired skills mandates the exclusion of neurodegenerative disorders and metabolic/storage disorders.

Parents' height and weight should be recorded; parents' height is the best predictor of ultimate stature.[43] An infant who was large at birth may not gain weight but rather "catch-down" to its genetic potential. This usually occurs in several months, and the infant's behavior remains appropriate. Family growth patterns should be examined, particularly if there is any history of constitutional delay of growth.[44]

Physical Examination

A global assessment of the infant's well-being should start the examination. The malnourished child has a wary, watchful appearance and avoids contact. When approached, the posture is one of avoidance. The infant appears apathetic and uninterested in the surroundings.[45] The child's general appearance should be examined for signs of neglect such as poor hygiene, severe diaper rash, unwashed skin, uncut fingernails, or filthy clothing. A flattened occiput and decreased hair suggest inadequate stimulation. The malnourished child has decreased subcutaneous fat, bony prominences, protuberant abdomen, flat buttocks, accentuated buccal sucking pads, muscle wasting, and poor tone.[46]

Anthropometric measurements must be carefully obtained and plotted. Weight is the first indicator to decline; weight loss with normal height and head circumference suggests acute malnutrition. Decline in height and head circumference indicates a chronic nutritional problem. It is useful to determine weight age and height age; these are obtained by taking the child's actual measurement and seeing at what age that represents the fiftieth percentile. The child's height and weight can be expressed as a percentage of the median for his or her age; this allows classification of the degree of malnutrition (Table 21–4).[47]

Table 21–4. ANTHROPOMETRIC MEASUREMENTS AND RISK

Weight/Age (%)	Height/Age (%)	Risk
<60	<70	Severe risk Hospitalize
61–75	70–80	Moderate risk Close outpatient evaluation
76–90	80–90	Low risk Outpatient follow-up

Determine weight/age and height/age by dividing the acutal measurement by the median value for age.

From Waterlow JC: Classification and definition of protein calorie malnutrition. Br Med J 1972; 3:566–569; with permission.

The child should be carefully examined for congenital malformations, especially minor anomalies such as body asymmetry and facial, ear, eye, and extremity malformations. The presence of one major anomaly or three minor anomalies increases the likelihood of a second major anomaly.[48]

Every organ system should be systematically examined. Signs of chronic pulmonary disease such as clubbing should be noted. The abdomen should be carefully palpated for organomegaly and masses; hepatomegaly may be present due to the fatty infiltration seen in malnutrition. Splenomegaly implies chronic disease, infection, or a storage disorder. A detailed neurologic examination must be performed, including a clinical assessment of sucking and swallowing. Oropharyngeal disorders are common, especially among infants with poor weight gain from lower socioeconomic groups, and they make feeding difficult[49] (Table 21–5).

Nutritional assessment should be part of the initial physical examination. Anthropometric measurements are helpful in defining the degree of nutritional deficit. The amount of subcutaneous tissue, the turgor and strength of the muscles, and any skin or mucous membrane lesions suggesting nutrient deficiency should be noted.

Laboratory Studies

The laboratory evaluation should be directed by the history and physical examination. Sills demonstrated that random laboratory investigations rarely uncover conditions unsuspected after the initial evaluation.[5] Homer and Ludwig confirmed that observation and demonstrated that the physical examination is the most sensitive indicator of organic disease.[6] The composite clinical history, physical examination, and psychosocial history are the most predictive indicators. Additionally, many laboratory studies, especially immunologic studies, are abnormal in cases of malnutrition.[50] A child with poor weight gain will develop immune deficiencies that lead to infections, loss of appetite, and further malnutrition. A better strategy is to nutritionally rehabilitate the child and then perform any indicated studies.

Useful screening studies include the complete blood count, looking for evidence of anemia. Anemia may be due to malnutrition, chronic blood loss, or chronic disease. A normal urinalysis and specific gravity greater than 1.015 exclude many serious renal problems. A lead level should also be obtained, since children with failure to thrive have increased lead levels. Malnutrition and iron deficiency also increase lead absorption.[51, 52]

Table 21–5. ORAL MOTOR ABNORMALITIES

Sucking, swallowing difficulties
Chewing difficulties
Tongue thrusting
Involuntary tonic biting
Excessive drooling
Intolerance for textures of developmentally appropriate foods

Modified from Mathisen B, Skuse D, Wolke D, et al: Oral-motor dysfunction and failure to thrive among inner city infants. Dev Med Child Neurol 1989; 31:293–302; with permission.

Although cystic fibrosis is a common cause of growth failure, the sweat chloride test should not be performed unless there are indications of pulmonary or gastrointestinal disease. Sweat electrolytes will be elevated in malnutrition; hence they should be tested after nutritional therapy.[53] Serum immunoreactive trypsinogen concentration has been proposed as a screening test, but there are many false positives, which may increase parental anxiety.[54]

Renal tubular acidosis may cause poor weight gain and is easily treated with citrate. Simultaneously measured serum electrolytes and urine pH will exclude this diagnosis.[55] Stool cultures should be obtained and examined for parasites if there is a history of chronic diarrhea or exposure to enteric pathogens such as in day care; in this setting, *Giardia lamblia* is a particular problem.[56] Serum albumin may be decreased because of malnutrition; however, the long half-life (21 days) makes rapid turnover proteins such as prealbumin and fibronectin better indicators of nutritional status.[57] Somatomedin C concentrations are also decreased, again a manifestation of nutritional status.[58] Serial determinations of these proteins are useful in gauging the response to nutritional therapy.[57, 59] The endocrine system is also affected by the degree of malnutrition: Growth hormone may be elevated, thyroid hormone is usually normal, but there is a decrease in T_4 and an increase in reverse T_3.[60]

Imaging should be based on the clinical history. A chest radiograph will help confirm suspected cardiac or pulmonary disease. The most common cause of vomiting in infants is gastroesophageal reflux; the upper gastrointestinal series is not sensitive or specific for the diagnosis of reflux.[61] The major benefit of the upper gastrointestinal series is to exclude anatomic abnormalities such as pyloric stenosis or malrotation.

A difficult question is when to test for human immunodeficiency virus (HIV) infection. Poor weight gain is a frequent feature of congenital HIV infection. Usually there are other symptoms such as chronic diarrhea, developmental delay, or opportunistic infections.[62] The decision to test should be based on the clinical findings, maternal risk factors, and the local epidemiology of HIV infection. Local regulations regarding consent for HIV testing must be followed.

Specific nutrient deficiencies are common in children with failure to grow—iron deficiency may be present in as many as half.[51] Iron deficiency itself may cause growth failure; it is also associated with neurodevelopmental sequelae.[63, 64] Rickets due to vitamin D deficiency has also been reported.[65]

Zinc deficiency also contributes to poor growth. Prassad and coworkers[66] demonstrated profound growth failure, anemia, and hypogonadism in adolescent Egyptian boys with severe zinc deficiency due to inadequate dietary zinc. Anorexia and altered taste are symptoms of zinc deficiency. It is uncertain whether inadequate dietary zinc causes the deficiency or whether some other factor, such as a prolonged diarrheal illness or impaired gastrointestinal absorption, is responsible. In any event,

Table 21–6. NUTRITIONAL PRINCIPLES

Nutritional assessment
Assessment of current dietary intake
Prescription of 1.5–2 RDA calories and protein to allow "catch-up" growth
Assessment of iron status
Multivitamin supplement; iron supplement if needed
Consideration of zinc supplementation
Close follow-up

RDA, recommended dietary allowance.

the resultant anorexia then perpetuates the problem. Walravens and associates showed zinc deficiency in a group of Head Start children with poor growth; in a double-blind controlled study, zinc supplementation resulted in increased energy and protein intake as well as improved growth.[67] Vanderkooy and Gibson[68] demonstrated lower height for age percentiles in boys with decreased hair zinc. Dietary zinc was inadequate, and the diets were rich in dairy products, which interfere with zinc absorption. This was interpreted as a growth-limiting mild zinc deficiency. Buzina and colleagues[69] demonstrated altered taste and zinc deficiency in children with delayed growth. Friel and associates[70] noted that premature infants with poor growth were more likely to have decreased zinc intake.

Zinc deficiency is difficult to determine biochemically; serum zinc concentrations give false positives and false negatives. Leukocyte or erythrocyte zinc is the best indicator of zinc status, but it is not readily available and is impractical to measure in small infants.[71] A trial of zinc sulfate (5 mg per day) can have dramatic results; changes in appetite and intake are usually apparent within several days.

THERAPY

Therapy is initially directed at the major medical problem: malnutrition and its complications. If present, fluid and electrolyte disturbances should be corrected. Nutritional principles are outlined in Table 21–6. Malnourished infants often require 110 to 200% of the normal dietary intake for catch-up growth.[72] This increased energy requirement will result in a large fluid intake, which may be beyond the infant's tolerance. In addition, there must be concern about the refeeding syndrome.[73] Infants and children with severe malnutrition may develop hypokalemia, hypophosphatemia, edema, and cardiac failure if refed too rapidly. Therefore, the caloric intake should be advanced slowly over 7 to 10 days and the child closely observed. The child may not be able to tolerate a lactose-containing formula if there has been any degree of intestinal injury. The volume and concentration of the formula are gradually increased until the calculated energy requirement is reached. One useful formula is:

$$\text{Energy Requirement for Catch-up (kcal/kg/day)} = \frac{\text{Calories Required for Weight Age} \times \text{Ideal Weight for Age (kg)}}{\text{Actual Weight (kg)}}$$

A similar calculation can be used for protein requirements. The ideal weight gain should be 30 gm per day in an infant and 60 to 90 gm per day in an older child.[74] Obviously several weeks will be required until there is significant weight gain.

Mildly malnourished patients can be treated as outpatients with close follow-up. Table 21–7 lists the indications for hospitalization. The nutritional rehabilitation can usually be provided by mouth. If the child is unable to consume adequate calories by mouth and the gastrointestinal tract is functioning, nutrition should be provided by the enteral route. Nasogastric feedings are the preferred method. If the child is intolerant to bolus feedings, continuous feedings via a small-bore nasoenteric tube may be helpful.[75] If vomiting is a major clinical concern, a nasojejunal tube can be inserted. Nasojejunal feedings should be administered continuously via a pump. If a more permanent enteric access is necessary, a gastrostomy tube can be placed surgically, endoscopically, or radiographically. Parenteral nutrition is rarely required for these conditions unless there is severe gastrointestinal compromise.

Therapy must include attention to the social and dietary factors that led to the poor growth. A nutritionist should be involved in family education. The nutritional advice given must be appropriate for the family's culture and economic means. For example, telling a single mother with three other children to give "three ounces of a powdered formula mixed with MCT oil every two hours" is guaranteed to fail. Basic nutritional information as well as specific feeding behavior guidelines should be provided.

Social workers and other mental health workers are necessary to deal with the numerous stresses present.[76] This multidisciplinary effort is crucial, since there are well-documented sequelae. It is difficult to separate environmental and nutritional factors, but poor nutrition and environmental deprivation frequently coexist. The goal of intervention is to prevent long-term growth and developmental disabilities. This requires adequate nutrition and restructuring of the environment to provide proper affective and cognitive stimulation.

Few of the published series have controlled for genetic growth potential, yet all have demonstrated some long-term physical, cognitive, or behavioral problems.[77–82] In several uncontrolled studies, 20 to 33% of children's weights and 5 to 33% of their heights were below the third to tenth percentile. Elmer and coworkers controlled for midparental height and found that 60% were at less than the third percentile at follow-up.[77] Chase and Martin, in a 3½-year follow-up, showed deficits in height, weight, and head circumference (68%, 53%, and

Table 21–7. CRITERIA FOR HOSPITALIZATION

Severe protein-calorie malnutrition, dehydration
Electrolyte abnormalities, especially hypokalemia, hypophosphatemia
Abused or seriously neglected children*
Failure of outpatient therapy

*Virtually all failure-to-thrive mortality is related to abuse.

37%, respectively).[78] Up to 50% of children may have some cognitive impairment, including school difficulties, and mild to moderate mental retardation.[79, 80] Teachers have rated these children as more difficult in the classroom. One quarter to one half have behavioral problems.[79] Mitchell and colleagues controlled for family problems and found no difference.[4] Chase and Martin[78] documented more difficult parent-child interactions, which might lead to further difficulties. Elmer and coworkers found that, at follow-up, approximately 60% of children suffered from anxiety or depression. Only two of the fifteen children were considered to be normal in growth, behavior, and intellectual ability.

The effects of malnutrition seem to be related to timing, duration, and etiology. Those whose malnutrition began after age 4 months had more cognitive problems than those who were malnourished in the first 4 months of life.[78] Expressive language is the most affected. Even mild medical illnesses can have a profound effect. Infants with pyloric stenosis who lost 10% of their body weight had increased learning problems, especially with attention and short-term memory.[80] Hufton and Oates[81] found that two thirds of the children they followed had abnormal personalities.

That only 13% of infants with failure to thrive are subsequently normal is a sobering statistic. Much more work is required in the early identification and prevention of this devastating condition. Altemeier and colleagues[82] have shown that antecedents for this syndrome can be identified prospectively. Risk factors include aberrant nurturing during the mother's childhood and conflicts between the parents of infants. Perinatal risk factors include pregnancy complications, short gestation, and residual minor medical problems.[82] By utilizing such data, we must begin to identify high-risk families and intervene before the morbidity and occasional mortality develop.

REFERENCES

1. Martin HP: Nutrition: Its relationship to children's physical, mental and emotional development. Am J Clin Nutr 1973; 26:766–775.
2. Stein Z, Susser M, Saenger G, et al: Nutrition and mental performance. Science 1978; 178:708–713.
3. Berwick DM: Non-organic failure to thrive. Pediatric Rev 1980; 1:265–270.
4. Mitchell W, Gorrell R, Greenberg R: Failure to thrive: A study in a primary care setting. Pediatrics 1980; 65:971–977.
5. Sills RH: Failure to thrive: The role of clinical and laboratory evaluation. Am J Dis Child 1978; 132:967–969.
6. Homer C, Ludwig S: Categorization of the etiology of failure to thrive. Am J Dis Child 1981; 135:848–851.
7. Cupoli JM, Hallock JA, Barness LA: Failure to thrive. Current Prob Pediatr 1980; 10:1–43.
8. Chapin HD: Are institutions for infants necessary? JAMA 1915; 64:1–3.
9. Bakwin H: Emotional deprivation in infants. J Pediatr 1949; 35:512–521.
10. Spitz RA, Wolff K: Anaclitic depression: An inquiry into the genesis of psychiatric conditions in early childhood. Psychoanal Study Child 1946; 2:313–339.
11. Widdowson EM: Mental contentment and physical growth. Lancet 1951; 1:1316–1318.
12. Talbot N: Dwarfism in healthy children: Its possible relation to emotional, nutritional and endocrine disturbances. New Engl J Med 1947; 236:783–793.
13. Coleman R, Provence S: Environmental retardation (hospitalism) in children living in families. Pediatrics 1957; 19:285–292.
14. Powell GR, Brasel JA, Blizzard RM: Emotional deprivation and growth retardation simulating idiopathic hypopituitarism. New Engl J Med 1967; 276:1271–1277, 1279–1283.
15. Whitten CR, Pettit MG, Fischoff J: Evidence that growth failure from maternal deprivation is secondary to undereating. JAMA 1969; 209:1675–1682.
16. Sameroff A, Chandler MJ: Reproductive risk and the continuum of caretaking casualty. *In* Horowitz PD, ed: Review of Child Development Research. Chicago, University of Chicago Press, 1978.
17. Rosenn D, Loeb L, Jura M: Differentiation of organic from non-organic failure to thrive syndrome in infancy. Pediatrics 1980; 66:698–704.
18. Gaensbauer TJ, Sands K: Distorted affective communications in abused/neglected infants and their potential impact on caretakers. J Am Acad Child Psychiatry 1979; 18:236–250.
19. Pugliese MT, Lifshitz F, Grad G, et al: Fear of obesity: A cause of short stature and delayed puberty. New Engl J Med 1983; 309:513–518.
20. Pugliese MT, Weyman-Daum M, Moses N, et al: Parental health beliefs as a cause of non-organic failure to thrive. Pediatrics 1978; 80:175–182.
21. Rathbun JM, Peterson KE: Nutrition in failure to thrive. *In* Grand RJ, Sutphen JL, Dietz WH, eds: Pediatric Nutrition: History and Practice. Boston, Butterworth Publishers, 1987.
22. Fomon SJ: Infant Nutrition. Philadelphia, WB Saunders, 1974.
23. Frank DA, Zeisel SH: Failure to thrive. Pediatr Clin North Am 1988; 35:1187–1206.
24. Karlberg PK, Engstrom I, Lichtenstein H, et al: The development of children in a Swedish urban community: A prospective longitudinal study. III. Physical growth during the first three years of life. Acta Paed Scand 1968; 187(Suppl):48–66.
25. Oates RK, Yu J: Children with non-organic failure to thrive: A community problem. Med J Australia 1971; 2:199–203.
26. Shaheen E, Alexander D, Truskowsky M, et al: Failure to thrive: A retrospective profile. Clin Pediatr 1986; 7:255–261.
27. Starret AL: Neurological and developmental disorders causing growth failure in infancy. *In* Accardo PJ, ed: Failure to Thrive in Infancy and Early Childhood: A Multidisciplinary Team Approach. Baltimore, University Park Press, 1982.
28. McJunkin JE, Bithoney WJ, McCormick MC: Errors in formula concentration in an outpatient population. J Pediatr 1987; 111:848–850.
29. Petersen KE, Washington J, Rathbun JM: Team management of failure to thrive. J Am Diet Assoc 1984; 84:810–815.
30. Williams EF, Woo P, Miller R, et al: The effects of adenotonsillectomy on growth in young children. Otolaryngol Head Neck Surg 1991; 104:509–514.
31. Culley WJ, Middleton TO: Caloric requirements of mentally retarded children with and without motor dysfunction. J Pediatr 1969; 75:380–384.
32. Gilmore HE, Rowland TW: Critical malnutrition in breast-fed infants. Am J Dis Child 1978; 132:885–887.
33. Davies DP, Evans TJ: Failure to thrive at the breast. Lancet 1976; 2:1194–1195.
34. Lawrence RA: Breastfeeding: A guide for the medical profession. 2nd ed. St. Louis, CV Mosby, 1985.
35. Hillervik-Lindquist C: Studies on perceived breast milk insufficiency: A prospective study in a group of Swedish women. Acta Paed Scand 1991; 376(Suppl):1–27.
36. Rowland TW, Zori RT, Lafleur WR, et al: Malnutrition and hypernatremic dehydration in breast-fed infants. JAMA 1982; 247:1016–1017.
37. Fraiberg S, Adelsen E, Shapiro V: Ghosts in the nursery. J Am Acad Child Psychiatry 1975; 14:387–422.
38. Pollit E, Eichler AW, Chan CK: Psychosocial development and behavior of mothers of failure to thrive infants. Am J Orthopsychiat 1975; 45:525–536.
39. Fischoff J, Whitten CF, Pettit MG: A psychiatric study of mothers of infants with growth failure secondary to maternal deprivation. J Pediatr 1971; 79:209–215.
40. Fosson A, Wilson J: Family interactions surrounding feedings on

infants with non-organic failure to thrive. Clin Pediatr 1987; 26:518–523.
41. Heptinstall E, Puckering C, Skuske D, et al: Nutrition and mealtime behavior in families of growth retarded children. Human Nutr: Appl Nutr 1987; 41A:309–402.
42. Sheridan MD. The intelligence of 100 neglectful mothers. Brit Med J 1956; 1:91–93.
43. Wingard J, Schoen EJ: Factors influencing length at birth and height at five years. Pediatrics 1974; 53:737–741.
44. Rallison ML: Growth disorders in infants, children and adolescents. New York, John Wiley and Sons, 1986.
45. Powell GF, Low J: Behavior in nonorganic failure to thrive. J Dev Behav Pediatr 1983; 4:26–33.
46. Barness LA: Manual of pediatric physical diagnosis. 5th ed. Chicago, Year Book Medical Publishers, 1981.
47. Waterlow JC: Classification and definition of protein calorie malnutrition. Brit Med J 1972; 3:566–569.
48. Marden PM, Smith DW, McDonald MJ: Congenital anomalies in the newborn infant, including minor variations. J Pediatr 1964; 64–357.
49. Mathisen B, Skuse D, Wolke D, et al: Oral-motor dysfunction and failure to thrive among inner city infants. Develop Med Child Neurol 1989; 31:293–302.
50. Chandra RK: Nutrition and immunity. Am J Clin Nutr 1991; 53:1087–1101.
51. Bithoney WG: Elevated lead levels in children with non-organic failure to thrive. Pediatrics 1986; 78:891–895.
52. Schwartz J, Angle C, Pitcher H: Relationship between childhood lead levels and stature. Pediatrics 1986; 77:281–288.
53. Christoffel KS, Lloyd-Still JD, Brown G, et al: Environmental deprivation and transient elevation of sweat electrolytes. J Pediatr 1985; 107:231–234.
54. Rock MJ, Mischler EH, Farrell PM, et al: Newborn screening for cystic fibrosis is complicated by age-related decline in immunoreactive trypsinogen levels. Pediatrics 1990; 85:1001–1007.
55. Santos O, Chan JCM: Renal tubular acidosis in children: Diagnosis, treatment and prognosis. Am J Nephrol 1986; 6:289–295.
56. Bartlett AV, Englender SJ, Jarvis BA, et al: Controlled trial of *Giardia lamblia:* Control strategies in day care centers. Am J Public Health 1991; 81:1001–1006.
57. Yoder MC, Anderson DC, Gopalakrishna GS, et al: Comparison of serum fibronectin, prealbumin and albumin concentrations during nutritional repletion in protein-calorie malnourished infants. J Pediatr Gastroenterol Nutr 1987; 6:84–88.
58. Clemmons RL, Klebanski A, Underwood LE, et al: Reduction of plasma immunoreactive somatomedin C during fasting in humans. J Clin Endocrinol Metab 1981; 53:1247–1250.
59. Clemmons DR, Underwood LE, Dickerson RN, et al: Use of plasma somatomedin C/insulin-like growth factor I measurements to monitor the response to nutritional repletion in malnourished patients. Am J Clin Nutr 1985; 41:191–198.
60. Smith IF, Latham MC, Azubuike JA, et al: Blood plasma levels of cortisol, insulin, growth hormone and somatomedin in children with marasmus, kwashiorkor and intermediate forms of protein-energy malnutrition. Proc Soc Exp Biol Med 1981; 167:607–611.
61. Sondheimer JM: Gastroesophageal reflux: Update on pathogenesis and diagnosis. Pediatr Clin North Am 1988; 35:103–116.
62. Scott GB, Buck BE, Leterman JG, et al: Acquired immunodeficiency syndrome in infants. New Engl J Med 1984; 301:76–80.
63. Lozoff B, Jimenez E, Wolf AW: Long-term developmental outcome of infants with iron deficiency. New Engl J Med 1991; 325:687–694.
64. Palti H, Maijer A, Adler B: Learning achievement and behavior at school of anemic and non-anemic infants. Early Human Develop 1985; 10:217–223.
65. Hayward I, Stein MT, Gibson MI: Nutritional rickets in San Diego. Am J Dis Child 1987; 141:1060–1062.
66. Prassad AS, Miale A, Farid Z, et al: Zinc metabolism in normals and patients with the syndrome of iron deficiency anemia, hypogonadism and dwarfism. J Clin Lab Med 1963; 61:537–549.
67. Walravens PA, Hambidge KM, Koepfter DM: Zinc supplementation in infants with a nutritional pattern of failure to thrive: A double blind, controlled study. Pediatrics 1989; 83:532–538.
68. Vanderkooy PD, Gibson RS: Food consumption patterns of Canadian preschool children in relation to zinc and growth status. Am J Clin Nutr 1987; 45:609–616.
69. Buzina R, Sapunar J, Milanovic N: Zinc nutrition and taste acuity in school children with impaired growth. Am J Clin Nutr 1980; 33:2262–2267.
70. Friel JK, Gibson RS, Kawash GF, et al: Dietary zinc intake and growth during infancy. J Pediatr Gastroenterol Nutr 1985; 4:747–751.
71. Gordon EF, Gordon TV, Passal DB: Zinc metabolism: Basic clinical and behavioral aspects. J Pediatr 1981; 99:341–349.
72. Ashworth A, Bell R, James WPT, et al: Calorie requirements of children recovering from protein calorie malnutrition. Lancet 1968; 1:600–602.
73. Mezoff AG, Gremse DA, Farrell MK: Hypophosphatemia in the nutritional recovery syndrome. Am J Dis Child 1989; 143:1111–1112.
74. Murray C, Glassman M: Nutrient requirements during growth and recovery from failure to thrive. *In* Accardo PJ, ed: Failure to Thrive in Infancy and Early Childhood: A Multidisciplinary Team Approach. Baltimore, University Park Press, 1982.
75. Parker P, Stroop S, Greene H: A controlled comparison of continuous versus intermittent feeding in the treatment of infants with intestinal disease. J Pediatr 1981; 99:360–364.
76. Accardo PJ, ed: Failure to Thrive in Infancy and Early Childhood: A Multidisciplinary Team Approach. Baltimore, University Park Press, 1982.
77. Elmer E, Gregg GS, Ellison P: Late results of the "failure to thrive" syndrome. Clin Pediatr 1969; 8:584–589.
78. Chase HP, Martin HP: Undernutrition and child development. N Engl J Med 1970; 282:933–939.
79. Pollitt E, Eichler A: Behavioral disturbances among failure to thrive children. Am J Dis Child 1976; 130:24–29.
80. Klein PS, Forbes GB, Nader PR: Effects of starvation in infancy (pyloric stenosis) on subsequent learning abilities. J Pediatr 1975; 87:8–15.
81. Hufton IW, Oates RK: Nonorganic failure to thrive: A long-term follow-up. Pediatrics 1977; 59:73–77.
82. Altemeier WA, O'Connor SM, Sherrod KB, et al: Prospective study of antecedents for nonorganic failure to thrive. J Pediatr 1985; 106:360–365.

Chapter 22

Abdominal Masses

PATRICK J. HEALEY and DONALD W. HIGHT

The discovery of an abdominal mass in a pediatric patient presents a complex challenge to both the pediatrician and the pediatric surgeon. Despite the fact that more than half of palpable abdominal masses are secondary to organomegaly and are of a nonsurgical nature, parents and treating physicians often anticipate the threat of incurable cancer or major surgery. A detailed clinical history including the family and maternal background must be obtained, and a thorough physical examination must be performed to generate a differential diagnosis suggesting the cause and the extent of disease. An expeditious work-up using pertinent laboratory studies and noninvasive imaging techniques is essential to assure prompt diagnosis and treatment.

The differential diagnosis and work-up vary according to the age of the patient. Most abdominal masses in the neonate are benign (87%) and are located in the retroperitoneum (90%). More than 50% of these benign conditions originate within the urinary tract, including hydronephrosis, multicystic dysplastic kidney, and renal vein thrombosis. Only 13% of abdominal masses in neonates are malignant, including sacrococcygeal teratoma, neuroblastoma, Wilms' and liver tumor, and lymphoma. Fewer than 10 to 15% of palpable abdominal masses in the neonate involve the gastrointestinal tract.[1] As the age of the patient increases, so does the likelihood of a solid mass being malignant. Retroperitoneal malignancy accounts for approximately 50% of abdominal masses in patients older than 1 year of age.[1] In later childhood, liver tumors, appendiceal abscesses, cysts of the omentum and bile duct, and ovarian tumors may present as palpable masses in the region of the epigastrium or pelvis.

DIAGNOSTIC IMAGING

Plain Abdominal Radiographs

Following physical examination, plain abdominal radiographs of the abdomen should be obtained. This technique is inexpensive and emits low ionizing radiation. As a single noninvasive examination, it permits evaluation of bowel gas pattern, bony abnormalities, and the presence of soft tissue densities or calcification. Displacement of the normal position of the kidney, liver, spleen, or bowel gas pattern may also suggest a retroperitoneal mass (Fig. 22–1). Stippled calcification is characteristic of neuroblastoma, whereas linear calcifications may suggest polycystic renal diseases or Wilms' tumor.

Ultrasound

Abdominal ultrasound has replaced excretory urography as the preferred study in the work-up of abdominal masses.[2] It is rapid and noninvasive and uses no ionizing radiation. Ultrasonography can quickly differentiate cystic from solid masses. It is readily available at most institutions and can usually be performed with minimal sedation or special preparation. Doppler ultrasound adds the capability of measuring blood flow in both the venous and arterial systems and is used when vascular lesions are suspected. Vascular flow rates are helpful in diagnosing hepatic lesions or when portal vein thrombosis or hemangiomas are suspected. Prenatal ultrasound has been helpful in detecting abdominal masses in the fetus, including renal and gastrointestinal masses as well as diaphragmatic hernia and congenital cardiac anomalies. Disadvantages of ultrasonography are its extreme operator dependency and limitations of imaging resulting from overlying bowel gas patterns or bone.

Computed Tomography

Computed tomography (CT) scans can provide serial cross-imaging of the abdomen and yield an excellent evaluation of intra-abdominal organs and retroperitoneal and pelvic masses. Resolution of objects down to 1 cm is enhanced with the use of intravenous or enteral contrast solution. Displacement of the kidney and ureter and caliceal dilatation are readily demonstrated (Fig. 22–2). Vascular tumors may demonstrate a peripheral region of contrast enhancement with central lucency. Because CT scan imaging requires a cooperative, motionless subject, sedation or general anesthesia is necessary in pediatric patients. The disadvantages of cost and exposure to ionizing radiation are outweighed by the accurate information gained, reducing the need for collaborative studies.

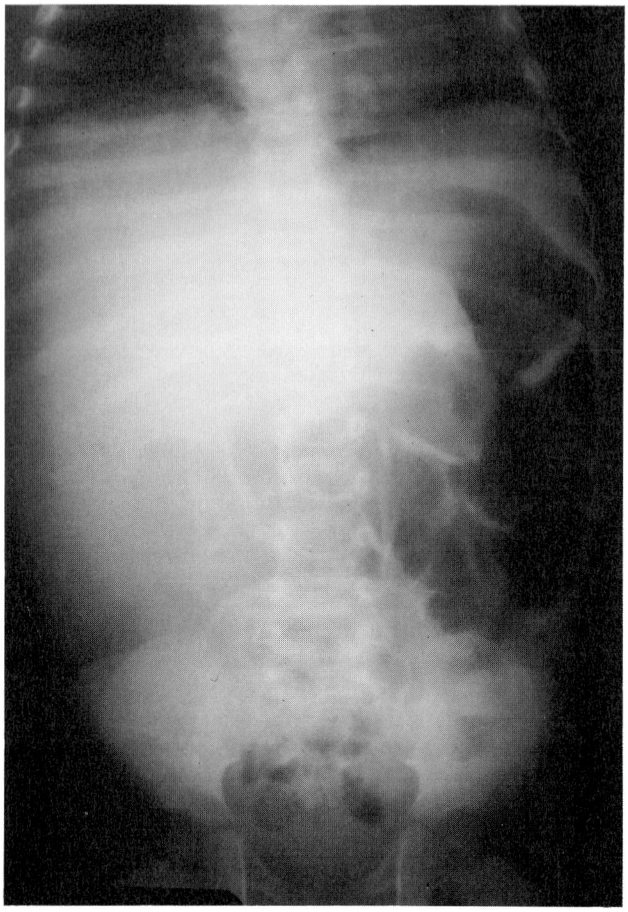

Figure 22–1. Plain radiograph of the abdomen showing a large right flank mass with visceral displacement.

Magnetic Resonance Imaging

Magnetic resonance (MR) imaging uses nonionizing radiation and yields high-resolution images in the axial and coronal planes.[3] It provides excellent tissue plane differentiation and does not require intravenous contrast. However, young children must be either sedated or administered general anesthesia to obtain high-resolution studies. As a relatively new technology, its exact role in the evaluation of pediatric abdominal masses has not been completely defined. MR imaging has proved to be as accurate as CT scans in the evaluation of solid lesions of the kidney, liver, and adrenal gland. It can define invasion of tissue planes, assess bone marrow, and show tumor involvement of the inferior vena cava, mediastinum, and spinal cord. MR imaging has also proved useful in evaluating resectability, preoperative staging of metastatic disease, and local extension of disease. Although there is an ever-expanding role for MR imaging, CT remains the procedure of choice for staging Wilms' tumor and defining the presence of intrapulmonary lesions.

Intravenous Urography

Dependence on intravenous urography to differentiate neuroblastoma from Wilms' tumor has been replaced by the use of either CT scan or MRI. Intravenous pyelograms are still useful in demonstrating the excretory function of the kidneys and in defining congenital renal anomalies such as obstructive ureteropelvic junction or renal ectopia. With the ever-present risk of anaphylactic reaction to the iodinated contrast material, one should strive to define abdominal masses by one of the alternative diagnostic imaging techniques.

ABDOMINAL MASSES IN NEONATES

Hydronephrosis

The most common cause of abdominal masses in the neonate, hydronephrosis is a dilatation of the renal pelvis and collecting system resulting from either mechanical or functional obstruction of the urinary outflow tract. Obstruction of the ureteropelvic junction often causes massive dilatation of the renal pelvis. The obstruction may be due to extrinsic compression from an aberrant accessory artery to the lower pole of the kidney or the result of a dysfunctional segment of the ureter. Chronic vesicoureteral reflux causes an elevated hydrostatic pressure and a functional obstruction of the ureter, leading to hydronephrosis and hydroureter. The inflammation caused by pyelonephritis may lead to ureteral strictures and subsequent hydronephrosis.

Bilateral hydronephrosis is found in 15% of infants and is associated with hydroureters and distention of the urinary bladder. In the male neonate this is most commonly due to posterior urethral valves (Fig. 22–3). These infants present with a distended abdomen, overflow incontinence, and bilateral flank masses. Such prolonged in utero renal obstruction may lead to renal failure and urinary ascites. Ultrasound demonstrates a dilated collecting system and renal pelvis along with a residual rim of renal parenchyma.

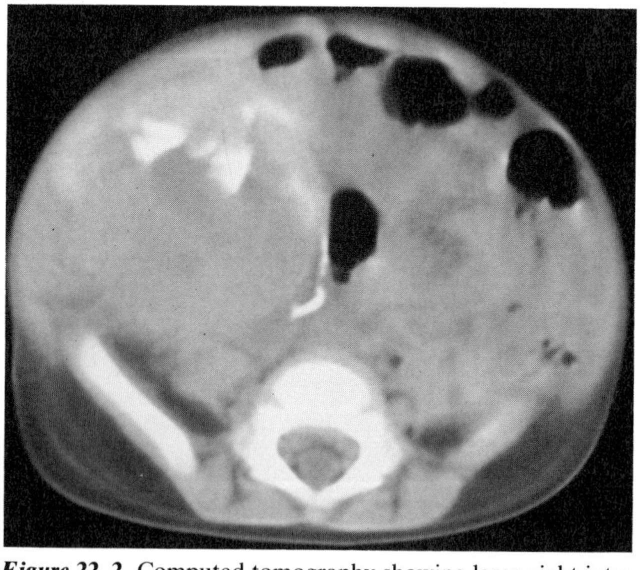

Figure 22–2. Computed tomography showing large right intrarenal mass with extension into and compression of adjacent structures.

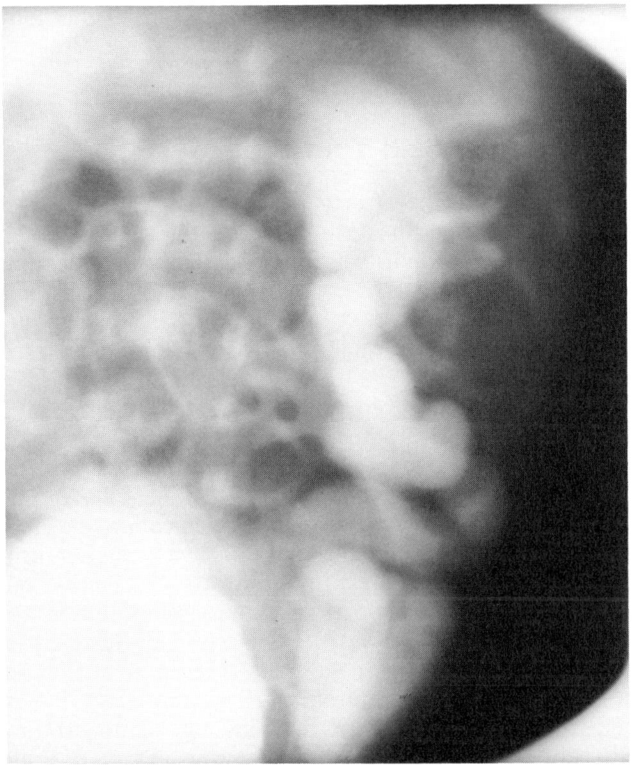

Figure 22–3. Voiding cystourethrogram showing severe ureteral dilatation associated with posterior urethral valves.

Multicystic Dysplastic Kidney

Multicystic dysplastic kidney (MCDK) comprises multiloculated cysts and a solid central core, with 60% discovered incidentally by the age of 1 year. The dysplastic collecting tubules become distended with urine after nephron formation is complete by the 20th week of gestation. A cycle of elevated hydrostatic pressure and tissue ischemia and hypoxia leads to necrosis and fibrosis of individual nephrons and subsequent loss of renal function.[4] A gradual involution of cysts then occurs. Macroscopically the proximal ureter is usually absent or atretic, and the renal artery is found to be hypoplastic. MCDK is frequently unilateral, but 15 to 20% occur bilaterally, with no sex or familial predilection. Plain roentgenograms show eggshell calcification in older patients. Renal ultrasound demonstrates grape clusters of multiloculated cysts. An intravenous pyelogram or renal scan may show little, if any, functional excretion. Retrograde pyelograms document an atretic or obstructed proximal collecting system.

In utero diagnosis may be made by 28 weeks of gestation using prenatal ultrasound. Unfortunately, involution of renal cysts in the developing fetus is not associated with improvement in renal function. Although nonoperative management has been suggested, nephrectomy in the neonate is usually recommended owing to the high likelihood of the subsequent onset of pain, infection, or hypertension or the chance of malignant tumor degeneration. Hydronephrosis or ureteropelvic obstruction has been reported in the contralateral kidney in as many as 20% of patients.[5] Preoperative ultrasonographic imaging and careful exploration at the time of surgery should be performed to exclude coexisting anomalies in the opposite kidney.

Renal Vein Thrombosis

Neonates presenting with a firm, smooth flank mass, abdominal distention, hypernatremia, and hematuria following stress or a septic period may have developed renal vein thrombosis. This entity follows hypoperfusion of the kidney due to shock, sepsis, or hemoconcentration. Antecedent gastrointestinal disease or perinatal sepsis may also produce this condition. Unless hemodynamic instability is rapidly corrected, venous thrombosis may then progress to renal arterial compromise and parenchymal infarction. Renal vein thrombosis has been associated with steroid and thiazide use during pregnancy,[6] maternal diabetes, and hypoglycemic seizures in the neonate.[1]

Findings on ultrasound show a diffusely enlarged, edematous kidney with increased echogenicity. Presence of thrombus in the inferior vena cava or encroachment of the contralateral renal vein may also be seen. The renal perfusion scan may range from nonvisualization to normal function, depending on the contralateral blood flow and the acuteness of the venous thrombosis.[1] Treatment should be supportive, with attention to underlying hypovolemia, resuscitation, and management of transient renal insufficiency. Anticoagulation is indicated if there is clinical evidence of pulmonary embolism or if there is high risk from embolism or clot in the inferior vena cava. Thrombectomy has been proposed in the older child with acute venous occlusion. Renal function generally improves with supportive measures, although nephrectomy may be necessary if uncontrollable sepsis or hypertension develops.[1] Thrombectomy of the renal vein is seldom indicated owing to the high rate of recurrent thrombosis.

Infantile Polycystic Kidney Disease

Infantile polycystic kidney disease (PKD), an autosomal-recessive disease, is usually discovered incidentally in the first few days of life. The excretory urogram outlines a cyst-filled kidney with a spongelike appearance. Ultrasound may demonstrate diffuse bilateral renal enlargement and increased echogenicity due to multiple small cysts. It is typically bilateral and may be associated with both cystic and fibrotic disease of the liver. Renal parenchymal cysts develop as a result of tubular ectasia. The clinical spectrum of infantile PKD may range from severe renal tubular disease with minimal hepatic involvement to scant renal disease with extensive hepatic fibrosis. A perfusion scan confirms nephromegaly with scant renal blood flow. Treatment is supportive and nonoperative in the neonatal period. Renal transplantation may be an option.

Mesoblastic Nephroma

Mesoblastic nephroma is the most common renal tumor in the neonate.[7] This benign neoplasm is a solid unencapsulated mass of disordered renal parenchyma. Bundles of connective tissue growing between intact nephrons may exhibit an infiltrative growth pattern at the interface of normal renal parenchyma.[8] This has been referred to as a fetal hamartoma or benign congenital Wilms' tumor. Recent studies have suggested a pathologic spectrum of disease, with classic benign nodular mesoblastic nephroma at one end and spindle cell sarcoma at the other.[9] Distention of the pelvocaliceal system as demonstrated by intravenous pyelography makes it indistinguishable from Wilms' tumor. Nephrectomy alone is curative in typical nodular disease, whereas adjuvant chemotherapy in older children is indicated if renal margins are grossly involved or histologically malignant.[9]

Nephroblastomatosis

A rare lesion of the neonatal kidney, nephroblastomatosis is characterized by small localized nodules along with bilateral subcapsule aggregates of persistent renal blastoma. This tissue is believed to be a precursor to Wilms' tumor. Multifocal nephroblastomatosis has been reported in 25% of patients with Wilms' tumor.[8] Ultrasound demonstrates solid echogenic or subcortical nodules along with bilateral renal enlargement. Intravenous pyelogram may show nephromegaly with pelvocaliceal distention resembling Wilms' tumor or adult PKD.[10] The treatment is controversial and requires a biopsy of renal parenchyma and a careful evaluation of bilateral renal function.

Adrenal Hemorrhage

Spontaneous hemorrhage into the adrenal gland produces an adrenal mass in the neonatal period. The incidence in neonates is 1.7 per 1,000; hemorrhage involves the right adrenal gland in 70%[7] of cases and is bilateral in 8 to 10%.[9] The etiology is related to sepsis, stress or associated birth trauma, asphyxia, or anoxic encephalopathy. These clinical conditions most frequently present during the first week of life. The neonate appears acutely ill, with an associated epigastric or flank mass. Spontaneous hemorrhage occurs within the gland, and ultrasound demonstrates an echoic suprarenal mass with variable compression and displacement of the kidney. Subsequent follow-up imaging may show a mixed echogenic pattern as the formed clot and calcification appear. Differentiation between hemorrhagic neuroblastoma and other associated benign masses may be difficult. Measurements of urinary catecholamines should be performed to rule out neuroblastoma. Treatment, once established, is generally supportive, nonoperative, and directed at correcting the underlying illness. Adrenal hemorrhage is usually resorbed with expectant management. Exploration is necessary only if the hematoma continues to expand or the clot liquifies, creating a large retroperitoneal cyst.

Sacrococcygeal Teratoma

Sacrococcygeal teratoma often presents at birth as a large external mass posterior to the anus (Fig. 22–4). It may also occur primarily as an abdominal or pelvic mass palpable by bimanual rectal examination. Intraspinal extension can produce symptomatic neurologic sequelae. The tumor is thought to arise from the coccyx, although the precise site of origin may vary. It is frequently detectable in utero by prenatal ultrasound. The majority of teratomas diagnosed at birth are benign (90%), whereas over 70% of those found at 4 months or later contain malignant neural elements.[9] Favorable features include the presence of calcification or large cystic elements. Malignant tumors have a higher proportion of solid tissue, with infiltrative elements and numerous areas of hemorrhage. Plain abdominal x-rays may show calcification. Although ultrasound is helpful in defining the extent of the mass relative to structures in the pelvis and the genitourinary system, the CT scan helps define the extent of the mass by demonstrating adjacent tissue invasion as well as the extent of solid and cystic components within the tumor mass. Calcification and the extent of vascularization or intraspinal extension[9] are best defined by intravenous contrast material enhancement of the CT scan examination. Treatment is complete surgical excision, including the removal of the coccyx. Less than 10% of these tumors require adjuvant chemotherapy if surgical excision is possible. Two-year postoperative follow-up examinations should include rectal examination to look for recurrent presacral tumor.

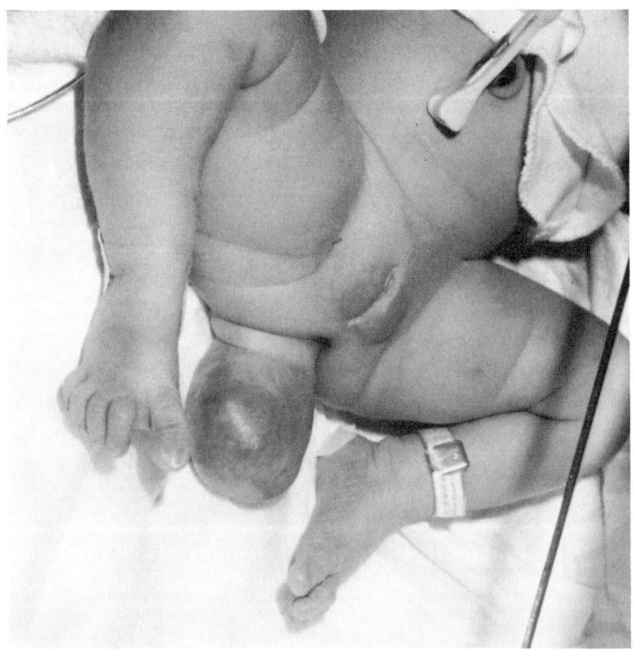

Figure 22–4. Infant with sacrococcygeal teratoma.

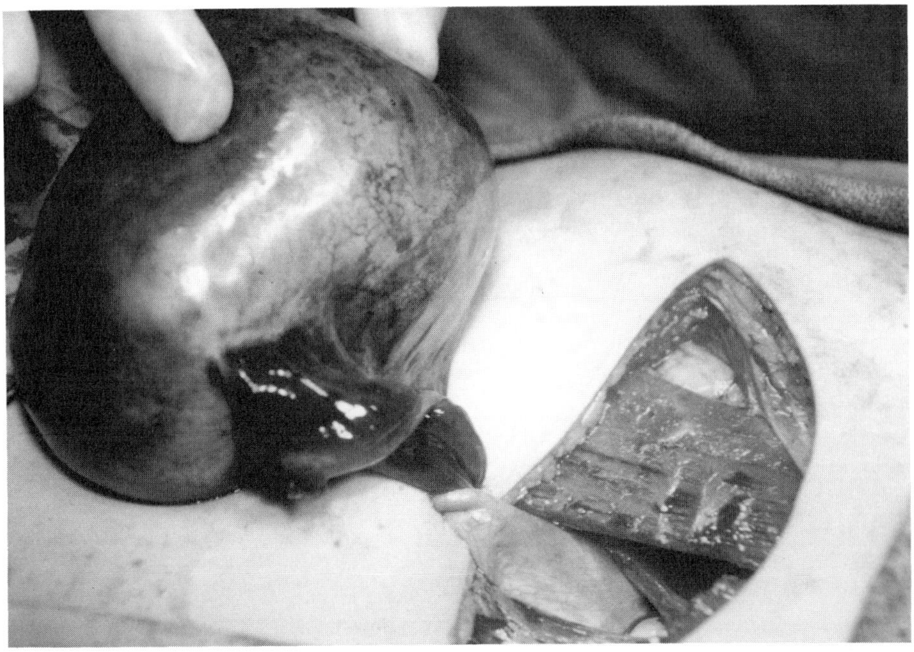

Figure 22–5. Ovarian mass associated with torsion and infarction.

Hydrometrocolpos

Hydrometrocolpos presents as a large lower midline mass arising from the pelvis of a female infant. The distended uterus or vagina is caused by an imperforate hymen or congenital cervical or vaginal stenosis.[1] Passage of transplacental maternal estrogens stimulates increased production of mucus from the cervix and uterus, resulting in massive distention of the vagina or uterus. Physical examination of the abdomen and lower perineum may reveal a bulging hymen or large suprapubic mass. Retrograde contrast studies of the genitourinary system should be performed to exclude renal anomalies. Treatment includes surgical incision and decompression of the obstructed uterus or vagina. Every effort should be made to preserve reproductive function and re-establish normal uterine anatomy.

If the vaginal introitus is patent on physical examination, associated anomalies including ectopic ureters, imperforate anus, and rectovaginal fistula should be excluded. Diagnostic work-up using ultrasound, barium enema, cystogram, and intravenous pyelogram may be necessary to complete the evaluation. Treatment remains surgical and directed at correcting anatomic defects, often requiring an abdominal perineal exposure.

The female patient may be undiagnosed until puberty, when a clinical history of developing secondary sexual characteristics, pelvic cramps, and primary amenorrhea emerges. The work-up begins with an ultrasound and MR imaging to confirm the presence of an obstructed genital system. A high incidence of endometriosis and secondary peritonitis with adhesions may result from reflux of endometrial secretions through the fallopian tubes.

Ovarian Masses

Follicular and theca lutein cysts stimulated by maternal estrogens or placental chorionic gonadotropins represent 3 to 5% of neonatal abdominal masses.[7] Small ovarian cysts are easily visualized on ultrasound. Most of these cysts will spontaneously resolve either prior to or shortly after delivery. Bilateral cysts are found 10% of the time and are associated with a history of maternal diabetes. Enlarging or symptomatic cysts secondary to hemorrhage, torsion, or adhesions to adjacent organs should be surgically excised, with preservation of residual ovarian tissue.

Tumors or cysts of the ovary may develop at any age, though they occur most frequently at puberty. Abdominal or pelvic pain secondary to traction, torsion, adhesions, hemorrhage, or rupture may occur, and a palpable lower abdominal mass is noted 50 to 80% of the time[1] (Fig. 22–5). Ascites is not common in the pediatric patient, but when it occurs it is associated with malignancy. The majority of pelvic masses are benign and cystic (85%). Solid masses have a higher incidence of malignancy. Ultrasound demonstrates the solid or cystic nature of the mass. Complex mixed echogenic masses, loss of definition of adjacent organs, ascites, and lymphadenopathy suggest malignancy. CT scan is most sensitive in identifying hemorrhage and necrosis and is excellent in determining the extent of disease.

Ovarian dermoid (teratoma) is the most common solid mass and contains derivation from two or three embryonic germ cell layers. Calcifications are common on abdominal x-ray. Malignant transformation of a single cell layer may occur (in 1 to 40% of cases).[1] Malignant teratoma is aggressive, bilateral 10% of the time, and may metastasize to the liver and lungs. Therefore, prompt surgical excision of ovarian dermoid is essential.

Tumors of the ovary represent 2% of childhood tumors, and more than 30% are malignant.[11] The majority (75–80%) are germ cell tumors, which include teratoma, dysgerminoma, and choriocarcinoma. Mesenchymal tumors and granulosa-theca cell tumors may produce estrogen and present clinically with precocious puberty and feminization. Androblastoma often presents with virilization and secondary androgen secretion. Epithelial cell tumors—cystadenocarcinoma, serous, or mucous—are rare prior to puberty.[12] Elevated human chorionic gonadotropin or alpha-fetoprotein is associated with embryonal carcinoma and is a useful screening and monitoring test. Surgery is the primary treatment and includes salpingo-oophorectomy of the involved side and careful inspection and evaluation of the contralateral ovary, as 10 to 15% of cases are bilateral. Extension beyond the ovary indicates total abdominal hysterectomy and bilateral salpingo-oophorectomy. Adjuvant chemotherapy and hormonal replacement may be necessary.

ABDOMINAL MASSES IN INFANTS AND CHILDREN

Gastrointestinal Masses

Approximately 20% of abdominal masses in infants arise from either the gastrointestinal tract (15%) or hepatobiliary system (5%).[10] If plain films demonstrate marked bowel gas displacement or an obstructive pattern, gastrointestinal contrast studies may help localize the site of the lesion. Duplications of the gastrointestinal tract are a common cause of a palpable mass in the infant, although malrotation, intestinal atresias, meconium ileus, meconium plug, and Hirschsprung's disease should be excluded. The clinical presentation of bowel obstruction with distention, vomiting, and pain may predominate. Cancers of the gastrointestinal tract are rare, constituting less than 1% of pediatric malignancies. Sarcomas of the gastrointestinal tract are more common than carcinomas. Lymphoma of the intestine, stomach, or colon may also present as an abdominal mass, though usually in the older patient[11] (see Chapter 52).

Intestinal Duplication

Duplications may be found at any point along the gastrointestinal tract and are a common cause of abdominal masses in the first several months of life. Sixty-six percent present by 1 year of age.[1] Characteristically, duplications arise in and along the mesenteric border and are located between the leaves of the mesentery (Fig. 22–6). Muscular layers lined with gastric or intestinal mucosa produce a round, tubular, or dilated mass. The anomalies and the involved intestine have a common muscular wall and blood supply, making resection of the duplicated segment difficult. Symptoms include pain, obstruction, or gastrointestinal hemorrhage. Intestinal perforation can result from occult intussusception, mucosal ulceration, volvulus, rupture, or cystic dilatation of an obstructed segment.

Duplications occur most commonly in the ileum, followed by the jejunum and colon. Colonic duplications often develop in the region of the presacral rectal space. Gastric duplications occur along the greater curvature of the stomach and rarely communicate with the gastric lumen.[6] A soft, mobile, compressible mass may be found high in the epigastrium on physical examination. Plain roentgenogram may suggest gastric dilatation or displacement of adjacent intestinal gas. Ultrasound shows a dilated cystic structure within the abdominal cavity. Upper gastrointestinal series or small bowel transient studies may demonstrate communication to a secondary lumen. Technetium scan may help define the presence of ectopic gastric mucosa within the duplicated segment. Division of the common wall or resection of a length of duplicated bowel may be required in order to completely remove the anomalous segment.

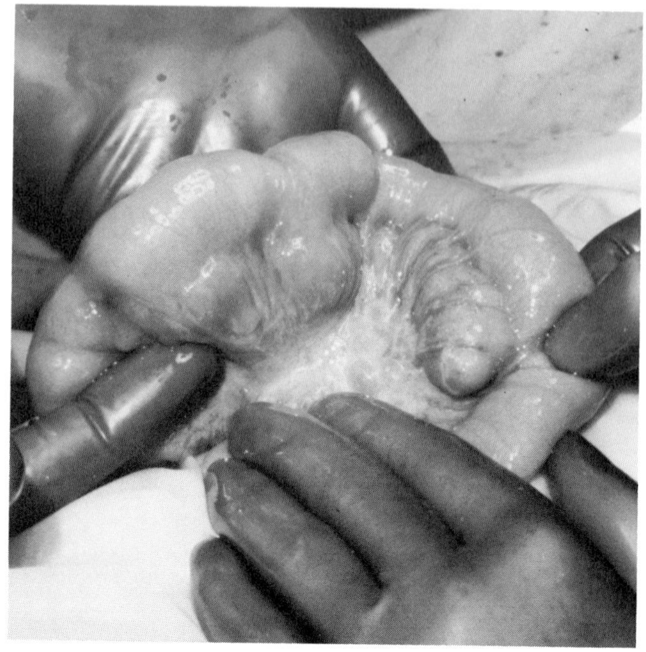

Figure 22–6. Ileal duplication noted on the mesenteric border of the bowel.

Midgut Volvulus

Incomplete rotation of the small bowel during development results in a narrow-based mesenteric pedicle, with the cecum frequently located either in the right upper quadrant or midepigastrium. Midgut volvulus occurs as a result of torsion of the malrotated segment around the vascular pedicle of the superior mesenteric artery. The resulting vascular occlusion of the small bowel leads to intestinal ischemia and proximal obstruction. Patients often present with the abrupt onset of abdominal pain, bilious vomiting, and a palpable mass. If the condition is not quickly recognized, dehydration, acidosis, septicemia, and hypovolemic shock ensue. A clinical history and physical examination suggest a catastrophic intra-abdominal event. A barium enema documents a displaced cecum. If clinical conditions permit, an upper gastrointestinal series outlines a tapering duodenal obstruction. Treatment consists of antibiotics, fluid resuscitation, and urgent laparotomy to reduce the midgut volvulus. Segmental resection or second-look operations are performed based on clinical stability and the condition of the bowel once the vascular circulation is restored (see Chapter 35).

Mesenteric Cysts

Cysts of the mesentery may occur anywhere along the length of the gastrointestinal tract. Thought to arise from congenitally obstructed ectopic lymphatic channels, mesenteric cysts are seen predominantly in older children. Most cysts appear in children 10 years of age or older (75%), peaking in incidence in the fourth decade of life.[1] Roughly 30% are asymptomatic and are discovered as incidental findings. Cysts cause gradual abdominal distention, chronic abdominal pain, or other nonspecific gastrointestinal complaints. Acute findings of hemorrhage, infection, or rupture develop in 60% of pediatric patients.[13, 14]

Mesenteric cysts are lined with endothelial cells and most commonly arise in the small bowel mesentery. An ultrasound demonstrates a large unilocular or septated echolucent mass. If palpable on physical examination, the cysts are soft, compressible, and quite mobile. Colonic cyst fluid is clear and serous in character, whereas small bowel mesenteric cysts are often chylous, containing fat globules and lymphocytes. Surgical excision is the treatment of choice, although the risks of recurrent cyst formation and infection remain long-term complications.

Omental Cysts

Less common than mesenteric cysts, omental cysts are similarly thought to arise in obstructed lymphatic channels within the omentum. Whether post-traumatic or congenital, most occur in older children, with 70% presenting by early adult life.[13, 14, 14a] Most (90%) are asymptomatic, although traction on the omentum may result in compression or torsion of the small bowel and symptoms of abdominal pain or partial small bowel obstruction.[11] Omental cysts are often flaccid, usually compressible and mobile, and, once found, should be excised with a surrounding rim of normal omentum.

Lymphangioma

Multicystic lymphatic collections seen in the neck as cystic hygromas may also arise within the abdomen. Simple capillary, cavernous, and cystic lymphangiomas have been described in the small bowel mesentery, mesocolon, omentum, retroperitoneum, pancreas, and spleen.[11] Usually asymptomatic and incidentally discovered, lymphangiomas may present with pain, occult infection, intestinal obstruction, ascites, and hemorrhage into dilated lymphatics. Ultrasound demonstrates multiloculated cystic masses with thin walls and variable echogenicity. Complete excision is often difficult, and the chance of recurrent cyst formation is high.

Appendiceal Abscess

Appendiceal abscess can be the cause of an abdominal mass in older children. A small localized perforation with periappendicitis and abscess formation occurs following a protracted period of abdominal pain or undiagnosed acute appendicitis. A right lower quadrant mass may be found on abdominal examination, and plain roentgenograms often demonstrate an appendicolith. Ultrasound shows the mixed echogenic right lower quadrant collection, which characterizes abscess formation. CT scan may confirm a periappendiceal collection, and a barium enema further supports the diagnosis of pericecal inflammation with partial obstruction of the cecum and failure to visualize the appendix. If the child has a stable clinical condition, initial treatment begins with intravenous antibiotics and is followed by an interval appendectomy several weeks later (see Chapter 53).

Liver Masses

In 5% of patients presenting with an abdominal mass, the origin is the liver or biliary tree.[6] Focal liver masses may be cystic or solid, benign or malignant, and may not be associated with systemic illness. Hepatomegaly in the infant or young child following traumatic subcapsular hematoma is an important cause of liver mass,[8] and the patient may present in shock. Liver cysts are rare and usually epidermoid, containing clear fluid; they may communicate with the biliary tree and are usually incidentally discovered on an ultrasound or CT scan obtained for a different reason. Symptoms of abdominal pain, nausea, jaundice, and hemodynamic instability are due to rupture, torsion, or hemorrhage of the cyst or compression of adjacent hepatic structures.

Polycystic liver disease is associated with renal cysts 75% of the time. Benign solid masses (35%) include hamartomas, nodular hyperplasia, and adenoma.[15] Mesenchymal hamartoma arises from connective tissue, contains liver cells and ductal and angiomatous elements (78%), and usually presents in the first year[1] involving the right lobe. Hamartomas increase in size with increased age. Ultrasound demonstrates a biphasic cystic lesion with solid components and no communication with the biliary tree. Technetium 99m scan exhibits little uptake in the mass, thus appearing as a cold nodule. Primary treatment is surgical excision due to symptomatic compression of adjacent liver, risk of hemorrhage, or malignant degeneration of the cyst epithelium.

Nodular hyperplasia represents areas of benign hepatocellular proliferation, which may be associated with micronodular cirrhosis or, in the neonate, secondary to maternal hormones. These regenerative nodules display increased uptake on radionuclide scan and may be symptomatic if mass effect, internal hemorrhage, or torsion occurs. Treatment is conservative, with observation and serial noninvasive studies.

Hepatic adenomas are benign, encapsulated, hypervascular masses of liver parenchyma that usually appear after puberty. The etiology is unclear, and the risk of malignant transformation is low. Twenty-five percent may infarct, leading to hemorrhage and emergent laparotomy and resection. There is a possible association with the use of oral contraceptives.

Hemangiomas are arteriovenous malformations of the liver that are usually seen in early childhood. Ninety to 95% of cavernous hemangiomas are solitary, small, and asymptomatic and may be associated with cutaneous hemangiomas. Spontaneous involution within five years is common; therefore, management is supportive and noninvasive. Percutaneous liver biopsy is contraindicated. A bruit over the mass may be heard on physical examination, and radionuclide scan of the liver is diagnostic in demonstrating a highly vascular lesion. If the hemangioma enlarges, risk of hemorrhage, thrombocytopenia secondary to platelet trapping, and congestive heart failure due to increased arteriovenous shunting is high and associated with increased mortality. Initial nonoperative treatment with transfusion, diuretics, digoxin, intravenous steroids, radiation therapy, hepatic artery embolization, or ligation may be necessary. If the patient remains hemodynamically unstable, surgical excision of the hemangioma with enucleation, wedge resection, or lobectomy/segmentectomy may be necessary and carries an approximate 9 to 10% mortality rate.[1] The classic triad of congestive heart failure, hepatomegaly, and cutaneous hemangiomas suggests the clinical diagnosis of cavernous hemangioma.

Sixty-five percent of solid liver masses in children are malignant, representing more than 6% of pediatric tumors discovered after the neonatal period.[10] Primary liver cancer, either hepatoblastoma or hepatocellular carcinoma, is the second most common gastrointestinal malignancy. Clinical presentation of a painless mass with hepatomegaly (40%), weight loss, and anorexia is common. Anemia, elevated aminotransferases, and bilirubin may also be noted, and the patient frequently presents with advanced disease.

Metastatic lesions to the liver include leukemia and lymphoma. Wilms' tumor is the most common solid tumor metastatic to the liver.[16] Liver metastasis may be single or multiple. Differences in echogenicity are noted on ultrasound, although MR imaging has become the imaging modality of choice in liver tumors. Inhomogeneous internal structure, adjacent nodules, and tumor extension into vascular structures all suggest malignancy.[16]

Hepatoblastoma is more common than hepatocellular carcinoma (4:1) and usually presents as a painless mass in the young patient less than three years old. Boys outnumber girls 3:1 and frequently present with unresectable liver disease or pulmonary metastases. Alphafetoprotein, an enzyme of fetal liver tissue, is often elevated in hepatoblastoma and is useful as a screening or monitoring test. The tumor is often a unifocal lobulated mass with areas of necrosis and calcification and surrounded by a pseudocapsule.[16] Venous invasion is common. Histology demonstrates epithelial or mixed mesenchymal-epithelial architecture and embryonal or fetal liver cytology. It is not associated with cirrhosis, and extramedullary hematopoiesis is common. Surgical resection of the tumor and/or metastasis is the mainstay of therapy, though chemotherapy and radiation therapy may reduce tumor burden. The overall cure rate is 20% at 5 years. If complete excision is possible, cure rates of up to 60% have been reported.

Hepatocellular carcinoma often presents as a single liver mass. Males outnumber females 4:1, and there are two peaks in incidence of the tumor: at age 4 years and 12–15 years. The incidence is higher in patients with pre-existing liver disease (e.g., tyrosinemia, chronic hepatitis, glycogen storage, cirrhosis), and the tumor is often invasive and multicentric at presentation. Hemorrhage and necrosis of the tumors are common.[16] The prognosis is poor, with an overall survival of 35% at 5 years. Microscopy demonstrates large hepatic cells with nuclear pleomorphism, tumor giant cells, and the absence of hematopoiesis. Paraneoplastic syndromes including hypercalcemia, hyperlipidemia, hypoglycemia, cirrhosis, virilization, and sexual precocity are associated. Survival is poor despite surgical excision (where possible), radiation, and chemotherapy.

Choledochal Cysts

Choledochal cysts (see also Chapter 71) are localized dilatations of the biliary tree and are generally discovered in older infants and children. Dilatation may be focal or fusiform, may involve the intrahepatic or extrahepatic bile ducts, or both, may be congenital or acquired, and may present with a palpable abdominal mass. Twenty to 30% present before age 1 year, and 60% by age 10; females outnumber males 4:1.

Clinical presentation with biliary obstruction includes fever, elevated bilirubin, hepatomegaly, and acholic stools (80%) in infants. In older children, however, symptoms of chronic low-grade biliary obstruction with biliary stasis are more frequent, and patients present with recurrent episodes of pain, jaundice, pancreatitis, and cholangitis. Liver abscesses, biliary stones, and portal hypertension may develop as the choledochal cyst becomes a nidus for infection and stone formation. The classic triad of abdominal pain, jaundice, and a palpable epigastric mass is seen in only a minority of patients.

Ultrasound has improved early diagnosis of choledochal cyst and demonstrates the cyst or associated ductal dilatation. Endoscopic retrograde cholangiopancreatography has an 80 to 90% accuracy in diagnosis and clearly demonstrates the anatomy of the biliary tree.[17] Complete excision of the choledochal cyst and establishment of adequate biliary drainage are essential.

Pancreatic Masses

Pancreatic masses are uncommon in children and rare in neonates. Benign processes include pseudocyst, duplication cyst, or focal phlegmonous regions of inflammation. Carcinomas are more frequent than sarcomas, and clinically the patient presents with abdominal or epigastric pain and fullness, weight loss, diarrhea, or evidence of endocrine effects. Jaundice is less common.

Von Hippel-Lindau disease, consisting of multiple

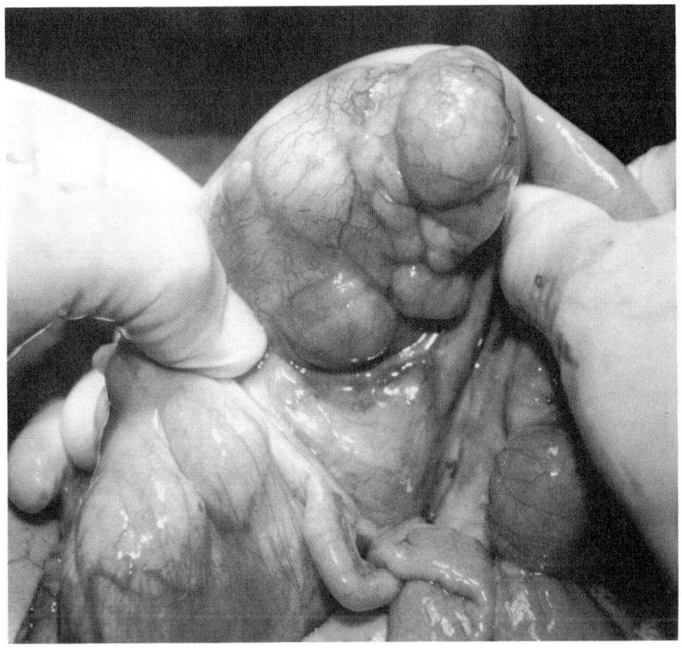

Figure 22–7. Burkitt's lymphoma involving the terminal ileum.

pancreatic and renal cysts with associated angiomata of the retina and cerebellum, is rare. Diagnostic imaging by ultrasound or CT scan guidance usually demonstrates the pancreatic or peripancreatic mass of homogeneous echogenicity.

Enlarged Spleen

Splenic enlargement in children is most often due to medical illness such as infection, portal hypertension, hemoglobinopathy, or malignancies such as lymphoma or leukemia. Primary splenic tumors are rare and often benign. Hamartomatous nodular aggregates of functioning splenic tissue often present asymptomatically with splenomegaly and may be solid or cystic in origin. Cavernous or diffuse hemangiomas may cause hypersplenism and result in a consumptive coagulopathy or spontaneous rupture, although the majority are asymptomatic.[11] Epidermoid and parasitic cysts of the spleen are usually incidental findings and asymptomatic. Post-traumatic pseudocysts or subcapsular hematomas are a common post-traumatic cause of splenic enlargement. The majority are successfully managed nonoperatively. Conservation of splenic tissue by splenorrhaphy or partial splenectomy is preferred when surgical intervention is required.

Rhabdomyosarcoma

Rhabdomyosarcoma is an aggressive infiltrating tumor that develops from primitive mesenchymal cells and frequently presents with prominent local infiltration and hematogenous lymphatic metastases. Primary sites include the head and neck (28%), bladder trigone and prostate (21%), extremities (18%), orbit (10%), and retroperitoneum (7%).[11] Intra-abdominal disease is usually secondary to extension from pelvis and retroperitoneum. Rhabdomyosarcoma is a poorly localized, diffuse mass and frequently presents with advanced local/regional disease and encasement of the superior mesenteric and celiac arteries. Clinical presentation is dependent on the primary tumor location and the extent of disease. On physical examination, a firm, fixed mass may be noted. Ultrasound demonstrates either a homogeneous echogenic mass similar to adjacent muscle or focal areas of decreased echogenicity secondary to necrosis and hemorrhage. CT scan is essential both for preoperative staging and to clearly delineate the local extent of disease. The primary treatment is surgical extirpation, with adjuvant chemotherapy and radiation for treatment of residual disease.

Lymphoma

Lymphoma of the small bowel, the most common malignant tumor of the gastrointestinal tract in children (see Chapter 52), arises most frequently in the distal ileum (Fig. 22–7). Patients may present with symptoms of partial small bowel obstruction, chronic crampy abdominal pain, anemia, or gastrointestinal bleeding. Differentiation includes leiomyosarcoma, rhabdomyosarcoma, and carcinoid tumors. A mobile mass may be palpable on physical examination, and ultrasound demonstrates a hypoechoic mass extending transmurally. Barium contrast of the small bowel shows irregular mucosal contour, suggesting ulceration and proximal aneurysmal dilatation.[10] A CT scan is necessary to stage the tumor and evaluate the retroperitoneum, liver, and adjacent organ structures for active disease. With lymphoma of the stomach, an ultrasound may demonstrate characteristic eccentric hyperechoic masses extending from the mucosal surface through the muscular wall.

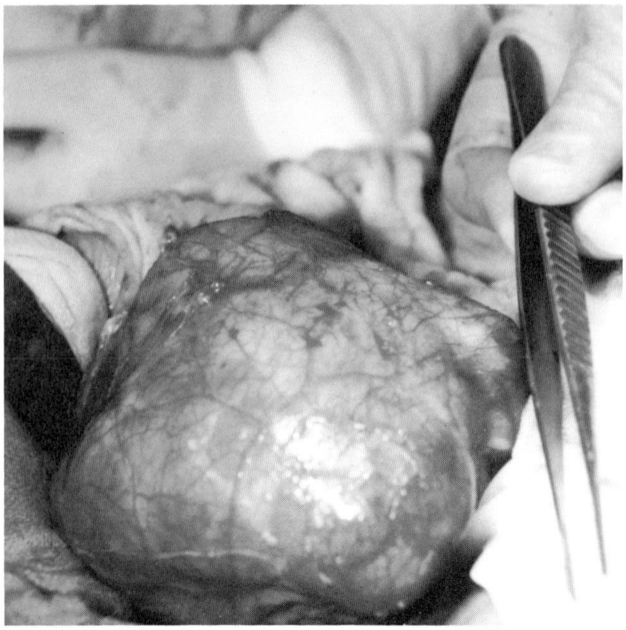

Figure 22–8. Operative view of a large, well-encapsulated Wilms' tumor.

Ulceration is evident on upper gastrointestinal endoscopy.

RETROPERITONEAL MASSES

Wilms' Tumor

Wilms' tumor (nephroblastoma) is an embryonal tumor of the kidney arising in rests of primitive mesodermal cells within the renal capsule (Fig. 22–8). It is the fourth most common abdominal tumor in childhood and presents in children averaging 3½ years of age. The tumor is usually palpable (90%), firm with distinct borders, and may present with pain (20%) and hematuria (15%).[1] Increasing pain in the region of an abdominal mass following trauma is suspicious of hemorrhage into a pre-existing tumor.

Nephroblastomas initially grow within the boundary of the renal capsule and invade the calyces and renal pelvis, ultimately extending into renal vessels and lymphatics. Extension of tumor into the renal vein occurs in 5 to 10% of patients. Invasion into the inferior vena cava is associated with distant pulmonary metastases in 60% of patients.[1] An additional 30% will develop metastases to the lymph nodes, liver, and bone within 2 years. The tumor is found to cross the midline in approximately half the patients. Bilateral Wilms' tumors arise in 5 to 10% of patients as a result of metachronous growth. Inheritance of Wilms' tumors is consistent with an autosomal dominant transmission and a deletion in the short arm of chromosome 11.[8] The bilateral disease is more common in familial Wilms' tumor, with 50 to 90% of patients developing renin-associated hypertension.[1] It may also be seen in syndromes of aniridia, mental retardation, hemihypertrophy, Down's syndrome, and Beckwith-Weidemann syndrome.[8]

Characteristic histology demonstrates small undifferentiated cells with primitive nephron formation. Ninety percent of tumors exhibit favorable triphasic histology consisting of tubular, epithelial, and stromal tissue. The remaining 10% exhibit sarcomatous, anaplastic, or rhabdoid histology and account for 50% of all Wilms' tumor deaths.[5]

Diagnostic evaluation includes a plain film of the chest to look for pulmonary metastases. Ultrasound outlines a characteristic complex intrarenal mass. Care should be directed at definition of the renal vena cava to exclude tumor involvement. An intravenous pyelogram documents function and caliceal distention, and the CT scan provides excellent definition of adjacent organ involvement and distant pulmonary metastases (Fig. 22–9). MR imaging has proved extremely accurate in evaluating the size and extent of Wilms' tumors, especially for details of the contralateral kidney. A limitation of MR imaging appears to be related to poor imaging of lung parenchyma to exclude metastatic disease. Treatment consists of surgical excision along with postoperative radiation and chemotherapy as determined by both histology and clinical staging. There is a 90% survival rate for stage I and stage II disease with favorable histology.[5] Preoperative chemotherapy may help downstage massive involvement and improve the possibility of subsequent surgical resection. Partial nephrectomies are indicated in order to conserve renal tissue in bilateral disease.

Neuroblastoma

Neuroblastoma is a highly malignant tumor arising in cells of neural crest origin. Although it is the third most common abdominal mass in the pediatric age group, it remains the most common malignancy in infancy. It may arise anywhere along the sympathetic chain within the chest (15%), abdomen (24%), pelvis (4%), or adrenal medulla (43%). Clinical prognosis is related to the size and site of the primary tumor, presence of metastatic disease, and production of metabolically active catecholamines. Weight loss, failure to thrive, ab-

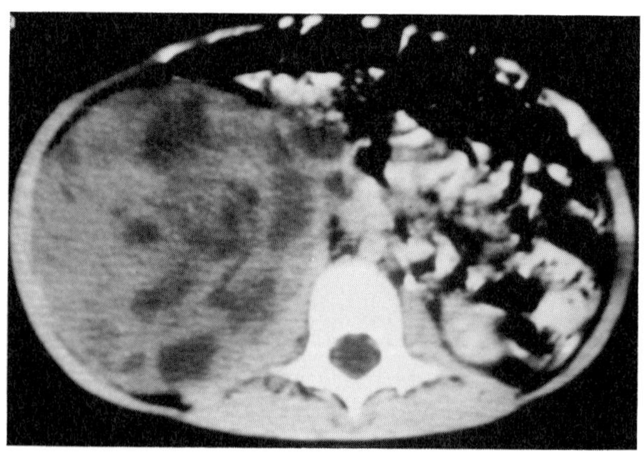

Figure 22–9. Computed tomography showing a well-demarcated Wilms' tumor of the right kidney.

dominal pain or distention, and anemia are frequently noted at presentation. Fifty to 75% of patients present with a palpable mass.[6] Intraspinal extension through intravertebral foramina may result in paralysis or paresis. Catecholamine production will cause hypertension, headaches, diarrhea, or diffuse sweating. The active metabolites of vanillylmandelic acid (VMA) or homovanillic acid (HVA) are detectable in 80% of patients.[6] Sixty to 70% of patients present with metastases involving lymph nodes, bone, bone marrow, liver, subcutaneous tissue, lungs, or brain.[1]

Physical examination may reveal a firm, poorly defined, immobile mass in the flank. Abdominal radiographs often suggest displacement of kidney and a mass stippled with calcifications. Chest radiography should be performed to exclude paraspinal or posterior mediastinal widening. Ultrasound confirms the solid external echogenic mass and its displacement of the kidney inferiorly and laterally. CT scan may be used to determine the extent of disease, delineate the tumor mass, and confirm the presence of calcification, retroperitoneal involvement, adjacent tissue extension, and evidence of distant metastatic disease (Fig. 22–10). MR imaging has become the imaging modality of choice equal to CT scan in accurately visualizing the retroperitoneum, great vessels, and intraspinal extension. Though unable to show calcifications, MR imaging is superior to the CT scan in evaluating bone marrow, which is involved in 50% of patients.[18] A bone scan is part of the evaluation to exclude metastatic disease, and I-131 metaiodobenzylguanidine (MIBG) scan is frequently used to exclude involvement of adjacent adrenal tissue.

Detection of urinary VMA or HVA is confirmatory of the diagnosis and is detectable on spot or 24-hour urine collection. Elevated levels of cystathionine, homoserine, neuron-specific enolase, and ferritin have been associated with a poor prognosis. Carcinoembryonic antigen levels are elevated in 25% of patients.[6] Favorable prognostic features include amplification of the n-*myc* oncogene, which is associated with mature neuroblastoma, diagnosis in infancy (younger than 2 years), favorable histology, stage IV-S disease, and thoracic location of the tumor.[1] Aggressive surgical excision should be employed whenever possible. Adjuvant chemotherapy and radiation therapy have added little to survival in advanced disease or in older children, in whom mortality approaches 80%.[7] New chemotherapeutic modalities that employ the adjunctive use of bone marrow transplantation have had promising results.

OTHER RENAL MASSES

Renal sarcomas are distinct from Wilms' tumor and constitute approximately 5% of pediatric renal tumors. Aggressive renal sarcomas demonstrate an infiltrative intrarenal growth pattern as opposed to the expansile pattern of Wilms' tumor. Metastatic disease to bones is common in more than 50% of cases.[8]

Multilocular cystic nephroma is an uncommon benign neoplasm presenting as an encapsulated mass containing multiple noncommunicating cysts. Ultrasound demonstrates multiloculated masses with septae. There is no communication with the collecting system when seen on intravenous pyelogram on CT scan.

Simple retention cysts may result from tubular obstruction or local vascular damage from inflammation within the collecting system. These lesions should be managed conservatively, as they are usually asymptomatic and rarely associated with hematuria or proteinuria. Further evaluation should include examination of the liver or the pancreas to exclude associated cystic disease.

Angiomyolipoma is a benign fatty tumor that is well visualized and most commonly causes pain and hemorrhage into the mass. Plain films demonstrate a charac-

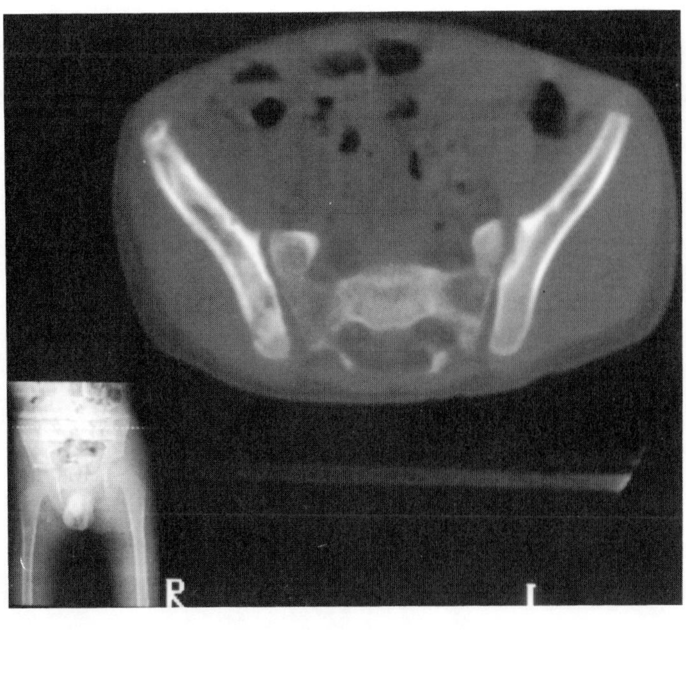

Figure 22–10. Computed tomography showing irregularity of the right iliac crest secondary to metastatic neuroblastoma.

teristic rim of the calcification. Treatment is surgical excision.

ADRENAL MASSES

Pheochromocytoma

Functionally active tumors of the adrenal gland occur in less than 50% of the pediatric population developing pheochromocytoma. Children, however, have a high incidence of tumors that occur bilaterally and arise in multiple extra-adrenal locations. Malignant transformation occurs in less than 2% of pheochromocytomas but is most common when arising in extra-adrenal locations. The majority of patients initially present with hypertension and associated disorders such as multiple endocrine adenopathy (MEA), von Hippel-Lindau disease, or neurofibromatosis. CT scan is excellent for staging of the disease, and an MIBG scan is useful for follow-up evaluation in demonstrating recurrent adrenal or metastatic disease.[18]

Adrenal Cortical Neoplasms

Although occurring in less than 1% of pediatric neoplasms, adrenal cortical tumors often produce symptoms of hyperadrenalism. Females outnumber males 5:1, with androgenic effects, virilization, and pseudoprecocious puberty suggestive of hyperfunctioning adrenal cortical secretion. Cushing's syndrome, feminization, and hyperaldosteronism are rare. Ultrasound demonstrates a solid adrenal mass with variable echogenicity within the tumor. Hemorrhage, necrosis, and calcifications are frequently noted. CT scan or MR imaging accurately assesses the extent of local disease and reveals metastatic disease in the liver, retroperitoneum, or inferior vena cava. Since invasion is present in 50% of patients, an evaluation for metastatic disease is mandatory. Surgery is the primary treatment when disease is localized. Chemotherapy may be used preoperatively to downstage large tumors or as an adjuvant to a postoperative treatment course.

REFERENCES

1. Stevenson RJ: Abdominal masses. Surg Clin North Am 1985; 65:1481–1504.
2. Teele RL, Share JC: The abdominal mass in the neonate. Semin Roentgenol 1988; 23:175–184.
3. Boechat MI, Kangarloo H: Magnetic resonance imaging of the abdomen in children. Am J Radiol 1989; 152:1245–1250.
4. Avni EF, Thoria Y, Lalmand B, et al: Multicystic dysplastic kidney: Natural history from in utero diagnosis and postnatal follow-up. J Urol 1987; 138:1420–1424.
5. Donaldson JS, Sholnik A: Pediatric renal masses. Semin Roentgenol 1988; 23:194–204.
6. Mahaffey SM, Rychman RC, Martin LW: Clinical aspects of abdominal masses in children. Semin Roentgenol 1988; 23:161–174.
7. Hartman GE, Shochat SJ: Abdominal mass lesions in the newborn: Diagnosis and treatment. Clin Perinat 1989; 16:123–135.
8. Bove KE: Pathology of selected abdominal masses in children. Semin Roentgenol 1988; 23:147–160.
9. Chan HS, Mancer K, Weitzman SS, et al: Congenital mesoblastic nephroma: A clinico-radiologic study of 17 cases representing the pathologic spectrum of the disease. J Pediatr 1987; 111:64–70.
10. Mertin DF, Kirks DR: Diagnostic imaging of pediatric abdominal masses. Pediatr Clin North Am 1985; 32:1397–1425.
11. Sty JR, Wells RG: Other abdominal and pelvic masses in children. Semin Roentgenol 1988; 23:216–231.
12. Ehren IM, Mahour GH, Isaacs H: Benign and malignant ovarian tumors in children and adolescents—a review of 63 cases. Am J Surg 1984; 147:339–344.
13. Vanck VN, Phillips AK: Retroperitoneal mesenteric and omental cysts. Arch Surg 1984; 119:838–842.
14. Molander ML, Mortensson W, Uden R: Omental and mesenteric cysts in children. Acta Paediatr Scand 1982; 71:272–279.

14a. Lawrence RA, Putnam TC, Webb SR: Omental cyst: Presentation in an infant with jaundice and increasing abdominal girth. J Pediatr Gastroenterol Nutr 1992; 15:97–99.

15. Ehren H, Mahour GH, Isaacs H: Benign liver tumors in infancy and childhood: Report of 48 cases. Am J Surg 1983; 145:325–329.
16. Boechet MI, Kangarloo HJ, Gilsang V: Hepatic masses in children. Semin Roengtenol 1988; 23:185–193.
17. Oldham KT, Hart MJ, White TT: Choledochal cysts presenting in late childhood and adulthood. Am J Surg 1981; 141:568–571.
18. Daneman A: Adrenal neoplasms in children. Semin Roentgenol 1988; 23:205–215.

Chapter 23

Jaundice

GLENN R. GOURLEY

INTRODUCTION

The term *jaundice* originates from the French word *jaune,* which means yellow. Jaundice, or icterus, refers to the yellow discoloration of the skin, sclerae, and other tissues owing to deposition of the bile pigment bilirubin. Jaundice is a sign that the serum bilirubin concentration has risen higher than normal levels (approximately 1.4 mg per dl after 6 months of age). The intensity of the yellow color is directly related to the elevation of the serum bilirubin and the related degree of deposition of bilirubin into the extravascular tissues. There are a wide variety of conditions associated with jaundice. Some of these states are so commonly recognized as to be termed *physiologic* (e.g., in the neonate) or are believed to be without significant health risk (e.g., Gilbert's syndrome). Alternatively, jaundice can be a manifestation of life-threatening hemolysis, infection, or liver failure. This chapter begins with a review of bilirubin metabolism. Thereafter, specific conditions associated with jaundice in neonates, infancy, and childhood are examined.

BILIRUBIN METABOLISM

The term *bilirubin* is derived from Latin (*bilis,* bile; *ruber,* red) and was used in 1864 by Städeler[1] to describe the red-colored bile pigment. Bilirubin is formed from the degradation of heme-containing compounds (Fig. 23–1). The largest source for the production of bilirubin is hemoglobin. However, other heme-containing proteins are also degraded to bilirubin, including the cytochromes, catalases, tryptophan pyrrolase, and muscle myoglobin.[2]

The formation of bilirubin is accomplished by cleaving the tetrapyrrole ring of protoheme (protoporphyrin IX), resulting in a linear tetrapyrrole. The first enzyme system involved in the formation of bilirubin is microsomal heme oxygenase, which is located primarily in the reticuloendothelial tissues[3] and, to a lesser degree, in tissue macrophages and intestinal epithelium.[4] This enzyme system results in a reduction of the porphyrin iron (Fe^{3+} to Fe^{2+}) and hydroxylation of the alpha carbon. This alpha-carbon is then oxidatively excised from the tetrapyrrole ring, yielding carbon monoxide. This excision opens the ring structure and is associated with oxygenation of the two carbons adjacent to the site of cleavage. The cleaved alpha-carbon is excreted as carbon monoxide, whereas the iron released can be reused by the body. The resultant linear tetrapyrrole is biliverdin IX-alpha. The *IX* designation is a result of Fischer's grouping of the protoporphyrin isomers, group IX being the physiologic source of bilirubin.[5] The stereospecificity of the enzyme produces cleavage almost exclusively at the alpha-carbon of the tetrapyrrole. This is unlike in vitro chemical oxidation, which results in cleavage at any of the four carbons (alpha, beta, gamma, and delta) linking the four pyrrole rings and produces an equimolar amount of the alpha, beta, gamma, and delta isomers.[6] The central (C–10) carbon on biliverdin IX-alpha is then reduced from a methene to a methylene group ($-CH_2-$), thus forming bilirubin IX-alpha. This is accomplished by the cytosolic enzyme biliverdin reductase.[7] The proximity of this enzyme results in little biliverdin ever being present in the circulation. Bilirubin formation can be assessed by the measurement of carbon monoxide production. Such assessments indicate that the daily production rate of bilirubin is 6 to 8 mg per kg per 24 hours in healthy term infants and 3 to 4 mg per kg per 24 hours in healthy adults.[8, 9] In mammals, approximately 80% of the bilirubin produced daily originates from hemoglobin.[10–13] The degradation of hepatic and renal heme appears to account for most of the remaining 20%, reflecting the rapid turnover of certain of these heme proteins. Although the precise fate of myoglobin heme is unknown, its turnover appears to be so slow as to be relatively insignificant.[14] The catabolism of hemoglobin occurs largely from the sequestration of erythrocytes at the end of their life span (120 days in adult humans, 90 days in neonates, and 50–60 days in rats). A small fraction of newly synthesized hemoglobin is degraded in the bone marrow. This process, termed *ineffective erythropoiesis,* normally represents less than 3% of daily bilirubin production but may be substantially increased in persons with hemoglobinopathies, vitamin deficiencies, and heavy metal intoxication.[15–17] Infants produce more bilirubin per unit of body weight because the red blood cell mass is greater and the red blood cell life span is shorter in infants. Additionally, hepatic heme

Supported in part by National Institutes of Health Grants HD 03352, HD29287, and HD28619 and a grant from the Madison General Hospital Medical and Surgical Foundation

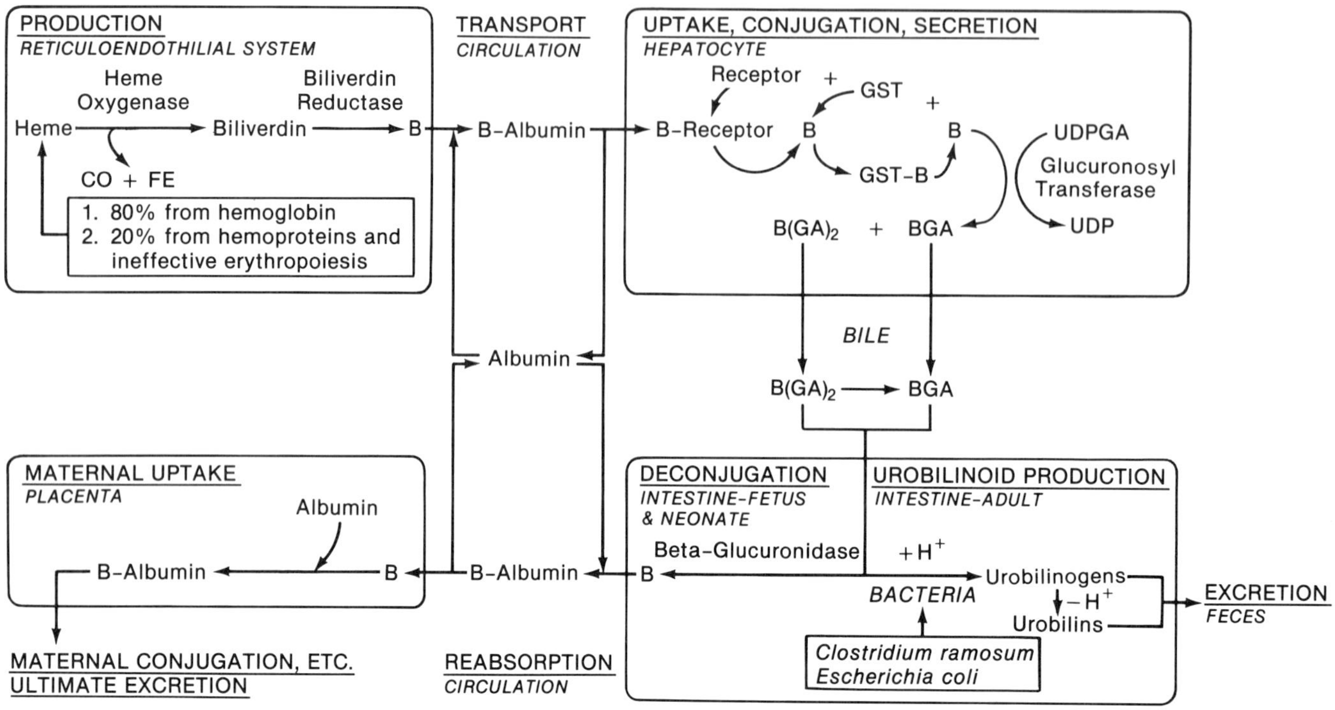

Figure 23–1. Metabolism of bilirubin (B) in the fetus, neonate and adult. GST, glutathione S-transferase; GA, glucuronic acid; UDP, uridine diphosphate.

proteins represent a larger fraction of the total body weight in infants.

Bilirubin requires a biotransformation to more water-soluble derivatives prior to its excretion from the body. This is explained by the structure of bilirubin.[18] Bilirubin is not linear but rather is extensively hydrogen bonded, as shown in Figure 23–2. The saturated middle carbon (C–10) allows rotation of the two halves of the bilirubin molecule. Thus, the pyrrole nitrogens and lactam oxygen of one half form hydrogen bonds with the carboxyl groups of the propionic acid side chain on the other half. The carbon-carbon double bonds at positions 4–5 and 15–16 can assume two different configurations, depending on whether the higher priority atoms or groups (based on atomic number) are on the same (Z, *zusammen,* German for *together*) or opposite (E, *entgegen,* German for *opposite*) sides of the double bond. The naturally occurring form of bilirubin is that shown in Figure 23–2, which is 4Z,15Z-bilirubin IX-alpha. Knowledge of this stereochemistry is important in understanding phototherapy, which will be discussed later. The internal hydrogen bonding of bilirubin makes the molecule extremely hydrophobic and insoluble in aqueous media.

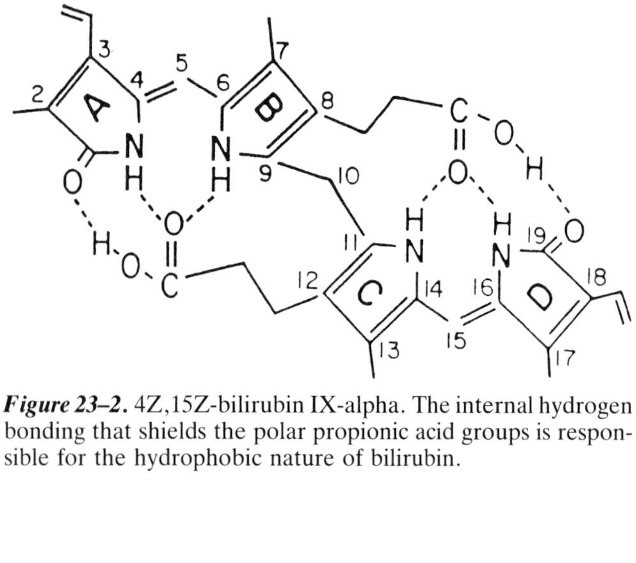

Figure 23–2. 4Z,15Z-bilirubin IX-alpha. The internal hydrogen bonding that shields the polar propionic acid groups is responsible for the hydrophobic nature of bilirubin.

Hence, when bilirubin is transported from its sites of production to the liver for excretion, a carrier molecule is necessary. Albumin serves this purpose.[19] Each albumin molecule is believed to possess a single high-affinity (7×10^7 M^{-1}) binding site for one molecule of bilirubin.[20] A binding affinity of this magnitude implies that essentially all bilirubin will be transported to the liver bound to albumin, with negligible amounts free to diffuse into other tissues. Secondary binding sites of lesser affinity also exist on albumin.

For the hepatocyte to take up bilirubin from the blood, a receptor of great affinity is required. The plasma membrane of the hepatocyte, adjacent to the sinusoid, has been shown to contain such a receptor carrier for bilirubin. This receptor facilitates the hepatocyte uptake of bilirubin[21] and is competitively inhibited by simultaneous exposure to bromsulfophthalein (BSP) and indocyanine green (ICG).

Once within the hepatocyte, bilirubin is bound by glutathione S-transferase B (GST), traditionally referred to as *ligandin.*[22–24] The affinity of purified GST for bilirubin ($K_a = 10^6$)[25] is less than that of albumin; however, GST is believed to be of importance in preventing bilirubin and its conjugates from refluxing into the circulation.[26]

Bilirubin is conjugated with glucuronic acid within the endoplasmic reticulum of the hepatocyte. The glucuronic acid donor is uridine diphosphate (UDP)–glucuronic acid. The enzyme responsible for this conjugation is bilirubin glucuronosyltransferase (BGT). Several different classes of glucuronosyltransferases, with different substrate specificity, have been described.[27, 28] The catalysis of bilirubin by BGT results in both monoglucuronides and diglucuronides of bilirubin.[29] BGT activity for bilirubin can be induced by narcotics, anticonvulsants, contraceptive steroids, and bilirubin itself.[30] Alternatively, BGT activity can be decreased by caloric and protein restriction.[31]

Following bilirubin conjugation, the bilirubin monoglucuronides and diglucuronides are secreted into bile via the biliary canaliculus. In normal adult duodenal bile, 70 to 90% of the bile pigments are bilirubin diglucuronides, and 7 to 27% are bilirubin monoglucuronides.[32–34] Smaller amounts of other bilirubin conjugates are also seen. After the first week of life, secretion of bilirubin conjugates by the hepatocyte is the rate-limiting step in bilirubin clearance.[35, 36] Canalicular secretion of bilirubin conjugates can be increased by choleretic agents (e.g., phenobarbital) and decreased by cholestatic agents (e.g., estrogens and anabolic steroids) or pathologic conditions (e.g., liver disease).[37]

In many circumstances bilirubin monoglucuronides and diglucuronides are not excreted from the hepatocyte fast enough to prevent reflux into the circulation. The subsequent elevation of serum bilirubin conjugate levels results in the spontaneous formation of delta-bilirubin. Delta-bilirubin, or bilirubin-albumin, is formed by the transesterification of the bilirubin glucuronide with an amino group on albumin producing a covalent bond between albumin and bilirubin.[38] Similar nonenzymatic reactions have been demonstrated between albumin and various drugs.[38–41] Delta bilirubin is not formed in hyperbilirubinemic conditions unless there is elevation of the conjugated bilirubin fraction.

Once bilirubin conjugates reach the intestine, several metabolic alternatives arise. In adults, the normal bacterial flora hydrogenate various carbon double bonds in bilirubin to produce assorted urobilinogens. Subsequent oxidation of the middle (C–10) carbon produces the related urobilins. These reduction-oxidation products of bilirubin are known collectively as *urobilinoids*[42] and are excreted in the feces. The bacterium most important in producing urobilinoids is *Clostridium ramosum*,[43] with which *Escherichia coli* has been shown to act synergistically.[44] The conversion of bilirubin conjugates to urobilinoids prevents the intestinal absorption of bilirubin known as the *enterohepatic circulation*.[45] Neonates lack an intestinal bacterial flora and thus are more susceptible to bilirubin reabsorption.

Alternatively, intestinal bilirubin conjugates can act as a substrate for either bacterial[46–48] or tissue[49] beta-glucuronidase. This ubiquitous enzyme cleaves the glucuronic acid moiety from bilirubin glucuronides, resulting in unconjugated bilirubin, which has been shown to be more easily absorbed from the intestine.[50] In the fetus, tissue beta-glucuronidase, which is detectable by 12 weeks of gestation, is believed to play an important role in facilitating intestinal bilirubin absorption that enables bilirubin to be cleared via the placenta. Lacking placental assistance, the neonate with increased intestinal beta-glucuronidase is at risk to experience higher serum bilirubin levels.[51]

JAUNDICE ASSESSMENT

Jaundice can be objectively quantified by the measurement of total serum bilirubin concentration. This includes two fractions: conjugated bilirubin (so-called "direct" reacting because color development takes place directly without the addition of methanol in the van den Bergh test) and unconjugated bilirubin ("indirect" fraction). Traditionally the terms *direct* and *indirect* are used interchangeably with conjugated and unconjugated bilirubin, although it is now recognized that this is not quantitatively correct. Jaundice can result from an elevation in either of these fractions. Serum bilirubin measurements are now most commonly made with automated laboratory methods and have been recently reviewed.[52] Erroneously elevated direct fractions have been reported when the total bilirubin level is high.[53]

A noninvasive method to assess jaundice is also available and is particularly useful in neonates. This transcutaneous jaundice meter (Minolta/Air-Shields Jaundice Meter 101) measures skin color, or "jaundice index," in an easy, painless manner. Measurements of jaundice index generally correlate with serum bilirubin levels with a correlation coefficient of $r > 0.9$.[54] Hence, use of the jaundice meter as a screening device is advocated.[54] Similarly, pressing an inexpensive Plexiglas color chart against the infant's nose (Ingram Icterometer) is also useful in assessing jaundice.[55, 56]

NEONATAL JAUNDICE

Infants are not jaundiced at birth, even if severe hemolysis existed in utero. This attests to the efficiency of placental clearance of bilirubin. However, during the first week of life, most, if not all, infants develop elevated serum bilirubin levels (>1.4 mg per dl). As the serum bilirubin rises the skin becomes more jaundiced in a cephalopedal manner. Icterus is first appreciated in the head and progresses caudally to the palms and soles. Kramer[57] found the following serum indirect bilirubin levels as jaundice progressed: head and neck, 4 to 8 mg per dl; upper trunk, 5 to 12 mg per dl; lower trunk and thighs, 8 to 16 mg per /dl; arms and lower legs, 11 to 18 mg per dl; and palms and soles, higher than 15 mg per dl. Hence, when the bilirubin was higher than 15 mg per dl, the entire body was icteric. Jaundice is best appreciated by blanching the skin with gentle digital pressure under well-illuminated (white-light) conditions. Visible jaundice will develop in at least one third of infants. Moderate jaundice (>12 mg per dl) occurs in at least 12% of breast-fed infants and 4% of formula-fed infants, whereas severe jaundice (>15 mg per dl) occurs in 2% and 0.3% of these respective feeding groups.[58]

Fundamentally, jaundice has only two causes: increased production or decreased excretion of bilirubin. These mechanisms are not mutually exclusive, and specific examples are listed in Table 23–1. One possible clinical approach to arrive at these diagnoses is presented in Figure 23–3.

The high incidence of jaundice in otherwise completely normal neonates, as described earlier, has resulted in use of the term *physiologic jaundice*. However, physiologic jaundice is merely the result of a number of factors involving increased bilirubin production and decreased excretion. Jaundice should always be considered to be a sign of a possible disease, and not routinely explained as physiologic. Specific characteristics of neonatal jaundice to be considered abnormal until proven otherwise include (1) development before 36 hours of age; (2) persistence beyond 10 days of age; (3) serum bilirubin higher than 12 mg per dl at any time; and (4) elevation of the conjugated fraction of bilirubin more than 2 mg per dl at any time.

There are a number of epidemiologic factors related to neonatal jaundice that have been reviewed elsewhere.[59, 60] Some of the factors associated with increased neonatal bilirubin levels are low birth weight, certain races (Asian, Native American, Greek), maternal medications (e.g., oxytocin), premature rupture of the membranes, increased weight loss after birth, delayed meconium passage, breast-feeding, and neonatal infection. Other factors are associated with decreased neonatal bilirubin levels and include maternal smoking, black race, and certain drugs given to the mother (e.g., phenobarbital).

Neonatal Jaundice Due to Increased Production of Bilirubin

The most common cause of severe early jaundice is fetal-maternal blood group incompatibility with resulting *isoimmunization*. Maternal immunization develops because of leakage of erythrocytes from the fetal to the maternal circulation. When the fetal erythrocytes carry different antigens, they are recognized as foreign by the maternal immune system, which forms antibodies against them (maternal sensitization). These antibodies (IgG immunoglobulins) cross the placental barrier into the fetal circulation and bind to fetal erythrocytes. In Rh incompatibility, sequestration and destruction of the antibody-coated erythrocytes takes place in the reticuloendothelial system of the fetus. In ABO incompatibility hemolysis is intravascular, complement mediated, and usually not as severe as in Rh disease.[61] Significant hemolysis can also result from incompatibilities between minor blood group antigens (e.g., Kell).[62] Although these conditions are predominantly associated with an elevation of unconjugated bilirubin, the conjugated fraction is occasionally elevated also.

Table 23–1. CAUSES OF NEONATAL HYPERBILIRUBINEMIA

Increased Production of Bilirubin
Fetal-maternal blood group incompatibilities
Extravascular blood in body tissues
Polycythemia
Red blood cell abnormalities (hemoglobinopathies, membrane and enzyme defects)
Induction of labor
Decreased Excretion of Bilirubin
Increased enterohepatic circulation of bilirubin
Breast-feeding
Inborn errors of metabolism
Hormones and drugs
Prematurity
Hepatic hypoperfusion
Cholestatic syndromes
Obstruction of the biliary tree
Combined Increased Production and Decreased Excretion of Bilirubin
Sepsis
Intrauterine infection
Congenital cirrhosis

Rh incompatibility usually does not develop until the second pregnancy. Thus, prenatal blood typing and serial testing of Rh-negative mothers for the development of Rh antibodies provide important information to guide possible intrauterine care. If maternal Rh antibodies develop during pregnancy, potentially helpful measures include serial amniocentesis (with bilirubin measurement),[63, 64] ultrasound assessment of the fetus,[65, 66] intrauterine transfusion,[67, 68] and premature delivery. The prophylactic administration of anti-D gamma globulin[69] has been most helpful in preventing Rh sensitization. The neonate with an Rh incompatibility presents with pallor, hepatosplenomegaly, and a rapidly developing jaundice in the first hours of life. If the problem is severe, the infant may be born with generalized edema (fetal hydrops). Laboratory findings in the neonate's blood include reticulocytosis, anemia, a positive direct Coombs' test, and a rapidly rising serum bilirubin level. Exchange transfusion continues to be an important therapy for seriously affected infants.[70]

ABO incompatibility usually presents clinically with the first pregnancy. ABO hemolytic disease is largely limited to blood group A or B infants born to group O mothers. ABO hemolytic disease is relatively rare in type A or B mothers. Development of jaundice is not as rapid as with Rh disease, and a serum bilirubin higher than 12 mg per dl on day 3 of life would be typical. Laboratory abnormalities include reticulocytosis (>10%) and a weakly positive direct Coombs' test, although this is sometimes negative. Anti-A or anti-B antibodies may be seen in the serum of the neonate if examined within the first few days of life before they rapidly disappear. Spherocytes are the most prominent feature seen in the peripheral blood smear with ABO incompatibility.

When *extravascular blood* is present within the body, the hemoglobin can be rapidly converted to bilirubin by tissue macrophages. Examples of this increased bilirubin production include cephalohematoma, ecchymoses, petechiae, and hemorrhage. Although diagnosis of this problem can often be made by physical examination, occult intracranial, intestinal, or pulmonary hemorrhage is associated with similar results. Similarly, swallowed blood can be converted to bilirubin by the heme oxy-

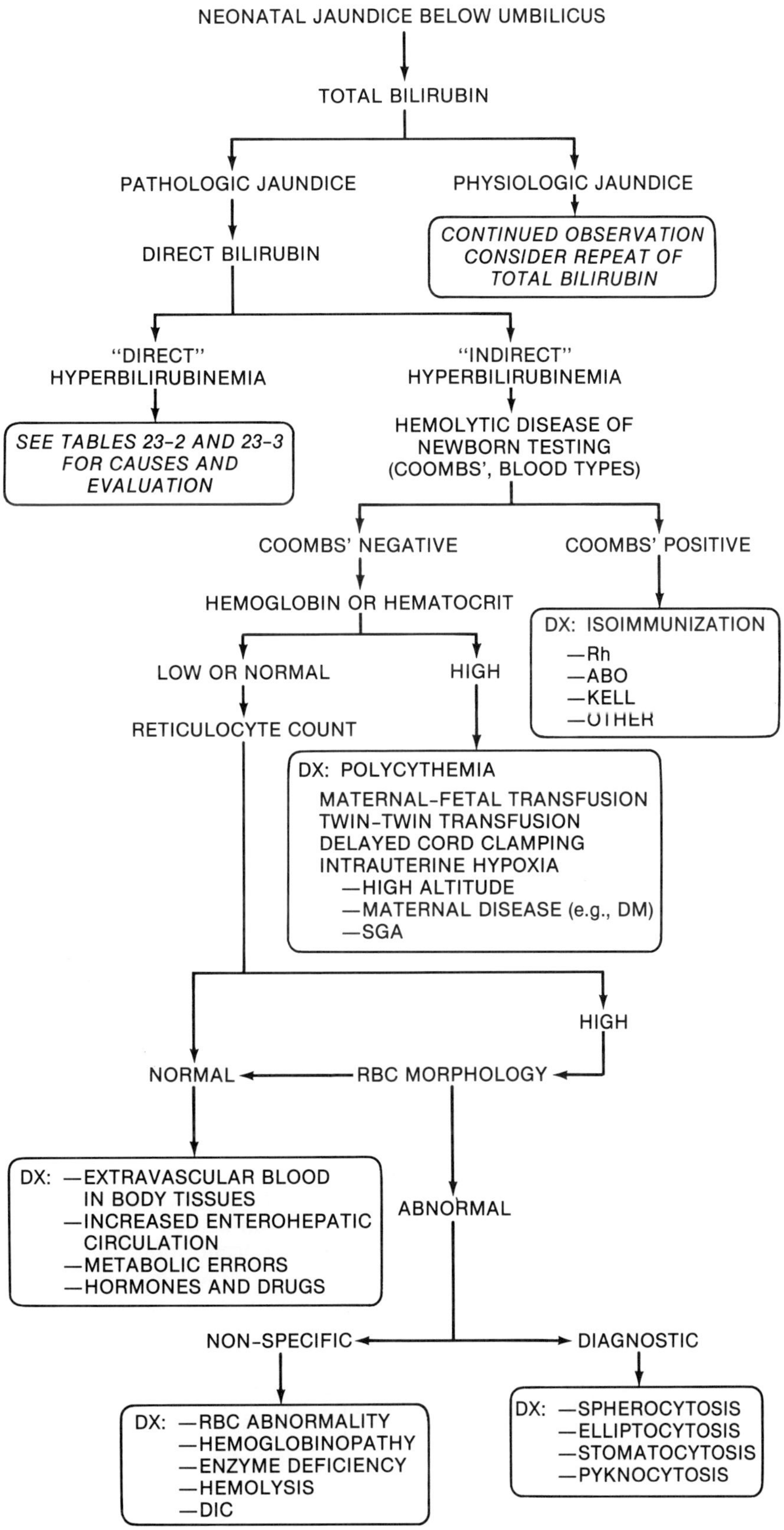

Figure 23–3. A clinical approach to the diagnosis of neonatal jaundice.

genase of intestinal epithelium. The Apt test can be used to distinguish blood of maternal or infant origin because of the differences in alkali resistance between fetal and adult hemoglobin.[71, 72]

Polycythemia can cause hyperbilirubinemia because the absolute increase in red blood cell mass results in an elevated bilirubin production through normal rates of erythrocyte breakdown. A number of mechanisms may result in neonatal polycythemia as reviewed by Danish,[73] and usually are distinguished by venipuncture hematocrit levels higher than 65%. During placental separation at the time of birth, bleeding may occur from the maternal circulation into the fetus (maternal-fetal transfusion) or because of a delay in cord clamping.[74] Twin-twin transfusions can also result in polycythemia. Similarly, intrauterine hypoxia and maternal diseases (e.g., diabetes mellitus[75]) can result in neonatal polycythemia. The therapy for symptomatic polycythemia is partial exchange transfusion, although treatment for asymptomatic polycythemia remains controversial.[74]

A number of specific abnormalities related to the red blood cell can result in neonatal jaundice, including hemoglobinopathies, and red blood cell membrane and enzyme defects. Hereditary spherocytosis is not usually a neonatal problem but hemolytic crises can occur and present with an increasing bilirubin level and a decreasing hematocrit level. A family history of spherocytosis, anemia, or early gallstone disease (before age 40) is helpful in suggesting this diagnosis. The characteristic spherocytes seen in the peripheral blood smear may be impossible to distinguish from those seen with ABO hemolytic disease. Other hemolytic anemias associated with neonatal jaundice include drug-induced hemolysis, deficiencies of the erythrocyte enzymes (glucose-6-phosphate dehydrogenase deficiency, pyruvate kinase deficiency, and others), and hemolysis induced by vitamin K or bacteria. Alpha-thalassemia can result in severe hemolysis and lethal hydrops fetalis.[76] Gamma-beta thalassemia may also present with hemolysis and severe neonatal hyperbilirubinemia.[77] There are a wide variety of clinical findings associated with the thalassemias, extending from profound intrauterine hydrops and death to mild neonatal jaundice and anemia or to neither jaundice nor anemia. Drugs or other substances responsible for hemolysis can be passed to the fetus or neonate across the placenta or via the breast milk, respectively.

Induction of labor with oxytocin has been shown to be associated with neonatal jaundice. There is a significant association between hyponatremia and jaundice in the infants of mothers who received oxytocin to induce labor.[78, 79] The explanation for this observation is not clear. It has been suggested that the 5% glucose in which the oxytocin is usually infused results in hypotonicity of the fetal circulation when the glucose is rapidly metabolized. This reaction is suggested to result in erythrocytes with increased osmotic fragility and accelerated destruction.

Neonatal Jaundice Due to Decreased Excretion of Bilirubin

Increased enterohepatic circulation of bilirubin is believed to be an important factor in neonatal jaundice. As previously reviewed, neonates are at risk for the intestinal absorption of bilirubin because (1) they lack an intestinal flora to convert bilirubin conjugates to urobilinoids; (2) they have significant amounts of beta-glucuronidase within the intestinal lumen that hydrolyzes bilirubin conjugates to bilirubin, which is more easily absorbed from the intestine; and (3) meconium, the intestinal contents accumulated during gestation, contains significant amounts of bilirubin.[80] Conditions that prolong meconium passage (e.g., Hirschsprung's disease, meconium ileus, or meconium plug syndrome) are associated with hyperbilirubinemia.[81, 82] Earlier passage of meconium has been shown to be associated with lower serum bilirubin levels.[83, 84] This may be facilitated by rectal temperature measurement during the neonatal period.[85] The enterohepatic circulation of bilirubin can be blocked by the enteral administration of compounds that bind bilirubin, such as agar,[45, 86, 87] charcoal,[88] and cholestyramine.[89]

Breast-feeding has been clearly identified as a factor related to neonatal jaundice,[58] and this subject has been reviewed elsewhere.[90, 91] Breast-fed infants have been shown to have significantly higher serum bilirubin levels than formula-fed infants on each of the first 5 days of life,[92] and this unconjugated hyperbilirubinemia can persist for weeks[93] to months.[94] During the first week of life, some clinicians distinguish this early jaundice as "breast-feeding jaundice" to differentiate it from the later "breast-milk jaundice syndrome" that occurs after the first week of life.[95–97] There is probably an overlap between these conditions and physiologic jaundice. Early reports linking breast milk and jaundice with a steroid (pregnane-3[α],20[β]-diol) in some samples[98] have not been confirmed by more recent larger studies using more sensitive methods.[99] There are also conflicting data regarding efforts to attribute this jaundice to increased lipase activity in the breast milk, resulting in elevated levels of free fatty acids, which could inhibit hepatic glucuronosyl transferase.[100–103] The enterohepatic circulation of bilirubin might be facilitated by the presence of beta-glucuronidase[51, 104, 105] or some other substance in human milk.[106] Other factors possibly related to jaundice in breast-fed infants include caloric intake, fluid intake, weight loss, delayed meconium passage, intestinal bacterial flora, and inhibition of bilirubin glucuronosyl transferase by an unidentified factor in the milk.[90] Lascari[96] suggests that a healthy breast-fed infant with unconjugated hyperbilirubinemia, normal hemoglobin concentration, reticulocyte count, and blood smear, no blood group incompatibility, and no other abnormalities found in physical examination may be presumed to have early breast-feeding jaundice. Because there is no specific laboratory test to confirm a diagnosis of breast-milk jaundice, it is important to rule out treatable causes of jaundice before ascribing the hyperbilirubinemia to breast milk. Maisels and Gifford[106] suggest waiting until the serum bilirubin level reaches 15 mg per dl before evaluating an otherwise well-appearing breast-fed infant.[107] The author believes that thorough evaluation should be performed when the serum bilirubin level reaches 12 mg per dl, thus allowing more time for intervention, should this prove necessary.

If the bilirubin level is increasing, published recommendations support encouraging mothers to breast-feed more frequently,[108, 109] with an average suggested interval between feeds of 2 hours and no feeding supplements.[59] More frequent nursing may not increase intake but has been suggested to increase peristalsis and stool frequency, thus promoting bilirubin excretion.[110] The point at which breast-feeding should be discontinued is controversial, and recommendations include bilirubin levels of 14,[111] 15,[96] 16 to 17,[109] and 18 to 20 mg per dl.[59] When breast-feeding is interrupted, formula feeding may be initiated for 24 to 48 hours, or breast- and formula-feeding can be alternated with each feeding. A decrease in the serum bilirubin levels of 2 to 5 mg per dl[110] is consistent with a diagnosis of breast milk jaundice. Breast-feeding may then be resumed, although serum bilirubin levels may increase for several days but gradually level off and decline.[96, 108] If breast-feeding is to be resumed following the interruption, it is important to preserve lactation with the use of a breast pump. In one study, interruption of breast-feeding for approximately 50 hours (during which time a formula was given) was shown to have the same bilirubin-lowering effect as a similar duration of phototherapy.[112]

Several *inborn errors of metabolism* can present with neonatal hyperbilirubinemia. Perhaps the most impressive of these is the *Crigler-Najjar syndrome,* or congenital nonhemolytic jaundice,[113] which is characterized by a hereditary deficiency of hepatic bilirubin glucuronosyltransferase.[114, 115] Without the ability to conjugate and hence excrete bilirubin, affected infants develop an intense, persistent jaundice in the first few days of life despite otherwise normal liver function tests. Serum bilirubin levels in the range of 25 to 35 mg per dl can result without treatment, and there is severe risk of kernicterus. Three types of Crigler-Najjar syndrome have been described. Types I and II are distinguished by treatment with phenobarbital. Type I shows no response to this therapy, and no bilirubin conjugates are seen in the bile.[116, 117] Type I patients require lifelong treatment with nocturnal phototherapy and blockage of the enterohepatic circulation. In type II, or Arias' syndrome,[118] phenobarbital produces an enhanced biliary excretion of bilirubin diglucuronide and monoglucuronide.[33, 119] Although this is associated with some decrease in the serum bilirubin level, significant jaundice persists (approximately 15 mg per dl). Recently described type III[120] resembles type I in that there is no biliary excretion of bilirubin glucuronide. However, type III patients do excrete monoglucoside and diglucoside conjugates of bilirubin. It has been speculated that type III patients lack the long-proposed permease[121] that has been hypothesized to transport UDP–glucuronic acid to the luminal side of the endoplasmic reticulum where glucuronosyltransferase is located. This absence forces the utilization of an inefficient substrate for conjugation to bilirubin, UDP-glucose.

Galactosemia is an autosomal-recessive disorder in which there is a deficiency of galactose–1-phosphate uridyltransferase, an enzyme necessary for the conversion of galactose to glucose. This deficiency results in the accumulation of galactose-1-phosphate, which is believed to be hepatotoxic. Conjugated or nonconjugated hyperbilirubinemia usually develops in the first week of life, once lactose is present in the diet. After consuming lactose, affected infants will excrete a non–glucose-reducing substance (galactose) in the urine. Although simple urinary tests can be helpful in suggesting this diagnosis, the diagnosis ultimately is made by demonstrating the enzyme deficiency in erythrocytes. Septicemia frequently develops in the first weeks of life. Treatment consists of complete elimination of galactose from the diet.

Hereditary fructose intolerance results from a deficiency of fructose–1-phosphate aldolase. Affected infants develop serious hepatocellular disease, hepatomegaly, and jaundice after the ingestion of anything containing fructose (e.g., sucrose). Diagnosis can be made with an intravenous fructose tolerance test or an enzyme assay of a liver specimen. Treatment consists of complete elimination of fructose from the diet.

Hereditary tyrosinemia, also known as tyrosinosis, tyrosinemia type I, or fumarylacetoacetate hydrolase (FAH) deficiency, is another rare autosomal-recessive disorder involving deficient metabolism of tyrosine and phenylalanine.[122] Tyrosine accumulates throughout the body, and progressive liver disease results. Infants can present in the first weeks to months of life with conjugated hyperbilirubinemia and hepatomegaly. Diagnosis is suggested by blood and urine amino acid analysis and established by tests for urinary or serum succinylacetone and tissue (e.g., lymphocyte) FAH.[122] Dietary restriction of phenylalanine and tyrosine are helpful while awaiting liver transplantation.[123] Hypermethioninemia can result from hereditary tyrosinemia but is not a specific disease entity.[124]

Alpha$_1$-antitrypsin deficiency can present with conjugated *hyperbilirubinemia* in the first months of life or liver disease in later childhood or adulthood. Alpha$_1$-antitrypsin, a protein made in the hepatocyte, is an important inhibitor of various proteases. There are more than 75 allelic variants,[125] which are classified with a Pi (protease inhibitor) phenotype according to the band position on isoelectric focusing of plasma proteins. The normal phenotype, PiMM, is found in 80 to 90% of the population.[126, 127] The most striking deficiency of alpha$_1$-antitrypsin is seen with the PiZZ phenotype in which serum alpha$_1$-antitrypsin levels are 5 to 15% of normal.[128] The people who are deficient in this phenotype have an increased incidence of neonatal hepatitis,[129, 130] early cirrhosis,[131] and liver malignancy[132] as well as pulmonary emphysema.[133] PiZZ alpha$_1$-antitrypsin deficiency is now believed to be the most common metabolic disease to cause neonatal hepatitis[134] and the most common metabolic disease prompting liver transplantation in the United States.[135] The prevalence of alpha$_1$-antitrypsin deficiency is approximately 1 in 2,000 people in the United States.[136] The pathophysiology of the tissue damage is not well understood, although one theory ascribes the liver injury to accumulation of alpha$_1$-antitrypsin within the liver cells.[137] There is considerable variability in the expression of this condition, as shown by the prospective studies of 200,000 newborn infants in Sweden by Sveger,[138] in which 127 PiZZ infants were identified and followed for 12 years. Fourteen infants developed obstructive jaundice in the first months of life, three of these dying with liver disease by the age of 8 years, with more than half showing persistently abnormal transaminase levels. At least 75% of the PiZZ infants showed no signs of liver disease by the age of 12 years. Diagnosis rests on determination of the Pi phenotype since alpha$_1$-antitrypsin is an acute-phase reactant, and serum levels can increase threefold to fourfold in response to inflammation.[139] Liver biopsy of PiZZ persons demonstrates distinctive periodic acid–Schiff-positive, diastase-resistant globules in hepatocytes, although this finding is occasionally seen in PiMM persons.[140, 141] The only effective therapy for end-stage liver disease due to alpha$_1$-antitrypsin deficiency is transplantation. Replacement therapy remains experimental.[142] Avoidance of smoking is important because of the pulmonary emphysema that ultimately develops in 60% of PiZZ persons.[143]

Various *hormones and drugs* may cause development of neonatal unconjugated hyperbilirubinemia. Congenital hypothyroidism can present with serum bilirubin levels higher than 12 mg per dl prior to the development of other clinical findings.[144] Similarly, hypopituitarism and anencephaly may be associated with jaundice due to inadequate thyroxine, which is necessary for hepatic clearance of bilirubin.

Infants of diabetic mothers have prolonged and higher serum bilirubin levels than do control patients.[145] Reasons for this hyperbilirubinemia might include prematurity, polycythemia, substrate deficiency for glucuronidation (secondary to hypoglycemia), poor hepatic perfusion (secondary to either respiratory distress, persistent fetal circulation, or cardiomyopathy), and beta-glucuronidase.[105]

The *Lucey-Driscoll syndrome*[146] consists of neonatal hyperbilirubinemia within families in whom there is an in vitro inhibition of glucuronosyltransferase by both maternal and infant serum. It is presumed that this is caused by gestational hormones.

Certain drugs may affect the metabolism of bilirubin and result in hyperbilirubinemia or displacement of bilirubin from albumin. Such displacement increases the risk of kernicterus and can be caused by sulfonamides[147] and ceftriaxone.[148] Pancuronium bromide[149] and chloral hydrate[150] have been suggested as causes of neonatal hyperbilirubinemia.

Prematurity is frequently associated with unconjugated hyperbilirubinemia in the neonatal period. Hepatic UDP-glucuronosyltransferase activity is markedly decreased in premature infants and increases steadily from 30 of weeks of gestation until reaching adult levels 14 weeks after birth.[151] In addition there may be deficiencies for both uptake[152] and secretion.[153] Bilirubin clearance improves rapidly following birth.[154]

Hepatic hypoperfusion can result in neonatal jaundice. Inadequate perfusion of the hepatic sinusoids may not allow sufficient hepatocyte uptake and metabolism of bilirubin. Causes of the hypoperfusion include patent ductus venosus (e.g., with respiratory distress syndrome), congestive heart failure, and portal vein thrombosis. *Obstruction of the biliary tree,* including such entities as biliary atresia, choledochal cyst, cholelithiasis, and cholangitis, may cause neonatal jaundice and are discussed elsewhere (see Chapter 71). Gallbladder sludge produced by ceftriaxone,[155] total parenteral nutrition,[156] or postsurgical fasting[157] can potentially progress to become symptomatic gallstones.[158]

Other *cholestatic syndromes* can result in jaundice due to decreased excretion of bilirubin. These syndromes present with elevation of the direct (conjugated) bilirubin fraction. There are many causes of neonatal cholestasis, some of which have already been mentioned. A brief list of causes of neonatal cholestasis is presented in Table 23–2. An exhaustive review is beyond the scope of this chapter and can be found elsewhere.[159–161] A suggested evaluation of neonatal conjugated hyperbilirubinemia is presented in Table 23–3.

Table 23–2. CAUSES OF NEONATAL CONJUGATED HYPERBILIRUBINEMIA

Defects in Anatomy
- Extrahepatic
  - Biliary atresia, choledochal cyst, neoplasm, choledocholithiasis
- Intrahepatic
  - Congenital hepatic fibrosis, nonsyndromatic paucity of the intrahepatic bile ducts, arteriohepatic dysplasia (Alagille's syndrome), cerebrohepatorenal syndrome (Zellweger's syndrome)

Defects in Metabolism
- Alpha$_1$-Antitrypsin deficiency, tyrosinemia, galactosemia, cystic fibrosis, hereditary fructose intolerance, cholestatic syndromes (e.g., Byler disease)

Infection
- Neonatal hepatitis
  - Viral: rubella, cytomegalovirus, herpes, varicella, coxsackie, hepatitis B, reo 3
  - Other: toxoplasmosis, syphilis, tuberculosis, listeriosis
- Sepsis
- Urinary tract infection with endotoxemia

Chromosomal Defects
- Down's syndrome, trisomy 13, trisomy 18

Toxic
- Total parenteral nutrition
- Chloral hydrate

Table 23–3. AN EVALUATION OF NEONATAL CONJUGATED HYPERBILIRUBINEMIA

- Liver function tests: alanine aminotransferase, gamma glutamyltransferase, bilirubin (total and direct), prothrombin time, albumin, serum bile acids
- Cultures: blood, urine, spinal fluid
- Eye examination: for chorioretinitis, posterior embryotoxon, cataracts
- Long bone films for evidence of congenital infection
- Serology for infection: immunoglobulin M, TORCH, VDRL, hepatitis B surface antigen
- Alpha$_1$-antitrypsin quantitation and phenotype
- Metabolic screen: urine and serum amino acids, urine-reducing substance
- Sweat chloride test
- Ultrasound examination of liver and biliary tree
- Hepatobiliary scintigraphy
- Percutaneous liver biopsy

Neonatal Jaundice Due to Both Increased Production and Decreased Excretion of Bilirubin

In neonatal diseases with jaundice due to decreased excretion and increased production of bilirubin, both conjugated and unconjugated bilirubin fractions can be elevated. Bacterial *sepsis* increases bilirubin production by producing erythrocyte hemolysis due to hemolysins released by bacteria. Endotoxins released by bacteria can also decrease canalicular bile formation.

Intrauterine infection is an important cause of neonatal jaundice. Organisms that can cause hepatitis and associated hyperbilirubinemia include the TORCH agents (toxoplasmosis, rubella, cytomegalovirus, herpes simplex), *Treponema, Listeria,* and *Mycobacterium tuberculosis* as well as hepatitis B, varicella, coxsackie, and probably reo 3 virus, which has been suggested to be a major cause of extrahepatic biliary atresia. Findings include hepatosplenomegaly with prominent extramedullary hematopoiesis in the liver, thrombocytopenia, chorioretinitis, and other abnormalities of the eye, central nervous system, and heart. Liver biopsy reveals characteristic giant cell hepatitis, although this finding is nonspecific and can be seen in liver disease unrelated to infection. Diagnosis is aided by specific IgM determinations and serologic tests.

Congenital cirrhosis and hepatic fibrosis have also been reported as causes of jaundice in neonates. Abnormal erythrocytes may contribute to bilirubin production. Diagnosis is generally made with liver biopsy.

Toxicity of Neonatal Jaundice

Kernicterus (in German, *kern* means *nucleus* and *icterus* means *yellow*) is the clinical condition associated with severe unconjugated hyperbilirubinemia and is named for the yellow staining of certain regions of the brain, particularly the basal ganglia, hippocampus, cerebellum, and nuclei of the floor of the fourth ventricle.[162, 163] Findings include a sluggish Moro reflex, opisthotonos, hypotonia, vomiting, high-pitched cry, hyperpyrexia, seizures, paresis of gaze ("setting sun sign"), oculogyric crisis, and death. Long-term findings include spasticity, choreoathetosis, and sensorineural hearing loss. Milder forms of bilirubin encephalopathy include cognitive dysfunction and learning disabilities.[164, 165] The mechanism of bilirubin toxicity is complex and has been reviewed elsewhere.[163] Although the neonatal period is the most common time for bilirubin-related brain damage, the neurotoxicity of bilirubin has also been documented in adults with Crigler-Najjar syndrome type I.[166] Recent speculation questions whether some mild degree of hyperbilirubinemia may be helpful because of the antioxidant capacity of bilirubin.[167]

The absolute level of serum bilirubin has not been a good predictor of the risk of severe neonatal jaundice, although it has long been known that kernicterus is likely with serum unconjugated bilirubin levels higher than 30 mg per dl and unlikely with levels lower than 20 mg per dl.[168, 169] Albumin concentration is an important variable because of the high-affinity binding with bilirubin. Drugs and organic anions also bind to albumin and can displace bilirubin, thereby increasing the free bilirubin that can diffuse into cells and cause toxicity.[170] The most notable example of this is the kernicterus that occurred with low bilirubin levels when sulfisoxazole was given to premature infants.[171] Walker[172] has reviewed neonatal bilirubin toxicity and drug-induced bilirubin displacement. There is considerable debate regarding the risk of hyperbilirubinemia to otherwise healthy full-term infants, with the suggestion that such infants are not at risk until the serum bilirubin level increases to well over 20 mg per dl.[173] Although it has been acknowledged that total serum bilirubin may not be the most important factor related to risk, there are, at present, no generally accepted tests of bilirubin binding or free bilirubin to prevent kernicterus or to avoid unnecessary therapy for jaundice.

Management of Neonatal Jaundice

The management of neonatal jaundice has been reviewed elsewhere.[110] The most important step in treatment of jaundice is the determination of the primary cause. In both conjugated (Tables 23–2 and 23–3) and unconjugated (see Fig. 23–3) hyperbilirubinemia, initial therapy should be directed at the primary cause of the jaundice. In addition, elevation of the unconjugated bilirubin fraction prompts concern about possible kernicterus independent of the cause of the jaundice. As recently reviewed,[172, 174] when the unconjugated bilirubin fraction is elevated, care must be given to avoid administration of agents that bind to albumin and, by displacing bilirubin, promote kernicterus. Although, historically, sulfonamides are the most well-known bilirubin-displacing agents, newer drugs such as ceftriaxone are also strong bilirubin displacers with a potential for inducing bilirubin encephalopathy.[148] Therapeutic options to decrease the unconjugated bilirubin concentration include phototherapy, exchange transfusion, enzyme induction, interruption of the enterohepatic circulation, and interruption of breast-feeding.

Phototherapy consisting of irradiation of the jaundiced infant with light has been recently reviewed.[175] Phototherapy changes the bilirubin molecule in two ways, allowing bilirubin to be excreted into the bile or the urine without the usual glucuronidation. One change involves a 180-degree twist around the double bonds between either the A and B or C and D rings,[176] converting the normal Z configuration to the E configuration. 4Z,15E bilirubin is preferentially formed and can spontaneously reisomerize to native bilirubin. More importantly a new seven-membered ring structure can be formed between rings A and B, resulting in "lumirubin,"[177] or "cyclobilirubin."[178] Both changes interfere with the internal hydrogen bonding of native bilirubin, and the lumirubin and E isomers can be excreted directly into bile. Lumirubin appears to be the major route to explain the success of phototherapy.[179] New phototherapy devices using woven fiberoptic pads are available.[180] Proposed guidelines for phototherapy have been published elsewhere.[110, 181] In general, phototherapy is used to prevent serum bilirubin concentrations from reaching levels necessitating exchange transfusion. Phototherapy is now frequently done at home.[182] Despite documented complications,[183] phototherapy is widely used and generally safe, but it should not be employed without prior diagnostic evaluation of the cause of the jaundice.

Exchange transfusion is the most rapid method to decrease acutely the serum bilirubin concentration. Indications for exchange transfusion vary and have been published elsewhere.[110, 183–186] Although there are many well-described risks with exchange transfusion, mortality should be low (<0.6%) if it is performed properly.[154, 187, 188]

There are a number of *pharmacologic* approaches to the prevention and treatment of neonatal hyperbilirubinemia that have been reviewed.[189] The enterohepatic circulation can be interrupted by the enteral administration of agents that bind bilirubin in the intestine and prevent reabsorption. Such agents include agar,[45, 87] cholestyramine,[89] and activated charcoal.[88] Increased intestinal peristalsis would be expected to allow less time for bilirubin absorption. Frequent feeding[190] and rectal stimulation[85] are associated with lower serum bilirubin levels. Enteral feeding of bilirubin oxidase, an enzyme that degrades bilirubin,[191] is an additional method to block the enterohepatic circulation that remains experimental.[192]

Since neonatal hepatic UDP-glucuronosyltransferase activity has been shown to be low,[151] it is not surprising that induction of hepatic UDP-glucuronosyltransferase results in lower serum bilirubin levels. Such induction in the neonate can be accomplished with prenatal maternal use of phenobarbital or diphenylhydantoin.[193, 194] In the postnatal period, use of phenobarbital by the neonate has the same bilirubin-lowering effect.[195]

An alternative approach is to block the first enzyme responsible for the production of bilirubin, heme oxygenase. This can be accomplished by several different metalloporphyrins, as recently reviewed.[196] Sn-protoporphyrin has been used successfully in the experimental management of jaundice in neonates with ABO incompatibility[197] and older patients with Crigler-Najjar syndrome.[197a] Treatment of neonatal jaundice with heme oxygenase inhibition remains experimental.

Table 23–4. CAUSES OF JAUNDICE IN INFANTS AND OLDER CHILDREN

Causes
Metabolic Disorders
Hereditary hyperbilirubinemias
Gilbert's syndrome
Dubin-Johnson syndrome
Rotor's syndrome
Crigler-Najjar syndrome
Wilson's disease
Alpha$_1$-antitrypsin deficiency
Cystic fibrosis
Viral Hepatitis
Hepatitis A, B, C, D, E; Epstein-Barr virus, cytomegalovirus
Chronic Active Hepatitis
Biliary Tract Disease
Cholecystitis, cholelithiasis, Caroli's disease, choledochal cyst
Tumor
Hepatic, biliary, pancreatic, peritoneal, duodenal
Red Blood Cell Abnormalities
Sickle cell disease, thalassemia, hemolysis
Drugs and Toxins
Acetaminophen, valproate, chlorpromazine, *Amanita* toxin, sepsis, and others
Sclerosing Cholangitis
Primary, secondary to inflammatory bowel disease
Veno-occlusive Disease
Pyrrolidizine alkaloids, bone marrow transplant
Impaired Delivery of Bilirubin to Liver
Congestive heart failure, cirrhosis

JAUNDICE IN INFANTS AND OLDER CHILDREN

A brief list of causes of jaundice in infants and older children is presented in Table 23–4. Several hereditary hyperbilirubinemia syndromes may present in infants or older children. These include Gilbert's, Dubin-Johnson, and Rotor's syndromes.

Gilbert's syndrome is generally not recognized until after puberty. It is characterized by a hereditary, chronic, mild unconjugated hyperbilirubinemia with otherwise normal liver function tests (for reviews, see references 198 and 199.) Gilbert's syndrome appears to be a heterogeneous group of disorders, all of which share at least a 50% decrease in hepatic bilirubin glucuronosyltransferase activity.[200–202] Based on plasma clearance of other organic anions (BSP and ICG), there appear to be at least four subtypes of Gilbert's syndrome.[203, 204] Mild hemolysis is not infrequent. Patients with this disorder show a pronounced increase of serum bilirubin concentration in response to fasting.[205] Odell and Gourley[198] speculate that some infants with neonatal jaundice are manifesting Gilbert's syndrome because of the transient hormonal milieu (estrogenization) of the fetus. Even though Gilbert's syndrome is usually not associated with negative implications for health or longevity, occasional patients complain of fatigue or abdominal pain.

Dubin-Johnson syndrome and Rotor's syndrome are two distinct but similar hyperbilirubinemia syndromes with autosomal-recessive inheritance. In both syndromes the direct and indirect fractions of bilirubin are elevated, although other liver function tests, including serum bile acid levels, are normal.[206–208] Both conditions can occur in males and females. Rotor's syndrome can be seen in early childhood,[209] whereas Dubin-Johnson syndrome presents from birth to 40 years of age. In both conditions total serum bilirubin levels usually range from approximately 2 to 7 mg per dl, with at least half present as conjugated bilirubin,[208, 210] but can reach 20 mg per dl under certain conditions, such as intercurrent illness.[210, 211]

Despite the many similarities between Dubin-Johnson and Rotor's syndromes, there are significant differences.

Dubin-Johnson syndrome occurs far more frequently than Rotor's syndrome, and the hyperbilirubinemia is often exacerbated by pregnancy and the use of oral contraceptives.[212] Liver histology is completely normal in Rotor's syndrome. However, in Dubin-Johnson syndrome, liver examination reveals a distinctive brown-black pigmentation visible grossly, with storage located in the lysosomes microscopically.[213] Currently, this pigment is believed to originate from melanin[214, 215] or metabolites of epinephrine.[216] Dubin-Johnson syndrome is more common in males, whereas there is no male predominance in Rotor's syndrome. Oral cholecystography is normal in Rotor's syndrome but often fails to visualize in Dubin-Johnson syndrome.

An important pathophysiologic finding in Rotor's syndrome is the marked reduction in hepatic anion storage.[217, 218] This observation is consistent with the finding of deficient GST activity in a patient with Rotor's syndrome.[219] This suggests that GST stores anions awaiting conjugation as well as those that have already been conjugated (see Fig. 23–1). Decreased storage allows both to reflux into the circulation, thus explaining the elevation of both direct and indirect bilirubin fractions. Hepatic anion storage is normal in Dubin-Johnson syndrome; however, there is a marked decrease in secretion by the biliary canaliculus,[212, 220] thus allowing reflux of conjugated bilirubin into the circulation.

An additional difference useful in differentiating these two syndromes can be seen in the total urinary excretion of coproporphyrins I and III. Urinary coproporphyrin excretion is 2.5 to 5 times elevated in Rotor's syndrome[221] but usually is normal or slightly elevated in Dubin-Johnson syndrome. Further, there are significant differences in the distribution of total urinary coproporphyrins I and III, with isomer I less than 80% of the total in Rotor's syndrome[222] and more than 80% of the total in Dubin-Johnson syndrome (normal is 25%).[223, 224]

Patients with Rotor's syndrome are asymptomatic and require no therapy. Although jaundice is lifelong, there is no associated morbidity or mortality. Although Dubin-Johnson syndrome is also associated with normal health and longevity, a significant number of patients have nonspecific abdominal complaints and hepatomegaly. Diagnosis can be made by confirming conjugated hyperbilirubinemia and otherwise normal liver function tests. Coproporphyrin excretion in the urine allows differentiation of the two syndromes.

Some additional diseases will be mentioned briefly. Jaundice has been shown to be a common presenting sign of *Wilson's disease*, which was present in 28% of 283 patients in one study.[225] The mean age of onset in this study by Saito[225] was 12 years, although this varies in other studies from the later teens to the early 20s. Hepatic symptoms have been reported in patients by the age of 3 years.[226] Wilson's disease is an inborn error of copper metabolism in which toxic amounts of copper accumulate in the liver, brain, kidney, and cornea. It is inherited in an autosomal-recessive fashion. Hemolytic crises and neurologic symptoms (dysarthria, clumsiness, and tremor) are less common presenting symptoms. More than 90% of patients demonstrate an abnormally low serum concentration of ceruloplasmin, a copper-transporting protein. Kayser-Fleischer rings, though pathognomonic in childhood, are rarely found in patients younger than 7 years of age. Urinary copper excretion and hepatic copper levels are both increased in Wilson's disease, although there is some overlap with other cholestatic conditions. The daily, lifelong use of penicillamine is the most effective therapy to decrease copper stores. Trientine is available for patients who develop a sensitivity to penicillamine.[227]

Many of the diseases described previously as causes of neonatal jaundice will also cause jaundice in infants and older children. *Viral hepatitis*[228] is a particularly large category that includes five known viruses (A through E) that cause a hepatitis primarily rather than a more widespread systemic disease with hepatitis. Epstein-Barr virus, cytomegalovirus, and other viruses can also cause hepatic dysfunction resulting in jaundice.

Chronic active hepatitis (CAH) is a heterogeneous syndrome distinguished by liver biopsy showing piecemeal necrosis and prominent plasma cell infiltration of the portal tracts and evidence of clinical disease for longer than 6 months.[229, 230] There are a variety of known causes for this syndrome, including hepatitis viruses B, C, and delta. CAH can also be seen as a manifestation of other liver diseases or as an adverse drug reaction.[231] In addition CAH can be detected when all known causes have been excluded. In this instance, if other immunologic features are present, including hyperglobulinemia (mainly IgG) and a variety of circulating autoantibodies, the term *autoimmune CAH* is used.[231] Autoimmune CAH is poorly understood, and a definite target antigen and pathogenetic antibody await identification. This disease is more common in females, and there is usually a favorable response to corticosteroid therapy.

ACKNOWLEDGMENTS

The author gratefully acknowledges the technical assistance of Bill Kreamer and Brenda Egan and thanks Dr. Gerard Odell for his comments during the preparation of the manuscript and Natty for his patience.

REFERENCES

1. Städeler G: Ueber die farbstoffe der galle. Justus Liebigs Ann Chem 1864; 132:323–354.
2. Schmid R, McDonagh AF: The enzymatic formation of bilirubin. Ann NY Acad Sci 1975; 244:533–552.
3. Tenhunen R, Marver HS, Schmid R: Microsomal heme oxygenase. Characterization of the enzyme. J Biol Chem 1969; 244:6388–6394.
4. Raffin SB, Woo CH, Roost KT, et al: Intestinal absorption of hemoglobin iron-heme cleavage by mucosal heme oxygenase. J Clin Invest 1974; 54:1344–1352.
5. Fischer H, Orth H: Die Chemie des Pyrrols. Leipzig, Akad. Verlagsges, 1937.
6. O'Carra P, Colleran E: Methine bridge selectivity in haem-cleavage reactions: Relevance to the mechanism of haem catabolism. Biochem Soc Trans 1976; 4:209–214.
7. Colleran E, O'Carra P: Enzymology and comparative physiology of biliverdin reduction. *In* Berk PD, Berlin NE, eds. International Symposium on Chemistry and Physiology of Bile Pigments. Washington, DC, US Goverment Printing Office, 1977, p 69.
8. Maisels MJ, Pathak A, Nelson NM, et al: Endogenous produc-

tion of carbon monoxide in normal and erythroblastotic infants. J Clin Invest 1971; 50:1–8.
9. Bloomer JR, Berk PD, Howe RB, et al: Comparison of fecal urobilinogen excretion with bilirubin production in normal volunteers and patients with increased bilirubin production. Clin Chim Acta 1970; 29:463.
10. Whipple GH, Hooper CW: Bile pigment metabolism: VII. Bile pigment output influenced by hemoglobin injections, anemia and blood regeneration. Am J Physiol 1917; 43:258–274.
11. London IM: Conversion of hematin to bile pigment. J Biol Chem 1950; 184:373–376.
12. Ostrow JD, Jandle JG, Schmid R: The formation of bilirubin from hemoglobin in vivo. J Clin Invest 1962; 41:1628–1637.
13. Coburn RF, Kane PB: Maximal erythrocyte and hemoglobin catabolism. J Clin Invest 1968; 47:1435–1446.
14. Daly JS, Little JM, Troxler RF, et al: Metabolism of ^{3}H-myoglobin. Nature 1967; 216:1030–1031.
15. London IM, West R: The formation of bile pigment in pernicious anemia. J Biol Chem 1950; 184:359–364.
16. Gray CH, Scott JJ: The effect of haemorrhage on the incorporation [α-C^{14}] glycine into stercobilin. J Biochem 1959; 71:38–42.
17. Robinson SH, Tsong M, Brown BW, et al: The sources of bile pigment in the rat: Studies of early labeled fraction. J Clin Invest 1966; 45:1569–1586.
18. Bonnett R, Davies JE, Hursthouse MB: Structure of bilirubin. Nature 1976; 262:327–328.
19. Bennhold H: Uber die vehikelfunktion der serumeiweisskorper. Ergeb Inn Med Kinderheilkd 1932; 42:273–375.
20. Jacobsen J. Binding of bilirubin to human serum albumin: Determination of the dissociation constants. FEBS Lett 1969; 5:112–114.
21. Scharschmidt BF, Waggoner JG, Berk PD: Hepatic organic anion uptake in the rat. J Clin Invest 1975; 56:1280–1292.
22. Levi AJ, Gatmaitan Z, Arias IM: Two hepatic cytoplasmic protein fractions, Y and Z, and their possible role in the hepatic uptake of bilirubin, sulfobromophthalein and other anions. J Clin Invest 1969; 48:2156–2167.
23. Fleischner G, Robbins J, Arias IM: Immunological studies of Y protein: A major cytoplasmic organic anion-binding protein in rat liver. J Clin Invest 1972; 51:677–684.
24. Habig WH, Pabst MJ, Fleischner G, et al: The identity of glutathione S-transferase B with ligandin, a major binding protein of liver. Proc Natl Acad Sci U S A 1974; 71:3879–3882.
25. Kamisaka K, Listowsky I, Arias IM: Circular dichroism studies of Y protein (ligandin), a major organic anion binding protein in liver, kidney and small intestine. Ann NY Acad Sci 1973; 226:148–153.
26. Wolkoff AW, Goresky CA, Sellin J, et al: Role of ligandin in transfer of bilirubin from plasma into liver. Am J Physiol 1979; 236:E638–E648.
27. Mackenzie PI, Joffe MM, Munson PJ, et al: Separation of different UDP glucuronosyltransferase activities according to charge heterogeneity by chromatofocusing using mouse liver microsomes: Three major types of aglycones. Biochem Pharmacol 1985; 34:737–746.
28. Koster AS, Schirmer G, Bock KW: Immunochemical and functional characterization of UDP-glucuronosyltransferases from rat liver, intestine and kidney. Biochem Pharmacol 1986; 35:3971–3975.
29. Hauser SC, Ziurys JC, Gollan JL: Regulation of bilirubin glucuronide synthesis in primate (*Macaca fascicularis*) liver: Kinetic analysis of microsomal bilirubin uridine diphosphate glucuronyltransferase. Gastroenterology 1986; 91:287–296.
30. Maddrey WC, Cukier JO, Maglalang AC, et al: Hepatic bilirubin UDP-glucuronyltransferase in patients with sickle cell anemia. Gastroenterology 1978; 74:193–195.
31. Duvaldestin P, Mahu JL, Berthelot P: Effect of fasting on substrate specificity of rat liver UDP-glucuronylsyltransferase. Biochim Biophys Acta 1976; 384:81–86.
32. Gourley GR, Siegel FL, Odell GB: A rapid method for collection and analysis of bile pigments in humans. Gastroenterology 1984; 86:1322.
33. Fevery J, Blanckaert N, Heirwegh KPM, et al: Unconjugated bilirubin and an increased proportion of bilirubin monoconjugates in the bile of patients with Gilbert's syndrome and Crigler-Najjar disease. J Clin Invest 1977; 60:970–979.
34. Goresky CA, Gordon ER, Shaffer EA, et al: Definition of a conjugation dysfunction in Gilbert's syndrome: Studies of the handling of bilirubin loads and of the pattern of bilirubin conjugates secreted in bile. Clin Sci 1978; 55:63–71.
35. Natzschka JC, Odell GB: The influence of albumin on the distribution and excretion of bilirubin in jaundiced rats. Pediatrics 1966; 37:51–61.
36. Arias IM, Johnson L, Wolfson S: Biliary excretion of injected conjugated and unconjugated bilirubin by normal and Gunn rats. Am J Physiol 1961; 200:1091–1094.
37. Zimmerman HJ: Hormonal derivatives and other drugs used to treat endocrine disease. *In* Hepatotoxicity: The Adverse Effects of Drug and Other Chemicals on the Liver. New York, Appleton, Crofts, 1978, pp 436–467.
38. Weiss JS, Guatam A, Lauff JJ, et al: The clinical importance of a protein-bound fraction of serum bilirubin in patients with hyperbilirubinemia. N Engl J Med 1983; 309:147–150.
39. Van Breemen RB, Fenselau C: Acylation of albumin by 1-O-acyl glucuronides. Drug Metab Dispos 1985; 13:318–320.
40. Stogniew M, Fenselau C: Electrophilic reactions of acyl-linked glucuronides-formation of clofibrate mercapturate in humans. Drug Metab Dispos 1982; 10:609–613.
41. Van Breemen RB: Electrophilic reactions of 1-O-acyl glucuronides (Dissertation). Baltimore, Johns Hopkins University, 1985.
42. Billing BH: Intestinal and renal metabolism of bilirubin including enterohepatic circulation. *In* Ostrow JD, ed. Bile Pigments and Jaundice. New York, Marcel Dekker, 1986, pp 255–269.
43. Midtvedt T, Gustafsson BE: Microbial conversion of bilirubin to urobilins *in vitro* and *in vivo*. Acta Pathol Microbiol Immunol Scand [B] 1981; 89:57–60.
44. Fahmy K, Gray CH, Nicholson DC: The reduction of bile pigments by faecal and intestinal bacteria. Biochim Biophys Acta 1972; 264:85–97.
45. Poland RL, Odell GB: Physiologic jaundice: The enterohepatic circulation of bilirubin. N Engl J Med 1971; 284:1–6.
46. Hawksworth G, Drasar BS, Hill MJ: Intestinal bacteria and the hydrolysis of glycosidic bonds. J Med Microbiol 1971; 4:451–459.
47. Kent TH, Fischer LJ, Marr R: Glucuronidase activity in intestinal contents of rat and man and relationship to bacterial flora. Proc Soc Exp Biol Med 1972; 140:590–594.
48. Nanno M, Morotomi M, Takayama H, et al: Mutagenic activation of biliary metabilites of benzo(a)pyrene by beta-glucuronidase–positive bacteria in human faeces. J Med Microbiol 1986; 22:351–355.
49. Musa BU, Doe RP, Seal US: Purification and properties of human liver β-glucuronidase. J Biol Chem 1965; 240:2811–2816.
50. Lester R, Schmid R: Intestinal absorption of bile pigments: I. The enterohepatic circulation of bilirubin in the cat. J Clin Invest 1963; 42:736–746.
51. Gourley GR, Arend RA: β-Glucuronidase and hyperbilirubinemia in breast-fed and formula-fed babies. Lancet 1986; 1:644–646.
52. Rutledge JC, Ou CN: Bilirubin and the laboratory: Advances in the 1980's, considerations for the 1990's. Pediatr Clin North Am 1989; 36:189–197.
53. Mair B, Klempner LB: Abnormally high values for direct bilirubin in the serum of newborns as measured with the DuPont aca. Am J Clin Pathol 1987; 87:642–644.
54. Schumacher RE: Noninvasive measurements of bilirubin in the newborn. Clin Perinatol 1990; 17:417–435.
55. Schumacher RE, Thornbery JM, Gutcher GR: Transcutaneous bilirubinometry: A comparison of old and new methods. Pediatrics 1985; 76:10–14.
56. Gossett IH, Oxon BM: A Perspex icterometer for neonates. Lancet 1960; 1:87–88.
57. Kramer LI: Advancement of dermal icterus in the jaundiced newborn. Am J Dis Child 1969; 118:454–458.
58. Schneider AP: Breast milk jaundice in the newborn—a real entity. JAMA 1986; 255:3270–3274.
59. Maisels MJ: Neonatal jaundice. *In* Avery GB, ed: Neonatalogy: Pathophysiology and Management of the Newborn. Philadelphia, JB Lippincott, 1987, pp 534–629.
60. Linn S, Schoenbaum SC, Monson RR, et al: Epidemiology of neonatal hyperbilirubinemia. Pediatrics 1985; 75:770–774.
61. Zipursky A: Mechanisms of hemolysis. Mead Johnson Symp Perinat Dev Med 1982; 17–24.

62. Wenk RE, Goldstein P, Felix JK: Kell alloimmunization, hemolytic disease of the newborn, and perinatal management. Obstet Gynecol 1985; 66:473–476.
63. Bevis DCA: The antenatal prediction of hemolytic disease of the newborn. Lancet 1952; 1:395–398.
64. Odell GB: Evaluation of fetal hemolysis. N Engl J Med 1970; 282:1204–1205.
65. Frigoletto FD, Greene MF, Benacerraf BR, et al: Ultrasonographic fetal surveillance in the management of the isoimmunized pregnancy. N Engl J Med 1986; 315:430–432.
66. Vintzileos AM, Campbell WA, Storlazzi E, et al: Fetal liver ultrasound measurements in isoimmunized pregnancies. Obstet Gynecol 1986; 62:162–167.
67. Grannum PA, Copel JA, Plaxe SC, et al: In utero exchange transfusion by direct intravascular injection in severe erythroblastosis fetalis. N Engl J Med 1986; 314:1431–1434.
68. Queenan JT: Erythroblastosis fetalis: Closing the circle. N Engl J Med 1986; 314:1448–1449.
69. Clarke CA: Prevention of Rh-hemolytic disease. Br Med J 1967; 4:484–485.
70. Allen FHJr, Diamond LK: Erythroblastosis fetalis, including exchange transfusion technique. Boston, Little, Brown, 1958, pp 1–155.
71. Apt L, Downey WS: Melena neonatorum: The "swallowed blood syndrome." J Pediatr 1955; 47:6–12.
72. Jacobs DS, Kasten BL, Demott WR, et al: APT test. *In* Laboratory Test Handbook with DRG Index. St. Louis, Mosby/Lexi-Comp, 1984, pp 277.
73. Danish EH: Neonatal polycythemia. *In* Brown EB, ed: Progress in Hematology. Vol. 14. New York, Grune and Stratton, 1986, pp 55–98.
74. Oh W: Neonatal polycythemia and hyperviscosity. Pediatr Clin North Am 1986; 33:523–532.
75. Mimouni F, Miodovnik M, Siddiqi TA, et al: Neonatal polycythemia in infants of insulin-dependent diabetic mothers. Obstet Gynecol 1986; 68:370–372.
76. Liang ST, Wong VCW, So WWK, et al: Homozygous α-thalassemia: Clinical presentation, diagnosis and management: A review of 46 cases. Br J Obstet Gynaecol 1985; 92:680–684.
77. Kan YW, Forget BG, Nathan DG: Gamma-beta thalassemia: A cause of hemolytic disease of the newborn. N Engl J Med 1972; 286:129–134.
78. Singhi S, Chookang E, Hall JSE: Intrapartum infusion of aqueous glucose solution, transplacental hyponatraemia, and risk of neonatal jaundice. Br J Obstet Gynaecol 1984; 99:1014–1018.
79. D'Souza SW, Lieberman B, Cadman J, et al: Oxytocin induction of labour: Hyponatraemia and neonatal jaundice. Eur J Obstet Gynecol Reprod Biol 1986; 22:309–317.
80. Odell GB: Normal metabolism of bilirubin during neonatal life. *In* Neonatal Hyperbilirubinemia. New York, Grune & Stratton, 1980, pp 35–49.
81. Boggs TR Jr, Bishop H: Neonatal hyperbilirubinemia associated with high obstruction of the small bowel. J Pediatr 1965; 66:349–356.
82. Porto SO: Jaundice in congenital malrotation of the intestine. Am J Dis Child 1969; 117:684–688.
83. Clarkson JE, Cowan JO, Herbison GP: Jaundice in full-term healthy neonates–a population study. Aust Pediatr J 1984; 20:303–308.
84. Rosta J, Makoi Z, Kertesz A: Delayed meconium passage and hyperbilirubinemia. Lancet 1986; 2:1138.
85. Cottrell BH, Anderson GC: Rectal or axillary temperature measurement: Effect on plasma bilirubin and intestinal transit of meconium. J Pediatr Gastroenterol Nutr 1984; 3:734–739.
86. Poland RL, Odell GB: The binding of bilirubin to agar. Proc Soc Exp Biol Med 1974; 146:1114–1118.
87. Odell GB, Gutcher GR, Whitington PF, et al: Enteral administration of agar as an effective adjunct to phototherapy of neonatal hyperbilirubinemia. Pediatr Res 1983; 17:810–814.
88. Ulstrom RA, Eisenklam E: The enterohepatic shunting of bilirubin in the newborn infant: I. Use of oral activated charcoal to reduce normal serum bilirubin values. J Pediatr 1964; 65:27–37.
89. Arrowsmith WA, Payne RB, Littlewood JM: Comparison of treatments for congenital nonobstructive nonhaemolytic hyperbilirubinemia. Arch Dis Child 1975; 50:197–201.
90. Gourley GR: The pathophysiology of breast milk jaundice. *In* Polin RA, Fox WW, eds: Fetal and Neonatal Physiology. New York, Grune & Stratton, 1992, 1173–1179.
91. Gartner LM, Auerbach KG: Breast milk and breastfeeding jaundice. *In* Barness LA, ed: Advances in Pediatrics. Vol 34. Chicago, Yearbook Medical Publishers, 1987, pp 249–274.
92. Saigal S, Lunyk O, Bennett KJ, et al: Serum bilirubin levels in breast- and formula-fed infants in the first 5 days of life. Can Med Assoc J 1982; 127:985–999.
93. Kivlahan C, James EJP: The natural history of neonatal jaundice. Pediatrics 1984; 74:364–370.
94. Gartner LM, Arias IM: Studies of prolonged neonatal jaundice in the breast-fed infant. J Pediatr 1966; 68:54–66.
95. Behrman RE, Kliegman JM. *In* Behrman RE, Vaughan VC III, Nelson WE, eds: Nelson Textbook of Pediatrics. 12th ed. Philadelphia, WB Saunders, 1983, pp 378–381.
96. Lascari AD: "Early" breast-feeding jaundice: Clinical significance. J Pediatr 1986; 108:156–158.
97. Orlowski JP: Breast milk jaundice—early and late. Cleve Clin Q 1983; 50:339.
98. Arias IM, Gartner LM, Seifter S, et al: Prolonged neonatal unconjugated hyperbilirubinemia associated with breast feeding and a steroid, pregnane–3(alpha), 20(beta)-diol in maternal milk that inhibits glucuronide formation in vitro. J Clin Invest 1964; 43:2037–2047.
99. Murphy JF, Hughs I, Verrier Jones ER, et al: Pregnanediols and breast-milk jaundice. Arch Dis Child 1981; 56:474–476.
100. Bevan BR, Holton JB: Inhibition of bilirubin conjugation in rat liver slices by free fatty acids, with relevance to the problem of breast-milk jaundice. Clin Chim Acta 1972; 41:101–107.
101. Poland RL, Schultz GE, Gayatri G: High milk lipase activity associated with breast-milk jaundice. Pediatr Res 1980; 14:1328–1331.
102. Hernell O: Breast-milk jaundice. J Pediatr 1982; 99:311–312.
103. Constantopoulos A, Messaritakis J, Matsaniotis N: Breast-milk jaundice: The role of lipoprotein lipase and the free fatty acids. Eur J Pediatr 1980; 134:35–38.
104. Gaffney PT, Buttenshaw RL, Ward M, et al: Breast milk β-glucuronidase and neonatal jaundice. Lancet 1986; 1:1161–2.
105. Sirota L, Ferrera M, Lerer N, et al: Beta glucuronidase and hyperbilirubinaemia in breast fed infants of diabetic mothers. Arch Dis Child 1992; 67:120–121.
106. Alonso EM, Whitington PF, Whitington SH, et al: Enterohepatic circulation of nonconjugated bilirubin in rats fed with human milk. J Pediatr 1991; 118:425–430.
107. Maisels MJ, Gifford K: Normal serum bilirubin levels in the newborn and the effect of breast-feeding. Pediatrics 1986; 78:837–843.
108. Gartner LM, Auerbach KG: Breast milk and breastfeeding jaundice. Adv Pediatr 1987; 34:249–274.
109. Gartner LM: Breast milk jaundice. *In* Hyperbilirubinemia in the Newborn: Report of the 85th Ross Conference on Pediatric Research. Columbus, OH, Ross Laboratories, 1983, pp 75–86.
110. Cashore WJ, Stern L: The management of hyperbilirubinemia. Clin Perinatol 1984; 11:339–357.
111. Osborn LM, Bolus R: Breast feeding and jaundice in the first week of life. J Fam Pract 1985; 20:475.
112. Amato M, Howald H, von Muralt G: Interruption of breast-feeding versus phototherapy as treatment of hyperbilirubinemia in full-term infants. Helv Paediatr Acta 1985; 40:127–131.
113. Crigler JF, Najjar VA: Congenital familial nonhemolytic jaundice with kernicterus. Pediatrics 1952; 10:169–180.
114. Blaschke TF, Berke PD, Scharschmidt BF, et al: Crigler-Najjar syndrome: An unusual course with development of neurological damage at age eighteen. Pediatr Res 1974; 8:573–590.
115. Duhamel G, Blanckaert N, Metreau JM, et al: An unusual case of Crigler-Najjar disease in the adult: Classification of types I and II revisited. J Hepatol 1985; 1:47–53.
116. Blumenschein SD, Kallen RJ, Storey B, et al: Familial nonhemolytic jaundice with late onset of neurologic damage. Pediatrics 1968; 42:786–792.
117. Bloomer JR, Berk PD, Howe RB, et al: Bilirubin metabolism in congenital nonhemolytic jaundice. Pediatr Res 1971; 5:256–264.
118. Arias IM, Gartner LM, Cohen M, et al: Chronic nonhemolytic unconjugated hyperbilirubinemia with glucuronyl transferase deficiency. Am J Med 1969; 47:395–409.

119. Gordon ER, Shaffer EA, Sass-Kortsak A: Bilirubin secretion and conjugation in the Crigler-Najjar syndrome type II. Gastroenterology 1976; 70:761–765.
120. Odell GB, Whitington PF: Crigler-Najjar syndrome, type III: A new variant of hereditary non-hemolytic, non-conjugated hyperbilirubinemia. Hepatology 1990; 12:871.
121. Berry C, Hallinan T: Summary of a novel, three-component regulatory model for uridine diphosphate glucuronyltransferase. Biochem Soc Trans 1976; 4:650–652.
122. Kvittingen EA: Hereditary tyrosinemia type I—an overview. Scand J Clin Lab Invest 1986; 46:27.
123. Starzl TE, Zitelli BJ, Shaw BW, et al: Changing concepts: Liver replacement for hereditary tyrosinemia and hepatoma. J Pediatr 1985; 106:604–606.
124. Scriver CR, Beaudet AL, Sly WS, et al: The Metabolic Basis of Inherited Disease. New York, McGraw-Hill, 1989, pp 697.
125. Brantly M, Nukiwa T, Crystal RG: Molecular basis of α_1-antitrypsin deficiency. Am J Med 1988; 84:13–31.
126. Fagerhol MK, Laurell CB: The Pi system—inherited variants of serum alpha-1-antitrypsin. Prog Med Genet 1970; 7:96–111.
127. Pierce JA, Eradio B, Dew TA: Antitrypsin phenotypes in St. Louis. JAMA 1975; 231:609–612.
128. Fagerhol MK: Quantitative studies on the inherited variants of serum alpha-1-antitrypsin. Scand J Clin Lab Invest 1969; 23:97–103.
129. Aagenas O, Matlary A, Elgio E, et al: Neonatal cholestasis in alpha-1-antitrypsin deficient children: Clinical, genetic, histological and immunohistochemical findings. Acta Paediatr Scand 1972; 51:632–642.
130. Porter CA, Mowat AP, Cook PJL, et al: Alpha-1-antitrypsin deficiency and neonatal hepatitis. Br Med J 1972; 3:435–439.
131. Sharp HL, Bridges RA, Krivit W, et al: Cirrhosis with alpha-1-antitrypsin deficiency: A previously unrecognized inherited disorder. J Lab Clin Med 1969; 73:434–439.
132. Berg NO, Eriksson S: Liver disease in adults with alpha-1-antitrypsin deficiency. N Engl J Med 1972; 287:1264–1267.
133. Eriksson S: Alpha-1-antitypsin deficiency and liver cirrhosis in adults. Acta Med Scand 1987; 221:461–467.
134. Moroz SP, Cutz E, Cox DW, et al: Liver disease associated with alpha-1-antitrypsin deficiency in childhood. J Pediatr 1976; 88:19–25.
135. Gartner JC, Zitelli BJ, Malatack JJ, et al: Orthotopic liver transplantation in children: Two-year experience with 47 patients. Pediatrics 1984; 74:140–145.
136. Silverman EK, Miletich JP, Pierce JA, et al: Alpha-1-antitrypsin deficiency: High prevalence in the St. Louis area determined by direct population screening. Am Rev Respir Dis 1989; 140:961–966.
137. Carrell RW: α_1-Antitrypsin: Molecular pathology, leukocytes and tissue damage. J Clin Invest 1986; 77:1427–1431.
138. Sveger T: The natural history of liver disease in α_1-antitrypsin deficient children. Acta Paediatr Scand 1988; 77:847–851.
139. Dickson I, Alper CA: Changes in serum proteinase inhibitor levels following bone surgery. Clin Chim Acta 1974; 54:381–385.
140. Carlson J, Eriksson S, Hagerstrand I: Intra- and extracellular alpha-1-antitrypsin in liver disease with special reference to PI phenotype. J Clin Pathol 1981; 34:1020–1025.
141. Bradfield JWB, Blenkinsopp WK: Alpha-1-antitripsin globules in the liver and PiM phenotype. J Clin Pathol 1977; 30:464–466.
142. Wewers MD, Casolaro A, Sellers SE, et al: Replacement therapy for alpha-1-antitrypsin deficiency associated with emphysema. N Engl J Med 1987; 316:1055–1062.
143. Janus ED, Phillips NT, Carrell RW: Smoking, lung function and α_1-antitrypsin deficiency. Lancet 1985; 1:152–154.
144. Thompson GN, McCrossin RB, Penfold JL, et al: Management and outcome of children with congenital hypothyroidism detected on neonatal screening in South Australia. Med J Aust 1986; 145:18–22.
145. Jahrig D, Jahrig K, Stiete S, et al: Neonatal jaundice in infants of diabetic mothers. Acta Paediatr Scand 1989; 360 (suppl):101–107.
146. Arias IM, Wolfson S, Lucey JF, et al: Transient familial neonatal hyperbilirubinemia. J Clin Invest 1956; 44:1442–1450.
147. Odell GB: Studies in kernicterus: I. Protein binding of bilirubin. J Clin Invest 1959; 38:823.
148. Brodersen R, Robertson A: Ceftriaxone binding to human serum albumin: Competition with bilirubin. Molec Pharmacol 1989; 36:478–483.
149. Freeman J, Lesko SM, Mitchell AA, et al: Hyperbilirubinemia following exposure to pancuronium bromide in newborns. Dev Pharmacol Ther 1990; 14:209–215.
150. Lambert GH, Muraskas J, Anderson CL, et al: Direct hyperbilirubinemia associated with chloral hydrate administration in the newborn. Pediatrics 1990; 86:277–281.
151. Kawade N, Onishi S: The prenatal and postnatal development of UDP-glucuronyltransferase activity towards bilirubin and the effect of premature birth on this activity in the human liver. Biochem J 1981; 196:257–260.
152. Obrinsky W, Denley ML, Brauer RW: Sulfobromophthalein sodium excretion test as a measure of liver function in premature infants. Pediatrics 1952; 9:421–438.
153. Vest M, Rossier R: Detoxification in the newborn: The ability of the newborn infant to form conjugates with glucuronic acid, glycine, acetate and glutathione. Ann NY Acad Sci 1963; 111:183–198.
154. Boggs TR Jr, Westphal MD Jr: Mortality of exchange transfusions. Pediatrics 1960; 26:745–755.
155. Lee SP, Lipsky BA, Teefey SA: Gallbladder sludge and antibiotics. Pediatr Infect Dis J 1990; 9:422–423.
156. Messing B, Bories C, Kunstlinger F, et al: Does total parenteral nutrition induce gallbladder sludge formation in lithiasis? Gastroenterology 1983; 84:1012–1019.
157. Bolondi L, Gaiani S, Testa S, et al: Gallbladder sludge formation during fasting after gastrointestinal tract surgery. Gut 1985; 26:734–738.
158. Lee SP, Maher K, Nicholls JF: Origin and fate of biliary sludge. Gastroenterology 1988; 94:170–176.
159. Heubi JE, Daugherty CC: Neonatal cholestasis: An approach for the practicing pediatrician. Curr Probl Pediatr 1990; 20:239–295.
160. Sokol RJ: Medical management of neonatal cholestasis. *In* Balistreri WF, Stocker JT, eds. Pediatric Hepatology. New York, Hemisphere, 1990, pp 41–76.
161. Balistreri WF: Neonatal cholestasis. J Pediatr 1985; 106:171–184.
162. Claireaux AE: Pathology of human kernicterus. *In* Sass-Kortsak A, ed: Kernicterus: A Report Based on a Symposium Held at the IX International Congress of Paediatrics. Toronto, University of Toronto Press, 1961, p 140.
163. Odell GB, Schutta HS: Bilirubin encephalopathy. *In* McCandless DW, ed: Cerebral Energy Metabolism and Metabolic Encephalopathy. New York, Plenum, 1985, pp 229–261.
164. Odell GB, Storey GNB, Rosenberg LA: Studies in kernicterus: III. The saturation of serum proteins with bilirubin during neonatal life and its relationship to brain damamge at five years. J Pediatr 1970; 76:12–21.
165. Isherwood DM, Fletcher KA: Neonatal jaundice: Investigation and monitoring. Ann Clin Biochem 1985; 22:109–128.
166. Gardner WA Jr, Konigsmark BW: Familial nonhemolytic jaundice: Bilirubinosis and encephalopathy. Pediatrics 1969; 43:365–376.
167. McDonagh AF: Is bilirubin good for you? Clin Perinatol 1990; 17:359–369.
168. Hsia DY-Y, Allen FH Jr., Gellis SS, et al: Erythroblastosis fetalis: VIII. Studies of serum bilirubin in relation to kernicterus. N Engl J Med 1952; 247:668.
169. Isherwood DM, Fletcher KA: Neonatal jaundice: Investigation and monitoring. Ann Clin Biochem 1985; 22:109–128.
170. Odell GB: The dissociation of bilirubin from albumin and its clinical implications. J Pediatr 1959; 55:268–279.
171. Harris RC, Lucey JF, MacLean JR: Kernicterus in premature infants associated with low concentrations of bilirubin in the plasma. Pediatrics 1958; 21:875–884.
172. Walker PC: Neonatal bilirubin toxicity—a review of kernicterus and the implications of drug-induced bilirubin displacement. Clin Pharmacokinet 1987; 13:26–50.
173. Newman TB, Maisels MJ: Does hyperbilirubinemia damage the brain of healthy full-term infants? Clin Perinatol 1990; 17:331–358.
174. Wadsworth SJ, Suh B: In vitro displacement of bilirubin by antibiotics and 2-hydroxybenzoylglycine in newborns. Antimicrob Agents Chemother 1988; 32:1571–1575.

175. Ennever JF: Blue light, green light, white light, more light: Treatment of neonatal jaundice. Clin Perinatol 1990; 17:467–481.
176. McDonagh AF, Lightner DA: "Like a shrivelled blood orange"— bilirubin, jaundice and phototherapy. Pediatrics 1985; 75:443–445.
177. McDonagh AF, Palma LA, Lightner DA: Phototherapy for neonatal jaundice: Stereospecific and regioselective photoisomerization of bilirubin bound to human serum albumin and NMR characterization of intramolecular cyclized photoproducts. J Am Chem Soc 1982; 104:6867–6869.
178. Itoh S, Onishi S, Manabe M, et al: Wavelength dependence of the geometric and structural photoisomerization of bilirubin bound to human serum albumin. Biol Neonate 1987; 51:10–17.
179. Onishi S, Isobe K, Itoh S, et al: Metabolism of bilirubin and its photoisomers in newborn infants during phototherapy. J Biochem (Toyko) 1986; 100:789–795.
180. Rosenfeld W, Twist P, Concepcion L: A new device for phototherapy. Pediatr Res 1989; 25:227A.
181. Fetus and Newborn Committee, Canadian Paediatric Society: Use of phototherapy for neonatal hyperbilirubinemia. Can Med Assoc J 1986; 134:1237–1245.
182. Grabert BE, Wardwell C, Harburg SK: Home phototherapy: An alternative to prolonged hospitalization of the full-term, well newborn. Clin Pediatr 1986; 25:291–294.
183. Gourley GR, Odell GB: Bilirubin metabolism in the fetus and neonate. *In* Lebenthal E, ed: Human Gastrointestinal Development. New York, Raven Press, 1989, pp 581–621.
184. Odell GB: Treatment of neonatal hyperbilirubinemia. *In* Neonatal Hyperbilirubinemia. New York, Grune & Stratton, 1980, p 117.
185. Gartner LM, Lee K-S: Jaundice and liver disease: I. Unconjugated hyperbilirubinemia. *In* Fanaroff AA, Martin RJ, eds: Behrman's Neonatal-Perinatal Medicine. 3rd ed. St. Louis, CV Mosby, 1983, pp 754–770.
186. Maisels MJ: Neonatal jaundice. *In* Avery GB, ed: Neonatology. 2nd ed. Philadelphia, JB Lippincott, 1981, pp 473–544.
187. Shapiro M: Safer exchange transfusions with ACD blood. Bibl Haematol 1965; Fasc 23:883–886.
188. Weldon VV, Odell GB: Mortality risk of exchange transfusion. Pediatrics 1968; 41:797–801.
189. Valaes TN, Harvey-Wilkes K: Pharmacologic approaches to the prevention and treatment of neonatal hyperbilirubinemia. Clin Perinatol 1990; 17:245–273.
190. DeCarvalho M, Klaus MH, Merkatz RB: Frequency of breastfeeding and serum bilirubin concentration. Am J Dis Child 1982; 136:737–738.
191. Wu T-W, Li GS: A new bilirubin-degrading enzyme from orange peels. Biochem Cell Biol 1988; 66:1248.
192. Johnson L, Dworanczyk R, Jenkins D: Bilirubin oxidase (BOX) feedings at varying time intervals and enzyme concentrations in infant Gunn rats. Pediatr Res 1989; 25:116A.
193. Gartner LM, Lee KS, Vaisman L, et al: Development of bilirubin transport and metabolism in the newborn rhesus monkey. J Pediatr 1977; 90:513–531.
194. Waltman R, Nigrin G, Bonura F, et al: Ethanol in prevention of hyperbilirubinaemia in the newborn. Lancet 1969; 2:1265–1267.
195. Stern L, Khanna NN, Levy G, et al: Effect of phenobarbital on hyperbilirubinemia and glucuronide formation in newborns. Am J Dis Child 1970; 120:26–31.
196. Rodgers PA, Stevenson DK: Developmental biology of heme oxygenase. Clin Perinatol 1990; 17:275–291.
197. Kappas A, Drummond GS, Manola T, et al: Sn-protoporphyrin use in the management of hyperbilirubinemia in term newborns with direct Coombs-positive ABO-imcompatibility. Pediatrics 1988; 81:485–497.
197a. Galbraith RA, Drummond GS, Kappas A: Suppression of bilirubin production in the Crigler-Najjar type I syndrome: Studies with the heme oxygenase inhibitor tin-mesoporphyrin. Pediatrics 1992; 89:175–182.
198. Odell GB, Gourley GR: Hereditary hyperbilirubinemia. *In* Lebenthal E, ed: Textbook of Gastroenterology and Nutrition in Infancy. 2nd ed. New York, Raven Press, 1989, pp 949–967.
199. Watson KJ, Gollan JL: Gilbert's syndrome. Baillieres Cun Gastroenterol 1989; 3:337–355.
200. Black M, Billing BH: Hepatic bilirubin UDP-glucuronyl transferase activity in liver disease. N Engl J Med 1969; 280:1266–1271.
201. Felsher BF, Craig JR, Carpio N: Hepatic bilirubin glucuronidation in Gilbert's syndrome. J Lab Clin Med 1973; 81:829–837.
202. Auclair C, Hakim J, Boivin H, et al: Bilirubin and paranitrophenol glucuronyl transferase activities of the liver in patients with Gilbert's syndrome. Enzyme 1976; 21:97–107.
203. Martin JF, Vierling JM, Wolkoff AW, et al: Abnormal hepatic transport of indocyanine green in Gilbert's syndrome. Gastroenterology 1976; 70:385–391.
204. Ohkubo H, Okuda K, Jida S: A constitutional unconjugated hyperbilirubinemia combined with indocyanine green intolerance: A new functional disorder. Hepatology 1981; 1:319–324.
205. Felsher BF, Richard D, Redeker AG: The reciprocoal relation between caloric intake and the degree of hyperbilirubinemia in Gilbert's syndrome. N Engl J Med 1970; 283:170–172.
206. Rotor AB, Manahan L, Florentin A: Familial nonhemolytic jaundice with direct van den Bergh reaction. Acta Med Phil 1948; 5:37–49.
207. Namihisa T, Yamaguchi K: The constitutional hyperbilirubinemia in Japan: Studies on 139 cases reported during the period 1963–1969. Gastroenterol Jpn 1973; 8:311–321.
208. Javitt NB, Kondo T, Kuchiba K: Bile acid excretion in Dubin-Johnson syndrome. Gastroenterology 1978; 75:931–932.
209. Vest MF, Kaufmann JH, Fritz E: Chronic nonhaemolytic jaundice with conjugated bilirubin in the serum and normal histology: A case study. Arch Dis Child 1960; 36:600–604.
210. Wolkoff AW: Inheritable disorders manifested by conjugated hyperbilirubinemia. Semin Liver Dis 1983; 3:65–72.
211. Gustein SL, Alpert L, Arias IM: Studies of hepatic excretory function. IV. Biliary excretion of sulfobromophthalein sodium in a patient with Dubin-Johnson syndrome and a biliary fistula. Isr J Med Sci 1968; 4:36–40.
212. Cohen L, Lewis C, Arias IM: Pregnancy, oral contraceptives and chronic familial jaundice with predominantly conjugated hyperbilirubinemia (Dubin-Johnson syndrome). Gastroenterology 1972; 62:1182–1190.
213. Muscatello U, Mussini I, Agnolucci MT: Dubin-Johnson syndrome: An electron microscopic study of the liver cell. Acta Hepatosplenol 1967; 14:162–170.
214. Ehrlich JC, Novikoff AB, Platt R, et al: Hepatocellular lipofuscin and the pigment of chronic idiopathic jaundice. Bull NY Acad Med 1960; 36:488–491.
215. Swartz HM, Sarna T, Varma RR: On the nature and excretion of the hepatic pigment in the Dubin-Johnson syndrome. Gastroenterology 1979; 76:958–964.
216. Arias IM, Blumberg W: The pigment in Dubin-Johnson syndrome. Gastroenterology 1979; 77:820–821.
217. Wolpert E, Pascasio FM, Wolkoff AW: Abnormal sulfobromophthalein metabolism in Rotor's syndrome and obligate heterozygotes. N Engl J Med 1977; 296:1099–1101.
218. Dhumeaux D, Berthelot P: Chronic hyperbilirubinemia associated with hepatic uptake and storage impairment. Gastroenterology 1975; 69:988–993.
219. Adachi Y, Yamamoto T: Partial defect in hepatic glutathionine S-transferase activity in a case of Rotor's syndrome. Gastroenterology 1987; 22:34–38.
220. Shani M, Gilon E, Ben-Ezzer J, et al: Sulfobromophthalein tolerance test in patients with Dubin-Johnson syndrome and their relatives. Gastroenterology 1970; 59:842–847.
221. Wolkoff AW, Wolpert E, Pascasio FN, et al: Rotor's syndrome: A distinct inheritable pathophysiologic entity. Am J Med 1976; 60:173–179.
222. Shimizu Y, Naruto H, Ida S, et al: Urinary coproporphyrin isomers in Rotor's syndrome: A study of eight families. Hepatology 1981; 1:173–178.
223. Ben-Ezzer J, Blonder J, Shani M, et al: Dubin-Johnson syndrome: Abnormal excretion of the isomers of urinary coproporphyrin by patients with Dubin-Johnson syndrome in Israel. Clin Sci 1971; 40:17–30.
224. Kondo T, Kuchiba K, Shimizu Y: Coproporphyrin isomers in Dubin-Johnson syndrome. Gastroenterology 1976; 70:1117–1120.
225. Saito T: Presenting symptoms and natural history of Wilson disease. Eur J Pediatr 1987; 146:261–265.

226. Odievere M, Vedrene J, Landrieu P, et al: Les fromes hepatiques "Pures" de la maladie de Wilson chey l'enfant. Arch Fr Pediatr 1974; 31:215.
227. Scheinberg IH, Jaffe ME, Sternlieb I: The use of trientine in preventing the effects of interrupting penicillamine therapy in Wilson's disease. N Engl J Med 1987; 317:209–213.
228. Ballistreri WF: Viral hepatitis. Pediatr Clin North Am 1988; 35:637–669.
229. De Groote J, Desmet VJ, Gedigk P, et al: A classification of chronic hepatitis. Lancet 1968; 2:626–628.
230. Leevy CM, Popper H, Sherlock S: Diseases of the Liver and Biliary Tract. Standardization of Nomenclature, Diagnostic Criteria and Diagnostic Methodology. Fogarty International Centre Proceedings No 22. Washington, DC, US Government Printing Office, 1976.
231. Johnson PJ, McFarlane IG, Eddleston ALWF: The natural course and heterogeneity of autoimmune-type chronic active hepatitis. Semin Liver Dis 1991; 11:187–196.

Section Three

THE ESOPHAGUS

Chapter 24

Anatomy and Physiology of the Esophagus

JOSEPH H. CLARK

Although the esophagus has traditionally been an overlooked and underappreciated organ in the gastrointestinal tract despite its accessibility to investigation, the past two decades have witnessed a resurgence of clinical interest in esophageal function and dysfunction. This chapter provides a basis for understanding normal esophageal anatomy and physiology.

The esophagus has two major functions: (1) to propel fluid or food from the mouth into the stomach and (2) to prevent the retrograde flow of gastric contents in between swallows. Since the precise anatomic components of the upper and lower esophageal sphincters remain controversial, they are considered in the section on physiology.

EMBRYOLOGY

The esophagus is first noted as a constriction separating the pharynx and stomach during the third week of gestation.[1] The fifth week of gestation is marked by migration of neuroblasts, elongation of the esophagus, and alteration of the esophageal epithelium into a bilayer. The circular muscle coat is first recognized at 6 weeks, followed by the longitudinal layer at 8 to 9 weeks. Vacuolization of the esophageal lumen occurs at 7 weeks, along with continued cephalad elongation. The esophageal epithelium is ciliated by 10 weeks, and striated muscle fibers begin to appear in the upper esophagus. Anticholinesterase reactivity is demonstrable at 10 weeks; differentiated ganglion cells are present by 13 weeks.

By the fifth month, the longitudinal and circular muscle layers of the upper esophagus are fully striated. The myenteric and submucosal plexuses are also well organized. Stratified squamous epithelium appears by the 25th week, and esophageal glands are seen by the 28th week.

ANATOMY

The esophagus is a distensible musculomucosal canal lined with stratified squamous epithelium. It extends from the pharynx at the level of C6 through the superior and posterior mediastinum and diaphragm before terminating at T11. The length is approximately 11 cm at birth gradually increasing to 24 to 30 cm in the adult by a rate of approximately 0.65 cm per year.[2] It extends approximately 40 cm from the incisors to the lower esophageal sphincter (LES) in adult men and is somewhat shorter in adult women. Esophageal length can be estimated in infants and children by the use of regression equations based on length.[3] The diameter at birth is 5 mm. The lateral diameter is eventually 30 mm, narrowing to 19 mm in the anteroposterior plane.

The esophagus begins in the midline at the cricopharyngeal muscle and deviates to the left along the lower trachea. After passing posteriorly to the left mainstem bronchus, it trends to the right until deviating to the left just above the diaphragm. The right aspect of the esophagus joins the stomach in a continuum, but the left side forms a sharp angle (incisura, or angle of His). The esophagus is frequently conceptualized as three anatomic segments: cervical, thoracic, and abdominal.

The *cervical esophagus* lies posteriorly to the membranous trachea, resting on the longus colli musculature and the prevertebral fascial plane. The recurrent laryngeal nerves lie in a groove between the esophagus and trachea bilaterally.

The *thoracic esophagus* maintains its relationship with the membranous trachea and prevertebral fascia until the level of T5 (tracheal bifurcation). It crosses posteriorly to the left mainstem bronchus and descends on the right side of the aorta until T9, where it passes in front of the aorta and through the diaphragmatic hiatus at T10. The left aspect of the superior mediastinum contains the left subclavian artery, the aortic arch, the thoracic duct, and the left parietal pleura. The right component includes the azygos vein and the right parietal pleura.

The distal thoracic esophagus relates to the pericardium anteriorly and the prevertebral fascia posteriorly. The vagus nerves form an esophageal plexus at the tracheal bifurcation that generates branches to the esophagus and tracheobronchial tree. The right posterior and left anterior vagus nerves coalesce from this plexus and descend along the esophagus into the abdomen.

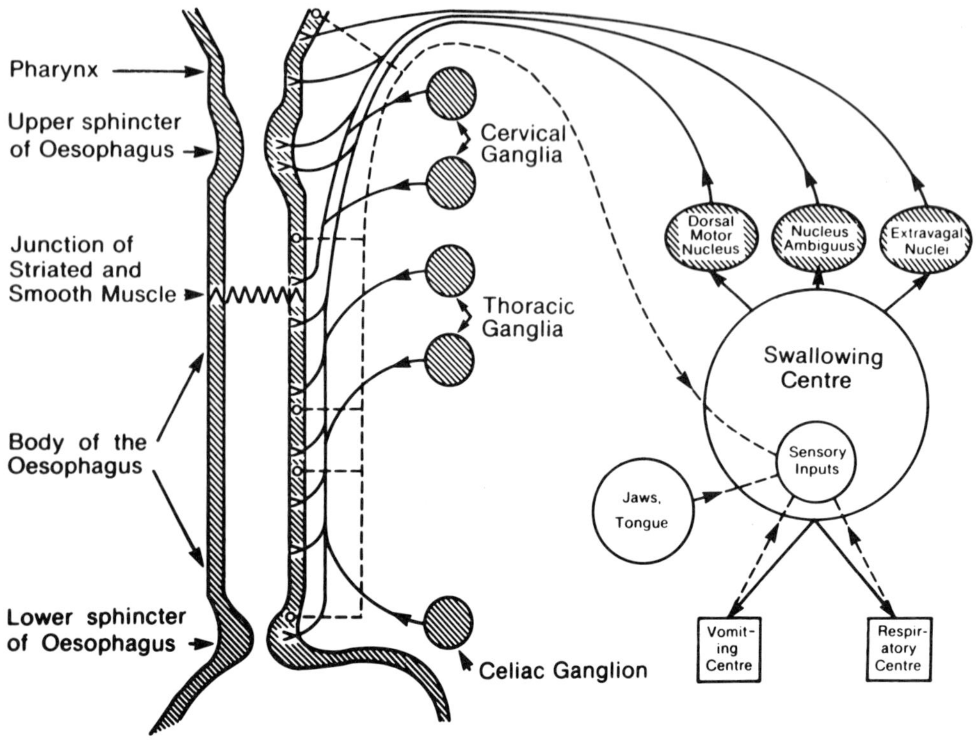

Figure 24–1. Diagrammatic representation of the extrinsic nerve supply to the esophagus. See text for complete explanation. (From Christensen J: The colon. *In* Christensen J, Wingate DL, eds: A Guide to Gastrointestinal Motility. Bristol, Wright- PSG, 1983, pp 198–214; with permission).

The *intra-abdominal esophagus* runs from the diaphragm to the gastroesophageal junction and is usually only 1.5 cm in length. It lies posterior to the left lobe of the liver and anterior to the diaphragmatic crura; it is the only part of the esophagus surrounded by serosa. The intra-abdominal esophagus is surrounded by positive pressure, which is in contrast with the negative intrathoracic pressure that surrounds the thoracic esophagus.

Vasculature

The arterial supply is variable but comprises three components.[4] The *cervical esophagus* is supplied from three segments of the inferior thyroid artery. The *thoracic esophagus* receives blood from the bronchial arteries (primarily left), direct branches of the descending aorta, and intercostal arteries in 20% of people. The *abdominal segment* is supplied from the left gastric artery, with a contribution from the left phrenic artery in 50% of people. Controversy remains about the degree of anastomoses between these three circuits, yet esophageal infarction is exceedingly rare.

Venous drainage begins in a submucosal plexus that passes through the esophageal wall into a periesophageal plexus. The inferior thyroid veins drain the cervical esophagus into the superior vena cava. The thoracic esophagus empties into the azygos and hemiazygos veins.

The distal thoracic and abdominal esophagus communicate with the portal system via the short gastric and the coronary veins. The differences in venous drainage account for the various causes of esophageal varices, depending on the area of involvement.

Lymphatic drainage is not as segmental as the arteriovenous supplies. Mucosal lymphatics drain into the submucosa and, subsequently, into longitudinal plexuses that pierce the esophageal wall. At least seven lymph node groups are involved, and drainage can become quite extensive, since the esophagus is not surrounded by serosa. Local groups include the paratracheal, parabronchial, paraesophageal, paracardial, and posterior mediastinal nodes. The superior and inferior deep cervical nodes are also involved.

Neurology

Parasympathetic and sympathetic innervation of the esophagus includes extrinsic and intrinsic components (Fig. 24–1). The extrinsic supply includes the swallowing center in the pons-oblongata, the vagus nerves, and the sympathetic fibers from the cervical and thoracic sympathetic ganglia. The intrinsic nerve supply involves Auerbach's myenteric plexus and Meissner's submucosal plexus.

The motor nerve supply arises in the nucleus of the spinal accessory nerve for the upper cervical esophagus and the dorsal motor nucleus of the vagus nerve for the remainder. The vagus nerve also supplies afferent fibers with cell bodies in the nodose ganglion, although specific details of this arrangement are lacking. The sympathetic supply is derived from the superior and inferior cervical sympathetic ganglia, the T4 and T5 ganglia, the preganglionic fibers from the greater and lesser splanchnic nerves, and the celiac plexus.

The myenteric plexus contains far more ganglia than does the submucosal plexus, and the concentration of ganglion cells is greatly increased in the smooth muscle segment, although no histologic differences are seen. The ganglion cells throughout demonstrate intense staining for vasoactive intestinal peptide and neuropeptide Y, although the clinical significance remains unclear.[5, 6]

The plexuses are believed to be primarily sensory in the striated muscle, since vagal postganglionic fibers innervate striated muscle fibers through cholinergic, nicotinic receptors. There are two types of effector neurons in the smooth muscle: One mediates cholinergic excitation of both longitudinal and circular muscles through muscarinic receptors, and the other mediates nonadrenergic, noncholinergic inhibition mainly of the circular layer. Sympathetic nerve fibers are also present but have only sparse contact with individual smooth muscle cells. It is believed that they provide only modulation of peristaltic events and sphincter tone through axosomatic and axoaxonic connections.

Histology

The esophagus consists of five distinct layers: mucosa, lamina propria, muscularis mucosae, submucosa, and muscularis propria.[7] These layers are surrounded by adventitia, except for the distal few centimeters that contain serosa arising from the phrenoesophageal ligament. The mucosa is a noncornified, stratified squamous epithelium that is a continuation of the pharynx. The squamous epithelium is replaced by columnar cells in the distal 1 to 3 cm (vestibule), although considerable variability in location may exist. This transition is marked by a change from pale esophageal mucosa to a deep red velvet gastric mucosa. The junctional boundary is irregular and is termed the *Z-line*.

Flat epithelial cells form the thicker superficial layer (stratified zone), and basophilic cells with pyknotic nuclei form the basal zone, which is 15% of the total thickness. Papillae from the lamina propria may normally extend into the stratified zone but not to exceed 50% of the thickness. Occasional mitotic figures may be seen. Reflux esophagitis is typified by hyperplastic thickening of the basal cell zone and extension of the papillae to the epithelial surface.

The lamina propria consists of loose areolar connective tissue containing lymphocytes, plasma cells, neurofibrils, and vessels. The superficial (cardiac) glands are located at either end of the esophagus. They secrete mucin and are variable in number. The muscularis mucosa extends the entire length of the esophagus in a longitudinal arrangement. The most proximal and distal segments have a spiral orientation.

The dense submucosa contains elastic and collagen fibers with scattered lymphocytes. It also contains the submucosal venous plexus, the Meissner's neurogenic plexus, and the deep esophageal glands. The deep esophageal glands predominate in the upper esophagus and may be considered a continuation of the minor salivary glands of the oropharynx. They are mucin-secreting tubuloaveolar glands of uncertain significance.

The muscularis propria is classically considered to include an inner circular layer, and an outer longitudinal layer although individual fibers may be arranged spirally in a variety of combinations extending from the adventitia to the submucosa. The esophageal smooth muscle layer is thinner than the longitudinal layer, which is unique to the gastrointestinal tract. The longitudinal fibers arise as three fascicles from the cricoid cartilage anteriorly and the lower esophageal constrictor bilaterally. The inner layer is an elliptical syncytium that ends 1 to 2 cm from the stomach and is replaced by the LES. The upper 5% of the esophagus contains only striated muscle fibers. A mixture of striated and smooth muscle exists for another 6 to 8 cm, until the lower half of the esophagus, which is exclusively smooth muscle.[8] Elastic fibers are abundant throughout, which contributes to the distensibility of this organ. Auerbach's myenteric plexus is sandwiched between the circular and the longitudinal layers.

PHYSIOLOGY

The physiology of swallowing is traditionally considered in three phases: the voluntary or oral phase, the involuntary or pharyngeal phase, and the esophageal phase. Swallowing occurs 70 times each hour during the wake state, 7 times each hour during sleep, and at a projected rate of 200 times per hour during eating.[9]

During the *oral phase,* food is voluntarily moved to the posterior part of the oropharynx by the tongue, which pulses backward and upward against the palate. The soft palate elevates and closes the nasopharynx. The epiglottis closes over the larynx while the hypopharynx narrows.

The *pharyngeal phase* begins as the presence of a food bolus stimulates afferent receptors that communicate with the swallowing center in the pons-oblongata. The respiratory center is inhibited briefly, and several involuntary responses occur: The soft palate closes the posterior nares, and the palatopharyngeal folds limit the pharyngeal width; the vocal cords close, and the epiglottis swings backward and downward; the larynx is pulled upward and forward by muscles attached to the hyoid bone, which effectively opens the esophageal orifice;[10] and the upper esophageal sphincter (UES) relaxes, and the superior pharyngeal constrictor muscle contracts, which initiates a peristaltic wave and propels food into the esophagus.

The *esophageal phase* involves transporting the food bolus by normal peristalsis into the stomach. This process takes between 7 and 10 seconds. The esophageal phase is the focus of the remainder of this chapter. The esophagus will be subdivided physiologically into three parts: UES, esophageal body, and LES.

Upper Esophageal Sphincter

The UES is defined as an area of increased pressure between pharynx and the esophageal body. It is located between C5 and C7 in adults and approximately 7 to 9 cm from the nares in infants.[11] The UES is present as early as 32 weeks of gestation and is fully functional in the immediate neonatal period. It varies between 0.5 and 1 cm in length in the neonate and 2 and 4 cm in the adult. The UES generally corresponds to the cricopharyngeal muscle, although the width of the muscle itself is only 1 cm, and the surgical myotomy of the cricopharyngeal muscle fails to abolish UES tone.[12–14] Normal UES pressure ranges between 18 and 44 cm H_2O in neonates studied with low-compliance perfusion catheters.[12]

The major functions of the UES involve prevention of esophageal distention during inspiration and protection against aspiration of regurgitated gastric contents. The sphincter is closed at rest. It demonstrates marked radial asymmetry with peak pressures in the posterior plane. The pressure may be reduced by as much as two thirds in the lateral direction. Axial asymmetry is also present since peak anterior pressures are generated 0.5 cm more proximal than are posterior forces in the adult. This corresponds with the inferior border of the cricopharyngeal muscle, which lies 0.5 cm below the hyoid cartilage. Laryngectomy abolishes both radial and axial asymmetry.

The UES receives extrinsic innervation from the vagus nerve exclusively. Nuclei originating in the nucleus ambiguus and the dorsal motor nucleus provide parasympathetic fibers. Sympathetic innervation appears to be clinically insignificant. Continuous tonic activity maintains closure of the UES at rest. The act of swallowing results in immediate cessation of continuous spike activity for 0.5 seconds, which results in UES relaxation (Fig. 24–2). Pharyngeal peristalsis and UES relaxation are finely coordinated by the swallowing center in the medulla, which transmits impulses via cranial nerves V, VII, IX, and XII. Animal studies indicate that a cholinergic, nicotinic-mediated mechanism is involved. UES function is dependent on bolus size.[14] Relaxation also occurs during gagging, retching, vomiting, and belching.[15] A spike burst of electrical activity subsequently occurs to increase UES pressure higher than baseline for 1 second before resting UES pressure returns.

UES pressure increases in response to intraluminal fluid boluses or balloon distention. It was believed originally that intraesophageal acid instillation increased UES pressure in adults and in infants older than 10 weeks of age, especially when instilled close to the UES.[12, 16] A more recent study in adults revealed no differences in UES pressure with or without acid exposure *but* a marked reduction during deep sleep.[17] The implication of UES pressure reduction for infants with gastroesophageal reflux remains unclear, since no specific abnormalities in pharyngeal or UES function have been identified.[12]

Esophageal Body

The resting pressure varies with inspiration from −5 to −15 mm Hg and from −2 to +5 mm Hg during expiration. The resting gastric pressure is +5 mm Hg. The act of swallowing is accompanied by a brief reduction in intraesophageal pressure presumably owing to a short inspiration immediately preceding deglutition. Esophageal peristalsis involves an orderly and progressive series of contractions that begin in the pharynx and advance aborally. The velocity is 3 cm per second in the proximal esophagus, 5 cm per second in the middle

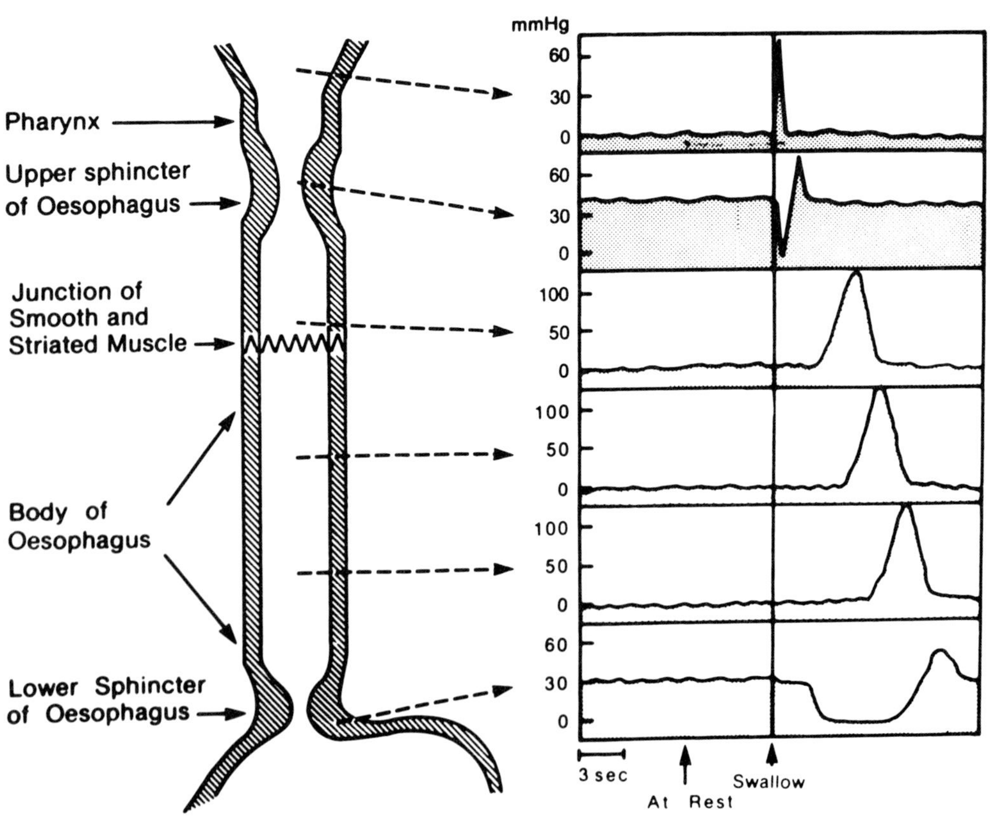

Figure 24–2. Pharyngeal and esophageal intraluminal pressures at rest and following deglutition. See text for complete explanation. (From Christensen J: The colon. *In* Christensen J, Wingate DL, eds: A Guide to Gastrointestinal Motility. Bristol, Wright-PSG, 1983, pp 198–214; with permission.)

esophagus, and 2 to 5 cm per second in the distal esophagus.[18] The duration of the pressure wave increases in the distal esophagus, and the amplitude may vary.

Swallowing has been observed in a 2-week-old fetus, and approximately 600 ml of amniotic fluid may be swallowed daily just prior to birth.[19] Coordination of swallowing and sucking may be poor in the first 12 hours of life or in infants weighing less than 1500 gm.[1, 11, 20] The velocity of distal esophageal contractions is 0.8 to 2 cm per second during the first week of life, which is considerably slower than that in the older child and adult.

Three types of esophageal contractions can occur. *Primary peristalsis* is initiated by swallowing and is associated with pharyngeal contraction and UES relaxation. *Secondary peristalsis* is originated by intraluminal distention (bolus or balloon) and is unaccompanied by pharyngeal or UES changes. It appears to be useful in esophageal clearance of refluxed gastric contents. *Tertiary peristalsis* refers to spontaneous contraction in the esophageal body; these are nonperistalitic and nonphysiologic.

The striated muscle in the upper esophagus is totally dependent on excitatory activity from the vagus nerve for primary and secondary peristalsis. Sequential activation of motor neurons is present. The smooth muscle is not innervated directly by the vagus nerve but rather through synapses in the submucosal and myenteric plexuses, which results in several important differences. Activation of the smooth muscle appears to be simultaneous rather than sequential, and intrinsic factors may be responsible for modulation of peristalsis. Further, vagotomy abolishes primary and secondary peristalsis in the striated musculature, but secondary smooth muscle peristalsis remains intact.[19]

Esophageal circular smooth muscle demonstrates an intrinsic latency of response to a stimulus that increases aborally. This latency manifests as peristalsis and is unrelated to delays in nerve conduction. There is a period of inhibition following vagal stimulation and prior to esophageal contraction that progressively lengthens throughout the esophageal body.[21] This contraction following the cessation of a stimulus is termed the *off response* and is nerve mediated but nonadrenergic, noncholinergic. The phrase *on response* refers to contractions that occur *during* stimulation. This is a cholinergic response and is mediated by M_2 muscarinic receptors. Cholinergic nerves predominate proximally, and noncholinergic nerves predominate distally, which could account for the intrinsic modulation of primary peristalsis.

The longitudinal muscle layer contracts during peristalsis, shortening the esophageal body. Longitudinal muscle contraction is more rapid in onset and velocity than is circular muscle. It has a peripherally mediated, aborally increasing gradient of contraction. The precise mechanism of coordination between longitudinal and circular smooth muscle is unknown. In a similar fashion, the coordination of peristalsis between striated and smooth muscle is not certain, although vagal efferent fibers may be involved.

Deglutition inhibition is a well-established phenomenon that remains poorly understood. If a second swallow occurs while the first swallow is still in the striated muscle segment, there will be an immediate and complete inhibition of the first swallow. If the first swallow is in the smooth muscle segment when the second swallow occurs, the initial swallow will progress for several seconds before dissipating. Conversely, the original swallow can alter the amplitude and velocity of subsequent swallows for as long as 10 seconds, depending on bolus size.[22] A series of rapid swallows results in a quiescent esophageal body and LES relaxation; the final swallow in the series will be followed by a solitary normal peristaltic wave. The precise mechanism is unclear, although an absence of vagal excitatory activity and vagal activation of nonadrenergic, noncholinergic inhibitory neurons have been postulated.

Esophageal evoked potentials following electrical stimulation and balloon distention of the esophagus have been described.[23, 24] These impulses are presumably conducted via nonmyelinated vagal afferents, based on the prolonged latency periods. The clinical significance of these observations is unclear but may play a role in psychosomatic disorders involving the esophagus.

Lower Esophageal Sphincter

The LES is a high-pressure zone between the esophagus and stomach. Its length gradually increases with age (approximately 1 cm in infants younger than 3 months, 1.6 cm in infants younger than 1 year, and 2 to 4 cm in adults).[15, 25, 26] LES pressure is well developed in the term neonate and may actually decrease with age.[26–30] Newell and associates[29] studied seven premature infants longitudinally and demonstrated a progressive increase in LES pressure. Although the LES pressures were initially low, they were consistently greater than the fundal pressure. This effective sphincter pressure increased from 7 mm Hg at 27 weeks of gestation to 18 mm Hg at 37 weeks. The LES lengthened during the same period from 6.5 to 10 mm.[29]

The LES prevents reflux of gastric contents into the lower esophagus and relaxes during swallowing to allow the passage of fluid or food into the stomach. The LES manifests radial asymmetry although not as great as does the UES. Peak pressures are obtained in the left posterior direction owing to the diaphragmatic crura. The LES remains closed except during swallowing, belching, and vomiting.[15] LES relaxation occurs within 2 seconds of the act of swallowing and lasts 8 to 10 seconds, allowing the peristaltic wave to pass through. LES relaxation results from activation of preganglionic vagal fibers. These fibers activate postganglionic neurons via nicotinic and muscarinic receptors. An unidentified noncholinergic, nonadrenergic compound is ultimately released.

Basal LES pressure is determined by three factors: intrinsic smooth muscle, neural control, and hormonal regulation. Intrinsic smooth muscle activity may be responsible for resting LES tone since the membrane potential is less than in the adjacent esophageal body or

Table 24–1. PHARMACOLOGIC AGENTS AFFECTING LES PRESSURE

Agents	LES Pressure *Increases*	LES Pressure *Decreases*
Hormones and peptides	Angiotensin Bombesin Gastrin Motilin Substance P Vasopressin Pancreatic polypeptide	Cholecystokinin Gastric inhibitory peptide Glucagon Neurotensin Progesterone Secretin Vasoactive intestinal peptide
Neurotransmitters	Alpha-adrenergic agonists Anticholinesterase Beta-adrenergic antagonists Cholinergic agonists	Alpha-adrenergic antagonists Anticholinergics Beta-adrenergic agonists Dopamine
Other	Cisapride Domperidone Histamine (H_1 receptor) Indomethacin Metoclopramide Prostaglandin F_2-alpha Serotonin (neural receptor)	Calcium channel blockers Cyclic adenosine monophosphate Diazepam Histamine (H_2 receptor) Lidocaine Morphine Prostaglandins E_1 and E_2 Serotonin (muscle receptor) Theophylline

stomach. The precise mechanism is unclear, although intracellular calcium may be involved.[25]

Autonomic neural regulation remains controversial. Sympathetic efferent fibers are provided by the thoracic greater splanchnic nerve. Alpha-adrenergic neurotransmitters and beta-blockade increase LES pressure; beta-agonists and alpha-blockade reduce LES pressure. Unfortunately, these effects are extremely short-lived. Parasympathetic innervation stems from the vagus nerves and produces LES relaxation during swallowing. It is unclear whether the cholinergic innervation has any effect on resting LES pressure, although bethanechol administration results in a brief increase in LES pressure.[26]

A variety of circulating hormones and other physiologic compounds have been investigated with regard to basal LES pressure. Table 24–1 summarizes the results to date, although a number of these effects may be pharmacologic rather than physiologic. Dietary protein raises LES pressure; dietary fat, ethanol, chocolate, caffeine, and peppermint reduce LES pressure. Smoking and pregnancy also lower LES pressure. Chloral hydrate (50 mg per kg) is recommended if sedation is required for manometric measurements, since it has no effect on LES pressure.[28]

REFERENCES

1. Grand RJ, Watkins JB, Torti FM: Development of the human gastrointestinal tract: A review. Gastroenterology 1976; 70:790–810.
2. Weaver TL: Anatomy and embryology. *In* Walker WA, Durie PR, Hamilton JR, et al, eds: Pediatric Gastrointestinal Disease. 1st ed, vol 1. Philadelphia, BC Decker, 1991, pp 195–216.
3. Strobel CT, Byrne WJ, Ament ME, et al: Correlation of esophageal lengths in children with height: Application to the Tuttle test without prior esophageal manometry. J Pediatr 1979; 94:81–84.
4. Swigart LL, Siekert RG, Hambley WC, et al: The esophageal arteries: An anatomic study of 150 specimens. Surg Gynecol Obstet 1950; 90:234–243.
5. Watchow DA, Furness JB, Costa M, et al: Distributions of neuropeptides in the human esophagus. Gastroenterology 1987; 93:1363–1371.
6. Christensen J, Williams TH, Jew J, et al: Distribution of vasoactive intestinal polypeptide—immunoreactive structures in the opposum esophagus. Gastroenterology 1987; 92:1007–1018.
7. Geboes K, Desmet V: Histology of the esophagus. Front Gastrointest Res 1978; 3:1–17.
8. Meyer GW, Castell DO: Anatomy and physiology of the esophageal body. *In* Castell DO, Johnson LF, eds: Esophageal Function in Health and Disease. New York, Elsevier, 1983, pp 1–15.
9. Castell DO: Physiology. *In* Hill L, Koyarek R, McCullum R, et al, eds: The Esophagus: Medical and Surgical Management. Philadelphia, WB Saunders, 1988, pp 25–32.
10. Jacobs P, Kahrilas PJ, Logemann JA, et al: Upper esophageal sphincter opening and modulation during swallowing. Gastroenterology 1989; 97:1469–1478.
11. Gryboski JD: The swallowing mechanism of the neonate: I. Esophageal and gastric motility. Pediatrics 1965; 35:445–452.
12. Sondheimer JM: Upper esohageal sphincter and pharyngoesophageal motor function in infants with and without gastroesophageal reflux. Gastroenterology 1983; 85:301–303.
13. Staiano A, Cucchiara S, Viia B, et al: Disorders of upper esophageal sphincter motility in children. J Pediatr Gastroenterol Nutr 1987; 6:892–898.
14. Kahrilas PJ, Dodds WJ, Dent J, et al: Upper esophageal sphincter function during deglutition. Gastroenterology 1988; 95:52–62.
15. Kahrilas PJ, Dodds WJ, Dent J, et al: Upper esophageal sphincter function during belching. Gastroenterology 1986; 91:133–140.
16. Gerhardt DC, Shuck TJ, Bordeaux RA, et al: Human upper esophageal sphincter: Response to volume, osmotic and acid stimuli. Gastroenterology 1978; 75:268–274.
17. Kahrilas PJ, Dodds WJ, Haeberle DB, et al: Effect of sleep, spontaneous gastroesophageal reflux, and a meal on upper esophageal sphincter pressure in normal human volunteers. Gastroenterology 1987; 92:466–471.
18. Humphries TJ, Castell DO. Pressure profile of esophageal peristalsis in normal humans as measured by direct intraesophageal transducers. Am J Dig Dis 1977; 22:641–645.
19. Goyal RK, Cobb BW: Motility of the pharynx, esophagus and esophageal sphincters. *In* Johnson LR, Christensen J, Grossman MI, et al, eds: Physiology of the Gastrointestinal Tract. 1st ed. New York, Raven Press, 1981, pp 359–391.

20. Gryboski JD, Thayer WR, Spiro HM: Esophageal motility in infants and children. Pediatrics 1963; 31:382–395.
21. Crist J, Giddo JS, Goyal RK: Intramural mechanism of esophageal peristalsis: Roles of cholinergic and non-cholinergic nerves. Proc Natl Acad Sci U S A 1984; 81:3595–3599.
22. Vanek AW, Diamant NE: Responses of the human esophagus to paired swallows. Gastroenterology 1987; 92:643—650.
23. Frieling T, Erick P, Wienbeck M: Cerebral responses evoked by electrical stimulation of the esophagus in normal subjects. Gastroenterology 1989; 97:475–478.
24. Castell DO, Wood JD, Frieling T, et al: Cerebral electrical potentials evoked by balloon distention of the human esophagus. Gastroenterology 1990; 98:662–666.
25. Gerhardt GC, Castell DO: Anatomy and physiology of the esophageal sphincters. *In* Castell DO, Johnson LE, eds: Esophageal Function in Health and Disease. New York; Elsevier, 1983, pp 17–29.
26. Moroz S, Espinoza J, Cumming W, et al: Lower esophageal sphincter function in children with and without gastroesophageal reflux. Gastroenterology 1976; 71:236–241.
27. Moroz SP, Beiko P: Relationship between lower esophageal sphincter pressure and serum gastrin concentration in the newborn infant. J Pediatr 1981; 99:725–728.
28. Vanderhoof JA, Rappaport PJ, Paxson CL: Manometric diagnosis of lower esophageal sphincter incompetence in infants: Use of a small, single lumen perfused catheter. Pediatrics 1978; 62:805–808.
29. Newell SJ, Sarkar PK, Durbin GM, et al: Maturation of the lower esophageal sphincter in the preterm baby. Gut 1988; 29:167–172.
30. Diamant NE: Development of esophageal function. Am Rev Respir Dis 1985; 131(suppl):S29–S32.

Chapter 25

Esophageal Atresia and Tracheoesophageal Fistula

SIGMUND H. EIN

INTRODUCTION

Esophageal atresia (EA), with or without a tracheoesophageal fistula (TEF), is "the epitome of modern surgery"[1] and the champagne of neonatal problems as far as pediatric surgeons are concerned. The variations in age and size of the patient, associated anomalies, pathologic types, operative approaches, and postoperative problems continue to challenge those clincians who have dedicated their working hours to the care of pediatric patients. W. J. Potts stated in 1957, "Congenital atresia of the eophagus with tracheoesophageal fistula is one of the most difficult deformities the pediatric surgeon is called upon to treat."[2] Thirty years later, J. G. Randolph noted, "Esophageal atresia is the anomaly which, by its urgency, its exacting requirements at the operating table, its demand for precise postoperative management and the long-term follow-up essential in the growing child, becomes the ultimate congenital abnormality for which pediatric surgeons prepare."[3]

The story of EA and TEF repairs reads like the gradual mastery of most other surgical problems.[4, 4a, 4b] Durston first described an infant with EA in 1670,[3] but not until the time of Vogt[5] (1929) and then Gross[6] (1953) was a classification of EA varieties developed. Various surgical attempts were made from the late 1800s until 1943, when Haight and Towsley[7] were the first successfully to repair EA and TEF. Before that event, all patients (including 32 reported by Lanman[8]) who had been primarily repaired had died. Two years before the first success of Haight and Towsley,[7] Leven[9] and Ladd[10] each had a survivor but had not achieved a primary repair.

EMBRYOLOGY AND PATHOGENESIS

EA and TEF occur in 1 in 3,000 to 5,000 live births[11–13] and are equally distributed according to sex. Embryologically, the esophagus, stomach, trachea, and lungs all are derived from the foregut.[14, 14a] The foregut is partitioned by a septum into two separate tubes (Fig. 25–1): (1) the trachea anteriorly, which then continues to develop cartilaginous rings and lung buds; and (2) the esophagus posteriorly, which stretches from the pharynx to the stomach. This process is complete by the fourth fetal week (when the embryo is 8 mm long). For unknown reasons, there is an incomplete tubular separation of the esophagus from top to bottom, causing an atresia,[15] and in most instances the posterior esophagus fails to separate completely from the trachea, creating a variety of TEFs or clefts, or both. Tracheal anomalies (atresias, stenoses, and clefts) may also occur in conjunction with esophageal defects.[16, 17]

Between the third and fourth fetal weeks (when

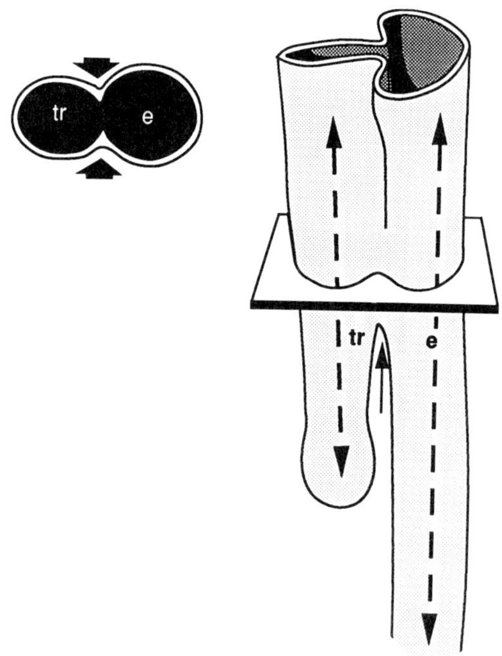

Figure 25–1. By the fourth fetal week (8-mm-long embryo), the foregut is partitioned into trachea anteriorly and esophagus posteriorly by a transverse septum; the septum also moves cephalad and caudally.

embryos are 3–4- and 8-mm long), the laryngotracheal sulcus is completed along with the segmentation of the parietal mesoderm on each side of the notochord and with the formation of sclerotomes, myotomes, and vertebrae. Segmentation of the embryo, therefore, happens at the same time that the tracheobronchial tree and esophagus separate.[18, 19]

Several questions have been raised about the standard embryologic theories just discussed. "The dominant role of the tracheoesophageal septum for differentiation of the foregut is highly hypothetical."[20] It has also been proposed that many of the unusual and rare types of EA and TEF, such as pure EA and pure TEF, have a pathogenesis different from that of combined EA and TEF.[20] Some embryologists believe that these "pure" defects develop not from a failure of foregut organogenesis but from secondary lesions (e.g., necrosis from local microcirculation[21]) of the already differentiated organs. Similarly, congenital bronchoesophageal fistulas cannot develop by faulty septal separation, because "the development of the bronchi and the differentiation of the esophagus and trachea are spatially independent procedures. Therefore, these fistulas can only develop after the organs have already differentiated."[22]

Half of the mothers of a fetus with an EA have polyhydramnios,[23] an association that may increase the chances for prenatal diagnosis. Neonates who have an EA with or without a TEF vary in weight from 800 to 4,000 gm (averaging 2,500 gm); 50% weigh more than 2,500 gm, and the remaining 50% are considered premature (weighing less than 2,500 gm). About 50% have other anomalies,[23a, 23b] with more than 40% having from one to four other defects[24]: cardiovascular,[24a, 24b] 25% (most common are patent ductus arteriosus and ventricular and atrial septal defects); gastrointestinal, 15% (imperforate anus and duodenal atresia); skeletal,[24c] 10% (digital and vertebral); genitourinary,[24d, 24e] 5% (hypospadias and undescended testis); and other congenital lesions, 15% (trisomy or lung agenesis or hypoplasia). As the number of systems with defects increases, the weight of the neonate decreases; 10% have defects incompatible with life (i.e., trisomy or complex cardiac defects).[18, 25, 25a] Aside from these groups of anomalies, the variety and complexity of abnormalities associated with EA and TEF mean that no specific combination will occur frequently, even in a large sample of patients. However, several syndromes are recognized in which there does appear to be a common denominator, including those defects referred to as VATER,*[26] VACTERL,†[27, 28] and CHARGE.‡[29, 29a] The occurrence of an extracardiac malformation should increase the suspicion that a child who has an EA with TEF also has a cardiac lesion (32%), and this likelihood increases twofold when there are two or more extracardiac abnormalities.[30] As with most common birth defects, the pathogenesis of an EA with or without TEF may be related to both genetic and environmental factors.[20, 30a] Most authors[3, 31] have reported normal karyotypes in infants with VATER syndrome.[26] It is likely that this malformation occurs early within the first trimester, when there is organ differentiation and septation (division). This possibility has led others to speculate that the developmental cause of EA and TEF may also affect other organ systems at the same time.[32] The fact that multiple anomalies and low birth weight often coexist suggests that these anomalies cause intrauterine growth retardation.[33] Families with these congenital esophageal defects have been reported.[34, 35]

*VATER, *v*ertebral defects, imperforate *a*nus, *t*racheoesophageal fistula, *r*adial and *r*enal dysplasia.

†VACTERL, *v*ertebral, *a*nal, *c*ardiac, *t*racheal, *e*sophageal, *r*enal, *l*imb.

‡CHARGE, *c*oloboma; *h*eart disease; choanal *a*tresia; *r*etarded growth and development; *g*enital hypoplasia; *e*ar anomalies and deafness.

CLASSIFICATION

Although there are many varieties and combinations of EA with and without TEF, the three most common are proximal EA and distal TEF (85%), pure EA (10%), and H-TEF (3%; see later discussion); the rest are rare (2%[36, 37, 37a]; Fig. 25–2). Acquired TEF in the pediatric patient is not common and is usually caused by a foreign body.[38, 39] Early recognition and treatment of the disease and its associated anomalies have greatly improved the survival rate.[24, 40, 41]

Esophageal Atresia with Distal Tracheoesophageal Fistula

Infants with EA and distal TEF (Fig. 25–2*A*) constitute about 85% of the total congenital esophageal defects; one half are premature, and one half have other anomalies. The esophageal gap is usually 1 to 2 cm, and the distal TEF most commonly joins the trachea at the carina. Variations can exist in these defects; the atretic gap can be millimeters to inches wide, and the fistula can join higher on the trachea or lower on the right main bronchus.

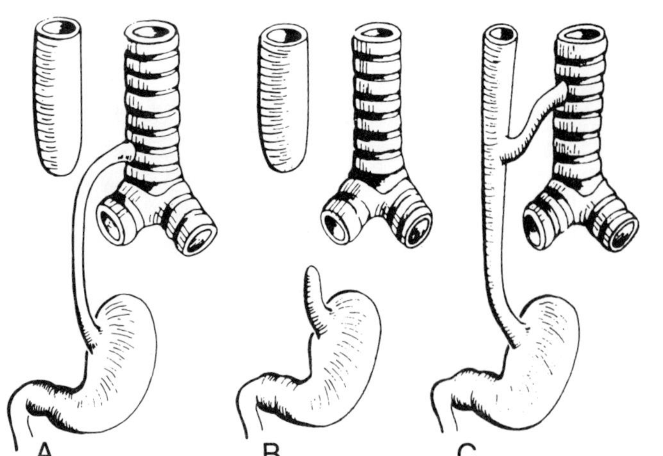

Figure 25–2. The three most common types of EA and TEF, accounting for 98% of cases. *A,* Proximal atresia and distal TEF (85%). *B,* Pure atresia (10%). *C,* H-TEF (3%).

Diagnosis

An EA and distal TEF should be diagnosed, as soon as the infant is delivered, by passage of a nasoesophageal radiopaque tube that stops 3 to 4 inches (6.25–10 cm) into the blind upper esophageal pouch (Fig. 25–3)[41a]; the tube should be left in place on suction, with hourly instillations of air, and a chest radiograph should be obtained. A tube smaller than 10-Fr will coil in the blind upper pouch and give a false sense of being in the stomach. If nasal obstruction (choanal atresia) exists, the tube can then be passed by mouth. If this simple, easy step is not carried out soon after birth, then the neonate will cough, choke, sputter, or turn blue on its saliva or with the first feeds. The latter situation is not rare but it should never occur. A false passage from the nasoesophageal tube occasionally happens; this possibility is signaled by a difficult tube passage and the presence of bloody mucus in the tube and the oropharyngeal area. A radiopaque water-soluble esophagram is then indicated. The treatment is the same as for an esophageal anastomotic leak.

The chest radiograph also shows the state of the lung fields. The commonest area of lung involvement from aspiration is the right upper lobe, and the prompt treatment of aspiration pneumonia with oxygen and antibiotics and the prevention of reaspiration are indicated. There is rarely any need to put contrast material into the upper pouch.[36, 42] However, should that become necessary, 0.25 to 0.5 ml of a water-soluble radiopaque solution is all that is required; an excessive amount will flood over into the tracheobronchial tree, creating acute respiratory problems (Fig. 25–4). If aspiration does occur, there will be a rapid onset of pulmonary edema, because of the high osmolarity of some of the water-soluble radiopaque contrast solutions. The proponents of the radiopaque solution approach believe that the rare upper esophageal pouch fistula will be found but that such an upper pouch fistula is never at the bottom of the pouch,[43] may not always be open,[36] and will almost certainly be found at surgery when the upper pouch is mobilized for anastomosis.[3] The chest radiograph usually reveals enough of the abdomen to determine whether any gas is present within the gastrointestinal tract, indicating a lower (distal) TEF (see Fig. 25–3). Rarely (in 15% of instances), the distal TEF is obliterated (without a long gap between the EA ends) so that there will be no gas in the bowel below the diaphragm.[44] Vertebral body defects (extra vertebrae or hemivertebrae; Fig. 25–5) and rib anomalies (extra ribs or hypoplastic ribs) raise the suspicion of an EA with

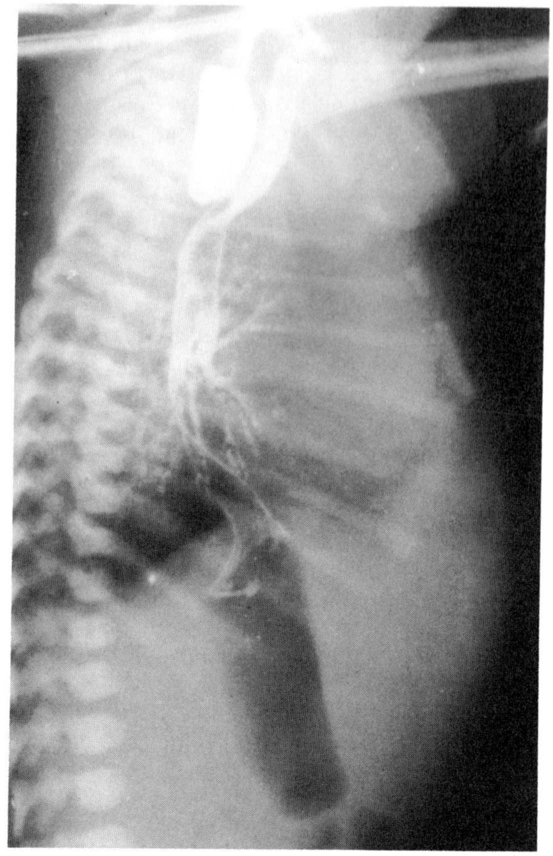

Figure 25–4. Excessive amount of radiopaque dye placed into a blind upper pouch, flooding over into the tracheobronchial tree and thereby into the distal TEF.

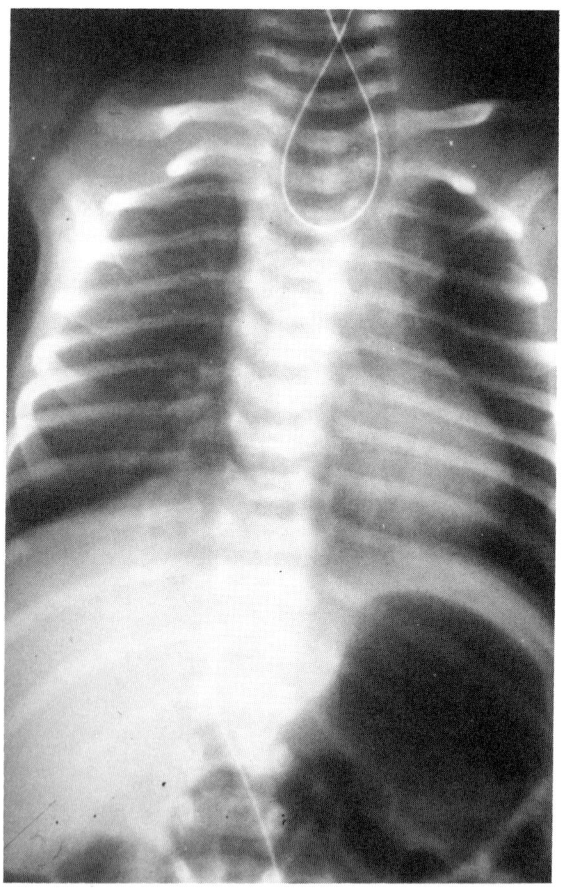

Figure 25–3. Coiled radiopaque nasogastric tube in blind upper pouch, giving a false impression of being in the stomach. Note the air in the gastrointestinal tract, indicating a distal TEF. Rarely, the TEF is so big that a large amount of air enters the stomach, and preliminary gastrostomy will be necessary to avoid gastric perforation.

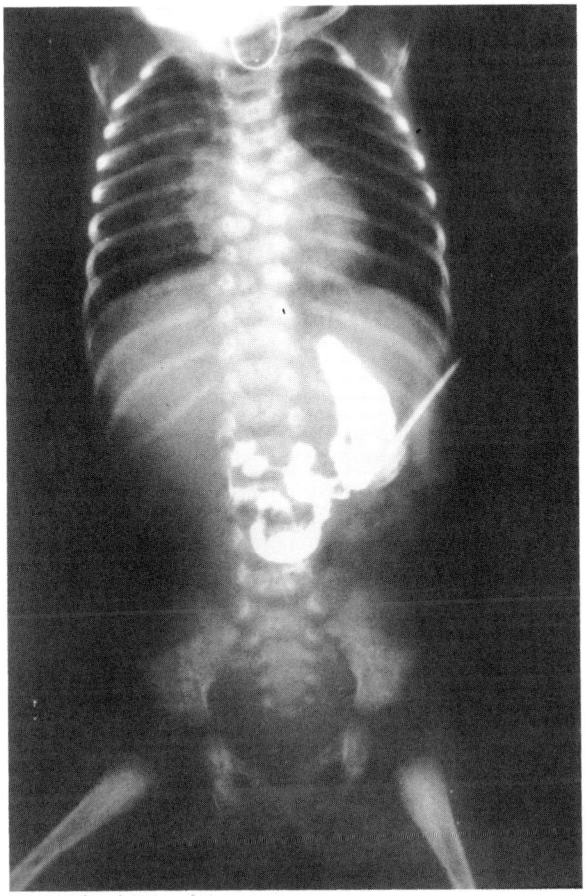

Figure 25–5. Thoracic vertebral body defects that often accompany the EA and TEF anomaly.

TEF. The incidence of these skeletal anomalies can be as high as 45%.[18, 19, 45] Heart size and the size of the descending aorta can be noted on chest radiograph. Cardiovascular abnormalities are diagnosed in 40% of patients by clinical examination, and in 60% by catheterization, autopsy, or both.[30] When the aorta is on the ipsilateral side, the repair of an EA is said to be more difficult; however, this occurrence is so unusual that it is often not even looked for, especially if there is no initial evidence of a congenital heart defect.[46] Dextrocardia usually signals that other congenital anomalies are present.

Most major associated defects, except for renal agenesis, require some form of surgical intervention early in the child's life. Surgery may not be indicated for the minor defects; the procedures that are performed are probably minimal and can be scheduled for a later date.[24] The commonest associated congenital anomalies are found in the cardiovascular system and include patent ductus arteriosus, ventricular and atrial defects, tetralogy of Fallot, and coarctation of the aorta. There is no known association between extracardiac malformation and the type of cardiac lesion (if any) that a neonate with EA and TEF may have.[30]

Most gastrointestinal anomalies require fairly urgent surgery and may seriously affect the treatment of EA and TEF.[24] In spite of the frequent coexistence of gastrointestinal lesions with cardiac abnormalities (with the former type often requiring several operations), endocarditis is not a problem[31] with appropriate antibiotic prophylaxis.[24] None of the skeletal defects requires immediate repair; therefore, routine screening of the spine in these neonates is unnecessary.[19, 47] Almost none of the genitourinary abnormalities requires immediate surgical intervention, although early identification is important.

Initial Management

The patient with EA and TEF must always be transported in the upright position to avoid gastroesophageal reflux of the highly acidic gastric juices. Intravenous fluids, electrolytes, and antibiotics are given.[48, 49, 49a] Intensive care nursing on a one-to-one basis is critical,[49b] and the oropharynx is suctioned frequently in spite of a properly functioning nasoesophageal tube in the upper pouch. By the next day, the neonate is usually well enough to be taken to the operating room for the definitive repair. If there is a delay for any reason, no harm will come from the wait as long as the stomach is not overdistended, or no gastroduodenal contents are refluxing into the distal esophagus through the TEF and into the tracheobronchial tree. Rarely, the fistula is so big that a large amount of air enters the stomach, and a preliminary gastrostomy is necessary to avoid gastric perforation (see Fig. 25–3). In the former situation a gastrostomy will help only as a means of gastric decompression, but if this is still unsatisfactory because of bile reflux into the distal esophagus and into the airway, transthoracic ligation and division of the TEF may be necessary (Fig. 25–6). This procedure eliminates the pulmonary soiling and allows the institution of gastrostomy feeds. Gastric division was tried as an alternative to the transthoracic TEF ligation, but it has not made the job easier.[50] Past teaching suggested that routine gastrostomy was necessary prior to (or simultaneous with) repair of an EA with TEF; however, it appears that this routine is being questioned, if not abandoned.[51, 52]

Surgical Approach

It is rarely necessary (and probably unwise) to embark on the primary repair of an EA and TEF in a neonate during the late night hours. The only surgery that seems to be indicated at that time is an emergency gastrostomy to prevent or treat gastric perforation. A right fourth interspace thoractomy approach is used most commonly, but once the incision is made, the number of variations from that point until the skin is closed is legion.[52a] If the aorta is found to be on the right (wrong) side at the time of thoracotomy, and if this hampers the exposure and repair, the chest can be closed and the repair carried out through a contralateral thoracotomy incision during the same anesthetic. Opinion is by no means unanimous as to which side is best in such rare situations.[46] Dextrocardia, per se, does not seem to hamper the usual right thoractomy approach. The first step of the operation is

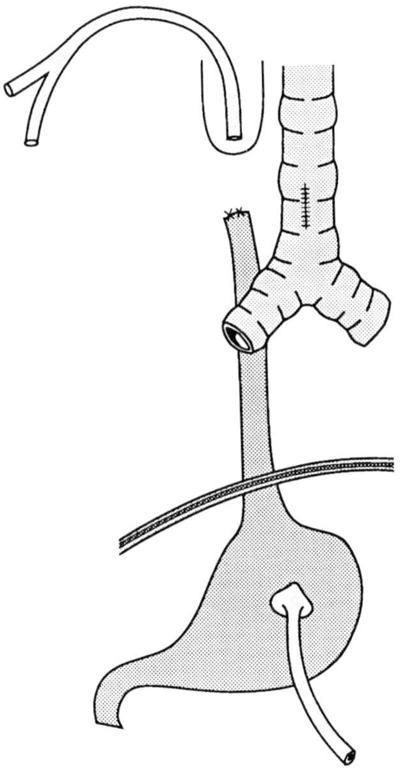

Figure 25–6. Transthoracic ligation and division of the TEF may be warranted to stop the gastroesophageal reflux from soiling the lungs and to allow the institution of gastrostomy feeds.

to ligate and divide the distal TEF (see Fig. 25–6); this will prevent gastroesophageal reflux into the tracheobronchial tree so that if an esophageal anastomosis cannot or should not be attempted, the neonate will still benefit from this operation. To leave the TEF only ligated (and undivided) invites refistulization in almost all instances.[53, 54] Although the trachea could be narrowed in the area of the TEF division and closure, this a rare occurrence. To the contrary, there is usually a small residual esophageal pouch or diverticulum that may cause problems if endotracheal intubation or endoscopy is done in the future. Occasionally, the TEF may enter the right main bronchus, or it may enter higher up on the trachea. This latter situation can cause some technical difficulty with the division and closure of the high TEF and the subsequent esophageal anastomosis, but the high anastomosis tends to have fewer stricture problems owing to the constant dilatation provided when food boluses project back and down during swallowing.

Most esophageal surgical pioneers would cringe at the constant pediatric surgical violation of the two basic principles of esophageal surgery: an adequate blood supply at both ends and a tension-free anastomosis. The usual anastomatic gap is about 1 to 2 cm, and any gap greater than that size increases the technical difficulty and the associated postoperative morbidity. Two basic principles should guide all pediatric surgeons in performing the esophageal anastomosis, and a point somewhere between the two must be achieved: (1) no neonate with an EA should die (all other things being equal) during an attempt to pull both the proximal and the distal esophageal pouches together; and (2) the neonate's own repaired esophagus (no matter what problems may be encountered) is better than any other tube or conduit that can be constructed. The anastomosis is usually between an upper esophageal pouch, which is the size of an adult's small finger, and a lower esophagus, which is usually smaller than a lead pencil. There are two types of anastomoses currently done (Fig. 25–7): (1) end-to-end, one layer and two layers[7] and (2) end-to-side, after the distal TEF is ligated in continuity.[55, 56] The first type is the commonest anastomosis performed by most pediatric surgeons. There are more leaks with a one-layer anastomosis but more strictures with a two-layer anastomosis,[57] and recurrent fistulas are commoner with an end-to-side anastomosis.[53, 54] If a rare (2%) proximal fistula is present (Fig. 25–8), it will be found (and divided) when the upper pouch is being mobilized.[36, 42]

Although Waterston and coworkers' 1962 classification[58] of the group of EA with the poorest prognosis (birth weight <2,500 gm, pneumonia, or other congenital anomalies) has been upgraded, there are some instances that preclude a primary anastomosis after the TEF has been ligated and divided. These include significant respiratory problems or a number of gross associated anomalies in severely ill premature infants[52a, 59]; a thin upper esophageal pouch usually found in the infant with cleft palate who is unable to swallow in utero; and an upper esophageal pouch that barely enters the chest. Corrective methods range from not performing a primary repair (staging)[60] to attempting to elongate the upper esophageal segment or committing the infant to an immediate neck esophagostomy and a later esophageal replacement. Staging does not preclude an anastomosis. The most popular method of elongation is the circular myotomy[61] (Fig. 25–9), which adds about 1 cm of length per myotomy. Other methods of upper and lower pouch elongation other than waiting a few months, repeated swallowing, and gastroesophageal reflux are an upper pouch bougienage,[62] electromagnetic bougienage,[63] the suture fistula technique,[64, 65] and an esophageal flap esophagoplasty.[66] When the anastomosis is

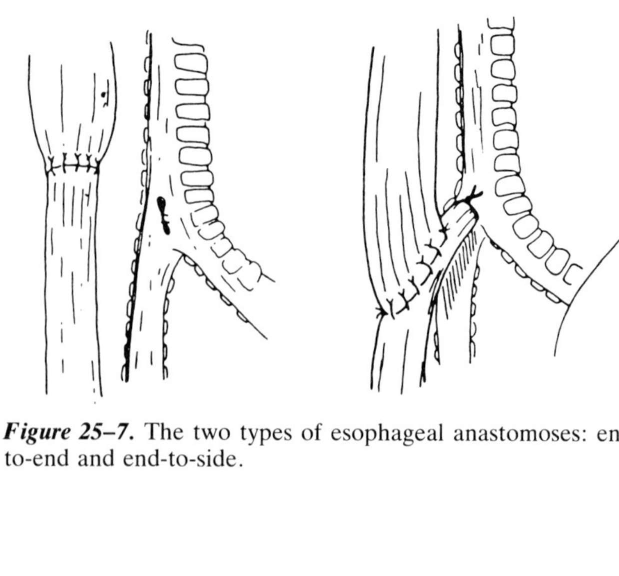

Figure 25–7. The two types of esophageal anastomoses: end-to-end and end-to-side.

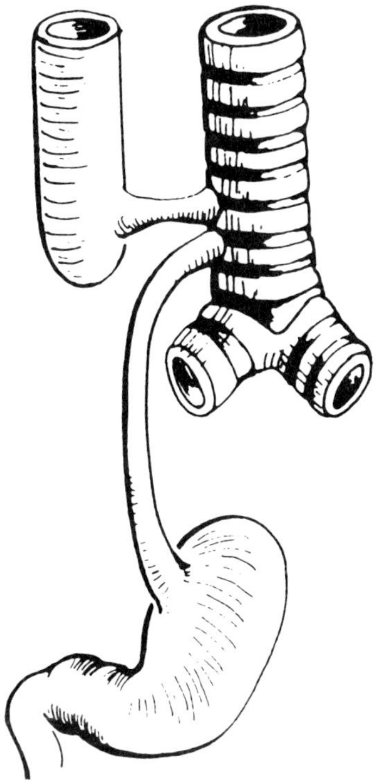

Figure 25–8. Rare proximal TEFs will be found when the upper pouch is mobilized.

completed, some surgeons place a small transanastomotic (nasogastric) feeding tube down the repaired esophagus into the stomach. This is done so that when an anastomotic leak occurs, the nasogastric tube can be used for enteral feeding for the 1 or 2 weeks needed for the leak to heal; otherwise, the infant would require a feeding gastrostomy or total parenteral nutrition (TPN).[51] Most often a chest tube is placed because of the thoracotomy and in the event of an anastomotic leak.

Early Postoperative Management

Weaning from ventilatory support occasionally may be prolonged.[67] Gastrostomy or nasogastric tube feeds can usually be started on the fourth postoperative day if there is no clinical evidence of an anastomotic leak.[67a] Any feeds put into the stomach by a gastrostomy or a feeding tube run the risk of refluxing into the repaired esophagus and threatening the integrity of the new anastomosis. Therefore, within the first week after esophageal surgery, only small amounts of feeds should be given slowly and in hourly drips. If the infant does vomit the feeds, the volume should be decreased. If no complications develop during the first postoperative week, a water-soluble radiopaque contrast esophagram is obtained; if there is no leak, all tubes are removed, and the infant is started on oral feeds. About 50% of the infants with a repaired EA do quite well and go home feeding normally within a few weeks after surgery.[52a] It is rare to view a postoperative radiopaque contrast esophagram and not see the anastomosis, which is always somewhat narrowed (Fig. 25–10). The most important aspect of an esophagram is not how narrow the anastomosis appears but how wide it can open.

The major worry about the neonatal esophageal anastomosis is a leak (Fig. 25–11). At least 50% of these EA anastomoses leak to some degree; the clinical manifestations depend on the size of the leak. The typical symptomatic anastomotic leak presents on the third or fourth postoperative day with some respiratory distress in an infant who becomes tachypneic, cyanotic, and septic; the chest radiograph typically shows a right pyopneumothorax. Ventilation may be necessary if the infant is seriously ill as well. Antibiotics and possibly another chest tube are required. The leak should be reassessed with an esophagram weekly until it heals, which should occur in several weeks. Nutrition can be maintained by tube feeds (provided that they do not reflux into the esophagus and out the anastomotic leak) or even TPN. Once the leak has closed, as determined both clinically and radiologically, the infant can be fed by mouth.

Many EA anastomotic leaks produce strictures,[57] and 30 to 40% of these strictures are symptomatic (with coughing, regurgitation, aspiration, and failure to gain weight; Fig. 25–12). The stricture may progress remarkably before the infant (on a fluid diet) becomes symptomatic. The diagnosis is confirmed by esophagram or esophagoscopy, or both. Most strictures will respond to one or more dilatations[53, 68]; however, these dilatations should not begin until 3 or 4 weeks after the anastomosis

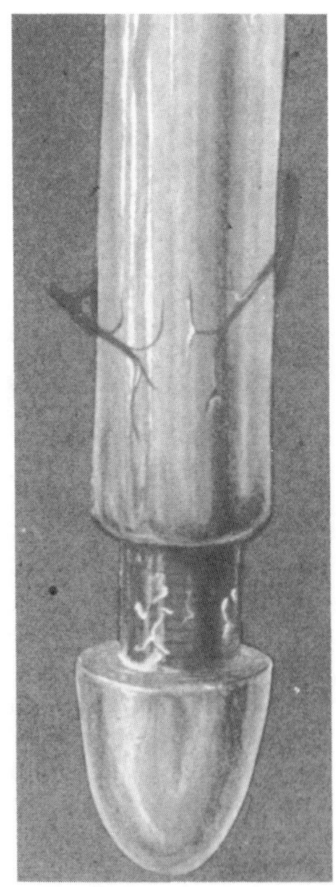

Figure 25–9. Circular myotomy of Livaditis near the distal part of the upper pouch; each myotomy adds 1 cm of length to the esophagus.

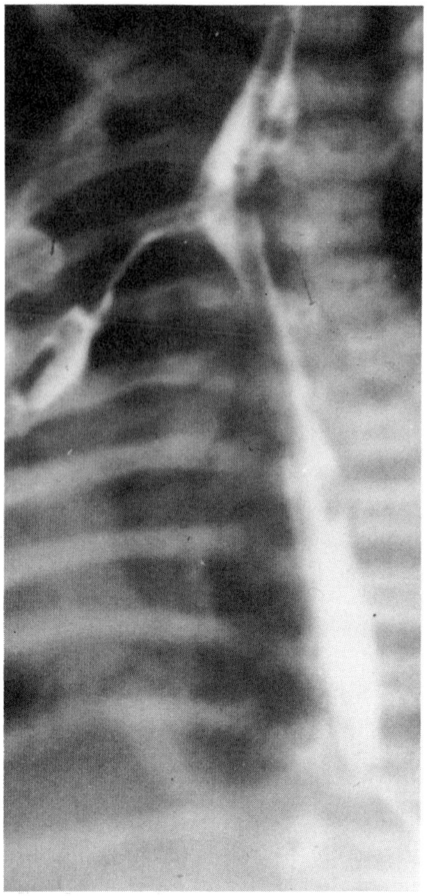

Figure 25–10. Esophagram 1 week after repair of the EA and distal TEF. Note the slight narrowing at the anastomosis.

was made. If prograde dilatation is impossible because of the severity of the stricture or angulation at the site of the stricture (as may be encountered with an end-to-side anastomosis or with a colon or gastric tube replacement neck anastomosis), then a gastrostomy should be made and a guide string passed like a nasogastric tube out of the gastrostomy back up to the nose. Dilatations can then be carried out along this string with graduated bougies. A gastrostomy postpones retrograde dilatations for 3 or 4 weeks until the stomach is well fixed to the anterior abdominal wall. Initially, dilatation of these short strictures may have to be carried out weekly, but after a few such procedures obvious improvement in symptoms and lumen size shoud be apparent, and the interval between dilatations may then be extended. If the stricture fails to respond to dilatations, or if the response is transient, the presence of gastroesophageal reflux must be ruled out.[69, 70] If the latter problem is not corrected, little permanent response to dilatations can be expected. Abnormal esophageal motility is evident on fluoroscopic examination of the repaired esophagus.[71, 71a] It is unusual that dilatations are required in patients older than 1 or 2 years of age, and it is rare to have to resect a persistent strictured EA anastomosis.

Late Postoperative Management

For about the first 3 months after surgical correction of an EA and distal TEF in an infant, there are usually no problems with swallowing because the newly joined esophagus does not have to handle more than fluids. Thereafter, the parents must slowly advance both the quantity and the quality of foods given until the anastomosis has matured and reached its maximum width and until the child can understand that he or she will always have to chew food well and eat slowly. Therefore, when baby foods are added, some dysphagia may become evident, and this warrants immediate investigation. A routine chest radiograph will show whether pneumonia is present, and a contrast study of the esophagus and stomach will detect any upper gstrointestinal tract disorder. The best method to demonstrate a recurrent TEF (10%) or a missed H-TEF (Fig. 25–13) is a prone pull-back tube esophagram. (A feeding tube is put into the lower esophagus of the prone patient, and as the tube is gradually pulled up the esophagus, water-soluble radiopaque contrast is injected under moderate pressure to dilate the esophagus and thus demonstrate the fistula.[72]) After the search for the fistula is complete, the infant should be given some contrast

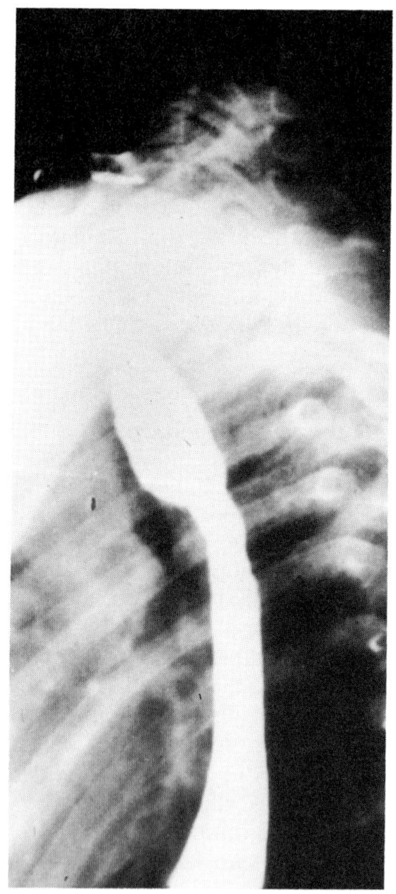

Figure 25–11. Anastomotic leak (seen on esophagram) usually occurs on the third or fourth postoperative day.

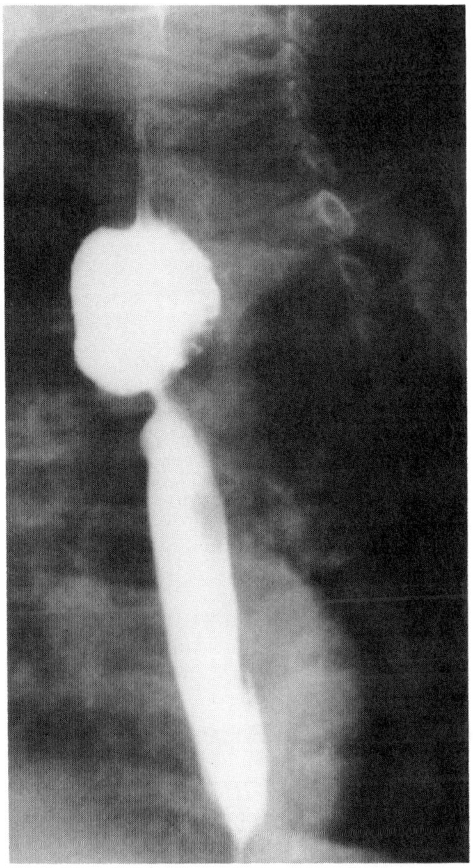

Figure 25–12. Symptomatic anastomotic stricture that occurs in 30 to 40% of EA repairs. Most strictures require and respond to several dilatations.

solution to swallow to reveal the presence of aspiration due to muscular incoordination (pharyngoesophageal dyskinesia) or fatigue, tracheomalacia, anastomotic stricture, gastroesophageal reflux, or pyloric stenosis.[73, 74] Gastroesophageal reflux is a significant problem in the postoperative EA and TEF infant. Half of these patients will have severe enough anastomotic, respiratory, or gastrointestional disturbances to require antireflux surgery. Even then, recurrent reflux may be a problem owing to the abnormal esophagal swallowing mechanism, short esophagus, or the surgeon's fear of wrapping the lower esophagus too tightly.[74–77]

There is well-documented evidence that squamous metaplasia[78] and tracheomalacia[78a] due to inadequately formed and missing cartilage are in the tracheal area of the TEF. Because of squamous metaplasia in the posterior muscular wall of the trachea and lateral and anterior walls of the trachea, there is an absence of respiratory ciliated columnar epithelium needed to clear the airway of mucus and secretions, leading to frequent respiratory infections during the first few years of life.[79, 80] The more easily collapsible trachea (tracheomalacia) adds to this problem and also accounts for the brassy, duck-like cough in these infants that is exacerbated by upper respiratory tract infections, especially during their early years. It is estimated that 25 to 50% of infants with EA and TEF will have tracheomalacia; 10 to 15%[81] of these infants (weeks or months after their repair) will have definite sudden respiratory symptoms ("dying spells") always associated with feeds. The cause of these arrests is said to be an obstructed or flattened trachea between the innominate artery and aortic arch anteriorly and the distended upper esophageal pouch posteriorly during feeds (Fig. 25–14). Whether this is actually mechanical tracheomalacia,[82] "reflex apnea,"[83] or the result of gastroesophageal reflux[84, 84a] is debated. A work-up must rule out neurologic, cardiovascular, or biochemical causes of these spells. The telltale radiograph sign is a narrow upper trachea just below the clavicles seen on a lateral chest radiograph (see Fig. 25–14). At bronchoscopy, the trachea is narrowed anteroposteriorly to a slit-like aperture that may completely obliterate with coughing, straining, or eating. Tracheostomy will keep the trachea open, but suspension of the innominate artery and aortic arch to the back of the sternum is easier and more successful, with no long-term side effects.[82, 85, 86]

It may require several years before some of these children can consume a normal unrestricted diet. During the toddler years, impacted foreign bodies (especially lumps of food) are frequently seen, because this is an age group in which food is often not well chewed; even a minor narrowing associated with a poorly coordinated distal esophagus will result in an impaction at the anastomosis.[71a]

Skeletal deformities (thoracic flattening and protru-

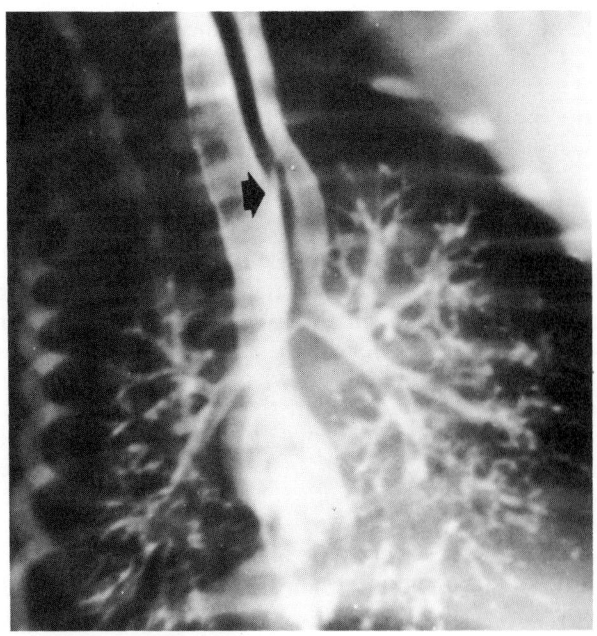

Figure 25–13. H-TEF *(arrow)* is best demonstrated by a prone pull-back esophagram using water-soluble radiopaque contrast solution. Note that the fistula is located just below the clavicles and runs upward from the esophagus to the trachea. A recurrent TEF is always seen at the anastomotic level.

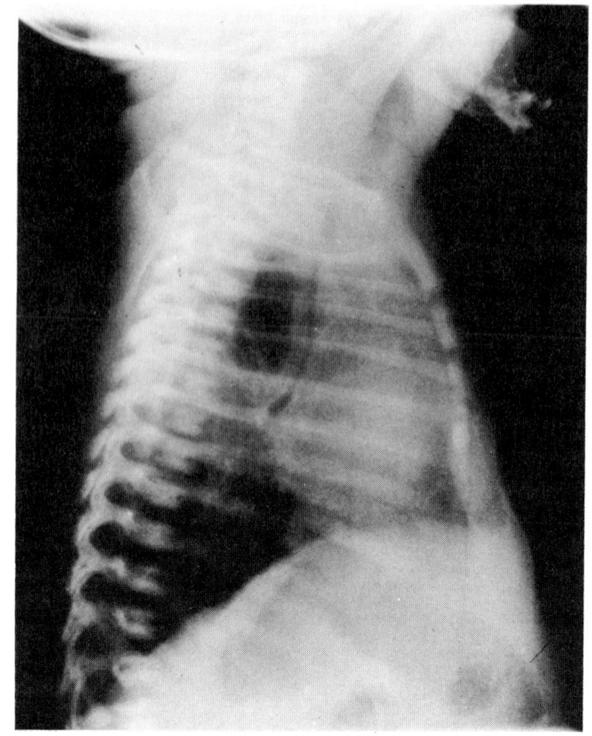

Figure 25–14. Tracheomalacia becomes symptomatic when the trachea is flattened between the aortic arch anteriorly and the distended proximal esophagus posteriorly (usually during feeds). If it is severe, suspending the aortic arch to the back of the sternum provides immediate relief.

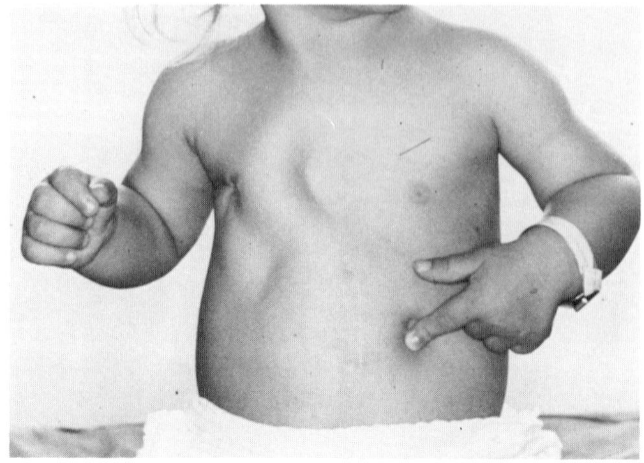

Figure 25–15. Thoracic flattening and protrusion that originate occasionally from the neonatal right thoracotomy incision to repair the EA and TEF.

sion [Fig. 25–15], shoulder elevation, and scoliosis) are abnormalities that originate with the thoracotomy incision and any postoperative problems within the pleural cavity; however, they are not obvious until the child is into the toddler age range and older. Their incidence may range from about 5% to as high as 50%. Appropriate orthopedic management is required.[87, 88]

Prognosis

In the past, much prognostic emphasis was placed on the weight of the neonate with EA and TEF; Waterston[58] and others[33, 40, 41, 57] believed that low birth weight alone (<2,500 gm) lowered the survival rate significantly. This correlation continues to exist,[24] but it is not nearly as strong as earlier. The consensus is that the surgeon should proceed with a primary anastomosis regardless of the patient's weight unless there are other complications.[89–91] Staging is now reserved for mitigating circumstances such as severe lung disease (respiratory distress syndrome, pneumonia) and other severe congenital anomalies.[40, 41]

About half the infants with an EA and distal TEF have no other anomalies, and they survive.[92, 92a–d] However, the problems begin when other anomalies are added to the other 50% of neonates with EA and TEF (Fig. 25–16).[40, 41, 92] The survival rates decrease proportionately with the presence of additional defects: 75% survival with one additional anomaly, and 60% survival with more than one.[24] The cardiovascular defects seem to be the most important in affecting the survival of these babies.

Pure Esophageal Atresia

Pure EA (see Fig. 25–2*B*) is much less common than the previously discussed EA with distal TEF. Forty percent of the patients are premature, and 50% have other anomalies.[43] Infants with this esophageal defect have their own set of problems, not so much with the immediate neonatal course but with surgical attempt to bridge the usual wide gap between esophageal ends.[92d]

The presentation of an infant with pure EA is usually not much different from that of an infant with both an EA and a distal TEF, so that the diagnosis should be made immediately after delivery when a nasogastric tube will not pass into the stomach. The same risk of a false passage made by the tube exists (as in the infant with EA and TEF).[93] The major difference in these infants, however, is that the threat of reflux aspiration of gastric acid into the distal esophagus and into the respiratory tract is nonexistent (because there is no TEF); the only concern is aspiration of saliva into the airway. The lack of a distal TEF can only be made radiologically by noting the absence of gas within the

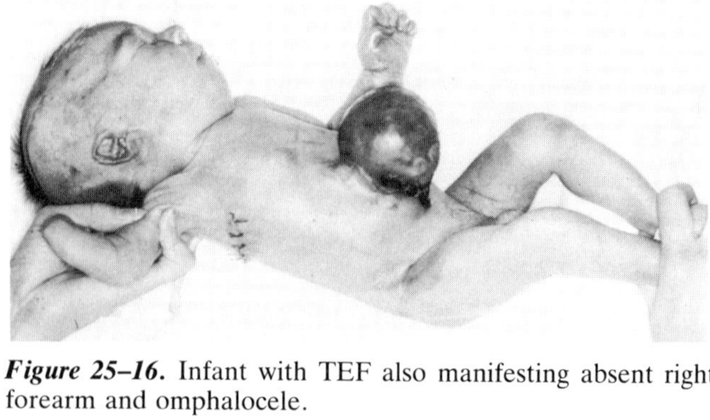

Figure 25–16. Infant with TEF also manifesting absent right forearm and omphalocele.

gastrointestinal tract in the abdomen (Fig. 25–17); this is not a fool-proof method, because about 15% of such atresias have an obliterated distal TEF without a long gap between the EA ends.[44] This lack of gastrointestinal air does not demonstrate any other intestinal atresias distally (e.g., duodenal atresia).

Although fewer neonates with pure EA are premature than in the group with a proximal EA and distal TEF, at least half have other anomalies in the same systems as do the infants with EA and TEF; one difference is that 20% have Down's syndrome.[43, 94] There are fewer cardiac anomalies than in the EA and TEF group but more gastrointestinal and skeletal defects.

There is no urgency to perform the esophageal reconstruction, which is seldom feasible, since the two blind esophageal ends are many centimeters apart initially. Therefore, the immediate focus of surgical attention (after the initial evaluation and stabilization) is on the feeding gastrostomy. In these neonates, the stomach is quite small and friable. Ideally, the gastrostomy tube should be placed in the middle of the anterior part of the stomach close to the lesser curvature, so that if the infant should need a gastric tube constructed from the greater curvature, the latter will be free. Sewing the stomach to the anterior abdominal wall is the safest approach to avoid intra-abdominal leakage of feeds from the gastrostomy site, but sometimes it cannot be done for anatomic reasons; therefore, extra caution is mandatory when introducing tube feeds postoperatively. Because there is an increased chance of associated duodenal atresia, the surgeon must check for this anomaly when making the gastrostomy by injecting some fluid into the stomach and watching it enter the jejunum past the ligament of Treitz. Feeds through the new gastrostomy in the infant with pure EA can be started in a few days, with small hourly amounts dripped slowly into the stomach rather than larger bolus feeds pushed in rapidly. This is to ensure a slow, progressive enlargement of the small stomach with less chance of perigastrostomy leakage into the peritoneal cavity or onto the abdominal wall. After a few weeks, the feeds can be safely increased in volume and spaced over 3 or 4 hours to stretch the stomach and to allow reflux into the lower esophageal segment. The gastrostomy tube must be open and upright after feeds so that gas can escape.

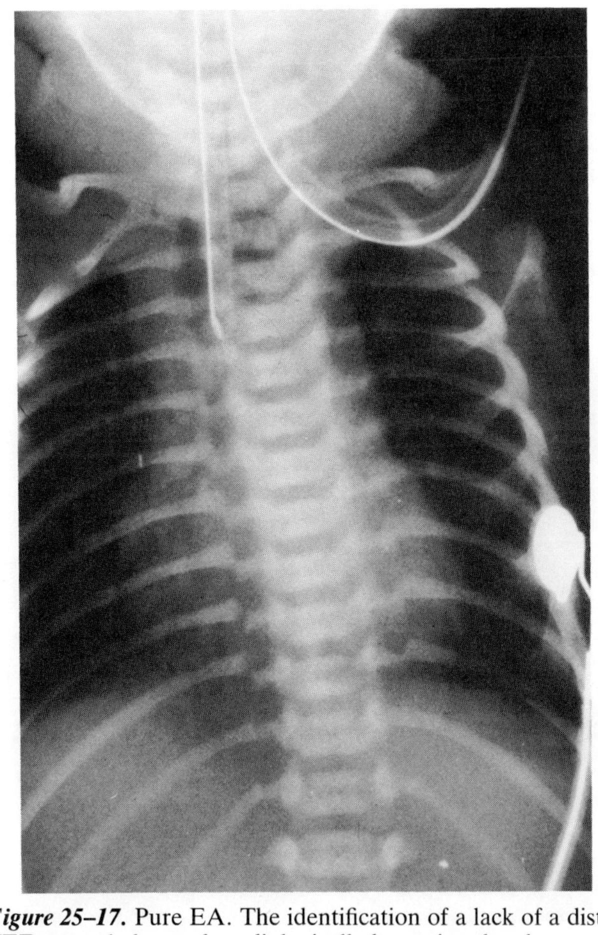

Figure 25–17. Pure EA. The identification of a lack of a distal TEF can only be made radiologically by noting the absence of gas within the gastrointestinal tract.

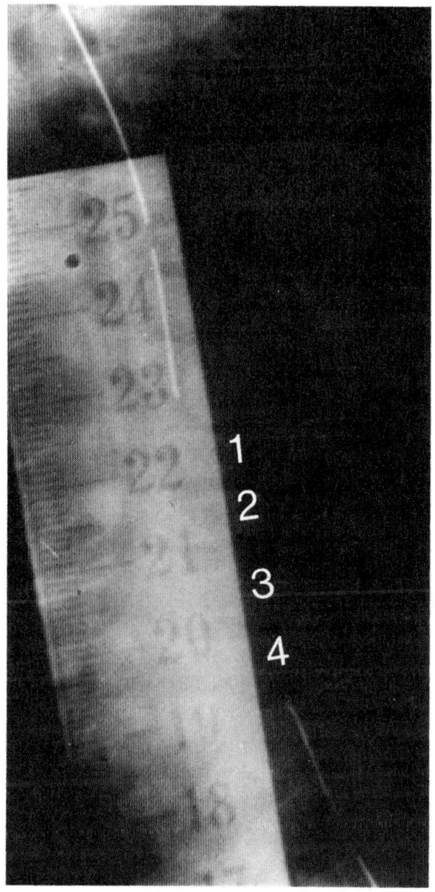

Figure 25–18. Gapogram without contrast material. Note that the two radiopaque tubes in each esophageal pouch are about 4 cm (vertebral bodies) apart.

The blind upper pouch must remain on constant suction. Ten to 20 ml of saliva (with its high salt content) is removed every 8 hours and should be returned to the infant in the form of normal saline and potassium to avoid salt depletion and hypokalemia; there is frequently one aspiration pneumonia per month, usually because the nasoesophageal suction tube plugs. At monthly intervals, the two esophageal pouches are assessed radiologically (by gapogram) to see how close they are (Fig. 25–18). If the gap is 3 cm or smaller (three

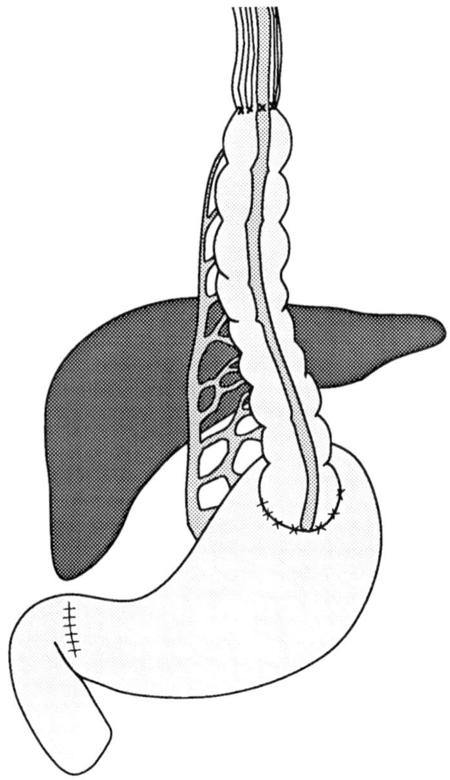

Figure 25–19. Colon replacement. It is usually accompanied by a pyloroplasty and also has three other anastomoses.

vertebral bodies), a primary repair is possible with the same technical aids used for bridging a wide gap for the infant with EA and distal TEF. The principle is the same as that with the common EA defect: the child's own esophagus (no matter what has to be safely done to bring it together) is infinitely better than any replacement that can be constructed

The immediate postoperative concerns for the infant with pure EA are related to the anastomosis (as with the EA and TEF group), except that there are no TEF problems; the anastomotic problems, however, are more significant because the tension, or pull, between the two esophageal pouches is greater in the pure EA group. After the repair has healed, there is the same constant radiologic dysfunction in the lower esophageal segment.[43, 71] If dysphagia develops after a few months, the same investigations must be undertaken to rule out virtually the same problems outlined for the EA with distal TEF group, except for a recurrent TEF. In spite of the unaffected trachea (no TEF), tracheomalacia may still occur. Gastroesophageal reflux is a significant problem in these infants with pure EA, possibly because of the greater pull upward on the lower esophageal pouch (including mobilization of the stomach[94]). It is estimated that as many as one third of these infants will require antireflux surgery within 3 months of their primary anastomosis, with a 30% recurrence rate.[76, 95]

Esophageal Replacement

If the gap between the two esophageal pouches is wider than 3 or 4 cm, the esophagus cannot be united for a primary anastomosis, and the infant will require an esophageal replacement.[95a] At a weight of 6 kg (15 lb), the time, age, and size are appropriate for the construction of a conduit to connect the two esophageal pouches. Options include colon[96] or gastric tube[97–99] replacement or the newly revived gastric transposition (pull-up).[94, 100, 101, 101a] The colon replacement is usually made isoperistaltic from any part of the colon (Fig. 25–19). It can be constructed with a primary anastomosis or staged, and it can be passed through the mediastinum, either via the pleural cavity or retrosternally. It is usually accompanied by a pyloroplasty and has three other anastomoses (esophagocolic, cologastric, and colocolic). The proximal (upper) anastomosis between the cervical esophagus and the upper end of the colon replacement does not create many problems. The major disadvantage of colon replacement is that it dilates and becomes tortuous with time (Fig. 25–20).

The gastric tube replacement can be made isoperistaltic or antiperistaltic (Fig. 25–21). It can be completed in one or two stages and can be passed through the mediastinum either via the pleural cavity or retrosternum. It does not need an accompanying pyloroplasty, and it has no other anastomoses past the stomach. The proximal (upper) anastomosis between the cervical esophagus and the upper part of the gastric tube is the source for most of the problems associated with the procedure, with 60% experiencing leakage, 40% stric-

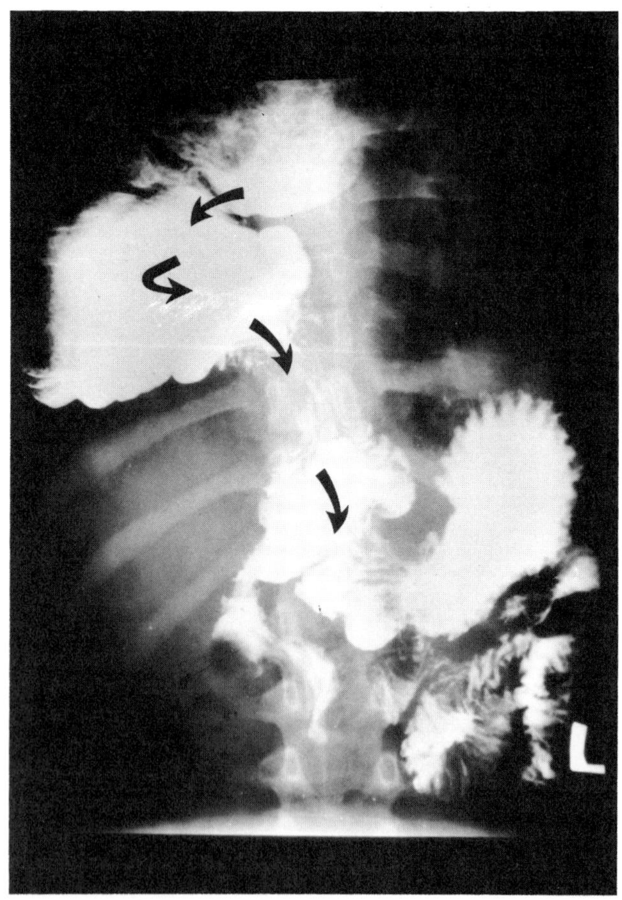

Figure 25–20. The major disadvantage of the colon replacement is that it dilates and becomes tortuous with time.

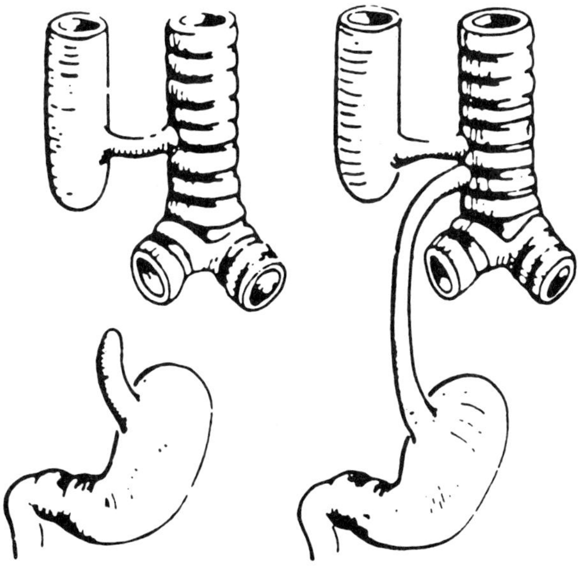

Figure 25–23. The major problem with the rare TEFs is that they are not recognized early. They may or may not be associated with an EA and may be single or multiple.

pleural cavity, or both. If technically feasible at the same time, the EA can be repaired, staged, or replaced at a later date (as described in the previous sections). The upper pouch TEF will always be encountered if the upper pouch is mobilized into the neck, whether the gap between the two esophageal segments is short or wide.[3] Once the TEF is recognized, division and closure are easily accomplised. The postoperative course, complications, and results are similar to the other types of EA and TEF.

Congenital esophagopulmonary fistulas are unusual in that many (24%) are not discovered until adult life,[109] when most of the patients have chronic irreversible pulmonary disease (Fig. 25–24). The same association with other congenital anomalies is seen as that in the more common EA with TEF group. The right bronchial tree is involved more than twice as often as the left (as in other types of bronchopulmonary anomalies). Patient age at diagnosis is older than that of TEFs, probably because the esophagopulmonary fistulas are smaller and more localized to smaller segments of the lung. The fistulous tract is lined by stratified squamous epithelium and becomes junctional with respiratory epithelium when it reaches the respiratory tract. Mucous glands, smooth muscle, and rudimentary tracheal rings all have been found in this fistulous tract. In 1954, the first esophagocystic pulmonary fistula was identified[109]; it is a rare variant of an esophagopulmonary fistula. In some instances numerous cysts are present throughout the lung, some of which are connected with bronchi; the cysts are lined by ciliated pseudostratified columnar epithelium. This entity is similar to the "ciliated epithelial cyst of the esophagus" that arises via a fistula from the lower esophagus also on the right side. In a few cases of aberrant lower lobes (extralobar and intralobar sequestration), there is a communication with the esophagus; occasionally, this communication is similar to a bronchus.[110] It has been proposed that "extralobar pulmonary sequestrations are derived from independent evaginations of cells with respiratory potential displaced on the esophagus."[111] Investigations must include radiology (the esophagram is positive in at least two thirds of cases)[112] and endoscopy. The surgical approach involves dividing the fistula and resecting the diseased lung; results are quite successful.

A *laryngotracheoesophageal cleft* is another rare variant of EA and TEF, except that the TEF runs more or less from the larynx all the way down to the carina.[113, 114] Three types are currently described: type 1, a laryngeal cleft; type 2, a partial cleft of the esophagus and the trachea; and type 3, a complete cleft from the larynx to the carina.[115] Richter first described this defect in 1792, but no further reports appeared in the literature until 1949.[3, 116] The first successful repair of a type 1 defect was in 1955.[115] The original foregut somehow fails to separate into two separate tubes by the fourth week, and it ends up as trachea in the anterior half and as esophagus in the posterior segment. It has been suggested that this cleft results from an arrest of the cephalad development of the tracheoesophageal septum.[117] Interruption of the septum formation extends the cleft upward into the larynx.[118] Twenty percent of infants with a laryngotracheoesophageal cleft also have an associated EA and TEF.[113]

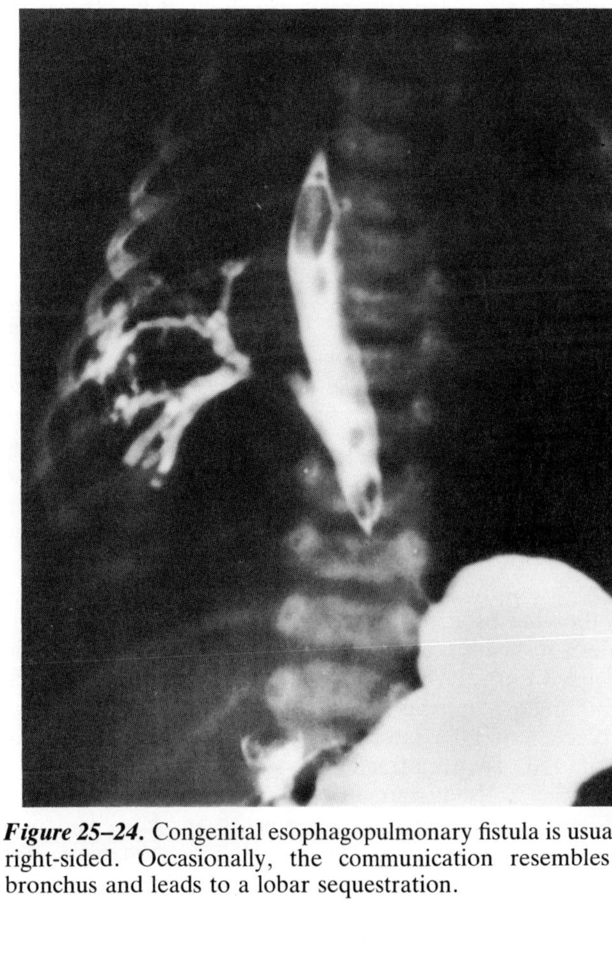

Figure 25–24. Congenital esophagopulmonary fistula is usually right-sided. Occasionally, the communication resembles a bronchus and leads to a lobar sequestration.

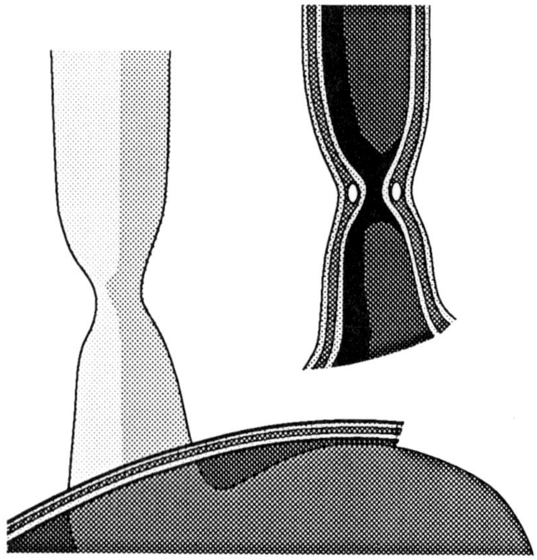

Figure 25–25. Most esophageal stenoses occur in the lower esophagus. Some stenoses may have an ectopic focus of respiratory tissue in the esophageal wall.

The clinical symptoms depend on the size of the cleft; they usually occur shortly after birth without feeds and include weak cry, coughing, choking, cyanosis, aspiration, pneumonia, apnea, and respiratory distress. Emergency intubation may be necessary.

Establishing the diagnosis is not always easy—the key is a high degree of suspicion. Swallow of water-soluble radiopaque contrast material shows an immediate massive aspiration from the pharyngoesophageal area into the trachea, so that the cleft cannot be seen easily.[119, 120] Even direct laryngoscopy and bronchoscopy may look normal until it is recognized that the bronchoscope or endotracheal tube can slip backward into the esophagus quite easily, creating an immediate moment of inadequate ventilation.[121]

Gastrostomy is necessary early in the treatment plan. Operative repair is not easy, nor is it often successful. If the cleft is laryngeal (type 1), repair is best approached from the neck (lateral or midline). The lower clefts (types 2 and 3) require either a right thoracotomy or both neck and chest incisions to approach the complete cleft. If the cleft is relatively short, a portion of the esophagus can be resected to repair the defect, and an end-to-end esophageal anastomosis made. For the complete cleft, the back of the trachea is closed using some of the posterior (esophageal) wall, hoping that there is enough esophagus remaining to make a significant-sized swallowing tube. If the esophageal remnant is not sufficient to fashion an adequate esophagus, then it should be used entirely for the trachea, a cervical esophagostomy made, and the infant committed to an esophageal replacement at a later date. All these infants end up intubated or with a tracheostomy, or both, usually for a long time. Recurrent TEFs are common; the repair effort is prolonged; and the results are fair. The first survivor of a complete laryngotracheoesophageal cleft (type 3) repair was reported only in 1984.[122]

Esophageal Stenosis and Web (Diaphragm)

Esophageal stenosis and web (diaphragm), variants of EA, are even rarer than those described in the previous section, occurring in 1:25,000 to 50,000 live births.[123] They were originally thought to be acquired inflammatory lesions due to gastroesophageal reflux[3] but have since been reclassified as true congenital lesions. There are different varieties of stenoses, including web (diaphragm) and fibromuscular stenosis.[123, 124] Tracheobronchial remnants in the wall of the esophagus were first reported in 1936.[125] After the tracheoesophageal septum forms, and both the esophagus and the tracheobronchial tree elongate, mesenchymal cells of the respiratory diverticulum become embedded in the esophageal wall in the form of respiratory epithelium, glands, and cartilage (Fig. 25–25). This ectopic focus can cause a stenosis that does not stretch. The development of an esophageal web (diaphragm) is similar to other gastrointestinal webs; it is a failure of the temporarily solid 10-week intestine to recanalize. The web may be associated with EA[125] or TEF,[126] or both (Fig. 25–26). Fibromuscular stenosis has been compared with pyloric stenosis in that the lower esophagus (with[127] or without[128–130] an accompanying EA, TEF, or both) has a localized segmental hypertrophy. Whether it is caused by a remnant of a perforated membrane (web) or a failure of the lumen to recanalize after being a temporary solid core is open to speculation. Microscopically, both the web and the segmental area have similar mucosal and submucosal components. Whereas the more common types of EA and TEF are associated with other anomalies in 50% of patients, this group has less than half of that association (imperforate anus or Down's syndrome).[124, 125]

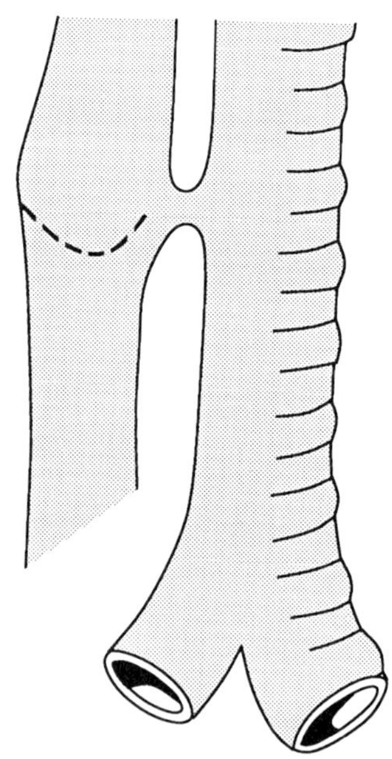

Figure 25–26. Most esophageal webs (diaphragms) are found in the mid-esophagus. They may or may not be associated with an EA or a TEF, or both.

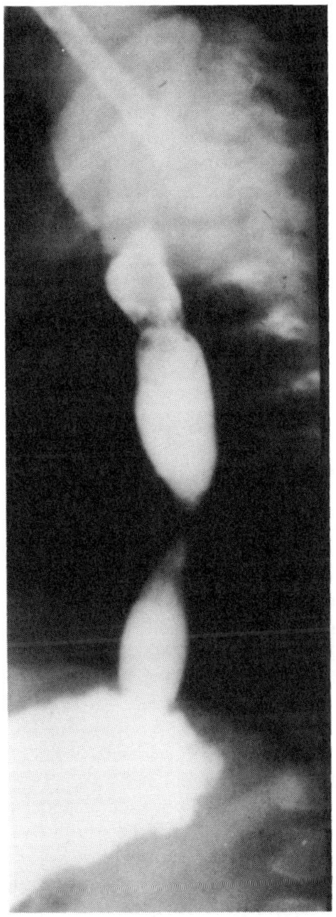

Figure 25–27. Lower esophageal congenital stenosis in an infant with a repaired EA and TEF. Gastroesophageal reflux has been ruled out.

The stenoses become apparent in infancy when the feeds are advanced to more solid components, and the resulting dysphagia leads to vomiting, failure to thrive, and aspiration. Esophageal webs (membranes) and their variations all present in neonates with symptoms and signs of EA.[125, 131, 132] All three of these pathologic entities require prompt radiologic or endoscopic evaluation, or both (Fig. 25–27). Gastroesophageal reflux for any reason (duodenal obstruction or malrotation) can be ruled out as a cause of this type of lesion by an upper gastrointestinal radiopaque contrast study. The exact location of the defect within the esophagus should be identified—most of the tracheobronchial remnant stenoses are in the distal part of the esophagus, whereas the webs (diaphragms) are in the middle. Endoscopy shows that the stenosis (due to tracheobronchial remnants) is more irregular and much firmer than the fibromuscular type[124]; the web (diaphragm) has a typical shelf-like appearance. Repair of the tracheobronchial remnant stenosis is best accomplished by thoracotomy and esophageal resection, since these stiff remnants make dilatation of the esophagus difficult and dangerous. The web (diaphragm) may be successfully treated by skilled endoscopy or by resection; the softer, more pliable fibromuscular stenosis can usually be successfully dilated. If esophageal resection is required for a low stenosis, and if it can be done through the abdomen, consideration should be given to an antireflux procedure to avoid iatrogenic gastroesophageal reflux.[124] The results of treatment are good.

REFERENCES

1. Myers NA: Oesophageal atresia: The epitome of modern surgery. Ann R Coll Surg Engl 1974; 54:277–287.
2. Potts WJ: The Surgeon and the Child. Philadelphia, WB Saunders, 1959, p 51.
3. Randolph JG: Esophageal atresia and congenital stenosis. *In* Welch KJ, Randolph JG, Ravitch MM, et al, eds: Pediatric Surgery. Chicago, Year Book Medical, 1986, pp 682–697.
4. Ashcraft KW, Holder TM: The story of esophageal atresia and tracheoesophageal fistula. Surgery 1969; 65:332–340.

4a. Myers NA: Evolution of the management of oesophageal atresia from 1948–1988. Pediatr Surg Int 1991; 6:407–411.

4b. Myers NA: The early history of esophageal atresia and tracheo-oesophageal fistula. *In* Beasley SW, Myers NA, Auldist AW, eds: Oesophageal Atresia. London, Chapman and Hall Medical, 1991, pp 1–16.

5. Vogt EC: Congenital esophageal atresia. Am J Roentgenol 1929; 22:463–465.
6. Gross RE: The Surgery of Infancy and Childhood. Philadelphia, WB Saunders, 1953, pp 75–102.
7. Haight C, Towsley HA: Congenital atresia of the esophagus with tracheoesophageal fistula: Extrapleural ligation of fistula and end-to-end anastomosis of esophageal segments. Surg Gynecol Obstet 1943; 76:672–688.
8. Lanman TH: Congenital atresia of the esophagus: A study of 32 cases. Arch Surg 1940; 41:1060–1083.
9. Leven NL: Congenital atresia of the esophagus with tracheoesophageal fistula: Report of successful extrapleural ligation of fistulous communication and cervical esophagostomy. J Thorac Surg 1941; 10:648–657.
10. Ladd WE: The surgical treatment of esophageal atresia and tracheoesophageal fistulas. N Engl J Med 1944; 230:625–637.
11. Haight C: Some observations on esophageal atresias and tracheoesophageal fistulas of congenital origin. J Thorac Surg 1959; 34:141–172.
12. Myers NA: Oesophageal atresia with distal tracheoesophageal fistulas: A long-term follow-up. Prog Pediatr Surg 1977; 10:5–18.
13. Sulamaa M, Gripenberg L, Alvenainen EK: Prognosis and treatment of congenital atresia of the esophagus. Acta Chir Scand 1951; 102:141–157.
14. Gray SW, Skandalakis JE: Embryology for Surgeons. Philadelphia, WB Saunders, 1972, pp 63–100.

14a. Beasley SW: Embryology. *In* Beasley SW, Myers NA, Auldist AW, eds: Oesophageal Atresia. London, Chapman and Hall Medical, 1991, pp 31–43.

15. Amoury RA: Structure and function of the esophagus in infancy and early childhood. *In* Ashcraft KW, Holder TM, eds: Pediatric Esophageal Surgery. Orlando, Grune & Stratton, 1986, pp 1–28.
16. Sankaran K, Bhagirath CP, Bingham WT, et al: Tracheal atresia, proximal esophageal atresia, and distal tracheoesophageal fistula: Report of two cases and review of the literature. Pediatrics 1983; 71:821–823.
17. Peison B, Levitsky E, Sprowls JJ: Tracheoesophageal fistula associated with tracheal atresia and malformation of the larynx. J Pediatr Surg 1970; 5:464–467.
18. Bond-Taylor W, Starer F, Atwell JD: Vertebral anomalies associated with esophageal atresia and tracheoesophageal fistula with reference to the initial operative mortality. J Pediatr Surg 1973; 8:9–13.
19. Dickens DRV, Myers NA: Oesophageal atresia and vertebral anomalies. Pediatr Surg Int 1987; 2:278–281.
20. Kluth D, Habenicht R: The embryology of usual and unusual types of esophageal atresia. Pediatr Surg Int 1987; 2:223–227.
21. Barnard C: The genesis of intestinal atresia. Surg Forum 1956; 7:393–396.

22. Smith EI: The early development of the trachea and the esophagus in relation to atresia of the esophagus and tracheoesophageal fistula. Contrib Embryol Carnegie Instit 1957; 36:41–57.
23. Scott JS, Wilson JK: Hydramnios as an early sign of esophageal atresia. Lancet 1957; 2:569–572.
23a. Myers NA, Beasley SW, Auldist AW: Oesophageal atresia and associated anomalies: A plea for uniform documentation. Pediatr Surg Int 1992; 2:97–100.
23b. Myers NA, Beasley SW, Auldist AW: Associated anomalies. *In* Beasley SW, Myers NA, Auldist AW, eds: Oesophageal Atresia. London, Chapman and Hall Medical, 1991, pp 211–228.
24. Ein SH, Shandling B, Wesson D, et al: Esophageal atresia with distal tracheoesophageal fistula: Associated anomalies and prognosis in the 1980's. J Pediatr Surg 1989; 24:1055–1059.
24a. Mee RBB, Beasley SW, Auldist AW, et al: Influence of congenital heart disease on management of oesophageal atresia. Pediatr Surg Int 1992; 2:90–93.
24b. Mee RBB: Congenital heart disease. *In* Beasley SW, Myers NA, Auldist AW, eds: Oesophageal Atresia. London, Chapman and Hall Medical, 1991, pp 229–239.
24c. Beasley SW, Phelan E, Kelly JH, et al: Urinary tract abnormalities in association with oesophageal atresia: Frequency, significance, and influence on management. Pediatr Surg Int 1992; 2:94–96.
24d. Phelan E, Kelly JH, Beasley SW: Urinary tract anomalies. *In* Beasley SW, Myers NA, Auldist AW, eds: Oesophageal Atresia. London, Chapman and Hall Medical, 1991, pp 241–248.
24e. Dickens DRV: Orthopaedic abnormalities. *In* Beasley SW, Myers NA, Auldist AW, eds: Oesophageal Atresia. London, Chapman and Hall Medical, 1991, pp 249–262.
25. Atwell JD, Beard RC: Congenital anomalies of the upper urinary tract associated with esophageal atresia and tracheoesophageal fistula. J Pediatr Surg 1974; 9:825–831.
25a. Campbell N: Case selection. *In* Beasley SW, Myers NA, Auldist AW, eds: Oesophageal Atresia. London, Chapman and Hall Medical, 1991, pp 287–301.
26. Quan L, Smith DW: The VATER association—vertebral defects, anal atresia, T-E fistula with esophageal atresia, radial and renal dysplasia: A spectrum of associated defects. J Pediatr 1973; 82:104–107.
27. Khoury MJ, Cordero JF, Greenberg F, et al: A population study of VACTERL association: Evidence for its etiologic heterogeneity. Pediatrics 1983; 71:815–820.
28. Temtanry SA, Miller JD: Extending the scope of the VATER association: Definition of the VATER syndrome. J Pediatr 1974; 85:345–349.
29. Valente A, Brereton RJ: Oesophageal atresia and the CHARGE association. Pediatr Surg Int 1987; 2:93–94.
29a. Kutiyanawala M, Wise RKH, Brereton L, et al: CHARGE and esophageal atresia. J Pediatr Surg 1992; 5:558–560.
30. Ein SH, Izukawa T, Su WJ, et al: The influence of cardiovascular malformations on the prognosis of esophageal atresia and distal tracheoesophageal fistula. Pediatr Surg Int 1989; 4:318–321.
30a. Bankier A, Brady J, Myers NA: Epidemiology and genetics. *In* Beasley SW, Myers NA, Auldist AW, eds: Oesophageal Atresia. London, Chapman and Hall Medical, 1991, pp 17–29.
31. Weber TR, Smith W, Grosfeld JL: Surgical experience in infants with the VATER association. J Pediatr Surg 1980; 15:849–854.
32. Holder TM, Ashcraft KW: Cardiac disease. *In* Welch KJ, Randolph JG, Ravitch MM, et al, eds: Pediatric Surgery. 4th ed. Chicago, Year Book, 1986, pp 1385–1389.
33. German JC, Mahour GH, Woolley MM: Esophageal atresia and associated anomalies. J Pediatr Surg 1976; 11:299–306.
34. Schimle RN, Leape LL, Holder TM: Familial occurrence of esophageal atresia: A preliminary report. *In* Birth Defects: Original Article Series. Vol 8. 1972, pp 22–23.
35. McIntosh D, Wright JE: Tracheo-oesophageal fistula in siblings. Pediatr Surg Int 1986; 1:246–248.
36. Cass D, Auldist A: Oesophageal atresia with proximal tracheo-esophageal fistula. Pediatr Surg Int 1987; 2:212–215.
37. Ashcraft KW, Holder TM: Esophageal atresia and tracheoesophageal malformations. *In* Holder TM, Ashcraft KW, eds: Pediatric Surgery. Philadelphia, WB Saunders, 1980, pp 266–283.
37a. Beasley SW: Anatomy. *In* Beasley SW, Myers NA, Auldist AW, eds: Oesophageal Atresia. London, Chapman and Hall Medical, 1991, pp 45–58.
38. Szold A, Udassin R, Seror D, et al: Acquired tracheoesophageal fistula in infancy and childhood. J Pediatr Surg 1991; 26:672–675.
39. Al-Arfah AL, Khwaja MS, El-Mouzan M: Acquired tracheo-esophageal fistula. Pediatr Surg Int 1991; 6:125–127.
40. Pohlson EC, Schaller RT, Tapper D: Improved survival with primary anastomosis in the low-birth-weight neonate with esophageal atresia and tracheoesophageal fistula. J Pediatr Surg 1988; 23:418–421.
41. Louhimo I, Lindahl H: Esophageal atresia: Primary results of 500 consecutively treated patients. J Pediatr Surg 1983; 18:217–229.
41a. Myers NA, Beasley SW: Diagnosis. *In* Beasley SW, Myers NA, Auldist AW, eds: Oesophageal Atresia. London, Chapman and Hall Medical, 1991, pp 77–92.
42. Van der Zee DC, Van der Staak FHT, Severijnen RSUM, et al: Proximal fistula in esophageal atresia: Pitfall in a routine procedure. Pediatr Surg Int 1988; 3:23–26.
43. Cumming WA: Esophageal atresia and tracheoesophageal fistula. Radiol Clin North Am 1975; 13:277–295.
44. Goh DW, Brereton RJ, Spitz L: Esophageal atresia with obstructed tracheoesophageal fistula and gasless abdomen. J Pediatr Surg 1991; 26:160–162.
45. Weigel W, Kaufman HJ: The frequency and types of other congenital anomalies in association with tracheoesophageal malformation. Clin Pediatr 1976; 15:819–834.
46. Stringel G, Coln D, Guertin L: Esophageal atresia and right aortic arch. Pediatr Surg Int 1990; 5:103–105.
47. Knight PJ, Clatworthy HW: Screening for latent malformations: Cost effectiveness in neonates with correctable anomalies. J Pediatr Surg 1982; 17:123–129.
48. Antimicrobial prophylaxis in surgery. Med Lett 1987; 29:91–94.
49. Bell MJ, Kosloske AM, Martin L, et al: Antimicrobial prophylaxis in pediatric surgical patients. Presented at the Meeting of the Surgical Section of the American Academy of Pediatrics, San Francisco, October 1983.
49a. Roy RND: Transport of the neonate with oesophageal atresia. *In* Beasley SW, Myers NA, Auldist AW, eds: Oesophageal Atresia. London, Chapman and Hall Medical, 1991, pp 93–102.
49b. Telfer HM, McDonnell GE: Nursing care. *In* Beasley SW, Myers NA, Auldist AW, eds: Oesophageal Atresia. London, Chapman and Hall Medical, 1991, pp 265–274.
50. Randolph JG, Tunell WP, Lilly J Jr: Gastric division in the critically ill infant with esophageal atresia and tracheoesophageal fistula. Surgery 1968; 63:496–502.
51. Kiely E, Satz L: Is routine gastrostomy necessary in the management of oesophageal atresia? Pediatr Surg Int 1987; 2:6–9.
52. Bishop PJ, Klein MD, Philippart AI, et al: Transpleural repair of esophageal atresia without a primary gastrostomy: 240 patients treated between 1951 and 1983. J Pediatr Surg 1985; 20:823–828.
52a. Beasley SW, Auldist AW: Oesophageal atresia with distal tracheo-oesophageal fistula. *In* Beasley SW, Myers NA, Auldist AW, eds: Oesophageal Atresia. London, Chapman and Hall Medical, 1991, pp 119–135.
53. Ein SH, Theman TE: A comparison of the results of primary repair of esophageal atresia with tracheoesophageal fistula using end-to-side and end-to-end anastomoses. J Pediatr Surg 1973; 8:641–645.
54. Poenaru D, Laberge J-M, Neilson IR, et al: A more than 25-year experience with end-to-end versus end-to-side repair for esophageal atresia. J Pediatr Surg 1991; 4:472–477.
55. Ty TC, Brunet C, Beardmore HE: A variation in the operative technique for the treatment of esophageal atresia and tracheo-esophageal fistula. J Pediatr Surg 1967; 2:118–125.
56. Touloukian RJ, Pickett LK, Spackman T: Repair of esophageal atresia by end-to-side anastomosis and ligation of the tracheo-esophageal fistula: A critical review of 18 cases. J Pediatr Surg 1974; 9:305–310.
57. Holder TM, Cloud DT, Lewis JE Jr, et al: Esophageal atresia and tracheoesophageal fistula: A survey of its members by the surgical section of the American Academy of Pediatrics. Pediatrics 1964; 34:542–549.
58. Waterston DJ, Bonham-Carter RE, Aberdeen E: Oesophageal atresia: Tracheo-oesophageal fistula. A study of survival in 218 infants. Lancet 1962; 1:819–822.

59. Abrahamson J, Shandling B: Esophageal atresia in the underweight baby: A challenge. J Pediatr Surg 1972; 7:608–613.
60. Koop CE, Hamilton JP: Atresia of the esophagus: Increased survival with staged procedures in the poor-risk infant. Ann Surg 1965; 162:389–401.
61. Livaditis A: Esophageal atresia: A method of overriding large segmental gaps. Z Kinderchir 1973; 13:298–306.
62. Howard R, Myers NA: Esophageal atresia: A technique for elongating the upper pouch. Surgery 1965; 58:725–727.
63. Hendren WH, Hale JR: Electromagnetic bougienage to lengthen esophageal segments in congenital esophageal atresia. N Engl J Med 1975; 293:428–432.
64. Rehbein F, Schweden N: Reconstruction of the esophagus without colon transplantation in cases of atresia. J Pediatr Surg 1971; 6:746–751.
65. Shafer AD, David TE: Suture fistula as a means of connecting upper and lower segments in esophageal atresia. J Pediatr Surg 1974; 9:669–673.
66. Davenport M, Bianchi A: Early experience with oesophageal flap oesophagoplasty for repair of oesophageal atresia. Pediatr Surg Int 1990; 5:332–335.
67. Davies MRQ, Beale PG: Protection of oesophageal anastomosis following uncomplicated repair of common-type oesophageal atresia by non-reversal of anaesthesia and graded withdrawal of respiratory support. Pediatr Surg Int 1991; 6:98–100.
67a. Auldist AW, Beasley SE: Oesophageal complications. *In* Beasley SW, Myers NA, Auldist AW, eds: Oesophageal Atresia. London, Chapman and Hall Medical, 1991, pp 305–329.
68. Chittmittrapap S, Spitz L, Kiely EM, et al: Anastomotic stricture following repair of esophageal atresia. J Pediatr Surg 1990; 25:508–511.
69. Pieretti R, Shandling B, Stephens CA: Resistant esophageal stenosis associated with reflux after repair of esophageal atresia: A therapeutic approach. J Pediatr Surg 1974; 9:355–357.
70. Gutierrez-Samroman C, Vila-Carbo J, Segarra-Llido V, et al: Long-term nutritional evaluation of 70 patients operated on for esophageal atresia. Pediatr Surg Int 1988; 3:123–127.
71. Desjardins JG, Stephens CA, Moes CAF: Results of surgical treatment of congenital tracheoesophageal fistula, with a note on cine-fluorographic findings. Ann Surg 1964; 160:141–145.
71a. Stokes KB: Pathophysiology. *In* Beasley SW, Myers NA, Auldist AW, eds: Oesophageal Atresia. London, Chapman and Hall Medical, 1991, pp 59–73.
72. Stringer DA, Ein SH: Recurrent tracheoesophageal fistula: A protocol for investigation. Radiology 1984; 151:637–641.
73. Glasson MJ, Bandrevics V, Cohen DH: Hypertrophic pyloric stenosis complicating esophageal atresia. Surgery 1973; 74:530–535.
74. Jolly SG, Johnson DG, Roberts CC, et al: Patterns of gastroesophageal reflux in children following repair of esophageal atresia and distal tracheoesophageal fistula. J Pediatr Surg 1980; 15:857–862.
75. Caniano D, Ginn-Pease E, King DR: The failed antireflux procedure: Analysis of risk factors and morbidity. J Pediatr Surg 1990; 25:1022–1026.
76. Ein SH: Pure esophageal atresia: A review of the 1980's. Unpublished data, 1991.
77. Lindahl H, Rintala R, Sariola H, et al: Cervical Barrett's esophagus: A common complication of gastric tube reconstruction. J Pediatr Surg 1990; 25:446–448.
78. Emery JL, Halladin J: Squamous epithelium in respiratory tract of children with tracheoesophageal fistula. Arch Dis Child 1971; 46:236–242.
78a. Spitz L, Phelan PD: Tracheomalacia. *In* Beasley SW, Myers NA, Auldist AW, eds: Oesophageal Atresia. London, Chapman and Hall Medical, 1991, pp 331–340.
79. Milligan DWA, Levison H: Lung function in children following repair of tracheoesophageal fistula. J Pediatr 1979; 95:24–27.
80. Dudley NE, Phelan PD: Respiratory complications in long-term survivors of esophageal atresia. Arch Dis Child 1976; 51:279–282.
81. Schwartz MZ, Filler RM: Tracheal compression as a cause of apnea following repair of tracheoesophageal fistula: Treatment by aortopexy. J Pediatr Surg 1980; 15:842–848.
82. Filler RM, Rossello PJ, Lebowitz RL: Life-threatening anoxic spells caused by tracheal compression after repair of esophageal atresia: Correction by surgery. J Pediatr Surg 1976; 11:738–748.
83. Fearon B, Shortreed R: Tracheobronchial compression by congenital cardiovascular anomalies in children: Syndrome of apnea. Ann Otolaryngol 1963; 72:949–969.
84. Ashcraft KW, Goodwin CD, Amoury RW, et al: Thal fundoplication: A simple and safe operative treatment for gastrointestinal reflux. J Pediatr Surg 1978; 13:643–647.
84a. Johnson DG, Beasley SW: Gastro-oesophageal reflux. *In* Beasley SW, Myers NA, Auldist AW, eds: Oesophageal Atresia. London, Chapman and Hall Medical, 1991, pp 341–358.
85. Mustard WT, Bayliss CD, Fearon B, et al: Tracheal compression by the innominate artery in children. Ann Thorac Surg 1969; 8:312–319.
86. Gross RE, Neuhauser EB: Compression of the trachea by an anomolous innominate artery: An operation for its relief. Am J Dis Child 1948; 75:570–574.
87. Freeman NV, Walkden J: Previously unreported shoulder deformity following right lateral thoracotomy for esophageal atresia. J Pediatr Surg 1969; 4:627–636.
88. Durning RP, Scoles PV, Fox OD: Scoliosis after thoractomy in tracheoesophageal fistula patients. J Bone Joint Surg 1980; 62:1156–1159.
89. Holder TM: Esophageal atresia and tracheoesophageal fistula. *In* Ashcraft KW, Holder TM, eds: Pediatric Esophageal Surgery. Philadelphia, Grune & Stratton, 1986, pp 29–52.
90. Randolph JG, Altman RP, Anderson KD: Selective surgical management based upon clinical status in infants with esophageal atresia. J Thorac Cardiovasc Surg 1977; 74:335–342.
91. Raffensperger JG: Discussion. *In* Randolph JG, Altman RP, Anderson KD: Selective surgical management based upon clinical status in infants with esophageal atresia. J Thorac Cardiovasc Surg 1977; 74:342.
92. Myers NA: Oesophageal atresia and/or tracheo-oesophageal fistula: A study of mortality. Prog Pediatr Surg 1979; 13:141–165.
92a. Beasley SW, Myers NA: Trends in mortality in oesophageal atresia. Pediatr Surg Int 1992; 2:86–89.
92b. Beasley SW, Myers NA: Trends in mortality. *In* Beasley SW, Myers NA, Auldist AW, eds: Oesophageal Atresia. London, Chapman and Hall Medical, 1991, pp 361–367.
92c. Beasley SW, Phelan PD, Chetcuti PAJ: Late results following repair of oesophageal atresia. *In* Beasley SW, Myers NA, Auldist AW, eds: Oesophageal Atresia. London, Chapman and Hall Medical, 1991, pp 369–394.
92d. Beasley SW: Oesophageal atresia without fistula. *In* Beasley SW, Myers NA, Auldist AW, eds: Oesophageal Atresia. London, Chapman and Hall Medical, 1991, pp 137–159.
93. Blair GK, Filler RM, Theodarescu D: Neonatal pharyngo-esophageal perforation mimicking esophageal atresia: Clues to diagnosis. J Pediatr Surg 1987; 22:770–774.
94. Myers NA, Beasley SW, Auldist AW, et al: Oesophageal atresia without fistula: anastomosis or replacement? Pediatr Surg Int 1987; 2:216–222.
95. Lindahl H, Rintala R, Louhimo I: Failure of Nissen fundoplication to control gastroesophageal reflux in esophageal atresia in patients. J Pediatr Surg 1989; 24:985–987.
95a. Myers NA, Beasley SW, Auldist AW: Oesophageal replacement. *In* Beasley SW, Myers NA, Auldist AW, eds: Oesophageal Atresia. London, Chapman and Hall Medical, 1991, pp 171–191.
96. German JC, Waterston DI: Colon interposition for the replacement of the esophagus in children. J Pediatr Surg 1976; 11:227–234.
97. Ein SH, Shandling B, Simpson JS, et al: A further look at the gastric tube as an esophageal replacement in infants and children. J Pediatr Surg 1973; 8:859–868.
98. Ein SH, Shandling B, Stephens CA: Twenty-one year experience with the pediatric gastric tube. J Pediatr Surg 1987; 22:77–81.
99. Anderson KD, Randolph JG: The gastric tube for esophageal replacement in children. J Thorac Cardiovasc Surg 1973; 6:333–342.
100. Spitz L: Gastric transposition via the mediastinal route for infants with long-gap esophageal atresia. J Pediatr Surg 1984; 19:149–154.
101. Spitz L: Gastric transposition for oesophageal substitution in children. Presented at the Meeting of the American Pediatric Surgical Association, Orlando, May 1991.

101a. Schärlz AF: Esophageal reconstruction in very long atresias by elongation of the lesser curvature. Pediatr Surg Int 1992; 2:101–105.
102. Lindahl H, Louhimo I, Virkola K: Colon interposition or gastric tube? Follow-up study of colon-esophagus and gastric tube–esophagus patients. J Pediatr Surg 1983; 18:58–63.
103. Myers NA, Egami K: Congenital tracheo-oeophageal fistula: "H" or "N" fistula. Pediatr Surg Int 1987; 2:198–211.
103a. Kent M, Myers NA, Beasley SW: Tracheo-oesophageal fistula: The "H" fistula. *In* Beasley SW, Myers NA, Auldist AW, eds: Oesophageal Atresia. London, Chapman and Hall Medical, 1991, pp 193–207.
104. Eckstein HB, Somasundaram K: Multiple tracheoesophageal fistulas without atresia: Report of a case. J Pediatr Surg 1966; 1:381–383.
105. Gans SL, Berci G: Inside tracheoesophageal fistula: New endoscopic approaches. J Pediatr Surg 1973; 8:205–211.
106. Ein SH, Stringer DA, Stephens CA, et al: Recurrent tracheoesophageal fistulas: Seventeen year review. J Pediatr Surg 1983; 18:436–441.
107. Hays DM, Woolley MW, Snyder WH Jr: Esophageal atresia and tracheoesophageal fistula: Management of the uncommon types. J Pediatr Surg 1966; 1:240–252.
108. Rodgers BM, Johnson AM, Minor GR, et al: Esophageal atresia with double fistula: The missed anomaly. Ann Thorac Surg 1984; 38:195–200.
108a. Auldist AW: Oesophageal atresia with proximal tracheo-oesophageal fistula. *In* Beasley SW, Myers, NA, Auldist AW, eds: Oesophageal Atresia. London, Chapman and Hall Medical, 1991, pp 161–170.
109. Blackburn WR, Amoury RA: Congenital esophago-pulmonary fistulas without esophageal atresia: An analysis of 260 fistulas in infants, children and adults. Rev Surg 1966; 23:153–175.
110. Hanna E: Broncho-esophageal fistula with total sequêstration of the right lung. Ann Surg 1963; 159:599–603.
111. Moscarella AA, Wyllie RH: Congenital communication between the esophagus and isolated ectopic pulmonary tissue. J Thorac Cardiovas Surg 1967; 55:672–676.
112. Paulin R, Longtin L: Congenital bronchoesophageal fistula in an adult. Can Med Assoc J 1970; 102:964–966.
113. Mahour GH, Cohen SR, Woolley MD: Laryngotracheo-esophageal cleft associated with esophageal atresia and multiple tracheoesophageal fistulas in a twin. J Thorac Cardiovasc Surg 1973; 65:223–226.
114. Zachary RB, Emery JL: Failure of separation of larynx and trachea from the esophagus: Persistent esophagotrachea. Surgery 1961; 49:525–529.
115. Petterson G: Laryngo-tracheo-esophageal cleft. Z Kinderchir 1969; 7:43–49.
116. Finlay HVL: Familial congenital stridor. Arch Dis Child 1949; 24:219–223.
117. Blumberg JB, Stevenson JK, Lemire RJ, et al: Laryngo-tracheoesophageal cleft, the embryologic complications: Review of the literature. Surgery 1965; 57:559–566.
118. Delahunty JE, Cherry J: Congenital laryngeal cleft. Ann Otolaryngol 1969; 78:96–106.
119. Frates RE: Roentgen signs in laryngotracheoesophageal cleft. Radiology 1967; 88:484–486.
120. Griscom NT: Persistent esophagotrachea: The most severe degree of laryngotracheoesophageal cleft. Am J Roentgenol 1966; 97:211–215.
121. Burroughs N, Leape LL: Laryngotracheoesophageal cleft: Report of a case successfully treated and review of the literature. Pediatrics 1974; 53:516–522.
122. Donahoe PK, Gee PE: Complete laryngotracheal cleft: Management and repair. J Pediatr Surg 1984; 19:143–147.
123. Wright VM: The esophagus: Congenital anomalies. *In* Walker WA, Durie PR, Hamilton JR, eds: Pediatric Gastrointestinal Disease. Philadelphia, Decker, 1991, p 369.
124. Nihoul-Fekete C, DeBacker A, Lortat-Jacob S, et al: Congenital esophageal stenosis: A review of 20 cases. Pediatr Surg Int 1987; 2:86–92.
125. Scherer LR, Grosfeld JL: Congenital esophageal stenosis, esophageal duplication, neurenteric cyst and esophageal diverticulum. *In* Ashcraft KW, Holder TM, eds: Pediatric Esophageal Surgery. Orlando, Grune & Stratton, 1986, pp 53–71.
126. Touloukian JR: Membranous esophageal obstruction simulating atresia with a double tracheoesophageal fistula in a neonate. J Thorac Cardiovas Surg 1972; 65:191–194.
127. Deiraniya AK: Congenital oesophageal stenosis due to tracheobronchial remnants. Thorax 1974; 29:720–725.
128. Paulino F, Roselli A, Aprigliano F: Congenital esophageal stricture due to tracheobronchial remnants. Surgery 1962; 53:547–550.
129. Ishida M, Tsuchida Y, Saito S, et al: Congenital esophageal stenosis due to tracheobronchial remnants. J Pediatr Surg 1969; 4:339–345.
130. Heyman MB, Berquist WE, Fonkalsrud EW, et al: Esophageal muscular ring and VACTERL association: A case report. Pediatrics 1981; 67:683–686.
131. Minnis JF Jr, Burko H, Brevetti G: Segmental duplication of the esophagus associated with esophageal atresia and tracheoesophageal fistula. Ann Surg 1961; 156:271–275.
132. Yahr WZ, Azzoni AA, Santulli TV: Congenital atresia of the esophagus with tracheoesophageal fistula: An unusual variant. Surgery 1962; 52:937–941.

Chapter 26

Gastroesophageal Reflux

SUSAN R. ORENSTEIN

Gastroesophageal reflux (GER) is one of the most common gastrointestinal problems in children. It produces a wide variety of symptoms and ranges in severity from physiologic regurgitation of infancy to a life-threatening disorder. This chapter reviews its pathophysiology, clinical manifestations, diagnostic evaluation, differential diagnosis, and therapy.

PATHOPHYSIOLOGY

The tonic pressure of the lower esophageal sphincter (LES) normally prevents the return of gastric material into the esophagus. However, swallowed material must move past the gastroesophageal junction into the stomach, and swallowed air or toxic materials occasionally must be eliminated retrogressively from the stomach. Thus, the LES is normally broached many times a day. It is remarkable that gastroesophageal competence is normally maintained so effectively, despite being overridden for such a diversity of reasons.

Reflux episodes do occur in normal children and adults. The episodes are brief, occurring about five times in the postprandial hour; their frequency decreases rapidly to a baseline near zero thereafter.[1]

Pathologic reflux, that which causes "reflux disease," occurs when reflux frequency is increased, when reflux clearance is decreased, when the refluxate is more noxious, when mucosal resistance is impaired, and perhaps when upper esophageal sphincter function or sleep-arousal control is disturbed; these aspects of pathophysiology are discussed later and outlined in Table 26–1. This discussion is based on pediatric studies when possible but often must rely on studies in adults and animals.

Increased Frequency of GER

Children with reflux disease manifest an increased frequency of reflux episodes compared with asymptomatic control subjects. This increased frequency of reflux is particularly notable during fasting periods, which may also correspond to periods of sleep.[2–4]

Lower Esophageal Sphincter: Hypotonia

Until recently, tonically low LES pressure—less than about 5 mm Hg[5]—was believed to be the main factor allowing increased frequency of reflux.[6–9] In adults, LES hypotonia has been found to be a more common mechanism for reflux episodes in patients with severe esophagitis, in whom it causes about 20% of episodes, than in those without esophagitis, in whom it causes about 1% of episodes.[10, 11] The question of whether the observed LES hypotonia might be an effect, rather than a cause, of the pathologic reflux was raised by animal studies that showed that LES hypotonia was induced by esophagitis and resolved when the esophagitis was treated.[12] However, studies using human subjects have not confirmed that healing of esophagitis reinstitutes LES tone.[13]

In contrast with the concept that LES hypotonia is the result of defective function of the sphincter itself is the concept that LES hypotonia is caused by abnormal control mechanisms.[13] Such abnormal controls have been postulated to lead to LES "pressure drifts" as part of the spectrum of LES hypotonia in patients with reflux disease.[11]

A controversial area is whether the LES tone increases in response to increased gastric pressure. Extrinsic abdominal compression increases LES pressure by being passively transmitted to the sphincter, which is intra-abdominal. Diaphragmatic contraction, such as during Valsalva maneuver or cough, will actively augment the LES tone (see later). Finally, it has been suggested that the LES tone itself increases reflexly in response to an increase in gastric pressure.[14] These three effects are aspects of normal LES function that might be disordered in children with reflux.

Lower Esophageal Sphincter: Transient Relaxations

Although absent LES pressure has been shown to be essential to the occurrence of a reflux episode,[15] at least half of the children with pathologic reflux have normal LES tone.[6–8, 16] Pediatric studies using the Dent sleeve[17] have demonstrated that a transient LES relaxation (TLESR), unassociated with swallowing, is a major

Table 26–1. PATHOPHYSIOLOGY OF REFLUX

Increased Frequency of Reflux Episodes
- LES hypotonia
- TLESRs
  - Increased in reflux disease?
    - Primarily—e.g., lack of supine suppression?
    - Secondarily—e.g., secondary to increased sleep arousals?
  - Result in reflux episodes more often in reflux disease?
    - Because of provocative positioning, delayed gastric emptying, etc.?
- Defective perisphincteric support
  - Non intra-abdominal LES (hiatal hernia)
  - Crural sphincteric dysfunction
  - Other—"mucosal rosette," cardioesophageal angle, phrenoesophageal ligament
- Increased gastric pressure
  - Decreased gastric compliance
  - Delayed gastric emptying
  - Externally applied increased abdominal pressure
- Increased gastric volume
  - Large meal
  - Gastric hypersecretion
  - Delayed gastric emptying

Decreased Esophageal Clearance of Refluxate
- Gravity effects—supine position
- Peristaltic dysfunction or infrequent swallowing
- Defective salivation

Increased Noxiousness of Refluxate
- Acid
- Pepsin
- Bile acids
- Trypsin

Defective Mucosal Resistance to Refluxate

Effects of Upper Esophageal Dysfunction

Effects of Sleep
- Gravity—noxious material at cardia and to pharynx; decreased clearance
- Decreased salivation and swallowing
- UES hypotonia

mechanism allowing a reflux episode to occur (Fig. 26–1).[18, 19] During a TLESR, the LES usually relaxes completely, to the level of gastric pressure, and remains atonic for 5 to 35 seconds.[13] Importantly, active inhibition of the crural diaphragm during a TLESR removes the diaphragm's contribution to gastroesophageal competence while the sphincter is relaxing.

TLESRs as Belches or Partial Swallows. TLESRs are probably a normal mechanism for venting air from the distended stomach via belching.[20–22] The aspects of gastric distention that lead to LES relaxation, in contrast with the aspects of gastric pressure that lead to LES contraction, are not known; perhaps stimulation of stretch receptors underlies the former response, and stimulation of pressure receptors underlies the latter.

An alternative view is that TLESRs that cause reflux are abortive swallows rather than dysfunctional belches. This view is supported by the finding of attenuated submental, pharyngeal, and esophageal motor activity at the onset of TLESRs.[11, 23, 24]

Rate of TLESRs. During wakefulness in normal, fasting, supine adults, TLESRs occur on average up to six times an hour[23, 25, 26]; during stable sleep, they occur rarely, if at all.[24] Studies differ on the issue of whether the TLESR rate increases postprandially in normal subjects.[23, 25, 26] One study of normal adults found that TSLERs did not increase after meals but that postprandial TLESRs were more likely to result in reflux.[23]

The postprandial TLESR rates of adults with pathologic reflux have been found to be the same as or greater than the rate in normal subjects.[24, 25] The authors who found similar postprandial TLESR rates in normal subjects compared with refluxers did, however, find that a greater proportion of TLESRs resulted in reflux in the reflux patients.[24]

Proportion of GER Episodes Associated with TLESRs. The percentage of reflux episodes that are associated with TLESRs is reported to be 94 to 100% in normal adults and 65 to 73% in adults with reflux disease.[10, 24] In one study of children with pathologic reflux, TLESRs caused only 34% of reflux episodes, with transient increases in abdominal pressure causing

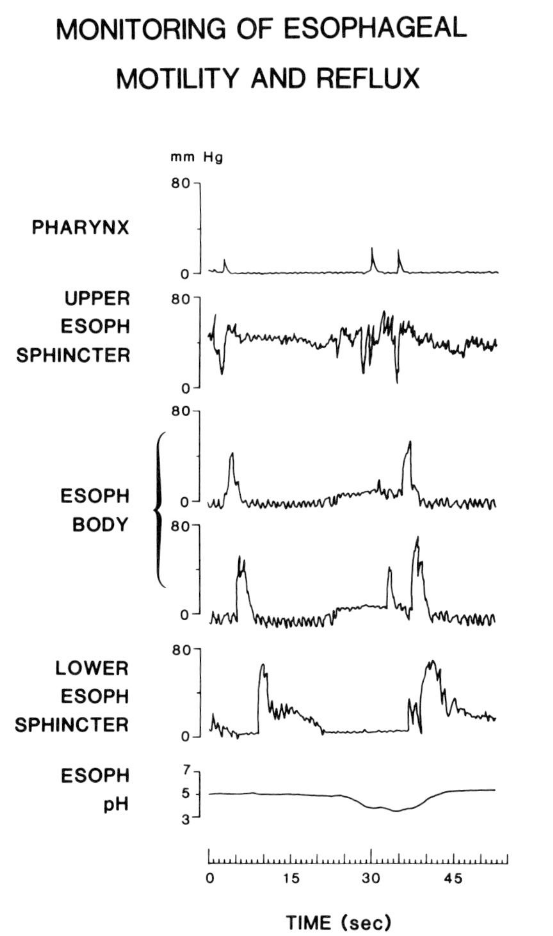

Figure 26–1. Transient lower esophageal sphincter relaxation (TLESR). A pH probe in the distal esophagus (bottom channel) records an episode of reflux due to a transient relaxation of the LES ("lower esoph sphincter" channel) unassociated with a swallow. The reflux causes a small pressure rise in the esophageal body, which is termed a *common cavity,* and is followed by two swallows that clear the refluxate. (From Orenstein SR: Gastroesophageal reflux. *In* Stockman JA II, Winter RJ, eds: Current Problems in Pediatrics. Chicago, Year Book Medical Publishers, May/June 1991, 21(5):195; with permission.)

most of the rest.[18] In another pediatric study, TLESRs caused 62% of reflux episodes in patients with esophagitis, LES hypotonia caused 14%, and increased gastric pressure caused 8%.[27]

Influences on TLESRs. LES relaxation is probably mediated by a vagal, noncholinergic, nonadrenergic neural inhibitory mechanism during TLESR and during swallowing.[28–30] In normal adults, TLESRs are suppressed in the supine position—a position more likely to result in reflux than in belching[23]—but it is unclear whether proprioception of gravitational postural effects or gastric cardia sensory distinction between gas and liquid is responsible for this difference.[13, 21, 31]

The role of TLESRs in reflux disease in children is just beginning to be explored. Important unanswered questions are: Do patients with reflux have more frequent TLESRs or merely TLESRs that are more frequently associated with reflux (because of frequent supine positioning or delayed gastric emptying, for example)? If they do have more frequent TLESRs, are they more frequent secondarily (due to a primary increase in sleep arousals,[32] for example) or because of a primary defect in their normal controls (such as lack of normal suppression in the supine position or when acid is at the cardia)?

Perisphincteric Factors

Periesophageal factors believed to contribute to gastroesophageal competence have included the intra-abdominal location of the LES, the sphincteric action of the diaphragmatic hiatus, the "mucosal rosette" at the gastroesophageal junction, the acute cardioesophageal angle of His, and the phrenoesophageal ligament.[13, 33, 34] The latter three contributions are probably minor.

The intra-abdominal location of the LES promotes sphincter competence by the passive transmission of intraperitoneal pressure elevations to the LES, thus countering the tendency of such pressure elevations to promote reflux.[34] Distortion of this normal relationship between the LES and the diaphragm, as in hiatal hernia, may thus predispose to reflux.[35]

Contraction of the crural diaphragm probably plays an active role in preventing reflux.[36–42] In contrast with the costal diaphragm, the crural diaphragm originates from the dorsal mesentery of the esophagus. Contraction of the crural diaphragm could prevent reflux from occurring during periods of increased intra-abdominal pressure caused by diaphragmatic contraction, such as straining, coughing, or deep inspiration. The fact that reflux episodes usually occur during expiration[42] supports this hypothesis, as does the fact that deep inspiration—a period of negative intraesophageal pressure and positive intragastric pressure—has been shown to provoke reflux episodes in patients with hiatal hernias[24] and in normal adults tested in an iron lung.[43] Hiatal herniation prevents the diaphragm's contraction from being applied to the esophagus, and the iron lung reveals the effects of inspiration without the protective effects of diaphragmatic contraction. The protective effects of crural contraction are also obliterated during a TLESR.[41]

Gastric Pressure

Transient increase in intra-abdominal pressure is an important mechanism for reflux episodes, accounting for as many as 54% of episodes in children.[10, 18] Since externally applied abdominal pressure may also be transmitted to the intra-abdominal LES, the expectation is that generalized increases in abdominal pressure would be less provocative for reflux than isolated increases in intragastric pressure of the same magnitude. Thus, gastric compliance and antegrade emptying would be important protections against retrograde movement of gastric contents. This area is controversial: Most investigators have noted both passive and active augmentation of LES pressure by increases in gastric pressure, but reduction of LES pressure has also been reported to follow isolated experimental elevation of intragastric pressure.[44]

Thus, although abdominal compression can increase reflux episodes, this effect may require the coincidence of a relaxed LES and a relaxed diaphragm[15] or other simultaneous impairments of the antireflux barrier.

Gastric Volume

Gastric volume is determined by the volume ingested, the volume secreted, and gastric emptying. Large meals and gastric hypersecretion have been implicated in some cases of GER disease. However, gastric emptying has received the most attention.

Similar to results in adult studies, delayed gastric emptying has been found in young children with reflux complicated by caloric insufficiency or by respiratory disease,[45, 46] but conflicting results are reported by others.[47, 48] In children younger than 3 years of age with uncomplicated reflux, normal gastric emptying has been described,[49, 50] but beyond that age, delayed emptying was found associated with low LES tone and esophagitis.[49] Gastric emptying is thus probably abnormal in at least a subset of refluxing children. Abnormalities of fundal or antral function have been proposed.[49, 51]

Extrinsic factors, such as the normal slowing of gastric emptying with increasing dietary osmolality and caloric density, are also important. In infants, late postprandial esophageal acid exposure was found to increase as the osmolality of a meal increased.[52]

There are three potential causal relationships between reflux and impaired gastric emptying: (1) more gastric material is available to reflux during TLESRs or episodes of increased abdominal pressure—i.e., delayed emptying causes increased reflux; (2) severe esophagitis may cause a vagal paresis leading to delayed emptying—i.e., increased reflux causes delayed emptying; or (3) both increased reflux and delayed gastric emptying are caused by a generalized foregut motor dysfunction.[34]

Decreased Esophageal Clearance of Refluxate

Patients with reflux disease often manifest prolonged reflux episodes, indicating dysfunction of esophageal clearance. Mechanisms that promote clearance, and thus reduce damage to the esophageal mucosa, are the bulk clearance of refluxate and the neutralization of the residual (Fig. 26–2).[53–55]

Gravitational Effects

Although gravity is the most obvious mechanism for esophageal clearance in the upright position, it probably plays only a minor role unless peristalsis is defective. Gravity allows a liquid bolus to precede the peristaltic wave in normal upright persons and contributes to bulk clearance in patients with severe esophageal dysmotility (e.g., achalasia) or following surgical esophageal replacement (e.g., with a gastric tube or colonic interposition). "Supine refluxers" are reported to have more severe esophagitis than "upright refluxers,"[56] but the esophagitis is more likely to be the result of peristaltic failure during sleep that accompanies recumbency than to gravitational effects of the recumbency itself.[57]

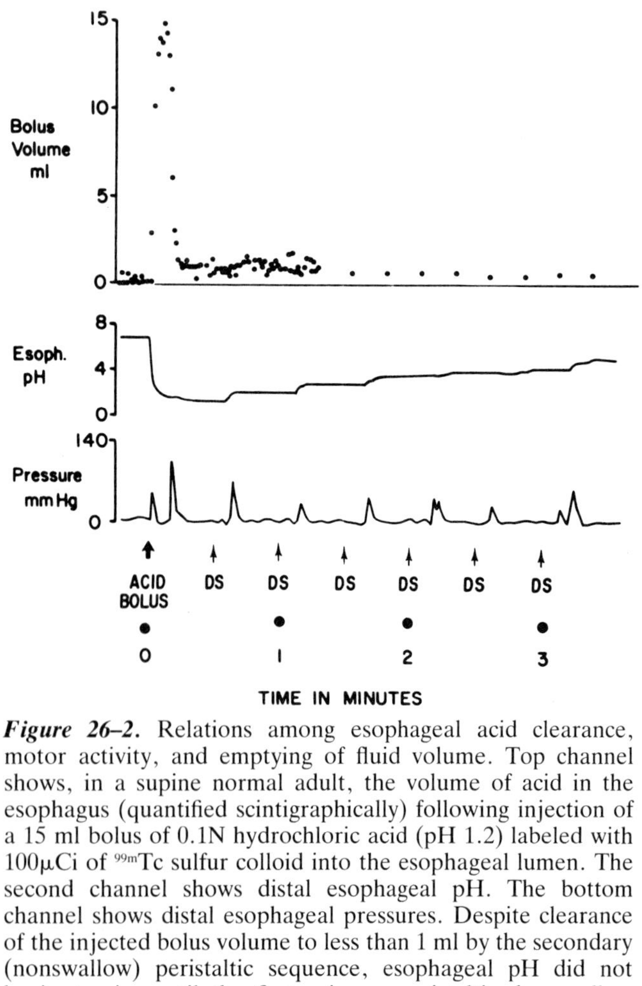

Figure 26–2. Relations among esophageal acid clearance, motor activity, and emptying of fluid volume. Top channel shows, in a supine normal adult, the volume of acid in the esophagus (quantified scintigraphically) following injection of a 15 ml bolus of 0.1N hydrochloric acid (pH 1.2) labeled with 100μCi of ^{99m}Tc sulfur colloid into the esophageal lumen. The second channel shows distal esophageal pH. The bottom channel shows distal esophageal pressures. Despite clearance of the injected bolus volume to less than 1 ml by the secondary (nonswallow) peristaltic sequence, esophageal pH did not begin to rise until the first primary peristaltic dry swallow (DS—without ingested material) wave. (Reprinted with permission from Helm JF, Dodds WJ, Pelc LR, et al. *The New England Journal of Medicine,* vol. 310, pp. 284–288, 1984.)

Peristalsis

Clearance of bolus of refluxate from the esophagus is chiefly by means of peristalsis, either primary—initiated by a swallow—or secondary—unassociated with a swallow (see Figs. 26–1 and 26–2).[54, 58] Esophageal acid or heartburn provokes primary peristalsis.[59, 60] Pressure or volume of a refluxed bolus in the esophagus provokes secondary peristalsis.[20, 61] Reflux in normal adults produces primary peristalsis more frequently than does secondary peristalsis.[58]

Normally, more than 90% of the refluxed volume is cleared by one or two normal peristaltic waves.[54] However, peristaltic abnormalities and delayed transit occur frequently in patients with esophagitis.[62, 63] These motor abnormalities have included simultaneous or repetitive contractions and failed or hypotensive peristalsis.[16, 62, 64, 65] The direction of causality between esophagitis and peristaltic dysfunction is uncertain, since normalization of peristalsis with treatment of the reflux has been inconsistent.[62, 63] Vicious cycles of esophagitis and peristaltic dysfunction may occur.

Saliva

After peristalsis has produced bulk clearance of refluxate, swallowing of saliva produces residual mechanical washdown of the lumen and neutralization of acid by salivary bicarbonate.[54, 56] "Water brash," the filling of the mouth with a large volume of salty fluid during episodes of reflux,[67, 68] is probably the symptomatic representation of the brisk salivary response to esophageal acidification.[69]

Increased Noxiousness of Refluxate

Acid

The degree of esophagitis correlates with acid exposure.[70, 71] Thus, gastric acid hypersecretion is associated with esophagitis,[72, 73] and prevention of acid secretion is associated with healing of esophagitis, even when reflux persists.[74] Acid secretion is low at birth but rises during the first month or two of life to a level comparable with that in adults.[75–78] Despite the ability of a meal to stimulate acid secretion, gastric pH remains high in infants for much of the day because of the buffering effect of frequent milk formula feedings.[79, 80] Whether esophagitis in infants depends more on other components of the refluxate is unknown.

Acid exposure inhibits Na^+, K^+, ATPase of epithelial cells, thus decreasing sodium exit and ultimately resulting in cell death.[81]

Pepsin

Although little is known about the role of pepsin in human esophagitis, one study found high esophageal pepsin concentrations in adults with strictures or Barrett's esophagus.[82] In infants, meal-stimulated pepsinogen secretion is much lower per kilogram than in adults,[78] reaching 50% of adult levels by 4 months of age and 100% by 2 years.[83] Furthermore, gastric pH may be too high in infants to support peptic activity.[79]

Pepsin may mediate epithelial cell shedding and induce worse injury than acid alone.[84, 85]

Bile Acids

For bile acids or trypsin to reach the esophagus during GER, duodenogastric reflux must occur first. Frequent duodenogastric reflux has been demonstrated in symptomatic adults.[86–88] Although human studies suggest that symptoms, but not esophagitis, may be worsened by duodenogastric reflux, an animal study demonstrated marked potentiation of acid injury to the esophagus when duodenogastric reflux was also present.[89] Bile acid concentrations in the duodenal lumen are low in the neonate, increasing gradually to adult levels during the first year of life.[90]

Bile acids' detergent property injures cell membranes and disrupts the mucosal barrier, thus facilitating acid injury to the esophagus, which is relatively impermeable to hydrogen ions.[84, 91, 92]

Trypsin

Trypsin is another possible duodenal contributor to reflux esophagitis.[93] Unlike the other injurious agents discussed and other pancreatic enzymes, trypsin secretion in newborns is comparable with that in older children and adults.[94]

In animals, trypsin potentiates bile acid–induced esophageal injury, producing more severe morphologic changes and hemorrhage than bile acids alone.[91, 95]

Mucosal Resistance to Refluxate

The role of mucosal resistance to injurious agents has been little explored in humans.[70] The mucous layer, the unstirred water layer, surface bicarbonate, and various aspects of the epithelium itself have been proposed as components of mucosal resistance to refluxate.[96] Interestingly, in contrast to its effect on gastric mucosa, indomethacin seems to augment esophageal cytoprotection.[85]

Upper Esophageal Sphincter Dysfunction

The upper esophageal sphincter (UES), largely consisting of the cricopharyngeal muscle, is the major barrier preventing material in the esophagus from being regurgitated or aspirated. It is thus a major defense against caloric loss and pulmonary complications. The UES has extremely variable tone, which rises with increasing states of arousal but is negligible during sleep.[97–99] Esophageal distention and acidification also increase UES pressure, particularly when they occur high in the esophagus.[100–103] The role of the UES in reflux has received attention only recently; it is likely that it will provide further insights in the future.

Arousal State: Sleep and Crying

There are a number of factors that make reflux during sleep particularly hazardous. Supine recumbency removes all the beneficial gravitational effects of the erect position. Noxious materials, rather than air, are positioned at the cardia and are available to move into the esophagus during TLESRs. A given volume of refluxate is also more likely to reach the pharynx in this position, and clearance of refluxate may be impaired, particularly in patients with infrequent swallowing or peristaltic dysfunction. Both salivation and swallowing frequency are markedly reduced during sleep, further impairing clearance.[57] UES atony also contributes to the hazard of reflux during sleep. Ameliorating these perils during sleep are the markedly reduced frequency of TLESRs and the resulting rarity of reflux episodes, at least in normal persons.

Crying has been suggested to provoke reflux episodes, presumably by a mechanism of augmented abdominal pressure[104]; however, preliminary study suggests that crying does not increase, and may even decrease, reflux.[105] Certainly the increased secretions swallowed during crying might improve acid clearance when reflux does occur in this state.

CLINICAL PRESENTATIONS

Infants Contrasted with Children and Adults

Older children and adults manifest GER disease similarly, but infants exhibit considerable differences from older patients. These differences include both the temporal course of reflux and its specific manifestations.

Whereas reflux disease in older children and adults tends to persist, in infants it tends to resolve during the first year or two of life.[106, 107] This is true for both the physiologic "spitting" of normal infants and pathologic infant reflux, which is responsible for considerable morbidity and occasional mortality while it persists.

Also in contrast with adults, symptoms of esophagitis are not the major manifestations of reflux in infants, although histologic esophagitis is common.[108–110] Prominent clinical manifestations in infants include malnutrition due to regurgitation, nonspecific irritability, and apnea. Rumination, stridor, lower respiratory disease, and neurobehavioral symptoms may also bring infants and young children to medical attention.

The fact that reflux differs in infants and adults suggests underlying developmental differences in the pathophysiology of reflux. These differences are only beginning to be explored.

Regurgitation

Regurgitant Versus Non-Regurgitant Reflux. Regurgitation is a far more frequent symptom in infants than it is in older children or adults. Regurgitant reflux received the earliest attention in children because it is evident without diagnostic testing. In studies of infants with reflux, less than 14% of scintigraphically detected reflux episodes and 17% of pH probe–detected reflux produced visible emesis.[111, 112] Another study of both children and infants demonstrated that fewer than 10% of scintigraphically detected episodes of reflux to the upper esophagus were regurgitated from the mouth.[113] It is unknown whether important differences underlie regurgitant and nonregurgitant reflux; abdominal muscle contraction may play a role in the former.[111]

Physiologic Infant Reflux. Inconsequential, physiologic "spitting up" occurs in normal infants, but do normal infants actually reflux more than do normal adults? Values for the frequency of reflux episodes derived from pH probe studies are similar in normal infants and adults when ordinary feedings are given (Fig. 26–3).[114, 115] However, meals increase reflux frequency and impair the ability of the pH probe to detect it, particularly in infants, because of the frequency and buffering capacity of their feedings and their lower acid secretion. More than three times as many episodes of reflux are detected in the two postprandial hours when acid feedings (apple juice, pH about 4) rather than cow's milk formula (pH about 6) are given.[116] Therefore, the normal reflux frequency range derived from studies using formula feedings may be disregarding 20 to 30 episodes per day. A rigorous definition of the normal frequency of reflux (during a normal diet but including nonacid reflux) is not yet available.

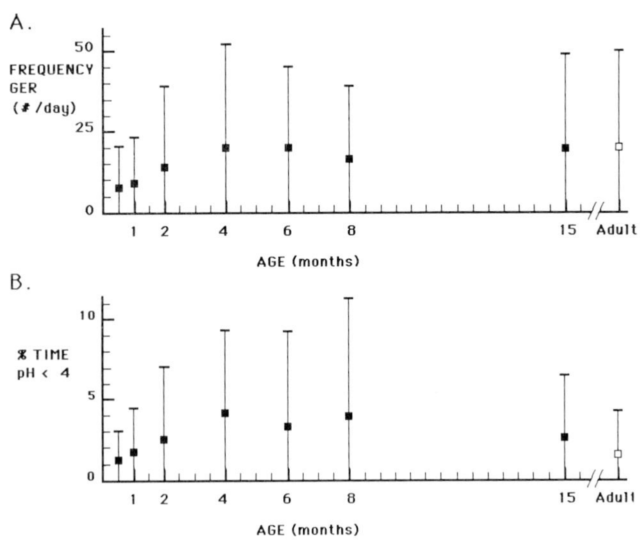

Figure 26–3. Physiologic reflux: Range of normal values during development. Graphic representation of normal ranges (mean ± 2 SD) for reflux in children of various ages (n = 285) and in adults (n = 15). *Top panel* depicts frequency of reflux episodes; *bottom panel* depicts total duration of esophageal acidification throughout the day, during normal activities and diet. (From Orenstein SR: Gastroesophageal reflux. *In* Stockman JA II, Winter RJ, eds: Current Problems in Pediatrics. Chicago, Year Book Medical Publishers, May/June 1991; 21(5):202; with permission.)

In contrast with the data for reflux frequency in infants, the data for total reflux time (a measure largely reflecting acid clearance) does show more reflux in infants than in adults (see Fig. 26–3). It is unknown whether normal infants have slower clearance because they have relatively impaired peristalsis or salivation or because they cannot voluntarily assume positions to profit from gravity.

Caloric Insufficiency. Regurgitation producing caloric insufficiency is an important manifestation of reflux in infants. A pathologic equivalent of physiologic spitting up, it can be severe enough to cause death if untreated. Regurgitant reflux in infants may consist of a small amount of material effortlessly drooling from the mouth or may be projectile and voluminous.

Poor intake, as well as regurgitation, may contribute to failure to thrive. Factors contributing to poor intake may include discomfort due to esophagitis or parents' hesitation to feed an infant whose response is regurgitation and irritability.[117]

Esophagitis

Esophagitis, identified histologically, occurs in 61 to 83% of infants with clinically important reflux.[108–110] Factors that increase the exposure of the esophagus to noxious material, particularly acid, make esophagitis more likely. Although esophagitis may present with symptoms suggesting pain, it can also be asymptomatic.

Chest Pain and Heartburn. Typical substernal burning, the "heartburn" (pyrosis) described by adults, also occurs in children suffering from esophagitis. Its burning quality, diffuse substernal location, exacerbation by citrus juices, and relief by liquid antacids are typical. Careful history taking may be needed to isolate such substernal discomfort from the epigastric pain that is more likely to represent gastric peptic disease and from vaguer "dyspeptic" symptoms recently associated with duodenogastric reflux in adults.[86] Odynophagia, pain on swallowing, usually represents esophageal inflammation; a subgroup of people with odynophagia will have reflux-mediated esophagitis.

In nonverbal infants, crying, irritability, sleep disturbance, "colic," and even rumination suggest esophagitis.[117] Infants may also display feeding difficulties, appearing avidly hungry for the bottle until their first swallows, then becoming irritable and refusing to take it.

Dysphagia. Dysphagia, the sensation of food "sticking" or "not going down right," is an important symptom of reflux.[118] Dysphagia has been linked to esophagitis,[119] to peristaltic dysfunction accompanying reflux disease,[62] and to peptic stricture. The response of dysphagia to therapy for reflux esophagitis has been variable[120, 121] (see Chapter 10).

Asymptomatic Esophagitis. In some ways, patients

whose esophagitis is asymptomatic are more problematic. Even severe esophagitis may remain asymptomatic, as demonstrated by children who present with peptic strictures without having experienced any discomfort attributable to esophagitis. The completely asymptomatic person will evade diagnosis, but there should be a high index of suspicion of esophagitis in patients with any symptoms suggesting reflux disease.

Complications of Reflux Esophagitis

Barrett's Esophagus. Barrett's columnar epithelium in the esophagus represents metaplastic changes in the squamous epithelium that is normally present.[122, 124] Its prevalence is 2 to 20% in adults with peptic esophagitis and as high as 44% in those with a stricture.[125–127] More than 170 cases have been reported in children.[128] Barrett's esophagus was found in 13% of children undergoing endoscopy for esophagitis symptoms,[129] and a male preponderance has been suggested.[130, 131]

Predisposing associations are gastric tube replacements of the esophagus,[132] probably because of the acid and pepsin exposure of the cervical esophageal remnant; antileukemic chemotherapy,[133] perhaps the result of nonspecific epithelial injury; and total gastrectomy,[134] possibly caused by the reflux of bile or trypsin. *Helicobacter pylori* has been described on the metaplastic gastric epithelium.[135–137]

Barrett's esophagus does not produce unique symptoms. It is diagnosed when endoscopic biopsy for symptoms of esophagitis or stricture reveals the columnar epithelium, suggested endoscopically by an unusually red color in areas of the esophageal mucosa. Radiography is inadequate to separate Barrett's esophagus from severe esophagitis, although deep esophageal ulcers and midesophageal strictures are radiographic signs often associated with Barrett's esophagus.[138–140]

Complications of Barrett's esophagus are esophageal ulcers, strictures, and adenocarcinoma. Barrett's ulcers are often deep, sometimes even leading to esophagotracheal fistulization, but they heal completely with aggressive antireflux therapy.[141–144] Two recent descriptions of a total of 24 cases of pediatric Barrett's esophagus documented esophageal strictures in more than 50% of them.[129, 131]

The most important complication of Barrett's esophagus is adenocarcinoma, which has an especially grim prognosis in the esophagus. Adenocarcinoma has a prevalence of 7 to 22% at diagnosis of Barrett's esophagus; its incidence has been estimated as one cancer in 52 to 441 patient-years of follow-up, 30 to 125 times higher than the rate in the general population.[145–148] These numbers are particularly ominous when pediatric patients are considered, because of the many anticipated years of increased susceptibility. Esophageal adenocarcinoma has been described in children with Barrett's esophagus.[149] Adenocarcinoma is particularly likely to arise in smokers, in patients with intestinal type metaplasia, and in patients with dysplasia.

Response of Barrett's esophagus to rigorous antireflux therapy is controversial. Regression of the abnormal epithelium and a return to normal squamous epithelium have been difficult to demonstrate with certainty.[130, 150–152] Adenocarcinoma has developed in Barrett's epithelium 8 years after competent fundoplication.[153] Nonetheless, vigorous antireflux therapy using fundoplication is recommended in the hope of arresting the transformation through dysplasia to adenocarcinoma. Yearly endoscopic and histologic surveillance of patients with Barrett's esophagus has been recommended to try to diagnose dysplasia before it progresses to adenocarcinoma.

Peptic Stricture. Another severe complication of reflux esophagitis is a peptic (reflux-associated) stricture (Fig. 26–4). The esophagitis that precedes such strictures may be asymptomatic. In a French series of 59 cases, 50% of the children were younger than 2 years of age, 25% were between 2 and 5, and the remainder were between 5 and 15.[154]

The primary symptom of a stricture is dysphagia. Regurgitation of undigested liquids and drooling of saliva suggest severe narrowing. Young infants taking a liquid diet may not be symptomatic until solids are added and the esophagus is obstructed above the stricture by a poorly chewed solid bolus. (Thus, a patient who suffers from an esophageal food impaction should

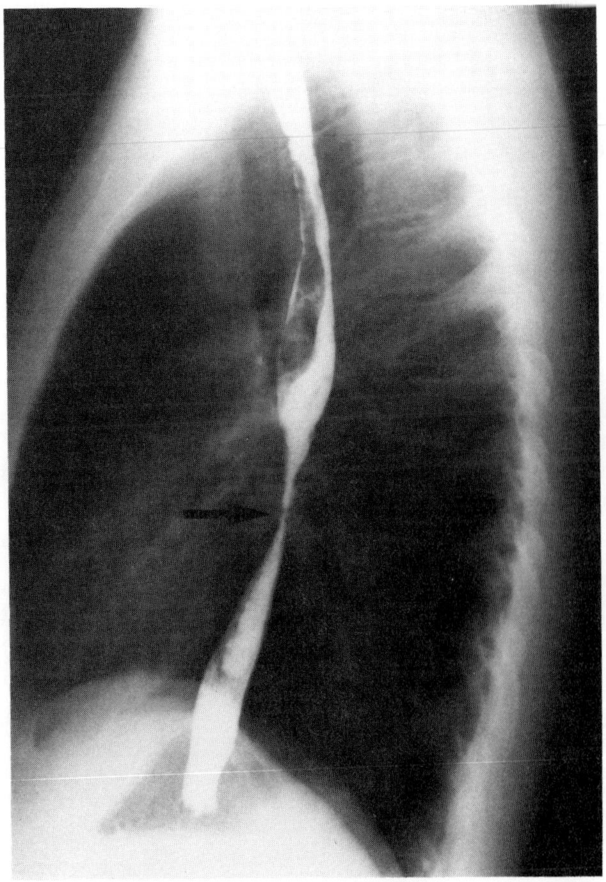

Figure 26–4. Barium esophagram demonstrating an esophageal stricture due to reflux (*arrow*). This 15-year-old boy is the same patient whose Barrett's-associated stricture is depicted endoscopically in Figure 10–10 of Chapter 10.

always be carefully studied for such a stricture.) More general signs that may be associated with a stricture are malnutrition, hematemesis, severe iron-deficiency anemia, and chest pain. The last three signs result from the underlying esophagitis.

Diagnosis of stricture is clearest radiographically. Pressure injection of barium may delineate the narrowed area better than simple swallowing, particularly in young infants who resist swallowing because of the dysphagia. Peptic strictures are usually about one third of the esophageal length above the diaphragm, between T6 and T10.

It is best to follow radiography with endoscopy for two purposes: diagnosis of the type of stenosis and treatment by balloon dilation. If the stricture is wide enough for the endoscope to be passed through it, biopsies should be taken just below it to confirm esophagitis and to evaluate for Barrett's epithelium. (If the stricture is initially too narrow, such biopsies can be done following dilation.) Most stenotic lesions in the esophagus are reflux related, but if esophagitis is absent, other stenotic lesions must be considered.

Treatment of peptic strictures has two goals: dilating the stricture and arresting the reflux. Dilation with the newer endoscopic balloon dilators has several advantages over bougienage with mercury-weighted rubber dilators.[155, 156] Balloon dilators are used during endoscopic visualization, and the radial forces they transmit to the stricture are probably safer than the shearing forces transmitted by the bougies. A single dilation is usually inadequate for permanent resolution of the stricture, and repeat dilations at intervals are usually required, particularly prior to elimination of reflux.[157, 158] Although esophageal dilations have most often been performed under general anesthesia in children, sedation is usually adequate for endoscopic dilations, and many children tolerate a program of recurrent bougienage while awake.[159] Esophageal dilation is not without risk: Perforation is the most common complication, and hemorrhage may also occur. Central nervous system infection (e.g., brain abscess) has also been reported, although none has followed dilation of a peptic stricture.[160]

The most definitive elimination of the reflux is by fundoplication, usually performed following one or several dilations. In the absence of fundoplication, nearly half of patients with chronic peptic strictures develop Barrett's esophagus.[127, 161]

Table 26–2. PREVENTION OF RESPIRATORY SEQUELAE DURING SWALLOW

Structures	Protective Functions
Mouth	Palate rise
Pharynx	Epiglottic tilt
Larynx	Cord closure
Esophagus	
Upper esophageal sphincter	Complete relaxation, coordinated with pharynx
Esophageal body	Primary peristalsis
Lower esophageal sphincter	Early, complete, prolonged relaxation

From Putnam PE, Ricker DH, Orenstein SR: Gastroesophageal reflux. *In* Beckerman R, Brouilette R, Hunt C, eds: Respiratory Control Disorders in Infants and Children. Baltimore, Williams & Wilkins, 1991, p 323; © 1991, the Williams & Wilkins Company; with permission.)

Respiratory Symptoms

When techniques to document nonregurgitant reflux were applied more widely to infants, it became evident that respiratory sequelae were among the most important and most complex manifestations of reflux in children.[162] Although aspiration causes some of these manifestations, particularly aspiration pneumonitis, it has become clear that reflex respiratory responses to refluxate that may remain intraesophageal are actually more common mechanisms. Both lower and upper respiratory tract symptoms may be caused by reflux.

Physiologic Protections

The routes of food and air intersect in the pharynx, mandating exquisite controls to prevent aspiration. Coordination of respiration with swallowing or with reflux is governed by brain stem nuclei, particularly in the area of the solitary tract nucleus. Protections against aspiration during swallowing and during reflux are listed in Tables 26–2 and 26–3.[163–166] Aspiration during swallowing must be distinguished from aspiration during reflux, since the management differs significantly.

Table 26–3. PREVENTION OF RESPIRATORY SEQUELAE DUE TO REFLUX

Structures	Protective Functions	Dysfunctions
Stomach	Antegrade emptying	Delayed gastric emptying
Esophagus		
Associated structures	Diaphragmatic hiatal tone	Hiatal hernia
LES	LES tone	Hypotensive LES
	Distinction of gas vs. liquid	Transient LES relaxations to liquid
Body	Secondary peristalsis	Impaired esophageal clearance
UES	UES tone	Hypotensive UES
Larynx, pharynx, mouth	Distinction of gas vs. liquid	Transient UES relaxations to liquid
	Swallow reflex	Impaired swallow reflex
	Cord closure	Impaired cord closure
	Arytenoid-epiglottic approximation	Impaired arytenoid-epiglottic approximation

From Putnam PE, Ricker DH, Orenstein SR: Gastroesophageal reflux. *In* Beckerman R, Brouillette R, Hunt C, eds: Respiratory Control Disorders in Infants and Children. Baltimore, Williams & Wilkins, 1991, p 323; © 1991, the Williams & Wilkins Company; with permission.)

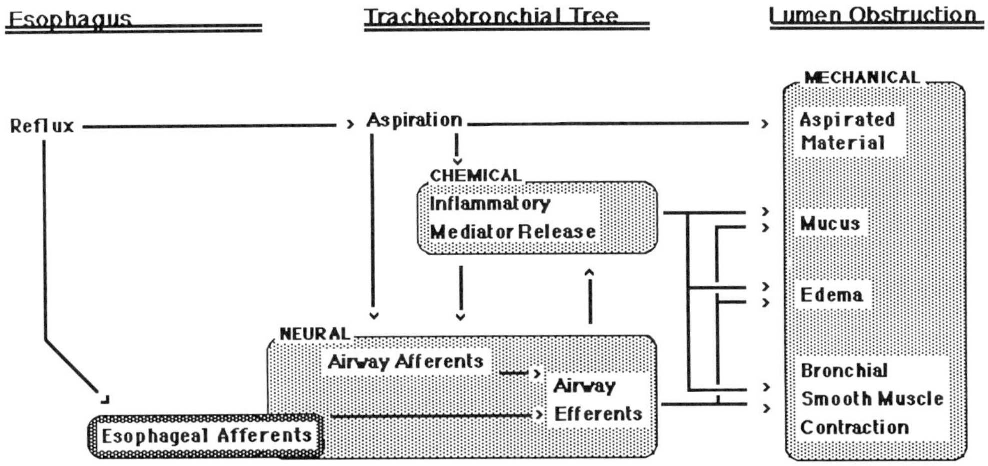

Figure 26–5. Mechanisms for reflux-associated respiratory dysfunction. Reflux may produce respiratory disease directly, by mechanical occlusion of the lumen with aspirated material, or indirectly. Reflux narrows the airway indirectly via neural or chemical induction of mucus secretion, edema, or muscle contraction. The neural mechanism can have local (airway) or distal (esophageal) afferents. (From Putnam PE, Ricker DH, Orenstein SR: Gastroesophageal reflux. *In* Beckerman R, Brouilette R, Hunt C, eds: Respiratory Control Disorders in Infants and Children. Baltimore, Williams & Wilkins, 1991, p 324. © 1991, The William & Wilkins Company; with permission.)

Pathologic Mechanisms: Reflux Causing Respiratory Disease

When physiologic protection fails (see Table 26–3), reflux causes respiratory disease. The mechanisms by which this occurs are diagramed in Figure 26–5.[165] When any of the three mechanisms (mechanical, neural, or chemical) involve the lower airway, bronchial obstruction results; when they involve the upper airway, laryngeal obstruction results. Bronchial obstruction—manifest as wheezing, for example—may have as its immediate cause aspirated material, locally produced secretions, mucosal edema, or smooth muscle contraction (Fig. 26–6).[167] The latter three immediate causes may be the end result of either airway stimulation by aspirated material or esophageal stimulation by refluxed material.

Aspiration. Aspiration of a large quantity of gastric material (macroaspiration) may lead to mechanical luminal obstruction and chemical pneumonitis.[9, 168–171] Macroaspiration of acidic material (pH <2.5) causes reflex airway closure, surfactant loss, epithelial damage, and pulmonary edema and hemorrhage, all resulting in severe hypoxemia.[172] Reflux rarely results in such severe aspiration, except perhaps in patients with depressed consciousness.

Aspiration insufficient to cause radiographic changes (microaspiration) may nevertheless stimulate upper airway neural elements or the release of inflammatory mediators, resulting in bronchospasm or laryngospasm.[165, 173–177] The role of microaspiration in reflux-associated respiratory disease is incompletely defined.

Reflex Response Without Aspiration (Neural Mediators from Esophagus). In contrast with the local reflexes described earlier, bronchoconstrictive reflexes with afferents in the esophagus have been demonstrated in animals[177] and in humans[178–184] and are blocked by vagal blockade or atropine.[183, 185, 186] Asthmatic children have shown evidence of bronchoconstriction during acid infusion into the esophagus but not during infusion of saline solution or antacid.[178]

It has been suggested that esophagitis uncovers vagal afferent receptors and is a prerequisite for this reflex bronchoconstriction. Adult asthmatic patients who complained of pyrosis during esophageal acid infusion (suggesting esophagitis) had a concomitant increase in respiratory system resistance, in contrast with nonasthmatic patients and to asthmatic patients who did not develop pyrosis.[179] However, no difference in lung resistance occurred after esophageal acid infusion in cats with or without esophagitis.[177] Both esophagitis and labile bronchial musculature may be necessary.

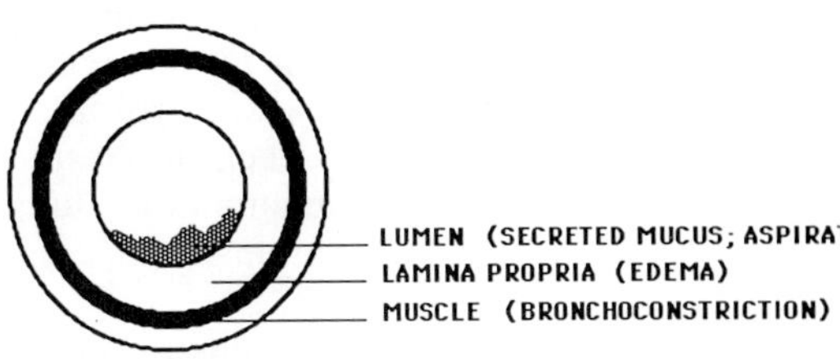

Figure 26–6. Four potential components of bronchial obstruction. Concentric loci of airway obstruction are the lumen, which can be narrowed by material from extrapulmonary or intrapulmonary sources; the lamina propria, which can be expanded at the expense of the lumen by edema; and the bronchial musculature, which can narrow the lumen by contracting. (From Putnam PE, Ricker DH, Orenstein SR: Gastroesophageal reflux. *In* Beckerman R, Brouilette R, Hunt C; eds: Respiratory Control Disorders in Infants and Children. Baltimore, Williams & Wilkins, 1991, p 325. © 1991, the Williams & Wilkins Company; with permission.)

Pathologic Mechanisms: Respiratory Disease Causing Reflux

Just as reflux can cause a multitude of respiratory symptoms, the converse is also true; vicious cycles aggravating the initial condition may ensue. Respiratory disorders or symptoms can provoke reflux if they alter any aspects of the "antireflux barrier." Thus, any respiratory functions that increase positive abdominal pressure, increase negative intrathoracic pressure, decrease the LES pressure, increase gastric acid production, or counteract gravity's pull of gastric contents caudad may worsen reflux (Table 26–4).

Thoracoabdominal Pressure Relationships. Positive abdominal pressure is increased by the forced expiration of coughing and wheezing, so that disorders with these symptoms, such as cystic fibrosis,[187–189] bronchopulmonary dysplasia,[190] asthma, and respiratory infections, may increase the frequency of reflux, particularly if the LES is hypotensive or herniated above the diaphragmatic hiatus. Negative intrathoracic pressure is increased by the forced inspiration of stridor and hiccups, so stridor and hiccups, both possibly caused by reflux, may in turn exacerbate reflux.

Lower Esophageal Sphincter Incompetence. Sudden, deep inspiration produces transient LES relaxation by a vagal reflex in cats.[191] Deep inspiration in humans would probably produce sphincter incompetence only when the contribution of diaphragmatic contraction is blocked, such as during mechanical ventilation or in the presence of hiatal hernia.

Table 26–4. REFLUX AND RESPIRATORY DISEASE: INTERACTIONS

Reflux Causing Respiratory Disorders
With aspiration (mechanical obstruction; local neural and chemical mediators)
Macroaspiration (aspiration pneumonia)
Microaspiration (chronic nonspecific lower respiratory disease? apnea?)
Without aspiration (neural mediation from esophageal afferents)
Reflex bronchospasm
Reflex laryngospasm (obstructive apnea; stridor)
Reflex central responses (central apnea; bradycardia)
Respiratory Disorders (activities/therapies) Causing Reflux
Thoracoabdominal pressure relationships
Forced expiration (cough, wheeze)
Forced inspiration (stridor, hiccups)
Lower esophageal sphincter incompetence
Reflexive
Smoking
Drugs
Nasogastric tube
Volume and noxiousness of gastric contents—due to drugs
Gravity—during chest physiotherapy, mechanical ventilation

Basic Respiratory Disorders and Reflux

Reflux may result in respiratory disease when the protective mechanisms fail (see Table 26–3). The ensuing disorders include those resulting from aspiration (e.g., pneumonia), from bronchial or laryngeal obstruction (e.g., asthma, apnea, or stridor), and perhaps from the central effects of reflux (e.g., apnea or bradycardia).

Pneumonia and Other Results of Aspiration. Pulmonary aspiration of gastric contents during reflux clearly causes some cases of pneumonia,[9, 192–194] although it is difficult to define inhalation of gastric contents as the cause in individual cases. This is because aspiration during reflux is infrequent and is difficult to distinguish hematogenously acquired pneumonitis from aspiration during swallowing. Aspiration has also been implicated in some instances of granulomatous pneumonia, lung abscess, obliterative bronchiolitis, pulmonary fibrosis, and chronic bronchitis.[168, 195–199]

Diagnosis of aspiration pneumonia remains problematic. In a patient with an abnormal chest radiograph,[200, 201] the diagnosis is suggested by a compatible history, including impairment of protective mechanisms by neurologic debility or depressed consciousness (see Table 26–3)[173, 192, 202–206] or choking and coughing during feeding or during emesis.[202, 207] Testing to support the diagnosis is discussed later.

Bronchial Obstruction. Clinical studies have shown abnormal reflux in 25 to 80% of children with asthma but in a smaller proportion of control children.[208–213] Quantitative reflux scores also correlated with measures of respiratory symptoms,[210, 211] and individual reflux episodes showed a temporal relationship to wheezing.[210] Finally, several studies have recorded an improvement in bronchospastic symptoms following therapy of reflux.[208, 211, 214, 215]

Nocturnal asthma symptoms, including cough, are especially suggestive of underlying reflux. Nocturnal reflux produces more prolonged esophageal acid exposure (because of a supine position and decreased salivation and swallowing) and a greater frequency of esophagitis, which may be important for reflux-provoked bronchospasm.[179, 210, 212, 213, 216] Nocturnal reflux may also occur at a time of increased vulnerability of the respiratory system, both because protective reflexes are depressed and because of reduced pulmonary oxygen reserves and depressed respiratory muscle responsiveness.[217, 218]

Several experimental studies in adults and children have shown evidence of bronchoconstriction in asthmatic patients during acid infusion into the esophagus but not during saline or antacid infusion (modified Bernstein test).[178–184] The bronchoconstriction occurred most reliably in asthmatic patients with evidence of peptic esophagitis. Esophageal acidification may induce bronchospasm directly or may potentiate bronchospasm induced by other stimuli.[184] This probably occurs by a vagal reflex and is inhibited by atropine.[183, 185, 186, 219]

Although contradictory clinical studies dispute a relationship between asthma and reflux,[209, 220–223] the evidence is best interpreted as showing that reflux exacerbates bronchospasm in at least a subgroup of patients. Reflux-related bronchial obstruction should be suspected in patients whose asthma is resistant to medical management, without an atopic basis, or accompanied by prominent nocturnal symptoms. The modified Bernstein test with associated pulmonary function testing is most useful in the diagnosis of reflux-related bronchospasm. Alternatively, if abnormal reflux is documented by pH probe, for example, response of the asthma to medical management of the reflux may be considered supporting evidence for this mechanism.

Questions regarding the afferent limb of this response are as yet unanswered: Are esophageal receptors "uncovered" by esophagitis? Does pain from heartburn contribute to the stimulus? Will nonacid reflux produce the response?

Laryngeal Obstruction—Apnea. Apnea is among the most serious effects of reflux. It occurs particularly during the first 6 months of life, especially in very young premature infants, and has probably been responsible for a proportion of the infant mortality designated *sudden infant death syndrome*. Apnea is characterized as obstructive (due to obstruction of the airway, as from laryngospasm) or central (due to cessation of respiratory efforts). Obstructive and central apnea may be pathologic elaborations of protective reflexes preventing aspiration.[224]

Laryngospasm can abruptly and completely block air movement into the entire respiratory tree, especially in infants, in whom both the cross-sectional area and the motor control of the upper airway may be limited. This obstructive apnea is manifest by cessation of air flow despite continuing respiratory efforts. Incomplete laryngospasm allows continuation of air flow, but the resistance of the narrowed larynx may be audible as stridor.

As with bronchospasm, early reports linking apnea to reflux implicated actual aspiration,[225] but other mechanisms are probably more common. Some infants with recurrent respiratory arrest become free of such episodes after medical or surgical treatment of reflux.[226–228] A temporal relationship between reflux and apnea can be documented using a nasal thermistor and thoracic impedance to identify obstructive apnea.[229–232] Although nonregurgitant reflux is demonstrated during testing, actual regurgitation may be infrequent. Reflux-related apnea in infants has been associated with a characteristic symptom complex suggesting obstructive apnea: A recently fed supine or seated infant with a prior history of regurgitation becomes rigid, apneic, staring, and plethoric, and then cyanotic or pale.[233] There may be no coughing, choking, or gagging. Parents may remember seeing respiratory efforts, suggesting obstructive apnea.

As with bronchospasm, acid (but not water or dilute formula) infused through a nasoesophageal tube has been documented to precipitate obstructive apnea in some infants with pathologic reflux.[228] The implication that reflux of early postprandial neutral gastric contents is incapable of provoking apnea is contrary to clinical experience and awaits further investigation.

Again, as with bronchospasm, some studies have disputed a causal relationship between reflux and apnea.[234–237] However, the evidence is best interpreted as indicating that reflux, even without aspiration, may cause apnea in a subgroup of infants. Most infants displaying this worrisome symptom of reflux will outgrow both their reflux and the propensity toward apnea during the first year of life, so the interim management becomes an essential issue, which has been controversial. Although some authors have advocated fundoplication for all such infants, others suggest a nonsurgical approach initially, combined with careful monitoring.[249, 250] Even in infants with life-threatening apnea, rigorous medical therapy, sometimes supplemented with cardiopulmonary monitoring, has proved adequate in most instances.

Laryngeal Obstruction—Stridor. Interesting analogies to the association of reflux and obstructive apnea are the few scattered reports associating reflux and stridor, in which stridor may be seen as a manifestation of incomplete laryngeal obstruction.[238–242] Chronic stridor may reflect laryngospasm if intermittent or laryngitis if continuous. Reflex laryngospasm manifest as stridor may require the presence of esophagitis, laryngitis, or an abnormal upper respiratory tract. It is possible that in some patients reflux-related stridor is produced by hyperventilation due to esophageal discomfort—a relative airway narrowing with no change in actual cross-sectional area.

Laryngeal obstruction, manifest as apnea or stridor, may thus result from reflux in some infants. The pathways involved in this response and the reason that not all infants exhibit this response are not clear. Whether esophageal or laryngeal receptors are involved, whether esophagitis is a prerequisite, whether acid material is necessary, and whether other predisposing abnormalities are required are unanswered questions. Symptomatic laryngospasm as a response to reflux generally occurs in younger children rather than bronchospasm. This may be because of the relatively small cross-sectional area of the upper airway, because of a tendency toward greater laxity of upper airway structures, or because of an immaturity of nervous control of the respiratory system.

Diagnosis of such reflux-induced laryngospasm may be achieved with pH probe and concurrent pneumogram (measuring both chest wall movement and air flow at the naris). For patients with stridor, either the modified Bernstein test or careful documentation of stridor during the pH probe test may be used.

Central Apnea and Bradycardia. Pathologic central apnea usually occurs during sleep, and it is unclear whether it is ever related to reflux.[243, 244] Studies in infants and immature animals suggest that episodes of central apnea may be produced by esophageal, laryngeal, or hypopharyngeal instillation of acid, cow's milk, or water, but not saline.[228, 245–247] Since the respiratory suppression was often associated with swallowing, it suggests that the response is an exaggeration of a normal protective reflex. The respiratory pauses during sucking and swallowing by normal term and preterm neonates may reach pathologic durations and provide further evidence for a central mechanism relating infant apnea to esophageal peristalsis.[243, 248] Laryngeal and nasopharyngeal receptors adjacent to the oropharynx may mediate such swallowing-associated central apnea.[250]

Bradycardia unrelated to apnea has been demonstrated to occur during feeding in preterm infants[243] and during esophageal acid infusion in piglets[244] and is yet another mechanism for reflux- or feeding-related cyanosis. In piglets the response required oropharyngeal acid and was not abolished by section of superior and recurrent laryngeal nerves and pharyngeal plexus.

Complex Respiratory Diseases and Reflux

In addition to the simple unidirectional causality between reflux and respiratory symptoms discussed earlier, bidirectional interactions may also play a role in more complex pulmonary disorders, several of which have received particular attention.

Bronchopulmonary Dysplasia. GER may prolong the course of bronchopulmonary dysplasia (BPD),[251] and an improvement in pulmonary status has been reported following fundoplication.[190, 252] Although a better understanding of the association of BPD and reflux is needed, the overinflation, wheezing, and airway reactivity that characterize BPD[253] mandate consideration of reflux in patient management.

Cystic Fibrosis. Hyperinflation and chronic cough may predispose to reflux in cystic fibrosis (CF).[187] Studies have found a greater incidence of reflux in patients with CF than in asymptomatic siblings,[188] an association between reflux and reduced pulmonary function,[254] and a positive response to medical or surgical management of reflux.[189]

As is the case for BPD, further work is needed before the role of reflux in CF is fully understood. In the meantime, reflux should be considered not only as a possible cause of the pulmonary disease in CF but also as a consequence of the pulmonary disease or its treatment.

Esophageal Atresia and Tracheoesophageal Fistula. Esophageal atresia occurs with tracheoesophageal fistula more than 90% of the time. Chronic respiratory disease following repair of esophageal atresia has long been noted.[255–257] It has been attributed to aspiration both during and between meals, the former due to anastomotic stricture[257] and the latter due to hypotensive lower esophageal sphincter with resultant reflux.[258, 259] Both are exacerbated by abnormal distal esophageal peristalsis.[255, 257, 260–264] These abnormalities of esophageal motility appear to be congenital, perhaps as the result of morphologic abnormalities of Auerbach's plexus in the distal esophagus.[265]

Respiratory Therapies and Reflux

Reflux may be worsened iatrogenically through pharmacologic and mechanical impairment of the antireflux barrier by respiratory therapies.

Pharmacologic Therapy. Xanthines (theophylline and caffeine), used to treat respiratory disorders such as asthma and apnea of prematurity, may exacerbate reflux by relaxing the LES and stimulating gastric acid secretion.[266–273]

Some beta-adrenergic agonists such as isoproterenol, metaproterenol, carbuterol, and terbutaline have also been implicated in LES hypotonia.[268, 274–277] Therefore, inhaled agents (beta$_2$ and cholinergic bronchodilators), with their low systemic absorption, have been recommended as first-line drug therapy in patients with asthma.[278]

Cigarette smoking, a respiratory "activity" rather than a respiratory therapy, also has pharmacologic effects. Smoking has been shown to provoke LES relaxation and increased frequency of reflux, probably mediated by nicotine or adrenergic stimulation, or both.[279–282] It is not known whether the passive smoking to which children are subjected has similar effects.

Nutritional Therapy. Nutritional repletion with nasogastric or gastrostomy tube has been used in patients malnourished because of CF or even because of reflux.[188, 283–286] Nasogastric tubes, however, have been reported to cause reflux severe enough to produce peptic stricture,[287] and intragastric feedings have been associated with increased reflux in a group of CF patients, although no increase in respiratory symptoms was detected.[188] Gastrostomy tube placement reduces LES pressure, which may worsen reflux.[286, 288, 289] Tube feedings are frequently given faster than a normal meal is taken, and these rapid, high-pressure bolus feedings may overwhelm the stomach's normal receptive relaxation. Therefore, in patients receiving intragastric tube feedings, it is prudent to infuse the feeding slowly and to employ prophylactic antireflux measures such as elevating the head of the bed and perhaps even adding pharmacologic antireflux therapy in some instances.

Mechanical Ventilation. Mechanically ventilated patients may suffer reflux-associated respiratory exacerbations due to intubation effects, positioning effects, and removal of the contribution of the crural diaphragm to gastroesophageal competence. Tracheal intubation impingement on nearby structures may impair both protective upper airway reflexes and UES opening during swallowing, resulting in aspiration.[290] Ventilated patients are also often kept supine, a position that increases reflux, slows gastric emptying, and worsens oxygenation.[291–293]

Chest Physiotherapy. Chest physiotherapy, used for many chronic lung diseases, including CF, may induce reflux through its provocative positioning and possibly the forced expiration and cough maneuvers that most methods of chest physiotherapy employ.[273] Routine chest percussion and postural drainage provoked reflux in eight of ten CF patients.[294]

Miscellaneous Respiratory Symptoms Related to Reflux

Belching (Eructation). Belching occurs during transient relaxations of the LES and is an important method of venting air from the stomach. When a fundoplication prevents the normal occurrence of TLESRs, the discomfort of "gas bloat" is the result. Belching requires not only TLESRs but also relaxation of the crural diaphragm[295] and the UES. The UES relaxes in response to esophageal body distention by gas, in contrast with its contractile response to esophageal body distention by fluid.[296] Like the gas bloat that occurs when LES relaxation to gastric distention is prevented, severe chest pain has been described in a patient whose UES failed to relax when gas was refluxed from her stomach into her esophagus.[297]

Hiccups (Singultus). Hiccups are an involuntary reflex contraction of the diaphragm followed by laryngeal closure. Hiccups have been temporally associated with spontaneous and induced esophageal acidification in both adults and infants.[241, 298, 299] Hiccups occurring with reflux may represent an involuntary reflex in the setting of esophagitis. Conversely, the increased gastroesophageal pressure gradient generated by the hiccups may produce the acid reflux. The response of hiccups to therapy for reflux has been variable.[298, 299]

Cough. Cough was the sole presenting manifestation of reflux in some adults, correlated with distal rather than proximal esophageal acidification, and responded to antireflux therapy.[300] Coughing has also been associated with acid reflux in infants.[241, 301] Reflux may cause cough (representing bronchospasm or reflex clearance of microaspiration); on the other hand, coughing may cause reflux by its effect on thoracoabdominal pressure relationships. Care is thus needed in interpretation when cough and reflux coexist (Fig. 26–7).

Hoarseness. Hoarseness has received attention as a possible consequence of reflux in adults.[302–306] The described characteristics of the reflux, response to therapy, and postulated mechanisms have varied.[302, 303, 305–308] Laryngoscopic findings have included normal mucosa; chronic arytenoid or vocal cord inflammation (edema, erythema), granulomata, or "contact ulcers"; and scarring, stenosis, or cancer.[303, 304, 306, 308, 309] As with other forms of reflux-related respiratory symptoms, postulated mechanisms have included direct acid injury and an indirect path mediated by reflexive chronic coughing and throat-clearing in response to reflux.[303] Hoarseness has also been linked to reflux in children.[310] Reflux should be considered in the occasional hoarse patient when evaluation, including laryngoscopy, suggests that reflux is responsible and eliminates other causes.

Pharyngonasal Regurgitation. The regurgitation of material into the nasopharynx or nose, either during swallowing or during reflux, is a little-explored phenomenon occurring largely in infants. A description of the findings in 57 infants and children who demonstrated pharyngonasal reflux during barium swallow has been published, as have occasional case reports.[311] Although it represents a failure of the normal airway protection, pharyngonasal regurgitation usually resolves without long-term consequence. It is most frequent in the first 3 months of life and may be associated with prematurity or with neuromuscular disease. It may produce apnea, since it may occlude the nose of infants who are obligate nose-breathers.

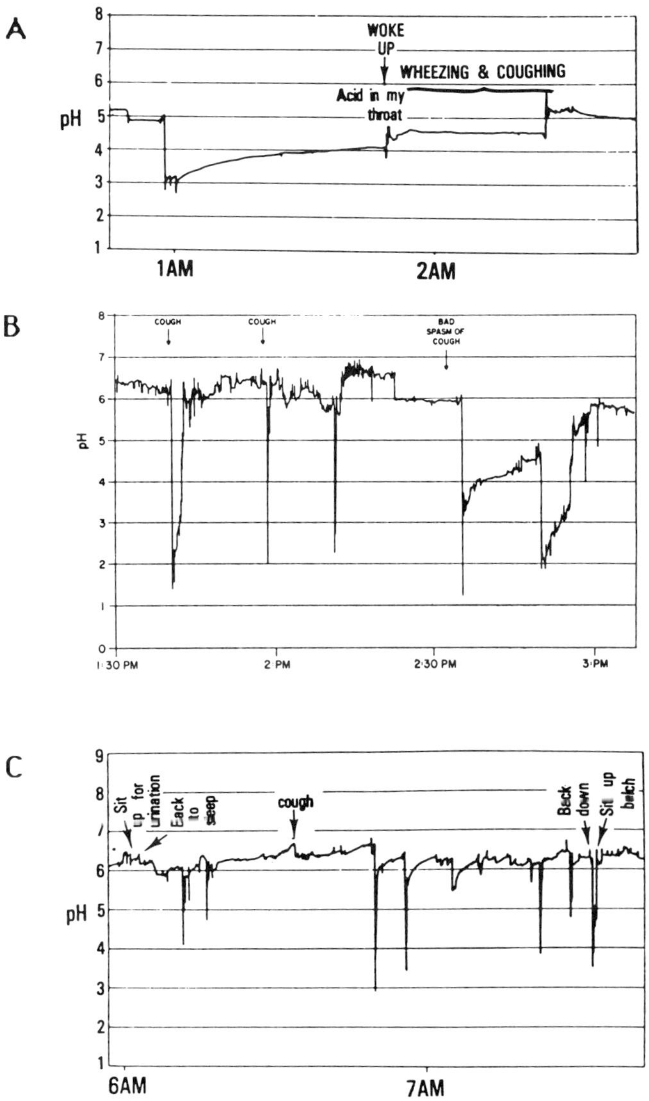

Figure 26–7. Three relationships between cough and reflux. pH probe tracings from three adults, showing (*A*) nocturnal supine reflux preceding cough in a patient with pathologic reflux, (*B*) cough preceding reflux in a patient with primary respiratory disease, and (*C*) no temporal relationship between cough and reflux in a third patient. These temporal relationships suggest causal ones. (Adapted from Pellegrini CA, DeMeester TR, Johnson LF, et al: Gastroesophageal reflux and pulmonary aspiration: Incidence, functional abnormality, and results of surgical therapy. Surgery 1979; 86:110–119; with permission.)

Neurobehavioral Response to Reflux

Sandifer's Syndrome

Neurobehavioral manifestations of reflux are exemplified by the posturing of Sandifer's syndrome.[312–315]

> The movements are of varying type and severity, involving the head and neck and sometimes the upper part of the trunk, but not the limbs. They usually consist primarily of a sudden extension of the head and neck into the position of opisthotonus. The head may be twisted continuously from side to side. The upper part of the trunk may become bent acutely to one side so that the head is pointing to the floor. The child may seem to be trying to turn himself upside down. A habitual position in some of the children has been lying supine on a bed with the head and neck hyper-extended over the side of the bed pointing to the floor. The head may be held inclined to one side for prolonged periods so that the abnormality might be described as an abnormal posture rather than movement. The movements sometimes continue no matter what other activity the child is engaged in. They may be accentuated during and immediately after meals. They cease during sleep.[316]

Interestingly, manometric evaluation of one child suggested that esophageal clearance may be improved by the posturing.[313]

Less Specific Neurobehavioral Manifestations

In infants, behaviors that seem to be attenuated versions of Sandifer's syndrome may suggest reflux. These include arching and staring associated with obstructive apnea, periods of cyanosis suggesting neonatal seizures, and irritable stretching or neck extension.

Rumination

The gagging, regurgitation, mouthing, and swallowing of refluxed material identified as rumination[317] may be either a cause of or a response to reflux. In individual infants, it may be difficult to determine whether a primary psychosocial cause exists for the behaviors, which have resulted in reflux, or whether the reflux is primary and the behaviors are merely a response to esophagitis. In either instance, vicious cycles may be initiated, and diagnosis and treatment of reflux and esophagitis may be important for resolution of the symptoms (see Chapter 10).

DIAGNOSIS

General Principles

Diagnostic evaluation of reflux is undertaken in patients suspected of having pathologic effects from reflux. Thus, infants with regurgitation but without nutritional or other sequelae are simply managed with the conservative antireflux measures described later. Even when nutritional effects (such as a drop in weight for length percentiles) are manifest, infants whose regurgitation does not suggest anatomic or metabolic disease may also have a trial of such nonpharmacologic therapy without further diagnostic measures if they are closely monitored for improvement during the early stages of therapy. Atypical emesis and emesis that does not clear during initial therapy should usually be evaluated radiographically. Infants with symptoms other than emesis should have a diagnostic evaluation tailored to their presentation before being considered for pharmacologic therapy.

For pediatric patients whose symptoms suggest esophagitis, the most efficient evaluation is probably esophageal biopsy, with or without endoscopy; endoscopy is useful (especially in older children) to exclude peptic ulcer disease elsewhere in the upper gastrointestinal tract. Evaluation for reflux in patients presenting with respiratory or neurobehavorial symptoms may begin with pH probe, with attention to documentation of synchrony of reflux episodes and discrete symptoms. Such documentation may include concurrent pneumogram or pulmonary function testing. Intraluminal acid infusion may be used in difficult cases and to sort out cause-and-effect relationships. Scintigraphy is useful, perhaps even in place of pH probe testing, in centers in which it has been refined to demonstrate even extremely brief episodes, and especially in patients in whom evaluation for aspiration or delayed gastric emptying is desirable or in those in whom it is important to detect reflux of neutralized postprandial gastric contents.

Radiology

In the pediatric age range, fluoroscopic evaluation is most useful in those children with emesis or feeding problems to eliminate other diagnoses from consideration.[318] Barium fluoroscopy can identify congenital or acquired structural causes for emesis, such as webs, stenoses, or malrotation of the upper gastrointestinal tract. Dysmotility of the esophagus causing feeding problems in the absence of pathologic reflux can also be suggested by the esophagram. Severe esophagitis or peptic strictures are reflux-related problems that are amenable to radiographic diagnosis (see Fig. 26–4). Air contrast (double contrast) radiography of the esophagus, a fairly specialized procedure, can delineate mucosal detail to a degree that is impossible with routine barium fluoroscopy, but it is not as sensitive as endoscopy.[319]

Scintigraphy

Technetium scintigraphy, although producing an image that is less sharp than that obtained in barium fluoroscopy, has several advantages over fluoroscopy for evaluation of reflux.[320] It can monitor for reflux following physiologic, nonacid meals; the monitoring can be prolonged for an hour or so (until the radionuclide has emptied from the stomach) without augmentation of the radiation exposure; and the radiation exposure is typically several-fold less than that from a routine barium study, an important consideration for young children. Its sensitivity for detection of reflux is reported to be 59 to 93%[321–323]; differences in sensitivity are likely to result from differences in technique, and regurgitant reflux is frequently missed.[324] Aspiration and quantitative gastric emptying[49] may be evaluated scintigraphically, although scintigraphy's sensitivity for the former is low,[325, 326] and scintographic evaluation of gastric emptying may be affected artifactually by superimposition of the distal duodenal image over that of the stomach.[327] Bulk esophageal clearance is also amenable to scintigraphic evaluation.[55] Optimal use of scintigraphy for evaluation of reflux demands that the radiologist take advantage of computer capabilities for continual monitoring in very brief time intervals rather than merely acquiring an occasional image on the gamma camera (Fig. 26–8).[328, 329] This technique is underused, and its capability is underdeveloped in most institutions.

Endoscopy, Biopsy, and Histology

Endoscopy and Biopsy

Endoscopy is useful to evaluate symptoms of pain, dysphagia, vomiting, or hematemesis to differentiate

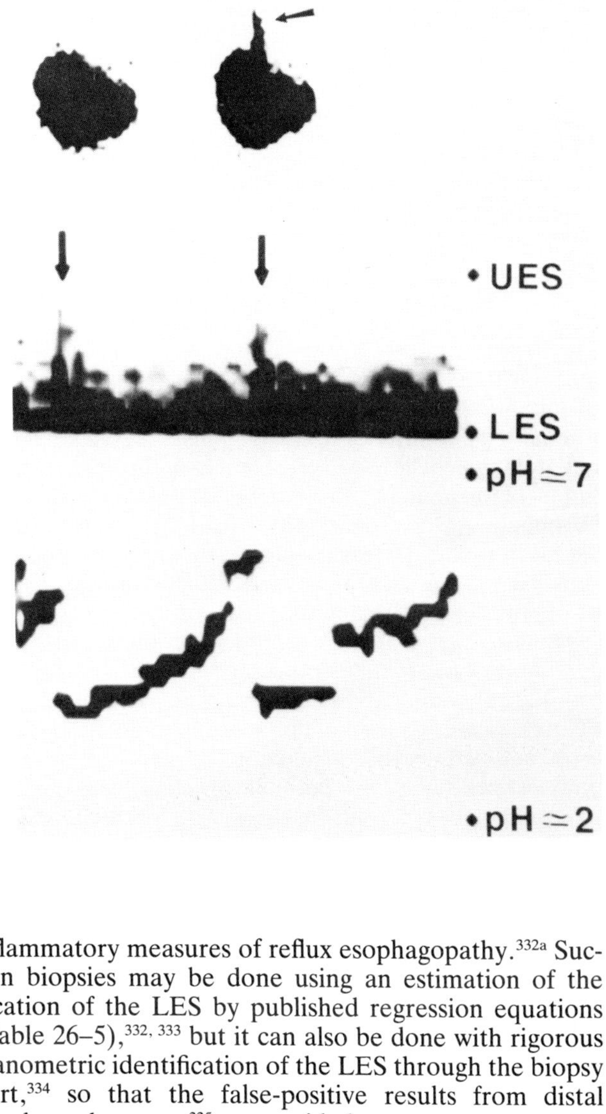

Figure 26–8. Scintigraphic respresentations of reflux. The top panel shows a posterior view of an infant's stomach filled with ^{99m}Tc sulfur colloid–labeled apple juice before (*left image*) and during (*right image*) gastroesophageal reflux (*arrow*). The middle panel shows, on a different occasion, a scintigraphic "condensed dynamic image" representation of two episodes of reflux (*arrow*) over a 10-minute period, depicted essentially continuously; the abscissa is time and the ordinate shows the spacial location of the refluxate in the esophagus, with markers for the upper (UES) and lower (LES) esophageal sphincters. The bottom panel is a pH probe recording from the distal esophagus at the same time as the scintigraphic representation above it; the abscissa is time and the ordinate shows the degree of acidification at one point in the distal esophagus, with markers indicating pH of 7 and 2. (Adapted from Rosenthal MS, Klein HA, Orenstein SR: Simultaneous acquisition of physiological data and nuclear medicine images. J Nucl Med 1988; 29:1848–1852; with permission.)

between reflux disease and other gastrointestinal disease with similar symptoms. Scoring systems for peptic esophagitis recognize a range of endoscopic signs—from erythema and hyperemia (which may be unreliable), through erosions and ulcerations, to strictures and Barrett's esophagus. Such endoscopic evidence should always be supported by histologic evidence from biopsies to identify nonreflux causes for the changes.

Because of the necessarily brief chronology of reflux in infants, reliable endoscopic manifestations of esophagitis are uncommon (despite the frequency of histologic esophagitis).[109, 330] In addition, other lesions of the upper gastrointestinal tract that may mimic inflammatory sequelae of reflux, such as peptic ulcers, are less frequent than as in adults. Furthermore, the small size of pediatric endoscopes makes histologic assessment of biopsies obtained through them insensitive for esophagitis, since basal layer hyperplasia and papillary elongation are usually impossible to evaluate.[110] Finally, reports of hypoxia due to the endoscope's impingement on the airway suggest that upper endoscopy in young infants may be more safely performed with airway maintenance ensured by intubation and general anesthesia.[331] Therefore, many infants may be most efficiently evaluated for peptic esophagitis using a suction biopsy instrument.

Suction esophageal biopsy requires no sedation, takes less than a minute in experienced hands, results in negligible morbidity, and produces a specimen adequate for evaluation of the morphometric as well as the inflammatory measures of reflux esophagopathy.[332a] Suction biopsies may be done using an estimation of the location of the LES by published regression equations (Table 26–5),[332, 333] but it can also be done with rigorous manometric identification of the LES through the biopsy port,[334] so that the false-positive results from distal esophageal mucosa[335] are avoided.

Histopathology

Morphometric parameters of the epithelium that are useful in the diagnosis of esophagitis are papillary height

Table 26–5. ESOPHAGEAL LENGTH REGRESSION EQUATIONS

Nose to Diaphragm (LES)*	Mouth to Diaphragm (LES)*
.252 (height in cm) + 5 (r = .93)†	.226 (height in cm) + 6.7 (r = .97)†
.24 (height in cm) + 5.2 (r = .96)‡	
.47 (crown-rump in cm) + .57 (r = .93)‡	

*pH probes and esophageal biopsies are generally performed at 87% of this distance.

†Data from Strobel CT, Byrne WJ, Ament ME, et al: Correlation of esophageal lengths in children with height: Application to the Tuttle test without prior esophageal manometry. J Pediatr 1979; 103:215–218; with permission.

‡Data from Putnam PE, Orenstein SR: Determining esophageal length from crown-rump length. Pediatr Res 1991; 29:111A; with permission.

Table 26–6. HISTOLOGIC MARKERS FOR ESOPHAGITIS

Histologic Marker	Normal Range	Sensitivity (%)	Negative Predictive Value (%)
Basal cell thickness	<25%*	89	73
Papillary height	<53%*	30	30
Epithelial eosinophils	0/mm†	26	29
Lamina propria eosinophils	<0.8/mm†	41	33
Epithelial neutrophils	0/mm†	15	26

*Expressed as percentage of total epithelial thickness.
†Expressed as number of cells per mm of muscularis mucosae length.
Adapted from Black DD, Haggitt RC, Orenstein SR, et al: Esophagitis in infants: Morphometric histologic diagnosis and correlation with measures of gastroesophageal reflux. Gastroenterology 1990; 98:1408–1414; with permission.

and basal cell thickness (Fig. 26–9).[108] Useful markers of inflammation include lamina propria eosinophils, epithelial eosinophils and neutrophils, "squiggle cells," and telangiectasias.[108, 336] Table 26–6 shows the upper limits of normal for the various parameters signifying esophagitis. Documentation of histologic esophagitis is useful in that it defines a child's reflux as pathologic and thus warranting treatment. It also prompts specific use of acid-reducing therapeutic measures.

Diagnosis of Barrett's esophagus requires histologic evaluation of specimens diligently identified as being of esophageal, rather than gastric, origin. The three types of metaplastic columnar epithelium found in Barrett's esophagus are cardiac ("junctional"—containing gastric mucous cells, but no parietal or chief cells); fundic (containing gastric mucous cells with parietal or chief cells); and intestinal ("specialized columnar"—containing goblet cells and often villi with brush borders (see Fig. 26–9). An "intermediate type," without any parietal, chief, goblet, or brush border cells and no cardiac glands, has also been described.[148] The cardiac epithelium and the intermediate type may be extremely difficult to distinguish from normal epithelium from the stomach adjacent to the esophagus, especially in the presence of a hiatal hernia. It seems that dysplasia and carcinoma occur almost exclusively in the intestinal and intermediate epithelium.[148]

A visually recognizable patch of gastric mucosa in the upper third of the esophagus (an "inlet patch") is considered to be a congenital lesion with an incidence of 4%. Usually asymptomatic, it has also been reported to cause upper esophageal stricture. Its presence in the upper esophagus and clear separation from normal gastric epithelium help to distinguish it from Barrett's esophagus.[337, 338]

Esophageal Manometry

The role of manometry is limited to those children with symptoms suggestive of esophageal dysmotility or those in whom antireflux surgery is contemplated. Infants with repaired esophageal atresia, for example, are a special group in whom reflux is common and often severe,[259] but in whom the frequent peristaltic dysfunction of the distal esophageal segment makes a tight fundoplication potentially hazardous.[339]

Intraluminal Esophageal Acid Perfusion

Intraluminal esophageal acid perfusion using chest pain (the Bernstein test) or other end points (the modified Bernstein test) has found expanded use recently, both in clinical practice and in research. It permits causal linkage of particular symptoms with esophageal acidification. In contrast with the spontaneous acidification accessible to pH probe, the timing and duration of acidification can be controlled, and complex observations can be precisely timed to periods of acidification and neutralization. This technique has been applied to respiratory symptoms (such as bronchospasm,[178, 180] stridor,[242] and hiccups[298]), to chest pain in children,[340] and to Sandifer's syndrome (unpublished data).

Esophageal pH Monitoring

Twenty-four–hour monitoring of intraluminal esophageal pH is regarded in children, as in adults, as the gold standard for diagnosing reflux.[341] Because children

Figure 26–9. Histologic sequelae of reflux. *A,* Normal esophageal squamous epithelium: The basal layer (*below long arrow*) is about 10% of the epithelial thickness, and papillae (*below short arrow*) are about 50%. Inflammatory cells are absent. *B,* Histologic esophagitis: The basal zone (*below long horizontal arrow*) is expanded to 70% of the epithelial thickness, and papillae (*below short horizontal arrow*) are elongated to 75% of the epithelial thickness. Degranulating eosinophils (*vertical arrows*) infiltrate the epithelium. *C,* Barrett's epithelium: Intestinal columnar epithelium with goblet cells (*arrows*) has replaced the normal squamous epithelium in this esophageal specimen. (Adapted from Orenstein SR: Gastroesophageal reflux. *In* Stockman JA II, Winter RJ, eds: Current Problems in Pediatrics. Chicago, Year Book Medical Publishers, May/June 1991; 21(5):218; with permission.)

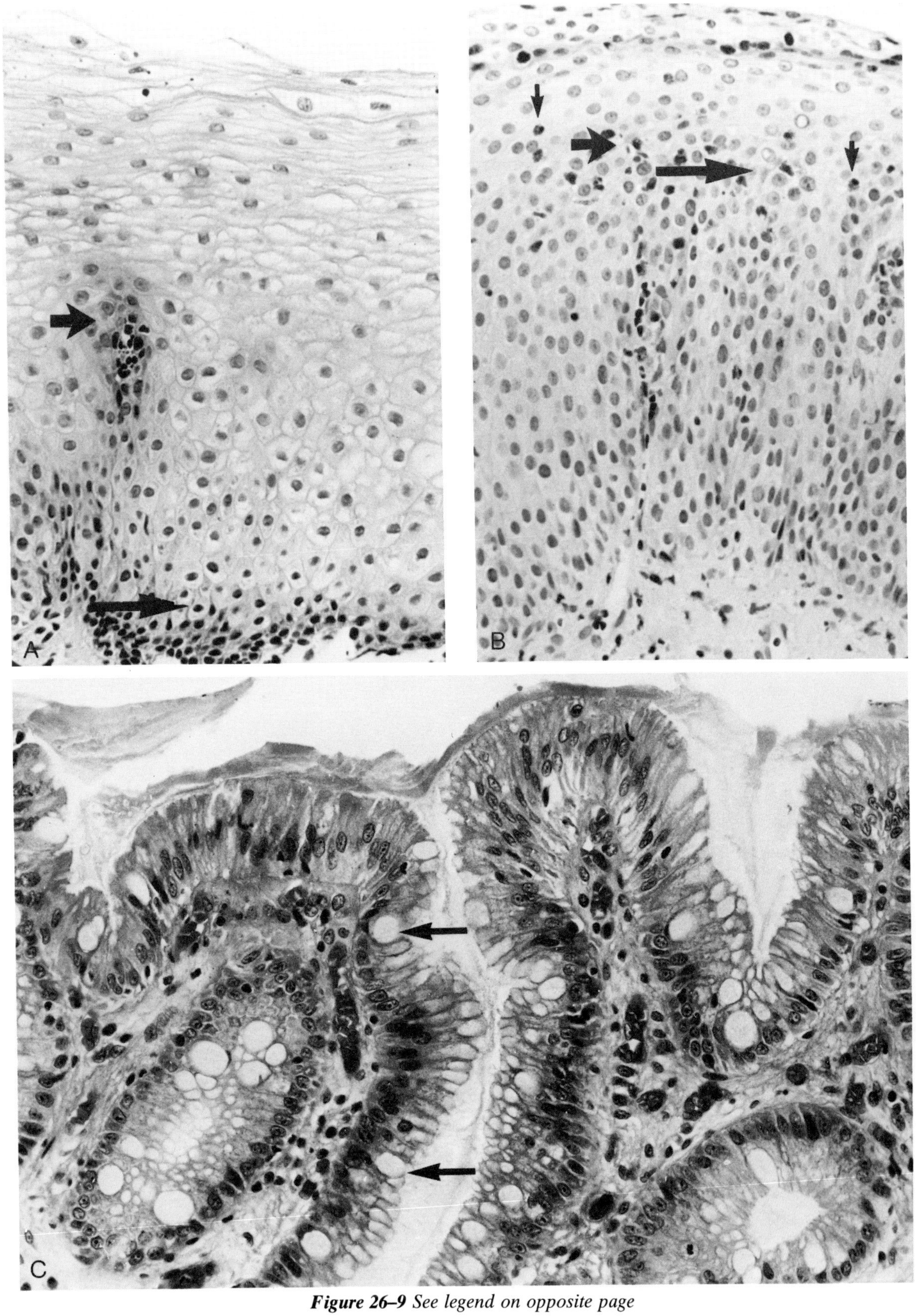

Figure 26–9 *See legend on opposite page*

can mimic their usual activities fairly well while hospitalized, and because they need close monitoring to ensure that they neither remove the probe nor destroy the equipment, pediatric pH probe studies are performed more often on inpatients than on outpatients. Assessment of whether monitoring periods briefer than 24 hours are valid measures of reflux has produced conflicting results; most centers still monitor for 24 hours. Although the pH probe can quantify frequency and duration of acid reflux, it cannot detect reflux for as long as 2 hours following infant formula feedings. Whether to use less physiologic feedings of acidic liquids (such as apple juice) to preserve the ability to detect postprandial reflux is an unresolved issue. The amount of reflux detected will vary greatly depending on technical points such as feeding type and position in which an infant is placed (Fig. 26–10),[342–344] details that contribute to the large day-to-day variability in pH probe results.[345] In addition to identifying patterns of normal or abnormal reflux (Fig. 26–11),[346] pH probe studies are scored to define reflux as quantitatively normal or abnormal. Scoring of pH probe studies generally includes quantification of the number of acid reflux episodes, of the average duration of such episodes, and of the total proportion of time during which the esophagus is acidified (Fig. 26–12).[116] The number of reflux episodes lasting longer than 5 minutes and the duration of the longest episode are other measures reflecting clearance. Age-related normal values for these parameters have been defined (see Fig. 26–3).[80, 114] Derived scores are used by some investigators to define reflux as pathologic or not[347, 348]; such derived scores have the disadvantage of obscuring the data on which they are based, and they tend to reduce the information obtained from the test to the simple identification of the child as normal or abnormal. A recently described computerized scoring system that quantifies the degree of acidification as well as its temporal aspects is intriguing but has not yet been completely evaluated.[71]

Perhaps more important than the quantity of reflux is the association of reflux episodes with the symptoms that prompted evaluation (see Fig. 26–7). This can be done during pH probe evaluation but requires careful monitoring, particularly in children. Apneic episodes, for instance, can be sought during concurrent pH probe and pneumocardiography, but the pneumocardiographic data must be temporally linked to the pH probe data with precision and must include nasal thermistor or end-

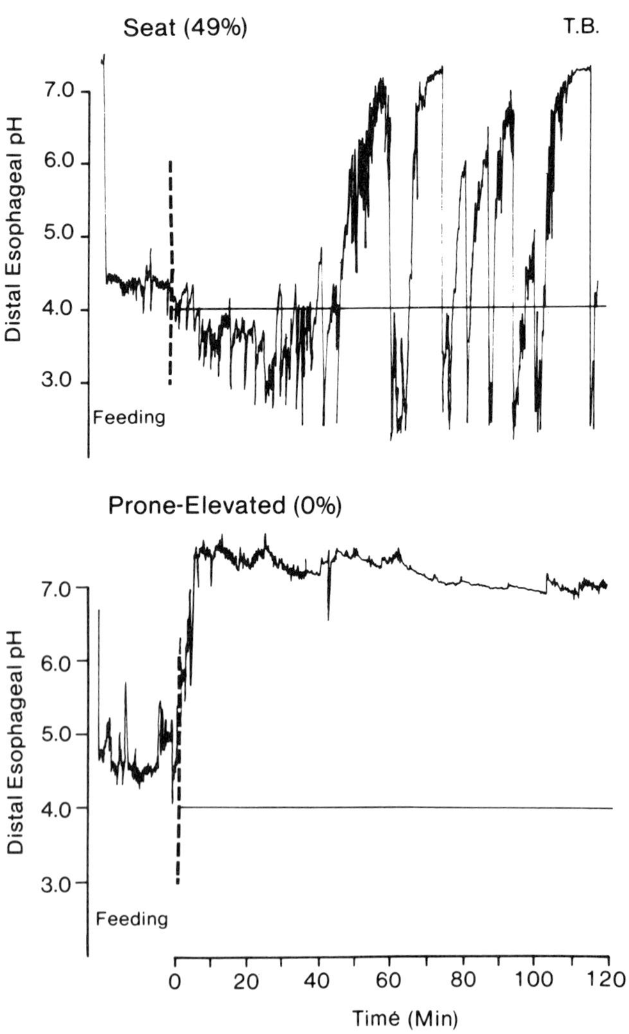

Figure 26–10. Effect of position on reflux quantity. An infant monitored in two different positions during two otherwise identical postprandial periods. In the seated position, the distal esophageal pH was below 4 for 49% of the time; in the prone, head-elevated position, the pH was never below 4.

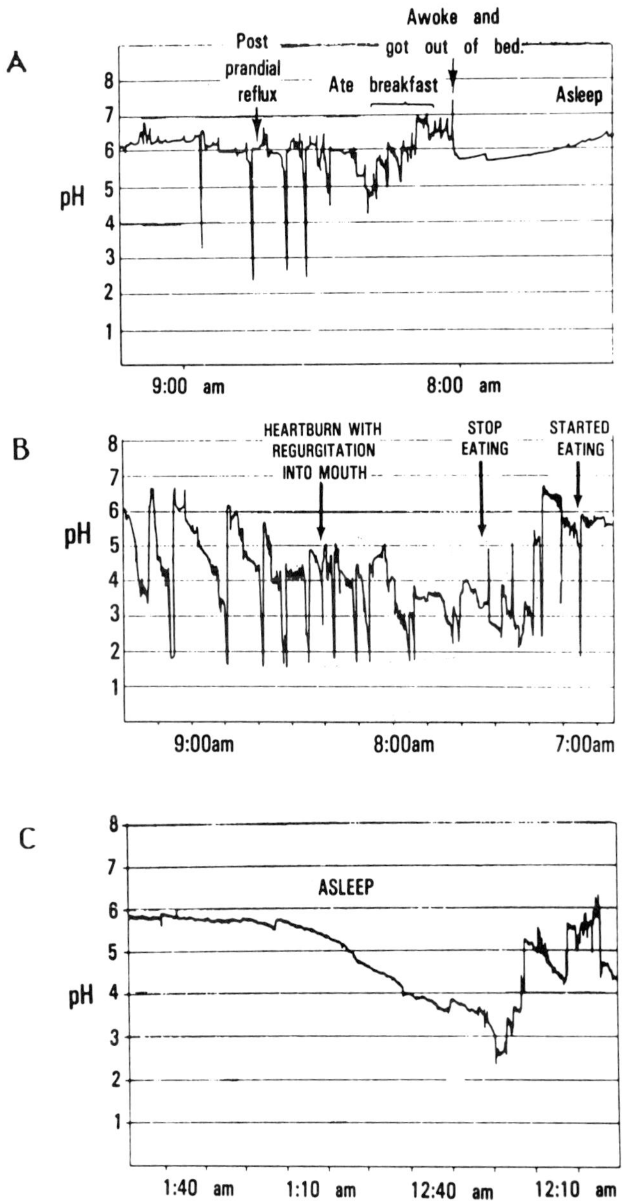

Figure 26–11. Patterns of reflux detected by pH probe. *A,* Occasional episodes of brief postprandial reflux are normal. *B,* Abnormal postprandial reflux may consist of more frequent episodes, which are nonetheless brief. *C,* Reflux during sleep is generally abnormal; even if infrequent, it may produce pathologic effects because it is poorly cleared during sleep. (Note that time is read from right to left on these tracings.) (Adapted from Johnson LF: New concepts and methods in the study and treatment of gastroesophageal reflux disease. Med Clin North Am 1981; 65:1195–1222; with permission.)

tidal carbon dioxide measurements to document obstructive apnea.

pH probe monitoring can be used to evaluate response to therapy. Antacids and other acid-reducing therapy should usually be stopped during such repeat pH probe studies, but whether to discontinue prokinetic agents depends on the question being addressed.

Miscellaneous Tests to Diagnose Aspiration

Methods to document aspiration of stomach contents include direct sampling of tracheobronchial secretions for detection of lipid-laden macrophages,[349, 350] lactose,[290] or dyes administered intragastrically.[351] These methods are invasive, requiring tracheal intubation or bronchoscopy, and are thus most suitable for patients requiring such instrumentation for other reasons. The intubation itself may affect the results.[352] Finally, a high incidence of false-positive results may limit the clinical utility of these tests.[353] Methods that do not require tracheal intubation or bronchoscopy are the upper gastrointestinal series[194, 200] and the more sensitive gastroesophageal scintigraphy[193, 194, 354, 355]; these methods involve radiation exposure, however, and are fairly insensitive because of the limited duration of monitoring possible. Variability of technique (including positioning, provocative maneuvers, radionuclide dose, and timing of imaging) is probably responsible for the marked variation in the frequency with which aspiration is detected by these methods. The bronchoscopic[356] and microscopic[357] characteristics of aspiration have been described and suggest the possibility of implicating aspiration by retrospective

GASTROESOPHAGEAL ACID – REFLUX MONITORING

FILE NUMBER

PATIENT NAME	UNIT NO.	DATE / /	REFERRING PHYSICIAN

HISTORY

PATIENT WEIGHT	PATIENT HEIGHT	DISTANCE FROM NARES/INCISORS	BY RADIOGRAPHY / MANOMETRY / CALCULATION .87 [5 + 0.252 (HT.)] =

pH PROBE STUDY

FEEDING NO. TYPE/VOL. CONDITIONS ★	TIME	TIME pH <4 (%)	#pH<4	#>5 MIN.	LONGEST	OTHER ★★
1.						
2.						
3.						
4.						
5.						
6.						
7.						
8.						

OVERALL STUDY

TOTAL						

FASTING	NORMAL	PATIENT
% TIME pH < 4	UP TO 2.2	
NO. EPISODES / HR.	UP TO 1	
LONGEST EPISODE (MIN.)	UP TO 12	
2 HOUR POST PRANDIAL	**NORMAL**	**PATIENT**
% TIME pH < 4	UP TO 10	
NO. EPISODES / HR.	UP TO 5	
LONGEST EPISODE (MIN.)	UP TO 12	

OVERALL REFLUX SCORE

# / d + 4 (# > 5′ / d) =	UP TO 50	

INTERPRETATION

★POSITION, MEDICATION, WAKEFULNESS, OTHER ★★VOMIT, WHEEZE, COUGH, APNEA, OTHER ASSOCIATED SX.

PHYSICIAN'S SIGNATURE	DATE

Figure 26–12 *See legend on opposite page*

evaluation soon after a suggestive episode; they may, however, be insensitive for microaspiration.

Summary of Diagnostic Evaluation

The approach to an individual patient may also be guided by the questions being asked.

Is There Pathologic Reflux? The presence of pathologic reflux can be defined endoscopically, histologically, by pH probe, radiographically, or scintigraphically. Reflux that produces endoscopic or (more sensitively) histologic esophagitis is certainly pathologic; thus, many clinicians use endoscopy with grasp biopsies or blind esophageal suction biopsies to diagnose pathologic reflux.[358] Reflux that may be pathologic in quantity or effect does not always produce esophagitis, so quantification of reflux and documentation of its temporal relationship to symptoms are often accomplished with intraluminal esophageal pH monitoring. The pH probe not only quantifies several parameters of reflux for which norms have been established[114] but also may be used to define a temporal association between acid reflux episodes and intermittent symptoms, such as respiratory or neurobehavioral ones. The pH probe does not detect reflux of nonacid material and thus may underestimate reflux frequency, particularly after neutral-pH feedings such as formula. Barium esophagram has often been used to diagnose reflux, but its lack of sensitivity (due to the brief monitoring time) and of specificity (due to the presence of physiologic reflux in normal people) makes it a poor choice for this purpose in most instances.[318] It is best used to observe anatomy and function and to eliminate other gastrointestinal disorders from consideration. Gastroesophageal scintigraphy produces less sharply detailed images than do barium contrast studies, but continuous monitoring throughout an entire postprandial period is possible. It is therefore likely that, with improved software and establishment of normal values, such nuclear medicine studies will be able to define pathologic quantities of reflux with a sensitivity between that of the barium esophagram and that of the pH probe and to avoid some of the nonphysiologic aspects of the pH probe.[359] Both scintigraphy and barium esophagram can also confirm pulmonary aspiration, although the false-negative rate may be high.

Documentation of reflux in pathologic quantities, even if pathologic effects have not been demonstrated with certainty, may be used as an excuse for treatment of reflux. If the symptoms that prompted therapy then resolve during treatment, that resolution is evidence that reflux may have caused the symptoms.

Is There a Temporal Relationship Between Reflux and a Particular Symptom? Documentation of a temporal association provides a more reliable indication that reflux caused the presenting symptom. Therefore, intermittent symptoms may be tested for temporal association with reflux using the pH probe and close observation for the symptom, as has been done for bronchospasm,[210] apnea,[229] and stridor.[240] This close observation may be supplemented by objective measurements, including pulmonary function testing, thermistor and cardiopneumogram, cutaneous monitoring for oxygen or carbon dioxide partial pressure, or video recording.[241]

Is Reflux Causing the Symptom? Showing a temporal association between intermittent symptoms and reflux episodes suggests causality, but a causal association and its direction are more conclusively demonstrated when simulation of reflux by esophageal acid infusion (modified Bernstein test) produces the symptom in question.[179–181, 228, 242] Again, observation of the symptom may be supplemented by objective measurements, such as those discussed earlier.

DIFFERENTIAL DIAGNOSIS

Because the symptoms with which pediatric patients can present vary considerably, and because their histories are brief and often secondhand, the differential diagnostic considerations may be fairly broad (Table 26–7). Emesis may represent metabolic or structural defects; irritability may represent many other causes of discomfort; respiratory symptoms may represent respiratory disease; and neurobehavioral signs may represent primary neurologic or metabolic disease. These considerations should prompt a broader evaluation than the evaluation for reflux-associated disease previously discussed.

THERAPY

General Principles

In contrast with adults and older children, most infants with symptomatic reflux will be free of pathologic reflux

Figure 26–12. pH probe scoring form. Form used at Children's Hospital of Pittsburgh for scoring pH probe studies. The calculation for insertion distance is near the top of the page. (From Strobel CT, Byrne WJ, Ament ME, et al: Correlation of esophageal lengths in children with height: Application to the Tuttle test without prior esophageal manometry. J Pediatr 1979; 103:215–218; with permission.) The composite score is found lower on the page. (From Euler AR, Byrne WJ: Twenty-four-hour esophageal intraluminal pH probe testing: A comparative analysis. Gastroenterology 1981; 80:957–961; with permission.) (Previously published in Orenstein SR: Gastroesophageal reflux. *In* Stockman JA II, Winter RJ, eds: Current Problems in Pediatrics. Chicago, Year Book Medical Publishers, May/June 1991; 21(5):221; with permission.)

Table 26–7. DIFFERENTIAL DIAGNOSIS OF REFLUX SYMPTOMS

Regurgitation, Vomiting (see Tables 10–8, 10–9, and 10–10 in Chapter 10)
Pain, Esophagitis Symptoms
- Cardiac pain
- Pulmonary or mediastinal pain; chest wall pain (e.g., costrochondritis)
- Nonesophagitis upper gastrointestinal inflammation (e.g., peptic ulcer disease)
- Nonesophagitis dysphagia
- Many possible causes of nonspecific irritability in infants
- Functional; malingering

Respiratory Symptoms (wheeze, stridor, cough, etc.)
- Extrinsic compression (e.g., vascular ring)
- Intrinsic obstruction (e.g., malformation, foreign body, cyst, tumor)
- Airways reactive to other stimuli (e.g., allergens, infection)
- Infection; inflammation; cystic fibrosis; pertussis; asthma; other
- "Central" events (e.g., central apnea; "cough tic")

Neurobehavioral Symptoms (Sandifer's syndrome, seizure-like spells)
- Seizures
- Dystonic reaction to drugs
- Vestibular disorders
- Early pertussis

Adapted from Orenstein SR: Gastroesophageal reflux. *In* Stockman JA II, Winter RJ, eds: Current Problems in Pediatrics. Chicago, Year Book Medical Publishers, May/June 1991; 21(5):223; with permission.

within a year or two. Thus, the use of antireflux measures and, when required, pharmacologic therapy will often result in the gratifying resolution of disease in these younger patients.

Stepwise augmentation of therapeutic intensity begins with conservative antireflux measures, and continues with a prokinetic agent if pathologic reflux is documented. Acid-reducing therapy is added in that majority of patients in whom esophagitis is present. Surgical management is reserved for serious manifestations unresponsive to maximal nonsurgical therapy or for intractable disease persisting beyond 18 to 24 months of age (Table 26–8).

Antireflux Measures

Initial treatment of reflux typically involves body positioning and dietary measures.

Positioning

Infants. In the past, the recommendation for infants as well as older patients was to remain upright to

Table 26–8. THERAPY FOR REFLUX

Conservative
- Position: prone or completely upright; avoid supine, semiseated
- Thicken infant feedings; 1 tbsp. dry rice cereal/oz formula (= 30cal/oz, if original formula is 20 cal/oz)
- Fast before bed
- Avoid large meals, obesity, tight clothing
- Avoid foods and medications that lower LES tone or increase gastric acidity: fatty foods, citrus, tomato, carbonated beverages, coffee, alcohol, smoke exposure, anticholinergics, adrenergics, xanthines including theophylline, caffeine and calcium channel blockers, prostaglandins

Pharmacologic*
- Prokinetic
  - Metoclopramide (0.1 mg/kg/dose qid: 0–30 min AC, HS) {restlessness, drowsiness, dystonic reactions—antidote: diphenhydramine} {{gastrointestinal obstruction, perforation, hemorrhage; pheochromocytoma; extrapyramidal risk}}
  - Bethanechol (0.1–0.3 mg/kg/dose tid or qid: 30–60 min AC, HS) {cholinergic: hypotension, flushing, headache, bronchospasm, salivation, abdominal cramping} {{urinary or gastrointestinal obstruction, perforation, hemorrhage, recent surgery, peritonitis; hypotension, bradycardia, epilepsy, asthma, hyperthyroidism, peptic ulcer}}
  - Domperidone (0.2–0.3–?0.6 mg/kg/dose tid or qid: AC, HS)—drug not available in United States
  - Cisapride (0.3 mg/kg/dose tid: AC)—drug not available in United States
- Antacid
  - Cimetidine (5–10 mg/kg/dose qid: AC, HS) {headache, confusion, pancytopenia, gynecomastia, cholestasis}
  - Ranitidine (2 mg/kg/dose tid) {similar to cimetidine; less gynecomastia, more hepatitis}
  - Famotidine, nizatidine (new, incompletely defined H_2 antagonists: adult, 40 mg HS, 300 mg HS, respectively)
  - Omepazole (new, incompletely defined H^+ pump blocker: adult, 20 mg HS)
  - Antacids (0.5–1 ml/kg/dose, 3–8× a day: 1–2 hr PC, HS) {diarrhea, constipation}
- Barrier or miscellaneous mechanism
  - Sucralfate slurry (1 gm in 5–15 ml solution, qid: PC, HS)—protects against bile salts, trypsin, acid {constipation, gastric concretions, potential binding of other medications}
  - Alaginic acid-antacid (2 gm 3–8× a day: PC)

Surgical
- Fundoplication: complete vs. loose wrap; ± gastrostomy, ± pyloroplasty
- Angelchik prosthesis

*Usual course is 8 weeks.
( )Common doses
{ }Partial list of side effects.
{{ }}Partial list of contraindications.
From Orenstein SR; Gastroesophageal reflux. *In* Stockman JA II, Winter RJ, eds: Current Problems in Pediatrics. Chicago, Year Book Medical Publishers, May/June 1991; 21(5):224; with permission.

minimize reflux. However, it has been established that poor truncal tone actually makes seated positioning detrimental[342]; thus, prone positioning is desirable whenever infants with reflux are not being held strictly vertical by their caretakers. Although elevation at the head of the bed has been recommended for infants in the prone position,[293, 343] a large controlled study failed to show a significant benefit of such head elevation when compared with a simple flat prone position.[360] In addition to decreasing reflux, a prone position improves gastric emptying,[291] decreases aspiration,[361] decreases energy expenditure,[362] decreases crying time,[363] and has numerous beneficial effects on respiratory disease; however, it does not change LES tone[364] compared with the supine position. The right-side-down lateral position has theoretical advantages, such as augmentation of gastric emptying as well as separating gastric contents from the gastroesophageal junction, but this position has not been definitively compared with prone position.

Children. For older children, optimal positioning is probably standing or sitting upright while awake and sleeping prone, possibly with the head of the bed elevated. At any age, the prone position is preferable to the supine during recumbency; supine positions, including supine-seated positions, worsen reflux, as do head-down positions.[227, 293, 342] Thus, chest physiotherapy that requires provocative positions is probably best performed fasting and perhaps with antacid pretreatment. Chronically ventilated patients may benefit from prone in preference to supine positioning, in spite of the technical difficulties with head positioning in such patients.

Diet

Thickening of Infant Formula. Thickening of formula has been recommended for years as therapy for infants with reflux. Usually rice cereal is added to milk formula in a concentration that requires enlarging the nipple to allow adequate flow. Although this therapy has not been shown by pH probe or by scintigraphic evaluation to decrease reflux,[112, 365] it does decrease the number and total volume of emeses.[112, 227] Since such thickening also diminishes crying (and therefore probably energy expenditure) and increases the caloric density of the formula, it is ideal therapy for infants with nutritional deficits due to regurgitant reflux.[112] Although infants are not able to retain all the extra energy and nitrogen supplied in the cereal,[366] infants with regurgitant reflux improve their weight accretion during such therapy. Whether it should also be used for nonregurgitant reflux, particularly that associated with respiratory symptoms, is not yet resolved.[112, 365] Although not observed in a very short-term study,[366] the main side effect is constipation.

Small and Frequent Feedings. Small, frequent meals are recommended because of the probable correlation between gastric volume and reflux quantity.[367] It is possible, however, that the frequency of feedings might counteract the benefits of the small feedings by converting more time to the postprandial period, in which most reflux occurs. This is a complex issue, with no clear answers at present. A reasonable approach is to recommend smaller, more frequent feedings for those infants who are being given unusually large volumes at infrequent feedings.

Fasting several hours before bedtime in the older child is relatively simple to implement and is uncontroversial, except perhaps in children with very poor nutrition.

Other Dietary Measures. In older pediatric patients, weight reduction in the obese and avoidance of foods known to have detrimental effects on LES tone or on gastric acidity are frequently suggested. These foods include fatty foods, acid foods (such as many citrus juices, carbonated beverages, and tomato products), coffee, and alcohol. Compliance with these recommendations is probably limited.

Other Conservative Measures

Additional measures that can be used in infants and children as well as in adults are avoidance of tight clothing and elimination of exposure to secondhand smoke and to unnecessary drugs that are known to exacerbate reflux.

Pharmacologic Therapy

Medications are usually not added to the treatment regimen unless pathologic reflux has been demonstrated. These drugs consist of prokinetic agents, which augment sphincter pressure and may also increase gastric emptying, and acid-reducing agents, which counteract the major known injurious component of gastric contents.

Prokinetic Agents

For children in whom pathologic gastroesophageal reflux has been demonstrated, the use of a prokinetic agent has theoretical support. Although, to date, no agent has been shown to decrease the frequency of LES relaxations (the major mechanism for the occurrence of reflux episodes), the abilities of prokinetic agents to raise tonic sphincter pressure, improve esophageal clearance, and speed gastric emptying are desirable.

Bethanechol. Bethanechol, a cholinergic drug, was the first such agent used in children.[6] Its augmentation of sphincter pressure,[6] esophageal peristaltic amplitude and duration,[367a] and salivary flow has obvious clinical relevance, although clinical results have been mixed.[368–371] Its potential for exacerbating bronchospasm limits its use in children with respiratory symptoms. It is probably not the best initial prokinetic agent to use.

Metoclopramide. Metoclopramide, a dopamine antagonist, raises LES pressure and improves gastric emptying as well as esophageal peristalsis, but does not increase salivation or bronchospasm. However, as with bethanechol, results of trials of metoclopramide in children have been mixed,[372–374] and the narrow margin of error between therapeutic effect and central nervous system side effects[375, 375a] mandates caution in its use. Nonetheless, many pediatric gastroenterologists currently use it as the initial prokinetic agent.

Domperidone. Published experience with domperidone, a peripheral dopamine antagonist, is even more limited in children than in adults, and this drug is unlikely to have advantages over other, more thoroughly studied agents.[376, 377]

Cisapride. Early experience with cisapride, a noncholinergic, nonantidopaminergic agent that enhances postganglionic acetylcholine release, has been favorable in children, and it may supersede the other agents as more familiarity with it is gained.[32, 378–381]

Acid-Reducing Agents

Because a relationship has been demonstrated between esophageal acid exposure and esophagitis in infants,[71] it is reasonable to treat infants who have esophagitis with acid-reducing therapies. Such therapies include antisecretory and acid-neutralizing drugs.

Antisecretory. Histamine-receptor (H_2) antagonists have been used successfully in children.[382] The most extensive experience is with cimetidine, but ranitidine and newer related drugs (famotidine and nizatidine) have also been used.[74] The less frequent dosing schedules of the latter drugs make them attractive alternatives to cimetidine.

Omeprazole, a new agent that blocks the proton pump in the acid-secreting parietal cell, results in far more complete blockage of acid secretion than do the histamine-receptor antagonists, which block only the histamine receptors on the parietal cell, leaving the gastrin receptors and cholinergic input unaffected. It has been effective in otherwise intractable esophagitis in adults, but problems of rapid relapse on withdrawal and concerns about safety limit its usefulness in children for the present.[383]

Acid-Neutralizing. Although it has been suggested that antacids are as efficacious as H_2-receptor antagonists for treatment of esophagitis in young children,[384] the reported frequency of administration (seven or more doses per day) makes compliance unlikely, and the large dose raises concern about potential side effects.[385, 386]

A good strategy is to use H_2-receptor blockade for children with demonstrated esophagitis. Antacids can be used as supplemental therapy for symptoms of pain, as primary therapy for children who would benefit from their constipating (aluminum) or stool-softening (magnesium) features, or as short-term empiric therapy when esophagitis has not been documented. The use of cimetidine as the antisecretory agent simplifies the dosing schedule for patients who are taking four daily doses of a prokinetic agent.

Mucosal Protective Agents

In tablet or suspension, sucralfate has been shown in one study involving children to be comparable with cimetidine, although the dose of the latter was low.[387] Sucralfate may prove to be a useful agent, particularly in children with severe esophagitis encompassing erosions or ulcerations, but data are still limited.

Explorations of the efficacy of alginic acid–antacid compounds in children are similarly scarce as well as contradictory.[388–390]

The intriguing suggestion that indomethacin may augment esophageal cytoprotection[85] implies a possible therapeutic role; its opposite effect on gastric mucosa, however, severely limits its potential utility.

Surgical Therapy

Fundoplication

Surgical therapy is used in children with severe or intractable symptoms. Fundoplication is the most reliable way to prevent reflux. Nissen fundoplication (Fig. 26–13)[391] increases LES pressure in children,[7, 392] but its efficacy in preventing reflux is not necessarily related to the rise in sphincter pressure.[393, 394] Function of the fundal wrap as a valve, for example, may also play a role.[395]

Older children. In neurologically normal older children with reflux-related respiratory symptoms or esophagitis, medical treatment of the reflux is usually effective, but the symptoms often recur when such therapy is discontinued. For such patients the alternatives of chronic medical therapy and surgical fundoplication can be debated if relapse occurs.

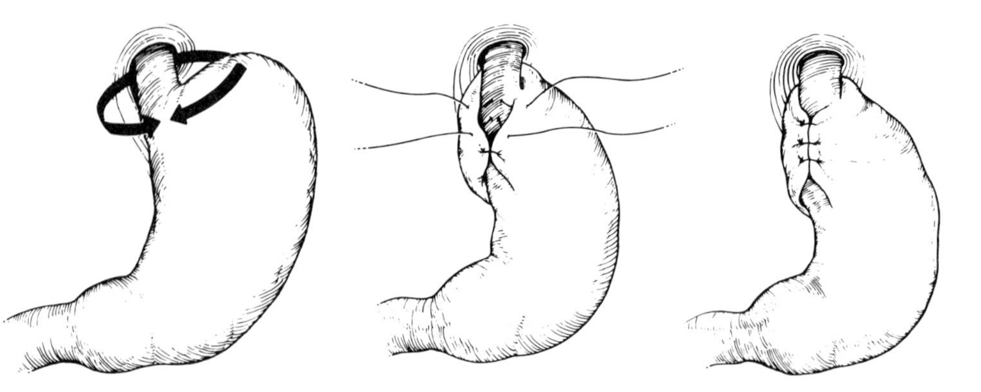

Figure 26–13. Diagram of a Nissen fundoplication. (From Schatzlein MH, Ballantine TVN, Thirunavukkarasu S, et al: Gastroesophageal reflux in infants and children. Arch Surg 1979; 114:505–510. Copyright 1979, American Medical Association; with permission.)

Groups Frequently Requiring Fundoplication. There are several groups of children with reflux disease who have been more likely to require fundoplication.[396–398] These include children with neurologic deficits, peptic strictures, or gastrostomy tube feedings.[399–402] Other children who frequently require surgery are those with respiratory symptoms associated with intractable reflux, such as those with repaired esophageal atresia or BPD.[190, 403, 404]

Neurologically devastated children with reflux are frequently chronically supine, have increased abdominal pressure due to spasticity, and have poor oropharyngeal handling of food. They are thus susceptible to aspiration during feeding as well as to reflux-induced respiratory symptoms. Although percutaneous gastrostomy feedings have been used for nutrition in such patients, a gastrostomy tube combined with fundoplication is often the optimal treatment. Infants with BPD may require fundoplication because their provocative positioning, chronic ventilator dependency, need for nasogastric feedings, disturbed thoracoabdominal pressure relationships, and aggravating medications make them resistant to medical managements of reflux.

Success Rate. Most pediatric series report the reduction or elimination of reflux in more than 90% of patients. Accurate preoperative identification of reflux as the cause of the symptoms is crucial: Some failures of surgical therapy have resulted from an incorrect assumption that reflux was the source of the symptoms in need of therapy.[397, 405]

Complications. Although surgical success rates are high, both short- and long-term complications are frequent and are more common in children with neurologic deficits or strictures.[396, 400, 402] Complications include herniation of the wrap through the hiatus, small bowel obstruction due to adhesions, and intraperitoneal leakage through an associated gastrostomy.[406–408] Long-term problems include gas bloat, inability to burp or vomit when necessary, and dysphagia.[409, 410] Problems related to gastric emptying include dumping (rapid emptying) and retching due to delayed emptying.[47]

Preventive strategies for these complications include the use of an intraluminal bougie during surgery; attention to crural closure and fixation of the wrap to the crura and diaphragm; pyloromyotomy in patients with preoperative gastric stasis; and avoidance of trauma to intestinal serosa or liver capsule.[406, 410]

"Loose" or Thal fundoplications are applicable in patients with esophageal dysmotility, such as esophageal atresia, but not in those with neurologic disability or feeding gastrostomies.[405, 411–413] A gastrostomy for feeding and venting is useful in those children in whom dysfunctional swallow contributes to respiratory disease and for those in whom gas bloat may be a problem; a gastrostomy is often performed in infants to protect the wrap postoperatively, even if its later closure is anticipated.

Crural Repair

Hiatal hernia is not repaired unless it is associated with complications, intractable reflux being the most common. Thus, crural repair is undertaken as part of an antireflux procedure, generally incorporating fundoplication.

Angelchik Antireflux Prosthesis

A decade ago, the Angelchik prosthesis, a C-shaped silicone-filled ring, was developed as an antireflux appliance for placement around the esophagus below the diaphragm. It was rigorously studied in children as small as 35 pounds several years ago, after having been used in more than 20,000 patients.[414] It produced improvement in reflux similar to Nissen fundoplication in the 22 patients who were randomized to receive it and required 30% less anesthesia time. Reported complications have included intra-abdominal migration and erosion through the stomach. Its role as therapy for pediatric reflux remains unclear.

REFERENCES

1. Jolley SG, Herbst JJ, Johnson DJ, et al: Postcibal gastroesophageal reflux in children. J Pediatr Surg 1981; 16:487–490.
2. Jolley SG, Johnson DJ, Herbst JJ, et al: The significance of gastroesophageal reflux patterns in children. J Pediatr Surg 1981; 16:859–865.
3. Vandenplas Y, DeWold D, Deneyer M, et al: Incidence of gastroesophageal reflux in sleep, awake, fasted, and postcibal periods in asymptomatic and symptomatic infants. J Pediatr Gastroenterol Nutr 1988; 7:177–180.
4. Dreizzen E, Escourrou P, Odievre M, et al: Esophageal reflux in symptomatic and asymptomatic infants: Postprandial and circadian variations. J Pediatr Gastroenterol Nutr 1990; 10:316–321.
5. Zaninotto G, DeMeester TR, Schwizer W, et al: The lower esophageal sphincter in health and disease. Am J Surg 1988; 155:104–111.
6. Moroz SP, Espinoza J, Cumming WA, et al: Lower esophageal sphincter function in children with and without gastroesophageal reflux. Gastroenterology 1976; 71:236–241.
7. Euler AR, Ament ME: Value of esophageal manometric studies in the gastroesophageal reflux of infancy. Pediatrics 1977; 59:58–61.
8. Euler AR, Ament ME: Decreased lower esophageal sphincter pressure in children with symptoms of gastroesophageal reflux. Am J Dis Child 1978; 132:528–529.
9. Christie DL, O'Grady LR, Mack DV: Incompetent lower esophageal sphincter and gastroesophageal reflux in recurrent acute pulmonary disease of infancy and childhood. J Pediatr 1978; 93:23–27.
10. Dodds WJ, Dent J, Hogan WJ, et al: Mechanisms of gastroesophageal reflux in patients with reflux esophagitis. N Engl J Med 1982; 307:1547–1552.
11. Dent J, Holloway RH, Toouli J, et al: Mechanisms of lower oesophageal sphincter incompetence in patients with symptomatic gastroesophageal reflux. Gut 1988; 29:1020–1028.
12. Eastwood GL, Castell DO, Higgs RH: Experimental esophagitis in cats impairs lower esophageal sphincter pressure. Gastroenterology 1975; 69:146–153.
13. Dent J: Recent views on the pathogenesis of gastro-esophageal reflux disease. Ballieres Clin Gastroenterol 1987;1:727–745.
14. Castell DO: The lower esophageal sphincter: Physiologic and clinical aspects. Ann Intern Med 1975; 83:390–401.
15. Dent J, Dodds WJ, Hogan WJ, et al: Factors that influence induction of gastroesophageal reflux in normal human subjects. Dig Dis Sci 1988; 33:270–275.
16. Hillemeier AC, Grill BB, McCallum R, et al: Esophageal and

gastric motor abnormalities in gastroesophageal reflux during infancy. Gastroenterology 1983; 84:741–746.
17. Dent J: A new technique for continuous sphincter pressure measurement. Gastroenterology 1976; 71:263–267.
18. Werlin SL, Dodds WJ, Hogan WJ, et al: Mechanisms of gastroesophageal reflux in children. J Pediatr 1980; 97:244–249.
19. Dent J, Davidson GP, Barnes BE, et al: The mechanism of gastro-oesophageal reflux in children. Aust Paediatr J 1981; 17:125
20. McNally EF, Kelly JE, Ingelfinger FJ: Mechanism of belching: Effects of gastric distension with air. Gastroenterology 1964; 46:254–259.
21. Wyman JB, Dent J, Heddle R, et al: Control of belching by the lower oesophageal sphincter. Gut 1990; 31:639–646.
22. Patrikios J, Martin CJ, Dent J: Relationship of transient lower esophageal sphincter relaxation to postprandial gastroesophageal reflux and belching in dogs. Gastroenterology 1986; 90:545–551.
23. Mittal RK, McCallum RW: Characteristics of transient lower esophageal sphincter relaxation in humans. Am J Physiol 1987; 252:G636-G641.
24. Mittal RK, McCallum RW: Characteristics and frequency of transient relaxations of the lower esophageal sphincter in patients with reflux esophagitis. Gastroenterology 1988; 95:593–599.
25. Holloway RH, Kocyan P, Dent J: Meals provoke gastroesophageal reflux by increasing the rate of transient lower esophageal sphincter relaxations. Gastroenterology 1989; 96:A214.
26. Freidin N, Fisher M, Boyd D, et al: Pattern of sleep and acid reflux in normal subjects and gastroesophageal reflux patients. Gastroenterology 1989; 96:A158.
27. Cucchiara S, Staiano A, DiLorenzo C, et al: Pathophysiology of gastroesophageal reflux and distal esophageal motility in children with gastroesophageal reflux disease. J Pediatr Gastroenterol Nutr 1988; 7:830–836.
28. Martin CJ, Patrikios J, Dent J: Abolition of gas reflux and transient lower esophageal sphincter relaxation by vagal blockade in the dog. Gastroenterology 1986; 91:890–896.
29. Holloway RH, Wyman JB, Dent J: Failure of transient lower oesophageal sphincter relaxation in response to gastric distention in patients with achalasia: Evidence for neural mediation of transient lower oesophageal sphincter relaxations. Gut 1989; 30:762–767.
30. Goyal RK, Paterson WG: Esophageal motility. *In* Wood JD, Schultz SG, eds: Handbook of Physiology, Section 6: The Gastrointestinal System, Vol 1: Motility and Circulation. New York, Oxford University Press, 1989, pp 865–908.
31. Cox MR, Martin CJ, Dent J: Postural suppression of transient lower esophageal sphincter relaxations is not mediated by gastric fluid receptors in the dog. Gastroenterology 1987; 92:1357.
32. Vandeplas Y, Deneyer M, Verlinden M, et al: Gastroesophageal reflux incidence and respiratory dysfunction during sleep in infants: Treatment with cisapride. J Pediatr Gastroenterol Nutr 1989; 8:31–36.
33. Cotton BR, Smith G: The lower oesophageal sphincter and anaesthesia. Br J Anaesth 1984; 56:37–46.
34. Altorki NK, Skinner DB: Pathophysiology of gastroesophageal reflux. Am J Med 1989; 86:685–689.
35. Santos GH: Is hiatus hernia responsible for reflux? Chest 1983; 84:242–244.
36. Boyle JT, Altschuler SM, Nixon TE, et al: Role of the diaphragm in the genesis of lower esophageal sphincter pressure in the cat. Gastroenterology 1985; 88:723–730.
37. Altschuler SM, Boyle JT, Nixon TE, et al: Simultaneous reflex inhibition of lower esophageal sphincter and crural diaphragm in cats. Am J Physiol 1985; 249:G586–591.
38. Mittal RK, Rochester DR, McCallum RW: Effect of the diaphragmatic contraction on lower oesophageal sphincter pressure in man. Gut 1987; 28:1564–1568.
39. Mittal RK, Rochester DF, McCallum RW: Electrical and mechanical activity in the human lower esophageal sphincter during diaphragmatic contraction. J Clin Invest 1988; 81:1182–1189.
40. Mittal RK, Rochester DF, McCallum RW: Sphincteric action of the diaphragm during a relaxed lower esophageal sphincter in humans. Am J Physiol 1989; 256:G139–G144.
41. Mittal RK, Fisher M, Sluss J: Electrical and mechanical inhibition of the crural diaphragm during transient relaxation of the lower esophageal sphincter. Gastroenterol 1989; 96:A347.
42. Dev NB, Boyle JT: Phasic contraction of the diaphragm during respiration impedes its role in the gastroesophageal antireflux barrier. Gastroenterology 1989; 96:A120.
43. Marino WD, Jain NK, Pitchumoni CS: Induction of lower esophageal sphincter (LES) dysfunction during use of the negative pressure body ventilator. Am J Gastroenterol 1988; 83:1376–1380.
44. Muler-Lissner SA, Blum AL: Fundic pressure rise lowers lower esophageal sphincter pressure in man. Hepato-gastroenterology 1982; 29:151–152.
45. Hillemeier AC, Lange R, McCallum R, et al: Delayed gastric emptying in infants with gastroesophageal reflux. J Pediatr 1981; 98:190–193.
46. Lin C-H, Tolia V, Kuhns LR, et al: Role of gastric emptying in infants with complicated gastroesophageal reflux. Pediatr Res 1989; 25:118A.
47. Jolley SG, Leonard JC, Tunnell WP: Gastric emptying in children with gastroesophageal reflux. I. An estimate of effective gastric emptying. J Pediatr Surg 1987; 22:923–926.
48. Euler AR, Byrne WJ: Gastric emptying times of water in infants and children: Comparison of those with and without gastroesophageal reflux. J Pediatr Gastroenterol Nutr 1983; 2:595–598.
49. DiLorenzo C, Piepsz A, Ham H, et al: Gastric emptying with gastro-oesophageal reflux. Arch Dis Child 1987; 62:449–453.
50. Jackson PT, Glasgow JFT, Thomas PS, et al: Children with gastroesophageal reflux with or without partial thoracic stomach (hiatal hernia) have normal gastric emptying. J Pediatr Gastroenterol Nutr 1989; 8:37–40.
51. Behar J, Ramsby G: Gastric emptying and antral motility in reflux esophagitis. Gastroenterology 1978, 74:253–256.
52. Sutphen JL, Dillard VL: Dietary caloric density and osmolality influence gastroesophageal reflux in infants. Gastroenterology 1989; 97:601–604.
53. Helm JF, Dodds WJF, Riedel DR, et al: Determinants of esophageal acid clearance in normal subjects. Gastroenterology 1983; 85:607–612.
54. Helm JF, Dodds WJ, Pelc LR, et al: Effect of esophageal emptying and saliva on clearance of acid from the esophagus. N Engl J Med 1984; 310:284–288.
55. Ferguson MK, Ryan JW, Little AG, et al: Esophageal emptying and acid neutralization in patients with symptoms of esophageal reflux. Ann Surg 1985; 201:728–735.
56. Little AG, DeMeester TR, Kirchner PT, et al: Pathogenesis of esophagitis in patients with gastroesophageal reflux. Surgery 1980; 88:101–107.
57. Sondheimer JM: Clearance of spontaneous gastroesophageal reflux in awake and sleeping infants. Gastroenterology 1989; 97:821–826.
58. Dent J, Dodds WJ, Friedman RH, et al: Mechanism of gastroesophageal reflux in recumbent asymptomatic human subjects. J Clin Invest 1980; 65:256–267.
59. Masden T, Wallin L, Boesby S, et al: Spontaneous peristaltic activity in the oesophagus after imitated acid gastro-oesophageal reflux: A study in normal subjects. Scand J Gastroenterol 1982; 17:811–815.
60. Carron DA, Massey BT, Dodds WJ, et al: Heartburn, but not esophageal acidification, per se, increases the rate of spontaneous swallowing. Gastroenterology 1989; 96:A74.
61. Masden T, Wallin L, Boesby S, et al: Oesophageal peristalsis in normal subjects: Influence of pH and volume during imitated gastro-oesophageal reflux. Scand J Gastroenterol 1983; 18:513–518.
62. Cucchiara S, Staiano A, DiLorenzo C, et al: Esophageal motor abnormalities in children with gastroesophageal reflux and peptic esophagitis. J Pediatr 1986; 108:907–910.
63. Allen ML, McIntosh DL, Robinson MG: Healing or amelioration of esophagitis does not result in increased lower esophageal sphincter contractile pressure. Am J Gastroenterol 1990; 85:1331–1334.
64. Kahrilas PF, Dodds WJ, Hogan WJ: Effect of peristaltic dysfunction on esophageal volume clearance. Gastroenterology 1988; 94:73–80.
65. Waters PF, DeMeester TR: Foregut motor disorders and their surgical management. Med Clin North Am 1981; 65:1235–1268.
66. Allen ML, Orr WC, Woodruff DM, et al: The effects of swallowing frequency and transdermal scopolamine on esophageal acid clearance. Am J Gastroenterol 1985; 80:669–672.
67. Pope CE II: Gastroesophageal reflux disease (reflux esophagitis).

In Sleisenger M, Fordtran, J, eds: Gastrointestinal Disease: Pathophysiology, Diagnosis, Management. Philadelphia, WB Saunders, 1983, p 453.
68. Helm JF, Dodds WJ, Hogan WJ: Salivary response to esophageal acid in normal subjects and patients with reflux esophagitis. Gastroenterology 1987; 93:1393–1397.
69. Sonnenberg A, Steinkamp U, Weise A, et al: Salivary secretion in reflux esophagitis. Gastroenterology 1982; 83:889–895.
70. Dodds WJ, Hogan WJ, Helm JF, et al: Pathogenesis of reflux esophagitis. Gastroenterology 1981; 81:376–394.
71. Vandenplas Y, Franckx-Goossens A, Pipeleers-Marichal M: Area under pH 4: Advantages of a new parameter in the interpretation of esophageal pH monitoring data. J Pediatr Gastroenterol Nutr 1989; 9:34–39.
72. Agha FP: Esophageal involvement in Zollinger-Ellison syndrome. AJR 1985; 144:721–725.
73. Collen MJ, Lewis JH, Benjamin SB: Gastric acid hypersecretion in refractory gastroesophageal reflux disease. Gastroenterology 1990; 98:654–661.
74. Klinkenberg-Knol EC, Jansen JM, Festen HP, et al: Double-blind multicentre comparison of omeprazole and ranitidine in the treatment of reflux oesophagitis. Lancet 1987; 1:349–351.
75. Yahav J: Development of parietal cells, acid secretion, and response to secretagogues. *In* Lebenthal E, ed: Human Gastrointestinal Development. New York, Raven Press, 1989, pp 341–351.
76. Cavell B: Postprandial gastric acid secretion in infants. Acta Paediatr Scand 1983; 72:857–860.
77. Hyman PE, Clarke DD, Everett SL, et al: Gastric acid secretory function in preterm infants. J Pediatr 1985; 106:467–470.
78. Agunod M, Yamaguchi N, Lopez R, et al: Correlative study of hydrochloric acid, pepsin, and intrinsic factor secretion in newborns and infants. Am J Dig Dis 1969; 14:400–414.
79. Sondheimer JM, Clark DA, Gervaise EP: Continuous gastric pH measurement in young and older healthy preterm infants receiving formula and clear liquid feedings. J Pediatr Gastroenterol Nutr 1985; 4:352–355,
80. Sutphen JL, Dillard VL: Effects of maturation and gastric acidity on gastroesophageal reflux in infants. Am J Dis Child 1986; 140:1062–1064.
81. Orlando RC, Bryson JC, Powell DW: Mechanisms of H^+ injury in rabbit esophageal epithelium. Am J Physiol 1984; 246:G718–G724.
82. Gotley DC, Ball D, Cooper MJ: Enzymatic activity in the refluxate of patients with gastro-oesophageal reflux disease (GORD). Gastroenterology 1989; 96:A178.
83. Yahav J, Carrion V, Lee PC, et al: Meal-stimulated pepsinogen secretion in premature infants. J Pediatr 1987; 110:949–951.
84. Salo JA, Lehto V-P, Kivilaakso E: Morphological alterations in esophagitis: Light microscopic and scanning and transmission electron microscopic study. Dig Dis Sci 1983; 28:440–448 .
85. Stein BE, Schwartzman ML, Carroll MA, et al: Role of arachidonic acid metabolites in acid-pepsin injury to rabbit esophagus. Gastroenterology 1989; 97:278–283.
86. Mattioli S, Pilotti V, Felice V, et al: Ambulatory 24-hr pH monitoring of esophagus, fundus, and antrum: A new technique for simultaneous study of gastroesophageal and duodenogastric reflux. Dig Dis Sci 1990; 35: 929–938.
87. Gowen GF: Spontaneous enterogastric reflux gastritis and esophagitis. Ann Surg 1985; 201:170–175.
88. Little AG, Martinez EL, DeMeester TR, et al: Duodenogastric reflux and reflux esophagitis. Surgery 1984; 96:447–454.
89. Evander A, Little AG, Riddell RH, et al: Composition of the refluxed material determines the degree of reflux esophagitis in the dog. Gastroenterology 1987; 93:280–286.
90. Suchy FJ: Development of bile formation and hepatic excretory function. *In* Lebenthal E, ed: Human Gastrointestinal Development. New York, Raven Press, 1989, 623–647.
91. Lillemoe KD, Johnson LF, Harmon JW: Alkaline esophagitis: A comparison of the ability of components of gastroduodenal contents to injure the rabbit esophagus. Gastroenterology 1983; 85:621–628.
92. Lalyre Y, Schmidt L, Buschmann R, et al: Early morphologic changes in the esophageal mucosa injured by bile salts. Gastroenterology 1984; 86:1149.
93. Salo JA, E Kivilaakso: Contribution of trypsin and cholate to the pathogenesis of experimental alkaline reflux esophagitis. Scand J Gastroenterol 1984; 19:875–881.
94. Lebenthal E, Lee PC: Development of functional response in human exocrine pancreas. Pediatrics 1980; 66:556–560.
95. Schulze-Delrieu K: Tryptic esophagitis. Gastroenterology 1984; 88:2004.
96. Orlando RC: Esophageal epithelial resistance. *In* Castell DO, Ott DJ, eds: Gastro-Esophageal Reflux Disease. Mount Kisco, NY, Futura Publishing, 1985, pp 55–79.
97. Cook IJ, Dent J, Shannon S, et al: Measurement of upper esophageal sphincter pressure: Effect of acute emotional stress. Gastroenterology 1987; 93:526–532.
98. Kahrilas PJ, Dodds WJ, Dent J, et al: Effect of sleep, spontaneous gastroesophageal reflux, and a meal on upper esophageal sphincter pressure in normal human volunteers. Gastroenterology 1987; 92:466–471.
99. Davidson GP, Dent J, Willing J: Monitoring of upper oesophaeal sphincter pressure in children. Gut 1991; 32:607–611.
100. Gerhardt DC, Shuck TJ, Bordeaux RA, et al: Human upper esophageal sphincter: Response to volume, osmotic, and acid stimuli. Gastroenterology 1978; 75:268–274.
101. Winship DH: Upper esophageal sphincter: Does it care about reflux? Gastroenterology 1983; 85:470–472.
102. Kahrilas PJ, Dent J, Dodds WJ, et al: A method for continuous monitoring of upper esophageal sphincter pressure. Dig Dis Sci 1987; 32:121–128.
103. Sondheimer JM: Upper esophageal sphincter and pharyngo-esophageal motor function in infants with and without gastroesophageal reflux. Gastroenterology 1983; 85:301–305.
104. Ulshen MH: Gastroesophageal reflux in infancy (selected summaries). Gastroenterology 1988; 95:534–539.
105. Orenstein SR: Effect of behavior state on infant gastroesophageal reflux frequency. Pediatr Res 1989; 25:121A.
106. Carre IJ: A historical review of the clinical consequences of hiatal hernia (partial thoracic stomach) and gastroesophageal reflux. *In* Gellis S, ed: Gastroesophageal Reflux: Report of the 76th Ross Conference on Pediatric Research. Columbus, OH, Ross Laboratories, 1979, pp 1–12.
107. Shepherd RW, Wren J, Evans S, et al: Gastroesophageal reflux in children: Clinical profile, course and outcome with active therapy in 126 cases. Clin Pediatr 1987; 26:55–60.
108. Black DD, Haggitt RC, Orenstein SR, et al: Esophagitis in infants: morphometric histologic diagnosis and correlation with measures of gastroesophageal reflux. Gastroenterology 1990; 98:1408–1414.
109. Shub MD, Ulshen MH, Hargrive CB, et al: Esophagitis: A frequent consequence of gastroesophageal reflux in infancy. J Pediatr 1985; 107:881–884.
110. Hyams JS, Ricci A Jr, Leichtner AM: Clinical and laboratory correlates of esophagitis in young children. J Pediatr Gastroenterol Nutr 1988; 7:52–56.
111. Orenstein SR, Deneault LG, Lutz JW, et al: Regurgitant reflux, in contrast to nonregurgitant reflux, is associated with rectus abdominus contraction in infants. Gastroenterology 1991; 100:A135.
112. Orenstein SR, Magill HL, Brooks P: Thickening of infant feedings for therapy of gastroesophageal reflux. J Pediatr 1987; 110:181–186.
113. Paton JY, Nanayakkhara CS, Simpson H: Vomiting and gastro-oesophageal reflux. Arch Dis Child 1988; 63:837–838.
114. Vandenplas Y, Sacre-Smits L: Continuous 24-hour esophageal pH monitoring in 285 asymptomatic infants 0–15 months old. J Pediatr Gastroenterol Nutr 1987; 6:220–224.
115. Johnson LF, DeMeester TR: Twenty-four-hour pH monitoring of the distal esophagus: A quantitative measure of gastroesophageal reflux. Am J Gastroenterol 1974; 62:325–332.
116. Sondheimer JM: Continuous monitoring of distal esophageal pH: A diagnostic test for gastroesophageal reflux in infants. J Pediatr 1980; 96:804–807.
117. Ryan P, Lander M, Ong TH, et al: When does reflux oesophagitis occur with gastro-oesophageal reflux in infants? A clinical and endoscopic study, and correlation with outcome. Aust Paediatr J 1983; 19:90–93.
118. Catto-Smith AG, Machida H, Butzner JD, et al: The role of gastroesophageal reflux in pediatric dysphagia. J Pediatr Gastroenterol Nutr 1991; 12:159–165.

119. Triadafilopoulos G: Nonobstructive dysphagia in reflux esophagitis. Am J Gastroenterol 1989; 84:614–618.
120. Gill RC, Bowes KL, Murphy PD, et al: Esophageal motor abnormalities in gastroesophageal reflux and the effects of fundoplication. Gastroenterology 1986; 91:364–369.
121. Marshall JB, Gerhardt DC: Improvement in esophageal motor dysfunction with treatment of reflux esophagitis: A report of two cases. Am J Gastroenterol 1982; 77:351–353.
122. Barrett NR: The lower esophagus lined by columnar epithelium. Surgery 1957; 41:881–894.
123. Berardi RS, Devaiah KA: Barrett's esophagus. Surg Gynecol Obstet 1983; 156:521–538.
124. Bozymski EM, Herlihy KJ, Orlando RC: Barrett's esophagus. Ann Intern Med 1982; 97:103–107.
125. Winters C Jr, Spurling TJ, Chobanian SJ, et al: Barrett's esophagus: A prevalent, occult complication of gastroesophageal reflux disease. Gastroenterology 1987; 92:118–124.
126. Zimbalist EH, Kurtz RC: Prevalence of Barrett's esophagus. Gastroenterology 1984; 86:369–370.
127. Spechler SJ, Sperber H, Doos WG, et al: The prevalence of Barrett's esophagus in patients with chronic peptic esophageal strictures. Dig Dis Sci 1983; 28:769–774.
128. Tudor RB: Barrett's esophagus in children: 170 cases. *In* Report no. 4, Childhood Disease Registry, Q & R Clinic, Sep 1, 1988.
129. Dahms BB, Rothstein FC: Barrett's esophagus in children: A consequence of chronic gastroesophageal reflux. Gastroenterology 1984; 86:318–323.
130. Skinner DB: Controversies about Barrett's esophagus. Ann Thorac Surg 1990; 49:523–524.
131. Hassall E, Weinstein WM, Ament ME: Barrett's esophagus in childhood. Gastroenterology 1985; 89:1331–1337.
132. Lindahl H, Rintala R, Sariola H, et al: Cervical Barrett's esophagus: A common complication of gastric tube reconstruction. J Pediatr Surg 1990; 25:446–448.
133. Dahms BB, Greco MA, Strandjord SE, et al: Barrett's esophagus in three children after antileukemic chemotherapy. Cancer 1987; 60:2896–2900.
134. Saul SH: The myths and realities of Barrett's esophagus. Endosc Rev 1987; 1987(Sept/Oct):21–37.
135. Talley NJ, Cameron AJ, Shorter RG, et al: *Campylobacter pylori* and Barrett's esophagus. Mayo Clin Proc 1988; 63:1176–1180.
136. Graham DY: *Campylobacter pylori* and Barrett's esophagus. Mayo Clin Proc 1988; 63:1258–1260.
137. DeGiacomo C, Fiocca R, Villani L, et al: Barrett's ulcer and *Campylobacter*-like organisms infection in a child. J Pediatr Gastroenterol Nutr 1988; 7:766–768.
138. Chen YM, Gelfand DW, Ott DJ, et al: Barrett's esophagus as an extension of severe esophagitis: Analysis of radiologic signs in 29 cases. AJR 1985; 145:275–281.
139. Chernin MM, Amberg JR, Kogan FJ, et al: Efficacy of radiologic studies in the detection of Barrett's esophagus. AJR 1986; 147:257–260.
140. Yulish BS, Rothstein FC, Halpin TC: Radiographic findings in children and young adults with Barrett's esophagus. AJR 1987; 148:353–357.
141. Kohler B, Kohler G, Riemann JF: Spontaneous esophagotracheal fistula resulting from ulcer in heterotopic gastric mucosa. Gastroenterology 1988; 95:828–830.
142. Pearson FG, Cooper JD, Patterson GA, et al: Peptic ulcer in acquired columnar-lined esophagus: Results of surgical treatment. Ann Thorac Surg 1987; 43:241–244.
143. Diehl JT, Thomas L, Bloom MB, et al: Tracheoesophageal fistula associated with Barrett's ulcer: The importance of reflux control. Ann Thorac Surg 1988; 45:449–450.
144. Kothari T, Mangla JC, Kalra TMS: Barrett's ulcer and treatment with cimetidine. Arch Intern Med 1980; 140:475–477.
145. Spechler SJ, Robbins AH, Bloomfield H, et al: Adenocarcinoma and Barrett's esophagus: An overrated risk? Gastroenterology 1984; 87:927–933.
146. Cameron AJ, Ott BJ, Payne WS: The incidence of adenocarcinoma in columnar-lined (Barrett's) esophagus. N Engl J Med 1985; 313:857–859.
147. Cameron AJ, Higgins JA, Linear gastric erosion: A lesion associated with large diaphragmatic hernia and chronic blood loss anemia. Gastroenterology 1986; 91:338–342.
148. Hameeteman W, Tytgat GNJ, Houthoff JH, et al: Barrett's esophagus: Development of dysplasia and adenocarcinoma. Gastroenterology 1989; 96:1249–1256.
149. Hoeffel JC, Nihoul-Fekete C, Schmitt M: Esophageal adenocarcinoma after gastroesophageal reflux in children. J Pediatr 1989; 115:259–261.
150. Brand DL, Ylvisaker JT, Gelfand M, et al: Regression of columnar esophageal (Barrett's) epithelium after anti-reflux surgery. N Engl J Med 1980; 302:844–848.
151. Williamson WA, Ellis FH Jr, Gibb SP, et al: Effect of antireflux operation on Barrett's mucosa. Ann Thorac Surg 1990; 49:537–542.
152. Conti Nabali S, Barresi G, Tuccari G, et al: Barrett's esophagus in an infant: A long standing history with final postsurgical regression. J Pediatr Gastroenterol Nutr 1988; 7:602–607.
153. Hamilton SR, Hutcheon DF, Ravich WJ, et al: Adenocarcinoma in Barrett's esophagus after elimination of gastroesophageal reflux. Gastroenterology 1984; 86:356–360.
154. Nihoul-Fekete C, Mitrofanoff P, Lortat-Jacob S: Les stenoses peptiques de L'oesophage chez l'enfant. Ann Pediatr 1979; 26:692–698.
155. Lindor KD, Ott BJ, Hughes RW Jr: Balloon dilatation of upper digestive tract strictures. Gastroenterology 1985; 89:545–548.
156. Johnsen A, Jensen LI, Mauritzen K: Balloon-dilatation of esophageal strictures in children. Pediatr Radiol 1986; 16:388–391.
157. Patterson DJ, Graham DY, Lacey Smith J, et al: Natural history of benign esophageal stricture treated by dilatation. Gastroenterology 1983; 85:346–350.
158. Glick ME: Clinical course of esophageal stricture managed by bougienage. Dig Dis Sci 1982; 27:884–888.
159. Orenstein SR, Whitington PF: Esophageal stricture dilatation in awake children. J Pediatr Gastroenterol Nutr 1985; 4(4):557–562.
160. Sharma BB, Donovan GK, Miller KA, et al: Central nervous system infections following esophageal dilatation in children. J Pediatr 1987; 110:572–574.
161. McCallum RW, et al: Progress report on the American College of Gastroenterology Barrett's esophagus study. American College of Gastroenterology Annual Meeting. Toronto, Ontario, 1984.
162. Orenstein SR, Orenstein DM: Gastroesophageal reflux and respiratory disease in children. J Pediatr 1988; 112:847–858.
163. Ogura JH, Kawasaki M, Takenouchi S: Neurophysiologic observations on the adaptive mechanisms of deglutition. Ann Otol Rhinol Laryngol 1964; 73:1062–1082.
164. Carpenter DO: Central nervous system mechanisms in deglutition and emesis. *In* Wood JD, Schultz SG, eds: Handbook of Physiology, Section 6: The Gastrointestinal System, Vol 1: Motility and Circulation. New York, Oxford University Press, 1989, pp 685–714.
165. Putman PE, Ricker DH, Orenstein SR: Gastroesophageal reflux. *In* Beckerman R, Brouilette R, Hunt C, eds: Respiratory Control Disorders in Infants and Children. Baltimore, Williams & Wilkins, 1991, pp 322–341.
166. Smith J, Wolkove N, Colacone A, et al: Coordination of eating, drinking, and breathing in adults. Chest 1989; 96:578–582.
167. Barnes PJ: Neural control of human airways in health and disease. Am Rev Respir Dis 1986; 134:1289–1314.
168. Danus O, Casar C, Larrain A, et al: Esophageal reflux: An unrecognized cause of recurrent obstructive bronchitis in children. J Pediatr 1976; 89:220–224.
169. Euler AR, Byrne WJ, Ament ME, et al: Recurrent pulmonary disease in children: A complication of gastroesophageal reflux. Pediatrics 1979; 63:47–51.
170. Henderson RD, Wolfe CR: Aspiration and gastroesophageal reflux. Can J Surg 1978; 21:352–354.
171. Pellegrini CA, DeMeester TR, Johnson LF, et al: Gastroesophageal reflux and pulmonary aspiration: Incidence, functional abnormality, and results of surgical therapy. Surgery 1979; 86:110–119.
172. Wynne JW, Modell JH: Respiratory aspiration of stomach contents. Ann Intern Med 1977; 87:466–474.
173. Huxley EJ, Viroslav J, Gray WR, et al: Pharyngeal aspiration in normal adults and patients with depressed consciousness. Am J Med 1978; 64:564–568.
174. Crausaz FM, Favez G: Aspiration of solid food particles into

lungs of patients with gastroesophageal reflux and chronic bronchial disease. Chest 1988; 93:376–378.
175. Widdicombe JG: Respiratory reflexes from the trachea and bronchi of the cat. J Physiol 1954; 123:55–70.
176. Boushey HA, Richardson PS, Widdicombe JG: Reflex effects of laryngeal irritation on the pattern of breathing and total lung resistance. J Physiol 1972; 224:501–513.
177. Tuchman DN, Boyle JT, Pack AL, et al: Comparison of airway responses following tracheal or esophageal acidification in the cat. Gastroenterology 1984; 87:872–881.
178. Davis RS, Larsen GL, Grunstein MM: Respiratory response to intraesophageal acid infusion in asthmatic children during sleep. J Allergy Clin Immunol 1983; 72:393–398.
179. Spaulding HS, Mansfield LE, Stein MR, et al: Further investigation of the association between gastroesophageal reflux and bronchoconstriction. J Allergy Clin Immunol 1982; 69:516–521.
180. Mansfield LE, Stein MR: Gastroesophageal reflux and asthma: A possible reflex mechanism. Ann Allergy 1978; 41:224–226.
181. Kjellen G, Tibbling L, Wranne B: Bronchial obstruction after oesophageal acid perfusion in asthmatics. Clin Physiol 1981; 1:285–292.
182. Perpina M, Pellicer C, Marco V, et al: The significance of the reflex bronchoconstriction provoked by gastroesophageal reflux in bronchial asthma. Eur J Respir Dis 1985; 66:91–97.
183. Andersen LI, Schmidt A, Bundgaard A: Pulmonary function and acid application in the esophagus. Chest 1986; 90:358–363.
184. Herve P, Denjean A, Jian R, et al: Intraesophageal perfusion of acid increases the bronchomotor response to methacholine and to isocapnic hyperventilation in asthmatic subjects. Am Rev Respir Dis 1986; 134:986–989.
185. Mansfield LE, Hameister HH, Spaulding HS, et al: The rose of the vagus nerve in airway narrowing caused by intraesophageal hydrochloric acid provocation and esophageal distention. Ann Allergy 1981; 47:431–434.
186. Denjean A, Herve P, Simonneau G, et al: Effects of acid infusion into the esophagus on airflow obstruction and bronchial hyperreactivity in adult asthmatic patients. Chest 1985; 5(suppl):201S–202S.
187. Bendig DW, Seilheimer DK, Wagner ML, et al: Complications of gastroesophageal reflux in patients with cystic fibrosis. J Pediatr 1982; 100:536–540.
188. Scott RB, O'Loughlin EV, Gall DG: Gastroesophageal reflux in patients with cystic fibrosis. J Pediatr 1985; 106:223–227.
189. Vinocur CD, Marmon L, Schidlow DV, et al: Gastroesophageal reflux in the infant with cystic fibrosis. Am J Surg 1985; 149:182–186.
190. Hrabovsky EE, Mullett MD: Gastroesophageal reflux and the premature infant. J Pediatr Surg 1986; 21:583–587.
191. Boyle JT, Altschuler SM, Patterson BL, et al: Reflex inhibition of the lower esophageal sphincter (LES) following stimulation of pulmonary vagal afferent receptors. Gastroenterology 1986; 90:1353.
192. Mendelson CL: The aspiration of stomach contents into the lungs during obstetric anesthesia. Am J Obstet Gynecol 1946; 52:191–205.
193. Chernow B, Johnson LF, Janowitz WR, et al: Pulmonary aspiration as a consequence of gastroesophageal reflux: A diagnostic approach. Dig Dis Sci 1979; 24:839–844.
194. McVeagh P, Howman-Giles R, Kemp A: Pulmonary aspiration studied by radionuclide milk scanning and barium swallow roentgenography. Am J Dis Child 1987; 141:917–921.
195. Perlman LV, Lerner E, D'Esopo N: Clinical classification and analysis of 97 cases of lung abscess. Am Rev Respir Dis 1969; 99:390–398.
196. Knoblich R: Pulmonary granulomatosis caused by vegetable particles. Am Rev Respir Dis 1969; 99:390–398.
197. Hardy KA, Schidlow DV, Zaeri N: Obliterative bronchiolitis in children. Chest 1988; 93:460–466.
198. Pearson JEG, Wilson RSE: Diffuse pulmonary fibrosis and hiatus hernia. Thorax 1971; 26:300–305.
199. Mays ED, Dubiois JJ, Hamilton GB: Pulmonary fibrosis associated with tracheobronchial aspiration: A study of the frequency of hiatal hernia and gastroesophageal reflux in interstitial pulmonary fibrosis of obscure etiology. Chest 1976; 69:512–515.
200. McCauley RGK, Darling DB, Leonidas JC, et al: Gastroesophageal reflux in children: A useful classification and reliable physiologic technique for its demonstration. Am J Roentgenol 1978; 130:47–50.
201. Darling DB, McCauley RGK, Leonidas JC, et al: Gastroesophageal reflux in infants and children: Correlation of radiological severity and pulmonary pathology. Radiology 1978; 127:735–740.
202. Sondheimer JM, Morris BA: Gastroesophageal reflux among severely retarded children. J Pediatr 1979; 94:710–714.
203. Epstein PE: Aspiration diseases of the lungs. *In* Fishman A, ed: Pulmonary Diseases and Disorders. New York, McGraw-Hill, 1988, pp 877–892.
204. Bannister WK, Sattilaro AJ: Vomiting and aspiration during anesthesia. Anesthesiology 1962; 23:251–264.
205. Dines DE, Baker WG, Scantland WA: Aspiration pneumonitis—Mendelson's syndrome. JAMA 1961; 176:229–231.
206. Arms RA, Dines DE, Tinstman TC: Aspiration pneumonia. Chest 1974; 65:136–139.
207. Lorber B, Swenson RM: Bacteriology of aspiration pneumonia. Ann Intern Med 1974; 81:329–331.
208. Berquist WE, Rachelefsky GS, Kadden M, et al: Gastroesophageal reflux-associated recurrent pneumonia and chronic asthma in children. Pediatrics 1981; 68:29–35.
209. Shapiro GG, Christie DL: Gastroesophageal reflux in steroid-dependent asthmatic youths. Pediatrics 1979; 63:207–212.
210. Martin ME, Grunstein MM, Larsen GL: The relationship of gastroesophageal reflux to nocturnal wheezing in children with asthma. Ann Allergy 1982; 49:318–322.
211. Hoyoux C, Forget P, Lambrechts L, et al: Chronic bronchopulmonary disease and gastroesophageal reflux in children. Pediatr Pulmonol 1985; 1:149–153.
212. Baer M, Maki M, Nurminen J, et al: Esophagitis and findings of long-term esophageal pH recording in children with repeated lower respiratory tract symptoms. J Pediatr Gastroenterol Nutr 1986; 5:187–190.
213. Gustafsson PM, Kjellman NIM, Tibbling L: Oesophageal function and symptoms in moderate and severe asthma. Acta Paediatr Scand 1986; 75:729–736.
214. Bernstein A: Gastro-oesophageal reflux and bronchial asthma. Br J Dis Chest 1980; 74:420.
215. Bancewicz J, Bernstein A, Pierry A, et al: Surgery for gastro-oesophageal reflux in asthmatic patients. Br J Dis Chest 1981; 75:320.
216. Jolley SG, Herbst JJ, Johnson DG, et al: Esophageal pH monitoring during sleep identifies children with respiratory symptoms from gastroesophageal reflux. Gastroenterology 1981; 80:1501–1506.
217. Henderson-Smart DJ, Read DJC: Reduced lung volume during behavioral active sleep in the newborn. J Appl Physiol 1979; 46:1081–1085.
218. Henderson-Smart DJ, Read DJC: Depression of intercostal and abdominal muscle activity and vulnerability to asphyxia during active sleep in the newborn. *In* Guilleminault C, Dement W, eds: Sleep Apnea Syndromes: Proceedings of the Kroc Symposium 1977. New York, AR Liss, 1978, pp 93–117.
219. Bray GW: Recent advances in the treatment of asthma and hay fever. Practitioner 1934; 133:368–379.
220. Hughes DM, Spier S, Rivlin J, et al: Gastroesophageal reflux during sleep in asthmatic patients. J Pediatr 1983; 102:666–672.
221. Perpina M, Ponce J, Marco V, et al: The prevalence of asymptomatic gastroesophageal reflux in bronchial asthma and in non-asthmatic individuals. Eur J Respir Dis 1983; 64:582–587.
222. Allen JL, Wohl MEB: Pulmonary function in older children and young adults with gastroesophageal reflux. Clin Pediatr 1986; 25:541–546.
223. Vraney GA, Pokorny C: Pulmonary function in patients with gastroesophageal reflux. Chest 1979; 76:678–680.
224. Widdicombe JG: Nervous receptors in the respiratory tract and lung. *In* Hornbein T, ed: Regulation of Breathing. New York, Marcel Dekker, 1981, pp 429–472.
225. Lilly JR, Randolph JG: Hiatal hernia and gastroesophageal reflux in infants and children. J Thorac Cardiovasc Surg 1968; 55:42–53.
226. Leape LL, Holder TM, Franklin JD, et al: Respiratory arrest in infants secondary to gastroesophageal reflux. Pediatrics 1977; 60:924–928.
227. Ramenofsky ML, Leape LL: Continuous upper esophageal pH

monitoring in infants and children with gastroesophageal reflux, pneumonia, and apneic spells. J Pediatr Surg 1981; 16:374–378.
228. Herbst JJ, Minton SD, Book LS: Gastroesophageal reflux causing respiratory distress and apnea in newborn infants. J Pediatr 1979; 95:763–768.
229. Herbst JJ, Book LS, Bray PF: Gastroesophageal reflux in the near miss sudden infant death syndrome. J Pediatr 1978; 92:73–75.
230. Menon AP, Schefft GL, Thach BT: Apnea associated with regurgitation in infants. J Pediatr 1985; 106:625–629.
231. Menon AP, Schefft GL, Thach BT: Frequency and significance of swallowing during prolonged apnea in infants. Am Rev Respir Dis 1984; 130:969–973.
232. MacFadyen UM, Hendry GMA, Simpson H: Gastro-oesophageal reflux in near-miss sudden infant death syndrome or suspected recurrent aspiration. Arch Dis Child 1983; 58:87–91.
233. Spitzer AR, Boyle JT, Tuchman DN, et al: Awake apnea associated with gastroesophageal reflux: a specific clinical syndrome. J Pediatr 1984; 104:200–205.
234. Walsh JK, Farrell MK, Keenen WJ, et al: Gastroesophageal reflux in infants: Relation to apnea. J Pediatr 1981; 99:197–201.
235. Sacre L, Vandenplas Y: Gastroesophageal reflux associated with respiratory abnormalities during sleep. J Pediatr Gastroenterol Nutr 1989; 9:28–33.
236. Ariango RL, Guilleminault C, Baldwin R, et al: Movement and gastroesophageal reflux in awake term infants with "near miss" SIDS, unrelated to apnea. J Pediatr 1982; 100:894–897.
237. Rosen CL, Frost JD, Harrison GM: Infant polygraphic studies and follow-up monitoring. Pediatrics 1983; 71:731–736.
238. Henry RL, Mellis CM: Resolution of inspiratory stridor after fundoplication: Case report. Aust Paediatr J 1982; 18:126–127.
239. Nielson DW, Heldt GP, Tooley WH: Stridor and gastroesophageal reflux in infants. Pediatrics 1990; 85:1034–1039.
240. Orenstein SR, Orenstein DM, Whitington PF: Gastroesophageal reflux causing stridor. Chest 1983; 84:301–302.
241. Feranchak AP, Orenstein SR, Cohn JF: Behaviors associated with gastroesophageal reflux episodes in infants: a study using pH probe and split-screen video. Pediatr Res 1990; 27:9A.
242. Orenstein SR, Kocoshis SA, Orenstein DM, et al: Stridor and gastroesophageal reflux: Diagnostic use of intraluminal esophageal acid perfusion (Bernstein test). Pediatr Pulmonol 1987; 3:420–424.
243. Guilleminault C, Coons S: Apnea and bradycardia during feeding in infants weighing >2000 gm. J Pediatr 1984; 104:932–935.
244. Kenigsberg K, Griswold PG, Buckley BJ, et al: Cardiac effects of esophageal stimulation: Possible relationship between gastroesophageal reflux (GER) and sudden infant death syndrome (SIDS). J Pediatr Surg 1983; 18:542–545.
245. Perkett EA, Vaughan RL: Evidence for a laryngeal chemoreflex in some human preterm infants. Acta Paediatr Scand 1982; 71:969–972.
246. Downing SE, Lee JC: Laryngeal chemosensitivity: A possible mechanism for sudden infant death. Pediatrics 1975; 55:640–649.
247. Harned HS Jr, Myracle J, Ferreiro J: Respiratory suppression and swallowing from introduction of fluids into the laryngeal region of the lamb. Pediatr Res 1978; 12:1003–1009.
248. Matthew OP, Clark ML, Pronske ML, et al: Breathing pattern and ventilation during oral feeding in term newborn infants. J Pediatr 1985; 106:810–813.
249. Farrell MK, Wolske S, Brocker D: Is surgery required for the infant with gastroesophageal reflux (GER) and apnea? A prospective study. Pediatr Res 1983; 17:187A.
250. Plaxico DT, Loughlin GM: Nasopharyngeal reflux and neonatal apnea. Am J Dis Child 1981; 135:793–794.
251. Lew C, Keens T, O'Neal M, et al.: Gastroesophageal reflux prevents recovery from bronchopulmonary dysplasia. Clin Res 1981; 29:149A.
252. Sindel BD, Maisels MJ, Ballantine TVN, et al: The effect of a Nissen fundoplication on infants with chronic lung disease. Pediatr Res 1985; 19:365A.
253. Motoyama EK, Fort MD, Klesh KW, et al: Early onset of airway reactivity in premature infants with bronchopulmonary dysplasia. Am Rev Respir Dis 1987; 136:50–57.
254. Stringer DA, Sprigg A, Juodis E, et al.: The association of cystic fibrosis, gastroesophageal reflux, and reduced pulmonary function. Can Assoc Radiol 1988; 39:100–102.
255. Dudley NE, Phelan PD: Respiratory complications in long-term survivors of oesophageal atresia. Arch Dis Child 1976; 51:279–282.
256. Milligan DWA, Levine H: Lung function in children following repair of tracheoesophageal fistula. J Pediatr 1979; 95:24–27.
257. Desjardins JG, Stephens CA, Moes CAF: Results of surgical treatment of congenital tracheal-esophageal fistula, with a note on cine-fluorographic findings. Ann Surg 1964; 160:141–145.
258. Whitington PF, Shermeta DW, Set DSY, et al: Role of lower esophageal sphincter incompetence in recurrent pneumonia after repair of esophageal atresia. J Pediatr 1977; 91:550–554.
259. Parker AF, Christie DL, Cahill JL: Incidence and significance of gastroesophageal reflux following repair of esophageal atresia and tracheoesophageal fistula and the need for anti-reflux procedures. J Pediatr Surg 1979; 14:5–8.
260. Lind JF, Blanchard RJ, Guyda H: Esophageal motility in tracheoesophageal fistula and esophageal atresia. Surg Gynecol Obstet 1966; 123:557–564.
261. Chrispin AR, Friedland GW, Waterston DJ: Aspiration pneumonia and dysphagia after technically successful repair of oesophageal atresia. Thorax 1966; 21:104–110.
262. Burgess JN, Carlson HC, Ellis FH: Esophageal function after successful repair of esophageal atresia and tracheoesophageal fistula. J Thorac Cardiovasc Surg 1968; 56:667–673.
263. Laks H, Wilkinson RH, Schuster SR: long-term results following correction of esophageal atresia with tracheoesophageal fistula: A clinical and cinefluorographic study. J Pediatr Surg 1972; 7:591–597.
264. Romeo G, Zuccarello B, Proietto F, et al: Disorders of the esophageal motor activity in atresia of the esophagus. J Pediatr Surg 1987; 22:120–124.
265. Nakazato Y, Landin BH, Wells TR: Abnormal Auerbach plexus in the esophagus and stomach of patients with esophageal atresia and tracheoesophageal fistula. J Pediatr Surg 1986; 21:831–837.
266. Stein MR, Towner TG, Weber RW, et al: The effect of theophylline on the lower esophageal sphincter pressure. Ann Allergy 1980; 45:238–241.
267. Berquist WE, Rachelefsky GS, Kadden M, et al: Effect of theophylline on gastroesophageal reflux in normal adults. J Allergy Clin Immunol 1981; 67:407–411.
268. Berquist WE, Rachelefsky GS, Rowshan N, et al: Quantitative gastroesophageal reflux and pulmonary function in asthmatic children and normal adults receiving placebo, theophylline, and metaproterenol sulfate therapy. J Allergy Clin Immunol 1984; 73:253–258.
269. Vandenplas Y, DeWolf D, Sacre L: Influence of xanthines on gastroesophageal reflux in infants at risk for sudden infant death syndrome. Pediatrics 1986; 77:807–810.
270. Johannesson N, Andersson KE, Joelsson B, et al: Relaxation of the lower esophageal sphincter and stimulation of gastric secretion and diuresis by antiasthmatic xanthines. Am Rev Respir Dis 1985; 131:26–31.
271. Goyal RK, Rattan S: Mechanism of the lower esophageal sphincter relaxation: Action of prostaglandin E_1 and theophylline. J Clin Invest 1973; 52:337–341.
272. Foster LJ, Trudeau WL, Goldman AL: Bronchodilator effects on gastric acid secretion. JAMA 1979; 241:2613–2615.
273. Newell SJ, Booth IW, Morgan MEI, et al: Gastroesophageal reflux in the pre-term infant. Pediatr Res 1987; 22:104.
274. Wong RK, Maydonovitch C, Garcia JE, et al: The effect of terbutaline sulfate, nitroglycerin, and aminophylline on lower esophageal sphincter pressure and radionuclide esophageal emptying in patients with achalasia. J Clin Gastroenterol 1987; 9:386–389.
275. Zfass AM, Prince R, Allen FN, et al: Inhibitory beta-adrenergic receptors in the human distal esophagus. Am J Dig Dis 1970; 15:303–310.
276. Christensen J: Effects of drugs on esophageal motility. Arch Intern Med 1976; 136:532–537.
277. DiMarino AJ, Cohen S: Effect of an oral $beta_2$-adrenergic agonist on lower esophageal sphincter pressure in normals and in patients with achalasia. Dig Dis Sci 1982; 27:1063–1066.
278. Mansfield LE: Gastroesophageal reflux and respiratory disorders: A review. Ann Allergy 1989; 62:158–163.

279. Dennish GW, Castell DO: Inhibitory effect of smoking on the lower esophageal sphincter. N Engl J Med 1971; 284:1136–1137.
280. Stanciu C, Bennett JR: Smoking and gastro-oesophageal reflux. Br Med J 1972; 3:793–795.
281. Rattan S, Goyal RK: Effect of nicotine on the lower esophageal sphincter. Gastroenterology 1975; 69:154–159.
282. Cryer PE, Haymond MW, Santiago JV, et al: Norepinephrine and epinephrine release and adrenergic mediation of smoking-associated hemodynamic and metabolic events. N Engl J Med 1976; 295:573–577.
283. Ferry GD, Selby M, Pietro TJ: Clinical response to short-term nasogastric feeding in infants with gastroesophageal reflux and growth failure. J Pediatr Gastroenterol Nutr 1983; 2:57–61.
284. Bertrand JM, Morin CL, Lasalle R, et al: Short-term clinical, nutritional, and functional effects on continuous elemental enteral alimentation in children with cystic fibrosis. J Pediatr 1985; 104:41–46.
285. Leroy LD, Durie PR, Pencharz PB, et al: Effects of long-term nutritional rehabilitation on body composition and clinical status in malnourished children and adolescents with cystic fibrosis. J Pediatr 1985; 107:225–230.
286. Berezin S, Schwarz SM, Halata MS, et al: Gastroesophageal reflux secondary to gastrostomy tube placement. Am J Dis Child 1986; 140:699–701.
287. Spiliopoulos A, Megevand R: Oesophagite peptique stenosante apres sondage oesogastrique. Helv Chir Acta 1980; 47:527–532.
288. Canal DF, Vane EW, Goto S, et al: Reduction of lower esophageal sphincter pressure with Stamm gastrostomy. J Pediatr Surg 1987; 22:54–57.
289. Jolley SG, Tunell WP, Hoelzer DJ, et al: Lower esophageal pressure changes with tube gastrostomy: A causative factor of gastroesophageal reflux in children? J Pediatr Surg 1986; 21:624–627.
290. Hopper AO, Kwong LK, Stevenson DK, et al: Detection of gastric contents in tracheal fluid of infants by lactose assay. J Pediatr 1983; 102:415–418.
291. Yu VYH; Effect of body position on gastric emptying in the neonate. Arch Dis Child 1975; 50:500–504.
292. Martin RJ, Herrel N, Rubin D, et al: Effect of supine and prone positions on arterial oxygen tension in the preterm infant. Pediatrics 1979; 63:528–531.
293. Meyers WF, Herbst JJ: Effectiveness of positioning therapy for gastroesophageal reflux. Pediatrics 1982; 69:768–772.
294. Foster AC, Voyles JB, Murphy SA: Twenty-four-hour pH monitoring in children with cystic fibrosis: Association of chest physical therapy to gastroesophageal reflux. Pediatr Res 1983; 17:118A.
295. Martin CJ, Dantas R, Dodds WJ, et al: Relaxation of the diaphragmatic hiatus is essential for GE reflux in the dog. Gastroenterology 1989; 96:A322.
296. Kahrilas PJ, Dodds WJ, Dent J, et al: Upper esophageal sphincter function during belching. Gastroenterology 1986; 91:133–140.
297. Kahrilas PJ, Dodds WJ, Hogan WJ: Dysfunction of the belch reflex: A cause of incapacitating chest pain. Gastroenterology 1987; 93:818–822.
298. Gluck M, Pope CE II: Chronic hiccups and gastroesophageal reflux disease: the acid perfusion test as a provocative maneuver. Ann Intern Med 1986; 105:219–220.
299. Shay SS, Myers RL, Johnson LF: Hiccups associated with reflux esophagitis. Gastroenterology 1984; 87:204–207.
300. Irwin RS, Zawacki JK, Curley FJ, et al: Chronic cough as the sole presenting manifestation of gastroesophageal reflux. Am Rev Respir Dis 1989; 140:1294–1300.
301. Berquist WE, Ament ME: Upper GI function in sleeping infants. Am Rev Respir Dis 1985; 131(Suppl):S29-S32.
302. Katz PO: Ambulatory esophageal and hypopharyngeal pH monitoring in patients with hoarseness. Am J Gastroenterol 1990; 85:35–40.
303. Wiener GJ, Koufman JA, Wu WC, et al: Chronic hoarseness secondary to gastroesophageal reflux disease: Documentation with a 24-hour ambulatory pH monitoring. Am J Gastroenterol 1989; 84:1503–1508.
304. Wilson JA, White A, vonHaacke NP, et al: Gastroesophageal reflux and posterior laryngitis. Ann Otol Rhinol 1989; 98:405–410.
305. McNally PR, Maydonovitch CL, Prosek RA, et al: Evaluation of gastroesophageal reflux as a cause of idiopathic hoarseness. Dig Dis Sci 1989; 34:1900–1904.
306. Pearlman NW, Stiegmann GV, Teter A: Primary upper aerodigestive tract manifestations of gastroesophageal reflux. Am J Gastroenterol 1988; 83:22–25.
307. Cherry J, Margulies SI: Contact ulcer of the larynx. Laryngoscope 1968; 78:1937–1940.
308. Hallewell JD, Cole TB: Isolated head and neck symptoms due to hiatus hernia. Arch Otolaryngol 1970; 92:499–501.
309. Chodosh PL: Gastro-esophago-pharyngeal reflux. Laryngoscope 1977; 87:1418–1427.
310. Putnam PE, Orenstein SR: Hoarseness and pediatric gastroesophageal reflux. Acta Paediatr Scand 1992 (in press).
311. Oestreich AE, Dunbar JC: Pharyngonasal reflux: Spectrum and significance in early childhood. AJR 1984; 141:923–925.
312. Kinsbourne M: Hiatus hernia with contortions of the neck. Lancet 1964; 1:1058–1061.
313. Puntis JWL, Smith HL, Buick RG, et al: Effect of dystonic movements on oesophageal peristalsis in Sandifer's syndrome. Arch Dis Child 1989; 64:1311–1313.
314. Bray PF, Herbst JJ, Johnson DG, et al: Childhood gastroesophageal reflux. Neurologic and psychiatric syndromes mimicked. JAMA 1977; 237:1342–1345.
315. Mandel H, Tirosh E, Berant M: Sandifer syndrome reconsidered. Acta Paediatr Scan 1989; 78:797–799.
316. Sutcliffe J. Torsion spasms and abnormal postures in children with hiatus hernia: Sandifer's syndrome. *In* Kaufmann HJ, ed: Progress in Pediatric Radiology. Vol 2: Gastrointestinal Tract. Basel, S. Karger Ag, 1969, pp 190–197.
317. Whitehead WE, Schuster MM: Behavioral approaches to the treatment of gastrointestinal motility disorders. Med Clin North Am 1981; 65:1397–1411.
318. Leonidas JC: Gastroesophageal reflux in infants: Role of the upper gastrointestinal series. AJR 1984; 143:1350–1351.
319. Ott DJ: Barium esophagram. *In* Castell D, Wu W, Ott D, eds: Gastro-Esophageal Reflux Disease: Pathogenesis, Diagnosis, Therapy. Mount Kisco, NY, Futura Publishing, 1985, pp 109–128.
320. Guillet J, Basse-Cathalinat B, Christophe E, et al: Routine studies of swallowed radionuclide transit in paediatrics: Experience with 400 patients. Eur J Nucl Med 1984; 9:86–90.
321. Seibert JJ, Byrne WJ, Euler AR, et al: Gastroesophageal reflux—the acid test: Scintigraphy or pH probe? AJR 1983; 140:1087–1090.
322. Heyman S, Kirkpatrick JA, Winter HS, et al: An improved radionuclide method for the diagnosis of gastroesophageal reflux and aspiration in children (milk scan). Radiology 1979; 131:479–482.
323. Rudd TG, Christie DL: Demonstration of gastroesophageal reflux in children by radionuclide gastroesophagography. Radiology 1979; 131:483–486.
324. Paton JY, Cosgriff PS, Nanayakkara CS: The analytical sensitivity of Tc99m radionuclide "milk" scanning in the detection of gastro-oesophageal reflux. Pediatr Radiol 1985; 15:381–383.
325. Fawcett HD, Hayden CK, Adams JC, et al: How useful is gastroesophageal reflux scintigraphy in suspected childhood aspiration? Pediatr Radiol 1988; 18:311–313.
326. Berdon WE, Mellins RB, Levy J: On the following paper by H. D. Fawcett, C. K. Hayden, J. C. Adams and L. E. Swischuk: How useful is gastroesophageal reflux scintigraphy in suspected childhood aspiration? Pediatr Radiol 1988; 18:309–310.
327. Seibert JJ, Byrne WJ, Euler AR: Gastric emptying in children: unusual patterns detected by scintigraphy. AJR 1983; 141:49–51.
328. Klein HA: Esophageal and other condensed dynamic images. Clin Nucl Med 1985; 10:530–531.
329. Rosenthal MS, Klein HA, Orenstein SR: Simultaneous acquisition of physiological data and nuclear medicine images. J Nucl Med 1988; 29:1848–1852.
330. Biller JA, Winter HS, Grand RJ, et al: Are endoscopic changes predictive of histologic esophagitis in children. J Pediatr 1983; 103:215–218.
331. Casteel HB, Fiedorek SC, Kiel EA: Arterial blood oxygen desaturation in infants and children during upper gastrointestinal endoscopy. Gastrointest Endosc 1990; 36:489–493.

331a. Putnam PE, Orenstein SR: Blind esophageal suction biopsy in children less than 2 years of age. Gastroenterology 1992; 102:A149.

332. Strobel CT, Byrne WJ, Ament ME, et al: Correlation of esophageal lengths in children with height: Application to the Tuttle test without prior esophageal manometry. J Pediatr 1979; 103:215–218.

333. Putnam PE, Orenstein SR: Determining esophageal length from crown-rump length. J Pediatr Gastroenterol Nutr 1991; 13:354–359.

334. Whitington PF, Orenstein SR: Manometric guidance in suction biopsy of the esophagus in children. J Pediatr Gastroenterol Nutr 1984; 3:535–538.

335. Weinstein WM, Bogoch ER, Bowes KL: The normal human esophageal mucosa: A histological reappraisal. Gastroenterology 1975; 68:40–44.

336. Dahms BB, Rothstein FC: Mucosal biopsy of the esophagus in children. Perspect Pediatr Pathol 1987; 11:97–123.

337. Steadman C, Kerlin P, Teague C, et al: High esophageal stricture: A complication of "inlet patch" mucosa. Gastroenterology 1988; 94:521–524.

338. Jabbari M, Goresky CA, Lough J, et al: The inlet patch: Heterotopic gastric mucosa in the upper esophagus. Gastroenterology 1985; 89:352–356.

339. Shepard R, Fenn S, Sieber WK: Evaluation of esophageal function in postoperative esophageal atresia and tracheoesophageal fistula. Surgery 1966; 59:608–617.

340. Berezin S, Medow MS, Glassman M, et al: Use of the intraesophageal acid perfusion test in provoking nonspecific chest pain in children. J Pediatr 1989; 115:709–712.

341. Davidson GP: Usefulness of oesophageal pH monitoring. Aust Paediatr J 1985; 21:243–244.

342. Orenstein SR, Whitington PF, Orenstein DM: The infant seat as treatment for gastroesophageal reflux. N Engl J Med 1983; 309:760–763.

343. Orenstein SR, Whitington PF: Positioning for prevention of infant gastroesophageal reflux. J Pediatr 1983; 103:534–537.

344. Tolia V, Kauffman RE: Comparison of evaluation of gastroesophageal reflux in infants using different feedings during intraesophageal pH monitoring. J Pediatr Gastroenterol Nutr 1990; 10:426–429.

345. Hampton FJ, MacFadyen UM, Simpson H: Reproducibility of 24 hour oesophageal pH studies in infants. Arch Dis Child 1990; 65:1249–1254.

346. Johnson LF: New concepts and methods in the study and treatment of gastroesophageal reflux disease. Med Clin North Am 1981; 65:1195–1222.

347. Jolley SG, Johnson DG, Herbst JJ, et al: An assessment of gastroesophageal reflux in children by extended monitoring of the distal esophagus. Surgery 1978; 84:16–22.

348. Euler AR, Byrne WJ: Twenty-four-hour esophageal intraluminal pH probe testing: A comparative analysis. Gastroenterology 1981; 80:957–961.

349. Williams HE, Freeman M: Milk inhalation pneumonia: The significance of fat filled macrophages in tracheal secretions. Aust Paediatr J 1973; 9:286–288.

350. Nussbaum E, Maggi JC, Galant SP: Association of lipid-laden alveolar macrophages and gastroesophageal reflux in children. Pediatr Res 1986; 20:475A.

351. Brand J, Brodsky N, Hurt H: No evidence of aspiration in intubated infants fed by orogastric (OG) or oroduodenal (OD) routes. Pediatr Res 1986; 20:405A.

352. Hurwitz AL, Duranceau A: Upper-esophageal sphincter dysfunction: Pathogenesis and treatment. Dig Dis 1978; 23:275–281.

353. Staugas R, Martin AJ, Binns G, et al: The significance of fat-filled macrophages in the diagnosis of aspiration associated with gastro-oesophageal reflux. Aust Paediatr J 1985; 21:275–277.

354. Fisher RS, Malmud LS, Roberts GS, et al: Gastroesophageal (GE) scintiscanning to detect and quantitate GE reflux. Gastroenterology 1976; 70:301–308.

355. Stein MR, Ghaed N: An isotope study of pulmonary aspiration by fiberoptic bronchoscopy. Chest 1976; 70:458–459.

356. Wolfe JE, Bone RD, Ruth WE: Diagnosis of gastric aspiration by fiberoptic bronchoscopy. Chest 1976; 70:458–459.

357. Wynne JW, Ramphal R, Hood CI: Tracheal mucosal damage after aspiration: A scanning electron microscope study. Am Rev Respir Dis 1981; 124:728–732.

358. Leape LL, Bhan I, Ramenofsky ML: Esophageal biopsy in the diagnosis of reflux esophagitis. J Pediatr Surg 1981; 16:379–384.

359. Orenstein SR, Klein HA, Rosenthal MS: Simultaneous comparison of pH probe and scintigraphy for gastroesophageal reflux (GER). Gastroenterology 1987; 92:1561.

360. Orenstein SR: Prone positioning in infant gastroesophageal reflux: Is elevation of the head worth the trouble? J Pediatr 1990; 117:184–187.

361. Hewitt VM: Effect of posture on the presence of fat in tracheal aspirate in neonates. Aust Paediat J 1976; 12:267–271.

362. Masterson J, Zucker C, Schulze K: Prone and supine positioning effect on energy expenditure and behavior of low birth weight neonates. Pediatrics 1987; 80:689–692.

363. Orenstein SR: Effects on behavior state of prone versus seated positioning for infants with gastroesophageal reflux. Pediatrics 1990; 85:765–767.

364. Byrne WJ, Euler AR, Campbell M: Body position and esophageal sphincter pressure in infants. Am J Dis Child 1982; 136:523–525.

365. Bailey DJ, Andres JM, Danek GD, et al: Lack of efficacy of thickened feeding as treatment for gastroesophageal reflux. J Pediatr 1987; 110:187–189.

366. Shulman RJ, Boutton TW, Klein PD: Impact of dietary cereal on nutrient absorption and fecal nitrogen loss in formula-fed infants. J Pediatr 1991; 118:39–43.

367. Sutphen JL, Dillard VL: Effect of feeding volume on early postcibal gastroesophageal reflux in infants. J Pediatr Gastroenterol Nutr 1988; 7:185–188.

367a. Sondheimer J, Arnold G: Early effects of bethanechol on the esophageal motor function of infants with gastroesophageal reflux. J Pediatr Gastroenterol Nutr 1986; 5:47–51.

368. Euler AR: Use of bethanechol for the treatment of gastroesophageal reflux. J Pediatr 1980; 96:321–324.

369. Strickland AD, Chang JH: Results of treatment of gastroesophageal reflux with bethanechol. J Pediatr 1983; 103:311–315.

370. Sondheimer JM, Mintz HL, Michaels M: Bethanechol treatment of gastroesophageal reflux in infants: Effect on continuous esophageal pH records. J Pediatr 1984; 104:128–131.

371. Orenstein SR, Lofton SW, Orenstein DM: Bethanechol for pediatric gastroesophageal reflux: A prospective, blind, controlled study. J Pediatr Gastroenterol Nutr 1986; 5:549–555.

372. Tolia V, Calhoun J, Kuhns L, et al: Randomized, prospective double-blind trial of metoclopramide and placebo for gastroesophageal reflux in infants. J Pediatr 1989; 115:141–145.

373. Machida HM, Forbes DA, Gall DG, et al: Metoclopramide in gastroesophageal reflux of infancy. J Pediatr 1988; 112:483–487.

374. Leung AKC, Lai PCW: Use of metoclopramide for the treatment of gastroesophageal reflux in infants and children. Curr Ther Res 1984; 36:911–915.

375. Hyams JS, Leichtner AM, Zamett LO, et al: Effect of metoclopramide on prolonged intraesophageal pH testing in infants with gastroesophageal reflux. J Pediatr Gastroenterol Nutr 1986; 5:716–720.

375a. Putnam PE, Orenstein SR, Wessel HB, et al: Tardive dyskinesia associated with metoclopramide use in a child. Pediatr Res 1992; 31:114A.

376. Grill BB, Hillemeier AC, Semeraro LA, et al: Effects of domperidone therapy on symptoms and upper gastrointestinal motility in infants with gastroesophageal reflux. J Pediatr 1985; 106:311–316.

377. Grill B, Rincon DM: Domperidone improves esophageal acid clearance and late post-prandial reflux time in infants with gastroesophageal reflux (GER). Pediatr Res 1986; 20:240A.

378. Cucchiara S, Staiano A, Capozzi C, et al: Cisapride for gastro-oesophageal reflux and peptic oesophagitis. Arch Dis Child 1987; 62:454–457.

379. Saye ZN, Forget PP, Geukbelle F: Effect of cisapride on gastroesophageal reflux in children with chronic bronchopulmonary disease: A double-blind cross-over pH-monitoring study. Pediatr Pulmonol 1987; 3:8–12.

380. Rode H, Stunden RJ, Millar AJ, et al: Esophageal pH assessment of gastroesophageal reflux in 18 patients and the effect of two prokinetic agents: Cisapride and metoclopramide. J Pediatr Surg 1987; 22:931–934.

381. Saye Z, Forget PP: Effect of cisapride on esophageal pH monitoring in children with reflux-associated bronchopulmonary disease. J Pediatr Gastroenterol Nutr 1989; 8:327–332.
382. Cucchiara S, Gobio-Casali L, Balli F, et al: Cimetidine treatment of reflux esophagitis in children: An Italian multicentric study. J Pediatr Gastroenterol Nutr 1989; 8:150–156.
383. Hetzel DJ, Dent J, Reed WD, et al: Healing and relapse of severe peptic esophagitis after treatment with omeprazole. Gastroenterology 1988; 95:903–912.
384. Cucchiuara S, Staiano A, Romaniello G, et al: Antacids and cimetidine treatment for gastro-oesophageal reflux and peptic oesophagitis. Arch Dis Child 1984; 59:842–847.
385. Sutphen JL, Dillard VL, Pipan ME: Antacid and formula effects on gastric acidity in infants with gastroesophageal reflux. Pediatrics 1986; 78:55–57.
386. Brand JM, Greer FR: Hypermagnesemia and intestinal perforation following antacid administration in a premature infant. Pediatrics 1990; 85121–124.
387. Arguelles-Martin F, Gonzalez-Fernande F, Gentles MG: Sucralfate versus cimetidine in the treatment of reflux esophagitis in children. Am J Med 1989; 86(Suppl 6A):73–76.
388. Buts JP, Leclercq V: Gaviscon and gastroesophageal reflux in children (letter). J Pediatr Gastroenterol Nutr 1987; 6:482–483.
389. Buts JP, Barudi C, Otte JB: Double-blind controlled study on the efficacy of sodium alginate (Gaviscon) in reducing gastroesophageal reflux assessed by 24 h continuous pH monitoring in infants and children. Eur J Pediatr 1987; 146:156–158.
390. Forbes D, Hodgson M, Hill R: The effects of Gaviscon and metoclopramide in gastroesophageal reflux in children. J Pediatr Gastroenterol Nutr 1986; 5:556–559.
391. Schatzlein MH, Ballantine TWN, Thirunavukkarasu S, et al: Gastroesophageal reflux in infants and children. Arch Surg 1979; 114:505–510.
392. Christie DL, Mack DV, Parker AF, et al: Use of intraoperative esophageal manometrics in surgical treatment of gastroesophageal reflux in pediatric patients. J Pediatr Surg 1978; 13:648–652.
393. Jolley SG, Tunell WP, Hoelzer DJ, et al: Intraoperative esophageal manometry and early postoperative esophageal pH monitoring in children. J Pediatr Surg 1989; 24:336–340.
394. Johnson DG, Herbst JJ, Oliveros MA, et al: Evaluation of gastroesophageal reflux surgery in children. Pediatrics 1977; 59:62–68.
395. Johnson DG, Jolley SG: Gastroesophageal reflux in infants and children: Recognition and treatment. Surg Clin North Am 1981; 61:1101–1115.
396. Spitz L, Kirtane J: Results and complications of surgery for gastro-oesophageal reflux. Arch Dis Child 1985; 60:743–747.
397. Leape LL, Ramenofsky ML: Surgical treatment of gastroesophageal reflux in children. Am J Dis Child 1980; 134:935–938.
398. Fonkalsrud EW, Berquist W, Vargas J, et al: Surgical treatment of the gastroesophageal reflux syndrome in infants and children. Am J Surg 1987; 154:11–18.
399. Jolley SG, Smith EI, Tunnell WP: Protective antireflux operation with feeding gastrostomy. Ann Surg 1985; 201:736–740.
400. Byrne WJ, Euler AR, Ashcraft E, et al: Gastroesophageal reflux in the severely retarded who vomit: Criteria for and results of surgical intervention in twenty-two patients. Surgery 1982; 91:95–98.
401. Mollitt DL, Golladay ES, Seibert JJ: Symptomatic gastroesophageal reflux following gastrostomy in neurologically impaired patients. Pediatrics 1985; 75:1124–1126.
402. Wilkinson JD, Dudgeon DL, Sondheimer JM: A comparison of medical and surgical treatment of gastroesophageal reflux in severely retarded children. J Pediatr 1981; 99:202–205.
403. Giuffre RM, Rubin S, Mitchell I: Antireflux surgery in infants with bronchopulmonary dysplasia. Am J Dis Child 1987; 141:648–651.
404. Ashcraft KW, Goodwin C, Amoury RA, et al: Early recognition and aggressive treatment of gastroesophageal reflux following repair of esophageal atresia. J Pediatr Surg 1977; 12:317–321.
405. Ashcraft KW, Holder TM, Amoury RA: Treatment of gastroesophageal reflux in children by Thal fundoplication. J Thorac Cardiovasc Surg 1981; 82:706–712.
406. Tunell WP, Smith EL, Carson JA: Gastroesophageal reflux in childhood: The dilemma of surgical success. Ann Surg 1983; 197:560–565.
407. Alrabeeah A, Giacomantonio M, Gillis DA: Paraesophageal hernia after Nissen fundoplication: A real complication in pediatric patients. J Pediatr Surg 1988; 23:766–768.
408. Dedinsky GK, Vane DW, Black CT, et al: Complications and reoperation after Nissen fundoplication in childhood. Am J Surg 1987; 153:177–183.
409. Harnsberger JK, Corey JJ, Johnson DJ, et al: Long-term follow-up of surgery for gastroesophageal reflux in infants and children. J Pediatr 1983; 102:505–508.
410. Fonkalsrud EW, Foglia RP, Ament ME, et al: Operative treatment for the gastroesophageal reflux syndrome in children. J Pediatr Surg 1989; 24:525–529.
411. Tunell WP: Gastroesophageal reflux in childhood: Implications for surgical treatment. Ped Ann 1989; 18:192–196.
412. Shepard R, Fenn S, Sieber WK: Evaluation of esophageal function in postoperative esophageal atresia and tracheoesophageal fistula. Surgery 1966; 59:608–617.
413. Tuggle DW, Tunell WP, Hoelzer DJ, et al: The efficacy of Thal fundoplication in the treatment of gastroesophageal reflux: The influence of central nervous system impairment. J Pediatr Surg 1988; 23:638–640.
414. Gourley GR, Pellett JR, Li BUK, et al: A prospective randomized double-blind study of gastroesophageal reflux surgery in pediatric-sized developmentally disabled patients: Nissen fundoplication versus Angelchik prosthesis. J Pediatr Gastroenterol Nutr 1986; 5:52–61.

Chapter 27

Portal Hypertension

ERIC HASSALL and DAVID ISRAEL

ANATOMY, PATHOPHYSIOLOGY, AND CLINICAL ASPECTS

Although bleeding from gastroesophageal varices accounts for only 10 to 15% of upper gastrointestinal bleeding in children,[1,2] variceal bleeding is often serious; varices and peptic ulcer disease together account for nearly all massive and potentially fatal hemorrhage in children. With rare exceptions, varices are the result of portal hypertension. An understanding of the hemodynamics of portal hypertension and subsequent vascular changes is important for a logical approach to diagnosis, management and specific treatment of variceal bleeding.

Definition of Portal Hypertension

The normal range of portal venous pressure is 5 to 10 mm Hg higher than the pressure present in the inferior vena cava. Portal hypertension is defined by an elevation of this pressure gradient to values above 10 to 12 mm Hg, and there is a strong correlation between portal pressures higher than 12 mm Hg and variceal bleeding.[3]

Normal Anatomy of the Portal Venous System

The portal venous system (Fig. 27–1) carries blood from the stomach, spleen, pancreas, gallbladder, and small and large intestine into the liver via the portal vein. The portal venous system is devoid of valves, and, therefore, the direction of blood flow is determined by pressure gradient and patency.

Etiology of Portal Hypertension

In adults, *intrahepatic portal hypertension* (IHPH) due to alcoholism and other causes of cirrhosis greatly overwhelms *extrahepatic portal hypertension* (EHPH) as the major cause of portal hypertension. In pediatric reports, the prevalence of etiology varies among different medical centers, depending on their referral base and expertise; for example, reports from liver transplant centers obviously show a prevalence of IHPH. However, a review of pediatric reports shows that in children, EHPH is at least 50% more prevalent as a cause of portal hypertension than is IHPH.[4–17] Table 27–1 describes the causes of portal hypertension in 398 children investigated at one institution from 1954 to 1983.[18]

The site of obstruction in EHPH may be prehepatic or posthepatic. *Prehepatic* refers to an obstruction anywhere in the portal venous system, that is, portal vein, splenic vein, or superior mesenteric vein, in any combination.[19, 20] Obstruction in the portal venous system is by far the commonest cause of EHPH (Table 27–2).[17–19, 21] Portal vein obstruction (PVO) alone is the commonest occurrence. PVO can be congenital or acquired secondary to infection, surgery, or trauma, but no clear cause can be found in about 50% of reported cases.[22] The presence of congenital anomalies associated with PVO has raised the possibility that PVO may be congenital in some cases.[20, 23] Congenital abnormalities of the heart, blood vessels, urinary tract, and biliary tree were found in 26% of children in one series of EHPH.[23] Umbilical vein catheterization is the commonest known cause of acquired PVO, but other conditions, such as local trauma, thrombosis, or endothelial damage, can cause PVO.[24]

Rarely, obstruction of the splenic vein may cause a localized form of portal hypertension known as *left-sided,* or *sinistral,* portal hypertension.[25] This condition is usually secondary to pancreatitis.

Posthepatic portal hypertension is usually due to Budd-Chiari syndrome. This disease results from obstruction anywhere from the intrahepatic branches of the hepatic vein to the entry of the inferior vena cava into the right atrium. The obstruction may be secondary to a congenital web or associated with various tumors, clotting disorders, trauma, and the use of contraceptives.[26, 27] Other posthepatic causes of portal hypertension include veno-occlusive disease and chronic constrictive pericarditis (see Table 27–1).

Of all the causes of IHPH in childhood, extrahepatic biliary atresia, congenital hepatic fibrosis, and alpha$_1$-antitrypsin deficiency are the commonest, accounting for about 30% of all cases with portal hypertension, whereas autoimmune chronic active hepatitis was found in 7%.[18] Although most cases of IHPH are associated with deterioration of liver function and poor outcome, congenital hepatic fibrosis is characterized by hepatomegaly and normal hepatocellular function. In Third

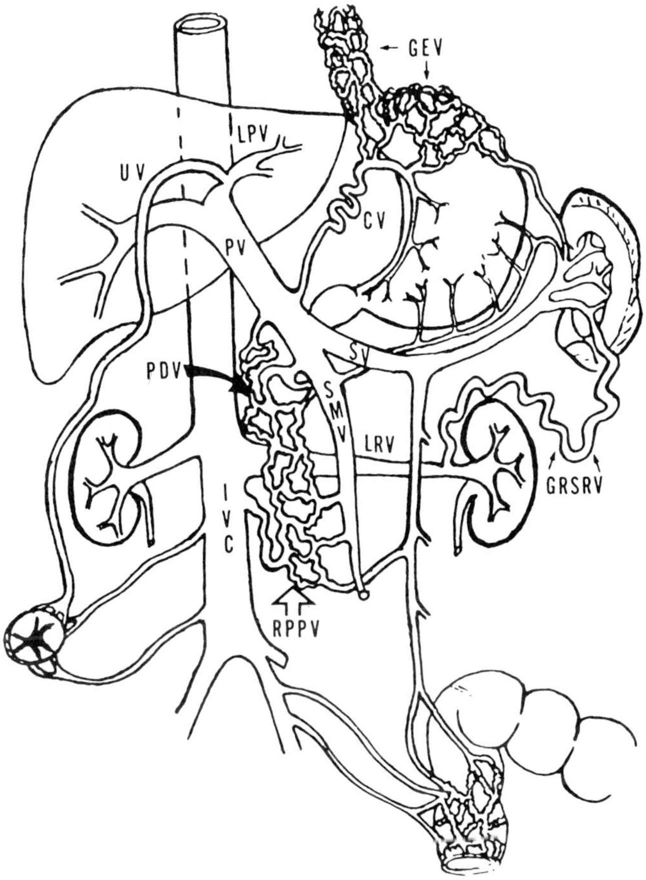

Figure 27–1. Diagram of the portal venous system and the common portosystemic collateral venous pathways in portal hypertension. GEV, gastroesophageal veins; UV, umbilical vein; LPV, left branch of portal vein; PV, portal vein; CV, coronary vein; PDV, pancreaticoduodenal veins; SV, splenic vein; SMV, superior mesenteric vein; LRV, left renal vein; IVC, inferior vena cava; GRSRV, gastrorenal-splenorenal veins; RPPV, retroperitoneal-paravertebral veins. (From Subramanyam BR, Balthazar EJ, Madamba MR, Raghavendra BN, Horii SC, Lefleur RS: Sonography of portosystemic venous collaterals in portal hypertension. Radiology 1983; 146:161–166; with permission.)

World countries, schistosomiasis causing so-called pipestem fibrosis is the most prevalent cause of IHPH, which is also associated with normal hepatocellular function.

Hemodynamic Considerations

Under normal conditions the liver offers low resistance to flow and can accommodate increased flow with minimal change in pressure. Portal hypertension usually occurs when there is increased resistance to flow. Classification of portal hypertension by the location and nature of increased resistance is logical for clinical purposes; therefore, the primary classification is into IHPH and EHPH.

In IHPH, the proposed mechanisms that may contribute to increased intrahepatic resistance are well summarized elsewhere.[28, 28a] These mechanisms include sphincterlike structures in the hepatic vein, as has been described in cats, regenerating nodules compressing hepatic venules and fibrous tissue deposits surrounding the terminal venules. Formation of a basement membrane in Disse's spaces and capillary transformation of sinusoids were also observed. Hepatocyte enlargement and sinusoid compression may occur with metabolic diseases, infections, or toxic injury to the liver.[28] In EHPH, the problem is a mechanical intraluminal obstruction to flow in extrahepatic blood vessels, most commonly obstruction of the portal vein itself. Normally, blood flow in the portal vein is toward the liver, so-called *hepatopetal* flow. In IHPH, as intrahepatic resistance to flow increases, blood will be diverted through portosystemic anastomoses, away from the liver. This component of blood flow is termed *hepatofugal.* In PVO some blood is diverted through portosystemic anastomoses, but some will bypass the obstruction via collaterals that develop around the obstructed portal vein, so-called *cavernous transformation*. In Budd-Chiari syndrome, there is initially marked liver congestion with an acute increase in liver size. This congestion is followed by hemodynamic changes similar to those described for IHPH. The development of hepatofugal flow represents a significant negative development, as deprivation of portal blood to the liver leads to damage of

Table 27–1. ETIOLOGY OF PORTAL HYPERTENSION IN 398 CHILDREN

Etiology	No. of Children*
EHPH	***(157)***
Prehepatic	
Portal vein obstruction	134
Posthepatic	
Budd-Chiari syndrome	18
Constrictive pericarditis	1
Veno-occlusive disease	4
IHPH	***(228)***
Congenital hepatic fibrosis	26
Cirrhosis including cholestatic cirrhosis	(202)
Extrahepatic biliary atresia	56
Alpha$_1$-antitrypsin deficiency	20
Byler's disease	13
Cystic fibrosis	8
Paucity of interlobular bile ducts	
Syndromatic	7
Nonsyndromatic	4
Sclerosing cholangitis	7
Extrahepatic bile duct lesion	7
Histiocytosis X	5
Unidentified	9
Postnecrotic cirrhosis	
Autoimmune chronic hepatitis	27
HB$_s$Ag positive	6
Seronegative	4
Wilson's disease	1
Idiopathic cirrhosis	28
Miscellaneous	***13***

*Numbers in parentheses are the total number of children in the particular category shown in the left column.

HB$_s$Ag, hepatitis B surface antigen.

Modified from Bernard D, Alvarez F, Brunelle F, et al: Portal hypertension in children. Clin Gastroenterol 1985; 14:33–55; with permission.

Table 27–2. CAUSES OF EXTRAHEPATIC PORTAL HYPERTENSION

Obstruction of Portal or Splenic Vein
Idiopathic
Congenital
Structural lesions
Omphalitis
Umbilical vein catheterization
Portal pyelophlebitis
Intra-abdominal sepsis
Surgery near the porta hepatis
Septicemia
Cholangitis
Trauma
Duodenal ulcer
Pancreatitis
Malignant disease
Lymph gland enlargement
Choledochal cyst
Increased Blood Flow
Arteriovenous fistula
Tropical splenomegaly

From Mowat AP, ed: Liver Disorders in Childhood. 2nd ed. London, Butterworth, 1987, pp 298–325; with permission.

hepatic parenchyma and predisposes to hepatic encephalopathy. This is discussed further in the section on the pathophysiology of surgical shunts.

Major portosystemic anastomoses that carry blood away from the liver are located at the gastroesophageal junction, hemorrhoidal plexus, falciform ligament, posterior abdominal wall draining into the inferior vena cava, left kidney or pulmonary vein (see Fig. 27–1). Collateral venous channels dilate and multiply to carry the increased blood flow, and the dilated veins in the submucosa and epithelium may bleed. Although the main varices that are likely to bleed are in the lower esophagus and proximal stomach, "ectopic varices" may occur throughout the gastrointestinal tract, peritoneum, biliary tree, vagina, and bladder.

In left-sided, or sinistral, portal hypertension, with segmental obstruction of the splenic vein, shunting of blood is through the short gastric veins,[25] with formation of esophageal and gastric varices and minimal vascular changes on the right side.

Portal hypertension secondary to increased blood flow into the portal system (high-flow portal hypertension) may occur secondary to an arteriovenous malformation[26] or post-traumatic arteriovenous fistula.[29] High-flow portal hypertension may also occur when splenomegaly of any cause leads to increased splenic blood flow which may perpetuate the portal hypertension. It is not clear, however, whether this factor alone can cause portal hypertension.[28]

Gastroesophageal Venous Anatomy and Varix Formation

Some studies[30–33] of the venous anatomy of the lower esophagus in normal subjects and in patients with portal hypertension have offered a model to explain the formation of varices and why bleeding preferentially occurs in the lower third of the esophagus. The veins of the lower esophagus and upper stomach are organized into four distinct layers in a continuum across the gastroesophageal junction (Fig. 27–2).

In portal hypertension, the deep intrinsic veins become quite dilated and displace the superficial venous plexus, thus coming closer to the epithelial surface. It is these dilated, deep intrinsic veins that constitute the main variceal channels, those bulging tortuous vessels seen at endoscopy. The model described by Kitano and coworkers[30] suggests that major variceal bleeding results from rupture of these vessels, whereas minor bleeds may occur from branches of the superficial plexus unconnected to a large varix or even from dilated intraepithelial channels. This model also suggests that the "cherry-red spots," "red wale markings," and "varix-on-varix" appearances at endoscopy probably represent large branches of the superficial venous plexus overlying large major varices. These varices may erode into the epithelium and initiate the bleeding episode.[30–33] Although this is a speculative interpretation of the venous anatomy, it is important, because these endoscopic signs may be predictive of impending variceal rupture.[21]

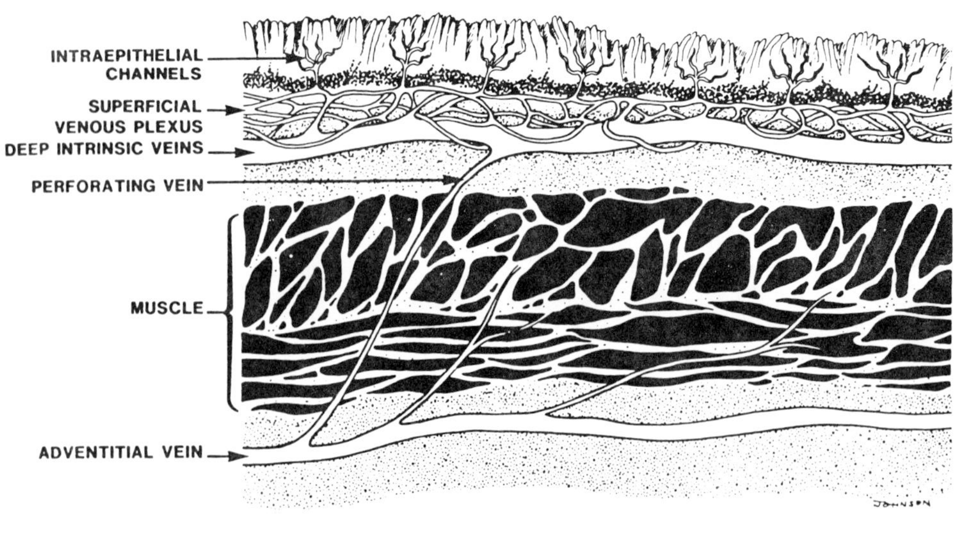

Figure 27–2. Diagrammatic representation of the venous drainage of the esophagus in normal humans. (From Kitano S, Terblanche J, Kahn D, et al: Venous anatomy of the lower esophagus in portal hypertension: Practical implications. Br J Surg 1986; 73: 525–531; by permission of the publishers Butterworth-Heinemann Ltd.)

Table 27–3. CLINICAL MANIFESTATIONS OF PORTAL HYPERTENSION

Splenomegaly	Internal hemorrhoids
Hematemesis	Small liver or hepatomegaly
Melena	Hypersplenism
Esophageal varices	Ascites
Malabsorption	Protein losing enteropathy
Caput medusae	Failure to thrive
Venous hum above umbilicus	Hepatic encephalopathy

Adapted from Mowat AT, ed: Liver Disorders in Childhood. 2nd ed. London, Butterworth, 1987, pp 298–325; with permission.

Perforating veins (see Fig. 27–2) occur predominantly just above the gastroesophageal junction. This fact may partly explain the prevalence of varices in this area as well as the recurrence of varices after sclerotherapy.

Rarely, esophageal varices can develop in the absence of portal hypertension, such as secondary to superior vena cava obstruction or benign giant lymphoma.[34] These varices are termed *downhill* to distinguish them from the more common *uphill* varices.

Why Do Varices Bleed?

From hemodynamic considerations, variceal bleeding is more likely to occur when variceal wall tension is high.[28] Wall tension is related to transmural pressure and vessel radius and inversely related to vessel wall thickness. Increased pressure within blood vessels leads to dilatation, with thinning of the vessel wall. These conditions are much more likely to result in variceal rupture when portal vein pressure is higher than 10 to 12 mm Hg; bleeding is rarely observed when the pressure is lower than this level.[3, 21] Vessels embedded in tissue have better support and a smaller radius at the same pressure, resulting in lower wall tension than that of similar vessels that are superficial. Thus, large varices, protruding into the esophageal lumen and lacking tissue support, are most likely to rupture and bleed.

Clinical Manifestations

The clinical manifestations of portal hypertension, per se, are similar regardless of the underlying cause, with the effects of increased venous pressure and engorgement present in different target organs (Table 27–3). Splenomegaly can be present as early as 1 month of age[20] and usually is seen before the age of 3 years.[12, 20] Splenomegaly is the commonest manifestation of portal hypertension, but gastrointestinal bleeding is a commoner presenting symptom (70% versus 25%).[17–20] Almost 40% of children with PVO will have a bleeding episode by 3 years of age, and almost all before 10 years of age (Table 27–4).[12, 20] In patients with EHPH, hematemesis or melena typically occurs in a previously healthy, thriving child spontaneously or following an acute upper respiratory tract infection treated with aspirin.

The presentation may also be with jaundice, palmar erythema, and vascular spider veins as manifestations of underlying liver disease. The liver size depends on the etiology; for example, a firm, small liver is usually found with cirrhosis, and firm hepatomegaly is seen with congenital hepatic fibrosis. A large liver is also seen in patients with Budd-Chiari syndrome.

One report[18] indicated that children with portal hypertension secondary to cirrhosis were less likely to bleed than were those with EHPH; only 30% of those with cirrhosis bled, in comparison with 80% with EHPH. This observation has to be cautiously interpreted, since patients with cirrhosis die at younger ages than do those with EHPH, and survival rates for each group were not available. However, one clear observation in children and adults is that when patients with chronic liver disease do bleed, bleeding is usually more severe, refractory to treatment, and poorly tolerated than it is in EHPH, and the morbidity and mortality are greater than they are in EHPH.

Ascites is often present in patients with advanced decompensated liver disease. It is seldom present in stable patients with EHPH but may occur in these patients with an acute gastrointestinal bleeding episode and sometimes with hypoalbuminemia, which is usually

Table 27–4. FEATURES OF PATIENTS WITH EXTRAHEPATIC PORTAL HYPERTENSION UNDERGOING SCLEROTHERAPY

Patient No.	Possible Factors Predisposing to EHPH	Age at First Bleeding (yr)	Age at Start of Sclerotherapy (yr)	Earliest Sign of Portal Hypertension, Age at Presentation (yr)
1	None known	6.3	7.5	Splenomegaly, 3
2	Sister (patient 3) has same condition	1.2	7.5	Bleeding, 1.2
3	Purulent omphalitis	2.8	9.0	Splenomegaly, 0.6
4	Kicked in abdomen 2 yr before first bleeding	10.0	15.0	Bleeding, 10
5	UV catheter, infant of diabetic mother	0.6	13.5	Bleeding, 0.6
6	UV catheter for exchange transfusion for Rh disease at 34 wk gestation	2.6	3.0	Splenomegaly, 0.3
7	None known	3.0	15.0	Splenomegaly, 0.5
8	None known	8.0	9.0	Bleeding, 8
9	Neonatal omphalitis, peritonitis	10.0	16.0	Bleeding, 10
10	None known	1.1	6.5	Bleeding, 1.1

UV, Umbilical vein.
From Hassall E, Berquist WE, Ament ME, et al: Sclerotherapy for portal hypertension in childhood. J Pediatr 1989; 115:69–74; with permission.

transient. Ascites may be the predominant feature in infants with EHPH,[35] who may present with gradual and progressive enlargement of the abdomen.

Rarely, primary pulmonary hypertension occurs in association with EHPH or IHPH,[36, 37] and presents with dyspnea on exertion, syncope, and chest pain. Primary pulmonary hypertension is usually first recognized in adulthood but may be seen in adolescence. Its prognosis is poor.

Diagnosis

History and physical examination may give important clues as to the presence of portal hypertension or its cause (see Table 27–3). The presence of unexplained splenomegaly as an incidental finding, or in a child who presents with hematemesis, is an indicator that portal hypertension may be present. Any child suspected of having portal hypertension should then undergo evaluation (Table 27–5).

The basic questions to be addressed are the following: Is portal hypertension present? If so, is it the result of underlying liver disease (IHPH) or of obstruction of the portal venous system (EHPH)?

The complete blood count will identify the presence and degree of hypersplenism, with thrombocytopenia and leukopenia. Serum aminotransferase levels are important indicators of liver disease, although they may be normal in compensated cirrhosis. Mild lowering of the serum albumin level in conjunction with normal coagulation studies might be an early sign of liver dysfunction, whereas abnormal coagulation studies in conjunction with cholestasis indicate more advanced liver damage. Appropriate studies are then called for to identify the cause of chronic liver disease (see Table 27–1) and should include liver biopsy.

Conventional ultrasound examination is often not accurate for liver or spleen size, nor are sonar changes in organ consistency diagnostic. Nevertheless, ultrasound is useful for evaluating portal vein size and tortuosity and may be helpful in detection and quantitation of ascites. Ultrasound also allows assessment of renal abnormalities as seen with congenital hepatic fibrosis. Doppler sonography is invaluable in assessing the presence and direction of blood flow through the portal vein (hepatopetal versus hepatofugal) and through the splenic and renal veins as well, as the presence of obstruction in posthepatic veins. The presence of collateral vessels around the portal vein (cavernous transformation) is a sign of extrahepatic portal vein obstruction, and convoluted, high-flow veins may be seen in the splenic hilum. Normally, with Doppler sonography, respiratory modulation of portal flow is present; loss of this sign is suggestive of portal hypertension, but the presence of the sign does not rule it out.[38–40]

Table 27–5. LABORATORY STUDIES IN THE EVALUATION OF PORTAL HYPERTENSION

Initial Steps
- CBC, differential, platelet count, PT/PTT
- Serum AST, ALT, alkaline phosphatase, bilirubin
- Serum total protein, albumin, ammonia
- Ultrasound of liver, biliary tree, portal venous system and kidneys, including Doppler sonography for venous flow pattern

Further Steps
- Investigation of causes of chronic liver disease (see Table 27–1)
- Upper gastrointestinal endoscopy
- Liver biopsy
- Angiography

CBC, complete blood count; PT/PTT, prothrombin time/partial thromboplastin time; AST, aspartate aminotransferase; ALT, alanine aminotransferase.

Barium swallow has a sensitivity of about 70% for detection of esophageal varices in adults[41]; however, with the availability of endoscopy, this examination is seldom indicated for this purpose, and it has no role in the patient with active upper gastrointestinal bleeding.

Upper gastrointestinal flexible endoscopy is now possible and safe in all pediatric age groups[1, 12, 42, 43] and is the most accurate and sensitive way of identifying gastric and esophageal varices. In the child with upper gastrointestinal bleeding, endoscopy should be performed as soon as the child is stable. Children with portal hypertension can bleed from a nonvariceal site,[18] and, for optimal management, it is vital to establish the bleeding site. The interventional role of endoscopic sclerotherapy is discussed separately (see section on treatment). Endoscopy may also be indicated in the asymptomatic child with portal hypertension if prophylactic treatment of varices is considered (see section on sclerotherapy).

In the asymptomatic or stable patient, endoscopy has also been used to predict the risk of bleeding from varices.[21, 44–46] This procedure may aid in better selection of patients and timing of sclerotherapy. Although in Europe and North America variceal size and tortuosity are used to predict the risk of variceal hemorrhage, more complex guidelines were compiled by the Japanese Research Society for Portal Hypertension.[45] Sarin and colleagues[21] studied the usefulness of all the different endoscopic signs, intravariceal pressure, and Child's grading in predicting the risk of variceal hemorrhage. They were able to identify the following variables, in decreasing importance: variceal size, intravariceal pressure, cherry-red spots, color of varices (blue or white), and red wale markings over the varices. Although all factors together could account for only 50% of the variability between the bleeding group and the nonbleeding group, variceal size alone explained 35% of the variability. Different grading systems for size of esophageal varices were found to be of comparable value.[21] Child's grading of liver disease was not an important factor in predicting variceal hemorrhage. The presence of esophagitis and its role in variceal bleeding is controversial[21, 45] but appears to be of minor importance.

Variceal wall thickness and tissue support are two important factors that cannot be evaluated directly by endoscopy. However, with devices attached to the endoscope tip, actual intravariceal pressure can be measured, making prediction of variceal hemorrhage more accurate.[38]

Endoscopy can also identify the presence of gastric

varices and portal hypertensive gastropathy, an important cause of nonvariceal bleeding.[47, 48] Gastric varices and portal hypertensive gastropathy are present in 60 to 80% of patients[20, 49, 50] and are the bleeding source in about half these patients. Angiography (Fig. 27–3) is invaluable in defining portal vascular anatomy precisely. It should be performed when the diagnosis of EHPH is suspected or made, as it clarifies future surgical or other therapeutic options (see section on treatment). It may also be helpful in identifying a site of active bleeding that is not within reach of the endoscope (i.e., small bowel) or if the patient is too ill to undergo endoscopy.[51–53] Angiography also has a valuable role in the treatment of portal hypertension (see the section on splenic embolization). Digital subtraction angiography allows a reduction in contrast material load and shortens the examination time.[54] Abdominal computed tomography (CT) can provide information about periesophageal varices but offers no advantage over Doppler ultrasound in the assessment of the portal system.[55]

Management of Acute Variceal Bleeding

Although most episodes of upper gastrointestinal bleeding in the pediatric age group are self-limited and can be managed conservatively, variceal bleeding can be massive and fatal. Regardless of the cause of gastrointestinal bleeding, the management of the unstable child with significant blood loss and hypovolemia is initial control of the airway, breathing, and circulation[56] (see Chapter 20). Two large-bore intravenous lines should be established, and blood drawn for complete blood count, platelet count, cross-match, prothrombin time, partial thromboplastin time, serum aminotransferases, alkaline phosphatase, electrolytes, creatinine, and urea. For children with resting tachycardia, initial volume replacement with crystalloid solution is indicated, with repeated intravenous boluses of 10 to 20 ml per kg given over 10 minutes even if initial hemoglobin and hematocrit levels are normal. Intravenous boluses should be repeated until the resting heart rate is within 10% of the normal heart rate for age. If more than 50 to 70 ml per kg is required over 4 to 6 hours, central vein pressure (CVP) might need to be monitored. Whole blood or packed red blood cells should be given if bleeding persists, with platelet transfusion planned if blood loss is more than 50% of total blood volume. A large-bore, well-lubricated nasogastric or orogastic tube should be passed to establish the presence of fresh or altered blood in the stomach. The presence of esophageal varices is not a contraindication to placement of a well-lubricated nasogastric tube. The absence of coffee grounds makes the diagnosis of variceal bleeding unlikely, but a duodenal ulcer may occasionally bleed only distal to the pylorus. With active bleeding, the gastric aspirate is likely to contain fresh blood, whereas the presence of coffee grounds indicates a slow bleeding rate or cessation of the hemorrhage. The nasogastric tube can be removed after lavage with 5 to 10 ml per kg of *room temperature* normal saline solution. The use of iced-saline lavage in children should be discouraged, since it may cause hypothermia in young children and has no demonstrable benefit over room temperature solution.[57] Patients with known liver disease and those with abnormal coagulation studies should be given vitamin K parenterally and fresh-frozen plasma (Table 27–6).

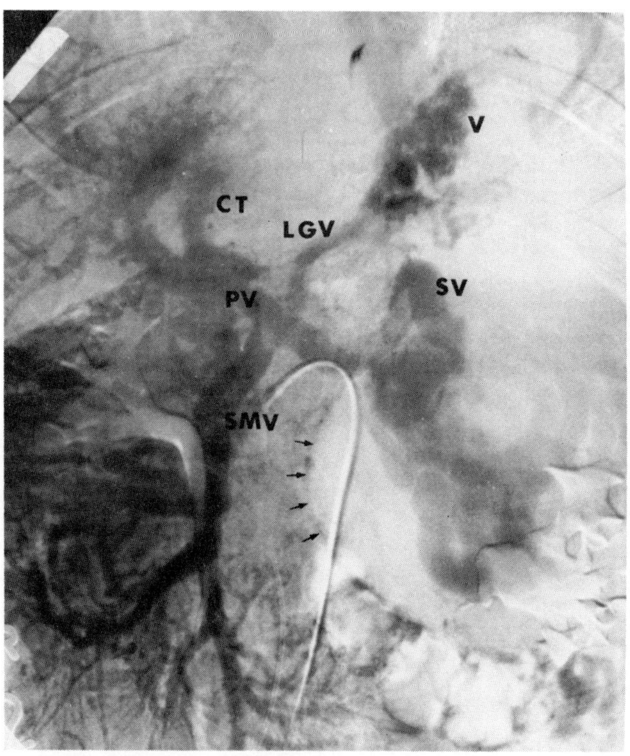

Figure 27–3. Delayed phase of superior mesenteric artery angiogram. This child had portal vein obstruction. Contrast material in the superior mesenteric vein (SMV) and portal vein (PV) up to the obstruction of PV. Cavernous transformation (CT) of the portal vein is demonstrated. Hepatofugal flow into dilated and tortuous splenic vein (SV), left gastric vein (LGV), and esophageal varices (V) is present. *Small arrows* indicate enlarged spleen. (Courtesy of Dr. Gordon Culham, BC Children's Hospital, Vancouver, BC.)

A resting heart rate within 10% of the normal range for age indicates an adequate volume replacement, and bleeding is assumed to have ceased if the resting heart rate remains in the normal range for age while the patient is receiving maintenance fluid volume. Further bed rest and close monitoring of vital signs and hemoglobin levels for at least 24 hours are mandatory. The patient should be kept NPO, with gradual introduction of clear fluids by mouth after 24 hours without active hemorrhage.

Pharmacologic Agents for Active Variceal Bleeding

Vasopressin is the most commonly used agent for variceal bleeding in children (see Table 27–6). It causes vasoconstriction of the precapillary arterioles of the gut, thus decreasing blood flow to the gut and lowering

Table 27–6. INITIAL PHASE OF MEDICAL TREATMENT

Agent	Dosage	Comments
Crystalloid blood	10–20 ml/kg normal saline or Ringer's lactate Whole blood/packed RBC	Continue until HR within 10% of normal range for age Monitor urine output
Vitamin K	1 mg/yr of age daily max 10 mg SC	Follow PT/PTT for correction
Fresh-frozen plasma	5 ml/kg	Over 15–30 min Repeat every 6–12 hr
Vasopressin	20 U/1.73 m^2 IV in 10–15 ml infusion of 5% D/W over 10 min followed by continuous IV 0.2 U/1.73 m^2/min in 5% D/W. Double the hourly dose every 1–2 hr if bleeding persists, max 0.8 U/1.73 m^2 min. If bleeding stops, continue treatment for 24 hr, then taper over 24–48 hr.	Bradycardia occurs with rapid IV push Follow for hypotension, water retention, dilutional hyponatremia Strict input-output records
Terlipressin	2 mg every 6 hr IV bolus	
Nitroglycerin	50–400 μg/min to maintain systolic blood pressure above 100 mm Hg	
Somatostatin	100–200 μg bolus followed by continuous 100–200 μg/hr	

RBC, red blood cells; SC, subcutaneous; IV, intravenous; D/W, dextrose in water; HR, heart rate; PT/PTT, prothrombin time/partial thromboplastin time.

portal flow. No data are available to support the efficacy of vasopressin in the pediatric age group, but it is standard treatment in children, and controlled studies in adults show an efficacy of 50% and recurrence of hemorrhage of 45%.[58] Vasopressin may cause hypotension, water retention, dilutional hyponatremia, and bradycardia. Although intra-arterial and selective mesenteric vein injections were tried in the past, the intravenous route is much simpler and as effective.[59]

Intravenous vasopressin is indicated for massive or persistent bleeding. This is initiated with a bolus dose of 20 U of vasopressin per 1.73 m^2 body surface area diluted in 10 to 15 ml per kg of 5% dextrose given over 10 minutes, which is followed by continuous intravenous infusion of 0.2 U per 1.73 m^2 per minute in 5% dextrose. Vasopressin dose may be doubled every 1 to 2 hours if active bleeding persists, to a maximum of 0.8 U per 1.73 m^2 per minute. Since it causes water retention, strict input and output fluid balance should be maintained. In the very ill child, CVP and urinary catheters are necessary for intravenous fluid management. Once bleeding has stopped, vasopressin infusion is maintained for 24 hours and then gradually tapered over 24 to 48 hours. The complete blood count should be monitored every 6 hours for unstable patients.

Endoscopy should be scheduled as soon as the patient is stable. The role of endoscopy is to identify the source of bleeding, since as many as 30 to 50% of patients with varices bleed from a nonvariceal source.[18, 60] In patients with active variceal bleeding not quickly responsive to medical treatment, sclerotherapy is indicated.

Where endoscopic sclerotherapy is available, there is little use for balloon tamponade. Although tamponade is effective in stopping acute bleeding in 90% of adults,[61, 62] there is a high rebleeding rate immediately after the balloon is deflated. Furthermore, the morbidity of balloon tamponade (aspiration, laryngeal or tracheal obstruction) is unacceptably high. Even with personnel experienced in its use,[62] tamponade should be considered only a temporizing measure prior to repeat sclerotherapy or to surgery.

Terlipressin (triglyceryl-vasopressin) has the same effect as vasopressin, with the advantages of prolonged, gradual release of active vasopressin, making every-6-hour dosing possible, and with fewer side effects than are reported with vasopressin.[63]

Somatostatin was also reported to exert a similar effect on portal blood flow with fewer side effects.[64] Nitroglycerin can decrease portal blood pressure by vasodilation and has been used in combination with vasopressin, with which it may ameliorate many of the vasoconstrictive side effects of vasopressin.[65, 66] There is limited experience with the use of these agents in children, and no clear indication for their use has been established in this age group.

Once active bleeding has stopped and the patient is hemodynamically stable, careful observation for 7 to 10 days is indicated, since there is a 30% recurrence of variceal bleeding within 6 weeks, with most episodes occurring in the first week following the initial bleed.[67] In the management of children with portal hypertension, it is important to avoid aspirin-containing products, which are a common precipitating cause of variceal bleeding. The patient or family is given a list of aspirin-containing products to be avoided (Table 27–7). Long-term therapy is planned as detailed in the treatment section.

TREATMENT OF PORTAL HYPERTENSION

Overview

Most acute variceal bleeding episodes respond to bed rest, blood transfusion, vasopressin infusion, and (increasingly rarely) balloon tamponade, as indicated. Occasionally, emergency sclerotherapy or surgery is re-

Table 27–7. PARENT INSTRUCTION SHEET: ASPIRIN-CONTAINING MEDICATIONS TO BE AVOIDED

We have determined that your child is at risk for bleeding from the upper digestive tract. Such bleeding may occur without obvious cause, but ingestion of aspirin and aspirin-containing medications will greatly increase the likelihood of bleeding.

THE FOLLOWING MEDICATIONS CONTAIN ASPIRIN AND SHOULD NOT BE GIVEN TO YOUR CHILD:

We suggest that you keep this list handy for easy reference, and that you make copies for your Doctor and your Pharmacist, plus any friends or relatives who may take care of your child periodically. If your child requires medication for fever or pain, give the recommended dose for age of acetaminophen—this drug is sold under many proprietary names including Tylenol, Panadol, Atasol, Campain, Exdol. Consult your Pharmacist to determine appropriate dose for age. New medications appear on the market periodically, therefore always check the label of the medication to ensure that it does not contain aspirin.

Preparations containing aspirin:

A.S.A. (Lilly) Equagesic (Wyeth)
A.S.A. Compound (Lilly)
Alka-Seltzer (Miles)
Alprine Bi Tabs (Ulmer)
*Anacin (Whitehall)
Anodynos-DHC Tablets (Tilden-Yates)
Ascodeen-30 (Burroughs-Wellcome)
Ascriptin (Rorer)
Aspirin
Bayer Aspirin (Glenbrook)
Buff-A Comp (Mayrand)
*Bufferin (Bristol-Myers)
Cirin (Zommer)
Codempiral (Burroughs-Wellcome)
Cope (Glenbrook)
Cordex preparations (Upjohn)
*Coricidin preparations (Schering)
Convangesic (Mallinckrodt)
Daprisal (SmithKline)
Daragesic (Meyer)
*Darvon Compound (Lilly)
Darvon w/A.S.A. (Lilly)
Demerol w/A.P.C. (Winthrop)
*Dristan (Whitehall)
Drocogesic No. 3 (Carrtone)
Ecotrin (SmithKline)
Empirin preparations (Burroughs-Wellcome)
Emprazil preparations (Burroughs-Wellcome)
*Excedrin (Bristol-Myers)
*Fiorinal preparations (Sandoz)
Monacet preparations (Rexall)
Nemu-gesic (Abbott)
Norgesic (Riker)
Novahistine w/A.P.C. (Pitman-Moore)
Pabirin Buffered Tablets (Dorsey)
Pentagesic (Kremers-Urban)
Percobarb preparations (Endo)
*Percodan preparations (Endo)
Persistin (Copper)
Phenaphen preparations (Robins)
Phenodyne preparations (Blue Line)
Predisal (Mallard)
Pyrroxate (Upjohn)
Robaxisal preparations (Robins)
Sigmagen (Schering)
Stero Darvon w/A.S.A. (Lilly)
Supac (Mission)
Synalgos preparations (Ives)
Synirin (Poythress)
Tetrex A.P.C. w/Bristamin (Bristol)
Trancogesic (Winthrop)
Vanquish (Glenbrook)
Vingesic (Amid)
Zactirin Compound-100 (Wyeth)

*Preparations in common use, whose aspirin content is not widely known. Note: aspirin is also called ACETYLSALICYLIC ACID, often abbreviated A.S.A.

Prepared by: Division of Gastroenterology
British Columbia Children's Hospital
Vancouver, BC, Canada

Reproduced with permission of Dr. Eric Hassall, Division of Gastroenterology, British Columbia Children's Hospital, Vancouver, BC, Canada.

quired to control acute bleeding unresponsive to medical measures, but by far the greatest challenge is the long-term prevention of variceal bleeding.

In approaching the treatment of variceal bleeding, the single most important consideration is the cause of the underlying portal hypertension. At the heart of the matter is that in obstruction of the portal venous system (EHPH), hepatic synthetic function is normal, whereas in hepatocellular disease with cirrhosis (IHPH), it is not. The two entities have different natural histories, and the prognosis in EHPH (good liver, bad veins) is far better than that in IHPH (bad liver, usually normal veins).

For children with IHPH, management of recurrent bleeding is usually a temporizing, stabilizing measure before the definitive treatment, liver transplantation, is performed. In EHPH, management of recurrent bleeding *is* the definitive treatment. This further defines the therapeutic approach, so it is helpful to consider each entity separately before specific treatment modalities are discussed.

Extrahepatic Portal Hypertension

Even though children with EHPH usually bleed recurrently and often massively, the acute bleeding episode usually stops spontaneously or with supportive therapy, as outlined earlier. Despite hypersplenism and thrombocytopenia, the platelets are functionally normal, and clotting factors and function are within normal limits. If the source of bleeding is proved to be variceal, and intravascular volumes are repleted promptly, bleeding is usually well tolerated, and mortality of the acute bleed is limited. Morbidity relates to multiple blood transfusions, recurrent hospitalizations, and the significant psychosocial consequences of repeated and unpredictable disruptions of home and school life. The natural history of childhood EHPH is one of recurrent episodes of bleeding, usually beginning before the age of 5 years, sometimes recurring more frequently during puberty, and decreasing after the age of 20 years.[68] In some authors' experience, some patients with EHPH will never bleed, and 20% or more of patients will not bleed at all after the age of 20 years[68]; this decrease may result from the formation of natural shunts that decompress the portal system in some patients. The formation of natural splenorenal shunts has been shown to be promoted by sclerotherapy of esophageal varices,[69] thus accelerating the natural history toward less bleeding.[12]

Intrahepatic Portal Hypertension

Hepatic cirrhosis with compromised hepatocellular function constitutes by far the majority of causes of IHPH in children (see Table 27–1). In these patients, spontaneous cessation of bleeding occurs less often, management of bleeding is more difficult, and complications of bleeding are more frequent. Even patients with compensated cirrhosis have much less hepatic and nutritional reserve than do children with EHPH, and they withstand bleeding less well. Therefore, patients with IHPH, as a group, have considerable morbidity and mortality resulting from variceal bleeding, higher with Child's class C than B and A.[70]

Drug Therapy

In 1980, Lebrec and associates[71] introduced the concept of beta-adrenergic blockade with oral propranolol for the long-term prevention of variceal bleeding. The rationale for use of beta-blockade is that decreases in portal pressure,[3] portocollateral flow, and variceal size all result from decreased cardiac output as well as from a possible direct action of the drug on the splanchnic bed and a decrease in intrahepatic portal vascular resistance. However, the precise mechanisms of action have not yet been proved.[72]

Although a large number of drugs decrease portal hypertension, only the following types have been evaluated for their long-term effects:

1. *Beta-adrenergic blockers*: The most widely used drug is propranolol, a nonselective blocker, taken in a dose sufficient to produce a sustained 25% decrease in resting heart rate. Nadolol,[73] a long-acting nonselective blocker, has also been used, as have selective beta$_1$-antagonists.[72] The latter have less effect on portal hypertension, because splanchnic vessels have no beta$_1$-receptors; therefore, reliance is placed on decreased cardiac output as the sole mechanism.
2. *Alpha-adrenergic agonists,* for example, clonidine.[72]
3. *5-Hydroxytryptamine antagonists,* for example, ketanserin.[72]

Combinations of vasoactive drugs have also been used, but of all the drugs, propranolol alone has been the most prevalently used and studied. Some trials have shown propranolol to be more effective than placebo in preventing variceal bleeding, especially in selected patients at low risk without hepatic decompensation.[3, 73–75] Poynard and associates[76] confirmed their earlier findings of the success of propranolol in preventing recurrent bleeding in these relatively healthy patients and also identified five factors that were independently associated with recurrent bleeding: noncompliance with treatment, absence of a persistently low heart rate, a history of bleeding, continued ingestion of alcohol, and the presence of hepatocellular carcinoma. Groszmann and coworkers[3] showed that the reduction by propranolol of the hepatic venous pressure gradient to less than 12 mm Hg protects from variceal bleeding and increases survival rate compared with a placebo-treated group. Both groups consisted of cirrhotic adults, largely with Child's class A or B disease. Because most bleeding events occurred during the first year, the protective effect appeared to be greatest in the period associated with the largest reduction in portal pressure. However, in unselected patients, other well-conducted randomized, controlled studies showed no benefit with the use of propranolol versus placebo.[77, 78] A controlled study comparing propranolol treatment with sclerotherapy showed that propranolol decreased variceal size significantly within 3 months and concluded that propranolol and sclerotherapy were equally successful for the long-term treatment of unselected cirrhotic patients.[79] However, another study concluded in favor of sclerotherapy.[80] Failures of propranolol have been attributed by some authors to the use of a dose that is too low.[72] For nonvariceal bleeding from portal hypertensive gastropathy, propanolol appears to be the only nonsurgical option,[47, 48] because these submucosal telangiectasias cannot be treated with injection sclerotherapy.

Relatively minor side effects of long-term beta-blockade include asthenia, which is common in the first weeks of therapy, and decreased libido. However, in the study by Burroughs and colleagues,[77] 15% of the propranolol-treated group stopped the medication because of the serious complication of hypotension, left ventricular failure, or hepatic encephalopathy.

What do the data just discussed mean for children, given that the findings are derived largely from adults with alcoholic cirrhosis? Although there are no controlled trials in children, there is some anecdotal experience with this therapy. Of 10 children with EHPH receiving sclerotherapy,[12] five failed a trial of propranolol of at least a year. However, the compliance with propranolol was not monitored closely.

Experience in children with long-term use of propranolol as a hypotensive agent for *systemic hypertension* has shown that, other than producing fatigue in some patients, it is usually well tolerated; serious adverse effects are unusual in the child with a healthy myocardium and in the absence of reactive airway disease. One theoretical risk of propranolol therapy is the possible inability to mount a compensatory increase in cardiac output in response to a major bleed. Children usually withstand volume loss better than do adults, and perhaps the use of propranolol will remove that "natural advantage."

Endoscopic Sclerotherapy

In the evolution of therapy for variceal bleeding, sclerotherapy was first described in Sweden in 1939,[81] antedating the development of surgical portosystemic shunts in 1945.[82, 83] The sporadic reports of success of sclerotherapy[84–87] were greatly overshadowed by the wide use of surgical shunts as the prevalent treatment of variceal bleeding from 1945 to the early 1970s. However, interest in sclerotherapy was renewed by further successful reports in 1973[88] and by developing disillusionment with standard portosystemic shunts.[89–91] The successful controlled trial of sclerotherapy by Terblanche and coworkers[92] led to a profusion of reports in adults but only a dozen or so pediatric reports in the last decade,[4–17] none of which were controlled.

Although varices at any portosystemic anastomosis may bleed (gastric, small bowel, or rectal), varices in the most distal 3 to 5 cm of esophagus are responsible for the greatest frequency, severity, and morbidity of bleeding. Endoscopic sclerotherapy blocks this particular superficial portosystemic shunt by directly injecting a sclerosing agent into or adjacent to the varices. Control of bleeding acutely may occur by spasm, thrombosis, or compression of vessels by edema. Thrombosis and tissue necrosis are demonstrable histologically within 24 hours, ulceration by 7 days, and fibrosis by 1 month; this process obliterates superficial, poorly supported vessels.[93] The high pressure is transmitted to other veins and results in the formation of deep veins in the muscularis propria, supported also by the fibrous tissue formed. Subepithelial varices (deep intrinsic veins) may also recanalize. If, in the process, perforating veins connecting superficial subepithelial veins to deeper veins are obliterated, subepithelial varices are less likely to re-form in the esophagus. The process is not curative but merely "plugs" the most vulnerable (and accessible) portion of the portosystemic system. Ingress of portal venous blood to the collaterals is blocked, thus elevating portal pressure, and varices may re-form in the esophagus or elsewhere. For this reason, sclerotherapy has been described as "irrational."[94] However, in EHPH, it has also been postulated[12] and shown[69] that sclerotherapy may accelerate the development of "natural" (i.e., nonsurgical) shunts at sites that tend not to bleed (splenorenal), thus protecting from rebleeding by portal decompression as well as by sclerosis of the susceptible veins.

Methods

Instruments and Anesthesia. Slotted, rigid endoscopes are said to have the advantage of ease of compression of a bleeding varix and rapid clearance of a bloody field. However, complications, particularly esophageal perforation, are commoner with rigid endoscopes[15, 17, 88, 92] than they are with flexible instruments.[8, 9, 95, 96] Flexible instruments can diagnose bleeding from sites other than the esophagus, which is an important advantage, since patients with portal hypertension may bleed fatally from sites other than varices, for example, gastric or duodenal ulcers. Furthermore, rigid endoscopy has the disadvantage of always requiring a general anesthetic.[97] Intravenous sedation has the advantage of avoiding the risks of repeated general anesthesia,[98] a consideration for patients with a chronic condition who may require many procedures over time. Flexible instruments (Fig. 27–4) have superseded rigid endoscopes in adults and children, and adults now rarely, if ever, undergo general anesthesia for the procedure. Although many pediatric exponents always use general anesthesia, more recently others have shown the advantages and safety of intravenous sedation for most pediatric cases[6, 12, 14] and general anesthesia for only a minority.[12] General anesthesia may be advantageous in certain pediatric patients, as for a child younger than 8 years of age or so, for an early sclerotherapy session in a patient with massive varices that may bleed actively, or for a patient who is bleeding rapidly. A sedated child with a stomach full of blood and without a protected airway in the last two circumstances is at risk for a poor-quality and possibly unsafe procedure. General anesthesia enables the use of a larger flexible endoscope in any given child, reducing the chance of occlusion of the suction channel, and if blood wells up in the esophagus, the airway is protected.[12, 99] Most investigators have not found the use of an overtube necessary to compress bleeding varices.

Sclerosing Agents. To be of use in sclerotherapy, an agent must produce a high sclerosis rate and a low incidence of esophageal damage. In childhood studies, British and Australian exponents have favored ethanolamine[9, 10, 13, 15, 17] and polidocanol (Aetoxisclerol). Most North American centers have switched from sodium morrhuate to tetradecyl sulfate, usually mixed with ethanol, saline,[7] or both (T.E.S.).[12] In animal studies, tetradecyl sulfate was more thrombogenic than was either sodium morrhuate or ethanolamine. Both 5% sodium morrhuate and undiluted 3% tetradecyl sulfate are excessively ulcerogenic; therefore, T.E.S. (1% tetradecyl sulfate) was developed.[100] Some clini-

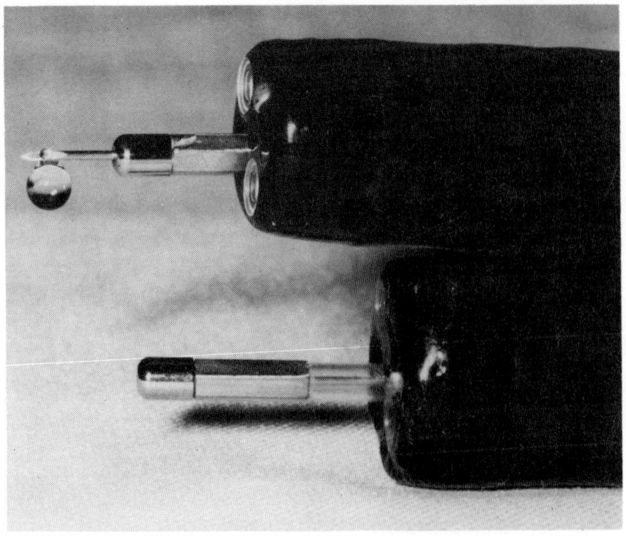

Figure 27–4. Tips of flexible fiberoptic endoscopes showing sclerotherapy needles retracted and extended.

cians have used ethanol either alone[11] or with polidocanol.[14] However, the use of a specific sclerosant may have less basis in science than in its availability in a particular country and in the authors' habit or bias. Many agents appear to be satisfactory.

Techniques. The goal of intravariceal injection is to induce variceal thrombosis, whereas paravariceal injection is said to thicken the mucosa overlying varices by inducing inflammation and fibrosis. Although one controlled trial suggested that intravariceal injection is superior to paravariceal,[101] Paquet,[6, 99] the main proponent of the latter technique, has longstanding favorable experience with paravariceal injection. In fact, intravariceal injection is often not directed purely into the varix, because some sclerosant may leak. Some clinicans deliberately use a combination technique. A description of our own technique follows, although it is clear that different techniques work, and endoscopists find the variations in technique that work best for them.

Gastroduodenoscopy is performed to exclude other potential sources of bleeding and to document the extent of gastric and duodenal varices. The site of the gastroesophageal junction is noted, as are the linear extent and size of varices. Varices are injected circumferentially, starting at the gastroesophageal junction and moving cephalad at the same session. Varices in only the distal 5 cm of esophagus are injected (only the distal 3 cm in children younger than 8 years old). It is neither necessary nor wise to aim to obliterate varices higher up the esophagus.[102] Intravariceal injections are performed until resistance is met or until the varix blanches. A sclerosant dose of 0.5 to 3 ml is given into each varix. Patent varices frequently bleed actively after needle withdrawal but usually stop bleeding after compression with the endoscope and observation. If not, the varix is reinjected at adjacent sites until hemostasis is observed. If active bleeding occurs, the head of the endoscopy table is elevated 30 degrees to prevent blood from welling up the esophagus. Blood from active bleeding should be washed into the stomach to clear the field for subsequent injection and later aspirated through the endoscope— this is easier than constantly suctioning the esophagus clean. One assistant suctions the pharynx to prevent aspiration. If oozing persists, a slow intravenous infusion of vasopressin is given during or immediately after the procedure. If all blood and clot cannot be aspirated from the stomach, a dose of metoclopramide is given intravenously to accelerate gastric emptying and lessen the possibility of vomiting or aspiration after the procedure. Metoclopramide, like vasopressin, has the additional benefit of increasing lower esophageal sphincter (LES) pressure and may be helpful in stopping variceal bleeding. For outpatient procedures, patients are monitored in a recovery area for 3 or 4 hours after endoscopy, then discharged. Patients are cautioned that mild dysphagia may occur for several days and that they should return immediately if an oral temperature higher than 38.5°C develops. Oral intake is restricted to liquids until the next morning. Sessions are scheduled to obliterate varices in the initial 4 to 8 weeks, with routine endoscopic re-evaluations at 2, 4, 8, and 12 months and every 6 to 8 months thereafter. If follow-up endoscopy shows that varices have recurred, sclerotherapy is repeated in as many sessions as necessary to reobliterate them. A recommended schedule and dosages of T.E.S. sclerosant mixture are given in Table 27–8. The timing of intravariceal sclerotherapy in adults has been examined in two controlled trials,[101, 103] both of which showed better results when injections were performed approximately weekly until varices had been eradicated rather than at longer intervals. The authors have not wanted to subject children to more than one procedure every 1 or 2 weeks, especially when a full dose of sclerosant had been used, and they want to allow some re-epithelialization of the esophageal ulcers to occur before reinjection.[12]

Different Indications

Sclerotherapy for the Control of Active Bleeding. Three controlled trials[104–106] and other uncontrolled studies[107–110] showed that sclerotherapy controls acute variceal bleeding in 90% of adult patients; it is more effective than either balloon tamponade or vasopressin alone, with which only 40 to 50% of patients are controlled.[111, 112] A single sclerotherapy session stops bleeding in 70% of patients,[103] and with the 30% who rebleed and require further injection, the percentage controlled can be increased to 90%. In the remaining 10% of patients who have further episodes of variceal bleeding after two sclerotherapy sessions during a single hospital admission, the mortality is 90% if the Child's class A patients (i.e., those who should survive anyway) are excluded.[113] This concept of the decreasing effectiveness of sclerotherapy is further supported by another study in which immediate sclerotherapy controlled bleeding in 88% of cases; when performed after 12 hours of vasopressin and nitroglycerin, that number was only 65%.[114] Thus, immediate sclerotherapy has the advantages of being incorporated into the diagnostic endoscopy and attaining early hemostasis in most patients. However, ongoing bleeding and transfusion, or the drug regimen itself, may adversely affect the efficacy of sclerotherapy as a salvage procedure.

About half of the pediatric studies had used sclero-

Table 27–8. RECOMMENDED GUIDELINES FOR SCLEROTHERAPY

Frequency
Sclerotherapy every 1 to 2 weeks until varices are obliterated. Usually three to six sessions are required, depending on size and number of varices.
Check endoscopy 1 month after last session to ensure variceal obliteration.
Repeat endoscopy every 6 to 8 months for first 2 years to detect early recurrence or inadequate sclerosis.
Annual endoscopy thereafter.
Dosage of T.E.S.
Use amount of sclerosant necessary to obliterate one fourth to one half of varices at each of initial sessions, fewer if patient has massive varices.
Use up to 0.8 ml/kg per session, not to exceed 30 ml per session.

From Hassall E, Berquist WE, Ament ME, et al: Sclerotherapy for portal hypertension in childhood. J Pediatr 1989; 115:69–74; with permission.

therapy for acute control of active bleeding in some patients (in addition to ongoing, long-term use in most); all those studies reported success in the control of active bleeding in 97 to 100% of patients, although all were uncontrolled studies, and many used vasopressin infusion simultaneously. Interpretation of these results is difficult, since they are generally not broken down by cause of portal hypertension. Most evaluated "all comers" ignoring the fact that bleeding stops spontaneously in 40 to 60% of all comers[115] and that the number climbs to 90% for those patients with EHPH.

Ongoing Sclerotherapy for Long-Term Prevention of Bleeding. Ongoing sclerotherapy refers to sclerotherapy performed after the initial hemorrhage has been controlled and is performed on a schedule to obliterate varices within a relatively short period, 2 months or so. This is followed by a long-term protocol of surveillance endoscopy to diagnose and treat recurrent varices. This is the commonest use of sclerotherapy, and it aims to prevent the high rate of rebleeding of varices. After cessation of an acute bleeding episode, 30% of adults will rebleed within 6 weeks, and an additional 40% will do so within a year, for a total of 70% within 12 months.[67, 116] Long-term sclerotherapy in adults showed decreased recurrence of bleeding in only two of five controlled studies, but the overall rebleeding rate in treated patients was still 50%.[117] Only one study actually showed improved survival in sclerotherapy-treated patients.[118] Thus, it is not clear whether sclerotherapy is the treatment of choice for IHPH in adults, particularly because esophageal complications, although not usually a major problem, do increase with time.[119]

The picture is quite different for EHPH. In a long-term follow-up study of sclerotherapy in children with EHPH,[12] 10 children each had four bleeding episodes requiring 11.3 units of blood per patient over a pre-sclerotherapy period of 5.6 years (all figures are means). Over a mean follow-up of 4.7 years (1.4–7.1), only two patients had recurrence of variceal bleeding; in one, variceal obliteration had not been completed, and the other had defaulted on sclerotherapy follow-up. Complications were few and easily managed. Once varices were eradicated by initial sclerotherapy sessions, no child missed school because of this illness, and all grew and developed normally. Furthermore, the frequency of sclerotherapy sessions and quantities of sclerosant decreased with time, suggesting that the natural history in EHPH of decreased bleeding (with time) might be accelerated by sclerotherapy.[12, 69] In a 44-month follow-up study of 39 teenage and adult patients with EHPH, similar excellent results led the authors to conclude that sclerotherapy was the treatment of choice for this disorder.[120]

Sclerotherapy for Preventing the First Episode of Bleeding. The rationale for so-called prophylactic sclerotherapy is that at least 30% of patients with cirrhosis will bleed from esophageal varices sometime in their lives, and almost 50% will die after the initial episode. The corollary to this argument is that some patients with cirrhosis or EHPH will never bleed from varices, so why risk precipitating a bleed resulting from complications with sclerotherapy?[121] Mortality is largely governed by functional hepatic reserve, as indicated by Child's grade. Only about 6% of those with the most hepatic reserve will die after the first bleed, and only 1 of 159 children and adults with EHPH died after the first bleed. Thus, the potential benefit of prophylactic sclerotherapy is low in those patients with the most hepatic reserve,[121] and the patient should have to "earn" therapy, with its potential problems. Furthermore, by the time a child with cirrhosis has recurrent variceal bleeding, the definitive therapy is more likely to be liver transplantation than it is sclerotherapy. Prophylactic sclerotherapy might be justified in patients with decreased hepatic reserve if endoscopic and hepatic criteria existed from which to select candidates, but as yet these have not been confirmed to be reliable.[121] The King's College group[13, 15] performed prophylactic sclerotherapy in children with IHPH but acknowledged its uncertain role, given potential complications and even spontaneous regression of varices in some children.[122] They advocate reserving it for children living where emergency treatment with safe blood transfusion (and vasopressin) is not quickly available or in those with "large extensive varices."

Sclerotherapy for Gastric Varices. Gastric varices are the bleeding source in 15 to 20% of acute bleeds in portal hypertension. Those varices on the lesser curve or in a hiatal hernia can be managed with sclerotherapy, but the results for actively bleeding fundal varices are poor, and the procedure may be hazardous.[117, 123] In many medical centers, bleeding gastric varices unresponsive to medical measures are managed surgically, with a portosystemic shunt or devascularizing surgery. However, injection of fundal varices with tissue adhesive agents has been successful in experienced hands.[117, 124]

Sclerotherapy for Rectal Varices. Rectal varices are not the same as hemorrhoids, or "piles,"[125] which are rare in children. They are dilated portosystemic submucosal veins formed between the high pressure superior hemorrhoidal vein of the portal system and the low-pressure middle and inferior hemorrhoidal veins of the systemic circulation. They are usually found in the mid or proximal rectum, as opposed to the more distal piles. The varices may bleed minimally or massively, and when they do not respond to supportive medical therapy with transfusion, vasopressin, and packing, and bleeding is recurrent or massive, they may be sclerosed successfully with T.E.S.[126, 127] There is not extensive experience with this procedure. Endoscopic variceal ligation, described later for esophageal varices, is gaining popularity for treatment of hemorrhoids and rectal varices.[124]

Complications

There are a wide variety of reported complications of sclerotherapy,[99, 128] but most are single case reports indicating that serious complications are very infrequent; in general, they appear to occur considerably less often in pediatric than in adult reports. Possible explanations include less intensive regimens used in children, fewer Child's class C patients, shorter follow-up, and the ability of children to better withstand the procedure.

Superficial ulceration within a week or so occurs

routinely as part of the process of injecting a substance that causes thrombosis as well as a chemical esophagitis. Mild pyrexia and transient minor chest pain or dysphagia are frequent and should not be regarded as complications.[99, 128] Bacterial sepsis occurs rarely but must be recognized early.[12, 128] A temperature higher than 39°C or a systemic illness within 24 to 36 hours of the procedure indicates the need for prompt evaluation. Asplenic patients are at high risk for bacterial sepsis and routinely should receive prophylactic antibiotics for sclerotherapy.[129] Transient hemoglobinuria in children has occurred, possibly owing to intravascular hemolysis by systemic escape of sclerosant[12, 16]; treated with increased fluid administration, it did not have sequelae. Shock lung has occurred with sodium morrhuate,[130] also likely owing to systemic escape. Paraplegia occurred in one child after mid-esophageal injection and presumed runoff to spinal cord vessels,[102] but this has never been described with a distal esophageal injection. Injection site leaks[107] may cause periesophagitis, pleural effusion, or mediastinitis. Patients with more than mild chest pain and fever should have a Gastrografin study, which may show a leak (localized and contained, in contrast with free perforation). These are usually managed nonsurgically. Sclerotherapy may[131] or may not[132] cause esophageal dysmotility on testing, and LES pressure is insignificantly decreased.[131, 132] Gastroesophageal reflux is prevalent before sclerosis and further increased after it, but symptoms or endoscopic evidence of esophagitis are rare.[131] Early, mild dysphagia following sclerosis is common, but esophageal motility is generally well preserved, and long-lasting disturbances of swallowing rarely result unless esophageal stricture occurs.[131, 132] Stricture complicates sclerotherapy in about 10% of cases and is usually easily managed with dilatation.[12, 16, 128] (Fig. 27–5).

Some factors may predictably predispose to certain complications. For example, free perforation, injection site leaks, and other complications are commoner with rigid endoscopy.[133] Repeated injections of the same bleeding varix may cause deep ulceration and rebleeding, false submucosal tract, or esophageal stricture,[12] as may the use of the more highly sclerosant solutions, such as 5% sodium morrhuate, 3% tetradecyl sulfate, undiluted alcohol, or polidocanol. More rapid obliteration of varices in a short time by multiple, early injections may do the same. Complications also appear to be more frequent in those studies in which sclerotherapy was used for control of active bleeding. In a 10-year follow-up study, it was found that the overall incidence of complications increased with time, since ongoing sclerotherapy is required, and the complication rate is cumulative for any given patient.[119] In the pediatric population, certain variables correlated with complications have been identified:[16] For early bleeding post-sclerotherapy, a platelet count lower than 100,000; for respiratory complications and formation of a false submucosal tract, weight less than 12 kg; for false tract alone, a need for more than six sclerotherapy sessions to eradicate varices. In general, sclerotherapy for children is a safe procedure.[9, 12, 16]

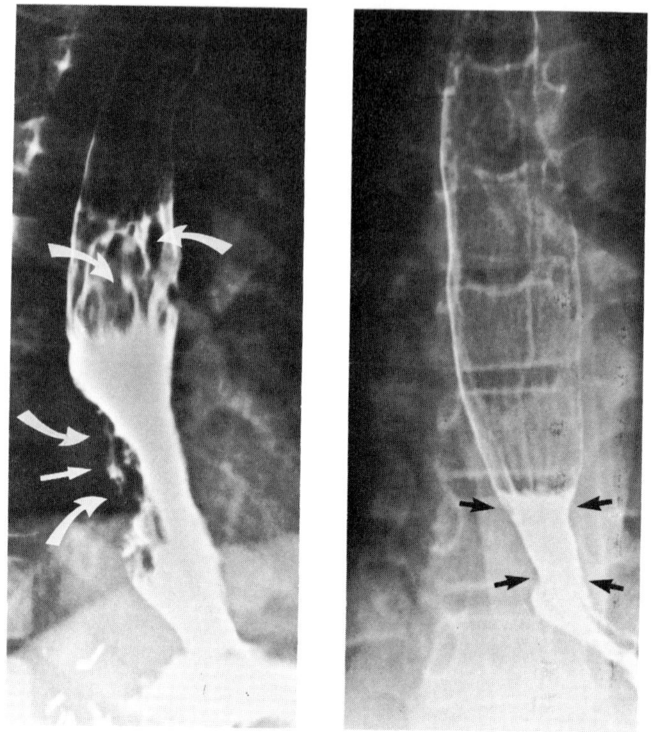

Figure 27–5. Barium esophagram. *Left,* Extensive esophageal varices *(white curved arrows). Right,* Absence of varices 6 months after initiation of sclerotherapy but with complication of distal esophageal stricture *(black arrows),* which responded easily to dilatation.

Percutaneous Transhepatic Obliteration of Varices

Percutaneous transhepatic obliteration of varices (PTOV) is performed by placing an angiographic catheter transhepatically into the portal vein and injecting a sclerosant or embolic substance into the coronary and short gastric veins, thereby interrupting flow into the varices.[94] In one large series,[134] this technique was effective in arresting acute variceal bleeding in 80% of procedures, with low morbidity and mortality. However, the rebleeding rate was high. The authors of that study suggested that PTOV may be indicated in patients with acute variceal bleeding who have not responded to conventional medical measures (vasopressin and balloon tamponade) and that once hemostasis is achieved, early elective surgery should be performed. If the patient is a poor surgical candidate, they suggest follow-up treatment with endoscopic sclerotherapy because repeat PTOV is more difficult technically, especially with new vessel formation. Thus, repeated PTOVs over a long period are not a viable option.

However, endoscopic sclerotherapy in the acutely bleeding patient[107, 114] has a higher success rate than PTOV, and skilled endoscopic therapy is probably more readily available in most medical centers than is skilled angiographic PTOV. Furthermore, in children and adults there is considerably more documented experience worldwide with endoscopic sclerotherapy than there is with PTOV[134, 135]; perhaps PTOV should be reserved for failure of both medical therapy and endoscopic sclerotherapy for acute variceal bleeding only.

Endoscopic Ligation of Varices

Endoscopic variceal ligation (EVL) is a technique recently developed by Stiegmann and coworkers[136, 137] as an alternative to endoscopic sclerotherapy. The therapy is based on the principles used in the elastic-banding technique for hemorrhoids. In the esophageal procedure, varices are mechanically ensnared and strangulated with small elastic "O" rings delivered onto the varix by a device on the end of a flexible fiberoptic endoscope. Studies in the canine variceal model and in humans show that EVL obliterates varices by necrosis, inflammation, and scar formation, which occur following banding. Venous channels in the esophageal lamina propria and submucosa are said to be eradicated, but the muscular wall is unaffected and therefore esophageal function is preserved.

The rationale for the use of EVL is that it is said to obliterate varices without the complications of injection sclerotherapy, that is, deep ulceration, esophageal strictures, perforation, or systemic sequelae, such as sepsis or pulmonary problems. Preliminary data suggest that its efficacy for acute bleeding of varices or for prevention of recurrent bleeding is similar to that of sclerotherapy.[137a]

The EVL technique itself is described in detail elsewhere.[136, 137] A disadvantage compared with sclerotherapy is that the endoscope must be removed after each ligation to reload a new elastic O ring onto the device at the tip of the endoscope. Because several ligations are necessary at one endoscopic session, an overtube is left in situ during the procedure to facilitate repeated removal, reloading, and passage of the endoscope.

Splenectomy and Splenic Embolization

In portal hypertension, splenomegaly may be of concern for several reasons. When very large, the spleen is at increased risk for rupture following trauma. Additionally, a very large spleen may cause a dragging sensation or pain in the left upper quadrant. Hypersplenism with thrombocytopenia can contribute to bleeding.

Splenectomy[138] or splenic artery embolization[139–141] has been used to treat portal hypertension with highly variable results. There has been a wide range of changes in the wedged hepatic vein pressure after these procedures, which may be explained by a study in which the splenic artery was partially occluded by a balloon catheter; splenic vein flow decreased greatly, but portal vein flow and pressure decreased relatively slightly because superior mesenteric flow showed a compensatory increase.[142]

As a management option for hypersplenism or variceal bleeding in portal hypertension, surgical splenectomy has many drawbacks. It does not cure variceal bleeding, except in the rare circumstance of left-sided, or sinistral, portal hypertension.[25] It jeopardizes future shunt options by removal of the splenic vein. For liver transplant candidates, it makes the definitive surgery more difficult. The incidence of postsplenectomy sepsis following splenectomy for trauma is 1 to 2%, some 50 times that in the general population.[143, 144] Children are particularly susceptible to this complication,[143, 144] especially those younger than 5 years of age.

Because of these concerns, complete splenic embolization was developed as an alternative to surgical splenectomy, but early reports showed a high rate of serious complications, including splenic abscess, pancreatitis, pneumonia, and sepsis. Later studies used only *partial* splenic embolization to produce a partial "medical splenectomy," aiming to treat hypersplenism and reduce spleen size but leave some functional splenic parenchyma intact to prevent postsplenectomy sepsis. The use of partial splenic embolization with careful sterile techniques, prophylactic antibiotics, and pneumococcal vaccine has virtually eliminated serious complications in adults and children.[140, 145]

The main indications for splenic management in portal hypertension are massive splenomegaly and hypersplenism. In the hands of an experienced angiographer, partial splenic embolization offers the most efficacious and safest approach. Decreased rates of variceal bleeding have occurred following this procedure, but whether this results from decreased portal pressure is questionable. Normalization of platelet counts may well be the reason.

Surgery

Portosystemic shunting was introduced in 1945, when Whipple[83] and Blakemore and Lord[82] applied the principles of the long-known Eck fistula[146] to the treatment of patients with portal hypertension. The rationale was that decompression of the high-pressure portal system would result in a decrease in bleeding from esophageal varices. Because of the enormous mortality of variceal bleeding, this promising surgical treatment was almost universally used for longer than a quarter of a century, until portacaval shunting was subjected to controlled study. Although variceal bleeding did decline dramatically, survival was not improved, and there was a high morbidity and mortality associated with hepatic encephalopathy.[90] Furthermore, when portacaval anastomosis was performed prophylactically in patients who had not yet bled, survival was shortened in the operated groups compared with the nonoperated groups.[89, 140] The disillusionment with standard portacaval shunts led to exploration of other portosystemic shunt techniques as well as renewed interest in sclerotherapy and, later, beta-blockade.

Pathophysiology of Surgical Shunts

The Importance of Portal Blood. In animal studies using split-liver perfusion, hepatic tissue with an intact splanchnic blood supply hypertrophies, whereas atrophy occurs in that perfused only by systemic blood.[90] Thus, splanchnic blood contains endogenous factors that are hepatotrophic, insulin being one likely such factor.

A problem with surgical shunt procedures is the resulting partial or complete diversion of portal blood away from the liver. Even though hepatic arterial blood flow may show a compensatory increase, at least a 20% overall reduction of blood flow occurs and hepatic arterial blood is qualitatively not comparable with portal blood. Diversion of portal blood has two major sequelae. A total diversion of portal blood results in hepatocyte atrophy, glycogen depletion, fatty infiltration, and disruption of organelles, but not cirrhosis. The changes are common to several species, including humans. These changes may occur in a previously normal liver or may be superimposed on pre-existing diseased liver. Second, hepatic encephalopathy may develop, and the risk depends on the severity of the underlying liver disease and the degree of hepatopetal flow remaining. Although rare, hepatic encephalopathy does develop in patients with noncirrhotic portal hypertension who have undergone a portacaval shunt (see later).

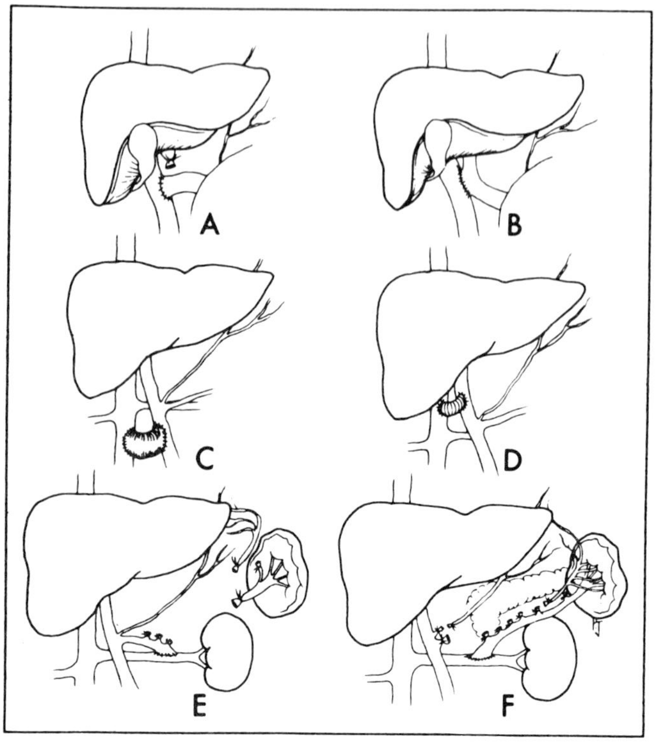

Figure 27–6. Portosystemic shunts used for emergency treatment of variceal bleeding: end-to-side portacaval shunt *(A);* side-to-side portacaval shunt *(B);* mesocaval interpositional H-graft *(C);* portacaval interpositional H-graft *(D);* central splenorenal shunt *(E);* and selective distal splenorenal shunt (Warren Shunt *[F]*). (From Terblanche J, Burroughs AK, Hobbs KEF: Controversies in the management of bleeding esophageal varices: I. N Engl J Med 1989; 320:1393–1398. Reprinted by permission of the New England Journal of Medicine [320; 1393, 1989].)

Types of Surgical Procedures

Surgical procedures for portal hypertension may be classified as follows:

1. Total portosystemic shunts
2. Selective portosystemic shunts
3. Makeshift portosystemic shunts
4. Angiographic portosystemic shunts
5. Portal nondecompressive operations

Procedures 1 through 4 are also referred to as *indirect procedures,* as they do not attack the varices themselves but aim to decompress them. The procedures referred to in the fifth item are also known as *direct procedures*, as they do surgically attack the varices themselves directly and do not decompress the portal circulation.

Total Portosystemic Shunts. Total portosystemic shunts divert most portal blood to the systemic circulation and include portacaval (PC), mesocaval (MC), and central splenorenal (CSR) shunts (Fig. 27–6). The CSR shunt is, of necessity, accompanied by splenectomy. There were considerations that shunts constructed more distally, that is, CSR, would allow only partial diversion, but angiographic and hemodynamic studies in cirrhotic patients showed these to be true total shunts. Franco and Smadja[147] obtained the following clinical results based on a summary of 17 studies involving more than 1,000 patients. Operative mortality averaged 9.5% (1–20%) and was related to Child's class but not liver histology. Better outcomes occurred in patients stabilized for several weeks after bleeding. Recurrent variceal bleeding averaged 6% (0–16%) and usually followed shunt thrombosis. Shunt thrombosis rates were 7% for end-to-side and 2% for side-to-side PC shunts, 10% for MC shunts, and 18% for CSR shunts. Total shunts were effective for treating ascites, when a side-to-side shunt is preferred to an end-to-side, which leaves high sinusoidal pressure and predisposes to ascites formation. The incidence of postshunt encephalopathy averaged 28% (9–46%) and chronic disabling encephalopathy 17% (7–25%). Successful treatment of this important complication by subtotal colectomy, colonic exclusion, or secondary liver arterialization is rare, but shunt takedown with restoration of hepatopetal flow does result in marked improvement. Four controlled studies failed to show significant prolongation of survival with therapeutic total shunts compared with nonoperated patients.[148–151]

Selective Portosystemic Shunts. Selective portosystemic shunts were developed in the hope of decreasing hepatic encephalopathy by maintaining portal blood flow. Blood is diverted from esophageal and gastric varices via the splenic vein to the left renal vein while the superior mesenteric contribution of venous blood to the liver is maintained (see Fig. 27–6).

The distal splenorenal (DSR) shunt developed by Warren and associates[152] diverts the distal end of the splenic vein into the left renal vein. Because the splenic vein also has collaterals to the portal and mesenteric veins, a disconnection procedure was performed with the DSR shunt to make it more selective, the whole procedure being known as the *Warren operation.* The second selective shunt is the coronocaval shunt, diverting the distal end of the left gastric vein into the inferior vena cava, as described by Inokuchi and the Cooperative Study Group.[153]

Clinical results of the Warren operation from several studies summarized by Franco and Smadja[147] and Terblanche and coworkers[154] showed a 15% average encephalopathy rate (4–32%), but severe disabling encephalopathy was seen in only 5% (0–11%). Operative mortality was initially higher than that for PC shunts owing to greater technical difficulties, but in practiced hands it was comparable with that for PC shunt. Prevention of recurrent variceal bleeding was similar to the rates for PC shunts, with an average shunt thrombosis rate of 8%.

Long-term selectivity has been evaluated by angiographic studies.[155–157] Preoperatively 87 to 94% of patients had good or fair portal perfusion of the liver. In late studies, as long as 3 years after surgery, 59 to 70% of patients had poor or no portal flow toward the liver. There was a progressive decrease in portal vein diameter and augmentation of collaterals from the mesenterico-portal to the gastrosplenic circulation.

The foregoing results were derived from studies up to 1982. In 1988, the largest randomized, controlled trial of DSR versus PC shunt after variceal bleeding dealt a severe blow to claims of success for the Warren operation.[158] This authoritative study in 303 cirrhotic patients with a mean 3.5-year follow-up showed similar operative mortality and cumulative survival and similar frequency and severity of hepatic encephalopathy for the two operations. Recurrent bleeding was more frequently prevented by PC than by DSR shunts. In contrast, in 1989 Paquet[159] performed the DSR shunt in patients highly selected on the basis of Child's class (no class C patients), liver volume (ultrasound), portal perfusion (scintigraphy), no activity or progression of liver disease (biopsy), no stenosis of hepatic artery, and suitable venous anatomy. Over a 5-year period, only 32 of 299 patients met these criteria. Preoperative endoscopic sclerotherapy was performed, and postoperative management included low-protein diet and lactulose. Five-year survival was 75%, and no rebleeding, encephalopathy, or shunt thrombosis occurred. This was not a controlled study.

Makeshift Portosystemic Shunts. Self-evidently, makeshift portosystemic shunts are shunts performed between any available portal and systemic veins when a conventional shunt is not possible, usually because of thrombosis in the portal system. Of necessity, these have often been performed in emergency situations, and their failure rate is high.[160, 161]

Angiographic Portosystemic Shunts. Angiographic portosystemic shunt procedure is known as TIPSS—transjugular intrahepatic portacaval stent shunt.[162, 162a] A stent is placed within the liver through hepatic parenchyma to connect intrahepatic branches of the portal and hepatic veins. The technique is performed by means of a combined percutaneous jugular and hepatic approach, with placement of a balloon expandable stent. The procedure has been shown to result in a significant decline in venous pressure gradient, cessation of variceal bleeding, and resolution of ascites, without a significant increase in blood ammonia levels. This intrahepatic portosystemic shunt has appeal for several reasons. A major advantage is that hepatopetal flow is maintained, thereby diminishing the risk of hepatic encephalopathy, the main morbidity of surgical shunts. Second, it may be feasible to increase the shunt lumen diameter by further balloon dilatation if necessary, or, in a case of excess shunting, to decrease the lumen by coaxial placement of new stents within the lumen. Third, it keeps options open—the patient may still go on to have a surgical shunt, if TIPSS fails, or a liver transplant. So far, the procedure has been used in patients too ill to undergo a surgical shunt, and at this time it is still in early clinical trials in adults. Issues of efficacy, cost, incidence of encephalopathy, duration of shunt patency, and the role of TIPSS relative to well-established procedures remain to be determined.[162b]

Portal Nondecompressive Operations. Boerema[163] and Crile[164] introduced the principle of transection of the lower esophagus to ligate varices and thereby achieve local devascularization. High operative complication rates were reduced by use of the stapling transection gun, but rebleeding rates were still high until more extensive intra-abdominal devascularization was performed.[165] Several procedures have been devised in which portal systemic connections are interrupted by esophageal or gastric transection, by ligation of periesophageal and perigastric veins, by splenectomy, and by combinations of these procedures, and in which hepatopetal flow is maintained. The procedures include the following:

1. Inokuchi's procedures[153]: esophageal and gastric transections, and cardiectomies, in which the lower esophagus and upper stomach are devascularized
2. Hassab procedure[166]: devascularization of stomach and lower esophagus with splenectomy
3. Sugiura procedure[167]: esophageal transection with paraesophagogastric devascularization and splenectomy.

These operations have an inherently transient effect, as they do not reduce portal pressure. And yet, in a controlled trial of prophylactic Inokuchi procedures versus a nonoperated control group, the operated patients did well—22% died over a 49-month follow-up (5% per year) versus 49% in the control group (16% per year). The most remarkable finding, however, was that liver failure was virtually eradicated as a cause of death in the operated group. Conn[168] suggests that the reason might be that eradication of portosystemic collaterals increases portal venous pressure and, therefore, hepatic blood flow. Prophylactic, nondecompressive surgery appears to have some merit, and controlled studies of the noncompressive surgery versus beta-blockers or sclerotherapy might be informative.

Surgical Procedures in Children

Although none of the surgical procedures has been subjected to controlled trials in children, there is extensive experience with surgery for portal hypertension in children. Most of the pediatric literature on surgical procedures refers to those performed for EHPH, in contrast with the adult studies, which are based largely on cirrhotic patients.

Although most of the types of surgery discussed in the previous section have been performed in children, shunts far outnumber direct procedures. Of the shunts, those most commonly performed in children have been CSR, MC, and makeshift shunts, in that order.[160, 161, 169–171] In a summary of several studies totaling 253 children with EHPH and 87 with IHPH, Fonkalsrud[161] suggested that the underlying disease determined the prognosis: Patients with EHPH did bettter than those with liver disease. MC shunts provided the best long-term relief from variceal bleeding. Direct operations were performed for patients otherwise unshuntable; they had a high rate of rebleeding (74%), but in general the procedures were not as extensive as those described earlier in adults. Makeshift shunts had a 90% rebleeding rate, whereas that for splenectomy alone was 88%. More recently, in 76 shunt procedures for EHPH, the French group of Alvarez and associates[169] used CSR shunt with splenectomy or MC shunts in most of their patients. In a mean 4-year follow-up, they reported no cases of fulminant infection in the 40 children who underwent splenectomy, although some patients were lost to follow-up. They all received daily oral penicillin prophylactically. However, because of the risks of splenectomy (performed with CSR shunts) and lower limb venous complications of MC shunts, they recently began to use MC shunts with jugular vein interposition. The jugular vein is large in young children, and this enables performance of a shunt operation even in children as young as 2 years old.

Surgery for Extrahepatic Portal Hypertension in Children. Most enthusiasm for the use of surgery has come from Alvarez and associates.[169] Their approach in using surgical shunting as first-line long-term therapy for children of all ages has been regarded by some authors as too aggressive,[172] given the following areas of concern.

Risk of Shunt Failure. In many surgical series there has been a high incidence of shunt thrombosis in children younger than 10 years of age or if the vessel to be decompressed is less than 10 mm in diameter.[161, 170, 172] However, Alvarez and associates[169] performed most of their 76 shunts in children between 1 and 8 years old. They were followed up for shunt patency early (15–30 days) or late (6–12 months), or both. Long-term follow-up was not reported and may have been incomplete as 12 of the 76 children were from countries outside of France; thus, their shunt patency number of 92% may be optimistic and may not represent long-term patency. Even in their expert hands, almost all shunt thromboses occurred in the children who were 6 years or age or younger. Shunt thrombosis following surgery in the young child has left many children "unshuntable" because of multiple vessels thrombosed.[12, 161, 172]

Risk of Hepatic Encephalopathy. Conventional wisdom has it that portosystemic encephalopathy (PSE) seldom occurs in adults with noncirrhotic livers and never occurs in children. However, several reports suggest otherwise. In 1964, one study reported PSE in 7 of 24 adults who had had shunts for EHPH.[173] Victor and coworkers[174] and Warren and colleagues[175] each reported two adults with PSE and normal liver following shunt procedures; in two patients the encephalopathy was reversed by takedown of the shunt. A disturbing report from Denmark found naturally formed portosystemic shunts at autopsy in 13 of 15 patients who had suffered severe mental disorders of previously unknown etiology; none of these shunts were found in the control group.[176] In 1973, a multidisciplinary study by Voorhees and coworkers[91] showed varying degrees of central nervous system impairment in 16 patients who had undergone portosystemic shunts 4 to 19 years previously. The manifestations in eight patients with normal livers were predominantly emotional, whereas those in eight with liver disease were largely neurologic. The severity of abnormalities in both groups was related to the duration of exposure to the shunt and the degree of hepatic impairment when present. In a subsequent review of 127 young patients (mid-teens to mid 20s), shunted for EHPH over a 30-year period, there was gross evidence of a central nervous system disorder in as many as 29% of patients, depending on the shunt used.[177]

In contrast, only one young child with a noncirrhotic liver has had well-documented PSE[178]; a 3-year-old child developed a severe behavior disorder followed by acute hepatic encephalopathy a year after end-to-side PC shunt for familial hypercholesterolemia. Of 70 children at risk for PSE in the study by Alvarez and associates,[169] none were known to have encephalopathy, but the number actually followed up is not clear, and the follow-up is short (mean 3–1/2 years).

Prophylactic Surgery. Alvarez and colleagues[169] have performed prophylactic portosystemic shunts in 12 children who had never bled or bled only after intake of aspirin. These children were from countries in which "proper medical care for gastrointestinal tract bleeding could not be ensured." When a child's home circumstances cannot ensure access to prompt resuscitation for gastrointestinal bleeding and safe blood products, there seems little option but to operate prophylactically, when special surgical expertise is available.

SUMMARY

Several new forms of treatment of portal hypertension in childhood have emerged. The precise role of many of the treatments has yet to be defined, but they all offer some advantages over surgical portosystemic shunts.

For EHPH in children, at present only the French group considers surgical shunting to be the first-line procedure. Most other authors consider sclerotherapy by injection to be the definitive treatment of choice and advocate surgical shunt for sclerotherapy failures rather than the reverse. Partial splenic embolization for hypersplenism has achieved excellent results as adjunctive therapy. Endoscopic variceal ligation may supersede injection sclerotherapy in the future.

For IHPH in children, the definitive therapy for those who bleed is usually liver transplantation, and control of bleeding is a temporizing measure. Sclerotherapy is useful for this purpose, and propranolol deserves trial. TIPSS has promise but is early in its development. Surgical shunting should be reserved only for those patients who fail other measures, as it may compromise transplantation surgery.

REFERENCES

1. Caulfield M, Wyllie R, Sivak MV, et al: Upper gastrointestinal tract endoscopy in the pediatric patient. J Pediatr 1989; 115:339–345.
2. Cox K, Ament ME: Upper gastrointestinal bleeding in children and adolescents. Pediatrics 1979; 63:408–413.
3. Groszmann RJ, Bosch J, Grace ND, et al: Hemodynamic events in a prospective randomized trial of propranolol versus placebo in the prevention of a first variceal hemorrhage. Gastroenterology 1990; 99:1401–1407.
4. Lilly JR, Stiegmann GV, Stellin G: Esophageal endosclerosis in children with portal vein thrombosis. J Pediatr Surg 1982; 17:571–575.
5. Atkinson JB, Woolley MM: Treatment of esophageal varices by sclerotherapy in children. Am J Surg 1983; 146:103–105.
6. Paquet KJ: Ten years' experience with paravariceal injection sclerotherapy of esophageal varices in children. J Pediatr Surg 1985; 20:109–112.
7. Vane DW, Boles ET, Clatworthy HW: Esophageal sclerotherapy: An effective modality in children. J Pediatr Surg 1985; 20:703–707.
8. Stray N, Fausa O: Injection sclerotherapy of bleeding esophageal varices. Scand J Gastroenterol 1985; 205:36–39.
9. Donovan TJ, Ward M, Shepherd RW: Evaluation of endoscopic sclerotherapy of esophageal varices in children. J Pediatr Gastroenterol Nutr 1986; 5:696–700.
10. Howard ER, Stringer MD, Mowat AP: Assessment of injection sclerotherapy in the management of 152 children with oesophageal varices. Br J Surg 1988; 75:404–408.
11. Sarin SK, Misra SP, Singal AK, et al: Endoscopic sclerotherapy for varices in children. J Pediatr Gastroenterol Nutr 1988; 7:662–666.
12. Hassall E, Berquist WE, Ament ME, et al: Sclerotherapy for portal hypertension in childhood. J Pediatr 1989; 115:69–74.
13. Stringer MD, Howard ER, Mowat AP: Endoscopic therapy in the management of esophageal varices in 61 children with biliary atresia. J Pediatr Surg 1989; 24:438–442.
14. Thapa BR, Mehta S: Endoscopic sclerotherapy of esophageal varices in infants and children. J Pediatr Gastroenterol Nutr 1990; 10:430–434.
15. Howard ER, Stamatakis JD, Mowat AP: Management of esophageal varices in children by injection sclerotherapy. J Pediatr Surg 1984; 19:2–5.
16. Proujansky R, Orenstein SR, Kocoshis SA: Patient and procedure variables associated with complications following variceal sclerotherapy in children. J Pediatr Gastroenterol Nutr 1991; 12:33–38.
17. Spence RAJ, Johnston GW, Odling-Smee GW, et al: Bleeding oesophageal varices with long-term follow-up. Arch Dis Child 1984; 59:336–340.
18. Bernard O, Alvarez F, Brunelle F, et al: Portal hypertension in children. Clin Gastroenterol 1985; 14:33–55.
19. Pinkerton JA, Holcomb GW, Foster JH: Portal hypertension in childhood. Ann Surg 1972; 175:870–886.
20. Alvarez F, Bernard O, Brunelle F, et al: Portal obstruction in children: I. Clinical investigation and hemorrhage risk. J Pediatr 1983; 103:696–702.
21. Sarin SK, Sundram KR, Ahuja RK: Predictors of variceal bleeding. Gut 1989; 30:1757–1764.
22. Mowat AP: Disorders of the portal and hepatic venous systems. *In* Mowat AP, ed. Liver Disorders in Childhood. 2nd ed. London, Butterworth, 1987; pp 298–323.
23. Odievre M, Pige G, Alagille D: Congenital abnormalities associated with extrahepatic portal hypertension. Arch Dis Child 1977; 52:383–385.
24. Brown KM, Kaplan MM, Donowitz M: Extrahepatic portal venous thrombosis: Frequent recognition of associated diseases. J Clin Gastroenterol 1985; 7:153–159.
25. Turrill FL, Mikkelsen WP: "Sinistral" (left-sided) extrahepatic portal hypertension. Arch Surg 1969; 99:365–368.
26. Sherlock S: Extrahepatic portal venous hypertension in adults. Clin Gastroenterol 1985; 14:1–20.
27. Capron JP, Lemay JL, Muir JF, et al: Portal vein thrombosis and fatal pulmonary thrombosis associated with oral contraceptive treatment. J Clin Gastroenterol 1981; 3:295–298.
28. Mahl TC, Groszmann RJ: Pathophysiology of portal hypertension and variceal bleeding. Surg Clin North Am 1990; 70:251–266.
28a. Bosch J, Pitcueta P, Feu F, et al: Pathophysiolgy of portal hypertension. Gastroenterol Clin North Am 1992; 21:1–14.
29. Donovan AJ, Reynolds TB, Mikkelsen WP, et al: Systemic-portal arteriovenous fistulas: Pathological and hemodynamic observations in two patients. Surgery 1969; 66:474–482.
30. Kitano S, Terblanche J, Kahn D, et al: Venous anatomy of the lower oesophagus in portal hypertension: Practical implications. Br J Surg 1986; 73:525–531.
31. Hashizume M, Kitano S, Yamaga H, et al: Angioarchitectural classification of esophageal varices and paraesophageal veins in selective left gastric venography. Arch Surg 1989; 124:961–966.
32. Butler H: The veins of the oesophagus. Thorax 1951; 6:266–296.
33. Spence RAJ: The venous anatomy of the lower oesophagus in normal subjects and in patients with varices. Br J Surg 1984; 71:739–744.
34. Shirakusa T, Iwasaki A, Okazaki M: Downhill esophageal varices caused by benign giant lymphoma. Scand J Thorac Cardiovasc Surg 1988; 22:135–138.
35. Clatworthy HW, Boles ET: Extrahepatic portal bed block in children: Pathogenesis and treatment. Ann Surg 1959; 150:371–385.
36. Robalino BD, Moodie DS: Association between primary pulmonary hypertension and portal hypertension: Analysis of the pathophysiology and clinical, laboratory and hemodynamics manifestations. J Am Coll Cardiol 1991; 17:492–498.
37. Lockhart A: Pulmonary arterial hypertension in portal hypertension. Clin Gastroenterol 1985; 14:123–138.
38. Lebrec D: Methods to evaluate portal hypertension. Gastroenterol Clin North Am 1992; 21:41–59.
39. Alpern MB, Rubin JM, Williams DM, et al: Porta hepatis: Duplex Doppler US with angiographic correlation. Radiology 1987; 162:53–56.
40. Sukigara M, Ohata M, Kamazuki T, et al: Assessment of the effect of respiration on the esophageal variceal blood flow using trans-esophageal real time two dimensional Doppler echocardiography. Hepatology 1988; 8:663–667.
41. O'Neill JA: Portal hypertension in childhood. *In* Dean RH, O'Neill JA, eds: Vascular Disorders of Childhood. Philadelphia, Lea & Febiger, 1983; pp 142–158.
42. Graham DY, Klish WJ, Ferry GD, et al: Value of fiberoptic gastrointestinal endoscopy in infants and children. South Med J 1978, 71:558–560.
43. Ament ME, Berquist WE, Vargas J, et al: Fiberoptic upper intestinal endoscopy in infants and children. Pediatr Clin North Am 1988; 35:141–155.
44. DeFranchis R, Primigrani M: Why do varices bleed? Gastroenterol Clin North Am 1992; 21:85–101.
45. Beppu K, Inokuchi K, Koyanagi N, et al: Prediction of variceal hemorrhage by esophageal endoscopy. Gastrointest Endosc 1981; 27:213–218.
46. Paquet KJ, Koussouris P: Is there an indication for prophylactic endoscopic injection sclerotherapy in patients with liver cirrhosis and portal hypertension? Endoscopy 1986; 18(suppl 2):32–35.
47. Smart HL, Triger DR: Clinical features of portal hypertensive gastropathy. Endoscopy 1991; 23:195–246.
48. Portal hypertensive gastropathy (editorial). Lancet 1991; 338:1045–1046.
49. Mathur SK, Dalvi AN, Someshwar V, et al: Endoscopic and radiological appraisal of gastric varices. Br J Surg 1990; 77:432–435.
50. Watanabe K, Kimura K, Matsutani S, et al: Portal hemodynamics

in patients with gastric varices. Gastroenterology 1988; 95:434–440.
51. Keller FS, Rosch J: Value of angiography in diagnosis and therapy of acute upper gstrointestinal hemorrhage. Dig Dis Sci 1981; 26(July suppl):78–89.
52. Durham JD, Kumpe DA, Van Stiegmann G, et al: Direct catheterization of the mesenteric vein. Radiology 1990; 177:229–233.
53. Afshani E, Berger PE: Gastrointestinal tract angiography in infants and children. J Pediatr Gastroenterol Nutr 1986; 5:173–186.
54. Foley WD, Stewart ET, Milbrath JR, et al: Digital subtraction angiography of the portal venous system. AJR 1983; 140:497–499.
55. Balthazar EJ, Naidich DP, Megibow AJ, et al: CT evaluation of esophageal varices. AJR 1987; 148:131–135.
56. Hassall E, Baldwin GA: Gastrointestinal bleeding. *In* Baldwin GA, ed: Handbook of Pediatric Emergencies. Boston, Little, Brown, 1989; pp 166–176.
57. Ponsky JL, Hoffman M, Swayngim DS: Saline irrigation in gastric hemorrhage: The effect of temperature. J Surg Res 1980; 28:204–205.
58. Grace ND: Variceal hemorrhage: Pharmacologic approach. *In* McDermott WV, ed: Surgery of the Liver. Boston, Blackwell Scientific Publications, 1988; pp 303–314.
59. Chojkier M, Groszmann RJ, Atterbury CE, et al: A controlled comparison of continuous intra-arterial and intravenous infusion of vasopressin in hemorrhage from esophageal varices. Gastroenterology 1979; 77:540–546.
60. Terblanche J, Burroughs AK, Hobbs KEF: Controversies in the management of bleeding esophageal varices. I. N Engl J Med 1989; 320:1393–1398.
61. Hunt PS, Korman MG, Hansky J, et al: An 8-year prospective experience with balloon tamponade in emergency control of bleeding esophageal varices. Dig Dis Sci 1982; 27:413–416.
62. Haddock G, Garden OJ, McKee RF, et al: Esophageal tamponade in the management of acute variceal hemorrhage. Dig Dis Sci 1989; 34:913–918.
63. Freeman JG, Cobden I, Lishman AH, et al: Controlled trial of terlipressin versus vasopressin in the early treatment of esophageal varices. Lancet 1982; 2:66–68.
64. Kravetz D, Bosch J, Teres J, et al: Comparison of intravenous somatostatin and vasopressin infusion in treatment of acute variceal hemorrhage. Hepatology 1984; 4:442–446.
65. Groszmann RJ, Kravetz D, Bosch J, et al: Nitroglycerin improves the hemodynamic response to vasopressin in portal hypertension. Hepatology 1982; 2:757–762.
66. Gimson AE, Westaby D, Hegarty J, et al: A randomized trial of vasopressin and vasopressin plus nitroglycerin in the control of acute variceal hemorrhage. Hepatology 1986; 6:410–413.
67. Graham DY, Smith JL: The course of patients after variceal hemorrhage. Gastroenterology 1981; 80:800–809.
68. Webb LJ, Sherlock S: The aetiology, presentation and natural history of extrahepatic portal venous obstruction. Q J Med 1979; 192:627–639.
69. Dilawari JB, Raju GS, Chawla YK: Developing large splenoadreno-renal shunt after endoscopic sclerotherapy. Gastroenterology 1989; 97:421–426.
70. Westaby D, Williams R: Portal hypertension. *In* Berk JE, Haubrich WS, Kalser MH, eds: Bockus Gastroenterology. Vol 5, 4th ed. Philadelphia, WB Saunders, 1985, pp 3062–3082.
71. Lebrec D, Corbic M, Nouel O, et al: Propranolol—a medical treatment for portal hypertension? Lancet 1980; 2:180–182.
72. Lebrec D: Current status and future goals of the pharmacologic reduction of portal hypertension. Am J Surg 1990; 160:19–25.
73. Lebrec D, Poynard T, Capron JP, et al: Nadolol for prophylaxis of gastrointestinal bleeding in patients with cirrhosis: A randomized trial. J Hepatol 1988; 7:118–125.
74. Conn HO, Grace ND, Bosch J, et al: Propranolol in the prevention of the first hemorrhage from esophagogastric varices: A multi-center, randomized clinical trial. Hepatology 1991; 13:902–912.
75. Poynard T, Cales P, Pasta L, et al: Beta-adrenergic antagonist drugs in the prevention of gastrointestinal bleeding in patients with cirrhosis and esophageal varices. N Engl J Med 1991; 324:1532–1538.
76. Poynard T, Lebrec D, Hillon P, et al: Propranolol for prevention of recurrent gastrointestinal bleeding in patients with cirrhosis: A prospective study of factors associated with rebleeding. Hepatology 1987; 7:447–451.
77. Burroughs AK, Jenkins WJ, Sherlock S, et al: Controlled trial of propranolol for the prevention of recurrent variceal hemorrhage in patients with cirrhosis. N Engl J Med 1983; 309:1539–1542.
78. Villeneuve JP, Pomier-Layrargues G, Infante-Rivard C, et al: Propranolol for the prevention of recurrent variceal hemorrhage: A controlled trial. Hepatology 1986; 6:1239–1243.
79. Fleig WE, Stange EF, Hunecke R, et al: Prevention of recurrent bleeding in cirrhotics with recent variceal hemorrhage: Prospective, randomized comparison of propranolol and sclerotherapy. Hepatology 1987; 7:355–361.
80. Alexandrino PT, Alves MM, Pinto Correia J: Propranolol or endoscopic sclerotherapy in the prevention of recurrence of variceal bleeding: A prospective, randomized controlled trial. J Hepatol 1988; 7:175–185.
81. Crafoord C, Frenckner P: Nonsurgical treatment of varicose veins of the esophagus. Acta Otolaryngol (Stockh) 1939; 27:422–429.
82. Blakemore AH, Lord TW: The technic of using vitallium tubes in establishing portacaval shunts for portal hypertension. Ann Surg 1945; 122:476–480.
83. Whipple AO: The problem of portal hypertension in relation to the hepatosplenopathies. Ann Surg 1945; 122:449–455.
84. Fearon B, Sass-Kortsak A: The management of esophageal varices in children by injection of sclerosing agents. Ann Otol Rhinol Laryngol 1959; 68:906–915.
85. Macbeth R: Treatment of esophageal varices in portal hypertension by means of sclerosing injections. Br Med J 1955; 2:877–880.
86. Moersch HJ: Treatment of esophageal varices by injection of a sclerosing solution. JAMA 1947; 135:754–757.
87. Patterson CO, Rouse MD: The injection treatment of esophageal varices. JAMA 1951; 130:384–386.
88. Johnston GW, Rodgers HW: A review of 15 years' experience in the use of sclerotherapy in the control of acute haemorrhage from oesophageal varices. Br J Surg 1973; 60:797–800.
89. Conn HO, Lindenmuth WW, May CJ, et al: Prophylactic portacaval anastomosis: A tale of two studies. Medicine 1972; 51:27–40.
90. Conn HO: Therapeutic portacaval anastomosis: To shunt or not to shunt. Gastroenterology 1974; 67:1065–1073.
91. Voorhees AB, Chaitman E, Schneider S, et al: Portal systemic encephalopathy in the non-cirrhotic patient: Effect of portal-systemic shunting. Arch Surg 1973; 107:659–663.
92. Terblanche J, Northover JMA, Bornman P, et al: A prospective controlled trial of sclerotherapy in the long term management of patients after esophageal variceal bleeding. Surg Gynecol Obstet 1979; 148:323–333.
93. Evans DMD, Jones JB, Cleary BK, et al: Oesophageal varices treated by sclerotherapy: A histopathological study. Gut 1982; 23:615–620.
94. Conn HO: Endoscopic sclerotherapy versus percutaneous transhepatic obliteration of varices: A conceptual approach. Gastroenterology 1989; 93:1428–1438.
95. Sivak MV, Stout PJ, Skipper G: Endoscopic injection sclerosis of esophageal varices. Gastrointest Endosc 1981; 27:52–57.
96. Lewis J, Chung RS, Allison J: Sclerotherapy of esophageal varices. Arch Surg 1980; 115:476–480.
97. Richardson VF, Robertson CF, Mowat AP, et al: Deterioration in lung function after general anaesthesia in patients with cystic fibrosis. Acta Pediatr Scand 1984; 73:75–79.
98. Hassall E, Gunasekaran T, Israel D, et al: Halothane hepatitis in children. J Pediatr Gastroenterol Nutr 1990; 11:553–557.
99. Paquet KJ, Fleig WE: Sclerotherapy of esophageal varices. *In* Papp JP, ed: Endoscopic Control of Gastrointestinal Hemorrhage. Boca Raton, CRC Press, 1981, pp 43–71.
100. Silpa ML, Jensen DM, Machicado GA, et al: Efficacy and safety of agents for variceal sclerotherapy. Gastrointest Endosc 1982; 28:152–153.
101. Sarin SK, Sachdev G, Nanda R, et al: Comparison of two time schedules for endoscopic scleotherapy: A prospective randomized controlled study. Gut 1986; 27:710–713.

102. Seidman E, Weber AM, Morin CL, et al: Spinal cord paralysis following sclerotherapy for esophageal varices. Hepatology 1984; 4:950–954.
103. Westaby D, Melia WM, Macdougall BRD, et al: Injection sclerotherapy for oesophageal varices: A prospective randomised trial of different treatment schedules. Gut 1984; 25:129–132.
104. Barsoum MS, Bolous FI, El-Rooby AA, et al: Tamponade and injection sclerotherapy in the management of bleeding oesophageal varices. Br J Surg 1982; 69:76–78.
105. Paquet K-J, Feussner H: Endoscopic sclerosis and esophageal balloon tamponade in acute hemorrhage from esophagogastric varices: A prospective controlled randomized trial. Hepatology 1985; 5:580–583.
106. Larson AW, Cohen H, Zweiban B, et al: Acute esophageal variceal sclerotherapy: Results of a prospective randomized controlled trial. JAMA 1986; 255:497–500.
107. Terblanche J, Yacoob HI, Bornman PC, et al: Acute bleeding varices: A five-year prospective evaluation of tamponade and sclerotherapy. Ann Surg 1981; 194:521–530.
108. Lewis JW: Survival and rebleed after acute and chronic injection sclerotherapy. *In* Sivak MV Jr, ed: Endoscopic sclerotherapy of esophageal varices. New York, Praeger, 1984, pp 89–97.
109. Paquet K-J: Endoscopic paravariceal injection sclerotherapy of the esophagus—indications, technique, complications: Results of a period of 14 years. Gastrointest Endosc 1983; 29:310–315.
110. Paquet K-J, Kalk J-F, Koussouris P: Immediate endoscopic sclerosis of bleeding esophageal varices: A prospective evaluation over five years. Surg Endosc 1988; 2:18–23.
111. Novis BH, Duys P, Barbezat GO, et al: Fiberoptic endoscopy and the use of the Sengstaken tube in acute gastrointestinal haemorrhage in patients with portal hypertension and varices. Gut 1976; 17:258–263.
112. Panes J, Teres J, Bosch J, et al: Efficacy of balloon tamponade in treatment of bleeding gastric and esophageal varices: Results in 15 consecutive episodes. Dig Dis Sci 1988; 33:454–459.
113. Bornman PC, Terblanche J, Kahn D, et al: Limitations of multiple injection sclerotherapy sessions for acute variceal bleeding. S Afr Med J 1986; 70:34–36.
114. Westaby D, Hayes PC, Gimson AES, et al: Controlled clinical trial of injection sclerotherapy for active variceal bleeding. Hepatology 1989; 9:274–277.
115. Fleischer D: Etiology and prevalence of severe persistent upper gastrointestinal bleeding. Gastroenterology 1983; 84:538–543.
116. Smith JL, Graham DY: Variceal hemorrhage: A critical evaluation of survival analysis. Gastroenterology 1989; 82:968–972.
117. Westaby D, Williams R: Status of sclerotherapy for variceal bleeding in 1990. Am J Surg 1990; 160:32–36.
118. Westaby D, Macdougall BRD, Williams R: Improved survival following injection sclerotherapy for esophageal varices: Final analysis of a controlled trial. Hepatology 1985; 5:627–631.
119. Kahn D, Jones B, Bornman PC, et al: Incidence and management of complications after injection sclerotherapy: A 10-year prospective evaluation. Surgery 1989; 105:160–165.
120. Kahn D, Terblanche J, Kitano S, et al: Injection sclerotherapy in adult patients with extrahepatic portal venous obstruction. Br J Surg 1987; 74:600–602.
121. Bullimore DW, Foster P: Prophylactic sclerotherapy for varices. Br Med J 1988; 297:370–371.
122. Odievre M: Long-term results of surgical treatment of biliary atresia. World J Surg 1978; 2:589–594.
123. Schubert TT, Schnell GA, Walden JM: Bleeding from varices in the fundus complicating sclerotherapy. Gastrointest Endosc 1989; 35:268–269.
124. Marcon N: Personal communication, 1991.
125. McCormack TT, Bailey HR, Simms JM, et al: Rectal varices are not piles. Br J Surg 1984; 71:163.
126. Wang M, Desigan G, Dunn D: Endoscopic sclerotherapy for bleeding rectal varices: A case report. Am J Gastroentrol 1985; 80:779–780.
127. Foutch PG, Sivak MV: Colonic variceal hemorrhage after endoscopic injection sclerosis of esophageal varices: A report of three cases. Am J Gastroenterol 1985; 79:756–760.
128. Sanowski RA, Waring JP: Endoscopic techniques and complications in variceal sclerotherapy. J Clin Gastroenterol 1987; 9:504–513.
129. Hassall E: Antibiotic prophylaxis during sclerotherapy for esophageal varices. J Pediatr 1990; 116:156–157.
130. Monroe P, Morrow CF, Millen JE, et al: Acute respiratory failure after sodium morrhuate esophageal sclerotherapy. Gastroenterology 1983; 85:693–699.
131. Greenholz SK, Hall RJ, Sondheimer JM, et al: Manometric and pH consequences of esophageal endosclerosis in children. J Pediatr Surg 1988; 23:38–41.
132. Cohen LB, Simon C, Korsten MA, et al: Esophageal motility and symptoms after endoscopic injection sclerotherapy. Dig Dis Sci 1985; 30:29–32.
133. Bornman PC, Kahn D, Terblanche J, et al: Rigid versus flexible endoscopic injection sclerotherapy: A prospective randomized controlled trial in patients with bleeding esophageal varices. Ann Surg 1988; 208:175–178.
134. Smith-Laing G, Scott J, Long RC, et al: Role of percutaneous transhepatic obliteration of varices in the management of hemorrhage from gastroesophageal varices. Gastroenterology 1981; 80:1031–1036.
135. Laing IA, Buist TAS, Fraser MS: Percutaneous transhepatic occlusion for bleeding oesophageal varices in polycystic disease. Arch Dis Child 1981; 56:954–963.
136. Stiegmann GV, Goff JS, Sun JH, et al: Endoscopic variceal ligation: An alternative to sclerotherapy. Gastrointest Endosc 1989; 35:431–434.
137. Stiegmann GV, Goff JS, Sun JH, et al: Endoscopy ligation of esophageal varices. Am J Surg 1990; 159:21–26.
137a. Stiegmann GV, Goff JS, Michaletz-Orody PA, et al: Endoscopic sclerotherapy as compared with endoscopic ligation for bleeding esophageal varices. N Engl J Med 1992; 326:1527–1532.
138. Miller EM, Hagedorn AB: Results of splenectomy. Ann Surg 1951; 134:815–821.
139. Alwmark A, Bengmark S, Gullstrand P, et al: Evaluation of splenic embolization in patients with portal hypertension and hypersplenism. Ann Surg 1982; 196:518–524.
140. Kumpe DA, Rumack CM, Pretorius DH, et al: Partial splenic embolization in children with hypersplenism. Radiology 1985; 155:357–362.
141. Goldman ML, Philip PK, Sarrafizadeh MS, et al: Intra-arterial tissue adhesive for medical splenectomy in humans. Radiology 1981; 140:341–349.
142. Nishida O, Moriyasu F, Nakamura T, et al: Interrelationship between splenic and superior mesenteric venous circulation manifested by transient splenic arterial occlusion using a balloon catheter. Hepatology 1987; 7:442–446.
143. Krivit W, Geibing GS, Leonard A: Overwhelming postsplenectomy infection. Surg Clin N Am 1979; 59:223–233.
144. Dickerman JD: Splenectomy and sepsis: A warning. Pediatrics 1979; 63:938–941.
145. Israel D, Hassall E, Culham G: Unpublished observations, 1985–1991.
146. Starzl TE, Porter KA, Francavilla A: The Eck fistula in animals and humans. Curr Probl Surg 1983; 20:688–752.
147. Franco D, Smadja C: Prevention of recurrent variceal bleeding: surgical procedures. Clin Gastroenterol 1985; 14:233–257.
148. Jackson FC, Perrin EB, Felix WR, et al: A clinical investigation of the portacaval shunt: V. Survival analysis of the therapeutic operation. Ann Surg 1971; 174:672–701.
149. Resnick RH, Iber FL, Ishihara AM, et al: A controlled study of the therapeutic portacaval shunt. Gastroenterology 1974; 76:843–857.
150. Reynolds TB, Donovan AJ, Mikkelsen WP, et al: Results of a 12-year randomized trial of portacaval shunt in patients with alcoholic liver disease and bleeding varices. Gastroenterology 1981; 80:1005–1011.
151. Rueff B, Prandi D, Degos F, et al: A controlled study of therapeutic portacaval shunt in alcoholic cirrhosis. Lancet 1976; 1:655–659.
152. Warren WD, Henderson JM, Millikan WJ, et al: Distal splenorenal shunt versus endoscopic sclerotherapy for long-term management of variceal bleeding: Preliminary report of a prospective, randomized trial. Ann Surg 1986; 203:454–462.
153. Inokuchi K, Co-operative Study Group of Portal Hypertension of Japan: Improved survival following prophylactic portal nondecompression surgery for esophageal varices. Hepatology 1990; 12:1–6.
154. Terblanche J, Burroughs AK, Hobbs KEF: Controversies in the management of bleeding esophageal varices. II. N Engl J Med 1989; 320:1469–1474.

155. Maillard JN, Flamant YM, Hay JM, et al: Selectivity of the distal splenorenal shunt. Surgery 1979; 86:663–671.
156. Nordlinger BM, Nordlinger DF, Fulenwider JT et al: Angiography in portal hypertension: Clinical significance in surgery. Am J Surg 1980; 139:132–141.
157. Belghiti J, Grenier P, Nouel O, et al: Long-term loss of Warren's shunt selectivity: Angiographic demonstration. Arch Surg 1981; 116:1121–1124.
158. Grace ND, Conn HO, Resnick RH, et al: Distal splenorenal vs. portal-systemic shunts after hemorrhage from varices: A randomized controlled trial. Hepatology 1988; 8:1475–1481.
159. Paquet K-J, Mercado MA, Koussouris P, et al: Improved results with selective distal splenorenal shunt in a highly selected patient population: A prospective study. Ann Surg 1989; 210:184–189.
160. Fonkalsrud EW, Myers NA, Robinson MJ: Management of extrahepatic portal hypertension in children. Ann Surg 1974; 180:487–493.
161. Fonkalsrud EW: Surgical management of portal hypertension in childhood: Long-term results. Arch Surg 1980; 115:1042–1045.
162. Richter GM, Noeldge G, Palmaz JC, et al: Transjugular intrahepatic portacaval stent shunt: Preliminary clinical results. Radiology 1990; 174:1027–1030.
162a. Zemel G, Katzen BT, Becker GJ, et al: Percutaneous transjugular portosystemic shunt. JAMA 1991; 266:390–393.
162b. Elta GH, Eckhauser FE: Portosystemic shunt without surgery. Hepatology 1992; 15:556–557.
163. Boerema I: Bleeding varices of the esophagus in cirrhosis of the liver and Banti's disease. Arch Chir Neerl 1949; 1:253–260.
164. Crile GS: Transesophageal ligation of bleeding esophageal varices: A preliminary report of seven cases. Arch Surg 1950; 61:654–660.
165. Johnston GW: Oesophageal transection and devascularization procedures. *In* Westaby D, Macdougall BRD, Williams R, eds: Variceal Bleeding. London, Pitman Medical, 1982.
166. Hassab MA: Gastroesophageal decongestion and splenectomy in the treatment of esophageal varices in bilharzial cirrhosis: Further studies with a report on 355 operations. Surgery 1967; 6K:169–176.
167. Sugiura M, Futugawa S: Further evaluation of the Sugiura procedure in the treatment of esophageal varices. Arch Surg 1977; 112:1317–1321.
168. Conn HO: Why is prophylactic portal nondecompressive surgery effective in preventing hemorrhage from esophageal varices? Hepatology 1990; 12:166–169.
169. Alvarez F, Bernard O, Brunelle F, et al: Portal obstruction in children: II. Results of surgical portosystemic shunts. J Pediatr 1983; 103:703–707.
170. Clatworthy HW: Extrahepatic portal hypertension. *In* Child CG, ed: Portal Hypertension. Philadelphia, WB Saunders, 1974, pp 257–261.
171. Mitra SK, Kumar V, Datta DV, et al: Extrahepatic portal hypertension: A review of 70 cases. J Pediatr Surg 1978; 13:51–54.
172. Fonkalsrud EW: Shunt operations for portal hypertension in children. J Pediatr 1983; 103:742–743.
173. Thompson EN, Williams R, Sherlock S: Liver function in extrahepatic portal hypertension. Lancet 1964; 1:352–356.
174. Victor M, Adams R, Cole M: The acquired (non-Wilsonian) type of chronic hepatocerebral degneration. Medicine 1965; 44:345–396.
175. Warren WD, Millikan WJ, Smith RB, et al: Non-cirrhotic portal vein thrombosis: Physiology before and after shunts. Ann Surg 1980; 192:341–349.
176. Kroll J, Fog R: Portal-systemic shunts and mental disorders. Acta Psychiatr Scand 1968; 44:255–260.
177. Voorhees AB, Price JB: Extrahepatic portal hypertension. Arch Surg 1974; 108:338–341.
178. Hassall E, Benson L, Hart M, et al: Hepatic encephalopathy in a non-cirrhotic child after portacaval shunt. J Pediatr 1984; 105:439–446.

Chapter 28

Achalasia and Other Motor Disorders

JOHN J. HERBST

NORMAL FUNCTION AND DEVELOPMENT

The esophagus is essentially a tube with sphincters at both ends. The lower esophageal sphincter (LES) protects the esophagus from gastric contents. The upper esophageal sphincter (UES) prevents air from entering the esophagus during negative intrathoracic pressure with inspiration and also protects the pharynx and the trachea from gastric material that may reflux into the esophagus. The normally exquisite coordination of motility in the esophagus and its upper and lower sphincters are discussed in this section (see also Chapter 24).

Upper Esophageal Sphincter

Although the lowest fibers of the pharyngeal constrictor muscles and possibly the highest striated muscle fibers of the esophagus mesh with the cricopharyngeal muscle to form the 2- to 4-cm-wide UES, the two terms (UES and cricopharyngeal muscle) are often used interchangeably. Physiologic modulation of sphincter pressure has been observed at 32 weeks of gestation.[1] UES pressures of 21.3 ± 7.4 mm Hg were noted by Sondheimer[2] in normal newborns. UES pressures in older children are higher than those in children younger than 1 year of age, and UES pressures in adults vary from 60 to 142 mm Hg, with pressures higher in the sagittal plane.[3, 4] Chronic stimulation by somatic nerves maintains UES pressure. Relaxation of the UES with a swallow is initiated in the swallowing center in the brain stem, and the programmed inhibition travels via the vagus nerve.[5]

Esophageal Body

The traditional assumption that the upper third of the esophagus is composed exclusively of striated muscle, and the distal third of smooth muscle was challenged by autopsy studies of 11 adults.[6] The authors found that the distal 62% of the circular muscle was exclusively smooth muscle, and only 4.2% of the most proximal circular muscle and 5.7% of the most proximal longitudinal muscle were exclusively striated muscle.

A *primary peristaltic wave* is initiated by a swallow and is coordinated by the swallowing center in the brain. The amplitude of the waves in the mid-esophagus is smaller than that in either end.[7] A swallow should initiate primary peristaltic waves 90% of the time in older patients. Coordination of peristaltic waves is poor in the first few days of life in term infants; this condition may persist for an extended period in premature infants.[8] Progression of peristalsis is slower in the first week of life (0.8–2 cm per second); it increases to approximately 4 cm per second in older children and adults.[9] Progressive *secondary peristaltic waves* may be induced by distention of the esophagus with food. *Tertiary peristaltic waves* are uncoordinated, random contractions of the esophagus. These waves commonly occur in the first week of life but are abnormal in older patients.[6, 8]

Lower Esophageal Sphincter

LES is a high-pressure zone in the most distal esophagus that abruptly relaxes with a swallow. Reports of LES pressure vary with time and respiration and among investigators, but it is generally agreed that pressure in older children and adults is approximately 20 mm Hg. Spontaneous relaxation is often associated with gastroesophageal reflux, whereas persistently depressed esophageal pressure is seen in reflux associated with severe esophagitis.[9, 10]

DISEASES OF ESOPHAGEAL MOTILITY

Symptoms

Dysphagia, chest pain, esophageal colic, and symptoms of aspiration and reflux occur most commonly in association with diseases of esophageal motility. Motility disorders occasionally produce distressing, life-threatening complications; but the symptoms usually are subtle and intermittent. The severity of radiologic, endoscopic, or manometric abnormalities does not correlate with the severity of the symptoms.

Dysphagia. A careful description of dysphagia often distinguishes motor disorders from anatomic obstruction. Motility disorders usually cause intermittent symptoms with the intake of liquids and solids. Warm liquids usually pass more easily, and ice-cold liquids often intensify the symptoms of motor disorders. If the symptoms are relieved by washing the material down with fluids, repeated swallowing, throwing back the head and shoulders, or a Valsalva maneuver, a motor disorder should be suspected. Emotional stress often exacerbates the symptoms of motor disorders.

Patients with dysfunction of the UES often experience a *transfer dysphagia,* which is an inability regularly to initiate the act of swallowing. The patient is aware that the bolus remains in the oropharynx, or the fluid may exit the nares or trachea. Choking occurs almost immediately on swallowing, and drooling is often constant. In less severe cases, the patient may have sensations of a constant fullness or of something stuck in the neck. The term *globus sensation*, or *globus hystericus*, does not signify a psychological disorder but rather a dysmotility of the upper esophageal or pharyngeal muscles.

Reflux Symptoms. Failure of the distal sphincter, coupled with poor clearance of acid from the esophagus, facilitates the development of esophagitis and heartburn. Patients with severe esophagitis from whatever cause have dysmotility and poor esophageal clearance.

Chest Pain. Perception of esophageal contractions is a sign of a motor disorder. Esophageal colic is thought to be due to extremely long or forceful contractions, but there is a poor correlation with strong contractions noted manometrically.[11] Esophageal pain is usually substernal, but it may radiate to the infrascapular area and occasionally into the neck, simulating coronary pain. The pain may last only a few seconds, or it may continue for several hours and even awaken the patient from sleep. Heartburn not associated with esophagitis is common.

Aspiration Symptoms. Ineffective peristalsis in the esophageal body may allow retrograde spilling into the airway. Some abnormality of UES function may be inferred in patients with relatively minor gastroesophageal reflux but severe respiratory symptoms.

DISORDERS OF THE STRIATED MUSCLE PORTION OF THE ESOPHAGUS

Primary Esophageal Disease

This section describes abnormal upper esophageal function caused by primary diseases of the esophagus. Similar abnormalities are caused by a multitude of systemic diseases, but only a few are discussed in detail (Table 28–1).

Table 28–1. MOTILITY DISORDERS OF ESOPHAGEAL STRIATED MUSCLE

Neurologic Diseases
Bulbar palsy
Cerebral palsy
Autonomic nervous system
Familial dysautonomia
Structural
Hemorrhage, thrombosis
Trauma
Tumor
Cyst
Neuromuscular Diseases
Myasthenia gravis
Botulism
Polio
Werdnig Hoffmann disease
Demyelinating disease
Multiple sclerosis
Muscular dystrophy
Myotonic dystrophy
Oculopharyngeal muscular dystrophy
Inflammatory Myopathy
Dermatomyositis
Polymyositis
Hypothyroidism

Upper Esophageal Hypertension and Achalasia. Dysphagia due to dysfunction of the UES is often diagnosed as cricopharyngeal spasm, when a prominent cricopharyngeal muscle is detected radiologically, or as cricopharyngeal achalasia, when cineradiographic studies demonstrate a failure of barium to pass the UES regularly. The implied hypertension is often not documented manometrically; patients with a large cricopharyngeal muscle on radiograph usually do not have elevated pressures.[12] A prominent muscle is often noted in normal children and in as many as 5% of adults having a barium swallow.[13, 14] Nevertheless, increased UES pressure was noted in some patients with a globus-type dysphagia, and sphincter biopsies revealed increased fibrosis.[14, 15] Incomplete cricopharyngeal relaxation with swallow is noted manometrically in some patients with UES achalasia but may not be detected in other patients with nonspecific UES myopathies and the corresponding symptoms and cineradiographic findings.[16] Symptoms of poor eating, choking, cough, nasal reflux, and sore throat were noted in 12 of 15 children with UES achalasia.[17] Cricopharyngeal achalasia has also been noted in patients with Down's syndrome.[18]

UES Hypotension. UES hypotension, which predisposes to aspiration of esophageal contents, may be seen in patients with a variety of myoneural diseases, including myasthenia gravis, poliomyelitis, and amyotrophic lateral sclerosis.

Upper Esophageal Incoordination

Premature UES Closure. This condition has been proposed as the main event in the pathogenesis of Zenker's diverticulum. Several studies have been able to document the classic manometric pattern in some but not all patients.[12] In one study, two patients were found to have premature relaxation of the UES, two patients had incomplete relaxation, and one had both premature and incomplete relaxation.[19]

Delayed Relaxation. This condition is associated with

gagging and aspiration. Patients with Riley-Day syndrome have delayed but complete relaxation of the UES and disordered motility in the esophagus.[19] Wyllie and associates described drooling and delayed relaxation of the UES due to nitrazepam.[20]

Miscellaneous. Several authors have described a poorly characterized pharyngeal incoordination associated with gagging and choking noted soon after birth.[21-23] Gavage feedings are usually needed for approximately 6 months until a spontaneous resolution occurs. In one fatal case there was a marked dilatation of the pharynx and a lack of ganglion cells in the proximal third of the esophagus.[21]

Secondary Esophageal Disease

Neurologic Diseases. Diffuse central nervous system dysfunction, for example, cerebral palsy, is often associated with dysphagia, presumably owing to disruption of the swallowing center and its neural afferent or efferent connections.

Poliomyelitis. Severe dysphagia, paralysis of the pharyngeal constrictors, cricopharyngeal dysfunction, and achalasia of the UES have been noted.[12] Onset of swallowing problems may be recognized as long as 30 years after the initial acute infection, possibly as a result of the normal attrition of nerve cells that occurs with aging in a patient who has already lost many motor neurons to an acute episode of poliomyelitis.[24]

Botulism. Botulism is characterized by an irreversible binding of toxin to cholinergic terminals, causing a reduction in UES pressure and in peristalsis in the proximal esophagus.[25]

Multiple Sclerosis. In one study,[12] 55% of patients had dysphagia with cricopharyngeal muscle problems being demonstrated.

Myasthenia Gravis. Dysphagia, choking, and aspiration are often the initial symptoms of myasthenia gravis. Characteristically, there is progressive dysphagia with repeated swallowing. A decreased amplitude of contraction may be detected only after repeated swallows, but it characteristically increases with edrophonium (Tensilon).[12]

Inflammatory Myopathy. Polymyositis, dermatomyositis, and scleroderma all have been associated with dysfunction of the proximal esophagus. Dysphagia is common in polymyositis and occasionally is the initial symptom.[12] Decreased UES pressure with normal or incomplete relaxation and poor amplitude of contractions in the pharyngeal constrictors and upper third of the esophagus have been reported. Improvement in dysphagia with steroid therapy occurs in some patients.

Treatment

Because symptoms due to cricopharyngeal achalasia improve with time in many children, a conservative approach to treatment with aggressive pulmonary and nutritional support is indicated. In adult patients with the clinical diagnosis of cricopharyngeal achalasia, myotomy is usually recommended, since improvement of symptoms with bougienage is short lasting.[12, 26] Following UES myotomy there is a decrease in sphincter pressure and clinical improvement, but increased aspiration with death has been reported. Children with both cricopharyngeal achalasia and esophageal incoordination have been successfully treated using bougienage, sometimes with a single dilatation.[16, 17, 27] In one series, 6 of 15 children with cricopharyngeal achalasia were managed conservatively with gavage feedings and positioning. Three of four patients with meningomyelocele improved after a shunt revision.[17] Dilatation for cricopharyngeal achalasia has been successful in infants as young as 5 months of age and has been successful for upper esophageal incoordination at the age of 2.5 years.[16, 41] Cricopharyngeal myotomy has been successful in children with cricopharyngeal incoordination and achalasia.[17, 28] An initial attempt at dilatation would seem reasonable, with myotomy reserved for those patients who do not respond to more conservative therapy.

DYSMOTILITY OF THE DISTAL ESOPHAGUS

Achalasia

The characteristic abnormalities of the distal esophagus demonstrated radiographically or manometrically include (1) increased LES pressure, (2) absent or incomplete relaxation of the LES with swallow, and (3) absence of progressive esophageal contractions.[28, 29] Table 28–2 lists some specific motility disorders of esophageal smooth muscle. The relative distal obstruction and the lack of proximal propulsive force result in a dilated esophagus, which may not be obvious early in the disorder. The contractions of the dilated esophagus are usually of low amplitude, but the term *vigorous achalasia* describes the rare patients with high-pressure tertiary contractions.[30]

The incidence of achalasia has been estimated as 1 in 10,000; fewer than 5% of those patients with symptoms are younger than 15 years of age.[29, 31, 32] These older estimates are similar to an epidemiologic study by Mayberry and Mayell,[33] who estimated an incidence rate varying from 1 in 1 million children in England to 3 in 1 million in Eire based on a study of 120 cases. Most cases of achalasia are sporadic, and there is no familial distribution. However, concordance of achalasia in monozygotic twins has been reported, the interval between the development of the disease in both being 12 years.[34] A number of cases of achalasia in siblings and close relatives have been reported.[32, 34-36]

Pathophysiology

Most cases of achalasia have no known cause, and there is no known animal model for achalasia. It is likely that there are subtle variations in the basic defect among different groups of patients, such as those occasional patients with familial disease, those with vigorous ach-

Table 28–2. MOTILITY DISORDERS OF ESOPHAGEAL SMOOTH MUSCLE

Primary Disorders
- Achalasia
- Diffuse esophageal spasm
- Nutcracker esophagus
- Nonspecific motor disorders

Secondary Disorders
- Intestinal diseases
  - Gastroesophageal reflux and esophagitis
  - Esophageal atresia
  - Scar formation
    - Sclerotherapy
    - Caustic ingestion
  - Intestinal pseudo-obstruction
  - Hirschsprung's disease
- Connective tissue diseases
  - Scleroderma
  - Dermatomyositis
  - Lupus erythematosus
  - CREST syndrome
  - Mixed connective tissue disease
  - Sjögren's syndrome
- Neuromuscular diseases
  - Muscular dystrophy
  - Degenerative disorders
  - Presbyesophagus
  - Autonomic nervous system
    - Postvagotomy syndrome
    - Riley-Day syndrome
    - Raynaud's phenomenon
- Psychiatric disorders
  - Bulimia
  - Depression
- Miscellaneous
  - Graft versus host disease
  - Diabetes
  - Thyroid dysfunction
  - Chagas' disease

alasia, those with various abnormalities in nerves and ganglia noted at autopsy, and those with minor variations in motility findings. The lack of relaxation of the LES is thought to be related to a partial or complete absence, functional impairment, or lack of central connections of postganglionic inhibitory nerves.[37]

Decreased numbers of ganglion cells are seen regularly in children and adults,[1] although muscle biopsies obtained at myotomy in several patients have been normal or have had adequate numbers of ganglion cells, with extensive perineural fibrosis.[38–40] Frequent but inconsistent pathologic findings on biopsy include chronic inflammatory infiltrate in the myenteric plexus and degenerative changes in the nerves or muscle fibers. A decrease in the number of ganglion cells, dissolution of nuclear material, and fragmentation of nerve cells have been noted in the dorsal motor nucleus of the vagus in addition to breaks in axon membranes and degeneration of myelin sheaths in the vagus nerve.[41, 42] Although the effects of neural degeneration have usually been isolated to the esophagus, Dooley and coworkers[43] detected decreased gastric acid production and pancreatic polypeptide release in 7 of 13 patients with achalasia.[43]

Methylcholine chloride (Mecholyl Cl), a synthetic acetylcholine, causes exaggerated, vigorous esophageal contractions in patients with achalasia (see Fig. 28–2*B*); the heightened response indicates denervation hypersensitivity.[44] Cholecystokinin (CCK) octapeptide causes a neurally mediated relaxation and a much weaker direct LES stimulation than can be demonstrated after pharmacologic nerve blockade. CCK causes a relaxation of LES pressure, but in patients with achalasia, a paradoxical increase in pressure consistent with denervation occurs.[45] Vasoactive intestinal peptide is thought to be an inhibitory neural transmitter involved in LES relaxation that is reduced or completely lacking in patients with achalasia.[46] Synaptic vesicles, especially large granular vesicles that are thought to contain vasoactive intestinal polypeptide, are rare in esophageal nerves in patients with achalasia.[47]

Clinical Picture

Fewer than 5% of all patients with achalasia manifest symptoms before the age of 15 years. A review of 167 pediatric cases indicated that 5.3% occurred in the first month of life, and 20% occurred during the first year.[1, 29, 32, 48] The overrepresentation of cases in the first year of life and the onset of symptoms in early life of many familial cases are circumstantial evidence that the basic pathophysiology of these cases may be different from those occurring later in life.

Symptoms often have an insidious onset, with a mean duration of symptoms prior to diagnosis of 23 months being noted in a recent review of 12 pediatric series.[49] Vomiting, dysphagia, weight loss, and failure to thrive are present in more than half of patients. Symptoms of dysphagia, vomiting, and slow eating tend to predominate in older children, whereas choking, cough, recurrent pneumonia, and failure to thrive tend to be more prominent in infants and toddlers. Dysphagia accompanies the ingestion of solids and liquids and may be worse during times of emotional stress or with rapid eating. Vomiting is an especially common symptom and may mimic bulimia, as patients induce vomiting to relieve a substernal fullness.[50, 51] The esophagus may become tremendously dilated and serve as a huge reservoir, with the patient vomiting food ingested hours earlier. In infants, vomited milk has not clotted and been soured by acid. The patient may be aware of a gurgling sound from food sloshing in the highly dilated esophagus. Aspiration may be a serious complication.

Diagnosis

Differential Diagnosis. The predominance of vomiting and weight loss in some patients necessitates consideration of gastroesophageal reflux, distal stricture, or other esophageal motility disorders. In Latin America, *Trypanosoma cruzi* infestation is common, and Chagas' disease must be considered.[39] Carcinoma of the stomach and other tumors have been associated with achalasia in adults, and two children with a clinical diagnosis of achalasia were subsequently shown to have leiomyomas of the distal esophagus.[38, 52] The autosomal-recessive syndrome of deafness, vitiligo, short stature, and muscle weakness as well as the syndrome of alacrima and corticotropin insensitivity has been associated with achalasia.[48, 53, 54]

Radiography. The lack of gastric air or the presence of an air-fluid level in the esophagus on a chest radiograph to evaluate a cough can suggest the diagnosis of achalasia.

Barium Swallow. Barium swallow shows an absence of relaxation of the LES and poor motility in the esophagus with an absence of progressive peristalsis.[29] The esophagus is usually dilated, and it may crowd the mediastinum and become tortuous, assuming a large sigmoid shape; however, dilation may be absent early in the disease (Fig. 28–1). Lack of relaxation of the LES results in a pinching-off of the distal esophagus, forming the classic birdlike beak appearance on an esophagogram.

Manometry. Manometry remains the preferred method of diagnosis. The function of the UES is normal in manometric studies, and a lack of propulsive peristalsis in the body of the esophagus is the most constant finding[28] (Fig. 28–2*A*). Resting pressure in the esophagus is usually mildly elevated over gastric pressure.[28] Failure of LES relaxation is considered a classic and constant finding in achalasia, but in a recent study of 23 adults with achalasia, complete relaxation of the LES was noted in 7 patients and confirmed with a Dent sleeve in

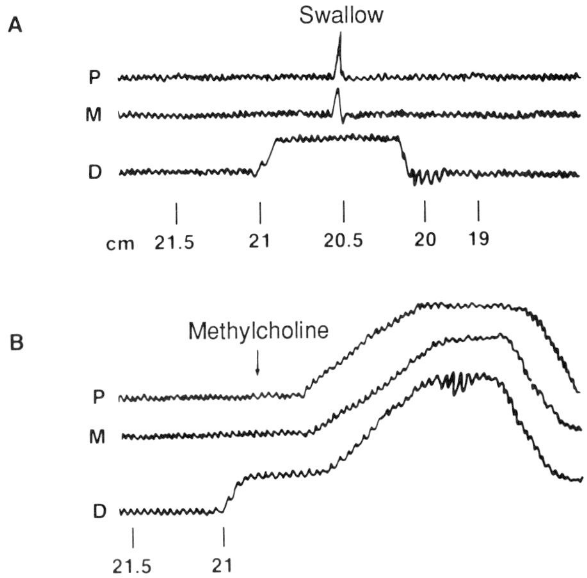

Figure 28–2. *A,* Typical motility tracing from a child with achalasia. The upper and middle tracings are 5 and 2.5 cm above the distal probe positioned in the LES. A swallow produces simultaneous contractions in the esophagus and no relaxation of the LES. Numbers indicate the distance from the distal port to the incisors. *B,* Motility tracing, as in *A,* demonstrating a marked increase in esophageal and LES pressure following methylcholine chloride (see text).

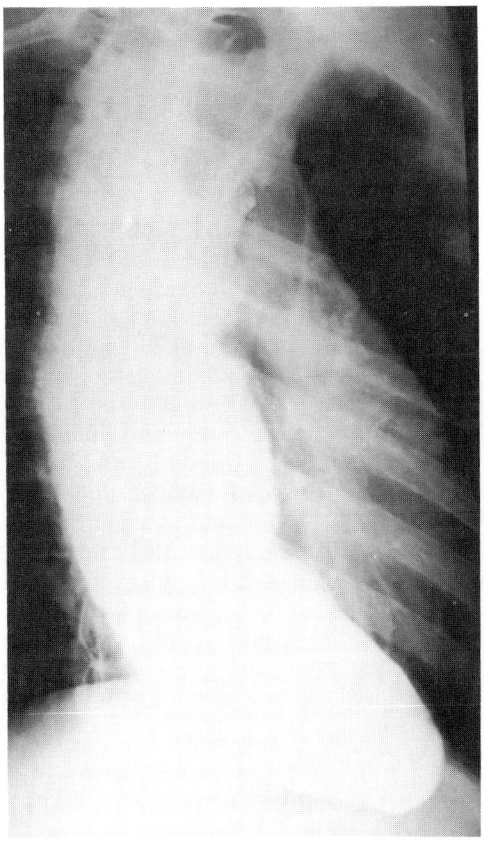

Figure 28–1. Barium esophagram demonstrating a dilated esophagus crowding the mediastinum in a patient with achalasia. Note the sigmoid shape of the distal segment that abruptly narrows at the LES.

2 of the 7 to rule out an artifact due to movement of the probe during a swallow.[55] The period of LES relaxation was shortened, and there was a functional obstruction at the LES. These seven patients had findings that may represent an early stage in the disease; they had symptoms for a shorter period and had less weight loss and less dilatation of the esophagus than the other 16 patients. Similar pressure changes occur in children and adults, and LES pressures of 40 mm Hg (twice the normal adult values) were noted in a neonate with achalasia.[56]

Provocative tests have been used during manometry to further define and confirm the diagnosis. An increase in esophageal pressure occurs after injection of methylcholine chloride (Fig. 28–2*B*). The test is usually painful and may exacerbate asthma or heart disease. The drug is not readily available, so it is seldom used.[44] CCK caused a contracture of the LES sphincter in 21 of 24 adults with achalasia, whereas it caused a relaxation in normal control subjects.[45] The test has not been shown to be specific and has not been used in children.

Endoscopy. Endoscopy is used mainly to exclude carcinoma or the rare leiomyoma that may mimic achalasia and to insert a guidewire for positioning of a balloon for LES dilatation. The esophagus appears patulous, and the LES does not dilate with insufflation of air. Occasionally, an esophagitis from stasis of food in the esophagus is noted.

Radionuclide Tests. Radionuclide tests using solids and liquids have been used to evaluate esophageal emptying. The value of the tests remains to be determined, but in the future they may provide an objective way of measuring esophageal emptying after therapy.[57]

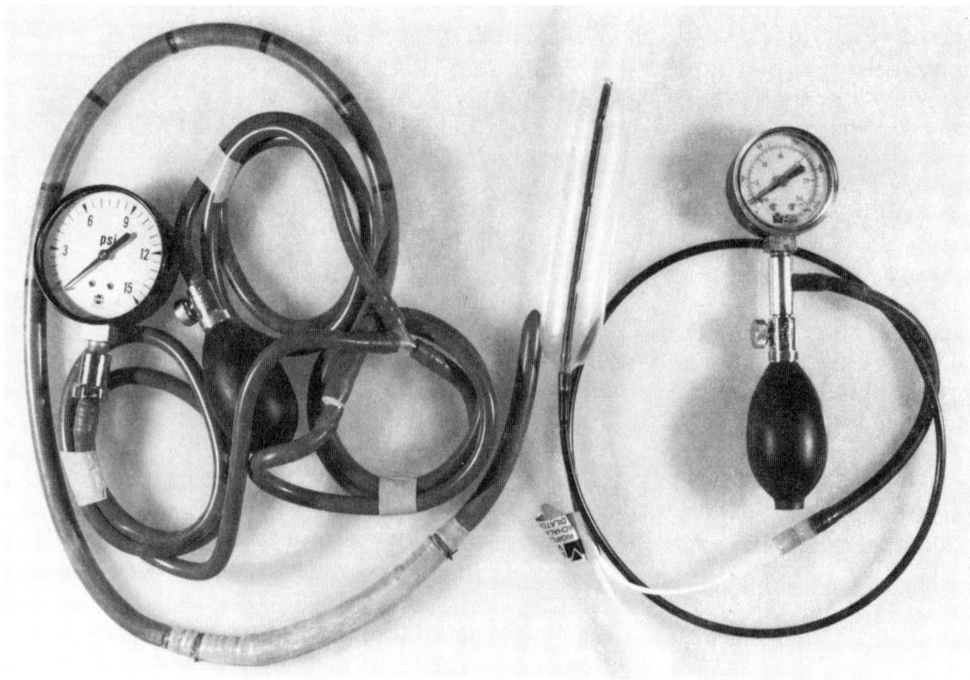

Figure 28–3. Pneumatic dilators for treatment of achalasia. *Left*, Browne-McHardy dilator using a latex balloon. *Right*, The more recently introduced Rigiflex dilator with a plastic balloon that inflates to a predetermined diameter.

Treatment

Relief of the functional obstruction of the LES is the cornerstone of therapy, whether drugs, dilatation, or surgery are used. Diet and nutrition play an additional role and are important in patients with failure to thrive and extreme weight loss. A soft diet encourages esophageal emptying, as does eating and snacking in an upright position and sleeping with the head of the bed elevated.

Drug Therapy. Isosorbide dinitrate, which decreases LES pressure, was used successfully to treat 15 adults for 8 to 15 months, but as many as half had significant side effects or became drug resistant.[58] Calcium channel blockers also lower LES pressure in achalasia. Although not quite as effective as isosorbide nitrate, the low incidence of side effects and the greater likelihood of some improvement now make nifedipine the drug of choice to treat achalasia.[58, 59] The experience with nifedipine in the treatment of children is quite limited, but it appears to be as effective as in adults.[40, 60] The major concerns are compliance with daily drug therapy and long-term effects of the drug. Its greatest value may be to allow a safe, symptom-free delay until definitive therapy is offered.

Dilatation. In older reports,[29, 32, 52, 61] dilatation with a bougie was associated with minor or short-term improvement and a high incidence of esophageal perforation. However, in one recent series, 10 of 20 patients responded to bougienage with mercury dilators sized 52 to 60 Fr without complications.[62] There are no recent reports in the use of such bougies for achalasia in children.

Balloon disruption of the sphincter has been employed for almost 80 years. Many different types of dilators have been used, and they have been inflated for varying periods[28, 29, 52] (Fig. 28–3). The specific techniques employed vary, but several basic principles have emerged.

Positioning of the balloon in the sphincter should be *confirmed* radiographically. In patients with a dilated, tortuous esophagus, passing the dilator over a wire inserted beyond the LES can ease insertion and prevent esophageal perforation. The diameter of the balloon after inflation should be known; the older dilators used latex balloons, and the diameter of the balloon varied with pressure. The Browne-McHardy dilator uses a net over the balloon that provides control over maximum diameter. The more recently introduced Rigiflex dilators use plastic balloons that are not elastic, and a specific diameter is ensured.[63] Pressure applied to the balloon varies, but a minimum pressure of 300 mm Hg is usually used. The bag is usually inflated once or twice per session, and the inflation period may last from 15 to 20 seconds to several minutes. Successful dilatation is usually associated with chest pain, and some blood will be noted on the dilator. Successful dilatation allows patients to eat a regular meal without dysphagia, and it should lead to a decrease in the amount of barium retained in the esophagus at follow-up. In adults, a success rate of 60 to 70% may be expected following a single dilatation.[64] Experience in several pediatric series was similar.[29, 32, 61, 65] A second dilatation can offer some improvement, but repeated dilatations are not warranted.

The main complications of balloon dilatations include esophageal perforation, noted in approximately 1.8%, and fever and pleural effusions in about 4%.[29, 64, 66] Rare complications include persistent pain, empyema, and oropharyngeal hematoma. Esophageal perforation is usually associated with severe pain, and there may be mediastinal emphysema or pleural effusion. Many clinicians, including this author, prefer a postoperative esophagram with a water-soluble contrast material to detect perforation. Most perforations are detected, but there may be a delayed appearance of the perforation.[67]

Treatment of the rare perforation varies from the use of total parental nutrition and antibiotics, especially with early detection, to thoracotomy and various surgical repairs.[64, 68] Wong and Johnson reported 53 perforations in adults in which 68% were treated conservatively with only a 4% mortality rate.[68] Although there are no case reports of perforation following balloon dilatation in children, there are reports of four children with fever, two with severe pain, one with aspiration pneumonia, and one with oropharyngeal hematoma.[32]

Surgery. Most modern surgical procedures are a variation of the Heller myotomy first performed in 1914.[69] The myotomy must be long enough to relieve the obstruction but not so long as to encourage excessive gastroesophageal reflux. The usual patients with achalasia require only a short myotomy in the area of the LES. Approximately 80% of adults will have satisfactory results, and similar results have been noted in children; however, there is a wide disparity in the reports of successful outcome in various series.[29, 32, 64, 70] A review of several pediatric series showed that death was not reported, but there was an overall morbidity of 7.1%, including perforation of the esophagus in 1.4% and rare cases of bleeding, postoperative intussusception, adhesion, atelectasis, and empyema.[64, 70]

Persistent dysphagia may be due to an insufficient myotomy[71] or an incompetent LES causing stricture and peptic esophagitis. An incomplete myotomy is the commonest condition, and manometry continues to reveal a high LES pressure.

The presence of a stricture or severe esophagitis seen at endoscopy indicates that gastroesophageal reflux is the cause of the dysphagia. The incidence of postmyotomy reflux ranges from 10 to 60%.[70, 72] In one prospective pediatric study, reflux was noted in 30% after myotomy, and some developed a peptic stricture.[72] The incidence of reflux increased with the time of follow-up—24% at 1 year, and 48% at 10 years.[73] A short myotomy has a lower risk of inducing gastroesophageal reflux than one that extends more than 1 cm below the gastroesophageal junction.[70] Some authors suggest performing an antireflux procedure at the time of surgery, but dysmotility of the esophagus continues, and obstructive symptoms secondary to an antireflux procedure have been reported.[54]

Myotomy Versus Balloon Dilatation. It is generally agreed that drugs are not recommended for long-term therapy; rather, the choice would be a surgical myotomy or balloon dilatation. This author believes that balloon dilatation should be the initial therapy in patients with no major contraindication. If the symptoms return, a second attempt is indicated, and if dysphagia continues, surgical myotomy is recommended. Although the success rate with balloon dilatation is slightly less than that with myotomy, the procedure is safe, and there is a rapid recovery with only an overnight hospital stay. Prior balloon dilatation does not decrease the subsequent success rate of a myotomy.[29, 70]

Esophageal Spasm

Primary and secondary spastic disorders have similar symptoms and therapeutic approaches. The relationship of pressure changes and symptoms is often uncertain, and similar pressure changes may occur with various systemic disorders.[74–77] As noted previously, symptoms may include chest pain, dysphagia, and respiratory problems as a result of aspiration.

Pathophysiology

The pathophysiology is not well understood. The most remarkable pathologic finding is a muscular hyperplasia of as much as 2 cm in the distal esophagus in some instances.[78] The myenteric neurons appear normal, but minor changes resembling wallerian degeneration have occasionally been noted in the vagus nerve.[79] Cholinergic stimulation often causes exaggerated esophageal contractions. Provocative tests in which cholinergic stimulants induce pain without motility change, motility changes without pain, or both, provide evidence of sensory motor dysfunction.[80, 81]

Distention of a small balloon in the distal esophagus causes pain in some patients without altering motility. Central factors play a role, since affective disorders are common and loud noises and stressful mental activity performed during motility studies can cause a mild increase in esophageal wave pressures.[82]

Motility Abnormalities. The changes in motility are restricted to the smooth muscle portion of the esophagus, most markedly in the distal 5 to 10 cm.[83] The abnormal contractions are interspersed among normal swallowing sequences. There are several types of abnormal contractions: (1) repeated esophageal contractions, usually nonpropulsive, following a single swallow, which may take the form of distinct contractions or multipeaked, prolonged contractions; (2) frequent variations in amplitude and duration of esophageal contractions (normal contractions last less than 7.5 seconds and do not exceed 140 mm Hg, even in adults, but pressures greater than 300 mm Hg may be noted in the distal esophagus); and (3) prolonged periods of repeated contractions with elevation of the baseline pressure, often associated with swallowing. All three types of abnormalities may be noted in the same patient at different times.[82]

A few patients have characteristic patterns of diffuse spasm or nutcracker esophagus, but most have a nonspecific pattern. With diffuse esophageal spasm, tertiary contractions follow more than one third of swallows. There are multiple hypertensive contractions per swallow, with pressures greater than 140 mm Hg and duration prolonged beyond 7.5 seconds.[83] LES pressures are usually normal. The term *nutcracker esophagus* describes a situation in which there are multiple nonperistaltic spastic contractions in the distal esophagus that cause segmentation of barium on a radiograph.

Clinical Features

Dysphagia is present in 30 to 60% of patients, and pain is noted in approximately 80% of older patient groups in which women predominate.[84] The pain is retrosternal, may radiate into the back, and lasts from minutes to hours. Heartburn is noted in as many as 20%, but it is not due to esophagitis and responds poorly to antacids. Symptoms of anxiety and depression are common, and 80% of patients will have a psychiatric disease during their lifetime. Although diffuse esophageal spasm is rare in childhood, a few infants present with apnea and bradycardia.[85] Nonspecific esophageal motility was also reported in four patients, with symptoms of "near miss" sudden infant death shortly after feeding. Esophageal strictures and dysmotility of the distal esophagus were noted during barium swallow and responded to intensive therapy for gastroesophageal reflux.

Diagnosis

Esophageal spasm should be suspected in children with dysphagia or suggestive chest pain. A barium study of the esophagus is usually performed initially. This examination may detect nonpropulsive contractions of the esophagus with poor propulsion of barium along the esophagus. Esophageal manometry usually defines the motor abnormalities in the distal esophagus and is the most useful test. Radionuclide studies can demonstrate the delayed clearance of the bolus from the esophagus but do not contribute enough information that they can be recommended for routine use.

Treatment

Treatment modalities are limited, nonspecific measures, such as avoiding extremely hot or cold food, and eating in an upright position in a relaxed atmosphere. Calcium channel blockers and nitrites improve symptoms.[22, 86] Cognizant of the high incidence of psychiatric problems, Clouse and associates[87] showed in a double-blind study in adults that low-dose therapy with the antidepressant trazodone hydrochloride improved symptoms. Esophageal dilatation with bougies is not effective. Pneumatic dilatation helps approximately 40% of patients with severe abnormalities noted at manometry and is especially effective in patients with incomplete relaxation of the LES.[64] Surgery should be considered a measure of last resort and usually consists of a long esophagomyotomy to the level of the aortic arch. This procedure probably should be reserved for patients with intractable, severe pain associated with intense contractions noted at manometry.[64]

Secondary Motility Disorders of the Distal Esophagus

Esophagitis. Nonspecific dysmotility problems are common in patients with peptic esophagitis. Kahrilas and colleagues[88] demonstrated that the percentage of adults failing to properly initiate peristaltic waves with a swallow increased from 3% with noninflammatory reflux disease to 30% with severe esophagitis, and 48% of patients with severe esophagitis had a regional peristaltic hypotension. Hillemeier and coworkers[89] showed that nonperistaltic contractions are commoner in infants with more severe reflux complicated by esophagitis than in uncomplicated reflux.[89] Cucchiara and associates[90] demonstrated a high incidence of tertiary contractions, double-peaked peristaltic waves, and decreased peristaltic pressure amplitude in children with severe esophagitis that improved after effective treatment of esophagitis. Following successful surgery for gastroesophageal reflux, there is an increase in peristaltic amplitude and an increase in LES pressure. The consensus is that the motility abnormalities are secondary to esophagitis and are not the primary event (see Chapter 26).

Esophageal Atresia and Tracheoesophageal Fistula. The commonest abnormalities associated with this condition are an absence of peristaltic waves in the proximal esophagus, frequent tertiary contractions with prolongation of acid clearance in the distal esophagus, normal to low LES pressure, and gastroesophageal reflux in approximately 60% of patients. Abnormal esophageal motility is present at birth and persists into adulthood (see Chapter 25).[91]

Connective Tissue Diseases

Scleroderma. Scleroderma is a systemic disease in which extensive deposits of connective tissue are found in the skin and intestine. Esophageal symptoms are more severe than with other collagen vascular diseases, being present in 50 to 75% of patients; occasionally, they are the presenting problem. In a series of seven children (mean age of 15 years), 72% had abnormalities similar to those in adults, including low-amplitude contractions, tertiary contractions, and LES hypotension.[92] Regurgitation, heartburn, and dysphagia are the commonest symptoms, and they tend to be worse in patients with Raynaud's phenomenon. With severe symptoms, abnormal esophageal contractions and gastroesophageal reflux are easily noted at cinefluoroscopy, in which an air-filled esophagus suggests esophageal atony. Esophageal manometry demonstrates the motility disorders, but similar findings can be seen in patients with severe gastroesophageal reflux. Scintiscan studies demonstrate poor clearance of the esophagus following deglutition in severe cases. Cimetidine, metoclopramide, and cisapride have improved symptoms.[93–95]

Other Connective Tissue Diseases. Similar, although usually less severe, problems have been reported in patients with other connective tissue diseases, including polymyositis, dermatomyositis, systemic lupus erythematosus, the CREST* syndrome, and mixed connective tissue disease, especially in patients with Raynaud's phenomenon. Esophagitis is usually not a major problem. Control of the systemic symptoms with steroid administration is often associated with some reduction in esophageal symptoms. Esophageal motility studies in patients with Sjögren's syndrome demonstrated decreased peristaltic contraction time and an increased rate of propulsion of peristaltic waves along the esoph-

---

*CREST is an acronym for *c*alcinosis, *R*aynaud's (phenomenon), *e*sophageal (dysfunction), *s*clerodactyly, *t*elangiectasia.

agus. The dysphagia noted in most of these patients may be related to a lack of saliva, which makes swallowing difficult.[96]

Graft Versus Host Disease. In one series, severe dysphagia, odynophagia, and retrosternal pain developed in 8 of 63 patients, including two children.[97] Severe desquamative esophagitis was noted in the upper and middle esophagus, and five of seven patients having esophageal manometry demonstrated tertiary contractions, aperistalsis following a swallow, and prolonged contractions of high amplitude.[97] Because only mucosal abnormalities were noted at autopsy, it is probable that the motility disorder initiated by the immunologic process was caused by severe esophagitis.

Hirschsprung's Disease. Although esophageal symptoms are absent, abnormal colon motility is accompanied by increases in tertiary contractions and double-peaked esophageal contractions that persist after surgical corrections of Hirschsprung's disease.[98]

Idiopathic Intestinal Pseudo-obstruction. Low or absent LES pressures and low-amplitude tertiary esophageal contractions occur.[99] Evaluation for these changes with esophageal manometry can serve as a screening test in patients suspected of having this disorder.

Diabetes Mellitus. More than half of patients with diabetic neuropathy have abnormal esophageal motility, although most do not have symptoms.[100] Failed contraction sequences, decreased amplitude, and duration of contractions as well as other nonspecific abnormalities have been noted.

Dysmotility Associated with Scar Formation. Patients who have swallowed lye or other toxic substances frequently have areas of increased fibrosis that require repeated dilatation. Dysphagia associated with esophageal narrowing may be caused by the stricture as well as by the lack of propulsive force across the area of esophageal narrowing.[101] Endoscopic injection therapy is effective in patients who have had hemorrhage from esophageal varices. Delayed development of dysphagia signals the development of abnormal motility and stricture formation.[101] Reduced LES pressure, decreased amplitude of peristalsis, and increased tertiary contractions have been noted. The changes may reflect the extent of fibrosis that developed after injections.

REFERENCES

1. Diamant NE: Development of esophageal function. Am Rev Respir Dis 1985; 131(Suppl):S29–S32.
2. Sondheimer JM: Upper esophageal sphincter and pharyngoesophageal motor function in infants with and without gastroesophageal reflux. Gastroenterology 1983; 85:301–305.
3. Moroz SP, Espinoza J, Cumming WA, et al: Lower esophageal sphincter function in children with and without gastroesophageal reflux. Gastroenterology 1976; 71:236–241.
4. Gerhardt DC, Castell DO: Anatomy and physiology of the esophageal sphincters. *In* Esophageal Function in Health and Disease. New York, Elsevier Biomedical, 1983, pp 17–30.
5. Weinstock LB, Clouse RE: Esophageal physiology: Normal and abnormal motor function. Am J Gastroenterol 1987; 81:399–405.
6. Meyer GW, Castell DO: Anatomy and physiology of the esophageal body. *In* Esophageal Function in Health and Disease. New York, Elsevier Biomedical, 1983, pp 1–15.
7. Humphries TJ, Castell DO: Pressure profile of esophageal peristalsis in normal humans as measured by direct intraesophageal transducers. Am J Dig Dis 1977; 22:641–645.
8. Gryboski JD: The swallowing mechanism of the neonate: I. Esophageal and gastric motility. Pediatrics 1965; 35:445–452.
9. Welch RW, Luckmann K, Ricks P, et al: Lower esophageal sphincter pressure in histologic esophagitis. Dig Dis Sci 1980; 25:420–426.
10. Dodds WJ, Dent J, Jogan WJ, et al: Mechanisms of gastroesophageal reflux in patients with reflux esophagitis. N Engl J Med 1982; 307:1547–1557.
11. Christensen J: Origin of sensation in the esophagus. Am J Physiol 1984; 246:G221–G225.
12. Kilman WJ, Goyal RK: Disorders of pharyngeal and upper esophageal sphincter motor function. Arch Intern Med 1976; 136:592–601.
13. Cattau EL Jr, Castell DO: Symptoms of esophageal dysfunction. *In* Esophageal Function in Health and Disease. New York, Elsevier Biomedical, 1983, pp 31–46.
14. Giedion A, Nolte K: The nonobstructive pharyngeo-esophageal cross roll. Ann Radiol 1973; 16:129–135.
15. Cruse JP, Edwards DA, Smith JF, et al: The pathology of cricopharyngeal dysphagia. Histopathology 1979; 3:223–232.
16. Dinari G, Danziger Y, Mimouni M, et al: Cricopharyngeal dysfunction in childhood: Treatment by dilatations. J Pediatr Gastroenterol Nutr 1987; 6:212–216.
17. Reichert TJ, Bluestone CD, Stool SE, et al: Congenital cricopharyngeal achalasia. Ann Otol Rhinol Laryngol 1977; 86:603–610.
18. Gelfand MD: Severe dysphagia due to an esophageal motility disorder associated with Down's syndrome (abstract). Gastroenterology 1981; 80:1154.
19. Staiano A, Cucchiara S, De Vizia B, et al: Disorders of upper esophageal sphincter motility in children. J Pediatr Gastroenterol Nutr 1987; 6:892–898.
20. Wyllie E, Wyllie R, Cruse RP, et al: The mechanism of nitrazepam-induced drooling and aspiration. N Engl J Med 1986; 314:35–38.
21. Gryboski JD, Walker AW: Suck and swallow. *In* Gastrointestinal Problems in the Infant. 2nd ed. Philadelphia, WB Saunders, 1983, pp 12–29.
22. Ardran GM, Benson PF, Butler NR, et al: Congenital dysphagia resulting from dysfunction of the pharyngeal musculature: A clinical and radiologic study. Dev Med Child Neurol 1965; 7:157–166.
23. Frank MM, Baghdassarian L, Gatewood OM: Transient pharyngeal incoordination in the newborn. Am J Dis Child 1966; 111:178–181.
24. Sonies BC, Dalakas MC: Dysphagia in patients with the postpolio syndrome. N Engl J Med 1991; 25:1162–1167.
25. Cannon RA: Differential effect of botulina toxin on esophageal motor function in infants. J Pediatr Gastroenterol Nutr 1985; 4:563–567.
26. Hurwitz AL, Duranceau A: Upper esophageal sphincter dysfunction: Pathogenesis and treatment. Am J Dig Dis 1978; 23:275–281.
27. Lernau OZ, Sherzer E, Mogle P, et al: Congenital cricopharyngeal achalasia: Treatment by dilatations. J Pediatr Surg 1984; 19:202–203.
28. Cohen S: Motor disorders of the esophagus. N Engl J Med 1979; 301:184–192.
29. Berquist WE, Byrne WJ, Ament ME, et al: Achalasia: Diagnosis, management, and clinical course in 16 children. Pediatrics 1983; 71:798–805.
30. Sanderson DR, Ellis FH Jr, Schlegel JF, et al: Syndrome of vigorous achalasia: Clinical and physiologic observations. Dis Chest 1967; 52:508–517.
31. Moersch HJ: Cardiospasm in infancy and childhood. Am J Dis Child 1929; 38:294–298.
32. Azizkhan RG, Tapper D, Eraklis A: Achalasia in childhood: A 20-year experience. J Pediatr Surg 1980; 15:452–456.
33. Mayberry JF, Mayell MJ: Epidemiological study of achalasia in children. Gut 1988; 29:90–93.
34. Stein DT, Knauer M: Achalasia in monozygotic twins. Dig Dis Sci 1982; 27:636–640.
35. Westely CR, Herbst JJ, Goldman S, et al: Infantile achalasia:

Inherited as an autosomal recessive disorder. J Pediatr 1975; 87:243–246.
36. Monnig PJ: Familial achalasia in children. Ann Thorac Surg 1990; 49:1019–1022.
37. Holloway RH, Dodds WJ, Helm JF, et al: Integrity of cholinergic innervation to the lower esophageal sphincter in achalasia. Gastroenterology 1986; 90:924–929.
38. Cassella RR, Brown AL Jr, Sayre GP, et al: Achalasia of the esophagus: Pathologic and etiologic considerations. Ann Surg 1964; 160:474–487.
39. Elder JB: Achalasia of the cardia in childhood. Digestion 1970; 3:90–96.
39a. Henderson RD, Marryat G: Cricopharyngeal myotomy as a method of treating cricopharyngeal dysphagia secondary to gastroesophageal reflux. J Thorac Cardiovasc Surg 1977; 74:721–725.
40. Buick RG, Spitz L: Achalasia of the cardia in children. Br J Surg 1985; 72:341–343.
41. Qualman SJ, Haupt HM, Yange P, et al: Esophageal Lewy bodies associated with ganglion cell loss in achalasia. Gastroenterology 1984; 87:848–856.
42. Cassella RR, Ellis FH Jr, Brown AL Jr: Fine-structure changes in achalasia of the esophagus: I. Vagus nerves. Am J Pathol 1965; 46:279–288.
43. Dooley CP, Taylor IL, Valenzuela JE: Impaired acid secretion and pancreatic polypeptide release in some patients with achalasia. Gastroenterology 1983; 84:809–813.
44. Kramer P, Ingelfinger FJ: Esophageal sensitivity to mecholyl in cardiospasm. Gastroenterology 1951; 19:242–251.
45. Dodds WJ, Dent J, Hogan WJ, et al: Paradoxical lower esophageal sphincter contraction induced by cholecystokinin-octapeptide in patients with achalasia. Gastroenterology 1981; 80:327–333.
46. Aggestrup S, Uddman R, Sundler F, et al: Lack of vasoactive intestinal polypeptide nerves in esophageal achalasia. Gastroenterology 1983; 84:924–927.
47. Friesen DL, Henderson RD, Hanna W: Ultrastructure of the esophageal muscle in achalasia and diffuse esophageal spasm. Am J Clin Pathol 1983; 79:319–325.
48. Nihoul-Fekete C, Bawab F, Lortat-Jacob S, et al: Achalasia of the esophagus in childhood: Surgical treatment in 35 cases with special reference to familial cases and glucocorticoid deficiency association. J Pediatr Surg 1989; 24:1060–1063.
49. Nurko S: Motor disorders. *In* Pediatric Gastrointestinal Disease. Vol 1. Philadelphia, BC Decker, 1991, pp 393–416.
50. Boyle JT, Cohen S, Watkins JB: Successful treatment of achalasia in childhood by pneumatic dilatation. J Pediatr 1981; 99:35–40.
51. Stacher G, Kiss A, Wiesnagrotki S, et al: Oesophageal and gastric motility disorders in patients categorized as having primary anorexia nervosa. Gut 1986; 27:1120–1126.
52. Payne WS, Ellis FH, Olsen AM: Treatment of cardiospasm (achalasia of the esophagus) in children. Surgery 1961; 50:731–735.
53. Rozychi DL, Ruben RJ, Ralpin I, et al: Autosomal recessive deafness associated with short stature, vitiligo, muscle wasting, and achalasia. Arch Otorhinolaryngol 1971; 93:194–197.
54. Nussinson LE, Hager H, Samara M: Familial achalasia with absent tear production. J Pediatr Gastroenterol Nutr 1988; 7:284–287.
55. Katz PO, Richter JE, Cowan R, et al: Apparent complete lower esophageal sphincter relaxation in achalasia. Gastroenterology 1986; 90:978–983.
56. Asch MJ, Liebman W, Lechman RS, et al: Esophageal achalasia: Diagnosis and cardiomyotomy in a newborn infant. J Pediatr Surg 1974; 9:911–912.
57. Holloway RH, Krosin G, Lange RC. Radionuclide esophageal emptying of a solid meal to quantitate results of therapy in achalasia. Gastroenterology 1983; 84:771–776.
58. Gelfond M, Rozen P, Gilat T: Isosorbide dinitrate and nifedipine treatment of achalasia: A clinical, manometric, and radionuclide evaluation. Gastroenterology 1982; 83:963–969.
59. Bortolloti M, Labo G: Clinical and manometric effects of nifedipine in patients with esophageal achalasia. Gastroenterology 1981; 80:39–44.
60. Maksimak M, Perlmutter DH, Winter HS: The use of nifedipine for the treatment of achalasia in children. J Pediatr Gastroenterol Nutr 1986; 5:883–886.
61. Nakayama DK, Shorter NA, Boyle JT, et al: Pneumatic dilatation and operative treatment of achalasia in children. J Pediatr Surg 1987; 22:619–622.
62. McJunkin B, McMillan WO Jr, Duncan HE Jr, et al: Assessment of dilation methods in achalasia: Large-diameter mercury bougienage followed by pneumatic dilation as needed. Gastrointest Endosc 1991; 37:18–21.
63. Stark GA, Castell DO, Richter JE, et al: Prospective randomized comparison of Brown-McHardy and microvasive balloon dilators in treatment of achalasia. Am J Gastroenterol 1990; 85:1322–1326.
64. Vantrappen G, Hellemans J: Treatment of achalasia and related motor disorders. Gastroenterology 1980; 79:144–154.
65. Fellows IW, Ogilvie AL, Atkinson MP: Pneumatic dilatation in achalasia. Gut 1983; 24:1020–1023.
66. Mandelstam P, Sugawa C, Silvis SE, et al: Complications associated with esophagogastroduodenoscopy and with esophageal dilatation. Gastrointest Endosc 1976; 23:16–19.
67. Ott DJ, Richter JE, Wu WC, et al: Radiographic evaluation of esophagus immediately after pneumatic dilatation for achalasia. Dig Dis Sci 1987; 32:962–967.
68. Wong RK, Johnson LF: Achalasia. *In* Esophageal Function in Health and Disease. New York, Elsevier Biomedical, 1983, pp 91–123.
69. Heller E: Extramukose Cardiaplastik beim chronischen Cardiospasmus mit Dilatation des Oesophagus. Mitt Grenzgeb Med Chir 1913; 27:141–149.
70. Okike N, Payne WS, Neufeld DM, et al: Esophagomyotomy versus forceful dilatation for achalasia of the esophagus: Results in 899 patients. Ann Thorac Surg 1979; 28:119–125.
71. Lemmer JH, Coran AG, Wesley JR, et al: Achalasia in children: Treatment by anterior esophageal myotomy (modified Heller operation). J Pediatr Surg 1985; 20:333–338.
72. Seo JK, Winter HS: Esophageal manometric and clinical response to treatment in children with achalasia (abstract). Gastroenterology 1987; 92:1634.
73. Jara FM, Toledo-Pereyra LH, Lewis JW, et al: Long-term results of esophagomyotomy for achalasia of the esophagus. Arch Surg 1979; 114:935–936.
74. McCallum RW: The spectrum of esophageal motility disorders. Hosp Pract 1987; 22:71–83.
75. Bennett JR, Hendrix TR: Diffuse esophageal spasm: A disorder with more than one cause. Gastroenterology 1970; 59:372–279.
76. Clouse RE, Lustman PJ: Psychiatric illness and contraction abnormalities of the esophagus. N Engl J Med 1983; 309:1337–1342.
77. Clouse RE, Staiano A: Contraction abnormalities of the esophageal body in patients referred for manometry: A new approach to manometric classification. Dig Dis Sci 1983; 28:784–791.
78. Ferguson TB, Woodbury JD, Roper CL, et al: Giant muscular hypertrophy of the esophagus. Ann Thorac Surg 1969; 8:209–218.
79. Cassella RR, Ellis FH Jr, Brown AL: Diffuse spasm of the lower part of the esophagus: Fine structure of the esophageal smooth muscle and nerve. JAMA 1965; 191:739–382.
80. Richter JE, Barish CF, Castell DO: Abnormal sensory perception in patients with esophageal chest pain. Gastroenterology 1986; 91:845–852.
81. Richter JE: Diffuse esophageal spasm. *In* Esophageal Motility Testing. New York, Elsevier Biomedical, 1987, p 118.
82. Richter JE, Dalton CB, Katz PO, et al: Stress: A modulator of esophageal contractions. Gastroenterology 1986; 90:1603.
83. Creamer B, Donoghue E, Code CF: Pattern of esophageal motility in diffuse spasm. Gastroenterology 1958; 34:782–796.
84. Reidel WL, Clouse RE: Variations in clinical presentation of patients with esophageal contraction abnormalities. Dig Dis Sci 1985; 30:1065–1071.
85. Schey WL, Replogie R, Campbell C, et al: Esophageal dysmotility and the sudden infant death syndrome. Radiology 1981; 140:67–71.
86. Richter JE, Dalton CB, Bradley LA, et al: Oral nifedipine in the treatment of noncardiac chest pain in patients with the nutcracker esophagus. Gastroenterology 1987; 93:21–26.
87. Clouse RE, Lustman PJ, Eckert TC, et al: Low-dose trazodone

for symptomatic patients with esophageal contraction abnormalities. Gastroenterology 1987; 92:1027–1036.
88. Kahrilas PJ, Dodds WJ, Hogan WJ, et al: Esophageal peristaltic dysfunction in peptic esophagitis. Gastroenterology 1986; 91:897–904.
89. Hillemeier AC, Grill BB, McCallum R, et al: Esophageal and gastric motor abnormalities in gastroesophageal reflux during infancy. Gastroenterology 1983; 84:741–746.
90. Cucchiara S, Staiano A, DiLorenzo C, et al: Esophageal motor abnormalities in children with gastroesophageal reflux and peptic esophagitis. J Pediatr 1986; 108:907–910.
91. Biller JA, Allen JL, Schuster SR, et al: Long-term evaluation of esophageal and pulmonary function in patients with repaired esophageal atresia and tracheoesophageal fistula. Dig Dis Sci 1987; 32:985–990.
92. Flick JA, Boyle JT, Tuchman DN, et al: Esophageal motor abnormalities in children and adolescents with scleroderma and mixed connective tissue disease. Pediatrics 1988; 82:107–111.
93. Petrokubi RJ, Jeffries GH: Cimetidine versus antacid in scleroderma with reflux esophagitis. Gastroenterology 1979; 77:691–695.
94. Ramirez-Mata M, Ibanez G, Alarcon-Segovia D: Stimulatory effect of metoclopramide on the esophagus and lower esophageal sphincter of patients with PSS. Arthritis Rheum 1977; 20:30–34.
95. Horowitz M, Maddern GJ, Maddox A, et al: Effects of cisapride on gastric and esophageal emptying in progressive systemic sclerosis. Gastroenterology 1987; 93:311–315.
96. Kjellen G, Fransson SG, Lindstrom F, et al: Esophageal function, radiography, and dysphagia in Sjögren's syndrome. Dig Dis Sci 1986; 31:225–229.
97. McDonald GB, Sullivan KM, Schuffler MD, et al: Esophageal abnormalities in chronic graft versus host disease in humans. Gastroenterology 1981; 80:914–921.
98. Staiano A, Corazziari E, Andreotti MR, et al: Esophageal motility in children with Hirschsprung's disease. Am J Dis Child 1991; 145:310–313.
99. Vargas JH, Sachs P, Ament ME: Chronic intestinal pseudo-obstruction syndrome in pediatrics: Results of a national survey by members of the North American Society of Pediatric Gastroenterology and Nutrition. J Pediatr Gastroenterol Nutr 1988; 7:323–332.
100. Clouse RE, Lustman PJ, Reidel WL: Correlation of esophageal motility abnormalities with neuropsychiatric status in diabetics. Gastroenterology 1986; 90:1146–1154.
101. Cadranel S, Lorenzo D, Rodesch P: Caustic ingestion and esophageal function. J Pediatr Gastroenterol Nutr 1990; 10:164–168.

Section Four

THE STOMACH

Chapter 29

Anatomy and Physiology of the Stomach

ALAN M. LAKE

The vertebrate stomach is a highly complex organ, adapting to the specific needs of the species. The only vertebrate lacking a glandular stomach is the duckbill platypus, a mammal so confused that it produces its young by laying eggs.[1]

Developmental Anatomy

The human fetal stomach evolves by 4 weeks of gestation as a fusiform dilatation of the primitive foregut. By 7 weeks, it has descended below the diaphragm. With maximal growth on the dorsal aspect, a greater curvature is created, which moves to the left with a 90-degree clockwise rotation at 6 to 8 weeks. In so doing, nerve derived from the left vagus supplies the anterior wall, and nerve from the right vagus innervates the posterior wall of the stomach. The stomach is divided into four regions: cardia, fundus, body, and antrum—the last region terminating in the pyloric sphincter (Fig. 29–1).

The initial primitive columnar cell lining of the stomach develops gastric pits or foveolae by 9 weeks, and by 13 weeks glandular epithelium is seen.[2] Smooth muscle development follows a cranial to caudal sequence, with muscularis mucosa differentiated in the proximal cardia of the stomach at 10 weeks, progressing to the distal pylorus by 18 weeks of gestation.

Arterial blood supply is derived from the celiac arterial trunk. The cardia receives arterial supply from the left gastric artery, with venous drainage to the portal vein. Fundic arterial supply is from the short gastric, and the body receives blood primarily from the left gastroepiploic. Venous return from these regions drains to the splenic vein. The antrum receives blood from the right gastric and right gastroepiploic arteries. Venous return from the right gastric enters the portal vein, and the right gastroepiploic returns to the superior mesenteric vein. Increases in local mucosal flow appear to result from the local vasodilating effects of adenosine, prostaglandin, and histamine. The lymphatic network of the stomach is less developed than that of the small bowel. Blind projections begin in the lamina propria, joining plexuses in the muscularis mucosa and mucosa.[3]

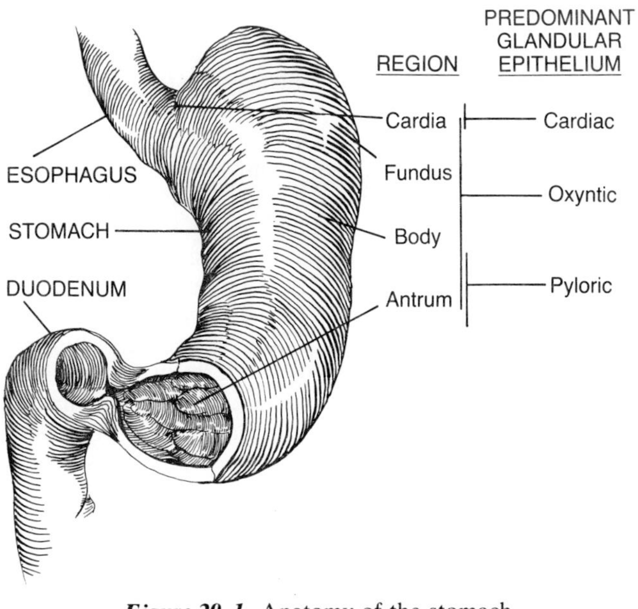

Figure 29–1. Anatomy of the stomach.

GASTRIC HISTOLOGY

The characteristic histologic feature of gastric epithelium is the gastric gland. There are three histologically and anatomically distinct types of gastric gland: cardiac, oxyntic, and pyloric. The oxyntic are the most prevalent, occupying the fundus and most of the body. In contrast, the surface epithelial mucous cells are uniformly similar in all four regions of the stomach.[4] The resulting mucous coat is 10 times thicker than the epithelial cell lining.

The cardiac glands contain predominantly mucus-secreting cells, though undifferentiated epithelial cells and enteroendocrine cells are also present. The cardiac glands occupy a small ring of gastric epithelium adjacent to the esophageal squamous epithelium and extend only a few millimeters into the cardia.

In contrast, the pyloric glands occupy the distal 10% of the gastric mucosal surface.[5] They are characterized by deep gastric pits. The two predominant cell types are the mucus-secreting cells and the gastrin-producing G cell.

Oxyntic glands extend from the cardia into the antrum. They contain a number of cell types: mucous neck cells, undifferentiated cells, intraepithelial lymphocytes, enteroendocrine cells, oxyntic or parietal cells, and the chief cell. The oxyntic cell is the major cell releasing hydrochloric acid,[6] and the chief cell is the major site of gastric synthesis and secretion of pepsinogen.[4] Figure 29–2, adapted from Ito,[4] depicts a simplified oxyntic gland. In vivo, one gastric pit may lead to as many as seven glands.[4] Although the distribution of cell types within a gland varies from one region to another, the chief cells are predominantly in the base, parietal cells are predominantly in the middle section (isthmus and neck), and enteroendocrine cells are distributed more randomly throughout the glandular epithelium.

The surface mucous cell appears by light microscopy to be a simple columnar epithelial cell extending from the surface into the gastric pits to the level of the isthmus. By special staining or electron microscopy, the apical mucous granules are usually densely packed below a lumenal surface characterized by short microvilli.[7] Below the mucous granules lies an active synthetic Golgi complex. The mechanism for secretion of mucus is incompletely understood, appearing to incorporate a slow steady exocytosis as well as possible transmembrane secretion or diffusion.[8, 9] Deeper within the gland, the mucous neck cells are in stages of differentiation. Surface mucous cells renew in about 72 hours, and neck mucous cells renew in about 1 week.[10, 11] When healing of resection margins is examined in animal models, the mucosa is rapidly regenerated from the isthmus region by undifferentiated cells at the margin in a manner that recapitulates embryonic development[12, 13] for all but the enteroendocrine cell, which appears to self-renew.

The oxyntic or parietal cells are most prevalent in the neck and isthmus region. A characteristic ultrastructural feature is a complex of canaliculi lined by microvilli coursing through the cytoplasm but in direct communication with the lumen. Two additional features are long, numerous microvilli (which lack a prominent glycocalyx) and large mitochondria. Within the apical microvilli lies maximal H^+, K^+ ATPase activity, the so-called proton pump.[14, 15] The outer surface of the microvilli is also the site of binding by anti-parietal cell autoantibodies.[16] The parietal cell is a convincing candidate for the synthesis and secretion of hydrochloric acid. Absence of parietal cells is associated with achlorhydria and the embryonic appearance of acid in the fetal stomach.

The chief or peptic cells reside primarily in the base of the oxyntic gland. This cell synthesizes, stores, and releases pepsinogen. Pepsinogen appears to be stored in zymogen granules in the apical cytoplasm and is released by exocytosis or merocrine secretion.[17]

Enteroendocrine cells appear to be less specific in their distribution within the gastric gland. Although the best characterized are the gastrin-producing G cell and the somatostatin-producing D cell of the pyloric gland, there are at least nine distinct enteroendocrine cell types producing a number of amines and peptides. In an effort to encompass all the cytochemical properties of the enteroendocrine cells, the concept of amine precursor uptake and decarboxylation (APUD) cells has been proposed.[18] In contrast to the parietal cell, the APUD cells differentiate from endodermal or neuroectodermal origins and appear to self-renew. Among the amines that appear to be synthesized are serotonin, histamine, and dopamine. Among the peptides synthesized are gastrin, somatostatin, vasoactive intestinal polypeptide (VIP), glucagon, and bombesin (gastrin-releasing peptide [GRP]).[19] Peptide hormone secretion from the enteroendocrine cell occurs at the basal and lateral cell membrane surface, not from the apical membrane. In so doing, the hormone is released to act locally within the glandular epithelium (termed *paracrine activation*) or systematically via the circulation (termed *endocrine activation*).[4, 20]

NEUROMUSCULAR FUNCTIONS

The stomach has three major functions dependent on intact neuromuscular integrity: storage of an ingested meal, mixing and grinding of the meal, and the controlled emptying of the meal into the duodenum. From the perspective of functional gastric motor activity, the stomach is divided into two parts: the proximal stomach consisting of cardia, fundus, and a portion of the body, and the antrum.

The proximal stomach regulates the accommodation of an ingested meal. This process of accommodation is mediated in large part by the inhibitory activity of the vagus nerve and allows the proximal stomach to distend without increasing intragastric pressure—a process termed *receptive relaxation*.[21, 22] As proximal gastric distention increases, a gentle contraction elevates the pressure gradient between the stomach and duodenum, facilitating the gastric emptying of liquids. Liquids are emptied from the stomach in an exponential fashion at a rate proportional to the amount ingested and the volume remaining in the stomach. At the cellular electrophysiologic level, the smooth muscle cells of the proximal stomach have a steady, nonfluctuating, transmembrane potential with contraction, resulting from small slow depolarization without spikes.[23]

In contrast, as solids reach the distal stomach, the antrum also contracts, allowing only the smallest particles and liquids to exit into the duodenum. The antral contractions drive the larger particles back into the body of the stomach by a retrograde propulsion generating a pressure exceeding 100 mm Hg.[24] This mechanical mixing and grinding combined with acid-peptic action reduce the solids to a size of 2 mm or less before entry into the duodenum is allowed. As a result, in contrast to the dynamics of liquids, solids are emptied in a linear fashion essentially unrelated to the amount of solid ingested with a meal. At the cellular electrophysiologic level, the distal gastric smooth muscle cells have slow cyclic changes in potential with high amplitude spike and pacemaker potential in response to both vagal and sympathetic stimulation.[23, 25]

In the fasting state, the distal stomach has continuous

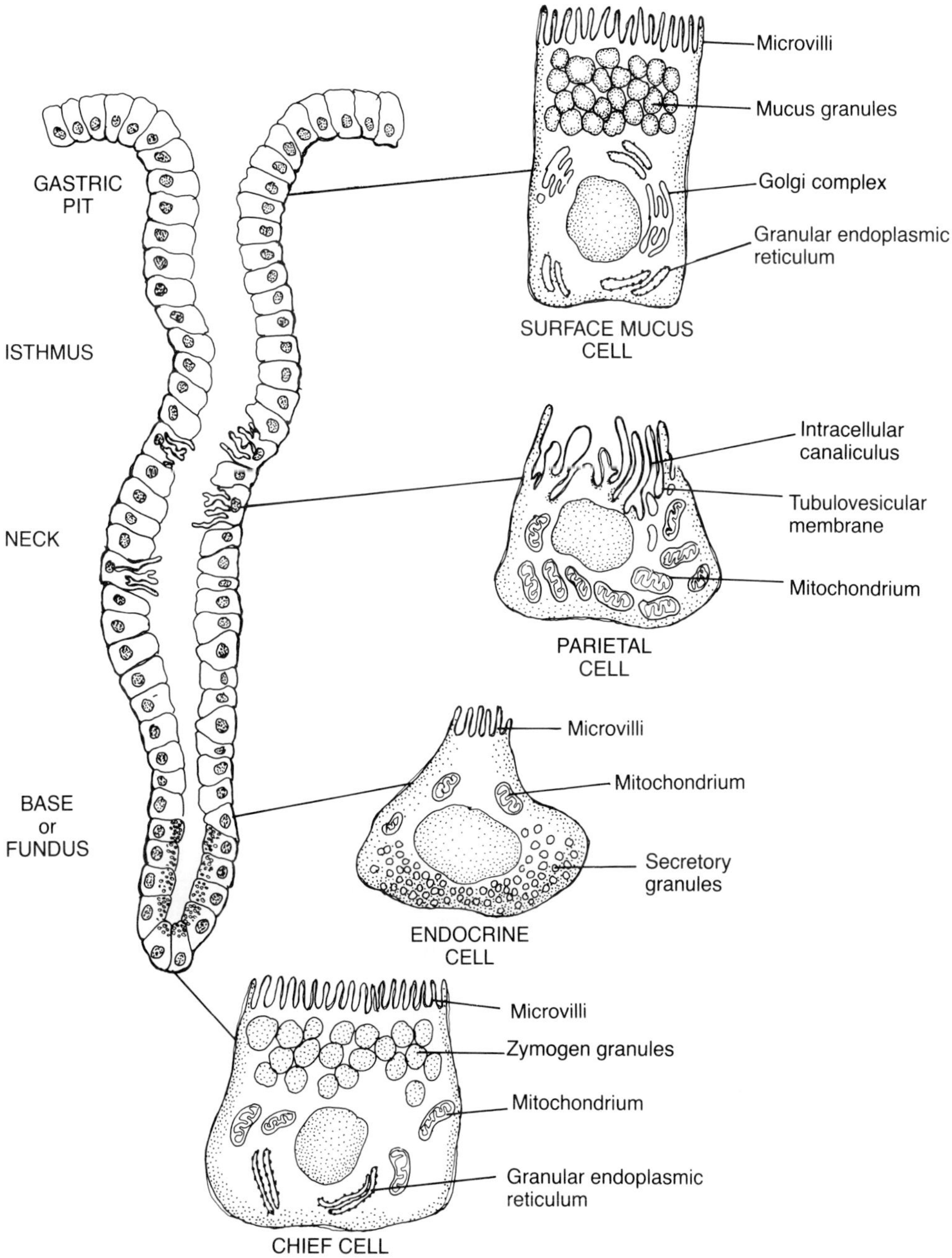

Figure 29–2. Schematic representation of a tubular oxyntic gland. (Modified from Ito S: Functional gastric morphology. *In* Johnson LR, ed: Physiology of the Gastrointestinal Tract. New York, Raven Press, 1987, pp 817–851; with permission.)

electrical activity of slow waves, with a maximal rate of three per minute, arising from a gastric pacemaker in the midbody of the greater curvature. This fasting electromechanical activity that migrates distally through the bowel is termed the *interdigestive myoelectric complex* (IMC).[26] Food ingestion inhibits the basal IMC; liquids induce irregular gastric contraction, and solids give rise to the vigorous antral contraction described above. The major polypeptide modulator of the IMC appears to be a motilin.[26] Recently, erythromycin has been found to be a motilin agonist, capable of facilitating gastric motility.

As noted above, the gastric emptying of ingested liquids is controlled primarily by the proximal stomach under vagal control. Hormonal stimulation of this process is induced by motilin and perhaps neurotensin. Inhibition of proximal gastric muscle function is achieved at physiologic levels by cholecystokinin and gastrin[27] and under laboratory conditions by somatostatin, VIP, gastrointestinal inhibitory peptide (GIP), and estrogen.[28, 29]

Distal gastric motility is heavily influenced by hormonal responses, often generated from antral and proximal small bowel receptors.[30] Stimulation of antral contraction is achieved with cholecystokinin, gastrin, bombesin, and motilin, and inhibition is encountered with calcitonin, secretin, glucagon, GIP, VIP, enkephalins, and somatostatin.[25] Although gastrin and cholecystokinin enhance antral contraction, they inhibit fundal contraction producing a net decrease in gastric emptying of liquids and mixed meals.

Gastric emptying is further influenced by the specific composition of the meal. The osmolality of the gastric effluent is one such factor, with rates of emptying slowed with either increases or decreases from isotonicity.[31] This is critical for the osmotically active carbohydrates and amino acids—with the exception of tryptophan, an amino acid with unique inhibiting properties. Increased duodenal content of fatty acids, especially 10–14 carbon chain fatty acids, also reduce the rates of gastric emptying.[32, 33] The influence of caloric density has been addressed in premature infants. Increased caloric density of the formula produces the expected reduction in rates of gastric emptying when expressed for volume; however, net caloric delivery to the duodenum actually increases.[34]

GASTRIC SECRETION

In 1770, Voltaire, in a letter to d'Alembert, stated: "Thought depends absolutely on the stomach, but in spite of that, those who have the best stomachs are not the best thinkers." Despite our subsequent best efforts, we have yet to identify the gastric origins of thought (or its inhibitors). We have made progress, however, extending our understanding of how the histologic glandular epithelium reviewed above produces such diverse products as hydrochloric acid, gastrin, pepsinogen, intrinsic factor, lipase, and mucus.

Hydrochloric Acid

Hydrochloric acid (HCl) is a simple electrolyte, produced by a single cell type in all species. It was first demonstrated in human gastric juice by Prout in 1824.[35] As noted previously, gastric HCl is secreted from the parietal cell via a complex system of canaliculi lined with microvilli. The human parietal cell is so efficient that it can concentrate the hydrogen ion levels in gastric juice to more than a millionfold the levels in plasma.

In the human newborn, acidification of gastric contents can be demonstrated almost immediately after birth by removal of the swallowed alkaline amniotic fluid and development of a gastric pH less than 4.[36, 37] The highest acid concentration occurs within 7 to 10 days, then it diminishes and achieves adult levels in 60 to 90 days.[38–40]

The control of gastric acid production in the immediate newborn period has been difficult to determine. In the first 2 days of life, full-term infants fail to increase acid secretion after stimulation with pentagastrin,[40] and the acid secretory response to the histamine analogue betazole hydrochloride (Histalog) is absent until 1 month of age.[41] Although basal acid output increases over the first four weeks of life, it does so on the basis of extrauterine age, not gestational age.[42] This suggests that extrauterine factors play a major role in the control of acid secretory function. Pentagastrin, although ineffective in the first 48 hours, does increase acid secretion by 1 week of age, with the magnitude of the response greater in term than preterm infants.[42, 43] In response to stimulation by meals, term newborns increase acid secretion for at least 2 hours.[44]

As all this suggests, acid secretion from the parietal cell is controlled by a complex system of stimulation and inhibition. There are three phases in the acid secretory cycle. The first is the cephalic phase, triggered by the sight, taste, and smell of food and mediated by the postganglionic cholinergic fibers of the vagus nerve. The second is the gastric phase, triggered by the ingestion of food and mediated in large part by the hormone gastrin. The third or intestinal phase is controlled by hormones released from stimulation of receptors in the proximal small bowel in response to the effluent from the stomach. In response to meal stimulation, the cephalic phase is felt to account for 30 to 50% of the acid response, the gastric phase for 40 to 50%, and the intestinal phase for less than 10%.

On the cellular level, agents acting on the parietal cell may be delivered by one or more of the following three mechanisms: (1) by release of a stimulating or inhibiting neurotransmitter such as acetylcholine from a nerve terminal (neurocrine secretion), (2) by delivery of a hormone such as gastrin via the circulation from a distant site of synthesis (endocrine secretion), and (3) by release into the interstitial fluid of a mediator such as somatostatin from a local synthetic site (paracrine secretion). Since intercellular and vascular transport are often critical to this process, data on the role of a specific mediator derived from isolated parietal cells, organ culture, or perfused in vivo pouches may be in conflict.

The gastric neuronal system consists of two main plexuses: the myenteric plexus, which innervates the muscle layers and regulates motor function; and the mucosal plexus, which innervates the mucosa and regulates gastric secretion. The vagus nerve communicates to each plexus with fibers that are 80 to 90% afferent and only 10 to 20% efferent. By immunohistochemical staining, the neurons of the mucosal plexus contain both nonpeptide transmitters such as acetylcholine, serotonin, and gamma aminobutyric acid (GABA) and peptide transmitters such as bombesin, VIP and substance K.[45]

In isolated parietal cells, separate receptors for histamine, acetylcholine, and gastrin have been documented.[46] The interactive processes involved are summarized in Figure 29–3. In isolated cells, postreceptor synergistic increases in acid release are noted for histamine with gastrin or acetylcholine.[46] A prereceptor synergistic response is also reported as both gastrin and acetylcholine enhance mast cell release of histamine.[45] In humans, histamine arises primarily from mast cells, and in animal systems it arises primarily from enterochromafin cells. Acetylcholine further enhances acid secretion by inhibiting the release of somatostatin from antral D cells, preventing somatostatin from inhibiting histamine release as well as G cell gastrin release.[47] Following vagotomy, increased gastric acidity stimulates release of somatostatin, and feedback inhibition of gastrin and histamine induces HCl secretion.[45]

Gastrin

Gastrin is synthesized and released from endocrine G cells located primarily in the gastric antrum. G cell secretion of gastrin is locally inhibited by somatostatin, derived from antral D cells located conveniently in close proximity to the G cell. There are two forms of gastrin: G–17 and G–34. Both are equally potent with regard to stimulation of parietal cell acid release, but G–34 has a longer plasma half-life.[48] Release of gastrin after a meal appears to be mediated by two neuronal processes. One is cholinergic, with induction of gastrin secretion and

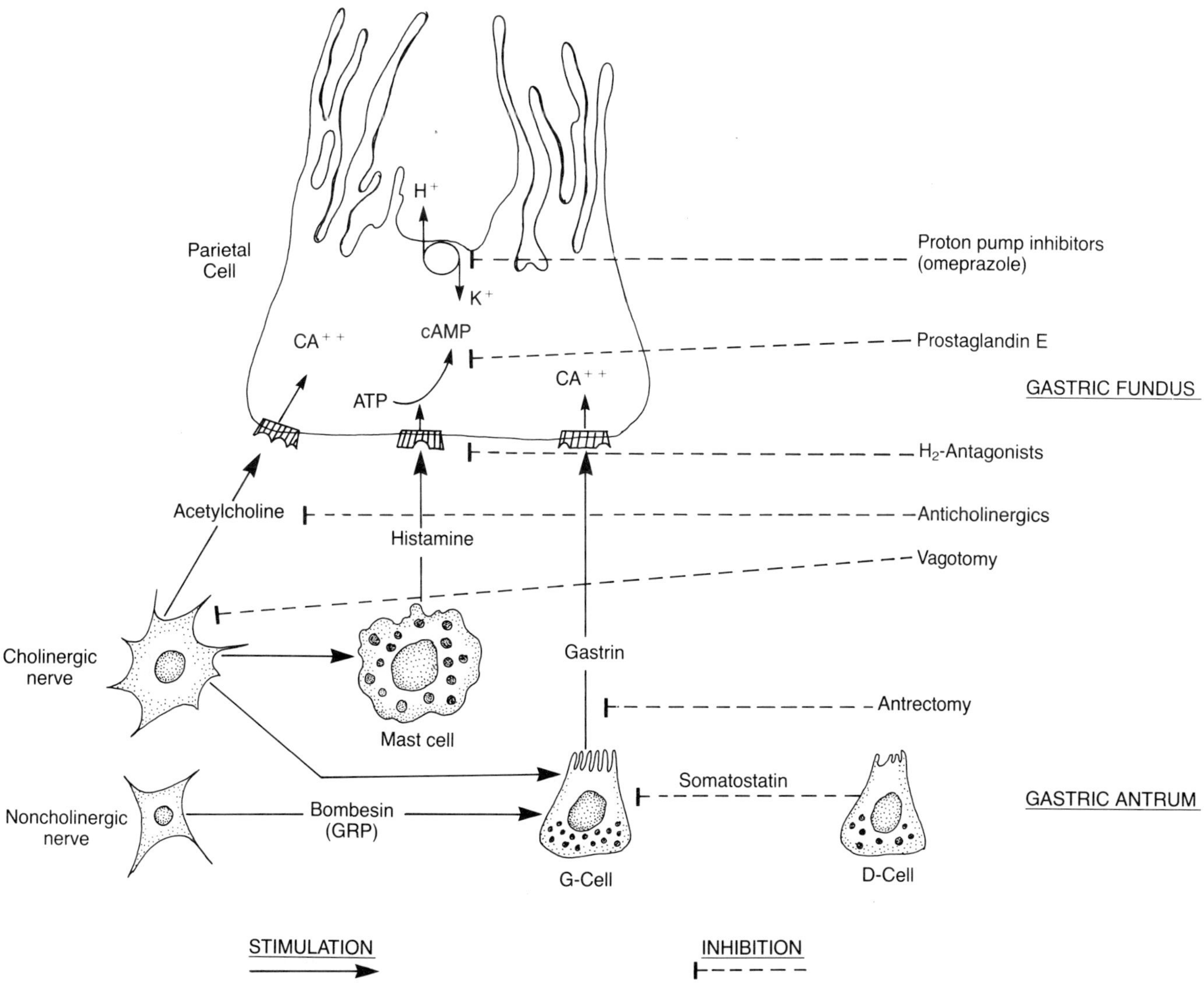

Figure 29–3. Stimulation and inhibition of parietal cell acid secretion.

somatostatin inhibition as reviewed above. The second is noncholinergic, with G cell proliferation and stimulated secretion following neuronal release of bombesin.[49]

Low-grade gastric distention, especially of the antrum, activates VIP neurons that inhibit gastrin secretion by releasing antral somatostatin and prostaglandin E. High-grade gastric distention, especially of the proximal stomach, stimulates vagal cholinergic gastric release. Partially digested intragastric and duodenal proteins, especially the amino acids tryptophan and phenylalanine, stimulate gastrin release.[50]

Inhibition of gastrin release is mediated not only by somatostatin but by secretin, neurotensin, GIP, and prostaglandin E. Somatostatin cells are distributed throughout the intestine, allowing action as an endocrine hormone as well as a paracrine inhibitor of G cell secretion. Intraintestinal fat is a major stimulus to somatostatin release, producing not only a substantial reduction in gastrin but a slowing of gastric emptying.[28, 29, 51, 52] Secretin is present mainly in the proximal small bowel and is released by intraduodenal acidification. Exogenous secretion also inhibits gastrin and acid secretion.[53] Neurotensin is synthesized in the ileum and released in response to intraintestinal fat to reduce gastric acidity.[45] Prostaglandin E, like somatostatin, interacts with inhibitory receptors coupled with adenylate cyclase to reduce parietal cell acid release.[54] It may also inhibit mast cell release of histamine to produce a net inhibition comparable to histamine H2 receptor antagonists.

In addition to its influence on gastric acidity, gastrin has a trophic effect on gastric epithelial maturity.[55] This may be relevant in two circumstances. First, the human neonate has transiently elevated gastrin at the time of low gastric acid secretion,[55] which may act to enhance mucosal epithelial maturation. Second, chronic pharmacologic inhibition of acid release, particularly with proton pump (H^+, K^+ATPase) inhibitors, is associated with marked hypergastrinemia and concern over possible long-term gastrin-induced dysplasia.[56]

Pepsinogen

In 1836, Schwann demonstrated that gastric digestion of protein required a "ferment" or "pepsin" in addition to HCl.[57] By 1881, Langley had defined a model for pepsin synthesis and secretion from the gastric chief cell that is the basis of our knowledge to this day.[58]

Pepsinogens are acidic proteinases and are also termed aspartic proteinases due to aspartate residues at the active site.[59, 60] The human gastric fundus elaborates, stores, and releases four acidic proteinases: pepsinogen I or A, pepsinogen II or C, cathepsin D, and cathepsin E. A fifth acidic proteinase—renin or chymosin—is elaborated by other mammals.[59, 61] All share the ability to hydrolyze protein at a pH below 5 and all are inhibited by pepstatins, although specific inhibitors have yet to be identified.

Pepsinogen A has a molecular weight of 43,500 and is synthesized by chief cells and mucous neck cells of the fundus, body, and cardia. Pepsinogen C is synthesized by the same cells as well as cells in the antrum, pylorus, Brunner gland, prostate, and seminal vesicle.[59, 62] At least four isomeric forms of pepsinogen are produced.

The glycoprotein cathepsin D is a lysosomal enzyme with a molecular weight of 42,000. It is synthesized by parietal cells, chief cells, mucous neck cells, pyloric gland cells, and macrophages. Cathepsin E (also called slow-moving protease) has a molecular weight of 84,000 with two subunits. It is elaborated by gastric surface and pit epithelial cells. It is not lysosomal, so it may have a role in intracellular proteolysis.[59]

The gastric chief cell contains zymogen granules that contain both pepsinogen A and pepsinogen C. On stimulation, the granules fuse with the apical cell membrane to initiate compound exocytosis, whereby each granule fuses to the membrane, with consecutive granules then fusing to the first.[63, 64] During maximal, prolonged stimulation, the granules disappear as pepsinogen secretion continues, suggesting a bypass of the need for storage zymogen granules.[64] Synthesis occurs as a prepepsinogen, containing a hydrophobic N-terminal sequence cleaved before secretion.[65]

The stimulation of pepsinogen secretion has been extensively studied in chief cell monolayers as well as organ culture and in vivo.[66] It would appear that both cholinergic and beta-adrenergic stimulation are important if not additive. Beta-adrenergic stimulation is probably mediated by cyclic adenosine monophosphate (cyclic AMP) and is inhibited by propranolol but not atropine or cimetidine.[66] Cholinergic stimulation is inhibited by atropine and seems to involve changes in intracellular calcium.[67]

Direct stimulation of pepsinogen secretion is also achieved with histamine, cholecystokinin (CCK), secretin, and VIP.[60] Furthermore, the actions are additive, suggesting separate peptide receptors. CCK probably acts through intracellular calcium release, and secretin and VIP act through cyclic AMP.[66] There is no direct stimulation achieved by gastrin or serotonin nor is inhibition seen with omeprazole. Somatostatin and prostaglandin E inhibit pepsinogen secretion probably by reduction in cyclic AMP. Since species-specific responses are common, generalizations for animal studies cannot be uniformly applied.[60]

Once secreted, pepsinogen is catalyzed to pepsin by the loss of an NH_2 terminal sequence. Pepsin activity is pH dependent. At an acid pH (<5), pepsin initiates the hydrolysis of most proteins and glycoproteins, including gastric mucus.[68] Pepsin is an endopeptidase preferentially cleaving peptide bonds formed by aromatic amino acids, thus exposing amino acids (tryptophan and phenylalanine) that are the most potent stimulants of acid release.[50, 59]

Pepsin activity is usually studied at a pH of 2 using a substrate such as bovine hemoglobin. At pH 5, pepsin loses hydrolytic activity but remains stable. Pepsin is irreversibly denatured above pH 7.2 or temperature greater than 65° C. In contrast, pepsinogen is resistent to denaturation by pH up to 10 or temperature up to 100° C.[69]

A number of studies have confirmed that pepsinogen A is not only electrophoretically heterogeneous but genetically polymorphic due to multiple genes and post-translational modifications of the gene product. There is thus great interest in its role in the genetic risk for peptic disease. It is evident that fasting serum levels of pepsinogens A and C are related to respective cell masses and rates of synthesis.[59] Following a meal, there is a rapid gastric secretion of pepsinogen and a slow rise in serum pepsinogen A. Marked elevation of serum pepsinogen I or A has been reported in chronic childhood peptic ulcer[70] and relapsing peptic ulcer in childhood[71] and may thus reflect increased peptic activity,[50] especially on a familial basis.[70] In contrast, in severe atrophic gastritis, serum levels of pepsinogen A are reduced and correlate with reduced gastric acidity, and serum levels of pepsinogen C are normal or increased.[50] Similar changes are seen in antral gastritis.

Pepsinogen has been identified by immunoelectrophoresis in the human fetal stomach by 8 weeks of gestation,[72] with peptic activity apparent by 16 weeks.[73] The peptic activity of 28-week, 1,000-gm premature infants is half that of term neonates.[74]

Intrinsic Factor

Intrinsic factor is a glycoprotein secreted by parietal cells in the oxyntic mucosa of the gastric body and fundus.[75] On the ultrastructural level, it is present on the tubulovesicular membrane, in the rough endoplasmic reticulum, and on the membrane of the perinuclear envelope.[76] By radioimmunoassay, intrinsic factor can be demonstrated in fetal gastric tissue by 11 weeks of gestation.[77]

Continuous low-grade secretion occurs under basal conditions by membrane-associated vesicular transport.[78] Increased secretion is stimulated by the same agents inducing parietal cell acid secretion: histamine, acetylcholine, and gastrin.[76] Peak release occurs in 15 to 30 minutes. Inhibition of intrinsic factor secretion is seen with H_2 receptor antagonists.

Studies in preterm and term infants confirm basal secretion of intrinsic factor, independent of gestation, acid secretion, or extent of enteral nutrition.[79] A dissociation of the stimulated release of acid and intrinsic factor has been documented well into the toddler years, with intrinsic factor secretion exceeding that of acid.[41, 80] Intrinsic factor secretion approaches adult levels by three months of age.[41] Congenital deficiency of intrinsic factor secretion has been reported as an autosomal recessive disorder occurring in the absence of any other gastric pathology.[81]

Following secretion, intrinsic factor competes for binding to vitamin B_{12} cobalamins with a second ligand termed *R protein* due to its rapid electrophoresis migration. In the stomach, vitamin B_{12} preferentially binds to R protein, however in the jejunum, pancreatic proteinases degrade R protein allowing intrinsic factor to bind nearly all of the vitamin B_{12}. In this bound form, vitamin B_{12} is then selectively absorbed in the terminal ileum.[82] Vitamin B_{12} remaining bound to R protein cannot be absorbed.

Gastric Lipase

Lipase activity was demonstrated in gastric juice in 1901; however, only recently has gastric epithelial secretion been demonstrated.[83] Lipase activity in humans of all ages is maximal in the gastric body and minimal in the antrum. Although the pH optimum is 5.5, lipase is active within an hour of birth, and its intragastric lipolytic release of long-chain fatty acids stimulates the secretion of CCK; release of medium-chain fatty acids allows rapid direct gastric absorption of lipid.[84] Gastric lipase can function in the absence of bile acids or other cofactors. It is inhibited by taurocholate.[83] A compensating increase in gastric lipase activity may be encountered when pancreatic insufficiency precludes release of pancreatic lipase.[83]

Gastric Mucus

The gastric epithelial and pit mucous cells secrete a water-insoluble mucous gel that forms a continuous protective layer approximately 180-μm thick. Mucin synthesis and total mucus volume increase after stimulation with histamine, acetylcholine, and gastrin, a pattern suggesting coupled secretion with acid.[85] The mucus acts as a diffusion barrier to lumenal pepsins and hydrochloric acid. Disruption of this mucous coat allows "back diffusion" of acid–peptic agents and loss of the pH gradient of bicarbonate, which is critical to maintaining epithelial integrity and renewal. Altered mucus synthesis and structure are obviously believed to contribute to the risk for peptic disease.

REFERENCES

1. Griffiths M: Digestion, growth and nitrogen balance in an egg-laying mammal, *Tachglossus aculeatus*. Comp Biochem Physiol 1965; 14:357–375.
2. Delemos C: The ultrastructure of endocrine cells in the corpus of the stomach of human fetuses. Am J Anat 1977; 148:359–384.
3. Rusznyak I: The gastrointestinal tract. *In* Youlten L, ed: Lymphatics and Lymph Circulation: Physiology and Pathology. Oxford, Pergamon Press, 1967, pp 92–97.
4. Ito S: Functional gastric morphology. *In* Johnson LR, ed: Physiology of the Gastrointestinal Tract. New York, Raven Press, 1987, pp 817–851.
5. Landboe-Christensen E: Extent of the pylorus zone in the human stomach. Acta Pathol Microbiol Scand 1944; 54:671–692.
6. Sachs G, Benglindh T: Physiology of the parietal cell. *In* Johnson LR, ed: Physiology of the Gastrointestinal Tract. New York, Raven Press, 1981, pp 567–602.
7. Helander HF: The cells of the gastric mucosa. Int Rev Cytol 1981; 70:217–290.
8. Kramer MF, Geuze JJ: Glycoprotein transport in the surface mucous cells of the rat stomach. J Cell Biol 1976; 73:533–547.
9. Ito S: Fine structure of the gastric mucosa. *In* Schnitka TK, Gilbert JAL, Hamini RC, eds: Gastric Secretion: Mechanisms and Control. Oxford, Pergamon Press, 1966, pp 3–24.
10. Stevens CE, LeBlond CP: Renewal of the mucous cells in the gastric mucosa of the rat. Anat Rec 1953; 115:231–245.

11. Lipkin M, Shenock P, Bell B: Cell proliferation kinetics in the gastrointestinal tract of man. II: Cell renewal in the stomach, ileum, colon, and rectum. Gastroenterology 1963; 45:721–729.
12. Blan H: Parietal cell regeneration in rat gastric mucosal wounds. A qualitative light and electron microscopical study. Umea Univ Med Dissertations 1982; 81:1–121.
13. Helander HF: Morphological studies on the margin of gastric corpus wounds in the rat. J Submicrosc Cytol 1983; 15:627–643.
14. Rubin W, Allasgharpour AA: Demonstration of a cytochemical difference between the tubulovescicular and plasmalemma of gastric parietal cells by ATPase and NPPase reaction. Anat Rec 1970; 184:251–264.
15. Saccomani G, Helander HF, Crago S, et al: Characterization of gastric mucosal membranes X: Immunological studies of gastric H^+K^+ATPase. J Cell Biol 1979; 83:271–283.
16. Hoedemaeker PJ, Ito S: Ultrastructural localization of gastric parietal cell antigen with peroxidase coupled antibody. Lab Invest 1970; 22:184–188.
17. Ito S, Winchester RJ: The fine structure of the gastric mucosa in the bat. J Cell Biol 1963; 16:541–578.
18. Pearse AGE, Taker T: Neuroendocrine embryology and the QPUD concept. Clin Endocrinol 1976; 5:229–244.
19. Grube D, Forssmann WG: Morphology and function of the enteroendocrine cells. Horm Metab Res 1979; 11:603–620.
20. Orci L: Morphologic events underlying the secretion of peptide hormones. *In* Jans VHT, ed: Endocrinology. Vol 2. Amsterdam, Excerpta Medica, 1977, pp 213–216.
21. Siegel JA, Urbain J-L, Adler LP: Biphasic nature of gastric emptying. Gut 1988; 29:85–89.
22. Read NW, Houghton LA: Physiology of gastric emptying and pathophysiology of gastroparesis. Gastroenterol Clin North Am 1988; 18:359–373.
23. Malagelada JR: Gastric motility disorders and their clinical implications. Scand J Gastroenterol 1989; 24:29–35.
24. Menomi H, McCallum RW: The physiology and pathophysiology of gastric emptying in humans. Gastroenterology 1984; 85:1592–1610.
25. Chaudhuri TK, Fink S: Gastric emptying in human disease states. Am J Gastroenterol 1991; 86:533–538.
26. Code CF, Marlett JA: The interdigestive myoelectric complex of the stomach and small bowel of dogs. J Physiol 1975; 246:289–309.
27. Debas HT, Farooq O, Grossman MI: Inhibition of gastric emptying as a physiological action of cholecystokinin. Gastroenterology 1975; 68:1211–1217.
28. Strunz UT, Code CF, Grossman MI: Effect of gastrin on electrical activity of antrum and duodenum of dogs. Proc Soc Exp Biol Med 1979; 161:25–27.
29. Hutson WR, Roehrkasse RL, Wald A: Influence of gender and menopause on gastric emptying and motility. Gastroenterology 1989; 96:11–17.
30. Rees WDW, Go VLW, Malagelada J-R: Antroduodenal motor responses to solid-liquid and homogenized meals. Gastroenterology 1979; 76:1438–1442.
31. Hunt JN, Pathak JD: The osmotic effects of some simple molecules and ions on gastric emptying. J Physiol 1960; 154:254–269.
32. Hunt JN, Knox MT: A relation between the chain length of fatty acids and the slowing of gastric emptying. J Physiol 1968; 194:327–336.
33. Stephens JR, Woolson RF, Cooke AR: Effects of essential and non-essential amino acids on gastric emptying in the dog. Gastroenterology 1975; 69:920–927.
34. Siegel M, Lebenthal E, Krantz B: Effect of caloric density on gastric emptying in premature infants. J Pediatr 1984; 104:118–122.
35. Prout W: On the nature of the acid and saline matters usually existing in the stomachs of animals. Philos Trans R Soc Lond 1824; 1:45–49.
36. Ebers DW, Smith DI, Gibbs GE: Gastric acidity in the first day of life. Pediatrics 1956; 18:800–802.
37. Avery GB, Randolph JG, Weaver T: Gastric acidity in the first day of life. Pediatrics 1966; 37:1005–1007.
38. Ames MD: Gastric acidity in the first ten days of life in the premature baby. Am J Dis Child 1960; 100:123–126.
39. Grand RJ, Watkins JB, Torti FM: Development of the human gastrointestinal tract. Gastroenterology 1976; 70:790–810.
40. Euler AR, Byrne WJ, Meis PJ, et al: Basal and pentagastrin stimulated acid secretion in newborn human infants. Pediatr Res 1979; 13:36–37.
41. Agunod M, Yamaguchi N, Lopez R, Luhby AL, Glass GBJ: Correlative study of hydrochloric acid, pepsin, and intrinsic factor secretion in newborns and infants. Am J Digest Dis 1969; 14:400–403.
42. Hyman PE, Clarke DP, Everett SL, et al: Gastric acid secretory function in preterm infants. J Pediatr 1985;106:467–471.
43. Euler AR, Byrne WJ, Campbell MF: Basal and pentagastrin stimulated gastric acid secretory rates in normal children and in those with peptic ulcer disease. J Pediatr 1983; 103:766–768.
44. Harada T, Hyman PE, Everett SL, Ament ME: Meal-stimulated gastric acid secretion in infants. J Pediatr 1984; 104:534–538.
45. Schubert ML, Shamburek RD: Control of acid secretion. Gastroenterol Clin North Am 1990; 19:1–25.
46. Soll AH: Secretagogue stimulation of ^{14}C-aminopyrine accumulation by isolated canine parietal cells. Gastroenterology 1982; 83:216–223.
47. Schubert ML, Edwards NF, Makhlouf GM: Neurally mediated gastric somatostatin secretion. Clin Res 1986; 34:445A.
48. Walsh JH, Isenberg JI, Ansfrell J: Clearance and acid stimulating action of human big and little gastrin in duodenal ulcer subjects. J Clin Invest 1976; 57:1125–1131.
49. Schubert ML, Makhlouf GM: Regulation of gastrin and somatostatin secretion by intramural neurons. Gastroenterology 1982; 83:626–632.
50. Taylor IL, Byrne WJ, Christie DL, et al: Effect of individual L-amino acids on gastric acid secretion and serum gastrin and pancreatic polypeptide release in humans. Gastroenterology 1982; 83:273–278.
51. Penman E, Wass JAH, Medbak S: Response of circulating immunoreactive somatostatin to nutritional stimuli in normal subjects. Gastroenterology 1981; 81:692–699.
52. Leth R, Lundell L, Olbe L: Effects of some gastrointestinal peptides on isolated human and rabbit gastric glands. Scan J Gastroenterol 1991; 26:89–96.
53. Mate L, Sakamoto T, Greeley GH. Regulation of gastric acid secretion by secretin and serotonin. Am J Surg 1985; 149:40–45.
54. Bunce KT: The effect of prostaglandins on the gastric parietal and nonparietal secretion on anaesthetized rat. J Pharm Pharmacol 1987; 39:825–831.
55. Lucas A, Aynsley-Green A, Bloom SR: Gut hormones. Clin Sci 1981; 60:349–353.
56. Creutzfeldt W, Lamberts R: Is hypergastrinemia dangerous to man? Scan J Gastroenterol 1991; 26:179–191.
57. Schwann T: Ueber das wesen des verdaungsprozesses. Poggndorf Ann Physik Chemie 1836; 38:358–364.
58. Langley JN: On the histology and physiology of pepsin forming glands. Philos Trans Soc Lond Ser B 1881;172:664–711.
59. Samloff IM: Peptic ulcer: The many proteases of aggression. Gastroenterology 1989; 96:586–595.
60. Muller MJ, Defize J, Hunt RH: Control of pepsinogen synthesis and secretion. Gastroenterol Clin North Am 1990; 19:27–39.
61. Kay J. Aspartic proteinases and their inhibition. *In* Kostka V, ed: Aspartic Proteinases and Their Inhibitors. Berlin, Walter de Gruyter, 1985, pp 1–17.
62. Samloff IM, Liebman WM: Cellular localization of the Group II pepsinogens in human stomach and duodenum by immunofluorescence. Gastroenterology 1973; 65:36–42.
63. Gibert AJ, Hersey SJ: Exocytosis in isolated gastric glands induced by secretagogues and hyperosmolarity. Cell Tissue Res 1982; 227:535–538.
64. Hirschowitz BI: Secretion of pepsinogen. *In* Code CF, ed. Handbook of Physiology: Alimentary Canal. Washington DC, American Physiology Society, 1967, pp 889–918.
65. Ichihara Y, Sogawa K: Takahashi K. Rat gastric pepsinogen in vitro synthesis and partial amino sequence. J Biochem 1982; 92:603–606.
66. Defize J, Meuwissen SGM: Pepsinogens: An update of biochemical physiological and clinical aspects. J Pediatr Gastroenterol Nutr 1987; 6:493–508.
67. Koelz HR, Hersey SJ, Sachs G, Ches GS: Cholinergic and beta-adrenergic pepsinogen release by isolated rabbit glands. Am J Physiol 1982; 243:218–225.
68. Pearson J, Allen A, Venables C: Gastric mucus: Isolation and

polymerase structure of the undergraded glycoprotein: Its breakdown by pepsin. Gastroenterology 1980; 78:709–715.
69. Hersey SJ: Pepsinogen secretion. *In* Johnson LR, ed. Physiology of the Gastrointestinal Tract. 2nd ed. New York, Raven Press, 1991, pp 947–955.
70. Tam PKH: Serum pepsinogen I in childhood duodenal ulcer. J Pediatr Gastroenterol Nutr 1987; 6:904–907.
71. Oderda G, Altare F, Dell'olio D, Ansaldi N: Prognostic value of serum pepsinogen I in children with peptic ulcer. J Pediatr Gastroenterol Nutr 1988; 7:645–650.
72. Hirsch-Marie H, Loisillier F, Touboul JP, Burtin P: Immunochemical study and cellular localization of human pepsinogen during ontogenesis and in gastric cancers. Lab Invest 1976; 34:623–632.
73. Keene MFL, Hewer EE. Digestive enzymes of the human fetus. Lancet 1929; 1:767–769.
74. Adamson I, Esangbedo A, Okolo AA, Omene JA: Pepsin and its multiple forms in early life. Biol Neonate 1988; 53:267–273.
75. Schepp W, Miederer SE, Ruoff HJ. Intrinsic factor secretion from isolated gastric mucosal cells of rat and man—two different patterns of secretagogue control. Agents Actions 1984; 14:522–528.
76. Donaldson RM: Intrinsic factor. *In* Johnson LR, ed: Physiology of the Gastrointestinal Tract. 2nd ed. New York, Raven Press, 1991, pp 976–988.
77. Schwartz M, Weber J: Gastric intrinsic factor in the human fetus. Scand J Gastroenterol 1971; 6:57–59.
78. Levine JS, Nkane PK, Allen RH: Human intrinsic factor secretion: Immunocytochemical demonstration of membrane-associated vesicular transport in parietal cells. J Cell Biol 1981; 90:644–655.
79. Marino LR, Bacon BR, Line JD, Halpin TC: Parietal cell function of full-term and premature infants: Unstimulated gastric acid and intrinsic factor secretion. J Pediatr Gastroenterol Nutr 1984; 3:23–27.
80. Rodbro P, Krasilnikoff PA, Christiansen PM. Parietal cell secretory function in early childhood. Scan J Gastroenterol 1967; 2:209–213.
81. Giorno JL, Dandine M, Gaudelis J, et al: Deficit congenital en factor intrinsique. Ann Pediatr (Paris) 1985; 32:277–280.
82. Allen RH, Seetharam B, Podel ER, Alpers DH. Effect of proteolytic enzymes on the binding of cobalamin to R protein and intrinsic factor. J Clin Invest 1978; 61:47–54.
83. DiPalma J, Kirk CL, Hamosh M, et al: Lipase and pepsin activity in the gastric mucosa of infants, children and adults. Gastroenterology 1991; 101:116–121.
84. Cohen M, Morgan GR, Hofmann AF: Lipolytic activity of human gastric and duodenal juice against medium and long chain triglycerides. Gastroenterology 1971; 60:115.
85. Shimamoto C, Takao Y, Asada S, et al: Regulation of human and rat gastric mucin synthesis: Assessment by histochemical and biochemical methods. Gastroenterology 1991; 100:A159.

Chapter 30

Pyloric Stenosis and Congenital Anomalies of the Stomach and Duodenum

FREDERICK ALEXANDER

Hypertrophic pyloric stenosis is the most frequent surgical disorder of the stomach and duodenum in infants and children. Although not of embryonic origin, it may share certain clinical manifestations with other malformations of the stomach and duodenum. Thus, it makes sense to consider these various disorders together to draw the proper clinical and pathophysiologic distinctions between them.

EMBRYOLOGY

Basic to an understanding of all these disorders is a knowledge of normal foregut embryology. The primitive foregut begins as a pharyngeal structure that elongates to form the primordia of the esophagus and the stomach.[1] The stomach first appears as a local dilatation between segments C3 and C5 at the fifth week of gestation. The next few weeks of gestation are a period of rapid elongation of the cranial foregut and intense mucosal proliferation of both the esophagus and the duodenum. At the end of the seventh week, the stomach is located at the level of T11 to L4, and there is differentiation of the greater and lesser curvature probably related to the differential growth of the opposite sides of the stomach. In classic view, the stomach then rotates clockwise about its vertical axis to bring the left vagus nerve anterior to the stomach and the right vagus posterior. Subsequent rotation on its anteroposterior axis allows the stomach to assume its final position. Finally, by the tenth week of gestation, rugae and longitudinal muscles are apparent in the stomach, and the lumen in both the esophagus and the duodenum has been formed by recanalization.[2]

PYLORIC STENOSIS

History

The first description of hypertrophic pyloric stenosis was made in 1788 by Hezekiah Beardsley, who described an obstructing scirrhosity in the pylorus at autopsy in a 5-year-old child.[3] Hirschsprung provided an accurate description of the condition in 1888 and first applied the name *congenital hypertrophic pyloric stenosis.*[4] Prior to the first attempt at extramucous pyloroplasty by Dufour and Fredette in 1908,[5] surgical options for this disorder consisted of gastroenterostomy, pyloric resection, jejunostomy, and intraluminal dilatation of the pyloric canal. Surgical mortality exceeded 60%, whereas 10 to 46% of infants died with conservative therapy. Extramucous pyloroplasty was only partially successful and often led to massive bleeding in that sutures cut through the pyloric muscle. In 1912, Ramstedt[6] took a decisive step by limiting the operative repair to splitting the pyloric muscle, which was subsequently proved to be curative and remains standard treatment today.

Incidence and Heredity

The incidence of pyloric stenosis is variable and may be increasing in males in certain parts of the United States and the United Kingdom. Laron and Horne[7] reported an incidence of 1 in 913 live births in the Pittsburgh area. They also found the incidence to be two and one half times greater in white infants as compared with black infants. Jed and associates[8] found that the incidence of pyloric stenosis in Olmsted County, Minnesota, increased in boys from 1.7 per 1,000 live births for the period 1950 to 1954, to 6.2 per 1,000 live births for the period 1980 to 1984, whereas rates for girls changed only from 0.6 to 0.9 per 1,000 live births during this period. Kerr[9] found an unprecedented rise in the incidence of pyloric stenosis in the central region of Scotland from an average of 2.2 per 1,000 live births for the period 1970 to 1977, to 8.8 per 1,000 live births in 1979. Knox and colleagues[10] found a similar increase in the incidence of pyloric stenosis in the West Midlands Health Region between 1974 and 1980, which correlated with a 31% increase in breastfeeding in Great Britain during the same period.[10, 11] It has been suggested that administration of dicyclomine hydrochloride (Bendectin) to the pregnant woman and seasonal variations may play a role in pyloric stenosis. However, there is currently no evidence to support this.

Pyloric stenosis is based on a polygenic mode of inheritance modified by sex.[12] The ratio of males to females with pyloric stenosis ranges between 4 and 6 to 1. Although believed to be more common in first-born children, pyloric stenosis has recently been shown to be more closely associated with smaller family size and higher socioeconomic class than with birth order.[13] Jed and associates[8] reported a positive family history in 13% of affected children. Other studies have shown that a mother who had pyloric stenosis has a four times greater chance of having a child with pyloric stenosis than does a similarly affected father.[14]

Pathogenesis

The exact cause of hypertrophic pyloric stenosis is unknown. In most instances, the condition presents with vomiting after 3 weeks of age; however, about 20% of patients with a classic type are symptomatic from birth.[15,16] Rollins and colleagues[17] showed prospectively, using sonography, that pyloric muscle hypertrophy is not present during the early newborn period in infants who later develop infantile pyloric stenosis. Sonography has also been used to show that subclinical disease may cause minor degrees of vomiting, with subsequent gradual resolution.[18] Late development of hypertrophic pyloric stenosis is rare but may occur in association with transpyloric feeding tubes.[19]

Lynn[20] proposed in 1960 that milk curds propelled by gastric peristalsis against a closed pyloric canal produce edema that narrows the pyloric canal and causes work hypertrophy of the pyloric and gastric musculature. Whether the initial cause is edema or an unexplained spasm of the antropyloric muscle, it seems clear that a vicious cycle is established that progresses to high-grade obstruction of the pyloric canal. Hypergastrinemia associated with hyperacidity has been suggested as a possible cause of pyloric stenosis.[21] In addition, elevations of prostaglandins E_2 and $F_{2\ alpha}$, both potent smooth muscle constrictors, have been found in infants with pyloric stenosis.[22] However, all these findings probably represent a secondary phenomenon caused by chronic gastric retention and distention.

Clinical Presentation

Nonbilious vomiting is the initial sign of infantile hypertrophic pyloric stenosis. The vomiting may or may not be projectile, is usually progressive, and may become brownish owing to gastritis in later stages. Prolonged vomiting may lead to dehydration, weight loss, and failure to thrive.

The onset of vomiting may occur as early as the first week or as late as 5 months of age.[23] As vomiting continues, hydrogen ion loss leads to an elevation of the serum bicarbonate followed by a decrease in serum chloride and the development of hypochloremic alkalosis.[24] Serum potassium levels usually remain normal; however, when potassium depletion does occur, it may lead to paradoxical aciduria owing to the preferential loss of hydrogen ions across the distal renal tubules in exchange for sodium reabsorption.[25]

Jaundice occurs in association with pyloric stenosis in approximately 2 to 5% of infants.[26,27] Approximately 50% of jaundiced infants with pyloric stenosis have a serum bilirubin level between 5 and 10 mg per dl that is mostly unconjugated.[28] Such elevations in the serum unconjugated bilirubin level have been seen in certain infants with neonatal bowel obstruction and have been ascribed in the past to the effects of acute starvation on an immature liver. Woolley and coworkers[29] found decreased levels of glucuronyl transferase in infants with hypertrophic pyloric stenosis. Labrune and colleagues[30] found abnormally low levels of glucuronyl transferase in several infants 4 to 5 months after pyloromyotomy, suggesting that the jaundice associated with pyloric stenosis may be an early manifestation of Gilbert syndrome. The role of caloric deprivation remains unclear, since a reduction in bilirubin levels occurs within 6 to 24 hours postoperatively, long before adequate caloric intake resumes.

Although there is no defined relationship between pyloric stenosis and other abnormalities, associated anomalies may be present in 6 to 20% of infants.[31] Many surgeons have noted a higher than expected occurrence of esophageal atresia and malrotation, which may occur in approximately 5% of infants with pyloric stenosis.[32]

Diagnostic Evaluation

The diagnosis of pyloric stenosis is best made by physical examination with the palpation of a pyloric mass. This firm, small, movable mass is similar to the size and shape of an olive and is located in the mid-epigastrium. A pyloric mass is pathognomonic and is palpable in 80% of cases by experienced examiners. To optimize the physical examination it is important first to empty the stomach of all air and fluid using a 10 Fr Replogle oral gastric tube. The catheter may then be removed, and the infant comforted with 5% glucose in water given orally. Occasionally, small doses of a sedative, such as morphine sulfate 0.1 mg per kg, may be given to facilitate the examination.

Imaging procedures should be reserved for infants with bilious vomiting or those with nonbilious vomiting in whom experienced examiners are unable to feel a pyloric mass. In the latter group of infants, the differential diagnosis includes gastroenteritis, gastroesophageal reflux, pylorospasm, allergic gastroenteropathy, and, rarely, antral or pyloric webs. To distinguish between them an upper gastrointestinal series (UGIS) may be performed. The characteristic findings of pyloric stenosis on UGIS are a constant elongation of the pyloric canal,[33] a double tract of barium along the pyloric canal

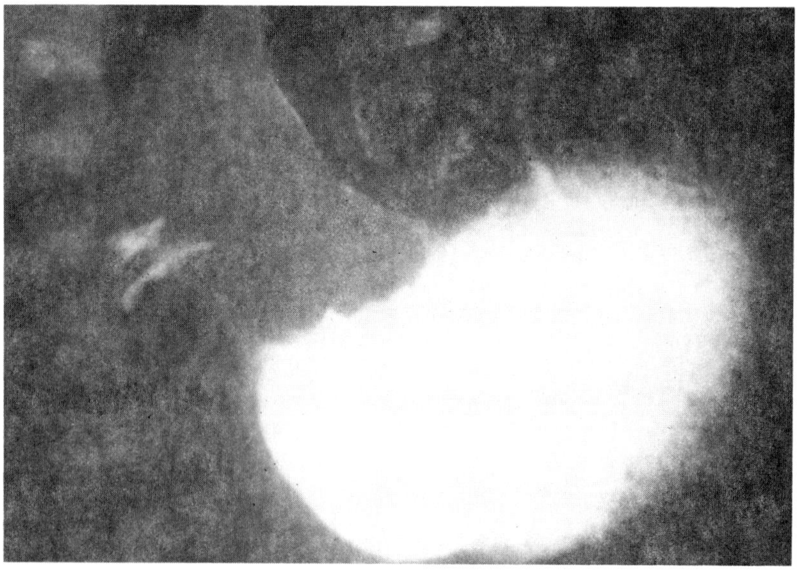

Figure 30–1. UGIS showing elongated pyloric channel and double-tract sign with shouldering of antrum characteristic of hypertrophic pyloric stenosis.

due to the folding of compressed mucosa,[34] and a prepyloric bulge into the distal antrum, producing an appearance that resembles shoulders or an umbrella[35] (Fig. 30–1). Delay in gastric emptying may not be used as a sign of pyloric stenosis because the pylorus may display a wide range of emptying times in normal infants.

Recently, sonography has been advocated as the imaging procedure of choice to confirm the diagnosis of pyloric stenosis.[36] First described by Teele and Smith,[37] sonography displays the hypertrophic pyloric musculature as a broad ring with a low echo density and an inner layer of high echo density corresponding to the mucosa. In addition to this characteristic overall appearance of the pylorus, strict criteria for hypertrophic pyloric stenosis have been developed that include a muscle thickness equal to or greater than 4 mm[38] or a pyloric length greater than 16 mm[39] or both (Fig. 30–2). Using these criteria, Forman and associates[40] found that sonography had a sensitivity of 89% and perfect specificity, whereas UGIS was found to have perfect sensitiv-

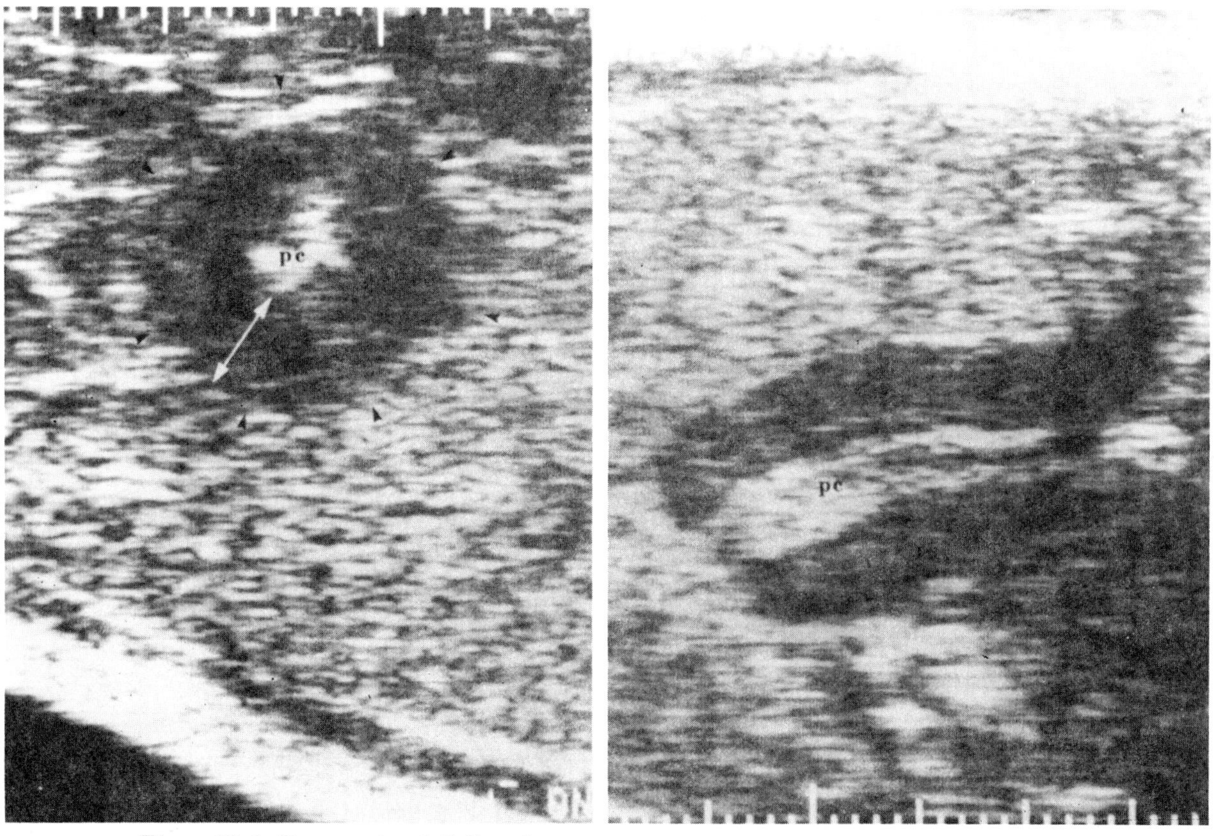

Figure 30–2. Cross-sectional *(left)* and transverse *(right)* sonogram of hypertrophic pyloric stenosis showing increased thickness and length of pyloric muscle. pc, pyloric channel.

ity and specificity. In their report, a palpable pyloric mass had a predictive value of 100%; but, in the absence of palpable mass, infants still had a 44% chance of pyloric stenosis. Further, while a positive sonogram indicated pyloric stenosis with 100% probability, a negative sonogram still left 8% of patients undiagnosed. The implication is that if sonography is used as the primary imaging modality in infants who do not have palpable pyloric mass or who have not been examined by a pediatric surgeon, then the number of patients requiring both sonography and UGIS may increase total costs. On the other hand, sonography limits radiation exposure and may facilitate the evaluation of nonbilious vomiting in infants.

Treatment

Initial treatment of pyloric stenosis is directed toward correction of dehydration and hypochloremic alkalosis. Although serum potassium levels are usually normal, it should be recognized that total body potassium may be markedly depleted before serum samples reflect hypokalemia. The degree of dehydration may be assessed according to the usual clinical parameters but is often reflected by the degree of hypochloremic alkalosis. Although most infants may be prepared for surgery within a 24-hour period, advanced dehydration and alkalosis may require preoperative preparation over several days.

For those infants with minimal dehydration and a normal electrolyte pattern, many surgeons advocate oral institution of a balanced electrolyte solution once the stomach has been lavaged with normal saline to remove obstructing milk curds and barium. Because vomiting may persist and the serum chloride and bicarbonate may be unreliable indices of the extent of the fluid and electrolyte losses, it is prudent to begin intravenous fluid using 5% dextrose and 0.33% saline with 5 mmol of potassium chloride added to each 250-ml intravenous bottle, even for those infants with apparent minimal dehydration.

Infants with moderate to severe fluid and electrolyte disturbances in whom serum bicarbonate may range from 25 to 60 mmol per L and serum chloride may range from 50 to 105 mmol per L are best treated with 5% dextrose in 0.45 to 0.9% saline given initially as a bolus of 10 to 20 ml per kg as required, and then at one and one half times maintenance for as long as required, until serum electrolytes have approached normal levels and total body water is judged to be sufficient. Once the stomach has been emptied, most infants stop vomiting. Only in rare cases is continued nasogastric drainage required, and then intravenous rates and electrolyte concentration must be adjusted to cover ongoing losses. Finally, after the infant has voided, it is important to add 5 to 10 mmol of potassium chloride to each 250-ml bottle to help correct the hypochloremic alkalosis.

Correction of alkalemia prior to surgery is essential to prevent postanesthetic apnea, which may occur as a result of alkalemic depression of the respiratory center.[41] Several reports have indicated the incidence of postoperative apnea to range between 1 and 3%.[42,43] Rapid induction of general endotracheal anesthesia is not required; however, the stomach should be drained with an oral gastric tube prior to induction to prevent aspiration.

The Ramstedt pyloromyotomy remains the surgical procedure of choice (Fig. 30–3). It is performed through a short right transverse incision placed at the liver edge.

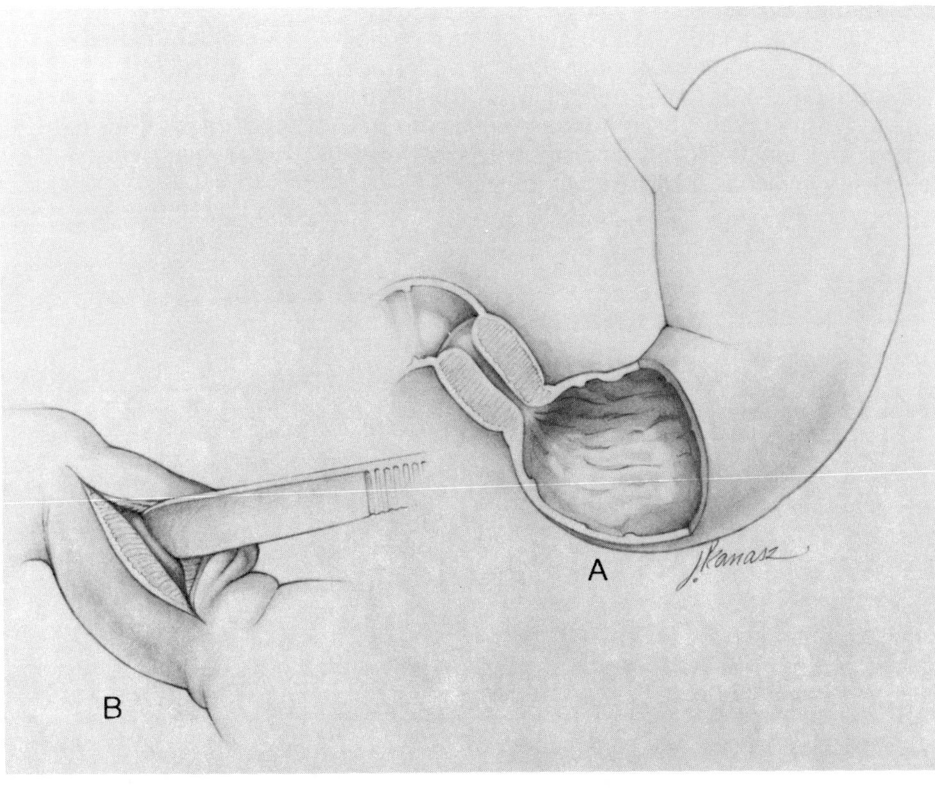

Figure 30–3. *A*, Cross-section of the elongated, narrow pyloric channel typical of pyloric stenosis. *B*, Pyloromyotomy is begun by bluntly separating muscle fibers on the anterior surface of the pylorus.

Whether the oblique muscles or the rectus abdominal muscles are split is a matter of personal preference. The pyloric mass is delivered into the wound and is then serosally incised, and the underlying muscle is bluntly split, allowing the mucosa to pout up into the cleft, indicating a release of the obstructive process. Important technical features of this operation include avoidance of a mucosal tear in the region of the pyloric vein, where the risk is greatest, and extension of the pyloromyotomy to the antrum, where recurrence is most likely. Mucosal disruption is inconsequential as long as it is recognized and treated by repair with absorbable suture and decompression of the stomach for 48 hours.

Postoperative vomiting is a well-recognized phenomenon, occurring in as many as 50% of the infants, and is most likely caused by persistent local edema along with inefficient gastric emptying.[44] In most cases, however, diluted feedings may be initiated within 12 to 24 hours after surgery, and most infants may be advanced to maintenance oral feedings within 36 to 48 hours after surgery. If vomiting continues, radiologic reassessment of persistent hypertrophic pyloric stenosis may be difficult. Serial sonograms taken postoperatively reveal initial swelling of the muscles with rapid involution over the next 3 weeks attaining normal thickness by 6 weeks.[45] Persistent hypertrophic pyloric stenosis due to an incomplete pyloromyotomy appears as persistent gastric outlet obstruction with muscle hypertrophy, but it may have a tapered appearance.[46]

Results

The surgical treatment of pyloric stenosis is curative,[47] and the prognosis for infants with pyloric stenosis depends on the associated anomalies. Reports[48–50] indicate a mortality rate between 0 and 0.5%, an incidence of recurrence near 1 and 3%, and an incidence of wound infection and adhesions between 1 and 5%. Postoperative bleeding is rare and transfusion is virtually never required. These percentages indicate the high degree of success and low morbidity and mortality that may be achieved with skilled pediatric surgical care.

CONGENITAL GASTRIC OUTLET OBSTRUCTION

History

Atresia limited to the pyloric antrum was first described by Calder in 1733.[51] Subsequently, Crooks[52] described the first pyloric membrane in 1828. Laudener in 1897 reported the first incomplete prepyloric membrane.[53] The first description of an antral web in the English literature was made by Parsons and Barding[54] in 1933. Since then, approximately 127 cases of congenital outlet obstruction have been reported involving the pylorus and antrum in three general forms, including complete segmental defects, fibrous cords, and webs.[55]

Incidence

Congenital gastric outlet obstruction due to pyloric atresia or prepyloric or antral webs is rare, representing fewer than 1% of all atresias and diaphragms of the alimentary tract.[56, 57] Cook and Rickham[53] reported an incidence of 0.003% during a period of 25 years at the Liverpool Regional Neonatal Center. Pyloric webs are by far the commonest of these reported; according to Bell and coworkers,[58] only 32 cases of antral webs were reported in children 16 years of age or younger. The rarity of these lesions notwithstanding, Tunnell and Ide Smith[59] state that the diagnosis of antral webs in infancy is being made with increasing frequency.

Etiology and Pathology

The etiology of these defects is unknown. However, because the antrum and pylorus do not undergo mucosal proliferation, the etiology is not related to failure of canalization. Instead, it is speculated that discontinuation of the endodermal tube before the eighth week of gestation leads to segmentation defects, and endodermal redundancy after the eighth week leads to antral web formation. Given early fixation and excellent collateral

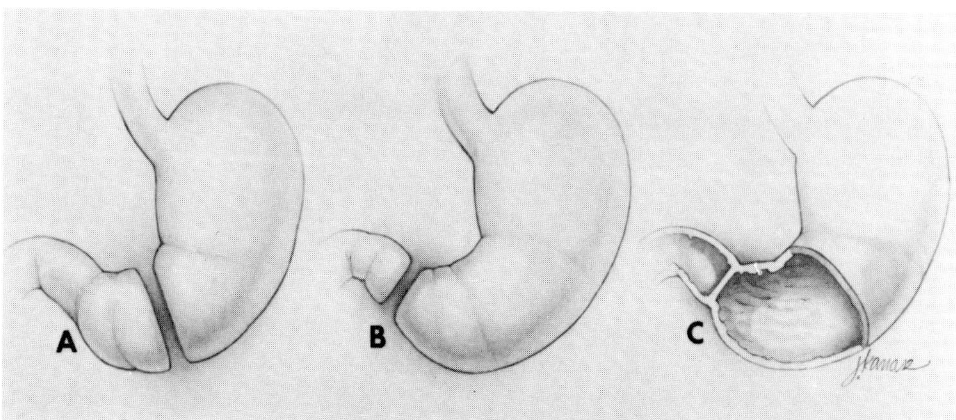

Figure 30–4. Congenital gastric outlet obstruction. *A*, Antral gap atresia: 1% of cases. *B*, Pyloric gap atresia: 27% of cases. *C*, Pyloric web: 67% of cases.

circulation of the stomach and duodenum, it is unlikely that in utero vascular accidents are causative factors.

Reports[60] indicate that the defects involving the antrum or pylorus may be of several types (Fig. 30–4). Antral defects are least common, with antral gap atresia occurring in 1% and antral membranes with partial openings occurring in 5% of patients. Pyloric gap atresias with complete or cord separation of the pylorus account for approximately 27% of the cases. Pyloric webs are commonest, occurring in 67% of cases, and include single and double membranes and solid atresias 1 to 2 cm in thickness.

Pyloric atresia may occur in an autosomal recessive mode in association with epidermolysis bullosa letalis.[61–63] Eighteen cases of pyloric atresia–epidermolysis bullosa syndrome have been reported since Korber and Glasson's initial report in 1977.[64] Gedde-Dahl and Lambrecht[65] have shown that families with pyloric atresia-epidermolysis bullosa syndrome are of two ethnic groups, American Indian and Lebanese-Turkish, thus favoring genetic linkage between two autosomal recessive genes.

Clinical Manifestations

Infants with antral or pyloric webs present quite differently from older children with the disorder.[55] Infants present with nonbilious vomiting, usually within the first days of life, along with feeding difficulties and distention of the stomach. Older children tend to present with epigastric pain, weight loss, nausea and vomiting, or symptoms compatible with peptic ulcer disease. Distribution by sex is nearly equal.[60] Polyhydramnios is reported in 61% of neonatal cases, and there is a high percentage of infants with low birth weight.[60,66,67] Rupture of the stomach in pyloric atresia may occur as early as 12 hours after birth.[68]

Diagnosis

The diagnosis of congenital outlet obstruction may be suggested by the nonspecific findings of a large dilated stomach with a single gas bubble. Since a dilated stomach with no gas in the distal bowel may also be seen in gastric hypotonia of the newborn,[69] it is important to proceed to UGIS. Bell and coworkers[58] report that the UGIS is 90% accurate in the diagnosis of congenital outlet obstruction. The typical UGIS findings of pyloric atresia are an absence of the beak sign seen with pyloric stenosis or duplication and the presence of a pyloric dimple sign formed by the shallow pyloric cavity at the proximal point of the atresia.[70] In pyloric atresia, sonographic examination may reveal an absence of the typical echolucent pattern of the pyloric muscle. An antral web may appear on an upper gastrointestinal radiograph as a thin septum projecting into the antral lumen perpendicular to its longitudinal axis several centimeters proximal to the pyloric canal (Fig. 30–5). In older infants and children, gastroscopy may be helpful when UGIS is unclear. Failure to pass the gastroscope into the duodenum is diagnostic of congenital gastric obstruction.

Treatment

As with hypertrophic pyloric stenosis, correction of dehydration and hypochloremic alkalosis is essential. Persistent vomiting should be treated with nasogastric suction and lavage if there has been previous feeding.

Operative repair should be approached through a transverse supraumbilical incision. The stomach is opened, and a Foley catheter is passed to exclude a wind sock diaphragm, which is a membranous septum that has prolapsed through the pyloric canal[71] (Fig. 30–6). Standard treatment of an antral web is simple excision. Pyloric webs or septa are best treated by

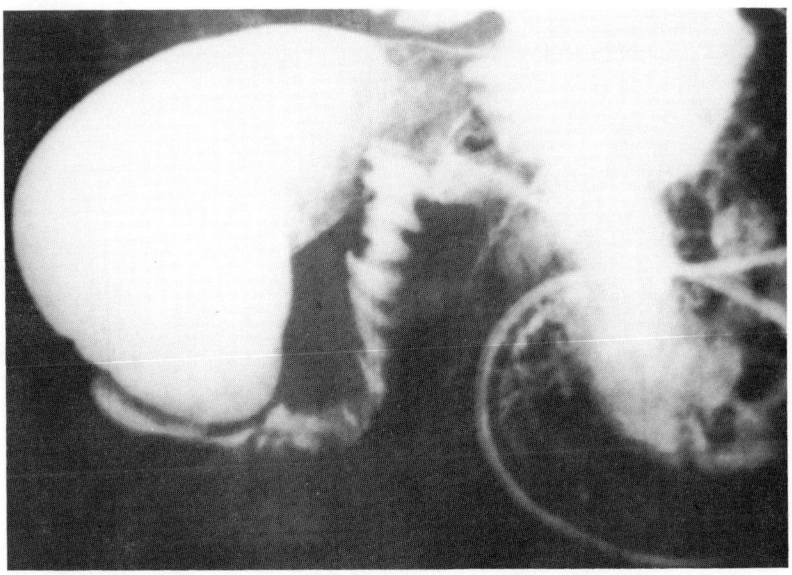

Figure 30–5. UGIS showing weblike filling defect of distal antrum and partial gastric outlet obstruction characteristic of antral web.

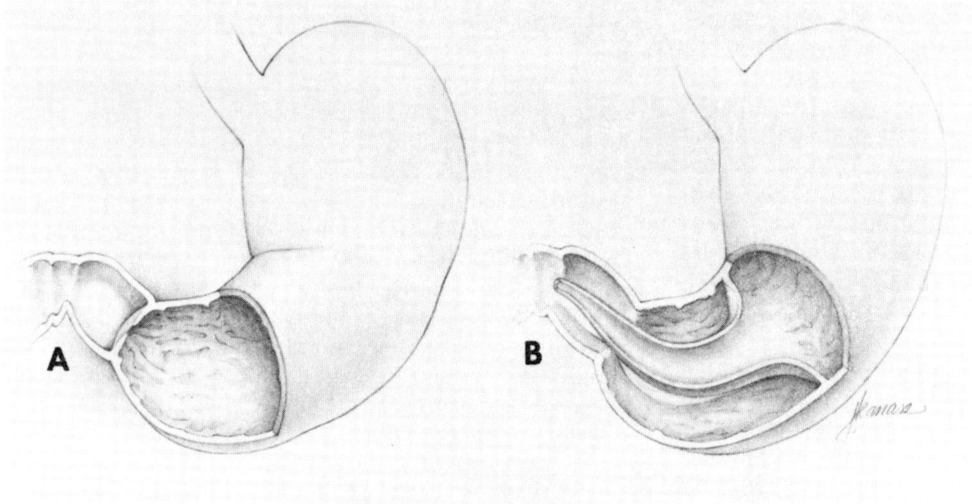

Figure 30–6. Prepyloric web *(A)* and wind sock deformity *(B)*. Antral webs with partial openings account for 5% of all cases of congenital outlet obstruction.

Heineke-Mikulicz pyloroplasty. For gap-type atresia, gastrojejunostomy and gastroduodenostomy both have been performed; however, gastroduodenostomy appears to offer superior results.[62,72]

Antral webs or membranes would seem to be ideal lesions for endoscopic management, since they consist mainly of mucosa and submucosa. A few such attempts have been reported, and one infant who underwent endoscopic resection of an antral web later developed stricture and required subsequent surgical management.[73] Endoscopic treatment should be reserved for selected older children and performed using radial incisions to prevent stenosis.[74]

Results

In his review of the literature, Moore[55] found an overall survival rate of 95% in infants and children undergoing excision of an antral web. The overall survival following pyloroplasty for pyloric membrane was 85%. Finally, the overall survival in infants with gap atresia was 84% following gastroduodenostomy versus 66% following posterior gastrojejunostomy.

GASTRIC VOLVULUS

History

Gastric volvulus was first described by Berti in 1866.[75] Subsequently, in 1904 Borchardt[76] described the classic triad of clinical manifestations: (1) sudden onset of violent epigastric pain, (2) intractable retching without production of vomitus, and (3) inability to pass a tube into the stomach. Gastric volvulus is rare and is encountered more frequently in adults than in children. Only five cases in children younger than 10 years of age were reported in a review of 260 cases between 1914 and 1971.[77] Gastric volvulus may be acute or chronic, but, according to Cole and Dickerson,[78] it is more likely to be acute in infants and young children.

Anatomy and Pathogenesis

The stomach is tethered in its longitudinal axis by the gastrohepatic, gastrosplenic, and gastrocolic ligaments (Fig. 30–7). It is tethered in its transverse axis by the gastrophrenic ligament and the retroperitoneal attachments of the second portion of the duodenum. For a volvulus to occur, these ligaments must be absent or stretched. In most cases there are associated mesenteric abnormalities, such as malrotation[79] and abnormal mobility at the hiatus.[80] Cole and Dickerson[78] reported eventration or herniation of the diaphragm to be present in 65% of patients with gastric volvulus up to 10 years

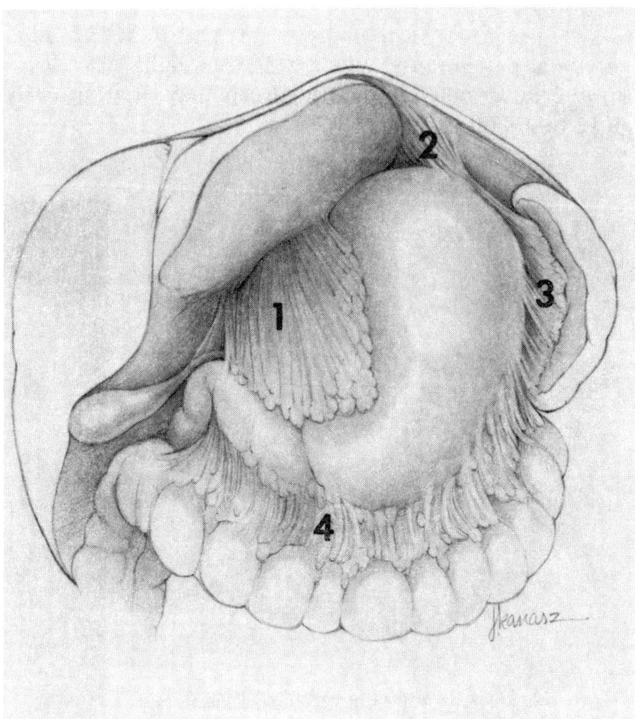

Figure 30–7. Peritoneal attachments of the stomach include (1) gastrohepatic ligament, (2) gastrophrenic ligament, (3) gastrosplenic ligament, and (4) gastrocolic ligament.

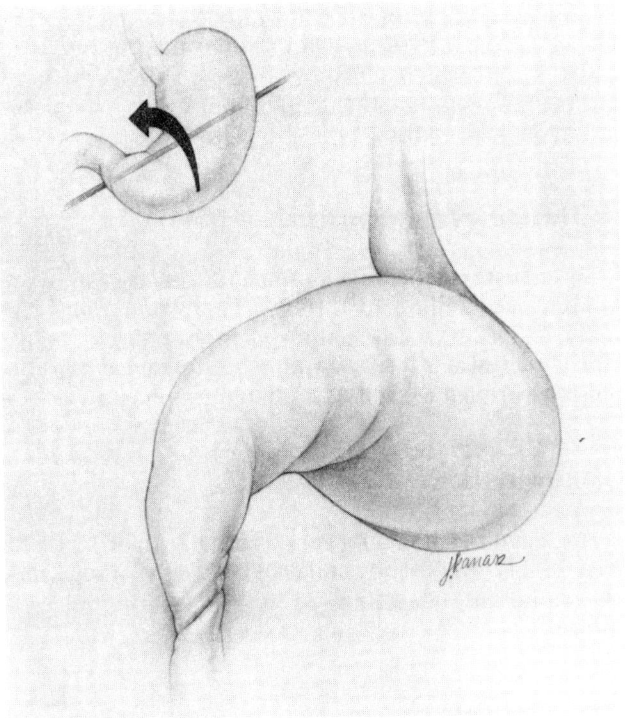

Figure 30–8. Organoaxial volvulus occurs in the longitudinal axis of the stomach.

of age. Idowu and colleagues[81] reported an even higher incidence of diaphragmatic abnormalities in infants up to 1 month of age with gastric volvulus. Recently, several cases of acute gastric volvulus have been reported in infants and smaller children with asplenia syndrome.[82] Approximately one third of patients with gastric volvulus have no associated abnormality, and in this group the etiology may be related to gastric distention.[79,80]

Gastric volvulus occurs when one part of the stomach rotates abnormally around another part. Rotation may occur along the longitudinal axis of the stomach to produce organoaxial volvulus (Fig. 30–8), or along the transverse axis to produce mesenteroaxial volvulus (Fig. 30–9). Organoaxial volvulus is commoner in children, occurring in approximately two-thirds of the reported cases.[80] Rarely, mixed volvulus may occur if the stomach is rotated in both plains. Torsion beyond 180 degrees results in complete gastric obstruction and strangulation of the vasculature.

Clinical Presentation

The clinical features of acute gastric volvulus are nonspecific but suggest high obstruction of the gastrointestinal tract.[83] The triad of Borchardt may not always apply in children. For example, pain in the newborn period is difficult to assess. Second, gastric volvulus in infants may produce bilious or nonbilious vomiting. Third, not all infants with gastric volvulus exhibit abdominal distention, and, in many infants, a nasogastric tube may be passed relatively easily.[78] Acute volvulus may advance rapidly to gastric strangulation, perforation, and cardiovascular collapse, and should be treated as a surgical emergency. Chronic gastric volvulus, commoner in older children, unusually presents with postprandial pain, belching, vomiting, and early satiety. Rarely does chronic volvulus lead to vascular compromise.

Gastric volvulus may be suggested on plain radiographs by a dilated stomach. In mesenteroaxial volvulus, erect radiographic films often show a double fluid level and a "beak" located near the esophagogastric junction, which is caused by gaseous distention of the inverted antrum.[79] In erect films, organoaxial volvulus shows just one air-fluid level and no characteristic beak. If a nasogastric tube is passed, the gastroesophageal junction is seen inferior to its normal position with respect to the fundus. On UGIS the gastroesophageal junction is in the normal position, and the stomach is visualized upside-down and often apparently located within the left chest when associated with a hiatal hernia or other diaphragmatic defect (Fig. 30–10).

Treatment

Acute gastric volvulus requires surgery as soon as adequate resuscitation has been performed. The stomach should be decompressed by nasogastric suction or, alternatively, by needle aspiration. Once the volvulus is reduced, predisposing causes should be investigated. Hiatal hernia, diaphragmatic eventration, or diaphragmatic hernia should be surgically corrected, and anterior gastrostomy along with gastropexy is usually curative. A fundoplication or other anti-reflux procedures should be performed only if there is evidence of severe reflux.[81]

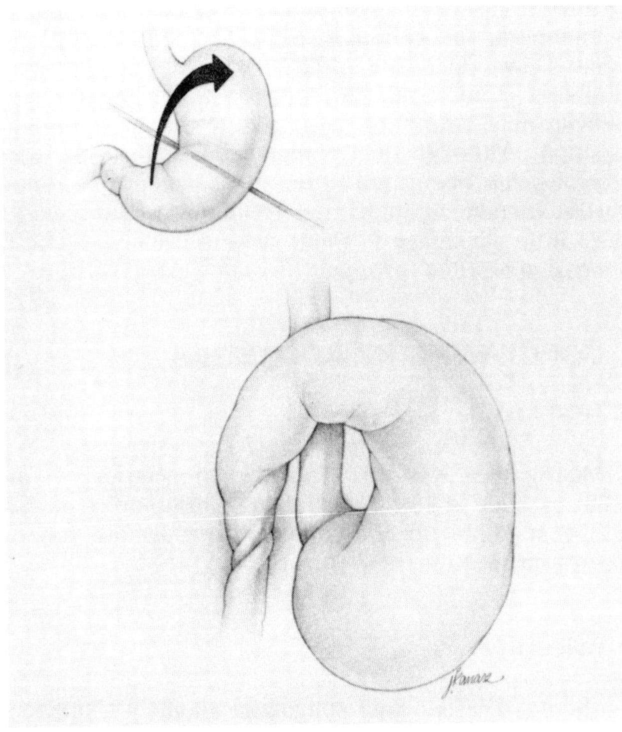

Figure 30–9. Mesenteroaxial volvulus occurs in the transverse axis of the stomach.

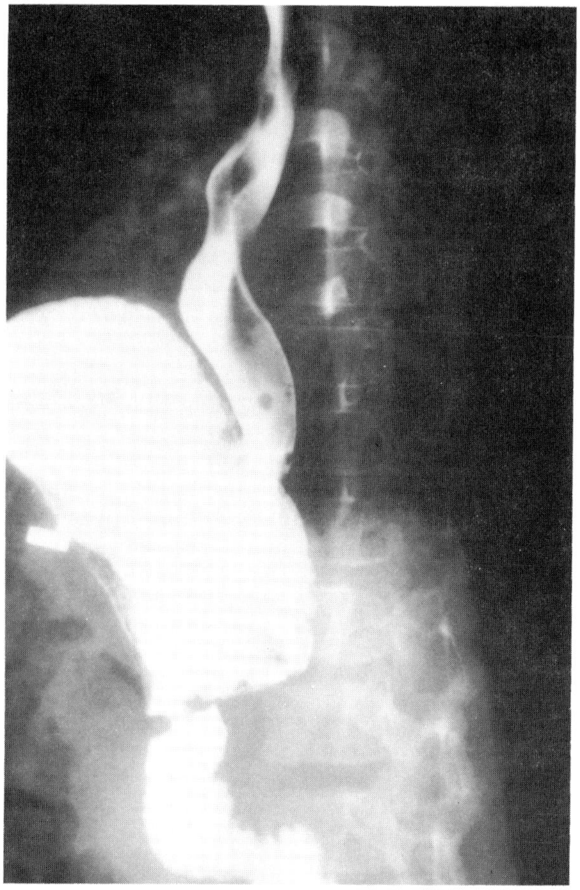

Figure 30–10. UGIS showing characteristic appearance of stomach in mesenteroaxial gastric volvulus.

In certain cases of chronic gastric volvulus, endoscopic correction has been advocated.[84] With air insufflation at a minimum, the endoscope is turned into a loop and rotated 180 degrees in a clockwise or anticlockwise direction. Endoscopic examination following this maneuver may reveal the stomach to be in a normal position. Although dual percutaneous endoscopic gastrostomy has been used in the management of chronic gastric volvulus in adults, this technique would seem to offer little advantage in children, who usually require a general anesthetic for repair of acute gastric volvulus.

CONGENITAL MICROGASTRIA

History

Microgastria was first described at necropsy of an adult by Dide in 1894.[85] Blank and Chisholm[86] reported a 26-year follow-up of a patient with congenital microgastria first seen in 1947.

Etiology

Microgastria is a rare congenital anomaly characterized by a small, tubular stomach, megaesophagus, and incomplete gastric rotation.[87] Multiple associated anomalies have been described, including malrotation, situs inversus, and asplenia.[88] Skeletal anomalies are common and include micrognathia, radial and ulnar hypoplasia, and hypoplastic nails.

Clinical Presentation

The most frequent symptoms of microgastria are vomiting and failure to thrive.[87] These symptoms generally result from associated gastroesophageal reflux, which may also cause aspiration, esophageal erosion, and hemorrhage as well as a dilated esophagus.

Diagnosis

The diagnosis of microgastria is usually made by UGIS (Fig. 30–11). Endoscopy and esophageal pH studies may be helpful in the setting of severe gastroesophageal reflux.

Treatment

Treatment is usually medical and consists of continuous gastrostomy or jejunostomy tube feedings. Gastroesophageal reflux should be treated conservatively with antacids and metoclopramide. When gastroesophageal reflux cannot be managed medically, antireflux procedures using the Hill or Thal repair may be considered. In most instances, the stomach will gradually dilate to accommodate oral feedings. In certain protracted cases, construction of a jejunal reservoir has been recommended.[89]

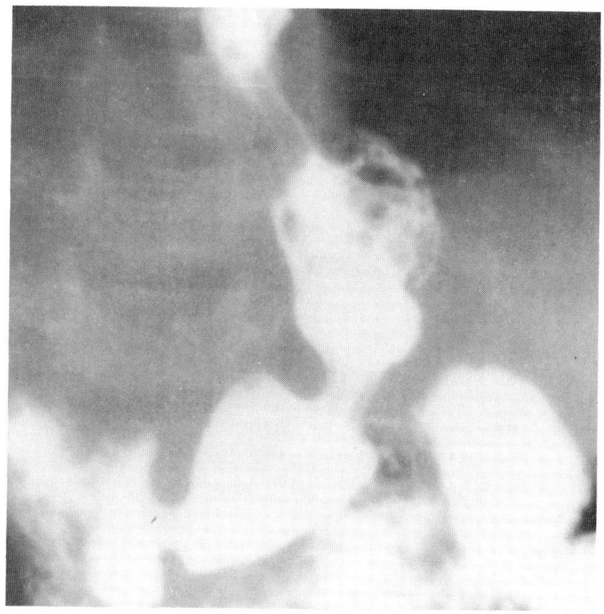

Figure 30–11. UGIS showing typical appearance of microgastria with gastroesophageal reflux.

GASTRIC AND DUODENAL DUPLICATION

History

Reginald Fitz[90] coined the word *duplication* to describe what he thought were cystic remnants of the omphalomesenteric duct. Various cystic abnormalities of the gastrointestinal tract were subsequently described, and in 1952 Gross and colleagues[91] suggested that the term *duplication* be used for all such anomalies, irrespective of their site, morphology, or embryologic derivations. Gastroduodenal duplications account for fewer than 10% of all alimentary tract duplications and were classified by Rowling in 1959[92] according to the following criteria: (1) the cyst wall is contiguous with the stomach wall; (2) the cyst is surrounded by smooth muscle contiguous with stomach muscle; and (3) the cyst wall is lined by alimentary epithelium. In 1979 Schwartz and coworkers[93] described a gastric duplication that was ectopic and separate from the stomach, taking issue with the requirement for continuity of the cyst wall with the stomach.

Embryogenesis and Pathology

Bremer[94] proposed that gastroduodenal duplications result from an error of recanalization in which there is coalescence of vacuoles within the embryonic duct wall or fusion of the longitudinal epithelial folds to form a hollow tube. Although this description may apply to duodenal duplications, the embryonic stomach does not go through a stage of mucosal proliferation and recanalization. McLetchie and associates[95] proposed an alternative theory in which abnormal adhesions between the notochord and the embryonic endoderm form a traction diverticulum, disorganizing endoderm as the embryo grows. Torma[96] points out that this theory may explain the frequent association of gastric duplications with esophageal and pancreatic duplications. Gastric duplications are closed, spherical structures on the greater curvature of the stomach and may be associated with enterogenous cysts in the posterior mediastinum, the esophagus, or the duodenum.[97–99] Gastric duplications may be tubular or cystic, and most are smaller than 12 cm in diameter. Wieczorek and colleagues[99] found that 82% of gastric duplications are cystic and do not communicate with the stomach, whereas 18% are tubular and do communicate. Several cases have been described in which etopic pancreatic tissue lines the cyst along with gastric mucosa.[96] Rarely, gastroduodenal duplications may be extensive tubular structures that traverse the diaphragm and are associated with anomalous upper cervical and thoracic vertebra.[100,101]

Associated congenital anomalies occur in 35% of patients with gastric duplications.[102] The commonest anomaly is another cyst, especially of the esophagus or duodenum, but vertebral anomalies and ectopic pancreas are frequently found.

Presentation

Gastric duplications are uncommon and are reported most frequently in children. Wieczorek and colleagues[99] reviewed the literature in 1984 and found a total of 109 reported gastric duplications. More than half of gastroduodenal duplications are diagnosed within the first year of life, and they are twice as common in females. The clinical presentation depends on the size and location of the cyst as well as the presence or absence of communication with the alimentary tract. The commonest presentation is that of gastric outlet obstruction, but in 65% of cases there is a palpable abdominal mass.[99] In many cases there is abdominal pain, weight loss, and failure to thrive. Occasionally, a large duplication cyst may perforate secondary to ulceration caused by stasis of gastric enzymes and hydrochloric acid with the cyst.[103] Noncommunicating duplications may cause gastric irritation, leading to gastritis or peptic ulceration. Thus, hematemesis or melena may be seen in approximately 30% of older children.[99] Finally, when there is a coexistent gastric and pancreatic duplication, pancreatitis or erosion into a contiguous viscus (e.g., the transverse colon) may occur.[104,105]

Diagnosis

Usually, a gastric duplication is revealed by UGIS as an extrinsic defect located on the greater curve of the stomach. A more distal cyst may distort the pyloric or duodenal channel, or both, and usually causes delayed gastric emptying. Sonography or computed tomographic scanning may be helpful in demonstrating contiguous cystic structures. Technetium-99m scanning can localize ectopic gastric mucosa but, because of overlapping uptake, is of little help in demonstrating structures adjacent to the stomach.[105]

Treatment

In most instances, the treatment of gastroduodenal duplications is excision of the cyst either by dissection from a common wall or by excision of the cyst with a margin of normal stomach and primary closure.[99,106] When there is a coexistent pancreatic duplication, the accessory pancreatic lobe can be ligated and transected at its origin.[104,105] When the aberrant pancreatic lobe is adherent to the stomach, an attempt should be made to dissect it free before a more extensive resection is undertaken. Similarly, it may be possible to avoid an extensive resection in the region of the gastroesophageal junction or pyloric channel by performing a partial excision of the gastroduodenal duplication and stripping the mucosa along the common wall to prevent subsequent ulceration.[107] The stomach should then be distended with air to detect any unsuspected perforation. When either complete resection or partial resection with mucosal stripping is not technically possible, marsupialization can be accomplished with internal drainage either into the duodenum or using a Roux-en-Y loop of jejunum.

Results

In their review, Wieczorek and colleagues[99] found an overall mortality of approximately 3%. In more than 10% of patients, perforation of the duplication cyst had occurred either freely into the peritoneal cavity or with fistula formation into adjacent structures. However, there has been only one reported death as a complication of cyst perforation.[108]

DUODENAL STENOSIS AND ATRESIA

History

Theremine[109] reported 11 cases of duodenal atresia in 1877. In 1901, Cordes[110] described the clinical manifestations of the anomaly and found 56 cases in the literature with no survivors. The first successful operation on a child with duodenal atresia was reported by Ernst[111] in 1916. By 1931 there were only nine survivors located by Webb and Wangensteen,[112] who refined the techniques of surgical repair. Finally, Ladd and Gross[113] developed the techniques that are still in use today.

Etiology and Pathology

Duodenal atresia is thought to arise from the failure of recanalization of the duodenal lumina or the persistence of epithelial proliferation that occurs between the fourth and the fifth weeks of gestation.[114] Less commonly, an annular pancreas causes external compression of the second portion of the duodenum. This may occur when the tip of the ventral pancreatic bud becomes fixed to the duodenal wall and, as rotation occurs, is drawn around the right side of the duodenum to fuse with the dorsal pancreas.[115] Duodenal stenosis usually occurs with annular pancreas but may also occur with extrinsic indentation of the duodenal wall caused by mesenteric bands or preduodenal portal veins. According to Gray and Skandalakis,[1] duodenal atresia may exist as an intact diaphragm or membrane formed of mucosa and submucosa (type 1), a short fibrous cord connecting two blind ends of duodenum (type 2), or a gap between blind duodenal ends (type 3). Type 1 atresia is most common and is located proximal to the ampulla of Vater in 15 to 30% of cases and at or distal to the ampulla of Vater in 70 to 85% of the cases.[116,117]

Incidence

Nixon[118] estimates the incidence of congenital duodenal obstruction to be about 1 in 10,000. About half of these infants are born prematurely, and several authors have found a female-to-male ratio of more than 2 to 1.[116,118] Spigland and Yazbeck[117] reported the relative incidence of various forms of congenital duodenal obstruction to be duodenal atresia in 42%, annular pancreas in 33%, and duodenal diaphragm in 23% of neonates.

Associated Anomalies

Down's syndrome occurs in 10 to 30% percent of infants with duodenal atresia.[116,118] More important, infants with duodenal atresia have a high risk of potentially life-threatening congenital anomalies, such as esophageal atresia in 10 to 20%, malrotation in 20%, congenital heart disease in 10 to 15%, and anorectal anomalies in approximately 5%.[116,117,119,120] Overall, about one third of infants with congenital duodenal obstruction have a life-threatening congenital anomaly, and half of those have multiple anomalies. The combination of duodenal atresia, esophageal atresia, and anorectal anomaly is almost always associated with anomalies of other systems and is almost always fatal.[120]

Clinical Presentation and Diagnosis

Bilious vomiting without abdominal distention is the most typical presentation of congenital duodenal obstruction. On the other hand, one third of patients may have nonbilious vomiting due to supra-ampullary atresia, and almost one half may have upper abdominal distention secondary to gastric dilatation. Meconium stools may be passed in the early stages; however, absence of meconium stools is not a dependable sign of complete intestinal obstruction in the neonate. Polyhydramnios occurs in approximately 50% of pregnancies in which there is congenital duodenal obstruction. This occurs because high intestinal obstruction prevents the normal absorption of amniotic fluid in the distal small intestine.[121]

The finding of a markedly distended stomach and first portion of duodenum without distal air on kidney, ureter, and bladder radiograph is known as the "*double bubble" sign* and is pathognomonic of duodenal atresia (Fig. 30–12). If nasogastric suction has already been instituted, it may be useful to instill 50 cc of air by nasogastric tube to demonstrate this finding. Prenatal diagnosis of duodenal atresia has become commoner with the increased use of prenatal sonography, which may also be used to detect associated anomalies.[122] If sonography is not obtained prenatally, it should be performed prior to surgery, along with echocardiography and radiography of the chest and spine.

A UGIS is usually not necessary to diagnose duodenal atresia and may be hazardous. On the other hand, the most important differential diagnosis to make is that of malrotation and volvulus, which may cause gangrene of the entire midgut within 6 to 12 hours. Thus, if plain films are not diagnostic, UGIS should be performed by

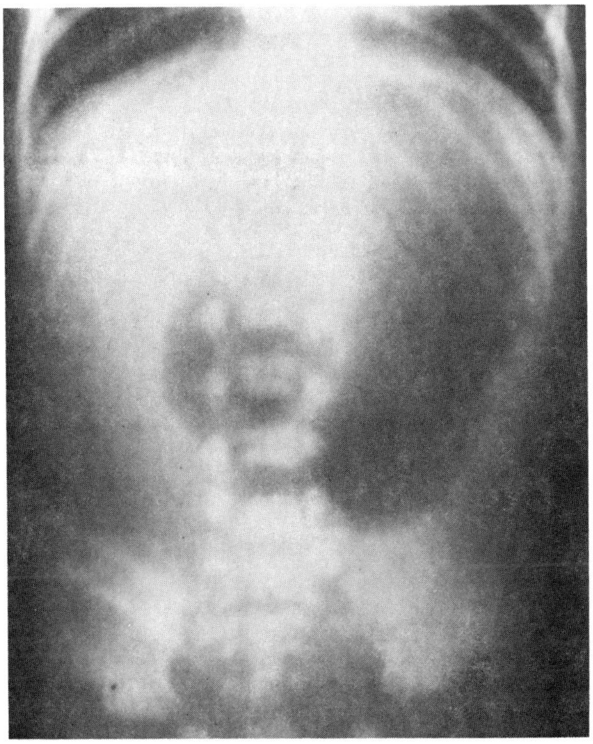

Figure 30–12. Double-bubble gas pattern characteristic of duodenal atresia.

an experienced radiologist with a nasogastric tube in place.

Treatment

The initial management of an infant with duodenal obstruction includes placement of a nasogastric or oral gastric tube, institution of intravenous fluids, and appropriate respiratory care. If malrotation and volvulus have been excluded, definitive surgery may be postponed to evaluate and treat life-threatening associated anomalies. In general, the repair of duodenal atresia is superseded by treatment of those life-threatening anomalies discussed previously.

The most frequently used surgical repair of all forms of intrinsic duodenal obstruction is the duodenoduodenostomy. This procedure is performed through a transverse supraumbilical incision through which the duodenum and ligament of Treitz are mobilized. A longitudinal incision is then made in the distal duodenum, through which a tube is passed to rule out secondary atresias. Then, either a longitudinal or a transverse incision is made in the proximal duodenum to fashion a side-to-side or a diamond-shaped anastomosis[123, 124] (Fig. 30–13) It has been recognized that anastomotic function may recover earlier when the dilated proximal duodenum is tapered.[125,126] This allows more effective coaptation of the opposing walls of the dilated intestines, leading to improved peristalsis.[127,128] Most surgeons prefer to leave a gastrostomy tube, since it drains more effectively and is less injurious to pulmonary status than is a nasogastric tube. Hyperalimentation is commonly used until the infant is feeding. Transanastomotic silicone tubes continue to be used by many surgeons for postoperative jejunal feedings; however, at least one study has shown that these tubes prolong the time until oral diet is tolerated and increase total length of hospitalization.[116]

Results

Survival following surgical repair of congenital duodenal obstruction ranges between 70 and 100% depending on the incidence of prematurity and associated anomalies. In most reports, the majority of deaths were directly attributable to associated anomalies. However,

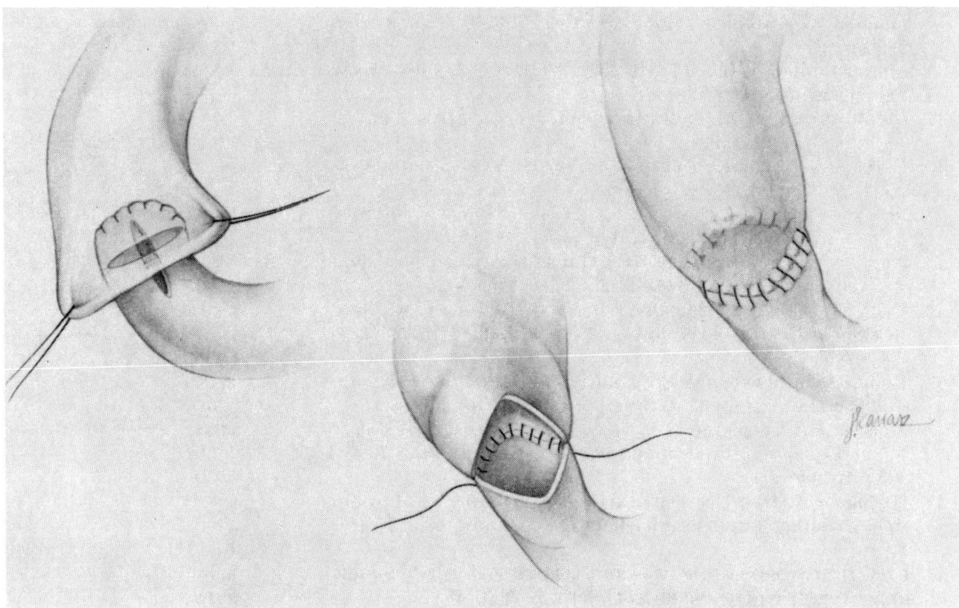

Figure 30–13. Diamond-shaped anastomosis developed by Kimura and associates,[124] which reduces time to initiation of oral feedings.

a large multi-institutional survey of duodenal atresia taken in 1969 showed that anastomotic problems were responsible for 16% of the deaths.[129] This percentage is operator dependent but, in experienced hands, currently is less than 5%. Although prolonged intravenous hyperalimentation was formerly required in many patients with megaduodenum, currently, most infants treated with duodenoduodenostomy may be started on feedings within 1 week and may be discharged from the hospital within 2 or 3 weeks.[130]

Attention has been focused on the late follow-up of duodenal atresia in which more than 25% of patients were symptomatic with abdominal pain as a result of chronic alkaline biliary reflux and blind loop syndrome secondary to a poorly emptying proximal duodenal pouch.[131] This complication may become less of an issue as more patients undergo tapering procedures. However, the importance of long-term follow-up of all patients for duodenal atresia cannot be overemphasized.

REFERENCES

1. Gray SW, Skandalakis JE: Embryology for Surgeons. Philadelphia, WB Saunders, 1972; pp 101–105.
2. Moutsouris C: The "solid stage" and congenital intestinal atresia. J Pediatr Surg 1966; 1:446–450.
3. Donovan EJ: Hezekiah Beardsley, congenital hypertrophic stenosis of the pyloris. Arch Pediatr 1958; 75:359.
4. Hirschsprung H: Falle von angeborener pylorusstenose: Beobachtet bie salingen. Jahrb Kinderhlk 1888; 27:61.
5. Dufour H, Fredette P: La steanose hypertrophique du pylore chez le noursson et son traitement chir surgical. Rev Chir 1908; 37:208.
6. Borgwardt G: Conrad Ramstedt—an appreciation. Z Kinderchir 1986; 41:195–200.
7. Laron Z, Horne LM: The incidence of infantile pyloric stenosis. Am J Dis Child 1957; 94:151.
8. Jed MB, Melton J, Griffin MR, et al: Factors associated with infantile hypertrophic pyloric stenosis. Am J Dis Child 1988; 142:334–337.
9. Kerr AM: Unprecedented rise in incidence of infantile hypertrophic pyloric stenosis. Br Med J 1980; 13:714–715.
10. Knox EG, Armstrong E, Hanes R: Changing incidence of infantile hypertrophic pyloric stenosis. Arch Dis Child 1983; 58:582–585.
11. Martin J, Monk J: Infant feeding in 1980. OPCS. London, Social Survey Division, HNSO, 1982.
12. Carter CO, Evans KA: Inheritance of congenital pyloric stenosis. J Med Genet 1969; 6:233–239.
13. Dodge JA: Infantile hypertrophic pyloric stenosis in Belfast. Arch Dis Child 1975; 50:171–178.
14. McKeown T, MacMahon B: Infantile hypertrophic pyloric stenosis in parent and child. Arch Dis Child 1955; 30:497.
15. Androssi RJ, Haff RC, Larsen GL: Infantile hypertrophic pyloric stenosis during the first week of life. Clin Pediatr 1977; 16:474.
16. Geer LL, Gaisie G, Mandell VS, et al: Evolution of pyloric stenosis in the first week of life. Pediatr Radiol 1985; 15:205–206.
17. Rollins MD, Shields, MD, Quinn RJM, et al: Pyloric stenosis: Congenital or acquired? Arch Dis Child 1989; 64:137–138.
18. Stunden RJ, LeQuesne GW, Little KET: The improved ultrasound diagnosis of hypertrophic pyloric stenosis. Pediatr Radiol 1986; 16:200–205.
19. Latchaw LA, Jacir NN, Harris BH: The development of pyloric stenosis during transpyloric feeding. J Pediatr Surg 1989; 24;823–824.
20. Lynn H: The mechanism of pyloric stenosis and its relationship to preoperative preparation. Arch Surg 1960; 81:453.
21. Spits L, Zail SS: Serum gastrin levels in congenital hypertrophic pyloric stenosis. J Pediatr Surg 1976; 11:33.
22. Laferla G, Watson J, Fyfe AHB, et al: The role of prostaglandins and $F\alpha_2$ in infantile hypertrophic pyloric stenosis. J Pediatr Surg 1986; 21:410–412.
23. Rendle-Short J, Zachary RB: Congenital pyloric stenosis in older babies. Arch Dis Child 1955; 30:70.
24. Touloukin RJ, Higgins E: The spectrum of serum electrolytes in hypertrophic pyloric stenosis. J Pediatr Surg 1983; 18:394–397.
25. Winters RW: Metabolic alkaloses of pyloric stenosis: The body fluid in pediatrics. Boston, Little, Brown, 1973, pp 402–414.
26. Benson CD: Infantile hypertrophic pyloric stenosis. *In* Welsh KJ, Randolph JG, Ravitch MM, et al, eds: Pediatric Surgery. 4th ed. Chicago, Yearbook Medical Publishers, 1986, pp 811–815.
27. Mackay AJ, Mackellar A: Infantile hypertrophic pyloric stenosis: A review of two-hundred and twenty-two cases. Aust NZ J Surg 1986; 56:131–133.
28. Chaves-Carbello E, Harris LE, Lynn HB: Jaundice associated with pyloric stenosis and neonatal small bowel obstruction. Clin Pediatr 1968; 7:198–202.
29. Woolley MM, Felsher BF, Asch MJ, et al: Jaundice, hypertrophic pyloric stenosis, and hepatic glucuronyl transferase. J Pediatr Surg 1974; 9:359–363.
30. Labrune T, Myara A, Huguet P, et al: Jaundice with hypertrophic pyloric stenosis: A possible early manifestation of Gilbert syndrome. J Pediatr 1989; 15:93–95.
31. Ahmed S: Infantile pyloric stenosis associated with major anomalies of the alimentary tract. J Pediatr Surg 1970; 5:660–666.
32. Ziedan B, Wyatt J, Mackersie A, et al: Recent results of treatment of infantile hypertrophic pyloric stenosis. Arch Dis Child 1988; 63:1060–1064.
33. Meuwissen T, Sloof JP: Roentgenologic diagnosis of congenital hypertrophic pyloric stenosis. Acta Pediatr 1932; 14:19–48.
34. Herran PJ, Darling DB, Sciamma F: The value of the double tract sign of the differentiating factor between pyloric spasm and hypertrophic pyloric stenosis. Radiology 1966; 86:723–725.
35. Shopfner CE, Kalmon EH, Coin CG: The diagnosis of hypertrophic pyloric stenosis. AJR 1964; 91:796–800.
36. Ball TI, Atkinson GO, Gay BB: Ultrasound diagnosis of hypertrophic pyloric stenosis: Real-time application and demonstration of new sonographic sign. Radiology 1983; 147:499–502.
37. Teele RL, Smith EH: Ultrasound and the diagnosis of idiopathic hypertrophic pyloric stenosis. N Engl J Med 1977; 296:1149–1150.
38. Blumhagen JD, Nobel HG: Muscle thickness in hypertrophic pyloric stenosis: Sonographic determination. Am J Roentgenol 1983; 140:221–223.
39. Wilson DA, VanHoutte JJ: The reliable sonographic diagnosis of hypertrophic pyloric stenosis. J Clin Ultrasound 1984; 12:201–204.
40. Forman HP, Leonida JC, Kronfeld GD: A rational approach to diagnosis of hypertrophic pyloric stenosis: Do the results match the claims? J Pediatr Surg 1990; 25:262.
41. Kumar V, Bailey WC: Electrolyte and acid-base problems in hypertrophic pyloric stenosis in infancy. Indian Pediatr 1935; 12:839.
42. Steven IM, Allen TH, Sweeny DB: Congenital hypertrophic pyloric stenosis—the anaesthetist's view. Anaesth Intensive Care 1973; 1:544–546.
43. Conn AW: Anaesthesia for pyloromyotomy in infancy. Can Anaes Soc J 1963; 10:18–29.
44. Scharli AF, Leditschke JF: Gastric motility after pyloromyotomy in infants: A reappraisal of postoperative feeding. Surgery 1968; 64:1133–1137.
45. Sauerbrei EE, Paloschi GGB: The ultrasonic features of hypertrophic pyloric stenosis, with emphasis on the postoperative appearance. Radiology 1983; 147:503–506.
46. Jamroz GA, Blocker SH, McAlister WH: Radiographic findings after incomplete pyloromyotomy. Gastrointest Radiol 1986; 11:139–141.
47. Scharli A, Sieber WK, Kiesewetter WB: Hypertrophic pyloric stenosis at the Children's Hospital of Pittsburgh from 1912 to 1967. J Pediatr Surg 1969; 4:108–114.
48. Bell MJ: Infantile pyloric stenosis: Experience with three hundred and five cases at the Louisville Children's Hospital. Surgery 1968; 64:983–989.
49. Benson CD: Infantile pyloric stenosis: Historical aspects and current surgical concepts. Prog Pediatr Surg 1971; 1:63–88.

50. Gibbs MK, vanHeerden JA, Lynn HB: Congenital hypertrophic pyloric stenosis: Surgical experience. Mayo Clin Proc 1975; 50:312–316.
51. Calder J: Two examples of children preternatural conformation of the guts. Med Essays and Obs (Edinburgh) 1733; 1:205.
52. Crooks. Estomac se terminant en cude sac. Arch Gen Med 1828; 17:264.
53. Cook RCM, Rickham PP: Gastric Outlet Obstruction in Neonatal Surgery. 2nd ed. London, Butterworth, 1978, pp 335–338.
54. Parsons LG, Barding S: Diseases of Infancy and Childhood. London, Oxford University, 1933.
55. Moore CM: Congenital gastric outlet obstruction. J Pediatr Surg 1989; 24:1242–1246.
56. Gerber BC, Aberdeen SO: Pre-pyloric diaphragm, an unusual abnormality. Arch Surg 1965; 90:472–475.
57. Simstein NL: Congenital gastric anomalies. Am Surg 1986; 52:264–268.
58. Bell MJ, Ternberg JL, McAlister W, et al: Antral diaphragm—a cause of gastric outlet obstruction in infants and children. J Pediatr 1977; 90:196–202.
59. Tunnell WP, Ide Smith E: Antral web in infancy. J Pediatr Surg 1980; 15:152–155.
60. Kume K, Ikeda K, Hayashida Y, et al: Congenital pyloric atresia: A report of three cases and review of the literature. J Pediatr Surg 1980; 16:259–268.
61. El Shafie M, Stidham LG, Klippel CH, et al: Pyloric atresia epidermolysis bullosa letalis: A lethal combination in two premature newborn siblings. J Pediatr Surg 1979; 14:446–449.
62. Bar-Maor JA, Nissan S, Nero S: Pyloric atresia. J Med Genet 1972; 9:70–72.
63. Pearson RW, Potter B, Strauss F: Epidermolysis bullosa hereditaria lethalis. Arch Dermatol 1974; 109:349–355.
64. Korber JS, Glasson MJ: Pyloric atresia associated with epidermolysis bullosa. J Pediatr 1977; 90:600–601.
65. Gedde-Dahl T Jr, Lambrecht LA: Principles and Practices in Medical Genetics. New York, Churchill-Livingstone, 1981.
66. Ducharma JC, Bensousson AL: Pyloric atresia. J Pediatr Surg 1975; 10:149–150.
67. Sloop RD, Montagne ACW: Gastric outlet obstruction due to congenital pyloric mucosal membrane. Am Surg 1967; 165:598–604.
68. Burnett HA, Halpert B: Perforation of the stomach of a newborn infant with pyloric atresias. Arch Pathol 1947; 44:318.
69. Franklin EA: Gastrointestinal Imaging in Pediatrics. 2nd ed. Philadelphia, Harper & Row, 1982, pp 131–142.
70. Gruenbaum M, Kornreich L, Ziv N: The imaging diagnosis of pyloric atresia. Z Kinderchir 1985; 40:308–311.
71. Bell MH, Ternberg JL, Keating JP, et al: Prepyloric gastric antral web: A puzzling epidemic. J Pediatr Surg 1978; 13:307–313.
72. Talwalker VC: Pyloric atresia: A case report. J Pediatr Surg 1967; 2:458–460.
73. Brandt LJ, Boley SJ, Dom F, et al: Endoscopic resection of an obstructing antral web in an infant. Dig Dis Sci 1978; 5:65–85.
74. Al-Kawas FH: Endoscopic laser treatment of an obstructing antral web. Gastrointest Endosc 1988; 34:349–351.
75. Berti A: Singolare attortigliamento dell' esofago duodeno sequito da rapida morte. Gass Med Ital 1866; 9:139.
76. Borchardt M: Zur Patologie und terapie des magenvolvuls. Arch Klin Chir 1904; 74:243.
77. Wastell C, Ellis H: Volvulus of the stomach: A review with a reported eight cases. Br J Surg 1971; 58:557–562.
78. Cole BC, Dickerson SJ: Acute volvulus of the stomach in infants and children. Surgery 1971; 70:707–717.
79. Ziprkowski MN, Teele RL: Gastric volvulus in childhood. AJR 1979; 132:921–925.
80. Cammeron AEP, Howard ER: Gastric volvulus in childhood. J Pediatr Surg 1987; 22:944–947.
81. Idowu J, Aitken DR, Gorgeson KE: Gastric volvulus in the newborn. Arch Surg 1980; 115:1046–1049.
82. Aoyama K, Tateishi K: Gastric volvulus in three children with asplenia syndrome. J Pediatr Surg 1986; 21:307–310.
83. Campbell JB: Neonatal gastric volvulus. AJR 1979; 132:723–725.
84. Eckhauser ML, Ferron JP: The use of dual percutaneous endoscopic gastrostomy in the management of chronic intermittent gastric volvulus. Gastrointest Endosc 1985; 31:340–342.
85. Dide M: Sur un estomac d'adulte type foetal. Bull Soc Anat Paris 1894; 69:669.
86. Blank E, Chisholm AJ: Congenital microgastria: A case report with a 26-year follow-up. Pediatrics 1973; 51:1037.
87. Campbell JR: Congenital microgastria. *In* Pediatric Surgery. Chicago, Yearbook Medical Publishers, 1986, pp 827–828.
88. Kessler H, Smulevicz JJ: Microgastria associated with agenesis of the spleen. Radiology 1973; 107:393.
89. Neifeld JP, Berman WF, Lawrence W Jr, et al: Management of congenital microgastria with a jejunal reservoir pouch. J Pediatr Surg 1980; 15:882.
90. Fitz RH: Persistent omphalo-mesenteric remains: Their importance in the causation of intestinal duplication, cyst formation, and obstruction. Am J Med Sci 1884; 88:30–57.
91. Gross RE, Holcomb GW Jr, Farber S: Duplications of the alimentary tract. Pediatrics 1952; 9:449–468.
92. Rowling JT: Some observations on gastric cysts. Br J Surg 1959; 46:441–445.
93. Schwartz DL, So HB, Becker JM: An ectopic gastric duplication arising from the pancreas and presenting with pneumoperitoneum. J Pediatr Surg 1979; 14:187–188.
94. Bremer JL: Diverticula and duplications of the intestinal tract. Arch Pathol Lab Med 1944; 38:132–140.
95. McLetchie NGB, Purves JK, Saunders RL: The genesis of gastric and certain intestinal diverticula and enterogenous cysts. Surg Gynecol Obstet 1954; 99:135–141.
96. Torma MJ: Of double stomachs. Arch Surg 1974; 109:155–157.
97. Alschibija T, Putnam TC, Yablin BA: Duplication of the stomach simulating hypertrophic pyloric stenosis. Am J Dis Child 1974; 127:120–122.
98. Bowmen M, Singh MP: Pyloric duplication in a preterm neonate. J Pediatr Surg 1984; 19:158–159.
99. Wieczorek RL, Seidman I, Ranson JH, et al: Congenital duplication of the stomach: Case report and review of the English literature. Am J Gastroenterol 1984; 79:597–602.
100. Lister J, Rickham PP: Neonatal surgery. *In* Rickham PP, Irving IM, eds: Neonatal Surgery. 2nd ed. London, Butterworth, 1978, pp 401–404.
101. Fitzgivens RJ Jr, Neugent FW, Ellis FH, et al: Unusual thoracoabdominal duplication associated with pancreatopleural fistula. Gastroenterology 1980; 79:344–347.
102. Bartels RJ: Duplication of the stomach: Case report and review of the literature. Ann Surg 1976; 33:747–752.
103. Sieunarine K, Manmohansingh E: Gastric duplication cysts presenting as an acute abdomen in a child. J Pediatr Surg 1989; 24:1152.
104. Rosenlund ML, Schnaufer L: Gastric duplications presenting as cyclical abdominal pain. Clin Pediatr 1978; 17:747–748.
105. Spence RK, Schnaufer L, Mahboubi S: Coexistent gastric duplication and accessory pancreas: Clinical manifestations, embryogenesis, and treatment. J Pediatr Surg 1986; 21:68–70.
106. Bishop HC, Koop CE: Surgical management of duplications of the alimentary tract. Am J Surg 1964; 167:434–442.
107. Holcomb GW, Gheissari A, O'Neill JA, et al: Surgical management of the alimentary tract duplications. Ann Surg 1988; 209:167–174.
108. Bower RJ, Silber WK, Kiesewetter WB: Alimentary tract duplication in children. Ann Surg 1978; 188:669–674.
109. Theremine: Veger kongenitale occlusionen des Duenndarms. Deutsche Ztschr Chir 1877; 8:34.
110. Cordes L: Congenital occlusion of the duodenum. Arch Pediatr 1901; 18:401.
111. Ernst NP: A case of congenital atresia of the duodenum treated successfully by operation. Br Med J 1916; 1:1644.
112. Webb CH, Wangensteen OH: Congenital intestinal atresia. Am J Dis Child 1931; 41:242.
113. Ladd WE, Gross RE: Abdominal Surgery of Infancy and Childhood. Philadelphia, WB Saunders, 1941.
114. Tandler J: Zur Entwicklungsgeschichte des menschlichen Duodenoms. Morphol JG 1902; 29:187.
115. Lecco TM: Zur Morphologie des Pankreas annulare Sitzungsb. Akad Wissensch Cl 1910; 119:391.
116. Mooney D, Lewis JE, Connors RH, et al: Newborn duodenal atresia: Improving outlook. Am J Surg 1987; 153:347–349.
117. Spigland N, Yazbeck S: Complications associated with surgical treatment of congenital intrinsic duodenal obstruction. J Pediatr Surg 1990; 25:1127–1130.

118. Nixon HH: Duodenal atresia. Br J Hosp Med 1989; 41:134–140.
119. Wayne ER, Burrington JD: Management of 97 children with duodenal obstruction. Arch Surg 1973; 107:857–861.
120. Danismend EN, Brown S, Frank JD: Morbidity and mortality in duodenal atresia. Z Kinderchir 1986; 41:86–88.
121. Lloyd JR, Clatworthy HW: Hydramnios as an aid to the early diagnosis of congenital obstruction of the alimentary tract. Pediatrics 1958; 21:903.
122. Hayden CK, Schwartz NZ, Davis M, et al: Combined esophageal and duodenal atresia: Sonographic findings. Am J Radiol 1983; 140:224.
123. Weitzman JJ, Prennin LP: An improved technique for the correction of congenital duodenal obstruction in neonates. J Pediatr Surg 1974; 9:385–388.
124. Kimura K, Mukohara N, Nishijima E, et al: Diamond-shaped anastomoses for duodenal atresia: An experience with forty-four patients over fifteen years. J Pediatr Surg 1990; 25:977–979.
125. Weisgerberg G, Boreau M: Resultats immediates et secondaires duodenoduodenostomies avec modelage dans le traitement de obstructions duodenales congenitales completes du nouveau-ne. Chir Pediatr 1982; 23:369–372.
126. Adzick NS, Harrison MR, deLorimier AA: Tapering duodenoplasty for megaduodenum associated with duodenal atresia. J Pediatr Surg 1986; 21:311–312.
127. deLorimier AA, Norman DA, Gooding CA, et al: Model for the cinefluoroscopic and manometric study of chronic intestinal obstruction. J Pediatr Surg 1973; 8:785–791.
128. Cloutier R: Intestinal smooth muscle response to chronic obstruction: Possible applications in jejunoileal atresia. J Pediatr Surg 1975; 10:3–8.
129. Fonkalsrud EW, deLorimier AA, Hayes D: Congenital atresia and stenosis of the duodenum. Pediatrics 1969; 43:79–82.
130. Weber TR, Lewis JE, Mooney D, et al: Duodenal atresia: A comparison of techniques of repair. J Pediatr Surg 1986; 21:1133–1136.
131. Kokkonen ML, Kalima T, Jaaskelainen J, et al: Duodenal atresia: Late follow-up. J Pediatr Surg 1988; 23:216–220.

Chapter 31

Helicobacter Pylori Gastroduodenal Disease in Infants and Children

STEVEN J. CZINN

INTRODUCTION

Gastroduodenal disease (gastritis, duodenitis, and peptic ulcer disease) is a significant health problem. Peptic ulcer disease alone affects nearly 4 million people in the United States annually, and the incidence is rising.[1, 2] With the advent of improved diagnostic tools, principally the small flexible fiberoptic endoscope, it is now recognized that gastroduodenal disease is present in children as well as in adults. The classic symptoms of peptic gastroduodenal disease are dyspepsia, vomiting, hematemesis, melena, and epigastric abdominal pain.[3] Because other diseases present with similar symptoms, the definitive diagnosis of peptic disease often requires esophagogastroduodenoscopy with biopsy.[4–9]

The pathogenesis of gastroduodenal disease has been extensively studied and reviewed elsewhere (see Chapter 33).[10–13] Despite this effort, the cause of gastroduodenal disease is not well understood. There is evidence that gastritis, gastric ulcers and duodenal ulcers are a continuum: gastritis or duodenitis develops at sites in which the mucosa is susceptible to damage by gastric acid and evolves into true ulcers.[14] According to this theory, gastroduodenal disease involves the interaction between gastric acid and mucosal cytoprotective mechanisms. In the stomach, mucus is the first line of defense against harmful exogenous agents; however, there are no data suggesting an abnormality in the quantity or quality of mucus in patients with gastroduodenal disease.[15, 16] Mucus, which is secreted by the gastric epithelial and neck cells in the gastric glands, permits the unidirectional flux of hydrogen ions and pepsinogen into the gastric lumen.[17] In addition, bicarbonate secreted by epithelial cells is retained in close proximity to the epithelium within the unstirred mucus layer, acting as an additional barrier to protect the mucosa from damage by acid and pepsin.[18] Mucus also contains other cytoprotective factors, including prostaglandin E_2 (PGE_2), which inhibits the release of gastrin and gastric acid secretion. PGE_2 also increases mucus secretion and enhances epithelial cell function, thereby serving to both prevent and heal peptic ulcers.[19] In the stomach, mucus, bicarbonate, and PGE_2 are the major cytoprotective factors. Impairment of any of these cytoprotective mechanisms promotes back-diffusion of hydrogen ions into the mucosa, thereby lowering the pH at the epithelial cell surface. At acid pH, pepsinogen is activated and autodigestion of gastric or duodenal mucosa is initiated.

The acid-secreting parietal cells possess specific histamine H_2 receptors that regulate acid secretion. H_2-receptor antagonists, such as cimetidine and ranitidine, are effective in the short-term symptomatic treatment of gastroduodenal disease. The temporary suppression of gastric acid allows for both resolution of symptoms and healing of the ulcer. However, most patients with peptic ulcer disease do not demonstrate hypersecretion of gastric acid, and the relapse rate for this therapy is as high as 85%.[20–24] The absence of hyperchlorhydria in ulcer patients and the high rate of relapse imply an underlying abnormality that persists despite therapy.

HISTORICAL BACKGROUND

Spiral-shaped microorganisms in the gastric mucosa have been the subject of many studies during the past century. It has been established that many animals, for example, cats, dogs, and monkeys, have upper gastrointestinal tract colonization with spiral-shaped bacteria,[25] and German investigators in the early twentieth century identified similar microorganisms in human gastric tissue.[26] This observation was confirmed in 1939 by Doenges,[27] who characterized "commensal" spirochetes in the "gastric glands" of humans and primates. These significant observations were quickly confirmed by other investigators, who identified spirochetal bacteria in gastric biopsies from approximately 50% of adults with gastritis, peptic ulcer disease, or both.[28] Despite the initial enthusiasm for a microbial etiology for human acid-peptic disease, skepticism surfaced following the publication of a large study by Palmer[29] involving more than 1,000 gastric biopsy specimens, which failed to confirm the previous reports. In 1975, Steer and Colin-Jones[30] unknowingly confirmed the previous association between spiral bacteria and human gastric tissue and erroneously concluded that these microorganisms represented contaminants, that is, *Pseudomonas aeruginosa*, and therefore bore no relationship to the associated gastritis or peptic ulcer disease. Subsequently, in Australia, Marshall and Warren[31] demonstrated *Campylobacter*-like organisms in human gastric tissue and, in an important study, were able to recover these pathogens in culture following prolonged incubation under microaerobic conditions.

This microorganism, initially named *Campylobacter pyloridis* or *Campylobacter pylori*, is now referred to as *Helicobacter pylori* and is routinely recovered from tissue specimens from adults and children with histologic evidence of gastritis, peptic ulcer disease, or both.[32] Thus, a relationship between this microorganism and human disease has been established. Evidence for a causal relationship between *H. pylori* and human illness was developed following novel experiments by two independent investigators who satisfied Koch's postulates by creating histologically confirmed gastritis with associated clinical signs and symptoms following consumption of a large inoculum of viable microorganisms.[33, 34] Similar studies have been performed in primates who develop histologic evidence of gastritis following oral challenge with *H. pylori*.[35]

MICROBIOLOGY AND BIOCHEMISTRY

Under light microscopy, *H. pylori* appears as a slender, S-shaped bacillus 2 to 5 μm long. Although the Gram stain is capable of identifying this microbial pathogen as a gram-negative rod, the pathogen stains poorly and is therefore difficult to identify in tissue specimens when this staining technique is used. Accordingly, most investigators have abandoned routine usage of the Gram stain in preference to other staining techniques, which include a silver-staining technique (Warthin-Starry stain), the acridine-orange stain, the Giemsa stain, and staining with hematoxylin-eosin.[36, 37] When the last histologic technique is used, these microorganisms can be visualized by experienced pathologists in the mucous coat overlying the gastric epithelium.

In addition to their morphologic appearance, *H. pylori* shares many other characteristics with human *Campylobacter*, including similar nutritional requirements, deoxyribonucleic acid (DNA) base composition, antibiotic sensitivity patterns, and the presence of the enzymes catalase and oxidase. However, important differences exist between this microorganism and *Campylobacter*, and these differences may play a role in the pathogenesis of human disease. Specifically, *H. pylori* has a smooth cell wall and four to six unipolar sheathed flagella, possesses a high urease content, is unable to reduce nitrate, and has a unique protein composition and fatty acid profile. Accordingly, the differences are great enough to justify a new genus, *Helicobacter*.[38–40]

DIAGNOSTIC METHODS

The definitive diagnosis of *H. pylori* gastritis or peptic ulcer disease requires recovery of the responsible pathogen from biopsy specimens. The endoscopic appearance can vary from normal-appearing gastric mucosa to erythema or frank ulcerations. Interestingly, most children with *H. pylori* have a nodular-appearing gastric antrum (Fig. 31–1).[41] *H. pylori* is rarely, if ever, recovered from histologically normal gastric tissue. Bacterial identification in biopsy specimens can be either direct or indirect. Direct bacterial identification in biopsy specimens initially used a silver-staining technique (Warthin-Starry) (Fig. 31–2); however, this cumbersome histologic method has been supplemented by other staining techniques. Recent studies in children have determined that the hematoxylin-eosin stain, when properly performed and viewed by an experienced pathologist is an effective means of identifying this microorganism in biopsy specimens obtained from infants and children.[42]

Recovery of *H. pylori* from biopsy specimens is now routine in most diagnostic microbiologic laboratories. A portion of the gastric biopsy specimen is homogenized with a mortar and pestle and diluted with brain-heart infusion broth prior to plating on Columbia agar plates containing 5% sheep's blood with and without antibiotic supplementation with vancomycin, nalidixic acid, and amphotericin B. The inoculated plates are incubated at 37°C under microaerobic conditions for an extended period (5–7 days). *H. pylori* grows on blood agar as small, translucent, nonhemolytic colonies. Confirmation of *H. pylori* is based on colony morphology and Gram stain, and the production of urease, catalase, and oxidase.

In addition to recovery of the responsible pathogen from tissue specimens, a number of indirect diagnostic techniques have been developed to overcome the diffi-

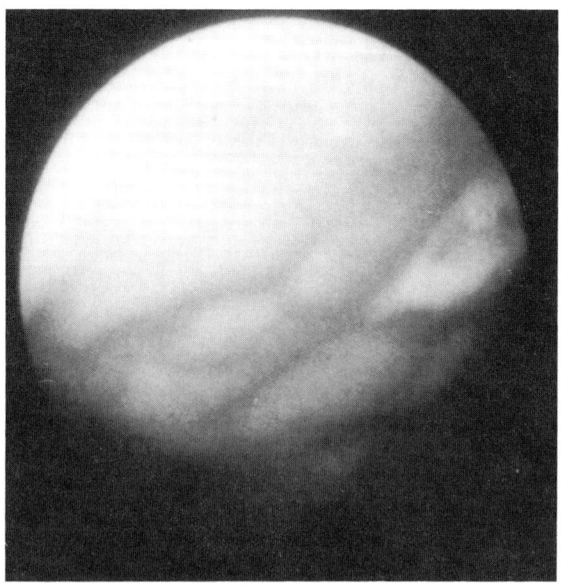

Figure 31–1. Endoscopic appearance of antral nodularity present in children with *Helicobacter pylori* gastritis.

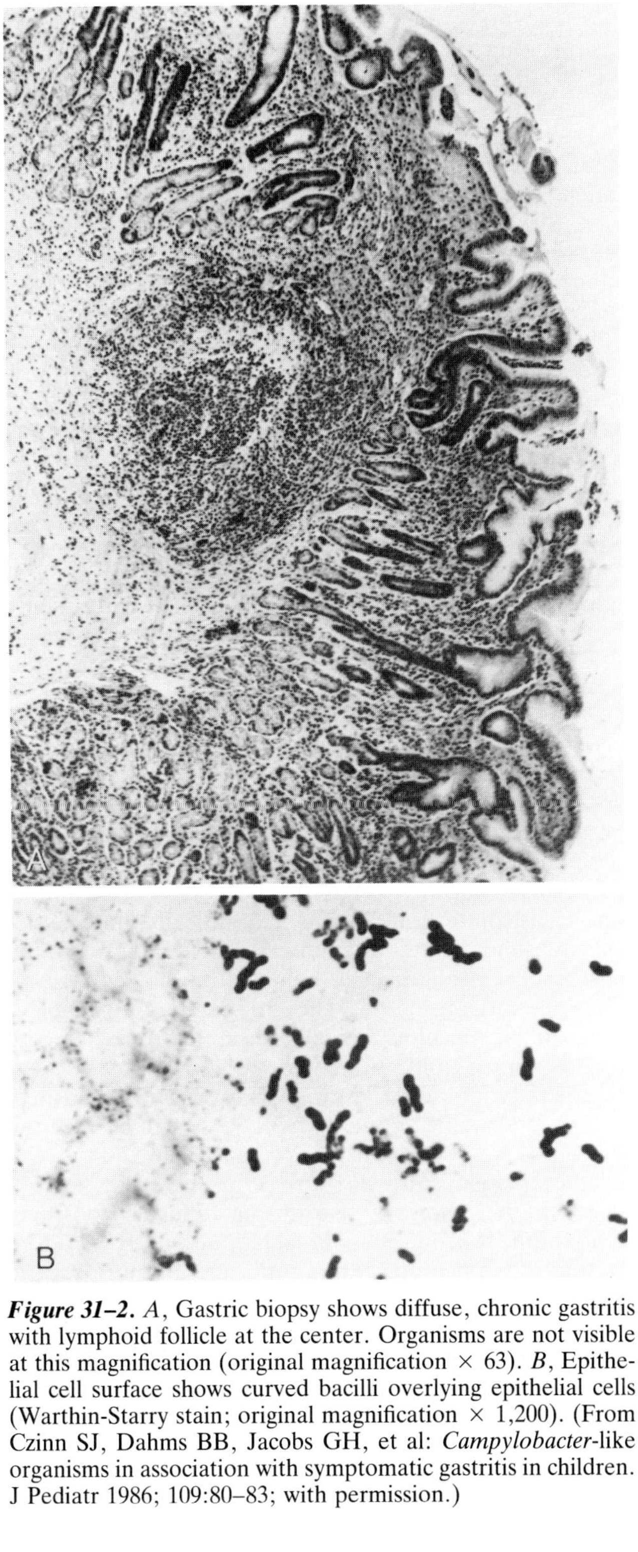

Figure 31–2. *A*, Gastric biopsy shows diffuse, chronic gastritis with lymphoid follicle at the center. Organisms are not visible at this magnification (original magnification × 63). *B*, Epithelial cell surface shows curved bacilli overlying epithelial cells (Warthin-Starry stain; original magnification × 1,200). (From Czinn SJ, Dahms BB, Jacobs GH, et al: *Campylobacter*-like organisms in association with symptomatic gastritis in children. J Pediatr 1986; 109:80–83; with permission.)

culties encountered in recovering this fastidious microorganism. Specifically, the placement of biopsy material into urea-containing transport broth prior to homogenization and plating is a useful diagnostic maneuver, as *H. pylori*–infected tissue yields an immediate color (from yellow to pink), reflecting a pH change due to the production of bicarbonate and ammonia following hydrolysis of urea.[43] False-negative results also occur owing to the concurrent use of topical anesthetics with antibacterial activity, improper handling and storage of biopsy specimens, overgrowth of commensal microorganisms, and inadequate duration of incubation.[44] Nevertheless, histologic examination of diseased tissue often demonstrates the presence of the responsible pathogen despite negative urease broth and culture results. Specifically, histologic examination of the diseased stomach characteristically reveals chronic inflammation with focal, acute glandular destruction. Unlike descriptions of *H. pylori* in adults, the predominant inflammatory cell in children is the lymphocyte. In addition, examination of the biopsy specimens under high magnification invariably demonstrates bacilli with a loose spiral configuration in the gastric mucous coat overlying the surface epithelial cells as well as a decrease in the mucous coat (see Fig. 31–2). False-positive results are extremely rare and have been observed only when the bacterial contaminants of biopsy material or the gastric biopsy material itself contains a urease-positive microorganism, such as *Proteus*.

Recent efforts have focused on the development of noninvasive diagnostic techniques for *H. pylori* infection to avoid the morbidity associated with endoscopic examination. Thus, the urea breath test, although not commercially available, has been demonstrated to be sensitive to and specific for *H. pylori* infection.[45–47] The test takes advantage of the high endogenous urease content of this microorganism. Specifically, the recovery of radiolabeled carbon dioxide in the exhaled air following ingestion of labeled urea (^{13}C) is indicative of *H. pylori* infection.

A number of investigators have demonstrated the usefulness of serologic diagnostic techniques. Thus, with the use of outer membrane proteins or whole cell lysates as the detecting antigen(s), it has been possible to document serologic evidence of *H. pylori* infection.[48–50] Children, like their adult counterparts, develop an immunoglobulin G (IgG) antibody response to *H. pylori*. The IgA antibody response in children is variable, and IgM antibodies have not been detected. Thus, a positive IgG enzyme-linked immunosorbent assay for antibody against *H. pylori* in the evaluation of children with chronic epigastric abdominal pain, vomiting, or both, strongly suggests the diagnosis of *H. pylori* gastroduodenal disease.[51–54]

PATHOGENESIS

The exact mechanism by which *H. pylori* produces gastroduodenal disease has not been established; however, several hypotheses have been proposed. The most popular explanations regarding the pathogenesis of *H. pylori* disease relate to the marked urease activity. Recent studies also suggest that urease is essential for colonization by *H. pylori*. A urease-negative mutant of *H. pylori* was unable to infect gnotobiotic pigs, whereas the parent strain infected 100% of challenged animals.[55] The large quantities of bicarbonate production following the hydrolysis of urea on the gastric mucosal surface result in an elevation of surface pH and an alteration in the Na^+,K^+–ATPase pump of the gastric epithelial cells, thereby permitting back diffusion of hydrogen ions and concomitant hyperchlorhydria.[56] Similarly, the production of high concentrations of ammonia, a potent cytotoxin, following the hydrolysis of urea at the gastric mucosal surface might result in gastric epithelial cell cytolysis and the resultant focal inflammation characteristic of *H. pylori* infection.[57–59] Two additional mechanisms that have been proposed to explain the pathogenesis of *H. pylori* disease are speculative. The first possibility is that cellular damage following *H. pylori* adhesions to gastric epithelial cells is not dissimilar from that proposed for enteropathogenic *Escherichia coli.*[60] Transmission electron microscopy studies have shown that this microorganism associates closely with a number of cell lines used in adherence assays.[61] In addition, partial fusion to surface epithelium and loss of microvilli have also been noted.[62] The mechanism by which *H. pylori* adheres to the gastric epithelium remains unclear. *H. pylori* has been shown to bind to a glycerolipid extracted from gastric tissue.[63] *H. pylori* has also been shown to contain a hemagglutinin with binding specificity to *N*-acetylneuraminyllactose and may be a colonization factor.[64] The second proposed mechanism concerns the proteolysis of gastric mucus and the resultant damage to underlying gastric epithelium.[65] Although both of these proposed pathogenic mechanisms acting alone or in combination may play a role in human *H. pylori* infection, a definitive understanding of the host-parasite interaction awaits the availability of a suitable animal model.

EPIDEMIOLOGY

Using the diagnostic techniques just discussed, an association between colonization with *H. pylori* and gastrointestinal disease has been established in both adults and children. Studies from many countries have confirmed that infection is a function of age, such that the colonization rate in adult patients undergoing endoscopy approaches 50%. Epidemiologic factors associated with colonization have not been established, but the geographic distribution of high colonization rates suggests that the standard of living may be an important predisposing factor. Specifically, colonization rates for both adults and children in developing countries far exceed those reported for adults and children from the United States and other industrialized countries.

Studies in pediatric patient populations have determined that 15% of all children undergoing endoscopy and gastric biopsy have evidence of *H. pylori* infection.[41, 42, 66–71] It is noteworthy that *H. pylori*–positive children have more severe gastritis than culture-negative children, who represented only 20% of moderate to severe, and 80% of the patients with mild gastritis. The mean age of this patient population was 12 years. In children with *H. pylori*–positive gastritis, presenting complaints included epigastric pain, vomiting, and hematemesis. In addition to the relationship between gastritis and *H. pylori*, several studies in adults and children have demonstrated an association between *H. pylori* infection-colonization and duodenal ulceration. In children, 90% of those with endoscopically proven duodenal ulcerations have *H. pylori* infection and associated gastritis. Studies in adults have documented that virtually all patients with duodenal ulcerations have *H. pylori* gastritis. Studies in adults have also shown a relationship between gastric ulceration and *H. pylori* gastritis, with some reports documenting colonization in 80% of this patient population. However, only 20% of our patients with endoscopically verified gastric ulceration had evidence of gastritis and *H. pylori* infection. Thus, in children, H. pylori is not a major causal factor for gastric ulcerations, and other causes must be considered. A relationship between this microorganism and other gastrointestinal diseases in children, that is, reflux esophagitis, celiac disease, protein-losing enteropathy, and hypertrophic gastritis, has been proposed but not confirmed. Similarly, the role of *H. pylori* in nonulcer dyspepsia in pediatric patients has not been determined.

Animal Model

The development of an animal model is necessary to determine with certainty the pathogenesis of *H. pylori* disease. Experimental infection has been produced in the rhesus monkey and gnotobiotic piglet; however, these models are extremely expensive to reproduce. Efforts have recently focused on the ferret, an animal whose gastrointestinal tract is anatomically and physiologically similar to the human gastrointestinal tract and, most important, subject to colonization with *Campylobacter*-like organisms.[73, 74] The isolates were morphologically similar but biochemically different from *H. pylori* isolated from children. Thus, unlike *H. pylori*, the ferret's microorganism is rapidly growing, with positive cultures detectable within 24 hours, and can be cultured at 37°C or 42°C on a variety of agar. The ferret *Campylobacter* organism is also urease positive but, in contrast with *H. pylori*, is also nitrate reductase positive. In addition, it produces beta-lactamase and is therefore resistant to most penicillins and cephalosporins. The endoscopic appearance of the ferret stomach revealed an antral nodularity not unlike that seen in pediatric patients. All infected animals have histologic evidence of chronic antral gastritis with infiltration of the lamina propria with mononuclear cells. Studies are currently under way to characterize the natural history of *Campylobacter*-associated gastritis in this animal. A murine model for *H. pylori* has also been reported. Germ-free mice can be infected with *Helicobacter felis*, a spiral organism isolated from the stomach of cats.[75] This model should allow investigators to clarify the role of *H. pylori* in the development of gastroduodenal disease.

TREATMENT

Laboratory studies have shown that *H. pylori* is susceptible to most antibiotics and bismuth-containing salts.[76, 77] To date, all adult studies attempting to treat gastritis by eradicating *H. pylori* with a single antimicrobial agent have been unsuccessful. This may be related to a number of factors, including the emergence of bacterial resistance. Most authorities currently recommend treating only adults with *H. pylori* in association with a duodenal ulcer and patients with gastritis who are symptomatic despite treatment with cytoprotective or acid-suppressing agents. The accepted recommendation for treatment of adults is bismuth subsalicylate, one tablet four times daily, tetracycline, 500 mg four times daily, and metronidazole, 400 mg three times daily for 2 to 4 weeks. No therapy is recommended for adults with asymptomatic *H. pylori* infection or nonulcer dyspepsia.

Pediatric patients have reportedly been successfully treated with amoxicillin, bismuth subsalicylate plus amoxicillin, or amoxicillin plus tinidazole.[54, 68, 72] However, many studies report significant relapse rates, and no long-term follow-up has been reported to confirm long-term eradication. To date, 6-month follow-up has reported a 17% relapse rate.[54] In addition, there is concern about the use of bismuth compounds in children, and metronidazole should be used with caution owing to the carcinogenic potential of this class of antibiotics. The author and colleagues have been unable consistently to eradicate *H. pylori* in their pediatric patients treated with amoxicillin, amoxicillin plus bismuth subsalicylate, or amoxicillin, bismuth subsalicylate, and metronidazole. Therefore, their approach to pediatric patients with symptoms consistent with peptic ulcer disease is to perform upper endoscopy and biopsy of the gastric antrum to document the presence of *H. pylori* or peptic ulcer disease, or both. If *H. pylori* gastroduodenal disease is confirmed, their initial therapy continues to be an H_2-receptor antagonist. Most of their patients became asymptomatic after a 6- to 8-week course with these agents, despite the continued presence of *H. pylori* colonization. Long-term follow-up (6 years) of these patients indicates that 50% remain asymptomatic, and the other half require chronic acid-suppressive therapy. The latter group would definitely benefit from treatment when a safe and effective therapy is available for the long-term eradication of *H. pylori*. Antimicrobial therapy for *H. pylori* remains extremely controversial, and no preferred therapy is available, since no prospective double-blind, long-term studies have been published. Therefore, only if a patient responds poorly to standard therapy does the author recommend a trial of antibiotics. If antimicrobial agents are used, patients should be advised that bacterial resistance to these agents may occur, making it virtually impossible to eradicate the organism. Although there is considerable evidence confirming the role of *H. pylori* in the pathogenesis of gastroduodenal disease, treatment with multiple antimicrobial agents for *H. pylori* infection should be used with caution until improved therapeutic agents are identified.

REFERENCES

1. Kurata JH, Haile EM, Elashoff JD: Sex differences in peptic ulcer disease. Gastroenterology 1985; 88:96–100.
2. Elashoff JD, Grossman JI: Trends in hospital admissions and death rates for peptic ulcer in the United States from 1970 to 1978. Gastroenterology 1980; 78:280–285.
3. Shepard MC, Holmes GKT, Cockel R: Clinical picture of peptic ulceration diagnosed endoscopically. Gut 1977; 18:524–530.
4. Misiewicz JJ: Peptic ulceration and its correlation with symptoms. Clin Gastroenterol 1978; 7:389–392.
5. Nelson RS, Urrea LH, Lanza FL: Evaluation of gastric ulcerations. Am J Dig Dis 1976; 21:389–392.
6. Kiel J, Anderson D: X-ray examination and/or endoscopy in the diagnosis of gastroduodenal ulcer and crater. Scand J Gastroenterol 1980; 15:39–43.
7. Tedesco FJ, Best WR, Littman A, et al: Role of gastroscopy in gastric ulcer patients. Gastroenterology 1977; 73:170–173.
8. Weinstein WM: Gastroscopy for gastric ulcers. Gastroenterology 1977; 73:1160–1162.
9. Rowland R, Durbridge T, Hecker R, et al: How many endoscopic biopsy specimens? Med J Aust 1976; 2:172–175.
10. Baron JH: Current views on pathogenesis of peptic ulcer. Gastroenterology 1982; 80:1–10.
11. Peters MN, Richardson CT: Stressful life events, acid hypersecretion, and ulcer disease. Gastroenterology 1983; 84:114–118.
12. McIntosh JH, Byth K, Pitper DW: Environmental factors in aetiology of chronic gastric ulcer. Gut 1985; 26:789–798.
13. Rhodes J: Etiology of gastric ulcer. Gastroenterology 1972; 63:171–182.
14. Kirk RM: Are gastric and duodenal ulcers separate diseases or do they form a continuum? Dig Dis Sci 1981; 26:149–152.
15. Allen A: Structure and function of gastrointestinal mucus. *In* Johnson LR, ed: Physiology of the Gastrointestinal Tract. New York, Raven Press, 1982, pp 617–639.
16. Schrager J, Oates MDG: Relation of human gastrointestinal mucus to disease states. Br Med Bull 1978; 34:79–82.
17. Venables CW: Mucus, pepsin and peptic ulcer. Gut 1986; 27:233–238.
18. Allen A, Garner A: Mucus and bicarbonate secretion in stomach and their possible role in mucosal protection. Gut 1980; 21:249–261.
19. Miller T: Protective effects of prostaglandins against gastric mucosal damage: Current knowledge and proposed mechanisms. Am J Physiol 1983; 245:G601–G621.
20. Gray GR, Smith IS, MacKenzie I, et al: Long-term cimetidine in the management of severe duodenal ulcer dyspepsia. Gastroenterology 1978; 74:397–401.
21. Korman MG, Hetzel DS, Hansky J, et al: Relapse rate of duodenal ulcer after cessation of long-term cimetidine treatment. Dig Dis Sci 1980; 25:88–91.
22. Bardhan KD, Cole DS, Hawkins BW, et al: Does treatment with cimetidine extended beyond initial healing of duodenal ulcer reduce the subsequent relapse rate? Br Med J 1982; 284:621–623.
23. Gough RR, Roman MG, Bardhan RD, et al: Ranitidine and cimetidine in prevention of duodenal ulcer relapse. Lancet 1984; 2:659–662.
24. Myrrick TJ, Misiewicz G: Histamine H_2-receptor antagonists in short- and long-term treatment of duodenal ulcers. Clin Gastroenterol 1984; 12:501–541.
25. Lee A, Hazell SL: *Campylobacter pylori* in health and disease: An ecological perspective. Microbiol Ecol Health Dis 1988; 1:1–16.
26. Krienitz W: Ueber das auftreten von mageninhalt bei carcinoma ventriculi. Dtsch Med Wochenschr 1906; 32:872.
27. Doenges LS: Spirochetes in the gastric glands of *Macacus rhesus* and of man without related disease. Arch Pathol 1939; 27:469–477.
28. Freedberg AS, Barron LE: The presence of spirochetes in human gastric mucosa. Am J Dig Dis 1940; 7:443–445.
29. Palmer ED: Investigation of the gastric mucosa spirochetes of the human. Gastroenterology 1954; 27:218–220.
30. Steer HW, Colin-Jones DG: Mucosal changes in gastric ulceration and their response to carbenoxolone sodium. Gut 1975; 16:59–597.
31. Marshall B, Warren JR: Unidentified curved bacilli in the stomach of patients with gastritis and peptic ulceration. Lancet 1984; 1:1311–1314.
32. Blaser MJ: Gastritis *Campylobacter*-like organisms, gastritis, and peptic ulcer disease. Gastroenterology 1987; 93:371–383.

33. Marshall BJ, Armstrong JA, McGechie DB, et al: Attempt to fulfill Koch's postulates for pyloric *Campylobacter*. Med J Aust 1985; 142:436–439.
34. Morris A, Nicholson G: Ingestion of *Campylobacter pyloridis* causes gastritis and raised fasting gastric pH. Am J Gastroenterol 1987; 87:192–198.
35. Baskerville A, Newell DG: Naturally occurring chronic gastritis and *C. pylori* infection in the rhesus monkey: A potential model for gastritis in man. Gut 1988; 29:465–472.
36. Rathbone BJ, Wyatt JI, Heatley RV: *Campylobacter pyloridis*—a new factor in peptic ulcer disease? Gut 1986; 27:635–641.
37. Madan E, Kemp J, Westblom TU, et al: Evaluation of staining methods for identifying *Campylobacter pylori*. Am J Clin Pathol 1988; 90:450–453.
38. Megraud F, Bonnet F, Garnier M, et al: Characterization of "Campylobacter pyloridis" by culture, enzymatic profile and protein content. J Clin Microbiol 1985; 22:1007–1010.
39. Czinn SJ, Speck WT: *Campylobacter pylori*: A new pathogen. J Pediatr 1989; 114(4 Pt 1):670.
40. Cadeput M, Lemoigne F, Megraud F: Cellular fatty acid composition of *Campylobacter pylori, ferret-clo,* and *wolinella* species. Presented at the Workshop on Gastroduodenal Pathology and *Campylobacter pylori*, Bordeaux, France, October 1988.
41. Hassall E, Dimmidk JE: Unique features of *Helicobacter pylori* disease in children. Dig Dis Sci 1991; 36:417–423.
42. Kilbridge PM, Dahms BB, Czinn J: *Campylobacter pylori*–associated gastritis and peptic ulcer disease in children. Am J Dis Child 1988; 142:1149–1152.
43. Czinn SJ, Carr H: Rapid diagnosis of *Campylobacter pyloridis*–associated gastritis. J Pediatr 1987; 110:569–570.
44. Czinn SJ, Carr HS, Speck WS: Topical anaesthetic agents and *Campylobacter pylori*. J Pediatr Gastroenterol Nutr 1989; 9:46–48.
45. Graham DY, Klein PD, Doyle JE, et al: *Campylobacter pylori* detected non-invasively by the ^{13}C-urea breath test. Lancet 1987; 1:1174–1177.
46. Graham DY, Klein PD, Opekun AR, et al: Effect of age on the frequency of active *Campylobacter pylori* infection diagnosed by the [^{13}C] urea breath test in normal subjects and patients with peptic ulcer disease. J Infect Dis 1988; 4:777–780.
47. Marshall BJ, Surveyor I: Carbon-14 urea breath test for the diagnosis of *Campylobacter pylori*–associated gastritis. J Nucl Med 1988; 29:11–16.
48. Jones DM, Eldridge J, Fox AJ, et al: Antibody to the gastric *Campylobacter*-like organism *("Campylobacter pyloridis")*: Clinical correlations and distribution in the normal population. J Med Microbiol 1986; 22:57–62.
49. Goodwin CS, Blincow E, Peterson G, et al: Enzyme-linked immunosorbent assay for *Campylobacter pyloridis*: Correlation with presence of *C. pyloridis* in the gastric mucosa. J Infect Dis 1987; 155:488–494.
50. Perez-Perez G, Dworkin BM, Chodos JE, et al: *Campylobacter pylori* antibodies in humans. Ann Intern Med 1988; 109:11–17.
51. Czinn S, Carr H, Sheffler L, et al: Serum IgG antibody against the outer membrane proteins of *Campylobacter pylori* in children with gastroduodenal disease. J Infect Dis 1988; 159:586–589.
52. Czinn SJ, Carr HS, Speck WT: The diagnosis of *Campylobacter pylori* gastritis using an enzyme-linked immunoassay. Rev Infect Dis 1991; 13:S700–S703.
53. Glassman MS, Dallal S, Berezin SH, et al: *Helicobacter pylori*–related gastroduodenal disease in children: Diagnostic utility of enzyme-linked immunosorbent assay. Dig Dis Sci 1990; 35:993–997.
54. Oderda G, Holton J, Altare F, et al: Amoxicillin plus tinidazole for *Campylobacter pylori* gastritis in children: Assessment by serum IgG antibody, pepsinogen 1, and gastrin levels. Lancet 1989; 1:690–692.
55. Eaton KA, Brooks CL, Morgan DR, et al: Essential role of urease in pathogenesis of gastritis induced by *Helicobacter pylori* in gnotobiotic piglets. Infect Immun 1991; 59:2470–2475.
56. Hazell SL, Lee A: *Campylobacter pyloridis*, urease, hydrogen ion back diffusion, and gastric ulcers. Lancet 1986; 2:15–17.
57. Leunk RD, Johnson PT, David BC, et al: Cytotoxic activity in broth-culture filtrates of *Campylobacter pylori*. J Med Microbiol 1988; 26:93–99.
58. Xu JK, Goodwin CS, Cooper M, et al: Intracellular vacuolization caused by the urease of *Helicobacter pylori*. J Infect Dis 1990; 161:1302–1304.
59. Cover TL, Puryear W, Perez-Perez GI, et al: Effect of urease on HeLa cell vacuolation induced by *Helicobacter pylori* cytotoxin. Infect Immun 1991; 59:1264–1270.
60. Neman-Simha V, Megraud F: In vitro model for *Campylobacter pylori* adherence properties. Infect Immun 1988; 59:3329–3333.
61. Tricottet V, Bruneval P, Vire O, et al: *Campylobacter*-like organisms and surface epithelium abnormalities in active, chronic gastritis in humans: An ultrastructural study. Ultrastruct Pathol 1986; 10:113–122.
62. Tricottet V, Bruneval P, Vire O, et al: *Campylobacter*-like organisms and surface epithelium abnormalities in active, chronic gastritis in humans: An ultrastructural study. Ultrastruct Pathol 1986; 10:113–122.
63. Lingwood CA, Law H, Pellizzari A, et al: Gastric glycerolipid as a receptor for *Campylobacter pylori*. Lancet 1989; 1:238.
64. Evans DJ, Evans DG, Smith KE, et al: Serum antibody responses to the *N*-acetylneuraminyllactose-binding hemagglutinin of *Campylobacter pylori*. Infect Immun 1989; 57:664–667.
65. Slomiany BL, Bilski J, Sarosiek J, et al: *Campylobacter pyloridis* degrades mucin and undermines gastric mucosal integrity. Biochem Biophys Res Comm 1987; 144:307–314.
66. Czinn SJ: *Helicobacter pylori*–induced gastritis in childhood. *In* Malfertheiner P: Proceedings of the Workshop on Gastroduodenal Pathology and *Campylobacter pylori*. Berlin, Springer-Verlag, 1990, pp 181–187.
67. DeGiacomo C, Lisato L, Negrini R, et al: Serum immune response to *Helicobacter pylori* in children: Epidemiologic and clinical applications. J Pediatr 1991; 119:205–210.
68. Oderda G, Dell'Olio D, Morra I, et al: *Campylobacter pylori* gastritis: Long-term results of amoxicillin therapy. Arch Dis Child 1988; 64:326–329.
69. Drumm B, Sherman P, Cutz E, et al: Association of *Campylobacter pylori* on the gastric mucosa with antral gastritis in children. N Engl J Med 1987; 316:1557–1561.
70. Glassman MS, Schwarz SM, Medow MS, et al: *Campylobacter pylori*–related gastrointestinal disease in children: Incidence and clinical findings. Dig Dis Sci 1989; 34:1501–1504.
71. Drumm B, O'Brien A, Cutz E, et al: *Campylobacter pyloridis*–associated primary gastritis in children. Pediatrics 1987; 80:192–195.
72. Drumm B, Sherman P, Chiasson D, et al: Treatment of *Campylobacter pylori*–associated antral gastritis in children with bismuth subsalicylate and ampicillin. J Pediatr 1988; 113:908–912.
73. Fox JG, Cabot EB, Taylor NS, et al: Gastric colonization by *Campylobacter pylori* subsp. *mustalea* in ferrets. Infect Immunol 1988; 56:2994–2996.
74. Fox JG, Correa P, Taylor NS, et al: *Campylobacter pylori*–associated gastritis and immune response in a population at increased risk of gastric carcinoma. Am J Gastroenterol 1989; 84:775–781.
75. Lee A, Fox JG, Otto G, et al: A small animal model of human *Helicobacter pylori* active chronic gastritis. Gastroenterology 1990; 99:1315–1323.
76. McNulty CAM, Dent JC, Wise R: Susceptibility of clinical isolates of *Campylobacter pyloridis* to 11 antimicrobial agents. Antimicrob Agents Chemother 1985; 28:837–838.
77. Lambert T, Megraud F, Gerbaud G, et al: Susceptibility of *Campylobacter pyloridis* to 20 antimicrobial agents. Antimicrob Agents Chemother 1986; 30:510–511.

Chapter 32

Gastritis

ARTHUR R. EULER

Until technologic advances enabled endoscopic equipment to become flexible and sufficiently small in diameter, the diagnosis of gastritis was almost universally made using surgical or suction biopsy specimens. Concurrently developed with the other advances in endoscopic design was the ability to obtain mucosal biopsies during endoscopy. Currently, gastritis is most frequently diagnosed by endoscopy. The increased use of endoscopic equipment has resulted in more frequent diagnosis of gastritis, but, unfortunately, the diagnosis is now often based on endoscopic appearance without the confirmation of a biopsy evaluation. Ideally, gastritis should be diagnosed histologically.

Gastritis is an important clinical entity. It has been documented as the commonest cause of upper gastrointestinal bleeding and the fifth commonest diagnosis made during outpatient consultations.[1, 2] In a Swedish survey, gastritis accounted for 30% of all gastrointestinal diagnosed disorders.[2] In that survey the diagnosis of gastritis was made 15 and 21 times more frequently than was peptic ulcer disease in male and female patients from birth to 19 years, respectively.[2]

Gastritis may be classified as primary or secondary, allowing a diagnosis based on the cause. Primary gastritis is most often associated with *Helicobacter pylori* infections (see Chapter 31) or with bile acid reflux.[3, 4] In primary gastritis, a chronic inflammatory process is often predominant and is frequently associated with duodenal ulcers.[5] *H. pylori*–associated antritis is believed to be a primary factor in this process.[6] Secondary gastritis more frequently has an acute inflammatory component and is usually associated with specific diseases, such as major-surface-area burns or head trauma; systemic illnesses, such as Henoch-Schönlein purpura, infections, and infestations; or ingested agents, such as corrosives or aspirin, that damage the gastric mucosa.

The exact pathophysiologic mechanisms that underlie the development of gastritis are not known. It is hypothesized that gastric inflammation develops when an imbalance occurs between aggressive factors, primarily hydrochloric acid and pepsin, and mucosal defense mechanisms, such as mucus and bicarbonate secretion, mucosal blood flow, surface hydrophobicity, and cell turnover.[7–10] Many of these mucosal defense parameters are associated with the action of endogenous prostaglandins whose production is decreased by aspirin or other nonsteroidal anti-inflammatory drugs (NSAIDs) that inhibit cyclooxygenase.[11] When the mucosal defense is compromised, back-diffusion of hydrogen ions occurs, which is the first step in a series of events resulting in inflammation.

CLINICAL PRESENTATION

The commonest clinical presentation is a constellation of signs and symptoms that usually includes epigastric pain and vomiting. The pain most often occurs during eating or in the immediate postprandial period. This pattern can result in decreased nutritional intake and subsequent inadequate growth or actual weight loss. Vomiting, if it occurs, also usually happens in the immediate postprandial period. Younger patients may have abdominal pain that they are unable to pinpoint to the epigastrium. Occasionally, only irritability and poor feeding are reported by the parents. Less frequently occurring symptoms are chest pain, anorexia fatigue, and nausea, and less frequent signs are hematemesis and melena. On physical examination epigastric tenderness is the commonest finding. Major upper gastrointestinal hemorrhage is rare, but documentation of fecal blood loss should be an integral part of every physical examination in the patient with a presumptive diagnosis of gastritis. These signs and symptoms are usually present, regardless of whether the gastritis is primary or secondary. Details of the signs and symptoms associated with specific causes are discussed later.

CAUSES

Stress-Induced Gastritis

A frequently diagnosed form of secondary gastritis is that associated with stress. Such gastritis usually occurs in patients admitted to the intensive care unit with significant problems involving many body systems. The mucosal lesions most often documented by endoscopy are erosions, and those less frequently are ulcers (Fig. 32–1). If the latter are associated with a severe burn, the ulcers are called *Curling's ulcers.*[12] If they are associated with central nervous system trauma or surgery, they are termed *Cushing's ulcers.*[13] The commonest presentation of patients with stress-associated gastric erosions and ulcers is a major upper gastrointestinal hemorrhage.

Idiopathic

The cause of diffuse varioliform gastritis, also termed *chronic erosive gastritis*, is unknown.[13–18] Multiple gastric erosions are found and are associated with epigastric pain, nausea, and vomiting. Few pediatric cases have been reported.[13, 15] A dosage of cromolyn sodium 200 mg once or twice daily has been associated with clinical and histologic improvement during a 3- to 4-month period in a few cases.[14, 15]

Gastric rugal fold enlargement associated with hypoproteinemia and anemia was first reported by Ménétrier in 1888.[19] There are rare reports of this disorder in infants, children, and adolescents.[20–23] The clinical presentation usually involves signs related to hypoproteinemia, such as ascites and edema, nausea, vomiting, and anorexia.[20–24] Diagnosis can be made by endoscopy and appropriate laboratory evaluations (Fig. 32–2). Therapy is symptomatic and supportive. The prognosis is generally good, and complete recovery is expected.[25]

Atrophic gastritis is uncommon in patients younger than 50 years of age and has been reported rarely in pediatric patients.[26, 27] Clinical presentation has included fatigue, dyspnea on exertion, and decreased activity levels.[28] Physical examination reveals only signs compatible with anemia. Maximal acid outputs are decreased, and antiparietal cell antibodies are usually present.[28] Therapy is supportive, usually consisting of vitamin B_{12} and ferrous sulfate.[28]

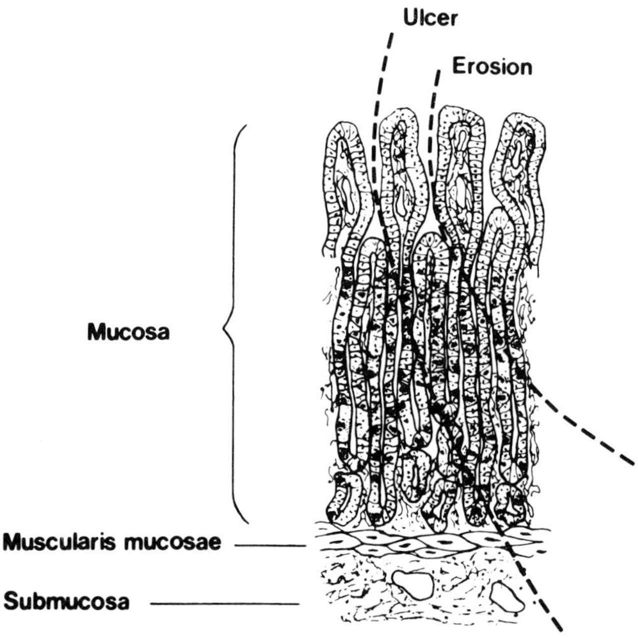

Figure 32–1. Erosion depth is confined to the mucosa. Ulcers involve the muscularis mucosa and the submucosa.

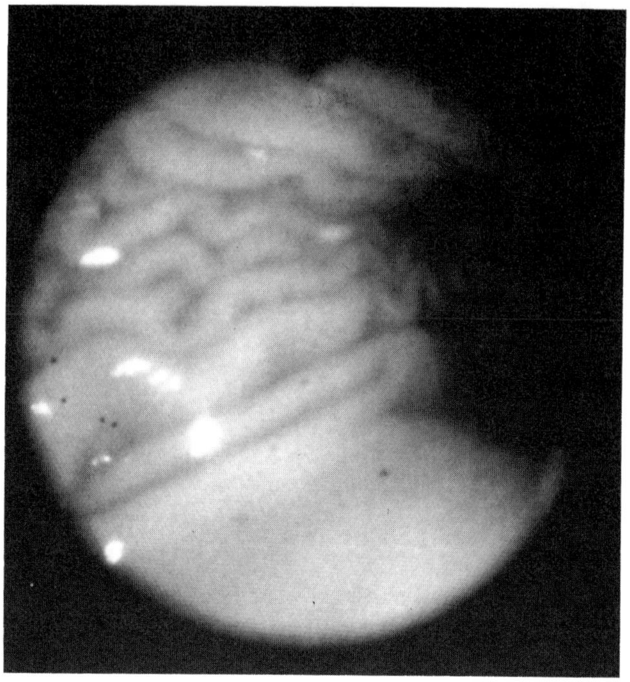

Figure 32–2. Endoscopic appearance of increased rugal folds in Ménétrier's disease.

Caustic Ingestions

Accidental ingestion of corrosive agents is a clinical problem unique to pediatrics. Suicide attempts with such agents most commonly occur among adolescents. The type of corrosive agent varies in different parts of the world. In the United States the commonest type is household lye, a strong alkali consisting primarily of sodium hydroxide.[29] Although strong alkalis such as lye usually cause significant esophageal damage, gastric damage can be extensive, with the prepyloric area being involved most frequently.[30, 31] In one series, all patients 15 to 20 years of age who ingested such alkalis had gastric and esophageal damage, whereas in most younger patients, only esophageal damage was found.[31] Antibiotics and steroids were used during the acute phase in that report, and a feeding jejunostomy was added in those cases with diffuse gastritis. Gastric obstruction secondary to prepyloric stricture formation often develops despite steroid use. Posterior gastrojejunostomy is the most frequent surgical approach for this complication.[31] Similar gastropathies had been documented after the ingestion of hydrochloric, sulfuric, or other strong acids.[32, 33] Treatment is similar to that described for alkali ingestion. Ferrous sulfate, commercial potash, pine oil cleaner, and calcium salts are among the other agents that are known to cause gastric damage.[34–36]

Drug-Induced Gastritis

Drug-related gastritis that occurs with over-the-counter or prescription medications is a poorly defined problem in pediatrics. NSAIDs, such as aspirin, ibuprofen, naproxen, and indomethacin, frequently cause gastropathy in adults.[37–39] Epidemiologic studies have documented a significant association with complications such as upper gastrointestinal hemorrhage and gastric perforation, often in asymptomatic adults.[40–42] In one of these studies involving 151 cases of gastroduodenal ulcers diagnosed by endoscopy, surgery, or autopsy, 21 of the 58 nonstress-related ulcers were associated with aspirin therapy.[43] More than one half (52%) of the aspirin-induced ulcers were gastric. Hemorrhage almost always accompanied the aspirin-associated ulcers. A similar correlation between hemorrhage and aspirin-associated gastric ulcers was also documented by Newman and associates.[44] Similar large-scale studies have not been performed in pediatric patients although smaller series have shown a correlation between these drugs and gastric problems similar to that documented in adults. The small number of series reported in the pediatric literature probably grossly underrepresents the magnitude of this problem (Figs. 32–3 and 32–4).

The pathophysiology underlying the gastric mucosal damage caused by aspirin and other NSAIDs is probably best understood by examining the effects of aspirin, which include a direct toxic effect on gastric epithelial cells and also a decrease in cyclooxygenase activity. The latter effect leads to a decrease in endogenous prostaglandin formation, which causes many effects, including decreased epithelial cell mucus and bicarbonate secretion, cell turnover, and mucosal blood flow.[8–11, 45] Subsequent to these changes, the mucosal defense barrier

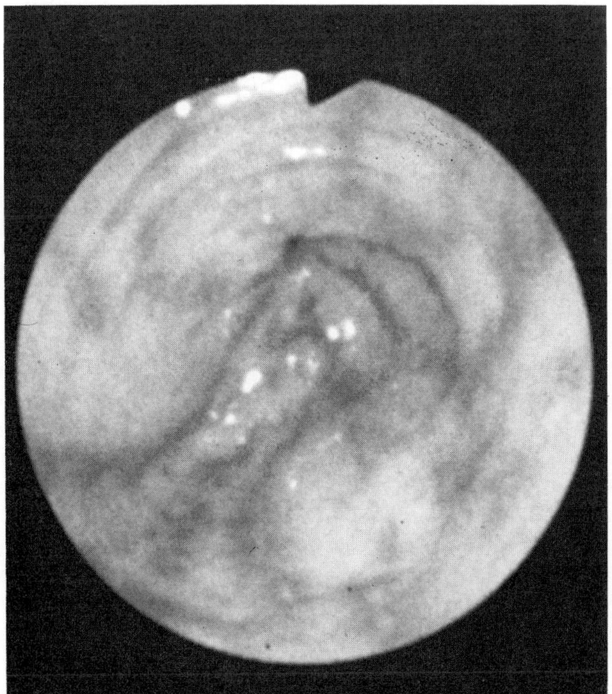

Figure 32–3. Antral linear hemorrhages and erosions in the prepyloric area in a child taking aspirin for rheumatoid arthritis.

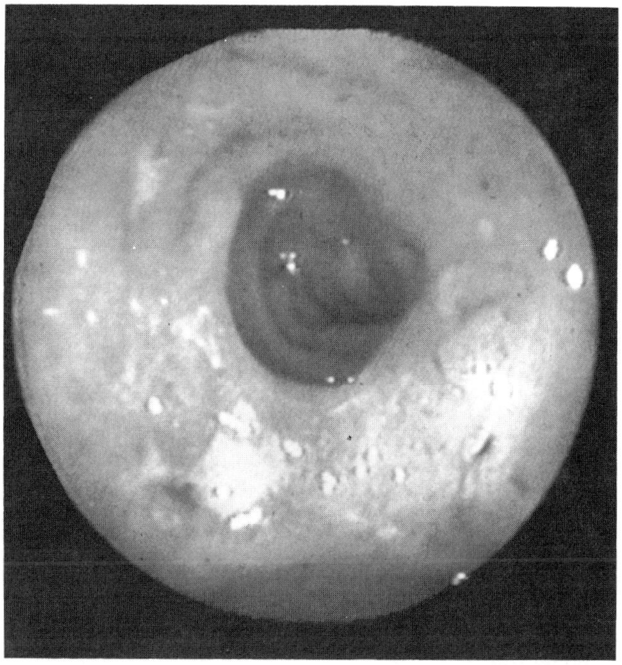

Figure 32–4. Antral ulcer in a patient taking aspirin.

is breached, with hydrogen ion back-diffusion being the initial step (Fig. 32–5).

Corticosteroids inhibit prostaglandin production by affecting a very early step in the prostaglandin metabolic pathway. In so doing, corticosteroids could theoretically influence all the gastric mucosal defense mechanisms affected by aspirin, but more profoundly than does aspirin. Conflicting clinical results, however, have been reported from various medical centers. A meta-analysis

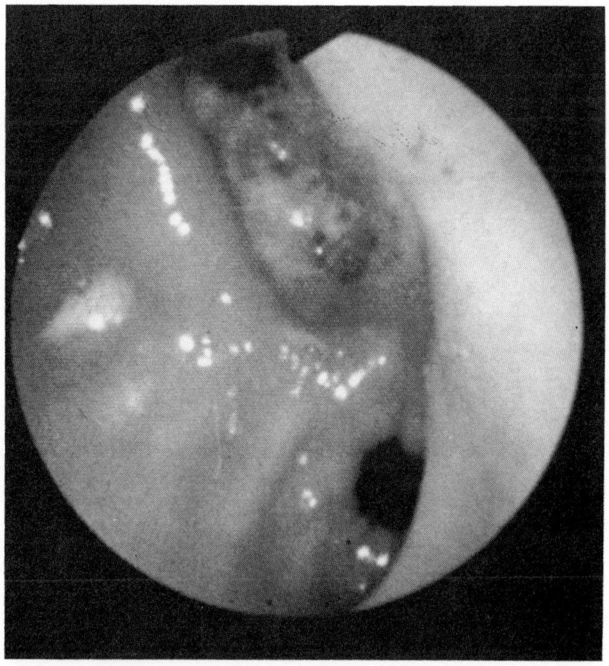

Figure 32–5. Antral ulcer and hemorrhages near the pylorus in a patient taking an NSAID for arthritis.

performed by Messer and coworkers[46] in adult patients examined the relationship between corticosteroid therapy and peptic ulceration or gastrointestinal hemorrhage. The data were pooled from 71 controlled clinical trials involving 3,064 patients. A relationship was found for both ulceration and hemorrhage, with the incidence varying directly with steroid dosage. No similar evaluations for pediatric patients have been reported, although there are statements in the literature that children experience gastric complications only rarely with corticosteroids.[47]

Other drugs reported to cause gastritis include penicillin, ampicillin, chloramphenicol, various cephalosporins, tetracycline, and valproic acid.[36, 48] The clinical presentation of gastritis with the latter two medications usually consists of feeding difficulties, particularly anorexia, refusal to eat, and vomiting. Gastritis is diagnosed by endoscopy, gastric biopsy, or both. Successful treatment has been undertaken with histamine H_2 receptor antagonists, antacids, or both. Valproate stimulation of central or peripheral gamma-aminobutyric acid (GABA)-ergic receptors, or both, is hypothesized to underlie the development of erosive gastritis in children through gastrin-stimulated increased gastric acid secretion.[48]

Ethanol can cause petechiae, hemorrhages, and erosions in humans (Fig. 32–6). In a volunteer study, Tarnawski and colleagues[49] showed that a single ingestion of 100 ml of 40% alcohol caused rapid endoscopic changes, specifically congestion and hemorrhages, within 5 minutes. Histology revealed epithelial cell exfoliation, lamina propria edema, and hemorrhagic changes associated with mucosal microvascular damage.[49] Laine and Weinstein[50] found subepithelial hemorrhages during endoscopy in 20 of 125 actively drinking alcoholic patients. Biopsies of these hemorrhagic lesions revealed superficial hemorrhage occurring primarily in the foveolar region, edema extending into the deeper gland region, and mild inflammatory infiltrates. Whether ingestion of less concentrated alcoholic beverages causes the gastric damage documented in these volunteers and patients is questioned by Kapzan and associates,[51] who found no correlation between gastric lesions and beer drinking.

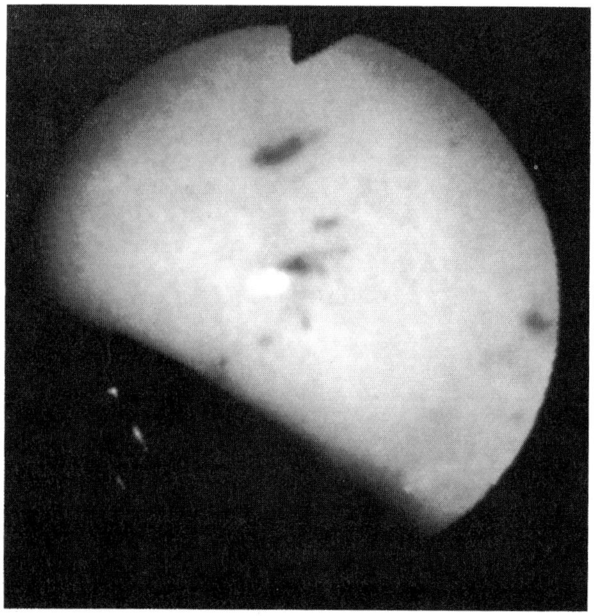

Figure 32–6. Submucosal hemorrhages in a patient ingesting 100 ml of 40% ethanol.

Ethanol has been shown in animal studies to have two distinct effects on the gastric mucosa. Extensive epithelial cell damage and exfoliation occur within 30 minutes of ethanol intake and are associated with a significant decrease in potential difference.[52, 53] Deeper mucosal layers also undergo damage involving the proliferative zone, deep mucosal necrosis, and vascular stasis.[54, 55]

Protein Sensitivity

Exogenous proteins can cause gastritis, particularly in infants who are fed cow's milk or cow's milk protein–based formulas. Erosive gastritis has been documented as the most frequent gastric pathologic condition.[56, 57] Chronic vomiting, failure to thrive, and gastrointestinal bleeding are the commonest components of the clinical presentation.[56–60] Kokkonen and coworkers[60] performed basal and maximal acid secretory studies in infants with cow's milk–associated antral gastritis. Maximal acid output was significantly decreased in milk-fed infants compared with control subjects (85 ± 78 versus 233 ± 66 μmol per kg per hour), and fasting serum gastrin levels were increased. When the offending protein was removed from the diet, the acid secretion parameters returned to normal levels. Therapy for cow's milk–induced gastritis consists primarily of removal of that protein from the diet plus additional nutritional support. Gastritis associated with soybean-based formula has also been reported.[61–63] Similar clinical presentations and pathologic conditions would be expected with other exogenous proteins. The exact pathophysiology underlying the relationship of gastritis with exogenous protein ingestion, although seemingly immunologic in nature, is unknown.

Eosinophilic Gastroenteritis

Eosinophilic gastroenteritis, a disease of unknown cause, may be associated with gastric inflammation (Figs. 32–7 and 32–8). The commonest clinical presentation is nausea, postprandial vomiting, abdominal pain, and failure to grow properly. An increase in serum immunoglobulin E (IgE) levels and peripheral eosinophilia are often present. Endoscopy usually discloses an erythematous, nodular gastric mucosal appearance, which is usually most prominent in the antrum. Histologic evaluation of the gastric mucosa usually reveals a dense eosinophilic infiltration. Disease severity is correlated with serum IgE levels.[63] Viral infections have been the most frequent source of infectious disease.[63] Specific therapy should be directed at infectious or dietary cause when these can be documented. Other therapeutic options include cromolyn sodium, cortico-

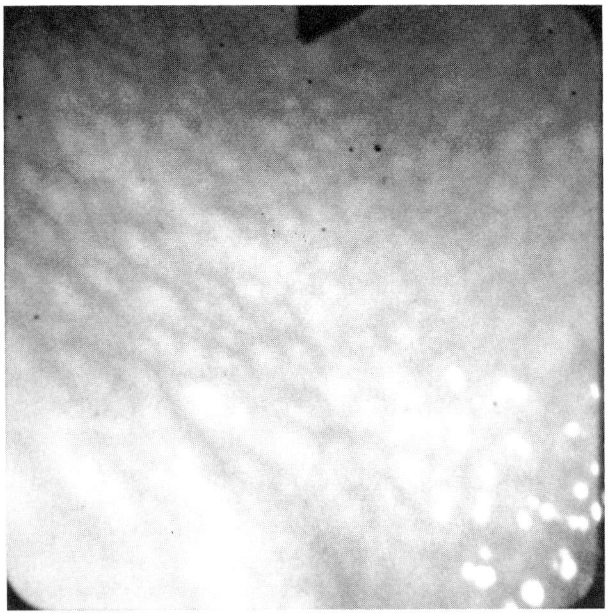

Figure 32–7. Appearance of erythematous nodular antral mucosa in an adolescent with eosinophilic gastroenteritis.

steroids, or both. The prognosis is relatively good, and mortality is rare, but prolonged treatment may be required.[61]

Infection

In adult patients, many gastric infections and infestations have been reported, including tuberculosis, syphilis, herpes simplex, cytomegalovirus, *Candida albicans*, histoplasmosis, mucormycosis, and parasites, such as *Anisakis* and *Strongyloides stercoralis*.[65–74] Most of these infections have been reported as a cause of gastritis in children, although the number of pediatric patients so involved is small in comparison with the number of adults so affected. Excluding *H. pylori* infections, gastric mucosal infections are rare, probably because of the antibacterial effect of hydrochloric acid and gastric motility. *Mycobacterium tuberculosis*, for example, has been the subject of a few isolated case reports and surveys.[75, 76] This organism, when it affects the gastrointestinal tract, tends to infect the ileum. It has been reported to affect the stomach in infants and preschool-aged children. The gastric lesions and the clinical presentation are similar to those in Crohn's disease. The diagnosis is dependent on a histologic study, in which acid-fast bacilli should be sought. Gastric washings are usually not diagnostic. Treatment is directed toward eradication of the bacillus. Syphilis, secondary or tertiary, has also been reported occasionally in pediatric patients.[76] The gastric mucosal appearance may vary from increased rugal folds to erosive gastritis and ulceration.[77–79] Since these mucosal appearances are not distinct, diagnosis is based on identification of *Treponema pallidum* in biopsy specimens and by appropriate serology. Treatment directed at eradication is associated with regression of the gastric lesions. Culture of *C. albicans* from the stomach has been reported in a number of pediatric populations, including neonates, severely burned children, and those with malnutrition.[80–82] These cultures were usually done on gastric aspirates. It is difficult to determine whether these organisms were pathogenic. In a group of elderly patients whose gastric ulcers had not healed after a therapeutic course of cimetidine, it was documented that the ulcer bases were colonized by *Candida*.[83] It was hypothesized that the organism was a pathogen in these cases, since all the ulcers healed after a subsequent 4-week course of nystatin. In contrast, in an Italian multicenter trial of 188 patients with gastric ulcers, 13 (6.9%) had ulcers considered to be colonized by *Candida*.[84] The healing of these ulcers was not affected by antifungal therapy. Similar therapeutic results were reported from a Danish study.[85] These conflicting results make the decision whether to use antifungal therapy a difficult one, particularly for the pediatrician, because similar clinical data in children are lacking. Such therapy should probably be reserved for the ill immunocompromised child who has not responded to conventional therapy. Fluconazole, a new fluorine-substituted, bistriazole antifungal compound, may be the agent of choice when such therapy is needed. It has the advantage over amphotericin B of being orally administered, with its absorption not being affected by food or high gastric pH.[86] The dosage used in immunocompromised children for candidiasis has been 6 mg per kg once daily.[87] Dosages as high as 12 mg per kg per day have been used, with increased hepatic transaminase levels in approximately 6% being the major side effect.[87]

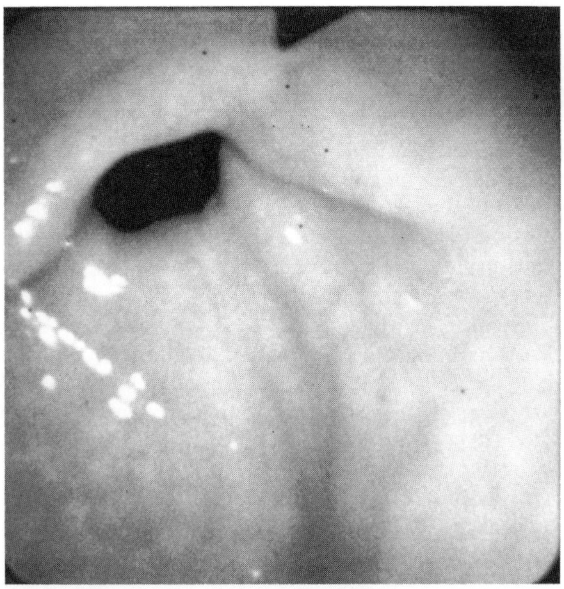

Figure 32–8. Erythematous nodular mucosa in the prepyloric area in a child with eosinophilic gastroenteritis.

Histoplasmosis as a cause of gastric mucosal damage has not been definitely established in either adult or pediatric patients. There have been no published reports of histoplasmosis in pediatric patients and only a few in adults. Orchard and associates[88] reported that any portion of the gastrointestinal tract can be involved, particularly the oral cavity. Hypertrophic gastric folds were reported by Fisher and Sanowski[89] as a manifestation of disseminated histoplasmosis. Culture of the organism from tissue is a requirement for diagnosis.

Mucormycosis associated with gastrointestinal disease is usually severe and often fatal.[90, 91] It is an invasive disease frequently associated with gangrenous lesions and perforations. Pediatric patients ranging in age from premature infants to children have been infected, with most of these being immunocompromised because of their age or primary diseases (leukemia). Therapy involves a combined surgical and chemotherapeutic approach.

Parasitic gastric infestations with *Anisakis* and *S. stercoralis* are rare, although the former infestation is becoming more frequently diagnosed in Japan, occasionally in association with bleeding gastric ulcers. There have been no published reports of either of these infestations with gastric mucosal abnormalities in children.

Several viruses, including varicella, cytomegalovirus, and herpes simplex, have also been documented as causes of gastric mucosal disease in pediatric patients. Published reports have also described isolated clusters of viral gastritis, such as the association of endoscopically documented hemorrhagic gastritis in seven children with hematemesis during an influenza A (H1N1) epidemic in Queensland, Australia.[92] The herpes zoster-varicella virus has been reported as a cause of gastritis in both adult and pediatric patients.[93–95] A case report from Houston, Texas, described a child presenting with fever, severe epigastric pain, anorexia, and a few vesicular lesions.[95] The child was receiving prednisone 45 mg per m^2 daily for treatment of nephrotic syndrome when the varicella eruptions began. Several shallow ulcers were noted on the soft palate. The vesicular lesions progressed over 36 hours to cover the entire face, trunk, and proximal extremities. The oral cavity also became more severely involved. An upper gastrointestinal series documented irregular serrations along the greater curvature and what was compatible with an ulcer in the prepyloric area. Anticholinergics and antacids relieved the symptoms within 96 hours. On the 10th day a repeat radiograph series was normal. The contribution of the corticosteroid to the gastrointestinal complication is unknown. That the herpes zoster-varicella virus can diffusely involve the gastrointestinal tract was reported in a Japanese study in which the virus was found in the liver, pancreas, esophagus, stomach, and intestine of two adult patients with leukemia.[96]

Herpes simplex can also involve the gastric mucosa,[96–99] although esophagitis is its commonest presentation. This infection most often occurs in patients who are immunocompromised. The clinical presentation usually includes epigastric pain, anorexia, nausea, and vomiting, in addition to odynophagia, dysphagia, or both. The gastric lesions are usually erosive.[97] Diagnosis is by biopsy, in which eosinophilic inclusion bodies are typical of this virus, and brush cytology. Specific antiviral therapy using acyclovir is indicated.[100]

Cytomegalovirus has been one of the most frequently reported viral causes of gastric mucosal abnormalities in children.[101–106] The infection seems to be commonest between the ages of 2 and 8 years. The clinical presentation is usually that associated with Ménétrier's disease: vomiting, ascites, and edema. The last two symptoms are secondary to the accompanying hypoalbuminemia. Radiography or endoscopy usually documents enlarged gastric rugal folds, although some studies have reported only gastritis.[103–105] Endoscopic biopsies reveal typical intranuclear inclusion bodies. The virus can also be cultured directly from these specimens. Therapy most often needs to be only supportive. The prognosis is usually excellent compared with the course in adults, with full recovery in 4 to 8 weeks.

Since no gastric mucosal lesion characteristic of human immunodeficiency virus infection has been found in adults, it is unlikely that any such lesion will be found in children, although no survey in pediatric patients has been reported. It is most likely that the lesions found will be secondary to infections with one or more of the following (as has been reported among adults with acquired immunodeficiency syndrome): *C. albicans*, cytomegalovirus, *H. pylori*, and herpes simplex.[107, 108] In these reports, nonspecific gastric lymphocytic inflammation was found when no pathogen was detected. Whether similar histologic findings would be present in pediatric patients without specific pathogens in the stomach is not known.

Crohn's Disease

Crohn's disease is an inflammatory process, histologically resembling tuberculosis, that can affect any portion of the gastrointestinal tract. Many publications have reported this disease's gastric manifestations.[109–112] Clinical presentation may range from no symptoms to epigastric pain when eating and postprandially, nausea, vomiting, and weight loss.[110–112] Hematemesis and melena are infrequently noted. Endoscopy may document mucosal inflammation, usually erosions and ulcerations.[109, 112] Mucosal biopsies are necessary for confirmation of the diagnosis and are often abnormal in patients with normal endoscopic findings.[109, 112] Histology reveals acute and chronic inflammation and, less frequently, noncaseating granulomas. In one study, 13 of 69 children with gastric Crohn's disease were diagnosed only following esophagogastroduodenoscopy and endoscopic mucosal biopsies, since the results of their barium upper gastrointestinal series were negative.[111] In this same study it was also determined that five children previously thought to have chronic ulcerative colitis did, in fact, have Crohn's disease. This change in diagnosis was based on the upper endoscopy and mucosal biopsies. It was recommended that such examinations be performed in all patients with ulcerative colitis before surgery is performed.[111] Therapy for Crohn's disease with gastric involvement does not differ from that usually employed for this disease (see Chapter 59).

Multisystem Disease

Gastric mucosal abnormalities have been reported in a number of multisystemic diseases that affect pediatric patients. A report of severe hemorrhagic gastritis in a 10-week-old boy with acute pancreatitis was made by Casaubon and coworkers.[113] This case is unusual, since the occurrence of major gastrointestinal hemorrhage accompanying acute pancreatitis is rare. An experimental prostaglandin (15-R–15 methyl PGE_2) was required to control the hemorrhage after H_2-receptor antagonists, antacids, sucralfate, and an elective vagotomy plus pyloroplasty failed to control the bleeding.

A number of diseases, hypothesized to be autoimmune in nature, have also been associated with gastritis. Four children with seronegative inflammatory arthritis developed persistent, severe nausea and abdominal pain.[114] Endoscopy with biopsies revealed antral gastritis and an increased number of mast cells in three patients. In the fourth patient, urinary histamine levels were increased. Gastric atrophy and atrophic gastritis in more than 30 adolescent patients with autoimmune thyroiditis (21) and nongoitrous juvenile hypothyroidism (10) have been reported.[115] Parietal cell antibodies were detected in eight of these patients, with achlorhydria being present in five. These patients also had many other possible autoimmune diseases, including atopy, diabetes mellitus, and collagen diseases. In an endoscopic biopsy study of 27 Russian children with systemic lupus erythematosus, Musaev and associates[115a] documented a high level of fibroblasts and inflammatory cells in the mucosa from the gastric body and antrum, pyloric bulb, and descending portion of the duodenum. Arteriolar walls in these areas exhibited IgG and IgM immune complexes during exacerbations, with decreased amounts during remissions. Inflammatory cell infiltrate increases were associated with progression of the primary disease. Henoch-Schönlein purpura is frequently accompanied by gastrointestinal symptoms such as epigastric or abdominal pain, vomiting, and rectal bleeding.[116] Tomomasa and colleagues[116] documented erosive gastritis and duodenitis, either alone or concurrent, in such patients. Vascular abnormalities similar to those found in the skin were documented in upper gastrointestinal mucosal biopsies.

Chronic Granulomatous Disease

Chronic granulomatous disease is often associated with a specific gastric abnormality—antral narrowing—in patients who develop upper gastrointestinal symptoms.[117, 118] This narrowing is associated with local granulomatous gastric wall thickening. Surgical resection was necessary in some patients, although others responded to antibiotics, corticosteroids or both. Some cases were associated with significant eosinophilic mucosal infiltrations, bringing into question whether these were some variant form of eosinophilic gastroenteritis. A case of subepithelial fibrosis involving the corpus was reported in a 15-year-old patient with chronic gastritis; this condition is in contradistinction to the antral involvement usually seen with granulomatous disease.[119] In this 15-year-old patient, erythema and nodularity were predominant in the corpus. Biopsies revealed chronic active gastritis with a strikingly thick collagenous band present immediately beneath the gastric epithelial cells. Treatment with H_2 receptor antagonists, sucralfate, and furazolidone was unsuccessful. Whether this disease process is similar to collagenous sprue is unknown.

Emphysematous Gastritis

Emphysematous gastritis, which is characterized by gas bubbles and thickening of the gastric wall, is a serious and often fatal condition caused by the presence of gas-forming bacteria.[120, 121] The condition is rare among adult and pediatric populations. Children usually present with significant symptomatology compatible with septicemia. The clinical significance of air within the gastric wall is great, with a mortality rate among adults exceeding 60%.[122] Treatment may include cessation of feedings, gastric decompression, broad-spectrum antibiotics, and nutritional support.

Bile Acid Reflux Gastritis

There continues to be ongoing debate regarding whether duodenogastric reflux of bile salts is a cause of gastritis in adult patients with an intact pyloric sphincter. Since there are few reports of bile acid reflux–associated gastritis in the pediatric literature, this review is based on published research involving adult patients. The association between bile acid reflux and gastritis development in the postoperative stomach is not discussed in this chapter; however, the mucosal changes associated with bile acid reflux found in the postoperative gastric remnant do provide valuable data for comparison with patients who have intact pyloric sphincters. The mucosal changes include foveolar hyperplasia, lamina propria edema and vasodilatation, and occasional acute and chronic inflammatory cells.[123] Using these criteria, Sobala and associates[124] evaluated 47 nonsurgical patients with similar, although less severe, histologic changes. Total fasting gastric bile salt concentrations were measured, and an assessment of cigarette, ethanol, and NSAID use was made. Gastric bile salt concentrations were not elevated, but increased NSAID use was documented. The conclusion was that the histologic findings were due to NSAID use, not bile acid reflux. In contrast, increased gastric bile salt concentration was documented in a Finnish study by Niemela.[125] In a symptom correlation study conducted by Meshkinpour and coworkers,[126] however, gastric bile salt levels were not increased. In this trial, symptoms were reproduced by infusion of the patient's own upper gastrointestinal contents into the stomach but were not reproduced by an infusion of bile salts alone. Nesland and coworkers[127] reported another study supporting the contention that bile acid reflux is not a significant clinical entity in patients with an intact pyloric sphincter.[127] In this study intragastric bile acids were measured in nonulcer dyspepsia patients and those with grade 2 or 3 antral erosive gastritis. There was no statistical difference found between these groups. Where do these conflicting data from adult patients leave the clinician who is dealing with a pediatric patient with the presumptive diagnosis of bile acid reflux–associated gastritis? The situation is far from satisfactory. A thorough histologic evaluation and complete history directed toward agents that might be causing the gastritis should be done. If no other cause is found, a fasting total gastric bile acid determination should be performed. If these acid levels are increased, a therapeutic trial should be undertaken with a compound known to bind bile salts. This approach may need significant revision if new data become available.

DIAGNOSIS

Upper gastrointestinal endoscopy has been shown to be a safe and accurate diagnostic technique for infants, children, and adolescents[128–133] (see Chapter 74). Many trials have documented this technique to be diagnostically superior to radiology, particularly for inflammatory lesions anywhere within the upper gastrointestinal tract.[129, 130, 134] These trials have also shown that erosive gastritis characterized by loss of vasculature pattern, hemorrhages, frank bleeding, and erosions is one of the commonest gastrointestinal diagnoses made in pediatric patients.[128, 130–132, 134] Although an endoscopic diagnosis of gastritis, particularly one erosive in nature, can be considered based on the findings discussed earlier, this diagnosis, as for all other types of gastritis, should be confirmed by histologic evaluation of endoscopic biopsies (Figs. 32–9 and 32–10).

Although not discussed in this chapter, such biopsies are also one critical method of establishing a diagnosis of *H. pylori* infection[135–137] (see Chapter 31). Multiple gastric biopsies should be obtained, regardless of the diagnosis being considered endoscopically. It is critical that all endoscopic diagnoses be confirmed by such histology, since studies have shown the correlation to be low between endoscopic and histologic diagnoses of gastroduodenal inflammatory lesions, except for perhaps severe cases.[138, 139] Newer techniques, such as radioisotope imaging and sonography, may prove to be useful adjuncts in the future but, currently, should be considered experimental.[140, 141]

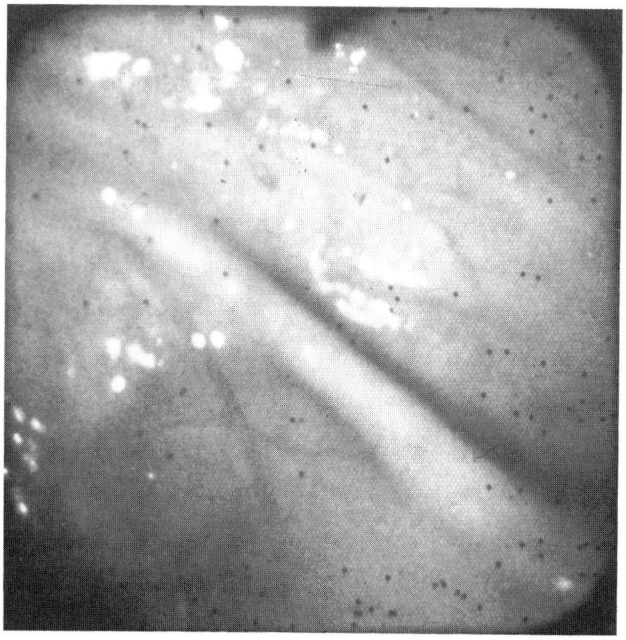

Figure 32–9. Normal antral and body mucosal appearance with a clearly discernible vascular pattern.

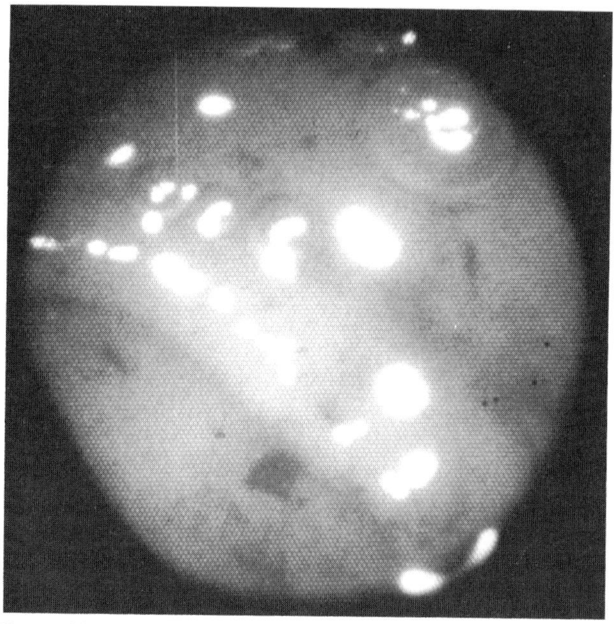

Figure 32–10. Gastritis of the antrum and the body with loss of vascular pattern, edema, and multiple mucosal hemorrhages.

Histologic evaluation of gastric biopsies, particularly those obtained by endoscopy, requires an excellent basic knowledge of normal gastric histology[142, 143] (see Chapter 29). Normal gastric mucosal histology involves two major glandular zones: (1) the fundus and body, containing fundic gland mucosa, and (2) the antrum, containing antral glands. Between these two major areas is a transitional zone, where glands of both types can be found.

In erosive gastritis, endoscopic biopsies usually do not provide specimens large enough to demonstrate the erosive lesions themselves and frequently contain only a nonspecific inflammatory component with a predominance of polymorphonuclear leukocytes. Specific diagnosis should be sought by looking for characteristic histologic patterns. With severe erosive prepyloric changes, the acute inflammatory element may be quite pronounced.[144] With increasing severity from grades 1 to 3, the incidence of acute inflammatory cells increases from 5 to 96%. Chronic inflammatory cells are also present in 50 to 90% of grades 1 and 3, respectively. Nonerosive gastritis can be classified into type A or B, depending on whether these changes are confined to the fundic or antral gland area, respectively.[145, 146] Often, the changes are found diffusely throughout both areas. The inflammatory component depends on the extent of involvement. In superficial gastritis there are chronic inflammatory cells throughout the glandular area and mild to severe gland loss. In gastric atrophy there is extensive gland loss but little inflammatory infiltrate. In all these nonerosive gastritis stages, the predominant inflammatory cell types are lymphocytes and plasma cells. Acute inflammatory cells are present in small numbers. Metaplasia resembling intestinal or pyloric mucosa may also be present in cases with severe nonerosive gastritis. It is therefore important that the endoscopist carefully assess the location from which the gastric biopsies are obtained and see that all specimens are accurately labeled.

TREATMENT

This section is limited to general principles of gastritis treatment. Therapy for *H. pylori*–associated gastritis is discussed in Chapter 31.

The treatment of stress-related erosive gastritis with major hemorrhage requires excellent supportive care, including intravenous fluids, blood products as needed, adequate nutritional support, and careful attention to hydration, electrolytes, systemic and central blood pressures, urine output, and respiratory function. As in most other areas of gastritis treatment in pediatric patients, clinical trials are limited, so extrapolation from adult data is needed. The specific goal of pharmacologic intervention is to maintain a gastric pH higher than 4 with antacids or H_2-receptor antagonists. The dosage used should be guided by frequent gastric pH measurements. Because of the decreased need for nursing intervention and accompanying reduction in costs, H_2-receptor antagonists have become the therapy of choice. Ranitidine and cimetidine have been evaluated most extensively in children. A ranitidine dose that achieves a serum range of 40 to 60 ng per ml suppresses gastric acid secretion by approximately 90%.[147] An adequate starting dose is 0.1 to 0.2 mg per kg per hour given as a continuous infusion.[148] Infusion adjustments should be made to achieve a satisfactory gastric pH ($\geq$4). A comparable dosage for initiation therapy with cimetidine would be 24 mg per kg daily. Adjustments should be made as described previously.[149] In children receiving other therapies involving metabolism by the cytochrome p-450 system, such as theophylline, consideration should be given to ranitidine use, since it has less effect on this system. With famotidine, a recommended initiation dose would be 0.3 to 0.4 mg per kg every 8 hours.[150] Prolonged intravenous use of famotidine may be associated with a decreased duration of maintaining intragastric pH lower than 4.[151] No similar nizatidine studies have been reported.

Oral antacid therapy for erosive gastritis has not been reported from any large clinical trials involving children. The palatability, constipation, and diarrhea problems with these agents make the H_2-receptor antagonists the preferable choice for oral therapy. Ranitidine and cimetidine given orally have been evaluated most extensively in pediatric patients. Cimetidine, at a dose of 20 to 40 mg per kg daily for 8 to 12 weeks, has been shown to be effective in healing inflammatory lesions of the upper gastrointestinal tract.[151–153] Ranitidine, at a dose of 4 to 6 mg per kg daily, has also been shown to be effective in healing such lesions.[147, 148, 154, 155] Ranitidine may be the drug of choice because of twice-daily dosing and less potential for drug interactions. Famotidine or nizatidine given orally for treatment of peptic disease of the upper gastrointestinal tract among pediatric patients has not been reported, except for famotidine's use in 17 severely handicapped Japanese children with reflux esophagitis, for whom an oral dose of 1 to 2 mg per kg daily was given in two episodes in patients weighing less than 10 kg and in three equal doses in others.[156] Reduction in vomiting, hematemesis, or both was documented in 15 patients within 3 weeks. The therapy was judged markedly effective in 29% and moderately effective in 41%. Five of 17 children so treated had transient mild elevations in aspartate aminotransferase and alanine aminotransferase.

Other general therapeutic measures include cessation of smoking and elimination of or decrease in ethanol ingestion. Removal of aspirin or other NSAIDs should be undertaken, if possible. Acetaminophen should be substituted to achieve pain relief. No dietary changes have been shown to be of benefit.

REFERENCES

1. Seneka BM, Sinha SN: Acute erosive gastritis in Port Moresby. P N G Med J 1984; 27:7–10.
2. Loof L, Adami HO, Agenas I, et al: The Diagnosis and Therapy Survey, October 1978–March 1983: Health care consumption and current drug therapy in Sweden with respect to the clinical diagnosis of gastritis. Scand J Gastroenterol 1985; 109 (Suppl):35–39.
3. Drumm B, Sherman P, Cutz E, et al: Association of *Campylobacter pylori* on the gastric mucosa with antral gastritis in children. N Engl J Med 1987; 316:1557–1561.
4. Meshkinpour H, Marks JW, Schoenfield LJ, et al: Reflux gastritis syndrome: Mechanism of symptoms. Gastroenterology 1980; 79:1283–1287.
5. Schrager S, Spink R, Mitra S: The antrum in patients with duodenal and gastric ulcers. Gut 1967; 8:497–508.
6. Blaser MJ: Gastric *Campylobacter*-like organisms, gastritis, and peptic ulcer disease. Gastroenterology 1987; 93:371–383.
7. Allen G, Garner A: Mucus and bicarbonate secretion in the stomach and their possible role in mucosal protection. Gut 1980; 21:249–262.
8. Leung FW, Robert A, Guth PH: Gastric mucosal blood flow in rats after 16, 16-dimethyl PGE_2 given at a cytoprotective dose. Gastroenterology 1985; 88:1948–1958.
9. Lichtenberger LM: Membranes and barriers with a focus on the gastric mucosal barrier. Clin Invest Med 1984; 51:573–583.
10. Lacy ER, Ito S: Rapid epithelial restitution of the rat gastric mucosa after ethanol injury. Lab Invest 1984; 51:573–583.
11. Robert A: Prostaglandins and the gastrointestinal tract. *In* Johnson LR, ed: Physiology of the Gastrointestinal Tract. New York, Raven Press, 1981, p 1407.
12. Curling TB: On acute ulceration of the duodenum in cases of burns. Med Surg Trans (London) 1842; 25:260.
13. Cushing H: Peptic ulcers and the interbrain. Surg Gynecol Obstet 1932; 55:1.
14. Couper R, Laski B, Drumm B, et al: Chronic varioliform gastritis in childhood. J Pediatr 1989; 115:441–444.
15. Caporali R, Luciano S: Diffuse varioliform gastritis. Arch Dis Child 1986; 61:405–407.

16. Green PHR, Fevre DI, Barrett PJ, et al: Chronic erosive (verrucous) gastritis. Endoscopy 1977; 9:74–78.
17. Lambert R, Andre C, Moulinier B, et al: Diffuse varioliform gastritis. Digestion 1978; 17:159—167.
18. Farthing MJG, Fairclough PD, Hegarty JE, et al: Treatment of chronic erosive gastritis with prednisolone. Gut 1981; 22:759–762.
19. Ménétrier P: Des polyadenomes Gastriques et de leurs Rapports Avec le Cancer de l'estomac. Arch Physiol Norm Pathol (Paris) 1888; 32:236–262.
20. Bloom RA, McQuaide JR: Benign hypertrophic gastropathy: Ménétrier's disease in childhood and adolescence. Clin Pediatr 1980; 19:533–535.
21. Marks MP, Lanza MV, Kahlstrom EJ, et al: Pediatric hypertrophic gastropathy. Am J Roentgenol 1986; 147:1031–1034.
22. Raic F, Votava A, Tambic L, et al: Hypertrophic gastritis in association with sepsis and death in a two-month-old infant. J Pediatr Gastroenterol Nutr 1988; 7:461–465.
23. Larsen B, Tarp U, Kristensen E: Familial giant hypertrophic gastritis (Ménétrier's disease). Gut 1987; 28:1517–1521.
24. Chouraqui JP, Roy CC, Brochu P, et al: Ménétrier's disease in children: Report of a patient and review of sixteen other cases. Gastroenterology 1981; 80:1042–1047.
25. Baker A, Volberg F, Sumner T, et al: Childhood Ménétrier's disease: Four new cases and discussion of the literature. Gastrointest Radiol 1986; 11:131–134.
26. Hebbel R: Chronic gastritis: Its relation to gastric and duodenal ulcer and to gastric carcinoma. Am J Pathol 1943; 19:43.
27. Kohli Y, Kato T, Suzuki K, et al: Incidence of atrophic gastritis with age in Japan and Canada. Jpn J Med 1987; 26:158–161.
28. Vaterlaws AL: Gastric atrophy in childhood. Arch Dis Child 1989; 44:710–714.
29. Postlethwait RW, Sealy WCL: Surgery of the Esophagus. Springfield, Il, Charles C. Thomas, 1961.
30. Dabadie A, Roussey M, Oummal M, et al: Accidental ingestion of caustics in children based on 100 cases. Arch Fr Pediatr 1989; 46:217–222.
31. Ragheb MI, Ramadan AA, Khalil MA: Corrosive gastritis. Am J Surg 1977; 134:343–345.
32. Poteshman NL: Corrosive gastritis due to hydrochloric acid ingestion. Am J Roentgenol 1967; 99:192–195.
33. Chong GC, Beahrs OH, Payne WS: Management of corrosive gastritis due to ingested acid. Mayo Clin Proc 1974; 49:861–865.
34. Gezernik W, Schmaman A, Chappel JS: Corrosive gastritis as a result of ferrous sulphate ingestion. S Afr Med J 1980; 57:151–154.
35. Brook MP, McCarron M, Mueller JA: Pine oil cleaner ingestion. Ann Emerg Med 1989; 18:391–395.
36. Cheili R, Perasso A, Giacosa A: Gastritis: A Critical Review. Berlin, Springer-Verlag, 1987.
37. Silvoso GR, Ivey KJ, Butt JH, et al: Incidence of gastric lesions in patients with rheumatic disease on chronic aspirin therapy. Ann Intern Med 1979; 91:517–520.
38. Aspirin Myocardial Infarction Study Research Group of National Heart, Lung, and Blood Institute: A randomized, controlled trial of aspirin in persons recovered from myocardial infarction. JAMA 1980; 243:661–669.
39. Lanza F, Royer G, Nelson R: An endoscopic evaluation of the effects of nonsteroidal anti-inflammatory agents on the gastric mucosa. Gastrointest Endosc 1975; 21:103–105.
40. Langman MJ: Ulcer complications and nonsteroidal anti-inflammatory drugs. Am J Med 1988; 84:15–19.
41. Laporte JR, Carne X, Vidal X, et al: Upper gastrointestinal bleeding in relation to previous use of analgesics and nonsteroidal anti-inflammatory drugs. Lancet 1991; 333:85–89.
42. Stodolnik E, Maurer P, Hoigne R, et al: Risk of acute upper gastrointestinal bleeding in patients with ulcerative disease and treatment with non-steroidal anti-inflammatory drugs (NSAIDs): Results from the Comprehensive Hospital Drug Monitoring Berne (CHDM). Euro J Clin Pharm 1990; 38:31–35.
43. Descos B, Hermier M, Foasso MF: Comparative study of four groups of gastroduodenal ulcers in children. Arch Fr Pediatr 1984; 41:399–404.
44. Newman LJ, Yu WY, Halata M, et al: Peptic ulcer disease in children: Aspirin induced. New York State J Med 1981; 81:1099–1101.
45. Ivey KJ: Gastrointestinal effects of antipyretic analgesics. Am J Med 1983; 75:53–64.
46. Messer J, Reitman D, Sacks HS, et al: Association of adrenocorticosteroid therapy and peptic ulcer disease. N Engl J Med 1983; 309:21–24.
47. Neidhardt MK: Monitoring of side effects in patients treated with corticosteroids or cytotoxic drugs. Monatsschr Kinderheilkd 1977; 125:53–60.
48. Marks WA, Morris MP, Bodensteiner JB, et al: Gastritis with valproate therapy. Arch Neurol 1988; 45:903–905.
49. Tarnawski A, Hollander D, Stachura J, et al: Alcohol injury to the normal human gastric mucosa: Endoscopic, histologic and functional assessment. Clin Invest Med 1987; 10:259–263.
50. Laine L, Weinstein WM: Histology of alcoholic hemorrhagic "gastritis": A prospective evaluation. Gastroenterology 1988; 94:1254–1262.
51. Kapzan B, Neumann P, Heilmann KL: Alcohol consumption and chronic gastritis. Leber Magen Darm 1985; 15:14–18.
52. Hollander D, Tarnawski A, Ivey KJ, et al: Arachidonic acid protection of rat gastric mucosa against ethanol injury. J Lab Clin Med 1982; 100:296–308.
53. Robert A, Nezamis JE, Lancaster C, et al: Cytoprotection by prostaglandins in rats: Prevention of gastric necrosis produced by alcohol, HCl, NaOH, hypertonic NaCl and thermal injury. Gastroenterology 1977; 77:433–443.
54. Tarnawski A, Stachura J, Ivey KJ, et al: Protection by prostaglandin against ethanol-induced gastric mucosal damage in man: An endoscopic and histologic assessment. Gastroenterology 1981; 80:1300.
55. Guth PH, Paulsen G, Nagata H: Histologic and microcirculatory changes in alcohol-induced gastric lesions in the rat: Effect of prostaglandin cytoprotection. Gastroenterology 1984; 87:1083–1090.
56. Coello-Ramirez P, Larrosa-Haro A: Gastrointestinal occult hemorrhage and gastroduodenitis in cow's milk protein intolerance. J Pediatr Gastroenterol Nutr 1984; 3:215–218.
57. El Mouzan MI, Al Quorain AA: Cow's milk–induced erosive gastritis in an infant. J Pediatr Gastroenterol Nutr 1990; 10:111–113.
58. Wilson JF, Heiner DC, Lahey ME: Milk-induced GI bleeding in infants with hypochromic, microcytic anemia. JAMA 1964; 189:122.
59. Walker-Smith J, Harrison M, Kilby A, et al: Cow's milk–sensitive enteropathy. Arch Dis Child 1978; 53:375–380.
60. Kokkonen J, Simila S, Herva R: Impaired gastric function in children with cow's milk intolerance. Eur J Pediatr 1979; 132:1–6.
61. Moss MH: Hypoprothrombinemic bleeding in a young infant. Am J Dis Child 1969; 117:540–542.
62. Tamir D, Levy J, Benderly A: Hypoprothrombinemia and bleeding in an infant on a soy bean diet. Harefuah 1972; 83:242–243.
63. Whitington PF, Whitington GL: Eosinophilic gastroenteropathy in childhood. J Pediatr Gastroenterol Nutr 1988; 7:379–385.
64. Konrad EA, Meister P: Fatal eosinophilic gastroenterocolitis in a two-year-old child. Virchows Arch [A] 1979; 329:347–353.
65. Sirk D: Primary tuberculosis of the stomach, caecum and appendix treated with antituberculous drugs. Br J Surg 1968; 55:230.
66. Butz WC, Watts JC, Rosales-Quintana S, et al: Erosive gastritis as a manifestation of secondary syphilis. Am J Clin Pathol 1975; 63:895–900.
67. Katzenstein AA, Maksen J: Candidal infection of gastric ulcers. Am J Clin Pathol 1979; 71:137–141.
68. Konok G, Haddad H, Strom B: Postoperative gastric mycosis. Surg Gynecol Obstet 1980; 150:337–341.
69. Orchard JL, Luparello F, Brunskill D: Malabsorption syndrome occurring in the course of disseminated histoplasmosis: Case report and review of gastrointestinal histoplasmosis. Am J Med 1979; 66:331–336.
70. Schulman A, Bornman P, Kaplan C, et al: Gastrointestinal mucormycosis. Gastrointest Radiol 1979; 4:385–388.
71. Campbell DA, Piercey JTA, Shnitka TK, et al: Cytomegalovirus-associated gastric ulcer. Gastroenterology 1977; 72:533–535.
72. Sperling HV, Reed WG: Herpetic gastritis. Dig Dis Sci 1977; 22:1033–1034.
73. Akasaka Y, Kizu M, Aoike A, et al: Endoscopic management of acute gastric anisakiasis. Endoscopy 1979; 2:158–162.

74. Milder JE, Walzer PD, Kilgore G, et al: Clinical features of *Strongyloides stercoralis* infection in an endemic area of the United States. Gastroenterology 1981; 80:1481–1488.
75. Vidal ML, Hortelano JG, del Castillo F: Abdominal tuberculosis in children. Med Clin (Barc) 1984; 83:650.
76. Singleton EB, King BA: Localized lesions of the stomach in children. Semin Roentgenol 1971; 6:220–234.
77. Anai H, Okada Y, Okubo K, et al: Gastric syphilis simulating linitis plastica type of gastric cancer. Gastrointest Endosc 1990; 36:624–626.
78. Beckman JW, Schuman BM: Antral gastritis and ulceration in a patient with secondary syphilis. Gastrointest Endosc 1986; 32:355–356.
79. Rosch W: Ulcerative processes of the stomach. Leber Magen Darm 1983; 13:194–200.
80. Kraeft H, Roos R: Bacterial colonization of the stomach in newborn infants with gastrostomy. Monatsschr Kinderheilkd 1983; 131:853–856.
81. Linares HA: A report of 115 consecutive autopsies in burned children. Burns Including Therm Injury 1982; 8:263–270.
82. Gracey M, Stone DE, Suharjono, et al: Isolation of *Candida* species from the gastrointestinal tract in malnourished children. Am J Clin Nutr 1974; 27:345–349.
83. Neeman A, Avidor I, Kadish U: Candidal infection of benign gastric ulcers in aged patients. Am J Gastroenterol 1981; 75:211–213.
84. DiFebo G, Miglioli M, Calo G, et al: *Candida albicans* infection of gastric ulcer frequency and correlation with medical treatment: Results of a multicenter study. Dig Dis Sci 1985; 30:178–181.
85. Gotlieb-Jensen K, Andersen J: Occurrence of *Candida* in gastric ulcers: Significance for the healing process. Gastroenterology 1983; 85:535–537.
86. Washton H: Review of fluconazole: A new triazole antifungal agent. Diagn Microbiol Infect Dis 1989; 12:229S–233S.
87. Viscoli C, Castagnola E, Fioredda F, et al: Fluconazole in the treatment of candidiasis in immunocompromised children. Antimicrob Agents Chemother 1991; 35:365–367.
88. Orchard JL, Luparello F, Brunskill D: Malabsorption syndrome occurring in the course of disseminated histoplasmosis: Case report and review of gastrointestinal histoplasmosis. Am J Med 1979; 66:331–336.
89. Fisher JR, Sanowski RA: Disseminated histoplasmosis producing hypertrophic gastric folds. Am J Dig Dis 1978; 23:282–285.
90. Michalak DM, Cooney DR, Rhodes KH, et al: Gastrointestinal mucormycoses in infants and children: A cause of gangrenous intestinal cellulitis and perforation. J Pediatr Surg 1980; 15:320–324.
91. Dennis JE, Rhodes KH, Cooney DR, et al: Nosocomial rhizopus infection (zygomycosis) in children. J Pediatr 1980, 96:824–828.
92. Armstrong KL, Fraser DK, Faoagali JL: Gastrointestinal bleeding with influenza virus. Med J Austr 1991; 154:180–182.
93. MacGregor GA: Herpes zoster of the stomach (letter). Lancet 1979; 2:1144.
94. Wislff F, Bull-Berg J, Myren J: Herpes zoster of the stomach (letter). Lancet 1979; 2:953.
95. Baker CJ, Gilsdorf JR, South MA, et al: Gastritis as a complication of varicella. South Med J 1973; 66:539–541.
96. Tashiro T, Masuda M, Saburi Y, et al: A clinical and pathological study on varicella-zoster virus pneumonia. Kansenschogaku Zasshi 1990; 64:224–230.
97. Howiler W, Goldber HI: Gastroesophageal involvement in herpes simplex. Gastroenterology 1976; 70:775–778.
98. Sperling HV, Reed WG: Herpetic gastritis. Am J Dig Dis 1977; 22:1033–1034.
99. Dahms BB, Rothstein FC: Mucosal biopsy of the esophagus in children. Perspect Pediatr Pathol 1987; 11:97–123.
100. Balfour HH Jr, Kelly JM, Suarez CS, et al: Acyclovir treatment of varicella in otherwise healthy children. J Pediatr 1990; 116:633–639.
101. Henderson SE, Sprague PL: A case of hypertrophic protein-losing gastropathy. Pediatr Radiol 1979; 8:261–262.
102. Stillman AE, Sieber O, Manthei U, et al: Transient protein-losing enteropathy and enlarged gastric rugae in childhood. Am J Dis Child 1981; 135:29–33.
103. Leonidas JC, Beatty EC, Wenner HA: Ménétrier disease and cytomegalovirus infection in childhood. Am J Dis Child 1973; 126:806–808.
104. Coad NA, Shah KJ: Ménétrier's disease in childhood associated with cytomegalovirus infection: A case report and review of the literature. Br J Radiol 1986; 59:615–620.
105. Floret D, Renaud H, Hage G, et al: Gastritis with hypoproteinemia in children: Relation to Ménétrier's disease and cytomegalic inclusion disease. Arch Fr Pediatr 1978; 35:82–89.
106. Roussel M, Dupont C, Sidibe T, et al: Benign hypertrophic gastritis associated with cytomegalovirus infection. Arch Fr Pediatr 1990; 47:271–273.
107. Sutherland LR, Church DL, Gill MJ, et al: Gastrointestinal function and structure in HIV-positive patients. Can Med Assoc J 1990; 143:641–646.
108. Hischel B: AIDS and gastrointestinal tract: A summary for gastroenterologists and surgeons. Schweiz Med Wochenschr 1990; 120:475–484.
109. Schmidt-Sommerfeld E, Kirschner BS, Stephens JK: Endoscopic and histologic findings in the upper gastrointestinal tract of children with Crohn's disease. J Pediatr Gastroenterol Nutr 1990; 11:448–454.
110. Mashako MN, Cezard JP, Navarro J, et al: Crohn's disease lesions in the upper gastrointestinal tract: Correlation between clinical, radiological, endoscopic, and histological features in adolescents and children. J Pediatr Gastroenterol Nutr 1989; 8:442–446.
111. Lenaerts C, Roy CC, Vaillancourt M, et al: High incidence of upper gastrointestinal tract involvement in children with Crohn's disease. Pediatrics 1989; 83:777–781.
112. Griffiths AM, Alemayehu E, Sherman P: Clinical features of gastroduodenal Crohn's disease in adolescents. J Pediatr Gastroenterol Nutr 1989; 8:166–171.
113. Casaubon PR, Vargas J, Ament ME: Protracted hemorrhagic gastritis in an infant recovering from acute pancreatitis. J Pediatr Gastroenterol Nutr 1987; 6:806–810.
114. Lindsley CB, Minter PB Jr: Seronegative juvenile rheumatoid arthritis and mast cell–associated gastritis. Arthritis Rheum 1991; 34:106–109.
115. Kuitunen P, Maenpaa J, Krohn K, et al: Gastrointestinal findings in autoimmune thyroiditis and non-goitrous juvenile hypothyroidism in children. Scand J Gastroenterol 1971; 6:336–341.
115a. Musaev SN, Novikova AV, Shershevskaia AIA, et al: The morphometric and immunohistochemical characteristics of the gastric and duodenal mucosa in systemic lupus erythematosus. Biull Eksp Biol Med 1991; 111:203–206.
116. Tomomasa T, Hsu JY, Itoh K, et al: Endoscopic findings in pediatric patients with Henoch-Schönlein purpura and gastrointesinal symptoms. J Pediatr Gastroenterol Nutr 1987; 6:725–729.
117. Griscom NT, Kirkpatrick JA Jr, Girdany BR, et al: Gastric antral narrowing in chronic granulomatous disease of childhood. Pediatrics 1974; 54:456–460.
118. Hirsch BZ, Whitington PF, Kirschner BS, et al: Isolated granulomatous gastritis in an adolescent. Dig Dis Sci 1989; 34:292–296.
119. Colletti RB, Trainer TD: Collagenous gastritis. Gastroenterology 1989; 97:1552–1555.
120. Udassin R, Aviad I, Vinograd I, et al: Isolated emphysematous gastritis in an infant. Gastrointest Radiol 1984; 9:9–12.
121. Rowen M, Myers M, Williamson RA: Emphysematous gastritis in a leukemic child. Med Pediatr Oncol 1976; 2:433–437.
122. Meyers HI, Parker JJ: Emphysematous gastritis. Radiology 1967; 89:426–431.
123. Dixon MF: Reflux gastritis. Acta Gastroenterol Belg 1989; 52:292–296.
124. Sobala GM, King RF, Axon AT, et al: Reflux gastritis in the intact stomach. J Clin Pathol 1990; 43:303–306.
125. Niemela S: Duodenogastric reflux in patients with upper abdominal complaints or gastric ulcer with particular reference to reflux-associated gastritis. Scand J Gastroenterol 1985; 115 (Suppl):1–56.
126. Meshkinpour H, Marks JW, Schoenfield LJ, et al: Reflux gastritis syndrome: Mechanism of symptoms. Gastroenterology 1980; 79:1283–1287.
127. Nesland AA, Rydning A, Berstad A: Intragastric bile acid concentrations in patients with erosive prepyloric changes. Scand J Gastroenterol 1957; 22:505–508.
128. Chang MH, Want TH, Hsu JY, et al: Endoscopic examination of the upper gastrointestinal tract in infancy. Gastrointest Endosc 1983; 29:15–17.

129. Gyepes MT, Smith LE, Ament ME: Fiberoptic endoscopy and upper gastrointestinal series: Comparative analysis in infants and children. Am J Roentgenol 1977; 128:53–56.
130. Cox K, Ament ME: Upper gastrointestinal bleeding in children and adolescents. Pediatrics 1979; 63:408–413.
131. Tam PK, Saing H: Pediatric upper gastrointestinal endoscopy: A 13-year experience. J Pediatr Surg 1989; 24:443–447.
132. Kochhar R, Misra VK, Tambi SS, et al: Upper gastrointestinal endoscopy in infants and children. Indian Pediatr 1989; 26:129–133.
133. Kato S, Saito Y, Harada Y, et al: Locations of peptic ulcers in children. Gastroenterol Jpn 1989; 24:476–480.
134. Tedesco FJ, Goldstein PD, Gleason WA, et al: Upper gastrointestinal endoscopy in the pediatric patient. Gastroenterology 1976; 70:492–494.
135. Kilbridge PM, Dahms BB, Czinn SJ: *Campylobacter pylori*–associated gastritis and peptic ulcer disease in children. Am J Dis Child 1988; 142:1149–1152.
136. Glassman MS, Schwartz SM, Medow MS, et al: *Campylobacter pylori*–related gastrointestinal disease in children. Dig Dis Sci 1989; 34:1501–1504.
137. Veereman-Wauters G, Ferrell L, Heyman MB: Trends in *Campylobacter pylori* in pediatric and adult antral biopsies: A 5-year retrospective analysis. West J Med 1989; 151:406–409.
138. Black DD, Haggitt RC, Whitington PF: Gastroduodenal endoscopic-histologic correlation in pediatric patients. J Pediatr Gastroenterol Nutr 1988; 7:353–358.
139. Elta GH, Appelman HD, Behler EM, et al: A study of correlation between endoscopic and histological diagnoses in gastroduodenitis. Am J Gastroenterol 1987; 82:749–753.
140. Stringer DA, Daneman A, Brunelle F, et al: Sonography of the normal and abnormal stomach (excluding hypertrophic pyloric stenosis in children). J Ultrasound Med 1986; 5:183–188.
141. Vasquez TE, Bridges RL, Braunstein P, et al: Gastrointestinal ulcerations: Detecting using a technetium-99m–labeled ulcer-avid agent. Radiology 1983; 148:227–231.
142. Owen DA: Normal histology of the stomach. Am J Surg Pathol 1986; 10:48–61.
143. Roca M, Truelove SC, Whitehead R: Proceedings: The histological state of the gastric and duodenal mucosa in healthy volunteers. Gut 1975; 16:404.
144. Nesland AA, Berstad A, Serck-Hanssen A: Histological findings in erosive prepyloric changes. Scand J Gastroenterol 1986; 21:239–245.
145. Whitehead R, Truelove SC, Gear MW: The histological diagnosis of chronic gastritis in fiberoptic gastroscope biopsy specimens. J Clin Pathol 1972; 25:1–11.
146. Weinstein WM: The diagnosis and classification of gastritis and duodenitis. J Clin Gastroenterol 1981; 3(Suppl 2):7–16.
147. Blumer JL, Rothstein FC, Kaplan BS, et al: Pharmacokinetic determination of ranitidine pharmacodynamics in pediatric ulcer disease. J Pediar 1985; 107:301–306.
148. De Angelis GL, Banchini G: Ranitidine in pediatric patients: Personal experience. Clin Trial J 1989; 26:370–375.
149. Chin TW, MacLeod SM, Fenje P, et al: Pharmacokinetics of cimetidine in critically ill children. Pediatr Pharmacol 1982; 2:285–292.
150. Kraus G, Krishna DR, Chmelarsch D, et al: Famotidine: Pharmacokinetic properties and suppression of acid secretion in pediatric patients following cardiac surgery. Clin Pharmacokinet 1990; 18:77–81.
151. Treem WR, Davis PM, Hyams JS: Suppression of gastric acid secretion by intravenous administration of famotidine in children. J Pediatr 1991; 118:812–816.
152. Thomson RB, Attenburrow AA, Goel KM: Cimetidine in primary duodenal ulcer in children. Scott Med J 1983; 28:164–167.
153. Somogyi A, Becker M, Gugler R: Cimetidine pharmacokinetics and dosage requirements in children. Eur J Pediatr 1985; 144:72–76.
154. Dimand RJ: Use of H_2-receptor antagonists in children. DICP 1990; 24:S42–S46.
155. Scorza A, Conti-Nibali S, Sferlazzas C, et al: Ranitidine in children with peptic ulcer and patients with pancreatic cystic fibrosis. Int J Clin Pharmacol Res 1990; 10:179–182.
156. Miyake S, Yamada M, Iwamoto H, et al: Effect of a new H_2-blocker, famotidine, in reflux esophagitis among severely handicapped children. Clin Ther 1987; 9:548–558.

Chapter 33

Peptic Ulcer in Children

JOYCE D. GRYBOSKI and MARY SUSAN MOYER

Although peptic ulcer disease may occur in 5 to 10% of the population at some time during life,[1] the incidence is far less in children. Estimates of ulcer frequency in children from large centers have increased two- or threefold over earlier figures.[2] This is due not only to increased suspicion of the disease but to the increased use of endoscopy in children.

Primary peptic ulcers are usually duodenal, and secondary peptic ulcers may be either gastric or duodenal. Primary ulcers may be associated with increases in certain hormones, particular disease states in which defense mechanisms are decreased, or increased gastric acidity, or they may result from direct injury to the mucosa. Although the symptoms differ, the end result is a circumscribed loss of tissue including mucosa, submucosa, and muscularis, which progresses to cause pain, bleeding, and even perforation.

Homeostasis of the gastric mucosa results from a fine balance between normal mucosal protective mechanisms and the aggressive forces of infection, injury, and acid and pepsin production (Table 33–1). In primary or chronic duodenal ulcer, pepsin and acid secretion is the major force contributing to acute and chronic ulceration. A discussion of the role of *Helicobacter pylori* in peptic disease is in Chapter 31.

ETIOLOGY AND PATHOGENESIS

Proteolytic Activity

Gastric function is initiated early; by the end of the first trimester the epithelium is differentiated into gastric pits and glands, which contain chief and parietal cells. Between 3 and 5 months' gestation, the fetal stomach is producing pepsin, cathepsin, renin, and acid, with enzyme activity greatest in the fundus. Enzyme activity increases throughout gestation, and after birth it rises sharply after the initiation of feedings.

Proteolytic activity arises from several enzymes of the aspartic-proteinase group: pepsinogens I and II and cathepsins D and E.[1–5] The inactive proenzymes are stored in the gastric mucosa and secreted as active enzymes, having optimal activity at a pH between 2 and 3. As endopeptidases the pepsins hydrolyze peptide bonds of proteins, particularly those formed by aromatic amino acids, which are the most potent stimuli of gastrin release.[6] Pepsinogen secretion is stimulated by cholinergic and beta-adrenergic pathways and by the gut hormones cholecystokinin, secretin, and vasoactive intestinal peptide. Secretion is inhibited by increased extracellular pepsin. Pepsinogen I is in greatest concentration in the fundus and body of the stomach and is increased in many patients with duodenal ulcer disease. Pepsinogen II is concentrated in the antrum, pylorus, and Brunner's glands of the duodenum and is elevated in antral gastritis.

In the neonate, although plasma pepsinogen is initially elevated, pepsin is present in only minute amounts in gastric secretion. During the first 4 months secretion increases until adult values are reached by age 2 years.[3, 4] The first study measuring mucosal pepsin in infants over 5 months, children, and adults showed no difference with age.[7] Highest levels are present in the body, but substantial levels are also present in the antrum. Duodenal mucosa contains pepsin, although in lower concentration than in the stomach. In the premature infant, stimulated pepsinogen secretion is dependent on gestational rather than postnatal age; meal-stimulated secretion is present in the first postnatal week in infants older than 31 weeks of gestation but does not appear until the third week in infants of 28 to 30 weeks' gestation.[8]

In addition to cleaving peptide bonds of dietary proteins, pepsin cleaves the glycoproteins of gastric mucus. If this barrier is disrupted, pepsin may attack gastric mucosa.[9, 10] It has been shown that the gastric juice of peptic ulcer patients contains more pepsin I in basal and stimulated samples than does that of controls.[11] Similarly, ulcer patients have high serum pepsinogen levels as well as increased total acid protease in the urine.[12, 13] Pepsin I has also been implicated in the etiology of gastric erosions induced by shock or by aspirin administration.[14, 15]

Gastric Acidity

Although hypersecretion of acid has long been considered a major factor in the etiology of peptic ulcer disease, it is also apparent that ulcers may develop in patients with normal or decreased acid secretion. A brief summary of gastric acid secretion is pertinent to

Table 33–1. HOMEOSTASIS OF THE GASTRIC MUCOSA

Defense Mechanisms	Aggressive Forces
Mucus-bicarbonate barrier	Alterations of gastric mucus
Mucus	Decreased duodenal mucus
Bicarbonate	Decreased duodenal bicarbonate
pH gradient	Disruption of pH gradient
Prostaglandins	Decreased prostaglandin synthesis
Inhibit gastric secretion	
Prevent deep tissue injury	
Increase bicarbonate secretion	
Preserve vascular flow	
Restore epithelial surface	
Other undefined cytoprotection	
Adaptive cytoprotection	
Epithelial resistance to mild injury	
Adequate circulatory flow	Decreased microcirculatory flow
	Bile reflux
	Increased pepsin
	Drugs, NSAIDs
	Stress
	Alcohol
	H. pylori infection

the understanding of normal and abnormal physiology.[16, 17]

Gastric secretion is constant in a basal state and is stimulated by the anticipation, taste, or smell of food. This *cephalic* phase of stimulation is mediated through the vagus nerve and provides one third to one half of the acid response to a meal. Activation of the second or *gastric* phase is by the presence of protein in the stomach, gastric stimulation, increased gastric pH, and distention. This constitutes one half of the acid response. The final or *intestinal* phase results from the presence of protein in the duodenum and contributes only 5% of total acid. Eventually, postprandial acidification of the stomach decreases acid secretion.

More than one billion parietal cells in the midsections of the oxyntic glands of the body and fundus of the stomach secrete acid. These cells contain the hydrogen ion pump, H^+, K^+ ATPase, which exchanges hydrogen for potassium ions across the apical membrane of the cell. Chloride ions move with potassium ions in exchange for secreted hydrogen ions. The parietal cell cytoplasm is stimulated through several pathways: neuroendocrine (acetylcholine) through muscarinic receptors, endocrine (gastrin) through gastrin receptors, and paracrine (histamine) through H_2 receptors. Stimuli may act synergistically.

Cholinergic agents and gastrin are effective in stimulating secretion by increasing cytosolic cell calcium. Histamine stimulates parietal cell function through stimulation of cyclic adenosine monophosphate (AMP), which in turn activates cyclic AMP–dependent protein kinases. Antral cell gastrin production is stimulated by cholinergic neurons and by noncholinergic neurons that release gastrin-releasing peptide. Assisting in the regulation of gastric secretion are the paracrine cells, which lie near the gastrin cells of the antrum and parietal cells of the fundus. These contain somatostatin, histamine, and serotonin receptors. Somatostatin inhibits gastric secretion, and its release is stimulated by low gastric acidity and by noncholinergic neurons. Somatostatin release is inhibited by cholinergic stimuli and by high gastric acidity. Serotonin (5-HT) activates cholinergic neurons and presynaptically inhibits release of acetylcholine.

Mucosal Protection

The major protective forces of the gastric mucosa are the mucus-bicarbonate barrier and prostaglandins.[18–30] The mucus-bicarbonate barrier is normally 10 to 20 times the depth of the epithelial layer. It serves as a barrier for the diffusion of high-molecular-weight pepsin, which is hindered by a gel-exclusion effect provided by mucous glycoprotein. The mucous cells of the stomach and Brunner's glands of the rat have been shown to contain subcellular organelles, which store hydrophobic material containing neutral lipids and phospholipids that are secreted into the mucous gel to provide a nonwettable lining for its surface to repel acid.[18] Bicarbonate is produced by the parietal cells at a rate approximating that of H^+ production and forms the alkaline tide of HCO_3.[22] The gastric and duodenal epithelium further secrete small amounts of bicarbonate.[20–22] In this mucous layer, protons diffuse toward the mucosa but are neutralized by bicarbonate to produce a pH gradient that remains functional until the pH falls below 2.[21] Mechanically the mucus protects the mucosa from lumenal trauma and protects it during re-epithelialization after it has been superficially damaged. In adults with peptic ulcer disease there is decreased polymerization of mucous glycoproteins as well as impaired duodenal mucosal bicarbonate production and an alteration of the pH gradient.[23–25] Bicarbonate production is normally stimulated by calcium and prostaglandins and is inhibited by nonsteroidal anti-inflammatory drugs, taurocholate, alcohol, and noradrenaline.

Prostaglandins, present in the gastric mucosa, inhibit histamine-stimulated gastric secretion.[16] They are also probably responsible for the phenomenon of mucosal adaptation in response to mild irritation.[22] Other functions are increase in mucus and bicarbonate production, prevention of mucosal barrier disruption, and, most important, maintenance of mucosal blood flow.[26, 27] Numerous studies have shown the protective effects of prostaglandins upon the gastric mucosa in preventing severe injury from ethanol, stress, aspirin, and indomethacin,[27–35] and it is possible that their synthesis is defective in ulcer patients.[30]

Gastric Secretion in Infants and Children

The gastric contents of the neonate are alkaline at the time of birth, probably due to the ingestion of amniotic contents, but acidify to pH 3.5 to 3.6 during the first hours of life.[36–43] Both basal and maximal acid outputs approximate 0.114 to 0.133 μg per kg per hour, respectively.[44] A few infants are achlorhydric or hypochlorhydric. By 48 hours the gastric pH varies between 1 and 3 but eventually stabilizes at 3.2. Early studies by Miller[40] showed a decrease in acidity at 10 days, which gradually rose during the third to fourth week of life. By 3 to 4 years of age, gastric secretion approximates adult values.

One third of premature infants have been shown to have alkaline gastric contents for at least 12 hours of life, and one fifth of these secrete little or no acid for the first 10 days.[41–43] Achlorhydria is most marked in the smallest prematures. Some studies have shown that the majority of prematures attain maximal acidity by 4 days, but others have shown a rapid increase in secretion at 6 hours followed by a gradual decrease over the next 14 weeks. Seabrook and colleagues[45] monitored 24-hour intragastric profiles in fed and fasted prematures (mean gestational age 31 weeks) at 40 days and showed the pH to be less than 4 the majority of the time and 2 or less for significant periods. Formula feeding elevated the pH for a mean of 72 minutes.

Stimulated acid secretion by betazole hydrochloride (Histalog) or pentagastrin provides a measure of cells available for maximal acid output.[38, 44] In term infants, Agunod and associates[38] showed low volumes of gastric juice, acid, and pepsin during the first day of life, which increased until the third week, declined briefly, and rose again after four weeks. In 1- and 2-day-old infants, the mean volume of gastric juice ranges between 6.9 and 7 ml per hour, with basal acid output (BAO) of 0.2 mmol per kg per hour.[37] This period of early low acid production has been further confirmed by studies using Histalog, which showed a decreased stimulated response persisting for four weeks.[38] Those using pentagastrin stimulation showed a failure of responsiveness only during the first 48 hours of life.[44] A secretory response to glucose and to formula feedings has been shown in one- and two-day-old term infants with BAO increasing from 0.038 to 0.064 mmol per kg per hour.[46] The response was weaker than that of older infants 6 to 31 months, who increased meal-stimulated output from 0.067 to 0.149 mmol per kg per hour.

Gastric acid output has been calculated largely as a function of age until 3 months, after which it correlates best with weight. In one study of 10 infants whose mean age was 21 months, maximal acid output (MAO) was 0.88 mEq per kg per hour for those of low weight and 1.62 and 2.02 mEq per kg per hour for those of medium and greater weight, respectively.[44] Studies of older infants and children show increases in MAO. Stimulated studies in prematures of mean birth weight of 1.9 kg have shown at 1 week, BAO of 12 μmol per kg per hour, which rose to 30 μmol per kg per hour by 4 weeks.[47] Pentagastrin-stimulated outputs were 21 μmol per kg per hour at 1 week, which increased to 44 μmol per kg per hour by 4 weeks. Acid secretion remained unchanged over the next 4 to 6 weeks. There was no difference in acid secretion between fed and unfed infants.

Gastrin

Gastrin is the hormone most intimately involved in the stimulation of gastric secretion.[48–51] Its release from gastric antral (G) cells is stimulated by dietary amino acids and proteins. Its release is inhibited by low intragastric pH, perhaps through somatostatin release by antral D cells.[52–55] Maternal gastrin levels at delivery (mean 67 pg per ml) are significantly higher than in the normal adult but fall to a mean of 50 pg per ml by 24 hours after delivery. Levels in the umbilical artery (105 pg per ml) and vein (107 pg per ml) are higher than values at 4 hours (76 pg per ml) and 8 hours (74 pg per ml) of life.[52] In another study, cord levels measured 135 pg per ml, with 13% being greater than 200 pg per ml. The authors were unable to correlate cord gastrin levels to type of delivery or Apgar score but found the highest levels in infants born to mothers with sickle-cell anemia.[54] In contrast to adults, in whom levels decrease after an 8-hour fast, levels of the neonate are not affected. Gemelli and coworkers[55] studied the contributions of gastrins 17 and 34 to this neonatal hypergastrinemia and found cord G-34 levels (163 pg per ml) to be higher than in adult controls and to increase at 12 hours to 225 pg per ml. Mean G-17 levels were similar to those of adult controls (29 versus 31 pg per ml) but increased significantly at 12 hours (48 pg per ml) and on day 4 (80 pg per ml). Several studies report increased gastrin levels after the first meal of glucose or breast milk, but others have not found such stimulation on days three and six of life.[57–61] Lucas and associates[58] have suggested that this initial hypergastrinemia accelerates mucosal growth and contributes to gut maturation.

In preterm infants, Hyman and colleagues[47] found serum gastrin levels at 1 week to be 64 pg per ml; these remained unchanged until 7 weeks, when they began to rise and reached to 157 pg per ml by 8 to 10 weeks. A similar course was reported in healthy term infants in whom levels measured 67 pg per ml at birth, 87 pg per ml at 1 month, and peaked to 162 pg per ml at 2 months, before decreasing over the third and fourth months. Over 22 months, levels gradually decreased but still remained higher than in adults.[61]

PRIMARY DUODENAL ULCER

Incidence

Although the true incidence is unknown, there is a suspicion that duodenal ulcer is on the increase in children. Eastham[62] has reviewed 16 publications involving more than 1,000 cases and states that large centers diagnose 3.5 new cases yearly. At his own center the detection rate has risen since 1970 from 1.5 to 5.4 per year.

Pathogenesis

As noted earlier, the combination of acid and pepsin is the major force in the development of peptic ulcer disease, although other factors such as psychological stress and hereditary predisposition are intimately involved in its genesis.

Table 33–2. GASTRIC ACID SECRETION IN CHILDREN WITH DUODENAL ULCER

	Concentration in mEq/hr			Concentration in mEq/kg/hr		
	BAO	*MAO*	*PAO*	*BAO*	*MAO*	*PAO*
Liebman[74]	2.3±0.8	17.1±2.8	18±3.3	0.06±0.024	0.53±0.09	0.571±0.098
Christie and Ament[6]	3.2±1.3	21.6±4.7	23.6±4.3	0.064±0.02	0.486±0.07	0.507±0.07
Euler et al[68]	2.1±0.58	9.58±1.7	—	0.08±0.01	0.86±0.28	—
Nord et al[115]	—	—	—	0.83	0.467	0.627
Tam and Saing[72]	—	—	—	0.165±12	0.55±0.16	—

Gastric Secretion. Although there is a good deal of overlap in the gastric acid secretion values of normal children and of those with duodenal ulcer (Table 33–2), most studies report an increase in maximal acid output (MAO).[63–70] Mohammed and colleagues[70] found the highest values for MAO and peak acid output (PAO) in those children requiring operation. Other studies suggest that although increased MAO often correlates with a poor prognosis, it does not always correlate with the severity of disease at the time of study. Although BAO is less often increased in ulcer patients, increases in BAO, MAO, and gastric volume have occasionally been found in children with ulcer, with BAO increased to 64 to 80 mEq per kg per hour.[68] In adults, increased nocturnal secretion of acid has been reported, but this has not been studied in children with ulcer. Causes of increased gastric acid secretion are noted in Table 33–3.

Gastrin. Mean fasting and postprandial gastrin levels may be normal or increased in children with peptic ulcer disease.[71–75] In one study of children with ulcer, fasting levels averaged 60.4 pg per ml as compared to 38 pg per ml in controls.[66] Stimulated values rose to 140 pg per ml in contrast to control values of 50 pg per ml or less.[73] Liebman[74] found fasting gastrin levels of children with duodenal ulcer to be comparable to those of controls, but postprandial levels of mean 68.7 pg per ml were significantly higher than those of children with gastric ulcer (50 pg per ml) or with recurrent abdominal pain (45 pg per ml).

Psychiatric Factors. Emotional stress is noted in the histories of 39 to 58% of children with chronic duodenal ulcer.[76–81] Several studies have examined the psychological traits of those with chronic duodenal ulcer and have found many children to be quiet, intelligent, overachieving, and passive, with underlying anger, frustration, and hostility. A poor interaction between family and peers was often identified. One study identified fear or loss of separation from an important figure, inadequacy, and over-reliance on a mother as important features in these children's lives. Actual loss of or separation from a loved one has been stressed as a precipitating factor in ulcer development in two reports involving 11 children.[79, 80] Ulcer may develop even in the mentally retarded who are asked to perform beyond their levels of capability. This has been a particular observation in two of our patients with Down's syndrome.

Genetics and Heredity. A family history of peptic ulcer disease is well recognized. In adult patients with ulcer, 20 to 50% report a family history of peptic ulcer disease. In children with ulcer the figures are even higher—25 to 62%—with first-degree relatives most often affected.[82–93] Males predominate, with 32% of fathers, 10.2% of grandparents, and only 8% of mothers having ulcer disease. In monozygotic twins there is a concordance of about 50%.[82, 83] Genetic studies suggest a higher heritability for children (0.91) than for adults (0.37).[84]

As in adults, children with ulcer have an increased incidence of blood group O, but unlike adults, do not have an increase in salivary nonsecretors of the blood group.[82, 83, 87] Histocompatibility antigen HLA B5 has been associated with ulcer in one study but has not been identified in others.[86]

In some patients peptic ulcer disease is associated with increases in certain biochemical or hormonal markers or with certain inherited diseases.[82–93] In one study of patients with early-onset duodenal ulcer and a strong family history of ulcer, two groups were identified: one with increased MAO and normal postprandial serum gastrin levels, and the other with normal acidity but an exaggerated postprandial gastrin response.[87]

Hyperpepsinogenemia I is another marker indicating genetic predisposition for ulcer disease. This was first described in a study of two large kindreds in which 50% of family members had hyperpepsinogenemia I.[88–90] In another study of 100 families with ulcer, 83% of the subjects were hyperpepsinogenemic, suggesting an autosomal dominant inheritance.[91] Tam measured serum pepsinogen in 14 patients with childhood duodenal ulcer, their parents, and 65 normal children.[92] In normals 3 to 16 years old, mean values were similar, averaging 53 to 60.9 ng per ml. Hyperpepsinogenemia (>90 ng per ml) occurred in 6 of 14 patients and 13 of 28 parents. All hyperpepsinogenemic patients had one or more affected parent. Although most hyperpepsinogenemic parents had affected children, not all did, suggesting an autosomal dominant inheritance with incomplete penetration.

Table 33–3. CAUSES OF GASTRIC ACID HYPERSECRETION

Zollinger-Ellison syndrome
Antral G cell hyperplasia or hyperfunction
Mastocytosis
Chronic renal failure
Hypertrophic gastropathy
Small intestinal resection—short gut
Hyperparathyroidism

Infection. See Chapter 31 for a discussion of *Helicobacter pylori.*

Pathology

The duodenal ulcer is a small circumscribed lesion extending through the muscularis mucosa, in contrast to an erosion that progresses only through the submucosa. Ulcers usually measure less than 1 cm in diameter and are located within the first centimeter or two from the pylorus. As described by Askanazy,[94] there are four layers of a peptic ulcer: (1) an outer layer comprising a superficial fibrinous coat of leukocytes and erythrocytes, (2) a zone of fibrinoid necrosis beneath this, (3) inflammatory granulation tissue containing blood vessels, and (4) the base, which is composed of fibrous tissue and extends beyond the margins of the mucosal defect. Immediately adjacent blood vessels show inflammation, endarteritis, medial hypertrophy, or even thrombosis. Ulcers may occur on the anterior or posterior walls of the duodenum. The former are more likely to cause free perforation, and the latter tend to penetrate into the pancreas.

Superficial injuries of the stomach are rapidly repaired by the upward migration of mucous neck cells; formation of a surface mucoid cap containing mucous glycoprotein, fibrin, and exfoliated cells; and the passive flux of bicarbonate-rich intestinal fluid. Healing of deep wounds requires both an inflammatory response and cell proliferation. Initially there are infiltration of macrophages and inflammatory cells, absorption of debris, synthesis of intracellular matrix, and new blood vessel formation. Active healing then occurs with epithelial cell migration over new granulation tissue and differentiation of epithelial cells. In chronic ulcer, healing often shows scarred mucosa with patches of atrophic epithelium and a few scattered glands. There is evidence that high acidity prolongs the initial phase of healing, but the trophic effects of gastrin accelerate it. Epidermal growth factor increases the mitogenic activity of the epithelial cells, as does gastrin.[22]

DISEASES ASSOCIATED WITH STIMULATION OF GASTRIC SECRETION

Antral G Cell Hyperplasia or Hyperfunction

It is becoming apparent that antral G cell hyperplasia and hyperfunction may well be two distinct entities: one with increased numbers of antral G cells, and the other with normal numbers of cells that are either hyperfunctioning or unusually sensitive to otherwise normal stimuli.[94–98] The results are similar, with somewhat elevated fasting serum gastrin levels and greatly increased postprandial levels, which may reach 200% or more of fasting values. Other findings are hyperchlorhydria and peptic ulcer. The hyperplastic form of the disease has been reported in several individual reports and in one describing four children who had only mild postprandial hypergastrinemia.[99] One child with the hyperfunctioning form had gastrointestinal bleeding at 10 and 11 months of age, and studies at three years showed normal numbers of G cells (112 ± 23.6 cells per mm mucosa) as compared with controls (82 to 141 cells per mm mucosa).[98] In this and in several other patients there was a strong family history of duodenal or gastric ulcer and an associated hyperpepsinogenemia I.

Zollinger-Ellison Syndrome

Zollinger-Ellison syndrome consists of marked gastric hypersecretion, peptic ulceration, and nonbeta islet cell tumor of the pancreas, with marked hypergastrinemia. The tumor, now termed a gastrinoma, may occur outside of the pancreas.[100]

The syndrome is rare in children, as indicated by a 1982 review in which data from 23 children were examined.[101] By 1984 Tudor's peptic ulcer registry had accumulated 38 cases of the disease in children, and it is estimated that approximately 50 patients have now been reported.[102] The disease is four times more common in boys than in girls. The symptoms are due to excessive gastric secretion stimulated by gastrin. The parietal cell mass of the stomach is increased three to six times, causing a marked increase in the basal acid output. Since the parietal cells are working maximally, there is little increase in acidity with stimulation. In the initial review of 28 children with the syndrome, most tumors were located in the pancreas, although two were in the stomach and one lay within the kidney.[101] In 12, a primary site of tumor was not identified. Metastases are usually to the liver. In preoperative studies in adults, computed tomography identified the tumor in fewer than half, but angiography identified it in 60%.

The symptoms are abdominal pain, vomiting, diarrhea, and even gastrointestinal hemorrhage.[100–103] The ulcers may be single or multiple and are located in the duodenum, jejunum, or both. A few may occur within the stomach. Endoscopic examination may reveal the conditions seen in a typical duodenal ulcer patient, but occasionally there are thickening of the gastric rugae and dilation of the duodenum. Any patient who responds poorly to conventional ulcer therapy or who has refractory disease or diarrhea should be evaluated by serum gastrin levels.

In a 21-year follow-up of 28 children, 14 had metastatic disease, and six of seven who had had less than total gastrectomy had died from complications of tumor growth and gastric hypersecretion.[101] Of the 16 who had had total gastrectomy, only one had died from tumor extension. This review suggests that in children, malignant gastrinomas are slow growing and compatible with relatively long life.

Systemic Mastocytosis

Systemic mastocytosis is a disease in which mast cells accumulate in the bone marrow, liver, spleen, gastrointestinal tract, and skin. In one review of 26 patients, 40% had abdominal pain and diarrhea, 28% had nausea and vomiting, and 24% had peptic ulcer disease.[104–106] Ulcer was presumably the result of histamine stimulation of the parietal cells. In a prospective study of 16 patients by Cherner and colleagues,[106] 80% had gastrointestinal symptoms of abdominal pain and/or diarrhea and nine had either a duodenal ulcer or duodenitis. Six patients had basal hypersecretion of acid, but maximal secretion was within normal range. Interestingly, plasma histamine levels did not correlate with the presence or absence of pain, and the quantitation of tissue mast cells also failed to correlate with symptoms. Pain disappeared in those treated with H_2 receptor antagonists, and follow-up endoscopy showed a decrease in disease activity. Serum gastrin levels were low, consistent with histamine-induced gastric stimulation.

Chronic Renal Disease and Transplantation

Renal insufficiency is associated with high levels of serum gastrin, since the kidney is the major site of gastrin degradation. Some patients have decreased gastric acid secretion, but others have hypersecretion and increases in serum cholecystokinin, glucagon, and gastric inhibitory polypeptide as well as increased gastrin levels.[107, 108] The majority of patients have normal basal and maximal acid output, although gastric acid secretion increases in some patients during dialysis. The incidence of peptic ulcer in adults with renal insufficiency approximates 10% but increases to 18% after renal transplantation. It has been speculated that this increase might be due to the combination of stress and corticosteroid therapy. Studies of 54 patients 6 weeks after transplantation have shown increased peak acid output and peptic ulcer symptoms in 30% of men and 10% of women. Four of six patients bled. Peptic ulcer did not correlate with blood urea nitrogen levels, hyperparathyroidism, or steroid dosage.[108]

Hyperparathyroidism

Hyperparathyroidism is a rare cause of peptic ulcer disease, and the association is due to the hypercalcemia that stimulates gastric secretion. Hypersecretion in patients with the multiple endocrine adenoma syndrome may also be due to gastrinoma.[109, 110]

Symptoms

As noted in an early review of peptic ulcer in children by Muggia and Spiro,[111] peptic ulcer symptoms vary with the age of the child and become more specific in adolescence.[111] Most primary ulcers in children under six years are gastric and affect boys and girls with equal frequency.[111–114] Later, duodenal ulcers predominate and there is a male predominance. One exception is a review of 27 children by Nord and coworkers[115] in which there was a male-female ratio of 1:1, with gastric ulcers predominating. In a study of 110 children with duodenal ulcer, the mean age at diagnosis was 11.3 years, with 46% having symptoms before age 10 and 15% having symptoms before age 6.[112] The average duration of symptoms before diagnosis is generally two years.

In the neonate the majority of ulcers are considered secondary to stress, although a few are considered primary with no identifiable cause. Nonspecific symptoms such as vomiting, feeding difficulties, and failure to thrive often herald the onset, but many infants present with upper gastrointestinal hemorrhage or perforation (usually along the greater curvature of the stomach) as the first sign of peptic disease. In infants several weeks to several months old, pyloric channel ulcer often mimics the symptoms of pyloric stenosis, beginning with vomiting that increases in severity until it becomes projectile. The disease may be complicated by the development of secondary pyloric stenosis.

The predominance of males is first noted in early childhood. The major symptoms of peptic ulcer disease in children are shown in Table 33–4. Recurrent abdominal pain is the major complaint of toddlers and young children. The pain may be generalized, periumbilical, or, rarely, in the right lower quadrant. Only a few children localize pain to the upper abdomen. It may occur at any time of day and is unrelated to eating or fasting. Nausea and vomiting are frequently associated complaints. In some children, upper gastrointestinal bleeding or even hematochezia may be the presenting complaint. We have seen several toddlers with feeding gastrostomies who developed fundal ulcers that were asymptomatic except for occult blood loss.

After the age of six, most ulcers are duodenal.[111–133] Pain becomes more typical with increasing age and is more often described as epigastric. It may be constant or intermittent and awakens the child from sleep during the night or early in the morning in up to 60% of cases. The pain usually appears within several minutes to an hour after meals and is relieved by food, milk, or antacid. The duration of pain is shorter than in the adult, often described as occurring in short bursts lasting less than 30 minutes at a time. Some children experience constant pain that is exacerbated rather than relieved by eating. Certain foods such as soda, spices, pickles, and spaghetti sauce are occasionally noted as particular irritants. One surgical series reported no preceding

Table 33–4. MAJOR SYMPTOMS OF PEPTIC ULCER DISEASE IN CHILDREN*

	Primary Ulcer (%)	Secondary Ulcer (%)
Abdominal pain	90	23
Nocturnal pain	51–60	—
Melena	37	82
Hematemesis	5	59
Vomiting	10	5
Perforation	0–2	28

*See references 2 and 111–130.

Table 33–5. MAJOR SYMPTOMS OF PEPTIC ULCER DISEASE IN CHILDREN ACCORDING TO AGE

	Neonate	Infancy	Early Childhood	Late Childhood
Hematemesis	+	+	+	+
Melena	+	+	+	+
Vomiting	+	+	+	
Abdominal pain			+	+
Failure to thrive		+		
Anorexia		+	+	

history of pain until presentation with bleeding, perforation, or gastric outlet obstruction.[72] Nausea is an important although less common symptom. Vomiting may occur immediately after eating but characteristically does not relieve the pain. Heartburn is a complaint in a few children, and headache has been mentioned in several reviews. Syncope from unrecognized anemia has been the first symptom in two of our adolescent females.

After evaluating data from 160 patients with ulcer-related signs and symptoms, Tomomasa and associates[132] found that epigastric pain and its relationship to eating, positive family history, vomiting, and bleeding were frequently found in ulcer patients, although no one symptom was statistically significant for predicting the diagnosis of ulcer.[132] The major symptoms according to age are listed in Table 33–5.

Differential Diagnosis

Many diseases mimic the symptoms of peptic ulcer disease (Table 33–6). Pneumonia can present as abdominal pain in the child. Giardiasis with its predilection for the duodenum and jejunum causes right upper quadrant or epigastric pain, with radiologic examination showing thickened duodenal folds. Distal esophagitis, gastritis, pancreatitis, and eosinophilic gastroenteritis often cause pain localized to the epigastrium. Right upper quadrant pain may also be due to biliary tract disease, ureteropelvic junction stricture, renal disease, and retrocecal appendix. Less frequent causes are spinal cord lesions, diabetes, Henoch-Schönlein purpura, and gastroduodenal Crohn's disease. Recurrent abdominal pain of childhood (see Chapter 14) can usually be differentiated from organic disease by its failure to awaken the child from sleep (with only 7% having nocturnal symptoms), its diffuseness throughout the abdomen, and the absence of vomiting or weight loss.[134] In contrast, the child with peptic ulcer disease frequently has tenderness to palpation of the epigastrium or right upper quadrant. Examination of the patient with his or her chin touching the chest tightens the rectus and differentiates muscular or functional pain from intra-abdominal pain, which lessens. Because the anorexia or vomiting associated with eating disorders must be differentiated from peptic ulcer disease, a detailed history of school or household stresses and weight concerns, as well as examination of teeth (for acid pitting) and knuckles (for excoriations induced by vomiting), should be undertaken.

Table 33–6 DISEASES THAT MAY MIMIC ULCER PAIN

Cholecystitis
Cholelithiasis
Crohn's disease
Ectopic pancreas
Eosinophilic gastroenteritis
Esophagitis
Giardiasis
Hepatitis
Pancreatitis
Pneumonia
Pyelonephritis
Spinal cord lesion
Ureteropelvic junction stricture

Primary Gastric Ulcer

Primary gastric ulcer is unusual, and undoubtedly many ulcers diagnosed in the past were associated with *Helicobacter pylori*[62, 135, 136] (see Chapter 31). In an extensive literature review, Eastham accumulated 317 cases of peptic ulcer, only 43 of which were gastric.[62] He notes that his group has seen only one chronic gastric ulcer in 500 endoscopic examinations.[62]

Gastric ulcers have been divided according to their location in the stomach: (1) those occurring in the antrum and often associated with duodenal ulcer, high acidity, and blood group O; and (2) those occurring in the acid-secreting portion of the stomach. It has been proposed that true gastric ulcers occur between the parietal cell area and the pyloric mucosa and are often associated with hyposecretion and blood group A.[135, 136] In adults, antral stasis with stimulation of gastrin and duodenogastric reflux are considered major factors in the development of gastric ulcer.

In children the symptoms of gastric ulcer are vague, with refusal of food, irritability, or anemia as the presenting features. In contrast with duodenal ulcer, epigastric or abdominal pain is unrelated to eating. Hemorrhage may occur in younger children.[137] The diagnosis is difficult by radiologic techniques, and endoscopy is usually required.

Complications of Peptic Ulcer

The major complications of peptic ulcer are hemorrhage and perforation. Hematemesis or melena are reported in more than half of reported cases, and bleeding can occur months to years after the onset of symptoms.[62] Perforation occurs in approximately 10% of patients: If anterior, it will result in peritonitis; if posterior, it will penetrate toward the pancreas, causing pancreatitis. Gastric outlet obstruction is an occasional complication in this country but is more often described in Indian children with ulcer disease.[133] Pyloric channel ulcer may cause a secondary pyloric stenosis. One 9-year-old patient with gastric outlet obstruction had failure to thrive and malabsorption that responded to medical therapy.[138]

Secondary Peptic Ulcer

Secondary peptic ulcers develop from decreased mucosal defense mechanisms or overaggression of one or more of the forces listed in Table 33–1. In children the majority of secondary ulcers are probably due to stress, although the increasing use of drugs, particularly the nonsteroidal anti-inflammatory drugs (NSAIDs), is causing an increase in drug-related ulcers. Since such ulcers are often silent until their presentation with perforation or hemorrhage and often occur in critically ill children, they are associated with increased morbidity and mortality. Half of these children require surgery. Complications are more often associated with acute duodenal than with acute gastric ulcers.

Acute or Stress Ulcer

In a survey of 29 hospitals in the United States and Canada, for which the diagnosis of peptic ulcer in children averaged 1.9 new cases per year, secondary ulcers were twice as common as primary ones, with acute gastric ulcers slightly more frequent than duodenal ulcers.[139] In infants, stress ulcers are related to sepsis, shock, traumatic delivery, respiratory or cardiac insufficiency, hypoglycemia, or dehydration. In older children they are more often due to life-threatening illness or follow trauma and often present as a terminal event. Ulcers may occur in the stomach, duodenum, or both. Generally they appear as a singular punched-out area with little surrounding reaction. Because of the rapidity with which they erode there is usually a lack of symptoms until the child develops a catastrophic hemorrhage or perforation.[140] In one series of infants younger than 11 weeks old, presentation in seven was hemorrhage or perforation, and nine had recurrent vomiting.[140] In a London review of 54 children, 30 had hemorrhage, 8 had perforation, 6 had shock, and 5 each had pain or vomiting.[139] In 34 of 54, ulceration was a terminal event.

Secondary ulcers occur with equal frequency in males and females. Death is most often related to the underlying disease, and the mortality is high, varying from 10 to 77%.[139–149] Ulcers within the duodenum are usually in the bulb but may occur in other locations. Krasna and colleagues[144] and Rosenlund and Koop[146] reported cases of duodenal ulcer confined to the second duodenum. Hsu and associates[142] described eight patients with irregularly shaped ulcers in both the first and second parts of the duodenum. All were infants or toddlers who had a preceding viral illness that was treated with antipyretics.

Curling's ulcer, which occurs in 0.5 to 13% of burned patients, may be the result of hemorrhagic gastritis, which occurs soon after a burn and is associated with normal gastric secretion.[150–152] Cushing's ulcer follows head trauma, encephalopathy, or surgery and is associated with gastric hypersecretion.[153, 154]

Because stress is associated with decreased microcirculation in the gastric mucosa as well as epithelial damage, new therapies using prostaglandins and the more potent antisecretory agents are being studied as replacements for conventional medical therapy.[155–157]

Drug-Related Ulcers

Infants with pulmonary hypertension and persistent fetal circulation who are treated with tolazoline are at risk for upper gastrointestinal bleeding from peptic ulcer, since the drug stimulates gastric and pepsin secretion through histamine release.[158] Increased gastric secretion may be associated with metabolic alkalosis through excessive gastric chloride losses.[159]

The relationship of corticosteroid therapy and ulcer disease remains controversial.[160, 161] Although a potential association was first noted in patients with rheumatoid arthritis, retrospective and prospective examinations of large numbers of patients have given conflicting results. Erosions or ulcerations have occasionally been reported in patients taking aminophylline and tetracycline.

Nonsteroidal Anti-inflammatory Drugs. Aspirin and other NSAIDs that cause gastritis and peptic ulceration in the adult also do so in the child. Implicated NSAIDs are indomethacin, naproxen, benoxaprofen, fenbufen, ibuprofen, piroxicam, tolmetin, and sulindac.[162–166] Although NSAID use is more often associated with gastric ulcers, it is a risk factor for bleeding duodenal ulcers as well. More than half of the carboxyl groups of aspirin are ionized at pH greater than 3.5, and all at pH 6.[163, 163a, 164] However, in acidic gastric juice, aspirin is not ionized and is rapidly absorbed and hydrolyzed to salicylic acid by esterases in the intestine, liver, and plasma. Aspirin and the other NSAIDs not only produce local injury but further affect the mucosa after absorption or when given systemically. Aspirin inhibits prostaglandin synthesis through inhibition of cyclo-oxygenase. It further decreases glycoprotein synthesis, changes the physicochemical nature of mucus and decreases it, and decreases bicarbonate secretion. Gastric secretion has been reported to be either increased or decreased. NSAIDs are further thought to increase production of inflammatory mediators such as platelet-activating factor, lipoxygenase products, and oxygen-free radicals through a shift of precursor fatty acids to certain metabolic pathways.

Animal studies have shown that gastric mucosal damage is dose dependent, with epithelial injury and hemorrhage occurring 4 hours after exposure; it becomes most pronounced at one week, but some changes are still present at four weeks. In response to injury, the mucus content of surface cells decreases, mitotic activity increases, and mucous and parietal cells migrate upward toward the lumenal surfaces while the epithelial cells exfoliate. Electron microscopy has shown disruption of the tight junctions of the mucosal cells. Salicylate injures the cell by decreasing mucosal adenosine triphosphate (ATP), causing cation fluxes, hydrogen back-diffusion, and a fall in transmucosal potential difference, but it does not inhibit cyclo-oxygenase.

There is vascular capillary damage, mast cell release of histamine, and plasma transudation into the lumen.

The mucosal blood flow, which is initially increased, later decreases. Epithelial proliferation is stimulated in the fundal but not in the antral mucosa. All these changes lead to the early development of petechiae, which clear within 1 week but are followed by the development of erosions. True ulcers do not develop until after one to three months of therapy. Of all patients taking NSAIDs, 20 to 29% develop gastric ulcers and 35 to 71% develop erosions.[162, 165] Diagnostically, McCarthy has attempted to distinguish NSAID ulcer from erosion, considering even a 5 mm lesion a true ulcer if it is three dimensional rather than flat.[165] In adults, a crude prevalence estimate is 13% for gastric ulcers and 11% for duodenal ulcers, as compared with 0.28% for the general population. In adults with rheumatoid arthritis, NSAID use is implicated in 20,000 hospitalizations and 2,600 deaths a years.[162] Adult patients taking 14 or fewer tablets of aspirin per week are not at risk, but those taking 22 or more are at increased risk for developing gastric ulcer. A similar dose responsiveness has been shown for ibuprofen and some other NSAIDs.[165] Impressively, Graham states that more than 10% of patients taking chronic NSAID therapy on any given day will have a gastric ulcer. It has further been shown that some NSAIDs delay healing of gastric lesions.[166, 167]

Tolerance develops in many patients with initial lesions and erosions. Clearing occurs despite continued therapy. NSAID-induced ulcers show only minimal inflammation or no evidence of gastritis adjacent to them in contrast to most other gastric ulcers.[166] It is suggested that patients with a previous history of ulcer or a family history of ulcer disease are at increased risk of developing NSAID ulcer. Since these ulcers are often silent, there may be no or few symptoms until they present catastrophically with life-threatening hemorrhage.

Ethanol Injury. Gastric injury by ethanol has been recognized since the nineteenth century. Ethanol in concentrations greater than 35% has been shown to cause focal areas of hyperemia, submucosal hemorrhage, edema, and necrosis.[168–171] Experimental studies in rats given 47% and 100% ethanol produced mucosal hyperemia within 1 minute of exposure.[168, 169] This was accomplished by dilation of submucosal arterioles, constriction of intramural venules, and mast cell degranulation. Specific microcirculatory studies have shown cessation of blood flow in the superficial microvessels, although they remained filled with blood cells, and there is an increase in microvascular permeability.[170] The reaction is thought to be due to release of leukotriene C4 and is inhibited by a lipoxygenase inhibitor and by prostaglandin E, although not by H_2 receptor antagonists.[171]

Duodenogastric Reflux. In the adult, duodenogastric reflux is considered a cause of gastritis and peptic ulcer disease, particularly when it is associated with delayed gastric emptying. Bile acids, lysolecithin, and trypsin are considered to be toxic to gastric epithelium.[172–175] In one study evaluating its significance in children, 1 hour fasting gastric juice from 49 children was analyzed for phospholipids (markers of bile), trypsin (marker of pancreatic reflux), and sialic acid (result of degradation of gastric mucus). Two children with gastritis and one with a prepyloric ulcer had elevated levels of one or more of the substances studied.[174]

OTHER DISEASES ASSOCIATED WITH PEPTIC ULCER

Several disease states common to children are associated with an increased incidence of peptic ulcer without documented hyperacidity.

Sickle-Cell Anemia. The most common cause of abdominal pain in children with sickle-cell anemia is vasoocclusion, with less frequent causes related to biliary disease, ischemic colitis, acute chest syndrome, functional abdominal pain, appendicitis, and duodenal ulcer. Perforated duodenal ulcer was first reported in a patient with illness in 1927,[176] and a 1973 review of 353 Jamaican patients noted duodenal ulcer in 7.6%, the majority of whom were males.[177] Studies have shown gastric acid secretion to be normal, with peak acid output lower than in ulcer patients without sickle-cell disease.[178] It is suggested that the etiology is actually vasoconstriction and occlusion with compromised healing of the resultant acute ulcer.[179]

Cystic Fibrosis. Although autopsy studies have shown an incidence of peptic ulceration in the stomach or duodenum in 8 to 44% of patients with cystic fibrosis, many were undoubtedly due to terminal stress ulceration.[180–182] Lloyd-Still[183] did not find an increased incidence in living children with cystic fibrosis despite decreased pancreatic bicarbonate production. A more likely estimate of ulcer approaches 2%. It has been suggested that ulcer is more common in black patients; Rosenstein and coworkers[184] reported ulcer in 3 of 25 black patients with cystic fibrosis. Gastric hypersecretion has been reported in one study but has not been substantiated in others.[185]

DIAGNOSIS OF PEPTIC DISEASE

The initial history and physical examination may suggest the diagnosis of peptic disease. Symptoms such as nausea, vomiting, early satiety, and pain that awakens the child at night as well as epigastric location, guarding, and occult blood in the stool on examination warrant further investigation. The two diagnostic options are radiographic imaging (upper gastrointestinal series) and upper gastrointestinal endoscopy. Flexible fiber-optic endoscopy can now be performed safely in infants and children[186, 187] and is particularly efficacious in diagnosing superficial lesions (gastritis, duodenitis, stress ulcerations) as well as localizing the site of upper gastrointestinal bleeding.[188] In one pediatric series of 89 patients with abnormal upper gastrointestinal series, 56 (63%) had normal upper endoscopies.[189] Conversely, in several other studies,[115, 188, 190] endoscopic evaluation of children with normal radiographic studies led to a pathologic diagnosis. In general, panendoscopy is diagnostically more sensitive and specific when compared to radiographic studies. Although a carefully performed upper gastrointestinal series may identify a significant proportion of duodenal ulcers, only about 50% of gastric ulcerations may be diagnosed radiographically compared to 80 to 95% with endoscopy.[115, 188]

Although endoscopy is the more sensitive study, an upper gastrointestinal series may be the initial procedure of choice in evaluating a child with chronic abdominal pain. The differential diagnosis of peptic disease in the pediatric patient is somewhat extensive, and the site of underlying pathology may be suggested on radiographic studies. A carefully performed upper gastrointestinal series may obviate the need for an invasive procedure, particularly in the case of duodenal ulcers. Certainly in the clinical setting of persistent symptoms and/or an equivocal or normal radiographic study, an upper endoscopy should be performed.

Diagnostic Radiography

A barium swallow with upper gastrointestinal series allows qualitative functional and anatomic evaluation of the upper gastrointestinal tract. A double contrast study, performed with air as well as barium, should increase sensitivity. A strict criterion for the diagnosis of an ulcer is persistent filling of the ulcer crater with barium (Fig. 33–1). In one series of 73 children with confirmed peptic ulcer disease, 64 (88%) were diagnosed radiographically; however 12 of 48 (25%) primary ulcers and 2 of 16 (12.5%) secondary ulcers required a repeat barium study for definitive diagnosis.[120] Again this supports an overall sensitivity of about 68% for initial radiographic diagnosis of gastroduodenal ulcers. Antral, pyloric, or duodenal spasm is suggestive but not diagnostic of peptic disease. In an anxious chid, a nondistensible or irritable duodenum may be normal. Deformity of the gastric antrum or duodenal bulb (Fig. 33–1) may indicate chronic disease but does not reliably differentiate active from quiescent irritation or ulceration. Gleason and associates[190] reported eight patients with histories of previous ulcer disease or surgery and antral, pyloric, or duodenal deformities on upper gastrointestinal studies. None of these patients had active ulceration documented on endoscopy.

Upper Endoscopy

Flexible fiber-optic upper endoscopy is more sensitive and, in most cases, more specific than radiographic studies. Not only can a specific lesion be identified and localized, but endoscopic biopsies may be taken as well. Particularly in the case of superficial lesions such as gastritis, visual assessment may not be sufficient to make a definitive diagnosis without histologic examination.[191] The patient should be stable and adequately sedated for this procedure. The only absolute contraindication to performing upper endoscopy is the presence of a perforation. Significant hemorrhage may hamper visualization, therefore, bleeding should be adequately controlled prior to undertaking endoscopy.

Endoscopically, primary ulcers are often single and appear as well-circumscribed craters with a diameter of 5 mm or more and are often surrounded by thickened and radiating mucosal folds (Fig. 33–2). They usually

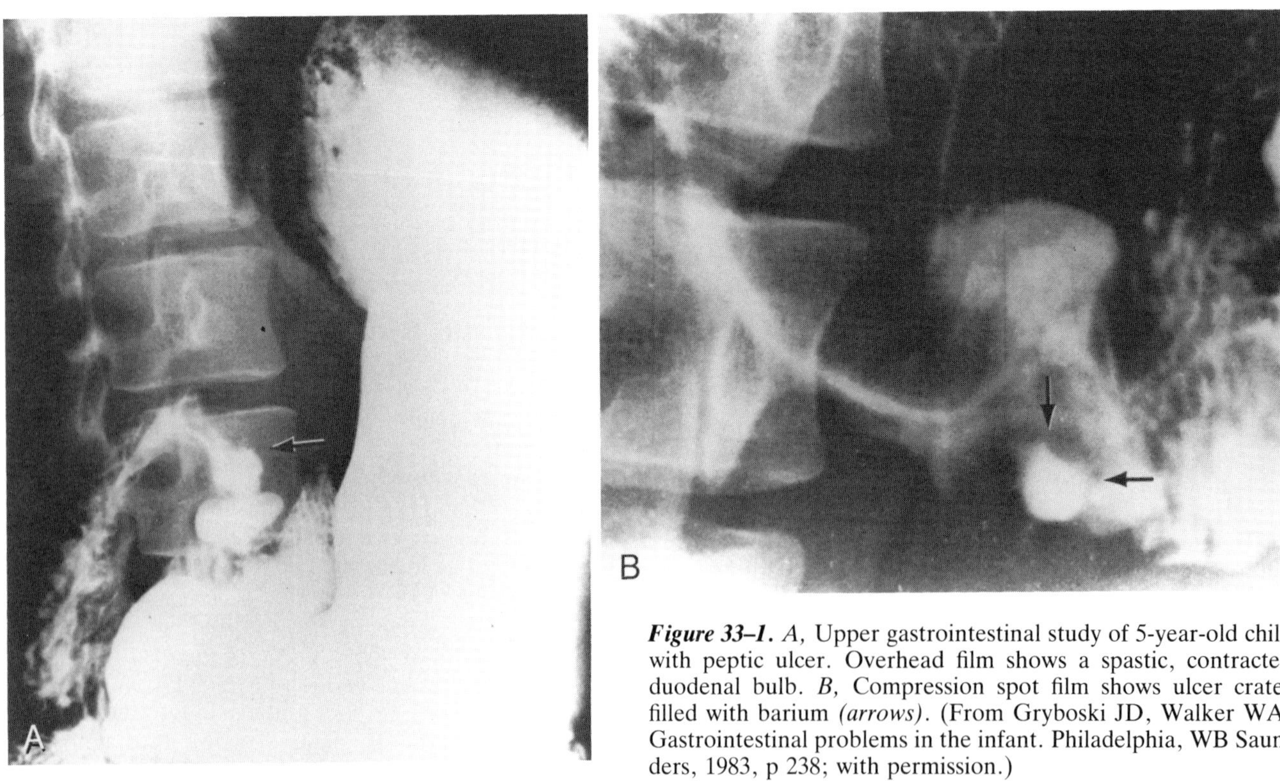

Figure 33–1. *A,* Upper gastrointestinal study of 5-year-old child with peptic ulcer. Overhead film shows a spastic, contracted duodenal bulb. *B,* Compression spot film shows ulcer crater filled with barium *(arrows)*. (From Gryboski JD, Walker WA: Gastrointestinal problems in the infant. Philadelphia, WB Saunders, 1983, p 238; with permission.)

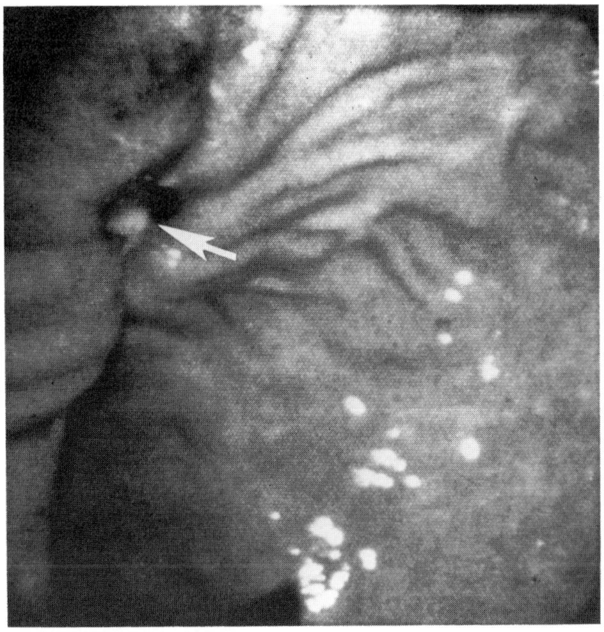

Figure 33–2. Primary peptic ulcer—proximal duodenum.

occur in the gastric antrum or proximal duodenum. Although the vast majority of primary ulcers in children are benign, some advocate biopsy of all gastric ulcers for a histologic diagnosis.[186, 192] Secondary ulcerations may be multiple and more superficial than primary ulcers (Fig. 33–3). Evidence of underlying gastritis or duodenitis is usually not present. Gastric erosions (Fig. 33–4) may also be identified as mucosal lesions that are somewhat smaller than frank ulcers and that are, on biopsy, superficial to the muscularis mucosae.

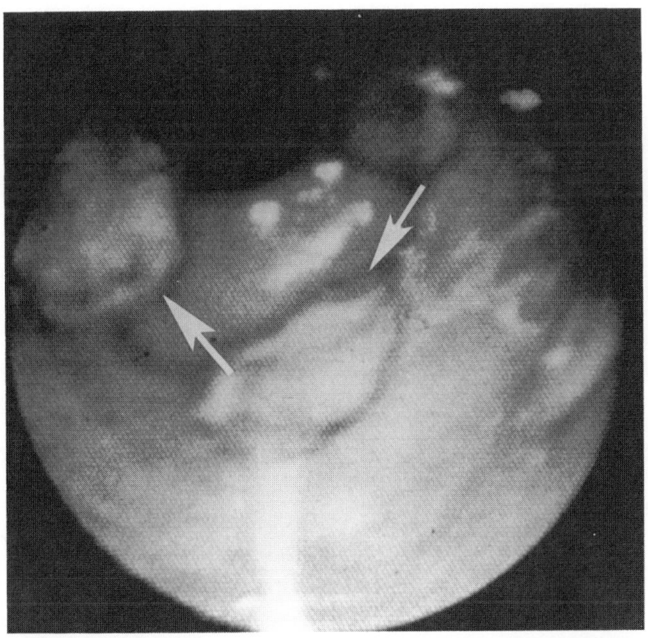

Figure 33–3. Secondary peptic ulcers—gastric antrum. (From Gryboski JD: Peptic ulcer disease in children. Pediatr Rev. Reproduced by permission of Pediatrics in Review, vol 12, p 16. Copyright 1990.)

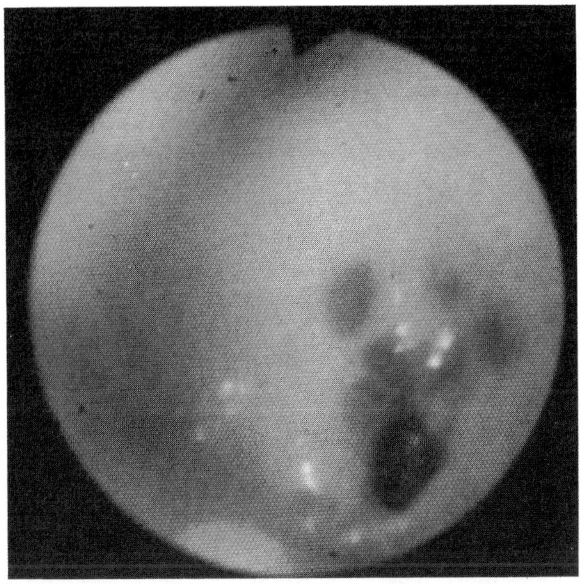

Figure 33–4. Aspirin-induced gastric erosions.

Endoscopy may also provide important prognostic information as well as allow therapeutic intervention in selected cases. In a series of adults,[193] the presence of a visible vessel in the ulcer crater was associated with a significant risk of rebleeding (56%) compared with those with oozing (8%) or those without signs of active hemorrhage (0%). Interventional procedures such as laser photocoagulation and electrocautery (bipolar) have been used with variable success in adult patients for control of bleeding or prevention of rebleeding.[194, 195] There are currently no published series on the efficacy or safety of these therapies in the pediatric population, and they should therefore be restricted to carefully selected situations or to well-controlled clinical trials.

Additional Evaluation

In the clinical setting of recurrent or persistent peptic ulcerations refractory to medical management or multiple ulcers identified in locations removed from the immediate pre- or postpyloric area, further evaluation is indicated. A baseline fasting serum gastrin can be obtained to identify patients with hypergastrinemia. Antacid medications should be discontinued prior to the test. Although there are several clinical situations of hyperchlorhydria in which serum gastrin may be elevated (see Table 33–3), most may be eliminated on the basis of history, physical examination, or routine laboratory evaluation. Those that require further testing are Zollinger-Ellison syndrome and antral G cell hyperfunction or hyperplasia.[95, 97, 196, 197] These conditions, though rare, have been reported in children,[98, 102, 103, 198] and the diagnosis should be pursued in the appropriate clinical setting.

In Zollinger-Ellison syndrome, fasting serum gastrin levels are usually greater than 150 pg per ml and may rise into the thousands. Antral G cell hyperplasia is

Table 33–7 FEATURES OF HYPERGASTRINEMIC CONDITIONS ASSOCIATED WITH INCREASED BASAL ACID OUTPUT[196]

	Zollinger-Ellison Syndrome	Antral G Cell Hyperplasia	Antral G Cell Hyperfunction
Serum gastrin level			
Fasting	↑↑↑	↑	↑
Postprandial	NC, ↓, ↑<50%	↑↑↑ (>100%)	↑↑↑ (>100%)
Secretin test	↑↑↑	NC, ↓, slight ↑	NC, ↓, slight ↑
Antral G cells		Increased	Normal
Hyperpepsinogenemia I	−	−	+
Gastrinoma	+	−	−

NC = no change.

suggested by an increased number of gastrin immunoreactive cells on biopsy, and antral G cell hyperfunction has been associated with hyperpepsinogenemia I, a familial condition with autosomal dominant inheritance.[90, 199, 200] Several provocative tests are currently in use that may help establish the diagnosis (Table 33–7).[196, 197] The calcium infusion test is administered over 3 hours in a dosage of 15 mg per kg.[201] Patients with a gastrinoma will have a threefold increase in gastrin levels or the levels will rise to greater than 500 pg per ml, whereas normal individuals will show little or no change. The secretin infusion test is probably even more sensitive and has largely replaced the calcium infusion test. After a dose of 3 μg per kg per hour, serum gastrin and gastric acidity will increase in the patient with a gastrinoma; in the duodenal ulcer patient, gastric acid output is inhibited by secretin.[202] In addition, patients with antral G cell hyperfunction or hyperplasia will also demonstrate no change, a decrease, or only a negligible increase in serum gastrin following secretin administration. Gastrin response to a standard meal may also aid in the differential diagnosis. The presence of antral G cell hyperfunction or hyperplasia will result in a very exaggerated postprandial rise (>100%) in serum gastrin, whereas patients with Zollinger-Ellison syndrome will have a decrease, no change, or no more than a 50% increase.[196, 197]

Formal basal and stimulated gastric acid output studies are difficult to perform in infants and young children and are rarely utilized outside of study protocols. However, monitoring gastric pH with an indwelling probe over a 12- to 24-hour period may be useful to assess therapeutic efficacy of a specific medical regimen in refractory or recurrent disease if no other etiology is identified.

MANAGEMENT OF PEPTIC DISEASE

Primary Ulcer Disease

Therapy in peptic ulcer disease is generally aimed at preventing further acid- and pepsin-related damage and thereby allowing the ulcer to heal. This may be accomplished by (1) neutralizing acid, (2) inhibiting acid secretion, (3) providing a protective barrier, or (4) enhancing the normal mucosal defense mechanisms (Table 33–8). The majority of treatment regimens have been modified from studies in adults, since well-controlled clinical trials in pediatric patients have not been performed. There are, however, several series that support the efficacy of similar therapeutic approaches in infants and children. Although pediatric doses are relatively well documented for a number of the frequently used medications, optimum dosing of others remains to be established (Table 33–9).

Acid Neutralization

Antacids. The therapeutic efficacy of antacids is based on their ability to decrease hydrogen concentration, thereby buffering gastric acidity. There are numerous antacids that vary in composition and potency.[203] The most commonly used preparations are a combination of magnesium and aluminum hydroxide. In general, calcium carbonate antacids are avoided because of the potential for acid rebound. When given in therapeutic doses, 1 and 3 hours after meals and at bedtime, antacids have been shown to be better than placebos in duodenal

Table 33–8 THERAPEUTIC AGENTS IN PEPTIC ULCER DISEASE: MECHANISMS OF ACTION

Acid Control
- Neutralization
  - Antacids
- Suppression
  - H_2 receptor blockers
    - Cimetidine
    - Ranitidine
    - Famotidine
    - Nizatidine
  - Anticholinergics
    - Pirenzepine
  - Proton pump inhibitors
    - Omeprazole
  - Prostaglandins
    - Misoprostol

Barrier/Binding
- Sucralfate
- Bismuth compounds
- (Prostaglandins)

Enhanced Mucosal Defense
- Prostaglandins
- (Sucralfate)
- (Bismuth compounds)

Parentheses indicate agents whose therapeutic effects may involve the mechanism of action listed.

Table 33–9 PEPTIC ULCER THERAPY: SELECTED AGENTS AND SUGGESTED ORAL DOSES

Medication	Adult Dose	Pediatric Dose
Antacids	30 ml (regular strength) 1 and 3 hr after meals and at bedtime	0.5–1 ml/kg/dose 1 and 3 hr after meals and at bedtime
Cimetidine	300 mg QID or 400 mg BID	20–40 mg/kg/day divided into QID or BID doses*
Ranitidine	150 mg BID	2–3 mg/kg/dose BID (children)† TID (infants)‡
Omeprazole	20–40 mg daily	No guidelines established
Sucralfate	1 gm QID	250 mg QID (infants)§ 0.5–1 gm QID (children)

*Efficacy of the BID dose has not been established in pediatric patients.
†May require TID dosing.
‡Neonates should be started on the lower dose.
§No pharmacokinetic studies in pediatric patients available.
From references 198, 206, 209, 210, 212, and 276.

ulcer disease.[204] They are also effective when used as maintenance therapy.[205] It has been suggested that liquid antacids have a better buffering capacity than tablets, but this has not been well established. Unfortunately, although antacids are generally well tolerated with few significant side effects, the need for frequent administration makes patient compliance difficult. They also may alter the bioavailability of other drugs either by directly binding the drug or by decreasing gastric acidity and modifying absorption of the drug (Table 33–10).

Reduction of Acid Secretion. Gastric acid production may be decreased by blocking either histamine receptors or parietal cells (anticholinergics), by inactivating intracellular mechanisms of acid production (prostaglandins), or by inhibiting the proton pump (omeprazole). Of these agents, H_2 receptor blockers have become the mainstay of ulcer therapy in both adult and pediatric patients with peptic ulcer disease.

Table 33–10 ANTACID INTERFERENCE WITH DRUG ABSORPTION[224]

Binding by Magnesium or Aluminum
Digoxin
Tetracycline
Ferrous sulfate
Aspirin
NSAIDs
Cimetidine
Ranitidine
Phenytoin
Quinidine
Chloroquine
Warfarin
Isoniazid
Effect of Decreased Acidity
Decreased Absorption
Tetracycline
Indomethacin
Chlorpromazine
Ketoconazole
Increased Absorption
Aspirin
Furosemide
Diazepam

H_2 Receptor Antagonists. A number of these agents are now available. They differ in their potency and effect on the cytochrome P450 system in the liver. These medications inhibit basal, nocturnal, and food-stimulated acid output.[206, 207] Cimetidine, the first agent available, has an imidazole ring structure and inhibits the cytochrome P450 system, which can affect the metabolism of other coadministered drugs metabolized by this system. Although initially prescribed on a q.i.d. dosing schedule, cimetidine has recently been shown to be effective if the daily dose is divided in two and administered twice a day, thus improving compliance.[208] Ranitidine has a furan ring structure and has significantly less effect on the P450 system. On a milligram basis it is more potent than cimetidine and is usually dosed twice a day. Pharmacokinetic studies in infants and younger children suggest that a three-times per day schedule may be more appropriate in these patients.[209] Other agents are available (famotidine, nizatidine), but their use in pediatric patients is limited and dosages have not been established. H_2 receptor blockers are effective in healing both duodenal (75–95% in 6–8 weeks)[200, 210–213] and gastric (80–90% in 8–12 weeks)[214–216] ulcers and can also prevent recurrence of ulcers when given as a single nighttime dose.[213a, 215, 215a] Suggested oral pediatric doses are given in Table 33–9. In general, treatment is continued for 6 to 8 weeks. If the ulcer recurs, the treatment regimen is repeated and followed by prophylactic nighttime administration of the drug for several months.

Anticholinergics. These agents decrease acid secretion by blocking the effect of acetylcholine on muscarinic receptors. Although their effect on acid production is more potent than the H_2 blockers, they are associated with more significant side effects (dizziness, dry mouth, constipation, blurred vision, urinary retention) at therapeutic doses, which limits their tolerance and therefore their usefulness.[217] Pirenzepine, an anticholinergic more selective for muscarinic receptors in the gastrointestinal tract,[218, 219] is now available but has limited use in children. Though effective, these drugs are rarely used alone as the primary antisecretory therapy and are not routinely necessary in the management of peptic ulcer disease.

Proton Pump Inhibitor. Omeprazole, a substituted benzimidazole, suppresses acid secretion by inhibiting the gastric proton pump (H^+, K^+ATPase) in the secretory membrane of the parietal cell. This drug is extremely effective in suppressing acid and can be given once or twice a day.[220, 221] It is currently recommended for severe, unresponsive gastroesophageal reflux disease and for pathologic hypersecretory states such as Zollinger-Ellison syndrome. Side effects are few; however, the results of long-term administration in animal studies have raised the concern of developing enterochromaffin-like (ECL) cell argyrophil carcinoid from dose-dependent stimulation and proliferation of these endocrine cells.[222] Whether this phenomenon is unique to omeprazole or reflects the capability of any antisecretory agent to elevate serum gastrin levels and thereby chronically stimulate these cells to varying degrees remains to be established. Until further studies can address this issue, use of omeprazole in pediatric patients should be reserved for selected clinical situations and should not be the drug of choice in treating peptic ulcer disease. However, when indicated, omeprazole can be effectively and safely used in children.[198] As in adults, long-term administration should be avoided except in cases of defined pathologic hypersecretion.

Therapeutic regimens with any of these agents will heal gastroduodenal ulcers with an efficacy correlating, to a certain degree, to the magnitude of their effect on acid secretion.[223] However, there are a number of potential side effects that are important to recognize in any patient on antisecretory therapy. The hypochlorhydria induced by these medications can affect the bioavailability of other coadministered drugs (Table 33–10)[224] and can predispose the patient to bacterial overgrowth. In addition, hypergastrinemia may develop in approximately 10% of those patients on long-acting antisecretory drugs.[225] The elevated serum gastrin, as previously mentioned, may have a trophic effect on the ECL cells in the gastric antrum, with resulting hyperplasia. It may therefore be advisable to obtain pre- and postprandial gastrin levels on patients requiring maintenance or long-term therapy with these agents.

Coating Agents

Sucralfate. Sucralfate is the aluminum salt of sulphated sucrose and, at an acidic pH, forms a paste that selectively adheres to damaged mucosa. By forming a complex with the proteinaceous exudate at the ulcer surface, this compound acts as a physical barrier to the damaging effects of acid, pepsin, and bile salts and inhibits peptic activity. Sucralfate has also been shown to buffer acid, bind pepsin and bile salts, increase the production of soluble mucus, and may stimulate prostaglandin production.[226, 227] Healing rates in duodenal ulcer disease are similar to those with H_2 antagonists in adults studies, and there may be fewer relapses.[226, 228] Chiang and colleagues[210] in a series of 17 children treated with 1 gm of sucralfate four times a day for eight weeks, reported a 92% rate of healing, with two of 16 patients (12.5%) on maintenance therapy relapsing. Efficacy in gastric ulcer is less well established. Side effects are few, although patients with renal disease may accumulate aluminum and, because sucralfate binds phosphate, hypophosphatemia is a theoretical possibility with prolonged use.[229] Because this agent must be administered four times a day and cannot be taken with food or other medications, compliance may be an issue. Although currently available only in tablet form, the pill can be crushed and mixed with water to form a slurry.

Bismuth Compounds. These substances have an action mechanism similar to sucralfate in that they coat the ulcer crater and protect the mucosa from further acid injury and proteolysis.[230] Like sucralfate, they also have various other effects on gastroduodenal function, including acid neutralization, enhanced mucus and prostaglandin production, and decreased gastric and intestinal motility. Although colloidal bismuth has been shown to be effective in the treatment of peptic ulcer disease, its primary therapeutic efficacy may be its ability to eradicate *Helicobacter pylori* from the gastric antrum.[231–233] This may also be the reason for the lower rate of relapse noted in ulcer patients treated with these compounds. This organism and its role in gastritis and peptic ulcer disease are discussed in Chapter 31. In general, bismuth compounds are not used in pediatric patients for the treatment of primary ulcer disease; their use is reserved for those documented cases of *Helicobacter*. Bismuth compounds are well tolerated, but side effects from bismuth intoxication have been reported;[234] therefore, judicious administration of long-term or repeated courses of therapy is suggested.

Cytoprotection

Prostaglandins. The role of prostaglandins (primarily of the E series) in cytoprotection of the gastrointestinal tract is now well established.[235] Proposed functions have previously been discussed and include stimulation of mucus and bicarbonate secretion, stimulation of macromolecular synthesis and surface-active phospholipids, enhancement of mucosal blood flow, stabilization of lysosomes, and inhibition of acid output. Several prostaglandin analogs including misoprostol, a recently released synthetic analog of prostaglandin E1, have been evaluated in therapeutic trials in adults. Some healing has been noted with doses that are too low to affect acid secretion and is presumably mediated by enhanced mucosal defense mechanisms.[236] However, other series suggest that therapeutic efficacy is related to the antisecretory properties of the prostaglandin.[237, 238] Side effects most commonly reported are diarrhea and abdominal pain. There is, to date, little information on the use of these agents in pediatric patients.

Other

Diet. Although at one time there was much interest in the contribution of diet to the development, exacerbation, or perpetuation of peptic ulcer disease, there have been no studies to substantiate any correlation between diet and disease. Alcohol should be avoided. Although certain foods may anecdotally contribute to symptoms, specific dietary restrictions do not play an important role in the medical management of peptic ulcer disease.

Smoking. Unlike diet, cigarette smoking does have a strong association with ulcer disease. In adults, patients who smoke have a higher incidence of ulcers as well as more ulcer recurrences. There are also more reported complications and a higher ulcer-related mortality.[239–242] Although this may not be an immediate issue in the management of the pediatric patient (other than adolescents) with ulcer disease, the fact that primary duodenal ulcers tend to be chronic in children as well as adults dictates counseling to patients and their parents about this risk factor.

Surgery. Indications for surgical intervention in the treatment of peptic ulcers in children are perforation, obstruction, severe bleeding, and intractable disease. Perforation is an absolute indication. Patients who initially present with partial gastric outlet obstruction from edema and spasm may respond to intensive medical therapy, including antisecretory medication and nasogastric tube decompression. A guideline for bleeding severe enough to require surgery is replacement of half the blood volume in 8 hours or a total exchange in 24 hours.[243, 244] Certainly massive bleeding (>85 ml per kg) within the first few hours of presentation necessitates emergency surgical intervention.[244] Intractable ulcer disease is somewhat more difficult to define. With the documented efficacy of prophylactic therapy in preventing recurrent ulcers, the definition proposed by Byrne[243] of endoscopically confirmed ulcers following two courses of H_2 blocking agents is no longer applicable. However, there are still those patients with persistent or recurrent disease despite optimum medical management[210] who may benefit from surgery. Prior to surgical referral these patients should be evaluated for hypergastrinemic syndromes, specifically Zollinger-Ellison syndrome and antral G cell hyperfunction or hyperplasia. In addition, the persistence or recurrence of ulcers, in spite of adequate medical management, should be verified endoscopically.

In general, emergency surgery may be limited to correction of the presenting complication, such as repair of the perforation, particularly in the patient who has not received medical therapy. The procedure of choice for more definitive surgical therapy is vagotomy and pyloroplasty,[188, 243, 245, 246] although some advocate antrectomy with vagotomy.[143] In adult series, truncal vagotomy alone is associated with a high recurrence rate; vagotomy with antrectomy, though resulting in a lower incidence of recurrent ulcer disease, is associated with significant side effects.[247] Highly selective vagotomies appear to be associated with fewer postoperative complications but are more difficult to perform, and experience in children is limited.

Zollinger-Ellison Syndrome

Medical therapy has utilized H_2 antagonists and more recently omeprazole.[196, 197] A somatostatin analog given twice daily by subcutaneous injection has been effective in decreasing gastrin levels and gastric acidity and in controlling symptoms.[248] Surgical alternatives include tumor excision if the tumor is located in the head of the pancreas or pancreatoduodenectomy if it lies in the tail. In some patients, gastrectomy has been associated with tumor regression. Chemotherapy for secondary hepatic tumors has utilized streptozotocin and 5-fluorouracil, but the overall 5-year survival rate is low, approximating 20%.[249, 250]

Secondary Ulcer Disease

The various etiologies of secondary peptic ulcers have been discussed. The same general therapeutic tenets of neutralizing or suppressing acid production or providing a mucosal barrier to acid back-diffusion and proteolysis hold for treatment of secondary ulcers as well. Two of the most common causes of secondary ulcers, those induced by stress or associated with the use of NSAIDs, warrant further comment.

Stress-Induced Ulcer. Titration of gastric acidity to a pH of 3.5 or greater with antacids has been shown to reduce the incidence of stress-related gastrointestinal bleeding in critically ill patients.[251] Although initial studies comparing H_2 receptor antagonist (cimetidine) therapy to antacids suggested that the antacids were superior,[252] this appeared to be related to administration of the intravenous cimetidine in boluses, allowing the gastric pH to fall between doses.[253] There is substantial support in the literature for the concept that maintaining the gastric pH at or above 4, either by antacids or by optimum dosing of H_2 blocking agents (frequent or continuous administration),[254, 255] decreases the incidence of stress-related erosions or ulcers and therefore reduces bleeding significantly.[206, 256]

Recently several studies have suggested that sucralfate is as effective as antacids or H_2 receptor blockers in preventing acute stress bleeding.[257–261] Alkalinization of the gastric pH with antacids or antisecretory medications can allow bacterial overgrowth and predispose to colonization of the airway as well.[262] This could potentially contribute to nosocomial pneumonia in these patients. Sucralfate may have an advantage in this clinical setting in view of its comparable efficacy in preventing stress-related ulcers and erosions without altering gastric pH. Indeed, in one study,[263] the incidence of nosocomial pneumonia was significantly less in patients who received sucralfate (10%) for prophylaxis compared to those receiving antacids (34%). However, in several other studies, prevalence rates were similar regardless of therapy.[257–259, 261] Therefore, further information is needed to support the theoretical advantage of sucralfate in this clinical setting, particularly in the pediatric patient population.

NSAID-Associated Ulcer. Ulcers or erosions that develop in patients taking NSAIDs may resolve with discontinuation of the drug or may even heal during therapy. Studies to date suggest that therapy for persistent ulcers with H_2 blockers, prostaglandin analogs, or omeprazole is superior to placebo in healing these drug-induced ulcers,[165, 264] although resolution may be slow. Omeprazole appears to be the most efficacious for refractory ulcers during continued administration of NSAIDs.[264] In clinical trials examining the efficacy of prophylactic treatment regimens, misoprostol, the prostaglandin E1 analog, was effective in preventing NSAID-associated gastric ulcers and acute duodenal damage.[265, 266] H_2 receptor antagonists were as efficacious as prostaglandins in preventing duodenal injury but did not prevent the development of gastric ulcers.[266–269] Sucralfate has been less effective in preventing NSAID-associated lesions than the other classes of drugs tested.[270] Ideally, the NSAID should be discontinued if gastroduodenal ulcers or erosions develop, since continuation of these medications may delay healing.[271] If the ulcers persist or the NSAID cannot be stopped, H_2 receptor antagonists or misoprostol can be used. Omeprazole should be reserved for refractory disease. The clinical benefit of general prophylactic administration of these medications with initiation of NSAID therapy has not been established.

PROGNOSIS IN CHILDREN WITH PEPTIC DISEASE

Children with gastric ulcer are not subject to recurrence once healing has occurred. Although Nord and associates[115] reported a 12% persistence or recurrence in their pediatric patients with gastric ulcer, it is possible that some of these patients were infected with *H. pylori*.

A few investigators have suggested a good prognosis for children with peptic ulcer disease, but the majority of studies provide evidence that the disease in children continues into adult life as a chronic or relapsing one.[200, 245, 272–275] Collins and coworkers[272] followed 31 children with duodenal ulcer for 13 to 29 years and found that 71% of the group had chronic or intermittent symptoms, primarily abdominal pain. Endoscopy was performed in only a few but showed persistent or recurrent ulcer in four. Odera and colleagues[273] reported relapse in 36% of 36 children, and White and associates[274] found 49% of their 41 patients to have recurrent ulceration. They noted that although cimetidine was helpful in controlling symptoms, it did not affect the long-term course of the disease. Murphy and Eastham[275] followed 19 patients for 14 to 27 years after diagnosis and found nine (47%) to have a proven ulcer in adult life and only six (31%) to have had a complete recovery. Ten (53%) had serious complications: eight had gastrointestinal bleeding, one had pyloric stenosis, and one had duodenal perforation. In a study comparing short- and long-term therapy upon the eventual course of disease Chiang and associates[210] found initial good response to antacids in 83%, to sucralfate in 94%, and to H_2 blockers in 87%. However, one year later, 12.5% of the sucralfate group, 28% of the H_2 blocker group, and 70% of the antacid-treated group had recurrent disease.

Elevated MAO and elevated serum pepsinogen have been associated with a poor prognosis and a more severe course of disease. Odera and coworkers[200] found a 41.9% recurrence of peptic ulcer one to five years after treatment, and all who relapsed had a pepsinogen I level above the normal limit of 56 ng per ml. No relapse occurred in children with lower values.

REFERENCES

1. Langaman MJS: Epidemiology of peptic ulcer disease. *In* Bockus HL, ed: Gastroenterology. London, WB Saunders, 1974, p 611.
2. Drumm B, Rhoads JM, Sringer DA, et al: Peptic ulcer disease in children: Etiology, clinical findings and clinical course. Pediatrics 1988; 82:410–414.
3. Rodbro P, Krasilnikoff PA, Bitsch V: Gastric secretion of pepsin in early childhood. Scand J Gastroenterol 1967; 2:257–260.
4. Waldum HL, Straume BK, Burhol PG, et al: Serum group I pepsinogens in children. Acta Paediatr Scand 1980; 69:215–218.
5. Defize J, Meuwissen SGM: Pepsinogens: An update of biochemical, physiologic and clinical aspects. J Pediatr Gastroenterol Nutr 1987; 6:493–508.
6. Taylor IL, Byrne WJ, Christie DL, et al: Effect of individual L-amino acids on gastric secretion and serum gastrin and pancreatic polypeptide release in humans. Gastroenterology 1982; 83:273–278.
7. DiPalma J, Kirk C, Hamosh M, et al: Lipase and pepsin activity in the gastric mucosa of infants, children and adults. Gastroenterology 1991; 101:116–121.
8. Yahav J, Weisselberg B, Reichman B, et al: Basal and meal-stimulated pepsinogen secretion in preterm infants: A longitudinal study. Gastroenterology 1991; 100:A554.
9. Samloff IM: Peptic ulcer disease: The many proteinases of aggression. Gastroenterology 1989; 96:586–595.
10. Pearson J, Allen A, Venables C: Gastric mucosa. Isolation and polymeric structure of undegraded glycoprotein: Its breakdown by pepsin. Gastroenterology 1980; 78:709–715.
11. Walker V, Taylor WH. Pepsin I secretion in chronic peptic ulceration. Gut 1980; 21:766–771.
12. Mirsky IA, Futterman P, Kaplan S: Blood plasma pepsinogen II. The activity of plasma from normal subjects and patients with duodenal ulcer. J Lab Clin Med 1952; 40:188–199.
13. Samloff IM, Liebman WM, Panitch NM: Serum group I pepsinogens by radioimmunoassay in control subjects and patients with peptic ulcer. Gastroenterology 1975; 769:83–90.
14. Ford TF, Grant DAW, Austen BM, et al: Intramucosal activation of pepsinogens in the pathogenesis of acute gastric erosions and their prevention by the potent semisynthetic amphipathic inhibitor pepstatinyl-glycyl-lysyl-lysine. Clin Chem Acta 1985; 145:37–47.
15. Ohe K, Ueno N, Yokoya H, et al: The activation of pepsinogen inside the gastric mucosa caused by the hydrogen back-diffusion during the course of aspirin ulceration. Hiroshima J Med Sci 1979; 29:1–11.
16. Wolfe MM, Soll AM: The physiology and strategies for drug therapy. N Engl J Med 1989; 319:1707–1715.
17. Feldman M: Peptic ulcer disease: Pathophysiology and strategies for drug therapy. Curr Concepts Gastroenterol 1985; 3:13–19.
18. Kao J-CJ, Lichtenberger LM: Phospholipid- and neutral lipid-containing organelles of rat gastroduodenal mucous cells. Gastroenterology 1991; 101:7–21.
19. Allen A, Leonard AJ, Sellers L. The mucus barrier: Its role in gastroduodenal mucosal protection. J Clin Gastroenterol 1988; 10(Suppl 1):S93–S98.
20. Flemstrom G, Garner A: Gastroduodenal HCO_3-transport: Characteristics and proposed role in acidity regulation and mucosal protection. Am J Physiol 1982; 242:G183–G193.
21. Takeuchi K, Magee D, Critchlow J, et al: Role of pH gradient of mucus in protection of gastric mucosa. Gastroenterology 1983; 84:331–340.
22. Matthews JB, Garner A: Stomach wars—a mucosal defense initiative. Aliment Pharmacol Therap 1991; 5:105–114.
23. Pearson JP, Ward R, Allen A, et al: Mucus degradation by pepsin: Comparison of mucolytic activity of human pepsin 1 and pepsin 3: Implications in peptic ulceration. Gut 1986; 27:243–248.

24. Younan F, Pearson J, Allen A, et al: Changes in the structure of the mucus gel in the mucosal surface of the stomach in association with peptic ulcer disease. Gastroenterology 1982; 82:827–831.
25. Isenberg JL, Selling JA, Hogan DL, et al. Impaired proximal duodenal mucosal bicarbonate secretion in patients with duodenal ulcer. N Engl J Med 1987; 316:347–349.
26. Holm L: Gastric mucosal blood flow and mucosal protection. J Clin Gastroenterol 1988; 10(Suppl 1):S114–S119.
27. Peterson WL: Pathogenesis and therapy of peptic ulcer. J Clin Gastroenterol 1990; 12(Suppl 2):S1–S6.
28. Malagelada JR, Ahlquist DA, Moore SC: Defects in prostaglandin synthesis and metabolism in peptic ulcer disease. Dig Dis Sci 1986; 31(Suppl 2):S20–S22.
29. Rachmilewitz D, Ligumsky M, Filch A, et al: Role of endogenous gastric prostanoids in the pathogenesis and therapy of duodenal ulcer. Gastroenterology 1986; 90:963–969.
30. Miller T: Protective effects of prostaglandins against gastric mucosal damage: Current knowledge and proposed mechanisms. Am J Physiol 1983; 245:601–623.
31. Robert A, Nezamis JE, Lancaster C, et al: Cytoprotection by prostaglandins in rats. Prevention of gastric necrosis produced by alcohol, HCl, NaOH, hypertonic NaCl and thermal injury. Gastroenterology 1979; 77:433–443.
32. Konturek P, Brzozowski T, Konturek SJ, et al: Role of epidermal growth factor, prostaglandin, and sulfhydryls in stress-induced gastric lesions. Gastroenterology 1990; 99:1607–1615.
33. Reinhard WH, Muller O, Halter F: Influence of long term 16, 16-dimethyl prostaglandin E_2 treatment on the rat gastrointestinal mucosa. Gastroenterology 1983; 85:1003–1010.
34. Inauen W, Wyss PA, Kayser S, et al: Influence of prostaglandins, omeprazole, and indomethacin on healing of experimental gastric ulcers in rats. Gastroenterology 1988; 95:636–641.
35. Yonei Y, Guth PH. Laparotomy stimulates an endogenous gastric mucosal protective mechanism in the rat: A microcirculatory and morphologic study of ethanol injury. Gastroenterology 1988; 95:600–611.
36. Ebers DW, Smith DI, Gibb GE: Gastric acidity on the first day of life. Pediatrics 1956; 18:800–804.
37. Thomson J: The volume and acidity of the gastric contents in the unfed newborn infant. Arch Dis Child 1951; 26:558–564.
38. Agunod M, Yamaguchi N, Lopez R, et al: Correlative study of hydrochloric acid, pepsin and intrinsic factor secretion in newborn infants. Am J Dig Dis 1969; 14:400–414.
39. Kopel FB, Barbero GJ: Gastric secretion in infancy and childhood. Gastroenterology 1967; 52:1101–1112.
40. Miller RA: Observations on the gastric acidity during the first month of life. Arch Dis Child 1942; 16:22–31.
41. Ames MD: Gastric acidity in the first ten days of life of the prematurely born baby. Am J Dis Child 1960; 100:122–126.
42. Harries JJ, Fraser AJ: The acidity of gastric contents of premature babies during the first fourteen days of life. Biol Neonate 1968; 12:186–194.
43. Wangel AG, Callender ST: Gastric secretion in the premature infant. Gut 1968; 9:249–256.
44. Euler AR, Byrne WJ, Meis PJ, et al: Basal and pentagastrin-stimulated gastric secretion in newborn infants. Pediatr Res 1979; 13:36–37.
45. Seabrook M, Amarnath RP, Amarnath M, et al: Twenty-four hour intragastric profiles in fed and fasted premature infants. Gastroenterology 1991; 100:A546.
46. Harada T, Hyman PE, Everett S, et al: Meal-stimulated gastric acid secretion in infants. J Pediatr 1984; 104:534–538.
47. Hyman PE, Clarke DD, Everett S, et al: Gastric acid secretory function in preterm infants. J Pediatr 1985; 106:467–470.
48. Walsh JH: Gastrointestinal hormones and peptides. *In* Johnson LR, ed: Physiology of the Gastrointestinal Tract. 2nd ed. Vol. 1. New York Raven Press, 1987, pp 181–253.
49. Walsh JH, Richardson CT, Fordtran JS: pH dependence of acid secretion and gastrin release in normal and ulcer patients. J Clin Invest 1975; 55:462–467.
50. Yamada T: Local regulatory actions of gastrointestinal peptides. *In* Johnson LR, ed: Physiology of the Gastrointestinal Tract. 2nd ed. Vol. 1. New York, Raven Press, 1987, pp 131–142.
51. Karnes WE Jr, Walsh JH: The gastrin hypothesis: Implications for anti-secretory drug selection. J Clin Gastroenterol 1990; 12(Suppl 2):S7–S12.
52. Rodgers BM, Dix PM, Talbert JM, et al: Fasting and postprandial serum gastrin in normal human neonates. J Pediatr Surg 1978; 13:13–17.
53. Eulcer SR, Byrne WJ, Cousins LM: et al. Increased serum gastrin concentration and gastric hyposecretion in the immediate newborn period. Gastroenterology 1977; 72:1271–1273.
54. Euler AR, Ament ME, Walsh JH: Human newborn hypergastrinemia: An investigation of prenatal and perinatal factors and their effect upon gastrin. Pediatr Res 1978; 12:652–656.
55. Gemelli M, Mami C, Mangara R, et al: Gastrin 17 and gastrin 34 before and after a meal in newborn infants. J Pediatr Gastroenterol Nutr 1987; 6:717–720.
56. Bloom SR: Hormonal response to first feeding in neonates. J Pediatr 1978; 93:900–901.
57. Aynsley-Green A, Bloom SR, Williamson DH, et al: Endocrine and metabolic response in the human newborn to first feed of breast milk. Arch Dis Child 1977; 52:291–295.
58. Lucas A, Bloom SR, Aynsley-Green A: Development of gut hormone responses to feeding in neonates. Arch Dis Child 1980; 55:678–682.
59. Magazzu G, Gemelli M, Pusturinos S, et al: Gastrinemia e secrezione acida gastrica durante i prima 5 giorni di vita. Minerva Pediatr 1981; 33:11–16.
60. Marchini G, Einberg J, Uynas-Moberg K: Plasma concentration of gastrin and somatostatin after breast feeding in 4 day old infants. Arch Dis Child 1988; 63:1218–1222.
61. Moazam F, Kirby WJ, Rodgers BM, et al: Physiology of serum gastrin production in neonates and infants. Ann Surg 1984; 199:389–405.
62. Eastham EJ: Peptic ulcer. *In* Walker WA, Durie P, Hamilton JR, et al, eds: Pediatric Gastrointestinal Disease: Pathophysiology, Diagnosis, Management. Vol 1. Philadelphia, BC Decker, 1991, pp 438–451.
63. Habbick BF, Melrose AG, Grant JC: Duodenal ulcer in children. Arch Dis Child 1968; 43:23–28.
64. Fieber M, Meschede R, Tolcmitt W: Aciditat und peptische aktivtat des magensafts bei gesunden und mucoviscidosis kranken kindern. Z Zinkerkeilkd 1975; 120:199–209.
65. Robb JDA, Thomas PS, Orszulok J, et al: Duodenal ulcer in children. Arch Dis Child 1972; 47:688–696.
66. Christie DL, Ament ME: Gastric acid hypersecretion in children with duodenal ulcer. Gastroenterology 1976; 71:242–244.
67. Christie DL, Ament ME: Diagnosis and treatment of duodenal ulcer in infancy and childhood. Pediatr Ann 1976; 5:672–677.
68. Euler AR, Byrne WJ, Campbell MF: Basal and pentagastrin-stimulated gastric acid secretory rates in normal children and in those with peptic ulcer disease. J Pediatr 1983; 103:766–768.
69. Ghai OP, Singh M, Walia BNS, et al: An assessment of gastric acid secretory response with "maximal" augmented histamine stimulation in children with peptic ulcer disease. Arch Dis Child 1965; 40:77–79.
70. Mohammed R, Hearns JB, Cream GP: Gastric acid secretion in children with duodenal ulceration. Scand J Gastroenterol 1982; 17:289–292.
71. Lari J, Lister J, Duthie HL: Response to gastrin pentapeptide in children. J Pediatr Surg 1968; 3:682–690.
72. Tam PKH, Saing H: Gastric acid secretion and emptying rates in children with duodenal ulcer. Pediatr Res 1986; 21:129–136.
73. Christie DL, Ament ME: Gastrin response to a protein meal in children with duodenal ulcer. Pediatr Res 1976; 10:353.
74. Liebman WM: Gastric acid secretion and serum gastrin levels in children with recurrent abdominal pain, gastric and duodenal ulcers. J Clin Gastroenterol 1980; 2:243–246.
75. Tam PKH: Hypergastrinemia in children: Duodenal ulcer. J Pediatr Surg 1988; 23:331–334.
76. Ackerman SH, Manaker S, Cohen MI: Recent separation and the onset of peptic ulcer disease in older children and adolescents. Psychosom Med 1981; 43:305–310.
77. Eberhard G: Peptic ulcer in twins—a study in personality, heredity and environment. Acta Psychiatr Scand 1968; 205(Suppl):18.
78. Taboroff LH, Brown WH: A study of the personality patterns of children and adolescents with peptic ulcer syndrome. Am J Pathopsychiatry 1954; 24:602–613.
79. Coddington RD: Peptic ulcer in children. Psychosomatics 1968; 9:38–43.

80. Wessel MA, McCullough AB: Bereavement—an etiologic factor on peptic ulcer in childhood and adolescence. J Adolesc Health Care 1982; 2:287–288.
81. Feldman M, Walker P, Green J, et al: Life events, stress and psychosocial factors on men with peptic ulcer disease. Gastroenterology 1986; 91:1370–1379.
82. Rotter JI: Peptic ulcer disease—more than one gene, more than one disease. Prog Med Genert 1980; 4:1–58.
83. Rotter JI: Genetic aspects of ulcer disease. Comp Ther 1981; 7:16–35.
84. Jackson RH: Genetic studies in peptic ulcer disease in childhood. Acta Paediatr Scand 1972; 61:493–497.
85. Fallstrom SP, Reinard T: Peptic ulcer disease in children. Acta Paediatr Scand 1961; 50:431–436.
86. O'Brien B, Thomson A, Dossetor J: HLA in peptic ulcer. Dig Dis Sci 1979; 24:314–315.
87. Lam SK, Ong GB: Identification of two subgroups of familial early-onset duodenal ulcers. Ann Intern Med 1980; 93:540–544.
88. Rotter JI, Peterson G, Samloff IM, et al: Genetic heterogeneity of hyperpepsinogenemia I and normopepsinogenemia I in duodenal ulcer disease. Ann Intern Med 1979; 91:373–377.
89. Rotter JI, Sones JQ, Samloff IM, et al: The genetics of peptic ulcer disease. Elevated serum group I pepsinogen concentrations in siblings and twins of ulcer probands. Gastroenterology 1977; 72:A1165.
90. Rotter JI, Sones JQ, Samloff IM, et al: Duodenal ulcer disease associated with elevated serum pepsinogen I. An inherited autosomal dominant disorder. N Engl J Med 1979; 300:63–69.
91. Habilbullah CM, Mujahid AM, Isham M, et al: Study of duodenal ulcer disease in 100 families using total serum pepsinogen as a genetic marker. Gut 1984; 25:1380–1383.
92. Tam PKH: Serum pepsinogen I in childhood duodenal ulcer. J Pediatr Gastroenterol Nutr 1987; 6:904–907.
93. Cown WK: Genetics of duodenal and gastric ulcer. Clin Gastroenterol 1973; 2:539–546.
94. Askanazy M: Uber Bau und Entstehung des chronischen Magengeschwurs sowie Soorpilzbefunde in ihm. Virchows Arch J Path 1921; 234:111–122.
95. Lewin KJ, Young K, Ulich T, et al: Primary gastrin cell hyperplasia: Report of 5 cases and review of the literature. Am J Surg Path 1984; 8:821–832.
96. Stave R, Brand T, Zaeg P: Immunohistochemical investigation of gastrin-producing cells (G cells): Estimation of antral density, mucosal distribution and total mass of G cells in resected stomachs from patients with peptic ulcer disease. Scand J Gastroenterol 1978; 13:199–203.
97. Friesen ST, Tomita T: Pseudo-Zollinger-Ellison syndrome: Hypergastrinemia, hyperchlorhydria without tumor. Ann Surg 1981; 194:481–493.
98. Zaatar R, Younoszai MK, Mitros F: Pseudo-Zollinger-Ellison syndrome in a child presenting with anemia. Gastroenterology 1987; 92:508–512.
99. Jaros W, Biller J, Flores A, et al: Significance of antral G cell hyperplasia in young patients. Gastroenterology 1985; 88:A1432.
100. Zollinger RM, Ellison EH: Primary peptic ulcerations of the jejunum associated with islet cell tumors of the pancreas. Ann Surg 1955; 142:709–713.
101. Wilson SD: The role of surgery in children with Zollinger-Ellison syndrome. Surgery 1982; 92:682–692.
102. Tudor R: Registry of peptic ulcers in children: Children with ZES. 1984 report no. 4. Bismark, ND.
103. Buchta RM, Kaplan JM: Zollinger-Ellison syndrome in a 9 year old child: Case report and review of this entity in childhood. Pediatrics 1971; 47:594–598.
104. Webb TA, Li CY, Yam LT: Systemic mast cell disease: A clinical and hematopathologic study of 26 cases. Cancer 1982; 49:927–938.
105. Miner PB: The role of the mast cell in clinical gastrointestinal disease with special reference to systemic mastocytosis. J Investig Dermatol 1991; 96(Suppl):S40–S44.
106. Cherner JA, Jensen RT, Dubois A, et al: Gastrointestinal dysfunction in systemic mastocytosis. Gastroenterology 1988; 95:657–666.
107. Meyers WC, Harris N, Stein S, et al: Alimentary tract complications after renal transplantation. Ann Surg 1979; 190:535–542.
108. Chisholm GD, Mee AD, Williams G, et al: Peptic ulceration, gastric secretion and renal transplantation. Brit Med J 1977; 1:1630–1632.
109. Snyder N, Scurry M, Sughes W: Hypergastrinemia in familial multiple endocrine adenomatosis. Ann Intern Med 1974; 80:321–325.
110. Snyder M, Scurry MT, Deiss WP: Five families with multiple endocrine adenomatosis. Ann Intern Med 1972; 76:53–58.
111. Muggia A, Spiro HM: Childhood peptic ulcer. Gastroenterology 1959; 37:715–724.
112. Murphy MS, Eastham EJ, Jiminez M, et al: Duodenal ulceration: Review of 100 cases. Arch Dis Child 1987; 62:544–548.
113. Netakhata ZN: Clinical picture and diagnosis of peptic ulcer in children. Pediatr Riya 1970; 72:67–71.
114. Nord KS: Peptic ulcer disease in the pediatric population. Pediatr Clin North Am 1988; 35:117–135.
115. Nord K, Rossi TM, Lebenthal E: Peptic ulcer in children: The predominance of gastric ulcers. Am J Gastroenterol 1981; 75:153–157.
116. Seagram CGF, Stephens CA, Cumming WA: Peptic ulceration at the Hospital for Sick Children, Toronto during the 20 year period 1949–1969. J Pediatr Surg 1973; 8:407–413.
117. Gryboski JD: Pain and peptic ulcer disease in children. J Clin Gastroenterol 1980; 2:277–279.
118. Gryboski JD: Peptic ulcer disease in children. Pediatr Rev 1990; 12:15–24.
119. Blodgett FD, Morris N, Lurie HJ: Children with peptic ulcers and their families. J Pediatr 1963; 62:280–281.
120. Deckelbaum RJ, Roy CC, Lussier-Lazaroff J, et al: Peptic ulcer disease: A clinical study in 73 children. Can Med Assoc J 1974; 111:225–228.
121. Tudor RB: Gastric and duodenal ulcers in children. Gastroenterology 1972; 62:823.
122. Singleton EB, Fayhus MH: Incidence of peptic ulcer as determined by radiologic examination in the pediatric age group. J Pediatr 1964; 65:858–862.
123. Goldberg HM: Duodenal ulcers in children. Br Med J 1957; 1:500–502.
124. Jewett TC Jr: Peptic ulcer in childhood. Comp Ther 1985; 11:55–61.
125. Krahauer LJ, Berry JR, Stewart JA: Peptic ulcer disease in children. Northwest Med 1967; 66:348–351.
126. Michener WM, Kennedy RJL, Dushane JW: Duodenal ulcer in childhood. Am J Dis Child 1960; 100:814–817.
127. Milliken JC: Duodenal ulceration in children. Gut 1965; 6:25–28.
128. Berg RM: Peptic ulcers in children. South Med J 1961; 54:325–331.
129. Nuss D, Lynn H: Peptic ulceration in children. Surg Clin North Am 1971; 51:945–953.
130. Tudor R: Peptic ulcerations in childhood. Pediatr Clin North Am 1967; 14:109–120.
131. Nord KS: Peptic ulcer disease in children and adolescents: Evolving dilemmas. J Pediatr Gastroenterol Nutr 1983; 2:397–399.
132. Tomomasa T, Hsu JY, Shigeta M, et al: Statistical analysis of symptoms and signs in pediatric patients with peptic ulcer. J Pediatr Gastroenterol Nutr 1986; 5:711–715.
133. Gahukamble DB, Fenn AS, Devadatta J, et al: Duodenal ulcer in South Indian children. Am J Surg 1983; 145:322–324.
134. Apley J: The child with abdominal pain. 2nd ed. Oxford, Blackwell Scientific Publications, 1975, pp 1–81.
135. Langman MS, Doll R: ABO blood groups and secretor status in relation to clinical characteristics of peptic ulcers. Gut 1965; 6:270–273.
136. Dodge J: The stomach. *In* Anderson C, Burke V, Gracey M, eds: Pediatric Gastroenterology. 2nd ed. Oxford, Blackwell Scientific Publications, 1987, pp 88–95.
137. Glynn PJU: Chronic gastric ulcer in an infant treated by gastrectomy. Aust NZ J Surg 1971; 40:256–258.
138. Benkov KJ, Becker H, Rose J, et al: Failure to thrive associated with chronic ulcer disease in a 9 year old boy. Am J Gastroenterol 1985; 80:524–526.
139. Kumar D, Spitz L: Peptic ulceration in children. Surg Gynecol Obstet 1984; 159:63–66.
140. Johnson D, L'Hereux P, Thompson T: Peptic ulcer disease in early infancy: Clinical presentation and roentgenographic features. Acta Paediatr Scand 1980; 69:753–760.

141. Cox K, Ament ME: Upper gastrointestinal bleeding in children. Pediatrics 1979; 63:408–413.
142. Hsu HY, Chang MH, Wang TH, et al: Acute duodenal ulcer. Arch Dis Child 1989; 64:774–779.
143. Curci M, Little K, Sieber WK, et al: Peptic ulcer disease in childhood reexamined. J Pediatr Surg 1976; 11:329–335.
144. Krasna IH, Schneider KM, Becker JM: Surgical management of stress ulcerations in childhood: Report of five cases. J Pediatr Surg 1971; 6:301–306.
145. Dunn S, Weber TR, Grosfeld JL, et al: Acute peptic ulcer in childhood: Emergency surgical therapy in 39 cases. Arch Surg 1983; 118:656–666.
146. Rosenlund ML, Koop CE: Diagnosis and treatment: Duodenal ulcer in childhood. Pediatrics 1970; 45:283–286.
147. Adeyami SD, Ein SH, Simpson JS: Perforated stress ulcer in infants. Ann Surg 1979; 190:706–708.
148. Morden RS, Schullinger JN, Mollitt DL, et al: Operative management of stress ulcers in children. Ann Surg 1982; 196:18–20.
149. Bell MJ, Keating JP, Ternberg JL, et al: Perforated stress ulcer in infants. J Pediatr Surg 1987; 16:998–1002.
150. Dimick S: Sixth National Burn Seminar: Gastrointestinal ulceration bleeding in children. J Trauma 1967; 7:119–120.
151. Pruitt BA Jr, Foley FD, Moncrieff JA: Curling's ulcer: A clinical pathologic study of 323 cases. Ann Surg 1970; 172:523–531.
152. Bruck HM, Pruitt BA: Curling's ulcer in children: A 12 year review of 63 cases. Trauma 1972; 12:490–496.
153. Schlumberger HG: Coexistent gastroduodenia and cerebral lesions in infancy and childhood. Arch Pathol 1951; 52:43–66.
154. Gottlieb G, Chu F, Sharlin HS: Perforation of a gastric ulcer associated with intracranial hemorrhage in a newborn infant. Radiology 1950; 54:595–598.
155. Vorder Bruegge WF, Peura DA:. Stress-related mucosal damage: Review of drug therapy. J Clin Gastroenterol 1990; 12(Suppl 2):S35–S40
156. Ohno T, Okabe S: Gastric surface epithelial cell damage induced by restraint and water immersion stress in rats. J Clin Gastroenterol 1988; 10:246–S52.
157. Kitajimo M, Otsuka S, Shimizu A, et al: Impairment of gastric microcirculation in stress. J Clin Gastroenterol 1988; 10:S120–S128.
158. Butt W, Auldist A, McDougall P, et al: Duodenal ulceration: A complication of tolazoline therapy. Aust Paediatr J 1986; 22:221–223.
159. Adams J, Hyde W, Procianoy R, et al: Hypochloremic metabolic alkalosis following tolazoline-induced gastric hypersecretion. Pediatrics 1980; 65:298–300.
160. Meltzer LE, Bockman AA, Kanenson W, Cohen A: The incidence of peptic ulcer among patients on longterm prednisone therapy. Gastroenterology 1958; 35:351–356.
161. Messer J, Reitman D, Sacks HS, et al: Association of adrenocorticoid therapy and peptic ulcer disease. N Engl J Med 1983; 309:21–24.
162. Guth P: The ulcer patient and nonsteroidal anti-inflammatory drugs: International perspectives on acid-peptic disorders. *In* Practical Gastroenterology. New York, Sugar Publications, 1988 (Suppl), pp 12–15.
163. Soll AH, Kurata J, McGuigan JE: Ulcers, nonsteroidal antiinflammatory drugs and related matters. Gastroenterology 1989; 96:561–568.
163a. Aabakken L: Non-steroidal anti-inflammatory drugs—the extending scope of gastrointestinal side effects. Aliment Pharmacol Ther 1992; 6:143–162.
164. Kauffman G: Aspirin-induced gastric mucosal injury: Lessons learned from animal models. Gastroenterology 1989; 96:606–614.
165. McCarthy DM: Nonsteroidal antiinflammatory drug-induced ulcers: Management by traditional therapies. Gastroenterology 1989; 96:662–674.
166. Graham DY, Smith JL: Aspirin and the stomach. Ann Intern Med 1986; 104:390–398.
167. Graham DY: Prevention of gastroduodenal injury induced by chronic nonsteroidal antiinflammatory injury. Gastroenterology 1989; 96:675–681.
168. Oates PJ, Hakkinen JP: Studies on the mechanism of ethanol-induced gastric damage in rats. Gastroenterology 1988; 94:10–21.
169. Yonei Y, Guth PH: Ethanol-induced gastric injury: Role of submucosal venoconstriction and leukotrienes. Dig Dis Sci 1991; 36:601–608.
170. Tarnawski A, Stachura J, Gergely H, et al: Microvascular endothelium—a major target for alcohol injury of the gastric mucosa. J Clin Gastroenterol 1988; 10(Suppl):S53–S64.
171. Tarnawski A, Stachura J, Hollander D, et al: Cellular aspects of alcohol-induced injury and prostaglandin protection of the human gastric mucosa. J Clin Gsatroenterol 1988; 10:S35–S45.
172. Ritchie WP: Alkaline reflux gastritis: A critical reappraisal. Gut 1984; 25:975–987.
173. Thomas WEG: Duodeno-gastric reflux: A common factor in pathogenesis of both gastric and duodenal ulcer. Lancet 1980; 20:1166–1168.
174. Mouterde O, Foucaud P, Vatier J, et al: Duodenogastric reflux in children: Measurement of phospholipids and trypsin in gastric contents. J Pediatr Gastroenterol Nutr 1990; 10:327–334.
175. Dewar EP, King RFG, Johnston D: Bile acid and lysolethicin concentration in the stomach of patients with gastric ulcer. Br J Surg 1983; 70:401–405.
176. Hein GE, McClla RL, Thorne GW: Sickle cell anemia with report of a case with autopsy. Am J Med Sci 1927; 173:763–772.
177. Serjeant GR, May H, Patrick A, et al: Duodenal ulceration in sickle cell anemia. Trans R Soc Trop Med Hyg 1973; 67:59–63.
178. Worsonu L, Konotey-Ahulu FID: Gastric acid secretion in sickle cell anemia. Gut 1971; 12:197–199.
179. Rao S, Royal JE, Conrad HA, et al: Duodenal ulcer in sickle cell anemia. J Pediatr Gastroenterol Nutr 1990; 10:117–120.
180. Anderson D: Pathology of cystic fibrosis. Ann NY Acad Sci 1962; 93:500–517.
181. Aterman K: Duodenal ulceration and fibrocystic disease of the pancreas. Am J Dis Child 1961; 101:210–215.
182. Oppenheimer EH, Esterly JR: Pathology of cystic fibrosis: Review of the literature and comparison with 146 autopsied cases. Perspect Pediatr Pathol 1975; 2:241–278.
183. Lloyd-Still JD: Growth, nutrition and gastrointestinal problems. *In* Lloyd-Still JD, ed: Textbook of Cystic Fibrosis. Boston, John Wright-PSG, 1983, p 252.
184. Rosenstein B, Perman JA, Kramer SS: Peptic ulcer disease in cystic fibrosis: An unusual occurrence in black adolescents. Am J Dis Child 1986; 140:9669.
185. Cox K, Isenberg JN: Hypersecretion of gastric acid in patients with pancreatic exocrine insufficiency due to cystic fibrosis. Gastroenterology 1978; 74:A1022.
186. Ament ME, Berquist WE, Vargas J, et al: Fiberoptic upper intestinal endoscopy in infants and children. Pediatr Clin North Am 1988; 35:141–155.
187. Caulfield M, Wiley R, Sivak MV, et al: Upper gastrointestinal tract endoscopy in the pediatric patient. J Pediatr 1989; 115:339–345.
188. Tedesco FJ, Goldstein DD, Gleason WA, et al: Upper gastrointestinal endoscopy in the pediatric patient. Gastroenterology 1976; 70:492–494.
189. Miller V, Doig CM: Upper gastrointestinal tract endoscopy. Arch Dis Child 1984; 59:1100–1102.
190. Gleason WA, Tedesco FJ, Keating JP, et al: Fiberoptic gastrointestinal endoscopy in infants and children. J Pediatr 1974; 85:810–813.
191. Black DB, Haggitt RC, Whitington PF: Gastroduodenal endoscopic-histologic correlation in pediatric patients. J Pediatr Gastroenterol Nutr 1988; 7:353–358.
192. Strobel CT, Smith LE, Eulcer AR: Primary gastric adenocarcinoma in the pediatric population. J Pediatr 1978; 92:850–851.
193. Storey DW, Brown SG, Swain CP, et al: Endoscopic prediction of recurrent bleeding in peptic ulcers. N Engl J Med 1981; 305:915–916.
194. Johnston JH, Jensen DM, Maunter W: Comparison of laser photocoagulation and electrocoagulation in endoscopic treatment of UGI bleeding. Gastroenterology 1979; 76:1162.
195. Peterson WL: Gastrointestinal bleeding. *In* Sleisenger MS, Fordtran JS, eds: Gastrointestinal Disease: Pathophysiology, Diagnosis, Management. 4th ed. Philadelphia, WB Saunders, 1989, pp 397–427.
196. Jensen RT, Gardner JD, Raufman JP, et al: Zollinger-Ellison syndrome: Current concepts and management. Ann Intern Med 1983; 98:59–75.

197. Maton PN, Gardner JD, Jensen RT: Diagnosis and management of Zollinger-Ellison syndrome. Endocrin Metab Clin North Am 1980; 18:519–543.
198. DeGiacomo C, Fiocca R, Villani L, et al: Omeprazole treatment of severe peptic disease associated with antral G cell hyperfunction and hyperpepsinogenemia I in an infant. J Pediatr 1990; 117:989–993.
199. Taylor IL, Calam J, Rotter JI, et al: Family studies of hypergastrinemic I duodenal ulcer. Ann Intern Med 1981; 95:421–425.
200. Odera G, Altare F, Dell'Olio D, et al: Prognostic value of serum pepsinogen I in children with peptic ulcer. J Pediatr Gastroenterol Nutr 1988; 7:645–650.
201. Sansenbacher LJ, Mekhjian HS, King DR, et al: Prognostic implication of calcium mediated gastrin levels in the ulcerogenic syndrome. Am J Surg 1973; 126:116–121.
202. Lamers C, van Tongeren J: Comparative study of the value of the calcium, secretin and meal-stimulated increased serum gastrin to the diagnosis of Zollinger-Ellison syndrome. Gut 1977; 18:128–135.
203. Drake D, Hollander D: Neutralizing capacity and cost effectiveness of antacids. Ann Intern Med 1981; 94:215–217.
204. Ippoliti AF, Sturdevant RAC, Isenberg JI, et al: Cimetidine vs. intensive acid therapy for duodenal ulcer. Gastroenterology 1978; 74:393–395.
205. Bardhan KD, Hunter JJO, Miller JP, et al: Antacid maintenance therapy in the prevention of duodenal ulcer relapse. Gut 1988; 29:1748–1754.
206. Feldman M, Burton ME: Histamine 2–receptor antagonists: Standard therapy for acid-peptic diseases: I. N Engl J Med 1990; 323:1672–1680.
207. Feldman M, Burton ME: Histamine 2–receptor antagonists: Standard therapy for acid-peptic diseases: II. N Engl J Med 1990; 323:1749–1755.
208. Kerr GD, Brown P, Lennon J, et al: Cimetidine: Twice daily administration in duodenal ulcer. A multicentre group study. Practitioner 1982; 226:978–980.
209. Sutphen JL, Dillard VL: Effect of ranitidine on twenty-four-hour gastric acidity in infants. J Pediatr 1989; 114:472–474.
210. Chiang BL, Chang MH, Lin MI, et al: Chronic duodenal ulcer in children: Clinical observation and response to treatment. J Pediatr Gastroenterol Nutr 1989; 8:161–165.
211. Denavit MF, Guerin J, Caldera R, et al: Ulcere duodenal chez un nourveaune. Ann Pediatr 1978; 25:494–498.
212. Tam PKH, Saing H: The use of H_2-receptor antagonist in the treatment of peptic ulcer disease in children. J Pediatr Gastroenterol Nutr 1989; 8:41–46.
213. Soll AH: Duodenal ulcer and drug therapy. *In* Sleisenger MH, Fordtran JS, eds: Gastrointestinal Disease: Pathophysiology, Diagnosis, Management. 4th ed. Philadelphia, WB Saunders, 1989, pp 814–879.
213a. Patel N, Ward U, Rogers MJ, et al: Nighttime or morning dosing with H_2-receptor antagonists: Studies on acid inhibition in normal subjects. Aliment Pharmacol Ther 1992; 6:381–388.
214. Legerton CW: Duodenal and gastric ulcer healing rates: A review. Am J Med 1984; 77(Suppl 5B):2–7.
215. Richardson CT: Gastric ulcer. *In* Sleisenger MH, Fordtran JS, eds: Gastrointestinal Disease: Pathophysiology, Diagnosis, Management. 4th ed. Philadelphia, WB Saunders, 1989, pp 879–909.
215a. Penston JG, Wormsley KG: Maintenance treatment with H_2-receptor antagonists for peptic ulcer disease. Aliment Pharmacol Ther 1992; 6:3–31.
216. Howden CW, Hunt RH: The relationship between suppression of acidity and gastric ulcer healing rates. Aliment Pharmacol Therap 1990; 4:25–33.
217. Grossman MI, Kurata JH, Rotter JI, et al: Peptide ulcer: New therapies, new disease. Ann Intern Med 1981; 95:609–627.
218. Feldman M: Inhibition of gastric acid secretion by selective and nonselective anticholinergics. Gastroenterology 1984; 86:361–366.
219. Texter ED Jr, Reilly PA: The efficacy and selectivity of pirenzepine: Review and commentary. Scand J Gastroenterol 1982; 72(Suppl):237–246.
220. Lindberg P, Brandstrom A, Bjorn W, et al: Omeprazole: The first proton pump inhibitor. Medicinal Research Reviews 1990; 10:1–54.
221. Walan A: Clinical utility and safety of omeprazole: The first proton pump inhibitor. Medicinal Research Reviews 1990; 10:1–54.
222. Ekman L, Hansson E, Havu N, et al: Toxicologic studies on omeprazole. Scand J Gastroenterol 1985; 108(Suppl):53–69.
223. Jones DB, Howden CW, Burget DW, et al: Acid suppression in duodenal ulcer: A meta-analysis to define optimal dosing with anti-secretory drugs. Gut 1987; 23:1120–1127.
224. Reynolds JC: Drug interactions and anti-ulcer therapy. J Clin Gastroenterol 1990; 12(Suppl 2):S54–S63.
225. Sharma B, Axelson M, Pounder RP, et al: Acid secretory capacity and plasma gastrin concentration after administration of omeprazole to normal subjects. Aliment Pharmacol Therap 1987; 1:67–76.
226. Brogden RN, Heel RC, Speight TM: Sucralfate: A review of its pharmacodynamic properties and therapeutic use in peptic ulcer disease. Drugs 1984; 27:194–209.
227. Szabo S, Hollander D: Pathways of gastrointestinal protection and repair: Mechanism of action of sucralfate. Am J Med 1989; 86(Suppl 6A):23–31.
228. Bolin TD, Davis AE, Duncombe VM, et al: Role of maintenance sucralfate in prevention of duodenal ulcer recurrence. Am J Med 1987; 83:91–94.
229. Leung ACT, Henderson IS, Halls DJ: Aluminum hydroxide vs sucralfate as phosphate binder in uraemia. Br Med J 1983; 286:1379–1381.
230. Wilson TR: The pharmacology of tri-potassium di-citrate bismuthate (TDB). Postgrad Med J 1975; 51:18–21.
231. Marshal BJ, Goodwin CS, Warren JR, et al: Prospective double-blind trial of duodenal ulcer relapse after eradication of *Campylobacter pylori.* Lancet 1988; 2:1437–1442.
232. Coughlan G, Gilligan D, Humphries H, et al: *Campylobacter pylori* and recurrence of duodenal ulcers—a 12-month follow-up study. Lancet 1987; 2:1109–1111.
233. Miller JP, Faragher EB: Relapse of duodenal ulcer—does it matter which drug is used in initial treatment? Br Med J 1986; 293:1117–1118.
234. Weller MP: Neuropsychiatric symptoms following bismuth intoxication. Postgrad Med J 1988; 64:308–310.
235. Robert A: Cytoprotection by prostaglandins. Gastroenterology 1979; 77:761–767.
236. Sontag SJ: Prostaglandins in peptic ulcer disease: An overview of current status and future directions. Drugs 1986; 32:445–457.
237. Agrawal NM, Saffouri B, Kruss D, et al: Healing of benign gastric ulcer: A placebo-controlled comparison of two dosage regimens of misoprostol, a synthetic analog of prostaglandin E1. Dig Dis Sci 1985; 30(Suppl):S164.
238. Kawkey CJ, Walt RP: Prostaglandins for peptic ulcer: A promise unfulfilled. Lancet 1986; 2:1084–1087.
239. Doll R, Jones FA, Pygott F: Effect of smoking on the production and maintenance of gastric and duodenal ulcers. Lancet 1958; 1:657–662.
240. McCarthy DM: Smoking and ulcers—time to quit. N Engl J Med 1984; 311:726–728.
241. Korman MG, Hansky J, Eaves ER, et al: Influence of cigarette smoking on healing and relapse in duodenal ulcer disease. Gastroenterology 1983; 85:871–874.
242. Eastwood GL: The role of smoking in peptic ulcer disease. J Clin Gsatroenterol 1988; 10(Suppl 1):S19–S23.
243. Byrne WJ: Diagnosis and treatment of peptic ulcer disease in children. Pediatr Rev 1985; 7:182–190.
244. Cox K, Ament ME: Upper gastrointestinal bleeding in children and adolescents. Pediatrics 1979; 63:408–413.
245. Puri P, Boyd E, Blake N, et al: Duodenal ulcer in childhood: A continuing disease in adult life. J Pediatr Surg 1978; 13:525–526.
246. Ravitch MM, Duremdas GD: Operative treatment of chronic duodenal ulcer in childhood. Ann Surg 1970; 171:641–646.
247. Meyer JH: Chronic morbidity after ulcer surgery. *In* Sleisenger MH, Fordtran JS, eds: Gastrointestinal Disease: Pathophysiology, Diagnosis, Management. Philadelphia; WB Saunders, 1989, pp 962–987.
248. Bonfils S, Ruszniewski P, Costil V, et al: Prolonged treatment of Zollinger-Ellison syndrome by long-acting somatostatin. Lancet 1986; 1:554–555.
249. Norton JA, Doppman JL, Collen MJ, et al: Prospective study of gastrinoma and resection in patients with Zolliner-Ellison syndrome. Ann Surg 1986; 204:468–479.

250. Williamson RCN: Endocrine and other unusual pancreatic tumors. Curr Opin Gastroenterol 1987; 3:749–755.
251. Hastings PR, Skillman JJ, Bushnell LS, et al: Antacid titration in the prevention of acute gastrointestinal bleeding. N Engl J Med 1978; 298:1041–1045.
252. Priebe JH, Skillman JJ, Bushnell LS, et al: Antacid titration in the prevention of acute gastrointestinal bleeding. N Engl J Med 1980; 302:426–430.
253. Ostro MJ, Russell JA, Soldin SJ, et al: Control of gastric pH with cimetidine: Boluses versus primed infusions. Gastroenterology 1985; 89:532–537.
254. Wiest DB, O'Neal W, Reigard JR, et al: Pharmacokinetics of ranitidine in critically ill infants. Dev Pharmacol Ther 1989; 12:7–12.
255. Lloyd CW, Martin WJ, Taylor BD, et al: Pharmacokinetics and pharmacodynamics of cimetidine and metabolites in critically ill children. J Pediatr 1985; 105:295–300.
256. Shuman RB, Shuster DP, Zuckerman GR: Prophylactic therapy for stress ulcer bleeding: A reappraisal. Ann Intern Med 1987; 106:562–567.
257. Driks MR, Craven DE, Celli BR, et al: Nosocomial pneumonia in intubated patients given sucralfate as compared to antacids or histamine type 2 blockers: The role of gastric colonization. N Engl J Med 1987; 317:1376–1382.
258. Cannon LA, Heiselman D, Gardner W, et al: Prophylaxis of upper gastrointestinal tract bleeding in mechanically ventilated patients: A randomized study comparing the efficacy of sucralfate, cimetidine and antacids. Arch Intern Med 1987; 147:2101–2106.
259. Tryba M, Zevounou F, Torok M, et al: Prevention of acute stress bleeding with sucralfate, antacids or cimetidine: A controlled study with pirenzepine as a basic medication. Am J Med 1985; 79(Suppl 2C):55–61.
260. Borrero E, Margolis IB, Bank S, et al: Antacid vs. sucralfate in preventing acute gastrointestinal bleeding: A randomized trial in 100 critically ill patients. Am J Surg 1984; 148:809–812.
261. Laggner AN, Lenz K, Base W, et al: Prevention of upper gastrointestinal bleeding in long-term ventilated patients: Sucralfate versus ranitidine. Am J Med 1989; 86(Suppl 6A):81–84.
262. Du Moulin GC, Paterson DG, Hedley-Whyte J, et al: Aspiration of gastric bacteria in antacid-treated patients: A frequent cause of postoperative colonization of the airway. Lancet 1982; 1:242–245.
263. Tryba M: Risk of acute stress bleeding and nosocomial pneumonia in ventilated intensive care unit patients: Sucralfate versus antacids. Am J Med 1987; 83(Suppl 3B):117–124.
264. Walan A, Bader J-P, Classen M, et al: Effect of omeprazole and ranitidine on ulcer healing and relapse rates in patients with benign gastric ulcer. N Engl J Med 1989; 320:69–75.
265. Graham DY, Agrawal NM, Roth SH: Prevention of NSAID-induced gastric ulcer with misoprostol: Multicentre, double-blind, placebo-controlled trial. Lancet 1988; 2:1277–1280.
266. Lanza FL, Aspinall RL, Swabb EA, et al: Double-blind, placebo-controlled endoscopic comparison of the mucosal protective effects of misoprostol versus cimetidine on tolmetin-induced mucosal injury to the stomach and duodenum. Gastroenterology 1988; 95:289–294.
267. Ehsanullah RSB, Page MC, Tildesley G, et al: Prevention of gastroduodenal damage induced by non-steroidal anti-inflammatory drugs: Controlled trial of ranitidine. Br Med J 1988; 297:1017–1021.
268. Robinson MG, Griffin JW Jr, Bowers J, et al: Effect of ranitidine on gastroduodenal mucosal damage induced by nonsteroidal antiinflammatory drugs. Dig Dis Sci 1989; 34:424–428.
269. Robinson MG, Mills RJ, Euler AR: Ranitidine prevents duodenal ulcers associated with non-steroidal antiinflammatory drug therapy. Aliment Pharmacol Therap 1991; 5:143–150.
270. Lanza F, Peace K, Gustitus L, et al: A blinded endoscopic comparative study of misoprostol versus sucralfate and placebo in the prevention of aspirin-induced gastric and duodenal ulceration. Am J Gastroenterol 1988; 83:143–146.
271. Stadler P, Armstrong D, Margalith D, et al: Diclofenac delays healing of gastroduodenal mucosal lesions: Double-blind placebo-controlled endoscopic study in healthy volunteers. Dig Dis Sci 1991; 5:594–600.
272. Collins JSA, Glasgow JFT, Trouton TG, et al: Twenty year review of duodenal ulcer. Arch Dis Child 1986; 61:407–409.
273. Odera G, Farina L, Ansaldi N: Peptic ulceration: Long-term outcome. Arch Dis Child 1986; 63:104–105.
274. White A, Carachi R, Young DG: Duodenal ulceration presenting in childhood: A long-term follow-up. J Pediatr Surg 1984; 19:6–8.
275. Murphy MS, Eastham EJ: Peptic ulcer disease in childhood: Long-term prognosis. J Pediatr Gastroenterol Nutr 1987; 6:721–724.
276. Shaw-Stiffel TA, Roberts EA: Treatment of acid-peptic disease. *In* Walker WA, Durie PR, Hamilton JR, et al, eds: Pediatric Gastrointestinal Disease: Pathophysiology, Diagnosis, Management. Vol 2. Philadelphia, BC Decker, 1991, pp 1702–1715.

Section Five

THE SMALL AND LARGE INTESTINE

Chapter 34

Anatomy and Physiology of the Small and Large Intestine

DEAN L. ANTONSON

Occupying the majority of the abdominal cavity and working in concert, the small and large intestine are responsible for the complex functions of nutrient digestion and absorption concomitant with fluid and electrolyte transport. Although digestion and absorption of nutrients, including vitamins and trace elements, are almost solely restricted to the small intestine, absorption and secretion of fluid and electrolytes occur with regional variability along both the small and large intestine. Additionally, both the small and large intestine serve important immunologic roles as well as provide a barrier to the potentially harmful external environment. The morphology of these organs is uniquely adapted to serve these purposes; cellular structure and function organize to provide remarkable efficiency. This chapter focuses on the morphology of the small and large intestine along with the physiologic roles of fluid and electrolyte transport. Discussions on the complex processes of nutrient digestion and absorption, gastrointestinal immunology, and overall neuronal and messenger-mediated gut motility and regulation are reserved for presentation elsewhere.

SMALL INTESTINE

Gross Anatomy

The small intestine is a tubular organ folded within the abdominal cavity into numerous loops (Fig. 34–1) and is divided into three segments: duodenum, jejunum, and ileum. Measured from its origin at the pylorus to its termination at the ileocecal valve, the small intestine averages between 250 and 300 cm in length in the newborn,[1–3] increasing to as much as 600 to 800 cm in the adult.[4] The duodenum constitutes approximately the first 25 cm of the small intestine, and the remaining length is arbitrarily divided into the proximal two fifths designated as jejunum and the distal three fifths designated as ileum. The transition from jejunum to ileum is arbitrary, as there is no histologic or gross anatomical demarcation that occurs between these segments. The duodenum is derived from the distal foregut during embryologic development, and the jejunum and ileum are derived from the endodermal midgut.[5] Although a distinct demarcation between jejunum and ileum is not apparent, structural differences are present with progression from proximal jejunum to distal ileum. In the proximal jejunum, the overall thickness of the abdominal wall is greatest, diminishing in size with distal progression. The diameter of the small intestine is also greatest in the jejunum, again diminishing distally. Lastly, the plicae circulares, which are platelike luminal protrusions of the submucosa covered by mucosa extending in a circular fashion along the inside diameter of the intestinal wall (but never running fully circumferentially), are most prominent in the distal duodenum and proximal jejunum (Fig. 34–2), decreasing in number and size with progression through the ileum. Surface area, as a consequence, is much greater in the distal duodenum and jejunum, with an estimated fourfold decrease in surface area occurring over the course of the small intestine.[6] Peyer's patches, which are small aggregates of lymphoid tissue containing four to five lymphoid follicles, are located along the antimesenteric border of the small intestine. They are present in greatest numbers from the mid-ileum distally to the level of the ileocecal valve. These lymphoid follicles, similar to other lymphoid tissue, are most prominent during childhood and regress in size with advancing age.

As a consequence of the need for propulsive peristaltic activity required for digestion, the majority of the small intestine is loosely suspended within the abdominal cavity on a thin, translucent mesentery. The mesentery begins as an anterior reflection of the posterior peritoneum, extending into the peritoneal cavity and circumferentially enveloping the small intestine, returning to become firmly attached to the posterior abdominal wall overlying the spine.[7] The proximal 2 to 5 cm of duodenum, including principally the pylorus, are occasionally supported on a short mesentery, and the remainder of the duodenum lies firmly fixed beneath the peritoneum in a retroperitoneal manner as it progresses in a

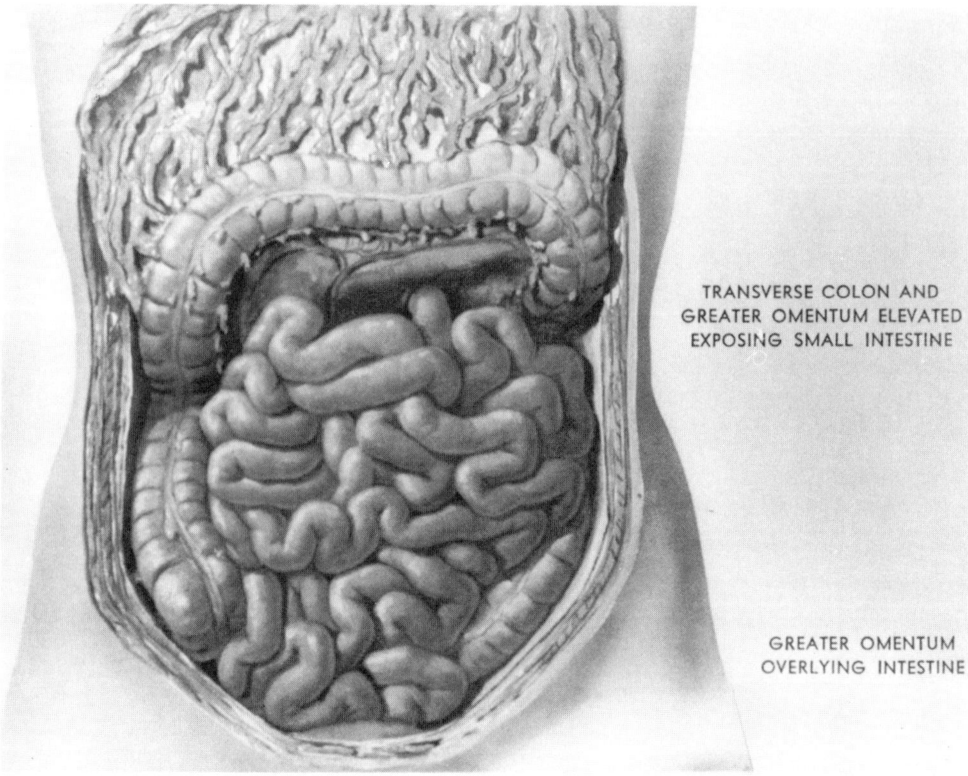

Figure 34–1. Gross anatomic arrangement of the small and large intestine within the abdominal cavity. The jejunal loops are normally situated upward to the left, and the ileal loops are lower to the right. (From Netter F: The CIBA Collection of Medical Illustrations. Vol 3, Part 2: Digestive System: Lower Digestive Tract. West Caldwell, NJ, CIBA Pharmaceutical, 1975, p 47; with permission.)

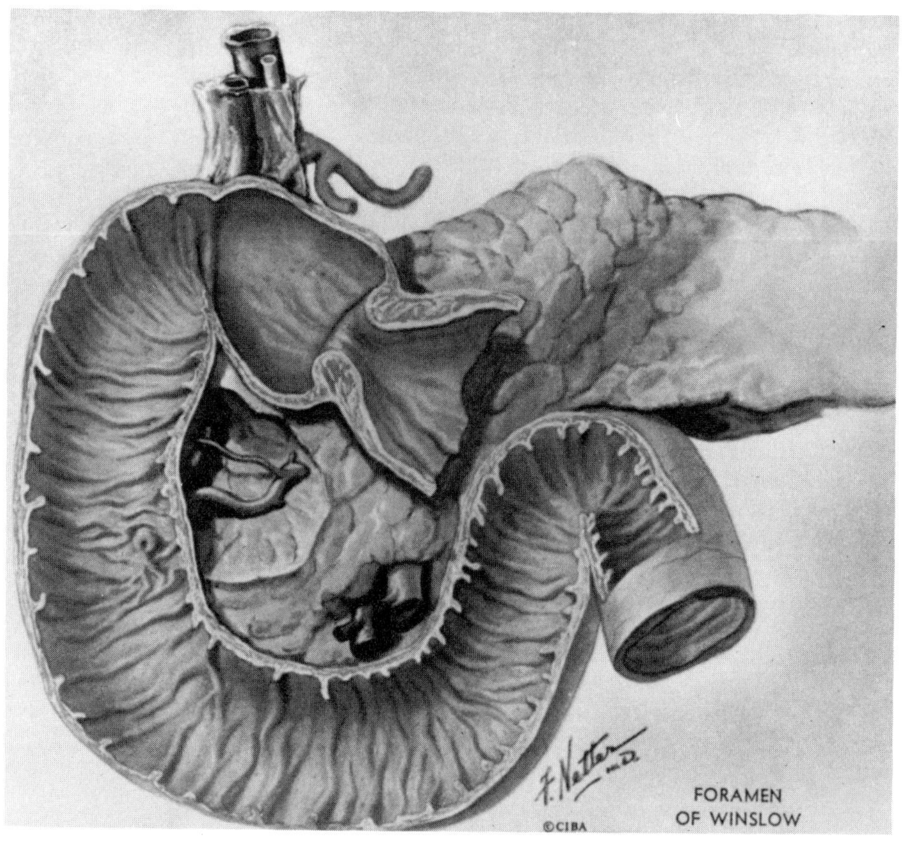

Figure 34–2. Gross anatomic configuration of the duodenum positioned in a horseshoe-shaped manner around the head of the pancreas. Note the prominent mucosal folds, the plicae circulares. (From Netter F: The CIBA Collection of Medical Illustrations. Vol 3, Part 1: Digestive System: Upper Digestive Tract. West Caldwell, NJ, CIBA Pharmaceutical, 1975, p 54; with permission.)

horseshoe-shaped configuration around the head of the pancreas (see Fig. 34–2). The duodenum emerges from this retroperitoneal location at the ligament of Treitz in the left upper quadrant. The entirety of the jejunum and ileum is thereafter suspended by this mesentery, with the exception of the very distal ileum, which is often located retroperitoneally, along with the cecum. The blood vessels, nerves, and lymphatics that supply and drain the small intestine course through the mesentery. The arterial arcades that course through the mesentery to supply the jejunum and ileum are derived from the superior mesenteric artery. The duodenum receives its arterial supply from various branches of the celiac trunk and superior mesenteric artery, including the supraduodenal artery, the gastroduodenal artery, the superior and inferior pancreatoduodenal arteries, and the right gastroepiploic artery.[8] Venous drainage of the small intestine occurs primarily through the portal vein and superior mesenteric vein, with a minor component flowing into the splenic vein.[8] Lymphatic drainage coursing through the mesentery from the villous lacteals and lymph follicles converges to preaortic lymph nodes around the superior mesenteric and celiac arteries. Lymphatic flow then progresses to the intestinal trunk (70%) or to the cisterna chyli (25%), continuing through the thoracic duct to drain into the left subclavian vein.[8] In contradistinction to the colonic mesentery, little fat is deposited in the mesentery of the small intestine, with the proximal mesentery being translucent in appearance and the mesentery of the more distal ileum being translucent to opaque, since minor fat deposition does occur here.[8] Normal embryologic rotation of the small intestine typically results in the proximal jejunal loops being located in the left upper quadrant of the abdomen, the distal jejunal and proximal ileal loops being located periumbilically, and the distal ileal loops being located in the right lower quadrant.

The duodenum is again arbitrarily divided into four segments: the proximal or first portion of the duodenum, including the pylorus and duodenal bulb; the second portion, defined as the descending portion; the third portion, which courses over the spine traversing laterally from right to left and lying just inferior to the origin of the superior mesenteric artery; and the fourth portion or ascending duodenum to the level of the ligament of Treitz (see Fig. 34–2). It is within the confines of the second portion of the duodenum that the pancreatic and biliary ducts drain. In the majority of children, the pancreatic and biliary ducts join together approximately 1 to 2 cm from the outer margins of the duodenal wall and then traverse the posteromedial aspect of the duodenal wall, entering this structure through the ampulla of Vater. In 5 to 10% of individuals, an accessory pancreatic duct also enters 1 to 2 cm proximal to this, as the duct of Santorini.[9]

Cellular Morphology

Four layers make up the wall of the small intestine. From outside inwardly, these consist of the serosa, the muscularis, the submucosa, and the mucosa. The mucosa is further subdivided into three distinctive regions and, again beginning from outside inwardly, are the muscularis mucosa, lamina propria, and epithelial cell layer (Fig. 34–3).

The serosa or outermost layer of the small intestine is a simple extension of the peritoneum and mesentery as it envelops this tubular organ. It consists of a single layer of flattened mesothelial cells supported by a small amount of loose connective tissue, the adventitia. A full serosal coat is present in all segments of the small intestine that are supported by a true mesentery. Those structures that are retroperitoneal, including the duodenum and very terminal portion of the ileum, have a serosal surface only on their anterior or anterolateral margins.

The muscularis comprises smooth muscle cells, which are divided distinctly into two separate layers: an outer longitudinal layer and an inner circular layer. The individual muscle cells are elongated and spindle shaped, possessing a single nucleus. The key histologic feature of these cells is the presence of numerous intercellular communications that are tightly adherent, termed *gap junctions.* This allows electrical as well as mechanical coupling to occur between cells. The cells are also surrounded by a noncontinuous thin septa and a thin basal lamina. The presence of intercellular coupling via the gap junctions along with noncontinuous septae functionally permits the uninterrupted proximal to distal integration required for progressive peristaltic contractions.[10] The muscular layers are heavily endowed with sympathetic and parasympathetic nerves arising primarily from the vagus and mesenteric nerves. This ganglionated nerve plexus, located between the longitudinal and circular layers of the muscle coat, is termed the *myenteric* or *Auerbach's plexus* and extends without discontinuity throughout the alimentary tract. From this plexus, small nerve fibrils ramify throughout the muscle layers to contact individual smooth muscle cells.

The submucosa is a band of dense connective tissue bounded below by the muscularis and above by the outermost layer of the mucosa, the muscularis mucosae. Lying adjacent to the mucosa, and given the specialized absorptive tasks of the mucosa, the submucosa is richly endowed with numerous arteries, veins, and lymphatic channels. Such a rich vascular supply is required to ensure adequate handling of absorbed fluids, nutrients, and electrolytes following a meal. Also lying within the submucosa is an extensive network of ganglion cells and nerve fibers constituting the *autonomic submucosal plexus,* or *Meissner's plexus,* which is again continuous along the entire length of the gastrointestinal tract. Prolific interdigitation occurs between both Meissner's and Auerbach's plexus, resulting in comprehensive neuroregulatory control of the small intestine. A sparse number of additional cells are also scattered within the submucosa, including macrophages, leukocytes, lymphocytes, plasma cells, mast cells, and occasional eosinophils.

Located primarily in the submucosa of the duodenum but extending for a variable length within the proximal jejunum are Brunner's glands (Fig. 34–4*A*). These are arrays of elaborately branched epithelial cells that con-

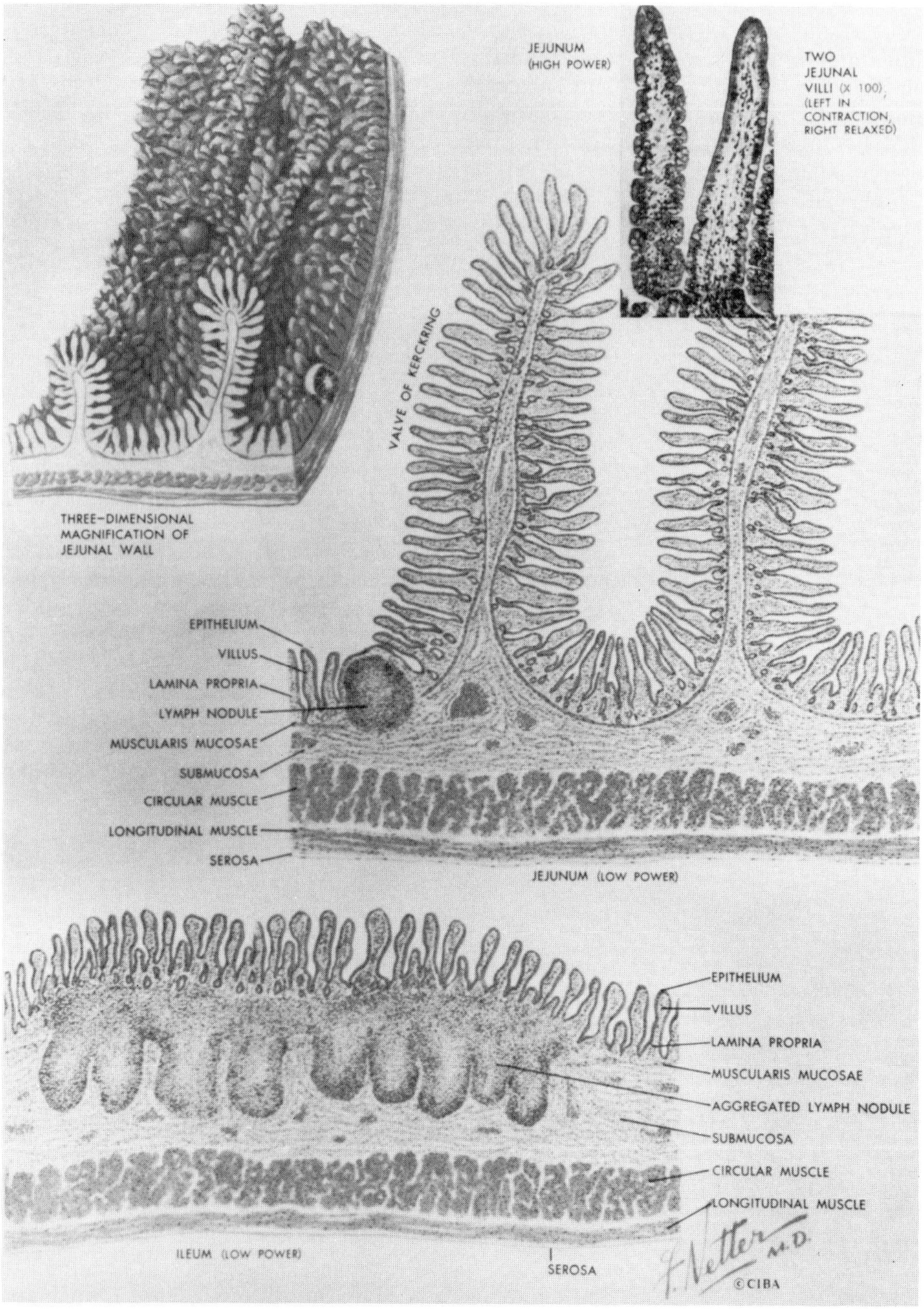

Figure 34–3. Schematic illustration of a cross-section of human jejunum and ileum. (From Netter F: The CIBA Collection of Medical Illustrations. Vol 3, Part 2: Digestive System: Lower Digestive Tract. West Caldwell, NJ, CIBA Pharmaceutical, 1975, p 49; with permission.)

tain both mucous and serous secretion. Brunner's glands interconnect and drain into the base of the duodenal crypts, where they secrete both mucous and bicarbonate.[11] The mucous secretion is believed to provide protection for the duodenum against acid peptic digestion. Although bicarbonate secretion was also believed to originate primarily from Brunner's glands, recent evidence suggests that this may occur from the duodenal epithelium as well.[12] Because of their submucosal location, Brunner's glands, when present in abundant numbers, may distort the architecture of the overlying mucosa. This is an important fact to be remembered by endoscopists during an upper gastrointestinal examination, so as not to be misled.

As indicated earlier, the innermost layer of the gastrointestinal tract, or mucosa, is composed of three distinct layers: the muscularis mucosae, lamina propria, and epithelial cell lining. The most striking morphologic and most important physiologic feature of the mucosa is the tremendous enhancement in surface area that is achieved via the mucosal formation of villi, which are small fingerlike or leaflike protrusions of the lamina propria covered by epithelium (see Fig. 34–4). The formation of intestinal villi, the presence of numerous microvilli on the surface of each enterocyte, and the previously mentioned mounding of the mucosa provided by the plicae circulares (also termed the *valves of Kerckring*) result in an overall 300- to 500-fold increase

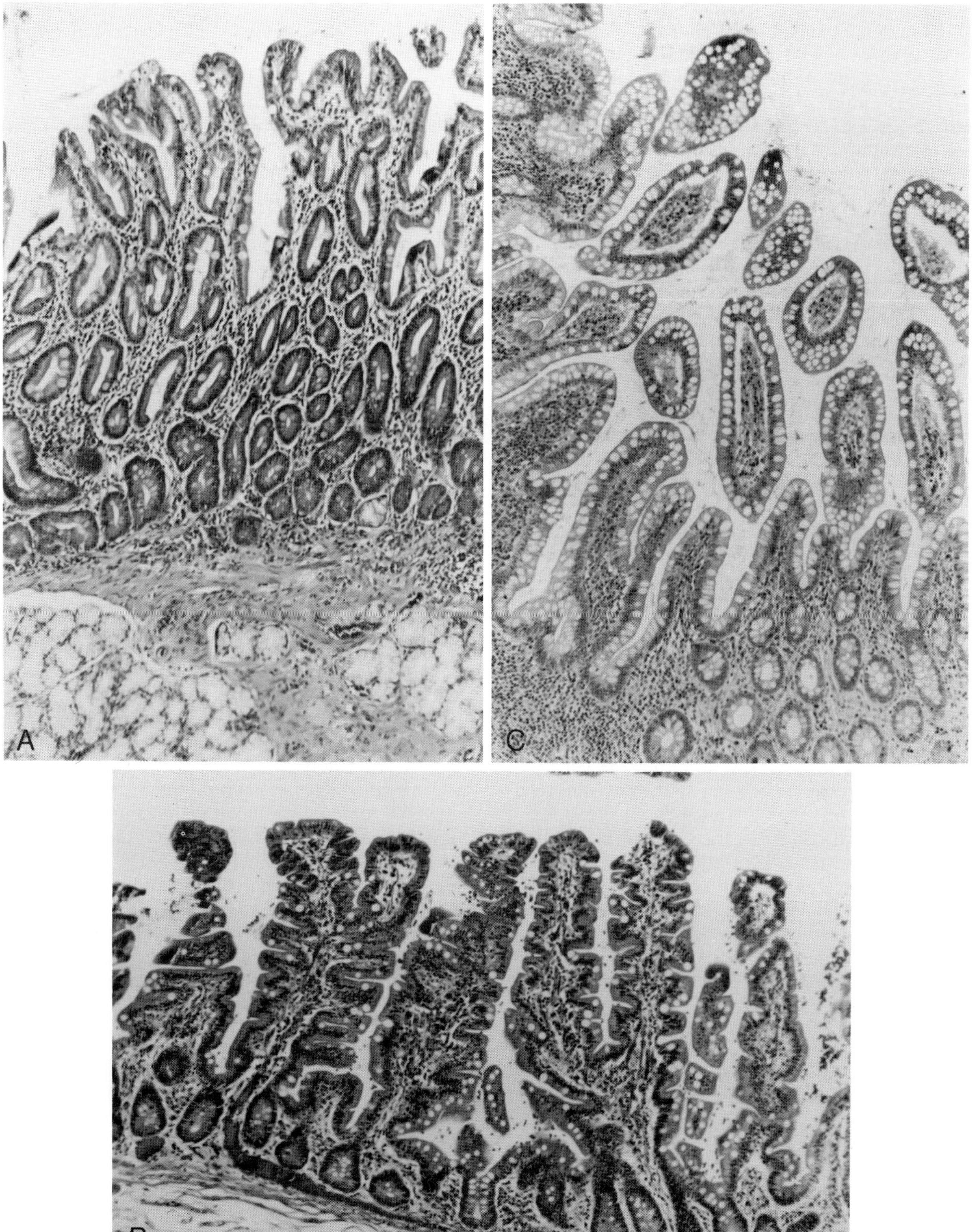

Figure 34–4. Light micrographs of normal human mucosa of the small intestine. *A,* Duodenal mucosa. Brunner's glands are readily identifiable within the submucosa. *B,* Jejunal mucosa. Villi are tall, thin, and most prominently developed within the jejunum. *C,* Ileal mucosa. Villi are broader and shorter, goblet cells are prominent, and the lamina propria contains more lymph follicles and lymphoid cells. Hematoxylin-eosin stain, × 100. (Courtesy of R. S. Markin, MD.)

in surface area.[13] In contrast, in the proximal duodenum, the villi are often fewer in number, wider, and ridged shaped. Duodenal villi are also shorter, increasing in size to a maximal height of approximately 1.5 mm in the proximal jejunum.[6] The villi in the distal duodenum and proximal jejunum are leaf shaped and only intermittently finger shaped, progressing to a more uniform finger shape in the distal jejunum. Thereafter, from the distal jejunum to the ileum, finger-shaped villi are predominant. Overall villous height decreases with progression distally through the ileum (see Fig. 34–4). Surrounding the base of each villi are several pitlike crypts, the crypts of Lieberkühn, which average in depth about one third to one fourth the height of the villus. The epithelium overlying the intestinal villi is continuous with that of the crypts. The intestinal villi are also variable in shape, with differences occurring between ethnic groups and among animal species. In several ethnic groups, including inhabitants of India, the Caribbean islands, and Southeast Asia, intestinal villi are shorter, and the crypts are somewhat deeper. The exact significance of these differences is as yet unknown.[12]

The deepest layer of the intestinal mucosa is the muscularis mucosae. This is a thin sheet of smooth muscle cells, averaging 3 to 10 cells thick, lying immediately above the submucosa.

Structurally supporting the epithelium and lying above the muscularis mucosae is the lamina propria. The lamina propria is composed of a thin layer of connective tissue that surrounds the crypts and extends into the fingerlike or leaflike villous protrusions. Arterioles, capillaries, veins, lacteals, small nerve fibrils, and numerous additional cellular elements are present within the lamina propria. A central artery rises within the center of each villus; at the villous tip it fans out in an umbrella-like capillary network that cascades down the sides of the villus in close proximity to the basal surfaces of the epithelial cells. The close proximity of the endothelial lining to the enterocytes allows for rapid transference of absorbed nutrients, fluids, and electrolytes. The capillary walls are fenestrated with diaphragmatic covers, which greatly facilitates the absorptive process.[14] Lymphatics as well as small nerve fibrils are present within the core of each villus, along with a scattering of plasma cells, macrophages, lymphocytes, eosinophils, fibroblasts, and mast cells. Regulation of intestinal transport is the result of the combined effects of cholinergic and adrenergic nerve fibrils, cytokines, histamine, and arachidonic acid released by the cellular elements above and the secretory products of the enteroendocrine cells within the mucosal epithelium. Overlying the surface of the lamina propria, and upon which are the columnar epithelial cells, is an approximate 30 nm amorphous sheet of basal lamina, containing lamina, heparin, sulfate, protoglycin, fibronectin, and type IV collagen.[12] The lamina propria is also the site of apparent immunoglobulin A (IgA) synthesis, providing significant immunologic protection to the host. The lamina propria contains numerous additional immunologic components, including helper and inducer T lymphocytes and other T lymphocyte subtypes.

Although the epithelial cell lining of the small intestine is continuous, cell populations differ between the crypts, the villi, and the epithelium overlying the lymphoid aggregates or Peyer's patches. Within the intestinal crypts, the most abundant cells are the undifferentiated columnar epithelial cells, with lesser amounts of goblet cells, enteroendocrine cells, Paneth cells, tuft cells, and occasional cuplike cells. The villous epithelium contains a similar population of cells, with maturing enterocytes replacing the undifferentiated cells; Paneth cells are uniformly absent. The epithelium overlying Peyer's patches similarly contains all these cellular elements plus one additional cell, the structurally distinctive M cell. Although the function of cells overlying the villi is absorption, crypt cells are responsible for water and ion secretion and cell renewal. Enteroendocrine cells function as regulatory cells both within the crypts and on the villous epithelium. The function of M cells appears to be that of assisting in antigen processing and sampling of luminal bacterial populations, but this is only speculation.[12]

Mitotic activity within the intestinal crypts is quite prolific. Undifferentiated crypt cells are multipotential, giving rise not only to intestinal absorptive cells but to all other cellular components, including goblet cells, enteroendocrine cells, Paneth cells, cup cells, tuft cells, and M cells. Following cell division, all cellular types, with the sole exception of the Paneth cell, migrate luminally along the intestinal crypt wall, differentiating as this progression occurs. Cells destined to become absorptive cells acquire the specialized structure and function needed for this process. Final acquisition to a mature cell type occurs on the sides of the villi, reaching maximum differentiation in the upper third of the villous tip. At the villous tip per se, an extrusion zone exists where senile cells degenerate and are sloughed into the intestinal lumen. Epithelial cellular migration and maturation occur on the average every 3 to 5 days, with the entire mucosal lining being replaced in somewhat less than a week. Overlying the Peyer's patches, epithelial cell differentiation produces a scattered number of M cells for suspected antigenic sampling. The orchestration of this whole process is likely the result of both luminal factors as well as autocrine, endocrine, and paracrine secretions from the surrounding cells.

Absorptive Cell

The major cellular component of both the crypts and the villi is the enterocyte, or absorptive cell, which is a tall columnar cell containing a basally located nucleus with one or several nucleoli. These cells rest tightly on their basal lamina and are attached at the apical pole to adjacent enterocytes by *tight junctions*. The luminal surface is thrown into numerous (1,000–2,000 per cell) fingerlike membrane extensions termed *microvilli* (Fig. 34–5), measuring approximately 1 mm in height.[6] The microvilli, therefore, are in direct contact with the luminal contents and contain the membrane-bound digestive proteins, transport proteins, and other elements necessary for nutrient absorption.[12] The microvillous membrane is 10 to 11 nm thick and is enriched with protein and glucoprotein.[6] The cholesterol and

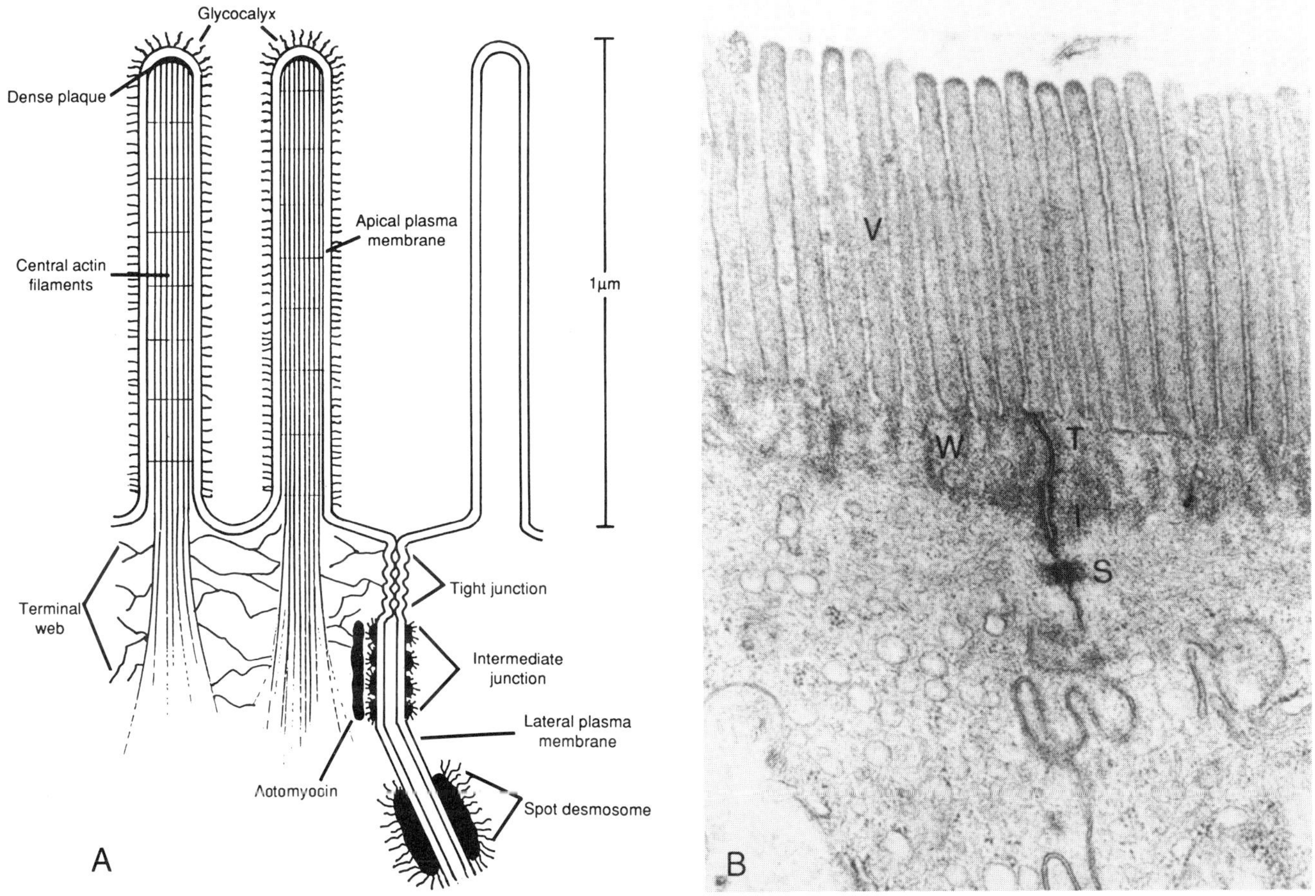

Figure 34–5. Microvillous membrane. *A,* Schematic illustration of the microvillous membrane and specialized supporting structures of the apical cytoplasm of adjacent intestinal absorptive cells. *B,* Electron micrograph of adjacent villous absorptive cells. The adjacent cells are tightly adherent through the formation of a junctional complex, containing a tight junction *(T),* intermediate junction *(I),* and spot desmosome *(S).* Thin supporting central filaments of actin are present within the microvillus *(V)* and terminate by embedding with filaments in the terminal web *(W).* × 15,000.

glycolipid content of this membrane is greater than that of the basolateral membrane, which is also somewhat thinner. Interposed between the microvilli and lying on top of the microvilli to a depth of approximately 0.5 µm is a filamentous glycoprotein coat called the *glycocalyx,* or the *fuzzy coat.* The glycoproteins making up this layer are firmly attached to the membrane surface and are resistant to removal by enzymatic activity.[4, 12] These proteins appear to be synthesized within the intestinal enterocytes, packaged by the Golgi apparatus, and secreted onto the surface of these cells. The microvilli are supported by an internal cytoskeleton located in the apical portion of the cells, called the *terminal web.* The terminal web also interdigitates with the junctional complexes, or *tight junctions.*

Adjacent enterocytes are tightly adherent at their apical pole through the formation of junctional complexes (see Fig. 34–5). These consist of three areas of tight membrane adherence: the most proximal tight junction or zonula occludens; an intermediate junction, or zonula adherens; and a deeper junction, the spot desmosome or macular adherence. Movement of fluid and ions through this intermembranous space is termed *paracellular transport.* The proximal and most tightly adherent section of the junction complex, the zonula occludens, measures approximately 100 to 600 nm in depth.[12] Discrete fusion sites are honeycombed within this junction, creating several barriers to the flow of water and electrolytes. The amount of molecular flow through this paracellular pathway is variable, being somewhat leakier in the proximal small intestine and somewhat tighter in the ileum. There is also evidence to suggest that the functional state of this junctional complex changes, maintaining a relatively high resistance between meals and a low resistance postprandially.[12] The intermediate junction lying just below the tight junction is less closely adherent, with cells being separated by a 15 to 20 nm gap. A fibrillar network is present between the cell membranes within this space, recently characterized as *uvomorulin.*[15] The main function of this area appears to be to provide support to the overall continuity of the junctional complex. The most distal element is that of the spot desmosome, where again adjacent lateral membranes are approximated to a space of between 30 and 50 nm.[12] Contrary to the zonula occludens, spot desmosomes are not continuous around the circumference of the cell, but are rather intermittently distributed. Again, the function of this area appears to be primarily to support the overall continuity and integrity of the tight junctions. The remainder of the lateral wall of the enterocyte below the spot desmosome is termed the *basolateral membrane.* This membrane differs both biochemically and structurally from the apical membrane. The basolateral membrane has smooth contours and broad folds, which likely interdigitate with adjacent lateral cellular membranes.[16] The disaccharidases and peptidases present on the apical membrane are not present in the basolateral membrane, but this membrane is heavily enriched with NA^+,K^+–ATPase, glycosyl transferases, and possibly adenyl cyclase.[12] Cholesterol is also less prominent in the basolateral membrane, and membrane fluidity is therefore higher than that of the apical membrane. The location of Na^+,K^+–ATPase in the basolateral membrane is the major energy-dependent mechanism controlling fluid and electrolyte transport.

In addition to the basally oriented nuclei, other cellular organelles are present within the enterocyte in anticipated polarity. Immediately above the nuclei lies the Golgi apparatus, responsible for the terminal glycosylation of synthesized proteins. Also scattered throughout the cell are free ribosomes, smooth and rough endoplasmic reticulum, microtubules, lysosomes, and mitochondria, all responsible and working in concert for the absorption, packaging, and subsequent extrusion of absorbed lipids, carbohydrates, and peptides.

Goblet Cell

Being present in far fewer numbers than the intestinal absorptive cells, the next most common cell populating the intestinal villi is the goblet cell. Goblet cells are again columnar in appearance. However, the apex of the cell is expanded with mucin-secreting granules and oval in configuration; the base of the cell remains narrowed, giving the cell the characteristic wineglass appearance. The nucleus and Golgi apparatus are basally oriented, and the remaining cellular organelles align themselves along the lateral margin of the cell, being compressed to these regions by the abundant mucin-secreting granules within the cell interior. Goblet cell mucus is largely composed of glycoprotein, is rich in carbohydrate,[17] and is discharged from the apical surface of the cell by apparent fusion of the apical membrane with the membrane of the granule by exocytosis.[18] Although the specific functions of goblet cell mucin remain speculative, it likely serves as a protective lubricant barrier to the epithelial surface, perhaps acts as a hydrating gel between the glycocalyx and unstirred water layer, and may bind specifically with bacterial surface antigens to inhibit their attachment to the epithelial cell surface.[12] There is mild disparity in cellular distribution along the axis of the gastrointestinal tract, with goblet cells being slightly more prominent in the distal ileum.[19] Goblet cells originate from undifferentiated crypt cells, with occasional further cell division occurring as they migrate up the crypts and onto the villous tips.[20]

Enteroendocrine Cell

Represented sparsely throughout the entire length of the small intestine, but present in both the crypt and villous regions, are the physiologically important enteroendocrine cells. These cells are again tall and columnar in appearance, have well-developed microvilli on the apical surface, and attach to adjacent enterocytes with typical tight junction formation. Endocrine cells have a basal to medially located large nucleus with a supranuclear Golgi apparatus. The most distinctive features of these cells are the neurosecretory granules contained within the cytoplasm, which tend to be distributed most prominently in the basilar region below the nucleus, with a scattering of granules also present along the lateral aspect of the nucleus and surrounding the Golgi apparatus.[21] By electron microscopy, the cytoplasm of the enteroendocrine cells is relatively less dense, compared to the surrounding enterocytes. The secretory granules of individual enteroendocrine cells appear to be relatively uniform in shape, size, and density, suggesting that the granules are relatively specific, secreting only a single or perhaps two biogenically active secretory amines or peptide hormones. Differing in their secretory products, a whole host of enteroendocrine cells are present along the length of the gastrointestinal tract, secreting such products as secretin, gastrin, vasoactive intestinal polypeptide (VIP), gastric inhibitory polypeptide (GIP), neurotensin, cholecystokinin, somatostatin, enteroglucagon, substance P, pancreatic polypeptide, and glycinin.[22, 23] The secretory products from the granules are discharged along the basilar to basolateral surface of the enteroendocrine cell and have both paracrine effects locally within the gastrointestinal tract and endocrine effects that modulate gastrointestinal function regionally as well as at distant organ sites. Several recent reviews detailing the classification of these cells and their secretory products are available for further review.[24–26]

Paneth Cell

Present in sparse numbers and located solely at the base of the crypts are the Paneth cells. These cells appear to be derived from undifferentiated crypt cells and are more pyramidal than columnar in shape, with the widest portion being at the base. The nucleus is basal in location, and numerous eosinophilic granules are present in the apical cytoplasm.[12] Microvilli are well developed over the narrowed surface membrane, but shorter in length. The secretory granules are believed to release their products through the surface membrane by exocytosis. The exact function of the Paneth cells and their secretory products remains in question, although a role in host protection is suggested by the cells' ability to phagocytize bacteria and protozoa,[27] as well as by the presence within the secretory granules of lysozyme[28] and trypsinlike activity.[29]

Cup Cell

Present in very sparse numbers within the crypts and on the villi of the small intestine are intestinal cup cells. These cells are tall and columnar, being somewhat narrower than the surrounding enterocytes. A distinctive feature of the cup cells is the microvillous surface, which contains shorter microvilli and a thickened glycocalyx coat.[30] This cell derives its name from the characteristic cuplike depression of the apical surface. The cell contains the normal array of cytoplasmic organelles; however, the mitochondria are unusual in configuration, being denser and having widened intracristal spaces.[31] The exact function of cup cells is unknown at present.

Tuft Cell

Another sparsely represented cell of the intestinal epithelium is the tuft or caveolated cell. This cell is characterized by the presence of tall, thick microvilli that protrude further into the gastrointestinal lumen than the surrounding microvillous membranes of the enterocytes. The cytoskeleton supporting the microvilli is also more prominent in these cells, extending deeper into the apical cytoplasm.[12] No known function is presently ascribed to these cells.

M Cell

Admixed with the normal mucosal cell population overlying intestinal Peyer's patches and present in sparse to moderate numbers are specialized M cells. M cells are easily recognized because of their distinctive shape, being more oval or globular in configuration, narrower at the apex, and widened at the base. The microvillous surface at the apex of the M cell is characterized by irregular shortened microvilli that are occasionally fused and, under electron microscopy, occasionally take on the appearance of ridges or folds rather than true microvilli.[32] Alkaline phosphatase activity of the microvillous membrane is decreased over levels found in the surrounding enterocytes.[33] The terminal web region is less well organized, and lysosomes are fewer in number.[12] The basal region of the M cells rests directly above the lymphoid follicles of the lamina propria, and it appears that these cellular characteristics allow M cells to function as antigen samplers of luminal contents. Endocytotic activity is located at the apical surface of the cell, likely arising from pitlike depressions over the apical membrane, allowing for the transport of larger molecular weight antigens from intestinal protozoa, bacteria, and viruses.[34] Transcellular transport of these antigens to the basilar surface with exocytotic presentation to the underlying lymphoid tissue is speculated to produce a secretory IgA response from within the crypts, which is then host protective.

Water Movement

The epithelial lining of the small intestine is an absorptive epithelium and is responsible for the isotonic transport of fluids across this cell layer. Fluid transported via this mechanism is then taken up by the intestinal capillaries, primarily as the result of Starling forces.[35] In general terms, the epithelium of the small intestine is a "leaky" epithelium, ideally suited for the isotonic transfer of fluids. The structural organization of the epithelial cells allows for this transfer, based primarily on the differing permeabilities of the apical and basolateral membranes and on the presence of tight junctions. Water can move through the intestinal epithelial by means of three pathways: (1) through the apical membrane into the cell and then through the basilar membrane, (2) through the apical membrane and then into the lateral intercellular space through the basolateral membrane, or (3) via the paracellular pathway, which results in water movement through the tight junctions into the lateral intercellular space. Although differences in opinion exist, the majority of water movement probably occurs through the apical membrane and then across the basolateral membrane, thereafter passing from the lateral intercellular space through the basal lamina for absorption by the intestinal capillaries. A comprehensive discussion of water movement through epithelial tissues is beyond the scope of this text, and the reader is referred to several recent reviews for further information on this topic.[35–37]

Although many questions remain unanswered regarding the specifics of water movement through the intestinal epithelium, a summary of the current understanding of osmotic water transfer is important. The three-compartment, two-membrane model for epithelial fluid transport that was developed by Curran and MacIntosh[38] still provides the best basis for understanding this phenomenon (Fig. 34–6). The principal tenets upon which this model is based are that the two membranes separating the three compartments have differing permeabilities to solutes, and that water moves from one compartment to another solely by physiochemical properties.[35, 39] Within the small intestine, water moves either by osmotic forces (a difference in solute concentration gradients) or by hydrostatic pressure. There is no strong evidence that any significant movement of water occurs by electrical potential difference gradients.[35] In terms of intestinal transport relative to this model, the outer compartment is considered to be equivalent to the luminal bulk phase, the middle compartment equivalent to the lateral intercellular space adjacent to the basolateral membrane, and the inner compartment equivalent to the interstitial space below the basal lamina. (Actually, for transcellular movement of water, three membranes must be passed: the apical surface membrane; the basolateral membrane; and the basal lamina, which is not a true membrane, but functions as a barrier through which fluid must move. However, since the apical and basolateral membranes are semipermeable membranes and the basal lamina is a permeable membrane,[35] the model still provides the

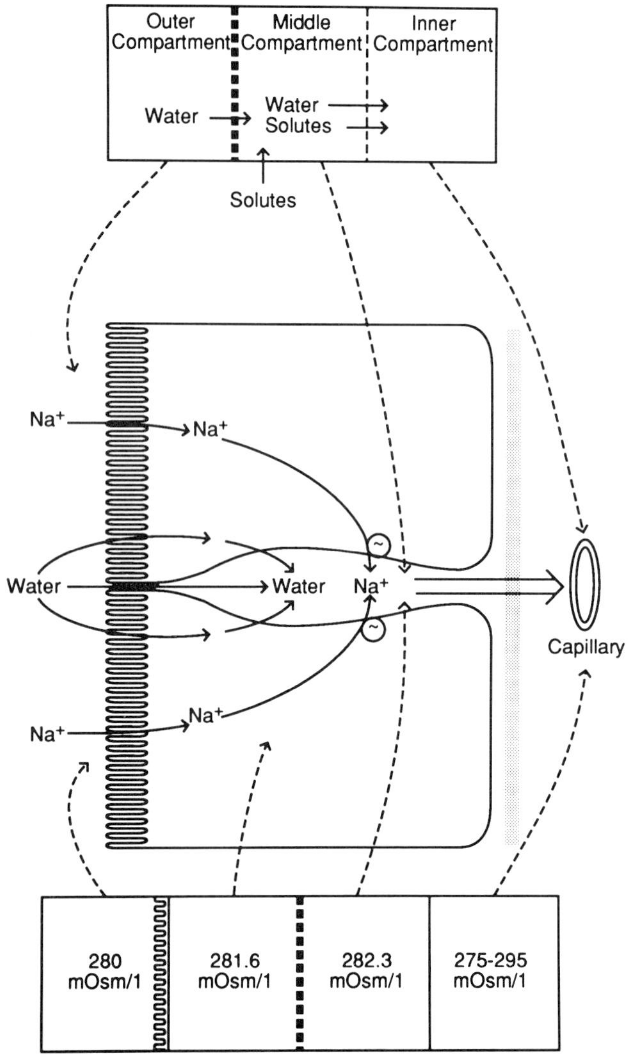

Figure 34–6. Schematic diagram of the proposed model for solute-coupled water transport. Upper panel depicts the three-compartment, two-membrane model developed by Curran and MacIntosh.[38] The lower panel further develops this model to reflect the three membranes through which the majority of water moves during absorption. The small osmolar differences noted between compartments in the lower panel are believed to be sufficient to account for the known rates of water transport. The semipermeable cell membrane has a high water permeability and a relatively lower solute permeability; the basal lamina has both high water and solute permeabilities. Water then moves across the apical and basolateral cell membranes by the osmolar gradients created as a result of solute transport and across the permeable basal lamina by the increased hydrostatic pressure generated in the lateral intercellular space. Since the force of the osmotic gradient across the basolateral membrane is greater than the force created by the increase in hydrostatic pressure, water will preferentially move across the basal lamina and not back into the cell.

necessary instruction to understand water movement. Exactly how these membranes function in series to move water by the transcellular route will be explained later in this chapter.) The membrane separating the outer compartment from the middle compartment is the apical cell membrane (ignoring for now the basolateral membrane), and the membrane separating the middle compartment from the inner compartment is the basal lamina and interstitial tissue. In this model, solutes entering the middle compartment create a relative degree of hypertonicity, which is followed by water movement across the semipermeable (apical) membrane by osmotic forces. The influx of water then increases hydrostatic pressure in the middle compartment, forcing both water and solutes out across the basal lamina. (Justification for the presence of increased hydrostatic forces consistent with this theory is provided by the known expansion of the lateral intercellular spaces that occurs during intestinal absorption of fluids.)[35] Since the apical membrane is semipermeable, solutes will not move back across this membrane, and since the osmotic force across this membrane exceeds the force generated by the small increase in hydrostatic pressure, water will not back diffuse through this membrane.[35] Since water and solutes can diffuse readily through the basal lamina, hydrostatic forces will direct that water and solutes move primarily from the middle compartment to the inner compartment (below the basal lamina for capillary absorption).

With this model in mind, the isotonic movements of water and solutes through the intestinal epithelium can then be understood. The differences in permeability between the apical membrane, basolateral membrane, and basal lamina are roughly analogous to this proposed model. Solute entry into the middle compartment is achieved primarily by active transport processes, which are the driving force for all fluid movement. The apical cell membrane, of course, contains the numerous active transport processes for solutes, including glucose and amino acids, which obligatorily transfer sodium in the process. The basolateral membrane contains the active transport process for sodium in the form of the Na^+, K^+–ATPase pump. During absorption, as solutes are actively transported across the apical membrane, a relative degree of hypotonicity develops in the unstirred layer above the apical membrane, concomitant with a cellular microenvironment of mild hypertonicity.[35] The osmotic forces generated by the osmolar difference across the apical membrane then account for water movement into the cell. Active transport of sodium across the basolateral membrane then results in a mild further increase in osmolarity across the basolateral membrane, with the lateral intercellular space now being slightly hypertonic as compared to the cell interior. This then results in the transference of water across the basolateral membrane into the intercellular space. Hydrostatic pressure increases within this space, which results in the further movement of solutes and water across the freely permeable basal lamina and interstitial space for absorption into the intestinal capillaries. Although the end result is that the transfer of fluid has occurred isotonically, relatively small differences in osmolality account for water movement across the apical and basolateral cell membranes. As can be anticipated, additional fluid is also transferred into the basolateral spaces across the tight junctions. As the tight junctions are less permeable than the basal lamina, fluid movement as defined by the above model is similarly present. Some differences in opinion exist, however, regarding the relative rates of transepithelial versus paracellular fluid movement, although current opinion favors the majority of fluid being absorbed via the transcellular route. Evidence for this is provided by the cross-sectional areas of these respective cellular components: the apical cross-sectional area is estimated to be 10^4 times greater than that of the cross-sectional area of the tight junctions.[35] For the paracellular route to account for the majority of fluid movement, water permeability through the tight junctions would have to exceed 10^4 times that present across the apical epithelium, which is not believed to be physiologically possible. That a certain component of fluid moves across the tight junctions, assisting in overall fluid absorption in the small intestine, is not in question.

Support for these hypotheses of water movement across the intestinal epithelial cells has recently been provided by analyses of fluid transport across the similarly leaky membranes of the Necturus gallbladder.[35, 40] Based on specific calculations obtained with this model, fluid movements through the intestinal epithelium can be achieved with osmotic differences of only 1.6 mOsm per L across the apical membrane, and of only an additional 0.7 mOsm per L across the basolateral membrane. In total, then, the osmotic difference between the luminal bulk phase and the lateral intercellular fluid needs to be only 2.3 mOsm per L to account for the normal rates of fluid transport known to occur.[40]

Ion Transport

In addition to absorbing required amounts of nutrients and water, the small intestinal mucosa is also responsible for the transportation of ions for the maintenance of normal physiologic homeostasis. To accomplish this task, the intestinal epithelium is endowed with specific absorptive as well as secretory mechanisms for the handling of luminal ions, including sodium, potassium, chloride, bicarbonate, and hydrogen, along with lesser amounts of polyvalent ions, including phosphate and sulfate. The intent of this section is not to provide the reader with an exhaustive overview of intestinal ion transport for monovalent and polyvalent ions, but rather to give a general overview of intestinal ion transport, focusing on the transport of the major constituents, including sodium, potassium, chloride, bicarbonate, and hydrogen.

Prior to embarking on such a review, some general principles about intestinal epithelial cell ion transport need to be presented:

1. The capacity for both absorption and secretion of intestinal ions is present along the entire length of the small intestine; however, variability does exist between the jejunum and ileum relative to the mechanisms that are primarily employed for ion transport.
2. Ion transport across the small intestinal epithelium occurs by three general mechanisms: passive diffusion, convention, or active transport. Passive diffusion of ions occurs either because of a difference in chemical concentration gradients or because of electrical potential differences. Convention, also termed *solvent drag,* results from the passive flow of solutes or ions secondary to water flow.[39] Active transport processes are carrier mediated and result from an energy-dependent process that moves ions against either an electrical or a chemical concentration gradient.
3. In all segments of the small intestine, the final common denominator resulting in the driving force for all active ion transport is the sodium-potassium pump (Na^+,K^+–ATPase) located along the basolateral membranes.[36]
4. Intestinal ion transport can occur across the small intestinal epithelium by either the transcellular or the paracellular route.
5. Absorption of ions is a function of the intestinal epithelium covering the villi, and secretion is a function of the crypt cells.[36]
6. The small intestinal epithelium of the jejunum and ileum is a "leaky" membrane, characterized by low electrical resistances, low transepithelial potential differences, high water permeabilities, and an inability to absorb sodium against significant concentration gradients.[35] There is a variable differentiation of this characteristic, with the jejunum being less restrictive to ion flow and with resistance increasing as progression occurs distally through the ileum and colon.
7. All ionic transport processes that move solutes against their electrochemical gradients are either primarily or secondarily linked to the active extrusion of sodium at the basolateral membrane via the Na^+,K^+–ATPase pump.[36]
8. Intestinal ion transport in any given segment of the small intestine is generally a reflection of several mechanisms, not solely the result of a single mechanism.

Changes in composition of the large volume of fluid and electrolytes presented to the intestine for absorption occur as fluids move from jejunum to ileum. The intestinal epithelium has adapted to this with mechanisms predominating in each segment that allow for the most efficient transport of ions. Although all the transport mechanisms are likely represented in the majority of enterocytes, their relative importance pertaining to function is variable, allowing for efficient fluid and ion absorption as the luminal contents are altered.

Sodium Absorption

The intestinal epithelium has adapted a number of mechanisms for sodium absorption. These include glucose- or amino acid–stimulated sodium absorption, electrogenic sodium absorption, sodium-hydrogen exchange, electroneutral sodium chloride absorption, and solvent drag.[36, 39, 41] In the jejunum, cotransport of sodium with amino acids and glucose, sodium-hydrogen exchange, and solvent drag are the primary mechanisms for sodium absorption. In the ileum, sodium absorption occurs primarily via electroneutral sodium chloride absorption (with a dual exchange of sodium for hydrogen and chloride for bicarbonate), bile salt–coupled sodium absorption, electrogenic sodium absorption, and questionably by means of a mechanism termed sodium-chloride symport.

Glucose- or Amino Acid–Stimulated Sodium Absorption

This is the major mechanism of sodium absorption within the proximal portion of the small intestine. Sodium accompanies the transport of both glucose and amino acid that are absorbed across the apical epithelium by active transport processes (Fig. 34–7). One to three sodium ions are transferred for each sugar molecule, and there are at least six amino acid carriers—four for neutral amino acids and one each for basic and acidic amino acids—all of which are coupled with inward sodium movement, with a stoichiometric relationship of 1:1.[42] Following absorption, sodium is removed from the enterocyte across the basolateral membrane via the Na^+, K^+–ATPase pump. Sodium (Na) is there joined by chloride (Cl), which has passed into the intercellular space by the paracellular route,[41] and both ions are then moved through the basal lamina by hydrostatic forces with water. Potassium (K) diffuses back out of the cell through special potassium-selective channels in the basal cell membrane.

Sodium-Hydrogen Exchange

As demonstrated by the elegant studies of Fordtran,[43, 44] when bicarbonate is present in the proximal jejunum, sodium appears to be absorbed via an exchange carrier for hydrogen (see Fig. 34–7). This process appears to result in a one-to-one exchange of sodium for hydrogen and can be inhibited by amiloride.[41]

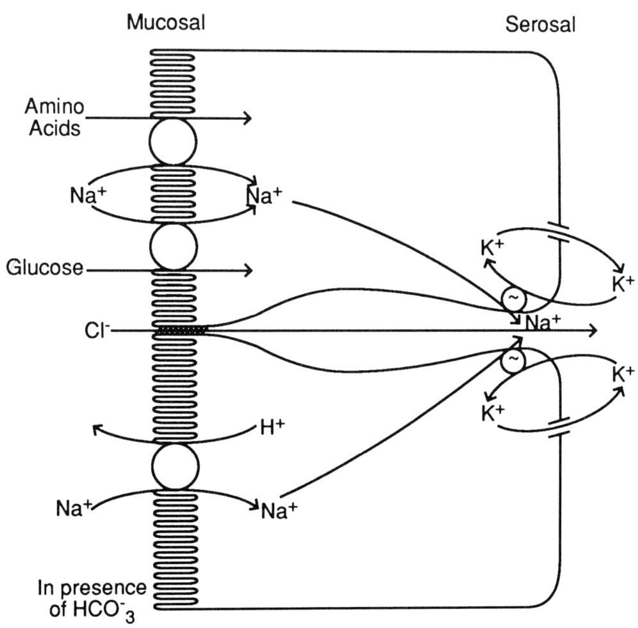

Figure 34–7. Schematic model of the predominant mechanisms of sodium and chloride absorption in the jejunum: glucose- or amino acid–stimulated sodium absorption and bicarbonate-dependent sodium-hydrogen exchange.

Some indirect stimulation of this sodium-hydrogen ion exchange also occurs with the active transport of amino acids. Protons rather than sodium accompany a portion of the amino acids transported across the apical membrane, resulting in an increased intracellular hydrogen ion pool, which can then be exchanged for sodium via this mechanism.[36, 41]

Solvent Drag

As indicated previously, large amounts of nutrients (including amino acids and sugars) and large volumes of fluid are absorbed across the proximal small intestine. Because of the large volume of fluid flow occurring across this "leaky" epithelium, some transport of ions, including primarily sodium, likely occurs by convectional forces, resulting in the absorption of sodium by the so-called solvent drag phenomenon.[39] Fordtran has suggested that as much as 85% of glucose-stimulated sodium absorption may occur via this mechanism.[45] In the human ileum, although the above-noted mechanisms are likely operational, they play a far less significant role in this segment. Ileal transport appears to be primarily the result of sodium-hydrogen and chloride-bicarbonate dual exchange, bile salt–coupled sodium absorption, and electrogenic sodium absorption.

Electrogenic Sodium Absorption

Electrogenic sodium absorption appears to be the primary means of sodium absorption in the distal colon, but it is also present to some extent in the ileum.[36, 41] The structural component that allows this mechanism to function efficiently is the presence of specialized sodium-selective channels within the ileal apical membrane. Sodium can then diffuse easily across this membrane, the driving force being the inwardly directed electrochemical gradient for sodium. Rapid removal of sodium across the basolateral membrane via the Na^+,K^+–ATPase pump maintains the electrochemical gradients favoring sodium absorption. Back diffusion of sodium across the tight junctions is more restriced than in jejunal segments, since resistance to sodium movement in ileal tight junctions is greater than in the jejunum. A greater potential difference can therefore be achieved across the ileal epithelial membrane, and sodium can be transported against greater osmolar differences. Sodium transport ceases in jejunal segments below luminal concentrations of approximately 133 mOsm per L, and the ileum can transport sodium down to luminal concentrations as low as 75 mOsm per L.[39]

Bile Salt–Coupled Sodium Transport

Bile salts are avidly absorbed in the terminal ileal regions of the small intestine, where greater than 95% of bile salts are reabsorbed for enterohepatic recirculation. Again sodium is coupled to bile salt absorption in a stoichiometric ratio of 1:1,[46] accounting for significant absorption of sodium via this mechanism (Fig. 34–8). Some component of solvent drag is also likely to be

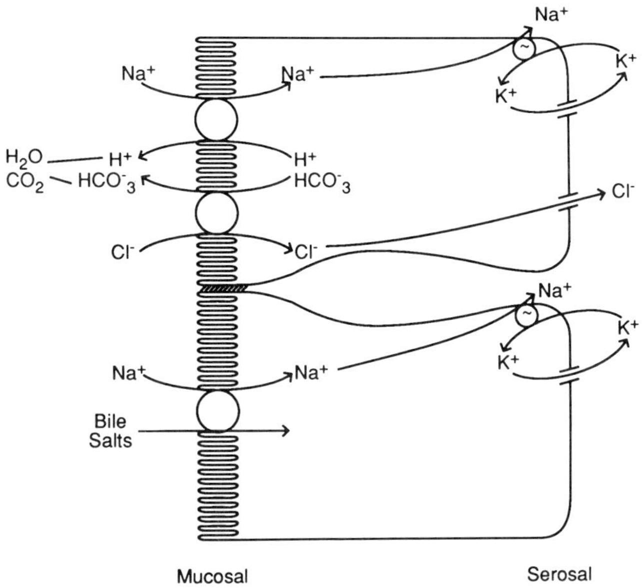

Figure 34–8. Schematic model of the predominant mechanisms of sodium and chloride absorption in the ileum: bile salt– or glucose-coupled sodium transport and sodium-hydrogen chloride-bicarbonate dual exchange. Chloride exits the cell through anion-selective channels.

operational, although much less prominent than in the jejunum.

Sodium-Hydrogen, Chloride-Bicarbonate Dual Exchange

Again, as detailed by the elegant experiments of Fordtran,[43, 47] this dual exchange mechanism appears to be a major factor in ileal ion transport. As a result of this transport mechanism, sodium appears to move into ileal epithelial cells in exchange for hydrogen, combined with the cotransport of chloride in exchange for bicarbonate (see Fig. 34–8). This process is electroneutral; during the exchange, sodium and chloride are absorbed across the apical membrane, and bicarbonate and hydrogen ions are secreted, combining in the luminal bulk phase to form water and carbon dioxide. Support for the ileal (as well as proximal colonic) predominance of this mechanism is provided by the rare diarrheal disorder, congenital chloridorrhea, in which the apparent absence of the chloride-bicarbonate exchanger leads to profuse, chloride-rich secretory diarrhea.[48]

This form of transport is inhibited by increased amounts of cyclic adenosine monophosphate (AMP), by changes in calcium concentration and by activation of protein kinase C.[36, 41] Also, almost all agents that result in intestinal secretion inhibit electroneutral sodium chloride absorption while stimulating active chloride secretion, the combined effects of which are likely responsible for most of the electrolyte secretion seen in diarrheal disorders.[36]

Sodium-Chloride Symport

In other animal species, additional carrier mechanisms appear to be present that allow for the electro-neutral transfer of sodium and chloride. These include sodium-chloride cotransport, 1 sodium, 1 potassium, 2 chloride cotransport, and cotransport of sodium-hydrogen and chloride-bicarbonate in which the bicarbonate may be replaced by hydroxyl, oxalate, or sulfate ions.[36, 41] To what extent these are operational in the human small intestine has not yet been fully elucidated.

Sodium Secretion and Potassium Absorption and Secretion

Both the secretion of sodium and the absorption and secretion of potassium appear to be strictly diffusional across the small intestinal epithelium.[41] Potassium-selective channels present in the basolateral membranes of intestinal epithelial cells allow for the rapid equilibration of potassium across this membrane during activation of the Na^+,K^+–ATPase pump. Potassium as well as sodium can also move through tight junctions via the paracellular route. The relatively small fixed negative charges present within the tight junctions favor cation movements over those of anions.

Chloride Absorption

Chloride absorption occurs across the small intestinal epithelium by two mechanisms. The first, already discussed, is chloride-bicarbonate exchange, which occurs primarily across the apical cell membrane in ileal tissue. The second route, most prominent in jejunal tissue, is passive chloride transfer through the paracellular pathway, which is responsible for the large volume of chloride absorbed proximally. In jejunal epithelium, as larger amounts of sodium are transported into the cell and extruded across the basolateral membrane, a potential difference develops, lumen negative, as well as a chemical gradient, both favoring the passage of chloride through the tight junctions and into the lateral intercellular spaces.[41] This mechanism is also responsible for some chloride movement in ileal epithelium. It is likely that a small amount of chloride is also transported via minor carriers such as sodium-chloride symport.

Chloride Secretion

Chloride secretion occurs in intestinal crypt cells because of the presence of two specific cell mechanisms (Fig. 34–9): apically located chloride-selective channels and a specific sodium-coupled cotransporter for chloride present in the basolateral membranes.[36, 41] The sodium-coupled cotransporter is a 1 sodium, 1 potassium, 2 chloride transporter, which is therefore electroneutral. Chloride carried across the basolateral membrane is then extruded from the cell through the specialized chloride-selective channels in the apical membrane, moving down both an electrical and a chemical gradient. The system is energized by the subsequent extrusion of sodium via the Na^+,K^+–ATPase pump, and potassium is recirculated through special potassium-selective chan-

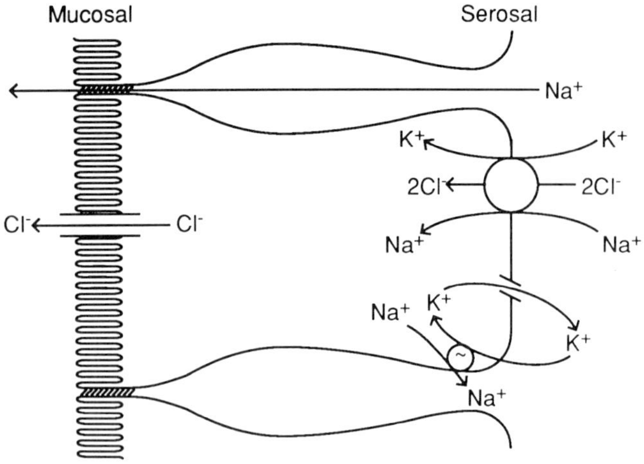

Figure 34–9. Schematic model for chloride secretion by intestinal crypt cells.

nels in the basolateral membranes. The chloride-selective channels are generally closed, but they can be opened by activating cyclic AMP, cyclic guanosine monophosphate (GMP), calcium, and likely protein kinase C. Cyclic AMP may be stimulated, as in the classic example with cholera toxin,[49] but it is also responsive to VIP,[50] adenosine,[51] and prostaglandins.[49] Cyclic GMP stimulation can result from *Escherichia coli* enterotoxin, calcium, and calcium ionophores.[36] The stimulation of chloride secretion is quite complex and is responsive to many secretagogues, including somatostatin, serotonin, neurotensin, substance P, and angiotensin. Concomitant with chloride secretion across the apical membrane, sodium diffuses through the paracellular pathway in response to the outwardly directed electrochemical gradient created.

Bicarbonate Secretion

Bicarbonate secretion is a function restricted solely to the ileum. As noted previously, in the presence of bicarbonate the jejunum secretes a hydrogen ion in exchange for sodium; the hydrogen ion and bicarbonate then likely combine within the intestinal bulk phase to form carbon dioxide and water.[44] No net absorption or secretion of bicarbonate is known to occur in the proximal small bowel. Ileal secretion of bicarbonate in exchange for chloride has previously been discussed, but the mechanism by which the ileum generates bicarbonate is not well identified. Research performed in the rabbit ileum suggests that bicarbonate is not generated by the presence of carbonic anhydrase within the cytosol, but rather is transported into the cell across the basolateral membrane from the interstitial fluid.[52] Several transport carriers for bicarbonate movement across the basolateral membrane have been proposed, but none has been fully identified.

LARGE INTESTINE

Gross Anatomy

The large intestine begins as a blind pouch hanging below the termination of the small intestine at the ileocecal valve, ends at the anus, and consists of the following segments: cecum; vermiform appendix; ascending, transverse, descending, and sigmoid colon; rectum; and anal canal (Fig. 34–10). The overall length of the large intestine in adults is approximately 120 to 150 cm, increasing from approximately 60 cm in the newborn. Although the wall of the colon remains relatively uniform in overall thickness throughout, the diameter of the colon diminishes as it progresses distally from cecum to anus. The cecum, ascending colon, and part of the transverse colon are derived from the embryonic midgut, and the distal transverse, descending, and rectosigmoid regions are derived from the hindgut. The lower third of the rectum is derived from the postallantoic gut.[53] Similar to the small intestine, the colon is enveloped by a mesentery extending as a reflection of the peritoneal lining. Only a portion of the colon, however, is fully suspended by this mesentery; the remaining portions remain fixed in a retroperitoneal manner, with the mesentery therefore being present over only the anterior or anterolateral surface. The appendix has a well-defined short mesentery, termed the *mesoappendix* (Fig. 34–11), and a portion of the cecum is also fully supported by mesentery. Additionally, the transverse colon and sigmoid colon are fully suspended by a mesentery, with the mesentery of the transverse colon being prominently developed as the *transverse mesocolon* (see Fig. 34–10). The proximal cecum, ascending colon, descending colon, and rectum have mesentery covering only a portion of their anterolateral surfaces. Being derived from the midgut, the cecum, ascending colon, and proximal two thirds of the transverse colon are supplied by blood from the superior mesenteric artery. The inferior mesenteric artery, arising from the distal aorta, supplies the remaining one third of the transverse colon, descending colon, and rectosigmoid region. The rectum and anal canal also receive a portion of their blood supply from the inferior mesenteric artery, in addition to branches from the internal iliac and median sacral arteries. The parasympathetic and sympathetic nerve supply to the colon follows in close juxtaposition to the arterial supply, with the proximal colon receiving its sympathetic neuronal innervation from the celiac and superior mesenteric ganglia and its parasympathetic supply from the vagus nerve. The distal colon receives sympathetic nerve supply from the lumbar segments of the sympathetic trunk, and parasympathetic nerves are derived from the pelvic splanchnic nerves.[53] Lymphatic drainage of the large intestine occurs through the mesentery in close approximation to the arterial and venous supplies, passing initially through small pericolic nodes adjacent to the medial aspect of the colon. Lymph flow then proceeds to the intermediate nodes lying within the mesentery, and finally to the terminal large colic nodes surrounding the superior and

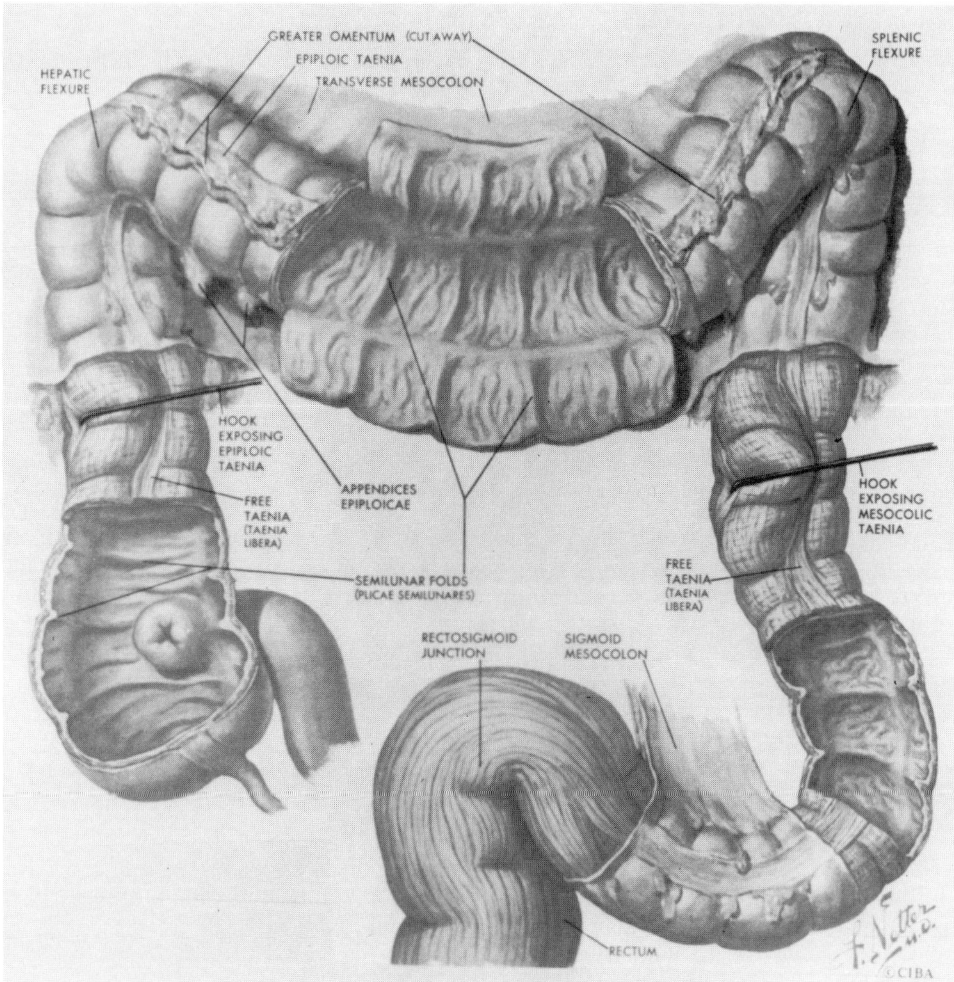

Figure 34–10. Gross anatomic configuration of the colon. (From Netter F: The CIBA Collection of Medical Illustrations. Vol 3, Part 2: Digestive System: Lower Digestive Tract. West Caldwell, NJ, CIBA Pharmaceutical, 1975, p 55; with permission.)

inferior mesenteric arteries. The rectum drains through perirectal nodes that lie in close contact with the rectal wall, draining both to the inferior mesenteric nodes and to the iliac nodes. Venous drainage of the colon is through the superior mesenteric vein, inferior mesenteric vein, and the superior, middle, and inferior rectal veins.[8]

The colon is characterized by several distinctive features. Although the muscular layer of the colon contains both circular and longitudinal muscles as is found in the small intestine, the outer longitudinal muscular layer is congregated into three distinct bands extending from the cecum to the rectum, termed the *teniae coli.* Outpouches of the colon occur between these longitudinal bands, termed *haustra,* giving the outer wall of the colon its characteristic sacculated appearance (see Fig. 34–10). Fatty outpouchings of the mesentery and serosa are also present, known as *appendices epiploicae*. These appendices epiploicae are found on the ascending, descending, transverse, and sigmoid segments, but are not present over the cecum, rectum, or anal canal. The luminal surface of the colon is thrown into intermittent irregular folds, termed the *plicae semilunares*.

The colon serves the primary functions of water and electrolyte absorption, along with the further processing, storage, and ultimate elimination of digested material. The colon is also capable of absorbing small amounts of volatile short-chain fatty acids, which result from anaerobic fermentation of nonabsorbed carbohydrates. The overall caloric contribution of these fatty acids is estimated to be approximately 7% of the total energy requirements,[53] with higher amounts likely being contributed during infancy.[54–56] The colon also functions as an important immunologic organ for the host.

Cecum

The cecum is defined as that segment of the proximal large intestine that extends from its pouchlike origin cephalad to the level of the ileocecal valve (see Fig. 34–11). The cecum is wider in diameter than it is long. In the adult the average length is approximately 6 cm and the width is 8 cm.[53] The ileocecal valve penetrates the cecum at its defined proximal end, passing through the wall in a perpendicular manner but directed slightly

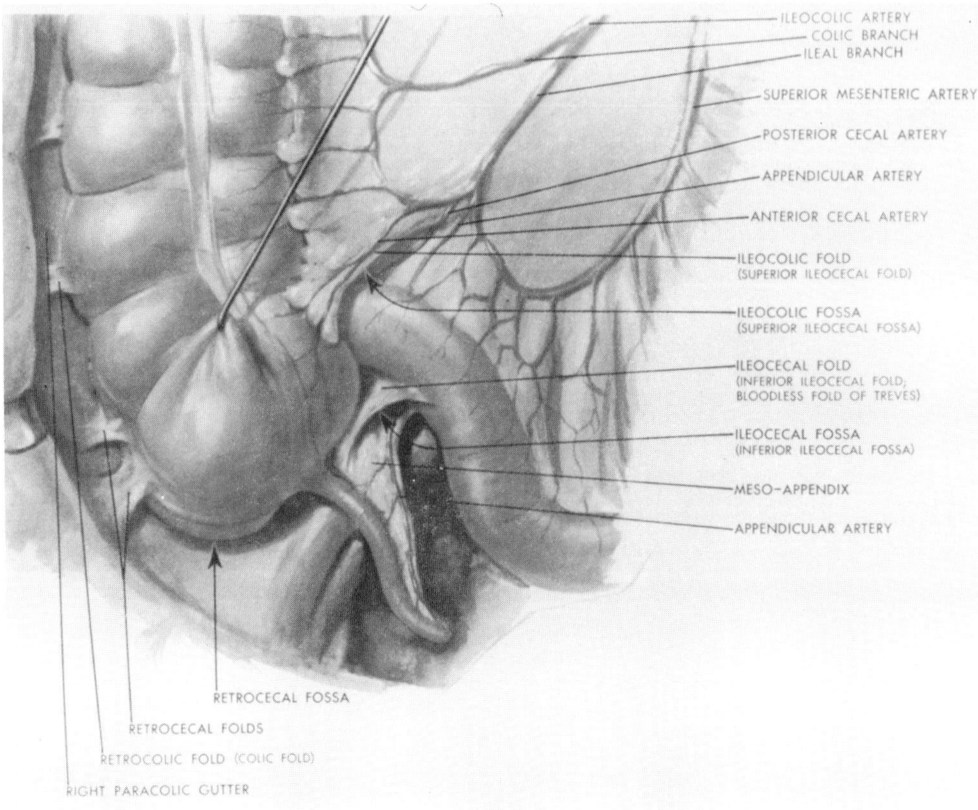

Figure 34–11. Gross anatomic configuration of the cecum. The appendix has a well-defined short mesentery, termed the mesoappendix. (From Netter F: The CIBA Collection of Medical Illustrations. Vol 3, Part 2: Digestive System: Lower Digestive Tract. West Caldwell, NJ, CIBA Pharmaceutical, 1975, p 5; with permission.)

downward. Two folds of approximating tissue are arranged in an elliptical manner over the orifice of the ileocecal valve, allowing the valve to function as a sphincter. The ileum generally enters the cecum along its posteromedial wall. The cecum, appendix, and the very last segment of terminal ileum are supported by a distinct mesentery and are mobile, resulting in the positional variability observed for these structures within the right lower quadrant.[53] In adults the resting pressure of the ileocecal valve is approximately 20 mm Hg above that of colonic pressure, with the length of this high-pressure zone extending for approximately 4 cm.[4] Integration of peristaltic activity and sphincteric relaxation is well-coordinated, generally allowing for the systematic passage of ileal contents into the cecum and precluding reflux back into the ileum.

Vermiform Appendix

Just inferior to the ileocecal valve is the normal location for the appendiceal opening (see Fig. 34–11). The appendix then descends inferiorly as a narrow tubular structure ranging in length from approximately 2 to 20 cm, being somewhat longer in children.[53] This organ functions as a lymphatic structure with many similarities to pharyngeal tonsils and Peyer's patches. The outer muscular layer of both the vermiform appendix and the cecum is circumferential, and the longitudinal muscular arrangement as teniae coli does not occur until the level of the ileocecal valve. The appendix may be located either dependently below the distal cecal pouch or behind the cecum anteriorly or posteriorly to the ileum.

Ascending Colon

The ascending colon originates at the level of the ileocecal valve and progresses in a cephalad manner to the inferior margin of the right lobe of the liver, where it takes a sharp angulation to the left, termed the *hepatic flexure*. The ascending colon is approximately 20 cm in length in the adult[4] and lies in a retroperitoneal location in approximately 75% of people.[53] In the remaining 25% of people, a short mesentery is present.

Transverse Colon

As the ascending colon angulates through the hepatic flexure and begins coursing anteriorly and medially, it arises from its retroperitoneal position to become fully enveloped in a well-developed extensive mesentery, termed the *transverse mesocolon*. The transverse colon then descends a variable distance into the pelvis as it courses medially across the abdomen, and has a length of approximately 40 to 50 cm.[53] The transverse colon lies anterior to the stomach and small intestine until its distal segment, where at the level of the 10th to 11th ribs it courses upward and posterior to lie under the inferior margin of the spleen, creating a second sharp angulation, the *splenic flexure*. A thickening of the peritoneum in this location, the *phrenicocolic ligament*, attaches the splenic flexure to the diaphragm. This suspension leaves the splenic flexure higher in location than the hepatic flexure.

Descending Colon

The descending colon extends from the splenic flexure distally to the level of the sigmoid colon near the left iliac crest. As the colon passes through the splenic flexure, it courses posteriorly and again takes up a retroperitoneal location covered only anteriorly by the peritoneum in the majority of people (65%).[53] The descending colon measures approximately 45 cm in length.

Sigmoid Colon

As the colon ascends over the pelvic brim, it again arises from its retroperitoneal location to be supported by a mesentery, termed the *sigmoid mesocolon*. The sigmoid colon ends as it joins the rectum at the level of the peritoneal reflection. The length of this segment is variable, and some redundancy is not uncommon. The sharpest angulation of this segment occurs where the sigmoid turns downward to unite with the rectum. In infants, this junction is approximately 9 cm from the anus, increasing to 15 cm in adults.[4]

Rectum

The rectum then extends from the sigmoid colon to the anal canal and measures approximately 15 cm in length in the adult.[53] The rectum generally follows a course along the sacral curvature, descending initially posteriorly and then anteriorly, joining the anus with a moderate inferior angulation at that level. The rectum is narrowest at the junction of the sigmoid, and expands into the rectal ampulla just before its junction with the anus (Fig. 34–12). The junction with the sigmoid is the point at which the peritoneum is reflected anteriorly; therefore, in the majority of people, the entire rectum lies below the peritoneum, with its outer surface of adventitia juxtaposed to the fascial structures within the pelvis. In some individuals, the peritoneal reflection does not occur until the midsection of the rectum. The outer muscular bands, teniae coli, converge to again circumferentially surround the colon approximately 5 to 6 cm proximal to the sigmoid junction.[53] As the outer muscle layer descends along the rectum, it becomes more prominently thickened into broad anterior and posterior bands. There are no haustra within the rectum; however, three readily identifiable curves are uniformly present. The upper and lower curves deviate to the right, and the middle curve deviates to the left (see Fig. 34–12).

Anal Canal

The anal canal begins at the distal end of the rectal ampulla and then passes inferiorly and outward as the anal opening. The rectum measures approximately 2 cm in length in the infant, increasing to 4.5 cm in the adult.[4] The junction of the rectal ampulla and anal canal occurs as the large intestine pierces the pelvic diaphragm, which is composed of the levator ani and coccygeus muscles. The space in which the anal canal lies is termed the *ischiorectal fossa,* the anal canal being supported within this space by a series of ligaments and muscular attachments.[53] That portion of the levator ani sling that surrounds the junction of the rectum and the anal canal is termed the *puborectalis muscle.* This muscle functions to pull the rectum forward in the resting state to assist in retaining stool, and relaxes to straighten the canal out and allow defecation to occur. At the junction between the anus and the rectum, the circular muscle layers thicken to become the internal anal sphincter, which circumferentially surrounds the anal canal to the level of the intersphincteric groove, which is the proximal margin of the external anal sphincter. The internal sphincter is composed of smooth muscle and is continuous with the circular muscular coat of the large intestine; the external sphincter is striated muscle. Internally, about midway within the anal canal, the mucosal folds are arranged in a longitudinal direction to form the anal columns, which converge distally to small flaps of tissue termed the *anal valves* (see Fig. 34–12). The level where the anal columns merge to form the anal valves is termed the *pectinate line.* Below the pectinate line, cell transition occurs from cuboidal to stratified squamous epithelium, which then continues to the anal opening and ends in an irregular or "white" zone termed the *zona alba.* Below this zone the lining becomes typically squamous epithelium of skin, containing sweat glands, sebaceous glands, and hair follicles.[53]

Cellular Morphology

The wall of the large intestine, similar to that of the small intestine, is composed of four layers: the serosa or adventitia, the muscularis, the submucosa, and the mucosa. The mucosa can be further subdivided into the epithelial cell lining, lamina propria, and muscularis mucosae. The outside lining of the large intestine is characterized by loose connective tissue termed the *adventitia,* which when covered by the peritoneal reflection containing squamous mesothelial cells is referred to as the *serosa.* Occasional, sparse numbers of macrophages, eosinophils, fibroblasts, and mast cells are found within the loose connective tissue constituting the adventitia. The muscularis of the colon consists again of two muscle layers: an inner circular layer and an outer longitudinal layer. The outer longitudinal muscle layer is condensed into three prominent muscular bands, the teniae coli, which run parallel to the longitudinal access of the large bowel. The teniae coli measure approximately 6 to 12 mm in width and thicken gradually with progression from the cecum to the sigmoid.[53] The longitudinal muscular layer is separated by a more prominent extracellular matrix than is present within the small bowel, containing increased amounts of collagen and elastin. The amount of collagen and elastin also increases with advancing age.[53] The septa dividing the

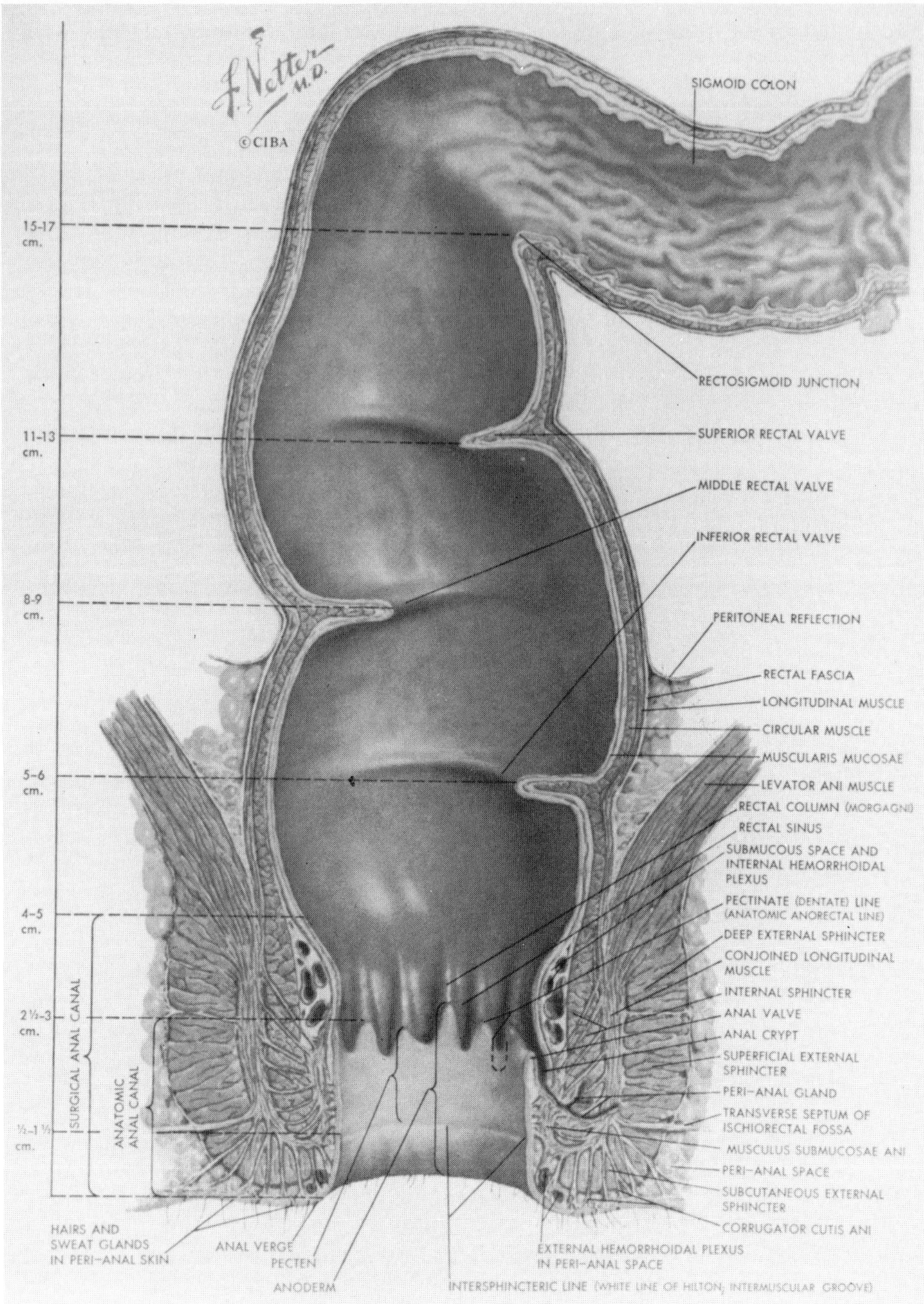

Figure 34–12. Gross anatomic configuration of the rectum and anus. Haustra are not present in the rectum; however, three readily identifiable curves are present: the upper and lower deviating to the right, and the middle deviating to the left. (From Netter F: The CIBA Collection of Medical Illustrations. Vol 3, Part 2: Digestive System: Lower Digestive Tract. West Caldwell, NJ, CIBA Pharmaceutical, 1975, p 58; with permission.)

muscular bundles are noncontinuous, allowing for full interdigitation of the various segments. Between the outer longitudinal and inner circular muscular layers run prominent nerve plexuses, which are continuous with the Auerbach's plexus of the small bowel. The inner circular muscle layer of the colon is not entirely oriented circumferentially but maintains a slight oblique posture with relation to the long axis of the colon.[53] Thin septa separate small groups of circular muscle fibers, which are noncontinuous, allowing for full muscular integration of peristaltic activity. The axons from Auerbach's plexus are numerous and ramify throughout the muscular layers to contact individual muscle cells. A similar arrangement of gap junctions as is present in the small intestine occurs in colonic smooth muscle cells.

Lying between the muscularis and the muscularis mucosae is the submucosa. This is a layer of loose connective tissue containing scattered cellular elements including fibroblasts, mast cells, macrophages, plasma cells, eosinophils, and lymphocytes. Meissner's submucosal plexus also courses through this layer in continuation from the small intestine. Large arteries and veins are also present to supply the muscularis and the mucosa.

The mucosa comprises three layers: the muscularis mucosae, lamina propria, and epithelial cell layer. The muscularis mucosae is a thin band of smooth muscle cells and fibers, averaging approximately 6 to 12 cells thick. This cell layer in the large intestine is slightly thicker than that present in the small intestine, and the thickness increases with progression from the cecum to the sigmoid.[53] The muscularis mucosae becomes most prominent in the rectum and anal canal, where it often appears as two separate thin layers rather than one. Lying above the muscularis mucosae is the lamina propria, a layer of loose connective tissue that extends up to the flat mucosal surface and interdigitates between the prominent crypts. Scattered cells including macrophages, eosinophils, lymphocytes, fibroblasts, and plasma cells are present within the lamina propria, plasma cells being the most prominent. Also scattered throughout the lamina propria are numerous lymphatic nodules, the cells of which are primarily IgA secreting.

The epithelial cell lining of the large intestine is a flat mucosa and does not contain the villi that are characteristic of the small intestine (Fig. 34–13). Prominent crypts of Lieberkühn are present that descend from the flat epithelial surface to lie just above the muscularis mucosa. The surface epithelium is a simple columnar epithelium composed of surface columnar cells, vacuolated cells, goblet cells, caveolated cells, and, restricted to the lower one third of the crypt, enteroendocrine cells and undifferentiated cells. The primary functions of the large bowel epithelium are water and electrolyte absorption and secretion of mucin.

Surface Epithelial Cell

Present in the upper regions of the crypts and the most prominent cell on the flat epithelial surface of the large intestine are the surface epithelial cells, also termed *principal cells*.[53] These cells are typical tall, slender, columnar epithelial cells whose primary function is that of fluid and electrolyte transport. These cells arise from undifferentiated "stem" cells at the base of the crypts from within the proliferative zone, which constitutes the distal one third of the crypt. Maturation and differentiation occur with upward migration along the lateral walls of the crypts. Vacuolated cells that line the lateral margins of the crypts are likely a transitional form of the fully mature surface epithelial cell.[53] Surface epithelial cells have a typical apical membrane containing numerous microvilli, supported by a well-developed terminal web. A prominent glycocalyx is also present above the microvillous membrane. Tight junctions are well developed, with an anatomic configuration similar to that present in small intestinal epithelial cells. Cytoplasmic organelles are typical of columnar absorptive cells, however, the nucleus is somewhat more centrally located and there is a scant amount of endoplasmic reticulum located both above and below the nucleus. The Golgi apparatus is more apical in location and is surrounded by secretory granules. A unique feature of the epithelial cells of the colonic surface is the presence of "R bodies," which are membrane-bound structures measuring approximately 0.2 to 1.5 μm in diameter scattered throughout the cytoplasm.[53, 57] Surface epithelial cells by light microscopy have a slightly eosinophilic cytoplasm.

Vacuolated Cell

Although some controversy exists, vacuolated cells derived from undifferentiated crypt cells are likely the percursors of the surface epithelial cells. Unlike other cells derived from the undifferentiated cells within the crypts, the vacuolated cells continue to demonstrate mitotic activity as they migrate upward along the lateral crypt wall.[53] The vacuoles contain material similar in composition to that of the glycocalyx, suggesting that endocytotic release of this material for glycocalyx formation occurs as these cells mature.

Goblet Cell

The second most common cell type present within the intestinal crypts and on the surface epithelium is the goblet cell, which is typical in shape, configuration, and

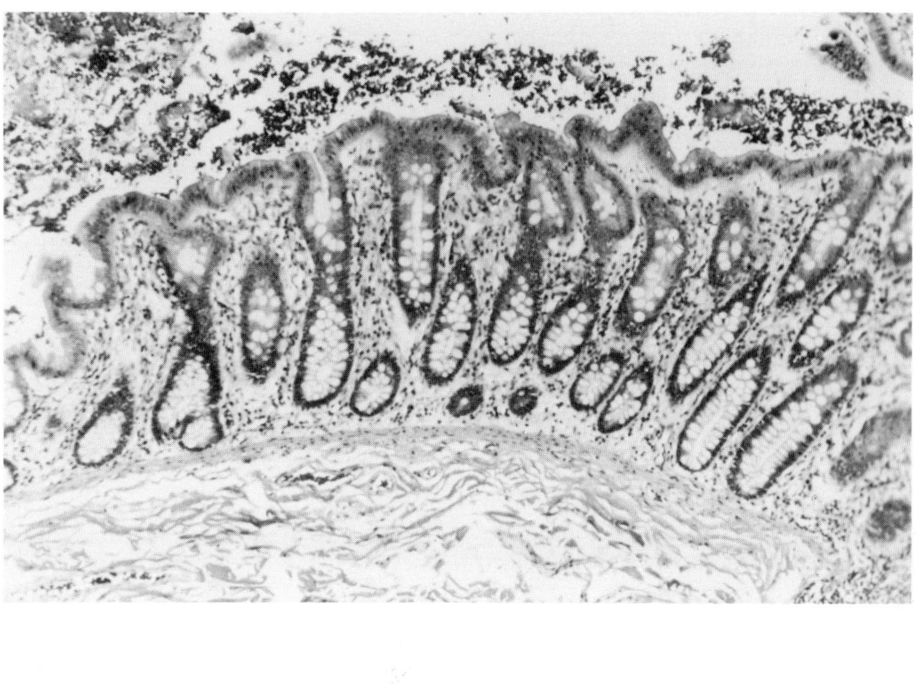

Figure 34–13. Light micrograph of human colonic mucosa. The surface of human colonic mucosa is flat, with prominent crypts of Lieberkühn descending to just above the muscularis mucosa. Hematoxylin-eosin stain, × 100. (Courtesy of R. S. Markin, MD.)

morphology to the goblet cells of the small intestine. The major secretory product of goblet cells is mucin, which is extruded from these cells to provide the surface mucous coat of the large intestine.

Enteroendocrine Cell

Enteroendocrine cells of the colonic epithelium are similar in structure to those of the small intestinal epithelium and arise from undifferentiated cells within the base of the crypts. Enteroendocrine cells are located within the crypts in the distal half to third, occasionally present in clusters. Differing cell populations are responsible for the production of numerous neuroregulatory peptides and hormones, including somatostatin, glucagon, cholecystokinin, GIP, motilin, neurotensin, PYY, and 5-hydroxytryptophan.

Caveolated Cell

Occasionally present in scant amounts within the large intestinal crypt, as well as on the surface epithelium, are caveolated cells. This cell type is similar in structure to that seen in the small intestine, having a teardrop shape with a narrowed apical surface. These cells constitute less than 1% of the total epithelial cell population.[53] Their function is currently unknown.

Undifferentiated Cell

Within the proliferative zone of the crypt are the undifferentiated stem cells, which are usually pyramidal in shape with a narrow apical surface. It is again proposed that all cell types populating the crypts and flat surface epithelium arise from these undifferentiated crypt (stem) cells.

Fluid and Electrolyte Transport

Water and ion transport across the colonic epithelium is quite similar to that of the small bowel epithelia previously discussed. Some regional specialization between the proximal and distal colon, however, does occur. The primary function of the large intestine is to absorb water and electrolytes, and the efficiency of the colon in removing water is quite impressive, operating at 80 to 90%. As is true for all epithelia, the driving forces for water movement are secondary to those for ion transport. The epithelial lining of the colon cannot be considered either "leaky" or "tight," but has permeability characteristics between these two, so is a moderately leaky membrane. This is reflected by the potential difference gradients that can be achieved across the large intestine compared to the small intestine. The large intestine is able to generate a potential difference of between –20 and –40 mv, but the jejunum and ileum can create a potential difference of only –3 and –6 mv, respectively.[4] The colon is therefore far more efficient in its ability to absorb water and electrolytes than is the small intestine.

The routes for water and ion transport are identical to those of the small intestine and involve both transepithelial and paracellular movements. Since mechanisms for water and ion transport have already been discussed, only the regional specialization that occurs in the colon is discussed in this section.

In the proximal colon, the major movements of sodium and chloride result from the apparent coupling of sodium and chloride absorption (Fig. 34–14). It is not known at the present time whether this coupled absorption is direct (sodium and chloride exchange occurring on a single carrier) or indirect (cotransport of sodium for hydrogen and chloride for bicarbonate).[58] The majority of studies to date, however, favor the indirect dual exchange, coupling sodium and chloride to hydrogen and bicarbonate as the most prominent mechanism involved in the proximal large intestine.[36, 58] As stated previously, since this process is electroneutral, large amounts of water and salt can be absorbed without the generation of steep concentration gradients.

In the distal large intestine, the most prominent mechanism for sodium absorption is electrogenic sodium absorption.[36, 58] In this epithelium, sodium-selective channels favor the apical movement of sodium into the cell, occurring down both an electrical and a chemical gradient (Fig. 34–15). Since this gradient can be readily maintained by the active extrusion of sodium across the basolateral membranes via the Na^+,K^+–ATPase pump, significant quantities of sodium can be absorbed against steep concentration gradients. Indeed, the distal colon is able to transport sodium with luminal concentrations as low as 30 mEq per L.[4] The basolateral membrane is more permeable to potassium than to sodium, therefore back diffusion of sodium does not occur to any significant extent. The electrical potential difference generated by the active absorption of sodium in the distal colon (with the lumen being negative) appears to be the driving force for potassium secretion, which is why potassium concentrations in stool are high.[36] In the distal small intestine, chloride is absorbed both through the

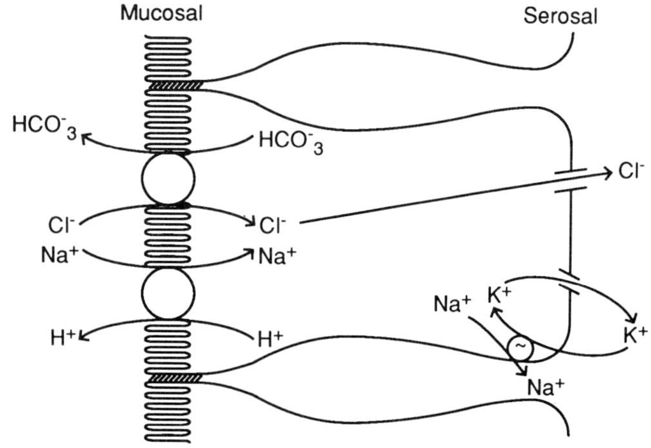

Figure 34–14. Schematic model of the predominant mechanism of sodium and chloride absorption in the proximal colon: sodium-hydrogen chloride-bicarbonate dual exchange. Chloride exits the cell through anion-selective channels.

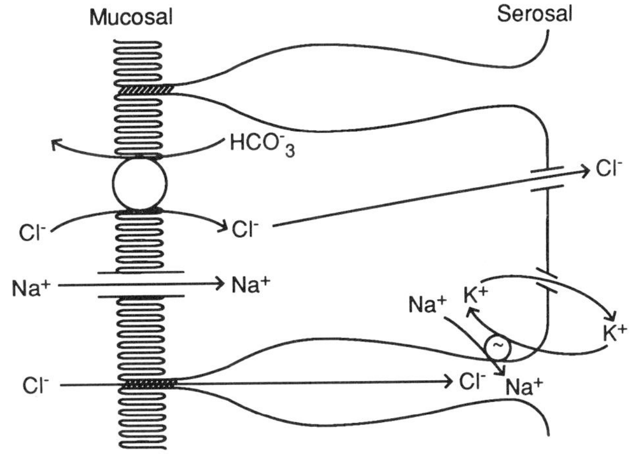

Figure 34–15. Schematic model of the predominant mechanism of sodium and chloride absorption in the distal colon: electrogenic sodium absorption. Chloride absorption occurs both through the paracellular route and across the apical membrane in exchange for bicarbonate.

paracellular pathway in response to electrogenic sodium uptake and across the apical membrane in exchange for bicarbonate. Hydrostatic forces are again operational within the lateral intercellular spaces, providing the driving force for water and ion movement across the basal lamina for capillary absorption.

Colonic handling of the remaining luminal ions, including chloride secretion, is quite similar to that of the small bowel epithelium, and the reader is referred to recent in-depth reviews for further discussion.[36, 58] Diarrheal states appear to be stimulated by the activation of chloride secretion in colonic tissue, similar to that previously discussed for small bowel epithelia. The colonic epithelium functions similar to the small bowel epithelium as well, in that the surface epithelial cells appear to be the major absorptive cells, and the crypt cells are secretory. Further evidence to support the morphologic view that the vacuolated cells lining the intestinal crypts are precursors to fully differentiated surface epithelial cells has recently been provided by in-depth studies. These studies have demonstrated that with secretory stimulation, vacuolated cells undergo membrane changes that result in the opening of chloride channels.[59] The fact that these secretory cells further differentiate as they move along the lateral aspects of the crypts to become absorptive surface cells is consistent with the overall general hypothesis of cell differentiation involving intestinal cell epithelia.

REFERENCES

1. Touloukian RJ, Walker-Smith GJ: Normal intestinal length in preterm infants. J Pediatr Surg 1983; 18:720–723.
2. Reiquam CW, Allen RP, Akers DR, et al: Normal and abnormal small bowel lengths. Am J Dis Child 1965; 109:447–451.
3. Walker-Smith JA: Massive resection of the small intestine. *In* Smith JW, ed: Diseases of the Small Intestine in Childhood. 3d ed. London, Butterworths, 1988, pp 380–381.
4. Trier JS, Winter HS: Anatomy, embryology, and developmental abnormalities of the small intestine and colon. *In* Sleisenger MH, Fordtran JS, eds: Gastrointestinal Disease. 4th ed. Philadelphia, WB Saunders, 1989, pp 991–1021.
5. Grand RJ, Watkins JB, Torti FM: Development of the human gastrointestinal tract. A review. Gastroenterology 1976; 70:790–810.
6. Weaver LT: Anatomy and embryology. *In* Walker WA, Durie PR, Hamilton JR, et al, eds: Pediatric Gastrointestinal Disease. Philadelphia, BC Decker, 1991, pp 195–216.
7. Clemente CD: The digestive system. *In* Clemente CD, ed: Gray's Anatomy of the Human Body. Philadelphia, Lea and Febiger, 1985, pp 1402–1514.
8. Woodburne RT: The abdomen. *In* Woodburne RT, ed: Essentials of Human Anatomy. 4th ed. New York, Oxford University Press, 1969, pp 359–459.
9. Dawson W, Langman J: An anatomical-radiological study of the pancreatic duct pattern in man. Anat Rec 1961; 139:59–68.
10. Gabella G: Structure of muscles and nerves in the gastrointestinal tract. *In* Johnson LR, ed: Physiology of the Gastrointestinal Tract. New York, Raven Press, 1981, pp 197–241.
11. Cooke AR: The glands of Brunner. *In* Code CF, ed: Handbook of Physiology, Section 6: The Alimentary Canal. Vol 2: Secretion. Baltimore, Williams & Wilkins, 1967, pp 1087–1095.
12. Madara JL: Functional morphology of epithelium of the small intestine. *In* Field M, ed: Handbook of Physiology, Section 6: The Gastrointestinal System. Vol 4: Intestinal Absorption and Secretion. New York, Oxford University Press, 1991, pp 83–120.
13. Wapnir RA, Fisher SE: Intestinal secretion and absorption. *In* Silverberg M, Daum F, eds: Textbook of Pediatric Gastroenterology. 2d ed. Chicago, Year Book Medical Publishers, 1988, pp 40–71.
14. Clementi F, Palade GE: Intestinal capillaries: I. Permeability of peroxidase and ferritin. J Cell Biol 1969; 41:33–58.
15. Boller K, Vestweber D, Kemler R: Cell-adhesion molecule uvomorulin is localized in the intermediate junctions of adult intestinal epithelial cells. J Cell Biol 1985; 100:327–332.
16. Vial J, Porter KR: Scanning microscopy of dissociated tissue cells. J Cell Biol 1975; 67:345–360.
17. Forstner JF, Jabbal I, Forstner GG: Goblet cell mucin of the rat small intestine: Chemical and physical characterization. Can J Biochem 1973; 51:1154–1166.
18. Specian RD, Neutra MR: Acceleration of secretion in colonic goblet cells by acetylcholine. J Cell Biol 1980; 85:626–640.
19. Moe H: On goblet cells, especially of the intestine of some mammalian species. Int Rev Cytol 1955; 4:299–334.
20. Merzel J, Leblond CP: Origin and renewal of goblet cells in the epithelium of the mouse small intestine. Am J Anat 1969; 124:281–306.
21. Sjolund K, Sanden G, Hakanson R, et al: Endocrine cells in human intestine: An immunocytochemical study. Gastroenterology 1983; 85:1120–1130.
22. Pearse AGE: The APUD cell concept and its implication in pathology. Pathol Annu 1974; 9:27–41.
23. Solcia E, Capella C, Buffa R, et al: The diffuse endocrine-paracrine system of the gut in health and disease: Ultrastructural features. Scand J Gastroenterol 1981; 16(Suppl 70):25–36.
24. Walsh JH: Gastrointestinal hormones. *In* Johnson LR, ed: Physiology of the Gastrointestinal Tract. 2d ed. New York, Raven Press, 1987, pp 181–253.
25. Solcia E, Capella C, Buffa R, et al: Endocrine cells of the digestive system. *In* Johnson LR, ed: Physiology of the Gastrointestinal Tract. 2d ed. New York, Raven Press. 1987, pp 111–130.
26. Polak JM: Endocrine cells of the gut. *In* Makhlouf GM, Schultz SG, eds: Handbook of Physiology, Section 6: The Gastrointestinal System. Vol 2: Neural and Endocrine Biology. New York, Oxford University Press, 1989, pp 79–96.
27. Erlandsen SL, Chase DG: Paneth cell function: Phagocytosis and intracellular digestion of intestinal microorganism: II. Spiral microorganism. J Ultrastruct Res 1972; 41:319–333.
28. Erlandsen SL, Parsons JA, Taylor TD: Ultrastructural immunocytochemical localization of lysozyme in the Paneth cells of man. J Histochem Cytochem 1974; 22:401–413.
29. Bohe M, Borgstrom C, Ohlsson K: Trypsin-like immunoreactivity in human Paneth cells. Digestion 1984; 30:271–275.
30. Madara JL, Carlson SL: Cup cells: Further structural characterization of the brush border and the suggestion that they may serve as an attachment site for an unidentified bacillus in guinea pig ileum. Gastroenterology 1985; 89:1374–1386.

31. Madara JL: Cup cells: Structure and distribution of a unique class of epithelial cells in guinea pig, rabbit, and monkey small intestine. Gastroenterology 1982; 83:981–994.
32. Owen RL, Jones AL: Epithelial cell specialization within human Peyer's patches: An ultrastructural study of intestinal lymphoid follicles. Gastroenterology 1974; 66:189–203.
33. Owen RL, Bhalla DK: Cytochemical analysis of alkaline phosphatase and esterase activities and of lectin-binding and anionic sites in rat and mouse Peyer's patch M cells. Am J Anat 1983; 168:199–212.
34. Madara JL, Bye WA, Trier JS: Structural features of and cholesterol distribution in M-cell membranes in guinea pig, rat, and mouse Peyer's patches. Gastroenterology 1984; 87:1091–1103.
35. Spring KR: Mechanism of fluid transport by epithelia. *In* Schultz SG, ed: Handbook of Physiology, Section 6: The Gastrointestinal System. Vol. 4: Intestinal Absorption and Secretion. New York, Oxford University Press, 1991, pp 195–207.
36. Field M: Intestinal ion transport mechanisms. *In* Field M, ed: Diarrheal Diseases. New York, Elsevier, 1991, pp 3–21.
37. Finkelstein A: Water Movement Through Lipid Bilayers, Pores, and Plasma Membranes. New York, Wiley, 1987.
38. Curran PF, MacIntosh JR: A model system for biological water transport. Nature Lond 1962; 193:347–348.
39. Binder HJ: Absorption and secretion of water and electrolytes by small and large intestine. *In* Sleisenger MH, Fordtran JS, eds: Gastrointestinal Disease. 4th ed. Philadelphia, WB Saunders, 1989, pp 1022–1045.
40. Spring KR: Fluid transport by gallbladder epithelium. J Exp Biol 1983; 106:181–194.
41. Sullivan SK, Field M: Ion transport across mammalial small intestine. *In* Field M, ed: Handbook of Physiology, Section 6: The Gastrointestinal System. Vol 4: Intestinal Absorption and Secretion. New York, Oxford University Press, 1991, pp 287–301.
42. Hopfer U: Membrane transport mechanisms for hexoses and amino acids in the small intestine. *In* Johnson LR, ed: Physiology of the Gastrointestinal Tract. 2d ed. New York, Raven Press, 1987, pp 1499–1526.
43. Fordtran JS, Rector FC, Carter NW: The mechanisms of sodium absorption in the human small intestine. J Clin Invest 1968; 47:884–900.
44. Turnberg L, Fordtran J, Carter N, et al: Mechanism of bicarbonate absorption and its relationship to sodium transport in human jejunum. J Clin Invest 1970; 49:548–556.
45. Fordtran JS: Stimulation of active and passive sodium absorption by sugars in the human jejunum. J Clin Invest 1975; 55:728–737.
46. Wilson FA: Intestinal transport of bile acids. Am J Physiol 1981; 241:G83–G92.
47. Turnberg L, Bieberdorf F, Morawski S, et al: Interrelationships of chloride, bicarbonate, sodium, and hydrogen transport in the human ileum. J Clin Invest 1970; 49:557–567.
48. Holmberg C, Perheentupa J, Launiala K, et al: Congenital chloride diarrhea: Clinical analysis of 21 Finnish patients. Arch Dis Child 1977; 52:255–267.
49. Kimberg DV, Field M, Johnson J, et al: Stimulation of intestinal mucosal adenyl cyclase by cholera enterotoxin and prostaglandins. J Clin Invest 1971; 50:1218–1230.
50. Schwartz CJ, Kimberg DV, Sheerin HE, et al: Vasoactive intestinal peptide stimulation of adenylate cyclase and active electrolyte secretion in intestinal mucosa. J Clin Invest 1974; 54:536–544.
51. Dobbins JW, Laurenson JP, Forrest JN: Adenosine and adenosine analogues stimulate adenosine cyclic 3′,5′-monophosphate-dependent chloride secretion in the mammalial ileum. J Clin Invest 1984; 74:929–935.
52. Smith PL, Cascairo MA, Sullivan SK: Sodium dependence of luminal alkalinization by rabbit ileal mucosa. Am J Physiol 1985; 249:G358–G368.
53. Lacy ER: Functional morphology of the large intestine. *In* Field M, ed: Handbook of Physiology, Section 6: The Gastrointestinal System. Vol 4: Intestinal Absorption and Secretion. New York, Oxford University Press, 1991, pp 121–194.
54. Potter GD, Lester R: The developing colon and nutrition. J Pediatr Gastroenterol Nutr 1984; 3:485–487.
55. Rechkemmer G: Transport of weak electrolytes. *In* Field M, ed: Handbook of Physiology, Section 6: The Gastrointestinal System. Vol 4: Intestinal Absorption and Secretion. New York, Oxford University Press, 1991, pp 371–388.
56. Bond JH, Levitt MD: Fate of soluble carbohydrate in the colon of rats and man. J Clin Invest 1976; 57:1158–1164.
57. Biempica L, Sternlieb I, Sohn HB, et al: R-bodies of human rectal epithelial cells. Arch Pathol Lab Med 1976; 100:78–80.
58. Halm DR, Frizzel RA: Ion transport across the large intestine. *In* Field M, ed: Handbook of Physiology, Section 6: The Gastrointestinal System. Vol. 4: Intestinal Absorption and Secretion. New York, Oxford University Press, 1991, pp 257–273.
59. Johnson RD, Halm DR, Krasny EJ, et al: Cellular specificity for chloride secretion in colonic crypt epithelium from the rabbit (abstract). J Cell Biol 1984; 99:292a.

Chapter 35

Congenital Anomalies of the Midgut

SOUHEIL GEBARA and HUGH V. FIROR

EMBRYOLOGY[1–3]

In a 2-week-old embryo, the bilaminar germ disk is located between the ectodermal amniotic cavity and the endodermal yolk sac, whereas the allantois represents a diverticulum in the caudad aspect of the yolk sac. The primitive streak appears with the primitive node at the cephalad end of the germinal disk during the third week of gestation. The mesodermal cells develop in this region by invagination of the epiblast cells that spread between the two layers to form the mesodermal layer. The process of folding transforms the embryo to a cylindrical shape (see Chapter 1, Fig. 1–1). At that time, the primitive gut is formed by two blind tubes—the foregut and hindgut–separated by the midgut, which communicates freely with the yolk sac. The endoderm comes in direct contact with the ectoderm at the blind ends of the foregut and the hindgut to form the buccopharyngeal and the cloacal membranes. The blood supply of the foregut, the midgut, and the hindgut is provided by the celiac axis and superior and inferior mesenteric arteries, respectively. The foregut gives rise to the pharynx, respiratory tract, esophagus, stomach, and duodenum proximal to the entry of the bile duct. The midgut forms the duodenum distal to the entry of the bile duct, jejunum, ileum, appendix, cecum, and colon proximal to its mid-transverse segment, as well as the liver and the pancreas. The hindgut evolves into the colon distal to its mid-transverse segment, rectum, and most of the urogenital system.

GROWTH AND ROTATION OF THE INTESTINE[1–7]

The duodenum is formed from the caudad part of the foregut and the cephalad part of the midgut (see Chapter 1, Fig. 1–2). The rotation of the stomach and the ventral pancreas drives the duodenum to rotate to the right and posteriorly. Thus, the duodenum takes its C shape and becomes fixed posteriorly. At the same time, the proximal end of the hindgut forms the fixed colic angle. The midgut grows and rotates between these two fixed points. The rapid growth of the midgut between the 5th and the 10th weeks forces it to make a U-shaped loop, with the superior mesenteric artery forming the axis and the yolk stalk attaching to the apex. The segment craniad to the superior mesenteric artery is called the *prearterial limb,* and the segment caudad to it is called the *postarterial limb.* Simultaneously, the liver grows rapidly and occupies a large part of the abdominal cavity. This process forces the midgut into the umbilical cord, forming the physiologic umbilical hernia. During this stage, the buds of the cecum and the appendix appear as a small local dilatation of the postarterial limb. Clinically, this helps distinguish the small from the large intestine. During its development, the midgut rotates in and out of the abdominal cavity. For descriptive purposes, the gut rotation is divided into three stages.

First Stage

The first stage of the midgut rotation (Fig. 35–1) is completed between the 5th and the 10th weeks of gestation while the loop is still in the umbilical cord. At this stage, the right lobe of the liver enlarges in the right caudad direction, pulling the left umbilical vein, which in turn pulls the prearterial loop to the right and caudad. This motion displaces the postarterial loop to the left and cephalad, achieving a 90-degree counterclockwise rotation. During this stage, the prearterial loop elongates rapidly while the cecum enlarges and becomes bulky.

Second Stage

During the second stage of midgut rotation (Fig. 35–2), liver growth slows and the abdominal cavity enlarges, making it possible for the bowel to return to the abdominal cavity at or about the beginning of the 10th week. The narrow umbilical orifice forces the bowel to retreat in an orderly fashion. The proximal portion of the prearterial loop first returns to the right of the superior mesenteric artery and then extends to the left

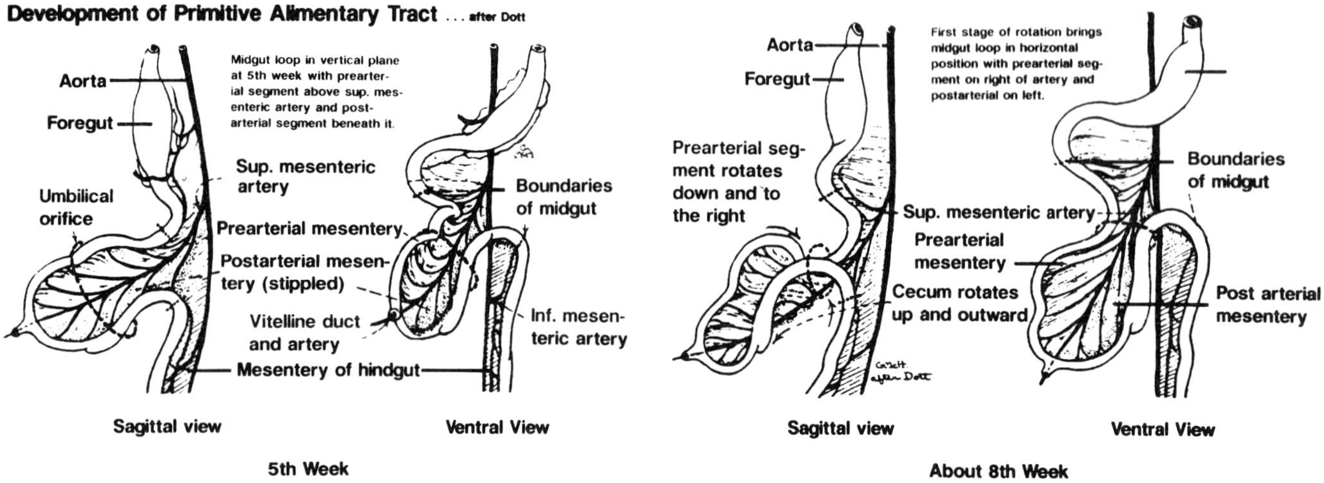

Figure 35–1. First stage of midgut rotation takes place between the 5th and the 10th weeks of gestation. (From Haymond HE, Dragstedt LR: Anomalies of intestinal rotation. Surg Gynecol Obstet 1931; 53:316–329; by permission of Surgery, Gynecology, and Obstetrics.)

under the pressure of the returning bowel. This movement forces the descending colon to occupy the left flank. The cecum returns last and lies in the right upper quadrant below the liver. At the end of the second stage, the midgut has completed a 270-degree counterclockwise rotation, with the duodenum lying posterior, and the colon anterior, to the superior mesenteric artery.

Third Stage

The third stage of midgut rotation starts during the 11th week and continues until shortly before birth. The cecum descends at this stage and reaches the right iliac fossa by the fifth month. The hepatic flexure then

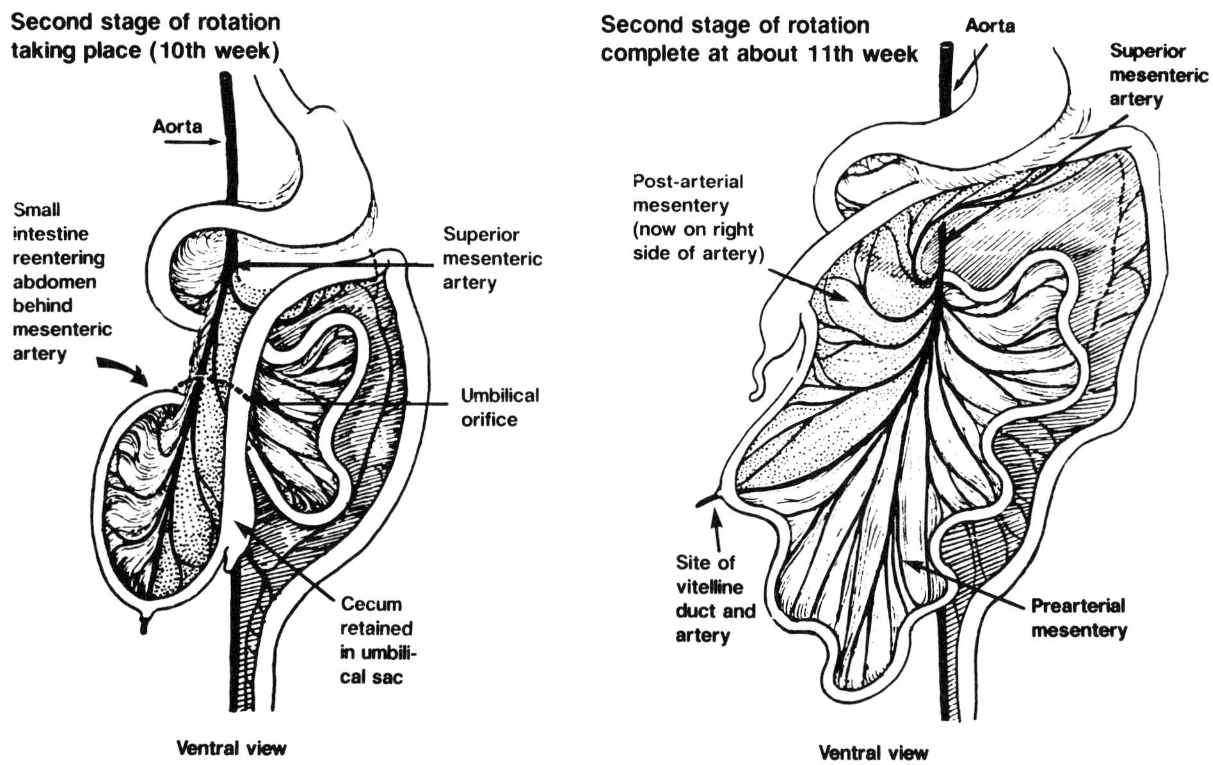

Figure 35–2. Second stage of gut rotation takes place between the 10th and the 11th weeks of gestation. (From Haymond HE, Dragstedt LR: Anomalies of intestinal rotation. Surg Gynecol Obstet 1931; 53:316–329; by permission of Surgery, Gynecology, and Obstetrics.)

appears, and the various parts of the gut are fixed in their permanent positions.

ANOMALIES OF INTESTINAL ROTATION

First-Stage Rotation

First-stage rotation anomalies[3–6] are rare conditions that occur in infants and result in extroversion of the cloaca. These anomalies include the underdevelopment of the postarterial limb and the nonrotation of the prearterial segment, leaving the small intestine in its primitive position.

Second-Stage Rotation

There are three major clinical anomalies that result from the abnormal movement during the second stage of rotation: nonrotation, reversed rotation, and malrotation.

In *nonrotation*[3–6, 8] (Fig. 35–3), the umbilical ring is lax and allows the midgut to return en masse to the abdominal cavity without rotation. The first and second parts of the duodenum (the foregut) are in a normal position, and the rest of the duodenum descends to the right of the superior mesenteric artery. The jejunum and the ileum occupy the right side of the midline; the ileum enters the cecum from the right side while the cecum is located in the left iliac fossa. The ascending colon is located left of the midline and continues with a U-shaped transverse colon that extends with a normally located hindgut. Failure of fixation is common, and in these instances the entire midgut loop is suspended by a narrow pedicle, called the *duodenocolic isthmus.* This failure of fixation predisposes to midgut volvulus.

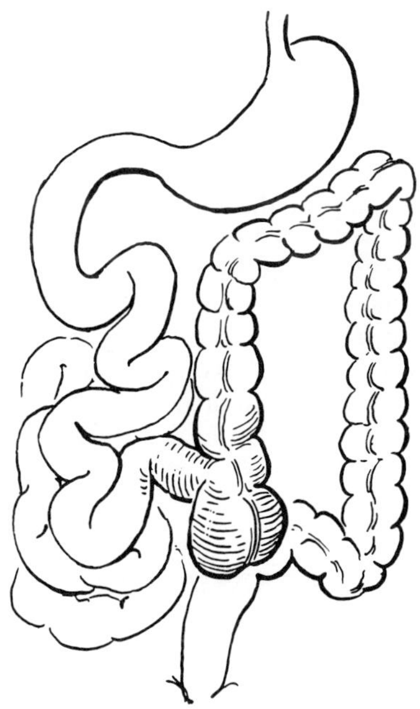

Figure 35–3. Nonrotation of the intestine. The jejunum and the ileum on the right side of the abdominal cavity, with the colon on the left. (From Wang C, Welch CE: Anomalies of intestinal rotation in adolescents and adults. Surgery 1963; 54:839–855; with permission.)

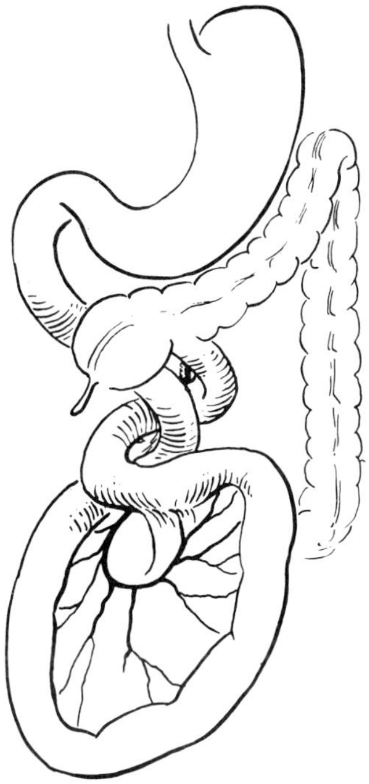

Figure 35–4. Malrotation, with the mesentery twisted on its pedicle. (From Wang C, Welch CE: Anomalies of intestinal rotation in adolescents and adults. Surgery 1963; 54:839–855; with permission.)

Reversed rotation[3–5, 9–14] is an uncommon condition that represents only 4% of reported cases of abnormal rotation. In this anomaly, the midgut rotates 90 to 180 degrees clockwise. The colon returns first to the abdominal cavity; the transverse colon lies posterior to the superior mesenteric artery and could be entrapped in a tunnel formed by a small intestinal mesenteric fixation. The duodenum passes anterior to the superior mesenteric artery and continues with the small bowel that occupies its normal position with a reversal of its anterior and posterior surfaces.

Malrotation[3–6, 15] (Fig. 35–4) is essentially an incomplete or deviated rotation and is the commonest form of abnormal rotation of the midgut. The cecum can be found in the subpyloric region anterior to the superior mesenteric artery, but, most commonly, it is located in the subhepatic region when the cecum fails to descend. When it fails to adhere to the posterior abdominal wall, the mesentery of the small bowel and the right colon forms a narrow pedicle at the level of the superior mesenteric artery, predisposing to midgut volvulus. Ladd's bands can complicate some cases of nondescent of the cecum. These bands may tightly connect either the cecum or the ascending colon to the duodenum, or extend from the cecum and the right colon to the right upper quadrant, crossing the duodenum. The bands can cause a variety of symptoms ranging from acute obstruction in neonates to chronic duodenal ileus in adults. Isolated incomplete rotation of the duodenum[16–19] is caused by the arrest of rotation of the duodenojejunal segment after it has rotated 180 degrees. In this abnormality, the duodenojejunal loop becomes fixed by adhesion along the superior mesenteric artery, predisposing to angulation, kinking, and obstruction.

Third Stage Rotation

The early fixation of the cecum or the failure in elongation of the colon can result in various degrees of an undescended cecum.[3–6] The failure of fixation of the cecum can leave it mobile, forming what Dott[4] termed the *mobile proximal colon*. The excessive elongation of the colon pushes the cecum into the pelvis, which makes the diagnosis of appendicitis difficult. The unattached duodenum results from its failure to adhere to the posterior abdominal wall and leaves it mobile, with a risk of acute kinking and acute or chronic obstruction. The failure of fixation of the mesentery of the small bowel and the right colon to the posterior abdominal wall leaves these organs hanging on the long narrow pedicle attached to the origin of the superior mesentery artery. This anomaly predisposes to volvulus.

Clinical Manifestations

Ten percent of intestinal obstruction in the neonate represent a complication of malrotation.[20] Intestinal obstruction affects more males than it does females by a ratio of 3 to 1.[4, 21, 22] Fifty to 80% of patients with rotation anomalies are symptomatic in infancy.[4, 21] Abnormal anatomy and fixation can cause kinks and compression of the bowel, as well as predisposition to ptosis, torsion, and volvulus.[4] The clinical presentation varies with the age at presentation.

Most infants present with recurrent episodes of bile-stained vomiting[21, 22] and acute small bowel obstruction.[3, 4, 21, 22] These symptoms usually present within the first week of life, represent surgical emergencies, and require prompt evaluation and treatment. Many patients present with symptoms misdiagnosed as colic and have had many changes in formula prior to diagnosis.[21] Abdominal distention may be found on physical examination but is more noticeable with volvulus.[21] Poor fluid intake can cause constipation, but, more often, when the course is complicated with volvulus, the patient passes bloody stool.[21, 22] Duodenal obstruction secondary to Ladd's bands mimics that of duodenal stenosis, with a double-bubble sign on plain abdominal radiograph.[3] Associated anomalies have been reported in approximately one third of patients and include omphalocele, duodenal atresia and stenosis, diaphragmatic hernia, congenital heart disease, and ileal or jejunal atresia.[21] The mortality rate among patients with associated anomalies is increased.[21]

Malrotation in older children may be asymptomatic or present as recurrent episodes of abdominal pain, vomiting, or both.[23] Many episodes are misdiagnosed as cyclic vomiting.[3, 21, 22] Symptoms can be caused by intermittent partial volvulus,[3] duodenal compression by Ladd's bands,[3, 21] fibrous bands at the level of duodenojejunal flexure,[3] or intestinal adhesion.[21] Chronic abdominal pain due to chronic, intermittent volvulus has been reported in patients with normal midgut rotation with nonfixation.[23] An unusual presentation of malrotation is that mimicking celiac disease with bouts of diarrhea and malabsorption.[21] An acute presentation with small bowel obstruction is usually the result of midgut volvulus. This serious, life-threatening complication of malrotation is the reason that symptoms suggestive of rotational abnormalities should be investigated.

An estimated 25 to 50% of adolescents and adults with malrotation are asymptomatic.[15, 22, 24] Acutely symptomatic adolescents and adults often present with acute bowel obstruction caused by volvulus or symptoms of chronic intestinal obstruction due to cecal torsion or pyloric obstruction.[15] A history of recurrent bouts of abdominal pain with occasional vomiting, diarrhea, or both may be elicited in most instances.[25] Ten to 25% of adolescents and adults with malrotation have symptoms related to peptic acid disease.[15, 22] Rees and Redo[22] postulated that chronic antral stasis due to partial duodenal obstruction may cause ulceration.

Confirmation of the diagnosis is usually made by radiographic studies. The plain film of the abdomen is usually nonspecific but can be helpful in the diagnosis of the symptomatic neonate.[26] Contrast studies are required to confirm the diagnosis. Barium enema may be helpful, but the normal position of the cecum does not exclude the possibility of a malrotation. An upper gastrointestinal examination will document the position of the ligament of Trietz and normal or abnormal bowel rotation.[26]

Surgical treatment of malrotation is indicated in symptomatic patients.[18, 27] The technique consists of the reduction of midgut volvulus, freeing the duodenum and the upper jejunum so that they remain in the right abdomen. The colon is freed in the left abdomen, with the cecum resting in the left lower quadrant. The appendix is removed at the same time. The surgical fixation of the bowel has been abandoned during the last 10 years. The duodenum should be checked for the presence of an intrinsic web. A Foley catheter is passed down into the jejunum through a gastrostomy, then is withdrawn after its balloon has been filled with saline to fill the intestinal lumen loosely. This technique helps identify the presence of a perforated web missed by inspection and palpation.[18, 27–30]

INTESTINAL ATRESIA AND STENOSIS

Atresia implies complete obstruction of the bowel, whereas *stenosis* refers to a partial obstruction of the lumen of the intestine. These anomalies are not rare, and they account for one third of all cases of neonatal intestinal obstruction, excluding anorectal malformation.[3]

Classification

Stenosis is caused by a partial diaphragm or other narrowing of the intestinal lumen.

Atresia can be divided into four types (Fig. 35–5).[3, 31] Type 1 is caused by the presence of an imperforate diaphragm with a normal length of the intestine. Type 2 consists of two blind ends connected by a band. Occasionally, a defect of the mesentery with or without a subnormal length of the bowel is also found. Type 3 is divided into two subtypes.

In type 3a, two blind ends are disconnected, with loss of the mesentery and the length of the bowel, whereas the blood supply to the unaffected bowel is normal. Type 3b is also termed the *apple peel* or *christmas tree atresia*, and the anomalies in this type include extensive jejunal atresia, loss of mesentery, and shortening of the bowel. The remaining ileum usually has an abnormal blood supply. Type 4 atresia is characterized by multiple intestinal occlusions with a loss of bowel length that can be extensive.

Causes

The causes of duodenal atresia differ from those of atresia in the rest of the small bowel.[3, 33–35] The duodenum passes through a solid stage, followed by recanalization through vacuolization between the fifth and the eighth weeks of gestation.[32, 33] Partial or complete failure of recanalization is thought to result in duodenal stenosis or atresia.[33–35] A generalized insult to the fetus might result in the arrest of duodenal development. This possibility would also explain the high incidence of associated anomalies with duodenal atresia. Louw and Barnard[36] were able to produce jejunoilial atresia by ligating the mesenteric vessels in fetal dogs. They concluded that at least a portion of intestinal atresia is caused by intrauterine vascular accidents. Intrauterine intestinal intussusception had also been reported to cause intestinal atresia.[37–42] Following experiments on lambs, Abrams[35] concluded that, except for duodenal atresia, most small bowel atresias are probably caused by vascular accidents during embryogenic development.

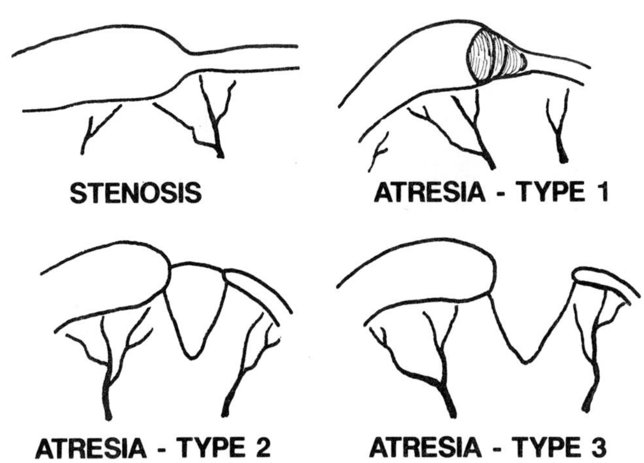

Figure 35–5. Types of intestinal atresia: Type 1, intraluminal diaphragm; type 2, two blind sacs connected by a band of tissue; and type 3, two blind sacs with loss of mesentery and distal bowel. (Adapted from Louw JH: Jejunal atresia and stenosis. J Pediatr Surg 1966; 1:8–23.)

Clinical Manifestations

The incidence of duodenal atresia is 0.5 to 1 in 10,000.[43] The disorder represents 45 to 50% of all cases of intestinal atresia[3, 44]; it affects males and females almost equally[44, 45] and is sporadic, although familial occurrences have been reported.[46] Most duodenal atresias are located in the second portion of the duodenum in the vicinity of the major ampulla.[33] Polyhydramnios during the last trimester of pregnancy is encountered in 30 to 45% of cases, and prematurity has been reported in 47 to 54%.[3, 44, 45] Associated malformations are identified in half of the patients and include Down's syndrome in approximately 30%, annular pancreas in 20%, malrotation in 20 to 32%, and congenital heart disease in 17 to 36%. Other reported malformations include tracheoesophageal fistula, imperforate anus, and renal anomalies. Multiple anomalies were seen in 24% of the reported cases.[44, 45] Symptoms develop during the first day of life in most patients.[45] A review by the surgical section of the American Academy of Pediatrics[45] found that the presenting symptom was vomiting in 85% of patients (75% have bile-stained emesis). Distention localized to the upper abdomen occurred in one third of the patients. Failure to pass meconium was seen in 48% of affected neonates, but this symptom did not discriminate between atresia and stenosis. Jaundice was noted in 37% of the infants.

In contrast with duodenal atresia, extragastrointestinal anomalies are less commonly found with atresia in the remaining intestine; the frequency of occurrence ranges between 7[47] and 52%.[48] Jejunoileal atresias are located in the proximal jejunum of 31% of affected infants, distal jejunum in 20%, proximal ileum in 13%, and distal ileum in 36%.[47] Multiple lesions have been reported in as few as 6.5%[47] and in as many as one third of the cases.[48] Polyhydramnios has been reported in 25% of the infants, prematurity in 25% of ileal atresias, and 38% of the patients with jejunal atresia.[47] Males and females are affected equally.[47, 52] Most patients with small bowel atresia are symptomatic during the first day of life.[47–49] In contrast with more proximal intestinal lesions, there is often a delay in the diagnosis of colon atresia, which accounts for fewer than 10% of all bowel atresias.[51] Bile-stained vomiting or nasogastric aspirate is the most frequent symptom found in 84 to 87% of the patients with small bowel atresia, followed by abdominal distention in 70 to 78%, and failure to pass meconium in 65 to 74% of the infants.[47, 49] Jaundice has been found in 32% of jejunal and 20% of ileal atresias.[47]

Diagnosis

Ultrasound studies are helpful in the prenatal diagnosis of atresia.[53] In addition, Deleze and coworkers[54] reported a high concentration of bile acid in the amniotic fluid with obstruction distal to the ampulla, which may be helpful if amniocentesis is performed. An upright plain abdominal radiograph will demonstrate the double-bubble sign in most cases of duodenal atresia,[50] and multiple air-fluid levels may be found in distal atresias.[3] The upper gastrointestinal contrast study is widely used,[44, 45] but its value has been questioned.[50] Barium enema examination can evaluate distal patency and possible malrotation.[55]

Treatment

Preoperative management should include stabilizing the patient with nasogastric tube decompression of the bowel, fluid and electrolyte administration, and respiratory support. Prenatal diagnosis allows earlier surgical intervention, with a lower incidence of metabolic complications.[56] The surgical treatment most often performed for duodenal atresia is primary duodenoduodenostomy or duodenojejunostomy.[45] In managing small bowel atresia, it is necessary to leave at least 75 cm of small bowel.[3, 55] Primary anastomosis is the most frequently used technique, although a two-stage technique may be performed in colonic atresia.[47–49, 57, 58]

Prognosis

The mortality rate associated with intestinal atresia has steadily declined,[55] owing, at least partially, to improvement in respiratory and intensive care,[50] as well as earlier diagnosis.[45, 58] The overall mortality rate for duodenal atresia was 40% in the survey by Fonkalsrud and associates,[45] and 42% and 38% in jejunal and ileal atresia, respectively.[47] Patients with low birth weights and associated anomalies have a higher mortality rate.[45, 47–49]

DUPLICATION OF THE GASTROINTESTINAL TRACT

Duplications are rare anomalies and consist of well-developed, tubular, or spherical structures with smooth muscle walls, firmly attached to the intestine and sharing a common blood supply. Duplications may communicate with the intestinal lumen and are located on the mesenteric border. Their mucosa resembles that of the gastrointestinal tract.[3, 59] Embryologically, these structures are classified as localized duplication, duplication associated with vertebral and spinal cord malformations, and duplication of the colon.[3]

Localized duplication has been attributed to failure of the vacuoles to coalesce properly[3, 59] or to localized anomalies in the development of the gut,[3] but neither of these hypotheses fully explains the location of these structures.[3] Localized duplications usually form cystic or tubular structures within the wall of the bowel or closely attached to it at its mesentery.[3, 59] Most are located in the ileum and produce symptoms by causing bowel obstruction, intussusception, volvulus, perforation or hemorrhage, or both.[3, 59–61] Abdominal pain, the presence of a mass or abdominal distention, and vomiting are common presenting symptoms.[3, 59–61] Respiratory distress is a frequent presenting symptom in infants.[62]

Duplication associated with vertebral and spinal cord malformations is thought to arise from the splitting of the notochord in the developing embryo.[3, 63–65] Spinal malformations range from a slight widening of the vertebrae to a complete anterior or posterior spina bifida.[64, 65]

Duplication of the colon is usually a part of exstrophy of the cloaca. Major anomalies of the lower urinary tract and genitalia accompany this malformation.[66] Associated duplication of the terminal ileum has been found in 25% of the patients reported by Ravitch.[66] An inadequate external opening predisposes to the distention of the colon,[66] with symptoms of acute or chronic lower intestinal obstruction.[67] Diarrhea and hematochezia may be the presenting symptoms.[68]

Diagnosis is suspected by the history and physical examination. Although helpful, radiologic studies are usually nonspecific[68] and may reveal a bowel obstruction, a mass effect with displacement of the normal intestine,[68] or a cystic mass on chest radiograph.[65] Many cases are discovered intraoperatively while the surgeon is trying to relieve a bowel obstruction.[61]

The treatment of choice is resection of the duplication with or without the adjacent bowel.[60, 62, 68] In long duplications that would require extensive bowel resection, a selective mucosal excision is recommended.[61] The mortality rate is high in patients with associated anomalies; Hocking and Young[68] reported an 18.9% mortality rate in their series.

ANNULAR PANCREAS

Embryology

The ventral and dorsal pancreatic buds are formed during the fourth week of fetal life. The ventral pancreatic bud migrates dorsally and comes to lie immediately below and behind the dorsal pancreas; then both buds fuse at approximately the seventh or eighth week of gestation.[1, 2, 72] (see Chapter 1, Fig. 1–3). Many hypotheses have been proposed to explain the development of annular pancreas, including the hypertrophy of normally disposed pancreatic primordia, the persistence of a left ventral bud, the failure of rotation of the ventral bud, and the fusion of aberrant pancreatic tissue.[69] The most accepted hypothesis is the failure of a complete rotation of the tip of the ventral bud to the right and posteriorly.[70] Histologically, annular pancreas is formed by normal pancreatic tissue partly or completely encircling the duodenum in ringlike fashion.[70] The anomaly is rare—only 15 cases were diagnosed at the Mayo Clinic during a 20-year period.[71] Annular pancreas was diagnosed in childhood in 52.5% of the cases, and the diagnosis was made during the neonatal period in 85.7% of these cases. Children presented with symptoms of duodenal obstruction or recurrent vomiting. Duodenal atresia or stenosis accompanied annular pancreas in most children. In the adult population, the most frequent symptom was abdominal pain in 69% of the patients, followed by nausea and vomiting in 60%.[71] Peptic ulcer disease was reported in 19% of adult patients, and hematemesis in 10.3%.[71] Annular pancreas is frequently associated with other congenital anomalies, such as Down's syndrome, cardiac defects, intestinal malrotation, duodenal atresia, and tracheoesophageal fistulas.[70, 71] The diagnosis is suspected by the history, but confirmation is difficult preoperatively.[70] Radiologically, the abdominal flat plate may reveal the double-bubble sign, and contrast studies may show the presence of a smooth annular filling defect with symmetric proximal dilatation and reverse peristalsis proximad to the obstruction.[70, 71] Endoscopic retrograde pancreatography, computed tomography scan, and ultrasound may be useful in formulating a diagnosis.[70] The treatment is surgical, and duodenoduodenostomy or duodenojejunostomy is the procedure usually performed.[71, 72] The prognosis depends on the age of the patient and the associated anomalies.[71]

REFERENCES

1. Sadler TW: Langman's Medical Embryology. 5th ed. Baltimore, Williams & Wilkins, 1985.
2. Corliss CE: Patten's Human Embryology: Elements of Clinical Development. New York, McGraw-Hill, 1976.
3. Louw JH, Cywes S: Embryology and anomalies of the intestine. *In* Berk JE, Haubrich WS, Kalser MH, et al, eds: Bockus Gastroenterology. 4th ed. Philadelphia, WB Saunders, 1985, pp 1439–1473.
4. Dott NM: Anomalies of intestinal rotation: Their embryology and surgical aspects with report of five cases. Br J Surg 1923; 11:251–286.
5. Snyder WH, Chaffin L: Embryology and pathology of the intestinal tract: Presentation of 40 cases of malrotation. Ann Surg 1954; 140:368–379.
6. Estrada RL: Anomalies of Intestinal Rotation and Fixation. Springfield, IL, Charles C Thomas 1958.
7. Haymond HE, Dragstedt LR: Anomalies of intestinal rotation. Surg Gynecol Obstet 1931; 53:316–329.
8. Berardi RS: Anomalies of midgut rotation in adult. Surg Gynecol Obstet 1980; 151:113–124.
9. Hunter JI: A mesenteric cyst of jejunal origin complicated by retrojejunal position of the transverse colon. Br Med J 1922; 11:800–802.
10. Amir-Jahed AK: Classification of reversed intestinal rotation. Surgery 1968; 64:1071–1074.
11. Scobie WG: A case of reversed rotation presenting as duodenal ileus. Br J Surg 1969; 56:709–711.
12. Stagg LH, Sheiner HJ: Reversed rotation of the gut incidental to cholecystitis in a left-sided gallbladder. Br J Surg 1973; 60:413–416.
13. Pearlman NW, Collins JS, Campbell DN, et al: Prearterial reversed midgut rotation. Arch Surg 1981; 116:1084–1087.
14. Borghol M, Holdsworth J: Reversed rotation of the midgut in an adult. Acta Chir Scand 1987; 153:395–397.
15. Wang C, Welch CE: Anomalies of intestinal rotation in adolescents and adults. Surgery 1963; 54:839–855.
16. Lewis E Jr: Partial duodenal obstruction with incomplete duodenal rotation. J Pediatr Surg 1966; 1:47–53.
17. Firor HV, Harris VJ: Rotational abnormalities of the gut: Re-emphasis of the neglected facet, isolated incomplete rotation of the duodenum. AJR 1974; 120:315–321.
18. Firor HV, Steiger E: Morbidity of rotational abnormalities of the gut beyond infancy. Cleve Clin Q 1983; 50:303–309.
19. Balthazar EJ: Intestinal malrotation in adults: Roentgenographic assessment with emphasis on isolated complete and partial nonrotations. Am J Roentgenol 1976; 126:358–367.
20. Long L: Intestinal obstruction in the newborn: review of 50 cases. Arch Surg 1967; 94:443–449.
21. Stewart DR, Colodney AL, Daggett WC: Malrotation of the bowel in infants and children: A 15-year review. Surgery 1976; 79:716–720.
22. Rees RJ, Redo FS: Anomalies of intestinal rotation and fixation. Am J Surg 1968; 116:834–841.
23. Janik JS, Ein SH: Normal intestinal rotation with nonfixation: A cause of chronic abdominal pain. J Pediatr Surg 1979; 14:670–674.
24. Findlay CW Jr, Humphreys GH: Collective reviews: Congenital anomalies of intestinal rotation in adults. Int Abstr Surg 1956; 103:417–438.
25. Devlin HB, Williams RSM, Pierce JW: Presentation of midgut malrotation in adults. Br Med J 1968; 1:803–807.
26. Simpson AJ, Leonidas JC, Krasna IH, et al: Roentgen diagnosis of midgut malrotation: Value of upper gastrointestinal radiographic study. J Pediatr Surg 1972; 7:243–252.
27. Gohl ML, DeMeester TR: Midgut nonrotation in adults: An aggressive approach. Am J Surg 1975; 129:319–323.
28. Ladd WE: Congenital obstruction of the duodenum in children. N Engl J Med 1932; 206:277.
29. Brennom WS, Bill AH: Prophylactic fixation of the intestine for midgut malrotation. Surg Gynecol Obstet 1974; 138:181–184.
30. Bill AH, Grauman D: Rationale and technic for stabilization of the mesentery in cases of nonrotation of the midgut. J Pediatr Surg 1966; 1:127–136.
31. Louw JH: Jejunal atresia and stenosis. J Pediatr Surg 1966; 1:8–23.
32. Tandler J: Zur Entwickelungsgeschichte des menschlichen duodenum in fruhen embryonalstadien. Morphol Jahrb 1900; 29:187–216.
33. Boyden EA, Cope JG, Bill AH Jr: Anatomy and embryology of congenital intrinsic obstruction of the duodenum. Am J Surg 1967; 114:190–202.
34. Louw JH: Investigation into the etiology of congenital atresia of the colon. Dis Colon Rectum 1964; 7:471–478.
35. Abrams JS: Experimental intestinal atresia. Surgery 1968; 64:185–191.
36. Louw JH, Barnard CN: Congenital intestinal atresia: Observations on its origin. Lancet 1955; 2:1065–1067.
37. Parkkulainen KV: Intrauterine intussusception as a cause of intestinal atresia. Surgery 1958; 44:1106–1111.
38. Gherardi GJ, Fisher JH: Atresia of the small intestine produced by intussusception in utero. N Engl J Med 1961; 264:229–231.
39. Grosfeld JL, Clatworthy HW: The nature of ileal atresia due to intrauterine intussusception. Arch Surg 1970; 100:714–717.
40. Todani T, Tabuchi K, Tanaka S: Intestinal atresia due to intrauterine intussusception: Analysis of 24 cases in Japan. J Pediatr Surg 1975; 10:445–451.
41. Pavri DR, Marshall DG, Armstrong RF, et al: Intrauterine intussusception: Case report and literature review. Can J Surg 1983; 26:376–378.
42. Reed DN, Polley TY, Rees MA: Jejunal atresia secondary to intrauterine intussusception, presenting as acute perforation. Can J Surg 1987; 30:203–204.
43. Nixon HH: Duodenal atresia. Br J Hosp Med 1989; 41:134–140.
44. Rescorla FJ, Grosfeld JL: Intestinal atresia and stenosis: Analysis of survival in 120 cases. Surgery 1985; 98:668–676.
45. Fonkalsrud EW, DeLorimier AA, Hays DM: Congenital atresia and stenosis of the duodenum: A review compiled from the members of the surgical section of the American Academy of Pediatrics. Pediatrics 1969; 43:79–83.
46. Best LG, Wiseman NE, Chudley AE: Familial duodenal atresia: A report of two families and review. Am J Med Genet 1989; 34:442–444.
47. DeLorimier AA, Fonkalsrud EW, Hays DM: Congenital atresia and stenosis of the jejunum and ileum. Surgery 1969; 65:819–827.
48. Paterson-Brown S, Stalewski H, Brereton RJ: Neonatal small bowel atresia, stenosis and segmental dilatation. Br J Surg 1991; 78:83–86.

49. Smith GHH, Glasson M: Intestinal atresia: Factors affecting survival. NZ J Surg 1989; 59:151–156.
50. Mooney D, Lewis JE, Connors RH, et al: Newborn duodenal atresia: An improving outlook. Am J Surg 1987; 153:347–349.
51. Coran AG, Eraklis AJ: Atresia of the colon. Surgery 1969; 65:828–831.
52. Pohlson EC, Hatch EI, Glick PL, et al: Individualized management of colonic atresia. Am J Surg 1988; 155:690–692.
53. Carrera JM: Prenatal diagnosis of gastrointestinal tract obstructions. Fetal Ther 1986; 1:96–97.
54. Deleze G, Sidiropoulos D, Paumgartner G: Determination of bile acid concentration in human amniotic fluid for prenatal diagnosis of intestinal obstruction. Pediatrics 1977; 59:647–650.
55. Hatch EI, Schaller RT Jr: Surgical management of multiple intestinal atresias. Am J Surg 1986; 151:550–552.
56. Miro J, Bard H: Congenital atresia and stenosis of the duodenum: The impact of prenatal diagnosis. Am J Obstet Gynecol 1988; 158:555–559.
57. Boles ET, Vassy LE, Ralston M: Atresia of the colon. J Pediatr Surg 1976; 11:69–75.
58. Benson CD, Lotfi MW, Brough AJ: Congenital atresia and stenosis of the colon. J Pediatr Surg 1968; 3:253–257.
59. Forshall I: Duplication of the intestinal tract. Postgrad Med J 1961; 37:570–589.
60. Bissler JJ, Klein RL: Alimentary tract duplications in children: Case and literature review. Clin Pediatr 1988; 27:152–157.
61. Ildstad ST, Tollerud DJ, Weiss RG, et al: Duplications of the alimentary tract. Ann Surg 1988; 208:184–189.
62. Pokorny WJ, Goldstein IR: Enteric thoracoabdominal duplications in children. J Thorac Cardiovasc Surg 1984; 87:821–824.
63. Alrabeeah A, Giacomantonio M, Lau H: Neurenteric cysts: A spectrum. J Pediatr Surg 1988; 23:752–754.
64. Bentley JFR, Smith JR: Developmental posterior enteric remnants and spinal malformations: The split notochord syndrome. Arch Dis Child 1960; 35:76–86.
65. Beardmore HE, Wiglesworth FW: Vertebral anomalies and alimentary duplications: Clinical and embryological aspects. Pediatr Clin North Am 1958; 5:457–474.
66. Ravitch MM: Hind gut duplication: Doubling of the colon and genital urinary tracts. Ann Surg 1953; 137:588–601.
67. Yousefzadeh DK, Bickers GH, Jackson JH Jr, et al: Tubular colonic duplication: Review of 1876–1981 literature. Pediatr Radiol 1983; 13:65–71.
68. Hocking M, Young DG: Duplications of the alimentary tract. Br J Surg 1981; 68:92–96.
69. Ikeda Y, Irving IM: Annular pancreas in a fetus and its three-dimensional reconstruction. J Pediatr Surg 1984; 19:160–164.
70. Volk BW, Allen RA: Embryology, anatomy, histology and anomalies of the pancrease. *In* Berk JE, Haubrich WS, Kalser MH, et al, eds: Bockus Gastroenterology. 4th ed. Philadelphia, WB Saunders, 1985, pp 3834–3843.
71. Kierman PD, ReMine SG, Kierman PC, et al: Annular pancreas. Arch Surg 1980; 115:46–50.
72. McGuigan JE, Ament ME: Anatomy, embryology, and developmental anomalies. *In* Sleisenger MH, Fordtran JS, eds: Gastrointestinal Disease: Pathology, Diagnosis, Management. 4th ed. Philadelphia, WB Saunders, 1989, pp 671–672.

Chapter 36

Inguinal Hernia and Hydrocele

FREDERICK ALEXANDER

Inguinal hernia is one of the commonest surgical problems of infancy and childhood, yet it continues to generate confusion and controversy. It occurs in 0.8 to 4.4% of children[1]; however, in premature infants the incidence may increase to 30%, depending on the age of gestation.[2] The peak incidence occurs in the neonatal period, when the defect is also most likely to cause symptoms usually related to incarceration and strangulation. The incidence subsequently declines with age but remains approximately six times commoner in boys than it is in girls.[3]

Inguinal hernia usually presents as an intermittent bulge in the groin that may extend into the scrotum or labia majora with crying or straining. These findings contrast with the fluctuant scrotal swelling that is characteristic of a hydrocele. On the other hand, because congenital inguinal hernias and hydroceles share a common origin, namely a patent processus vaginalis, they may be difficult to distinguish clinically or may occur in conjunction with each other. Further, their management relative to the timing of surgery and contralateral exploration remains a point of controversy.

HISTORY

Hernias were described in ancient times, but not until the early nineteenth century was the anatomy of the inguinal canal accurately described. Bassini[4] in 1887 was the first author to describe the successful use of high ligation of the hernia sac in combination with anatomic repair. This concept was modified in 1899 by Ferguson,[5] who advocated incision of the external oblique fascia to improve surgical exposure. In 1950, Potts and coworkers[6] recommended simple high ligation and removal of the hernia sac for routine hernia repair in children, which has become the standard of care.

EMBRYOLOGY AND PATHOGENESIS

The processus vaginalis is a tubular extension of the peritoneal membrane that passes through the internal ring and into the scrotum during the third month of gestation. This membrane surrounds the testis and gubernaculum and probably contributes to testicular descent in the seventh month of gestation by downward transmission of intra-abdominal pressure.[7] The processus vaginalis usually obliterates some time after testicular descent is complete, although the timing and mechanism of closure are unknown. Failure of the processus vaginalis to obliterate is the commonest cause of inguinal hernia and hydrocele in infants and children. However, autopsy studies have shown that the processus vaginalis may remain patent in a large number of asymptomatic children and adults,[8,9] suggesting that other factors also may be involved. For example, an increase in abdominal pressure or fluid may play an important role in the clinical development of a hernia or a hydrocele. Placement of a ventriculoperitoneal shunt or a peritoneal dialysis catheter in a formerly asymptomatic patient frequently leads to the rapid development of a clinical hernia or hydrocele.

CLINICAL PRESENTATION

Incomplete obliteration of the processus vaginalis may lead to a variety of clinical presentations (Fig. 36–1). For example, closure of the processus may occur at any point between the internal ring and the scrotum, leading to various degrees of herniation into the inguinal canal. The processus vaginalis may remain open into the scrotum, forming a complete inguinal hernia. On the other hand, the processus vaginalis may close incompletely along its longitudinal axis, leading to fluid accumulation in the scrotum or a hydrocele. If the processus remains open sufficiently to allow bidirectional movement of fluid, a *communicating hydrocele* may result, which usually fluctuates in size. Late obliteration of the processus may entrap fluid within the tunica vaginalis surrounding the testis, resulting in a *noncommunicating hydrocele.*

Usually the child with a hernia presents with a history of intermittent pain or swelling of the groin. An incarcerated hernia is often associated with bilious vomiting and obstipation and is the commonest cause of small bowel obstruction in infants and children who have not

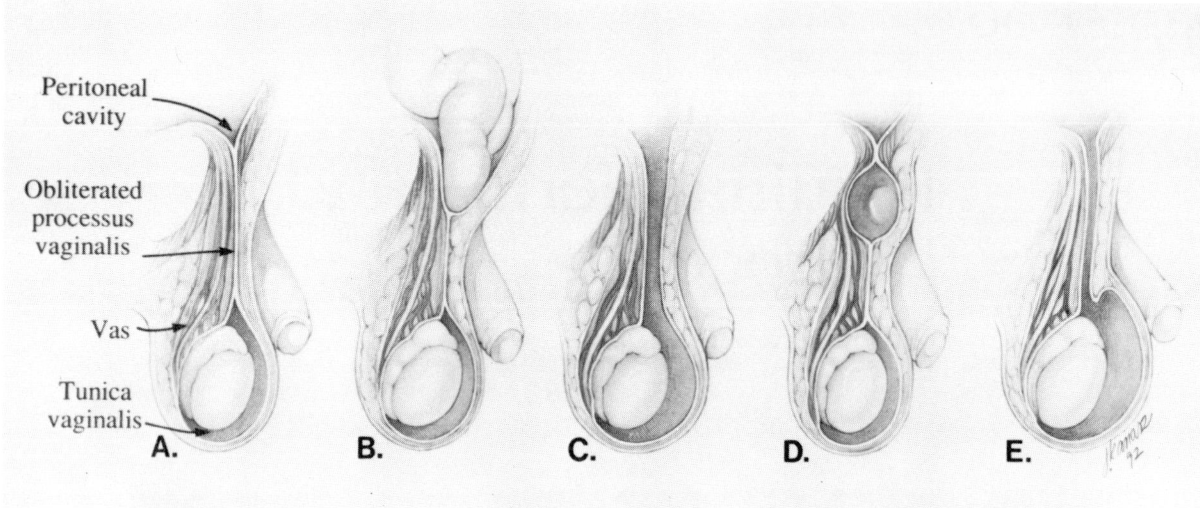

Figure 36–1. Spectrum of anatomic abnormalities of the processus vaginalis. *A,* Normal anatomy. *B,* Inguinal hernia. *C,* Complete hernia. *D,* Hydrocele of the cord. *E,* Communicating hydrocele.

had prior surgery. Therefore, an incarcerated inguinal hernia should be highly suspected in any child with signs of intestinal obstruction. When incarceration leads to diminished circulation in the herniated viscus, ischemic necrosis or a strangulated hernia may result. In contrast, children with hydroceles usually present with asymptomatic scrotal swelling.

Examination of a child for inguinal hernia or hydrocele may be facilitated by extending the child's hips in a supine position to encourage straining or crying. Manual palpation of the groin and scrotum often reveals the significant findings described previously. It is important to palpate both testicles within the scrotum, since an undescended or retractile testis may often pose as an inguinal hernia. Usually, gentle pressure applied manually in a cephalad and posterior direction will result in a sudden reduction of an inguinal hernia. Reduction of the hernia may be confirmed by simultaneous palpation of the contralateral groin, which should feel absolutely symmetric following reduction of the hernia. Transillumination is the hallmark of a hydrocele, and hydroceles frequently fluctuate in size, becoming less prominent at night when the infant is sleeping. If swelling of the inguinal canal may be reduced by gentle caudal pressure, leaving the inguinal canal flat and symmetric with the contralateral groin, then the presence of a hydrocele has been confirmed. Communicating hydroceles are unique in that they may be "reduced" in both directions. Occasionally it may be difficult to distinguish between an incarcerated hernia and a loculated hydrocele of the cord, particularly in premature or neonatal infants. Both conditions may transilluminate and may be irreducible; however, a hydrocele of the cord is otherwise asymptomatic as opposed to an incarcerated hernia, which is generally tender and associated with intestinal symptoms. Failure to reduce a hernia after administration of intramuscular morphine sulfate or meperidine, or a plain radiographic film of the abdomen that reveals signs of small bowel obstruction or a gas bubble below the inguinal ligament, also indicates an incarcerated hernia. If the clinician is unable to distinguish an incarcerated hernia (Fig. 36–2) from a loculated hydrocele, surgical exploration is recommended.

In some instances, a bulge in the groin may be seen by the parents or pediatrician but may not be demonstrated by examination. In this setting, the finding of thickening of the cord at the level of the internal ring may suggest the presence of a hernia. Otherwise, the surgeon may accept the diagnosis based on the description or may re-evaluate the child during a second visit.

MANAGEMENT

Inguinal hernias should be repaired promptly after the diagnosis is made to prevent incarceration. Although the overall risk of incarceration is unknown, this risk is much higher during the first year of life. Rowe and Clatworthy[10] found that two thirds of incarcerated hernias occur in children younger than 1 year of age and that two thirds of these children required surgical reduction. Given proper technique and adequate sedation, most children may now undergo manual reduction and thus avoid the anesthetic hazards of emergent surgical reduction. If manual reduction is easily and promptly accomplished, the child may be discharged and scheduled for elective outpatient surgery. In the more difficult cases, successful manual reduction should be followed by admission and subsequent hernia repair prior to discharge from the hospital. In those infants and children who are hospitalized for unrelated severe or life-threatening problems and are found to have an inguinal hernia, repair is best deferred until their condition stabilizes. In premature infants, repair is often deferred until just prior to discharge from the neonatal intensive

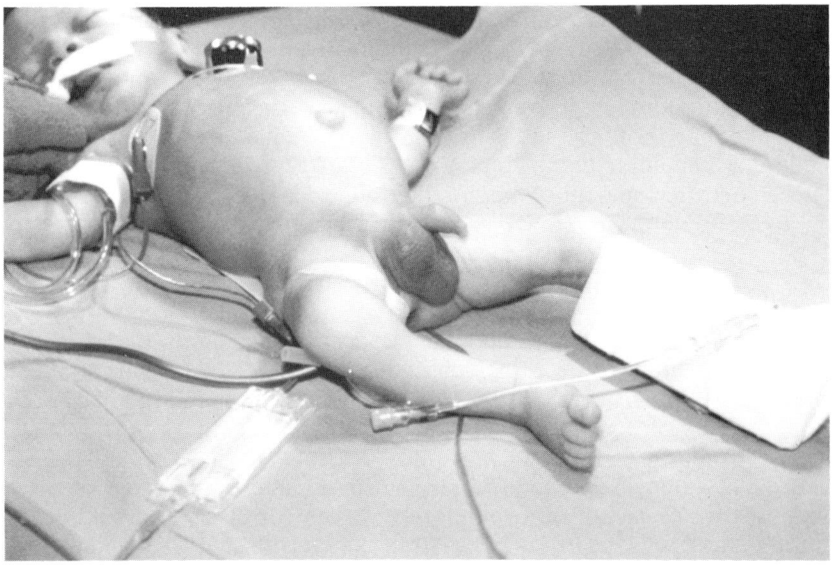

Figure 36–2. Typical appearance of an incarcerated hernia in a premature infant prior to surgical reduction and repair.

care unit, so that they may be closely observed postoperatively.

Hydrocele, in contrast with inguinal hernia, frequently resolves spontaneously, particularly during the first 2 years of life. Noncommunicating hydroceles in infancy usually resolve spontaneously, and even communicating hydroceles often resolve during the first 12 to 18 months of life (Fig. 36–3). Thus, in the absence of a hernia, it is prudent to observe a hydrocele for at least 18 months before recommending surgical repair. If the hydrocele shows no signs of resolution between 18 and 24 months of life, then surgical repair should be recommended. Since a persistent hydrocele in this setting is most likely to be communicating, the repair must be performed through the groin and must include high ligation of the processus vaginalis. The distal portion of the hydrocele sac should be trimmed with care so as not to injure the testis or structures of the cord.

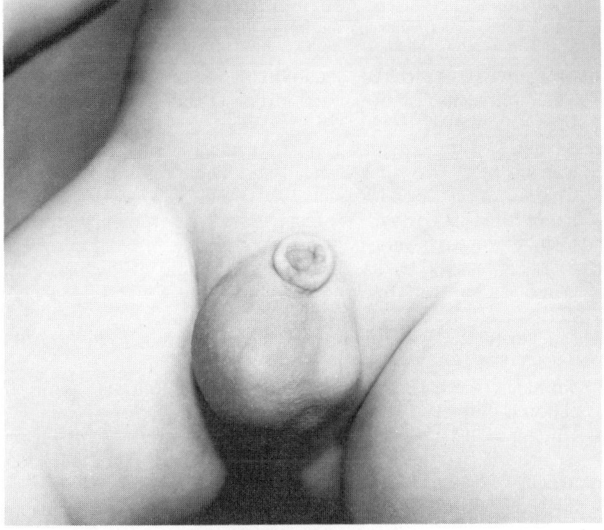

Figure 36–3. Typical appearance of a hydrocele, which frequently regresses by 2 years of age.

Surgical repair of hernias and hydroceles in children is usually performed as an outpatient procedure under general anesthesia. A transverse skin incision is made within the skin crease midway between the symphysis pubis and the anterior iliac crest. This incision is carried down through Scarpa's fascia, exposing the external oblique fascia. The external oblique fascia may then be opened, exposing the inguinal canal and the structures of the cord. At this point, the cremasteric muscle is gently separated, exposing the hernia sac, which always lies anterior to the structures of the cord. The hernia sac is gently dissected away from the structures of the cord and is then divided and traced to its origin at the internal ring, where it is ligated and amputated. The distal sac may be trimmed but not completely removed, since this is unnecessary and even hazardous. In a premature infant, or indeed in any child with an associated undescended testicle, the repair must be performed in conjunction with an orchiopexy. Sliding hernias are rare in children and may infrequently include the appendix or Meckel's diverticulum (Littre's hernia) as part of the hernia sac. In this situation, the appendix or Meckel's diverticulum may be carefully dissected away from the wall of the sac and then excised in the usual fashion. This will allow adequate separation and exposure of these structures to allow a purse-string closure of the sac. When exploration is carried out for incarceration, the incarcerated viscera should be carefully inspected for signs of ischemia and, if none are found, subsequently reduced. As a general rule, if an incarcerated hernia may be successfully reduced manually, it is unnecessary to inspect the intestine at the time of the subsequent hernia repair.

There has been considerable controversy over the issue of contralateral exploration. Many surgeons[11–13] have reported a high incidence of contralateral inguinal hernia or patent processus vaginalis when routine contralateral groin exploration is carried out in children with a unilateral, clinically apparent inguinal hernia. Thus, Gilbert and Clatworthy[14] concluded that it was justifiable to perform a bilateral inguinal hernia repair in any healthy infant or child with a unilaterally apparent hernia, irrespective of age, sex, or side involved.

On the other hand, Sparkman,[15] in a large review, found that although a contralateral patent processus vaginalis may be found in 50 to 60% of all infants and children, unilateral hernia repair was followed by the subsequent devlopment of a contralateral hernia in only 15 to 20% of the operated group. Bock and Sobye[16] reported only a 15% incidence of contralateral hernia in a group of 174 children who underwent unilateral hernia repair and were followed for 27 to 36 years. In a review of 2,764 infants and children, Rowe and colleagues[17] found a 63% incidence of patency of the processus vaginalis in the first 2 months, with a decline until 2 years of age when the incidence leveled off to 41%. From these reports, it would appear that the processus vaginalis obliterates near birth in approximately 40% of cases, with obliteration of another 20% during the first 2 years of life. After 2 years of age, nearly 40% of children still have a patent processus vaginalis, but fewer than half of these children develop a clinically apparent hernia.

The major advantage of routine contralateral exploration is the avoidance of a second operation with its cost and its risk of anesthesia. The major disadvantages of routine contralateral exploration include the possibility of a technical mishap leading to infertility, which is a minimal risk in experienced hands, as well as the increase in postoperative pain. Also, routine contralateral exploration with only a 15 to 20% expected incidence of hernia may raise the issue of unnecessary surgery. To reduce the number of unnecessary explorations and yet avoid reoperation, a number of studies[16, 18–21] have examined whether age, sex, or the side of the clinically apparent hernia could be used to determine the need for contralateral exploration. Of these factors, only age has any relationship to the risk of development of a contralateral hernia. Bock and Sobye[16] found that 47% of children whose primary hernia was repaired before the age of 1 year developed a contralateral hernia, compared with only 11% of those whose primary hernia was repaired after the first year of life. These data suggest that routine contralateral exploration may be justified during the first year or two of life, but not in older infants and children. Several studies[16, 18] have shown a slightly increased risk of contralateral hernia when the clinically apparent hernia appears on the left side as compared with the right; however, these findings are disputed by other studies in which little or no difference was found.[19, 20] Finally, Bock and Sobye[16] found that the incidence of contralateral hernia in girls who underwent unilateral repair of a clinical hernia was only 8%. Thus, the major reason for contralateral exploration in girls appears to be the low risk of damage to the reproductive organs.[21]

COMPLICATIONS

According to Rowe and Lloyd,[22] the overall rate of complications after elective hernia repair is approximately 2%, which increases to 19% following repair of incarcerated hernia. In fact, with continued technical improvements as well as with advances in pediatric anesthesia and neonatal intensive care, the incidence of perioperative complications should approach 0 to 1%. The risk of postoperative complications is higher in the premature infant, in whom intraoperative and postoperative respiratory complications are directly related to anesthetic care. Postoperative apnea caused by immaturity of the diaphragm or the intercostal muscle or abnormal responses to hypoxia and hypercapnia is not uncommon in premature infants. Therefore, the authors[22] recommended that premature infants with inguinal hernias undergo repair prior to discharge from the neonatal unit, allowing them to be closely monitored following surgery. Premature infants younger than 1 year of age who develop inguinal hernias while at home should be admitted for overnight observation following inguinal hernia repair, and the use of apnea monitors in this group of patients is highly recommended. Finally, the incidence of recurrence following repair of inguinal hernia should be minimal but may be slightly higher in premature infants. A plicated layer of oblique fascia buttressed to the internal ring may further reduce the risk of recurrence.

REFERENCES

1. Bronsther B, Abrams MW, Elboim C: Inguinal hernias in children: A study of 1,000 cases and review of the literature. J Am Med Wom Assoc 1972; 27:522–525.
2. Harper RG, Garcia A, Sia C: Inguinal hernia: A common problem of premature infants weighing 1,000 grams or less at birth. Pediatrics 1975; 56:112–115.
3. Holder TM, Ashcraft KW: Groin hernias and hydroceles. *In* Holder TM, Ashcraft KW, eds. Pediatric Surgery. Philadelphia, WB Saunders, 1980; pp 594–608.
4. Bassini E: Nuovo metodo per la cura radicale dell'ernia inguinale. Atti Congr Assoc Med Ital Pavia 1889; 2:179–182.
5. Ferguson AH: Oblique inguinal hernia: Typical operation for its radical cure. JAMA 1899; 33:6–14.
6. Potts WJ, Riker WL, Lewis JE: The treatment of inguinal hernia in infants and children. Ann Surg 1950; 132:566–576.
7. Shrock P: The processus vaginalis and gubernaculum. Surg Clin North Am 1971; 51:1263–1268.
8. Morgan EH, Anson BJ: Anatomy of region of inguinal hernia: The internal surface of parietal layers. Q Bull Northwestern Univ Med School 1942; 16:20–37.
9. Snyder WH Jr, Greaney EM Jr: Inguinal hernia. *In* Welch KJ, Ravitch MM, O'Neill JA, et al, eds: Pediatric Surgery, 2nd ed. Chicago, Year Book Medical, 1969; pp 692–700.
10. Rowe MI, Clatworthy HW: Incarcerated and strangulated hernias in children. Arch Surg 1970; 101:136–139.
11. McLaughlin CW Jr, Kleager C: Management of inguinal hernia in infancy and early childhood. AMA J Dis Child 1956; 92:266–271.
12. Mueller B, Rader G: Inguinal hernia in children. Arch Surg 1956; 73:595–596.
13. Rothenberg RE, Barnett T: Bilateral herniotomy in infants and children. Surgery 1955; 37:947–950.
14. Gilbert M, Clatworthy HW Jr: Bilateral operations for inguinal hernia and hydrocele in infancy and childhood. Am J Surg 1959; 97:255–259.
15. Sparkman RS: Bilateral exploration in inguinal hernia in juvenile patients. Surgery 1962; 51:393–406.
16. Bock JE, Sobye JV: Frequency of contralateral hernia in children. Acta Chir Scand 1970; 136:707–709.

17. Rowe MI, Copelson LW, Clatworthy HW: The patent processus vaginalis and the inguinal hernia. J Pediatr Surg 1969; 4:102–107.
18. Clausen EG, Jake RJ, Bingley FM: Contralateral inguinal exploration of unilateral hernia in infants and children. Surgery 1958; 44:735–740.
19. Kiesewetter WB, Parenzan L: When should hernia in the infant be treated bilaterally? JAMA 1959; 171:287–290.
20. Fischer R, Mumenthaler A: 1st bilaterale herniotomic bei Saiiglingen und Klein Kindern mit einseitiger Leistenhernia angezeigt? Helv Chir Acta 1957; 24:346–350.
21. Wright JE: Inguinal hernia in girls: Desirability and dangers of bilateral exploration. Aust Paediatr 1982; 18:55–57.
22. Rowe MI, Lloyd DA: Inguinal hernia. *In* Welch KJ, Randolph JA, Ravitch MM, et al, eds: Pediatric Surgery. 3rd ed. Chicago, Year Book Medical, 1986; pp 779–793.

Chapter 37

Anterior Abdominal Wall Defects

FREDERICK ALEXANDER

INTRODUCTION

Defects of the anterior abdominal wall may be classified according to their umbilical or extraumbilical location. Although the embryology and pathogenesis are still unclear, these malformations are readily distinguished by their clinical presentation.

Umbilical defects are commonest and include congenital umbilical hernia, hernia of the cord, and omphalocele. An umbilical hernia (Fig. 37–1) is usually discovered within a few days following separation of the cord, and it appears as a skin-covered sac overlying a dilated umbilical ring that contains only small intestine. It occurs most frequently in black children and often closes spontaneously by 4 years of age. Hernia of the cord and omphalocele are recognized at birth as umbilical defects covered by a peritoneal and an amniotic membrane. *Hernia of the cord* refers to umbilical defects smaller than 4 cm in diameter in which loops of intestine herniate into the peritoneal sac (Fig. 37–2). Omphalocele applies to umbilical defects larger than 4 cm in diameter in which the peritoneal sac may contain intestine and other viscera (Fig. 37–3). Rarely, the overlying membrane may rupture during the delivery, exposing normal-appearing intestine surrounded by remnants of the sac. Omphaloceles occur in 1 in 4,200 live births[1] and, less commonly, may involve defects of the sternum or the diaphragm or exstrophy of the bladder. Omphaloceles of all kinds are frequently associated with other anomalies, including cardiovascular malformations; trisomies 13, 18, and 21; and Beckwith-Wiedemann syndrome (macroglossia, gigantism, and transient hypoglycemia).

Extraumbilical defects, called *gastroschisis,* occur in 1 in 12,300 live births,[2] although their incidence appears to be increasing. Gastroschisis is most often located to the right of the umbilical cord and is frequently separated from it by a skin bridge. Apart from its extraumbilical location, gastroschisis is readily distinguished from omphalocele by the lack of a peritoneal sac and the absence of herniated solid viscera (Fig. 37–4). The eviscerated mass of bowel is covered by a thick and densely adherent peel that renders it prone to volvulus. In contrast with omphalocele, gastroschisis is rarely associated with extra-abdominal malformations. Finally, gastroschisis is usually characterized by a well-developed abdominal wall, as opposed to omphalocele in which the abdominal wall is often deficient in somatic elements.

HISTORY

Omphalocele was first described in Lycosthenes' *Chronicon* in 1557[3] and subsequently in Ambroise Pare's classic text of 1634.[4] In 1733, James Couder described a newborn with gastroschisis in whom the intestine was lying on the abdomen with an intact navel one and one-half inches below the defect.[5] Uncertainty regarding the embryology and clinical presentation of these anomalies has existed until the past several decades. Moore and

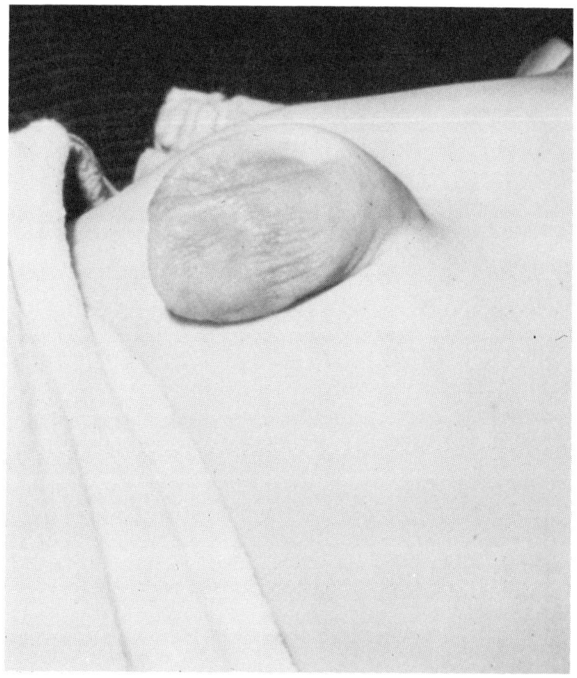

Figure 37–1. Typical appearance of an umbilical hernia that may close spontaneously by 4 years of age.

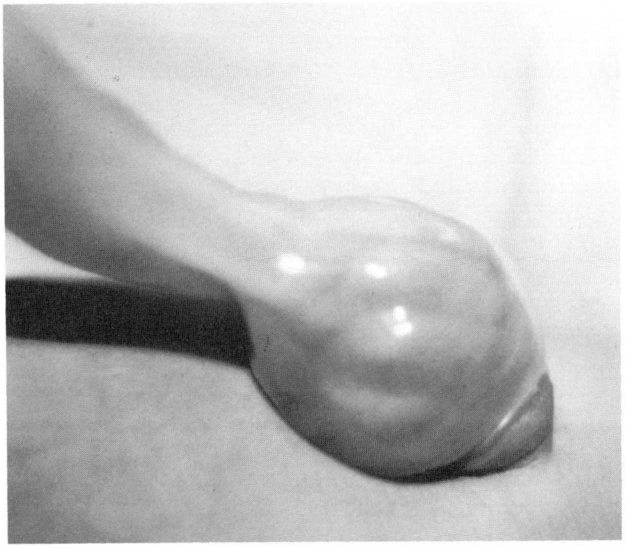

Figure 37–2. Typical appearance of a hernia of the cord in which small intestine only is visible through an intact peritoneal sac.

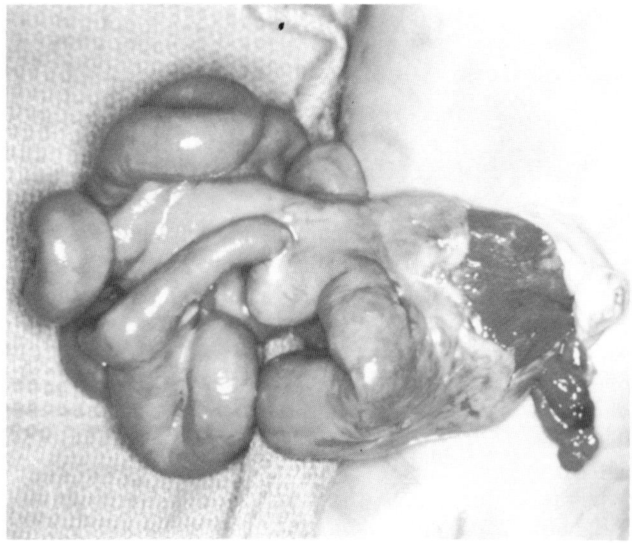

Figure 37–4. Typical gastroschisis defect located to the right of the umbilicus with thin intervening skin bridge and no remnant of peritoneal sac.

Stokes[6] in 1953 were among the first authors to distinguish between gastroschisis and omphalocele based on the location and the presence or the absence of a membranous sac. In 1963, Duhamel[7] emphasized the difference in embryologic origin between these two anomalies and postulated a teratogenic event affecting development. More recently, Shaw[8] and DeVries[9] postulated that gastroschisis may be caused by a mechanical rather than a teratogenic event, explaining the relative infrequency of extra-abdominal congenital malformations.

Although spontaneous closure of small omphaloceles was observed in the eighteenth and nineteenth centuries, the mortality of large omphaloceles and gastroschisis

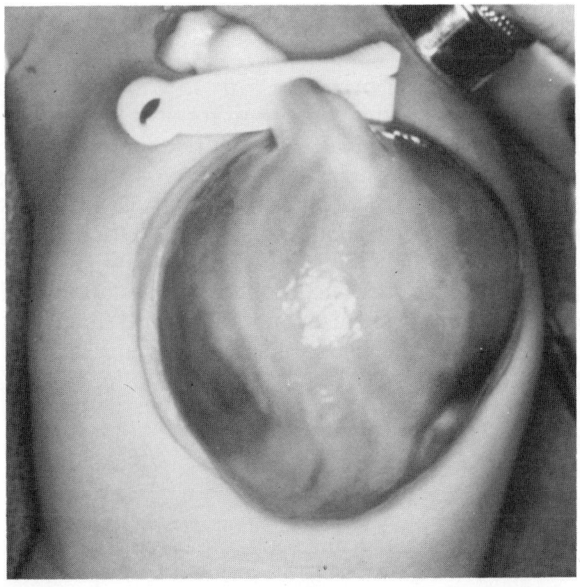

Figure 37–3. Typical omphalocele. Note the relative paucity of lateral abdominal wall.

remained nearly 100%. Surgical closure of a small omphalocele was first reported in 1803 by Hey,[10] but primary operative closure was hampered by increased intra-abdominal pressure with diaphragmatic elevation and caval compression, leading to respiratory and cardiovascular collapse. Successful treatment of omphalocele by topical application of alcohol was reported by Ahlfeld in 1899.[11] This form of treatment was lengthy, requiring 2 to 5 months of hospitalization and subsequent correction of the resultant ventral hernia, yet suggested the advantages of staged operative closure later applied to both omphalocele and gastroschisis.

In 1948, Gross[12] reported a two-stage closure of large omphaloceles in which flaps of widely mobilized skin were closed over intact amnion, and abdominal reconstruction with fascial closure was accomplished later. This technique resulted in a mortality rate as high as 60%; nevertheless, it represented a major advance in the treatment of these abdominal wall defects. The concept of staged repair was further advanced by Schuster,[13] who used a reef of Teflon mesh sewn to the abdominal wall under which polyethylene film temporarily covered the exposed viscera prior to the closure of the abdominal wall. This technique was modified in 1969 by Allen and Wrenn,[14] who used silicone sheeting to create a pouch that contained the exposed viscera, which were gradually reduced into the abdomen. At the same time, the development of total parenteral nutrition[15] helped decrease the mortality of staged repair in patients with large omphalocele and gastroschisis to the current levels of 15 to 30% and 10%, respectively.[16, 17] Subsequent improvements in neonatal mechanical ventilation along with the use of paralytic agents and stretching of the abdominal wall[18] have stimulated an increased interest in primary fascial closure of large omphalocele and gastroschisis. Primary fascial closure of gastroschisis was first reported by Watkins in 1943[19] but, for reasons stated previously, was slow to gain acceptance. It is apparent that current techniques and supportive care may allow primary fascial closure for all but the most difficult abdominal wall defects.

EMBRYOLOGY AND PATHOGENESIS

The intra-abdominal wall is derived from cephalic, caudal, and lateral folds that are well demarcated by the third week of gestation. Each of these folds is composed of somatic layers, which form the abdominal wall, and splanchnic layers, which enclose the foregut, midgut, and hindgut. During the third and fourth weeks of gestation, the midgut enlarges more rapidly than does the body of the embryo, filling the yolk sac in the extraembryonic coelom. A large opening in the midgut, which is connected to the yolk sac and referred to as the *omphalomesenteric duct,* continues to decrease in size throughout this gestational period. By the 10th and 11th weeks of gestation, development of the abdominal wall is sufficient to allow the return of the midgut into the embryonic coelom, where rotation and subsequent fixation take place.

Developmental failure of the lateral embryonic folds is most likely caused by a teratogenic event occurring within the first 3 weeks of gestation that prevents the return of the midgut into the abdomen and results in an omphalocele.[7] Failure of formation of the cephalic folds results in an epigastric abdominal wall defect that is frequently associated with sternal separation, diaphragmatic and pericardial defects, and intracardiac anomalies (Cantrell's deformity). Since the allantois, or primitive bladder, is enclosed by the somatic layer of the caudal fold, failure of formation of this layer results in exstrophy of the urinary bladder combined with a hypogastric omphalocele. Splanchnic deficiencies of the caudal fold result in anorectal agenesis (imperforate anus) and, when combined with somatic deficiencies of the same layer, result in cloacal exstrophy.

The cause of omphalocele is unknown. However, because omphaloceles are frequently associated with severe extra-abdominal anomalies, a teratogenic cause is most likely. Cardiac manifestations occur in 30 to 50%, and chromosomal defects in 10 to 40% of infants with omphaloceles.[17] Other defects frequently associated with omphalocele that support a catastrophic teratogenic event are genitourinary malformations and Beckwith-Wiedemann syndrome.[20] Omphalocele may occasionally occur in familial maternal twins and has no known mode of genetic transmission.

By contrast, gastroschisis is associated with a low incidence of extra-abdominal malformations, suggesting a mechanical rather than a teratogenic cause. Early descriptions of the embryogenesis of gastroschisis invoke a developmental failure of one of the lateral folds of the somatopleure. Duhamel[7] proposed that gastroschisis may result from a failure of differentiation of the mesenchymal framework of one of the lateral folds, with resorption of the ectodermal layer in that region. Gray and Skandalakis[22] stated that gastroschisis results from an arrest of migration of the embryonic musculature from the dorsal myotomes into the framework of the splanchnopleure. Hoyme and coworkers[23] postulated that gastroschisis results from premature regression of one of the two omphalomesenteric arteries, leading to ischemic changes of the developing abdominal wall. This hypothesis could also explain the relatively high incidence of intestinal atresia associated with gastroschisis. On the other hand, investigation of human embryos with gastroschisis whose gestational ages vary from 6 to 30 weeks reveals no evidence of ischemia of the developing abdominal wall.[24] Currently, the most plausible explanation for gastroschisis has been made by Shaw,[8] who postulated that gastroschisis results from an early tear of the umbilical cord that occurs after complete enfolding of the lateral somatic layers of the abdominal wall but before complete closure of the umbilical ring. Thus, gastroschisis may result from a mechanical rather than a teratogenic event occurring between the fourth and eighth weeks of gestation. This assumption is supported both by studies of aborted human embryos[25] and by antenatal sonographic studies of human embryos with gastroschisis.[26] Further, it explains the relative infrequency of associated extra-abdominal anomalies and the variability of the condition of exposed bowel, depending on the gestational age at which the tear occurs.

Although it is acknowledged that the severity of the fibrous peel in gastroschisis is related to the duration of exposure of intestine to amniotic fluid, the pathogenesis of this process is unknown. Studies in the chick embryo reveal that amniotic fluid peritonitis and progressive serosal fibrosis occur after the 15th day of incubation, corresponding with the 30th week of gestation in the human embryo, when renal function begins.[27–29] At this specific developmental age, there is a decrease in amniotic osmolality and sodium level coupled with an increase in urea, creatinine, and uric acid levels. The fibrous peel that subsequently develops causes intestinal foreshortening and malfunction but is not associated with abnormalities of the muscularis layer or ganglion cells.[30–32] Resolution of the peel is observed within 2 or 3 weeks after replacement of the intestine within the abdominal cavity.

Intestinal atresia occurs in 5 to 15% of infants with gastroschisis[33, 34] and is thought to result from a pinching effect of the abdominal wall on the mesentery or a torsion of the prolapsed intestine (Fig. 37–5).[35, 36] Atresia associated with gastroschisis may be single or multiple and involve large or small intestine.[37, 38] Often, there is sonographic evidence of bowel dilatation and mural thickening as early as the 23rd week of gestation, which correlates with intestinal dysmorphia and dismotility.[27, 39] In the most extreme cases, torsion or volvulus associated with gastroschisis may lead to fetal loss (Fig. 37–6).

DIAGNOSIS

Prenatal screening using sonography and serum alphafetoprotein level assessment has made it possible to diagnosis abdominal wall defects in utero. Sonographic detection of omphalocele and gastroschisis is operator

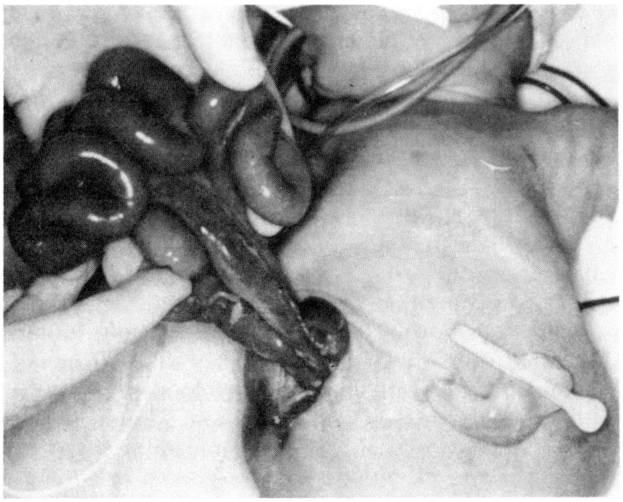

Figure 37–5. Gastroschisis with wide separation from umbilicus and evidence of mesenteric pinching by the fascial defect.

dependent and may yield an overall sensitivity of approximately 75%.[40, 41] The specificity of sonography in distinguishing between these two defects based on location of the defect with respect to the cord and on the presence or absence of a membranous sac may approach 100%.[39]

The impact of antenatal diagnosis of abdominal wall defects is unclear; however, it does allow prenatal pa-

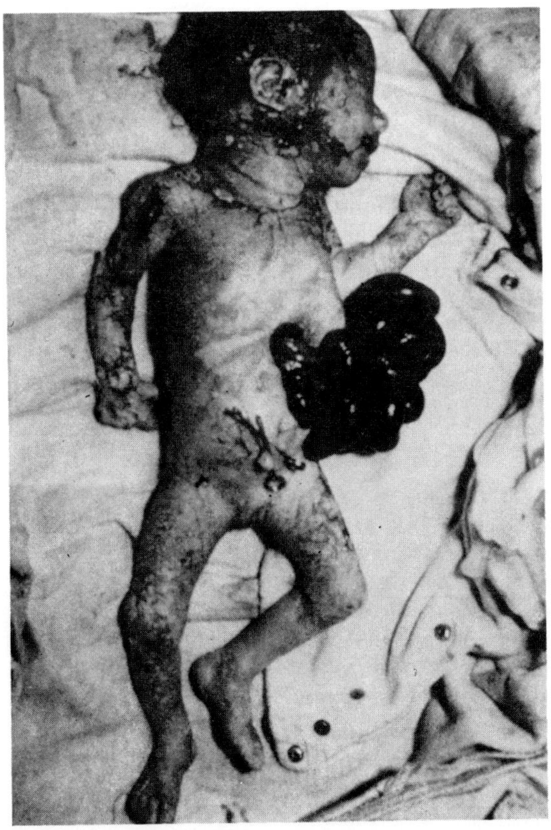

Figure 37–6. Stillborn infant with gastroschisis and midgut volvulus.

rental counseling and maternal transport to specialized centers.[39, 40, 42] Prenatal diagnosis of omphalocele may be particularly important because of the frequent association of chromosomal and congenital anomalies, allowing specialized prenatal or postnatal care or elective termination of pregnancy in certain highly selective cases. Recent reports[39, 43] suggest that sonography may be useful in detecting antenatal volvulus in cases of gastroschisis in which there is a sudden development of bowel distention. There are no known sonographic findings that may predict volvulus or ischemic damage of the bowel. Therefore, weekly sonography of the fetus with gastroschisis in the last trimester and daily sonography in the last few weeks before birth may be indicated.

Postnatally, omphalocele and cord hernias may be distinguished from gastroschisis by the presence of a peritoneal membrane that encompasses the umbilical cord. Hernias of the cord are umbilical defects smaller than 4 cm in diameter that contain only loops of intestine. Omphaloceles are larger than 4 cm in diameter and often contain liver in addition to hollow viscera. Rarely, the omphalocele sac may rupture during delivery, leaving a circumferential residue of peritoneal and amniotic membrane. Sternal cleft, imperforate anus, or exstrophy may be readily appreciated in association with omphalocele. Other associated malformations, such as esophageal atresia and cardiac, renal, and upper urinary tract anomalies, should be excluded by expeditious diagnostic studies, including chest radiograph with nasogastric intubation, echocardiography, and abdominal sonography. Finally, other findings, such as hypotonia, low-set ears, weak cry, microphthalmia, and micrognathia, may suggest associated chromosome abnormalities.

Gastroschisis may be recognized as an extra-abdominal defect that is usually separated from the cord by a bridge of skin. The defect usually lies to the right of the umbilical cord and is never enclosed by a sac. The intestine is usually herniated without liver and is markedly thickened, adherent, and covered by a dense, fibrous peel. Because of the relative absence of associated extra-abdominal anomalies, routine ancillary radiologic studies are rarely required.

TREATMENT

Although it is generally agreed that the route of delivery has little effect on the morbidity and the survival in infants with either omphalocele or gastroschisis,[43–45] it has been suggested that the timing of delivery may have an impact on the outcome of infants with gastroschisis. Fitzsimmon and associates[46] have advocated elective cesarean delivery of infants with gastroschisis at 36 weeks of gestation to reduce the fibrous peel and to facilitate primary closure. Using this approach, they achieved primary closure in more than 90% of infants with gastroschisis, with a markedly reduced hospital stay. On the other hand, Crabbe and colleagues[47] and Roberts and Burge[40] could find no correlation between gestational age at delivery and outcome. Thus, elective cesarean delivery currently cannot be recommended for either gastroschisis or omphalocele, unless sonographic evidence of sudden bowel distention indicates an antenatal volvulus.

The postnatal management of abdominal wall defects begins in the delivery room with placement of a nasogastric sump tube that is put on low, continuous suction or is aspirated every 15 minutes. With gastroschisis or ruptured omphalocele it is crucial to recognize torsion of the bowel, indicated by a bluish discoloration of the bowel or mesenteric twist, that might have occurred during the delivery process. Every effort must be made to ensure proper positioning and support of the bowel prior to transport to prevent vascular compromise. The exposed bowel or membrane should be wrapped in a warm, sterile dressing that may be soaked with 0.25% povidone-iodine or neomycin solution and covered with a plastic film or bowel bag to prevent hypothermia and evaporative fluid loss. Intravenous access should be obtained through an upper extremity, and an initial infusion of 10 to 20 ml per kg of a balanced salt solution (e.g., 10% dextrose with 0.45% sodium chloride) should be given in addition to broad-spectrum antibiotics. Oxygen supplementation and mechanical ventilation should be instituted as indicated, and the infant placed in a neutral thermal environment. Hypothermia and relative dehydration leading to metabolic acidosis are preventable yet have been reported in as many as 40% of infants with gastroschisis transported to major referral centers.[48, 49] Metabolic disturbances in this setting are potentially hazardous and should be corrected prior to surgical repair.

The surgical treatment of abdominal wall defects must be individualized based on the type of defect and the size of the defect as well as the presence of associated anomalies. Omphalocele and gastroschisis differ markedly in terms of their pathophysiology; however, both conditions involve a relative loss of intestinal domain within the abdominal cavity. Thus, depending on the size of the defect, the repair of both conditions may create potential diaphragmatic and caval compressions. Other anomalies, such as intestinal atresia associated with gastroschisis and VACTERL* abnormalities associated with omphalocele, may further complicate the treatment of these defects.

The ideal surgical repair of abdominal wall defects is primary closure without compromise of the infant's respiratory status, venous return, and intestinal blood supply.[50–52] This repair may be accomplished easily with smaller defects and is greatly facilitated by the use of paralytics, such as pancuronium bromide, mechanical stretching of the abdominal wall, and, particularly for gastroschisis, the use of preoperative irrigations via a rectal tube using warm saline or 1% acetylcystine to loosen and remove viscid, impacted meconium. Overall, primary surgical repair may be accomplished in 30 to 90% of patients[53–55] and is more frequently reported with gastroschisis than with omphalocele. Of course, the major limiting factor is increased abdominal pressure potentially leading to cardiopulmonary compromise and multisystem organ failure. When attempts at primary closure cause undue pressure, other measures must be taken to achieve closure of the abdominal wall. Moreover, following abdominal closure, persistent acidosis and general deterioration should raise the suspicion of necrotic bowel that may result from excessive intra-abdominal pressure.[56]

Many experimental studies have been conducted to demonstrate the effect of increased intra-abdominal pressure on general and regional blood flow. Lynch and associates[57] demonstrated that acute elevations in intra-abdominal pressure to a level higher than 20 mm Hg resulted in significant decreases in blood pressure and cardiac output. Masey and coworkers[58] found a 20 to 40% reduction in renal and gastrointestinal blood flow following acute elevations in intra-abdominal pressure higher than 15 to 20 mm Hg in newborn lambs. Harmon and colleagues[59] demonstrated in dogs that renal blood flow remains depressed with acute elevations in intra-abdominal pressure higher than 20 mm Hg despite normalization of cardiac output using volume expanders.

Prospective clinical studies have shown that elevated intra-abdominal pressure resulting from primary closure of abdominal wall defects leads predictably to clinical deterioration. Yaster and associates[60] reported oliguria and poor peripheral perfusion requiring reoperation in 4 of 11 infants who developed intragastric pressures higher than 20 mm Hg with primary closure of the abdominal wall. In a subsequent study, the same group[61] found no postoperative complications related to increased intra-abdominal pressure when intragastric pressure was monitored during a trial of fascial closure, and a prosthetic pouch was placed on any infant who experienced an intragastric pressure higher than 20 mm Hg. Intragastric pressure monitoring has been used since it was first suggested by Wesley and coworkers[62] in 1981; however, there is more recent evidence that vesical and inferior vena caval pressures are more closely correlated with intra-abdominal pressure than is intragastric pressure.[63] Finally, inspiratory pressure may not always correlate with intra-abdominal pressure, specifically in the presence of pulmonary hypoplasia[64] or hyaline membrane disease. Nevertheless, an increase in inspiratory pressure higher than 30 mm Hg may frequently indicate an elevation in intra-abdominal pressure higher than 20 mm Hg.

When an elevation in intra-abdominal pressure higher than 20 mm Hg prevents primary fascial closure, staged closure using skin flaps or a temporary Silastic pouch is generally advocated. In 1980 Fonkalsrud[65] reported a 94% survival rate using extensive skin flaps in infants with gastroschisis and coincident large disparity in size between eviscerated intestine and the abdominal cavity. Skin closure is generally followed by second-stage repair of the large ventral hernia at 6 to 12 months. When skin closure is used for omphalocele, the amniotic membrane may be left intact to facilitate closure and return of normal bowel function.

The major difficulty with skin flap repair is that second-stage closure may result in ventilatory failure requiring mechanical support or bowel dysfunction re-

*Abnormalities of the *v*ertebrae, *a*nus, *c*ardiovascular system, *t*rachea, *e*sophagus, *r*enal system, and *l*imb.

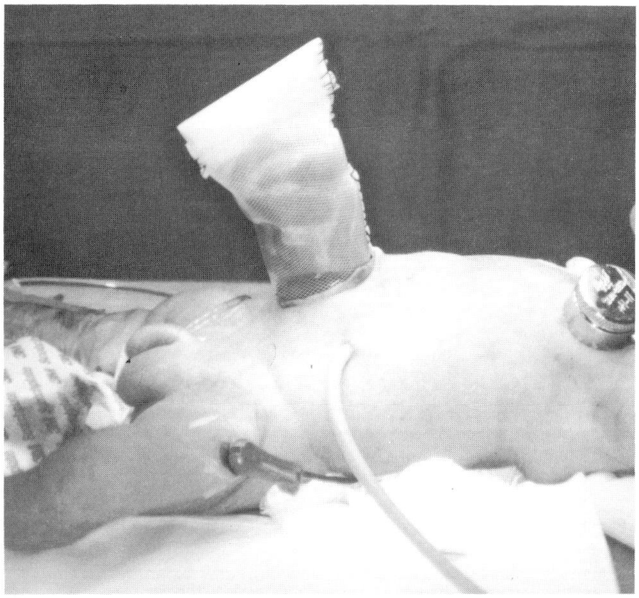

Figure 37–7. Silastic pouch allows delayed closure of giant omphalocele and gastroschisis without caval or diaphragmatic compression.

quiring prolonged hyperalimentation. Alternatively, reinforced Silastic sheeting (0.2–1 mm thickness) may be sutured to both sides of the fascial defect and to itself, forming a pouch (Fig. 37–7). It is important that the pouch has parallel sides to function properly, and this is usually accomplished by enlarging the fascial defect.

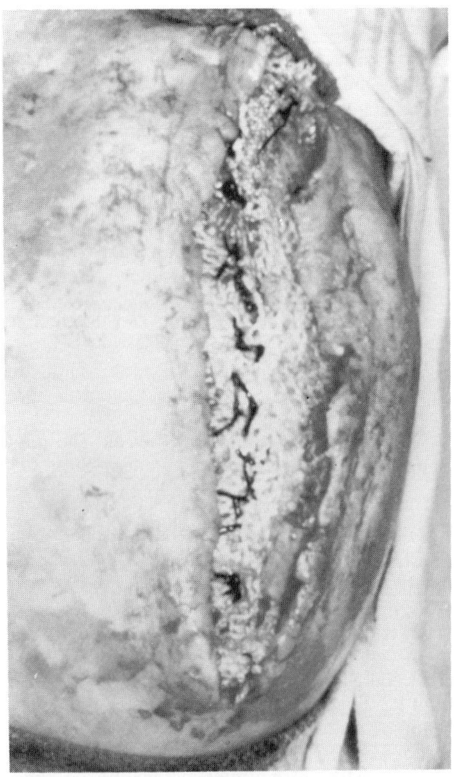

Figure 37–8. Last stage of Silastic pouch closure showing frequent occurrence of wound sepsis.

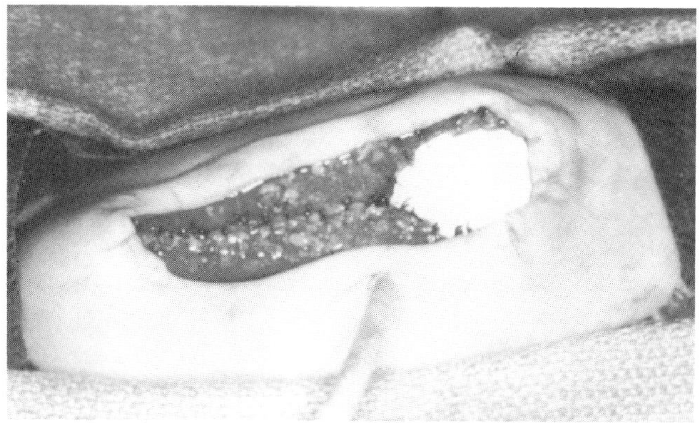

Figure 37–9. Primary fascial closure of giant omphalocele with Gore-Tex patch repair of epigastric component.

The pouch is covered with povidone-iodine ointment and dry gauze, and at least once daily the contents of the pouch are manually reduced and held in place with a row of sutures. Ideally, complete reduction of the eviscerated contents is accomplished and the fascia closed within 1 week. As with skin closure of omphalocele, the pouch may be applied over an intact amnion to reduce the duration of ileus following fascial closure.[66]

Closure of the pouch with reduction of the eviscerated bowel may often require more than 1 week and is associated with an increased incidence of sepsis and intestinal necrosis (Fig. 37–8).[67] Thus, although both Silastic pouch and skin flaps may be used to repair abdominal wall defects with severe visceroabdominal disproportion, both techniques may incur serious problems. Another technique first advocated by Stone[68] is an immediate primary repair using a prosthetic patch to keep intra-abdominal pressure less than 20 mm Hg. Gore-Tex is particularly useful, since it is incorporated into tissue and need not be removed. This technique has been used by the author in five cases of gastroschisis or giant omphalocele with severe visceroabdominal disproportion (Fig. 37–9). Overall, cosmetic and functional results have been excellent, and complete enteral feedings have been established within a mean of 2 weeks following repair.[69]

Intestinal dysfunction or ileus may occur for variable periods following repair of abdominal wall defects using any technique previously described. The infants who are most likely to have prolonged ileus are those with ischemic compromise of the intestine or gastroschisis with severely thickened peel or atresia. Many studies have shown a reduction in the length of postoperative ileus when primary closure is used[17, 34, 55] compared with staged closure using skin flaps or pouch; however, these results may reflect the selection of patients with less severe visceroabdominal disproportion. When prolonged ileus is anticipated, central venous access is generally achieved during the first operative procedure. Central venous hyperalimentation has been particularly useful when gastroschisis is associated with intestinal atresia. In such instances, the atretic bowel may be returned to the abdomen and repaired in a delayed fashion,[70] temporarily exteriorized,[71] or anastomosed primarily when a proximal segment of intestine is involved,[72] depending on the surgeon's judgment. Central hyperalimentation makes possible any of these options, with a reasonable expectation of success.

RESULTS

The survival rate of infants with abdominal wall defects has steadily increased, boosted by the advent of the Silastic pouch, hyperalimentation, and high-frequency, pressure-regulated ventilators. Following the introduction of skin flaps by Gross[12] in 1948 for large omphalocele with severe visceroabdominal disproportion, overall survival barely approached 40%. Currently, survival of infants with omphalocele ranges between 70 and 85%.[18, 23, 55] Complications of omphalocele closure depend on the method of repair used. Common complications following omphalocele closure include wound sepsis associated with the Silastic pouch repair and ischemic bowel caused by overzealous primary fascial closure. However, these complications are only a minor cause of mortality compared with associated cardiac and chromosomal anomalies, which are the principal cause of death in infants with omphalocele. Other malformations associated with omphalocele that lead to high mortality are diaphragmatic hernia with or without Cantrell's pentalogy and cloacal exstrophy.[73]

Prematurity occurs in approximately 25% of infants with omphalocele and is significantly correlated with increased mortality. However, a large proportion of premature or low-birth-weight infants with omphalocele have other life-threatening anomalies that account for the observed increase in mortality. Thus, prematurity is a less important risk factor in omphalocele than are associated anomalies. The size of the omphalocele defect is also a relatively minor risk factor, one that has more impact on morbidity than mortality in infants with omphalocele who had either a large defect or herniation of the liver.

In contrast, the current mortality of gastroschisis is approximately 10%. Gastroschisis is associated with a lower incidence of associated malformations than is omphalocele, with jejunoileal and colonic atresia accounting for most of the associated anomalies. Prematurity or low-birth-weight occurs in approximately 60% of infants with gastroschisis[18, 73] but does not correlate with increased mortality. As with omphalocele, the size of the defect is not an important factor in survival. On the other hand, intestinal complications related to closure of the defect are the most important cause of death. Volvulus, intestinal necrosis, and fistula have been encountered with the use of both Silastic pouch and primary fascial closure. Long-term intestinal dysfunction requiring total parenteral nutrition is more likely following Silastic pouch rather than primary fascial closure of gastroschisis. Hyperalimentation-associated intrahepatic cholestasis and cirrhosis, although uncommon, are therefore more likely to occur following Silastic pouch closure than following primary fascial closure.

REFERENCES

1. Baird PA, MacDonald EC: An epidemiologic study of congenital malformation of the anterior abdominal wall in more than half a million consecutive live births. Am J Hum Genet 1981; 33:470–478.
2. Rangarathnam CS, Lal RB, Swenson O: Gastroschisis. Arch Surg 1969; 98:742–748.
3. Ballantyne JW: Manual of Antenatal Pathology and Hygiene: The Embryo. Edinburgh, 1904.
4. Pare A: The Works of That Famous Chirurgeon. *In* Cotes TH, Young R, eds: London, Book 24. 1634, p 59.
5. Bernstein P: Gastroschisis: A rare teratologic condition in the newborn. Arch Pediatr 1940; 505:13.
6. Moore TC, Stokes GE: Gastroschisis: Report of two cases treated by a modification of the gross operation for omphalocele. Surgery 1953; 33:112.
7. Duhamel B: Embryology of exomphalos and allied malformations. Arch Dis Child 1963; 33:142.
8. Shaw A: The myth of gastroschisis. J Pediatr Surg 1975; 10:235.
9. DeVries PA: The pathogenesis of gastroschisis and omphalocele. J Pediatr Surg 1980; 15:245–251.
10. Hey W: Practical Observations in Surgery. London, Cadell and Davies, 1803, p 266.
11. Ahlfeld F: Alkohol bei der behandlung inoperabiler Brauchbruchen. Monatsschr Geburtshilfe Gynakol 1899; 10:124.
12. Gross RE: A new method for surgical treatment of large omphaloceles. Surgery 1948; 24:277.
13. Schuster SR: A new method for the stage repair of large omphaloceles. Surg Gynecol Obstet 1967; 125:837.
14. Allen RG, Wrenn EL Jr: Silon as a sac in the treatment of omphalocele and gastroschisis. J Pediatr Surg 1969; 4:3–8.
15. Wilmore DW, Groff DB, Bishop HC, et al: Total parenteral nutrition in infants with catastrophic gastrointestinal anomalies. J Pediatr Surg 1969; 4:189–199.
16. Schwaitzberg SD, Pokorny WJ, McGill CW, et al: Gastroschisis and omphalocele. Am J Surg 1982; 144:650–654.
17. Mayer T, Black R, Matlack ME, et al: Gastroschisis and omphalocele. Ann Surg 1980; 192:783–787.
18. Raffensperger JG, Jona JZ: Gastroschisis. Surg Gynecol Obstet 1974; 138:230–234.
19. Watkins DE: Gastroschisis. Va Med Month 1943; 78:42.
20. Knight PJ, Sommer A, Clatworthy HW: Omphalocele: A prognostic classification. J Pediatr Surg 1981; 16:599–604.
21. Havalad S, Noblett H, Speidel BD: Familial occurrence of omphalocele suggesting sex-linked inheritance. Arch Dis Child 1979; 54:142–151.
22. Gray SW, Skandalakis JE: Embryology for Surgeons. Philadelphia, WB Saunders, 1972.
23. Hoyme HE, Higginbottom MC, Jones KL: The vascular pathogenesis of gastroschisis: Intrauterine interruption of the omphalomesenteric artery. J Pediatr 1981; 98:228–231.
24. Tibboel D, Raine P, McNee M, et al: Developmental aspects of gastroschisis. J Pediatr Surg 1986; 21:865–869.
25. Tibboel D, Vermey-Keers C, Kluck P, et al: The natural history of gastroschisis during fetal life: Development of fibrous coating on bowel loops. Teratology 1986; 33:267–272.
26. Glick PG, Harrison MR, Adzick NS, et al: The missing link in the pathogenesis of gastroschisis. J Pediatr Surg 1985; 20:406–409.
27. Kluck P, Tibboel D, Van Der Kamp AMW, et al: The effect of fetal urine on the development of the bowel in gastroschisis. J Pediatr Surg 1983; 18:47–50.
28. Eskestka B: Amniotic Fluid. Amsterdam, Elsevier North-Holland, 1978, pp 35–36.
29. Tibboel D, Kluck P, Van Der Camp AMW, et al: The development of the characteristic anomalies found in gastroschisis: Experimental and clinical data. Z Kinderchir 1985; 40:355–360.
30. Touloukin RJ, Spackman TJ: Gastrointestinal function and radiographic appearance following gastroschisis repair. J Pediatr Surg 1971; 6:423–434.
31. O'Neill JA Jr, Grosfeld JL: Intestinal malfunction after antenatal exposure of viscera. Am J Surg 1974; 127:129–132.
32. Amoury RA, Beatty EC, Wood WG, et al: Histology of the

intestine in human gastroschisis—relationship to intestinal malfunction: Dissolution of the "peel" and its ultrastructural characteristics. J Pediatr Surg 1988; 23:950–956.
33. Shah R, Woolley MM: Gastroschisis and intestinal atresia. J Pediatr Surg 1991; 26:788–790.
34. Mayer T, Black R, Matlak ME, et al: Gastroschisis and omphalocele: An 8-year review. Ann Surg 1980; 192:783–787.
35. Santulli TV, Blank WA: Congenital atresia of the intestine: Pathogenesis and treatment. Ann Surg 1961; 154:939–948.
36. Tibboel D, Van Der Kamp AMW, Molenaar JC: The effect of experimentally induced intestinal perforation at an early developmental stage. J Pediatr Surg 1981; 16:1017–1020.
37. Pokorny WJ, Harberg FJ, McGill CW: Gastroschisis complicated by intestinal atresia. J Pediatr Surg 1981; 16:261–263.
38. Amoury RA, Ashkraft KW, Holder TM: Gastroschisis complicated by intestinal atresia. Surgery 1977; 82:373–381.
39. Bond SJ, Harrison MR, Philly RA, et al: Severity of intestinal damage in gastroschisis: Correlation with prenatal sonographic findings. J Pediatr Surg 1988; 23:520–525.
40. Roberts J, Burge DM: Antenatal diagnosis of abdominal wall defects: A missed opportunity? Arch Dis Child 1990; 20:687–689.
41. Sermer M, Benzie RJ, Pitson L, et al: Prenatal diagnosis and management of congenital defects of the anterior abdominal wall. Am J Obstet Gynecol 1987; 156:308–312.
42. Harris BA Jr, Wirtschafter DD, Huddleston JF, et al: In utero versus neonatal transportation of high-risk perinates: A comparison. Obstet Gynecol 1981; 57:496–499.
43. Bethel CAI, Seashore JH, Touloukian RJ: Caesarean section does not improve outcome in gastroschisis. J Pediatr Surg 1989; 24:1–4.
44. Kirk EP, Wahr M: Obstetric management of the fetus with omphalocele or gastroschisis: A review and report of 112 cases. Am J Obstet Gynceol 1983; 146:512–516.
45. Hasan S, Hermansen MC: The prenatal diagnosis of ventral abdominal wall defects. Am J Obstet Gynecol 1986; 155:842–845.
46. Fitzsimmon SJ, Nyberg DA, Dale RC, et al: Prenatal management of gastroschisis. Obstet Gynecol 1988; 71:910–913.
47. Crabbe DCG, Thomas DFM, Beck T, et al: Prenatally diagnosed gastroschisis: A case for preterm delivery? Pediatr Surg Int 1991; 6:108–110.
48. Muragi T, Tsugawa C, Nishijima E, et al: Gastroschisis: A 17-year experience. J Pediatr Surg 1989; 24:343–345.
49. King DR, Savrin R, Boles ET: Gastroschisis update. J Pediatr Surg 1980; 15:553–557.
50. Schuster SR: Omphalocele and gastroschisis. *In* Welch KJ, Randolph JG, Ravitch MM, et al, eds: Pediatric Surgery. 2nd ed. Chicago, Yearbook Medical Publishers, 1986; pp 740–763.
51. Swartz KR, Harrison MW, Campbell TJ, et al: Selective management of gastroschisis. Ann Surg 1986; 203:214–218.
52. Campbell TJ, Campbell JR, Harrison MW: Selective management of omphalocele. Am J Surg 1982; 143:572–574.
53. Schwartz MZ, Tyson KR, Milliorn K, et al: Staged reduction using Silastic sac is the treatment of choice for large congenital abdominal wall defects. J Pediatr Surg 1983; 18:713–719.
54. Luck SR, Sherman JO, Raffensperger JG, et al: Gastroschisis in 106 consecutive newborn patients. Surgery 1985; 98:677–683.
55. Canty TG, Collins DL: Primary fascial closure in infants with gastroschisis and omphalocele: A superior approach. J Pediatr Surg 1983; 18:707–712.
56. Ein SH, Superina R, Bagwell C, et al: Ischemic bowel after primary closure for gastroschisis. J Pediatr Surg 1988; 23:728–730.
57. Lynch FP, Ochi T, Scully JM, et al: Cardiovascular effects of increased intra-abdominal pressure in newborn piglets. J Pediatr Surg 1974; 9:621–626.
58. Masey SA, Koehler RC, Buck JR, et al: Effect of abdominal distention on central and regional hemodynamics in neonatal lambs. Pediatr Res 1985; 19:1244–1249.
59. Harmon PK, Kraw IL, McLachlan HD, et al: Elevated intra-abdominal pressure and renal function. Ann Surg 1982; 196:594–597.
60. Yaster M, Buck JR, Dudgeon DL, et al: Hemodynamic effects of primary closure of omphalocele/gastroschisis in human newborns. Anesthesiology 1988; 69:84–88.
61. Yaster M, Scherer TLR, Stone MM, et al: Prediction of successful primary closure of congenital abdominal wall defects using intraoperative measurements. J Pediatr Surg 1989; 24:1217–1220.
62. Wesley J, Drongowski R, Coran AG: Intragastric pressure measurement: A guide for reduction and closure of the Silastic chimney in omphalocele and gastroschisis. J Pediatr Surg 1981; 16:28–30.
63. Lacey SR, Bruce J, Brooks SP, et al: The relative merits of various methods of indirect measurement of intra-abdominal pressure as a guide to closure of abdominal wall defects. J Pediatr Surg 1987; 22:1207–1211.
64. Hershenson MB, Brouillett RT, Clemka L, et al: Respiratory insufficiency in newborns with abdominal wall defects. J Pediatr Surg 1985; 20:348–353.
65. Fonkalsrud EW: Selective repair of neonatal gastroschisis based on degree of visceroabdominal disproportion. Ann Surg 1980; 191:139–144.
66. DeLorimier AA, Adzick NS, Harrison MR: Amnion inversion in the treatment of giant omphalocele. J Pediatr Surg 1991; 26:804–807.
67. Ein SH, Rubin SZ: Gastroschisis: Primary closure or Silon pouch. J Pediatr Surg 1980; 15:549–552.
68. Stone HH: Immediate permanent fascial prosthesis for gastroschisis and massive omphalocele. Surg Gynecol Obstet 1982; 153:221–224.
69. Alexander F: Immediate repair of giant omphalocele and gastroschisis with Gore-Tex patch. (Submitted).
70. Shaw R, Wolley MM: Gastroschisis and intestinal atresia. J Pediatr Surg 1991; 26:788–790.
71. Pokorny WJ, Harbert FJ, McGill CW: Gastroschisis complicated by intestinal atresia. J Pediatr Surg 1981; 16:261–263.
72. Gornall P: Management of intestinal atresia complicating gastroschisis. J Pediatr Surg 1989; 24:522–524.
73. Stringel G, Filler RM: Prognostic factors in omphalocele and gastroschisis. J Pediatr Surg 1979; 14:515–519.

Chapter 38

Maldigestion and Malabsorption

STEVEN H. ERDMAN and JOHN N. UDALL, JR.

The gastrointestinal tract receives ingested nutrients, digests them, and absorbs the simple constituents. Normal intestinal digestion and absorption can be divided into sequential stages: (1) luminal hydrolysis and solubilization, (2) hydrolysis at the enterocyte membrane, (3) absorption across the enterocyte membrane and cellular processing, and (4) uptake from the enterocyte into blood and lymph. In the luminal stage, proteins, carbohydrates, and lipids are hydrolyzed by enzymes released from salivary glands, the stomach, and the pancreas. Bile from the liver helps this process by creating a solubilizing organic environment in which lipids can be digested. Digestion continues at the level of the intestinal cell membrane, where hydrolysis of peptides and disaccharides by brush border enzymes takes place. This is followed by the cellular absorption of amino acids, small peptides, monosaccharides, monoglycerides, and fatty acids. Once inside the enterocyte, nutrients are processed. (It should be noted that water and small molecules may also be absorbed by a paracellular route.) Absorbed nutrients are then transported into blood and lymph and carried into distant organs for storage or metabolism. Diseases that interrupt any of these stages may lead to inefficient digestion and absorption.

PATHOPHYSIOLOGIC MECHANISMS

A list of maldigestive and malabsorptive disorders is shown in Table 38–1. They are reviewed in this chapter, and an approach to diagnosis and management of these disorders is presented.

Digestion in the Lumen

Mouth

Although there are obvious differences between the mouth and the rest of the gastrointestinal tract, there are similarities in terms of exocrine secretion.[1] The exocrine secretion present in the mouth, the saliva, is important for normal digestion. Three pairs of salivary glands help in elaborating the fluid: the parotid, submandibular, and sublingual glands. The contribution of these three glands to the total amount of saliva is 20, 60, and 20%, respectively.[2] Numerous smaller glands are localized in the lips, palate, tongue, and cheeks; these glands also contribute to the exocrine fluid. Saliva contains amylase and lipase; both hydrolytic enzymes are important to digestion. The amylase is almost entirely derived from the parotid glands. Lingual lipase is secreted by the serous glands (von Ebner) under the circumvallate papillae of the tongue. Also present in the saliva is a carrier protein for vitamin B_{12}. This carrier protein, or haptocorrin, is known as R binder protein.[3]

One disease that may have an unexpected effect on digestion in the mouth is cystic fibrosis (CF). Cystic fibrosis is now recognized to be a generalized abnormality of the exocrine glands of the body secondary to a dysfunctional cystic fibrosis transmembrane conductance regulator protein[4] (see Chapter 66). In CF the submandibular glands may enlarge, with an associated reduction in salivary fluid volume. However, parotid glands and amylase production seem less affected.[1] Studies of lingual lipase in CF patients suggest that salivary lipase activity is higher in these patients than in controls. This results in an increased intragastric lipolysis of a triglyceride test meal.[5] It is also of interest that in Sjögren's syndrome there is little or no saliva, yet maldigestion does not seem to be a feature of this disease.[6]

Stomach

The stomach is essential for normal digestion. Gastric acid, pepsinogen, lipase, and intrinsic factor produced by the gastric mucosa all participate in the intraluminal stage of digestion. The production of hydrochloric acid by parietal cells is important, since a low pH facilitates the conversion of pepsinogen to pepsin.[2] Gastric lipase, produced by chief cells of the fundus, is necessary for complete digestion of the fat present in human milk.[7, 8] In addition, intrinsic factor, a protein elaborated by the gastric mucosa, binds vitamin B_{12} in the duodenum after it is released from an R binder. Vitamin B_{12} bound to intrinsic factor is protected from luminal hydrolysis.[3, 9, 10]

When acid production of the stomach is decreased

Table 38–1. GASTROINTESTINAL DISEASES ASSOCIATED WITH MALDIGESTION AND MALABSORPTION

Disease/Condition	Pathophysiology
	Intraluminal Digestion
Stomach	
Protein-calorie malnutrition	Decreased acid production, hypochlorhydria[11, 12]
Zollinger-Ellison syndrome	Inactivation of pancreatic enzymes at a low duodenal pH, and decreased ionization of conjugated bile salts[14]
Pernicious anemia	Decreased intrinsic factor secretion, vitamin B_{12} malabsorption
Dumping syndrome	Rapid emptying of stomach contents into the small intestine, dilution of enzymes[17–19]
Pancreas	
Cystic fibrosis	Impaired secretion of enzymes and bicarbonate
Shwachman-Diamond syndrome	Impaired secretion of enzymes
Acute/chronic pancreatitis	Impaired secretion of enzymes and bicarbonate
Protein-calorie malnutrition	Impaired secretion of enzymes[93]
Trypsinogen deficiency	Impaired secretion of enzyme[20–22]
Lipase deficiency	Impaired secretion of enzyme[24]
Amylase deficiency	Impaired secretion of enzyme[25, 26]
Liver	
Cholestasis syndromes	Impaired secretion of bile salts with deficient micelle formation (see Tables 38–2 and 38–3)
Ileal disease or surgery	Intestinal malabsorption of bile salts, deficient bile salt pool
Intestine	
Enterokinase deficiency	Impaired activation of luminal pancreatic enzymes[27, 28]
Protein-calorie malnutrition	Bacterial overgrowth with consumption of nutrients, toxin production, and deconjugation of bile acids[29–32]
Anatomic duplication	Bacterial overgrowth with consumption of nutrients; altered mucosal blood flow[33]
Blind loop syndrome	
Short bowel syndrome	
Pseudo-obstruction	
	Digestion at the Enterocyte Membrane
Congenital disaccharidase deficiency	Impaired digestion of a specific disaccharide leading to bacterial fermentation in the colon
Lactase[35–39]	
Sucrase-isomaltase[41–45]	
Trehalase[47]	
Acquired/late-onset disaccharidase deficieny	Loss of enzyme activity due to mucosal injury or loss of activity with age
Lactase	
Sucrase-isomaltase	
Glucoamylase[46]	
	Enterocyte Absorption
Protein-calorie malnutrition	"Damage" vs. "adaptive regulation," altered mucosal architecture[93]
Hartnup's disease	Transport defect of neutral amino acids[48–50]
Lysinuric protein intolerance	Transport defect of dibasic amino acids in intestine and kidney[48, 51, 52]
Blue diaper syndrome	Isolated transport defect of tryptophan[48, 54]
Oast-house syndrome	Isolated transport defect of methionine in intestine and kidney[55, 56]
Lowe's syndrome	X-linked trait with defect in transport of lysine and arginine[57]
Glucose-galactose malabsorption	Selective defect in glucose and galactose sodium cotransport system[58–63]
Congenital chloride diarrhea	Selective defect in chloride transport by the intestine[124–126]
Abetalipoproteinemia	Absent production of apolipoprotein B, lipoproteins, and chylomicrons absent[64]
Hypobetalipoproteinemia	Impaired production of apolipoprotein B[48]
Celiac disease	Damage to absorptive/digestive surface
Short bowel syndrome	Loss of absorptive/digestive surface, abnormal transit
Mucosal injury syndromes	Damage to digestive/absorptive surface
Milk/soy protein intolerance	
Postenteritis syndrome	
Tropical sprue	Damage to digestive/absorptive surface
Whipple's disease	Lymphatic obstruction, impaired lipid transport(?), patchy enteropathy
Bacterial infection	Damage to digestive/absorptive surface, abnormal motility
Shigella	
Salmonella	
Campylobacter	
Cholera	Secretory water and electrolyte loss
Giardiasis	Disruption of epithelial function secondary to adhesion or toxin(?)
Crohn's disease/regional enteritis	Damage to digestive/absorptive surface, chronic gastrointestinal blood loss
Acrodermatitis enteropathica	Impaired absorption of zinc

Table continued on following page

Table 38–1. GASTROINTESTINAL DISEASES ASSOCIATED WITH MALDIGESTION AND MALABSORPTION *Continued*

Disease/Condition	Pathophysiology
	Uptake into Blood and Lymph
Congestive heart failure	Venous distention, bowel wall edema[65]
Intestinal lymphangiectasia	Obstructed lymphatic transport of lipid and fat-soluble vitamins, intestinal protein loss[66–70]
Intestinal lymphoma	Obstructed lymphatic transport of lipid and fat-soluble vitamins
Carcinoid syndrome	Obstructed lymphatic transport of lipid and fat-soluble vitamins
	Miscellaneous Disorders
Immune deficiency syndromes	Altered bacterial flora
Allergic gastroenteropathy	Unknown immune mechanism
Eosinophilic gastroenteropathy	Unknown immune mechanism
Drugs	
Methotrexate	Damage to mucosal surface by interfering with enterocyte replication
Cholestyramine	Blocked reabsorption of bile salts in the ileum by drug; malabsorption of calcium, fat, bile acids, and fat-soluble vitamins
Phenytoin	Calcium, folic acid malabsorption
Sulfasalazine	Folic acid malabsorption
H_2 receptor antagonists	Impair the acid/proteolytic liberation of vitamin B_{12}

due to malnutrition,[11, 12] disease,[13] or medication, the conversion of pepsinogen to pepsin is retarded. With decreased levels of pepsin, protein digestion may be compromised. The production of excessive quantities of acid, as occurs in Zollinger-Ellison syndrome, depresses the luminal pH in the duodenum and thus inactivates hydrolytic enzymes of the pancreas important for digestion.[14]

Pernicious anemia is a chronic disease characterized by the absence of intrinsic factor. Normally, vitamin B_{12} binds stoichiometrically with intrinsic factor. The intrinsic factor–B_{12} complex is resistant to digestion in the small intestine, and the vitamin is then absorbed by receptor-mediated endocytosis in the ileum.[15, 16] This sequence does not occur when there is no intrinsic

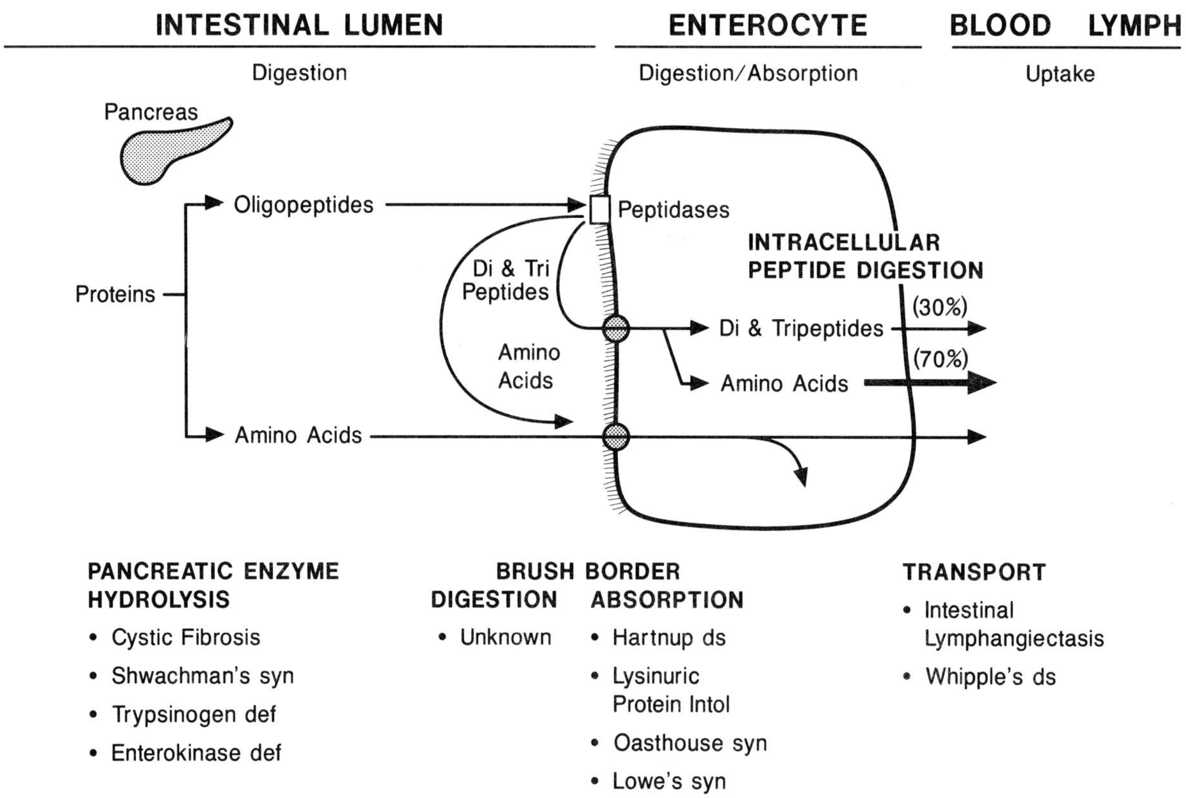

Figure 38–1. Digestion and absorption of dietary proteins. Major events in the digestive and absorptive process are shown with some of the associated disease states that result in the maldigestion and malabsorption of proteins. (Modified from Silverman A, Roy CC: Pediatric Clinical Gastroenterology. 3rd ed. St. Louis, CV Mosby, 1983; with permission.)

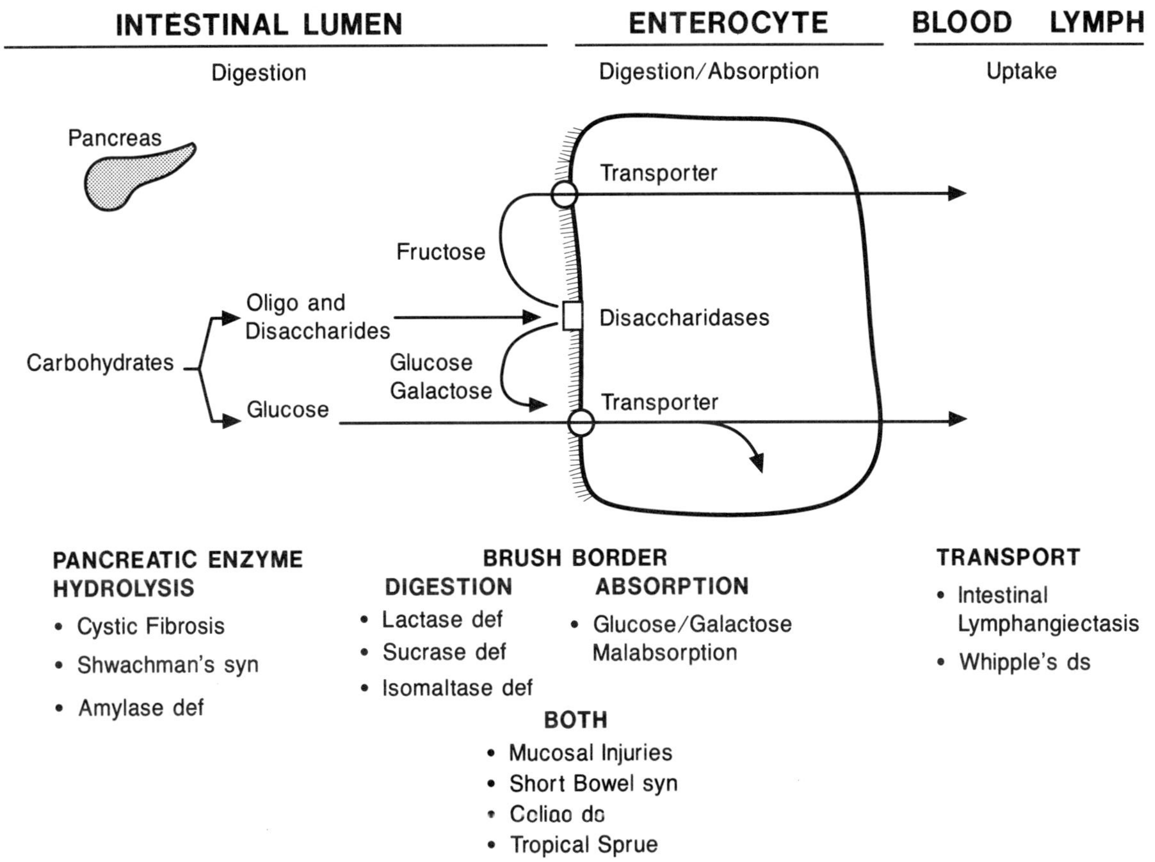

Figure 38–2. Digestion and absorption of dietary carbohydrates. Major events in the digestive and absorptive process are shown with some of the associated disease states that result in the maldigestion and malabsorption of carbohydrates. (Modified from Silverman A, Roy CC: Pediatric Clinical Gastroenterology. 3rd ed. St. Louis, CV Mosby, 1983; with permission.)

factor, as is the case in pernicious anemia. The disease, however, is not common in infancy and childhood.

Hemigastrectomy for peptic ulcer disease may decrease gastric mass and result in the dumping syndrome. Other surgical procedures more common in childhood, such as the Nissen fundoplication, may also result in the dumping syndrome.[17–19] The syndrome is the result of pyloric sphincter malfunction and altered digestion and motility, leading to the rapid emptying of a meal into the duodenum. This results in hyperglycemia, which triggers insulin release. Later, hypoglycemia, pallor, diaphoresis, and diarrhea can develop.

Pancreas

The pancreas is both an exocrine and an endocrine organ. The exocrine portion of the pancreas elaborates pancreatic juice and delivers the fluid to the duodenum. These processes are essential for normal digestion. Pancreatic juice has two functionally important constituents: bicarbonate ions and digestive enzymes. The digestive enzymes play a major role in the digestion of ingested nutrients, i.e., protein (Fig. 38–1), carbohydrates (Fig. 38–2), and lipids. It is of interest that protein and carbohydrate hydrolysis requires only the enzymes of the gastrointestinal tract. However, complete digestion and solubilization of dietary triglycerides require not only colipase-dependent lipase, but also gastric lipase and bile salt–stimulated lipase (Fig. 38–3).[8]

Diseases of the pancreas, such as cystic fibrosis, Shwachman-Diamond syndrome, and acute and chronic pancreatitis, may be associated with a decrease in hydrolytic enzyme secretion, which is important in digestion. A deficiency of pancreatic enzymes also occurs in severe protein-calorie malnutrition. In addition, pancreatic proteases are important for vitamin B_{12} absorption. These enzymes help release vitamin B_{12} from R or binder proteins, allowing the vitamin to bind intrinsic factor.[3, 15, 16] Although there may be a failure to degrade R proteins and free vitamin B_{12} for binding to intrinsic factor in diseases of the pancreas, vitamin B_{12} deficiency is very rare in exocrine pancreatic dysfunction.[3]

Deficiencies of pancreatic trypsinogen, lipase, and amylase have been described. In 1965, Townes reported a six-week-old white male infant with chronic diarrhea, failure to gain weight, hypoproteinemia, and edema. The infant was unable to hydrolyze dietary protein due to a singular deficiency of pancreatic trypsinogen.[20] Morris and Fisher reported a second child with trypsinogen deficiency disease in 1967.[21] Since then, an additional patient has been reported.[22] The diagnosis of trypsinogen deficiency in these three patients was made

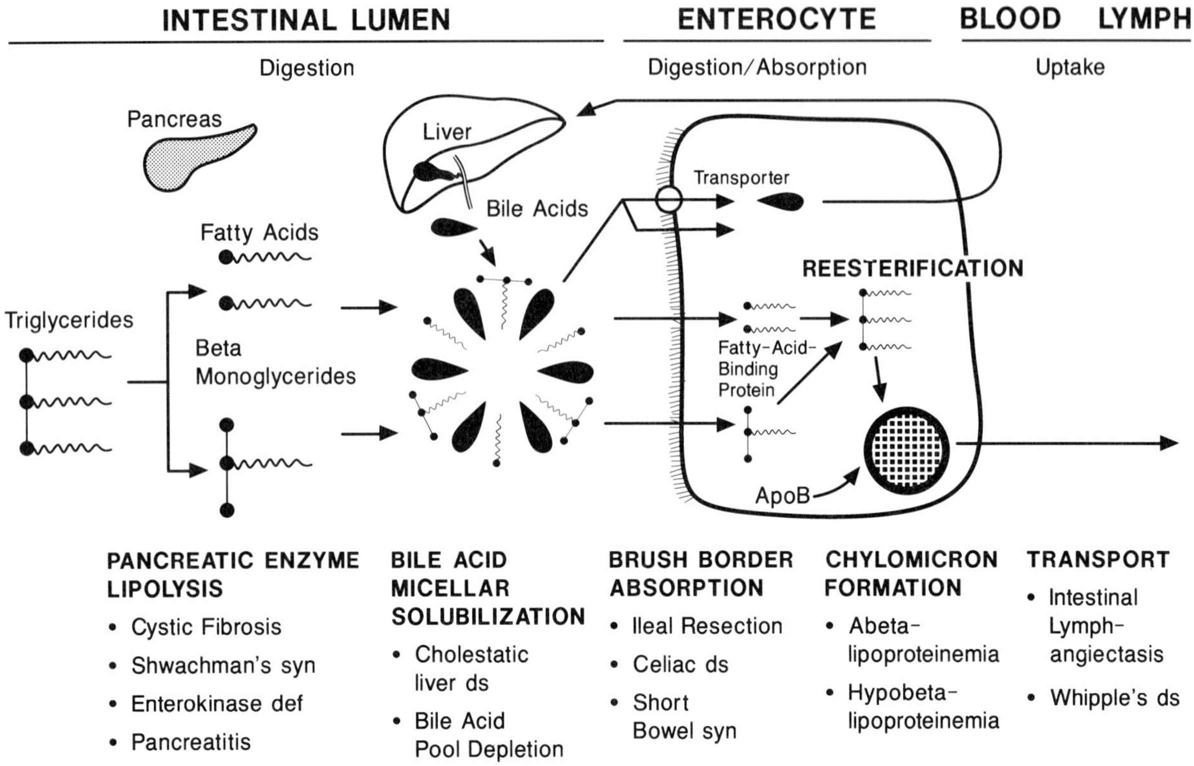

Figure 38–3. Digestion and absorption of dietary triglycerides. Major events in the digestive and absorptive process are shown with some of the associated disease states that result in the maldigestion and malabsorption of triglycerides. (Modified from Silverman A, Roy CC: Pediatric Clinical Gastroenterology. 3rd ed. St. Louis, CV Mosby, 1983, p 250; with permission.)

on the basis of undetectable tryptic activity in duodenal juice. It has been suggested that these three children may have had low trypsin activity on the basis of enteropeptidase (enterokinase) deficiency and not trypsinogen deficiency, since enteropeptidase was not measured in the three reported cases.[23] In 1964, Sheldon described five children with congenital pancreatic lipase deficiency.[24] All five had decreased lipase in duodenal fluid aspirates. He suggested that the deficiency was attributable to an autosomal recessive gene. Pancreatic amylase deficiency has also been described. Lowe and May reported a 13-year-old boy whose duodenal juice showed a persistent absence of amylase with a decreased level of trypsin but a normal amount of lipase.[25] Another case of amylase deficiency was reported by Lilibridge and Townes.[26] They described a two-year-old child who showed poor weight gain on a diet containing starch, despite a more than adequate caloric intake. Weight gain and growth improved when starch was eliminated from the diet and replaced by disaccharides.

Liver

The products of triglyceride hydrolysis, fatty acids and monoglycerides, are solubilized by bile salts to form micelles (see Chapter 2). The fatty acids and monoglycerides are then absorbed in the small intestine. Disorders that interrupt the delivery of bile salts to the small intestine, or interrupt the enterohepatic circulation of bile salts, result in impaired micelle formation and fat maldigestion. These diseases are also usually associated with malabsorption of fat-soluble vitamins (vitamins A, D, E, and K), which can lead to clinical manifestations of vitamin deficiencies. Tables 38–2 and 38–3 list the numerous diseases that can impair hepatic function and result in maldigestion and malabsorption of nutrients.

Small Intestine

Biochemical and anatomic abnormalities of the small intestine may contribute to maldigestion. Congenital enterokinase deficiency is a condition that is associated with decreased amounts of enterokinase in the brush border. The enzyme is necessary for the activation of trypsinogen and other luminal proteases. It was first reported by Hadorn and associates, and its occurrence in siblings supports an autosomal recessive mode of inheritance.[27] Individuals with the disease present with diarrhea, edema, severe growth retardation, and hypoproteinemia. In the Hadorn report, it was noted that the lipase concentration in unstimulated duodenal fluid was normal, but fat was still malabsorbed; this may have been related to failure of activation of pro-colipase to colipase. The specific diagnosis of enterokinase deficiency rests on the addition of exogenous enterokinase to duodenal juice, resulting in generation of normal tryptic activity. Pancreatic enzyme supplementation in children with this deficiency generates normal proteolytic activity in the duodenum, and clinical problems appear to resolve.[28]

Availability of ingested nutrients for absorption may also be compromised by overgrowth of the bowel with bacteria, as occurs in malnutrition,[29–32] the blind loop syndrome,[33] short bowel syndrome, and pseudo-obstruction. In addition, substances present in the diet in high concentrations may bind and inhibit the efficient absorption of certain nutrients, such as the binding of oxalates or fatty acids to calcium and the binding of phytates to iron.

Table 38–2. NEONATAL CHOLESTATIC DISORDERS AT RISK FOR MALABSORPTION

Anatomic
Extrahepatic disorders
  Biliary atresia
  Biliary hypoplasia or duct stenosis
  Sclerosing cholangitis[95]
Mixed extrahepatic/intrahepatic disorders
  Congenital hepatic fibrosis/infantile polycystic disease
  Caroli's disease

Idiopathic
Intrahepatic disorders
  "Idiopathic" neonatal hepatitis
  Arteriohepatic dysplasia—Allagille's syndrome
  Nonsyndromic paucity of intrahepatic bile ducts
  Byler's disease
  Familial benign recurrent cholestasis
  Hereditary cholestasis with lymphedema

Metabolic Diseases Affecting the Hepatocyte
Tyrosinemia
Wolman's disease
Niemann-Pick disease
Gaucher's disease
Galactosemia
Fructosemia
Glycogen storage diseases type III or IV
Alpha-1-antitrypsin deficiency
Cystic fibrosis
Neonatal iron storage disease
Multiple acyl-CoA dehydrogenation deficiency

Inflammatory/Hepatitis
Viral infections
  Cytomegalovirus (CMV)
  Hepatitis B virus
  Hepatitis C virus—suspected[96–98]
  Varicella virus
  Rubella virus
  Herpes virus
Bacterial and parasitic infections
  Tuberculosis
  Listeriosis
  Syphilis
  Toxoplasmosis
Toxin
  Total parenteral nutrition–associated cholestasis
  Sepsis with an infection at a distant site; endotoxin mediated(?)
  Drugs
  Breast milk–secreted drugs[99]

Miscellaneous
Histiocytosis syndromes
Neonatal lupus

Modified from Balistreri WF: Neonatal cholestasis. J Pediatr 1985; 106:171–189.

Table 38–3. CHOLESTATIC DISORDERS IN CHILDREN AND YOUNG ADULTS THAT MAY BE ASSOCIATED WITH MALABSORPTION

Anatomic
Extrahepatic disorders
  Choledochal cyst
  Bile duct stenosis
  Biliary tract neoplasms[102]
  Cholelithiasis with obstruction[103]
  Primary sclerosing cholangitis[104, 105]
Mixed extrahepatic/intrahepatic disorders
  Congenital hepatic fibrosis
  Infantile polycystic disease of liver and/or kidney
  Caroli's disease

Idiopathic
Intrahepatic disorders
  Hepatic tumor[106]
  Familial benign recurrent cholestasis—Summerskill's syndrome
  Hereditary cholestasis with lymphedema—Aagenaes' syndrome
  Arteriohepatic dysplasia—Alagille's syndrome
  Nonsyndromatic paucity of intrahepatic bile ducts
  Indian childhood cirrhosis[107]

Metabolic Diseases Affecting the Hepatocyte
Gaucher's disease
Alpha$_1$-antitrypsin deficiency
Cystic fibrosis
Hepatolenticular degeneration—Wilson's disease[108]
Porphyria[109]

Infectious/Drug Induced
Viral infections
  Cytomegalovirus (CMV)
  Hepatitis B virus
  Chronic active hepatitis
  Hepatitis C virus[110]
  Herpes virus
  Varicella virus
Bacterial and parasitic infections
  Tuberculosis
  Syphilis
  Leptospirosis
  Malaria[111]
Toxin/drug induced
  Parenteral nutrition associated
  Sepsis with an infection at a distant site-endotoxin mediated(?)
  Pregnancy, estrogen, progesterone[112–120]
  Drug

Miscellaneous
Inflammatory bowel disease[121]
Histiocytoses syndromes
Autoimmune liver disease[122]
Graft-vs-host liver disease[123]

Modified and reprinted with permission from Balistreri WF: Semin Liver Dis 1987; 7:1–7, Thieme Medical Publishers, Inc.; and Alagille D, Odievre M: Liver and Biliary Tract Disease in Children. New York, John Wiley & Sons, 1979, pp 163–252. Copyright © 1979, John Wiley & Sons, Inc.

Digestion at the Enterocyte Membrane

A continuous sheet of epithelial cells (enterocytes) covers the surfaces of the villi and crypts. Other cells are interspersed in this epithelial carpet, including goblet cells, endocrine cells, intraepithelial lymphocytes, paneth cells, caveolated cells, and mucous cells.[2] Some of the cell types are common to both villous and crypt epithelium, and others are exclusively found in either the villous region or the crypt region.

At the surface of the epithelium, aminopeptidases present in the brush border hydrolyze most, but not all, of the remaining oligo- and dipeptides produced by luminal digestion of proteins. In addition, there are specific hydrolysis-transport proteins for dipeptides, which simultaneously hydrolyze dipeptides and transport them into the enterocyte.

Carbohydrates are also hydrolyzed by membrane-associated enzymes. It is of interest that the pattern of carbohydrate ingestion changes with age.[34] During infancy the disaccharide lactose accounts for most of the dietary carbohydrate. However, in older children and adults starch makes up about 60% of ingested carbohydrate, with sucrose and lactose constituting the remainder.[34] The complex carbohydrates present in the diet of the older child and adult are hydrolyzed to disaccharides and monosaccharides. The disaccharides are hydrolyzed to monosaccharides by specific disaccharidases located in the brush border membrane of intestinal epithelial cells. Monosaccharides are then transported across the enterocyte membrane. When there is a deficiency of a brush border disaccharidase, the maldigested disaccharide moves with luminal contents into the colon, where it is metabolized by colonic bacteria. Carbon dioxide, hydrogen, and other gases and organic acids are produced with consequent abdominal distention, flatulence, and diarrhea. Although a number of disaccharidase deficiencies have been described, the most common is lactase deficiency.

There are several types of lactase deficiency. Congenital lactase deficiency is rare and is associated with symptoms occurring a short time after birth when lactose is present in the diet.[35–39] The largest group of patients with this disorder is from Finland, where 16 cases have been recently described.[39] No more than 40 cases have been reported altogether. Adult-onset lactase deficiency, or primary adult-type hypolactasia, is due to the physiologic decline in lactase that occurs with age in mammals. The persistence of the enzyme in Caucasian groups should be considered the exception. Some racial groups with adult-onset lactase deficiency begin losing the enzyme in very early childhood; in others the loss of the disaccharide occurs later.[40] A third type of lactase deficiency may occur when there is loss or destruction of small intestinal epithelial cells as the result of intestinal disease or inflammation.

Congenital sucrase-isomaltase deficiency is a less common form of disaccharide deficiency. It was first described in 1961 by Weijers and coworkers.[41] Although it is generally considered to be a rare condition, the heterozygote frequency in white American subjects is 2%,[42] and the homozygote frequency in Eskimos is as high as 10%.[43–45] Symptoms vary from severe diarrhea in infancy to intermittent, bothersome symptoms in the older child. The correct diagnosis may, therefore, be missed for several months or years, with symptoms being attributed to conditions such as "toddler diarrhea" or "maternal anxiety." The diagnosis is established by the demonstration of deficient sucrase and isomaltase activities in a morphologically normal jejunal biopsy. Maltase activity is also reduced, since sucrase accounts for a large proportion of the total maltase activity. As with the other congenital disorders of carbohydrate digestion, dietary withdrawal of the offending sugars results in prompt symptomatic improvement.

Glucoamylase, or maltase, is a brush border enzyme important in hydrolyzing linear alpha-1-4 glucose polymers. Glucose is produced in this process. All the alpha-glucosidases except trehalase can hydrolyze maltose to yield glucose and are therefore called *maltases*. A deficiency of maltase activity has been described in patients with severe mucosal injury.[46] Theoretically, it may lead to carbohydrate maldigestion, although its clinical significance appears to be minimal. Congenital glucoamylase deficiency has not been described.

Trehalose (alpha-D-glucopyranoside) is a nonreducing disaccharide that occurs in plants such as mushrooms, in some microorganisms, and in many insects. Trehalase deficiency has been documented in a family who developed symptoms following the ingestion of mushrooms.[47] An autosomal dominant type of inheritance has been suggested.

Absorption into the Enterocyte

Amino Acids

Amino acids are rapidly absorbed by a group of sodium-coupled co-transport systems, similar to those present in the proximal tubular cell of the kidney. Absorption of some dipeptides is more rapid than absorption of the constituent amino acids. Amino acids, once absorbed, pass through the enterocyte rapidly, with only a small fraction being used for protein synthesis within the enterocyte. The small fraction of di- and tripeptides that enter the enterocyte is mostly hydrolyzed within the enterocyte. Carrier proteins for amino acid exit from the enterocyte are likely located on basolateral membranes, but they have not been well characterized.

Defective protein absorption because of impaired dipeptide or amino acid transport by the enterocyte is extremely rare, perhaps because of the redundancy of substrate specificity. A generalized defect in protein absorption would be fatal. However, there are several diseases of amino acid transport worth mentioning.

Hartnup's disease is a condition that results from a defect in the transport of free neutral amino acids in the small intestine and the proximal renal tubule.[48] The first realization that Hartnup's disease was an inherited disorder is told best by Dr. Harvey Levy.[49] In 1951, a 12-year-old boy, E. Hartnup (E. H.), was admitted to the Middlesex Hospital, London, England, with mild cerebellar ataxia and a red, scaly rash on the exposed areas of his body. His mother avowed that he had pellagra, for her eldest daughter (P. H.) had identical symptoms and had been treated at the hospital in 1937 for that disease. Although the rash in E. H. was quite consistent with pellagra, other findings were not, and a diagnosis of pellagra as a dietary deficiency was untenable. Apart from variable cerebellar signs and retarded mental development, the only abnormality detected at that time was in the urinary excretion of free amino acids. Paper chromatography of the urine disclosed an excretion pattern of amino acids quite unlike that seen in any other disease. At the same time, P. H., then age 19, had a recurrence of ataxia (without a rash), similar to that which she had had in childhood when the pellagra-like rash was most severe. The excretion pattern of amino acids in her urine was identical to that of her brother E. H. It was then clear that these two siblings were affected by the same disease. An inherited condition seemed probable when it was learned that the parents were first cousins.[49] The disease was not fully described in the medical literature, however, until 1956.[50]

The onset of Hartnup's disease occurs in early childhood with attacks of cerebellar ataxia and a pellagra-like rash appearing after exposure to sunlight. Mental retardation and/or a dementing psychiatric disturbance similar to that seen in pellagra can occur. These clinical manifestations are, however, intermittent and variable, with the skin rash being the primary cause of most referrals. The pellagra results from the abnormally small proportion of dietary tryptophan available for the nutritionally important kynurenine-nicotinamide pathway. Unabsorbed free tryptophan is metabolized by intestinal bacteria to produce metabolites such as indoles, some of which may be potent inhibitors of the kynurenine-nicotinamide pathway and may, therefore, further decrease the already diminished production of nicotinamide. As tryptophan can be absorbed in the form of di- and tripeptides, it is perhaps surprising that clinical symptoms occur at all. However, all clinical attacks are associated with an inadequate or irregular diet, and this may well result in insufficient absorption of peptide-bound tryptophan. The metabolism of the other neutral amino acids in this disorder does not seem to present the same difficulties. There is no specific treatment for the condition other than supplements of nicotinamide (25–150 mg every 24 hours). The ultimate prognosis is good, with some amelioration of the condition in later life.[48, 49]

Lysinuric protein intolerance (LPI) presents with severe symptoms that include marked failure to thrive, diarrhea, vomiting, protein intolerance, hepatic splenomegaly, and often mental retardation.[51, 52] The defect is in the transport of dibasic amino acids and is inherited as an autosomal recessive trait. The transport defect has been demonstrated in the small intestine, the liver, and the proximal renal tubules.[48, 51, 52] Onset is in infancy, commencing at the time of weaning from the breast to a cow's milk formula. After the first year of life, protein aversion is common, and symptoms ameliorate with a decreased protein intake. If a high protein intake is maintained, hyperammonemia, hepatosplenomegaly, and sometimes coma develop. The cornerstone of treatment is a low-protein diet in the range of 1.5 gm per kg body weight or less. Early attempts at preventing hyperammonemia with arginine or ornithine supplements have not been entirely successful, presumably because of poor intestinal absorption. Diarrhea occurs if more than 22 gm of arginine is ingested. However, the use of this urea cycle intermediate will allow the use of a low-protein diet and results in catch-up growth.[48, 51] Rajantie and colleagues[53] have shown that another urea cycle intermediate, citrulline, is absorbed entirely normally and is capable of preventing the ornithinopenic hyperammonemia in LPI. This may allow a higher intake of dietary protein.

Blue diaper syndrome results from the isolated malabsorption of tryptophan. The disease is also associated with an increased absorption of calcium.[48] Thier and Alpers[54] have suggested that a specific tryptophan transport system is defective in blue diaper syndrome, rather than a group-specific transport system, which is affected in Hartnup's disease. The disease is inherited as an autosomal recessive trait and presents in the neonatal period with failure to thrive, recurrent pyrexia, irritability, constipation, and a blue discoloration of the diapers.[48] The stools contain large quantities of indoles, tryptophan, tryptamine, and indolic acid. The blue discoloration results from the presence of indigotin (indigo blue), an oxidation product of urinary indicans.

Oast-house syndrome (methionine malabsorption) is a very rare condition. It was first described by Smith and Strang.[55] They described a neonate who was developmentally retarded, had recurrent episodes of edema, and had excessive urinary excretion of alpha-hydroxybutyric acid (a bacterial breakdown product of methionine), which gave the infant an unusual odor similar to that of an oast-house. (Oast is the British word for a kiln for drying hops or malt.) Later, Hooft and associates[56] described a similar child who malabsorbed methionine and excreted large amounts of alpha-hydroxybutyric acid in the urine, which gave the child an oast-house odor. The infant they described presented with convulsions, diarrhea, and severe mental retardation. On treating the patient with a methionine-free diet, the symptoms improved.

Lowe's syndrome, unlike the other conditions mentioned above, is inherited as a sex-linked trait and is characterized by mental retardation, cataracts, and renal tubular acidosis with aminoaciduria. Defective absorption of lysine and arginine has been demonstrated,[57] but the significance of this is not clear.

Monosaccharides

Monosaccharides produced by the action of brush border oligosaccharidases are small hydrophilic molecules that do not penetrate cell membranes rapidly. Simple diffusion of these compounds across membranes is slow, but diffusion is an important means of uptake when the monosaccharide is at high luminal concentrations. For the most part, however, specific sodium-coupled transport systems mediate efficient transport or absorption of monosaccharides, including glucose. These transport systems are presumably integral membrane proteins and use energy to transport glucose and other monosaccharides. The monosaccharides glucose, galactose, xylose, and fructose may also enter enterocytes by means of a third mechanism, facilitated diffusion. In this type of transport, a molecule to be transported, such as fructose, couples with its carrier on the external side of the membrane and the complex either diffuses or rotates within the membrane. At the inner side of the membrane the transported molecule dissociates from its carrier. An important difference exists between simple diffusion and facilitated diffusion. Facilitated diffusion depends on a fixed number of carrier protein sites, therefore, this process is saturable, unlike simple diffusion.[2]

Glucose-galactose malabsorption was first described in 1962 by Lindquist and Meeuwisse.[58] In vivo[59, 60] and in vitro[61, 62] studies have shown markedly impaired or absent sodium-coupled mucosal uptake of glucose. In many patients, clinical tolerance to the offending carbohydrates improves with age, despite the fact that the enzyme deficiency and transport defect persist. Wozniak and coworkers[63] have shown that there are at least two molecular variants of the transport defect. One results from deletion of the transport site, which does not change with age. In the other there is a reduced number of normally functioning transport sites, which appear to increase in number with age. Absorption of fructose, xylose, leucine, and alanine is intact. The finding that amino acid absorption and Na^+,K^+–ATPase activity are normal suggests that alterations of the sodium gradient are not involved in the pathophysiology of this condition.

Fatty Acids and Monoglycerides

The products of lipid digestion, including fatty acids, monoglycerides, cholesterol, sterol vitamins, and other lipids, pass from the intestinal lumen through the intestinal water into the enterocyte cytoplasm. Lipolysis products move through the intestinal aqueous milieu and across the peripheral unstirred water layer and mucous gel by diffusion of large liposomes and mixed micelles, extension of a viscous hydrocarbon phase, or diffusion of lipid monomers in free solution. All these processes occur, although the first two are quantitatively more important than the third in view of the substantial thickness of the intestinal unstirred water layer and the low aqueous solubility of most lipolysis products.[2] Medium-chained triglycerides, 6 to 12 carbon units in length, are rapidly and completely hydrolyzed by pancreatic lipase to fatty acids and glycerol, both of which are rapidly taken up by enterocytes.

Abetalipoproteinemia is a rare disorder of lipid processing within the enterocyte. Lipids once absorbed as monoglycerides and fatty acids into the enterocyte are reassembled as triglycerides and incorporated into chylomicrons, which are then transported into the blood. In abetalipoproteinemia there is inefficient or defective chylomicron formation. The triglyceride in the affected cells does not appear to receive the normal apoprotein coating. The defect is presumed to involve the synthesis of apo B or intracellular assembling of apo B with lipid.[64] In order to explain all the manifestations of the disease, which affects a number of organ systems, the hypothesis of some generalized defect in cell membranes has been put forward. The disease is characterized by malformed erythrocytes (acanthocytes), retinitis pigmentation, and a form of Friedreich's ataxia. Biochemically there is profound hypocholesterolemia and a total absence of low-density lipoproteins from the plasma. The mode of inheritance is autosomal dominant, and it appears more predominantly in males (70%). Treatment consists of dietary restriction of triglycerides. Medium-chain triglycerides should be substituted for long-chain triglycerides, and adequate fat-soluble vitamins and linoleic acid should be provided.[64]

Familial hypobetalipoproteinemia is similar to abetalipoproteinemia. In the heterozygote state of this condition, the intestinal mucosa and fat absorption are probably normal.[48] In homozygotes, the intestinal tract findings mimic those of abetalipoproteinemia, including fat malabsorption and extensive neutral fat accumulation in enterocytes. Various forms of hypobetalipoproteinemia have been described, indicating that the intestinal transport of triglyceride to the plasma is under complex genetic control.

Uptake into Blood and Lymph

Cardiac failure can cause bowel edema and lead to malabsorption.[65] Another disease that results in malabsorption at the level of uptake into blood and lymph is intestinal lymphangiectasia.[66–69] This is a condition in which the subepithelial lymph ducts are dilated and functionally obstructed. Consequently, removal of chylomicrons in the lymph is abnormally slow. A small bowel biopsy may not help in the diagnosis of this disease process.[70] Treatment is a low-fat diet in which predominantly medium-chain triglycerides are ingested. Infiltrative diseases of the small intestine—for example, tuberculous enteritis, intestinal lymphoma, and Whipple's disease—may compress lymphatic vessels in the small intestinal wall and retard chylomicron removal. In addition, enlargement of regional lymph nodes such as occurs in tuberculosis, lymphoma, metastatic carcinoma, and metastatic carcinoid disease may produce obstruction and fat malabsorption.

DIAGNOSIS

Obtaining a good history, performing a physical examination, and judiciously using laboratory studies will generally provide the information necessary to diagnose a maldigestion or malabsorption disorder.

History

The symptoms of diarrhea, weight loss, and poor growth are not unique to malabsorption. Many nongastrointestinal disorders such as urinary tract infections or central nervous system disorders produce similar symptoms. However, with other clues from a complete and accurate clinical history, an etiology can often be implicated. Important aspects of the history include:

1. A chronological description of all symptoms (fever, diarrhea, abdominal pain, etc.), the relationship of

symptoms to changes in life style or stress, and the introduction of antibiotics or other medications should be obtained. Exacerbation of chronic medical problems should also be considered.

2. Assessment of appetite, activity, and sleeping habits prior to the onset of the symptoms is important.

3. A dietary history is necessary to assess intake in terms of nutritional type and quantity. Note should be made of the dietary manipulations employed in an attempt to resolve symptoms. The physician should ascertain whether there has been prolonged dietary restriction initiated to control diarrhea. Dietary restrictions can all too frequently result in malnutrition.

4. A perinatal history should be obtained. Signs and symptoms present from birth suggest a congenital disorder but do not rule out acquired causes of malabsorption. A history of prior abdominal surgery can suggest an anatomic cause for malabsorption such as intestinal stricture or partial small bowel obstruction.

5. A history of serial infections can implicate cystic fibrosis or an immune deficiency syndrome as a possible cause of maldigestion or malabsorption.

6. Inquire about recent travel on the part of the patient or immediate family members to tropical or underdeveloped areas. If a child is cared for in a day-care nursery, this might implicate infections such as giardia as a cause of malabsorption.

7. Many maldigestive and malabsorptive disorders affect organ systems other than the intestinal tract. Systemic complaints not directly related to the digestive tract such as malaise, edema, fever, delayed onset of menses, secondary amenorrhea, or weight loss may suggest inflammatory bowel disease or early liver disease. Evidence of bleeding, bruising, or rashes may be secondary to a deficiency state that accompanies malabsorption.

8. A family history should be obtained since other family members may have similar signs and symptoms. This can suggest a genetically determined or infectious disorder.

Physical Examination

The number and prominence of physical findings may parallel the severity and chronicity of the malabsorptive disorder. The physical examination may be unremarkable or show subtle abnormalities known to be associated with mild malabsorption. During the examination it may be noticed that the child is depressed and passive in response. This is common in moderate to severe malnutrition. Many chronically malnourished children also show evidence of developmental delay. Accurate measurement of height, weight, and head circumference; calculation of weight for length; and construction of a growth curve are fundamental parts of the physical examination. The plotted growth curves for weight and length can provide invaluable information in the assessment of growth problems secondary to the nutritional inadequacies of chronic maldigestive and malabsorptive disorders.[71] Examination of the head, face, and neck may reveal evidence of fat-soluble or water-soluble vitamin deficiencies (e.g., xerophthalmia in vitamin A deficiency, or cheilitis and smooth tongue in vitamin B complex deficiencies). Examination of the trunk, buttocks, and extremities can give a subjective impression of muscle wasting or decreased fat stores. A more accurate measurement of muscle mass and fat stores can be provided by skin fold thickness measurements (see Chapter 81). The cardiac examination may reveal a rapid heart rate from anemia, or bradycardia secondary to protein-calorie malnutrition. Abdominal distention may be detected, reflecting fatty infiltration of the liver, laxity of abdominal musculature, or both. This can be associated with protein-calorie malnutrition. Tenderness of the liver may be secondary to fatty infiltration or congestive heart failure. A prominent abdominal venous pattern, a palpable spleen, or a noticeable fluid wave on abdominal examination may herald chronic liver disease with portal hypertension and ascites. The absence of, or delay in the appearance of, secondary sex characteristics is common with chronic malabsorption in older children. Nail bed pallor from decreased blood hemoglobin and clubbing of the nail beds can occur in both celiac disease[72] and inflammatory bowel disease.[73,74] Joint pain, swelling, and erythremia can be extraintestinal manifestations of inflammatory bowel disease. Abnormalities of color and texture in the skin and hair can be seen in fat soluble vitamin and trace element deficiency states. The neurologic examination may reveal the abnormal reflexes of Chvostek's or Trousseau's sign from hypocalcemia.

Laboratory Testing

Laboratory studies can help confirm the presence of maldigestion and malabsorption and, more importantly, help identify the cause. They can elucidate specific vitamin or trace element deficiency states as well as document adequate serum levels during supplemental vitamin therapy. Studies can be divided into three categories based on availability, expense, and invasiveness (Table 38–4).

Initial Screening Tests

Stool Examination. The identification of occult blood and fecal leukocytes in a stool specimen would suggest an inflammatory condition of the lower colon. Decreased stool pH can reflect carbohydrate maldigestion and malabsorption in the small intestine and subsequent fermentation by colonic bacteria. Overt carbohydrate malabsorption will show positive reducing substances in the stool. A test for qualitative fecal fat excretion or stain for fat globules can be a quick and simple way to screen for fat malabsorption.[75] If there is a suspicion of a gastrointestinal pathogen, stool samples should be obtained for bacterial culture and examination for ova and parasites.

The diagnostic value of fecal testing is lost if the stool is not taken to the laboratory quickly and tested immediately. Collection of a stool sample can be a challenge

Table 38–4. DIAGNOSTIC STUDIES IN THE EVALUATION OF MALDIGESTION AND MALABSORPTION

Initial Studies
Stool examination for blood, leukocytes, reducing substances, and *C. difficile* toxin. Stool examination for ova and parasites and cultures for infectious bacterial pathogens.
Complete blood count
Serum electrolytes, blood urea nitrogen, creatinine, calcium, phosphorus, albumin, total protein
Urinalysis and culture
Second-Phase Studies
Sweat chloride test
Breath analysis
D-Xylose test
Serum carotene, folate, B_{12}, and iron levels
Fecal alpha-1-antitrypsin level
Fecal fat studies or coefficient of fat absorption studies
Fatty test meal,[80] Lundh test meal[79]
Third-Phase Studies
Fat-soluble vitamin levels: A, 25-hydroxy D, and E
Contrast radiographic studies: upper gastrointestinal series, or barium enema
Small intestinal biopsy for histology, and mucosal enzyme determination
Specialized Studies
Bentiromide excretion test
Schilling test
Serum/urine bile acid determination
Endoscopic retrograde pancreatography
Provocative pancreatic secretion testing

for the mother of a child with liquid stools. Rectal aspiration using an 8–10 Fr feeding tube and a 20 ml syringe may be tried.[75] Other techniques include lining a disposable diaper with plastic wrap to prevent absorbance or utilizing a urine collection bag that has been placed over the anus. Stool samples that cannot be processed immediately and examined for bacterial pathogens, ova, and parasites can be placed in an appropriate preservative or transport medium for later analysis.

Complete Blood Count. Anemia is common in malabsorption syndromes, including celiac disease, cystic fibrosis, and inflammatory bowel disease. The microcytic, hypochromic anemia of iron deficiency is prevalent and may be due to either chronic blood loss through the gastrointestinal tract or iron malabsorption. Less commonly, megaloblastic anemia can occur. In untreated celiac disease, this can be due to reduced serum and red blood cell folate levels.[76] The chronic malabsorption of folate and vitamin B_{12} may also produce megaloblastic anemia.[77] In cystic fibrosis, iron deficiency anemia with low serum ferritin is seen frequently, even in stable patients.[78] In cystic fibrosis patients with advanced pulmonary disease, polycythemia is seen less frequently than with other pulmonary disorders of comparable severity. The anemia associated with inflammatory bowel disease can present as iron deficiency anemia, megaloblastic anemia, or the anemia of chronic disease.

Additional Blood Tests. In patients with malabsorption, the chronic loss of electrolytes and base can be reflected by low serum levels of sodium, potassium, chloride, and bicarbonate. Depending on the degree of malnutrition present in the patient, total serum proteins, including albumin, can be depressed. Due to its relatively long half-life, serum albumin may not reflect current nutritional status. Serum proteins with a relatively shorter half-life may be used as nutritional markers. These include prealbumin (transthyretin), somatomedin c, retinol-binding protein, and transferrin (see section on nutritional management).

Second-Phase Testing

Serum concentrations of carotene, folate, and vitamins B_{12}, A, and E have also been used to assess maldigestive and malabsorptive states. Monitoring absorbed lipids following a standardized meal can be helpful in assessing maldigestion and malabsorption.[79, 80]

In mild to moderate malabsorption, quantitative fat excretion measured in a 72-hour stool collection will provide the most accurate estimation of fat malabsorption. This information along with a 72-hour dietary history can be used to calculate a coefficient of fat absorption. A fecal fat excretion study does not identify the pathophysiologic cause of malabsorption; it documents only the presence of fat maldigestion and/or malabsorption. In addition, a 72-hour stool collection is difficult to obtain from a small child. For these reasons, quantitative fecal fat excretion studies are not commonly used.

The steatocrit is a newer measurement to assess fat malabsorption.[81] It is based on the principle that when a stool sample is homogenized and centrifuged at 15,000 rpm for 15 minutes, the lipid portion will rise to the top and the solid aqueous portion will gravitate to the bottom. If this is done in a hematocrit tube, one can estimate the amount of fat in a given stool sample. This will provide a crude estimate of fat malabsorption.[81]

Breath Test. The specific applications of breath analysis are outlined in Chapter 77. Breath hydrogen testing is performed principally for the investigation of lactose malabsorption or bacterial overgrowth of the small intestine, although other applications show promise. Abundant data support its use as an accurate indirect test of lactase insufficiency. Similarly, sucrase deficiency or small intestinal bacterial overgrowth can be diagnosed using breath hydrogen testing.

D-Xylose Test. The absorption of D-xylose is thought to be a passive process that reflects the functional surface area of the bowel and is independent of bile salts, pancreatic exocrine secretion, or intestinal brush border enzymes. A standard dose is given by mouth. It is based on body surface area (14.5 gm per m^2 up to a maximum dose of 25 gm as a 10% oral water solution). Approximately 50% of the absorbed dose is metabolized in the liver with the remaining being excreted in the urine. The 1-hour D-xylose can be used to assess D-xylose absorption after the standard dose. The serum level should exceed 25 mg per dl. A timed urine collection following the standard oral dose can also be used to approximate D-xylose absorption. The sensitivity and specificity of this test is somewhat controversial.[82–87] However, it does remain a relatively noninvasive screen for malabsorption.

Third-Phase Testing

Intestinal Biopsy. The diagnostic value of small intestinal biopsy varies with the disease process. Capsule biopsy specimens are obtained from the area of the duodenojejunal junction, and endoscopic biopsies are usually obtained from the proximal to mid duodenum. Serial biopsy specimens from other areas of the proximal small bowel can be considered when intermittent or patchy disease distribution is suspected. The careful mounting of the biopsy sample prior to fixation allows for proper orientation. The diagnostic ability of intestinal biopsy varies with the disease entity (see Chapters 73 and 79).

Finally, a variety of specific tests exists for assessment of pancreatic secretory function (see Chapter 65).

MANAGEMENT

Only selected management principles are outlined here, since treatment principles have been noted elsewhere in the chapter and text.

Therapy for malabsorptive disorders is based on first identifying the disease process and applying specific treatment principles for the disease. Second, if protein-calorie malnutrition is present, this should be vigorously treated enterally, parenterally, or both. The goal of nutritional support in pediatric practice is to provide adequate protein, calories, and lipids for catch-up growth and maintenance of normal growth.

Maldigestion

For altered luminal digestion, specific therapies can be initiated, depending on the cause. Supplemental enzymes can be provided to augment depressed enzyme secretion by the pancreas, as is the case in cystic fibrosis and Shwachman-Diamond syndrome. These can be given along with a histamine$_2$ receptor antagonist to help minimize the acid-mediated degradation of enzymes in the stomach. Fat-soluble vitamin supplements can be provided in an attempt to overcome disorders of absorption. New pharmacologic strategies have been developed to enhance the absorption of vitamin E by incorporation of the vitamin with polyethylene glycol.[88, 89] The majority of dietary medium-chain triglycerides can improve fat absorption in patients with impaired triglyceride digestion and absorption. Liver disease and cholestasis can occur with cystic fibrosis. Recently, Cotting and colleagues showed that when eight cystic fibrosis patients were treated with ursodeoxycholic acid, their liver function and nutritional status improved.[90]

As noted earlier, the dumping syndrome has been shown to be a complication of the Nissen fundoplication. Recently, the symptoms that occurred with the dumping syndrome were alleviated with the use of uncooked starch.[91]

Malabsorption

In patients with mild to moderate malabsorption, a slow continuous infusion of nutrients by way of a nasogastric tube or through a gastrostomy may increase absorption. The slow rate increases the contact time between nutrients and the absorptive surface. This form of therapy is ideal for nocturnal feedings, but an enteral infusion pump will be necessary. Other modalities, such as the use of taurine, may improve fat absorption in patients with cystic fibrosis.[92]

Patients with severe malabsorption that has resulted in significant protein-calorie malnutrition may require parenteral nutritional support, which can provide the necessary nutrients, including minerals, vitamins, and iron (see Chapter 84).

REFERENCES

1. Basu MK, Chisholm DM: Oral manifestation of gastrointestinal disease. *In* Bouchier IAD, Allan RN, Hodgson HJF, et al, eds: Textbook of Gastroenterology. London, Bailliere Tindall, 1984, pp 1–10.
2. Granger DN, Barrowman JA, Kvietys PR: Eating: Salivation, mastication, and deglutition. *In* Clinical Gastrointestinal Physiology: A Saunders Monograph in Physiology. Philadelphia, WB Saunders, 1985, pp 31–51.
3. Gueant JL, Champigneulle B, Gaucher P, et al: Malabsorption of vitamin B_{12} in pancreatic insufficiency of the adult and of the child. Pancreas 1990; 5:559–567.
4. Cheng SH, Gregory RJ, Marshall J: Defective intracellular transport and processing of CFTR is the molecular basis of most cystic fibrosis. Cell 1990; 63:827–834.
5. Fredrikzon B, Blackberg L: Lingual lipase: An important lipase in the digestion of dietary lipids in cystic fibrosis? Pediatr Res 1980; 14:1387–1390.
6. Talal N: Sjögren's syndrome. *In* Samter M, ed: Immunological Diseases. 4th ed. Boston, Little, Brown & Co., 1988, pp 1501–1507.
7. Moreau H, Bernadac A, Gargouri Y, et al: Immunocytolocalization of human gastric lipase in chief cells of the fundic mucosa. Histochemistry 1989; 91:419–423.
8. Bernback S, Blackberg L, Hernell O: The complete digestion of human milk triacylglycerol in vitro requires gastric lipase, pancreatic colipase-dependent lipase, and bile-salt stimulated lipase. J Clin Invest 1990; 85:1221–1226.
9. Allen RH, Seetharam B, Podell E, et al: Effect of proteolytic enzymes on the binding of cobalamin to R protein and intrinsic factor. J Clin Invest 1978; 61:47–54.
10. Allen RH, Seethadam B, Allen NC, et al: Correction of cobalamin malabsorption in pancreatic insufficiency with a cobalamin analogue that binds with high affinity to R protein but not to intrinsic factor. J Clin Invest 1978; 61:1628–1634.
11. Adesola AO: The influence of severe protein deficiency (kwashiorkor) on gastric acid secretion in Nigerian children. Br J Surg 1968; 55:866.
12. Gracey M, Cullity GJ, Suharjono, et al: The stomach in malnutrition. Arch Dis Childhood 1977; 52:325–327.
13. Verner JV, Morrison AB: Endocrine pancreatic islet disease with diarrhea: Report of a case due to diffuse hyperplasia of non-beta islet tissue with a review of 54 additional cases. Arch Intern Med 1974; 133:492–500.
14. Isenberg JI, Walsh JH, Grossman MI: Zollinger-Ellison syndrome. Gastroenterology 1973; 65:140–165.
15. Robertson JA, Gallagher ND: In vivo evidence that cobalamin is absorbed by receptor-mediated endocytosis in the mouse. Gastroenterology 1985; 88:908–912.
16. Gueant JL, Gerard A, Monin B, et al: Radioautographic localization of iodinated human intrinsic factor in the guinea pig ileum using electron microscopy. Gut 1988; 29:1370–1378.
17. Meyer S, Deckelbaum RJ, Lax E, et al: Infant dumping syn-

drome after gastroesophageal reflux surgery. J Pediatr 1981; 99:235–237.
18. Caulfield ME, Wyllie R, Firor HV, et al: Dumping syndrome in children. J Pediatr 1987; 110:212–215.
19. Rivkees SA, Crawford JD: Hypoglycemia pathogenesis in children with dumping syndrome. Pediatrics 1987; 80:937–942.
20. Townes PL: Trypsinogen deficiency disease. J Pediatr 1965; 66:275–285.
21. Morris MD, Fisher DA: Trypsinogen deficiency disease. Am J Dis Child 1967; 114:203–208.
22. Townes PL, Bryson MF, Miller G: Further observations on trypsinogen deficiency disease: Report of a second case. J Pediatr 1967; 71:220–224.
23. Green JR, Bender SW, Posselt HG, et al: Case report: Primary intestinal enteropeptidase deficiency. J Pediatr Gastroenterol Nutr 1984; 3:630–633.
24. Sheldon W: Congenital pancreatic lipase deficiency. Arch Dis Child 1964; 39:268–271.
25. Lowe CV, May DC: Selective pancreatic deficiency: Absent amylase, diminished trypsin, and normal lipase. Am J Dis Child 1951; 82:459–464.
26. Lilibridge CB, Townes PL: Physiologic deficiency of pancreatic amylase in infancy: A factor in iatrogenic diarrhea. J Pediatr 1973; 82:279–282.
27. Hadorn B, Tarlow MJ, Lloyd JK, et al: Intestinal enterokinase deficiency. Lancet 1969; 1:812–813.
28. Ghishan FK, Lee PC, Lebenthal E, et al: Isolated congenital enterokinase deficiency: Recent findings and review of the literature. Gastroenterology 1983; 85:727–731.
29. Mata LJ, Jimenez F, Cordon M, et al: Gastrointestinal flora of children with protein-calorie malnutrition. Am J Clin Nutr 1972; 25:1118–1126.
30. Heyworth B, Brown J: Jejunal microflora in malnourished Gambian children. Arch Dis Child 1975; 50:27–33.
31. Gracey M, Suharjono, Sunoto, et al: Microbial contamination of the gut: Another feature of malnutrition. Am J Clin Nutr 1973; 26:1170–1174.
32. Gilman RH, Partanen R, Brown KH, et al: Decreased gastric acid secretion and bacterial colonization of the stomach in severely malnourished Bangladesh children. Gastroenterology 1988; 94:1308–1314.
33. Toskes PP, Donaldson RM: The blind loop syndrome. *In* Sleisenger MH, Fordtran JS, eds: Gastrointestinal Disease: Pathophysiology, Diagnosis, Management. 4th ed. Philadelphia, 1989, WB Saunders, 1989, pp 1289–1297.
34. Burke V: Mechanisms of intestinal digestion and absorption. *In* Anderson CM, Burke V, Gracey M, eds: Paediatric Gastroenterology. 2d ed. Melbourne, Blackwell Scientific Publications, 1987, pp 137–184.
35. Holzel A, Schwarz V, Sutcliffe KW: Defective lactose absorption causing malnutrition in infancy. Lancet 1959; 1:1126–1128.
36. Lifshitz F: Congenital lactase deficiency. J Pediatr 1966; 66:229–237.
37. Launiala K, Kuitunen P, Visakorpi JK: Disaccharidases and histology of duodenal mucosa in congenital lactose malabsorption. Acta Paediatr Scand 1966; 55:257–263.
38. Levin B, Abraham JM, Burgess EA, et al: Congenital lactose malabsorption. Arch Dis Child 1970; 45:173–177.
39. Savilahti E, Launiala K, Kuitunen P: Congenital lactase deficiency: A clinical study on 16 patients. Arch Dis Child 1983; 58:246–252.
40. Koldovsky O. Digestion and absorption of carbohydrates, protein and fat in infants and children. *In* Walker WA, Watkins JB, eds: Nutrition in Pediatrics: Basic Science and Clinical Application. Boston, Little, Brown & Co., 1985, pp 253–277.
41. Weijers HA, Van de Kamer JH, Dicke WK, et al: Diarrhoea caused by deficiency of sugar splitting enzymes I. Acta Paediatr Scand 1961; 50:55–71.
42. Welsh JD, Poley JR, Bhatia M, et al: Intestinal disaccharidase activities in relation to age, race, and mucosal damage. Gastroenterology 1978; 75:847–855.
43. Ellestad-Sayed JJ, Haworth JC: Disaccharide consumption and malabsorption in Canadian Indians. Am J Clin Nutr 1977; 30:698–703.
44. Ellestad-Sayed JJ, Haworth JC, Hildes JA: Disaccharide malabsorption and dietary patterns in two Canadian Eskimo communities. Am J Clin Nutr 1978; 31:1473–1478.
45. Gudmand-Hoyer E: Sucrose malabsorption in children: A report of thirty-one Greenlanders. J Pediatr Gastroenterol Nutr 1985; 4:873–877.
46. Lebenthal E, Lee PC: Glucoamylase and disaccharidase activities in normal subjects and in patients with mucosal injury of the small intestine. J Pediatr 1980; 97:389–393.
47. Madzarovova-Nohejlova J: Trehalase deficiency in a family. Gastroenterology 1973; 65:130–133.
48. Muller DPR, Milla PJ: Selective inborn errors of absorption. *In* Milla PJU, Muller DPR, eds: Harrises' Paediatric Gastroenterology. Edinburgh, Churchill Livingstone, 1988, pp 211–238.
49. Levy HL: Hartnup disorder. *In* Scriver CR, Beaudet AL, Sly WS, et al, eds: The Metabolic Basis of Inherited Disease. New York, McGraw-Hill, 1989, pp 2515–2527.
50. Baron DN, Dent CE, Harris H, et al: Hereditary pellagra-like skin rash with temporary cerebellar ataxia. Constant renal aminoaciduria and other bizarre biochemical features. Lancet 1956; 2:421–428.
51. Rajantie J, Simell O, Perheentupa J: Lysinuric protein intolerance. Basolateral transport defect in renal tubuli. J Clin Invest 1981; 67:1078–1082.
52. Rajantie J, Simell O, Perheentupa J: Lysinuric protein intolerance: Basolateral transport defect in renal tubuli. J Clin Invest 1981; 67:1078–1082.
53. Rajantie J, Simell O, Perheentupa J: Intestinal absorption in lysinuric protein intolerance: Impaired for diamino acids, normal for citrulline. Gut 1980; 21:519–524.
54. Thier SO, Alpers DH: Disorders of intestinal transport of amino acids. Am J Dis Child 1969; 117:13–23.
55. Smith AJ, Strang LB: An inborn error of metabolism with the urinary excretion of alpha-hydroxy-butyric acid and phenylpyruvic acid. Arch Dis Child 1958; 33:109–113.
56. Hooft C, Timmermans J, Snoeck J, et al: Methionine malabsorption in a mentally defective child. Lancet 1964; 2:20.
57. Bartsocas CS, Levy HL, Crawford JD, et al: A defect in intestinal amino acid transport in Lowe's syndrome. Am J Dis Child 1969; 117:93–95.
58. Lindquist B, Meeuwisse GW: Chronic diarrhea caused by monosaccharide malabsorption. Acta Paediatr 1962; 51:674–685.
59. Hughes WS, Senior JR: The glucose-galactose malabsorption syndrome in a 23-year-old woman. Gastroenterology 1975; 68:142–145.
60. Fairclough PD, Clark ML, Dawson AM, et al: Absorption of glucose and maltose in congenital glucose-galactose malabsorption. Pediatr Res 1978; 12:1112–1114.
61. Stirling CE, Schneider AJ, Wong MD, et al: Quantitative radioautography of sugar transport in intestinal biopsies from normal humans and a patient with glucose-galactose malabsorption. J Clin Invest 1972; 51:438–451.
62. Booth IW, Patel PB, Sule D, et al: Demonstration of defective jejunal brush border Na^+-coupled glucose transport in congenital glucose-galactose malabsorption (abstract). Pediatr Res 1987; 22:98.
63. Wozniak E, Fenton TR, Walker-Smith JA, et al: Glucose absorption in congenital glucose-galactose malabsorption: A kinetic basis for clinical remission (abstract). Pediatr Res 1984; 18:1063.
64. Havel RJ, Kane JP: Structure and metabolism of plasma lipoproteins. *In* Scriver CR, Beaudet AL, Sly WS, et al, eds: The Metabolic Basis of Inherited Disease. New York, McGraw-Hill, 1989, pp 1129–1164.
65. Davidson JD, Waldmann TA, Goodman DS, et al: Protein-losing gastroenteropathy in congestive heart-failure. Lancet 1961; 1:899–902.
66. Pomerantz M, Waldman TA: Systemic lymphatic abnormalities associated with gastrointestinal protein loss secondary to intestinal lymphangiectasia. Gastroenterology 1963; 45:703–711.
67. Mistilis SP, Skyring AP, Stephen DD: Intestinal lymphangiectasia: Mechanism of enteric loss of plasma-protein and fat. Lancet 1965; 1:77–80.
68. Vardy PA, Lebenthal E, Schwachmann H: Intestinal lymphangiectasia: A reappraisal. Pediatrics 1975; 55:842–851.
69. Bolton RP, Cotter KL, Losowsky MS: Impaired neutrophil function in intestinal lymphangiectasia. J Clin Pathol 1986; 39:876–880.
70. Hart MH, Vanderhoof JA, Antonson DL: Failure of blind small bowel biopsy in the diagnosis of intestinal lymphangiectasia. J Pediatr Gastroenterol Nutr 1987; 6:803–805.

71. Silverman A, Roy CC: Physical signs. *In* Pediatric Clinical Gastroenterology. 3d ed. St. Louis, CV Mosby Co., 1983, pp 38–43.
72. Benson GD, Kowlessar OD, Sleisenger MH: Adult celiac disease with emphasis upon response to the gluten-free diet. Medicine (Baltimore) 1964; 43:1–40.
73. Fielding JF, Cooke WT: Finger clubbing and regional enteritis. Gut 1971; 12:442–444.
74. Hamilton JR, Bruce GA, Abdourhaman M, et al: Inflammatory bowel disease in children and adolescents. Adv Pediatr 1979; 26:311–341.
75. Sondheimer JM: Office stool examination: A practical guide. Contemporary Pediatrics 1990; 7(2):63–82.
76. Dormandy KM, Waters AH, Mollin DL: Folic acid deficiency in celiac disease. Lancet 1963; 1:632–635.
77. Hoffbrand AV, Douglas AP, Fry T, et al: Malabsorption of dietary folate (pteroylglutamates) in adult coeliac disease and dermatitis herpetiformis. Br Med J 1970; 4:85–89.
78. Ater JL, Herbst JJ, Landaw SA, et al: Relative anemia and iron deficiency in cystic fibrosis. Pediatrics 1983; 71:810–814.
79. Lundh G: Pancreatic exocrine function in neoplastic and inflammatory disease. A simple and reliable new test. Gastroenterology 1962; 42:275–280.
80. Goldstein R, Blodheim O, Levy E, et al: The fatty meal test: An alternative to stool fat analysis. Am J Clin Nutr 1983; 38:763–768.
81. Columbo C, Maiavacca R, Ronchi M, et al: The steatocrit: A simple method for monitoring fat malabsorption in patients with cystic fibrosis. J Pediatr Gastroenterol Nutr 1987; 6:926–930.
82. Rolles CJ, Nutter S, Kendal MJ, et al: One-hour blood-xylose screening-test for coeliac disease in infants and young children. Lancet 1973; 2:1043–1045.
83. Christie DL: Use of the one-hour blood xylose test as an indicator of small bowel mucosal disease. J Pediatr 1978; 92:725–728.
84. Buts JP, Morin CL, Roy CC, et al: One-hour blood xylose test: A reliable index of small bowel function. J Pediatr 1978; 90:729–733.
85. Levine JJ, Seidman E, Walker WA: Screening tests for enteropathy in children. Am J Dis Child 1987; 141:435–438.
86. Urban E: The A, B, C of d-xylose absorption. Gastroenterology 1989; 97:512–513.
87. Lifschitz CH, Polanco I: The d-xylose test in pediatrics: Is it useful? Gastroenterology 1989; 97:246–247.
88. Sokol RJ, Henbi JE, Butler-Simon N: Treatment of vitamin E deficiency during chronic childhood cholestasis with oral d-alpha-tocopheryl polyethylene glycol-1000 succinate. Gastroenterology 1987; 93:975–985.
89. Sokol RJ: Vitamin E and neurologic deficits. Adv Pediatr 1990; 37:119–148.
90. Cotting J, Lentze MJ, Reichen J: Effects of ursodeoxycholic acid treatment on nutrition and liver function in patients with cystic fibrosis and longstanding cholestasis. Gut 1990; 31:918–921.
91. Girtzelmann R, Hirsig J: Infant dumping syndrome: Reversal of symptoms by feeding uncooked starch. Eur J Pediatr 1986; 145:504–506.
92. Belli DC, Levy E, Darling P, et al: Taurine improves the absorption of a fat meal in patients with cystic fibrosis. Pediatrics 1987; 80:517–523.
93. Solomons NW, Molina S, Bulux J: Effect of protein-energy malnutrition on digestive and absorptive capacities of infants and children. *In* E. Lebenthal, ed: Textbook of Gastroenterology and Nutrition in Infancy. 2d ed. New York, Raven Press, 1989, pp 517–533.
94. Balistreri WF: Neonatal cholestasis. J Pediatr 1985; 106:171–189.
95. Amedee-Manesme O, Bernard O, Brunelle F, et al: Sclerosing cholangitis with neonatal onset. J Pediatr 1987; 111:225–229.
96. Tong MJ, Thursby M, Rakela J, et al: Studies on the maternal-infant transmission of the viruses which cause acute hepatitis. Gastroenterology 1981; 80:999–1004.
97. Giovannini M, Tagger A, Ribero ML, et al: Maternal-infant transmission of hepatitis C virus and HIV infections: A possible interaction (letter). Lancet 1990; 335:1166.
98. Wejstal R, Hermodsson S, Iwarson S, et al: Mother to infant transmission of hepatitis C virus infection. J Med Virol 1990; 30:178–180.
99. Frey B, Schubiger G, Musy JP: Transient cholestatic hepatitis in a neonate associated with carbamazepine exposure during pregnancy and breast-feeding. Eur J Pediatr 1990; 150:136–138.
100. Balistreri WF: Foreword: Neonatal cholestasis—lessons from the past, issues for the future. Semin Liver Dis 1987; 7:1–7.
101. Alagille D, Odievre M: Liver and Biliary Tract Disease in Children. New York, John Wiley & Sons, 1979, pp 163–252.
102. Akers DR, Needham ME: Sarcoma botryoides (rhabdomyosarcoma) of the bile ducts with survival. J Pediatr Surg 1971; 6:474–479.
103. Shaffer EA: Gallbladder disease. *In* Walker WA, Durie PR, Hamilton JR, et al, eds: Pediatric Gastrointestinal Disease. Philadelphia, BC Decker, 1991, pp 1152–1170.
104. Classen M, Gotze H, Richter HJ, et al: Primary sclerosing cholangitis in children. J Pediatr Gastroenterol Nutr 1987; 6:197–202.
105. Spivak W, Grand RJ, Eraklis A: A case of primary sclerosing cholangitis in childhood. Gastroenterology 1982; 82:129–132.
106. Horowitz ME, Etcubanas E, Webber BL, et al: Hepatic undifferentiated (embryonal) sarcoma and rhabdomyosarcoma in children. Cancer 1987; 59:396–402.
107. Bhave SA, Pandit AN, Pradhan AM, et al: Liver disease in India. Arch Dis Child 1982; 57:922–928.
108. Perman JA, Welin SL, Grand RJ, et al: Laboratory measures of copper metabolism in the differentiation of chronic active hepatitis and Wilson disease in children. J Pediatr 1979; 94:564–568.
109. Meyer UA: Hepatic porphyrias: New findings on the nature of metabolic defects. *In* Popper H, Schaffner F, eds: Progressive Liver Diseases. New York, Grune & Stratton, 1976, pp 280–293.
110. Sherlock S: Hepatitis C viral infection—an update. Supplement to Diseases of the Liver and Biliary System. 8th ed. Oxford, Blackwell, 1990, pp 1–9.
111. Davenport M. Neonatal malaria and obstructive jaundice. Arch Dis Child 1986; 61:515–517.
112. Orellana-Alcalde JM, Dominguez JP: Jaundice and oral contraceptive drugs. Lancet 1966; 2:1278–1280.
113. Stoll BA, Andrews JT, Motteram R: Preliminary communications: Liver damage from oral contraceptives. Brit Med J 1966; 1:960–961.
114. Ockner RK, Davidson CS: Hepatic effects of oral contraceptives. N Engl J Med 1967; 276:331–334.
115. Davis RA, Kern F Jr, Showalter R, et al: Alterations of hepatic Na^+,K^+-ATPase and bile flow by estrogen: Effects on liver surface membrane lipid structure and function. Proc Natl Acad Sci 1978; 75:4130–4134.
116. Kern F Jr, Everson GT, DeMark B, et al: Biliary lipids, bile acids, and gallbladder function in the human female: Effects of contraceptive steroids. J Lab Clin Med 1982; 99:798–805.
117. Royal College of General Practitioners Oral Contraception Study. Oral contraceptives and gallbladder disease. Lancet 1982; 2:957–959.
118. Lieberman DA, Keeffe EB, Stenzel P: Severe and prolonged oral contraceptive jaundice. J Clin Gastroenterol 1984; 6:145–148.
119. Frezza M, Pozzato G, Chiesa L, et al: Reversal of intrahepatic cholestasis of pregnancy in women after high dose S-adenosyl-1-methionine administration. Hepatology 1984; 4:274–278.
120. Vose M: Estrogen cholestasis: Membranes, metabolites or receptors? Gastroenterology 1987; 93:643–649.
121. Schrumpf E, Fausa O, Kolmannskog F, et al: Sclerosing cholangitis in ulcerative colitis: A follow-up study. Scand J Gastroenterol 1982; 17:33–39.
122. Mieli-Vergani G, Mowat AP: The immunology of autoimmune chronic active hepatitis. *In* Branski D, Dinari G, Rosen P, et al, eds: Paediatric Gastroenterology: Aspects of Immunology and Infections. Basel, Karger, 1986, pp 256–265.
123. Ferrara JLM, Deeg HJ: Graft-versus-host disease. N Engl J Med 1991; 324:667–674.
124. Gamble JL, Fahey KR, Appleton J, et al: Congenital alkalosis with diarrhea. J Pediatr 1945; 26:509–518.
125. Darrow DC: Congenital alkalosis with diarrhea. J Pediatr 1945; 26:149–152.
126. Holmberg C: Electrolyte economy and its normal regulation in congenital chloride diarrhea. Pediatr Res 1978; 12:82–86.

Chapter 39

Bacterial Overgrowth in the Small Bowel

MAUREEN M. JONAS

Small bowel bacterial overgrowth is a condition in which the microflora of the upper small bowel, or a localized section of it, resembles that of the distal ileum or colon, containing large numbers of coliforms and anaerobic bacteria (greater than 10^6 organisms per ml). Synonyms for this condition include blind loop syndrome, stagnant loop syndrome, and stasis syndrome. The clinical significance of bacterial overgrowth syndrome is twofold: it is often a sequela of an underlying disorder predisposing to the disturbed pattern of flora, and it may have profound clinical consequences, such as chronic diarrhea or severe malnutrition. Study of this entity has led to an understanding of the normal intestinal microflora, natural mechanisms for its control, and the effects of changes in diet, medications, surgery, and gastrointestinal illness.

NORMAL INTESTINAL MICROFLORA

The human infant is born with a sterile gastrointestinal tract. During the first few days of life, colonization with a variety of microorganisms occurs, and a complex pattern of aerobic and anaerobic flora develops. It is known that the intestinal tract becomes infected via the oral route, since infants born with intestinal obstruction acquire the usual colonic flora proximal to the obstruction.[1] The rate and proportion of anaerobic colonization has been shown to be partially determined by the route of delivery and the type of feeding.[2] The presence of gram-positive bacteria in stool was found to be influenced by the type of feeding in young infants,[3] but the evolution to an adult microflora has not been extensively studied. The bacterial flora in the adult population has been been well characterized during the last 25 years.

Each section of the gastrointestinal tract contains a unique type and number of bacteria (Table 39–1). The stomach is virtually sterile, containing less than 10^3 organisms per ml, most of which are gram-positive and aerobic, such as streptococci, staphylococci, and lactobacilli. The normal microflora of the proximal small bowel is similar to that of the stomach, with up to 10^4 organisms per ml. Some fungal species may be detected, as well as small numbers of coliforms and anaerobic bacteria. In the distal ileum, gram-negative organisms predominate. Coliforms and anaerobes, such as *Bacteroides, Bifidobacterium, Fusobacterium,* and *Clostridium,* are found in total concentration as high as 10^5 or 10^6 per ml. Distal to the ileocecal valve, bacterial concentration is 10^{10} to 10^{12} per ml, with 1,000 times more anaerobic than aerobic organisms.[4]

Limitation of the bacterial population of the small intestine and control of the types of organisms present are accomplished by several mechanisms: normal peristalsis, gastric acid secretion, bacterial growth inhibition by bile, intraluminal pH and oxidation-reduction potential, and, possibly, metabolic interactions among the bacteria themselves.[5] When one or more of these mechanisms are disrupted, quantitative and qualitative changes in upper small bowel flora occur, resulting in the syndrome of small bowel bacterial overgrowth.

PREDISPOSING CONDITIONS

Maintenance of the normal numbers and types of intestinal flora is accomplished by the mechanisms enumerated above. The most important of these is intestinal motility, since disorders leading to stasis of intestinal contents are those most frequently associated with small bowel bacterial overgrowth.[6] Table 39–2 lists the most common anatomic causes and motor disorders causing

Table 39–1. PREDOMINANT GASTROINTESTINAL FLORA IN NORMAL SUBJECTS

	Stomach	Upper Small Bowel	Distal Ileum/ Colon
Organisms per ml	$<10^3$	10^{3-4}	$10^{5-6}/10^{10-12}$
Aerobes	Streptococci Staphylococci Lactobacilli Fungi	Streptococci Staphylococci Lactobacilli Fungi Coliforms (few)	Coliforms
Anaerobes		Rare	Bacteroides Bifidobacteria Fusobacteria Clostridia

Table 39–2. FACTORS ASSOCIATED WITH SMALL BOWEL BACTERIAL OVERGROWTH

Anatomic Causes of Small Intestinal Stasis
Diverticuli
Surgical loops
End-to-side anastomosis
Side-to-side anastomosis
Continent ileostomy
Ileo-anal pouch anastomosis
Partial small bowel obstruction
Stricture
Mass
Adhesions
Motor Disorders Causing Small Intestinal Stasis
Intestinal pseudo-obstruction (neuropathic, myopathic, idiopathic)
Autonomic neuropathy (diabetic)
Absent or abnormal migrating motor complex
Anatomic Causes of Small Bowel Contamination
Enterocolic fistula
Loss of ileocecal valve
Abnormality in Host Defenses
Achlorhydria or hypochlorhydria
Immune deficiency
Malnutrition
Miscellaneous
Chronic pancreatitis
Cirrhosis
Feeding tubes

small intestinal stasis. Some, such as diverticula, continent ileostomies, and diabetic autonomic neuropathy, are uncommon in pediatric patients. Others, such as small bowel strictures seen after bouts of necrotizing enterocolitis in neonates, intestinal pseudo-obstruction syndromes, and ileoanal pouch anastomosis after colectomy, are encountered in infants and children with some frequency. Adults have been identified with abnormalities in the interdigestive motor complex of the small intestine—the "intestinal housekeeper"; some of these patients had evidence of bacterial overgrowth.[7] Abnormalities in this migrating myoelectric complex have not been well characterized in children.

In addition to stasis, there are other factors, also listed in Table 39–2, that may cause bacterial overgrowth. The small bowel may become contaminated by anatomic abnormalities, such as an enterocolonic fistula, or by surgical loss of the ileocecal valve.[8] Abnormalities in host defenses, such as achlorhydria, malnutrition, and panhypogammaglobulinemia, are associated with an increased frequency of bacterial overgrowth, but these associations are less clear-cut. For example, overgrowth has long been known to occur after gastric ulcer surgery. However, overgrowth is much more likely in the setting of antrectomy or Billroth II anastomosis than with parietal cell vagotomy alone,[9] indicating that it is not simply the decrease in gastric acid output, but disruption of normal anatomy and/or innervation that is responsible for the increased colonization.

Patients with hypogammaglobulinemia or agammaglobulinemia have an increased incidence of small bowel bacterial overgrowth, yet those with a deficiency of immunoglobulin A (IgA) alone (the immunoglobulin class most abundant in the intestine) do not.[10, 11] In one study of adults with chronic lymphocytic leukemia, some had overgrowth without achlorhydria or stasis and were found to have absent secretory piece in jejunal aspirates (secretory piece is a component of intestinal IgA).[12] One adult with selective IgA deficiency developed overgrowth only after treatment with high-dose steroids.[13] These cases suggest that local regulation of immunity may be more important than systemic regulation in the control of luminal flora.

Patients with acquired immune deficiency syndrome (AIDS) commonly have diarrhea with wasting and malabsorption. Many gastrointestinal lesions have been identified in these patients, including an increased incidence of common bacterial infections, opportunistic infections, and mucosal injury unrelated to infection. Small bowel bacterial overgrowth has not been commonly reported in this patient population, yet in one study of adults, duodenal cultures were positive in 12 of 14 patients, and none of seven controls.[14] In another study, gastric and duodenal cultures were commonly positive in AIDS patients, but in association with hypochlorhydria.[15] One pediatric AIDS patient with a necrotizing jejunitis was found to have overgrowth of *Klebsiella*.[16] It is not clear whether clinically significant bacterial overgrowth is truly uncommon in patients with AIDS, whether other factors must be present in order for it to develop, or whether it is overshadowed by the numerous other gastrointestinal disorders seen in this patient group.

Small bowel bacterial overgrowth has been reported in protein-calorie malnutrition in childhood.[17] Most commonly, these studies have been done in tropical climates among populations from poor socioeconomic backgrounds, making their interpretation difficult.[18, 19] One study of Nigerian children clearly showed qualitative and quantitative differences in the duodenal flora of malnourished subjects versus controls from the same population,[20] indicating a significant association with malnutrition. However, it is known that generalized malnutrition may be accompanied by changes in gastric acid output,[17, 18] decreased intestinal motility,[21] and aberrations in immune function,[22] any of which might increase the propensity for bacterial proliferation in the upper small bowel. Moreover, overgrowth can cause severe malabsorption (by mechanisms that will be discussed later), leading to profound malnutrition and thus creating a self-sustaining process.

Bacterial overgrowth has been described sporadically in other conditions, such as chronic pancreatitis and cirrhosis,[23] but the pathophysiology in these disorders has not been totally elucidated. Antibacterial activity has been demonstrated in normal pancreatic fluid,[24] but its physiologic role remains speculative. A recent animal study demonstrated delayed intestinal transit as an effect of portal hypertension,[25] which may explain the occasional finding of overgrowth in cirrhosis. Increased numbers of abnormal flora have been found in infants fed by intragastric or intrajejunal tubes[26, 27]; the implications of this finding have not been well studied.

PATHOPHYSIOLOGY OF MALABSORPTION

The predominant pathophysiologic mechanisms operative in small bowel bacterial overgrowth are summarized in Table 39–3. The initial reports of patients with bacterial overgrowth described individuals presenting with megaloblastic anemia, secondary to vitamin B_{12} deficiency, and massive steatorrhea.[28, 29] Investigation of these defects led to demonstration of intraluminal abnormalities secondary to the bacterial proliferation.[30] It was not until much later that significant intestinal mucosal injury, with its attendant absorptive and secretory defects, was described in this syndrome. It is known that a wide spectrum of absorptive derangements may occur from bacterial overgrowth.

Steatorrhea was one of the earliest described consequences of bacterial overgrowth in humans and of artificially created blind loops in animals.[31, 32] Normally, ionized, water-soluble conjugated bile salts are found in the duodenum and jejunum, where they are needed for micellarization of the products of fat digestion to allow transmucosal absorption. Some bacteria, particularly *Bacteroides* species, are capable of hydrolysis of these compounds into free, unconjugated bile acids, which are then quickly reabsorbed into intestinal mucosa[31] and might then be of insufficient concentration for effective fat absorption. This was the presumed mechanism for steatorrhea in bacterial overgrowth, until it was demonstrated that supplementation with oral bile salts did not correct the malabsorption.[33] In addition, the steatorrhea seen in animals with experimental blind loops was greater than that seen with experimental biliary diversion, with no bile salts available for micellarization.[34] Thus, other mechanisms were sought, including the potential toxicity or inhibitory effects of intraluminal free bile acids.[35] Subsequently, several workers demonstrated the previously unrecognized intestinal mucosal injury present in bacterial overgrowth[36–38] and attempted to determine its pathogenesis; putative causes have included bacterial proteases,[39] lectins,[40] and acetaldehyde,[41] among others.

Ament and coworkers[36] examined 212 biopsies from three patients and found a patchy mucosal lesion in each patient. The light microscopic findings ranged from normal to severely abnormal, with varying degrees of villous atrophy and lamina propria infiltrate. Electron microscopy of 60 biopsies demonstrated abnormalities that correlated with the severity of clinical illness and included evidence of decrease in enterocyte fat absorption and transcellular transport after feeding. Subsequently, other investigators have demonstrated functional correlates of these histologic abnormalities, including monosaccharide[42] and disaccharide[39] malabsorption and abnormal electrolyte transport.[43]

Megaloblastic anemia and vitamin B_{12} deficiency were among the earliest recognized features of bacterial overgrowth, and the earliest to be explained pathophysiologically. The primary cause is avid uptake of vitamin B_{12} by the abnormal bacterial flora, especially anaerobes.[44, 45] These organisms were found to bind the cyanocobalamin, whether or not is was already bound to intrinsic factor or gastric mucosa.[46] One group of workers has demonstrated production of analogues of vitamin B_{12} in patients with overgrowth,[47] but the clinical significance of this finding has not been elucidated. Contrary to vitamin B_{12}, folic acid levels (serum and red blood cell) are normal or elevated in patients with bacterial overgrowth.[48] This is because the bacteria synthesize folate, which becomes available for uptake by the host.[49]

Four mechanisms of protein malabsorption or net loss have been enumerated:[50] impaired utilization of dietary nitrogen secondary to bacterial competition for substrate,[51, 52] impaired transport of amino acids and peptides across damaged mucosal surfaces,[37, 53] loss (secretion) of endogenous proteins,[54, 55] and decreased levels of enterokinase with subsequent decrease in release in pancreatic proteases.[56]

Similarly, carbohydrate malabsorption in small bowel bacterial overgrowth is multifactorial. Production of short-chain fatty acids (which interfere with fat absorption, as discussed above) attests to utilization of dietary carbohydrate by the bacteria.[57] The mucosal injury that has been described previously is associated with loss of disaccharidase activity, primarily lactase.[37, 58, 59] Impaired absorption of monosaccharides was shown to be a consequence of bacterial small bowel contamination many years ago.[42] At that time, it was suggested that this defect was caused by the high intraluminal concentrations of deconjugated bile salts seen in overgrowth, since in vitro experiments had demonstrated this phenomenon.[60] However, in a series of infants with acquired monosaccharide intolerance, it was shown that the flora of duodenal fluid is often normal at the onset of monosaccharide malabsorption, and anaerobes appear only after several days in some patients.[61] This finding argues against small bowel bacterial overgrowth as a primary cause of monosaccharide intolerance and raises the question of whether this intolerance is simply another nonspecific consequence of the intestinal mucosal injury.

Aberrations in active transport of sodium and chloride have been identified in the animal model for bacterial overgrowth, the self-filling blind loop in the rat.[43] These workers demonstrated decreases in sodium and chloride

Table 39–3. PATHOPHYSIOLOGY OF SMALL BOWEL BACTERIAL OVERGROWTH

Steatorrhea
- Luminal—deconjugation of bile salts
  - Below critical micellar concentration
  - Toxic effect
- Mucosal—decreased mucosal uptake and transport

Vitamin B_{12} Deficiency
- Uptake by the abnormal bacterial flora

Protein Malabsorption/Loss
- Bacterial competition for ingested nitrogen
- Impaired cellular transport
- Secretion (protein-losing enteropathy)
- Decreased enterokinase and pancreatic proteases

Carbohydrate Malabsorption
- Luminal—utilization by bacteria
- Mucosal
  - Decreased disaccharidase activity
  - ? Monosaccharide intolerance

Fluid and Electrolyte Loss
- Changes in glucose-dependent sodium reabsorption
- Abnormal chloride flux
- Increased mucosal surface area
- Increased depth of tight junctions between crypt cells

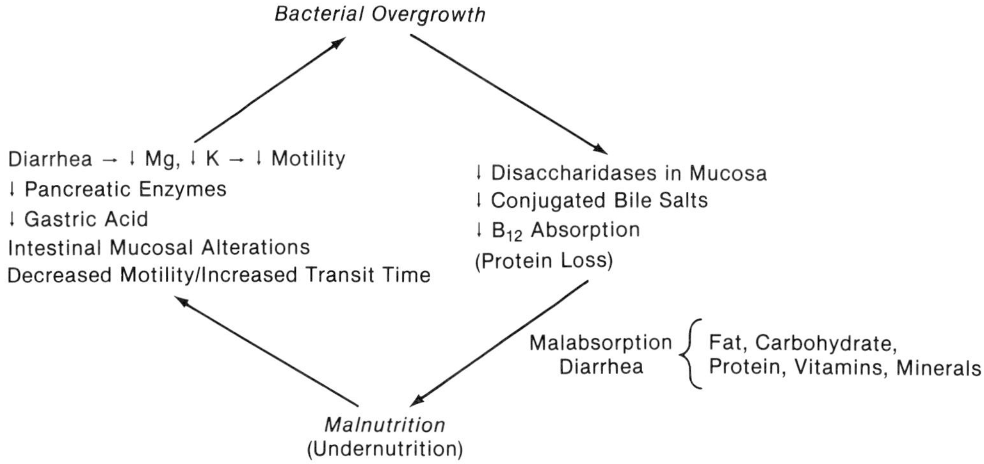

Figure 39–1. Interrelationship between malnutrition and bacterial overgrowth. (From Heyman MB, Perman JA: Nutrition in bacterial overgrowth syndromes of the gastrointestinal tract. *In* Grand RJ, Sutphen JL, Dietz WH, eds: Pediatric Nutrition: Theory and Practice. Stoneham, MA, Butterworth-Heinemann, 1987, p 449; with permission.)

fluxes, increase in epithelial resistance, and alterations in both glucose-dependent sodium absorption and chloride homeostatic mechanisms. The morphologic correlates of these abnormalities include increases in the mucosal surface area and, ultrastructurally, increased depth in crypt tight junctions.[62] The authors speculate that these changes represent an adaptive response to minimize the fluid and electrolyte loss of cellular injury. In vivo studies of this process have not been reported.

Absorption of other micronutrients may also be affected by small bowel bacterial contamination. In the presence of steatorrhea, impairment in the absorption of fat-soluble vitamins may occur. Although isolated patients with clinical vitamin deficiencies have been reported,[34] they are not common in this disorder. In experimental animals, gastrointestinal bleeding with a compensatory increase in iron absorption has been noted in the bacterial overgrowth model.[63]

DRUG METABOLISM

It has been established that intestinal flora participates in the metabolism of some pharmacologic agents.[64–66] Examples include the deconjugation of digitalis and chloramphenicol conjugates, allowing enterohepatic circulation and increased bioavailability, and the transformation of parent compounds, such as sulfasalazine and L-dopa, into metabolites with different permeability characteristics and target organs. The theoretical effect of bacterial proliferation in the upper small bowel on these processes has been discussed,[34] but clinical correlation is lacking.

MALNUTRITION

As alluded to earlier, there is a complex relationship between nutritional status and bacterial flora in the upper small intestine. There is no doubt that bacterial overgrowth can lead to severe malnutrition by causing fat, protein, and carbohydrate malabsorption. It is less often appreciated that malnutrition can cause bacterial proliferation in the upper small bowel by a number of mechanisms. This interrelationship is shown schematically in Figure 39–1. Undernutrition can cause changes in intestinal motility, and the resultant stasis may lead to overgrowth.[21] Malnutrition has also been shown to be associated with decreased gastric acid output[18, 67] and decreased pancreatic enzyme secretion,[68] both of which may increase the likelihood of overgrowth. The villous injury seen in protein-calorie malnutrition can cause carbohydrate malabsorption, which in turn may provide additional substrate for bacterial proliferation. Finally, improvement in nutritional status is associated with increased absorption and resolution of overgrowth.[55]

CLINICAL FEATURES

Patients with bacterial overgrowth may exhibit a spectrum of clinical findings, as shown in Table 39–4. In some patients, abnormal flora populating the upper small bowel have no manifestations, but in others, the signs and symptoms may be masked by underlying intestinal or systemic disease, such as Crohn's disease or AIDS. The classic presentation is that of chronic diarrhea, steatorrhea with wasting, and vitamin B_{12}-deficiency anemia. Bacterial overgrowth with its subsequent disaccharide malabsorption has been implicated as a cause of isolated recurrent abdominal pain in toddlers.[69] Two reports have documented production of lactic acid by abnormal intestinal flora, with resultant

Table 39–4. CLINICAL FEATURES OF SMALL BOWEL BACTERIAL OVERGROWTH

Signs and Symptoms
None
Related to underlying disease
Chronic diarrhea
Steatorrhea
Wasting
Recurrent abdominal pain
Megaloblastic anemia
Associated Disorders
Lactic acidosis
Arthritis-dermatitis syndrome
Hepatobiliary disease

systemic metabolic acidosis.[70, 71] Two clinical syndromes first reported in adults after jejunoileal bypass surgery have now been reported in patients with overgrowth. The first is the arthritis-dermatitis syndrome, in which there is a necrotizing vasculitis in the skin and polyarthritis or polyarthralgia.[72–74] The pathogenesis is felt to be deposition of immune complexes formed from bacterial peptidoglycans, immunoglobulins, and complement.[75] The second syndrome is hepatic steatosis and/or hepatobiliary inflammation. In a recent study using the experimental rat model, hepatic injury was shown to be unrelated to infection in the mesenteric lymph nodes, portal vein, or systemic circulation. The hepatic lesion was prevented by or treated with metronidazole, which was effective in decreasing the numbers of *Bacteroides* species in the blind loops. The authors speculate that, based on other experimental evidence, the cell wall peptidoglycan-polysaccharide polymers of these organisms are the toxic components.[76]

DIAGNOSIS

The first step in making the diagnosis of bacterial overgrowth is clinical suspicion in the setting of an underlying condition known to predispose to it, such as a motility disorder, a stricture from prior inflammatory disease, or previous gastrointestinal surgery (see Table 39–2). Table 39–5 lists the tests that have been shown to be of value in making the diagnosis of small bowel bacterial overgrowth. Contrast radiographs of the small intestine may disclose anatomic abnormalities such as strictures, diverticula, or dilated loops, but a normal small bowel series does not exclude the presence of overgrowth. Tests for the most common absorptive defects may be suggestive, such as measurement of the coefficient of fat absorption or a Schilling test with intrinsic factor, which should both be abnormal by the mechanisms discussed above.

Duodenal aspiration and culture is the most direct and sensitive method of diagnosing small bowel contamination, but this method has several drawbacks. First, duodenal intubation is an invasive procedure and, in children, may require sedation, restraint, and technical expertise. In addition, culture of strict anaerobes is not possible in many routine microbiology laboratories. This latter difficulty is somewhat bypassed by the almost universal finding of large numbers (10^6 per ml) of aerobic and facultative anaerobic organisms present in the upper small bowel of patients with anaerobic bacterial overgrowth,[77] as opposed to the 10^3 to 10^4 organisms per ml found in the duodenal fluid of normal individuals.

Table 39–5. DIAGNOSTIC TESTS IN SMALL BOWEL BACTERIAL OVERGROWTH

Test
Contrast radiography
Measurement of fecal fat excretion
Schilling test with intrinsic factor
Duodenal aspirate and culture
Duodenal fluid concentrations of:
Deconjugated bile salts
Short-chain fatty acids
Serum unconjugated bile acids
Breath tests
$^{14}CO_2$ production after:
$^{14}CO_2$-cholyl-glycine
$^{14}CO_2$-D-xylose
H_2 production after:
Fasting
Lactulose
Lactose
Glucose

Some indirect methods employ the search for metabolic products of the abnormal flora in duodenal fluid, such as deconjugated bile salts[78] or short-chain fatty acids.[57] Although the presence of these by-products not usually found in the upper small bowel is suggestive of bacterial overgrowth, the necessity for duodenal intubation and sophisticated laboratory procedures such as gas chromatography-mass spectrometry (GC-MS) or high-pressure liquid chromatography makes these methods less clinically practical.

In the past, urinary excretion of indican was used as an indirect sign of overgrowth, since luminal bacteria convert dietary tryptophan to indican,[79] but this test is not specific for bacterial overgrowth. Subsequently, it was demonstrated that patients with overgrowth have abnormal bile acid profiles in serum, with large amounts of unconjugated bile acids, predominantly deoxycholic acid.[80, 81] Other researchers showed that the greatest discrimination between normal subjects and patients with bacterial overgrowth could be made when primary or unconjugated bile acids were measured in 2-hour postprandial sera by GC-MS.[82] Again, the availability of these methods may be limited.

Because of the cumbersome nature of these tests, investigators have explored the use of breath tests as an aid in diagnosis. Breath testing entails administration of a test substance and measurement of a product of its bacterial catabolism in the individual's expired air. Again taking advantage of bacterial deconjugation of bile salts in the small bowel lumen, early work described increased breath $^{14}CO_2$ production after administration of cholyl-^{14}C-glycine in patients with overgrowth.[83] The primary drawback of this test was its inability to distinguish overgrowth from ileal malabsorption of the bile acid secondary to underlying intestinal disease. Several years later, after demonstration of catabolism of orally administered D-xylose into CO_2 by abnormal intestinal flora,[84] a $^{14}CO_2$-D-xylose test was devised and, when modified to avoid the osmotic effect of unabsorbed xylose, was shown to discriminate well between healthy individuals or patients with miscellaneous gastrointestinal disorders and patients with bacterial overgrowth.[85] The superiority of this test over the bile acid breath test was demonstrated,[86] but, over the years, different groups of investigators have disagreed about its sensitivity and specificity.[87–89]

These tests, although less invasive and difficult than those previously described, are not well suited for use in children, since radioactive materials must be used. In 1979, Rhodes and coworkers[90] reported the use of the lactulose hydrogen breath test to detect bacterial overgrowth. This test was found to have similar specificity

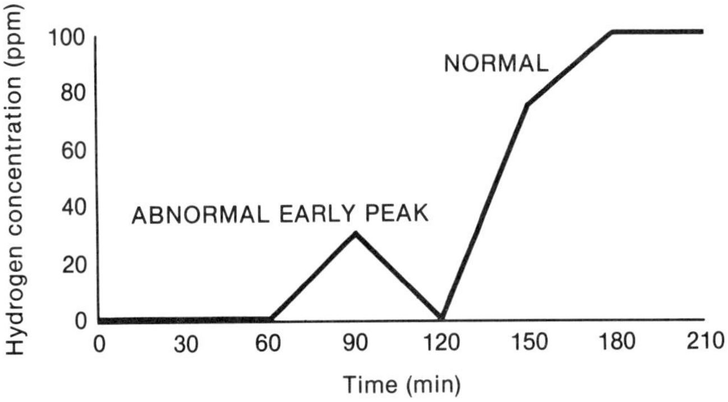

Figure 39–2. Lactulose breath H_2 test in a patient with small bowel bacterial overgrowth, demonstrating the early peak of H_2 produced when the sugar is catabolized by the bacteria in the proximal intestine, and the late peak seen in all subjects as the substrate reaches colonic flora.

and sensitivity to the bile acid breath test, with the added ability to distinguish overgrowth from ileal disease. The diagnosis of small bowel contamination is made by this method when there is an early peak in breath H_2 concentration, produced by catabolism of the lactulose by bacteria in the small intestine. This early peak is in addition to the large peak seen in normal subjects at 2 to 3 hours (Fig. 39–2), when the nonabsorbable sugar reaches the colonic flora. With similar methodology, fasting breath H_2 production and H_2 production after lactose administration were measured in infants and children with small bowel bacterial overgrowth after intestinal operations.[91] Affected patients were distinguished from healthy controls by both criteria: elevated fasting breath H_2 production and an early, sustained increase in H_2 production after lactose administration. In addition, infants with lactose malabsorption were distinguished from overgrowth patients, with a later peak in H_2 excretion, 2 to 3 hours after loading. The simple determination of fasting breath H_2 concentration was shown to be helpful in the detection of bacterial overgrowth in both children and adults presenting with chronic diarrhea.[92] Finally, the combination of elevated fasting breath H_2 level and increased H_2 excretion after glucose administration was found to be quite specific for the diagnosis of bacterial overgrowth.[93] Although many of these methods can provide valuable information, the optimal conditions, substrate, and timing of breath testing for the diagnosis of overgrowth are not yet clear.

Table 39–6. TREATMENT STRATEGIES FOR SMALL BOWEL BACTERIAL OVERGROWTH

Correction of Predisposing Condition, if Possible
Surgical repair
Prokinetic drugs
Nutritional Rehabilitation
Correction of global malnutrition
Correction of isolated nutrient deficiencies
Antibiotics
Drugs with action against anaerobes
Broad-spectrum antibiotics

TREATMENT

Treatment strategies for small bowel bacterial overgrowth are outlined in Table 39–6. The therapeutic approach has three facets. The first is correction of the predisposing condition, if possible. Anatomic causes may require surgical therapy, such as repair of strictures or fistulae or resection of diverticula. Motility disorders resulting in stasis may be more difficult to treat, but they may be amenable to prokinetic agents currently being evaluated, such as domperidone and cisapride. Patients on histamine–2 antagonists for peptic disease may benefit from regimens using higher doses with lower frequency, allowing some gastric acid to be secreted. Often, however, it is impossible to eradicate the underlying condition, and other therapeutic options must be considered.

The second component of therapy is nutritional rehabilitation. As discussed, patients with overgrowth may have profound global malnutrition or isolated micronutrient deficiencies. Evidence of this must be sought, and replacement therapy instituted. If severe underlying intestinal disease is present, nutritional therapy may involve parenteral alimentation. In many patients, however, the intestinal tract may be used. Low-fat diets supplemented with medium-chain triglycerides may be helpful[34] but are probably not necessary in most patients.[50] Because of the continued interaction between malnutrition and bacterial overgrowth, nutritional repletion may be associated with better response to the third component of therapy, antibiotics.[77]

The optimal antimicrobial therapy for small bowel bacterial overgrowth has not been elucidated. Some authors strongly recommend direct duodenal fluid culture and determination of antibiotic sensitivities as a method of determining therapy[77]; others find this invasive maneuver of little value.[94] Success is most commonly measured by improvement in clinical symptoms, such as diarrhea, or in indicators of malabsorption, such as steatorrhea and carbohydrate intolerance, rather than by repetitive culture of intestinal fluid. Since anaerobes, especially *Bacteroides,* have been implicated in most of the pathophysiologic processes of overgrowth,[32] use of antibiotics with some activity against anaerobes, such as metronidazole and chloramphenicol, has been somewhat successful[95, 96]; use of aminoglycosides, to which *Bacteroides* are usually resistant, has not.[97, 98] Alternatively, use of broad-spectrum antibiotics, such as tetracycline, ampicillin, or lincomycin, has also been successful in treatment of this syndrome.[69, 99] The mechanisms for this response are believed to be reversal of the changes in the microenvironment in the intestinal lumen caused by the aerobes, such as decreases in oxygen tension and oxidation-reduction potential, and generalized alterations in the bacterial microecology.[77]

The optimal length of antibiotic therapy has not been defined. Most investigators recommend a course of 2 to 4 weeks, since this duration of treatment has been associated with prolonged remission of symptoms in many patients.[100] Sometimes a longer second course is necessary, and, less commonly, continuous antibiotic administration with a rotating schedule of agents is necessary.

REFERENCES

1. Bishop RF, Anderson CM: Bacterial flora of the stomach and small intestine in children with intestinal obstruction. Arch Dis Child 1960; 35:487–491.
2. Long SS, Swenson RM: Development of anaerobic fecal flora in healthy newborn infants. J Pediatr 1977; 91:298–301.
3. Baberto GJ, Runge G, Fischer D, et al: Investigations on the bacterial flora, pH, and sugar content in the intestinal tract of infants. J Pediatr 1952; 40:152–163.
4. Simon GL, Gorbach SL: The human intestinal microflora. Dig Dis Sci 1986; 31(Suppl):147S–162S.
5. Simon GL, Gorbach SL: Intestinal flora in health and disease. Gastroenterology 1984; 86:174–193.
6. Gorbach SL: Population control in the small bowel. Gut 1967; 8:530–532.
7. Vantrappen G, Janssens J, Hellemans J, et al: The interdigestive motor complex of normal subjects and patients with bacterial overgrowth of the small intestine. J Clin Invest 1977; 59:1158–1166.
8. Griffen WO, Richardson JD, Medley ES: Prevention of small bowel contamination by ileocecal valve. South Med J 1971; 64:1056–1058.
9. Greenlee HB, Gelbart SM, DeOrio AJ, et al: The influence of gastric surgery on the intestinal flora. Am J Clin Nutr 1977; 30:1826–1833.
10. Brown WR, Savage DC, Dubois RS, et al: Intestinal microflora of immunoglobulin-deficient and normal human subjects. Gastroenterology 1972; 62:1143–1152.
11. McLoughlin GA, Hede JE, Temple JG, et al: The role of IgA in the prevention of bacterial colonization of the jejunum in the vagotomized subject. Br J Surg 1978; 65:435–437.
12. Smith GM, Chesner IM, Asquith P, Leyland MJ: Small intestinal bacterial overgrowth in patients with chronic lymphocytic leukaemia, J Clin Pathol 1990; 43:57–59.
13. Denison H, Wallerstedt S: Bacterial overgrowth after high-dose corticosteroid treatment. Scand J Gastroenterol 1989; 24:561–564.
14. Budhraja M, Levendoglu H, Kocka F, et al: Duodenal mucosal T cell subpopulation and bacterial cultures in acquired immune deficiency syndrome. Am J Gastroenterol 1987; 82:427–431.
15. Lake-Bakaar G, Quadros E, Beidas S, et al: Gastric secretory failure in patients with the acquired immunodeficiency syndrome (AIDS). Ann Intern Med 1988; 109:502–504.
16. McLoughlin LC, Nord KS, Joshi VV, et al: Severe gastrointestinal involvement in children with the acquired immunodeficiency syndrome. J Pediatr Gastroenterol Nutr 1987; 6:517–524.
17. Mata LJ, Jimenez F, Cordon M, et al: Gastrointestinal flora of children with protein-calorie malnutrition. Am J Clin Nutr 1972; 25:1118–1126.
18. Gracey M, Suharjono J, Sunoto W, et al: Microbial contamination of the gut: Another feature of malnutrition. Am J Clin Nutr 1973; 26:1170–1174.
19. Heyworth B, Brown J: Jejunal microflora in malnourished Gambian children. Arch Dis Child 1975; 50:27–33.
20. Omòike IU, Abiodun PO: Upper small intestinal microflora in diarrhea and malnutrition in Nigerian children. J Pediatr Gastroenterol Nutr 1989; 9:314–321.
21. Gracey M, Stone DE, Suharjono J, et al: Isolation of *Candida* species from the gastrointestinal tract in malnourished children. Am J Clin Nutr 1974; 27:345–349.
22. Chandra RK: Immunocompetence in undernutrition. J Pediatr 1972; 81:1194–1200.
23. Martini GA, Phear EA, Ruebner B, et al: The bacterial content of the small intestine in normal and cirrhotic subjects: Relation to methionine toxicity. Clin Sci 1956; 16:35–51.
24. Rubinstein E, Mark Z, Haspel J, et al: Antibacterial activity of the pancreatic fluid. Gastroenterology 1985; 88:927–932.
25. Reilly JA, Quigley EMM, Forst CF, et al: Small intestinal transit in the portal hypertensive rat. Gastroenterology 1991; 100:670–674.
26. Challacombe DN, Richardson JM, Anderson CM: Bacterial microflora of the upper gastrointestinal tract in infants without diarrhea. Arch Dis Child 1974; 49:264–269.
27. Challacombe D: Bacterial microflora in infants receiving nasojejunal tube feeding (letter). J Pediatr 1974; 85:113.
28. Watson GM, Witts LJ: Intestinal macrocytic anaemia. Br Med J 1952; 1:13–17.
29. Badenoch J: Steatorrhoea in the adult. Br Med J 1960; 1:963–974.
30. Donaldson RM: Role of enteric microorganisms in malabsorption. Fed Proc 1967; 26:1426–1431.
31. Drasas BS, Hill MJ, Shiner M: The deconjugation of bile salts by human intestinal bacteria. Lancet 1966; 1:1237–1238.
32. Kim YS, Spritz N, Blum M, et al: The role of altered bile acid metabolism in the steatorrhea of experimental blind loop. J Clin Invest 1966; 45:956–962.
33. Shimoda SS, O'Brien TK, Saunders DR: Fat absorption after infusing bile salts into the human small intestine. Gastroenterology 1974; 67:7–18.
34. King CE, Toskes PP: Small intestine bacterial overgrowth. Gastroenterology 1979; 76:178–186.
35. Wanitschke R, Ammon HV: Effects of dihydroxy bile acids and hydroxy fatty acids on the absorption of oleic acid in the human jejunum. J Clin Invest 1978; 61:178–186.
36. Ament ME, Shimoda SS, Saunders DR, et al: Pathogenesis of steatorrhea in three cases of small intestinal stasis syndrome. Gastroenterology 1972; 63:728–747.
37. Giannella RA, Rout WR, Toskes PP: Jejunal brush border injury and impaired sugar and amino acid uptake in the blind loop syndrome. Gastroenterology 1974; 67:965–974.
38. Toskes PP, Giannella RA, Jervis HR, et al: Small intestinal mucosal injury in the experimental blind loop syndrome. Gastroenterology 1975; 68:1193–1203.
39. Jonas A, Krishnan C, Forstner G: Pathogenesis of mucosal injury in the blind loop syndrome. Gastroenterology 1978; 75:791–795.
40. Banwell JG, Boldt DH, Meyers J, et al: Phytohemagglutinin derived from red kidney bean (*Phaseolus vulgaris*): A cause for intestinal malabsorption associated with bacterial overgrowth in the rat. Gastroenterology 1983; 84:506–515.
41. Baraona E, Julkunen R, Tannenbaum L, et al: Role of intestinal bacterial overgrowth in ethanol production and metabolism in rats. Gastroenterology 1986; 90:103–110.
42. Gracey M, Burke V, Oshin A, et al: Bacteria, bile salts, and intestinal monosaccharide malabsorption. Gut 1971; 12:683–692.
43. Schulzke J-D, Fromm M, Menge H, et al: Impaired intestinal sodium and chloride transport in the blind loop syndrome of the rat. Gastroenterology 1987; 92:693–698.
44. Donaldson RM Jr: Malabsorption of Co60-labeled cyanocobalamin in rats with intestinal diverticula. Gastroenterology 1962; 43:271–281.
45. Giannella RA, Broitman SA, Zamcheck N: Vitamin B_{12} uptake by intestinal microorganisms: Mechanism and relevance to syndromes of intestinal bacterial overgrowth. J Clin Invest 1971; 50:1100–1107.
46. Giannella RA, Broitman SA, Zamcheck N: Competition between bacteria and intrinsic factor for vitamin B_{12}: Implications for vitamin B_{12} malabsorption in intestinal bacterial overgrowth. Gastroenterology 1972; 62:255–260.
47. Brandt LJ, Bernstein LH, Wagle A: Production of vitamin B_{12} analogues in patients with small-bowel bacterial overgrowth. Ann Intern Med 1977; 87:546–551.
48. Hoffbrand AV, Tabaqchali S, Mollin DL: High serum-folate levels in intestinal blind loop syndrome. Lancet 1966; 1:1339–1342.
49. Hoffbrand AV, Tabaqchali S, Booth CC: Small intestinal bacterial flora and folate status in gastrointestinal disease. Gut 1971; 12:27–33.
50. Sherman P, Lichtman S: Small bowel bacterial overgrowth syndrome. Dig Dis 1987; 5:157–171.
51. Jones EA, Craigie A, Tavill AS, et al: Protein metabolism in the intestinal stagnant loop syndrome. Gut 1968; 9:466–469.
52. Miller B, Mitchison R, Tabaqchali S, et al: The effects of excessive bacterial proliferation on protein metabolism in rats with self-filling jejunal sacs. Eur J Clin Invest 1971; 2:23–31.

53. Mazzacca G, Musella S, Andria G, et al: Brush border peptidases and arylamidases in the experimental blind loop syndrome of the rat. Acta Hepato-gastroenterol 1977; 24:364–367.
54. Nygaard K, Rootwelt K: Intestinal protein loss in rats with blind segments of the small bowel. Gastroenterology 1968; 54:52–55.
55. King CE, Toskes PP: Protein-losing enteropathy in the human and experimental rat blind loop syndrome. Gastroenterology 1981; 80:504–509.
56. Rutgeerts L, Mainguet P, Tytgat G, Eggermont E: Enterokinase in contaminated small-bowel syndrome. Digestion 1974; 10:249–254.
57. Hoverstad T, Bjorneklett A, Fausa O, et al: Short-chain fatty acids in the small-bowel bacterial overgrowth syndrome. Scand J Gastroenterol 1985; 20:492–499.
58. Jonas A, Flanagan PR, Forstner GG: Pathogenesis of mucosal injury in the blind loop syndrome. Brush border enzyme activity and glycoprotein degradation. J Clin Invest 1977; 60:1321–1330.
59. Sherman P, Wesley A, Forstner G: Sequential disaccharidase loss in rat intestinal blind loops: Impact of malnutrition. Am J Physiol 1985; 248:G626–G632.
60. Gracey M, Burke V, Oshin A: Reversible inhibition of intestinal active sugar transport by deconjugated bile salt in vitro. Biochim Biophys Acta 1971; 225:308–314.
61. Kilby AM, Dolby JM, Honour P, et al: Duodenal bacterial flora in early stages of transient monosaccharide intolerance in infants. Arch Dis Child 1977; 52:228–234.
62. Schulzke J-D, Fromm M, Bentze CJ, et al: Adaptation of the jejunal mucosa in the experimental blind loop syndrome: Changes in paracellular conductance and tight junction structure. Gut 1987; 28(S1):159–164.
63. Giannella RA, Toskes PP: Gastrointestinal bleeding and iron absorption in the experimental blind loop syndrome. Am J Clin Nutr 1976; 29:754–757.
64. Scheline RR: Metabolism of foreign compounds by gastrointestinal microorganisms. Pharmacol Rev 1973; 25:451–523.
65. Goldman P, Peppercorn MA, Goldin BR: Metabolism of drugs by microorganisms in the intestine. Am J Clin Nutr 1974; 27:1348–1355.
66. Lindenbaum J, Rund DG, Butler VP, et al: Inactivation of digoxin by the gut flora: Reversal by antibiotic therapy. N Engl J Med 1981; 305:789–794.
67. Viteri FE, Schneider RE: Gastrointestinal alterations in protein-calorie malnutrition. Med Clin North Am 1974; 58:1487–1505.
68. Gyr K, Felsenfeld O, Zimmerli-Ning M: The effect of oral pancreatic enzymes on the intestinal flora of protein-deficient vervet monkeys challenged with *Vibrio Cholerae.* Am J Clin Nutr 1979; 32:1592–1596.
69. Davidson GP, Robb TA, Kirubakanan CP: Bacterial contamination of the small intestine as an important cause of chronic diarrhea and abdominal pain: Diagnosis by breath hydrogen test. Pediatrics 1984; 74:229–235.
70. Schoorel EP, Giesberts MAH, Blom W, et al: D-lactic acidosis in a boy with short bowel syndrome. Arch Dis Child 1980: 55:810–812.
71. Stolberg L, Rolfe R, Gitlin N, et al: D-lactic acidosis due to abnormal gut flora. Diagnosis and treatment of two cases. N Engl J Med 1982; 306:1344–1348.
72. Jorizzo JL, Apisarnthanarx P, Subrt P, et al: Bowel-bypass syndrome without bowel bypass. Bowel-associated dermatosis-arthritis syndrome. Ann Intern Med 1983; 143:457–461.
73. Klinkhoff AV, Stein HB, Schlappner OLA, Boyko WB: Post-gastrectomy blind loop syndrome and the arthritis-dermatitis syndrome. Arth Rheum 1985; 28:214–217.
74. Fairris GM, Ashworth J, Cotterill JA: A dermatosis associated with bacterial overgrowth in jejunal diverticula. Br J Dermatol 1985; 112:709–713.
75. Clegg DO, Zone JJ, Samuelson CO Jr, Ward JR: Circulating immune complexes containing secretory IgA in jejunoileal bypass disease. Ann Rheum Dis 1985; 44:239–244.
76. Lichtman SN, Keku J, Schwab JH, Sartor RB: Hepatic injury associated with small bowel bacterial overgrowth in rats is prevented by metronidazole and tetracycline. Gastroenterology 1991; 100:513–519.
77. Goldstein F, Mandle RJ, Schaedler RW: The blind loop syndrome and its variants: Microbiologic aspects of diagnosis and treatment. Am J Gastroenterol 1973; 60:255–264.
78. Northfield TC, Drasar BS, Wright JT: Value of small intestinal bile acid analysis in the diagnosis of the stagnant loop syndrome. Gut 1973; 14:341–347.
79. Aarbakke J, Schjonsby H: Value of urinary simple phenol and indican determinations in the diagnosis of the stagnant loop syndrome. Scand J Gastroenterol 1976; 11:409–414.
80. Setchell KDR, Harrison DL, Gilbert JM, et al: Serum unconjugated bile acids: Qualitative and quantitative profiles in ileal resection and bacterial overgrowth. Clin Chim Acta 1985; 152:297–306.
81. Masclee A, Tangerman A, Van Schaik A, et al: Unconjugated serum bile acids as a marker of small intestinal bacterial overgrowth. Eur J Clin Invest 1989; 19:384–389.
82. Bolt MJG, Stellaard F, Sitrin MD, et al: Serum unconjugated bile acids in patients with small bowel bacterial overgrowth. Clinica Chimica Acta 1989; 181:87–102.
83. Sherr HP, Sasaki Y, Newman A, et al: Detection of bacterial deconjugation of bile salts by a convenient breath-analysis technic. N Engl J Med 1971; 285:656–661.
84. Toskes PP, King CE, Spivey JC, et al: Xylose catabolism in the experimental rat blind loop syndrome. Gastroenterology 1978; 74:691–697.
85. King CE, Toskes PP, Spivey JC, et al: Detection of small intestine bacterial overgrowth by means of a ^{14}C-D-xylose breath test. Gastroenterology 1979; 77:75–81.
86. King CE, Toskes PP, Guilarte TR, et al: Comparison of the one-gram d-[^{14}C] bile acid breath test in patients with small-intestine bacterial overgrowth. Dig Dis Sci 1980; 25:53–58.
87. Rumessen JJ, Gudmand-Hoyer E, Bachmann E, et al: Diagnosis of bacterial overgrowth of the small intestine. Comparison of the ^{14}C-D-xylose breath test and jejunal cultures in 60 patients. Scand J Gastroenterol 1985; 20:1267–1275.
88. King DE, Toskes PP: Comparison of the 1-gram [^{14}C]xylose, 10-gram lactulose-H_2 and 80-gram glucose-H_2 breath tests in patients with small intestine bacterial overgrowth. Gastroenterology 1986; 91:1447–1451.
89. Suhr O, Danielsson A, Horstedt P, et al: Bacterial contamination of the small bowel evaluated by breath tests, 75Se-labelled homocholic-tauro acid, and scanning electron microscopy. Scand J Gastroenterol 1990; 25:841–852.
90. Rhodes JM, Middleton P, Jewell DP: The lactulose hydrogen breath test as a diagnostic test for small-bowel bacterial overgrowth. Scand J Gastroenterol 1979; 14:333–336.
91. Nose O, Kai H, Harada T, et al: Breath hydrogen test in infants and children with blind loop syndrome. J Pediatr Gastroenterol Nutr 1984; 3:364–367.
92. Perman JA, Modler S, Barr RG, et al: Fasting breath hydrogen concentration: Normal values and clinical application. Gastroenterology 1984; 87:1358–1363.
93. Kerlin P, Wong L: Breath hydrogen testing in bacterial overgrowth of the small intestine. Gastroenterology 1988; 95:982–988.
94. Isaacs PET, Kim YS: Blind loop syndrome and small bowel bacterial contamination. Clin Gastroenterol 1983; 12:395–414.
95. Bjorneklett A, Fausa O, Midtvedt T: Small-bowel bacterial overgrowth in the postgastrectomy syndrome. Scand J Gastroenterol 1983; 18:277–287.
96. Hammond-Gavvaden C, Heinkens GT, Jackson AA: Small bowel overgrowth in malnourished children as measured by breath hydrogen test. West Indian Med J 1985; 34:48–49.
97. Barry RE, Chow AW, Billesdon J: Role of intestinal microflora in colonic pseudo-obstruction complicating jejunoileal bypass. Gut 1977; 18:356–359.
98. Welkos SL, Toskes PP, Baer H, et al: Importance of anaerobic bacteria in the cobalamin malabsorption of the experimental rat blind loop syndrome. Gastroenterology 1981; 80:313–320.
99. Sarna SK: Cyclic motor activity: Migratory motor complex. Gastroenterology 1985; 89:894–913.
100. Banwell JG, Kistler LA, Giannella RA, et al: Small intestinal bacterial overgrowth syndrome. Gastroenterology 1981; 80:834–845.

Chapter 40

Protein-Losing Enteropathy

WALLACE A. GLEASON, JR.

Gastrointestinal protein loss was found to be responsible for "idiopathic catabolic hypoproteinemia" by Gordon[1] in 1959, who described the process as "exudative enteropathy," implying an active protein secretion localized to the intestine. Since lesions in the esophagus (gastroesophageal reflux) and stomach (hypertrophic gastropathy) may also cause enteric protein loss, the term *gastrointestinal protein loss* proposed by Waldmann[2, 3] seems more accurate, reflecting a wider distribution of lesions and the transudative nature of the protein loss accompanying lymphatic obstruction. Nonetheless, the term most commonly used to describe this situation is *protein-losing enteropathy*.

PATHOPHYSIOLOGY

The gastrointestinal tract may be responsible for as much as 10% of total body protein catabolism. Normally, less than 2% of circulating serum albumin is lost per day. Gastrointestinal protein catabolism, in which circulating proteins are imported into cells and degraded in lysosomes, is different from protein-losing enteropathy, in which proteins are spilled into the lumen of the gastrointestinal tract. The highly impermeable barrier to gastrointestinal protein loss consists of the cell membranes of enterocytes joined at apical tight junctions. Compromise of this barrier, allowing serum proteins to enter the intestinal lumen, results from (1) mucosal erosion or ulceration; (2) obstruction of the thoracic duct transmitted back to the lacteals, the thin lymphatic channels within the core of the small intestinal villi, resulting in rupture and loss of the constituents of lymph (fluid, proteins, lymphocytes); or (3) surface cell loss or damage, with disruption of the mucosal barrier.[4]

Many types of circulating proteins may be lost during this process. Since albumin is responsible for most of the oncotic pressure holding fluid within the vascular space, loss of albumin into the intestine decreases plasma oncotic pressure, with subsequent leakage of fluid out of capillaries. This results in edema, which is frequently the most dramatic sign of protein-losing enteropathy. Loss of immunoglobulin can result in recurrent infections.

The hypoalbuminemia depends on at least three variable factors: (1) the rate of albumin loss, (2) the liver's ability to increase the rate of synthesis to replace the deficit and keep up with ongoing losses, and (3) the decrease in nonenteric catabolism in response to lower serum levels.

DIAGNOSIS

Protein-losing enteropathy is not a specific disease, but a pathophysiologic process.[5] Successful treatment therefore requires precise diagnosis of the underlying disease with its extensive differential diagnosis.[6] This discussion is limited to those disorders that have been associated with protein-losing enteropathy in children.

Symptoms of the underlying illness may include diarrhea, abdominal pain, and allergic phenomena and may be elicited in the medical history. Edema, usually positional, is a frequent complaint and finding. In infants, edema frequently manifests as facial and periorbital swelling. Older children, who spend more time erect, are more likely to develop ankle and leg edema. Asymmetric lymphedema may be a clue to an underlying disorder of lymphatic channels such as primary intestinal lymphangiectasia.

The goal of initial laboratory investigations is to ascertain and explain the hypoalbuminemia, taking into account the lower normal values for serum albumin in infants and children (Table 40–1) and other possible etiologies (e.g., renal or liver disease or malnutrition).

Anthropometric criteria for height for age (length in infants), weight for age, and weight for height are readily determined. These are reliable data that can rule out malnutrition of a degree required to produce hypoalbuminemia. Routine urinalysis can rule out proteinuria, and normal levels of transaminases exclude hepatic dysfunction. A convenient and reliable estimate of hepatic synthetic function is provided by the prothrombin time, although vitamin K deficiency due to intestinal malabsorption can lead to an abnormal result. Prothrombin time should become normal promptly after a

Table 40–1. AGE-RELATED NORMAL VALUES IN GM PER DL (RANGE) FOR SERUM PROTEINS

Age	Total	Albumin	Globulin
Premature	5.5 (4–6)	3.7 (2.5–4.5)	1.8 (1.2–2)
Neonate (term)	6.4 (5–7.1)	3.4 (2.5–5)	3.1 (1.2–4)
1–3 months	6.6 (4.7–7.4)	3.8 (3–4.2)	2.5 (1–3.3)
3–12 months	6.8 (5–7.5)	3.9 (2.7–5)	2.6 (2–3.8)
1–15 years	7.4 (6.5–8.6)	4.0 (3.2–5)	3.1 (2–4.4)

From Cole CH, ed: The Harriet Lane Handbook: A Manual for Pediatric House Officers. 10th ed. Chicago, Year Book Medical Publishers, 1984, p 354; with permission.

parenteral dose of vitamin K if it is due to vitamin K deficiency.

DEMONSTRATION OF PROTEIN-LOSING ENTEROPATHY

The demonstration of protein-losing enteropathy requires the detection in stool of a circulating macromolecule that is not absorbed, secreted, or degraded in the gastrointestinal tract. The easier it is to measure the marker, the more useful the test will be. Most such techniques involve identification of markers that have either been injected or secreted into the blood compartment.

The original demonstration of exudative enteropathy used ^{131}I-labeled polyvinyl pyrrolidone.[1] Since the rate of protein loss could theoretically be affected by the size, shape, and charge of the labeled macromolecule, the use of ^{131}I-albumin soon followed as a more physiologic marker. Although the technique for iodination of macromolecules was straightforward and the iodinated macromolecules were easy to detect, thyroid uptake of the ^{131}iodine, luminal digestion of the radiolableled albumin, and reabsorption of ^{131}I-labeled peptides confounded interpretation.[7] Most of these problems were solved with the introduction of ^{51}Cr-labeled albumin,[2] which became the most widely used radiolabeled macromolecule for studying protein-losing enteropathy.[3]

Radiolabeled macromolecules impose hazards and inconveniences, limiting their attractiveness for use in children. Exposure to ionizing radiation prohibits their use in pediatric clinical research. Six to ten days of hospitalization are required, as is a 48- to 72-hour stool collection with meticulous avoidance of urine contamination—a difficult task in infants and children. These inconveniences, and the emergence of better techniques, have made interest in these techniques largely historical.

Extensive clinical experience using sodium pertechnitate ^{99m}Tc-labeled human serum albumin for scintigraphy has revealed that less than 0.5% of an intravenous dose normally appears in stool or urine within 24 hours.[8] Based on this observation, scintigraphic imaging has been used to demonstrate gastrointestinal protein loss.[9–11] Unlike other techniques, scintigraphic imaging localizes the site of gastrointestinal protein loss, but it is not yet clear how that information is useful. Exposure to radiation limits its utility in pediatrics. Although this technique may be helpful in documenting protein-losing enteropathy, experience is too limited to allow such a judgment at present.

FECAL EXCRETION OF ALPHA$_1$-ANTITRYPSIN

In 1977, Crossley and Elliott showed that children with gastrointestinal protein loss documented by ^{51}Cr-labeled albumin had levels of fecal alpha-1-antitrypsin (FA$_1$-AT), measured by radial immunodiffusion, that were 10-fold higher than were levels from adults and children with no evidence of protein-losing enteropathy.[12] FA$_1$-AT was independent of serum levels of alpha$_1$-antitrypsin (A$_1$-AT) and fecal water content. Random samples varied no more than twofold, validating the use of random samples as a screening test for protein-losing enteropathy.

FA$_1$-AT fulfills the criteria as a marker for protein-losing enteropathy and has the following additional advantages:

1. It is a serum protein.
2. It is not present in the diet; thus fecal levels reflect only protein entering the intestine from the intravascular space.
3. Its molecular weight of 50,000 daltons is similar to that of albumin.
4. As a protease inhibitor, it resists intraluminal proteolysis and is excreted without degradation in the stool.
5. Urine contamination of the stool specimen will not invalidate the result—a feature particularly helpful in pediatric patients.

The original description of this technique emphasized its simplicity.[12] Further studies in which FA$_1$-AT clearance (FA$_1$-AT times the weight of stool per 24 hours divided by serum A$_1$-AT) was determined provide no convincing evidence that the increase in precision to be gained justifies the inconvenience of prolonged stool collection. These studies, however, are useful in validating the use of random samples. For example, there is a linear correlation between the clearances of radiolabeled serum albumin and FA$_1$-AT[13–15] and little day-to-day variation in the excretion of FA$_1$-AT during several consecutive days of stool collection.[14, 16, 17] FA$_1$-AT is excreted in two forms: alone and complexed with enzyme.[18] As a result, radial immunodiffusion slightly underestimates the total amount of FA$_1$-AT present and may account for the slight differences noted between the clearances of FA$_1$-AT and radiolabeled serum albumin.[13, 19]

Levels of FA$_1$-AT in stool are stable. Ninety-three percent of the FA$_1$-AT remained after 72 hours of incubation at 37°C, allowing transport of specimens prior to assay. A$_1$-AT is undetectable in gastric juice, and

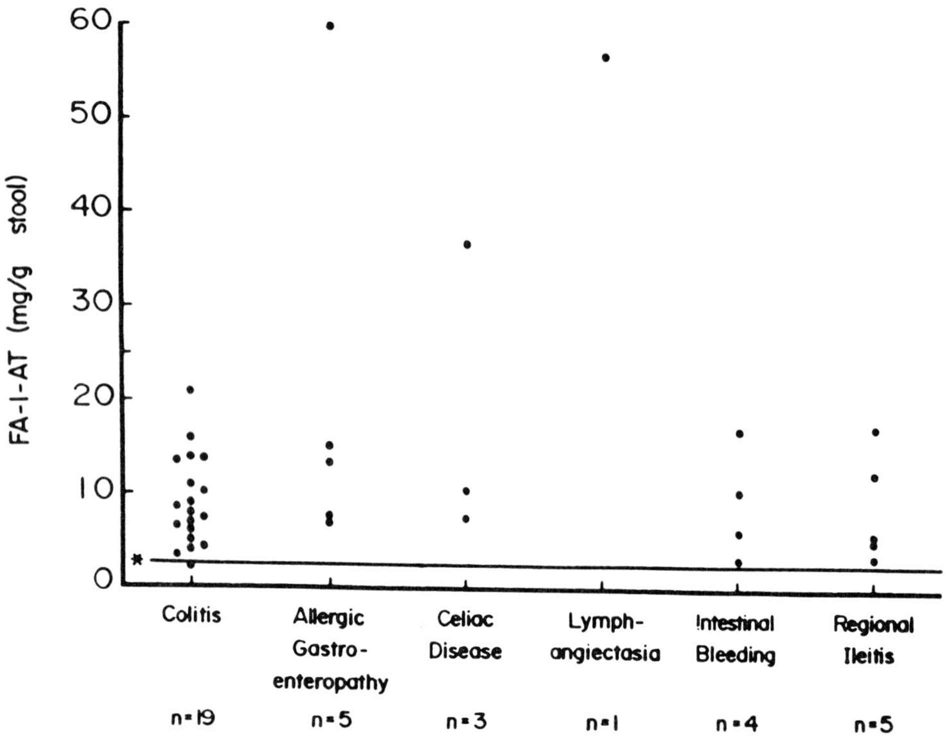

Figure 40–1. Random FA_1-AT concentrations in children with various gastrointestinal disorders. (From Thomas DW, Sinatra FW, Merritt RJ: Random fecal alpha$_1$-antitrypsin concentration in children with gastrointestinal disease. Gastroenterology 1981; 80:776–782; with permission.)

exogenous A_1-AT is destroyed in vitro after 1-hour incubation at 37°C, in gastric juice but not in duodenal juice.[13] The reliability of FA_1-AT in detecting esophageal or gastric protein loss is therefore questionable.

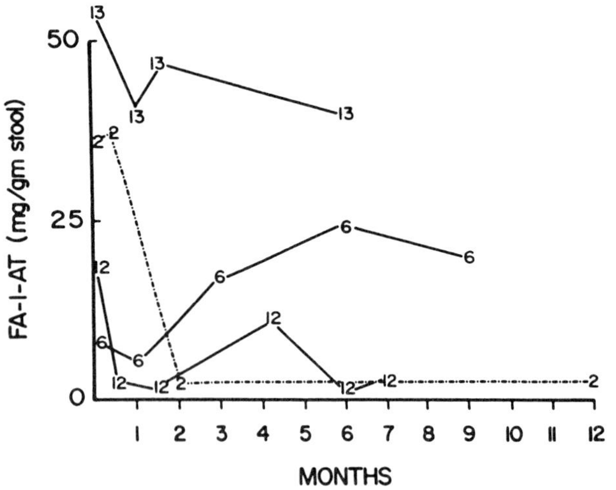

Figure 40–2. Serial random FA_1-AT concentrations in four children. Case 2, Falling level in response to introduction of a gluten-free diet in a child with celiac disease. Case 6, Initial response to an elemental diet in a child with allergic gastroenteropathy with subsequent relapse after reintroduction of solid foods. Case 12, Response to ileal resection for regional ileitis followed by relapse 4 months after surgery and subsequent response to corticosteroid therapy. Case 13, Lymphangiectasia after cardiac surgery unresponsive to total parenteral nutrition, elemental diet, and dietary fat restriction. (From Thomas DW, Sinatra FW, Merritt RJ; Random fecal alpha$_1$-antitrypsin concentration in children with gastrointestinal disease. Gastroenterology 1981; 80:776–782; with permission.)

Since meconium contains higher levels of A_1-AT than does stool,[20] this technique is not recommended in neonates younger than 1 week of age. Although one might expect that patients with low levels of circulating A_1-AT may have falsely low levels of FA_1-AT, increased levels of FA_1-AT has been reported in patients with homozygous P_iZZ A_1-AT deficiency. Although the mechanism of excretion of FA_1-AT in these patients is unclear and is not related to the presence of liver disease, it is not thought to contribute to the low circulating levels of A_1AT.[21]

With the wide use of this simple, accurate test, subclinical protein-losing enteropathy has been found in many disorders in which it was unexpected (Figs. 40–1, 40–2). This discovery has broadened the scope and expanded the differential diagnosis of protein-losing enteropathy to include disorders other than those presenting with hypoalbuminemia (e.g., normal serum albumin values in 24% of children in one series).[22] Although this may reflect the insensitivity of serum albumin as a test for protein-losing enteropathy, it also questions the clinical importance of gastrointestinal protein loss of this extent. These disorders rarely, if ever, present with hypoalbuminemia and edema, and the magnitude of protein loss is only two to four times normal, considerably less than in children presenting with hypoalbuminemia.

SPECIFIC ENTITIES

Infections

Protein-losing enteropathy is seen in a number of gastrointestinal infections characterized by mucosal erosion or ulceration (Table 40–2). Forty percent of children with acute diarrheal illnesses have elevated levels of FA_1-AT. The levels can be up to four times the upper limit of normal, and elevated levels commonly accompany inflammatory conditions such as salmonellosis and parasitic infections.[23–26] Increased levels of FA_1-AT occur in enterocolitis due to *Clostridium dificile*[27] and *Clostridium perfringens*.[28] FA_1-AT is transiently increased in rotavirus diarrhea,[23–26] although studies on this point are not unanimous.[25] Increased FA_1-AT excretion rarely persists longer than 5 days in these infections, an important point in the commonly encountered clinical problem of distinguishing between an acute, self-limited infection and a chronic enteric disorder.[26] These diagnoses are best approached by microbiologic studies identifying the agents in stool specimens. Cytomegalovirus and *Helicobacter pylori* have been implicated in the pathogenesis of hypertrophic gastropathy (see later).

The observation that measles commonly precipitates kwashiorkor in children in developing nations led to studies demonstrating protein-losing enteropathy in malnourished African children with measles infection.[29, 30] According to a recent study in Bangladesh, enteric infections, a major problem in malnourished children recovering from measles, are more likely to be complicated by protein-losing enteropathy in children within 2 weeks of recovering from measles than in those with an absent or remote history of measles.[31]

The clinical importance of the relatively small gastrointestinal loss of protein in these children is uncertain. Gastrointestinal protein loss in enteric infections may be important in the development of malnutrition in children with diarrhea,[23–26] but increased gastrointestinal protein loss in children with marasmus and marasmic kwashiorkor without enteric infection[32, 33] also suggests a self-perpetuating abnormality of intestinal function due to mucosal edema regardless of the inciting factor.

Unlike the conditions described earlier, giardiasis[34–36] and strongyloidiasis[37] can cause gastrointestinal protein loss in sufficient quantity to result in hypoalbuminemia and edema. Both conditions are diagnosed by identifying the parasites or their cysts or ova in stool or, more dependably, by duodenal intubation or a string test, such as the Enterotest (see Chapter 49).

Table 40–2. PROTEIN-LOSING ENTEROPATHY IN INFANTS AND CHILDREN

Mucosal Erosion or Ulceration

Infectious

- *Clostridium dificile*[27]
- *Clostridium perfringens*[28]
- Cytomegalovirus[89]
- *Giardia lamblia*[34–36]
- *Helicobacter pylori*[37, 91–93]
- Hypertrophic gastropathy (Ménétrier's disease)[83–90]
- Measles[29–31]
- Rotavirus[23–26]
- Salmonellosis[24]
- *Strongyloides stercoralis*[37]

Noninfectious

- Allergic gastroenteropathy[38]
- Anastomotic ulceration/ischemia[42–44]
- Atopic dermatitis[40, 41]
- Burns[65]
- Cow's milk feeding[58]
- Gastroesophageal reflux[54]
- Gluten-sensitive enteropathy[16, 55]
- Graft-vs-host disease[45]
- Henoch-Schönlein purpura[39]
- Inflammatory bowel disease[22, 47–51]
- Malakoplakia[64]
- Malnutrition[32, 33]
- Multiple polyposis[59–63]
- Necrotizing enterocolitis[56]
- Phenobarbital hypersensitivity[46]
- Systemic lupus erythematosus[52, 53]

Lymphatic Obstruction

Intestinal lymphangiectasia

- Arsenic poisoning[73]
- Familial[67–69]
- Heart disease[74–80]
- Inflammatory[70]
- Nephrotic syndrome[81]
- Noonan's syndrome[71, 72]
- Primary[66–73]

Noninfectious Inflammatory Disorders

In 1967, Waldmann and colleagues described six children presenting with edema, growth retardation, extreme hypoalbuminemia (1.5–2.4 gm per dl), hypogammaglobulinemia, anemia, eosinophilia, and other manifestations of allergy, such as asthma, eczema, and allergic rhinitis.[38] Although most of these patients were infants, one was 14 years old. Normal absorption of D-xylose and the absence of steatorrhea excluded gluten-sensitive enteropathy, cystic fibrosis, and intestinal lymphangiectasia. All had protein-losing enteropathy that responded to an elimination diet or corticosteroids. These patients were determined to be allergic to cow's milk, based on the reversal of gastrointestinal protein loss when it was excluded from the diet and the development of vomiting and diarrhea and exacerbation of the gastrointestinal protein loss when it was reintroduced—leading to the designation "allergic gastroenteropathy." A similar steroid-responsive protein-losing enteropathy has been encountered in patients with Henoch-Schönlein purpura.[39]

Although protein-losing enteropathy has been indirectly implicated in the mechanism of hypoalbuminemia in a child with atopic dermatitis,[40] a more formal assessment found no greater increase in the incidence of gastrointestinal protein loss in children with atopic dermatitis than was found in normal children.[41]

Anastomotic ulceration after distal small bowel resection causes recurrent iron deficiency[42, 43] and protein-losing enteropathy with or without persistent hypoalbuminemia.[43] A similar picture can be seen as a repercussion of intestinal ischemia.[44]

Twenty-five percent of patients undergoing bone-marrow transplantation develop graft versus host disease involving the intestine, a disorder with hypoproteinemia that is due, in part, to protein-losing enteropathy. This disorder is more common in children older than 13 years of age and is heralded by the development of diarrhea more than 20 days after bone-marrow transplantation.[45] A similar clinical syndrome has been ascribed to phenobarbital hypersensitivity.[46]

Inflammatory bowel disease is an important cause of protein-losing enteropathy (see Figs. 40–1, 40–2). In general, the severity of hypoalbuminemia and the degree of protein loss are greater in patients with Crohn's disease than in those with ulcerative colitis, and greater in those with diffuse small bowel disease than in those with limited small bowel or colonic disease.[22, 47, 48] Classically, 50 to 60% of children with Crohn's disease have mild to pronounced hypoalbuminemia.[49–51] An even greater proportion, 70 to 80%, have protein-losing enteropathy without hypoalbuminemia when studied with radiolabeled serum albumin. In mild cases with normal levels of serum albumin, there is little correlation between measures of severity or extent of disease and the amount of gastrointestinal protein loss.

In young women, systemic lupus erythematosus can present with hypoalbuminemia and edema due to gastrointestinal protein loss,[52] and this has also been recorded in a child.[53]

In a curious syndrome of gastroesophageal reflux, protein-losing enteropathy, and finger clubbing, the mechanism of protein-losing enteropathy was presumably exudation from the inflamed esophageal mucosa, since it was accompanied by bleeding and resolved completely after successful surgical treatment by fundoplication.[54]

Children with untreated celiac disease have elevated levels of FA_1-AT that are approximately three times normal at diagnosis and decrease with the duration of dietary gluten elimination (see Figs. 40–1, 40–2).[16, 55] Elevated levels of FA_1-AT are also seen in neonatal necrotizing enterocolitis.[56] Although a correlation between blood in the stools and levels of FA_1-AT might be expected in inflammatory intestinal disorders such as these, none has been found in several studies,[22, 47, 48, 56, 57] probably because the mass ratio of hemoglobin to A_1-AT in plasma is roughly 160 to 1 at normal levels of both proteins.[18]

Infants fed cow's milk–based formulas have higher levels of FA_1-AT than do exclusively breast-fed infants or breast-fed infants whose feedings are supplemented with cow's milk–based formula. Although it is tempting to speculate that this is evidence of a subtle enteropathy associated with cow's milk, again there was no correlation between FA_1-AT and hemoglobin in the stools of these infants.[58]

Juvenile colonic polyps are usually solitary, histologically benign lesions with no premalignant potential that cause painless hematochezia or, less commonly, intussusception. A syndrome of multiple juvenile polyps with chronic gastrointestinal bleeding and protein-losing enteropathy can lead to inanition. Unlike solitary juvenile colonic polyps, which are seen most commonly in preschool-aged children, these lesions present in infancy.[59–61] Macrocephaly, in one case due to intracranial cysts, has been reported in several cases.[62, 63] The mechanism of gastrointestinal protein loss is unknown, but inflammation has been incriminated in the pathogenesis of both solitary and multiple juvenile polyps. The prognosis is poor because of the hundreds of polyps throughout the stomach, small bowel, and colon. Malakoplakia of the colon produces a similar clinical picture, with chronic gastrointestinal bleeding and gastrointestinal protein loss as a result of polypoid lesions throughout the colon. These lesions have the characteristic histiocytic infiltration and Michaelis-Guttman bodies when examined histologically.[64]

FA_1-AT levels are increased in burned children. Claimed to be caused by an alteration in intestinal mucosal permeability demonstrable in burned patients, FA_1-AT correlates with the surface area of the burn.[65] The levels in even the most severely burned children are only slightly elevated, and the clinical significance is unclear.

Since fecal excretion of FA_1-AT tends to decrease as inflammatory gastrointestinal disorders resolve, FA_1-AT may be a convenient, noninvasive way to provide follow-up for infants and children with such illnesses.

Lymphatic Obstruction

The term *intestinal lymphangiectasia* describes a group of disorders in which dilatation of the lacteals—the fine, thin-walled lymphatic channels extending up into the small bowel villi—results from obstruction of the flow of lymph through the thoracic duct and into the superior vena cava.[66] Fat intake leads to further distention and rupture of lacteals, resulting in steatorrhea and drainage of lymph into the intestine. The resulting loss of protein, lymphocytes, and immunoglobulins ultimately results in hypoalbuminemia, lymphopenia, and hypogammaglobulinemia, respectively. These findings can represent important clues to the diagnosis, and the presence of all three is virtually pathognomonic.

Intestinal lymphangiectasia may be primary or secondary to other causes of lymphatic obstruction. Familial forms, with different patterns of inheritance, have been described,[67–69] and Fleisher and associates described a patient with intestinal lymphangiectasia thought to be caused by an inflammatory disorder because of its response to corticosteroid therapy.[70] The intestine may be the only site of lymphatic obstruction, or it may coexist with multifocal lymphatic dysplasia, such as Noonan's syndrome.[71, 72] Intestinal lymphangiectasia has been described as a manifestation of arsenic poisoning.[73]

Cardiac disorders or surgical procedures resulting in transmission of elevated pressure from the right atrium into the superior vena cava and thoracic duct, including clinically silent constrictive pericarditis,[74] have been complicated by the development of intestinal lymphangiectasia (see Fig. 40–2).[75–78] More recently, resolution of protein-losing enteropathy with corticosteroid therapy has been reported in patients with intestinal lymphangiectasia due to right atrial hypertension after a Fontan procedure for congenital heart disease.[79, 80] The response of some of these patients, who have been seriously ill with severe diarrhea, anasarca, and inanition, after 15 days of intravenous corticosteroids indicates that patience and persistence are important in dealing with this difficult clinical situation. These observations imply that corticosteroid responsiveness of some forms of secondary intestinal lymphangiectasia may be due to effects other than the anti-inflammatory effect of these agents. Postulated mechanisms include stabilization of lymphatic and capillary membranes and a decrease in the volume of lymphatic tissue.

Gastrointestinal protein loss occurs in the acute phase of idiopathic nephrotic syndrome. Its cause is unknown, but histologic features of intestinal lymphangiectasia have been found in intestinal biopsies of some children.[81] Perhaps the known variability of the extent and severity of the intestinal lesion in patients with intestinal lymphangiectasia explains why it can be demonstrated only in some nephrotic patients.[82] The reader is referred to the detailed discussion of intestinal lymphangiectasia in Chapter 45.

Hypertrophic Gastropathy (Ménétrier's Disease)

A syndrome of gastrointestinal protein loss and giant hypertrophy of the gastric rugae has been recognized to have radiologic, endoscopic, and histologic features suggestive of Ménétrier's disease.[83, 84] However, since Ménétrier's disease in adults is not transient, as the disorder seems to be in children and adolescents, a better term is *transient hypertrophic gastropathy*.[85, 86] These children present with abdominal pain and vomiting and with the gradual development of edema and ascites. The cause is unknown, but an allergic cause has been suggested by several cases in children with a history of atopy.[87] Some cases have been associated with evidence of infection with cytomegalovirus.[88, 89] The ultrastructural finding of increased width of tight junctions between the plasma membranes of gastric epithelial cells, recently cited as responsible for gastrointestinal protein loss, seems equally plausible as a result of edema.[90] Recovery of *H. pylori* from children with hypertrophic gastropathy[91–93] and the observation of severe gastrointestinal protein loss in children with *H. pylori* gastritis[37] have engendered the speculation that this organism is responsible for transient hypertrophic gastropathy in childhood. All reports emphasize that transient hypertrophic gastropathy is benign and self-limited, requiring no specific therapy. The distinctions between true Ménétrier's disease, as it is encountered in adults, taken together with the association of hypertrophic gastropathy with infectious agents, serve as the rationale for classifying it in the category of infections in Table 40–2.

TREATMENT

As previously stated, the treatment of protein-losing enteropathy is the treatment of the underlying disease. The reader is therefore referred to sections of this text in which specific diagnostic entities are discussed.

REFERENCES

1. Gordon RS: Exudative enteropathy. Abnormal permeability of the gastrointestinal tract demonstrable with labeled polyvinyl pyrrolidone. Lancet 1959; 1:325–327.
2. Waldmann TA: Gastrointestinal protein loss demonstrated by ^{51}Cr-labeled albumin. Lancet 1961; 2:121–123.
3. Waldmann TA: Gastrointestinal protein loss in pediatrics. *In* James AE, Wagner HN, Cooke RE, eds: Pediatric Nuclear Medicine. Philadelphia, WB Saunders, 1974, pp 442–445.
4. Perrault J, Markowitz H: Protein-losing gastroenteropathy and the intestinal clearance of serum alpha$_1$-antitrypsin. Mayo Clin Proc 1984; 59:278–279.
5. Parfitt AM: Familial neonatal hypoproteinemia with exudative enteropathy and intestinal lymphangiectasis. Arch Dis Child 1966; 41:54–62.
6. Colon AR, Sandberg DH: Protein-losing enteropathy in children. South Med J 1973; 66:641–644.
7. Freeman T, Gordon AH: Measurement of albumin leak into the gastrointestinal tract using I-131 albumin and ion exchange resins by mouth. Gut 1964; 5:155–157.
8. McAfee JG, Stern GF, Fueger MS, et al: Tc-99m labeled serum albumin for scintillation scanning of the placenta. J Nucl Med 1964; 5:936–946.
9. Divgi CR, Lisann NM, Yeh SDJ, et al: Technetium-99m albumin scintigraphy in the diagnosis of protein-losing enteropathy. J Nucl Med 1986; 27:1710–1712.
10. Lan JA, Chervu LR, Marans Z, et al: Protein-losing enteropathy detected by ^{99m}Tc-labeled human serum albumin abdominal scintigraphy. J Pediatr Gastroenterol Nutr 1988; 7:872–876.
11. Kashiwagi T, Fukui H, Jyoku T, et al: Imaging diagnosis of protein- losing enteropathy by 99m Tc-labeled serum albumin. Kaku-Igaku 1990; 27:1361–1368.
12. Crossley JR, Elliot RB: Simple method for diagnosing protein-losing enteropathies. Lancet 1977;1:428–429.
13. Florent C, L'Hirondel C, Desmazures C, et al: Intestinal clearance of alpha-antitrypsin: A sensitive method for the detection of protein-losing enteropathy. Gastroenterology 1981; 81:777–780.
14. Hill RE, Hercz A, Corey ML, et al: Fecal clearance of alpha$_1$-antitrypsin: A reliable measure of enteric protein loss in children. J Pediatr 1981; 99:416–418.
15. Karbach U, Ewe K, Bodenstein H: Alpha$_1$-antitrypsin, a reliable endogenous marker for instestinal protein loss and its application in patients with Crohn's disease. Gut 1983; 24:718–723.
16. Dinari G, Rosenbach Y, Zahavi I, et al: Random fecal alpha$_1$-antitrypsin excretion in children with intestinal disorders. Am J Dis Child 1984; 138:971–973.
17. Maggazzu G, Jacono G, DiPasquale G, et al: Reliability and usefulness of random fecal alpha$_1$-antitrypsin concentration: Further simplification of the method. J Pediatr Gastroenterol Nutr 1985; 4:402–407.
18. Buffone GJ, Shulman RJ: Characterization and evaluation of immunochemical methods for the measurement of fecal alpha$_1$-antitrypsin. Am J Clin Pathol 1985; 83:326–330.
19. Perrault J, Markowitz H: Protein-losing gastroenteropathy and the intestinal clearance of serum alpha$_1$-antitrypsin. Mayo Clin Proc 1984; 59:288–289.
20. Ryley HC, Lynne N, Brogan TD, et al: Plasma proteins in meconium from normal infants and from babies with cystic fibrosis. Arch Dis Child 1974; 49:901–904.
21. Grill BB, Tinghitella T, Hillemeier AC, et al: Increased intestinal clearance of alpha$_1$-antitrypsin in patients with alpha$_1$-antitrypsin deficiency. J Pediatr Gastroenterol Nutr 1983; 2:95–98.
22. Thomas DW, Sinatra FR, Merritt RJ: Random fecal alpha$_1$-antitrypsin concentration in children with gastrointestinal disease. Gastroenterology 1981; 80:776–782.
23. Maki M, Harmionen A, Vesikari T, et al: Fecal excretion of alpha$_1$-antitrypsin in acute diarrhea. Arch Dis Child 1982; 57:154–156.
24. Fontana M, Zuin G, Galli L, et al: Fecal alpha$_1$-antitrypsin excretion in acute diarrhea: Relationship with causative pathogens. Helv Pediatr Acta 1988; 43:211–218.
25. Hoffman H Du, Hanekom C: Random fecal alpha$_1$-antitrypsin excretion in children with acute diarrhea. J Trop Pediatr 1987; 33:299–301.

26. Zuin G, Fontana M, Nicoli S, et al: Persistence of protein loss in acute diarrhea—a follow-up study by fecal alpha$_1$-antitrypsin measurement. Acta Paediatr Scand 1991; 80:961–993.
27. Rybolt AH, Bennett RG, Laughon BE, et al: Protein-losing enteropathy with *Clostridium dificile* infection. Lancet 1989; 1:1353–1355.
28. Ehringhaus C, Dominick H-C, Schuller M: Protein-losing enteropathy associated with *Clostridium perfringens*. Lancet 1989; 2:268–269.
29. Dossetor JFB, Whittle HC: Protein-losing enteropathy and malabsorption in acute measles enteritis. Br Med J 1975; 2:592–593.
30. Axton JHM: Measles: A protein-losing enteropathy. Br Med J 1975; 2:79–80.
31. Sarker SA, Wahed MA, Rahaman MM, et al: Persistent protein-losing enteropathy in post measles diarrhea. Arch Dis Child 1986; 61:739–743.
32. Lunn PG, Whitehead RG, Coward WA: Two pathways to kwashiorkor? Trans Roy Soc Trop Med Hyg 1979; 73:438–444.
33. Madina EH, Soliman AT, Morsi MR: Protein-losing enteropathy in the different forms of protein-energy malnutrition. J Trop Pediatr 1987; 33:254–256.
34. Sherman P, Liebman WM: Apparent protein-losing enteropathy associated with giardiasis. Am J Dis Child 1980; 134:893–894.
35. Sutton DL, Kamath KR: Giardiasis with protein-losing enteropathy. J Pediatr Gastroenterol Nutr 1985; 4:56–59.
36. Korman SH, Bar-Oz B, Mandelberg A, et al: Giardiasis with protein-losing enteropathy: Diagnosis by fecal alpha$_1$-antitrypsin determination. J Pediatr Gastroenterol Nutr 1990; 10:249–252.
37. Sullivan PB, Thomas JE, Eastham EJ, et al: *Helicobacter pylori* and protein-losing enteropathy. Arch Dis Child 1990; 65:332–333.
38. Waldmann TA, Wochner RD, Laster L, et al: Allergic gastroenteropathy: A cause of excessive protein loss. N Engl J Med 1967; 276:761–769.
39. Reif S, Jain A, Santiago J, et al: Protein-losing enteropathy as a manifestation of Henoch-Schönlein purpura. Acta Pediatr Scand 1991; 80:482–485.
40. Jenkins HR, Walker-Smith JA, Atherton DJ: Protein-losing enteropathy in atopic dermatitis. Pediatr Dermatol 1986; 3:125–129.
41. Pike MG, Riches P, Atherton DJ: Fecal alpha$_1$-antitrypsin concentration and gastrointestinal permeability to oligosaccharides in atopic dermatitis. Pediatr Dermatol 1989; 6:10–12.
42. Parashar K, Kyawhla S, Booth IW, et al: Ileocolic ulceration: A long-term complication following ileocolic anastomosis. J Pediatr Surg 1988; 23:226–228.
43. Couper RTL, Durie PR, Stafford SE, et al: Late gastrointestinal bleeding and protein loss after distal small-bowel resection in infancy. J Pediatr Gastroenterol Nutr 1989; 9:454–460.
44. Thompson JF, Levy J, Stolar CJH, et al: Protein-losing enteropathy in prolonged post-ischemic ileitis. J Pediatr Gastroenterol Nutr 1986; 5:504–507.
45. Weisdorf SA, Salati LM, Longsdorf JA, et al: Graft-versus-host disease of the intestine: A protein losing enteropathy characterized by fecal alpha$_1$-antitrypsin. Gastroenterology 1983; 85:1076–1081.
46. Knutsen AP, Shah M, Schwarz KB, et al: Graft versus host–like illness in a child with phenobarbital hypersensitivity. Pediatrics 1986; 78:581–584.
47. Grill BB, Hillemeier AC, Gryboski JD: Fecal alpha$_1$-antitrypsin clearance in patients with inflammatory bowel disease. J Pediatr Gastroenterol Nutr 1984; 3:56–61.
48. Thomas DW, Sinatra FR, Merritt RJ: Fecal alpha$_1$-antitrypsin excretion in young people with Crohn's disease. J Pediatr Gastroenterol Nutr 1983; 2:491–496.
49. Silverman A, Roy CC: Pediatric clinical gastroenterology. 3d ed. St. Louis, CV Mosby, 1983, p 377.
50. Beeken WL, Busch HJ, Sylvester DL: Intestinal protein loss in Crohn's disease. Gastroenterology 1972; 62:207–215.
51. Beeken WL: Absorptive defects in young people with Crohn's disease. Pediatrics 1973; 52:69–74.
52. Perednia DA, Corosh NA: Lupus-associated protein-losing enteropathy. Arch Intern Med 1990; 150:1806–1810.
53. Tsukahara M, Matsuo K, Kojima H: Protein-losing enteropathy in a boy with systemic lupus erythematosus. J Pediatr 1980; 97:778–779.
54. Herbst JJ, Johnson DG, Oliveros MA: Gastroesophageal reflux with protein-losing enteropathy and finger clubbing. Am J Dis Child 1976; 130:1256–1258.
55. Catassi C, Cardinali E, D'Angelo G, et al: Reliability of random fecal alpha-antitrypsin determination on nondried stools. J Pediatr 1986; 109:500–502.
56. Shulman RJ, Buffone G, Wise L: Enteric protein loss in necrotizing enterocolitis as measured by fecal alpha-1-antitrypsin excretion. J Pediatr 1985; 107:287–289.
57. Woodruff C, Fabacher D, Latham C: Fecal alpha$_1$-antitrypsin and infant feeding. J Pediatr 1985; 106:228–232.
58. Morrow RJ, Lawson N, Hussaini SH, et al: The usefulness of fecal hemoglobin, albumin and alpha$_1$-antitrypsin in the detection of gastrointestinal bleeding. Ann Clin Biochem 1990; 27:208–212.
59. Arbeter AM, Courtney RA, Gaynor MF: Diffuse gastrointestinal polyposis associated with chronic blood loss, hypoproteinemia, and anasarca in an infant. J Pediatr 1970; 76:609–611.
60. Soper RT, Kent TH: Fatal juvenile polyposis in infancy. Surgery 1971; 69:692–698.
61. Gourley GR, Odell GB, Selkurt J, et al: Juvenile polyps associated with protein-losing enteropathy. Dig Dis Sci 1982; 27:941–945.
62. Schwartz AM, McCauley RKG: Juvenile gastrointestinal polyposis. Radiology 1976; 121:441–444.
63. Scharf GM, Becker JHR, Laage NJ: Juvenile gastrointestinal polyposis or the infantile Cronkhite-Canada syndrome. J Pediatr Surg 1986; 21:953–954.
64. Satti MB, Abu-Melha A, Taha OMA, et al: Colonic malakoplakia and abdominal tuberculosis in a child: Report of a case with review of the literature. Dis Colon Rectum 1985;28:353–357.
65. Matoth I, Granot E, Gorenstein A, et al: Gastrointestinal protein loss in children recovering from burns. J Pediatr Surg 1991; 26:1175–1178.
66. Waldmann TA, Steinfeld JL, Dutcher TF, et al: The role of the gastrointestinal system in idiopathic hypoproteinemia. Gastroenterology 1961; 41:197–207.
67. Bronspiegel N, Zelnick N, Rabinowitz H, et al: Aplasia cutis congenita and intestinal lymphangiectasia: An unusual complication. Am J Dis Child 1985; 139:509–513.
68. Mucke J, Hoepffner W, Scheerschmidt G, et al: Early onset lymphedema, recessive form—a new form of genetic lymphedema syndrome. Eur J Pediatr 1986; 145:195–198.
69. Hennekam RCM, Geerdink RA, Hamel BCJ, et al: Autosomal recessive intestinal lymphangiectasia and lymphedema, with facial anomalies and mental retardation. Am J Med Genet 1989; 34:593–600.
70. Fleisher TA, Strober W, Muchmore AV, et al: Corticosteroid-responsive intestinal lymphangiectasia secondary to an inflammatory process. N Engl J Med 1979; 300:605–606.
71. Vallet HL, Holtzapple PG, Eberlein WR, et al: Noonan syndrome with intestinal lymphangiectasis: A metabolic and anatomic study. J Pediatr 1972; 80:269–274.
72. Herog DB, Logan R, Kooistra JB: The Noonan syndrome with intestinal lymphangiectasia. J Pediatr 1976; 88:270–272.
73. Kobayashi A, Ohbe Y: Protein-losing enteropathy associated with arsenic poisoning. Am J Dis Child 1972; 121:515–517.
74. Vesin P, Cattan D: Constrictive pericarditis with protein-losing enteropathy: Role of the lymphatic system. *In* Dirke G, Norberg R, Plantin L, eds: Physiology and Pathophysiology of Plasma Protein Metabolism. London, Pergamon Press, 1968, pp 115–162.
75. Sondheimer JM, Hamilton JR: Intestinal function in infants with severe congenital heart disease. J Pediatr 1978; 92:572–578.
76. Gleason WA, Roodman ST, Laks H: Protein-losing enteropathy and intestinal lymphangiectasia after superior vena cava-right pulmonary artery (Glenn) shunt. J Thorac Cardiovasc Surg 1979; 77:843–846.
77. Hess J, Kruizinga K, Bijleveld CMA, et al: Protein-losing enteropathy after Fontan operation. J Thorac Cardiovasc Surg 1984; 88:606–609.
78. Kirk CR, Gibbs JL, Wilkinson JL, et al: Protein-losing enteropathy caused by baffle obstruction after Mustard's operation. Br Heart J 1988; 59:69–72.
79. Rothman A, Snyder J: Protein-losing enteropathy following the Fontan operation: Resolution with prednisone therapy. Am Heart J 1991; 121:618–619.
80. Rychik J, Piccoli DA, Barber G: Usefulness of corticoid steroid therapy for protein-losing enteropathy after the Fontan procedure. Am J Cardiol 1991; 68:819–821.
81. Salazar De Sousa J, Guerreiro O, Cunha A, et al: Association of nephrotic syndrome with intestinal lymphangiectasia. Arch Dis Child 1968; 43:245–248.

82. Vardy PA, Lebenthal E, Schwachman H: Intestinal lymphangiectasia: A reappraisal. Pediatrics 1975; 55:842–851.
83. Sandberg DH: Hypertrophic gastropathy (Ménétrier's disease) in childhood. J Pediatr 11971; 78:866–868.
84. Tokatli A, Ozsoylu S: Ménétrier disease in a child. J Pediatr Gastroenterol Nutr 1991; 12:404–406.
85. Lachman RS, Martin DJ, Vawter GF: Thick gastric folds in childhood. Am J Radiol 1971; 112:83–92.
86. Pesce F, Barbino A, Dufour C, et al: Hypertrophic gastropathy with transient sessile polyps. J Pediatr Gastroenterol Nutr 1992; 14:323–326.
87. Marks MP, Lanza MV, Kahlstrom EJ, et al: Pediatric hypertrophic gastropathy. Am J Radiol 1986; 147:1031–1034.
88. Stillman AE, Sieber O, Manthei U, et al: Transient protein-losing enteropathy and enlarged gastric rugae in childhood. Am J Dis Child 1981; 135:29–33.
89. Leonidas JC, Beatty EC, Wenner HA: Ménétrier's disease and cytomegalovirus infection in childhood. Am J Dis Child 1973; 126:806–808.
90. Oderda G, Cinti S, Cangiotti AM, et al: Increased tight junction width in two children with Ménétrier's disease. J Pediatr Gastroenterol Nutr 1990; 11:123–127.
91. Hill ID, Sinclair-Smith C, Lastovica AJ, et al: Transient protein losing enteropathy associated with acute gastritis and *Campylobacter pylori*. Arch Dis Chid 1987; 62:1215–1219.
92. *Campylobacter pylori* and protein losing enteropathy in children (editorial). Lancet 1988; 1:865–866.
93. Cohen HA, Shapiro RP, Frydman M, et al: Childhood protein-losing enteropathy associated with *Helicobacter pylori* infection. J Pediatr Gastroenterol Nutr 1991; 13:201–203.

Chapter 41

Celiac Disease

RICCARDO TRONCONE and SALVATORE AURICCHIO

Celiac disease (CD), also called *gluten-sensitive enteropathy*, is a permanent intestinal intolerance to the dietary wheat gliadin and related proteins that produces lesions in genetically susceptible persons.

HISTORICAL BACKGROUND

CD was first described by Samuel Gee in 1888, but it was not until the early 1950s that Dicke in Holland established the role of wheat and rye flour in the pathogenesis of the disease and identified the protein known as *gluten* as the harmful factor in those cereals.[1] Additional understanding of the disease followed the development of peroral biopsy techniques of the small bowel. A characteristic mucosal lesion, villous atrophy,[2] was identified and led to the development of criteria for the diagnosis of celiac disease by the European Society for Paediatric Gastroenterology and Nutrition (ESPGAN)[3] in 1969.

CEREAL PROTEINS AND OTHER ENVIRONMENTAL FACTORS

The cereals that are toxic for people with celiac disease are wheat, rye, barley, and probably oats. Rice and maize are nontoxic and are usually used as wheat substitutes in the diet of celiac patients. Cereal grains belong to the grass family (Gramineae). Grains other than wheat that are toxic for celiac patients (e.g., rye, barley, and oats) bear a close taxonomic relationship to wheat (Fig. 41–1).[4] Wheat seed endosperm contains heterogeneous protein classes differentiated according to their extractability and solubility in different solvents into albumins, globulins, gliadins, and glutenins. The wheat toxicity results from the gliadin protein fraction,[5] and the toxicity of other cereals is most likely associated with prolamin fractions equivalent to gliadins in the grain of these other species.[6]

Gliadins are single polypeptide chains ranging in molecular weight from 30 to 75 kd. Gliadins have a low charge and a high glutamine and proline content. They have been classified according to their electrophoretic mobilities into groups designated alpha, beta, gamma, and omega. More recently they have been classified on the basis of their N-terminal amino acid sequences into alpha, gamma, and omega types. A-gliadin is the major alpha gliadin component that is associated with celiac disease. Its primary amino acid sequence has been determined,[7] and in vitro studies based on the effect of specific A-gliadin peptides of known amino acid sequences on the organ culture of atrophic celiac mucosa have led to the identification of some putatively toxic sequences. The largest amino acid sequences that are common to in vitro toxic peptides and absent in the nontoxic peptides are pro-ser-gln-gln and gln-gln-gln-pro.[8] It is difficult to assess how the results obtained by in vitro models apply to the in vivo situation. The identification of the peptide amino acid sequences responsible for toxicity in celiac patients must ultimately rely on in vivo studies based on gluten challenge.

The influence of environmental factors other than gluten in CD is suggested by changes in the incidence of the disease over time and in various locations, and by the reported discordance in about 30% of monozygotic twins. Feeding practices seem to be relevant; the protective effect of breast feeding has been well documented.[9] More recently, Scandinavian studies have suggested that the type and amount of cereals introduced in infant diets have a profound effect on the clinical features and incidence of the disease.[9a]

Among environmental factors that could play a role in CD are infective agents. Adenovirus serotype 12 (Ad 12) is of particular interest because one of its proteins (E1b protein) shows significant amino acid sequence homology with an antigenically active gluten peptide.[10] Viral infection and subsequent exposure to gliadin might trigger the development of the enteropathy as a result of immunological cross-reactivity. Although serological evidence of past exposure to Ad12 is present in a higher percentage of celiac patients than healthy subjects,[11] and T cell responses to the viral dodecapeptide sharing homology with A-gliadin have been found in celiac patients,[12] no antibodies to the specific adenovirus 12 E1b 58 kd protein cross-reacting with A-gliadin have been demonstrated in patients with CD.[13]

GENETICS OF CELIAC DISEASE

Family Studies

The occurrence of celiac disease in multiple family members has been well documented. In a recent multi-

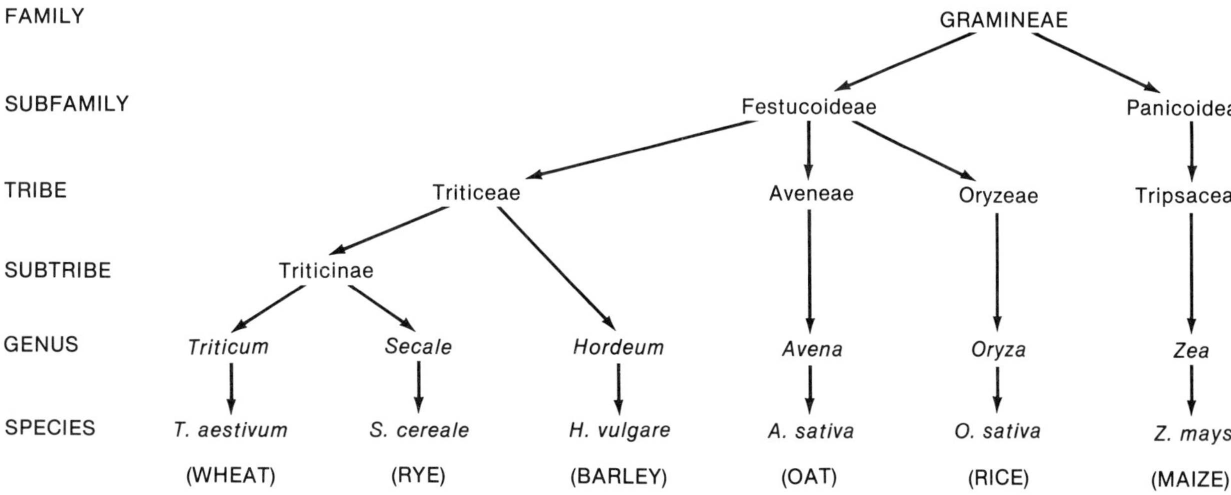

Figure 41–1. Taxonomic relationships of major cereal grains. (From Kasarda DD, Qualset CO, Mecham DK, et al: A test of toxicity of bread made from wheat lacking alpha-gliadins coded for by the 6A chromosome. *In* McNicholl B, McCarthy CF, Fottrell PF, eds: Perspectives in Celiac Disease. Lancaster, MTP Press, 1978, pp 55; with permission.)

center study, the prevalence of celiac disease among first-degree relatives of celiac patients was 8.7%. Most of the newly diagnosed patients were asymptomatic,[14] but most of them could be identified by immunoglobulin A (IgA) antireticulin antibody determination. When nonaffected relatives of patients with celiac disease were compared to a control population, they exhibited an increased serum level of gliadin antibodies.[15] In vitro proliferation of lymphocytes suggested a primed cell-mediated immunity to gliadin.[16] The importance of genetic factors in celiac disease is also suggested by a concordant rate of 75% in monozygotic twin pairs with the disease.[17]

Genetic Markers

The major genetic association of celiac disease is with genes and gene products of the major histocompatibility complex (MHC) locus on chromosome 6. The human MHC includes three subregions: class I (HLA-A, -B, -C), class II (HLA-DR, -DQ, -DP), and class III (properdin Bf, complement C2 and C4, and 21 hydroxylase). The strongest association of CD is with the HLA class II D region markers; class I and class III region gene association are secondary to linkage disequilibrium between specific markers (alleles) in those regions and in the class II D region. HLA-DR3 and HLA-DQw2 specificities are present in more than 90% of celiac patients.[18] The joint segregation of HLA-DP genes with those encoding serologic specificities HLA-DR3 and HLA-DQw2 suggests that the class II HLA haplotype associated with celiac disease is extended throughout the entire HLA D region.[19] The interest in an association between CD and MHC class II genes is that these genes code for molecules whose predominant function is to bind selected antigens and to make them recognizable by T cells. Each subregion of the HLA class II region (HLA-DR, -DQ, and -DP) contains A and B genes, which encode the respective alpha and beta chains of the alpha-beta heterodimer molecule expressed on the surface of the antigen presenting cells. It is now suggested that the association leading to disease susceptibility is not with a structural variant in a particular class II gene, but with a novel molecule created by transcomplementation of alpha and beta chains (Fig. 41–2).[20]

EPIDEMIOLOGY

The reported prevalence of CD ranges from 12 to 203 per 100,000, with a mode around 90 per 100,000.[21] The prevalence in women appears to be greater than that in men. High prevalence rates have been reported in European countries (Fig. 41–3), but CD is uncommon in the United States, even in those population groups with the same genetic background as European populations. CD has been well documented in other geographic areas such as the Indian subcontinent, North Africa, the Middle East, and South America. Significant changes in prevalence have also been noted over time.

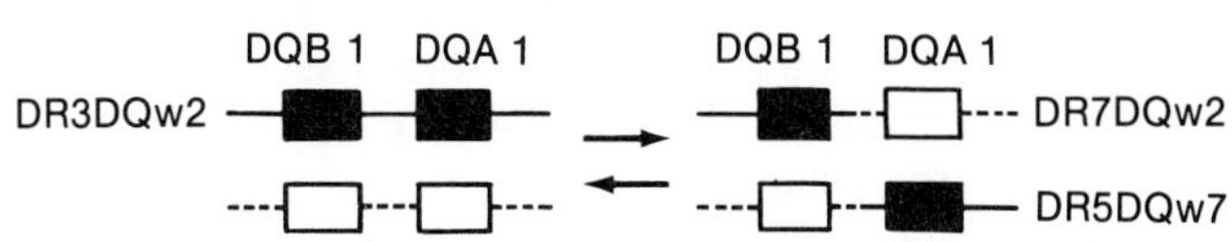

Figure 41–2. Schematic representation of structural relationships between MHC genes. Boxes with equivalent shading represent identical genes. Most CD patients share a particular combination of a DQA1 and a DQB1 gene. These genes are arranged in cis position on the DR3DQw2 haplotype and in trans position in DR5DQw7/DR7DQw2 heterozygous individuals. Thus, the great majority of CD patients share the same HLA DQ alpha/beta heterodimer involved in antigen presentation. (From Sollid ML, Markussen G, Ek J, et al: Evidence for a primary association of celiac disease to a particular HLA-DQ alpha/beta heterodimer. J Exp Med 1989; 169:345–350; by copyright permission of the Rockefeller University Press.)

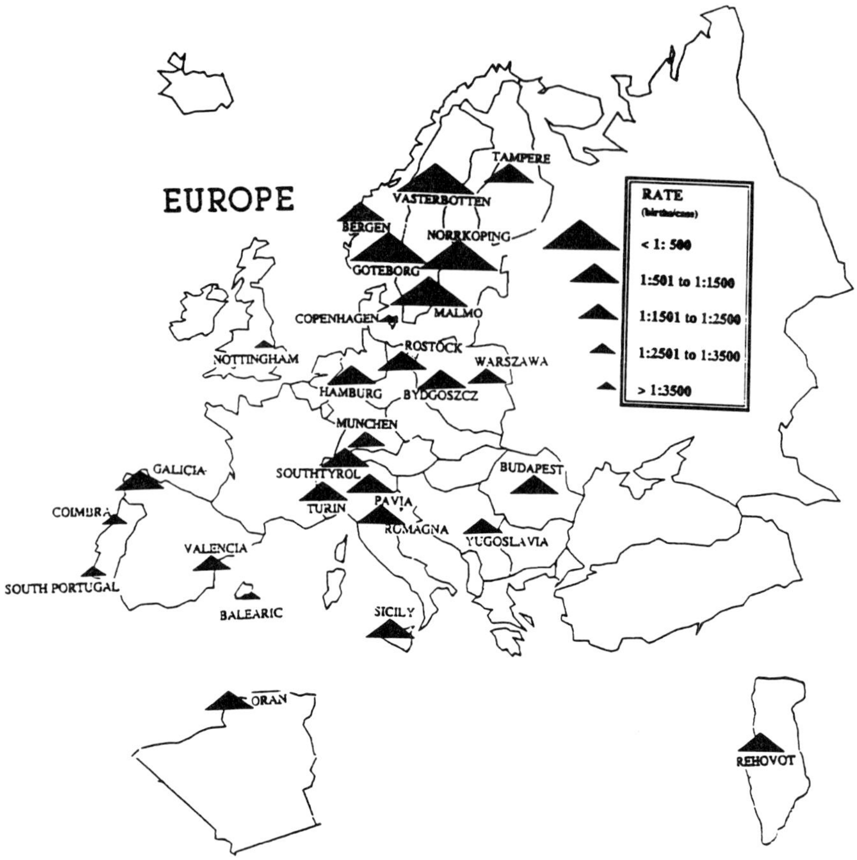

Figure 41–3. Incidence of CD in Europe. Results from the Working Group on Epidemiology of CD of ESPGAN. (Courtesy of Dr. L. Greco.)

Some of these variations may be consequences of environmental factors other than dietary gluten. Changes in infant feeding practices, such as prolonged breast feeding,[9] lower antigenicity of the formulas used, and later introduction of gluten into the diet, have all been considered to explain the reported decline in the incidence of CD.[21, 22] Nevertheless, it is now becoming clear that in the countries where a decreasing incidence of CD has been found, the disease is not really disappearing, but only changing in clinical presentation. In Finland, CD is rarely diagnosed under the age of five years, presenting in the majority of cases in school-aged children and adolescents.[23] Recently, a significantly higher incidence of CD has been reported in Sweden—one in 300 people—and has been attributed to the earlier introduction of gluten-containing formulas.

A precise estimate of the prevalence of CD is difficult because of the paucity of symptoms in some patients with a characteristic biopsy. Asymptomatic cases have been identified in screening programs of high-risk populations (e.g., first-degree relatives of CD patients and patients affected by diseases known to be associated with CD) and even in healthy people. Among blood donors, the prevalence of asymptomatic celiac disease has been found to be as high as one in 266.[24] This finding, along with the recent figures of prevalence in Sweden, suggests that the true prevalence of the disease is much higher than supposed, and probably approaches one in 300 people.

Finally, it is now becoming clear that an even greater proportion of individuals has a latent form of gluten sensitivity with apparently normal small intestinal mucosa despite exposure to moderate amounts of gluten (preceliac disease). In some of these individuals, increasing the amount of gluten in the diet will precipitate the enteropathy.[25, 26] The true prevalence of latent celiac disease remains unknown.

PATHOGENESIS

Theories of Pathogenesis

The earliest theory of the pathogenesis of CD is based on the "missing peptidase" hypothesis elaborated in the 1950s. Despite intensive investigation, this hypothesis has not been validated. Several authors have shown that the pattern of gliadin digestion is no different in celiacs as compared to normal subjects, and that peptidase activities are normal, or almost normal, in the mucosa of celiacs on a gluten-free diet.

Another theory proposed to explain the pathogenesis of the mucosal lesion in CD is based on a direct nonimmunomediated cytotoxic activity of gliadin peptides on the small intestine. Evidence for a cytotoxic mechanism of injury is supported by studies showing that gliadin peptides inhibit improvement of the in vitro cultured atrophic celiac mucosa, cause reversible inhibition of the in vitro development of fetal rat intestine, and are able to agglutinate undifferentiated human

K562(S) cells.[27] A nonimmunomediated, lectin-like effect of gliadin related to this ability to bind glycoproteins with high mannose glycans has been proposed following the demonstration of in vivo induction of gliadin-mediated enterocyte damage in rats treated with swainsonine, a substance that induces the expression of high-mannose-type glycoproteins on enterocytes.[28]

Alternatively, it has been suggested that CD, like other food-protein-sensitive enteropathies, has an immunologic basis. The immunologic theory is supported by data at the systemic and mucosal level. The presence of high titers of serum IgG and IgA antibodies to gliadin in patients with active disease has been recognized for a long time and has been used for diagnostic purposes.[29] In untreated CD, a striking increase of jejunal IgA, IgM, and IgG immunocytes has been noted,[30] and in intestinal secretions raised levels of immunoglobulins IgA, IgM, and IgG and of antigliadin antibody have been demonstrated.[31] Recently it has been reported that this characteristic pattern of intestinal humoral immunity in celiac patients with enteropathy persists after mucosal recovery on a gluten-free diet, suggesting that there is permanent abnormality of mucosal immunity.[31]

Evidence of a cell-mediated reaction to gliadin in the peripheral blood and jejunal mucosa of celiac patients has been observed.[32] Reactivity to gluten in the peripheral blood is decreased in patients on a gluten-containing diet in comparison to those who are treated, suggesting that gliadin-reactive lymphocytes may be specifically sequestered in the gut mucosa.[33] However, the most striking evidence for involvement of cell-mediated mechanisms in the mucosa of celiac patients comes from analogies with animal models in which intestinal delayed-type hypersensitivity has been induced. Villous atrophy, hyperplasia of the crypts of Lieberkuhn, and raised numbers of intraepithelial lymphocytes are all features observed in models of activation of gut cell-mediated immunity, such as allograft rejection, graft-versus-host reaction, or infection with nematodes.[34] The parallels between such models and CD suggest a common immunopathogenic mechanism. In CD, crypt enterocytes have an increased mitotic rate; a role played by lymphokines has been hypothesized, but the actual lymphokine has not been identified, although interleukin 2 and gamma interferon seem to be excluded. The cellularity of the celiac mucosa is significantly increased, both in the lamina propria and in the intraepithelial compartments. Although the CD4 to CD8 lymphocyte ratio is unchanged both in the epithelium and in the lamina propria, many more CD4+ cells show signs of activation as they express the CD7 phenotype.[35] Furthermore, the percentage of CD3+ intraepithelial lymphocytes expressing the CD45RO marker is increased, suggesting an accumulation of antigen-primed memory T cells in the celiac epithelium.[36] Increased numbers of "double negative" intraepithelial T cells (CD3+ CD4− CD8−), most of these cells expressing the T cell receptor gamma delta, have also been demonstrated.[37] Such an increase has been reported to be specific for celiac disease; furthermore, the finding of an increased proportion of gamma/delta+ T cells in patients on a gluten-free diet seems to suggest a primary abnormality.[38] The function of this cell subset remains obscure, although it has been suggested that these cells may primarily be directed against intestinal microorganisms or are perhaps specialized for elimination of transformed, infected, or otherwise "stressed" autologous cells. Also mediated by soluble factors (e.g., gamma interferon) is the increased epithelial expression of MHC class II determinants: In the normal human small intestine, HLA-DR is expressed by the villous enterocytes, and epithelial cells in the Lieberkuhn crypts do not express this marker; in patients with untreated celiac disease, any enhanced HLA-DR expression occurs in the crypt epithelium.[39] The latter phenomenon has recently been reproduced in vitro in the celiac mucosa from patients in remission cultured in the presence of gliadin peptides. This model could prove useful for the identification of unknown epitopes of gliadin that might trigger the T cell-mediated mucosal immune response.[40] Finally, a marked upregulation of the expression of intercellular adhesion molecule 1 (ICAM 1) has been noted in the cells infiltrating the lamina propria of CD patients.[41] ICAM 1 is a cell surface sialoglycoprotein induced in response to proinflammatory cytokines and is crucial for the cell-cell interactions in the early phases of the immune response.

Spectrum of Cell-Mediated Intestinal Damage

It should be noted that structural features of cell-mediated intestinal damage represent a spectrum. Marsh[42] has demonstrated, by sequential challenge and clinical history, that a mucosal lesion evolves from an early phase characterized by an infiltrative pattern, through a hyperplastic lesion, to the destructive picture of the flat mucosa. The mucosa in the earlier phase is characterized by normal villi whose epithelium is filled with numerous small nonmitotic lymphocytes. This occurs in patients challenged orally with a low dose of gliadin, in some first-degree relatives of celiac patients, and in many cases of dermatitis herpetiformis. Increasing the dose of gliadin used for the challenge and the time of observation has made it possible to observe the evolution of the lesion to a hyperplastic phase, essentially characterized by crypt hyperplasia, which precedes villous flattening and does not represent a compensatory response. The end stage of such a process is the classical flat lesion characterized by villous atrophy, crypt hyperplasia, and large highly mitotic intraepithelial lymphocytes (see Chapters 73 and 79). This is the picture that can be observed in untreated celiacs and some dermatitis herpetiformis patients. The evolution of the lesion is presumably dependent on the degree and the duration of the antigenic load, but other unknown environmental factors (e.g., concurrent infections) as well as the genetic background are likely to play a role in determining the progression to a more severe lesion.

The process leading to sensitization to gliadin rather than tolerance could be triggered at different levels. Abnormal permeability of the epithelium and defective gliadin handling at the mucosal level could play a significant role, as well as antigen presentation in the context of a peculiar assortment of products of the MHC. Finally, abnormality of T cells could be implicated.

In general, information about the mucosal handling of gliadin is scanty. The intracellular processing of gliadin is a phenomenon relevant for the induction of an appropriate immune response. The first step in the induction of an immune response is the uptake of antigen by cells that process and then present the antigen to T cells. In rodents and in humans, enterocytes have been shown to function as antigen-presenting cells (APC). Limited data are available about the processing of gliadin by epithelial cells in CD. Gliadin fed to mice is processed during the absorption across the gut mucosa and rendered tolerogenic; transfer of serum-containing, gut-absorbed gliadin produces a state of specific immunological unresponsiveness in recipient animals.[43]

The association of CD with genes and gene products of the MHC locus on chromosome 6 is probably involved in the development of an abnormal immune response to gliadin. The interest of such an association is that these genes code for molecules whose predominant function is to bind selected antigens and to make them recognizable by T cells. A molecule associated with CD has already been identified,[20] but the precise sequence of gliadin that interacts with it is not known.

Two-Stage Model

It has recently been suggested[44] that inappropriate immunity to gliadin, probably genetically restricted, is a condition not only expressed in the gut but also in the skin, mouth (as recurrent aphthae), kidneys (as IgA nephropathy), and joints (as arthritis). Proposed pathologic markers include raised levels of secretory antibodies to gliadin and changes of mucosal architecture, such as increased number of intraepithelial lymphocytes and an increased number of intraepithelial T lymphocytes expressing the gamma-delta receptor.[45] According to the two-stage model of CD, the condition called latent celiac disease would require a second insult to allow full evolution of gluten-induced intestinal damage. Factors favoring progression in some individuals might include a temporary increase in intestinal permeability, an increased gluten intake, or the adjuvant effect of intestinal infection.

In conclusion, evidence suggests that mucosal cell-mediated immunity plays a crucial role in the pathogenesis of the celiac lesion. The primary immune-effect theory is, in principle, not in contrast with the direct cytotoxic activity of gliadin peptides suggested by in vitro studies. Such toxic effect, which seems to be exerted against immature, poorly differentiated cells, could find a target in the intestinal epithelium undergoing a rapid turnover, as in the case of a cell-mediated mucosal immune reaction.

CLINICAL PRESENTATION

Clinical features of CD differ considerably, depending on the age at presentation. Intestinal symptoms are common in children diagnosed within the first two years of life. Failure to thrive, chronic diarrhea, abdominal distention, muscle wasting, anorexia, and irritability are often present. Vomiting may occur in a third of the early presenting patients. The clinical history reveals normal growth in the first months of life, but within weeks or months following the introduction of wheat into the diet, stools become foul, greasy, and bulky and the abdomen becomes distended. The rate of growth diminishes as the appetite wanes, and the child usually becomes irritable. A small number present with fulminant diarrhea leading to dehydration and shock (celiac crisis). Presentation of the disease later in childhood is characterized by the prevalence of extraintestinal symptoms, similar to the adult type of onset. In the Tampere region of Finland, celiac disease is rarely diagnosed under the age of five years, manifesting itself mostly with minor abdominal symptoms, short stature, delayed puberty, anemia, and joint complaints.[46] Among extraintestinal symptoms, short stature has long been recognized as a presenting symptom of celiac disease; approximately 10% of patients with isolated short stature undergoing jejunal biopsy have been found to have villous atrophy.[47] Recently, arthritis[48, 49] and chronic cryptogenetic hepatitis[50] have been associated with CD; in all cases symptoms resolved on a gluten-free diet. An association between CD and epilepsy in patients with bilateral occipital calcifications has been proposed (L. Greco and E. Del Giudice, personal communication). Dental abnormalities have been described in children with CD, including severe enamel hypoplasia in 30% of untreated CD children.[51] The enamel defect is related to the presence of gluten in the diet and rapidly heals on gluten withdrawal. Gluten challenge tends to reproduce the enamel defect. Therefore, it has been suggested that diagnostic challenge be delayed until after the age of seven years, when most crowns of permanent teeth have developed, to reduce potential dental damage.

Family studies demonstrate that CD may also be clinically silent.

ASSOCIATED DISEASES

Dermatitis herpetiformis is characterized by a symmetrical pruritic skin rash with subepidermal blisters and granular subepidermal deposits of IgA in remote, uninvolved skin. Most patients with dermatitis herpetiformis have abnormal small intestinal biopsy pathology that is histologically indistinguishable from that of celiac disease, although usually less severe. In children with DH, approximately 50% have been reported to have subtotal villous atrophy, and 30% have partial villous atrophy on jejunal biopsy.[52] The histology returns to normal after dietary exclusion of gluten. In some patients with dermatitis herpetiformis, villous flattening developed when they were given additional dietary gluten.[25] The pattern of secretory IgA is virtually identical to that reported in celiac patients and in those patients with dermatitis herpetiformis with a normal jejunal histology.[44] It has been hypothesized that intestinal sensitivity is present in all cases, with a variable requirement of dietary gluten for its expression. Therapy with dapsone usually leads to prompt clinical improvement; a strict gluten-free diet permits a reduction or discontinuation of dapsone over a period of months. Improvement of skin lesions also seems to occur on a gluten-free diet in patients with no evident mucosal abnormality. Interestingly, in the same patients the rash recurs when rechallenged with gluten.

Some diseases, many with an autoimmune pathogenesis,[53–55] are found with a higher than expected frequency in celiac patients; among these are thyroid diseases,[56] sarcoidosis,[57] and insulin-dependent diabetes mellitus (IDDM).[58]

Another disease reported to be associated with CD is IgA nephropathy (IgAN),[59] which is also associated with dermatitis herpetiformis. IgA and complement deposits similar to those typically found in IgAN patients have been found in the glomeruli of DH patients who had no previous signs or symptoms of renal disease.

High levels of gliadin antibodies have been described in Down's syndrome.[60] In a recent review from Queen Elizabeth Hospital in London, an increased incidence of Down's syndrome has been found in CD patients, compared to the general population.[61]

Selective IgA deficiency is also a condition associated with celiac disease. In an evaluation of 26 children with IgA deficiency, small intestinal biopsy demonstrated subtotal villous atrophy in three cases.[62] Screening tests other than those based on the measurement of IgA isotype antibodies must be adopted if celiac disease is suspected in IgA-deficient patients.

Finally, there are reports of associations between celiac disease and other diseases of the gastrointestinal tract, such as cystic fibrosis[63] and cow's milk protein intolerance.[64] There is no increased prevalence of atopy in CD children.[65]

LABORATORY FINDINGS

Tests for Malabsorption

Tests for malabsorption are usually helpful in approaching the diagnosis of celiac disease. Determination of hemoglobin, serum iron, calcium, phosphorus, alkaline phosphatase, magnesium, and proteins may be indicative of malabsorption. In particular, red blood cell folate levels have been found to be a sensitive index.[14] Prothrombin levels should be checked before performing intestinal biopsy.

Quantitative fat studies remain the best method of demonstrating lipid malabsorption. A coefficient of fat absorption is determined by measuring grams of fecal fat excreted in 72 hours divided by grams of fat intake during the same time interval. The product is multiplied by 100 to give a percentage, normal being greater than 94%. Among absorption tests, however, the 1-hour blood xylose test has been used most often.[66] An oral dose of 5 gm of xylose for children below 30 kg in weight, or 14.5 gm per square meter to a maximum of 25 gm followed by a 60-minute blood level determination, leads to the best separation between untreated patients and controls. Nevertheless, the rate of false-positive and false-negative results limits the test's usefulness.

Permeability Test

Over the last few years, tests based on intestinal permeability to sugars have been found of value as a noninvasive screening tool. Most are based on the differential intestinal absorption of two nonmetabolized substrates. In untreated CD, the absorption of the smaller probe (mannitol or rhamnose) is reduced due to the loss of intestinal surface area, and that of the larger one (lactulose or cellobiose) is increased, because paracellular pathways are "leakier" and/or increased in number. Expression of the results as a ratio of disaccharide-monosaccharide recovery gives a good separation between normal cases and patients with celiac disease.[67, 68] Although this test has a sufficient sensitivity for abnormalities of jejunal mucosa, it is also characterized by a low specificity for CD. False positives occur mainly in patients with mucosal abnormalities due to other causes (e.g., Crohn's disease, atopic eczema, food allergy, and damage induced by nonsteroidal anti-inflammatory agents).

Antigliadin Antibody Test

Among noninvasive screening tests, the measurement of serum antigliadin antibodies (AGA) has found great application over the last few years.[29] The sensitivity of the test is high, although it does not reach 100%. When IgG and IgA isotypes are considered separately, IgG AGA show a higher sensitivity than IgA, but at the cost of many false-positive results (Table 41–1). Postinfection malabsorption, Crohn's disease, and cow's milk protein intolerance are the most common diagnoses among the false-positive subjects. In dermatitis herpetiformis,[69] a positive correlation has been found between IgG and IgA AGA titers and the severity of gluten-sensitive enteropathy. Nongastrointestinal disorders have been associated with elevated AGA levels. High levels of IgG AGA have been reported in atopic eczema,[70] pemphigus,[71] and pemphigoid.[72] High levels of total AGA have also been reported in patients affected by Sjögren's syndrome,[73] and high levels of IgG AGA have been found in patients affected by rheumatoid arthritis[74] and sarcoidosis.[75] A practical problem in relation to the use of IgA AGA in diagnosis of CD is the high prevalence of IgA deficiency (about one in 50) in celiac disease. Age is also important; the sensitivity of both assays is higher in infants than in older children and adults with CD. After the introduction of a gluten-free diet, there is a gradual decline in the levels of serum AGA, but high levels persist in intestinal secretions. After the reintroduction of gluten in the diet, AGA titers rise in most patients, but it is unclear whether this rise is an early predictor of mucosal relapse or whether it only represents an anamnestic response.

Table 41–1. CLINICAL STUDIES OF SERUM IgG AND IgA ANTIGLIADIN ANTIBODIES (AGA) IN UNTREATED CELIAC PATIENTS AND CONTROL SUBJECTS

Author	Year	Number of Celiacs (Normal Diet)	Number of Controls	Antigen (if Specified)	Method Used	Expression of Results	IgG + IgA AGA		IgG AGA		IgA AGA	
							sens	*spec*	*sens*	*spec*	*sens*	*spec*
Studies in Children												
Unsworth	1981	32	152	Crude gliadin	Immuno-fluorescence	Number of positive	100	85				
Burgin Wolff	1983	72	114	Crude gliadin	Fluorescent immuno-sorbent	Titer reciprocal value			100	84		
Savilahti	1983	19 (<2 years)	36	Crude gliadin	ELISA	% of positive serum			100		100	
		13 (>2 years)							55		64	
Unsworth	1983	66	249	Crude gliadin	ELISA	Titer reciprocal value	100	80			100	86
Volta	1983	50	166		ELISA				100	95	86	100
Kilander	1983	8	8	Crude gliadin	DIG ELISA	Diameter of reaction			100	100	100	100
Blazer	1984	28	89	Crude gliadin	Immuno-fluorescence	Titer reciprocal value			100	76		
Stennhamar	1984	30	58	Crude gliadin	DIG ELISA	Diameter of reaction	100	97			100	97
Arranz	1986	37	24	Crude gliadin	ELISA	% of positive serum	91	74			61	81
Stahlberg	1986	31	278		ELISA	% of positive serum			94	67	90	86
Koninckx	1986	19	103		ELISA	% of positive serum					100	95
Kelly	1987	20	57		ELISA	Ratio $\frac{\text{OD test}}{\text{OD background}}$			95	98		
Dias	1987	43			Immuno-fluorescence				91			
Tucker	1988	17	114	Crude gliadin	ELISA	OD test			88	90	73	65
Burgin Wolff	1989	331	255	Crude gliadin	Fluorescent immuno-sorbent	Titer reciprocal value			100	83	89	96
Guandalini	1989	359	880	Crude gliadin	ELISA (most)	Not reported			98	78	91	97
Rich	1990	15	45	Crude gliadin	ELISA	% of positive serum			100	58	53	93
Calabaig	1990	50	138	Crude gliadin	ELISA	% of positive serum			94	42	73	84
Studies in Adults												
O'Farrelly	1983	44	46	A-gliadin	ELISA	Ratio $\frac{\text{OD test}}{\text{OD background}}$	82	87				
Kilander	1983	36	54	Crude gliadin	DIG ELISA	Diameter of reaction			78	94	67	94
Friis	1985	69	205		DIG ELISA	Diameter of reaction	95	98				

DIG, diffusion in gel; OD, optical density; sens, sensitivity; spec, specificity.
From Troncone R, Ferguson A: Antigliadin antibodies. J Pediatr Gastroenterol Nutr, 1991; 12:150–158; with permission.

Other Antibodies in the Serum of Patients with Celiac Disease

AGA are not the only antibodies present in elevated titers in the serum of celiac patients. Raised levels of antibodies to other cereal proteins, both toxic and nontoxic,[76] and to noncereal dietary antigens have been found;[77] they are likely to be the result of increased mucosal permeability. Among nondietary antibodies, reticulin antibodies are of special interest. Several types have been described with the immunofluorescent method, using rodent tissue as antigens—the R1-type for celiac disease. Antibodies belonging to the IgG class are of limited diagnostic value in celiac disease, but IgA antibodies show high sensitivity and specificity for the diagnosis of celiac disease.[78] A new group of connective tissue antibodies, IgA antiendomysium antibodies (EMA), also determined with immunofluorescence, seems to be closely related to reticulin antibodies. Both reticulin and endomysium antibodies are directed against reticulin-like, silver-stain positive fibers in connective tissue. EMA react only with the connective tissue around smooth muscle fibers in the esophagus of primates. They also are quite characteristic of celiac disease.[79] Recently, a binding to human jejunum of serum IgA antibody (JAB) from children with celiac disease has been reported. Tissue absorption studies have shown that JAB and EMA are probably identical.[80] All these antibodies disappear on gluten-free diet and rise on gluten challenge, and they tend to reflect the extent of mucosal damage.

No test has so far proved sensitive and specific enough to replace the jejunal biopsy. Normal results of any such tests should not dissuade a suspicious clinician from performing a biopsy in a patient whose clinical history and physical findings suggest celiac disease. Nevertheless, some of them (permeability tests, immunologic tests) remain useful tools for screening subjects in at-risk groups (e.g., first-degree relatives of celiac patients). These tests may also be of value in assessing compliance with a gluten-free diet and, during challenge, as early predictors of relapse, with the aim of obtaining a definitive diagnosis in the shortest time and with minimum side effects.

DIAGNOSIS

In 1969, ESPGAN recommended three intestinal biopsies for the diagnosis of celiac disease in childhood: one performed at the time of presentation; a second after the patient has been on a gluten-free diet, when the mucosa is expected to have returned to normal; and the final biopsy after the patient has been rechallenged with gluten, when villous atrophy is expected to have recurred.[3]

Twenty years later, a working group from the ESPGAN reconsidered such diagnostic criteria.[81] The two requirements mandatory for the diagnosis of celiac disease remain: (1) the finding of villous atrophy, with hyperplasia of the crypts and abnormal surface epithelium, while the patient is eating adequate amounts of gluten (see Chapters 73 and 79); and (2) a full clinical remission after withdrawal of gluten from the diet. The finding of circulating IgA antibodies to gliadin, reticulin, and endomysium at the time of diagnosis and their disappearance on a gluten-free diet add weight to the diagnosis. A control biopsy to verify the effect of the gluten-free diet on the mucosal architecture is considered mandatory only in patients with equivocal clinical response to the diet and in patients who were asymptomatic at first presentation (as is often the case with patients diagnosed through screening programs).

Gluten challenge is not considered mandatory, but it may be indicated when there is any doubt about the initial diagnosis—for example, when no initial biopsy was done or when the biopsy specimen was inadequate or not typical of celiac disease. The diagnostic challenge may also be helpful when differentiating other causes of intestinal disease that could be responsible for the flat mucosa (e.g., cow's-milk-sensitive enteropathy, postenteritis syndrome, giardiasis). Since most of these disorders occur in the first two years of life, gluten challenge is usually recommended in patients diagnosed within the first two years of life.

Age is a factor in determining when the challenge should be performed. It is not advisable to challenge children within 1 year after the first biopsy. Children challenged before the age of 3 years showed enamel defects in their permanent central incisors. Furthermore, growth is affected by gluten challenge. Older children may also be easier to biopsy, since they are able to swallow a biopsy capsule. Rechallenge should also be discouraged during the pubertal spurt.

Gluten challenge should be performed under strict medical supervision. It should be preceded by an assessment of mucosal histology and performed with a standard dose of at least 10 gm gluten without disrupting established dietary habits. A further biopsy is taken when there is a noticeable clinical relapse or, in any event, after 3 or 6 months. Laboratory tests (IgA gliadin, reticulin, and endomysium antibodies; absorptive and permeability tests), more than clinical symptoms, can be of help in assessing the timing of the biopsy in order to shorten the duration of the challenge.[82] If no changes of mucosal architecture, or only minimal changes, become evident, patients should be strictly followed up and a further biopsy obtained in the absence of symptoms or altered laboratory tests after two years. If the histological picture is still unchanged, long-term follow-up into adult life is vital, with further biopsies taken if symptoms recur or if an antibody test becomes abnormal.

THERAPY

Gluten-Free Diet

Since the identification of gluten as an etiologic factor in celiac disease, a strict gluten-free diet has become the cornerstone of the management of such patients. Their diet should exclude wheat, oats, rye, and barley; rice and maize are nontoxic and are usually used as wheat substitutes.

The clinical response to withdrawal of gluten is often dramatic, but it must be stressed that the gluten-free diet is recommended for both symptomatic and asymptomatic CD patients. Normalization of the jejunal histology occurs after about 6 months. The most likely cause of lack of response is failure to adhere strictly to the diet, but the possibilities of sensitivity to other dietary proteins, lymphoma, and immune deficiency should also be considered. The most serious potential complication from long-standing CD is malignancy. Cancer develops in adulthood and seems to be related to the consumption of gluten in celiac patients.

Holmes and colleagues have demonstrated that the risk of developing a small intestinal lymphoma is increased only in patients on a reduced-gluten or normal diet. In patients on a gluten-free diet for five years or more, the risk of developing malignancies over all sites (increased morbidity for cancer of the mouth, pharynx, and esophagus has also been noted in celiac patients) is not increased when compared to the general population.[83] The role of a gluten-free diet in protecting against malignancies was also suggested in a series from Scotland, where the mortality rate in celiacs diagnosed in childhood and maintaining a gluten-free diet was similar to that of the general population, with no deaths from malignancies.[84] Therefore, it is strongly recommended that the restriction of gliadin and related prolamines be complete and for life in all CD patients.

Other Therapeutic Measures

Specific vitamin, mineral, and trace element deficiencies should be corrected. Replacement therapy can generally be discontinued after clinical and histologic recovery on a gluten-free diet has been documented.

Other dietary measures are rarely needed. The disaccharidase activity is greatly depressed in atrophic celiac mucosa, but it is advisable to remove milk and lactose-containing products only if intolerance is clinically manifest. Secondary lactase deficiency resolves rapidly after institution of a gluten-free diet, and milk can usually be tolerated after 2 to 4 weeks of the diet.

When patients present in celiac crisis, rapid correction of volume depletion and fluid and electrolyte abnormalities is crucial, and steroid therapy is helpful. Short-term administration of steroids (1–2 mg per kg of prednisone every 24 hours for 1–2 weeks) may be used in severely ill infants in whom anorexia and malabsorption do not rapidly respond to the gluten-free diet.

REFERENCES

1. Dicke WM, Weijers HA, Van de Kramer JK: Coeliac disease: The presence in wheat of factor has a deleterious effect in cases of coeliac disease. Acta Pediatr 1953; 42:34–42.
2. Shiner M, Doniach I: Histopathologic studies in steatorrhoea. Gastroenterology 1960; 38:419–440.
3. Meeuwisse G: Diagnostic criteria in celiac disease. Acta Pediatr Scand 1970; 59:461–463.
4. Kasarda DD, Qualset CO, Mecham DK, et al: A test of toxicity of bread made from wheat lacking alpha-gliadins coded for by the 6A chromosome. *In* McNicholl B, McCarthy CF, Fottrell PF, eds: Perspectives in Celiac Disease. Lancaster, MTP Press 1978, pp 55–61.
5. Van de Kamer JH, Weijers HA, Dicke WK: An investigation into the injurious constituents of wheat in connection with their action on patients with celiac disease. Acta Pediatr 1953; 42:223–231.
6. Auricchio S, Cardelli M, De Ritis G, et al: An in vitro animal model for the study of cereal components toxic in celiac disease. Pediatr Res 1984; 18:1372–1378.
7. Kasarda DD, Okita TW, Bernardin JE, et al: Nucleic acid (cDNA) and amino acid sequences of alpha-type gliadins from wheat (*Triticum aestivum L.*). Proc Natl Acad Sci USA 1984; 81:4712–4716.
8. De Ritis G, Auricchio S, Holly WJ, et al: In vitro (organ culture) studies of the toxicity of specific A-gliadin peptides in celiac disease. Gastroenterology 1988; 94:41–49.
9. Auricchio S, Follo D, De Ritis G, et al: Working hypothesis. Does breast feeding protect against the development of clinical symptoms of celiac disease in children? J Pediatr Gastroenterol Nutr 1983; 2:428–433.

9a. Maki M, Holm K, Ascher E, et al: Factors affecting clinical presentation of coeliac disease: Role of type and amount of gluten-containing cereals in the diet. *In* Auricchio S, Visakorpi JK (eds): Common Food Intolerances: I. Epidemiology of Coeliac Disease. Dyn Nutr Res, Basel, Karger, 1992; 2:76–82.

10. Kagnoff MF, Austin RK, Hubert JJ, Kasarda DD: Possible role for a human adenovirus in the pathogenesis of celiac disease. J Exp Med 1984; 160:1544–1557.
11. Kagnoff MF, Patterson YJ, Kumar PJ, et al: Evidence for the role of a human intestinal adenovirus in the pathogenesis of celiac disease. Gut 1987; 28:995–1001.
12. Mantzaris GJ, Karagiannis JA, Priddle JD, Jewell DP: Cellular hypersensitivity to a synthetic dodecapeptide derived from human adenovirus 12 which resembles a sequence of A-gliadin in patients with celiac disease. Gut 1990; 31:668–673.
13. Howdle PD, Blair Zajdel ME, Smart CJ, et al: Lack of serological response to an E1b protein of adenovirus 12 in celiac disease. Scand J Gastroenterol 1989; 24:282–286.
14. Auricchio S, Mazzacca G, Tosi R, et al: Celiac disease as a familial condition: Identification of asymptomatic celiac patients within family groups. Gastroenterology International 1988; 1:25–31.
15. Stern M, Bender SW, Gruttner R, et al: Serum antibodies against gliadin and reticulin in a familial study of celiac disease. Eur J Pediatr 1980; 135:31–36.
16. Auricchio S, Buffolano W, Ciccimarra F, et al: In vitro proliferation of lymphocytes from celiac children and their first-degree relatives in response to wheat gliadin-derived peptides. J Pediatr Gastroenterol Nutr 1982; 1:515–524.
17. Polanco I, Biemond I, van Leeuwen A, et al: Gluten sensitive enteropathy in Spain: Genetic and environmental factors. *In* McConnell RB, ed: Genetics of Celiac Disease. Lancaster, MTP Press, 1981, pp 211–231.
18. Tosi R, Vismara D, Tanigaki N, et al: Evidence that celiac disease is primarily associated with DC locus allelic specificity. Clin Immunol Immunopathol 1983; 28:395–404.
19. Kagnoff MF, Harwood JI, Bugawan TL, Erlich HA: Structural analysis of the HLA-DR, -DQ and -DP alleles on the celiac disease-associated -DR3 (DRw17) haplotype. Proc Natl Acad Sci USA 1989; 86:6274–6278.
20. Sollid ML, Markussen G, Ek J, et al: Evidence for a primary association of celiac disease to a particular HLA-DQ alpha/beta heterodimer. J Exp Med 1989; 169:345–350.
21. Logan RFA, Rifkind EA, Busuttil A, et al: Prevalence and "incidence" of celiac disease in Edinburgh and the Lothian region of Scotland. Gastroenterology 1986; 90:334–342.
22. Simila S, Kokkonen J, Voulukka P, Kouvalainen K: Childhood celiac disease. Lancet 1981; 1:494–495.
23. Maki M, Holm K: Incidence and prevalence of celiac disease in Tampere. Celiac disease is not disappearing. Acta Pediatr Scand 1990; 79:380–382.
24. Hed J, Lieden G, Ottosson E, et al: IgA anti-gliadin antibodies and jejunal mucosal lesions in healthy blood donors. Lancet 1986; 2:215.
25. Ferguson A, Blackwell JN, Barnetson RStC: Effect of additional

dietary gluten on the small intestinal mucosa of volunteers and of patients with dermatitis herpetiformis. Scand J Gastroenterol 1987; 22:543–549.

26. Doherty M, Barry RE: Gluten-induced mucosal changes in subjects without overt small-bowel disease. Lancet 1981; 1:517–520.
27. Auricchio S, Troncone R: In vitro methods for the study of celiac disease. Front Gastrointest Res 1992; 19:44–51.
28. Kottgen E, Beiswenger M, James LF, Bauer CH: In vivo induction of gliadin-mediated enterocyte damage in rats by the mannosidase inhibitor swainsonine: A possible animal model for celiac disease. Gastroenterology 1988; 95:100–106.
29. Troncone R, Ferguson A: Antigliadin antibodies. J Pediatr Gastroenterol Nutr 1991; 12:150–158.
30. Scott H, Ek J, Baklien K, Brandtzaeg P: Immunoglobulin-producing cells in jejunal mucosa of children with celiac disease on a gluten free diet and after gluten challenge. Scand J Gastroenterol 1980; 15:81–88.
31. O'Mahony S, Arranz E, Barton JR, Ferguson A: Dissociation between systemic and mucosal humoral immune responses in celiac disease. Gut 1991; 32:29–35.
32. Holmes GKT, Asquith P, Cook WT: Cell mediated immunity to gluten fraction III in adult celiac disease. Clin Exp Immunol 1976; 24:259–265.
33. Howdle PD, Bullen AW, Losowski MS: Cell-mediated immunity to gluten within the small intestinal mucosa in celiac disease. Gut 1982; 23:115–122.
34. Ferguson A: Models of immunologically driven small intestinal damage. *In* Marsh MN, ed: Immunopathology of the Small Intestine. New York, Wiley, 1987, pp 225–252.
35. Malizia G, Trejdosiewicz LK, Wood GM, et al: The microenvironment of celiac disease: T cell phenotypes and expression of the T2 "T blast" antigen by small bowel lymphocytes. Clin Exp Immunol 1985; 60:437–446.
36. Halstensen TS, Scott H, Brandtzaeg P: Human CD8+ intraepithelial lymphocytes are mainly CD45RA-RB+ and show increased co-expression of CD45RO in celiac disease. Eur J Immunol 1990; 20:1825–1830.
37. Spencer J, Isaacson PG, Diss TC, MacDonald TT: Expression of disulfide-linked and non-disulfide-linked forms of the T cell receptor gamma/delta heterodimer in human intestinal intraepithelial lymphocytes. Eur J Immunol 1989; 19:1335–1338.
38. Savilahti E, Arato A, Verkasalo M: Intestinal gamma/delta receptor-bearing T lymphocytes in celiac disease and inflammatory bowel diseases in children. Constant increase in celiac disease. Pediatr Res 1990; 28:579–581.
39. Arnaud-Battandier F, Cerf-Bensussan N, Amsellem R, Schmitz J: Increased HLA-DR expression by enterocytes in children with celiac disease. Gastroenterology 1986; 91:1206–1212.
40. Fais S, Maiuri L, Pallone F, et al: Gliadin-induced changes in the expression of MHC-class II antigens by human small intestinal epithelium: Organ culture studies with coeliac disease mucosa. Gut 1992; 33:472–475.
41. Sturgess RP, Macartney JC, Makgoba MW, et al: Differential upregulation of intercellular adhesion molecule-1 in celiac disease. Clin Exp Immunol 1990; 82:489–492.
42. Marsh MN: Studies of intestinal lymphoid tissue. XI. The immunopathology of cell-mediated reactions in gluten sensitivity and other enteropathies. Scanning Microsc 1988; 2:1663–1684.
43. Troncone R, Maiuri L, Raia V, et al: Intestinal absorption and gut processing of gliadin in mice. J Pediatr Gastroenterol Nutr 1991; 13:322.
44. O'Mahony S, Vestey JP, Ferguson A: Similarities in intestinal humoral immunity in dermatitis herpetiformis without enteropathy and in celiac disease. Lancet 1990; 335:1487–1490.
45. Maki M, Holm K, Collin P, Savilahti E: Increase of gamma/delta T cell receptor bearing lymphocytes in normal small bowel mucosa of a patient with latent celiac disease. Gut 1991; 32:1412–1414.
46. Maki M, Kallonen K, Lahdeaho ML, Visakorpi JK: Changing pattern of childhood celiac disease in Finland. Acta Pediatr Scand 1988; 77:408–412.
47. Cacciari E, Salardi S, Lazzari R, et al: Short stature and celiac disease: A relationship to consider even in patients with no gastrointestinal tract symptoms. J Pediatr 1983; 103:708–711.
48. Pinals RS: Arthritis associated with gluten-sensitive enteropathy. J Rheumatol 1986; 13:201–204.
49. Bourne JT, Kumar P, Huskisson EC, et al: Arthritis and celiac disease. Ann Rheumatic Dis 1985; 44:592–598.
50. Leonardi S, Bottaro G, Patane R, Musumeci S: Hypertransaminasemia as the first symptom in infant celiac disease. J Pediatr Gastroenterol Nutr 1990; 11:404–406.
51. Ainne L, Maki M, Collin P, Keyrilainen O: Dental enamel defects in celiac disease. J Oral Pathol Med 1990; 19:241–245.
52. Reunala T, Kosnai T, Karpati S, et al: Dermatitis herpetiformis: Jejunal findings and skin response to gluten free diet. Arch Dis Child 1984; 59:517–522.
53. Reunala T, Salmi J, Karvonen J: Dermatitis herpetiformis and celiac disease associated with Addison's disease. Arch Dermatol 1987; 123:930–932.
54. Stene-Larsen G, Mosvold J, Ly B: Selective vitamin B_{12} malabsorption in adult celiac disease. Report on three cases with associated autoimmune diseases. Scand J Gastroenterol 1988; 23:1105–1108.
55. Stenhammar L, Ljunggren CG: Thrombocytopenic purpura and celiac disease. Acta Paediatr Scand 1988; 77:764–766.
56. Mulder CJJ, Tytgat GNJ, Groenland F, Pena AS: Combined celiac disease and thyroid disease; a study of 17 cases. J Clin Nutr Gastroenterol 1988; 3:89–92.
57. Douglas JD, Gillon J, Logan RFA, et al: Sarcoidosis and celiac disease: An association. Lancet 1984; 2:13–14.
58. Savilahti E, Simell O, Koskimes S, et al: Celiac disease in insulin-dependent diabetes mellitus. J Pediatr 1986; 108:690–693.
59. Helin H, Mustonen J, Reunala T, Pasternack A: IgA nephropathy associated with celiac disease and dermatitis herpetiformis. Arch Pathol Lab Med 1983; 107:324–327.
60. Storm W: Prevalence and diagnostic significance of gliadin antibodies in children with Down syndrome. Eur J Pediatr 1990; 149:833–834.
61. Amil Dias J, Walker-Smith J: Down's syndrome and celiac disease. J Pediatr Gastroenterol Nutr 1990; 10:41–43.
62. Savilahti E, Pelkonen P, Visakorpi JK: IgA deficiency in children. A clinical study with special reference to intestinal findings. Arch Dis Child 1971; 46:665–670.
63. Goodchild MC, Nelson R, Anderson CM: Cystic fibrosis and celiac disease: Co-existence in two children. Arch Dis Child 1973; 48:684–691.
64. Watt J, Pincott JR, Harries JT: Combined cow's milk protein and gluten-induced enteropathy: Common or rare? Gut 1983; 24:165–170.
65. Greco L, De Seta L, D'Adamo G, et al: Atopy and celiac disease: Bias or true relation? Acta Paediatr Scand 1990; 79:670–674.
66. Rolles CJ, Nutter S, Kendall MJ, et al: One-hour blood xylose screening-test for coeliac disease in infants and young children. Lancet 1973; 2:1043–1045.
67. Juby LD, Rothwell J, Axon ATR: Lactulose/mannitol test: An ideal screen for celiac disease. Gastroenterology 1989; 96:79–85.
68. Juby LD, Rothwell J, Axon ATR: Cellobiose/mannitol sugar test: A sensitive tubeless test for celiac disease: Results on 1,010 unselected patients. Gut 1989; 30:476–480.
69. Unsworth DJ, Leonard JN, McMinn RMH, et al: Anti-gliadin antibodies and small intestinal mucosal damage in dermatitis herpetiformis. Brit J Dermatol 1981; 105:653–658.
70. Finn R, Harvey MM, Johnson PM, et al: Serum IgG antibodies to gliadin and other dietary antigens in adults with atopic eczema. Clin Exp Dermatol 1985; 10:222–228.
71. Kumar V, Jain N, Beutner EH, Chorzelski TP: Detection of antigliadin antibodies in bullous diseases and their recognition of similar antigenic polypeptides. Arch Allergy Appl Immunol 1987; 83:155–159.
72. Kieffer M, Barnetson RStC: Increased gliadin antibodies in dermatitis herpetiformis and pemphigoid. Br J Dermatol 1983; 108:673–678.
73. Teppo AM, Maury CPJ: Antibodies to gliadin, gluten and reticulin glycoprotein in rheumatic diseases: Elevated levels in Sjogren's syndrome. Clin Exp Immunol 1984; 57:73–78.
74. O'Farrelly C, Marten D, Melcher D, et al: Association between villous atrophy in rheumatoid arthritis and a rheumatoid factor and gliadin-specific IgG. Lancet 1988; 2:819–822.
75. McCormick PA, Feighery C, Dolan C, et al: Altered gastrointestinal immune response in sarcoidosis. Gut 1988; 29:1628–1631.
76. Troncone R, Auricchio S, DeVincenzi M, et al: An analysis of cereals which react with serum antibodies in patients with celiac disease. J Pediatr Gastroenterol Nutr 1987; 6:346–350.
77. Scott H, Fausa O, Ek J, Bradtzaeg P: Immune response patterns

in celiac disease. Serum antibodies to dietary antigens measured by an enzyme linked immunosorbent assay (ELISA). Clin Exp Immunol 1984; 57:25–32.

78. Maki M, Hallstrom O, Vesikari T, Visakorpi JK: Evaluation of serum IgA-class reticulin antibody test for the detection of childhood celiac disease. J Pediatr 1984; 105:901–905.
79. Chorzelski TP, Beutner EH, Suley J, et al: IgA antiendomysium antibody. A new immunological marker of dermatitis herpetiformis and celiac disease. Br J Dermatol 1984; 111:395–402.
80. Karpati S, Buzgin-Wolff A, Krieg T, et al: Binding to human jejunum of serum IgA antibody from children with celiac disease. Lancet 1990; 336:1335.
81. Walker-Smith JA, Guandalini S, Schmitz J, et al: Revised criteria for the diagnosis of celiac disease. Arch Dis Child 1990; 65:909–911.
82. Mayer M, Greco L, Troncone R, et al: Early prediction of relapse during gluten challenge in childhood celiac disease. J Pediatr Gastroenterol Nutr 1989; 8:474–479.
83. Holmes GKT, Prior P, Lane MR, et al: Malignancy in celiac disease. Effect of a gluten free diet. Gut 1989; 30:333–338.
84. Logan RFA, Rifkind EA, Turner ID, Ferguson A: Mortality in celiac disease. Gastroenterology 1989; 97:265–271.

Chapter 42

Allergic Gastroenteropathy

A. WESLEY BURKS

DEFINITIONS AND PREVALENCE

Adverse gastrointestinal reactions to food components have been reported for several hundred years. Hippocrates noted that cow's milk could cause gastric upset and urticaria.[1] In the twentieth century, the number of cases of adverse gastrointestinal reactions to foods has increased partially because of the increased awareness of both physicians and patients. Only in the last 15 years has much scientific work been done to better understand the pathophysiology of these adverse reactions.

In 1984, the National Institutes of Health defined the terms used to describe adverse reactions to food.[2] The utilization of these terms has allowed better communication in the scientific literature regarding various reactions to food components.

Adverse reaction (sensitivity) to a food is a general term that can be applied to a clinically abnormal response attributed to an ingested food or food additive.

Food hypersensitivity (allergy) is an immunologic reaction resulting from the ingestion of a food or food additive. This reaction occurs only in some patients, may occur after only a small amount of the substance is ingested, and is unrelated to any physiologic effect of the food or food additive. To most investigators, the term is synonymous with reactions that involve the immunoglobulin E (IgE) mechanism, of which anaphylaxis is the classic example.

Food intolerance is a general term describing an abnormal physiologic response to an ingested food or food additive; this reaction has not been proved to be immunologic and can include idiosyncratic, metabolic, pharmacologic, or toxic responses to food or food additives. This term has often been overused and, like the term food hypersensitivity, has been applied incorrectly to all adverse reactions to foods.

The proper use of the above terms will alleviate some of the confusion regarding adverse reactions to foods that has arisen over the years.

Today's consumer marketplace reflects widespread interest and concern about adverse reactions to certain foods and food ingredients. Heavy advertising has drawn attention to the potential for allergic reactions to a wide array of household products. In 1983, the *Federal Register* reported that "some 15% of the population may be allergic to some food ingredients or ingredient."[3] Twenty-two percent of people responding to a consumer survey avoided particular foods based on the mere possibility that the food might contain an allergen.[4]

Because of different diagnostic criteria, it has been difficult to ascertain the exact prevalence of adverse reactions to various food items. Adverse reactions to cow's milk are reported to be from 0.3 to 7.5%.[1, 5] In a prospective study of 500 consecutively born children, Bock and Martin reported that at the end of three years, 142 (28%) of the children were suspected of having an adverse reaction to one or more foods.[6] When these patients were subjected to a double-blind placebo-controlled food challenge to confirm the reaction, only 27 (5%) had positive challenges. Most of the early reactions allegedly caused by foods were diarrheas and rashes that did not recur on reinstitution of the same food. In studies of children with atopic dermatitis, children with severe disease have an approximately 60% chance of having a significant food hypersensitivity reaction.[7, 8] From other studies, children with less severe atopic dermatitis appear to have a 33% incidence of food hypersensitivity reactions.[9]

The natural history of adverse food reactions depends on the nature of the reaction and the particular food one is sensitive to. Patients with food hypersensitivity reactions to soy and wheat tend to outgrow their sensitivity within the first several years after diagnosis; those who react to milk, peanuts, eggs, and fish tend not to lose this sensitivity over time.[10] In comparison, children who have either milk or soy intolerance often outgrow this adverse reaction within the first two years of life.[11]

GASTROINTESTINAL IMMUNITY

The gastrointestinal tract has an intricate immune system that acts as a barrier against foreign antigens, i.e., microbes or food products.[12] This gastrointestinal immune system has a nonspecific and specific immunologic barrier in which molecules are properly handled. The gut lumen allows macromolecules to be absorbed intact. Normally, oral tolerance to the antigen is induced, but in some cases a local and then systemic immune reaction may lead to sensitization.

Antigens may pass through the mucosal surface through the M cells overlying Peyer's patches, through the enterocytes via endocytosis and exocytosis, or through intracellular gaps (Fig. 42–1). Different food antigens have been shown to cross the mucosal barrier to different degrees during postnatal maturation.[13]

The normal gastrointestinal tract is protected by a number of host defense mechanisms, both immunologic and nonimmunologic.[14] Bacterial and viral populations that inhabit the gastrointestinal tract are important in preventing overgrowth of pathogenic organisms and thus are important in maintaining normal gastrointestinal function.[15] Several substances produced and secreted in the gastrointestinal epithelial mucosal and submucosal glands and in the liver play a major role in maintaining normal intestinal function. Glycoproteins in the mucous coat covering the gastrointestinal surface are thought to provide a number of defense mechanisms. Included among these mechanisms are the prevention of parasitic, bacterial, and viral attachment to the epithelium and interaction with allergens and enterotoxins to deter their epithelial penetration.[16, 17] Another nonspecific defense mechanism is the mucosal lining of the gastrointestinal tract, in which the epithelial cells are constantly being renewed.

Immunologically, the gastrointestinal tract provides a defense by means of the reticuloendothelial cells (Kupffer's cells) of the liver, immunoglobulin production, cell-mediated immunity, and mast cell activation. The humoral immune system of the gastrointestinal tract involves the local production of primarily IgA and IgM. In adults, IgA-producing cells predominate, with IgM-, IgG-, IgE-, and IgD-producing cells occurring less often.[18] The immunoglobulins in intestinal secretions increase with the individual's exposure to bacterial and food antigens. Measurements of fecal IgA antibodies in bottle-fed, healthy infants suggest that the intestinal IgA-producing cell system may reach maturity as early as 1 to 2 months.[19]

The humoral immune response appears to be induced primarily in the Peyer's patches. Here the antigen penetrates the epithelium into the subepithelial zone, where lymphocyte sensitization occurs. Primed lymphocytes then leave through the efferent lymphatics, pass through the mesenteric nodes and thoracic duct to the systemic circulation into the spleen and other organs, and return to the lamina propria, where B lymphocytes differentiate into plasma cells (see Fig. 42–1).[20, 21] The functions of gut-associated immunoglobulins include defense against microorganisms and control of antigen absorption.

In the gastrointestinal tract, cell-mediated immunity is independent of a comparable systemic cell-mediated immunity.[22] Priming of T cells to antigens in the lumen can take place in the Peyer's patches. These cells travel through the thoracic duct to the blood stream and return to the lamina propria as T effector cells.

Mast cells in the mucosa reside primarily in the lamina propria, occasionally within the epithelial layer, and in the submucosa near small blood and lymphatic vessels. In animal models, mast cells in the lamina propria differ from mast cells in the submucosa, skin, and other organs.[23] Both the mucosal mast cell and the connective

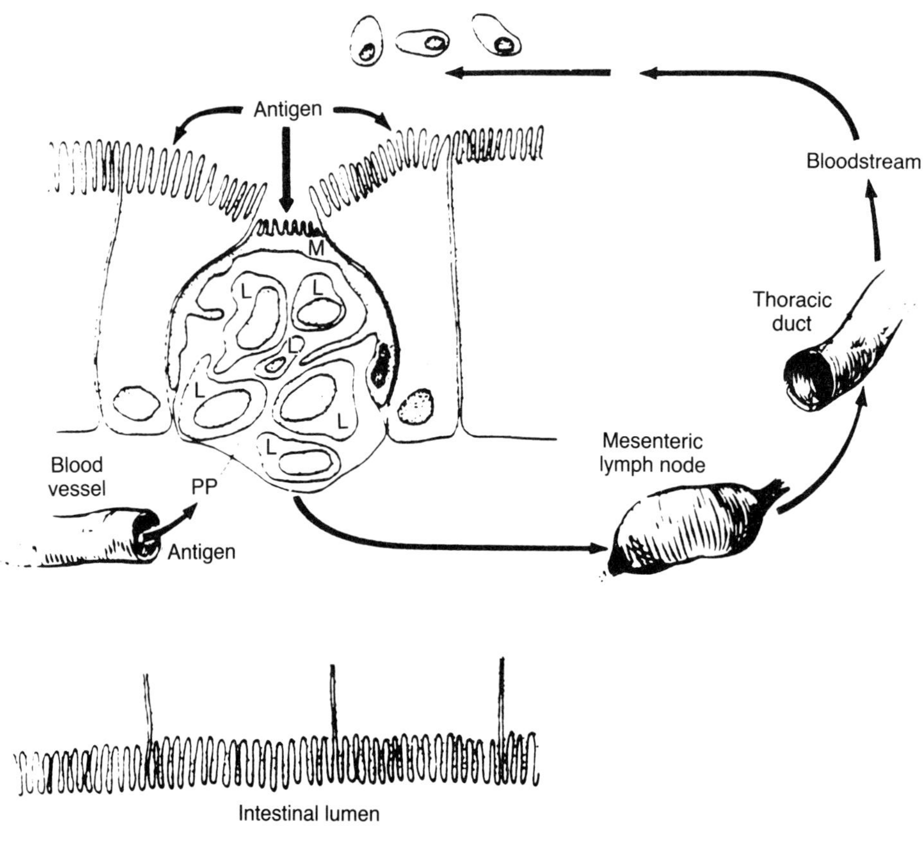

Figure 42–1. Schematic representation of cell cycle for plasma cells populating the intestinal mucosa. Lymphocytes (L) within the gut-associated lymphoid tissues are stimulated by antigens entering the intestinal lumen via specialized epithelium (M cells), across absorptive cells, or from the systemic circulation. These lymphoblasts then migrate to the mesenteric nodes and then enter the systemic circulation as plasmoblasts to redistribute along mucosal surfaces to differentiate into plasma cells. (Adapted from Stern M, Walker WA: Food allergy and intolerance. Pediatr Clin North Am 1985; 32:471–492; with permission.)

tissue–type mast cell contain IgE and histamine.[24, 25] Mast cell degranulation results in the release of preformed mediators such as histamine and chemotactic factors and generates secondary mediators such as leukotrienes. The consequences of the release of these mediators include a local change in vasopermeability, stimulation of mucus production, increased muscle contraction, stimulation of pain fibers, and recruitment of inflammatory cells.

FOOD ANTIGENS

Only a limited number of food allergens have been studied in an attempt to isolate, purify, and characterize the allergens (Table 42–1). These foods include milk, soy, egg, peanuts, and fish. Some foods appear to be major allergens because of the frequency with which they are consumed; other foods are important allergens most likely because of their structure. These proteins generally range in size from 10 kd to 65 kd.[26] The codfish allergen Gad c I (Allergen M) is the best characterized food allergen.[27] This allergen contains 113 amino acids and is relatively resistent to proteases, heat, and denaturants.

Food antigens appear to be modified by gastrointestinal absorption and degradation.[28] The difference in allergenicity following this process remains to be fully elucidated. Food technology processing such as heat treatment, homogenization, and spray drying may alter the antigenicity of the food proteins.[29]

Recent studies have shown that human breast milk contains foreign food proteins that the mother is ingesting. These proteins can elicit an allergic response in an infant who is being breast-fed.[30, 31]

Cow's Milk Proteins

Cow's milk proteins are consumed in large amounts during the first several months of life by most infants. Even breast-fed infants are exposed to cow's milk proteins because of the transfer of these proteins through the breast milk. There are both casein (80%) and whey (20%) proteins in cow's milk.[2] Although not entirely substantiated, the whey protein beta-lactoglobulin appears to be the most allergenic of all the cow's milk proteins.[2] Lactalbumin, bovine gamma globulin, and bovine serum albumin are also noted to be allergens in cow's milk.

Cow's milk proteins have been implicated in a number of different clinical diseases, from milk hypersensitivity to milk protein intolerance. In sensitive assays, virtually 100% of individuals who consume milk make IgG and IgM antibodies to the milk proteins.[32] There does not appear to be any relationship between the level of serum antibody and adverse reactions to milk. There does appear to be a reasonable correlation between the presence of specific IgE to cow's milk proteins and milk hypersensitivity.[32] Milk proteins appear susceptible to proteolytic cleavage, with possible formation of new allergens.[33]

Table 42–1. FOOD ANTIGENS

Cow's Milk Proteins	**Egg**
Beta-lactoglobulin	Egg white—ovalbumin
Lactalbumin	**Other**
Bovine gamma globulin	Peanuts
Bovine serum albumin	Fish
Soybean Proteins	Nuts
2, 7, 11, 15S proteins	Beef, chicken, pork
Soybean trypsin inhibitor	Shellfish

Soy

Much is known about the soybean protein and its fractions, but little has been done to examine their allergenicity.[34] Approximately 90% of the seed proteins in soybeans are salt-soluble albumins, which comprise a broad range of molecular sizes and display four major sedimentation components in the ultracentrifuge—2, 7, 11, and 15S.[35] Soybean proteins have been noted to cause IgE-mediated symptoms as well as soy protein intolerance symptoms. Soy protein formulas have been used as secondary formulas in children who have adverse reactions to milk protein formulas. Recent data suggest that at least 50% of children who have milk protein intolerance will have soy protein intolerance.[36] Previous assumptions that soy protein is less allergenic than cow's milk protein are unlikely to be substantiated. It is not known which of the soy protein fractions is the most allergenic. One study found the 2S fraction to be the most allergenic, but another study could not substantiate this.[34, 37] A soybean trypsin inhibitor has been identified and documented by skin testing, passive transfer skin test, and an in vitro specific IgE assay to be an allergen that causes IgE-mediated reactions.[38]

Egg

Eggs are one of the three primary foods that cause IgE-mediated reactions in children.[7, 8] Egg white contains the protein that most often causes the IgE-mediated reactions.[2] The majority of egg white is composed of ovalbumin, which is easily denaturated by heating. Other egg proteins include egg lysozyme and ovomucoid.

Other Food Antigens

There are numerous other food antigens that are encountered throughout life. Peanuts, fish, nuts, shellfish, wheat, fruits, and various meats have all been studied to some extent as allergens. In peanuts, several allergens have been identified and characterized, including Peanut 1 (with major protein bands at 20 kd and 30 kd) and a concanavalin A-reactive glycoprotein (with a protein band at 65 kd).[39, 40] Recent work has identified a major allergen with two closely migrating protein bands at 63.5 kd.[41] Fish, particularly cod, is an important allergen, causing IgE-mediated symptoms in children and adults. Various symptoms from asthma to anaphylaxis have been noted to be caused by fish. Symptoms are seen in some individuals following inhalation of steam from cooking fish.

PATHOGENESIS

Genetic Predisposition

Development of IgE-mediated allergic disease is for the most part genetically determined.[42] A child with one atopic parent has approximately a 30% chance of developing allergic disease; a child with two parents who are atopic has approximately a 60% chance of developing allergic disease.[43] The concentration of IgE in cord blood appears to correlate well with the later development of IgE-mediated disease.[44] Children with cord blood IgE levels above 0.5 IU per ml have a significant likelihood of developing IgE-mediated disease.[42, 45]

Sensitization to many foods occurs during the first year of life. Milk, eggs, and peanuts are common allergens during this time period. Fish and nuts do not typically cause IgE-mediated problems until later in childhood or in adulthood.

The effect of delayed feeding of certain foods to prevent allergic disease has received much attention in the past several years. The most recent comprehensive study found that maternal avoidance of certain foods during the last trimester of pregnancy and the child's avoidance of certain foods for the first year of life only delayed the onset of allergic diseases.[42] When examined at 12 months, the group avoiding certain foods did not have as much allergic disease, but by 24 months of age there were no differences in the amount of allergic disease between the two groups.

Food-Specific Antibodies

The formation of specific IgG, IgA, and IgM antibodies to a food protein is a natural phenomenon that indicates exposure rather than sensitization.[46] Serum IgG antibodies specific for cow's milk, soy, ovalbumin, and other foods have been documented to rise after initial introduction of these foods and then fall after infancy.[47] The role of food-specific antibodies (including IgG_4), other than IgE, in causing adverse food reactions is highly speculative. The IgG specific for milk proteins tends to be higher in children with documented IgE-mediated symptoms to milk, but there is no direct correlation.[48] There is, however, a role for IgE-specific antibodies in children with IgE-mediated adverse reactions.[48] It has been shown that in children with atopic dermatitis, the presence of food-specific IgE signifies that there is a 20 to 30% chance of having a positive double-blind placebo-controlled food challenge.[7, 8] In comparison, in children who have a negative screening for food-specific IgE, the likelihood of having an adverse reaction to that food is minuscule.

The role of serum antibodies in food protein intolerance is still unknown. One study has shown elevation of specific IgG and IgA antibody titers in the study group compared with the nonfood-sensitive patients.[49] The researchers showed an increase in specific IgA antibodies and a decrease in specific IgM antibodies on challenge with soy. Subsequent articles on a similar group of patients found the difference in serum-specific IgG and IgE antibodies not to be statistically different between the group with a positive food challenge and the group with a negative food challenge.[50]

Several recent studies have tried to identify a group of children who have late reactions to milk protein.[51] These authors devised a protocol where children receive a milk challenge on three consecutive days with increasingly larger amounts of milk protein given on each day. Children who have an adverse reaction on the initial day are said to be immediate reactors, and those who do not react until the third day are said to be late reactors. These studies are confusing because they do not take into consideration children who react to only larger amounts of protein.

Serum food-specific antibodies have been investigated extensively in children who have adverse reactions to foods. Other than the IgE-specific antibodies in food hypersensitivity, the role of these antibodies has not been fully elucidated.[52] Therefore, the utility of measuring food-specific antibodies, other than IgE, is of doubtful diagnostic significance.

Food Hypersensitivity

By definition, food hypersensitivity is an immunologic reaction resulting from the ingestion of a food or food additive. For the most part, this term is synonymous with IgE-mediated reactions to foods. Children with food hypersensitivity usually have evidence of specific IgE to the food in question. This food-specific IgE will then bind to the mast cells in the gastrointestinal mucosa as well as in other tissues. After subsequent exposure to that particular food, there exists the potential for mast cell activation, which will then cause the various clinical symptoms. This process is influenced by a number of factors, including the age of the patient, the digestive process, the gastrointestinal permeability, the antigenic structure of that food, and the patient's genetic predisposition.[53]

Children with food hypersensitivity most often have symptoms within 2 hours after ingesting the food. Symptoms are usually related to the gastrointestinal tract, respiratory tract, and skin. Gastrointestinal symptoms may include nausea, cramping, pain, abdominal distention, vomiting, flatulence, and diarrhea. Respiratory symptoms may include wheezing, coughing, hoarseness, and rhinitis. Skin reactions are evidenced by urticaria and/or angioedema, exacerbations of atopic dermatitis, and cutaneous erythema.

A typical patient will have a family history of allergic diseases, an elevated serum IgE (though not always), and evidence of specific IgE to the food in question.[54, 55] Evidence of specific IgE to a food may be obtained by prick skin testing (in vitro).[54] Skin testing measures mast cell–bound IgE, and the radioallergosorbent test (RAST) measures serum-specific IgE.[53] The presence of food-specific antibodies has a very poor predictive accuracy (only 20 to 30% will actually have positive food challenges) but a good negative predictive accuracy (those with negative results are extremely unlikely to have food hypersensitivity).[7, 8] There is some indirect correlation in that the larger the positive skin test or the higher the RAST score, the more likely the patient is to have a food hypersensitivity reaction to that particular food.

The mechanism of IgE-mediated symptoms has been partially elucidated. After exposure to the specific food allergen, the multivalent antigen then bridges two IgE molecules and the mast cell releases a variety of mediators. These mediators include histamine, proteases, eosinophil chemotactic factors, and neutrophil chemotactic factors.[53] These substances then influence capillary permeability, smooth muscle contractility, mucus secretion, and chemotaxis. Studies of the gastrointestinal mucosa have examined the end result of this IgE-mediated phenomenon. Intragastric provocation under endoscopic control produced edema, erythema, and petechial bleeding after food challenge.[56, 57] Histamine,[58] eosinophil major basic protein,[59] and histamine-releasing factors[60] have all been shown to be involved in immediate hypersensitivity reactions to foods.

Non-IgE-Mediated Immunologic Reactions

Several studies have examined the role of cytotoxic (type II) or immune complex (type III) mediated adverse reactions to foods. The various studies in which these mechanisms have been examined have not produced specific results. The local deposition of IgG and complement C3 in the subepithelial connective tissue has been shown but not confirmed.[61] In addition to possible local deposition, immune complexes containing food antigens (cow's milk and egg proteins) and immunoglobulins (IgG and IgE) have been described in the sera of possibly food-allergic patients.[62, 63] Another study identified IgG and IgE immune complexes in supposedly food-sensitive patients.[64]

The studies on non-IgE adverse food reactions that may be immunologic in nature are diverse and not well documented. The evidence that there are such clinical reactions remains very much in doubt.

Protein Intolerance

Food protein intolerance is often manifest as milk or soy-protein intolerance during the first several years of life. Numerous studies have examined the possible immunologic mechanism present in this disease. The significance of food-specific antibodies in the pathogenesis of food protein intolerance is frequently debated. Recent studies that have examined children with documented milk and soy protein intolerance have found no differences between challenge-positive and challenge-negative groups with regard to serum IgG or IgE-specific antibodies to either milk or soy.[37, 50]

Aside from antibody production, other immunologic factors have been thought to play a role in food protein intolerance. One study found evidence for lymphocyte sensitization in children with documented milk and soy protein intolerance.[65] The results indicated a significant difference in the mean geometric stimulation index to various milk and soy proteins when comparing the challenge-positive and challenge-negative groups. Another mechanism was postulated when investigators found evidence for an increase in nonspecific concanavalin A-induced suppressor cell activity in patients with milk protein intolerance.[66] They postulated that the delayed maturation of a suppressor cell population might be the cause of the intolerance. Depressed neutrophil chemotaxis was noted in one group of patients with milk or soy protein intolerance.[67] Increased production of a lymphokine, leukocyte-migration-inhibition factor has been linked to food protein intolerance.[68]

In animal models using gastrointestinal parasitic infection and graft-versus-host disease, a linkage between cell-mediated immune reactions and enterocyte damage has been postulated.[69] The changes noted in these animal models include the finding that increased numbers of intraepithelial lymphocytes were connected with increased crypt mitotic activity and with decreased villous enterocyte height. Some clinical studies have noted that in children with apparent food protein intolerance the relative number of intraepithelial lymphocytes is increased[70]—thus the link between cell-mediated immune reactions and enterocyte damage.

CLINICAL MANIFESTATIONS

A wide variety of symptoms have been described secondary to food hypersensitivity or food protein intolerance in children of different ages (see Tables 42–2 and 42–3). Many of these clinical symptoms have been reproduced by double-blind, placebo-controlled food challenges.[71] Other symptoms that have been noted only in case reports or in poorly controlled studies include joint swelling and pain, headache, apathy, irritability, and hyperkinesis.

Table 42–2. FOOD HYPERSENSITIVITY SYMPTOMS

Gastrointestinal: nausea, cramping, pain, abdominal distention, vomiting, flatulence, diarrhea
Respiratory: wheezing, coughing, hoarseness, rhinitis
Skin: urticaria and/or angioedema, cutaneous erythema, exacerbations of atopic dermatitis
Cardiovascular: arrhythmias, hypotension

Table 42–3. FOOD PROTEIN INTOLERANCE SYMPTOMS

Vomiting	Gross or occult blood
Diarrhea	Irritability or colic (?)
Malabsorption	

The gut functions not only as the target organ but as the vehicle for delivery of the food antigens to other target organs such as the skin, respiratory tract, and cardiovascular system. Most often, patients have simultaneous reactions from multiple organ systems. Depending on the type of medical clinic studied, one can find various frequencies for the most common end-organ system affected. For example, in studies of patients with severe atopic dermatitis, the most common site for the adverse food reaction is the skin.[7, 8] But in studies of children taken from other clinics, gastrointestinal symptoms may predominate.

The clinical symptoms of adverse food reactions are best thought of in terms of which organ or organs are affected. The time frame for the reaction is also important to note. Food hypersensitivity reactions most often occur within 2 hours of ingesting the food antigen, although anaphylaxis has occurred up to 4 hours later.[72] Patients with challenges for food protein intolerance are often monitored for up to 24 hours after the challenge begins (although the symptoms usually occur within the first 6 to 8 hours).

Food Hypersensitivity

Immediate hypersensitivity reactions to food antigens are expressed clinically by a diversity of signs and symptoms ranging from abdominal pain to anaphylaxis (see Table 42–2). The clinical expression is influenced by many factors, including the age and awareness of the patient, the quantity of food ingested, and the presence of other medical problems.[53]

Food hypersensitivity may be expressed in one or more extraintestinal target tissues. The basis for preferential reactivity of one target organ over another is unknown. It is not uncommon for a child to have different clinical manifestations for each food he or she is sensitive to. For example, a child may have urticaria and wheezing after ingesting peanuts, but vomiting after ingesting eggs. Skin reactions include urticaria and/or angioedema, cutaneous erythema, and exacerbations of atopic dermatitis. Respiratory symptoms may include wheezing, coughing, hoarseness, and rhinitis.

Patients with severe food hypersensitivity may experience food anaphylaxis. Systemic anaphylaxis may involve multiple target organs as evidenced by abdominal pain, nausea, emesis, diarrhea, dyspnea, cyanosis, chest pain, urticaria, angioedema, arrhythmias, hypotension, and shock.[53] The first anaphylactic episode may be unexpected or may be preceded by minor symptoms such as abdominal discomfort or urticaria on previous exposure to the food. Milk, peanuts, and fish are not uncommon causes of systemic anaphylaxis in children. Systemic anaphylaxis generally occurs within 30 minutes after ingesting the food but has been reported to occur later.[72]

Food Protein Intolerance

Food intolerance is often manifested during the first several years of life as milk or soy protein intolerance.[11] This disease appears to be transient, but it often results in damage to the intestinal mucosa and causes mucosal dysfunction. The best studied food protein intolerance is cow's milk intolerance.[73] Soy protein has been similarly studied as well as intolerances to egg, fish, rice, and chicken.[74, 75]

Symptoms can be acute or may begin insidiously (see Table 42–3). The predominant symptoms may include vomiting, diarrhea, malabsorption resulting in growth failure, and gross or occult blood in the stool, resulting in anemia. Subtle symptoms may be irritability or colic during the first several months of life. The later symptom is not a common manifestation of protein intolerance.

Morphologic studies of the small intestine in individuals with cow's milk intolerance have shown different degrees of villous atrophy with a nonhomogeneous, patchy distribution.[76] In severe cases, the gastrointestinal biopsies may be indistinguishable from those found in celiac disease.[77] The clinical course and enteropathy caused by cow's milk is fully reversible after its elimination from the diet. A morphologic definition of the diagnosis based on small intestine biopsy has not been accepted by most investigators.

Acute gastroenteritis has been thought to predispose to the development of cow's milk intolerance, but this has not been proved.[78] Often disaccharidase (lactase) deficiency occurs along with cow's milk protein intolerance and may make the diagnosis difficult by perpetuating the symptoms.

A separate gastrointestinal entity related to foods has been described, called *food-induced colitis*.[79] The main clinical symptoms are chronic bloody diarrhea, anemia, and abdominal pain. Proctosigmoidoscopy has revealed mucosal erythema and aphthous lesions; histologically there is gross eosinophilic infiltration and focal ulceration. The differentiation between this clinical entity and severe milk protein intolerance is often difficult to make. In the few reported cases of this entity there was a family history of allergic diseases, peripheral blood eosinophilia, elevated total serum IgE levels, and elevated specific IgE levels. These cases responded well to elimination of cow's milk.

Other Nongastrointestinal Manifestations

Inflammatory joint disease has been speculated to be caused by cow's milk in one report.[80] There were increases in milk-specific IgG antibodies and IgG-milk immune complexes in this patient. Current evidence would suggest that dietary elimination is not of proven benefit in rheumatoid disease. Migraine headaches have been linked to adverse food reactions in some patients.[81] It appears that foods may cause migraine headaches in some but certainly not the majority of cases. Studies that linked hyperactivity, hyperkinesis, and other related problems to adverse food reactions have been around for a number of years.[82] The results are anecdotal, and the conclusions are not justified. There appears to be no reason to assume that adverse food reactions play a part in this symptom complex.

DIAGNOSIS

The cornerstone of diagnosis of adverse food reactions is a complete history and physical examination and a positive oral challenge. Laboratory tests may be helpful, particularly in children with suspected food hypersensitivity reactions. Goldman and colleagues originally set forth criteria for the diagnosis of cow's milk allergy.[73] For patients suspected of having food protein intolerance, most investigators follow the guidelines of Powell (Table 42–4).[11] In patients who are suspected of having food hypersensitivity reactions, double-blind, single-blind, or open challenges should be performed.

In the oral food challenge to confirm food protein intolerance, the patient is given 0.6 gm of protein per kilogram of body weight. The patient is then monitored for the following criteria: (1) symptoms of vomiting or diarrhea, (2) an increase in the peripheral neutrophil count of more than 3,500 per mm^3 between blood drawn immediately before oral challenge and 6 to 8 hours after challenge, (3) the appearance of blood in the stool, (4) the appearance of leukocytes in Wright's-stained fecal mucus, and (5) the appearance of Charcot-Leyden crystals or eosinophilic debris in the stool by Hansel's stain. The challenge is considered positive if three or more manifestations are present, equivocal if two are observed, and negative if one or none are observed.[11]

For patients with possible food hypersensitivity reactions, double-blind, single-blind, or open challenges are recommended. Double-blind, placebo-controlled food challenges are indicated for clinical research studies and for difficult cases when other challenges have produced confusing results. It is preferable for patients to have been on a diet free from the suspected food for at least 3 to 4 weeks prior to any challenge. Double-blind, placebo-controlled food challenges can be done in either an outpatient or inpatient setting. Up to 10 gm of dehydrated food is administered in opaque capsules or juice over 1 hour.[83] Two challenges are performed each day: one with the suspected food and the other with a placebo (sucrose or corn starch). The sequence of challenges should be determined by someone other than the physician or person doing the challenge, preferably a nutritionist. The patient is followed closely for at least 2 hours after the challenge to watch for related skin, respiratory, or gastrointestinal symptoms. If both challenges are negative, the food should then be given openly to ensure that the patient can tolerate the food. In single-blind challenges, the patients or parents do not know what food is being challenged. In open challenges, everyone involved knows what food is being consumed.

Table 42–4. CHALLENGE CRITERIA—FOOD PROTEIN INTOLERANCE

Symptoms of vomiting or diarrhea
Increase in peripheral neutrophil count of more than 3,500/mm^3 between prechallenge and 6–8 hours postchallenge
Blood in the stool
Leukocytes in Wright's stained fecal mucus
Charcot-Leyden crystals or eosinophils debris in the stool (Hansel's stain)

For children, the foods implicated in over 90% of documented food hypersensitivity reactions are milk, egg, peanut, soy, wheat, and fish.[71]

Laboratory procedures performed to support the clinical diagnosis of food hypersensitivity are based on the identification of antigen-specific IgE. Skin tests identify mast cell–specific IgE, and blood tests (e.g., RAST) identify antigen-specific IgE in the serum. Laboratory tests such as total IgE determinations and eosinophil counts do not reliably correlate with immediate hypersensitivity reactions to foods.[84] Skin testing with foods involves the application of food antigen extracts to the dermis and is the most direct and reliable method of demonstrating specific IgE antibodies.[85] The usual method is the puncture or prick skin test, in which a drop of food extract is placed on the skin. The skin is then punctured through the drop with a sterile needle. Extracts for testing are usually supplied as 1:20 wt per vol extracts in 50% glycerine. Intradermal skin testing is discouraged because it produces clinically irrelevant positive results.[86] Food hypersensitivity reactions to foods are unusual in the face of negative skin tests.[87] As stated earlier, positive skin tests carry only a 20 to 30% chance of predicting a positive food challenge.[7, 8]

The RAST and the enzyme-linked immunosorbent assay (ELISA) are directed at an in vitro demonstration of IgE directed to specific antigens. The RAST is the most commonly used in vitro test. The RAST and ELISA have proved useful as research tools in the identification of food antigens and in the standardization of allergenic extracts. Clinically, the in vitro tests are more expensive and time-consuming, but they may be used when skin testing with extracts may pose a hazard, such as in someone who has experienced anaphylaxis to that particular antigen. They may also be used in patients with severe skin disease, such as eczema that is so extensive as to preclude skin testing, or in patients with severe dermatographism. In research settings, peripheral blood basophils from individuals with suspected food hypersensitivity can be examined in vitro to determine whether they degranulate to dilute suspensions of food antigen (histamine release assay). Degranulation requires the presence of IgE on the basophil specific to the suspected food. Such degranulation is monitored by histamine released into the supernatant fluid. Basophil degranulation tests correlate with skin tests but still do not establish a definite diagnosis of food hypersensitivity.

Numerous tests to confirm or refute the diagnosis of food hypersensitivity have been suggested. Several studies have used IgG specific for foods to aid in the diagnosis. As previously discussed, IgG specific for certain food appears to be only a sign of exposure and not true sensitivity. Recent assays have tried to correlate IgG subclasses specific for certain foods as good predictors for food hypersensitivity. IgG_4 has been touted as the best predictor. Unfortunately, like total specific IgG, the reliability of these tests has not proved to be beneficial in diagnosis. The detection of immune complexes with food antigens and antibodies through a modified radioimmunoassay or C1q binding has not proved to be beneficial in the diagnosis of food hypersensitivity.

In the diagnosis of food protein intolerance, several investigators have used cell-mediated assays as research tools to examine the pathogenesis of this disorder, but its usefulness as a clinical diagnostic tool has not been validated. Similarly, the leukocyte migration-inhibiting factor has not proved to be a generally helpful diagnostic aid.[88]

There are a multitude of additional tests that have been used over the years to try to establish a diagnosis of an adverse food reaction. These tests include leukocytotoxic testing, subcutaneous and sublingual provocation, and neutralization testing. A recent study showed quite nicely the strong placebo effect of subcutaneous provocation testing.[89] These techniques have been reviewed and have not been approved by the American Academy of Allergy and Immunology as diagnostic aids for adverse food reactions.[90]

Intestinal Biopsy and Function

In order to establish diagnostic criteria, the gastrointestinal tract has been investigated from a morphologic and functional standpoint. At present, no specific gastrointestinal functional tests or specific biopsies have been able to replace the clinical and immunologic methods previously discussed.[91]

Several studies from one group have used intragastric provocation under endoscopic control to examine patients with possible adverse food reactions.[56, 57] The clinical findings appeared to agree with the mast cell degranulation assay employed in patients diagnosed with immediate food reactions. These studies are not likely to be applied widely to children. Without confirmation of the diagnosis by means of a double-blind, placebo-controlled food challenge, the results of these studies must be left in doubt.

Due to the different means of diagnosis from various investigators and the lack of good challenge studies, there have been no consistent mucosal biopsy findings in children. Children with eosinophilic gastroenteropathy have had gastric biopsies, and children with food protein intolerance have had small bowel biopsies done in multiple studies.[91, 92] One study tried to correlate pre- and postchallenge biopsy results with diagnosis, with mixed results.[93]

For children with food protein intolerance or food hypersensitivity with only gastrointestinal manifestations, small intestinal biopsy may be necessary to differentiate these diseases from such illnesses as celiac disease, lymphangiectasia, or microvillous atrophy. In patients with possible food-induced colitis, biopsy may be an important part of the diagnosis when finding IgE-containing mucosal plasma cells.

Recent studies have applied gut function tests as noninvasive screening tests for malabsorption.[94, 95] The utility of these tests is still in question for the diagnosis of adverse food reactions.

TREATMENT

The treatment of allergic disease is threefold: avoidance, medical therapy, and immunotherapy, if necessary.[2] A diet in which the offending food is eliminated is the treatment of choice for adverse food reactions. Nutritional counseling for the management of elimination diets is often helpful. A child's fish-free diet may be comparatively simple compared to a diet in which several foods must be eliminated. As noted by many, the routine and indiscriminate use of elimination diets without a firm diagnosis is widespread.[96] Patients have been noted to have malnutrition and symptoms of protein, calorie, and trace element deficiencies.[97]

For patients with food hypersensitivity, a diet free of the offending food is the treatment of choice. Almost all patients will have only one or two foods that must be eliminated.[71] It is now known that patients who follow the elimination diet often lose their sensitivity within the first 1 to 2 years after diagnosis.[10] Soy and wheat sensitivity appears to be lost much sooner than sensitivity to foods such as eggs, milk, peanuts, and fish.[10] For infants and toddlers who have milk hypersensitivity, soy formulas can be substituted for the milk protein in most cases. For patients who have both milk and soy hypersensitivity—a small minority of patients—a protein hydrolysate may be necessary. Recent reports have documented that a very small percentage of patients will react to hydrolysate formulas, so caution should be used even with these formulas.[98] The patient and parents must be aware of the different names for the foods they are sensitive to. For example, sodium caseinate is a common term used to denote milk proteins in various foods. Many drinks are labeled milk-free, which often means that they do not have lactase, not that they do not contain milk proteins. The routine use of oligoantigenic or elemental diets in the diagnosis of food hypersensitivity should be strongly discouraged.

For patients with food protein intolerance, such as milk or soy protein intolerance, the treatment of choice again is elimination of the suspected substance from the diet. For infants and toddlers, this means placing them on a protein hydrolysate formula. There are several excellent casein and whey hydrolysate formulas on the market now. In patients with documented milk protein intolerance, the formula of choice should be the protein hydrolysate, since over 50% of these children have documented soy protein intolerance in challenge studies.[36] Milk formulas that have been partially hydrolyzed should not be used for these diseases. Most hydrolysates have a bitter taste but are tolerated when used consistently. Milk and soy protein intolerance is normally lost within the first two years of life, so hydrolysate formulas will not have to be used for long.

Medical Therapy

The pharmacologic treatment of adverse food reactions is directed toward any systemic effects the reaction may have on its target organ. Medical therapy should never be directed toward primary treatment of the reaction. Patients may need antihistamines, bronchodilators, or steroids in the case of significant reactions.

For primary therapy of food hypersensitivity, several medications have been tried unsuccessfully, including oral cromolyn. Oral cromolyn has been investigated in a number of studies.[99–101] As stated in a recent review from data obtained in appropriately double-blind studies, oral cromolyn has no place in the treatment of food hypersensitivity.[102] Other medications such as oral ketotifen, aspirin, and indomethacin have been suggested as possible medications for treatment of this disorder.[100] To date, there is no therapeutic reason for use of these medications.

An option to reduce clinical symptoms for many allergic diseases is immunotherapy with the offending allergen. However, oral, sublingual, and subcutaneous immunotherapy has no place in the treatment of any adverse food reaction.[53]

PREVENTION

There are numerous studies on the possible preventive effects of avoidance diets on the development of adverse food reactions and other allergic problems.[103–105] These studies have sought to either prevent or postpone atopic disease by breast-feeding or delayed introduction of solid foods. Recent investigations[42] involving patients with either one or two family members who had previous allergic disease have shown that maternal avoidance during the last trimester of pregnancy and a diet free from these foods for the first several months of life will only postpone the allergic symptoms but not prevent them. At age 12 months the infants on the avoidance diet did have fewer atopic symptoms, but by 24 months there were no differences between the two groups. Studies other than this one have not been able to control for environmental factors such as smoking, pets, and house dust allergens.

The routine use of protein hydrolysate formulas for allergy prevention has been advocated by some, but for most patients its use should be discouraged.[106] The widespread use of either soy or protein hydrolysate formulas for infants at risk to develop atopy or adverse food reactions lacks substantial and rational evidence.[96]

REFERENCES

1. Bahna SL, Heiner DC: Allergies to Milk. New York, Grune & Stratton, 1980, pp 1–3.
2. Anderson JA, Sogn DD: Adverse Reactions to Foods. National Institute of Allergy and Infectious Diseases, NIH Publication No. 84-2442. 1984.
3. Federal Register. 1983; 48:32749.
4. Sloan AE, Powers ME: A perspective on popular perceptions of adverse reactions to foods. J Allergy Clin Immunol 1986; 78:125.
5. Gerrard JW, Mackenzie JWA, Goluboff N, et al: Cow's milk allergy: Prevalence and manifestations in an unselected series of newborns. Acta Paediatr Scand 1973; 234 (Suppl):1–21.
6. Bock SA, Martin M: The incidence of adverse reactions to foods—a continuing study (abstract). J Allergy Clin Immunol 1983; 71(2):98.
7. Sampson HA: Role of immediate food hypersensitivity in the pathogenesis of atopic dermatitis. J Allergy Clin Immunol 1983; 71:473–480.
8. Sampson HA, McCaskin CC: Food hypersensitivity in atopic dermatitis: Clinical relevance of food hypersensitivity reactions. J Pediatr 1988; 113:447–451.
9. Burks AW, Mallory SB, Williams LW, et al: Atopic dermatitis: Clinical relevance of food hypersensitivity reactions. J Pediatr 1988; 113:447–451.
10. Sampson HA, Scanlon SM: Natural history of food hypersensitivity in children with atopic dermatitis. J Pediatr 1989; 115:23–27.
11. Powell GK: Milk- and soy-induced enterocolitis of infancy: Clinical features and standardization of challenge. J Pediatr 1978; 93:553–560.
12. Walker WA: Transmucosal passage of antigens. *In* Schmidt E, Reinhardt MC, eds: Food Allergy. New York, Raven Press, 1988, p 15.
13. Müller G, Bernsau I, Müller W, et al: Cow milk protein antigens and antibodies in serum of premature infants during the first 10 days of life. J Pediatr 1986; 109:869–873.
14. Walker WA: Host defense mechanisms in the gastrointestinal tract. Pediatrics 1976; 47:901–916.
15. Tennant B, Malm OJ, Horowitz RE, et al: Response of germ-free , conventional, conventionalized and *E. coli* monocontaminated mice to starvation. J Nutr 1968; 94:151–160.
16. Springer GF: Importance of blood-group substances in interactions between man and microbes. Ann NY Acad Sci 1970; 169:134–152.
17. Strombeck DR, Harrold D: Binding of cholera toxin to mucins and inhibition by gastric mucin. Infect Immun 1976; 10:1266–1272.
18. Brandtzaeg P: The humoral immune systems of the human gastrointestinal tract. Monogr Allergy 1981; 17:195–221.
19. Haneberg B, Aarshog D: Human faecal immunoglobulins in healthy infants and children, and in some with diseases affecting the intestinal tract or the immune system. Clin Exp Immunol 1975; 22:210–222.
20. Parrott DMV: The gut as a lymphoidal organ. Clin Gastroenterol 1976; 5:211–228.
21. Gowans JL, Knight EJ: The route of re-circulation of lymphocytes in the rat. Proc R Soc Lond [Ser B] 1974; 159:257–282.
22. Galindo B, Myrvick QN: Migratory response of granulomatous alveolar cells from BCG-sensitized rabbits. J Immunol 1970; 105:227–237.
23. Enerbäck L: Mast cells in the rat gastrointestinal mucosa. II. Dye-binding and metachromatic properties. Acta Pathol et Microbiol Scand 1966; 66:303–312.
24. Mohri K, Reimann HJ, Lorenz W, et al: Histamine content and mast cells in human gastric and duodenal mucosa. Agenta Actions 1978; 8:372–375.
25. Enerbäck L: Mast cell heterogeneity: The evaluation of the concept of a specific mucosal mast cell. *In* Befus AD, Bienenstock J, Denburg JA, eds: Mast Cell Differentiation and Heterogeneity. New York, Raven Press, 1986, p 1.
26. Chapman MD: Purification of allergens. Curr Opin Immunol 1989; 1;647–653.
27. Aas K: Antigens and allergens of fish. Int Arch Allergy Appl Immunol 1969; 36:152–155.
28. Stern M, Walker WA: Food proteins and gut mucosal barrier. I. Binding and uptake of cow's milk proteins by adult rat jejunum in vitro. Am J Physiol 1984; 246:G556–562.
29. Coombs RR, McLaughlan P: Allergenicity of food proteins and its possible modification. Ann Allergy 1984; 53:592–596.

30. Can A, Marsden RA, Kilshaw PJ: Egg and cow's milk hypersensitivity in exclusively breast fed infants with eczema, and detection of egg protein in breast milk. Br Med J 1985; 291:932–935.
31. Machtinger S, Moss R: Cow's milk allergy in breast-fed infants: The role of allergen and maternal secretory IgA antibody. J Allergy Clin Immunol 1986; 77:341–347.
32. Metcalfe DD: Food allergens. Clin Rev Allergy 1985; 3:331–349.
33. Spies JR, Stevan MA, Stein WJ, et al: The chemistry of allergens. XX. New antigens generated by pepsin hydrolysis of bovine milk protein. J Allergy 1970; 45:208–219.
34. Shibasaki M, Suzuki S, Tajima S, et al: Allergenicity of major component proteins of soybean. Int Arch Allergy Appl Immun 1980; 61:441–448.
35. Naismith WEF: Ultracentrifuge studies on soybean protein. Biochem Biophys Acta 1955; 16:203–210.
36. Burks AW, Casteel HB, Fiedorek SC, et al: A prospective food challenge study of two different types of soy protein isolates in patients with possible milk or soy protein intolerance (abstract). J Allergy Clin Immunol 1991; 87:175.
37. Burks AW, Brooks JR, Sampson HA: Allergenicity of major component proteins of soybean determined by enzyme linked immunosorbent assay (ELISA) and immunoblotting in children with atopic dermatitis and positive soy challenges. J Allergy Clin Immunol 1991; 87:175.
38. Moroz LA, Yang WH: Kunitz soybean trypsin inhibitor: A specific allergen in food anaphylaxis. N Engl J Med 1980; 302:1126–1128.
39. Sachs MI, Jones RT, Yunginger JW: Isolation and partial characterization of a major peanut allergen. J Allergy Clin Immunol 1981; 67:27–34.
40. Barnett D, Howden MEH, Bonham B, et al: Aspects of legume allergy research. Proc Sydney Allergy Group 1985; 4:104–118.
41. Burks AW, Williams LW, Helm RM, et al: Identification of a major peanut allergen, Arah I, in patients with atopic dermatitis and positive peanut challenges. J Allergy Clin Immunol 1991; 88:172–179.
42. Zeiger RS, Heller S, Mellon MH, et al: Effect of combined maternal and infant food-allergen avoidance on development of atopy in early infancy: A randomized study. J Allergy Clin Immunol 1989; 84:72–89.
43. Kjellman NIM: Epidemiology of food allergy. *In* Schmidt E, Reinhardt MC, eds: Food Allergy. New York, Raven Press, 1988, p 301.
44. Hattevig G, Kjellman B, Bjorksen B: Clinical symptoms and IgE responses to common food proteins and inhalants in the first 7 years of life. Clin Allergy 1987; 17:571–578.
45. Fölth-Magnusson K, Kjellman NIM: Development of atopic disease in babies whose mothers were receiving exclusion diet during pregnancy—a randomized study. J Allergy Clin Immunol 1987; 80:868–875.
46. Gunther M, Aschaffenburg R, Matthews RH, et al: The levels of antibodies to the proteins of cow's milk in the serum of normal infants. Immunology 1960; 3:296–306.
47. May CD, Fomon SJ, Remigio L: Immunologic consequences of feeding infants with cow's milk and soy products. Acta Paediatr Scand 1982; 71:43–51.
48. Dannaeus A, Johansson SGO, Foucard T, et al: Clinical and immunological aspects of food allergy in childhood. I. Estimation of IgG, IgA and IgE antibodies to food antigens in children with food allergy and atopic dermatitis. Acta Paediatr Scand 1977; 66:31–37.
49. McDonald PJ, Goldblum RM, van Sickle GJ, et al: Food protein-induced enterocolitis: Altered antibody response to ingested antigen. Pediatr Res 1984; 18:751–755.
50. Burks AW, Casteel HB, Brooks JR, et al: Enzyme linked immunosorbent assay and immunoblotting determination of antibody response to major component proteins of soybeans in patients with soy protein intolerance. J Pediatr Gastroenterol Nutr 1988; 8:195–203.
51. Hill DJ, Fiser MA, Shelton MJ, et al: Manifestations of milk allergy in infancy: Clinical and immunologic findings. J Pediatr 1986; 109:270–276.
52. Nakagawa T, Mukoyama T, Baba M, et al: Egg white-specific IgE and IgG_4 antibodies in atopic children. Ann Allergy 1986; 57:359.
53. Kettelhut BV, Metcalfe DD: Adverse reactions to foods. *In* Middleton E, et al, ed: Allergy: Principles and Practice. 3d ed. St. Louis, CV Mosby Company, 1988, pp 1481–1502.
54. Dannaeus A, Johansson SGO: A follow-up study of infants with adverse reactions to cow's milk. I. Serum IgE, skin test reactions and RAST in relation to clinical course. Acta Paediatr Scand 1979; 68:377–382.
55. Björksten B, Ahlstedt S, Björksten F, et al: Immunoglobulin E and immunoglobulin G4 antibodies to cow's milk in children with cow's milk allergy. Allergy 1983; 38:119–124.
56. Reimann HJ, Ring J, Ultsch B, et al: Intragastral provocation under endoscopic control (IPEC) in food allergy: Mast cell and histamine changes in gastric mucosa. Clin Allergy 1985; 15:195–202.
57. Selbekk BH: A comparison between in vitro jejunal mast cell degranulation and intragastric challenge in patients with suspected food intolerance. Scand J Gastroenterol 1985; 20:299–303.
58. Sampson HA, Jolie PL: Increased plasma histamine concentrations after food challenges in children with atopic dermatitis. N Engl J Med 1984; 311:372–376.
59. Leiferman KM, Ackerman SJ, Sampson HA, et al: Dermal deposition of eosinophil granule major basic protein in atopic dermatitis: Comparison with onchocerciasis. N Engl J Med 1985; 313:282–285.
60. Sampson HA, Broadbent KR, Broadbent JB: Spontaneous release of histamine from basophils and histamine-releasing factor in patients with atopic dermatitis and food hypersensitivity. N Engl J Med 1989; 321:228–232.
61. Shiner M: Ultrastructural features of allergic manifestations in the small intestine of children. Scand J Gastroenterol 1981; 70 (Suppl):49–64.
62. Frick OL: B-lactoglobulin in immune complexes in milk-sensitive children (abstract). J Allergy Clin Immunol 1982; 69:157.
63. Leary HL Jr, Halsey JF: An assay to measure antigen-specific immune complexes in food allergy. J Allergy Clin Immunol 1984; 74:190–195.
64. Cunningham-Rundles C, Brandeis WE, Good RH: Bovine antigens and the formulation of circulating immune complexes in selective immunoglobulin A deficiency. J Clin Invest 1979; 64:272–279.
65. Van Sickle GJ, Powell GK, McDonald PJ, et al: Milk- and soy protein-induced enterocolitis: Evidence for lymphocyte sensitization to specific food proteins. Gastroenterology 1985; 88:1915–1921.
66. Weil S, Kuperman O, Ilfeld D, et al: Non-specific suppressor cell activity and lymphocyte response to beta-lactoglobulin in cow's milk protein hypersensitivity. J Pediatr Gastroenterol Nutr 1982; 1:389–393.
67. Butler HL, Byrne WJ, Marmer DJ, et al: Depressed neutrophil chemotaxis in infants with cow's milk and/or soy protein intolerance. Pediatrics 1981; 67:264–268.
68. Ashkenazi A, Levin S, Idar D, et al: In vitro cell-mediated immunologic assay for cow's milk allergy. Pediatrics 1980; 66:399–402.
69. Kay RA, Ferguson A: Intestinal T cells, mucosal cell-mediated immunity and their relevance to food allergic disease. Clin Rev Allergy 1984; 2:55–68.
70. Kosnai I, Kuitunen P, Savilahti E, et al: Cell kinetics in the jejunal crypt epithelium in malabsorption syndrome with cow's milk protein intolerance and in coeliac disease. Gut 1980; 21:1041–1046.
71. Sampson HA: IgE-mediated food intolerance. J Allergy Clin Immunol 1988; 81:495–504.
72. Sampson HA, Mendelson L, Rosen JP: Fatal and near-fatal food anaphylaxis reactions in children (abstract). J Allergy Clin Immunol 1991; 87(2):176.
73. Goldman AS, Anderson DW, Sellers WA, et al: Milk allergy. I. Oral challenge with milk and isolated milk proteins in allergic children. Pediatrics 1963; 32:425–433.
74. Iyngkaran N, Abidin Z, Meng LL, et al: Egg protein-induced villous atrophy. J Pediatr Gastroenterol Nutr 1982; 1:29–33.
75. Vitoria JC, Camarero C, Sojo A, et al: Enteropathy related to fish, rice, and chicken. Arch Dis Child 1982; 57:44–48.
76. Manuel PD, Walker-Smith JA, France NE: Patchy enteropathy in childhood. Gut 1979; 20:211–215.

77. Kosnai I, Kuitunen P, Savilahti E, et al: Cell kinetics in the jejunal crypt epithelium in malabsorption syndrome with cow's milk protein intolerance and in coeliac disease. Gut 1980; 21:1041–1046.
78. Walker-Smith JA: Cow's milk intolerance as a cause of postenteritis diarrhea. J Pediatr Gastroenterol Nutr 1982; 1:163–173.
79. Gryboski JD, Burkle F, Hillman R: Milk-induced colitis in an infant. Pediatrics 1966; 38:299–302.
80. Panush RS, Stroud RM, Webster EM: Food-induced (allergic) arthritis. Inflammatory arthritis exacerbated by milk. Arthritis Rheum 1986; 29:220–226.
81. Mansfield LE, Vaughan TR, Waller SF, et al: Food allergy and adult migraine: Double-blind and mediator confirmation of an allergic etiology. Ann Allergy 1985; 55:126–129.
82. Feingold B: Why your child is hyperactive. New York, Random House, 1975.
83. Bock SA, Atkins FM, Zeiger RS, et al: Double-blind, placebo-controlled food challenge (DBPCFC) as an office procedure: A manual. J Allergy Clin Immunol 1988; 82:986–997.
84. Atkins FM, Steinberg SS, Metcalfe DD: Evaluation of immediate adverse reactions to foods in adult patients. I. Correlation of demographic, laboratory, and prick skin test data with response to controlled oral food challenge. J Allergy Clin Immunol 1985; 75:348–355.
85. Yunginger JW: Proper application of available laboratory tests for adverse reactions to foods and food additives. J Allergy Clin Immunol 1986;78:220–223.
86. Bock SA, Buckley J, Holst A, et al: Proper use of skin tests with food extracts in diagnosis of hypersensitivity to food in children. Clin Allergy 1977; 7:375–383.
87. Bock SA, Lee Y, Remigio LK, et al: Studies of hypersensitivity reactions to foods in infants and children. J Allergy Clin Immunol 1978; 62:327–334.
88. David TJ: Anaphylactic shock during elimination diets for severe atopic eczema. Arch Dis Child 1984; 59:983–986.
89. Jewett DL, Fein G, Greenberg MH: A double-blind study of symptom provocation to determine food sensitivity. N Engl J Med 1990; 323:429–433.
90. Atkins FM, Metcalfe DD: The diagnosis and treatment of food allergy. Ann Rev Nutr 1984; 4:233–255.
91. Brostoff J, Challacombe SJ: Food allergy and intolerance. London, Bailliere Tindall, 1987.
92. Katz AJ, Twarog FJ, Zeiger RS, et al: Milk-sensitive and eosinophilic gastroenteropathy: Similar clinical features with contrasting mechanisms and clinical course. J Allergy Clin Immunol 1984; 74:72–78.
93. Berg NO, Jakobsson I, Lindberg T: Do pre- and post-challenge small intestinal biopsies help to diagnose cow's milk protein intolerance? Acta Paediatr Scand 1979; 68:657–661.
94. Ford RP, Barnes GL, Hill DJ: Gastrointestinal hypersensitivity to cow's milk protein: The diagnostic value of gut function tests. Aust Paediatr J 1986; 22:37–42.
95. Flick JA, Sampson HA, Perman JA: Intestinal permeability to carbohydrates in children with atopic dermatitis (AD) and food hypersensitivity (abstract). Ped Research 1988; 23:303.
96. Stern MA: Gastrointestinal allergy. *In* Walker WA, et al, eds: Pediatric Gastrointestinal Disease: Pathophysiology, Diagnosis, Management. Philadelphia, BC Decker, 1991, pp 557–574.
97. How necessary are elimination diets in childhood? (editorial). Br Med J 1980; 1:138.
98. Bock SA: Probable allergic reaction to casein hydrolysate formula. J Allergy Clin Immunol 1989; 84:272.
99. Businco L, Benincori N, Nini G, et al: Double-blind crossover trial with oral sodium cromoglycate in children with atopic dermatitis due to food allergy. Ann Allergy 1986; 57:433–438.
100. Osvath P, Kelenhegyi K, Micskey E: Comparison of ketoifen and DSCG in treatment of food allergy in children. Allergol Immunopathol 1986; 14:515–518.
101. Burks AW, Sampson HA: Double-blind placebo-controlled trial of oral cromolyn sodium in children with egg hypersensitivity. J Allergy Clin Immunol 1988; 81:417–423.
102. Sogn D: Medications and their use in the treatment of adverse reactions to foods. J Allergy Clin Immunol 1986; 78:238–243.
103. Halpern SR, Sellers WA, Johnson RB, et al: Development of childhood allergy in infants fed breast, soy, or cow milk. J Allergy Clin Immunol 1973; 51:139–151.
104. Saarinen UM, Backman A, Kajosaari M, et al: Prolonged breast-feeding as prophylaxis for atopic disease. Lancet 1979; 2:163–166.
105. Kajosaari M, Saarinen UM: Prophylaxis of atopic disease by six months' total solid food elimination. Evaluation of 135 exclusively breast-fed infants of atopic families. Acta Paediatr Scand 1983; 72:411–414.
106. Hamburger RN: Diagnosis of food allergies and intolerances in the study of prophylaxis and control groups in infants. Ann Allergy 1984; 53:673–677.

Chapter 43

Eosinophilic Gastroenteritis

ROY PROUJANSKY

In 1967, Waldmann and coworkers[1] described six children with a clinical syndrome characterized by edema, growth failure, gastrointestinal protein loss, and peripheral and intestinal mucosal eosinophilia. Two of these patients responded to elimination of milk from their diet and subsequently outgrew their illness, being able to tolerate milk ingestion without a recurrence of symptoms. The remaining patients had a more chronic disorder requiring corticosteroid therapy on an intermittent or continuous basis to control their symptoms. Subsequent studies further clarified the similarities and differences between the protein-sensitive and idiopathic forms of eosinophilic gastroenteritis.[2] The idiopathic form of eosinophilic gastroenteritis is a relatively uncommon disorder, usually affecting the upper gastrointestinal tract, which may present at any age and which often requires steroid therapy for the control of symptoms. Protein-sensitive eosinophilic gastroenteritis is a much more frequent clinical occurrence, affecting the upper or lower gastrointestinal tract of children, which responds to dietary therapy and ultimately resolves as the patient gets older. Both conditions share the frequent occurrence of prominent and significant mucosal eosinophilia, suggesting similarities in pathogenesis.

In this chapter, we review the clinical manifestations, diagnostic approach, and treatment of each of these conditions as well as briefly discuss our current understanding of relevant pathophysiology.

CLINICAL PRESENTATION

Idiopathic Eosinophilic Gastroenteritis

The idiopathic form of eosinophilic gastroenteritis presents a highly variable clinical picture, depending on the anatomic and histologic distribution of the eosinophilic process. Tissue eosinophilia can be mucosal, muscular, or serosal and has been described to affect the esophagus, stomach, intestine, or colon alone or in combination (Table 43–1).[3] Despite this variation in anatomic and histologic involvement, certain clinical patterns are more frequent than others.

Mucosal Form

The most commonly encountered presentation, resulting from mucosal involvement of the stomach and variable degrees of the small intestine, is similar to Waldmann's original patients with prominent protein-losing gastroenteropathy. These patients often have growth failure, or weight loss, and edema. Gastrointestinal symptoms such as abdominal pain, vomiting, and diarrhea may occur, and in some patients, these symptoms may be exacerbated by the ingestion of specific foods. Many patients, however, have no gastrointestinal symptoms at all despite significant mucosal inflammation resulting in malabsorption or an enteric protein-losing state. Associated atopic symptoms, such as urticaria, eczema, or asthma, are often present. Anemia, hypoalbuminemia, and peripheral eosinophilia are nearly uniformly present, and patients with an atopic history may have elevated serum levels of total or food-specific gamma E immunoglobulin (IgE) or positive skin tests to a variety of dietary antigens.[4] Quantitative immunoglobulin levels may also be significantly reduced owing to the protein-losing state. Fecal occult blood may be present, and enteric protein loss may be demonstrable by enhanced excretion of fecal alpha$_1$-antitrypsin. Abnormal absorption of D-xylose or steatorrhea may also occur depending on the extent of small intestinal mucosal involvement.

Although the mucosal form of idiopathic eosinophilic gastroenteritis most commonly affects the upper gastrointestinal tract, there have also been reported cases of patients with an idiopathic eosinophilic colitis.[5] Similar to those patients with upper gastrointestinal involvement, these patients may also have prominent protein loss and associated atopic features in association with bloody diarrhea and other colitic symptoms.

Muscular Form

More prominent obstructive symptoms may also be seen in patients with idiopathic eosinophilic gastroenteritis depending on the extent of muscular involvement of the bowel wall. Muscular hypertrophy, resulting in some degree of gastric outlet obstruction, is the most common presentation of the muscular form of idiopathic eosino-

Table 43–1. CLINICAL PRESENTATIONS OF EOSINOPHILIC GASTROENTERITIS

Disorder	Clinical Presentation
Mucosal disease (idiopathic and protein-sensitive)	Malabsorption syndromes Diarrhea Weight loss Failure to thrive Chronic blood loss Anemia Guaiac-positive stools Protein-losing enteropathy Edema Hypoalbuminemia Colitis Bloody diarrhea
Muscular disease (idiopathic and protein-sensitive)	Gastric outlet obstruction Abdominal pain Vomiting Anorexia Intestinal obstruction Abdominal pain
Serosal disease (idiopathic)	Ascites

Adapted from references 3, 16, and 54.

philic gastroenteritis and often occurs in association with prominent gastrointestinal mucosal involvement, as noted earlier.[6] Obstructive lesions of the small bowel are somewhat less frequent, as are hypertrophic ileocolonic and colonic lesions. Atopic features appear to be a less prominent association in the muscular form of eosinophilic gastroenteritis unless significant mucosal disease is also present.

Serosal Form

The third and least common presentation of idiopathic eosinophilic gastroenteritis is that of eosinophilic ascites.[7, 8] This usually results from serosal and subserosal involvement of the small intestine and colon and is often associated with no other gastrointestinal symptoms. Occasionally, however, the eosinophilic process is transmural with symptoms reflecting the involvement of all three layers. Eosinophilic ascites usually presents with the insidious onset of peritoneal fluid accumulation without significant gastrointestinal symptoms. Paracentesis of the ascitic fluid usually reveals a predominantly eosinophilic cellularity, although occasionally this may evolve over time with the degree of ascitic fluid eosinophilia being less notable at the onset of symptoms. In addition to mucosal, muscular, and serosal involvement of the gastrointestinal tract by the eosinophilic process, one can occasionally see involvement of extraintestinal organs such as the spleen,[9] gallbladder,[10] liver,[11] and pancreas.[12]

Protein-Sensitive Eosinophilic Gastroenteritis

The protein-sensitive forms of eosinophilic gastroenteritis usually occur in infants and children below the age of 2 years and most commonly result from a reaction to cow's milk or soy proteins or, infrequently, breast milk. For clinical purposes, these conditions can be divided into those that result from upper gastrointestinal involvement and protein-sensitive colitis.

Protein-Sensitive Gastroenteritis

An immunologic reaction to dietary proteins, which results in significant enteritis or gastroenteritis, is usually seen at any age from the newborn period up to approximately 2 years of age. Many of the symptoms and signs of these patients are similar to those that occur in the mucosal form of idiopathic eosinophilic gastroenteritis. These patients can usually be distinguished, however, by their younger age and their clinical response to dietary modification. The clinical presentation of these patients can be quite variable, and several syndromes have been described that may occasionally have some overlap. In children less than 6 months of age, vomiting, diarrhea, and failure to thrive are quite common.[13–16] Many of these infants may also have colitic features, as described later. These patients can usually be shown to have some degree of mucosal malabsorption, varying degrees of hypoalbuminemia and enteric protein loss, and frequently gastrointestinal blood loss. The severity of these symptoms can be highly variable, ranging from infants with poor weight gain and mild anemia to those with severe diarrhea and significant malnutrition.[17] Similar to the muscular form of idiopathic eosinophilic gastroenteritis, pyloric narrowing simulating pyloric stenosis has been described.[18] Beyond 6 months of age, inflammation of the upper gastrointestinal tract, resulting from milk or soy protein, appears to be associated with fewer gastrointestinal symptoms. A typical patient is the cow's milk–fed infant with significant anemia or mild edema, resulting from gastrointestinal blood or protein loss with few or no gastrointestinal symptoms.

At presentation, many of these infants will have undergone multiple formula changes, usually from a cow's milk protein formula to a variety of soy protein formulas. Occasionally these formula changes are associated with transient improvement followed by a recurrence of symptoms, leading to confusion about the cause of the patient's symptoms. Less commonly, unusual and inappropriate dietary regimens have been implemented in an attempt to resolve the patient's symptoms.[19]

Protein-Sensitive Colitis

Protein-sensitive colitis tends to occur in young infants, ingesting cow's milk, soy formula, or breast milk, and is characterized by variable degrees of bloody stools or bloody diarrhea.[20–22] These infants are usually relatively healthy in appearance unless they have significant upper gastrointestinal symptoms as well. On occasion, they are described as "colicky" babies. Their stools are often described as mucousy in appearance or are noted to contain mucous with flecks or streaks of blood throughout the stool. Laboratory investigation may reveal anemia and peripheral eosinophilia. Hypoalbuminemia is usually not present. Sigmoidoscopic evaluation may reveal edema, erythema, punctate hemorrhage, and mucosal ulceration, frequently in a patchy distribution in the rectosigmoid and descending colon.[23]

PATHOPHYSIOLOGY

The hallmark of the idiopathic and protein-sensitive forms of eosinophilic gastroenteritis is prominent tissue eosinophilia. A variety of factors have been thought to play a role in the recruitment of eosinophils to the mucosa and in the pathophysiology of these disorders. Because of the often prominent atopic features present clinically, a great deal of interest has focused on the role of mast cells and IgE-dependent mechanisms in eosinophil recruitment and tissue damage. Experimentally it can be demonstrated that IgE-dependent, mucosal mast cell activation can lead to protein exudation across the gastric mucosa.[24] Mucosal mast cell activation can also be shown to produce a late-phase inflammatory response in the gastric mucosa, suggesting that IgE-mediated reactions could explain both the acute symptoms associated with specific food ingestion and the more chronic symptoms resulting from a sustained inflammatory reaction.[25] Although these mechanisms may be important in some patients, eosinophilic gastroenteritis also occurs in patients without atopic features. In addition to mast cell–derived mediators, a variety of factors of lymphocyte origin have been described that may play a primary role in tissue eosinophil recruitment and activation.[26] It is thus possible that eosinophilic gastroenteritis may be the end result of a variety of different pathophysiologic processes, explaining some of the clinical heterogeneity present in this group of disorders.

Independent of the mechanisms responsible for eosinophil recruitment, a great deal of circumstantial evidence has accumulated to suggest that eosinophil granule proteins and other constituents play a significant role in the tissue damage and altered gastrointestinal physiology that occur in these conditions. Eosinophil granules contain a variety of potentially cytotoxic proteins, and extracellular release of these proteins and activation of tissue eosinophils have been observed in sections of affected mucosa from patients with eosinophilic gastroenteritis.[26–28] Eosinophils are capable of producing a number of mediators, which may be proinflammatory (leukotrienes), may alter gastrointestinal motility (substance P), or are capable of altering epithelial cell kinetics (transforming growth factor-alpha).[29–31] Release of a number of these proinflammatory proteins and mediators has been shown to be possible by both IgE-dependent and IgA-dependent activation.[32, 33] Thus it is quite likely that following recruitment to the gastrointestinal tract, eosinophils play an important role in the ensuing tissue damage.

In spite of accumulating information regarding the mechanisms that may be responsible for eosinophil recruitment to tissues and subsequent tissue damage, the initial events resulting in the idiopathic forms of eosinophilic gastroenteritis remain to be elucidated. The age-related decline in the incidence of the protein-sensitive forms of this disorder, however, suggests that developmental factors may be important. The neonatal period is a time when the gastrointestinal mucosa may be particularly vulnerable to mounting an abnormal response to dietary antigens. In experimental studies in mice, both humoral and cellular immune responses to dietary antigens can be demonstrated in mice exposed to new antigens during the first week of life.[34, 35] After this, an immune response cannot be elicited to these antigens following oral exposure. Similarly, in human infants with milk-induced or soy protein–induced enterocolitis, one can demonstrate evidence of systemic humoral and cellular immune responses to milk or soy proteins.[36, 37] Thus oral tolerance may be more easily disrupted in the newborn infant predisposing to protein sensitivity.

DIAGNOSIS AND DIFFERENTIAL DIAGNOSIS

The diagnosis of eosinophilic gastroenteritis should be suspected when any of the previously mentioned clinical features occur in association with significant peripheral blood eosinophilia. When mucosal involvement is suspected, initial evaluation may be aimed at demonstrating gastrointestinal blood loss, loss of serum proteins, and evidence of malabsorption. Subsequent investigations should include radiographic and histologic demonstration of the extent of gastrointestinal involvement. Contrast studies of the upper gastrointestinal tract may demonstrate prominent gastric folds, antral mucosal nodularity, and thickened folds in the small bowel. Air contrast study of the gastric antrum may be particularly effective at demonstrating the irregular mucosal surface.[38] When muscular features are present, significant narrowing of the antrum or pylorus may be noted (Fig. 43–1). Muscular involvement beyond the stomach may produce radiographic evidence of small intestinal or ileocolonic strictures simulating Crohn's disease.[39]

Confirmation of a suspected diagnosis of eosinophilic gastroenteritis requires histologic evidence of an eosinophilic inflammatory reaction in the affected portion of the gastrointestinal tract. When the upper gastrointestinal tract is affected, the gastric antrum is the area most consistently involved, and biopsy procedures should include sampling from this location (Fig. 43–2).[40] Involvement of the duodenal and jejunal mucosa may be more patchy, requiring multiple biopsies with careful histologic evaluation of multiple sections to identify eosinophilic infiltrates (Fig. 43–3). In the idiopathic form of this disorder, significant mucosal eosinophilia can also occasionally be found in esophageal and colonic mucosa. When the muscular form of the disease is present, mucosal biopsy may demonstrate the eosinophilic lesion. Occasionally, however, a diagnosis of the muscular form of eosinophilic gastroenteritis is not made until a surgically resected stricture is available for histologic evaluation.

Because of the protean manifestations and varied

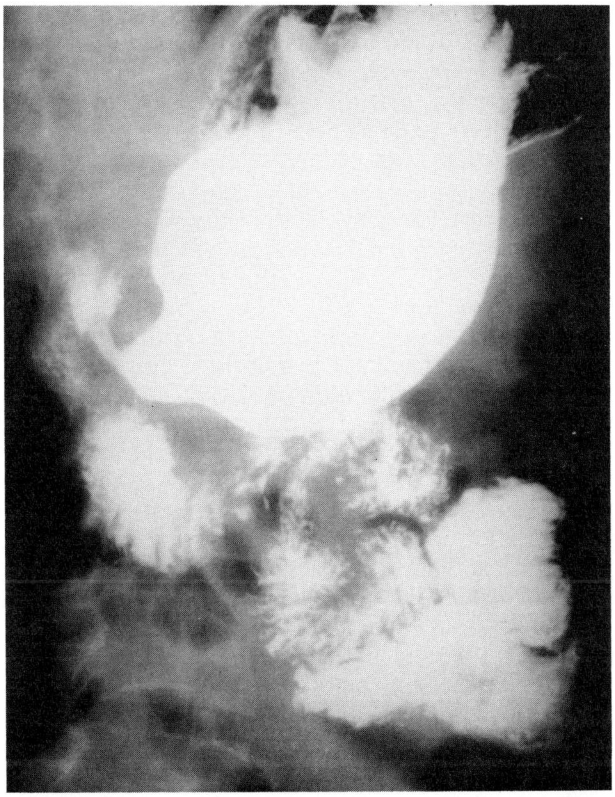

Figure 43–1. Contrast study of the upper gastrointestinal tract in a patient with the muscular form of eosinophilic gastroenteritis revealing marked narrowing of the antrum and pylorus. (Courtesy of R. Teele.)

presentations of eosinophilic gastroenteritis, it should be included in the differential diagnosis of a variety of symptoms and signs resulting from protein-losing enteropathy, malabsorption, partial gastric outlet obstruction, and colitis. Diseases such as Ménétrier's disease and Crohn's disease may also produce a protein-losing state in association with radiographic evidence of thickened gastric folds or a nodular gastric antrum. Ménétrier's disease may be distinguished by its predilection for involvement of the body and the fundus of the stomach, and both Ménétrier's disease and Crohn's disease should be discernible by histologic assessment.[41] Chronic granulomatous disease may also produce antral narrowing in association with a mucosal lesion with a predominantly eosinophilic infiltrate and may be suspected by the presence of the appropriate history of recurrent infections and disease in other organ systems.[42] Significant mucosal eosinophilia can also be seen in parasitic infection, with oral gold therapy, during the course of several vasculitic diseases, and occasionally early in the course of relapsing inflammatory bowel disease.[43–46] Eosinophilic gastroenteritis may also be seen as part of a more generalized disorder such as the hyper-IgE syndrome or the idiopathic hypereosinophilic syndrome.[47, 48]

The diagnosis of the protein-sensitive forms of eosinophilic gastroenteritis requires two separate steps. First, an initial diagnostic evaluation must demonstrate that an eosinophilic inflammatory lesion is responsible for the patient's symptoms. Second, it must be shown that this lesion results from a reaction to a specific dietary antigen by rechallenging the patient.[49]

Proof that any of these eosinophilic inflammatory processes are the result of formula or milk protein sensitivity requires showing that the patient's symptoms improve on antigen withdrawal and that they recur with subsequent rechallenge. The way in which formula withdrawal and rechallenge are performed should be individualized depending on the character and the severity of the patient's initial presentation.

For patients who were initially being fed a cow's milk protein formula, one can remove cow's milk protein from the diet and substitute a soy protein formula. Approximately one third of patients who are sensitive to cow's milk protein, however, will also be sensitive to soy protein. Thus some patients may have persistent symptoms or develop a recurrence of symptoms on soy formula. The remaining alternative for these patients is to use one of several elemental formulas to allow the patient's symptoms to resolve. For the exclusively breast-fed infant, there are several alternatives. Occasional successes have been achieved by restricting the cow's milk intake of the patient's mother.[22] If this is not successful at resolving the patient's symptoms, one can additionally restrict the mother's intake of soy protein. The widespread distribution of cow's milk and soy proteins in a variety of foods, however, makes this type

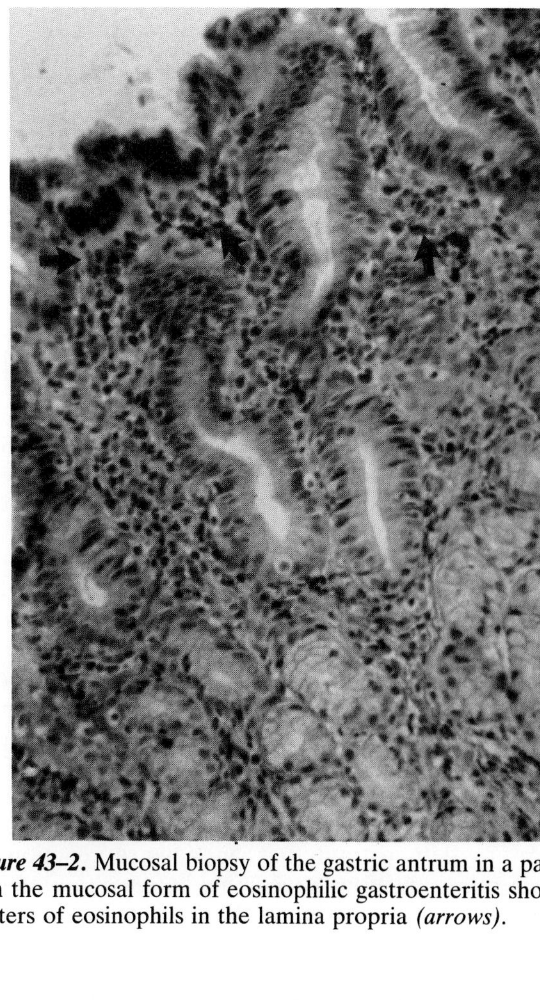

Figure 43–2. Mucosal biopsy of the gastric antrum in a patient with the mucosal form of eosinophilic gastroenteritis showing clusters of eosinophils in the lamina propria *(arrows).*

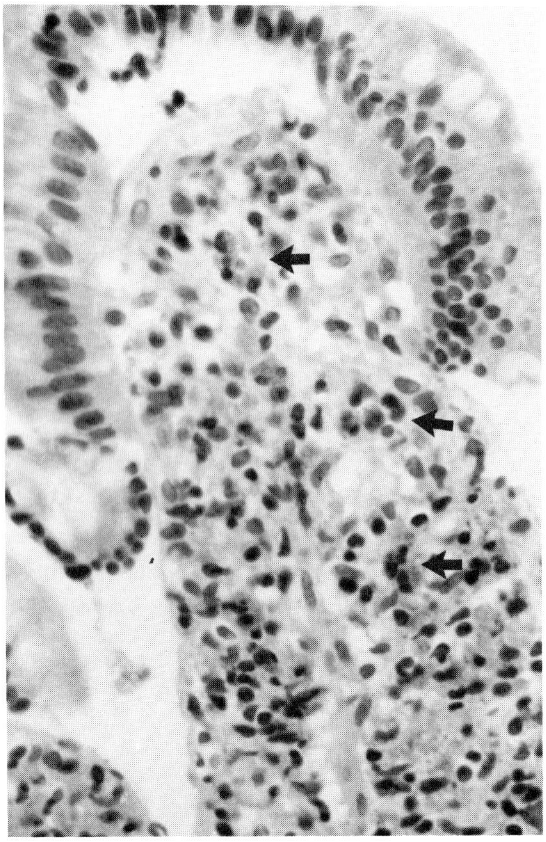

Figure 43–3. Mucosal biopsy of the proximal small bowel in a patient with the mucosal form of eosinophilic gastroenteritis. *Arrows* denote clusters of eosinophils throughout the lamina propria.

of maternal dietary restriction potentially unsafe for the lactating woman. Breast-fed patients who do not respond to alteration of the maternal diet should be changed over to an elemental formula. For the slightly older child who is receiving cow's milk and a variety of other solids and liquids, one can simply restrict the milk intake to obtain an initial remission of symptoms. Patients who respond partially or not at all to antigen withdrawal should be carefully evaluated for their adherence to the recommended dietary restriction. If dietary restriction has been adhered to and no clinical response has occurred, it is unlikely that the patient has a protein-sensitive component to the inflammatory disease.

The timing and the mechanism for rechallenging a patient who has improved with milk or formula withdrawal are dependent on a number of factors. First, it is important to assess how sick the patient is at initial presentation. The patient who presented initially with severe diarrhea requiring hospitalization and a prolonged course of parenteral nutrition is going to need to be challenged more carefully than the thriving infant who had bloody, mucousy stools while on soy formula. Second, when rechallenge is performed, one should attempt to demonstrate that an adverse reaction to formula reintroduction is recurring before the patient's symptoms become as severe as they were initially. Third, the prolonged use of elemental formulas can be quite costly. Because some patients will outgrow their sensitivity quite rapidly, one should not be arbitrary about the length of time that these formulas need to be used without using rechallenge as a guide.

For the patient with protein-sensitive gastroenteritis, the challenge protocol should be symptom specific. One should look for vomiting or diarrhea as a reaction to formula reintroduction for the patient who had these symptoms initially. Evidence of a recurrence of blood in the stool should be sought for the colitis patient being rechallenged. These symptoms may recur immediately or may take several days to develop. For the patient who presented initially with significant edema and hypoalbuminemia without significant gastrointestinal symptoms, however, one needs to use additional diagnostic techniques to demonstrate that a reaction is occurring before the patient's development of edema. If at presentation the patient had enhanced fecal $alpha_1$-antitrypsin excretion documenting enteric protein loss, one may wish to use prechallenge and postchallenge fecal $alpha_1$-antitrypsin levels to document a positive challenge before the patient's becoming symptomatic. Similarly, prechallenge and postchallenge D-xylose levels may be useful for demonstrating a positive challenge before the onset of severe symptoms for the patient who had a severe malabsorptive process initially.[50] This approach can also be taken one step further using prechallenge and postchallenge small intestinal mucosal biopsies to guide further therapy.[51] The prechallenge biopsy is to document that the intestinal mucosa is completely normal, before challenge, to avoid subsequent confusion. Although this approach may be useful for demonstrating that mucosal injury is recurring before the onset of severe symptoms, several authors have noted patients with abnormal postchallenge biopsies who remain asymptomatic in spite of continued rechallenge.[52, 53] For these patients, careful follow-up to determine that no adverse effects are occurring may allow them to remain on an unrestricted diet.

MANAGEMENT

The alternatives available for treating the patient with eosinophilic gastroenteritis are dependent on whether or not they have the protein-sensitive or idiopathic form of the disease. For those with the protein-sensitive disorder, management is dietary, using repeated rechallenge to assess when and if the patient has outgrown the sensitivity. For patients who have had relatively mild symptoms at initial diagnosis, rechallenge can often be performed within a few weeks. Some infants resolve the protein sensitivity quickly, allowing them to return to a less restrictive, less costly diet fairly rapidly. Patients who have a positive reaction at the time of rechallenge should resume the dietary approach that allowed them to remain symptom-free. They can then be rechallenged again at regular intervals until it is clear that sensitivity has resolved. Most patients will have resolved sensitivity by 1 year of age. It may be prudent to avoid rechallenge until this time for the patients who had severe symptoms initially. Ultimately when such patients are re-evaluated for protein sensitivity, challenge should be done initially with minute amounts of antigen, increasing slowly while observing for a response. Occasionally, positive reactions in this setting have been severe, suggesting that selected patients should be rechallenged under controlled conditions.[15]

The treatment options for the management of a patient with the idiopathic form of eosinophilic gastroenteritis are more limited and vary to some extent depending on which form of the disease is present. For patients with predominantly mucosal disease, there have been a number of treatment approaches designed to remove multiple antigens from the diet using an exclusively elemental formula as the sole dietary nutrient. Some successes have been reported with this approach; however, some of these patients have been younger patients who, in fact, have had a more self-limited disease process. For patients with prominent atopic symptoms, skin testing or the demonstration of food-specific IgE antibodies may be useful for determining which dietary antigens may be worth eliminating.

For the majority of patients, however, a fairly prompt and effective remission can be obtained with the use of steroids.[54] Many patients have a rapid response to oral prednisone, in a dosage of 1 to 2 mg per kg per day, and can rapidly be tapered to low-dose, every-other-day steroid therapy. It is often possible to maintain partial or complete remissions of the disease process with a dosage of prednisone that produces no observable side effects and that has no significant suppressive effects on linear growth. Exacerbations can then frequently be controlled with brief, high-dose pulses of steroid therapy, with rapid return to the low-dose, alternate-day schedule. The effectiveness of this approach makes it a preferable alternative for many patients to severe dietary restriction and the use of an exclusive elemental diet. Several investigators have noted the often striking sensitivity of eosinophilic ascites to steroid therapy and the maintenance of remission on dosages that one might think were homeopathic.

A remaining alternative for medical therapy for this disorder is the use of mast cell–stabilizing agents such as oral cromolyn and ketotifen. Both of these agents have been described to be effective for selected patients with eosinophilic gastroenteritis, and in a few cases, these agents have had efficacy when other immunosuppressive therapy has failed.[55–57] They can also be combined with low-dose steroid therapy in an attempt to maintain remission at a reduced steroid dosage.

REFERENCES

1. Waldmann TA, Wochner RD, Laster L, et al: Allergic gastroenteropathy: A cause of excessive gastrointestinal protein loss. N Engl J Med 1967; 276:761–769.
2. Katz AJ, Twarog FJ, Zeiger RS, et al: Milk-sensitive and eosinophilic gastroenteropathy: Similar clinical features with contrasting mechanisms and clinical course. J Allergy Clin Immunol 1984; 74:72–78.
3. Klein NC, Hargrove RL, Sleisenger MH, et al: Eosinophilic gastroenteritis. Medicine 1970; 49:299–319.
4. Caldwell JH, Sharma HM, Hurtubise PE, et al: Eosinophilic gastroenteritis in extreme allergy: Immunopathological comparison with nonallergic gastrointestinal disease. Gastroenterology 1979; 77:560–564.
5. Tedesco FJ, Huckaby CB, Hamby-Allen M, et al: Eosinophilic ileocolitis: Expanding spectrum of eosinophilic gastroenteritis. Dig Dis Sci 1981; 26:943–948.
6. Caldwell JH, Mekhjian HS, Hurtubise PE, et al: Eosinophilic gastroenteritis with obstruction: Immunologic studies of seven patients. Gastroenterology 1978; 74:825–829.
7. McNabb PC, Fleming CR, Higgins JA, et al: Transmural eosinophilic gastroenteritis with ascites. Mayo Clin Proc 1979; 54:119–122.
8. Hyams JS, Treem WR, Schwartz AN: Recurrent abdominal pain and ascites in an adolescent. J Pediatr 1988; 113:569–574.
9. Robert F, Omura E, Durant JR: Mucosal eosinophilic gastroenteritis with systemic involvement. Am J Med 1977; 62:139–143.
10. Kerstein MD, Sheahan DG, Gudjonsson B, et al: Eosinophilic cholecystitis. Am J Gastroenterol 1976; 66:349–351.
11. Everett GD, Mitros FA: Eosinophilic gastroenteritis with hepatic eosinophilic granulomas. Am J Gastroenterol 1980; 74:519–521.
12. Smith PM, Morgans ME, Clark CG, et al: Lipodystrophy, pancreatitis and eosinophilia. Gut 1975; 16:230–234.
13. Iyngkaran N, Robinson MJ, Prathap K, et al: Cow's milk protein-sensitive enteropathy: Combined clinical and histological criteria for diagnosis. Arch Dis Child 1978; 53:20–26.
14. Kuitunen P, Visakorpi JK, Savilahti E, et al: Malabsorption syndrome with cow's milk intolerance: Clinical findings and course in 54 cases. Arch Dis Child 1975; 50:351–356.
15. Powell GK: Milk- and soy-induced enterocolitis of infancy: Clinical features and standardization of challenge. J Pediatr 1978; 93:553–560.
16. Goldman H, Proujansky R: Allergic proctitis and gastroenteritis in children. Am J Surg Pathol 1986; 10:75–86.
17. Ament ME, Rubin CE: Soy protein—another cause of the flat intestinal lesion. Gastroenterology 1972; 62:227–234.
18. Snyder JD, Rosenblum N, Wershil B, et al: Pyloric stenosis and eosinophilic gastroenteritis in infants. J Pediatr Gastro Nutr 1987; 6:543–547.
19. Sinatra FR, Merritt RJ: Iatrogenic kwashiorkor in infants. Am J Dis Child 1981; 135:21–23.
20. Jenkins HR, Pincott JR, Soothill JF, et al: Food allergy: The major cause of infantile colitis. Arch Dis Child 1984; 59:326–329.
21. Halpin TC, Byrne WJ, Ament ME. Colitis, persistent diarrhea, and soy protein intolerance. J Pediatr 1977; 91:404–407.
22. Lake AM, Whitington PF, Hamilton SR: Dietary protein-induced colitis in breast-fed infants. J Pediatr 1982; 101:906–910.
23. Berezin S, Schwarz SM, Glassman M, et al: Gastrointestinal milk intolerance of infancy. Am J Dis Child 1989; 143:361–362.
24. Wershil BK, Wang Z-S, Galli SJ: The gastric late-phase response: Fibrin deposition and neutrophil infiltration in an IgE-dependent reaction. Pediatr Res 1990; 27:119A.
25. Wershil BK, Wang Z-S, Galli SJ: Evidence of mast-cell dependent neutrophil infiltration during IgE-dependent gastric inflammation in the mouse: Does this represent a gastric late phase reaction? Gastroenterology 1991; 100:A625.
26. Weller PF: The immunobiology of eosinophils. N Engl J Med 1991; 324:1110–1118.
27. Keshavarzian A, Saverymuttu SH, Tai P-C, et al: Activated eosinophils in familial eosinophilic gastroenteritis. Gastroenterology 1985; 88:1041–1049.
28. Torpier G, Colombel JF, Mathieu-Chandelier C, et al: Eosinophilic gastroenteritis: Ultrastructural evidence for a selective release of eosinophil major basic protein. Clin Exp Immunol 1988; 74:404–408.
29. Weller PF, Lee CW, Foster DW, et al: Generation and metabolism of 5-lipoxygenase pathway leukotrienes by human eosinophils: Predominant production of leukotriene C4. Proc Natl Acad Sci USA 1983; 80:7626–7630.
30. Aliakbari J, Sreedharan SP, Turck CW, et al: Selective localization of vasoactive intestinal peptide and substance P in human eosinophils. Biochem Biophys Res Comm 1987; 148:1440–1445.
31. Wong DTW, Weller PF, Galli SJ, et al: Human eosinophils express transforming growth factor alpha. J Exp Med 1990; 172:673–681.

32. Capron M, Capron A, Dessaint J-P, et al: Fc receptors for IgE on human and rat eosinophils. J Immunol 1981; 126:2087–2092.
33. Abu-Ghazaleh RI, Fujisawa T, Mestecky J, et al: IgA-induced eosinophil degranulation. J Immunol 1989; 142:2393–2400.
34. Hanson DG. Ontogeny of orally induced tolerance to soluble proteins in mice. I. Priming and tolerance in newborns. J Immunol 1981; 127:1518–1524.
35. Strobel S, Ferguson A: Immune responses to fed protein antigens in mice. 3. Systemic tolerance or priming is related to age at which antigen is first encountered. Pediatr Res 1984; 18:588–594.
36. McDonald PJ, Goldblum RM, Van Sickle GJ, et al: Food protein-induced enterocolitis: Altered antibody response to ingested antigen. Pediatr Res 1984; 18:751–755.
37. Van Sickle GJ, Powell GK, McDonald PJ, et al: Milk- and soy protein-induced enterocolitis: Evidence for lymphocyte sensitization to specific food proteins. Gastroenterology 1985; 88:1915–1921.
38. Teele RL, Katz AJ, Goldman H, et al: Radiologic features of eosinophilic gastroenteritis (allergic gastroenteropathy) of childhood. AJR 1979; 132:575–580.
39. Haberkern CM, Christie DL, Haas JE. Eosinophilic gastroenteritis presenting as ileocolitis. Gastroenterology 1978; 74:896–899.
40. Katz AJ, Goldman H, Grand RJ: Gastric mucosal biopsy in eosinophilic (allergic) gastroenteritis. Gastroenterology 1977; 73:705–709.
41. Chouraqui JP, Roy CC, Brochu P, et al: Ménétrier's disease in children: Report of a patient and review of sixteen other cases. Gastroenterology 1981; 80:1042–1047.
42. Griscom NT, Kirkpatrick JA, Girdany BR, et al: Gastric antral narrowing in chronic granulomatous disease of childhood. Pediatrics 1974; 54:456–460.
43. Kuipers FC, van Thiel PH, Rodenberg W, et al: Eosinophilic phlegmon of the alimentary canal caused by a worm. Lancet 1960; 2:1171–1173.
44. Martin DM, Goldman JA, Gilliam J, et al: Gold-induced eosinophilic enterocolitis: Response to oral cromolyn sodium. Gastroenterology 1981; 80:1567–1570.
45. Suen KC, Burton JD: The spectrum of eosinophilic infiltration of the gastrointestinal tract and its relationship to other disorders of angiitis and granulomatosis. Hum Pathol 1979; 10:31–43.
46. Rutgeerts P, Geboes K, Vantrappen G, et al: Natural history of recurrent Crohn's disease at the ileocolonic anastomosis after curative surgery. Gut 1984; 25:665–672.
47. Donabedian H, Gallin JI. The hyperimmunoglobulin E recurrent-infection (Job's) syndrome. Medicine 1983; 62:195–208.
48. Alfaham MA, Ferguson SD, Sihra B, et al: The idiopathic hypereosinophilic syndrome. Arch Dis Child 1987; 62:601–613.
49. Goldman AS, Anderson DW, Sellers WA, et al: I. Oral challenge with milk and isolated milk proteins in allergic children. Pediatrics 1963; 32:425–443.
50. Morin CL, Buts J-P, Weber A, et al: One-hour blood-xylose test in diagnosis of cow's milk protein intolerance. Lancet 1979; 1:1102–1104.
51. Shiner M, Ballard J, Brook CGD, et al: Intestinal biopsy in the diagnosis of cow's milk protein intolerance without acute symptoms. Lancet. 1975; 2:1060–1063.
52. Sumithran E, Iyngkaran N: Is jejunal biopsy really necessary in cow's milk protein intolerance? Lancet 1977; 2:1122–1123.
53. Iyngkaran N, Yadav M, Boey CG, et al: Effect of continued feeding of cows' milk on asymptomatic infants with milk protein sensitive enteropathy. Arch Dis Child 1988; 63:911–915.
54. Steffen RM, Wyllie R, Petras RE, et al: The spectrum of eosinophilic gastroenteritis. Report of six pediatric cases and review of the literature. Clin Pediatr 1991; 30:404–411.
55. Moots RJ, Prouse P, Gumpel JM: Near fatal eosinophilic gastroenteritis responding to oral sodium cromoglycate. Gut 1988; 29:1282–1285.
56. Heatley RV, Harris A, Atkinson M: Treatment of a patient with clinical features of both eosinophilic gastroenteritis and polyarteritis nodosa with oral sodium cromoglycate. Dig Dis Sci 1980; 25:470–472.
57. Melamed I, Feanny SJ, Sherman PM, et al: Benefit of ketotifen in patients with eosinophilic gastroenteritis. Am J Med 1991; 90:310–314.

Chapter 44

Short Bowel Syndrome

William R. Treem

Management of the child with short bowel syndrome (SBS) is one of the greatest challenges facing the pediatric gastroenterologist and requires a thorough knowledge of the potential consequences of massive bowel resection. Providing adequate nutrition and avoiding complications are critical, since clinical experience has confirmed the remarkable capacity of most of these patients to achieve normal enteral feeding over a sufficient period of time. Two major developments have dramatically altered the prognosis for even the most severely affected infants and children. More than 20 years ago, the first patient given total parenteral nutrition was an infant with SBS.[1] Since then, parenteral nutrition has become an indispensable part of the acute and chronic management of SBS. More recently, limited success with small bowel transplantation has offered hope to those without sufficient intestinal adaptation to support enteral feedings.[2]

This chapter reviews the etiology, pathophysiology, clinical evaluation, and management of patients with SBS. Emphasis is placed on factors that mediate intestinal adaptation and complications that inhibit this process. Special consideration is given to the unique nutritional needs of these patients. Recent experience with newer medical and surgical therapies, including small bowel transplantation, is explored.

DEFINITION

SBS is defined as malabsorption, fluid and electrolyte loss, and malnutrition following massive small bowel resection. As much as half of the small intestine may be lost without significant long-term problems in sustaining normal nutrition, provided the duodenum, distal ileum, and ileocecal valve (ICV) are spared. In contrast, distal ileal resections that include the ICV may induce severe diarrhea even though only 25% of the small bowel has been resected. Resection of more than 75% of the small intestine with preservation of the ICV invariably produces initial intractable malabsorption and diarrhea. Wilmore[3] reviewed the case histories of 50 infants under two months of age and defined SBS as less than 75 cm of residual small intestine. Since the length of the small intestine is estimated to be 200 to 300 cm at birth in a full-term neonate,[4] these infants underwent a greater than 50% resection. This definition may not be applicable in preterm infants because the total intestinal length normally doubles from the 26th to 38th week of gestation.[5] Thereafter the length of the small intestine increases to 600 to 800 cm in the adult; intestinal diameter also changes from 1.5 cm to 3 to 4 cm.[6] These changes and the development of the plicae circulares, villi, and microvilli combine to enlarge the absorptive surface area from approximately 950 cm^2 at birth to 7,500 cm^2 in the adult.[7] The infant does not tolerate massive small bowel resection as well as the adult because of a lack of intestinal reserve. Conversely, the infant has a more favorable long-term prognosis because of a greater residual capacity for growth and development.[8]

ETIOLOGY

Table 44–1 summarizes the causes of SBS in infants collated from several published series.[3, 9–14] The most common causes include necrotizing enterocolitis, volvulus, jejunoileal atresia(s), and gastroschisis. Midgut volvulus and diffuse small bowel Crohn's disease predominate in the older child.[15] Less frequent etiologies of SBS include trauma to the gastrointestinal tract[16] and total colonic aganglionosis with proximal extension into the small bowel.[12]

The majority of infants with necrotizing enterocolitis respond to medical therapy or require less than one fourth of their small intestines resected.[17] SBS has been reported in 7 to 38% of infants surviving surgical therapy for necrotizing enterocolitis[18–21] Several authors have stressed the importance of differentiating areas of complete transmural necrosis from potentially viable bowel in an effort to avoid massive small bowel resections.[22] At present, there is no accurate method for making this distinction, though some have advocated intraoperative fluorescein dye angiography or Doppler ultrasound.[12] Rather than creating a short bowel initially, many surgeons perform a "second-look operation" within 24 to 48 hours to determine whether any areas that appeared necrotic at first are actually viable.

Midgut volvulus resulting in SBS is most often the result of congenital malrotation of the colon and malfixation of the intestine. The damaged area corresponds to the intestine supplied by the superior mesenteric artery, and infarction results in a loss of almost all the small

Table 44–1. SUMMARY OF SERIES ON THE ETIOLOGY OF SHORT BOWEL SYNDROME IN INFANTS

	No. of Subjects						
Etiologic Disorder	***Wilmore***[3] ***(1972)***	***Bohane et al***[9] ***(1979)***	***Cooper et al***[16] ***(1984)***	***Dorney et al***[11] ***(1985)***	***Grosfeld et al***[12] ***(1986)***	***Caniano et al***[13] ***(1989)***	***Goulet et al***[14] ***(1991)***
Volvulus	30	2	6	6	5	1	22
Atresia(s)	14	6	3	3	13	5	36
Gastroschisis	5	3	2	1	5	5	10
Necrotizing enterocolitis	0	4	5	2	24	2	11
Other*	1	0	0	1	7	1	8
Total	50	15	16	13	54	14	87

*Meconium peritonitis, extensive intestinal angioma, complicated intussusception, congenital short bowel syndrome.

bowel except for a few centimeters of proximal jejunum and distal ileum. These areas are sustained by collateral circulation from the celiac axis and inferior mesenteric artery. Other congenital anomalies resulting in volvulus include a twist of a heavy intestinal loop secondary to meconium ileus or a twist about a congenital remnant of the omphalomesenteric duct. Midgut volvulus may present acutely in older children with bilious vomiting or insidiously after several intermittent episodes of unexplained abdominal pain and vomiting. In one recent series, SBS acquired between the ages of 2 and 16 years was secondary to midgut volvulus in 10 to 13 patients.[15] Volvulus may also be related to previous surgery and adhesive bowel obstruction.[12]

Two other important congenital causes of SBS are jejunoileal atresia(s) and gastroschisis. In several series, these two etiologies account for 30 to 60% of the cases.[3, 9–14] Atresias result from ischemic necrosis of the fetal intestine due to a vascular catastrophe. Multiple etiologies of in utero vascular occlusion have been documented, including volvulus of the small intestine, intussusception, internal hernia with strangulation, and constriction of the mesentery in a tight gastroschisis or omphalocele defect.[23, 24] Adjacent surviving intestinal segments may sustain incomplete ischemic damage with important implications for altered function in the remaining bowel. Most often, infants with intestinal atresia present with bilious vomiting, abdominal distention, and failure to pass meconium. Polyhydramnios and jaundice are also common clinical findings.

Familial apple peel jejunal atresia is a particularly severe form of congenital intestinal atresia that frequently results in SBS.[25] This distinct anatomic malformation is characterized by proximal intestinal atresia, absence of the distal superior mesenteric artery and the dorsal mesentery, and retrograde blood supply to the surviving distal small bowel from the right colic vessels. Many of these patients are premature and have a malrotated microcolon, and a significant proportion have evidence of healed meconium peritonitis. A rare familial syndrome affecting multiple siblings has been described with the features of a congenital short small bowel, malrotation, pyloric stenosis, and features of pseudo-obstruction.[26]

Rarely, infants with Hirschsprung's disease have aganglionosis that involves the entire colon and a substantial portion or all of the small intestine. Prior to the advent of total parenteral nutrition, these patients died with persistent intestinal obstruction and secondary malnutrition and infection. In spite of the motor abnormality, aganglionic ileum and colon maintain normal absorptive function.[27] With newer surgical techniques, these children may overcome their functional SBS.

PATHOPHYSIOLOGY

The basic defect of SBS is a markedly decreased intestinal surface area for absorption of fluid, electrolytes, and nutrients coupled with a rapid and often disordered transit of intestinal contents, which compromises intraluminal digestion. The effect of the intestinal resection depends on six main factors: (1) the amount of remaining small intestine, (2) whether it is proximal (jejunal) or distal (ileal), (3) whether the ileocecal valve has been resected, (4) whether the colon has been resected as well, (5) the degree of intestinal adaptation over time, and (6) the presence of residual bowel disease or surgical complications. These factors influence the fluid, electrolyte, and nutrient requirements for each individual patient and determine the time required until full intestinal adaptation.

SITE-SPECIFIC PATHOPHYSIOLOGY

It is rare that the duodenum must be resected with other segments of the small bowel. Duodenal resection or bypass will result in malabsorption of iron, folate, and calcium and put the patient at risk for anemia and osteopenia. A lack of coordinated mixing of bile and pancreatic secretions with duodenal contents may also affect intraluminal digestion and absorption of fat- and lipid-soluble vitamins.

Selective proximal jejunal resections generally result in little chronic diarrhea because the intact ileum and colon adapt to reabsorb nutrients and excess fluid and electrolytes.[28] However, duodenal and jejunal mucosa is also the site of secretin and cholecystokinin synthesis and, theoretically, extensive loss of jejunum should result in decreased hormonal stimulation of pancreatic and biliary secretion. This hypothesis is open to question, since recent studies in animals have shown that pancreatic enzyme synthesis and secretion are well maintained after major small bowel resection.[29] Extensive jejunal resection may lead to a reduction in intestinal lactase (or other disaccharidase) activity. Undigested lactose undergoes bacterial fermentation, with production of lactate and other volatile short-chain fatty acids, and contributes to an osmotic diarrhea. Nonhydrolyzed and nonabsorbed sugars also provide a fertile milieu for bacterial overgrowth and the production of potentially toxic metabolic by-products of bacterial metabolism such as D-lactate. Measurements of carbohydrate excretion in children with large resections of both jejunum and ileum show fecal loss of up to 65% of dietary carbohydrate and a direct correlation between stool weight and fecal carbohydrate excretion.[30]

In the jejunum, there is back diffusion of fluid and electrolytes into the lumen due to leaky epithelial junctions, and the luminal contents remain isotonic even as the bulk of nutrients is being absorbed. Conversely, in the ileum, the tight junctions are less permeable; there is less back diffusion and an increased concentration of the luminal contents. Thus, resection of the ileum has more profound effects on the volume and tonicity of intestinal contents reaching the colon.

Moderate loss of the terminal ileum and right colon may also contribute to diarrhea because of a reduced capacity to absorb sodium chloride. Only the ileum and colon can absorb sodium chloride against a steep concentration gradient.[31] Sodium chloride absorption against electrochemical gradients is a prerequisite to continued fluid absorption in this area, since most sodium chloride has been absorbed proximally, and poorly absorbed solutes (such as potassium, divalent cations, and carbohydrates) become concentrated in luminal fluid within the lower ileum and colon. Total gut perfusion studies of adults after ileocolic resections confirm a reduced capacity to absorb sodium chloride and water, which is exacerbated when patients are studied with a hypotonic sodium chloride solution.[32]

Resection of the ileum also causes diarrhea and steatorrhea secondary to the malabsorption of bile salts. After entry into the intestinal tract, the large majority (95 to 98%) of conjugated bile salts are absorbed either passively in the proximal small intestine or actively in the distal ileum.[33] The bulk of intestinal reabsorption takes place in the terminal ileum via an active carrier-mediated system that is sodium dependent. Active ileal absorption is necessary to maintain the bile salt pool, and resection of the ileum can lead to loss of bile salts at a rate that cannot be compensated by increased liver synthesis.

The main determinant of the degree of passive diffusion of bile acids in the small intestine and colon is the polarity of the bile salt species. Nonpolar compounds such as free bile salts can readily diffuse through the "unstirred" water layer and intestinal mucosal membrane; as polarity increases with the addition of hydroxyl, glycine, or taurine groups, diffusion decreases dramatically.[34] Under normal circumstances, the concentration of free bile acids is very low in the proximal small bowel, since there are few anaerobic bacteria to deconjugate or dehydroxylate primary bile salts, and passive small bowel absorption is a minor pathway for total enterohepatic recirculation of bile acids. In patients with SBS and bacterial overgrowth, passive diffusion assumes more importance and, as a result, the intraluminal bile salt concentration may be sufficiently reduced to impede micelle formation in the proximal small bowel.[35]

Figure 44–1 summarizes the consequences of the malabsorption of bile salts in SBS. In an adult, if less than 100 cm of distal ileum is resected, watery diarrhea (termed *cholerrheic diarrhea*) will result without signifi-

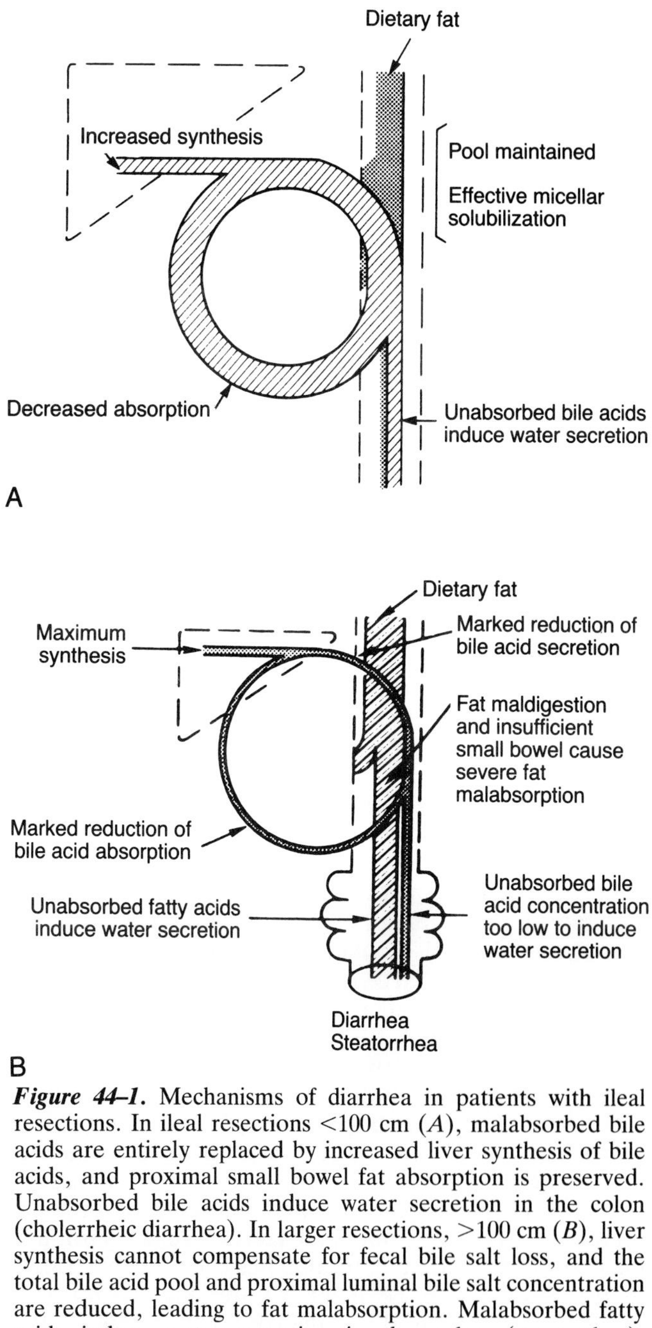

Figure 44–1. Mechanisms of diarrhea in patients with ileal resections. In ileal resections <100 cm (*A*), malabsorbed bile acids are entirely replaced by increased liver synthesis of bile acids, and proximal small bowel fat absorption is preserved. Unabsorbed bile acids induce water secretion in the colon (cholerrheic diarrhea). In larger resections, >100 cm (*B*), liver synthesis cannot compensate for fecal bile salt loss, and the total bile acid pool and proximal luminal bile salt concentration are reduced, leading to fat malabsorption. Malabsorbed fatty acids induce water secretion in the colon (steatorrhea). (Adapted from Hofman AF, Poley JR: Role of bile acid malabsorption in pathogenesis of diarrhea and steatorrhea in patients with ileal resection: I. Response to cholestyramine or replacement of dietary long-chain triglyceride by medium-chain triglyceride. Gastroenterology 1972; 62:931; with permission.)

cant steatorrhea. Increased amounts of bile salts reach the colon and are lost in the feces, but the liver compensates by increasing bile acid synthesis up to 20-fold.[36] Intraluminal concentrations of bile salts are maintained, and there is normal fat digestion and absorption in the proximal small bowel. In the colon, the high concentration of secondary bile acids produced by bacterial deconjugation and dehydroxylation induces reversible secretion of sodium and water via mechanisms of increased mucosal cyclic adenosine monophosphate (cAMP) levels and direct damage by bile salts to the colonic epithelium.[37, 38] The bile acid concentration in the fecal aqueous phase may exceed the concentration of 3 mmol per L sufficient to produce water and electrolyte secretion from the colon.[39]

If more than 100 cm of ileum has been resected, massive bile salt loss, which overwhelms the liver's ability to compensate, will result in steatorrhea. The resultant drop below the critical micellar concentration (CMC) of intraluminal bile acids necessary for absorption of dietary fat and fat-soluble vitamins leads to an increase in fatty acids entering the colon. In some patients, duodenal bile salt concentrations may be near normal during the first meal of the day; however, subsequent meals may be accompanied by intraluminal concentrations below the CMC.[40] Fatty acids, like bile acids, impair colonic water and ion absorption, stimulate colonic fluid secretion (especially when they are hydroxylated by colonic bacteria), and lower stool pH. Bile acids entering the colon are less important in this scenario, since the bile salt pool is markedly reduced, and bile salts are diluted by the large intraluminal volume and precipitated at the lower intracolonic pH. Following ileal resection, children also have interruption of the enterohepatic circulation of bile acids, increased fecal bile acid excretion, accelerated disappearance of isotopically labeled bile acids from the duodenal bile, reduced pool sizes after an overnight fast, and a reduced magnitude of rise in postprandial serum bile acid concentrations.[41]

Resection of the ileocecal valve (ICV) is associated with increased severity of disease and prolonged reliance on nutritional supplementation. An intact ICV prevents reflux of colonic bacteria and bacterial overgrowth. Without the ICV, bacterial colonization of the ileum will not only impair bile salt reabsorption but also aggravate the malabsorption of vitamin B_{12}.

Patients who have undergone a partial or total colectomy in addition to extensive small bowel resection (particularly ileal) are more prone to develop severe dehydration, hypovolemia, hypokalemia, hypomagnesemia, and hyponatremia, or the "end-jejunostomy syndrome."[42] The large potential reserve capacity of the intact healthy adult human colon has been demonstrated by the absorption of six liters of water and 800 mEq of sodium slowly perfused into the cecum.[43] The colon also salvages malabsorbed carbohydrate by bacterial fermentation to short-chain fatty acids (SCFA), which are absorbed and utilized as fuel by colonic epithelial cells. A recent study comparing adults with SBS and an intact colon versus those with SBS and no colon demonstrated marked carbohydrate malabsorption in all patients with SBS but increased bacterial fermentation and reclamation of malabsorbed carbohydrate by those patients with an intact colon preventing a loss of energy in the feces.[44] The uptake of SCFA also stimulates colonic reabsorption of sodium and water.[45] In patients with combined ileal and colonic resections, the severity of diarrhea and fecal electrolyte composition is more closely related to the amount of residual colon than to the degree of ileal resection.[46]

The presence of an intact colon can have a detrimental effect under certain circumstances. In general, patients with small bowel resection and an intact colon will not lose an excessive amount of fluid and electrolytes unless the fluid load in the colon exceeds its absorptive capacity or malabsorbed bile salts and fatty acids stimulate colonic fluid secretion. Excessive production of volatile short-chain fatty acids secondary to bacterial fermentation of massive amounts of malabsorbed carbohydrate contributes to the osmotic load and resulting diarrhea. The presence of a functional colon may also allow for increased colonic absorption of oxalate (described below), leading to kidney stone formation.

MOTILITY DISTURBANCES

Intestinal resection can have profound effects on small bowel motility, disrupting the normal patterns necessary for effective intraluminal contact of nutrients with enzymes or absorptive surfaces. Motility disturbances depend once again on the site and extent of resection. The consequence of proximal small bowel resection is primarily a decrease in the inhibition of gastric emptying by intestinal chyme.[42] The faster emptying rate appears to correlate directly with the remaining jejunal length, suggesting a loss of a small intestinal brake on gastric emptying.[47] Despite an increase in the rate of gastric emptying in patients with proximal small bowel resections, small bowel transit remains normal because of slow transit through the intact ileum.

The interdigestive migrating motor complex (MMC) is normally faster in the duodenum and jejunum, averaging 4 to 6 cm per minute during phase III and slower in the ileum, decreasing to 1 to 2 cm per minute in the terminal ileum.[48] At any given time, phase III activity is present over a 25- to 35-cm segment in the proximal duodenum, but only over a 5- to 15-cm segment in the terminal ileum. When the distal bowel is resected, the slowing effect of the ileum is lost. There are experimental data showing that an intact ICV prolongs transit time of luminal contents within the small bowel.[49] Total intestinal transit is also correlated with the length of remaining colon in patients with colonic resection.[50]

MALABSORPTION OF SPECIFIC ELECTROLYTES, VITAMINS, AND TRACE ELEMENTS

Deficiencies of divalent cations are not uncommon after intestinal resection, leading to symptoms of tetany, osteopenia, osteomalacia, and spontaneous fracture. Even though the rate of absorption of iron, calcium, and magnesium is maximal in the duodenum, these cations are absorbed throughout the small bowel. Luminal availability of calcium may be decreased by sequestration as insoluble calcium soaps in patients with steatorrhea. Calcium absorption may be further compromised by fat-soluble vitamin D malabsorption, since intestinal calcium transport is dependent on adequate levels of active vitamin D.[51] Magnesium and zinc can also form complexes with unabsorbed fatty acids, preventing normal transport.[52] Hypomagnesemia may further aggravate calcium homeostasis because of the role of magnesium as a cofactor for parathormone, which stimulates bone resorption and renal hydroxylation of vitamin D to its active form. Zinc deficiency also develops in the setting of fat malabsorption. In addition to the clinical consequences, zinc-deficiency may have a detrimental effect on small bowel adaptation after bowel resection. Rats subjected to a 70% bowel resection and fed a zinc-deficient diet prior to surgery showed adaptive hyperplasia but decreased mucosal protein and DNA content of the small bowel and a reduction in zinc-dependent intestinal metalloenzyme activity compared to rats fed a zinc-replete diet.[53]

Malabsorption of the fat-soluble vitamins increases with increasing steatorrhea and deficiencies of vitamins A, D, E, and K have all been described in patients with SBS. Iron deficiency also occurs due to a loss of the proximal small bowel absorptive surface area. Some patients also develop small intestinal mucosal blood loss from chronic stasis, mucosal injury, and even mucosal ulceration, especially at the site of a previous anastomosis.[54] Recently, a syndrome of noninfectious colitis and hematochezia has been described in infants with SBS, which may contribute to iron deficiency.[55]

Vitamin B_{12} malabsorption is almost invariably present when more than 100 cm of terminal ileum has been resected. Because B_{12} receptors are restricted to the ileum, there is no adaptation of vitamin B_{12} absorption after a large ileal resection. Less extensive resections will not result in decreased absorption, provided there is no residual ileal disease and no bacterial overgrowth. In the setting of bacterial overgrowth, there is competitive uptake of intrinsic factor–bound vitamin B_{12} by anaerobic bacteria[56] and/or conversion of some of the ingested vitamin B_{12} by bacterial flora (especially *Bacteroides*) to vitamin B_{12} analogues, making less active vitamin available to the host.[57] Vitamin B_{12} deficiency may also affect small bowel adaptation, since it alters both small bowel mucosal cell morphology and transport functions.[58, 59] Deficiencies of other water-soluble vitamins are uncommon in all except those patients with minimal remaining small bowel. Folate is normally absorbed in the proximal small intestine after deconjugation of dietary folates by the mucosa to pteroylmonoglutamates. Conservation of body folate stores is enhanced by a significant enterohepatic recirculation.[60] In the setting of proximal small bowel bacterial overgrowth and extensive duodeno-jejunal resection, absorption and the enterohepatic circulation may be sufficiently impaired to result in significant folate malabsorption.

SPECIFIC CLINICAL CONSEQUENCES OF BOWEL RESECTION

Although the primary causes of deficient absorption in SBS are a loss of absorptive surface and disruption of normal motility patterns, there are also major secondary effects of small bowel resection that exacerbate the malabsorption, may delay small bowel adaptation, and complicate the management of patients with SBS.

Gastric Acid Hypersecretion

Gastric acid hypersecretion occurs after massive small bowel resection in both experimental animals[61] and approximately 50% of adult patients.[62] It is a transient phenomenon, returning to normal in most patients within one year of the resection.[63] Gastric acid hypersecretion may interfere with intraluminal digestion by lowering the pH of the duodenum, inactivating pancreatic enzymes, and impairing micelle formation and lipolysis.[64] The increased secretion of acid can also cause direct mucosal damage, including peptic ulcer disease in the proximal small bowel. The high solute load of excessive gastric secretions may add to the diarrhea by presenting the small intestinal remnant with an increased fluid and electrolyte load and by stimulating peristalsis.[65]

Gastric hypersecretion after massive resection has been attributed to hypergastrinemia and an increase in parietal cell mass due to either a loss of small bowel tissue responsible for gastrin degradation[66] or a decrease in levels of an intestinal gastrin inhibitory factor.[63] Candidate hormonal inhibitors include secretin, cholecystokinin (CCK), vasoactive intestinal polypeptide (VIP), gastric inhibitory peptide, or enteroglucagon. However, elevated gastrin levels do not always correlate with an increase in acid secretion. Hypergastrinemia may persist months or years after small bowel resection, long after basal acid secretion has returned to normal.[63] In both adult and pediatric studies, the presence and magnitude of gastric acid hypersecretion appear to be proportional to the length of intestine resected, becoming more prevalent in patients with less than one third of the small bowel remaining.[67]

Bacterial Overgrowth

Chronic bacterial overgrowth is a frequent complication of SBS and may play a large role in perpetuating malabsorption. Factors that promote bacterial overgrowth include (1) absence of the ICV; (2) presence of a partial small bowel obstruction from a tight anastomosis, an ischemic stricture, or an adhesion; (3) presence of a dilated, hypotonic bowel segment with disordered motility; (4) presence of an entero-enteral fistula secondary to an underlying inflammatory disease such as Crohn's disease or a surgical complication; and (5) relative achlorhydria secondary to the prolonged use of histamine H_2 receptor antagonists to prevent gastric acid hypersecretion.

In addition to the previously mentioned profound effects of bacterial overgrowth on fat and vitamin B_{12} absorption, there are other wide-ranging consequences for the patient with SBS.[68] Abnormalities or complete absence of phase III activity of the MMC has been described in patients with bacterial overgrowth.[69] Antibiotic therapy restored phase III activity as the overgrowth was reversed. Abnormalities of the small bowel mucosa in patients with bacterial overgrowth have been demonstrated by both light and electron microscopy and are characterized by patchy areas of blunting and broadening of the villi and damage to the jejunal enterocyte brush border.[70]

A number of biochemical and functional abnormalities are recognized as consequences of the mucosal injury. Patients with bacterial overgrowth may have depressed levels of maltase, sucrase, lactase, and enterokinase in jejunal biopsies.[71] Depressed serum protein levels are also seen. In addition to the effect on brush border peptidases, there is evidence to suggest that small bowel bacteria deaminate dietary protein moieties,[72] interrupting normal uptake of peptides and amino acids. Protein-losing enteropathy and even a flat-villous lesion resembling celiac sprue have been documented in occasional patients with bacterial overgrowth.

D-Lactic Acidosis

D-Lactic acidosis is a rare complication of SBS and intestinal bypass surgery.[73, 74] Patients present with symptoms of confusion, slurred speech, unsteady gait, stupor, and even coma and physical findings of dysarthria, nystagmus, and Kussmaul breathing. In some cases, milder episodes of behavioral changes, dizziness, and incoordination may precede the more serious episode. The patients have a metabolic acidosis with an increased anion gap, elevated plasma levels of D-lactate, and normal levels of L-lactate. Prerequisites for this syndrome are small bowel bacterial overgrowth and exposure of these bacteria to fermentable carbohydrate. In some reports, lactobacillus species have been implicated as the major producers of D-lactate,[75] and in an early case report, ingestion of *Lactobacillus acidophilus* tablets was incriminated as a precipitating factor.[76] In general, colonic fecal flora in these patients shows a reduction in anaerobes such as *Bacteroides* and a predominance of gram-positive anaerobes, especially *Lactobacillus, Eubacterium*, and *Bifidobacterium* species. In several children, D-lactic acidosis has followed liberalization of their diet to include more carbohydrate including lactose,[73, 77] and in one patient, the syndrome followed a lactose breath hydrogen test. Malabsorption of lactose leads to bacterial generation of progressively larger amounts of lactic acid. Accumulation of lactic acid in the lumen results in a drop in luminal pH, which favors the growth of acid-producing and acid-tolerant bacteria, such as *Lactobacillus*, at the expense of the normally predominant gut bacteria.

Although enteric microorganisms produce both optical isomers L-lactate and D-lactate from sugars, mammals produce predominantly L-lactate and only minimal quantities of D-lactate. In some cases, neurologic symptoms are correlated with rises in serum D-lactate concentration, however, it is not clear whether it is the D-lactate or some other toxin produced in parallel with it that causes the encephalopathy.[78] The possibility of an as yet undiscovered toxin is supported by a study that found that approximately 3% of a control symptom-free hospital population (60% of whom had undergone previous intestinal surgery) had raised serum D-lactate concentrations.[79]

Effective treatment consists of correction of the acidosis with bicarbonate infusion, cessation of enteral carbohydrate, and reduction of the colonic flora with antibiotics such as oral vancomycin, neomycin, or metronidazole. One recent report suggests that reduction of monosaccharides and disaccharides and substitution of carbohydrate in the polymeric form is effective prophylaxis for D-lactic acidosis, avoiding the need for multiple courses of oral antibiotics.[80]

Renal Stones and Gallstones

Dietary oxalate reacts with calcium within the lumen to form highly insoluble complexes of calcium oxalate that are not absorbed. In patients with fat malabsorption, dietary calcium binds with unabsorbed fatty acids, is unavailable to complex with dietary oxalate, and frees oxalate to be absorbed primarily in the colon and eventually excreted in the urine.[81] Patients with SBS, large ileal resections, and an intact colon are at risk of hyperoxaluria.[82]

The incidence of gallstones in adult patients who have undergone ileal resection may be as much as threefold greater than the normal population.[83] This is presumably secondary to depletion of the bile salt pool, giving rise to lithogenic bile.[84] Early studies documented cholesterol gallstones in adults with ileal resections[85] and suggested that interruption of the enterohepatic circulation was responsible for cholelithiasis in children with SBS.[86] A recent study of 21 children receiving long-term total parenteral nutrition has shown that nine of 14 patients with previous ileal resection or ileal disorders developed cholelithiasis, whereas none of seven children without ileal involvement had gallstones.[87] While confirming the importance of ileal pathology, this study raised questions about the mechanism underlying stone formation, since analysis revealed black pigment gallstones consisting mainly of calcium bilirubinate, and unsaturated with cholesterol.

In both animal models and humans, biliary stasis and obstruction have been associated with the formation of biliary sludge and pigment stones in the gallbladder and common duct.[88, 89] Analysis of biliary sludge has shown predominantly calcium bilirubinate granules, few cholesterol crystals, and a high proportion of unconjugated bilirubin.[90] Gallstones in adults treated with prolonged total parenteral nutrition are pigment stones and have a very high calcium bilirubinate content, suggesting that stasis is a factor in their formation.[91] Fasting, lack of hormonal stimuli that regulate gallbladder emptying, and prolonged sequestration of gallbladder bile appear to be important factors leading to the formation of sludge and pigment gallstones in children with SBS maintained on total parenteral nutrition.

In four recent reviews of SBS in infancy and childhood, 20 of 174 patients (12%) developed cholelithiasis and 16 of the 20 required cholecystectomy for acute cholecystitis, biliary colic, or both.[11–14] Because of the high incidence of this complication in children with significant ileal resections, some centers perform cholecystectomy routinely during the initial bowel resection or at the time of reestablishment of intestinal continuity.[14]

SMALL BOWEL ADAPTATION

Modern techniques of parenteral nutrition have allowed time for adaptation to take place, improving the prospects for survival with normal growth and eventual enteral feedings in children with as little as 11 cm of small bowel and an intact ICV or 25 cm of small bowel without an ICV.[11, 92, 93] Many factors stimulate the intestinal epithelium to become hyperplastic and increase its absorptive capacity. A proposed scheme of interwoven stimuli is outlined in Figure 44–2. Results that support this framework derive largely from animal investigations. A discussion of mechanisms of bowel adaptation can be divided into the role of (1) luminal nutrients, (2) endogenous fuels for the gut, (3) pancreatic secretions, (4) circulating hormones, (5) growth factors, and (6) intracellular modulators.

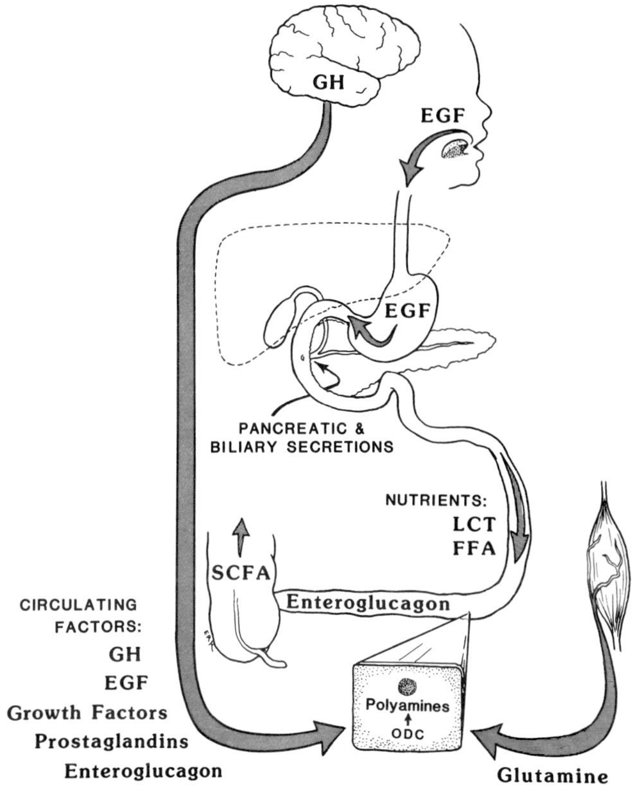

Figure 44–2. Multifactorial schematic of influences on small bowel adaption, including (a) luminal nutrients, (b) gastrointestinal and systemic hormones, (c) growth factors, (d) pancreatic and biliary secretions, (e) substrates for enterocyte metabolism, and (f) intracellular mediators of DNA and protein synthesis. GH, growth hormone; EGF, epidermal growth factor; LCT, long-chain triglycerides; FFA, free fatty acids; SCFA, short-chain fatty acids; ODC, ornithine decarboxylase.

General Evidence for Intestinal Adaptation

Before discussing trophic factors, it is important to review the research models used to demonstrate the morphologic and functional changes of bowel adaptation. Resection of the small bowel in animals results in mucosal hyperplasia of the remaining small intestine, provided the animal is fed orally. These changes are particularly striking in the residual ileum after jejunectomy and are less dramatic in the jejunum remaining after ileal resection.[94] The major morphologic change is increased height of the villi and elongation of the crypts (Fig. 44–3), resulting from increased numbers of cells but not increased size of individual cells.[95] There is an increased rate of cell renewal and an increase in the rate of cell migration up the villus. In the rat, the maximal rate of cell renewal is established by 12 days after small bowel resection and is correlated with the amount of intestine resected.[96] Mucosal hyperplasia persists for several months in this model, during which time functional improvement continues due to lengthening of the remnant bowel.[97] Measurements of mucosal ribonucleic acid (RNA), deoxyribonucleic acid (DNA), and tritiated thymidine radioactivity show rapid intense epithelial cell proliferation throughout the colon as well, after both jejunal and ileal resection.[98] Exclusion of a part of the small intestine in animals either as a self-emptying blind loop or a Thiry-Vella fistula results in mucosal hyperplasia in the remaining bowel, similar in continuity to that seen after partial resection, and mucosal hypoplasia in the excluded segment.[99, 100] The structural and functional atrophy of the bypassed small bowel can be rapidly reversed by restoration of normal intestinal continuity.

The morphologic changes are accompanied by functional increases in the absorption of most nutrients. An increase in nutrient absorption per centimeter of remaining bowel has been shown for fat, protein, glucose, galactose, sucrose, maltose, sodium, water, bile acids, vitamin B_{12}, calcium, and zinc.[101] However, when rates of absorption are expressed in terms of mucosal weight or protein content, there is either no change or a decrease in absorption. Several studies have shown that disaccharidase and peptidase activities are normal or decreased after resection, suggesting a relative metabolic immaturity of individual enterocytes in the hyperplastic mucosa.[102, 103] However, other investigations reveal that

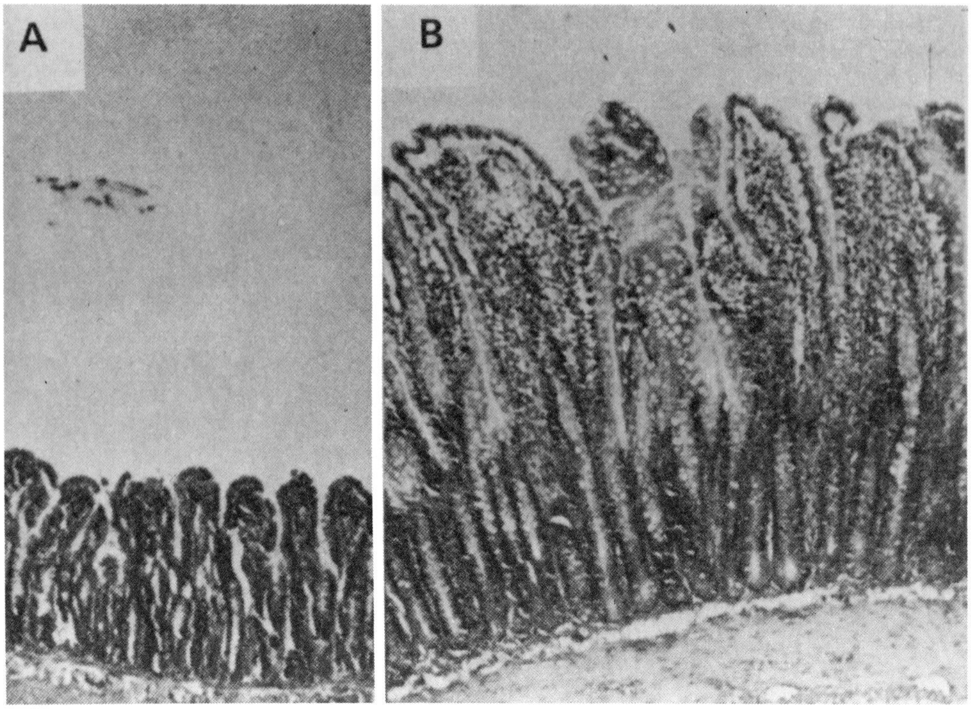

Figure 44–3. Ileal hyperplasia 1 month after jejunal resection in a rat maintained on a chow diet. *A*, Normal ileum. *B*, Ileum after jejunal resection. Hematoxylin and eosin × 1,400. (From Weser E: Nutritional aspects of malabsorption: Short gut adaptation. Am J Med 1979; 67:116; with permission.)

individual enterocytes can develop enhanced enzyme activity of certain disaccharidases, enterokinase, and Na^+, K^+–ATPase, probably related to increased exposure to their respective substrates.[104] Three weeks after rats have undergone a 60% proximal small bowel resection, ileal enterocytes develop four times the alpha-glucosidase activity of control cells. Presumably, the trigger to the postresectional increments in alpha-glucosidase activity is the sudden exposure of the ileum to carbohydrates that were previously absorbed in the now resected jejunum.[105] The discrepancy between some of these studies may be related to the timing of the evaluation of enterocyte enzyme or transport activity, since it appears that functional adaptation may lag behind morphologic changes.

There are few studies that document similar morphological changes of adaptation in the human small intestine. Studies of patients with jejunoileal bypass surgery have shown that the jejunoileum left in continuity becomes elongated and the villi increase in height both in the jejunum (24 to 40%) and in the ileum (38 to 70%).[106, 107] These data confirm the animal work cited above, showing greater adaptation in the distal bowel.

The Importance of Luminal Nutrients

Nutrients in the lumen of the small intestine are essential for the maintenance of mucosal mass. Not only starvation, but even the provision of adequate protein and calories exclusively via total parenteral nutrition (TPN), results in mucosal hypoplasia in humans, and experimental animals. After 21 days of TPN therapy in patients, there are significant decreases in the height of the microvilli, and all disaccharidase activities decline compared to pre-hyperalimentation values.[108] The decreased enzyme activities are rapidly restored after oral feeding is resumed. The weight, protein, and DNA contents of enteric mucosa are 20 to 35% lower in rats maintained with parenteral nutrition for 1 to 3 weeks compared with controls receiving normal or elemental diets by mouth.[109] Disaccharidase activity and glucose uptake are also decreased. Even after as little as 24 hours of fasting, total small intestinal sucrase and maltase decline 50% in the rat, and pancreatic enzyme content and secretion are impaired.[110, 111]

Nutrients may stimulate mucosal adaptation by several interrelated mechanisms, including (1) direct contact with and uptake by the mucosal surface, (2) stimulus of local gut and extraintestinal hormones, and (3) release of pancreatic secretions and other potential growth factors. The direct stimulatory effect of nutrients on growth of the absorptive mucosa is thought to be responsible for the normal proximal to distal absorptive gradient; proximal jejunal villi are taller and have greater absorptive capacity because of abundant exposure to nutrients, most of which are depleted by the time intestinal chyme reaches the distal small bowel. Jejunectomy results in increased exposure of the ileum to nutrients and marked hyperplasia. Similarly, when a segment of ileum is transplanted proximally and exposed to the jejunal nutrient environment, that segment becomes hyperplastic and takes on the morphologic and functional absorptive characteristics of proximal intestine.[112] Conversely, a jejunal segment transposed to the ileal environment undergoes opposite changes and decreases its mucosal mass.[113] Thus, the proximal intestine may normally function at a level close to the limit of its capacity to differentiate and adapt. The distal intestine, as a result of proximal absorption, may receive fewer nutrients ordinarily and function at less than full potential. Numerous studies in animals have demonstrated that even in the presence of small bowel resection (the most potent trigger of small intestinal mucosal hyperplasia), no adaptation will take place unless luminal nutrients are provided. In spite of adequate calories and a positive nitrogen balance, both rats and dogs maintained on total parenteral nutrition after small bowel resection failed to demonstrate intestinal adaptation compared to controls fed the same solution via the oral route.[114, 115] These findings suggest that after intestinal resection, parenteral nutrition should be supplemented with enteral nutrients as soon as possible to stimulate adaptation.

An attempt has been made to determine the specific nutrients responsible for stimulating the adaptive response by infusing single nutrients into the gastrointestinal tract while the experimental animal is otherwise nourished with total parenteral nutrition. Among the micronutrients, long-chain triglycerides (LCT) given intragastrically to rats after resection promote intestinal adaptation to a greater extent than proteins and polysaccharides.[116] The same effect is not seen with medium-chain triglycerides (MCT),[117] which are often used to provide a major source of fat calories to patients with SBS because they do not require digestion by pancreatic enzymes and colipase and are not as dependent on bile acids for micellar solubilization and absorption. Free fatty acids have been found to be a more potent stimulator of small bowel adaptation than LCT.[118] A recent attempt has been made to further characterize the nature of the fatty acid stimulus by showing that omega-3 fatty acids in menhaden fish oil stimulate mucosal hyperplasia after massive small bowel resection more than either safflower oil (omega-6 fatty acids) or beef tallow (saturated and mono-unsaturated fatty acids).[119] It is not known if the effect of fatty acids is mediated by direct exposure of the ileum to high concentrations of luminal fat or to stimulation of circulating hormones. The importance of fatty acids is further emphasized by findings that dietary induction of essential fatty acid deficiency in the rat prior to surgical resection leads to a significantly impaired adaptive response.[120]

The effects of individual infusions of sugars on small bowel adaptation have also been studied in experimental animals. Glucose and fructose are more effective in maintaining intestinal mass when fed orally to rats otherwise nourished exclusively with TPN than the nonmetabolizable sugar analogue, 3-0 methyl glucose.[121] However, when infusions of 5% sucrose, maltose, and lactose are given, significantly greater mucosal growth is seen throughout the small bowel than with equal concentrations of glucose, fructose, and galactose.[122] These studies have given rise to the concept that the functional work of hydrolysis of disaccharides, which is necessary for their absorption, is more important to small bowel adaptation than simply luminal contact of the substrate with the enterocyte or even mucosal metabolism by the enterocyte of the resulting monosaccharides.[123] Further support for this concept comes from studies that show no intestinal hyperplasia in response to the nonhydrolyzed disaccharide lactulose or to sucrose when acarbose, an alpha-glucosidase inhibitor, is administered simultaneously.[122]

Proteins also contribute to adaptive changes in the small intestine after resection. Some studies suggest that whole proteins such as casein are more potent than hydrolysates in inducing mucosal hyperplasia in rats undergoing small bowel resection.[124] However, even amino acids infused into the ileum have been shown to produce significant hyperplasia in rats maintained on TPN and to prevent hypoplasia of the jejunum when infused into the proximal small bowel.[125]

Recently, attention has centered on the contribution of nucleotides to small bowel growth and maturation. Nucleotides constitute as much as 5% of the total nitrogen in human milk. They can be synthesized endogenously; however, tissues with rapid turnover, such as the small intestine, may rely on exogenous dietary nucleotides and conservation of purines and pyrimidines via an intracellular salvage pathway to maintain their nucleotide pool. A purine-deficient diet induces increased de novo nucleotide synthesis in the small intestine, but not to the same extent as in the liver or the colon.[126] A purine-free diet also decreases activity of the rate-limiting enzyme in the purine salvage pathway in the small intestinal epithelial cell. Thus, the small intestine may be particularly susceptible to a nucleotide-deficient diet. Developing rats given a diet supplemented with nucleotides showed increased disaccharidase activity and gut protein content, and an increased villous height in the proximal small bowel compared to their counterparts fed a nucleotide-free diet.[127]

The Role of Metabolic "Fuels" for the Enterocyte

Information about the origin and nature of substrates for energy production in the small intestine and colon has led to renewed interest in their potential clinical usefulness as supplements in patients undergoing small bowel adaptation. The roles of glutamine and short-chain fatty acids in colonic and small bowel adaptation are being actively investigated.

Glutamine

Glutamine is the preferred substrate for small bowel oxidative metabolism. In the fed rat, small bowel metabolism of circulating glutamine released from skeletal muscle accounts for 46% of the CO_2 produced by the small intestine, and glucose and ketone bodies contribute 10% and 11%, respectively.[128] Glutamine release by skeletal muscle is markedly increased during catabolic states such as trauma, sepsis, burns, and surgery. In these situations there is striking enhancement of glutamine uptake by intestinal epithelial cells, reflecting an increased metabolic need.[129, 130] Progressively decreasing plasma concentrations and decreasing skeletal muscle concentrations of glutamine reflect the severity of the illness and suggest that over time, glutamine release from muscle may not be adequate to meet small bowel metabolic requirements.[131, 132]

The effects of providing glutamine-supplemented nutrition on small intestinal growth and function have been investigated in a number of animal models. When rats are fed with a standard formula lacking in glutamine, mucosal atrophy takes place.[133] Oral diets supplemented with glutamine result in greater mucosal hyperplasia after 60% small bowel resection compared to isocaloric, isonitrogenous diets.[134] The provision of glutamine-enriched parenteral solutions as the sole source of nutrition is associated with relative preservation of small bowel mucosa in rats.[135] In these formulations, glutamine is substituted for other nonessential amino acids, and a direct correlation is found between glutamine intake and intestinal DNA content, mucosal web weight, sucrase, maltase, and villous height.

Glutamine is absent from all but a few currently available elemental diets. No amino acid preparation for use in TPN contains glutamine because of poor stability and spontaneous degradation to pytoglutamic acid and ammonia. In order to overcome these problems, peptide analogues of glutamine have been developed.[136, 136a]

Short-Chain Fatty Acids

Short-chain fatty acids (SCFA), including primarily acetate, propionate, and butyrate, are produced by bacterial fermentation of dietary carbohydrates and fiber in the colon.[137] They are avidly absorbed by the colonic mucosa and, at the same time, stimulate colonic sodium and water absorption.[45, 138] SCFA, especially butyrate, have been shown to be the preferred substrate for energy metabolism in isolated colonocytes.[139] Depending on the quantity of fiber and complex polysaccharides in the diet, colonic absorption of SCFA may normally supply 5 to 10% of the daily energy requirements.[140] The small intestine also has the capacity to absorb SCFA. Although normal SCFA concentrations within the small bowel are low, small intestinal mucosal absorption is as efficient as colonic absorption when SCFA are available.[141]

Numerous animal studies have documented that removal of fiber from the diet results in reversible ileal and colonic mucosal atrophy.[142, 143] Either feeding a fiber-supplemented diet or infusing SCFA into the proximal colon of rats that had undergone cecectomy to deprive them of their normal production of SCFA in the cecum results in increased colonic, ileal, and jejunal mucosal DNA content and weight compared to controls fed the same fiber-free elemental diet.[144, 145] The adaptive effect of a fiber-supplemented diet is inhibited by antibiotics, suggesting that it is due to bacterial fermentation of available fiber and the production of SCFA.[146]

Since butyrate is the preferred oxidative fuel for colonocytes in vitro, it is likely that the provision of SCFA directly stimulates colonic mucosal growth. However, the mechanism by which SCFA infusion in the colonic lumen or intraperitoneal injection of SCFA stimulates small intestinal mucosal proliferation is unknown.[147, 148] One possibility is that it releases a trophic hormone. Fermentable fiber refed to starved rats stimulates the crypt cell production rate in the colon and distal small intestine, and elevated levels of plasma enteroglucagon correlate with the proliferative response.[149] Inert bulk and poorly fermentable fiber do not have the same effect. Immunohistochemical studies have located enteroglucagon-producing cells in the distal ileum, cecum, and proximal colon.[150] It is possible that SCFA normally generated in the cecum are physiologic stimulators of enteroglucagon release. Extraintestinal metabolism of SCFA by the liver may also contribute to small intestinal adaptation by generation of the preferred oxidative fuels of the small bowel enterocyte; portal blood concentrations of SCFA are four to 10 times higher than systemic levels, and hepatic metabolism of butyrate and acetate results in the production of glutamine and ketone bodies.[151, 152]

Preliminary investigations of the effect of SCFA or fermentable fiber supplementation in animal models of short bowel syndrome have recently been published. In rats undergoing an 80% small bowel resection, pectin supplementation of an elemental diet resulted in increases in mucosal weight, DNA, RNA, and protein in the colon and small bowel compared with resected rats fed an elemental diet alone. Villus height, crypt depth, and mucosal thickness in the ileum were all significantly greater in the pectin-supplemented rats.[153] The addition of SCFA to TPN following massive small bowel resection in the adult rat prevented the usual small intestinal mucosal atrophy seen in rats maintained on SCFA-free TPN.[154]

Trophic Effects of Enteric Hormones

The stimulus of mucosal adaptation in the proximal small bowel after infusion of nutrients into the distal segments, or the amelioration of mucosal atrophy in segments not in continuity with the nutrient stream, suggests that circulating gut hormones released by nutrient exposure play an important role.[155] Additional evidence for humoral regulation comes from studies in pairs of parabiotic rats that share a common circulation. When one member of the pair undergoes intestinal resection, intestinal hyperplasia occurs in both rats.[156] Sorting out the relative contributions of various hormones has been the subject of intense study.

Enteroglucagon

Interest in the hormone enteroglucagon was stimulated by the observation that a patient with an enteroglucagon-producing tumor of the kidney had intestinal mucosal hyperplasia that disappeared when the tumor was resected.[157] In animal models of bowel resection, plasma enteroglucagon levels are increased and correlate with the degree of resection and the crypt cell production rate in the remaining segment.[158, 159] No other hormone except for peptide tyrosine tyrosine (PYY) is elevated in a similar pattern. Other indirect evidence of the role of enteroglucagon includes:

1. Increased enteroglucagon messenger RNA levels in rat ileum soon after massive small bowel resection,

with further stimulation by the provision of enteral nutrients.[160]

2. Decreased plasma enteroglucagon levels and reduced evidence of small bowel mucosal hyperplasia after combined small bowel resection and diversion of pancreatic secretions (which would be expected to divert the preproglucagon precursor of small bowel enteroglucagon).[161]

3. Lack of adaptive hyperplasia of the isolated small bowel in rats with a Thiry-Vella fistula and ileal resection compared to rats with an equivalent resection of the jejunum proximal to the fistula, suggesting that adaptation is modulated by factors localized to the distal small intestine, where cells producing enteroglucagon are predominantly located.[162]

4. Increased plasma enteroglucagon levels and mucosal proliferation in response to small bowel resection when bombesin is given, which stimulates enteroglucagon release, and the opposite response to somatostatin, which suppresses release of enteroglucagon.[163]

Direct evidence linking infusion of enteroglucagon with small intestinal mucosal adaptation has not yet been obtained.

Cholecystokinin, Secretin, and Pancreaticobiliary Secretions

Diversion of pancreaticobiliary secretions into the ileum stimulates ileal mucosal growth, suggesting a role in small bowel adaptation.[164, 165] The degree of ileal hyperplasia after transplantation of the papilla into the ileum is greater in rats fed regular diets than in those fed elemental diets or nourished parenterally.[164] These observations are consistent with the fact that elemental diets and TPN are less effective in stimulating endogenous pancreatic secretions than complex diets. Studies in rats and dogs have shown that parenteral injections of cholecystokinin (CCK) combined with secretin can prevent hypoplasia of intestinal mucosa associated with TPN.[166, 167] Continuous intravenous infusion of octapeptide-CCK in rats maintained on TPN after jejunal resection results in significant mucosal hyperplasia compared to rats maintained on TPN alone but does not stimulate mucosal growth to the extent seen in enterally fed animals.[167] In the presence of normal enteral nutrition, CCK may have little effect on small intestinal adaptation, since the removal of pancreaticobiliary secretions does not adversely influence the adaptive response to short bowel in rats fed regular chow,[168] and the administration of a dose of CCK sufficient to cause hyperplasia of the pancreas does not stimulate mucosal hyperplasia beyond that which normally occurs with regular chow feeding.[169] It is more likely that the trophic effects of CCK seen in the TPN model are secondary to hormonal stimulation of pancreaticobiliary secretions. In rats undergoing jejunoileal bypass, CCK causes no mucosal proliferation in the bypassed intestine, whereas increased intestinal mass is observed in the bowel in continuity with endogenous pancreaticobiliary secretions.[170]

Prostaglandins

Prostaglandin E_2 (PGE_2) induces a proliferative response in the duodenum and proximal jejunum, particularly in suckling rats.[171] These observations have stimulated studies of proximal small intestinal adaptation after massive distal small bowel resection in rats treated with 16,16-dimethyl-PG-E_2 or prostaglandin analogues.[172, 173] Treatment with subcutaneous PGE_2 increases mucosal hyperplasia, mucosal maltase concentrations, and leucine uptake in the remaining proximal segment.[172] Although crypt cell mass is increased, production rates are not, suggesting that prostaglandins act by prolonging cell survival rather than by increasing cell production.

Growth Factors

Epidermal growth factor (EGF) is a polypeptide hormone that is secreted directly into the small intestine by Brunner's glands and produces stimulation of DNA synthesis throughout the gastrointestinal tract.[174] EGF stimulates ornithine decarboxylase activity, the rate-limiting enzyme for polyamine synthesis, which is necessary for rapid growth of tissues.[175] When administered parenterally, EGF causes precocious development of the small intestine in suckling rats.[176] Parenteral administration of EGF significantly reduces the hypoplasia produced throughout the gastrointestinal tract by 10 days of TPN in adult rats and stimulates crypt cell production rates.[177] Direct intraluminal administration of EGF into the ileum of adult rats markedly increases ornithine decarboxylase activity, DNA synthesis, and crypt cell proliferation both in the ileum and, to a lesser extent, in the nonexposed jejunum.[178] A greater rise in DNA synthesis can be elicited in the jejunum by direct infusion of EGF. Saliva, duodenal secretions, and bile are rich sources of EGF, and this hormone may be an important factor in the maintenance of mucosal mass in the proximal small bowel and the mucosal proliferation in the ileum exposed to proximal intestinal contents after jejunectomy. Growth hormone has been implicated in the response to small bowel resection because hypophysectomized animals do not undergo mucosal hyperplasia following enterectomy in spite of the provision of sufficient enteral calories.[179] Growth hormone releasing factor stimulates epithelial cell proliferation in the rat jejunum.[180] An analogue of human growth hormone, plerocercoid growth factor, increases the duodenal and jejunal mucosal proliferative response to 70% after jejunoileal resection in young rats fed normal chow.[181]

Other unidentified growth factors have been extracted from the proximal intestinal mucosa of rats two to four days after small bowel resection.[182] The extracts augment DNA synthesis of mouse jejunal explants. This stimulatory activity is destroyed by protease treatment, is specific for intestinal cells, and is not abolished by diversion of the pancreaticobiliary secretions away from the proximal intestine. Rats nourished intravenously after small bowel resection do not demonstrate this extractable proximal small bowel mucosal activity.[183]

The role of other growth factors such as insulin-like growth factor (IGF-1) and transforming growth factor alpha (TGF) is currently under investigation.[184–186]

Polyamines in Intestinal Adaptation

Rapid tissue and cell growth is associated with the rapid accumulation of tissue polyamines. Ornithine is the starting substrate for the biosynthesis of the polyamines: putrescine, spermidine, and spermine. Decarboxylation of ornithine to form putrescine is the rate-limiting step in polyamine biosynthesis catalyzed by ornithine dicarboxylase (ODC). An increase in ODC activity is one of the earliest events that occurs during the transition of cells from dormancy to active proliferation.[187] Polyamines have been shown in vitro to facilitate nearly all aspects of DNA, RNA, and protein synthesis.

Polyamine biosynthesis and ODC activity have been investigated in the rat intestinal resection model of small bowel adaptation. Marked increases in ODC and S-adenosylmethionine decarboxylase (SAM-DC) activity and their synthetic products putrescine and spermidine are found in rat ileal mucosa immediately after 50% jejunectomy[188] (Fig. 44–4). Rates of mucosal cell proliferation are highly significantly correlated with the ODC activity. Increased mucosal ODC activity and polyamine synthesis are also found in other models of functional intestinal adaptation, including intestinal maturation in newborn rats,[189] intestinal response during lactation,[190] and intestinal response to starvation and refeeding.[191] The central role of polyamines in mediating intestinal proliferation and maturation is further supported by studies that show that corticosterone and epidermal growth factor, both known maturation-inducing factors, increase ODC activity and polyamine synthesis.[175, 192] Alpha-difluoromethyl ornithine (DFMO), a specific irreversible ODC inhibitor, given to rats three days prior to jejunectomy completely suppresses increases in ODC activity and polyamine content in the intestinal mucosa and results in the abolition of any signs of intestinal adaptation.[193, 194] Thus, the increases in ODC activity and subsequent polyamine biosynthesis are critical for proliferative activity of the intestinal crypt cell compartment in response to bowel resection, but at present it is unclear how various luminal nutrients, hormones, and growth factors interact with the enterocyte to trigger polyamine synthesis.

The question of the benefit of exogenously administered polyamines is raised by studies showing that spermine and spermidine given orally to neonatal rats induce precocious mucosal structural and biochemical changes characteristic of postweaning maturation.[195] One recent study in patients with short bowel syndrome correlated postprandial jejunostomy fluid polyamine levels with intestinal remnant length and carbohydrate absorp-

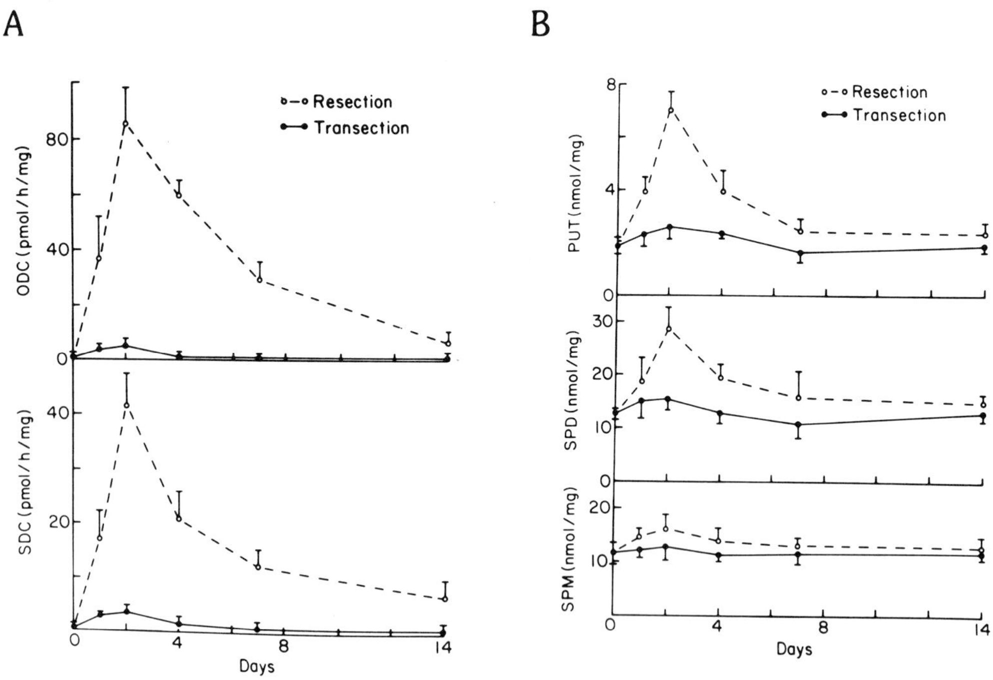

Figure 44–4. *A*, Mucosal activities of polyamine biosynthetic enzymes ornithine decarboxylase (ODC) and S-adenosylmethionine decarboxylase (SDC) after intestinal resection, showing significant differences between resected animals (*open circles*) and transected controls (*closed circles*). *B*, Mucosal levels of polyamines putrescine (PUT), spermidine (SPD), and spermine (SPM) after intestinal resection, showing significant differences in putrescine and spermine during days 1–4 postresection. (From Luk GD, Baylin SB: Polyamines and intestinal growth: Increased polyamine biosynthesis after jejunectomy. Am J Physiol 1983; 24:G658–G659; with permission.)

Table 44–2. FLUID AND ELECTROLYTE COMPOSITION OF INTESTINAL LUMINAL CONTENTS OF INFANTS

Type of Fluid	Amount (ml/kg/24 hr)	Ion Concentration (mEq/L)		
		Na+	*K*+	*Cl*−
Dietary	100	30	20	30
Saliva	70	3	25	20
Gastric juice	50	50	7.5	140
Pancreaticobiliary secretions	45	100	3	30
Duodenum	285	—	—	—
Distal ileum*	60 (new)	—	—	—
	25 (established)	100	26	—
Rectum	5–10	22	54	21

*Data from new ileostomies and established ileostomies.
Adapted from Rhodes JM, Powell DW: Diarrhea. *In* Walker WA, Durie PR, Hamilton JR, et al, eds: Pediatric Gastrointestinal Disease: Pathophysiology, Diagnosis, Management. Philadelphia, BC Decker, 1991, p 63; with permission.

tion,[196] suggesting that polyamine content might serve as an indicator of mucosal hyperplasia and prove useful in assessing the response to specific diets.

MANAGEMENT OF THE PATIENT WITH SHORT BOWEL SYNDROME

The management of infants and children with massive intestinal resections can be divided into acute and chronic phases. The acute phase encompasses the stabilization of fluid and electrolyte needs, the early provision of parenteral nutrition to reverse catabolism, the judicious use of pharmacologic agents to combat gastric acid hypersecretion and loss of luminal fluid and electrolytes, and the limited provision of enteral glucose and electrolyte solutions and elemental diets to stimulate small bowel adaptation. The chronic phase includes the gradual transition from parenteral to enteral nutrition; determination of supplemental enteral fluid, electrolyte, divalent cation, trace element, and vitamin needs; and specific treatment of complications of SBS. Long-term management involves careful monitoring of growth and nutritional parameters and close surveillance for the potential complications of parenteral nutrition, including catheter-related sepsis, cholestatic liver disease, and gallstones. Loss of oral motor skills and aversion to oral feeding are particular problems in infants with SBS that must be addressed early, long before any substantial intake of nutrients by the oral route.

Total Parenteral Nutrition and Fluid and Electrolyte Therapy

Infants and children undergoing massive intestinal resection require the immediate placement of a nutritional central venous catheter to allow for the management of their fluid, electrolyte, and nutritional needs in the postoperative period. In patients with less extensive resections, usually those with a remaining long jejunal segment, an intact ileocecal valve, and a colon in continuity, enteral feedings may be well tolerated after the initial brief postoperative ileus and period of anastomotic and wound healing. The purpose of the initial phase of therapy is to assess fluid and electrolyte losses and replace them in the parenteral fluid, and to provide adequate amino acids to maintain the synthesis of essential proteins and avoid excessive muscle catabolism. Solutions used include dextrose at a range of 20 to 30 gm per dl and amino acids at a concentration designed to provide 2.5 to 3.0 gm per kg per day. Intravenous lipids should be administered a minimum of twice a week to provide at least 8% of total calories as fat and to prevent essential fatty acid deficiency. In practice, most infants with massive small bowel resections who are entirely reliant on parenteral nutrition receive as much as 20 to 40% of their total calories as fat to provide additional calories without exceeding their fluid or glucose tolerance.

Table 44–2 provides the approximate fluid and electrolyte composition of intestinal luminal contents at various segments. A key tenet of managing patients with SBS is to individualize their care by assessing and anticipating their specific needs. Excessive fluid losses via gastrostomy, jejunostomy, ileostomy, enterocutaneous fistula, or feces should be quantified by measuring the volume and electrolyte composition at each site. A comparable mixture of fluid and electrolytes can then be replaced prophylactically on a volume per volume basis. In the initial phases of acute management, when stool and ostomy output may be rapidly changing, the use of a second pump may be necessary, with a reassessment of the composition of the infused solution more than once a day. Measurement of serum sodium, potassium, calcium, and magnesium is a relatively insensitive way of diagnosing early electrolyte deficiencies, and quantitative urine collections may enhance their detection. Later, when losses are more predictable, appropriate electrolytes can be added to the TPN solution to account fully for the proper balance. In addition to extra sodium and potassium, acetate (over and above the acetate salts of amino acids contained in many TPN solutions) will often be included to compensate for excessive losses of bicarbonate. Ostomy losses may change with time and must be periodically reviewed. An infant with a newly created ileostomy absorbs approximately 80% of the small bowel fluid load,[197] whereas a child with an established ileostomy absorbs more than 90% of the same volume.[198] This may be secondary to recruitment of an ileal amiloride-inhibitable sodium channel, which is normally present only in the distal colon and is stimulated by increased intestinal fluid losses and resulting mineralocorticoid excess.[199]

Patients with large volume and electrolyte losses will benefit from early reanastomosis of the small intestine to the colon. In some patients with all or part of the colon bypassed, colonic infusion of fluid and electrolytes via a mucous fistula may be useful in maintaining plasma volume and positive fluid and electrolyte balance.[200] Reinfusion of secretions from the proximal stoma into the mucous fistula may allow reabsorption of up to 70% of the reinfused secretions and also prevent hypoplasia of the unused distal segment, thereby facilitating the eventual reanastomosis.[201, 202]

Standard quantities of vitamins and trace minerals are added to the parenteral nutrition solution and usually are sufficient. In patients with high-output proximal fistulas, and in premature infants, additional zinc may be required. Deficiencies of zinc, copper, chromium, manganese, selenium, and molybdenum have all been described in patients receiving prolonged TPN.[203] Prevention of the cardiomyopathy, macrocytosis, and depigmentation of skin and hair associated with selenium deficiency[204, 205] requires the addition of 20 μg per L of selenium to the TPN solution.[206] Monitoring blood levels of the above trace elements, iron, biotin, B_{12}, folate, and fat-soluble vitamins every three to six months is mandatory in patients dependent on total parenteral nutrition.[207]

Enteral Feedings

Enteral feedings are of primary importance in stimulating the adaptive response to bowel resection. In recent years, there has been a trend away from a prolonged period of "bowel rest" and toward earlier introduction of luminal nutrients in patients with SBS. In preparation for early feeding, a gastrostomy tube is often surgically placed at the time of the original intestinal resection. This facilitates enteral feeding in patients who may be too sick or unwilling to take appropriate formulas by mouth. The placement of a long-term nasogastric feeding tube may exacerbate upper respiratory problems or lead to the development of aversive feeding behavior and is a less attractive alternative. Regardless of the technique used to deliver nutrients, sucking behavior in infants should be encouraged to ease the eventual transition to oral feeding and contribute to more complete digestion of formula by stimulating the elaboration of lingual lipase and salivary amylase.[208] In general, continuous infusion is preferred over bolus administration of nutrients because of documentation of improved fat, nitrogen, calcium, zinc, and copper absorption in infants with SBS.[209] A significant increase in body weight during continuous feeding as compared to intermittent feeding has also been demonstrated in patients with SBS, chronic diarrhea, and congenital heart disease.[209, 210]

Glucose-containing fluid and electrolyte solutions are often the earliest enteral feedings employed. This first step in enteral feedings permits an assessment of the possible response to a more complex meal. A high sodium-containing solution (approximately 85 mEq per L) used in conjunction with glucose or glucose polymers is well absorbed.[42, 211, 212] In a recent study, patients with high jejunostomies were given an oral rehydration solution in which glucose was replaced with complex carbohydrate (maltodextrin), and the sodium concentration was raised without changes in osmolality. With these modifications, patients showed improvements in sodium absorption without increases in fluid loss.[213]

The optimal nutrient composition of enteral feedings in short bowel patients is controversial. Recent studies have challenged previously held views that low-fat, elemental diets are best tolerated. Increased knowledge of small bowel adaptation has prompted investigation of new formulations designed to enhance mucosal hyperplasia and nutrient absorption.[214] In an effort to supply the gut with some luminal nutrients, the initial feeding is most often an elemental formula supplying less than 10% of the total daily caloric intake via constant intragastric feedings. Stool volume, pH, and reducing substances are closely monitored for signs of severe malabsorption, which would compromise fluid and electrolyte balance and mitigate against continued increases in enteral feeding. Advances must be slow, and parenteral nutrition must be reduced concurrently without compromising total protein and caloric intake. There is no evidence that diluting an enteral formula helps, and this practice will only substitute hypocaloric fluid for an equivalent volume of more complete parenteral nutrition. If marked carbohydrate intolerance is documented, a carbohydrate-free elemental formula can be used to supply some stimulus for mucosal adaptation. Glucose polymers or fructose may be added in graded concentrations as tolerated.

Previous studies in patients with SBS documented the efficacy of elemental diets with protein hydrolysates or amino acids, glucose polymers, and medium-chain triglycerides in the early adaptive stages of short bowel syndrome.[215–217] These formulas were thought to be more easily absorbed and to stimulate less endogenous gastrointestinal secretions. However, more recent studies have shown that elemental diets are no better absorbed than polymeric ones even in the early phases of enteral feeding.[202, 218] In patients with jejunostomies, there is no difference in caloric absorption, stomal output, and electrolyte losses between an elemental and polymeric diet. Potential disadvantages of an elemental diet are the high cost, the high osmolality, and the lack of stimulation of colonic mucosal proliferation.[219]

Protein hydrolysates are typically used for the protein source. There is no clear indication that hydrolysates are better at inducing small bowel adaptation than intact proteins, but the former are more rapidly absorbed[220] and result in improved nitrogen balance in patients with end jejunostomies.[221] Since protein absorption occurs predominantly by intact dipeptide and tripeptide absorption, free amino acids are not necessary.

Carbohydrate is generally provided in the form of

glucose polymers or sucrose. Lactose is poorly tolerated in most patients in the early phase after significant small bowel resection and should be avoided until adequate documentation of lactose tolerance. With increasing time for mucosal adaptation, carbohydrate absorption increases, improving to approximately 70% of the total carbohydrate ingested.[222, 223] Increased absorption is found in patients with a colon in continuity, where salvage of carbohydrate by bacterial fermentation appears to be important in overall gut conservation of carbohydrate-derived energy.[224] In these patients, restriction of dietary lactose and sucrose and provision of some carbohydrate as complex polysaccharide (starch) or in the form of nonstarch fermentable fiber may improve overall energy utilization from carbohydrate, reduce colonic luminal osmolality, and facilitate colonic reabsorption of water. The addition of the fermentable fiber pectin to a diarrhea-inducing polymeric formula that was tube-fed to normal subjects reversed diarrhea and normalized low levels of fecal short-chain fatty acids.[225] The potential role of complex polysaccharide or fiber in the enteral feeding of patients with SBS has not been systematically investigated.

Documentation of the contribution of carbohydrate malabsorption to diarrhea has led to a reevaluation of earlier observations that a high-carbohydrate, low-fat diet of predominantly medium-chain triglycerides was better for patients with SBS.[226, 227] Low-fat diets theoretically decrease the possibility that malabsorption of long-chain fatty acids will cause colonic water secretion and contribute to poor absorption of divalent cations. Recent studies have contradicted these assumptions. In patients with jejunostomies, a high-fat diet induced a linear increase in the fat absorbed, an increased caloric intake, no increase in ostomy fluid output, but an increased loss of divalent cations.[228, 229] In a controlled crossover study of a high-fat versus a high-carbohydrate diet in adults with greater than 50% small bowel resection, there were no differences in the calcium, magnesium, and zinc absorbed, the volume of stool or ostomy output, urine volume, or electrolyte excretion between the dietary periods regardless of whether the patient had a jejunostomy, ileostomy, or enterocolonic anastomosis. Although the fecal fat excretion was three times higher on the high-fat than on the high-carbohydrate diet, the proportion of ingested fat absorbed was unchanged, and the mean percentage of total calories absorbed averaged 65% of intake on both diets.[230] A recent study of six infants with intractable diarrhea, including four with SBS, also demonstrated satisfactory weight gain and no differences in stool weight, electrolyte losses, and the enteral absorption of fat in infants fed a lower carbohydrate, higher fat formula.[231] The preponderance of fecal energy loss was from carbohydrate-derived energy irrespective of formula consumed. These studies and the increased palatability of higher-fat diets suggest that many patients with SBS need not be relegated to low-fat diets for a prolonged period of time.

The transition to oral bolus feedings from parenteral nutrition and constant enteral tube feedings is often very gradual and may take months or even years. The rapidity of this transition depends not only on the length and health of the remaining intestine but also on the avoidance of medical and surgical complications. With the advent of home parenteral nutrition, it is routine for the patient to be sent home on some combination of cycled parenteral and enteral nasogastric or gastrostomy feedings even while the transition to oral formula and solid foods is being made. Several recent studies have assessed the absorptive capacity of stable short-bowel patients in an attempt to define their nutritional needs and predict the eventual transition to a full oral diet.[222, 223] Stable adults with SBS ingesting an ad libitum oral diet absorb approximately two thirds of total ingested calories and up to three quarters of dietary protein. These studies dictate that in planning for eventual autonomy from parenteral nutrition, the patient must have the capacity to ingest at least 150% of expected kilocalories per kilogram and 130% of expected grams per kilogram protein for ideal body weight in order to counteract the increased losses of nutrients. Adaptive hyperphagia has been observed in several studies of ambulatory patients allowed ad libitum oral intake.[232, 233] Compensatory hyperphagia would only be expected to develop in infants and children with no active bowel disease, no stricture or severe motility disturbance, and no aversion to oral feedings.

It is important for the clinician to predict whether a patient is likely to need long-term parenteral nutrition. Recently, energy absorption from 300 ml of a polymeric liquid formula was used as a measure of "intestinal failure" in adult patients with SBS.[234] Figure 44–5 shows the fraction of ingested calories absorbed from a liquid test meal in three groups of patients. With one exception, the patients with the shortest remaining small bowel segments who were dependent on parenteral nutrition absorbed less than 35% of test meal energy. This simple noninvasive test of energy absorption measured by bomb calorimetry may be useful in identifying patients who will continue to require supplemental parenteral nutrition.

Poor absorption of fat-soluble vitamins, calcium, magnesium, and zinc is common in children with SBS. Without supplementation, complications of rickets or tetany may accompany calcium, magnesium, and vitamin D malabsorption, especially in infants and children with less than 50 cm of remaining small intestine at the time of the original surgery.[235] Oral administration of most minerals and vitamins is usually sufficient to maintain serum levels, although intermittent parenteral administration of vitamins K and D may occasionally be necessary. Availability of newer preparations of vitamins E and D complexed with polyethylene-glycol succinate enhance absorption even in a bile salt–deficient luminal environment.[236] In patients with ileal resections greater than 100 cm, B_{12} malabsorption is invariably present. Periodic screening of blood counts, blood smears, and serum B_{12} levels is important, and, if necessary, a Schilling's test can be performed. Replacement of calcium is often mandatory, especially in patients consuming a lactose-free diet. Parenteral injections of magnesium sulfate or citrate may be necessary because oral magnesium supplements often lead to increased diarrhea.

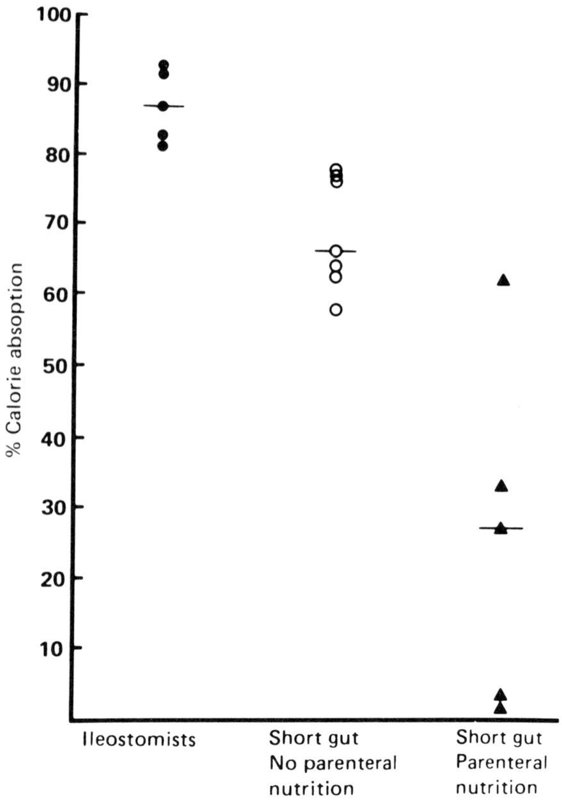

Figure 44–5. Energy absorption (percentage of calories ingested) from 300 ml Ensure in three groups of patients: those with ileostomies; those with SBS without parenteral nutrition; and those with SBS with a long-term need for parenteral nutrition. Horizontal bars represent median values. The three groups are significantly different at the $P < .01$ level. (From Rodrigues CA, Lennard-Jones JE, Thompson DG, et al: Energy absorption as a measure of intestinal failure in the short bowel syndrome. Gut 1989; 30:181; with permission.)

Oxalate excretion should be monitored in those with steatorrhea and an intact colon. If hyperoxaluria is demonstrated (urinary oxalate excretion greater than 50 mg per day), a low-oxalate diet is instituted eliminating chocolate, tea, cola, and vegetables such as spinach, celery, and carrots. The addition of oral elemental calcium supplements may also help decrease oxalate absorption and excretion in the urine, decreasing the risk of oxalate renal stones. Inability to achieve therapeutic blood levels with oral antibiotics may also be a problem in children with SBS. Absorption appears to be proportional to the length of the remaining bowel, and significant malabsorption is common in infants who have undergone greater than a 50% small bowel resection.[237] In these patients, parenteral antibiotics are necessary for even routine infections such as otitis media.

PHARMACOLOGIC THERAPY

The goals of drug therapy in patients with SBS are to reduce incapacitating diarrhea, help control fluid and electrolyte loss, and treat intervening complications. Pharmacologic manipulations cannot compensate for lack of absorption and may be detrimental if used indiscriminately, but judicious use of drugs may permit the patient to control symptoms sufficiently to leave the hospital. Both cimetidine and ranitidine effectively suppress gastric acid hypersecretion and reduce gastric secretory volume after massive small bowel resection.[238, 239] Cimetidine and more recently omeprazole also decrease jejunostomy fluid volume and excretion of sodium and potassium in adults with severe SBS.[240] Cimetidine prevents marked drops in jejunal pH and enhances fatty acid absorption in adults with massive small bowel resection and a jejunocolostomy.[64] Intravenous administration of an H_2 receptor antagonist should start immediately after the bowel resection. Oral treatment is rarely necessary for longer than one year postresection.

Several antidiarrheal drugs including codeine, diphenoxylate, and anticholinergic agents have been used in patients with SBS. In children, the only drug of this kind that has gained widespread acceptance is loperamide because of its lack of extraintestinal opiate effects at therapeutic doses. Loperamide is a synthetic opiate, a calmodulin inhibitor, and a calcium channel blocker that antagonizes the effects of substance P and neurotensin in vitro.[241, 242] In normal adults, loperamide increases the frequency of the small intestinal migrating motor complexes but greatly shortens phase two and lengthens phase one, resulting in a reduction of propulsive activity and a slower transit.[243] Loperamide decreases ileal output in patients with ileostomies.[244] In patients with SBS, loperamide has similarly been shown to shorten the duration of the characteristic postprandial motility pattern (phase two), although it significantly increased the motility index and frequency of peaks.[245] Other factors such as the known antisecretory activity, or effects on colonic motility may play a role in the drug's antidiarrheal activity.[246] Doses from 0.1 to 1.0 mg per kg per day have been used in children with SBS. Some caution must be exercised in those patients with risk factors for bacterial overgrowth, since delay in intestinal transit would be expected to promote proliferation of small bowel flora.

Cholestyramine, an ion-exchange resin that binds intraluminal dihydroxy bile acids, is often given to reduce the effects of malabsorbed bile salts on the colon.[247] In children, an appropriate dose is 100 to 400 mg per kg per day in three divided doses. Cholestyramine also binds dietary oxalate and prevents its absorption. Disadvantages of cholestyramine therapy include further depletion of an already shrunken bile salt pool in those patients with steatorrhea. In these cases, the drug may actually worsen the diarrhea and steatorrhea. With this concern in mind, some clinicians will use cholestyramine only in conjunction with high medium-chain triglyceride formulas or a low-fat diet.[14, 36] A therapeutic trial may be necessary to determine the drug's potential benefit in the individual patient. Cholestyramine also binds vitamin D and may exacerbate malabsorption of other fat-soluble vitamins as well as folate.[248] In large doses, cholestyramine can cause a hyperchloremic metabolic acidosis. Aluminum hydroxide antacids also bind bile salts but are associated with depletion of phosphorus and calcium and resultant osteomalacia.[249, 250]

Octreotide is an octapeptide somatostatin analogue that has been used successfully to partially control diarrhea associated with vasoactive intestinal polypeptide–secreting tumors and carcinoid syndrome in adults,[251–253] and with idiopathic secretory diarrhea and congenital microvillous atrophy in children.[254, 255] Somatostatin is known to inhibit exocrine secretions from the stomach, pancreas, and small intestine, and to reduce splanchnic blood flow and slow gastrointestinal motility.[256, 257] Octreotide can be administered subcutaneously. The clinical effect peaks 2 hours after injection and lasts for up to 12 hours. Recently, the use of intravenous and subcutaneous octreotide has been investigated in patients with SBS.[258] In a five-year-old patient, octreotide reduced massive ileostomy fluid losses by two thirds and prolonged transit time from mouth to ileostomy from 20 to 360 minutes.[259] In adult patients with high-output proximal jejunostomies, octreotide reduces stomal fluid losses and sodium output and improves urine output while reducing but not eliminating the need for intravenous fluid and electrolyte supplementation.[260–262] In small bowel perfusion studies in fasted subjects, octreotide has no direct effect on jejunal absorption of sodium and water.[263] Since the majority of luminal sodium in the proximal jejunum derives from gastrointestinal and pancreaticobiliary secretions, and octreotide is known to reduce pancreatic secretion in patients with high jejunostomies by 63% after stimulation with CCK,[264] it is likely that the reduction of stomal fluid losses is a consequence of suppression of upper gastrointestinal and pancreatic secretions. In contrast to its effect on fluid and sodium, octreotide does not influence net absorption of potassium, calcium, magnesium, zinc, fat, nitrogen, or total calories.[265, 266]

In the few long-term studies of octreotide in the management of patients with SBS, drug tolerance has been good, with no significant changes in glucose homeostasis, thyroid function, or fat malabsorption. Data on growth hormone secretion and growth velocity in children treated with long-term octreotide are not available. In short-term studies in normal adults, twice-daily injections of 50 μg octreotide given at 8:00 AM and 5:30 PM delayed spontaneous daytime peaks of growth hormone secretion for 6 hours after dosing but did not significantly alter nocturnal and total 24-hour growth hormone secretion.[267] At present, it appears that octreotide may reduce stomal or fecal water and sodium loss and decrease reliance on parenteral supplementation or oral rehydration solutions.

Treatment of chronic bacterial overgrowth may result in profound improvement of diarrhea. The diagnosis should be suspected in the child with SBS whose intolerance to enteral feedings is out of proportion to the residual length of small intestine or whose diarrhea significantly worsens with excessive bloating, eructation, and flatulence. Megaloblastic anemia is typically present. Folate levels are usually normal or even high, since intestinal bacteria produce folic acid, but serum vitamin B_{12} levels are low, and vitamin B_{12} absorption with or without added intrinsic factor is abnormal. Less commonly, iron-deficiency anemia or a mixed picture results from mucosal damage and chronic blood loss secondary to bacterial overgrowth. Deficiencies in fat-soluble vitamins may appear with the patient presenting with purpura, osteomalacia, or night blindness. Hypoproteinemia is common and may reflect a protein-losing enteropathy. Small bowel barium roentgenograms should be performed in any patient with these findings to show the site and extent of any structural lesion (Fig. 44–6). Enteroclysis can better delineate a discrete stricture or mucosal disease.

The gold standard for the diagnosis of bacterial overgrowth has been proximal small bowel intubation and the demonstration of the presence of a complex flora of strict anaerobes and coliforms in numbers greater than 10^6 organisms per ml.[268] Because of the difficulty performing this test on infants and small children, the possible contamination with mouth and upper respiratory flora, and the requirement for strict anaerobic culture techniques, other less invasive tests have been developed. A single elevated fasting breath hydrogen sample[269] or a combination of a high fasting breath hydrogen and a rise in breath hydrogen 2 hours after a 50 gm oral glucose challenge has been advocated as an indicator of bacterial overgrowth.[270] Many of these breath tests suffer from difficulty in separating patients with massive small bowel resection (whose rapid transit and subsequent colonic bacterial action on the fermentable or labeled substrate would be expected to yield an early peak) from those with true proximal small bowel bacterial overgrowth. In this respect, the ^{14}C D-xylose breath test may have an advantage, since a small dose should be totally absorbed even in a short proximal bowel, provided the mucosa is intact.[271]

The choice of antimicrobial therapy has largely been empiric. Tetracycline enjoys popularity in adult patients because of its effectiveness against *Bacteroides* species. In pediatric patients, combinations of metronidazole and trimethoprim-sulfamethoxazole or oral vancomycin and gentamicin have been used with success. Cyclic treatment of 1 week every 1 to 2 months may be necessary. Surgical procedures to resect a stricture or taper a dilated hypotonic segment have been reported to be effective in small numbers of cases (see later). Prokinetic agents such as metaclopromide and cisapride may be useful in patients with dilated proximal segments, bile reflux, pseudo-obstruction, and bacterial overgrowth.[272]

LONG-TERM PARENTERAL NUTRITION THERAPY

The development of total parenteral nutrition is the most important technical advance in improving growth, development, and survival in infants and children with SBS. The advent of home parenteral nutrition has revolutionized long-term care and allowed children and families to enjoy a more normal life in spite of severe gastrointestinal pathology. Often, the parenteral nutri-

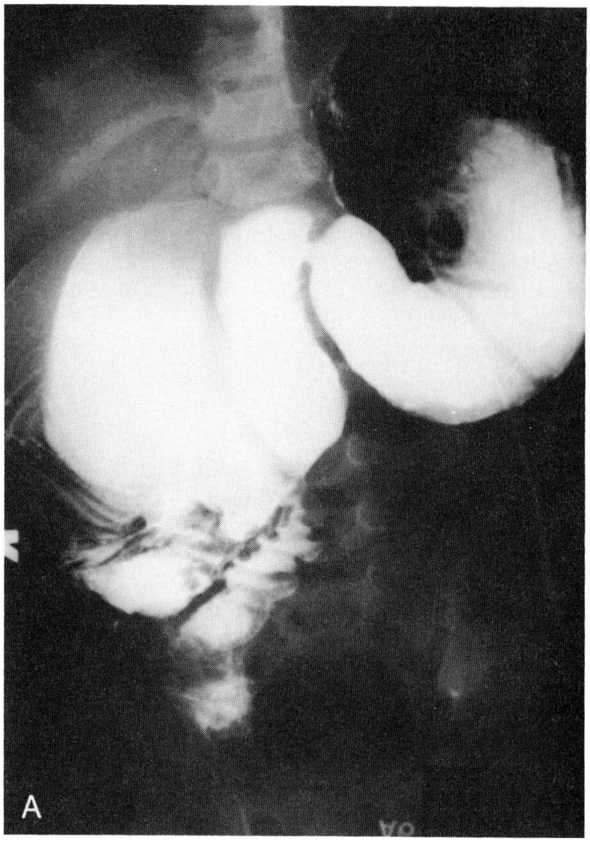

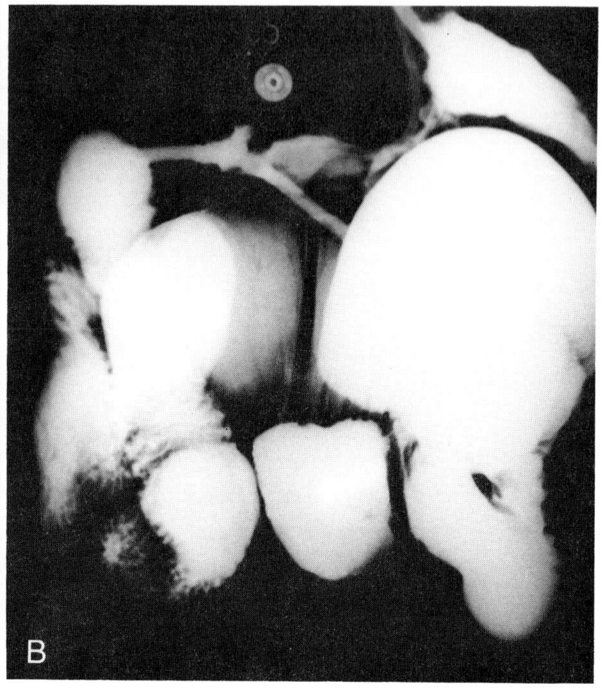

Figure 44–6. Two examples of proximal small bowel dilated loops giving rise to stasis, mucosal injury, bacterial overgrowth, and malabsorption. *A*, The duodenum is massively dilated secondary to an adhesion. *B*, There is a dilated hypotonic large midjejunal loop in which the barium demonstrates retrograde as well as antegrade peristalsis.

tion infusion can be limited to the nighttime hours, allowing routine daily activities and school attendance. Several recent studies have demonstrated that children with SBS receiving home TPN therapy can achieve normal growth rates, anthropometric measurements, and visceral protein levels.[273, 274] However, with prolonged use of TPN has come the recognition of major complications. Morbidity and mortality are most commonly related to central venous catheter infections and progressive liver disease, which accounted for 11 deaths in 102 patients over a 10-year period in a recent review.[272]

Catheter-Related Infections

In 104 infants and children collated from three recent published series of neonatal SBS patients who were receiving TPN at home, the rate of catheter-related sepsis approximated 2.0 episodes per 1,000 days.[11, 13, 14] Gram-positive cocci dominate the list of organisms responsible for Broviac catheter sepsis, accounting for approximately 60 to 75% of all isolates.[276] Coagulase-negative *Staphylococcus* is the most common isolate in our experience. *Staphylococcus aureus* and streptococcal species are also important pathogens, and gram-negative rods including pseudomonas species account for about 25% of blood isolates. Fungal infections are uncommon but result in a high degree of mortality. We currently prescribe oral antifungal prophylaxis to all patients with SBS maintained on home TPN. Antibiotic prophylaxis should also be considered prior to dental work, gastrointestinal endoscopies or cystoscopies, incision and drainage of abscesses, and after any episode of catheter breakage and repair.

Every patient with SBS and a fever, no obvious focal infection, and a central venous catheter should be treated for potential catheter-related sepsis. A high white blood count is suggestive but is not always present. New onset of glucose intolerance and glycosuria may be helpful clues. In many cases, eradication of the organism causing sepsis can be accomplished without removal of the catheter.[277, 278] A response to therapy with resolution of fever is usually seen within a five-day period, and lack of response has been associated with the presence of an abscess, endocarditis, septic venous thrombosis, immunocompromised status, and the organisms *Pseudomonas aeruginosa* and *Candida albicans*.[276] Infections with these organisms are absolute indications to remove the catheter. If blood cultures remain positive for 48 hours after isolation of an organism and treatment with appropriate antibiotics, strong consideration should be given to removing the catheter. Because of the high incidence of infections with non-aureus staphylococcal species, treatment should be initiated with vancomycin and an aminoglycoside antibiotic.

TPN-Associated Liver Disease

The etiology of progressive cholestatic liver disease associated with prolonged TPN is not fully elucidated.[280] Retrospective studies of premature neonates receiving TPN have found that intestinal resection for necrotizing enterocolitis and other congenital abnormalities is a strong risk factor for the development of cholestasis.[281–283] Adults with severe Crohn's disease and those undergoing extensive small bowel resections for other reasons develop severe cholestasis, bile ductular proliferation, and fibrosis several months after the resection and initiation of TPN.[284, 285] Colonization of the excluded segment by aerobic and anaerobic organisms has been well documented in patients with jejunoileal bypass surgery who develop similar hepatic lesions.[286] Treatment with metronidazole at the onset of TPN administration to patients with Crohn's disease[287, 288] and at the time of jejunoileal bypass surgery[289] prevents liver enzyme abnormalities and hepatic steatosis characteristically seen in such patients not treated with antibiotics. These observations suggest that intestinal bacterial proliferation, particularly of anaerobic organisms, is involved in the pathogenesis of cholestatic liver injury in patients with SBS.[289a]

Mechanisms postulated to link hepatic disease with intestinal bacterial proliferation include bacterial deconjugation of bile salts and production of hepatotoxic bile acids,[290] release of bacterial endotoxin,[291] or release of bacterial cell wall components such as peptidoglycan-polysaccharide polymers directly into the portal circulation.[292] Lithocholic acid, a secondary bile acid normally formed by bacterial metabolism of chenodeoxycholic acid, produces severe liver damage with cholestasis in several animal species similar to that seen in patients receiving TPN.[293] In patients with Crohn's disease treated with TPN, an increase in the percentage of biliary lithocholate correlates with elevated levels of serum alkaline phosphatase and aminotransferase.[294] Using a rat blind-loop model of small bowel bacterial overgrowth, Lichtman and colleagues[292] have reproduced a hepatic lesion similar to that described in patients after chronic TPN therapy, jejunoileal bypass surgery, and chronic inflammatory bowel disease. They have also demonstrated that bacteria themselves are not found in the injured liver but speculate that translocation of intestinal bacterial cell wall polymers may be responsible for the liver damage. Further experiments in the same model have demonstrated that metronidazole and tetracycline eliminate *Bacteroides* species from the blind loop and prevent or reverse liver injury, but gentamicin and polymyxin B (which binds bacterial endotoxin) do not.[295] These investigators conclude that continued exposure to luminal anaerobic bacteria and their cell wall products is necessary for the progression of chronic experimental hepatobiliary inflammation. Peptidoglycan-polysaccharide has been implicated, since there are increased circulating antibodies to peptidoglycans and since mutanolysin, an enzyme whose only known function is to degrade peptidoglycan-polysaccharides, prevents hepatic injury in this model.

Recent work in rat models of TPN and small bowel bacterial overgrowth has implicated tumor necrosis factor (TNF-alpha) in the chronic hepatic damage produced. Continuous infusion of TNF-alpha plus TPN resulted in marked liver enlargement, bile ductular hyperplasia, and moderate fatty change compared to rats infused with TPN alone or rats infused with TNF-alpha but fed orally.[296] Intraperitoneal injection of peptidoglycan-polysaccharide results in marked uptake by Kupffer cells in the liver and stimulates their production of TNF.[297] Pentoxifylline interferes with TNF release from Kupffer cells and prevents hepatic injury in rats with small bowel bacterial overgrowth.

Death from severe progressive liver disease was documented in 10 out of 190 pediatric patients with SBS on long-term TPN.[10–14] Early institution of enteral feedings to promote intestinal motility, avoidance of iron overload,[289a] and attention to the treatment of bacterial overgrowth with antibiotics, prokinetic agents, and surgical procedures may significantly reduce the morbidity and mortality associated with this complication.

SURGICAL THERAPY

Surgical therapy should be reserved for patients with specific complications such as strictures or partial obstruction with resulting dilatation, stasis, and bacterial overgrowth; or those whose anatomy precludes sufficient adaptation to allow autonomy from parenteral nutrition.[298, 299] The risk of making the patient worse by further resection or creation of new adhesions or strictures must be balanced against the risk of recurrent catheter-related sepsis, progressive liver disease, or loss of available sites for nutritional catheters. Though some of the procedures described below have shown remarkable anecdotal success, controlled prospective long-term studies are lacking, and firm conclusions about their merits are difficult to reach.

Intestinal Interpositions

Based on studies in animals, reversal of short segments of small intestine (3 to 15 cm) or interposition of isoperistaltic or antiperistaltic segments of colon has been advocated in order to delay gastric emptying, slow intestinal transit, and increase absorption.[300–303] Warden and Wesley reversed 3-cm segments of distal ileum in five infants with greater than 25 cm of residual small bowel at the time of the reversal. All patients had at least initial improvements, with two showing an increase in mouth to anus transit time; however, diarrhea recurred in one, and another died of overwhelming pneumonia soon after surgery.[304] Other reports also describe initial improvement followed by a return to the preoperative status.[299]

Glick and coworkers[305] reported the interposition of 8 to 14 cm of isoperistaltic colon, just distal to the ligament of Treitz, in six infants with SBS. It was not clear why only three of the infants responded and were able to discontinue parenteral nutrition. The major disadvantage of interposition of both small intestinal and colonic reversed segments is that they cause an element of functional obstruction that may favor stasis and an increased tendency for bacterial overgrowth.

Intestinal Lengthening and Tapering Procedures

In 1980, Bianchi[306] devised a method in pigs that had undergone massive small bowel resection for doubling the length of the dilated remaining small bowel based on the arrangement of the blood vessels of the mesentery. These vessels divide into anterior and posterior branches, permitting longitudinal splitting of the gut between them, reconstruction of the split gut into narrower tubes, and reanastomosis of these tubes in continuity. Four children underwent the tube intestinal lengthening procedure, increasing their small bowel length from 30 to 54 cm to 42 to 101 cm. All were able to wean from TPN to full enteral feedings. However, one required a second laparotomy for intestinal obstruction, and in three of the children, the operation was performed before full intestinal adaptation had taken place.[307] Tapering the dilated segment of small bowel is as important as, if not more important than, lengthening it to restore coaptation of the walls and more normal peristalsis in patients with stasis and bacterial overgrowth (Fig. 44–7).[308] Tapering enteroplasty is effective at the time of an original operation for intestinal atresia as well.[309] Other strategies to preserve intestinal length include stricture plasty and serosal patching,[310] particularly in those with Crohn's disease in whom discrete strictures or perforations may develop, otherwise necessitating multiple small bowel resections.

Artificial Enteric Sphincters

The importance of a functioning ileocecal valve (ICV) to prolong small bowel transit and prevent bacterial overgrowth has prompted efforts to construct an artificial ICV. Studies have shown benefits of surgically constructed valves in experimental animals[311, 312]; however, attempts in humans have yielded inconclusive results and, in certain cases, have led to obstruction.[313, 314] Most artificial valves are created by deliberately fashioning a short jejunocolic or colojejunal intussusception or fashioning a small bowel to colon anastomosis via a submucosal tunnel in the receiving colon.

Other experimental surgical procedures include the formation of neomucosa by interposing colonic serosa [315, 316] or abdominal wall muscle[317] between small bowel segments to allow new mucosa to grow over the patch. Retrograde electrical pacing at a distal small bowel site has been tried in dogs with SBS to slow the flow of intestinal chyme and increase absorption.[318] These procedures have shown some promising results in animal models of SBS[319] but have not been successfully applied to humans.[299]

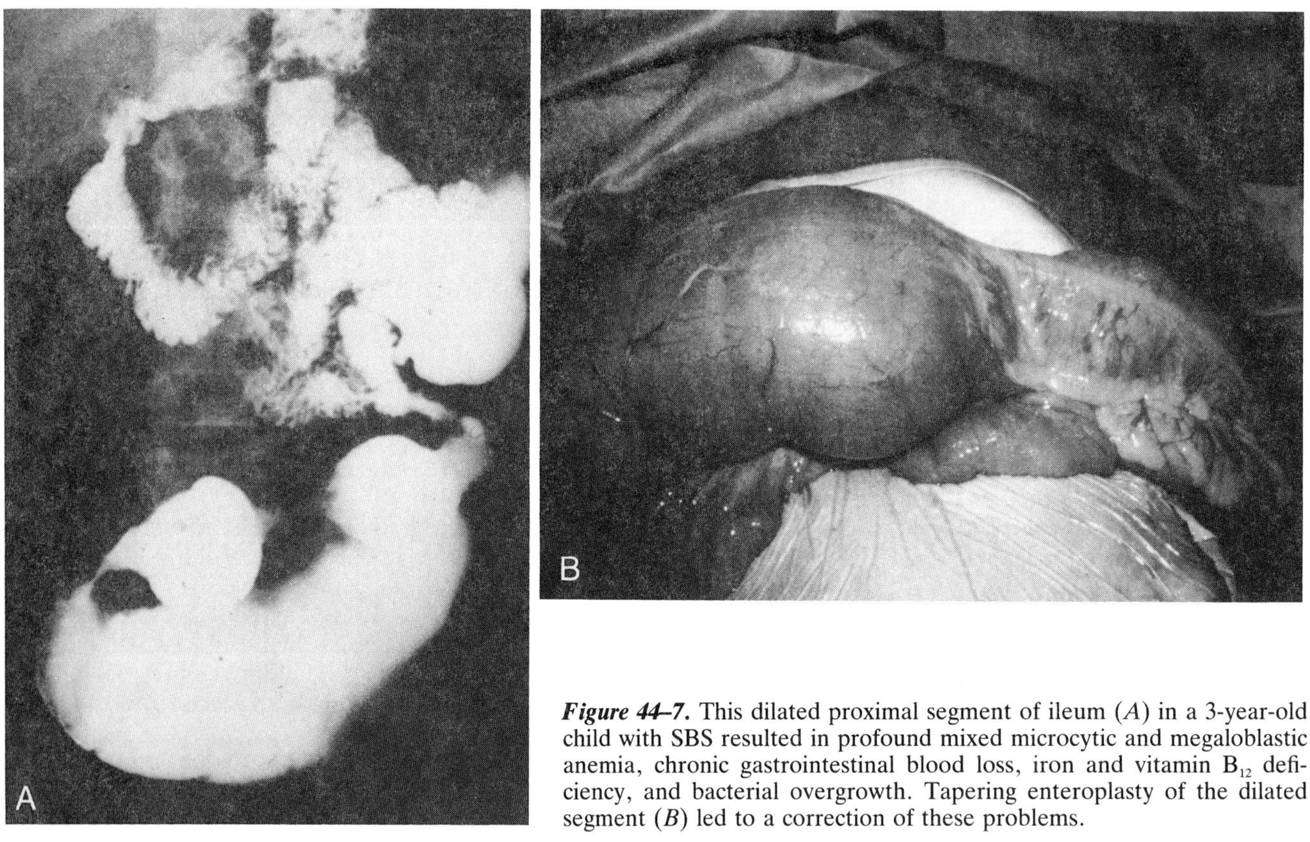

Figure 44–7. This dilated proximal segment of ileum (*A*) in a 3-year-old child with SBS resulted in profound mixed microcytic and megaloblastic anemia, chronic gastrointestinal blood loss, iron and vitamin B_{12} deficiency, and bacterial overgrowth. Tapering enteroplasty of the dilated segment (*B*) led to a correction of these problems.

SMALL BOWEL TRANSPLANTATION

In 1959, Lillihei and associates[320] demonstrated that small bowel transplantation (SBT) was technically possible in a canine model. At the time, available immunosuppressive agents were unable to control the fulminant rejection that developed within days of the surgery. Between 1964 and 1970, seven transplant patients died because of technical failure, graft rejection, or sepsis all within 2.5 months of surgery.[321] In addition to the problem of rejection, it became clear that unlike other solid organ grafts, SBT created the potential for significant graft-versus-host disease (GVHD) because the graft includes large amounts of lymphoid tissue in the form of mucosal and submucosal lymphocytes, Peyer's patches, and mesenteric lymph nodes.[322, 323] The advent of cyclosporine and other newer, potent, selective immunosuppressive agents stimulated renewed interest in SBT. In the past decade, work has progressed from successful transplants in rats, pigs, and primates[324–327] to small clinical trials. Ongoing clinical trials can be justified on the basis of the limited options that are available for patients who develop severe complications while receiving TPN, the improved results in animal studies, the recent success of pancreatoduodenal transplantation,[328] and the demonstrated ability to detect rejection and remove the graft without mortality.[329] A full discussion of SBT is beyond the scope of this chapter. The reader is referred to several excellent recent reviews of the subject.[330–332]

A summary of the recent experience with small bowel transplantation through 1991 is shown in Table 44–3. Experience with isolated small bowel transplantation has been only partially successful,[329, 333–336] but combined liver–small bowel transplantation appears more promising, and more centers are preparing to undertake this procedure.[337–339] Operative procedures include a mixture of partial and total donor small bowel segments and porto-portal or portal-systemic venous anastomoses. In most cases the distal end of graft and the native ileum

Table 44–3. PARTIAL SUMMARY OF RECENT PUBLISHED EXPERIENCE WITH SMALL BOWEL TRANSPLANTATION THROUGH MID-1991

Center	Reference No.	Patient Identification No.	Age of Patient	Type of Transplant	Duration of Graft Survival (Graft Status or Cause of Death)	Outcome
Paris	329	1	9 mo	Intestine	3 hr (Necrosis)	Alive (TPN)
			3 yr	Intestine	2 mo (Rejection)	Alive (TPN)
		2	9 yr	Intestine	6 mo (Renal failure)	Death
		3	6 yr	Intestine	17 mo (Rejection)	Alive (TPN)
		4	5 mo	Intestine	30 mo	Alive (fed)
		5	9 mo	Intestine	12 d (Rejection)	Alive (TPN)
Kiel	333	6	5 yr	Intestine	12 d (Rejection)	Alive (TPN)
	335	7	42 yr	Intestine	23 mo	Alive (fed)
Ontario	334	8	8 yr	Intestine	15 d (Rejection)	Alive (TPN)
	337	9	41 yr	Liver-intestine	30 mo	Alive (fed)
	337a	10	47 yr	Liver-intestine	3 mo (Stroke)	Death
		11	37 yr	Liver-intestine	18 mo	Alive
		12	27 yr	Liver-intestine Stomach-pancreas	7 mo (Lymphoma)	Death
		13	32 yr	Liver-intestine Stomach-pancreas	3 mo	Alive
Europe	2	14	Adult	Liver-intestine Stomach-pancreas	8 mo (Recurrent pancreatic cancer)	Death
Sweden	337b	15	14 mo	Intestine	2 mo (Rejection, sepsis)	Death
Chicago	338	16	17 mo	Liver-intestine Stomach-pancreas	4 d	Death
		17	9 mo	Liver-intestine Stomach-pancreas	3.5 mo (Lymphoma)	Death
Pittsburgh	339	18	3.5 yr	Liver-intestine Stomach-pancreas	6 mo (Lymphoma)	Death
	328, 328a	19	4 yr	Liver-intestine	9 mo	Alive (fed)
		20	2 yr	Liver-intestine	13 mo	Alive (fed)
		21	27 yr	Liver-intestine	13 mo	Alive (fed)
		22	31 yr	Intestine	16 mo	Alive (TPN)
		23	3 yr	Liver-intestine	5 mo	Alive (TPN)
Wisconsin	339a	24	14 mo	Liver-intestine	2 mo (Pulmonary failure)	Death
Austria	339b	25	49 yr	Liver-intestine Stomach-pancreas	8 mo (Recurrent pancreatic cancer)	Death

(if applicable) are exteriorized as ostomies to allow monitoring for rejection and GVHD via serial mucosal biopsies.

All patients with isolated small bowel transplants experienced acute rejection in spite of treatment with immediate large intravenous doses of cyclosporine and methylprednisolone, and in many cases antilymphocyte globulin and azathioprine as well. The use of FK506 in some cases did not prevent rejection, which presented with fever, dysmotility (ileus or diarrhea) of the graft, and malabsorption.[340a] Additional strategies to reduce acute rejection and GVHD include treatment of the donor with intravenous OKT3 or other monoclonal antibodies and methylprednisolone[337, 340, 341] or in vitro treatment of the harvested small bowel graft with radiation or a vascular washing solution that includes cyclosporine and antilymphocyte globulin.[329, 342] In view of the sensitivity of the small bowel to rejection damage and the potential for GVHD, it seems certain that good tissue typing will be a prerequisite for long-term success.[343] Support for this premise comes from a successful SBT in which the patient was a 42-year-old female who received a 60-cm graft from a half-sister who was homozygous for one-haplotype of the A, B, and DR antigens of the recipient.[335]

Other investigators have proposed that the success of SBT will be enhanced by simultaneous orthotopic liver transplantation.[323, 338] Experimental work has shown that in both the rat and the pig a hepatic allograft induces tolerance to subsequent skin grafts from the liver donor strain but not from other sources.[344, 345] Simultaneous liver transplantation also appears to prevent kidney graft damage by cytotoxic antibodies in humans.[346, 347] Rats with combined liver–small bowel transplants are less likely to undergo rejection than those with isolated small intestinal transplants,[348] and the onset of rejection can be delayed in the recipients of multivisceral grafts.[349] Many children with SBS and dependence on TPN have sustained severe hepatic injury and require simultaneous liver-bowel transplantation to prevent liver failure and ensure long-term survival.

Numerous questions remain to be answered before SBT becomes an acceptable therapeutic alternative. Pretransplantation immunosuppression of the graft and post-transplantation immunosuppression of the recipient must be refined. The balance between rejection and GVHD is delicate. Experimental work supports the concept that the GVH reaction can induce a state of permanent suppression of cell-mediated and humoral responses. The immunosuppressive effect of subclinical GVHD may actually be beneficial to the survival of small bowel allografts.[350] Cyclosporine may adversely affect the microvasculature of the small intestine similar to its effect on the kidney.[351] FK506 is a neutral macrolide that, on a molar basis, is a more potent inhibitor of T helper cell function than cyclosporine and may be superior in preventing rejection in a rat model of orthotopic SBT.[352]

Technical aspects of SBT also require further investigation. In ideal circumstances, the venous drainage of the small bowel graft should be connected to the recipient portal system, but in many instances, the portal vein may be inaccessible or thrombosed. Although total diversion of portal flow in rats and dogs invariably results in significant liver atrophy and precipitates hyperammonemia and amino acid imbalances,[353, 354] recent studies suggest that systemic drainage in the pig model of SBT results in no significant long-term metabolic or functional hepatic deterioration.[355] In this animal model, portal blood flow is only partially diverted because venous flow from the stomach, duodenum, pancreas, spleen, and large bowel continues to flow through the liver. The optimum length of the graft is also unknown. Longer segments of intestine have a greater potential to cause GVHD.[356] Another concern vital to the postoperative management of patients undergoing SBT is prevention of bacterial translocation from the gut to the blood stream.[357] Recent experimental work shows that bacterial counts of enteric organisms rise rapidly in the mesenteric lymph nodes and spleen in association with episodes of rejection.[358] Early attempts at SBT were plagued by fatal episodes of gram-negative sepsis thought to be secondary to ischemic damage to the preserved small bowel graft and translocation of enteric organisms into the systemic circulation during reperfusion. Optimal methods of pre- and post-transplantation selective bowel decontamination with antibiotics remain to be determined.

PROGNOSIS OF INFANTS AND CHILDREN WITH SHORT BOWEL SYNDROME

The prognosis of SBS has dramatically improved since the advent of TPN. With the possibility that small bowel transplantation may become a viable therapeutic option, even those infants with intestinal loss so massive as to make the possibility of enteral nutrition unlikely may be candidates for support with TPN.[359] Decisions about rational treatment must be made on an individual basis. Most infants are currently treated with lifesaving surgery and prolonged nutritional support to buy time for further development and refinement of clinical small bowel transplantation (Figure 44–8).

Table 44–4 summarizes the most recent collected series of infants with SBS. Prior to the routine use of long-term TPN, Wilmore and Dudrick collected much of the published pediatric experience through 1972.[1] The survival rate was 95% in 20 infants with a jejunoileal length of 38 to 75 cm, both with and without an ICV. Infants with 15 to 38 cm of jejunoileum survived 50% of the time, provided the ICV was intact; those without an ICV all died. All infants with less than 15 cm of small intestine with or without an ICV died. Overall survival was 52%.

Since that time, survival has improved, and the length of viable residual jejunoileum deemed necessary for survival and eventual small bowel adaptation has decreased. Most recent series have documented greater than 80% overall survival.[10–14] In infants with only 0 to 30 cm of residual jejunoileum, the survival rate was still 69%.[11] Goulet and colleagues recently documented a

Table 44–4. PROGNOSIS OF SHORT BOWEL SYNDROME IN INFANTS

	Wilmore[3]	Bohan[9]	Cooper[10]	Dorney[11]	Grosfeld[12]	Caniano[13]	Goulet[14]	
Total no. of patients	50	15	16	13	54	14	87	
Residual length of jejunoileum (cm)	0–75	25–150	15–105	0–30	13–120	15–53	<40	40–80
No. (%) of patients who survived	26 (52)	13 (86)	13 (81)	9 (69)	45 (83)	12 (86)	24 (67)	47 (92)
No. reaching full adaptation*	26 (52%)	12/13	13/13	5/9	?	8/12	18/24	44/47
Time (mean or range) to full adaptation (mo)	?	2–10	14	4–32	13/14	18	27m	14m
No. (%) of deaths	24 (48)	2 (14)	3 (19)	4 (31)	9 (17)	2 (14)	16 (18)	
Causes of death								
Sepsis	?	2/2	0/3	2/4	3/9	0/2	12/16	
Hepatic failure	?	0/2	3/3	2/4	5/9	2/2	0/16	
Gallstones and cholangitis	?	?	?	6/13	2/54	3/14	9/87	

*Full adaptation is defined as complete autonomy from parenteral nutrition and full enteral feedings.

94% survival rate in infants with less than 40 cm of small bowel born after 1980 (when home parenteral nutrition was introduced) compared to a 65% survival rate for those treated prior to 1980.[14] Survival continues to be correlated with the length of remaining jejunoileum; 92% of infants with 40 to 80 cm of residual small intestine survived, versus 66% of those with less than 40 cm.[14]

The prognosis for small bowel adaptation and total autonomy from parenteral nutrition is also related to residual jejunoileal length. In the era of prolonged TPN, as little as 10 cm with an ICV and 20 cm without an ICV may allow eventual conversion to full enteral nutrition.[11] The duration of dependence on parenteral nutrition appears to be inversely proportional to the length of residual small bowel, but it is also dependent on the presence or absence of an ICV.[13, 14] Patients with less than 40 cm of small bowel and no ICV required more than twice as much time to complete adaptation compared to those who retained their ICV. Extensive colon resection also appears to delay full enteral nutrition.[14]

Adult patients also show a statistically significant correlation between the length of the remaining small bowel and the necessary duration of intestinal support.[360] However, neither adult patients with 10 to 30 cm of remaining small intestine plus their ICV and colon nor those with less than 60 cm minus the ICV and colon were able to achieve autonomy from parenteral nutrition. These data suggest that increased capacity for adaptation exists in neonates undergoing massive resection compared to adults. The functional and adaptive capability of the residual intestine is adversely affected by the primary disease, which may continue to be active, as in patients with Crohn's disease; or it may be influenced by the presence of surgical complications such as strictures or adhesions, which affect motility and promote bacterial overgrowth.

The main causes of morbidity and mortality in children with severe SBS are chronic progressive liver disease with complications of hepatic failure, portal hypertension, gastrointestinal bleeding, and peritonitis or sepsis related to bacterial translocation from the gut or colonization of the nutritional catheter. Further clinical research into strategies to prevent or retard these sequelae of chronic TPN and bacterial overgrowth is necessary. Small bowel transplantation may soon be a reasonable therapeutic option for those patients whose residual small intestine is incapable of full adaptation and who have progressively developed life-threatening complications precluding continued intravenous nutritional support.

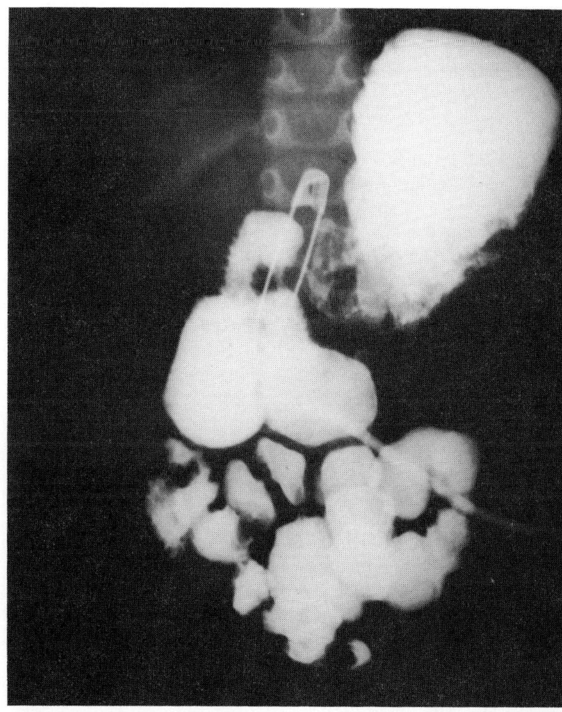

Figure 44–8. This child was born with massive jejunoileal and right colonic atresia, with approximately 12 cm of viable small bowel and a left colon. Two subsequent procedures—resection of further necrotic small bowel and resection of stenotic sigmoid colon—have left him with a dilated duodenum and minimal jejunum anastomased to the left colon. The child is now 5 years old and has cirrhosis. He underwent a cholecystectomy for cholelithiasis and cholecystitis, has mild renal damage from multiple courses of nephrotoxic antibiotics for bacterial and fungal sepsis, and has had multiple central catheter replacements. He is now a candidate for combined liver–small bowel transplant.

REFERENCES

1. Wilmore DW, Dudrick SJ: Growth and development of an infant receiving all nutrients exclusively by vein. JAMA 1968; 203:860–864.
2. Schroeder P, Goulet O, Lear PA: Small bowel transplantation: European experience. Lancet 1990; 336:110–111.
3. Wilmore DW: Factors correlating with a successful outcome following extensive intestinal resection in newborn infants. J Pediatr 1972; 80:88–95.
4. Siebert JR: Small-intestine length in infants and children. Am J Dis Child 1980; 134:593–595.
5. Touloukian RJ, Walker Smith GJ: Normal intestinal length in pre-term infants. J Pediatr Surg 1983; 18:720–723.
6. Trier JS, Winter HS: Anatomy, embryology, and developmental abnormalities of the small intestine and colon. *In* Sleisenger MH, Fordtran JS, eds: Gastrointestinal Disease: Pathophysiology, Diagnosis, and Management. Philadelphia, WB Saunders, 1989, pp 991–1021.
7. Klish WJ, Putnam TC: The short gut. Am J Dis Child 1981; 135:1056–1061.
8. Ziegler MM: Short bowel syndrome in infancy: Etiology and management. Clinics in Perinatology 1986; 13:163–173.
9. Bohane TD, Haka-Ikse K, Biggar WD, et al: A clinical study of young infants after small intestinal resection. J Pediatr 1979; 94:552–558.
10. Cooper A, Floyd TF, Ross AJ, et al: Morbidity and mortality of short-bowel syndrome acquired in infancy: An update. J Pediatr Surg 1984; 19:711–717.
11. Dorney SFA, Ament ME, Berquist WE, et al: Improved survival in very short small bowel of infancy with use of long-term parenteral nutrition. J Pediatr 1985; 107:521–525.
12. Grosfeld JL, Rescorla FJ, West JW: Short bowel syndrome in infancy and childhood. Am J Surg 1986; 151:41–46.
13. Caniano DA, Starr J, Ginn-Pease ME: Extensive short-bowel syndrome in neonates: Outcome in the 1980's. Surgery 1989; 105:119–124.
14. Goulet OJ, Revillon Y, Jan D, et al: Neonatal short bowel syndrome. J Pediatr 1991; 1991:18–23.
15. Ricour C, Duhamel JF, Arnaud-Battandier F, et al: Enteral and parenteral nutrition in the short-bowel syndrome in children. World J Surg 1985; 9:310–315.
16. Grosfeld JL, Rescorla FJ, West KW: Gastrointestinal injuries in childhood: Analysis of 53 patients. J Pediatr Surg 1989; 24:580–583.
17. Abbasi S, Pereira GR, Johnson L, et al: Long-term assessment of growth, nutritional status, and gastrointestinal function in survivors of necrotizing enterocolitis. J Pediatr 1984; 104:550–554.
18. Kliegman RM, Fanaroff AA: Neonatal necrotizing enterocolitis: A nine-year experience. II. Outcome assessment. Am J Dis Child 1981; 135:608–611.
19. Ricketts RR: Surgical therapy for necrotizing enterocolitis. Ann Surg 1984; 200:653–657.
20. Cikrit D, West KW, Schreiner R, et al: Long-term follow-up after surgical management of necrotizing enterocolitis: Sixty-three cases. J Pediatr Surg 1986; 21:533–535.
21. Jackman S, Brereton RJ, Wright VM: Results of surgical treatment of neonatal necrotizing enterocolitis. Br J Surg 1990; 77:146–148.
22. Kliegman RM, Fanaroff AA: Necrotizing enterocolitis. N Engl J Med 1984; 310:1093–1103.
23. Haller JA, Tepas JJ, Pickard LR, et al: Intestinal atresia: Current concepts of pathogenesis, pathophysiology, and operative management. Am Surgeon 1983; 49:385–391.
24. Grosfeld JL, Ballantine TVN, Shoemaker R: Operative management of intestinal atresia and stenosis based on pathologic findings. J Pediatr Surg 1979; 14:368–375.
25. Seashore JH, Collins FS, Markowitz RI, et al: Familial apple peel jejunal atresia: Surgical, genetic, and radiographic aspects. Pediatrics 1987; 80:540–544.
26. Sansaricq C, Chen WJ, Manka M, et al: Familial congenital short small bowel with associated defects. Clin Pediatr 1983; 23:453–455.
27. Ziegler MM, Ross AJ, Bishop HC: Total intestinal aganglionosis: A new technique for prolonged survival. J Pediatr Surg 1987; 22:82–83.
28. Appleton GVN, Bristol JB, Williamson RCH: Proximal enterectomy provides a stronger systemic stimulus to intestinal adaption than distal enterectomy. Gut 1987; 28(S1):165–168.
29. Gelinas MD, Morin CL, Morrisset J: Exocrine pancreatic function following proximal small bowel resection in rats. J Physiol 1982; 322:71–82.
30. Ameen VZ, Powell GK, Jones LA: Quantitation of fecal carbohydrate excretion in patients with short bowel syndrome. Gastroenterology 1987; 92:493–500.
31. Fordtran JS, Rectror FC, Carter NW: The mechanisms of sodium absorption in the human intestine. J Clin Invest 1968; 47:884–900.
32. Arrambide KA, Santa Ana CA, Schiller LR, et al: Loss of absorptive capacity for sodium chloride as a cause of diarrhea following partial ileal and right colon resection. Dig Dis Sci 1989; 34:193–201.
33. Schiff ER, Small NC, Dietschy JM: Characterization of the kinetics of the passive and active transport mechanisms of bile acid absorption in the small intestine and colon of the rat. J Clin Invest 1972; 51:1351–1362.
34. Dietschy MJ, Wilson FA: Characterization of bile acid absorption across the unstirred water layer and brush border of the rat jejunum. J Clin Invest 1972; 51:3015–3025.
35. Schreiber AJ, Simon FR: Overview of clinical aspects of bile salt physiology. J Pediatr Gastroenterol Nutr 1983; 2:337–345.
36. Hofmann AF, Poley JR: Role of bile acid malabsorption in pathogenesis of diarrhea and steatorrhea in patients with ileal resection: I. Response to cholestyramine or replacement of dietary long-chain triglyceride by medium chain triglyceride. Gastroenterology 1972; 62:918–934.
37. Chadwick VS, Gaginella TS, Carlson GL, et al: Effect of molecular structure on bile acid-induced alterations in absorptive function, permeability and morphology in the perfused rabbit colon. J Lab Clin Med 1979; 94:661–674.
38. Saunders DR, Hedges JR, Sillery J, et al: Morphological and functional effects of bile salts on rat colon. Gastroenterology 1975; 68:1236–1245.
39. Mekhjian HS, Phillips SF, Hofmann AF: Colonic secretion of water and electrolytes induced by bile acids: Perfusion studies in man. J Clin Invest 1971; 50:1569–1577.
40. Poley JR, Hofmann AL: Role of fat maldigestion in pathogenesis of steatorrhea in ileal resection. Gastroenterology 1976; 71:38–44.
41. Heubi JE, Balistreri WF, Partin JC, et al: Enterohepatic circulation of bile acids in infants and children with ileal resection. J Lab Clin Med 1980; 95:231–240.
42. Allard JP, Jeejeebhoy KN: Nutritional support and therapy in the short bowel syndrome. Gastroenterol Clin 1989; 18:589–601.
43. Debongnie JC, Phillips SF: Capacity of the human colon to absorb fluid. Gastroenterology 1978; 74:698–703.
44. Royall D, Wolever TM, Jeejeebhoy KN: Colonic salvage of malabsorbed carbohydrate in short bowel syndrome (abstract). Gastroenterology 1990; 98:A429.
45. Binder HJ, Mehta P: Short-chain fatty acids stimulate active sodium and chloride absorption in vitro in the rat distal colon. Gastroenterology 1989; 96:989–996.
46. Mitchel JE, Breuer RI, Zuckerman L, et al: The colon influences ileal resection diarrhea. Dig Dis Sci 1980; 25:33–41.
47. Nightingale JMD, van der Sijp JRM, Kamm MA: Disturbed gastric emptying in short bowel syndrome. Correlation with jejunal length and evidence for a "colonic brake" (abstract). Gastroenterology 1991; 100:A235.
48. Sarna SK: Cyclic motor activity; migrating motor complex: 1985. Gastroenterology 1985; 89:894–913.
49. Gazet JC, Kopp J: The surgical significance of the ileocecal junction. Surgery 1964; 56:565–573.
50. Cummings JH, James WPT, Wiggins HS: Role of the colon in ileal-resection diarrhea. Lancet 1973; 1:344–347.
51. Weser E, Fletcher JT, Urban E. Short bowel syndrome. Gastroenterology 1979; 77:572–579.
52. Ladefoged K, Nicolaidou P, Jarnum S: Calcium, phosphorus, magnesium, zinc and nitrogen balance in patients with severe short bowel syndrome. Am J Clin Nutr 1980; 33:2137–2144.
53. Vanderhoof JA, Park JHY, Grandjean CJ: Effect of zinc deficiency on mucosal hyperplasia following 70% bowel resection. Am J Clin Nutr 1986; 44:670–677.

54. Couper RTL, Durie PR, Stafford SE, et al: Late gastrointestinal bleeding and protein loss after distal small-bowel resection in infancy. J Pediatr Gastroenterol Nutr 1989; 9:454–460.
55. Taylor SF, Sondheimer JM, Sokol RJ, et al: Non-infectious colitis associated with short gut syndrome in infants. J Pediatr 1991; 119:24–28.
56. Welkos SL, Toskes PP, Baer H: Importance of anaerobic bacteria in the cobalamin malabsorption of the experimental rat blind loop syndrome. Gastroenterology 1981; 80:313–320.
57. Schjonsky H: Vitamin B_{12} absorption and malabsorption. Gut 1989; 30:1686–1691.
58. Arvanitakis C: Functional and morphologic abnormalities of the small intestinal mucosa in pernicious anemia. Acta Hepatogastroenterol 1978; 25:313–318.
59. Joshi M, Hyams JS, Treem WR: Cytoplasmic vacuolization of enterocytes: An unusual histopathologic finding in juvenile nutritional megaloblastic anemia. Modern Pathol 1991; 4:62–65.
60. Steinberg SE, Campbell CL, Hellman RS: Kinetics of the normal folate enterohepatic cycle. J Clin Invest 1979; 64:83–88.
61. Landor JH, Baker WK: Gastric hypersecretion produced by massive small bowel resection in dogs. J Surg Res 1964; 4:518–522.
62. Straus E, Gerson GD, Yalow RS: Hypersecretion of gastrin associated with short bowel syndrome. Gastroenterology 1974; 66:175–180.
63. Williams NS, Evans P, King RFGJ: Gastric acid secretion and gastrin production in the short bowel syndrome. Gut 1985; 26:914–919.
64. Cortot A, Fleming CR, Malagelada JR: Improved nutrient absorption after cimetidine in short-bowel syndrome with gastric hypersecretion. N Engl J Med 1979; 300:79–81.
65. Dubois A, van Eerdewegh P, Gardner JD: Gastric emptying and secretion in Zollinger-Ellison syndrome. J Clin Invest 1977; 59:255–263.
66. Becker HD, Reeder DD, Thompson JC: Extraction of circulating endogenous gastrin by the small bowel. Gastroenterology 1973; 65:903–906.
67. Hyman PE, Everett SL, Harada T: Gastric acid hypersecretion in short bowel syndrome in infants: Association with extent of resection and enteral feeding. J Pediatr Gastroenterol Nutr 1986; 5:191–197.
68. Isaacs PT, Kim YS: Blind loop resection and small bowel bacterial contamination. Clinics in Gastroenterology 1983; 12:395–414.
69. Vantrappen G, Janssens J, Hellemans J, et al: The inter-digestive motor complex of normal subjects and patients with bacterial overgrowth of the small intestine. J Clin Invest 1977; 59:1158–1166.
70. Ament ME, Shimoda SS, Saunders DP, et al: Pathogenesis of steatorrhea in three cases of small intestinal stasis syndrome. Gastroenterology 1972; 63:728–747.
71. King CE, Toskes PP: Small intestine bacterial overgrowth. Gastroenterology 1979; 76:1035–1055.
72. Curtis KJ: Protein digestion and absorption in the blind-loop syndrome. Dig Dis Sci 1979; 24:923–929.
73. Perlmutter DH, Boyle JT, Campos JM, et al: D-lactic acidosis in children: An unusual metabolic complication of small bowel resection. J Pediatr 1983; 102:234–238.
74. Carr DB, Shih VE, Richter JM, et al: D-lactic acidosis simulating a hypothalamic syndrome after bowel bypass. Ann Neuro 1982; 11:195–197.
75. Stolberg L, Rolfe R, Gitlin N, et al: D-lactic acidosis due to abnormal gut flora; diagnosis and treatment of two cases. N Engl J Med 1982; 306:1344–1348.
76. Oh MS, Phelps KR, Traube M, et al: D-lactic acidosis in a man with short bowel syndrome. N Engl J Med 1979; 301:249–252.
77. Rosenthal P, Pesce M: Long-term monitoring of D-lactic acidosis in a child. J Pediatr Gastroenterol Nutr 1985; 4:674–676.
78. Hudson M, Pocknee R, Mowat NAG: D-lactic acidosis in short bowel syndrome: An examination of possible mechanisms. Quart J Med 1990; 274:157–163.
79. Thurn JR, Pierpont GL, Ludvigsen CW, et al: D-lactate encephalopathy. Am J Med 1985; 79:717–721.
80. Mayne AJ, Handy DJ, Preece MA, et al: Dietary management of D-lactic acidosis in short bowel syndrome. Arch Dis Child 1990; 65:229–231.
81. Chadwick VS, Modha K, Dowling RH: Mechanism for hyperoxaluria in patients with ileal dysfunction. N Engl J Med 1973; 289:172–176.
82. Dobbins JW, Binder HJ: Importance of the colon in enteric hyperoxaluria. N Engl J Med 1977; 296:298–300.
83. Heaton KW, Read AF: Gallstones in patients with disorders of the terminal ileum and disturbed bile salt metabolism. Br Med J 1969; 3:494–496.
84. Hill GL, Mair WSJ, Golligher JC: Gallstones after ileostomy and ileal resection. Gut 1975; 16:932–936.
85. Cohen S, Kaplan M, Gottleib L, Patterson J: Liver disease and gallstones in regional enteritis. Gastroenterology 1971; 60:237–245.
86. Pellorin D, Tertin P, Nihoul-Fekete C, et al: Cholelithiasis and ileal pathology in childhood. J Pediatr Surg 1975; 10:35–41.
87. Roslyn JJ, Berquist WE, Pitt HA, et al: Increased risk of gallstones in children receiving total parenteral nutrition. Pediatrics 1983; 71:784–789.
88. Bernhoft RA, Pellegrini CA, Broderick WC, et al: Pigment sludge and stone formation in the acutely ligated dog gallbladder. Gastroenterology 1983; 85:1166–1171.
89. Boonyapisit ST, Trotman BW, Ostrow DW: Unconjugated bilirubin and the hydrolysis of conjugated bilirubin in gallbladder bile of patients with cholelithiasis. Gastroeterology 1978; 24:70–74.
90. Allen B, Bernhoft R, Blanckaert N, et al: Sludge is calcium bilirubinate associated with bile stasis. Am J Surg 1981; 141:51–56.
91. O'Brien CB, Berman JM, Fleming CR, et al: Total parenteral nutrition gallstones contain more calcium bilirubinate than sickle cell gallstones (abstract). Gastroenterology 1986; 90:1752.
92. Postuma R, Moroz S, Friesen F: Extreme short-bowel syndrome in an infant. J Pediatr Surg 1983; 18:264–268.
93. Kurz R, Sauer H: Treatment and metabolic findings in extreme short bowel syndrome with 11 cm jejunal remnant. J Pediatr Surg 1983; 18:257–263.
94. Weser E, Hernandez MH: Studies of small bowel adaptation after intestinal resection in the rat. Gastroenterology 1971; 60:69–75.
95. Weser E: Nutritional aspects of malabsorption. Short gut adaptation. Am J Med 1979; 67:1014–1020.
96. Hanson WR, Osborne JW, Sharp JG: Compensation by the residual intestine after intestinal resection in the rat. II. Influence of the amount of tissue removed. II. Influence of post-operative tissue interval. Gastroenterology 1977; 72:692–700, 701–705.
97. Williamson RCN: Intestinal adaptation: Structural, function and cytokinetic changes. N Engl J Med 1978; 298:1393–1402.
98. Nundy S, Malamud D, Obertop H, et al: Onset of cell proliferation in the shortened gut. Colonic hyperplasia after ileal resection. Gastroenterology 1977; 72:263–266.
99. Gleeson MH, Cullen J, Dowling RH: Intestinal structure and function after small bowel by-pass in the rat. Clin Sci 1972; 43:731–742.
100. Keren DF, Elliot HL, Brown GD, et al: Atrophy of villi with hypertrophy and hyperplasia of Paneth cells in isolated (Thiry-Vella) ileal loops in rabbits: Light-microscopic studies. Gastroenterology 1975; 68:83–93.
101. Weser E: Nutritional aspects of malabsorption: Short-gut adaptation. Clinics in Gastroenterology 1983; 12:443–461.
102. Bury KD: Carbohydrate digestion and absorption after massive resection of the small intestine. Surg Gynecol Obstet 1972; 135:177–187.
103. Urban E, Michel AM: Separation of adaptive mucosal growth and transport after small bowel resection. Am J Physiol 1983; 7:G295–300.
104. McCarthy DM, Kim YS: Changes in sucrase, enterokinase, and peptide hydrolase after intestinal resection. The association of cellular hyperplasia and adaptation. J Clin Invest 1973; 52:942–951.
105. Chaves M, Smith MW, Williamson RCH: Increased activity of digestive enzymes in ileal enterocytes adapting to proximal small bowel resection. Gut 1987; 28:981–987.
106. Iverson BM, Schjonsby H, Skagen DW, et al: Intestinal adaptation after jejuno-ileal bypass operation for massive obesity. Eur J Clin Intest 1976; 6:355–360.
107. Dudrick SJ, Daly JM, Castro G, et al: Gastrointestinal adaptation following small bowel bypass for obesity. Ann Surg 1977; 185:642–648.
108. Guedon C, Schmitz J, Lerebours E, et al: Decreased brush

border hydrolase activities without gross morphologic changes in human intestinal mucosa after prolonged total parenteral nutrition of adults. Gastroenterology 1986; 90:373–378.

109. Levine GM, Deren JJ, Steiger E, et al: Role of oral intake in maintenance of gut mass and disaccharidase activity. Gastroenterology 1974; 67:975–982.
110. Deren JJ, Brotman SA, Zamcheck N: Effect of diet upon intestinal disaccharidases and disaccharide absorption. J Clin Invest 1967; 46:186–194.
111. Lee PC, Brooks S, Lebenthal E: Effect of fasting and refeeding on pancreatic enzymes and secretagogue responsiveness in rats. Am J Physiol 1982; 242:G215–221.
112. Mienge H, Robinson JWL: Functional and structural characteristics of the rat intestinal mucosa following ileojejunal transposition. Acta Hepatogastroenterol 1978; 25:150–154.
113. Gronqvist B, Engstrom B, Grimelius L: Morphologic studies of the rat small intestine after jejuno-ileal transposition. Acta Chiurgica Scand 1975; 141:208–217.
114. Feldman EJ, Dowling RH, McNaughton J, et al: Effects of oral versus intravenous nutrition on intestinal adaptation after small bowel resection in the dog. Gastroenterology 1976; 70:712–719.
115. Morin CL, Ling V, VanCaillie M: Role of oral intake on intestinal adaptation after small bowel resection in growing rats. Pediatr Res 1978; 12:268–271.
116. Lentze MJ: Intestinal adaptation in short-bowel syndrome. Eur J Pediatr 1989; 148:294–299.
117. Vanderhoof JA, Grandjean CJ, Kaufman SS, et al: Effect of high percentage medium-chain triglyceride diet on mucosal adaptation following massive bowel resection in rats. J. Parenter Enter Nutr 1984; 8:685–698.
118. Grey VL, Garofolo C, Greenberg GR, et al: The adaptation of the small intestine after resection in response to free fatty acids. Am J Clin Nutr 1984; 40:1235–1242.
119. Vanderhoof JA, Adrian TE, Blackwood DI, et al: Effect of high fat diets on mucosal adaptation following massive bowel resection (abstract). Gastroenterology 1991; 100:A552.
120. Hart MH, Grandjean CJ, Park JHY, et al: Essential fatty acid deficiency and post resection mucosal adaptation in the rat. Gastroenterology 1988; 94:682–687.
121. Weser E, Tawil T, Fletcher JT: Stimulation of small bowel mucosal growth by gastric infusion of different sugars in rats maintained on total parenteral nutrition. *In* Robinson JWL, Dowling RH, Riecken EO, eds: Mechanisms of Intestinal Adaptation. Falk Symposium 30. Lancaster, England, MTP Press, 1982, pp 141–149.
122. Weser E, Babbitt J, Hoban M: Intestinal adaptation: Different growth responses to disaccharides compared with monosaccharides in rat small bowel. Gastroenterology 1986; 91:1521–1527.
123. Clark RM: "Luminal nutrition" versus "functional work load" as controllers of mucosal morphology and epithelial replacement in rat small intestine. Digestion 1977; 15:411–424.
124. Vanderhoof JA, Grandjean CJ, Burkley KT, et al: Effect of casein versus casein hydrolysate on mucosal adaptation following massive bowel resection in infant rats. J Pediatr Gastroenterol Nutr 1984; 3:262–267.
125. Spector MH, Levine GM, Deren JJ: Direct and indirect effects of dextrose and amino acids on gut mass. Gastroenterology 1977; 72:706–710.
126. Leleiko NS, Bronstein AD, Baliga S, Munro HN: De novo purine nucleotide synthesis in the rat small and large intestines. Effect of dietary protein and purines. J Pediatr Gastroenterol Nutr 1983; 2:313–319.
127. Uauy R, Stringel G, Thomas R, Quan R: Effect of dietary nucleotides on growth and maturation of the developing gut in the rat. J Pediatr Gastroenterol Nutr 1990; 10:497–503.
128. Windmueller HG: Glutamine utilization by the small intestine. Adv Enzymol 1982; 53:201–237.
129. Souba WW, Scott TE, Wilmore DW: Intestinal consumption of intravenously administered fuels. J Parenter Enter Nutr 1985; 9:18–22.
130. Souba WW, Wilmore DW: Postoperative alteration of arteriovenous exchange of amino acids across the gastrointestinal tract. Surgery 1983; 94:342–350.
131. Roth E, Funovics J, Muhlbacher F, et al: Metabolic disorders in severe abdominal sepsis; glutamine deficiency in skeletal muscle. Clin Nutr 1982; 1:25–41.
132. Askanazi J, Carpentier YA, Michelson CB, et al: Muscle and plasma amino acids following injury. Influence of intercurrent infection. Ann Surg 1980; 193:78–85.
133. Smith RJ, O'Dwyer S, Wang XD, et al: Glutamine nutrition and the gastrointestinal tract. *In* The Gastrointestinal Response to Injury, Starvation and Enteral Nutrition. Report of the 8th Ross Conference in Medical Research. Columbus, Ohio, 1988, pp 76–78.
134. Jacobis DO, Evans DA, Mealy K, et al: Combined effects of glutamine and epidermal growth factor on the rat intestine. Surgery 1988; 104:358–364.
135. Hwang TL, O'Dwyer ST, Smith RJ, et al: Preservation of small bowel mucosa using glutamine enriched parenteral nutrition. Surg Forum 1986; 37:56–58.
136. Magnusson I, Kihlberg R, Alvestrand A, et al: Utilization of intravenously administered N-acetyl-L-glutamine in humans. Metabolism 1989; 38:82–88.
136a. Tamada H, Nezu R, Imamura I, et al: The dipeptide alanyl-glutamine prevents intestinal mucosal atrophy in parenterally fed rats. JPEN J Parenter Enteral Nutr 1992; 16:110–116.
137. Roediger WEW: Role of anaerobic bacteria in the metabolic welfare of the colonic mucosa in man. Gut 1980; 21:793–798.
138. Ruppin H, Bar-Meir S, Soergel KH, et al: Absorption of short-chain fatty acids by the colon. Gastroenterology 1980; 78:1500–1507.
139. Roediger WEW: Utilization of nutrients by isolated epithelial cells of the rat colon. Gastroenterology 1982; 83:424–429.
140. Cummings JH, Branch WJ: The importance of short-chain fatty acids in man. Scand J Gastroenterol 1984; 20:88–99.
141. O'Dwyer ST, Smith RJ, Kripke SA, et al: New fuels for the gut. In Rombeau JL, Caldwell MD, eds: Clinical Nutrition: Enteral and Tube Feeding. 2d ed. Philadelphia, WB Saunders, 1990, pp 540–555.
142. Ecknauer R, Sircar B, Johnson LR: Effect of dietary bulk on small bowel intestinal morphology and cell renewal in the rat. Gastroenterology 1981; 81:781–786.
143. Jacobs LR, Lupton JR: Effect of dietary fibers on rat large bowel mucosal growth and cell proliferation. Am J Physiol 1984; 246:G378–G385.
144. Kripke SA, Fox AD, Berman JM, et al: Stimulation of intestinal mucosal growth with intracolonic infusion of short-chain fatty acids. J Parenter Enter Nutr 1989; 13:109–116.
145. Kelberman I, Cheetham B, Levine G, et al: Dietary fiber promotes colonic adaptation (abstract). Gastroenterology 1991; 100:A527.
146. Kelberman I, Cheetham B, Rosenthal J, et al: Short-chain fatty acids overcome antibiotic inhibition of colonic adaptation (abstract). Gastroenterology 1991; 100:A527.
147. Tutton PJM, Barkla DH: Further studies on the effect of adenosine cyclic monophosphate derivatives on cell proliferation in jejunal crypts of rat. Clin Exp Pharmacol Physiol 1982; 9:671–674.
148. Skakata T, Yajima T: Influence of short chain fatty acids on the epithelial cell division of the gastrointestinal tract. Q J Exp Physiol 1984; 69:639–648.
149. Goodlad RA, Lenton W, Ghatel MA: Proliferative effects of fibre on the intestinal epithelium: Relationship to gastrin, enteroglucagon and PYY. Gut 1987; 28(S1):221–226.
150. Bloom SR: Gut and brain-endocrine connections. The Gaulstonian lecture, 1979. J R Coll Physicians Lond 1980; 14:51–57.
151. Dankert J, Zijlstra JB, Wolthers BG: Volatile fatty acids in human peripheral and portal blood. Quantitative determination by vacuum distillation and gas chromatography. Clin Chim Acta 1981; 110:301–307.
152. Cross TA, Pall C, Oberhansli R, et al: Ketogenesis in the living rat followed by 13C NMR spectroscopy. Biochemistry 1984; 23:6398–6402.
153. Koruda MU, Rolandelli RH, Settle RG: The effect of a pectin supplemented elemental diet on intestinal adaptation to massive small bowel resection. J Parenter Enter Nutr 1986; 10:343–350.
154. Koruda MJ, Rolandelli RH, Settle RG, et al: Effect of parenteral nutrition supplemented with short chain fatty acids on intestinal adaptation to massive small bowel resection. J Parenter Enter Nutr 1986; 10:343–350.
155. Dworkin LD, Levine GM, Farber NJ, et al: Small intestinal mass of the rat is partially determined by indirect effects of intraluminal nutrition. Gastroenterology 1976; 71:626–630.

156. Williamson RCH, Malt RA: Humoral modulation of compensatory intestinal hyperplasia. *In* Robinson JWL, Dowling RH, Riecken EO, eds: Mechanisms of Intestinal Adaptation. Lancaster, England, MTP Press, 1982, pp 215–224.
157. Gleeson MH, Bloom SR, Polak JM, et al: An endocrine tumor in kidney affecting small bowel structure, motility and absorptive function. Gut 1971; 12:733–742.
158. Jacobs LR, Polak JM, Bloom SR, et al: Intestinal mucosal and fasting plasma levels of immunoreactive enteroglucagon in three animal models of intestinal adaptation: Resection, hypothermic hyperphagia, and lactation in the rat. *In* Robinson JWL, Dowling RH, Riecken EO, eds: Mechanisms of Intestinal Adaptation. Lancaster, England, MTP Press, 1982, pp 231–240.
159. Bloom SR: Gut hormones in adaptation. Gut 1987; 28(S1):31–35.
160. Taylor RG, Verity K, Fuller PJ: Ileal glucagon gene expression: Ontogeny and response to massive small bowel resection. Gastroenterology 1990; 99:724–729.
161. Al-Mukhtar MY, Sagor GR, Ghatel MA, et al: The role of pancreatic-biliary secretions in intestinal adaptation after resection and its relationship to plasma enteroglucagon. Br J Surg 1983; 70:398–400.
162. Appleton GVN, Bristol JB, Williamson RCH: Proximal enterectomy provides a stronger systemic stimulus to intestinal adaptation than distal enterectomy. Gut 1987; 28(S1):165–168.
163. Sagor GR, Ghatei MA, O'Shaughnessy DJ, et al: Influence of somatostatin and bombesin on plasma enteroglucagon and cell proliferation after intestinal resection in the rat. Gut 1985; 26:89–94.
164. Weser E, Drummond A, Tawil T: Effect of diverting bile and pancreatic secretions into the ileum on small bowel mucosa in rats fed a liquid formula diet. J Parenter Enter Nutr 1982; 6:39–42.
165. Aiman GC: Influence of bile and pancreatic secretions on the size of the intestinal villi in the rat. Am J Anat 1971; 132:167–178.
166. Hughes CA, Bates T, Dowling RH: Cholecystokinin and secretin prevent the intestinal mucosal hypoplasia of total parenteral nutrition in the dog. Gastroenterology 1987; 75:34–41.
167. Weser E, Bell D, Tawil T: Effects of octapeptide cholecystokinin, secretin and glucagon on intestinal mucosal growth in parenterally nourished rats. Dig Dis Sci 1981; 26:409–416.
168. Ulshen MH, Herbst CA: Effect of removal of pancreaticobiliary secretions on adaptation to short bowel in orally nourished rats. Am J Clin Nutr 1984; 39:762–770.
169. Vanderhoof JA, Park JHY, Mohammadpour H, et al: Effect of cholecystokinin on mucosal hyperplasia following massive intestinal resection (abstract). Gastroenterology 1991; 100:A552.
170. Fine H, Levine GM, Shiau YF: Effects of cholecystokinin and secretin on intestinal structure and function. Am J Physiol 1983; 245:G358–G363.
171. Koetz HR, Lentz MJ, Muller OM, et al: Effect of 16,16-dimethyl prostaglandin E_2 on small intestinal mucosa in suckling rats. Eur J Clin Invest 1987; 17:293–300.
172. Vanderhoof JA, Grandjean CJ, Baylor JM, et al: Morphological and functional effects of 16,16 dimethyl prostaglandin-E_2 on mucosal adaptation after massive distal small bowel resection in the rat. Gut 1988; 29:802–808.
173. Hollworth ME, Granger DN, Ulrich-Baker MG, et al: Pharmacologic enhancement of adaptive growth after extensive small bowel resection. Pediatr Surg Int 1988; 3:55–61.
174. Marti U, Burwen SJ, Jones AL: Biological effects of epidermal growth factor with emphasis on the gastrointestinal tract and liver: An update. Hepatology 1989; 9:126–138.
175. Fehlman EJ, Anres D, Grossman MI: Epidermal growth factor stimulates ornithine decarboxylase activity in the digestive tract of mouse. Proc Soc Exp Biol Med 1978; 159:400–402.
176. Malo C, Menard D: Influence of epidermal growth factor on the development of suckling mouse intestinal mucosa. Gastroenterology 1982; 83:28–35.
177. Goodlad RA, Wilson TJG, Lenton W, et al: Proliferative effects of urogastrone-EGF on the intestinal epithelium. Gut 1987; 28(S1):37–43.
178. Ulshen MH, Lynn-Cook LE, Raasch RH: Effects of intraluminal epidermal growth factor on mucosal proliferation in the small intestine of adult rats. Gastroenterology 1986; 91:1134–1140.
179. Taylor B, Murphy GM, Dowling RH: Effect of food intake and the pituitary on intestinal structure and function after resection (abstract). Gut 1975; 16:397–398.
180. Lehy T, Accary JP, Dubrasquet M, et al: Growth hormone releasing factor (somatocrinin) stimulates epithelial cell proliferation in the rat digestive tract. Gastroenterology 1986; 90:646–653.
181. Hart MH, Phares CK, Erdman SH, et al: Augmentation of post resection mucosal hyperplasia by plerocercoid growth factor (PGF). Dig Dis Sci 1987; 32:1275–1280.
182. Grey VL, Morin CL: Evidence for a growth-stimulating fraction in the rat proximal intestine after small bowel resection. Gastroenterology 1985; 89:1305–1312.
183. Grey VL, Morin CL: Role of food in appearance of growth-stimulating activity in rat proximal intestine after small bowel resection. Dig Dis Sci 1988; 33:78–82.
184. Vanderhoof JA, Clark R, McCuskar RH: Effects of IGF-1 and DES-(1-3)-IGF1 on mucosal adaptation after jejunoileal resection in rats (abstract). Gastroenterology 1991; 100:A552.
185. Selub SE, Lund PK, Jin C, et al: Effect of intraluminal EGF infusion on jejunal and ileal expression of IGF-mRNA in adult rats (abstract). Gastroenterology 1991; 100:A546.
186. Selub SE, Roundtree DB, Ulshen MH, et al: Transforming growth factor mRNA abundance in massive small bowel resection (abstract). Gastroenterology 1991; 100:A547.
187. Luk GD, Yang P. Polyamines in intestinal and pancreatic adaptation. Gut 1987; 28(S1):95–101.
188. Luk GD, Baylin SB: Polyamines and intestinal growth-increased polyamine biosynthesis after jejunectomy. Am J Physiol 1983; 245:G656–G660.
189. Luk GD, Marton LJ, Baylin SB: Ornithine decarboxylase is important in intestinal mucosal maturation and recovery from injury in rats. Science 1980; 21:195–198.
190. Luk GD, Baylin SB: Polyamines and intestinal growth: Absolute requirement for ODC activity in adaptation during lactation. Am J Physiol 1984; 247:G553–G557.
191. D'Agostino L, Danielle B, Pignata S, et al: Modifications in ornithine decarboxylase and diamine oxidase in small bowel mucosa of starved and refed rats. Gut 1987; 28(S1):135–138.
192. Malo C, Menard D: Synergistic effect of insulin and thyroxin on the differentiation and proliferation of epithelial cells of suckling mouse small intestine. Biol Neonate 1983; 44:177–184.
193. Luk GD, Baylin SB: Inhibition of intestinal epithelial DNA synthesis and adaptive hyperplasia after jejunectomy in the rat by suppression of polyamine biosynthesis. J Clin Invest 1984; 74:698–704.
194. Hosomi M, Lirussi F, Stace HN, et al: Mucosal polyamine profile in normal and adapting (hypo and hyperplastic) intestine: Effects of DFMO treatment. Gut 1987; 28(S1):103–107.
195. Dufour C, Dandrifosse G, Forget P, et al: Spermine and spermidine induce intestinal maturation in the rat. Gastroenterology 1988; 95:112–116.
196. Thompson JS, Laughlin BS: Relationship of jejunostomy and urine polyamine content to refeeding and intestinal structure and function. J Parenter Enter Nutr 1989; 13:13–17.
197. Ho TF, Yip WCL, Tay JSH, et al: Rice water and milk: Effect on ileal fluid osmolality and volume. Lancet 1982; 1:169.
198. Schwartz KB, Ternberg JL, Bell MJ, et al: Sodium needs of infants and children with ileostomy. J Pediatr 1983; 102:509–513.
199. Will PC, Cortright RN, Grosedose RG, et al: Amiloride-sensitive salt and fluid absorption in small intestine of sodium-depleted rats. Am J Physiol 1985; 248:G133–G141.
200. Rodgers JB, Bernard HR, Balint JA: Colonic infusion in the management of the short bowel syndrome. Gastroenterology 1976; 70:186–189.
201. Puppala BL, Mangurtan HH, Kraut JR, et al: Distal ileostomy drip feedings in neonates with short bowel syndrome. J Pediatr Gastroenterol Nutr 1985; 4:489–494.
202. Levy E, Frileux P, Sandrucci S, et al: Continuous enteral nutrition during the early adaptive stage of the short bowel syndrome. Br J Surg 1988; 75:549–553.
203. Purdum PP, Kirky DF: Short-bowel syndrome: A review of the role of nutrition support. J Parenter Enter Nutr 1991; 15:93–101.
204. Van Rij AM, Thomson CD, McKenzie JM: Selenium deficiency in total parenteral nutrition. Am J Clin Nutr 1970; 32:2076–2085.
205. Reeves WC, Marcuard SP, Willis SE, et al: Reversible cardiomyopathy due to selenium deficiency. J Parenter Enter Nutr 1989; 13:663–665.

206. Dahlstrom KA, Ament ME, Medhin MG, et al: Serum trace elements in children receiving long-term parenteral nutrition. J Pediatr 1986; 109:625–630.
207. Mock DM, Baswell DL, Baker H, et al: Biotin deficiency complicating parenteral alimentation: Diagnosis, metabolic repercussions, and treatment. J Pediatr 1985; 106:762–769.
208. Hamosh M, Scanlon JW, Ganot D, et al: Fat digestion in the newborn: Characterization of lipase in gastric aspirates of premature and term infants. J Clin Invest 1981; 67:838–846.
209. Parker P, Stroop S, Greene H: A controlled comparison of continuous versus intermittent feeding in the treatment of infants with intestinal disease. J Pediatr 1981; 99:360–364.
210. Schwartz SM, Gewitz MH, Sec CC, et al: Enteral nutrition in infants with congenital heart disease and growth failure. Pediatrics 1990; 86:368–373.
211. Griffin GE, Fagan EF, Hodgson HJ, et al: Enteral therapy in the management of massive gut resection complicated by chronic fluid and electrolyte depletion. Dig Dis Sci 1982; 27:902–908.
212. MacMahon RA: The use of the World Health Organization oral rehydration solution in patients on home parenteral nutrition. J Parenter Enter Nutr 1984; 8:720–723.
213. Beaugerie L, Cosnes J, Verwaerde F, et al: Isotonic high sodium oral rehydration solution (ORS) for increasing sodium reabsorption in short bowel syndrome (abstract). Gastroenterology 1990; 98:A158.
214. Young EA, Cioletti LA, Winborn WB, et al: Comparative study of nutritional adaptation to defined formula diet in rats. Am J Clin Nutr 1980; 33:2106–2110.
215. Voitk AJ, Echave V, Brown RA, et al: Use of elemental diet during the adaptive stage of short gut syndrome. Gastroenterology 1973; 65:419–426.
216. Simko V, Linscheer WG: Absorption of different elemental diets in short bowel syndrome lasting 15 years. Dig Dis Sci 1976; 21:419–425.
217. Christie DS, Ament ME: Dilute elemental diet and continuous infusion technique for management of short bowel syndrome. J Pediatr 1975; 87:705–708.
218. McIntyre PB: The short bowel. Br J Surg 1985; 72:592–593.
219. Janne P, Carpentier Y, Williems G, et al: Colonic mucosal atrophy induced by a liquid elemental diet in rats. Am J Dig Dis 1977; 22:808–812.
220. Vanderhoof JA, Grandjean CJ, Burkley KT, et al: Effect of casein versus casein hydrolysate on mucosal adaptation following massive bowel resection in growing rats. J Pediatr Gastroenterol Nutr 1984; 3:262–267.
221. Cosnes J, Evard D, Beaugerie JG, et al: Prospective randomized trial comparing small peptides vs whole proteins in patients with a high jejunostomy (abstract). Gastroenterology 1990; 98:A165.
222. Messing B, Pigot F, Rongier M, et al: Intestinal absorption of free oral hyperalimentation in the very short bowel syndrome. Gastroenterology 1991; 100:1502–1508.
223. Woolf GM, Miller C, Kurian R, et al: Nutritional absorption in short bowel syndrome. Evaluation of fluid, calorie, and divalent cation requirements. Dig Dis Sci 1987; 32:8–15.
224. Bond JH, Currier BE, Buchwald H, et al: Colonic conservation of malabsorbed carbohydrate. Gastroenterology 1980; 78:444–447.
225. Zimmaro DM, Rolandelli RH, Koruda MJ, et al: Isotonic tube feeding formula induces liquid stool in normal subjects: Reversal by pectin. J Parenter Enter Nutr 1989; 13:117–123.
226. Bochenek W, Rodgers JB, Balint JA: Effects of changes in dietary lipids on intestinal fluid loss in the short-bowel syndrome. Ann Intern Med 1970; 72:205–213.
227. Andersson H, Isaksson B, Sjogren B: Fat-reduced diet in the symptomatic treatment of small bowel disease. Gut 1974; 15:351–359.
228. Simko V, McCarroll AM, Goodman S, et al: High-fat diet in the short-bowel syndrome: Intestinal absorption and gastroenteropancreatic hormone responses. Dig Dis Sci 1980; 25:333–339.
229. Oveson L, Chu R, Howard L: The influence of dietary fat on jejunostomy output in patients with severe short bowel syndrome. Am J Clin Nutr 1983; 38:270–277.
230. Woolf GM, Miller C, Kurian R, et al: Diet for patients with a short bowel: High fat or high carbohydrate. Gastroenterology 1983; 84:823–828.
231. Galeano NF, Leroy C, Belli D, et al: Comparison of two special infant formulas designed for the treatment of protracted diarrhea. J Pediatr Gastroenterol Nutr 1988; 7:76–83.
232. DeCecco S, Nelson J, Burnes J, et al: Nutritional intake of gut failure patients on home parenteral nutrition. J Parenter Enter Nutr 1987; 11:529–532.
233. Cosnes J, Lamy PH, Beaugerie L, et al: Adaptive hyperphagia in patients with post surgical malabsorption. Gastroenterology 1990; 99:1814–1819.
234. Rodrigues CA, Lennard-Jones JE, Thompson DG, et al: Energy absorption as a measure of intestinal failure in the short bowel syndrome. Gut 1989; 30:176–183.
235. Ohkohchi N, Igarashi Y, Tazawa Y, et al: Evaluation of the nutritional condition and absorptive capacity of nine infants with short bowel syndrome. J Pediatr Gastroenterol Nutr 1986; 5:198–206.
236. Sokol RJ, Heubi JE, Butler-Simon N, et al: Treatment of vitamin E deficiency during chronic childhood cholestasis with oral d-d tocopheryl polyethylene glycol-1000 succinate. Gastroenterology 1987; 93:975–985.
237. Menardi G, Guggenbichler JP: Bioavailability of oral antibiotics in children with short-bowel syndrome. J Pediatr Surg 1984; 19:84–86.
238. Murphy JP, King DR, Dubois A: Treatment of gastric hypersecretion with cimetidine in the short-bowel syndrome. N Engl J Med 1979; 300:80–81.
239. Hyman PE, Garvey TQ, Harada T: Effect of ranitidine on gastric acid hypersecretion in an infant with short bowel syndrome. J Pediatr Gastroenterol Nutr 1985; 4:316–319.
240. Nightingale JMD, Walker ER, Burnham WR, et al: Omeprazole reduces secretory diarrhea in some patients with the short bowel syndrome (SBS) (abstract). Gut 1989; 30:A179.
241. Chang EB, Brown DR, Wang NS, et al: Secretagogue-induced changes in membrane calcium permeability in chicken and chinchilla ileal mucosa: Selective inhibition by loperamide. J Clin Invest 1986; 78:281–287.
242. O'Brien JD, Thompson DG, McIntyre A, et al: Effect of codeine and loperamide on upper intestinal transit and absorption in normal subjects and patients with post vagotomy diarrhea. Gut 1988; 29:312–318.
243. Schiller LR, Santa Ana CA, Morawski SG, et al: Mechanism of the anti-diarrheal effect of loperamide. Gastroenterology 1984; 86:1475–1480.
244. Tytgat GN, Hiubregtse K, Dagevor J, et al: Effect of loperamide on fecal output and composition in well-established ileostomy and ileo-rectal anastomosis. Am J Dig Dis 1977; 22:669–676.
245. Remington M, Malagelada JR, Zinsmeister A, et al: Abnormalities in gastrointestinal motor activity in patients with short bowels: Effect of a synthetic opiate. Gastroenterology 1983; 85:629–636.
246. Sandhu BK, Tripp JH, Candy DCA, et al: Loperamide studies on its mechanism of action. Gut 1981; 22:658–662.
247. Hofmann AF, Poley JR: Cholestyramine treatment of diarrhea associated with ileal resection. N Engl J Med 1969; 281:397–402.
248. West RJ, Lloyd JK: The effect of cholestyramine on intestinal absorption. Gut 1975; 16:93–98.
249. Sali A, Murray WR, Mackay C: Aluminum hydroxide in bile-salt diarrhea. Lancet 1977; 2:1051–1053.
250. Spencer H, Kramer L: Antacid-induced calcium loss. Arch Intern Med 1983; 143:657–659.
251. Matron PN, O'Dorisio TM, Howe BA: Effect of a long-acting somatostatin analogue (SMS 201–995) in a patient with pancreatic cholera. N Engl J Med 1985; 312:17–21.
252. Kvols LK, Moertel CG, O'Connell MJ, et al: Treatment of the malignant carcinoid syndrome: Evaluations of a long-acting somatostatin analogue. N Engl J Med 1986; 315:663–666.
253. Vinik AI, Tasi ST, Moattari AR: Somatostatin analogue (SMS 201–995) in the management of gastroenteropancreatic tumors and diarrhea syndromes. Am J Med 1986; 81(Suppl 6B):23–40.
254. Jaros W, Biller J, Green S, et al: Successful treatment of idiopathic secretory diarrhea of infancy with the somatostatin analogue SMS 201–995. Gastroenterology 1988; 94:189–193.
255. Couper RTL, Berzen A, Berall G, et al: Clinical response to the long acting somatostatin analogue SMS 201–995 in a child with congenital microvillus atrophy. Gut 1989; 30:1020–1024.
256. Krejs GJ: Physiological role of somatostatin in the digestive tract: Gastric acid secretion, intestinal absorption, and motility. Scand J Gastroenterol 1986; 21 (Suppl 119):47–53.
257. Reichlin S: Somatostatin. N Engl J Med 1983; 309:1495–1501, 1556–1563.

258. Williams NS, Cooper JC, Axon AT, et al: Use of a long acting somatostatin analogue in controlling life threatening ileostomy diarrhea. Br Med J 1984; 289:1027–1028.
259. Ohlbaum PH, Galperine RI, Demarquez JL, et al: Use of a long-acting somatostatin analogue (SMS 201–995) in controlling a significant ileal output in a five year old child. J Pediatr Gastroenterol Nutr 1987; 6:466–470.
260. Nightingale JMD, Lennard-Jones JE, Walker ER, et al: Jejunal efflux in short bowel syndrome. Lancet 1990; 336:765–768.
261. O'Keefe SJD, Burnes JU, Peterson ME: Octreotide in the long-term management of home parenteral nutrition patients with massive stomal losses of fluid and electrolytes (abstract). Gastroenterology 1991; 100:A540.
262. Shaffer JL, O'Hanrahan T, Rowntree S, et al: Does somatostatin analogue (SMS 201–995) reduce high output stoma effluent? A controlled trial (abstract). Gut 1988; 29:A1432.
263. Dueno MI, Bai JC, Santangelo WE, et al: Effect of somatostatin analogue on water and electrolyte transport and transit time in human small bowel. Dig Dis Sci 1987; 32:1092–1096.
264. O'Keefe SJD, Bennett WM, Burton DD, et al: Measurement of pancreatic and gastric secretion, pancreatic and mucosal protein synthesis in normal subjects and patients with short bowel syndrome by ^{14}C leucine and stimulatory hormone infusion (abstract). Gastroenterology 1990; 98:A229.
265. Ladefoged K, Christensen KC, Hegnhoj J, et al: Effect of a long acting somatostatin analogue SMS 201–995 on jejunostomy effluents in patients with severe short bowel syndrome. Gut 1989; 30:943–949.
266. deMontigny S, Maki S, Lemann M, et al: Effect of a long acting analog of somatostatin (SMS 201–995) on water and electrolyte losses, nutrient absorption and gastrointestinal transit in short bowel syndrome (abstract). Gastroenterology 1991; 100:A519.
267. Davies RR, Miller M, Turner SJ, et al: Effects of somatostatin analogue SMS 201–995 in normal man. Clin Endocrinol 1986; 24:665–674.
268. Corazza GR, Menozzi MG, Strocchi A, et al: The diagnosis of small bowel bacterial overgrowth: Reliability of jejunal culture and inadequacy of breath hydrogen testing. Gastroenterology 1990; 98:302–309.
269. Perman JA, Modler S, Barr RG, et al: Fasting breath hydrogen concentration: Normal values and clinical application. Gastroenterology 1984; 87:1358–1363.
270. Kerlin P, Wong L: Breath hydrogen testing in bacterial overgrowth of the small intestine. Gastroenterology 1988; 95:982–988.
271. Craig RM, Atkinson AJ: D-xylose testing: A review. Gastroenterology 1988; 95:223–231.
272. Puntis JWL, Booth IW, Buick R: Cisapride in neonatal short gut. Lancet 1986; 2:108–109.
273. Dahlstrom KA, Strandvik B, Kopple J, et al: Nutritional status in children receiving home parenteral nutrition. J Pediatr 1985; 107:219–224.
274. Lin CH, Rossi TM, Heitlinger LA, et al: Nutritional assessment of children with short-bowel syndrome receiving home parenteral nutrition. Am J Dis Child 1987; 141:1093–1098.
275. Vargas JH, Ament ME, Berquist WE, et al: Long-term home parenteral nutrition in pediatrics: Ten years experience in 102 patients. J Pediatr Gastroenterol Nutr 1987; 6:24–32.
276. Decker MD, Edwards KM: Central venous catheter infections. Pediatr Clin North Am 1988; 35:579–612.
277. Wang EEL, Prober CG, Ford-Jones L: The management of central intravenous catheter infections. Pediatr Infect Dis 1984; 3:110–113.
278. Prince A, Heller B, Levy J, et al: Management of fever in patients with central venous catheters. Pediatr Infect Dis 1986; 5:20–24.
279. Nahata MC, King DR, Powell DA, et al: Management of catheter-related infections in pediatric patients. J Parenter Enter Nutr 1988; 12:58–59.
280. Merritt RJ: Cholestasis associated with total parenteral nutrition. J Pediatr Gastroenterol Nutr 1986; 5:9–22.
281. Pereira GR, Sherman MS, DiGiacomo J, et al: Hyperalimentation-induced cholestasis. Increased incidence and severity in premature infants. Am J Dis Child 1981; 135:842–845.
282. Dahms BB, Halpin TC: Serial liver biopsies in parenteral nutrition-associated cholestasis of early infancy. Gastroenterology 1981; 81:136–144.
283. Postuma R, Trevenen CL: Liver disease in infants receiving total parenteral nutrition. Pediatrics 1979; 63:110–115.
284. Craig RM, Neumann T, Jeejeebhoy KN, et al: Severe hepatocellular reaction resembling alcoholic hepatitis with cirrhosis after massive small bowel resection and prolonged total parenteral nutrition. Gastroenterology 1980; 79:131–137.
285. Stanko RT, Nathan G, Mendelow H, et al: Development of hepatic cholestasis and fibrosis in patients with massive loss of intestine supported by prolonged parenteral nutrition. Gastroenterology 1987; 92:197–202.
286. Hocking MP, Duerson MC, O'Leary JP, et al: Jejunoileal bypass for morbid obesity. N Engl J Med 1983; 308:995–999.
287. Capron JP, Gineston JL, Herve MA, et al: Metronidazole in prevention of cholestasis associated with total parenteral nutrition. Lancet 1983; 1:446–447.
288. Lambert JR, Thomas SM: Metronidazole prevention of serum liver enzyme abnormalities during total parenteral nutrition. J Parenter Enter Nutr 1985; 9:501–503.
289. Drenick EJ, Fisler J, Johnson D: Hepatic steatosis after intestinal bypass. Prevention and reversal by metronidazole, irrespective of protein-caloric malnutrition. Gastroenterology 1982; 82:535–548.
289a. Colomb V, Goulet O, Rambaud C, et al: Long-term parenteral nutrition in children: Liver and gallbladder disease. Transplant Proc 1992; 24:1054–1055.
290. Palmer RH: Bile acids, liver injury and liver disease. Arch Intern Med 1972; 130:606–617.
291. Nolan JP: Endotoxin, reticuloendothelial function, and liver injury. Hepatology 1981; 5:458–465.
292. Lichtman SN, Sartor RB, Keku J, et al: Hepatic inflammation in rats with experimental small intestinal overgrowth. Gastroenterology 1990; 98:414–423.
293. Kakis G, Yousef IM: Pathogenesis of lithocholate and taurolithocholate-induced intrahepatic cholestasis in rats. Gastroenterology 1978; 75:595–607.
294. Folin-Fortunet H, LeQuernec L, Erlinger S, et al: Hepatic alternations during total parenteral nutrition in patients with inflammatory bowel disease: A possible consequence of lithocholate toxicity. Gastroenterology 1982; 82:932–937.
295. Lichtman SN, Keku J, Schwab JH, et al: Hepatic injury associated with small bowel bacterial overgrowth in rats is prevented by metronidazole and tetracycline. Gastroenterology 1991; 100:513–519.
296. Matsui J, Cameron RG, Kuo GC, Jeejeebhoy KN: Liver enlargement and proliferation of bile ductular cells during cachectin/TNF-alpha infusion with total parenteral nutrition. Gastroenterology 1991; 100:A536.
297. Lichtman SN, Okoruwa E, Currin RT, Lemasters JJ: Kupffer cells (KC) have a role in hepatic injury associated with small bowel bacterial overgrowth (abstract). North American Society Pediatric Gastroenterology and Nutrition meeting, 1991.
298. Thompson JS, Rikkers LF: Surgical alternatives for the short bowel syndrome. Am J Gastroenterol 1987; 82:97–106.
299. Devine RM, Kelly KA: Surgical therapy of the short bowel syndrome. Gastroenterol Clin North Am 1989; 18:603–618.
300. Barros D'Sa AB: An experimental evaluation of segmental reversal after massive small bowel resection. Br J Surg 1979; 66:493–500.
301. Tanner WA: The effect of reversed jejunal segments on the myoelectrical activity of the small bowel. Br J Surg 1978; 65:567–571.
302. Hutzer NE, Salzberg AM: Pre-ileal transposition of colon to prevent the development of short bowel syndrome in puppies with 90% small intestinal resection. Surgery 1971; 70:189–197.
303. Sidhu GS, Narasimharao KL, Rani VU, et al: Absorptive studies after massive small bowel resection and antiperistaltic colon interposition in Rhesus monkey. Dig Dis Sci 1985; 30:483–488.
304. Warden MJ, Wesley JR: Small bowel reversal procedure for treatment of the "short gut" body. J Pediatr Surg 1978; 13:321–323.
305. Glick PL, deLorimier AA, Adzick NS, et al: Colon interposition: An adjuvant operation for short-gut syndrome. J Pediatr Surg 1984; 19:719–725.
306. Bianchi A: Intestinal loop lengthening: A technique for increasing small intestinal length. J Pediatr Surg 1980; 15:145–151.
307. Bianchi A: Intestinal lengthening: An experimental and clinical review. J R Soc Med 1984; 77:35–41.

308. Thompson JS, Vanderhoof JA, Antonson DL: Intestinal tapering and lengthening for short bowel syndrome. J Pediatr Gastroenterol Nutr 1985; 4:495–497.
309. Weber TR, Vane DW, Grosfeld JL: Tapering enteroplasty in infants with bowel atresia and short gut. Arch Surg 1982; 117:684–688.
310. Thompson JS: Strategies for preserving intestinal length in the short-bowel syndrome. Dis Col Rec 1986; 30:208–213.
311. Vinograd I, Merguerian P, Udassin R, et al: An experimental model of a submucosally tunneled valve for the replacement of the ileocecal valve. J Pediatr Surg 1984; 19:726–731.
312. Lopez-Perez GA, Martinez AJ, Machuca J, et al: Experimental antireflux intestinal valve. Am J Surg 1981; 141:597–600.
313. Waddell WR, Kern F, Halgrimson CG, et al: A simple jejunocolic valve for relief of rapid transit and the short bowel syndrome. Arch Surg 1970; 100:438–444.
314. Ricotta J, Zuidema GD, Gadacz TR, et al: Construction of an ileocecal valve and its role in massive resection of the small intestine. Surg Gynecol Obstet 1981; 151:310–314.
315. Thompson JS: Growth of neomucosa after intestinal resection. Arch Surg 1987; 122:316–319.
316. Thompson JS, Harty RJ, Saigh JA, et al: Morphologic and nutritional responses to intestinal patching following intestinal resection. Surgery 1988; 103:79–86.
317. Lillemoe KD, Berry WR, Harmon JW, et al: Use of vascularized abdominal wall pedicle flaps to grow small bowel neomucosa. Surgery 1982; 91:293–300.
318. Gladen HE, Kelly KA: Enhancing absorption in the canine short bowel syndrome by intestinal pacing. Surgery 1980; 87:281–286.
319. Gladen HE, Kelly KA: Electrical pacing for the short-bowel syndrome. Surg Gynecol Obstet 1981; 153:697–700.
320. Lillihei R, Goot B, Miller F: The physiological response of the small bowel of the dog to ischemia including prolonged in vitro preservation of the bowel with successful replacement and survival. Ann Surg 1959; 150:543–560.
321. Grant D: Intestinal transplantation: Current status. Transplant Proc 1989; 21:2869–2871.
322. Monchik GJ, Russell PS: Transplantation of small bowel in the rat: Technical and immunological considerations. Surgery 1971; 70:693–702.
323. Kirkman RL: Small bowel transplantation. Transplantation 1984; 37:429–433.
324. Lee KK, Schraut WH: Structure and function of orthotopic small bowel allografts in rats treated with cyclosporine. Am J Surg 1986; 151:55–59.
325. Diliz-Perez HS, McClure J, Bedetti C, et al: Successful small bowel allotransplantation in dogs with cyclosporine and prednisone. Transplantation 1984; 37:126–129.
326. Kimura K, LaRosa CA, Blank MA, et al: Successful segmental transplantation in enterectomized pigs. Ann Surg 1990; 211:158–163.
327. Hale DA, Waldorf KA, Kleinschmidt J, et al: Small intestinal transplantation in non-human primates. J Pediatr Surg 1991; 26:914–920.
328. Starzl TE, Todo S, Tzakis A: The many faces of multivisceral transplantation. Surg Gynecol Obstet 1991; 172:335–344.
328a. Todo S, Tzakis A, Reyes J, et al: Clinical small bowel or small bowel plus liver transplantation under FK 506. Transplant Proc 1991; 23:3093–3095.
329. Goulet O, Revillon Y, Brousse JN, et al: Small-bowel transplantation in children. Transplant Proc 1990; 22:2499–2500.
330. Schraut WH: Current status of small-bowel transplantation. Gastroenterology 1988; 94:525–538.
331. Watson AJM, Lear PA: Current status of intestinal transplantation. Gut 1989; 30:1771–1782.
332. Wood RFM: International symposium on small-bowel transplantation. Transplant Proc 1990; 22:2423–2426.
333. Hansmann ML, Deltz E, Gundlach M, et al: Small bowel transplantation in a child: Morphologic, immunohistochemical, and clinical results. Am J Clin Pathol 1989; 92:686–692.
334. Grant D, Wall W, Zhong R, et al: Experimental clinical intestinal transplantation: Initial experience of a Canadian centre. Transplant Proc 1990; 22:2497–2498.
335. Deltz E, Schroeder P, Gebhardt H, et al: Successful clinical small bowel transplantation. Clin Transpl 1989; 3:89–91.
336. Cohen Z, Silverman RE, Wassef R, et al: Small intestinal transplantation using cyclosporine. Report of a case. Transplantation 1986; 42:613–621.
337. Grant D, Wall W, Mimeault R, et al: Successful small-bowel/liver transplantation. Lancet 1990; 335:181–184.
337a. McAlister V, Wall W, Ghent C, et al: Successful small intestine transplantation. Transplant Proc 1992; 24:1236–1237.
337b. Wallender J, Ewald U, Lackgren G, et al: Extreme short bowel syndrome, in neonates: An indication for small bowel transplantation? Transplant Proc 1992; 24:1230–1235.
338. Williams JW, Sankary HN, Foster PF: Splanchnic transplantation: An approach to the infant dependent on parenteral nutrition who develops irreversible liver disease. JAMA 1989; 261:1458–1462.
339. Stangl TE, Rowe MI, Todo S, et al: Transplantation of multiple abdominal viscera. JAMA 1989; 261:1449–1457.
339a. D'Alessandro AM, Kalayogh M, Sollinger HW, et al: Liver-intestinal transplantation: Report of a case. Transplant Proc 1992; 24:1228–1229.
339b. Margreiter R, Konigsrainer A, Schmidt Koller J, et al: Successful multivisceral transplantation. Transplant Proc 1992; 29:1226–1227.
340. Diflo T, Shaffer DS, Maki T, et al: The effect of antilymphocyte globulin and cyclosporine on orthotopic small bowel allografts in the rat. Transplant Proc 1988; 20:200–202.
340a. Tzakis AG, Todo S, Reyes J, et al: Clinical intestinal transplantation: Focus on complications. Transplant Proc 1992; 24:1238–1240.
341. Stangl MJ, Lee KKW, Lee TK, et al: Graft retreatment with monoclonal antibodies prior to small-bowel transplantation. Transplant Proc 1990; 22:2483–2484.
342. Williams JW, McClellan T, Peters TG, et al: Effect of pretreatment graft irradiation in canine intestinal transplantation. Surg Gynecol Obstet 1988; 167:197–204.
343. Gundlach M, Schmidt P, Hell K, et al: The influence of major histocompatability complex subloci differences on graft rejection in small-bowel transplantation. Transplant Proc 1990; 22:2474–2475.
344. Kamada N, Davies HS, Roser B: Reversal of transplantation immunity by liver grafting. Nature 1981; 292:840–842.
345. Calne RY, Sells RA, Pena JR, et al: Induction of immunological tolerance by porcine liver allografts. Nature 1969; 223:474–476.
346. Gonwa Ta, Nery JR, Husberg BS, et al: Simultaneous liver and renal transplantation in man. Transplantation 1988; 46:690–693.
347. Fung JJ, Makowka L, Griffin M, et al: Successful sequential liver-kidney transplantation in patients with preformed lymphocytotoxic antibodies. Clin Transplant 1987; 1:187–194.
348. Zhong R, He G, Skai Y, et al: Combined small bowel and liver transplantation in the rat: Possible role of the liver in preventing intestinal allograft rejection. Transplantation (in press).
349. Murase N, Demetris AJ, Kim DG, et al: Rejection of multivisceral allografts in rats. A sequential analysis with comparison to isolated orthotopic small bowel and liver grafts. Surgery 1990; 108:880–889.
350. Saat RE, deBruin E, Heineman E, et al: Irradiation of the donor combined with cyclosporin A treatment of the recipient prevents graft-versus-host disease and leads to prolonged survival of small-bowel allografts. Transplant Proc 1990; 22:2465–2466.
351. Crane PW, Clark C, Sowter RL, et al: Cyclosporine toxicity in the small intestine. Transplant Proc 1990; 22:2432.
352. Lee KKW, Todo S, Langrehr JM, et al: Comparison of short-term immunosuppressive therapy with cyclosporine and FK 506 in small-bowel transplantation. Transplant Proc 1990; 22:2485–2486.
353. Lauterberg BH, Sautter V, Preisig R, et al: Hepatic functional deterioration after porta caval shunt in the rat. Gastroenterology 1976; 71:221–227.
354. Starzl TE, Francavilla A, Halgrimson CG, et al: The origin, hormonal nature, and action of hepatotrophic substances in portal venous blood. Surg Gynecol Obstet 1973; 137:179–199.
355. Kaneko H, Fischman MA, Buckley TM, et al: A comparison of portal versus systemic venous drainage in the pig small-bowel allograft recipient. Surgery 1991; 109:663–670.
356. Deltz E, Muller-Hermelink HK, Ulrich K, et al: Development of graft versus host reaction in various target organs after small intestinal transplantation. Transplant Proc 1981; 13:1215–1216.
357. Toledo-Pereyra LH, Raij L, Simmons RL, et al: Role of endo-

toxin and bacteria in the long-term survival of preserved small bowel allografts. Surgery 1974; 73:474–481.
358. Grant D, Hurlbutt D, Zhong R, et al: Intestinal permeability and bacterial translocation following small bowel transplantation in the rat. Transplantation 1991; 52:221–224.
359. Caniano DA, Kanoti GA: Newborns with massive intestinal loss: Difficult choices. N Engl J Med 1988; 318:703–707.
360. Gouttebel MC, Saint-Aubert B, Astre C, et al: Total parenteral nutrition needs in different types of short bowel syndrome. Dig Dis Sci 1986; 31:718–723.

Chapter 45

Defects in Fat Transport

ANUPAMA CHAWLA and FREDRIC DAUM

Defects in fat transport include (1) an inability to synthesize chylomicrons (abetalipoproteinemia [ABL] and homozygous hypobetalipoproteinemia [HBL]); (2) an inability to transport chylomicrons (chylomicron retention, or Anderson's disease); and (3) defects in lymphatic transport due to obstruction of the intestinal lymphatics (lymphangiectasia).

PATHOPHYSIOLOGY

A knowledge of the physiology of fat absorption and transport is essential to understanding the pathophysiology underlying the diseases of fat transport (see Chapter 2).[1]

Lipolytic products of dietary fats cross the enterocyte membrane by passive diffusion. These products are then transported to the endoplasmic reticulum, where triglyceride synthesis takes place and chylomicron formation is initiated. The surface of the triglyceride droplets is stabilized by a monolayer of phospholipids, cholesterol, and apoproteins, mainly apolipoprotein B (Apo B), Apo A-II, and Apo A-IV.

Subsequently, chylomicrons accumulate in the Golgi apparatus, where glycosylation is completed and final assembly takes place. Golgi vesicles filled with chylomicrons then migrate under the control of the microtubular apparatus toward the basolateral aspect of the cell. After fusion of the Golgi vesicles with the plasmalemma, there is bulk exocytosis of the chylomicrons in the intercellular spaces and into the lymphatics through gaps between the endothelial cells. Alterations in these processes lead to the accumulation of fat in the enterocytes or the intestinal lymphatics.

ABETALIPOPROTEINEMIA AND HOMOZYGOUS HYPOBETALIPOPROTEINEMIA

ABL[2] and homozygous HBL[3] are phenotypically almost indistinguishable.[4] Both these inherited conditions involve defects in lipid transport and plasma lipoprotein deficiency. Apo B is the main protein component of low-density lipoprotein (LDL) and constitutes about 24% of the LDL particle. Apo B is the ligand for the cellular recognition and the catabolism of LDL by the LDL receptors. The LDL receptor–Apo B interaction and subsequent catabolism mediate the clearance of LDL from plasma and regulate cellular cholesterol biosynthesis. Apo B seems to be important for lipoprotein assembly and secretion. Thus, the absence of Apo B in ABL and homozygous HBL abolishes the secretion of chylomicrons and very-low-density lipoprotein (VLDL).[5, 6]

Genetically, ABL and HBL appear to be different from each other. ABL has an autosomal recessive inheritance pattern, whereas HBL is an autosomal dominant disease. Biochemically, both homozygous ABL and homozygous HBL result in the absence of Apo B in plasma. ABL heterozygotes have normal levels of Apo B and Apo B–containing lipoprotein, whereas HBL heterozygotes have half-normal plasma levels[7] (which further supports the premise that ABL and HBL are transmitted as autosomal recessive and dominant diseases, respectively).

Some studies have attempted to differentiate between these two diseases at the molecular level.[7, 8] Analysis by immunohistochemistry reveals a normal to increased concentration of hepatic Apo B protein in ABL patients and reduced concentrations in those with HBL. Hepatic Apo B messenger ribonucleic acid (mRNA) is significantly increased in ABL but is decreased to 8 to 14% of control values in HBL subjects. Deoxyribonucleic acid from both HBL and ABL subjects shows no abnormality as detected by Southern blot analysis. The defect in HBL is believed to be a translation defect; this is suggested by the finding of reduced quantities of mRNA and intracellular immunologically reactive Apo B in comparison with complete absence of Apo B in the plasma. On the other hand, the molecular defect in ABL is thought to be secondary to defective cellular Apo B secretion,[9] since hepatic Apo B mRNA is increased in the presence of decreased plasma levels. Previously, intestinal Apo B (Apo B_{48}) was believed to be absent in both ABL and HBL; however, a recent report[10] suggests that patients with ABL synthesize Apo B_{48}. This study demonstrated detectable but low levels of Apo B_{48}, markedly increased Apo B mRNA, and evidence of Apo B degradation products, indicating that the defect in patients with ABL may be in the degradation of Apo B_{48} and not in its synthesis.[10]

Clinical Features

ABL was first described in 1950 by Bassen and Kornzweig[2] in an 18-year-old Jewish girl with neuromuscular disturbances, retinitis pigmentosa, and "thorny-appearing" erythrocytes. The disease usually presents in infancy with fat malabsorption, failure to thrive, and acanthocytosis on peripheral blood smear.[11, 12] The diagnosis may be delayed until adult life, when retinal and neurologic abnormalities become more apparent. The presence of steatorrhea, demyelinating neurologic disease, atypical retinitis pigmentosa, severe acanthocytosis when associated with a biochemical profile of low serum cholesterol and plasma triglycerides, as well as absent betalipoprotein, are suggestive of ABL and homozygous HBL. In ABL, the parents are normal, whereas in HBL heterozygous parents have phenotypic and biochemical changes.

The retinal and neurologic abnormalities that occur in children usually between 5 and 10 years of age are progressive and lead to severe ataxia and visual impairment. Typical features include pigmentary retinopathy, dysarthria, ataxia, areflexia, extensor plantar reflex, and dorsal column sensory loss.[12] Athetoid movements may also be noted,[12] and peripheral sensory neuropathy has been described.[13, 14] There is increasing evidence that most, if not all, of the neurologic dysfunction is attributable to a profound deficiency of fat-soluble vitamins A and E and that early treatment may prevent or reverse neurologic changes.[15–18]

The presence of acanthocytes in the peripheral blood smear is typical of ABL (Fig. 45–1), although this is not specific.[19] Fifty to 70% of the erythrocytes are abnormal. Acanthocytes are not detected in the bone marrow, and the membrane distortion is presumed to be acquired after release into the peripheral circulation. Acanthocytosis has also been reported with other neurologic syndromes. Reversible acanthocytosis has been reported in children with severe malnutrition[20] and anorexia nervosa.[21, 22] Acanthocytes have decreased membrane fluidity and increased microviscosity, and these abnormalities are not corrected by dietary vitamin E supplementation.[23] Hemolytic anemia, thought to be secondary to autohemolysis secondary to vitamin E deficiency, is also noted in these patients.

Ocular manifestations have been reported in patients as young as 5 to 10 years of age. Diminished vision is usually the initial complaint. Other ocular defects include problems with dark adaptation, nystagmus, ophthalmoplegia, ptosis, cataracts, and anisocoria.[24] Vitamin A supplementation may reverse the electroretinographic abnormalities but does not prevent the development of pigmentary retinopathy.[25–27] The use of vitamin E to prevent pigmentary retinopathy has been suggested.[15]

The extent and severity of hepatic damage in ABL are variable. Steatosis, fibrosis, and micronodular cirrhosis have been described (Fig. 45–2). Partin and associates[28] reported histochemical and ultrastructural findings from four serial biopsies obtained from a boy between 10 and 30 months of age with ABL. The initial biopsy showed large fat droplets, which became smaller and less numerous on a medium-chain triglyceride (MCT) diet. However, there was a progression of the initial mild hepatic fibrosis to advanced micronodular cirrhosis with the appearance of alcoholic hyalin in the hepatocytes.

Collins and associates[29] speculated that the alcoholic hyalin may be related to the accumulation of 2-carbon fragments derived from MCT in the presence of defective hepatic triglyceride secretion. Hepatic light microscopy and ultrastructural studies appear to be similar before and after vitamin E therapy.[29] However, after 1 month of daily vitamin E therapy, the transaminase levels have been reported to return to normal.

A variant of ABL (normotriglyceridemic ABL) has been reported in three patients,[30] including the presence of Apo B_{48} in the plasma after a fatty meal.

Diagnosis

A serum cholesterol level lower than 50 mg per dl and a barely detectable triglyceride level in the presence

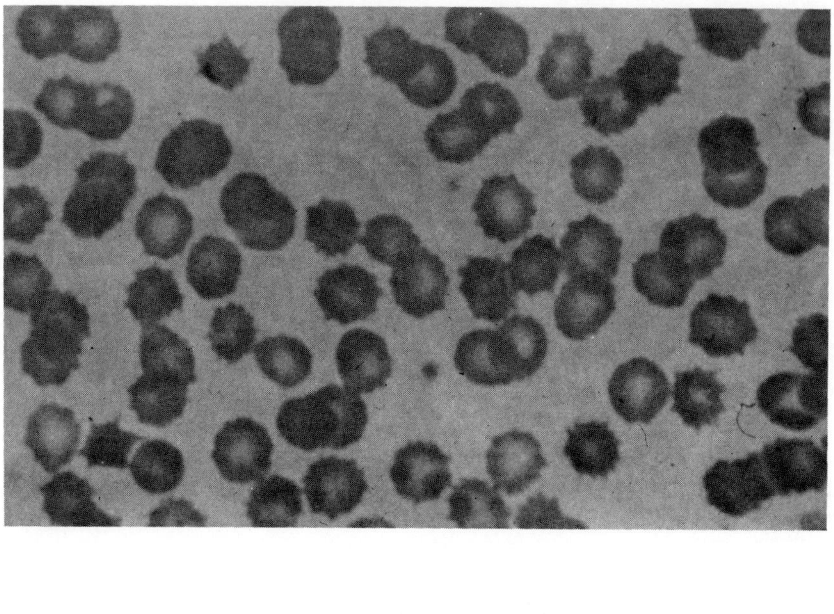

Figure 45–1. Acanthocytes in the peripheral blood smear in ABL (50–70% of the erythrocytes).

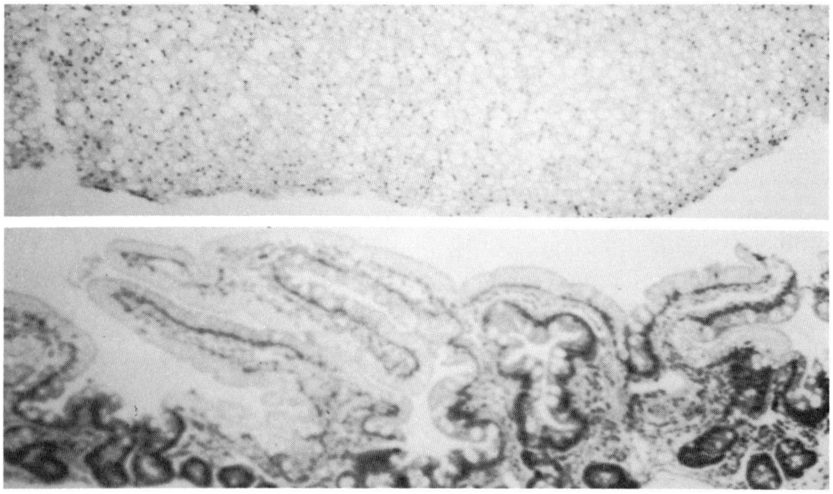

Figure 45–2. *Top panel*, Percutaneous liver biopsy from a 15-month-old boy with ABL revealing diffuse steatosis. *Bottom panel*, Small bowel biopsy from the same patient showing lipid-laden enterocytes. (Courtesy of Jeffrey Hyams, MD.)

of acanthocytes is suggestive of HBL and ABL. The diagnosis is confirmed by the absence of betalipoprotein and a small bowel biopsy that reveals villi of relatively normal appearance but with marked foamy vacuolation of the enterocytes covering the upper two thirds of the villus; the vacuoles stain for neutral lipid (Figs. 45–2 and 45–3). Endoscopically, there may be a cream–yellow appearance, which represents fat within the mucosa.

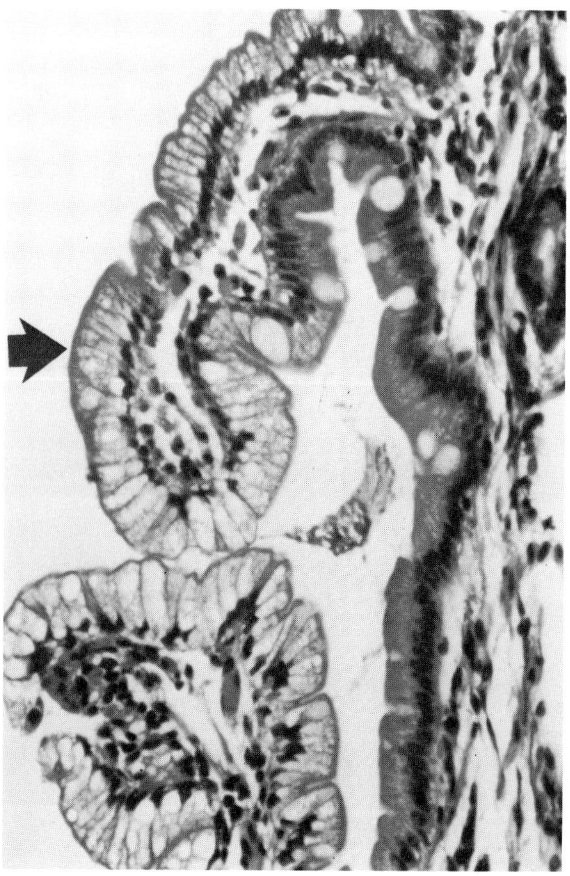

Figure 45–3. Biopsy specimen from a patient with ABL showing vacuolated villus cells (*arrow*). Hematoxylin-eosin stain, × 500. (Courtesy of Ellen Kahn, MD.)

Management

With early modification of the diet with restriction of long-chain fats and supplementation with MCT and fat-soluble vitamins, there is evidence that normal physical growth potential can be achieved, and the neurologic and ophthalmologic deterioration minimized.[15] The use of MCT is suggested because MCT bypasses both the acylglycerate synthesis step and the chylomicron formation by the intestinal epithelium.[31] Fat-soluble vitamins A, E, and K should be provided in adequate doses. Vitamin dosage should be tailored to maintain normal plasma levels of vitamins A and E and to maintain normal prothrombin time with vitamin K.

ANDERSON'S DISEASE (CHYLOMICRON RETENTION DISEASE)

In 1961, Anderson and coworkers[32] described a 7-month-old girl whose presentation resembled that of a patient with ABL but without acanthocytosis, retinitis pigmentosa, or neurologic abnormalities. The patient also had abetalipoproteins in her plasma, although in reduced concentrations. Other patients with features similar to those described by Anderson and coworkers have also been reported.[33–36]

The cause of the disease is unknown. The existence of an isolated defect of Apo B production by the intestine (Apo B_{48}) has been speculated, with an autosomal recessive inheritance pattern.[37]

Clinical Features

Features typical of Anderson's disease include diarrhea, steatorrhea, decreased serum cholesterol and phospholipid levels, decreased serum alphalipoprotein and betalipoprotein levels (50% of normal), absence of circulating chylomicrons postprandially, and enterocytes filled with chylomicrons.

In contrast with ABL, plasma cholesterol levels in Anderson's disease are higher than 50 mg per dl and serum triglyceride levels may be normal.[36] Some of the contrasting features among Anderson's disease, ABL, and HBL are outlined in Table 45–1. The presence of serum LDLs and the absence of acanthocytosis, retinitis pigmentosa, and ataxia also help distinguish this disease from ABL and homozygous HBL. Neuromuscular manifestations appear to be less severe and may even be absent. Ocular abnormalities are subclinical and usually require electrophysiologic studies for detection.

After a fat load, the enterocytes contain large numbers of fat particles in the endoplasmic reticulum and within dilated vesicles in the Golgi zone. These particles are morphologically similar to chylomicrons. The presence of numerous oil red O-positive lipid droplets in the jejunal mucosa suggests that intestinal absorption of fatty acids with esterification into triglycerides does take place, but triglycerides are not seen in the intercellular spaces and lacteals. Absence of chylomicrons and intestinal VLDL further attests to a defect in exocytosis from the intestinal cells.

Ultrastructural studies of fat absorption in jejunal biopsies suggest features of normal fat absorption as well as those associated with ABL. Few large lipid droplets similar to those found in ABL are seen, although most of the fat droplets gorging the cells are much smaller and more uniform in size. The chylomicron-sized lipid droplets are bound by membranes of the smooth endoplasmic reticulum in the supranuclear region of the cell and cluster within vesicular structures, whereas in ABL the lipid droplets are not enclosed within smooth endoplasmic reticulum membranes.

There is no indication of fat transport from the cells with complete juxtaposition of cell membranes and the absence of fat particles exterior to the basement membrane.

Management

Roy and colleagues[36] have reported success in treating eight patients with typical features of Anderson's disease by restricting long-chain fat intake and supplementing the diet with MCT. Supplements of vitamins A and E were prescribed, and plasma levels were maintained at the lower limit of the normal range. Electrophysiologic ophthalmologic abnormalities were significantly corrected, and neuromuscular defects did not progress in these patients. These data are encouraging, although long-term outcome in these patients remains to be seen.

INTESTINAL LYMPHANGIECTASIA

Intestinal lymphangiectasia encompasses any disorder that impairs lymphatic flow from the intestine, resulting in excessive enteric loss of plasma proteins.[38] Documented causes of lymphangiectasia are listed in Table 45–2.

Etiology

Primary intestinal lymphangiectasia (PIL) is caused by a disturbance in the lymphatic system, probably congenital in origin. Secondary intestinal lymphangiectasis (SIL) is a result of, or coexists with, associated pathologic conditions (see Table 45–2). In PIL, abnormal lymphatic vessels are located primarily at the level of the small intestine, although the entire lymphatic system below the diaphragm may be abnormal, and flow toward the thoracic duct is obstructed.[39] PIL has been described in a patient with Noonan's syndrome,[40] but whether PIL actually was present remains conjecture, since this patient also had complex heart disease with right-sided heart failure, which can result in SIL. PIL has also been associated with lymphedema of the limbs, the genitalia, and the face. Cases with moderate mental

Table 45–1. CHARACTERISTICS OF ABL, HBL, AND ANDERSON'S DISEASE

	ABL	Homozygous or Heterozyous HBL	Anderson's Disease
Inheritance	Autosomal recessive	Autosomal dominant	Autosomal recessive
Growth failure	+ + +	+ + to normal	+ +
Neurologic findings	Constant	Constant to mild (rarely milder)	Less severe to absent
Ocular lesions	Constant	Constant to subclinical	Subclinical
Acanthocytes (% of erythocytes)	50–70%	50–70% to rarely	Absent or mild (<5%)
Anemia	Mild to severe	Mild to severe or normal	
Intestinal apoprotein B_{48}	Reduced, 15% of normal	? Absent	Reduced
Hepatic apoprotein B_{100}	Increased	Decreased	Decreased
Cholesterol	Reduced <50 mg/dl	Reduced to ½ normal	Low but >50 mg/dl
Triglycerides (VLDL)	Barely detectable	Barely detectable to normal or low	Low to normal
Electron microscopy	Lipid droplets in enterocytes are large, not enclosed within smooth endoplasmic reticulum membranes		Lipid droplets much smaller, uniform in size, bound by smooth endoplasmic reticulum

+ + = mild; + + + = moderate to severe.

Table 45–2. INTESTINAL LYMPHANGIECTASIA

Intestinal Lymphangiectasia
Functional[43]
Associated with enteric protein loss, lymphopenia, and hypoalbuminemia
Primary Intestinal Lymphangiectasia
Isolated
Associated with lymphatic abnormalities elsewhere in the body[39–42]
Secondary Intestinal Lymphangiectasia
Cardiovascular Anomalies
Congestive heart failure[44]
Constrictive pericarditis[45]
Budd-Chiari syndrome[46]
Glenn shunt[47]
Fontan procedure[48]
Superior vena cava thrombosis
Mesenteric Lymphatic Involvement
Lymphomas[49]
Tuberculosis[50]
Sarcoidosis[51, 52]
Radiation therapy[53]
Volvulus
Intestinal Inflammatory Diseases
Systemic lupus erythematosus[54]
Tuberculosis[50]
Behçet's syndrome[55]
Crohn's disease[56, 57]
Drugs
Arsenic[58]
Chemotherapeutic agents[53]
Thoracic Duct Obliteration
Iatrogenic
Mediastinal tumor

retardation have also been described.[41] PIL has been known to occur in families.[42]

Clinical Features

PIL usually occurs in early childhood or infancy but has been diagnosed in adolescence. SIL has been reported to occur at all ages, depending on the underlying cause. Since the advent of flexible esophagogastroduodenoscopy, with biopsies directed at the affected sites, the diagnosis of PIL or SIL is being made with increasing frequency. The sex incidence appears to be equal in both conditions. Symptoms and signs range from abdominal pain to hypoproteinemic edema and chylous ascites.[59, 60] Recently, a patient has been described as having chylous reflux into the abdominal skin resembling lymphangioma circumscriptum in a patient with PIL.[61] In SIL, the signs and symptoms of the underlying disease may be the primary presentation. Intestinal lymphangiectasia noted in the absence of clinical manifestations has been called *functional lymphangiectasia*.[43]

Hypoalbuminemia and hypogammaglobulinemia, hypolipidemia, and lymphopenia are characteristic of intestinal lymphangiectasia. Diarrhea, hypoproteinemia, edema, and growth retardation are usual clinical features. Rarely, hypocalcemia may be severe enough to cause tetany.[60] Low serum ceruloplasmin concentrations have also been reported.[62] Enteric protein loss can be documented by measuring the fecal alpha$_1$-antitrypsin clearance. Fecal alpha$_1$-antitrypsin clearance is a reliable and inexpensive method of determining enteric protein losses without the use of radioactive tracers and correlates well with ^{51}Cr-albumin clearance.[63, 64]

Intestinal lymphangiectasia and other disorders of the lymphatic circulation have been associated with several immunologic aberrations, including lymphopenia, reduced peripheral blood T cells, diminished responses to mitogens, negative delayed hypersensitivity by skin testing, and hypogammaglobulinemia.[65, 66] Although not common, systemic immunodeficiency has been demonstrated with decreased cell-mediated immunity and systemic infections with atypical *Mycobacterium*, warts, and cellulitis.[67, 68]

Lymphocyte subpopulations have been evaluated in a small group of children with abnormal lymphatic circulation.[69] The percentage and absolute numbers of helper-inducer (CD4) lymphocytes were markedly reduced in all patients, whereas the percentage of suppressor-cytotoxic (CD8) lymphocytes was normal or increased. The abnormal cellular immunity in intestinal lymphangiectasia may be attributed to low levels of circulating CD4 lymphocytes and marked hypogammaglobulinemia, a consequence of the loss of immunoglobulins and lymphocytes into the intestine. To evaluate the local mucosal immune system in intestinal lymphangiectasia, two parameters of cell-mediated and humoral immunity have been studied. Immunoglobulin-producing plasma cells within the lamina propria were normal, suggesting normal local antibody and secretory immunoglobulin production, but intraepithelial lymphocytes were significantly reduced,[70] even though gastrointestinal immunity appeared to be intact clinically. Impaired neutrophil function has also been reported in three patients with intestinal lymphangiectasia.[71]

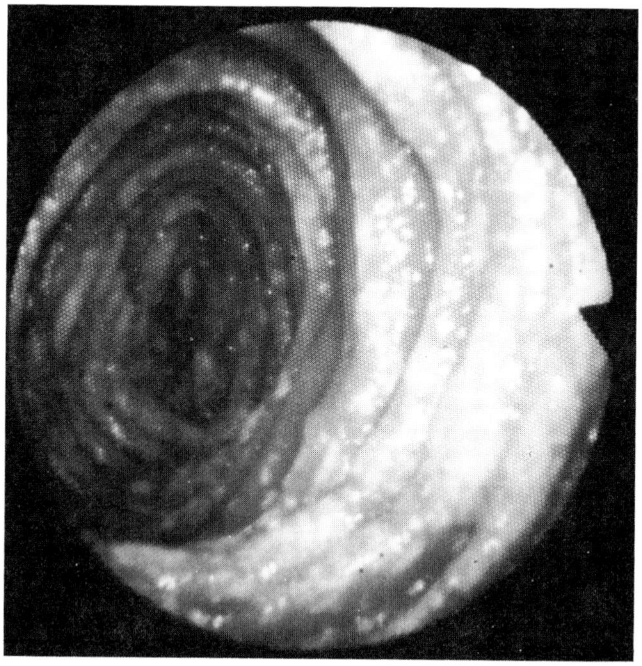

Figure 45–4. Endoscopic picture of the duodenum showing snowflake-like lesions, which histologically represent lacteals dilated with fat.

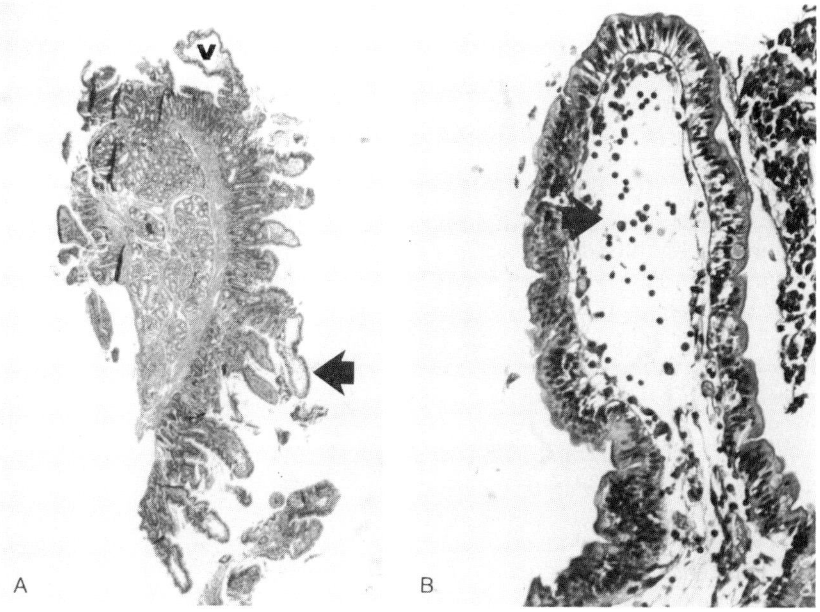

Figure 45–5. Lymphangiectasia. *A,* Low-power magnification of expanded villi (*V*) with dilated lymphatic channels (*arrow*). Hematoxylin-eosin × 50. *B*, Higher magnification of a villus with dilated lacteal (*arrow*). Hematoxylin-eosin, × 200. (Courtesy of Ellen Kahn, MD.)

Diagnosis

The presence of stool lymphocytes, lymphopenia, hypoalbuminemia, and hypolipidemia is suggestive of intestinal lymphangiectasia. The diagnosis is confirmed by endoscopic and histologic findings that are characteristic of this disorder.[72, 73]

Endoscopic visualization of the mucosa may show scattered white spots which have been described as having a snowflake-like appearance (Fig. 45–4). When biopsies of these spots are performed and the tissues observed under a dissecting microscope, milky-white substances are seen in the stroma of the villi. Histologically (Fig. 45–5*A* and *B*), there are markedly dilated lymphatics in the lamina propria, the submucosa, or both. On electron microscopic evaluation, there are dilated lymphatic vessels filled with chylomicrons and precipitated lymph proteins. These findings are also present in the dilated intraepithelial gaps extending from the basal membrane to the luminal part of the epithelium. The lymphatic vessels, especially in PIL, exhibit prominent endothelial membranes in comparison with the normal vessels and usually closed cell junctions.[74] A high-fat meal during the evening before endoscopic evaluation may make the diagnosis more apparent.[75] Other histologic findings include mild to moderate lymphoplasmacytic inflammation and villous injury with blunting and edema.

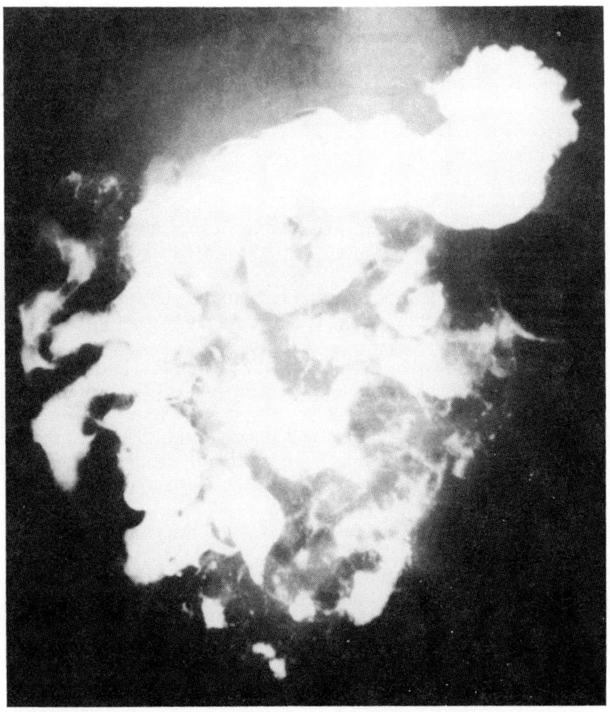

Figure 45–6. Intestinal lymphangiectasia. Prominent valvulae conniventes are present throughout the small bowel, as well as scalloped circular defects, which represent enlarged lymphatic channels. (Courtesy of Micha N. Ziprkowski, MD.)

Small bowel contrast studies show thickened, nodular mucosal folds that simulate the stacking of coins (Fig. 45–6).[60] The lymphatic system may be imaged by lymphangiography using radiopaque contrast material via a pedal injection, which enables visualization of both the peripheral lymphatic channels and the lymph nodes. Lacteals in the bowel wall in intestinal lymphangiectasia fill in the delayed phase of a peripheral lymphangiogram and appear as punctate densities.[37]

Management

The mainstay of treatment in PIL is dietary modification. A high-protein, low-fat diet with MCT supplementation (C 6:0 to C 12:0) is recommended. The rationale for the use of MCT is that MCT bypasses the intestinal lymphatic system and directly enters the portal venous system. In infancy, therapy may be achieved by the use of a ready-made formula, including Pregestimil and Alimentum, which contain MCT as well as long-chain triglyceride. In older children, a low-fat diet can be supplemented with MCT oil.[76]

Varying degrees of success resulting from dietary modification have been described, ranging from transient, partial reversal of lymphopenia to complete correction of the blood profile.[60, 77, 78] Increase in linear growth with dietary management alone has also been reported. Spinocerebellar symptoms due to intestinal lymphangiectasia have been reported, with findings typical of vitamin E deficiency.[79] Vitamin supplementation is recommended according to guidelines similar to those for ABL.

In SIL, correction of the underlying cause is the most effective treatment. Recently, antiplasmin therapy with tranexamic acid (4[aminomethyl]cyclohexanecarboxylic acid) was shown to be effective in an adult with intestinal lymphangiectasia and increased plasma fibrinolytic activity.[80] Antiplasmin therapy successfully decreased intestinal protein loss and corrected the serum protein concentration in this patient. Corticosteroids have been shown to be effective in patients with intestinal lymphangiectasia secondary to an inflammatory process (increased sedimentation rates and normal or increased immunoglobulin levels).[81] More recently, in a patient with SIL after a Fontan procedure, corticosteroid therapy was shown to be beneficial, with clinical improvement and normalization of the serum albumin level.[82]

ACKNOWLEDGMENT

The authors thank Mrs. Debra Syper for secretarial help in the preparation of this manuscript.

REFERENCES

1. Friedman HI, Nylund B: Intestinal fat digestion, absorption, and transport. Am J Clin Nutr 1980; 33:1108–1139.
2. Bassen FA, Kornzweig A: Malformation of the erythrocytes in a case of typical retinitis pigmentosa. Blood 1950; 5:381–392.
3. Mars H, Lewis LA, Robertson AL, et al: Familial hypo-beta-lipoproteinemia. Am J Med 1969; 46:886–892.
4. Cottrill C, Glueck CJ, Leuba V, et al: Familial homozygous hypobetalipoproteinemia. Metabolism 1974; 23:779–791.
5. Zannis VI, Hussain MM, Cladaras M, et al: Molecular biology of human apolipoprotein B and related diseases. Adv Exp Med Biol 1988; 243:107–121.
6. Herbert PN, Assmann G, Gotta AM, et al: Familial lipoprotein deficiency; Abetalipoproteinemia, hypobetalipoproteinemia and Tangier disease. *In* Stanbury JB, Wyngaarden JB, Fredrickson DS, eds: The Metabolic Basis of Inherited Disease, 4th ed. New York, McGraw-Hill, 1982; pp 589–621.
7. Ross RR, Gregg RE, Law SW, et al: Homozygous hypobetalipoproteinemia: A disease distinct from abetalipoproteinemia at the molecular level. J Clin Invest 1988; 81:590–595.
8. Lackner KJ, Monge JC, Gregg RE, et al: Analysis of the apolipoprotein B gene and messenger ribonucleic acid in abetalipoproteinemia. J Clin Invest 1986; 78:1707–1712.
9. Blackhardt BD, Ludwig EM, Pierolti BR, et al: Structure of the apolipoprotein B gene. J Biol Chem 1986; 261:15364–15367.
10. Glickman RM, Glickman JN, Magun A, et al: Apolipoprotein synthesis in normal and abetalipoproteinemic intestinal mucosa. Gastroenterology 1991; 101:749–755.
11. Lloyd JK, Muller DPR: Management of abetalipoproteinemia in childhood. *In* Peeters H, ed: Protides of Biological Fluids: 19th Colloquium. Oxford, Pergamon Press, 1972, p 331.
12. Hardie RJ: Acanthocytosis and neurological impairment—a review. Q J Med 1989; 264:291–306.
13. Traber MG, Sokol RJ, Ringel SP, et al: Lack of tocopherol in peripheral nerve of vitamin E–deficient patients with peripheral neuropathy. N Engl J Med 1987; 317:262–265.
14. Muller DPR, Lloyd JK, Bird AC: Long-term management of abetalipoproteinemia. Arch Dis Child 1977; 52:209–214.
15. Muller DPR: Vitamin E: Its role in neurological function. Postgrad Med J 1986; 62:107–112.
16. Muller DPR, Lloyd JK, Wolff OH: The role of vitamin E in the treatment of neurological features of abetalipoproteinemia and other disorders of fat absorption. J Inherited Metab Dis 1985–8 (Suppl 1):88–92.
17. Harding AE: Vitamin E and the nervous system. CRC Crit Rev Neurobiol 1987; 3:89–103.
18. Gracey M, Hilton HB: Acanthocytes and hypobetalipoproteinemia. Lancet 1973; 1:679.
19. Singer K, Fisher B, Perlstein MA: Acanthocytosis: A genetic erythrocyte malformation. Blood 1952; 7:577–591.
20. Mant MJ, Faragher BS: The hematology of anorexia nervosa. Br J Haematol 1972; 23:737–749.
21. Myers TJ, Perkerson MD, Witter BA, et al: Hematologic findings in anorexia nervosa. Conn Med 1981; 45:14–17.
22. Biemer JJ: Acanthocytosis—biochemical and physiological considerations. Ann Clin Lab Sci 1980; 10:238–249.
23. Dieckert JP, White M, Christmann, et al: Angioid streaks associated with abetalipoproteinemia. Ann Ophthalmol 1989; 21:173–179.
24. Gouras P, Carr RE, Gunkel RD: Retinitis pigmentosa in abetalipoproteinemia: Effects of vitamin A. Invest Ophthalmol Vis Sci 1971; 10:784.
25. Sperling MA, Hiles DA, Kennerdell JS: Electroretinographic responses following vitamin A therapy in abetalipoproteinemia. Am J Ophthalmol 1972; 73:342.
26. Wolff OH, Lloyd JK, Tonks EL: Abetalipoproteinemia with special reference to the visual defect. Exp Eye Res 1964; 3:439.
27. Azizi E, Zaidman JL, Eschar J, et al: Abetalipoproteinemia treated with parenteral and oral vitamins A and E, and with medium chain triglycerides. Acta Paediatr Scand 1978; 67:797.
28. Partin JS, Partin JC, Schubert WK, et al: Liver ultrastructure in abetalipoproteinemia: Evolution of micronodular cirrhosis. Gastroenterology 1974; 67:107–118.
29. Collins JC, Scheinberg IH, Giblin DR, et al: Hepatic peroxisomal abnormalities in abetalipoproteinemia. Gastroenterology 1989; 97:766–770.
30. Malloy MJ, Kane JP, Hardman DA, et al: Normotriglyceridemic abetalipoproteinemia. J Clin Invest 1981; 67:1441–1450.
31. Isslebacher KJ, Scheig R, Plotkin GR, et al: Congenital beta-lipoprotein deficiency: An hereditary disorder involving a defect in the absorption and transport of lipids. Medicine 1964; 43:347–361.
32. Anderson CM, Townley RR, Freeman M: Unusual causes of steatorrhea in infancy and childhood. Med J Aust 1961; 11:617–622.
33. Silverberg M, Kessler J, Neumann PZ, et al: An intestinal lipid transport defect: A possible variant of hypo-B-lipoproteinemia. Gastroenterology 1968; 54:1271.
34. Partin JC, Schubert WK: Jejunal mucosal biopsy studies in two new types of hypobetalipoproteinemia: Light, electron microscopical, and biochemical analysis (abstract). Gastroenterology 1970; 58:1022.
35. Polonovski C, Navarro J, Fontaine JL, et al: Maladie d'Anderson. Ann Pediatr 1970; 17:342–354.
36. Roy CC, Levy E, Green PH, et al: Malabsorption, hypocholesterolemia, and fat-filled enterocytes with increased intestinal apoprotein B. Gastroenterology 1987; 92:390–399.
37. Bouma ME, Beucler I, Aggerneck LP, et al: Hypobetalipoproteinemia with accumulation of an apoprotein B–like protein in intestinal cells. J Clin Invest 1986; 78:398–410.
38. Waldmann TA, Steinfeld JL, Dutcher TF: The role of the gastrointestinal system in "idiopathic hypoproteinemia." Gastroenterology 1961; 41:197–207.
39. Levine C: Primary disorders of the lymphatic vessels—a unified concept. J Pediatr Surg 1989; 24:233–240.

40. Vallet HL, Holtzapple PG, Eberlein WR, et al: Noonan syndrome with intestinal lymphangiectasis. J Pediatr 1972; 80:269–274.
41. Hennekam RCM, Geerdink RA, Hamel BCJ, et al: Autosomal recessive intestinal lymphangiectasia and lymphedema, with facial anomalies and mental retardation. Am J Med Genet 1989; 34:593–600.
42. Shani M, Theodor EM, Frand M, et al: A family with protein-losing enteropathy. Gastroenterology 1974; 66:433–445.
43. Patel AS, DeRidder PH: Endoscopic appearance and significance of functional lymphangiectasia of the duodenal mucosa. Gastrointest Endosc 1990; 36:376–378.
44. Davidson JD, Goodman DS, Waldmann TA, et al: Protein-losing gastroenteropathy in congestive heart failure. Lancet 1961; 1:899–902.
45. Nelson DL, Blaese RM, Strober W, et al: Constrictive pericarditis, intestinal lymphangiectasia, and reversible immunologic deficiency. J Pediatr 1975; 86:548–554.
46. Tsuchiya M, Oshio C, Asakura H, et al: Budd-Chiari syndrome associated with protein-losing enteropathy. Gastroenterology 1978; 75:114–117.
47. Gleason WA, Roodman ST, Laks H: Protein-losing enteropathy and intestinal lymphangiectasia after superior vena cava–right pulmonary artery (Glenn) shunt. J Thorac Cardiovasc Surg 1979; 77:843–846.
48. Hess J, Kruizinga K, Bijleveld MA, et al: Protein-losing enteropathy after Fontan operation. J Thorac Cardiovasc Surg 1984; 88:606–609.
49. Douglas AP, Weetman AP, Haggith JW: The distribution and enteric loss of ^{51}Cr-labelled lymphocytes in normal subjects and in patients with coeliac disease and other disorders of the small intestine. Digestion 1976; 14:29.
50. Ploddi A, Atisook K, Hargrove NS: Intestinal lymphangiectasia in intraabdominal tuberculosis. J Med Assoc Thailand 1988; 71:518–523.
51. Levinson JD, Kirsner JB: Infiltrative diseases of the small bowel and malabsorption. Dig Dis 1970; 15:741–766.
52. Van Tilburg AJP, Van Blankenstein M, Verschog L: Intestinal lymphangiectasia in systemic sclerosis. Am J Gastroenterol 1988; 83:1418–1419.
53. Rao SSC, Dundas S, Holdsworth CD: Intestinal lymphangiectasia secondary to radiotherapy and chemotherapy. Dig Dis Sci 1987; 32:939–942.
54. Edworthy SM, Fritzler MJ, Kelly JK, et al: Protein-losing enteropathy in systemic lupus erythematosus associated with intestinal lymphangiectasia. Am J Gastroenterol 1990; 85:1398–1402.
55. Asakura H, Morita A, Morishita T, et al: Histopathological and electron microscopic studies of lymphangiectasia of the small intestine in Behçet's disease. Gut 1973; 14:196–203.
56. Kahn E, Daum F: Pseudopolyps of the small intestine in Crohn's disease. Hum Pathol 1984; 15:84–86.
57. Gad A: The diagnosis of gastroduodenal Crohn's disease by endoscopic biopsy. Scand J Gastroenterol 1989; 24(Suppl 167):23–28.
58. Kobayashi A, Ohbe Y: Protein-losing enteropathy associated with arsenic poisoning. Am J Dis Child 1971; 121:515–517.
59. Van der Meer SB, Forget PP, Willebrand D: Intestinal lymphangiectasia without protein loss in a child with abdominal pain. J Pediatr Gastroenterol Nutr 1990; 10:246–248.
60. Vardy PA, Lebenthal E, Schwachman H: Intestinal lymphangiectasia: A reappraisal. Pediatrics 1975; 55:842–851.
61. O'Driscoll JB, Chalmers RJ, Warnes TW: Chylous reflux into abdominal skin simulating lymphangioma circumscriptum in a patient with primary intestinal lymphangiectasia. Clin Exp Dermatol 1991; 16:124–126.
62. O'Donnell D, Myers AM: Intestinal lymphangiectasia with protein-losing enteropathy. Aust NZ J Med 1990; 20:167–169.
63. Karbach U, Ewe K: Enteric protein loss in various gastrointestinal diseases determined by intestinal alpha$_1$-antitrypsin clearance. Z Gastroenterol 1989; 27:P362–P365.
64. Karbach U, Ewe K, Bodenstein H: Alpha$_1$-antitrypsin, a reliable endogenous marker for intestinal protein loss and its application in patients with Crohn's disease. Gut 1983; 24:718–723.
65. Strober W, Wochner RD, Carbone PP, et al: Intestinal lymphangiectasia: A protein-losing enteropathy with hypogammaglobulinemia, lymphocytopenia and impaired homograft rejection. J Clin Invest 1967; 46:1643–1656.
66. Garty BZ, Levinson AI, Danon YL, et al: Lymphocyte subpopulations in children with abnormal lymphatic circulation. J Allergy Clin Immunol 1989; 84:515–520.
67. Ward M, Small WP, LeRoux A, et al: Malignant lymphoma and extensive viral wart formation in a patient with intestinal lymphangiectasia and lymphocyte depletion. Postgrad Med J 1977; 53:753–757.
68. Ross JD, Reid KDG, Ambujakshan VP: Recurrent pleural effusion, protein-losing enteropathy, malabsorption, and mosaic warts associated with generalized lymphatic hypoplasia. Thorax 1971; 26:119–124.
69. Yamamoto H, Tsutsui T, Mayumi M, et al: Immunodeficiency associated with selective loss of helper/inducer T cells and hypogammaglobulinaemia in a child with intestinal lymphangiectasia. Clin Exp Immunol 1989; 75:196–200.
70. Myszor MF, Davidson A, Hodgson HJF: The local mucosal immune system in intestinal lymphangiectasia. J Clin Lab Immunol 1988; 26:1–3.
71. Bolton RP, Cotter KL, Losowsky MS: Impaired neutrophil function in intestinal lymphangiectasia. J Clin Pathol 1986; 39:876–880.
72. Asakura H, Miura S, Morishita T, et al: Endoscopic and histopathological study on primary and secondary intestinal lymphangiectasis. Dig Dis Sci 1981; 26:312–320.
73. Abramowsky C, Hupertz V, Kilbridge P, et al: Intestinal lymphangiectasia in children: A study of upper gastrointestinal endoscopic biopsies. Pediatr Pathol 1989; 9:289–297.
74. Riemann JF, Schmidt H: Synopsis of endoscopic and other morphological findings in intestinal lymphangiectasia. Endoscopy 1981; 13:60–63.
75. Veldhuyzen van Zanten SJO, Bartelsman JFWM, Tytgat GNJ: Endoscopic diagnosis of primary intestinal lymphangiectasia using a high-fat meal. Endoscopy 1986; 18:108–110.
76. Jeffries GH, Chapman A, Sleisenger MH: Low-fat diet in intestinal lymphangiectasia. N Engl J Med 1964; 270:761–766.
77. Holt PR: Dietary treatment of protein loss in intestinal lymphangiectasia. Pediatrics 1964; 34:629–635.
78. Tift WL, Lloyd JK: Intestinal lymphangiectasia. Arch Dis Child 1975; 50:269–276.
79. Gutmann L, Shockcor W, Gutmann L, et al: Vitamin E–deficient spinocerebellar syndrome due to intestinal lymphangiectasia. Neurology 1986; 36:554–556.
80. Mine K, Matsubayashi S, Nakai Y, et al: Intestinal lymphangiectasia markedly improved with antiplasmin therapy. Gastroenterology 1989; 96:1596–1599.
81. Fleisher TA, Strober W, Muchmore A, et al: Corticosteroid-responsive intestinal lymphangiectasia secondary to an inflammatory process. N Engl J Med 1979; 11:605–606.
82. Rothman A, Snyder J: Protein-losing enteropathy following the Fontan operation: Resolution with prednisone therapy. Am Heart J 1991; 121:618–619.

Chapter 46

Infectious Diarrhea

D. WAYNE LANEY, JR., and MITCHELL B. COHEN

Despite the myriad advances in modern medicine, diarrheal disease remains a major global problem, especially among pediatric patients. Even in a country as well developed as is the United States, an estimated 21 million to 37 million episodes of diarrhea occur annually in children younger than 5 years of age.[1] Of that number, 10% of children are seen by a physician, more than 200,000 children are hospitalized, and between 300 and 400 children die from the illness. Worldwide, the number of childhood deaths as a result of diarrhea is higher than 4 million per year.[2]

Knowledge of diarrheal disease has increased remarkably during the past few decades.[3, 4] Numerous bacterial pathogens and an increasing number of viral pathogens have been demonstrated to cause diarrhea. This increased understanding of pathogenic mechanisms has led to improvements in therapy. This chapter discusses the major viral and bacterial agents of infectious diarrhea, including their epidemiology, pathogenesis, clinical manifestations, diagnosis, and therapy.

VIRAL GASTROENTERITIS

Diarrheal disease caused by viral agents occurs far more frequently than does similar disease of bacterial etiology. In fact, viral gastroenteritis is the second commonest illness in the United States; first is the common cold.[5] Despite the frequent occurrence of viral enteritides, identification of specific viruses as causative agents is a relatively recent development. The first published description of a gastroenteritis-producing virus came in 1972, with the identification of the Norwalk virus.[6] Rotavirus and the enteric adenoviruses were subsequently identified as bona fide enteric viral pathogens. The discussion focuses on these established pathogens, then continues with a brief summary of calicivirus and astrovirus and the current status of several candidate pathogens.

MECHANISMS OF VIRAL DISEASE PRODUCTION

The first step in the induction of diarrhea is exposure to the virus, usually via person-to-person contact with contaminated feces. In developing nations, spread via contaminated water is also likely.[7] In a prospective study by Santosham and colleagues,[8] in an Apache Indian population, the pattern of spread of rotavirus was believed to be most consistent with a respiratory route, yet these investigators were unable to isolate rotavirus from nasal secretions of affected patients.

Transmissible gastroenteritis, caused by a coronavirus, produces a disease in piglets that is similar in many respects to human rotavirus infection. It has thus been accepted as a model for the mechanism of enteric viral diarrheal illness. After introduction into the intestinal lumen, the transmissible gastroenteritis agents simultaneously invade villous enterocytes along the entire span of the small bowel.[9] The crypt enterocytes are spared, suggesting the possibility of virus-specific attachment mechanisms in the more differentiated villous cells.[9] The infected villous cells are then shed, accounting for the blunted villi and the mucosal irregularities that are apparent histologically.[10] Hyperplasia of the mucosal crypts is possible, and there can be an increase in inflammatory cells in the lamina propria.[11] As infected cells are shed from the villi, immature cells migrate upward from the crypts. These immature cells have been shown to be deficient in lactase and sucrase.[11] The deficiency in these brush border membrane hydrolases may contribute to an osmotic diarrhea. In addition, there is decreased active sodium transport in the jejunum and the ileum in the presence of an invasive viral enteritis. Cyclic adenosine monophosphate (AMP) has been shown *not* to be stimulated by the process of viral invasion and is therefore not believed to be involved in the observed alteration in fluid balance.[11]

Rotavirus

Rotavirus was first identified as a specific viral pathogen in duodenal cells of children with diarrhea by Bishop and associates in 1973.[12] Subsequent studies indicated that rotavirus is responsible not only for more cases of diarrheal disease in infants and children than is any other single cause but also for a significant portion of deaths caused by diarrhea in both developed and developing countries throughout the world.[13]

Virology

Rotavirus is classified as a member of the family Reoviridae of the RNA viruses. Rotaviruses are round particles 68 nm in diameter and are composed of two separate shells (capsids). The capsids surround a 38-nm icosahedral core structure, which in turn encloses the double-stranded ribonucleic acid (RNA) core. This structure gives the virus its characteristic appearance of a wide-rimmed wheel with spokes radiating from a hub, from which its name was derived (*rota* is Latin for wheel).

Rotaviruses are classified based on antigenic properties of various proteins found in the capsid structure. The first major classification is the "group" that is determined by the antigenic makeup of a protein identified as VP6 on the inner capsid of the virus.[6] Most viruses infecting humans are classified as group A, although rotaviruses from groups B and C have occasionally been associated with human diarrheal disease as well. The next level of classification is the subgroup, which is determined by other antigenic differences among the VP6 proteins. At least two subgroups are known to exist.[6] Subgroup typing has proved important in studying patients who experience more than one episode of rotaviral infection. In these patients, recurrent infections usually but not necessarily involve agents of different subgroups, which suggests that subgroup antigens are not sufficient for inducing the production of protective antibodies.[14] Finally, the rotaviruses are classified into a variety of serotypes based on the antigenic differences of the VP4 or VP7 proteins that are found in the outer capsid.[4]

Epidemiology

Rotavirus infection appears to occur throughout the world. In temperate climates, a sharp increase in incidence of cases occurs during the winter months.[13] This seasonal variance is not typically seen in the tropics.[15]

Although the virus may affect all age groups, it most commonly produces disease in children between 6 and 24 months of age. Within this age group, rotavirus is the most commonly identified cause of diarrheal disease.[13] A study in Washington, D.C., found that most children have developed rotavirus antibodies by age 2, which helps explain the observed decreased incidence of rotaviral infection in later childhood.[16] The disease does occur in the adult population, however, and has even been known to produce epidemics.[17, 18] A prospective study by Wenman and coworkers[19] found that rotavirus infection occurs in adult populations with approximately half the frequency of that seen in children. Those adults whose children had rotavirus were more likely to be infected than were adults without infected children. Most adults found to have rotavirus infection were asymptomatic; if symptoms were present, they were generally mild. This would seem to indicate that the antibody acquired earlier in life provides protective benefit.

The other age group that appears to have protection from rotavirus infection is the neonate. The virus can be found in stool samples from asymptomatic neonates.[20] Neonatal epidemics of rotavirus excretion have been described in which approximately half of the nursery patients examined were found to have rotavirus. Many of these infants were asymptomatic, and those with disease had only mild symptoms.[21, 22] Breast-fed infants have been shown to be less likely to be infected, and, when infected, these infants are apparently less likely than their bottle-fed counterparts to suffer symptoms of disease. This may reflect the protective effect of maternal antibodies in colostrum and breast milk.[23] Nosocomial spread of rotaviral illness among hospitalized infants has also been documented.[24]

Clinical Manifestations

Once a susceptible patient has come in contact with rotavirus, a 48- to 72-hour incubation period occurs before the onset of symptoms.[15] Illness typically begins with the sudden onset of diarrhea and vomiting. The diarrhea is usually watery and may occasionally be associated with gross or occult blood in the stool.[25] The fluid loss from diarrhea and vomiting is often severe enough to cause dehydration. Fever is present in most of the patients as well.[15] A comparison of rotaviral symptoms with those caused by other enteric viral illnesses is presented in Table 46–1.

Diarrhea caused by rotavirus usually lasts from 2 to 8 days.[26] Shedding of viruses into the intestinal lumen begins about 3 days after infection and may persist for as long as 3 weeks.[27, 28]

In addition to gastrointestinal symptoms, patients with rotavirus often have respiratory tract symptoms.[15] Of 150 patients hospitalized with acute gastroenteritis, 26% were found to have rhinitis, 8% had abnormal breath sounds, 49% had pharyngeal erythema, and 18% had palpable cervical adenopathy.[29] In addition, 19% had signs of otitis media. None of these nongastrointestinal manifestations associated with rotavirus infection, however, seemed helpful in the recognition of rotaviral disease, because the non–rotavirus-infected group had similar signs and symptoms. The clinical symptoms of rotavirus infection are more severe in patients with underlying malnutrition. In the malnourished murine

Table 46–1. VIRAL ENTERIC PATHOGENS

	Predominant Age Group Affected	Seasonality	Duration of Symptoms
Rotavirus	6–24 months	↑ in winter months	2–8 days
Norwalk virus	Older children, adults	Winter and summer	12–48 hours
Enteric adenovirus	<2 years	↑ in summer months	up to 14 days
Calicivirus	3 months–6 years	Unknown	2–8 days
Astrovirus	1–3 years	Unknown	1–4 days

rotavirus model, a smaller inoculum is required for infection, less time is required for incubation, and the symptoms are more severe.[30]

Pathophysiology

Rotavirus invades the intestinal epithelial cells and replicates, causing cell death and sloughing. Histologically, this is manifest as blunting of the intestinal villi.[31] In response to the loss of villous cells, there is crypt hypertrophy. An increase in the number of inflammatory cells may also be present in the lamina propria. Disease effects are apparently limited to the duodenum and the proximal jejunum,[15] since studies in patients with known rotavirus disease have yielded normal gastric and rectal biopsies.[32]

Diagnosis

Rotavirus was initially linked to acute gastroenteritis through electron microscopic evidence of viral particles in biopsy specimens of affected patients.[12] This technique continues to be useful in rotavirus detection, especially in correlation with monoclonal or polyclonal antibodies (immunoelectron microscopy [IEM]).[26] Many other detection methods have been developed using antirotavirus antibodies. These include enzyme-linked immunosorbent assay (ELISA) (Fig. 46–1), radioimmunoassay, latex particle agglutination (LA), and immunofluorescence. Many antigenic detection systems are commercially available, offering relative ease in evaluating large numbers of specimens. They are limited, however, to detection of rotaviruses of group A.[26] The polymerase chain reaction (PCR) has also been applied to the detection of rotavirus in stool.[28] Rotavirus may be cultured from stool; however, isolation rates higher than 70% have not been achieved.[33]

Treatment and Prevention

Currently, supportive care with oral or intravenous rehydration is the mainstay of therapy. No antiviral agents effective against rotavirus have yet been developed.

Vaccines effective in preventing rotavirus infection are being developed.[34] Both attenuated bovine strains (RIT 4237) and rhesus monkey strains (RRV) of rotavirus have been used to prepare vaccines currently being investigated in field trials.[35, 36] A double-blind, randomized field study using both vaccines failed to show that either vaccine was effective in preventing rotaviral diarrhea.[37] A vaccine prepared from a naturally attenuated human strain is also being evaluated.[38]

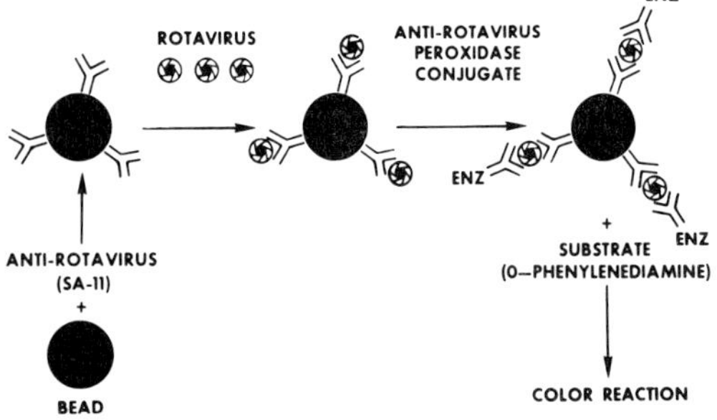

Figure 46–1. Graphic representation of ELISA for rotavirus (Rotazyme, Abbott Laboratories). (Reprinted with permission of Ross Laboratories, Columbus, OH 43216. From Acute Diarrhea in Infants and Children: Update, © 1984 Ross Laboratories.)

Norwalk Virus

The Norwalk virus is named after the community of Norwalk, Ohio, where, in 1968, a major epidemic of acute infectious, nonbacterial gastroenteritis occurred. Using bacteria-free stool filtrates from patients in this and other similar outbreaks, investigators were able to produce acute gastroenteritis in a volunteer population and to establish the existence of the Norwalk agent as an infectious entity.[39] In 1972, Kapikian and coworkers,[6] using IEM, identified small viral particles in stool filtrates of patients from the Norwalk outbreak. Their findings were the first definitive association of a specific virus with acute gastroenteritis.

Virology

The Norwalk virus is a 27-nm nonenveloped round virus. It was initially thought to be a DNA virus and classified as "parvoviruslike."[40] More recent investigations have shown this to be an RNA virus, structurally similar to the caliciviruses.[41] At least three distinct serotypes of the Norwalk virus have been identified.[42] Several other viruses are similar to the Norwalk virus in structure and are described collectively as Norwalklike viruses. These organisms are also named for the communities in which they were first isolated and include Montgomery County, Hawaii, Snow Mountain, Taunton, Otofuke, and Sapporo viruses.[43]

Epidemiology

Although the Norwalk virus has been most extensively studied in the United States, it is apparently worldwide in distribution.[40] In the developed world, this virus typically affects a population ranging from older children to adults. In less developed countries, a younger age group is typically involved.[40] Of patients exposed to the Norwalk virus either naturally or experimentally, approximately 50% develop clinical symptoms.

Studies evaluating the prevalence of anti-Norwalk antibody among populations of various age groups demonstrate a biphasic age distribution. From birth to 3 months, 20% have anti-Norwalk antibody. This is presumed to be of maternal origin and to have been acquired either transplacentally or through breast milk. The group from 3 months to 12 years of age has only a 5% antibody-positive rate, reflecting both the loss of maternally acquired antibody and the relative infrequency of infection in this age group. During the adolescent years, the antibody prevalence increases dramatically, reaching the 50% level by age 18 years. The adult population also exhibits a 50% positive rate.[44] This age distribution of antibody positivity parallels the characteristic distribution of clinical disease owing to the Norwalk virus, with older children and adults being most often affected.

Transmission of the Norwalk virus is most often fecal-oral. Unlike rotavirus, this usually involves the spread of infection to a large population through a common source rather than from direct person-to-person contact.[45] In one outbreak, an infected bakery employee transmitted the virus through food products to approximately 3,000 people.[46] Outbreaks have also been related to ingestion of raw oysters and clams[47] and to contaminated water supplies. Nosocomial spread of this disease has been documented.[41] In addition to its fecal-oral spread, there is some evidence that the Norwalk virus is transmitted through a respiratory route in the form of aerosolized particles from vomitus.[48] Although previously referred to as "winter vomiting disease,"[49] the Norwalk agent produces outbreaks of disease that can occur throughout the year.

Pathophysiology

The histologic changes induced by the Norwalk virus in an infected host have been studied in small bowel biopsies from infected volunteers.[50] Those volunteers who remained free of clinical symptoms had normal biopsy specimens, whereas those with symptoms exhibited marked, but nonspecific, changes, including focal areas of villous flattening and disorganization of epithelial cells. On electron microscopy, microvilli were shortened, and there was dilatation of the endoplasmic reticulum. These volunteers had repeat biopsies 2 weeks after the illness, and normal histology was again present. Other investigators have demonstrated the presence of normal gastric and rectal histology in patients suffering the effects of the Norwalk agent, as is typical of viral gastroenteritis.[40]

Clinical Manifestations

The clinical manifestations of disease produced by the Norwalk virus include nausea, vomiting, and cramping abdominal pain (see Table 46–1). Diarrhea is said to be a less consistent feature of this illness. In the original outbreak, only 44% of patients experienced diarrhea, whereas 84% had vomiting.[49] Other studies, however, have found that diarrhea occurs in most children who become ill from this virus.[51, 52] Fever occurs in approximately one third of affected patients. Respiratory symptoms are not typically a part of this illness, in contrast with rotaviral disease. An incubation period of approximately 48 hours has been noted before the onset of symptoms.[49] Symptoms persist from 12 to 48 hours, and following their resolution, no sequelae have been noted.

Diagnosis and Treatment

Development of techniques for diagnosis of the Norwalk virus has been difficult owing to the lack of methods for culturing the virus in vitro and the lack of an appropriate animal model. The identification of a protein-coding region of the Norwalk virus genome by Matsui and colleagues[53] may facilitate future research efforts in improving diagnostic and epidemiologic tools.

The treatment for Norwalk illness is supportive, using oral rehydration solutions if necessary. Significant dehydration is uncommon, and the need for hospitalization is rare.

Enteric Adenovirus

The enteric adenoviruses are among the most recently recognized viral pathogens that cause acute gastroenteritis. Adenoviruses are a large group of viruses long recognized for their role in the pathogenesis of respiratory infections and keratoconjunctivitis. Most of the 41 serotypes are known to be shed in the feces of infected patients. In patients with predominantly gastrointestinal symptoms, the organisms are detectable by electron microscopy of stool samples; however, they fail to grow using standard tissue culture conditions.[27] Their unique cell culture requirements allow for the differentiation of nonenteric adenoviruses from the enteric serotypes (Ad40 and Ad41), which are recognized to be the second commonest viral cause of childhood gastroenteritis.[54, 55]

Infection with enteric adenoviruses apparently occurs throughout the year, although a slight increase in incidence during the summer months has been noted.[56] This disease tends to affect predominantly younger children, with most patients being younger than 2 years of age.[57] Enteric adenovirus is spread by the fecal-oral route. Transmission of the disease to family contacts is unusual.

Diarrhea is the most commonly reported symptom from enteric adenoviral infection. In contrast with diarrhea from other viral enteritides, diarrhea from enteric adenovirus typically persists for a prolonged period, sometimes as long as 14 days. Viruses may be excreted in the feces of infected patients for 1 to 2 weeks.[56] Vomiting frequently occurs but is usually mild and of a much shorter duration than is the diarrhea. Dehydration has been seen in approximately half of affected patients, and hospitalization is sometimes necessary. The frequency of association of respiratory symptoms to infection with enteric adenovirus is unclear.[57]

The diagnosis of enteric adenovirus is best made by electron microscopy or IEM of stool samples or from intestinal biopsy specimens. ELISA[58] and PCR[59] techniques have also been used successfully in enteric adenovirus diagnosis. Treatment is mainly supportive, with oral rehydration solutions useful in cases of dehydration.

Calicivirus

Caliciviruses are grouped with the small, round structured viruses, which also include the Norwalk virus and astrovirus. Calicivirus, named for the cup-shaped depressions on its surface (from the Greek *calyx,* or cup), has been found to be responsible for approximately 3% of cases of diarrhea in studies evaluating a hospitalized population and a group of children in day care centers.[60, 61] This organism most commonly infects children in the 3-month to 6-year age group, and most children aged 12 years or older have developed calicivirus antibody.[62] Symptoms caused by calicivirus include vomiting and diarrhea, with fever and upper respiratory symptoms possible as well. Transmission occurs through person-to-person spread or through contamination of food or water.[62] There is evidence that an asymptomatic carrier state exists and that such persons may periodically excrete viruses.[63]

Astrovirus

Astrovirus, similar to calicivirus, is a single-stranded RNA virus grouped with the small, round structured viruses. Astrovirus is worldwide in distribution and tends to infect mainly children in the 1- to 3-year age group. Most children infected with astrovirus develop symptoms.[64] Vomiting, diarrhea, abdominal pain, and fever all are commonly seen with infection owing to this agent, and symptoms typically last 1 to 4 days.[62] Spread of the virus may occur via the fecal-oral route from person-to-person contact or through contaminated food or water. Asymptomatic shedding of astrovirus has also been reported.[65]

Other Viruses

A variety of other viruses are currently being studied to determine what role, if any, they may play in the pathogenesis of human enteric infections. Many candidate pathogens are loosely grouped under the title "small round viruses" (SRV). Caul and Appleton[43] have suggested a further division of this group into (1) featureless (or smooth) SRVs, including enteroviruses, parvoviruses, and "probable parvoviruses" (cockle, Ditchling, Parramatta, and Wollan agents) and (2) structured SRVs, including astrovirus, calicivirus, and the Norwalk virus and its relatives. With the exception of those viruses previously discussed in detail, insufficient data are available to ascertain clinical and epidemiologic differences, if any, among the various SRVs.

Pestivirus, a single-stranded RNA virus of the togavirus family, has been found in the feces of 24% of children living on an American Indian reservation who had diarrhea attributable to no other infectious agent.[66] These children experienced only mild diarrhea but had more severe respiratory complaints.

Coronavirus is known to cause an upper respiratory illness in humans and has been shown to cause diarrhea in some animals.[62] The role of this agent in human diarrheal disease is unclear, and at least one study found coronavirus more commonly in children without diarrhea than in those who were ill.[67] Interestingly, coronavirus has been implicated in an outbreak of necrotizing enterocolitis in a Dallas nursery.[68]

Toroviruses are pleomorphic viruses recognized to cause enteric illness in a variety of animals.[69] Members of this group, originally described in Berne, Switzerland, and Breda, Iowa, and named for those cities, have been seen in the feces of humans with diarrheal disease.[70] Their causative role in human disease, however, remains unproved. Similarly, picobirnavirus is known to cause disease in animals and has been isolated from stools of humans with diarrheal illness.[71]

Cytomegalovirus has been associated with enteritis and colitis, but this seems to occur almost exclusively among immunocompromised patients. In this population, cytomegalovirus causes a viremia and is carried by the blood stream to a variety of sites, including organs of the gastrointestinal tract.

BACTERIAL GASTROENTERITIS

Host-Defense Factors

For an infecting bacterial agent to cause diarrhea, it must first overcome the following gastrointestinal tract defenses: (1) gastric acidity, (2) intestinal motility, (3) mucus secretion, (4) normal intestinal microflora, and (5) specific mucosal and systemic immune mechanisms. Gastric acidity is the first barrier encountered by infecting organisms.[72] Many studies have demonstrated the bactericidal properties of gastric juice at pH less than 4.[73] In patients with achlorhydria or decreased gastric acid secretion, the gastric pH is higher, and this bactericidal effect is diminished. Gastric acidity then serves to decrease the number of viable bacteria that proceed to the small intestine.

Organisms surviving the gastric acidity barrier are trapped within the mucus layer of the small intestine, facilitating their movement through the intestine by peristalsis. If motility in the intestine is abnormal or absent, organisms are more readily able to initiate the infectious process. Some organisms can elaborate toxic substances that impair intestinal motility.[74] Increased intestinal peristalsis, which occurs during some enteric infections, may be an attempt by the host to rid itself of infective organisms.

In addition to its role in conjunction with intestinal motility, mucus also serves to provide a nonspecific barrier to bacterial proliferation and mucosal colonization.[75] This barrier has been shown to be effective in preventing toxins from exerting their effects. Exfoliated mucosal cells trapped in the mucus layer may trap invading microorganisms. Mucus also contains carbohydrate analogues of surface receptors, which may prevent invading organisms from binding to actual receptors.[76]

The normal endogenous microflora of the gut serves as its next line of defense. Anaerobes, which are a large component of the normal flora, elaborate short-chain fatty acids and lactic acid, which are toxic to many potential pathogens. In breast-fed infants, this line of defense is enhanced by the presence of anaerobic lac-

Table 46–2. BACTERIAL PATHOGENS GROUPED BY PATHOGENIC MECHANISM

Invasive	Cytotoxic	Toxigenic	Adherent
Shigella	*Shigella*	*Shigella*	Enteropathogenic *E. coli*
Salmonella	Enteropathogenic *Escherichia coli*	Enterotoxigenic *E. coli*	Enterohemorrhagic *E. coli*
Yersinia enterocolitica	Enterohemorrhagic *E. coli*	*Y. enterocolitica*	
Campylobacter jejuni	*Clostridium difficile*	*Aeromonas*	
Vibrio parahaemolyticus		Cholera and non-O1 vibrios	

From Cohen MB: Etiology and mechanisms of acute infectious diarrhea in infants in the United States. J Pediatr 1991; 118:S34–43; with permission.)

tobacilli, which produce fermentative products that act as toxins to foreign bacteria. Further evidence in support of the importance of endogenous microflora is the increase in susceptibility to infection after one's normal flora has been reduced by antibiotic administration, as is seen with *Clostridium difficile* infection.

The most complex element in the host-defense armamentarium involves the mucosal and systemic immune systems. Both serum and secretory antibodies may exert their protective effects at the intestinal level, even though the serum components are produced outside the gut. An immune response may be *specific* to a particular infective agent or *generalized* to a common group of bacterial antigens.

MECHANISMS OF BACTERIAL DISEASE PRODUCTION

Bacteria have developed a variety of virulence factors (Table 46–2) to overcome host-defense mechanisms: (1) *invasion* of the mucosa, followed by intraepithelial cell multiplication or invasion of the lamina propria; (2) production of *cytotoxins,* which disrupt cell function via direct alteration of the mucosal surface; (3) production of *enterotoxins,* polypeptides that alter cellular salt and water balance yet leave cell morphology undisturbed; and (4) *adherence* to the mucosal surface with resultant flattening of the microvilli and disruption of normal cell functioning. Each of the bacterial virulence mechanisms acts on specific regions of the intestine. Enterotoxins are primarily effective in the small bowel, whereas the effects of cytotoxin and direct epithelial cell invasion occur more commonly in the colon. Enteroadhesive mechanisms appear to function in both the small intestine and the colon.

Salmonella

Members of the species *Salmonella* are currently recognized as the commonest cause of bacterial diarrhea among children in the United States. Surveillance data from the Centers for Disease Control indicate that the incidence of disease caused by this bacteria is increasing.[77] Infection owing to *Salmonella* may present in one of several different clinical syndromes, including (1) acute gastroenteritis; (2) focal, nonintestinal infections; (3) bacteremia; (4) asymptomatic carrier state; and (5) enteric fever (including typhoid fever). Each of these entities may be caused by any of the commonly recognized species of *Salmonella.*

Microbiology

Salmonella is a motile, gram-negative bacillus of the family Enterobacteriaceae. It can be identified on selective media because it does not ferment lactose. Three distinct species of *Salmonella* are now recognized: *Salmonella enteritidis, Salmonella choleraesuis,* and *Salmonella typhi. S. enteritidis* is further subdivided into approximately 1,700 serotypes. Each serotype is referred to by its genus and serotype names (e.g., *Salmonella typhimurium*) rather than the formally correct *S. enteritidis,* serotype *typhimurium. S. choleraesuis* and *S. typhi* are known to have only one serotype each.

Epidemiology

Salmonella is estimated to cause 1 to 2 million gastrointestinal infections each year in the United States.[77] At Children's Hospital Medical Center, Cincinnati, salmonellae are the most commonly isolated bacterial enteropathogens (Fig. 46–2). The highest attack rate for salmonellosis is in infancy, with a lower incidence of symptomatic infection in patients older than 6 years[77, 78] (Fig. 46–3). Nontyphoidal *Salmonella* is usually spread via contaminated water supplies or foods, with meat and fowl, eggs, and raw milk frequently implicated. Although it is possible that any of these food sources might become contaminated through contact with an infected

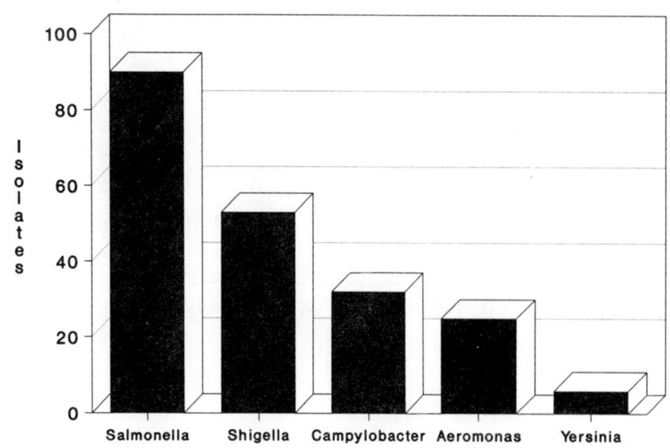

Figure 46–2. Bacterial enteropathogens isolated at Children's Hospital Medical Center, 1989. (Data from the Infection Control Office, Children's Hospital Medical Center, Cincinnati, Ohio.)

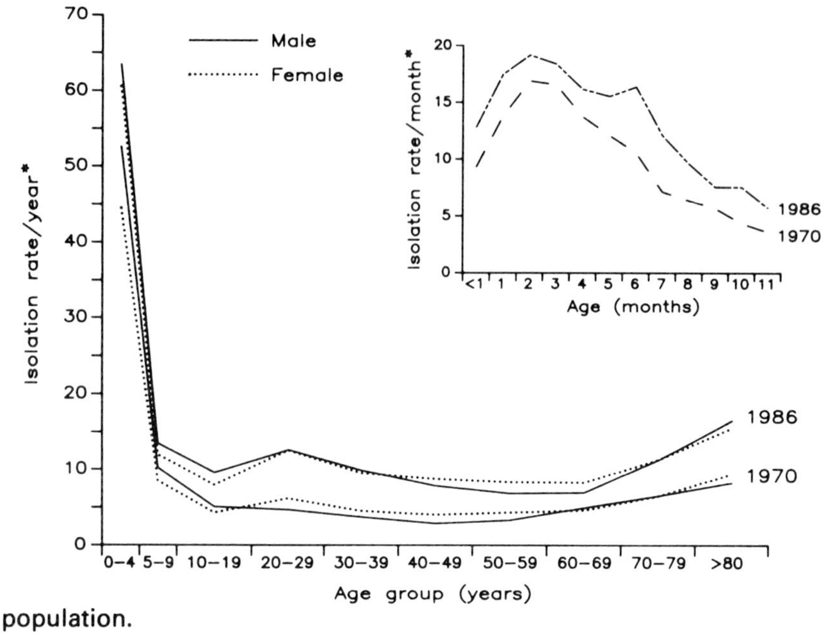

Figure 46–3. *Salmonella* isolation rates, by age and sex of patient, United States, 1970 and 1986. (From Hargrett-Bean NT, Pavia AT, Tauxe RV: *Salmonella* isolates from humans in the United States, 1984–1986. MMWR 1988; 37[SS-2]:25–31; with permission.)

food handler, the farm animals themselves are often infected. Pets, notably cats and turtles, may also harbor *Salmonella*. Person-to-person spread of infection also occurs and is especially common in cases involving infants.[79]

Pathogenesis

Inocula of less than 10^3 salmonellae are probably sufficient to cause disease.[79] Patients in whom host defenses are diminished are more likely to develop clinical manifestations of disease. This has been demonstrated in patients who have reduced levels of gastric acid.[72] Patients with lymphoproliferative diseases and hemolytic diseases, especially sickle cell anemia, are more likely to experience severe disease and develop complications from *Salmonella* infection. The mechanisms for this increased susceptibility may involve altered macrophage function,[80] defective complement activation,[81] or damage to the bones from thromboses.

Having overcome host defenses, *Salmonella* produces disease through a process that begins with colonization of the ileum and the colon. The organisms next invade enterocytes and colonocytes and proliferate within epithelial cells and in the lamina propria. From the lamina propria, *Salmonella* may then move to the mesenteric lymph nodes and eventually to the systemic circulation, causing bacteremia. Because these organisms invade enterocytes and colonocytes, both gastroenteritis, with watery diarrhea, and colitis, with bloody diarrhea, may result.

Clinical Manifestations

Following an incubation period of 12 to 72 hours, *Salmonella* usually produces a mild, self-limited illness characterized by fever and watery diarrhea. Blood or mucus or both are commonly present in the stool. Bacteremia occurs in approximately 6% of *Salmonella* infections in children but occurs much less frequently in adults.[82] Patients may develop sequelae following *Salmonella* infection, including pneumonia, meningitis, and osteomyelitis.

Even in those patients in whom no sequelae occur, excretion of the organisms may persist for several weeks. In patients younger than 5 years of age, the median time of excretion has been shown to be 7 weeks, with 2.6% of patients continuing to shed organisms for 1 year or longer.[83] Studies have also shown a higher incidence of the development of the carrier state among children who develop salmonellosis than is seen in adults.[83] Localization of *Salmonella* organisms in chronic carriers is often in the biliary tract and is frequently associated with cholelithiasis.

Diagnosis and Treatment

Diagnosis of *Salmonella* infection can be made through stool or blood culture. Culture of material from freshly passed stools, rather than culture from rectal swab, and use of enriched media increase the likelihood of recovering the organism.[83] Owing to the increased risk of developing the carrier state, antimicrobial treatment of uncomplicated cases of *Salmonella* gastroenteritis is not recommended.[84] Treatment is recommended in patients at high risk for the development of disseminated disease, including those who are immunocompromised, those with hematologic disease, patients with artificial implants, and pregnant women. Treatment is also recommended for patients at any age who appear toxic.

Treatment of children younger than 1 year of age with salmonellosis remains controversial because of the risk of bacteremia and secondary infections. Antimicrobial therapy is recommended for infants with *Salmonella* bacteremia. Parenteral antibiotics are recommended for any infant (younger than 3 months of age) with a stool culture that is positive for *Salmonella.*[85]

Most *Salmonella* are sensitive to a wide variety of antibiotics, including ampicillin (35 mg per kg [maximum 1 gm] per dose, given every 4 hours, intravenously, for 14 days), chloramphenicol (20 mg per kg [maximum 1 gm] per dose, given every 6 hours, intravenously or orally, for 14 days), trimethoprim-sulfamethoxazole (trimethoprim, 5 mg per kg [maximum 160 mg], plus sulfamethoxazole, 25 mg per kg [maximum 800 mg], given every 12 hours, orally, for 14 days), and the third-generation cephalosporins.[86] The emergence of antibiotic-resistant strains may reflect, in part, the widespread use of prophylactic antibiotics in the routine feeding of farm animals.[87]

A follow-up stool culture is generally not warranted unless a patient is employed in the preparation of food.[87] If evidence of a "cure" is necessary, two to three consecutive negative stool cultures, obtained 1 to 3 days apart, are sufficient.[87]

Typhoid Fever

Although uncommon in the United States, typhoid fever, caused by *S. typhi,* commonly affects children in developing countries. *S. typhi* differs from other salmonellae in that it requires a human host. The disease it causes also differs in severity from the typically mild gastroenteritis caused by other members of the genus and has a case fatality rate of 12 to 32%.[87]

Typhoid fever typically begins with a period of fever lasting approximately 1 week. Patients then complain of headache and abdominal pain. Diarrhea is not usually a manifestation of typhoid fever, and many patients experience constipation. Hepatomegaly and splenomegaly have also been frequently noted.[88] The characteristic "rose spots" (palpable, erythematous lesions) typical in adult cases of typhoid fever occur with far less frequency in pediatric patients.[88] Patients may become chronic carriers.

Diagnosis of typhoid fever is made on the basis of positive blood cultures. *S. typhi* is sensitive to several antimicrobial agents, including ampicillin, chloramphenicol, trimethoprim-sulfamethoxazole, and the third-generation cephalosporins. Ampicillin is the current drug of choice, and resistant strains are not typically encountered.[86]

A live oral vaccine from an attenuated strain of *S. typhi* (Ty21a) has been available in the United States since 1989; one recommended dosing schedule is four doses given every other day.[34] Current efforts are directed toward development of other attenuated strains, which may provide successful immunization in single-dose therapy.[89] Vaccine based on the Vi antigen from the *S. typhi* polysaccharide capsule is undergoing field trials.[34]

Shigella

Bacillary dysentery, an illness caused by *Shigella,* was described in ancient Greece. Osler,[90] in 1892, referred to the disease as "one of the four great epidemic diseases of the world." He further stated: "In the tropics it destroys more lives than cholera, and it has been more fatal to armies than powder and shot." Despite our increased knowledge of the pathogenesis and treatment of shigellosis, this organism continues to be a significant cause of diarrheal disease.

Microbiology

Shigella is a gram-negative, nonmotile, non–lactose-fermenting aerobic bacillus, closely related to members of the genus *Escherichia.* The organisms are classified into four species or groups known as *Shigella dysenteriae, Shigella flexneri, Shigella boydii,* and *Shigella sonnei* (groups A, B, C, and D, respectively). Members of groups A, B, and C exist in numerous serotypes, but only one serotype of group D is known.[91] *S. sonnei* is the most commonly recovered *Shigella* species in the developed world, accounting for 70% of isolates in the United States.[87] *S. dysenteriae* and *S. flexneri* are the most commonly recovered species of *Shigella* in the developing world.[91]

Epidemiology

Shigella is worldwide in its distribution, and the incidence and severity of shigellosis span an equally broad range. In Highland Mayan Indian children, the incidence of shigellosis was 1,900 cases per 1,000 children per year in the third year of life.[92] In the developed world, *Shigella* occurs much less frequently. Approximately 20% of the bacterial enteropathogens isolated at Children's Hospital Medical Center, Cincinnati, were *Shigella* (see Fig. 46–2). These data are in agreement with other studies that have found *Shigella* to be the second commonest pathogen identified in cases of bacterial diarrhea in children aged 6 months to 10 years.[93] It may also be the most common bacterial cause of outbreaks of diarrhea in day care settings.[94] Outbreaks of shigellosis have also been described in residential institutions. This disease is endemic on American Indian reservations in the Southwest.

Shigella is predominantly spread via the fecal-oral route, with person-to-person contact the most likely method. Secondary spread to household contacts may occur.[94] The infection may be spread through contamination of food and water, as often occurs in areas of poor sanitation and inadequate personal hygiene.[95] Spread of *Shigella* has also been documented to occur venereally among homosexual men.[96]

Clinical Manifestations

Patients infected with *Shigella* may experience a mild, self-limited watery diarrhea that is clinically indistinguishable from gastroenteritis caused by a variety of other agents. The more classic form of shigellosis, however, is bacillary dysentery. This illness usually begins with fever and malaise, followed by watery diarrhea and cramping abdominal pain. By the second day of illness, blood and mucus are usually present in the stools, and tenesmus has become a prominent symptom. At this point, in approximately 50% of affected patients, the stool volume decreases, with only scant amounts of blood and mucus being passed.[91] This pattern of bloody, mucus-containing stools is referred to as *dysentery*. Bacteremia is an uncommon feature of this illness[86]; however, several other complications have been reported, including seizures (in children), arthritis, purulent keratitis,[91] and the hemolytic uremic syndrome.[97] Nonsuppurative arthritis is the most commonly occurring extraintestinal complication of shigellosis.[98] Patients who carry the histocompatibility locus HLA-B27 may be predisposed to the development of this complication as well as to the development of Reiter's syndrome.[99] The association of seizures with shigellosis was earlier attributed to the neurotoxic effect of the *Shigella* toxin (Shiga toxin). It now seems likely, however, that the seizures may simply represent a subgroup of common febrile seizures and have no direct relationship to the effects of Shiga toxin.[95]

Pathogenesis

Shigella has been found to cause disease only in humans and in the higher apes.[91] The organisms are potent, with as few as 10 organisms being able to cause disease in a healthy adult.[100] Patients infected with *Shigella* may excrete 10^5 to 10^8 organisms per gr of feces.[95] This high rate of excretion and the relatively low number of organisms required to produce disease make possible the widespread distribution of disease.

For *Shigella* to exert its pathologic effects on a host, it is thought to require two factors: (1) the ability to invade cells, an attribute that is encoded for by a large invasiveness plasmid, and (2) the ability to multiply intracellularly.[101] Shiga toxin is elaborated by all species, although in greater amounts by *Shigella dysenteriae* than by other species,[91] and may also play a role in the pathogenesis of *Shigella* infection. The toxin has neurotoxic, enterotoxic, and cytotoxic effects.[78] Structurally, it is composed of an active, or A, subunit (molecular weight 32 Kd) surrounded by five binding, or B, subunits (77 Kd).[102] The B subunits bind to cell-specific receptors and are taken up by endocytosis.[95] Within the cell, the B subunits are cleaved away, and the remaining A subunit is shortened by proteolysis. This molecule is thought then to bind to the 60s ribosome and inhibit protein synthesis, leading to cell death and sloughing.[102] This is the presumed mechanism for the cytotoxic effect. An enterotoxic effect of Shiga toxin in the ileum may account for the early watery diarrhea.

Diagnosis and Treatment

In patients with signs and symptoms of colitis, the diagnosis of shigellosis should be considered. Stool culture provides the only definitive means to differentiate this organism from other invasive pathogens. *Shigella* may be cultured from stool specimens or rectal swabs, especially if mucopus is present, but there may be a delay of several days from the onset of symptoms to the recovery of organisms. Sigmoidoscopy or colonoscopy typically reveals a friable mucosa, possibly with discrete ulcers. Rectal biopsy may be useful to differentiate shigellosis from ulcerative colitis.[103]

In addition to rehydration, antimicrobial therapy has been recommended for *Shigella* (1) to shorten the course of the disease; (2) to decrease the period of excretion of the organisms[104]; and (3) to decrease the secondary attack rate, since humans provide the only reservoir for the organism. Those clinicians who advise against the routine treatment of shigellosis with antibiotics argue that (1) the disease is most often self-limited and (2) the use of antibiotics may facilitate the development of resistant strains[105] and may increase the likelihood of developing the hemolytic uremic syndrome as a sequela.[97] The authors recommend antibiotic therapy for patients who are severely ill at the time of diagnosis or who remain ill at the time of identification of *Shigella* in a stool culture.

A wide range of antibiotics has been used to treat *Shigella,* necessitated by the development of resistant strains. Currently, the agent of choice is trimethoprim-sulfamethoxazole (trimethoprim, 5 mg per kg [maximum 160 mg], plus sulfamethoxazole, 25 mg per kg [maximum 800 mg] per dose, given every 12 hours, orally or intravenously, for 5 days). Ampicillin (20 mg per kg [maximum 500 mg] per dose, given every 6 hours, orally or intravenously, for 5 days) may also be used if local strains are typically susceptible.[86] Amoxicillin is ineffective against *Shigella.*[106] Nalidixic acid (55 mg per kg per day given every 6 hours for 5 days) has also proved effective. Tetracycline, ciprofloxacin, and norfloxacin have been used successfully for the treatment of *Shigella,* but these agents should be used only in adult patients.[86]

Development of a vaccine for shigellosis is currently underway. These efforts include vaccines using a modified *Escherichia coli* strain; one employing a mutant strain of *S. flexneri,* which lacks the ability to proliferate intracellularly; and one based on a strain with mutations in its virulence genes.[34]

Campylobacter

Microbiology

Campylobacter is a gram-negative, motile, curved or spiral-shaped rod, exhibiting a "seagull" appearance when identified in stained stool smears.[107] Multiple species of *Campylobacter* have been recognized, including *Campylobacter jejuni, Campylobacter fetus, Campylobacter coli,* and *Campylobacter laridis,* with *C. jejuni* being the one most commonly associated with disease in humans.[108] *Campylobacter upsaliensis* has been reported as another member of this group that causes diarrhea,[109] and it seems probable that still others may be identified.

Epidemiology

Campylobacter is recognized to be worldwide in distribution. In developing countries, *Campylobacter* is a significant bacterial cause of diarrhea in children younger than 2 years of age, yet it rarely occurs in those same areas in older children and adults.[87] When infection does occur in the population older than 2 years of age, it tends to be asymptomatic.[110] It is likely that patients in these countries are infected with *Campylobacter* early in life and then develop immunity, thus making asymptomatic infection more typical in older children and adults.

In the industrialized world, most patients infected with *Campylobacter* develop symptoms.[110] The number of *Campylobacter* infections in these countries is now recognized to be quite high, with some studies finding this organism to be the commonest cause of bacterial diarrhea.[87] Interestingly, *Campylobacter* tends to infect people in two distinct age groups: children in the first year of life and young adults (Fig. 46–4).[111]

Campylobacter may be spread by direct contact or through contaminated sources of food and water. Milk, meat, and eggs, especially if undercooked, have been implicated in outbreaks. These sources may be contaminated from human fecal shedding, or the organisms may be harbored in the asymptomatic farm animals.[112] *Campylobacter* is commonly spread among populations of children in day care centers.

Pathogenesis

The mechanisms through which *Campylobacter* produce disease are not fully understood. Walker and coworkers[108] have identified three potential mechanisms: (1) adherence to the intestinal mucosa followed by the elaboration of toxin; (2) invasion of the mucosa in the terminal ileum and colon; and (3) "translocation," in which the organisms penetrate the mucosa and replicate in the lamina propria and mesenteric lymph nodes. The variety of pathogenic mechanisms may account for the spectrum of disease caused by *Campylobacter*. It is also conceivable that different strains or serotypes of *Campylobacter* may demonstrate different pathogenic mechanisms,[87] as is seen with *E. coli*.

Clinical Manifestations

Campylobacter may cause disease ranging from mild diarrhea to frank dysentery. Typically, patients experience fever and malaise followed by diarrhea, nausea, and abdominal pain that may mimic appendicitis[78] or inflammatory bowel disease. The symptoms usually resolve in less than 1 week.[113] Bacteremia may rarely occur, with some species implicated more often than are others.[114] *Campylobacter* is also known to cause meningitis, abscesses, septic abortions, pancreatitis, and pneumonia. Guillain-Barré syndrome and Reiter's syndrome are documented to occur as sequelae of *Campylobacter* infection.[87] Following the resolution of symptoms, patients may continue to shed organisms for as long as 7 weeks.[115]

Diagnosis and Treatment

Campylobacter can be recognized by microscopic examination of a Gram-stained stool smear or by darkfield microscopy. Methylene blue examination of stool smears for fecal leukocytes has also proved useful in the diagnosis of *Campylobacter* infection.[116] Culture of the organisms, the gold standard for diagnosis, is routinely accomplished in most laboratories if selective media are used and cultures are incubated at 42°C. Because disease caused by *Campylobacter* is usually mild and self-limited, supportive treatment alone should suffice. In cases of severe disease, erythromycin (10 mg per kg [maxi-

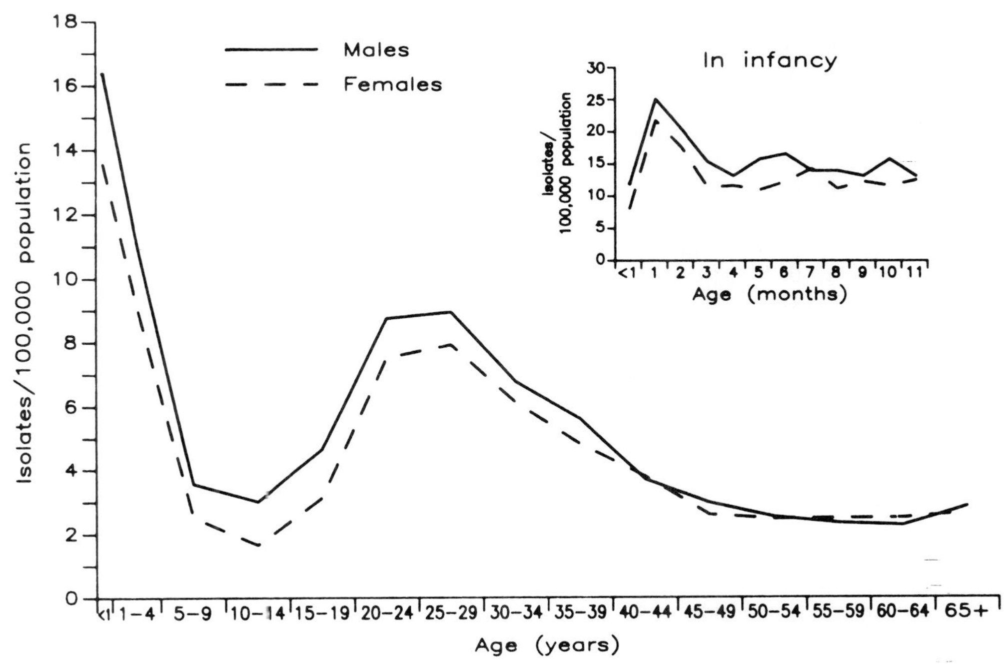

Figure 46–4. Annual isolation rates of *Campylobacter* by age and sex, United States, 1982–1986. (From Tauxe RV, Hargrett-Bean N, Patton CM, et al: *Campylobacter* isolates in the United States, 1982–1986. MMWR 1988; 37[SS-2]:1–13.)

mum 500 mg] per dose, given every 6 hours for 5 to 7 days) has been recommended.[86] The need for antibiotic therapy has been questioned, based in part on several studies that demonstrated a decrease in the duration of excretion of *Campylobacter* following antibiotic treatment but no decrease in the duration of symptoms. In general, in these studies, antimicrobial therapy was begun late in the course of the illness. In a placebo-controlled, double-blind trial, Salazar-Lindo and colleagues[117] demonstrated a shortened duration of illness, from 4.2 to 2.5 days, in patients who received erythromycin by day 4 of their illness. For cases of *Campylobacter* septicemia, gentamicin (1.5 to 2.5 mg per kg per dose, intramuscularly or intravenously, given every 8 hours) is recommended, with chloramphenicol and erythromycin acceptable as alternatives. Tetracycline (250 to 500 mg per dose, intravenously, given every 6 to 12 hours) may be used in patients older than 8 years of age.[86] Antibiotic treatment is recommended for outbreaks of *Campylobacter* in day care settings because treatment has been shown to eliminate fecal shedding of organisms within 48 hours.[108]

Yersinia

Microbiology

The genus *Yersinia* includes the species *Yersinia pestis,* which causes plague; *Yersinia pseudotuberculosis,* known to cause pseudoappendicitis, mesenteric adenitis, and gastroenteritis; and *Yersinia enterocolitica,* recognized with increasing frequency as a cause of bacterial diarrhea. *Yersinia* is a gram-negative, coccoid bacillus that is facultatively anaerobic. It is non–lactose-fermenting and is observed to be motile at temperatures of 25°C but nonmotile at 37°C.

Epidemiology

Yersinia was initially thought to occur with greater frequency in countries with cooler climates[118] but is now recognized to be worldwide in distribution. Although the true incidence and prevalence of this organism are not known, in some areas yersiniosis occurs more frequently than does shigellosis.[119] Outbreaks due to *Yersinia* have been associated with spread through contaminated water and foods, including bean sprouts, tofu, and chocolate milk.[119, 120] Pork has also been implicated as a source, as in the Fulton County, Georgia, outbreak in 1990, in which chitterlings were found to be the vehicle of infection.[121, 122] The organism tends to cause disease more frequently in young children, with 24 months the median age in one study.[123] *Yersinia* may also be spread among household contacts. In addition, there may be an increased incidence in the summer months.[119, 123]

Pathogenesis

Y. enterocolitica produces disease through an invasive route. After penetrating the mucosal epithelium, primarily in the ileum, organisms replicate in Peyer's patches and accumulate in the mesenteric lymph nodes.[119] Most serotypes produce an enterotoxin similar to the *E. coli* heat-stable toxin but only at temperatures higher than 30°C; therefore, it may *not* have an important role in disease production by *Yersinia* in the human intestine. There is speculation on the role of preformed toxin in causing disease, because toxin may be produced when the organisms are present in refrigerated foods.[119]

The virulence of *Y. enterocolitica* has been shown to be plasmid related. Different serotypes exhibit different degrees of virulence. Serotypes O:3, O:8, and O:9 are the ones most frequently associated with diarrheal disease.[119]

Clinical Manifestations

The most frequent clinical syndrome caused by *Y. enterocolitica* is gastroenteritis, which typically affects young children. After an incubation period of 1 to 11 days, patients develop diarrhea, fever, and abdominal pain.[119] A marked increase in white blood cell count is common. The symptoms usually resolve in 5 to 14 days but have been known to persist for several months. Excretion of organisms occurs for about 6 weeks.[123] Several complications, including appendicitis, have been documented following *Y. enterocolitica* infection.

In older children and young adults, *Yersinia* is more likely to produce the pseudoappendicular syndrome, in which signs and symptoms mimic appendicitis.[119] In this same age group, there has also been an association of *Y. enterocolitica* with nonspecific abdominal pain.[124] Radiographic changes in the terminal ileum more often associated with Crohn's disease, namely mucosal thickening and aphthous ulcers, have been seen with yersiniosis in young adults.[78]

Yersinia bacteremia occurs, and despite therapy with appropriate antibiotics, has a case fatality rate of 34 to 50%. The finding of *Yersinia* in blood from asymptomatic donors, however, makes the possibility of transient bacteremia seem likely as well.[119]

Sequelae following *Yersinia* infection include erythema nodosum and reactive arthropathy. This arthropathy tends to involve the weight-bearing joints of the lower extremities and has been noted to occur most often in *Yersinia* patients who carry the histocompatibility antigen HLA-B27.[125]

Diagnosis and Treatment

Yersinia may be cultured using selective media, preferably with "cold enrichment." Despite the best of methods, culture of *Yersinia* may require as long as 4 weeks. In addition to diagnosis by culture, *Yersinia* may also be detected serologically, through the use of agglutinin titers. These measurements appear to be useful only in conjunction with cultures, because agglutinin titers may be affected by a number of factors, including the patient's age and underlying disease and the previous use of antibiotics and immunosuppressive agents.[126]

Antibiotics have not been proved effective in alleviating symptoms of *Yersinia* or in shortening the period of its excretion.[119] Pai and associates[127] compared the efficacy of trimethoprim-sulfamethoxazole versus placebo in the treatment of *Yersinia* gastroenteritis and found no significant difference. It should be noted, however, that therapy was not begun until near the end of the course of the illness.[127] In cases of severe disease or in patients with underlying illness, treatment is recommended. Trimethoprim-sulfamethoxazole, aminoglycosides, chloramphenicol, and third-generation cephalosporins are generally recommended. Tetracycline and quinolones are alternative choices for adult patients.[86] Gentamicin or chloramphenicol is recommended for treatment of septicemia.

Cholera

Although cholera is a disease rarely encountered in developed countries, it remains an important entity. Investigation of the pathogenesis of cholera led to the recognition and the understanding of the mechanism of action of cholera toxin, which remains the prototype for bacterial enterotoxins. Cholera is also important, from a therapeutic perspective, in that initial efforts in the use of oral rehydration solutions were carried out in patients with cholera. Finally, cholera remains a disease capable of epidemic spread through parts of the world in which sanitation is poorly developed, as evidenced by the epidemic that began in Peru in early 1991.[128]

Microbiology

Vibrio cholerae is a gram-negative, motile, curved bacillus that is free-living in bodies of salt water.[129] *V. cholerae* is classified on the basis of antigens into group O1 and non-O1. Non-O1 *V. cholerae* are also referred to as *nonagglutinable* ("NAG") *vibrios*. Group O1 is further subdivided into two biotypes: classic and El Tor. The classic biotype was traditionally the agent responsible for epidemic cholera. In the current pandemic, however, the El Tor biotype has replaced the classic biotype in all areas except in southern Bangladesh.[130] The El Tor biotype is also responsible for sporadic cases of cholera and has been shown to have a significantly lower infection to case ratio than does the classic biotype.[131] Several other vibrios produce diarrheal disease, including *Vibrio parahaemolyticus, Vibrio mimicus,* and *Vibrio fluvialis.*

Epidemiology

V. cholerae is spread via contamination of food and water supplies. There is no evidence of an animal reservoir, but humans may serve as transient carriers.[131] On rare occasions, humans may chronically carry the organism, with the gallbladder identified as the site of carriage.[132]

Owing to the nature of its spread, persons living in areas with adequate sanitation are at minimal, if any, risk for encountering cholera. Travel to endemic areas has been of concern; however, if normal precautions are taken, such as drinking bottled water and eating no raw or undercooked foods, the risk to American travelers in endemic areas is less than one in 500,000.[133] Cholera has for centuries been endemic to Asia and the Indian subcontinent. The United States Gulf Coast is now also recognized as an endemic area.[134]

Pathogenesis

V. cholerae enters its potential host through the oral route, usually in contaminated food or water. Volunteer studies have shown that a relatively large number of organisms—approximately 1 million—must be ingested to produce symptoms.[135] Similar to other ingested organisms, *V. cholerae* must survive the acidic gastric environment. The importance of this as a host-protective factor is borne out by the increased occurrence of cholera in patients with absent or reduced gastric acidity.[72, 135]

The organisms travel to the small intestine, where they adhere to the epithelium. This process may be aided by production of mucinase.[135] The intestinal epithelium remains intact with normal morphology.[136] *Vibrio* species produce a toxin that is composed of a central subunit (A) surrounded by five B subunits; the latter bind to a ganglioside, GM_1, which serves as the toxin receptor. This binding facilitates the transfer of the A subunit across the cell membrane, where it is cleaved into two components denoted A_1 and A_2. The disulfide linkage between A_1 and A_2 is reduced to liberate an active A_1 peptide, which acts as a catalyst to facilitate the transfer of adenosine diphosphate–ribose from nicotinamide adenine dinucleotide to a guanylnucleotide-binding regulatory protein (G_s). G_s then stimulates adenylate cyclase, located on the basolateral membrane, thereby increasing cyclic AMP. This result in turn leads to chloride secretion and a net flux of fluid into the intestinal lumen.[137]

Although this mechanism of toxin action adequately explains the clinical symptoms of cholera, similar symptoms have been noted in patients infected with strains that do *not* produce the classic cholera toxin. This finding has led to the speculation that multiple toxins, or other forms of the classic toxin, may be involved in the pathogenesis of cholera.[129]

Clinical Manifestations

After an incubation period, which ranges from 5 hours to 6 days,[129] the symptoms of cholera usually begin abruptly with vomiting and profuse, watery diarrhea. The stool soon becomes clear, with bits of mucus giving it the so-called rice-water appearance. Patients do not experience tenesmus but rather a sense of relief with defecation.[129] Fever is typically not present. The rate of fluid loss with cholera is remarkable, with rates in excess of 1 L per hour reported in adult patients.[136]

Diagnosis and Treatment

V. cholerae may be easily grown from culture of fecal material in 6 to 10 hours. It is a "most unfastidious

Table 46–3. DIARRHEOGENIC *ESCHERICHIA COLI*

Name	Abbreviation	Pathogenic Mechanisms	Illness	Diagnosis
Enteropathogenic *E. coli*	EPEC	Adherence to enterocytes	Infantile diarrhea in underdeveloped countries	Serotype Biopsy Enterocyte adherence factor gene probe
Enterotoxigenic *E. coli*	ETEC	Enterotoxin elaboration	Infantile diarrhea in underdeveloped countries Traveler's diarrhea	Bioassay Immunoassays Gene probe for toxins
Enteroinvasive *E. coli*	EIEC	Invasion of epithelial cells	Dysenterylike symptoms	Bioassay Gene probe
Enterohemorrhagic *E. coli*	EHEC	Cytotoxin elaboration	Hemorrhagic colitis	Serotyping Gene probe
Diffuse adhering *E. coli*	DAEC	?Adherence	?Childhood diarrhea ?Traveler's diarrhea	Adherence pattern to specific cell culture lines
Enteroaggregative *E. coli*	EAggEC	?Enterotoxin elaboration	Persistent diarrhea in underdeveloped countries	Adherence pattern to specific cell culture lines Gene probe

pathogen," requiring only standard bacteriologic media.[131] The mainstay of cholera treatment is rehydration. In cases in which the disease is less severe and recognized early, oral rehydration solutions are appropriate and effective. When purging is excessive (>10 ml per kg per hr) intravenous rehydration is required.

Antibiotics have been shown to cause a decrease in the duration of diarrhea, the total amount of fluid lost, and the length of time organisms are excreted.[129] Tetracycline (250 to 500 mg per dose, given every 6 hours for 3 to 5 days) has been recommended as an appropriate antibiotic for adults,[136] and furazolidone (1.25 mg per kg [maximum 100 mg] per dose, given every 6 hours for 10 days) has been suggested for children[138] and pregnant patients. Ampicillin, chloramphenicol, trimethoprim-sulfamethoxazole, and doxycycline may also be used. Cholera vaccines, available for a number of years, provide only limited protection for a brief period and are therefore not currently recommended.

Other Vibrios

The noncholera vibrios, *V. parahaemolyticus, V. fluvialis, V. mimicus,* and several others, have been shown to cause gastrointestinal illnesses as well as wound infections and septicemia. Although each organism has its own characteristics, most noncholera vibrios produce a protein toxin identical to the classic cholera toxin.[129] Some species also produce a heat-stable toxin similar to *E. coli* heat-stable toxin.[139, 140] Although these organisms produce a choleralike illness, the stool may sometimes contain blood and leukocytes. This has led to speculation that some members of this group, namely *V. parahaemolyticus,* may be capable of invasiveness as well as toxin production.[129] In the United States, gastroenteritis caused by these vibrios is most often associated with the ingestion of raw oysters.[141]

Gastroenteritis caused by non-O1 vibrios tends to be far milder than that caused by *V. cholerae.* In severe cases of diarrhea or septicemia, antibiotics may be helpful, with the agents used for *V. cholerae* recommended.

Escherichia Coli

E. coli is a gram-negative bacteria of the family Enterobacteriaceae. The species constitutes a diverse group of organisms, including *nonpathogenic* strains, which are among the most common bacteria in the normal flora of the human intestine, and *pathogenic* strains, which are the most commonly identified gram-negative pathogens. Pathogenic *E. coli* strains that cause diarrheal illnesses have been recognized since the 1940s.[142, 143]

These diarrheogenic *E. coli* have been studied extensively and are currently classified, on the basis of serogrouping or pathogenic mechanisms, into four major groups[142]: (1) *enteropathogenic E. coli* (EPEC), an important cause of diarrhea in infants in underdeveloped countries; (2) *enterotoxigenic E. coli* (ETEC), a cause of diarrhea in infants in poorly developed areas of the world and a cause of traveler's diarrhea in adults; (3) *enteroinvasive E. coli* (EIEC), which cause a dysentery-like illness; and (4) *enterohemorrhagic E. coli* (EHEC), which cause hemorrhagic colitis. Each of these groups of *E. coli* has its own unique properties (Table 46–3). Two other provisional categories of diarrheogenic *E. coli* are defined on the basis of their ability to produce distinctive patterns of adherence in tissue culture: (1) *diffuse adhering E. coli* (DAEC), which may cause diarrhea in children[144] and travelers; and (2) *enteroaggregative E. coli* (EAggEC), which may cause persistent diarrhea in children in developing countries.[145]

Enteropathogenic Escherichia Coli

The high frequency of occurrence of EPEC is limited to areas in which sanitary conditions are suboptimal.[142] In the United States, EPEC infection is now uncommon. EPEC have been associated with community outbreaks of disease and have also been described as causing sporadic cases of protracted diarrhea.[146–148]

EPEC have been shown to cause disease as a result of adherence to the brush border membrane of enterocytes, which causes destruction of microvilli, evident by electron microscopy, and resultant loss of cell function.[142] An enterocyte adherence factor is encoded by a specific plasmid.[142] This plasmid has been shown to be specifically responsible for the pathogenicity of EPEC strains.[149] EPEC generally does not produce toxins and does not invade host cells.

Patients with symptomatic EPEC infection typically experience diarrhea, vomiting, malaise, and fever. The stool may contain mucus but does not usually contain blood. Symptoms with EPEC infection are more severe than with some other enteric infections and may persist for 2 weeks or longer.[142] In some patients, EPEC have caused protracted diarrhea with dehydration, malnutrition, and zinc deficiency as complications; treatment with parenteral hyperalimentation has been required.[147] EPEC can be detected by serotyping of isolated *E. coli*[145, 146] or by demonstrating the presence of the enterocyte adherence factor by gene probe technology.[150] Diagnosis of EPEC may be made by demonstrating the presence of adherent organisms on small intestinal or rectal biopsy.[145–147]

Although controlled studies of antibiotic therapy for EPEC have been few, the significant morbidity associated with this agent argues for treatment with antibiotics in most cases. Trimethoprim-sulfamethoxazole (trimethoprim, 5 mg per kg [maximum 160 mg], plus sulfamethoxazole, 25 mg per kg [maximum 800 mg], given every 12 hours) has been used with some success, as have oral neomycin and gentamicin.

Enterotoxigenic Escherichia Coli

ETEC are recognized as an important cause of diarrhea in infants in less-developed areas of the world. In endemic areas, children in the first few years of life may be infected several times each year.[151] In the United States, cases of ETEC among children are uncommon.[87, 152]

The production of disease by ETEC begins with colonization of the small intestine. There the bacteria depend on fimbriae (also called *pili*) to facilitate attachment to the mucosal surface and overcome the forward motion of peristalsis.[142] This attachment process causes no detectable structural changes in the architecture of the brush border membrane but does allow the bacteria to release their enterotoxins, heat-labile toxin (LT) and heat-stable toxin (ST), in close proximity to the enterocyte brush border membrane where toxin receptors are present.[153] These toxins in turn stimulate either adenylate cyclase (in the case of LT) or guanylate cyclase (in the case of ST), and both ultimately result in a net fluid secretion from the intestine.[154]

Clinically ETEC infection causes nausea, abdominal pain, and watery diarrhea.[142] Stools typically contain neither mucus nor leukocytes. ETEC can be diagnosed by the use of bioassays such as the suckling mouse assay,[155] immunoassays, or gene probes specific for either ST[156] or LT.[157] There are currently no widely available practical assays for the diagnosis of ETEC.

Supportive measures are sufficient therapy for most cases of ETEC diarrhea, with oral rehydration a mainstay of therapy. Antibiotics, including trimethoprim-sulfamethoxazole, have been shown to decrease the duration of diarrhea due to ETEC and to shorten the duration of fecal excretion of the organisms.[158] Possibly of greater importance in the future management of ETEC-associated disease is the development of vaccines against the organism. Clinical trials involving prototype vaccines of several types, including live oral vaccines and nonliving antigen vaccines, have been undertaken with encouraging results.[34]

Enteroinvasive Escherichia Coli

EIECs differ from most members of the species in that they are often nonmotile and are unable to ferment lactose. These properties are similar to those observed with shigellae. EIEC and shigellae also share common virulence mechanisms. These organisms preferentially colonize the colon and invade and replicate within epithelial cells, where they cause cell death.[142]

In light of the fact that EIEC produces disease in a manner similar to *Shigella,* it is not surprising that these organisms cause symptoms of dysentery. Patients experience cramping abdominal pain and tenesmus. Watery diarrhea occurs initially, later progressing to stools mixed with mucus and leukocytes. Gross blood is not always present in the stool,[159] and bacteremia does not occur.

Infection due to EIEC is uncommon, but outbreaks of disease have occurred in the United States. Diagnosis is dependent on bioassay (the Sérény test), serotyping, ELISA, or deoxyribonucleic acid probe techniques.[160] EIEC should be considered in the differential diagnosis of dysentery-like illnesses. Treatment is currently limited to supportive measures, although ampicillin given intramuscularly has been associated with bacteriologic cure and clinical improvement.[159]

Enterohemorrhagic Escherichia Coli

EHEC have been recognized to cause a syndrome of hemorrhagic colitis. In some studies, this organism is found to be the commonest cause of acute bloody diarrhea.[161]

EHEC may occur in sporadic cases but has also been associated with outbreaks of disease in nursing homes, day care centers, and other institutions.[142] Food-borne spread is often implicated in these disease outbreaks, with hamburger and unpasteurized milk both documented as vehicles.[162, 163]

EHEC may cause disease through the production of cytotoxins, similar if not identical to those produced by shigellae. These toxins have also been shown to have a cytopathic effect on HeLa and Vero cells. For these reasons, the toxins are known alternatively as *Shigalike toxins* or *verotoxins.*[142] Certain Shigalike toxins bind to a globotriosylceramide receptor on the intestinal cell surface. This stimulates a sequence of events leading to disruption of the 60s ribosome with consequent interruption of cellular protein synthesis.[164]

Clinically EHEC may produce a wide range of symptoms ranging from relatively mild watery diarrhea to bloody diarrhea to a potentially severe hemorrhagic colitis.[165] Patients usually experience cramping associated with diarrhea, but fever is atypical.[165] Symptoms may persist from a few days to 2 weeks. Endoscopic examination in cases of hemorrhagic colitis may reveal diffuse mucosal edema, with areas of hemorrhage especially likely in the ascending and proximal transverse colon.[162] Histologic findings may range from normal to the presence of pseudomembranes.

Hemolytic uremic syndrome, characterized by microangiopathic hemolytic anemia, uremia, and thrombocytopenia, has been shown to occur as a sequela of approximately 10% of cases of hemorrhagic colitis due to EHEC.[165, 166] Thrombotic thrombocytopenic purpura is another, albeit less frequent, sequela of EHEC infection. Both hemorrhagic colitis due to EHEC and the sequelae of hemolytic uremic syndrome have been observed to occur with greater frequency in younger patients.

Diagnosis of EHEC may be made by serotyping, with the serotype O157:H7 frequently responsible.[167] Immunoassays and gene probe techniques are also available for diagnosis.[168]

Treatment of EHEC disease is currently limited to supportive measures. Antibiotics have not been proved to be beneficial. The most important aspect of therapy is making the correct diagnosis and thereby avoiding other diagnostic procedures or surgery for the bloody diarrhea. In all cases of bloody diarrhea in which EHEC is suspected, the astute clinician should be aware of the possible sequelae, especially hemolytic uremic syndrome, and monitor the patient accordingly.

Clostridium Difficile

C. difficile is a gram-positive anaerobic bacillus. Disease caused by this organism may manifest itself in a variety of ways, ranging from asymptomatic carriage to potentially life-threatening pseudomembranous colitis. This organism has been primarily, but not exclusively, associated with illness following disruption of the normal intestinal flora by antibiotics.

Epidemiology

Of great interest in the study of *C. difficile* is the difference in the incidence of isolation of the organism and its toxin in various age groups. *C. difficile* toxin has been found in the feces of 10% of normal-term neonates and 55% of those in a neonatal intensive care unit (NICU).[169] The substantially higher incidence of toxin excretion in the NICU patients has been interpreted by some authors as evidence for nosocomial spread of *C. difficile.* Most infants found to have toxin in their stools were asymptomatic. A small group of toxin-positive infants had signs and symptoms of necrotizing enterocolitis, but no clear relationship to *C. difficile* or its toxin could be demonstrated. The presence of *C. difficile* toxin in these asymptomatic infants may indicate the coexistence of some protective antitoxic substance,[170] or may reflect a lack of appropriate toxin receptors in patients in this age group.[171]

The incidence of *C. difficile* toxin positivity decreases beyond the neonatal period. In one group of children younger than 2 years of age admitted for evaluation of diarrhea, only 4.9% were found to have *C. difficile* organisms, and not all of those had *C. difficile* toxin.[172] Groups of healthy adults examined for the presence of *C. difficile* have been found to have a 3% positivity rate.[169] Adults who develop disease owing to *C. difficile* are also more likely than children to experience severe colitis symptoms.

Pathogenesis

The pathogenesis of *C. difficile* diarrhea is not fully understood, but the organism is known to elaborate two cytotoxins, A and B. Toxin A also exhibits enterotoxin activity. Only those strains of *C. difficile* that produce toxins are known to cause disease. The presence of toxins themselves is apparently not sufficient to provoke clinical symptoms, and host response factors must be invoked to explain asymptomatic infection in infants. Pantosti and colleagues[173] demonstrated that different strains may be involved in asymptomatic and symptomatic infections. In adults, the presence of both *C. difficile* and toxin is almost always coexistent with disease.[169]

Clinical Manifestations

C. difficile may cause an illness that is in many ways indistinguishable from that caused by other common enteric pathogens. Patients experience mild, watery diarrhea, which lasts only a few days and spontaneously resolves. Most of these patients clear the bacteria within 21 days.[174] In some patients, however, symptoms may persist for weeks to months. Sigmoidoscopic examination in these patients has occasionally revealed ulcerated mucosal lesions more commonly seen with pseudomembranous colitis.

Pseudomembranous colitis is the disease that is classically associated with *C. difficile.* Patients with this disease are often extremely ill with high fever, leukocytosis, and hypoalbuminemia. Stools from these patients are mixed with blood and leukocytes.

Diagnosis and Treatment

C. difficile should be suspected in cases of colitis or in cases of mild diarrhea in which blood and leukocytes are noted in the stool. Concurrent or recent exposure (within several weeks) to antibiotics should increase the suspicion of *C. difficile* as the causative agent of colitis or mild diarrhea. It should be remembered that the use of virtually all antibiotics may predispose to *C. difficile* disease.[87]

Diagnosis of *C. difficile* can be made by culture of the organism and examination for the presence of toxin in feces. Current laboratory detection of *C. difficile* toxin requires the use of a tissue culture system, with demonstration of a cytopathic effect that can be neutralized by specific antitoxin. Other assays, including a latex agglutination test, show promise as more rapid clinical tools. There is some evidence to suggest a correlation between higher toxin levels and symptoms of increased severity.[175] Sigmoidoscopy in cases of pseudomembranous colitis typically reveals friable white exudate overlying multiple ulcerated areas.[176] The histologic findings of such lesions are depicted in Figure 46–5. Pseudomembranes may not be found in the rectosigmoid but may be present in the more proximal colon.

In cases of mild diarrheal illness due to *C. difficile*, discontinuation of any antibiotics the patient is receiving may be sufficient therapy. In cases of severe illness and especially in cases of pseudomembranous colitis, treatment should also include oral vancomycin (5–10 mg per kg [maximum 500 mg] given every 6 hours for 7 days)[86, 177] or metronidazole (5–10 mg per kg [maximum 500 mg] every 8 hours for 7 days).[178]

There is a fairly high rate of relapse of illness—nearly 40% in some series—following treatment of *C. difficile*.[179] These relapses usually occur within 1 month of completion of therapy and have been thought possibly to result from the activation of *C. difficile* spores remaining from the primary infection.[179] Most of these cases of relapse are responsive to a second course of vancomycin or metronidazole. There are reports of multiple relapses in which cholestyramine, given as a slurry (120 mg per kg per dose every 8 hours) for 4 weeks and tapered over the following 3 weeks, was effective in eradication of the organism.[179] Intravenously administered gamma globulin is an alternative therapy for chronic *C. difficile* enterocolitis.[180]

Aeromonas and *Plesiomonas*

Within the past few years, several organisms not previously recognized as enteric pathogens have been linked to diarrheal disease. This includes organisms of the genus *Aeromonas* and the closely related bacterium *Plesiomonas shigelloides* (previously classified as *Aeromonas shigelloides*). These organisms are gram-negative, facultatively anaerobic bacilli classified in the family Vibrionaceae. They are oxidase positive, differentiating them from members of the Enterobacteriaceae.[181]

Aeromonas

Several members of the genus *Aeromonas,* including *Aeromonas hydrophila,* are common inhabitants of fresh and brackish water in the United States.[181] These organisms were initially recognized as opportunistic pathogens in immunocompromised hosts, especially those with malignant hematologic diseases. The organisms also have been known to cause disease in patients with underlying hepatobiliary disease.[181] *Aeromonas* has been isolated from healthy persons as well and has therefore been thought to be part of the normal flora. Despite initial studies that yielded conflicting results,[182] it is now generally accepted that *A. hydrophila* is an enteric pathogen.

Studies in Australian children with diarrhea have found *Aeromonas* species present in 10% of patients.[183] Infection appears to occur most frequently in children younger than 2 years of age.[184] Of patients with *Aeromonas* isolated from stool cultures at Children's Hospital Medical Center, Cincinnati, in 1990, approximately 50% were younger than 3 months (Fig. 46–6). *Aeromonas* infection occurs more often in the summer months.[181]

It is known that not all *Aeromonas* species are pathogenic. The method of pathogenesis remains unclear.[87] Both cytotoxic[184] and enterotoxic[181] properties have been observed, but neither these nor other pathogenic mechanisms are found consistently in strains isolated from patients with *Aeromonas*-associated disease.[182] *Aeromonas caviae,* a commonly isolated species, demonstrates both adherence and cytotoxin production.[185]

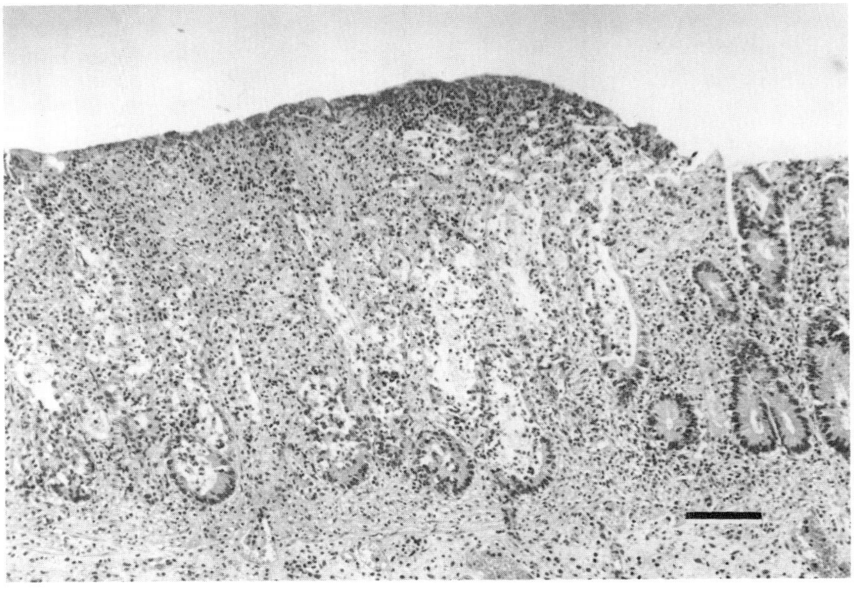

Figure 46–5. Photomicrograph of biopsy tissue demonstrating pseudomembranous colitis. Leukocytes and cellular debris are apparent in the material that overlies the inflamed, superficially necrotic crypts and forms the pseudomembrane. Note the intact epithelium on the right side of the illustration. (Bar = 0.1 mm.) (Courtesy of the Department of Pathology, Children's Hospital Medical Center, Cincinnati, Ohio.)

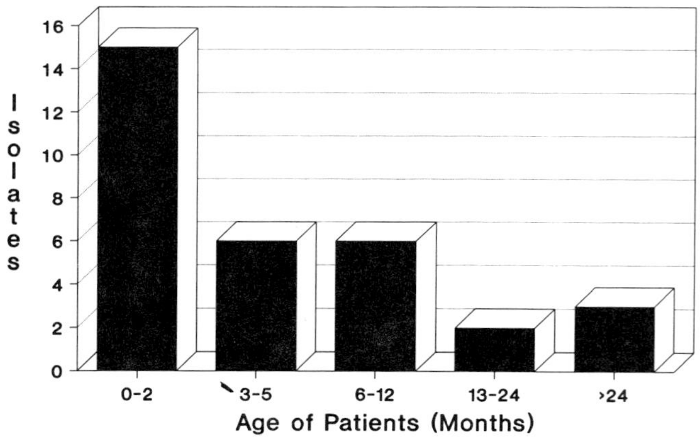

Figure 46–6. *Aeromonas* isolates at Children's Hospital Medical Center, 1990. (Data from the Infection Control Office, Children's Hospital Medical Center, Cincinnati, Ohio.)

Clinical symptoms attributed to *Aeromonas* can be grouped into three categories: (1) acute watery diarrhea, the most common syndrome; (2) dysentery, which is usually self-limited; and (3) persistent watery diarrhea. Cramping abdominal pain and vomiting may also occur.[184] Fecal leukocytes have been observed in some cases.[182] It is important to note that symptoms may occasionally be severe and especially when dysentery is present, have been incorrectly diagnosed as ulcerative colitis.[183]

In mild cases of *Aeromonas* infection, supportive treatment should suffice. In patients who are immunocompromised, are otherwise acutely ill, or have persistent illness, treatment with antibiotics is recommended. Trimethoprim-sulfamethoxazole is usually effective (trimethoprim, 5 mg per kg [maximum 160 mg], plus sulfamethoxazole, 25 mg per kg [maximum 800 mg], every 12 hours for 14 days), as are tetracycline, chloramphenicol, and the aminoglycosides.[181] Most strains of *Aeromonas* are resistant to the penicillins, including ampicillin.[181]

Plesiomonas

P. shigelloides, similar to *Aeromonas,* is commonly found in the environment, especially in bodies of water.[186] In 1988, a case of *Plesiomonas* was linked to aquarium water harboring the organism.[187] Unlike *Aeromonas,* however, *Plesiomonas* has been reported to occur in epidemics, with contaminated water often found to be the cause.[186] *Plesiomonas* is also known to be spread through improperly cooked seafood.[188]

The pathogenesis of disease due to *P. shigelloides* is not well understood. A cytotoxin has been found in some strains[186] but not in others. An invasive mechanism is also suspected owing to the colitis symptoms.[188] In addition to small-volume stools with leukocytes and possible blood, patients may also experience severe abdominal pain. Fever has been seen in approximately one third of patients.[188] In one group of adult patients, symptoms persisted longer than 2 weeks in 75% and longer than 4 weeks in 32%.[188]

Diagnosis of *P. shigelloides* is made by stool culture. Although this illness is usually self-limited, treatment with antimicrobial agents has been shown to decrease the duration of symptoms,[188] with trimethoprim-sulfamethoxazole or aminoglycosides suggested as appropriate choices. There are no controlled trials of antimicrobial treatment of gastroenteritis caused by this organism.

Mycobacterium Avium–Intracellulare

Mycobacterium avium and *Mycobacterium intracellulare,* known collectively as *Mycobacterium avium–intracellulare* or *Mycobacterium avium* complex (MAC), are acid-fast bacilli that have been recognized primarily for their role in cases of atypical tuberculosis. These organisms are now recognized as causative agents of diarrheal symptoms as well. In a review of pediatric cases of atypical mycobacterial infections, Lincoln and coworkers[189] described two immunocompetent patients whose clinical findings included diarrhea and colonic ulceration.

Of even greater significance than these sporadic cases of MAC infections in immunocompetent hosts is their occurrence among immunocompromised patients. In patients with the acquired immunodeficiency syndrome, MAC is the most commonly isolated agent causing systemic bacterial infections.[190] These patients may also suffer symptoms of chronic diarrhea and abdominal pain.[191, 192] MAC has also been noted to cause diarrhea in bone marrow transplantation patients[193] and in a patient with cystic fibrosis.[194]

The MAC organisms may be cultured from gastric and duodenal aspirates obtained endoscopically and from the stool, the bone marrow, and the blood.[190] Endoscopic examination in patients with MAC may reveal findings similar to those seen in Whipple's disease with minute superficial ulcerations in the small bowel.[192] Treatment of MAC infections with conventional antituberculosis agents is usually unsuccessful in eradicating the organisms or alleviating symptoms.[190]

CONCLUSION

Despite this chapter's extensive catalog of both bacterial and viral infectious agents, from 40 to 60% of cases of diarrhea are currently not attributable to any known cause.[55] Doubtless, as techniques for identification and culture become more sophisticated, other causative agents will be identified, and the percentage of diarrheal illnesses described as idiopathic or nonspecific will continue to decline. Advances in the widespread use of improved oral rehydration solutions have led to a decline in the morbidity and mortality due to diarrhea. One can hope that preventive measures will advance as well, leading to a reduction in the incidence of diarrheal disease.

REFERENCES

1. Glass RI, Lew JF, Gangarosa RE, et al: Estimates of morbidity and mortality rates for diarrheal diseases in American children. J Pediatr 1991; 118:S27–33.
2. Snyder JD, Merson MH: The magnitude of the global problem of acute diarrhoeal disease: A review of active surveillance data. Bull WHO 1982; 60:605–613.
3. Guerant RL, Bobak DA: Bacterial and protozoal gastroenteritis. N Engl J Med 1991; 325:327–340.
4. Blacklow NR, Greenberg HB: Viral gastroenteritis. N Engl J Med 1991; 325:252–264.
5. Blacklow NR, Cukor G: Viral gastroenteritis. N Engl J Med 1981; 304:397–406.
6. Kapikian AZ, Wyatt RG, Dolin R, et al: Visualization by immune electron microscopy of a 27-nm particle associated with acute infectious nonbacterial gastroenteritis. J Virol 1972; 10:1075–1081.
7. Ramia S: Transmission of viral infections by the water route: Implications for developing countries. Rev Infect Dis 1985; 7:180–188.
8. Santosham M, Yolken RH, Wyatt RG, et al: Epidemiology of rotavirus diarrhea in a prospectively monitored American Indian population. J Infect Dis 1985; 152:778–783.
9. Shepherd RW, Butler DG, Cutz E, et al: The mucosal lesion in viral enteritis: Extent and dynamics of the epithelial response to virus invasion in transmissible gastroenteritis of piglets. Gastroenterology 1979; 76:770–777.
10. Hamilton JR, Gall DG, Butler DG, et al: Viral gastroenteritis: Recent progress, remaining problems. *In* Elliot K, Knight J, eds: Acute Diarrhoea in Childhood. Amsterdam, Elsevier, 1975, pp 209–222.
11. Shepherd RW, Gall DG, Butler DG, et al: Determinants of diarrhea in viral enteritis: The role of ion transport and epithelial changes in the ileum in transmissible gastroenteritis in piglets. Gastroenterology 1979; 76:20–24.
12. Bishop RF, Davidson GP, Holmes IH, et al: Virus particles in epithelial cells of duodenal mucosa from children with acute nonbacterial gastroenteritis. Lancet 1973; 2:1281–1283.
13. Ho MS, Glass RI, Pinsky PF, et al: Rotavirus as a cause of diarrheal morbidity and mortality in the United States. J Infect Dis 1988; 158:1112–1116.
14. Simhon A, Chrystie IL, Totterdell BM, et al: Sequential rotavirus diarrhoea caused by virus of same subgroup. Lancet 1981; 1:1174.
15. Steinhoff MC: Rotavirus: The first five years. J Pediatr 1980; 96:611–622.
16. Yolken RH, Wyatt RG, Zissis G, et al: Epidemiology of human rotavirus types 1 and 2 as studied by enzyme-linked immunosorbent assay. N Engl J Med 1978; 299:1156–1161.
17. Lycke E, Blomberg J, Berg G, et al: Epidemic acute diarrhoea in adults associated with infantile gastroenteritis virus. Lancet 1978; 2:1056–1057.
18. Meurman OH, Laine MJ: Rotavirus epidemic in adults. N Engl J Med 1977; 296:1298–1299.
19. Wenman WM, Hinde D, Feltham S, et al: Rotavirus infection in adults: Results of a prospective family study. N Engl J Med 1979; 301:303–306.
20. Banatvala JE, Chrystie IL, Totterdell BM: Rotaviral infections in human neonates. J Am Vet Med Assoc 1978; 173:527–530.
21. Totterdell BM, Chrystie IL, Banatvala JE: Rotavirus infections in a maternity unit. Arch Dis Child 1976; 51:924–928.
22. Bishop RF, Hewstone AZ, Davidson GP, et al: An epidemic of diarrhea in human neonates involving a reovirus-like agent and "enteropathogenic" serotypes of *E. coli.* J Clin Pathol 1976; 29:46–49.
23. Chrystie IL, Totterdell BM, Banatvala JE: Asymptomatic endemic rotavirus infections in the newborn. Lancet 1978; 1:1176–1178.
24. Ryder RW, McGowan JE, Hatch MH, et al: Reovirus-like agent as a cause of nosocomial diarrhea in infants. J Pediatr 1977; 90:698–702.
25. Delage G, McLaughlin B, Berthiaume L: A clinical study of rotavirus gastroenteritis. J Pediatr 1978; 93:455–457.
26. Bartlett AV III, Bednarz-Prashad AJ, DuPont HL, et al: Rotavirus gastroenteritis. Annu Rev Med 1987; 38:399–415.
27. Flewett TH, Bryden AS, Davies H, et al: Epidemic viral enteritis in a long-stay children's ward. Lancet 1975; 1:4–5.
28. Wilde J, Yolken R, Willoughby R, et al: Improved detection of rotavirus shedding by polymerase chain reaction. Lancet 1991; 337:323–326.
29. Rodriguez WJ, Kim HW, Arrobio JO, et al: Clinical features of acute gastroenteritis associated with human reovirus-like agent in infants and young children. J Pediatr 1977; 91:188–193.
30. Riepenhoff-Talty M, Offor E, Klossner K, et al: Effect of age and malnutrition on rotavirus infection in mice. Pediatr Res 1985; 19:1250–1253.
31. Davidson GP, Barnes GL: Structural and functional abnormalities of the small intestine in infants and young children with rotavirus enteritis. Acta Paediatr Scand 1979; 68:181–186.
32. Middleton PJ, Szymanski MT, Abbott GD, et al: Orbivirus acute gastroenteritis of infancy. Lancet 1974; 1:1241–1244.
33. Urasawa T, Urasawa S, Taniguchi K: Sequential passages of human rotavirus in MA-104 cells. Microbiol Immunol 1981; 25:1025–1035.
34. Levine MM: Vaccines and milk immunoglobulin concentrates for prevention of infectious diarrhea. J Pediatr 1991; 118:S129–136.
35. Clark HF, Borian FE, Bell LM, et al: Protective effect of WC3 vaccine against rotavirus diarrhea in infants during a predominantly serotype 1 rotavirus season. J Infect Dis 1988; 158:570–587.
36. Christy C, Madore HP, Pichichero ME, et al: Field trial of Rhesus rotavirus vaccine in infants. Pediatr Infect Dis J 1988; 7:645–650.
37. Santosham M, Letson GW, Wolff M, et al: A field study of the safety and efficacy of two candidate rotavirus vaccines in a Native American population. J Infect Dis 1991; 163:483–487.
38. Flores J, Perez-Schael I, Blanco M, et al: Comparison of reactogenicity and antigenicity of M37 rotavirus vaccine and rhesus-rotavirus-based quadrivalent vaccine. Lancet 1990; 336:330–334.
39. Dolin R, Blacklow NR, DuPont H, et al: Transmission of acute infectious nonbacterial gastroenteritis to volunteers by oral administration of stool filtrates. J Infect Dis 1971; 123:307–312.
40. Cukor G, Blacklow NR: Human viral gastroenteritis. Microbiol Rev 1984; 48:157–179.
41. Spender QW, Lewis D, Price EH: Norwalk like viruses: Study of an outbreak. Arch Dis Child 1986; 61:142–147.
42. Kapikian AZ, Yolken RH, Greenberg HB, et al: Gastroenteritis viruses. *In* Lennette EH, Schmidt NJ, eds: Diagnostic Procedures for Viral, Rickettsial and Chlamydial Infections. Washington, DC, American Public Health Association, 1978, pp 927–995.
43. Caul EO, Appleton H: The electron microscopical and physical characteristics of small round human fecal viruses: An interim scheme for classification. J Med Virol 1982; 9:257–265.
44. Blacklow NR, Cukor G, Bedigian MK, et al: Immune response and prevalence of antibody to Norwalk enteritis virus as determined by radioimmunoassay. J Clin Microbiol 1979; 10:903–909.
45. Jenkins S, Horman JT, Israel E, et al: An outbreak of Norwalk-related gastroenteritis at a boys' camp. Am J Dis Child 1985; 139:787–789.
46. Kuritsky JN, Osterholm MT, Greenberg HB, et al: Norwalk gastroenteritis: A community outbreak associated with bakery product consumption. Ann Intern Med 1984; 100:519–521.
47. Morse DL, Guzewich JJ, Hanrahan JP, et al: Widespread outbreaks of clam- and oyster-associated gastroenteritis: Role of Norwalk virus. N Engl J Med 1986; 314:678–681.
48. Greenberg HB, Wyatt RG, Kapikian AZ: Norwalk virus in vomitus. Lancet 1979; 1:55.
49. Adler JL, Zickl R: Winter vomiting disease. J Infect Dis 1969; 119:668–673.
50. Agus SG, Dolin R, Wyatt RG, et al: Acute infectious nonbacterial gastroenteritis: Intestinal histopathology. Ann Intern Med 1973; 79:18–25.
51. Storr J, Rice S, Phillips AD, et al: Clinical associations of Norwalk-like virus in the stools of children. J Pediatr Gastroenterol Nutr 1986; 5:576–580.
52. Kjeldsberg E, Ånestad G, Greenberg H, et al: Norwalk virus in Norway: An outbreak of gastroenteritis studied by electron microscopy and radioimmunoassay. Scand J Infect Dis 1989; 21:521–526.
53. Matsui SM, Kim JP, Greenberg HB, et al: The isolation and

characterization of a Norwalk virus-specific cDNA. J Clin Invest 1991; 87:1456–1461.
54. Wadell G, Allard A, Johansson M, et al: Enteric adenoviruses. *In* Bock G, Whelan J, eds: Novel Diarrhoea Viruses. CIBA Foundation Symposium 128. Chichester, England, John Wiley, 1987, pp 63–91.
55. Kotloff KL, Losonsky GA, Morris Jr JG, et al: Enteric adenovirus infection and childhood diarrhea: An epidemiologic study in three clinical settings. Pediatrics 1989; 84:219–225.
56. Uhnoo I, Wadell G, Svensson L, et al: Importance of enteric adenoviruses 40 and 41 in acute gastroenteritis in infants and young children. J Clin Microbiol 1984; 20:365–372.
57. Wood DJ: Adenovirus gastroenteritis. Br Med J 1988; 296:229–230.
58. Martin AL, Kudesia G: Enzyme linked immunosorbent assay for detecting adenoviruses in stool specimens: Comparison with electron microscopy and isolation. J Clin Pathol 1990; 43:514–515.
59. Allard A, Girones R, Juto P, et al: Polymerase chain reaction for detection of adenoviruses in stool samples. J Clin Microbiol 1990; 28:2659–2667.
60. Ellis ME, Watson B, Mandal BK, et al: Micro-organisms in gastroenteritis. Arch Dis Child 1984; 59:848–855.
61. Matson DO, Estes MK, Glass RI, et al: Human calicivirus–associated diarrhea in children attending day care centers. J Infect Dis 1989; 159:71–78.
62. Viral agents of gastroenteritis: Public health importance and outbreak management. MMWR 1990; 39:(RR-5)1–23.
63. Cubitt WD: The candidate caliciviruses. *In* Bock G, Whelan J, eds: Novel Diarrhoea Viruses. CIBA Foundation Symposium 128. Chichester, England, John Wiley 1987, pp 126–143.
64. Kurtz JB, Lee TW: Astroviruses: Human and animal. *In* Bock G, Whelan J, eds: Novel Diarrhoea Viruses. CIBA Foundation Symposium 128. Chichester, England, John Wiley 1987, pp 92–107.
65. Ashley CR, Caul EO, Paver WK: Astrovirus-associated gastroenteritis in children. J Clin Pathol 1978; 31:939–943.
66. Yolken R, Dubovi E, Leister F, et al: Infantile gastroenteritis associated with excretion of pestivirus antigens. Lancet 1989; 1:517–520.
67. Flewett TH, Beards GM, Brown DWG, et al: The diagnostic gap in diarrhoeal aetiology. *In* Bock G, Whelan J, eds: Novel Diarrhoea Viruses. CIBA Foundation Symposium 128. Chichester, England, John Wiley 1987, pp 238–249.
68. Resta S, Luby JP, Rosenfeld CR, Siegel JD: Isolation and propagation of a human enteric coronavirus. Science 1985; 229:978–981.
69. Woode GN: Breda and Breda-like viruses: Diagnosis, pathology and epidemiology. *In* Bock G, Whelan J, eds: Novel Diarrhoea Viruses. CIBA Foundation Symposium 128. Chichester, England, John Wiley 1987, pp 175–191.
70. Horzinek MC, Weiss M, Ederveen J: Toroviridae: A proposed new family of enveloped RNA viruses. *In* Bock G, Whelan J, eds: Novel Diarrhoea Viruses. CIBA Foundation Symposium 128. Chichester, England, John Wiley, 1987, pp 162–174.
71. Pereira HG, Fialho AM, Flewett TH, et al: Novel viruses in human faeces. Lancet 1988; 2:103–104.
72. Giannella RA, Broitman SA, Zamcheck N: Influence of gastric acidity on bacterial and parasitic enteric infections. Ann Intern Med 1973; 78:271–276.
73. Giannella RA, Broitman SA, Zamcheck N: Gastric acid barrier to ingested microorganisms in man: Studies in vivo and in vitro. Gut 1972; 13:251–256.
74. Justus PG, Martin JL, Goldberg DA, et al: Myoelectric effects of *Clostridium difficile:* Motility-altering factors distinct from its cytotoxin and enterotoxin in rabbits. Gastroenterology 1982; 83:836–843.
75. Forstner G, Sherman P, Forstner J: Mucus: Function and structure. *In* Boedeker EC, ed: Attachment of Organisms to the Gut Mucosa. Vol 2. Boca Raton, FL, CRC Press, 1985, p 13.
76. Boedeker EC: Enterocyte adherence of *Escherichia coli:* Its relation to diarrheal disease. Gastroenterology 1982; 83:489–492.
77. Hargrett-Bean NT, Pavia AT, Tauxe RV: *Salmonella* isolates from humans in the United States, 1984–1986. MMWR 1988; 37(SS-2):25–31.
78. Bishop WP, Ulshen MH: Bacterial gastroenteritis. Pediatr Clin North Am 1988; 35:69–87.
79. Blaser MJ, Newman LS: A review of human salmonellosis: I. Infective dose. Rev Infect Dis 1982; 4:1096–1106.
80. Kaye D, Gill FA, Hook EW: Factors influencing host resistance to *Salmonella* infections: The effects of hemolysis and erythrophagocytosis. Am J Med Sci 1967; 254:205–215.
81. Hand WL, King NL: Serum opsonization of *Salmonella* in sickle cell anemia. Am J Med 1978; 64:388–395.
82. Torrey S, Fleisher G, Jaffe D: Incidence of *Salmonella* bacteremia in infants with *Salmonella* gastroenteritis. J Pediatr 1986; 108:718–721.
83. Buchwald DS, Blaser MJ: A review of human salmonellosis: II. Duration of excretion following infection with nontyphi *Salmonella.* Rev Infect Dis 1984; 6:345–356.
84. Aserkoff B, Bennett JV: Effect of antibiotic therapy in acute salmonellosis on the fecal excretion of salmonellae. N Engl J Med 1969; 281:636–640.
85. St. Geme HW III, Hodes HL, Marcy SM, et al: Consensus: Management of *Salmonella* infection in the first year of life. Pediatr Infect Dis J 1988; 7:615–621.
86. Pickering LK: Therapy for acute infectious diarrhea in children. J Pediatr 1991; 118:S118–128.
87. Blaser MJ: Bacterial gastrointestinal infections. Gastroenterol Ann 1986; 3:317–340.
88. Colon AR, Gross DR, Tamer MA: Typhoid fever in children. Pediatrics 1975; 56:606–609.
89. Levine MM, Hone D, Stocker BAD, et al: Vaccines to prevent typhoid fever. *In* Woodrow G, Levine MM, eds: New-Generation Vaccines. New York, Marcel Dekker, 1990, pp 269–287.
90. Osler W: The Principles and Practice of Medicine. New York, D. Appleton & Company, 1892.
91. Levine MM: Bacillary dysentery: Mechanisms and treatment. Med Clin North Am 1982; 66:623–638.
92. Mata LJ: The children of Santa Maria Caugué: A prospective field study of health and growth. Cambridge, MA, MIT Press, 1978.
93. Cohen MB: Etiology and mechanisms of acute infectious diarrhea in infants in the United States. J Pediatr 1991; 4:S34–39.
94. Weissman JB, Gangarosa EJ, Schmerler A, et al: Shigellosis in day-care centres. Lancet 1975; 1:88–90.
95. Keusch GT, Donohue-Rolfe A, Jacewicz M: *Shigella* toxin(s): Description and role in diarrhea and dysentery. Pharmacol Ther 1982; 15:403–438.
96. Mildvan D, Gelb AM, William D: Veneral transmission of enteric pathogens in male homosexuals: Two case reports. JAMA 1977; 238:1387–1389.
97. Butler T, Islam MR, Azad MAK, Jones PK: Risk factors for development of hemolytic uremic syndrome during shigellosis. J Pediatr 1987; 110:894–897.
98. Barrett-Connor EB, Connor JB: Extraintestinal manifestations of shigellosis. Am J Gastroenterol 1970; 53:234–245.
99. Calin A, Fries JF: An "experimental" epidemic of Reiter's syndrome revisited. Follow-up evidence on genetic and environmental factors. Ann Intern Med 1976; 84:564–566.
100. Levine MM, DuPont HL, Formal SB, et al: Pathogenesis of *Shigella dysenteriae* 1 (Shiga) dysentery. J Infect Dis 1973; 127:261–270.
101. Hale TL: Genetic basis of virulence in *Shigella* species. Microbiol Rev 1991; 55:206–224.
102. O'Brien AD, Holmes RK: Shiga and shiga-like toxins. Microbiol Rev 1987; 51:206–220.
103. Surawicz CM, Belic L: Rectal biopsy helps to distinguish acute self-limited colitis from idiopathic inflammatory bowel disease. Gastroenterology 1984; 86:104–113.
104. Tong MJ, Martin DG, Cunningham JJ, Gunning J: Clinical and bacteriological evaluation of antibiotic treatment in shigellosis. JAMA 1970; 214:1841–1844.
105. Ross S, Controni G, Khan W: Resistance of shigellae to ampicillin and other antibiotics. JAMA 1972; 221:45–47.
106. Nelson JD, Haltalin KC: Amoxicillin less effective than ampicillin against *Shigella* in vitro and in vivo: Relationship of efficacy to activity in serum. J Infect Dis 1974; 129:S222–227.
107. Williams EK, Lohr JA, Guerrant RL: Acute infectious diarrhea: II. Diagnosis, treatment and prevention. Pediatr Infect Dis J 1986; 5:458–465.
108. Walker RI, Caldwell MB, Lee EC, et al: Pathophysiology of *Campylobacter* enteritis. Microbiol Rev 1986; 50:81–94.

109. Goosens H, Vlaes L, DeBoeck M, et al: Is *"Campylobacter upsaliensis"* an unrecognised cause of human diarrhoea? Lancet 1990; 335:584–586.
110. Sjögren E, Ruiz-Palacios G, Kaijser B: *Campylobacter jejuni* isolations from Mexican and Swedish patients, with repeated symptomatic and/or asymptomatic diarrhoea episodes. Epid Infect 1989; 102:47–57.
111. Tauxe RV, Hargrett-Bean N, Patton CM, et al: *Campylobacter* isolates in the United States, 1982–1986. MMWR 1988; 37(SS-2):1–13.
112. Jones LV, Rodríguez RS: Bacterial-induced diarrhea. Drugs 1988; 36(Suppl 4):6–17.
113. Blaser MJ, Reller LB: *Campylobacter* enteritis. N Engl J Med 1981; 305:1444–1452.
114. Spelman DW, Davidson N, Buckmaster ND, et al: *Campylobacter* bacteraemia: A report of 10 cases. Med J Aust 1986; 145:503–505.
115. Karmali MA, Fleming PC: *Campylobacter* enteritis in children. J Pediatr 1979; 94:527–533.
116. Thorson SM, Lohr JA, Dudley S, et al: Value of methylene blue examination, dark-field microscopy, and carbol-fuchsin Gram stain in the detection of *Campylobacter* enteritis. J Pediatr 1985; 106:941–943.
117. Salazar-Lindo E, Sack RB, Chea-Woo E, et al: Early treatment with erythromycin of *Campylobacter jejuni*-associated dysentery in children. J Pediatr 1986; 109:355–360.
118. Mollaret HH, Bercovier H, Alonso JM: Summary of the data received at the WHO reference center for *Yersinia enterocolitica.* Contr Microbiol Immunol 1979; 5:174–184.
119. Cover TL, Aber RC: *Yersinia enterocolitica.* N Engl J Med 1989; 321:16–24.
120. Black RE, Jackson RJ, Tsai T, et al: Epidemic *Yersinia enterocolitica* infection due to contaminated chocolate milk. N Engl J Med 1978; 298:76–79.
121. Lee LA, Gerber AR, Lonsway DR, et al: *Yersinia enterocolitica* O:3 infections in infants and children, associated with the household preparation of chitterlings. N Engl J Med 1990; 322:984–987.
122. Lee LA, Taylor J, Carter GP, et al: *Yersinia enterocolitica* O:3: An emerging cause of pediatric gastroenteritis in the United States. J Infect Dis 1991; 163:660–663.
123. Marks MI, Pai CH, Lafleur L, et al: *Yersinia enterocolitica* gastroenteritis: A prospective study of clinical, bacteriological, and epidemiologic features. J Pediatr 1980; 96:26–31.
124. Attwood SEA, Mealy K, Cafferkey MT, et al: *Yersinia* infection and acute abdominal pain. Lancet 1987; 1:529–533.
125. Dequeker J, Jamar R, Walravens M: HLA-B27, arthritis and *Yersinia enterocolitica* infection. J Rheumatol 1980; 7:706–710.
126. Bottone EJ, Sheehan DJ: *Yersinia enterocolitica:* Guidelines for serologic diagnosis of human infections. Rev Infect Dis 1983; 5:898–906.
127. Pai CH, Gillis F, Tuomanen E, Marks MI: Placebo-controlled double-blind evaluation of trimethoprim-sulfamethoxazole treatment of *Yersinia enterocolitica* gastroenteritis. J Pediatr 1984; 104:308–311.
128. Update: Cholera outbreak—Peru, Ecuador, and Colombia. MMWR 1991; 40:225–227.
129. Morris Jr JG, Black RE: Cholera and other vibrioses in the United States. N Engl J Med 1985; 312:343–350.
130. Siddique AK, Baqui AH, Eusof A, et al: Survival of classic cholera in Bangladesh. Lancet 1991; 337:1125–1127.
131. Finkelstein RA: Cholera. Crit Rev Microbiol 1973; 2:553–623.
132. Azurin JC, Kobari K, Barua D, et al: A long-term carrier of cholera: Cholera Dolores. Bull WHO 1967; 37:745–749.
133. Snyder JD, Blake PA: Is cholera a problem for US travelers? JAMA 1982; 247:2268–2269.
134. Shandera WX, Hafkin B, Martin DL, et al: Persistence of cholera in the United States. Am J Trop Med Hyg 1983; 32:812–817.
135. Carpenter CCJ: Clinical and pathophysiologic features of diarrhea caused by *Vibrio cholerae* and *Escherichia coli. In* Field M, Fordtran JS, Schutz SG, eds: Secretory Diarrhea. Bethesda, MD, American Physiological Society, 1980, pp 66–73.
136. Carpenter CCJ: Cholera and other enterotoxin-related diarrheal diseases. J Infect Dis 1972; 126:551–564.
137. Moss J, Burns DL, Hsia JA, et al: Cyclic nucleotides: Mediators of bacterial toxin action in disease. Ann Intern Med 1984; 101:653–666.
138. Karchmer AW, Curlin GT, Huq MI, Hirschhorn N: Furazolidone in paediatric cholera. Bull WHO 1970; 43:373–378.
139. Honda T, Arita M, Takeda T, et al: Non-O1 *Vibrio cholerae* produces two newly identified toxins related to *Vibrio parahaemolyticus* hemolysin and *Escherichia coli* heat-stable enterotoxin. Lancet 1985; 2:163–164.
140. Nishibuchi M, Seidler RJ: Medium-dependent production of extracellular enterotoxins by non-O1 *Vibrio cholerae, Vibrio mimicus,* and *Vibrio fluvialis.* Appl Environ Microbiol 1983; 45:228–231.
141. Wilson R, Lieb S, Roberts A, et al: Non-O group 1 *Vibrio cholerae* gastroenteritis associated with eating raw oysters. Am J Epidemiol 1981; 114:293–298.
142. Levine MM: *Escherichia coli* that cause diarrhea: Enterotoxigenic, enteropathogenic, enteroinvasive, enterohemorrhagic and enteroadherent. J Infect Dis 1987; 155:377–389.
143. Levine MM: *Escherichia coli* infections. N Engl J Med 1985; 313:445–447.
144. Girón JA, Jones T, Millán-Vellasco F, et al: Diffuse-adhering *Escherichia coli* (DAEC) as a putative cause of diarrhea in Mayan children in Mexico. J Infect Dis 1991; 163:507–513.
145. Bhan MK, Raj P, Levine MM, et al: Enteroaggregative *Escherichia coli* associated with persistent diarrhea in a cohort of rural children in India. J Infect Dis 1989; 159:1061–1064.
146. Sherman P, Drumm B, Karmali M, Cutz E: Adherence of bacteria to the intestine in sporadic cases of enteropathogenic *Escherichia coli*–associated diarrhea in infants and young children: A prospective study. Gastroenterology 1989; 96:86–94.
147. Rothbaum R, McAdams AJ, Giannella R, Partin JC: A clinicopathologic study of enterocyte-adherent *Escherichia coli:* A cause of protracted diarrhea in infants. Gastroenterology 1982; 83:441–454.
148. Neto UF, Ferreira VC, Patricio FRS, et al: Protracted diarrhea: The importance of the enteropathogenic *E. coli* (EPEC) strains and *Salmonella* in its genesis. J Pediatr Gastroenterol Nutr 1989; 8:207–211.
149. Levine MM, Nataro JP, Karch H, et al: The diarrheal response of humans to some classic serotypes of enteropathogenic *Escherichia coli* is dependent on a plasmid encoding an enteroadhesiveness factor. J Infect Dis 1985; 152:550–559.
150. Baudry B, Savarino SJ, Vial P, et al: A sensitive and specific DNA probe to identify enteroaggregative *Escherichia coli,* a recently discovered diarrheal pathogen. J Infect Dis 1990; 161:1249–1251.
151. Black RE, Brown KH, Becker S, et al: Longitudinal studies of infectious diseases and physical growth of children in rural Bangladesh: II. Incidence of diarrhea and association with known pathogens. Am J Epidemiol 1982; 115:315–324.
152. Gorbach SL, Kean BH, Evans DG, et al: Traveler's diarrhea and toxigenic *Escherichia coli.* N Engl J Med 1975; 292:933–936.
153. Cohen MB, Guarino A, Shukla R, et al: Age-related differences in receptors for *Escherichia coli* heat-stable enterotoxin in the small and large intestine of children. Gastroenterology 1988; 94:367–373.
154. DeJonge HR: The mechanism of action of *Escherichia coli* heat-stable toxin. Biochem Soc Trans 1984; 12:180–184.
155. Giannella RA: The suckling mouse model for the detection of heat-stable *Escherichia coli* enterotoxin: Characteristics of the model. Infect Immunol 1976; 14:95–99.
156. Moseley SL, Hardy JW, Huq MI, et al: Isolation and nucleotide sequence determination of a gene encoding a heat-stable enterotoxin of *Escherichia coli.* Infect Immunol 1983; 39:1167–1174.
157. Moseley SL, Echeverria P, Seriwatana J, et al: Identification of enterotoxigenic *Escherichia coli* using three enterotoxin gene probes. J Infect Dis 1982; 145:863–869.
158. Black RE, Levine MM, Clements ML, et al: Treatment of experimentally induced enterotoxigenic *Escherichia coli* diarrhea with trimethoprim, trimethoprim-sulfamethoxazole, or a placebo. Rev Infect Dis 1982; 4:540–545.
159. DuPont HL, Formal SB, Hornick RB, et al: Pathogenesis of *Escherichia coli* diarrhea. N Engl J Med 1971; 285:1–9.
160. Taylor DN, Echeverria P, Sethabutr O, et al: Clinical and microbiologic features of *Shigella* and enteroinvasive *Escherichia coli* infections detected by DNA hybridization. J Clin Microbiol 1988; 26:1362–1366.
161. Pai CH, Gordon R, Sims HV, et al: Sporadic cases of hemor-

rhagic colitis associated with *Escherichia coli* O157:H7: Clinical, epidemiologic and bacteriologic features. Ann Intern Med 1984; 101:738–742.

162. Remis RS, MacDonald KL, Riley LW, et al: Sporadic cases of hemorrhagic colitis associated with *Escherichia coli* O157:H7. Ann Intern Med 1984; 101:624–626.
163. MacDonald KL, O'Leary MJ, Cohen ML, et al: *Escherichia coli* O157:H7, an emerging gastrointestinal pathogen: Results of a one-year, prospective, population-based study. JAMA 1988; 259:3567–3570.
164. Obrig TG, Moran TP, Colinas RJ: Ribonuclease activity associated with the 60S ribosome-inactivating proteins ricin A, phytolaccin and Shiga toxin. Biochem Biophys Res Comm 1985; 130:879–884.
165. Ostroff SM, Kobayashi JM, Lewis JH: Infections with *Escherichia coli* O157:H7 in Washington state: The first year of statewide surveillance. JAMA 1989; 262:355–359.
166. Cleary TG: Cytotoxin-producing *Escherichia coli* and the hemolytic uremic syndrome. Pediatr Clin North Am 1988; 35:485–501.
167. Neill MA, Tarr PI, Clausen CR, et al: *Escherichia coli* O157:H7 as the predominant pathogen associated with the hemolytic uremic syndrome: A prospective study in the Pacific Northwest. Pediatrics 1987; 80:37–40.
168. Cohen MB, Giannella RA: Hemorrhagic colitis associated with *Escherichia coli* O157:H7. Adv Intern Med 1991; 37:163–183.
169. Donta ST, Myers MG: *Clostridium difficile* toxin in asymptomatic neonates. J Pediatr 1982; 100:431–434.
170. Rolfe RD: Binding kinetics of *Clostridium difficile* toxins A and B to intestinal brush border membranes from infant and adult hamsters. Infect Immunol 1991; 59:1223–1230.
171. Eglow R, Pothoulakis C, Itzkowitz S, et al: Diminished *Clostridium difficile* toxin A (TxA) receptors in newborn rabbit ileum correlates with reduced biological effect. Gastroenterology 1991; 100(pt. 2):A521.
172. Ellis ME, Mandal BK, Dunbar EM, et al: *Clostridium difficile* and its cytotoxin in infants admitted to hospital with infectious gastroenteritis. Br Med J 1984; 288:524–526.
173. Pantosti A, Cerquetti M, Gianfrilli PM: Electrophoretic characterization of *Clostridium difficile* strains isolated from antibiotic-associated colitis and other conditions. J Clin Microbiol 1988; 26:540–543.
174. Tvede M, Schiøtz PO, Krasilnikoff PA: Incidence of *Clostridium difficile* in hospitalized children. Acta Paediatr Scand 1990; 79:292–299.
175. Chang TW, Gorbach SL: Rapid identification of *Clostridium difficile* by toxin detection. J Clin Microbiol 1982; 15:465–467.
176. Schwarz RP, Ulshen MH: Pseudomembranous colitis presenting as mild, chronic diarrhea in childhood. J Pediatr Gastroenterol Nutr 1983; 2:570–573.
177. Fekety R, Silva J, Kauffman C, et al: Treatment of antibiotic-associated *Clostridium difficile* colitis with oral vancomycin: Comparison of two dosage regimens. Am J Med 1989; 86:15–19.
178. Teasley DG, Gerding DN, Olson GM: Prospective randomized trial of metronidazole versus vancomycin for *Clostridium difficile*-associated diarrhoea and colitis. Lancet 1983; 2:1043–1046.
179. Pruksananonda P, Powell KR: Multiple relapses of *Clostridium difficile*-associated diarrhea responding to an extended course of cholestyramine. Pediatr Infect Dis J 1989; 8:175–178.
180. Leung DYM, Kelly CP, Boguniewicz M, et al: Treatment with intravenously administered gamma globulin of chronic relapsing colitis induced by *Clostridium difficile* toxin. J Pediatr 1991; 118:633–637.
181. Holmberg SD, Farmer JJ III: *Aeromonas hydrophila* and *Plesiomonas shigelloides* as causes of intestinal infections. Rev Infect Dis 1984; 6:633–639.
182. Challapalli M, Tess BR, Cunningham DG, et al: *Aeromonas*-associated diarrhea in children. Pediatr Infect Dis J 1988; 7:693–698.
183. Gracey M, Burke V, Robinson J: *Aeromonas*-associated gastroenteritis. Lancet 1982; 2:1304–1306.
184. Agger WA, McCormick JD, Gurwith MJ: Clinical and microbiological features of *Aeromonas hydrophila*-associated diarrhea. J Clin Microbiol 1985; 21:909–913.
185. Namdari H, Bottone EJ: Microbiologic and clinical evidence supporting the role of *Aeromonas caviae* as a pediatric enteric pathogen. J Clin Microbiol 1990; 28:837–840.
186. Olsvik O, Wachsmuth K, Kay B, et al: Laboratory observations on *Plesiomonas shigelloides* strains isolated from children with diarrhea in Peru. J Clin Microbiol 1990; 28:886–889.
187. Aquarium-associated *Plesiomonas shigelloides* infection—Missouri. MMWR 1989; 38:617–619.
188. Kain KC, Kelly MT: Clinical features, epidemiology, and treatment of *Plesiomonas shigelloides* diarrhea. J Clin Microbiol 1989; 27:998–1001.
189. Lincoln EM, Gilbert LA: Disease in children due to mycobacteria other than *Mycobacterium tuberculosis*. Am Rev Resp Dis 1972; 105:683–714.
190. Young LS: *Mycobacterium avium* complex infections. J Infect Dis 1988; 157:863–867.
191. Hawkins CC, Gold JWM, Whimbey EW, et al: *Mycobacterium avium* complex infections in patients with the acquired immunodeficiency syndrome. Ann Intern Med 1986; 105:184–188.
192. Gillin JS, Urmacher C, West R, et al: Disseminated *Mycobacterium avium–intracellulare* infection in acquired immunodeficiency syndrome mimicking Whipple's disease. Gastroenterology 1983; 85:1187–1191.
193. Ozkaynak MF, Lenarsky C, Kohn D, et al: *Mycobacterium avium–intracellulare* infections after allogeneic bone marrow transplantation in children. Am J Pediatr Hematol Oncol 1990; 12:220–224.
194. Kinney JS, Little BJ, Yolken RH, et al: *Mycobacterium avium* complex in a patient with cystic fibrosis: Disease vs. colonization. Pediatr Infect Dis J 1989; 8:393–396.

Chapter 47

Intussusception

KAREN W. WEST and JAY L. GROSFELD

Intussusception is a frequent cause of bowel obstruction in children younger than 2 years of age and remains one of the commonest surgical emergencies in infancy and childhood. The initial description of the invagination of one segment of bowel into another was made by Paul Barbette in the late 1600s,[1] and the first successful surgical reduction was described by Sir Jonathan Hutchinson in 1871. Hutchinson's detailed report,[2] presented to the Medico-Chirurgical Society, described a toddler's symptoms of crampy, intermittent abdominal pain that had lasted a month and had been associated with vomiting, bloody stools, and the eventual prolapse of the ileum out of the rectum. Attempts at reduction using chloroform anesthesia, dangling the child by the feet, and simultaneous enemas were unsuccessful. When laparotomy was pursued in spite of the moribund condition of the child, however, the bowel was found to be viable and was safely reduced.

A few reports of hydrostatic reduction continued to appear in the literature, but it was only in the 1930s that Ravitch and McCune[3] standardized and popularized the hydrostatic barium reduction techniques. Early diagnosis and therapeutic intervention were aimed at preventing the patient morbidity and mortality noted in these early reports.

ETIOLOGY

Intussusception is a process that occurs when a proximal segment of bowel (intussusceptum) telescopes into a more distal segment (intussuscipiens), dragging the associated mesentery with it. As edema develops, venous and lymphatic congestion lead to "currant-jelly stools" (blood mixed with mucus), and vascular compromise is possible. Ultimately, ischemia, perforation, and peritonitis are possible sequelae if the diagnosis is delayed.

Seventy-five to 90% of the cases of ileocolic intussusception are idiopathic, with no identifiable lead point observed. Most episodes occur in otherwise healthy and well-nourished children, with a male predominance. Sixty percent of the patients are younger than 1 year of age, and 80% of the cases occur before the patient's second birthday.[3–5] Seasonal variation has been reported corresponding with the peak season for gastroenteritis, although this observation varies in large series. Thirty percent of the children may experience otitis media, flu-like illness, or an upper respiratory tract infection prior to the onset of intussusception. Viremia is thought to accentuate the lymphatic tissues in the intestinal tract, resulting in hypertrophy of Peyer's patches in the lymphoid-rich terminal ileum, which may act as a lead point for ileocolic intussusception. Although adenovirus and rotavirus have been implicated in the etiology of intussusception, the results of viral studies vary from one institution to another and may depend on methods of detection.[6–9]

In 2 to 5% of cases, a pathologic lead point is identified (Table 47–1). This tends to occur more commonly in the older child (older than 5 years of age) and can include small bowel lymphomas, Meckel's diverticulum, duplication cysts, various polyps (e.g., Peutz-Jeghers syndrome), juvenile vascular malformations, such as hemangiomas (Fig. 47–1), inverted appendiceal stumps, and even *Ascaris lumbricoides*.[10–12] Small bowel intussusception may follow an episode of Henoch-Schönlein purpura, with the bowel wall hematoma acting as the lead point.[12] Patients with cystic fibrosis have an increased risk of developing an intussusception, particularly following an episode of dehydration and meconium ileus–equivalent syndrome.[13] In these latter cases, the thick, inspissated stool may act as the lead point for the process. Additionally, the older child with repeated episodes of upper respiratory tract infections and a concomitant intussusception should have a sweat chloride determination as part of the evaluation.

Table 47–1. PATHOLOGIC LEAD POINTS IN 13 OF 120 PATIENTS WITH IDIOPATHIC INTUSSUSCEPTION*

Lead Point	No. of Patients
Bowel wall hematoma	3
Non-Hodgkin's lymphoma	2
Hamartomatous polyps	2
Submucosal hemangioma	1
Carcinoid tumor	1
Juvenile polyp	1
Ascaris lumbricoides	1
Meckel's diverticulum	1
Appendix (cystic fibrosis)	1

*From the J. W. Riley Hospital for Children, Indianapolis.

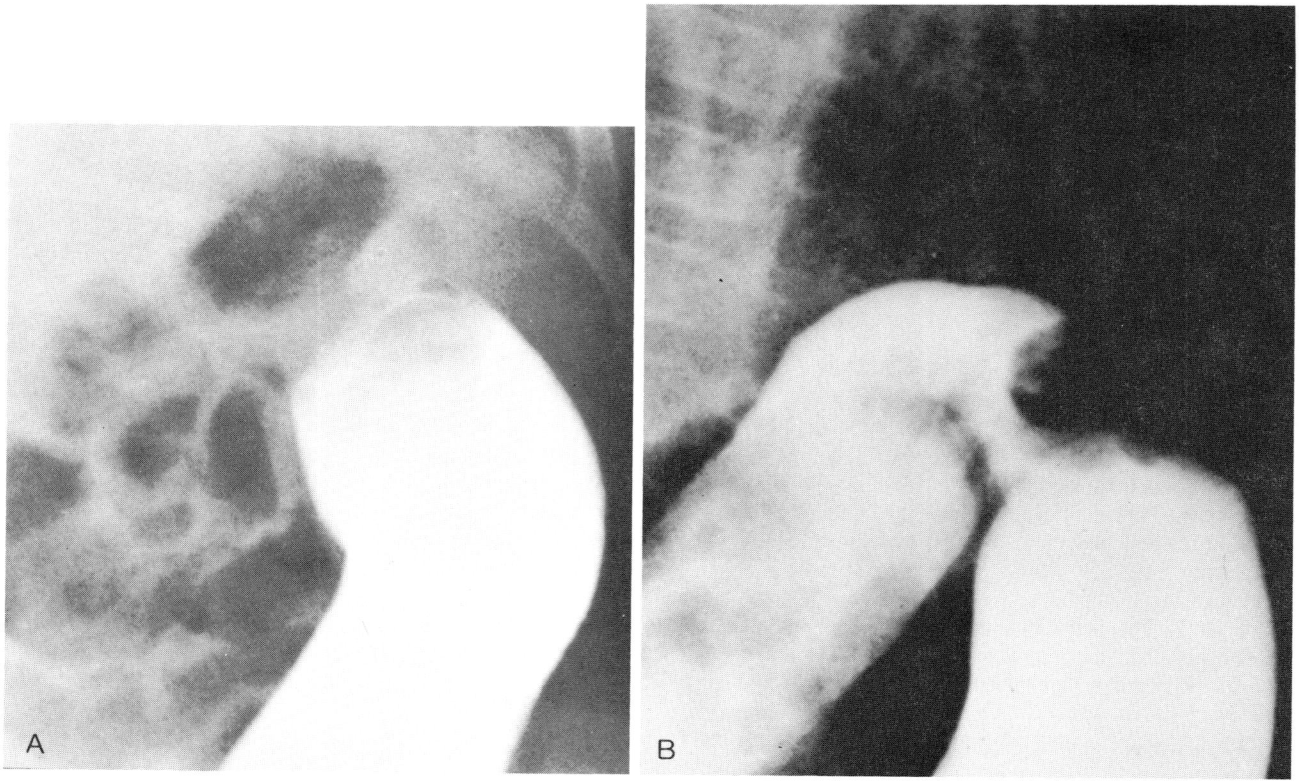

Figure 47–1. This 6-month-old infant with a recurring colocolic intussusception *(A)* was noted to have a submucosal hemangioma *(B)* as the pathologic lead point when complete reduction was achieved.

Rarely, nonobstructive small bowel–small bowel intussusceptions may be associated with celiac disease and may be related to the disordered motility, excessive secretions, or bowel wall weakness found in this entity.[14, 15] Additionally, obstructing intussusceptions have been identified in patients with Crohn's disease who developed abdominal pain and bilious emesis.[16, 17]

CLINICAL PRESENTATION AND PHYSICAL EXAMINATION

Intussusception usually is characterized by the sudden onset of intermittent, crampy abdominal pain accompanied by screaming, inconsolable crying and a "drawing up" of the legs toward the abdomen. The episodes become more frequent and may be followed by initially clear gastric emesis. Bilious emesis may develop as the obstruction progresses. In between the painful episodes the child may act in an age-appropriate manner. Sixty percent of the authors' patients had been evaluated for gastroenteritis by an office-based physician or in an emergency department setting at least once prior to referral for diagnosis.[4, 12] As the symptoms progress, increasing lethargy may develop and can be mistaken for meningitis until clear spinal fluid is obtained following lumbar puncture. The classically described triad of pain, a palpable sausage-shaped abdominal mass, and currant-jelly stools is seen in only 15% of patients at the time of presentation.[4, 12] In the authors' series of 120 patients, the most frequent symptoms initiating referral included emesis (82%), abdominal pain (75%), rectal bleeding (currant-jelly stools, gross blood, or Hematest-positive stool) (75%), palpable abdominal mass (65%), and lethargy or sepsis (40%). The sausage-shaped abdominal mass can usually be palpated in the right upper quadrant, with an empty void noted in the right lower quadrant. In three of these patients, the intussusceptum could be palpated on rectal examination at the time of admission. Abdominal tenderness is caused by distended loops of bowel irritating the peritoneum. Evidence of peritonitis is rare, because the potentially necrotic intussusceptum is surrounded by viable distal bowel.

DIAGNOSIS AND NONSURGICAL TREATMENT

A high index of suspicion, coupled with early diagnosis of intussusception, may obviate the need for surgical intervention. The electrolyte pattern depends on the duration of symptoms, the degree of dehydration, and the frequency of vomiting. Laboratory findings usually show an elevated white blood cell count (usually >10,000 per mm^3). Erect and recumbent plain abdominal radiographs are obtained and often demonstrate a

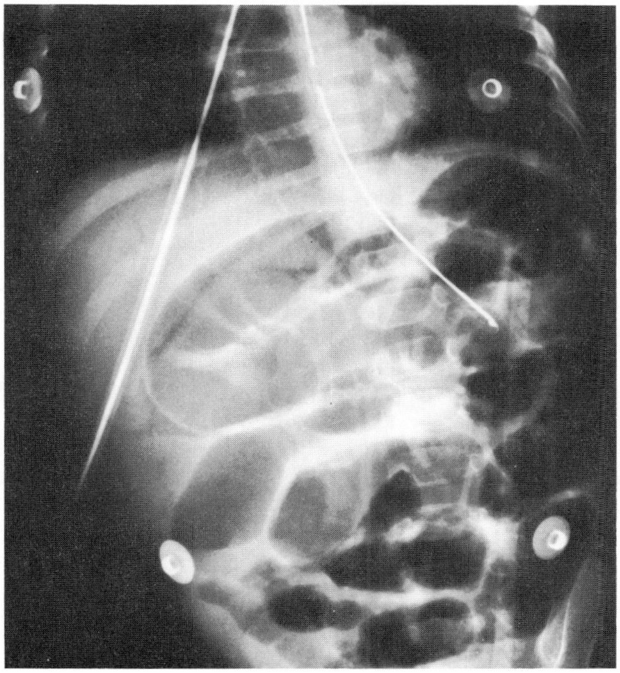

Figure 47–2. Multiple air-fluid levels are noted on the admitting radiographs in a child with symptoms of an intussusception for 5 days prior to admission.

variety of findings, including a nonspecific bowel gas pattern, air-fluid levels, or, rarely, free air consistent with a bowel perforation in cases with delayed diagnosis (Fig. 47–2).

A nasogastric tube is inserted, and intravenous fluid resuscitation is initiated prior to obtaining a radiologic diagnosis and attempting a reduction of the intussusception. Once the infant's condition is stable and adequate hydration is ensured, sedation may be safely used prior to an attempted reduction (Table 47–2). Because intussusception represents an intestinal obstruction, most surgeons routinely administer broad-spectrum antibiotics prior to any reduction attempts. When possible, the surgeon should be present in the radiology suite to observe the actual procedure. During this time the operating room is also notified about the case so that the transition from the radiology suite to the operating room is a smooth one in instances in which the hydrostatic barium enema reduction fails.

Table 47–2. SUGGESTED SEDATION PROTOCOLS FOR REDUCTION ATTEMPTS

Agent	Dose	Route
1. Secobarbital	1 mg/kg	Intramuscular
or		
2. Morphine (>1 year of age)	0.1 mg/kg	Intramuscular
or		
3. Meperidine	1 mg/kg	Intramuscular
Promethazine	0.5 mg/kg	Intramuscular
Chlorpromazine	0.5 mg/kg	Intramuscular

The standard procedure for diagnosis and treatment of ileocolic intussusception remains the hydrostatic barium enema. The risk of bowel perforation during the procedure varies from 1 to 3%, depending on the series reviewed.[3, 4, 12, 18, 19] Precautions include maintaining the height of the barium column at no more than 3 feet higher than the chest, limiting the constant hydrostatic pressure to no longer than 5 minutes, and avoiding abdominal manipulation during the procedure. The presence of an intraluminal mass and the "coiled spring" sign confirms the diagnosis of intussusception. A satisfactory reduction is noted when the intussusception passes retrograde through the ileocecal valve, and there is free reflux of barium into the last 2 feet of the terminal ileum (Fig. 47–3). If significant progress in moving the intussusceptum proximally is noted, reduction can be attempted again. The supplemental use of glucagon, which relaxes colonic smooth muscle, has not been effective in a randomized, multicenter, double-blinded study of 30 patients.[20, 21] This study reported no difference between the successful rate of reduction in children receiving a placebo and those receiving glucagon.[20, 21] Hydrostatic barium enema reduction is successful in 50 to 80% of cases, depending largely on the duration of symptoms and the referral pattern of the institution.[5, 9, 12, 22, 23] The success rate is reduced if symptoms are present longer than 48 hours (50%) versus less than 48 hours (70%). Bowel perforations are documented in 0.5 to 2.4% of the attempted reduction studies.[12, 23–25] When perforation is noted, it often occurs at the point of uninvolved intussuscipiens (usually the transverse colon) and when no excessive pressure has been used during the procedure (Fig. 47–4). The mesenteric vascular arcade system between the ileocolic and the right colic vessels may be incomplete in some children, and the arterial supply to the transverse colon may be compromised before the region becomes involved as the actual intussusceptum. As the back pressure from the venous and the lymphatic obstruction exceeds the arterial inflow pressure, full-thickness necrosis of the surrounding bowel wall can occur with minimal hydrostatic pressure during the radiologic studies. This group of children tends to be younger than 6 months of age, are ill for longer than 72 hours, and have evidence of a complete bowel obstruction noted on the initial abdominal radiographs.[12, 24, 25] In these high-risk cases, the barium study should be used only to confirm the diagnosis, and no attempt at therapeutic reduction should be undertaken. In the authors' last 120 patients seen with intussusception, three perforations occurred during the reduction attempts: one presented with free intraperitoneal air, and two had transverse colon perforations with barium extravasation noted at the time of laparotomy.

Hydrostatic reduction of the intussusception under ultrasound guidance has gained popularity as well.[23] In this method, water-soluble media is used, and satisfactory reduction is noted with the disappearance of the intussusceptum at the ileocecal valve, the retrograde flow of contrast medium into the small bowel, and the collapse of the previously distended right colon.

In recent years, air reduction techniques have gained popularity as an alternative to the barium or water-

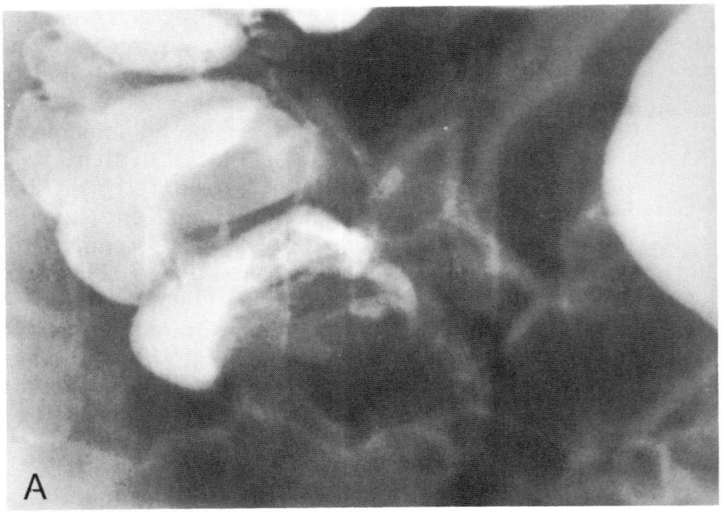

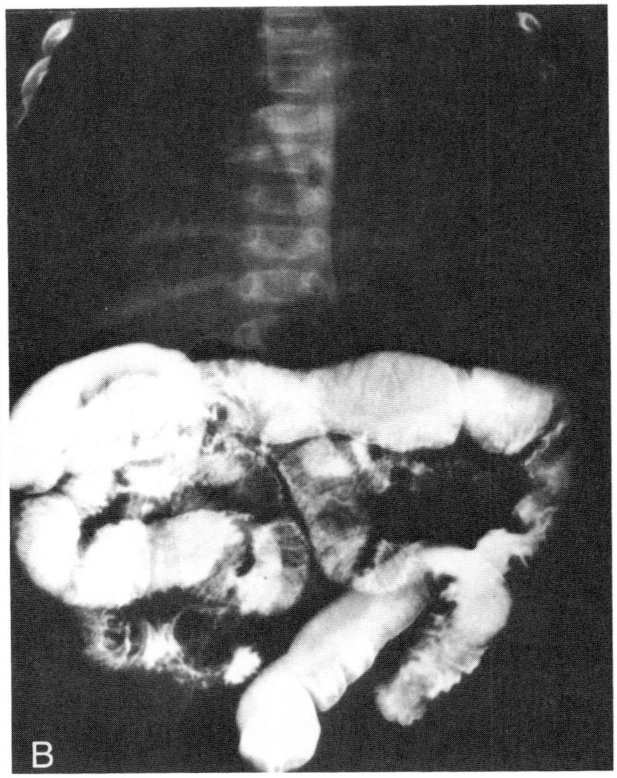

Figure 47–3. *A,* As an example of incomplete reduction of the intussusception, there is no free flow of barium into the small bowel noted in this study. *B,* Complete reduction is assured, with free flow of contrast flowing into the several feet of terminal ileum.

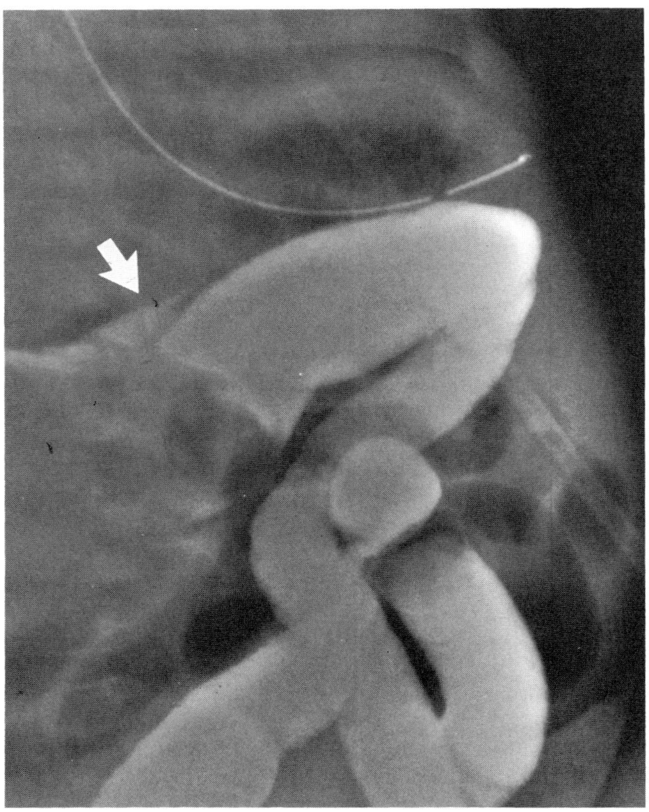

Figure 47–4. Although excessive hydrostatic pressure was not used during this barium study, a mid-transverse colon perforation occurred *(arrow)*.

soluble hydrostatic methods.[26] The initial reports concerning air reduction were published in 1897, but large series were not reported until 1959.[27] With this method, the buttocks are securely taped together, and a catheter with an anal seal device allows for the controlled inoculation of the colon with air under fluoroscopic guidance. Precautions during the process include maximum insufflation pressures of 120 mm Hg, attempts limited to 3 minutes, and no more than three successive attempts. Reflux of air into the terminal ileum and the disappearance of the mass at the ileocecal valve document a successful reduction. If the completeness of reduction is questioned, the air study can be repeated, or water-soluble contrast material can be instilled to confirm the free flow of material into the small bowel.[28] Using this technique in more than 6,000 patients, Chinese clinicians have reported the successful reduction of intussusception in 95% of cases, with other reports ranging from 73 to 95%.[29–31] The perforation rate varies from 0.14 to 0.2% (compared with 0.5–2.4% with hydrostatic techniques).[28–31] Additional advantages of air reduction modalities include lower radiation exposure and decreased patient cost.[32] When perforations are noted (on an upright or lateral decubitus abdominal radiograph obtained at the end of the procedure) with the air reduction method, the colonic wall tears are smaller than those observed with the hydrostatic barium techniques, peritoneal spillage tends to be minimal, and barium peritonitis is avoided. If the amount of air in the peritoneal cavity compromises the cardiorespiratory status of the patient during the transfer to surgery, needle decompression of the abdomen can be safely accomplished.

Following the successful reduction of an ileocolic intussusception, temperatures higher than 38°C are often noted. Fever may result from the release of endotoxin, cytokines (tumor necrosis factor, interleukin-1, and interleukin-6), or bacterial translocation. Nasogastric suction is maintained until bowel function has returned and a normal bowel movement has been passed. Feedings are advanced as tolerated, and most patients may be discharged from the hospital within 36 hours after reduction. Recurrent intussusception may be noted in 8 to 12% of patients following radiologic reduction and may occur during the initial hospitalization or months later (4 hours to 2 years in the authors' series).[12]

SURGICAL THERAPY

In children who have evidence of free peritoneal air on admitting abdominal radiographs, signs of peritoneal irritation, and prolonged symptoms (>5 days) at the time of clinical presentation, no attempt at hydrostatic barium reduction is made, and an operation is planned following an appropriate intravenous fluid resuscitation and the administration of broad-spectrum antibiotics.[12] Endotracheal intubation for general anesthesia is performed with the patient awake to minimize the risk of aspiration due to the obstructed intestinal tract. Following adequate skin preparation and wound draping, a transverse right lower quadrant incision is performed. In some patients in whom the radiologic reduction techniques have been unsuccessful, a complete reduction of the intussusception is noted at the time of laparotomy in 7 to 10% of reported cases.[12, 22, 33, 34] This outcome may result from the relaxation of smooth muscles during the induction of general anesthesia, which spontaneously reduces the intussusception. In these cases, the appendix is removed, and the abdomen closed. If the mass is still present, the bowel is mobilized to allow identification of the site of the intussusception. Manual reduction is attempted, with the intussusceptum being carefully milked proximally. The mass may reach a point of obstruction at the ileocecal valve. Gentle handling of the tissues is important to avoid serosal splitting of the colonic wall at this point (Fig. 47–5). Once the reduction is complete, an appendectomy is performed and, if present, Jackson's veil (a thickened band of peritoneum that often appears to draw the terminal ileum into the cecum) is divided. If the mass cannot be completely reduced, a right hemicolectomy with end-to-end anastomosis is performed. Bowel resection may be necessary in 15 to 41% of cases in various reported series. When a pathologic lead point is identified, resection of the lesion is accomplished (Fig. 47–6). When colonic perforations are encountered, the decision to perform a primary bowel anastomosis or temporary double-barrel ostomies depends on the hemodynamic status of the patient, the extent of fecal soiling, and the surgeon's preference. In cases of barium peritonitis, the barium should be débrided from the peritoneal surfaces. If an

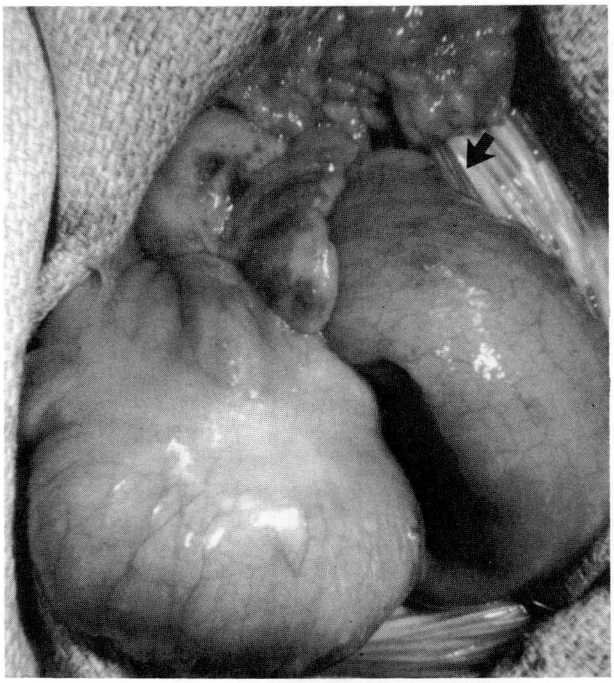

Figure 47–5. Typical appearance of an idiopathic ileocolic intussusception after the right colon has been mobilized to assist manual reduction *(arrow)*.

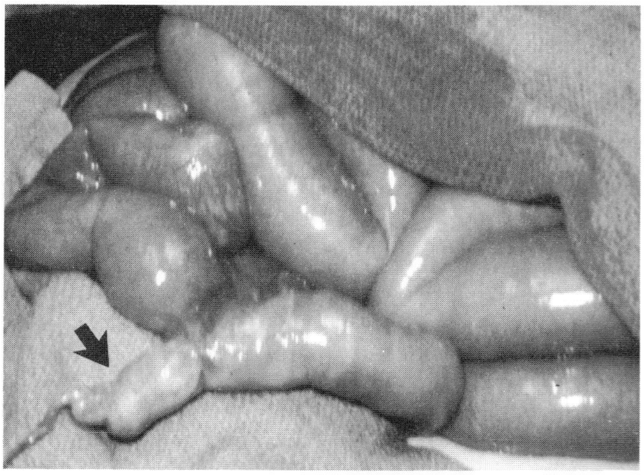

Figure 47–6. A Meckel's diverticulum *(arrow)* was the lead point for an intussusception that occurred in this child following a severe closed head injury.

enterostomy is performed, the stoma may be closed as soon as the patient's condition warrants (10–94 days in the authors' experience). Postoperative complications encountered include fever, prolonged ileus, wound infection, and intra-abdominal abscess (in cases of transverse colon perforations) (Table 47–3).

The incidence of recurrent intussusception following surgical reduction is extremely low, varying from 0 to 3%.[12, 33, 34] Although there have been no deaths related to intussusception reported at the J. W. Riley Hospital for Children, significant patient morbidity, extended length of stay, and hospitalization costs resulting from delay in diagnosis and referral for definitive treatment were observed (Table 47–4). When death occurs with intussusception, it is related to sepsis, peritonitis, and hemodynamic instability.

Postoperative Intussusception

Postoperative intestinal obstruction is a well-recognized complication of abdominal surgery and is usually caused by the formation of adhesions. A less well-recognized cause is postoperative intussusception (POI), which differs from its idiopathic counterpart in its clinical presentation.[33–44] In the patient with POI, the most frequently encountered symptoms include bilious emesis, abdominal distention, and irritability. Most episodes occur in the first postoperative week (in contrast with 14 days or longer when the obstruction is secondary to adhesions), and 75% of the children have a return of bowel function after their initial procedure when the symptoms of an obstruction develop (Table 47–5). The abdominal radiographs reveal multiple air-fluid levels and a stepladder bowel pattern consistent with a mechanical small bowel obstruction. During a 21-year period at J. W. Riley Hospital, 41 patients with POI were encountered (Table 47–6). Seventeen of the children underwent the initial operative procedure for complications of gastroesophageal reflux or disordered esophageal motility. Fifteen of these children were neurologically impaired and included infants with Smith-Lemli-Opitz and Cornelia de Lange's syndromes. As in most other series concerning POI, pathologic lead points were rarely found and constituted only 3% of cases.[35, 36, 38, 41] Although the causes of POI are unknown, postulated causes of invagination include a suture line, tumor implants on the bowel wall, appendiceal stumps, and Miller-Abbott tubes being removed with the balloon inflated. Other proposed causes of this form of intussus-

Table 47–3. POSTOPERATIVE COMPLICATIONS IN 120 CASES OF IDIOPATHIC INTUSSUSCEPTION*

Condition	No. of Patients
Fever >38.5° C	75
Ileus >7 days	9
Wound infection	8
Pneumonia	4
Urinary tract infection	2
Ostomy stenosis	2
Wound dehiscence	2
Intra-abdominal abscess	2

*From the J. W. Riley Hospital for Children, Indianapolis.

Table 47–4. LENGTH OF HOSPITALIZATION RELATED TO TYPE OF THERAPY FOR INTUSSUSCEPTION*

Method	Average No. of Days	Range
Air reduction	1.5	1–2
Hydrostatic barium reduction	1.5	1–4
Intraoperative manual reduction	6.8	3–29
Bowel resection	10	4–47

*From the J. W. Riley Hospital for Children, Indianapolis.

Table 47–5. INITIAL SURGICAL PROCEDURES PRECEDING POSTOPERATIVE INTUSSUSCEPTION*

Procedure	No. of Patients
Foregut motility	
Nissen fundoplication	15
Gastropexy	1
Heller myotomy	1
Neurocrestopathy	
Neuroblastoma	5
Hirschsprung's disease	3
Small bowel resection	4
Inguinal herniorrhaphy	3
Urinary tract reconstruction	3
Thoracic procedures	2
Ventral hernia	1
Nephrectomy	1
Hepatic resection	1
Ventriculoatrial shunt	1
Total	41

*From the J. W. Riley Hospital for Children, Indianapolis.

Table 47–6. LOCATION OF LESION IN VARIOUS FORMS OF INTUSSUSCEPTION*

Location	No. of Patients	
	Idiopathic	*Postoperative*
Ileocolic	109	5
Ileoileal	3	28
Colocolic	5	0
Jejunojejunal	3	6
Jejunoileal	0	2
Total	120	41

*From the J. W. Riley Hospital for Children, Indianapolis.

ception include serosal damage during the previous operative procedure that can lead to lymph node hypertrophy, which may then act as a subsequent lead point for the process.[37, 45] Perhaps the serosal exudate may become fixed as an adhesion and prevent the spontaneous reduction of the small bowel intussusception, which is often observed to occur spontaneously at the time of laparotomy.[43] Children with underlying conditions associated with disordered esophageal motility (e.g., gastroesophageal reflux and achalasia) may be at higher risk for POI.[35, 36, 41] A central nervous system component has also been implicated in this process with the observation that stimulation of the premotor cortex in the brain of a *Macaca mulatta* primate model can induce the occurrence of a small bowel intussusception.[46] Other neuroendocrine factors have also been suggested, since children with neural crest abnormalities (Hirschsprung's disease, achalasia of the esophagus, and neuroblastoma) also appear to be at higher risk for the occurrence of POI.[35, 36, 44]

Unlike in infants and children with idiopathic ileocolic intussusception, diagnostic contrast studies are not as helpful in this group of patients, since most cases of POI occur in the small bowel (see Table 47–6).[35, 36] In the authors' experience, only five of the patients had the intussusceptum at the ileocecal valve, and the hydrostatic barium enema was successful in reducing the lead point in only three children. One child with Hirschsprung's disease had a right-sided colostomy, in which the contrast studies are not helpful unless the diagnosis is uncertain and can be used to differentiate adynamic ileus from mechanical obstruction. Laparotomy performed early in the clinical course of POI can obviate the need for segmental bowel resection and bowel anastomosis, since most lesions can be manually reduced (Fig. 47–7). Four of 41 children in this series required resection. The patients had a duration of symptoms ranging from 10 to 21 days (mean 17 days) and had associated bacteremia or required mechanical ventilatory support and muscular paralysis following their initial surgical procedure. The postoperative complications encountered in POI patients included fever higher than 38.5°C (10), wound infection (4), pneumonia (4), prolonged ileus (4), urinary tract infection (2), and bacteremia (1). There were no deaths in this group of patients. As in the treatment of the commoner idiopathic variety of intussusception, a prompt laparotomy prevents bowel necrosis and reduces the overall morbidity and mortality.

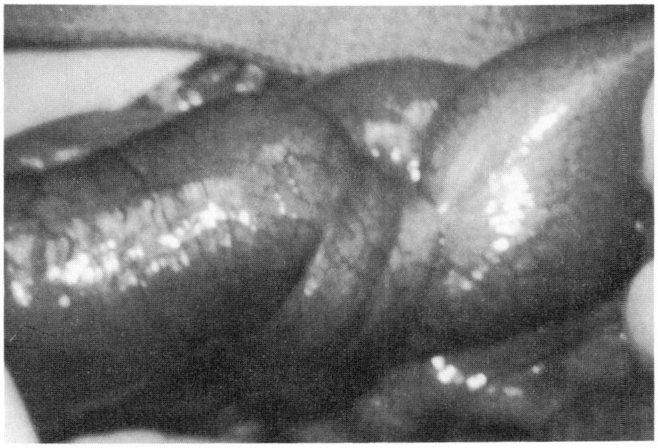

Figure 47–7. Intraoperative view of a jejunal-ileal intussusception that occurred 1 week following a Nissen fundoplication procedure.

REFERENCES

1. Barbette P: Oeuvres Chirurgiques et Anatomiques. Geneva, Francois Miege, 1674, p 522.
2. Hutchinson J: A successful case of abdominal section for intussusception. Proc R Med Chir Soc 1873; 7:195–196.
3. Ravitch MM, McCune RM: Reduction of intussusception by hydrostatic pressure: An experimental study. Bull Johns Hopkins 1948; 82:550–552.
4. Ravitch MM: Intussusception in infancy and childhood. N Engl J Med 1958; 259:1058–1064.
5. Rosenkrantz JG, Cox JA, Silverman FN, et al: Intussusception in the 1970's: Indication for operation. J Pediatr Surg 1977; 12:367–373.
6. Konno T, Suzuki H, Kutsuzawa T, et al: Human rotavirus infection in infants and young children with intussusception. J Med Virol 1982; 2:265–269.
7. Mulcahy DL, Kamath KR, deSilva LM, et al: A two-part study of the aetiological role of rotavirus in intussusception. J Med Virol 1982; 9:51–55.
8. Nicholas JC, Ingrand D, Fortier B, et al: A one-year virological survey of acute intussusception in childhood. J Med Virol 1982; 9:267–271.
9. Freund H, Hurvitz H, Schiller M: Etiologic and therapeutic aspects of intussusception in childhood. Am J Surg 1977; 134:272–274.
10. Danis RK: Lymphoid hyperplasia of the ileum—always a benign disease? Am J Dis Child 1974; 127:656–658.
11. Ein SH: Leading points in childhood intussusception. J Pediatr Surg 1976; 11:209–211.
12. West KW, Stephens B, Vane DW, et al: Intussusception: Current management in infants and children. Surgery 1987; 102:781–787.
13. Holsclaw DS, Rocmans C, Shwachman H: Intussusception in patients with cystic fibrosis. Pediatrics 1971; 48:51–58.
14. Ruoff M, Lindner AE, Marshak RH: Intussusception in sprue. Am J Roentgenol 1968; 104:525–528.
15. Valletta EA, Mastella G: Incidence of celiac disease in a cystic fibrosis population. Acta Paediatr Scand 1989; 78:784–785.
16. Cohen DM, Conard FU, Treem WR, et al: Jejuno-jejunal intussusception in Crohn's disease. J Pediatr Gastroenterol 1992; 14:101–103.
17. Knowles MC, Fishman EK, Kuhlman JE, et al: Transient intus-

susception in Crohn's disease: CT evaluation. Radiology 1989; 170:814.
18. Ravitch MM, McCune RM: Intussusception in infants and children. J Pediatr 1950; 37:153–173.
19. Hirschsprung H: Et Tilfaelde at Subakut Tarminvagination. Hospitals-Tidende 1976; 3:321–322.
20. Hoy GR, Dunbar D, Boles ET Jr: The use of glucagon in the diagnosis and management of ileocolic intussusception. J Pediatr Surg 1977; 12:939–944.
21. Franken EA, Smith WL, Chernish SM, et al: The use of glucagon in hydrostatic reduction of intussusception. Radiology 1983; 146: 687–689.
22. Lynn HB: Intussusception. *In* Holder TM, Ashcraft KW, eds: Pediatric Surgery. 5th ed. Philadelphia, WB Saunders 1980, pp 438–444.
23. Bolia A: Case report: Diagnosis and hydrostatic reduction of an intussusception under ultrasound guidance. Clin Radiol 1985; 36:655–657.
24. Mercer S, Carpenter B: Mechanism of perforation occurring in the intussusception. Can J Surg 1982; 25:481–483.
25. Ein SH, Mercer S, Humphrey A, et al: Colon perforation during attempted barium enema reduction of intussusception. J Pediatr Surg 1981; 16:313–315.
26. Guo JB, Ma X, Ahou Q: Results of air pressure enema reduction of intussusception: 6,396 cases in 13 years. J Pediatr Surg 1986; 12:1201–1203.
27. Fiorito ES, Recalde Cuestas LA: Diagnosis and treatment of acute intestinal intussusception with controlled insufflation of air. Pediatrics 1959; 24:241.
28. Stringer DA, Ein SH: Pneumatic reduction: Advantages, risks, and indications. Pediatr Radiol 1990; 20:475.
29. Jinzhe Z, Yenxia W, Linchi W: Rectal inflation reduction of intussusception in infants. J Pediatr Surg 1986; 21:30.
30. Hedlund GL, Johnson FJ, Strife JS: Ileocolic intussusception: Extensive reflux of air preceding pneumatic reduction. Radiology 1990; 174:187.
31. Shiels WE, Bisse GS, Kirks DR: Simple device for air reduction of intussusception. Pediatr Radiol 1990; 20:472.
32. Palder SB, Ein SH, Stringer DA et al: Intussusception: Barium or air? J Pediatr Surg 1991; 26:271–275.
33. Ein SH, Stephens CA: Intussusception: 354 cases in 10 years. J Pediatr Surg 1971; 6:16–27.
34. Wayer ER, Campbell JB, Burrington JD, et al: Management of 344 children with intussusception. Radiology 1973; 107:597–601.
35. Mollitt DL, Ballantine TVN, Grosfeld JL: Postoperative intussusception in infancy and childhood: Analysis of 119 cases. Surgery 1979; 86:402–408.
36. West KW, Stephens B, Rescorla FJ, et al: Postoperative intussusception: Experience with 36 cases in children. Surgery 1988; 104:781–787.
37. Ein SH, Ferguson JN: Intussusception: The forgotten postoperative obstruction. Arch Dis Child 1982; 57:788–790.
38. McGovern JB, Gross RE: Intussusception as a postoperative complication. Surgery 1968; 63:507–513.
39. Cox JA, Martin CW: Postoperative intussusception. Arch Surg 1973; 106:263–266.
40. Stevenson EO, Hays DM, Snyder WH: Postoperative intussusception in infants and children. Am J Surg 1967; 113:562–567.
41. Jolley SG, Tunell WP, Hollinger DT: Postoperative small bowel obstruction in infants and children. Am J Surg 1967; 113:562–567.
42. Dudgeon DL, Hays DM: Intussusception complicating the therapy of malignancy in childhood. Arch Surg 1972; 105:52–56.
43. Shaw A, Francois E: An unusual case of postoperative intussusception. Surgery 1966; 59:455–457.
44. Cohen MO, Baker M, Grosfeld JL, et al: Postoperative intussusception in children with neuroblastoma. Br J Radiol 1982; 55:197–200.
45. Nissan S, Levy E: Intussusception in infancy caused by hypertrophic Peyer's patches. Surgery 1966; 59:1108–1110.
46. Watts JW, Fulton JF: Intussusception—the relationship of the cerebral cortex to intestinal motility in the monkey. N Engl J Med 1934; 210:883–896.

Chapter 48

Chronic Intestinal Pseudo-obstruction

PAUL E. HYMAN and CARLO DiLORENZO

Chronic intestinal pseudo-obstruction is a clinical diagnosis based on phenotype. It may be defined as the presence of signs and symptoms characteristic of intestinal blockage in the absence of an anatomic obstruction. The most common signs are abdominal distention and failure to thrive. The most common symptoms are abdominal pain, vomiting, and constipation or diarrhea. The term *chronic idiopathic intestinal pseudo-obstruction* was first used to organize an approach to the care of children with this group of unexplained symptoms.[1] More recently, chronic intestinal pseudo-obstruction has come to represent a number of different conditions that vary widely in terms of their cause, severity, course, and response to therapy (Table 48–1). Examples of genetic heterogeneity in pseudo-obstruction include, but are not limited to, descriptions of a wide spectrum of abnormal gastric, small intestinal, and colonic myoelectric activity and contractions as well as abnormalities in nerve and muscle from tissue samples. Preliminary classification systems are used in an attempt to organize the variety of nerve and muscle disorders that cause the symptoms into a heuristic model. In some ways, chronic intestinal pseudo-obstruction is an obsolete term, because it is now possible to employ sophisticated pathologic and physiologic techniques to distinguish among many disorders that cause the symptoms.

Although these diseases have distinctive pathophysiologic characteristics, they are considered together because of their clinical and therapeutic similarities. There is sometimes disagreement and sometimes confusion among physicians concerning precisely what constitutes a diagnosis of chronic intestinal pseudo-obstruction. For individual communications, it may be better to provide a description of the patient and the clinical course. On the other hand, grouping may be useful for increasing physician awareness of these rare conditions as well as for issues of diagnosis and management.

ETIOLOGY

Pseudo-obstruction may occur as a primary disease or as a secondary manifestation of a large number of other conditions that may transiently (e.g., hypothyroidism or phenothiazines) or permanently (e.g., scleroderma or amyloidosis) alter bowel motility (Table 48–2).

Most primary congenital forms of both neuropathic and myopathic pseudo-obstruction are apparently sporadic. That is, there is no family history of pseudo-obstruction, no associated syndrome, and no evidence of other predisposing factors such as toxins, infections, ischemia, or autoimmune disease.

In a few cases, chronic intestinal pseudo-obstruction may result from a familial inherited disease. There are reports of autosomal dominant[2, 3] and recessive[4–6] neuropathic, and dominant[7–9] and recessive[10, 11] myopathic, patterns of inheritance. In the autosomal dominant diseases, there is variability in expressivity and penetrance; some of those affected die in childhood, but those less handicapped are able to reproduce.

Pseudo-obstruction may result from exposure to toxins during critical developmental periods in utero. A few children with fetal alcohol syndrome and a few with narcotic-abusing mothers have neuropathic forms of pseudo-obstruction. Presumably any substance that alters neuronal migration or maturation might affect the

Table 48–1. HETEROGENEITY OF CHRONIC INTESTINAL PSEUDO-OBSTRUCTION IN PEDIATRIC PATIENTS

Onset	**Symptoms**
Congenital	Constant or intermittent
Acquired	Vary in intensity
Acute	Cyclic
Gradual	
	Areas of Involvement
Presentation	Entire gastrointestinal tract
Acute bowel obstruction	Segmental
Gastroesophageal reflux	Megaduodenum
Constipation	Small bowel
Chronic abdominal pain	Colon
Chronic abdominal distention	
	Pathology
Etiology	Myopathy
Sporadic	Neuropathy
Familial	Absent neurons
Toxic	Immature neurons
Ischemic	Degenerating neurons
Viral	No microscopic abnormality
Autoimmune	

Table 48–2. CAUSES OF CHRONIC PSEUDO-OBSTRUCTION IN CHILDREN

Primary Pseudo-Obstruction
Visceral myopathy
Sporadic
Familial
Visceral neuropathy
Sporadic
Familial
Secondary Pseudo-Obstruction (Related to or Associated with Recognized Causes)
Muscular dystrophies
Scleroderma and other connective tissue diseases
Postischemic neuropathy
Postviral neuropathy
Generalized dysautonomia
Hypothyroidism
Diabetic autonomic neuropathy
Drugs—anticholinergics, opiates, Ca^{2+} channel blockers
Severe inflammatory bowel disease
Postorgan transplantation
Amyloidosis
Chagas disease
Fetal alcohol syndrome
Chromosome abnormalities
Multiple endocrine neoplasia 2B
Radiation enteritis

development of the myenteric plexus and cause pseudo-obstruction.

Children with chromosomal abnormalities or syndromes may suffer from pseudo-obstruction. It is known that children with Down's syndrome may have abnormal esophageal motility,[12] neuronal dysplasia in the myenteric plexus, and a higher incidence of Hirschsprung's disease than the general population. A few children with Down's syndrome have a myenteric plexus neuropathy so generalized and so severe that they present with pseudo-obstruction. Children with neurofibromatosis, multiple endocrine neoplasia, type 2B (MEN 2B), Russell-Silver syndrome, and other chromosomal aberrations and autonomic neuropathies may suffer from severe neuropathic constipation. Children with Duchenne's muscular dystrophy sometimes develop pseudo-obstruction,[13] especially in the terminal stages of life. Esophageal manometry (A. Staiano, personal communication) and gastric emptying[14] are abnormal in Duchenne's dystrophy, suggesting that the myopathy includes gastrointestinal smooth muscle, even in asymptomatic children.

Acquired pseudo-obstruction may be a rare complication of viral acute gastroenteritis, presumably resulting from viral injury to neurons of the myenteric plexus.[15] Cytomegalovirus infection of the myenteric plexus can cause pseudo-obstruction.[16] Preliminary observations implicate Epstein-Barr virus[17] and rotavirus[18] as well. Many of the acquired cases of pseudo-obstruction might be a result of myenteric plexus neuritis from viral infection.

Very preterm infants often have prolonged feeding difficulties. These difficulties may be related in part to immature motility patterns or to ischemia induced by the failure to meet the increased need for blood flow following feeding. Some infants with bronchopulmonary dysplasia appear to have severe gastrointestinal motility abnormalities. Their preterm birth and stormy courses of chronic hypoxemia and ischemia are consistent with the development of pseudo-obstruction due to myenteric plexus injury or maturation arrest. Children may develop pseudo-obstruction following necrotizing enterocolitis[19] or gastroschisis, presumably for similar reasons of local ischemia and neuronal injury or maturational arrest.

There is speculation that some cases of pseudo-obstruction may be mediated by an abnormality of the immune system. Many affected infants and toddlers have food allergies. A few older children have pseudo-obstruction associated with autoimmune features such as persistently positive antinuclear antibodies or systemic rhabdomyolysis.

PATHOLOGY

There may be histologic abnormalities in the muscle or nerve or, rarely, both.[20, 21] Normal histology is found in about 10% of cases that are studied appropriately. In such cases there may be an abnormality in some biochemical aspect of stimulus-contraction coupling.

When laparotomy is imminent for a child with pseudo-obstruction, there must be timely communication between the surgeon and the pathologist. It is generally agreed that a laparotomy is not indicated for biopsy alone,[22] perhaps because a pathologic diagnosis usually does not alter the clinical management or the clinical course. When surgery is indicated (e.g., for cholecystectomy or creation of a feeding jejunostomy), a plan should be made to obtain a biopsy of full thickness bowel, at least 2 × 2 cm in diameter. The tissues should be processed for histology, histochemistry for selected peptides and enzymes, electron microscopy, and silver stains.

Muscle disease may be inflammatory but is more often noninflammatory. In light microscopy of both familial and sporadic forms of hollow visceral myopathy, the muscularis appears thin. The external longitudinal muscle layer is more involved than the internal circular muscle, and there may be extensive fibrosis within the muscle tissue. By electron microscopy there is vacuolar degeneration and disordered myofilaments (Fig. 48–1A and B).

Neuropathic disease is best examined with silver stains of the myenteric plexus[23, 24] as well as routine histology. The presence of neurons in the submucous plexus of a suction biopsy eliminates Hirschsprung's disease as a diagnostic possibility but is inadequate for the evaluation of other neuropathies.

There may be maturational arrest of the myenteric plexus (Fig. 48–2A and B). This hypoganglionosis is characterized by fewer neurons, and the neurons may be smaller than normal. Maturational arrest may be a primary congenital disorder or may occur secondary to ischemia or infection. Changes may be patchy or generalized.

Intestinal neuronal dysplasia,[25] or hyperganglionosis, is characterized histologically by hyperplasia of the para-

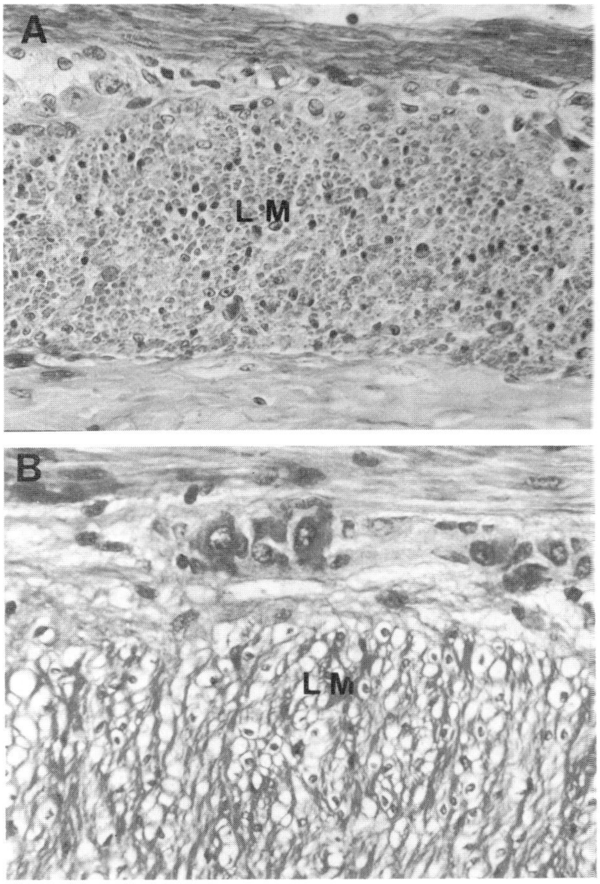

Figure 48–1. Visceral myopathy. *A*, Longitudinal muscle cut in cross section from the small intestine of a control infant. *B*, Longitudinal muscle from an infant with visceral myopathy showing classic vacuolar degeneration. Note the normal neurons in the myenteric plexus above the longitudinal muscle. Magnification × 136. (Courtesy of Dr. Michael D. Schuffler.)

sympathetic neurons and fibers of the myenteric and sometimes submucous plexuses. Children with intestinal neuronal dysplasia are a heterogeneous group even within pseudo-obstruction. Children with primary pseudo-obstruction due to neuronal dysplasia may have disease that is limited to the colon or disseminated. Other children may have neuronal dysplasia associated with prematurity, protein allergy, chromosomal abnormalities, MEN 2B, and neurofibromatosis.

CLINICAL FEATURES

Presentation

More than half the affected children develop symptoms at or shortly after birth. A few children are diagnosed in utero, with ultrasound findings of polyhydramnios and megacystis and marked abdominal distention (Fig. 48–3). About two thirds of children with congenital symptoms were born preterm. Intestinal malrotation is found in both neuropathic and myopathic congenital forms of pseudo-obstruction. Of children presenting at birth, about 40% have a malrotation. In the most severely affected infants symptoms of acute bowel obstruction appear within the first hours of life. Less severely affected infants present months later with symptoms of vomiting and diarrhea and failure to thrive. More than three quarters of the children develop symptoms by the end of the first year of life, and the remainder present sporadically through the first two decades.

Although there is great individual variation in the number and intensity of signs and symptoms, it may be useful to note the relative frequencies within this pop-

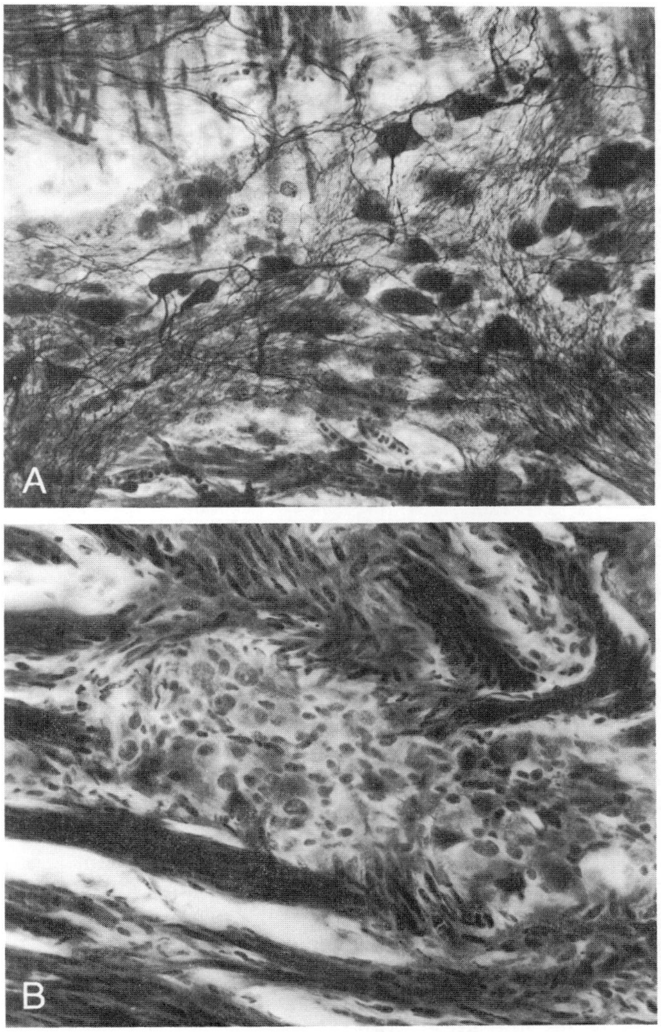

Figure 48–2. Maturational arrest of myenteric plexus. *A*, Ganglionic area of myenteric plexus from the small intestine of a control infant. Note the numerous argyrophilic neurons and axons. *B*, Ganglionic area of myenteric plexus from the small intestine of an infant with chronic intestinal pseudo-obstruction caused by maturational arrest. Note the absence of argyrophilic neurons and axons. The ganglion is filled with numerous cells, which are probably glial cells and immature neurons. Magnification × 544. (Courtesy of Dr. Michael D. Schuffler.)

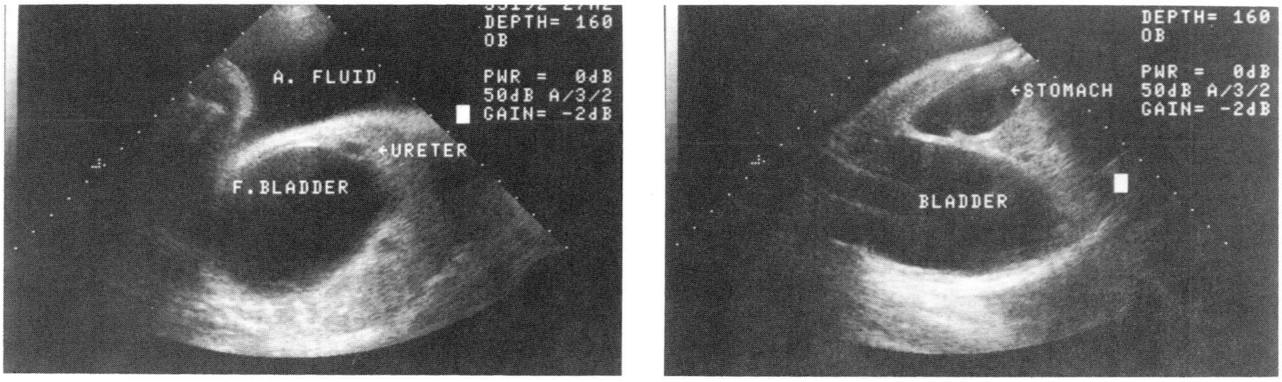

Figure 48–3. Ultrasound of infant with pseudo-obstruction diagnosed in utero. There is polyhydramnios as well as distention of the stomach and urinary bladder. (Courtesy of Radha Cherukuri, M.D.)

ulation. Abdominal distention and vomiting are the most common features, with complaints in about three quarters of the patients. Constipation, abdominal pain, and poor weight gain are features in about 60%. Diarrhea is a complaint in one third. Urinary tract smooth muscle is affected in those with both hollow visceral neuropathy and hollow visceral myopathy—about one fifth of all pseudo-obstruction patients. Often these children are severely affected and present at birth with the descriptive diagnosis of megacystic-microcolon intestinal hypoperistalsis syndrome.

The majority of children experience a clinical course characterized by relative remissions and exacerbations. Many are able to identify factors that precipitate deteriorations, including intercurrent infections, general anesthesia, psychological stress, and poor nutritional status.

The radiographic signs are those of intestinal obstruction, with air fluid levels (Fig. 48–4), dilated small intestine in one third of children, and microcolon in those studied because of obstruction at birth.[26] There may be prolonged stasis of contrast material placed into the affected bowel, so it is prudent to plan a means to evacuate the contrast fluid, or to use a nontoxic, isotonic water-soluble contrast in order to prevent barium from solidifying and presenting a true anatomic obstruction. Children may feel well but still show radiographic evidence of bowel obstruction. The greater problem arises when children develop an acute deterioration. Radiographs may demonstrate the same patterns of bowel obstruction that are seen when the child feels well. In children who had previous surgery, it can be difficult to discriminate between physical obstruction related to adhesions and an episodic increase in the symptoms of pseudo-obstruction.

Diagnosis

Chronic intestinal pseudo-obstruction is a clinical diagnosis, based on the signs and symptoms delineated above, in the absence of an anatomic obstruction. However, pseudo-obstruction is a commonly misdiagnosed disease in infants and children.[27] Despite the early and dramatic clinical presentation in many children, the time between the onset of disease and diagnosis has averaged about 3 years, as physicians mistakenly attribute the symptoms to more common conditions.

Further diagnostic testing may provide additional information about the nature and severity of the patho-

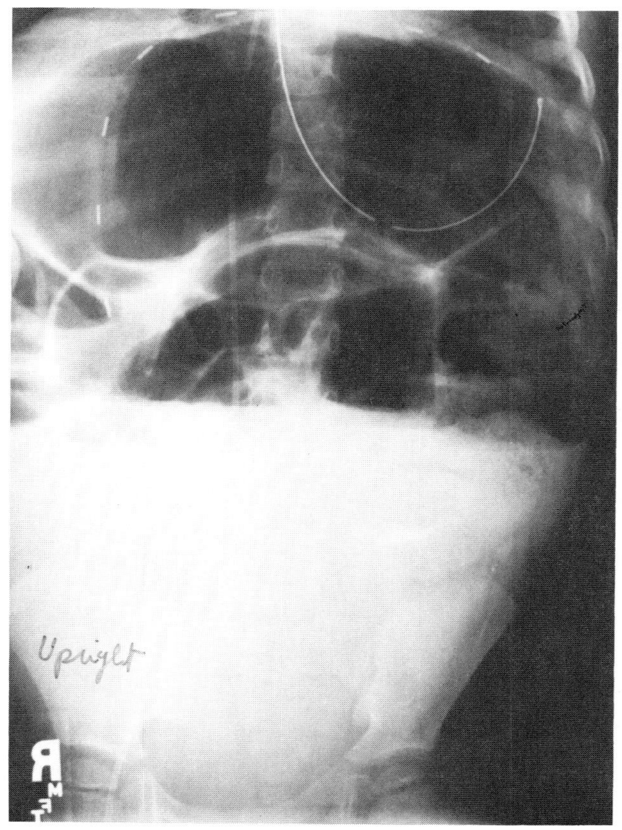

Figure 48–4. Upright abdominal radiograph in a 4-year-old boy with hollow visceral myopathy. Note massive bowel dilatation and air-fluid levels, central venous catheter in the inferior vena cava, and antroduodenal manometry catheter in the stomach and the duodenum.

physiology. Manometric studies are much more sensitive than radiographic tests to evaluate the strength and coordination of contraction and relaxation in the esophagus, gastric antrum, small intestine, colon, and anorectal area.

Gastric emptying of a solid nutrient meal is the best screening test for mild gastroparesis. In severely affected children there may be very delayed gastric emptying of solids or liquids and reflux of intestinal contents back into the stomach.

Esophageal motility abnormalities can be demonstrated with manometry in about half those affected by pseudo-obstruction. In children with myopathy, contractions are low amplitude but coordinated in the distal two thirds of the esophagus. Lower esophageal sphincter pressure is low, and relaxation of the sphincter is complete. When the esophagus is affected by neuropathy, contraction amplitude in the esophageal body may be high, normal, low, or absent. There may be simultaneous, spontaneous, or repetitive contractions. There may be incomplete relaxation of the lower esophageal sphincter.

Antroduodenal manometry is always abnormal in intestinal pseudo-obstruction involving the upper gastrointestinal tract. However, manometry is often abnormal in partial or complete small bowel obstruction. Although the manometric patterns of true obstruction may differ from those of pseudo-obstruction in adults,[28, 29] such distinction was not clear in children we have studied. Antroduodenal manometry should not be used as a test to differentiate true bowel obstruction from pseudo-obstruction. Manometry should be done after a diagnosis of pseudo-obstruction is established, in order to determine the physiologic correlates for the symptoms, to assess drug responses, and for prognosis. Contrast radiography and, as a last resort, exploratory laparotomy, are best for differentiating true obstruction from pseudo-obstruction.

Increases in intraluminal pressure are inversely proportional to the bowel diameter (Laplace's law). Therefore, in dilated bowel it is possible that no contractions are recorded, and the test is uninterpretable because tension developed by the muscle is insufficient to raise the pressure. Acute pseudo-obstruction is usually associated with ileus, so that patterns of antroduodenal contractions may not reflect the underlying abnormality. As in the esophagus, intestinal myopathy causes low-amplitude coordinated contractions, and neuropathy causes uncoordinated contractions. Interpretation of antroduodenal manometry requires recognition of normal and abnormal features (Table 48–3). Although sophisticated mathematics and computer software may be employed to calculate motility indices and analyze results, the abnormalities in pseudo-obstruction are commonly discrete and easily interpreted by eye[30, 31] (Fig. 48–5A–E). They contrast markedly with normal features of antroduodenal manometry (Fig. 48–6A and B).

In most cases the manometric disorganization correlates with the clinical severity and the anatomic lesion. For example, children with total aganglionosis have contractions of normal amplitude that are never organized into migrating motor complexes (MMCs), fed patterns, or even bursts or clusters of contractions, but are simply a monotonous pattern of random events. Children with such a pattern are dependent on total parenteral nutrition (TPN). In contrast, there are children with normal MMCs and a normal phase 2–like pattern after meals who have abnormal nonpropagating bursts of contractions. These children usually eat by mouth, although they complain of bloating, pain, vomiting, and constipation. Greater than 80% of children with MMCs are enterally nourished, but greater than 80% of children without MMCs require partial or total parenteral nutrition. Discrete abnormalities in the organization of intestinal contractions are listed in Table 48–3.

Table 48–3. ANTRODUODENAL MANOMETRIC FEATURES FROM STUDIES IN 300 CHILDREN*

Normal Features
Migrating motor complex (fasting)
Postprandial (phase 2–like) pattern
Abnormal Features in Duodenum
Short, nonpropagating clusters
Tonic contractions
Retrograde propagation of phase 3
Giant single-propagating contractions
Absent phase 2 (with increased MMC frequency)
Persistently low-amplitude or absent contractions
Long bursts
Postprandial Abnormalities
Antral hypomotility after a solid nutrient meal
Absent or decreased motility
Failure to induce a fed pattern (MMC persists)

*From Hyman, unpublished data. Each of these features is easily recognized by visual inspection of the recording.

Colonic manometry is abnormal in colonic pseudo-obstruction. There is no postprandial gastrocolonic response[32, 33] in those with neuropathic disease. That is, contractions are normal in amplitude, but the expected postprandial increase in motility index is lacking. In those with myopathy there are usually no colonic contractions. There is often a decrease in transit of luminal contents.

Anorectal manometry is normal in chronic intestinal pseudo-obstruction. There is an absence of the rectoinhibitory reflex only in Hirschsprung's disease.

Electrogastrography is in its formative stages of development but may prove to be a useful, noninvasive diagnostic tool for the evaluation of children with pseudo-obstruction.[34] Skin electrodes are placed over the stomach, just as surface electrodes are placed over the heart to perform electrocardiography. The electrical slow wave rhythms of the gastric body and antrum are recorded. Gastric slow waves normally occur at a rate of 3 per minute. Gastric neuropathies are characterized by decreases (bradygastria) or increases (tachygastria) in slow wave frequency.

The sensory afferent neurons of the gut link pain to motility.[35] It seems likely that pain and stress alter motility, just as abnormal motility results in pain. Methods to measure the contribution of sensory afferent neurons to the control of gastrointestinal motility are limited largely to animals and laboratories. Further

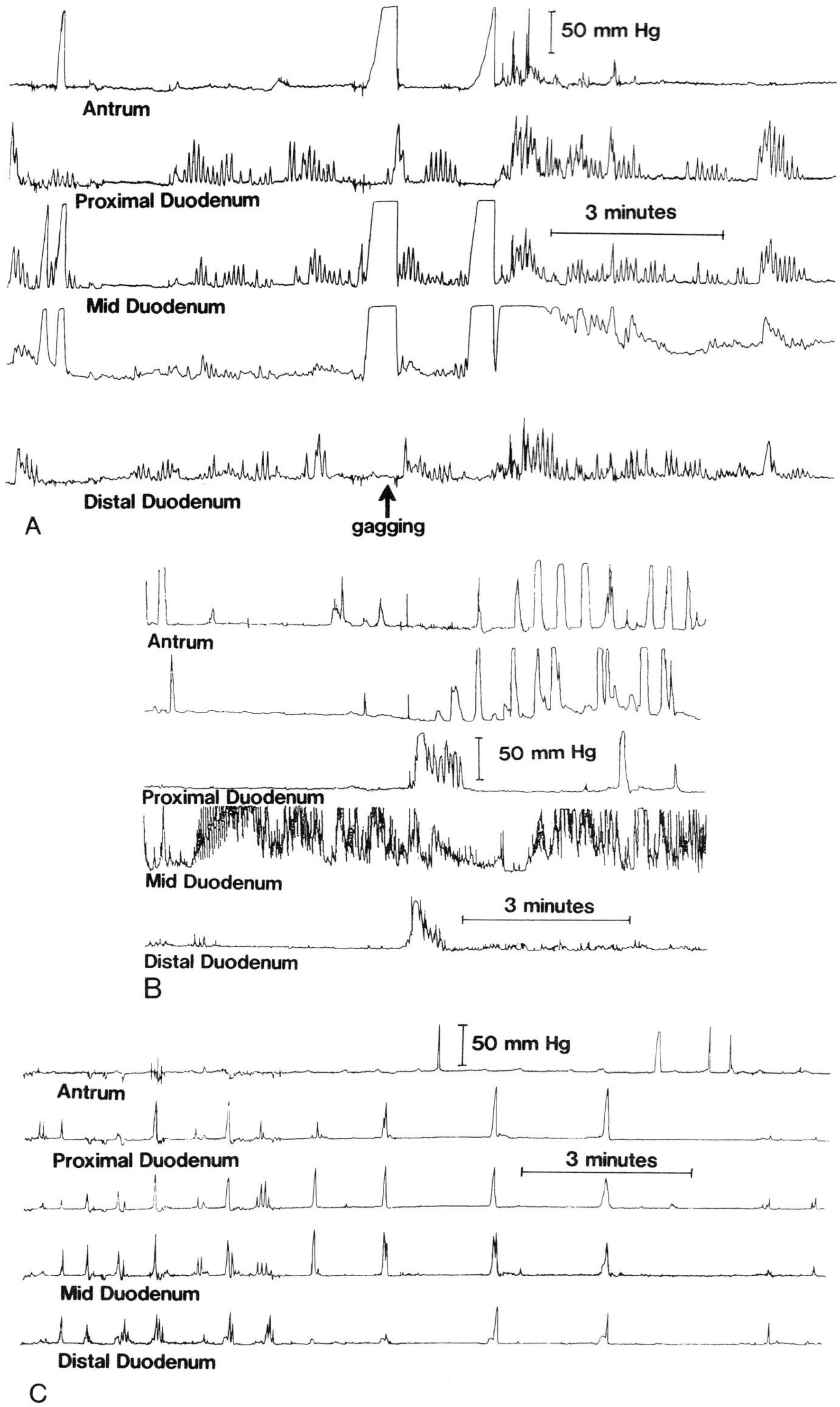

Figure 48–5. Discrete abnormalities in antroduodenal manometry. *A,* Giant retrograde duodenal contractions, propagating into the antrum. *B,* Tonic contractions in the mid-duodenum. *C,* Single propagating high-amplitude duodenal contractions. These "single ring" contractions are associated with irritable bowel disorders when the MMC is present.

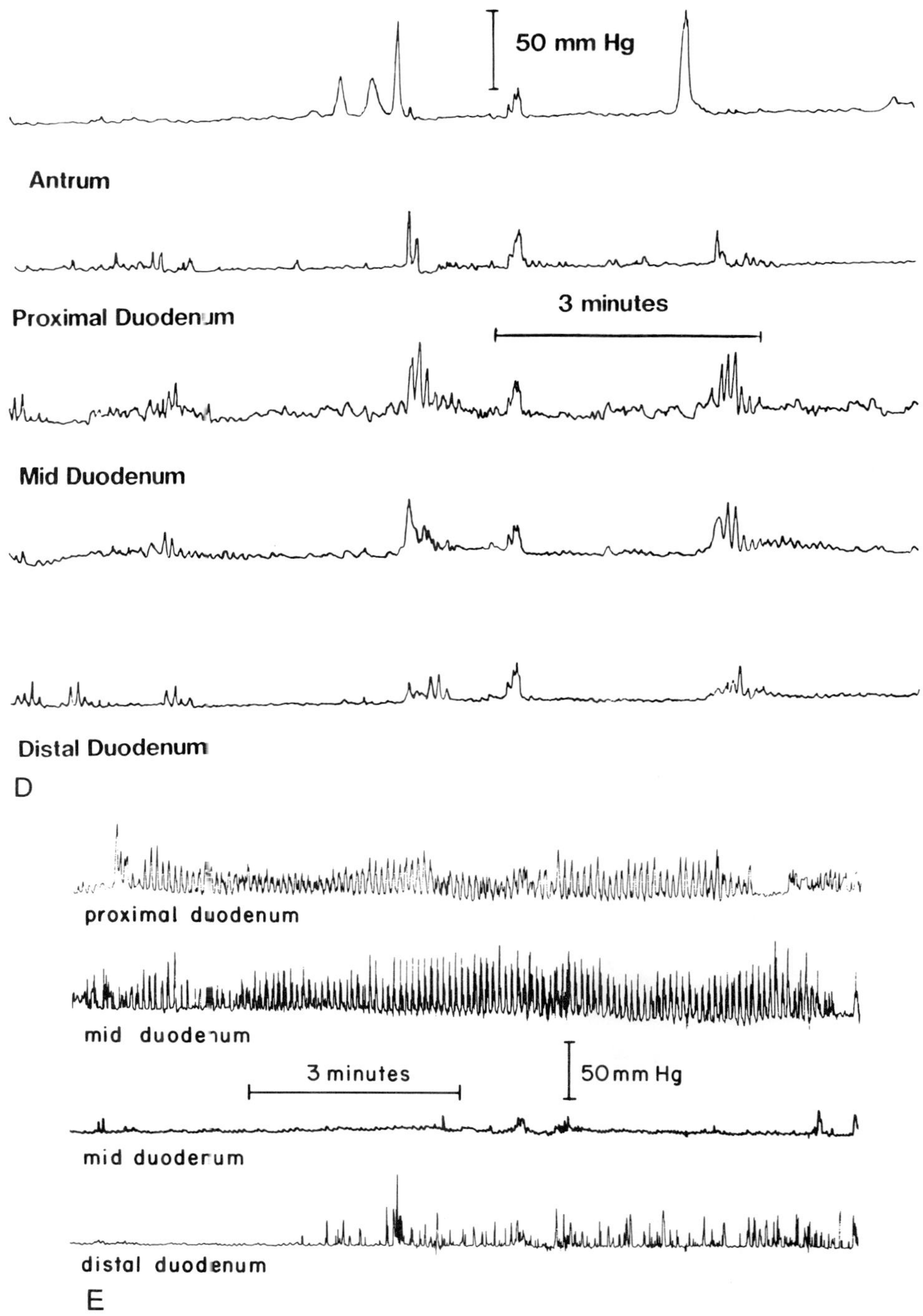

Figure 48–5 Continued D, Nonpropagating, simultaneous, short clusters in monotonous pattern continuing uninterrupted for a 6-hour study. *E,* Long burst of nonpropagating duodenal contractions.

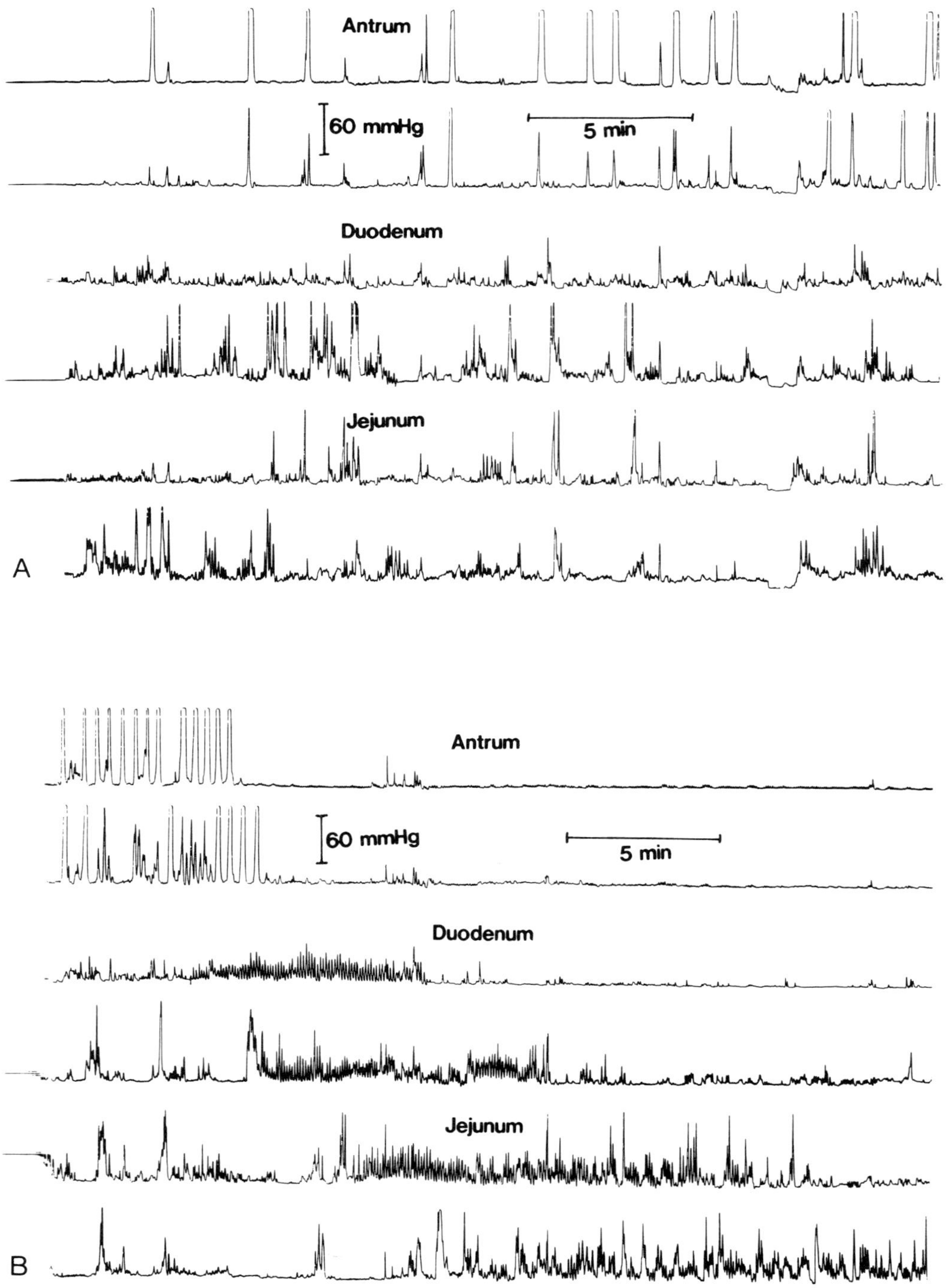

Figure 48–6. *A,* Phase 2-like activity, consisting of random, intermittent, variable-amplitude contractions in the gastric antrum and the duodenum. This is also the postprandial pattern that interrupts the MMC. *B,* Phase 3 of the MMC.

investigations into this area may provide insight into the pathophysiology of pseudo-obstruction in some of the affected children.

TREATMENT

Nutrition Support

The goal of nutrition support is to achieve normal growth and development with the fewest possible complications and greatest patient comfort. In children with pseudo-obstruction, motility improves as nutritional deficiencies resolve and worsens as malnutrition recurs.

Roughly a third of children require partial or total parenteral nutrition. One third require total or partial tube feedings, and a third eat by mouth. TPN is the least desirable means of achieving nutritional sufficiency because of its high rate of complications. In the absence of enteral nutrients, the gastrointestinal tract does not grow or mature normally.[36] In the absence of the postprandial rise in trophic and stimulant gastrointestinal hormones, there is bile stasis and liver disease.[37] TPN-associated cholelithiasis[38] and progressive liver disease are important causes of morbidity and mortality in children with pseudo-obstruction. The minimal volume, composition, and route of enteral support required to reverse or prevent the progression of gastrointestinal complications have not been determined. It seems likely that a complex liquid formula containing protein and fat, given by mouth or gastrostomy tube, and contributing 10 to 25% of the child's total caloric requirement would be sufficient to stimulate postprandial increases in splanchnic blood flow and the plasma concentrations of gastrin and other trophic factors. Every effort should be extended to maximize enteral nutritional support in parenteral nutrition–dependent children.

Continuous enteral feeding via gastrostomy or jejunostomy may be effective when bolus feedings fail. Most children with visceral myopathy and a few with neuropathy have an atonic stomach and almost no gastric emptying. In these children, a feeding jejunostomy may be helpful for the administration of medications and for drip feedings. Care must be taken to place a jejunostomy into an undistended bowel loop.

Bolus intragastric feedings may be useful for infants and toddlers on TPN who will not suck or drink or for the administration of unpalatable nutrition supplements for older children.

Drugs

Prokinetic drugs are helpful in a minority of children with pseudo-obstruction. Bethanechol, neostigmine, metoclopramide, and domperidone have not been useful. The 5-HT_3 receptor antagonist cisapride has been a helpful adjunct in a minority of children. Cisapride's mechanism of action is to facilitate the release of acetylcholine and to stimulate gastrointestinal smooth muscle contraction directly. Cisapride is most likely to work in children with MMC but without dilated bowel. Cisapride increases the number and strength of contractions in the duodenum of children with pseudo-obstruction but does not initiate the MMC in patients without it or inhibit discrete abnormalities.[39]

A trial of cisapride is appropriate for every child with pseudo-obstruction. For children on TPN, the trial should be initiated when there is no acute illness and no malnutrition, coincident with initiation of enteral feedings. Liquid suspension (1 mg per ml) or tablet (5 or 10 mg) is administered 0.1 to 0.3 mg per kg per dose three or four times daily. Side effects include gastrointestinal complaints and irritability, observed in about 5% of children.

Erythromycin, a motilin receptor agonist, appears to facilitate gastric emptying in those with neuropathic gastroparesis by stimulating high-amplitude 3-minute antral contractions, relaxing the pylorus, and inducing antral phase 3 episodes at low, nonantibiotic doses of 1 to 3 mg per kg intravenously or 3 to 5 mg orally. Erythromycin does not appear to be effective for more generalized motility disorders.

Antibiotics are used for bacterial overgrowth. Bacterial overgrowth is associated with steatorrhea, fat-soluble vitamin malabsorption, and malabsorption of the intrinsic factor–vitamin B_{12} complex. It is possible that bacterial overgrowth contributes to bacteremia and frequent episodes of central venous catheter–related sepsis and to TPN-associated liver disease. Further, bacterial overgrowth, mucosal injury, malabsorption, fluid secretion, and gas production may contribute to chronic dilatation of the intestine. Chronic use of antibiotics may result in the emergence of resistant strains of bacteria or overgrowth with fungi. Thus, the advisability of treatment of bacterial overgrowth cannot be generalized, but should be considered on an individual basis.

About a third of children with neuropathic pseudo-obstruction have some evidence of gastric acid hypersecretion or peptic disease. However, excessive gastrostomy drainage may result from retrograde flow of intestinal contents into the stomach, and not from gastric acid hypersecretion. Gastric secretory function or gastric pH should be tested before beginning antisecretory drugs. Histamine H_2 receptor antagonists may be used to suppress gastric acid hypersecretion. Tolerance develops after a few months of intravenous use,[40] so the drug should be given orally when possible. When a drug is added to TPN, gastric pH should be assessed at regular intervals to monitor drug efficacy. Induction of achlorhydria is inadvisable, because it will facilitate bacterial overgrowth in the stomach.

Constipation is treated with mineral oil, suppositories, or enemas. An enteral lavage solution works well in those with disease confined to the colon but will cause massive distention in children with more proximal disease.

Pain control is often a serious management problem. Visceral pain is relatively subjective. Chronic narcotic administration is inadvisable, because narcotic withdrawal may simulate the visceral pain of pseudo-obstruction. Consultation with pain management specialists is advisable for patients who complain of chronic pain.

Electromechanical Pacing

Electromechanical pacing of the bowel is in its infancy. Surgically placed wires on the gastric serosa are used to deliver a paced series of electrical impulses that stimulate coordinated ringlike contractions through the gastric antrum. It is possible to treat gastric arrhythmias and improve gastric emptying in patients with gastroparesis.[41] It will take a much greater feat of electrical engineering to pace a segment of small bowel, which requires complex coordination for digestion and propulsion during fasting and after meals.

Surgery

One of the management challenges in pseudo-obstruction is the evaluation and re-evaluation of the newborn and child with episodic acute obstructive episodes. Although most acute episodes are pseudo-obstruction, it is important to intervene with surgery if the episode is a true bowel obstruction, appendicitis, or other surgical condition. Many children with episodes of acute pseudo-obstruction undergo repeated exploratory laparotomies. It is especially important to avoid unnecessary abdominal surgery in children with pseudo-obstruction for several reasons: (1) They often suffer from very prolonged postoperative ileus; (2) adhesions develop, creating a diagnostic problem each time there is a new obstructive episode; and (3) adhesions following laparotomy may distort normal tissue planes and make future surgeries much riskier in terms of bleeding and organ perforation. After several laparotomies with no evidence of mechanical obstruction, the surgeon may choose a more conservative management plan for subsequent episodes, including pain management, nutritional support, and abdominal decompression.

Gastrostomy was the only procedure reducing the number of hospitalizations in adults with pseudo-obstruction,[42] and the experience with children seems to be similar. Gastrostomy provides a quick and comfortable means of evacuating gastric contents, relieving pain and nausea related to gastric and bowel distention. Continued "venting" may decompress more distal regions of small bowel, eliminating the need for nasogastric intubation or pain medication. Gastrostomy is used for enteral feeding and the administration of enteral medication. Gastrostomy placement should be considered for those receiving parenteral nutrition and for children who will need tube feedings for longer than 2 months. In many patients, endoscopic gastrostomy placement is ideal. In those with contraindications to endoscopic placement, surgical placement is appropriate. Care must be taken to place the ostomy in a suitable position, well above the gastric antrum in the midbody.

Fundoplication is rarely indicated in pseudo-obstruction. Following fundoplication, symptoms may change from vomiting to repeated retching due to outlet obstruction at the lower esophageal sphincter.[43] In children with pseudo-obstruction, vomiting is reduced by venting the gastrostomy. Acid reflux is controlled with antisecretory medication.

Results of pyloroplasty or Roux-en-Y gastrojejunostomy to improve gastric emptying in pseudo-obstruction have been poor; gastric emptying remains delayed. Altering the anatomy rarely improves the function of the dilated fundus and body.

Small bowel resections or tapering operations may provide relief for months or even years. However, if the pathophysiologic condition was present in other areas of bowel, then these areas gradually dilate and symptoms recur.

Colectomy is sometimes necessary in congenital forms of generalized pseudo-obstruction to decompress an abdomen so distended that respiration is impaired. In general, colon diversions are inadvisable because of a high incidence of diversion colitis.[44] Diversion colitis may cause symptoms of abdominal pain and tenesmus, signs of hematochezia, and predispose to bacteremia.

Colectomy may be curative in a small group of children with neuropathic pseudo-obstruction confined to the colon. These children are able to eat normally and grow, but they are unable to defecate spontaneously. Their pathology may show neuronal dysplasia or maturational arrest, and their colon manometry is abnormal, with an absence of a postprandial rise in motility index. Before surgery, antroduodenal manometry should be done to determine whether the asymptomatic upper gastrointestinal tract is involved. Abnormal antroduodenal manometry is a relative contraindication to colectomy because upper gastrointestinal disease, usually with pain as a prominent symptom, often follows colon resection. A major difficulty is the possibility of normal duodenal manometry but ileal neuropathy. A second surgery may be required to resect the ileum in those with ileocolonic neuropathy.

An ileostomy or cecostomy may be placed for regular infusion of an enteral lavage solution. The infusion ostomy using a small "button" ostomy appliance has not yet been thoroughly evaluated. It may prove to be an important mode of therapy in patients with colonic pseudo-obstruction.

The failure of medical management may signal a need for total bowel resection. Rarely a mucosal secretory disorder complicates the management of pseudo-obstruction. Several liters of intestinal secretions drain from the available orifices each day. When secretions cannot be controlled with opiates, anticholinergics, antibiotics, steroids, or somatostatin analogue, it may be necessary to resect the entire bowel to avoid electrolyte abnormalities and nutritional disturbances caused by the large volume of losses. Total bowel resection may be used for intractable pain or repeated life-threatening central venous catheter infections due to bacterial contamination of the stagnant loops of bowel. Total bowel resection should be considered alone or in combination with small bowel transplantation.

Small bowel or combined liver/bowel transplants have the potential to cure children with pseudo-obstruction. Intestinal transplantation is in its infancy, but offers great promise for the future.

REFERENCES

1. Byrne W, Cipel L, Euler A, et al: Chronic idiopathic intestinal pseudo-obstruction syndrome in children: Clinical characteristics and prognosis. J Pediatr 1977; 90:585–589.
2. Roy AD, Bharucha H, Nevin NC, et al: Idiopathic intestinal pseudo-obstruction: A familial visceral neuropathy. Clin Genet 1980; 18:291–297.
3. Mayer EA, Schuffler MD, Rotter JI, et al: Familial visceral neuropathy with autosomal dominant transmission. Gastroenterology 1986; 91:1528–1535.
4. Schuffler MD, Bird TD, Sumi SM, et al: A familial neuronal disease presenting as intestinal pseudo-obstruction. Gastroenterology 1978; 75:889–898.
5. Haltia M, Somer H, Palo J, et al: Neuronal intranuclear inclusion disease in identical twins. Ann Neurol 1984; 15:316–321.
6. Patel H, Norman MG, Perry TL, et al: Multiple system atrophy with neuronal intranuclear hyaline inclusions. Report of a case and review of the literature. J Neurol Sci 1985; 67:57–65.
7. Faulk DL, Anuras S, Gardner D: A familial visceral myopathy. Ann Intern Med 1987; 89:600–606.
8. Schuffler MD, Pope CE: Studies of idiopathic intestinal pseudo-obstruction. II. Hereditary hollow visceral myopathy: Family studies. Gastroenterology 1977; 73:339–344.
9. Schuffler MD, Lowe MC, Bill AH: Studies of idiopathic intestinal pseudo-obstruction: I. Hereditary hollow visceral myopathy: Clinical and pathological studies. Gastroenterology 1977; 73:327–328.
10. Anuras S, Mitros FA, Nowak TV, et al: A familial visceral myopathy with external ophthalmoplegia and autosomal recessive transmission. Gastroenterology 1983; 84:346–353.
11. Ionasescu V, Thompson SH, Ionasescu R, et al: Inherited ophthalmoplegia with intestinal pseudo-obstruction. J Neurol Sci 1983; 59:215–228.
12. Hillemeier C, Buchin PJ, Gryboski J: Esophageal dysfunction in Down syndrome. J Pediatr Gastroenterol Nutr 1982; 1:101–104.
13. Leon SH, Schuffler MD, Kettler M, et al: Chronic intestinal pseudoobstruction as a complication of Duchenne's muscular dystrophy. Gastroenterology 1986; 90:455–459.
14. Barohn RJ, Levine EJ, Olson JO, et al: Gastric hypomotility in Duchenne's muscular dystrophy. N Engl J Med 1988; 319:15–18.
15. Oh JJ, Kim CH: Gastroparesis after presumed viral illness: Clinical and laboratory features and natural history. Mayo Clin Proc 1990; 65:636–642.
16. Sonsino E, Movy R, Foucaud P, et al: Intestinal pseudo-obstruction related to cytomegalovirus infection of the myenteric plexus. N Engl J Med 1984; 311:196–197.
17. Vassallo M, Camilleri M, Caron BL, et al: Intestinal pseudo-obstruction from selective cholinergic dysautonomia due to infectious mononucleosis. Gastroenterology 1990; 98:A400.
18. Amarnath RP: Post infectious transient gastroparesis. Gastroenterol Nutr 1991; 4:A570.
19. Vanderwinden JM, Dassonville, VanderVeken E, et al: Post-necrotizing enterocolitis pseudo-obstruction treated with cisapride. Z Kinderchir 1990; 45:282–285.
20. Krishnamurthy S, Schuffler MD: Pathology of neuromuscular disorders of the small intestine and colon. Gastroenterology 1987; 93:610–639.
21. Lake BD: Observations on the pathology of pseudo-obstruction. *In* Milla PJ, ed: Disorders of Gastrointestinal Motility in Childhood. Chichester, John Wiley & Sons, 1988, pp 81–90.
22. Schuffler MD: Chronic intestinal pseudo-obstruction: Progress and problems. J Pediatr Gastroenterol Nutr 1990; 10:157–163.
23. Smith B: The Neuropathology of the Alimentary Tract. London, Edward Arnold, 1972.
24. Schuffler MD, Jonak Z: Chronic idiopathic intestinal pseudo-obstruction caused by a degenerative disorder of the myenteric plexus: The use of Smith's method to define the neuropathology. Gastroenterology 1982; 82:476–486.
25. Schofield ED, Yunis EJ: Intestinal neuronal dysplasia. J Pediatr Gastroenterol Nutr 1991; 12:182–189.
26. Vargas JH, Sachs P, Ament ME: Chronic intestinal pseudo-obstruction syndrome in pediatrics: Results of a national survey by members of the North American Society of Pediatric Gastroenterology and Nutrition. J Pediatr Gastroenterol Nutr 1988; 7:323–332.
27. Glassman M, Spivak W, Mininberg D, et al: Chronic idiopathic intestinal pseudo-obstruction: A commonly misdiagnosed disease in infants and children. Pediatrics 1989; 83:603–608.
28. Summers RW, Anuras S, Green J: Jejunal manometry patterns in health, partial intestinal obstruction, and pseudo-obstruction. Gastroenterology 1983; 85:1301–1306.
29. Camilleri M: Jejunal manometry in distal subacute mechanical obstruction: Significance of prolonged simultaneous contractions. Gut 1989; 30:468–475.
30. Hyman PE, McDiarmid SV, Napolitano JA, et al: Antroduodenal motility in children with chronic intestinal pseudo-obstruction. J Pediatr 1988; 112:899–905.
31. Hyman PE, Napolitano JA, Diego A, et al: Antroduodenal manometry in the evaluation of chronic functional gastrointestinal symptoms. Pediatrics 1990; 86:39–44.
32. Snape WJ Jr, Sullivan MA, Cohen S: Abnormal gastrocolic response in patients with intestinal pseudoobstruction. Arch Intern Med 1980; 140:386–387.
33. DiLorenzo C, Reddy SN, Villanueva-Meyer J, et al: Simultaneous colonic manometry and transit in children. Gastroenterology 1990; 98:A435.
34. Bisset WM, Devan SP, Milla PJ: Gastric antral dysrhythmia in children with congenital idiopathic intestinal pseudo-obstruction. J Gastroenterol Int Mot 1989:1: A53.
35. Mayer EA, Raybould HE: Role of visceral afferent mechanisms in functional bowel disorders. Gastroenterology 1990:99:1688–1704.
36. Hyman PE, Feldman EJ, Ament ME, et al: Effect of enteral feeding on the maintenance of gastric acid secretory function. Gastroenterology 1983; 84:341–345.
37. Dahms BB, Halpin TC Jr: Serial liver biopsies in parenteral nutrition-associated cholestasis of early infancy. Gastroenterology 1981:81:136–144.
38. Roslyn JJ, Berquist WE, Pitt HA, et al: Increased risk of gallstones in children receiving total parenteral nutrition. Pediatrics 1983; 71:784–789.
39. DiLorenzo C, Reddy SN, Villanueva-Meyer J, et al: Cisapride in children with chronic intestinal pseudo-obstruction: An acute, double-blind crossover placebo controlled trial. Gastroenterology 1991; 101:1564–1570.
40. Hyman PE, Garvey TQ, Abrams CE: Tolerance to intravenous ranitidine. J Pediatr 1987; 110:794–796.
41. Courtney TL, Schirmer BD, Bellahsene BE, et al: Gastric electrical stimulation as a possible new therapy for patients with severe gastric stasis. Gastroenterology 1991; 100:A822.
42. Pitt HA, Mann LL, Berquist WE, et al: Chronic intestinal pseudo-obstruction: Management with total parenteral nutrition and a venting enterostomy. Arch Surg 1985; 120:614–618.
43. DiLorenzo C, Flores A, Hyman PE: Intestinal motility in symptomatic children with fundoplication. J Pediatr Gastroenterol Nutr 1991; 12:169–173.
44. Ordein J, DiLorenzo C, Flores A, Hyman PE: Diversion colitis in children with pseudo-obstruction. Am J Gastroenterol 1992; 87:88–90.

Chapter 49

Enteric Parasites

STANLEY H. KORMAN and RICHARD J. DECKELBAUM

Intestinal parasitic diseases are a major cause of morbidity and mortality worldwide. Until recently, most Western physicians needed to be familiar with only a few of these organisms such as *Giardia lamblia, Entamoeba histolytica*, and *Enterobius vermicularis*, which may be endemic in developed countries. What were previously regarded as exotic tropical diseases are now increasingly encountered as a result of international travel to and immigration from Third World countries. Furthermore, the growing population of patients with immunodeficiency due to human immunodeficiency virus (HIV) infection, malignancy, or immunosuppressive therapy is particularly susceptible to a number of parasitic infections that may be innocuous in healthy populations.

The development of in vitro cultivation techniques and the application of immunologic and molecular biology techniques have significantly expanded our understanding of the basic biology and pathogenetic mechanisms of many of these parasites. This chapter presents a general approach to the epidemiology, clinical manifestations, diagnosis, and treatment of intestinal parasitoses and to an understanding of pathogenetic mechanisms and the interrelationship of nutritional and immune status and parasitic disease. A classification of the intestinal parasites and a list of abbreviated names used in the text are presented in Table 49–1A (helminths) and B (protozoa). The major clinical manifestations, appropriate diagnostic investigations, and recommended chemotherapeutic agents for each parasite are summarized in Table 49–2. Drug dosage regimens, precautions, and side effects are presented in Table 49–3. Apart from several organisms of particular significance to Western pediatric practice—namely, *E. histolytica, Cryptosporidium* species, *G. lamblia*, and *Strongyloides stercoralis*—an in-depth discussion of individual organisms is beyond the scope of this chapter. The reader should consult the articles in the references, especially the excellent descriptions of parasite life cycles by Katz and associates.[1]

PREDISPOSING FACTORS

Social and Environmental Conditions. Substandard hygiene practices, inadequate sanitation facilities, and contaminated food and water supplies are the major factors responsible for the high prevalence of parasitic diseases in developing countries. Human excreta are often used as crop fertilizers, thereby ensuring perpetuation of the parasite life cycle. Climatic conditions in tropical countries favor the transmission of parasites. Within such communities, children with low socioeconomic status and from overcrowded urban slum environments have a much higher risk of parasite infection.[2, 3]

Travelers and Immigrants from Endemic Regions. High prevalence rates of single or multiple parasitic infections have been described in immigrant and refugee populations arriving in Western countries[4]; many of these infections may then be transmitted to susceptible contacts. Illegal immigrants constitute a particular problem, as they may be missed by special screening programs for new immigrants.

Day-Care Centers. The increasing use of day-care facilities has been recognized as a major factor in the spread of enteric pathogens, including parasites, in Western countries.[5] *G. lamblia* and *Cryptosporidium* have been associated with outbreaks of diarrhea as well as with high rates of asymptomatic infection. Conditions in day-care centers are often ideal for person-to-person transmission of enteropathogens: frequent direct physical contact between large numbers of susceptible children, especially before the age of toilet training; handling and mouthing of shared toys; frequent hands-on child contact by staff, who often have little understanding of basic hygiene principles; and lack of isolation facilities for sick children. Siblings and parents of day-care attendees are also at risk of infection.

Institutions. Children residing in institutions, particularly those for the mentally retarded, are at risk of several parasitic infections, including *G. lamblia, Cryptosporidium, E. histolytica,* and *Str. stercoralis*. High prevalence rates of *Str. stercoralis* may be found even in areas where it is not endemic. *E. histolytica* isolates commonly belong to a pathogenic zymodeme.

Dietary Practices. Eating raw or undercooked fish predisposes to infection with *Diphyllobothrium latum* and *Capillaria philippinensis*. Similarly, *Taenia saginata* may be acquired from inadequately cooked beef, and *Taenia solium* and *Trichinella spiralis* from pork. Children who practice geophagia (earth eating) are prone to a variety of parasitic infections as a result of ingesting cysts or larvae in fecal-contaminated soil.[6] The pica may

Table 49–1. CLASSIFICATION OF THE MAJOR PARASITIC CAUSES OF INTESTINAL DISEASE

Organism	Abbreviated Name	Common Name* or Classification†	Disease	Infective Stage	Route of Infection
A. Helminths					
Nematodes (roundworms)					
Ancylostoma duodenale	*An. duodenale*	hookworm	uncinariasis	filariform larvae	feces-soil-skin
Ascaris lumbricoides	*As. lumbricoides*	roundworm	ascariasis	embryonated eggs	feces-soil-mouth
Capillaria philippinensis	*C. philippinensis*	none	capillariasis	larvae	eating raw fish
Enterobius vermicularis	*Es. vermicularis*	pinworm	enterobiasis	embryonated eggs	perineum-hands-mouth
Necator americanus	*N. americanus*	hookworm	uncinariasis	filariform larvae	feces-soil-skin
Strongyloides stercoralis	*Str. stercoralis*	threadworm	strongyloidiasis	filariform larvae	feces-soil-skin/mouth
Trichinella spiralis	*Ta. spiralis*	none	trichinosis	larvae	undercooked meat
Trichuris trichiura	*Ts. trichiura*	whipworm	trichuriasis	embryonated eggs	feces-soil-mouth
Cestodes (tapeworms)					
Diphyllobothrium latum	*D. latum*	fish tapeworm	diphyllobothriasis	pleurocercoid larvae	eating raw fish
Hymenolepis nana	*H. nana*	dwarf tapeworm	hymenolepiasis	embryonated egg	fecal-oral
Taenia saginatum	*Tae. saginatum*	beef tapeworm	taeniasis	cysticerci	undercooked beef
Taenia solium	*Tae. solium*	pork tapeworm	taeniasis	cysticerci	undercooked pork
Trematodes (flukes)					
Schistosoma mansoni	*Sch. mansoni*	—	schistosomiasis	cercariae	feces-water-snail-water-skin
Schistosoma japonicum	*Sch. japonicum*	—	schistosomiasis	cercariae	feces-water-snail-water-skin
B. Protozoa					
Balantidium coli	*Ba. coli*	Ciliophora (ciliate)	balantidiasis	cyst	
Blastocystis hominis	*Bl. hominis*	Sarcodina (pseudopodia)	blastocytosis	cyst	
Cryptosporidium species	*Cryptosporidium* spp.	Coccidia	cryptosporidiosis	oocyst	
Entamoeba histolytica	*E. histolytica*	Sarcodina (pseudopodia)	amebiasis	cyst	
Giardia lamblia	*G. lamblia*	Mastigophora (flagellate)	giardiasis	cyst	
Isospora belli	*I. belli*	Coccidia	isosporiasis	oocyst	

*For helminths, common name is shown.
†For protozoa, classification is shown.

be secondary to iron deficiency or an accepted cultural practice.

Contact with Livestock or Domestic Animals. There is a potential for zoonotic transmission of several of the human enteric parasites that have a reservoir in a variety of animals, including *Cryptosporidium* (calves, sheep, domestic pets), *E. histolytica* (dogs), *Balantidium coli* (pigs), *G. lamblia* (beavers, domestic pets), and *Str. stercoralis* (dogs, primates). Zoonotic transmission has been definitively established for all of these except *G. lamblia* and *Str. stercoralis*.

Individual Predisposition. Community surveys of helminth prevalence reveal that certain individuals have very high worm burdens (and therefore greater morbidity). After deworming, this pattern of heavy infestation often recurs in the same individuals, with several parasite-prone individuals often being clustered within a household.[7] This phenomenon might reflect host genetic susceptibility or may be related to environmental exposure and risk factors.

Malnutrition and Immunosuppression. These risk factors are discussed in depth later.

PATHOGENESIS

Some human enteric parasites are nonpathogenic commensals and never cause disease, such as *Entamoeba coli* and *Chilomastix mesnili*. For others such as *Dientamoeba fragilis*, controversy exists about whether they can ever cause disease or are instead "innocent bystanders" to which a multitude of symptoms are falsely attributed. Another example is *Blastocystis hominis*, which has been the subject of a number of recent studies either attesting to[8] or denying[9] its pathogenicity. For many of the enteric parasites whose capacity to cause disease is unquestioned—for example, *G. lamblia, E. histolytica*, and *Str. stercoralis*—most infections are, nevertheless, asymptomatic. Factors that determine the expression of asymptomatic to severely symptomatic disease are in general poorly understood, as are the mechanisms of pathogenesis.

Parasite Factors. Parasite-related determinants of pathogenicity are best illustrated by *E. histolytica*. All *E. histolytica* isolates capable of causing invasive disease

Table 49–2. CLINICAL FEATURES, DIAGNOSIS, AND TREATMENT OF INTESTINAL PARASITIC DISEASES

Parasite	Major Clinical Features	Method of Diagnosis	Recommended Therapy
Protozoa			
Ba. coli	Watery diarrhea, colitis	Stool O & P, rectoscopy scrapings	Tetracycline or metronidazole
Bl. hominis	Diarrhea (debatable)	Stool O & P	Metronidazole
Cryptosporidium	Immunocompetent: self-limiting diarrhea Immunocompromised: intractable diarrhea, hepatobiliary involvement	Stool: acid-fast stain, immunofluorescence, ELISA Small intestinal sample	Spiramycin, hyperimmune bovine colostrum (the role of these therapies is not yet clear)
E. histolytica	Asymptomatic cyst excretors Rectocolitis (dysentery) Liver or other organ abscess	Stool: O & P, ELISA; rectoscopy; serology Abdominal ultrasound, CT scan	Luminal amebicide for noninvasive disease: diiodohydroxyquin or diloxanide or paromomycin Invasive disease: metronidazole, (dehydro)emetine in severe cases, plus a luminal amebicide
G. lamblia	Asymptomatic carriers Acute/chronic diarrhea, malabsorption	Stool: O & P, ELISA Small intestinal sample	Metronidazole/tinidazole/ornidazole or furazolidone or quinacrine; although widely used, metronidazole is not approved for giardiasis in the U.S.A.
Isospora belli	As for *Cryptosporidium*	Stool: acid-fast stain; small intestinal sample	Cotrimoxazole
Nematodes			
An. duodenale *N. americanus*	Anemia ± hypoproteinemia, rash, Löfflerlike syndrome, eosinophilia	Stool O & P	Mebendazole or albendazole
As. lumbricoides	Intestinal and hepatobiliary obstruction, Löfflerlike syndrome, eosinophilia	Stool O & P	Mebendazole or albendazole, gastrograffin for bowel obstruction
C. philippinensis	Intractable diarrhea, malabsorption	Stool O & P	Mebendazole or albendazole
Es. vermicularis	Nocturnal anal pruritus	Cellophane tape test	Mebendazole or pyrantel pamoate or piperazine or pyrvinium pamoate
Str. stercoralis	Diarrhea, malabsorption, rash, Löfflerlike syndrome, eosinophilia, hyperinfection syndrome	Stool: O & P, agar-plate culture; small intestinal sample; serology	Thiabendazole or albendazole, Ivermectin(?)
Ta. spiralis	Transient diarrhea, myalgia, fever, periorbital edema, eosinophilia	Serology, elevated CPK and LDH	Thiabendazole; must be given within 24 hr of ingesting trichinous meat
Ts. trichiura	Rectal prolapse, anemia rarely	Stool O & P	Mebendazole or albendazole
Cestodes			
D. latum	Vitamin B_{12} deficiency	Stool O & P	Niclosamide or praziquantel, vitamin B_{12} and folic acid
H. nana	Cramps, diarrhea	Stool O & P	Niclosamide or praziquantel
Tae. saginatum	Vague abdominal symptoms rarely	Stool O & P	Niclosamide or praziquantel
Tae. solium	Vague abdominal symptoms rarely; cysticercosis (neural or other organs)	Stool O & P CT scan, serology	Niclosamide or praziquantel Praziquantel
Trematodes			
Schistosoma	Rash, swimmer's itch, acute fever with eosinophilia, intestinal ulcers, polyps, strictures, liver fibrosis, portal hypertension	Stool O & P, rectal snips	Praziquantel

Stool O & P, Microscopic examination of stools for ova and parasites; CPK, creatine phosphokinase; LDH, lactic dehydrogenase.

can be identified by possession of specific markers, including characteristic isoenzyme electrophoresis profiles (zymodemes). However, even *E. histolytica* expressing these determinants of pathogenicity may be isolated from asymptomatic carriers, so additional, as yet unidentified, factors must be involved. Biochemical properties of *E. histolytica* responsible for its capacity to adhere, invade, and lyse host cells include a galactose-inhibitable adherence lectin, several proteases, phospholipase A, and an enterotoxin activity.[10] An adherence-mediating lectin has also been identified in *G. lamblia.*[11] *Str. stercoralis* secretes a potent histolytic metalloprotease with elastase activity, which facilitates its migration at speeds of up to 10 cm per hour through host tissues; similar proteases have been identified in other invasive helminths.[12]

The parasite burden or load of infection appears to be a major determinant of symptomatic disease for many of the helminths. For example, development of anemia in hookworm infection is directly related to the number of worms in the gut and the consequent volume of blood lost. Most helminths do not multiply in the host (the autoinfectious cycles of *Str. stercoralis* and *C. philippinensis* are exceptions), and the worm burden depends on the degree of continuing exposure to infection. For protozoa there is often no clear correlation between parasite burden and symptomatology: *G. lamblia* trophozoites may be extremely difficult to find in biopsy specimens from some of the most severe giardiasis cases.

Host Factors. Immune response is probably the most important host-related determinant of symptomatic disease. Asymptomatic *Str. stercoralis* carriers may develop

Table 49–3. DRUGS USED IN THE TREATMENT OF INTESTINAL PARASITIC INFECTIONS

Drug Name	Indications	Route	Pediatric Dose	Adult Dose	Doses per Day	Days of Therapy	Precautions	Side Effects
Albendazole*	All nematodes except strongyloidiasis:	Oral	400 mg (>2-yr-old)	400 mg	1	1	Teratogenic and mutagenic in experimental studies	As for mebendazole; side effects rare in single-dose therapy
	uncomplicated hyperinfection	Oral Oral	400 mg 400 mg	400 mg 400 mg	1 1	3 15	Hepatic disease	
Dehydroemetine*†	A synthetic, less toxic derivative of emetine (see below)							
Diiodohydroxyquin (Iodoquinol)	Luminal amebicide	Oral	13.3 mg/kg	650 mg	3	20	Iodine sensitivity; hepatic, renal, or thyroid disease; optic neuropathy	GI disturbance, fever, chills, headache, pruritus ani, goiter, hypersensitivity; subacute myelo-optic neuropathy only with prolonged, high doses
Diloxanide furoate	Luminal amebicide	Oral	25 mg/kg	500 mg	3	10	None	Flatulence, vomiting, pruritus, urticaria
Emetine HCl	Fulminating amebic dysentery and amebic liver abscess	Deep subcutaneous or intramuscular (not intravenous)	0.5 mg/kg; maximum total daily dose: <8 yr, 10 mg; >8 yr, 20 mg	0.5 mg/kg; maximum per day: 65 mg	2	5 Maximum 10 days; at least 6 weeks between courses	Cardiac disease, renal disease, neuromuscular disease; use in children only with severe amebiasis unresponsive to other drugs	Injection site pain, weakness, abscess, degenerative myocarditis, arrhythmias, chest pain, heart failure, flatulence, vomiting, pruritus, urticaria
Furazolidone	Giardiasis	Oral	1.25 mg/kg	100 mg	4	7–10	Disulfiram-like reaction with alcohol, mild G6PD hemolysis, neonatal hemolysis, MAO inhibitor properties, oncogenic in rodents	Yellow-brown urine, GI disturbance, headache, hypersensitivity, leukopenia
Ivermectin*†	Strongyloidiasis, ascariasis, trichuriasis	Oral	200 μg/kg		1	1	None	Few side effects documented as yet
Mebendazole	Enterobiasis‡ Ascariasis, hookworm, trichuriasis, capillariasis, trichinosis	Oral Oral	100 mg 100 mg	100 mg 100 mg	1 2	1 3	Liver disease, inflammatory bowel disease, hypersensitivity to mebendazole	GI disturbance, hypersensitivity (fever, rash), neutropenia, alopecia, headache, dizziness
Metronidazole	Amebiasis (invasive) Balantidiasis Giardiasis	Oral or IV Oral Oral	15 mg/kg 15 mg/kg 5 mg/kg	750 mg 750 mg 250 mg	3 3 3	5–10 5 10	Carcinogenic in rodents, mutagenic in bacteria, disulfiram-like reaction with alcohol, liver disease	GI disturbance, dizziness, headache, dry mouth, metallic taste, dark urine, seizures, peripheral neuropathy, hypersensitivity, leukopenia
Niclosamide			<34 kg / >34 kg					GI disturbance, rash, pruritus ani, drowsiness, headache, dizziness, unpleasant taste in mouth
	Taeniasis, diphyllobothriasis	Oral	1 gm / 1.5 gm	2 gm	1	1	None	
	Hymenolepiasis	Oral		2 gm	1	7		
			1 gm / 1.5 gm followed by		1	1		
			0.5 gm / 1 gm		1	6		
Ornidazole*	Amebiasis (invasive) Giardiasis	Oral Oral	40 mg/kg 40 mg/kg	1.5 gm 1.5 gm	1 1	3 1	As for metronidazole	
Piperazine	Ascariasis Enterobiasis‡	Oral Oral	75 mg/kg 65 mg/kg	3.5 g 2.5 g	1 1	2 7	Not to be used concurrently with pyrantel	GI disturbance, CNS disturbance, hypersensitivity
Praziquantel	Diphyllobothriasis, taeniasis Hymenolepiasis Schistosomiasis	Oral Oral Oral	10–20 mg/kg 25 mg/kg 40 mg/kg	Same Same Same	1 1 1	1 1 1	Ocular cysticercosis, liver disease, hypersensitivity	Dizziness, malaise, headache, drowsiness, fever, sweating, GI disturbance, bad taste in mouth
Pyrantel pamoate	Enterobiasis‡ Ascariasis Hookworm	Oral Oral Oral	11 mg/kg 11 mg/kg 11 mg/kg	Same Same Same	1 1 1	1 1 3	Not to be used concurrently with piperazine, pyrantel hypersensitivity	Dizziness, drowsiness, headache, insomnia, GI disturbance, hypersensitivity
Pyrvinium*	Enterobiasis‡	Oral	150 mg/m^2	5 mg/kg; max 350 mg	1	1	Inflammatory bowel disease, pyrvinium hypersensitivity	Red stools, hypersensitivity (rash), GI disturbance

Table continued on following page

Table 49–3. DRUGS USED IN THE TREATMENT OF INTESTINAL PARASITIC INFECTIONS *Continued*

Drug Name	Indications	Route	Pediatric Dose	Adult Dose	Doses per Day	Days of Therapy	Precautions	Side Effects
Thiabendazole	Strongyloidiasis:						May elevate serum levels of theophylline, renal disease, hepatic disease	Dizziness, drowsiness, headache, tinnitus, seizures, confusion, GI disturbance, dry eyes and mouth, hypersensitivity Stevens-Johnson syndrome, crystalluria; blurred or yellow vision
	uncomplicated	Oral	25 mg/kg	1.5 g	2	3		
	hyperinfection	Oral	25 mg/kg	1.5 g	2	5–15		
	Capillariasis	Oral	25 mg/kg	1.5 g	1	30		
	Trichinosis (within 24 hr of ingesting trichinous pork)	Oral	25 mg/kg	1.5 g	2	2–4		
Tinidazole*	Amebiasis (invasive)	Oral	50 mg/kg	2 g	1	3–5	As for metronidazole	
	Giardiasis	Oral	50 mg/kg	2 g	1	1 or 2		

*Not commercially available in the United States.
†Available from the Centers for Disease Control (CDC); telephone (404) 639-3670; (404) 639-2888 (emergency after-hours service).
‡In treatment of enterobiasis, a repeat dose should be given 10–14 days after the first dose.
G6PD, glucose-6-phosphate dehydrogenase deficiency; MAO, monoamine oxidase.

fatal "hyperinfection" syndrome after immunosuppressive therapy. Certain immune deficiency states (congenital hypogammaglobulinemia) but not others (AIDS) predispose to chronic symptomatic giardiasis. Immunity acquired as a result of prior exposure to a parasite may not prevent reinfection but may protect against development of symptomatic disease. This mechanism may account for travelers' diarrhea occurring in visitors to regions endemic for *G. lamblia* (e.g., St. Petersburg) who, not having previously encountered the pathogen, are immunologically "naive," whereas infection in local inhabitants is almost always asymptomatic. Nutritional status of the host is another potential factor; it may act directly, as in development of anemia in *Trichuris trichiura* or hookworm infections, or indirectly, by suppression of immunity.

Microenvironmental Factors. The importance of the parasite's microenvironment within the intestine is being increasingly appreciated. *E. histolytica* may acquire virulence when associated with certain enteric bacteria but not with others.[13] Symptomatic giardiasis may be related to *Candida*[14] or bacterial[15] overgrowth of the small intestine.

IMMUNOLOGIC AND NUTRITIONAL STATUS

Parasitic infections interact with the host's immunologic and nutritional status by a series of complex and interdependent mechanisms illustrated in Figure 49–1.

The susceptibility to and severity of parasitic infections may be influenced by the host's nutritional and immunologic status. For example, malnutrition predisposes to massive, invasive *Str. stercoralis* infection (hyperinfection syndrome), and *Cryptosporidium* infections may be more severe and prolonged in malnourished children.[16] Primary immunodeficiencies such as congenital hypogammaglobulinemia and selective immunoglobulin A (IgA) deficiency are associated with persistent giardiasis. Increasingly important today are secondary immunodeficiency states (whether due to AIDS, cancer

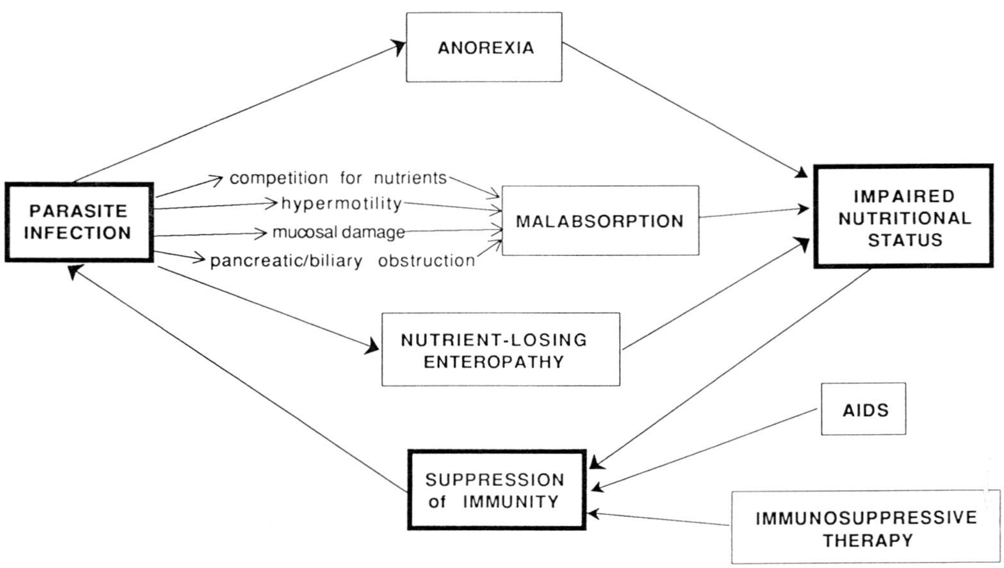

Figure 49–1. Interrelationships of intestinal parasitic infections with host nutritional and immune status.

chemotherapy, or immunosuppressive therapy for autoimmune diseases and transplantation). *Cryptosporidium,*[17] *Isospora belli,*[18] *Str. stercoralis,*[19] *G. lamblia,*[20, 21] and *E. histolytica* may be particularly hazardous in these situations.

Parasites can in turn exert adverse effects on host nutritional status by a variety of mechanisms. The anorexia associated with heavy parasitic infestations can significantly reduce caloric intake. Malabsorption may result from competition for specific nutrients (e.g., *D. latum* and vitamin B_{12} deficiency), hypermotility, structural or ultrastructural damage to the mucosa[22] (e.g., *G. lamblia*), and disturbance of pancreatic and biliary function by invading parasites (e.g., *Ascaris lumbricoides, Cryptosporidium*). The nutritional impact of parasitic infections is well illustrated by studies showing improved growth[23] and physical fitness[24] in children after deworming. The nutritional implications of giardiasis have been reviewed[25]; studies of Guatemalan village children have demonstrated deleterious effects of *G. lamblia* infection on growth[26] and increased growth associated with decreased prevalence of *G. lamblia* after mass treatment with metronidazole.[27] The number and intensity of parasitic infestations in pregnant malnourished Guatemalan women have been associated with intrauterine growth retardation in their offspring.[28]

PRESENTING FEATURES

Gastroenteritis. Diarrhea with or without vomiting is associated with a number of helminth infections—*Str. stercoralis, C. philippinensis*, and occasionally *Hymenolepis nana*—and with all the pathogenic intestinal protozoa. Persistent diarrhea is suggestive of *G. lamblia, Cryptosporidium, Str. stercoralis*, and *C. philippinensis.* Bloody diarrhea is found with *E. histolytica* and *Balantidium coli* infections and in intestinal schistosomiasis. Voluminous watery diarrhea occurs in cryptosporidiosis in the immunocompromised.

Abdominal Pain. Abdominal pain is a common symptom of many of the intestinal parasitoses; even in the absence of other gastrointestinal symptoms, children presenting with significant abdominal pain warrant screening by stool microscopy for parasitic infection. Intestinal or biliary obstruction due to *Ascaris* may produce severe symptoms; symptoms mimicking peptic ulcer have also been described. Milder abdominal pain may be associated with strongyloidiasis, capillariasis, hymenolepiasis, and hookworm infection. All the pathogenic intestinal protozoa can produce abdominal pain; tenesmus occurs in amebic dysentery.

Failure to Thrive. Giardiasis[29] and strongyloidiasis[30] are the main parasitic causes of malabsorption with failure to thrive. For many other parasites, a causal relationship between infection and nutritional impairment is difficult to prove in the setting of polyparasitism and underlying malnutrition.

Abdominal Complications. The capacity of several of the gastrointestinal parasites to migrate or invade from their usual intestinal habitat may result in acute abdominal emergencies or subacute complications. Acute appendicitis may be caused by *Enterobius, E. histolytica,* and *Str. stercoralis.* Toxic megacolon may complicate fulminating amebic colitis, and ileus, shock, and sepsis occur in disseminated strongyloidiasis. *Str. stercoralis* can also produce massive upper gastrointestinal bleeding. Bowel obstruction is characteristic of ascariasis, and bowel perforation may be caused by *Ascaris lumbricoides, E. histolytica,*[31] and rarely *Balantidium coli.* Rectal prolapse suggests *Trichuris trichiura.* Granulomatous intestinal polyps and fibrotic strictures may occur in schistosomiasis.

Invasion of the biliary tree by *Ascaris* may present as biliary colic or acute cholecystitis, cholangitis, pancreatitis, or liver abscess.[32] Biliary tract invasion by *Cryptosporidium* in the immunocompromised host can produce acute cholecystitis and sclerosing cholangitis.[33] Hepatobiliary involvement by *E. histolytica* results in liver abscess and occasionally cholecystitis. Hepatic fibrosis in schistosomiasis produces portal hypertension and its attendant complications. Genitourinary involvement occurs with *Ascaris, E. histolytica,* and *Enterobius.*

Passage of Worms. Sighting by the patient or parent of part or all of a worm may be the first clue to helminth infection. The female pinworm (*Enterobius vermicularis*) emerges at night and may be observed in the perineal region or on the outside of the stool as a white, threadlike worm a little less than a centimeter in length. *Ascaris lumbricoides* may be regurgitated during vomiting or passed in the stools. It is a pink-yellow round worm about 15 to 35 cm in length, resembling an earthworm. Tapeworm gravid proglottids (egg-containing worm segments) may be passed in the stool or may exit spontaneously through the anal sphincter. The proglottids of *Tae. saginata* and *Tae. solium* and *Diphyllobothrium latum* can be distinguished microscopically by the number of their lateral uterine branches. Rarely, a large strip of the entire worm, several feet in length, may be passed.

Pulmonary Manifestations. During their larval migratory phase, *Ascaris*, hookworm, and *Strongyloides* may produce a Löfflerlike pneumonitis associated with transient respiratory symptoms, pulmonary infiltrates, and eosinophilia. In *E. histolytica* infection, pleuropulmonary abscesses and pleural effusion may result from hematogenous seeding of the lungs or by direct extension from a liver abscess. Cryptosporidial infection may involve the respiratory tract, producing chronic cough, dyspnea, bronchiolitis, and pneumonitis, especially in immunodeficient individuals.[34] Transient respiratory symptoms have been reported in immunocompetent children.[35] Cor pulmonale is an occasional complication of schistosomiasis. Giardiasis has occasionally been reported as a cause of asthma.

Itch. Itching in hookworm, *Strongyloides*, and *Schistosoma* infection is related to larval penetration of the skin. Nocturnal perianal itching is highly suggestive of enterobiasis. Tapeworm proglottids emerging from the anus produce a tingling sensation as they crawl down the thigh.

Skin Eruptions. Hookworm infection may be associated with an erythematous, papulovesicular rash at the site of larval penetration. Similarly, *Strongyloides* infection can produce a transient urticarial rash known as "larva currens," which begins perianally and migrates to the abdomen and thighs. The papular rash of "swimmer's itch" in schistosomiasis is a hypersensitivity response. Several reports have described chronic urticaria that resolves after eradication of *Giardia* infection.

Anemia. Hypochromic iron-deficiency anemia may occur in hookworm infection. The development of anemia is determined not only by the amount of blood loss, which in turn depends on the worm burden, but also by the availability of iron in the diet and the capacity of the small intestine to reabsorb the lost iron. It is therefore not surprising that anemia is not usually observed in otherwise healthy Western individuals with hookworm, in contrast to the situation in Third World countries. The relationship of *Trichuris trichiura* to anemia is similar; since the adult worm sucks only about 0.005 ml of blood per day, anemia is likely to develop only with extremely heavy infestations associated with poor diet and polyparasitism. Causes of anemia in schistosomiasis include bleeding from esophageal varices or intestinal ulcerations and hypersplenism. Megaloblastic anemia and associated neurologic syndromes due to vitamin B_{12}, folate deficiency, or both, develop in less than 2% of *D. latum* infections. Anemia in giardiasis is related to the generalized malabsorptive process, which may include hematinic factors such as iron, folate, vitamin B_{12}, and vitamin E.

Eosinophilia. Eosinophilia in association with gastrointestinal symptoms is suggestive of parasitic, particularly helminthic, infection but needs to be differentiated from allergy, eosinophilic gastroenteritis, inflammatory bowel disease, and rarely polyarteritis and lymphoma. Very high peripheral eosinophil counts are characteristic of strongyloidiasis, although in the hyperinfection syndrome this response is often absent. High eosinophil counts are seen in acute schistosomiasis. Significant eosinophilia occurs also in hookworm and *Ascaris* infection, particularly during the larval migration phase. In *Trichinella spiralis* infection, the eosinophil count may rise to high levels after the tenth day; by this time, the transient intestinal symptoms have resolved. Mild eosinophilia may occasionally be seen in tapeworm infections and in some cases of trichuriasis. Protozoan infections are typically not associated with eosinophilia, although mild elevations are occasionally reported. An exception is *Isospora*, which may produce eosinophil counts of up to 20%.

DIAGNOSTIC APPROACH

Stool Microscopy

Microscopic examination of the stools for protozoan trophozoites and cysts and helminth eggs and larvae is the basic, first-line method for diagnosis of intestinal parasitoses.[36] Although the standard methodologies have remained virtually unchanged for decades, the procedure is fraught with pitfalls. Accuracy of the examination depends both on the experience of the microscopist and on the extent to which the following principles of specimen collection, preservation, and examination are adhered to.

Specimen Collection. Stools should be collected without contamination by water or urine, which may destroy trophozoites. Barium and mineral oil laxatives interfere with the examination and should not be administered for 7 days prior to collection. Two or three specimens should be examined at intervals of 2 to 3 days apart to account for intermittent excretion, especially for *E. histolytica, G. lamblia, D. latum*, and *Taenia*.

Preservation. Stool specimens for microscopy diagnosis of parasitic infections should be examined fresh, preferably within 1 to 2 hours of being passed. The reason for this is that protozoan trophozoites are highly labile and rapidly lose their characteristic morphology and motility. The trophozoite rather than cyst forms are particularly likely to be found in diarrheal stools. If the specimen cannot be examined fresh, one part of stool should be thoroughly mixed with three parts of polyvinyl alcohol (PVA) fixative, which preserves the trophozoites. Protozoan cysts and helminth eggs and larvae can be reliably detected in unpreserved stools for up to 48 hours, provided the specimen has been refrigerated; if a longer delay before examination is unavoidable, an additional aliquot of the specimen should be preserved in 5 or 10% formalin.

Merthiolate iodine formaldehyde (MIF), sodium acetate-formalin (SAF), and phenol ethanol formalin (PAF) preserve trophozoites as well as cysts, eggs, and larvae and obviate the need for using two separate fixatives.

Microscopy. Fresh stools are initially examined using a direct saline wet mount. Motile trophozoites are most easily detected in this preparation. An iodine-stained mount facilitates detection of protozoan cysts. If negative, a concentration procedure (e.g., formalin-ether sedimentation or zinc-sulfate flotation) is essential to enable detection of protozoan cysts and helminth eggs and larvae present in small numbers. A fecal smear stained with trichrome or iron-hematoxylin is useful for detection and confirmatory identification of protozoa and provides a permanent record. For preserved specimens, the formalin-fixed portion is used for the wet mount and concentration procedure, and the PVA-fixed portion for the permanent record.

Small Intestinal Sample

Duodenal Aspirate and Biopsy. Some cases of intestinal parasitic infections may be missed by routine stool microscopy for a variety of reasons: low numbers or intermittent excretion of the organism, difficulty in obtaining appropriate specimens, or technical inexperience. For those parasites that inhabit the small intestine, diagnosis may require examination of a specimen of fluid and tissue from this region. An aspirate and biopsy may be obtained by endoscopy or a jejunal biopsy procedure. Organisms may be difficult to detect in the histologic sections themselves and may be more easily identified in an impression smear made by touching the luminal surface of the biopsy tissue against a glass slide.[37] Endoscopic brushings are also useful for this purpose.[38, 39] Immunoperoxidase staining of biopsied tissues using specific antibodies against *G. lamblia*[40] and *Cryptosporidium*[41] may facilitate the histologic detection of these organisms.

Duodenal String Test. A simple, cheap, and safe alternative to these more invasive procedures is the duodenal string test[42] (Entero-Test, HDC Corporation, San Jose, CA). A weighted gelatin capsule in pediatric and adult sizes containing an absorbent nylon line (90 or 140 cm in length, respectively) is swallowed after the free protruding end of the string has been taped to the cheek. Four hours later the string is withdrawn, and the absorbed small intestinal fluid is squeezed from the distal, bile-stained (alkaline) portion of the string onto a glass slide for microscopic examination. This procedure has been used successfully for diagnosis of giardiasis, cryptosporidiosis, isosporiasis, ascariasis, and hookworm infection.

Proctoscopy

In dysentery cases with suspected *E. histolytica* or *Balantidium coli* infection but negative stool microscopy results, trophozoites may be found in scrapings or biopsies taken from ulcerated tissue during a cautiously performed proctosigmoidoscopy. For diagnosis of schistosomiasis, rectal biopsies ("snips") are squashed immediately between two glass slides (without having been fixed in formalin) and examined microscopically under low power.

Immunodiagnosis

Stool Antigen Detection. A promising new approach to the diagnosis of intestinal parasitic infections is the detection of parasite antigen in the stools by immunologic methods such as enzyme-linked immunosorbent assay (ELISA), immunofluorescence (IF), or counterimmunoelectrophoresis (CIE). Diagnostic tests have been described for *G. lamblia*,[43] *E. histolytica*,[44] and *Cryptosporidium*.[45] The most common approach is a "double sandwich" ELISA analogous to the commonly used stool test for rotavirus. The capture antiserum may be directed against preparations of whole organisms or against a single, specific parasite antigen such as GSA 65, a stable *G. lamblia*–specific antigen utilized in a commercially available kit for diagnosis of giardiasis (ProSpecT/*Giardia*, Alexon Inc., Mountain View, CA).[46]

These methods offer several advantages over diagnosis by routine stool microscopy. Large numbers of specimens can be easily processed in a relatively short time, making such tests eminently suited to large-scale epidemiologic studies. The commercial *Giardia* diagnostic test, for example, requires no special instrumentation and, because a positive result is read simply as the development of any color change in the reaction, the test can be performed by a technician without any particular skills or training. Increasingly, there is evidence to suggest that the immunodiagnostic methods can detect cases missed by stool microscopy while retaining a high degree of specificity.[47] Presumably, parasite antigen is still excreted in the stools even when whole organisms are present in low numbers or absent due to cyclical parasite excretion. The need for collection and examination of multiple specimens may be obviated by these techniques. Their major drawback, particularly in areas where multiple parasitoses are common, is that microscopy is still required to detect other parasite infections. Future development of kits containing a panel of reagents for multiple parasites may overcome this problem.

Serology. An alternative approach applicable to those parasites against which the host mounts an immune response is the detection of specific antibodies in serum. Serologic methods are particularly useful for screening or for seroprevalence surveys. Specific and sensitive tests have been described for *Str. stercoralis*,[48] *G. lamblia*,[49] *E. histolytica*,[50] and *Cryptosporidium*[51] using gel-diffusion ELISA, CIE, IF, complement fixation (CF), or hemagglutination (HA). Simple and rapid slide agglutination tests have been reported for *E. histolytica*[52] and *G. lamblia*.[53] Serology is particularly useful for diagnosing invasive amebiasis[54]; asymptomatic cyst excretors usually give negative results with the standard assays available. The highest titers are found in extraintestinal disease; serology is the definitive test in diagnosing cases of amebic liver abscess, the majority of which have negative stool examinations. According to a recent report, a serologic method allows the differentiation between infection with virulent and nonvirulent *E. histolytica* strains by detecting specific antibodies to the *E. histolytica* adherence-mediating lectin required for pathogenicity.[55] Measurement of IgA antibodies in saliva was found to be useful in diagnosing *E. histolytica* infection in children; the salivary IgA titer correlated with the level of parasite antigen excreted in the stools.[56]

One drawback in interpreting serologic assays is that serum antibody titers may persist for months or years after cure or spontaneous clearing of the infection, making differentiation of present and past infection difficult. This is particularly so for giardiasis, although according to one report, measurement of specific anti-*Giardia* IgM rather than IgG overcame this problem.[57]

Miscellaneous Procedures

Techniques for parasite cultivation are available for *E. histolytica*[36] and *G. lamblia*,[58] but are not used for routine diagnostic purposes. DNA hybridization probes that identify parasite-specific DNA sequences can be used as a sensitive diagnostic test permitting analysis of large numbers of specimens; such a test has been described for detection of *E. histolytica* in stool samples directly applied to nylon membranes.[59] A culture of feces performed in a modified agar plate allows *Str. stercoralis* and hookworm to be identified by the characteristic furrows they leave.[60] The Cellotape test is used for the diagnosis of enterobiasis.

THERAPY

Adequate if less than ideal treatment is available for most intestinal parasitic infections; an important exception is *Cryptosporidium*. The recommended chemotherapeutic agents for specific infections are listed in Table 49–2, and drug dosage schedules, precautions, and side effects are in Table 49–3.

When a parasite is identified in a patient suffering from symptoms consistent with the infection, the decision to treat is clear-cut. However, most parasitic infestations are not associated with any apparent symptoms or other ill effects. The question of whether to treat such asymptomatic carriers is far more complex. Arguments proposed in favor of treating asymptomatic infections include (1) carriers pose a risk to the environment and to their immediate contacts and family members; (2) occult, subclinical effects of the infection may be present despite the absence of overt disease; and (3) the asymptomatic carrier state may convert to symptomatic disease in the future. Opponents of routine treatment of asymptomatic carriers argue that (1) these infections have no clinical consequence and therefore do not warrant treatment by drugs that have significant side effects and are expensive; (2) many infections resolve spontaneously without treatment; and (3) in endemic regions, there is a high likelihood that the patients will be reinfected within a short time after treatment.

The decision whether or not to treat asymptomatic infection must therefore be made on an individual case basis, taking into account the prevalence of the parasite in the area and other local conditions, the financial resources available, and the risks associated with the specific parasite. Although widespread treatment of asymptomatic carriers may not be warranted, treatment may be indicated in selected high-risk situations such as very young or malnourished infants, food handlers, individuals exposed to immunosuppressed patients, or asymptomatic carriers with a family member who suffers from recurring symptomatic disease with the same parasite (e.g., *G. lamblia, Enterobius vermicularis*). The specific issues relating to treatment of asymptomatic *E. histolytica* and *G. lamblia* infections are discussed in the descriptions of the individual parasites.

CONTROL OF PARASITE INFECTIONS

Achieving control of enteric parasitic diseases in developing countries remains a priority. Vaccines are not yet available for any of these agents, although progress toward their development is being made for some, such as the purified *E. histolytica* adherence lectin.[61] Improving water supplies and sanitation standards is a laudable goal but one that is expensive, difficult to achieve, and not necessarily effective.

A novel and exciting approach to the control of helminth disease is the use of mass or targeted chemotherapy. Most helminths do not multiply in the human host (*Str. stercoralis* is an important exception), and the intensity of infection varies considerably. Symptoms occur only in the minority of individuals (mostly school age) with the highest worm burdens. Mass chemotherapy of whole communities or of targeted populations (e.g., schoolchildren) can eliminate morbidity by reducing the worm burden to below the disease-producing threshold, even if infection is not totally eradicated. It has been proposed that three broad-spectrum antihelminthics administered in a single low dose at intervals of 1 to 4 years could control more than 90% of the major helminth infections of children: albendazole or other benzimadoles for hookworm, ascariasis, and trichuriasis; ivermectin for strongyloidiasis and filaria; and praziquantel for cestodes and trematodes.[62]

In the developed countries, efforts are directed toward control of the endemic protozoa: *G. lamblia, Cryptosporidium,* and *E. histolytica.* Prevention of waterborne transmission requires adequate filtration of water supplies in view of the resistance of the cyst forms of these organisms to chlorination. Education of day-care center attendants regarding the importance of hand washing can have a significant impact on person-to-person transmission in this setting.

PROTOZOA

Entamoeba Histolytica

E. histolytica is estimated to infect more than 10% of the world's population. Its distribution is worldwide, but its greatest prevalence is in developing countries. Endemic infection in both temperate and tropical regions is directly related to standards of sanitation and hygiene. Although 90 to 99% of infections are asymptomatic, it is a major cause of morbidity and mortality, accounting for at least 40,000 deaths a year.

Transmission is by fecal-oral spread of the cyst form via contaminated water or food or by direct person-to-person contact. The mature cyst measures 10 to 15 μm in diameter, contains four nuclei, and is resistant to hostile environmental conditions. After ingestion, excystation occurs in the small intestine, yielding eight uninuclear trophozoites that establish infection in the large intestine, either remaining in the lumen or invading the mucosa. The anaerobic, motile, pseudopod-forming trophozoites range in size from 10 to 60 μm; their cytoplasm may contain ingested erythrocytes. Encystment occurs in the large bowel to complete the life cycle.

Pathogenesis. Mechanisms of pathogenicity are better understood for *E. histolytica* than for any other intestinal parasite. Sargeaunt analyzed thousands of clinical isolates using thin-layer starch gel electrophoresis and demonstrated that all isolates from cases of invasive disease belonged to selected zymodemes (electrophoretic motility profiles).[63] Isolates with these "pathogenic" zymodemes induce liver abscess formation in hamsters and contact-dependent cell lysis in tissue culture. A prerequisite for the cytopathic effect is a galactose-specific lectin (carbohydrate-binding protein) that mediates adherence of *E. histolytica* trophozoites to human colonic mucins or mammalian target cells.[64] Pathogenic isolates can also be discriminated from nonpathogenic isolates by (1) hybridization with specific DNA probes,[65, 66] (2) possession of a 30 kilo-Dalton surface antigen,[67] and (3) identification of specific antigenic epitopes on the adherence-mediating lectin.[64]

The accepted view that zymodemes (isoenzyme profiles) are a fixed, stable characteristic of pathogenic and nonpathogenic isolates has recently been challenged by Mirelman[13] and others.[68] They observed that by changing the conditions and bacterial associates in the culture, a cloned isolate with a nonpathogenic zymodeme could convert to a pathogenic zymodeme and acquire virulence factors. Furthermore, the isolate reverted to a nonpathogenic zymodeme when recultured with the bacterial flora accompanying the original isolate but not with that from a pathogenic isolate. These findings raise the possibility that determinants in the intestinal microenvironment such as bacterial flora may trigger a switching between nonpathogenic and pathogenic states, although this hypothesis has yet to be proved in vivo.

Clinical Features. Noninvasive intestinal infection in cyst passers is characterized by heme-negative stools, absence of hematophagous trophozoites, and normal colonic mucosa. Although a multitude of gastrointestinal and other symptoms have been attributed to this state, it is doubtful that the association is more than coincidental.

Invasive intestinal disease typically presents as dysenteriform rectocolitis with abdominal pain, tenesmus, and bloody diarrhea. Rectal bleeding without diarrhea may occur in children. Rectosigmoidoscopy reveals hyperemic, edematous mucosa with punctate hemorrhages and small ulcers. The typical flask-shaped ulcers are not always present. Amebic dysentery may be distinguished from shigellosis by its more gradual onset, lack of a fever, and paucity of leukocytes in the heme-positive stools due to lysis of neutrophils by *E. histolytica*. Complications include toxic megacolon, especially after inappropriate corticosteroid therapy; fulminant colitis with colonic perforation; and pseudotumoral amebomas, producing colonic masses or constricting lesions. The existence of a more chronic, nondysenteriform colitis that may mimic inflammatory bowel disease is less well defined. Certainly the possibility of invasive amebiasis should always be excluded in suspected inflammatory bowel disease before instituting corticosteroid therapy.[69]

Extraintestinal invasive disease may involve any organ, but most commonly the liver. In most cases of amebic liver abscess, there is no history of antecedent intestinal disease, and *E. histolytica* cysts and trophozoites cannot be detected in stool or colonoscopy specimens. Acute presentation is with right upper quadrant abdominal and shoulder pain, fever, and cough. Weight loss may be the most prominent manifestation in subacute presentations. Physical examination reveals extreme hepatic tenderness, and there may be signs of a sympathetic serous effusion and atelectasis at the right lung base. Laboratory findings include a normocytic anemia, leukocytosis without eosinophilia, elevated erythrocyte sedimentation rate, hypoalbuminemia, moderate elevation of alkaline phosphatase, and slight transaminase elevation. Major complications are intra-abdominal rupture and pleuropulmonary involvement by direct or hematogenous extension.

Diagnosis. Diagnosis of intestinal amebiasis depends on demonstration of *E. histolytica* organisms in stools. The finding of hematophagous trophozoites is pathognomonic of invasive disease. In suspected cases with negative microscopy, examination of colonoscopy aspirates, scrapings, or biopsies from ulcer margins may be diagnostic.

Ultrasound and computerized tomography are invaluable for localizing a liver abscess (usually in the right lobe, with multiple lesions in some cases) and differentiating it from other space-occupying lesions, in particular a tumor, pyogenic abscess, or hydatid cyst. In view of the negative stool findings, definitive diagnosis usually requires demonstration of specific serum anti-*E. histolytica* antibodies[54]; serology may be falsely negative in the early days of the illness. In exceptional cases, it may be necessary to perform a fine needle aspiration under imaging guidance, which yields a creamy, yellowish, or bloodstained material (anchovy sauce). On microscopic examination, leukocytes are scarce and *E. histolytica* trophozoites can be detected in only a minority of cases; an indirect immunofluorescent antibody stain may improve their detection.[70]

Therapy. Invasive intestinal and extraintestinal amebiasis is treated with metronidazole or a related derivative (tinidazole, ornidazole). In severe, fulminating cases, parenteral emetine (or its less toxic derivative dehydroemetine, if available) may be added for the first few days. In order to prevent a possible relapse of symptomatic disease, an intraluminal amebicide (diloxanide furoate, paromomycin, or diiodohydroxyquin) should be administered concurrently with or following completion of treatment with the tissue amebicide, which by itself does not eradicate the intraluminal encysted organisms. For asymptomatic cyst passers, treatment with a luminal amebicide alone is sufficient.

The issue of treatment for asymptomatic *E. histolytica* cyst excretors is particularly controversial.[71] In a study from India, no clinical symptoms or histologic abnormalities could be ascribed to the *E. histolytica* carrier state, which resolved spontaneously without development of invasive disease in 15 subjects followed long term. It was concluded that treatment of cyst passers was not justified, considering the high carrier rate and enormous expense involved.[72] In another study, however, two of 20 asymptomatic excretors of cysts belonging to pathogenic zymodemes developed amebic dysentery. These investigators advocated treating all carriers of pathogenic zymodemes—defined by isoenzyme electrophoresis of cultured trophozoites or, more simply, by a strongly positive serologic response on the gel-diffusion test.[73] Furthermore, if there is indeed an in vivo counterpart to the in vitro observations of Mirelman and others that nonpathogenic *E. histolytica* strains cultured with certain bacteria can convert to a pathogenic zymodeme with virulence factors, there may be a case for treating all asymptomatic *E. histolytica* carriers.[13]

Cryptosporidium Species

Cryptosporidium[74] is a coccidian parasite that has long been familiar to veterinarians as a cause of diarrhea in young livestock animals. It came into prominence only in the early 1980s, when it was associated with life-threatening gastroenteritis in AIDS and other immunocompromised patients. It was subsequently recognized as a major cause of acute, self-limited gastroenteritis in healthy populations, particularly in 1- to 5-year-old children. In many reports from laboratories in both developing and developed countries throughout the world, *Cryptosporidium* ranks between the first and fourth most commonly identified enteropathogen.[75]

Most *Cryptosporidium* infections in humans and livestock animals are probably caused by *C. parvum,* a smaller-sized species; however, because the taxonomic description of *Cryptosporidium* is not yet clear, human isolates are usually referred to as *Cryptosporidium* species (spp). The complex life cycle is initiated by ingestion of the environmentally resistant oocysts. The mature, sporulated oocyst undergoes excystation, yielding four motile sporozoites that implant at the brush border just under the enterocyte cell membrane, forming an intracellular but extracytoplasmic parasitophorous vacuole. Further development involves asexual (merogeny) and sexual (gamogeny) multiplication, resulting eventually in oocyst formation. The oocyst may be shed in the feces to infect new hosts or may sporulate and excyst in situ; such autoinfectious recycling permits very heavy infection to develop.

Transmission.[75] Infection is generally acquired via the fecal-oral route, although transmission via sputum or vomitus and acquisition by inhalation have been proposed. Many human infections are zoonotic, derived predominantly from contact with cattle or sheep but also possibly from cats. Consumption of unpasteurized milk may be responsible for some cases. Contamination of water supplies is responsible for cryptosporidial travelers' diarrhea and for well-documented outbreaks; considering the resistance of oocysts to chemical disinfectants, adequate filtration is required to eliminate this threat. Foodborne transmission is also described. Direct person-to-person transmission accounts for secondary cases in family members, outbreaks in day-care centers, and nosocomially acquired infections. Indirect transmission via contaminated endoscopes is a significant risk. A protective effect from breast-feeding has been suggested.[76]

Clinical Features. An asymptomatic carrier state for *Cryptosporidium* has been identified in adults undergoing endoscopy[77] and in infants in southern India.[78]

The duration and severity of symptomatic cryptosporidiosis depend on the immune competence of the patient. In otherwise healthy individuals, the infection produces an acute, self-limiting watery diarrhea lasting 4 to 14 days, which may be accompanied by abdominal cramps and flu-like symptoms including headache and cough.

Immunocompromised patients typically suffer from voluminous cholera-like diarrhea, severe abdominal pain, and profound weight loss lasting for months; in this population it is often fatal. Attacks of abdominal cramps and diarrhea may be precipitated by eating. Malabsorption of lactose, fat, xylose, and vitamin B_{12} as well as protein-losing enteropathy have been well documented. Biliary tract involvement presents as severe right upper quadrant pain and vomiting with elevated alkaline phosphatase and gamma-glutamyl transpeptidase levels; radiologic findings resemble sclerosing cholangitis.[33] Not all cases conform with these extremes of the clinical spectrum. Some immunodeficient patients may inexplicably have mild, self-limiting disease. Malnourished children may develop chronic, severe diarrhea, resulting in exacerbation of their malnutrition.

Diagnosis. Although initial reports of diagnosis of human cryptosporidiosis were based on small intestinal or rectal biopsy specimens, these invasive procedures are unnecessary; diagnosis is most easily made by microscopic examination of a specially stained fecal smear for detection of oocysts. Yeast cells resemble *Cryptosporidium* oocysts morphologically and can easily be confused with them. A modified acid-fast stain allows the acid-fast and therefore red-staining oocysts to be differentiated from the colorless yeast cells. Oocysts are found in large numbers in liquid stools, especially from immunodeficient patients, but may be few in number in semiformed or formed stools. In such cases, sensitivity of detection may be improved by using a concentration procedure such as formalin-ether sedimentation, zinc sulfate, or Sheather's sucrose flotation. A highly specific and sensitive immunofluorescent antibody stain based on a monoclonal antibody to the oocyst wall is commercially available (Meridian Diagnostics, Cincinnati, OH). It is particularly useful in cases with few or rare oocysts in the stool, or for confirmation of the identity of oocysts by laboratories with limited experience in this diagnosis.[79] A double-sandwich ELISA technique for detection of *Cryptosporidium* antigen in stools has been reported.[45] Immunofluorescence and ELISA assays have been used to detect specific IgG and IgM antibody responses in serum[51]; AIDS patients may have very low titers. These serologic tests are mainly of value in epidemiologic studies rather than for diagnosis of individual cases.

Therapy. A consistently effective anticryptosporidial agent for immunosuppressed patients with cryptosporidiosis is sorely needed but yet to be identified. A large number of antimicrobial agents tried singly and in combination have proved to be ineffective. Spiramycin has been the subject of conflicting reports, both in immunocompromised patients and in controlled trials in immunocompetent infants.[80, 81] Eflornithine has recently been reported to induce complete remission or palliation in some AIDS patients with debilitating diarrhea.[82] Immunotherapy offers an alternative approach. Discontinuing or delaying corticosteroid or cytotoxic therapy may allow spontaneous resolution of the infection.

Treatment with bovine hyperimmune colostrum appears promising in AIDS patients.[83] A dialyzable extract from lymph node lymphocytes of immunized calves has produced sustained symptomatic improvement in AIDS patients.[84]

Nonspecific antidiarrheals (opiates, loperamide, cholestyramine) have generally been ineffective in controlling fluid losses. At present, the mainstay of treatment remains adequate fluid and electrolyte replacement therapy and parenteral alimentation in selected cases.

Giardia Lamblia

G. lamblia exists in two forms. The motile, flagellated, binucleated pear-shaped trophozoite is found in the proximal small bowel attached to the brush border. Adherence is mediated both by mechanical forces related to the ventral "suction" disc and by a mannose-binding lectin that is activated by trypsin.[11] Ellipsoid cysts form in the lumen of the small intestine and are passed in the stools; they are resistant to a range of environmental conditions. The life cycle is completed when the quadrinucleated cysts are ingested, pass through the stomach, and excyst, yielding two trophozoites in the upper small bowel. The life cycle can be reproduced in vitro by mimicking the conditions that exist in vivo: excystation of cysts is stimulated by hydrochloric acid, and encystation of trophozoites by a high bile salt concentration.[85] *G. lamblia* trophozoites may be cultured in a special medium enriched with serum and bile salts. Cultures may be established by acid-induced excystation of cysts purified from stool specimens, or more directly from trophozoites in duodenal juice obtained by aspiration or using the string test.[58]

Epidemiology. *G. lamblia* is found throughout the world and is the most commonly identified intestinal parasite in the developed world. Ingestion of as few as 10 cysts may be sufficient to produce infection. Indirect fecal-oral transmission may occur via food or, more commonly, via water, which accounts for most outbreaks of giardiasis and cases of travelers' diarrhea in reports ranging from Leningrad to U.S. national parks. Children may acquire infection from swimming pools or water slides, as the cysts of *G. lamblia* are resistant to chlorination. Direct person-to-person transmission accounts for the very high prevalence rates described in many day-care center studies over the past decade. Although outbreaks of symptomatic disease have been described in the day-care setting, the more usual pattern is asymptomatic carriage; this may be maintained for many months.[86] Day-care centers have been identified as a major factor in maintaining endemic levels of *G. lamblia* infection in a community.[87] High prevalence rates of *G. lamblia* have recently been reported in patients with cystic fibrosis[88] as well as Crohn's disease.[89]

Pathology and Pathogenesis. The light microscope appearance of the mucosa in cases of giardiasis ranges from completely normal to subtotal villous atrophy with crypt hyperplasia and proliferation of intraepithelial and lamina propria lymphocytes.[29] The grading of the mucosal abnormality may or may not correlate with the clinical severity. Trophozoites may be difficult to identify, particularly if the pathologist is not familiar with their characteristic *S*-like curled shape when seen sectioned longitudinally rather than face on. Ultrastructural studies may reveal microvillous disruption as well as circular imprints from the "suction" disc of the trophozoite and the presence of a mucoid pseudomembrane, which may play a role in causing malabsorption.[90]

The determinants of symptomatic versus asymptomatic infection and the mechanisms of pathogenicity are poorly understood for *G. lamblia,* although many theories have been proposed. A role for parasite-related factors is suggested by studies of experimental *G. lamblia* infections in human volunteers[91] and animal models, which provide some limited evidence for the existence of strains varying in pathogenicity, perhaps analogous to the situation for *E. histolytica.* In contrast to *E. histolytica,* however, no markers of virulence have yet been identified in *G. lamblia* isolates, which have been differentiated by a variety of techniques including isoenzyme electrophoresis,[92] surface antigen analysis,[93] DNA restriction fragment length polymorphisms,[94] and karyotype analysis.[94a] The role of endosymbiotic microorganisms identified in *Giardia* species, including bacteria and mycoplasmalike organisms[95] and a double-stranded RNA virus,[96] remains to be determined.

Possible host-related factors include a suggestion of genetic predisposition related to possession of blood group A or certain human leukocyte antigen alleles.[97] Participation of humoral and cell-mediated mechanisms in the host immune response to *Giardia* infection has been well documented in human studies and experimental animal models,[98] and persistent symptomatic giardiasis may be a problem in certain human immunodeficiency states. Nevertheless, most cases of symptomatic giardiasis occur in otherwise healthy individuals with no discernible immune deficiency. Previous exposure to *G. lamblia* infection may be a factor in preventing the development of symptomatic disease; however, first *G. lamblia* infections documented in infants followed from birth may also be asymptomatic (Dr. R. Dagan, personal communication, 1991).

Luminal factors possibly related to pathogenesis include (1) bacterial[15] or fungal[14] overgrowth of the small intestine, (2) deconjugation of intraluminal bile salts,[15] and (3) presence of breast milk, which has giardicidal properties related to free fatty acids cleaved from milk triglyceride by a bile salt–stimulated lipase present in human milk.[99]

Clinical Features. Symptomatic giardiasis may present as an acute onset of watery diarrhea with abdominal cramps and bloating, or as an ill-defined onset with a chronic or relapsing course over weeks or many months associated with weight loss or failure to thrive, abdominal distention, anorexia, abdominal discomfort, and flatulence. A full-blown malabsorption syndrome clinically resembling celiac disease may include steatorrhea; secondary lactase deficiency; malabsorption of xylose; deficiencies of iron, folic acid, and vitamins A, B_{12}, and E; and a protein-losing enteropathy. Rare extraintestinal manifestations include urticaria and arthralgia.

Diagnosis. The initial approach is stool microscopy for detection of cysts and/or trophozoites. The latter are more likely to be found in watery, diarrheal stools. The sensitivity of stool microscopy varies considerably, depending on the skill of the microscopist and the degree to which the previously outlined principles of stool collection, preservation, and concentration are adhered to. In addition, because the prepatency period (time from infection until appearance of organisms in the stool) of 2 to 3 weeks may be longer than the incubation period (time from infection until onset of symptoms) of 1 to 2 weeks, stool examinations may be falsely negative early in the disease.[100] If giardiasis is still suspected clinically despite three negative stool examinations, a small intestinal sample should be obtained: The string test is the simplest and least invasive of the alternatives. There is increasing evidence that a commercial ELISA test for detection of *G. lamblia* antigen in stools can correctly diagnose many cases in which stool microscopy is negative[101]; it may become the method of choice in this situation. With the availability of these safe and sensitive diagnostic procedures, there is little justification for an empiric trial of anti-*Giardia* therapy for suspected but unconfirmed giardiasis.

A diagnostic predicament occurs when *G. lamblia* trophozoites are unexpectedly discovered at a biopsy procedure performed in a child with clinical and histologic features of celiac disease. On occasion, *G. lamblia* may produce such changes; alternatively, *G. lamblia* may be acting as an "innocent bystander" in a genuine case of celiac disease. In such cases, a decision regarding a gluten-free diet should be deferred until the response to a course of anti-*Giardia* therapy has been evaluated. A clear-cut and sustained improvement indicates giardiasis. A temporary response suggests a combined etiology, or associated bacterial overgrowth responding to metronidazole. If there is no response, a gluten-free diet is instituted. In regions where *G. lamblia* is endemic, this situation can be avoided by routinely using the string test to exclude giardiasis before small bowel biopsy is performed in the evaluation of suspected celiac disease.

Therapy. Of the presently available drugs (see Table 49–2), metronidazole is probably the most effective and best tolerated,[102] but it is not approved for use in giardiasis in the United States. The single-dose nitroimidazoles are not available in the United States either. Quinacrine is often poorly tolerated by children; furazolidone has a lower efficacy but is better tolerated and is available as a liquid suspension. Culture techniques for *G. lamblia* are being applied to in vitro drug sensitivity testing in a search for more effective and better tolerated chemotherapeutic agents; the lipophilic tetracycline derivatives doxycycline and thiacycline[103] and the benzimadoles mebendazole and albendazole[104] appear promising.

Occasionally, stools may remain positive for *G. lamblia* or symptoms may persist despite a course of anti-*Giardia* therapy. The possible causes of and approach to this clinical situation are outlined in Table 49–4. Combination therapy with two drugs (metronidazole and quinacrine) may be successful when repeated courses of a single drug have been unsuccessful.[105]

Table 49–4. APPROACHES TO FAILED THERAPY OF *GIARDIA* INFECTION

Possible Causes	Solution
Stools Remain Positive Despite Treatment	
Poor compliance	Discussion with patient or parent; consider metronidazole 50 mg/kg/day for 3 days or tinidazole* 50 mg/kg single dose
Reinfection	Examine family members and close contacts; consider treating whole family, close contacts
Immune deficiency	Check immune function, especially IgA; combination therapy: metronidazole and quinacrine
Resistant strain	*Giardia* isolation and sensitivity testing*; higher dose or alternative drug; combination therapy: metronidazole and quinacrine
Stools Are Negative but Symptoms Persist	
Occult infection	String test; if positive, manage as above for failed therapy with stools positive
Secondary lactase deficiency	Lactose breath hydrogen test; lactose-free diet if positive
Alternative etiology	Another enteropathogen; other gastrointestinal disease (celiac disease, cow's-milk allergy)

*If available.

The question of treating asymptomatic *G. lamblia* carriers remains controversial. *G. lamblia* differs from *E. histolytica* in that conversion from an asymptomatic carrier state to symptomatic disease has not been described. In a prospective study of healthy children in day care, long-term *G. lamblia* carriers showed no ill effects in terms of growth achievement, hemoglobin level, and occurrence of gastrointestinal and respiratory symptoms when compared to uninfected controls.[85] Therefore, in the absence of risk factors (see earlier discussion on therapy), there is no compelling justification for treating otherwise healthy carriers of *G. lamblia.*

Isospora Belli

I. belli is a coccidian parasite of intestinal epithelial cells; unlike *Cryptosporidium,* however, it has no known animal reservoir. Its clinical features are almost identical to those of *Cryptosporidium,* depending on whether the infection occurs in immunocompetent or immunocompromised individuals. A mild eosinophilia, unusual in other protozoan infections, is common. Diagnosis is by a modified acid-fast stool examination for detection of oocysts, which are ovoid and much larger than *Cryptosporidium* oocysts. Isosporiasis responds readily to treatment with cotrimoxazole. Relapses are common in AIDS patients but can be prevented by long-term prophylaxis with cotrimoxazole or sulfadoxine-pyrimethamine.[18]

Balantidium Coli

Infection with *Ba. coli*[106] cysts is often related to contact with pigs. The large, ciliated trophozoites may invade the colonic mucosa, facilitated by secretion of hyaluronidase, to produce a colitis that must be differentiated from amebic and bacillary dysentery. Intestinal perforation may occur in severe cases, but hepatic involvement is rare. The trophozoites can be identified in fresh stools or scrapings from an ulcer margin. Response to treatment (see Table 49–2) is satisfactory.

Blastocystis Hominis

Bl. hominis is a frequently found anaerobic protozoan that may be observed in vacuolated, granular, and ameboid forms. Debate continues whether it is a cause of acute or chronic gastroenteritis and abdominal pain[8] or an "innocent bystander" identified fortuitously in patients with an additional enteropathogen or noninfectious cause for their gastrointestinal symptoms.[9]

HELMINTHS

Strongyloides Stercoralis

Infection is usually acquired through penetration of intact skin by filariform larvae after contact with soil contaminated by feces; skin invasion may produce a pruritic, papular erythematous rash. The larvae migrate via the blood stream to the lungs; at this stage a Löfflerlike syndrome with eosinophilia may occur. From the alveolar spaces, the larvae crawl up the airway passages to the pharynx and are swallowed. In the small intestine they become embedded in the mucosa and mature into adult female worms. Intestinal involvement presents with abdominal pain, watery or mucousy diarrhea, and eosinophilia, and may be complicated by malabsorption and protein-losing enteropathy. It is a recognized cause of intractable diarrhea of infancy syndrome.[107]

Embryonated eggs from the hermaphroditic adult worm hatch in the submucosa, producing rhabditidiform larvae that are excreted in the feces, allowing the free-living (nonparasitic) phase of the cycle to be completed in the soil. Alternatively, the rhabditidiform larvae can transform prematurely into filariform larvae while still in the colon and then directly invade the colorectal mucosa or the perianal skin and migrate to the lungs or elsewhere. This "autoinfection" cycle allows the infection to persist in a quiescent manner for the rest of the individual's life even in the absence of ongoing external infection.

In situations in which the host's nutritional or immunologic status is disturbed, however, the autoinfection cycle may be massively amplified, leading to an overwhelming larval invasion known as the hyperinfection syndrome. Larvae can disseminate into virtually every organ of the body, and secondary bacterial sepsis may be produced by enteric bacteria adhering to the invading larvae. Clinical features include severe abdominal pain, diarrhea, pneumonitis, ileus, shock, and generalized or focal gram-negative sepsis. Eosinophilia may be absent. Development of the syndrome has been associated with malnutrition, steroid or chemotherapy, solid organ transplantation, HIV infection, lymphoma, and other malignancy. It is less common than might be expected in AIDS patients in endemic areas. Because of the risk of hyperinfection syndrome, candidates for immunosuppressive therapy who have a history of visiting or residing in an endemic area should be thoroughly screened for occult *Str. stercoralis* infection and treated appropriately.[108] Endemic areas include Southeast Asia, Eastern Europe, West Africa, the Caribbean, and southern United States.

Microscopic examination of stools for detection of rhabditidiform larvae often misses low-grade infections, even when a concentration procedure is used; examination of a small intestinal sample (particularly the string test[41]) is more reliable. Specific and sensitive serologic assays have been described but are not yet widely available.[48] Antigens that may be useful for stool immunodiagnosis have been identified. A simple agar-plate method for fecal culture allows *Str. stercoralis* to be detected by the characteristic furrows it leaves.[59]

Thiabendazole is the best treatment available but has a significant failure rate, and side effects are common. Ivermectin, a new broad-spectrum antihelminthic, has shown very promising results.[109]

Ascaris Lumbricoides

Ascariasis is the most common helminth infection worldwide and is usually asymptomatic. Its major manifestations are pneumonitis and intestinal or biliary tract obstruction.[32] Therapeutic options in obstructive complications include piperazine, which paralyzes the worms; gastrografin, which dehydrates and shrinks the worms; and endoscopic or surgical removal.

Capillaria Philippinensis

C. philippinensis[110] is a 2- to 4-mm-long roundworm found in the small intestinal mucosa and must therefore be differentiated from *Str. stercoralis*. Infection is acquired by eating uncooked fish containing the larvae, which then mature into egg-laying adult worms. As in strongyloidiasis, production of autoinfective larvae allows a massive worm burden to develop. The life cycle is completed by excretion of eggs in the stool and their ingestion by fish. Fish-eating birds are an alternative definitive host. Migratory birds have the potential to spread the disease, which was first described nearly 30 years ago in the Philippines but has since been reported in Thailand, Japan, Taiwan, Iran, and Egypt.

Clinical manifestations include intractable diarrhea, abdominal pain, borborygmi, progressive weight loss and cachexia, steatorrhea, protein-losing enteropathy, and hypokalemia. Untreated disease has a high mortality. Diagnosis is by identification in the stools of the characteristic peanut-shaped 20- to 40-μm eggs with flat bipolar plugs. Larvae and adult worms may also be found in the stools. Treatment with mebendazole or albendazole achieves complete cure, but relapses may occur if the course of therapy is not completed.

Enterobius Vermicularis

Enterobiasis is the most common helminth infection in the United States, the highest prevalence being in school-age children. Migration of the female worm to lay its eggs at night produces perianal and perineal pruritus. Aberrant migration can result rarely in dysuria, salpingitis, and appendiceal colic. A piece of cellotape applied to the perineal region and affixed to a glass slide allows the eggs to be easily detected. Treatment (see Table 49–2) is most effective when a second dose is given after 10 to 14 days in order to kill worms that have hatched from eggs ingested after the first dose. Treatment of household members should be considered.

Hookworm

The adult worms of *Necator americanus* and *Ancylostoma duodenale* attach to the duodenal and jejunal mucosa and cause blood loss amounting to about 0.03 and 0.2 ml per worm per day, respectively.[111] Protein loss also occurs. Development of anemia and occasionally hypoproteinemia is therefore dependent on the worm load and on the dietary intake and body stores of iron and protein. The characteristic ovoid, thin-shelled eggs are easily identified in the stools.

Trichinella Spiralis

Transient gastroenteritis may follow ingestion of trichinous pork; adult worms can be found at the base of villi and may produce a mild partial villous atrophy. The major features of the infection, however, are related to systemic larval invasion.

Trichuris Trichiura

The adult worms embed themselves in the mucosa of the proximal colon,[112] but may sometimes be found more distally at proctoscopy. Only the heaviest infections are associated with symptoms, which may include mucousy or even blood-stained diarrhea, rectal prolapse, anemia, clubbing, and poor growth. It is difficult to prove to what extent these symptoms are due to the infection itself or to commonly associated enteric infections (especially hookworm, ascariasis, amebiasis, and shigellosis) and malnutrition. The lemon-shaped eggs are easily identified in the stool, and treatment is straightforward.

Cestodes

The adult tapeworms that inhabit the human intestine consist of a head, or scolex, for attachment and multiple proglottids, which are hermaphroditic egg-producing segments. *Taenia solium* and *saginata* may reach a length of 20 and 30 feet, respectively, but produce minimal or no symptoms except when a gravid proglottid or an entire strip of worm exits through the anus. *D. latum* may reach 50 feet in length and occasionally causes vitamin B_{12} deficiency. *Hymenolepis nana* is only 1 to 2 inches long.

Cestode eggs passed in the stool are ingested by the intermediate host and develop into larvae, which migrate to various organs and produce encysted forms. Humans can become the intermediate as well as the definitive host for *Tae. solium* either by ingestion of eggs in food or water contaminated with human feces or by autoinfection in a subject already harboring an adult worm. Cysticerci (fluid-filled larval cysts) may then develop in virtually any organ, but particularly in the central nervous system. Humans are the only intermediate host for *H. nana;* cysticercoid larvae develop within the villi. Autoinfection may produce a heavy worm load, with development of abdominal cramps and diarrhea.

Schistosoma Species[113]

Infection is acquired when cercariae liberated from the intermediate snail hosts penetrate the skin, sometimes producing "swimmers itch." After migration through the lungs and liver, they mature into adult worms and lodge in the superior *(Sch. japonicum)* or inferior *(Sch. mansoni)* mesenteric venules. An acute, typhoid-like illness with eosinophilia (Katamaya fever) may develop at this stage. Chronic disease in individuals with a heavy worm burden results from a granulomatous inflammatory response by the host to the parasite eggs in the intestine and liver, with eventual fibro-obstructive sequelae. Bowel lesions produce ulceration and bleeding, and occasionally polyp or stricture formation. Liver function is usually preserved in hepatic fibrosis, but portal hypertension may result in massive splenomegaly, variceal bleeding, and hypersplenism. The availability of praziquantel has revolutionized the therapy of schistosomiasis.

REFERENCES

1. Katz M, Despommier DD, Gwadz RW: Parasitic Diseases. New York, Springer Verlag, 1989.
2. Holland CV, Taren DL, Crompton DW, et al: Intestinal helminthiases in relation to the socioeconomic environment of Panamanian children. Soc Sci Med 1988; 26:209–213.
3. Kan SP, Guyatt HL, Bundy DA: Geohelminth infection of children from rural plantations and urban slums in Malaysia. Trans R Soc Trop Med Hyg 1989; 83:817–820.
4. Salas SD, Heifetz R, Barrett-Connor E: Intestinal parasites in Central American immigrants in the United States. Arch Int Med 1990; 150:1514–1516.

5. Bartlett AV, Moor M, Gary GW, et al: Diarrheal illness among infants and toddlers in day care centers. I. Epidemiology and pathogens. J Pediatr 1985; 107:495–502.
6. Robinson BA, Tolan W, Golding-Beecher O: Childhood pica. Some aspects of the clinical profile in Manchester, Jamaica. West Indian Med J 1990; 39:20–26.
7. Forrester JE, Scott ME, Bundy DA, et al: Predisposition of individuals and families in Mexico to heavy infection with *Ascaris lumbricoides* and *Trichuris trichiura.* Trans R Soc Trop Med Hyg 1990; 84:272–276.
8. Miller RA, Minshew BH: *Blastocystis hominis*: An organism in search of a disease. Rev Infect Dis 1988; 10:930–938.
9. Doyle PW, Helgason MM, Mathias RG, et al: Epidemiology and pathogenicity of *Blastocystis hominis.* J Clin Microbiol 1990; 28:116–121.
10. Ravdin JI: *Entamoeba histolytica:* From adherence to enteropathy. J Infect Dis 1989; 159:420–429.
11. Ward HD, Keusch GT, Pereira EA: Induction of a phosphomannosyl binding lectin activity in *Giardia.* Bioessays 1990; 12:211–215.
12. McKerrow JH, Brindley P, Brown M, et al: *Strongyloides stercoralis:* Identification of a protease that facilitates penetration of skin by the infective larvae. Exp Parasitol 1990; 70:134–143
13. Mirelman D: Effect of culture conditions and bacterial associates on the zymodemes of *Entamoeba histolytica.* Parasitol Today 1987; 3:37–40.
14. Naik SR, Rau NR, Vinayak VK, et al: Presence of *Candida albicans,* in normal and in *Giardia lamblia* infected human jejunum. Ann Trop Med Parasitol 1978; 72:493–494.
15. Tandon BN, Tandon RK, Satpathy BK, et al: Mechanism of malabsorption in giardiasis: A study of bacterial flora and bile salt deconjugation in upper jejunum. Gut 1977; 18:176–181
16. Sallon S, Deckelbaum RJ, Schmid II, et al: *Cryptosporidium,* malnutrition and chronic diarrhea in children. Am J Dis Child 1988; 142:312–315.
17. Soave R: Cryptosporidiosis and isosporiasis in patients with AIDS. Infect Dis Clin North Am 1988; 2:485–493.
18. Pape JW, Verdier RI, Johnson WD Jr: Treatment and prophylaxis of *Isospora belli* infection in patients with the acquired immunodeficiency syndrome. N Engl J Med 1989; 320:1044–1047.
19. DeVault GA Jr, King JW, Rohr MS, et al: Opportunistic infections with *Stronglyoides stercoralis* in renal transplantation. Rev Infect Dis 1990; 12:653–671.
20. Bromiker R, Korman SH, Or R, et al: Severe giardiasis in two patients undergoing bone marrow transplantation. Bone Marrow Transplant 1989; 4:701–703.
21. Korman SH, Granot E, Ramu N: Severe giardiasis in a child during cancer therapy. Am J Gastroenterol 1989; 84:450–451.
22. Buret A, Gall DG, Nation PN, et al: Intestinal protozoa and epithelial cell kinetics, structure and function. Parasitol Today 1990; 6:375–380.
23. Stephenson LS, Latham MC, Kurz KM, et al: Treatment with a single dose of albendazole improves growth of Kenyan schoolchildren with hookworm, *Trichuris trichiura,* and *Ascaris lumbricoides* infections. Am J Trop Med Hyg 1989; 41:78–87.
24. Stephenson LS, Latham MC, Kinoti SN, et al: Improvements in physical fitness of Kenyan schoolboys infected with hookworm, *Trichuris trichiura* and *Ascaris lumbricoides* following a single dose of albendazole. Trans R Soc Trop Med Hyg 1990; 84:277–282.
25. Solomons NW: Giardiasis: Nutritional implications. Rev Infect Dis 1982; 4:859–869.
26. Farthing MJG, Mata L, Urrutia JJ, et al: Natural history of *Giardia* infection of infants and children in rural Guatemala and its impact on physical growth. Am J Clin Nutr 1986; 43:395–405.
27. Gupta MC, Urrutia JJ: Effect of periodic antiascariasis and antigiardia treatment on nutritonal status of preschool children. Am J Clin Nutr 1982; 36:79–86.
28. Villar J, Klebanoff M, Kestler E: The effect on fetal growth of protozoan and helminthic infection during pregnancy. Obstet Gynecol 1989; 74:915–920.
29. Kay R, Barnes GL, Townley RRW: *Giardia lamblia* infestation in 154 children. Aust Paediatr J 1977; 13:98–104.
30. O'Brien W: Intestinal malabsorption in acute infection with *Strongyloides stercoralis.* Trans R Soc Trop Med Hyg 1975; 69:69–77.
31. Balikian JP, Bitar JG, Rishani KK, et al: Fulminant necrotizing amebic colitis in children. Am J Proctol 1977; 28(1):69–73.
32. Khuroo MS, Zargar SA, Mahajan R: Hepatobiliary and pancreatic ascariasis in India. Lancet 1990; 335: 1503–1506.
33. Schneiderman DJ, Cello JP, Laing FC: Papillary stenosis and sclerosing cholangitis in the acquired immunodeficiency syndrome. Ann Intern Med 1987; 106:546–549.
34. Travis WD, Schmidt K, MacLowry D, et al: Respiratory cryptosporidiosis in a patient with malignant lymphoma: Report of a case and review of the literature. Arch Pathol Lab Med 1990; 114:519–522.
35. Egger M, Mäusezahl D, Odermatt P, et al: Symptoms and transmission of intestinal cryptosporidiosis. Arch Dis Child 1990; 65:445–447.
36. Melvin DM, Brooke MM: Laboratory procedures for the diagnosis of intestinal parasites: US Department of Health and Human Services. HHS Publication No. (CDC) 85-8282, 1985.
37. Kamath KR, Murugasu R: A comparative study of four methods for detecting *Giardia lamblia* in children with diarrheal disease and malabsorption. Gastroenterology 1974; 66:16–21.
38. Marshall JB, Kelley DH, Vogele KA: Giardiasis: Diagnosis by endoscopic brush cytology of the duodenum. Am J Gastroenterol 1984; 79:517–519.
39. Silverman JF, Levine J, Finley JL, et al: Small intestinal brushing cytology in the diagnosis of cryptosporidiosis in AIDS. Diagn Cytopathol 1990; 6:193–196.
40. Fleck SL, Hames E, Warhurst DC: Detection of *Giardia* in human jejunum by the immunoperoxidase method: Specific and non-specific results. Trans R Soc Trop Med Hyg 1985; 79:110–113.
41. Bonnin A, Petrella T, Dubremetz JF, et al: Histopathological method for diagnosis of cryptosporidiosis using monoclonal antibodies. Eur J Clin Microbiol Infect Dis 1990; 9:664–666.
42. Korman SH: The duodenal string test: A simple multipurpose diagnostic tool in clinical pediatrics. Am J Dis Child 1990; 144:803–805.
43. Green EL, Miles MA, Warhurst DC: Immunodiagnostic detection of *Giardia* antigen in faeces by a rapid visual enzyme-linked immunosorbent assay. Lancet 1985; 2:691–693.
44. Merino E, Glender W, del Muro R, et al: Evaluation of the ELISA test for detection of *Entamoeba histolytica* in feces. J Clin Lab Anal 1990; 4:39–42.
45. Ungar BL: Enzyme-linked immunoassay for detection of *Cryptosporidium* antigens in fecal specimens. J Clin Microbiol 1990; 28:2491–2495.
46. Rosoff JD, Sanders CA, Sonnad SS, et al: Stool diagnosis of giardiasis using a commercially available enzyme immunoassay to detect *Giardia*-specific antigen 65 (GSA 65). J Clin Microbiol 1989; 27:1997–2002.
47. Janoff EN, Craft JC, Pickering LK, et al: Diagnosis of *Giardia lamblia* infections by detection of parasite-specific antigens. J Clin Microbiol 1989; 27:431–435.
48. Genta RM: Predictive value of an enzyme-linked immunosorbent assay (ELISA) for the serodiagnosis of strongyloidiasis. Am J Clin Pathol 1988; 89:391–394.
49. Miotti PG, Gilman RH, Santosham M, et al: Age-related rate of seropositivity of antibody to *Giardia lamblia* in four diverse populations. J Clin Microbiol 1986; 24:972–975.
50. Lin TM, Schubert CM, Kiefer DJ, et al: Two rapid and simple enzyme immunoassays for human antibodies to *Entamoeba histolytica.* J Immunoassay 1989; 10:301–313.
51. Ungar BL, Soave R, Fayer R, et al: Enzyme immunoassay detection of immunoglobulin M and G antibodies to *Cryptosporidium* in immunocompetent and immunocompromised persons. J Infect Dis 1986; 153:570–578.
52. Robert R, Mahaza C, Bernard C, et al: Evaluation of a new bicolored latex agglutination test for immunological diagnosis of hepatic amoebiasis. J Clin Microbiol 1990; 28:1422–1424.
53. Sherman RA, Moody AH: *Giardia* antigen and antibody detection using coagglutination. Serodiagn Immunother Infect Dis 1990; 4:231–241.
54. Healy GR: Immunologic tools in the diagnosis of amebiasis: Epidemiology in the United States. Rev Infect Dis 1986; 8:239–246.
55. Ravdin JI, Jackson TF, Petri WA Jr, et al: Association of serum antibodies to adherence lectin with invasive amebiasis and symp-

tomatic infection with pathogenic *Entamoeba histolytica.* J Infect Dis 1990; 162:768–772.
56. del Muro R, Acosta E, Merino E, et al: Diagnosis of intestinal amebiasis using salivary IgA antibody detection. J Infect Dis 1990; 162:1360–1364.
57. Goka AKJ, Rolston DDK, Mathan VI, et al: Diagnosis of giardiasis by specific IgM antibody enzyme-linked immunosorbent assay. Lancet 1986; 2:184–186.
58. Korman SH, Hais E, Spira DT: Routine in vitro cultivation of *Giardia lamblia* using the string test. J Clin Microbiol 1990; 102:249–252.
59. Samuelson J, Acuna-Soto R, Reed S, et al: DNA hybridization probe for clinical diagnosis of *Entamoeba histolytica.* J Clin Microbiol 1989; 27:671–676.
60. Arakaki T, Iwanaga M, Kinjo F, et al: Efficacy of agar-plate culture in detection of *Strongyloides stercoralis* infection. J Parasitol 1990; 76:425–428.
61. Petri WA Jr, Ravdin JI: Protection of gerbils from amebic liver abscess by immunization with the galactose-specific adherence lectin of *Entamoeba histolytica.* Infect Immun 1991; 59:97–101.
62. Warren KS: An integrated system for the control of the major human helminth parasites. Acta Leidensia 1990; 59:443–452.
63. Sargeaunt PG: The reliability of *Entamoeba histolytica* zymodemes in clinical diagnosis. Parasitol Today 1987; 3:40–44.
64. Petri WA Jr, Jackson TF, Gathiram V, et al: Pathogenic and nonpathogenic strains of *Entamoeba histolytica* can be differentiated by monoclonal antibodies to the galactose-specific adherence lectin. Infect Immun 1990; 58:1802–1806.
65. Tannich E, Horstmann RD, Knobloch J, et al: Genomic DNA differences between pathogenic and nonpathogenic *Entamoeba histolytica.* Proc Natl Acad Sci USA 1989; 86:5118–5122.
66. Bracha R, Diamond LS, Ackers JP, et al: Differentiation of clinical isolates of *Entamoeba histolytica* by using specific DNA probes. J Clin Microbiol 1990; 28:680–684.
67. Blakely P, Sargeaunt PG, Reed SL: An immunogenic 30-kDa surface antigen of pathogenic clinical isolates of *Entamoeba histolytica.* J Infect Dis 1990; 162:949–954.
68. Andrews BJ, Mentzoni L, Bjorvatn B: Zymodeme conversion of isolates of *Entamoeba histolytica.* Trans R Soc Trop Med Hyg 1990; 84:63–65.
69. Patel AS, DeRidder PH: Amebic colitis masquerading as acute inflammatory bowel disease: The role of serology in its diagnosis. J Clin Gastroenterol 1989; 11:407–410.
70. Yang SJ: Detection of *Entamoeba histolytica* trophozoites in liver pus by the indirect fluorescent antibody test for the aetiological diagnosis of amoebic liver abscess. Ann Trop Med Parasitol 1989; 83:253–255.
71. Jackson TFHG: *Entamoeba histolytica* cyst passers—to treat or not to treat? S Afr Med J 1987; 72:657–658.
72. Nanda R, Baveja U, Anand BS: *Entamoeba histolytica* cyst passers: Clinical features and outcome in untreated subjects. Lancet 1984; 2:301–303.
73. Gathiram V, Jackson TFHG: A longitudinal study of asymptomatic carriers of pathogenic zymodemes of *Entamoeba histolytica.* S Afr Med J 1987; 72:669–672.
74. Crawford FG, Vermund SH: Human cryptosporidiosis. CRC Crit Rev Microbiol 1988; 16:113–159.
75. Casemore DP: Epidemiological aspects of human cryptosporidiosis. Epidemiol Infect 1990; 104:1–28.
76. Mata L: *Cryptosporidium* and other protozoa in diarrheal disease in less developed countries. Ped Infect Dis 1986; 5 (Suppl):S17–S129.
77. Roberts WG, Green PH, Ma J, et al: Prevalence of cryptosporidiosis in patients undergoing endoscopy: Evidence for an asymptomatic carrier state. Am J Med 1989; 87:537–539.
78. Mathan M, Venkatesan S, George R, et al: *Cryptosporidium* and diarrhoea in southern Indian children. Lancet 1985; 2:1172–1175.
79. Rusnak J, Hadfield TL, Rhodes MM, et al: Detection of *Cryptosporidium* oocysts in human fecal specimens by an indirect immunofluorescence assay with monoclonal antibodies. J Clin Microbiol 1987; 27:1135–1136.
80. Saez-Llorens X, Odio CM, Umana MA, et al: Spiramycin vs. placebo for treatment of acute diarrhea caused by *Cryptosporidium.* Pediatr Infect Dis J 1989; 8:136–140.
81. Wittenberg DF, Miller NM, van den Ende J: Spiramycin is not effective in treating *Cryptosporidium* diarrhea in infants: Results of a double-blind randomized trial. J Infect Dis 1989; 159:131–132.
82. Rolston KV, Fainstein V, Bodey GP: Intestinal cryptosporidiosis treated with eflornithine: A prospective study among patients with AIDS. J Acquir Immune Defic Syndr 1989; 2:426–430.
83. Nord J, Ma P, DiJohn D, et al: Treatment with bovine hyperimmune colostrum of cryptosporidial diarrhea in AIDS patients. AIDS 1990; 4:581–584.
84. McMeeking A, Borkowsky W, Klesius PH, et al: A controlled trial of bovine dialyzable leukocyte extract for cryptosporidiosis in patients with AIDS. J Infect Dis 1990; 161:108–112.
85. Gillin FD, Boucher SE, Rossi SS, et al: *Giardia lamblia*: The roles of bile, lactic acid, and pH in the completion of the life cycle in vitro. Exp Parasitol 1989; 69:164–174.
86. Ish-Horowicz M, Korman SH, Shapiro M, et al: Asymptomatic giardiasis in children. Pediatr Infect Dis J 1989; 8:773–779.
87. Sealy DP, Schuman SH: Endemic giardiasis and day care. Pediatrics 1983; 72:154–158.
88. Roberts DM, Craft JC, Mather FJ, et al: Prevalence of giardiasis in patients with cystic fibrosis. J Pediatr 1988; 112:555–559.
89. Scheurlen C, Kruis W, Spengler U, et al: Crohn's disease is frequently complicated by giardiasis. Scand J Gastroenterol 1988; 23:833–839.
90. Poley JR, Rosenfield S: Malabsorption in giardiasis: Presence of a luminal barrier (mucoid pseudomembrane): A scanning and transmission electron microscopic study. J Pediatr Gastroenterol Nutr 1982; 1:63–80.
91. Nash TE, Herrington DA, Losonsky GA, et al: Experimental human infections with *Giardia lamblia.* J Infect Dis 1987; 156:974–984.
92. Korman SH, LeBlancq SM, Spira DT, et al: *Giarda lamblia:* Identification of different strains from man. Parasitol Res 1986; 72:173–180.
93. Nash TE, Conrad JT, Merritt JW Jr: Variant specific epitopes of *Giardia lamblia.* Mol Bioch Parasitol 1990; 42:125–132.
94. Nash TE, McCutchan T, Keister D, et al: Restriction-endonuclease analysis of DNA from 15 *Giardia* isolates obtained from humans and animals. J Infect Dis 1985; 152:64–73.
94a. Korman SH, LeBlancq SM, Deckelbaum RJ, et al: Investigation of human giardiasis by karyotype analysis. J Clin Invest 1992; 89:1725–1733.
95. Feely DE, Chase DG, Hardin EL, et al: Ultrastructural evidence for the presence of bacteria, viral-like particles and mycoplasma-like organisms associated with *Giardia* spp. J Protozool 1988; 35:151–158.
96. Miller RL, Wang AL, Wang CC: Purification and characterization of the *Giardia lamblia* double-stranded RNA virus. Mol Bioch Parasitol 1988; 28:189–196.
97. Pettoello Mantovani M, Guandalini S, Cosentini E, et al: ABO blood-group distribution and HLA typing in children with giardiasis. Trans R Soc Trop Med Hyg 1990; 84:380–381.
98. denHollander N, Riley D, Befus D: Immunology of giardiasis. Parasitol Today 1988; 4:124–131.
99. Gillin FD: *Giardia lamblia:* The role of conjugated and unconjugated bile salts in killing by human milk. Exp Parasitol 1987; 63:74–83.
100. Jokipii AMM, Jokipii L: Prepatency of giardiasis. Lancet 1977; 1:1095–1097.
101. Schieven BC, Hussain Z: Evaluation of an enzyme-immunoassay test kit for diagnosing infections with *Giardia lamblia.* Serodiagn Immunother Infect Dis 1990; 4:109–113.
102. Davidson RA: Issues in clinical parasitology: The treatment of giardiasis. Am J Gastroenterol 1984; 79:256–261.
103. Edlind TE: Tetracyclines as antiparasitic agents: Lipophilic derivatives are highly active against Giardia lamblia in vitro. Antimicrob Agents Chemother 1989, 33:2144–2145.
104. Edlind TD, Hang TL, Chakraborty PR: Activity of the antihelminthic benzimadoles against *Giardia lambia* in vitro. J Infect Dis 1990; 162:1408–1411.
105. Smith PD, Gillin FD, Spira WM, et al: Chronic giardiasis: Studies on drug sensitivity, toxin production, and host immune response. Gastroenterology 1982; 83:797–803.
106. Cross JH: Balantidiasis and other intestinal protozoa. *In* Warren KS, Mahmoud AAF, eds: Tropical and Geographic Medicine. New York, McGraw Hill, 1990, pp 349–352.

107. Granot E, Deckelbaum RJ, Heldenberg D, et al: Strongyloidiasis in infancy. Isr J Med Sci 1983; 19:1089–1093.
108. Genta RM: Global prevalence of strongyloidiasis: Critical review with epidemiologic insights into the prevention of disseminated disease. Rev Infect Dis 1989; 11:755–767.
109. Maquira C, Jiminez G, Guerra JG, et al: Ivermectin for human strongyloidiasis and other intestinal helminths. Am J Trop Med 1989; 40:304–309.
110. Cross JH: Intestinal capillariasis. Parasitol Today 1990; 6:26–28.
111. Miller TA: Hookworm infection in man. Adv Parasitol 1979; 17:315–383.
112. Gilman RH, Chong YH, Davis C, et al: The adverse consequences of heavy *Trichuris* infection. Trans R Soc Trop Med Hyg 1983; 77:432–438.
113. Mahmoud AAF, Wahab MFA: Schistosomiasis. *In* Warren KS, Mahmoud AAF, eds: Tropical and Geographic Medicine. New York, McGraw Hill, 1990, pp 458–473.

Chapter 50

Meckel's Diverticulum and Other Omphalomesenteric Duct Remnants

MARSHALL Z. SCHWARTZ and IVA SMOLENS

Remnants of the embryonic yolk sac, also referred to in utero as the *omphalomesenteric duct,* or *vitelline duct,* are the most common postnatal anomalies of the gastrointestinal tract. The most frequently occurring residual of the yolk sac is a diverticulum arising from the antimesenteric border of the distal ileum, which has come to be known as Meckel's diverticulum. The complications related to remnants of the embryonic yolk sac are numerous and may be life threatening.

HISTORY

An unusual diverticulum of the small intestine was first described in 1658 by Hildanus[1] and again in 1672 by Lavater.[2] Ruysch illustrated this anomaly in 1701.[3] However, it was not until the early nineteenth century that Sir Johann Freidrich Meckel[4] first published his observations about the anatomy and the embryology of this ileal diverticulum. As a result of this landmark paper, this anomaly bears his name.

INCIDENCE

A remnant of the embryonic yolk sac remains in 1 to 3% of all infants, thus making this the most common congenital gastrointestinal anomaly.[5–9]

The distribution and frequency of omphalomesenteric duct remnants are shown in Table 50–1. When a Meckel's diverticulum is found incidentally at surgery or at autopsy, the sex ratio is approximately equal.[5] However, it appears that males develop pathology related to a Meckel's diverticulum more frequently than females, in a ratio of 3:1.[5, 10] This is related, in part, to a male preponderance for intussusception from a Meckel's diverticulum acting as the lead point. Although the incidence of omphalomesenteric duct remnants (especially Meckel's diverticulum) is high, the risk for development of symptoms from these anomalies is relatively low. According to Soltero and Bill,[7] the risk of developing a complication from a Meckel's diverticulum is approximately 4%. Development of symptoms from a Meckel's diverticulum appears more likely to occur in childhood; 80% of all surveyed patients requiring surgery were under 10 years of age, and nearly half of the patients were under two years of age.[11, 12]

EMBRYOLOGY AND ANATOMY

During the first and second weeks following fertilization, the yolk sac arises from and dominates the ventral surface of the embryo. The embryo is sustained by the nutrient-filled yolk sac until the placental unit is established. A portion of the yolk sac becomes incorporated into the ventral wall of the primitive gut. Shortly thereafter the connection between the embryo and the yolk sac narrows and lengthens to develop into the omphalomesenteric or vitelline duct. Between the fifth and seventh weeks of gestation, the omphalomesenteric duct attenuates, involutes, and separates from the intestine.[5] Just prior to this separation, the epithelium of the yolk sac develops an appearance similar to that of the gastric

Table 50–1. DISTRIBUTION AND FREQUENCY OF OMPHALOMESENTERIC DUCT REMNANTS IN TWO STUDIES

	Frequency (%)	
Type of Remnant	***Moses*[9] *(1,605 cases)***	***Söderlund*[6] *(413 cases)***
Meckel's diverticulum	82	96
Patent omphalomesenteric duct	6	2.4
Solid cord	10	—
Umbilical remnant	1	1.2
Cystic remnant	1	0.24

lining.[5] Partial or complete failure of involution of the omphalomesenteric duct results in various residual structures, depending on the stage at which this process fails to progress. That portion of the omphalomesenteric duct that does not become atretic will persist and grow and develop along with the remainder of the gastrointestinal tract. Persistent patency of the omphalomesenteric duct is determined by the tenth week of gestation.[5] If the distal end of the omphalomesenteric duct remains attached to the umbilical cord, a fistula will result (Figs. 50–1*A* and 50–2). If the distal end retracts from the umbilicus, a diverticulum will result (Fig. 50–1*D*). The diverticulum may remain attached to the undersurface

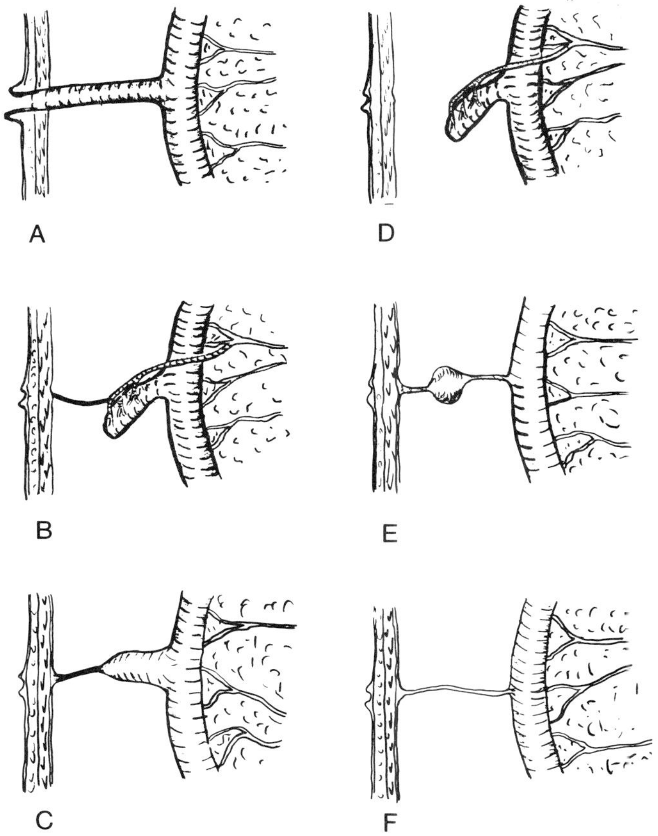

Figure 50–1. Some of the commoner abnormalities that result from the embryonic yolk sac are shown. *A*, Patent omphalomesenteric duct representing a communication from the terminal ileum to the umbilicus. *B*, Meckel's diverticulum with a patent right vitelline artery as blood supply to the Meckel's diverticulum and a residual of the vitelline artery illustrated as a cord to the undersurface of the umbilicus. *C*, Meckel's diverticulum with a cord connecting the tip of the Meckel's diverticulum to the undersurface of the umbilicus. The cord (band) represents the distal residual of the omphalomesenteric duct. *D*, Typical appearance of a Meckel's diverticulum with persistence of the vitelline artery. *E*, Involution of the proximal and distal ends of the omphalomesenteric duct with residual cord or band and central preservation of the omphalomesenteric duct, resulting in a mucosa-lined cyst. *F*, Intraperitoneal band from the ileum to the undersurface of the umbilicus, representing involution without resolution of the omphalomesenteric duct.

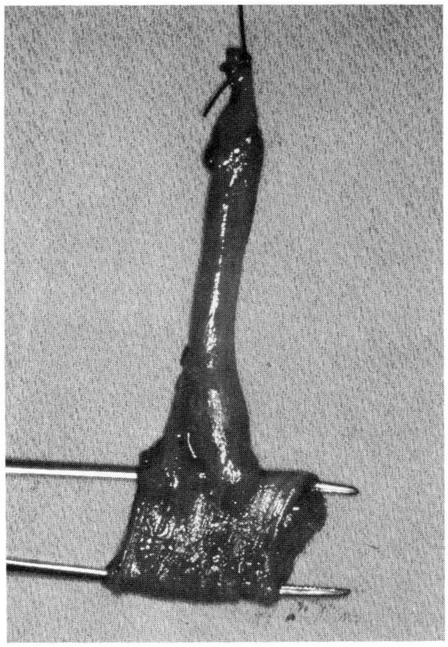

Figure 50–2. Operative specimen showing a segment of the terminal ileum (with forceps through the lumen) and a patent omphalomesenteric duct with a tie around the distal portion that extended through the umbilicus.

of the umbilicus by a solid cord, as a residual from either the yolk sac (Fig. 50–1*C*) or the vitelline vessels (Fig. 50–1*B*).

There are many abnormalities that result from remnants of the embryonic yolk sac. The numerous variations can be generally categorized as discussed in the following sections.

Patent Omphalomesenteric (Vitelline) Duct

The vitelline duct represents a persistent connection between the distal ileum and umbilicus and accounts for 2.5 to 6% of omphalomesenteric duct remnants.[6, 9] Of interest is that males predominate by a ratio of 5 to 1.[6] Also of importance is that ectopic gastric mucosa is identified in approximately one third of the patients with a complete fistula.[6] Clinical presentation of this anomaly usually occurs in the first one to two weeks of life. Following the natural atrophy and separation of the umbilical cord stump, drainage from the umbilicus occurs, having the appearance of intestinal contents. Inspection of the umbilicus reveals either an opening or a polypoid mass, which represents a limited prolapse of the patent omphalomesenteric duct. Confirmation of the diagnosis can be made by injection of contrast material into the sinus tract and demonstrating that it drains into the distal small intestine. Complications of a patent omphalomesenteric duct include prolapse through the umbilicus of the patent duct or the ileum via the omphalomesenteric duct. Partial prolapse of the duct or

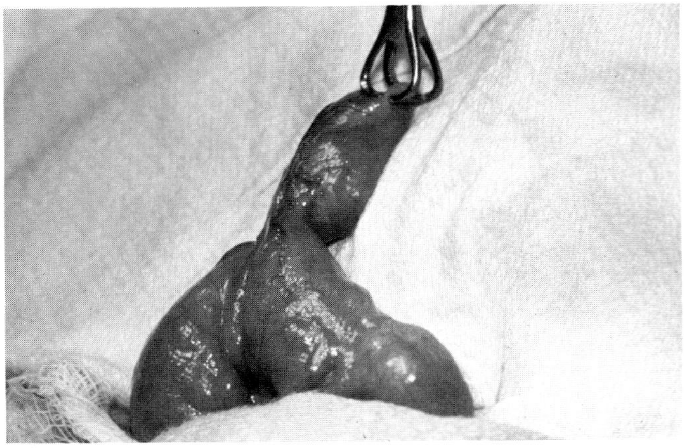

Figure 50–3. Typical appearance of a Meckel's diverticulum.

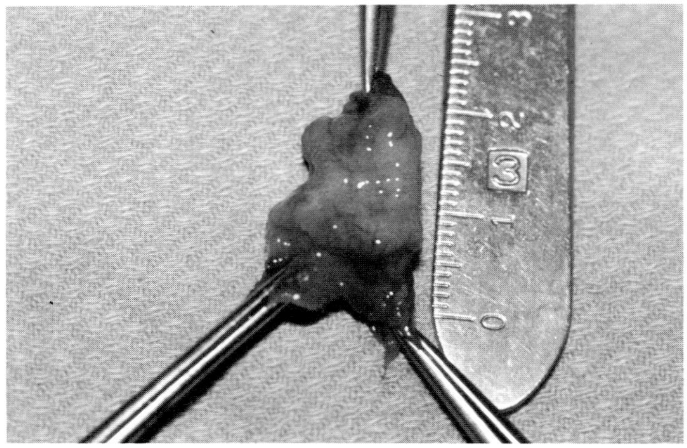

Figure 50–5. Meckel's diverticulum opened with the upper two thirds containing ectopic gastric mucosa and the lower two thirds containing typical ileal mucosa. An area of ulceration at the junction of the gastric mucosa and ileal mucosa could be seen at the time of surgery, but it is difficult to see in the operative photograph.

ileum has been mistaken for an umbilical polyp and amputated with significant adverse sequelae.

Meckel's Diverticulum

Meckel's diverticulum is a congenital abnormality that is the most common of the embryonic yolk sac remnants and represents at least 80% of all these anomalies.[6, 9] The diverticulum contains all three layers of the intestinal wall and is typically located 40 to 50 cm from the ileocecal valve.[13] However, this distance is related to the age of the patient at the time of diagnosis. Meckel's diverticulum presents in a variety of shapes and lengths. The diverticulum originates from the antimesenteric border of the bowel and is typically 3 to 6 cm in length and slightly smaller than the diameter of the small intestine (Figs. 50–3 and 50–4). Occasionally a Meckel's diverticulum is attached to the undersurface of the umbilicus or to another portion of the abdominal wall or bowel by a fibrous cord. Of considerable significance is the presence of ectopic tissue within a Meckel's diverticulum (Fig. 50–5). Although the majority of Meckel's diverticula are lined with ileal mucosa, gastric, duodenal, and colonic mucosa have been described.[13] In addition, bile duct mucosa and ectopic pancreatic tissue have also been demonstrated in Meckel's diverticula.[13] Numerous studies have indicated that 40 to 80% of symptomatic Meckel's diverticula contain ectopic tissue.[14–17] In the majority of these cases the ectopic tissue is gastric mucosa or pancreatic tissue.

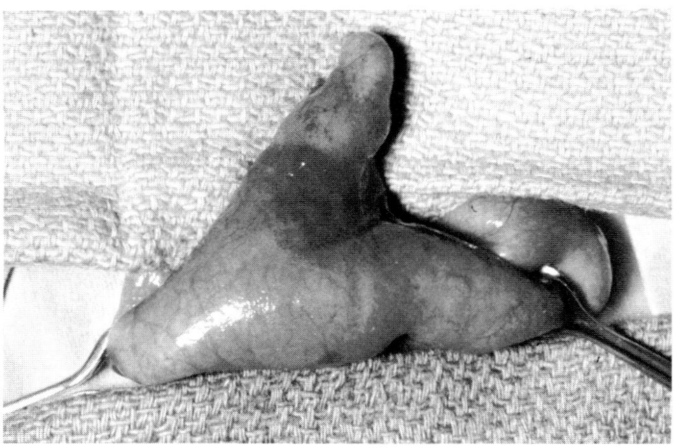

Figure 50–4. Meckel's diverticulum with gastric mucosa in the distal portion and inflammation near its base, indicative of ulceration.

Omphalomesenteric Cyst

Involution of the omphalomesenteric duct at the umbilicus and at the ileal end can result in a mucosa-lined cystic mass in either the intraperitoneal (Fig. 50–1*E*) or the preperitoneal space. These cysts contain all three layers of the small intestine. Presentation of these cysts is from either infection (particularly preperitoneal cysts) or obstruction (intraperitoneal cysts).

Omphalomesenteric Duct Remnants at the Umbilicus

Remnants at the umbilicus are uncommon, but when present they are usually identifiable within the first one to two weeks of life. Their presence is usually not evident until the umbilical stalk has atrophied and fallen off. What remains is a polypoid mass covered by mucosa at the umbilicus or a limited sinus that ends blindly. Umbilical polyps are frequently confused with umbilical granulomas. Umbilical sinuses usually become evident because of persistent drainage at the umbilicus. However, this drainage is small in amount and does not have the typical appearance of intestinal contents. Treatment for both lesions is excision.

Omphalomesenteric Band

An omphalomesentric band results from involution of the omphalomesenteric duct but without disappearance of the tissue. As a result, a solid cord connecting the ileum to the undersurface of the umbilicus can result (Fig. 50–1*F*). This abnormality usually becomes evident as the cause of an intestinal obstruction. Diagnosis of these bands is generally made at the time of surgical exploration.

Vitelline Blood Vessel Remnants

Occlusion but failure of involution of the vitelline blood vessel can also result in a fibrous cord within the peritoneal cavity. It may extend from the ileum or a Meckel's diverticulum to the undersurface of the umbilicus (see Fig. 50–1*B* and *F*). This remnant becomes clinically evident by producing intestinal obstruction as a result of a segment of a small intestine twisting around the band.

CLINICAL PRESENTATION

Hemorrhage

Intermittent and painless bleeding from the rectum is the most common presentation of a Meckel's diverticulum, and, therefore, the most common presentation of all the variations of yolk sac remnants. The etiology of the bleeding is from peptic ulceration at the junction of the ectopic gastric mucosa and normal ileal mucosa. Acid production by the gastric mucosal parietal cells is not neutralized because of the absence of duodenal bicarbonate. Therefore, the pathophysiology exists to develop a "marginal" ulcer at the junction of the gastric and ileal mucosa. The bleeding can be excessive and dramatic if the erosion is at the site of the embryonic vitelline artery (see Fig. 50–1*B*). Although this bleeding may be massive, it is usually self-limiting because of contraction of the splanchnic vessels in response to hypovolemia. According to a study by Rutherford and Akers,[18] children younger than 2 years of age presenting with hemorrhage secondary to a Meckel's diverticulum had an average hemoglobin level of 6.6 mg per dl, whereas older children had an average hemoglobin level of 8.8 mg per dl. The stool of patients with a bleeding Meckel's diverticulum typically contains bright red blood, characterized as "currant jelly" or "brick red" in appearance. Bleeding from a Meckel's diverticulum can also present with intermittent and less dramatic bleeding as evidenced by tarry stools.

Intestinal Obstruction

Complete or partial small bowel obstruction is the next most common clinical manifestation of a Meckel's diverticulum or other intraperitoneal omphalomesenteric duct remnants. The mechanism of obstruction can be by intraperitoneal bands, intussusception, internal herniation, or volvulus. The most common mechanism of obstruction is from intussusception of the Meckel's diverticulum, the clinical presentation of which is similar to that of idiopathic intussusception. Of significance is that most patients with this phenomenon are males, and it is most likely to appear in older children.[6] Other causes of intestinal obstruction are usually a result of intraperitoneal bands as a residual of the omphalomesenteric duct itself or the vessels associated with the duct. As noted previously, this fibrous band or cord can extend from a Meckel's diverticulum or from the antimesenteric border of the ileum itself. The presentation is typical of any with small bowel obstruction. The onset of bilious vomiting and abdominal distention are usually the heralding signs. Rarely will the cause of the partial or complete intestinal obstruction be determined preoperatively in these patients.

Meckel's Diverticulitis

A Meckel's diverticulum can become the sight of acute inflammation. The clinical presentation is nearly identical to acute appendicitis. Rarely is the diagnosis of Meckel's diverticulitis made preoperatively. It is usually made at the time of exploration for acute appendicitis when a normal appendix is found, but only if the surgeon searches for a Meckel's diverticulum. As is the case with appendicitis, perforation in Meckel's diverticulitis occurs in approximately one third of the cases (Fig. 50–6).[7, 19] The mechanism of Meckel's diverticulitis is usually obstruction similar to appendicitis, but may also be from peptic ulceration resulting in perforation.

DIAGNOSIS

Diagnosis of omphalomesenteric duct remnants depends on the clinical presentation. As noted previously, diagnosis of umbilical abnormalities can generally be made by physical examination. In the absence of symptoms, diagnosis of a Meckel's diverticulum is generally not indicated. It is only when a Meckel's diverticulum

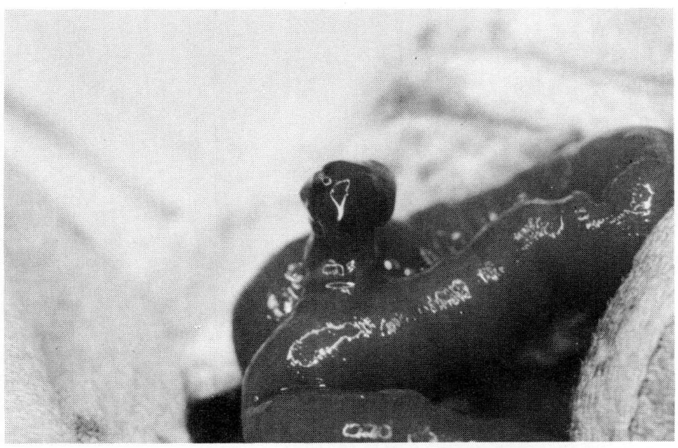

Figure 50–6. Perforation of a Meckel's diverticulum with marked inflammation of the ileum in the area of the Meckel's diverticulum.

or other intraperitoneal remnants of an omphalomesenteric duct produce symptoms that diagnosis becomes relevant. In an infant or child who presents with significant painless rectal bleeding, the presence of a Meckel's diverticulum should always be considered. Unfortunately, confirmation of the presence of a Meckel's diverticulum can be difficult. Standard abdominal radiographs are of no value in the diagnosis of bleeding from a Meckel's diverticulum. Barium contrast studies such as an upper gastrointestinal series with a small bowel follow-through rarely make the diagnosis of a Meckel's diverticulum.

In 1967 Harden and coworkers[20] described a technique, and in 1970 Jewett and associates[14] utilized the technique, of intravenous technetium-99m pertechnetate to visualize ectopic gastric mucosa. It had been known that gastric mucosa had an affinity for this isotope. Because the cause of bleeding from a Meckel's diverticulum is most often due to ectopic gastric mucosa, it was reasoned that this might be a way of visualizing a Meckel's diverticulum under these conditions (Fig. 50–7). This study has now come to be known as a *Meckel's Scan*. The technique has since been further refined by noting that certain substances can enhance the visualization of the ectopic gastric mucosa, including pentagastrin, glucagon, and cimetidine.[21, 23] It was initially thought that the uptake of the ^{99m}Tc isotope was by the gastric parietal cells. However, subsequently it has been demonstrated that the mucus-secreting cells of the gastric mucosa are responsible for the uptake.[24, 25] The availability of the Meckel's scan has significantly aided in the diagnosis of painless rectal bleeding in infants and children. Unfortunately, this study has limitations because it is sensitive in only 85% of cases and specific in 95% of cases.[21, 24] Therefore, a bleeding Meckel's diverticulum will not always be visualized using this technique.

Superior mesenteric angiography has been utilized in patients with suspected bleeding from a Meckel's diverticulum.[25] The diagnosis is based on the demonstration of a branch of the ileocolic artery that represents a remnant of the right vitelline artery (see Fig. 50–1*B*). In our opinion, this study is rarely if ever indicated in the diagnosis of a Meckel's diverticulum.

An additional study that has been used in certain cases has been ^{99m}T-labeled red blood cells. This nuclear medicine technique is not specific for Meckel's diverticulum, but it can be used for localizing the site of bleeding in patients with intermittent and relatively low rates of bleeding.[27]

In patients who present with intestinal obstruction from an omphalomesenteric duct remnant, the etiology of the obstruction is rarely determined preoperatively. In fact, there is no great advantage in determining the etiology preoperatively. These patients require prompt surgical exploration to relieve the obstruction. Similarly, patients with inflammation of a Meckel's diverticulum require prompt surgical exploration. Most often these patients undergo abdominal exploration with the preoperative diagnosis of appendicitis. However, one differentiating factor may be the presence of significant free intraperitoneal air. This radiographic finding is exceptionally rare in patients with a perforated appendix. However, it is not unusual to see free air radiographically with perforation of a Meckel's diverticulum.

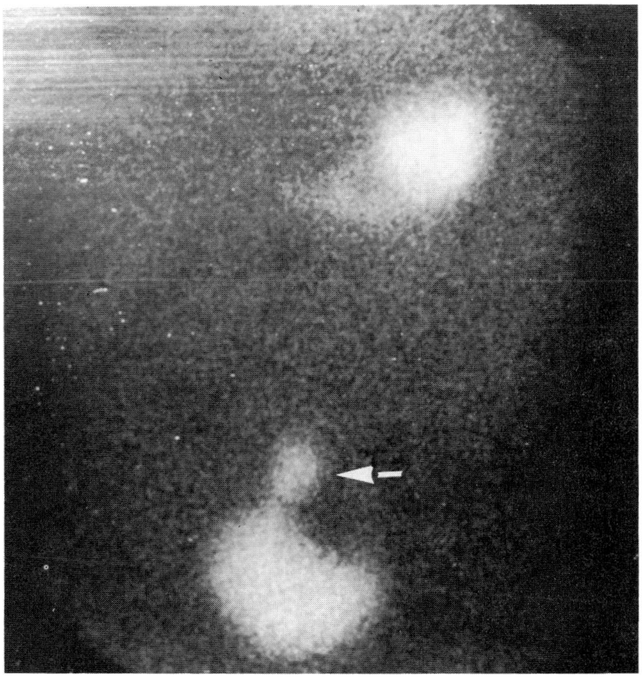

Figure 50–7. Typical appearance of a positive Meckel's scan with an area of increased uptake above the area of the bladder in the lower midabdomen (*arrow*).

TREATMENT

Meckel's Diverticulum

A Meckel's diverticulum causing symptoms should always be removed. The surgical approach is generally through a right lower quadrant transverse incision. Adequate preoperative resuscitation with intravenous fluid and (if indicated) packed red blood cell transfusions is necessary. If the presenting problem is hemorrhage, the extent of the resection will depend on the extent of ectopic gastric mucosa within the Meckel's diverticulum. In general, the ectopic gastric mucosa is limited to the distal portion of the Meckel's diverticulum (see Fig. 50–5). However, in some circumstances the ectopic mucosa extends to the junction of the ileum and may even extend into the ileum. When excising a Meckel's diverticulum it is important to remove all ectopic tissue and to be sure that closure of the bowel wall does not result in narrowing of the ileal lumen (Fig. 50–8). Numerous surgical techniques have been described to avoid these potential complications. If the ectopic gastric mucosa extends far enough into the ileum so that excision of the Meckel's diverticulum along with a portion of the ileal wall would result in narrowing of the ileum, then it is appropriate to perform a limited small bowel

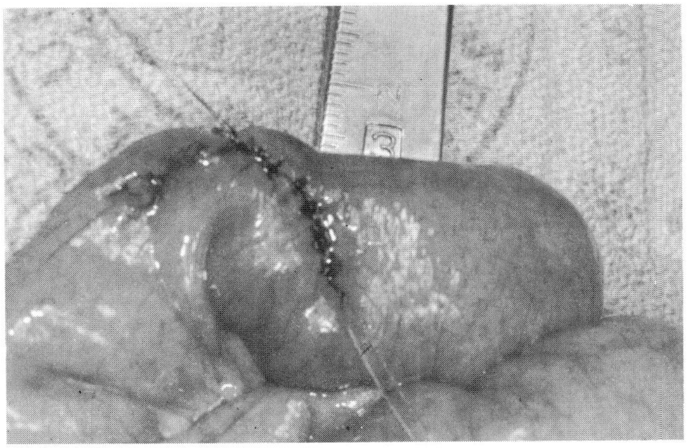

Figure 50–8. Typical closure of the ileum following resection of a Meckel's diverticulum. The resection has been done in an oblique fashion across the antimesenteric border of the ileum to avoid narrowing the lumen.

resection, which would include the Meckel's diverticulum, and construct an end-to-end anastomosis.

The surgical approach for intussusception induced by a Meckel's diverticulum is similar to that for the idiopathic variety. In fact, it is unlikely that the cause of the intussusception would be known prior to laparotomy. The index of suspicion should increase that a "lead point" exists in children older than 2 to 3 years of age. If at exploration a Meckel's diverticulum is identified as the lead point, it should be excised.

Postoperative complications are uncommon following excision of a Meckel's diverticulum. Although a leak at the sight of ileal closure and infection (either intraperitoneal or wound) can occur, these complications should not exceed 2%.

An area of ongoing controversy is the approach to a Meckel's diverticulum found incidentally at the time of laparotomy for another reason. Some authors believe that a Meckel's diverticulum should always be removed when found.[5, 18] This is based on the potential risks of the complications of perforation, obstruction, and the development of neoplasms. Those authors opposed to incidental diverticulectomy argue that there is a low lifetime risk of developing symptoms related to the presence of a Meckel's diverticulum.[11] Soltero and Bill[7] calculated the incidence of complications related to a Meckel's diverticulum to be 4.2%. These authors calculated that it would take 800 incidental Meckel's diverticulectomies to avoid one death, and in their experience, there was a 9% postoperative complication rate following Meckel's diverticulectomy.[7] Their patient review demonstrated a considerably lower complication rate from a Meckel's diverticulum than initially cited by Meckel and in subsequent studies.[28]

It is the bias of this chapter's authors to individualize each circumstance. If a Meckel's diverticulum is discovered at laparotomy, then careful palpation should be undertaken to determine the presence of ectopic gastric mucosa or pancreatic tissue. This would be evident as either thickening or a mass within the wall of the diverticulum. Under these circumstances it would be appropriate to remove the Meckel's diverticulum. Another circumstance that may warrant incidental Meckel's diverticulectomy is if the base of the diverticulum is narrow, thus increasing the risk of obstruction and perforation. If a Meckel's diverticulum is encountered that does not present any of the features noted above, then there is probably little basis for its removal. Another factor that should be taken into consideration is whether opening the small intestine and creating a potentially contaminated operative field would jeopardize the outcome of the primary operation. When peritoneal bands extending from a Meckel's diverticulum are encountered, they should be removed.

Patent Omphalomesenteric Duct

A patent omphalomesenteric duct should always be surgically excised from the junction of the umbilicus to its junction with the ileum. Care should be taken to remove all portions of the communication at the umbilicus to avoid subsequent complication.

Omphalomesenteric Cyst

Frequently, omphalomesenteric cysts present as an infected mass beneath the umbilicus. As previously noted, these are either preperitoneal or intraperitoneal. These cystic remnants can become quite large during the course of an infection, and an effort at excision may be inappropriate. Incision and drainage followed by cyst excision after the infection has resolved would be more appropriate.

SUMMARY

Omphalomesenteric duct remnants are common in the population at large with Meckel's diverticulum representing most of these anomalies. Most Meckel's diverticula are asymptomatic, but when they are symptomatic the symptoms are usually rectal hemorrhage or obstruction from intussusception. Symptomatic Meckel's diverticula should be removed with care to avoid narrowing the ileal lumen. In the absence of ectopic tissue or a narrow base, an asymptomatic Meckel's diverticulum should not be incidentally removed.

REFERENCES

1. Hildanus F: Opera observationum et curationum, medico-chirurgicarum, quae extant omnia, etc. Francof, J Beveri, 1646.
2. Lavater JH: De Εντεροπεριστολη seu intestinorum compressione. Basilae, 1672.
3. Ruysch F: Opera Omnia. Amsterdam, Jansson-Waesberg, 1757.
4. Meckel JF: Ueber die Divertikel am Darmkanal. Arch Physiol 1809; 9:421–453.

5. Gray SW, Skandalakis JE: Embryology for Surgeons. Philadelphia, WB Saunders, 1972, pp 156–167.
6. Söderlund S: Meckel's diverticulum, a clinical and histologic study. Acta Chir Scand 1959; 118(suppl):1–233.
7. Soltero MJ, Bill AH: The natural history of Meckel's diverticulum and its relation to incidental removal. Am J Surg 1976; 132:168–173.
8. Collins DC: A study of 50,000 specimens of the human vermiform appendix. Surg Gynecol Obstet 1955; 101:137–145.
9. Moses WR: Meckel's diverticulum. N Engl J Med 1947; 237:118–122.
10. Androulakis JA, Gray SW, Lionakis B, et al: The sex ratio of Meckel's diverticulum. Am Surg 1969; 35:455–460.
11. Amory RA: Meckel's diverticulum. *In* Welch KJ, et al: Pediatric Surgery. 4th ed. Chicago, Year Book Medical Publishers, 1986, pp 859–867.
12. Gross RE: The Surgery of Infancy and Childhood. Philadelphia, WB Saunders, 1953, pp 212–220.
13. Yamaguchi M, Takeuchi S, Awazu S: Meckel's diverticulum: Investigation of 600 patients in Japanese literature. Am J Surg 1978; 136:247–249.
14. Jewett TC Jr, Duszynski DO, Allen JE: The visualization of Meckel's diverticulum with ^{99m}Tc-pertechnetate. Surgery 1970; 68:567–570.
15. Wansbrough RM, Thomson S, Leckey RG: Meckel's diverticulum: A 42-year review of 273 cases at the Hospital for Sick Children, Toronto. Can J Surg 1957; 1:15–20.
16. Kiesewetter WB: Meckel's diverticulum in children. Arch Surg 1957; 75:914–919.
17. Lüdtke FE, Mende V, Köhler H, et al: Incidence and frequency of complications and management of Meckel's diverticulum. Surg Gynecol Obstet 1989; 169:537–542.
18. Rutherford RB, Akers DR: Meckel's diverticulum: A review of 148 pediatric patients, with special reference to the pattern of bleeding and to mesodiverticular vascular bands. Surgery 1966; 59:618–626.
19. Seagram CGF, Louch RE, Stephens CA, et al: Meckel's diverticulum: A 10-year review of 218 cases. Can J Surg 1968; 11:369–373.
20. Harden RM, Alexander WD, Kennedy I: Isotope uptake and scanning of stomach in man with ^{99m}Tc-pertechnetate. Lancet 1967; 1:1305–1307.
21. Anderson GF, Sfakianakis G, King DR, et al: Hormonal enhancement of technetium-99m pertechnetate uptake in experimental Meckel's diverticulum. J Pediatr Surg 1980; 15:900–905.
22. Khettery J, Effmann E, Grand RJ, et al: Effect of pentagastrin, histologic, glucagon, secretin, and perchlorate on the gastric hording of ^{99m}Tc pertechnetate in mice. Radiology 1976; 120:629–631.
23. Treves S, Grand RJ, Eraklis AJ: Pentagastrin stimulation of technetium^{99m} uptake by ectopic gastric mucosa in a Meckel's diverticulum. Radiology 1978; 128:711–712.
24. Cooney DR, Duszynski DO, Camboa E, et al: The abdominal technetium scan (a decade of experience). J Pediatr Surg 1982; 17:611–619.
25. Keramidas DC, Coran AG, Zaleska RW: An experimental model for assessing the radiopertechnetate diagnosis of gastric mucosa in Meckel's diverticulum. J Pediatr Surg 1974; 9:879–883.
26. Okazaki M, Higashihara H, Yamasaki S, et al: Arterial embolization to control life-threatening hemorrhage from a Meckel's diverticulum. Am J Roentgen 1990; 154:1257–1258.
27. Winzelberg GG, McKusick KA, Strauss HW, et al: Evaluation of gastrointestinal bleeding by red blood cells labeled in vivo with technetium 99m. J Nuclear Med 1979; 20:1080–1086.
28. Mackey WC, Dineen P: A fifty year experience with Meckel's diverticulum. Surg Gynecol & Obstet 1983; 156:56–64.

Chapter 51

Pseudomembranous Colitis

THOMAS M. ROSSI

DEFINITION

Although the terms *pseudomembranous colitis* (PMC), *antibiotic-associated diarrhea* (AAD), *antibiotic-associated colitis* (AAC), Clostridium difficile *diarrhea* (CDD), and Clostridium difficile–*associated colitis* (CDAC) are frequently used interchangeably, there are distinctions. As in many clinical diseases, understanding the evolution of the pathophysiology of the disorder helps explain the overlap in terms. In a broad sense, there is some justification in using the above terms interchangeably. Strictly speaking, the diagnosis of pseudomembranous enterocolitis requires either endoscopic or histologic evidence of pseudomembranes, which may be present in the small bowel, colon, or both. In this condition, the mucosa is red, edematous, and friable, with multiple raised yellow-white plaques (Fig. 51–1). Microscopic examination reveals necrotic cells and fibrinous material arranged in a pattern that simulates a volcanic eruption covering a section of lamina propria that contains polymorphonuclear leukocytes (Fig. 51–2).[1, 2]

Clarification of the association of PMC with antibiotic usage is worth mentioning. For the cause of the diarrhea to be attributed to antibiotics, the illness should occur within 6 weeks of antibiotic usage. The diarrheal illness that follows antibiotic usage, antibiotic-associated diarrhea, can be of several varieties; PMC represents the most severe form. In most instances, AAD is usually mild and self-limited. It is frequently ascribed to alterations in the intestinal flora. When associated with evidence of *C. difficile*, it is referred to as CDD. The term Clostridium difficile–*associated diarrhea* describes diarrhea associated with the identification of *Clostridium difficile (C. difficile)* in the absence of pseudomembranes. It is estimated that about 10% of cases of AAD progress to colitis, which may be either PMC or a nonspecific colitis characterized by focal necrosis and polymorphonuclear infiltration in the lamina propria. Although the absolute incidence of *C. difficile* as the cause of antibiotic-associated diarrhea of the self-limited variety is unknown, its link to colitis and PMC is definitive. The terms *PMC* and *antibiotic-associated colitis* (AAC) are therefore used interchangeably with C. difficile–*associated colitis*. It is now generally accepted that *C. difficile* is the etiologic agent in virtually all cases of PMC and AAC and in approximately 25% of cases of AAD in humans. Most patients with AAD, therefore, have neither colitis, PMC, or evidence of *C. difficile* and do not respond to treatment with vancomycin or metronidazole.[3]

ETIOLOGY

Although PMC is most commonly associated with antibiotic usage and, since the late 1970s has been linked to *C. difficile* isolation from the stools,[4, 5] pseudomembranes have been found in other clinical settings. In the past, prior to the availability of antibiotics, PMC occurred in the postoperative period following intestinal surgery. Intestinal obstruction and colonic carcinoma were judged to be risk factors.[6] Other nonintestinal and nonantibiotic-associated instances of PMC were reported following severe burns, shock, ischemia, leukemia, and uremia, as well as in patients with Hirschsprung's disease.[7–10]

Furthermore, PMC has occasionally been encountered in healthy persons exhibiting none of the above risk factors.[2, 11] Following discovery of its link to intestinal surgery, PMC was noted in many patients who received broad-spectrum antibiotics preoperatively and, in this situation, was attributed to enterotoxin produced by *Staphylococcus aureus*.[12, 13] Antibiotic-resistant strains were isolated from some patients. Interestingly, in the 1950s and 1960s, vancomycin was recognized to be effective in the treatment of PMC.[14] However, in many instances staphylococci were not identified in either stool cultures or cultures of pseudomembranes obtained at postmortem examinations.[15] Nevertheless, until recently, PMC was considered synonymous with staphylococcal colitis. Cases of PMC have also been attributed to organisms such as *Salmonella*, *Clostridium perfrin-*

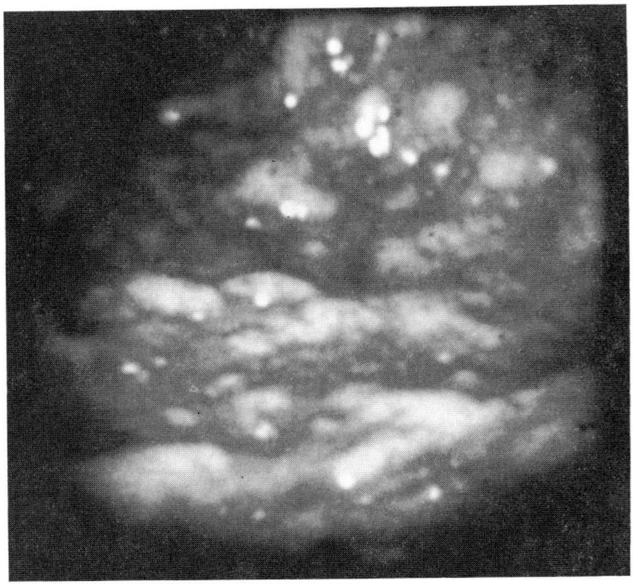

Figure 51–1. Pseudomembranous colitis. Endoscopic features demonstrate exudative plaques adherent to colonic mucosa.

gens type C, *Plesiomonas shigelloides*, and other clostridia.[3, 16, 17]

To better understand the relationship of infection and antibiotics to the development of colitis, animal models were developed. Using *Staphylococcus*, the disease could not be produced in animals. However, the administration of a wide variety of parenteral and enteral antibiotics to Golden Syrian hamsters produced a fatal form of enterocolitis. Following the discovery of a cytotoxin of *Clostridium sordellii* in the stool of a patient with PMC, reports of isolates of *C. difficile* and its toxin in the animal model and in patients with enterocolitis and PMC appeared.[3, 18, 19] *C. difficile* was found to produce a similar toxin that was neutralized by *C. sordellii* antitoxin.[20] The link to *C. difficile* was further strengthened when it was subsequently discovered that hamsters that were passively immunized with *C. sordellii* antitoxin did not develop colitis following antibiotic administration.[21]

The antibiotic susceptibility of the *C. difficile* isolates indicated susceptibility to vancomycin and metronidazole. Pretreatment of hamsters with either of these drugs protected them from enterocolitis.[3, 22] PMC in humans was then successfully treated by either oral vancomycin or metronidazole.[3, 17, 23]

The true incidence of PMC developing with enteric infections other than *C. difficile* is unknown, but it is certainly considered rare. In cases in which *C. difficile* is not demonstrated, it is still highly suspected by clinicians as the etiology.[3] It is now generally accepted that the vast majority of, if not all, cases of PMC are associated with toxin-producing *Clostridium difficile* infection following antibiotic usage.[3]

Nearly all antimicrobial agents have been implicated in PMC, including antifungal, antiviral, and antimicrobial agents to which *C. difficile* is susceptible, for example, vancomycin and metronidazole.[3] Oral, parenteral, or topical antibiotics may precipitate the condition. The risk appears to be independent of the dosage or duration of treatment. The lack of a dose relationship may reflect the fact that even low concentrations have a significant impact on susceptible organisms in the flora of the intestinal tract. Most cases in the past have been associated with clindamycin or lincomycin. The incidence of PMC in adults treated with clindamycin has been reported to be greater than one in 10,000 cases.[3] Some initial reports described the incidence of diarrhea associated with the drug to be 20%, with 10% and 2% of these cases documented to have either colitis or PMC, respectively.[24, 25]

More recently, ampicillin and the cephalosporins have been recognized to produce this complication.[2, 26] However, the incidence with these agents is probably less

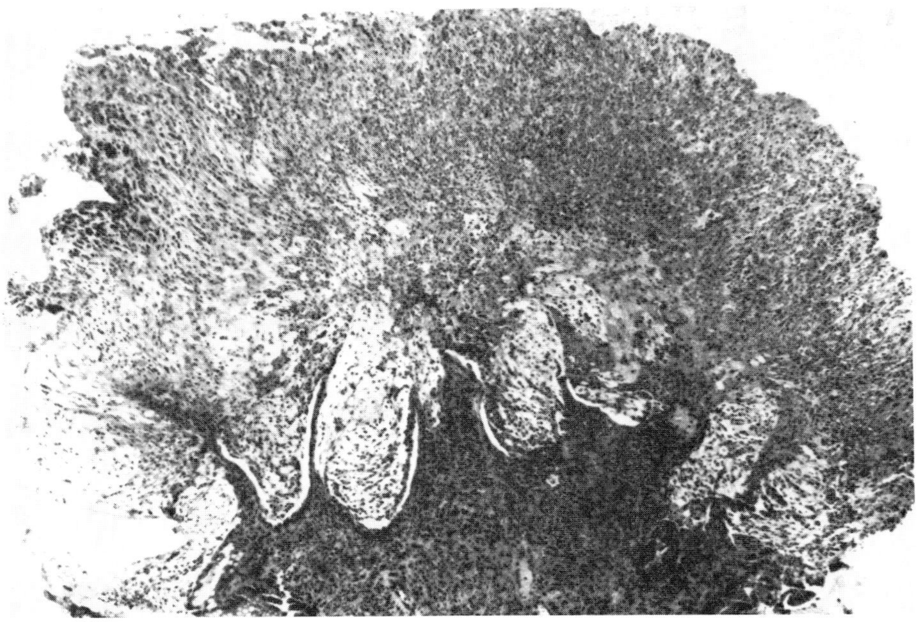

Figure 51–2. Pseudomembranous colitis. Microscopic features exhibit intense polymorphonuclear infiltration and exudate adherent to surface mucosa.

than that with clindamycin. In prospective studies in adults, ampicillin induced diarrhea in 5 to 17% of patients, but PMC developed in only one of 315 and one of 138 patients.[22, 27]

PATHOPHYSIOLOGY

Disruption in the resistance to *C. difficile* proliferation provided by the normal intestinal flora following antibiotic exposure is an important factor influencing the development of disease. Anaerobic organisms are believed to be more likely to exert suppressive effects against the growth of *C. difficile*. Antibiotics such as penicillins, clindamycin, and cephalosporins inhibit the colonic anaerobic population. In animal studies, as the counts of anaerobic bacteria fall, the susceptibility to *C. difficile* disease increases.[28]

C. difficile is a sporulating organism that survives well in the environment. The organism is found in soil, water, and the stools of healthy dogs, cats, and wild animals. The spores are resistant to the usual quaternary ammonium compounds and phenolics and require alkaline glutaraldehyde or phosphate-buffered hypochlorite solutions for eradication.[3, 28] This factor is important and may explain the in-hospital acquisition risk stated below.

Toxins account for the pathogenicity of the organism. About 25% of *C. difficile* isolates do not produce toxins and are therefore not considered causative agents for diarrhea or colitis.[3] Colitis develops from toxin production within the intestinal lumen. *C. difficile* produces five toxic factors, the most important of which are toxin A, an enterotoxin, and toxin B, a cytotoxin.[3, 28] Toxin A binds to receptors on the mucosal surface. Binding of toxin to the epithelial membrane microfilaments produces contraction, hemorrhage, necrosis, and inflammation.[3, 29] Toxin A is believed to be the major factor for virulence. Structural changes in the intercellular tight junctions enhance permeability to fluids and loss of protein into the lumen.[28, 30] Enterotoxin injected into ligated rabbit ileal loops elicits severe epithelial damage, with hemorrhage and increased fluid secretion.[28] Toxin B induces alteration in cell shape by acting on intracellular actin microfilaments. The other toxins of *C. difficile* may increase intestinal myoelectric responses and peristalsis. Isolates producing either toxin A or toxin B almost invariably produce the other toxin as well, but not necessarily to the same degree. This variability may account for the observed variation in the manifestations and the severity of the illness.

It is generally agreed that the amount of toxin B detected in an individual's stools does not correlate well with the severity of the illness[31]; however, when groups of patients are studied, higher titers tend to be associated with more severe disease.[3] It is unclear whether the toxins can induce secretion of fluid and electrolytes by purely biochemical mechanisms without the production of colitis. Diarrhea associated with *C. difficile* toxins is almost always associated with inflammatory mucosal lesions.[3]

Another factor that affects pathogenicity of *C. difficile* is the resistance of the host. Patients at higher risk of infection appear to be the elderly, immunocompromised, or neutropenic patients receiving chemotherapeutic agents or those with long hospital stays.[3, 28, 32]

CLOSTRIDIUM DIFFICILE IN INFANTS AND CHILDREN

In the pediatric age group the link between *C. difficile* and disease is less clear. *C. difficile* was initially described in 1935 as a component of the normal fecal flora of newborn infants.[33] Colonization of normal newborns is high—estimated to be 52%—reaching 78% of infants in neonatal intensive care units.[34, 35] In adults, a range of 3 to 7% exists.[32]

Most infants with evidence of *C. difficile* and its toxin in their stools are asymptomatic. Several mechanisms have been proposed to account for the apparent resistance of newborns' intestines to the adverse effects of these toxins. Passively acquired serum antibody does not seem to be the explanation. Antibodies or some other factor in colostrum may play a role.[3] A glycoprotein found in milk (fetulin), or a subunit of it, may interfere with the action of these toxins on the cecum.[3, 36] In addition, these toxins do not bind well to the still immature intestinal mucosa, presumably because of a lack of receptors for the toxins.[37] As newborn infants acquire their normal intestinal flora, the rate of isolation of *C. difficile* and its toxins from their stools declines toward the rate characteristic of adults. Loss of the organism and increase in susceptibility to the toxins appear highly variable, since PMC, although uncommon, can occur in infants and children.[3, 38, 39]

Infants with failure to thrive, chronic diarrhea, and stools containing *C. difficile* and its toxin have been found to have cryptitis on rectal biopsy. Treatment with oral vancomycin led to improvement in symptoms, suggesting that the organism was pathogenic in these instances.[39, 40] In such cases, a therapeutic trial may be the only diagnostic criteria to determine whether the presence of *C. difficile* is coincidental or pathogenic in symptomatic infants.[3]

There is a link in both infants and adults to nosocomial acquisition of the organism. Indeed, most colonization and infection among hospitalized patients appear to be nosocomial in origin.[32] The organism is highly prevalent in the hospital environment. Isolation of the organism from the hands of hospital staff and in the rooms of patients as well as from items such as bedding, mops, and floors has been documented.[41, 42] The environment appeared to harbor the strains found in infants in one study, and also to be the main source of the organism.[43]

In addition to environmental contamination, evidence for person-to-person transmission exists. Transmission of organisms from infant to infant by hands of nursery personnel seemed responsible for the high rates of colonization in one study.[44] The introduction into a nursery of a heavily colonized infant formerly in an intensive care unit was followed by spread of that infant's strain to other infants in the nursery. Twenty-one per cent of adults with negative cultures on admission to hospitals have subsequently become positive during their hospital stay. In one third of these cases, diarrhea occurred. About 63% of patients acquiring *C. difficile* are silent carriers who shed constantly and contaminate the hospital environment.[32] Since these carriers are not treated for *C. difficile*, they continue to spread the organism. Acquisition from contaminated material may therefore explain clustering of cases and those not associated with antibiotic usage.

Clinical Features

The spectrum of disease induced by enteric *C. difficile* infection varies widely. The severity of the symptoms can range from mild diarrhea to fulminant colitis. The diarrhea ascribed to antibiotic usage usually consists of loose or watery stools, sometimes containing mucus, but rarely with evidence of gross blood.[2, 3, 45] The diarrhea usually begins within 3 to 9 days after initiation of antibiotics. In about 20% of patients, diarrhea does not begin until up to 6 weeks after antibiotics have been discontinued. Most patients with antibiotic-associated diarrhea have a benign, self-limited course in which symptoms resolve within 5 to 10 days following discontinuation of the antibiotic.[2, 3, 45] The diarrhea, however, can be more severe. Occasionally, bowel movements can occur 30 times a day, and the duration of the diarrhea can be 4 to 6 weeks.[46]

Subgroups of patients with AAC exhibiting no diarrhea have been identified. Some patients do not have frank diarrhea, but have an increased frequency of formed stools. Also, some patients with antibiotic-associated colitis have no history of diarrhea but exhibit an acute abdomen with toxic megacolon, colonic perforation, or peritonitis.[3, 47] Recently, six cases presenting with acute abdomen in the absence of diarrhea were described.[48] The clinical picture mimicked small bowel ileus, Ogilvie's syndrome, volvulus, and ischemia. Colonoscopy was performed safely in these patients. Other patients with AAC and no diarrhea may present with a fever of unknown origin following antibiotic exposure.[2]

Pseudomembranous enterocolitis can be a catastrophic disease. Patients may present with high fever, abdominal pain, and ileus leading to irreversible shock and death within 2 to 3 days.[2] If unrecognized and untreated, mortality rates of 10 to 20% are quoted. The most frequent causes of death include hypovolemic shock secondary to excessive electrolyte, fluid, and protein loss; colonic perforation; sepsis; and hemorrhage. High fever, marked abdominal tenderness, bloody diarrhea (5 to 10% of cases of PMC), leukocytosis, and hypoalbuminemia are indicative of severe colitis. Fecal leukocytes are present in 50% of cases and help confirm the diagnosis in a patient suspected of having AAC. Hypoalbuminemia may be severe enough to induce anasarca. The fulminant colitis picture described may be similar to the toxic megacolon of inflammatory bowel disease. PMC may cause symptoms that may be interpreted as an acute exacerbation of an underlying chronic inflammatory bowel disease. Polyarthritis has been reported with PMC.[49] It should be suspected when patients with inflammatory bowel disease develop diarrhea after receiving antibiotics.

The colitis of PMC may even be restricted to the transverse or right colon.[50] In such instances, the abdominal symptoms and signs may be localized to the specific site of involvement. The clinical picture may also be confused with Ogilvie's syndrome, that is, colonic pseudo-obstruction.[51]

DIAGNOSIS

The diagnosis of PMC is rapidly established by the visualization of inflammation signifying colitis and by identifying pseudomembranes on sigmoidoscopy. Biopsies aid in the confirmation of the visual findings of erythema, friability, or ulcerations. They may reveal pseudomembranes that are too small to visualize endoscopically. Isolated proximal colonic lesions may be present in about 10% of cases. In such cases, colonoscopy is required for establishing the diagnosis. Although the preferred method of diagnosis consists of direct visualization of the colonic mucosa, plain films of the abdomen may show a markedly edematous colon, distorted haustral markings, and distention of the entire colon. Air-contrast barium enemas must be performed with caution in any patient suspected of having severe colitis for fear of precipitation of perforation or toxic megacolon. Rounded filling defects may be demonstrated in PMC. Computerized tomography (CT) scan may show thickened bowel wall and peritonitis.[52]

Nonspecific laboratory findings that also support the diagnosis of severe colitis in PMC include leukocytosis, presence of fecal leukocytes, elevation of sedimentation rate, and hypoproteinemia. Protein-losing enteropathy can be confirmed by the detection of elevated levels of fecal alpha-one-antitrypsin concentrations.[53]

The most useful laboratory test consists of culture of the stool for *Clostridium difficile* and determination of the presence of its toxins. Anaerobic cultures using selective media can detect as few as 100 colony-forming units of *C. difficile* per gm of stool.[3, 54] Patients with PMC usually have organisms in the range of 10^4 to 10^8 per gm of stool. Almost all patients with PMC (85 to 95%), therefore, have positive cultures. The isolation of *C. difficile* from the stools, however, does not signify disease. As mentioned above, asymptomatic carriers exist. Also, in one study, 22% of patients with cystic fibrosis and 11% of patients with other conditions and no history of diarrhea were positive for *C. difficile*.[55]

The preferred method to establish the diagnosis of *C. difficile*–induced disease is toxin detection. The best clinical correlations appear to be with the toxin. The standard toxin assay requires tissue cultures to demonstrate a cytopathic toxin. Tests to detect *C. difficile* toxin B usually employ monolayer cultures of fibroblast cell lines to detect the characteristic cytopathogenic effect.[56] The clinical experience with the tissue culture assay shows 95 to 100% of patients with a confirmed diagnosis of antibiotic-associated PMC have positive tests.

Counterimmunoelectrophoresis has been used as a rapid method for detection of toxin B in fecal extracts. The nonspecific antisera used in these tests may detect other proteins produced by *C. difficile* and are subject to false-positive and false-negative results.[3, 57] An inexpensive latex agglutination test is rapidly gaining application.[3, 58] It has been found to detect a nonpathogenic protein that is distinct from toxin A. Unfortunately, nontoxigenic isolates of *C. difficile* can produce this protein.

Additionally, several other species of organisms can also produce a cross-reactive organism.[59] The sensitivity and specificity of the latex test have been estimated at about 90%, but its positive predictive value ranged from a low of 17% when the prevalence of the disease was low to a high of 95% when the prevalence was high.[60] Its main use, therefore, is in acting as a rapid screening test. Enzyme-linked immunosorbent assays for toxin A are also now commercially available.

TREATMENT

Therapy of PMC, AAC, and CDD depends on the severity of symptoms. Discontinuation of the implicated antibiotic may be the only necessary therapeutic intervention in a patient with uncomplicated mild diarrhea. Diarrhea will usually abate within 7 to 10 days. Corticosteroids and antiperistaltic agents may prolong and exacerbate the diarrhea and should also be discontinued. In more advanced cases, fluid and electrolyte support and total parenteral nutrition may be required. In patients with signs of colitis, including PMC, oral treatment with vancomycin (40 mg per kg per day divided into three daily doses) or metronidazole (20–30 mg per kg per day divided into three daily doses) is begun and continued for 7 to 10 days. Vancomycin is the "gold standard" against which other treatments are measured. It is relatively nontoxic and poorly absorbed when given orally. Stool concentrations greater than 16 μg per ml are easily achieved. *C. difficile* is readily inhibited at vancomycin concentrations less than 5 μg per ml. Patients unable to receive vancomycin orally should be given the drug via nasogastric tube. A formidable problem is posed by those patients who have advanced ileus and are unable to receive any enteral therapy. The use of intravenous vancomycin for the treatment of this disorder is not recommended because concentrations within the bowel lumen will not reach satisfactory levels. Seriously ill patients have failed to respond using intravenous vancomycin. When parenteral therapy must be given, experienced investigators advise trying intravenous vancomycin in combination with intravenous metronidazole.[3] Parenteral therapy should be given only when oral therapy is not likely to be possible, and even then attempts at administering oral therapy should be made. Consideration may also be given to rectal instillation of vancomycin in concentrations of 125 to 500 mg per 0.5 L of solution. In advanced cases, colectomy may be required and may be lifesaving.[3]

Metronidazole has been found to offer a cure rate of 92% (versus 100% with vancomycin) in patients with diarrhea or colitis, or both.[61] It is well absorbed systemically in the small intestine; therefore, concerns are raised about its ability to reach the colonic lumen in adequate concentrations. This is of particular concern in patients with advanced ileus, in whom slow intestinal transit may result in complete absorption from the small bowel.[3] Evidence for the transport of intravenously administered metronidazole into the intestinal lumen is not yet totally convincing.[3] Metronidazole is considerably less expensive than oral vancomycin.

Empiric therapy should be started while awaiting results of stool examinations in patients who are seriously ill. This may prevent the progression of the most severe complications of PMC. Discontinuation of the inducing antibiotic, although desirable, is not absolutely necessary if specific therapy is provided. If the inducing antibiotic is required, as in the case of life-threatening infections, specific oral therapy in addition to supportive care should be started promptly.[3] Vancomycin can suppress the disease in hamsters despite the continuation of antimicrobials. Continuation of clindamycin or other therapy in patients treated with oral vancomycin has not been harmful.[3]

Failure to respond to either vancomycin or metronidazole in 3 to 4 days should prompt the switch to the other drug. Thus far, *C. difficile* has been very susceptible to vancomycin or metronidazole. Most isolates are also susceptible to rifampin. Alternative therapies have included cholestyramine, teicoplanin, or bacitracin. Teicoplanin is a glycopeptide that resembles vancomycin and is effective against *C. difficile* but does not offer any advantage over vancomycin. Cholestyramine, an anion-exchange resin, binds *C. difficile* toxin B. It may also bind vancomycin, so the simultaneous administration of both should be avoided. Bacitracin is an alternative to vancomycin. However, further reports are necessary before general usage is recommended.

Relapses following treatment with vancomycin or metronidazole occur in as many as 10 to 20% of cases at a mean of 7 days.[62] Persistence of the organism or its spores appears to be more common than reinfection. Most relapses occur within a few weeks of cessation of therapy. Some patients suffer more than one relapse. There are no general satisfactory recommendations regarding the treatment of relapses. Longer courses of treatment followed by gradual tapering have been found to be successful anecdotally. Pulsed doses given every 4 to 5 days also may be tried.[28]

REFERENCES

1. Price AB, Davies DR: Pseudomembranous colitis. J Clin Pathol 1977; 30:1–12.
2. Bartlett JG: The pseudomembranous enterocolitides. *In* Sleisenger M, Fordtran J, eds: Gastrointestinal Disease: Pathophysiology, Diagnosis, Management. 4th ed. Philadelphia, WB Saunders, 1989, pp 1307–1320.
3. Fekety R: Antibiotic-associated diarrhea. *In* Field M, ed: Current Topics in Gastroenterology: Diarrheal Diseases. New York, Elsevier Science Publishing Company, 1991, pp 293–317.
4. Bartlett JG, Chang TW, Gurwith M, et al: Clindamycin-associated

colitis due to toxin producing species of *Clostridium* in hamsters. J Infect Dis 1977; 136:701–705.
5. Larson HE, Price AB, Hanour P, et al: *Clostridium difficile* and the aetiology of pseudomembranous colitis. Lancet 1978; 1:1063–1066.
6. Penner A, Bernheim A: Acute postoperative enterocolitis. Arch Pathol 1939; 27:966.
7. Kelber M, Ament ME: *Shigella dysenteriae*. I: A forgotten cause of pseudomembranous colitis. J Pediatr 1976; 89:595–596.
8. Cudmore MA, Silva J, Fekety R, et al: *Clostridium difficile* colitis associated with cancer chemotherapy. Arch Intern Med 1982; 142:333–335.
9. Thomas GFM, Fernie DS, Bayston R, et al: Enterocolitis in Hirschsprung's disease: A controlled study of the etiologic role of *Clostridium difficile*. J Pediatr Surg 1986; 21:22–25.
10. Thomas GFM, Fernie DS, Malone M, et al: Association between *Clostridium difficile* and enterocolitis in Hirschsprung's disease. Lancet 1982; 1:78–79.
11. Wald A, Mendelow H, Bartlett JG: Nonantibiotic associated pseudomembranous colitis due to toxin-producing clostridia. Ann Intern Med 1980; 92:798–799.
12. Azar H, Drapanas T: Relationship of antibiotics to wound infection and enterocolitis in colon surgery. Am J Surg 1968; 115:209–217.
13. Altemeier WA, Hummell RP, Hill EO: Staphylococcal enterocolitis following antibiotic therapy. Ann Surg 1963; 157:847–858.
14. Kahn MY, Hall WH: Staphylococcus enterocolitis treatment with oral vancomycin. Ann Intern Med 1966; 65:1–7.
15. Dearing WH, Baggenstoss AH, Weed LA: Studies on the relationship of *Staphylococcus aureus* to pseudomembranous enteritis and to post-antibiotic enteritis. Gastroenterology 1960; 38:441–451.
16. Hovius SER, Rietra PJ: Salmonella colitis clinically presenting as a pseudomembranous colitis. Neth J Surg 1982; 34:81–82.
17. Schwartz JN, Hamilton JP, Fekety R, et al: Ampicillin-induced enterocolitis: Implication of toxigenic *Clostridium perfringes* type C. J Pediatr 1980; 97:661–663.
18. Lusk RH, Fekety FR, Silva J, et al: Clindamycin-induced enterocolitis in hamsters. J Infect Dis 1978; 137:464–475.
19. Rifkin GD, Fekety FR, Silva J, et al: Antibiotic-induced colitis: Implication of a toxin neutralized by *Clostridium sordellii* antitoxin. Lancet 1977; 2:1103–1106.
20. Bartlett JG: Antibiotic-associated pseudomembranous colitis. Rev Infect Dis 1979; 1:530–539.
21. Allo M, Silva J, Fekety FR, et al: Prevention of clindamycin-induced colitis in hamsters by *Clostridium sordellii* antitoxin. Gastroenterology 1979; 76:351–355.
22. Fekety R, Silva J, Toshniwal R, et al: Antibiotic-associated colitis: Effects of antibiotics upon *Clostridium difficile* and the disease in hamsters. Rev Infect Dis 1979; 1:386–397.
23. Pashby NL, Bolton RP, Sherriff RJ: Oral metronidazole in *Clostridium difficile* colitis. Br Med J 1979; 1:1605–1606.
24. Gurwith MJ, Rabin HR, Love K: Diarrhea associated with clindamycin and ampicillin therapy. J Infect Dis 1977; 135:104–110.
25. Swartzberg JE, Maresca RM, Remington JS: Clinical study of gastrointestinal complications associated with clindamycin therapy. J Infect Dis 1977; 135:99–103.
26. Aronsson B, Mollby R, Nord CE: Antimicrobial agents and *Clostridium difficile* in acute enteric disease: Epidemiological data from Sweden, 1980–1982. J Infect Dis 1985; 151:476–481.
27. Lusk RH, Fekety FR, Silva J, et al: Gastrointestinal side effects of clindamycin and ampicillin therapy. J Infect Dis 1977; 135:111–119.
28. McFarland LV: The epidemiology of *Clostridium difficile* infections. Viewpoints on Digestive Diseases 1990; 22:20–24.
29. Thelestam M, Bronnegard M: Interaction of cytopathogenic toxin from *Clostridium difficile* with cells in tissue culture. Scand J Infect Dis 1980; 22:16–29.
30. Hecht G, Pothoulakis C, LaMont JT, et al: *Clostridium difficile* toxin A perturbs cytoskeletal structure and tight junction permeability of cultured human intestinal epithelial monolayers. J Clin Invest 1988; 82:1516–1524.
31. Burdon DW, George RH, Mogg G, et al: Faecal toxin and severity of antibiotic-associated pseudomembranous colitis. J Clin Pathol 1981; 34:548–555.
32. McFarland LV, Mulligan ME, Kwok RYY, et al: Nosocomial acquisition of *Clostridium difficile* infection. N Engl J Med 1989; 320:204–210.
33. Hall IC, O'Toole E: Intestinal flora in newborn infants with description of a new pathogenic anaerobe, *Bacillus difficilis*. Am J Dis Child 1935; 49:390.
34. Fekety R, Kim K-H, Brown D, et al: Epidemiology of antibiotic-associated colitis. Isolation of *Clostridium difficile* from the hospital environment. Am J Med 1981; 70:906–908.
35. Welch DF, Marks MI: Is *Clostridium difficile* pathogenic in infants? J Pediatr 1982; 100:393–395.
36. Griffin GE, Heath J, Knox P: The action of *Clostridium difficile* cytotoxin is inhibited by specific glycoproteins. *In* Abstracts of the 22d Interscience Conference on Antimicrobial Agents and Chemotherapy. Washington, DC, American Society for Microbiology, 1982, abstract 596.
37. Chang TW, Sullivan NM, Wilkins TD: Insusceptibility of fetal intestinal mucosa and fetal cells to *Clostridium difficile* toxins. Acta Pharmacol Sin 1986; 7:448–453.
38. Buts JP, Wever AM, Roy CC, et al: Pseudomembranous colitis in childhood. Gastroenterology 1977; 73:823–827.
39. Scapa E: Pseudomembranous colitis in a 5 week old infant. Br Med J 1982; 284:824.
40. Batts DH, Martin D, Holmes R, et al: Treatment of antibiotic-associated *Clostridium difficile* diarrhea with oral vancomycin. J Pediatr 1980; 97:151–153.
41. Mulligan ME, Folfe RD, Finegold SM, et al: Contamination of a hospital environment by *Clostridium difficile*. Curr Microbiol 1979; 3:173–175.
42. Kim KH, Fekety R, Batts DH, et al: Isolation of *Clostridium difficile* from the environment and contact of patients with antibiotic-associated colitis. J Infect Dis 1981; 143:42–50.
43. Delmee M, Verellen G, Avesani V, et al: *Clostridium difficile* in neonates: Serogrouping and epidemiology. Eur J Pediatr 1988; 147:36–40.
44. Bacon A, Fekety R, Schaberg DS, et al: Epidemiology of *Clostridium difficile* colonization in newborns: Results using a bacteriophage and bacteriocin typing system. J Infect Dis 1988; 158:349–354.
45. Neu HC, Prince A, Neu CO, et al: Incidence of diarrhea and colitis associated with clindamycin therapy. J Infect Dis 1977; 135:S120–S125.
46. Tedesco FJ, Barton RW, Alpers HD: Clindamycin-associated colitis. Ann Intern Med 1974; 81:429–433.
47. Drapkin MS, Worthington MG, Chang TW, et al: *Clostridium difficile* colitis mimicking acute peritonitis. Arch Surg 1985; 120:1321–1322.
48. Triadafilopoulos G, Hallstone AE: Acute abdomen as the first presentation of pseudomembranous colitis. Gastroenterology 1991; 101:685–691.
49. Atkinson MH, McLeod BD: Reactive arthritis associated with *Clostridium difficile* enteritis. J Rheumatol 1988; 15:520–522.
50. Arber N, Vdassin R, Amir G, et al: Localized pseudomembranous colitis simulating carcinoma of the cecum. Am J Gastroenterol 1987; 82:1193–1195.
51. Sloyer AF, Panella VS, Demas BE, et al: Ogilvie's syndrome: Successful management without colonoscopy. Dig Dis Sci 1988; 33:1391–1396.
52. Yankes JR, Baker ME, Cooper C, et al: CT appearance of fecal pseudomembranous colitis. J Comput Assist Tomogr 1988; 12:394–395.
53. Rybolt AH, Laughon BE, Greenough WB, et al: Protein-losing enteropathy associated with *Clostridium difficile* infection. Lancet 1989; 1:1353–1355.
54. Levett PN: *Clostridium difficile* in habitats other than the human gastrointestinal tract. J Infect 1986; 12:253–263.
55. Welkon CJ, Long SS, Thompson CM, et al: *Clostridium difficile* in patients with cystic fibrosis. Am J Dis Child 1985; 139:805–808.
56. Chang TW, Lauermann M, Bartlett JG: Cytotoxicity assay in antibiotic-associated colitis. J Infect Dis 1979; 140:765–770.
57. Levine HG, Kennedy M, LaMont JT: Counterimmunoelectrophoresis vs. cytotoxicity assay for the detection of *Clostridium difficile* toxin. J Infect Dis 1982; 145:398.
58. Sherman ME, Defirolami PC, Thorne G, et al: Evaluation of a latex agglutination test for diagnosis of *Clostridium difficile* associated colitis. Am J Clin Pathol 1988; 89:228–233.

59. Lyerly DA, Ball DW, Toth J, et al: Characterization of cross-reactive proteins detected by culturette brand rapid latex test for *Clostridium difficile*. J Clin Microbiol 1988; 26:397–400.
60. Bennett RG, Laugon BE, Mundy LM, et al: Evaluation of a latex agglutination test for *Clostridium difficile* in two nursing home outbreaks. J Clin Microbiol 1989; 27:889–893.
61. Teasley DG, Gerding DN, Olson MN, et al: Prospective randomized trial of metronidazole versus vancomycin for the treatment of *Clostridium difficile* associated diarrhea and colitis. Lancet 1983; 2:1043–1046.
62. Bartlett JG: *Clostridium difficile*: Clinical considerations. Rev Infect Dis 1990; 12:S243–S251.

Chapter 52

Neoplasms of the Gastrointestinal Tract

STEVEN J. WEISMAN and STEVEN K. BERGSTROM

Although tumors of the gastrointestinal tract are uncommon in childhood, a wide spectrum of pathology is seen. The lesions range from benign, isolated polyps of the colon to more aggressive lymphomas, carcinomas, and soft tissue tumors. They may be seen as an isolated occurrence or as a component of syndromes such as familial polyposis coli. Although children do not usually present with the typical gastrointestinal tumors seen in adults, the symptoms of disease are somewhat generic. There may be a palpable mass, bleeding, pain, intestinal obstruction, or even failure to thrive. Once evaluation points to a mass lesion somewhere in the gastrointestinal system, consultation with the pediatric oncologist and pathologist is essential. Even though 5% or less of the tumors prove to be malignant, careful handling of any biopsy or solid-mass tissues may prove to be a critical component in the diagnostic evaluation. Samples of a lymphoma, for example, should be processed for cell surface markers, cytogenetics, routine histology, and electron microscopy. Similar studies may be required for other malignancies as well. Such an evaluation will not only contribute to the staging workup of the child but may also significantly influence the choice of a specific treatment plan.

This chapter discusses tumors of the gastrointestinal tract based upon both pathology and anatomic location.

LYMPHOID TUMORS

Benign Lymphoid Hyperplasia

Lymphoid hyperplasia is generally a reactive process that results in enlargement of the normal lymphoid follicles of the intestinal submucosa. Histologic examination shows these to be normal, polyclonal cell populations, which retain the normal architecture of the nodule. Focal disease has been described in the small intestine, particularly the distal ileum and the appendix, and the rectum in children.[1] More extensive involvement of the stomach or the small intestine may be associated with dysgammaglobulinemia, in which the lymphoid hyperplasia appears to be compensatory. Patients may present with infectious complications, including giardiasis. Lymphoid hyperplasia of the small intestine and the rectum has been associated with intussusception and prolapse, respectively.[2, 3] Treatment is generally symptomatic and related to the extent of pathology induced by the presence of the hyperplasia.

Lymphomas

Malignant lymphoid disease, whether it be Hodgkin's disease or non-Hodgkin's lymphoma, frequently involves the abdomen. Hodgkin's disease rarely presents with symptoms associated with the gastrointestinal tract, although enlargement of the aortic and mesenteric nodes may displace the bowel. Non-Hodgkin's lymphomas, particularly of the small, noncleaved cell type, have frequently been associated with the gastrointestinal tract and warrant special consideration. The evaluation of a child with a lymphoma is detailed in Table 52–1.

Non-Hodgkin's Lymphoma

Non-Hodgkin's lymphoma accounts for about 7% of all malignancies in children.[4] Of these, the great majority involve the small, noncleaved cell type of tumor, which may or may not express B cell characteristics (Table 52–

Table 52–1. EVALUATION OF CHILD WITH LYMPHOMA

Complete blood count
Liver and renal chemistries
Lactate dehydrogenase
Uric acid
Calcium and phosphorous
Serum electrolytes
Quantitative immunoglobulins
Tissue biopsy
Immunologic surface markers
Hematoxylin and eosin slides
Electron micrographs
Bone marrow aspirate and biopsy
Lumbar puncture with cytology
Chest radiograph and (if abnormal) computed tomography scan
Abdominal-pelvic ultrasound
Gallium-67 scan

2). Advances in our understanding of these tumors, coupled with improvements in the therapy available for these patients, have made them a model for our understanding of tumors in general, and lymphoid disease in particular.

Primary non-Hodgkin's lymphomas can arise in any of several locations in the gastrointestinal tract. Gastric Burkitt's lymphoma with pancreatic infiltration, but no local lymph node involvement, has been described in an adolescent boy.[5] Ileocolic lymphoma appears to be the commonest site in the gastrointestinal tract in children. Fifty-four of 58 primary gastrointestinal lymphomas reported by Fleming and colleagues were localized to this area.[6] A case of what appeared to be a classic benign rectal polyp that instead was a localized non-Hodgkin's lymphoma has also been described.[7]

Burkitt's lymphoma, or small, noncleaved cell lymphomas, represents the overwhelming majority of abdominal lymphomas of childhood. Much of the current understanding of these tumors began in equatorial Africa, where Burkitt observed that the occurrence of these tumors among native Africans coincided with the distribution of malaria-causing mosquitoes.[8] Further observations led to an association with Epstein-Barr viral (EBV) infections and an association with a chromosomal abnormality, the t(8;14) translocation.[9]

The nature of small, noncleaved cell lymphomas seen in American children differs in many respects from those seen in Africa. Both frequently present with abdominal involvement, but the familiar jaw presentation seen in African children is rare among the sporadic cases seen in the Western world. Also, treatment of sporadic disease appears to be more complicated than in Africa, where single-agent therapy over a short time appears to be effective. Probably these remain distinct, though closely related, disease entities.

The t(8;14) translocation has proved seminal in our understanding of the underlying mechanisms of cell dysregulation in Burkitt's lymphoma. This brings the immunoglobulin heavy chain gene enhancer, found on chromosome 14, into juxtaposition with the c-myc oncogene, found on chromosome 8.[10, 11] Changes in the expression of the c-myc gene are thought to result in the malignancy. The contribution of stimulatory influences such as malaria or EBV infection has not been completely delineated, but ongoing B lymphocyte stimulation probably plays a role.

Therapy and Outcome. Treatment and survival rates in patients with non-Hodgkin's lymphoma, particularly B cell–related disease, have undergone revolutionary changes since the 1970s. Irrespective of tissue histology, localized abdominal lymphoma appears to have an excellent prognosis. Thirty-two of 58 cases reported by Fleming and colleagues underwent complete resection.[6] All but one of the youngsters was alive without disease recurrence after one year. On the other hand, only 13 of 26 children survived with residual lymphoma after surgery.

The success achieved by application of multiagent chemotherapy to Hodgkin's disease stimulated interest in multiagent regimens for non-Hodgkin's lymphoma. The use of cyclophosphamide, methotrexate, and vincristine in patients with Burkitt's lymphoma resulted in a significant increase in long-term survival.[12] Further intensification of the multidrug treatment regimen resulted in the LSA_2-L_2 protocol of the Sloan-Kettering Cancer Center.[13] Following the success of similar intensive regimens of chemotherapy, recent studies have looked at decreasing the severity and duration of therapy. The Pediatric Oncology Group piloted a protocol in which patients with limited-stage disease received multiagent chemotherapy over a total of 8 months versus traditional therapy, including radiation, lasting for 15 months.[14] Disease-free survival in the brief treatment schedule, 87.9%, was comparable with that in the traditional group (87.3%). The study also raised questions concerning the value of radiotherapy in treatment of localized disease, since there was no demonstrable difference between those who received radiation treatment and those who did not.

Table 52–2. COMMON TYPES OF CHILDHOOD NON-HODGKIN'S LYMPHOMA

Lymphoblastic
Usually T (thymocyte)
Some pre-B
Small Noncleaved Cell
Usually B
Diffuse Large Cell
Usually B (immunoblastic)
Some B (follicular)
Rare T

POLYPS

Benign polyps represent, overall, the most common tumors of the lower gastrointestinal tract in children (see Chapter 58). These may be divided into four groups: juvenile polyps, hamartomatous polyps, inflammatory fibroid polyps, and lymphoid polyps.

Malignant adenomas of the colon, either solitary or multiple, have been described, usually in connection with familial polyposis. Although three separate clinical syndromes have been described (familial polyposis coli, Gardner's syndrome, and Turcot's syndrome), they share many clinical and pathologic features that make them difficult to distinguish. All three represent autosomal dominant inherited diseases, and adenomatous polyposis is a common feature of them all.

Gastrointestinal involvement with von Recklinghausen's disease is not unusual. Tumors, as well as hyperplasia of the neuronal elements of the gastrointestinal tract, have been described in these patients and may be the cause of abdominal symptoms.[15] Other rare tumors, including those associated with the multiple endocrine neoplasia syndromes, may involve the intestine.

CARCINOID TUMORS

Carcinoid tumors of the gastrointestinal tract have been reported in children. Most of these tumors represent benign tumors of the appendix, where they are generally discovered as an incidental finding following surgery for acute appendicitis (Table 52–3). A large series of patients with appendiceal carcinoid tumors reported by Ryden and coworkers showed a strong preponderance in females among children.[16] Although invasion of the muscularis was noted in some of these cases, no metastatic disease was seen, and follow-up showed no recurrence. Field and associates reviewed 19 cases of carcinoid tumor, 16 involving the appendix.[17] A single case of a 15-year-old patient with a 2 cm lesion in the ileum and multiple hepatic nodules was included in this series. This patient also had symptoms of carcinoid syndrome, with flushing and respiratory difficulties. Chow and colleagues reported four cases of malignant carcinoid tumors in children.[18] The primary site of the tumor was reported in two of these cases: ileum and transverse colon. Three showed evidence of widespread metastases, and the fourth exhibited invasion of the bowel wall. None of these patients had symptoms associated with carcinoid syndrome, nor were elevated serotonin metabolites detected. Three succumbed to their disease, and a fourth remained alive at the time of the report. Among the patients who received therapy, doxorubicin, cyclophosphamide, actinomycin D, and vincristine were used.

Table 52–3. LOCATIONS AND TYPES OF GASTROINTESTINAL TUMORS

	Common	Uncommon
Carcinoid	Appendix	Ileum Colon Stomach
Tongue and mouth	Benign remnants Thyroid Hemangioma Cyst	Carcinoma Rhabdomyosarcoma
Esophagus	Benign lesions Cyst Duplication Lipoma Hamartoma	Leiomyoma Carcinoma
Stomach	Benign lesions Polyps Duplication Teratoma Lipoma	Leiomyoma Leiomyosarcoma Leiomyoblastoma Rhabdomyosarcoma Adenocarcinoma
Small intestine	Lymphoma	Leiomyoma Leiomyosarcoma Carcinoma
Large intestine	Colorectal carcinoma	Leiomyoma Leiomyosarcoma Hemangioma Lymphoma
Pancreas	Endocrine tumors Insulinoma Vipoma Glucagonoma Gastrinoma	Serous adenoma Mucinous adenoma Pancreaticoblastoma Pancreatic carcinoma
Biliary tract	Rhabdomyosarcoma	Carcinoma
Retroperitoneum	Rhabdomyosarcoma Wilms' tumor Lymphoma Neuroblastoma Ovarian germ cell tumor Primitive neuroectodermal tumor	—

TUMORS OF THE TONGUE AND MOUTH

Tumors in the tongue and mouth are uncommon in children and infants (see Table 52–3). Carcinoma of the tongue has been reported in an adolescent as well as in a neonate.[19, 20] A series of 23 children with squamous cell lesions of the lips or tongue was published by Moore, but almost all cases were in adolescents.[21] Two infants with rhabdomyosarcoma of the tongue presented as newborns with botryoid-type lesions.[22, 23] It appears that the majority of lesions in this location are benign and often represent embryologic remnants, including lingual thyroid glands, hemangiomas, or cysts. If lesions are large enough, even the benign ones can lead to compromise of the airway. Nasopharyngeal carcinomas may certainly present with extension into the oral cavity. These tumors appear to be the second most common carcinoma of childhood, but because they arise outside of the gastrointestinal tract, they are not covered in this discussion.[24, 25]

ESOPHAGEAL TUMORS

Benign rather than malignant tumors predominate in the esophagus. Intramural cysts are most common; only rarely have intramural or intraluminal solid lesions been reported.[26, 27] More commonly, duplications, lipomas, or hamartomas have been noted (see Table 52–3).

Recently leiomyoma of the esophagus was reported by Bourque and associates in two children.[28] The authors were also able to locate a total of 18 other cases with a combined mean age of 14 years. Over 35% of these children had involvement of the entire esophagus. As expected, patients presented with dysphagia, vomiting, dyspnea, retrosternal pain, or coughing. Simple radiographic studies may be misleading and misdiagnose achalasia. Endoscopy is essential and helps plan for a difficult surgical procedure, which usually involves surgical resection.

Carcinomas of the esophagus may rarely occur in children. Attempts have been made to associate these lesions with caustic ingestion, as has been done in adults.[29–31] These squamous cell lesions have been diagnosed anywhere from 13 to 71 years after the initial ingestion. Two fatal cases of adenocarcinoma in older children with Barrett's esophagus were reported by Hoeffel and colleagues.[32] Other examples of similar carcinomatous lesions were not associated with specific esophageal disorders.[33–36]

STOMACH TUMORS

A vast array of benign tumors of the stomach have been seen in children (see Table 52–3). Various types of polyps, duplications, ectopic pancreatic tissue, leiomyomas, hemangiopericytomas, carcinoid tumors, and lipomas can be found in children of various ages.[37–40] Benign gastric teratomas are well documented in the pediatric literature. They are most commonly discovered in newborns and have remarkable male predominance.[41–45] Although teratomas in other locations are frequently found to contain malignant components, it appears that in all but two out of more than 50 gastric lesions, such tissues have been absent.[46] All these tumors may present with similar clinical signs, including a mass effect, bleeding, or gastric obstruction.

Muscle tumors of the stomach range from the benign leiomyoma to the malignant rhabdomyosarcoma or leiomyosarcoma.[47] Over half of the smooth muscle tumors reported by these authors were malignant. The leiomyosarcomas can invade locally as well as distantly to locations such as the liver.[39, 48] This lesion in particular may be difficult for pathologists to distinguish from benign leiomyomas. Therefore, generously wide surgical margins that may require subtotal gastrectomy are preferred. Several children with epithelioid leiomyomas (leiomyoblastoma) who were successfully treated with surgery have also been reported recently.[49–51] None of these children had associated pulmonary chondrohamartomas, which have been associated with these tumors and may be incorrectly interpreted as distant metastases.[52] Reports of two fatal cases of gastric rhabdomyosarcoma, which had associated neck metastases, emphasize the need to consider the stomach as a potential primary site in this malignancy.[53, 54]

Although two newborn infants have been reported with adenocarcinoma of the stomach, this tumor, so common in adults, is a very rare entity in children.[55, 56] There may be an association between several immunodeficiency syndromes and adenocarcinoma of the stomach. These include ataxia-telangiectasia, common variable immunodeficiency, and isolated immunoglobulin A (IgA) deficiency.[55, 57, 58] Most cases, however, appear to be sporadic in the older child.[59–61] Surgical management must be aggressive for these malignant tumors. The precise role, if any, for chemotherapy and radiation therapy remains to be determined.

SMALL INTESTINAL TUMORS

As previously mentioned, gastrointestinal lymphomas occur most commonly in the small intestine (see Table 52–3). It is also true that in children, lymphomas are the commonest tumor in this location. Lymphoid hyperplasia and carcinoid tumors are the second most frequently seen lymphomas. As one would expect, tumors in this location may commonly lead to intussusception, intestinal obstruction, and bleeding, as well as cause nonspecific symptoms, such as abdominal pain, vomiting, and diarrhea.

Smooth muscle tumors are found in this location as well as in the stomach. These lesions include duodenal and jejunal leiomyomas and duodenal and ileal leiomyosarcomas.[62–66] It would appear, as expected, that complete surgical resection is the most reliable form of therapy for the malignant tumors; most children with subtotal surgical treatment of these tumors eventually succumb to the sarcomatous lesions. A relationship of these tumors to infection with human immunodeficiency virus (HIV) has been described.[67, 68] The precise relationship of this viral infection with the cause of the tumors remains to be determined.

A case of granulocytic sarcoma of the ileum with local lymph node metastases was recently treated with allogeneic bone marrow transplantation.[69] This approach may play a role in the other difficult to treat gastrointestinal malignancies. Other malignancies that have been treatment enigmas include the adenocarcinomas; however, these tumors appear in the small bowel less commonly than in the stomach or colon.[24, 70] Gastric tumors may be associated with the various polyposis syndromes (see Chapter 58). Several cases of hemangiomas in the small intestine have been noted, with expected bleeding complications.[71, 72]

COLONIC AND RECTAL TUMORS

Tumors of the large bowel and rectum follow the same general histologic patterns discussed in the sections covering the more proximal anatomic sites (see Table 52–3). Colorectal carcinoma is not only the most commonly found carcinoma in children but, after primary liver tumors, it is the most common true gastrointestinal malignancy.[24, 73] Ulcerative colitis, familial polyposis, Turcot's syndrome, and Gardner's syndrome are predisposing conditions to colonic carcinoma.[74–78] Children who have undergone ureterocolic anastomoses for conditions such as exstrophy of the bladder have a several thousandfold greater risk of developing adenocarcinoma at the surgical site.[79]

Colorectal carcinoma is more common in males than females. It may occur more frequently in the Mississippi Valley in the United States, where investigators have attempted to correlate the incidence with exposure to herbicides and pesticides.[80, 81] In addition, there may be a higher incidence in young African-Americans.[73] These tumors often produce increased amounts of the carcinoembryonic antigen (CEA) or CA 19–9 (another carcinoma membrane marker), which thereby allows easier follow-up during or after therapy. Children infrequently have lesions in the rectum; in fact, there appears to be a shift from lesions on the left side of the colon (seen in adults) to a more even distribution throughout the colon in children.[24, 82] Abdominal pain, which may be vague, is often the presenting complaint. Sometimes there may be signs of obstruction or bleeding. In adults, anemia may be the initial finding. Children and adolescents tend to present with more advanced disease than adults.[83, 84, 84a] In fact, the majority have Dukes' stage D disease. It is not uncommon for there to be peritoneal, lymph node, omental, liver, ovary, or even far distant metastases. Almost one third of these young patients have the mucinous variant of adenocarcinoma, which may represent a more poorly differentiated form with a worse prognosis.[84]

Surgery should attempt complete resection. If lesions are too large or involve critical structures, preoperative radiotherapy with chemotherapy may be indicated. Various agents have been used in adults with limited to variable success. However, inadequate tumor removal has been associated with a grim ultimate prognosis.[24, 73]

Other tumors that may be encountered in the large intestine or rectum are those of smooth muscle or vascular origin. Leiomyosarcomas have been reported, including several in neonates.[85–87] In addition, leiomyomas and leiomyosarcomas have been seen in HIV-infected children.[67, 68] Finally, intestinal hemangiomas presenting both as a single mass lesion and as diffuse colonic hemangiomatosis have been reported in young infants.[88, 89]

PANCREATIC TUMORS

Pancreatic tumors are, fortunately, rare in children.[90, 91] These tumors may be of endocrine origin, benign cystic origin, or malignant (see Table 52–3). Because of their retroperitoneal location, some of these tumors can become rather extensive before diagnosis. The functioning endocrine tumors may produce insulin, vasoactive peptide, glucagon, gastrin, or somatostatin.[92–95] Most of these tumors are small, solitary, nonmalignant lesions that present because of associated endocrine symptoms. Even the malignant varieties present because of the overproduction of substances such as insulin rather than because of mass effect or metastatic disease[91] (see Chapter 70). Benign cysts of the pancreas are also rare.[91, 96] These lesions can be rather large and may result in symptoms from compression of surrounding structures. The serous adenomas are truly benign and do not require aggressive surgical removal. On the other hand, the mucinous cysts have malignant potential and must be resected.[97] Benign pseudocysts occur in children.

Pancreatoblastoma (infantile carcinoma of the pancreas) usually arises in the head of the pancreas and is an encapsulated tumor that must be distinguished from true pancreatic carcinoma.[98, 99] The undifferentiated appearance of the tumors may suggest the presence of a neuroblastoma or even an islet-cell tumor. These tumors may produce alpha-fetoprotein, CEA, or alpha$_1$-antitrypsin.[100–102] These tumors may represent fetal rests from the ventral anlage of the pancreas. Surgical removal is often possible and leads to an excellent prognosis. One case of a recurrence in the liver has been noted.[91]

Pancreatic carcinoma, which is rare in children, may have the same grim prognosis as in adults.[103, 104] This tumor has been diagnosed in an infant as young as three weeks of age,[105] but in a series of 38 cases reviewed by Welch,[106] the mean age was just over 9 years. The tumors tend to arise in the head or body of the pancreas.[107] There may be lymph node or liver involvement. Surgery usually necessitates pancreaticoduodenectomy. In the few cases in which surgery was subtotal and adjunctive chemotherapy and radiotherapy were employed, the experience has been similar to that in adults, with fatal outcome.[91, 108]

BILIARY TUMORS

Biliary tract tumors have been described in children (see Table 52–3).[109–113] When such lesions are discovered, they usually have already spread to the liver or adjacent lymph nodes. Such a diagnosis should be considered in all patients who present with extrahepatic biliary obstruction. Adenocarcinoma may develop in the wall of a choledochal cyst[110] (see Chapter 71). The prognosis for carcinomatous tumors of the biliary tree is, unfortunately, thought to be similar to that in adults. Unless there can be surgical removal of all tumor, survival is very poor.

In children and adolescents, the most common tumor in these locations is a rhabdomyosarcoma. Lesions may be specifically in the biliary ducts or in the gallbladder itself.[111, 112] In a review of 33 total cases reported in the literature, only seven were alive 7 to 42 months after diagnosis.[112] Most children had tumors originating in the common bile duct. Ruymann and colleagues reported on 10 additional cases of this tumor that were collected from almost 1,700 children enrolled in the Intergroup Rhabdomyosarcoma Study during an 11-year period.[113] Seven of the patients had common bile duct disease; three had extension into the liver, and three had lymph node spread. These patients were all treated with combined modality therapy involving extirpating or debulking surgery (7 patients), chemotherapy (10 patients), and radiotherapy (7 patients). Four children were long-term survivors. Thus, aggressive multimodal therapy may play a critical role in this rare tumor.

RETROPERITONEAL TUMORS

Sarcomas, usually rhabdomyosarcoma, are the most frequently encountered tumors involving the retroperitoneum.[114, 115] These tumors are often quite large at diagnosis, and over one third of patients already have distant metastatic disease. Critical vascular or organ structures are often caught in the large primary tumor, making complete resection difficult or impossible. The prognosis with chemotherapy and radiation therapy remains dismal if primary surgical treatment is less than complete. The use of aggressive second-look procedures after cytoreduction with these other modalities may serve to improve survival in these difficult to treat children. Other retroperitoneal tumors are listed in Table 52–3.

REFERENCES

1. Byrne WJ, Jimenez JF, Euler AR: Lymphoid polyp (focal lymphoid hyperplasia) of the colon in children. Pediatrics 1982; 69:598–600.
2. Ranchod M, Lewin KJ, Dorfman RF: Lymphoid hyperplasia of the gastrointestinal tract: A study of 26 cases and review of the literature. Am J Surg Pathol 1978; 2:383–400.

3. Rambaud JC, De Saint-Louvent P, Marti R, et al: Diffuse follicular lymphoid hyperplasia of the small intestine without primary immunoglobulin deficiency. Am J Med 1982; 73:125–132.
4. Young JL, Ries LG, Silverberg E, et al: Cancer incidence, survival and mortality for children younger than 15 years. Cancer 1986; 58:598–602.
5. Olinici CD, Vasiu R: Gastric Burkitt's lymphoma: Case report and review of the literature. Morphol Embryol (Bucur) 1990; 36:39–41.
6. Fleming ID, Turk PS, Murphy SB, et al: Surgical implications of primary gastrointestinal lymphoma of childhood. Arch Surg 1990; 125:252–256.
7. Paris RC, Hammami A, Kim H, et al: Non-Hodgkin's lymphoma presenting as a rectal polyp in a child. J Pediatr Surg 1990; 25:1280–1282.
8. Burkitt DP: Geographical distribution. *In* Burkitt DP, Wright DH, eds: Burkitt's Lymphoma. Edinburgh, Churchill Livingstone, 1970, pp 186–197.
9. Zech L, Haglund U, Nilsson K: Characteristic chromosomal abnormalities in biopsies and lymphoid cell lines from patients with Burkitt and non-Burkitt lymphomas. Int J Cancer 1976; 17:47–56.
10. Taub R, Kirsh I, Morton C: Translocation of the C-*myc* gene into the immunoglobulin heavy chain locus in human Burkitt lymphoma and murine plasmacytoma cells. Proc Natl Acad Sci USA 1982; 79:7837–7841.
11. Dalla-Favera R, Bregni M, Erikson J: Human C-*myc* oncogene is located on the region of chromosome 8 that is translocated in Burkitt lymphoma cells. Proc Natl Acad Sci USA 1982; 79:7824–7827.
12. Ziegler JL: Treatment results of 54 American patients with Burkitt's lymphoma are similar to the African experience. N Engl J Med 1977; 297:75–80.
13. Wollner N, Burchenal JH, Lieberman PH: Non-Hodgkin's lymphoma in children: A comparative study of two modalities of therapy. Cancer 1976; 37:123–134.
14. Link MP, Donaldson SS, Berard CW, et al: Results of treatment of childhood localized non-Hodgkin's lymphoma with combination chemotherapy with or without radiotherapy. N Engl J Med 1990; 322:1169–1174.
15. Feinstat T, Tesluk H, Schuffler MD: Megacolon and neurofibromatosis: A neuronal intestinal dysplasia. Case report and review of the literature. Gastroenterology 1984; 86:1573–1579.
16. Ryden SE, Drake RM, Franciosi RA: Carcinoid tumors of the appendix in children. Cancer 1975; 36:1538–1542.
17. Field JL, Adamson LF, Stoeckle HE: Review of carcinoids in children. Pediatrics 1962; 29:953–960.
18. Chow CW, Sane S, Campbell PE: Malignant carcinoid tumors in children. Cancer 1982; 49:802–811.
19. Frank LW, Enfield CD, Miller AJ: Carcinoma of the tongue in a newborn child: Report of a case. Am J Cancer 1936; 26:775–777.
20. Patel DD, Dave RI: Carcinoma of the anterior tongue in adolescence. Cancer 1976; 37:917–921.
21. Moore C: Visceral squamous cancer in children. Pediatrics 1958; 21:573–581.
22. Telleschi S: Unusual pathology and cytological peculiarities of the so-called botryoid sarcoma (congenital botryoid sarcoma of the tongue and infantile uterine botryoid sarcoma with rupture of the organ and hemoperitoneum). Arch Vecchi Anat Pathol 1970; 56:671.
23. Leibert PS, Stool SE: Rhabdomyosarcoma of the tongue in an infant. Results of combined radiation and chemotherapy. Ann Surg 1973; 178:621–624.
24. Pratt CB, George SL, Green AA, et al: Carcinomas in children: Clinical and demographic characteristics. Cancer 1988; 61:1046–1050.
25. McWhirter WR, Stiller CA, Lennox EL: Carcinomas in childhood: A registry-based study of incidence and survival. Cancer 1989; 63:2242–2246.
26. Totten RS, Stout AP, Humphreys GH, et al: Benign tumors and cysts of the esophagus. J Thorac Surg 1953; 25:606–622.
27. Watson RR, O'Connor TM, Weisel W: Solid benign tumors of the esophagus. Ann Thorac Surg 1967; 4:80–91.
28. Bourque MD, Spigland N, Bensoussan AL, et al: Esophageal leiomyoma in children: Two cases and review of the literature. J Pediatr Surg 1989; 24:1103–1107.
29. Kinnam J, Shin HI, Wetteland P: Carcinoma of the esophagus after lye corrosion. Acta Chir Scand 1968; 134:489–493.
30. Appelqvist P, Salmo M: Lye corrosion carcinoma of the esophagus. Cancer 1980; 45:2655.
31. Leape LI, Ashcraft KW, Scarpelli DG, et al: Hazard to health-liquid lye. N Engl J Med 1971; 284:578–581.
32. Hoeffel JC, Nihoul-Fekete C, Schmitt M: Esophageal adenocarcinoma after gastroesophageal reflux in children. J Pediatr 1989; 115:259–261.
33. Al Hilou R, Atkins J, Matthews HR: Oesophageal adenocarcinoma in a boy of fifteen years. J Laryngol Otol 1984; 98:643–646.
34. Soni NK, Chatterji P: Carcinoma of the esophagus in an eight-year-old child. J Laryngol Otol 1980; 94:327–329.
35. Stephan BH: Zur Casuistik der dysphagie bei kindern (Sarcoma oesphagei bei einem 4 jahrigen knaben). Jahrb Kinderheikd 1990; 30:354–359.
36. Shahi UP, Sudarsan, Dattagupta S, et al: Carcinoma of the oesophagus in a 14-year-old child: Report of a case and review of the literature. Tropical Gastroenterol 1989; 10:224–228.
37. Landing BH, Martin LW: Tumors of the gastrointestinal tract and pancreas. Pediatr Clin North Am 1959; 6:413–426.
38. MacKinnon D, Nash FW: Pyloric obstruction due to pancreatic heterotopia in a child. Br Med J 1957; 1:87–88.
39. Yannopoulos K, Stout AP: Smooth muscle tumors in children. Cancer 1962; 15:958–971.
40. Quinn FM, Brown S, O'Hara D: Hemangiopericytoma of the stomach in a neonate. J Pediatr Surg 1991; 26:101–102.
41. Nandy AK, Sengupta P, Chatterjee SK, et al: Teratoma of the stomach. J Pediatr Surg 1974; 9:563–564.
42. Cairo MS, Grosfeld JL, Weetman RM: Gastric teratoma: Unusual cause for bleeding of the upper gastrointestinal tract in the newborn. Pediatrics 1981; 67:721–724.
43. Purvis JM, Miller RC, Blumenthal BI: Gastric teratoma: First reported case in a female. J Pediatr Surg 1979; 14:86–87.
44. Senocak ME, Kate G, Buyukpamukcu N, et al: Gastric teratoma in children including the third reported female case. J Pediatr Surg 1990; 25:681–684.
45. Matias IC, Huang YC: Gastric teratoma in infancy: Report of a case and review of world literature. Ann Surg 1973; 178:631–636.
46. Balik E, Tyncyurek M, Sayan A, et al: Malignant gastric teratoma in an infant. Zeitschrift Fur Kinderchirurgie 1990; 45:383–385.
47. Wurlitzer FP, Mares AJ, Isaacs H, et al: Smooth muscle tumors of the stomach in childhood and adolescence. J Pediatr Surg 1973; 3:421–427.
48. Johnson H, Hutter JJ, Paplanus SH: Leiomyosarcoma of the stomach: Results of surgery and chemotherapy in an eleven-year-old girl with liver metastases. Med Pediatr Oncol 1980; 8:137–142.
49. Rogers BB, Grishaber JE, Mahoney DH, et al: Gastric leiomyoblastoma (epithelioid leiomyoma) occurring in a child: A case report. Pediatr Pathol 1989; 9:79–85.
50. Luzzatto C, Galligioni A, Candiani F, et al: Gastric leiomyoblastoma in childhood—a case report and review of the literature. Z Kinderchir 1989; 44:373–376.
51. Hamazoe R, Shimizu N, Nishidoi H, et al: Gastric leiomyoblastoma in childhood. J Pediatr Surg 1991; 26:225–227.
52. Tisell LE, Angervall L, Dahl I, et al: Recurrent and metastasizing gastric leiomyoblastoma (epithelioid leiomyosarcoma) associated with multiple pulmonary chrondro-hamartomas. Cancer 1978; 41:259–265.
53. Templeton AW, Heslin DJ: Primary rhabdomyosarcoma of the stomach and esophagus. Am J Roentgenol 1961; 86:896–899.
54. Mahour GH, Isaacs H, Chang L: Primary malignant tumors of the stomach in children. J Pediatr Surg 1980; 15:603–608.
55. Siegel SE, Hays DM, Romansky S, et al: Carcinoma of the stomach in childhood. Cancer 1976; 2:253.
56. Cullingworth CJ: Case of cancer of the stomach in an infant five weeks old. Br Med J 1977; 2:253.
57. Haerer AF, Jackson JF, Evers CG: Ataxia-telangiectasia with gastric adenocarcinoma. JAMA 1969; 210:1884–1887.
58. Fraser KJ, Rankin JG: Selective deficiency of IgA immunoglob-

ulins associated with carcinoma of the stomach. Aust Ann Med 1970; 19:165–167.
59. McNeer G: Cancer of the stomach in the young. Am J Roentgenol Radium Ther Nucl Med 1941; 45:537–550.
60. Goto S, Ikeda K, Ishli E, et al: Carcinoma of the stomach in a 7-year-old boy: A case report and a review of the literature on children under 10 years of age. Z Kinderchir 1984; 39:137–140.
61. Schwartz MG, Spaglione NA: Gastric carcinoma in the young: Overview of the literature. Mt Sinai J Med 1984; 51:720–723.
62. Freeman J: Leiomyoma of small bowel: A case report. J Pediatr Surg 1979; 14:477–478.
63. Riggle KP, Boeckman CR: Duodenal leiomyoma: A case report of hematemesis in a teenager. J Pediatr Surg 1988; 23:850–851.
64. Monheit DB, Degenshein GA: Leiomyosarcoma of the small bowel in a child. Ann Intern Med 1955; 43:903–907.
65. Marshall DG, Kim F: Leiomyosarcoma of the duodenum. J Pediatr Surg 1987; 22:1007–1008.
66. McGrath PC, Neifeld JP, Kay S, et al: Principles in the management of pediatric intestinal leiomyosarcomas. J Pediatr Surg 1988; 23:939–941.
67. Chadwick EG, Connor EJ, Hanson IC, et al: Tumors of smooth-muscle origin in HIV-infected children. JAMA 1990; 263:182–184.
68. McLoughlin LC, Nord KS, Joshi VV, et al: Disseminated leiomyosarcoma in a child with acquired immune deficiency syndrome. Cancer 1991; 67:2618–2621.
69. Kowal-Vern A, Johnson FL, Trujillo Y, et al: Granulocytic sarcoma of the ileum treated by bone marrow transplantation. Am J Pediatr Hem Oncol 1991; 13:34–38.
70. Kabra SK, Kumar CL, Mathur M, et al: Adenocarcinoma of small bowel. Indian Pediatr 1990; 27:987–989.
71. Basaklar AC: Haemangiomas of the gastrointestinal tract in children. Z Kinderchir 1990; 45:114–116.
72. Hansen U, Boesgaard S, Anderson J: Cavernous hemangioma of the jejunum: Long-standing anaemia in a child. Acta Paediatr Scand 1990; 79:1124–1127.
73. Rao BN, Pratt CB, Fleming ID, et al: Colon carcinoma in children and adolescents: A review of 30 cases. Cancer 1985; 55:1322–1326.
74. Wilcox HR, Beattie JL: Carcinoma complicating ulcerative colitis during childhood. Am J Clin Pathol 1956; 26:778–786.
75. Kottmeier PK, Clatworthy HW: Intestinal polyps and associated carcinomas in childhood. Am J Surg 1975; 110:709–716.
76. Sherlock P, Lipkin M, Winauer SJ: Predisposing factors in carcinoma of the colon. Adv Intern Med 1975; 20:121–150.
77. Turcot J, Despies JP, St. Pierre F: Malignant tumors of the central nervous system associated with familial polyposis of the colon: Report of two cases. Dis Colon Rectum 1959; 2:465–468.
78. Gardner EJ: Follow-up study of a family group exhibiting dominant inheritance for a syndrome including intestinal polyps, osteomas, fibromas, and epidermal cysts. Am J Hum Genet 1962; 14:376–390.
79. Eraklis AJ, Folkman MJ: Adenocarcinoma at the site of ureterosigmoidostomies for exstrophy of the bladder. J Pediatr Surg 1978; 13:730–734.
80. Pratt CB, Rivera G, Shanks E, et al: Colorectal carcinoma in adolescents: Implications regarding etiology. Cancer 1977; 40(Suppl):2464–2472.
81. Caldwell GC, Cannon SB, Pratt CB, et al: Serum pesticide levels in childhood colorectal carcinoma patients. Cancer 1981; 48:774–778.
82. Abrams JS, Reines HD: Increasing incidence of right-sided lesions in colorectal carcinoma. Am J Surg 1979; 137:522–526.
83. Hoerner MT: Carcinoma of the colon and rectum in persons under twenty years of age. Am J Surg 1958; 96:47–53.
84. Griffin PM, Liff JM, Greenberg RS, et al: Adenocarcinomas of the colon and rectum in persons under 40 years old. Gastroenterology 1991; 100:1033–1040.
84a. Brown RA, Rode H, Millar AJW, et al: Colorectal carcinoma in children. J Pediatr Surg 1992; 27:919–921.
85. Ein SH, Beck AR, Allen JE: Colon sarcoma in the newborn. J Pediatr Surg 1979; 14:455–457.
86. Kriss N: Leiomyosarcoma of the colon in an infant: Case report and review. Am J Roentgenol Radium Ther Nucl Med 1960; 84:540–545.
87. Nagaya M, Tsuda M, Ishiguro Y: Leiomyosarcoma of the transverse colon in a neonate: A rare cause of meconium peritonitis. J Pediatr Surg 1989; 19:504–508.
88. Leighton DM, Benghanem T, Montagne JP, et al: A case of rectal bleeding in infancy. Aust Radiol 1990; 34:89–90.
89. Ibarguen E, Sharp HL, Snyder CL, et al: Hemangiomatosis of the colon and peritoneum: Case report and management discussion. Clin Pediatr 1988; 27:425–430.
90. Grosfeld JL, Clatworthy HW, Hamoudi AB: Pancreatic malignancy in children. Arch Surg 1970; 101:370–375.
91. Grosfeld JL, Vane DW, Rescoria FJ, et al: Pancreatic tumors in childhood: Analysis of 13 cases. J Pediatr Surg 1990; 25:1057–1062.
92. Rich RH, Dehner LP, Okinaga K, et al: Surgical management of islet-cell adenoma in infancy. Surgery 1978; 84:519–526.
93. Garces LY, Drash A, Kenny FM: Islet cell tumors in the neonate. Pediatrics 1968; 41:796.
94. Brenner RW, Sank LI, Kerner MB, et al: Resection of a vipoma of the pancreas in a 15-year-old girl. J Pediatr Surg 1986; 21:983–985.
95. Wilson SD, Ellison EH: Total gastric resection in children with the Zollinger-Ellison syndrome. Arch Surg 1965; 91:165–173.
96. Gundersen AE, Janis JF: Pancreatic cystadenoma in childhood: Report. J Pediatr Surg 1969; 4:478–481.
97. Logan SE, Voet RL, Tompkins RT: The malignant potential of mucinous cysts of the pancreas. West J Med 1982; 136:157–162.
98. Becker WF: Pancreatoduodenectomy for carcinoma of the pancreas in an infant: Report of a case. Ann Surg 1957; 145:864–872.
99. Horie A, Yano Y, Kotoo Y, et al: Morphogenesis of pancreatoblastoma, infantile carcinoma of the pancreas. Cancer 1977; 39:247–254.
100. Iseki M, Suzuki T, Koizumi Y, et al: Alpha-fetoprotein-producing pancreatoblastoma. Cancer 1986; 57:1833–1835.
101. Ohaki Y, Misugi K, Fukuda J, et al: Immunohistochemical study of pancreatoblastoma. Acta Pathol Jpn 1987; 37:1581–1590.
102. Buchino JJ, Castello FM, Nagaraj HS: Pancreatoblastoma, a histochemical and ultrastructural analysis. Cancer 1984; 53:963–969.
103. Moynan RW, Neerhout RC, Johnson TS: Pancreatic carcinoma in childhood. J Pediatr 1964; 65:711–720.
104. Tsukimoto I, Watanabe K, Lin JB, et al: Pancreatic carcinoma in children in Japan. Cancer 1973; 31:1203–1207.
105. Robey G, Daneman A, Martin DJ: Pancreatic carcinoma in a neonate. Pediatr Radiol 1983; 13:284–286.
106. Welch KJ: The pancreas. *In* Ravich MM, Randolph JG, Rowe MI, et al, eds: Pediatric Surgery. 3rd ed. Chicago, Year Book Publishers, 1984, pp 1090–1096.
107. Taxy JB: Adenocarcinoma of the pancreas in childhood. Cancer 1976; 37:1508–1518.
108. Carmprodon R, Quentanilla E: Successful long-term results with resection of pancreatic carcinoma in children: Favorable prognosis for an uncommon neoplasm. Surgery 1984; 95:420–426.
109. Kelly TR, Chamberlain TR: Carcinoma of the gallbladder. Am J Surg 1982; 143:737–741.
110. Fujiwara Y, Ohizumi T, Kakizaki G, et al: Case of a congenital choledochal cyst associated with carcinoma. J Pediatr Surg 1976; 11:587–588.
111. Nagaraj HS, Kmetz DR, Leitner C: Rhabdomyosarcoma of the bile ducts. J Pediatr Surg 1977; 12:1071–1074.
112. Mihara S, Matsumoto H, Tokunaga F, et al: Botryoid rhabdomyosarcoma of the gallbladder in a child. Cancer 1982; 49:812–818.
113. Ruymann FB, Raney RB, Crist WM, et al: Rhabdomyosarcoma of the biliary tree in childhood. A report from the Intergroup Rhabdomyosarcoma Study. Cancer 1985; 56:575–581.
114. Crist WM, Raney RB, Tefft M, et al: Soft tissue sarcomas arising in the retroperitoneal space in children: A report from the Intergroup Rhabdomyosarcoma Study (IRS) Committee. Cancer 1985; 56:2125–2132.
115. Jaques DP, Coit DG, Hajdu SI, et al: Management of primary and recurrent soft-tissue sarcoma of the retroperitoneum. Ann Surg 1990; 212:51–59.

Chapter 53

Appendicitis

JUDAH FOLKMAN and DENNIS P. LUND

Appendicitis is the commonest condition requiring emergency surgery in children. It is also the most frequently misdiagnosed illness in children. In most institutions, the rate of "negative appendectomy" varies from 10 to 30%. The rate of perforated appendixes, however, which results in part from delays in diagnosis, is also 30%. Despite the fact that the clinical findings of appendicitis were well described more than a century ago,[1] this disease continues to confound medical practitioners. Prompt and accurate diagnosis of appendicitis requires clinical acumen based on a thorough history and physical examination (there is no single laboratory test or pathognomonic sign for appendicitis).

DIAGNOSIS

It is important to establish the time of onset of symptoms with some accuracy, because in children, the appendix commonly perforates about 36 hours after pain begins. The parent may first have been aware that the child awoke at 3 AM with abdominal pain. However, a more precise history is obtained by dividing time into segments between meals. With this approach, the parent may now recall that the child first started to look unwell between lunch and dinner on the previous day, that the child "picked" at dinner. Thus, if the clinician is examining the child the following afternoon, the disease has been under way for at least 24 hours. Anorexia itself is not a discriminating sign: half of the appendicitis patients the authors have seen have said they were hungry. Approximately 80% of children with appendicitis will have perforated appendixes within 48 hours of the development of symptoms.

Pain

The first symptom of appendicitis is periumbilical pain. There are almost no exceptions. Stretch receptors embedded in the small blood vessels of the appendix transmit the first signs of inflammation along mesenteric nerve fibers, eventually to the T10 spinal nerve that supplies the dermatome at the level of the umbilicus (see Chapter 17). In fact, most diseases affecting the small intestine begin with a display of pain in this dermatome.

After a few hours the patient may vomit, but the absence of vomiting is meaningless. Many cases of appendicitis progress to perforation without the occurrence of vomiting. The importance of the vomiting, if it does occur, is that is usually *follows* the periumbilical pain. By contrast, in gastroenteritis, vomiting often *precedes* abdominal pain. The mechanism of vomiting is thought to depend, again, on the stretch receptors in the appendix itself. This has been observed during operations performed on elderly patients under local anesthesia. Although the abdominal wall can be made completely insensitive by the local anesthetic, traction on the appendix may induce vomiting.

After a few more hours, the periumbilical pain usually shifts to the right lower quadrant. Right lower quadrant pain is probably induced by a small amount of inflammatory fluid traveling from the appendix to the parietal peritoneum. The inflamed appendix itself does not usually touch the underside of the parietal peritoneum. In fact, in the more than 30 conditions causing acute abdominal pain that require emergency operation, in most instances, by the time the pain has finally shifted to the parietal peritoneum, it is being transmitted by a fluid. Except for an inflamed gallbladder or liver, the affected organ itself does not touch the parietal peritoneum. Once this concept is clearly understood, it is easier to diagnose unusual patterns of abdominal pain that appendicitis may present. Fluids that may be present in the abdomen, and those that transmit pain in most "acute abdomens," are listed in Table 53–1.[2]

Table 53–1. RELATION OF INTRAPERITONEAL FLUIDS TO ABDOMINAL PAIN

Ascitic fluid	Not painful
Chyle	Not painful
Urine	Painful if infected or concentrated
Blood	Pain for a few hours, but may subside if bleeding stops and blood diluted
Pancreatic enzymes	Continuous pain
Hydrochloric acid	Very painful, unremitting
Inflammatory fluid or pus	Very painful
Fecal material	Very painful
Bile	Worse than others

From Folkman MJ: Appendicitis. *In* Ravitch MM, Welch KJ, Benson CD, et al, eds: Pediatric Surgery. 3rd ed. Chicago, Year Book Medical Publishers, 1979, pp 1004–1009; with permission.

If inflammatory fluid, and not the appendix itself, induces right lower quadrant pain, why was McBurney able to write in 1889 that in most instances the point of maximal tenderness was localized to an area two thirds of the way between the umbilicus and the anterior iliac spine? Why would inflammatory fluid not spread randomly around the whole abdominal cavity? It appears that the fluid is traveling by capillary action between the thin planes that exist among coils of intestine in the unopened abdomen. That this process happens is suggested by the tracking of radiopaque dye in similar planes after the dye has been injected into the peritoneal cavity, as, for example, during an intrauterine transfusion. A good way of illustrating this is to consider how blue dye might travel if it were poured into a transparent plastic sandwich bag into which other plastic bags had previously been stuffed.

The irritation of the parietal peritoneum is more localized and more intense than is the referred pain in the periumbilical region. For this reason the periumbilical pain is suppressed, just as a counterirritant applied to the chest suppresses the tickle of a cough. This observation may not apply if the appendix lies behind the cecum. In retrocecal appendicitis, the periumbilical pain may persist for days and may never shift to the right lower quadrant, even after perforation.[3]

Physical Signs

Physical signs usually begin to appear after pain has shifted to the right lower quadrant. At first, there is "wincing" tenderness in the right lower quadrant. Younger children may use their own hands to find the spot or place their hand under the examiner's hand. The examiner may use the stethoscope to listen simultaneously with palpation. The most reliable diagnostic sign of appendicitis is *localized tenderness* in the right lower quadrant. As the peritoneal irritation progresses, there is guarding (voluntary rigidity of the muscle) and, finally, rebound tenderness. Stretch receptors in the parietal peritoneum respond to the rate of stretch, not to direction. Therefore, rebound tenderness is elicited by the examiner pressing down slowly, holding for a few seconds while the patient is comfortable, and then removing the hands quickly. If the patient suddenly winces, this is true rebound tenderness, which is a reliable sign of peritoneal irritation. (There are only a few situations that do not require operation when rebound tenderness is present, for example, severe gastroenteritis, pneumonia, lead poisoning, and Henoch-Schönlein purpura.) The patient who experiences abdominal pain on the way to the hospital when the car goes over small bumps (the parents may say that they had to drive slowly because the patient could "feel" every pebble on the road) is demonstrating referred rebound tenderness. So, too, are the patients who feel abdominal pain when they step or jump from the examining table, or wince when they cough. Alternatively, patients who can hop up and down on one foot without pain will seldom have appendicitis.

Most medical students, when asked to name the signs of peritoneal irritation, will respond, "tenderness, guarding, spasm, and rebound tenderness." But these signs come only from the anterior abdominal wall. Unfortunately, many students progress far into their postgraduate years conceiving of the abdomen as having only an anterior surface. In fact, it is a six-sided cavity. The subdiaphragmatic peritoneum, the pelvic peritoneum, and the posterior and lateral aspects of the abdomen have signs unique from those of the anterior abdominal wall.

Rectal examination may reveal tenderness on the right side. The authors usually perform the rectal examination by asking the child to try to have a bowel movement while lying on the examining table on his or her back, and they ask the parents to explain that to the child with whatever euphemism is used by the family. Both the parent and the examining physician continuously encourage the child to keep pushing down during the rectal examination, and then the physician congratulates the child on the success, so that the child reinterprets the examining gloved finger as a bowel movement. This works well because the sphincter automatically dilates, and there is no expression of pain or discomfort on the child's face unless the fingertip actually compresses an inflamed area within the pelvis.

Temperature is usually elevated by 1°F in the child with nonperforated appendix. Therefore, fever is not a reliable sign of appendicitis.

Laboratory Aids

Urinalysis is the most important laboratory test used to establish the diagnosis of appendicitis. If the diagnosis is not clearly appendicitis, and if a boy has more than 15 white blood cells per high-power field, then a Gram stain should be done and the urine sent to the laboratory for culture. If there is evidence of a urinary tract infection, the child may be treated with intravenous antibiotics for a few hours. In a girl, more than 30 white blood cells per high-power field would have the same significance, but only if the urine is collected either from a midstream specimen while the labia have been spread or by catheterization of the bladder. Urine obtained from a collecting bag applied to the patient may have many white blood cells from the vagina and cannot be interpreted reliably.

The white blood cell count is less helpful. Most children who have been vomiting have an increased white blood cell count. Although there is usually an increase in polymorphonuclear neutrophils, and the total count does not usually exceed 20,000 per mm^3 in a patient with a nonperforated appendix, the total white blood cell count is influenced by so many factors that it is not dependable in arriving at the diagnosis. It is common in a child without toxicity to see a white blood cell count lower than 5,000 per mm^3 when the appendix is not perforated. Such children may have suffered an upper respiratory tract viral infection with leukopenia 2 weeks before the appendicitis. One can surmise (but not prove) that this leukopenia has persisted, despite the bacterial infection within the appendix.

Radiographs

Plain radiographs may be helpful if the diagnosis is in doubt but are otherwise not obtained routinely, except in infancy. The commonest indicator of appendicitis is a curvature of the spine concave to the right. A dilated cecum containing an air-fluid level is also common. A calcified fecalith can sometimes be seen if the film is well exposed and if two or three films are taken with the child in different positions to portray the fecalith unobscured by bony structures. Fifty per cent of children with a fecalith and abdominal pain can be expected to have a perforated appendix. When the appendix is perforated (especially in infants), there may be a paucity of bowel gas in the right lower quadrant and an increase in the thickness of the lateral abdominal wall owing to soft tissue edema and evidence of free peritoneal fluid.[4] The appendix has usually perforated by the time a child younger than 2 years of age is brought to the physician. Although only about 2% of all children treated for appendicitis are younger than 2 years, the abdominal film assumes greater value because the diagnosis is difficult at this age. Common radiographic abnormalities in these infants are listed in Table 53–2.

A chest film may also be helpful when the diagnosis is in doubt, because lower lobe pneumonia may refer pain to the midabdomen.

The use of ultrasound in the diagnosis of appendicitis has gained popularity, but the data provided are operator dependent and easily misinterpreted. This caveat makes effective communication between the surgeon and the ultrasonographer of paramount importance; in fact, the authors prefer to be present for the ultrasound examination when possible. The normal appendix is usually not visualized on ultrasound. However, a thickened or noncompressible appendix may be seen (Fig. 53–1), as well as periappendiceal fluid, a fecalith, or even a periappendiceal abscess.[5] Ultrasound should be reserved for the difficult diagnostic cases, since it delays surgery. However, in selected cases with an experienced sonographer, the authors have found this test to be valuable, especially in girls, for whom gynecologic pathology may confuse the issue. It is important to remember that negative results from an ultrasound scan do not rule out the diagnosis of appendicitis but must be considered as factors in the overall clinical picture.

Table 53–2. RADIOGRAPHIC ABNORMALITIES IN 25 INFANTS WITH APPENDICITIS

	No. of Patients	%
Abnormal gas pattern	21	87
Free peritoneal fluid	21	84
Scoliosis	18	72
Psoas obscuration	14	56
Thickened abdominal wall	8	32
Fecalith	8	32
Abscess	5	20
No diagnostic abnormality	3	12

From Wilkinson RH, Bartlett RH, Eraklis AJ: Diagnosis of appendicitis in infancy: The value of abdominal radiographs. Am J Dis Child 1969; 118:687–690; with permission. Copyright 1969, American Medical Association.

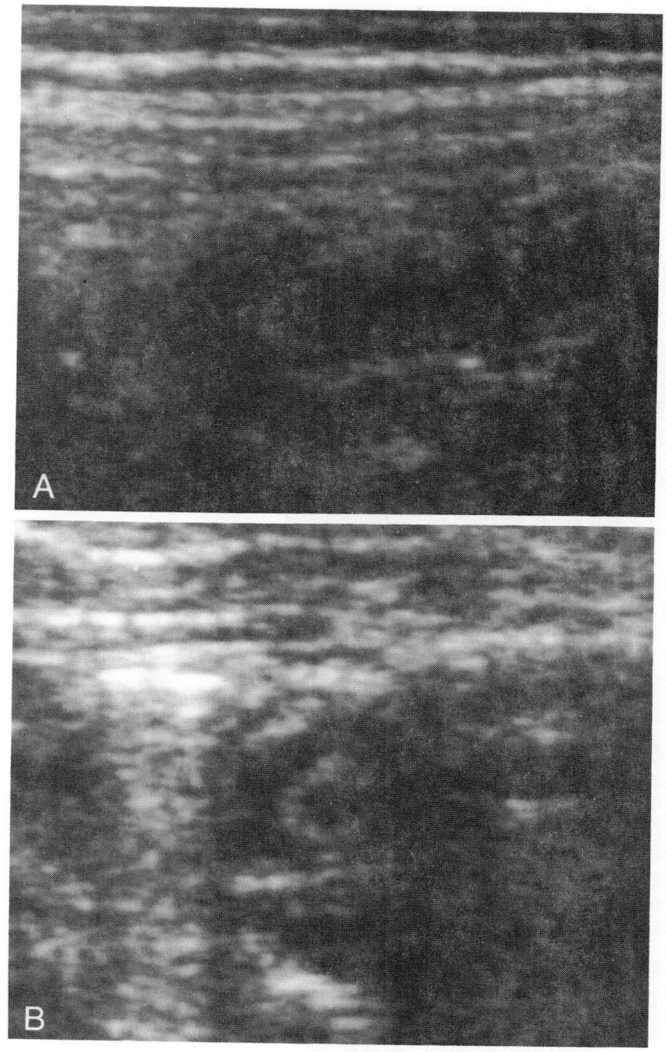

Figure 53–1. Ultrasound scans showing a thickened, noncompressible appendix in longitudinal *(A)* and transverse *(B)* views in a 13-year-old girl with a 12-hour history of abdominal pain and nausea. Findings at operation were acute appendicitis without perforation or fecalith.

Other radiologic tests, such as a barium enema and an intravenous pyelogram, may provide useful information, such as demonstrating a partially obstructed ureter or an extrinsic impression on the cecum (Fig. 53–2). These tests are reserved for more chronic cases that present as diagnostic dilemmas.

The Child with a Perforated Appendix

Once the appendix has perforated, the child lies still. The right leg may be drawn up. In several of the authors' patients, the right hip flexion was so marked that osteomyelitis or pyarthrosis of the hip had to be ruled out. The child often breathes with an open mouth because of slight tachypnea. The end of each inspiration may be stopped short because of abdominal pain. There may

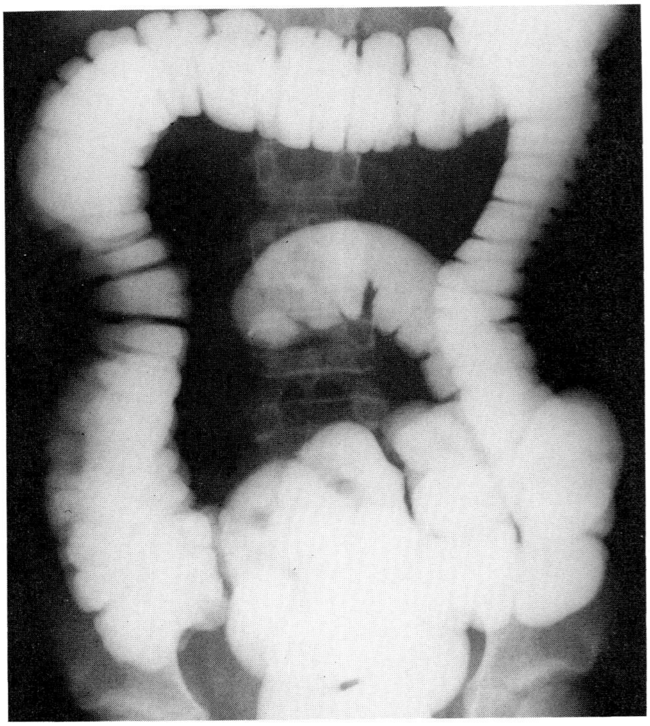

Figure 53–2. Barium enema from a 12-year-old girl with a history of intermittent abdominal pain and nausea of many months' duration. She presented this time with nausea, and plain radiographs suggested small bowel obstruction. This examination shows an extrinsic compression of the cecum and an abrupt cut-off of contrast material refluxing through the terminal ileum. At operation, she was found to have an inflamed appendix, with phlegmon in the right lower quadrant and multiple adhesions with small bowel obstruction.

be a change in the vomiting pattern. Although a child with early appendicitis vomits once or twice or not at all, after perforation occurs vomiting is more frequent, and the vomitus may contain small bowel contents because of paralytic ileus. The child is hot and dry, with a temperature of 101 to 104°F. In infants, pain and muscle spasm may be detected over the entire abdominal wall, whereas in older children the signs of perforation may remain localized to the right lower quadrant or lower abdomen for awhile. Retrocecal perforated appendix is the exception, because palpation of the anterior abdomen may elicit few or no signs. The patient may complain only of periumbilical pain.

Many children with a perforated appendix have "diarrhea," and the physician then makes the erroneous diagnosis of gastroenteritis. However, the diarrhea accompanying perforated appendicitis is only a small amount of mucus or slime that is the result of irritation of the rectosigmoid colon by inflammatory fluid; it is not a high-volume diarrhea. The child is dehydrated owing to plasma loss within the abdominal cavity from the inflamed peritoneum. In contrast, the dehydrated appearance of a child with true gastroenteritis is due mainly to high-volume losses of fluid from diarrhea and vomiting.

The child who has been "sick for a week" probably harbors a large appendiceal abscess, walled off from the peritoneal cavity. When the abscess begins to leak into the abdominal cavity, the child shows signs of extreme toxicity, oliguria, mottling of the skin, evidence of gram-negative septicemia, and a decreasing platelet count.

Peristalsis is infrequent or absent. Occasional high-pitched sounds may be heard over a dilated intestinal loop. Radiographs show signs of paralytic ileus or partial obstruction of the small intestine. Rectal tenderness is marked. If rectal tenderness is absent, the ruptured appendix may reside high in the right retroperitoneal space.

DIFFERENTIAL DIAGNOSIS

Appendicitis is a common disease with many uncommon presentations. The authors have seen appendicitis present as a subphrenic abscess, an incarcerated hernia, an intermittent small bowel obstruction, and diverticulitis. Appendicitis must be included in the differential diagnosis of any patient who presents with abdominal pain. Children younger than 2 years of age and obese patients, particularly premenarchal girls, represent the most difficult diagnostic groups, in the authors' experience. Obesity interfers with the physical examination by making it difficult to elicit direct tenderness and guarding. Very young children are unable to give a history. More than 70% of very young children with appendicitis will have perforated appendix by the time of presentation.[6, 7]

Gastroenteritis. Gastroenteritis is the commonest cause of abdominal pain in children who arrive at an emergency department. The commonest error is to diagnose gastroenteritis in a child who actually has retrocecal appendicitis. Some signs that distinguish the two conditions are outlined in Table 53–3.

Urinary Tract Infection. If a urinary tract infection is present, the fever and the leukocytosis may be increased

Table 53–3. DIFFERENTIAL DIAGNOSIS OF APPENDICITIS AND GASTROENTERITIS

	Gastroenteritis	Appendicitis
Onset of periumbilical pain	Coexistent with or after vomiting	Before vomiting
Diarrhea	High-volume, frequent	Mucous or low-volume, "irritative" type of diarrhea; infrequent
Peristalsis	High-frequency, low-pitch	Low-frequency or absent; high-pitch if paralytic ileus
Rectal tenderness	Usually absent	Usually present
Rebound tenderness (or referred rebound tenderness, such as "painful ride to hospital")	Usually absent	Often present, especially in cases of perforation

From Folkman MJ: Appendicitis. *In* Ravitch MM, Welch KJ, Benson CD, et al, eds: Pediatric Surgery. 3rd ed. Chicago, Year Book Medical Publishers, 1979, pp 1004–1009; with permission.

out of proportion to the abdominal signs, in contrast with the usual signs of appendicitis. If there is pyuria and the urine has been collected correctly, and the signs are not clearly consistent with appendicitis, then it is permissible to treat the patient with intravenous antibiotics for a few hours. However, if the patient does not improve rapidly, or if the diagnosis is still in doubt, the authors proceed with an appendectomy.

Constipation. Constipation is a common cause of abdominal pain in older children. The right lower quadrant pain persists or may be intermittent in a constipated child, but it rarely progresses. If an abdominal film shows a colon filled with feces, the authors give a small Fleet's enema. If all symptoms clear after a large bowel movement, they allow the child to return home.

Bacterial Enteritis. It is common for children with infectious enteritis, particularly from *Yersinia* or *Salmonella*, to present with abdominal pain. Usually, there is more than the expected amount of diarrhea, but right lower quadrant pain is common, and there may even be a shift of pain from the periumbilical region to the right lower quadrant. These patients often appear quite toxic, and leukocytosis is prominent. Cramps and high fever also are frequent. At operation, the appendix is not inflamed. Culture of lymph nodes or stool may yield *Salmonella*, and *Yersinia* may be diagnosed from stool cultures or serology. *Campylobacter* can also cause a similar picture. Typically, there are cramps, fever, watery diarrhea, and, frequently, blood per rectum. The diagnosis is made by culture of the organism from stool (see Chapter 46).

Crohn's Disease. Regional enteritis has a more protracted course than does appendicitis. Often, the child with regional enteritis has had bowel symptoms for a year or more, including crampy abdominal pain, diarrhea, and failure to thrive. Occasionally, however, the presentation is similar to that of appendicitis, and the first discovery of the disease is during appendectomy. At operation, the bowel, usually the terminal ileum, is thickened with mesenteric fat creeping over the bowel wall. A biopsy specimen of an ileocolic mesenteric lymph node often shows granulomas. If the cecum is uninvolved, and a secure closure of the appendiceal stump can be achieved, it is recommended to remove the appendix in this instance. Primary resection of the affected bowel should not be undertaken (see Chapter 59).

Pelvic Inflammatory Disease. Pelvic inflammatory disease (PID) is also a diagnostic consideration. The onset of abdominal pain is often preceded by the menstrual period. The pain usually begins in the lower quadrants rather than in the periumbilical area, as it does in appendicitis. Pain on motion of the cervix is the hallmark of PID, and there may be bilateral adnexal tenderness. Gram stain of the purulent cervical discharge may reveal gram-negative intracellular diplococci. The sedimentation rate is usually higher than 15 mm per hour in most cases, whereas in appendicitis, the sedimentation rate is almost always normal (1–10 mm per hour). If the differential diagnosis is in doubt, or if the signs persist after initiation of treatment, it is wise to do an appendectomy. The authors performed surgery on young adolescents with appendicitis who were originally thought to have gonorrhea, because the cervical smear revealed gram-negative diplococci. Culture in these patients showed these were only the saprophytic *Neisseria* that may be present normally in the vagina.

Ovarian Cyst. Pathology in the ovary can mimic appendicitis. The commonest cause is rupture of an ovarian cyst. The pain is usually quite abrupt in onset and begins in the right lower quadrant. There is frequently tenderness. If the girl is menstruating, the pain often occurs in midcycle, but ovarian cysts are frequent at menarche as well. Ultrasound may aid in delineating free fluid or other cysts in the ovary, or it may indicate a recently ruptured follicular cyst. If the diagnosis is in doubt, laparoscopy may help define the pathologic state, but this test does not rule out appendicitis unless the appendix is fully visualized.

Iliac Adenitis. Again, the pain associated with iliac adenitis begins in the right lower quadrant or inguinal area and not in the periumbilical region. The symptoms usually extend over many more days than in most cases of appendicitis. There may be a history of some small injury to the foot a few weeks before the inguinal pain. A careful examination of the lower extremities is essential. There may be an inguinal mass or obliteration of the inguinal crease.

Pneumonia. Right lower lobe pneumonia may refer pain to the abdomen through the T10 and T11 nerves. A chest film, presence of abnormal respiratory signs (flaring, grunting, tachypnea), and increased toxicity should help confirm the diagnosis. Every other year or so the authors see a child in whom the right lower lobe infiltrate and the fever do not resolve after 2 days of antibiotic treatment, and the underlying process turns out to be a localized rupture of a high retrocecal appendix with a collection of fluid beneath the right diaphragm.

Mesenteric Adenitis. Mesenteric adenitis is most likely caused by a viral infection or other inflammation of the lymph nodes clustered in the mesentery of the terminal ileum. The authors' policy is not to make this diagnosis until after appendectomy.

The Cost of Diagnostic Error. The sequelae of perforation are so dangerous that if the diagnosis appears to be appendicitis, even if one is not absolutely certain, it is always preferable to remove the appendix before perforation and accept the occasional error of removing a normal appendix. This course is preferable to the opposite diagnostic error of waiting so long that perforation occurs. If the diagnosis is in doubt, the authors prefer to admit the child *for repeated observation by the same physician.* Sending the child home to return the next day only ensures that the child will be seen by a different physician, who cannot accurately judge whether the signs have progressed. There continues to be a small but definite mortality associated with appendicitis in the United States, and almost all these deaths are associated with a delay in diagnosis. The average length of hospital stay for the child with acute appendicitis at Children's Hospital—Boston is 2 or 3 days, whereas the child with a perforated appendix will stay for 10 days and incur much higher costs.

TREATMENT

Appendectomy on the day of diagnosis is the ideal treatment. Even in a sick child who must be prepared with rehydration, antibiotics, correction of electrolyte imbalance and ketosis, and reduction of fever, the authors have always been able to perform the operation the same day. If the child is toxic, or if perforation is suspected, acetaminophen per rectum is given to reduce fever, and antibiotics, usually ampicillin, clindamycin, and gentamicin, are started intravenously. A nasogastric tube is inserted to empty the stomach. If an experienced pediatric anesthetist is available, he or she may prefer to place the tube after the child is asleep. The child may be comforted preoperatively by morphine, 0.1 mg per kg. However, atropine is withheld until just before induction of anesthesia and is then given intravenously to avoid additional elevation of temperature.

Operative Technique

A transverse muscle-splitting incision is used, more lateral to the midline in a child than in an adult, because the rectus muscle is relatively wider in a child. Peritoneal fluid cultures are obtained on first entering the abdomen. It is always possible to remove the appendix, even in the presence of an abscess or a severe perforation with peritonitis. Only rarely have the authors resorted to mere drainage of the abscess, followed by later appendectomy. It is important not to leave behind a fecalith that may have fallen out of a perforated appendix during the procedure. The safest approach is to mobilize the anterior cecal wall out of the abdomen, so that the entire appendix lies above the abdominal wall. Rarely, one has to enlarge the incision slightly and carry the dissection along the lateral gutter of the right colon for a few centimeters (as in the beginning of a right colectomy) to deliver a difficult retrocecal appendix. At the completion of the appendectomy, copious amounts of saline or dilute cefazolin solution are used to irrigate the abdomen, being sure to remove all the irrigant prior to closure. The authors always leave two small Penrose drains in place if the appendix has perforated or is severely gangrenous. One drain is left in the pelvis, and one is led up the right gutter; both drains exit at the lateral side of the incision. These drains are then removed over a 3-day period, beginning on postoperative day 7.

On extremely rare occasions, the appendiceal stump is so gangrenous or the cecum so edematous that the stump cannot be inverted or closed safely. In this situation, it is wisest to do a limited ileocecal resection with an end-to-end, two-layer ileo–right colic anastomosis. The authors attempt to position the anastomosis away from the abscess cavity and to separate the two with omentum.

The authors occasionally see a child with such diffuse right lower quadrant tenderness or induration of the abdominal wall that is is difficult to distinguish between an appendiceal abscess or an abscess in the inguinal lymph nodes secondary to inguinal adenitis. In these instances, they first remove the appendix through a low McBurney incision. If the appendix is normal, the peritoneum and transverse fascia are then closed, and an extraperitoneal dissection is continued inferiorly toward the iliac nodes. If pus is obtained by needle aspiration, drainage is established through the same incision.

Antibiotics

Antibiotics are begun preoperatively for a child who appears toxic and has evidence of perforation. The child with uncomplicated acute appendicitis receives intravenous cefazolin for 24 hours perioperatively. If a perforated appendix is found at the time of operation, then three antibiotics (ampicillin, gentamicin, and clindamycin) are begun intravenously in the recovery room and continued for 10 days. Gentamicin dosage is adjusted based on blood peak and trough levels. If resistant organisms, particularly *Pseudomonas*, grow from intraoperative peritoneal cultures, antibiotics are changed appropriately. This treatment regimen has been used at the Children's Hospital—Boston for the past 10 years. Obviously, this regimen may have to be changed in the future, because the anaerobic flora change their sensitivity to antibiotics. However, compared with any other approach, this course of therapy has resulted in a low incidence of postoperative abdominal or pelvic abscess.[8]

COMPLICATIONS

Intestinal Obstruction. Paralytic ileus may persist for 3 to 5 days following removal of a perforated appendix. Occasionally, this ileus is followed by a few days of normal intestinal function and then by mechanical obstruction with cramping pain. Most of the patients with obstruction can be managed with nasogastric tube decompression until the inflammatory adhesions subside. Repeat laparotomy at this time is meddlesome, unless there is evidence of strangulation or closed-loop obstruction. In contrast, obstructions that occur more than 4 weeks postoperatively may require prompt operation. Surgeons who are not experienced with young children often are confused about the appropriate timing for re-exploration. Recently, a child was transferred to the Children's Hospital—Boston from another hospital, where a surgeon had performed a re-exploration for intestinal obstruction 5 days after the removal of a perforated appendix. No distinct point of obstruction was found, although many inflammatory adhesions were present. After a number of postsurgical wound complications, the intestine began to function. However, 1 month later, there was a new episode of intestinal obstruction. This complication was treated with insertion of a nasogastric tube, but after a few days the child's condition deteriorated, and at operation, a loop of gangrenous bowel was found to be tethered by a single strong adhesive band. The initial reoperation was too early, and the second was too late.

Abscess. Many abdominal or pelvic abscesses subside

spontaneously while patients are receiving antibiotic therapy and probably represent a phlegmon or cellulitis with agglutinated loops of bowel rather than a true abscess (see Chapter 18). The progress of these masses can be followed by repeat rectal examinations or with computed tomography (CT) scans. If the mass is not enlarging and the child, treated with antibiotics, is not toxic, it is safe to wait as long as necessary for the abscess to point and be drained. With the use of ultrasound and CT scanning, it is frequently possible to drain such abscesses percutaneously, leaving a small drain in the cavity. This procedure can usually be done with sedation and local anesthesia.

The authors have seen one patient with bilateral ureteral obstruction secondary to retroperitoneal inflammation after removal of a perforated appendix at another institution. This condition responded to percutaneous drainage of the kidneys and intravenous antibiotics and subsequently resolved completely.

Operative intervention is necessary when the child remains toxic and tender, despite percutaneous drainage and appropriate antibiotic coverage, or if the abscess cavity looks too complex to drain using the percutaneous approach. If fever and leukocytosis persist in the absence of pelvic inflammation, a chest film, ultrasound, or CT scan may reveal subphrenic inflammation. These symptoms may still subside with antibiotics. A true subphrenic abscess, however, requires drainage in the appropriate manner. A subphrenic abscess is almost always accompanied by a sympathetic pleural effusion.

The commonest organism found in appendiceal pelvic abscess is *Bacteroides*. The use of clindamycin when the appendix has perforated has markedly reduced the incidence of abscess formation.

Nutritional Complications. If paralytic ileus is prolonged, a variety of insidious secondary complications may appear, such as low-grade fever, malabsorption, chronic diarrhea, and poor wound healing. A cachectic child may require intravenous hyperalimentation.

Sterility. Sterility may be a complication of a perforated appendix in the girl who has developed a pelvic abscess or pelvic peritonitis. Although the literature is controversial on this topic,[9] women of childbearing age who have a previous diagnosis of perforated appendix and pelvic abscess may have an increased rate of infertility.[10]

Appendicitis in Leukemia. Patients with leukemia who are in symptomatic relapse suffer a number of complications after appendectomy that may be fatal. They may have recurrent hemorrhage, wound separation, and slough of intestinal closures resulting in septicemia. In a leukemic child with appendicitis, one may try to induce a rapid remission before attempting appendectomy, because the mortality from operation during relapse probably outweighs the risk of nonoperative therapy carried out while trying to produce a remission of the leukemia.

Perforated Appendix in Children Younger Than One Year of Age. In neonates or infants with a perforated appendix, the major postoperative complication is gram-negative septicemia. The authors have learned to follow the platelet count as an indicator of the severity of the septicemia. Animal experiments by Das and associates[11] indicate that the platelet count decreases because the platelets absorb (and inactivate) endotoxin that is diffusing into the blood stream from the peritoneal cavity. In addition to vigorous antibiotic therapy, platelet transfusions are given as necessary to keep the platelet count at least as high as 100,000 per mm^3 or higher. The rationale is not to prevent bleeding, but to try to reduce the amount of unbound circulating endotoxin. Any neonate or infant younger than 1 year of age presenting with a perforated appendix should be investigated for Hirschsprung's disease.

SUMMARY

Appendicitis is noteworthy for the diagnostic problems it may present. The guideposts to successful management include awareness of the time sequence and pace of developing clinical symptoms; a clear understanding of the physiology of abdominal pain and its shifts in location; and, finally, perhaps a willingness to ensure that the puzzling patient is observed at frequent intervals by the same physicians as the clinical picture emerges.

REFERENCES

1. Fitz RJ: Perforating inflammation of vermiform appendix with special reference to its early diagnosis and treatment. Am J Med Sci 1886; 92:321–345.
2. Folkman MJ: Appendicitis. *In* Ravitch MM, Welch KJ, Benson CD, et al, eds: Pediatric Surgery. 3rd ed. Chicago, Year Book Medical Publishers, 1979, pp 1004–1009.
3. Poole GV: Anatomic basis for delayed diagnosis of appendicitis. South Med J 1990; 83:771–773.
4. Zona JG, Selke AC, Bellin RP: Radiologic aids in the diagnosis of appendicitis in children. South Med J 1975; 68:1373–1376.
5. Teele RL, Share JC: Ultrasonography of infants and children. Philadelphia, WB Saunders, 1991; pp 346–356.
6. Wilkinson RH, Bartlett RH, Eraklis AJ: Diagnosis of appendicitis in infancy: The value of abdominal radiographs. Am J Dis Child 1969; 118:687–690.
7. Rappaport WD, Peterson M, Stanton C: Factors responsible for the high perforation rate seen in early childhood appendicitis. Am Surg 1989; 55:602–605.
8. Schwartz MZ, Tapper D, Solenberger RI: Management of perforated appendicitis in children: The controversy continues. Ann Surg 1983; 197:407–411.
9. Puri P, McGuinness EP, Quiney EJ: Fertility following perforated appendicitis in girls. J Pediatr Surg 1989; 24:547–549.
10. Mueller BA, Daling JR, Moore DE, et al: Appendectomy and risk of tubal infertility. N Engl J Med 1986; 315:1506–1508.
11. Das J, Schwartz AA, Folkman J: Intraperitoneal platelets: Protective role in rats with endotoxemia of peritoneal origin. Surg Forum 1974; 25:37.

Chapter 54

Hirschsprung's Disease

SYLVAIN KLEINHAUS and SCOTT J. BOLEY

Hirschsprung's disease, or congenital aganglionic megacolon, is the commonest cause of lower intestinal obstruction in neonates. The classic clinical manifestations were first described and recognized as being a separate entity in 1887 by Harold Hirschsprung,[1] but the basic pathophysiologic defect was first described in the 1940s, and the first curative operation was presented by Swenson and Bill in 1948.[2] Since that time, progress has been made in the understanding of Hirschsprung's disease, but much remains to be learned.

PATHOPHYSIOLOGY

The main defect in Hirschsprung's disease is an abnormal innervation of the bowel beginning at the anus, including the internal sphincter, and extending proximally for a variable distance. The commonest transition from abnormal to normal bowel is in the rectosigmoid area. The basic histologic finding is the absence of Meissner's and Auerbach's plexuses, and where these ganglia are absent there are hypertrophied nerve bundles between the circular and the longitudinal muscles and in the submucosa (Fig. 54–1*A* and *B*). These are the parasympathetic ganglia and nerves that control normal contraction and relaxation, and they can be best visualized by the use of an acetylcholinesterase stain (Fig. 54–2*A* and *B*). In addition, there are adrenergic and nonadrenergic modulators that contribute to normal function. The exact role of these modulators is uncertain, and the concentration of these elements varies from case to case and from level to level within the bowel, which may help explain the variation in severity of symptoms from one patient to the next, even when the level of aganglionosis may be the same.

INCIDENCE AND DISTRIBUTION

In the survey by the American Academy of Pediatrics (AAP) Surgical Section,[3] the overall ratio of male to female patients was 3.8 to 1. The ratio was 2.8 to 1 in long segment disease and 2.2 to 1, male to female, in total colonic aganglionosis. There was no reported difference between blacks and whites in incidence of Hirschsprung's disease. Family incidence becomes a factor only in very long segment disease involving the entire colon; there was a 21% incidence of aganglionosis in a family member in these patients. In the same AAP survey, the extent of aganglionosis showed the commonest levels to be the rectosigmoid and the sigmoid areas (Table 54–1).

In most cases of Hirschsprung's disease, the zone of aganglionosis extends proximally from the anus to a certain point above which the bowel is normal. A small number of substantiated cases have been reported with skip areas, that is, an area of normal bowel between two areas of aganglionosis. In any case in which postoperative intestinal dysfunction is encountered, the presence of a skip area must be considered.[4]

Hirschsprung's disease is not classically associated with other congenital anomalies; however, in a report from Japan[5] there was a greater than expected incidence of Down's syndrome (2.9%) and cardiac anomalies (2.5%), especially in the cases with longer segment disease.

CLINICAL FEATURES

Ninety percent or more of normal neonates pass meconium within the first 24 hours of life, and 99% by 48 hours of life. Any infant who does not pass meconium by 48 hours of age should be considered as having Hirschsprung's disease until proved otherwise. Some patients with Hirschsprung's disease pass meconium within the first day of life but subsequently have infrequent stools. Normally, the gastrocolic reflex is well developed in neonates, and they stool after each feeding, four to six times daily. Infants with Hirschsprung's disease stool less frequently, in some instances only once or twice a week, and often do not come to the pediatrician's attention until the first postnatal visit. At that time, the infant will probably have a distended abdomen, unless seen immediately after a bowel movement, and even then will have stool palpable in the colon. Sometimes the child presents with diarrhea as the predominant sign. A rectal examination should be performed; in most instances, sphincter tone will be normal, not extra tight as some clinicians might suspect. Care should be taken to stand at the head of the examining table, since removal of the examining finger is almost

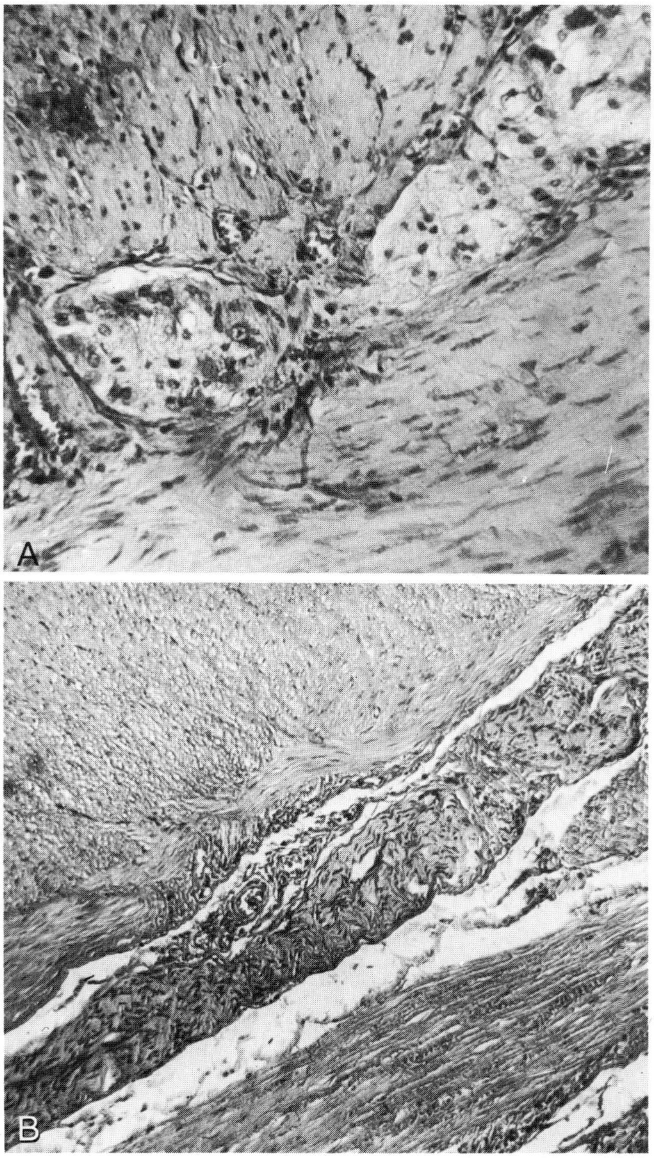

Figure 54–1. A, Normal histology of intermuscular ganglia. Hematoxylin and eosin stain. *B*, Hirschsprung's disease with hypertrophied nerve bundles and absence of ganglion cells. Hematoxylin and eosin stain.

certain to be followed by an explosive discharge of foul-smelling liquid stool. This is almost pathognomonic of Hirschsprung's disease with early enterocolitis. The early diagnosis of Hirschsprung's disease, before the onset of enterocolitis, has been shown to be essential in reducing the morbidity and mortality of Hirschsprung's disease,[3] and any neonate in whom there is a suspicion of Hirschsprung's disease should have a diagnostic investigation as soon as possible. It is the authors' policy not to discharge from the hospital any neonate in whom Hirschsprung's disease is suspected until the diagnosis has been either established or excluded. Whereas in the not so distant past, Hirschsprung's disease went frequently unrecognized until the second or third year of life, and sometimes even later, this is no longer common, and the child with a protuberant potbelly, chronic constipation, and stunted growth is rarely seen. However, in those populations that shun medical advice, these children can still be found.

DIAGNOSIS

In the past, the mainstays in establishing the diagnosis of Hirschsprung's disease were the barium enema and a full-thickness rectal biopsy. The barium enema, although still used widely, has several shortcomings. First, it is not usually diagnostic before 7 to 14 days of age. The barium enema diagnosis is based primarily on the presence of a "transition zone," which is a funnel-shaped area of intestine with a normal distal area and a dilated proximal area (Fig. 54–3). This dilatation is the result of a functional obstruction in the distal bowel caused by the nonrelaxation of the aganglionic bowel. The proximal bowel proceeds with its normal contractions and forces more and more stool distally against this functional obstruction. The most proximal portion of the aganglionic bowel distends, as does the normal bowel above it. In addition, the normal bowel hypertrophies in an attempt to overcome the obstruction. This process does not occur in utero, since the defecatory process normally does not begin before delivery, and the transition zone develops in the first weeks of life and is rarely seen prior to 1 week of age. Barium enemas also require a delayed film at 24 or 48 hours to document colonic emptying. If a substantial portion of the instilled barium is still present in the colon on the delayed films, there is increased suspicion of Hirschsprung's disease even in the absence of a transition zone. It is also important to take lateral views of the pelvis with the contrast material in place, but with the instilling catheter removed, so that low transition zones can be observed (Fig. 54–4). All these signs, although suggestive, are usually followed by a full-thickness rectal biopsy for absolute confirmation of Hirschsprung's disease prior to the performance of a colostomy.

The full-thickness biopsy is not a benign procedure in a neonate. General anesthesia is required, and the procedure itself entails a certain morbidity. The biopsy must be taken at least 1.5 cm above the dentate line, since the distal 1 to 2 cm of bowel are normally hypoganglionic or aganglionic, and the specimen should be at least 2 cm long. It is important that the surgeon orient the specimen for the pathologist so that the critical

Table 54–1. EXTENT OF AGANGLIONOSIS

Area	Percentage
Rectum-rectosigmoid	30
Sigmoid	44
Left colon	11
Splenic flexure	4
Transverse colon	2
Right colon	1
Total colonic and above	8

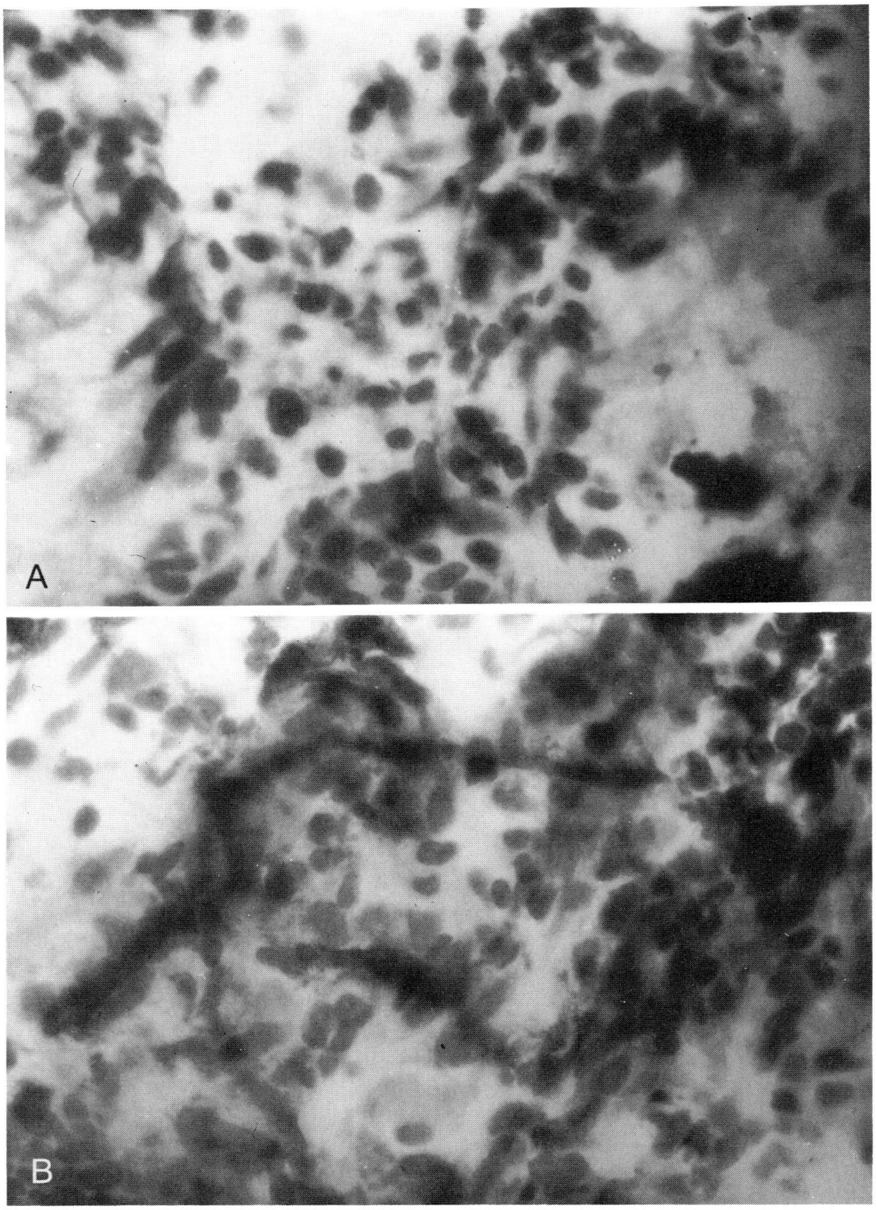

Figure 54–2. *A,* Suction biopsy with acetylcholinesterase stain demonstrating normal histology. *B,* Acetylcholinesterase stain with obvious neurofibrils typical of Hirschsprung's disease.

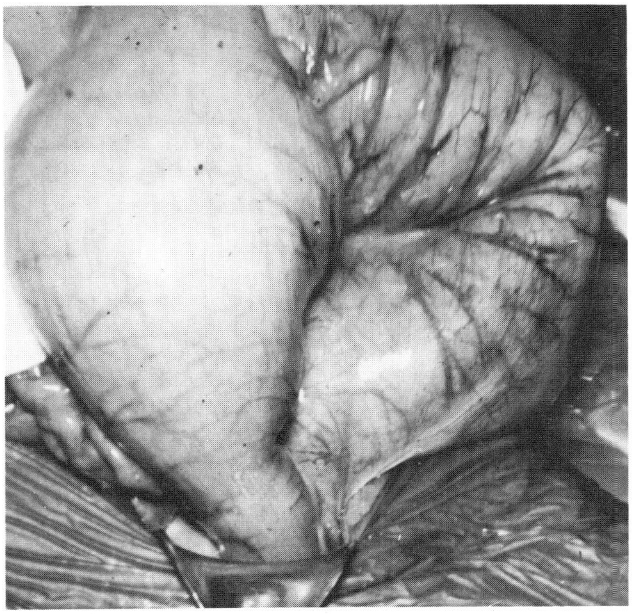

Figure 54–3. Hirschsprung's disease. Distended proximal sigmoid colon demonstrating funnel-shaped transition zone tapering down to normal-sized (but aganglionic) distal rectosigmoid.

interfaces between the muscle layers and the submucosa can be properly examined and interpreted. A full-thickness rectal biopsy also makes the performance of the major procedure more difficult, regardless of the operation or technique employed. The postbiopsy scarring makes dissection within the pelvis more time consuming and obscures the tissue planes, the identification of which is crucial for optimal results.

The authors believe that anorectal manometry and suction biopsies are, currently, the most reliable indicators of Hirschsprung's disease. Manometry can be done at any age and should be diagnostic. When the rectal balloon is inflated, there should be reflex relaxation of the internal sphincter. The manometry, when properly done and interpreted, has been specific; if relaxation is seen, the patient almost certainly does not have Hirschsprung's disease (Fig. 54–5*A* and *B*). Immediately following the manometry, the authors insert the suction biopsy apparatus and get two biopsy specimens, one at 2 cm and one at 3 cm above the dentate line. An adequate biopsy specimen has enough submucosa for the pathologist to identify ganglion cells, if present (see Fig. 54–1). In addition, the specimen is stained for acetylcholinesterase.[6] The presence of large numbers of positively stained neurofibrils is suggestive of Hirschsprung's disease and, in the absence of ganglion cells, is considered diagnostic (see Fig. 54–2). Again, the level of the biopsy, its depth, and the expertise of the pathologist are of paramount importance for proper interpretation.

If there is a discrepancy among the results of the anorectal manometry, the suction biopsies, and the barium enema, the first two tests are repeated. If there is still some doubt about the exact diagnosis, a full-thickness biopsy is performed.

ENTEROCOLITIS ASSOCIATED WITH HIRSCHSPRUNG'S DISEASE

The entercolitis associated with Hirschsprung's disease carries a significantly increased morbidity and mortality rate, and every effort must be made to prevent the occurrence of enterocolitis. Although its exact cause is unknown, it is believed that a combination of factors acts in concert to result in the enterocolitis of Hirschsprung's disease. The lack of relaxation of the distal bowel causes the stool to stagnate in the rectum or more proximal bowel, resulting in an increased number and quantity of fecal breakdown products. As the bowel distends, the intraluminal pressure increases. The resultant decrease in intramural capillary blood flow adversely affects the protective mucosal barrier, allowing the fecal breakdown products, bacteria, and toxins to attack the bowel wall itself and eventually enter the blood stream. Clinically, the picture is one of abdominal distention, foul-smelling diarrhea that is frequently bloody, and an elevated temperature and sepsis. Treatment consists of nasogastric decompression, intravenous fluid resuscitation, broad-spectrum antibiotics, and warm saline enemas for colonic decompression. Re-

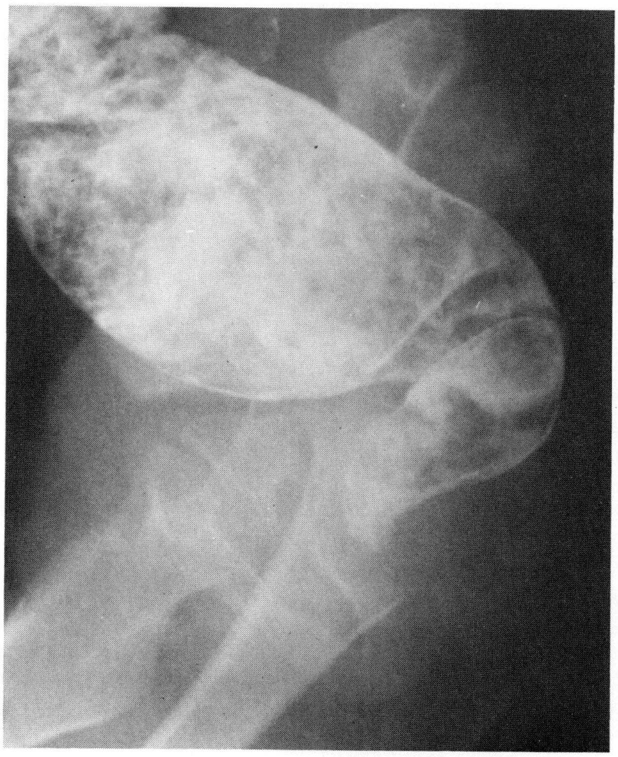

Figure 54–4. Barium enema examination (lateral view of pelvis) demonstrating dilated proximal colon and transition zone. The diameter of the rectum is usually larger than that of the sigmoid.

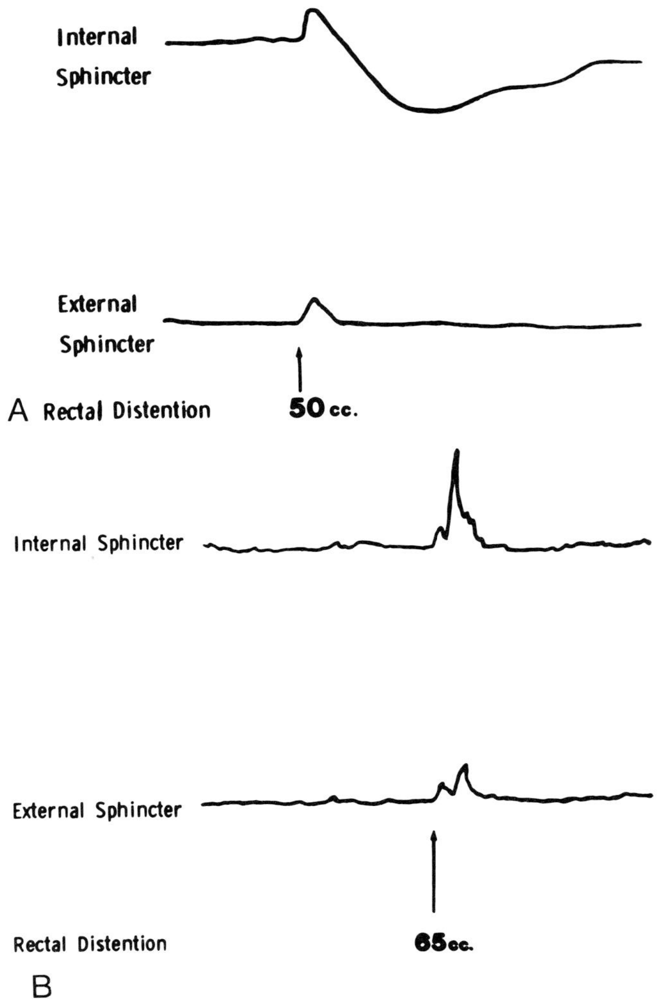

Figure 54–5. Anorectal manometry. *A*, Normal pattern showing internal sphincter relaxation after stimulation by inflation of rectal balloon. *B*, Hirschsprung's disease manometry with no relaxation of internal sphincter after distention by rectal balloon.

peated roentgenograms of the abdomen are necessary for monitoring bowel distention and possible perforation. A proximal colostomy is performed as soon as the child's condition permits.

Prevention of enterocolitis can best be accomplished by the early detection of Hirschsprung's disease. It has been shown that if the diagnosis can be made in the first month of life, especially within the first 2 weeks of life, the incidence of enterocolitis can be significantly reduced, but unfortunately, not eliminated.[3, 7]

Even with the colostomy in place, enterocolitis may persist or recur,[8] and following the definitive operations, there is a recurrent enterocolitis rate as high as 15%, depending on the operation.[3] Persistent anorectal spasm or stricture is often implicated in these postoperative bouts of enterocolitis, but this is certainly not the only cause. Disturbed immune function and mucin production may also play a role in the persistence of this serious complication. Severe small bowel mucosal injury and intractable diarrhea requiring long-term nutritional support may be seen following marked bouts of enterocolitis.[9]

TREATMENT

Once the diagnosis has been confirmed, the only definitive treatment of children with Hirschsprung's disease is operative relief of the functional obstruction produced by the abnormally innervated lower bowel. However, the choice of operation, its timing, and the extent of staging are not unanimous. The options are to perform the operation of choice as soon as convenient in the neonatal period, or to wait until the infant is 6 months to a year old and weighs at least 15 pounds. If the definitive operation is to be delayed, a temporary colostomy is usually performed. There is also a difference of opinion as to where this temporary colostomy should be placed: sigmoid, or left or right transverse colon. Some surgeons, especially in Europe, individualize their treatment and attempt to manage the infants with enemas, suppositories, and dilatations without a colostomy before the definitive procedure. A colostomy is performed only if these measures are unsuccessful in maintaining the child distention free with regular bowel movements and preventing the onset of enterocolitis. The prevention of enterocolitis is essential in minimizing the morbidity and mortality of Hirschsprung's disease.

If the diagnosis of Hirschsprung's disease is confirmed in a child prior to the development of enterocolitis, the authors create a temporary colostomy and perform the definitive operation when the child is between 6 and 12 months of age, weighs at least 15 pounds, or both. The colostomy is performed as soon as feasible after confirmation of the diagnosis to avoid the hazards of enterocolitis and sudden deterioration of the child's condition, which can develop rapidly, regardless of an apparent benign clinical picture.

If enterocolitis is already present at the time of diagnosis, the authors first decompress the bowel with warm saline irrigations through a rectal tube and resuscitate the child with intravenous fluids, electrolytes, and blood products. Broad-spectrum antibiotic coverage is also administered intravenously. A large-sized nasogastric tube is passed and placed on constant low suction. The authors defer the colostomy until the patient's general condition improves and stabilizes, except in those cases in which the colon cannot be adequately decompressed by nonoperative means or perforation has occurred. All children who have had enterocolitis are maintained with the colostomy for at least 1 year before the definitive operation is undertaken. This delay allows maximum healing to take place in the defunctionalized colon and facilitates the later dissection.

In those infants in whom there has been no enterocolitis, the authors usually place the colostomy in the most distal, easily accessible ganglionic colon above the transition zone, so that the colostomy may be easily included in the excised specimen at the time of the definitive operation. The presence of normal ganglion cells at the colostomy site must be confirmed by frozen section. Thus, in the commonest form of Hirschsprung's disease, involving the rectum and lower rectosigmoid only, the sigmoid loop is brought out as a colostomy in the left lower quadrant of the abdomen. In those cases in which there is longer segment disease, more proximal sites are selected, for example, in the terminal ileum, where the entire colon is aganglionic.

In the neonate it is especially advantageous to place the colostomy as low as possible, because this allows the ganglionic bowel to develop and function normally with appropriate elongation of the vessels and the bowel itself, resulting in the desired length and mobility required for the pull-through operation.

In the critically ill infant with enterocolitis, the authors do not start with seromuscular frozen section biopsy specimens at the peritoneal reflexion, as they would in the child without enterocolitis to find the lowest ganglionic bowel, but rather it is their practice to perform a right transverse colostomy with frozen-section confirmation of normal ganglia. Of course, if the extent of the aganglionic segment is more proximal, another appropriate site is chosen, for example, the terminal ileum, if the entire colon is aganglionic. Sometimes the right transverse colon is chosen for the colostomy even in cases of short segment Hirschsprung's disease when the decision is made to maintain the colostomy after the definitive procedure to protect the endorectal anastomosis.

Several procedures have been successfully employed as the definitive operations for Hirschsprung's disease. Each of these techniques has its proponents, and all have been used with acceptable results. The basic goal of these operations is to relieve the functional obstruction produced by the aganglionic nonpropulsive distal segment without damaging any of the adjacent pelvic structures while affording the child the best chance for normal defecation and continence.

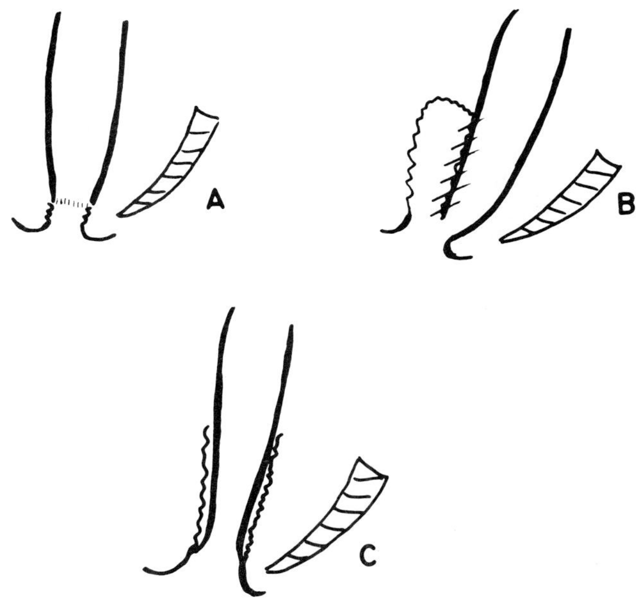

Figure 54–6. Surgical procedures for Hirschsprung's disease. *A*, Swenson procedure. The aganglionic rectum is excised, and the normal colon *(heavy black line)* is anastomosed to the distal 1 to 2 cm of the aganglionic rectum *(wavy line)*. *B*, Duhamel procedure. The normal colon is brought down behind the aganglionic rectum, anastomosed to it, and the contiguous walls incised and anastomosed to each other with a stapler. *C*, Endorectal procedure. The aganglionic rectum is stripped of its mucosa, and the normal colon is brought down within the muscularis of the rectum and anastomosed about 1 to 1.5 cm above the dentate line.

Endorectal Pull-Through Procedure

The authors perform the endorectal pull-through procedure with a primary anastomosis, as described by Boley,[10] for all children with Hirschsprung's disease. In the latest survey conducted by the AAP Surgical Section,[3] this operation is also the one preferred by most North American pediatric surgeons. The technique of the endorectal pull-through was developed by adapting the procedure described by Ravitch and Sabiston[11] for familial polyposis. The basic principle of this operation is to strip the aganglionic rectum of its mucosa and then to bring normally innervated colon through the residual rectal muscular cuff, in effect, bypassing the abnormal bowel from within. This technique permits normally propulsive bowel to be brought to the anocutaneous junction without interfering with sphincter function and minimizing the danger of injury to any pelvic structures, since the entire dissection is done within the lumen of the rectum (Fig. 54–6*C*).

The rectum is transected at the level of the peritoneal reflexion. Any remaining colon above this level that is aganglionic, as determined by frozen-section biopsy specimens at the time of operation, is resected. The mucosa of the rectum is stripped to about 1 cm above the dentate line by a combined abdominal and perineal approach. If the child had a sigmoid colostomy, it is taken down and the bowel prepared for the pull-through. It is essential that the mesentery be long enough for the normal bowel to be brought down to the anus without any tension. If there has been any foreshortening of the mesentery, dissection and careful pruning of the vascular arcades can usually provide an adequate length of tension-free bowel for a comfortable pull-through. This ganglionic bowel is then brought down through the rectal aganglionic cuff. Soave,[12] who first applied this principle in children with Hirschsprung's disease, employs a staged nonanastomotic technique by leaving the stump of the colon protruding from the anus to allow a spontaneous anastomosis to occur. About 3 weeks later, the excess colon is trimmed off, and several sutures are placed to anchor the bowel. In the endorectal pull-through with primary anastomosis, as described by Boley,[10] the colon is anastomosed to the rim of anorectal mucosa at the time of the pull-through. The primary anastomosis obviates the need for prolonged hospitalization and frequent dilatations necessary after the nonsutured anastomosis, as described by Soave.[12] In addition, the primary anastomotic technique has been associated with fewer early and late complications, especially enterocolitis.

Rectosigmoidectomy

The first successful operation for Hirschsprung's disease, the rectosigmoidectomy, was described by Swenson and Bill in 1948.[2] The basic principle of this technique is the resection of all but the most distal aganglionic bowel and restoration of bowel continuity with preservation of anal continence. The aganglionic rectum is mobilized through an abdominal approach and is meticulously dissected and separated from all pelvic structures to within 2 cm of the dentate line (see Fig. 54–6*A*). The proximal normal bowel is pulled through the pelvis, and an anastomosis is performed to the most distal 1.5 to 2 cm of rectum above the dentate line. For many years this was the only operation available, and it is still the yardstick against which all other operations are measured. The operation is technically difficult to perform properly, and the significant complication rate has stimulated the search for better alternatives.

Retrorectal Transanal Pull-Through Procedure

In 1956 Duhamel,[13] in France, described the first widely accepted alternative to Swenson's operation for Hirschsprung's disease—the retrorectal transanal pull-through procedure. The rationale of this procedure is the bringing down of normally innervated bowel behind the abnormally innervated rectum to about 1 to 2 cm above the dentate line and performing a long anastomosis between the two (see Fig. 54–6*B*). This procedure creates a neorectum with an anterior half with normal sensory receptors, and a posterior half with normal propulsion. Duhamel's original operation has been modified and refined by himself and others. In the procedure as it is performed currently, the upper end of the rectum is divided, and any proximal remaining aganglionic bowel is resected. A tunnel is created behind the remaining rectum by careful blunt dissection, and a transverse incision is made in the posterior half of the rectum approximately 1 cm above the dentate line. The normal bowel is pulled through the tunnel to the rectal incision, and its posterior wall is sutured to the lower edge of the rectal incision. Using a crushing instrument or, more recently, a stapler, the opposed anterior wall of the pull-through bowel and the posterior wall of the rectum are incised and stapled. The proximal end of the rectum is joined to the pull-through bowel, creating the previously mentioned neorectum with normal sensory innervation in front and normal ganglionic propulsive bowel behind.

The Duhamel operation reduces pelvic dissection to a minimum and retains the sensory side of the rectal reflexes. It is simpler and safer than is Swenson's procedure but shares with it the problems associated with retention of a portion of aganglionic colon and sphincter. If the anastomosis posteriorly is too low, incontinence becomes a problem; if it is too high, and too long a portion of aganglionic rectum is left in continuity, the risk of recurrent obstructive symptoms becomes significant.

Anorectal Myectomy

Anorectal myectomy as first popularized by Lynn[14] consists of the excision of a 1-cm wide strip of the rectal muscle starting at 1 cm above the anocutaneous junction and then extending cephalad for at least 5 cm. This maneuver removes the upper portion of the internal sphincter as well as the circular muscle of the rectum. This procedure has been advocated for use in ultrashort segment Hirschsprung's disease and has been used successfully by some surgeons in combination with a low anterior resection. However, there have been few series with long-term results following the myectomy, and its use has been limited to a combination of diagnostic and treatment procedure in questionable cases of Hirschsprung's disease. It has also been used as a secondary procedure in children whose primary operations have given less than optimal results.

Total Colonic Aganglionosis

Long segment Hirschsprung's disease involving at least the entire colon and often some portion of the distal small bowel presents an especially difficult problem. Diagnosis is often delayed, since on barium enema the colon appears normal, and a small bowel transition zone is difficult to document. Manometry and suction biopsies confirm the presence of Hirschsprung's disease, but the extent of aganglionosis is ascertained only at laparotomy with serial seromuscular biopsies. Although total colectomy and ileostomy for ileoanal aganglionosis with or without a pouch has been performed with satisfactory results in adults with polyposis or ulcerative colitis, it is not clear that normal growth and development would occur if these procedures were performed in infants. Martin[15] proposed the first operation specifically for long segment disease, which consisted essentially of an extended Duhamel procedure with a long side-to-side anastomosis of retained sigmoid and left colon to the normal small bowel, which is passed retrorectally and anastomosed near the dentate line.

The latest operation for total colonic aganglionosis is that proposed by Boley.[16] The cecum and ascending colon are anastomosed as an on-lay patch graft to the most distal normal small bowel, which is then pulled through the amputated rectum that has been stripped of its mucosa, and a primary anastomosis is performed. The authors have treated several cases using this technique, with excellent results.

Long-Term Results

The Swenson procedure has been used for 40 years, and the long-term results have been acceptable, but the problems of recurrent enterocolitis and difficulties with defecatory control have led to minor modifications and, ultimately, the search for a better procedure. The first of these was the Duhamel procedure. Its early problems with fecalomas in the anterior residual rectum also led to technique modifications and better results. The endorectal pull-through procedure with primary anastomosis as proposed by Boley subsequently became the most widely used procedure for Hirschsprung's disease. This procedure and that of Duhamel have yielded the lowest rates of recurrent enterocolitis, about 5%, and the best continence according to several large series.[3, 17] The morbidity and mortality rates should be low, and the long-term results have been excellent, although by no means perfect.

SUMMARY

The recognition of Hirschsprung's disease before any enterocolitis has occurred is the single most important factor in reducing the morbidity and mortality of Hirschsprung's disease, and it cannot be stressed enough that any infant who has not passed meconium in the first 24 to 48 hours of life must undergo manometry and suction biopsies before being allowed to leave the hospital. Early recognition and prompt effective treatment will reduce problems to a minimum and improve long-term results.

REFERENCES

1. Hirschsprung H: Jahrb Kinderh 1887; 27:1.
2. Swenson O, Bill AH: Resection of rectum and rectosigmoid with preservation of the sphincter for benign spastic lesions producing megacolon: An experimental study. Surgery 1948; 24:212–216.
3. Kleinhaus S, Boley SJ, Sheran M, et al: Hirschsprung's disease: A survey of the members of the Surgical Section of the American Academy of Pediatrics. J Pediatr Surg 1979; 14:588–597.
4. Martin LW, Buchino JJ, LeCoultre C, et al: Hirschsprung's disease with skip area (segmental aganglionosis). J Pediatr Surg 1979; 14:686–688.
5. Ikeda K, Goto S: Additional anomalies in Hirschsprung's disease: An analysis based on the nationwide survey in Japan. Kinderchirgie 1986; 41:279–281.
6. Meier-Ruge W, Lutterbeck PM, Herzog B, et al: Acetylcholinesterase activity in suction biopsies of the rectum in the diagnosis of Hirschsprung's disease. J Pediatr Surg 1972; 7:11–18.
7. Teitelbaum DH, Qualman SJ, Caniano DA: Hirschsprung's disease, identification of risk factors for enterocolitis. Ann Surg 1988; 207:240–244.
8. Fujimoto T, Puri P: Persistence of enterocolitis following diversion of fecal stream in Hirschsprung's disease. Pediatr Surg Int 1988; 3:141–146.
9. Branski D, Lebenthal E: Small intestinal changes in enterocolitis complicating Hirschsprung's disease. J Clin Gastroenterol 1979; 1:237–240.
10. Boley SJ: New modification of the surgical treatment of Hirschsprung's disease. Surgery 1964; 56:1015–1019.
11. Ravitch MM, Sabiston DC Jr: Anal ileostomy with preservation of the sphincter. Surg Gynecol Obstet 1947; 84:1095–1099.
12. Soave F: Hirschsprung's disease: A new surgical technique. Arch Dis Child 1964; 39:116–120.
13. Duhamel B: Retrorectal and transanal pull-through procedure for the treatment of Hirschsprung's disease. Dis Colon Rectum 1964; 7:455–460.
14. Lynn HB: Rectal myectomy in Hirschsprung's disease, a decade of experience. Arch Surg 1975; 110:991–994.
15. Martin LW: Surgical management of total colonic aganglionosis. Ann Surg 1972; 176:343–350.
16. Boley SJ: A new operative approach to total colonic aganglionosis. Surg Gynecol Obstet 1984; 159:481–484.
17. Holschneider AM: Complications after surgical treatment of Hirschsprung's disease. *In* Heberer G, Denecke H, eds: Colo-Rectal Surgery. New York, Springer-Verlag, 1982.

Chapter 55

Imperforate Anus

SYLVAIN KLEINHAUS and SCOTT J. BOLEY

Imperforate anus is the name applied to a group of congenital malformations involving the perineal area, the most prominent feature of which is an abnormal or absent anus. Although several different classifications of these disorders have been suggested, the one proposed by Stephens and Smith[1] is the most widely accepted. Their classification divides the anomalies into three categories—high, intermediate, and low—and subdivides each according to gender. The anatomic differences between the male and the female pelvis become important in determining the degree of severity and the treatment options in this series of malformations (Table 55–1).

EMBRYOLOGY

By the fourth week of fetal development, the cloaca has formed, and it has become separated from the exterior of the embryo by the cloacal membrane. Under normal circumstances, this membrane slowly atrophies until it is essentially absent by the end of the sixth week of development. During the same period, a series of septa subdivide the cloaca into anterior urogenital and posterior rectal portions (Fig. 55–1). The first of these septa migrates caudally and fuses with two lateral septa, which grow medially. In the female, the urogenital tract is again subdivided in the coronal plane, which results in the interposition of the vagina between the urethra and the rectum. If there is any disturbance in this migration, the exact location or the nonfusion of these septa will determine the height of the rectourethral or the rectovaginal fistula.

Table 55–1. ANATOMIC CLASSIFICATION OF IMPERFORATE ANUS

Category	Female	Male
High	Rectovaginal fistula (upper half of vagina)	Rectovesical fistula Rectourethral fistula (prostatic level)
Intermediate	Rectovaginal fistula	Rectourethral fistula
Low	Rectovestibular fistula Rectofourchette fistula Rectoperineal fistula Covered anus	Rectoperineal fistula Covered anus

INCIDENCE

Most large series and collections of series of cases of imperforate anus report an incidence of about 1 in 5,000 births.[1–3] Overall, the ratio of males to females is roughly 3 to 2. However, this ratio is 2 to 1 in high lesions but only 1 to 1 in low lesions. In males, more than 85% of high lesions have a fistula to the urethra or bladder, whereas in females with high lesions, about 80% have a fistula to the vagina. More than 90% of low lesions, in both males and females, have a fistula to the perineum or a potential opening covered with a thin membrane.

CLASSIFICATION

The basic division of imperforate anus anomalies is into categories of high and low lesions. The dividing line is the levator ani muscle—if the rectum ends above the levator ani muscle, the anomaly is considered high; if the rectum passes through the levator ani muscle, the anomaly is low. In the past, an invertogram, or upside-down radiograph, as proposed by Wangensteen and Rice,[4] was used to determine the level—if the air column passed caudad to a line between the back of the pubis and the coccyx, it was considered low; if the air did not pass the line, it was considered high. Many false-high readings with the invertogram have led to the adoption of a clinical assessment of the level of imperforate anus. Any male child in whom the fistulous opening is not visible is considered as having a high imperforate anus. A female child in whom the fistula opens in the perineum, the fourchette, the vestibule, or the lower one-third of the vagina has a low fistula; if the fistula opens above the lower third of the vagina, it is considered a high fistula. In the female child, there is an intermediate level in which the rectum ends high but the fistula extends lower in the vagina or the vestibule. Despite the low opening, this last type must be treated in the same fashion as is a high lesion.

ASSOCIATED ANOMALIES

The differentiation and development of the cloacal area into male and female phenotypes and the separa-

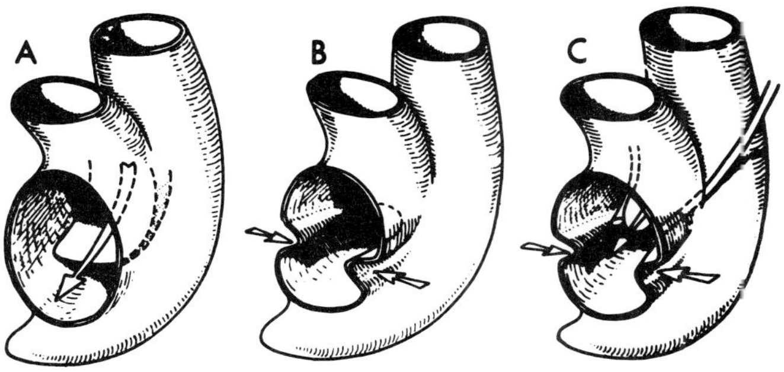

Figure 55–1. Embryologic development of the anorectum and the urogenital septa. Eponymous terms denoting the means of subdivision of the cloaca. *A,* Craniocaudad descent of Tourneux fold. *B,* Lateral plicae of Rathke dividing the lumen from side to side. *C,* Combination of the folds of Tourneux and Rathke. (From Duhamel B: Morphogenese Pathologique Des Monstruosities aux Malformations. Paris, Masson and Cie, 1966; with permission.)

tion of the rectum from the genitourinary apparatus occur during the earliest stages of embryonic growth. Therefore, it is not surprising that imperforate anus is associated with many other anomalies, because at this crucial time any untoward influence on development may simultaneously affect other organ systems. In a series from Toronto Children's Hospital,[5] 51% of 162 patients had associated anomalies in organ systems other than the genitourinary system. The commonest abnormalities were skeletal, cardiac, sacral, neurologic (central nervous system), and intestinal, including tracheoesophageal fistula. Although many of these anomalies were inconsequential, others were life threatening and incompatible with life. Some of these coexistent anomalies are easy to identify, whereas others are difficult, and it is incumbent on the neonatal surgical team to evaluate the patient prior to focusing on any single problem. In particular, a nasogastric tube must be passed to rule out an esophageal atresia; an electrocardiogram, sonocardiogram, or both, should be performed to evaluate heart function, and a chest roentgenogram to reveal any vertebral or rib defects. An abdominal sonogram and a clean-catch urine specimen help delineate any renal anomalies and may disclose the presence of a rectourinary tract fistula. Many of these anomalies have been grouped in the VACTER or VACTERL acronyms,* the importance of which is to emphasize the need to investigate for the presence of other anomalies when one or two elements of the constellations have been identified (see Chapter 25).

ANATOMIC CONSIDERATIONS

Male Gender

Because the anatomic differences between male and female infants are so important in the case of imperforate anus, the discussion focuses on each group separately.

Low Lesions

In male infants, the basic definition of a low lesion is a rectal pouch that is below the pubococcygeal line, with an abnormal anal opening. The simplest form of this anomaly is the *covered anus,* which consists of an anus in the normal position but with a membranous occlusion. Embryologically, this tissue is a remnant of the membrane that separates the internal from the external cloaca. Usually this membrane is quite thin and translucent, and meconium is visible through it (Fig. 55–2). The treatment consists of making a cruciate incision through the membrane and gently dilating the orifice, which is sometimes stenotic. Care must be taken when the incision is made not to injure the external sphincter fibers that are immediately adjacent to and underlying the borders of the membrane. The dilatations usually must be repeated several times to ensure an adequate anal orifice. Some authors consider congenital anal stenosis to be a form of imperforate anus, and the treatment is simple dilatation, continuing until the infant stools normally without straining. Covered anus and anal stenosis are usually local abnormalities and are rarely associated with sacral anomalies or the other abnormalities discussed previously.

The other low anomaly in the male is the *rectocutaneous* or *anocutaneous fistula.* In some instances, the orifice of the fistula is easily visible in the midline, anterior to where the anus should be normally. In other patients, the opening is small, barely admitting the tip of a No. 22 angiocatheter (Fig. 55–3). In any child without a normal anal orifice, a careful search must be made along the median raphe from the perineal body up to, and including, the scrotum. It may take 24 to 48 hours for the subcutaneous fistulous tract to become discolored by the meconium and even longer for a little

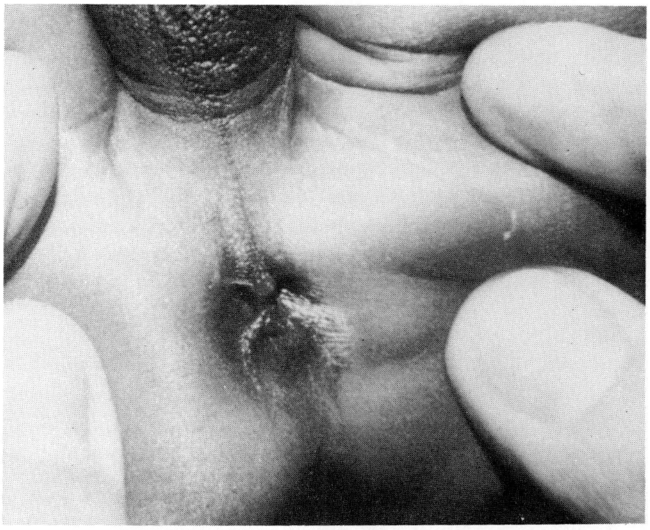

Figure 55–2. Covered anus in a male neonate. A small drop of mucus is visible at the anterior border of the anus.

*VACTER, *v*ertebral, *a*nal, *c*ardiac, *t*racheal, *e*sophageal, *r*enal. VACTERL includes the same terms, except for the addition of *l*imbs.

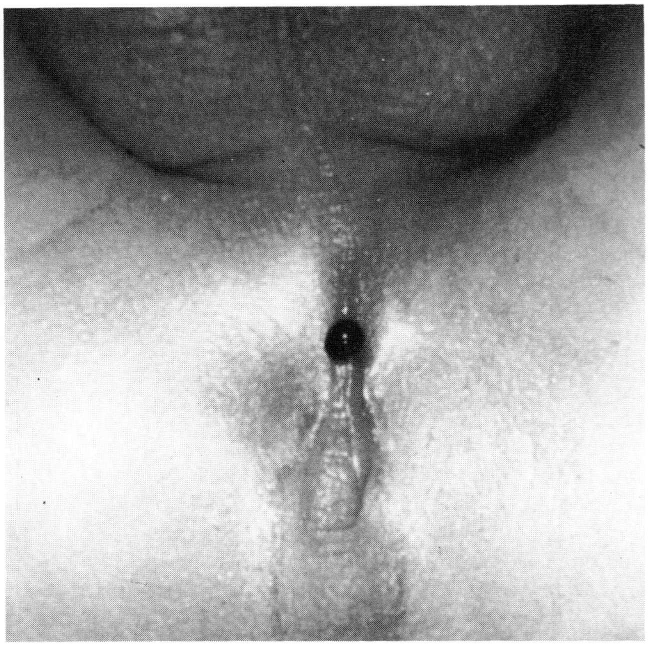

Figure 55–3. Anocutaneous fistula. The bead of meconium became visible only at 36 hours of life.

bead of meconium to become visible at the orifice of the fistula. This time is the most crucial period for the infant. If a fistulous opening is found, the procedure required is relatively simple: A fistulogram with contrast medium will define the anatomy in most instances. If available, a magnetic resonance imaging study will provide additional information on the relationship between the pelvic muscular anatomy and the rectal pouch. Although these roentgenologic tests are not essential in most instances, the information they provide is invaluable when the child has an intermediate-type imperforate anus with a perineal fistula.

The distinction between a low and an intermediate fistula can be made clinically at the time of examination. When a probe or a clamp is gently inserted into the fistula, it is possible to determine the direction of the tract. In a low lesion, the tract follows a posterior course and can usually be felt in the perineum. The fistula is opened surgically and followed back to the point where the anus would normally be found, and an anoplasty is performed. The results are uniformly satisfactory with essentially normal continence. In an intermediate lesion, the tract courses cephalad to join the rectal pouch above the levator sling, in which case a colostomy is performed. If there is no fistula, the infant must be assumed to have a high imperforate anus, and the first step in the surgical treatment is a colostomy.

High Lesions

The high type of imperforate anus in the male consists of a rectal pouch that is above the pubococcygeal line and the puborectalis muscle and, in most instances, of a fistula to the genitourinary tract. The commonest of these fistulas ends in the urethra in the area of the prostate. The bulbous urethra is the second commonest fistulous site; less commonly, the fistula ends in the bladder. The urinalysis in patients with rectourethral or bladder fistulas frequently reveals the presence of meconium epithelial cells, which is diagnostic of a fistula. Less frequently, the urine contains air bubbles originating from the distended rectal pouch. However, the absence of these epithelial cells or air, or both, does not guarantee the absence of a fistula, since the fistula may be quite narrow and clogged with inspissated meconium. If, after careful examination no perineal opening is found, a colostomy is performed. This procedure is not performed on an emergency basis at the time of birth, but, as discussed earlier, a waiting period of 48 to 72 hours is allowed to give the patient every opportunity to push meconium through a fistula, if present. The colostomy should be a double-barrel type, with separated stoma, because recurrent urinary tract infections commonly occur in patients with nondiverting colostomies owing to the constant leakage of meconium or stool through the fistula. These recurrent infections may lead to permanent renal damage; therefore, it is imperative that the fecal stream be diverted. It is the authors' preference to perform a right transverse double-barreled colostomy. The alternative is a sigmoid-diverting colostomy. The advantages of the right transverse colostomy are several. It allows the surgeon to do whatever is necessary at the time of the definitive procedure without having to disturb the colostomy. At the same time, the procedure does not endanger the vascular supply of the rectosigmoid, so that no matter what approach is used for the definitive repair, there should be no threat of devascularization of the pull-through or the colostomy. This consideration is especially important in the higher lesions with a shorter rectal pouch and a bladder fistula.

Prior to the definitive procedure, the authors perform a contrast enema through the distal limb of the colostomy to visualize the distal bowel and the fistula. The fistula is sometimes difficult to delineate, and a voiding cystourethrogram can be helpful. The two studies are often performed simultaneously for optimal visualization and localization of the fistula (Fig. 55–4).

The definitive procedure is performed when the infant weighs 15 to 20 pounds, or at about the age of 1 year. There are three main operations currently in use for the definitive repair of these anomalies, and all are based on the pioneering work of Stephens and Smith,[1] stressing the importance of the puborectalis muscle in maintaining continence. The first group of operations involves the identification of the levator ani apparatus through a posterior approach between the coccyx and the sacrum. Once this structure has been identified, a perineal approach is used to create an anal orifice within the external sphincter muscle. The abdomen is then entered, normal rectosigmoid is passed through the puborectalis sling, and an anastomosis with the neoanus completes the procedure. The exact techniques are those of Stephens,[6] Swenson and Donnellan,[7] and Rehbein.[8] Kiesewetter[9] combined the sacral and the perineal techniques of the aforementioned approaches and used an abdominal endorectal procedure to bring the colon down through the puborectalis muscle. Mollard and associates[10] described an anterior perineal approach to

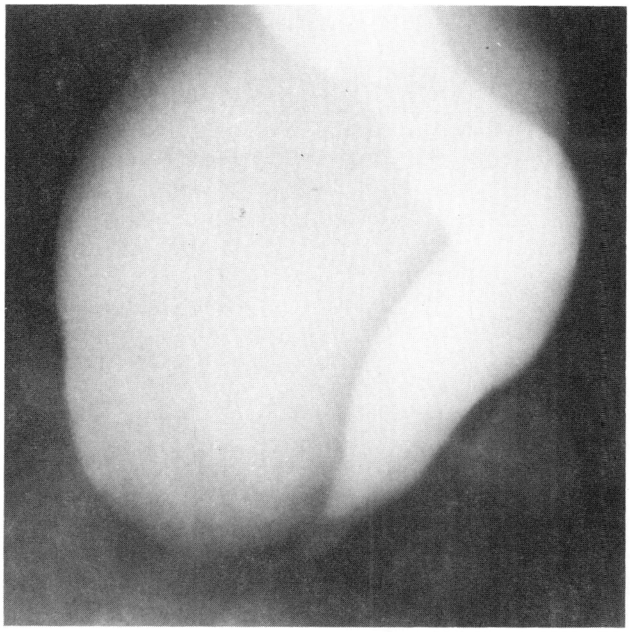

Figure 55–4. Opacification study of the bladder and the distal colon showing a fistula into the bladder.

the puborectalis muscle that then uses Rehbein's[8] endorectal technique for bringing the colon down to the anus. The most recent operation is that described by DeVries and Pena,[11] called the *posterior sagittal anorectoplasty*. The principles described by Stephens[6] are adhered to, but the approach is different: As the name implies, a posterior sagittal incision is made below the sacrum, and all the structures are divided in the midline. This approach allows all the anatomic landmarks to be identified and the colon to be brought down and placed in the appropriate position with great precision. This last procedure requires repeated and frequent dilatations of the anorectal canal during the postoperative period.

Female Gender

Low Lesions

The low lesions in female infants can have their openings anywhere along the midline anterior to the normal anal orifice. The fistulas that open into the perineal body may have a large or a small diameter. If fecal flow is adequate with no straining at stool and no constipation, no immediate treatment is necessary. If the orifice is too small for normal passage of stools, gentle, repeated dilatations are all that is required at this time. The more posterior orifices do not require any further treatment once defecation is normal. The more anterior perineal lesions are best treated by a cutback procedure, which consists of incising the posterior superficial wall of the perineal fistula back to the superficial anal sphincter fibers and then suturing the mucosa to the skin. This procedure redirects the fecal stream to its normal exit point, does not injure any important structures, and has proved to give excellent functional results. There is minimal scarring in the perineum and many women have had uncomplicated vaginal deliveries after this operation. The perineal body grows in early adolescence, and the appearance after puberty is essentially normal.

If the lesion is more anterior and opens in the fourchette (Fig. 55–5), the primary concern is adequate defecation. Again, if the opening of the fistula is too small, dilatation will usually give satisfactory results in the neonatal period. Although, in the past, some patients were left with a fourchette fistula, and even though they had adequate defecatory function, the situation was not esthetically pleasing. In addition, the vaginal and the urethral orifices were often contaminated by feces, and urinary tract infections and vaginitis occurred frequently. For these reasons, the authors perform anal transplantations in these patients. The fistula is cored out, the normal anal position within the external sphincter identified, and the fistulous tract brought back down within the fibers of the sphincter. This procedure recreates the normal anatomic structure and removes the cause of recurrent genitourinary infections. However, it does result in some perineal scarring, and extra care must be taken at the time of vaginal delivery.

The rectovaginal fistulas that open at the lower one third of the vagina are considered low lesions and are treated the same way as are fourchette fistulas, but even more care must be taken at the time of the anal transplantation to be absolutely certain that the pubo-

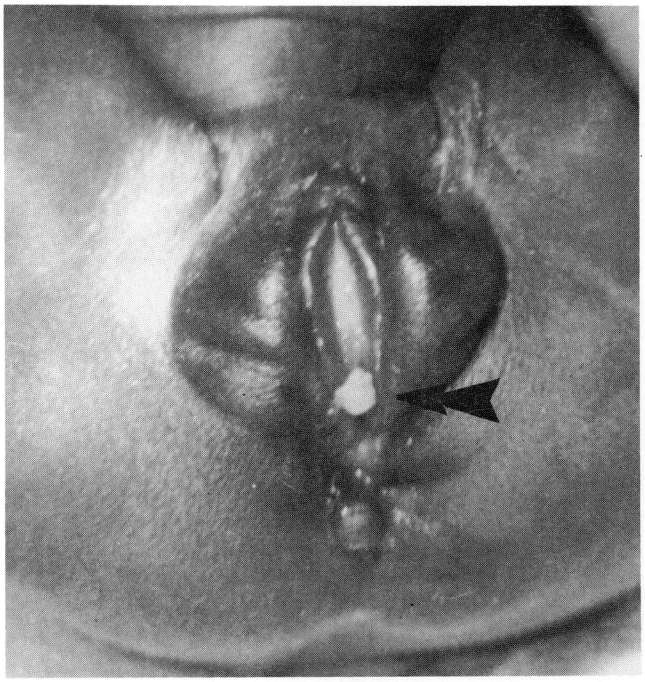

Figure 55–5. Rectofourchette fistula *(arrow)* in one identical twin; the other twin was normal. The *arrow* points to fecal material at the orifice of the fistula.

rectalis muscle is not injured. This precaution is not always simple to follow, since the fistula may not be devascularized so the tube cannot be ultra thin. At the same time the surrounding nerves and muscles must be preserved. A posterior sagittal anoplasty may be used to repair this lesion.

Intermediate Lesions

Any rectovaginal fistula that opens above the lowest portion of the vagina but below that portion of the vagina that is at the level of the cervix is considered an intermediate fistula. In these cases, the fistulous tract passes through the puborectalis muscle, but just barely. The opening is always on the posterior wall of the vagina and can be visualized only by using a small nasal speculum. The constant presence of stool in the vagina results in vaginitis and urinary tract infections in all of these cases, and it is the authors' practice to perform a right transverse colostomy in the early neonatal period. This procedure reduces the frequency of (but does not eliminate) urinary tract infections and prevents fecal vaginitis. Unnecessary delay in performance of the colostomy may also result in fecal impaction above the fistula. The authors usually do not dilate these intermediate lesions, because of the difficulty in visualization and the fragility of the surrounding tissues. One must also be aware of the intermediate type of imperforate anus, which opens at the fourchette or the perineum. The level of the rectal pouch is above the puborectalis muscle, but the fistula is long and reaches the area commonly associated with low fistulas. Investigation of associated anomalies is pursued, and corrective measures are taken when appropriate. The definitive surgical treatment of these intermediate anomalies is the use of the pull-through technique or the posterior sagittal anoplasty method.

High Lesions

Rectovaginal fistulas that open into the upper third of the vagina or above are categorized as high. In female infants, a fistula into the bladder is exceptional, because the reproductive organs separate the urinary tract from the rectum. Inspection of the perineum and vagina reveals stool in the vagina and the orifice of the fistula in the upper vagina or posterior fornix. It is also important to examine the introitus and look for the presence of a normal hymen. If these anatomic aspects are abnormal, the patient should be categorized as having a cloacal anomaly, and further investigation is necessary to determine the extent of the malformation. All these lesions require a colostomy during the neonatal period to prevent the complications described earlier. Any associated cardiovascular, renal, and skeletal abnormalities must be identified and treated, when indicated.[12, 13] The exact anatomy of the cloaca is defined by the use of a voiding cystourethrogram, and ultrasound and magnetic resonance imaging techniques have recently been added to the investigative armamentarium.[14, 15]

SURGERY

All patients with intermediate or high anomalies should have a diverting colostomy within 48 to 72 hours of birth. As previously discussed, the authors prefer a right transverse colostomy with separated stomas. The basic principle of the definitive operation is the identification and preservation of the puborectalis portion of the levator sling, with passage of the pulled-through colon anterior to this muscle.

The first of the classic operations that resulted in acceptable continence was that proposed by Stephens[6, 16] and then modified by Rehbein[8] and Kiesewetter.[9] These authors used posterior perineal approaches to identify the puborectalis muscle and then an abdominal approach to bring the colon down through the sling to the preselected and prepared neoanus. In 1978, Mollard and associates[10] described an anterior perineal approach to identifying the puborectalis muscle and creating the neoanus. The latest approach is that described by DeVries and Pena[11] in which the entire perineum is opened in the sagittal plane, all the structures are identified, and the colon, which may or may not need to be prepared by an abdominal approach, is precisely placed in its proper position. The posterior sagittal anoplasty seems to be especially useful for the reconstruction of cloacal anomalies.[17]

OUTCOME

The long-term results of all low lesions should be excellent. The levator ani and puborectalis muscle mechanisms should not have been disturbed, and gross continence should be normal. In most instances, only a knowledgeable examiner will be able to recognize the signs of any intervention. In female patients with a cutback, the perineal body grows at puberty, so that the anatomic configuration of the perineum is essentially normal.

The results are not so successful in the correction of high or intermediate lesions.[18, 19] Even for skilled surgeons, the procedures described earlier give varying results. Although most patients will be grossly continent and can control the frequency of defecation, some patients will have unexpected accidents. Many of these patients have sacral anomalies and neurologic deficits resulting in sensory and motor defects that preclude normal continence. Unsatisfactory early results sometimes ameliorate with time; some patients' defecatory control will improve as they approach adolescence, when social pressures increase and accessory muscles are used to a greater degree. The puborectalis muscle sling is always small in high imperforate anus lesions and must be dilated to enable the rectum or the colon to be pulled through during the repair. Several years may be required for the sling to provide adequate continence, so parents should be informed not to expect toilet training at the usual time. For cases in which the puborectalis muscle sling does not exert enough forward traction on the lower rectum, the authors have successfully employed the Kottmeier procedure to release the levator ani muscle and reinforce the puborectalis muscle.[20] This procedure often improves the patient's ability to distinguish between gas and stool and also to control their egress.

Most patents with high imperforate anus, regardless of the type of operation they undergo, have so-called "2-cm incontinence." Because the normal anal orifice is absent and the neoanus does not have normal sensory innervation, the patients are not aware of the presence of any residual fecal material in the distal portion of the anal canal after defecation. More important, the fibers of the external sphincter are rudimentary at best, so that the normal final stage of defecation—the strong contraction of the external sphincter—which forces all residual fecal material out of the distal 2 cm of the anal canal, is extremely weak. These factors result in staining of the undergarments and objectionable odors if not properly attended to. Instructions on how digitally to clean this last 2 cm segment contribute to the parents' and the patients' satisfaction with the results of treatment.

Some patients who have more frequent staining of the undergarments may benefit from dietary regulation. The patients and the families learn which foods provoke accidents and which foods are well tolerated. Judicious use of enemas may make the patient more able to control defecation. It is common for these children to have an anal mucosal prolapse requiring secondary anoplasty. A few of these patients will be unable to control their bowel movements, despite all medical and surgical measures. This situation is usually the result of a severe congenital deficiency of the neurologic control and the muscular structure of the sphincter complex. Under these circumstances, it is sometimes necessary to perform a permanent colostomy. Although certainly not an ideal situation, a properly constructed abdominal wall colostomy is easier to care for and results in a better quality of life than does an incontinent anorectum with perianal excoriation and pain.

In summary, imperforate anus comprises a number of anomalies that differ greatly in severity and outcome. The more benign, low type of anomalies are repaired relatively easily and can be expected to yield defecatory control that is essentially normal and esthetic results that are satisfactory. The higher group of anomalies, in which the rectal pouch lies at or above the level of the puborectalis sling, and for which complicated reconstruction is required, are more problematic. The long-term results, although adequate, are not perfect and frequently require patience and perseverance on the part of both the patient and the physician.

REFERENCES

1. Stephens FD, Smith ED: Anorectal Malformations in Children. Chicago, Year Book Medical Publishers, 1971.
2. Santulli TV, Schullinger JN, Kiesewetter WB, et al: Imperforate anus: A survey from the members of the Surgical Section of the American Academy of Pediatrics. J Pediatr Surg 1971; 6:484.
3. Smith EI, Tunell WP, Williams GR: A clinical evaluation of the surgical treatment of anorectal malformations. Ann Surg 1978; 187:583.
4. Wangensteen OH, Rice CO: Imperforate anus. Ann Surg 1930; 92:77.
5. Fleming SE, Hall R, Gysler M, et al: Imperforate anus in females: Frequency of genital tract involvement, incidence of associated anomalies, and functional outcome. J Pediatr Surg 1986; 21:146–150.
6. Stephens FD: Malformation of the anus. Aust NZ J Surg 1953; 23:9.
7. Swenson O, Donnellan WL: Preservation of the puborectalis sling in imperforate anus repair. Surg Clin North Am 1967; 47:173–178.
8. Rehbein F: Imperforate anus: Experiences with abdomino-perineal and abdomino-sacroperineal pull-through procedures. J Pediatr Surg 1967; 2:99.
9. Kiesewetter WB: Imperforate anus: The rationale and technique of the sacroabdomino-perineal operation. J Pediatr Surg 1967; 2:106.
10. Mollard P, Marechal JM, Jaubert de Beauje M: Surgical treatment of high imperforate anus with definition of the puborectalis sling by an anterior perineal approach. J Pediatr Surg 1978; 13:499–504.
11. DeVries PA, Pena A: Posterior sagittal anorectoplasty. J Pediatr Surg 1982; 17:638.
12. Teixeira OHP, Malhotra K, Sellers J, et al: Cardiovascular anomalies with imperforate anus. Arch Dis Child 1983; 58:747–749.
13. Tunell WP, Austin JG, Barnes PD, et al: Neuroradiologic evaluation of sacral abnormalities in imperforate anus complex. J Pediatr Surg 1987; 22:58–61.
14. Donaldson JS, Black CT, Reynolds M, et al: Ultrasound of distal pouch in infants with imperforate anus. J Pediatr Surg 1989; 24:465–468.
15. Sato Y, Pringle KC, Bergman RA, et al: Congenital anorectal anomalies: MRI imaging. Radiology 1988; 168:157–162.
16. Stephens FD: Congenital imperforate rectum, rectourethral and rectovaginal fistulae. Aust NZ J Surg 1953; 22:161.
17. Pena A: The surgical management of persistent cloaca: Results in 54 patients treated with a posterior sagittal approach. J Pediatr Surg 1989; 24:590–598.
18. Iwai N, Hashimoto K, Goto Y, et al: Long-term results after surgical correction of anorectal anomalies. Z Kinderchir 1984; 39:35–39.
19. Ditesheim JA, Templeton JM Jr: Short-term versus long-term quality of life in children following repair of high imperforate anus. J Pediatr Surg 1987; 22:581–587.
20. Kottmeier PK: A physiologic approach to the problem of anal incontinence through the use of the levator ani as a sling. Surgery 1966; 60:1262–1266.

Chapter 56

Gastrointestinal Aspects of Acquired Immunodeficiency Syndrome in Children

KEITH J. BENKOV

During the first decade since the description of acquired immunodeficiency syndrome (AIDS),[1–3] much has been learned, investigated, and implemented in its diagnosis, epidemiology, and treatment. What was initially thought to be a disease limited to homosexual men and intravenous drug abusers was soon discovered also to be a disease that could be contracted by transfusion of infected blood products, by heterosexual activity, and by vertical transmission from mother to neonate.[4, 5] More recently, the incidence of infection with the human immunodeficiency virus (HIV) has decreased among homosexual groups and increased among heterosexual groups. By the end of 1990, almost 3,000 infected children younger 13 years of age had been reported to the Centers for Disease Control, which represented almost 2% of all cases in the United States. During 1990, there was a 21% increase in reported cases compared with the preceding year.[6] However, estimates suggest that there may be from 2 to 10 times as many infected asymptomatic people.[7] Estimates indicate that, worldwide, by the end of 1992, 4.5 million infants would have been born to HIV-infected women, among whom roughly one third will develop AIDS.[8]

As AIDS has become more prevalent and its protean nature more appreciated, medical management has changed significantly. Initially, most efforts were directed toward terminally ill patients with severe respiratory disease who had little chance of extended survival. It is now recognized that the course of AIDS may be protracted, with a long period from the infection, to the onset of symptoms, and to eventual death.[9] Newer medications, such as zidovudine (formerly named AZT) and dideoxycytidine (ddC), have altered the course of the infection and dramatically prolonged survival.[10] Increasing interest has now focused on prophylaxis of infection by opportunistic organisms and maintenance of the quality of life.

IMMUNOLOGIC ASPECTS OF HIV

HIV has a marked affinity for the CD4 molecule, principally expressed on helper T lymphocytes. Once the virus binds the CD4 region, it becomes internalized, uncoated, and transcribed by reverse transcriptase to a proviral deoxyribonucleic acid (DNA) that becomes incorporated into the host DNA. It can remain dormant for long periods or reproduce in great numbers at any time. This rapid replication is usually provoked by an immunologic stimulus, such as another viral infection. Infection of the T lymphocyte with the virus destroys the cell and eventually results in a defect in cellular immunity.[9] A summary of immunologic abnormalities seen in patients with AIDS is shown in Table 56–1.

Other cells also contain the CD4 surface molecule, but in lower amounts. These cells include monocytes, macrophages, dendritic cells, glial cells, and possibly certain intestinal endothelial cells.[11] HIV infection of these cells does not seem as cytotoxic as infection of lymphocytes. Abnormalities in humoral immunity can also be profound,[12] and polyclonal hypergammaglobulinemia is frequently seen, despite defective antibody response to foreign antigens.[13]

GASTROINTESTINAL TRACT

Gastrointestinal disease is an important feature of HIV infection (Table 56–2).[9, 14, 15, 15a] Since gastrointestinal dysfunction frequently leads to malnutrition, it has a particularly profound effect on growth and development in the pediatric population. The subsequent discussion focuses on HIV-associated infection and dysfunction of the gastrointestinal tract and hepatobiliary system, as well as the overall nutritional management of HIV-infected patients.

Table 56–1. IMMUNE SYSTEM ABNORMALITIES IN AIDS

T Lymphocyte
Total lymphopenia
Decreased T4 (helper) cells
Elevated, normal, or decreased T8 (suppressor) cells
Decreased delayed-type hypersensitivity, anergy
Clinical susceptibility to infections, neoplasms
Decreased help for B cells in vitro
Decreased proliferative responses to mitogens in vitro
Decreased cytotoxic responses in vitro
B Lymphocyte
Elevated serum immunoglobulins and immune complexes
Inadequate serologic response to immunizations
Elevated spontaneous proliferation in vitro
Decreased response to signals for B cell activation in vitro
Increased response to B cell growth factors in vitro
Monocyte-Macrophage
Decreased granulomatous response
Increased susceptibility to infections
Decreased chemotaxis in vitro
Decreased monocyte-dependent T cell proliferation in vitro
Decreased Fc receptor function in vitro
Decreased C3-receptor–mediated clearance in vitro
Decreased expression of HLA-DR
Other Cells
Decreased natural killer cell activity in vitro

Mouth, Esophagus, and Stomach

Oral candidiasis is frequently a presenting feature in children eventually diagnosed with AIDS; it frequently coexists with esophageal candidiasis as well.[16] Although nystatin is frequently used to treat these children, it is often ineffective. Older children can be allowed to suck on clotrimazole vaginal suppositories, but in most patients with refractory disease, fluconazole or ketoconazole can be used.[17] Although rare, ketoconazole-resistant *Candida* infections have been described.[18] Ketoconazole-associated hepatotoxicity is unusual in children. Unless stomatitis is treated aggressively, it will diminish the oral intake of these children and contribute to malnutrition.

Noninfectious lesions are also found in the oral cavity in HIV-infected patients. Hairy leukoplakia (white lesions on the lateral edges of the tongue), first described in homosexual patients, has also been described in children.[19] The histologic appearance of epithelial hyperplasia is thought to be secondary to Epstein-Barr virus and was never described prior to the HIV epidemic. Kaposi's sarcoma, which can occur anywhere in the gastrointestinal tract, can originate in the mouth, with red, blue, or purple lesions that can be flat or raised and singular or multiple in number. Histologically, the lesions are thought to arise from either blood or lymphatic vessels.[20]

The same organisms that cause stomatitis also can infect the esophagus, with more profound symptoms noted. Localized pain is typical of herpes simplex stomatitis, whereas dysphagia occurs with esophageal involvement. Cytomegalovirus (CMV) may also be associated with esophagitis. Diagnosis of these infections can be made by viral culture of material obtained at endoscopy as well as by cytologic smears and immunohistochemical stains of biopsy material.[21] Treatment of herpesvirus infection is generally with acyclovir, whereas ganciclovir has been used to treat CMV infection.[22] *Cryptosporidium,* an agent more commonly found in the small intestine, has also been reported to be associated with esophagitis.[23]

Gastric infection tends to occur less frequently in persons with HIV infection. Although *Helicobacter pylori* infection has been found in patients with AIDS, it is unclear whether the incidence is higher than in the general population.[24] CMV infection has been associated with pyloric channel thickening and evidence of gastric outlet obstruction.[25]

Upper gastrointestinal endoscopy is generally used to confirm and delineate upper gastrointestinal infection. Blind brushing of the esophagus has also been suggested as a diagnostic tool.[26] One general practice is to treat apparent dysphagia empirically with oral antifungal agents and reserve endoscopic examinations for refractory cases. Endoscopy has the advantage of allowing inspection of the entire upper gastrointestinal tract, whereas the brushing is limited to the esophagus.

Small Intestine

The hallmark of small intestinal disease is diarrhea, which is seen in as many as two thirds of adults and children with AIDS.[4, 27, 28] Specific treatment is provided following delineation of the causes of diarrhea, usually infection, malabsorption, or both. At times the presentation may mimic inflammatory bowel disease.[29]

An identifiable enteric pathogen can be found in slightly fewer than half of adult AIDS patients, although not all these patients have diarrhea.[15a, 27, 30] Pathogens

Table 56–2. GASTROINTESTINAL MANIFESTATIONS OF AIDS IN CHILDREN

Oral Cavity
Thrush
Stomatitis
Hairy leukoplakia
Kaposi's sarcoma
Esophagus and Stomach
Esophagitis: *Candida,* herpes
Cytomegalovirus, cryptosporidiosis of stomach and esophagus
Helicobacter gastritis
Small and Large Intestine
Bacterial: *Shigella, Salmonella, Yersinia, Campylobacter*
Parasitic: *Entamoeba, Giardia, Strongyloides, Cryptosporidium, Isospora, Microsporidium*
Viral: CMV, HIV, herpes
Mycobacteria: *Mycobacterium tuberculosis, M. avium-intracellulare*
Fungal: *Candida, Cryptococcus*
Appendicitis
Pseudomembranous colitis
Necrotizing enterocolitis
Potential Malignancies
Kaposi's sarcoma
Lymphoma
Leiomyosarcoma
Burkitt's lymphoma

are more frequently associated with diarrhea, but these patients do not necessarily represent a sicker group as determined by weight loss or serum albumin levels. Although opportunistic infections of the intestinal tract play a large role in the clinical status of many patients, even "routine" pathogens tend to be more virulent and more refractory to treatment. The organisms most commonly found include *Cryptosporidium,* CMV, *Mycobacterium avium-intracellulare, Entamoeba histolytica, Giardia, Campylobacter, Salmonella, Isospora,* and *Strongyloides.*[31]

AIDS patients with diarrhea and no isolated pathogen show a higher incidence of inflammation on small intestinal biopsy compared with AIDS patients without diarrhea. There is a 25% incidence of acid-fast–stained organisms in biopsy specimens in patients with diarrhea and negative stool examinations.[28]

In homosexual men with AIDS who have negative stool examinations for enteric or parasitic pathogens, CMV, herpesvirus, and adenovirus may be found on small intestinal biopsy even in the absence of diarrhea.[31] This observation suggests that some of the opportunistic organisms isolated from this population may be present without causing symptoms.

Patients with diarrhea frequently have abnormal biopsies and decreased xylose absorption. Abnormalities of the jejunal biopsy specimens include partial villus atrophy, crypt hyperplasia, and increased intraepithelial lymphocytes. This type of diarrhea is not always secondary to infectious agents, be they enteric pathogens, opportunistic organisms, or parasites. There is a nonspecific inflammatory response of the small intestinal epithelium that may be related to the HIV itself or, perhaps, secondary to undetected viral infections.

With the use of techniques involving immunohistologic staining, HIV antigen has been detected in mucosal biopsy specimens of HIV-infected patients with gastrointestinal symptoms.[32] The exact site of the intestinal HIV infection is not clear; some reports have isolated HIV from the endothelial cells[33] as compared with mucosal monocytes. In those patients with HIV antigen isolated from small intestinal mucosa (Fig. 56–1), inflammatory changes and lower levels of disaccharidases have been found. Thus, a low-grade enteropathy with inflammation and a maturational defect in enterocyte development may be caused by HIV.[32]

Malabsorption and HIV Infection

Malabsorption is not universal in AIDS patients but should always be a consideration, especially in the presence of diarrhea or weight loss. In a recent report,[34] 28 children with HIV infection were studied for carbohydrate malabsorption. Twenty-two of these children met the criteria for failure to thrive, and 20 of them met the criteria for some degree of malnutrition, 12 of whom were classified as moderate to severe. Eleven patients had diarrheal symptoms, of whom five had documented infections with either *Cryptosporidium, Giardia,* or CMV. Of the total group tested, there was a 40% incidence of lactose malabsorption, and 39% of xylose absorption test results were abnormal (with a high correlation with enteric infections). Only nine children had small bowel biopsies: four biopsy specimens were abnormal, three of which were associated with intestinal infections.

In another series,[35] 17 HIV-infected infants were examined for lactose malabsorption. Nine infants had gastrointestinal symptoms, and no pathogens were isolated; nine weighed at the fifth percentile or lower; however, only six had diarrhea. Again, there was a strong correlation between lactose malabsorption and gastrointestinal symptoms.[35]

In an adult series of HIV patients with diarrhea

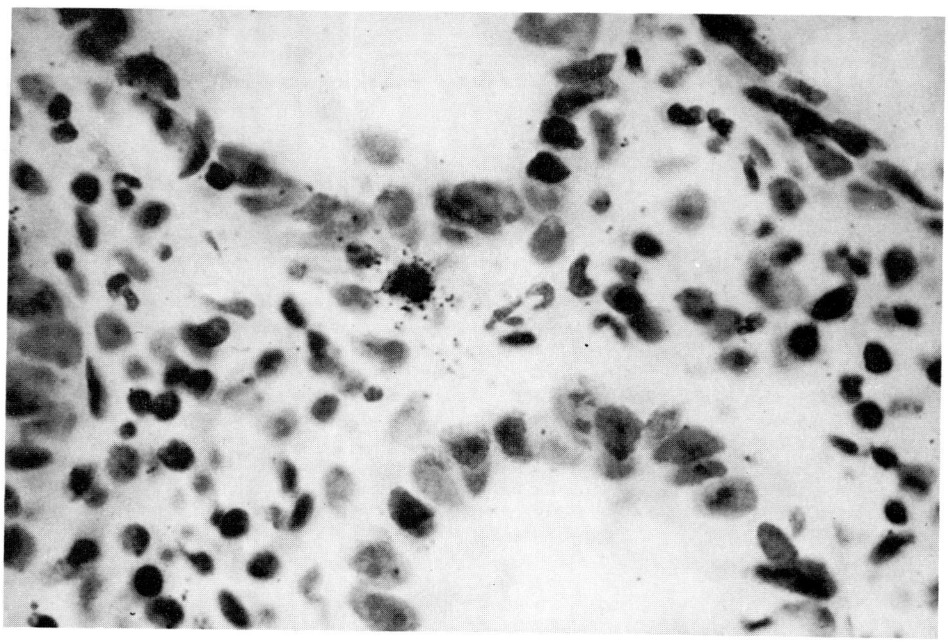

Figure 56–1. In situ hybridization staining of small intestinal biopsy specimen revealing human immunodeficiency virus. (Courtesy of Donald Kotler, MD.)

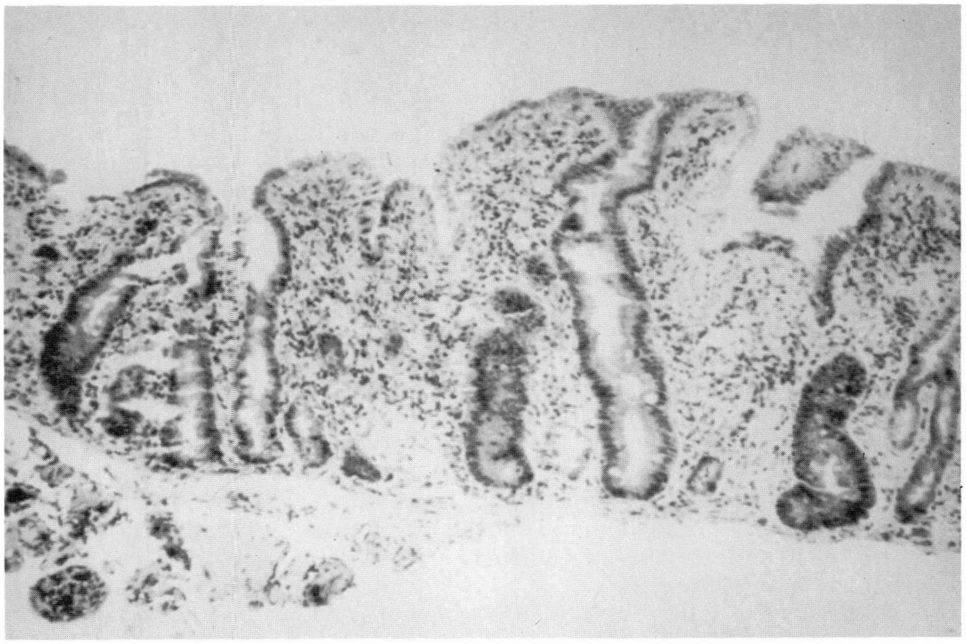

Figure 56–2. Subtotal villus atrophy associated with infection with *Cryptosporidium.* (Courtesy of Donald Kotler, MD.)

investigated for malabsorption, 88% had fat malabsorption, and the mean 1-hour xylose level was 19.3 ± 10.8 mg per dl.[28]

Specific Infections of the Large and Small Intestine

Cryptosporidium. *Cryptosporidium* infects predominantly the small intestine and tends to be found in microvilli (Figs. 56–2 and 56–3). Infection can cause a secretory diarrhea that can be quite refractory to treatment and can possibly be associated with anorexia, vomiting, weight loss, and malnutrition. Diagnosis is made by isolation of the organism via a stool flotation method and a modified Ziehl-Neelsen stain.[36] Biopsy material has a particularly high yield of recovering the organism. Antibiotic therapy is usually ineffective in this population, and the cysts are virtually never eradicated.[37] Zidovudine can often produce improvement in the diarrhea, occasionally eliminating the organism from the stool.[38] Hyperimmune bovine colostrum has been used to treat refractory *Cryptosporidium*-associated diarrhea in an adult AIDS patient.[39] Trials with diclazural, letrazural, and paromomycin are now in progress.

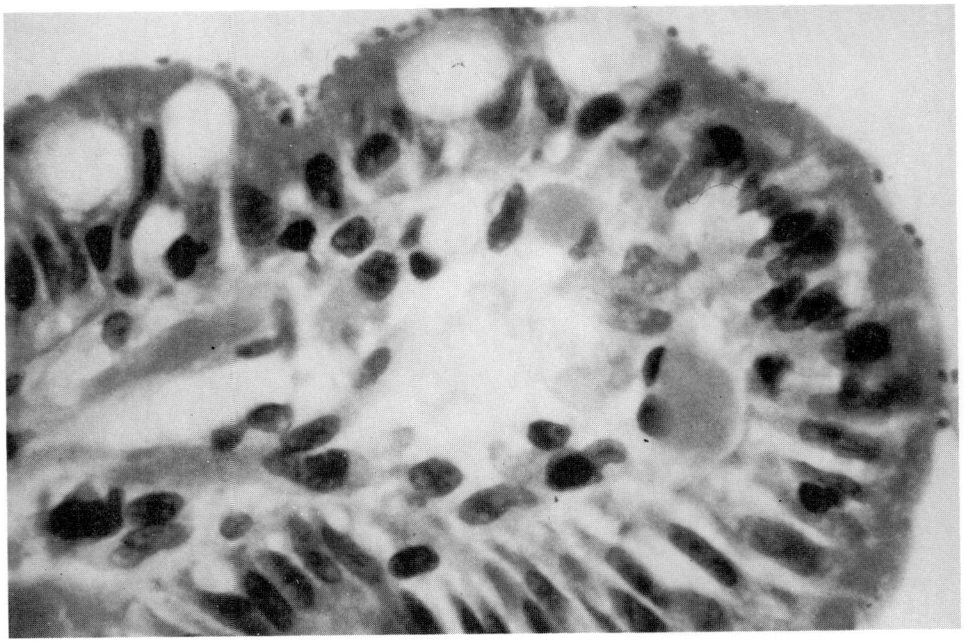

Figure 56–3. *Cryptosporidium* seen along a villus tip. (Courtesy of Donald Kotler, MD.)

Isospora Belli. *Isospora belli* is another opportunistic coccidian parasitic infection similar to *Cryptosporidium* that is found more typically in adult patients (Fig. 56–4).[40] It forms a larger cyst than does *Cryptosporidium* and usually results in a self-limited diarrheal illness in immunocompetent hosts. It is endemic in warm climates, and in AIDS patients causes a chronic, wasting diarrhea. Unlike *Cryptosporidium,* effective treatment is available with trimethoprim-sulfamethoxazole, which can also be used for prophylaxis.[41]

Other Parasitic Infections. Interestingly, *Entamoeba histolytica* is not as frequently identified in AIDS patients in the United States compared with an incidence as high as 25% in healthy homosexual groups. Symptoms may be variable, but in many patients the isolation from stool may merely represent a commensal organism. Dysenteric symptoms do occur, but invasive amebiasis is not readily seen.[42–45] Treatment for asymptomatic infections can consist of iodoquinol, diloxamide foveate, or puromycin. More severe infections are treated with metronidazole and iodoquinol.[15]

Giardia lamblia infections are also common and, similarly, can vary in presentation. *G. lamblia* probably represents the commonest nonopportunistic protozoan parasite, identified in 4 to 15% of all symptomatic AIDS patients in the United States.[42, 43] These infections are generally treated with quinacrine, metronidazole, or furazolidone.[15] *Blastocystis hominis* occasionally causes gastrointestinal illness in immunocompetent hosts but can cause significant diarrhea in children with AIDS. Unlike in *Cryptosporidium,* metronidazole is one of several drugs that can eradicate this infection.[46]

Intestinal Microsporidia may be associated with diarrhea in AIDS patients[47] (Fig. 56–5). The causative organism, *Enterocytozoon bieneusi,* seems to be identified in patients with AIDS and diarrhea with increasing frequency.[48, 48a, 48b] *Strongyloides stercoralis* has been found in AIDS patients with diarrhea and seems to be related to geographic location.[38]

Bacterial Infections. Probably the commonest bacterial enteritis in patients with HIV is *Salmonella,* which is frequently accompanied by bacteremia and disseminated infection.[38] Presumed *Salmonella* gastroenteritis should be treated in AIDS patients with the appropriate antibiotics, usually ampicillin, trimethoprim-sulfamethoxazole, or chloramphenicol, pending cultures. Extraintestinal *Salmonella* infection requires parenteral antibiotics.[15] *Shigella* gastroenteritis usually responds to trimethoprim-sulfamethoxazole. *Campylobacter* infections can present similarly, but erythromycin may not affect the clinical course, merely decrease shedding.[15] *Yersinia enterocolitica* infections may cause focal infections and bacteremia in the immunosuppressed patient. Isolation by the laboratory requires special techniques. *Aeromonas hydrophila* infections usually cause acute gastroenteritis but may also cause extraintestinal infections.[44]

***Mycobacterium* Infections.** One of the more refractory infections of the intestinal tract is caused by *Mycobacterium,* which is quite rare in healthy children. *Mycobacterium tuberculosis* gives the typical right-sided pain that can mimic Crohn's disease.[29, 29a] The atypical species, *M. avium-intracellulare,* usually causes a more diffuse infection of the small intestine. Histologic findings can range from minimal changes to total villus atrophy, with an appearance close to that of Whipple's disease.[49] No effective treatment is currently available for this infection.

The most readily available location to obtain atypical *Mycobacterium* is the duodenum, either by culture or histologic staining. There is a high incidence of finding additional involvement, in the esophagus, the rectum, or the liver. There is also an 85% incidence of finding the organism in the blood. Malabsorption is frequent, but not universal, among infected patients, and approximately 50% have decreased xylose absorption.[50]

Fungal Infections. Fungal infections with *Candida albicans, Cryptococcus neoformans, Histoplasma capsulatum,* and *Coccidioides immitis* also occur and rarely are invasive.[15]

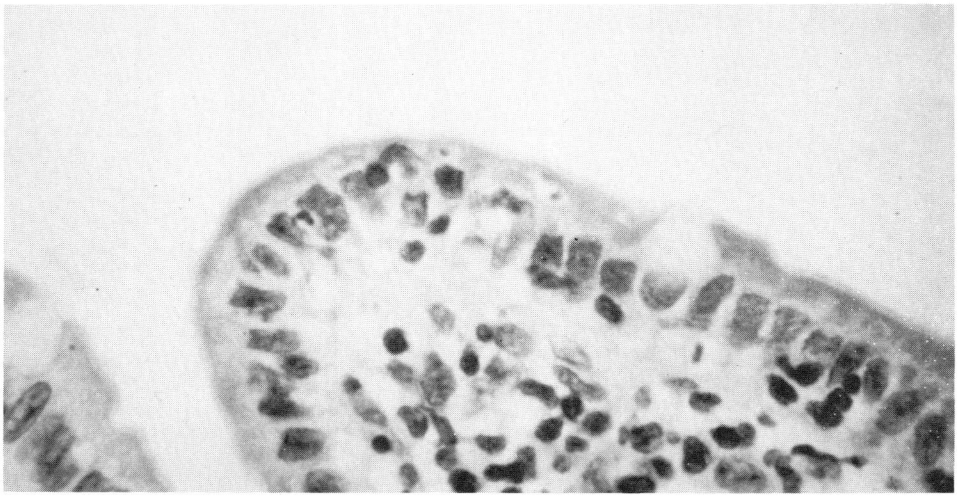

Figure 56–4. *Isospora belli* macrogametocytes seen within apical cytoplasm in the small intestine. (Courtesy of Donald Kotler, MD.)

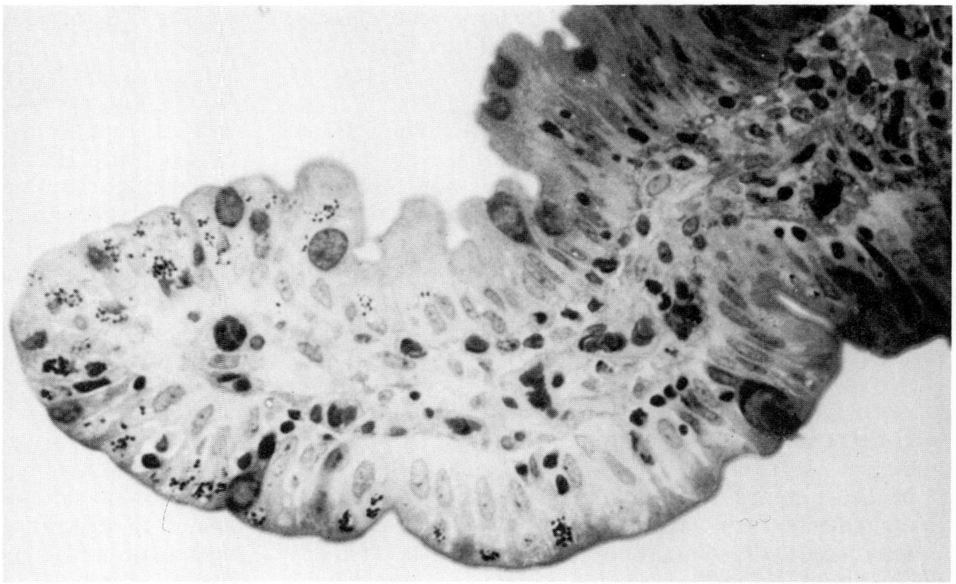

Figure 56–5. *Microsporidium* noted invading the surface epithelium of the small intestine. (Courtesy of Donald Kotler, MD.)

Large Intestine

Manifestations of large intestine involvement of patients with AIDS generally appear colitis-like and are usually secondary to the infectious agents noted earlier. The signs and symptoms usually consist of frequent bloody diarrhea, tenesmus, fever, and abdominal pain and distention.

Viral Infections. As many as 70% of adults with AIDS may develop CMV infection, and their symptoms reflect a wide clinical spectrum. The virus may be recovered from noninflamed colonic mucosa from asymptomatic patients and from those with presumed CMV-associated colitis (Fig. 56–6). It also may be absent from colonic mucosa from extremely ill patients, where it is being shed in the stool. Colonic dilatation may be seen, which can improve with or without treatment. Necrotizing lesions leading to perforation of the bowel also can occur.[51] Ganciclovir therapy for the lesions has been used.[18] The major toxicity with this drug, similar to many other agents used to treat this syndrome, is bone marrow suppression. Relapse of infection occurs in as many as one third of patients within 2 months.[52]

Herpes simplex virus can cause an infection of the colon similar to that of the mouth and the esophagus. More typically, the virus causes perianal disease and proctitis, although mild diarrhea can be present. Treatment is generally with acyclovir.[43]

Another consideration for bloody diarrhea in these patients is pseudomembranous colitis from *Clostridium*

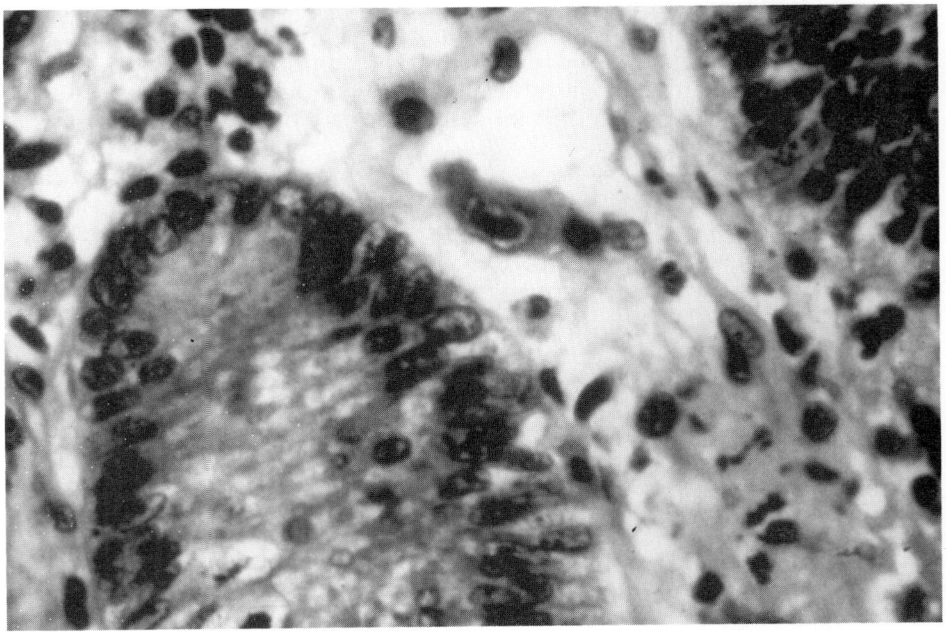

Figure 56–6. Colonic biopsy revealing an inclusion body typical of cytomegalovirus infection. (Courtesy of Donald Kotler, MD.)

difficile. Many children with AIDS have received frequent courses of antibiotics. Treatment consists of oral metronidazole or vancomycin, with a relapse rate as high as 20%.[15]

Infections with various organisms may mimic other clinical conditions. *M. avium-intracellulare* has caused appendicitis.[53] Pneumatosis intestinalis as well as massive gastrointestinal hemorrhage may result from necrotizing infections.[54, 55] Because enteric infection in HIV-infected patients may be severe, empiric therapy pending diagnostic results has been recommended.[56, 57] Lastly, colitis associated with toxoplasma infection has been described.[57a]

Gastrointestinal Neoplasms

In direct contrast with adult patients, gastrointestinal malignancy is rarely reported in children with AIDS. Adults eventually diagnosed with AIDS may first develop either Kaposi's sarcoma or non-Hodgkin's lymphoma as the primary presentation. The lymphomas are usually B-cell derived and are usually not seen in young children. Burkitt's lymphoma affecting the pancreas has been described in a child.[58] The diagnosis of unusual manifestations of AIDS may require multiple imaging studies.[59]

Kaposi's sarcoma does occur in children, especially those who contract AIDS after infancy from blood products. Two infants have been reported, both of Haitian mothers, who, after their death from respiratory infections, incidentally had Kaposi's sarcoma in lymph nodes and spleen on autopsy.[60] Disseminated leiomyosarcoma in a child also has been seen.[61]

LIVER DISEASE IN AIDS

The occurrence of hepatomegaly and elevated transaminase levels in children with AIDS is common (Table 56–3). Hepatosplenomegaly has been reported in 93% of infants, whereas 57% had elevated transaminase levels.[14] Mild hepatosplenomegaly may represent an activation of the reticuloendothelial system as part of the diffuse lymphadenopathy seen in childhood AIDS.[12] Most severe liver disease is secondary to various infectious agents.[62–64] Several drugs used in the treatment of AIDS, notably zidovudine, may be associated with increased aminotransferase levels. Primary infection of the liver with HIV may occur.[65]

Table 56–3. HEPATOBILIARY MANIFESTATIONS OF AIDS IN CHILDREN

Hepatitis
- Viral hepatitis: A, B, C, CMV
- *Mycobacterium*
- Other: *Candida, Cryptococcus, Histoplasma, Coccidioides, Pneumocystis*
- Drug toxicity

Cholecystitis
- Acalculous: CMV, *Cryptosporidium*

Cholangitis
- CMV
- *Cryptosporidium*
- *Cryptococcus*
- Primary sclerosing

Pancreatitis

The major problem in attempting to correlate liver pathologic changes between adult and pediatric patients is related to the different risk factors found in different populations of AIDS patients. Homosexual men encounter different infections than do intravenous drug abusers as compared with infants who acquire HIV vertically. In addition, some reports provide autopsy data that no doubt will differ from the pathology reports from percutaneous liver biopsies done antemortem.

Liver biopsy specimens often show a relative lack of histologic inflammatory activity in view of the high incidence of increased transaminase levels and the exposure to hepatitis-causing viruses.[66] This finding has been attributed to impaired cell-mediated immunity that fails to initiate the inflammatory and subsequent fibrotic process. In one series of 34 patients evaluated for either increased transaminase levels, hepatomegaly, or unexplained fever, 13 had granulomas, seven of which had *Mycobacterium* on either staining or culture[67] (Fig. 56–7). Portal inflammation was seen in only 11 patients, with piecemeal necrosis in only 1 and minimal portal fibrosis in 8.[67] This series of patients was fairly evenly represented by Haitian, homosexual, and drug abuser patients and a few patients with venereal and maternally acquired HIV infections. Peliosis hepatis has been found in several series of patients.[67a]

In another series of 44 patients, more than 80% of whom were intravenous drug abusers with either AIDS or AIDS-related complex (ARC), 36% had granulomas, of which 82% were secondary to *Mycobacterium.*[62] Chronic active hepatitis was seen in 27%. The other findings in this series included 25% of patients with either mild nonspecific or chronic persistent hepatitis and 6% with alcoholic cirrhosis. In a similar population of 21 patients with AIDS who underwent liver biopsy, 48% had granulomas, most from *Mycobacterium,* but the biopsies of the other patients also revealed either CMV or histoplasmosis.[63] The other diagnoses made were probable CMV hepatitis with inclusion bodies and chronic hepatitis. Forty-three percent of the biopsy specimens were labeled nondiagnostic, although many of them had fatty changes. In still another series of 36 patients with AIDS, 60% of whom were intravenous drug abusers, granulomas were found in 61%. Two thirds of the granulomas were secondary to *Mycobacterium,* and the remainder were secondary to either CMV or schistosomiasis or were undetermined. Fourteen percent had cirrhosis of an undetermined cause, and only one patient had chronic active hepatitis.[64] In a series of patients that was fairly evenly distributed between intravenous drug abusers and homosexuals, the commonest finding was macrovesicular steatosis.[66]

Less information is available regarding hepatic pathologic changes in children. The largest series consisted of 30 children with AIDS or ARC. Pathologic reports from 26 of them were derived from autopsy, whereas 4 had

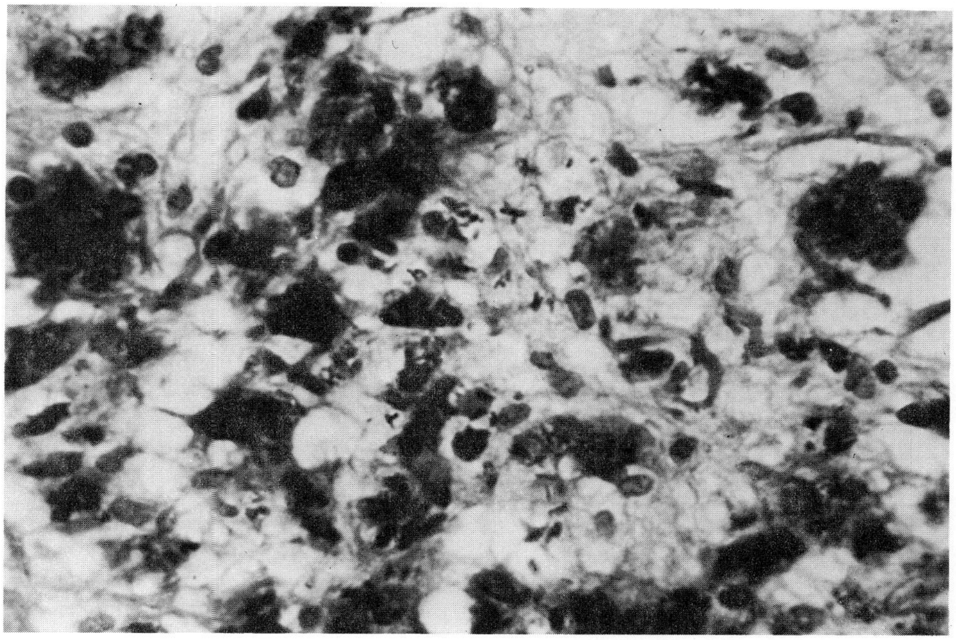

Figure 56–7. Acid-fast stain of liver biopsy specimen demonstrating *Mycobacterium avium-intracellulare.* (Courtesy of Donald Kotler, MD.)

percutaneous biopsies antemortem.[68] Most (21) of these children had been born to Haitian women, whereas 4 were children of intravenous drug abusers, and 5 had no known risk factors. Only two biopsy specimens were classified as normal, whereas 12 had only one finding; 16 cases had two or more findings, and the pathologic changes were more varied. Giant cell transformation was seen in seven specimens. Five had isolated CMV, with or without giant cell transformation; Kaposi's sarcoma was found in four cases, and lymphoma in one. Lymphoplasmocytic infiltrate was found in two cases, and granulomas were isolated in only one. The nonspecific findings included 14 cases with steatosis, 7 with portal inflammation, and 3 with paracentral necrosis. The infrequent finding of granulomas in children with AIDS compared with adult AIDS patients probably reflects the decreased exposure to the infectious agents associated with this finding.[68]

One child with AIDS and increased transaminase levels for longer than 6 months had a percutaneous liver biopsy showing chronic active hepatitis and portal fibrosis.[69] In a series of nine children with AIDS who underwent percutaneous liver biopsy, four had granulomas with *M. avium-intracellulare* isolated.[70] Another series of four children with hepatitis and AIDS showed that all had signs of chronic active hepatitis with portal fibrosis, inflammatory infiltrate, piecemeal necrosis, and bridging fibrosis.[71] Immunocytology performed on the tissue revealed an increase in cytotoxic-suppressor cells. The cause of the chronic active hepatitis was not clear.

Specific Hepatic Infections in AIDS

Viral Hepatitis

There is an almost 95% prevalence of hepatitis B antibodies present in adult AIDS patients, although only 10% of these patients are positive for hepatitis B surface antigen. Children have a variable risk based on the different mechanisms for the acquisition of HIV.[72] The incidence of chronic active hepatitis and cirrhosis from hepatitis B is no higher than that of the general population and immunocompetent hosts. The clinical course of hepatitis B appears to be mild, and long-term sequelae are rare.[73]

Hepatitis A. There is probably an increased incidence of hepatitis A in homosexual patients, but the infection does not seem to have any different clinical course in this population.[73] There does not appear to be an increased incidence in children.

Hepatitis C. Serologic testing for hepatitis C has been available only recently. Preliminary results show an increased incidence in intravenous drug abusers, with or without HIV infection. Patients with AIDS who are not intravenous drug abusers have an incidence of hepatitis C antibodies similar to that of the general population.[74] It is unclear whether those AIDS patients with hepatitis C infection have a more protracted course.[73] A report published before the serologic testing was available indicated that patients with non-A, non-B hepatitis and HIV infection had a higher incidence of chronic active hepatitis on liver biopsy.[75]

Mycobacterium. Of all the opportunistic infections of the liver, *Mycobacterium* appears to be the most commonly detected pathogen, found in 10 to 30% of adults studied with liver biopsies.[62–66] Most cases are caused by *M. avium-intracellulare,* but there are cases of *M. tuberculosis* as well. Characteristic pathologic changes include poorly differentiated, noncaseating granulomas in both hepatocytes and Kupffer's cells. Hepatic infection is almost always associated with disseminated disease and fever. Jaundice is variable, and hepatomegaly is generally present with markedly increased alkaline phosphatase levels.[72]

Cytomegalovirus. The second commonest opportunistic infection of the liver is CMV.[62–66] Although this is not as common a finding on antemortem liver biopsy, it is detected in 30 to 40% of all autopsies on AIDS patients.[72, 76] Histologically, intranuclear and cytoplasmic inclusion bodies with periportal inflammation and some hepatic necrosis are found.[72] CMV of the liver also usually represents disseminated infection. Serum aminotransferase levels are frequently increased out of proportion to increases in alkaline phosphatase levels.

Fungal and Parasitic Infections. Hepatic involvement represents disseminated infections, with *C. neoformans* being the commonest pathogen, but *H. capsulatum, C. albicans,* and *C. immitis* have also been reported.[63, 76] *Pneumocystis carinii* has also been documented in the liver, but as part of disseminated infection.[77]

Biliary and Pancreatic Involvement in AIDS

Most reports of biliary disease involve adult AIDS patients, usually presenting with right upper quadrant pain and fever, with or without jaundice. Several cases of acalculous cholecystitis have been thought to be caused by CMV or *Cryptosporidium,* although other infectious agents probably contribute.[73] Whether these cases represent primary infection of the gallbladder or the biliary tree is not certain. Cases of cholangitis secondary to *Cryptococcus, Candida,* and *Salmonella* have also been reported.[78, 79] Some consideration has been given to the theory that these cases of cholangitis may also represent immune dysfunction, because cases of sclerosing cholangitis have been associated with other immunodeficiencies in children.[78, 80]

Clinical evidence of pancreatic disease may be found in patients with AIDS. Various infections and infiltrative malignancies have been coincidentally reported on autopsies.[81, 82] CMV-induced pancreatitis and subsequent complications seem to have contributed to the demise of two patients; however the diagnosis was made only postmortem.[83]

Reports regarding acute pancreatitis detected antemortem are brief and conflicting. Some authors have indicated that cases of pancreatitis are only drug related,[84] whereas others claim an incidence as high as 46% when amylase and lipase levels were monitored routinely in a group of 35 patients.[85] A larger group of adult AIDS patients admitted over a 4-year period showed an incidence of 3.7%.[86] The development of insulin-dependent diabetes has also been described in adult AIDS patients.[87] In one report, 17% of a large group of children with HIV infection developed pancreatitis over a several-year period.[88] The use of pentamidine was significantly associated with pancreatitis in these children. Serum amylase levels were not always a good predictor of the development of pancreatitis.

A unified approach to the evaluation of hepatobiliary and pancreatic disease in AIDS is necessary. Hepatosplenomegaly accompanied by increased transaminase levels should not be the sole indication for liver biopsy, unless also accompanied by fever. The liver biopsy becomes a useful tool when specific treatment is available for an infection and when there is a need to isolate an organism. As noted previously, it is rare to document a "new" infection that is limited solely to the liver. More commonly, a disseminated disease affects the liver.[73]

NUTRITION AND AIDS

The nutritional management of children with AIDS is similar to the management of any other child with chronic illness (see Chapter 83). These children have many reasons to be at risk nutritionally, most of which involve pathologic changes in gastrointestinal tract (Table 56–4). The role of malnutrition as it contributes to the progression of the illness is an area of ongoing investigation.[89] The clinical management of malnutrition in children with AIDS is important because there appears to be a detrimental effect of malnutrition on neurologic development.[90]

Children with any chronic illness frequently have a diminished oral intake. In children with AIDS, specific causes for decreased intake include mouth pain related to fungal or viral infections of the oral cavity and esophagitis causing odynophagia.[91] Increases in cachectin and tumor necrosis factor, both associated with anorexia in other chronic illnesses, have been found in AIDS patients.[92] Various medications used in the treatment of AIDS and its associated infections can also cause anorexia.[65] Early satiety may occur with massive hepatosplenomegaly or infiltrative lesions of the gastrointestinal tract.[93]

Caloric requirements can also be increased based on clinical status. There appears to be some conservation of lean body mass in adult AIDS patients who are clinically stable.[94] Recurrent fevers increase metabolic requirements, as does the extra respiratory effort associated with pneumonia and other respiratory infections. Metabolic rates have been shown to increase by 20 to 60% in these settings.[94] These acutely ill patients often need nutritional intervention, especially if the clinical course is marked by repeated hospitalizations.

Table 56–4. FACTORS CONTRIBUTING TO MALNUTRITION IN CHILDREN WITH AIDS

Factor
Decreased Intake
Pain secondary to stomatitis
Dysphagia secondary to esophagitis
Anorexia from medications
Vomiting due to gastrointestinal tract infections
Generalized anorexia from chronic disease, cachectin
Early satiety from organomegaly, infiltrative lesions
Increased Caloric Requirements
Fever
Increased respiratory effort
Malabsorption
Villus atrophy secondary to infectious agents
Loss of brush border enzymes
Pancreatic insufficiency secondary to malnutrition
Cholestasis from liver disease

Table 56–5. IMMUNOLOGIC DEFICITS ASSOCIATED WITH PRIMARY MALNUTRITION

Lymphopenia
Decreased T cells
Decreased cell-mediated immunity
Anergy
Decreased secretion of immunoglobulins
Decreased serum complement
Decreased phagocytosis
Decreased killer cell activity

The incidence of malabsorption has been described earlier. Contributing to the malabsorption are infectious agents, inflammation of the absorptive surface of the small intestine, and malnutrition itself. Even in the face of malabsorption, these children can usually be managed by supplying extra calories either orally or nasogastrically.

Malnutrition itself affects the immune status (Table 56–5). A cellular immunodeficiency state similar to the effects described in AIDS may occur.[95] The signs include lymphopenia, anergy, reversed T4:T8 ratios, and abnormal macrophage function.[96] Micronutrient deficiencies can also cause specific immunodeficiencies.[97]

There have been isolated reports of specific nutrient needs in children with AIDS, mostly focusing on vitamin and mineral deficiencies.[98] Zinc deficiency has been described in AIDS,[99] but this is also a frequent occurrence in any child with chronic diarrhea. Folate deficiency has been described in relation to neurologic disease and AIDS.[100] Selenium deficiency has been associated with the cardiomyopathy of AIDS.[101]

The commonest nutritional deficiency in these children remains one of total calories. Nutritional assessments should be done periodically on all infants and children with AIDS.[102] Routine formulas may be used in most situations, unless severe malabsorption is present. Although oral supplemental feedings should always be attempted first, enteral tube feedings have proved to be successful in promoting weight gain.[103] Some consideration should be given to the type of tube feedings used. Nasoduodenal feedings may prevent reflux in children with respiratory compromise or who are on ventilators.[104] Soft Silastic nasogastric tubes can be used for long periods, and gastrostomies have also been useful, although some authors believe that the gastrostomy site does not heal well in these children. In some instances, parenteral nutrition is required. There are obvious disadvantages to the placement of central venous catheters in these immunocompromised patients.[105] Parenteral and enteral nutritional support also may be performed in the home, if capable caretakers are available.

REFERENCES

1. Gotlieb MS, Schroff R, Schanker HM, et al: *Pneumocystis carinii* pneumonia and mucosal candidiasis in previously healthy homosexual men. N Engl J Med 1981; 305:1426–1431.
2. Masur H, Michelis MH, Green JB, et al: An outbreak of community-acquired *Pneumocystis carinii* pneumonia. N Engl J Med 1981; 305;1431–1438.
3. Siegal FP, Lopez C, Hammer GS, et al: Severe acquired immunodeficiency in male homosexuals, manifested by chronic perianal ulcerative herpes simplex lesions. N Engl J Med 1981; 305:1439–1444.
4. Rubinstein A, Sicklick M, Gupta A, et al: Acquired immunodeficiency with reversed T4/T8 ratios in infants born to promiscuous and drug-addicted mothers. JAMA 1983; 249:2350–2356.
5. Oleske J, Minnefor A, Cooper R, et al: Immune deficiency syndrome in children. JAMA 1983; 249:2345–2350.
6. The HIV/AIDS epidemic: The first 10 years. MMWR 1991; 40:337–359.
7. Update: Acquired immunodeficiency syndrome–United States, 1989. MMWR 1990; 39:81–86.
8. Chin J: Current and future dimensions of the HIV/AIDS pandemic in women and children. Lancet 1990; 336:221–224.
9. Falloon J, Eddy J, Wiener L, et al: Human immunodeficiency virus infection in children. J Pediatr 1989; 114:1–30.
10. Krasinski K: Retroviral therapy and clinical trials for HIV-infected children. J Pediatr 1991; 119:S63-S68.
11. Fauci A: The human immunodeficiency virus: Infectivity and mechanisms of pathogenesis. Science 1988; 239:617–622.
12. Bernstein LJ, Ochs HD, Wedgewood RJ, et al: Defective humoral immunity in pediatric acquired immunodeficiency. J Pediatr 1985; 107:352–357.
13. Iochim HL: Immunopathogenesis of human immunodeficiency virus infection. Cancer Res 1990; 54:5612S–5617S.
14. Scott GB, Buck BE, Leterman JG, et al: Acquired immunodeficiency syndrome in infants. N Engl J Med 1984; 310:76–81.
15. Powell KR: Approach to gastrointestinal manifestations in infants and children with HIV infection. J Pediatr 1991; 119:S34-S40.

15a. Ullrich R, Heise W, Bergs C, et al: Gastrointestinal symptoms in patients infected with human immunodeficiency virus: Relevance of infective agents isolated from gastrointestinal tract. Gut 1992; 33:1080–1084.

16. Tavitian A, Raufman JP, Rosenthal LE, et al: Oral candidiasis as marker for esophageal candidiasis in patients with the acquired immunodeficiency syndrome. Ann Intern Med 1986; 104:54–55.
17. DeWit S, Weerts D, Goossens H, et al: Comparison of fluconazole and ketoconazole for oropharyngeal candidiasis in AIDS. Lancet 1989; 1:746–748.
18. Tavitian A, Raufman JP, Rosenthal LE, et al: Ketoconazole-resistant *Candida* esophagitis in patient with AIDS. Gastroenterology 1986; 90:443–445.
19. Greenspan JS, Mastrucci MT, Leggot PJ, et al: Hairy leukoplakia in child (letter). AIDS 1988; 2:143.
20. Greenspan D, Greenspan JSS: The oral clinical features of HIV infection. Gastroenterol Clin North Am 1988; 17:535–543.
21. Rabeneck L, Bokyo WJ, McClean DM, et al: Unusual esophageal ulcers containing enveloped virus-like particles in homosexual men. Gastroenterology 1986; 90:1882–1889.
22. Erice A, Jordan C, Chace BA, et al: Ganciclovir treatment of cytomegalovirus disease in transplant recipients and other immunocompromised hosts. JAMA 1987; 257:3082–3087.
23. Kazlow PG, Shak K, Benkov KJ, et al: Esophageal cryptosporidiosis in a child with acquired immune deficiency syndrome. Gastroenterology 1986; 91:1301–1303.
24. Logan RPH, Polson RJ, Rao G, et al: *Helicobacter pylori* and HIV infection (letter). Lancet 1990; 1:1456.
25. Victoria MS, Nangia BS, Jindrak K: Cytomegalovirus pyloric obstruction in a child with acquired immunodeficiency syndrome. Pediatr Infect Dis 1985; 4:550–552.
26. Bonacini M, Laine L, Gal AA, et al: Prospective evaluation of blind brushing of the esophagus for *Candida* esophagitis in patients with human immunodeficiency virus infection. Am J Gastroenterol 1990; 85:385–389.
27. Dworkin B, Wormser GP, Rosenthal WS, et al: Gastrointestinal manifestations of the acquired immunodeficiency syndrome: A review of 22 cases. Am J Gastroenterol 1985; 80:774–778.
28. Gillin JS, Shike M, Alcock N, et al: Malabsorption and mucosal abnormalities of the small intestine in acquired immunodeficiency syndrome. Ann Intern Med 1985; 102:619–622.
29. Benkov KJ, Stawski C, Sirlin SM, et al: Childhood AIDS

mimicking Crohn's disease. Am J Gastroenterol 1985; 80:260–265.

29a. Bargallo N, Nicolav C, Luburich P, et al: Intestinal tuberculosis in AIDS. Gastrointest Radiol 1992; 17:115–118.

30. Rene E, Marche C, Regnier AG, et al: Intestinal infections in patients with acquired immunodeficiency syndrome: A prospective study in 132 patients. Dig Dis Sci 1989; 34:773–780.

31. Kotler DP, Gaetz HP, Lange M, et al: Enteropathy associated with the acquired immunodeficiency syndrome. Ann Intern Med 1984; 101:421–428.

32. Ulrich R, Zeitz M, Heise W, et al: Small intestinal structure and function in patients infected with human immunodeficiency virus (HIV): Evidence for HIV-induced enteropathy. Ann Intern Med 1989; 111:15–21.

33. Nelson JA, Wiley CA, Reynolds-Kohler C, et al: Human immunodeficiency virus detected in bowel epithelium from patients with gastrointestinal symptoms. Lancet 1988; 1:259–262.

34. Miller TL, Orav EJ, Martin SR, et al: Malnutrition and carbohydrate malabsorption in children with vertically transmitted human immunodeficiency virus 1 infection. Gastroenterology 1991; 100:1296–1302.

35. Yolken RH, Hart W, Oung I, et al: Gastrointestinal dysfunction and disaccharide intolerance in children infected with human immunodeficiency virus. J Pediatr 1991; 118:359–363.

36. Garcia LS, Bruckner DA, Brewer TC, et al: Techniques for the recovery of *Cryptosporidium* oocysts from stool specimens. J Clin Microbiol 1983; 18:185–190.

37. Whiteside M, MacLeod C, Fischl M, et al: Update: Treatment of cryptosporidiosis in patients with AIDS. JAMA 1984; 251:1661–1662.

38. Gazzard BG: HIV disease and the gastroenterologist. Gut 1988; 29:1497–1505.

39. Ungar BL, Ward DJ, Fayer R, et al: Cessation of *Cryptosporidium*-associated diarrhea in an acquired immunodeficiency syndrome patient after treatment with hyperimmune bovine colostrum. Gastroenterology 1990; 98:486–488.

40. DeHovitz JA, Pape JW, Boncy M, et al: Clinical manifestations and therapy of *Isospora belli* infection in patients with the acquired immunodeficiency syndrome. N Engl J Med 1986; 315:87–90.

41. Pape JW, Verdier RI, Johnson WD: Treatment and prophylaxis of *Isospora belli* infection in patients with the acquired immunodeficiency syndrome. N Engl J Med 1989; 320:1044–1047.

42. Laughon BE, Druckman DA, Vernon A, et al: Prevalence of enteric pathogens in homosexual men with and without acquired immunodeficiency syndrome. Gastroenterology 1988; 94:984–993.

43. Smith PD, Lane C, Gill VJ, et al: Intestinal infections in patients with the acquired immunodeficiency syndrome (AIDS). Ann Intern Med 1988; 108:328–333.

44. Quinn TC, Slamm WE, Goodell SE, et al: The polymicrobial origin of intestinal infections in homosexual men. N Engl J Med 1983; 309:576–582.

45. Connolly GM, Shangor DC, Hawkins DA, et al: Noncryptosporidial diarrhoea in human immunodeficiency virus (HIV) infected patients. Gut 1989; 30:195–200.

46. Narkewicz MR, Janoff EN, Sokol RJ, et al: *Blastocystis hominis* gastroenteritis in a hemophiliac with acquired immune deficiency syndrome. J Pediatr Gastroenterol Nutr 1989; 8:125–128.

47. Modigliani R, Bories C, le Charpentier Y, et al: Diarrhoea and malabsorption in acquired immune deficiency syndrome: A study of four cases with special emphasis on opportunistic protozoan infestations. Gut 1985; 26:179–187.

48. Rijpstra AAC, Canning EU, Van Ketel RJ, et al: Use of light microscopy to diagnose small intestinal microsporidiosis in patients with AIDS. J Infect Dis 1988; 157:827–831.

48a. Blanshard C, Hollister WS, Peacock CS, et al: Simultaneous infection with two types of intestinal Microsporidia in a patient with AIDS. Gut 1992; 33:418–420.

48b. Orenstein JM, Tenner M, Kotler DP: Localization of infection by the Microsporidium *Enterocytozoon bieneusi* in the gastrointestinal tract of AIDS patients with diarrhea. AIDS 1992; 6:195–197.

49. Gillin JS, Urmacher C, West R, et al: Disseminated *Mycobacterium avium-intracellulare* infection in acquired immunodeficiency syndrome mimicking Whipple's disease. Gastroenterology 1983; 85:1187–1191.

50. Gray JR, Rabeneck L: Atypical mycobacterial infection of the gastrointestinal tract in AIDS patients. Am J Gastroenterol 1989; 84:1521–1524.

51. Rene E, Marche C, Chevalier T, et al: Cytomegalovirus colitis in patients with acquired immunodeficiency syndrome. Dig Dis Sci 1988; 33:741–750.

52. Chachoua A, Dieterich D, Krasinski K, et al: 9-(1,3-Dihydroxy-2-propoxymethyl) guanine (ganciclovir) in the treatment of cytomegalovirus gastrointestinal disease with the acquired immunodeficiency syndrome. Ann Intern Med 1987; 107:133–137.

53. Patrick CC, Hawkins EP, Guerra C, et al: Clinical conference: A patient with leukemia in remission and acute abdominal pain. J Pediatr 1987; 111:624–629.

54. Balbi JH, McAbee G, Annunziato D, et al: Fatal gastrointestinal hemorrhage in a child with AIDS (letter). JAMA 1989; 262:1470.

55. Dolgin SE, Larsen JG, Shah KD, et al: CMV enteritis causing hemorrhage and obstruction in an infant with AIDS. J Pediatr Surg 1990; 25:696–698.

56. McLoughlin LC, Nord KS, Joshi VV, et al: Severe gastrointestinal involvement in children with the acquired immunodeficiency syndrome. J Pediatr Gastroenterol Nutr 1987; 6:517–524.

57. Johanson JF, Sonnenberg A: Efficient management of diarrhea in the acquired immunodeficiency syndrome (AIDS). Ann Intern Med 1990; 112:942–948.

57a. Pauwells A, Meyohas MC, Eliaszewicz M, et al: Toxoplasma colitis in the acquired immunodeficiency syndrome. Am J Gastroenterol 1992; 87:518–519.

58. Graif M, Kessler A, Neumann Y, et al: Pancreatic Burkitt lymphoma in AIDS: Sonographic appearance. AJR 1987; 146:1290–1291.

59. Haney PJ, Yale-Leohr AJ, Nussbaum AR, et al: Imaging of infants and children with AIDS. AJR 1989; 152:1033–1041.

60. Buck BE, Scott GB, Valdes-Dapena M, et al: Kaposi sarcoma in two infants with acquired immune deficiency syndrome. J Pediatr 1983; 103:911–913.

61. McLoughlin LC, Nord KS, Joshi VV, et al: Disseminated leiomyosarcoma in a child with acquired immune deficiency syndrome. Cancer 1991; 67:2618–2621.

62. Comer GM, Mukherjee S, Scholes JV, et al: Liver biopsies in the acquired immune deficiency syndrome: Influence of endemic disease and drug abuse. Am J Gastroenterol 1989; 84:1525–1531.

63. Kahn SA, Saltzman BR, Klein RS, et al: Hepatic disorders in the acquired immune deficiency syndrome: A clinical and pathologic study. Am J Gastroenterol 1986; 81:1145–1148.

64. Cappell MS, Schwartz MS, Biempica L: Clinical utility of liver biopsy in patients with serum antibodies to the human immunodeficiency virus. Am J Med 1990; 88:123–130.

65. Dubin G, Braffman MN: Zidovudine-induced hepatotoxicity. Ann Intern Med 1989; 110:85–86.

65a. LaFon ME, Kirn A: Human immunodeficiency virus infection of the liver. Semin Liv Dis 1992; 12:197–204.

66. Lebovics E, Thung SN, Schaffner F, et al: The liver in the acquired immunodeficiency syndrome: A clinical and histologic study. Hepatology 1985; 5:293–298.

67. Gordon SC, Reddy KJ, Gould EE, et al: The spectrum of liver disease in the acquired immunodeficiency syndrome. J Hepatol 1986; 2:475–484.

67a. Bach N, Theise ND, Schaffner F: Hepatic histopathology in the acquired immunodeficiency syndrome. Semin Liv Dis 1992; 12:205–212.

68. Jonas MM, Roldan EO, Lyons HJ, et al: Histopathologic features of the liver in pediatric acquired immune deficiency syndrome. J Pediatr Gastroenterol Nutr 1989; 9:73–81.

69. Thung SN, Gerber MA, Benkov KJ, et al: Chronic active hepatitis in a child with human immunodeficiency virus infection. Arch Pathol Lab Med 1988; 112:914–916.

70. Collins JC, Rubinstein A, Morecki R: *Mycobacterium avium-intracellulae* (M. ai) infection is readily diagnosed by liver biopsy in children with AIDS. Gastroenterology 1985; 88:1654.

71. Duffy LF, Daum F, Kahn E, et al: Hepatitis in children with acquired immune deficiency syndrome: Histopathologic and immunocytologic features. Gastroenterology 1986; 90:173–181.

72. Schneiderman DJ, Arenson DM, Cello JP, et al: Hepatic disease in patients with acquired immune deficiency syndrome (AIDS). Hepatology 1987; 7:925–930.
73. Schneiderman DJ: Hepatobiliary abnormalities of AIDS. Gastroenterol Clin North Am 1988; 17:615–630.
74. Polywka S: Hepatitis C virus antibodies among different groups at risks and patients with suspected non-A, non-B hepatitis. Infection 1991; 19:81–84.
75. Martin P, DiBisceglie AM, Kassianides C, et al: Rapidly progressive non-A, non-B hepatitis in patients with human immunodeficiency virus infection. Gastroenterology 1989; 97:1559–1561.
76. Reichert CM, O'Leary TJ, Levens DL, et al: Autopsy pathology in the acquired immune deficiency syndrome. Am J Pathol 1983; 112:357–382.
77. Sachs JR, Greenfield SM, Sohn M, et al: Disseminated *Pneumocystis carinii* infection with hepatic involvement in a patient with the acquired deficiency syndrome. Am J Gastroenterol 1991; 86:82–85.
78. Routlet D, Valla D, Brun-Vezinet F, et al: Cholangitis in the acquired immunodeficiency syndrome: Report of two cases and review of the literature. Gut 1987; 28:1653–1660.
79. Bucuvalas JC, Bove KE, Kaufman RA, et al: Cholangitis associated with *Cryptococcus neoformans*. Gastroenterology 1985; 88:1055–1059.
80. Naveh Y, Mendelsohn H, Spira G, et al: Primary sclerosing cholangitis associated with immunodeficiency. Am J Dis Child 1983; 137:114–117.
81. Hui AN, Koss MN, Meyer RR: Necropsy findings in acquired immunodeficiency syndrome: A comparison of premortem diagnoses with postmortem findings. Hum Pathol 1984; 15:670–676.
82. Klatt EC, Shibata D: Cytomegalovirus infection in the acquired immunodeficiency syndrome: Clinical and autopsy findings. Arch Pathol Lab Med 1988; 112:540–544.
83. Wilcox CM, Forsmark CE, Grendell JH, et al: Cytomegalovirus-associated acute pancreatic disease in patients with acquired immunodeficiency syndrome: Report of two patients. Gastroenterology 1990; 99:263–267.
84. Brivet F, Coffin B, Bedossa P, et al: Pancreatic lesions in AIDS (letter). Lancet 1987; 1:570–571.
85. Zazzo J-F, Pichon F, Regnier B: HIV and the pancreas (letter). Lancet 1987; 1:1212–1213.
86. Bernal A, del Junco G, Pinoit G, et al: Acute pancreatitis in patients with AIDS (abstract). *In* Proceedings of the Fifth International Conference on AIDS. Montreal, Canada, International Development Research Centre, June 1989, p 261.
87. Vendrel J, Nubiola A, Goday A, et al: HIV and the pancreas (letter). Lancet 1987; 1:1212.
88. Miller TL, Winter HS, Luginbuhl LM, et al: Pancreatitis in pediatric human immunodeficiency virus infection. J Pediatr 1992; 120:223–227.
89. Singer P, Katz DP, Dillon L, et al: Nutritional aspects of the acquired immunodeficiency syndrome. Am J Gastroenterol 1992; 87:265–273.
90. Belman AL, Ultmann MH, Horoupian D, et al: Neurological complications in infants and children with acquired immune deficiency syndrome. Ann Neurol 1985; 18:560–566.
91. Ghiron L, Dwyer J, Stollman LB: Nutrition support of the HIV-positive, ARC, and AIDS patient. Clin Nutr 1989; 8:103–113.
92. Lahdevirta J, Maury CPJ, Teppo A-M, et al: Elevated levels of circulating cachectin/tumor necrosis factor in patients with acquired immunodeficiency syndrome. Am J Med 1988; 85:289–291.
93. Greene JB: Clinical approach to weight loss in the patient with HIV infection. Gastroenterol Clin North Am 1988; 17:573–586.
94. Kotler DP: Protein-energy malnutrition in AIDS. Nutr Clin Pract 1990; 5:41–42.
95. Gray RH: Similarities between the acquired immunodeficiency syndrome and protein calorie malnutrition. Am J Public Health 1983; 73:1332.
96. Chandra RK: Nutrition, immunity and infection: Present knowledge and future directions. Lancet 1983; 1:688–691.
97. Beisel WR, Edelman R, Nauss K, et al: Single-nutrient effects on immunologic functions: Report of a workshop sponsored by the Department of Food and Nutrition and its nutrition advisory group of the American Medical Association. JAMA 1981; 245:53–58.
98. Nicholas SW, Leung J, Fennoy I: Guidelines for nutritional support of HIV-infected children. J Pediatr 1991; 119:S59–S62.
99. Fabris N, Mocchegiani E, Galli M, et al: AIDS, zinc deficiency and thymic hormone failure. JAMA 1988; 259:839–840.
100. Smith I, Howells DW, Kendall B, et al: Folate deficiency and demyelination in AIDS. Lancet 1987; 2:215.
101. Dworkin BM, Antonechia PP, Smith F: Reduced selenium content in the acquired immunodeficiency syndrome. J Parenter Enteral Nutr 1989; 13:644–647.
102. Bentler M, Stanish M: Nutrition support of the pediatric patient with AIDS. J Am Diet Assoc 1987; 87:488–491.
103. Fennoy I, Leung J: Refeeding and subsequent growth in the child with AIDS. Nutr Clin Pract 1990; 5:54–58.
104. Wilkinson JD, Greenwald BM: The acquired immuno-deficiency syndrome: Impact on the pediatric intensive care unit. Crit Care Clin 1988; 4:831–844.
105. Shannon KM, Ammann AJ: Acquired immune deficiency syndrome in children. J Pediatr 1985; 106:332–342.

Chapter 57

Irritable Bowel Syndrome

ADAM G. MEZOFF

The term *irritable bowel syndrome* (IBS) describes a constellation of intestinal symptoms that include (1) abdominal distention and pain, (2) relief of abdominal pain with bowel movements, (3) increasingly frequent bowel movements with onset of pain, and (4) looser stools with onset of pain.[1] In adults, more than 90% of patients with IBS have at least two of these symptoms; only 30% of patients with an underlying organic disease have two or more of these symptoms.[2] Patients with IBS may also complain of constipation, mucus in their stools, or a feeling of incomplete evacuation. Recently, guidelines for the diagnosis of IBS based on symptomatic criteria have been published.[3] They include (1) abdominal pain relieved by defecation, (2) disturbed defecation, and (3) bloating or abdominal distention (Table 57–1).

Many terms have been used in the past to describe this symptom complex: *spastic colon, nervous colon, unstable colon*, and *spastic colitis*. The term *colitis*, however, should not be included in the description of this disorder, because it implies histologic evidence of colonic inflammation. This is clearly absent in patients with IBS.

The purpose of this chapter is to review the epidemiology, pathophysiology, signs and symptoms, and treatment of IBS. Much of the information presented is gleaned from studies in adults, as little data are available on this subject in the pediatric literature. This may reflect either a significant difference in the incidence of this disorder in adults as opposed to children or perhaps, simply a difference in terminology used to describe a similar entity.

EPIDEMIOLOGY

In Western cultures, IBS is thought to occur in 15 to 30% of the general population.[4] It occurs more often in whites than in nonwhites, and more often among Jews than non-Jews. In adults, IBS accounts for a significant amount of absenteeism from work. It is the seventh commonest cause for visits to a primary care physician[5] and the commonest cause for referral to a gastroenterologist.[6, 7] Psychological and cultural factors play a significant role in determining which persons seek help from their physicians, and only about one in four patients with symptoms of bowel dysfunction seek medical attention. It has been suggested that females with IBS seek medical attention more often than males, and this may explain the ratio of females to males (2 to 1) with this disorder.[5] Symptoms begin before age 35 in 50% of adults with IBS, and as many as 33% of adult patients trace the onset of their complaints to childhood. Currently, it is unclear what symptoms suggest the diagnosis of IBS in children and what the spectrum of this disorder represents. It has been hypothesized that infantile colic as well as chronic nonspecific diarrhea of childhood are forms of IBS.[8] However, the symptom complex in children that is most consistent with this diagnosis is chronic abdominal pain. Other terms used to describe this disorder include *recurrent abdominal pain* or *functional abdominal pain* (see Chapter 14). Although some children with chronic abdominal pain may experience this symptom as a result of somatization of a significant psychological problem, many parents point out that their child's pain is unrelated to any apparent psychological triggers. As in IBS in adults, this disturbance is exacerbated by stress and anxiety but not necessarily caused by these stimuli. In these patients, the term *irritable bowel* legitimizes the pain to some degree by implying that the locus of the problem is in the stomach or intestine, not the psyche.

Appley and Naish, in their classic study in children,

Table 57–1. SYMPTOMATIC CRITERIA FOR IBS

Continuous or Recurrent Symptoms of:
1. Abdominal pain, relieved with defecation, or associated with a change in frequency or consistency of stool
2. Disturbed defecation (two or more of):
   (a) Altered stool frequency
   (b) Altered stool form (hard or loose/watery)
   (c) Altered stool passage (straining or urgency, feeling of incomplete evacuation)
   (d) Passage of mucus, usually with stools
3. Bloating or feeling of abdominal distention

From Thompson WG, Dotevall G, Drossman DA, et al: Irritable bowel syndrome: Guidelines for the diagnosis. Gastroenterol Int 1989; 2:92–95; with permission.

defined chronic abdominal pain as at least three bouts of pain severe enough to affect the child's activities over a period of not less than 3 months, with attacks occurring during the year preceding the examination.[9] They surveyed 1,000 school-aged children and their mothers and found that, on average, 10.8% of children in this age range fulfilled these criteria. Girls were affected more often than boys (12.3% versus 9.5%), with a peak incidence between 8 and 10 years of age. Although patients younger than 5 years of age generally did not complain of chronic abdominal pain, in retrospect, many patients with chronic abdominal traced the onset of their symptoms to before age five. There was a strong tendency for abdominal and "nervous" disorders to occur in the parents of these children. Faull and Nicol[10] noted a greater prevalence of chronic abdominal pain in 6-year-old patients than did Appley and Naish. They surveyed 494 6-year-old children and found the prevalence of chronic abdominal pain to be between 24.5 and 26.9%.

Based on these epidemiologic studies, chronic abdominal pain in children parallels IBS in adults in many ways. The incidence of chronic abdominal pain, as well as the differences in the incidence of this complaint between the sexes, support this theory. The changes in bowel habits commonly seen in adults with IBS may be a developmental phenomenon, with problems becoming apparent at older ages. Regardless, it remains a matter of speculation whether these two disorders are indeed one and the same.

PATHOPHYSIOLOGY

IBS is thought to be a problem of gastrointestinal motility, perhaps of both the upper and the lower tract. However, since there are no histologic, microbiologic, or biochemical abnormalities associated with this symptom complex, the possibility that IBS merely represents an altered perception of normal gastrointestinal functions has also been entertained. Heaton and coworkers[11] addressed this issue by studying 26 unselected adult females with IBS and comparing them with 27 women with recurrent colonic pain who had not consulted a physician (noncomplainers) and 27 healthy control subjects. They found that abdominal pain was six times more frequent and was more often considered severe in the IBS patients. Defecation was more frequent, more erratic in timing, and more likely to produce stools of extreme form in patients with IBS, and bloating was three times commoner in these patients than in their healthy counterparts. Noncomplainer subjects were intermediate between control subjects and patients previously diagnosed with IBS. IBS patients clearly had higher anxiety and depressive scores than the noncomplainer group, and in every parameter of bowel dysfunction the patients diagnosed with IBS were more severely affected than the noncomplainer group or healthy control group.

Sawyer and associates[12] studied chronic abdominal pain in children and focused on their responsiveness to pain in general. They speculated that children with nonorganic recurrent abdominal pain would perceive pain during routine phlebotomy as more intense than their counterparts with an organic cause of their abdominal pain. The children's perception of pain was quantitated by means of a visual analogue scale. However, no difference between normal children and those diagnosed with functional abdominal pain was found. These studies suggest that there is indeed a physiologic abnormality associated with IBS.

Studies evaluating the electrical response of the colon to various stimuli suggest a difference between normal patients and those with an irritable bowel. IBS patients have a different basal frequency of myoelectric slow waves, different myoelectric and motor response to meals, and a different effect of anticholinergic medication on meal-induced colonic activity.[1]

Motility studies performed in adults with IBS yield varying results, depending on the predominant complex the patient experiences. A pattern of hypermotility exists during symptomatic periods in patients with a pain-predominated symptom complex. High-amplitude pressure waves are found 10 times more commonly in patients with this form of IBS than normal.[13] Balloon dilatation of the rectosigmoid and rectum induces more spastic contractions in IBS patients than in their normal counterparts.[14] Pineiro-Carrero and colleagues[15] studied gastroduodenal motility in eight adolescents with recurrent abdominal pain and seven age-matched controls. They found that the motility pattern of patients with abdominal pain differed from that of the normal patients in four ways: (1) short duration of the activity front of the migrating motor complex, with poor antral contractility; (2) high-pressure, nonpropagating duodenal contractions; (3) disrupted activity fronts of the migrating motor complex; and (4) prominent duodenal contractions before the activity front, with multiple propagating single-ring contractions.

It has been postulated that these disturbances in colonic motility represent a problem with smooth muscle function and that this problem may not be limited to the gastrointestinal tract. There are several studies that suggest that IBS represents a more global smooth muscle dysfunction. Whorell and colleagues[16] and Watier and coworkers[17] have demonstrated abnormal urodynamics in patients with IBS. Whorell and associates[18] have shown an increase in the incidence of orthostatic hypotension in patients with IBS when compared with healthy control subjects. Fielding and Regan[19] described an increase in blood pressure response to a "cold pressor" test in patients with IBS when compared with their normal counterparts. White and coworkers[20] investigated smooth muscle function in the lungs of patients with IBS by airway responsiveness to an inhaled methacholine challenge. They found a decrease in the forced expiratory volume of 20% or more in all 11 patients with IBS they studied, compared with 6 of 11 patients with organic bowel disease (duodenal ulcer, short gut, Crohn's disease, etc.) and only 4 of 11 normal patients. They suggested, as did Read,[21] that IBS may represent the "asthma of the gut."

Incidental reports of resolution of symptoms in IBS

patients placed on fructose-free diets[22] prompted Rumessen and coworkers[23] to postulate that fructose-sorbitol malabsorption may play a significant role in the development of IBS. Nelis and coworkers[24] tested this hypothesis by comparing the incidence of fructose-sorbitol malabsorption in 73 patients with IBS to that in 83 healthy age-matched control subjects. They found that 30.1% of IBS patients and 40.2% of healthy controls had evidence of fructose-sorbitol by breath hydrogen testing. Although this suggests that fructose-sorbitol malabsorption may be one of many triggering events in patients with IBS, it does not support the contention that it is of etiologic significance.

Issenman and coworkers[25] studied 149 healthy children at 22, 40, and 74 months of age. They employed a 24-hour dietary record in an attempt to determine the prevalence of chronic digestive complaints and the relationship to intake of fluid, fiber, or carbohydrate-fat ratio. They found that of all the factors studied, excessive fluid intake (1,470 ± 600 ml per day versus 840 ± 300 ml per day) correlated most strongly with children experiencing abdominal pain or alternating diarrhea and constipation (7 of 22 children). They postulated that this excessive fluid intake may provoke symptoms of IBS in these children.

Thus, experimental evidence points to some functional physiologic difference between patients with IBS and their healthy counterparts. The nature of this disturbance, be it a motility disorder or a global smooth muscle dysfunction, has yet to be elucidated.

CLINICAL FEATURES

Gastrointestinal Manifestations

Abdominal Pain

Abdominal pain is the commonest symptom in patients with IBS. The pain may be crampy or sharp, dull or burning, or a nondescript fullness. The pain may occur any place in the abdomen, but it is often periumbilical or lower abdominal. Pain is often precipitated by meals and rarely awakens patients from sleep. If the pain seems to wake the patient from sleep, care must be taken in eliciting the history to ensure that the patient indeed wakes up because of the pain rather than for some other reason and then notices the pain. In the study by Appley and Naish[9] of chronic abdominal pain in children, two thirds of those studied complained of discomfort around their umbilicus. Most of the remainder complained of pain in the midepigastrium. Faull and Nicol[10] determined the characteristics of abdominal pain in 50 6-year-old children suffering with chronic abdominal pain.[10] The pain in these children was of varying duration (5 minutes to 24 hours per day) and was usually felt in the periumbilical region. Abdominal pain was often associated with other symptoms such as pallor (76%), nausea (52%), anorexia (58%), and tiredness (66%). Most parents (82%) described their children as miserable or listless during an episode of pain. Children ceased to have pain during school holidays about 30% of the time, and 42% of children missed some school because of their pain, although regular absence was uncommon. There was no generalized pattern to the onset of pain in the group as a whole, although some children had a specific time of onset that was typical for them.

Abdominal Distention

Adults with IBS commonly complain about abdominal distention and increased belching or flatulence. Patients may even be unable to tolerate wearing a belt at the end of the day because of this feeling of distention, which is thought to represent a heightened awareness of or sensitivity to their distention rather than an increase in abdominal girth. No comparable symptoms have been regularly described in children, although clinical experience has suggested similarities.

Bowel Habits

Change in bowel habits is frequently part of the IBS symptom complex, often beginning in adolescence. The problem with bowel movements is often progressive and leads to bouts of alternating diarrhea and constipation. Either constipation or diarrhea can predominate, and each patient often has predominance of one of these symptoms. There is often a great deal of patient-to-patient variability, although young children typically have less alterations in their bowel movements than older patients.

Patients with predominantly constipation may go for days or more than a week without defecating. Abdominal pain may increase with prolonged episodes of obstipation. When defecation finally occurs, it leads to relief, but often with a sense of incomplete evacuation. This leads to hours of straining during attempts to have a bowel movement.

Patients with a predominance of diarrhea may have loose, small-volume stools. The initial bowel movement may seem somewhat normal but, subsequently, increasingly loose movements are noted. Abdominal pain preceding and relieved by the movement is common. Often diarrhea is a postprandial event, correlating with the amount rather than with the type of food ingested.

Excess mucus may be a finding in IBS, the cause of which is unknown. Blood in bowel movements is seen in IBS only with associated anorectal disease, such as fissures from constipation.

Upper Intestinal Symptoms

As many as one half of adults with IBS may experience symptoms of upper intestinal involvement, such as dyspepsia, nausea, vomiting, and heartburn. These symptoms are variably found in children.

Extraintestinal Manifestations

Urinary frequency occurs in as many as 65% of adults with IBS, and dysmenorrhea has been noted in as many as 90% of affected adult women. Headache, often migraine-like, is a common accompanying symptom in children with chronic abdominal pain.

Psychological Manifestations

Chaudhary and Truelove[26] noted abnormal psychological manifestations that influenced the onset of symptoms or exacerbated previously existing symptoms in as many as 80% of the 130 IBS patients they studied. Depression, anxiety, and substitution of somatic complaints for anxiety or depression (somatization) were the commonest psychological manifestations noted. Other authors have found that between 54 and 100% of patients with IBS experience some form of mood or anxiety disorder.[27–29] Walker and coworkers[30] compared the psychological profiles of 28 patients with IBS and compared these patients with 19 controls with inflammatory bowel disease. They found that patients with IBS had intermittent *DSM-III-R** anxiety and depressive disorders and that even between major episodes they retained a substantial but subclinical psychological distress. The lifetime prevalence of psychiatric disorders in the IBS patients they studied was 93%, with a 61% lifetime prevalence of depression. A large percentage of patients with IBS also had a prior diagnosis of anxiety disorders. The authors speculated that these anxiety disorders were due to a dysregulation of autonomic nervous system function, which could be associated with the development of a disorder of enteric nervous system motility.

Whitehead and associates[31] found that IBS patients, compared with peptic ulcer and healthy patients, reported more frequent minor illnesses (such as colds), experienced trivial illnesses as more serious, and were more disabled by them. Patients with IBS reported pain from colonic balloon inflation sooner than normal controls,[32, 33] suggesting either more severe upset with minor physiologic alterations or more sensitivity to these upsets. In their study in children, Appley and Naish[9] noted that patients with chronic abdominal pain had a typical psychological profile. He described them as "timid, nervous, anxious, or overconscientious." He stated that in children with this underlying predisposition, school or other difficulties seemed to be the trigger for evoking abdominal pain.

Hodges and coworkers[34] attempted to define the pattern of life events in children with recurrent abdominal pain by means of standardized psychological testing with the Coddington Life Events Inventory.[35] They compared 30 children with recurrent abdominal pain to 67 with behavioral disorders, as well as 42 normal control subjects. They found that children with recurrent abdominal pain and behavioral problems were experiencing high levels of stress, with a Coddington Life Events score between one and two standard deviations above the normative mean for age. Children in different groups experienced different types of life events, with the recurrent abdominal pain group more likely to have experienced events related to illness, hospitalization, and death.

Robinson and coworkers[36] found that adolescents with functional complaints in general (chest pain, recurrent abdominal pain, limb pain, and hyperventilation syndrome) had lower self-esteem, more psychophysiologic symptoms, and a lower self-evaluation than did patients coming for physical examination or routine health maintenance.

*Diagnostic and Statistical Manual of Mental Disorders (Third Edition—Revised). Published by the American Psychiatric Association, Washington, DC, 1987.

Inciting Events

Clearly, there may be an association between exacerbations of IBS and stressful or anxiety-provoking experiences. Food intolerances may also play a role, and individual patients often note the association of abdominal pain with the ingestion of specific foods, such as wheat and milk products, as well as alcohol or caffeine-containing beverages. Cigarette smoking may exacerbate the symptoms of IBS, and women with IBS report an exacerbation of their symptoms with menses.[37]

In the study in children by Faull and Nicol,[10] there were three major groups of precipitants: (1) "nerves" or school-related worries, (2) overeating or eating problems, and (3) use of abdominal pain to "get out of something."

DIAGNOSIS

IBS is a clinical constellation of symptoms and, to a large extent, remains a diagnosis of exclusion. Patients ultimately diagnosed with IBS must therefore have other causes of abdominal pain considered (Table 57–2), including lactose intolerance, inflammatory bowel disease, giardiasis, and somatization of a particular psychological event. Other less common disorders causing chronic abdominal pain include acid-peptic disease, dysmenorrhea, hemolytic anemia, constipation, ureteropelvic junction obstruction, and hepatitis. Lactose intolerance is often suggested by history, but it can be unsuspected because of abundant nonmilk sources of lactose and delayed symptoms, up to several hours after ingestion. Lactose intolerance has been diagnosed in up to a third of patients with chronic abdominal pain.[38] Diets high in sorbitol may also produce symptoms of an irritable bowel. Inflammatory bowel disease is generally accompanied by other symptoms such as hematochezia, fever, and weight loss, as well as laboratory parameters such as increased sedimentation rate. *Giardia* can cause significant abdominal pain, flatus, and diarrhea, much like IBS. Sometimes a travel history or recent camping expedition suggests this possibility. Specific stressful psychological events must be sought to exclude significant somatization due to a particular event, without an irritable bowel in addition.

In general, IBS begins during the first two or three decades of life, is essentially found in the waking state, has recurrent but intermittent symptoms, and is unac-

Table 57–2. CAUSES OF CHRONIC ABDOMINAL PAIN

Psychogenic
Functional
- Constipation
- Irritable bowel syndrome
- Carbohydrate malabsorption (e.g., lactose, sucrose, fructose, sorbitol)

Idiopathic
- Inflammatory bowel disease
- Celiac disease

Urinary Tract Disorders
- Ureteropelvic junction obstruction
- Urinary tract infection
- Kidney stones
- Hydronephrosis

Peptic Disorders
- Esophagitis
- Gastritis
- Duodenitis
- Peptic ulcer

Reproductive System Dysfunction
- Endometriosis
- Dysmenorrhea
- Mittelschmerz

Hemolytic Anemias
- Sickle-cell anemia

Masses and Tumors
Medications
- Aspirin
- Nonsteroidal anti-inflammatory drugs
- Antibiotics (e.g., erythromycin)
- Bronchodilators

Pancreatic Disorders
- Chronic pancreatitis
- Cystic fibrosis

Hepatobiliary Disorders
- Gallstones
- Chronic hepatitis
- Biliary tract infection or dysfunction
- Choledochal cyst

Miscellaneous
- Porphyria
- Hyperlipoproteinemia
- Diskitis
- Parasites

Anatomic
- Duplication cysts
- Mesenteric cysts

Neurologic
- Abdominal migraine
- Abdominal epilepsy
- Transverse myelitis

companied by significant systemic complaints, such as fever, weight loss, and anorexia.[39] To further aid in the differentiation between functional and organic disease, Talley and coworkers[40] devised a self-reporting questionnaire. When employed in 399 test subjects, this questionnaire helped differentiate functional (IBS, functional dyspepsia) versus organic gastrointestinal disease. Functional gastrointestinal disease was also distinguished from organic disease, somatoform disorders, and health.

After a careful history and physical examination, clinicians who suspect IBS will often need to perform some screening tests to reassure the parents and themselves that organic illness is unlikely. A complete blood count and erythrocyte sedimentation rate, as well as a urinalysis, are often helpful. Patients whose abdominal symptoms are associated with milk products should receive a lactose breath hydrogen test. This test should also be considered for children with pain in the late morning, even if in school, since many children have a bowl of cereal with milk for breakfast.

TREATMENT

Perhaps the most important treatment for IBS is reassurance of both the parents and the child. Patients should be told that although their symptoms may be significant, they are not dangerous. Many different modalities have been tried to help alleviate the suffering of patients with IBS, including fiber supplementation, medications, and psychotherapy.

Fiber

The initial therapy for adults with IBS is often a trial of increased fiber by dietary means or fiber supplements

Table 57–3. DIETARY FIBER CONTENT OF SELECTED FOODS AND FIBER SUPPLEMENTS

Amount	Weight (gm)	Food Item	Dietary Fiber (gm)
		Fruits	
Medium	138	Apple, raw	2.8
Medium	166	Pear, raw	4.1
1 cup	160	Grapes, raw	2.6
1 cup	155	Pineapple, raw	2.4
1 cup	149	Strawberries, raw	2.8
		Vegetables	
½ cup	92	Broccoli, frozen spears, boiled	2
7½ in. stalk	40	Celery, raw	0.4
½ cup	82	Corn, frozen, boiled	1.7
½ cup	52	Cucumber, raw	0.3
½ cup	80	Peas, green	3
		Grains	
1 waffle	39	Common Sense Oat Bran	2
1 waffle	39	Nutrigrain	2
1 slice	35	Freihoffer's Stone Ground 100% Whole Wheat Bread	3
½ cup	27	Uncle Ben's Whole Grain Brown Rice	1
1 slice	28	Pepperidge Farm Five Star Fiber Harvest Wheat Bread	2.5
⅔ cup	28	Multi-Bran Chex	4
1 cup	28	Heartwise	6
½ cup	28	Kellogg's Cracklin' Oat Bran	4
½ cup	28	Fruit & Fibre	4
½ cup	28	Fiber One	12
		Fiber Supplements	
1 level tbsp		Citrucel, regular	2
1 heaping tbsp		Citrucel, orange	2
1 rounded tsp		Metamucil, regular	3.4
1 rounded tbsp		Metamucil, orange	3.4
1 rounded tbsp		Metamucil, strawberry	3.4
2 wafers		Metamucil, fiber wafers	3.4
4 cookies		Fibermed, miniatures	5

Data from Bowes & Church, Food Values of Portions Commonly Used. 15th ed. Philadelphia, JB Lippincott, 1989, and from manufacturers' labels.

Table 57–4. MEDICATIONS USED IN THE TREATMENT OF IRRITABLE BOWEL SYNDROME

Anticholinergics and/or Antispasmodics
Dicyclomine (Bentyl)
Trycyclamol and/or phenobarbital
5 anticholinergic
Hyoscyamine (Levsin)
Hyoscyamine, phenobarbital, atropine, scopolamine (Donnatal)
Mebeverine
Trimebutine
Antidepressants
Amitriptyline
Desipramine
Trimipramine
Carminatives
Peppermint oil
Dopamine Antagonists
Domperidone
Opioids
Loperamide (Imodium)
Tranquilizers
Fluphenazine and nortriptyline
Lorazepam
Mepiprazole
Phenaglycodol or meprobamate
Other
Diltiazem
Phenytoin
Timolol

(Table 57–3). Fiber may prolong stool transit time, allowing more time for water and electrolyte absorption, as well as increase stool water content in persons with constipation. Fiber has also been shown to help reduce fasting and postprandial rectosigmoid pressures.[41] Fiber supplementation has proven effective in several studies[42, 43]; however, in rigorously controlled double-blind studies, the results are less impressive.[44–46] Feldman and coworkers[47] studied the effect of fiber on children with recurrent abdominal pain. Fifty-two patients were recruited from the private practices of community physicians in a randomized, double-blind, placebo-controlled trial. They found that by supplementing the diet of these children with at least 10 gm of fiber, they could significantly lessen their abdominal pain. In fact, 13 of 26 patients in the treated group (versus 7 of 26 in the placebo group) had a 50% decrease in frequency of attacks of abdominal pain. However, this trial lasted only 6 weeks, and studies in adults suggest that declining treatment efficacy over time is not unusual. Klein[48] suggests 8 to 12 weeks as the minimum treatment time necessary to ensure that declining treatment efficacy over time does not occur.

Medications

There is a long list of medications that have been studied and continue to be used in the treatment of patients with IBS (Table 57–4). In 1988, Klein[48] reviewed previous studies suggesting that these medications may be efficacious and found that none of the reports, when critically reviewed, offered convincing evidence that any therapy was more effective than was placebo in treating patients with IBS. He had concerns about the methodology used in these studies, particularly the lack of a generally agreed on definition and an accurate means of monitoring the response to therapy. Subsequently Thompson and colleagues[2] published their consensus opinion on the definition of IBS (see Table 57–1), and Svedlund and associates[49] published a clinical rating scale for use in patients with IBS and peptic ulcer disease. These tools may prove useful in future studies of patients with IBS. Currently, however, there is no strong evidence supporting one therapy over another or any therapy over placebo.

In practice, many gastroenterologists find the use of anticholinergics helpful in alleviating the symptoms of their IBS patients. It would seem preferable, however, for the initial therapy in children with IBS to address the possible dietary (sorbitol, caffeine, etc.) as well as psychological triggers of this disorder. A high-fiber diet could be implemented while exploring the contribution of psychological factors to the patient's symptoms. If this initial approach is not successful in providing significant relief from symptoms, and there is no evidence for an underlying organic cause for the patient's symptoms, then a trial of medication might be considered.

Psychological Treatment

Guthrie and coworkers[50] attempted to study the effect of psychotherapy in a controlled trial of patients with IBS. They enrolled only patients who had not improved with standard medical therapy during the previous 6 months. Three months after the start of therapy, the treatment group showed significantly greater improvement than the controls on both the gastroenterologist's and the patient's ratings of diarrhea and abdominal pain. Problems with constipation changed little. Good prognostic factors included overt psychiatric symptoms on entry and intermittent pain clearly exacerbated by stress. Those patients with constant abdominal pain did not tend to improve with psychotherapy.

Bury[51] reported a retrospective study of 111 children referred to a consultative pediatric practice for recurrent abdominal pain. He stressed the importance of firm reassurance with a psychosomatic approach, although the details of the psychosomatic approach were not given. This study was not controlled, and although long-term follow-up was available for several patients, it was not available for all. He stated that at follow-up, 35% of children were completely pain free, 42% were "somewhat better" (although the definition of "somewhat better" is unclear), and 21% were no better.

SUMMARY

The diagnosis of IBS in children remains enigmatic because (1) there are no universally accepted criteria for diagnosis, although efforts are being made in this direction;[2] (2) the diagnosis is based on a constellation of clinical findings in adults that may not always be apparent in children (such as changes in bowel habit); and (3) although certain motility disturbances may be common, there is no standard objective test available to confirm or exclude the diagnosis. Future studies aimed at discovering a unifying pathophysiologic phenomenon, such as smooth muscle dysfunction, will greatly aid in the diagnosis of this entity.

From a practical standpoint, the diagnosis of IBS (as opposed to functional abdominal pain) does not preclude the investigation of possible psychological factors associated with the patient's abdominal pain. Parents tend to be more receptive to pursuing these psychological triggers in the context of an underlying somatic complaint, and if a large psychological component is discovered in pursuit of these "triggers," it can be dealt with appropriately. Stickler and coworkers,[52] in their long-term follow-up study of children with chronic abdominal pain, described appropriate treatment of this problem. They emphasized the need for patients with this disorder, particularly those missing school, to be given a clean bill of health. In addition, they stressed the importance of providing the child with a face-saving device, an excuse, that can explain prolonged absences to peers (e.g., prolonged stomach flu). The diagnosis of IBS may well be technically correct and can serve as this face-saving device. It also provides a means to defuse the anger some parents feel at the trouble and concern their children, without an "organic" cause to their abdominal pain, have caused them.

Undoubtedly there is a subgroup of patients with primarily psychogenic reasons for abdominal pain. However, there are many patients with abdominal pain for whom no organic cause is apparent and who do not clearly demonstrate solely psychogenic triggers. It is perhaps these patients who are most appropriately diagnosed as having IBS.

REFERENCES

1. Schuster MM: Irritable bowel syndrome *In* Sleisenger MH, Fordtran JS, eds: Gastrointestinal Diseases: Pathophysiology, Diagnosis, Management. 4th ed. Philadelphia, WB Saunders, 1989, pp 21–52.
2. Thompson WG, Dotevall G, Drossman DA, et al: Irritable bowel syndrome: Guidelines for the diagnosis. Gastroenterol Int 1989; 2:92–95.
3. Manning AP, Thompson WG, Heaton KW, et al: Towards positive diagnosis of the irritable bowel. Br Med J 1978; 2:653–654.
4. Thompson WG, Heaton KW: Functional bowel disorders in apparently healthy people. Gastroenterology 1982; 79:283–288.
5. Everhart JE, Renault PF: Irritable bowel syndrome in office-based practice in the United States. Gastroenterology 1991; 100:998–1015.
6. Ferguson A, Sircus W, Eastwood MA: Frequency of "functional" gastrointestinal disorders (letter). Lancet 1977; 2:613–614.
7. Harvey RF, Salih SY, Read AE: Organic and functional disorders in 2,000 gastroenterology outpatients. Lancet 1983; 1:632–634.
8. Davidson M, Wasserman R: The irritable colon of childhood (chronic nonspecific diarrhea syndrome). J Pediatr 1966; 69:1027–1038.
9. Appley J, Naish N: Recurrent abdominal pains: A field survey of 1,000 school children. Arch Dis Child 1958; 33:165–170.
10. Faull C, Nicol AR: Abdominal pain in six-year-olds: An epidemiological study in a new town. J Child Psychiat 1986; 27:251–260.
11. Heaton KW, Ghosh S, Braddon FEM: How bad are the symptoms and bowel dysfunction of patients with the irritable bowel syndrome? A prospective, controlled study with emphasis on stool form. Gut 1991; 32:73–79.
12. Sawyer MG, Davidson GP, Goodwin D, et al: Recurrent abdominal pain in childhood: Relationship to psychological adjustment of children and families: A preliminary study. Aust Paediatr J 1987; 23:121–124.
13. Wangle AG, Deller DJ: Intestinal motility in man: III. Mechanisms of constipation and diarrhea with particular reference to the irritable colon syndrome. Gastroenterology 1965; 48:69–84.
14. Mitra R, Chura C, Rajendra GR, et al: Abnormal response to rectal distension in irritable bowel syndrome. Gastroenterology 1974; 66:A770.
15. Pineiro-Carrero VM, Andres JM, Davis RH, et al: Abnormal gastroduodenal motility in children and adolescents with recurrent functional abdominal pain. J Pediatr 1988; 113:820–825.
16. Whorell PJ, Lupton EW, Erduran D, et al: Bladder smooth muscle dysfunction in patients with irritable bowel syndrome. Gut 1986; 27:1014–1017.
17. Watier A, Devroede G, Duranceau A, et al: Constipation with colonic inertia: A manifestation of systemic disease? Dig Dis Sci 1983; 28:1025–1033.
18. Whorell PJ, McCallum M, Creed FH, et al: Non-colonic features of irritable bowel syndrome. Gut 1986; 27:37–40.
19. Fielding JF, Regan R: Excessive cold pressor response in the irritable colon syndrome. Ir J Med Sci 1984; 153:348–350.
20. White AM, Stevens WH, Upton AR, et al: Airway responsiveness to inhaled methacholine in patients with irritable bowel syndrome. Gastroenterology 1991; 100:68–74.
21. Read NW: Irritable bowel syndrome (IBS)—definition and pathophysiology. Scand J Gastroenterol 1987; 130(Suppl):1–7.
22. Anderson DEH, Nygren A: Four cases of long-standing diarrhea and colic pains cured by fructose-free diet: A pathogenetic discussion. Acta Med Scand 1978; 203:87–92.
23. Rumessen JJ, Gudmand-Hoyer E: Functional bowel disease: Malabsorption and abdominal distress after ingestion of fructose, sorbitol and fructose-sorbitol mixtures. Gastroenterology 1988; 95:694–700.
24. Nelis GF, Vermeeren MAP, Jansen WIM: Role of fructose-sorbitol malabsorption in the irritable bowel syndrome. Gastroenterology 1990; 99:1016–1020.
25. Issenman RM, Hewson S, Pirhonen D, et al: Are chronic digestive complaints the result of abnormal dietary patterns? Am J Dis Child 1987; 141:679–682.
26. Chaudhary NA, Truelove SC: The irritable colon syndrome. Q J Med 1962; 31:307–323.
27. Wender PH, Kalm M: Prevalence of attention deficit disorder, residual type, and other psychiatric disorders in patients irritable colon syndrome. Am J Psychiatry 1983; 140:1579–1582.
28. Young SJ, Alpers DH, Norland CC, et al: Psychiatric illness and the irritable bowel syndrome. Gastroenterology 1976; 70:162–166.
29. Hislop IG: Psychological significance of the irritable colon syndrome. Gut 1971; 12:452–457.
30. Walker EQ, Roy-Byrne PP, Katon WJ, et al: Psychiatric illness and irritable bowel syndrome: A comparison with inflammatory bowel disease. Am J Psychiatry 1990; 147:1656–1661.
31. Whitehead WE, Winget C, Fedaravicius AS, et al: Learned illness behavior in patients with irritable bowel syndrome and peptic ulcer. Dig Dis Sci 1982; 27:202–208.
32. Swabrick ET, Hegarty JE, Bat L, et al: Site of pain from the irritable bowel. Lancet 1980; 2:443–446.
33. Ritchie J: Pain from distention of the pelvic colon by inflating a balloon in the irritable colon syndrome. Gut 1973; 14:125–132.
34. Hodges K, Kline JJ, Barbero G, et al: Life events occurring in families of children with recurrent abdominal pain. J Psychosom Res 1984; 28:185–188.
35. Coddington RD: The significance of life events as etiologic factors in the diseases of children. I. A survey of professional workers. J Psychosom Res 1972; 16:7–18.
36. Robinson DP, Greene JW, Walker LS: Functional somatic complaints in adolescents: Relationship to negative life events, self-concept, and family characteristics. J Pediatr 1988; 113:588–593.
37. Whitehead WE, Cheskin LJ, Heller BR, et al: Evidence for

exacerbation of irritable bowel syndrome during menses. Gastroenterology 1990; 98:1485–1489.
38. Liebman WM: Recurrent abdominal pain in children: Lactose and sucrose intolerance. Pediatrics 1979; 64:43–45.
39. Friedman G: Irritable bowel syndrome: I. A practical approach. Am J Gastroenterol 1989; 84:863–867.
40. Talley NJ, Phillips SF, Wiltgen CM, et al: Assessment of functional gastrointestinal disease: The bowel disease questionnaire. Mayo Clin Proc 1990; 65:1456–1479.
41. Cook IJ, Irvine EJ, Campbell D, et al: Effect of dietary fiber on symptoms and rectosigmoid motility in patients with irritable bowel syndrome. Gastroenterology 1990; 98:66–72.
42. Prior A, Whorell PJ: Double-blind study of isphaghula in irritable bowel syndrome. Gut 1987; 28:1510–1513.
43. Thompson WG: A strategy for management of the irritable bowel. Am J Gastroenterol 1986; 81:95–100.
44. Longstreth GF, Fox DD, Youkeles L, et al: Psyllium therapy in the irritable bowel syndrome: A double-blind trial. Ann Intern Med 1981; 95:53–56.
45. Soltoft J, Gudmand-Hoyer E, Krag B, et al: A double-blind trial of the effect of wheat bran on symptoms of irritable bowel syndrome. Lancet 1976; 1:270–272.
46. Lucey MR, Clark ML, Lowndes J, Dawson AM: Is bran efficacious in irritable bowel syndrome? A double-blind placebo controlled crossover study. Gut 1987; 28:221–225.
47. Feldman W, McGrath P, Hodgson C, et al: The use of dietary fiber in the management of simple, childhood, idiopathic, recurrent, abdominal pain. Am J Dis Child 1985; 139:1216–1218.
48. Klein KB: Controlled treatment trials in the irritable bowel syndrome: A critique. Gastroenterology 1988; 95:232–241.
49. Svedlund J, Sjodin I, Dotevall G: GSRS—A clinical rating scale for gastrointestinal symptoms in patients with irritable bowel syndrome and peptic ulcer disease. Dig Dis Sci 1988; 33:129–134.
50. Guthrie E, Creed F, Dawson D, et al: A controlled trial of psychological treatment for the irritable bowel syndrome. Gastroenterology 1991; 100:450–457.
51. Bury RG: A study of 111 children with recurrent abdominal pain. Aust Paediatr J 1987; 23:117–119.
52. Stickler GB, Murphy DB: Recurrent abdominal pain. Am J Dis Child 1979; 133:486–489.

Chapter 58

Polyps and Polyposis Syndromes

REGINO P. GONZALEZ-PERALTA and JOEL M. ANDRES

Intestinal polyps are tumors that protrude into the lumen of the bowel. They are characterized by their gross appearance, location, number per unit area of intestinal surface, presence or absence of a stalk (pedunculated versus sessile), association with extraintestinal lesions, and histologic features that determine their relative risk of malignant transformation.

In adults, most intestinal polyps are either true *neoplastic* polyps, that is, adenomatous lesions, or *benign hyperplastic* polyps. These polyps rarely occur in children and are not discussed in this chapter, except for the adenomas associated with the inherited polyposis syndromes—familial polyposis coli, Gardner's syndrome, and Peutz-Jeghers syndrome.

Juvenile polyps are the most common type of intestinal tumor in children and are a common cause of rectal bleeding. Generally, polyps are asymptomatic; the greatest concern is the propensity of certain polyps to become malignant. Juvenile polyps may be classified as *hamartomatous* polyps, but some authors refer to them as *inflammatory* or *retention* polyps. Most of the inherited polyposis syndromes are autosomal dominant diseases, except for Turcot's syndrome, which is probably autosomal recessive. These inherited conditions are either hamartomatous or adenomatous polyposis syndromes (Table 58–1). Carcinomas generally do not evolve from the hamartomatous syndromes, whereas malignant change is a major concern in the adenomatous syndromes. *Mixed juvenile-adenomatous polyps* have also been reported. The *noninherited polyposes* may include nodular lymphoid hyperplasia, inflammatory polyps, and the rare syndromes described by Cronkhite-Canada and Ruvalcaba-Myhre-Smith.

JUVENILE POLYPS

Clinical Characteristics

The origin and the genetic predisposition of juvenile polyps are unknown; they are believed to have either a hamartomatous or an inflammatory etiology. Juvenile polyps, also referred to as *retention* polyps, are the most common polypoid lesion of the colon in children, accounting for nearly 90% of colorectal polyps. These polyps are rarely discovered in children younger than 1 year of age and are usually diagnosed between the ages of 2 and 10 years. Early precolonoscopy reports indicated that juvenile polyps were usually solitary and invariably were located in the rectosigmoid colon. In the past few years, however, new findings have emerged. In one study, the incidence of multiple polyps substantially increased. Further, more juvenile polyps were noted to occur in the right colon. None were described proximal to the descending colon in the period from 1974 to 1975, whereas the incidence was 44% in the period from 1982 to 1984.[1] Similar results were reported by other investigators,[2] who noted that 58% of patients had more than one polyp and that 26% of the polyps were located proximal to the transverse colon. The differences in these findings probably represent more extensive use of colonoscopy in the evaluation of rectal bleeding in children during the later periods.

Children with juvenile polyps characteristically present with asymptomatic hematochezia, usually mild, although the associated rectal bleeding can be profuse. As many as one third of affected children can experience microcytic, hypochromic anemia related to chronic blood loss.[2] Diarrhea and tenesmus can occur, especially if the polyps are located in the distal colon. Similarly, rectal prolapse or prolapse of a rectal polyp is occasion-

Table 58–1. CLASSIFICATION OF POLYPS AND POLYPOSIS SYNDROMES

Juvenile Polyp(s)
Inherited Hamartomatous Polyposis Syndromes
Juvenile polyposis
Peutz-Jeghers syndrome
Cowden's syndrome
Inherited Adenomatous Polyposis Syndromes
Familial polyposis coli
Gardner's syndrome
Turcot's syndrome
Noninherited Polyposis
Lymphoid polyposis
Inflammatory polyposis
Cronkhite-Canada syndrome
Ruvalcaba-Myhre-Smith syndrome

ally seen. Colocolonic intussusception associated with pedunculated polyps is rare. Juvenile polyps have been noted at ureterosigmoidostomy anastomotic sites.[3]

Pathology

Grossly (Fig. 58–1*A*), juvenile polyps are large (0.5–3 cm) and usually erythematous, which contrasts with the normal pink colonic mucosa. The polyp surface glistens, and large fluid-filled cystic areas are typically noted on cut-section examination. They are often friable and bleed easily when manipulated by the colonoscope. Most juvenile polyps are pedunculated; sessile polyps are rare. Histologically (Fig. 58–1*B*), they are mucosal lesions that consist of dilated, mucus-filled, tortuous cystic glands and inflammatory cells in a prominent lamina propria. The glands are composed of well-formed mucous-secreting cells. Occasionally, dilated glands rupture into the stroma, eliciting a foreign giant cell reaction.[4]

Juvenile Polyps, Adenoma, and Cancer

Recent reports have documented adenomatous changes in juvenile polyps.[2, 3, 5–12] Juvenile polyps are not neoplastic, per se, but focal adenomatous areas[2, 5–8a] and epithelial dysplasia[13] in these polyps may confer a risk of carcinoma, even in children.[6–8a] Most if not all colorectal carcinomas arise from pre-existing adenomas of the colon.[10] In addition, relatives of patients with juvenile polyposis are at risk of developing cancer.[6, 9] Because of these facts, it has been suggested that juvenile polyposis (versus isolated juvenile polyps) should be considered as seriously as the familial adenomatous polyposis syndromes, except that regular colonoscopic surveillance may obviate the need for prophylactic colectomy.[12, 13] Even though the degree of association between juvenile polyps and gastrointestinal carcinoma is probably low, this pathogenetic sequence needs to be studied more carefully.

Diagnosis and Management

Specific guidelines for the management of children with juvenile polyps are difficult to establish, because the natural history of this common problem is not clearly understood. Unfortunately, there is a paucity of literature to support the general belief that most juvenile polyps outgrow their vascular supply, become necrotic, and subsequently autoamputate. However, because of significant anemia and the possibility that adenomatous polyps may be more common in children than was previously believed, the diagnosis by colonoscopy and removal of all juvenile polyps may be warranted. After conscious sedation, colonoscopy and polypectomy can be safely accomplished with snare electrocauterization[2]; general anesthesia is rarely required. After the removal of mixed juvenile-adenomatous polyps, children should be carefully monitored. Although the precise recommendation regarding the frequency of endoscopic evaluation is not known in such instances, surveillance colonoscopy is suggested at least every 2 years, or earlier if rectal bleeding recurs. For the newly referred child, a colonoscopy to the cecum is prudent when polyps are noted by barium contrast study (Fig. 58–2) or suspected because of prolapse of a rectal mass, and in the presence of unexplained rectal bleeding.[2] After removal of an isolated juvenile polyp, a child does not require any further evaluation unless there is a recurrence of rectal bleeding.

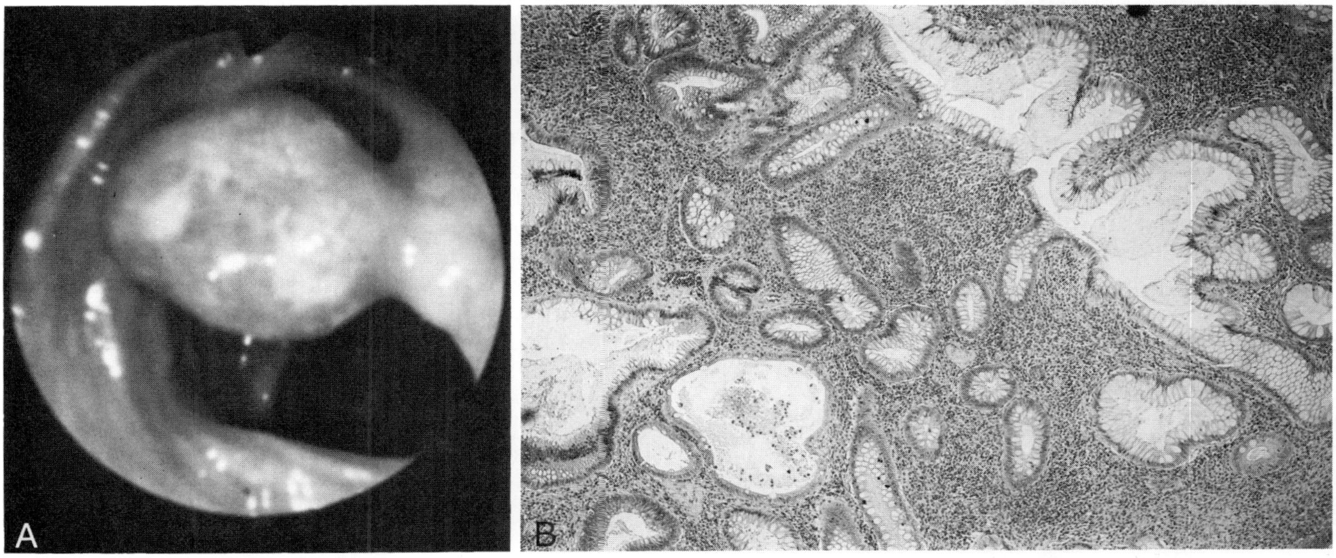

Figure 58–1. Juvenile polyp. *A,* Large pedunculated polyp in distal colon as seen through the colonoscope (Courtesy of William R. Treem, MD). *B,* This lowpower (× 63) photomicrograph of a juvenile polyp demonstrates the typical cystic, mucus-filled glands and prominent lamina propria with inflammatory cells.

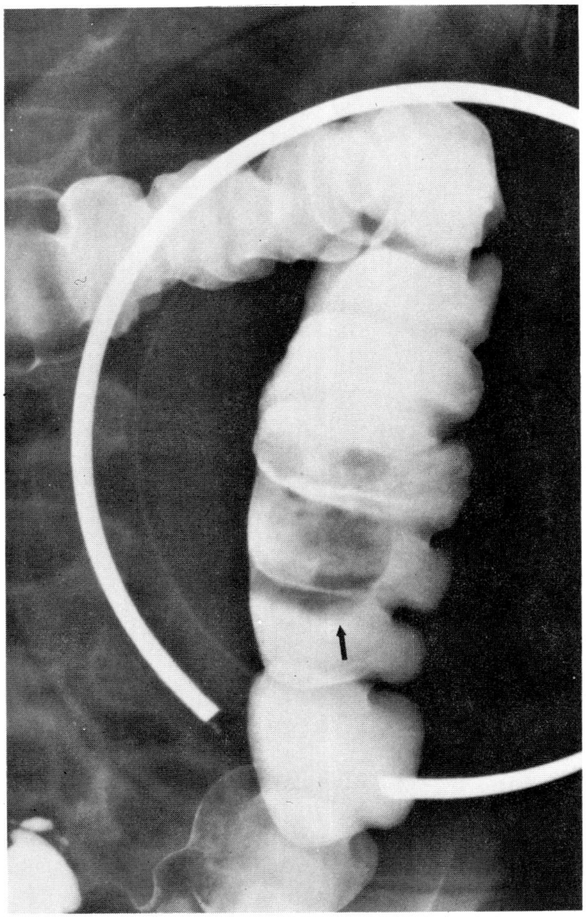

Figure 58–2. This barium enema spot film of the distal colon demonstrates a large juvenile polyp *(arrow)*.

INHERITED HAMARTOMATOUS POLYPOSIS SYNDROMES

There are familial syndromes that are characterized by hamartomatous polyps of the gastrointestinal tract. These include juvenile polyposis, Peutz-Jeghers syndrome, and Cowden's syndrome (Table 58–2).

Juvenile Polyposis

This group of rare familial syndromes includes (1) juvenile polyposis, (2) juvenile polyposis of infancy, and (3) generalized gastrointestinal polyposis.[14, 15]

The commonest of these polyposis syndromes is juvenile polyposis, in which children with multiple colonic polyps are usually diagnosed in the first decade of life.[14, 15] An autosomal dominant gene is suspected but not proved, as approximately 50% of affected persons have a positive family history. The diagnosis of juvenile polyposis is likely when five or more juvenile polyps are discovered in the colorectum or throughout the gastrointestinal tract, *or* with the presence of any number of juvenile polyps plus a family history of juvenile polyposis.[13, 16] Associated anomalies include hypertelorism, intestinal malrotation, hydrocephalus, undescended testis, and Meckel's diverticulum.[14] Similar findings characterize juvenile polyposis of infancy, in addition to involvement of the stomach and the small intestine. Bloody or mucoid diarrhea usually occurs in the first few weeks of life. Rectal prolapse and intussusception may develop, the latter leading to death in a few instances.[17] In these children, diarrhea and intestinal protein losses lead to severe malnutrition and failure to thrive. There is some evidence that this form of juvenile polyposis represents autosomal recessive inheritance.[18] In generalized juvenile polyposis, there are multiple polyps throughout the gastrointestinal tract,[19] but sometimes they are confined exclusively to the stomach.[20]

Peutz-Jeghers Syndrome

Clinical Characteristics

Peutz[21] first noted the association of mucocutaneous pigmentation with intestinal polyposis in three generations of a Dutch family. Twenty-eight years later, Jeghers and associates[22] reported 10 similar cases, and Peutz-Jeghers syndrome became widely recognized. By 1969, Peutz-Jeghers syndrome was described in 321 patients of wide ethnic and geographic distribution.[23] A Mendelian dominant mode of inheritance was first suggested by Jeghers and associates.[22] In one study of five generations of a family, only three persons were free of abnormal pigmentation or polyps.[24] However, only 50% of people with Peutz-Jeghers syndrome provide a positive family history. This probably represents an incomplete diagnosis of the disorder in relatives. Moreover, it is estimated that fewer than 5% of people with polyposis do not have hyperpigmentation, and fewer than 5% have hyperpigmentation without gastrointestinal polyps.[16] These variations suggest an autosomal dominant gene with high penetrance and variable expression.[23]

The abnormal pigmentation (Fig. 58–3) consists of

Table 58–2. INHERITED HAMARTOMATOUS POLYPOSIS SYNDROMES: CLINICAL CHARACTERISTICS

Syndrome	Location of Polyps	Extraintestinal Abnormalities	Risk of Cancer
Juvenile polyposis	Mainly colon; also small intestine	—	Colon—small
Peutz-Jeghers syndrome	Small intestine; also colon and stomach	Pigmented spots of lips, mouth, and hands	Gastrointestinal cancer and ovarian tumors
Cowden's syndrome	Colon and stomach	Lipomas, papillomas, multiple other hamartomas	Breast and thyroid cancer

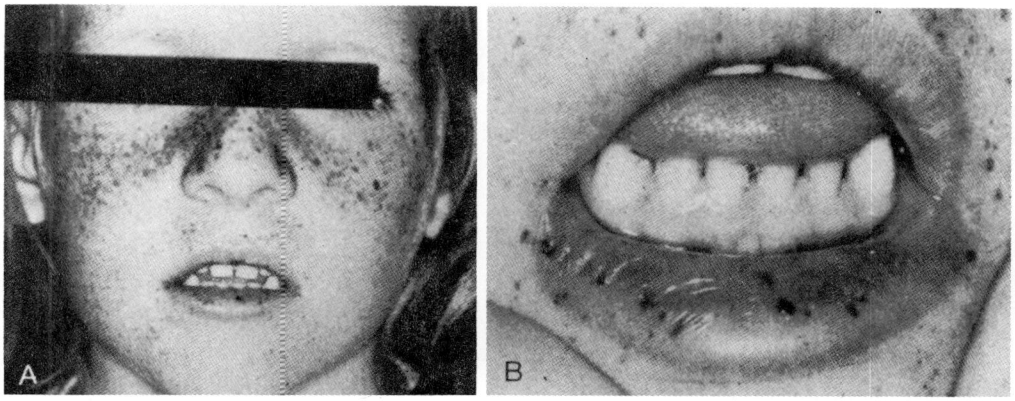

Figure 58–3. Mucocutaneous pigmentation in Peutz-Jeghers syndrome. *A,* Brown-black macules are distributed over the face and lips of a 5-year-old patient. *B,* The pigmented lesions are seen involving the lips and crossing the vermillion border. (From Yosowitz P, Hobson R, Ruymann F. Am J Dis Child 1974; 128:709–712; with permission. Copyright 1974, American Medical Association.)

brown-black macules, 1 to 5 mm in diameter, which look like freckles and vary in number and distribution. They usually appear during infancy or early childhood and commonly involve the lips and oral mucosa; they may be also found on the hands, feet, digits, tongue, eyelids, or perineum.[25, 26] Although the hyperpigmentation on the lips is the most reliable finding, these, like cutaneous lesions, tend to fade over time. In addition, lip pigmentation is not uncommonly found in persons without Peutz-Jeghers syndrome. Unlike the skin pigmentation, mucosal lesions like those involving the gingiva persist and are thus more helpful for diagnosis.[16]

Multiple polyps are found in more than 90% of cases,[26] especially in older persons, although solitary polyps have been described. They vary in number and distribution, sometimes involving the entire gastrointestinal tract. The tumors are frequently present in the small bowel, particularly in the jejunum. In decreasing order of frequency, they can be found in the colon, stomach, duodenum, and appendix.[26] Rarely, polyps occur in the nasopharynx and the urinary bladder.[21]

Pathology

The polyps in patients with Peutz-Jeghers syndrome are sessile or pedunculated, varying in size from 1 to 3 cm. Histologically (Fig. 58–4), the polyps are hamartomatous and consist of a glandular epithelium with prominent branching bands of smooth muscle within the lamina propria.[4] Unlike juvenile polyps, the lamina propria of Peutz-Jeghers syndrome polyps appears normal.

Diagnosis and Management

Approximately one third of persons with Peutz-Jeghers syndrome are diagnosed during childhood and adolescence.[26] The commonest presenting complaint is abdominal pain, which has been reported to occur in as many as 87% of pediatric patients.[25] Symptoms usually appear during adolescence, although they have been reported in young children[27] and infants.[28] The abdominal pain is commonly colicky, intermittent, and related

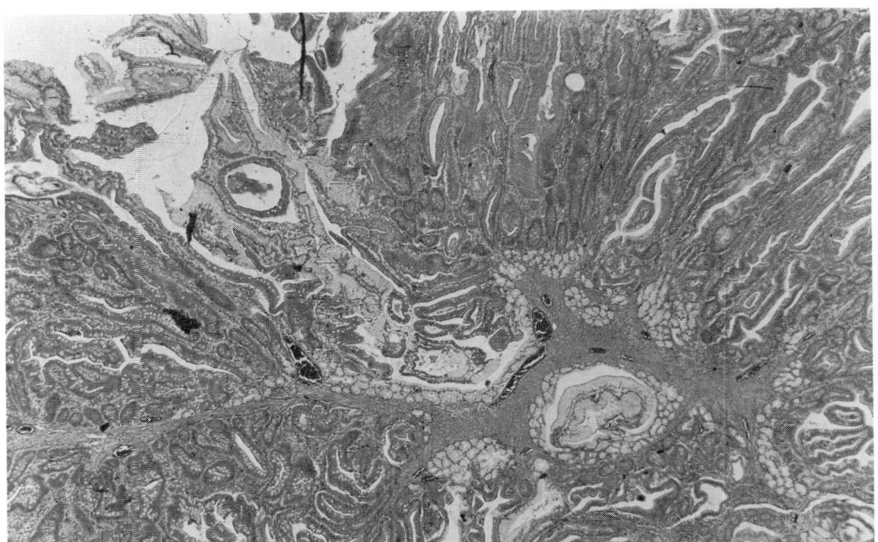

Figure 58–4. Peutz-Jeghers syndrome. Low-power photomicrograph (× 25) of Peutz-Jeghers polyp demonstrates the typical branching bands of smooth muscle surrounded by glandular epithelium.

to recurrent intussusception, which rarely causes complete obstruction and usually reduces spontaneously.[29] Microcytic, hypochromic anemia secondary to chronic gastrointestinal blood loss is encountered. However, in contrast with children with juvenile polyposis, anemia is a far more common finding.[26]

The potential of polyps in Peutz-Jeghers syndrome to undergo malignant transformation has been much debated. Earlier literature probably overestimated malignant transformation because of the unusual histologic findings, especially the admixture of glandular tissue with smooth muscle elements interpreted as tumor invasion. As the hamartomatous nature of these tumors was recognized, the cancerous potential was considered negligible.[30] Although this is now generally accepted, hamartomatous polyps in patients with Peutz-Jeghers syndrome have been discovered to contain areas of adenoma and carcinoma.[31] In addition, gastrointestinal cancer has been reported in patients with Peutz-Jeghers syndrome, usually in those with stomach or duodenal involvement.[23] Small intestinal and colonic adenocarcinoma have also been noted.[32] Moreover, breast cancer,[33, 34] ovarian tumors,[35] sex cord tumors,[36, 37] and Sertoli cell tumors[38] have been described. It was recently reported that malignancy developed in 15 patients with Peutz-Jeghers syndrome (gastrointestinal carcinoma, 4; nongastrointestinal, 10; and multiple myeloma, 1). With the use of relative risk analysis, it was concluded that persons with Peutz-Jeghers syndrome have a risk that is 18 times greater for cancer than is expected in the general population.[33] Thus, although the risk is considerably less than is seen with other inherited polyposis syndromes, the risk of malignancy is substantial in Peutz-Jeghers syndrome.[33, 39]

When the diagnosis of Peutz-Jeghers syndrome is considered based on family history and clinical findings, the gastrointestinal tract must be thoroughly investigated. Upper gastrointestinal contrast studies may identify larger polyps in the stomach, the duodenum, and the small intestine (Fig. 58–5). Similarly, air contrast barium enema or flexible colonoscopy delineates polyps in the large bowel. Conservative management is advocated in the treatment of patients with Peutz-Jeghers syndrome.[16, 23] Bed rest, mild sedation, and nasogastric suction usually suffice during an episode of intussusception. If bowel obstruction is suspected, surgical intervention should not be delayed. Since the subsequent development of polyps may require further surgical procedures, as many polyps as possible should be removed. Surgery should be considered also in patients with significant gastrointestinal bleeding or with frequent episodes of abdominal pain. Because of the apparent higher risk for malignant transformation, surgical or endoscopic removal of gastric and duodenal polyps is recommended.[23, 27] Moreover, female patients should undergo regular pelvic examinations.

Cowden's Syndrome

Cowden's syndrome is characterized by multiple hamartomatous lesions of ectodermal, mesodermal, and endodermal origin. The mucocutaneous lesions are the most characteristic extraintestinal feature of this syndrome and include hyperkeratotic papillomas of the lips, tongue, and nares.[40] This polyposis syndrome with orocutaneous hamartomas is considered an autosomal dominant disorder that usually presents in the second or third decade of life.[41] Polyps occur throughout the gastrointestinal tract, but are commonest in the colon and stomach.[41] All colonic polyps have been characterized as hamartomatous.[42] The frequency of gastrointestinal cancer is apparently not increased in patients with this disorder. There is a high incidence of breast involvement in women; most of the lesions are fibrocystic or fibroadenomatous, but ductal carcinomas have been reported.[43] Thyroid disease is present in many patients, usually in the form of nodular hyperplasia or follicular adenoma of the thyroid.[43]

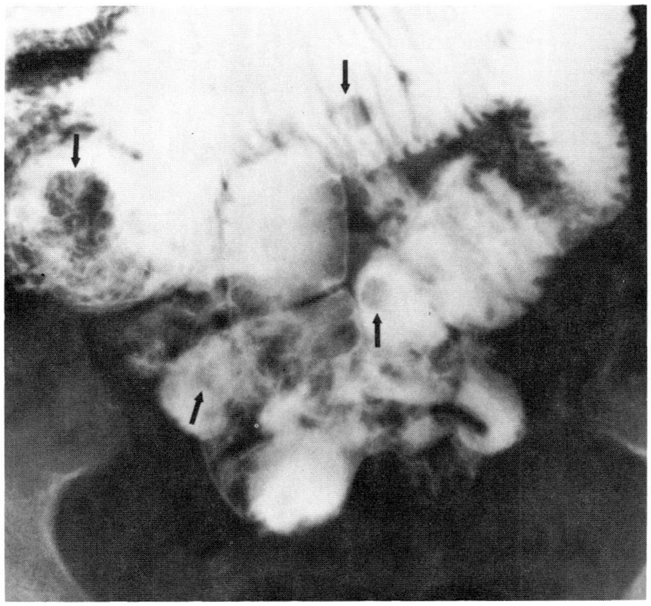

Figure 58–5. This barium contrast study demonstrates the presence of several polyps in the intestine *(arrows)* of a child with Peutz-Jeghers syndrome.

INHERITED ADENOMATOUS POLYPOSIS SYNDROMES

The inherited adenomatous polyposis syndromes include familial polyposis coli, Gardner's syndrome, and Turcot's syndrome (see Table 58–1). They all have an autosomal dominant mode of inheritance, except Turcot's syndrome, and are characterized by the development of hundreds of gastrointestinal polypoid lesions that invariably undergo malignant transformation. The syndromes are distinguished by the location of the polyps and the presence of extraintestinal abnormalities.

Familial Polyposis Coli

Familial polyposis coli is an autosomal dominant disease that occurs in approximately 1 in 10, 000 live births. The term *polyposis coli* is a misnomer, since polyps

Table 58–3. INHERITED ADENOMATOUS POLYPOSIS SYNDROMES: CLINICAL CHARACTERISTICS

Syndrome	Location of Polyps	Extraintestinal Abnormalities	Risk of Cancer
Familial polyposis coil	Colon; also ileum, duodenum, ampulla, and gastric antrum	Osteomas of mandible	Colon, small intestine—marked
Gardner's syndrome	Colon; small intestine, ampulla, and stomach	Osteomas of mandible, skull, and long bones; lipomas; fibromas; desmoid tumors	Colon, small intestine—marked
Turcot's syndrome	Colon	Brain tumors	Colon—marked; medulloblastoma, glioma

have been discovered in the stomach and the small intestine.[44]

Clinical Characteristics

The adenomatous polyps usually appear in the second or third decade of life. Younger patients initially have a small number of polyps, but familial polyposis coli is characterized by the gradual development of thousands of sessile colonic polyps throughout its length (Table 58–3). As it is in Gardner's syndrome, colorectal cancer should be considered inevitable in the natural history of familial polyposis coli. Malignant change occurs in polyps, but also can develop in surrounding mucosa that may appear normal to the endoscopist.[45]

The adenomatous polyposis syndromes cannot always be categorized exclusively as either familial polyposis coli or Gardner's syndrome. When carefully sought, even extraintestinal manifestations, such as mandibular osteomas and upper gastrointestinal polyps, can be seen in most patients with familial polyposis coli.[46] Adenomatous polyps may be found in the ileum, duodenum, periampullary region, papilla of Vater, and antrum.[47, 48, 48a] Thus, it has become difficult to argue that familial polyposis coli and Gardner's syndrome are not variable expressions of a single disease entity.

Pathology

In familial polyposis coli, the polyps are small, usually less than 5 mm in diameter (Fig. 58–6*A*), and histologically identical to the polyps noted in patients with Gardner's syndrome. Their surface is often divided into "lobules" by interconnecting clefts in the apex of the polyp. The glands are lined by elongated epithelial cells with hyperchromatic nuclei, and mucin content is generally diminished (Fig. 58–6*B*). Numerous mitotic figures are commonly noted.[4]

Genetics and Cancer

Recently, alteration of gene structure and expression has been noted in familial polyposis coli and Gardner's syndrome; specifically, there is allelic deletion in a small region on the long arm of chromosome 5.[49, 50] Allelic deletions and mutations may occur on several chromosomes, suggesting mutational activation of an oncogene and loss of tumor suppressor genes in the development of colon cancer.[51, 52] In general, findings suggest that an inherited susceptibility to colonic adenomas and colorectal cancer is responsible for the adenoma-dysplasia-carcinoma sequence.[53] Research advances, such as gene carriage, will eventually be used clinically to identify persons at risk for colon cancer.[52]

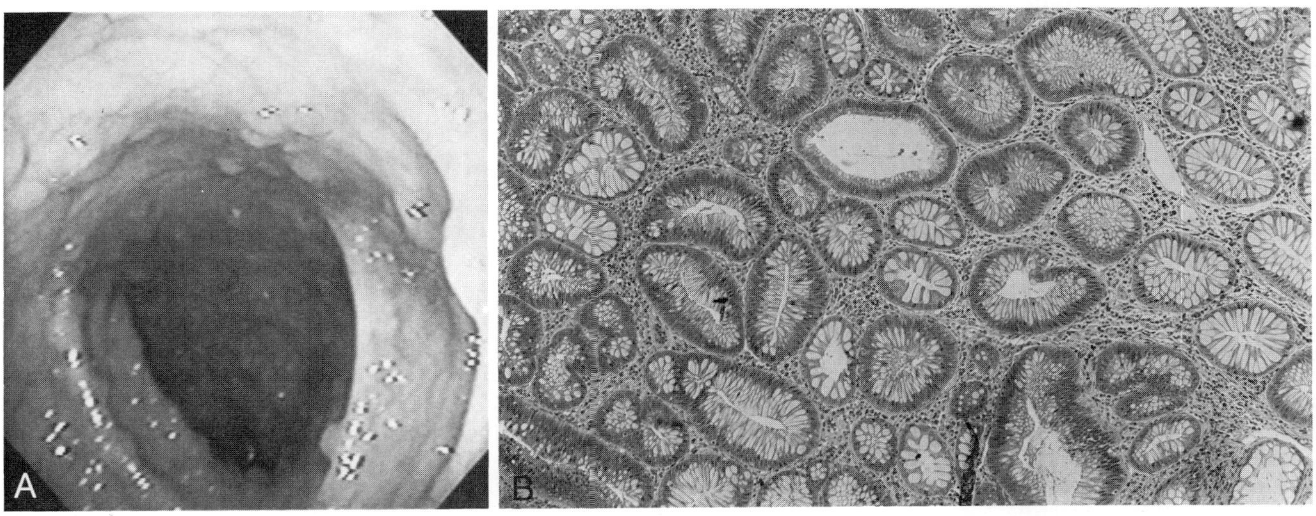

Figure 58–6. Familial polyposis coli. *A*, Multiple, small, sessile polyps noted at the time of colonoscopy. *B*, This photomicrograph (× 100) of a polyp demonstrates the tightly packed, proliferating adenomatous epithelium with hyperchromatic nuclei and mucin depletion. The small amount of lamina propria is free of inflammation.

Diagnosis and Management of Adenomatous Polyposis

No consensus exists in the literature as to the identification and monitoring of adults and children at risk for malignancy. Many authors believe that surveillance of patients with asymptomatic familial polyposis should begin during adolescence.[54] However, other authors advocate a more aggressive approach and recommend an evaluation of the gastrointestinal tract by the end of the first decade of life.[55] This recommendation is based on the fact that malignant changes in patients with multiple colonic polyposis have been reported prior to 9 years of age. Moreover, the incidence of colon cancer in children with adenomatous polyposis younger than 13 years of age was reported to be 6.5%.[56] In a large review of 75 patients, 4 children (5.3%) were documented to have carcinomatous changes at the time of initial evaluation.[57] Diagnosis of familial polyposis coli is based on the presence of more than 100 adenomatous polyps in the colon. Surgery is generally required for polyps larger than 5 mm in diameter, because the risk of advanced cancer is higher in polyps of that size compared with those smaller than 5 mm.[58] When there are six to nine polyps per square centimeter, the malignant potential of familial adenomatous polyposis is highly significant. Children in this category should be operated on prior to 15 years of age[58]; otherwise, the timing of colectomy is controversial, and no markers are available to predict malignant transformation of adenomas. All family members should be carefully examined.

Colonoscopy is completed early in the evaluation, because it allows for identification of these small sessile lesions that may be overlooked by barium studies and provides tissue acquisition for histologic review. Children with documented adenomatous polyposis should be examined at least annually. Patients who manifest the polyposis gene require total colectomy; this usually occurs in late adolescence or young adulthood.

The ileal pouch–anal anastomosis is considered superior to the ileoanal or ileorectal anastomosis, although some surgeons believe the latter two procedures are satisfactory for children.[59] Ideally, the procedure should eliminate the need for ileostomy and ensure intestinal continuity and continence. Ileoanal anastomosis is preferable to the ileorectal anastomosis procedure, especially because the risk for future carcinoma is eliminated, and there is no need for regular sigmoidoscopic reexaminations. The advantages of the ileorectal procedure include the higher possibility of anorectal continence and a shorter convalescence after major surgery. Some investigators advocate the ileorectal anastomosis if no adenomatous polyps are discovered in the rectum.

Finally, because of the possibility of carcinoma of the ampulla of Vater, duodenum, and antrum in patients with familial adenomatous polyposis, it is imperative to conduct regular surveillance of the upper gastrointestinal tract in all of these patients, even after surgical extirpation of the large intestine.[60]

Gardner's Syndrome

Clinical Characteristics

Gardner's syndrome is characterized by the triad of gastrointestinal polyps, osteomas, and soft tissue tumors. The polyps are numerous (usually more than 1,000) and at times appear to carpet the intestinal mucosa. They are almost exclusively small (2–5 mm) and sessile, although occasional pedunculated lesions are encountered. The polyps were initially reported to involve only the colon; however, recent studies have demonstrated that they often occur in the stomach, the duodenum, and, less commonly, other parts of the small intestine.[61, 62] The upper gastrointestinal polyps are usually asymptomatic until they are large, when bleeding and bowel obstruction can become manifest. Histologically, adenomas are typically found in the gastric antrum and the duodenum, especially in the periampullary region. Jejunal and ileal polyps are, histologically, adenomas or focal lymphoid hyperplasia. In general, the risk of malignant transformation of gastric and small intestinal polyps is negligible; however, duodenal tumors have a high proclivity for malignancy.[54]

Bony abnormalities include osteomas, which do not develop until the second decade of life, and thickening of the long bones. The osteomas most commonly involve the skull, including the calvaria, the maxilla, and the mandible. The soft tissue lesions are usually epidermoid cysts, which are often misdiagnosed as sebaceous cysts. They are usually found on the head, neck, and trunk. Subcutaneous fibromas, which commonly involve the scalp, shoulders, arms, and back, and desmoid tumors are sometimes noted. The desmoid tumors, also referred to as *diffuse mesenteric fibromatosis*, are a particularly serious complication, because they occur intra-abdominally and lead to intestinal, vascular, and ureteral obstruction.[63]

Other extraintestinal malformations of Gardner's syndrome include dental abnormalities, such as odontomas, dentiginous cysts, and supernumerary teeth. These lesions are usually detected by panoramic radiography of the teeth and mandible. Recently, hyperpigmentation of the retinal epithelium was reported in patients with Gardner's syndrome.[64] The retinal pigmentation was found to be a specific and sensitive early clinical marker for Gardner's syndrome in persons at risk for the development of the disease.[64, 65] This syndrome has also been associated with carcinoma of the pancreas and the ampulla of Vater,[66] in addition to hepatoblastoma.[67]

Diagnosis

Many patients initially seek medical attention because of known affected relatives. However, when the syndrome is not suspected, rectal bleeding, diarrhea, and abdominal pain are frequent presenting complaints; mucoid rectal discharge occurs less frequently. Interestingly, and in contrast with the familial hamartomatous polyposis syndromes, intussusception is rarely a problem in Gardner's syndrome.[68] Constitutional symptoms and signs, such as anorexia, weight loss, and weakness, may be the presenting manifestations of occult malignancy. Although colonic polyps generally appear during the first two decades of life, they have been documented from 8 months to 72 years of age.[55] Polyps usually do not produce symptoms until 10 years after their appearance, a fact that underscores the importance of identifying people at risk. The significance of adenomatous polyposis syndromes, including Gardner's syndrome, relates to the inevitable malignant transformation, which is usually not detected until 10 years after polyps are identified and approaches 100% by age 55 years in untreated cases.[54]

Turcot's Syndrome

Turcot's syndrome represents the association between familial adenomatous polyposis and neural tumors. The initial report described two cases of familial polyposis in siblings who both developed cerebral tumors, a medulloblastoma and a glioblastoma.[69] This syndrome is a rare autosomal recessive disorder[70]; the diagnosis should be restricted to patients with familial polyposis associated with medulloblastomas or gliomas.[71] It is an example of a pluripotential gene mutation that also predisposes to neural malignancy.[71] Patients with Turcot's syndrome are frequently adolescents, and they present with symptoms attributable to either intestinal or neural tumors. In general, colon cancer may occur at an earlier age in this syndrome.[72] Already described in patients with the other familial adenomatous polyposis syndromes, hypertrophy of the retinal pigment epithelium was recently reported in a young patient with Turcot's syndrome.[72a]

NONINHERITED POLYPOSIS DISORDERS

Lymphoid Polyposis

Clinical Characteristics

Nodular lymphoid hyperplasia, or aggregates of lymphoid follicles, gives rise to submucosal nodules in the intestine of children (Table 58–4). These lymphoid polyps are small (1–5 mm), sessile, umbilicated protrusions that typically are noted in the distal colon, although they may be seen throughout the intestinal tract. They probably represent a response of intestinal lymphoid tissue to chemical, infectious, or traumatic stimulation.[73] An association has been described with dysgammaglobulinemia,[74] especially when the lymphoid polyps are limited to the small intestine. It has also been noted in Hirschsprung's disease complicated by enterocolitis[75] and in children with inflammatory bowel disease.[76]

Lymphoid hyperplasia is generally considered a benign, self-limited entity, probably representing a normal response of lymphoid tissue in children. Although controversial, it may be a source of rectal bleeding when the lymphoid polyps are friable and associated with overlying ulcers.[77]

Diagnosis and Management

The radiologic and endoscopic appearance of nodular lymphoid hyperplasia may be confused with the familial polyposis syndromes. The lymphoid polyps are distinguished from adenomatous polyps by their central umbilication. Histologically, nodular lymphoid hyperplasia consists of lymphoid follicles with enlarged germinal centers composed of mature lymphocytes. Lymphoid polyps involving the terminal ileum have been reported in association with familial polyposis coli and Gardner's syndrome, and they may lead to confusion with the diagnosis of Crohn's disease of the ileum. Symptoms associated with lymphoid polyps usually regress spontaneously, unless the polyps are a lead point for intussusception.

Inflammatory Polyposis

Inflammatory polyps, or pseudopolyps, are noted in any form of severe colitis, especially during the regenerative and healing phase of inflammation. They are small, usually less than 1 cm in diameter, although they may be large, irregular, and solitary, mimicking a malignant mass. Inflammatory polyps should always be differentiated from colon carcinoma, especially in patients who have had ulcerative colitis for more than 10 years.[78] Histologically, inflammatory cells and granulation tissue are noted first; later, the polyp may consist

Table 58–4. NONINHERITED POLYPOSIS: CLINICAL CHARACTERISTICS

Disorders	Location of Polyps	Extraintestinal Abnormalities	Risk of Cancer
Nodular lymphoid polyposis	Colon: lymphoid hyperplasia	—	—
Inflammatory polyposis	Colon: pseudopolyps	—	Colon, e.g., with ulcerative colitis
Cronkhite-Canada syndrome	Colon, small intestine: hamartomas	Skin hyperpigmentation, alopecia, dystrophic nails	Gastrointestinal cancer—small
Ruvalcaba-Myhre-Smith syndrome	Colon: hamartomas	Pigmentation of glans penis, mental retardation, macrocephaly	—

of normal mucosa. Other diseases that may give rise to inflammatory polyps include amebiasis[79] and chronic bacterial infections.

Cronkhite-Canada Syndrome

Juvenile polyps occur throughout the gastrointestinal tract in the Cronkhite-Canada syndrome. This noninherited syndrome is rare in children; extraintestinal signs include alopecia, onychodystrophy, and brown macular lesions of the skin.[80] Severe malabsorption is present in most of the adult patients, and the prognosis is poor because of complications of protein-losing enteropathy and malnutrition.[80] A child with infantile Cronkhite-Canada syndrome was recently reported, who after removal of multiple polyps, died following surgery for intussusception.[81]

Adenomatous epithelium has been reported in the hamartomatous polyps of these patients with Cronkhite-Canada syndrome, which may confer a risk of malignant transformation. Gastrointestinal carcinomas have occurred in 5% of these patients.[82]

Ruvalcaba-Myhre-Smith Syndrome

The Ruvalcaba-Myhre-Smith syndrome is a rare entity characterized by macrocephaly, pigmented penile lesions, and intestinal polyps.[83] Additional associated features include café au lait spots; ocular abnormalities, for example, posterior embryotoxon; subcutaneous lipomas; psychomotor retardation; and a unique lipid storage disease.[84–86] The intestinal polyps primarily involve the colon, although they are also found in the terminal ileum. Upper gastrointestinal polyps have not been reported. These polyps occur during childhood, initially manifested by rectal bleeding and abdominal pain related to intussusception. Recurrent intussusception, just as in Peutz-Jeghers syndrome, has required subtotal colectomy in some patients.[86] Histologically, the polyps are hamartomatous; malignant transformation has not been observed.[85]

REFERENCES

1. Mestre JR: The changing pattern of juvenile polyps. Am J Gastroenterol 1986; 81:312–314.
2. Cynamon HA, Milov DE, Andres JM: Diagnosis and management of colonic polyps in children. J Pediatr 1989; 114:593–596.
3. Van Driel MF, Zwiers W, Grond J, et al: Juvenile polyps at the site of a ureterosigmoidostomy: Report of five cases. Dis Colon Rectum 1988; 31:553–557.
4. Cooper HS: Intestinal neoplasms. *In* Sternberg SS, ed: Diagnostic Surgical Pathology. New York, Raven Press, 1989, pp 1017–1026.
5. Friedman CJ, Fechner RE: A solitary juvenile polyp with hyperplastic and adenomatous glands. Dig Dis Sci 1982; 27:946–948.
6. Stemper TC, Kent TH, Summers RW: Juvenile polyposis and gastrointestinal carcinoma: A study of a kindred. Ann Intern Med 1975; 83:639–646.
7. Beacham CH, Shields HM, Raffensperger EC, et al: Juvenile and adenomatous gastrointestinal polyposis. Dig Dis 1978; 23:1137–1143.
8. Goodman ZD, Yardley JH, Milligan FD: Pathogenesis of colonic polyps in multiple juvenile polyposis. Cancer 1979; 43:1906–1913.

8a. O'Riordain DS, O'Dwyer PJ, Cullen AF, et al: Familial juvenile polyposis coli and colorectal cancer. Cancer 1991; 68:889–892.

9. Rosen P, Baratz M: Familial juvenile colonic polyposis with associated colon cancer. Cancer 1982; 49:1500–1503.
10. Morson BD: Genesis of colorectal cancer. Clin Gastroenterol 1976; 5:505–525.
11. Baptist SJ, Sabatini MT: Coexisting juvenile polyps and tubulovillous adenoma of colon with carcinoma in situ: Report of a case. Hum Pathol 1985; 16:1161–1163.
12. Longo WE, Touloukian RJ, West AB, et al: Malignant potential of juvenile polyposis coli. Dis Colon Rectum 1990; 33:980–984.
13. Jass JR, Williams CB, Bussey HJ, et al: Juvenile polyposis: A precancerous condition. Histopathology 1988; 13:619–630.
14. Gathright, JB, Cofer TW: Familial incidence of juvenile polyposis coli. Surg Gynecol Obstet 1974; 138:185–188.
15. Grotsky HW, Rickert RK, Smith WD, et al: Familial juvenile polyposis coli: A clinical and pathologic study of a large kindred. Gastroenterology 1982; 82:494–501.
16. Erbe RW: Current concepts in genetics: Inherited gastrointestinal-polyposis syndromes. N Engl J Med 1976; 294:1101–1104.
17. LeLuyer B, LeBihan M, Metayer P, et al: Generalized juvenile polyposis in an infant: Report of a case and successful management by endoscopy. J Pediatr Gastroenterol Nutr 1985; 4:128–134.
18. Sachatello CR, Hahn IS, Carrington CB: Juvenile gastrointestinal polyposis in a female infant: Report of a case and review of the literature of recently recognized syndrome. Surgery 1974; 75:107–114.
19. Sachatello CR, Pickren JW, Grace JT: Generalized juvenile gastrointestinal polyposis. Gastroenterology 1970; 58:699–708.
20. Watanabe A, Nagashima H, Motoi M, et al: Familial juvenile polyposis of the stomach. Gastroenterology 1979; 77:148–151.
21. Peutz JLA: On a very remarkable case of familial polyposis of the mucous membranes, of the intestinal tract and nasopharynx accompanied by peculiar pigmentations of the skin and mucous membrane. Ned Tijdschr Geneeskd 1921; 10:134–146.
22. Jeghers H, McKusick VA, Katz KH: Generalized intestinal polyposis and melanin spots of the oral mucosa, lip and digits: A syndrome of diagnostic significance. N Engl J Med 1949; 241:1031–1036.
23. Dozois RR, Judd ES, Dahlin DC, et al: The Peutz-Jeghers syndrome: Is there a predisposition to development of intestinal cancer? Arch Surg 1969; 98:509–517.
24. McAllister AJ, Richards KF: Peutz-Jeghers syndrome: Experience with 20 patients in 5 generations. 1977; 134:717–720.
25. Wenzl JE, Bartholomew LG, Hallenbeck GA, et al: Gastrointestinal polyposis with mucocutaneous pigmentation in children (Peutz-Jeghers syndrome). Pediatrics 1961; 28:655–661.
26. Bartholomew LG, Dahlin DC, Waugh JM: Intestinal polyposis associated with mucocutaneous melanin pigmentation (Peutz-Jeghers syndrome). Gastroenterology 1957; 32:434–451.
27. Yosowitz P, Hobson R, Ruyman F: Sporadic Peutz-Jeghers syndrome in early childhood. Am J Dis Child 1974; 128:709–712.
28. Morens DM, Garvey SP: An unusual case of Peutz-Jeghers syndrome in an infant. Am J Dis Child 1975; 129:973–976.
29. MGH Case Records (Case 24–1975). N Engl J Med 1975; 292:1340–1345.
30. Bussey HJR, Veale AMO, Morson BC: Genetics of gastrointestinal polyposis. Gastroenterology 1978; 74:1325–1330.
31. Miller LJ, Bartholomew LG, Dozois RR, et al: Adenocarcinoma of the rectum arising in a hamartomatous polyp in a patient with Peutz-Jeghers syndrome. Dig Dis Sci 1983; 28:1047–1051.
32. Dodds WJ, Schulte WJ, Hensley GT, et al: Peutz-Jeghers syndrome and gastrointestinal malignancy. Am J Roentgenol 1972; 115:374–377.
33. Giardiello FM, Welsh SB, Hamilton SR, et al: Increased risk of cancer in the Peutz-Jeghers syndrome. N Engl J Med 1987; 316:1511–1514.
34. Trau H, Schewach-Millet M, Fisher BK, et al: Peutz-Jeghers syndrome and bilateral breast carcinoma. Cancer 1982; 50:788–792.
35. Dozois RR, Kempers RD, Dahlin DC, et al: Ovarian tumors associated with the Peutz-Jeghers syndrome. Ann Surg 1970; 172:233–238.

36. Dubois RS, Hoffman WH, Krishnan TH, et al: Feminizing sex cord tumor with annular tubules in a boy with Peutz-Jeghers syndrome. J Pediatr 1982; 101:568–571.
37. Solh HM, Azoury RS, Najjar SS: Peutz-Jeghers syndrome associated with precocious puberty. J Pediatr 1983; 103:593–595.
38. Cantu JM, Rivera H, Ocampo-Campos R, et al: Peutz-Jeghers syndrome with feminizing Sertoli cell tumors. Cancer 1980; 46:223–228.
39. Spigelman AD, Murday V, Phillips RK: Cancer and the Peutz-Jeghers syndrome. Gut 1989; 30:1588–1590.
40. Lloyd KM, Dennis M: Cowden's disease: A possible new syndrome complex with multiple system involvement. Ann Intern Med 1963; 58:136–143.
41. Weinstock JV, Kawanishi H: Gastrointestinal polyposis with orocutaneous hamartomas (Cowden's disease). Gastroenterology 1978; 74:890–895.
42. Carlson GJ, Nivatvongs S, Snover DC: Colorectal polyps in Cowden's disease (multiple hamartoma syndrome). Am J Surg Pathol 1984; 8:763–770.
43. MGH Case Records (Case 24–1987). N Engl J Med 1987; 316:1531–1540.
44. Bulow S: Colorectal polyposis syndromes. Scand J Gastrenterol 1984; 19:289–293.
45. Deschner EE, Lipkin M: Proliferative patterns in colonic mucosa in familial polyposis. Cancer 1975; 35:413–418.
46. Utsunomiya J, Nakamura T: The occult osteomatous changes in the mandible in patients with polyposis coli. Br J Surg 1975; 62:45–51.
47. Tonelli F, Nardi F, Bechi P, et al: Extracolonic polyps in familial polyposis coli and Gardner's syndrome. Dis Colon Rectum 1985; 28:664–668.
48. Iida M, Yao T, Itoh H, et al: Endoscopic features of adenoma of the duodenal papilla in familial polyposis of the colon. Gastrointest Endosc 1981; 27:6–8.
48a. Sarre RG, Frost AG, Jagelman DG, et al: Gastric and duodenal polyps in familial adenomatous polyposis: A prospective study of the nature and prevalence of upper gastrointestinal polyps. Gut 1987; 28:306–314.
49. Bodmer WF, Bailey CJ, Bussey HJR, et al: Localization of the gene for familial adenomatous polyposis on chromosome 5. Nature 1987; 328:614–616.
50. Leppert M, Dobbs M, Scambler P, et al: The gene for familial polyposis coli maps to the long arm of chromosome 5. Science 1987; 238:1411–1412.
51. Vogelstein B, Fearon ER, Hamilton SR, et al: Genetic alterations during colorectal-tumor development. N Engl J Med 1988; 319:529–532.
52. Ahnen DJ: Lessons from the genetics of colon cancer. Scand J Gastroenterol 1990; 175:(Suppl)166–176.
53. Cannon-Albright LA, Skolnick MH, Bishop T, et al: Common inheritance of susceptibility to colonic adenomatous polyps and associated colorectal cancers. N Engl J Med 1988; 319:533–537.
54. Boman BM, Levin B: Familial polyposis. Hosp Pract 1986; 21:155–170.
55. Naylor EW, Lebenthal E: Early detection of adenomatous polyposis coli in Gardner's syndrome. Pediatrics 1979; 63:222–225.
56. Reed TE, Neel JV: A genetic study of multiple polyposis of the colon. Am J Hum Genet 1955; 7:236–263.
57. Abramson DJ: Multiple polyposis in children: A review and a report of a case in a six year old child who had associated asthma and nephrosis. Surgery 1967; 61:288–301.
58. Bartram CL, Thornton A: Colonic polyp patterns in familial polyposis. Am J Roentgenol 1984; 142:305–308.
59. Odigwe L, Sherman PM, Filler R, et al. Straight ileoanal anastomosis and ileal pouch–anal anastomosis in the surgical management of idiopathic ulcerative colitis and familial polyposis in children: Follow up and comparative analysis. J Pediatr Gastroenterol Nutr 1987; 6:426–429.
60. Jagelman DG, DeCosse JJ, Bussey HJR: Upper gastrointestinal cancer in familial adenomatous polyposis. Lancet 1988; 1:1149–1150.
61. Watanabe H, Enjoji M, Yao T, et al: Gastric lesions in familial adenomatosis coli. Hum Pathol 1978; 9:269–283.
62. Burt RW, Rikkers LF, Gardner EJ: Villous adenoma of the duodenal papilla presenting as necrotizing pancreatitis in a patient with Gardner's syndrome. Gastroenterology 1987; 92:532–535.
63. Richards RC, Rogers SW, Gardner EJ: Spontaneous mesenteric fibromatosis in Gardner's syndrome. Cancer 1981; 47:597–601.
64. Traboulsi EI, Krush AJ, Gardner EJ, et al: Prevalence and importance of pigmented ocular fundus lesions in Gardner's syndrome. N Engl J Med 1987; 316:661–667.
65. Traboulsi EI, Maumenee IH, Krush AJ, et al: Congenital hypertrophy of the retinal pigment epithelial predicts colorectal polyposis in Gardner's syndrome. Arch Ophthalmol 1990; 108:525–526.
66. Schnur PL, David E, Brown PW, et al: Adenocarcinoma of the duodenum and the Gardner syndrome. JAMA 1973; 223:1229–1232.
67. Krush AJ, Traboulsi EI, Offerhaus JA, et al: Hepatoblastoma, pigmented ocular fundus lesions and jaw lesions in Gardner's syndrome. Am J Med Genet 1988; 29:323–332.
68. Bussey HJR: Familial polyposis coli: Family studies, histopathology, differential diagnosis, and results of treatment. Baltimore, Johns Hopkins University Press, 1975, p 69.
69. Turcot J, Despres J-P, St Pierre F: Malignant tumors of the central nervous system associated with familial polyposis of the colon. Dis Colon Rectum 1959; 2:465–468.
70. Baughman FA, List CF, Williams JR, et al: The glioma-polyposis syndrome. N Engl J Med 1969; 281:1345–1346.
71. Jarvis L, Bathwist N, Mohan D, et al: Turcot's syndrome: A review. Dis Colon Rectum 1988; 31:907–914.
72. Itoh H, Ohsato K: Turcot's syndrome and its characteristic colonic manifestation. Dis Colon Rectum 1985; 28:399–402.
72a. Munden PM, Sobol WM, Weingeist TA: Ocular findings in Turcot syndrome (glioma-polyposis). Ophthalmology 1991; 98:111–114.
73. McNicholas T, Brereton RJ, Raafat F: Lymphoid polyps of the rectum. J Pediatr Gastroenterol Nutr 1985; 4:297–302.
74. Hermans PE, Huizenga KA, Hoffman HN, et al: Dysgammaglobulinemia associated with nodular lymphoid hyperplasia of the small intestine. Am J Med 1966; 40:78–89.
75. Shannon R, Vickers TH: Multiple colonic polyposis and Hirschsprung's disease. Aust J Surg 1967; 37:108–113.
76. Ament ME, Ochs HD, Davis SD: Structure and function of the gastrointestinal tract in primary immune deficiency syndrome. Medicine 1973; 52:227–248.
77. Kaplan B, Benson J, Rothstein F, et al: Lymphonodular hyperplasia of the colon as a pathologic finding in children with lower gastrointestinal bleeding. J Pediatr Gastrenterol Nutr 1984; 3:704–708.
78. Teague RH, Read AE: Polyposis in ulcerative colitis. Gut 1975; 16:792–795.
79. Berkowitz O, Bernstein LH: Colonic pseudopolyps in association with amebic colitis. Gastroenterology 1975; 68:786–789.
80. Daniel ES, Ludwig SL, Lewin KJ, et al: The Cronkhite-Canada syndrome: An analysis of the pathologic features and therapy in 55 patients. Medicine 1982; 61:293–309.
81. Schart GM, Becker JHR, Laage NJ: Juvenile gastrointestinal polyposis or the infantile Cronkhite-Canada syndrome. J Pediatr Surg 1986; 21:953–954.
82. Katayama Y, Kimura M, Konn M: Cronkhite-Canada syndrome associated with a rectal cancer and adenomatous changes in colonic polyps. Am J Surg Pathol 1985; 9:65–71.
83. Ruvalcaba RHA, Myhre S, Smith DW. Sotos syndrome with intestinal polyposis and pigmentary changes of the genitalia. Clin Genet 1980; 18:413–416.
84. DiLiberti JH, Weleber RG, Budden S: The Ruvalcaba-Myhre-Smith syndrome. Am J Med Genet 1983; 15:491–495.
85. DiLiberti JH, D'Agostino AN, Ruvalcaba RHA, et al: A new lipid storage myopathy observed in individuals with the Ruvalcaba-Myhre-Smith syndrome. Am J Med Genet 1984; 18:163–167.
86. Gretzula JC, Hevia O, Schachner LS, et al: Ruvalcaba-Myhre-Smith syndrome. Pediatr Dermatol 1988; 5:28–32.

Chapter 59

Crohn's Disease

JEFFREY S. HYAMS

> We propose to describe, in its pathologic and clinical details, a disease of the terminal ileum, affecting mainly young adults, characterized by a subacute or chronic necrotizing and cicatrizing inflammation. The ulceration of the mucosa is accompanied by a disproportionate connective tissue reaction of the remaining walls of the involved intestine, a process which frequently leads to stenosis of the lumen of the intestine, associated with the formation of multiple fistulas.
>
> Crohn B, Ginzburg L, Oppenheimer G. JAMA 1932; 99:1323–1329

With these words, written more than half a century ago, Crohn, Ginzburg, and Oppenheimer presented a pithy summary of a disease whose cause is still obscure and whose occurrence in many populations appears to have increased significantly in the ensuing years. Yet these investigators appreciated only part of the clinical spectrum of Crohn's disease, which they thought was confined to the distal small bowel. In 1960, Crohn's disease was shown by Lockhart-Mummery and Morson[1] to affect the colon unequivocally, and subsequent clinical and pathologic observations have revealed that Crohn's disease can affect any part of the alimentary tract from the mouth to the anus. It is a disease that has similar clinical and pathologic manifestations in children and adults, but in the former group, it may also have a major impact on growth and development. Its clinical course is difficult to predict, with variable responses to medical therapy and a strong tendency to recur despite removal of all obvious disease at the time of surgery.

EPIDEMIOLOGY

Epidemiologic studies of inflammatory bowel disease in children are limited. Data from Scandanavia suggested an overall incidence of Crohn's disease in the population of 5.3 per 100,000, with the age-specific incidence for individuals 15 to 19 years of age being 16.0 per 100,000, and for those less than 15 years of age 2.5 per 100,000.[2, 3] In Scotland, the incidence of Crohn's disease in children less than 16 years of age in 1983 was 2.3 per 100,000.[4] The prevalence of Crohn's disease at that time in Scotland was estimated at approximately 9.5 per 100,000 Scottish children,[4] whereas in a survey performed by the British Pediatric Gastroenterology Group, the prevalence of Crohn's disease was 11 per 100,000 British children up to age 18.[5] Although the incidence of Crohn's disease in most Western populations strikingly increased in the 1950 through 1980 period,[6, 7] more recent observations have shown a modest decline in new cases.[8] A birth cohort analysis performed in Sweden suggested an increased risk for Crohn's disease for individuals born from 1945 through 1954 compared with other decades, particularly those born in the early part of each year.[9]

Crohn's disease is more common in whites than nonwhites. Males and females are equally affected. Approximately 25% of new cases of Crohn's disease occur in individuals less than 20 years of age. The peak incidence of Crohn's disease appears to be in the second and third decades of life. Fewer than 5% of pediatric cases occur in individuals less than 5 years of age.[10]

Crohn's disease appears to be more common in Jews than non-Jews, and in the Jewish population, the disease is more common in families of middle European origin relative to those of Polish or Russian origin.[11] In a study from the United States, Crohn's disease appeared to be more frequent in northern compared with southern areas as well as urban compared with rural areas.[12]

ETIOLOGY

Despite intensive investigation, the etiology of Crohn's disease, similar to that of ulcerative colitis, remains unknown. Because it is clear that inflammatory bowel disease tends to be more common in first-degree relatives of affected individuals, a genetic predisposition to these disorders has been suggested. Additional hypotheses have been put forward to suggest that infectious agents, environmental toxins, abnormal immune regulation, dietary factors, neuroendocrine abnormalities, and psychological factors may be integral to the pathogenesis of inflammatory bowel disease (Fig. 59–1).

Genetic Observations

Familial aggregation of inflammatory bowel disease has been amply demonstrated.[13–18] At the time of diagnosis of either ulcerative colitis or Crohn's disease, the likelihood of finding inflammatory bowel disease in a first-degree relative of the proband is 5 to 25%.[14, 16, 17, 17a] Siblings of patients with Crohn's disease are 17 to

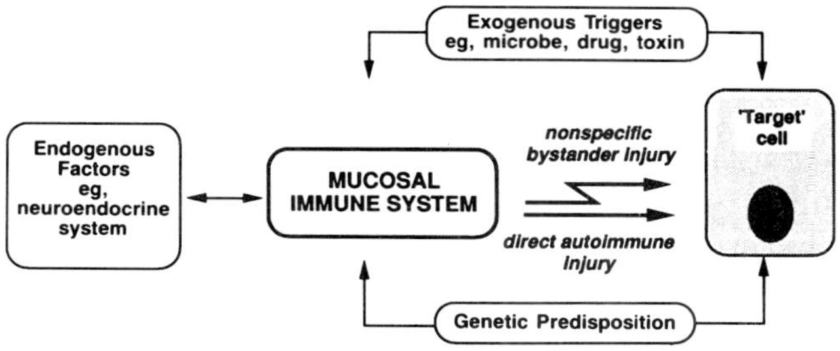

Figure 59–1. Overview of the elements that might contribute to the pathogenesis of inflammatory bowel disease. (From Shanahan F: Pathogenesis of inflammatory bowel disease: A perspective [Autoimmunity Forum]. Gastroenterology 1989; 1:3; with permission.)

35 times more likely to develop the disease than others in the general population. Parents of patients with Crohn's disease are 35 to 70 times more likely to develop Crohn's disease than is the general population.[15] The likelihood of a sibling developing Crohn's disease is approximately 7%, whereas the risk for offspring is about 9%.[14] Although it is more common for the inflammatory bowel disease aggregation in a family to stay disease specific (e.g., Crohn's disease begets Crohn's disease), in a substantial number of families there may be the development of either Crohn's disease or ulcerative colitis in relatives. The concordance for Crohn's disease in monozygotic twins is quite high,[19] and the disease has been reported in monozygotic triplets, who all became ill within a 1-year period.[20]

Attempts to apply simple mendelian genetic principles to inflammatory bowel disease have been unsuccessful, and no specific genetic marker of either ulcerative colitis or Crohn's disease has been validated, although it has been suggested that human leukocyte antigen (HLA) B44 and Cw5 may play a role in the development of Crohn's disease.[21] It has been presumed that a "predisposition" to inflammatory bowel disease might be inherited but that other factors (e.g., environmental, infectious, immunologic) must be involved in pathogenesis as well. Conflicting data have been published regarding increased intestinal permeability to a variety of macromolecular markers in individuals with Crohn's disease as well as in some of their relatives.[22–24] It has been hypothesized that this increased intestinal permeability might lead to increased gut uptake of dietary or microbial antigens, which could then initiate a chronic inflammatory state.

Infection

Initially Crohn's disease was considered likely to be caused by an infection because of many similarities to intestinal tuberculosis. Considerable effort has been made to establish mycobacterial infection in the pathogenesis of Crohn's disease. This effort has partly been spurred by the observations of a chronic granulomatous inflammation in the bowel of ruminants, Johne's disease,[25] and the report of goats developing a granulomatous enteritis after being fed a mycobacterium isolated from Crohn's disease tissue.[26] Unfortunately more recent serologic observations[27] as well as culture[28] and various immunologic techniques[29] have not supported a role for mycobacteria in Crohn's disease.

Although different types of bacteria *(Salmonella, Shigella, Campylobacter, Yersinia, Aeromonas, Clostridium difficile, Escherichia coli)* may cause a clinical illness resembling either Crohn's disease or ulcerative colitis, none has been regularly isolated from stool or tissue of patients subsequently determined to have inflammatory bowel disease. L-form bacteria (cell wall defective) have been suggested as putative causative agents,[30] whereas others have postulated that abnormal mucosal absorption of bacterial cell wall peptidoglycans from endogenous flora might be important.[31, 32] To date, no convincing evidence has been reported to implicate a particular virus or *Chlamydia* as an etiologic factor, and serologic studies have not supported a role for these agents.[33, 34]

Immunologic Mechanisms

The immune system has long been suspected of playing a significant role in the pathogenesis of inflammatory bowel disease. Evidence supporting such an association has been based on the histopathology of intestinal lesions, the response of the disease to immunosuppressive medications, the systemic complications of presumed immune etiology, and numerous laboratory observations. The report of complete remission of gastrointestinal symptoms in a man with a history of severe Crohn's disease who then developed human immunodeficiency virus infection has suggested that CD4 T cells and a competent immune system are important to the pathogenesis of Crohn's disease.[35] Involved tissue revealing infiltration with lymphocytes, plasma cells, macrophages, and other inflammatory cells seems to implicate the immune system in at least the final common pathway for the development of bowel inflammation.

Lymphoid cells constitute about one fourth of the cells present in the intestine, and therefore gut-associated lymphoid tissue (GALT) represents a major component of the body's immune system.[36] GALT is organized in several interconnecting components, including Peyer's patches, lamina propria lymphoid cells, and intraepithelial lymph cells (Fig. 59–2). This lymphoid system is constantly being stimulated by dietary and microbial antigens. M cells, in Peyer's patch lymphoid follicles, appear to be a major site of antigen entry and processing.[36] Although not specific to Crohn's disease, aphthous lesions or ulceration of the epithelium covering Peyer's patch lymphoid follicles may be one of the earliest definable abnormalities present in Crohn's disease. This observation has implied that antigen uptake from the bowel lumen may be important in the etiology of Crohn's disease. It is possible that a defect in antigen processing or immunoregulation could result in a chronic inflammatory state.[37] Subsequent events might include chronic stimulation and proliferation of lymphocytes, release of cytokines, recruitment of neutrophils and

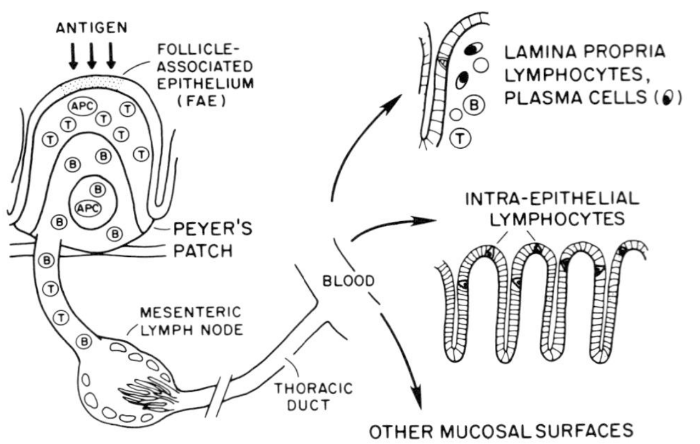

Figure 59–2. The organization of gut-associated lymphoid tissue (GALT). (From Elson CO: The immunology of inflammatory bowel disease. *In* Kirsner JB, Shorter RG, eds: Inflammatory Bowel Disease. 3rd ed. Philadelphia, Lea & Febiger, 1988, p 122; with permission.)

other effector cells, and eventual tissue injury.[38–43] Nonlymphoid intestinal cells would then be "innocent bystanders" and would be injured as a result of abnormal immunoregulation.[44] It has also been suggested that abnormal or enhanced antigen presentation by intestinal epithelial cells might contribute to tissue damaging immunologic responses.[45, 45a] In this regard, recent data have shown that diversion of the fecal stream at the time of ileal resection greatly decreases the likelihood of recurrent disease in the "neoterminal" ileum.[46] This finding has suggested that stimulation by the fecal stream is important to the pathogenesis of recurrent disease at the anastomotic site.

An alternative hypothesis has proposed that intestinal injury in Crohn's disease is based on an autoimmune response. This hypothesis has been fueled by the findings of antibodies to intestinal epithelial cells[37, 47] as well as mucosal and peripheral blood lymphocyte cytotoxicity against these cells.[37, 48, 49] What has not been clear from any study to date is whether this autoreactivity represents a primary phenomenon in the causation of Crohn's disease or a secondary development following gut inflammation on another basis. A potential schema for involvement of the immune system in the development of Crohn's disease is shown in Figure 59–3.

Allergy and Diet

Stimulation of the enteric immune system by dietary antigens has been proposed as a potential contributing factor to Crohn's disease.[50] Conflicting data exist as to whether immunoglobulin E (IgE)-mediated events might be important.[37] Serum antibodies to cow's milk proteins have been found to be higher in patients with Crohn's disease compared with those with ulcerative colitis or controls, suggesting either increased uptake of dietary antigens or enhanced immunologic response in these patients.[51, 52] Breast-feeding, which has been suggested to decrease macromolecular uptake by the im-

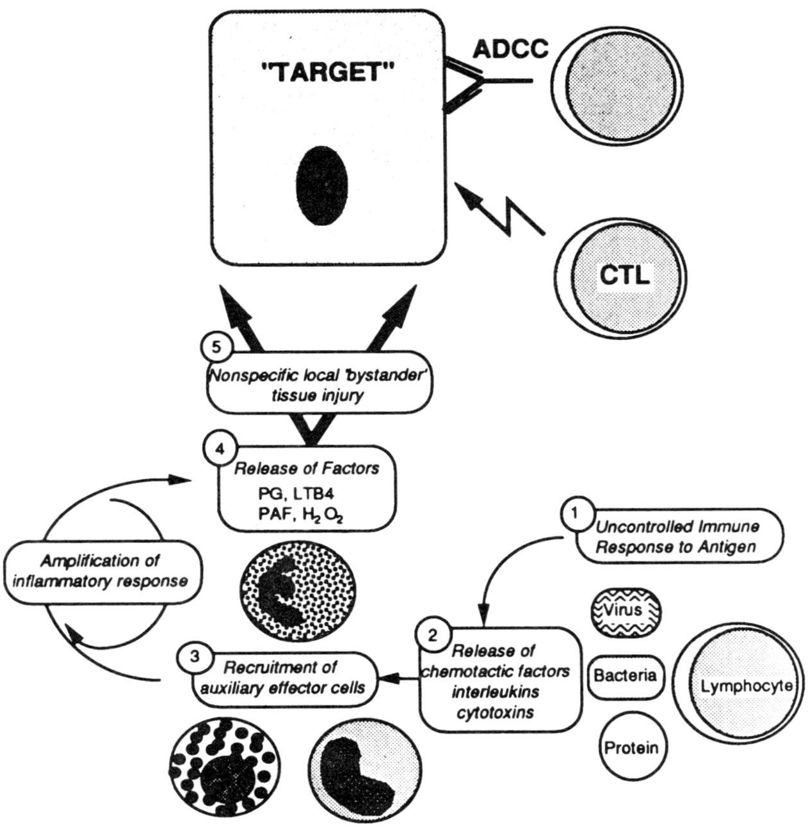

Figure 59–3. Potential immune mechanisms leading to tissue injury in inflammatory bowel disease. These might include direct autoimmune attack on a putative target cell such as the epithelial cell by (1) antibody-dependent cellular cytotoxicity (ADCC) and cytotoxic T lymphocytes or (2) nonspecific "innocent bystander" injury as an indirect result of a defect in mucosal immunoregulation. Uncontrolled reactivity to a variety of antigens leads to lymphocyte proliferation, cytokine release, and recruitment of auxiliary effectors such as neutrophils. Neutrophil products, particularly LTB4, and reactive oxygen metabolites amplify the inflammatory response and lead to local tissue injury. (From Shanahan F: Pathogenesis of inflammatory bowel disease: A perspective [Autoimmunity Forum]. Gastroenterology 1989; 1:3; with permission.)

mature gut,[53] has been linked in one study to a protective effect against the development of Crohn's disease.[54] Another large study of almost 500 children with inflammatory bowel disease from several countries, however, found no association between disease development and frequency of breast-feeding or other dietary factors.[55]

Psychological Factors

Emotional factors have long been thought to be important in the pathogenesis of inflammatory bowel disease, but no causal relationship has ever been demonstrated, and major stressful life events occurring before the onset of disease are no more common in inflammatory bowel disease patients than in controls.[55] In addition, there is no evidence that stressful life events or depressed mood precipitates exacerbation of disease.[56] More intriguing, however, may be the potential relationship between neuropeptides and modulation of the immune system.[57] Profound effects on immune function have been demonstrated for substance P (enhanced T cell proliferation, increased monocyte chemotaxis),[58] vasoactive intestinal peptide (increased natural killer [NK] cell cytotoxicity),[59] beta-endorphin and enkephalin (increased NK cell cytotoxicity),[60] and somatostatin (decreased lymphocyte proliferation, alteration of mast cell function).[61, 62] Although not causing Crohn's disease, it is conceivable that alterations in emotional state might influence the immune system and therefore modulate disease activity.

PATHOLOGY

An appreciation of the clinical manifestations of Crohn's disease can be complete only after a thorough understanding of the pathology of this disorder.

Macroscopic Appearance

Gross inspection of bowel in cases of well-established Crohn's disease reveals marked wall thickening as a result of transmural edema and chronic inflammation. Mural thickening is often accompanied by narrowing of the bowel lumen, which may be severe enough to cause clinical obstruction. The mesentery is thickened with edematous, indurated fat that migrates over the serosal surface of the bowel. Mesenteric lymph nodes are also frequently enlarged. The bowel mucosa may reveal small aphthous lesions, which may coalesce into larger irregular and deeper ulcers. Bowel inflammation and ulceration may be confluent; however, more characteristically it is punctuated by "skip areas" of grossly and even microscopically normal mucosa. *Cobblestoning* of the surface lining may occur as a result of extensive linear and serpiginous mucosal ulceration with associated regeneration and hyperplasia, in addition to marked submucosal thickening (Fig. 59–4). Stricture formation may then occur in this setting of chronic granulomatous inflammation as a result of fibrous tissue proliferation involving first the submucosa and then the deeper layers of bowel wall. The production of several cytokines in inflamed tissue may act as a stimulus to local collagen synthesis.[63]

Loops of adjacent bowel may become matted together because of serosal and mesenteric inflammation. Fistulas are thought to arise when transmural bowel inflammation extends through the serosa into adjacent structures, such as bowel, abdominal wall, bladder, vagina, or perineum. Frequently a fistulous tract may end blindly in an inflammatory mass (phlegmon) adjacent to the bowel and involves the bowel itself as well as mesentery, lymph nodes, and occasionally a chronic active abscess cavity.

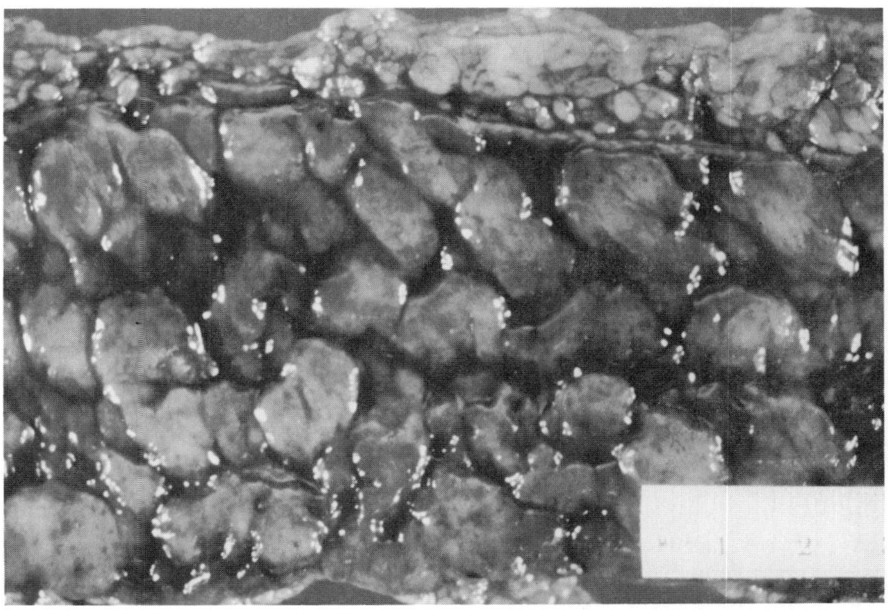

Figure 59–4. Resection specimen from patient with Crohn's colitis revealing marked bowel wall thickening with cobblestoning.

Microscopic Appearance

The findings on histologic examination of the bowel in Crohn's disease are highly dependent on the duration of disease involvement[63a, 64]; however, the classic Crohn's lesion is that of transmural enterocolitis (Figure 59–5*A*). Early disease may manifest as superficial aphthoid lesions of the mucosa, usually overlying a lymphoid follicle (Fig. 59–5*B*). Granulomas are frequently reported at this early stage. As disease progresses, mucosal ulcers may become confluent, producing broad depressed ulcer beds. Subsequently there is sequential progression from mucosal disease to profound transmural infiltration of the bowel with lymphocytes, histiocytes, and plasma cells. The inflammation is characteristically extensive in the submucosa and is also characterized by edema, lymphatic dilatation, and collagen deposition (Fig. 59–5*C*). The last-mentioned feature is responsible for obliteration of the submucosa, which results in stricture, obstruction, or both. Deep fissuring ulceration into the muscularis propria frequently occurs and when prominent is highly characteristic of Crohn's disease even in the absence of granulomas. Crypt abscesses and goblet cell depletion are common but may not be as marked as in ulcerative colitis. Pyloric metaplasia and neuronal hyperplasia of the myenteric plexus are common concomitant histologic findings, although they are not specific. Not infrequently mucosa that was thought to be normal grossly reveals abnormalities such as edema and an increase in mononuclear cell density in the lamina propria.[65]

Although thought to be classic histologic findings in Crohn's disease, granulomas may not be found in up to 40% of surgically resected specimens and 60 to 80% of mucosal biopsies.[66–68] Granulomas may be found in any layer of the bowel wall, although most commonly in the superficial submucosa (Fig. 59–5*D*). They may also be present in extraintestinal structures such as lymph nodes, mesentery, and peritoneum. Some observations have suggested that these characteristic granulomas may be a secondary phenomenon owing to breaks in mucosal integrity and subsequent host inflammatory response to bacterial antigens.[69]

ANATOMIC DISTRIBUTION

Previous reports of patterns of anatomic gastrointestinal involvement in children and adults with Crohn's disease have primarily been based on radiographic evaluation[70–72] and thus may seriously underestimate the true extent of involvement. We now appreciate the fact that careful endoscopic and histologic evaluation of radiographically normal bowel may frequently reveal signs of inflammation.[73, 74] If the extent of anatomic involvement is based on gross involvement detectable radiographically, several patterns of involvement emerge. The majority of affected individuals (50–60%) have involvement of the terminal ileum and variable segments of the colon, although most commonly the ascending colon. Approximately 30 to 35% have small intestinal involvement only, with most of these individuals displaying disease in the terminal ileum. Ten percent to 15% of patients have disease limited to the large bowel. Involvement of the esophagus, stomach, or duodenum, which historically had been considered rare (<5%)[75] based on radiologic examination, has now been shown to affect 30 to 40% of children when careful endoscopic and biopsy techniques are applied.[76, 77]

PATHOPHYSIOLOGY OF GASTROINTESTINAL SYMPTOMS

The presence of active inflammation in the small and large intestine leads to a number of physiologic derangements which culminate in diarrhea, gastrointestinal bleeding, and abdominal pain (Fig. 59–6). Extensive jejunal and ileal disease may lead to malabsorption. Malabsorbed fatty acids entering the colon impair electrolyte and water absorption.[78] Abnormal terminal ileal function may result in bile acid loss, with an eventual decrease in luminal bile acid concentration worsening steatorrhea.[79] Bile salts also may significantly impair colonic absorption of electrolytes.[80] Bacterial overgrowth in the small bowel associated with obstruction and stasis or enteroenteric fistula may lead to mucosal damage and bile salt deconjugation, further worsening symptoms.

The normal function of the colon to absorb the large fluid and electrolyte load presented by the small bowel is significantly decreased in the presence of colitis.[81] Inflammatory mediators such as prostaglandins and leukotrienes may alter bowel permeability and electrolyte transport.[82] Diffuse mucosal disease leads to exudation of serum proteins and frank bleeding. Abdominal pain results either from gut distention usually associated with obstruction or inflammation or irritation of the serosa resulting from transmural inflammation. Abnormal motility as well as gut distention may also lead to abdominal cramping.[83]

CLINICAL FEATURES

The presenting clinical features of children and adolescents with Crohn's disease are shown in Table 59–1.[70, 84–87] As can be seen, abdominal pain and diarrhea

Table 59–1. PRESENTING CLINICAL FEATURES OF 325 CHILDREN WITH CROHN'S DISEASE

Feature	Percent
Abdominal pain	75
Diarrhea	65
Weight loss	65
Growth retardation	25
Nausea/vomiting	25
Rectal bleeding	20
Perirectal disease	15
Extraintestinal manifestations	25

Data compiled from Gryboski and Spiro[70]; Burbige, Huang, and Bayless[84]; Posthuma and Moroz[85]; Raine[86]; and Barton and Ferguson.[87]

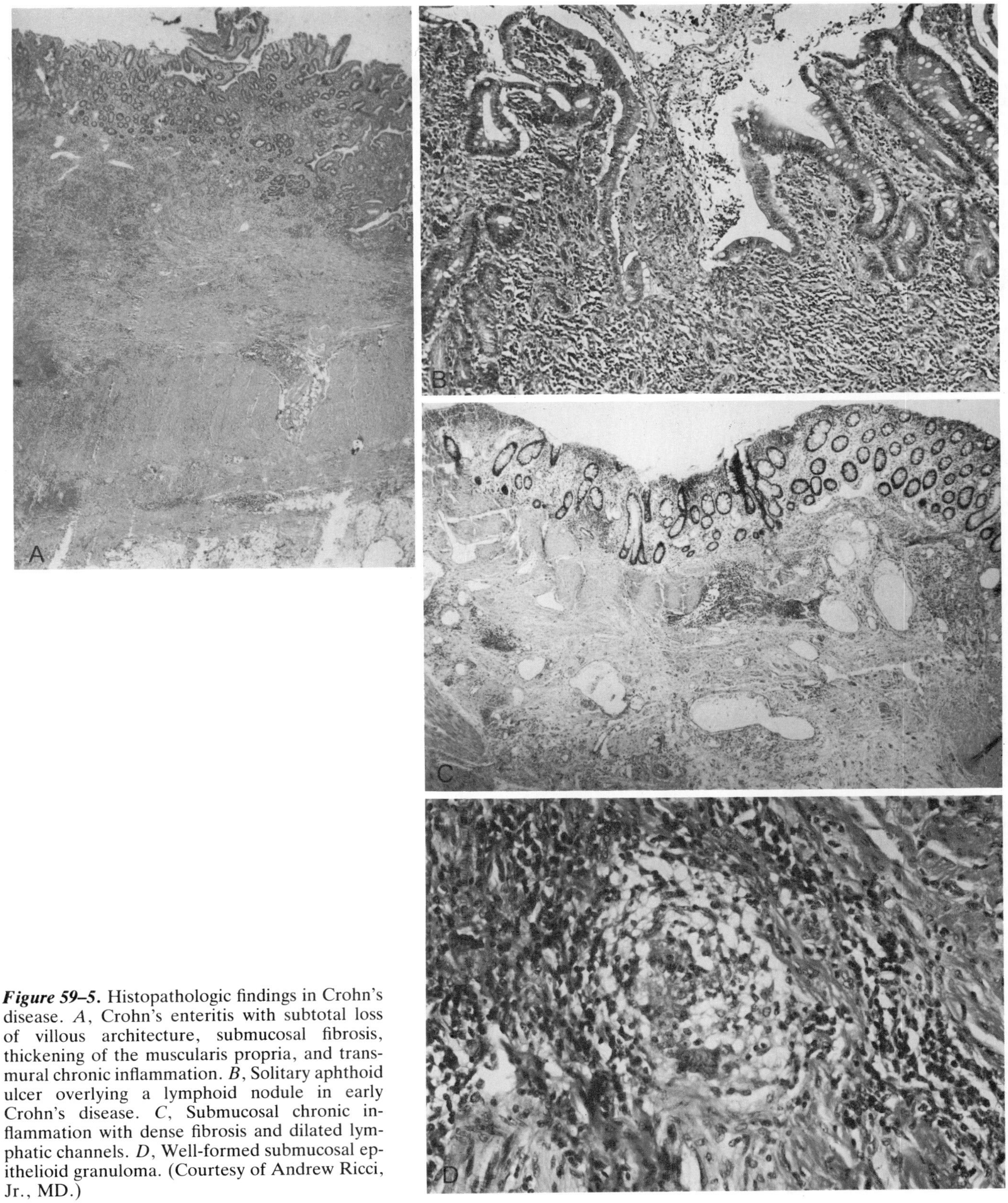

Figure 59–5. Histopathologic findings in Crohn's disease. *A*, Crohn's enteritis with subtotal loss of villous architecture, submucosal fibrosis, thickening of the muscularis propria, and transmural chronic inflammation. *B*, Solitary aphthoid ulcer overlying a lymphoid nodule in early Crohn's disease. *C*, Submucosal chronic inflammation with dense fibrosis and dilated lymphatic channels. *D*, Well-formed submucosal epithelioid granuloma. (Courtesy of Andrew Ricci, Jr., MD.)

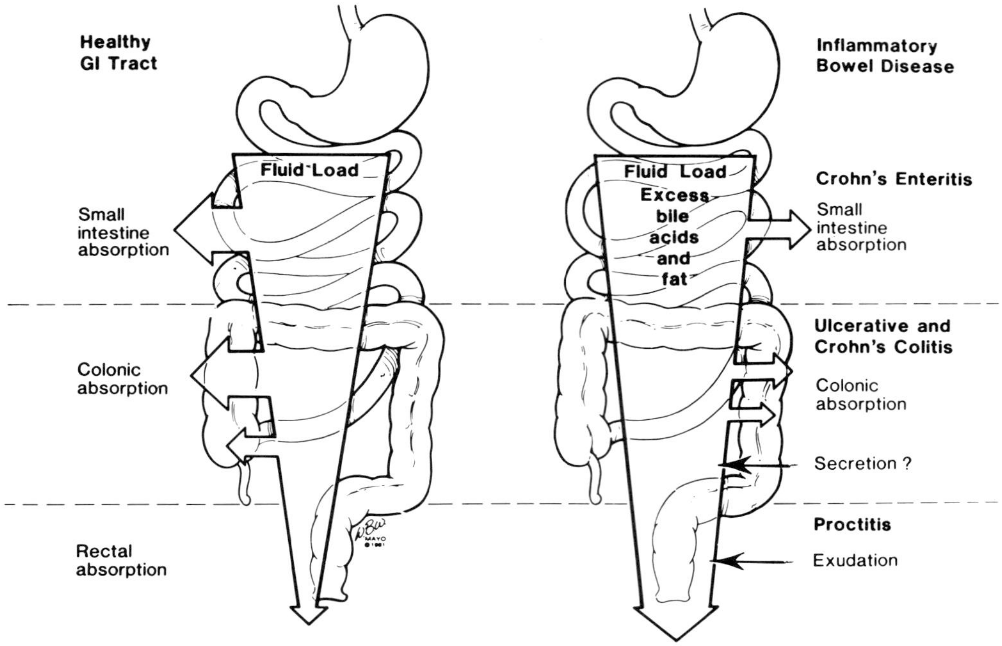

Figure 59–6. Summary of major pathophysiologic factors resulting in diarrhea in inflammatory bowel disease. (From Phillips SF: Pathophysiology of symptoms and clinical features of inflammatory bowel disease. *In* Kirsner JB, Shorter RG, eds: Inflammatory Bowel Disease. 3rd ed. Philadelphia, Lea & Febiger, 1988, p 247; with permission.)

are prominent. The characteristics of the abdominal pain may be variable depending on the site of bowel involvement. Right lower quadrant discomfort is common with terminal ileum or cecal disease and is frequently associated with tenderness on abdominal palpation. Not infrequently a fullness or distinct mass is noted in this area. Periumbilical pain is common with colonic disease or more diffuse small bowel disease. Epigastric pain is seen in 70% of children with gastroduodenal involvement,[88] whereas odynophagia and dysphagia are observed in most patients with Crohn's disease of the esophagus.[89] The abdominal pain associated with Crohn's disease tends to be persistent, is often severe, and frequently awakens the child from sleep. It is often made worse by eating and may increase during defecation if the colon is involved. At times, the acute development of right lower quadrant pain without a well-established previous history of illness will suggest a diagnosis of appendicitis, but at laparotomy findings consistent with Crohn's disease are discovered.

Diarrhea is seen in two thirds of children and may range from two to three loose movements per day to a marked increase (>8 to 10 movements per day) in stooling with nocturnal defecation. Diarrhea that awakens a patient at night is virtually always a pathologic finding. Gross blood in the stools is unusual with isolated small bowel disease and more common when the colon is involved. Severe hemorrhage, however, may be seen in the setting of small bowel disease when bowel ulceration extends deeply into the bowel wall and involves a larger blood vessel.

Fever, observed in approximately 50% of patients, may be low grade or may be spiking (to 40°C) and may persist for extended periods before a diagnosis is made. Nausea and vomiting are frequent and may be seen with involvement of any part of the bowel, although more frequently with upper tract involvement. Fatigue is also a common complaint. Anorexia, weight loss, and diminution in growth velocity may be seen in 20 to 60% of children (see later).

Not infrequently children develop perirectal inflammation with fissures, fistulas, or tags and are given diagnoses of hemorrhoids or perianal condyloma before a diagnosis of Crohn's disease is established.[90] Drainage from these fistulas may be impressive, but perirectal pain is unusual unless there is actual abscess formation.

Extraintestinal Manifestations

Signs and symptoms outside of the gastrointestinal tract are frequently observed in Crohn's disease and may be seen in the absence of obvious gastrointestinal disease.[91–93]

Joint Symptoms. Arthralgias and arthritis are observed in up to 15% of children with Crohn's disease[70, 84, 94–97] and may be present for several years before the development of gastrointestinal symptoms. Although any joint may be involved, the large joints of the leg are more commonly affected. Arthritis is generally nondeforming, transient, and asymmetric. It is more common when there is colonic involvement rather than isolated small bowel disease. Ankylosing spondylitis, often associated with HLA-B27 positivity, is found in 2 to 6% of patients with Crohn's disease.[97] Although the course of ankylosing spondylitis is usually independent of that of the bowel disease, the activity of peripheral joint findings usually parallels the activity of bowel disease.[93] Clubbing, a form of hypertrophic osteoarthropathy, is common in children with Crohn's disease, particularly when the small bowel is affected.[70]

Musculoskeletal Symptoms. Myalgias are occasionally

reported by patients, particularly when receiving high doses of corticosteroids. Granulomatous myositis and myopathy associated with Crohn's disease of the colon has been reported.[98] This author has seen dermatomyositis develop in a teenager with Crohn's disease.

Skin Manifestations. Cutaneous manifestations associated with Crohn's disease include erythema nodosum, pyoderma gangrenosum, epidermolysis bullosa acquisita, polyarteritis nodosa, and "metastatic" Crohn's disease.[99, 99a] The first two conditions may be seen in 1 to 4% of patients. Metastatic Crohn's disease, granulomatous dermatitis at sites remote from the gastrointestinal tract, has rarely been reported in the pediatric population.[100]

Oral Mucosa Manifestations. Canker sores are a frequent complaint of individuals with inflammatory bowel disease. Although most often painless, they may at times be associated with marked discomfort and are usually more prominent during periods of increased bowel activity. Histologically these lesions may show lymphedema of the lamina propria and occasionally non-caseating granulomas.[101, 102]

Ocular Symptoms. Up to 10% of patients may have ocular complications, including iritis, episcleritis, uveitis, and orbital pseudotumor.[103–105] Posterior subcapsular cataracts may be seen with prolonged corticosteroid therapy.

Vascular Symptoms. Thrombocytosis, elevations in fibrinogen, factor V, and factor VIII, and depression in antithrombin III level have been associated with a hypercoagulable state in some patients with inflammatory bowel disease.[106–108] Vascular complications have included deep vein thrombosis, pulmonary emboli, and neurovascular disease with accompanying seizures and encephalopathy.[109, 110] Vasculitis involving the aorta and subclavian artery has been described.[111]

Renal Disease. Ureteral obstruction and hydronephrosis may be seen with ileocolic inflammation when an inflammatory mass encases the right ureter.[112–114] Severe hypertension may be seen in this setting [114] Additional urinary complications may include enterovesical fistulas, perivesical infection, perinephric abscess, and nephrolithiasis.[115, 116] A predisposition to renal stones may occur in the setting of large fluid and bicarbonate losses in patients with an ileostomy as well as in individuals with extensive ileal disease or following ileal resection. Oxalate, urate, and phosphate stones have been found.[116]

Amyloidosis is an unusual complication of Crohn's disease that has been observed in children and may be associated with renal failure.[117–119] The development of proteinuria or elevated creatinine in a patient with longstanding Crohn's disease should suggest this entity.

Hepatobiliary Manifestations. Abnormalities of the liver and biliary system may include fatty liver,[120] pericholangitis,[120] sclerosing cholangitis,[121] chronic hepatitis,[120] cirrhosis,[120] hepatic granuloma,[93] hepatic abscess,[122, 123] cholelithiasis,[124, 125] granulomatous cholecystitis,[126] and acalculous cholecystitis.[127] Hepatic steatosis is most common in the setting of malnutrition and may be made worse by concomitant corticosteroid therapy. Pericholangitis is now generally regarded as part of the spectrum of sclerosing cholangitis.[128, 129] Approximately 10% of patients with sclerosing cholangitis have Crohn's disease.[121] Terminal ileal resection or significant inflammation is associated with increased enteric bile acid loss and an interruption of the enterohepatic circulation of bile acids.[130] Bile may then become supersaturated with cholesterol, leading to gallstone formation.

Gastrointestinal Complications

Significant gastrointestinal complications that may be seen in the course of Crohn's disease include massive acute hemorrhage, obstruction, perforation, abscess formation, fistula formation, toxic megacolon, and cancer.

Hemorrhage. Massive acute gastrointestinal hemorrhage is seen in approximately 1% of patients with Crohn's disease.[131] As noted previously, it is secondary to ulceration into a larger vessel and generally requires operative intervention.

Obstruction. Intestinal obstruction may occur secondary to severe bowel wall inflammation with or without localized phlegmon or abscess formation, stricture formation associated with chronic inflammation, or adhesions associated with previous surgery. With the exception of the last-mentioned cause, obstruction is more frequently partial than complete.[132] More rare causes of obstruction have included giant pseudopolyposis,[133] gallstone ileus,[134] and carcinoma.[135] Undigested food occluding the lumen of a strictured bowel may also cause a blockage. Chronic low-grade obstruction may lead to proximal bacterial overgrowth.

Perforation. Free perforation (i.e., that not accompanying an abscess or chronic fistula) has been considered to be a relatively unusual finding in Crohn's disease. It most commonly occurs in the ileum, although other areas of the bowel may be affected.[136] Rarely it may be the initial presentation of the disease. No relationship to perforation has been established among corticosteroid therapy, duration of disease, toxic dilatation, or obstruction.[136] Classic signs of peritonitis may be masked in the presence of high doses of corticosteroids.

Abscess. Transmural bowel inflammation with fistulization and perforation may lead to the formation of abscesses. These abscesses may be enteroperitoneal, interloop, intramesenteric, retroperitoneal-ileopsoas, hepatic, splenic, or subdiaphragmatic.[137] Fever and abdominal pain are invariably present, although it may be difficult to differentiate clinically between an abscess and an exacerbation of the underlying disease with phlegmon formation.[138] Fecal flora is found when these abscesses are cultured. At times, right hip pain may indicate the development of an iliopsoas abscess.

Fistula Formation. Fistula formation is common during the course of Crohn's disease. Although perianal and perirectal fistulization is most common, additional types of fistulas include enteroenteric, enterovesical, enterovaginal, and enterocutaneous ones. The most common enteroenteric fistula is between the ileum and the sigmoid colon. Enterocolic fistulas may lead to bacterial overgrowth of the proximal bowel as well as short-circuiting of nutrient exposure to small bowel surface for absorption.

Toxic Megacolon. The exact frequency of toxic megacolon in Crohn's disease in children is unknown but is considered to be quite low. In adult series, it has ranged from 2 to 11%.[139, 140]

Carcinoma. Although not as great as seen in ulcerative colitis, the risk of bowel carcinoma in Crohn's disease is still considerably greater than (approximately 20 times) that found in the general population.[141] Carcinoma occurring in excluded bowel segments following a diversionary procedure has been a particular concern in the past[142] and has led to the abandonment of this type of procedure.

Malnutrition

The cause of malnutrition in Crohn's disease is usually multifactorial and includes suboptimal dietary intake, increased gastrointestinal losses, malabsorption, and increased requirements associated with marked inflammatory activity (Figure 59–7). Anorexia is an important feature and may be severe enough in some cases to be confused with anorexia nervosa.[143] At times, affected children do not eat because of a fear of abdominal cramping or increased stooling, but more frequently the anorexia cannot be explained. Delayed gastric emptying noted in some children with Crohn's disease[144] may affect oral intake. Elevated levels of tumor necrosis factor (cachectin), which have been associated with anorexia in other chronic inflammatory states, have been observed in one study[145] but not in another.[145a] Marked mucosal inflammation leads to the loss of cellular constituents and hematochezia, with the development of severe protein-losing enteropathy[146] and iron-deficiency anemia. Fecal calcium and magnesium losses may be increased.[147]

Malabsorption of multiple dietary components has been demonstrated in Crohn's disease.[148] Fat malabsorption may be associated with (1) a decreased bile acid pool secondary to bile salt malabsorption from ileal disease or ileal resection; (2) extensive small bowel mucosal disease; or (3) bacterial overgrowth of the proximal bowel.[84, 149] Although lactose malabsorption has been demonstrated in up to 30% of children with Crohn's disease,[150] this figure is similar to an age-matched and ethnically matched control population. Increased fecal nitrogen excretion has been demonstrated[151] but may more reflect active loss rather than malabsorption. Hypoalbuminemia is common.[152] Deficiency states for iron,[153] folic acid,[153] vitamin B_{12},[154] nicotinic acid,[155] vitamin D,[156] vitamin K,[153] calcium,[157] magnesium,[158] and zinc[159] have been demonstrated. Medications may interfere with the absorption of certain nutrients (e.g., sulfasalazine and folic acid).

Few data are available regarding actual energy requirements in children with Crohn's disease and whether they are different from similarly aged healthy children. In one study, basal metabolic rates were not different in adolescents with Crohn's disease compared with controls.[160] In adults with Crohn's disease, energy expenditure is similar to a control population.[161, 162] In poorly nourished adults with Crohn's disease, an increased energy expenditure per unit body mass was observed compared with those patients who were more than 90% of ideal body weight.[161, 162] The activity of the Crohn's disease did not affect energy expenditure.[161]

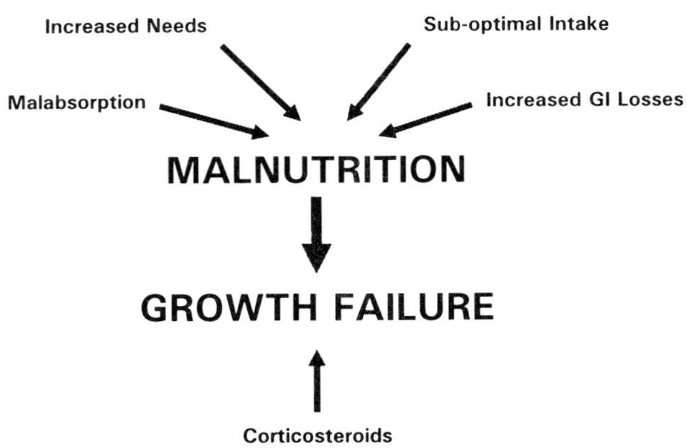

Figure 59–7. Contributing factors to the development of malnutrition and growth failure in children and adolescents with inflammatory bowel disease.

Growth Failure

A decrease in normal growth parameters is the eventual consequence of chronic undernutrition in children and adolescents with Crohn's disease. Ideally serial measurements over an interval of at least 6 to 12 months are available to calculate growth velocity, and then comparison can be made to expected norms for height velocity for age and sex.[163] Although a decrease of 2 standard deviations establishes significant growth failure, any decrease from expected values should alert the clinician to a potential serious problem. Retardation of bone age by 2 standard deviations or more below the chronologic age (usually more than 2 years) is a frequent finding in children with growth delay, as is delayed sexual maturation[164, 165] in the adolescent. Care should be taken in interpreting a patient's absolute height value and percentile in light of parental heights.

Insulin-like growth factor I (IGF-1) (somatomedin C) levels have been noted to be low in some children with growth failure[166] and most likely reflect poor nutrition rather than any intrinsic abnormality in the IGF–1 system. Growth hormone levels are generally normal in children with Crohn's disease.[167] High-dose chronic corticosteroid therapy is associated with significantly decreased growth velocity independent of disease activity.[168]

Growth delay may precede clinical illness by months or years.[169] In addition, continued growth problems may be observed even during periods of relatively quiet gastrointestinal symptoms after the diagnosis has been established and appropriate therapy started. Intensive nutritional supplementation can usually improve growth parameters (see later).

Psychological Disturbances

Considerable attention has been paid to the psychological implications of inflammatory bowel disease in children and adolescents.[170–175] The major abnormality found in most studies[172, 175] has been depression, which may be present at the time of diagnosis or develop during the course of the illness. Neither disease activity nor the use of corticosteroid therapy has correlated with the development of depression.[173, 175] Life events, although not necessarily related to the onset of inflammatory bowel disease, appear to relate to the development of depression.[175]

DIAGNOSIS

The diagnosis of Crohn's disease is usually established by a combination of clinical and laboratory observations as well as radiologic, endoscopic, and histologic findings (Table 59–2). Because the clinical findings may involve many systems outside of the gastrointestinal tract, the diagnosis may be delayed for months to years before appropriate diagnostic studies are performed. Even when the presenting symptoms are primarily gastrointestinal, other diagnoses are often initially invoked.

Physical Examination

Physical examination in a child suspected of having Crohn's disease should include careful abdominal examination, with particular attention to tenderness, fullness, or mass. A gentle attempt to elicit peritoneal signs should be made. Careful inspection of the perirectal area and perineum should be performed. The presence of stomatitis, clubbing, arthritis, erythema nodosum, or pyoderma gangrenosum is suggestive of inflammatory bowel disease. Height and weight should be recorded and compared with previous values to calculate rates of change.

Table 59–2. CLINICAL AND LABORATORY FINDINGS USED TO ESTABLISH A DIAGNOSIS OF CROHN'S DISEASE

History	**Laboratory Tests**
Abdominal pain	Anemia
Diarrhea	Elevated ESR
Rectal bleeding	Hypoalbuminemia
Fever	Thrombocytosis
Arthritis	Positive guaiac
Rash	**Radiography**
Family history of IBD	Nodularity
Physical Examination	Skip areas
Abdominal tenderness	String sign
Mass	Fistula
Perirectal disease	Ulceration
Clubbing	**Endoscopy**
Stomatitis	Ulcers
Erythema nodosum	Cobblestoning
Pyoderma gangrenosum	Rectal sparing
Growth Data	
Height and weight velocity decreases for age	

IBD, inflammatory bowel disease; ESR, erythrocyte sedimentation rate.

Laboratory Evaluation

The clinician evaluating a child or adolescent with suspected Crohn's disease frequently performs a battery of hematologic and biochemical studies for screening purposes before embarking on a series of more expensive and invasive studies. Abnormalities frequently found include anemia (70% of cases), elevated erythrocyte sedimentation rate (80%), hypoalbuminemia (60%), and guaiac-positive stools (35%).[176] Although thrombocytosis is also common (60%), total leukocyte count is commonly normal. Anemia is most frequently secondary to iron deficiency associated with blood loss, and serum iron and ferritin levels are low. Macrocytosis suggests folate or vitamin B_{12} deficiency.

Serum zinc, magnesium, calcium, and phosphorus levels may occasionally be low, particularly in the nutritionally depleted patient. Serum aminotransferases are abnormal in approximately 10% of patients at the time of diagnosis. Although xylose absorption tests and 72-hour fecal fat excretion may be abnormal, they are rarely needed in the evaluation of most patients. Breath hydrogen testing for lactose malabsorption may be helpful in subsequent dietary management.

Careful examination of multiple stool specimens should be made for bacterial enteric pathogens and parasites. Fecal alpha$_1$-antitrypsin, although not commonly measured, is abnormal in almost 90% of cases at presentation.[176] Urinalysis should be performed to exclude pyuria or infection associated with enterovesical fistula.

Radiographic Evaluation

In most cases of presumed inflammatory bowel disease, radiographic evaluation of the gastrointestinal tract will be performed to confirm the diagnosis, evaluate the extent of disease, and help distinguish between Crohn's disease and ulcerative colitis. It is important that all appropriate stool studies be completed before the introduction of barium into the gastrointestinal tract. In an acutely ill patient with suspected severe colitis, barium enema should be deferred because of the risk of perforation or toxic megacolon. Although barium enema has historically been a primary tool to evaluate colonic disease, it has been increasingly replaced by colonoscopic studies. This largely represents greater technical expertise in the performance of these studies in children, an awareness of the significantly increased sensitivity of endoscopic evaluation compared with contrast studies in finding colonic inflammation, and the ability to obtain tissue for histologic evaluation. When possible, double-contrast (air-barium) enemas are preferable to single-contrast studies in defining mucosal detail. Evaluation of fistulas emanating from the colon is best performed with barium enema.

Because small bowel involvement is seen in 80 to 90% of cases of Crohn's disease, the performance of an upper gastrointestinal series with small bowel follow-through is essential. It can be performed with oral ingestion of contrast material or by enteroclysis. A plain abdominal radiograph before the ingestion of contrast material may suggest partial obstruction associated with narrowed intestinal segments. Careful fluoroscopy and abdominal palpation are used to identify irregular, nodular (cobblestoned), and thickened bowel loops as well as stenotic areas (string sign), deep ulcers, and fistulas (Fig. 59–8). Terminal ileal nodularity is common in Crohn's disease and may be difficult to distinguish from nodular lymphoid hyperplasia (NLH),[177] although in NLH the nodules are usually 3 mm or less in diameter. Inflammation, edema, fibrosis, and spasm may give a mass effect, and differentiation from lymphoma may be difficult. At times, enteroclysis may be helpful in overcoming spasm and providing better detail to distinguish between the two entities. Antegrade filling of the colon may help identify areas of gross colonic involvement (Fig. 59–9).

The presence of a tender mass in the right lower quadrant in a patient with Crohn's disease suggests the presence of an inflammatory phlegmon or abscess. Ultrasound examination may help reveal bowel wall thickening (Fig. 59–10) as well as extraluminal fluid collections suggesting abscess. Computed tomography (CT) is helpful in delineating extramural extension of inflammation by fistulization to adjacent structures and in diagnosing abdominal and pelvic abscesses (Fig. 59–11).[178, 179] Nuclear medicine studies with leukocytes labeled with indium-111 have been used in adults to identify involved intestinal segments as well as to help identify abscesses.[180, 181] It has been suggested that this technique may have particular value in differentiating between fibrous and inflammatory strictures as well as in a post–ileal resection patient with diarrhea in attempting to demonstrate recurrent inflammation. In children indium-111 scintigraphy appears to be considerably less sensitive and specific than colonoscopy and biopsy for detecting colonic inflammatory bowel disease,[182] and because indium has a relatively long half-life (3 days), its use in children will most likely be limited.

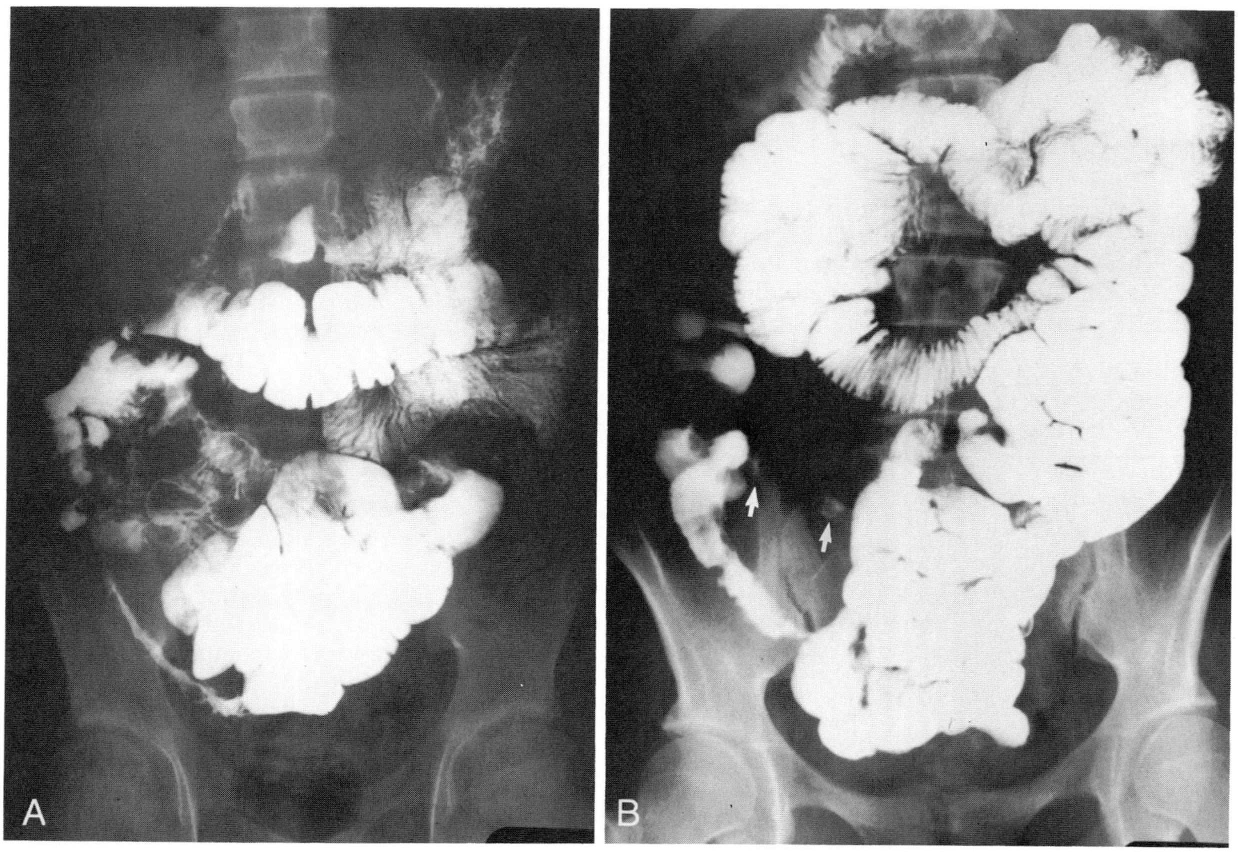

Figure 59–8. Radiographic findings in Crohn's disease involving the terminal ileum. *A*, "String sign" with marked terminal ileal narrowing and irregular mucosal pattern. *B*, Separation of terminal ileum from more proximal ileum associated with inflammatory phlegmon/abscess. Note extravasation of barium *(arrows)* into an interloop abscess. (Courtesy of Stuart Markowitz, MD.)

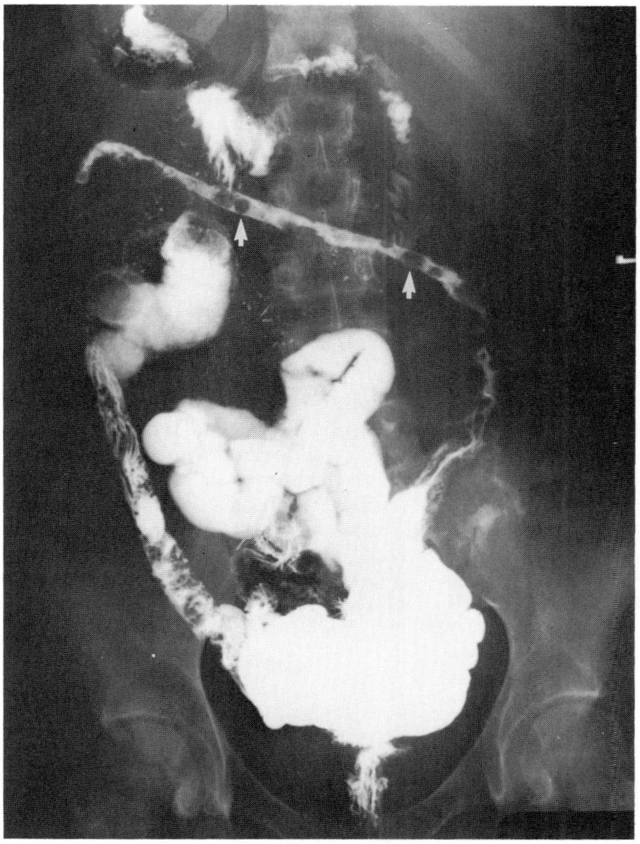

Figure 59–9. Antegrade cologram revealing marked narrowing of ascending and transverse colon with loss of normal mucosal pattern and multiple filling defects *(arrows)* representing pseudopolyps. (Courtesy of Stuart Markowitz, MD.)

Endoscopic and Histologic Evaluation

Endoscopic and histologic evaluation of the gastrointestinal tract are invaluable in the diagnosis of Crohn's disease and its differentiation from ulcerative colitis. The presence of a normal rectum and sigmoid colon on flexible sigmoidoscopy and biopsy in a patient with persistent bloody diarrhea excludes a diagnosis of ulcerative colitis and in the presence of negative cultures for enteric pathogens is highly suggestive of Crohn's disease. The finding of focal or segmental involvement of the colon with histologic documentation of skip areas of normal mucosa, fissures or sinuses, sarcoid-like granuloma, or ulceration of the terminal ileum supports a diagnosis of Crohn's disease.[183] The ability to perform a biopsy of the terminal ileum during colonoscopy greatly increases the sensitivity of this procedure to help establish a diagnosis of Crohn's disease.[184] Granulomas are found in approximately one third of cases with endoscopic biopsies of the colon and are more likely to be found with multiple biopsies and serial sectioning.[67, 68] Macroscopically normal bowel may still reveal signs of significant inflammation as well as granuloma and may help establish colonic disease despite normal colonoscopy grossly as well as normal radiographic evaluation of the colon.[65, 185] Phospho-soda enemas and bisacodyl suppositories may occasionally cause nonspecific inflammatory changes in the rectal mucosa and should probably be avoided in preparation of the patient for sigmoidoscopic examination.[186] Esophagogastroduodenoscopy and biopsy are more sensitive than radiologic evaluation for detecting Crohn's disease of the upper gastrointestinal tract.[187]

DIFFERENTIAL DIAGNOSIS

The varied modes of presentation of Crohn's disease may lead to a long differential diagnosis (Table 59–3). Right lower quadrant pain may suggest appendicitis,[188] infection (e.g., *Campylobacter, Yersinia*), neoplasm (particularly lymphoma), ovarian pathology, intussusception, mesenteric adenitis, and Meckel's diverticulum–related problems (torsion, diverticulitis). More chronic periumbilical or epigastric abdominal pain is often considered to represent irritable bowel syndrome, constipation, lactose intolerance, peptic disease, or urinary tract pathology. When bloody diarrhea occurs, it is more commonly regarded as infectious, and this is

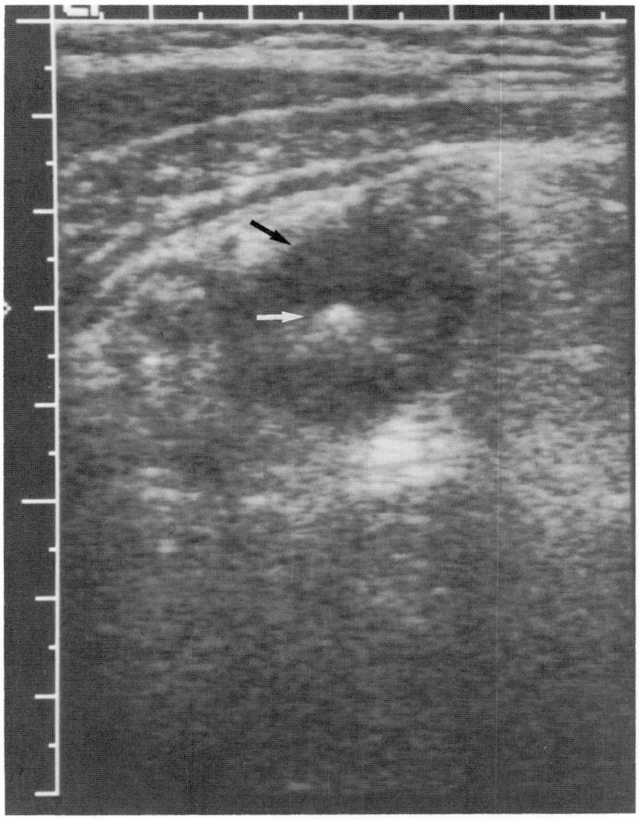

Figure 59–10. Cross-sectional ultrasound study through terminal ileal loop revealing markedly thickened bowel wall. The bright central echo *(white arrow)* represents luminal gas, and the *black arrow* represents the serosal bowel surface. (Courtesy of Frederick Conard, MD.)

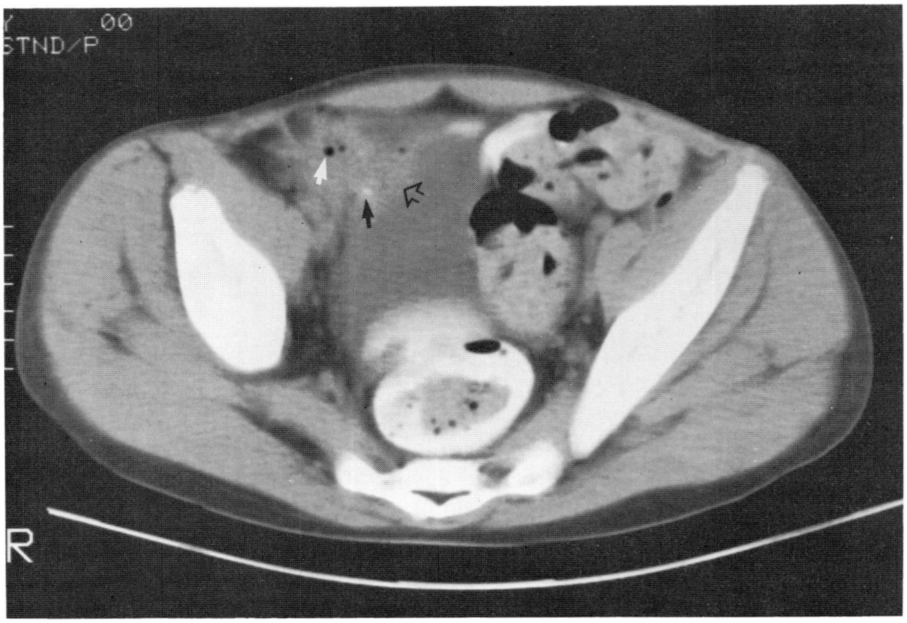

Figure 59–11. Computed tomographic scan of patient with terminal ileal disease and pneumaturia revealing thickened bladder wall *(open arrow)* and perivesical abscess containing air *(white arrow)*. Extraluminal contrast material *(black arrow)* is noted in the inflammatory mass. (Courtesy of Stuart Markowitz, MD.)

usually the case. Hemolytic-uremic syndrome may mimic inflammatory bowel disease quite closely,[189, 190] as can Henoch-Schönlein purpura.[191] More chronic watery diarrhea may be considered to represent irritable bowel syndrome, lactose intolerance, giardiasis, or the ingestion of excessive amounts of sorbitol-containing products. Perirectal inflammation or fissures or tags may be confused with perianal streptococcal infection, hemorrhoids, and condyloma. Short stature and delayed pubertal development may often initially be evaluated as an endocrinopathy before consideration of Crohn's disease is made. Anorexia and weight loss may be confused with anorexia nervosa. Likewise, persistent joint symptoms and particularly frank arthritis are often considered to represent juvenile rheumatoid arthritis if gastrointestinal symptoms are not present at presentation. Crohn's disease is an important consideration in the differential diagnosis of chronic hepatitis.

THERAPY

No available therapy is curative in patients with Crohn's disease. Rather, current interventional techniques are directed toward controlling symptoms and addressing complications. It must be emphasized that treatment should be directed primarily toward symptoms and not abnormal laboratory tests, biopsies, or radiographs. It is clear that there may be considerable dissociation between abnormal tests and clinical activity.[192–194] Assessment of disease activity in children must include not only the usual signs and symptoms of Crohn's disease, but also growth parameters. The impact of disease activity and types of treatment are of considerable importance in devising treatment strategies. A pediatric Crohn's disease activity index (PCDAI) has been formulated to standardize assessment of disease activity.[195]

Table 59–3. DIFFERENTIAL DIAGNOSIS OF PRESENTING SYMPTOMS OF CROHN'S DISEASE

Primary Presenting Symptom	Diagnostic Considerations
Right lower quadrant abdominal pain, with or without mass	Appendicitis, infection (e.g., *Campylobacter, Yersinia*), lymphoma, intussusception, mesenteric adenitis, Meckel's diverticulum, ovarian cyst
Chronic periumbilical or epigastric abdominal pain	Irritable bowel, constipation, lactose intolerance, peptic disease
Rectal bleeding, no diarrhea	Fissure, polyp, Meckel's diverticulum, rectal ulcer syndrome
Bloody diarrhea	Infection, hemolytic-uremic syndrome, Henoch-Schönlein purpura, ischemic bowel, radiation colitis
Watery diarrhea	Irritable bowel, lactose intolerance, giardiasis, cryptosporidium, sorbitol, laxatives
Perirectal disease	Fissure, hemorrhoid (rare), streptococcal infection, condyloma (rare)
Growth delay	Endocrinopathy
Anorexia, weight loss	Anorexia nervosa
Arthritis	Collagen vascular disease, infection
Liver abnormalities	Chronic hepatitis

Treatment of Crohn's disease can be divided into four basic categories: pharmacologic, nutritional, surgical, and psychosocial. Each has its limitations, and most frequently a combination of several therapeutic modalities is appropriate for selected patients.

Pharmacologic Treatment

Although several types of medications have been shown to be effective in inducing remission in active Crohn's disease, none has clearly demonstrated prophylactic value. Therefore once remission is achieved, it is customary to attempt to taper medication dosages gradually. Most efficacy data have been derived in adults, and current treatment strategies in children are extrapolated from these studies. Dosing schedules and indications for therapy are shown in Table 59–4.

Corticosteroids. Several large clinical studies have shown that corticosteroids are significantly more effective than placebo in inducing remission in patients with active small bowel[196, 196a] or large bowel disease.[196a] Proposed mechanisms of action have included inhibition of neutrophil- and monocyte-mediated activity by inhibition of leukotriene and prostaglandin production as well as by direct action on lymphocyte cellular activity.[197] Once remission is achieved, the medication is tapered over weeks to months. Prednisone absorption may be poor, and some patients may require parenteral administration initially.[198] Although "sicker" patients are frequently hospitalized and receive corticosteroids parenterally, no study has shown that this method of administration is superior to oral dosing. Corticosteroid therapy should be used with caution in the patient with Crohn's disease and intra-abdominal sepsis. High-dose corticosteroid therapy may mask signs of intra-abdominal infection or even perforation.

Side effects associated with chronic corticosteroid therapy can be serious and include growth suppression, posterior subcapsular cataracts and glaucoma,[199] aseptic necrosis of the femoral head, vertebral collapse, hypertension, and depression. Cosmetic side effects, particularly troubling to the adolescent, include acne, facial puffiness, hirsutism, and striae. Peptic disease is rare in the author's experience. Because of these problems, there should be an active attempt to use the minimum corticosteroid dose necessary to control symptoms and continually try to wean the dosage. Alternate-day therapy (0.2–0.5 mg/kg prednisone) is associated with minimal side effects and does not appear to depress growth velocity.[16] Long-term, low-dose daily therapy in adults has not been shown to prevent relapse or decrease progression of disease.[200] Fluticasone propionate, a topically active corticosteroid of low systemic bioavailability after oral administration, has shown promise in the treatment of individuals with mild to moderate Crohn's disease.[201] Use of this type of medication has particular appeal because of the possibility of avoiding many of the serious side effects associated with corticosteroid use.

Sulfasalazine. Although sulfasalazine has been shown to treat colonic Crohn's disease effectively and has not demonstrated significant efficacy in small bowel involvement,[196] it nonetheless is still frequently used to treat small bowel disease. The role of newer aminosalicylic acid (5-ASA) agents in the treatment of Crohn's disease in children has not been established, although preliminary observations in adults have suggested a potential role for delayed release 5-ASA compounds. A delayed-release form of 5-ASA (Asacol) may be superior to placebo in the maintenance treatment of Crohn's ileitis.[202] The author has used 5-ASA enemas (mesalamine) effectively in treating distal colonic disease in a small number of patients with Crohn's colitis. The anti-inflammatory activity of sulfasalazine and its analogs is thought to be due to decreased prostaglandin and leukotriene synthesis by inhibition of the cyclooxygenase and lipoxygenase pathways of arachidonic acid metabolism (see Chapter 60).[202a]

Common side effects at the initiation of sulfasalazine therapy include nausea, abdominal pain, and headache. These generally subside after several days to a week or two. More serious side effects of sulfasalazine include a hypersensitivity rash, bone marrow depression, pancreatitis, and reversible male infertility.[203]

Antibiotics. Broad-spectrum antibiotic therapy is fre-

Table 59–4. PHARMACOLOGIC TREATMENT OF CROHN'S DISEASE

Drug	Daily Dose	Indications	Comment
Prednisone	1–2 mg/kg q.d.–b.i.d. Maximum 40–60 mg	Small or large bowel disease	Once remission achieved, lower by 5 mg every week Attempt to achieve q.o.d. schedule. Continue to taper and then stop
Sulfasalazine	30–50 mg/kg b.i.d.–t.i.d. Maximum 3 gm	Large bowel disease	In allergic or intolerant patient, consider use of 5-ASA compounds
Metronidazole	15–20 mg/kg b.i.d.–t.i.d. Maximum 1.5 gm	Perirectal or colonic disease	May require prolonged use Neurotoxicity important
6-Mercaptopurine or azathioprine	1–2 mg/kg q.d. Maximum 100 mg	Severe disease Corticosteroid toxicity	Effect may be delayed for 3–6 months Need careful monitoring

q.d., every day; b.i.d., twice a day; t.i.d., three times a day, q.o.d., every other day.

quently required to treat intraabdominal abscess formation in Crohn's disease. Triple therapy with ampicillin, gentamicin, and clindamycin or metronidazole is most frequently given. This type of antibiotic therapy is also frequently administered in the febrile patient even in the absence of documented intra-abdominal sepsis often because of the presumption of "microfistulization" and localized infection.

Considerable attention has also focused on the role of metronidazole as either primary therapy or in the treatment of perirectal disease. Metronidazole has been shown to be more effective than placebo and slightly more effective than sulfasalazine as primary therapy in adults and as with sulfasalazine, appears to be more helpful in colonic than small bowel disease.[204, 204a] Perirectal disease improves in some patients treated with long courses of metronidazole, but even in those successfully treated only approximately 25% can have the drug discontinued without recurrence of disease.[205] The mechanism of action of metronidazole is unclear and has been postulated to relate to its potent antianaerobic bacterial activity as well as suppressing cell-mediated immunity.[206]

Peripheral neuropathy is the most common significant side effect of metronidazole therapy. In children treated chronically (4–11 months), 85% developed a sensory peripheral neuropathy or reduced nerve conduction velocity.[207] Paresthesias have been described in 50% of adults treated for 6 or more months.[205] Fortunately, the neuropathy is generally reversible in most patients on decreasing dosage or discontinuation of the medication. A disulfiramlike effect has been observed with metronidazole. Potential carcinogenicity has been a concern in laboratory animals but has not been documented in humans.

Immunosuppressive Therapy. Although no double-blind, placebo-controlled studies have examined the utility of immunosuppressive therapy in children with Crohn's disease, two nonblinded studies have suggested a role for azathioprine[208] or 6-mercaptopurine[209] in these patients. Both studies examined particularly ill patients, many of whom were dependent on high doses of corticosteroids. In both reports, the addition of immunosuppressive therapy to existing medication regimens resulted in improvement in symptoms in about 75% of patients and allowed a decrease in corticosteroid dosage. In most patients, no significant improvement in symptoms was noted before 3 to 4 months of therapy. Toxicity was negligible in both these studies.

In large adult studies examining the role of 6-mercaptopurine in treating Crohn's disease, side effects have included pancreatitis (3%), bone marrow depression (2%), allergic reactions (2%), and drug-induced hepatitis (<1%).[210, 210a] Pancreatitis usually resolves promptly on discontinuation of therapy.[211] One case of a brain lymphoma possibly associated with 6-mercaptopurine therapy has been reported.[210] Use of 6-mercaptopurine in Crohn's disease has been suggested when high-dose corticosteroid therapy cannot be withdrawn, in the presence of severe perirectal or internal fistulization, and before panproctocolectomy and ileostomy in patients with intractable symptoms.[210]

Additional immunosuppressive medications have been used in treating severe Crohn's disease. Cyclosporine was found to be more effective than placebo in reducing symptoms in a group of adults with severe disease.[212] Efficacy of therapy was observed as early as 2 weeks into treatment, and no significant toxicity was noted during the 3 months of therapy. A short course of cyclosporine therapy, however, does not appear to result in long-term improvement in chronic active disease.[213] Potential roles for methotrexate,[214] plasmapheresis,[215] and intravenous gammaglobulin[216] have also been suggested. In all these studies, the rationale for the use of these potent medications has been the belief that the body's immune system is central to the perpetuation of intestinal inflammation.

Although the use of immunosuppressive medication in the treatment of Crohn's disease in children is now common, the potential long-term toxicity is not clear. Until long-term safety data are available, its clinical use should still be restricted to the most severely ill patients. Whether it may have a role as primary therapy in a broader range of patients must await controlled clinical trials.

Other Agents. Additional therapeutic modalities are also available that diminish symptoms while not actually decreasing bowel inflammation. Antimotility agents such as loperamide may be helpful in controlling nocturnal diarrhea. Dicyclomine may provide relief from cramping in those patients who also have irritable bowel syndrome–like symptoms. This problem is occasionally seen in adolescents. Cholestyramine, a bile acid binding resin, may control diarrhea in those patients who have had terminal ileal resection or extensive ileal disease and who have significant bile acid loss into the colon stimulating colonic secretion.

Nutritional Therapy

The recognition of the profound micronutrient and macronutrient deficiencies in patients with Crohn's disease has spurred considerable interest in investigating the role of nutritional therapy in the management of this disorder. Assessment of nutritional status by measurement of height, weight, growth velocity, anthropometric data, and serum protein determinations is a critical element in devising treatment strategy. Any mineral or vitamin deficiencies (iron, folic acid, vitamin B_{12}, calcium, magnesium, and zinc) should be treated with specific therapy. The use of nutritional therapy can be directed in several ways, including primary therapy without accompanying pharmacologic intervention, adjunctive therapy with concomitant medications (especially to treat growth failure), and in preoperative preparation.

Primary Therapy. Several early studies suggested that remission rates in patients with active Crohn's disease were similar when patients were treated with elemental diets compared with corticosteroids.[217–219] A more recent study suggested significantly improved and faster remission rates in patients treated with corticosteroid and sulfasalazine compared with those receiving enteral nutrition solely with an oligopeptide diet.[220] Complete bowel rest with total parenteral nutrition does not appear to be more effective than an elemental diet in inducing remission.[221] Polymeric diets may not be as effective as elemental diets in treating active disease.[222] It has been postulated that elemental diets may decrease intestinal inflammation by decreasing antigenic stimuli to the gut. Duration of remission induced by elemental diets appears to be less in those patients with colonic involvement, fistula, and perianal disease.[223] Concern has been raised that elemental diets, lacking fermentable fiber, may not provide adequate substrate for the generation of short-chain organic acids (acetic, proprionic, butyric), which are important energy sources for colonic epithelial cells.[224, 225] Occasionally, pediatric patients who have profound growth failure but minimal gastrointestinal symptoms can be managed with long-term nutritional supplementation alone and do not require drug therapy.

Adjunctive Therapy. Intensive nutritional support has been used as adjunctive therapy in addition to pharmacologic agents in several clinical situations. In patients with severe disease and clinical evidence of malnutrition, total parenteral nutrition is useful in improving body protein stores.[226] The efficacy of bowel rest and total parenteral nutrition in promoting clinical improvement has been supported in some reports[227, 228] but not in others.[221, 229] The course of perianal or internal fistula does not appear to be changed by bowel rest and parenteral nutrition. Rarely, patients with extensive bowel resection require long-term parenteral nutritional support for treatment of short gut syndrome. In children and adolescents, intensive nutritional support has been shown to be effective in reversing growth retardation in most patients.[160, 230–232] It is *imperative* that nutritional support be started in these patients well before physiologic bone maturation and fusion of epiphyses if catch-up growth is to be expected. Intervention has been provided as total parenteral nutrition, oral supplements, and continuous elemental diet infusions. In some patients, these types of therapy have been used for extended periods, and in others they have been given as defined courses at regular intervals.

Preoperative Therapy. It is common clinical practice to replete nutritional deficiencies before major resectional surgery in patients with Crohn's disease. Whether this decreases postoperative problems in these individuals is not clear.

Administration of Nutritional Therapy

Details of nutritional support are reviewed in Chapters 83 and 84. In children with Crohn's disease, the ideal form of nutritional support is an increase in oral intake. This frequently occurs following the institution of corticosteroid therapy. Restrictive low-residue diets are not associated with a better outcome than normal unrestricted diets,[233] and patients should generally be allowed to eat ad libitum. Lactose may occasionally need to be restricted if lactose intolerance is documented. Oral supplements given at times that will not interfere with meals are helpful in increasing daily protein and caloric intake. Nocturnal tube feedings of an elemental formula are generally well accepted if patients are given adequate emotional support and encouragement. Once an adolescent starts to see a marked improvement in energy level and body habitus following the institution of this therapy, he or she is usually willing to continue it as long as necessary.

Surgery

Approximately 50 to 70% of children or adults with Crohn's disease require surgery within the first 10 to 15 years after diagnosis.[234–236] Indications for surgery in children and adolescents with Crohn's disease are shown in Table 59–5. Most frequently.intractable symptoms despite medical therapy and corticosteroid toxicity represent the primary reasons for surgical intervention. Patients with ileal disease tend to have a higher frequency of obstructive symptoms requiring surgery than patients with colonic disease.[70]

Because resectional therapy is not curative, patients and their families must be fully informed of the risks of recurrent disease. Following terminal ileal resection, endoscopic evidence of disease is present at the neoterminal ileum in more than 70% of adults at 1 year postsurgery, although only 35% are symptomatic.[237] Approximately 80% of children with terminal ileal or ileocecal resection are clinically well 4 years after surgery.[235] More extensive colonic resection in patients with ileocolitis or segmental colitis is often followed by relapse in up to 70% of cases within 5 years of surgery.[235] In children, the recurrence rate after panproctocolectomy and ileostomy appears to depend partly on the

Table 59–5. INDICATIONS FOR SURGERY IN CROHN'S DISEASE

Failure of medical therapy
Intractable symptoms
Corticosteroid toxicity
Social invalidism
Obstruction—acute or chronic
Gastroduodenal
Small bowel
Large bowel
Hemorrhage
Small bowel lesion
Large bowel lesion
Fulminant colitis, with or without toxic megacolon
Perforation
Free
Closed, with abscess
Fistula
Intractable perirectal disease
Enteroenteric
Enterocutaneous
Enterovesical
Enterovaginal
Growth retardation
Carcinoma
Obstructive uropathy

presence of ileal disease at the time of surgery. Patients who required surgery for ileocolitis had a 70% relapse rate within 5 to 10 years compared with a 15% rate for those with colitis alone.[238] Children undergoing intestinal resection within 1 year of onset of symptoms have been noted to have delayed recurrence of active disease compared with patients whose preoperative duration of symptomatic disease was greater.[239]

Newer surgical techniques have attempted to decrease the need for bowel resection in patients who have previously undergone surgery and in whom recurrent disease is characterized by stricture formation. Several strictured areas may be present, and resection of each would entail loss of considerable bowel length. Several convincing reports have now appeared that document the use of strictureplasty to treat these localized recurrences.[240, 241] In this procedure, a longitudinal incision is made through the stenotic bowel and the opening is then closed transversely. This procedure can generally be done only if there is no acute severe inflammation, abscess, or phlegmon at the strictured site.[240]

Severe perirectal disease continues to be a vexing problem and may require surgical therapy. Fecal diversion with an ileostomy or colostomy has generally not proved effective in controlling perianal disease,[242] although in this author's experience, some patients have had resolution of perirectal fistula and abscess following diversion and have subsequently had reanastomosis without recurrence. It may be difficult to distinguish between recurrent or ongoing Crohn's colitis and diversion colitis in the excluded rectosigmoid in patients with a diverting colostomy. For most patients, suppurative complications of perirectal disease can be addressed with conservative measures such as abscess drainage, anal fistulotomy, and partial internal sphincterectomy.[243, 244] Proctectomy is required in 10 to 15% of patients with severe perirectal disease.[243]

Despite intensive medical and nutritional therapy, growth failure persists in some children and adolescents with Crohn's disease. Convincing evidence exists that improved growth in children after surgery may occur provided that at the time of surgery the child is either prepubertal or in early puberty.[235, 245, 246] Marked increases in growth velocity (catch-up growth) are usually seen in these patients provided that postoperative nutritional state is not compromised and corticosteroid therapy can be discontinued or tapered to alternate-day therapy.

Psychiatric Therapy

Monitoring the effects of chronic illness on psychological and social functioning is crucial in dealing with the child or adolescent with inflammatory bowel disease. Psychiatric symptoms, particularly depression, may be seen and should be addressed by skilled consultants. Children should be encouraged to participate in age-appropriate activities as much as possible. Adolescents may have a particularly difficult time as they try to achieve independence from their family at a time that their illness makes this especially difficult. Patients facing surgery often benefit greatly from having an age-matched and sex-matched peer who has undergone similar surgery visit them and discuss what it is "really like" in the preoperative period. Most pediatric patients consider that the quality of their lives significantly improves after surgery.[238, 247]

PROGNOSIS

At present, Crohn's disease is a chronic incurable illness marked by periods of exacerbation and remission. Only 1% of patients with well-documented Crohn's disease do not suffer at least one relapse following diagnosis and initial therapy.[248] Certain subgroups of patients, defined by anatomic extent of disease, may fare better or worse than others. In general, patients with ileocolitis have a poorer response to medication and a greater need for surgery than do patients with limited small bowel disease.[70, 71] One study has suggested that the presence of granuloma on rectosigmoid biopsy at the time of diagnosis portends a poorer prognosis with more extensive intestinal involvement and perianal disease.[249] Having other family members affected by inflammatory bowel disease does not appear to affect the course of a child with Crohn's disease.[250]

Considerable attention has been paid to trying to identify specific factors associated with relapse of disease once remission has been established. Although a number of enteric infections have been suggested as causing disease relapse, this has not been documented in a convincing way.[251] Anecdotally, parents often relate that their child recently suffered from a viral respiratory infection before a relapse of disease. One study suggested that up to 40% of exacerbations in childhood inflammatory bowel disease might be associated with an antecedent or concomitant viral illness, particularly Epstein-Barr virus or adenovirus.[252] It has been postulated that viral infection may affect the body's immune system and indirectly affect the course of bowel inflammation.[251]

In examining large populations of adults with Crohn's disease, about 45% are well at a point in time, 30% have mild disease activity, and 25% have moderate to severe disease activity.[248] Similar data are not available for children, but in this author's experience, these percentages appear to be applicable to children and adolescents as well. The majority of pediatric patients with Crohn's disease function well and are able to participate in age- appropriate activities, albeit with modification at times of increased disease activity.

Mortality rates in Crohn's disease have varied in different studies, with estimates ranging from no increased mortality[248] to a twofold increased risk of dying compared with a matched group drawn from the general population.[253] Death from Crohn's disease in the pediatric population is extremely rare.

SUMMARY

The care of the child or adolescent with Crohn's disease requires a multidisciplinary approach with attention devoted to medical, nutritional, surgical, and psychological issues. An understanding of how the disease has impact on normal growth and development (both physical and emotional) is essential to optimizing therapy. Considerable attention should be devoted to educating the child or adolescent and family regarding the disease process and rationale behind as well as complications of therapy. An optimistic and supportive attitude is essential. Age-appropriate support groups can be of significant value in helping individuals with Crohn's disease cope with their illness.

ACKNOWLEDGMENT

The author is deeply indebted to Andrew Ricci, Jr., M.D., for his contribution to the pathology section of this chapter, and to Stuart Markowitz, M.D., for his contribution to the discussion of radiographic evaluation.

REFERENCES

1. Lockhart-Mummery H, Morson B. Crohn's disease (regional enteritis) of the large intestine and its distinction from ulcerative colitis. Gut 1960; 1:87–105.
2. Haug K, Schrumpf EH, Halvorsen JF, et al, and the Study Group of Inflammatory Bowel Disease in Western Norway: Epidemiology of Crohn's disease in Western Norway. Scand J Gastroenterol 1989; 24:1271–12.
3. Olafsdottir EJ, Gjermund F, Haug K: Chronic inflammatory bowel disease in children in western Norway. J Pediatr Gastroenterol Nutr 1989; 8:454–458.
4. Barton JR, Gillon S. Ferguson A: Incidence of inflammatory bowel disease in Scottish children between 1968 and 1983: Marginal fall in ulcerative colitis, three-fold rise in Crohn's disease. Gut 1989; 30:618–622.
5. Ferguson A, Rifkind EA, Doig CM: Prevalence of chronic inflammatory bowel disease in British children. *In* McConnell RB, Rozen P, Langman MJS, Gilat T, eds: The Genetics and Epidemiology of Inflammatory Bowel Disease (Front Gastrointest Res 11). Basel, Karger, 1986; pp 68–72.
6. Garland CF, Lilienfeld AM, Mendeloff AI, et al: Incidence rates of ulcerative colitis and Crohn's disease in fifteen areas of the United States. Gastroenterology 1981; 81:1115–1124.
7. Rose JDR, Roberts GM, Williams G, et al: Cardiff Crohn's disease jubilee: The incidence over 50 years. Gut 1988; 29:346–351.
8. Stowe SP, Redmond SR, Stormont JM, et al: An epidemiologic study of inflammatory bowel disease in Rochester, New York. Hospital incidence. Gastroenterology 1990; 98:104–110.
9. Ekbom A, Helmich C, Zack M, Adami HO: The epidemiology of inflammatory bowel disease: A large, population based study in Sweden. Gastroenterology 1991; 100:350–358.
10. Grand RJ, Homer DR: Approaches to inflammatory bowel disease in childhood and adolescence. Pediatr Clin North Am 1975; 22:835–850.
11. Roth MP, Peterson GM, McElree C, et al: Geographic origins of Jewish patients with inflammatory bowel disease. Gastroenterology 1989; 97:900–904.
12. Sonnenberg A, McCarty DJ, Jacobsen SJ: Geographic variation of inflammatory bowel disease within the United States. Gastroenterology 1991; 100:143–149.
13. Mayberry JF, Rhodes J, Newcombe RG: Familial prevalence of inflammatory bowel disease in relatives of patients with Crohn's disease. Br Med J 1980; 280:84.
14. Farmer RG, Michener WM, Mortimer EA: Studies of family history among patients with inflammatory bowel disease. Clin Gastroenterol 1980; 9:271–277.
15. Fielding JF: The relative risk of inflammatory bowel disease among parents and siblings of Crohn's disease patients. J Clin Gastroenterol 1986; 8:655–657.
16. Bennett RA, Rubin PH, Present DH: Frequency of inflammatory bowel disease in offspring of couples both presenting with inflammatory bowel disease. Gastroenterology 1991; 100:1638–1643.
17. Lashner BA, Evans AA, Kirsner JB, Hanauer SB: Prevalence and incidence of inflammatory bowel disease in family members. Gastroenterology 1986; 91:1396–1400.

17a. Meucci G, Vecchi M, Torgano G, et al: Familial aggregation of inflammatory bowel disease in Northern Italy: A multicenter study. Gastroenterology 1992; 103:514–519.

18. Erholm M, Munkholm P, Langholz E, et al: Familial occurrence of inflammatory bowel disease. N Engl J Med 1991; 324:84–88.
19. Klein GL, Ament ME, Sparkes RS: Monozygotic twins with Crohn's disease: A case report. Gastroenterology 1980; 79:931–933.
20. Purrmann J, Bertrams J, Borchard F, et al: Monozygotic triplets with Crohn's disease of the colon. Gastroenterology 1986; 91:1533–1539.
21. Purrmann J, Bertrams J, Knapp M, et al: Gene and haplotype frequencies of HLA antigens in 269 patients with Crohn's disease. Scand J Gastroenterol 1990; 25:981–985.
22. Hollander D, Vadheim CM, Brettholz E, et al: Increased intestinal permeability in patients with Crohn's disease and their relatives. A possible etiologic factor. Ann Intern Med 1986; 105:883–885.
23. Murphy MS, Eastham EJ, Nelson R, et al: Intestinal permeability in Crohn's disease. Arch Dis Child 1989; 64:321–325.
24. Teahon K, Smethurst P, Levi AJ, et al: Intestinal permeability in patients with Crohn's disease and their first-degree relatives. Gut 1992; 33:320–323.
25. Morgan KL: Johne's and Crohn's. Chronic inflammatory bowel diseases of infectious etiology. Lancet 1987; 1:1017–1019.
26. Chiodini RJ, VanKruiningen HJ, Thayer et al: Possible role of mycobacteria in inflammatory bowel disease. I. An unclassified mycobacterium species isolated from patients with Crohn's disease. Dig Dis Sci 1984; 29:1073–1079.
27. Kobayashi K, Brown WR, Brennan PJ, Blaser MJ: Serum antibodies to mycobacterial antigens in active Crohn's disease. Gastroenterology 1988; 94:1404–1411.
28. Graham DY, Markesich DC, Yoshimura HH: Mycobacteria and inflammatory bowel disease. Results of culture. Gastroenterology 1987; 92:436–442.
29. Tanaka K, Wilks M, Coates PJ, et al: Mycobacterium paratuberculosis and Crohn's disease. Gut 1991; 32:43–45.
30. Belsheim MR, Darwich RZ, Watson WC, Schieven B: Bacterial L-form isolation from inflammatory bowel disease patients. Gastroenterology 1983; 85:364–369.
31. Sartor RB, Cromartie WJ, Powell DW, Schwab JH: Granulomatous enterocolitis induced in rats by purified bacterial cell wall fragments. Gastroenterology 1985; 89:587–595.
32. Sartor RB, Compton KY, Cleland DR, Schwab JH: Serum antibody response indicates intestinal absorpton of bacterial cell wall peptidoglycan. Gastroenterology 1986; 90:1615A.
33. Greenberg HB, Gebhard RL, McClain CJ, et al: Antibodies to viral gastroenteritis viruses in Crohn's disease. Gastroenterology 1979; 76:349–350.
34. Elliott PR, Forsey T, Darougar S, et al: Chlamydiae and inflammatory bowel disease. Gut 1981; 22:25–27.
35. James SP: Remission of Crohn's disease after human immunodeficiency virus infection. Gastroenterology 1988; 95:1667–1669.
36. Kagnoff MF: Immunology and disease of the gastrointestinal tract. *In* Sleisinger MH, Fordtran JS, eds: Gastrointestinal Disease. Pathophysiology, Diagnosis, Management. 4th ed. Philadelphia, WB Saunders, 1989; pp 114–144.
37. Elson CO: The immunology of inflammatory bowel disease. *In* Kirsner JB, Shorter RG, eds: Inflammatory Bowel Disease. 3rd ed. Philadelphia, Lea and Febiger, 1988; pp 97–164.
38. Ligumsky M, Simon PL, Karmfeli F, Rachmilewitz D: Role of interleukin 1 in inflammatory bowel disease-enhanced production during active disease. Gut 1990; 31:686–689.
39. Holte H, Spjeldnaes N, Kruse A, Windelborg B: Histamine release from gut mast cells from patients with inflammatory bowel disease. Gut 1990; 31:791–794.

40. Brynskov J, Tvede N, Andersen CB, et al: Increased concentrations of interleukin 1β, interleukin-2, and soluble interleukin-2 receptors in endoscopical mucosal biopsy specimens with active inflammatory bowel disease. Gut 1992; 33:55–58.
40a. Stevens C, Walz G, Singaram C, et al: Tumor necrosis factor-α, interleukin-1β, and interleukin-6 expression in inflammatory bowel disease. Dig Dis Sci 1992; 37:818–826.
40b. Mullin GE, Lazenby AJ, Harris ML, et al: Increased interleukin-2 messenger RNA in the intestinal mucosal lesions of Crohn's disease but not ulcerative colitis. Gastroenterology 1992; 102:1620–1627.
40c. Ruthlein J, Ibe M, Burghardt W, et al: Immunoglobulin G (IgG), IgG1, and IgG2 determinations from endoscopic biopsy specimens in control, Crohn's disease, and ulcerative colitis subjects. Gut 1992; 33:507–512.
41. Wallace JL, MacNaughton WK, Morris GP, Beck PL: Inhibition of leukotriene synthesis markedly accelerates healing in a rat model of inflammatory bowel disease. Gastroenterology 1989; 96:29–36.
42. Donowitz M: Arachidonic acid metabolites and their role in inflammatory bowel disease. An update requiring addition of a pathway. Gastroenterology 1985; 88:580–587.
43. Ahrenstedt O, Knutson L, Nilsson B, et al: Enhanced local production of complement components in the small intestines of patients with Crohn's disease. N Engl J Med 1990; 322:1345–1349.
44. Shanahan F: Pathogenesis of inflammatory bowel disease: A perspective. Autoimmun Forum Gastroenterology 1989; 1:2–4.
45. Bland P: MHC class II expression by the gut. Immunol Today 1988; 9:174–176.
45a. Mayer L, Shlien R: Evidence for function of Ia molecules on gut epithelial cells in man. J Exp Med 1987; 166:1471–1483.
46. Rutgeerts P, Goboes K, Peeters M, et al: Effect of faecal stream diversion on recurrence of Crohn's disease in the neoterminal ileum. Lancet 1991; 337:771–774.
47. Strober W, James SP: The immunologic basis of inflammatory bowel disease. J Clin Immunol 1986; 6:415–432.
48. Shorter RG, McGill DB, Bahn RC: Cytotoxicity of mononuclear cells for autologous colonic epithelial cells in colonic disease. Gastroenterology 1984; 86:13–22.
49. Roche JK, Fiocchi C, Youngman K: Sensitization to epithelial antigens in chronic mucosal inflammatory disease. Characterization of human intestinal mucosa-derived mononuclear cells reactive with purified epithelial cell-associated components in vitro. J Clin Invest 1985; 75:522–530.
50. Saavedra-Delgado AM, Metcalfe DD: Interaction between food antigens and the immune system in the pathogenesis of gastrointestinal diseases. Ann Allergy 1985; 55:694–702.
51. Lerner A, Rossi TM, Park B, et al: Serum antibodies to cow's milk proteins in pediatric inflammatory bowel disease. Crohn's disease versus ulcerative colitis. Acta Paediatr Scand 1989; 78:384–389.
52. Frieri M, Claus MM, Boris M, et al: Preliminary investigation on humoral and cellular immune responses to selected food proteins in patients with Crohn's disease. Ann Allergy 1990; 64:345–351.
53. Seidman E, Walker WA: Intestinal defenses. *In* Kirsner JB, Shorter RG, eds: Inflammatory Bowel Disease. 3rd ed. Philadelphia, Lea & Febiger, 1988; pp 65–74.
54. Koletzko S, Sherman P, Corey M, et al: Role of infant feeding practices in development of Crohn's disease in childhood. Br Med J 1989; 298:1617–1618.
55. Gilat T, Hacohen D, Lilos P, Langman MJS: Childhood factors in ulcerative colitis and Crohn's disease. An international cooperative study. Scand J Gastroenterol 1987; 22:1009–1024.
56. North CS, Alpers DH, Helzer JE, et al: Do life events or depression exacerbate inflammatory bowel disease? Ann Interm Med 1991; 114:381–386.
57. Shanahan F, Anton P: Neuroendocrine modulation of the immune system. Possible implications for inflammatory bowel disease. Dig Dis Sci 1988; 33:41S–49S.
58. Ruff MR, Wahl SM, Pert CB: Substance P receptor-mediated chemotaxis of human monocytes. Peptides 1985; 6(Suppl):107–11.
59. Rola-Pleszcynski M, Bolduc D, St-Pierre S: The effects of VIP on natural killer cells. J Immunol 1985; 135:2569–2573.
60. Mathews PM, Froehlich CJ, Sibbit WL, Bankhurst AD: Enhancement of natural cytotoxicity by beta-endorphin. J Immunol 1983; 130:1658–1662.
61. Stanisz AM, Befus D, Bienenstock J: Differential effects of vasoactive intestinal polypeptide, substance P, and somatostatin on immunoglobulin synthesis and proliferations by lymphocytes from Peyer's patches, mesenteric lymph nodes, and spleen. J Immunol 1986; 136:152–156.
62. Goetzl EJ, Payan DG: Inhibition by somatostatin of the release of mediators from human basophils and rat leukemic basophils. J Immunol 1984; 133:3255–3259.
63. Stallmach A, Schuppan D, Riese H, et al: Increased collagen type III synthesis by fibroblasts isolated from strictures of patients with Crohn's disease. Gastroenterology 1992; 102:1920–1929.
63a. Morson BC, Dawson IMP: Inflammatory disorders. *In* Gastrointestinal Pathology. 2nd ed. London, Blackwell Scientific Publications, 1979; pp 272–336.
64. Rickert RR, Carter HW: The "early" ulcerative lesion of Crohn's disease: Correlative light and scanning electron microscopic studies. J Clin Gastroenterol 1980; 2:11–19.
65. Goodman MJ, Skinner JM, Truelove SC: Abnormalities in apparently normal bowel mucosa in Crohn's disease. Lancet 1976; 1:275–278.
66. Riddell RH. Pathology of idiopathic inflammatory bowel disease. *In* Kirsner JB, Shorter RG, eds: Inflammatory Bowel Disease. 3rd ed. Philadelphia, Lea & Febiger, 1988; pp 329–350.
67. Chong SKF, Blackshaw AJ, Boyle S, et al: Histologic diagnosis of chronic inflammatory bowel disease in childhood. Gut 1985; 26:55–59.
68. Surawicz CM, Meisel JL, Ylvisaker T, et al: Rectal biopsy in the diagnosis of Crohn's disease: Value of multiple biopsies and serial sectioning. Gastroenterology 1981; 81:66–71.
69. Cartun RW, VanKruinigen HJ, Berman MM: An immunohistochemical search for infectious agents in Crohn's disease. Modern Pathol 1990; 3:16A.
70. Gryboski JD, Spiro HM: Prognosis in children with Crohn's disease. Gastroenterology 1978; 74:807–817.
71. Farmer RG, Whelan G, Fazio VW: Long-term follow-up of patients with Crohn's disease. Relationship between the clinical pattern and prognosis. Gastroenterology 1985; 88:1818–1825.
72. Mekhjian HS, Switz DM, Melnyk CS, et al: Clinical features and natural history of Crohn's disease. Gastroenterology 1979; 77:898–906.
73. Elliott PR, Lennard-Jones JE, Bartram GI, et al: Colonoscopic diagnosis of minimal change colitis in patients with a normal sigmoidoscopy and normal air-contrast barium enema. Lancet 1982; 1:650–651.
74. Heyman MB, Perman JA, Ferrell LD, Thaler MM: Chronic nonspecific inflammatory bowel disease of the cecum and proximal colon in children with grossly normal-appearing colonic mucosa: Diagnosis by colonoscopic biopsies. Pediatrics 1987; 80:255–261.
75. Fielding JF, Toye DKM, Beton DC, Cooke WT: Crohn's disease of the stomach and duodenum. Gut 1970; 11:1001–1006.
76. Lenaerts C, Roy CC, Vaillancourt M, et al: E. High incidence of upper gastrointestinal tract involvement in children with Crohn disease. Pediatrics 1989; 83:777–781.
77. Mashako MNL, Cezard JP, Navarro J, et al: Crohn's disease lesions in the upper gastrointestinal tract: Correlation between clinical, radiological, endoscopic, and histological features in adolescents and children. J Pediatr Gastroenter Nutr 1989; 8:442–446.
78. Rhoads JM, Powell DW. Diarrhea. *In* Walker WA, Durie PR, Hamilton JR, et al, eds: Pediatric Gastrointestinal Disease. Pathophysiology, Diagnosis, Management. Philadelphia, BC Decker, 1991; pp 62–78.
79. Hofman AF: Bile acid malabsorption caused by ileal resection. Arch Intern Med 1972; 130:597–605.
80. Phillips SF, Gaginella TS: Intestinal secretion as a mechanism in diarrheal disease. *In* Jerzy Glass GB, ed: Progress in Gastroenterology. Vol III. New York, Grune & Stratton, 1977; pp 481–504.
81. Head LH, Heaton JW, Kivel RM: Absorption of water and electrolytes in Crohn's disease of the colon. Gastroenterology 1969; 56:571–579.
82. Phillips SF: Pathophysiology of symptoms and clinical features

of inflammatory bowel disease. *In* Kirsner JB, Shorter RG, eds: Inflammatory Bowel Disease. 3rd ed. Philadelphia, Lea & Febiger, 1988; pp. 239–256.

83. Summers RW, Anuras S, Green J: Jejunal manometry patterns in health, partial intestinal obstruction, and pseudo-obstruction. Gastroenterology 1983; 85:1290–1300.
84. Burbige EJ, Huang SS, Bayless TM: Clinical manifestations of Crohn's disease in children and adolescents. Pediatrics 1975; 55:866–871.
85. Posthuma R, Moroz SP: Pediatric Crohn's disease. J Pediatr Surg 1985; 20:478–482.
86. Raine PAM: BAPS collective review. Chronic inflammatory bowel disease. J Pediatr Surg 1984; 19:18–23.
87. Barton JR, Ferguson A: Clinical features, morbidity and mortality of Scottish children with inflammatory bowel disease. Q J Med 1990; 75:423–439.
88. Griffiths AM, Alemayehu E, Sherman P: Clinical features of gastroduodenal disease in adolescents. J Pediatr Gastroenterol Nutr 1989; 8:166–171.
89. Treem WR, Ragsdale BD. Crohn's disease of the esophagus: A case report and review of the literature. J Pediatr Gastroenterol Nutr 1988; 7:451–455.
90. Markowitz J, Daum F, Aiges H, et al: Perianal disease in children and adolescents with Crohn's disease. Gastroenterology 1984; 86:829–833.
91. Greenstein AJ, Janowitz HD, Sachar DB: The extraintestinal complications of Crohn's disease and ulcerative colitis: A study of 700 patients. Medicine 1976; 55:401–412.
92. Kirsner JB. The local and systemic complications of inflammatory bowel disease. JAMA 1979; 242:1177–1183.
93. Danzi JT: Extraintestinal manifestations of idiopathic inflammatory bowel disease. Arch Intern Med 1988; 148:297–302.
94. Lindsley CB, Schaller JG: Arthritis associated with inflammatory bowel disease. J Pediatr 1974; 84:16–20.
95. Passo MH, Fitzgerald JF, Brandt KD: Arthritis associated with inflammatory bowel disease in children. Relationship of joint disease to activity and severity of bowel lesion. Dig Dis Sci 1986; 31:492–497.
96. Weiner SR, Clarke J, Taggart NA, et al: Rheumatic manifestations of inflammatory bowel disease. Semin Arthr Rheumat 1991; 20:353–366.
97. Moll JM: Inflammatory bowel disease. *In* Panayi GS, ed: Clinics in Rheumatic Disease. Philadelphia, WB Saunders, 1985; pp 87–105.
98. Menard D, Haddad H, Blain JG, et al: Granulomatous myositis and myopathy associated with Crohn's colitis. N Engl J Med 1976; 295:819.
99. Paller AS: Cutaneous changes associated with inflammatory bowel disease. Pediatr Dermatol 1986; 3:439–445.
99a. Levitt MD, Ritchie JK, Lennard-Jones JE, et al: *Pyoderma gangrenosum* in inflammatory bowel disease. Br J Surg 1991; 78:676–678.
100. Sutphen JL, Cooper PH, Mackel SE, Nelson DL: Metastatic cutaneous Crohn's disease. Gastroenterology 1984; 86:941–944.
101. Scully C, Cochran KM, Russell RI, et al: Crohn's disease of the mouth: An indicator of intestinal involvement. Gut 1982; 23:198–201.
102. Plauth M, Jenss H, Meyle J: Oral manifestations of Crohn's disease. An analysis of 79 cases. J Clin Gastroenterol 1991; 13:29–37.
103. Hopkins DJ, Horan E, Burton EI, et al: Ocular disorders in a series of 332 patients with Crohn's disease. Br J Ophthalmol 1974; 58:732–737.
104. Salmon JF, Wright JP, Murray ADN: Ocular inflammation in Crohn's disease. Ophthalmology 1991; 98:480–484.
105. Young RSK, Hodes BL, Cruse RP, et al: Orbital pseudotumor and Crohn disease. J Pediatr 1981; 99:250–252.
106. Talbot RW, Heppell J, Dozois RR, Beart RW Jr: Vascular complications of inflammatory bowel disease. Mayo Clin Proc 1986; 61:140–145.
107. Lake AM, Stauffer JQ, Stuart MJ: Hemostatic alterations in inflammatory bowel disease. Dig Dis Sci 1978; 23:897–902.
108. Lam A, Borda IT, Inwood MJ, Thomson S: Coagulation studies in ulcerative colitis and Crohn's disease. Gastroenterology 1975; 68:245–251.
109. Lloyd-Still JD, Tomasi L: Neurovascular and thromboembolic complications of inflammatory bowel disease in childhood. J Pediatr Gastroenterol Nutr 1989; 9:461–466.
110. Mezoff AG, Cohen MB, Maisel SK, Farrell MK: Crohn disease in an infant with central nervous system thrombosis and protein-losing enteropathy. J Pediatr 1990; 117:436–439.
111. Yassinger S, Adelman R, Cantor D, et al: Association of inflammatory bowel disease and large vascular lesions. Gastroenterology 1976; 71:844–846.
112. Hyams JA, Weinberg SR, Alley JL: Chronic ileitis with concomitant ureteritis. Am J Surg 1943; 61:117–120.
113. Present DH, Rabinowitz JG, Banks PA, Janowitz HD: Obstructive hydronephrosis—a frequent but seldom recognized complication of granulomatous disease of the bowel. N Engl J Med 1969; 280:523–528.
114. Kent GG, McGowan GE, Hyams JS, Leichtner AM: Hypertension associated with unilateral hydronephrosis as a complication of Crohn's disease. J Pediatr Surg 1987; 22:1049–1050.
115. Shield DE, Lytton B, Weiss RM, Schiff M Jr: Urologic complications of inflammatory bowel disease. J Urol 1976; 115:701–776.
116. Deren JJ, Porush JG, Levitt MF, Khilnani MT: Nephrolithiasis as a complication of ulcerative colitis and regional enteritis. Ann Intern Med 1962; 56:843–853.
117. Kirschner BS, Samowitz WS: Secondary amyloidosis in Crohn's disease of childhood. J Pediatr Gastroenterol Nutr 1986; 5:816–821.
118. Kahn E, Markowitz J, Simpser E, et al: Amyloidosis in children with inflammatory bowel disease. J Pediatr Gastroenterol Nutr 1989; 8:447–453.
119. Gitkind MJ, Wright SC: Amyloidosis complicating inflammatory bowel disease. A case report and review of the literature. Dig Dis Sci 1990; 35:906–908.
120. Dew MJ, Thompson H, Allan RN: The spectrum of hepatic dysfunction in inflammatory bowel disease. Q J Med 1979; 189:113–135.
121. Porayko MK, Wiesner RH, LaRusso NF, et al: Patients with asymptomatic primary sclerosing cholangitis frequently have progressive disease. Gastroenterology 1990; 98:1594–1602.
122. Watts HD: Multiple hepatic abscesses complicating regional enteritis. The importance of prior surgery or corticosteroid therapy. Dig Dis 1978; 23:41S–47S.
123. Mir-Madjlessi SH, McHenry MC, Farmer RG: Liver abscess in Crohn's disease. Report of four cases and review of the literature. Gastroenterology 1986; 91:987–993.
124. Baker AL, Kaplan MM, Norton RA, Patterson JF: Gallstones in inflammatory bowel disease. Dig Dis 1974; 19:109–112.
125. Cohen S, Kaplan M, Gottlieb L, Patterson J: Liver disease and gallstones in regional enteritis. Gastroenterology 1971; 60:237–245.
126. McClure J, Banerjee SS, Schofield PS: Crohn's disease of the gall bladder. J Clin Pathol 1984; 37:516–518.
127. Hyams JS, Baker E, Schwartz AN, et al: Acalculous cholecystitis in Crohn's disease. J Adoles Health Care 1988; 10:151–154.
128. Wee A, Ludwig J: Pericholangitis in chronic ulcerative colitis: Primary sclerosing cholangitis of the small bile ducts. Ann Intern Med 1985; 102:581–587.
129. LaRusso NF, Weisner RH, Ludwig J, MacCarty RL: Primary sclerosing cholangitis. N Engl J Med 1984; 310:899–903.
130. Rutgeerts P, Ghoos Y, Vantrappen G, Fevery J. Biliary lipid composition in patients with nonoperated Crohn's disease. Dig Dis Sci 1986; 31:27–32.
131. Robert JR, Sachar DB, Greenstein AJ: Severe gastrointestinal hemorrhage in Crohn's disease. Ann Surg 1991; 213:207–211.
132. Glotzer DJ: Indications for operation in inflammatory bowel disease—a surgeon's opinion. *In* Kirsner JB, Shorter RG, eds: Inflammatory Bowel Disease. 3rd ed. Philadelphia, Lea & Febiger; 1988; pp 549–584.
133. Difebo G, Gizzi G, Cappello IP: Unusual case of colonic subobstruction by giant pseudopolyposis in Crohn's colitis. Endoscopy 1981; 13:90–92.
134. Highman L, Jagelman DG: Gallstone ileus complicating terminal ileal Crohn's disease. Br J Surg 1981; 68:201–202.
135. Kirchmann HMA, Bender SW: Intestinal obstruction in Crohn's disease in childhood. J Pediatr Gastroenterol Nutr 1987; 6:79–83.
136. Katz S, Schulman N, Levin L: Free perforation in Crohn's

disease. A report of 33 cases and review of the literature. Am J Gastroenterol 1986; 81:38–43.
137. Huizenga KA, Schroeder KW: Gastrointestinal complications of ulcerative colitis and Crohn's disease. *In* Kirsner JB, Shorter RG, eds: Inflammatory Bowel Disease. 3rd ed. Philadelphia, Lea & Febiger, 1988; pp 257–280.
138. Biller JA, Grand RJ, Harris BH: Abdominal abscesses in adolescents with Crohn's disease. J Pediatr Surg 1987; 22:873–876.
139. Grant CS, Dozois RR: Toxic megacolon: Ultimate fate of patients after successful medical management. Am J Surg 1984; 147:106–110.
140. Grieco MD, Bordan DL, Geiss AC, Beil AR Jr: Toxic megacolon complicating Crohn's colitis. Ann Surg 1980; 191:75–80.
141. Weedon DD, Shorter RG, Ilstrup DM, et al: Crohn's disease and cancer. N Engl J Med 1973; 289:1099–1103.
142. Greenstein AJ, Sachar D, Pucillo A, et al: Cancer in Crohn's disease after diversionary surgery. A report of 7 carcinomas occurring in excluded bowel. Am J Surg 1978; 135:86–90.
143. Jenkins AP, Treasure J, Thompson RP: Crohn's disease presenting as anorexia nervosa. Br Med J 1988; 296:699–700.
144. Grill BB, Lange R, Markowitz R, et al: Delayed gastric emptying in children with Crohn's disease. J Clin Gastroenterol 1985; 7:216–226.
145. Murch SH, Lamkin VA, Savage MO, et al: Serum concentrations of tumor necrosis factor-alpha in childhood chronic inflammatory bowel disease. Gut 1991; 32:913–917.
145a. Hyams JS, Treem WR, Eddy E, et al: Tumor necrosis factor alpha not elevated in children with inflammatory bowel disease. J Pediatr Gastroenterol Nutr 1991; 12:439–447.
146. Thomas DW, Sinatra FR, Merritt RJ: Fecal alpha-1-antitrypsin excretion in young people with Crohn's disease. J Pediatr Gastroenterol Nutr 1983; 2:491–496.
147. Motil KJ, Altschuler SI, Grand RJ: Mineral balance during nutritional supplementation in adolescents with Crohn disease and growth failure. J Pediatr 1985; 107:473–479.
148. Jeejeebhoy KN, Ostro MJ: Nutritional consequences and therapy in inflammatory bowel disease. *In* Kirsner JA, Shorter RG, eds: Inflammatory Bowel Disease. 3rd ed. Philadelphia, Lea & Febiger, 1988; pp 513–528.
149. Beeken W: Absorptive defects in young people with regional enteritis. Pediatrics 1973; 52:69–74.
150. Kirschner BS, DeFavaro MV, Jensen W: Lactose malabsorption in children and adolescents with inflammatory bowel disease. Gastroenterology 1981; 81:829–832.
151. Beeken W, Busch HJ, Sylwester DL: Intestinal protein loss in Crohn's disease. Gastroenterology 1972; 62:207–215.
152. Kirschner BS: Nutritional consequences of inflammatory bowel disease on growth. J Am Coll Nutr 1988; 7:301–308.
153. Motil KJ, Grand RJ: Nutritional management of inflammatory bowel disease. Pediatr Clin North Am 1985; 32:447–469.
154. Filipson S, Hultean L, Lindstedt G: Malabsorption of fat and vitamin B12 before and after ileal resection for Crohn's disease. Scand J Gastroenterol 1978; 13:529–536.
155. Pollach S, Enat R, Haim S, et al: Pellagra as the presenting manifestation of Crohn's disease. Gastroenterology 1982; 82:948–952.
156. Harries AD, Brown R, Heatley RV, et al: Vitamin D status in Crohn's disease: Association with nutrition and disease activity. Gut 1985; 26:1197–1203.
157. Krawitt EL, Beeken WL, Janney CD: Calcium absorption in Crohn's disease. Gastroenterology 1976; 71:251–254.
158. Grand RJ, Colodny AH: Increased requirement for magnesium during parenteral therapy for granulomatous colitis. J Pediatr 1972; 81:788–790.
159. Hendricks KM, Walker WA: Zinc deficiency in inflammatory bowel disease. Nutr Rev 1988; 46:401–408.
160. Kelts DG, Grand RJ, Shen G, et al: Nutritional basis of growth failure in children and adolescents with Crohn's disease. Gastroenterology 1979; 76:720–727.
161. Chan ATH, Fleming CR, O'Fallon WM, Huizenga KA: Estimated versus measured basal energy requirements in patients with Crohn's disease. Gastroenterology 1986; 91:75–78.
162. Kushner RF, Schoeller DA: Resting and total energy expenditure in patients with inflammatory bowel disease. Am J Clin Nutr 1991; 53:161–165.
163. Tanner JM, Davies PSW: Clinical longitudinal standards for height and height velocity for North American children. J Pediatr 1985; 107:317–329.
164. Kleinman RE, Balistreri WF, Heyman MB, et al: Nutritional support for pediatric patients with inflammatory bowel disease. J Pediatr Gastroenterol Nutr 1989; 8:8–12.
165. Grand RJ, Motil KJ: Growth failure in inflammatory bowel disease. *In* Bayless TM, ed. Current Therapy in Gastroenterology and Liver Disease. 2nd ed. Toronto, BC Decker, 1986; pp 223–229.
166. Kirschner BS, Sutton MM: Somatomedin-C levels in growth-impaired children and adolescents with chronic inflammatory bowel disease. Gastroenterology 1986; 91:830–836.
167. Tenore A, Berman WF, Parks JS, Bongiovanni AM: Basal and stimulated growth hormone concentrations in inflammatory bowel disease. J Clin Endocr Metab 1977; 44:622–628.
168. Hyams JS, Moore RE, Leichtner AM, et al: Relationship of type I procollagen to corticosteroid therapy in children with inflammatory bowel disease. J Pediatr 1988; 112:893–898.
169. Kanof ME, Lake AM, Bayless TM: Decreased height velocity in children and adolescents before the diagnosis of Crohn's disease. Gastroenterology 1988; 95:1523–1527.
170. Bruce T: Emotional sequelae of chronic inflammatory bowel disease in children and adolescents. Clin Gastroenterol 1986; 15:89–104.
171. Schwarz SP, Blanchard EB: Inflammatory bowel disease: A review of the psychological assessment and treatment literature. Ann Behav Med 1990; 12:95–105.
172. Burke P, Meyer V, Kocoshis S, et al: Depression and anxiety in pediatric inflammatory bowel disease and cystic fibrosis. J Am Acad Child Adolesc Psychiatry 1989; 28:948–951.
173. Wood B, Watkins JB, Boyle JT, et al: Psychological functioning in children with Crohn's disease and ulcerative colitis: Implications for models of psychobiological interaction. J Am Acad Child Adolesc Psychiatry 1987; 26:774–781.
174. Wood B, Boyle JT, Watkins JB, et al: Sibling psychological status and style as related to the disease of their chronically ill brothers and sisters: Implications for models of biopsychosocial interaction. J Dev Behav Pediatr 1988; 9:66–72.
175. Burke P, Kocoshis SA, Chandra R, et al: Determinants of depression in recent onset pediatric inflammatory bowel disease. J Am Acad Child Adolesc Psychiatry 1990; 29:608–610.
176. Thomas DW, Sinatra FR: Screening laboratory tests for Crohn's disease. West J Med 1989; 150:163–164.
177. Stringer DA: Imaging inflammatory bowel disease in the pediatric patient. Radiol Clin North Am 1987; 25:93–113.
178. Gore RM, Cohen MI, Vogelzang RL, et al: Value of computed tomography in the detection of complications of Crohn's disease. Dig Dis Sci 1985; 30:701–709.
179. Cohen HL, Brill PW, Winchester P, et al: Imaging of psoas muscle abscess in adolescents with Crohn's disease. Am J Dis Child 1985; 139:1223–1225.
180. Saverymuttu SH, Camilleri M, Rees H, et al: 111-Indium granulocyte scanning. Comparison with colonoscopy, histology and faecal 111-indium excretion in assessing disease extent and activity in colitis. Gastroenterology 1986; 90:1121–1128.
181. Rothstein RD, Alavi A: The role of scintigraphy in the management of inflammatory bowel diease. J Nucl Med 1991; 32:856–859.
182. Tolia V, Kuhns LR, Chang CH, Slovis TL: Comparison of Indium–111 scintigraphy and colonsocopy with histologic study in children for evaluation of colonic chronic inflammatory bowel disease. J Pediatr Gastroenterol Nutr 1991; 12:336–339.
183. Goldman H, Antonioli DA: Mucosal biopsy of the rectum, colon, and distal ileum. Human Pathol 1982; 13:981–1012.
184. Lipson A, Bartram CI, Williams CB, et al: Barium studies and ileoscopy compared in children with suspected Crohn's disease. Clin Radiol 1990; 41:5–8.
185. Hyams JS, Goldman H, Katz AJ: Differentiating small bowel Crohn's disease from lymphoma. Role of rectal biopsy. Gastroenterology 1980; 79:340–343.
186. Meisel JL, Bergman D, Graney D, et al: Human rectal mucosa: Proctoscopic and morphological changes caused by laxative. Gastroenterology 1977; 72:1274–1279.
187. Mashako MNL, Cezard JP, Navarro J, et al: Crohn's disease lesions in the upper gastrointestinal tract: Correlation between clinical, radiological, endoscopic, and histological features in

adolescents and children. J Pediatr Gastroenterol Nutr 1989; 8:442–446.
188. Ruiz V, Unger SW, Morgan J, Wallack MK: Crohn's disease of the appendix. Surgery 1990; 107:113–117.
189. Whitington PF, Friedman AL, Chesney RW: Gastrointestinal disease in the hemolytic-uremic syndrome. Gastroenterology 1979; 76:728–733.
190. Loirat C, Sonsino E, Moreno AV, et al: Hemolytic-uremic syndrome: An analysis of the natural history and prognostic features. Acta Paediatr Scand 1984; 73:505–514.
191. Allen DM, Diamond LK, Howell DA: Anaphylactoid purpura in children (Schonlein-Henoch syndrome). Review with a follow-up of the renal complications. Am J Dis Child 1960; 99:833–854.
192. Modigliani R, Mary JY, Simon JF, et al, the Groupe d'Etude Therapeutique des Affections Inflammatoires Digestives: Clinical, biological, and endoscopic picture of attacks of Crohn's disease. Evolution on prednisolone. Gastroenterology 1990; 98:811–818.
193. Holmquist L, Ahren C, Fallstrom SP: Clinical disease activity and inflammatory activity in the rectum in relation to mucosal inflammation assessed by colonoscopy. A study of children and adolescents with chronic inflammatory bowel disease. Acta Paediatr Scand 1990; 79:527–534.
194. Holmquist L, Ahren C, Fallstrom SP: Relationship between results of laboratory tests and inflammatory activity assessed by colonoscopy in children and adolescents with ulcerative colitis and Crohn's colitis. J Pediatr Gastroenterol Nutr 1989; 9:187–193.
195. Hyams JS, Ferry GD, Mandel FS, et al: Development and validation of a pediatric Crohn's disease activity index. J Pediatr Gastroenterol Nutr 1991; 10:439–447.
196. Summers RW, Switz DM, Sessions JT Jr, et al: National Cooperative Crohn's Disease Study: Results of drug treatment. Gastroenterology 1979; 77:847–869.
196a. Malchow H, Ewe K, Brandes JW, et al: European Cooperative Crohn's Disease Study (ECCDS): Results of drug treatment. Gastroenterology 1984; 86:249–266.
197. Routes J, Claman HN: Corticosteroids in inflamatory bowel disease. J Clin Gastroenterol 1987; 9:529–535.
198. Shaffer JA, Williams SE, Turnberg LA, et al: Absorption of prednisolone in patients with Crohn's disease. Gut 1983; 24:182–186.
199. Tripathi RC, Kirschner BS, Kipp M, et al: Corticosteroid treatment for inflammatory bowel disease in pediatric patients increases intraocular pressure. Gastroenterology 1992; 102:1957–1961.
200. Smith RC, Rhodes J, Heatley RV, et al: Low dose steroids and clinical relapse in Crohn's disease: A controlled trial. Gut 1978; 19:606–610.
201. Carpani de Kaski M, Peters AM, Lavender JP, Hodgson HJF: Fluticasone propionate in Crohn's disease. Gut 1991; 32:657–661.
202. Prantera C, Pallone F, Bruneti G, et al: Oral 5-aminosalicylic acid (Asacol) in the maintenance treatment of Crohn's disease. Gastroenterology 1992; 103:363–368.
202a. Dreyling KW, Hoppe V, Peskar BA, et al: Leukotrienes in Crohn's disease: Effect of sulfasalazine and 5-aminosalicylic acid. Adv Prostaglandin Thrombaxane Leukotriene Res 1987; 17:339–343.
203. Peppercorn M: Advances in drug therapy for inflammatory bowel disease. Ann Intern Med 1990; 112:50–60.
204. Ursing B, Alm T, Barany F, et al: A comparative study of metronidazole and sulfasalazine for active Crohn's disease: The cooperative Crohn's disease study in Sweden. II. Result. Gastroenterology 1982; 83:550–562.
204a. Sutherland I, Singleton J, Sessions J, et al: Double-blind, placebo-controlled trial of metronidazole in Crohn's disease. Gut 1991; 32:1071–1075.
205. Brandt LJ, Bernstein LH, Boley SJ, Frank MS. Metronidazole therapy for perineal Crohn's disease: a follow-up study. Gastroenterology 1982; 83:383–387.
206. Myers S, Sachar DB: Medical therapy of Crohn's disease. *In* Kirsner JB, Shorter RG, eds. Inflammatory Bowel Disease. 3rd ed. Philadelphia, Lea & Febiger, 1988, pp 477–502.
207. Duffy LF, Daum F, Fisher SE, et al: Peripheral neuropathy in Crohn's disease patients treated with metronidazōle. Gastroenterology 1985; 88:681–684.
208. Verhave M, Winter HS, Grand RJ: Azathioprine in the treatment of children with inflammatory bowel disease. J Pediatr 1990; 117:809–814.
209. Markowitz J, Rosa J, Grancher K, et al: Long-term 6-mercaptopurine treatment in adolescents with Crohn's disease. Gastroenterology 1990; 99:1347–1351.
210. Present DH, Meltzer SJ, Krumholz MP, et al: 6-mercaptopurine in the management of inflammatory bowel disease: Short- and long-term toxicity. Ann Intern Med 1989; 111:641–649.
210a. O'Brien JJ, Bayless TM, Bayless JA: Use of azathioprine or 6-mercaptopurine in the treatment of Crohn's disease. Gastroenterology 1991; 101:39–46.
211. Haber CJ, Meltzer SJ, Present DH, Korelitz BI: Nature and course of pancreatitis caused by 6-mercaptopurine in the treatment of inflammatory bowel disease. Gastroenterology 1986; 91:982–986.
212. Brynskov J, Freund L, Rasmussen SN, et al: A placebo-controlled, double-blind, randomized trial of cyclosporine therapy in active chronic Crohn's disease. N Engl J Med 1989; 321:845–850.
213. Brynskov J, Freund L, Norby Rasmussen S, et al: Final report on a placebo-controlled, double blind, randomized, multicentre trial of cyclosporin treatment in active chronic Crohn's disease. Scand J Gastroenterol 1991; 26:689–695.
214. Kozarek RA, Patterson DJ, Gelfand MD, et al: Methotrexate induces clinical and histologic remission in patients with refractory inflammatory bowel disease. Ann Intern Med 1989; 110:353–356.
215. Holdstock GE, Fisher JA, Hamblin TJ, Loehry C: Plasmapheresis in Crohn's disease. Digestion 1979; 19:197–201.
216. Levine DS, Fischer SH, Christie DL, et al: Intravenous immunoglobulin therapy for active, extensive and medically refractory idiopathic ulcerative or Crohn's colitis. Am J Gastroenterol 1992; 87:91–99.
217. Sanderson IR, Udeen S, Davies PSW, et al: Remission induced by an elemental diet in small bowel Crohn's disease. Arch Dis Child 1987; 61:123–127.
218. Morin CL, Roulet M, Weber A, Lapointe N: Continuous elemental alimentation in the treatment of children and adolescents with Crohn's disease. JPEN 1982; 6:194–199.
219. O'Morain C, Segal AW, Levi AJ: Elemental diet as primary treatment of acute Crohn's disease: A controlled trial. Br Med J 1984; 288:1859–1862.
220. Lochs H, Steinhardt HJ, Klaus-Wentz B, et al: Comparison of enteral nutrition and drug treatment in active Crohn's disease. Results of the European cooperative Crohn's disease study IV. Gastroenterology 1991; 101:881–888.
221. Greenberg GR, Fleming CR, Jeejeebhoy KN, et al: Controlled trial of bowel rest and nutritional support in the management of Crohn's disease. Gut 1988; 29:1309–1315.
222. Giaffer MH, North G, Holdsworth CD: Controlled trial of polymeric versus elemental diet in treatment of active Crohn's disease. Lancet 1990; 1:816–819.
223. Teahon K, Bjarnason I, Pearson M, Levi AJ: Ten years' experience with an elemental diet in the management of Crohn's disease. Gut 1990; 31:1133–1137.
224. Roediger WE. The colonic epithelium in ulcerative colitis: An energy-deficient disease? Lancet 1980; 2:712–715.
225. Harig JM, Soergel KH, Komorowski RA, Wood CM: Treatment of diversion colitis with short-chain fatty acid irrigation. N Engl J Med 1989; 320:23–28.
226. Christie PM, Hill GL: Effect of intravenous nutrition on nutrition and function in acute attacks of inflammatory bowel disease. Gastroenterology 1990; 99:730–736.
227. Dickinson RJ, Ashton MG, Axon ATR, et al: Controlled trial of intravenous hyperalimentation and total bowel rest as an adjunct to the routine therapy of acute colitis. Gastroenterology 1980; 79:1199–1204.
228. Sitzmann JV, Converse RL Jr, Bayless TM: Favorable response to parenteral nutrition and medical therapy in Crohn's colitis. A report of 38 patients comparing severe Crohn's and ulcerative colitis. Gastroenterology 1990; 99:1647–1652.
229. McIntyre PB, Powell-Tuck J, Wood SR, et al: Controlled trial

of bowel rest in the treatment of severe acute colitis. Gut 1986; 27:481–485.
230. Kirschner BS, Klich JR, Kalman SS, et al: Reversal of growth retardation in Crohn's disease with therapy emphasizing oral nutritional restitution. Gastroenterology 1981; 80:10–15.
231. Morin CL, Roulet M, Roy CC, Weber A: Continuous elemental enteral alimentation in children with Crohn's disease and growth failure. Gastroenterology 1980; 79:1205–1210.
232. Belli DC, Seidman E, Bouthillier L, et al: Chronic intermittent elemental diet improves growth failure in children with Crohn's disease. Gastroenterology 1988; 94:603–610.
233. Levenstein S, Prantera C, Luzi C, D'Ubaldi A: Low residue or normal diet in Crohn's disease: A prospective controlled study in Italian patients. Gut 1985; 26:989–993.
234. Agrez MV, Valente RM, Pierce W, et al: Surgical history of Crohn's disease in a well-defined population. Mayo Clin Proc 1982; 57:747–752.
235. Davies G, Evans CM, Whand WS, Walker-Smith JA: Surgery for Crohn's disease in childhood: Influence of site of disease and operative procedure on outcome. Br J Surg 1990; 77:891–894.
236. Farmer RG, Michener WM: Prognosis of Crohn's disease with onset in childhood or adolescence. Dig Dis Sci 1979; 24:752–757.
237. Rutgeerts P, Gebhoes K, Vantrappen G, et al: Predictability of the postoperative course of Crohn's disease. Gastroenterology 1990; 99:956–963.
238. Hyams JS, Grand RJ, Colodny AH, et al: Course and prognosis after colectomy and ileostomy for inflammatory bowel disease in childhood and adolescence. J Pediatr Surg 1982; 17:400–405.
239. Griffiths AM, Wesson DE, Shandling B, et al: Factors influencing postoperative recurrence of Crohn's disease in childhood. Gut 1991; 32:491–495.
240. Fazio VW, Galandiuk S, Jagelman DG, Lavery IC: Strictureplasty in Crohn's disease. Ann Surg 1989; 210:621–625.
241. Dehn TCB, Kettlewell MGW, Mortensen NJM, et al: Ten-year experience of strictureplasty for obstructive Crohn's disease. Br J Surg 1989; 76:339–341.
242. Orkin BA, Telander RL: The effect of intra-abdominal resection or fecal diversion on perianal disease in pediatric Crohn's disease. J Pediatr Surg 1985; 20:343–347.
243. Fry RD, Shemesh EI, Kodner IJ, Timmcke A: Techniques and results in the management of anal and perianal Crohn's disease. Surg Gynecol Obstetr 1989; 168:42–48.
244. Sohn N, Korelitz BI, Weinstein MA: Anorectal Crohn's disease: Definitive surgery for fistulas and recurrent abscesses. Am J Surg 1980; 139:394–397.
245. Hyams JS, Moore RE, Leichtner AM, et al: Longitudinal assessment of type I procollagen in children with inflammatory bowel disease subjected to surgery. J Pediatr Gastroenterol Nutr 1989; 8:68–74.
246. McLain BI, Davidson PM, Stokes KB, Beasley SW: Growth after gut resection for Crohn's disease. Arch Dis Child 1990; 65:760–762.
247. Lask B, Jenkins J, Nabarro L, Booth I: Psychosocial sequelae of stoma surgery for inflammatory bowel disease in childhood. Gut 1987; 28:1257–1260.
248. Binder V, Hendriksen C, Kreiner S: Prognosis in Crohn's disease based on results from a regional patient group from the county of Copenhagen. Gut 1985; 26:146–150.
249. Markowitz J, Kahn E, Daum F: Prognostic significance of epitheliod granulomas found in rectosigmoid biopsies at the initial presentation of pediatric Crohn's disease. J Pediatr Gastroenterol Nutr 1989; 9:182–186.
250. Rosa J, Grancher K, Markowitz J, et al: Lack of effect of having a parent or sibling with inflammatory bowel disease on severity and course of the disease in a child. J Pediatr 1988; 113:710–711.
251. Blumberg RS: Relapse of chronic inflammatory bowel disease. A riddle wrapped in a mystery inside an enigma. Gastroenterology 1990; 98:792–796.
252. Kangro HS, Chong KSF, Hardiman A, et al: A prospective study of viral and mycoplasma infections in chronic inflammatory bowel disease. Gastroenterology 1990; 98:549–553.
253. Prior P, Gyde S, Cooke WT, et al: Mortality in Crohn's disease. Gastroenterology 1981; 80:307–312.

Chapter 60

Ulcerative Colitis

MAUREEN E. CAULFIELD and WILLIAM MICHENER

> The term colitis is sometimes used as though synonymous with dysentery. Our usual language has been indeed too indefinite made incorrect in speaking of all afflictions of the large intestine as dysentery; for the true dysenteric process, although in many features like simple ulcerative colitis . . . is a disease having certain definite characters. . . . For example, we have seen a case attended by discharge of mucus and blood where, after death, the whole internal surface of the colon presented a highly vascular, soft, red surface, covered with tenacious mucus and adherent lymph, and here and there showing a few points of ulcerations; the coats, also were much swollen by exudation into the mucous and submucous tissues. In other examples there has been extensive ulceration, commencing in the follicles, and spreading from them to destroy the tissue around, thus producing a ragged ulcerated surface.
>
> Wilks S, Moxon W, 1875[1]

It has been more than a century since Wilks and Moxon recognized ulcerative colitis as a distinct idiopathic inflammatory bowel disease confined to the mucosa of the colon and rectum. Great strides have been made in our understanding of the clinicopathologic features, natural history, and complications of this disease. Ulcerative colitis may affect a young population, with approximately 20% of those afflicted diagnosed before the age of 20 years. Increased efficiency and accuracy of diagnosis as well as refinement of medical and surgical therapeutic options have improved the outlook for children with ulcerative colitis.

EPIDEMIOLOGY

Epidemiologic studies of ulcerative colitis attempt to estimate incidence and prevalence of the disease as well as demographic characteristics. Most of the epidemiologic reports are limited because of the difficulties inherent in gathering complete, unbiased data about a chronic disease in large populations.

Disease incidence provides a direct estimate of the risk of developing ulcerative colitis in a defined population each year and is reported as the number of new cases per 100,000 of the population per year. There is marked geographic variation in incidence rates for this disease from country to country. Ulcerative colitis is most common in the developed countries of North America, Scandinavia, and Europe and is also seen with increased frequency in southern Europe and developing countries of other continents.[2] Reported incidence rates vary between 2 and 14 per 100,000 population, with the age-specific incidence for those 10 to 19 years of age being 2.3 cases per 100,000.[2, 3] Compared with Crohn's disease, the incidence rate of ulcerative colitis appears to be stable or declining in many parts of the world, such as the United Kingdom, Denmark, Finland, and Sweden.[4]

Disease prevalence, or the number of cases per 100,000 of population at any point in time, measures the burden of the illness in that population. Most studies are limited and report only symptomatic patients who contact the health care system over a defined period of time. The prevalence of ulcerative colitis ranges from 6 to 100 patients per 100,000 depending on the geographic area surveyed. Most reports estimate the prevalence of the disease in northern Europe and the United States to be 50 to 75 per 100,000.[2, 5]

Ulcerative colitis affects males and females equally. It is relatively uncommon below the age of 5 years, although onset in infancy has been reported.[6] In children and young adults, the disease most frequently has its onset between the ages of 15 and 25 years.[5, 7] Ulcerative colitis occurs more commonly in whites, especially those of Jewish origin. The incidence of ulcerative colitis among South African Jewish whites is twice that of non-Jewish whites and seven times that of nonwhites.[8]

Familial aggregation of ulcerative colitis is well known, with the occurrence ranging from 5 to 29%.[9–14] Overall, more first-degree relatives than second- or third-degree relatives with a positive family history of ulcerative colitis were found,[13] and in children with the disease, one third had a first-degree relative identified with inflammatory bowel disease.[11] The predominant family members afflicted are siblings. Twin studies have shown a much higher concordance for Crohn's disease (44%) than for ulcerative colitis (6.3%).[15] An ambitious study using complex segregation analysis in over 100 pedigrees with two or more members with ulcerative colitis suggests that familial ulcerative colitis may be caused by a rare additive major gene.[16]

Several environmental factors such as smoking, contraceptive pills, and dietary factors have been implicated as affecting the relative risk of developing ulcerative colitis. In an international case control study, however, 197 patients with onset of disease in childhood were compared with two age- and sex-matched controls for each patient. No significant differences were found between patients and controls in relation to environmental contacts during childhood.[17]

ETIOLOGY

The etiology of ulcerative colitis remains obscure despite the rapid accumulation of experimental data. Many theories have been proposed and investigated such as genetic factors, alterations of immunity, infection, allergy and diet, and psychological factors.

Genetic Influences

Epidemiologic studies showing increased prevalence of ulcerative colitis in first-degree family members support the theory that genetic factors contribute to the pathogenesis of the disease. Associations with the major histocompatibility antigen system are inconclusive because studies from different countries show clustering of haplotypes that are ethnically or geographically related rather than disease-specific. That is, ulcerative colitis was found to be associated with human leukocyte antigen (HLA)-B5 and HLA-DR-2 in Japan, with HLA-A2, BW35, and BW40 in Ashkenazi Jews in Israel, and with HLA-A11 in the Netherlands.[18, 19] By contrast, the association of HLA-B27 with ankylosing spondylitis and colitis appears to be more universal.

Immunity

Antineutrophil cytoplasmic antibodies in patients with ulcerative colitis have been identified that are distinct from those found in Wegener's granulomatosis and are present in the majority of patients with ulcerative colitis but not Crohn's disease.[20] A blinded study that compared the specificity of antineutrophil cytoplasmic antibodies for ulcerative colitis with other colitides found the presence of the antibodies to be 60% sensitive and 94% specific for ulcerative colitis.[21] These antibodies have also been linked to primary sclerosing cholangitis[22]; identification of the target antigens may facilitate understanding of the underlying immune response and development of a disease marker assay for ulcerative colitis. The specific role, if any, for antineutrophil antibodies in the pathogenesis of ulcerative colitis is unclear.

Infectious Agents

At present, no solid evidence has been found to support an infectious agent directly responsible for the intestinal inflammation of ulcerative colitis. A number of agents have been investigated including numerous bacteria and viral organisms.

Allergy and Diet

Allergy to dietary antigens was among the earliest theories put forth to explain the etiology of ulcerative colitis. Cow's milk protein has been most widely studied and was given early support from Truelove,[23] who showed symptomatic improvement when patients were placed on a milk-free diet and relapse with its reintroduction. In addition, high titers of antibodies to milk protein were found in the serum of ulcerative colitis patients; however, these antibodies were later found in patients with Crohn's disease and in normal controls.[24, 25]

Reports of early infant feeding and weaning practices have been conflicting. Studies of infant feeding showed 18 to 30% of ulcerative colitis patients and 7 to 12% of healthy controls were not breast-fed, suggesting a role for dietary influences.[26, 27] In addition, a retrospective review showed a significantly greater incidence of infantile cow's milk protein sensitivity in patients who later developed ulcerative colitis compared with healthy controls.[28] The results of a large, multicenter, international study, however, did not find any relationship between early feeding practices or the occurrence of cow's milk protein sensitivity and the development of ulcerative colitis.[17]

There is evidence that colonic mucosal cells require short-chain fatty acid nutrients derived from the fecal stream and that intestinal diversion or decreased utilization of these fatty acids by mucosal cells (demonstrated in patients with ulcerative colitis) results in inflammation.[29] Preliminary studies in patients with diversion colitis and ulcerative colitis showed that irrigation with short-chain fatty acids resulted in amelioration of symptoms and endoscopic inflammation.[30, 31]

Psychological Factors

The relationship of psychological factors to the etiology of ulcerative colitis has been questioned for many decades. One report reviewed all known English language literature on this subject and found the majority of the 138 studies were flawed in research design, such as lack of control subjects, unspecified manner of data collection, and absence of diagnostic criteria. Methodologic flaws were significantly related to the finding of a positive association between psychiatric factors and ulcerative colitis. Seven well-designed studies showed no such association.[32]

PATHOLOGY

Macroscopic Findings

The pathologic findings in ulcerative colitis vary depending on the severity and duration of the disease. The disease characteristically is confined to the colon and rectum, rarely extending into the terminal ileum. The affected area is continuous from the rectum proximally without intervening normal mucosa. Rectal sparing of the disease is unusual but does occur[33]; therapeutic suppositories and enemas may decrease rectal inflammation, giving the appearance of normal rectal mucosa.

The earliest phases of colonic injury are manifested by an increase in surface blood flow resulting in a macroscopic and endoscopic picture of diffuse erythema. With increased inflammation, the vascular architecture is disrupted, resulting in edema recognized as "granularity." The granular appearance results from multiple reflections of light from individual mounds of edema punctuated by the colon crypts. As the inflammation increases and the crypt abscesses expand, the mucosal margins are undermined, and superficial sloughing leads to numerous small surface ulcerations on a background of erythema causing spontaneous bleeding. The ulcers may be covered with inflammatory exudate. As the injury progresses, crypt abscesses rupture and become confluent at the level of the crypt bases, dissecting off the superficial mucosa from just above the muscularis mucosa. The resulting large, flat, deep mucosal ulcers are separated by the inflamed nonulcerated areas appearing as nodular, polypoid, or filamentous pseudopolyps. Mucosal bridges may form by fusion of one polyp to another or to adjacent mucosa. Because ulcerative colitis is primarily a mucosal disease, the serosa usually appears normal but may show varying degrees of hyperemia. Occasionally active inflammation may penetrate the colonic wall producing small pericolic abscesses.

With remission, the vascularity subsides and the ulcers heal, but the pseudopolyps remain as well as residual fibrosis and thickening of the wall. The chronically diseased colon may be foreshortened and show thickening of the wall and narrowing of the lumen.

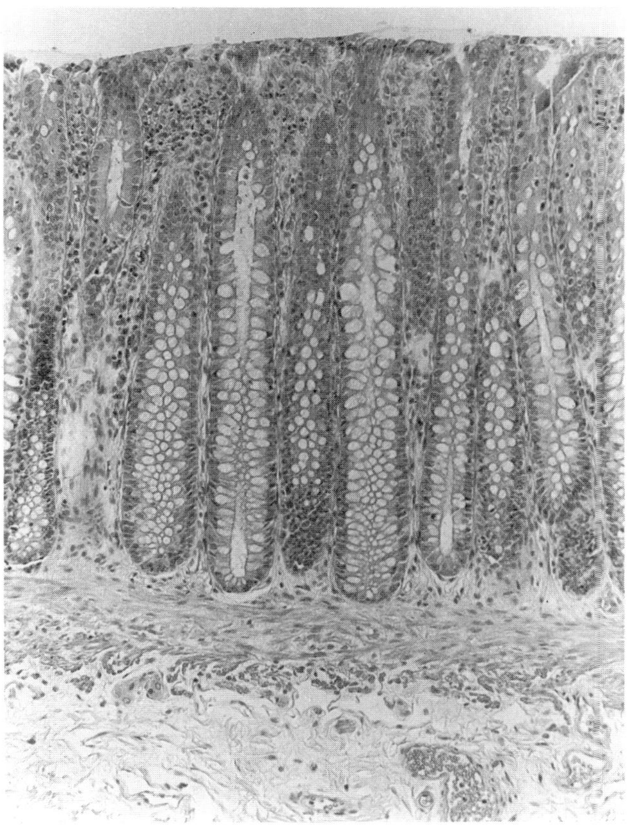

Figure 60–1. Colonic biopsy. Normal colonic mucosa with a smooth luminal surface and straight, parallel, tightly packed crypts. (Courtesy of Robert Petras, MD.)

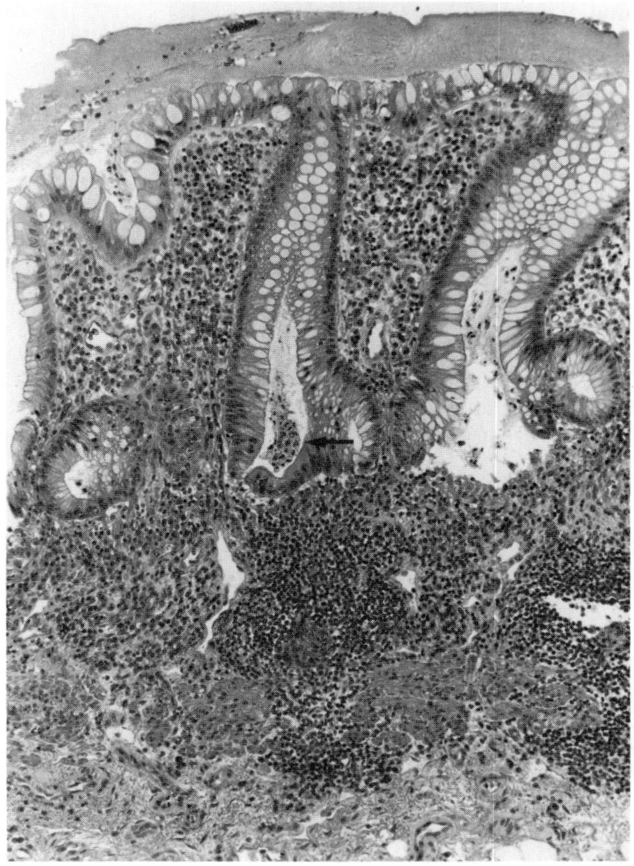

Figure 60–2. Colonic biopsy. Chronic ulcerative colitis in the active phase. There is a background of atrophy and crypt distortion with crypt abscess formation (*arrow*). (Courtesy of Robert Petras, MD.)

Microscopic Findings

Histologically acute ulcerative colitis is characterized by the presence of inflammation in the crypts, depletion of goblet cell mucin, and the presence of a chronic inflammation in the lamina propria (Figs. 60–1 and 60–2). The earliest histologic features are edema of the lamina propria and congestion of the mucosal vessels, occurring throughout the area of involvement. The earliest feature that is specifically suggestive of ulcerative colitis is the presence of scattered focal collections of polymorphonuclear cells in the lamina propria near the base of the crypt. Aggregations of lymphocytes, eosinophils, and mast cells are seen in the lamina propria in acute ulcerative colitis, which also helps to exclude other causes of acute colitis. Neutrophilic infiltration ranges from small aggregations within the crypt epithelium (cryptitis) to invasion of the crypt lumen (crypt abscesses). As the disease progresses, the abscesses spread into adjacent crypts and enlarge, and mucosal ulcerations appear. In addition, the epithelium of the crypt shows histologic depletion of mucus-secreting cells, which reflects the degree of acute inflammation; goblet-cell depletion of mucus is most pronounced in crypts with intense inflammation. The lesions of ulcerative colitis are generally confined to the mucosa, although some extention into the submucosa is seen in more severe cases. In acute fulminating ulcerative colitis, the inflammatory process may extend through all layers, including the serosa.[34]

Resolution of the inflammatory process can produce a variety of appearances (Fig. 60–3). Generally, as healing occurs, the mucin content in the superficial portions of the crypts begins to increase and return to normal levels. The bases of the regenerating crypts may fall short of the muscularis mucosa despite having regained a relatively normal appearance. Quiescent ulcerative colitis shows architectural distortion of the mucosa with Paneth's cell metaplasia, enteroendocrine cell hyperplasia, and a low-grade lymphoid infiltrate but without neutrophilic infiltration, cryptitis, crypt abscesses, or epithelial injury.[35]

CLINICAL FEATURES

Presentation

Most pediatric patients are diagnosed with ulcerative colitis during adolescence (Table 60–1). The commonest presenting symptom of ulcerative colitis in childhood is diarrhea. Of 125 pediatric patients evaluated at the time of diagnosis, 93% had diarrhea, 86% had rectal bleeding or abdominal pain, 67% experienced weakness, 51% experienced weight loss, 42% had nausea and vomiting, and 37% had fever.[36] At least one half of pediatric and adolescent patients have an insidious onset, with intermittent low-grade fever usually accompanied by mild diarrhea and rectal bleeding.[37] These patients most often have mild abdominal pain without weight loss or hypoalbuminemia. The onset is more dramatic in approximately one third of patients, who have bloody diarrhea, tenesmus, urgency, low-grade fever, weight loss, and mild anemia. A more fulminant presentation occurs in 10% of children, characterized by more than six bloody stools per day, fever, weight loss, and tachycardia. Laboratory studies may demonstrate hypoproteinemia, anemia, leukocytosis, thrombocytosis, and elevated acute-phase reactants. The most extreme presentation is toxic megacolon characterized by abdominal distention, fever, and tachycardia. Other signs include hypotension, dehydration, and mental status changes.

Table 60–1. AGE AT THE TIME OF DIAGNOSIS IN 455 PEDIATRIC PATIENTS WITH ULCERATIVE COLITIS

Age at Diagnosis (years)	Number (n = 455)	Percent
<5	4	0.6
6–10	56	12
11–15	153	34
16–20	242	53

From Michener WM, Caulfield ME, Wyllie RW, Farmer RG: Management of inflammatory bowel disease: 30 years of observation. Cleve Clin J Med 1990; 58:686; with permission.

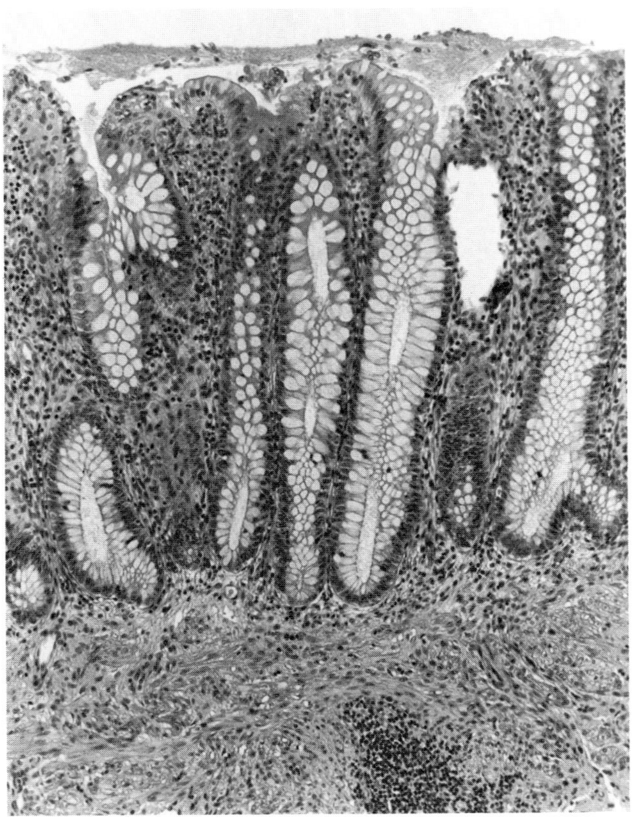

Figure 60–3. Colonic biopsy. Chronic ulcerative colitis in the quiescent phase. There is hypertrophy of the muscularis mucosa accompanied by mild crypt distortion with branching and budding of the colonic crypts. (Courtesy of Robert Petras, MD.)

Diagnosis

The diagnosis of most patients with inflammatory bowel disease is based on the information synthesized from the history, physical examination, laboratory values, endoscopic studies, barium radiographs, and histopathology.

Laboratory Values

Approximately 50% of children with ulcerative colitis have a hypochromic anemia at the time of diagnosis. More often acute-phase reactants such as an elevated erythrocyte sedimentation rate or thrombocytosis may be demonstrated. Hypoalbuminemia is more common in patients with advanced ulcerative colitis and usually correlates with the severity of mucosal disease. Stool examination typically reveals the presence of leukocytes and blood. Stools should be sent for microbiologic evaluation looking for the presence of ova, parasites, bacterial pathogens, and *Clostridium difficile* toxin.

Endoscopic Studies

Despite the many differences in clinical and radiologic findings among ulcerative colitis, Crohn's disease, and other specific colitides, differentiation may be difficult. Endoscopic evaluation of the colonic mucosa affords direct visualization of normal and diseased bowel as well as the means to perform directed tissue biopsies and can assist in making the correct diagnosis. The major indications for endoscopic evaluation of inflammatory bowel disease are listed in Table 60–2.

Endoscopically, the earliest manifestation of colonic injury by ulcerative colitis is an increase in mucosal blood flow resulting in diffuse erythema. Loss of the normal vascular pattern and disruption of the normal light reflections, resulting in the granular mucosal appearance, are due to thickening of the mucosa from edema (Fig. 60–4). The engorged mucosa may demonstrate contact bleeding or friability. Small surface ulcerations together with the engorged mucosa lead to spontaneous bleeding. Small ulcers may coalesce into large ulcerations; these ulcers are never surrounded by normal mucosa and always occur on a background of inflammation.

The typical ulcer in Crohn's disease originates in the submucosa, creating the endoscopic appearance of an aphthous ulcer in an area of normal mucosa. These ulcers tend to enlarge but encroach on normal-appearing mucosa. True cobblestoning, caused by submucosal inflammation, is pathognomonic of Crohn's disease and has a spectrum of endoscopic features ranging from a uniform nodularity to furrowed ulcerations demarcating areas of inflammation. Severe cobblestoning may be confused with pseudopolyp formation; pseudopolyps are generally tall and slender, and the adjacent mucosa is usually flat, unlike the wide nodules of cobblestoning, which are distinctly contiguous. Many mucosal abnormalities are common to both diseases, including pseudopolyp formation, mucosal bridging, loss of the shape of interhaustral septa, and the presence of fibrotic strictures and linear mucosal scars. In the late stages of both diseases, the endoscopic findings may resemble each other and differentiation may not be possible.

Table 60–2. INDICATIONS FOR ENDOSCOPY IN INFLAMMATORY BOWEL DISEASE

Differential diagnosis
Ulcerative colitis
Crohn's disease
Other specific colitis
Investigation of radiographic abnormalities
Mass lesion
Stricture
Dysplasia
Extent of disease
Perioperative evaluation

Although nonspecific, there are endoscopic features more common to infectious colitis than to inflammatory bowel disease. These include a yellowish exudate that partially covers the mucosal surface, the absence of ulcerations, the intense hyperemia of the mucosa (in contrast with the deeper red color seen with inflammatory bowel disease), and a patchiness within the same colonic segment with multiple areas of involvement adjacent to normal mucosa.

When colonoscopy or sigmoidoscopy is used to make a specific diagnosis, biopsies should be obtained and labeled as to location in the colon. Identifying patterns of inflammation may help to unravel diagnostic problems if specific histopathology is equivocal.

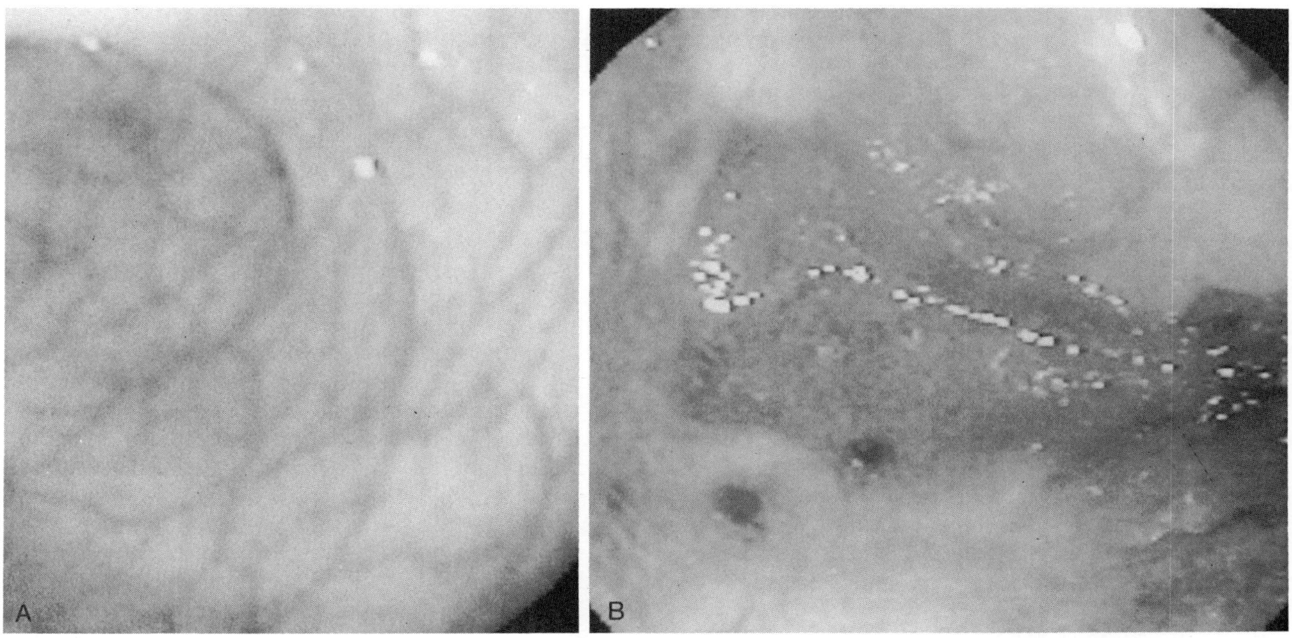

Figure 60–4. Endoscopic views of the colon. *A*, Normal vascular pattern, mucosa smooth and glistening. *B*, Moderately severe ulcerative colitis with loss of vascular pattern, granularity, and exudate. (Courtesy of Jeffrey Hyams, MD.)

Radiographs

Plain films of the abdomen in mild to moderate disease are usually normal. Patients with severe colitis may have thumbprinting resulting from mucosal edema, abnormal dilation of the colon (>8 cm), or both.

Barium enema may demonstrate a number of abnormalities. The double-contrast study is preferred, because single column studies are less sensitive, missing an abnormality 20 to 30% of the time. The earliest finding is the granular appearance resembling fine or coarse sandpaper. As the injury progresses, ulcerations give the bowel contour an irregular, serrated appearance. "Collar button" ulcerations are seen when the ulcers are deep and penetrate the submucosa. Polypoid lesions may be identified and usually represent pseudopolyp formation. As the disease becomes chronic, loss of haustration progresses from the left colon to the cecum, and in time, the colon becomes shortened and resembles a narrow "stove pipe" tube.

Ultrasound examinations correlate with the radiographic and endoscopic findings but are not helpful in making a differential diagnosis.[37a]

Differential Diagnosis

The predominant symptoms of ulcerative colitis in children are diarrhea, rectal bleeding, and abdominal pain. Infectious colitis caused by *Salmonella, Shigella, Campylobacter, Yersinia,* enterohemorrhagic *Escherichia coli, Aeromonas,* or ameoba may present with similar symptoms and can usually be identified by stool culture. The bloody diarrhea of hemolytic uremic syndrome may resemble ulcerative colitis. *C. difficile* colitis may also mimic ulcerative colitis; identification of the toxin in the stool and the presence of pseudomembranes on endoscopic examination are helpful in confirming the diagnosis. If colitic symptoms persist or relapse despite treatment for an identified infectious colitis, the diagnosis of ulcerative colitis should be considered.

Irritable bowel syndrome may present with diarrhea and abdominal pain but not rectal bleeding. Normal physical examination, laboratory studies, and proctosigmoidoscopy exclude ulcerative colitis. Allergic colitis is generally a disease of infancy, which resolves when the patient is placed on an elemental diet. In older children, eosinophilic colitis should be regarded as suspicious for ulcerative colitis. In children who may have been victims of sexual abuse or in adolescents engaging in homosexual activity, other atypical infectious agents should be considered, including herpes simplex virus and lymphogranuloma venereum.

Differentiation of Crohn's colitis from ulcerative colitis may not always be possible. Granulomas are found in only 10% of patients with Crohn's colitis, and endoscopic appearance may be equivocal.[38] If disease is identified in other parts of the bowel or if it is noncontinuous in the colon, Crohn's disease is likely.

EXTRAINTESTINAL MANIFESTATIONS

More than 100 systemic complications involving almost every organ system of the body have been described in inflammatory bowel disease. Extraintestinal manifestations may precede, accompany, or follow inflammatory bowel disease. The pathogenesis of these symptoms remains speculative.

Musculoskeletal Symptoms

Arthralgias and monoarticular large joint arthritis are the most common extraintestinal manifestations of ulcerative colitis.[39] In approximately 10% of children with ulcerative colitis, a "colitic" type of arthritis is described as a migratory, asymmetric arthritis affecting the large joints of the lower extremities.[40, 41] Flares of this type are generally associated with active inflammatory bowel disease, but deformity of the joint rarely occurs. Ankylosing spondylitis occurs in approximately 6% of those with ulcerative colitis.[42] Those with spondylitis have progression of the spinal disease independent of flares of ulcerative colitis.[40, 41]

Dermatologic Symptoms

Erythema nodosum is described as red, raised, firm, tender nodules ranging in size from 1 to several centimeters, which are usually located on the extensor surfaces of the lower and upper extremities. It is seen with greater frequency (<5%) than pyoderma gangrenosum (<1%) in patients with ulcerative colitis.[39] Pyoderma gangrenosum is an ulcerative cutaneous lesion that classically has been associated with ulcerative colitis but is also seen in Crohn's disease.[43, 43a] As with erythema nodosum, its presence usually coincides with active bowel disease. Most patients with pyoderma gangrenosum have pancolitis.[43] These lesions generally resolve with treatment of the underlying bowel disease.

Hepatobiliary Symptoms

The reported incidence of hepatobiliary problems in patients with ulcerative colitis varies widely but is thought to occur in 5 to 10% of these patients.[44] The nature of the relationship between inflammatory bowel disease and hepatobiliary disease remains unclear. There does not appear to be any correlation between the incidence and type of liver disease and the severity, duration, and extent of the underlying bowel disease.[44]

Many hepatobiliary lesions have been reported in these patients, including fatty liver, pericholangitis, sclerosing cholangitis, cirrhosis, and chronic hepatitis. Fatty infiltration is a macrovesicular, nonspecific, reversible lesion that does not progress to permanent liver damage.

Patients may present with hepatomegaly but are otherwise asymptomatic. Pericholangitis is the most common abnormality seen in biopsy specimens from patients with inflammatory bowel disease.[44] With the use of endoscopic retrograde cholangiopancreatography (ERCP), many adult patients with pericholangitis have been shown to have sclerosing cholangitis, leading to speculation that it may represent the small duct lesion of sclerosing cholangitis.[45] The incidence of cirrhosis associated with ulcerative colitis varies with the selection of patients for study but is thought to be 1 to 5%. These patients often have significant colitis[46]; if colectomy is necessary, an ileoanal anastomosis is preferred because of the risk of developing peristomal varices.[47] Chronic hepatitis has also been described, but many characteristics of the disease remain undefined. Treatment with corticosteroids has been reported in small groups of patients, but results have been inconsistent.[48, 49] One small study showed improvement in the biochemical parameters of the hepatitis after colectomy.[50]

Primary sclerosing cholangitis is a chronic cholestatic syndrome characterized by fibrosing inflammation of the biliary radicals, resulting in bile duct obliteration, biliary cirrhosis, and hepatic failure (see Chapter 71). It occurs in approximately 4% of patients with inflammatory bowel disease, with the majority of cases associated with ulcerative colitis.[51, 52] There is no relationship between this disease and the onset, duration, activity, or extent of the underlying bowel disease. Presenting symptoms include fatigue, weight loss, jaundice, and pruritus; a cholestatic biochemical profile is seen with an elevated alkaline phosphatase level. The diagnosis of primary sclerosing cholangitis may predate that of inflammatory bowel disease in children.[53] ERCP is the diagnostic method of choice. There is no proved palliative or curative treatment except for liver transplantation for those patients in the terminal stage. In those patients who have had liver transplantation without colectomy, intestinal symptoms due to ulcerative colitis appear to improve, presumably because of immunosuppressive therapy with cyclosporine and prednisone.[53a] Colectomy does not appear to influence the course of the disease.[44]

Hematologic Symptoms

Iron-deficiency anemia is the most common hematologic manifestation of ulcerative colitis and results from excessive blood loss from the gastrointestinal tract. Patients taking sulfasalazine may have macrocytic anemia related to malabsorption of folate or less frequently, a hemolytic, Coombs-positive anemia.[46]

Vascular Symptoms

The incidence of thromboembolic complications in inflammatory bowel disease has been reported to be 1.3%; deep venous thrombosis, pulmonary embolism, arterial thrombosis, and cerebral vasculitis have been described.[54] The Mayo Clinic saw 92 patients in 11 years with vascular complications, mainly thromboembolism of the deep peripheral and pulmonary veins. Twenty-five percent of the patients died from the acute thrombotic episode, and 14% had recurrent episodes concurrent with active bowel disease.[54] The cause of these thrombotic events is unknown, although a variety of clotting abnormalities have been identified.

Ocular Symptoms

There is a wide range of ocular manifestations reported with ulcerative colitis, but these problems are rarely encountered in children. Asymptomatic uveitis has been described in children with Crohn's disease and ulcerative colitis.[55] Other problems include episcleritis, cataracts, keratopathy, marginal corneal ulcerations, and central serous retinopathy.[46] Posterior subcapsular cataracts may develop after long-term, high-dose corticosteroid therapy.

Renal Symptoms

Renal calculi occur in approximately 5% of patients with ulcerative colitis and are composed of calcium oxalate or uric acid.[56] Lithogenic factors include chronic dehydration, oliguria, decreased water absorption, and infection.

Growth Failure

Growth retardation is less commonly found in children and adolescents with ulcerative colitis than with Crohn's disease. Severe growth failure (height below the third percentile) has been reported to occur before the initiation of corticosteroid therapy in approximately 2% of pediatric patients with the disease.[57] Motil and coworkers[58] described consecutive pediatric patients with ulcerative colitis who were prospectively evaluated for growth failure by Waterlow's criteria, and height-for-age deficiencies were found in 19% of ulcerative colitis patients compared with 56% of Crohn's disease patients.[58]

COMPLICATIONS

Bleeding

Rectal bleeding is a common sign of ulcerative colitis. Massive hemorrhage, however, is rare, with an incidence of approximately 3%.[59] These patients typically have severe disease with sudden bleeding that requires urgent blood transfusion or continued heavy bleeding that necessitates multiple transfusions. In contrast to Crohn's disease, most often a single bleeding site cannot be identified, and only large areas of eroded, ulcerated mucosa are seen. Most cases are treated by conservative measures. The decision to operate in this clinical situation, however, may be influenced by other coexisting factors.

Perforation

Free perforation of the colon is potentially the most serious complication of ulcerative colitis because it often results in generalized peritonitis, which was fatal in 75% of the patients reviewed in 1964.[59] It often occurs in the clinical setting of toxic megacolon or severe fulminant colitis, but it can also occur in moderately severe disease. First episodes of colitis are more likely to lead to free perforation as evidenced by the series of Edwards and Truelove[59] (13 of 20 patients who perforated developed the complication with their first episode of colitis). Most perforations occur in the left colon, and multiple sites can be involved.

The presenting features of perforation include generalized abdominal pain, rebound tenderness, distention, rigidity, and absent bowel sounds. High-dose corticosteroid therapy may mask signs of perforation, and in patients receiving such therapy who clinically deteriorate, a plain film of the abdomen to detect the presence of free air should be performed. Emergent colectomy is then indicated.

Stricture

The development of a colonic stricture may complicate chronic ulcerative colitis at any time. In the series of Edwards and Truelove[59] one third occurred within the first 5 years of the onset of the disease, with most between 5 and 25 years. It is unclear how often this complication occurs; Goulston and McGovern[60] found strictures in 12% of their surgical specimens obtained from patients with extensive, chronic, continuous disease. The histology did not show extensive fibrosis but hypertrophy and thickening of the muscularis mucosae. The strictures were commonest in the rectum and sigmoid but were found in all segments of the colon. Generally, they were 2 to 3 cm in length, but longer strictures were seen (up to 15 to 30 cm).

Management of the patient with a colonic stricture usually results in a surgical procedure. The finding of a stricture automatically raises the possibility of carcinoma, and these lesions should be examined colonoscopically with biopsies to try to exclude malignancy. These tools may not be definitive in differentiating benign from malignant strictures, especially in those patients who have had ulcerative colitis for 7 to 10 years, and surgical excision may be indicated. Patients who have symptoms of partial or complete obstruction are also surgical candidates. A limited trial of medical therapy may be attempted in those with ulcerative colitis for less than 5 years who are asymptomatic, with careful follow-up provided.[61]

Toxic Megacolon

Toxic megacolon refers to the acute life-threatening dilatation of the colon that occurs as a relatively uncommon but potentially devastating complication of acute colitis. The exact incidence of this complication in patients with ulcerative colitis is difficult to assess accurately but is believed to be in the range of 3 to 5%.[62] Although it was thought that toxic megacolon was a complication of only ulcerative colitis, it is now clear that this condition appears in a variety of other illnesses that predispose to colitis such as infection and Crohn's disease.[63, 64] In a series of 615 patients with Crohn's disease, the overall incidence of toxic megacolon was 3.7%. If the cases of Crohn's disease limited to the colon were selected, the incidence of toxic megacolon was 11%.[65]

Factors predisposing to the development of toxic megacolon include duration of disease less than 5 years (25–40% of patients who develop toxic megacolon do so with the first attack of colitis), the presence of pancolitis, the severity of the disease process, concurrent use of opiates or anticholinergic medication, and recent barium enema or colonoscopy.[66–68] The latter two factors appear to have a direct effect on the neuroganglion cell function.

The pathophysiology of toxic megacolon is not completely understood. The universal pathologic finding is severe transmural inflammation with muscle destruction and serosal inflammation. It has been postulated that crypt abscesses erupt with subsequent development of submucosal, intramuscular, and serosal fistulas. The muscle layers become inflamed, and the cellular infiltrate penetrates into the deeper layers of the colonic wall, thereby disrupting smooth muscle function. Aperistalsis ensues with dilatation of the colon. The barrier function of the colon then breaks down, with development of local peritonitis, leakage of toxins, release of bacterial antigens, and finally systemic toxemia.[34]

The criteria most often used to diagnose toxic megacolon are those developed by Jalan and colleagues[69] in a review of 399 consecutive patients with ulcerative colitis yielding 55 cases of toxic megacolon. Two clinical diagnostic criteria were formulated. First, evidence of colonic dilatation must be shown either clinically (abdominal distention or peritoneal signs) or radiographically (segmental or total colonic distention). Second, evidence of toxicity, including fever, tachycardia, leukocytosis, and anemia, should be present. Other signs include dehydration, mental status changes, electrolyte imbalance, hypoalbuminemia, and hypotension. It should be emphasized, however, that toxic megacolon is a bedside diagnosis, in which one finds a "toxic" patient who may be confused, dehydrated, and hypotensive with a distended, tender abdomen. It is also important to appreciate that "toxic megacolon" usually develops over a period of hours or days. Frequent examination of the patient looking for evidence of changing or decreasing bowel sounds or gradual distention of the abdomen will alert the physician to the impending development of toxic megacolon.

Of note is that the clinical case definition does not include the frequency or character of stools. Although toxic megacolon usually develops during severe attacks of colitis, many patients will actually have a *decrease* in stool frequency, volume, or blood content as toxic megacolon develops. The inexperienced observer may erroneously interpret this change in stool pattern as a sign of clinical improvement. The distending abdomen may be only mildly tender or even nontender, especially if perforation has not yet occurred; this may lead the examiner to underestimate the severity of the patient's illness.

The management of toxic megacolon includes initial medical therapy and consideration of the various surgical options. As with most medical management, it is always prudent to begin with prevention. Toxic megacolon should be anticipated in every case of inflammatory bowel disease, especially in those patients with severe pancolitis, first episode of colitis, or a history of toxic megacolon. If a particularly severe episode of colitis does not respond to the usual measures in 2 to 3 days, the patient should be admitted to the hospital. Once admitted, close attention should be directed toward the development of abdominal distention, evidence of toxicity, and the amount of gas on abdominal films. Radiographically, the dilatation is often segmental, with the transverse colon and splenic flexure being the most common sites. Loss of colonic haustrations is also a feature. Linear serrations representing colonic wall ulcerations may be seen. In Fazio's series,[70] a mean diameter of the colon at the point of maximal dilatation was 9.2 cm, with a range of 5 to 16 cm.

Because the main prognostic factor is the presence of perforation, the goal of medical management is to avoid this complication. With this in mind, the patient may be admitted to the intensive care unit for close monitoring of vital signs, serial examinations, and surgical consultation. The patient should not take anything by mouth, and a nasogastric tube should be placed to low intermittent suction. Some investigators have recommended the use of an intestinal tube or a rectal tube. These methods are cumbersome and carry the risk of perforation, and thus these tubes are not routinely used. Frequent turning of the patient, particularly into the prone position, has been recommended by some to facilitate passage of colonic gas.[71] The patient should be aggressively rehydrated with correction of electrolyte abnormalities and transfused as needed. All anticholinergic medication and narcotics should be discontinued. The stool should be sent for culture, ova and parasite examination, and *C. difficile* toxin. A complete blood count and abdominal films should be followed twice daily; physical examinations are performed four to six times daily at a minimum. Because of the potential for perforation and peritonitis, broad-spectrum antibiotics with adequate gram-negative and anaerobic coverage are considered standard therapy. Total parenteral nutrition may be employed, but no controlled trials have been done showing an improvement in outcome. The usefulness of corticosteroids remains in question because no controlled trials have been performed in patients with toxic megacolon. Signs of toxicity may be masked by the use of these medications. Studies reviewing the incidence of perforation and mortality in patients with toxic megacolon in the pre-corticosteroid era and those treated with corticosteroids do not show any disadvantage.[66, 69] Despite the lack of data, intravenous corticosteroids are usually given routinely at a dose of 1 to 2 mg per kg per day.

Because prolonged medical therapy only increases the risk of colonic perforation with its consequent high mortality,[68] the standard of care has shifted toward earlier surgical intervention. The majority of the literature to date recommends immediate maximal medical therapy with delay of surgery no longer than 24 to 72 hours if there has not been significant improvement.[66–68, 70]

Carcinoma

For patients with ulcerative colitis, the risk of developing a colonic malignancy is significant. Most long-term studies of patients with longstanding ulcerative colitis, when subjected to statistical analysis, yield similar estimates of cancer risk; after one decade of ulcerative colitis, the yearly risk of cancer is 0.5 to 1%.[72, 73] The lifetime risk of developing colon cancer in patients with ulcerative colitis is approximately 15% compared with 5% in the general population. These rates are much higher than in any age- and sex-matched control population and are much more striking in younger patients. The frequency of colon cancer in patients under 21 years of age diagnosed with ulcerative colitis varies from 9 to 20% at 20 years; the youngest patient with colon cancer was 16 years old, and the earliest cancer occurred 11 years after diagnosis.[11, 74]

Total duration of ulcerative colitis is recognized as an important risk factor in the development of carcinoma. There is no detectable increase in the incidence of cancer in the first 8 to 10 years of the disease. Anatomic extent of disease is also a risk factor, although patients with less than pancolitis (excluding limited proctosigmoiditis and proctocolitis) are also at significant risk. Patients with left-sided colitis develop colon cancer 10 years later than those with extensive disease.[75] In most studies, the severity of the onset, age of the onset, or the difficulty of the clinical course do not correlate with increased cancer risk.[73, 76–81] One population-based study of 3,117 patients with ulcerative colitis, however, showed that the age at diagnosis and extent of disease were strong independent risk factors for colorectal cancer.[82]

The colorectal carcinomas that arise in the background of ulcerative colitis are adenocarcinomas. They differ from those that arise in patients without ulcerative colitis in that they tend to be more infiltrative and less exophytic. The tumors are typically flat or slightly elevated lesions and do not arise from adenomatous polyps but arise directly from flat mucosa, and they are evenly distributed throughout the colon (unlike those found in the general population, who tend to have left colon lesions). Multifocal or synchronous lesions have been found in 10 to 20% of the patients with ulcerative colitis and carcinoma compared with 3% of those found in the general population.[83, 84] The long-term survival with colitis-associated cancer is similar to other colorectal cancers of the same stage.

Colitis-associated cancer is absolutely preventable if the patient has a colectomy within the first decade of the disease. Because this recommendation is difficult for most patients and physicians to accept, an attempt is made to identify high-risk patients and place them in a surveillance program that will reliably detect precancerous lesions. Currently the most accepted approach is colonoscopic surveillance with random biopsies looking for dysplasia.[85–88] The validity of the dysplasia/carcinoma sequence has been suggested but unproved. Riddell and colleagues[86] reported that high-grade dysplasia occurs after 13 to 16 years of the disease, early cancer after 19 years, and advanced cancer after 24 years, suggesting a temporal relationship between dysplasia and cancer. It is not clear if all patients who develop high-grade dysplasia go on to develop cancer, but a significant number of patients with high-grade dysplasia have a concurrent colonic malignancy. The advantage of screening for dysplasia is that it is distributed in a more widespread pattern than the malignancy itself. Problems using high-grade dysplasia as the marker of cancer development are that false-positive results are common, and a significant number of patients with high-grade dysplasia are not found to have cancer. Worse, there is an appreciable rate of false-negative results. In one autopsy series, more than 50% of the colon specimens containing malignancy had no evidence of high-grade dysplasia.[89] In addition, the significance of low-grade versus high-grade dysplasia is unclear, especially when found in the setting of flat mucosa. The finding of low-grade or high-grade dysplasia in association with a mass suggests coexisting carcinoma, and colectomy should be advised.[90]

Colonoscopic surveillance is begun yearly after 7 to 10 years for those patients with universal disease and after 15 to 20 years for those with left-sided disease. Two to four biopsy specimens are taken every 10 cm from the cecum to the rectum. Once dysplasia is found, the following guidelines outlined by Korelitz[91] and others[92] seem warranted (Fig. 60–5):

1. If high-grade or low-grade dysplasia is found in conjunction with a "mass lesion," colectomy is indicated.
2. If high-grade dysplasia is found in flat mucosa on more than one occasion and there are no extenuating circumstances, colectomy is indicated.
3. If low-grade dysplasia is found on three or more consecutive examinations, colectomy is indicated.
4. If dysplasia does not lead to immediate surgery, the frequency of subsequent colonoscopy should not extend beyond 3 months.
5. When the classification of dysplasia is not absolute and the degree and severity would influence the decision, a second experienced pathologist should be consulted.
6. If dysplasia is found at multiple sites, even when low grade, this should add support to recommend a colectomy.

MEDICAL THERAPY

The goals of medical therapy in ulcerative colitis are to induce remission of colonic inflammation, maintain the quiescent state by controlling exacerbations, and prevent complications of the disease. A variety of therapeutic modalities are available, although none are specific in action nor predictable in achieving the desired result.

Sulfasalazine

Sulfasalazine (S.A.S.P.) was originally developed by Svartz more than four decades ago for the treatment of rheumatoid arthritis. Subsequent uncontrolled studies suggested efficacy in patients with ulcerative colitis. It was not until 1962 that the first controlled trial showed its superiority over placebo in patients with mild, relapsing ulcerative colitis.

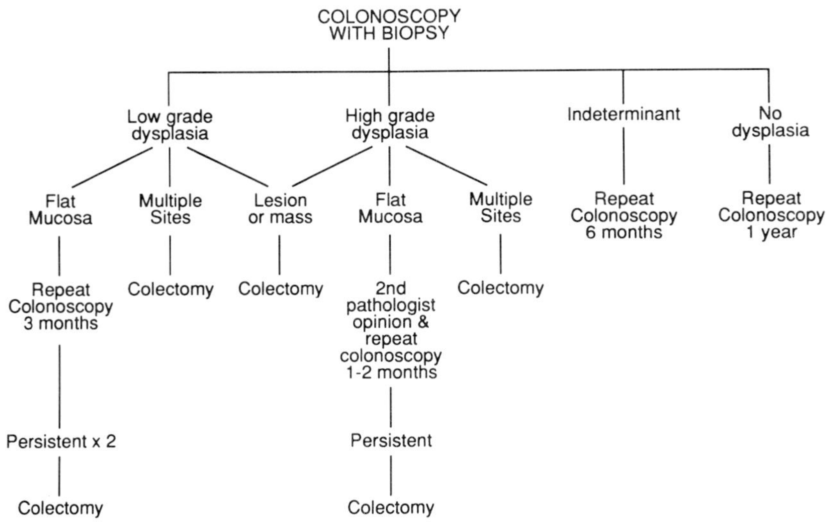

Figure 60–5. Algorithm for dysplasia screening.

Sulfasalazine is classified as a prodrug because the azo-bond between 5-aminosalicylic acid (5-ASA) and sulfapyridine (SP) must be cleaved to liberate the active moiety of 5-ASA.[93] Sulfasalazine is poorly absorbed from the stomach and small intestine, with only 10% of the oral dose reaching the systemic circulation. It is extensively protein-bound, with an average serum concentration of 18 µg per ml in those receiving 3 to 6 gm daily. Once absorbed systemically, a small percentage is excreted unchanged either in urine or bile.[94] Most of the drug is delivered to the distal small bowel and colon.

Sulfasalazine is metabolized mainly in the colon to SP and 5-ASA by anaerobic bacteria, which possess an intracellular azo-reductase enzyme. The amount of 5-ASA released depends on the rate of colonic transit of sulfasalazine and the integrity of the colonic flora. Most of the SP is absorbed and subsequently metabolized by the liver by means of acetylation, glucuronidation, and hydroxylation. The main route of elimination is via the acetylation pathway. There is a bimodal distribution of "slow" and "fast" acetylators, which is genetically controlled. "Slow" acetylators have higher circulating levels of SP, which may contribute to unwanted side effects.[95]

Compared with SP, 5-ASA is not absorbed as readily from the colon, resulting in low serum and urine levels. Virtually all of 5-ASA recovered from stool and urine is acetylated. The primary site of acetylation is not the liver but the colonic mucosa; once acetylated in the colon, the product does not appear to cross colonic epithelium.[96] Approximately one half of the absorbed 5-ASA is bound to plasma proteins, and no correlation exists between the acetylator phenotype of the individual and the rate of acetylation of 5-ASA.[97]

The precise mechanism of action of sulfasalazine and its metabolites remains unknown. Sulfasalazine and 5-ASA have been shown to have several actions on the metabolism of eicosanoids[98] and folate[99] as well as on leukocyte motility and bacterial flora.[100] These actions lead to inhibition of prostaglandin and leukotriene synthesis and decreased chemotactic activity of formylated bacterial peptides, thereby preventing recruitment of activated lymphocytes and neutrophils and amplification of the inflammatory response. More recently, 5-ASA and sulfasalazine have been found to scavenge and to inhibit generation of reactive oxygen species.[101, 102] In addition, sulfasalazine and 5-ASA both appear to suppress production of platelet activating factor in vitro by incubated ulcerative colitis mucosa.[103]

Early placebo-controlled studies of sulfasalazine showed efficacy in treating mild to moderate colitis using doses of 4 to 6 gm daily.[104] The drug has not been studied as a single agent for acute severe colitis. Once remission occurs, continued therapy beyond 1 year with sulfasalazine (2 gm per day) is superior to placebo in maintaining remission and preventing relapse.[105] Although higher doses of 4 gm per day are associated with a decreased rate of relapse in adults, most patients cannot tolerate the side effects and are maintained on 2 gm per day.[106] Duration of maintenance therapy is generally long term, most often 1 or more years. For patients with chronic colitis or frequently relapsing disease, the drug can be continued indefinitely.

Table 60–3. ADVERSE EFFECTS OF SULFASALAZINE

Hypersensitivity
Fever
Rash
Arthritis
Pericarditis
Pleuritis
Pancreatitis
Hepatitis
Autoimmune anemia
Bloody diarrhea
Acute colitis
Reversible
Oligospermia
Interference with Folate Absorption
Megaloblastic anemia
Dose-related
Dyspepsia
Headache
Anorexia
Myalgia
Arthralgia

No studies are available in children regarding the efficacy of sulfasalazine. Most authors recommend a daily dose of 40 to 60 mg per kg to a maximum of 2 to 4 gm per day.[107, 108] To minimize side effects, patients are usually started on 25 mg per kg daily and advanced to a maintenance dose over 7 to 10 days.

Unfortunately, approximately 15 to 30% of patients who are placed on sulfasalazine have at least one side effect (Table 60–3).[109, 110] Nausea, vomiting, anorexia, headache, and myalgias are the commonest dose-related side effects, which are usually controlled by gradual titration of the dose, administration with meals, the use of an enteric-coated preparation, or reduction of the dose.[97] More serious hypersensitivity reactions such as fever, rash, arthritis, hepatitis, pleuritis, and various autoimmune abnormalities are generally reversible with discontinuation of the drug. Absorption of folate is abnormal and may lead to hematologic abnormalities. Reversible oligospermia has been reported in adult men.[111] Animal studies in prepubertal rats suggest that fertility is normal once the animals are withdrawn from the drug and undergo sexual maturation. Persistent abnormalities, however, may be detected in the chromatid bodies.[112] Another complication of sulfasalazine is the development of bloody diarrhea, which was first described in children. The bloody stools abated with discontinuation of the drug and reemerged when the drug was readministered.[113]

Aminosalicylates

The hypothesis that toxicity of sulfasalazine could be attributed to SP and clinical efficacy to 5-ASA (mesalamine, mesalazine) has resulted in a concerted pharmacologic effort to develop new ASA agents for the treatment of ulcerative colitis and Crohn's disease. These efforts have resulted in new agents, both topical and systemic, that may expand the scope of medical therapy of inflammatory bowel disease.

Oral Formulations of 5-ASA

Because 5-ASA is fully absorbed in the stomach, it must be protected and delivered to the intestinal site of inflammation. Three mechanisms have been developed: (1) a carrier molecule linked to 5-ASA; (2) a pH-dependent, delayed-release acrylic coating of the drug; and (3) a time-dependent slow-release outer coating (Table 60–4). Coupling the 5-ASA molecule to a carrier is the mechanism underlying the efficacy of sulfasalazine. Owing to the high incidence of side effects from the SP carrier molecule, new carriers have been developed. Olsalazine (Dipentum), which couples two molecules of 5-ASA together via an azo-bond, has been shown to be better than placebo in controlling active disease and to have a relapse rate comparable with that of sulfasalazine.[114–116] At present, there does not appear to be any therapeutic advantage of olsalazine over sulfasalazine except for the sulfasalazine-intolerant patient. Mesalamine, when coated with an acrylic polymer that dissolves at a particular pH, can be delivered to the distal small bowel and colon, thus decreasing the incidence of unwanted side effects and possibly providing some therapeutic benefit to those with small bowel Crohn's disease. Controlled studies in patients with ulcerative colitis have shown relapse rates comparable with that of sulfasalazine for Asacol and Claversal.[117, 118] In addition, Asacol may have increased efficacy in the treatment of mild to moderate ulcerative colitis compared with sulfasalazine.[119] The pH-independent slow-release mesalamine (Pentasa) has 5-ASA in small ethylcellulose beads that gradually release the drug throughout the gastrointestinal tract. In a report of 400 adult patients with ulcerative colitis, a dose of 4 gm per day was superior to a 2-gm dose (both superior to placebo) with regard to producing remissions or significant improvement.[120] Data are also available that demonstrate the efficacy of oral 5-ASA (Dipentum, Asacol, Pentasa) in preventing relapse of ulcerative colitis.[97]

As anticipated, the oral 5-ASA preparations have fewer side effects than sulfasalazine. As many as 15% of patients intolerant of sulfasalazine, however, are also intolerant of the newer preparations. Reversible watery diarrhea occurs in 10 to 30% of patients treated with oral 5-ASA[121]; this may be secondary to a secretory effect on the small bowel.[122] Nephrotoxicity is a potential side effect of systemically absorbed 5-ASA; serum concentrations of the drug and its metabolites are lower than those necessary to induce interstitial nephritis in animals.[123]

Experience with olsalazine in children with ulcerative colitis is limited.[124–126] Fifty-nine children with mild to moderate ulcerative colitis were randomized to receive olsalazine (30 mg/kg/day) or sulfasalazine (60 mg/kg/day) for 6 months.[126] Children receiving olsalazine required the addition of corticosteroids more often than those receiving sulfasalazine ($P = 0.0014$). A higher percentage of sulfasalazine-treated patients were asymptomatic or improved at 2, 3, 6, and 12 months. Side effects attributed to the drugs were frequent in both groups.

Olsalazine has become available in the United States, but the appropriate pediatric dose is unclear. Sanberg-Gertzen and Jarnerot[124] report plasma levels similar to adult levels in children 6 to 16 years old and state that no special pediatric dosing is required. Ferry and associates[126] gave 30 mg per kg daily of olsalazine with a maximum of 2 gm daily. Olsalazine is available in 250-mg capsules, with a recommended adult daily dosage of 1 gm per day for maintenance of remission. Asacol is supplied as a 400-mg tablet, with a recommended daily adult dosage of 2.4 gm.

Topical Aminosalicylic Acid Derivatives

Topical mesalamine preparations have been studied for the treatment of distal colitis and proctosigmoiditis. Numerous trials have assessed the therapeutic efficacy of this drug given as either an enema or suppository. Mesalamine enema (4 gm) is superior to placebo and topical hydrocortisone (100 mg) for the treatment of active distal ulcerative colitis over a 2- to 6-week period as measured by clinical, endoscopic, and histologic criteria.[127–129] 5-ASA suppositories (500 mg) are well tolerated and superior to placebo for the treatment of active proctosigmoiditis.[130] Mesalamine enemas and suppositories may have some role in the maintenance of remission. Biddle and colleagues[131] assessed relapse in

Table 60–4. ORAL FORMULATIONS OF 5-AMINOSALICYLIC ACID

Generic Name	Trade Name	Configuration or Coating	Delivery Site
"Carrier" Drugs			
Sulfasalazine	Azulfidine	5-ASA–Sulfapyridine	Colon
Olsalazine	Dipentum	5-ASA–5-ASA	Colon
Balsalizide	Colazide	5-ASA–4-Aminobenzoyl alanine	Colon
Ipsalazide		5-ASA–4-Aminobenzoyl glycine	
Enteric Coated (Slow and Delayed Release)			
Mesalamine	Asacol	Eudragit S	Distal ileum
	Asacolon	(pH >7)	Colon
Mesalamine	Mesasal	Eudragit L	Ileum
	Claversal	(pH >6)	Colon
	Salofalk		
Mesalamine	Pentasa	Ethylcellulose-coated microgranules	Duodenum
		(pH independent)	Jejunum
			Ileum
			Colon

Table 60–5. TOPICAL FORMULATIONS OF 5-AMINOSALICYLIC ACID

Generic Name	Trade Name	Dosage*	Delivery Site
5-ASA enemas	Rowasa	4 gm at bedtime	Left colon
5-ASA suppository	Rowasa	500 mg twice daily	Rectum

*Recommended adult dose.

25 patients who had achieved remission with nightly enemas and randomized them to receive 5-ASA enemas (1 gm) or placebo; there was a significantly lower incidence of relapse in the 5-ASA group compared with those taking placebo. Similar results were obtained using mesalamine suppositories.[132] The reported use of topical 5-ASA in children is limited. In a group of nine children (8 to 21 years), mesalamine enemas (4 gm) were given to treat acute distal ulcerative colitis over a 6-week period. Seven patients improved clinically and endoscopically; no adverse effects were reported.[133]

Topical mesalamine appears to be well tolerated, although anal irritation and pancreatitis have been reported.[134] The drug is available in the United States as Rowasa (Reid-Rowell) and comes in a 60-ml, 4-gm enema or 500-mg suppository. Recommended adult dosage is 4 gm as a nightly enema for acute distal ulcerative colitis or 500 mg twice daily as a suppository for acute proctitis (Table 60–5).

Corticosteroids

Corticosteroids are useful agents for the treatment of active inflammatory bowel disease because of their multiple, although not clearly specified, effects on the inflammatory response. Systemic bioavailability is excellent, and the drug is bound by corticosteroid-binding globulin (transcortin) and albumin; increasing doses and hypoalbuminemia increase the unbound fraction, leading to increased toxicity.[97] The elimination of the drug occurs by various metabolic pathways and urinary excretion; barbiturates, phenytoin, and rifampin increase the clearance of these agents, whereas oral contraceptives raise transcortin levels and decrease clearance.[97]

Corticosteroids are thought to act by controlling the rate of synthesis of immunomodulating proteins. At the cellular level, glucocorticoids bind with specific receptors within the cytosol of nucleated cells. The steroid-receptor complex undergoes an allosteric change and is transported into the nucleus, where it directs the genetic message to transcribe RNA, resulting in the synthesis of inflammatory-modulating proteins. These proteins ameliorate intestinal inflammation and its clinical manifestations in a variety of ways.[135] In ulcerative colitis, prednisolone has been shown to inhibit colonic mucosal production of eicosanoids by inducing synthesis of inhibitors of phospholipase A_2 and cyclooxygenase.[136–139] In vitro, corticosteroids inhibit production of growth factors such as platelet activating factor (PAF) and lymphokines such as interleukin-1 (IL-1) and interleukin-2 (IL-2).[103] Under the influence of glucocorticoids, absorption of water and electrolytes is facilitated. Unfortunately, the entire cascade of the anti-inflammatory response to corticosteroids remains obscure.

A number of structural modifications have been made to the cortisone molecule with the goal of increasing potency and decreasing adverse effects.[140] The anti-inflammatory effects of corticosteroids depend on their binding to the glucocorticoid receptor. At least two sites are required for binding: a double bond in the 4–5 position and a ketone at the C3 position. Prednisone and prednisolone have a double bond at the 1–2 position, resulting in a less pronounced mineralocorticoid effect. More potent compounds (triamcinolone and beclomethasone) were developed by adding a halogen at the 9 position thereby blocking the binding of the corticosteroid to the transcortin receptor, which is responsible for detoxification. Because these compounds are not readily degradable, they remain in the systemic circulation longer, resulting in increased potency. Topical preparations were modified by altering side chains, resulting in enhanced tissue binding and greater affinity for the glucocorticoid receptor. Newer topical compounds such as budesonide have approximately 15 times the potency of prednisolone and approximately 100 times that of hydrocortisone when applied topically. Formulations with fewer side effects have been developed, which are either poorly absorbed from the gut or rapidly metabolized after absorption. If the halogen is removed from the 9 position, the binding site to the transcortin receptor is unblocked. The result is an agent that is not only very active topically because of the side chains, but also is rapidly detoxified if it gains access to the systemic circulation. This is the underlying mechanism for compounds such as fluticasone and tixocortol. These topical agents have undergone preliminary studies, and no adrenal suppression has been documented. Efficacy has been equal to or better than topical prednisolone preparations.[141–143]

Toxic effects of corticosteroids are observed, resulting from continued use of large doses. Acute adrenal insufficiency results from too rapid withdrawal after prolonged therapy. The characteristic withdrawal syndrome includes fever, myalgia, arthralgia, nausea, vomiting, and malaise. Recurrent diarrhea may result from relapse of colitis as the drug is withdrawn. Pseudotumor cerebri with papilledema is a rare reaction that may occur during reduction or withdrawal from steroids. Generally the use of corticosteroids for days or a few weeks does not lead to adrenal insufficiency on reduction of the dose.

The principal complications from prolonged therapy are hyperglycemia and glycosuria, increased vulnerability to infections, gastrointestinal abnormalities, osteoporosis, osteonecrosis, myopathy, posterior subcapsular cataracts, growth retardation, and Cushing's habitus.

Acne is a frequent side effect that often leads to noncompliance. Controversy exists regarding the incidence and cause of peptic ulcers in individuals treated with corticosteroids; Conn and Blitzer[144] concluded that the evidence does not support an association between peptic ulcers and corticosteroid treatment. Weakness of the proximal musculature of the arms and legs is a serious complication and an indication to discontinue the drug; recovery may be slow and incomplete. Development of posterior subcapsular cataracts as well as osteoporosis and aseptic necrosis of the femoral head has been reported in patients receiving prolonged corticosteroids and mandates discontinuation of the medication.[145] Growth retardation can be a serious problem in children but can be lessened by the use of alternate-day therapy.[146]

The efficacy of systemic corticosteroid therapy over placebo for mild to severe ulcerative colitis was proved more than 35 years ago by Truelove and Witts.[147] One prospective study demonstrated that adrenocorticotropic hormone (ACTH) was more effective than intravenous hydrocortisone in patients who had been exposed to prior corticosteroid therapy.[148] Prolongation of intravenous corticosteroid therapy beyond 2 weeks increases operative mortality without increasing the number of patients who improve on medical therapy alone.[149] Most systemic corticosteroid therapy is given in the form of oral prednisone or intravenous methylprednisolone. The optimum oral and intravenous doses of these drugs remain obscure; most authors recommend an oral or systemic dose of 1 to 2 mg per kg daily to a maximum of 40 to 60 mg.[37, 107, 108] After 2 to 3 weeks, when the patient's symptoms are improving, the daily dosage may be reduced slowly over a period of 4 to 6 weeks. No difference in efficacy was demonstrated between a single oral daily dose and divided doses.[150] Alternate-day corticosteroid therapy greatly reduces the frequency of side effects in children.[146] In contrast with SASP, systemic corticosteroids alone do not appear to maintain remission. Controlled trials have shown an equal relapse rate in corticosteroid-treated and placebo groups.[147, 151]

Topical hydrocortisone in left-sided ulcerative colitis is effective compared with placebo.[97] Preparations are available commercially in a liquid (100 mg) or foam (80 mg) enema form. The amount of systemic absorptions is determined by the degree of colonic inflammation and length of time the enema is retained. The degree of mucosal absorption is less than that of an equivalent oral dose, but 75% of a rectal dose may be absorbed, leading to adrenal suppression and other side effects.[152]

Immunosuppressive Medication

6-Mercaptopurine and Azathioprine

6-Mercaptopurine (6-MP) is a purine analog that interferes with nucleic acid synthesis. Azathioprine was developed to decrease the rate of inactivation of 6-MP by reacting with sulfhydryl compounds and thus serving as a prodrug, permitting the slow liberation of 6-MP in the tissues.[153] Although the exact mechanism is unknown, both of these drugs decrease lymphocyte toxicity and suppress amplification of cell-mediated immunity.[154]

These drugs appear to have their major benefit as a corticosteroid-sparing agent in the treatment of chronic, active ulcerative colitis. No response to azathioprine (2.5 mg/kg) was demonstrated in a placebo-controlled study of patients with acute ulcerative colitis.[155] Subsequent studies demonstrated a corticosteroid-sparing effect of azathioprine (1.5–2.5 mg per kg) in patients with chronic active disease compared with placebo.[156, 157] Korelitz and associates[158] reported their retrospective results of 13 children with incapacitating ulcerative colitis treated with 6-MP: 9 had "some response" to the adjunctive medication, and 5 children had reversal of growth failure.[158] Nine pediatric patients with corticosteroid-dependent chronic ulcerative colitis who received azathioprine (2 mg per kg) were studied prospectively.[159] Six of the children had a complete response to therapy over 3 months as measured by improvement in symptoms, weight gain, improvement in laboratory parameters, and reduction of the corticosteroid dose. These studies suggest that 6-MP and azathioprine may have a role in a subgroup of patients with intractable chronic disease.

The short-term side effects of azathioprine at doses of 2 mg per kg appear to be minimal. Mild symptoms include nausea, hair loss, and mild, transient peripheral neuropathy. In a review of 400 patients on azathioprine therapy for a mean of 5 years, the major complications of therapy were pancreatitis (3%), bone marrow depression (2%), allergic reactions (2%), and drug-induced hepatitis (0.5%).[160] Infections developed in 7% of the patients and neoplasms in 3% (only one malignancy was thought to be related to the drug). In a retrospective review of 28 patients treated for a mean of 12 months, however, a significant number of side effects were noted, including five patients with leukopenia and one patient with acute lymphoblastic leukemia.[161] The risk of teratogenesis is unknown, but this effect has not been reported. The frequency of side effects necessitates close supervision, with regular monitoring of the complete blood count weekly for the first month of therapy and monthly thereafter.

Cyclosporin A

Cyclosporin A is a suppressor of cell-mediated immunity. It acts primarily by blocking the production of lymphokines from helper T cells (gamma-interferon and IL-2), by inhibiting T cell–dependent B cell activation and expansion of helper and cytotoxic T cell subsets and by promoting antigen-specific suppressor T cells.[162] Limited data have been published on the use of cyclosporine in ulcerative colitis. The initial case report was that of an elderly patient with proctocolitis who received cyclosporine (12 mg/kg), resulting in clinical and histologic improvement during 6 weeks of therapy.[163]

Administration of cyclosporine in the acutely ill patient with fulminant colitis may hold some promise. A small group of five patients with severe acute colitis were given cyclosporine (10 mg per kg): None of the patients required a colectomy, although the follow-up period was only 1 to 4 months.[164] In a pilot study by Lichtiger and Present,[165] 20 patients with acute ulcerative colitis who were failing after 7 days of intensive steroid therapy were given intravenous cyclosporine (4 mg/kg) for 2 weeks. Those who avoided colectomy were placed on oral cyclosporin A (6–8 mg/kg/day) for 6 months. Of the 20 patients, four failed treatment and required colectomy, and one had an anaphylactic reaction to the drug. Fifteen patients avoided an initial colectomy, but only eight patients had completed 6 months of the study and were doing well off corticosteroids. Three patients relapsed, two underwent colectomy, and one was treated with 6-MP and has avoided colectomy.[165] Experience in pediatric patients is limited. Six pediatric patients with fulminant ulcerative colitis were placed on oral cyclosporine (to maintain a trough level of 200–250 ng/ml by whole blood radioimmunoassay).[166] All six patients responded with decreased cramping and disappearance of blood in the stool over a period of 4 to 14 days. Five of the six patients were discharged from the hospital; one patient elected to have a colectomy at day 20 of cyclosporine treatment. Overall, four of six children underwent colectomy within 8 months. Complications included mild hypertension, hirsutism, and mild increase in serum creatinine level. Oral cyclosporine appears to be of benefit as short-term therapy for children with severe ulcerative colitis to avoid precipitous colectomy but does not appear to result in long-term remission in the majority of patients.[166] There are no comparison data with other immunosuppressive drugs and none with the newer 5-ASA compounds.

Cyclosporine toxicity may be acute or chronic. Nephrotoxicity is dose-related and is reversible with a reduction of the medication. There is a risk of developing neoplasia, especially monoclonal lymphoma. Other side effects such as hirsutism, tremors, gingival hyperplasia, hypertension, paresthesias, and headache occur commonly. The role of cyclosporine in ulcerative colitis has not yet been determined, although it appears at least to have a short-term beneficial effect. Its chronic use in a surgically curable disease is currently being debated. Experience with topical administration is lacking but theoretically may be of benefit in patients with resistant proctitis. Toxicity is common, and the patients must be monitored frequently. At present, its use should be confined to protocol studies in tertiary referral centers.

Methotrexate

Methotrexate is a folic acid antagonist studied in patients with inflammatory bowel disease. Kozarek and coworkers[167] reported an open-label study of the effectiveness of 25 mg per week of intramuscular methotrexate in 21 patients with refractory Crohn's disease or ulcerative colitis. Five of seven patients with ulcerative colitis demonstrated clinical improvement. Diarrhea, nausea, hair loss, elevated transaminase levels, and transient leukopenia were seen in a few patients. Phase 2 studies are in progress; however, even if methotrexate is proved to be as efficacious as azathioprine, its use may be limited by long-term side effects such as pneumonitis and hepatic fibrosis.

Supportive Therapy

Antidiarrheal medications may improve symptoms without affecting the inflammatory response in patients with mild to moderate ulcerative colitis. Patients with ileostomies or ileoanal anastomoses may also obtain benefits from antidiarrheal medications, such as diphenoxylate with atropine, loperamide, paregoric, or dehydrated tincture of opium. Loperamide is considered the safest and best tolerated drug.[168] The main contraindication for its use is the presence of severe or unstable disease because these patients are at higher risk to develop toxic megacolon. Side effects include nausea, vomiting, drowsiness, dizziness, and mental status changes.

Nutrition

The results of parenteral nutrition as therapy for patients with acute ulcerative colitis are unpredictable, and long-term remission is uncommon. Werlin and Grand[169] reported 14 adolescents with severe colitis. Initial improvement occurred in 32% receiving total parenteral nutrition but only one patient maintained the remission at 2 years. Seashore and coworkers[170] studied eight children with ulcerative pancolitis who were also placed on parenteral nutrition. Half of the children improved (three of the four within 1 week), and the other four patients deteriorated and required surgery. Parenteral nutrition cannot be recommended as primary treatment of acute colitis. Rather, in selected cases it may have an auxilliary role in nutritionally depleted patients.

Antimicrobial Agents

The use of metronidazole in the treatment of uncomplicated ulcerative colitis has not been proved. Gilat and associates[171] have shown an effect in the maintenance of remission of ulcerative colitis. Negative results were obtained when it was studied as single-agent therapy for ulcerative proctitis and as adjunctive therapy (with corticosteroids) for severe ulcerative colitis.[172, 173]

Investigational Agents

Encouraging preliminary results have been reported with the following agents: eicosapentaenoic acid (EPA from fish oil),[174, 174a] superoxide dismutase,[175] chloroquine,[176] intravenous immunoglobulin,[177] clonidine,[178] and short-chain fatty acids.[31]

SURGICAL THERAPY

Surgical removal of the entire colon and rectum provides the only cure for ulcerative colitis. Advancements in surgical technique and stomal care in the 1950s firmly established panproctocolectomy and permanent ileostomy as the standard surgical treatment for patients with acute complicated or chronic disease. The biggest advantage of this procedure is that it can be performed as a one-stage operation. It can be life-saving and restore the child's good health, but there is a substantial psychological and social price to pay. Despite eventual adaptation to and acceptance of a permanent ileostomy, most patients would, if given the opportunity, seriously consider a change to a continent ileostomy.[179] Continence-preserving operations have evolved over the past 20 years and have expanded the options to those patients facing colectomy.

Indications for Surgery

Table 60–6 lists the indication for surgery in ulcerative colitis.

Urgent Indications

Most patients with ulcerative colitis have mild to moderate disease, which can usually be managed with medical therapy alone. Approximately 5 to 10% require acute surgical intervention secondary to progressive colitis unresponsive to medical therapy or because of a life-threatening complication of the disease (i.e., hemorrhage, perforation, or toxic megacolon).

The operation of choice must be individualized to the clinical situation. In general, colectomy, ileostomy, and mucus fistula of the retained rectum is one of the quickest and safest operations for acute fulminating colitis. The patient generally recovers quickly and over a few months returns to good health. A second operation that preserves continence can then be done safely. In some cases of toxic megacolon, in which the risk of perforation during colectomy is high, a diverting loop ileostomy and decompressive colostomy ("blow hole") may be performed.

Table 60–6. INDICATIONS FOR SURGERY

Acute
Failure of medical therapy for acute colitis
Hemorrhage
Perforation
Toxic megacolon
Elective
Chronic ill health
Chronic steroid dependence
High-grade dysplasia or malignancy

Elective Indications

Patients with chronic ill health, corticosteroid dependence, or dysplasia should be considered for elective colectomy. In the past, elective surgery was delayed as long as possible to spare the child or adolescent an ileostomy. Physicians, patients, and families are now more accepting of surgery as a therapeutic option because most children with chronic ulcerative colitis can now be offered a continence-preserving operation. These operations are being done earlier in the course of the disease, avoiding complications of the disease (i.e., fulminant colitis, chronic ill health, dysplasia) and its therapy.

Surgical Options

Figure 60–6 shows the surgical options for ulcerative colitis.

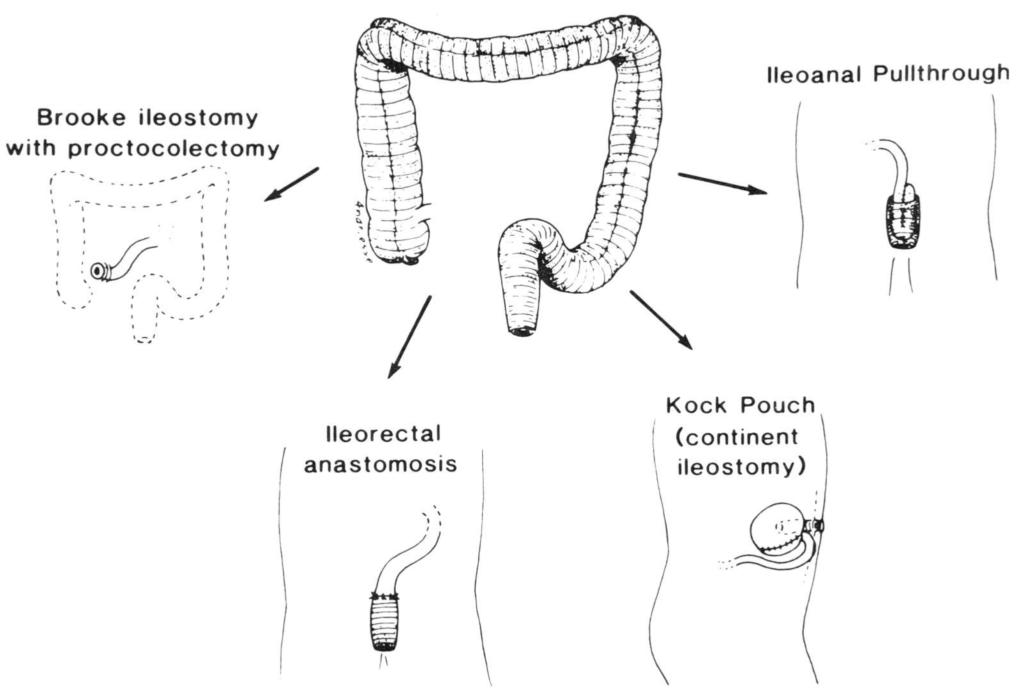

Figure 60–6. The surgical options for ulcerative colitis are diagrammed. (From Shamberger RC, Lillihei CW, Winter HS: Surgical management of ulcerative colitis in children and adolescents. Prog Inflammat Bowel Dis 1991; 12:5; with permission.)

Proctocolectomy and Ileostomy

Despite the proved efficacy of proctocolectomy with ileostomy for the treatment of ulcerative colitis, most children are offered alternative operations that preserve continence. The advantages of proctocolectomy with permanent ileostomy are the patient is cured of colitis without the risk of recurrence, the risk of subsequent colorectal malignancy is eliminated, and only a single operation is required. The child is left with a permanent ileostomy with the resulting psychosocial challenges, and the possibility of future ileorectal or ileoanal anastomosis is unlikely. Rarely, autonomic nerve injury from pelvic dissection may result in sexual or bladder dysfunction. Despite the advancements in the techniques and materials used for stomal care, most patients and their families favor a continence-preserving procedure.

Continent Ileostomy (Kock Pouch)

Since the advent of the ileal pouch anastomosis, the indications for this operation are dwindling. It may be an option for patients with a failed permanent ileostomy who wish to convert to a continent stoma, patients with a failed ileo-anal anastomosis who want to avoid a permanent ileostomy, or patients in whom anal sphincter function is poor. After removal of the entire colon and rectum, a pouch and stoma are created from the distal ileum. A nipple valve is constructed to store stool inside the pouch until it is convenient to drain the pouch with a small catheter. The stoma is often placed lower than a conventional stoma, and it is flush with the skin. Most patients cover the stoma with a small piece of gauze and do not require any kind of appliance. The major disadvantages of the continent ileostomy include malfunction of the nipple valve (which requires surgical revision in 9% of the patients), pouchitis, and the fact that an ostomy is still present. Limited data are available for the pediatric population; Orkin and colleagues[180] refer to nine children who had this operation before 1980, but the group's data were not reported separately. Enthusiasm for this procedure has been tempered by experience and the development of the ileal pouch–anal anastomosis and is not considered an initial option for pediatric patients faced with colectomy.

Ileorectal Anastomosis

Ileorectal anastomosis is a one-stage operation in which the entire colon is removed and the ileum is connected to the rectum. The rectum must be free of moderate or severe disease and dysplasia. Rectal compliance must be adequate because it functions as a reservoir for stool.

A small pediatric series was published of 36 patients with ulcerative colitis who underwent ileorectal anastomosis.[181] Six patients went on to have a proctectomy for intolerable number of bowel movements (3), progressive disease (1), rectovaginal fistula (1), or dysplasia (1). One patient died of rectal carcinoma 14 years after the operation.

Functionally, patients have an average of four to six bowel movements per day and are generally continent. Disadvantages of the operation include the continued risk of developing carcinoma and the possibility of continuing proctitis. The long-term results of ileorectal anastomosis for 60 children and adults with ulcerative colitis showed the cumulative probability of having a functional anastomosis at 10 years to be 51%.[182] Proctectomy was most often required because of dysplasia or cancer or recurrent inflammation in the retained rectum. When compared with the ileoanal anastomosis, proponents of the ileorectal anastomosis point to the relative technical ease of the operation, the absence of a second procedure, and the lower incidence of complications related to pelvic dissection.

Ileoanal Anastomosis

The concept that continence could be preserved in patients with ulcerative colitis led to the popularity of the continent ileostomy in the 1970s. The technical difficulty and the number of complications associated with this procedure led to the development of the ileoanal anastomosis (IAA). In 1977, Martin and colleagues[183] reported the results of colectomy and mucosal proctectomy (mucosectomy) in 17 children and adolescents with ulcerative colitis. Fifteen patients obtained acceptable continence, although many had difficulty with frequent stools and perianal skin irritation. The outcome of a subsequent series of young patients showed that all patients had occasional nocturnal encopresis that improved with balloon dilatation of the distal ileum.[184] Almost one third of these patients required conversion to lateral side-to-side pouch or a J pouch because of stool frequency associated with small capacity and low ileal compliance.[180] Another determinant of continence was the level at which the ileoanal anastomosis was made. Initially, rectal mucusectomy was done with anastomosis at the dentate line. This led to injury to the anal sphincter mechanisms in some patients, but the risk of recurrent disease was very low. Others placed the anastomosis 1 to 2 cm above the columns of Morgagni, thereby preserving some columnar epithelium; continence was well preserved, but the incidence of recurrent anorectal inflammation increased. If the anastomosis is placed at the top of the columns of Morgagni, transitional epithelium is retained, but there is little risk of damaging the sphincter mechanism; these patients have nocturnal continence and a low incidence of recurrent disease.[185]

The importance of ileal compliance as well as a functioning anal sphincter in maintaining continence led to the development of a pelvic reservoir in the form of an ileal pouch. The operation, ileal pouch–anal anastomosis (IPAA), involves removal of the entire colon and rectum, thereby curing the disease (Fig. 60–7). The reservoir is constructed from the distal ileum and anastomosed to the proximal portion of the anus. A variety of different shaped pouches can be designed depending on the anatomy of the patient and the preference of the surgeon, but the most common and easiest to construct is the J pouch. A temporary ileostomy is fashioned (either a loop ileostomy or an end ileostomy) and 2 to

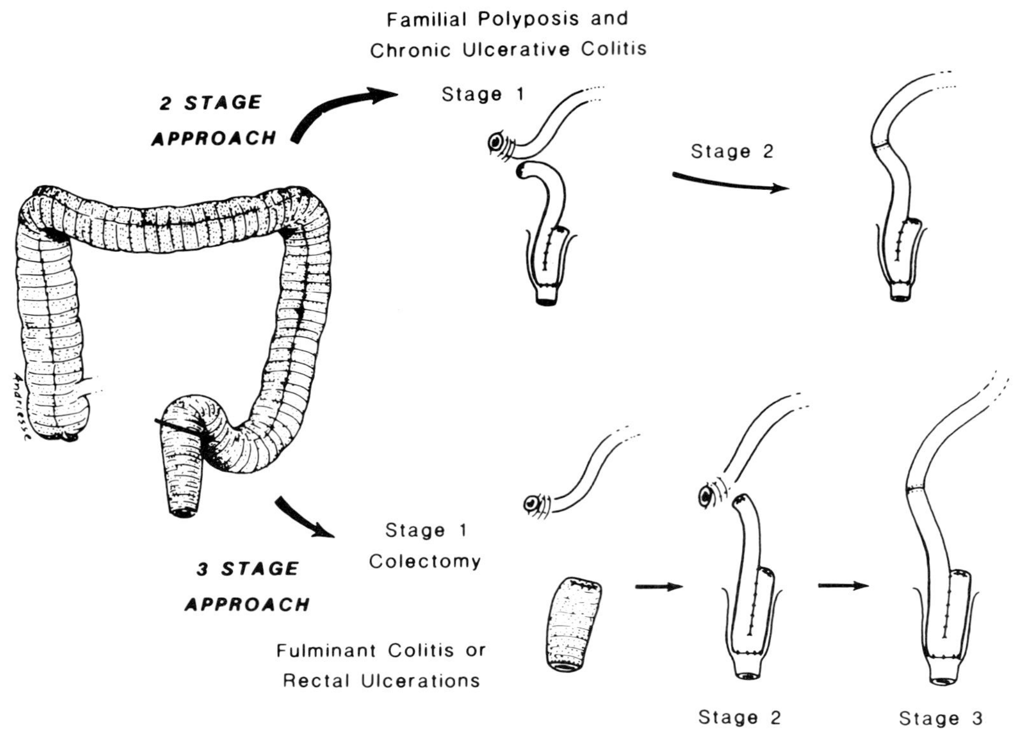

Figure 60–7. Depiction of the surgical sequences for the ileal-pouch anal anastomosis depending on the clinical situation. (From Shamberger RC, Lillihei CW, Winter HS: Surgical management of ulcerative colitis in children and adolescents. Prog Inflammat Bowel Dis 1991; 12:6; with permission.)

3 months later is taken down and the bowel is put back into circuit.

The pooled results of multiple retrospective reports of more than 1000 patients who have had this operation show an overall mortality of 0.3%, which is similar to that of conventional proctocolectomy.[186] Postoperative morbidity, however, is much higher, with more than one third of the patients experiencing at least one complication. A significant proportion of the morbidity occurs after ileostomy closure. The occurrence of pelvic sepsis, reported in approximately 10% of the patients, has been reduced in later series because of improvements in technique (i.e., using a shorter cuff of denuded rectum and better drainage of the presacral space).[187] Other important complications include obstruction (13%), stricture formation (12%), pouchitis (30%), unrecognized Crohn's disease, and unacceptable functional results.[186] In one pediatric series[186a] reviewing 82 patients (67 with ulcerative colitis) who had either a lateral ileal reservoir (76) or straight pull-through (6), complications were noted in 52% of patients. Most of these were early in this series. Only 3 of the last 40 patients required reoperation.

In the Mayo Clinic series of 982 patients,[188] 144 required reoperation because of pouch-related complications (i.e., patients operated on for small bowel obstruction were not included). More than 50% of the 144 patients required more than one operation, but overall salvage was 70%. Patients with pelvic sepsis accounted for the bulk of the pouch excisions. Interestingly, no patient in this series required reoperation for pouchitis.

Daytime continence in a mixed group of children (straight IAA and IPAA) approached 90%.[180] Mean stool frequency was five stools per day and 1.3 stools per night. Stool frequency gradually decreased over 1 year and generally remained constant thereafter. Theoretically, the larger pouches (i.e., the S and W) should decrease the frequency of stool when compared with the lower capacity J and lateral pouches. Volume of stool passed over 24 hours and motility of the ileal pouch, however, are more important determinants of stool frequency over the long term.[189]

Nonspecific inflammation of the ileal reservoirs or pouchitis may be seen in approximately one third of these patients postoperatively. The cause is unclear, although patients who had IPAA for ulcerative colitis have a much higher incidence of pouchitis compared with those who were operated for familial polyposis. One etiologic theory relates pouchitis to alterations in bacterial flora owing to stasis within the pouch. Microbiologic as well as motility studies have been done in these IPAA patients, but no distinguishing differences have been found between those with good results and those with recurrent pouchitis.[190] Another theory suggests that pouchitis may be a form of inflammatory bowel disease. Pouch biopsies usually show the presence of acute and chronic inflammation. O'Connell and associates[190] obtained biopsy specimens from 20 patients, six with pouchitis and 14 without. All biopsy specimens showed increased number of plasma cells and lymphocytes within the lamina propria, with no crypt abscesses seen. Neither the presence of colonic metaplasia nor the degree of inflammation correlated with the incidence of pouchitis. No factors were found to predict the future occurrence of pouchitis. No correlation was found between the severity of colitis at the time of colectomy and the development of pouchitis. The most common presenting features are diarrhea (73%), abdominal cramping (59%), bloody effluent (59%), and rectal or peristomal pain (52%).[191] Endoscopic features are nonspecific and include edema, erythema, and friability. Ulceration, exudate, and hemorrhage are found less frequently. Oral metronidazole therapy, alone or in combination with pouch drainage, is the most common therapeutic modality. Systemic corticosteroid therapy and hydrocortisone enema instillation into the reservoir are utilized less frequently. After an average of 22 days of therapy, approximately one half of patients are asymptomatic off all therapy.[191]

Carcinoma of the ileal pouch has been reported.[191a] This cancer was thought to arise from remnants of rectal mucosa left in the muscular rectal cuff. Despite the frequency of morbidity following the IPAA, it is now the surgical procedure routinely performed when patients with ulcerative colitis or familial polyposis are faced with a colectomy. The patient, parents, and physicians must be aware of the advantages and disadvantages before undertaking the operation. Young, otherwise healthy, informed and motivated patients generally achieve continence and improved quality of life following the IPAA.

PROGNOSIS

Based on the follow-up of 292 pediatric patients with ulcerative colitis,[11] 10% had a single episode of colitis and no further symptoms, whereas 20% of the children had intermittent problems. One half of the patients had chronic symptoms that were not incapacitating, whereas 20% of the children had chronic incapacitating symptoms. Approximately one third of the 121 patients with ulcerative colitis studied between 1975 and 1984 underwent colectomy[39]; those with pancolitis at the time of diagnosis were more likely to have surgery than those with limited disease. The natural history of proctosigmoiditis in children is somewhat different than that in adults and is characterized by the tendency toward proximal extension (usually within the first 5 years from diagnosis) in approximately one third of patients.[192] Death from ulcerative colitis in children is rare[39]; most deaths occur from unrelated or unknown causes, with a small number caused by postoperative complications or colonic carcinoma. Approximately 20% of pediatric patients with ulcerative colitis describe their quality of life as "good" (less than three bowel movements per day, regular school attendance, considers self healthy).[11] Only a small number (6%) are unable to attend school and have abdominal pain and diarrhea; most patients describe their quality of life as "fair." No differences in activity level were noted in the nonoperated versus the operated groups of patients with ulcerative colitis.[39]

Children and adolescents with ulcerative colitis must be followed longitudinally. Recognizing relapse, controlling the disease, and monitoring its complications require regular follow-up, support, and education from the physician. Transition from adolescence to young adulthood is a particularly critical time; the patient must be well educated about the disease and transfer ongoing care to an adult gastroenterologist.

REFERENCES

1. Wilks S, Moxon W: Lectures on Pathological Anatomy. 2nd ed. London, J & A Churchill, 1875.
2. Pena AS, Shivananda S, Mayberry JF: Epidemiology of ulcerative colitis. *In* O'Morain C, ed: Ulcerative Colitis. Ann Arbor; CRC Press, 1991, pp 1–8.
3. Caulkins BM, Lilienfeld AM, Garland CF, et al: Trends in incidence rates of ulcerative colitis and Crohn's disease. Dig Dis Sci 1984; 29:913–920.
4. Whelen G: Epidemiology of inflammatory bowel disease. Med Clin North Am 1990; 74:1–12.
5. Mendeloff AI: The epidemiology of inflammatory bowel disease. Clin Gastroenterol 1980; 9:257–270.
6. Chong SKF, Blackshaw AJ, Morson BC, et al: Prospective study of colitis in infancy and early childhood. J Pediatr Gastroenterol Nutr 1986; 5:352–358.
7. Grand RI, Homer DR: Approaches to inflammatory bowel disease in childhood and adolescence. Pediatr Clin North Am 1975; 22:835–850.
8. Wright JP, Frogatti J, O'Keffe EA, et al: The epidemiology of inflammatory bowel disease in Cape Town 1980–1984. S Afr Med J 1986; 70:10–15.
9. Lashner BA, Evans AA, Kirsner JB, et al: Prevalence and incidence of inflammatory bowel disease in family members. Gastroenterology 1988; 91:1396–1400.
10. Farmer RJ, Michener MM, Mortimer EA: Studies of family history among patients with inflammatory bowel disease. Clin Gastroenterol 1980; 9:271–277.
11. Michener WM, Farmer RG, Mortimer EA: Long-term prognosis of ulcerative colitis with onset in childhood or adolescence. J Clin Gastroenterol 1979; 1:301–305.
12. Monsen U, Brostrom O, Nordenvall B, et al: Prevalence of inflammatory bowel disease. Scand J Gastroenterol 1987; 22:214–218.
13. Orholm M, Munkholm P, Langholz E, et al: Familial occurrence of inflammatory bowel disease. N Engl J Med 1991; 324:84–88.
14. Michener WM, Caulfield M, Farmer RG, et al: Genetic counselling and family history in IBD: 30 years' experience at the Cleveland Clinic. Can J Gastroenterol 1990; 4:350–354.
15. Tysk C, Lindberg E, Jarnerot G, et al: Ulcerative colitis and Crohn's disease in an unselected population of monozygotic and dizygotic twins: A study of heritability and the influence of smoking. Gut 1988; 29:990–996.
16. Monsen U, Iselius L, Johansson C, et al: Evidence for a major additive gene in ulcerative colitis. Clin Genet 1989; 36:411–414.
17. Gilat T, Hacohen D, Lilos P, et al: Childhood factors in ulcerative colitis and Crohn's disease: An international cooperative study. Scand J Gastroenterol 1987; 22:1009–1024.
18. Nahir M, Gicconi D, Eidelman S, et al: HLA antigens in ulcerative colitis. Lancet 1976; 2:573.
19. Asakura H, Tsuchiya M, Aiso S, et al: Association of human lymphocyte DR2 antigen with Japanese ulcerative colitis. Gastroenterology 1982; 82:413–418.
20. Rump JA, Scholmerich J, Gross V, et al: A new type of perinuclear anti-neutrophil cytoplasmic antibody (p-ANCA) in active ulcerative colitis but not in Crohn's disease. Immunobiology 1990; 181:406–413.
21. Duerr RH, Targan SR, Landers CJ, et al: Anti-neutrophil antibodies in ulcerative colitis. Comparison with other colitides/diarrheal illnesses. Gastroenterology 1991; 100:1590–1596.
22. Duerr RH, Targan SR, Landers CJ, et al: Neutrophilic cytoplasmic antibodies: A link between primary sclerosing cholangitis and ulcerative colitis. Gastroenterology 1991; 100:1385–1391.
23. Truelove SC: Ulcerative colitis provoked by milk. Br Med J 1961; 1:154–160.
24. Jewell DP, Truelove SC: Circulating antibodies to cow's milk proteins in ulcerative colitis. Gut 1972; 13:796.
25. Taylor KB, Truelove SC: Circulating antibodies to milk proteins in ulcerative colitis. Br Med J 1961; 2:924.
26. Acheson ED, Truelove SC: Early weaning in the aetiology of ulcerative colitis. A study of feeding in infancy in cases and controls. Br Med J 1961; 2:929–933.
27. Whorwell PJ, Holdstock G, Whorwell GM, et al: Bottle feeding,

early gastroenteritis and inflammatory bowel disease. Br J Med 1979; 1:382.
28. Glassman MS, Newman LJ, Berezin S, et al: Cow's milk protein sensitivity during infancy in patients with inflammatory bowel disease. Am J Gastroenterol 1990; 85:838–840.
29. Roediger WE: The colonic epithelium in ulcerative colitis: An energy-deficiency disease? Lancet 1980; 2:712–715.
30. Harig JM, Soergel KH, Komorowski RA, et al: Treatment of diversion colitis with short-chain fatty acid irrigation. N Engl J Med 1989; 320:23–28.
31. Breuer RI, Buto SK, Christ ML, et al: Short chain fatty acids for distal ulcerative colitis. Gastroenterology 1990; 98:A161.
32. North CS, Clouse RE, Spitznagel EL, et al: The relation of ulcerative colitis to psychiatric factors: A review of findings and methods. Am J Psychiatry 1990; 147:974–981.
33. Spiliadis CA, Lennard-Jones JE: Ulcerative colitis with relative sparing of the rectum: Clinical features, histology, and prognosis. Dis Colon Rectum 1987; 30:334–336.
34. Riddell RH: Pathology of idiopathic inflammatory bowel disease. *In* Kirsner JB, ed: Inflammatory Bowel Disease. Philadelphia, Lea & Febiger, 1988; pp 329–350.
35. Whitehead R: Mucosal Biopsy of the Gastrointestinal Tract. 2nd ed. Philadelphia, WB Saunders, 1979, p 241.
36. Michener WM: Ulcerative colitis in children. Pediatr Clin North Am 1967; 14:159–163.
37. Motil KJ, Grand RJ: Ulcerative colitis and Crohn's disease in children. Pediatr Rev 1987; 9:109–120.
38. Waye JD: Endoscopy in inflammatory bowel disease: Indications and differential diagnosis. Med Clin North Am 1990; 74:51–65.
39. Michener WM, Caulfield ME, Wyllie RW, et al: Management of inflammatory bowel disease: 30 years of observation. Cleve Clin J Med 1990; 57:685–691.
40. Passo MH, Fitzgerald JF, Brandt KD: Arthritis associated with inflammatory bowel disease in children: Relationship of joint disease to activity and severity of bowel lesion. Dig Dis Sci 1986; 31:492–497.
41. Lindsley CB, Schaller JG: Arthritis associated with inflammatory bowel disease in children. J Pediatr 1974; 84:16–20.
42. Greenstreet AJ, Janowitz HD, Sachar DB: The extra-intestinal complications of Crohn's disease and ulcerative colitis: A study of 700 patients. Medicine 1976; 55:401–412.
43. Mir-Madjlessi SH, Taylor JS, Farmer RG: Clinical course and evolution of erythema nodosum and pyoderma gangrenosum in chronic ulcerative colitis: A study of 42 patients. Am J Gastroenterol 1985; 80:615–620.
43a. Levitt MD, Ritchie JK, Lennard-Jones JE, et al: Pyoderma gangrenosum in inflammatory bowel disease. Br J Surg 1991; 78:676–678.
44. Vierling JM: Hepatobiliary complications of ulcerative colitis and Crohn's disease. *In* Zakim D, Boyer TD, eds: Hepatology: A Textbook of Liver Disease. Philadelphia, WB Saunders, 1990, pp 1126–1158.
45. Wee A, Ludwig J: Pericholangitis in chronic ulcerative colitis: Primary sclerosing cholangitis of the small bile ducts. Ann Intern Med 1985; 102:581–587.
46. Rankin GB: Extraintestinal and systemic manifestations of inflammatory bowel disease. Med Clin North Am 1990; 74:39–50.
47. Wiesner RH, LaRusso NF, Dozois RR, et al: Peristomal varices after proctocoloectomy in patients with primary sclerosing cholangitis. Gastroenterology 1986; 90:316–322.
48. Czaja AJ, Wolf AM: Immunopathic disease associated with severe chronic active liver disease: Determinants of treatment response? Gastroenterology 1980; 78:A1152.
49. Gray N, MacKay IR, Taft LI, et al: Hepatitis, colitis, and lupus manifestations. Am J Dig Dis 1958; 3:481–491.
50. Olsson R, Hulten L: Concurrence of ulcerative colitis and chronic active hepatitis: Clinical courses and results of colectomy. Scand J Gastroenterol 1975; 10:331–335.
51. Christophi C, Hughes ER: Hepatobiliary disorders in inflammatory bowel disease. Surg Gynecol Obstet 1985; 160:187–193.
52. Desmet VJ, Geboes K: Liver lesions in inflammatory bowel disorders. J Pathol 1987; 151:247–255.
53. Kane W, Miller K, Sharp HL: Inflammatory bowel disease presenting as liver disease during childhood. J Pediatr 1980; 97:775–778.
53a. Gavaler JS, Delemos B, Bell SH, et al: Ulcerative colitis disease activity as subjectively assessed by patient-completed questionnaires following orthotopic liver transplantation for sclerosing cholangitis. Dig Dis Sci 1991; 36:321–328.
54. Talbot RW, Heppell J, Dozois RR, et al: Vascular complications of inflammatory bowel disease. Mayo Clin Proc 1986; 61:140–145.
55. Daum F, Gould HB, Gold D, et al: Asymptomatic transient uveitis in children with inflammatory bowel disease. Am J Dis Child 1979; 133:170–171.
56. Banner MP: Genitourinary complications of inflammatory bowel disease. Radiol Clin North Am 1987; 25:199–209.
57. McCaffery TD, Nasr K, Lawrence AM, et al: Severe growth retardation in children with inflammatory bowel disease. Pediatrics 1970; 45:386–393.
58. Motil KJ, Grand RJ, Davis-Kraft E: The epidemiology of growth failure in children and adolescents with inflammatory bowel disease. Gastroenterology 1983; 84:A1254.
59. Edwards FC, Truelove SC: Factors in the long-term prognosis of ulcerative colitis. Part III: Complications. Gut 1964; 75:97–103.
60. Goulston SJ, McGovern VJ: The nature of benign strictures in ulcerative colitis. N Engl J Med 1969; 281:290–295.
61. Huizenga KA, Schroeder KW: Gastrointestinal complications of ulcerative colitis and Crohn's disease. *In* Kirsner JB, Shorter RG, eds: Inflammatory Bowel Disease. Philadelphia, Lea & Febiger, 1988, pp 257–280.
62. McInerney GT, Sauer WG, Baggenstoss AH, et al: Fulminating ulcerative colitis with marked colonic dilatation: A clinicopathologic study. Gastroenterology 1962; 42:2944–2957.
63. Greico MB, Bordan DL, Geiss AC, et al: Toxic megacolon complicating Crohn's colitis. Ann Surg 1980; 191:75–80.
64. Cone JB, Wetzel W: Toxic megacolon secondary of pseudomembranous colitis. Dis Colon Rectum 1982; 25:478–482.
65. Farmer RG, Hawk WA, Turnbull RB: Clinical patterns in Crohn's disease: A statistical study of 615 cases. Gastroenterology 1975; 68:627–635.
66. Norland CC, Kirsner JB: Toxic dilatation of the colon (toxic megacolon): Etiology, treatment and prognosis in 42 patients. Medicine 1969; 48:229–250.
67. Heppell J, Farouk E, Dube S, et al: Toxic megacolon: An analysis of 70 cases. Dis Colon Rectum 1986; 29:789–792.
68. Binder SC, Patterson JF, Glotzer DJ: Toxic megacolon in ulcerative colitis. Gastroenterology 1974; 66:909–915.
69. Jalan KN, Sircus W, Card WI, et al: An experience of ulcerative colitis: Toxic dilatation in 55 cases. Gastroenterology 1969; 57:68–82.
70. Fazio VW: Toxic megacolon in ulcerative colitis and Crohn's colitis. Clin Gastroenterol 1980; 9:271–278.
71. Present DH, Wolfson D, Gelernt IM, et al: Medical decompression of toxic megacolon by "rolling": A new technique of decompression with favorable long-term follow-up. J Clin Gastroenterol 1988; 10:485–490.
72. Prior P, Gyde SN, McCartney JC, et al: Cancer morbidity in ulcerative colitis. Gut 1982; 23:490–497.
73. Katzka I, Brody RS, Morris E, Katz S: Assessment of colorectal cancer risk in patients with ulcerative colitis: Experience from a private practice of gastroenterology. Gastroenterology 1983; 85:22–29.
74. Devroede GJ, Taylor WF, Sauer J, et al: Cancer risk and life expectancy of children with ulcerative colitis. N Engl J Med 1973; 289:491–495.
75. Sugita A, Sachar DB, Bodian C, et al: Colorectal cancer in ulcerative colitis. Influence of anatomical extent and age of onset on colitis-cancer interval. Gut 1991; 32:167–169.
76. Dobbins W: Dysplasia and malignancy. Ann Rev Med 1984; 35:33–48.
77. Gilat T, Fireman Z, Morris E, et al: Colorectal cancer in patients with ulcerative colitis: A population study in Central Israel. Gastroenterology 1983; 294:870–877.
78. Kvist N, Jacobsen O, Kvist HK, et al: Malignancy in ulcerative colitis. Scand J Gastroenterol 1989; 24:497–506.
79. Lennard-Jones JE, Ritchie JK, Morson BC, et al: Cancer surveillance in ulcerative colitis. Lancet 1983; 2:149–152.
80. Greenstein AJ, Sachar DB, Smith R, et al: Cancer in universal

and left-sided ulcerative colitis: Factors in determining risk. Gastroenterology 1979; 77:290–294.

81. Sachar DB, Greensterin AJ: Cancer in ulcerative colitis: Good news and bad news. Ann Intern Med 1981; 95:642–644.
82. Ekbom A, Helmick C, Zack M, et al: Ulcerative colitis and colorectal cancer. A population-based study. N Engl J Med 1990; 323:1228–1232.
83. Greenstein AJ, Heimann TM, Sachar DB, et al:A comparison of multiple synchronous colorectal cancer in ulcerative colitis, familial polyposis coli, and de novo cancer. Ann Surg 1986; 203:123–128.
84. Mir-Madjlessi SH, Farmer RG, Easley KA, et al: Colorectal and extracolonic malignancy in ulcerative colitis. Cancer 1986; 58:1569–1574.
85. Rosenstock E, Farmer RG, Petras R, et al: Surveillance for colitis-associated carcinoma in ulcerative colitis. Gastroenterology 1985; 89:1342–1346.
86. Riddell RH, Goldman H, Ransohoff DF, et al: Dysplasia in inflammatory bowel disease: Standarized classification with provisional application. Hum Pathol 1983; 14:931–968.
87. Nugent FW, Haggitt RC, Gilpin PA: Cancer surveillance in ulcerative colitis. Gastroenterology 1991; 100:1241–1248.
88. Lashner BA, Kane SV, Hanauer SB: Colon cancer surveillance in chronic ulcerative colitis: Historical cohort study. Am J Gastroenterol 1990; 85:1083–1087.
89. Ransohoff DF, Riddell RH, Levin B: Ulcerative colitis and colonic cancer: Problems of assessing the diagnostic usefulness of mucosal dysplasia. Dis Colon Rectum 1985; 28:383–388.
90. Manning AP, Bulgium OR, Dixon MF, et al: Screening by colonoscopy for colonic epithelial dysplasia and inflammatory bowel disease. Gut 1987; 28:1489–1494.
91. Korelitz BI: Considerations of surveillance, dysplasia, and carcinoma of the colon in the management of ulcerative colitis and Crohn's disease. Med Clin North Am 1990; 74:189–199.
92. Lennard-Jones JE, Melville DM, Morson BC, et al: Precancer and cancer in extensive ulcerative colitis: Findings among 401 patients over 22 years. Gut 1990; 31:800–806.
93. Azad Kahn AK, Piris J, Truelove SC: An experiment to determine the active moiety of SASP. Lancet 1977; 2:892–895.
94. Hanauer SB, Kirsner JB: Medical therapy in ulcerative colitis. *In* Kirsner JB, ed. Inflammatory Bowel Disease. Philadelphia, Lea & Febiger, 1988, pp 431–475.
95. Das KM, Eastwood MA, McManus JPA, et al: Adverse reactions during salicylazosulfapyridine therapy and the relation with drug metabolism and acetylator phenotype. N Engl J Med 1973; 289:491–495.
96. Ireland A, Jewell DP: Mechanism of action of 5-aminosalicylic acid and its derivatives. Clin Sci 1990; 78(2):119–125.
97. Hanauer SB, Stathopoulos G: Risk-benefit assessment of drugs used in the treatment of inflammatory bowel disease. Drug Safety 1991; 6:192–219.
98. Rampton DS, Hawkey CJ: Prostaglandins in ulcerative colitis. Gut 1984; 25:1399–1413.
99. Baum CL, Selhub J, Rosenberg IH: Antifolate actions of sulphasalazine on intact lymphocytes. J Lab Clin Med 1981; 97:779–784.
100. Rhodes JM, Bartholomew TC, Jewell DP: Inhibition of leukocyte motility by drugs used in ulcerative colitis. Gut 1981; 22:642–647.
101. Ahnfelt-Ronne I, Neilsen OH, Christensen A, et al: Clinical evidence supporting the radical scavenger mechanism of 5-aminosalicylic acid. Gastroenterology 1990; 98(5):1162–1169.
102. Miyachi Y, Yoshioka A, Imamura S, Niwa Y: Effect of sulphasalazine and its metabolites on the generation of reactive oxygen species. Gut 1987; 28:190–195.
103. Eliakim R, Karmeli F, Razin E, et al: Role of platelet activating factor in ulcerative colitis. Gastroenterology 1988; 95:1167–1172.
104. Dick AP, Grayson MJ, Carpenter RG, et al: Controlled trial of sulphasalazine in the treatment of ulcerative colitis. Gut 1964; 5:437–442.
105. Dissanayake AS, Truelove SE: A controlled therapeutic trial of long–term maintenance treatment of ulcerative colitis with sulfasalazine. Gut 1973; 14:923–926.
106. Azad Kahn AK, Howes DT, Piris J, et al: Optimum dose of sulphasalazine for maintainence treatment in ulcerative colitis. Gut 1980; 21:232–240.
107. Kirschner BS: Inflammatory bowel disease in children. Pediatr Clin North Am 1988; 35:189–205.
108. Michener WM, Wyllie R: Management of children and adolescents with inflammatory bowel disease. Med Clin North Am 1990; 74:103–114.
109. Neilson OH: Sulfasalazine intolerance. A retrospective survey of the reasons for discontinuing treatment with sulfasalazine in patients with chronic inflammatory bowel disease. Scand J Gastroenterol 1982; 17:389–393.
110. Singleton JW, Summers RW, Kern FJ, et al: A trial of sulfasalazine as adjunctive therapy in Crohn's disease. Gastroenterology 1979; 77:870–882.
111. O'Morain C, Smethurst P, Dore CJ, et al: Reversible male infertility due to sulphasalazine: Studies in man and rat. Gut 1984; 25:1078–1084.
112. Hadziselimovic F, Keller B, Hennes U, et al: Toxic effect of sulphasalazine on prepubertal testes. *In* Hadziselimovic F, Herzog B, Burgin-Wolff A, eds: Inflammatory Bowel Disease and Coeliac Disease in Children. Boston, Kluwer Academic Publishers, 1990, pp 99–115.
113. Werlin SL, Grand RJ: Bloody diarrhea— a new complication of sulfasalazine. J Pediatr 1978; 92:450–451.
114. Ireland A, Mason CH, Jewell DP: A controlled trial comparing olsalazine and SASP for the maintenance treatment of ulcerative colitis. Gut 1988; 29:835–837.
115. Robinson M, Gitnick G, Balart L, et al: Olsalazine in the treatment of mild-moderate ulcerative colitis. Gastroenterology 1988; 94:A380.
116. Selby WS, Barr GD, Ireland A, et al: Olsalazine in active ulcerative colitis. Br Med J 1985; 291:1373–1375.
117. Rutgeerts P: Mesalazine is as effective as SASP in maintaining ulcerative colitis in remission. Int Congress Rome 1988; 1:A166.
118. Dew MJ, Hughes P, Harries AD, et al: Maintenance of remission in ulcerative colitis with an oral preparation of 5-ASA. Br Med J 1982; 285:1012.
119. Riley SA, Mani V, Goddman MJ, et al: Comparison of delayed-release 5-ASA and SASP in the treatment of mild to moderate ulcerative colitis. Gut 1988; 29:669–674.
120. Hanauer SB, Schwartz J, Roufail W, et al: Dose-ranging study of oral mesalamine capsule (Pentasa) for active ulcerative colitis. Gastroenterology 1989; 96:A195.
121. Austin CA, Cann PA, Jones TH, et al: Exacerbation of diarrhea and pain in patients treated with 5-ASA for ulcerative colitis. Lancet 1984; 1:917–918.
122. Ireland A, Jewell DP: Sulphasalazine and the new salicylates. Eur J Gastroenterol Hepatol 1989; 1:43–50.
123. Bilyard KG, Joseph EC, Metcalf R: Mesalazine: An overview of key preclinical studies. Scand J Gastroenterol 1990; 25:52–55.
124. Sandberg-Gertzen H, Jarnerot G: Dipentum in children with ulcerative colitis: Tolerance and pharmacokinetic experience. Gastroenterology 1990; 98:A201.
125. Tolia V, Massous N, Klotz U: Oral 5-aminosalicylic acid in children with colonic chronic inflammatory bowel disease: Clinical and pharmacokinetic experience. J Pediatr Gastroenterol Nutr 1989; 8:333–338.
126. Ferry G, Grand R, Kirschner B, et al: Results of the pediatric gastroenterology collaborative research group (PGCRG) clinical trial comparing olsalazine with sulfasalazine in mild to moderate childhood ulcerative colitis. Gastroenterology 1990; 98:A169.
127. Campieri M, Lanfrachi GA, Bertoni F, et al: Treatment of ulcerative colitis with high-dose 5-aminosalicylic acid enemas. Lancet 1981; 2:270–271.
128. Friedman LS, Richter JM, Kirkham SE, et al: 5-Aminosalicylic acid enemas in refractory distal ulcerative colitis: A randomized, controlled trial. Am J Gastroenterol 1986; 81:412–417.
129. Sutherland LR, Martin F, Jewell DP, et al: 5-Aminosalicylic acid enemas in the treatment of remission in distal ulcerative colitis, proctosigmoiditis, and proctitis. Gastroenterology 1987; 92:1894–1898.
130. Williams CN, Haber G, Aquino JA: Double-blind placebo-controlled evaluation of 5-ASA suppositories in active distal proctitis and measurement of extent of spread using 99m Tc-labelled 5-ASA suppositories. Dig Dis Sci 1987; 32(Suppl):71–75.
131. Biddle WL, Greenberger NJ, Swan JT, et al: 5-ASA enemas:

Effective agent in maintaining remission in left-sided ulcerative colitis. Gastroenterology 1988; 94:1075–1079.
132. D'Arienzo A, Panarese A, D'Armiento FP, et al: 5-Aminosalicylic acid suppositories in the maintenance of remission in idiopathic proctitis or proctosigmoiditis: A double-blind placebo-controlled clinical trial. Am J Gastroenterol 1990; 85:1079–1082.
133. Caulfield M, Wyllie R, McKinney M, et al: 5-Aminosalicylic acid enemas in the treatment of distal ulcerative colitis in children. Gastroenterology 1989; 6:A490.
134. Isaacs KL, Murphy D: Pancreatitis after rectal administration of 5-aminosalicylic acid. J Clin Gastroenterol 1990; 12:198–199.
135. Claman HN: Anti-inflammatory effects of corticosteroids. Clin Immunol Allergy 1984; 4:317.
136. Ligumsky M, Karmeli F, Sharon P, et al: Enhanced thromboxane A_2 and prostacyclin production by cultured rectal mucosa in ulcerative colitis and its inhibition by steroids and sulfasalazine. Gastroenterology 1981; 80:444–449.
137. Lauritsen K, Laursen LS, Bukhave K, et al: Effects of topical 5-ASA and prednisolone on prostaglandin E_2 and leukotriene B_4 levels determined by equilibrium in vivo dialysis of rectum in relapsing ulcerative colitis. Gastroenterology 1986; 91:837–844.
138. Flower RJ, Blackwell GJ: Anti-inflammatory steroids induce biosynthesis of a phospholipase A_2 inhibitor which prevents prostaglandin generation. Nature 1979; 278:456–459.
139. Hawkey CJ: Evidence that prednisolone is inhibitory to the cyclooxygenase activity of human rectal mucosa. Prostaglandins 1982; 23:397–409.
140. Haynes RC, Murad F: Adrenocorticotropic hormone; adrenocortical steroids and their synthetic analogs; inhibitors of adrenocortical steroid biosynthesis. *In* Gilman A, Goodman LS, Rall TW, Murad F, eds: The Pharmacological Basis of Therapeutics. New York, Macmillan, 1985, pp 1459–1489.
141. Van der Heide H, Mulder CJ, Witnik EH: Comparison of enema containing beclomethasone dipropionate or prednisone–21-phosphate in the treatment of distal ulcerative colitis. Gastroenterology 1987; 92:349–355.
142. Danielsson A, Hellers A, Lyrenas E, et al: A controlled randomized trial of budesonide versus prednisolone retention enemas in active distal ulcerative colitis. Scand J Gastroenterol 1987; 22:987–992.
143. Hanauer SB, Kirsner JB, Barrett WE: The treatment of left-sided ulcerative colitis with tixocortol pivalate. Gastroenterology 1986; 90:A1449.
144. Conn HO, Blitzer BL: Non-association of adrenocorticosteroid therapy and peptic ulcer. N Engl J Med 1976; 294:473–479.
145. Goldstein MJ, Gelzayd EA, Kirsner JB: Some observations on the hazards of corticosteroid therapy in patients with inflammatory bowel disease. Trans Am Acad Ophthalmol Otolaryngol 1967; 71:254–261.
146. Sedeghi-Nejad A, Senior B: The treatment of ulcerative colitis with alternate-day corticosteroids. Pediatrics 1969; 43:840–845.
147. Truelove SC, Witts LJ: Cortisone in ulcerative colitis: Final report on a therapeutic trial. Br Med J 1955; 2:1041.
148. Meyers D, Sacher DB, Goldberg JD, Janowitz HD: Corticotropin versus hydrocortisone in the intravenous treatment of ulcerative colitis: A prospective, randomized, double-blind clinical trial. Gastroenterology 1983; 85:351–357.
149. Schjonsby H, Heinmann P, Kremer D, et al: Intensive treatment in severe attacks of ulcerative colitis. Acta Med Scand 1977; 603(Suppl):43.
150. Powell-Tuck J, Bown RL, Lennard-Jones JE: A comparison of oral prednisolone given as single or multiple daily doses for active proctocolitis. Scand J Gastroenterol 1978; 13:833–837.
151. Lennard-Jones JE, Misiewicz JJ, Connell AM, et al: Prednisone as maintenance treatment for ulcerative colitis. Lancet 1965; 2:188–189.
152. Halvorsen S, Myren J, Aakvaag A: On the absorption of prednisone and prednisolone disodium phosphate after rectal administration. Scand J Gastroenterol 1969; 4:581–584.
153. Calabresi P, Parks RE: Chemotherapy of neoplastic diseases. *In* Gilman A, Goodman LS, Rall TW, Murad F, eds: The Pharmacological Basis of Therapeutics. New York, Macmillan, 1985, pp 1272–1274.
154. Campbell AC, Skinner JM, Hersey P, et al: Immunosuppression in the treatment of inflammatory bowel disease: II. The effects of azathioprine on lymphoid cell populations in a double-blind trial in ulcerative colitis. Clin Exp Immunol 1976; 24:248–258.
155. Jewell DP, Truelove SC: Azathioprine in ulcerative colitis: Final report on controlled therapeutic trial. Br Med J 1974; 4:627–630.
156. Kirk AP, Lennard-Jones JE: Controlled trial of azathioprine in chronic ulcerative colitis. Br Med J 1982; 284:1291–1292.
157. Rosenberg JL, Wall AJ, Levin B, et al: A controlled trial of azathioprine in the management of chronic ulcerative colitis. Gastroenterology 1975; 69:96–99.
158. Korelitz BI, Glass JL, Wisch N: Long-term observations of children with ulcerative colitis treated with an immunosuppressive (6-mercaptopurine). Gastroenterology 1977; 72:A1083.
159. Verhave M, Winter HS, Grand RJ: Azathioprine in the treatment of children with inflammatory bowel disease. J Pediatr 1990; 117:809–814.
160. Present DH, Meltzer SJ, Krumholtz MP, et al: 6-Mercaptopurine in the management of inflammatory bowel disease: Short- and long-term toxicity. Ann Intern Med 1989; 111:641–649.
161. Lobo AJ, Foster PN, Burke DA, et al: The role of azathioprine in the management of ulcerative colitis. Dis Colon Rectum 1990; 33:374–377.
162. Hess AD, Colombani PM: Cyclosporin: Mechanism of action. Prog Allergy 1986; 38:198–221.
163. Gupta S, Keshavarzian A, Hodgson HJ: Cyclosporin in ulcerative colitis. Lancet 1984; 2:1277–1278.
164. Bianchi PA, Porro G, Panza E, et al: Cyclosporin A in acute ulcerative colitis. Ital J Gastroenterol 1987; 9:40–41.
165. Lichtiger S, Present DH: Preliminary report: Cylcosporin in treatment of severe active ulcerative colitis. Lancet 1990; 336(8706):16–19.
166. Treem WR, Davis PM, Hyams JS: Cyclosporine treatment of severe ulcerative colitis in children: Immediate and long-term follow-up. J Pediatr 1991; 119:994–997.
167. Kozarek RA, Patterson DJ, Ball TJ, et al: Methotrexate induces clinical and histologic remission in patients with refractory inflammatory bowel disease. Ann Intern Med 1989; 110:353–356.
168. Barrett KE, Dharmasathaphorn K: Pharmacological aspects of therapy in inflammatory bowel diseases: Anti-diarrheal agents. J Clin Gastroenterol 1988; 10:57–63.
169. Werlin SL, Grand RJ: Severe colitis in children and adolescents. Gastroenterology 1977; 73:828–832.
170. Seashore JH, Hillemeier AC, Gryboski JD: Total parenteral nutrition in the management of inflammatory bowel disease in children: A limited role. Am J Surg 1982; 143:504–507.
171. Gilat T, Leichtman G, Delpre G, et al: A comparison of metronidazole and sulfasalazine in the maintenance of remission in patients with ulcerative colitis. J Clin Gastroenterol 1989; 11:392–395.
172. Chapman RW, Selby WS, Jewell DP: Controlled trial of intravenous metronidazole as an adjunct to corticosteroids in severe ulcerative colitis. Gut 1986; 27:1210–1212.
173. Davies PS, Rhodes J, Heatley RV, et al: Metronidazole in the treatment of chronic proctitis: A controlled trial. Gut 1977; 18:680–681.
174. McColl T, O'Leary J, Bloomfield J, et al: Eicosapentaenoic acid. Gastroenterology 1988; 94:A294.
174a. Aslan A, Triadafilopoulos G: Fish oil fatty supplementation in active ulcerative colitis: A double-blind, placebo-controlled crossover study. Am J Gastroenterol 1992; 87:432–437.
175. Petkau BM: Scientific basis for the clinical use of superoxide dismutase. Cancer Treat Rev 1986; 13:17–44.
176. Mayer L, Sachar DB: Efficacy of chloroquine in the treatment of inflammatory bowel disease. Gastroenterology 1988; 94:A293.
177. Fischer SH, Levine DS, Haggitt RC, et al: Immunoglobulin therapy for active and extensive idiopathic ulcerative and Crohn's colitis. Gastroenterology 1990; 98:A170.
178. Lechin F, Van der Dijs B, Insausti CL, et al: Treatment of ulcerative colitis with clonidine. J Clin Pharmacol 1985; 25:219–226.
179. Pemberton JH, Philips SF, Ready RR, et al: Quality of life after Brooke ileostomy and ileal pouch-anal anastomosis: Comparison of performance status. Ann Surg 1989; 209:620–628.
180. Orkin BA, Telander RL, Wolff BG, et al: The surgical management of children with ulcerative colitis: The old vs. the new. Dis Colon Rectum 1990; 33:947–955.

181. Lavery IC, Michener WM, Jagelman DC: Ileorectal anastomosis for inflammatory bowel disease in children and adolescents. Surg Gynecol Obstet 1983; 157:553–556.
182. Leijonmarck CE, Logberg R, Ost A, et al: Long-term results of ileorectal anastomosis in ulcerative colitis in Stockholm County. Dis Colon Rectum 1990; 33:195–200.
183. Martin LW, LeCoultre C, Schubert WK: Total colectomy and mucosal proctectomy with preservation of continence. Ann Surg 1977; 186:477–480.
184. Telander RI, Perrault J: Colectomy with rectal mucusectomy and ileal-anal anastomosis in young adults: Its use for ulcerative colitis and familial polyposis. Arch Surg 1981; 116:623–629.
185. Martin LW, Torres AM, Fischer JE, et al: The critical level for preservation of continence in the ileoanal anastomosis. J Pedatr Surg 1985; 20:664–667.
186. O'Connell PR, Keane FB: Surgery for ulcerative colitis. *In* O'Morain C, ed: Ulcerative Colitis. Ann Arbor: CRC Press, 1991, pp 153–168.
186a. Fonkalsrud EW, Loar N: Long-term results after colectomy and endorectal pull-through procedure in children. Ann Surg 1992; 215:57–62.
187. Taylor BA, Dozois RR: The J ileal pouch-anal anastomosis. World J Surg 1987; 11:727–734.
188. Galandiuk S, Scott NA, Dozois RR, et al: Ileal pouch-anal anastomosis: Reoperation for pouch-related complications. Ann Surg 1990; 212:446–452.
189. O'Connell PR, Pemberton JH, Kelly KA: Determinants of stool frequency after ileal pouch-anal anastomosis. Am J Surg 1987; 153:157.
190. O'Connell PR, Rankin DR, Weiland RH, et al: Enteric bacteriology, absorption, morphology, and emptying after ileal pouch anastomosis. Br J Surg 1986; 73:909–914.
191. Zuccaro G, Fazio VW, Church JM, et al: Pouch ileitis. Dig Dis Sci 1989; 34:1505–1510.
191a. Puthu D, Rajan N, Rao R, et al: Carcinoma of the rectal pouch following restorative proctocolectomy: Report of a case. Dis Colon Rectum 1992; 35:257–260.
192. Mir-Madjlessi SH, Michener WM, Farmer RG: Course and prognosis of idiopathic ulcerative proctosigmoiditis in young patients. J Pediatr Gastroenterol Nutr 1986; 6:194–199.

Chapter 61

Neonatal Necrotizing Enterocolitis

ROBERT M. KLIEGMAN

Neonatal necrotizing enterocolitis (NEC) is a disease of unknown etiology that predominantly affects premature infants in level II or III neonatal intensive care units during the infants' convalescence from the common cardiopulmonary disorders associated with prematurity.[1–6] NEC is the most common and most serious acquired gastrointestinal disorder among hospitalized preterm neonates and is associated with significant acute and chronic morbidity and mortality.[1] Indeed, NEC is the most common cause of gastrointestinal perforation and acquired short bowel syndrome among patients in the neonatal intensive-care unit.[1, 7] It has been estimated that in the United States there are approximately 2,000 to 4,000 cases of NEC annually.[1] Furthermore, between 1960 and 1980 the proportion of infectious disease–related deaths due to NEC increased from 4 to 33%.[8]

EPIDEMIOLOGY

NEC is a disease affecting premature infants during their convalescence from other diseases of immaturity.[1, 9] It is unusual to see NEC during the acute phase of respiratory distress syndrome, hypoxic-ischemic encephalopathy (birth asphyxia), heart failure from congenital heart disease or a patent ductus arteriosus, and other acute neonatal disease processes.[1, 10] Although NEC is noted predominantly in premature neonates, approximately 10% of cases occur in nearly full-term or full-term infants whose preceding risk factors have included polycythemia, cyanotic heart disease (usually with angiographic catheterization studies), chronic diarrhea, or a prior anatomic obstructive gastrointestinal malformation (volvulus or gastroschisis).[1, 11]

NEC occurs predominantly in neonates after the onset of enteral alimentation, as 95% of affected infants have been fed for various amounts of time.[1, 12, 13] NEC usually develops during the first 2 weeks of life in relatively well neonates who have been fed normally, but may be delayed for 90 days in low-birth-weight infants kept NPO for prolonged periods.[1] NEC tends to develop later among infants whose birth weights were less than 1,000 gm. Thus the more immature the infant at birth the later the possible onset of NEC. Such data suggest that immaturity of gastrointestinal function is a major risk factor.[1, 9, 14] Many case-controlled studies have suggested that immaturity is the only readily identifiable risk factor for the development of NEC.[1, 6] Immature function of host defense, gastrointestinal motility, digestion, healing, and mucosal integrity (permeability), and circulation may contribute to the pathogenesis of NEC (see later).[14–16]

The incidence of NEC varies among neonatal intensive-care units; some units have no cases of NEC. The overall incidence varies from 3 to 5% of all neonatal intensive-care admissions.[1] The incidence among very low birth weight (less than 1,500 gm) infants who survive long enough to be fed approaches 10 to 15%. The incidence is greatest among infants between 500 and 750 gm at birth (13 to 20%); it declines to approximately 1 to 3% among infants larger than 1,750 gm.[1, 4] The baseline incidence is influenced by periodic outbreaks or epidemics of NEC that become superimposed on an endemic case background. Because infants between 500 and 750 gm at birth represent a very small proportion of infants in neonatal intensive-care units (less than 10% of all births), the mean birth weight of infants affected with NEC is between 1,350 and 1,500 gm and the mean gestational age is between 30 and 32 weeks postconception.

There is no association between the occurrence of NEC and sex, race (other than the increased incidence of low-birth-weight status among blacks), and inborn or transport status.[1] NEC has very rarely been reported in successive pregnancies and among siblings in multiple gestations. Because twins and triplets are often born prematurely, they seem to be over-represented among cases of NEC.[1, 17] In contrast to what would be expected, the incidence of NEC among twins appears to be higher in the well, first-born twin rather than in the second twin, who usually has a lower Apgar score and a more complicated hospital course.

NEC is a disease of surviving neonates. Most affected patients are considered "gainers and growers" who, prior to the onset of NEC, had few if any manifestations of gastrointestinal dysfunction and few apparent sequelae of the previous diseases of prematurity from which they had been recovering.[9, 10] In most instances the majority of such preterm infants had respiratory distress syndrome days to weeks prior to the onset of NEC. With the advent of surfactant therapy for respiratory distress syndrome, there may be more infants who survive this disorder and are now at risk for NEC during their convalescence.[10]

Because NEC is seen in premature infants, many factors associated with prematurity were thought to be risk factors for NEC. These risk factors were related to diseases, procedures, or complications that may produce gastrointestinal ischemia, infection, or altered digestion. Mucosal injury following a combination of these risk factors was thought to produce NEC. Ischemic risk factors included birth asphyxia, respiratory distress syndrome, hypoxia, hypotension, patent ductus arteriosus, polycythemia, anemia, the presence of umbilical arterial catheters, and exchange transfusion. Because these risk factors were identified as part of a profile among affected infants, they were thought to contribute to the pathogenesis of NEC. Although each may contribute to mucosal injury, new case-controlled studies suggest that these processes are equally present among affected patients and unaffected controls.[1] Therefore these risk factors merely describe the low-birth-weight population and are no longer thought to be direct contributing factors in the pathogenesis of NEC (see later). New epidemiologic investigations emphasize that the predominant risk factor is prematurity, with associated immature host defense and gastrointestinal function.

PATHOLOGY

Traditionally, the pathologic appearance of NEC has demonstrated varying features of inflammation and coagulation necrosis.[18] The latter has been interpreted as being due to ischemia, but more recent evidence suggests that inflammatory mediators can produce lesions with coagulation necrosis similar to that following ischemia.[19, 20]

Most tissue specimens from patients with NEC are obtained at autopsy in fatal cases or by surgical resection following gastrointestinal perforation.[18] There are a few studies that examined rectal mucosal biopsies in patients with mild NEC (not fatal, not requiring resection).[1] These latter studies, however, may not reveal a complete picture because (1) more severe NEC is a transmural process, involving all three layers of the bowel wall; (2) mild cases may not represent more severe disease in terms of etiology (mild NEC may represent an allergic-inflammatory process characterized by epithelial or lamina propria eosinophilic infiltration, a finding not usually observed in surgical pathology); and (3) NEC often involves the terminal ileum, ileocecal area, and ascending colon, and rarely just the rectal mucosa. Alternatively, the eosinophilia noted in the rectal mucosal biopsies may represent the early-initiation phase of the illness, which later becomes masked by complicating peritonitis, secondary bacterial invasion, and neutrophilic infiltration. In addition, eosinophilic infiltrates may not always suggest allergic processes and may be a nonspecific gastrointestinal response of an immature host.

Superficial inspection of affected resected surgical or autopsy tissue reveals mucosal ulceration, hemorrhage, edema, and the presence of the submucosal or subserosal gas-filled cysts typical of pneumatosis intestinalis (Fig. 61–1). Approximately 50% of infants have involvement of both the small and large intestine (distal ileum and proximal colon), 25% have just colonic disease, and 25% have only ileal lesions.[1, 18] Involvement of the jejunum, the stomach, or the entire length of bowel from the ligament of Treitz to the rectum is less common; the latter is present in fatal cases of NEC. Approximately equal numbers of infants have either continuous segments of involvement or skipped lesions.

Histologic examination of resected tissue reveals coagulation necrosis in approximately 90%, inflammation in approximately 90%, and the presence of eosinophils (15%), ulceration (75%), hemorrhage (75%), peritonitis (70%), bacterial overgrowth (70%), and reparative process (70%).[18] Pneumatosis intestinalis is present in only 50% of pathologic specimens.

Coagulation necrosis is the predominant pathology in

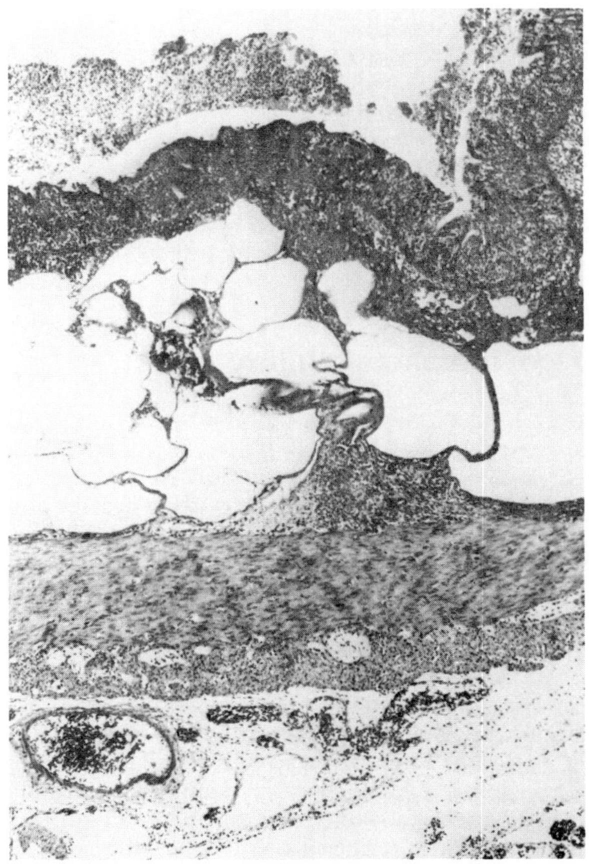

Figure 61–1. Microscopic evidence of severe submucosal gas-filled cysts (pneumatosis intestinalis) in a preterm infant with NEC. Note the marked hemorrhage throughout the bowel wall and the inflammatory exudate on the surface of the mucosa. Hematoxylin-eosin stain, ×56. (Courtesy of Beverly Dahms, MD.)

most specimens.[1,18] Coagulation necrosis, when present with inflammatory lesions, is often observed in an alternating manner in adjacent microscopic fields. Inflammatory changes include acute and chronic signs of inflammation, including serositis, peritonitis, inflammatory pseudomembranes, crypt abscesses, and bacterial or fungal overgrowth. When coagulation necrosis is present with signs of inflammation, the coagulative process is often the dominant lesion.

Large-vessel thrombi are unusual autopsy findings in the mesenteric arteriole system of patients with NEC.[1, 18] Small-vessel thrombi are present in 30% but may represent secondary phenomena or autopsy artifacts.

Interestingly, reparative processes of both acute and chronic types are noted in over 50% of cases.[18] Such reparative changes include focal epithelial regeneration, granulation tissue formation, and fibrosis. The latter two processes are usually noted in the mucosal and submucosal layers but may occasionally extend into the muscularis. Such fibrotic processes may be associated with the later development of strictures in the recovering infant.

PATHOGENESIS

Early theories related to the pathogenesis of NEC proposed a relationship between gastrointestinal ischemia, enteral alimentation, and microorganisms.[1] Although the precise contributions of these variables remain ill defined, a multifactorial pathogenesis involving these risk factors plus immature gastrointestinal function and immature host defense mechanisms seems possible for the initiation and subsequent propagation of NEC (Figs. 61–2, 61–3).[1, 2]

Hypoxic-Ischemic Injury

Alterations of mesenteric blood flow may occur at the large-vessel arterial level and may be associated with redistribution of systemic blood flow or may be within the gastrointestinal system itself with redistribution of local mucosal blood flow.[1, 2, 21–24] The systemic alterations may be associated with global hypoxia, asphyxia, exchange transfusion, arterial runoff lesions such as a patent ductus arteriosus, shock, or anemia. The local alterations of the mucosal circulation may be associated with less severe perturbations of these systemic factors plus those local changes occurring during enteral alimentation, polycythemia, intestinal distention, or luminal exposure to bacterial toxins or inflammatory mediators. Some events may be initiated during the prenatal period (cocaine exposure, placental insufficiency with intrauterine growth retardation) or may occur after birth.[23, 24] Infants exposed to cocaine prenatally may be at higher risk for the development of NEC. Although they tend to have higher birth weights and greater gestational age than others at risk for NEC, they develop NEC sooner and have fewer traditionally identifiable risk factors. This suggests some circulatory role of in utero gastrointestinal ischemia secondary to cocaine's known vascular effects, which may produce fetal vasoconstriction.[23] Further evidence linking prenatal intestinal ischemia and NEC among intrauterine growth–retarded infants can be demonstrated by reduced blood flow detected by fetal Doppler ultrasonography.[24] In most cases this reduced blood flow would not have been identified without ultrasonography, suggesting that fetal mesenteric ischemia often goes undetected.

The regulation of postnatal mesenteric blood flow is complex and not well studied. Autoregulation of regional blood flow is determined by responses to nutrients and autocrine effects of various locally produced gut hormones.[1, 16] These effects may be modified by disease states, the autonomic and central nervous systems, and systemic processes producing vasoconstriction or hypotensive reduction of local tissue blood flow.

Regional intestinal hyperemia in response to local enteral nutrients is associated with increased local mucosal blood flow, oxygen delivery, oxygen consumption, and oxygen extraction. Oxygen-derived metabolic processes support aerobic energy–requiring intestinal mechanisms such as mucosal active transport, secretion, motility, digestion, macromolecule synthesis, and cell growth.[1, 16, 21] The postprandial intestinal mucosal hyperemia in adults is due to selective vasodilation of the mesenteric artery and is regulated by central and local mechanisms (local hormones, nutrients). It is possible that an imbalance between oxygen delivery and oxygen consumption, together with an inability to augment oxygen extraction (flow-dependent model), predisposes the immature intestine to hypoxic mucosal injury during alimentation. Such hypoxic mucosal injury may alter energy-dependent processes, produce malabsorption,

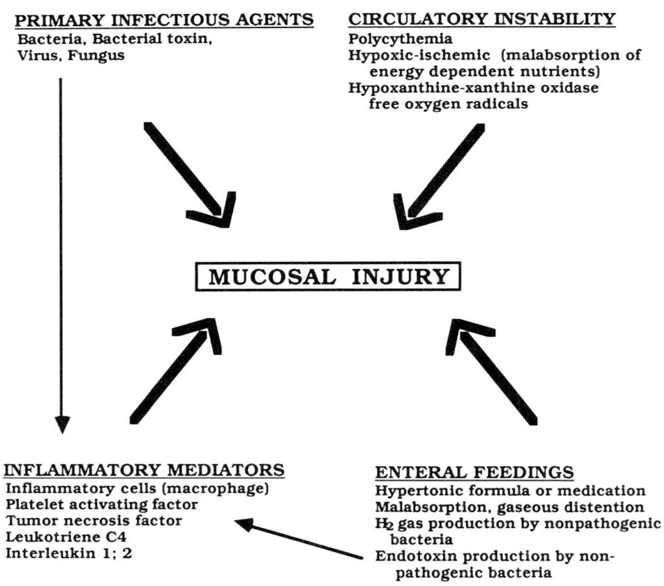

Figure 61–2. Hypothetical contributory variables that may initiate intestinal mucosal injury leading to necrotizing enterocolitis. (From Polin R, Fox W: Neonatal and Fetal Medicine: Physiology and Pathophysiology. Philadelphia, WB Saunders, 1992; with permission.)

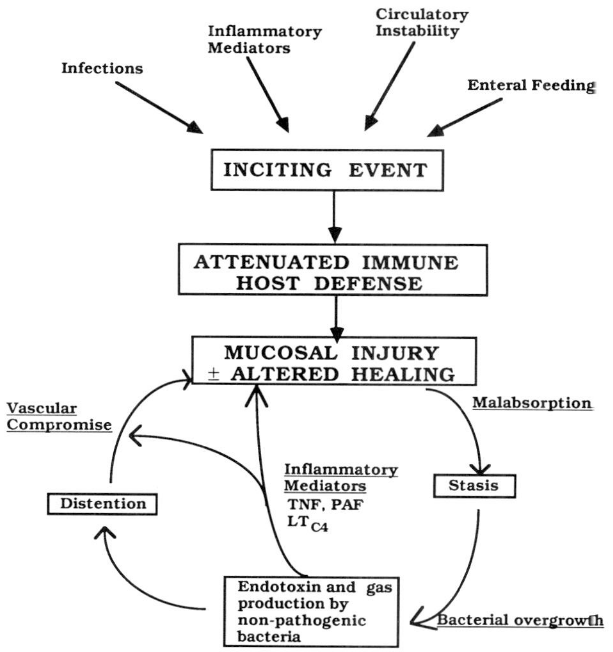

Figure 61–3. Hypothetical cycles of primary events and secondary propagating factors for neonatal intestinal mucosal injury that may produce necrotizing enterocolitis. (Adapted from Polin R, Fox W: Neonatal and Fetal Medicine: Physiology and Pathophysiology. Philadelphia, WB Saunders, 1992; with permission.)

mucosal ulceration, and increased mucosal permeability, and predispose to secondary bacterial invasion. Alternatively, postischemia reperfusion injury may further embarrass mucosal integrity and function, thus perpetuating the mucosal injury.

Experimental models in mature and immature models support each of these hypotheses as possible mechanisms for mucosal injury.[1] Nonetheless there is a paucity of evidence to suggest that episodes of identifiable hypoxic-ischemic events contribute to the pathogenesis of NEC in most infants.[1] Of all the suggested ischemic risk factors for NEC, only polycythemia, exchange transfusion, and possibly exposure to cocaine are associated with the later development of NEC.[1]

Enteral Alimentation

Because 95% of infants with NEC have been enterally fed prior to its onset, enteral alimentation has been proposed as a contributing factor in the pathogenesis of NEC.[12, 13] Various hypotheses propose that it is the composition of the milk, the rate of milk volume increments, the immaturity of gastrointestinal absorptive or host defense processes, or other variables (osmolality) that contribute to the pathogenesis of NEC.[1, 12, 13]

One hypothesis proposes that human milk reduces the risk for NEC.[25, 26] Animal models support a role for the breast milk macrophage, but human data suggest that immunoglobulins, specifically IgA, may have a protective advantage. Indeed, both enterally administered IgA and human milk may reduce the incidence of NEC.[26] Human milk may also reduce allergic reactions while enhancing digestion and absorption of normal nutrients. Although most studies have not demonstrated a protective effect of human milk, many have been confounded by milk preparation methods that may destroy the immunoprotective components of the milk. Recent evidence suggests that pasteurized human milk is effective in reducing the incidence of NEC in premature infants.[25]

The volume of milk fed to infants may also predispose the patient to NEC.[12, 13] Excessively rapid increments of milk feeding may overcome the infant's intestinal absorptive ability, resulting in malabsorption. Malabsorbed carbohydrates contribute to enhanced intestinal bacterial gas production, resulting in abdominal distention.[1, 27] High intraluminal pressure from gaseous distention may reduce mucosal blood flow, producing secondary intestinal ischemia.[9] In addition, dissection of bacterial gas products from the intestinal lumen may produce pneumatosis intestinalis or, if gas enters the portal venous system, hepatic venous gas may be evident. Analysis of gas from the intestinal lumen and cysts of pneumatosis intestinalis reveals a profile typical of intestinal bacterial fermentation of malabsorbed carbohydrates (e.g., hydrogen, methane, carbon dioxide).[1] Breath hydrogen excretion has been proposed as a method to support the diagnosis of NEC.[28]

Earlier hypotheses had suggested that maintaining at-risk patients NPO may reduce the incidence of NEC. Delayed feeding for asphyxiated infants or those with umbilical arterial or venous catheters and respiratory distress syndrome has not consistently reduced the incidence of NEC.[1] In fact, delayed feeding may do more harm than good by increasing the risk of intestinal mucosal atrophy, cholestatic jaundice, osteopenia of prematurity, and hyperalimentation-related complications.[1]

Large volumes of milk feedings, increased too rapidly during the feeding schedule, may place undue stress on a previously injured or immature intestine. Feeding increments in excess of 20 to 30 ml per kg per 24 hours have been associated with an increased risk of NEC in at least two studies.[12, 13] Such information should temper enthusiasm for excessively rapid feeding protocols for low-birth-weight infants. It suggests that daily increments should be based on the clinical examination, evidence of feeding intolerance, and a recommended volume increment below 20 to 30 ml per kg per 24 hours.

Hypertonic formula and enteric medications may have direct adverse effects on mucosal blood flow and intestinal motility. Subsequent injury may predispose to NEC.[1] Alternatively, direct pharmacologic effects of an agent on systemic host defense (vitamin E) or regional blood flow (indomethacin) may result in mucosal injury, increasing the risks for NEC in susceptible neonates.[22]

Infectious-Inflammatory Agents

There are multiple epidemiologic investigations that have provided circumstantial or direct evidence to suggest that NEC is associated with one or more microbiologic agents.[1] NEC has been reported to occur in epidemics or clustered episodes due to an identifiable enteric pathogen; more often no identifiable agent is discovered.[1, 9] The suspicion of a transmittable agent is corroborated by the observation that epidemics abate following the institution or reinforcement of specific infectious disease–control measures (gowning, gloving, nurse cohorts, and especially careful hand washing).[1] Epidemics have been associated with recovery of no specific agent or with the recovery of a single pathogen such as *Escherichia coli*, *Klebsiella*, *Salmonella*, *Staphylococcus epidermidis*, *Clostridium butyricum*, coronavirus, rotavirus, and enteroviruses.[1, 4] In the future, the more sensitive molecular bioiogy techniques such as the polymerase chain reaction may be helpful in identifying agents. This method detects small amounts of viral or bacterial DNA or RNA that other culture and antigen (enzyme-linked immunosorbent assay) methods have failed to identify.[29] For example, reverse transcriptase-polymerase chain reaction identifies rotavirus RNA when standard antigen immunoassays are negative in many older children with rotavirus diarrhea.[29]

Additional evidence suggesting that NEC is due to an infectious agent includes the observation of related infantile diarrheal illnesses within a community or among personnel in the neonatal intensive-care unit.[1] Furthermore, there are many similarities between NEC (pathology, symptoms, immature susceptibility) and many enterotoxemias in young animals and humans. Such enteric toxin-mediated illnesses may be due to *Clostridium*, *S. epidermidis,* or other toxin-producing enteric pathogens.[30, 31] Alternatively, endotoxin production by the "normal" gram-negative enteric flora may predispose the immature intestine to mucosal injury if endotoxin production exceeds its elimination.[9, 20, 32] Endotoxin stimulates host inflammatory cells to produce various mediators such as tumor necrosis factor and platelet activating factor.[20] Both of these and other inflammatory cytokines can initiate or propagate the pathologic process characterized by coagulation necrosis, inflammation, increased vascular permeability, edema, hemorrhage, local thrombosis, and platelet consumption. The resulting cytokine mediator–induced thrombocytopenia, neutropenia, hypotensive-hypovolemic shock (third space fluid losses), metabolic acidosis, and hemorrhagic diarrhea are quite similar to the clinical manifestations of NEC in human neonates.

The blood culture is positive in 20 to 30% of patients with NEC.[1, 4] Reports of the responsible bacteremic pathogens before 1980 demonstrated a predominance of *E. coli* and *Klebsiella.*[1] Current reports of agents producing bacteremia in patients with NEC suggest that *S. epidermidis* is the most common blood isolate, followed by the gram-negative organisms noted in earlier studies.[4] It remains to be determined whether the organisms recovered in blood or peritoneal cultures are the primary pathogens or secondary invading organisms that gain access to the circulation or peritoneum through a markedly compromised and damaged mucosa.

Unifying Hypothesis of Pathophysiology

The predominant risk factor for NEC is prematurity and not the associated diseases of premature infants. Nonetheless, multiple potentially adverse events may produce mucosal injury, with the net result being manifest as NEC. Figure 61–2 provides potential initiating events, and Figure 61–3 identifies additional pathologic factors that may propagate NEC once mucosal injury exceeds the immature host's ability to repair the process. Although it is hoped that one microbiologic agent or other process will be found to be responsible for NEC, it is more probable that NEC is a final common pathway for an immature intestinal response to injury.[9, 10] If pneumonia may be caused by different bacteria, fungi, parasites, and viruses, it is equally tenable that NEC is caused by a select group of neonatal enteric pathogens or other pathologic processes all acting on an immature intestine.

CLINICAL MANIFESTATIONS

Early signs and symptoms of NEC are often nonspecific and include subtle signs of the "sepsis syndrome" and more specific but equally subtle signs of gastrointestinal disease.[1] Nonspecific nongastrointestinal manifestations include apnea, bradycardia, lethargy, temperature instability (hypothermia or the need to increase the Isolette temperature to maintain normal body temperature), cyanosis, mottling, cool extremities, and acidosis.[1] More specific but not diagnostic gastrointestinal manifestations are related to ileus, third space fluid losses, local coagulopathy, and intestinal hemorrhage. Gastrointestinal signs and symptoms include abdominal distention, abdominal tenderness, emesis, increased gastric residual volume, hematemesis, hematochezia, bright red blood from the rectum, absent bowel sounds, abdominal guarding, and diarrhea. The latter is an uncommon isolated manifestation of NEC. As the disease progresses in severity, there is disseminated intravascular coagulation, hypotensive (septic and hypovolemic) shock, ascites, peritonitis, and intestinal perforation. Focal findings may include erythematous streaking of the anterior abdominal wall around the umbilicus and the course of the subcutaneous umbilical vein, and erythema with a mass in the right lower quadrant, representing a local perforation, with matted bowel forming a local abscess.

Disease stage should be classified as noted in Table 61–1 (modified Bell criteria). Stage I represents subclinical (no diagnostic radiographic or ultrasonographic signs) NEC or other gastrointestinal or systemic disturbances. Stages II and III NEC are documented disease. Progression from one stage to another usually occurs within 24 to 48 hours after the onset of symptoms. Once stabilized, patients with NEC rarely progress to another stage; most episodes of perforation occur at presentation (stage IIIB) or among patients with stage IIIA that

Table 61–1. MODIFIED BELL'S STAGING CRITERIA FOR NEONATAL NECROTIZING ENTEROCOLITIS

Stage	Systemic Signs	Intestinal Signs	Radiologic Signs	Treatment
IA—Suspected NEC	Temperature instability, apnea, bradycardia, lethargy	Elevated pregavage residuals, mild abdominal distention, emesis, guaiac-positive stool	Normal or intestinal dilation, mild ileus	Nothing by mouth, antibiotics for 3 days pending cultures
IB—Suspected NEC	Same as above	Bright red blood from rectum	Same as above	Same as above
IIA—Definite NEC, mildly ill	Same as above	Same as above *plus* diminished or absent bowel sounds with or without abdominal tenderness	Intestinal dilation, ileus, pneumatosis intestinalis	Nothing by mouth, antibiotics for 7–10 days if examination is normal in 24–48 hr
IIB—Definite NEC, moderately ill	Above *plus* mild metabolic acidosis and mild thrombocytopenia	Above *plus* definite abdominal tenderness, with or without abdominal cellulitis, or right lower quadrant mass, absent bowel sounds	Same as stage IIA with or without portal vein gas, with or without ascites	Nothing by mouth, antibiotics for 14 days, $NaHCO_3$ for acidosis
IIIA—Advanced NEC, severely ill, bowel intact	Same as stage IIB *plus* hypotension, bradycardia, severe apnea, combined respiratory and metabolic acidosis, disseminated intravascular coagulation, neutropenia, anuria	Above *plus* signs of generalized peritonitis, marked tenderness, distention of abdomen, and abdominal wall erythema	Same as stage IIB, definite ascites	Same as above plus as much as 200+ ml/kg fluids, fresh frozen plasma, inotropic agents, intubation, ventilation therapy, paracentesis, surgical intervention if patient fails to improve with medical management within 24–48 hr
IIIB—Advanced NEC, severely ill, bowel perforated	Same as stage IIIA	Same as stage IIIA	Same as stage IIB *plus* pneumoperitoneum	Same as above *plus* surgical intervention

Adapted from Bell MJ, Ternberg JL, Feigin RD, et al: Neonatal necrotizing enterocolitis: Therapeutic decisions based upon clinical staging. Ann Surg 1978; 187:1–7.

progresses to stage IIIB. Perforation usually occurs within 48 to 72 hours of the onset of disease manifestations in patients with stage IIIA NEC. The modified Bell staging criteria are also useful in comparing cases of NEC in the literature.

DIAGNOSIS

The diagnosis of NEC is confirmed by the radiographic presence of pneumatosis intestinalis or hepatic venous gas (Figs. 61–4 and 61–5). Gastrointestinal perforation (pneumoperitoneum; Figs. 61–6 and 61–7) is strong evidence for NEC, but the diagnosis must then be confirmed by histopathologic evidence (see section on pathology).

Hepatic venous gas and ascites may also be demonstrated by abdominal ultrasonography, and inapparent pneumatosis intestinalis may become more evident by performing a contrast enema.[1, 33–35] Nonetheless, except under unusual circumstances (to rule out a volvulus), contrast studies are not needed to determine the diagnosis of NEC. Ancillary laboratory evaluations may reveal thrombocytopenia with or without evidence of disseminated intravascular coagulation, anemia, neutropenia, metabolic acidosis from septic or hypovolemic shock, respiratory acidosis from increased intra-abdominal pressure and poor diaphragm excursion, elevated breath hydrogen excretion, and radiographic signs of an ileus, an isolated dilated intestinal loop, or ascites.[1, 20]

The differential diagnosis of NEC is outlined in Table 61–2.

PREVENTION

NEC may not be completely eliminated, but certain interventions have been demonstrated to lower the incidence of NEC.

Oral administration of an IgA-IgG preparation has been demonstrated to lower the incidence of NEC; however, intravenous administration of IgG (IVIG) has not affected the incidence of NEC.[26] The oral preparation (73% IgA, 26% IgG) reduced the incidence of NEC among recipients to zero cases, whereas control patients had an incidence of 7%. Further study is needed to determine whether this protocol can be generalized to other neonatal intensive-care units.

Administration of human milk was demonstrated to reduce the incidence of NEC among preterm infants in

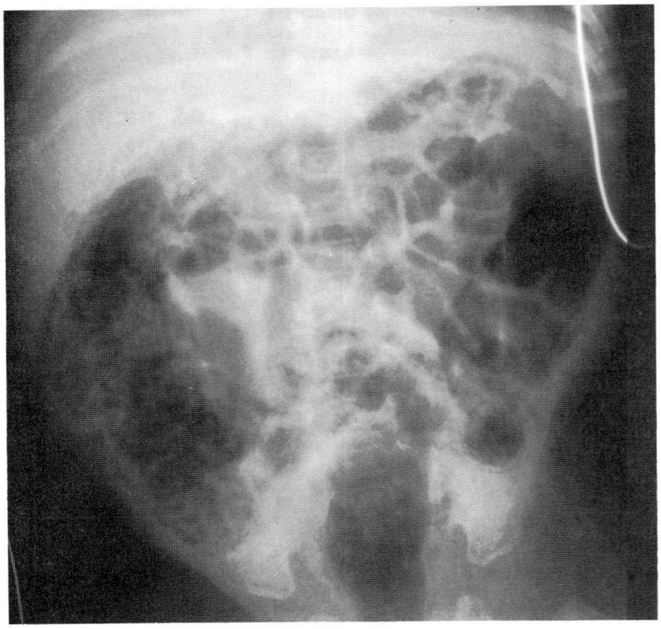

Figure 61–4. Abdominal roentgenogram demonstrating distended loops of small and large bowel, the bubble appearance of pneumatosis intestinalis predominantly in the right lower quadrant, and portal venous gas over the liver. (Courtesy of Stuart Morrison, MD.)

one study.[25, 36] This investigation employed pasteurized human milk and demonstrated a significant reduction of NEC. Other studies, however, were unable to demonstrate a reduction in the incidence or elimination of NEC with human milk feeding among low-birth-weight infants.[1] Again, further studies are needed to determine the protective efficacy of human milk feedings to preterm neonates.

Prenatal and postnatal administration of corticosteroids has been demonstrated to lower the incidence of NEC.[37] Steroids enhance lung maturation and are also thought to accelerate intestinal maturation, thus potentially reducing the "immaturity" factor in the pathogenesis of NEC. Neonates received 2 mg per kg of dexamethasone every 12 hours for two doses. Postnatal steroids, independent of antenatal steroids, were effective in reducing the incidence of NEC in one investigation.[37]

Finally, although never demonstrated in a randomized trial, judicious slow enteral feeding protocols (no vol-

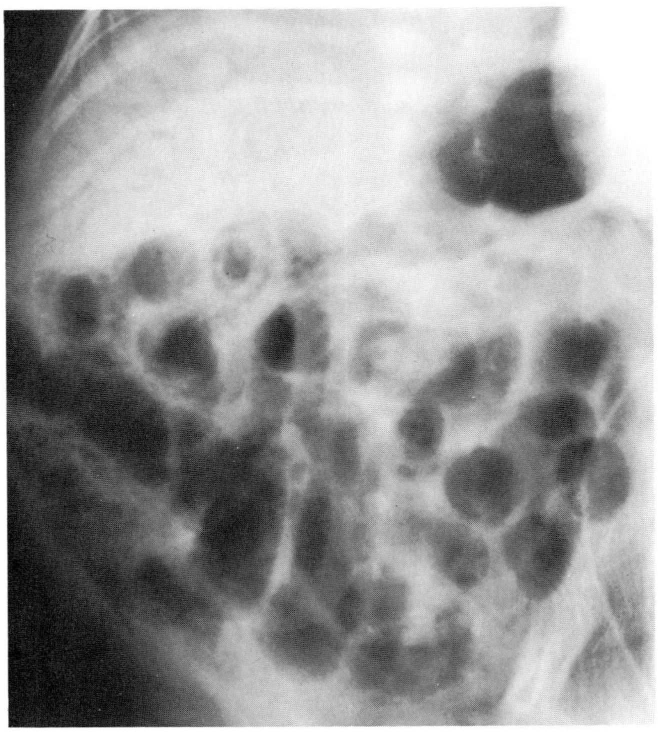

Figure 61–5. Abdominal roentgenogram demonstrating distention, pneumatosis intestinalis, and marked hepatic venous gas. (Courtesy of Stuart Morrison, MD.)

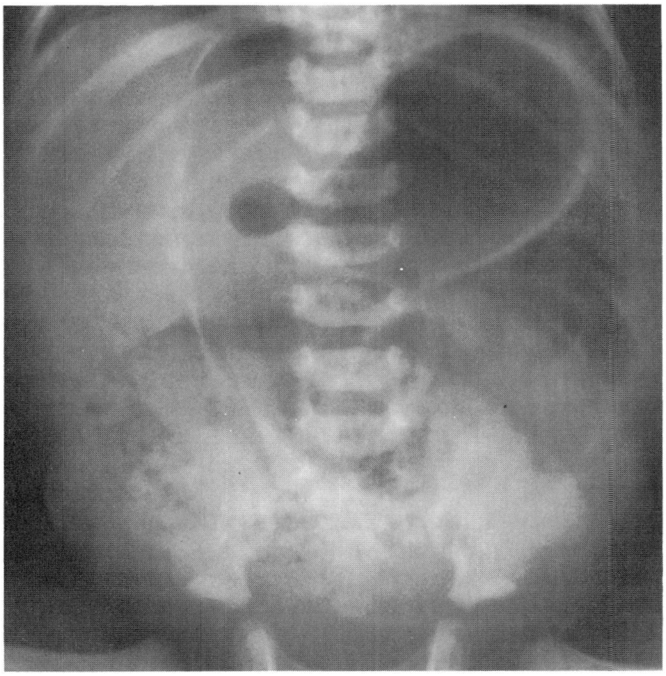

Figure 61–6. Abdominal roentgenogram demonstrating less pneumatosis intestinalis, marked distention, and pneumoperitoneum as evident by the line appearing between the liver and lower midline region depicting the falciforme ligament of the umbilical vein. Note hazy, less clear area over the liver representing free gas in the abdomen. Pneumoperitoneum in patients with NEC represents intestinal perforation. (Courtesy of Stuart Morrison, MD.)

ume increments exceeding 20 to 30 ml per kg per 24 hours) may reduce the occurrence of NEC.[12, 13] There is sufficient circumstantial evidence from multiple case-controlled studies to suggest that slow feeding protocols are associated with a lower incidence of NEC. Furthermore, careful attention to the clinical appearance of the child and to signs of feeding intolerance (distention, hematochezia, larger gastric residuals, emesis) also may be beneficial in identifying infants in earlier stages of NEC.[1]

Table 61–2. DIFFERENTIAL DIAGNOSIS OF NEC

Systemic Disease
Sepsis with ileus
Pneumothorax dissecting to the abdomen, producing pneumoperitoneum
Hemorrhagic disease of the newborn
Swallowed maternal blood
Postasphyxial bowel necrosis
Gastrointestinal Disease
Volvulus
Malrotation
Pseudomembranous colitis
Hirschsprung's colitis
Intussuception
Umbilical arterial thromboembolism
Spontaneous bowel perforation
Hepatic-splenic-adrenal hemorrhage
Stress ulcer
Meconium ileus
Milk protein allergy[1, 11]

THERAPY

NEC may present in a wide spectrum of severity. The mildest enteritis form manifests as a hemorrhagic colitis; the more fulminant state is similar to that noted in patients with gram-negative septic shock, commonly referred to as sepsis syndrome.

Abdominal distention is a universal feature of NEC. Significant abdominal distention may reduce the mes-

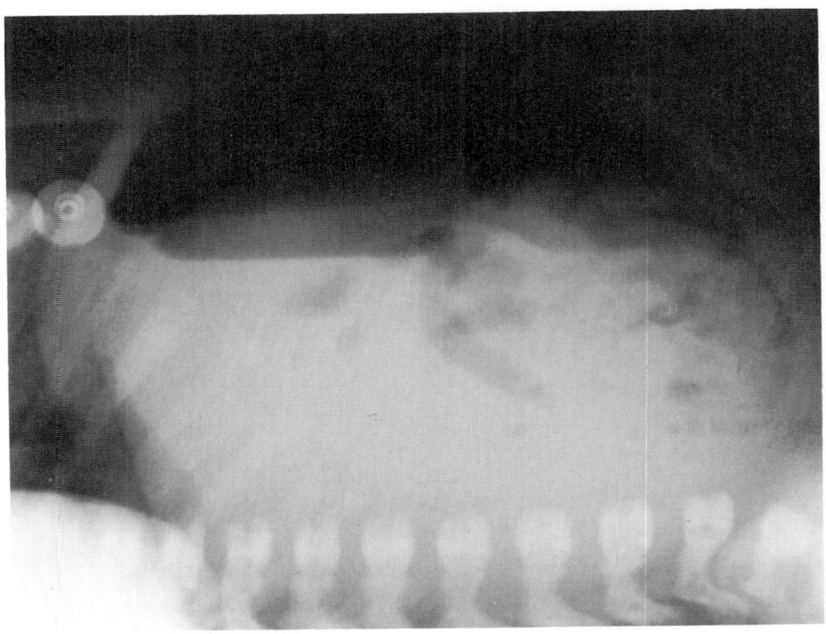

Figure 61–7. Cross-table lateral view most often employed to demonstrate pneumoperitoneum due to intestinal perforation in patients with NEC. Note the free gas in the abdomen above the liver and beneath the anterior abdominal wall. (Courtesy of Stuart Morrison, MD.)

enteric arterial perfusion pressure, thus exacerbating a previously compromised intestinal blood flow. Models of the effects of increased intra-abdominal pressure have reported such adverse consequences as increased systemic vascular resistance, decreased cardiac output, decreased urine output, and "apparent" hypovolemia.[38–40] Surgical decompression of increased intra-abdominal pressure in human adults restores systemic arterial oxygenation, cardiac output, and urine production within 15 minutes of the procedure.[38]

Increased intra-abdominal pressure in patients with NEC is due to the development of tense ascites, marked intestinal gas production, stasis (ileus), and inflammatory fluid exudation with hemorrhage into the lumen of the small and large intestine. It is imperative to reduce abdominal distention with nasogastric tube placement and no further formula feeding (NPO). The decompression tube should be the largest that the patient can tolerate. On occasion, paracentesis or placement of an intra-abdominal drain under local anesthesia has been helpful in stage III disease. Finally, if the patient fails to respond to medical management within 24 to 48 hours of the start of the illness, an exploratory laparotomy can result in abdominal decompression by removal of necrotic tissue and inflammatory exudate.

The bacteremia associated in approximately 20 to 30% of patients with NEC is probably not the primary cause of the disease. Nonetheless, appropriate antimicrobial therapy must be directed against these bacteria even if the bacteremia is due to bowel injury and secondary bacterial invasion. Patients with both NEC and bacteremia usually have more severe disease and a higher mortality.[1] Although the precise antibiotic regimen for the treatment of NEC has not been determined, there is evidence that the clinician must remain flexible, as there has been an apparent change in the pathogens recovered in patients with NEC.[1, 4, 41, 42] This may reflect a bacterial shift in the fecal colonization of premature infants during the last two decades. Nonetheless, the changing pattern of the agents recovered during bacteremia requires close scrutiny and appropriate modification of antimicrobial therapy. Traditional antimicrobial treatment of NEC employs systemic administration of a semisynthetic penicillin (ampicillin, ticarcillin) and an aminoglycoside (gentamicin, kanamycin). Recent evidence suggests a beneficial response with the use of vancomycin and cefotaxime.[43] Vigilant attention to the microbiology of blood, fecal, and peritoneum cultures in patients with NEC is needed for appropriate modification of antibiotic therapy (see Table 61–1 for duration of antimicrobial therapy).

The treatment of severe NEC manifest as septic shock is not unlike that of other causes of bacteremia-associated hypotension noted in the sepsis syndrome. Endotoxin-stimulated production of inflammatory mediators such as bradykinin, tumor necrosis factor, or platelet activating factor results in increased vascular permeability, large transcapillary loss of fluid, increased pulmonary artery pressure with hypoxia, lactic acidosis, and hypotension. Hypermetabolism increases oxygen requirements. Once stabilized from the septic shock state, all patients require parenteral nutrition while NPO. Fluid losses plus the initial vasodilation increase water and electrolyte requirements. Despite rapid killing of bacteria by antibiotics, the diverse effects of bacterial products (endotoxin, etc.) are still evident. The net result is a markedly reduced cardiopulmonary ability to meet the oxygen requirements of the peripheral tissues.[44–46]

Septic shock progresses through two important phases. The early phase is characterized by a pink warm state with hyperventilation, increased cardiac output, decreased systemic vascular resistance, and a narrow arteriovenous oxygen difference. The latter observation is due to a maldistribution of oxygen to tissue beds; those tissues with a greater oxygen requirement remain hypoxic. The second phase of septic shock is characterized by cyanosis, mottling, cold extremities, oliguria, narrow pulse pressure, and decreased cardiac output with markedly increased systemic vascular resistance.

The decreased cardiac output in septic shock (and NEC) may be due to pooling of blood and fluid in the capacitance peripheral vessels and loss of fluid in third spaces as well as a specific myocardial dysfunction characteristic of severe bacteremic states. The myocardial depression is not due to ischemia but rather to various mediators released as a response to inflammation and hypotension. Circulatory failure results in a flow-limited ability to provide the oxygen necessary to support energy metabolism (local tissue oxygen consumption). Circulatory failure causes tissue hypoxia and metabolic (lactic) acidosis. Some of the cellular defects of oxygen utilization may not be due to hypoxia-ischemia alone. Tumor necrosis factor released during endotoxemia has various metabolic consequences that may interfere with mitochondrial oxygen utilization.[44]

Methods used to treat septic shock must take into consideration the linear relationship between oxygen delivery and local tissue oxygen consumption.[44] This flow-dependent relationship can be improved by restoring the circulating blood volume (preload) with fluid resuscitation and by improving myocardial contractility with inotropic-sympathomimetic agents.

An acute "adult" respiratory distress–like syndrome (ARDS) may be present in patients with NEC. This is due in part to inflammatory or vasoactive mediators producing noncardiogenic pulmonary edema. Hypoxia is exacerbated by increased pulmonary artery pressure, abdominal distention with reduced diaphragmatic excursion, and myocardial contractile failure. Adequate oxygen delivery is closely dependent on appropriate ventilator management of patients with NEC. Methods that improve oxygen delivery also reduce local lactate production and improve metabolic acidosis. A successful outcome in patients with septic shock is related to the ability of the therapeutic measures to improve cardiac output. In addition to support for the failing circulation, careful attention must be given to the pulmonary problems associated with NEC.

The application of these principles to the therapy of NEC must emphasize judicious use of fluid resuscitation. If fluid administration is unsuccessful in restoring perfusion and urine production or correcting the metabolic acidosis, pharmacologic therapy with inotropic agents (dopamine, dobutamine) can be used to improve oxygen delivery by improving myocardial contractility and occasionally by vasodilation. The administration of inotropic, vasodilator, or vasopressor agents must be carefully titrated against peripheral perfusion, blood pressure, urine production, metabolic acidosis, and central venous pressure if available. The therapeutic balance between vasopressor (myocardial contractility) agents and vasodilation (afterload reduction) is often difficult to achieve but may be benefited by additional fluid therapy.

Future therapy of NEC or septic shock–like states may need to take into consideration the effects of the various inflammatory mediators (e.g., cytokines, prostaglandins) associated with tissue injury. Various blocking agents of these mediators and anti-inflammatory drugs have produced encouraging results in experimental models of endotoxemia or septic shock. Nonetheless, it is possible that the mediator-induced damage is already irreversible by the time the patient presents with hypotensive septic shock. It is most likely that therapy directed against these mediators must be initiated early in the course of the disease before irreversible tissue injury has occurred.

REFERENCES

1. Kliegman RM, Walsh MC: Neonatal necrotizing enterocolitis: Pathogenesis, classification and spectrum of disease. Curr Prob Pediatr 1987; 17:213–288.
2. Kosloske AM: A unifying hypothesis for pathogenesis and prevention of necrotizing enterocolitis. J Pediatr 1990; 117:S68–S74.
3. Holman RC, Stehr-Green JK, Zelasky MT: Necrotizing enterocolitis mortality in the United States, 1979–85. Am J Publ Health 1989; 79:987–989.
4. Palmer SR, Biffin A, Gamsu HR: Outcome of neonatal necrotising enterocolitis: Results of the BAPM/CDSC surveillance study, 1981–1984. Arch Dis Child 1989; 64:388–394.
5. Ricketts RR, Jerles ML: Neonatal necrotizing enterocolitis: Experience with 100 consecutive surgical patients. World J Surg 1990; 14:600–605.
6. Walther FJ, Verloove-Vanhorick SP, Brand R, et al: A prospective survey of necrotising enterocolitis in very low birthweight infants. Pediatr Perinatal Epidemiol 1989; 3:53–61.
7. Bell MJ: Perforation of the gastrointestinal tract and peritonitis in the neonate. Surg Gynecol Obstet 1985; 160:20–26.
8. Jason JM: Infectious disease-related deaths of low birth weight infants, United States, 1968 to 1982. Pediatrics 1989; 84:296–303.
9. Kliegman RM: Models of the pathogenesis of necrotizing enterocolitis. J Pediatr 1990; 117:S2–S5.
10. Kliegman RM: Neonatal necrotizing enterocolitis: Bridging the basic science with the clinical disease. J Pediatr 1990; 117:833–835.
11. Eggli KD, Loyer E, Anderson K: Neonatal pneumatosis cystoides intestinalis caused by volvulus of the mid intestine. Arch Dis Child 1989; 64:1189–1190.
12. Anderson DM, Kliegman RM: The relationship of neonatal alimentation practices to the occurrence of endemic necrotizing enterocolitis. Am J Perinatol 1991; 18:62–67.
13. Zabielski PB, Groh-Wargo SL, Moore JJ: Necrotizing enterocolitis: Feeding in endemic and epidemic periods. J Parenteral Enteral Nutr 1989; 13:520–524.
14. Udall JN: Gastrointestinal host defense and necrotizing enterocolitis. J Pediatr 1990; 117:S33–S43.
15. Morriss FH, Moore M, Gibson T, et al: Motility of the small intestine in preterm infants who later have necrotizing enterocolitis. J Pediatr 1990; 117:S20–S23.
16. Aynsley-Green A, Lucas A, Lawson GR, et al: Gut hormones and regulatory peptides in relation to enteral feeding, gastroenteritis, and necrotizing enterocolitis in infancy. J Pediatr 1990; 117:S24–S32.
17. Powell RW, Dyess DL, Luterman A, et al: Necrotizing enterocolitis in multiple-birth infants. J Pediatr Surg 1990; 25:319–321.
18. Ballance WA, Dahms BB, Shenker N, et al: Pathology of neonatal necrotizing enterocolitis: A ten-year experience. J Pediatr 1990; 117:S6–S13.
19. Tracey KJ, Beutler B, Lowry SF, et al: Shock and tissue injury induced by recombinant human cachectin. Science 1986; 234:470–474.
20. Caplan MS, Hsueh W: Necrotizing enterocolitis: Role of platelet activating factor, endotoxin, and tumor necrosis factor. J Pediatr 1990; 117:S47–S51.
21. Nowicki P: Intestinal ischemia and necrotizing enterocolitis. J Pediatr 1990; 117:S14–S19.
22. Coombs RC, Morgan MEI, Durbin GM, et al: Gut blood flow velocities in the newborn: Effects of patent ductus arteriosus and parenteral indomethacin. Arch Dis Child 1990; 65:1067–1071.
23. Downing GJ, Horner SR, Kilbride HW: Characteristics of perinatal cocaine-exposed infants with necrotizing enterocolitis. Am J Dis Child 1991; 145:26–27.
24. Hackett GA, Campbell S, Gamsu H, et al: Doppler studies in the growth retarded fetus and prediction of neonatal necrotising enterocolitis, haemorrhage, and neonatal morbidity. Brit Med J 1987; 294:13–16.
25. Hoy C, Millar MR, MacKay P, et al: Quantitative changes in faecal microflora preceding necrotising enterocolitis in premature neonates. Arch Dis Child 1990; 65:1057–1059.
26. Eibl MM, Wolf HM, Furnkranz H, et al: Prevention of necrotizing enterocolitis in low-birth-weight infants by IgA-IgG feeding. N Engl J Med 1988; 319:1–7.
27. Clark DA, Miller MJS: Intraluminal pathogenesis of necrotizing enterocolitis. J Pediatr 1990; 117:S64–S67.
28. Cheu HW, Brown DR, Rowe MI: Breath hydrogen excretion as a screening test for the early diagnosis of necrotizing enterocolitis. Am J Dis Child 1989; 143:156–158.
29. Wilde J, Yolken R, Willoughby R, et al: Improved detection of rotavirus shedding by polymerase chain reaction. Lancet 1991; 337:323–326.
30. Scheifele DW: Role of bacterial toxins in neonatal necrotizing enterocolitis. J Pediatr 1990; 117:S44–S46.
31. Rotbart HA, Johnson ZT, Reller LB: Analysis of enteric coagulase-negative staphylococci from neonates with necrotizing enterocolitis. Pediatr Infect Dis J 1989; 8:140–142.
32. Fink MP, Cohn SM, Lee PC, et al: Effect of lipopolysaccharide on intestinal intramucosal hydrogen ion concentration in pigs: Evidence of gut ischemia in a normodynamic model of septic shock. Crit Care Med 1989; 17:641–646.
33. Buras R, Guzzetta P, Avery G, et al: Acidosis and hepatic portal venous gas: Indications for surgery in necrotizing enterocolitis. Pediatrics 1986; 78:273–277.
34. Brill PW, Olson SR, Winchester P: Neonatal necrotizing enterocolitis: Air in Morison pouch. Radiology 1990; 174:469–471.
35. Weinberg B, Peralta VE, Diakoumakis EE et al: Sonographic findings in necrotizing enterocolitis with paucity of abdominal gas as the initial symptom. Mt Sinai J Med 1989; 56:330–333.
36. Dugdale AE: Breast milk and necrotising enterocolitis. Lancet 1991; 337:435.
37. Halac E, Halac J, Begue EF, et al: Prenatal and postnatal corticosteroid therapy to prevent neonatal necrotizing enterocolitis: A controlled trial. J Pediatr 1990; 117:132–138.
38. Cullen DJ, Coyle JP, Teplick R, et al: Cardiovascular, pulmonary, and renal effects of massively increased intra-abdominal pressure in critically ill patients. Crit Care Med 1989; 17:118–121.
39. Richards WO, Scovill W, Baekhyo S, et al: Acute renal failure associated with increased intra-abdominal pressure. Ann Surg 1983; 197:183–187.

40. Celoria G, Steingrub J, Dawson JA, et al: Oliguria from high intraabdominal pressure secondary to ovarian mass. Crit Care Med 1987; 15:78–79.
41. Rotbart H, Levin M: How contagious is necrotizing enterocolitis? Pediatr Infect Dis 1983; 2:406–413.
42. Scheifele DW, Bjornson GL, Dyer RA, et al: Delta-like toxin produced by coagulase-negative staphylococci is associated with neonatal necrotizing enterocolitis. Infect Immun 1987; 55:2268–2273.
43. Scheifele DW, Ginter GL, Olsen E, et al: Comparison of two antibiotic regimens for neonatal necrotizing enterocolitis. J Antimicrobial Chemotherapy 1987; 20:421–429.
44. Rackow EC, Astiz ME, Weil MH: Cellular oxygen metabolism during sepsis and shock: The relationship of oxygen consumption to oxygen delivery. JAMA 1988; 259:1989–1993.
45. Natanson C, Danner RL, Elin RJ, et al: Role of endotoxemia in cardiovascular dysfunction and mortality: *Escherichia coli* and *Staphylococcus aureus* challenges in a canine model of human septic shock. J Clin Invest 1989; 83:243–251.
46. Carcillo JA, Pollack MM, Ruttimann UE, et al: Sequential physiologic interactions in pediatric cardiogenic and septic shock. Crit Care Med 1989; 17:12–16.

Chapter 62

Protracted Diarrhea

JOHN T. BOYLE

Pediatric gastroenterology continues to use a list of vague "traditional" adjectives to classify a variety of specific and nonspecific disorders. *Intractable* and *protracted* are two such adjectives. When applied to the description of diarrhea, the term *intractable* was originally used to describe all known and unknown causes of chronic noninfectious diarrhea.[1] More recently, both adjectives have been used interchangeably to classify all infectious and noninfectious causes of chronic diarrhea resulting from or causing chronic malnutrition, including those that respond to specific dietary, pharmacologic, or surgical therapy and those that are refractory to any kind of therapy.[2, 3] The downside of this all-encompassing terminology has been a confusing literature regarding the differential diagnosis, treatment, and prognosis.

A redefinition of terminology is needed to streamline differential diagnosis, characterize pathophysiology, evaluate treatment outcomes, and better understand prognosis. The adjective *protracted* means prolonged or chronic but connotes severe, mysterious, or out of the ordinary. The adjective *intractable* implies resistant to all forms of therapy, fatal. The term *protracted* is more appropriate to describe a classification of severe chronic diarrhea distinct from the common infectious, dietary, and functional causes of chronic diarrhea; distinct from disorders of maldigestion (e.g., pancreatic insufficiency, disaccharidase deficiency); and distinct from short bowel syndrome. The differential diagnosis includes disorders that dramatically alter the processes that normally regulate the balance between intestinal absorption and secretion. In this chapter, *protracted diarrhea* is defined as severe diarrhea (greater than 20 ml per kg per day) that begins any time after birth, persists for more than 2 weeks, and requires change in not only the composition but also the mode of delivery of nutrition. The most frequent causes of protracted diarrhea are idiopathic and produce both osmotic and secretory diarrhea because of severe mucosal injury. Present evidence suggests that severe mucosal injury may be caused by genetic defects in epithelial proliferation and differentiation or by disorders of immune regulation. Other disorders causing protracted diarrhea include congenital mucosal ion transport defects, tumors that produce high circulating levels of intestinal secretagogues, functional or mechanical bowel obstruction, and certain uncommon intraluminal infections.

CLINICAL PRESENTATION

Protracted diarrhea is primarily a disorder of infancy. In the majority of patients reported in the United States, the onset of symptoms is before 3 months of age. In contrast, in third world countries, onset of protracted diarrhea is as likely to occur between 6 and 12 months of age in patients with antecedent chronic malnutrition. In the United States, two patterns of presentation are observed. Rarely, fulminant diarrhea may begin at birth or during the first few days of life. In such infants, prematurity and polyhydramnios are common. More commonly—especially today with early postpartum discharge—diarrhea begins at home in the first few weeks of life and is often associated with anorexia and vomiting. Because the symptoms are suggestive of viral gastroenteritis or milk protein allergy, the initial therapeutic approach is most often dietary manipulation, which many times seems to result in transient improvement. Routine stool cultures are usually not performed at the onset of diarrhea. Usually within a period of days, symptoms recur or exacerbate. Recurrent use of oral hydration fluids or persistent attempts to find a formula that an infant will tolerate delay diagnosis and are probably the major reasons that evidence of malnutrition may be present by the time of hospitalization. In fact, chronic poor weight gain is usually the stimulus for hospitalization rather than acute dehydration. In the hospital, introduction of intravenous feedings and complete bowel rest may cause the diarrhea and vomiting to lessen or even disappear, suggesting that the symptoms are indeed related to food intake. However, attempts at refeeding, most often with one of the commercial formulas containing hydrolyzed casein and glucose polymers (Pregestimil, Nutramigen, Alimentum), are again associated with exacerbation of the diarrhea. Although not emphasized in the literature, persistent anorexia and vomiting may also limit the ability to provide adequate nutrition via the oral route. In many infants anorexia and vomiting, and not diarrhea, are the initial impetus to beginning supplemental nasogastric feeding after initial intravenous nutritional rehabilitation. Over time, persistence of the diarrhea becomes the major factor determining management. In patients in whom a treatable entity is not discovered, evidence of both osmotic and secretory diarrhea becomes obvious in that diarrhea persists despite total intravenous feedings.

DIFFERENTIAL DIAGNOSIS

Table 62–1 suggests a differential diagnosis of protracted diarrhea. It does not include common enteric infections, dietary protein-induced enteropathies such as cow's milk protein allergy or celiac disease, or congenital disorders of carbohydrate digestion and transport such as congenital lactase deficiency, sucrase-isomaltase deficiency, or glucose-galactose malabsorption. The development of chronic severe diarrhea following primary enteric bacterial, viral, or parasitic infection is rare without antecedent mucosal injury from malnutrition, cow's or soy milk protein allergy, bacterial overgrowth, or immunodeficiency.[2, 4–9] Similarly, by their very definition, dietary protein-induced enteropathies and disorders of carbohydrate digestion and transport should respond to withdrawal of the offending antigen or substrate from the diet.[10, 11] No direct data exist to link dietary protein-induced enteropathy to a protracted hypersensitivity disorder once the suspected antigen has been removed from the diet. Although enteric infection or acquired protein intolerance should not be classified as entities responsible for protracted diarrhea, they may act as the stimulus that unmasks a genetic disorder of immune regulation or epithelial renewal.

Congenital Transport Defects

To date, there have only been a few congenital transport defects associated with protracted diarrhea. *Congenital chloride diarrhea* (chloridorrhea) is a rare autosomal recessive disorder resulting from a selective defect in the Cl, HCO_3 exchange transport system in the epithelium of the ileum and colon.[12–15] The net effect is high chloride concentration in the stool. Prematurity and polyhydramnios are common. Abdominal distention and severe secretory diarrhea are present from birth. Electrolyte disturbances in untreated patients include hyponatremia, hypochloremia, and alkalosis. Treatment consists of initial intravenous rehydration and electrolyte replacement followed by daily oral replacement of ongoing diarrheal losses of Na^+, Cl^-, and water. This can be accomplished with a commercial oral rehydration fluid plus supplemental NaCl and KCl titrated to maintain normal serum electrolytes. Normal growth and development can be expected despite lifelong diarrhea.

Two patients have been reported with evidence of a specific *defect in Na^+,H^+exchange* in ileal and colonic epithelium.[16, 17] The clinical presentation resembled congenital chloride diarrhea in that the patients had evidence of polyhydramnios, abdominal distention, and secretory diarrhea beginning at birth. In contrast to congenital chloride diarrhea, however, the patients became acidotic and stool electrolytes showed high Na^+, in excess of Cl^-. Daily oral replacement of ongoing diarrheal losses of Na^+, Cl^-, and water with a commercial glucose-based oral rehydration fluid plus supplemental sodium citrate corrected serum electrolytes and allowed for normal growth, suggesting that uncoupled Na^+ transport and Na^+ coupled with organic solutes remain intact.

Two patients have been reported with suspected *primary bile acid malabsorption* as a cause of protracted diarrhea.[18, 19] Both had onset of profuse osmotic diarrhea at 2 days of age with introduction of feedings. Diagnostic evaluation revealed carbohydrate and fat malabsorption despite evidence of normal pancreatic function and normal histology and electron microscopy of the proximal jejunum and ileum. Because in vitro studies indicated a defect in bile acid transport, the authors speculated that primary bile acid malabsorption was the primary cause of both patients' diarrhea. The failure of cholestyramine to significantly reduce stool weight in either patient, together with subsequent adult studies that have shown that most patients with idiopathic chronic diarrhea have bile acid malabsorption, suggests that the abnormality in the above patients could as likely be a manifestation of an underlying intestinal motility or absorptive defect rather than the primary cause of diarrhea.[20]

Transport defects such as congenital enterokinase deficiency,[21] acrodermatitis enteropathica,[22] and Menkes' disease[23] may be associated with chronic diarrhea, vomiting, and failure to thrive. Rarely is there a secretory component to the diarrhea. The patients may fulfill criteria for protracted diarrhea because the diarrhea persists despite elemental diets, often necessitating parenteral nutrition.

Table 62–1. DIFFERENTIAL DIAGNOSIS OF PROTRACTED DIARRHEA

Congenital Transport Defects
Congenital chloride diarrhea
Congenital sodium diarrhea
Primary bile acid malabsorption
Intestinal Obstruction
Hirschsprung's disease
Congenital or acquired small bowel obstruction
Enteric fistula
Secretory Tumors
Neural crest tumors
Primary Infection
Adherent *E. coli*
Bacterial overgrowth
Drug Induced
Laxatives
Iatrogenic
Idiopathic Villus Atrophy
Congenital microvillus atrophy
Associated with immunodeficiency
Severe combined immunodeficiency
Common variable immunodeficiency
AIDS
Autoimmune enteropathy

Intestinal Obstruction

The basis for intestinal obstruction as a cause of protracted diarrhea comes from anecdotal case reports describing chronic secretory diarrhea in patients with enterocolitis complicating Hirschsprung's disease,[24] or in patients with partial bowel obstruction from stenosis of the small intestine.[25] Such patients have significant abdominal distention but may not always have vomiting. Evidence of rectal bleeding is rare. Protracted diarrhea has even been reported in ultrashort-segment Hirschsprung's disease.[26] The exact mechanisms for the protracted diarrhea are unknown. Distended bowel proximal to an intestinal stenosis (e.g., congenital stenosis following necrotizing enterocolitis or complicating severe small bowel inflammation) or an adynamic segment of bowel (e.g., Hirschsprung's disease) may result in neuroimmunomodulation of intestinal transport processes or motor programs, perhaps triggered by bacterial stasis. From animal experiments it is known that powerful bursts of contractions recur at frequent intervals proximal to an intestinal obstruction, presumably as the bowel attempts to overcome the obstruction.[27] Animal experiments also suggest that mucosal inflammation and secretion may develop in the distended bowel.[28, 29] Surgical treatment of stenosis or Hirschsprung's disease usually results in resolution of the diarrhea. Enterocolitis complicating Hirschsprung's disease, however, may recur at any age and time postoperatively, suggesting permanent alteration in the factors that modulate transport and motility in the proximal bowel (see Chapter 54).[30]

Secretory Tumors

Protracted diarrhea (associated with hypokalemia, flushing spells, and occasionally achlorhydria) may be the predominant clinical manifestation of neural crest tumors in children, including ganglioneuroma, ganglioneuroblastoma, and neuroblastoma.[31–36] The earliest reported age at presentation has been 6 months. The retroperitoneum, posterior mediastinum, and pancreas are the most likely areas of tumor origin. Such tumors have been found to contain cells capable of secreting catecholamines, glucagon, gastrin, secretin, gastric inhibitory polypeptide, and vasoactive intestinal polypeptide (VIP). Because of elevated plasma levels of VIP in most reported patients, the polypeptide has been incriminated as the secretagogue mediating the diarrhea. Circumstantial evidence to support this hypothesis is provided by prolonged VIP IV infusion studies in animals and healthy volunteers in which increased plasma VIP levels produced profuse secretory diarrhea.[37, 38] Although levels of catecholamines and related metabolites in the urine are elevated in most patients, there has been no observed correlation between the level of these substances and development of protracted diarrhea, suggesting that they are unlikely causative agents for the diarrhea. Neural crest tumors are the only tumors reported to produce VIP and protracted diarrhea in children. Surgical removal of the VIP-secreting tumor results in resolution of the secretory diarrhea.

Secretory diarrhea associated with somatostatinoma, glucagonoma, multiple endocrine neoplasia, and carcinoid syndrome has not been reported to date in children. It is important to emphasize that elevation of plasma VIP levels in patients with protracted diarrhea is not diagnostic for a polypeptide-secreting tumor. Elevated plasma VIP levels have also been reported in patients with protracted diarrhea associated with severe mucosal injury[39] and nonspecific hyperplasia of non-beta islet cells in the pancreas[40] (see Chapter 70).

Infection

As stated above, viral gastroenteritis and enterotoxin-producing bacteria are rarely primary causes of protracted diarrhea without antecedent mucosal injury from malnutrition, cow's or soy milk protein allergy, or bacterial overgrowth.[2, 4–9] Chronic enteric infections are also well-described complications of primary or secondary immunodeficiency states.[41–46] Protracted severe diarrheal illness may be caused by opportunistic pathogens such as *Cryptosporidium*, Microsporida, cytomegalovirus (CMV), *Isospora belli, Mycobacterium avium-intracellulare*, or coccidiosis in patients with acquired immunodeficiency[47–49] (see Chapter 56).

It is controversial whether bacterial overgrowth of the proximal small bowel can be a primary cause of protracted diarrhea in children.[9] Protracted diarrhea has been reported to result from sporadic colonization of the small bowel by enteropathogenic strains of *Escherichia coli*. These strains are neither enterotoxigenic nor enteroinvasive, but exhibit localized attaching and effacing adherence to enterocyte brush borders.[50–54] The pathogenesis of the diarrhea has been hypothesized to be related to enterocyte damage, perhaps related to damage to the glycocalyx, microvillus borders, and terminal webs at the sites of bacterial adherence.[54] Diagnosis is suspected by culturing reported strains from duodenal aspirates and is confirmed by small bowel histology showing patchy villus atrophy and electron microscopy showing enterocyte-adherent organisms. The best evidence that adherent *E. coli* is a primary cause of protracted diarrhea is anecdotal reports of prompt resolution of the diarrhea following intravenous gentamicin therapy.[50, 53] In other reports, diarrhea may persist for several months, particularly in malnourished patients, suggesting the possibility of opportunistic infection.[54]

Drug-Induced Diarrhea

Protracted diarrhea in children may be a clinical manifestation of child abuse or Munchausen's syndrome.[55] In this scenario a parent surreptitiously induces diarrhea in the child by giving laxatives, a well-recognized pathogenesis of secretory diarrhea in adults.[56–58] Diagnosis should be suspected if past, family, or social history indicates a potential for abuse. The clinical picture of surreptitious laxative ingestion includes abdominal pain, vomiting, muscle weakness, lassitude, hypokalemia, and nonspecific inflammation and/or melanosis on rectal biopsy. The latter finding of mild colitis often confuses the diagnostic picture by suggesting an organic disorder.[59] Diagnosis of laxative abuse is dependent on a high index of suspicion, the stool electrolyte pattern, and chemical testing of the stool and urine (see below).

Protracted diarrhea may also be iatrogenic. A case of protracted diarrhea has been reported in which the vehicle for suspending an active drug for oral preparation was responsible for apparent secretory diarrhea.[60] A comatose adolescent developed apparent secretory diarrhea when he was receiving no enteral feedings except nasogastric administration of hydralazine hydrochloride, furosemide, diphenylhydantoin, propranolol hydrochloride, and hydrocortisone. The physicians caring for the patient were unaware that the hydralazine was prepared by mixing hydralazine hydrochloride injection with a 70% solution of sorbitol. The osmotic nature of the diarrhea was suspected by the sodium and chloride concentrations within the stool, which were consistently less than 50 mEq per L. The case points out the importance of determining the vehicle of any enteral medication being given to a patient with protracted diarrhea.

Idiopathic Villus Atrophy

The majority of cases of protracted diarrhea in the United States are associated with severe mucosal injury of unknown etiology. Atrophy of the mucosa may occur with or without inflammation in the lamina propria and epithelium. The mucosal lesion probably represents the final common pathway for a number of pathogenic mechanisms. Three distinct diagnostic subgroups have been differentiated to date under this classification.

Congenital Microvillus Atrophy.[61–66] Protracted diarrhea in this autosomal recessive disorder begins at birth or within the first week of life. All patients require total parenteral nutrition for survival. Small bowel biopsies show total villus atrophy (Fig. 62–1). The length of the crypts appears normal, but there is no evidence of mitotic activity. The lamina propria appears normal or has a mild nonspecific increase in cellularity. Although the enterocytes retain their columnar shape, electron microscopy reveals shortened and irregular microvilli. The apical cytoplasm of the enterocytes contains a mixture of round to oval electron-dense lysosomal inclusions or cystic structures, suggestive of invaginated brush borders. Although intact, terminal webs of villus cells are distorted. In contrast to the villus cells, the ultrastructure of the crypt cells is preserved. Ultrastructural abnormalities have also been demonstrated in colonic, biliary, and renal epithelium.

Although unproven, the restriction of the abnormality to the absorptive cells suggests a failure of normal maturation and differentiation of crypt cells. To date, no effective therapy is available.

Immunologic Deficiency. When the literature is examined critically, protracted diarrhea is a predominant clinical manifestation only in patients with primary combined immunodeficiencies, including severe combined immunodeficiency (SCID) and common variable immunodeficiency (CVID), and in patients with acquired immunodeficiency syndrome (AIDS).[41, 42, 46–48, 66, 67] Protracted diarrhea is rarely associated with disorders of antibody production (agammaglobulinemia, selective immunoglobulin A [IgA] deficiency, defects of phagocytic function, or complement deficiencies), unless there is evidence of concomitant T cell deficiency. Isolated reports of intractable diarrhea with flat jejunal mucosa and selective IgA deficiency, unresponsive to a gluten-free diet, have not included detailed studies of T cell function.[68]

A primary immunodeficiency state or AIDS should be suspected in patients with chronic diarrhea who have (1) persistently positive cultures for viral or bacterial agents that normally cause self-limited diarrhea; (2) recurrent otitis media, sinusitis, or bronchopulmonary infection; (3) opportunistic infections with pathogens such as *Candida albicans*, CMV, *Cryptosporidium*, Microsporida, *I. belli*, *Mycobacterium avium-intracellulare*, or coccidiosis; (4) skin lesions such as generalized erythema, desquamation, eczema, seborrhea, telangiectasia, or abnormal hair; or (5) recurrent hematologic abnormalities, including aplastic anemia, hemolytic anemia, neutropenia, or thrombocytopenia.

SCID is actually used to describe multiple hereditary syndromes characterized by a functional deficiency of both cellular and humoral immunity, with clinical symptoms beginning in the first few months of life.[69] In most cases the underlying molecular defect is unknown. Two notable exceptions are SCID associated with a deficiency of an enzyme of purine metabolism[70] and class I–II major histocompatibility complex (MHC) deficiency syndrome, in which there is an absence of MHC antigens on the cell membranes of lymphocytes.[71] CVID is primarily distinguished from SCID by later onset of combined immune dysfunction.[67]

SCID or CVID should be considered the primary mechanisms facilitating protracted diarrhea in infants with or without a positive family history if there is (1) the clinical phenotype described above; (2) evidence of B cell dysfunction, including low or fluctuating levels of immunoglobulins and absence of specific antibodies directed against exogenous antigens; and (3) evidence of T cell dysfunction, including variable lymphopenia, cutaneous anergy, and evidence of abnormal in vitro lymphocyte response to mitogens or encountered antigens (CMV, *Candida*). Small bowel biopsies may or may not be helpful. Absence of plasma cells in the lamina propria and "foamy" macrophages in the intestinal villi suggest immunodeficiency.[46]

A distinct subset of children with combined immunodeficiency syndromes may manifest autoimmune disorders.[67] In fact, the autoimmune manifestations and not infections may be the major clinical problems. A primary immune disorder may not be recognized because some patients have fluctuating serum concentrations of immunoglobulins, and T cell abnormalities may be mild and nonspecific. Manifestations of autoimmune disease in CVID may include idiopathic thrombocytopenia, autoimmune hemolytic anemia, neutropenia, chronic active hepatitis, parotiditis, arthritis, or Guillain-

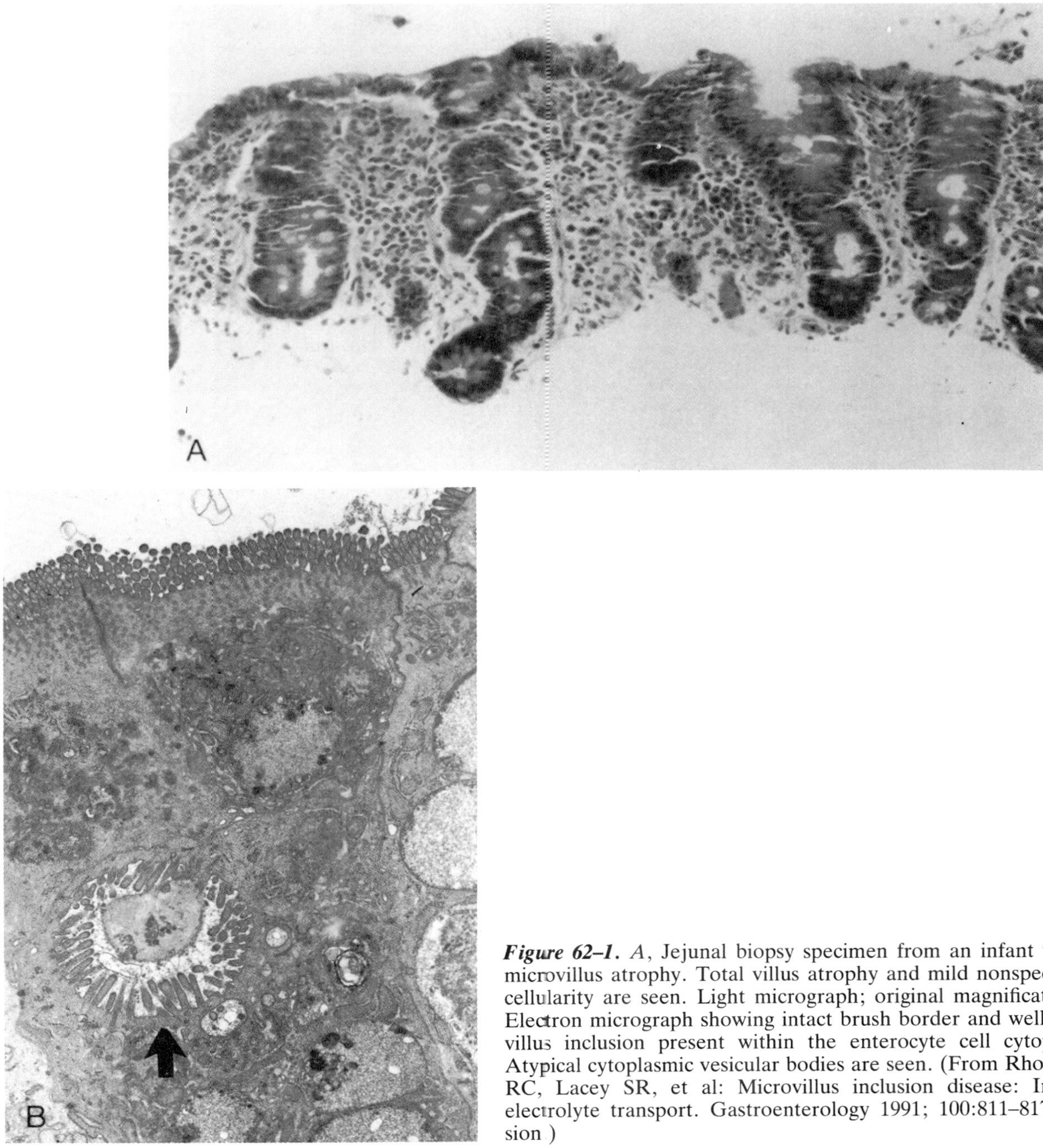

Figure 62–1. *A*, Jejunal biopsy specimen from an infant with congenital microvillus atrophy. Total villus atrophy and mild nonspecific increase in cellularity are seen. Light micrograph; original magnification × 100. *B*, Electron micrograph showing intact brush border and well-formed microvillus inclusion present within the enterocyte cell cytoplasm (*arrow*). Atypical cytoplasmic vesicular bodies are seen. (From Rhoads JM, Vogler RC, Lacey SR, et al: Microvillus inclusion disease: In vitro jejunal electrolyte transport. Gastroenterology 1991; 100:811–817; with permission.)

Barré syndrome. In patients reported to date, laboratory studies reveal an increase in the ratio of T cells expressing the T helper phenotype to T cells expressing the T suppressor phenotype and markedly diminished in vitro antibody production by B cells. The prognosis for such patients is poor, although the clinical course may be improved by immunosuppressive therapy. So-called refractory sprue (enteropathy beginning after 1 year of age that is histologically identical to celiac disease but responds to immunosuppressive therapy rather than a gluten-free diet) may indeed be CVID presenting as an autoimmune phenomenon.[72]

AIDS has become important in the differential diagnosis of immunodeficiency disease in infants and children. The human immunodeficiency virus (HIV) produces a generalized disturbance of regulatory pathways in the immune system. AIDS should be suspected in any infant with protracted diarrhea and evidence of T cell immune deficiency. The distinctive immunologic profile of T cell immunodeficiency (reduced helper-suppressor cell ratio), polyclonal hypergammaglobulinemia, and antibodies to HIV is not found in other primary or secondary immunodeficiency disorders.

Autoimmune Enteropathy.[66, 73–80] A number of reports have described a subgroup of patients with protracted diarrhea who have features of autoimmune disease including circulating enterocyte autoantibodies and concurrent extraintestinal disease. Both familial and sporadic cases have been described. The preponderance of cases reported to date have been in males. The diarrhea usually begins between 2 and 4 weeks of age, but initially it is not fulminant. Rarely is a precipitating infectious disorder identified. Short-lived improvement may follow sequential dietary changes, but the overall course is progressive. The onset of a secretory component to the diarrhea may be delayed until after 2 months of age. Histology reveals evidence of a generalized inflammatory disorder affecting both the small intestine and colonic mucosa (Fig. 62–2). Small bowel biopsy reveals villus atrophy and diffuse nonspecific inflammation in the lamina propria. In most cases, there is crypt hyperplasia with increased mitoses similar to celiac disease. The finding of crypt abscesses, crypt hypoplasia, or decreased crypt mitoses is considered a poor prognostic sign.[66] Electron microscopy reveals shortened, disrupted microvilli, swollen mitochondria, and lysosomal bodies. Colonic biopsy specimens reveal variable degrees of inflammation in the lamina propria, goblet cell depletion, and crypt distortion. Rarely, colonic inflammation may be severe enough to cause gross rectal bleeding. Tests of T and B cell function are characteristically normal. Serum immunoglobulin concentrations may reflect the degree of protein-losing enteropathy with decreases in IgG and normal IgA and IgM. The immunologic marker of this disorder that suggests an autoimmune phenomenon is the detection of circulating antienterocyte antibodies by indirect immunofluorescence. IgG, IgA, and IgM autoantibodies have been reported in individual patients. Circulating antibodies against renal epithelial cells, anti–smooth muscle antibodies, antinuclear antibodies, and antithyroid microsomal antibodies have also been described in individual cases. Most patients at some time in their clinical course develop evidence of at least one concurrent extraintestinal autoimmune disorder, including membranous glomerulonephritis, interstitial nephritis, hypothyroidism, hemolytic anemia, thrombocytopenia, type 1 diabetes mellitus, Sjögren's syndrome, and polyarthritis. In many cases reported to date, immunosuppressive treatment with a variety of agents allowed partial improvement of the diarrhea. A relapsing pattern of the clinical course is characteristic, and patients are rarely able to be weaned off the immunosuppressive therapy. Response to therapy and long-term prognosis seem to depend on the severity of the diarrhea and histologic lesions. A relatively favorable evolution was reported in patients who had a fecal output lower than 80 ml per kg per day, villus atrophy without crypt damage, and only mild colonic inflammation.[66]

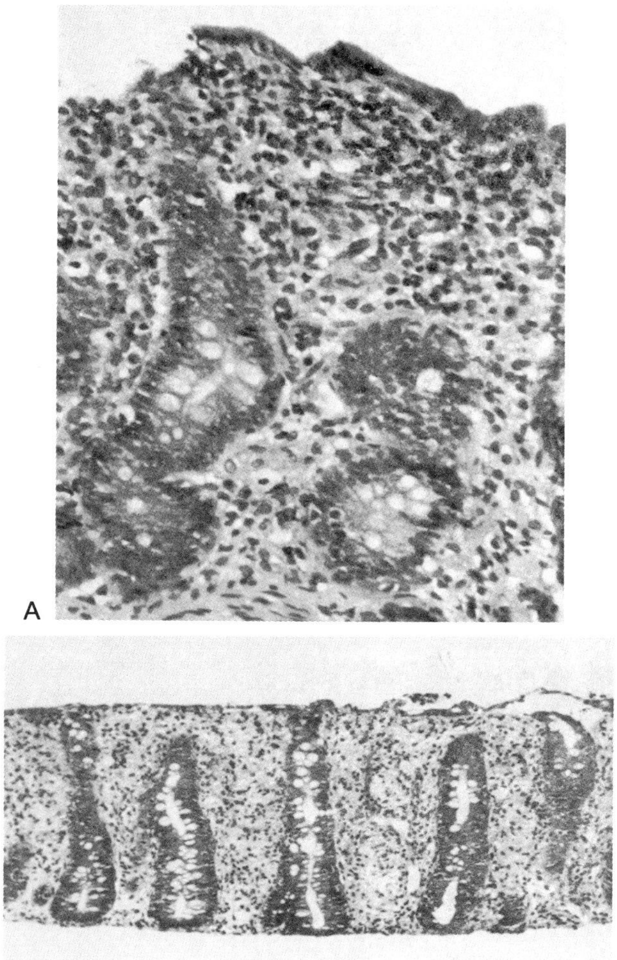

A

B

Figure 62–2. *A*, Jejunal biopsy specimen from an infant with autoimmune enteropathy. Severe villus atrophy and crypt hyperplasia are present. Original magnification × 250. (From Colletti RB, Guillot AP, Rosen S, et al: Autoimmune enteropathy and nephropathy with circulating autoantibodies. J Pediatr 1991; 118:853–864; with permission.) *B*, Histologic appearance of typical autoimmune colitis. Note preservation of crypt architecture, irregularity of surface epithelium, and increased cellularity of the lamina propria. Original magnification × 250. (From Hill SM, Milla PJ, Bottazzo GF, et al: Autoimmune enteropathy and colitis: Is there a generalized autimmune gut disorder? Gut 1991; 32:36–42; with permission.)

The pathogenesis of autoimmune enteropathy is unknown. No specific human leukocyte antigen (HLA) genotype has been identified. It has been speculated that the enterocyte autoantibodies are cytotoxic, since they have been reported to fix complement. To date, however, autoantibodies have not been demonstrated in situ. Moreover, it is not clear whether the appearance of autoantibodies precedes or follows the intestinal lesion. An alternative hypothesis is that activated mucosal T cells directed toward a "self antigen" are responsible for the mucosal injury either by direct cytotoxicity against epithelial cells or by secretion of lymphokines.[66] Defective expression of HLA class II molecules in the crypt epithelium of both the small and large intestine has been reported in this disorder, suggesting a regulatory gene defect.[81] These aberrant products may favor presentation of epithelial surface autoantigens that may initiate or sustain abnormal intestinal T cell activation. It may be that in the initial stages of the disease, intestinal bacterial or dietary foreign protein may be the stimulus for activated mucosal T cells. Alternatively, as a consequence of the initial inflammatory process, local tissue antigens may be released, which may be the stimulus for a subsequent autoimmune response in genetically susceptible individuals.

Autoimmune enteropathy resembles Crohn's disease in that both small and large bowels are involved, there are similar features of immune activation, and there may be a similar response to immunosuppressive therapy. However, in autoimmune enteropathy, no granuloma has been identified in biopsies of either the small bowel or colon. Crohn's disease has been reported in infancy in patients presenting with partial small bowel obstruction (occasionally associated with secretory diarrhea).[82] At surgery, localized segments of small bowel have been resected that contain transmural inflammation, but no granuloma. In some cases, disease has not recurred; in others, a more diffuse mucosal inflammatory process develops, requiring immunosuppressive therapy. The exact mechanism of the inflammatory process in these patients is not clear.

Autoimmune enteropathy may indeed be associated with a heterogeneous group of disorders. Even without knowledge of the exact pathogenesis, the presence of circulating enterocyte autoantibodies or the presence of extraintestinal autoimmune disease justifies immunosuppressive therapy with or without evidence of primary immunodeficiency.

Pathogenesis of Diarrhea in Idiopathic Villus Atrophy

Three factors contribute in variable degrees to the production of protracted diarrhea: alteration of mucosal morphology, active intestinal secretion, and altered intestinal motility (Table 62–2).

Alteration of Mucosal Morphology. The digestive tract of healthy mammals is an organ of conservation as well as assimilation.[83–85] Not only does the gastrointestinal tract receive, mix, digest, and absorb widely variable and unpredictable amounts of food with remarkable efficiency, but it allows considerable quantities of fluid and electrolytes from the extracellular fluid to pass across the mucosa into the gut lumen and be reabsorbed. Paramount to understanding the movements of fluid in the gut is an appreciation that both active absorptive and secretory processes function simultaneously in both the small intestine and the colon. In the adult human, the total load of water and electrolytes that is presented daily to the intestines approximates the extracellular fluid compartment of the body (8 to 10 L of water, and more than 1,000 mEq of electrolytes).[83] The contribution of the diet is small (approximately 20%) compared with that of endogenous salivary, gastric, biliary, pancreatic, and small intestinal secretions. Since the normal adult excretes only approximately 0.2 L of fecal water per day, the overall efficiency of reabsorption approaches 98%.[83] Although there are no comparable studies in infants and children, data compiled from a number of studies suggest a comparable efficiency of conservation and assimilation.[85]

Table 62–2. PATHOGENESIS OF DIARRHEA IN IDIOPATHIC VILLUS ATROPHY

Alteration of Mucosal Morphology
Reduced absorptive surface area
Altered epithelial turnover
Altered mucosal permeability
Expanded crypts
Loss of colonic salvaging function
Active Intestinal Secretion
Exaggeration of normal physiology caused by increased production or release of multiple neurohumoral paracrine substances by the enteric nervous system and immune system
Altered Intestinal Motility

Altered mucosal morphology results in a reversal of net fluid and electrolyte absorption to net intraluminal fluid electrolyte accumulation. Accumulation of intraluminal fluid and electrolytes results from malabsorption of dietary constituents and bile acids, imbalance of normal ion transport processes, and loss of colonic salvage capacity.

Malabsorption results from loss of intestinal absorptive surface area and functional changes in absorptive capacity along the villus-crypt unit. Cytodifferentiation of the normal gastrointestinal epithelium is largely completed by birth.[86] The epithelial surface area of the gastrointestinal tract is increased three times (relative to a cylinder) by the small intestinal valvulae conniventes. The villus-crypt units increase the surface area another tenfold. The microvilli that coat the luminal surface of the epithelial cells increase the surface area another twentyfold. The net result is that the surface area is increased some 600 times relative to a cylinder. Villus atrophy or microvillus shortening or destruction may dramatically reduce effective absorptive area not only for dietary constituents but also for bile acids.

Evidence also suggests that enterocytes mature both morphologically and biochemically while migrating from the crypts to become digestive-absorptive cells of the villus. The enzyme distribution patterns on the villus-crypt unit suggest a high degree of functional differentiation associated with enterocyte maturity. Lactase, fatty acid esterification activity, and lipid esterifying enzymes are primarily localized to the apical villus.[87, 88] Evidence has also been found for sequential development of transport systems along the villus-crypt axis. Autoradiography suggests that only the enterocytes in the top third of the villus transport sugars and amino acids in vivo.[89] This functional differentiation of the villus-crypt unit may be adversely affected by disorders that affect enterocyte differentiation such as may occur in congenital microvillus atrophy as well as by disorders that result in mucosal injury in which compensatory attempts at epithelial renewal may result in increased rates of cell migration up the villus-crypt unit so that immature cells populate the apical villus. Such aberrations may reduce absorptive function independent of absorptive surface area and contribute significantly to carbohydrate, fat, and protein malabsorption.

Water movement in the intestine is passive and, therefore, governed by osmotic gradients created by transport of solute from one side of the mucosa to the other. Evidence suggests that simultaneous absorptive and secretory processes are carried out by two separate epithelial cell types on the villus-crypt unit.[90] Villus cells are primarily absorptive, and crypt cells are primarily secretory. Net absorption of solute and water depends on the efficient transport properties of the brush border and basolateral membranes of the surface epithelial cells and on the ionic permeability of the pericellular or "shunt" pathway (the tight junction between epithelial cells and the intercellular space) of the villus to absorb water and chloride actively secreted in the basal state in the crypts.[91] Clearly, this balance is affected by immune mediators that activate cells that destroy enterocytes from the villi and increase intestinal permeability, resulting in "leaky membranes." Crypt cell hyperplasia, in an attempt to renew the epithelium in response to injury, may compound the problem by increasing the capacity of active chloride secretion.

Colonic function is often the critical determinant for the development of diarrhea.[92] Active sodium absorption is more effective in the colon, and passive pericellular permeability is markedly decreased compared with that of the proximal bowel. The colon also plays an important role in salvaging calories and decreasing the osmotic gradient from malabsorbed sugars and dietary fiber by passively absorbing short-chain fatty acids resulting from the metabolism of malabsorbed carbohydrate by colonic flora.[93] In the healthy adult, the maximum capacity of the colon to absorb water may be two to three times the normal ileocecal flow.[94] As long as ileocecal flow is less than colonic absorptive capacity, significant alterations in small intestinal fluid movement (even net secretion) may be present, but diarrhea will not occur. In children, ileostomy and stool output studies indicate that this reserve of absorptive capacity may not be as great due to higher ileocecal flow per body weight.[95] Thus, in infants and children, when small intestinal absorption and ileocecal flow are normal, a relatively small decrease in colonic absorption resulting from mucosal injury will produce significant increases in stool water output. If net colonic secretion is present due to "leaky membranes" or increased intracellular messenger concentration resulting from release of neurohumoral-paracrine substances, there will be even greater volumes of stool water.

Active Intestinal Secretion. Absorptive and secretory transport properties are regulated by intracellular messengers including free Ca^{2+}, cyclic adenosine monophosphate, and cyclic guanosine monophosphate.[90] Increased concentrations of these messengers alter conductance channels and protein carriers to inhibit coupled NaCl entry into the villus absorptive cells of the small intestine and proximal colon and stimulate secretion from the crypt epithelium of both the small and large intestine. Stimulators of active secretion in patients with idiopathic villus atrophy include intraluminal factors such as bile acids and hydroxy fatty acids that result from malabsorption[96, 97] and many neurohumoral-paracrine substances (Table 62–3) released or produced by the enteric nervous system and the immune system.[98, 99] Most of the neurohumoral-paracrine substances probably participate in the normal physiology of intestinal secretion and absorption. These substances promote secretion by binding to membrane receptors and increasing the concentrations of the intracellular messengers. The gut most likely is converted into a secretory organ by exaggerations of normal physiology. Particularly important in exaggerating secretion may be the mediators of the inflammatory process, including arachidonic acid metabolites, cytokines, bacterial products (endotoxin and chemotactic peptide made by bacteria), and immune mediators released by many of the inflammatory cells, such as tumor necrosis factor, interferon, platelet-activating factor, and oxygen radicals.[98, 99] Neurohumoral-paracrine substances can also affect release of other neurohumoral or paracrine stimulators, alter motility, and change blood flow, all of which could potentially affect electrolyte transport.

Table 62–3. NEUROHUMORAL-PARACRINE REGULATORS THAT CAUSE SECRETION

Neurotransmitters	Hormones
Acetylcholine	Angiotensin
Vasoactive intestinal peptide	Cholecystokinin
ATP	Secretin
Serotonin	Bombesin
Substance P	Gastrin
Paracrine Substances	Gastric inhibitory polypeptide
Bradykinin	Motilin
Serotonin	Calcitonin
Neurotensin	Glucagon
Histamine	Vasopressin
Cyclooxygenase pathway products	
Arachidonic acid	
Prostaglandins of E series	

ATP, adenosine triphosphate.

Altered Intestinal Motility. Most authors believe that abnormal motility coexists with disturbed transport in protracted diarrhea because agents that impede motility (opioids and their derivatives) are often helpful in reducing the number and volume of stools. Quantitative data to support this belief, however, are lacking. The nature of the motility changes may be multifactorial.[100, 101] Certainly many of the neurohumoral-paracrine substances that mediate intestinal secretion also affect intestinal motility. To date, however, there are no reports that describe specific alterations in intestinal smooth muscle or the enteric nervous system in protracted diarrhea. Increased intestinal motor activity in the small intestine may also be secondary to distention of the bowel caused by accumulation of intraluminal contents by the mechanisms described above. In animal studies, rapid infusion of saline or hypertonic mannitol into the gut lumen evokes an abnormal motor pattern associated with extremely rapid transit through the intestines. Finally, increased frequency of colonic mass movements or sigmoid hypomotility may allow the unrestrained flow of intestinal contents to gain access to the rectum.

DIAGNOSTIC EVALUATION

Classification of the Diarrhea

Any infant who presents with diarrhea in the first week of life, or any child who is admitted with severe diarrhea of greater than 2 weeks duration associated with weight loss should be given nothing by mouth and started on intravenous nutrition. If the diarrhea ceases within 24 to 48 hours, secretory diarrhea is not present. Rather, a disorder of carbohydrate absorption or protein intolerance is most likely. In such cases, further workup is dictated by age, current diet, and previous dietary manipulation.

Onset of profuse osmotic diarrhea in the first week of life in a breast-fed infant or an infant fed a cow's milk formula suggests congenital lactase deficiency[102] or glucose-galactose malabsorption.[103] Symptoms that persist after a switch to a soy formula (all contain glucose polymers with or without sucrose) suggest the latter diagnosis. Onset of profuse osmotic diarrhea in the first week of life in an infant initially fed a soy formula containing sucrose suggests the possibility of autosomal recessive sucrase-isomaltase deficiency.[104] A presumptive diagnosis can be made by appropriate breath hydrogen testing. Measurement of disaccharidase activities in small intestinal biopsies can be done to confirm the diagnosis. Older infants fed lactose-containing formulas who have sucrase-isomaltase deficiency usually develop diarrhea when sucrose-containing solids are added to the diet.

Today it is rare for an infant or child to be hospitalized for diagnosis and management of severe chronic diarrhea without a previous trial of a formula containing a protein hydrolysate to treat dietary protein intolerance (cow's milk or soy). All such formulas in the United States (Nutramigen, Pregestimil, Alimentum) currently contain glucose polymers as their carbohydrate source. Resolution of diarrhea within 24 to 48 hours of instituting complete bowel rest in such patients suggests the possibility of acquired polymeric glucose intolerance or acquired monosaccharide intolerance. If diarrhea recurs on refeeding with a formula containing a protein hydrolysate and glucose polymers, a trial of a carbohydrate-free formula with added dextrose is recommended.[105] If symptoms still persist, tolerance of fructose as the carbohydrate source suggests a diagnosis of acquired monosaccharide intolerance.[106]

Persistence of diarrhea after instituting complete bowel rest suggests a secretory component to the diarrhea. Active intestinal secretion can be confirmed by measurement of stool osmolality and electrolytes.[107] Freshly assayed diarrheal stool samples have an osmolality between 280 and 330 mOsm per L regardless of whether the diarrhea is osmotic or secretory. An elevated stool osmolality (greater than 330 mOsm per L) indicates ongoing bacterial metabolism due to improper stool storage or severe dehydration. The latter can be differentiated by finding an elevated serum osmolality. A low stool osmolality (less than 280 mOsm per L) implies that water has been added to the stool. One should always measure osmolality on a fresh stool specimen when there is a suspicion of possible factitious diarrhea. If one assumes a constant stool osmolality of 290 mOsm per L in diarrheal stool, the osmotic gap can be estimated by measurement of stool electrolyte concentration. Stool electrolyte concentrations are not affected by bacterial metabolism. Since sodium (Na) and potassium (K) are the major cations in stool, osmolality can be calculated by multiplying by two the stool concentration of Na and K. The osmotic gap then equals 290 − 2(Na + K). In osmotic diarrhea (specific or generalized malabsorption), diarrheal stool has a low Na (less than 50 mEq per L) and an increased osmotic gap (greater than 160 osmole). In secretory diarrhea, the diarrheal stool has a high Na (greater than 90 mEq per L), and the osmotic gap is less than 20 osmole and frequently negative. Stool electrolytes are diagnostic in only one disorder, congenital chloride diarrhea, in which chloride concentration exceeds the sum of Na^+ and K^+.[12]

Evaluation for Infection

All patients should be evaluated for antibodies to HIV. Although infections are rarely the primary cause of protracted diarrhea, routine evaluation for infection is indicated in all patients, including bacterial and viral stool cultures, rotavirus antigen assay, *Clostridium difficile* toxin assay, and stool ova and parasites, including *Cryptosporidium*. Prolonged enteric infection with any of these agents should suggest underlying immunodeficiency.

Biochemical Evaluation

Biochemical evaluation often gives hints to the severity of the diarrheal disorder or to the presence of complications such as small intestinal bacterial overgrowth.[108] The two most helpful tests are the serum albumin test and 1-hour D-xylose test (measurement of blood concentration of D-xylose 1 hour after oral administration of 14.5 gm per m^2). Hypoalbuminemia, attributed to protein-losing enteropathy, indicates a significant disturbance in intestinal mucosal integrity. Abnormal D-xylose may indicate disordered mucosal integrity, disordered gastric emptying, or bacterial overgrowth. An elevated fasting breath H_2 concentration may also indicate bacterial overgrowth.[108] Typical standard tests of malabsorption (breath tests, fecal fat, duodenal trypsin, and lipase) add little as diagnostic tests, since early evaluation of intestinal morphology is indicated in all these patients (see below).

Evaluation of Anatomy

A normal plain flat plate and upright film of the abdomen should not be viewed as sufficient to rule out intestinal obstruction. Partial intestinal obstruction should be excluded by an upper gastrointestinal series with follow-through examination of the small bowel. Barium is the agent of choice unless perforation is suspected. The idea that barium should not be used in partial small bowel obstruction is a myth and has been discredited by numerous investigators.[109] Water-soluble agents become diluted to such an extent that they are of less value in small bowel obstruction. Distended loops of bowel filled with fluid are easily identified when opacified with barium and are the primary indication of an obstructive process. Segmentation and flocculation of barium, thickening of the mucosal folds, and nodular indentation in the mucosa are nonspecific signs that may be caused by a number of disorders and are of little diagnostic value.

Evaluation of Secretory Tumor

Serum VIP levels and urinary vanilmandelic acid (VMA) assay are sufficient to screen for possible secretory tumor.[31–40] Elevations should generate a search for a tumor by ultrasonography, computed tomography (CT) scan, and possibly magnetic resonance imaging (MRI).

Evaluation of Immune Status

Selected tests of immune function should be performed soon after initial intravenous nutritional rehabilitation. Waiting too long runs the risk that secondary factors such as malnutrition, infection, and transfusions will cloud interpretation of the results. The goal of testing is to determine whether an individual patient has any evidence of combined T and B cell immunodeficiency.[110]

Tests for B Cell Deficiency. Quantitative immunoglobulin levels should be compared with those of age-matched control subjects. In general, immunoglobulin levels within 2 standard deviations for age-matched controls are considered normal. An IgG level less than 200 mg per dl or a total immunoglobulin level less than 400 mg per dl usually indicates significant antibody deficiency. Caution must be exercised in interpreting an isolated decrease in serum IgG in patients with severe hypoalbuminemia. A decrease in IgG with normal IgA and IgM is typical of protein-losing enteropathy. Screening tests of antibody function are recommended. IgM antibody function is estimated by isoagglutinin titers (anti-A and/or anti-B). In the immunized subject, antibody titers to poliovirus, tetanus antigen, or diphtheria antigen can be used to estimate IgG function. If unimmunized, antibody titers before and 2 weeks after tetanus or killed poliovirus immunizations should be obtained. An inadequate response (less than a fourfold rise in titer) is suggestive of antibody deficiency regardless of immunoglobulin levels. Antibody response to antigens to which the patient has been exposed (e.g., CMV) also yield evidence of antibody function. IgG subclass determinations are indicated if IgG levels are normal or near normal but antibody function is deficient. Abnormalities of IgG and IgE (both high and low levels) are not uncommon in incomplete antibody deficiency syndromes. IgE levels may be high in chemotactic disorders, partial T cell deficiencies, allergic disorders, and parasitic infection.

Tests for T Cell Deficiency. The presence of lymphopenia ($<2,000$ cells per mm^3) is suggestive of T cell immunodeficiency. An absent thymic shadow in the newborn period also suggests T cell immunodeficiency. Monoclonal antibodies can be used to enumerate T cell numbers and subsets. In most cellular immunodeficiencies, T cells are reduced in proportion to the degree of cellular immune impairment. The ratio between helper and suppressor T cells, normally 2:1, is characteristically reduced in AIDS. T cell function can be screened by delayed hypersensitivity skin tests (*Candida* antigen, tetanus toxoid). The proliferative response of T cells to mitogens (e.g., phytohemagglutinin, pokeweed mitogen, concanavalin A), or antigens to which the patient has previously been exposed (e.g., *Candida*, tetanus, CMV), should be determined when skin tests yield negative or equivocal results. Special procedures are also available to assess production of lymphokines, cytotoxic (natural killer, antibody dependent, or cytotoxic T cell) function, or enzyme (adenosine deaminase [ADA] or nucleoside phosphorylase [PNP]) deficiency.

Indicators of Autoimmune Enteropathy. The most specific indicator of autoimmune enteropathy reported to date is the presence of circulating antiepithelial cell antibodies measured by indirect immunohistology.[75–80] Unfortunately, most hospital and commercial laboratories do not routinely perform this test at this time. Other measures of autoantibody production that are routinely available in most hospital laboratories include antinuclear antibody (ANA), anti-DNA antibody, anti–smooth muscle antibody, antimitochondrial antibody, and rheumatoid factor. A direct Coombs' test should be performed in any patient with evidence of hemolytic anemia. Antiadrenal, anti–glomerular basement membrane, anti–renal tubular, anti–islet cell, antiparietal, antireticulum, antithyroid microsomal, and antithyroglobulin antibody measurements are available from commercial laboratories. However, "fishing" expeditions are rarely fruitful without direct evidence of organ dysfunction outside the gastrointestinal tract.

Although tests of phagocytic and complement deficiencies are often included as part of an immune evaluation, there is no direct evidence that these types of disorders play a primary role in the pathogenesis of protracted diarrhea. Similarly, HLA phenotyping to date has not aided in predicting diagnosis or prognosis. The value of tests for serum immune complexes (Clq binding, conglutinin solid phase assay, polyethylene glycol [PEG] assay, and Raji cell assay) has not been evaluated.[111]

EVALUATION OF INTESTINAL MORPHOLOGY

Small bowel and colonic rectal biopsies are essential to aid in the diagnosis and management of protracted diarrhea. The best chance at establishing a diagnosis requires that the biopsy be performed early in the diagnostic evaluation before the inevitable confounding variables of chronic malnutrition, bacterial overgrowth, or secondary infection ensue. Normal biopsies or mild nonspecific inflammatory changes that do not significantly alter villus-crypt architecture support aggressive evaluation and management of cellular transport defects, secretory tumors, obstruction, or factitious diarrhea. A small bowel biopsy that shows total villus atrophy, normal-appearing or hypoplastic crypts with little evidence of mitotic activity, and a lamina propria that appears normal or has a mild nonspecific increase in cellularity suggests a diagnosis of congenital microvillus atrophy. Routine histology of colonic biopsies in the latter condition is normal. A small bowel biopsy with total or subtotal villus atrophy, normal-appearing or hyperplastic crypts with definite mitotic activity, and mononuclear infiltrate in the lamina propria with or without increased numbers of polymorphonuclear cells or eosinophils suggests immunoadherent *E. coli*, bacterial overgrowth, immunodeficiency, or autoimmune enteropathy. Duodenal fluid should be obtained at the time of small bowel biopsy for aerobic and anaerobic culture. Electron microscopy should be performed on all small bowel biopsies, looking for adherent bacteria, microvillus atrophy, and microvillus inclusions. Evidence of microscopic colitis suggests an immunodeficiency or autoimmune enteropathy.

Intestinal morphology not only aids in diagnosis but directs management by identifying those patients with inflammatory lesions who, in the absence of identifiable enteric infections, become candidates for immunosuppressive therapy. There is no evidence that the degree of mucosal inflammation predicts ultimate clinical prognosis.[112, 113] There is also no evidence that small bowel morphology can be used as an index of a child's ability to tolerate a particular enteral formula. Similarly, quantitation of disaccharidase levels in small bowel biopsies adds little to diagnosis or predicting the clinical response to specific enteral formulas.

MANAGEMENT

Management and diagnosis of protracted diarrhea are concurrent exercises. Specific therapy is instituted if a correctable etiology is found. Management of idiopathic villus atrophy usually requires a nutritional and pharmacologic approach.

Nutritional Management

The first goal of management is to reverse the ongoing catabolic state. In patients with documented secretory diarrhea, intravenous nutrition and complete bowel rest should be instituted while diagnostic evaluation proceeds. It is critical to avoid iatrogenic prolongation of disease by irrational dietary trials. Early placement of a Broviac catheter facilitates nutritional rehabilitation and allows for frequent monitoring of appropriate laboratory studies. Refeeding of patients with secretory diarrhea should be postponed until the patient's expected weight based on height is back at the fiftieth percentile. Refeeding at that point is mandatory because of the proven beneficial effects of enteral nutrients on mucosal growth.[114–117] One should always work from a base of full nutrition provided by parenteral nutrition, reducing parenteral calories only as tolerance of increasing enteral nutrition is demonstrated. Although some gastroenterologists have suggested that the results of tests of mucosal function, such as the 1-hour D-xylose, be used to help predict tolerance of enteral feedings,[118] refeeding is, in practice, a process of trial and error. In most cases, oral intake is limited by anorexia and vomiting. Nasogastric feedings may be given for extended periods through small-bore polyurethane or Silastic rubber catheters. It has been shown that patients with protracted diarrhea are often able to tolerate continuous intragastric feeding when intermittent bolus feeding results in continuing diarrhea and nutritional deprivation.[119] Therefore, a conservative approach is to initiate a refeeding program with continuous feeds. The initial refeeding formula should be isotonic and contain glucose polymers. If not tolerated, a glucose- or fructose-based formula may be tried. Ideally, one should begin enteral feedings with small volumes of full-strength elemental formula, gradually increasing volume as tolerated. For reasons that remain unclear, some patients will tolerate only nasogastric feedings of diluted elemental formulas. In some patients, reinstitution of nasogastric feedings unmasks a significant disorder of gastric emptying, which may necessitate progression to nasojejunal feeding. Tolerance of enteral feedings may be improved by aggressive administration of intravenous albumin in patients with serum albumin concentrations below 2.5 gm per dl.[118] The beneficial effects of oncotic reconstitution by albumin administration have been speculated to result from improved mucosal function because of decreased mucosal edema.[120] It has been suggested that aggressive use of enteral nutrition can be utilized in protracted diarrhea without sacrificing nutritional rehabilitation if increased stool volume, electrolyte, and bicarbonate losses are replaced by intravenous fluids.[118] This author believes that such an approach is cumbersome, prone to frequent shifts in intravascular fluid balance, and hard to incorporate into home-based therapy. It is not indicated except in cases of progressive hyperalimentation-induced cholestasis.

Recent animal investigations have suggested that specific dietary substrates including L-glutamine,[121] dietary nucleotides,[122] polyamines,[123] and epidermal growth factor[124, 125] may play important roles in intestinal recovery and adaptation. To date, none of these factors have been critically studied as therapeutic agents in patients with protracted diarrhea. Many gastroenterologists have fed patients breast milk, speculating that it may provide some unknown trophic factor.[126] There are no reports of proven efficacy. Moreover, problems of availability, storage, and possible transmission of infectious agents, such as CMV, are factors that make widespread treatment trials with human milk products difficult to accomplish.

The major long-term risks of parenteral nutrition include catheter-related sepsis and cholestasis.[127] In fact, death of patients with protracted diarrhea in the United States is far more likely to be the result of secondary infection or progressive hyperalimentation-induced liver disease than progressive malnutrition. Another long-term risk of both parenteral and nasogastric enteral nutrition that is not given much attention in the literature is aversive behavior toward oral feeding. Even if a patient can be completely weaned off parenteral nutrition over a period of time, it may be months before that patient accepts oral bolus feedings. Ability to offer a variety of oral foods is also restricted by the standard practice of avoiding introduction of milk and soy protein back into the diet for months after improvement of the diarrhea. If a long period of feeding therapy is contemplated, placement of a percutaneous gastrostomy may facilitate ongoing provision of enteral calories.[128]

Pharmacologic Therapy

Table 62–4 lists the pharmacologic options available in the management of idiopathic villus atrophy based on specific pathophysiologic mechanisms believed to be involved in an individual patient. None of these approaches is completely effective in eradicating the diarrhea, and their use is generally empiric.

Therapy of Altered Intestinal Morphology. As stated above, enteral nutrition must be viewed as a drug because of the proven efficacy of luminal nutrients to promote intestinal growth and adaptation.[114–117] It is essential to begin some enteral nutrition as soon as possible after initial intravenous nutritional rehabilitation, even in the presence of ongoing diarrheal losses.

A major decision point in management is whether to institute immunosuppressive therapy. Although carefully controlled studies have not been performed to evaluate the efficacy of agents such as corticosteroids, azathioprine, cyclophosphamide, or cyclosporine, there are enough anecdotal reports of partial resolution of the diarrhea with such agents to justify their use in patients with clinical manifestations or laboratory evidence that suggests autoimmune enteropathy.[72, 73, 78, 79] It would also seem that a trial of immunosuppressive therapy would be justified in patients with documented evidence of immunodeficiency if small bowel biopsy revealed an inflammatory enteropathy without evidence of an infectious etiology, especially if there are clinical manifestations or laboratory indications of an autoimmune process.[67] One consideration would be to use cyclosporine as the immunosuppressive agent of choice because of the usual poor response to corticosteroids.[78] Furthermore, preliminary reports suggest that the time from onset of therapy to obvious clinical response is short, often in terms of weeks. A reasonable initial dose is 10 mg per kg per day given orally or by nasogastric tube two or three times daily, then gradually increasing or decreasing the dosage as required to achieve a whole blood level of 150 to 200 ng per ml measured by radioimmunoassay.[78]

Table 62–4. PHARMACOLOGIC THERAPY OF IDIOPATHIC VILLUS ATROPHY

Therapy of Altered Intestinal Morphology
Enteral nutrition
Immunosuppressive therapy
Cholestyramine
"Bowel cocktail"
Antisecretory Therapy
Somatostatin
Bismuth subsalicylate
Adrenergic agonists
Chlorpromazine
Lithium carbonate
Propranolol
Drugs That Alter Motility
Opioid drugs

There is little evidence that intravenous immunoglobulin is beneficial in patients with low levels of IgG from ongoing protein-losing enteropathy unless there is an ongoing active infection.[129] The only clear indication for replacement therapy with immunoglobulin is severe impairment in antibody-forming or functional capacity. An intriguing but unexplored therapy in protracted diarrhea is IgA-IgG feeding.[130] Such therapy may prevent the development of necrotizing enterocolitis in low-birth-weight infants.[131] Binding of an intact immunoglobulin to alimentary, bacterial, or viral antigens may reduce contact with the gut mucus and facilitate elimination.

Cholestyramine is a strongly basic anion exchange resin that binds tightly to bile acids in the intestinal lumen and may protect against direct bile acid–induced injury of the upper small bowel mucosa and bile acid–induced secretion in the colon.[132] Cholestyramine in doses of 4 to 20 gm has been reported to be effective in dramatically reducing diarrheal output in selected patients with protracted diarrhea.

The empiric use of a bowel cocktail has been advocated in patients with immunodeficiency or severe malnutrition or in patients with suspected bacterial overgrowth.[133] Hill and colleagues[133] have proposed a combination of oral or nasogastric gentamicin (50 mg per kg per day every 4 hours for 3 days), cholestyramine (1 gm every 6 hours for 5 days), and metronidazole (100 mg every 8 hours for 5 days).

Antisecretory Therapy. A somatostatin analogue (octreotide, Sandostatin) has been reported to significantly decrease the secretory diarrhea caused by neuroendocrine tumors.[134–136] The subcutaneous administration of somatostatin has also been reported to reduce stool output in idiopathic villus atrophy in which no high concentration of a circulating secretagogue can be identified.[137] The latter effect may be because of its antimotility effect rather than its antisecretory effect. The initial dose reported was 0.7 μg per kg twice a day. The dosage was increased by steps of 0.3 μg per kg per dose twice a day at 3-day intervals until further increases in dosage failed to produce significant additional decreases in stool output. Other than the need for twice-daily injections, the only side effect reported was irritability.

Nonsteroidal anti-inflammatory agents, including indomethacin and salicylates (bismuth subsalicylate, sulfasalazine, 5-aminosalicylate), have been reported to decrease diarrhea in inflammatory bowel disorders.[138] Since these agents are prostaglandin synthetase inhibitors, it has been proposed that they exert their antisecretory effect by inhibiting release of prostaglandin mediators in inflamed intestine. To date, there has been no critical evaluation of the effect of these agents in patients with protracted diarrhea. It is obvious from anecdotal clinical experience that they are at best only partially effective. Bismuth subsalicylate also binds bile acids that may contribute to protracted diarrhea.

Based on continued advancement in our understanding of mechanisms of intestinal ion transport, a number of novel therapeutic agents are now being studied that alter these mechanisms at various points in the absorptive and secretory process.[139] Adrenergic agonists, such as clonidine, are potential agents to treat protracted diarrhea since they stimulate absorption of water and electrolytes and inhibit HCO_3 and Cl secretion in both the small and large intestine. In animal and human studies, clonidine has been reported to reduce diabetic diarrhea, diarrhea associated with opiate withdrawal, and secretory diarrhea in a patient with bronchogenic adenocarcinoma.[140] Despite these antisecretory effects under experimental conditions, the centrally mediated hypotensive and sedative side effects of clonidine have thus far limited its use as an antidiarrheal agent. Lidamidane, a newer agent with alpha$_2$-adrenergic agonist properties, may prove to have more clinical use since it does not cross the blood-brain barrier. Other potentially useful agents currently being studied include chlorpromazine derivatives, lithium carbonate, beta-adrenergic blockers, calcium channel blockers, enkephalin analogues, and Cl channel blockers.[139]

Antimotility Agents. Most of the antisecretory agents described above also possess antimotility activity. To date, however, the most commonly used agents to decrease fluid transit through the gut are opiates or opiate derivatives.[141] Loperamide is the agent of choice because it has the highest antidiarrheal specificity.[142] Loperamide is initiated at a dose of 0.5 mg per kg per day given three times a day and then increased according to the effect on stool volume 0.5 mg per kg per day every 48 hours up to a maximal dose of 3 mg per kg per day.

PROGNOSIS

Adequate follow-up data on infants with protracted diarrhea (as defined previously) are lacking. Most reports to date have included heterogeneous patient populations and have depicted variable outcomes regarding both the duration of severe diarrhea and the response to nutritional and pharmacologic therapy. It is clear that research efforts must continue to be directed toward improving our knowledge of intestinal permeability, enterocyte differentiation, the intestinal immune response, and the effect of intestinal injury on motility. A strong argument can also be made for development of a central registry to track diagnosis, management, and outcome of these rare diarrheal syndromes.

REFERENCES

1. Avery GB, Villavicencio O, Lilly JR, et al: Intractable diarrhea in early infancy. Pediatrics 1968; 41:712–722.
2. Lo CW, Walker WA: Chronic protracted diarrhea of infancy: A nutritional disease. Pediatrics 1983; 72:786–800.
3. Vanderhoof JA: The protracted diarrhea syndrome. *In* Balistreri WF, Vanderhoof JA, eds: Pediatric Gastroenterology and Nutrition. London, Chapman and Hall Medical, 1990, pp 123–131.
4. Guerrant RL, Bobar DA: Bacterial and protozoal gastroenteritis. N Engl J Med 1991; 325:327–340.
5. Blacklow NR, Greenberg HB: Viral gastroenteritis. N Engl J Med 1991; 325:252–264.
6. Khoshoo V, Raj P, Srivastava R, et al: Salmonella typhimurium associated severe protracted diarrhea in infants and children. J Pediatr Gastroenterol Nutr 1990; 10:33–36.
7. Dutta P, Lahiri M, Sen D, et al: Prospective hospital based study on persistent diarrhea. Gut 1991; 32:787–790.
8. Iyngkaran N, Robinson MH, Sumithron E: Cow's milk protein-sensitive enteropathy: An important factor in prolonging diarrhoea of acute infective enteritis in early infancy. Arch Dis Child 1978; 53:150–153.
9. Challacombe DN, Richardson JM, Rowe B, et al: Bacterial microflora of the upper gastrointestinal tract in infants with protracted diarrhea. Arch Dis Child 1974; 49:270–277.
10. Lebenthal E: Cow's milk allergy. Pediatr Clin North Am 1975; 22:827–833.
11. Stern M, Walker WA: Food allergy and intolerance. Pediatr Clin North Am 1985; 32:471–492.
12. Holmberg C: Congenital chloride diarrhea. Clin Gastroenterol 1986; 15:583–602.
13. Norio N, Perheentupa J, Launiala K, et al: Congenital chloride diarrhea, an autosomal recessive disease. Genetic study of 14 Finnish and 12 other families. Clin Genet 1971; 2:182–192.
14. Turnberg LA: Abnormalities in intestinal electrolyte transport in congenital chloridorrhea. Gut 1971; 12:544–551.
15. Bieberdorf FA, Gorden P, Fordtran JS: Pathogenesis of congenital alkalosis with diarrhea. J Clin Invest 1972; 51:1958–1968.
16. Holmberg C, Perheentupa J: Congenital Na^+ diarrhea: A new type of secretory diarrhea. J Pediatr 1985; 106:56–61.
17. Booth IW, Murer H, Stang G, et al: Defective jejunal brush border Na^+/H^+ exchange: A cause of congenital secretory diarrhea. Lancet 1985; 1:1066–1069.
18. Heubi JE, Balistreri WF, Partin JC: Refractory infantile diarrhea due to primary bile acid malabsorption. J Pediatr 1979; 94:546–551.
19. Heubi JE, Balistreri WF, Fondacaro JD, et al: Primary bile acid malabsorption: Defective in vitro ileal active bile acid transport. Gastroenterology 1982; 83:804–811.
20. Schiller LR, Hogan RB, Morawski SG, et al: Studies of the prevalence and significance of radiolabeled bile acid malabsorption in a group of patients with idiopathic chronic diarrhea. Gastroenterology 1985; 92:151–160.
21. Ghishan FK, Lee PC, Lebenthal E, et al: Isolated congenital enterokinase deficiency. Gastroenterology 1983; 85:727–731.
22. Moynahan EJ: Acrodermatitis enteropathica: A lethal inherited human zinc-deficiency disorder. Lancet 1974; 11:399–400.
23. Danks DM, Campbell PE, Stevens BJ, et al: Menkes' kinky hair syndrome: An inherited defect in copper absorption with widespread effects. Pediatrics 1972; 50:188–201.
24. Nixon HH: Hirschsprung's disease in the newborn. *In* Holschneider AM, ed: Hirschsprung's Disease. New York, Thieme-Stratton, 1982, pp 103–113.
25. Agarwala B: Persistent diarrhea in a two month old infant. Hosp Prac 1983; 18:100E–100K.
26. Cox KL: Persistent diarrhea, colitis in a malnourished infant. Hosp Prac 1985; 20:64–68.
27. Wingate DL: The small intestine. *In* Christensen J, Wingate DL, eds: A Guide to Gastrointestinal Motility. London, Wright PSG, 1983, pp. 128–155.
28. Shields R: Surgical aspects of the absorption of water and electrolytes by the intestine. Monograph Surg Sci 1964; 1:119–172.
29. Mirkovitch V, Menge H: Movements of water and ions across dog ileal mucosa following ischemia or occlusion. *In* Robinson JWL, ed: Intestinal Ion Transport. Lancaster, PA, MTP, 1975, pp 251–260.
30. Joppich I: Late complications of Hirschsprung's disease. *In* Holschneider AM, ed: Hirschsprung's Disease. New York, Thieme-Stratton, 1982, pp 251–262.

31. Kaplan SJ, Holbrook CT, McDaniel HG, et al: Vasoactive intestinal peptide secreting tumors in childhood. Am J Dis Child 1980; 134:21–24.
32. Socha J, Dobrazanska A, Rowecka K, et al: Chronic diarrhea due to vipoma in two children. J Pediatr Gastroenterol Nutr 1984; 3:143–148.
33. Funato M, Fujimura M, Shimada S, et al: Rapid changes of serum vasoactive intestinal peptide after removal of ganglioneuroblastoma with watery-diarrhea-hypokalemia-achlorhydria syndrome in a child. J Pediatr Gastroenterol Nutr 1982; 1:131–135.
34. Hansen LP, Lund HT, Fahrenkrug J, et al: Vasoactive intestinal polypeptide (VIP)-producing ganglioneuroma in a child with chronic diarrhea. Acta Pediatr Scand 1980; 69:419–424.
35. Jansen-Goemans A, Engelhardt J: Intractable diarrhea in a boy with vasoactive intestinal peptide-producing ganglioneuro-blastoma. Pediatrics 1977; 59:710–716.
36. Mitchell CH, Sinatra FR, Crast FW, et al: Intractable watery diarrhea, ganglioneuroblastoma and vasoactive intestinal peptide. J Pediatr 1976; 89:593–595.
37. Schwartz CJ, Kimberg DV, Sheerin HE, et al: Vasoactive intestinal peptide stimulation of adenylate cyclase and active electrolyte secretion in intestinal mucosa. J Clin Invest 1974; 54:536–544.
38. Kane MG, O'Dorisio TM, Krejs GJ: Production of secretory diarrhea by intravenous infusion of vasoactive intestinal polypeptide. N Engl J Med 1983; 309:1482–1485.
39. Udall JN, Singer DB, Huang CTL, et al: Watery diarrhea and hypokalemia associated with increased plasma vasoactive intestinal peptide in a child. J Pediatr 1976; 88:819–821.
40. Ghishan FK, Soper RT, Nassif EG, et al: Chronic diarrhea in infancy: Non-beta islet cell hyperplasia. Pediatrics 1979; 64:46–49.
41. Ament M: Immunodeficiency syndrome and gastrointestinal disease. Pediatr Clin North Am 1975; 22:807–825.
42. Walker WA: Host defense mechanisms in the gastrointestinal tract. Pediatrics 1976; 57:901–916.
43. Arbo A, Santos JI: Diarrheal diseases in the immunocompromised host. Pediatr Infect Dis J 1987; 6:894–906.
44. Levinsky RJ, Marshall WC, Pincott J, et al: Protracted diarrhea, immunodeficiency and viruses. Eur J Pediatr 1982; 138:271–272.
45. Saulsbury FT, Winkelstein JA, Yolken RH: Chronic rotavirus infection in immunodeficiency. J Pediatr 1980; 97:61–65.
46. Horowitz S, Lorenzsonn VW, Olsen WA, et al: Small intestinal disease in T cell deficiency. J Pediatr 1980; 97:61–65.
47. Kotler DP, Gaetz HP, Lange M, et al: Enteropathy associated with acquired immunodeficiency syndrome. Ann Intern Med 1984; 101:421–428.
48. Weber J: Gastrointestinal disease in AIDS. Clin Immunol Aller 1986; 6:519–541.
49. McLoughlin LC, Nord KS, Joshi VV, et al: Severe gastrointestinal involvement in children with the acquired immunodeficiency syndrome. J Pediatr Gastroenterol Nutr 1987; 6:517–524.
50. Ulshen MH, Rollo JL: Pathogenesis of *Escherichia coli* gastroenteritis in man—another mechanism. N Engl J Med 1980; 302:99–101.
51. Clausen CR, Christie DL: Chronic diarrhea in infants caused by adherent enteropathogenic *Escherichia coli*. J Pediatr 1982; 100:358–361.
52. Sherman P, Drum B, Karmali M, et al: Adherence of bacteria to the intestine in sporadic cases of enteropathogenic *Escherichia coli*-associated diarrhea in infants and young children. A prospective study. Gastroenterology 1989; 96:86–94.
53. Hill SM, Phillips AD, Walker-Smith JA: Enteropathogenic *Escherichia coli* and life-threatening chronic diarrhea. Gut 1991; 32:154–158.
54. Rothbaum R, McAdams AJ, Giannella R, et al: A clinicopathologic study of enterocyte adherent *Escherichia coli*: A cause of protracted diarrhea in infants. Gastroenterology 1982; 83:441–454.
55. Ackerman NB, Strobel CT: Polle syndrome: Chronic diarrhea in Munchausen's child. Gastroenterology 1981; 81:1140–1142.
56. Morris AI, Turnberg LA: Surreptitious laxative abuse. Gastroenterology 1979; 77:780–786.
57. Powell DW, Lawrence BA, Morris SM, et al: Effect of phenolphthalein on in vitro rabbit ileal electrolyte transport. Gastroenterology 1980; 78:454–463.
58. Ewe K: Effect of laxatives on intestinal water and electrolyte transport. Eur J Clin Invest 1972; 2:282.
59. Meisel JL, Bergman D, Saunders DR, et al: Human rectal mucosa: Proctoscopic and morphologic changes caused by laxatives. Gastroenterology 1976; 70:918.
60. Charney EB, Bodurtha JN: Intractable diarrhea associated with the use of sorbitol. J Pediatr 1981; 98:157–158.
61. Davidson GP, Cutz E, Hamilton JR, et al: Familial enteropathy: A syndrome of protracted diarrhea from birth, failure to thrive, and hypoplastic villus atrophy. Gastroenterology 1978; 75:783–790.
62. Cutz E, Rhoads JM, Drumm B, et al: Microvillus inclusion disease: An inherited defect of brush border assembly and differentiation. N Engl J Med 1989; 320:646–651.
63. Phillips AD, Jenkins P, Raafat F, et al: Congenital microvillus atrophy: Specific diagnostic features. Arch Dis Child 1985; 60:135–140.
64. Carruthers L, Phillips AD, Dourmashkin R, et al: Biochemical abnormality in brush-border membrane protein of a patient with congenital microvillus atrophy. J Pediatr Gastroenterol Nutr 1985; 4:1–6.
65. Rhoads JM, Vogler RC, Lacey SR, et al: Microvillus inclusion disease: In vitro jejunal electrolyte transport. Gastroenterology 1991; 100:811–817.
66. Cuenod B, Brousse N, Goulet O, et al: Classification of intractable diarrhea in infancy using clinical and immunological criteria. Gastroenterology 1990; 99:1037–1043.
67. Conley ME, Park CL, Douglas SD: Childhood common variable immunodeficiency with autoimmune disease. J Pediatr 1981; 108:915–922.
68. Anderson KE, Finlayson NDC, Deschner EE: Intractable malabsorption with flat jejunal mucosa and selective IgA deficiency. Gastroenterology 1974; 67:709–716.
69. Rosen FS, Cooper MD, Wedgwood RJP: The primary immunodeficiencies. N Engl J Med 1984; 311:235–241, 298–310.
70. Martin DW, Gelfand EW: Biochemistry of diseases of immunodevelopment. Annu Rev Biochem 1981; 50:845–877.
71. Touraine JL: The bare lymphocyte syndrome: Report on the registry. Lancet 1981; 1:319–320.
72. Bernstein EF, Whitington PF: Successful treatment of atypical sprue in an infant with cyclosporine. Gastroenterology 1988; 95:199–124.
73. Fisher SE, Boyle JT, Holtzapple P: Chronic protracted diarrhea and jejunal atrophy in an infant. Dig Dis Sci 1981; 26:181–186.
74. Ellis D, Fischer SE, Smith LI, et al: Familial occurrence of renal and intestinal disease associated with tissue autoantibodies. Am J Dis Child 1982; 132:323–326.
75. Unsworth J, Hutchins P, Mitchell J, et al: Flat small intestinal mucosa and autoantibodies against gut epithelium. J Pediatr Gastroenterol Nutr 1982; 1:503–513.
76. Walker-Smith JA, Unsworth DJ, Hutchins P, et al: Autoantibodies against gut epithelium in child with small intestinal enteropathy. Lancet 1982; 1:566–567.
77. Savage MO, Mirakian R, Wozniak ER, et al: Specific autoantibodies to gut epithelium in two infants with severe protracted diarrhoea. J Pediatr Gastroenterol Nutr 1985; 4:187–195.
78. Seidman EG, Lacaille F, Russo P, et al: Successful treatment of autoimmune enteropathy with cyclosporine. J Pediatr 1990; 117:929–932.
79. Colletti RB, Guillot AP, Rosen S, et al: Autoimmune enteropathy and nephropathy with circulating autoantibodies. J Pediatr 1991; 118:853–864.
80. Hill SM, Milla PJ, Bottazzo GF, et al: Autoimmune enteropathy and colitis: Is there a generalized autoimmune gut disorder? Gut 1991; 32:36–42.
81. Mirakian R, Hill S, Richardson A, et al: HLA product expression and lymphocyte subpopulation in jejunum biopsies of children with idiopathic protracted diarrhoea and enterocyte autoantibodies. J Autoimmun 1988; 1:263–277.
82. Miller RC, Larsen E: Regional enteritis in early infancy. Am J Dis Child 1971; 122:301–311.
83. Phillips SF, Wingate DL: Fluid and electrolyte fluxes in the gut. Adv Intern Med 1979; 24:429–453.
84. Phillips SF: Diarrhea: A current view of the pathophysiology. Gastroenterology 1972; 63:495–518.
85. Rhoads JM, Powell DW: Diarrhea. *In* Walker WA, Durie PR,

Hamilton JR, et al, eds: Pediatric Gastrointestinal Disease. Pathophysiology, Diagnosis, Management. Philadelphia, BC Decker, 1991, pp 62–78.
86. Madara JL, Trier JS: Functional morphology of the mucosa of the small intestine. *In* Johnson LR, ed: Physiology of the Gastrointestinal Tract. 2d ed. New York, Raven Press, 1987, pp 1209–1249.
87. Boyle JT, Celano P, Koldovsky O: Demonstration of a difference in expression of maximal lactase and sucrase activity along the villus in the adult rat jejunum. Gastroenterology 1980; 79:503–507.
88. Shiau YF, Boyle JT, Umstetter C, et al: Apical distribution of fatty acid esterification capacity along the villus-crypt unit of the rat jejunum. Gastroenterology 1980; 79:47–53.
89. Kinter WP, Wilson TH: Autoradiographic study of sugar and amino acid absorption by everted sacs of hamster small intestine. J Cell Biol 1965; 25:19–39.
90. Donowitz M, Welsh MJ: Regulation of mammalian small intestine electrolyte secretion. *In* Johnson LR, ed: Physiology of the Gastrointestinal Tract. 2d ed. New York, Raven Press, 1987, pp 1351–1388.
91. Fordtran J. Stimulation of active and passive sodium absorption by sugars in the human jejunum. J Clin Invest 1975; 55:728–737.
92. Binder HJ, Sandle GI: Electrolyte absorption and secretion in the mammalian colon. *In* Johnson LR, ed: Physiology of the Gastrointestinal Tract. 2d ed. New York, Raven Press, 1987, pp 1389–1418.
93. Ruppin H, Bar-Meir S, Soergel KH, et al: Absorption of short-chain fatty acids by the colon. Gastroenterology 1980; 78:1500–1507.
94. Debongie JL, Phillips SF: Capacity of the human colon to absorb fluid. Gastroenterology 1978; 74:698–703.
95. Schwartz KB, Ternberg JL, Bell MJ, et al: Sodium needs of infants and children with ileostomy. J Pediatr 1983; 102:509–513.
96. Bright-Asare P, Binder HJ: Stimulation of colonic secretion of water and electrolytes by hydroxy fatty acids. Gastroenterology 1978; 64:81–88.
97. Mekhjian HS, Phillips SF, Hofmann AF: Colonic secretion of water and electrolytes induced by bile acids: Perfusion studies in man. J Clin Invest 1971; 50:1569–1577.
98. Cooke HJ: Neural and humoral regulation of small intestinal electrolyte transport. *In* Johnson LR, ed: Physiology of the Gastrointestinal Tract. 2d ed. New York, Raven Press, 1987, pp 1307–1350.
99. Bern MJ, Sturbaum CW, Karayalcin SS, et al: Immune system control of rat and rabbit colonic electrolyte transport: Role of prostaglandins and enteric nervous system. J Clin Invest 1989; 83:1810–1820.
100. Read N: Intestinal motility in the pathogenesis of diarrhea. Pract Gastroenterol 1984; 8:32–35.
101. Summers RW: Role of motility in infectious diarrhea (editorial). Gastroenterology 1981; 80:1070–1071.
102. Lifshitz F: Congenital lactase deficiency. J Pediatr 1966; 69:229–237.
103. Evans L, Grasset E, Heyman M, et al: Congenital selective malabsorption of glucose and galactose. J Pediatr Gastroenterol Nutr 1985; 4:878–886.
104. Antonovicz I, Lloyd JD, Khaw KT, et al: Congenital sucrase-isomaltase deficiency. Observation over a period of 6 years. Pediatrics 1972; 49:847–853.
105. Fisher SE, Leone G, Kelly RH: Chronic protracted diarrhea; intolerance to dietary glucose polymers. Pediatrics 1981; 67:271–273.
106. Clark JH, Bullock L, Fitzgerald JF: Dietary fructose in the management of intractable diarrhea of infancy. J Pediatr Gastroenterol Nutr 1986; 5:81–86.
107. Shiau YF, Feldman GM, Fesnick MA, et al: Stool electrolyte and osmolality measurements in the evaluation of diarrheal disorders. Ann Intern Med 1985; 102:773–775.
108. Perman JA, Modler S, Barr RG, et al: Fasting breath hydrogen concentrations: Normal values and clinical applications. Gastroenterology 1984; 87:1358–1363.
109. Franken EA Jr: Small bowel. *In* Gastrointestinal Radiology in Pediatrics. Hagerstown, MD, Harper & Row, 1975, pp 95–156.
110. Stiehm ER: Clinical and laboratory evaluation of the child with suspected immunodeficiency. Pediatr Rev 1985; 7:53–61.
111. Lawley TJ, James SP, Jones EA: Circulating immune complexes: Their detection and potential significance in some hepatobiliary and intestinal diseases. Gastroenterology 1980; 78:626–641.
112. Rossi TM, Lebenthal E, Nord KS, et al: Extent and duration of small intestinal mucosal injury in intractable diarrhea of infancy. Pediatrics 1990; 66:730–735.
113. Goldgar CM, Vanderhoof JA: Lack of correlation of small bowel biopsy and clinical course of patients with intractable diarrhea of infancy. Gastroenterology 1986; 90:527–531.
114. Williamson RCN: Intestinal adaptation. N Engl J Med 1978; 198:1393–1402, 1444–1450.
115. Eastwood GL: Gastrointestinal epithelial renewal. Gastroenterology 1977; 72:962–975.
116. Weser E: Luminal nutrients and intestinal adaptation. J Pediatr Gastroenterol 1985; 4:165–166.
117. Green HL, McCabe DR, Merenstein GB: Protracted diarrhea and malnutrition in infancy: Changes in intestinal morphology and disaccharidase activities during treatment with total intravenous nutrition or oral elemental diets. J Pediatr 1975; 87:695–704.
118. Orenstein SR: Enteral versus parenteral therapy for intractable diarrhea of infancy: A prospective, randomized trial. J Pediatr 1986; 109:277–286.
119. Parker P, Stroop S, Greene H: A controlled comparison of continuous versus intermittent feeding in the treatment of infants with intestinal disease. J Pediatr 1981; 99:360–364.
120. Doweiko JP, Nompleggi DJ: The role of albumin in human physiology and pathophysiology. Part III: Albumin and disease states. JPEN 1991; 476–483.
121. Windmueller HG, Spaeth AE: Identification of ketone bodies and glutamine as the major respiratory fuels in vivo for post-absorptive rat small intestine. J Biol Chem 1978; 253:69–76.
122. Nunez MC, Ayuoarte MJ, Morales D, et al: Effect of dietary nucleotides on intestinal repair in rats with experimental chronic diarrhea. JPEN 1990; 14:598–604.
123. Wang JY, McCormack SA, Viar MJ, et al: Stimulation of proximal small intestinal mucosal growth by luminal polyamines. Am J Physiol 1991; 261:G504-G511.
124. Oka Y, Ghishan FK, Green HL, et al: Effect of mouse epithelial growth factor-urogastrone on the functional maturation of rat intestine. Endocrinology 1983; 112:940–944.
125. Thornburg W, Matrisian L, Magun B, et al: Gastrointestinal absorption of epidermal growth factor in suckling rats. Am J Physiol 1984; 246:G80–G85.
126. Shulman RJ, Lifschitz CH, Langston C, et al: Human milk and the rate of small intestinal mucosal recovery in protracted diarrhea. J Pediatr 1989; 114:218–224.
127. Sandler RH, Kleinman RE: Cholestasis associated with parenteral nutrition. *In* Walker WA, Durie PR, Hamilton JR, et al, eds: Pediatric Gastrointestinal Disease: Pathophysiology, Diagnosis, Management. Philadelphia, BC Decker, 1991, pp 1065–1074.
128. Ponsky JL, Gauderer MWL: Percutaneous endoscopic gastrostomy: A nonoperative technique for feeding gastrostomy. Gastrointest Endosc 1981; 27:9–11.
129. Buckley RH, Schiff RI: The use of intravenous immune globulin in immunodeficiency disease. N Engl J Med 1991; 325:110–117.
130. Losonsky GA, Johnson JP, Winkelstein JA, et al: Oral administration of human serum immunoglobulin in immunodeficient patients with viral gastroenteritis. J Clin Invest 1985; 76:2362–2367.
131. Eibl MM, Wolf HM, Furnkranz H, et al: Prevention of necrotizing enterocolitis in low birth weight infants by IgA-IgG feeding. N Engl J Med 1988; 319:1–7.
132. Tamer MA, Santora TR, Sandberg DH: Cholestyramine therapy for intractable diarrhea. Pediatrics 1974; 53:217–220.
133. Hill ID, Mann MD, Househam KC, et al: Use of oral gentamicin, metronidazole, and cholestyramine in the treatment of severe persistent diarrhea in infants. Pediatrics 1986; 77:477–481.
134. Ruskone A, Rene E, Chayvialle JA, et al: Effect of somatostatin on diarrhea and on small intestinal water and electrolyte transport in a patient with pancreatic cholera. Dig Dis Sci 1982; 27:459–466.
135. Dharmsathaphorn K, Sherwin RS, Cataland S, et al: Somatostatin inhibits diarrhea in the carcinoid syndrome. Ann Intern Med 1980; 92:68–69.

136. Maron PN, O'Dovisio TM, Howe BA, et al: Effects of a longacting somatostatin analogue (SMS 201–995) in a patient with pancreatic cholera. N Engl J Med 1985; 312:17–21.
137. Jaros W, Biller J, Greer S, et al: Successful treatment of idiopathic secretory diarrhea of infancy with somatostatin analogue SMS 201995. Gastroenterology 1988; 94:189–193.
138. Soriano-Brucher H, Avendano P, O'Ryan M, et al: Bismuth subsalicylate in the treatment of acute diarrhea in children: A clinical study. Pediatrics 1991; 87:18–26.
139. Fedorak RN, Field M: Anti-diarrheal therapy. Prospects for new agents. Dig Dis Sci 1987; 32:195–205.
140. Dharmsathaphorn K: Adrenergic agonists: A newer class of antidiarrheal drug. Gastroenterology 1986; 91:769–770.
141. Synder SH, Childers SR: Opiate receptors and opioid peptides. Ann Rev Neurosci 1979; 2:35–64.
142. Schiller LR, Santa Ana CA, Morawski SG, et al: Mechanism of the antidiarrheal effect of loperamide. Gastroenterology 1984; 86:1475–1480.

Chapter 63

Other Diseases of the Small Intestine and Colon

SAMUEL A. KOCOSHIS

ISCHEMIC BOWEL DISEASE

Etiology and Pathogenesis

Arteriosclerotic peripheral vascular disease virtually never appears in children. Nonetheless, small intestinal and/or colonic ischemia may result from a wide variety of pediatric conditions. As shown in Table 63–1, these conditions cause ischemia by obstructing superior mesenteric arterial flow, restricting superior mesenteric venous return, or impeding superior and inferior mesenteric flow to the colon. Regardless of the underlying condition, ischemia occurs only when a combination of factors interact to overcome the abundant collateral blood flow that supplies both the small and large intestine. Generally, rapid occlusion of a single large vessel leads to almost immediate opening of collaterals.[1] However, after prolonged obstruction, persistent, generalized small vessel vasoconstriction may worsen vascular insufficiency.[2] Important, if poorly understood, factors altering intestinal blood flow include preferential flow to higher-priority organs during conditions of low cardiac output,[3] local changes in vasoactive peptide levels,[4] and alterations in sympathetic nervous system tone.[4, 5]

In addition to endogenous factors, certain exogenous pharmacologic agents may predispose to intestinal ischemia. Chief among them are digoxin,[6] ergot alkaloids,[7] and estrogens.[8]

Clinical Manifestations

The patient with chronic mesenteric arterial insufficiency may experience classical abdominal angina.[9, 10] Long pain-free periods are present during fasting, but 20 to 30 minutes after meals, crampy or colicky periumbilical abdominal pain occurs and lasts for as long as several hours. Weight loss ensues despite lack of diarrhea or steatorrhea. A striking paucity of positive abdominal findings belies the seriousness of the condition.

Bowel subjected chronically to arterial insufficiency tends to heal with stricture formation.[10, 11] When strictures have formed, symptoms of partial or complete bowel obstruction appear.

Acute interruption of mesenteric flow leads to much more catastrophic consequences.[12] The patient initially experiences colicky, periumbilical pain that rapidly worsens, becomes generalized, and eventually leads to peritoneal findings, including exquisite abdominal pain with movement. The pain is accompanied by ileus and bilious vomiting. Patients experience hematemesis or pass "currant jelly" stools if mucosal necrosis is severe. Fever (often rising to 39° or 40°C) and vascular collapse appear in advanced cases.

Patients with mesenteric venous thrombosis commonly experience abdominal pain, but the pain is nonspecific and localizes poorly.[10, 13] Most patients experience vomiting, diarrhea, and occult rectal bleeding. Because enteric protein loss may be profound, these patients may present with peripheral edema or ascites. When the thrombosis is acute, progression to peritonitis may be rapid.

Signs and symptoms of ischemic colitis are no different from those of ulcerative colitis. The patient experiences crampy, left lower quadrant abdominal pain with concomitant bloody diarrhea. Classically, the volume of blood loss is insufficient to produce adverse hemodynamic or hematologic consequences.

Laboratory, Radiographic, Endoscopic, and Histologic Diagnosis

No specific laboratory findings accompany arterial or venous insufficiency. Patients may experience leukocytosis or anemia, and acute phase markers may appear in serum.[14] Chronic insufficiency may lead to protein-losing enteropathy reflected by hypoproteinemia, hypoalbuminemia, and elevated fecal $alpha_1$-antitrypsin concentrations.[11] Steatorrhea and carbohydrate malabsorption may sometimes be present.[11]

Sickle cell disease, thrombocytosis, liver disease,

Table 63–1. DISORDERS ASSOCIATED WITH ISCHEMIC BOWEL DISEASE IN CHILDREN

Mesenteric Arterial Insufficiency		Mesenteric Venous Thrombosis	Ischemic Colitis
Large Vessel Disease	***Small Vessel Disease***		
Congenital constrictive mesenteric bands	Amyloidosis	Antithrombin III deficiency	Ascariasis
Congenital mesenteric artery aneurysm or arteriovenous malformation		Ascariasis	Drug induced Digoxin Ergot alkaloids Oral contraceptives
	Repair of coarctation of aorta	Hepatic cirrhosis	
Septic emboli from bacterial endocarditis		Intra-abdominal sepsis	
Ehlers-Danlos syndrome	Drug induced Digoxin Ergot alkaloids Oral contraceptives Thiazides	Oral contraceptives	Necrotizing enterocolitis of infancy
Pancreatitis		Pancreatectomy	Schistosomiasis
Liver transplantation with hepatic artery "steal"		Pancreatitis	Sigmoid volvulus
		Paroxysmal nocturnal hemoglobinuria	
Mycotic emboli from fungal sepsis	Necrotizing enterocolitis of infancy	Protein C deficiency	Strangulated hernia
Umbilical artery catheterization	Vasculitis Degos' disease Dermatomyositis Hemolytic-uremic syndrome Henoch-Schönlein purpura Hepatitis Inflammatory bowel disease Periarteritis nodosa Polymyositis Systemic lupus erythematosus	Schistosomiasis	Surgical compromise of inferior mesenteric artery
		Sickle cell anemia	Vasculitis Degos' disease Dermatomyositis Hemolytic-uremic syndrome Henoch-Schönlein purpura Hepatitis Inflammatory bowel disease Periarteritis nodosa Polymyositis Systemic lupus erythematosus
		Splenectomy	
		Thrombocytosis	
		Variceal sclerotherapy	

schistosomiasis, and abdominal sepsis are clinically obvious causes of pediatric mesenteric venous thrombosis. If these diagnoses have been excluded, patients should undergo evaluation for paroxysmal nocturnal hemoglobinuria and deficiency of antithrombin III, protein C, or protein S.

The plain abdominal film is usually not helpful in patients with mesenteric arterial insufficiency.[15] However, the small bowel series may show thickened small bowel folds and a "herringbone" pattern of ulceration.[16] Long-standing insufficiency may lead to single or multiple discrete strictures. Small bowel mucosa will also be thickened and may show evidence of intramural hemorrhage in patients with mesenteric venous thrombosis. In ischemic colitis, "thumbprinting" of the colon is often quite evident.[16] Abnormalities are most commonly found at the splenic flexure and sigmoid colon, which are watershed areas farthest from the superior and inferior mesenteric arterial supplies.

Early angiography has been advocated for adults with mesenteric atherosclerotic disease,[10] but it may be meddlesome in children who are much more likely to have small vessel disease than large vessel occlusion. In the patient with suspected mesenteric venous thrombosis, angiography may reveal a venous thrombosis during the delayed phase or simply delayed emptying of arterial arcades. Again, angiography is a very insensitive tool in pediatric practice, and the clinician should not delay laparotomy when indicated. In addition, angiography is seldom helpful in patients with colonic ischemia.[10]

Upper or lower endoscopy reveals patchy mucosal hemorrhage and ulcerations that extend into the submucosa when the process is long-standing. The rectum is spared in 94% of patients with ischemic colitis.[10]

Histologic changes encompass a range of severity and bowel wall depth according to the type and severity of ischemia present.[17] Acute, complete obstruction produces superficial necrosis quickly followed by full-thickness necrosis. In nonocclusive ischemia, necrosis may be confined to mucosa and submucosa, with sparing of muscularis propria. Edema and vascular congestion are quite prominent in venous occlusion but also occur in arterial occlusion. Specimens from patients with vasculitis due to collagen-vascular disease may reveal arteritis with or without medial fibrosis or medial necrosis.[17] Fibrin thrombi may occlude the vessel walls. Leukocytoclasis is also characteristic.[17] Iron stains reveal extensive mucosal iron deposition in ischemic colitis when the vascular insult occurred remotely and a reparative process is taking place.

Treatment

Vasodilators such as papaverine, though used in adults with large vessel disease,[10] probably have no place in the management of children whose ischemia is usually due to vasculitis. However, a course of anticoagulants should be considered for children with venous thrombosis and hypercoagulable states.

Of course, correction of dehydration and acidosis and treatment of underlying predisposing conditions should be attempted, but patients with peritoneal signs are candidates for laparotomy and possible segmental bowel resection. If the viability of bowel is in question, the surgeon may elect to perform diverting enterostomies and a subsequent "second-look" operation.

RADIATION ENTERITIS

Radiation Biology and Epidemiology

Radiation-induced enteropathy has been recognized since 1897.[18] Despite refinements in delivery of ionizing radiation over the past century, the disorder persists to this day. Some authors even contend that the incidence is increasing,[19] though incidence and prevalence figures are difficult to calculate. Authors vary in their diagnostic criteria for radiation enteritis, and many series fail to include those children who die early in the course of radiation therapy. These impediments notwithstanding, the prevalence figures generally quoted are approximately 2 to 25%.[20–22] However, one series suggests that 70% of patients suffer change in bowel habits following pelvic irradiation.[23]

The total doses of radiation required to produce clinical damage in 5% of adult patients in 5 years (TD 5/5) or 50% of adult patients in 5 years (TD 50/5) range from 6,000 to 7,500 centigrays (equal to rads) for esophagus, 4,500 to 5,000 for stomach, 4,500 to 6,500 for small bowel and colon, and 5,500 to 8,000 for rectum.[24] Factors that predispose to chronic enteropathy include high radiation dosage, ongoing chemotherapy, large quantities of intestine residing within the pelvis (as seen in females and the elderly), previous surgery, and peripheral vascular disease.[25]

Some authors suggest that children are more resistant to chronic enteritis than are adults.[26, 27] Instead, the paucity of complications in children may be due to the lower radiation doses they receive. In contrast to adults with relatively radioresistant carcinoma, most pediatric patients with neuroblastoma, Wilms' tumor, or Hodgkin's lymphoma receive less than 3,600 centigrays.[24] Pediatric patients with pelvic rhabdomyosarcoma may receive a maximum of 6,000 centigrays to the pelvis.[24]

Pathogenesis

The adverse effects of radiation on the bowel may be categorized as acute and chronic injuries. Acute injury is a direct cytotoxic effect on replicating epithelial cells.[28] The mechanism of cell destruction begins with free-radical generation and subsequent alterations in DNA structure. DNA transcription and protein synthesis subsequently cease.[29] Generally, the small bowel is more sensitive than the colon to acute injury.[29] Chronic damage is the result of submucosal fibrosis that leads to obliteration of small blood vessels and lymphatics.[30] In many respects, this entity resembles chronic ischemic enteritis.

Clinical Features

During radiation therapy, acute injury produces abdominal cramps, diarrhea, and vomiting in 67 to 100% of patients.[22, 23] Symptoms resolve within 6 weeks of cessation in most patients, but damage is severe enough in 20% to mandate reduction in radiation dose.[31] The severity of acute symptoms is directly related to the development of chronic enteritis.[32]

Symptoms of chronic enteritis usually appear within 6 to 24 months after therapy.[33] However, a number of patients develop their first symptoms many years later. The most common mode of presentation is small bowel obstruction, and patients experience bilious vomiting, abdominal distention, and abdominal pain.[34] Fistulae, leading to diarrhea, may also develop. Free or confined perforation with abscess formation may complicate the course. A separate entity, radiation proctocolitis, produces bloody diarrhea, crampy abdominal pain, and tenesmus.[35]

Laboratory, Radiographic, and Histologic Diagnosis

Laboratory findings are neither diagnostically sensitive nor specific, but lactose malabsorption,[36] steatorrhea, vitamin B_{12} malabsorption, and bile salt wasting are common in acute injury.[37]

The above laboratory findings may be present in chronic injury; in addition, the patient often experiences small intestinal bacterial overgrowth due to stasis or fistula.[37] Secondary lymphangiectasia results in protein-losing enteropathy characterized by depressed serum proteins, lymphopenia, elevated fecal $alpha_1$-antitrypsin levels, and lymphocytes in stool.

Contrast radiography may reveal thickened folds, adhesions, mucosal effacement, fistulas, and luminal narrowing.[38]

Histologic changes include subtotal villus atrophy,[28] mucosal ulceration, bowel wall necrosis, and lymphangiectasia.[39]

Vasculitis may also be seen, and vascular morphology may be altered by hyaline-ring thickening of arteriolar walls.[28] Inflammatory cells may infiltrate the intima of vessels, and intraluminal thrombi may form.[30]

Treatment

During the acute phase, low-residue, low-lactose diets are often helpful.[40] Some authors have also successfully employed prostaglandin synthetase inhibitors,[41] corticosteroids,[42] sulfasalazine,[43] and elemental diets.[42]

Chronic enteritis is more difficult to control, and trials

of elemental diets, steroids, sulfasalazine, cholestyramine, and other antibiotics have met with variable results.[37, 39] Patients with malnutrition despite adequate intake should receive parenteral nutrition.

Surgical resection and fistulectomy are often necessary. Wide resection, rather than limited surgery, is recommended by Galland and Spencer.[33] Ideally, anastomoses should be between segments of bowel that have escaped the radiation field. Some surgeons bypass rather than resect involved bowel loops.[44] However, others feel just as strongly that, when possible, excision is preferable to bypass because bypassed bowel is still at risk for perforation and fistulization.[33]

HEMOLYTIC-UREMIC SYNDROME

Epidemiology

First described by von Gasser and colleagues[45] in 1955, the triad of microangiopathic hemolytic anemia, thrombocytopenia, and acute renal failure, known as *hemolytic-uremic syndrome*, has a worldwide distribution. It is the most common cause of acute renal failure in children.[46] It usually appears in children less than 10 years old, has a peak incidence in children 1 to 2 years of age,[47–50] and is rarely seen in older children and adults.[51] It appears to be endemic in Argentina,[52] South Africa,[53] and the Pacific coast of North America,[47, 54] but the overall incidence seems to be increasing in many other geographic regions.[47–50]

Prognosis tends to be better in the "epidemic" form[48] than the sporadic form.[55] The worst prognosis is in the autosomal recessive familial form.[56] An extraordinarily high percentage of cases is preceded by infection with verotoxin-producing *Escherichia coli* 0157:H7.[47, 51, 57–61] Recent epidemiologic studies document infection with *E. coli* 0157:H7 among 64% of patients with hemolytic-uremic syndrome from Vancouver, Canada[58]; 58% from Seattle, Washington[59]; 23% from Great Britain[60]; 7.5% from Toronto, Canada[57]; and 2% from Buenos Aires, Argentina.[61] Other bacteria,[61] viruses,[62] or parasites are also associated. For example, 55% of Argentinian children with hemolytic-uremic syndrome have evidence of antecedent shigella infection.[61] Other predisposing factors include administration of antiviral vaccines to children[63] and cancer chemotherapeutic agents to adults.[64]

Many of the bacteria associated with hemolytic-uremic syndrome produce cytotoxins. Indeed, there is a striking similarity between *E. coli* 0157:H7 verotoxin and Shiga toxin produced by *Shigella dysenterii*.[65]

Blood group P1 predisposes to postenteropathic hemolytic-uremic syndrome because the terminal disaccharide on the P1 antigen acts as a verotoxin receptor.[66]

Pathogenesis

The pathologic events of "typical" hemolytic-uremic syndrome are initiated by intravascular platelet activation that, in turn, is precipitated by endothelial cell damage. Evidence supporting platelet activation includes loss of platelet nucleotide into plasma,[67] hyporesponsiveness to platelet-aggregating agents,[68] and alterations in platelet-produced growth factors.[69]

Endothelial damage may occur by direct bacterial cytotoxin-induced cytolysis,[65] by systemic endotoxin release,[70] by cell membrane lipid peroxidation,[71] or by immune complex–mediated damage.[72]

Release of platelet-aggregating factor[73] or factor VIII multimers[74] is probably a secondary process.

Prostacyclin depletion is commonly observed in hemolytic-uremic syndrome,[75] but this may be an epiphenomenon. A schematic diagram of the proposed pathogenic mechanism is shown in Figure 63–1.

Clinical Features

A prodromal gastroenteritis precedes about 95% of epidemic hemolytic-uremic syndrome cases.[46, 51–53] In 75% of those cases, diarrhea is bloody.[46, 51–53] Diffuse abdominal pain and vomiting are also common. At times, peritoneal signs are prominent, leading to exploratory laparotomy.[76, 77] Resolution of gastrointestinal symptoms is accompanied by sudden onset of extreme pallor, easy bruising, oliguria, and sometimes anasarca.[52]

Radiologic, Endoscopic, and Laboratory Findings

Barium enemas are frequently requested in the emergency department at the time of presentation to rule out intussusception. Findings including thumbprinting (Fig. 63–2), mucosal irregularity, and ulceration are consistent with an ischemic process.[75]

Endoscopic findings are nonspecific, and mucosa usually appears hyperemic, edematous, and friable.[78]

Histologic appearance may vary from that of nonspecific colitis to that of ischemic bowel disease.[78]

Stool culture may reveal enteric pathogens such as *Campylobacter, Yersinia, Salmonella,* or *Shigella.* Of these four, shigella is the most likely to be found.[61]

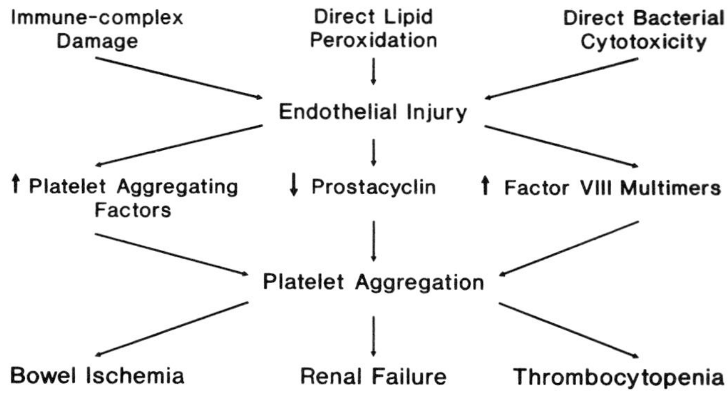

Figure 63–1. Proposed pathogenesis of hemolytic-uremic syndrome. Increased platelet aggregation precedes the development of thrombocytopenia, ischemic bowel disease, and renal failure, which characterize this disorder.

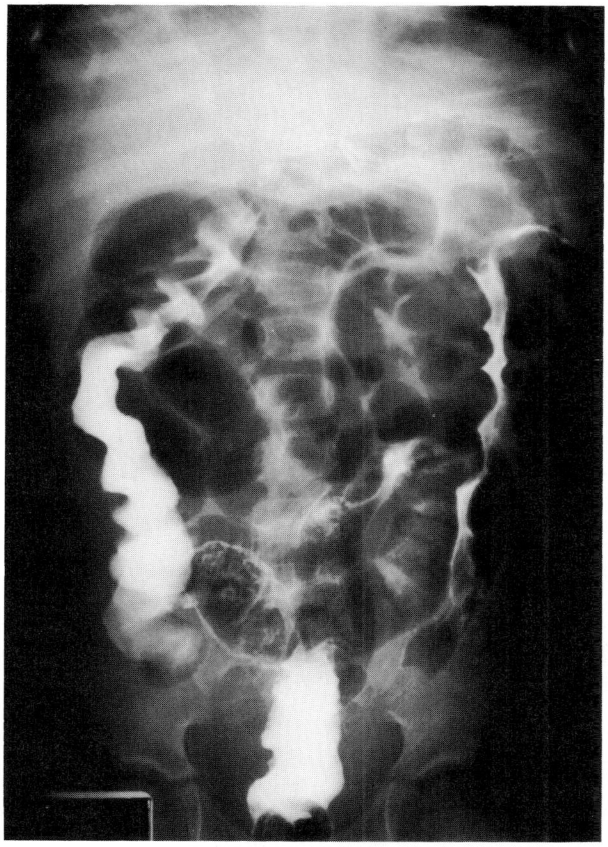

Figure 63–2. Extensive colonic "thumbprinting" in a patient who presented with bloody diarrhea associated with *E. coli* 0157:H7 infection. The "thumbprints" represent submucosal hemorrhages throughout the colon. (Courtesy of Richard Towbin, MD.)

Stools should also be cultured for coliforms—specifically strains that do not ferment sorbitol. *E. coli* 0157:H7 is the only strain of these associated with hemolytic-uremic syndrome.[47–51, 57–61] Cultures taken during the first 6 days of enteritis are more likely to be positive than those taken afterward.[79] Searching for fecal verotoxin by DNA probes also improves yield.[61]

As the enteritis improves, hemoglobin concentration falls precipitously to the range of 5 to 6 gm per dl, and red cells are morphologically abnormal. Fragments, burr cells, helmet cells, and other bizarre forms appear. Thrombocytopenia is present in 92% of patients, and coagulopathy in 85%.[46, 52, 53]

Oliguric acute renal failure occurs in 64 to 92% of patients who sometimes develop hypertension or azotemia.[46, 52, 53] Elevation of serum aminotransferases has been reported in over half of patients, and pancreatitis affects 21%.[80]

Complications

Small bowel and colonic perforation (often during peritoneal dialysis) are recognized complications.[76] Intussusception has also been reported. Intestinal strictures or fistulas are potential late complications. Severe pancreatitis may lead to exocrine or endocrine pancreatic insufficiency.[80] Renal thrombotic microangiopathy produces glomerulosclerosis and chronic renal failure in 6% of children with the epidemic form and 60% with the sporadic form.[46, 52, 53] Central nervous system complications such as encephalopathy, seizures, and stroke may be seen.

Treatment

Patients with severe gastrointestinal symptoms should receive bowel rest and parenteral nutrition. Use of broad-spectrum antibiotics should be considered in children with fulminant colitis. Red cell transfusions, fluid restriction, and diuretic use are the cornerstones of supportive therapy.

Azotemia or electrolyte imbalance may necessitate peritoneal dialysis or hemodialysis. The risks of hemodialysis in the face of coagulopathy should be weighed against the risks of peritoneal dialysis in the face of bowel ischemia.[76]

A large, controlled series has failed to show benefit from anticoagulant therapy,[81] but some data favor the use of plasmapheresis[82] or plasma transfusions[83] in selected patients. Caution in transfusing anti-T negative plasma is mandated by the high incidence of circulating T (Thomas-Friedenreich) antigen among patients with hemolytic-uremic syndrome.[84]

HENOCH-SCHÖNLEIN PURPURA

History and Epidemiology

Henoch-Schönlein purpura is a systemic vasculitis characterized by a purpuric rash that was probably first described in 1801 by Heberden.[85] Thirty-one years later, Schönlein carefully described the rash as purpura and recognized that the rash and associated arthritis constituted a distinct clinical syndrome.[86] In 1874, Henoch, one of Schönlein's students, noted that gastrointestinal symptoms accompany the rash.[87] Later he reported the association between nephritis and the syndrome.[88]

This entity is distributed worldwide and can affect individuals of any age.[89] However, 75% of patients are less than 7 years of age, and the median age of onset is 4 years.[90] There is a 2:1 male predominance, and the majority of cases occur in winter and early spring.[90] Almost all pediatric cases are preceded by a viral[91–93] or bacterial illness[94] or by a vaccination.[95] Some adult cases are associated with lymphoma,[96] prostatic cancer,[97] and other neoplasms.[98] Drugs such as salicylates, phenacetin, penicillin, erythromycin, and quinidines have also been implicated.[95]

Pathogenesis

Central to the pathogenic process is deposition of immunoglobulin A (IgA) immune complexes upon post-capillary venules throughout the body following presentation of some unknown antigen.[99] The alternate complement pathway is activated, resulting in depletion of plasma C_3 and deposition of C_3 in immune complexes. The fact that classical pathway activation does not occur is proved by the development of Henoch-Schönlein purpura in C_2-deficient individuals.[100] Whether excessive IgA production or diminished degradation takes place is uncertain.

Clinical Features

Skin involvement is universally present.[90] Discrete, red "palpable purpura" develop primarily on the buttocks, lower extremities, and distal upper extremities (Fig. 63–3). Rarely, the rash may involve the face and upper trunk as well. Lower extremity edema is quite common, with scrotal, facial, or scalp edema less common.[90]

Gastrointestinal involvement is also very common and usually appears no sooner than 1 week before the rash or 1 week afterward.[90, 101–103] However, it may occasionally precede the rash by several weeks. Patients usually experience diffuse abdominal pain, vomiting, and hematochezia.

Joint pain and overt pauciarticular arthritis occur in over half of affected patients. The knees and ankles are the most commonly involved joints.[90]

Renal manifestations such as overt hematuria and proteinuria occur in 30 to 40% of patients.[90] At times the renal involvement may be severe enough to produce hypertension or the nephrotic syndrome.

Central nervous system vasculitis may produce headaches and personality changes ranging from emotional lability to stupor and seizures.[104]

Pancreatitis,[105] cholecystitis,[106] pulmonary hemorrhage,[107] ureteral obstruction,[108] orchitis,[103] and myocardial infarction[109] have all been reported.

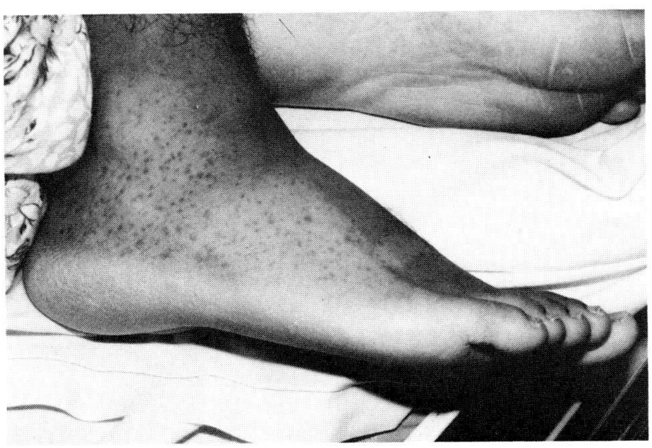

Figure 63–3. Showers of 2- to 4-mm palpable purpura that appeared on the lower extremities of a teenager who had been complaining of diffuse abdominal pain and diarrhea for 1 week prior to their appearance. The presence of purpura in this distribution confirmed the diagnosis of Henoch-Schönlein purpura.

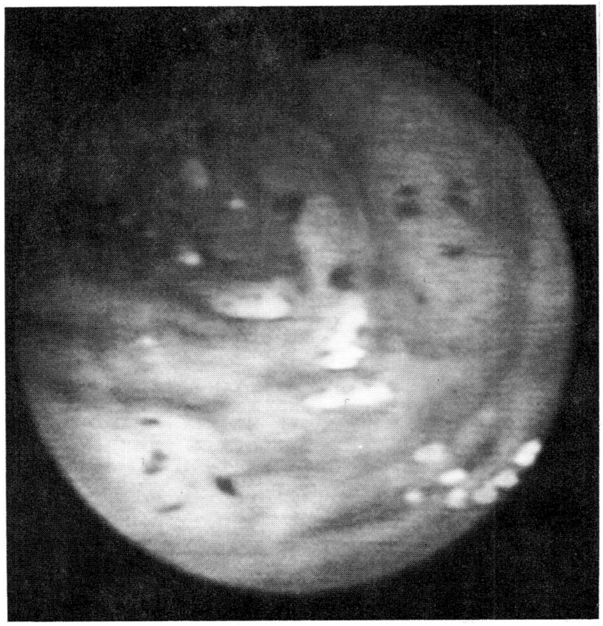

Figure 63–4. Endoscopic photograph revealing patchy hyperemia of duodenal mucosa in a patient later shown to have Henoch-Schönlein purpura.

Intussusception occurs in about 10% of children with abdominal pain.[90, 102, 103] Bowel perforation and small bowel stricture are much less common.[110]

Laboratory, Radiographic, Endoscopic, and Histologic Findings

About 75% of patients have leukocytosis and an elevated sedimentation rate, but gastrointestinal bleeding is rarely severe enough to produce anemia.[90] Platelet counts are generally normal despite the presence of purpura. Microscopic hematuria and proteinuria are seen in nearly half of patients.[90] Immunologic abnormalities include elevation of serum IgA, deficiency in serum C_3, and presence of circulating immune complexes in serum.[99, 100] Additionally, circulating antineutrophil cytoplasmic antibodies are present in a large percentage of patients.[111] An important indicator of poor prognosis is depletion of circulating factor VIII.[112]

Barium enema or small bowel series may reveal findings identical to those of any ischemic process—namely, coarsening of folds, spiculations of bowel wall, and thumbprinting.[113]

Endoscopy displays purpuric lesions of the small bowel and colon that are similar to those of the skin.[114] In addition, punctate hemorrhages and aphthoid lesions may be seen (Fig. 63–4).

Biopsy of bowel or skin reveals leukocytoclastic vasculitis (Fig. 63–5). Immunohistochemical stains show selective IgA and C_3 deposition on the wall of venules and the mesangium of renal glomeruli, a finding that differentiates Henoch-Schönlein purpura from other

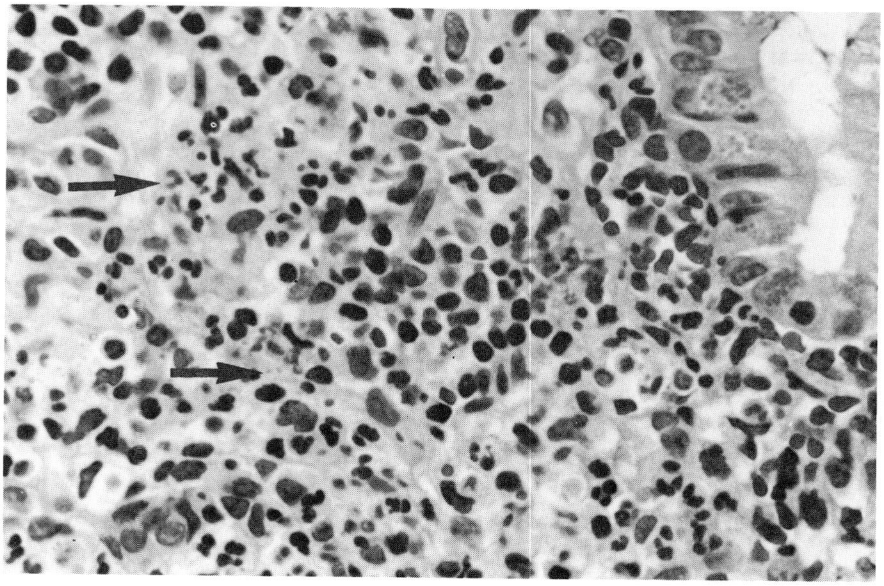

Figure 63–5. Duodenal biopsy in Henoch-Schönlein purpura showing extravasation of red cells and polymorphonuclear infiltrate of lamina propria. This field also shows leukocytoclasis or fragmentation of neutrophil nucleii producing "nuclear dust" (*arrows*). Hematoxylin-eosin stain, × 400.

vasculitides.[99] Renal biopsies traverse a spectrum of severity from focal glomerulonephritis to glomerular crescent formation and necrotizing arteriolitis, which carry a poor prognosis.[90]

Treatment and Prognosis

Corticosteroids do not alter the course of either the skin disease or the renal process, but an anecdotal report from 1960 suggests a salutary effect upon gastrointestinal symptoms.[90] More recent retrospective analysis casts doubt upon the efficacy of corticosteroids. At best, steroids seem to shorten the gastrointestinal course by only 1 to 2 days.[102] The decision to embark upon a course of corticosteroids should be tempered by the concern that symptoms of perforation or intussusception may be masked by the medication.

Though corticosteroids do not alter the course of renal insufficiency, case reports have suggested that azathioprine may be effective therapy.[115] Results of renal transplantation have been disappointing because at least 75% of patients experience a relapse in the transplanted kidney.[116]

Plasmapheresis may induce a temporary fall in serum IgA levels with symptomatic improvement, but symptoms tend to reoccur within a few days following cessation of therapy.[117]

Administration of factor VIII to those patients with depressed serum levels seems to ameliorate symptoms and shorten the symptomatic period.[118, 119]

Generally, Henoch-Schönlein purpura carries a good prognosis with complete resolution of central nervous system, gastrointestinal, and renal disease in more than 90% of patients.[90] Rarely, signs and symptoms will wax and wane. Two to 4% of children will develop renal insufficiency warranting dialysis.[116]

AMYLOIDOSIS

Nomenclature

The archaic classification categorized amyloidosis of heart, gastrointestinal tract, tongue, skin, and nerves as primary, whereas renal, splenic, hepatic, and adrenal amyloidosis were termed secondary. This system failed to consider whether an underlying infection, inflammation, or tumor was responsible for the amyloid deposits or whether the deposition was independent of any coexisting disease. Accordingly, the old classification has been replaced by the following six categories: (1) primary (lacking a coexisting disease), (2) associated with myeloma, (3) secondary (associated with infection or collagen-vascular disease), (4) familial, (5) local (confined to one organ), and (6) amyloidosis of aging.[120] This classification takes into account the pathogenesis of the disorder and the biochemical structure of individual amyloids.

Epidemiology

The overall prevalence of primary and secondary amyloidosis is probably less than 0.15%, and most cases are seen in adults.[121] However, amyloidosis may occasionally appear in children on hemodialysis[122] or with familial Mediterranean fever,[123] long-standing juvenile rheumatoid arthritis,[124] cystic fibrosis,[125] Crohn's disease,[126] autoimmune enteropathy,[127] and glycogenosis.[128] In developing countries, it has been seen in young people with long-standing tuberculosis[129] or leprosy.[130]

Pathogenesis and Biochemistry

The pathogenesis of amyloidosis remains unknown, but many data are available regarding the biochemistry of amyloid. A working hypothesis can therefore be proposed for amyloid deposition. Amyloid A (AA) predominates in inflammatory diseases and in familial Mediterranean fever.[131] It is composed of 76 amino acids and has a molecular weight of 8,500 daltons. A soluble protein (SAA) of 160,00 daltons displays N-terminal homology with AA, and its production is markedly enhanced during inflammation.[132] However, elevated SAA does not always lead to amyloidosis.[133] A second substance, amyloid enhancing factor, also produced by inflammation in susceptible individuals, catalyzes the proteolytic conversion of SAA to AA.[134] The site of synthesis is unknown, but electron microscopy suggests that reticuloendothelial cells both synthesize and degrade amyloid.[134]

Clinical Findings

Though amyloidosis may produce peripheral neuropathy, respiratory disease, cardiac conduction defects or cardiac failure, renal failure, or hepatomegaly with portal hypertension, this discussion is confined to gastrointestinal manifestations.

Seventy to 85% of patients with secondary amyloidosis have gastrointestinal involvement.[135, 136] Symptoms may be produced by one of three mechanisms. First, amyloid deposits may produce gastric outlet or small bowel obstruction.[137] Second, diffuse infiltration of the bowel wall may impair motility.[135] Finally, infiltration around blood vessels produces bowel ischemia.[135] The symptoms of gastrointestinal amyloidosis may therefore be those of obstruction (vomiting and abdominal distention), steatorrhea (copious and frequent stools, weight loss, and nutrient deficiencies), or intestinal ischemia (abdominal pain and gastrointestinal bleeding).

Radiographic, Endoscopic, and Histologic Findings

Though single-contrast radiography may miss subtle findings, double-contrast small bowel series may reveal innumerable 1- to 3-mm granularities, larger 3- to 4-mm nodules, or 4- to 10-mm polypoid lesions.[138] Irregular folds or multiple erosions may also be seen.

Endoscopy also reveals excrescences or erosions in any region of the gastrointestinal tract from tongue to rectum. Endoscopic abnormalities are most common in the duodenum (75%) and least common in the esophagus (16%).[136] Gastric lesions are present in 70% of patients, and colonic lesions in 54%.[136]

Histologic examination is more sensitive than endoscopy, revealing submucosal and mucosal amyloid deposits in 100% of duodenal biopsies, 95% of gastric biopsies, 91% of colonic biopsies, and 72% of esophageal biopsies.[136] Histologic sensitivity can be increased by staining specimens with Congo red and inspecting them under a polarizing microscope to display the green birefringence of amyloid.[139]

Treatment

A variety of therapeutic agents have been employed in an attempt to decrease antigenic stimulation, inhibit amyloid synthesis, prevent amyloid deposition, or enhance amyloid mobilization. None has been unequivocally successful. Corticosteroids appear to have no effect upon the progression of disease.[140] The use of alkylating agents in primary amyloidosis is controversial,[141, 142] and they have not been systematically studied in secondary amyloidosis. Results of vitamin C therapy are also disappointing.[143]

The only form of amyloidosis in which pharmacotherapy unquestionably alters the course is familial Mediterranean fever. Colchicine reduces the frequency of pain episodes and prevents amyloid deposition.[144]

Surgery to resect ischemic bowel may be necessary if amyloidosis has produced mesenteric vascular occlusion.[145]

BEHÇET'S DISEASE

History and Epidemiology

Behçet, a Turkish dermatologist, first described the constellation of oral ulceration, genital ulceration, and iritis in 1937.[146] Following his original report, gastrointestinal ulceration, central nervous system vasculitis, arthritis, thrombophlebitis, skin lesions, and cardiovascular abnormalities have been recognized as components of the same entity.[147] The prevalence is 0.3 to 10 per 100,000, and there is a 3:1 male predominance.[148] The disorder is much more common in Japan and Turkey than in the United States or Europe.[149] The most common age of presentation is in the third decade of life, but pediatric cases are being recognized with greater frequency. Human leukocyte antigen (HLA) type B27 is associated with the arthritis of Behçet's disease, B12 with the mucocutaneous lesions, and B5 with the iritis.[146] No association with any particular DR antigen has been found.[150]

Pathogenesis

The pathogenesis of Behçet's disease is unknown, but infectious etiologies have been proposed. The presence of circulating immune complexes and complement activation provides evidence for an autoimmune process.[151]

Clinical Features

Aphthous ulceration of the mouth and genitalia is present in 60 to 98% of patients with Behçet's disease.[148] Mouth ulcers are quite small. They are covered by pseudomembrane and surrounded by a red margin. The genital ulcers are identical to mouth ulcers in appearance, and they are located on the scrotum or vulva. Skin lesions include erythema nodosum or sterile pustules. Although 80% of adults have anterior and posterior uveitis, only 21% of pediatric patients have this finding.[152] Superficial thrombophlebitis, deep vein thrombosis, and arterial occlusion may affect any extremity. The arthritis is a nonmigratory, nondeforming polyarthritis.[148]

Neurologic symptoms include peripheral neuropathies, cranial nerve palsies, dementia, or seizures. Meningoencephalitis with cerebrospinal fluid pleocytosis may occur.[153]

Gastrointestinal symptoms are identical to those of inflammatory bowel disease. Gastrointestinal involvement includes the right colon in 50% of children, ileum in 25%, and distal colon in 25%.[152] Patients have pain, diarrhea, and sometimes hematochezia. Fistulas and perforation are common. The 12% of patients with esophageal ulceration experience dysphagia.[152]

Diagnosis

There are no pathognomonic biochemical, radiographic, endoscopic, or histologic findings. Indeed, many cases described in the literature share features with Crohn's disease, including discontinuous distribution of lesions, ileal involvement, and giant cell granulomata.[152] However, the gastrointestinal ulcers of Behçet's disease tend to be deep and flask shaped.[154, 155] They are devoid of giant cell change.

The Japanese Behçet Disease Research Committee has defined clinical criteria for the diagnosis.[156] The presence of four major criteria (iritis, oral ulceration, genital ulceration, and skin changes) satisfies the requirement for complete Behçet's disease. The presence of two major criteria and two of the three minor criteria (arthritis, bowel disease, and neurologic findings) constitutes a diagnosis of incomplete Behçet's disease.

Treatment

Corticosteroids and other immunosuppressants, such as chlorambucil and cyclosporine, have been employed with some success.[153] Successful therapy with colchicine has also been reported.[153]

DEGOS' DISEASE

History and Epidemiology

Kohlmeier first described this disorder in 1941, but he considered it an atypical form of thromboangiitis obliterans.[157] Degos, Delort, and Tricot, in their publications of 1942[158] and 1948,[159] characterized it as a distinct clinicopathologic entity. Slightly more than 100 cases have been reported.[160] Most have been in their second or third decade of life, but the age range is 3 weeks to 65 years of age.[161, 162] The male-to-female ratio is 3:1,[161, 162] and it has been reported in a family.[163]

Pathogenesis

Degos' disease is a unique obliterative (but not necrotizing) endarteritis that affects small- to medium-sized vessels. The pathogenesis is unknown, and all attempts to implicate a particular virus or specific immunologic event have been unsuccessful.[161] However, the discovery of anticardiolipin antibodies and circulating lupus anticoagulant links it to other collagen-vascular diseases.[164] Additionally, there is evidence for increased platelet adhesiveness that can be corrected by antiplatelet drugs.[165, 166]

Clinical Features

The hallmark of Degos' disease is the development of 1- to 3-mm cutaneous papules that appear singly or in crops of up to several dozen.[161] They are found predominantly over the upper trunk and arms. Face, scalp, hands, and feet are generally spared. They begin as pinkish, round papules that umbilicate and become depressed within a few days. Finally, the lesions atrophy to become depressed, porcelain-white ovals that may be covered by a fine scale. The margin is often telangiectatic. Most patients develop skin lesions before abdominal symptoms, but occasionally abdominal symptoms antedate the rash.[156, 167]

Identical lesions appear throughout the gastrointestinal tract and can be identified on the mucosal surface by endoscopy or on the serosal surface by laparoscopy or laparotomy.[162] At least two thirds of patients experience intermittent bouts of diffuse, severe abdominal pain that tends to improve spontaneously if perforation has not occurred.[161] However, there is a strong propensity for spontaneous, minute perforations that sometimes can be seen endoscopically.[162] Regardless of multiple intestinal surgeries, the majority of patients die of abdominal sepsis or peritonitis within 2 years after diagnosis.[168]

Other viscera such as heart, kidneys, bladder, liver, pancreas, and lungs may be affected, but seldom produce symptoms.[161]

Seventeen percent of patients experience neurologic involvement, with multiple small infarctions eventually leading to encephalomalacia.[167, 169] Approximately 8% of patients develop severe, progressive dementia.[169]

Histologic Diagnosis

Skin biopsies reveal hyperkeratotic, atrophic epidermis; dyscellular basal layer; and avascular, acellular dermis.[161] The margins of lesions possess numerous ectatic blood vessels.

Arteriolar changes seen in the skin are also present in intestine and other organs.[162] Arteriolar lumens are occluded by proliferating endothelial cells and thrombi.[161] The vessel walls are thickened by edema, but do not necrose.

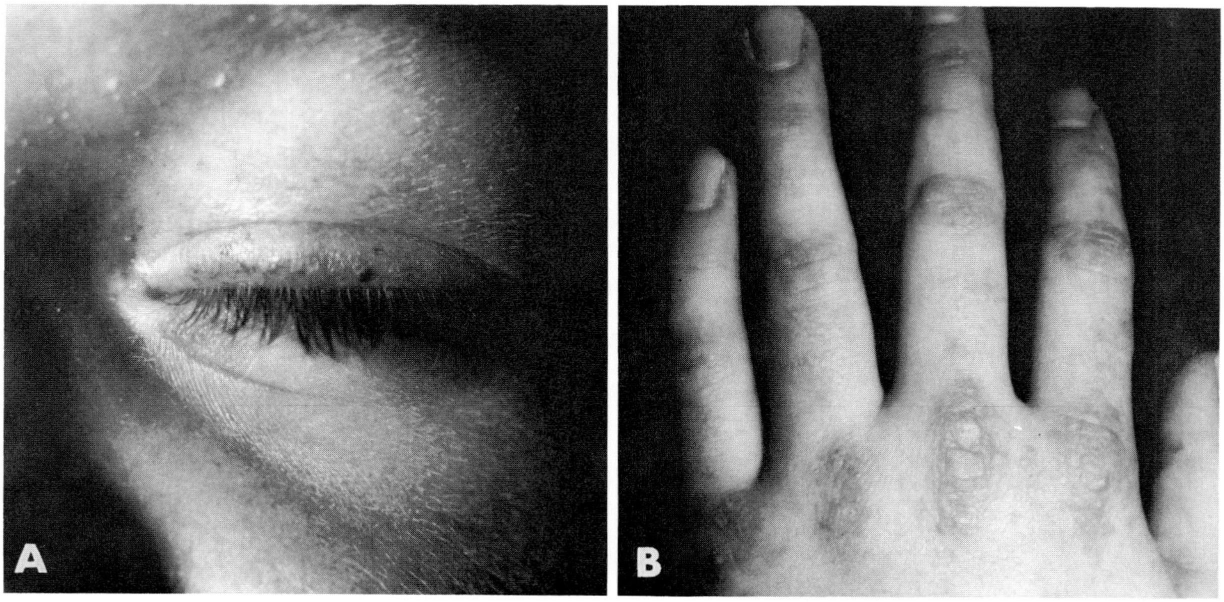

Figure 63–6. *A*, Heliotrope rash of dermatomyositis with violaceous discoloration of eyelids. *B*, Gottron's patches, which are erythematous, scaly areas overlying metacarpophalangeal joints of both hands. (Courtesy of Bernard Cohen, MD.)

Therapy

A variety of agents such as corticosteroids, cyclophosphamide, sulfanilamides, iodohydroxyquinolone, and other antibiotics have been used without success.[161]

Heparin, phenformin, and ethylestrenol have been employed to increase fibrinolysis, but these also appear ineffective.[161] Two case reports suggest efficacy of aspirin and dipyridamole in the face of increased platelet adhesiveness.[165, 166]

DERMATOMYOSITIS

Epidemiology

The incidence of dermatomyositis ranges from 1 per million[170] to 2.2 per 100,000 (in Israel).[171] The incidence is 7 to 10 times higher in North American or South African blacks than among Caucasians.[170] The disorder has a worldwide distribution, and its greatest incidence among children is in 10 to 14 year olds.[170, 171] A second peak is seen in 45 to 64 year olds.[170, 171] One report suggests that most cases present in late winter and early spring,[172] but those results have been disputed.[173] A few reports of familial dermatomyositis have appeared.[174] HLA types B8 and DR3 are present in greater than expected frequency among children with dermatomyositis.[175]

Pathogenesis

The etiology of dermatomyositis is unknown, but the current working hypothesis is that affected patients experience an immunologic response to a virus. Serologic evidence implicates coxsackie B[172] and other enteroviruses,[176] but data are far from convincing.

A variety of autoantibodies are present, but none are specific for the disorder.[177]

Clinical Features

The rash is the most consistent finding in the majority of cases, but muscle weakness may predominate in others.[178] The skin rash has three salient features.[179] First a heliotrope facial rash may be quite prominent. This rash consists of periorbital erythroderma with swollen eyelids resembling a sunburn (Fig. 63–6*A*). The second prominent feature is the Gottron patch—an elevated, bluish-red papule overlying knuckles. Several papules may overlie fingers (Fig. 63–6*B*) or toes. The third feature is the presence of telangiectasia overlying the proximal nailfolds.

Calcinosis of soft tissues accompanies long-standing disease.[180]

Muscle weakness is symmetric and involves the proximal muscles. Subtle difficulty appears in motor skills such as placing objects on high shelves, phonating, or climbing steps.[181] Progression is slow, but eventually the weakness becomes quite apparent to the casual observer.

Gastrointestinal symptoms are prominent in up to one third of patients.[180, 182–184] Most complain of dysphagia due to weakness of esophageal striated muscle.[180, 182] Furthermore, mesenteric vasculitis may produce intestinal ulcerations and multiple gastrointestinal perforations.[183, 184] Abdominal pain may be a prominent symptom in this subset of patients. A malabsorption syndrome has also been reported in occasional patients.[185]

Laboratory Findings

No specific laboratory tests exist, but several are extremely helpful. Serum muscle enzymes (creatine phosphokinase, lactic dehydrogenase, aldolase, and aspartate aminotransferase) are likely to be moderately elevated.[181–186]

Electromyographic abnormalities are also present.[186] Muscle irritability and spontaneous activity at rest are common. In addition, about half of the patients display fibrillation and early full recruitment with moderate activity. High-frequency discharges are seen in about 20% of patients.

Muscle biopsy reveals a focal inflammatory myopathy, but if unaffected muscles are biopsied, pathologic findings will be absent.[181, 186]

The vasculitis of this disorder affects capillaries, arterioles, and venules. Inflammation may be absent or present, and the most consistent finding is the presence of reticulotubular endothelial inclusions.[187]

Treatment and Prognosis

Corticosteroids at a dose of 1 to 2 mg per kg unquestionably improve the course of childhood dermatomyositis.[180] For corticosteroid-refractory or steroid-dependent cases, azathioprine,[188] cyclophosphamide,[189] methotrexate,[190] and hydroxychloroquine[191] have been employed with positive results.

The outcome is favorable in the majority of cases.[177, 180, 181, 186] Seventy-five percent of patients are left with no sequelae, and only 15 to 25% experience long-term muscle weakness or loss of function.[177, 180, 181] Only 5 to 10% of patients die of complications, but bowel perforation is a common cause of death and must be diagnosed early to permit a satisfactory surgical outcome.[183, 184]

SOLITARY RECTAL ULCER SYNDROME AND COLITIS CYSTICA PROFUNDA

History and Pathogenesis

Solitary rectal ulcer syndrome and colitis cystica profunda were thought to be unrelated processes throughout the eighteenth, nineteenth, and first half of the twentieth centuries. However, in 1967, Wayte and Helwig[192] noted a striking histologic similarity between biopsies of nine patients with colitis cystica profunda and those of four additional patients with solitary rectal ulcers reported by Haskell and Rovner in 1965.[193] Madigan and Morson[194] confirmed the histologic similarity of the two disorders.

Recently, visualization of external or internal rectal prolapse in a high percentage of patients with both disorders has led to a working pathogenic theory.[195, 196] Presumably, mucosal prolapse of the anterior rectum leads to stretching of blood vessels, trauma to the mucosa, thickening of the muscularis mucosae, ulceration, and (in colitis cystica profunda) implantation of surface epithelium into the submucosa. Recent rectal electromyographic and manometric studies have confirmed that patients with both disorders frequently experience abnormal expulsion dynamics.[197] They contract rather than relax their external sphincters with voluntary defecatory effort. This abnormality leads to excessive intrarectal pressure during defecation. Presumably the increased pressure initiates the sequence of events delineated above.

Epidemiology

In Ireland, where the most extensive epidemiologic studies have been performed, the incidence is 1 case per 100,000.[198] Though most patients reported in the literature are adults, children are unquestionably affected. Females appear to be at somewhat greater risk than males.

Clinical Features

Symptoms are variable, but 70 to 89% of patients pass bright-red blood from the rectum.[199, 200] Other symptoms include mucoid rectal discharge, diarrhea, constipation, crampy abdominal pain, tenesmus, and proctalgia. Bleeding may be severe enough to require transfusion. Rare patients may also experience rectal obstruction.

Endoscopic Features

The anus may be patulous, and Valsalva's maneuver may produce internal prolapse of the anterior rectal wall.[200] The mucosa may be hyperemic, edematous, or friable.[200]

The solitary ulcer syndrome is a misnomer, for over half of patients have multiple ulcers.[199, 201] The ulcer or ulcers range from a few millimeters to several centimeters in diameter. Most are located between 5 and 18 cm from the anal verge. Polypoid lesions are seen in some patients with the solitary rectal ulcer syndrome. Patients with colitis cystica profunda should, by definition, lack ulcers. However, solitary rectal ulcer and colitis cystica profunda are probably the same entity in different phases of evolution, and ulceration may coexist with multiple firm nodules studding the bowel wall in colitis cystica profunda.[202]

Histologic Features

Because many diagnostic entities may explain the sigmoidoscopic findings of solitary rectal ulcer and colitis cystica profunda, all patients should undergo biopsies of ulcerated areas and of intact mucosa in search of the pathognomonic histologic features of these syndromes. Biopsies will reveal "fibromuscular obliteration" of the lamina propria[199, 200] (Fig. 63–7). This finding rules out idiopathic inflammatory bowel disease even in the face of acute and chronic inflammation. A second feature of solitary rectal ulcer/colitis cystica profunda that distinguishes it from inflammatory bowel disease is the presence of submucosal mucus-filled cysts up to 2 cm in diameter.[199, 200]

Treatment

Conservative medical management with stool softeners or mineral oil will sometimes reduce bleeding.[199, 200] However, refractory cases may require one of the many surgical options available, including anterior proctopexy, posterior proctopexy, or mucosal sleeve resection with rectal wall plication. In the unlikely event of severe bleeding or obstruction, diverting colostomy may be necessary.[203]

MALAKOPLAKIA

History and Epidemiology

This rare disorder was first described in the urinary tract by Michaelis and Gutmann in 1902.[204] Subsequently, extraurinary involvement was identified, and in 1965, Terner and Lattes reported a case of gastrointestinal malakoplakia.[205] Since that time, only a handful of gastrointestinal cases have been reported,[206–210] but despite the rarity of this disorder, some generalizations can be made. It occurs with equal frequency in males and females, and the age range is 6 weeks to 88 years of age. It may be confined to the gastrointestinal tract or may also involve testis, prostate, epididymis, endometrium, broad ligament, vagina, retroperitoneum, adrenal gland, brain, bone, tonsil, or conjunctiva.[211] It may be a primary phenomenon or associated with other pathologic entities such as ulcerative colitis, adenocarcinoma, or immunodeficiency.[209]

Clinical Features

Most patients experience diarrhea, gross rectal bleeding, and abdominal pain.[206, 210] Weight loss and fever may predominate, or the lesions may produce intestinal obstruction. Some patients develop fistulas or confined perforations with pelvic abscesses.[210] Occasional patients may be asymptomatic, with the lesion being found incidentally.[208]

The lesions may be unifocal, multinodular, or masslike, with involvement of adjacent organs.[207] Sixty percent of cases are located in the left colon, but others may be confined to right colon, cecum, or ileocecal region.[207] The stomach is affected in about 10% of cases, and the most common type of fistula is gastrocolic.[207]

Endoscopic and Histologic Appearance

Grossly, the lesions are soft, slightly raised, umbilicated, bright-yellow plaques.[208] A multinodular variant consists of multiple 3- to 4-mm polypoid nodules.

The histologic lesions are composed of sheets of histiocytes with small eccentric nuclei.[208] They contain pathognomonic, target-shaped, calcified cytoplasmic inclusions called Michaelis-Gutmann bodies.[208] Numerous coliform bacteria and digested bacterial remnants are present within lysosomes.[208]

Pathogenesis

Though the pathogenesis remains unknown, work by Lou and Teplitz[212] and by Abdou and coworkers[213]

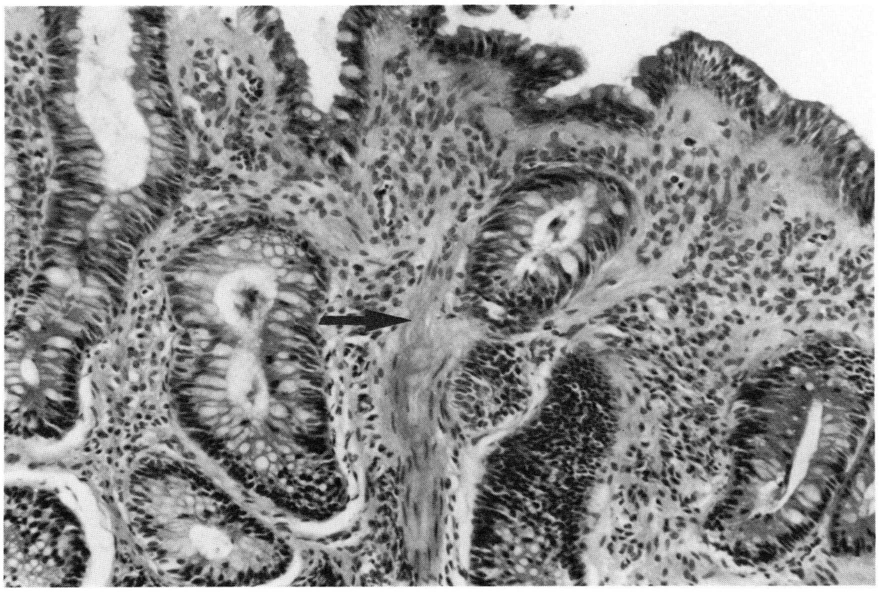

Figure 63–7. Rectal biopsy taken just peripheral to a "solitary rectal ulcer." Though the mucosal surface is intact, a smooth muscle fascicle extends into the lamina propria (*arrow*). Fibrosis also widens the lamina propria. These features are typical of the solitary rectal ulcer syndrome and colitis cystica profunda. Hematoxylin-eosin stain, × 100.

suggests that phagocyte bacterial killing is impaired. Therefore, gram-negative bacteria aggressively attack the epithelium of a number of tubular organs.

Treatment

Some patients have responded symptomatically to trimethoprim-sulfate[210] and to bethanechol (which facilitates bacterial killing).[213] However, those patients with fistulae require surgical excision and bowel resection. Patients with associated malignancy usually succumb, but isolated malakoplakia is sometimes compatible with long-term survival.[210]

TYPHLITIS

History and Epidemiology

The term *typhlitis* was first employed by Wagner and associates[214] in 1970 to describe a necrotizing colitis that involves the cecum and possibly the ileum or several regions of the colon. It is synonymous with the ileocecal syndrome or with neutropenic enteropathy. Most reported cases are neutropenic pediatric patients with leukemia,[214, 215] but it has also been seen in patients with other forms of neutropenia[216] or immune deficiency[216] and after solid organ transplantation.[217] Though considered rare by some, it is present at the time of death in 10 to 25% of leukemic patients who come to autopsy.[214, 215] Therefore, it may be the terminal event in a significant number of fatal leukemias. The prevalence is no different between lymphocytic and myelocytic leukemia, and the sex distribution appears to be approximately equal.[215] The majority of cases have been reported in children, but as chemotherapy regimens for adults become more aggressive, its incidence in adults also appears to be increasing.[218]

Pathogenesis

The pathogenesis of this disorder is unknown, but Prolla and Kirsner[219] have postulated that the sequence of events is initiated by a breakdown in the mucosal barrier due to chemotherapy or to leukemic infiltrates. Subsequently, bacteria invade the bowel wall, proliferate due to neutropenia, and produce endotoxin that leads to further mucosal damage.

Clinical Features

According to Katz and colleagues,[215] 78% of patients have abdominal pain and distention. The pain is usually in the right lower quadrant but may be more diffuse. Bright-red rectal bleeding was not observed in early reports,[214] but more recent reports describe it in about one third of patients.[215] Vomiting, diarrhea, and upper gastrointestinal bleeding are seen less frequently. Fever is seen in nearly all patients, and 14% of patients experience respiratory distress.

Anatomic Distribution

At autopsy, disease is confined to the cecum and appendix in only 22% of patients, whereas the cecum is involved in conjunction with the ileum and sometimes the ascending colon in 51%.[215] Discrete ulcerations extending throughout the colon are seen in 27% of autopsy specimens.[215]

Laboratory Findings

Almost all patients have absolute neutrophil counts less than 1,500 per mm^3, and 78% have counts less than 500 per mm^3.[214, 215]

Blood cultures taken when the patient is symptomatic are almost always positive for gram-negative bacteria or *Staphylococcus aureus*.[215] Fungal sepsis is also quite common, with 16% of premortem blood cultures growing *Candida, Aspergillus*, or *Cryptococcus*.[215]

Radiographic, Endoscopic, and Histologic Findings

Plain films and barium enema may show evidence of ileus, small bowel obstruction, pneumatosis coli, thickened bowel wall, cecal deformity, or nonfilling of the cecum.[220, 221] However, the preferred diagnostic modalities are ultrasonography[222] or computed tomography.[223] Thickened bowel wall may be visualized, and the progression or regression of the process can be followed with serial sonographic or tomographic examinations.

Endoscopy may reveal multiple colonic ulcers or a large, discrete area of cecal necrosis and ulceration. Though coagulopathy and neutropenia significantly increase the risk of colonoscopy and biopsy, these procedures should strongly be considered (if coagulopathy can be corrected) to rule out cytomegalovirus enteritis, whose clinical features are nearly identical.[224] Biopsy material should be sent not only for microscopy but also for bacterial, fungal, and viral culture.

A histologic picture of superficial cecal ulceration and hemorrhagic mucosal necrosis is characteristic.[214, 215] Blood vessels may be infiltrated by bacteria or fungal elements. Adjoining tissue is histologically normal.

Treatment

Typhlitis is not uniformly fatal if aggressive antibiotic treatment and supportive care are provided.[215] Fluid depletion and electrolyte imbalance should be corrected. Antibiotics with a broad enough spectrum to cover *S. aureus*, coliforms, and anaerobes should be administered. If a patient fails to defervesce after 72 hours of antibacterial therapy, antifungal coverage should be considered.[215]

Authors differ in the timing of surgery and the type of operation to perform in this group of patients. Some would operate when patients experience local peritoneal irritation[225] or when pneumatosis intestinalis is radiographically evident; others would await the onset of generalized peritonitis.[226] Even some cases of severe gastrointestinal hemorrhage have been managed nonoperatively.[227] Surgical techniques cover a spectrum from cecostomy and drainage to right hemicolectomy and ileocolostomy. Operative mortality ranges from 8 to 50%.[225, 226]

REFERENCES

1. Boley SJ, Treiber W, Winslow PR, et al: Circulatory response to acute reduction of superior mesenteric arterial flow (abstract). The Physiologist 1969; 12:180.
2. Boley SJ, Regan JA, Tunick PA, et al: Persistent vasoconstriction—a major factor in nonocclusive mesenteric ischemia. Curr Top Surg Res 1971; 3:425–433.
3. Haglund U, Abe T, Ahren C, et al: The intestinal mucosal lesions in shock. I. Studies on the pathogenesis. Eur Surg Res 1976; 8:435–447.
4. Granger D, Richardson P, Kvietys P, Mortillaro N: Intestinal blood flow. Gastroenterology 1980; 78:837–863.
5. Nowicki PT, Caniano DA, Szaniazlo K: Effect of intestinal denervation on intestinal vascular response to severe arterial hypoxia in newborn swine. Am J Physiol 1987; 253:G201–G205.
6. Shanbour LL, Jacobson ED: Digitalis and the mesenteric circulation. Am J Dig Dis 1972; 17:826–828.
7. Stillman A, Weinberg M, Mast W, Palpant S: Ischemic bowel disease attributable to ergot. Gastroenterology 1977; 72:1336–1337.
8. Bernardino M, Lawson T: Discrete colonic ulcers associated with oral contraceptives. Dig Dis Sci 1976; 21:503–506.
9. Hertzer N, Beven E, Humphries A: Chronic intestinal ischemia. Surg Gynecol Obstet 1977; 145:321–328.
10. Reinus JF, Brandt LJ, Boley SJ: Ischemic diseases of the bowel. Gastroenterol Clin North Am 1990; 19:319–343.
11. Huizinga WK, Nirmul D, Domingo Z, Ngakane H: Late presentation of small-bowel injury—hypoproteinemia, anaemia and obstruction. A report of 2 cases. South Afr Med J 1988; 73:251–252.
12. Ottinger L: Mesenteric ischemia. N Engl J Med 1982; 307:535–537.
13. Anane-Sefah JC, Blair E, Reckler S: Primary mesenteric venous occlusive disease. Surg Gynecol Obstet 1975; 141:740–742.
14. DeLaney HM: Prognostic factors in infarction of the intestine. Surg Gynecol Obstet 1972; 135:253–256.
15. Tomchik S, Wittenberg J, Ottinger LW: The roentgenographic spectrum of bowel infarction. Radiology 1970; 96:249–260.
16. O'Connell TX, Kadell B, Tompkins RK: Ischemia of the colon. Surg Gynecol Obstet 1976; 142:337–342.
17. Morson BC, Dawson IMP: Gastrointestinal Pathology. 2nd ed. Oxford, Blackwell, 1979, pp 380–398.
18. Walsh D: Deep tissue traumatism from roentgen ray exposure. Br Med J 1897; 2:272–273.
19. Allen-Mersh TG, Wilson EJ, Hope-Stone HF, Mann CV: Has the incidence of radiation-induced bowel damage following treatment of uterine carcinoma changed in the last 20 years? J R Soc Med 1986; 79:387–390.
20. Manson GR, Guernsey JM, Hanks, GE, Nelson TS: Surgical therapy for radiation enteritis. Oncology 1968; 22:241–257.
21. Roswit B, Malsky SJ, Reid CB: Severe radiation injuries of the stomach, small intestine, colon and rectum. Am J Roentgenol Radium Ther Nucl Med 1972; 114:460–475.
22. Donaldson SS, Jundt S, Ricour C, et al: Radiation enteritis in children. A retrospective, clinicopathologic correlation, and dietary management. Cancer 1975; 35:1167–1178.
23. Newman A, Katsaris J, Blendis LM, et al: Small intestinal injury in women who have had pelvic radiotherapy. Lancet 1973; 2:1471–1473.
24. Rubin P, Casarett G: A direction for clinical radiation pathology: The tolerance dose. *In* Vaeth JM, ed: Frontiers of Radiation Therapy and Oncology. Vol. 16. Baltimore, University Park Press, 1972, pp 1–16.
25. DeCosse JJ, Rhodes RS, Wentz WB, et al: The natural history and management of radiation induced injury of the gastrointestinal tract. Ann Surg 1969; 170:369–384.
26. Loughlin KR, Retik AB, Weinstein HJ, et al: Genitourinary rhabdomyosarcoma in children. Cancer 1989; 63:1600–1606.
27. Mauch P, Tarbell N, Weinstein H, et al: Stage IA and IIA supradiaphragmatic Hodgkin's disease: Prognostic factors in surgically staged patients treated with mantle and paraaortic irradiation. J Clin Oncol 1988; 6:1576–1583.
28. Trier JS, Browning TH: Morphological response of the mucosa of the human small intestine to x-ray exposure. J Clin Invest 1966; 45:194–204.
29. Quastlar H: The nature of intestinal radiation death. Radiation Res 1956; 4:303–320.
30. Carr ND, Pullen BR, Haselton PS, et al: Microvascular studies in human radiation bowel disease. Gut 1984; 25:448–454.
31. Joslin CA, Smith CW, Malik A: The treatment of cervix cancer using high activity Co-60 sources. Br J Radiol 1972; 45:257–270.
32. Buchler DA, Kline JC, Peckham BM, et al: Radiation reactions in cervical cancer therapy. Am J Obstet Gynecol 1971; 111:745–750.
33. Galland RB, Spencer J: Natural history and surgical management of radiation enteritis. Br J Surg 1987; 74:742–747.
34. Galland RB, Spencer J: The natural history of clinically established radiation enteritis. Lancet 1985; 1:1257–1258.
35. Bosch A, Frias Z: Complications after radiation therapy for cervical carcinoma. Acta Radiol (Ther) (Stockh) 1977; 16:53–62.
36. Strykker JA, Mortel R, Hepner GW: The effect of pelvic irradiation on lactose absorption. Radiat Oncol Biol Phys 1978; 4:859–863.
37. Yeoh E, Horowitz M: Radiation enteritis. Brit J Hosp Med 1988; 39:498–504.
38. Mendelson RM, Nolan DJ: The radiological features of chronic radiation enteritis. Clin Radiol 1985; 36:141–148.
39. Wellwood JM, Jackson BT: The intestinal complications of radiotherapy. Br J Surg 1973; 60:814–818.
40. Bounous G, LeBel E, Shuster J, et al: Dietary protection during radiation therapy. Strahlentherapie 1975; 149:476–483.
41. Mennie AT, Dalley VM, Dinneen LC, et al: Treatment of radiation-induced gastrointestinal distress with acetylsalicylate. Lancet 1975; 2:942–943.
42. Loiudice TA, Lang JA: Treatment of radiation enteritis: A comparison study. Am J Gastroenterol 1983; 78:481–487.
43. Rauch K, Weiland H: Behandlung der radiogenen kolitis mit salicylazosulfapyridin (Azulfidine). Strahlungtherapie 1972; 143:660–663.
44. Swan RW, Fowler WC, Boronow RC: Surgical management of radiation injury to the small intestine. Surg Gynecol Obstet 1976; 142:325–327.
45. von Gasser C, Gautier E, Steck A, et al: Hamolytisch-uramische syndrome. Bilaterale Nierenrindennekrosen bei akuten erworbenen hamolytischen Anamien. Schweiz Med Wschr 1955; 85:905–909.
46. Kaplan BS, Proesmans W: The hemolytic uremic syndrome of childhood and its variants. Semin Hematol 1987; 24:148–160.
47. Kinney JS, Gross TP, Porter CC, et al: Hemolytic-uremic syndrome: A population-based study in Washington, DC and Baltimore, Maryland. Am J Public Health 1988; 78:64–65.
48. Tarr PL, Neill MA, Allen J, et al: The increasing incidence of the hemolytic-uremic syndrome in King County, Washington: Lack of evidence for ascertainment bias. Am J Epidemiol 1989; 129:582–586.
49. Martin DL, MacDonald KL, White KE: The epidemiology and clinical aspects of the hemolytic-uremic syndrome in Minnesota. N Engl J Med 1990; 323:1161–1167.
50. Rowe PC, Orrbine E, Wells GA, et al: Epidemiology of hemolytic-uremic syndrome in Canadian children from 1986 to 1988. J Pediatr 1991; 119:218–224.
51. Neill MA, Agosti J, Rosen H: Hemorrhagic colitis with *Esche-*

richia coli 0157:H7 preceding adult hemolytic uremic syndrome. Arch Intern Med 1985; 145:2215–2217.
52. Gianantonio CA, Vitacco M, Mendilaharzu F, et al: The hemolytic-uremic syndrome. Nephron 1973; 11:174–192.
53. Kaplan BS, Katz J, Krawitz S, et al: An analysis of the results of therapy in 67 cases of the hemolytic-uremic syndrome. J Pediatr 1971; 78:420–425.
54. Lieberman E: Hemolytic-uremic syndrome. J Pediatr 1972; 80:1–16.
55. Drummond KN: Hemolytic uremic syndrome—then and now. N Engl J Med 1985; 312:116–118.
56. Kaplan BS, Chesney RW, Drummond KN: Hemolytic uremic syndrome in families. N Engl J Med 1975; 292:1090–1093.
57. Karmali MA, Petric M, Lim C, et al: The association between hemolytic uremic syndrome and infection by verotoxin-producing *Escherichia coli*. J Infect Dis 1985; 151:775–782.
58. Gransden WPR, Damm MAS, Anderson JD, et al: Further evidence associating hemolytic uremic syndrome with infection by verotoxin-producing *Escherichia coli* 0157:H7. J Infect Dis 1986; 154:522–524.
59. Neill MA, Tarr PI, Clausen C, et al: *Escherichia coli* 0157:H7 as the predominant pathogen associated with the hemolytic uremic syndrome: A prospective study in the Pacific Northwest. Pediatrics 1987; 80:37–40.
60. Scotland SM, Rowe B, Smith HR, et al: Vero cytotoxin-producing strains of *Escherichia coli* from children with haemolytic uraemic syndrome and their detection by specific DNA probes. J Med Microbiol 1988; 25:237–243.
61. Lopez EL, Diaz M, Grinstein S, et al: Hemolytic uremic syndrome and diarrhea in Argentine children: The role of Shiga-like toxins. J Infect Dis 1989; 160:469–475.
62. Ray C, Tucker VL, Harris DJ, et al: Enterovirus associated with the hemolytic-uremic syndrome. Pediatrics 1970; 46:378–388.
63. Mathieu H, LeClerc F, Habib R, et al: Etude clinique et biologique de 37 observations de syndrome hemolytique et uremique. Arch Franc Pediat 1969; 26:369–390.
64. Gradishar WJ, Vokes EE, et al: Chemotherapy-related hemolytic-uremic syndrome after the treatment of head and neck cancer. Cancer 1990; 66:1914–1918.
65. O'Brien AD, Holmes RK: Shiga and shiga-like toxins. Microbiol Rev 1987; 51:206–220.
66. Taylor CM, Milford DV, Rose PE, et al: The expression of blood group P1 in post-enteropathic haemolytic uraemic syndrome. Pediatr Nephrol 1990; 4:59–61.
67. Walters MDS, Levin M, Smith C, et al: Intravascular platelet activation in the hemolytic uremic syndrome. Kidney Int 1988; 33:107–115.
68. Fong JSC, Kaplan BS: Impairment of platelet aggregation in the hemolytic uremic syndrome. Evidence for platelet "exhaustion." Blood 1982; 60:564–569.
69. Levin M, Stroobant P, Walters MDS, et al: Platelet derived growth factors as possible mediators of vascular proliferation in the sporadic haemolytic uremic syndrome. Lancet 1986; 2:830–833.
70. Koster F, Levin J, Walker L, et al: Hemolytic uremic syndrome after shigellosis: Relation to endotoxemia and circulating immune complexes. N Engl J Med 1978; 298:927–933.
71. O'Regan S, Chesney RW, Kaplan BS, et al: Red cell membrane phospholipid abnormalities in the hemolytic uremic syndrome. Clin Nephrol 1980; 15:14–17.
72. Furase A, Hattori S, Matusda I: A case hemolytic uremic syndrome with high concentration of circulating immune complexes in the initial stage. Int J Pediatr Nephrol 1983; 4:123–126.
73. Monnens L, Van de Meer W, Langenhuysen C, et al: Platelet aggregating factor in the epidemic form of hemolytic uremic syndrome in childhood. Clin Nephrol 1985; 24:135–137.
74. Moake JL, Byrnes JJ, Troll JH, et al: Abnormal VIII: von Willebrand factor patterns in the plasma of patients with the hemolytic uraemic syndrome. Blood 1984; 64:592–598.
75. Remuzzi G, Misiani R, Marchesi D, et al: Haemolytic uraemic syndrome: Deficiency of plasma factor(s) regulating prostacyclin activity? Lancet 1978; 2:871–872.
76. Whitington PF, Friedman AL, Chesney RW: Gastrointestinal disease in the hemolytic-uremic syndrome. Gastroenterology 1979; 76:728–733.
77. Brandt ML, O'Regan S, Rousseau E, et al: Surgical complications of the hemolytic-uremic syndrome. J Pediatr Surg 1990; 25:1109–1112.
78. Berman W Jr: The hemolytic-uremic syndrome: Initial clinical presentation mimicking ulcerative colitis. J Pediatr 1972; 81:275–278.
79. Tarr PI, Neill MA, Clausen CR, et al: *Escherichia coli* 0157:H7 and the hemolytic uremic syndrome: Importance of early cultures in establishing the etiology. J Infect Dis 1990; 162:553–556.
80. Grodinsky S, Telmesani A, Robson WL, et al: Gastrointestinal manifestations of hemolytic uremic syndrome: Recognition of pancreatitis. J Pediatr Gastroenterol Nutr 1990; 11:518–524.
81. Van Damme Lombaerts R, Proesmans W, Van Damme B, et al: Heparin plus dipyridamole in childhood hemolytic-uremic syndrome: A prospective, randomized study. J Pediatr 1988; 113:913–918.
82. Defreyn G: Plasmapheresis in the haemolytic-uraemic syndrome in children. Br Med J 1981; 282:1667–1668.
83. Loirat C, Sonsino E, Hinglais N, et al: Treatment of the childhood haemolytic uraemic syndrome with plasma. Pediatr Nephrol 1988; 2:279–285.
84. McGraw ME, Lendon M, Stevens RF, et al: Haemolytic uraemic syndrome and the Thomsen Friedenreich antigen. Pediatr Nephrol 1989; 3:135–139.
85. Heberden W cited by Rook A: Heberden's cases of anaphylactoid purpura. Arch Dis Child 1958; 33:271–272.
86. Schönlein JL: Allgemeine und specielle pathologie und therapie. Freiburg: Etlinger, 1837, pp 48–49.
87. Henoch E: Uber eine eigenthumliche form von purpura. Klin Wchnschr 1874; 11:641–643.
88. Henoch E: Neunter Aschnitt III. Die hamorrhagische diatheses purpura. Vorlesung uber kinderdrandkeiten. Berlin, Hirschwald, 1895, pp 847.
89. Cream JJ, Gumpel JJ, Peachey RDG: Schönlein-Henoch purpura in the adult. Q J Med 1970; 39:461–484.
90. Allen DM, Diamond LK, Howell DA: Anaphylactoid purpura in children (Schönlein-Henoch syndrome). Am J Dis Child 1960; 99:833–854.
91. Maggiore G, Martini A, Grifco D: Hepatitis B virus infection and Schönlein-Henoch purpura. Am J Dis Child 1984; 138:681–682.
92. Garty BZ, Danon YL, Nitzan M: Schönlein-Henoch purpura associated with hepatitis A infection (letter). Am J Dis Child 1985; 139:547.
93. LeFrere J, Courouce A, Soulier J, et al: Henoch-Schönlein purpura and human parvovirus infection. Pediatrics 1986; 78:183–184.
94. Bywaters EG, Isdale I, Kempton JJ: Schönlein-Henoch purpura: Evidence for a group A beta-hemolytic streptococcal aetiology. Q J Med 1957; 26:161–175.
95. Ackroyd MD: Allergic purpura, including purpura due to foods, drugs, and infections. Am J Med 1953; 14:605–632.
96. Gagliano RS, Costanzi JJ, Beathard GA, et al: The nephrotic syndrome associated with neoplasia: An unusual paraneoplastic syndrome. Report of a case and review of the literature. Am J Med 1976; 60:1026–1031.
97. Garcias VA, Herr HW: Henoch-Schönlein purpura associated with cancer of the prostate. Urology 1982; 19:155–158.
98. Mitchell DM: Relapse of Henoch-Schönlein disease associated with lung carcinoma. J R Soc Med 1979; 72:614–615.
99. Stevenson JA, Leong LA, Cohen AH, et al: Henoch-Schönlein purpura: Simultaneous demonstration of IgA deposits in involved skin, intestine, and kidney. Arch Pathol Lab Med 1982; 106:192–195.
100. Fauci AS, Haynes BF, Katz P: The spectrum of vasculitis: Clinical, pathologic, immunologic and therapeutic considerations. Ann Intern Med 1978; 89:660–676.
101. Glasier CM, Siegel MK, McAlister WH, et al: Henoch-Schönlein syndrome in children: Gastrointestinal manifestations. Am J Roentgenol 1981; 136:1081–1085.
102. Rosenbloom ND, Winter HS: Steroid effects on the course of abdominal pain in children with Henoch-Schönlein purpura. Pediatrics 1987; 79:1018–1021.
103. Katz S, Borst M, Seekri I, et al: Surgical evaluation of Henoch-Schönlein purpura: Experience with 110 children. Arch Surg 1991; 126:849–854.
104. Belman A, Leicher C, Moshe S, et al: Neurologic manifestations

of Schönlein-Henoch purpura: Report of three cases and review of the literature. Pediatrics 1985; 75:687–692.
105. Branski D, Gross V, Gross-Kieselstein E, et al: Pancreatitis as a complication of Henoch-Schönlein purpura. J Pediatr Gastroenterol 1982; 1:275–276.
106. Case 14-1980. Case records of the Massachusetts General Hospital: Weekly clinicopathological exercises. N Engl J Med 1980; 302:853–858.
107. Olson JC, Kelly KJ, Pan CG, et al: Pulmonary disease with hemorrhage in Henoch-Schönlein purpura. Pediatrics 1992; 89:1177–1181.
108. Powell JM, Ware H, Williams G: Recurrent ureteric obstruction in association with Henoch-Schönlein purpura. Postgrad Med J 1987; 63:699–701.
109. Delhumeau A, Cavellat JF, Granry JC, et al: Cardiac tamponade in rheumatoid purpura. Ann Francaises d'Anesthesie et de Reanimation 1982; 1:183–185.
110. Lombard KA, Shah PC, Thrasher TV, et al: Ileal stricture as a later late complication of Henoch-Schönlein purpura. Pediatrics 1986; 77:396–398.
111. Wall Bake AWL, Lobatto SS, Jonges L et al: IgA antibodies directed against cytoplasmic antigens of polymorphonuclear leukocytes in patients with Henoch-Schönlein purpura. Adv Exp Med Biol 1987; 216B:1593–1598.
112. Kamitsuji H, Tani K, Yasui M, et al: Activity of blood coagulation factor XIII as a prognostic indicator in patients with Henoch-Schönlein purpura. Eur J Pediatr 1987; 146:519–523.
113. Rodriguez-Erdmann F, Levitan R: Gastrointestinal and roentgenological manifestations of Henoch-Schönlein purpura. Gastroenterology 1968;54:260–264.
114. Tomomasa T, Hsu JY, Itoh K, et al: Endoscopic findings in pediatric patients with Henoch-Schönlein purpura and gastrointestinal symptoms. J Pediatr Gastroenterol Nutr 1987; 6:725–729.
115. Dosa S, Caerns SA, Mallick NP, et al: Relapsing Henoch-Schönlein syndrome with renal involvement in a patient with an IgA monoclonal gammopathy—a study of the results of immunosuppressant and cytotoxic therapy. Nephron 1980; 26:145–148.
116. Hasegawa A, Kawamura T, Ito H, et al: Fate of renal grafts with recurrent Henoch-Schönlein purpura nephritis in children. Transplant Proc 1989; 21:2130–2133.
117. Kauffmann RH, Houwert DA: Plasmaphoresis in rapidly progressive Henoch-Schönlein glomerulonephritis and the effect on circulating IgA immune complexes. Clin Nephrol 1981; 16:155–160.
118. Utani A, Ohta M, Shinya A, et al: Successful treatment of adult Henoch-Schönlein purpura with factor XIII concentrate. J Am Acad Dermatol 1991; 24:438–442.
119. Fukui H, Kamitsuji H, Nagao T, et al: Clinical evaluation of a pasteurized factor XIII concentrate administration in Henoch-Schönlein purpura. Thromb Res 1989; 56:667–675.
120. Kyle R, Bayrd E: Amyloidosis. Medicine 1975; 54:271–299.
121. Cohen AS: Amyloidosis. *In* McCarthy DJ, ed: Arthritic and Allied Conditions. 4th ed. Philadelphia, Lea and Febiger, 1989, pp 1273–1293.
122. Bardin T, Zingraff J, Shirahame T, et al: Hemodialysis-associated amyloidosis and beta-2 microglobulin: A clinical and immunohistochemical study. Am J Med 1987;83:419–424.
123. Kocak H, Besbas N, Saatci U, et al: Amyloidosis in children with familial Mediterranean fever. Turk J Pediatr 1989; 31:281–287.
124. David J: Amyloidosis in juvenile chronic arthritis. Clin Exp Rheumatol 1991; 9:73–78.
125. Travis WD, Castile R, Vawter G, et al: Secondary (AA) amyloidosis in cystic fibrosis. A report of three cases. Am J Clin Pathol 1986; 85:419–424.
126. Kahn E, Markowitz J, Simpser E, et al: Amyloidosis in children with inflammatory bowel disease. J Pediatr Gastroenterol Nutr 1989; 8:447–453.
127. Pearson RD, Swenson I, Schenk EA, et al: Fatal multisystem disease with immune enteropathy heralded by juvenile rheumatoid arthritis. J Pediatr Gastroenterol Nutr 1989; 8:259–265.
128. Kikuchi M, Haginoya K, Miyabayashi S, et al: Secondary amyloidosis in glycogen storage disease type Ib. Eur J Pediatr 1990; 149:344–345.
129. Looi LM: The pattern of amyloidosis in a Malaysian patient population. Histopathology 1991; 18:133–141.
130. Ponce P, Ramos A, Ferreira ML, et al: Renal involvement in leprosy. Nephrol Dial Transplant 1989; 4:81–84.
131. Husby G, Sletten K, Michaelson TE, et al: Amyloid fibril protein subunit, "protein AS": Distribution in tissue and serum in different clinical types of amyloidosis including that associated with myelomatosis and Waldenstrom's macroglobulinemia. Scand J Immunol 1973; 2:395–404.
132. Linke RP, Sipe JD, Pollock PS, et al: Isolation of low-molecular-weight serum component antigenically related to an amyloid fibril protein of unknown origin. Proc Natl Acad Sci USA 1975; 72:1473–1475.
133. Sipe JD, Vogel SN, Sztein MB, et al: The role of interleukin I on acute phase serum amyloid A (SAA) and serum amyloid P (SAP) biosynthesis. Ann NY Acad Sci 1982; 389:137–150.
134. Kisilevsky R, Boudreau L: Kinetics of amyloid deposition I. The effects of amyloid-enhancing factor and splenectomy. Lab Invest 1983; 48:53–59.
135. Gilat T, Revach M, Sohar E: Deposition of amyloid in the gastrointestinal tract. Gut 1969; 10:98–104.
136. Tada S, Iida M, Iwashita A, et al: Endoscopic and biopsy findings of the upper digestive tract in patients with amyloidosis. Gastrointest Endosc 1990; 36:10–14.
137. Jensen K, Raynor S, Rose SG, et al: Amyloid tumors of the gastrointestinal tract: A report of two cases and review of the literature. Am J Gastroenterol 1985; 80:784–786.
138. Tada S, Iida M, Matsui T, et al: Amyloidosis of the small intestine: Findings on double-contrast radiographs. Am J Roentgenol 1991; 156:741–744.
139. Bennhold H: Eine spezifische Amyloidfarbung mit Kongorot. Munchen Med Wochenschr 1922; 69:1537–1538.
140. Stoeber E: Corticosteroid treatment of juvenile chronic polyarthritis over 22 years. Eur J Pediatr 1976; 121:141–147.
141. Buxbaum JN, Hurley ME, Chuba J, et al: Amyloidosis of the AL type. Clinical, morphologic and biochemical aspects of the response to therapy with alkylating agents and prednisone. Am J Med 1979; 67:867–878.
142. Gertz MA, Kyle RA, Greipp PR: Response rates and survival in primary systemic amyloidosis. Blood 1991; 77:257–262.
143. Baltz ML, Caspi D, Glatthaar B, et al: The failure of ascorbic acid therapy to alter the induction or remission of murine amyloidosis. Clin Exp Immunol 1984; 57:657–662.
144. Zemer D, Pras M, Sohar E, et al: Colchicine in the prevention and treatment of the amyloidosis of familial Mediterranean fever. N Engl J Med 1986; 314:1001–1005.
145. O'Doherty DP, Neoptolemos JP, Wood VF: Place of surgery in the management of amyloid disease. Br J Surg 1987; 74:83–88.
146. Behçet H: Uber rezidivierende aphthose, durch ein Virus verusaschte Geschwure am Mund, am Auge und an den Genitalien. Dermatol Wochenschr 1937; 105:1152–1157.
147. Mason RM, Barnes CG: Behçet's syndrome with arthritis. Ann Rheum Dis 1969; 28:95–102.
148. Chajek T, Fainaru M: Behçet's disease. Report of 41 cases and a review of the literature. Medicine 1975; 54:179–196.
149. O'Duffy JD: Summary of international symposium on Behçet's disease. J Rheum 1978; 5:229–233.
150. Lehner T, Batchelor JR, Challacombe SJ, et al: An immunogenetic basis for tissue involvement in Behçet's syndrome. Immunology 1979; 37:895–900.
151. Valesini GV, Picardo M, Pastore R, et al: Circulating immune complexes in Behçet's syndrome: Purification, characterization and cross reactivity studies. Clin Exp Immunol 1981; 44:522–529.
152. Stringer DA, Cleghorn GJ, Durie PR, et al: Behçet's syndrome involving the gastrointestinal tract—a diagnostic dilemma in childhood. Pediatr Radiol 1986; 16:131–134.
153. Arbesfeld SJ, Kurban AK: Behçet's disease. New perspectives on an enigmatic syndrome. J Am Acad Dermatol 1988; 19:767–779.
154. Watanabe I, Kuwabara N, Fukada Y: Histopathological studies in intestinal Behçet's disease. Stomach Intest 1979; 7:903–913.
155. Chong SKF, Wright VM, Nishigame T, et al: Infantile colitis: A manifestation of intestinal Behçet's syndrome. J Pediatr Gastroenterol Nutr 1988; 7:622–627.
156. Lakhanpal S, Tani K, Lie JT, et al: Pathological features of Behçet's syndrome. A review of Japanese autopsy registry data. Hum Pathol 1985; 16:790–795.

157. Kohlmeier W: Multiple Hautnekrosen bei thrombangiitis obliterans. Arch Dermatol Syphil 1941; 181:783–792.
158. Degos R, Delort J, Tricot R: Dermatite papulo-squameuse atrophiante. Bull Soc Franc Dermatol Syphil 1942; 49:148–150.
159. Degos R, Delort J, Tricot R: Papulose atrophiante maligne (syndrome cutaneo-intestinal). Bul Memoir Soc Medicale Hopit Paris 1948; 64:803–806.
160. Burg G, Vieluf D, Stolz W, et al: Maligne atrophische papulose (Morbus Kohlmeier-Degos). Hautarzt 1989; 40:480–485.
161. Degos R: Malignant atrophic papulosis. Br J Dermatol 1979; 100:21–135.
162. Casparie MK, Meyer JWR, van Huystee BEW, et al: Endoscopic and histopathologic features of Degos' disease. Endoscopy 1991; 23:231–233.
163. Habbema L, Kisch LS, Starink TM: Familial malignant atrophic papulosis (Degos' disease)—additional evidence for heredity and a benign course (letter). Br J Dermatol 1986; 114:134–135.
164. Englert HJ, Hawkes CH, Boey ML, et al: Degos' disease: Association with anticardiolipin antibodies and the lupus anticoagulant. Br Med J 1984; 289:576.
165. Stahl D, Thomsen K, Hou-Jensen K: Malignant atrophic papulosis. Arch Dermatol 1978; 114:1687–1689.
166. Drucker CR: Malignant atrophic papulosis: Response to antiplatelet therapy. Dermatologica 1990; 180:90–92.
167. Case 44-1980. Case records of the Massachusetts General Hospital: Weekly clinicopathologic exercises. N Engl J Med 1980; 303:1103–1111.
168. Black MM: Malignant atrophic papulosis (Degos' disease). Int J Dermatol 1976; 15:405–411.
169. Horner FA, Myers GJ, Stumpf DA, et al: Malignant atrophic papulosis (Kohlmeier-Degos disease) in childhood. Neurology 1976; 26:317–321.
170. Medsger TA Jr, Dawson WN, Masi AT: The epidemiology of polymyositis. Am J Med 1970; 48:715–723.
171. Benbassat J, Geffel D, Zlotnick A: Epidemiology of polymyositis-dermatomyositis in Israel. Isr J Med Sci 1980; 16:197–200.
172. Christensen ML, Pachman LM, Maryjowski MC: Antibody to coxsackie-B virus: Increased incidence in sera from children with recently diagnosed juvenile dermatomyositis (abstract). Arthritis Rheum 1983; 26:S24.
173. Koch MJ, Brody JA, Gillespie MM: Childhood polymyositis: A case-control study. Am J Epidemiol 1976; 104:627–631.
174. Harati Y, Niakan E, Bergman EW: Childhood dermatomyositis in monozygotic twins. Neurology 1986; 36:721–723.
175. Friedman JM, Pachman LM, Maryjowski ML, et al: Immunogenetic studies of juvenile dermatomyositis: HLA-DR antigen frequencies. Arthritis Rheum 1983; 26:214–216.
176. Rosenberg NL, Rotbart HA, Abzug MJ, et al: Evidence for a novel picornavirus in human dermatomyositis. Ann Neurol 1989; 26:204–209.
177. Pachman LM, Friedman JM, Maryjowski-Sweeney ML, et al: Immunogenetic studies of juvenile dermatomyositis: III. Study of antibody to organ-specific and nuclear antigens. Arthritis Rheum 1985; 28:151–157.
178. Spenser CH, Hanson V, Singsen BH, et al: Course of treated juvenile dermatomyositis. J Pediatr 1984; 105:399–408.
179. Everett MA, Curtis AC: Dermatomyositis. Arch Int Med 1957; 100:70–76.
180. Miller LC, Michael AF, Kim Y: Childhood dermatomyositis: Clinical course and long-term follow-up. Clin Pediatr 1987; 26:561–566.
181. Norins AL: Juvenile dermatomyositis. Med Clin North Am 1989; 73:1193–1209.
182. Metheny JA: Dermatomyositis: A vocal and swallowing disease entity. Laryngoscope 1978; 88:147–161.
183. Magill HL, Hixson SD, Whitington D, et al: Duodenal perforation in childhood dermatomyositis. Pediatr Radiol 1984; 14:28–30.
184. Schullinger JN, Jacobs JC, Berdon WE: Diagnosis and management of gastrointestinal perforations in childhood dermatomyositis with particular reference to perforations of the duodenum. J Pediatr Surg 1985; 20:521–524.
185. Transfeldt EE, Morley JE, Segal F, et al: Polymyositis as a cause of malabsorption. A case report. S Afr Med J 1977; 51:176–178.
186. Pachman LM: Juvenile dermatomyositis. Pediatr Clin North Am 1986; 33:1097–1117.
187. Boylan RC, Sokoloff L: Vascular lesions in dermatomyositis. Arthritis Rheum 1960; 3:379–386.
188. Benson MD, Aldo MA: Azathioprine therapy in polymyositis. Arch Intern Med 1973; 132:547–551.
189. Miller G, Heckmatt JZ, Dubowitz V: Drug treatment of juvenile dermatomyositis. Arch Dis Child 1983; 58:445–450.
190. Metzger AL, Bohan A, Goldberg LS: Polymyositis and dermatomyositis: Combined methotrexate and corticosteroid therapy. Ann Intern Med 1974; 81:182–189.
191. Olson NY, Lindsley CB: Adjunctive use of hydroxychloroquine in childhood dermatomyositis. J Rheumatol 1989; 16:1545–1547.
192. Wayte DM, Helwig EB: Colitis cystica profunda. Am J Clin Pathol 1967; 48:159–169.
193. Haskel B, Rovner H: Solitary ulcer of the rectum. Dis Colon Rectum 1965; 8:333–336.
194. Madigan MR, Morson BC: Solitary ulcer of the rectum. Gut 1969; 10:871–881.
195. Kuijpers MC, Schreve RH, Hoedemakers HTC: Diagnosis of functional disorders of defecation causing the solitary rectal ulcer syndrome. Dis Colon Rectum 1986; 29:126–129.
196. Goei R, Baeten C, Arends JW: Solitary rectal ulcer syndrome: Findings at barium enema study and defecography. Radiology 1988; 168:303–306.
197. Womack NR, Williams NS, Mist JHH, et al: Anorectal function in the solitary rectal ulcer syndrome. Dis Colon Rectum 1987; 30:319–323.
198. Martin CJ, Parks TG, Biggart JD: Solitary rectal ulcer syndrome in Northern Ireland 1971–1980. Br J Surg 1981; 68:744–747.
199. Levine DS: "solitary" rectal ulcer syndrome: Are "solitary" rectal ulcer syndrome and "localized" colitis cystica profunda analogous syndromes caused by rectal prolapse? Gastroenterology 1987; 92:243–253.
200. Niv Y, Bat L: Solitary rectal ulcer syndrome—clinical, endoscopic, and histological spectrum. Am J Gastroenterol 1986; 48:486–491.
201. Hershfield NB, Langevin JE, Kelly JK: Endoscopic and histologic features of the solitary rectal ulcer syndrome (SRUS). Gastointest Endosc 1984; 30:162.
202. Guest CB, Reznick RK: Colitis cystica profunda: Review of the literature. Dis Colon Rectum 1989; 32:983–988.
203. Stavorovsky M, Weintraub S, Ratan J, et al: Successful treatment of a benign solitary rectal ulcer by temporary diverting sigmoidostomy: Report of a case. Dis Colon Rectum 1977; 20:347–350.
204. Michaelis L, Gutmann C: Ueber Einschlusse in Blasentumoren. Ztschr Klin Med 1902; 47:208–215.
205. Terner JY, Lattes R: Malakoplakia of colon and retroperitoneum. Am J Clin Pathol 1965; 44:20–31.
206. Sanusi ID, Tio FO: Gastrointestinal malacoplakia: Report of a case and a review of the literature. Am J Gastroenterol 1974; 62:356–365.
207. Nakabayashi H, Ito T, Izutsu K: Malakoplakia of the stomach: Report of a case and review of the literature. Arch Pathol Lab Med 1978; 102:136–139.
208. Chaudhry AP, Saigal KP, Intengan M, et al: Malakoplakia of the large intestine found incidentally at necropsy: Light and electron microscopic features. Dis Colon Rectum 1979; 22:73–81.
209. McClure J: Malakoplakia of the gastrointestinal tract. Postgrad Med J 1981; 57:95–103.
210. Harfi HA, Akhtar M, Subayti YA, et al: Gastrointestinal malacoplakia in children. Clin Pediatr 1985; 24:423–428.
211. Scheiner C, Dor AM, Basbous D, et al: La malacoplasie: Formes anatomo-cliniques, revue de la litterature, a propos de 15 observations personnelles. Arch Anat Pathol 1975; 23:199–208.
212. Lou TY, Teplitz C: Malakoplakia: Pathogenesis and ultrastructural morphogenesis—a problem of altered macrophage response. Hum Pathol 1974; 5:191–207.
213. Abdou NI, NaPombejara C, Sagawa A, et al: Malakoplakia: Evidence for monocyte lysosomal abnormality correctable by cholinergic agonist in vitro and in vivo. N Engl J Med 1977; 297:1413–1419.
214. Wagner ML, Rosenberg HS, Fernbach DJ, et al: Typhlitis: A complication of leukemia in childhood. Am J Roentgenol 1970; 109:341–350.
215. Katz JA, Wagner ML, Gresik MV, et al: Typhlitis: An 18-year experience and postmortem review. Cancer 1990; 65:1041–1047.

216. Merine DS, Fishman EK, Jones B, et al: Right lower quadrant pain in the immunocompromised patient: CT findings in 10 cases. Am J Roentgenol 1987; 149:1177–1179.
217. Matalo NM, Garfinkle SE, Wolfman EF Jr: Intestinal necrosis and perforation in patients receiving immunosuppressive drugs. Am J Surg 1976; 132:753–754.
218. Keidan RD, Fanning J, Gatenby RA, et al: Recurrent typhlitis: A disease resulting from aggressive chemotherapy. Dis Colon Rectum 1989; 32:206–209.
219. Prolla JC, Kirsner JB: The gastrointestinal lesions and complications of leukemias. Ann Intern Med 1964; 61:1084–1103.
220. Abramson SJ, Berdon WE, Baker DH: Childhood typhlitis: Its increasing association with acute myelogenous leukemia. Radiology 1983; 146:61–64.
221. Taylor AJ, Dodds WJ, Gonyo JE, et al: Typhlitis in adults. Gastrointest Radiol 1985; 10:363–369.
222. Teefey SA, Montana MA, Goldfogel GA, et al: Sonographic diagnosis of neutropenic typhlitis. Am J Radiol 1987; 149:731–733.
223. Williams GW, Rauch RF, Kelvin FM, et al: CT detection of typhlitis. J Comput Assist Tomogr 1985; 9:363–365.
224. Proujansky R, Orenstein SR, Kocoshis SA, et al: Cytomegalovirus gastroenteritis after liver transplantation. J Pediatr 1988; 113:700–703.
225. Skibber JM, Matter GJ, Pizzo PA, et al: Right lower quadrant pain in young patients with leukemia. Ann Surg 1987; 206:711–716.
226. Shaked A, Shinar E, Freund H: Neutropenic typhlitis: A plea for conservation. Dis Colon Rectum 1983; 26:351–352.
227. Meyerovitz MF, Fellows KE: Typhlitis: A cause of gastrointestinal hemorrhage in children. Am J Radiol 1984; 143:833–835.

Section Six

THE PANCREAS AND BILE DUCTS

Chapter 64

Anatomy and Physiology of the Pancreas

LEO A. HEITLINGER and H. JUHLING McCLUNG

In the first portion of this chapter, the anatomy, embryology, and congenital anomalies of the pancreas are presented in an attempt to integrate basic concepts into a framework that will be useful to the clinician. The anatomy of the retroperitoneal pancreas has become more comprehensible as imaging studies have improved. With ultrasonography and computed tomography in routine use and more widespread use of magnetic resonance imaging on the horizon, the clinician has a greater opportunity to define the "state of the pancreas."

EMBRYOLOGY

The pancreas is a foregut derivative that develops from dorsal and ventral pancreatic buds (Fig. 64–1 and Table 64–1). The dorsal bud is the larger, appears first, and grows rapidly into the dorsal mesentery. The ventral bud is intimately associated with the duodenum and follows it as the duodenum rotates to the right to form the C-loop. Most of the pancreas is derived from the dorsal bud, whereas the head and part of the uncinate process are derived from the ventral bud. The organogenesis of the pancreas is complete by the eighth week of gestation, and the pancreatic parenchyma is differentiated to endocrine and exocrine units at approximately 20 weeks of gestation.[1] The complex regulation of pancreatic organogenesis and differentiation is beyond the scope of this chapter. The literature is extensive and is reviewed elsewhere.[2, 3]

ANATOMY

The pancreas is situated in the upper abdomen in a retroperitoneal location bounded by the C-loop of the duodenum, spleen, and stomach, at its medial, superior and inferior, lateral, and anterior borders, respectively (Fig. 64–2). Posteriorly the vertebral column traverses the midportion of the pancreas. Between the stomach and pancreas is the potential space, Morrison's pouch or lesser sac, which may become prominent when ascites, pancreatitis, or surgical conditions of the abdomen are present. The opening to the lesser sac lies medial to the pancreas and is known as the epiploic foramen. Vascular supply to the pancreas is via multiple branches of the celiac and superior mesenteric arteries. Venous drainage is via the portal vein. Lymphatics are numerous, although they are rarely appreciated except during pancreatitis. Neural innervation is supplied by both branches of the vagal and of the sympathetic systems[4] (Table 64–2).

The adult pancreas is between 85 and 100 gm in weight; the newborn pancreas weighs approximately 5 gm. Macroscopically the gland is divided into four portions: head, neck (overlying the vertebral column), body, and tail. On a weight basis, the head is the largest portion. Within each portion, the tissue appears to be lobular in organization. The exocrine secretions are drained by numerous ductules that join together, forming the main pancreatic duct (Fig. 64–3). The main duct (of Wirsung) drains with the biliary secretions into the duodenum at an oblique angle through the ampulla of Vater. In some individuals, a minor papilla, which drains the minor duct of Santorini, is located approximately 2 cm superior to the ampulla of Vater.[4]

Table 64–1. EMBRYOLOGY OF THE PANCREAS

Foregut derivation
Ventral and dorsal buds form by 4th week
Head and uncinate process derived from ventral bud
Body and tail derived from dorsal bud
Organogenesis complete by 8th week
Endocrine and exocrine tissue differentiated by 20th week

Table 64–2. ANATOMY OF THE PANCREAS

Arterial supply from celiac axis and superior mesenteric artery branches
Venous drainage via portal vein
Vagal and sympathetic innervation
Major and minor pancreatic ductular drainage variable

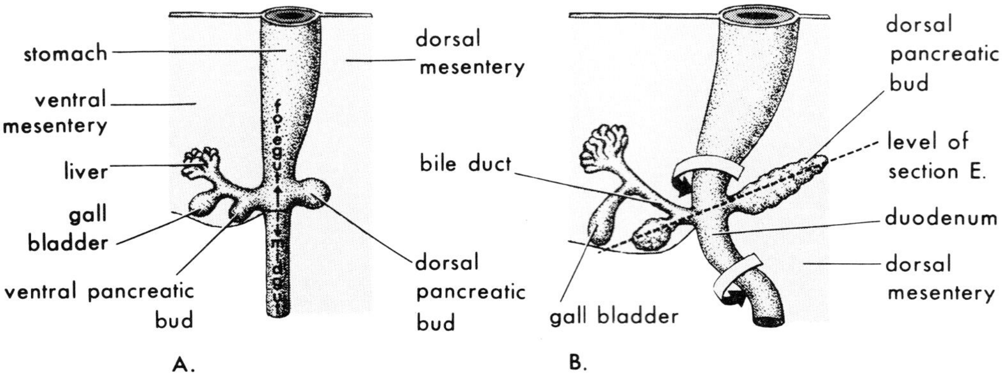

Figure 64–1. Embryology of the pancreas. *A*, The pancreas forms from two evaginations from the primitive foregut. *B*. As the duodenum lengthens and elongates, the pancreatic buds attain their adult relationships. (From Moore KL: The Developing Human. Philadelphia, WB Saunders, 1982, p 226; with permission.)

Histology and Ultrastructure

Histologically the unit of organization of the exocrine pancreas is the lobule. Within each lobule of the pancreas is the functional exocrine unit, the acinus; the functional unit of the endocrine pancreas, the islets of Langerhans; and intercalated and interlobular ducts (Table 64–3 and Fig. 64–4).

The acinus is composed of many secretory cells. The acinar cells are highly polarized with basal nucei, an extensive network of rough endoplasmic reticulum and Golgi, whereas zymogen granules are near the apical aspect of the cell. The cellular apical surface is populated by a lush microvillus membrane. Cellular junctions are highly specialized to prevent retrograde flow of enzymes from the acinar lumen to the interstitial space. The

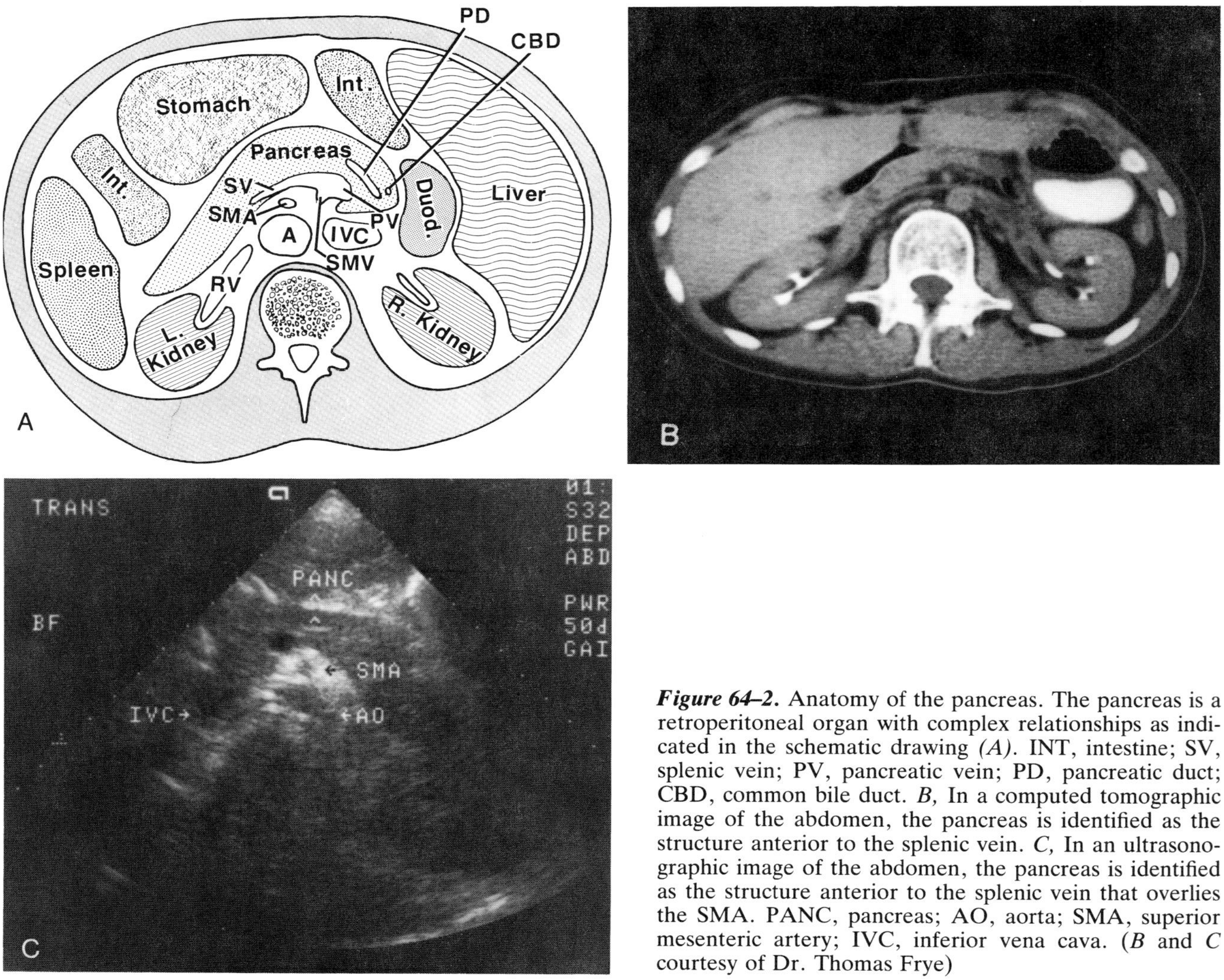

Figure 64–2. Anatomy of the pancreas. The pancreas is a retroperitoneal organ with complex relationships as indicated in the schematic drawing *(A)*. INT, intestine; SV, splenic vein; PV, pancreatic vein; PD, pancreatic duct; CBD, common bile duct. *B,* In a computed tomographic image of the abdomen, the pancreas is identified as the structure anterior to the splenic vein. *C,* In an ultrasonographic image of the abdomen, the pancreas is identified as the structure anterior to the splenic vein that overlies the SMA. PANC, pancreas; AO, aorta; SMA, superior mesenteric artery; IVC, inferior vena cava. (*B* and *C* courtesy of Dr. Thomas Frye)

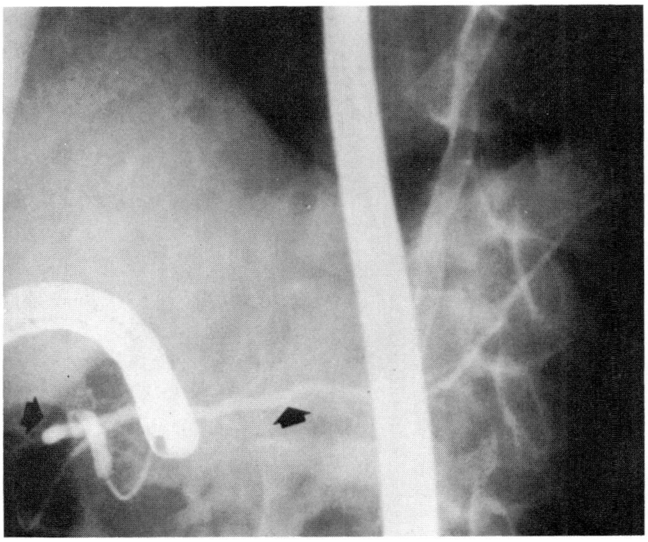

Figure 64–3. Normal ductular anatomy. On injection of the main pancreatic duct at the ampulla *(left arrow)*, the course of the duct *(right arrow)* from head to tail is smooth and gradually tapering as the tail is reached. No nodularity or areas of narrowing are evident. (Courtesy of Dr. John Fromkes)

zymogen granules are electron-dense secretory vesicles that contain the many enzymes produced by the pancreas to assist in the digestion of food and turnover of the epithelial surface of the gut. The release of enzymes from the zymogen granule to the acinar lumen occurs by fusion of the membrane of the granule with the apical membrane and exocytosis of the contents of the granule. In this fashion, the membranous portion of the granules is largely conserved for later use by the acinar cell.[5]

The islets contain the endocrine cells of the pancreas. The composition, function, and regulation of the endocrine portion of the pancreas is not the focus of this chapter, but suffice it to say, with endocrine cells in close proximity to the exocrine cells of the pancreas, both insulin and glucagon are significant regulators of pancreatic enzyme synthesis and secretion.[3]

The ductular network of the pancreas has two major functions. First, ductular epithelium is the site of water and electrolyte secretion in response to a meal or to secretagogue stimulus. Second, the network acts as a conduit for the fluid, enzymes, and electrolytes secreted by the exocrine cells for their passage to the duodenum, which is their site of action in health. The fine structure of the ductular epithelium differs from that of the acinar cells in two ways. First, the apical surface is not populated by microvilli. Second, no secretory granules are present near the apical surface. The cytoplasm is populated by numerous mitochondria to support their high metabolic rate. The intercellular junctions are also highly specialized to prevent the entry of fluid and enzymes into the interstitial spaces of the pancreas. The latter is of obvious importance for the prevention of spillage of enzymes into the parenchyma of the pancreas, which thereby avoids the potential for spontaneous activation of zymogens.

Table 64–3. HISTOLOGY AND ULTRASTRUCTURE

Acinus is the functional unit of exocrine pancreas.
Acinar cells produce and secrete enzymes.
Enzymes and inactive precursors are stored in zymogen granules.
Centroacinar and ductular epithelia secrete fluid and electrolytes.
Islet of Langerhans is the functional unit of the endocrine pancreas.

Table 64–4. CONGENITAL ANOMALIES OF THE PANCREAS

Most are the result of a failure of rotation, fusion of pancreatic buds, or both
Pancreatic agenesis or hypoplasia
Heterotopic pancreatic tissue
Annular pancreas
Ductular anomalies: pancreas divisum
Congenital cysts: isolated pancreatic, choledochocele, choledochal cyst, Caroli's disease

Congenital Anomalies

Although the total number of types of congenital anomalies affecting the pancreas is large, each individual anomaly is rare. Typically, anomalies represent failures of rotation, fusion, or both (Table 64–4). The mechanisms contributing to the genesis of failures of rotation or fixation remain obscure.

Complete *pancreatic agenesis and hypoplasia* have both been reported. Only one long-term survivor of functional pancreatic agenesis has been reported.[6] As would be expected, treatment of both exocrine and endocrine pancreatic insufficiency was required in this case. Fewer than 12 cases of partial agenesis of the pancreas have been reported in the literature; the data are predominantly reported from autopsy series.[7]

Heterotopic pancreas, or normal pancreatic tissue in an abnormal location, is among the more common of the pancreatic anomalies, occurring in as many as 15% of all autopsy specimens.[8] Stomach, duodenum, and jejunum are among the most common locations for heterotopias. Tissue can be implanted in any portion of the bowel and has been reported in the lung as well.[7] The tissue usually is present as a small nodule less than 5 mm in diameter and located in the submucosa. The mechanism underlying the anomaly is unknown. Although most heterotopias are asymptomatic, they can cause difficulties dependent on location by giving rise to obstruction, pain, intussusception, and other similar symptoms. The lesions are approached only if symptomatic; because the lesions are usually in the submucosa, endoscopic biopsies often are insufficient in making the diagnosis; therefore, surgical biopsy, and excision when indicated, is often needed to exclude more ominous diagnoses.

Annular pancreas is included in the differential diagnosis of all infants with persistent bilious vomiting in the newborn period. The lesion consists of a "band-like" constriction surrounding the duodenum. The band

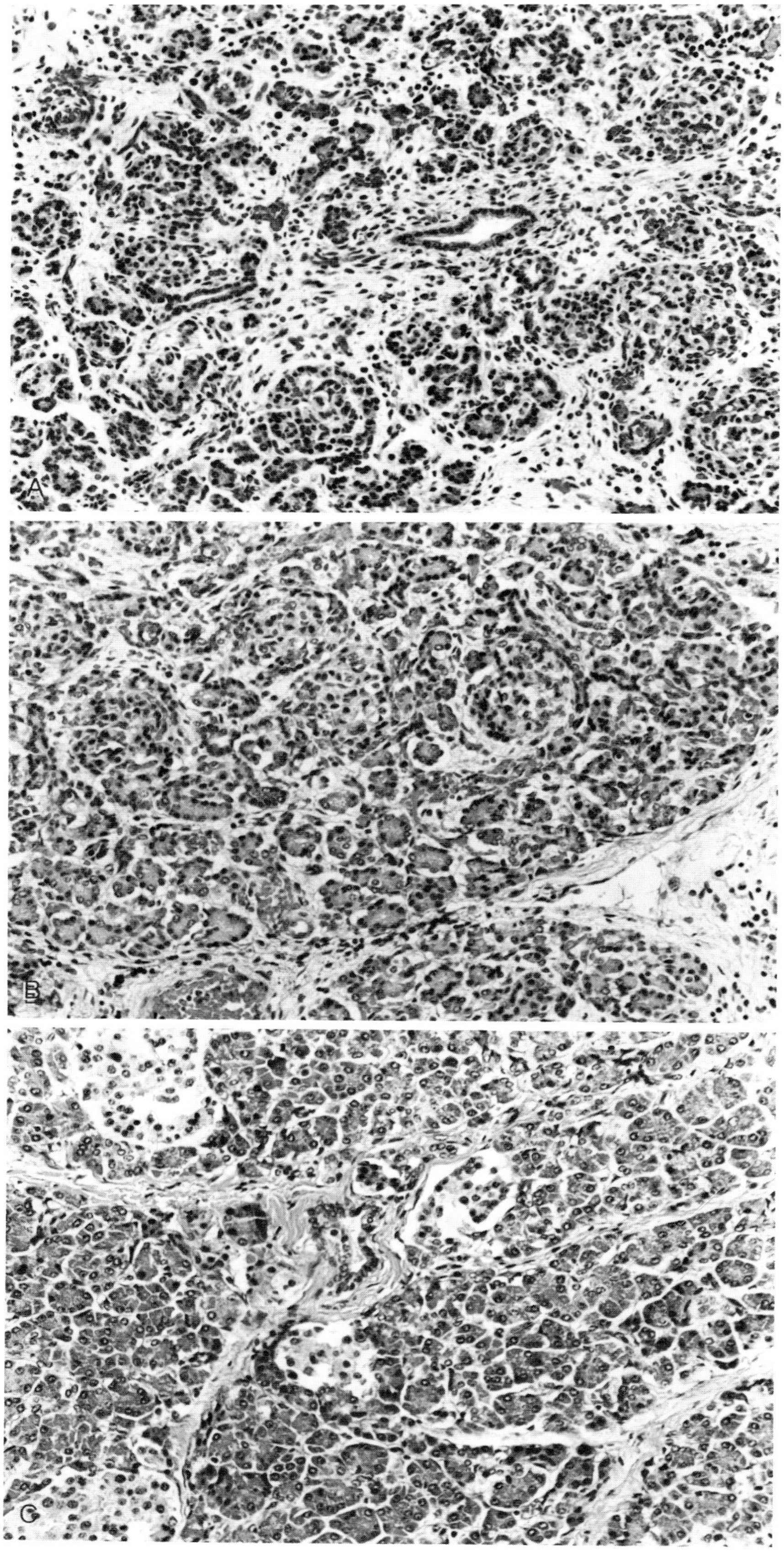

Figure 64–4. Histology of the pancreas. At 20 weeks' gestation *(A)*, the ductular and glandular structures are rudimentary. At 28 weeks *(B)*, ductular, acinar, and islet structures are readily identified and have an appearance similar to that of a 16 year old *(C)*. (Courtesy of Dr. Carl Boesel)

typically will have significant vascular connections and a functional ductular system. The pathogenesis of the lesion is controversial, but the lesion clearly represents an error of rotation or fixation (or both) of the pancreatic anlagen.[9] The lesion most often presents in the newborn period but can present as late as adulthood. Annular pancreas presenting in infancy is often associated with other anomalies; adults have most commonly presented with the single lesion.[10] The approach to diagnosis in infancy has been the performance of the plain abdominal radiograph. The classic double-bubble pattern of duodenal obstruction is present, indicating that exploration is required. The search for additional anomalies is made at that time, and the segment is bypassed with a duodenoduodenostomy as the procedure of choice.[7] In contrast, the evaluation of the older child or the adult is in general more extensive, with contrast radiography the initial study. Rarely, endoscopic retrograde cholangiopancreatography or computed tomography has been required to confirm the diagnosis. Treatment in the older child or adult also involves a drainage procedure. Morbidity and mortality are most often associated with the presence and severity of associated congenital anomalies.

The significance of *abnormalities of the pancreatic ducts* has been an area of controversy. The majority of individuals have one or two arrangements: drainage of pancreatic secretions through the major duodenal papilla or drainage of the secretions through both the major and minor papillae with communication between the two ducts. In the former case, many individuals will have an identifiable minor papilla with no secretions draining through that site. These two variations account for nearly 85% of all individuals. Less common variations include drainage through both major and minor papillae without communication between the two ducts, i.e., pancreas divisum; drainage through the minor duct and major duct with insertion of the major duct several millimeters proximal to the major papillae, i.e., common channel; and drainage through both the major and minor papillae with the common bile duct entering the duodenum distal to the major pancreatic duct. Each of these less common variants accounts for approximately 5% of autopsy specimens.[11]

The controversy about the variation of anatomy of pancreatic drainage has been centered around the importance of pancreas divisum and common channel in the genesis of pancreatitis. Although relatively small percentages of individuals appear to have one of these anatomic variants, in autopsy series a greater percentage of patients with chronic pancreatitis have pancreas divisum or common channel than expected by chance alone. A more complete discussion of this controversy is presented in Chapters 68 and 69.

Congenital cysts of the pancreatic ductular system and bile ducts have been described. Solitary pancreatic cysts are uncommon and rarely give rise to symptoms. When symptoms are present, drainage procedures have been advocated. Cystic anomalies of the biliary tree include choledochal cyst, choledochocele, and Caroli's disease. These disorders are discussed more fully in Chapter 71.

PHYSIOLOGY

The main function of the exocrine pancreas is to manufacture and deliver enzymes required for the digestion of dietary fuels to their site of action. A large number of pancreatic enzyme precursors are synthesized in substantial quantities each day. The healthy adult pancreas produces approximately 2 to 6 gm that are delivered to the duodenum in approximately 2.5 L of fluid.[12] The synthesis and secretion of these enzymes are carefully orchestrated and are under complex neural and hormonal control.

Pancreatic Enzymes

The pancreas secretes a series of enzymes that relate to the major components of the human diet: proteins, fats, and carbohydrates (Table 64–5). Many of the enzymes are secreted as an inactive precursor, i.e., zymogen, whereas others are secreted in their active form. These zymogens and active enzymes for the digestion of foodstuffs are secreted in response to meals or neural or hormonal signals. After synthesis in rough endoplasmic reticulum, post-translational modifications in the Golgi complex, and condensation into secretory granules, the enzymes and zymogens reside in the zymogen granules located at the apex of the acinar cells. In response to a stimulus, the contents of the granules are discharged into the acinar lumen by exocytosis.[13] Scheele and Palade[14] have suggested that zymogen enzymes are mixed in the granules and are therefore discharged in a quantal or parallel fashion. Other investigators have suggested that individual enzymes can be released preferentially in response to secretogogues.[15] This area remains controversial.

Nearly all of the secreted enzymes are glycoproteins with neutral to alkaline isoelectric points and molecular weights in the 20,000 to 50,000 kd range. The pH optima are in the neutral range; many of the enzymes are irreversibly inactivated at acid pH. The specific charac-

Table 64–5. PANCREATIC ENZYMES

Endopeptidases
Trypsin(ogen)* (anionic, mesotrypsin, cationic isozymes)
Chymotrypsin(ogen) A and B
(Pro)elastase A and B
Exopeptidases
(Pro)carboxypeptidase A and B
Lipases
Lipase
Colipase
(Pro)phospholipase A_2
Carbohydrases
Amylase
Other
RNase
DNase
Lysosomal enzymes

*Enzymes secreted as inactive precursors have a suffix or prefix in parentheses to indicate correct nomenclature.

teristics of each enzyme have been reviewed in detail by Rinderknecht.[12] The magnitude of secretion of enzymes is in sizeable excess of that required for the digestion of dietary substrates; approximately a 90% reduction in enzyme secretion is required for steatorrhea to develop.[16]

Pancreatic proteases include both endopeptidases and exopeptidases. Endopeptidases cleave internal bonds within protein chains; the several endopeptidases differ in the specific bonds within a peptide chain that are attacked. Exopeptidases attach the bond adjacent to either the amino or carboxyl terminus. Trypsin, chymotrypsin, and elastase are endoproteases that are classified as serine proteases; i.e., they attach bonds adjacent to serine residues. Each of these enzymes is secreted as a zymogen that is inactive until a terminal peptide is cleaved. Trypsinogen, chymotrypsinogen, and proelastase are the precursors of trypsin, chymotrypsin, and elastase. The carboxypeptidases A and B are exopeptidases that cleave the residues adjacent to the amino terminus of peptides. Like the endopeptidases listed, the carboxypeptidases are secreted as inactive precursors named procarboxypeptidase A and B.

Several enzymes responsible for the digestion of neutral lipids are present in the pancreatic secretions. Pancreatic lipase is the principle enzyme responsible for the hydrolysis of dietary triglycerides. Gastric- and bile salt–stimulated breast milk lipases also contribute significantly to the digestion of dietary lipids. Lipase hydrolyzes triglycerides on the surface of fat droplets; therefore, emulsification of dietary fat by bile salts is crucial for rapid rates of lipolysis. Clearly, reduced surface areas available for attack by the enzyme will result in lowered rates of hydrolysis of triglyceride. Bile salts act as inhibitors of pancreatic lipase; for optimal rates of hydrolysis, colipase, a second enzyme of pancreatic origin, is required to counteract the inhibition of pancreatic lipase that would be present in the absence of bile salts. Lipase appears to be secreted in its active form; it is unknown whether colipase is secreted in the active form or as a zymogen. Phospholipase A_2 is an enzyme present in pancreatic secretions that hydrolyzes phospholipids present in micelles and biologic membranes. The latter property may be important in the pathogenesis of pancreatitis (see Chapter 68). The enzyme is secreted as a zymogen designated prophospholipase A_2.

Dietary starches are primarily hydrolyzed to glucose oligomers, predominantly DP_2 through DP_5, and alpha-limit dextrins by pancreatic amylase. Amylase is secreted in its active form by the pancreatic acinar cells. Salivary and mammary amylases can assist in the digestion of dietary starch and are probably important in the adaptation of individuals with pancreatic insufficiency to starch-containing diets. Glucoamylase, an intestinal brush border enzyme, represents an alternate site of starch digestion before intestinal absorption of glucose from starch. Finally, colonic salvage of malabsorbed carbohydrate has been proposed as a mechanism to retrieve carbohydrate calories in the amylase-deficient individual.

Enzymes to hydrolyze nucleic acids are also present in pancreatic secretions. Ribonuclease and deoxyribonuclease are present both in the pancreatic parenchyma and in the secretions. These enzymes may not be synthesized for secretion but may serve a "housekeeping function," i.e., the degradation of nucleic acids required for the synthesis of secretory enzymes. The physiologic function of these enzymes is a matter of ongoing debate.[12]

Enterokinase, or enteropeptidase, is critical to the activation of pancreatic zymogens. Although trypsinogen can spontaneously be activated to trypsin, the process is slow and inefficient.[17] Catalysis by enterokinase is several orders of magnitude more rapid. This peptidase is present in duodenal fluid and is assumed to be secreted by duodenal enterocytes. The enzyme specifically removes an N-terminal peptide from trypsinogen[18] and has no other known native substrate. Active trypsin is then able to initiate a cascade of events ending in the activation of the other zymogens.

Enzymes of lysosomal origin are also secreted. The lysosomal enzymes differ from those discussed earlier in that they function at significantly lower pHs and are not packaged in zymogen granules. Similar to the enzymes in zymogen granules, lysosomal enzymes are secreted in response to native or pharmacologic stimuli.[19]

Secretion of Enzymes

Pancreatic exocrine secretion appears to be complex and under neural and hormonal control. In animal models, four classic phases of secretion have been described: cephalic, gastric, intestinal, and postabsorptive (Table 64–6). The cephalic phase refers to secretion stimulated by the sight, smell, or taste of food. The gastric phase refers to secretion in response to distention of the stomach. The intestinal phase refers to stimulation of secretion by the entry of acid or nutrients into the duodenum. The postabsorptive phase is the means by which secreted enzymes exert feedback inhibition on further secretion by the pancreas.

In humans, enzyme secretion seems to correlate with motility in the upper intestine. Diurnal patterns contain interdigestive and postprandial phases. In the adult human, the postprandial phase is of long duration, and meals occur frequently during the day; consequently, pancreatic exocrine secretion is in the interdigestive period from midnight to morning and only briefly during

Table 64–6. SECRETION OF ENZYMES AND FLUID

Four Classic Phases:
Cephalic—in response to sight, smell, or taste of food
Gastric—in response to distention
Intestinal—in response to entry of HCl and food into duodenum
Postabsorptive—feedback inhibition, enzymes in duodenum
Mediators for Secretion
Enzymes—CCK and ACh
Fluid and electrolytes—secretin and VIP

the day.[20] The native stimuli for the secretion of pancreatic enzymes are the entry of acid, fat, protein, or carbohydrate into the duodenum. Saline and other nonnutritive stimuli that distend the duodenum are much less potent stimuli for secretion of enzymes.[21] Cephalic and gastric phases of secretion have not been clearly defined in humans. The putative signals for secretion of the enzymes in response to entry of acid or food into the duodenum are cholecystokinin and acetylcholine. Other hormones and cholinergic agents have been studied in variety of in vivo and in vitro systems. Feedback inhibition of pancreatic secretion by luminal trypsin has been proposed to occur; but pharmacologic concentrations of trypsin appear to be required to reduce further secretion of enzymes.[22]

Secretion of Fluid and Electrolytes

Pancreatic juice contains the enzymes reviewed earlier in an isotonic, colorless solution. Osmolality appears to be independent of flow rate; pH is generally above 8. Cationic concentrations are similar to those found in plasma. Bicarbonate and chloride concentrations in sum approximate 115 mEq per L and are inversely proportional to one another. Basal fluid exhibits high chloride and low bicarbonate concentrations (<20 mEq per L); the reverse is demonstrated in stimulated fluids with bicarbonate concentrations in excess of 60 mEq per L.[23] Centroacinar and duct cells appear to be the source of pancreatic bicarbonate secretion.[24] Support of this original hypothesis by Hollander was provided by Dreiling and colleagues,[25] who demonstrated that a carbonic anhydrase inhibitor was able to attenuate bicarbonate secretion without affecting enzyme secretion. More recent studies have elucidated the mechanisms of fluid and electrolyte secretion by the pancreatic ductular epithelium and identified the putative native and pharmacologic stimuli that regulate secretion.

Significant interspecies differences in the signals for pancreatic fluid and electrolyte secretion have been identified. In humans, the native stimulus for fluid and electrolyte secretion appears to be secretin that is released by endocrine cells of the duodenum in response to feeding.[26] This response can be amplified by the presence of cholinergic stimuli or cholecystokinin; these stimuli in the absence of secretin elicit modest fluid and bicarbonate secretion. Neither gastric distention[27] nor sham feeding[28] result in bicarbonate secretion in humans. Despite extensive searches for other signals for secretin release to the circulation, intraduodenal acidification is the only established putative signal. The vagus appears to have no role in secretin release.[29]

Receptors for Secretagogues on Pancreatic Exocrine Cells

The development of isolated acinar preparations and plasma membranes from acinar cells has facilitated study of the receptors to which secretagogues bind to effector cells of the exocrine pancreas. The postreceptor mechanisms that translate the signal to the observed effect have also been studied with these techniques. Similar studies to elucidate the mechanisms of fluid and electrolyte secretion by ductular epithelium have been hampered by the difficulty in obtaining an isolated ductular preparation.

The binding of a ligand to its receptor is both necessary and sufficient to initiate a sequence of events that ultimately results in enzyme secretion. The development of radiolabeled ligands with high specific activity was required to demonstrate that the binding of substances was a specific signal to initiate enzyme secretion. Both agonist and antagonist analogs of native compounds have been prepared to demonstrate the specificity of the binding process.[30]

Receptors on acinar cells have been divided into two classes defined by the postreceptor events that follow the binding of ligand to receptor[30] (Table 64–7). The first group of receptors is represented by the cholecystokinin (CCK) receptors. Ligand occupation of CCK receptors is followed by mobilization of calcium and subsequent enzyme release. Receptors for the following agonists all mobilize calcium as part of the postreceptor cascade preceding enzyme release: bombesin, physalemin, and muscarinic/cholinergic agents such as carbachol. The second group of receptors is represented by secretin receptors. Ligand occupation of secretin receptors is followed by increased intracellular concentrations of cyclic adenosine monophosphate (cAMP) and subsequent enzyme release. Receptors for the following agonists stimulate cAMP generation as a postreceptor event that precedes enzyme secretion: vasoactive intestinal polypeptide (VIP) and cholera toxin. Although the postreceptor effects differ, occupation of a receptor of either class is associated with discharge of the contents of zymogen granules in a specific, dose-dependent fashion.

Receptors for CCK and structurally related peptides share several characteristics other than identical postreceptor events. First, concentrations associated with maximal enzyme release are broad and in the nanomolar range. Concentrations in excess of those associated with maximal enzyme release have been shown to reduce enzyme efflux. Several hypotheses have been generated to explain these observations; both multiple receptor models and several binding sites on a single peptide

Table 64–7. RECEPTORS ON ACINAR CELLS

Associated with Calcium Mobilization
Cholecystokinin
Bombesin
Physalemin
Muscarinic agonists
Associated with cAMP Elaboration
Secretin-preferring*
VIP-preferring*
Cholera toxin

*The secretin-preferring receptor binds both secretin and VIP but has a higher affinity for secretin; the converse is true for the VIP-preferring receptor.

have been proposed.[31, 32] Second, CCK receptors appear to be localized to the basolateral membrane of the acinar cells. Third, the C-terminal portion of the ligand binds to the receptor. Binding to the receptor also depolarizes the cells, reduces plasma membrane resistance, and increases cyclic guanosine monophosphate (cGMP).[33]

The properties of the muscarinic receptors on acinar cells have also been characterized. The lower affinities of the muscarinic agonists for binding have led to a greater reliance on inhibition data with selective muscarinic antagonists. Nonetheless, binding of muscarinic agonists is associated with calcium mobilization and release of enzyme in a fashion similar to that for the CCK receptors. The receptors have not been localized to the basolateral membrane, but that is their presumed location.[34]

The properties of receptors that lead to the generation of cAMP is much more complicated than for the agents that mobilize calcium. Both VIP and secretin appear to share two sets of receptors. The first has a higher affinity for VIP, the second a higher affinity for secretin.[35] Occupation of either receptor is closely related to increased intracellular cAMP. In contrast to the ligands that bind to receptors associated with calcium mobilization, the N-terminal portion of the ligand binds to the receptor. No changes in the electrophysiology of the acinar cells has been detected after binding of ligands of this class. The location of the receptors has not been definitively documented; they are clearly in the cell membrane and presumed to be in a basolateral location.[36]

Table 64–8. STIMULUS-SECRETION COUPLING

Calcium Mobilization
Binding of ligand to receptor (CCK, cholinergic agonists)
Generation of IP_3 and DAG
Mobilization of calcium from ER and mitochondria
Release of zymogen granules
Generation of cAMP
Binding of ligand to receptor (secretin, VIP)
Activation of adenylate cyclase
Phosphorylation of regulatory proteins
Release of zymogen granules

IP_3, inositoltriphosphate; DAG, diacylglycerol; ER, endoplasmic reticulum.

Stimulus-Secretion Coupling

The occupation of receptors on the surface of acinar cells by ligands results in a series of intracellular events that ultimately lead to the secretion of enzymes and fluid. In the pancreatic acinar cell, two intracellular messengers that stimulate secretion after binding of ligand to receptors have been mentioned: calcium and cAMP (Table 64–8).

Calcium is mobilized in response to the occupation of CCK or muscarinic receptors. Calcium is required for enzyme secretion. The initial evidence was supplied by conducting enzyme release experiments in Ca^{2+}-free media. Enzyme release was markedly attenuated under these conditions.[37] More recent studies with calcium ionophore have supported the concept that mobilization of calcium from several sources, i.e., intracellular and extracellular, results in enzyme release even in the absence of binding of a ligand to a receptor.[38] The latter study supports the concept that calcium movement is an event that is distal to receptor binding but proximal to enzyme release.

The mechanism of calcium mobilization appears to involve phosphatidylinositol and its polyphosphate derivatives. The generation of inositol triphosphate and diacylglycerol by the hydrolysis of phosphatidylinositol-4,5-biphosphate, a membrane-bound phospholipid, follows the binding of ligand to either CCK or muscarinic receptors.[39] This reaction could be coupled to calcium mobilization by two processes. First, calcium could be bound to negatively charged inositol groups on the inner surface of the plasma membrane and released in response to hydrolysis of the inositide. Second, the inositides and diacylgycerol could act as messengers to other intracellular sites of calcium storage and thereby mediate its release. Diacylglycerol has been shown to activate protein kinase C directly.[40] These possibilities have been extensively reviewed by William and Hootman.[41]

The generation of cAMP after the binding of ligand to either the secretin or the VIP receptors has also been implicated as a precursor to enzyme secretion. First, substances known to activate adenylate cyclase without occupation of the receptors have been shown to induce enzyme release.[42] Second, synthetic analogs of cAMP when delivered to acinar cells can induce enzyme release. Finally, agents that induce secretion of enzymes by binding to the secretin or VIP receptors increase intracellular concentrations of cAMP.[43]

The mechanisms by which calcium and cAMP mediate enzyme release have also been extensively investigated. Calcium binds to calmodulin; the calcium calmodulin complex is then able to activate a series of protein kinases.[44] cAMP appears to exert its effects by binding to the regulatory subunit of protein kinase C; this results in the activation of the enzyme.[45] The activation of these protein kinases results in the phosphorylation of a series of regulatory proteins in the cytosol and in organelles. These phosphorylated proteins have a variety of functions, including activation of ion channels and the discharge of enzymes from zymogen granules at the apex of the acinar cell.

Development of Pancreatic Secretion

Despite structural maturity of the pancreas at term, the newborn is known to secrete markedly lower amounts of pancreatic enzymes than older children or adults. The magnitude of reduction, timing of maturation, and candidate mechanisms that explain these observations are partially defined (Table 64–9).

Balance studies performed on infants suggest that pancreatic function is markedly reduced in normal human infants. The digestive capacity for dietary protein

Table 64–9. DEVELOPMENT OF ENZYME SECRETION

Human Newborns: Absorption of Nutrients
Physiologic steatorrhea
Limited capacity to hydrolyze protein
Carbohydrates tolerated owing to colonic salvage
Attains normal levels by 6–12 months
Enzyme Concentration in Pancreas of Neonates
Proteases near normal
Lipase markedly diminished
Amylase absent
Enzyme Secretion
No response to meals or secretagogues in neonates
Attenuated responses from 1–6 months of age
Candidate mechanisms
Reduced enzyme content
Altered receptor number or affinity
Postreceptor defects

was reported to be approximately two thirds of that observed in 6-month-old infants.[46] Coefficients of absorption of dietary lipid have been reported to vary from 58.3 to 88.7% for preterm and from 71.7 to 95.3% for full-term infants.[47] The wide variation is due in part to differences in lipid source. Non–breast-fed infants rarely appear to retain more than 90% of ingested lipid.[48] Absorption of dietary cereals from the small bowel is also limited in newborns. Shulman and associates[49] demonstrated that nearly all of a cereal meal was absorbed by term newborns and used for energy. Concordance of hydrogen and carbon dioxide peaks demonstrated that the majority of cereal-derived carbon was absorbed from the colon after fermentation by colonic flora.[49] The reduction in the absorption of macronutrients cited here continues for approximately the first year after birth.[50]

A failure to secrete enzymes in response to a meal or secretogogues is one candidate mechanism to explain the absorptive deficits cited earlier. Neonates have been shown to be unresponsive to administration of cholecystokinin or secretin.[51] This lack of responsiveness to secretogogues is short-lived, approximately 1 to 2 months in duration.[51] The lack of responsiveness to CCK has been suggested to be due to a receptor defect; this is supported by the intact response to calcium ionophore in the rat pancreas.[52] An alternate mechanism, not yet addressed in the literature, is that receptor kinetics may be altered by membrane composition and hence fluidity. Stimulus-secretion coupling following occupation of secretin receptors has also been shown to be immature in the rat.[53] The lack of responsiveness of the neonatal pancreas appears to be due to changes at both receptor and postreceptor sites.

After the infant pancreas becomes responsive to secretogogues, the magnitude of enzyme secretion has been shown to be less than that observed in older children or adults.[54] Mature concentrations of lipase and amylase are not attained in the duodenum until more than 1 year of age.

The observation that the infant secretes less pancreatic enzymes than the adult appears to be explained in part by reduced enzyme content of the pancreatic parenchyma. Lipase was markedly reduced and amylase undetectable in all specimens.[55] Autopsy data confirm that the same pattern persists for most of infancy.[56] It is unknown whether diminished enzyme synthesis, increased enzyme degradation, or both are the mechanisms by which reduced enzyme contents are maintained in the infant pancreas.

The human infant exhibits a number of compensatory pathways to adapt to the relative deficiencies of pancreatic lipase and amylase. Gastric lipolysis has been documented to occur in humans and in several animal species. This process is mediated by a gastric lipase and, in the rat, a lingual lipase. Bile salt–stimulated lipase of human milk is an additional alternate pathway of lipase available to the breast-fed infant.[57] Salivary and mammary amylases are enzymes shown to be of potential importance in the digestion of starch.[58, 59] Colonic fermentation of carbohydrates is an additional efficient mechanism to retrieve energy from dietary carbohydrate.[49]

SUMMARY

The exocrine pancreas is an organ of extreme complexity, the nuances of which have been elucidated in recent years. The major function of the exocrine pancreas is to deliver digestive enzymes and fluid to the duodenum, where they assist in the digestion of dietary substrates. The release of enzymes and fluid is under exquisite neural and hormonal control. The binding of neurotransmitters and hormones to receptors on secretory cells initiates a cascade of events that culminate in the release of enzyme from zymogen granules, which are a site of storage within the acinar cell. The secretory apparatus of the pancreas is immature at birth, but despite diminished enzyme secretion by infants, compensatory pathways for relative pancreatic amylase and lipase deficiency are able to contribute to digestion and absorption of dietary starch and lipid under most circumstances. The developmental regulation and control of pancreatic secretion remain areas of fertile investigation with many questions remaining to be answered in the laboratory.

REFERENCES

1. Moore KL: The Developing Human. Philadelphia, WB Saunders, 1982.
2. Githens S: Differentiation and development of the exocrinepancreas in animals. *In* Go VWL, Gardner JD, Brooks FP, et al, eds: The Exocrine Pancreas: Biology, Pathobiology, and Diseases. New York, Raven Press, 1986, pp 21–31.
3. Lebenthal E, Lev R, Lee PC: Prenatal and postnatal development of the human exocrine pancreas. *In* Go VLW, Gardner JD, Brooks FP, et al, eds: The Exocrine Pancreas: Biology, Pathobiology, and Diseases. New York, Raven Press, 1986, pp 33–44.
4. Bockman DE: Anatomy of the pancreas. *In* Go VLW, Gardner JD, Brooks FP, et al, eds: The Exocrine Pancreas: Biology, Pathobiology, and Diseases. New York, Raven Press, 1986, pp 1–7.
5. Kern HF: Fine structure of the human exocrine pancreas. *In* Go

VWL, Gardner JD, Brooks FP, et al, eds: The Exocrine Pancreas: Biology, Pathobiology, and Diseases. New York, Raven Press, 1986, pp 9–19.
6. Howard CP, Go VLW, Infante AJ: Long-term survival in a case of functional pancreatic agenesis. J Pediatr 1980; 97:786–789.
7. Newman BJ, Lebenthal E: Congenital anomalies of the exocrine pancreas. *In* Go VWL, Gardner JD, Brooks FP, et al, eds: The Exocrine Pancreas: Biology, Pathobiology, and Diseases. New York, Raven Press, 1986, pp 773–782.
8. Busard JM, Walters W: Heterotopic pancreatic tissue. Arch Surg 1950, 60:674–682.
9. Gray SW, Skandalakis JE: Embryology for Surgeons. Philadelphia, WB Saunders, 1972, pp 263–282.
10. Kiernan PD, ReMine SG, Kiernan PC, et al: Annular pancreas: Mayo Clinic experience from 1957 to 1976 with a review of the literature. Arch Surg 1980; 115:46–50.
11. Berman LG, Prior JT, Abramow SM, et al: A study of the pancreatic duct system in man by the use of vinyl acetate casts of postmortem preparations. Surg Gynecol Obstet 1960; 110:391–403.
12. Rinderknecht H; Pancreatic secretory enzymes. *In* Go VWL, Gardner JD, Brooks FP, et al, eds: The Exocrine Pancreas: Biology, Pathobiology, and Disease. New York, Raven Press, 1986, pp 163–183.
13. Palade G: Intracellular aspects of the process of protein synthesis. Science 1975; 189:347–358.
14. Scheele GA, Palade GE: Studies of the guinea pig pancreas: Parallel discharge of enzyme activities. J Biol Chem 1975; 250:2660–2670.
15. Rothman SS: The digestive enzymes of the pancreas: A mixture of inconstant proportions. Annu Rev Physiol 1977; 39:373–389.
16. De Magno EP, Go VLW, Summerskill WHJ: Relations between pancreatic enzyme outputs and malabsorption in severe pancreatic insufficiency. N Engl J Med 1973; 288:813–815.
17. Kassell B, Kay J: Zymogens of proteolytic enzymes. Science 1973; 180:1022–1027.
18. Maroux S, Baratti J, Desnuelle P: Purification and specificity of porcine enterokinase. J Biol Chem 1971; 246:5031–5039.
19. Rinderknecht H, Renner IG, Koyama HH: Lysosomal enzymes in pure pancreatic juice from normal healthy volunteers and chronic alcoholics. Dig Dis Sci 1979; 24:180–186.
20. Brunner H, Northfield TC, Hofmann AF, et al: Gastric emptying and secretion of bile acids, cholesterol, and pancreatic enzymes during digestion: Duodenal perfusion studies in healthy subjects. Mayo Clin Proc 1974; 49:851–860.
21. Go VLW, Hofmann AF, Summerskill WHJ: Pancreozymin bioassay in man based on pancreatic enzyme secretion: Potency of specific amino acids and other digestive products. J Clin Invest 1970; 9:1558–1564.
22. Slaff J, Jacobson D, Tillman CR, et al: Protease-specific suppression of pancreatic exocrine secretion. Gastroenterology 1984; 87:44–52.
23. Dreiling DA, Janowitz HD: The secretion of electrolytes by the human pancreas. Gastroenterology 1956; 30:382–390.
24. Hollander F, Birnbaum D: The role of carbonic anhydrase in pancreas. Trans NY Acad Sci 1952; 15:56–58.
25. Dreiling DA, Janowitz HD, Halpern M: The effect of a carbonic anhydrase inhibitor, Diamox, on human pancreatic secretion. Gastroenterology 1955; 29:262–279.
26. Chey WY, Lee YH, Hendricks JG, et al: Plasma secretin concentrations in fasting and postprandial state in man. Am J Dig Dis 1978; 23:981–988.
27. Cargill JM, Wormsley KG: Effect of gastric distension on human pancreatic secretion. Acta Hepato-Gastroenterol 1979; 6:235–238.
28. Defilippi C, Solomon TW, Valenzuela JE: Pancreatic secretory response to sham feeding in humans. Digestion 1982; 23:217–223.
29. Case RM, Argent BF: Bicarbonate secretion by pancreatic duct cells: Mechanisms and control. *In* Go VWL, Gardner JD, Brooks FP, et al, eds: The Exocrine Pancreas: Biology, Pathobiology, and Diseases. New York, Raven Press, 1986, pp 213–243.
30. Gardner JD, Jensen JT: Secretagogue receptors on pancreatic acinar cells. *In* Johnson LCR, Christensen JC, Jackson MJ, et al, eds: Physiology of the Gastrointestinal Tract. New York, Raven Press, 1987, pp 1109–1127.
31. Sankaran H, Goldfine ID, Bailey H, et al: Relationship of cholecystokinin receptor binding to regulation of biological functions in pancreatic acini. Am J Physiol 1982; 242:G250–257.
32. Collins SM, Abdelmoumene S, Jensen RT, et al: Cholecystokinin-induced persistent stimulation of enzyme secretion from pancreatic acini. Am J Physiol 1981; 240:G459–465.
33. Peterson OH: Electrophysiology of exocrine gland cells. *In* Johnson LR, Christensen JC, Jackson MJ, et al, eds: Physiology of the Gastrointestinal Tract. New York, Raven Press, 1981, pp 749–772.
34. Larose L, Dumont Y, Asselin J, et al: Muscarinic receptor of rat pancreatic acini: [^{3}H] QNB binding and amylase secretion. Eur J Pharmacol 1981; 76:247–254.
35. Jensen RT, Gardner JD: Identification and characterization of receptors for secretagogues on pancreatic acinar cells. Fed Proc 1981; 40:2486–2496.
36. LeMeuth V, Farjaudon N, Bawab W, et al: Characterization of binding sites for VIP-related peptides and activation of adenylate cyclase in developing pancreas. Am J Physiol 1991; 260:G265–274.
37. Hokin LE: Effects of calcium omission on acetylcholine-stimulated amylase secretion and phospholipid synthesis in pigeon pancreas slices. Biochim Biophys Acta 1966; 115:219–221.
38. Eimerl S, Savion N, Heichal O, et al: Induction of enzyme secretion in rat pancreatic slices using the ionophore A23187 and calcium: An experimental bypass of the hormone receptor pathway. J Biol Chem 1974; 249:3991–3993.
39. Orchard JL, Davis JS, Larson RE, et al: Effects of carbachol and pancreozymin (cholecystokinin-octapeptide) on polyphosphoinositide metabolism in rat pancreas in vitro. Biochem J 1984; 217:281–287.
40. Nishizuka Y: The role of protein kinase C in cell surface signal transduction and tumor production. Nature 1984; 308:693–698.
41. William JA, Hootman SR: Stimulus-secretion coupling in pancreatic acinar cells. *In* Go VWL, Gardner JD, Brooks FP, et al, eds: The Exocrine Pancreas: Biology, Pathobiology, and Diseases. New York, Raven Press, 1986, pp 123–139.
42. Heisler S: Forskolin potentiates calcium-dependent amylase secretion from rat pancreatic acinar cells. Can J Physiol Pharmacol 1983; 61:1168–1176.
43. Robberecht P, Conlon TP, Gardner JD: Interaction of porcine vasoactive intestinal peptide with dispersed pancreatic acinar cells from guinea pig. J Biol Chem 1976; 251:4635–4639.
44. Vandermeers A, Vandermeers-Piret MC, Rathe J, et al: A calcium-dependent protein activator of guanosine-3-5-monophosphate phosphodiesterase in bovine and rat pancreas. Eur J Biochem 1977; 81:377–386.
45. Jensen RT, Gardner JD: Cyclic nucleotide-dependent protein kinase activity in acinar cells from guinea pig pancreas. Gastroenterology 1978; 75:806–817.
46. Hirata Y, Matsuo P, Kobuku H: Digestion and absorption of milk protein in infants' intestine. Kobe J Med Sci 1965; 11:103–109.
47. Katz L, Hamilton JR: Fat absorption in infants of birth weight less than 1300 gm. J Pediatr 1974; 85:608–614.
48. Fomon SJ, Ziegler EE, Thomas LN, et al: Excretion of fat by normal full-term infants fed various milks and formulas. Am J Clin Nutr 1970; 23:1299–1333.
49. Shulman RJ, Wong WW, Irving CS, et al: Utilization of dietary cereal by young infants. J Pediatr 1983; 103:23–28.
50. Lebenthal E, Lee PC, Heitlinger LA: Impact of the development of the gastrointestinal tract on infant feeding. J Pediatr 1983; 102:1–9.
51. Lebenthal E, Lee PC: Development of functional response in human exocrine pancreas. Pediatrics 1980; 66:556–560.
52. Doyle CM, Jamieson JD: Development of secretogogue response in rat pancreatic acinar cells. Dev Biol 1978; 65:11–27.
53. Shimizu K, Lebenthal E, Lee PC: Immature stimulus-secretion coupling of the developing exocrine pancreas and ontogenic

changes for protein kinase C. Biochim Biophys Acta 1988; 968:186–191.

54. Delachaume-Salem E, Sarles H: Evolution en fonction de la age de la sécrétion pancreatique humaine normale. Biol Gastroenterol (Paris) 1970; 2:135–146.
55. Track NS, Creutzfeldt C, Bokermann M: Enzymatic, functional, and ultrastructural development of the exocrine pancreas. II. The human pancreas. Comp Biochem Physiol 1975; 51:95–100.
56. Lebenthal E, Lev R, Lee PC: Prenatal and postnatal development of the human exocrine pancreas. *In* Go VWL, Gardner JD, Brooks FP, et al, eds: The Exocrine Pancreas: Biology, Pathobiology, and Diseases. New York, Raven Press, 1986, pp 33–43.
57. Jensen RG, Clark RM, deJong FA, et al: The lipolytic triad: Human lingual, breast milk, and pancreatic lipase—physiological implications of their characteristics in digestion of dietary fats. J Pediatr Gastroenterol Nutr 1982; 1:243–255.
58. Heitlinger LA, Lee PC, Dillon WP, Lebenthal E: Mammary amylase: A possible alternate pathway of carbohydrate digestion in infancy. Pediatr Res 1983; 17:15–18.
59. Hodge C, Lebenthal E, Lee PC, Topper W: Amylase in the saliva and in the gastric aspirates of premature infants: Its potential role in glucose polymer hydrolysis. Pediatr Res 1983; 17:998–1001.

Chapter 65

Pancreatic Function Testing

HINDA R. KOPELMAN

The exocrine pancreas is a complex organ whose function is to secrete digestive enzymes, fluid, and bicarbonate into the duodenum to help digest intraluminal nutrients and facilitate their absorption. Pancreatic function can, therefore, be examined by methods that assess either the ability of the pancreas to secrete digestive enzymes or the efficacy of nutrient digestion and absorption. Because pancreatic function may be perturbed by a number of pathologic processes, recognition of the presence of pancreatic functional abnormalities may be instrumental in the diagnosis of specific diseases. Because pancreatic pathology may perturb function to varying degrees, quantitation of the degree of functional impairment and the remaining pancreatic functional reserve is mandatory in determining the need for therapeutic intervention and, in some instances, may also be extremely helpful in prognosis.

The exocrine pancreas has a tremendous functional reserve capacity. It was apparent from adult studies published in 1973 that pancreatic maldigestion causing measurable steatorrhea and creatorrhea did not occur until pancreatic trypsin and lipase secretion fell below 10% of control values.[1] Using more sensitive enzyme assays, it has now been demonstrated that loss of 98 to 99% of pancreatic lipase and colipase secretory activity is necessary (Fig. 65–1) before clinical malabsorption, detected by steatorrhea, occurs.[2] Unfortunately, this means that assessment of pancreatic function by recognizing the presence of maldigestion and malabsorption will detect only severe impairment. More sensitive methods are required to detect and quantitate impairment resulting in less than 98% loss of enzyme secretory capacity. This reality helps to define the two most frequent clinical problems that pancreatic function testing may help resolve and the rationale for choosing any particular tool:

1. Does the patient have pancreatic insufficiency (maldigestion and malabsorption) requiring therapeutic intervention with digestive enzyme and vitamin replacement?
2. Does the patient have pancreatic disease, despite sufficient functional reserve to escape malabsorption (pancreatic sufficiency), and, if so, how severe is it?

The wide array of available tools to assess pancreatic function attests to the lack of one ideal method that can respond to these clinical questions in a specific, sensitive, quantitative, and noninvasive manner. The choice of testing for any given clinical situation depends in part on the question being asked; the need for specificity, sensitivity, and quantitation in the particular clinical situation; the degree of invasiveness acceptable; and the availability of local expertise. This chapter reviews the methods used to assess pancreatic function in the pediatric population, attempting to emphasize the advantages and disadvantages of each test, and the clinical situations in which each may be most applicable.

DOES THE PATIENT HAVE PANCREATIC INSUFFICIENCY?

Because of the importance of recognizing patients unable to digest and absorb nutrients adequately to institute appropriate therapy, this clinical question may be the most frequent reason for pancreatic function testing. Pancreatic insufficiency has been defined functionally as the excretion in stool of more than 7% of dietary fat intake owing to severe pancreatic impairment,[3] resulting from the loss of at least 98% of pancreatic lipase and colipase secretory capacity.[2] In patients known to have pancreatic disease (e.g., patients with cystic fibrosis [CF] or chronic pancreatitis), pancreatic function testing is required to determine if the disease process has caused impairment severe enough to have resulted in pancreatic insufficiency. For this purpose, a number of noninvasive tests are available that detect maldigestion and malabsorption in stool. Because they are not specific for pancreatic malabsorption, they may be complemented or replaced by one of several tests that diagnose pancreatic impairment as the cause of the malabsorption when this is clinically not known. In addition, some of these latter tests, performed on samples of blood, urine, or breath instead of stool, are preferred by some centers because of ease and convenience of both collection and processing of samples. None of the tests discussed in this section are

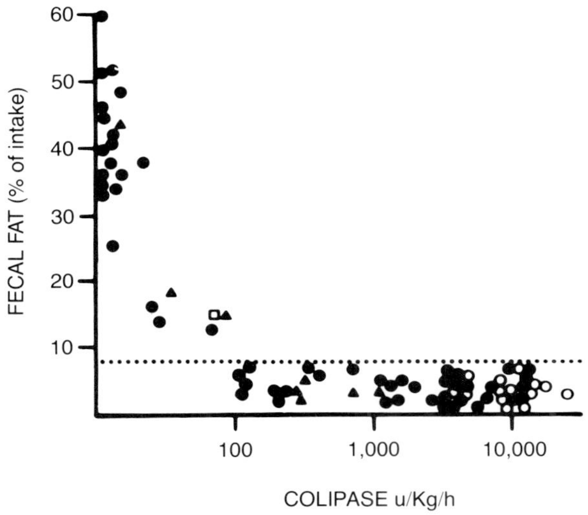

Figure 65—1. Fecal fat excretion is plotted against pancreatic colipase secretory capacity in patients with CF (●), Shwachman's syndrome (▲), pancreatic hypoplasia (□), and normal subjects (○). An abnormal fecal fat excretion is not evident until colipase secretion falls below 120 U per kg per hour or 1 to 2% of mean normal values.

sensitive enough to detect pancreatic disease in the absence of pancreatic insufficiency. Further, only a few can be used quantitatively to assess therapeutic response.

Nonspecific Tests of Pancreatic Insufficiency

72-Hour Stool Fat Balance

This test has become the gold standard in the diagnosis of malabsorption. Steatorrhea is used to define malabsorption when the amount of fat excreted in the stool over a period of 3 to 5 days exceeds 7% of the recorded dietary fat intake during the same period of time for infants and children more than 6 months of age. Infants under 6 months may normally excrete up to 15% of dietary fat intake as a result of physiologic immaturity of hepatobiliary and pancreatic secretory capacity.[4]

This test is reliable and can be used to quantitatively assess responses to therapeutic intervention in patients with malabsorption, provided that attention is paid to a number of important details.

1. Patients must be on a stable and adequate dietary fat intake for at least 3 days before beginning the balance study and must continue this intake throughout the duration of the balance study. The study is invalid if it is performed during inadequate dietary fat intake, if it includes periods of fasting, vomiting of intake, or changes in intake of fat. In adults, a diet containing 100 gm of fat per day is required. In infants, we recommend a dietary fat intake of *no less than* 3 gm per kg per day. Rather than adhering to a strict diet, pediatric patients are required to have all intake carefully recorded, under supervision of a dietician, to allow the calculation of dietary fat intake from these food records. Dietary assessment before initiating the balance study is advisable to ensure adequate fat intake and appropriate recordkeeping of intake.
2. All stools must be collected during the period of study, into preweighed containers, and must include any oil or fat passed with bowel movements. It is inadequate to scoop stools from the toilet bowl, as significant fat excretion may be lost.
3. During the period of collection, and until assay for fat content, stools must be kept refrigerated or frozen to minimize bacterial degradation of fat.
4. Patients with constipation or delayed transit may give erroneous results. This problem may be partially overcome by extending the collection period from 3 to 5 days.
5. The method used by the laboratory to extract and measure fat is important. Some methods, such as the van de Kamer method,[5] will not extract and detect medium-chain triglycerides (MCT) and are therefore inadequate for patients receiving formulas or supplements with MCT. Methodology to detect both long-chain triglycerides (LCT) and MCT in stool are available.[6] Alternatively, testing should be performed before initiating the use of MCT.

When used appropriately, the 72-hour stool fat balance is a useful tool to assess the presence of pancreatic insufficiency in patients with pancreatic disease. It can determine the degree of response of malabsorption to therapy and the need for more aggressive investigation or therapy if responses prove inadequate. It can be performed at home provided that adequate teaching and supervision are supplied. The experience in some centers suggests superior compliance and success with this approach compared with balance studies performed in the hospital.[7]

Although both fecal nitrogen and fecal carbohydrate excretion may be used as indices of pancreatic insufficiency, they do not provide further diagnostic information and may be less accurate than fecal fat determination as a result of the variable degree of colonic absorption of these nutrients and their degradation and utilization by colonic flora.

Stool Smear for Fat

In an attempt to avoid the inconvenience of a 3- to 5-day collection of stool and dietary intake record, spot stool samples have been examined microscopically for undigested or neutral fat droplets. Although fat droplets can be seen quite easily as clear globules under the 40 × power light microscope lens, staining with Sudan for neutral fat enhances their visualization. The identification of multiple fat droplets on a slide prepared with a thin smear of stool examined under the light microscope is a useful screening tool, suggesting the presence of steatorrhea. Although crude, it identifies patients who should have fecal fat losses documented and quantified.

Steatocrit

Attempting to detect and quantify steatorrhea, Colombo and colleagues[8] reported their experience with the steatocrit test for monitoring fat malabsorption in patients with CF. Using this simple method, a sample of homogenized stool is centrifuged in a hematocrit tube at 15,000 rpm for 15 minutes. Stool lipid separates to the top of the liquid and can be quantitated. Further experience with this test is warranted before it can be fully evaluated. Although a single random sample of stool may not accurately reflect the capability for fat digestion and absorption, this technique could be performed on multiple samples to improve reliability. Provided that expectations of sensitivity are not unrealistic, this method may prove useful in crudely detecting the response of malabsorption to the institution of therapy.

Oral Tolerance Tests

Oral tolerance tests compare the rise in serum of a substance that has been ingested to the rise in normal subjects. These tests are not specific for pancreatic disease but rather detect digestive and absorptive defects of pancreatic, hepatobiliary, or intestinal origin. They may be made somewhat more specific by repeating the protocol after the administration of pancreatic enzymes to detect any improvement in serum profile of the administered substance.

The most recent version of such a test has been the report of an oral fat loading test.[9] The ingestion of a standard meal containing a total of 50 gm of fat, equal amounts of butter and margarine, emulsified in 70 ml of water, was followed by serum measurements of triglycerides and chylomicrons at 2, 3, and 5 hours. An abnormal result was defined as a rise in serum triglycerides of less than 100% above fasting levels, a rise of less than 1.13 mmol per L, or the appearance of less than 7% chylomicrons.

Specific Tests of Pancreatic Insufficiency

The tests described in this section are used to differentiate pancreatic insufficiency from malabsorption caused by intestinal or hepatobiliary disease. They are, however, not sensitive enough to discriminate the presence of pancreatic disease without insufficiency from normal pancreatic functional capacity.

Stool Trypsin and Chymotrypsin

Earlier experience with assays of trypsin and chymotrypsin activity in stool for the detection of pancreatic insufficiency was associated with significant false-positive and false-negative results.[10, 11] Variability in intestinal transit time, degradation of enzyme activity in stool by both pancreatic and bacterial proteases, and variable binding of enzyme activity to insoluble fecal residue interfered with the reliability of the test. Further, the time-consuming titrimetric assay used was not popular with clinical laboratories.

A new photometric assay has become available that is more convenient.[12] It assays fecal chymotrypsin, which is more resistant to fecal bacterial degradation than trypsin and is relatively stable in stool. Chymotrypsin is now solubilized in stool using this method, overcoming yet another source of previously unreliable results. Fecal chymotrypsin can be measured on an aliquot of stool obtained during a 3-day fat balance study[13] or on three random stool samples.[14] Both methods have shown good correlation between stool chymotrypsin activity and stimulated duodenal output of chymotrypsin. Clearly, however, patients receiving pancreatic enzyme supplementation must discontinue their therapy for at least 5 days before sampling. In the presence of constipation or delayed intestinal transit, this period may not be sufficient.

Bentiromide

This is the first of a number of tests to be described that obviate the need to collect and assay fecal material. It relies on the principles presented diagrammatically in Figure 65–2. Bentiromide (*N*-benzoyl-L-tyrosyl-*p*-aminobenzoic acid) is a nonabsorbable synthetic peptide.[15] When specifically cleaved by chymotrypsin, the moiety, p-aminobenzoic acid (PABA), is released, rapidly absorbed across intact intestinal mucosa, conjugated in the liver, and excreted in the urine. It can, therefore, be detected and quantitated in either blood or urine. Assuming normal intestinal, hepatic, and renal function, urinary PABA excretion is dependent on pancreatic function; plasma PABA determinations are a reflection of pancreatic function, assuming only an intact intestinal mucosal surface.

A number of variations of this test have been described with varying degrees of complexity to correct for potential defects in intestinal, hepatic, and renal

N-Benzoyl-L-tyrosyl-p-aminobenzoic acid

(BENTIROMIDE)

|

hydrolysis by chymotrypsin

|

p-aminobenzoic acid

(PABA)

|

intestinal absorption

hepatic conjugation

urinary excretion

Figure 65–2. The principle of the bentiromide test.

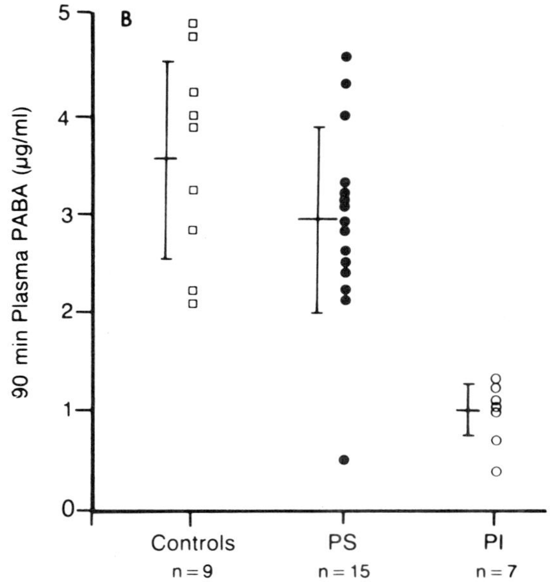

Figure 65–3. The 90-minute plasma PABA value discriminated patients with pancreatic insufficiency (PI) from controls with no overlap. It was unable to discriminate patients with pancreatic sufficiency (PS) from controls.

function; to simplify the test; or to improve sensitivity and specificity. In its simplest form, the test was recommended in adults as a 6-hour urinary collection after the ingestion of 500 mg of bentiromide.[16] When adequate diuresis was maintained, recovery in the urine of less than 50% of the ingested dose reflected pancreatic insufficiency. To improve the sensitivity of the test, by correcting for intestinal, hepatic, or renal impairment, an equivalent dose of free PABA (170 mg of PABA) was recommended as a second step, followed by a 6-hour urine collection and expression of urinary PABA recovery/free PABA recovery.[17]

To avoid the need for a second test with free PABA, investigators reported on the simultaneous administration with bentiromide of C^{14} free PABA,[18] unsuitable for pediatric use, or p-aminosalicylic acid (PAS), a structural analog of free PABA.[19] The latter has been used in pediatrics to improve the sensitivity of this test.[20] The introduction of a plasma PABA assay[21, 22] not only improved the sensitivity and specificity but also obviated the need for timed urine collections. Using bentiromide, 15 mg per kg per dose, discrimination between normal controls and older children with pancreatic insufficiency was optimized at 90 and 120 minutes (Fig. 65–3) with virtually no overlap in values.[23] Unfortunately, the test was unable to detect CF patients with pancreatic sufficiency and as little as 5% of normal chymotrypsin secretory capacity nor patients with Shwachman's syndrome and pancreatic sufficiency with as little as 1% of normal secretory capacity. In infants, the test was found to discriminate CF from controls if a higher dose (30 mg per kg) and a liquid meal were used.[23a]

Attempts to improve sensitivity further have included providing a liquid or standard meal during bentiromide administration to stimulate pancreatic secretion, increasing the dose of bentiromide administered to 30 mg per kg per dose, developing more sensitive high-pressure liquid chromatography (HPLC) methodology to detect serum PABA, and altering the chemical structure of the synthetic peptide as substrate. Reports of the use of 4-*N*-acetyl-L-tyrosyl aminobenzoic acid instead of bentiromide suggest this may be promising.[24, 25] Problems with specificity include the chymotrypsin-like activity present in intestinal brush border and intestinal bacterial flora[26, 27] as well as a number of foods and drugs that interfere with PABA determinations.[28] To date, no refinements have permitted the bentiromide test to quantitate pancreatic function beyond the identification of pancreatic insufficiency.

Pancreolauryl Test

Similar to the bentiromide test, the pancreolauryl test consists of the oral administration of a synthetic compound and its subsequent specific cleavage by a pancreatic enzyme, absorption, conjugation, and excretion of a measurable moiety in the urine (Fig. 65–4). Ingested fluorescein dilaurate (0.5 mmol in adults) is hydrolyzed by pancreatic cholesterol esterase, producing fluorescein, which can easily be measured by either spectrophotometric or fluorometric techniques in urine or serum.[29]

The recommended test consists of the ingestion of 0.5 mmol of fluorescein dilaurate in adults with a standard meal and maintenance of diuresis, followed by a 10-hour urine collection. A second test using equimolar free fluorescein is required to correct for individual differences in intestinal, hepatic, and renal function.[30] A serum test has been described with maximal discriminatory power between 240 and 300 minutes.[31]

Sensitivity and specificity are probably comparable to the bentiromide test. This test can also detect only pancreatic insufficiency and is not sensitive enough to quantitate less severe pancreatic impairment. Bacterial degradation of fluorescein dilaurate, like bentiromide, can occur. Falsely abnormal test results can be obtained in patients with biliary disease or inflammatory bowel

Fluorescein dilaurate

|

hydrolysis by cholesterol ester hydrolase

|

Fluorescein

|

intestinal absorption

hepatic conjugation

urinary excretion

Figure 65–4. The principle of the pancreolauryl test.

disease and patients on zinc therapy.[32] Brush border enzymes are not active on this compound, however, and there is less interference with exogenous drugs (niacin and sulfasalazine need to be avoided). In addition, analysis of fluorescein is easier than its rival, PABA.[30]

Stable Isotope–Labeled Breath Tests

To develop simple and accurate screening tests for steatorrhea to replace the 72-hour fecal fat test, the ingestion of radioactively labeled triglycerides was followed by measurement of the label in carbon dioxide excreted in the breath.[33] The appearance of labeled carbon dioxide in the breath depended on the intraluminal digestion of lipids. The use of nonradioactively labeled ^{13}C substrates has made this technology suitable for application in pediatrics.

In the initial study reported in children, the ^{13}C-labeled triglyceride, triolein, provided 100% sensitivity and 89% specificity in detecting fat malabsorption.[34] The inability of patients with steatorrhea owing to pancreatic insufficiency to digest the ^{13}C-MCT, trioctanoin, differentiated them from patients with either mucosal intestinal or biliary disease (Fig. 65–5). To obviate the need for sequential testing with these two different substrates, a synthetic "mixed" triglyceride substrate, with a medium-chain fatty acid labeled with ^{13}C, was evaluated.[35] In this test, the ^{13}C oxygen breath excretion depends on the hydrolysis of the medium-chain moiety by pancreatic lipase. Although this test was abnormal in most patients with pancreatic disease and mean results were lower than mean values in patients with nonpancreatic steatorrhea, the test failed to differentiate pancreatic insufficiency from other causes of malabsorption in all cases.

Although sensitivity appears quite good, attempts to improve specificity for pancreatic disease continue. Repeating the test after administration of pancreatic enzymes might improve specificity. Newer substrates, such as cholesteryl octanoate, which is hydrolyzed by the pancreatic-specific cholesterol esterase, may be promising.[36] Finally, techniques of adapting expensive stable isotope technology for routine clinical use are required before this noninvasive approach can be introduced widely.

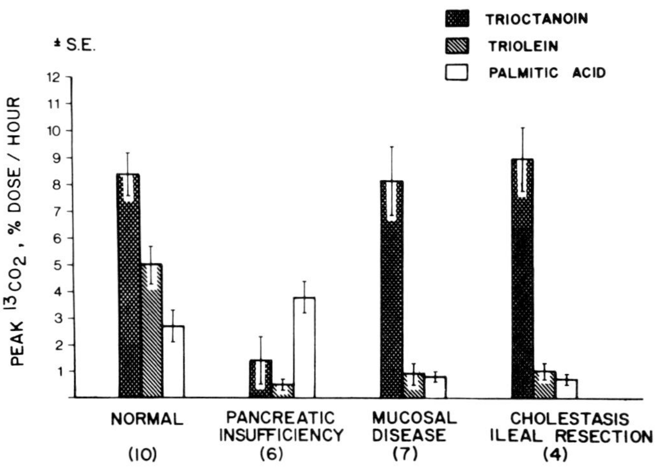

Figure 65–5. The ^{13}C breath test differentiated patients with pancreatic insufficiency from normal subjects and those with steatorrhea owing to other causes by a low response to both triolein and trioctanoin (MCT) substrates.[34]

Serum Pancreatic Enzymes

Immunoassay techniques are now available for the specific detection of various pancreatic enzymes in serum. Pancreatic enzymes are detectable in the sera of normal individuals, concentrations varying normally with age. Some enzymes, such as amylase and lipase, tend to increase from early infancy owing to the maturation of pancreatic enzyme levels, whereas trypsin(ogen) levels are present in mature amounts early on and change little with age in the pediatric population.[37] In the absence of acute pancreatitis, ductal obstruction as is seen in CF or pancreatic stones, and impaired renal function, all conditions in which serum pancreatic enzymes are pathologically elevated, the serum levels of pancreatic enzymes reflect the amount of functional acinar tissue. Thus, serum pancreatic enzyme determinations can be specific tests for the detection of pancreatic insufficiency, with the caveats already mentioned. Unfortunately, they are all unable to quantitate pancreatic function in the range of pancreatic sufficiency.

Low pancreatic isoamylase determinations can be used to detect pancreatic insufficiency in older children. The test is of little use in infancy because pancreatic amylase values are normally low. In addition, assays of total serum amylase concentrations and enzymatic activity assays are of no value because they do not differentiate pancreatic from salivary amylase.[38, 39]

Serum lipase can now be detected using a sensitive and specific enzyme-linked immunosorbent assay (ELISA), which is available commercially.[40] Because pancreatic lipase secretion increases during the first 3 to 6 months of age, this test would not be expected to discriminate patients with pancreatic insufficiency in early infancy. It has been evaluated in patients with CF.[41, 42] Not surprisingly, values were elevated in the first years of life, presumably secondary to pancreatic ductal obstruction, and therefore could not provide a reliable assessment of the amount of functional pancreatic tissue.[41] Beyond 5 years of age, however, immunoreactive serum pancreatic lipase levels proved to be both sensitive (95%) and specific (85%) in detecting pancreatic insufficiency.[42]

Serum immunoreactive trypsin(ogen) has been the pancreatic enzyme most studied as a test of pancreatic function. Specific radioimmunoassays[43, 44] and, more recently, an ELISA using a monoclonal antibody specific for trypsinogen[45] have been developed. In adult patients, the level of serum immunoreactive trypsinogen (IRT) was able to differentiate patients with pancreatic insufficiency from those with steatorrhea of nonpancreatic origin (Fig. 65–6) with no overlap.[46] This test was unable to quantitate pancreatic function in patients with impairment of lesser degrees (pancreatic sufficiency). Serum IRT has now also been evaluated extensively in

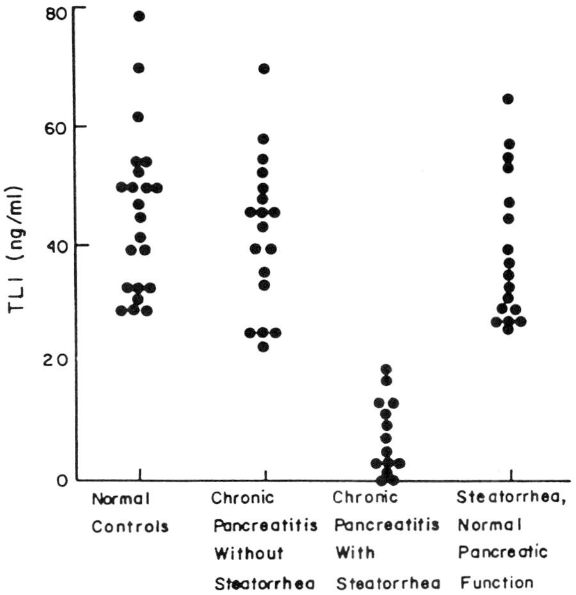

Figure 65–6. The IRT value discriminated patients with pancreatic steatorrhea from those with steatorrhea owing to other pathology.[46]

the pediatric population, both with[47] and without CF.[48] Because serum levels vary little with age, even in early infancy, it is the serum pancreatic enzyme of choice for function testing. In patients with pancreatic diseases other than CF, this test was able to identify pancreatic insufficiency secondary to Shwachman's syndrome, insulin-dependent diabetes mellitus, and chronic pancreatitis from nonpancreatic steatorrhea. In CF, patients over the age of 7 years with pancreatic insufficiency could be detected using low IRT values, with a predictive rate of 94%.

DOES THE PATIENT HAVE PANCREATIC DISEASE, AND HOW SEVERE IS IT?

Because of the tremendous enzyme secretory capacity of the exocrine pancreas, extensive loss of functional acinar tissue must occur before pancreatic insufficiency manifests clinically.[2, 49] The pancreatic function tests discussed thus far are capable of detecting this degree of pancreatic functional impairment. They are, however, not sensitive enough to detect important degrees of pancreatic functional impairment in patients without malabsorption. Direct tests of pancreatic secretory capacity in response to exogenous stimulation are presently the only means of detecting pancreatic disease and quantitating the functional loss in these patients.

Pharmacologic Pancreatic Stimulation Tests

Many variations have been used to study the response of the exocrine pancreas to standard exogenous stimulation with pharmacologic doses of hormones. In principle, maximal or near-maximal stimulation with standard doses of intravenously administered pancreatic secretagogues forces the pancreas to secrete fluid, HCO_3, and digestive enzymes at maximal capacity. By collecting these secretions in a quantitative manner from the duodenum, the secretory capacity of these parameters can be assessed as a percent of the response seen in normal or control subjects. Because of the variation in choice of hormones, doses, bolus versus continuous infusion, methods of collection, and assays used in quantitation of enzyme activities, patient data must be interpreted relative to the range of normal values established for the particular techniques used.

The technique used at the Hospital for Sick Children in Toronto has been responsible for providing a great deal of valuable information on pancreatic function in large numbers of pediatric patients[2, 49–52] and is described in detail (Fig. 65–7). Modified from the method originally described by Go and coworkers at the Mayo Clinic,[53] it requires placement of a nasoduodenal double-lumen tube under fluoroscopic control such that the proximal port opens near the ampulla of Vater, and several ports open 5 to 12 cm distally near the ligament of Treitz. A nonabsorbable marker solution of sulfobromophthalein sodium (Bromsulphalein) in 5% mannitol is infused at a constant rate through the proximal port, allowed to mix with pancreatic secretions in the duodenum, and aspirated distally by intermittent low suction into closed flasks maintained on ice. The first 20 to 30 minutes are allowed for equilibration of the system, washout of the duodenum, and gastric aspiration via a separate nasogastric tube, to avoid contamination of duodenal contents with gastric acid and pepsin. During the subsequent three 20-minute collection periods, pancreatic secretions are aspirated from the duodenum during continuous intravenous infusion of both secretin and cholecystokinin (CCK). Nasogastric suction is maintained throughout. Determinations of fluid, electrolyte, and enzyme activity are assessed and corrected for the amount of marker recovered in secretions.

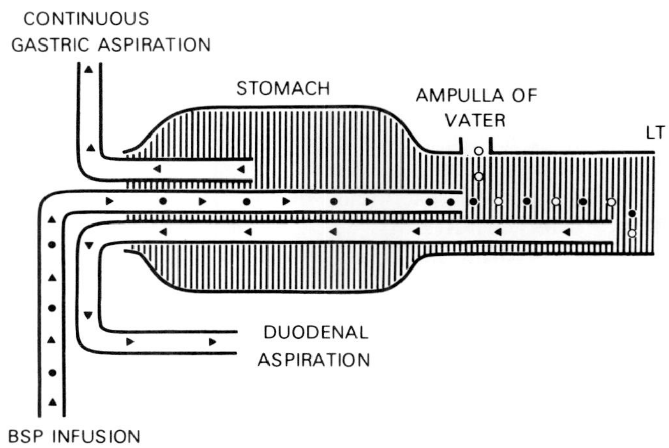

Figure 65–7. Diagrammatic representation of the pharmacologic pancreatic stimulation test as it is performed at the Hospital for Sick Children in Toronto. BSP, Bromsulphalein; LT, ligament of Treitz.

A variety of assays are available for assessment of secretory capacity. In Toronto, the enzyme activities measured routinely by titrimetric assays are trypsin,[54] colipase, and total lipase.[49] Fluid, electrolyte, and HCO_3 outputs are also assessed. Although other enzymes are amenable to measurement, it is worth noting that amylase secretion in particular is very dependent on patient age and therefore difficult to use as a standard parameter in the pediatric population.

This form of pancreatic function test is clearly invasive and labor-intensive and requires a degree of expertise not always available. Unfortunately, it is currently the only means of assessing and quantitating pancreatic function in the group of patients with more than 1 to 2% of pancreatic residual secretory capacity. It may be mandatory in the detection of pancreatic disease, and thus in the establishment of the diagnosis, in patients with Shwachman's syndrome in the absence of steatorrhea or in patients suspected of having CF in whom the diagnosis is difficult because of mild involvement, equivocal sweat chloride results, or both. It may also provide important prognostic information in patients with known pancreatic disease and pancreatic sufficiency in whom the pathology is progressive (CF, chronic pancreatitis). These patients may have a very wide spectrum of residual pancreatic function, from 2 to 100% of normal secretory capacity. Patients who, on testing, are at the lower end of this spectrum are at much greater risk of developing pancreatic insufficiency with disease progression than those at the upper end of the functional reserve spectrum. Patients at increased risk can be followed more closely, counseled on symptoms and signs to report, and prepared with the appropriate expectations.

Nutrient Pancreatic Stimulation Tests

Using a more physiologic approach to the stimulation of pancreatic secretion, a variety of tests have been described that involve the ingestion or infusion of intraluminal nutrients into the duodenum and the determination of pancreatic enzyme activities recovered from the duodenum. Although essential amino acids are probably the most potent nutrient stimuli[55] and their presence in the duodenum does not interfere with enzymatic or electrolyte determinations on duodenal contents, they have not been used to assess pancreatic function clinically in the pediatric age group.

The most used test meal, the Lundh meal, is composed of intact nutrients, with 5% protein, 6% fat, and 15% carbohydrate in 300 ml of total volume for adults.[56] Although it is far more physiologic than the secretin/CCK stimulation test, it is burdened with a number of disadvantages, making interpretation rather qualitative. Salivary and gastric secretions contaminate duodenal contents; no marker perfusion technique or balloon occlusion is included to make measurements more quantitative; and the presence of nutrient substrate in the duodenal contents makes the enzymatic determinations of lipase, protease, and amylase activities difficult.

SUMMARY

Pancreatic function testing is a potentially valuable tool in the assessment, diagnosis, prognosis, and overall management of pancreatic disease in pediatrics. Because of the array of different tests available, it is important to understand the clinical question being asked and the information required as well as the advantages and disadvantages of the different tests to choose the tool likely to provide the most benefit.

REFERENCES

1. Di Magno EP, Go VLW, Summerskill WJH: Relations between pancreatic enzyme outputs and malabsorption in severe pancreatic insufficiency. N Engl J Med 1973; 288:813–815.
2. Gaskin KJ, Durie PR, Lee L, et al: Colipase and lipase secretion in childhood-onset pancreatic insufficiency. Gastroenterology 1984; 86:1–7.
3. Forstner G, Durie P: Cystic fibrosis. *In* Walker WA, Durie PR, Hamilton JR, et al, eds: Pediatric Gastrointestinal Disease. Philadelphia, BC Decker, 1991, pp 1179–1197.
4. Fomon SJ, Ziegler ER, Thomas LN, et al: Excretion of fat by normal full-term infants fed various milks and formulas. Am J Clin Nutr 1970; 23:1299–1313.
5. van de Kamer JK, ten Bokkel Huinink H, Weyers HA: Rapid method for the determination of fat in feces. J Biol Chem 1949; 177:347–355.
6. Jeejeebhoy KN, Ahmed S, Kozak G: Determination of fecal fats containing both medium and long chain triglycerides and fatty acids. Clin Biochem 1970; 3:157–163.
7. Ellis L, Kalnins D, Durie P: Stool collections can be successfully performed at home—the Toronto experience. Pediatr Pulm 1990; 5(Suppl):261.
8. Colombo C, Maiavacca R, Ronchi M, et al: The steatocrit: A simple method for monitoring fat malabsorption in patients with cystic fibrosis. J Pediatr Gastroenterol Nutr 1987; 6:926–930.
9. Goldstein R, Blondheim O, Levy E, et al: The fatty meal test: An alternative to stool fat analysis. Am J Clin Nutr 1983; 38:763–768.
10. Haverbach BJ, Dyce VJ, Gutentag PJ, et al: Measurement of trypsin and chymotrypsin in stool: A diagnostic test for pancreatic exocrine function. Gastroenterology 1963; 44:588–597.
11. Ammann RW, Tagwercher E, Kashiwagi H, et al: Diagnostic value of fecal chymotrypsin and trypsin assessment for detection of pancreatic disease. Am J Dig Dis 1968; 13:123–126.
12. Kaspar P, Moller G, Wahlefeld A: New photometric assay for chymotrypsin in stool. Clin Chem 1984; 30:1753–1757.
13. Bonin A, Roy CC, Lasalle R, et al: Fecal chymotrypsin: A reliable index of exocrine pancreatic function in children. J Pediatr 1973; 83:594–600.
14. Brown GA, Sule D, Williams J, et al: Faecal chymotrypsin: A reliable index of exocrine pancreatic function. Arch Dis Child 1988; 63:785–789.
15. Imondi AR, Stradley RP, Wolgemuth R: Synthetic peptides in the diagnosis of exocrine pancreatic insufficiency in animals. Gut 1972; 13:726–731.
16. Toskes PP: Bentiromide as a test of exocrine pancreatic function in adult patients with pancreatic exocrine insufficiency: Determination of appropriate dose and urinary collection interval. Gastroenterology 1983; 85:565–569.
17. Mitchell CJ, Humphrey CS, Bullen AW, et al: Improved diagnostic accuracy of a modified oral pancreatic function test. Scand J Gastroenterol 1979; 14:737–741.
18. Mitchell CJ, Field HP, Simpson FG, et al: Preliminary evaluation of a single day tubeless test of pancreatic function. Br Med J 1981; 282:1751–1753.

19. Hoek FJ, van den Berg FA, Klein Elhorst JT, et al: Improved specificity of the PABA test with *p*-aminosalicylic acid (PAS). Gut 1987; 28:468–473.
20. Puntis JWL, Berg JD, Buckley TM, et al: Simplified oral pancreatic function test. Arch Dis Child 1988; 63:780–784.
21. Dockter G, Nacu I, Kohlberger E: Determination of protease-cleaved p-aminobenzoic acid (PABA) in serum after oral administration of *N*-benzoyl-L-tyrosyl p-aminobenzoic acid (PABA-peptide) in children. Eur J Pediatr 1981; 135:277–279.
22. Delchier J-C, Soule J-C: BT-PABA test with plasma PABA measurements: Evaluation of sensitivity and specificity. Gut 1983; 24:318–325.
23. Weizman Z, Forstner GG, Gaskin KJ, et al: Bentiromide test for assessing pancreatic dysfunction using analysis of paraaminobenzoic acid in plasma and urine: Studies in cystic fibrosis and Shwachman's syndrome. Gastroenterology 1985; 89:596–604.
23a. Laufer D, Cleghorn G, Forstner G, et al: The bentiromide test using plasma *p*-aminobenzoic acid for diagnosis of pancreatic insufficiency in young children: The effect of two different doses and a liquid meal. Gastroenterology 1991; 101:207–213.
24. Malis F, Fric P, Kasahrek E, Slaby J: Comparative study of the estimation of exocrine pancreatic function using p-(N-acetyl-L-tyrosyl) and p-N-benzoyl-L-tyrosyl) aminobenzoic acid. Acta Hepatogastroenterol 1983; 30:99–101.
25. Malis F, Fric P, Kasahrek E, et al: A paroral test of pancreatic insufficiency with 4-(N-acetyl-L-tyrosyl) aminobenzoic acid in children with cystic fibrosis. J Pediatr 1979; 94:942–944.
26. Sterchi EE, Green JR, Lentz MJ: Non pancreatic hydrolysis of N-benzoyl-L-tyrosyl-p-aminobenzoic acid (PABA-peptide) in the human small intestine. Clin Sci 1982; 62:557–560.
27. Gyr K, Felsenfeld O, Imondi AR: Chymotrypsin-like activity of some intestinal bacteria. Dig Dis Sci 1978; 23:413–416.
28. Heyman MB: The bentiromide test; how good is it? Gastroenterology 1985; 89:685–687.
29. Lankisch PG, Brauneis J, Otto J, Goke B: Pancreolauryl and NBT-PABA tests: Are serum tests a more practicable alternative to urine tests in the diagnosis of exocrine pancreatic insufficiency? Gastroenterology 1986; 90:350–354.
30. Scharp S, Iliano L: Two indirect tests of exocrine pancreatic function evaluated. Clin Chem 1987; 33:5–12.
31. Cummings JGR, Forsyth JS, Boyd EJS, et al: Diagnosis of exocrine insufficiency in cystic fibrosis by use of fluorescein dilaurate test. Arch Dis Child 1986; 61:573–575.
32. Reddy NK, Kaur U, Bambery P, et al: Pancreolauryl pancreatic function test (letter). Gastroenterology 1989; 96:1377–1378.
33. Newcomer AD, Hormann AF, DiMagno EP, et al: Triolein breath test: A sensitive and specific test for fat malabsorption. Gastroenterology 1979; 76:6–13.
34. Watkins JB, Klein PD, Schoeller DA, et al: Diagnosis and differentiation of fat malabsorption in children using 13C-labelled lipids: Trioctanoin, triolein and palmitic acid breath tests. Gastroenterology 1982; 82:911–917.
35. Van trapper GR, Rutgeerts PJ, Ghoos YF, et al: Mixed triglyceride breath test: A noninvasive test of pancreatic lipase activity in the duodenum. Gastroenterology 1989; 96:1126–1134.
36. Cole SG, Rossi S, Stern A, Hofmann AF: Cholesteryl octanoate breat test: Preliminary studies on a new noninvasive test of human pancreatic exocrine function. Gastroenterology 1987; 93:1372–1380.
37. Lebenthal E, Lee PC: Development of functional response in human exocrine pancreas. Pediatrics 1980; 66:556–560.
38. O'Donnell MD, Miller NJ: Plasma pancreatic and salivary type amylase and immunoreactive trypsin concentrations: Variations with age and reference ranges for children. Clin Chim Acta 1980; 104:265–273.
39. Davidson GP, Koheil A, Forstner GG: Salivary amylase in cystic fibrosis: A marker of disordered autoimmune function. Pediatr Res 1978; 12:967–970.
40. Grenner G, Deutsch G, Schmidtberger R, et al: A highly sensitive enzyme immunoassay for the determination of pancreatic lipase. J Clin Chem Clin Biochem 1982; 20:515–520.
41. Cleghorn G, Benjamin L, Corey M, et al: Age-related alterations of immunoreactive pancreatic lipase and cationic trypsinogen in young children with cystic fibrosis. J Pediatr 1985; 107:377–381.
42. Cleghorn G, Benjamin L, Corey M, et al: Serum immunoreactive pancreatic lipase and cationic trypsinogen for the assessment of exocrine pancreatic function in older patients with cystic fibrosis. Pediatrics 1986; 77:301–306.
43. Borgstrom A, Ohlsson K: Radioimmunological determination and characterization of cathodal trypsin-like immunoreactivity in normal human plasma. Scand J Clin Lab Med 1976; 36:809–814.
44. Geokas MC, Largman C, Brodrick JW, Johnston DH: Determination of human pancreatic cationic trypsinogen in serum by radioimmunoassay. Am J Physiol 1979; 236:E77–E83.
45. Bowling FG, Watson ARA, Rylatt DB, et al: Monoclonal antibody-based enzyme immunoassay for trypsinogen in neonatal screening for cystic fibrosis. Lancet 1987; 1:826–827.
46. Jacobson DG, Curington C, Connery K, et al: Trypsin-like immunoreactivity as a test for pancreatic insufficiency. N Engl J Med 1984; 310:1307–1309.
47. Durie PR, Forstner GG, Gaskin KJ, et al: Age-related alterations of immunoreactive pancreatic cationic trypsinogen in sera from cystic fibrosis patients with and without pancreatic insufficiency. Pediatr Res 1986; 20:209–213.
48. Moore DJ, Forstner GG, Largman C, et al: Serum immunoreactive cationic trypsinogen; a useful indicator of severe exocrine dysfunction in the pediatric patient without cystic fibrosis. Gut 1986; 27:1362–1368.
49. Gaskin KJ, Durie PR, Hill RE, et al: Colipase and maximally activated pancreatic lipase in normal subjects and patients with steatorrhea. J Clin Invest 1982; 69:427–434.
50. Gaskin KJ, Durie PR, Corey M, et al: Evidence for a primary defect of pancreatic HCO_3^- secretion in cystic fibrosis. Pediatr Res 1982; 16:554–557.
51. Kopelman H, Durie P, Gaskin Z, et al: Pancreatic fluid secretion and protein hyperconcentration in cystic fibrosis. N Engl J Med 1985; 313:329–334.
52. Kopelman H, Corey M, Gaskin K, et al: Impaired chloride secretion, as well as bicarbonate secretion, underlies the fluid secretory defect in the cystic fibrosis pancreas. Gastroenterology 1988; 95:349–355.
53. Go VLW, Hofmann AF, Summerskill WHJ: Simultaneous measurements of total pancreatic, biliary and gastric outputs in man using a perfusion technique. Gastroenterology 1970; 58:321–328.
54. Dyck WP: Titremetric measurements of fecal tryspin and chymotrypsin in cystic fibrosis with pancreatic exocrine insufficiency. Am J Dig Dis 1967; 12:310–317.
55. Go VLW, Hofmann AF, Summerskill WHJ: Pancreozymin bioassay in man based on pancreatic enzyme secretion: Potency of specific amino acids and other digestive products. J Clin Invest 1970; 49:1558–1564.
56. Lundh G: Pancreatic exocrine function in neoplastic and inflammatory disease: A simple and reliable new test. Gastroenterology 1962; 42:275–280.

Chapter 66

Cystic Fibrosis

HINDA R. KOPELMAN

Cystic fibrosis (CF) is an inherited disease, occurring in one in 2,000 to one in 2,500 live births among whites. It was first recognized as a distinct entity in the 1930s because of characteristic pathologic findings affecting both the pancreas and the lungs.[1] It remains the most frequent cause of pancreatic insufficiency and chronic lung disease in the pediatric age group. Although pulmonary and pancreatic manifestations are the most frequent and most prominent clinical problems, CF is a multisystem disease, affecting virtually all exocrine glands and organs lined by epithelial cells (Fig. 66–1). The universal involvement of the sweat glands is the basis for the diagnostic test, the sweat test, used worldwide in the identification of affected individuals. Involvement of the pancreas, the intestinal tract, and the hepatobiliary system increasingly demands the expertise of the gastroenterologist. Further, it has become apparent that some patients with CF develop significant malnutrition refractory to conservative nutritional management, and more aggressive approaches have become part of the standard of care offered by gastrointestinal and nutritional consultants.

Over the past 50 years, since the original description of this disorder, increasing knowledge and understanding have altered approaches to management. Improvements in choice and routes of administration of antibiotics, chest physiotherapy, replacement of pancreatic enzymes, vitamins, and nutritional supplementation; earlier recognition of complications; and more aggressive management have been associated with an increase in life expectancy. Median survival has gone from 4 years of age, in the 1960s, to 25 years of age in the 1980s, and almost 80% of affected individuals live beyond their twentieth birthday.[2] With the increasing expertise and availability of organ transplantation technology to correct lung and liver failure, survival data are likely to continue to improve. The advent of newer approaches to correct the basic physiologic or genetic (or both) defect in the pulmonary epithelium in the future will also favorably alter long-term prognosis and survival. As life expectancy increases and advances in the correction of pulmonary pathology are made, the gastrointestinal and nutritional aspects of the care of these patients will take on an ever greater importance in the overall management of CF.

DIAGNOSIS

The diagnosis of CF should be suspected in the presence of at least one of the major manifestations of this disease; involvement of the pancreas, lungs, or both; any of the other findings documented in Figure 66–1; a positive family history of the disorder; or some combination of these findings. In the appropriate clinical setting, a sweat chloride concentration of greater than 60 mEq per L on two occasions in a sweat sample of at least 100 mg confirms the diagnosis of CF.[3, 4] Sweat testing should be performed in a center experienced in the administration and interpretation of this technique because erroneous results may be obtained owing to inaccuracies in the technique itself. Although the simpler Orion sweat chloride electrode may be used as a screening test, a diagnosis should be made based only on the results of a sweat chloride determination from a weighed sample of sweat, obtained after pilocarpine iontophoresis (Gibson-Cooke method). It should also be remembered that a variety of conditions may result in false-positive and false-negative values. The most frequent clinically relevant of these are the falsely elevated sweat chloride result seen in malnutrition and the falsely normal result seen in the presence of hypoalbuminemia and edema.[5] In both instances, sweat testing should be repeated after resolution of the malnutrition or edema to verify the results.

CF in infancy may also be detected by measuring serum trypsinogen values. In contrast to the situation in pancreatic insufficiency in older individuals, serum trypsinogen levels are elevated in CF in early infancy,[6] probably reflecting ductal obstruction, subclinical pancreatitis, or both. Neonatal screening for elevated serum trypsinogen values in heel-prick blood samples has been performed in a number of communities. It has been demonstrated to shorten the mean time to diagnosis, allowing earlier intervention, and appears to be able to identify the majority of CF patients, including those with pancreatic sufficiency.[7, 8] It is important to recognize that this screening test identifies individuals requiring further diagnostic investigation, including a repeat serum trypsinogen, a sweat test, and appropriate clinical evaluation, before a definitive diagnosis is established. The majority of infants with elevated serum trypsinogen values on screening will not have CF.

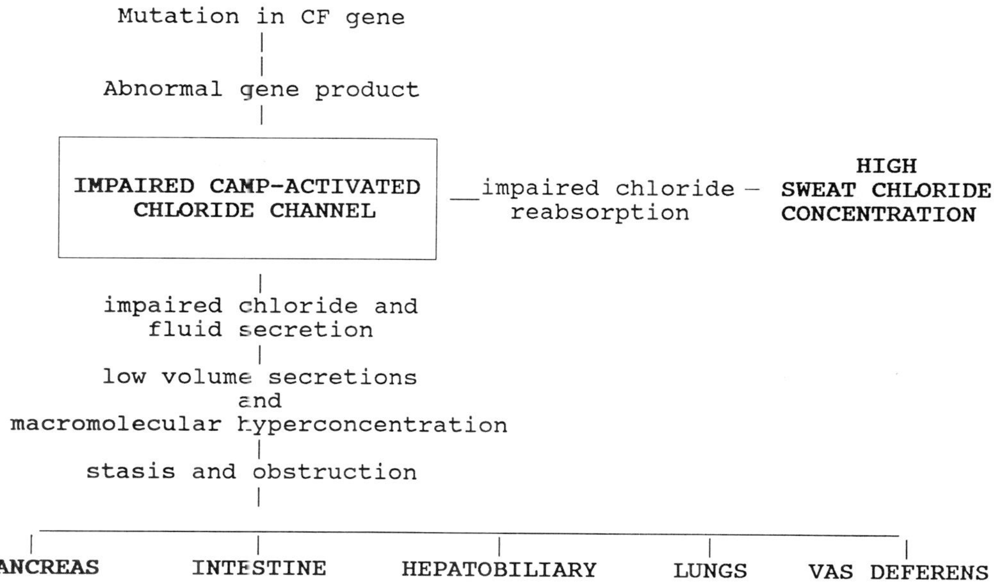

Figure 66–1. The pathogenesis of CF.

GENETICS

CF is an autosomal recessive disorder, largely occurring in the white population. It is rare in Asians, black African populations, and native Americans, but racial intermixing has increased the frequency of the disease in these populations. The high carrier frequency, approximately 5%, in the white population suggested some survival advantage to heterozygotes. It has been proposed that the CF gene conferred protection to infants during epidemics of cholera, a cyclic adenosine monophosphate (cAMP)-dependent diarrheal illness, in the past.[9]

The CF gene has now been localized to the long arm of chromosome 7[10, 11] cloned and sequenced.[12] The most common mutation (F508), accounting for approximately 70% of all CF genes, has been identified as a 3 base pair deletion, responsible for the absence of a phenylalanine at position 508 in the translated protein.[12] A number of other, less common mutations in the CF gene have now been described, but not all mutations have yet been identified. As a result, mutation analysis cannot yet be used for purposes of population screening for CF, and this has been discouraged.[13, 14] On the other hand, probes of DNA polymorphism are available, and testing for carriers, using blood samples, and prenatal diagnosis, using either amniotic cell DNA or chorionic villus sampling, are virtually 100% informative. Provided that a DNA sample is available from the affected individual in the family, it is mandatory to offer prenatal screening and carrier screening to couples with a family history of CF. The associated professional genetic counseling is an integral part of the education and management of this disorder.

PATHOGENESIS

The past decade has seen a rapid advance in our appreciation of the basic genetic, biochemical, and physiologic defect in CF. Even as new information emerges, attempts are underway to develop newer diagnostic and treatment approaches to CF using the cellular and molecular understanding that is accumulating.

It is now clear that the CF gene product, cystic fibrosis transmembrane regulator (CFTR),[12] is a protein made up of 1,428 amino acids. It is expressed in epithelial cells and is often, although not exclusively, associated with the apical cell membrane of tissues affected pathologically in CF. Insertion of the correct (nonmutated) genetic material into CF cells in vitro has corrected the physiologic defect expressed.[15, 16] It is now well accepted that the protein plays a central role in the regulation of anion transport in epithelial cells, but whether that role is as a regulatory molecule, a transporter, or the chloride channel itself is still speculative.[17] Whether it may function in other capacities besides anion transport within cells is also unknown.

The basic physiologic defect in CF appears to be abnormal regulation of epithelial cell chloride transport.[18–20] The first demonstration of defective chloride permeability in the CF sweat duct in 1983[21] was supported by similar findings in CF respiratory epithelium,[22] in sweat secretory coil,[23] tracheal cells,[24] intestinal epithelium,[25] and pancreatic cells.[26, 27] Apical chloride channels in these CF epithelia fail to open in response to stimulation by cAMP-dependent pathways, thus interfering with the appropriate movement of chloride across cell membranes. In the sweat duct, failure to open apical chloride channels interferes with the normal reabsorption of chloride and accounts for the high chloride concentration in CF sweat, diagnostic of the disease. In the other organs affected in CF, apical chloride channels are an important component of the membrane transport pathways involved in the epithelial secretion of fluid (Fig. 66–2). The transport of anions, such as chloride, is required to move water across membranes and into secretions.[20] The failure to secrete sufficient amounts of fluid onto the luminal surfaces of the bronchi and intestine may predispose to the gel formation of respiratory

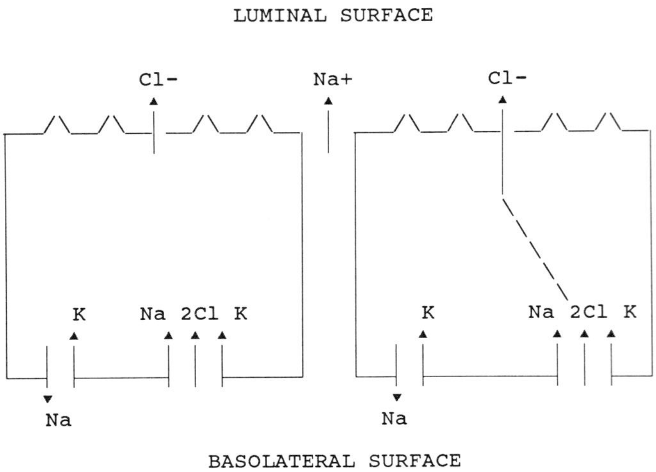

Figure 66–2. Model of a fluid-secreting and chloride-secreting epithelial cell. The basolateral Na^+, K^+–ATPase removes Na^+ from cells in exchange for K^+. Na^+ re-enters the cell down a favorable electrochemical gradient along with K^+ and Cl^-, thus allowing Cl^- to build up inside the cell. When the apical chloride channels open in response to cellular signals, Cl^- leaves the cell down its electrochemical gradient. Paracellular movement of Na^+ follows to maintain electroneutrality, and osmotically obliged water moves into the lumen. In CF, the chloride channel fails to open in response to the cellular signal cAMP.

and intestinal mucin, increasing viscosity, decreasing clearance, and promoting obstruction. The inspissation of secretions causing distention and obstruction of ducts in pancreatic, biliary, and salivary tissue may similarly be explained by the high concentrations of macromolecules, tendency to precipitation, and poor flow owing to impaired fluid secretion of these organs. The study of CF pancreatic secretions provided strong evidence in support of this hypothesis.[28]

PULMONARY DISEASE

This chapter does not focus in depth or on the pulmonary problems of CF. Pulmonary involvement, however, is the most common clinical manifestation of the disease and one of the hallmarks in its diagnosis. The lungs are unaffected in utero but become involved to varying degrees in approximately 95% of patients. Pulmonary presentations may range from severe ventilatory failure in infancy to recurrent pneumonias, bronchiectasis, chronic cough, and chronic or recurrent wheezing. Patients are characteristically infected and colonized by *Staphylococcus aureus* and *Pseudomonas aeruginosa* in the pulmonary tree for reasons not as yet completely clarified. The routine approach to pulmonary management includes regular chest physiotherapy and oral or inhaled antibiotics, parenteral antibiotics for unresponsive pulmonary exacerbations, and bronchodilator therapy when necessary. Controversy exists concerning the use of anti-inflammatory agents and nocturnal home oxygen therapy. Newer modalities such as aerosol $alpha_1$-antitrypsin treatment,[29] DNase I inhaled agents to alter ion transport and improve luminal hydration,[29a, 29b] amiloride,[30] nucleotides,[31] and ultimately inhaled genetic material to correct the CF defect are all still experimental approaches not yet in routine clinical use.

Pulmonary complications of CF include atelectasis, bronchiectasis, hemoptysis, and pneumothorax. Progressive chronic obstructive pulmonary disease eventually results in hypoxemia, carbon dioxide retention, and cor pulmonale. The respiratory failure secondary to end-stage CF lung disease has now been successfully managed by heart-lung or double lung transplantation in a growing number of centers with good results.[33, 34]

PANCREATIC DISEASE

In contrast to the pulmonary disease of CF, pancreatic pathology begins in utero. An arrest of acinar development has been documented before birth, and the earliest pancreatic lesion evident is the presence of dilated acini and ductules, filled with secretory material occluding the lumen.[35] Subsequent tissue damage, presumed to result from acinar release of lytic enzymes, leads to the progressive loss of functioning acini and their replacement by fibrous tissue and fat. The extent of tissue damage and destruction is highly variable, accounting for the differences in clinical presentation and severity of pancreatic manifestations. This spectrum of clinical disease is the result, in part, of the genetic heterogeneity seen in this disorder.[36]

Pancreatic Insufficiency

The majority of patients with CF (80 to 85%) have virtually complete loss of acinar tissue, resulting in an inability to secrete sufficient digestive enzymes for nutrient digestion and absorption. Pancreatic insufficiency is one of the hallmarks of CF and together with pulmonary disease and elevated sweat electrolyte concentrations completes the clinical triad of findings diagnostic of the disease. Genetically these patients are most often homozygous for the common gene mutation, delta F508, thought to cause the expression of this typical and clinically more severe phenotype.

As a result of maldigestion and malabsorption, these individuals may present clinically with large, frequent, greasy stools; poor weight gain or frank weight loss; manifestations of fat-soluble vitamin deficiencies; and, in infants less than 6 months of age, with hypoalbuminemia, edema, and anemia.[37] The presence of malabsorption cannot always be assessed from the history of abnormal stool pattern. Parents and patients may describe stools as normal. Further, an increased appetite and intake may adequately compensate for malabsorption, at least early in the disease process, allowing these patients to maintain weight and gain weight. A high index of suspicion, based on the history, physical examination, and other presenting features, should encourage a diagnostic investigation to identify the presence of pancreatic insufficiency (see Chapter 65).

The management of pancreatic insufficiency includes appropriate dietary counseling and supplementation with pancreatic enzyme preparations and fat-soluble vitamins. The use of special infant formulas, containing hydrolyzed proteins and medium-chain triglycerides (Pregestimil, Portagen, Alimentum), is usually unnecessary. These formulas are more expensive, less palatable, and do not obviate the need for pancreatic enzyme supplementation.[38] In fact, most infants will thrive on any infant formula or on breast milk,[39] provided that adequate energy intake and enzyme supplementation are prescribed appropriately. Low-fat diets are now considered inappropriate in the management of pancreatic insufficiency because they tend to limit the intake of total energy as well as essential fatty acids.

Successful management of pancreatic insufficiency can usually be achieved by administration of commercial preparations of pancreatic enzymes. Enteric-coated enzyme preparations are preferred. Their resistance to acid denaturation in the stomach makes them more effective, requiring fewer pills to achieve optimal digestion and absorption. The enzyme dose required is empiric and depends on a number of variables, including dietary fat intake and gastric acidity. Infants are usually prescribed 1 capsule of powdered enzyme (not enteric coated) per 120 ml infant formula. The enzyme should be mixed with a few teaspoons of strained food, rather than being added to the formula. Older children are prescribed 12,000 to 18,000 units of lipase per meal and 4,000 to 6,000 per snack of an enteric-coated preparation as an empiric starting dose. This dose should be increased to achieve optimal clinical and biochemical digestion and may reach 30,000 to 40,000 units per meal and 10,000 to 18,000 per snack.

Frequently, steatorrhea in CF patients is not completely corrected despite enzyme supplementation. A number of mechanisms have been proposed to explain this phenomenon. Excessive gastric acid secretion in CF[40] coupled with inadequate bicarbonate secretion[26] to buffer duodenal acidity may alter the intraluminal intestinal milieu in the CF patient. The resultant low intestinal pH may interfere with the complete dissolution of enteric-coated enzyme preparations and inhibit maximal enzyme activation. Low pH may also precipitate secreted bile salts,[41] rendering them unavailable for fat digestion. This latter problem may be particularly evident in some CF patients who are taurine deficient[42, 43] and therefore more likely to conjugate their secreted bile salts with glycine rather than taurine. Glycine-conjugated bile salts are less resistant to precipitation in the duodenal milieu than are the predominately taurine-conjugated bile salts of the individual without CF. In the presence of adequate growth and weight gain, it is not clear that aggressive attempts to correct stool pattern or biochemical malabsorption of stool fat is necessary. In some individuals, however, uncorrected malabsorption may contribute to clinical problems such as poor weight gain. Additional enzyme supplementation beyond the high doses already prescribed is ineffective. In this small number of patients, several "enhancers" of enzyme efficacy have been advocated and shown to be of clinical benefit. Pharmacologic attempts to counteract gastric acid inhibition of enzyme activity and enteric-coating dissolution have been effective, using the H_2 antagonists,[44] and the proton pump inhibitor, omeprazole.[45] The prostaglandin analog, misoprostil, has also demonstrated a positive effect on fat digestion when added to the regimen of pancreatic enzymes in patients with CF.[46, 47] In addition, oral taurine supplementation (30 mg per kg per day) of these refractory patients has demonstrated some benefit in isolated reports. Because the long-term effects of all of these agents in CF are unknown, they should be used judiciously and their beneficial effects on absorption documented. The search for other modalities to enhance digestion and absorption in these patients may include acid or lingual lipases, which may be more active in the lower pH and bile salt milieu of the CF intestine than currently used pancreatic lipases.

Pancreatic Sufficiency

In approximately 15 to 20% of CF patients, pancreatic damage and destruction have not been extensive enough to result in maldigestion and malabsorption. These CF patients are identifiable by their normal fat digestion on fecal balance studies or normal bentiromide or fluorescein dilaurate test results. This CF group is distinguished by a number of clinically important features. As a result of their normal digestion and absorption, they do not require pancreatic enzyme supplementation. They do not usually develop the gastrointestinal complications of meconium ileus, hepatobiliary disease, or distal intestinal obstruction syndrome. Also, their prognosis, both nutritionally and from the perspective of pulmonary function, is far better.[48] Interestingly, these patients are usually not homozygous for the F508 gene mutation,[36] suggesting a genetic basis, at least in part, for their clinically "less severe" disease.

These patients do, however, have CF. In one large reported series,[48] 75% of pancreatic-sufficient patients had some evidence of pulmonary disease; 39% had clubbing; 30% had nasal polyps; 4% had rectal prolapse. Sweat chloride levels were elevated, although mean values were lower than in pancreatic-insufficient patients, and pulmonary function deteriorated with age, although less markedly than in the group of patients with insufficiency. These patients tend to present clinically at a later age unless detected by either routine neonatal screening using trypsinogen or sweat testing because of a family history of CF.

Because of their more limited disease, this group of patients has been invaluable in allowing us to learn about pancreatic function in general and the primary pathophysiology of the pancreatic lesion in CF. They continue to provide the opportunity to unravel the correlations between phenotype and genotype in this genetically heterogeneous disorder. By the use of duodenal intubation, marker perfusion, and exogenous pancreatic stimulation, pancreatic function has been quantitated sensitively in this group of patients.[49] The variability in residual pancreatic exocrine secretory capacity among pancreatic sufficient patients is perhaps one of the most striking features to emerge from such studies. One half of the patients demonstrated a normal enzyme secretory capacity, implying limited destruction of acinar tissue. These subjects provided the opportunity to examine CF secretion for primary abnormalities unhindered by effects secondary to pancreatic damage. Secretions were highly concentrated in protein as a result of defective pancreatic fluid secretion, supporting the hypothesis that inadequate macromolecular solubilization, stasis, and poor clearance predisposed to obstruction in CF.[28] Further, it was evident that diminished fluid secretion was due to diminished secretion of both bicarbonate and chloride ions[27] and was consistent with the findings of abnormal anion transport in both sweat and respiratory epithelia in CF.

The remaining individuals with pancreatic sufficiency demonstrated variable loss of residual pancreatic secretory capacity, ranging from 2 to 100% of normal values. Only when secretory capacity dropped below 2% of normal colipase/lipase values did malabsorption occur.[49] This extreme variability raises a clinically relevant issue. It is clear that at least some individuals with CF and pancreatic sufficiency develop progressive loss of pancreatic function with time,[50] presumably from continual or recurrent ductal obstruction and exocrine tissue damage. Some of these patients eventually require enzyme supplementation. The likelihood of developing insufficiency may certainly relate to the degree of functional pancreatic reserve, making quantitative pancreatic testing a useful prognostic tool.

Pancreatitis

Pancreatitis occurs in 2 to 3% of patients with CF and may be the presenting feature of the disease.[51, 51a] It occurs only in patients with pancreatic sufficiency, presumably because of residual acinar function capable of causing such a pancreatic response. In one series, 8% of sufficient CF patients experienced clinical pancreatitis.[48] Because of the milder clinical course and absence of malabsorption in pancreatic sufficient patients, the diagnosis of CF may not be suspected. Pancreatitis, especially if recurrent, should be an indication for sweat testing, despite the absence of other findings of the disease.[51]

Diabetes Mellitus

CF patients with pancreatic exocrine insufficiency have pancreatic endocrine dysfunction of alpha, beta, and pancreatic polypeptide cells.[52] At least 30% have abnormal glucose tolerance when challenged with glucose loads,[53] and 1 to 13% develop adult-onset type diabetes mellitus,[54, 55] requiring insulin, dietary manipulation, or both. Although the exocrine deficiency may be responsible for endocrine dysfunction, it has generally been assumed that the extensive pancreatic fibrosis ultimately disrupts islet cell function as well. The development of diabetes mellitus in a CF patient may occasionally account for poor weight gain, and its recognition and appropriate management frequently correct the problem. The diagnosis of diabetes mellitus does not appear to affect survival in CF patients.[56]

INTESTINAL DISEASE

The intestinal manifestations are associated with and result from the tendency to partial or complete obstruction of the lumen of the gastrointestinal tract. Clinically relevant pathology may occur in utero or at any time during the patient's life and includes meconium ileus and peritonitis, intestinal atresias, distal intestinal obstruction, and rectal prolapse. A number of pathologic, radiologic, and functional abnormalities of little clinical significance have been described in CF and merit mention to put them into an appropriate clinical perspective.

Pathologic, Radiologic, and Functional Findings

Increased numbers of mucin-filled goblet cells, dilated crypts filled with mucin, and eosinophilic casts are pathologic features of the intestinal mucosa characteristic of CF and may be helpful, if present on pathologic specimens, in raising suspicion of the diagnosis.[57–59] Common radiologic findings in CF patients such as thickened duodenal folds and nodular filling defects[60, 61] have little clinical significance and should not be interpreted as signs of inflammatory or infiltrative disease without further confirmation. Intramural intestinal gas on abdominal radiograph, pneumatosis intestinalis, may be present in CF patients with advanced pulmonary disease.[62] It is of no medical threat to the patient and requires no intervention. Intestinal villous structure in CF is intact, D-xylose absorption is normal,[63] and intestinal lactase activity is normal or increased. Lactose intolerance, if it occurs, reflects the ethnic and age-related prevalence in the normal population and is unrelated to CF.[64] Selective intestinal absorptive defects in amino acids and bile acids have been reported but remain unconfirmed.

Meconium Ileus

Meconium ileus is the first clinical manifestation of CF and occurs in approximately 10 to 15% of patients. It may be associated with polyhydramnios in utero and presents at birth or within the first 48 hours after birth as a bowel obstruction. Meconium causes obstruction in the terminal ileum, and these infants fail to pass meconium, developing progressive abdominal distention and bilious vomiting. The radiographic findings are typical, demonstrating distended small bowel loops on abdominal radiograph, associated with bubbles of gas and stool trapped within the bowel and described as a ground-glass appearance (Fig. 66–3). A barium enema reveals an unused and therefore collapsed "microcolon" (Fig. 66–4).

Meconium ileus is frequently complicated by intestinal perforation in utero, volvulus, and intestinal atresias. Perforation, causing a meconium peritonitis, may be associated with ascites, adhesions, and intra-abdominal calcifications. Meconium ileus is virtually pathognomonic of CF, although isolated reports of its occurrence in the absence of CF exist.[65–67] The presence of meconium peritonitis or intestinal atresias should be indications for sweat testing to diagnose CF because 30% of patients with peritonitis and 20% with atresias have been found to have CF.[68] A distinction has been made in the past between meconium plug and meconium ileus in CF. It is now apparent that meconium plugs in the colon, whether passed spontaneously or causing obstruction, may indeed be the first manifestation of CF.[69] Although not all patients with meconium plug have CF, this condition probably represents one end of a spectrum of CF meconium disease.[70]

The cause of meconium disease in CF has been debated. Pancreatic insufficiency probably plays a major role in its pathogenesis, as it is seen almost exclusively in CF patients with insufficiency and occasionally in patients with pancreatic disease but without CF. CF patients have been reported with meconium disease and pancreatic sufficiency, but on quantitative testing, these patients had severely impaired pancreatic enzyme secretion, consistent with a role for pancreatic dysfunction in the pathogenesis.[71] It is presumed that the impairment of pancreatic proteolytic digestion of intestinal luminal protein, particularly albumin and mucin glycoprotein, increases the viscosity of meconium and its tendency to obstruct. With the demonstration of defective chloride transport in CF epithelia, including the intestinal epithelium,[25, 72, 73] an important role has also been proposed for the chloride transport defect and inadequate intestinal fluid secretion, causing poor luminal solvation of proteins and mucin. Patients with meconium ileus are homozygous for the common F508 mutation associated with the clinically more severe phenotype of CF.[12]

For uncomplicated meconium ileus, intestinal obstruction may be relieved by the administration of water-soluble hypertonic contrast enemas (Gastrografin or Hypaque) under fluoroscopic control. If unsuccessful or in the presence of peritonitis, volvulus, or suspected atresia, operative intervention is mandatory. Enterotomy, removal of the plug, and intestinal irrigation are frequently sufficient. A limited ileal resection may be necessary in the presence of atresia, volvulus, perforation, or difficulty in relieving obstruction. The prognosis for these patients in the first year of life is over 90% survival and beyond 1 year, no different from that of the overall CF population.[73a]

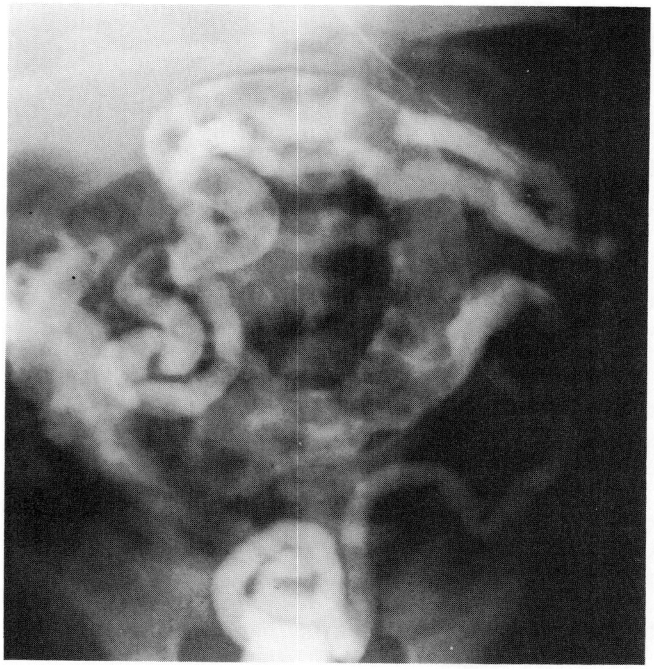

Figure 66–4. Meglumine diatrizoate (Gastrografin) enema of the same infant with meconium ileus. The unused colon (microcolon) is of thin caliber, and multiple filling defects can be seen in the ileum.

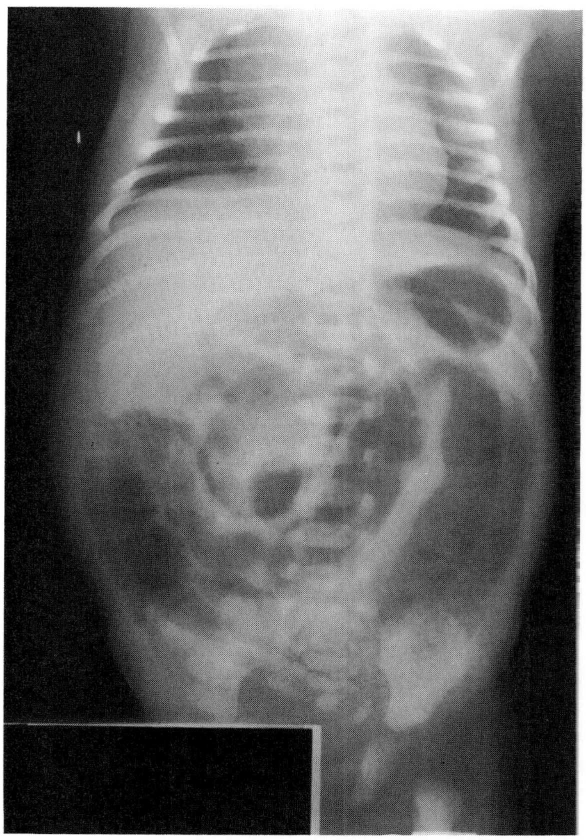

Figure 66–3. Abdominal radiograph of an infant with meconium ileus. Distended small bowel loops are filled with material that gives a bubbly, "ground-glass" appearance on the film.

Distal Intestinal Obstruction Syndrome

About 10 to 20% of patients beyond the neonatal period develop a spectrum of symptoms attributable to partial or complete intestinal obstruction by inspissated secretions. In the adult CF population, this figure may be even higher. The pathophysiology of distal intestinal obstruction syndrome (DIOS) may have some similarities to that described for meconium disease of the newborn. Pancreatic insufficiency accounts for decreased proteolytic degradation of macromolecules. Defective epithelial chloride and fluid secretion contribute to poor clearance of concentrated, viscid luminal secretions. Disordered intestinal motility has also been suggested as a factor in the pathogenesis of this disorder.[74]

Although the clinical spectrum is wide, DIOS is most often a chronic condition, presenting with recurrent crampy abdominal pain, and may cause decreased appetite and even weight loss. Although patients may report daily passage of stool, large amounts of stool may be palpable on abdominal examination, especially in the right lower quadrant, and are evident on abdominal radiograph. On occasion, acute or subacute episodes of intestinal obstruction may present with vomiting, abdominal distention, and tenderness. Particularly when associated with fever and elevated white blood cell count, these episodes need to be differentiated from the far less common conditions requiring surgical intervention, such as appendicitis, abscess, and neoplasm. Intussusception has been reported to occur in 1% of CF patients with DIOS.

Surgical intervention for DIOS is rarely necessary. In the presence of acute intestinal obstruction, intravenous hydration and nasogastric suction are indicated. Relief of the obstruction is first attempted with the administration of N-acetylcysteine (Mucomist), a mucolytic agent sufficiently irritating to the intestinal mucosa to be effective in dislodging the obstructing fecal mass. Mucomist in a 10% solution may be administered by mouth, nasogastric tube, or enema. Refractory cases may require the administration of hypertonic enemas (Gastrografin, Hypaque) under fluoroscopic control to reduce the obstruction. In the absence of complete intestinal obstruction, balanced isotonic electrolyte lavage solutions (Colyte, Golytely) have been used either orally or by nasogastric tube with excellent results.[75] Medical management in the chronic situation should include the administration of adequate pancreatic enzymes and may necessitate an increase in the dose previously administered; stool softeners such as mineral oil or psyllium hydrophilic mucilloid (Metamucil), and a high-fiber diet. The use of cisapride, a prokinetic agent, in treating chronic DIOS was disappointing.[76] Patients' subjective sense of well-being improved, but no objective evidence of clearance of obstruction, decrease in symptoms, or decreased need for intestinal lavage was apparent.

Rectal Prolapse

Rectal prolapse occurs in approximately 20% of CF patients, and in about half, it is the presenting feature. It usually begins in the first few years of life, when it is frequently recurrent, may improve on initiation of pancreatic enzyme therapy, and often spontaneously resolves by 5 years of age.[77, 78] In patients in whom prolapse persists, it can frequently be reduced and controlled by the child and family at home and only occasionally does it require surgical correction. Although the cause is often ascribed to the passage of large, bulky, frequent stools; malnutrition; or both; it occurred in 4% of CF patients with pancreatic sufficiency in one series,[48] suggesting that other factors, perhaps chronic cough, must play a role.

Constipation

Constipation occurs in CF patients far more frequently than the typical DIOS.[79] It may be interpreted as "an improvement in malabsorption" because it frequently occurs in older patients, and it is often tempting to manage it by reducing enzyme supplementation and thereby inducing a malabsorption with subsequent increased stooling. This approach to management should be avoided. Not only does this compromise energy and fat-soluble vitamin absorption but it may also precipitate an episode of DIOS. Constipation in CF should be managed as it is in the general population, with enemas, stool softeners, and a high-fiber diet.

OTHER GASTROINTESTINAL PROBLEMS

Other gastrointestinal problems occur in patients with CF. Some may be related to the disease and its management. Others are probably unrelated to CF but have been reported in CF patients.

Symptoms of regurgitation and heartburn were found in more than 20% of CF patients over the age of 5 years in one study, and confirmation of reflux by esophageal pH probe recordings was demonstrated.[80] CF patients are probably at increased risk for gastroesophageal reflux in view of their chronic pulmonary disease: Hyperinflation and chronic cough increase intra-abdominal pressure, and medications such as bronchodilators may decrease the lower esophageal sphincter pressure. Anemia, anorexia, and even weight loss may be caused, or exacerbated, by reflux esophagitis, so attention to this diagnostic possibility,[81] its identification, and appropriate management are warranted.

Patients with CF develop peptic ulcer disease.[82, 83] One report in a small number of patients suggested that CF patients secreted increased gastric acid.[40] In addition, the inability to secrete normal amounts of bicarbonate[26] may account for increased unbuffered acid, which may predispose to mucosal injury. This problem should be considered in the differential diagnosis of upper abdominal pain in these patients.

Crohn's disease has now been described in a number of patients with CF.[84] Its diagnosis may be difficult and delayed in the presence of CF owing to the underlying inflammatory, nutritional, biochemical, and radiographic features of CF, which may mimic or mask the disease. Pathologic confirmation of inflammatory bowel disease, however, in the presence of fistulas and abscesses confirms the diagnosis. Celiac disease has been described in several patients with CF,[85] including in family studies.[86]

HEPATOBILIARY DISEASE

Hepatobiliary disease in CF represents a spectrum of disorders of varying frequency and clinical significance. In general, the more frequent abnormalities have little or no effect on overall health and well-being, whereas the most significant clinical disorder, multilobular hepatobiliary cirrhosis,[87–90] has been estimated to occur in 2 to 5% of the CF population.

Liver

Symptoms of liver disease in CF are rare and can be subtle, and test results of hepatic function or liver enzymes are frequently normal until pathology is advanced. Therefore, the clinical findings of hepatomegaly and hepatosplenomegaly are of considerable diagnostic importance. Enlargement of the liver in CF must be differentiated from displacement of the liver owing to lung hyperinflation. If truly enlarged, the liver contour and consistency should be assessed. A firm, smooth, rounded liver contour may suggest the presence of hepatic congestion secondary to cor pulmonale in the appropriate clinical setting of advanced pulmonary disease. More frequently, it represents hepatic steatosis and suggests the presence of significant nutritional deficiency. Fatty liver is probably the most common finding on liver biopsy specimens in CF, occurring in some 15 to 40% of patients examined,[1, 88] and it is frequently encountered in infants and children with CF.[91] In contrast, the palpation of a hard, irregular, or nodular liver contour in a patient with CF, with or without splenomegaly, deserves further attention. It is often the presenting sign of significant liver pathology.

Focal Biliary Fibrosis

The characteristic pathologic findings in the liver of patients with CF consist of small bile duct obstruction by eosinophilic plugs, dilatation of ductules with bile duct proliferation, inflammation, and fibrous tissue formation in and around portal tracts. Generally, there is preservation of hepatocytes and parenchymal architecture.[92, 93] These findings may be present in up to 50% of autopsy cases, including infants dying early with meconium disease. The lesion is frequently patchy in nature and may be missed on percutaneous liver biopsy. This lesion represents the primary obstructive pathophysiology of CF in the liver. Patients with CF, including those with normal pancreatic enzyme secretion, secrete significantly less bile salt on pharmacologic stimulation than do controls.[94] This may suggest a primary biliary anion transport defect, either in bile salts themselves or in biliary chloride or bicarbonate. Improvement in bile flow, using choleretic agents such as ursodeoxycholic acid,[95, 95a] holds some promise.

Multilobular Biliary Cirrhosis

Most frequently detected because of hepatomegaly or hepatosplenomegaly, this entity is often asymptomatic, yet it may be associated with significant morbidity and mortality.[90, 96] Clinical assessment often reveals mildly elevated or normal transaminases; an elevated gamma glutamyltranspeptidase may be the first biochemical abnormality; and ultrasonography of the liver may demonstrate an echogenic organ, consistent with either fatty liver or cirrhosis. Functional abnormalities are infrequent owing to hepatocellular preservation, so hyperbilirubinemia, coagulopathy uncorrectable by vitamin K administration, ascites, and encephalopathy are uncommon.[90, 96] These patients, however, frequently progress to portal hypertension and esophageal varices. Clinically they present with variceal bleeding and hypersplenism. Liver biopsy may be misleading in this condition owing to sampling error.

The occurrence of liver disease as a result of another cause in patients with CF warrants consideration. Several patients with CF have been reported to have an abnormal Pi phenotype.[97] Chronic active hepatitis, a treatable lesion, as well as chronic infectious hepatitis should be considered.

The pathogenesis of cirrhosis in CF has been presumed to represent the progression of focal biliary fibrosis as it involves increasing areas of liver tissue. Although a familial tendency was initially reported in CF patients who developed liver disease,[98] and it has been noted to occur largely in patients with F508, no CF genotype has been specifically linked to the development of liver disease in CF.[98a] Whether other genetic predisposing factors may subsequently be identified to contribute to this phenotypic presentation remains to be seen. It has been proposed that multilobular cirrhosis may develop secondary to extrahepatic biliary obstruction.[100] CF patients with significant liver pathology have been identified with common bile duct stenosis secondary to pancreatic fibrosis and both intrahepatic[100a] and extrahepatic biliary tract abnormalities[100] similar to sclerosing cholangitis. This hypothesis awaits confirmation by long-term prospective studies and support by several centers.

No effective treatment is currently available to halt or reverse the pathologic processes of biliary fibrosis or cirrhosis. Experimental approaches, however, with taurine, ursodeoxycholic acid, or both, are being tried to minimize putative toxic effects and enhance bile flow. Results of short-term trials are promising.[95, 95a, 101, 101a] Management of biliary cirrhosis remains supportive. Hepatic failure is rarely the cause of morbidity or mortality. Rather, variceal hemorrhage secondary to portal hypertension is being encountered with increasing frequency, presumably as life expectancy increases. Owing to the effectiveness and relative ease of performing esophageal sclerotherapy, this modality has come into wide use for the management of esophageal varices after the first significant bleeding episode. The use of injection sclerotherapy in CF is no different from its use for other conditions associated with esophageal variceal bleeding. Prophylactic treatment, before any bleeding episode, is not generally encouraged. Portosystemic shunting is rarely entertained in view of the degree of pulmonary disease and the ultimate availability of liver transplantation should sclerotherapy prove inadequate. Hepatic transplantation has now successfully been accomplished in patients with CF.[102]

Gallbladder and Biliary Tree

Anatomic and functional abnormalities of the gallbladder and cystic duct are seen in as many as 30 to 45% of CF patients, unrelated to age.[103–106] "Microgallbladders," which are contracted or atrophic and filled with thick mucus; atrophic, occluded cystic ducts; and nonfunctioning gallbladders do not cause symptoms or clinical problems. Prolonged neonatal jaundice, lasting weeks and mimicking biliary atresia, has been associated with CF, is probably secondary to biliary plugging, and may often be associated with meconium ileus.[107] It usually resolves in the first 3 months of life and does not appear to be associated with an increased risk for more significant hepatobiliary pathology later in life. Mild cholestasis without jaundice, beyond infancy, appears to be quite common in CF, based on the prevalence of elevated fasting serum bile salt values.[108, 109] Because these values do not correlate with the type or severity of hepatobiliary pathology, occurring with steatosis as well as cirrhosis, nor with other tests assessing the liver, their significance is currently unknown.

Patients with CF have an increased incidence of biliary stones, with a prevalence of gallstones of 10% according to one study.[106] These are cholesterol stones and are thought to occur as a result of excessive intestinal bile salt losses,[110] diminishing the bile salt pool available for secretion.[111] Fecal losses of bile salts may be partially corrected by improving steatorrhea with pancreatic enzyme supplements.[110] Most biliary stones are detected by ultrasonography in asymptomatic individuals and require no treatment. Symptomatic cholelithiasis, however, requires intervention. The introduction of laparoscopic cholecystectomy may significantly diminish the risks of prolonged anesthesia and laparotomy in CF patients with advanced pulmonary disease.

Extrahepatic biliary tract obstruction was found in a large number of CF patients with hepatomegaly.[100] The lesion, most often a distal common bile duct stricture, was detected by hepatobiliary scintigraphy and percutaneous cholangiography. In those patients presenting with recurrent right abdominal pain, associated with meals and fatty foods, correction of the strictures, confirmed at laparotomy, led to complete symptomatic relief. Of note, not all patients presented with jaundice, nor did they have dilated bile ducts on ultrasonography. The authors suggested that this lesion might be involved in the pathogenesis of multilobular cirrhosis. Until further study, it seems prudent to investigate CF patients with hepatomegaly and right upper quadrant pain for biliary strictures with a scintiscan, follow up suggestive abnormalities by percutaneous cholangiography, and provide surgical correction for symptomatic strictures. The prevalence of common bile duct strictures in the general CF population is not known.

NUTRITION

Patients with CF are at increased risk for developing protein-energy malnutrition and specific micronutrient deficiencies. The deleterious effects of inadequate nutrition on growth and development, school performance, daily activities, body image, emotional well-being, and immune function have been well documented in other settings. Because CF children are now living into adulthood, these factors take on increased significance. The increased life expectancy in the better nourished Toronto CF clinic[2] and the association of better nutritional status with improved pulmonary function and prognosis[48] are additional justification for attention to the nutritional status of these patients. Data from aggressive nutritional intervention programs have suggested improved patient well-being,[112, 113] slower pulmonary function deterioration,[112, 113] and improved exercise capacity and respiratory muscle strength.[114] With the advent of lung transplantation, the need to maintain or improve nutrition to optimize the perioperative and postoperative course has increased.

The pathogenesis of nutritional deficiencies in CF can be divided into three major contributing factors: increased losses secondary to malabsorption, increased energy expenditure, and inadequate energy intake (Fig. 66–5).

Increased Losses

Malabsorption affects most patients with CF, and is caused by a variety of problems. The primary factor is inadequate pancreatic secretion of lipolytic, proteolytic,

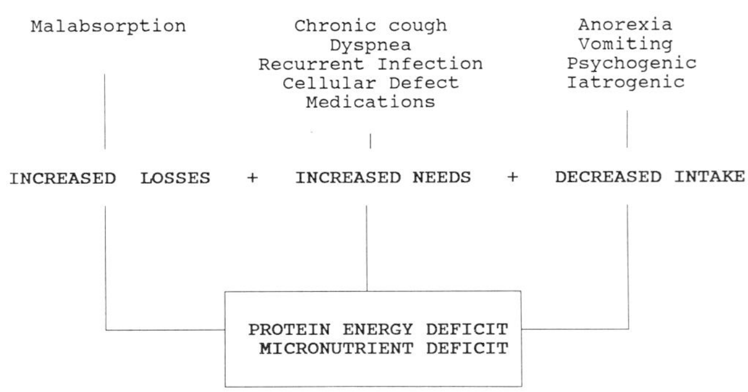

Figure 66–5. The pathogenesis of malnutrition in CF.

and amylolytic enzymes required for the digestion of dietary fats, proteins, and carbohydrates. The lower intraluminal intestinal pH in CF may interfere with uncoating and activation of supplemental enzymes and tends to precipitate bile salts, making them unavailable for lipolysis and fat digestion. Excessive fecal bile salt losses from acid precipitation, binding to undigested nutrients, and impaired reabsorption further compromise fat digestion by shrinking the bile salt pool available for secretion and diminishing available taurine for bile salt conjugation. An increased and less permeable unstirred water layer, owing to intestinal mucin and undigested albumin, also interferes with absorption of macronutrients and micronutrients.

Because of the impairment in digestion and absorption of fat, protein, and carbohydrate, excessive losses of total energy intake, essential fatty acids, fat-soluble vitamins, and minerals may occur. These losses may be greatly diminished by the introduction of pancreatic enzyme supplements. Losses are often not completely corrected, however, and management depends on the ability to compensate for smaller degrees of loss by increasing intakes of these nutrients.

Increased Energy Expenditure

Studies have now clearly documented that, in addition to energy losses through malabsorption, patients with CF have increased energy requirements.[115–117] A mild increase in resting energy expenditure has been suggested by several investigators to be related to the underlying genetic and metabolic defect in CF.[116, 117] If so, this probably accounts only for a small proportion of the increase in energy requirements of CF patients, as young CF patients or those with mild pulmonary involvement are able to maintain normal weight gain, growth, and nutrition on 100 to 120% of the recommended dietary allowance for age.[118] Of far more clinical significance, CF patients with dyspnea, chronic cough, or both, have been shown to have resting energy expenditures of 85 to 153% of predicted values for age, sex, and weight, during periods when they were free of pulmonary exacerbations.[115] In this group, patients with more severe pulmonary function and nutritional status had greater energy expenditures. During pulmonary exacerbations, energy expenditures increased even further, and studies have now demonstrated that the use of long-term beta-adrenergic agonist bronchodilator therapy itself is associated with increased energy expenditure.[119]

Decreased Intake

Although the classic presentation of an infant or young child with CF includes the presence of a voracious appetite, this characteristic is unfortunately not universal, nor does it persist. Despite long-term efforts to encourage the intake of a high-energy diet, one study of medically stable CF adolescents demonstrated energy intakes equivalent to, and not in excess of, peers without CF.[120] Unfortunately, a number of factors conspire to compromise the intake of CF patients. Acute respiratory exacerbations are probably the most common cause of decreased intake. Anorexia, perhaps associated with elevated circulating levels of tumor necrosis factor,[121] and vomiting with coughing spells interfere with intake at the very time that energy requirements are increased, and together these factors account for the characteristic weight loss associated with pulmonary exacerbations. Once treatment is initiated, weight gain is usually recovered. As disease progresses and exacerbations are more frequent, however, a cycle of catabolism and energy deficit may interfere with the recovery and maintenance of normal nutritional status. As nutrition deteriorates, further anorexia, fatigue, and decreased taste, perhaps associated with zinc deficiency, interfere with intake.

In the past, energy intakes of CF patients were often restricted because of recommendations for low-fat diets, to limit stool bulk and frequency; unpalatable hydrolyzed formulas; and the well-intentioned notions of parents and health care professionals about the avoidance of "junk" foods, consumed by adolescent peers. Unfortunately, many of these unnecessary restrictions only limited energy intakes. Finally, some adolescents, particularly females, conscious of body image and products of our society's "thin is beautiful" culture, may use CF as a means of controlling weight gain and further limit dietary intake. In our experience, however, this is infrequent.

Finally, it should be remembered that CF patients have a variety of organic reasons for decreased intake and vomiting, related to the gastrointestinal manifestations of this disorder. Esophagitis secondary to gastroesophageal reflux, DIOS, constipation, peptic ulcer, hepatobiliary complications, pancreatitis, and partial obstructions secondary to previous intestinal surgery may all be associated with decreased appetite and intake.

Consequence of Malnutrition

The result of increased losses, increased requirements, and decreased intake is a significant energy deficit, which accounts for poor weight gain and growth, pubertal delay, significant loss of subcutaneous adipose tissue, and muscle wasting. It may frequently be associated with deficiencies of vitamins, minerals, essential fatty acids, taurine, and perhaps other, as yet unrecognized nutrients.

Protein-Energy Deficit

The risk of protein energy deficiency in CF is real and clinically manifested in a variety of ways. Fatty liver and hypoproteinemia, edema, and anemia in CF infants are presentations of nutritional deficiency. Poor weight gain, height/weight discrepancies, and eventually, poor growth causing nutritional stunting may all occur in CF secondary to prolonged uncorrected protein energy deficits. With attention to the treatment of steatorrhea and dietary advice regarding high-energy intakes, most infants and children, once diagnosed with CF, attain good weight gain, growth, and development.[122] Unfortunately, the risk of deficiency appears to increase again in the preadolescent and early adolescent years. Girls seem to be affected more than boys, but both demonstrate decreased weight gain, growth, and delay in pubertal development, which may be severe.[123] These preadolescents are frequently beginning to experience worsening pulmonary disease in association with falling away from weight and eventually height curves. They are frequently thin, with pronounced loss of subcutaneous fat and muscle, and as the process advances, they may fall well below two standard deviations for weight and height for age. None of these findings is a primary phenotypic manifestation of CF, nor are they secondary to endocrine deficiencies. Rather, they may be entirely reversed, or prevented, if treated early and aggressively with nutritional rehabilitation.

Vitamin Deficiencies

Fat-soluble vitamin deficiencies are often present biochemically in patients with CF if inadequate supplementation is provided. Clinical signs of vitamin A deficiency are rare but may occur.[124, 125] In addition, associated zinc and protein energy deficiency may interfere with the transport of vitamin A from liver stores and manifest as a low serum vitamin A level.[126] The effects of longstanding vitamin E deficiency, including ataxia, loss of deep tendon reflexes and position and vibration senses, and peripheral nerve conduction defects have been reported.[127–129] Osteopenia, owing to both vitamin D deficiency and protein energy deficiency, has been reported.[130–132] Vitamin K deficiency may present with overt bleeding,[133, 134] particularly in patients on prolonged antibiotics, and is correctable with supplemental vitamin K.

Mineral Deficiencies

It has been observed that CF patients with advanced pulmonary disease are less likely to develop polycythemia than patients with similarly severe pulmonary failure but without CF. It has therefore been suggested that these CF patients have anemia, relative to their hypoxemia, despite normal hemoglobin levels.[135] Iron-deficiency anemia and low serum ferritin levels are seen in CF. Low serum zinc levels in CF may be seen in patients with protein energy malnutrition and vitamin A deficiency.[136] Because zinc deficiency, presumably secondary to poor intakes, can be associated with altered taste and anorexia, its contribution to poor intake should be evaluated, and, if necessary, zinc supplementation should be initiated. Hypomagnesemia may occur in CF as a result of malabsorption and increased stool losses and increased urine losses associated with the administration of aminoglycosides.[137] In addition, nutritional rehabilitation may be associated with the development of hypokalemia, hypomagnesemia, and hypophosphatemia. Although uncommon, clinical presentations consistent with these deficiencies should be recognized.

Essential Fatty Acid Deficiency

Although clinical essential fatty acid (EFA) deficiency, with skin rash, growth retardation, poor immunity, poor wound healing, and thrombocytopenia, may occasionally occur in CF,[138] abnormalities in EFA composition of plasma and tissues in CF have frequently been recognized.[139, 140] Decreased linoleic acid and increased palmitoleic, oleic, and eicosatrienoic acids in CF are particularly seen in patients with malabsorption, protein energy malnutrition, or both. Linoleic acid supplementation alone may fail to improve EFA status, particularly if malnutrition and malabsorption are not improved. Supplemental calories and an increase in body weight, however, improved EFA deficiency,[141] supporting the view that patients unable to meet energy requirements because of increased needs and decreased intake may use EFA as energy sources, thus contributing to deficiency.

Nutritional Management

An aggressive approach to nutritional management in CF is crucial. Because dietary preferences and prejudices are established early and may be difficult to change, parents and patients must be taught and encouraged to follow a high-energy diet, liberal in fat, with larger portions than other children at meals, and high-energy snacks between meals and at bedtime. Although energy requirements in CF vary greatly, they have empirically been estimated as 120 to 150% of the recommended nutrient intake for age. Pancreatic enzyme and fat-soluble vitamin supplementation should be maximized to achieve normal growth, weight gain, and serum vitamin and mineral levels (vitamin A, E, 25-hydroxyvitamin D, PT/PTT, zinc). Patients are usually begun on a multivitamin preparation at twice the recommended daily dose (providing vitamin A, 8000 IU; vitamin D, 800 IU) and on vitamin E, 100 to 200 IU. Vitamin K, zinc, and increased vitamin A or E can be provided as necessary.

When growth and weight gain are not optimal, assessments of dietary intake at home, compliance with pancreatic supplemental enzymes, and 72-hour fecal fat excretion as a percent of dietary fat intake are mandatory. Malabsorption should be minimized and energy intake maximized. Oral liquid energy supplements, milkshakes, and supplemental polysaccharide or medium-chain triglycerides can be encouraged when diet does not meet energy requirements. Gastrointestinal complications interfering with intake or absorption should be considered, and psychosocial issues interfering with optimal compliance and management should be dealt with as directly as possible.

Unfortunately, as the disease progresses, a proportion of patients become increasingly more malnourished as their intakes fail to meet requirements. Under these circumstances, long-term approaches to nutritional therapy in CF have been successfully used at home, including parenteral nutrition[142] and night-time enteral feedings of high-energy liquid supplements by nasogastric,[80] gas-

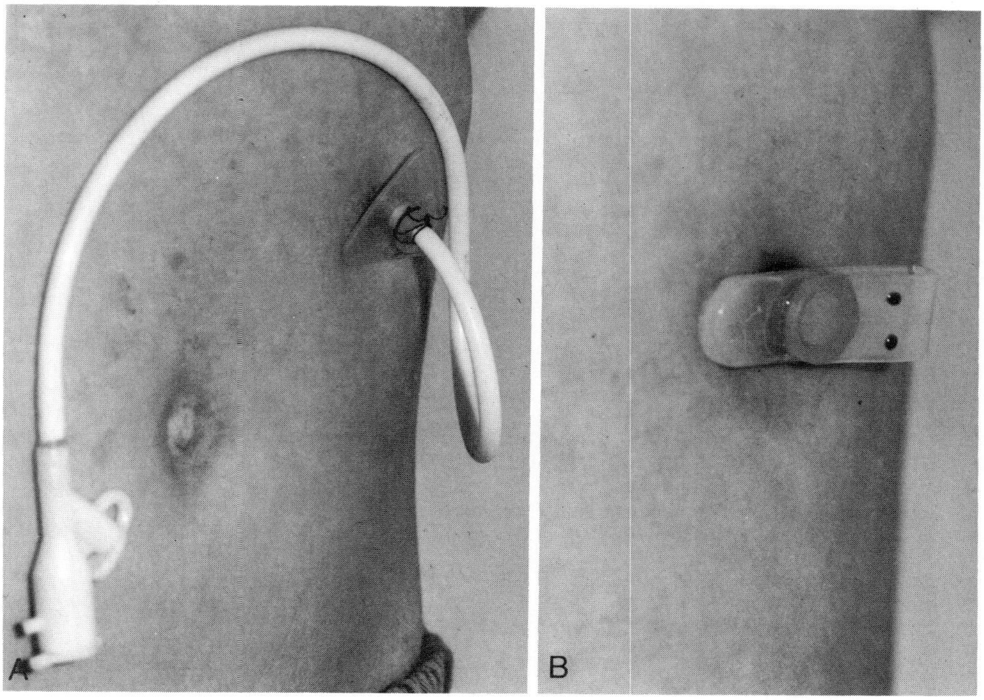

Figure 66–6. *A*, A percutaneous gastrostomy feeding tube in a patient with CF. *B*, The same patient has just had the gastrostomy tube removed, and a gastrostomy button has been inserted in its place.

trostomy,[112] and jejunostomy[113] tubes. In general, the higher financial cost and risk of complications of parenteral nutrition have increasingly favored the use of enteral feedings in most centers. Elemental preparations ensure maximum absorption without the need for pancreatic enzyme supplementation overnight and are usually well tolerated. It is frequently possible to administer 1,200 to 2,400 calories overnight to supplement daytime oral consumption. Nasogastric feeding requires the individual's sustained commitment to insert and remove the tube daily and may be hampered by the presence of nasal polyps, congestion, and frequent coughing up of the tube. Percutaneous gastrostomy tubes may be inserted without general anesthetic or laparotomy and provide easy access for long-term nightly feedings (Fig. 66–6*A*). Patients are frequently happier when gastrostomy tubes are subsequently replaced by the less cumbersome and more esthetically pleasing gastrostomy button (Fig. 66–6*B*). Despite the frequency of occult gastroesophageal reflux in CF, nasogastric and gastrostomy feedings are usually well tolerated. The head of the bed should be elevated during feeds, feeds should be completed at least 1 to 2 hours before physiotherapy or nasogastric tube removal, and prokinetic agents such as domperidone or cisapride may be used to enhance gastric emptying. Some centers have used jejunostomy tubes to avoid difficulties with gastroesophageal reflux.

All patients receiving supplemental feedings demonstrate weight gain and growth, provided that both compliance and management are optimal. In addition to weight gain, growth, and pubertal development, nutritional rehabilitation improves patient well-being and general level of activity, improves exercise capacity and respiratory muscle strength, and may slow the deterioration of pulmonary function. On theoretical grounds, increased respiratory muscle strength and immunity as well as an improved micronutrient environment should have beneficial long-term effects on pulmonary status and ultimately on prognosis. Although retrospective cross-sectional studies have documented a correlation between good nutrition and improved lung function and survival, the long-term prospective effect of nutritional rehabilitation on pulmonary status and prognosis is still being evaluated.

REFERENCES

1. Anderson D: Cystic fibrosis of the pancreas and its relation to celiac disease. Am Dis Child 1938; 56:344–399.
2. Corey M, McLaughlin FJ, Williams M, et al: A comparison of survival, growth, and pulmonary function in patients with cystic fibrosis in Boston and Toronto. J Clin Epidemiol 1988; 41:583–591.
3. DiSant'Agnese P, Darling R, Perera G, et al: Abnormal electrolyte composition of sweat in cystic fibrosis of the pancreas. Pediatrics 1953; 12:549–563.
4. Shwachman H, Mahmoodrai A: Pilocarpine iontophoresis sweat testing: Results of seven years' experience. Med Probl Pediatr 1967; 10:158–182.
5. MacLean W, Tripp R: Cystic fibrosis with edema and falsely negative sweat test. J Pediatr 1973; 83:85–90.
6. Crossley JR, Smith PA, Edgar BW, et al: Neonatal screening for cystic fibrosis, using immunoreactive trypsin assay in dried blood spots. Clin Chim Acta 1981; 113:111–121.
7. Wilcken B: An evaluation of screening for cystic fibrosis in genetics and epithelial cell dysfunction. *In* Riordan JR, Buchwald M, eds: Cystic Fibrosis. New York, Alan R. Liss, 1987, p 201.
8. Waters D, Dorney S, Gruca M, et al: Pancreatic function in infants identified as having cystic fibrosis in a neonatal screening programme. N Engl J Med 1990; 322(5):303.
9. Baxter PS, Goldhill J, Hardcastle J, et al: Accounting for cystic fibrosis. Nature 1988; 335:211.
10. Mainwright BJ, Scambler PJ, Schmidtke J, et al: Localization of

cystic fibrosis locus to human chromosome 7 cen-q22. Nature 1985; 318:384–385.

11. Knowlton RG, Cohen-Haguenauer O, Nguyen VC, et al: A polymorphic DNA marker linked to cystic fibrosis is located in chromosome 7. Nature 1985; 318:380–381.
12. Kerem B, Rommens JM, Buchanan JA, et al: Identification of the cystic fibrosis gene: Genetic analysis. Science 1989; 245:1073–1079.
13. Caskey CT, Kaback MM, Beaudet AL: The American Society of Human Genetics statement on cystic fibrosis screening. Am J Hum Genet 1990; 46:393.
14. Statement from the National Institutes of Health Workshop on population screening for the cystic fibrosis gene. N Engl J Med 1990; 323:70–71.
15. Rich DP, Anderson MP, Gregory RJ, et al: Expression of cystic fibrosis transmembrane conductance regulator corrects defective chloride channel regulation in cystic fibrosis airway epithelial cells. Nature 1990; 347:358–363.
16. Drumm ML, Pope HA, Cliff WH, et al: Correction of the cystic fibrosis defect in vitro by retro-virus-mediated gene transfer. Cell 1990; 62:1227–1233.
17. Quinton PM: Righting the wrong protein. Nature 1990; 347:226.
18. Quinton P: Cystic fibrosis: A disease in electrolyte transport. FASEB J 1990; 4:2709–2717.
19. Welsh M: Abnormal regulation of ion channels in cystic fibrosis epithelia. FASEB J 1990; 4:2718–2725.
20. Frizzell RA: Cystic fibrosis: A disease of ion channels? Trends Neurosci 1987; 10:190–193.
21. Quinton PM: Chloride impermeability in cystic fibrosis. Nature 1983; 301:421–422.
22. Knowles MR, Gatzy JAT, Boucher RC: Relative ion permeability of normal and cystic fibrosis epithelium. J Clin Invest 1983; 71:1410–1417.
23. Sato K, Sato F: Defective beta adrenergic response of cystic fibrosis sweat glands in vivo and in vitro. J Clin Invest 1984; 73:1763–1771.
24. Widdicombe JH, Welsh MH, Finkbeiner WE: Cystic fibrosis decreases the apical membrane chloride permeability of monolayers cultured from cells of tracheal epithelium. Proc Natl Acad Sci 1985; 82:6167–6171.
25. Berschneider HM, Knowles MR, Azizkhan RG, et al: Altered intestinal chloride transport in cystic fibrosis. FASEB J 1988; 2:2625–2629.
26. Kopelman H, Corey M, Gaskin K, et al: Impaired chloride secretion, as well as bicarbonate secretion, underlies the fluid secretory defect in the cystic fibrosis pancreas. Gastroenterology 1988; 95:349–355.
27. Schoumacher RA, Ram J, Iannuzzi MC, et al: A cystic fibrosis pancreatic adenocarcinoma cell line. Proc Natl Acad Sci 1990; 87:4012–4016.
28. Kopelman H, Durie P, Gaskin K, et al: Pancreatic fluid secretion and protein hyperconcentration in cystic fibrosis. N Engl J Med 1985; 312:329–334.
29. McElvaney NG, Hubbard RC, Birrer P, et al: Aerosal α-1-antitrypsin treatment for cystic fibrosis. Lancet 1991; 337:392–394.
29a. Shak S, Capon DJ, Hellmiss R, et al: Recombinant human DNase I reduces the viscosity of cystic fibrosis sputum. Proc Natl Acad Sci USA 1990; 87:9188–9192.
29b. Hubbard RC, McElvaney NG, Birrer P, et al: Preliminary study of aerosolized recombinant human deoxyribonuclease I in the treatment of cystic fibrosis. N Engl J Med 1991; 326:812–815.
30. Knowles MR, Church NL, Waltner WE, et al: A pilot study of aerosolized amiloride for the treatment of lung disease in cystic fibrosis. N Engl J Med 1990; 322:1189–1194.
31. App EM, King M, Helfesrieder R, et al: Acute and longterm amiloride inhalation in cystic fibrosis lung disease. A rational approach to cystic fibrosis therapy. Am Rev Respir Dis 1990; 141:605–612.
32. Knowles MR, Clarke LL, Boucher RC: Activation by extracellular nucleotides of chloride secretion in the airway epithelia of patients with cystic fibrosis. N Engl J Med 1991; 325:533–538.
33. Leval MR, Smyth RS, Whitehead B, et al: Heart and lung transplantation for terminal cystic fibrosis. J Thoracic Cardiovasc Surg 1991; 101:633–642.
34. Frist WH: North American results: Cystic fibrosis treated with heartlung transplant. Transplant Proc 1991; 23:1205–1206.
35. Imrie J, Fagan D, Sturgess J: Quantitative evaluation of the development of the exocrine pancreas in CF and control infants. Am J Pathol 1979; 95:697–707.
36. Kerem B, Buchanan JA, Durie P, et al: DNA marker haplotype association with pancreatic sufficiency in cystic fibrosis. Am J Hum Genet 1989; 44:827–834.
37. Dolan T, Rowe D, Gibson L: Edema and hypoproteinemia in infants with cystic fibrosis. Clin Pediatr 1970; 9:295–297.
38. Durie PR, Newth CJ, Forstner GG, et al: Malabsorption of medium-chain triglycerides in infants with cystic fibrosis: correction with pancreatic enzyme supplements. J Pediatr 1980; 96:862–864.
39. Holliday KE, Allen JR, Waters DL, et al: Growth of human milk-fed and formula-fed infants with cystic fibrosis. J Pediatr 1991; 118(1):77–79.
40. Cox KL, Isenberg JN, Ament ME: Gastric acid hypersecretion in cystic fibrosis. J Ped Gastroenterol Nutr 1982; 16:554–557.
41. Zentler-Munro PL, Fine DR, Batten JC, et al: Effect of cimetidine on enzyme inactivation, bile acid precipitation and lipid solubilisation in pancreatic steatorrhea due to cystic fibrosis. Gut 1985; 26:892–901.
42. Darling PB, Lepage G, Leroy C, et al: Effect of taurine supplements on fat absorption in cystic fibrosis. Pediatr Res 1985; 19(6):578–582.
43. Belli DC, Levy L, Darling P, et al: Taurine improves the absorption of a fat meal in patients with cystic fibrosis. Pediatrics 1987; 80:517–523.
44. Durie PR, Bell L, Linton W, et al: Effect of cimetidine and sodium bicarbonate on pancreatic replacement therapy in cystic fibrosis. Gut 1980; 21:778–786.
45. Heijerman HG: Omeprazole enhances the efficacy of pancreatin in cystic fibrosis. Ann Intern Med 1991; 114(3):200–201.
46. Robinson P, Sly PD: Placebo-controlled trial of misoprostol in cystic fibrosis. J Pediatr Gastro Nutr 1990; 11:37–40.
47. Cleghorn GJ, Shepherd RW, Holt TL: The use of a synthetic prostaglandin E1 analogue as an adjunct to pancreatic enzyme replacement in cystic fibrosis. Scand J Gastroenterol 1988; 143(Suppl):142–147.
48. Gaskin K, Gurwitz D, Durie PR, et al: Improved respiratory prognosis in patients with cystic fibrosis with normal fat absorption. J Pediatr 1982; 100:857–862.
49. Gaskin KJ, Durie PR, Lee L, et al: Colipase and lipase secretion in childhood onset pancreatic insufficiency: Delineation of patients with steatorrhea secondary to relative colipase deficiency. Gastroenterology 1984; 86:1–7.
50. Durie P, Kopelman H, Corey M, et al: Pathophysiology of the exocrine pancreas in cystic fibrosis. *In* Matella G, Quinton PM, eds: Cellular and Molecular Basis of Cystic Fibrosis. San Francisco, San Francisco Press, 1988, pp 186–190.
51. Schwachman H, Lebenthal E, Khaw K: Recurrent acute pancreatitis in patients with cystic fibrosis with normal pancreatic enzymes. Pediatrics 1975; 55:86–94.
51a. Atlas AB, Orenstein DM: Pancreatitis in young children with cystic fibrosis. J Pediatr 1992; 120:756–759.
52. Moran A, Diem P, Klein DJ, et al: Pancreatic endocrine function in cystic fibrosis. J Pediatr 1991; 118:715–723.
53. Handwerger S, Roth J, Gordon P, et al: Glucose intolerance in cystic fibrosis. N Engl J Med 1969; 281:451–461.
54. DiSant'Agnese P, Davis PB: Cystic fibrosis in adults: Seventy-five cases and a review of 232 cases in the literature. Am J Med 1979; 66:121–132.
55. Finkelstein SM, Wielinski CL, Elliott GR, et al: Diabetes mellitus associated with cystic fibrosis. J Pediatr 1988; 112:373–377.
56. Reisman J, Corey M, Canny G, et al: Diabetes mellitus in patients with cystic fibrosis: Effect on survival. Pediatrics 1990; 86:374–377.
57. Shwachman H, Holsclaw D: Examination of the appendix at laparotomy as a diagnostic clue in cystic fibrosis. N Engl J Med 1972; 286:1300–1301.
58. Freye H, Kurtz S, Spock A, et al: Light and electron microscopic examination of the small bowel of children with cystic fibrosis. J Pediatr 1964; 64:575–579.
59. Rubin C, Dobbins W: Peroral biopsy of the small intestine. A review of its diagnostic usefulness. Gastroenterology 1965; 49:676–697.

60. Grossman H, Berdon W, Baker D: Gastrointestinal findings in cystic fibrosis. Am J Roentgenol 1966; 97:227–238.
61. Taussig L, Saldino R, DiSant'Agnese P: Radiographic abnormalities of the duodenum and small bowel in cystic fibrosis of the pancreas (mucoviscidosis). Radiology 1973; 106:369–376.
62. Wood R, Herman C, Johnson K, et al: Pneumatosis coli in cystic fibrosis: clinical, radiological and pathological features. Am J Dis Child 1975; 129:246–248.
63. Buts JP, Morin CL, Roy CC, et al: One-hour blood xylose test: A reliable index of small bowel function. J Pediatr 1978; 92:729–733.
64. Lebenthal E, Antonowicz I, Shwachman H: Correlation of lactase activity, lactose intolerance and milk consumption in different age groups. Am J Clin Nutr 1975; 28:595–600.
65. Hurwitt E, Arnheim E: Meconium ileus associated with stenosis of the pancreatic ducts. Am J Dis Child 1942; 64:443–454.
66. Auburn R, Feldman S, Gadacz T, et al: Meconium ileus secondary to partial aplasia of the pancreas; report of a case. Surgery 1969; 65:689–693.
67. Dolan T, Touloukian R: Familial meconium ileus not associated with cystic fibrosis. J Pediatr Surg 1974; 9:821–824.
68. Noblett H: Meconium ileus. *In* Ravitch M, Welsh K, Benson C, et al, eds: Pediatric Surgery. Chicago, Year Book Medical Publishers, 1979, p 943.
69. Rosenstein BJ: Cystic fibrosis presenting with meconium plug syndrome. Am J Dis Child 1978; 132:167–169.
70. Olsen MM, Luck SR, Lloyd Still J, et al: The spectrum of meconium disease in infancy. J Pediatr Surg 1982; 17(5):479–481.
71. Lands L, Zinman P, Wise M, et al: Pancreatic function testing or meconium ileus in cystic fibrosis: two case reports. J Pediatr Gastroenterol Nutr 1988; 7:276–279.
72. Taylor CJ, Baxter PS, Handcastle J, et al: Failure to induce secretion in jejunal biopsies from children with cystic fibrosis. Gut 1988; 29:957–962.
73. Baxter PS, Wilson AJ, Read NW, et al: Abnormal jejunal potential difference in cystic fibrosis. Lancet 1989; 1:464–465.
73a. Del Pin CA, Czyrko C, Ziegler MM, et al: Management of survival of meconium ileus: A 30-year review. Ann Surg 1992; 215:179–185.
74. Durie P: Gastrointestinal motility disorders in cystic fibrosis. *In* Milla PJ, ed: Disorders of Gastrointestinal Motility in Childhood. Chichester, Wiley, 1988, pp 91–99.
75. Cleghorn GJ, Stringer DA, Forstner G, et al: Treatment of the distal intestinal obstruction syndrome in cystic fibrosis with a balanced intestinal lavage solution. Lancet 1986; 1:8–11.
76. Koletzko S, Corey M, Ellis L, et al: Effects of cisapride in patients with cystic fibrosis and distal intestinal obstruction syndrome. J Pediatr 1990; 117(5):815–822.
77. Kulczycki LL, Shwachman H: Studies in cystic fibrosis of the pancreas: Occurrence of rectal prolapse. N Engl J Med 1958; 259:409–412.
78. Stern R, Izant RJ, Boat TF, et al: Treatment and prognosis of rectal prolapse in cystic fibrosis. Gastroenterology 1986; 82:707–710.
79. Rubinstein S, Moss R, Lewiston N: Constipation and meconium ileus equivalent in patients with cystic fibrosis. Pediatrics 1986; 78:473–479.
80. Scott RB, O'Laughlin EV, Gall DG: Gastroesophageal reflux in patients with cystic fibrosis. J Pediatr 1985; 106:223–227.
81. Feigelson J, Girault F, Pecau Y: Gastroesophageal reflux and esophagitis in cystic fibrosis. Acta Paediatr Scand 1987; 76:989–990.
82. Anderson D: Pathology of cystic fibrosis. Ann NY Acad Sci 1962; 93:500–517.
83. Aterman K: Duodenal ulceration and fibrocystic pancreas disease. Am J Dis Child 1961; 101:210–215.
84. Ojeda VJ, Levitt S, Ryan G, et al: Cystic fibrosis, Crohn's colitis, and adult meconium ileus equivalent. Dis Colon Rectum 1986; 29:567–571.
85. Katz A, Falchuk M, Shwachman H: The coexistence of cystic fibrosis and celiac disease. Pediatrics 1976; 57:715–721.
86. Franklin J, Asquith P, Rosenberg I: The occurrence of cystic fibrosis and celiac sprue within a single sibship. Am J Dig Dis 1974; 19:149–155.
87. DiSant'Agnese P, Blanc W: A distinctive type of biliary cirrhosis of the liver associated with cystic fibrosis of the pancreas. Pediatrics 1956; 18:387–409.
88. Craig M, Haddad H, Shwachman H: The pathological changes in the liver in cystic fibrosis of the pancreas. Am J Dis Child 1957; 93:357–369.
89. Webster R, Williams H: Hepatic cirrhosis associated with fibrocystic disease of the pancreas. Am J Dis Child 1953; 28:343–350.
90. Stern R, Stevens D, Boat T, et al: Symptomatic hepatic disease in cystic fibrosis: Incidence, course, and outcome of portal systemic shunting. Gastroenterology 1976; 70:645–649.
91. Wilroy R, Crawford S, Johnson W: Cystic fibrosis with extensive fat replacement of the liver. J Pediatr 1966; 68:67–73.
92. Farber S: Pancreatic function and disease in early life: V. Pathological changes associated with pancreatic insufficiency in early life. Arch Pathol 1944; 37:238–250.
93. Oppenheimer E, Esterly J: Hepatic changes in young infants with cystic fibrosis: Possible relation to focal biliary cirrhosis. J Pediatr 1975; 86:683–689.
94. Weizman Z, Durie P, Kopelman H, et al: Bile acid secretion in cystic fibrosis—evidence for a primary defect. Gut 1986; 27:1362–1368.
95. Colling J, Lentze MJ, Reiden J: Effects of ursodeoxycholic acid treatment on nutrition and liver function in patients with cystic fibrosis and longstanding cholestasis. Gut 1990; 31:918–921.
95a. de Caestecker JS, Jazrawi RP, Petroni ML, et al: Ursodeoxycholic acid in chronic liver disease. Gut 1991; 32:1061–1065.
96. Kopel F: Gastrointestinal manifestations of cystic fibrosis. Gastroenterology 1972; 62:483–491.
97. Tanner MS: Current clinical management of hepatic problems in cystic fibrosis. J R Soc Med 1986; 79(Suppl 12):38–43.
98. Shuster S, Shwachman H, Toyama W, et al: The management of portal hypertension in cystic fibrosis. J Pediatr Surg 1977; 12:201–206.
98a. Duthie A, Doherty DG, Williams C, et al: Genotype analysis for AF508, G551D, R553X mutations in children and young adults with cystic fibrosis with and without chronic liver disease. Hepatology 1992; 15:660–664.
99. Ferrari M. Colombo C, Sebastio G, et al: Cystic fibrosis patients with liver disease are not genetically distinct. Am J Hum Genet 1991; 48(4):815–816.
100. Gaskin KJ, Waters DLM, Howman-Giles R, et al: Liver disease and common bile duct stenosis in cystic fibrosis. N Engl J Med 1988; 318:340–346.
100a. O'Brien S, Keogan M, Casey M, et al: Biliary complications of cystic fibrosis. Gut 1992; 33:387–391.
101. Colombo C, Setcheff KD, Podda M, et al: Effects of ursodeoxycholic acid therapy for liver disease associated with cystic fibrosis. J Pediatr 1990; 117(3):482–489.
101a. Colombo C, Castellani MR, Balistreri WF, et al: Scintigraphic documentation of an improvement in hepatobiliary excretory function after treatment with ursodeoxycholic acid in patients with cystic fibrosis and associated liver disease. Hepatology 1992; 15:677–684.
102. Mieles LA, Orenstein D, Teperman L, et al: Liver tranplantation in cystic fibrosis. Lancet 1989; 1:1073.
103. Feigelson J, Pecau Y, Sauvegrain J: Liver function studies and biliary tract investigations in mucoviscidosis. Acta Pediatr Scand 1970; 59:539–544.
104. Esterly J, Oppenheimer E: Observations in cystic fibrosis. I. The gallbladder. Johns Hopkins Med J 1962; 110:247–254.
105. Isenberg J, L'Heureux P, Warwick W, et al: Clinical observations on the biliary system in cystic fibrosis. Am J Gastroenterol 1976; 65:134–141.
106. L'Heureux P, Isenberg J, Sharp H, et al: Gallbladder disease in cystic fibrosis. Am J Roentgenol 1977; 128:953–956.
107. Valman H, France N, Wallis P: Prolonged neonatal jaundice in cystic fibrosis. Arch Dis Child 1971; 46:805–809.
108. Davidson GP, Corey M, Hassel FM, et al: Immunoassay of serum conjugates of cholic acid in cystic fibrosis. J Clin Pathol 1980; 35:390–394.
109. Robb TA, Davidson GP, Kirubakaran C: Conjugated bile acids in serum and secretions—response to cholecystokinin/secretin stimulation in children with cystic fibrosis. Gut 1985; 26:1246–1256.
110. Weber A, Roy C, Morin C, et al: Malabsorption of bile acids in children with cystic fibrosis. N Engl J Med 1973; 289:1001–1005.

111. Watkins J, Tercyac A, Szczepanik P, et al: Bile salt kinetics in cystic fibrosis: Influence of pancreatic enzyme replacement. Gastroenterology 1977; 73:1023–1028.
112. Levy LD, Durie PR, Pencharz PB, et al: Effects of long-term nutritional rehabilitation on body composition and clinical status in malnourished children and adolescents with cystic fibrosis. J Pediatr 1985; 107:225–230.
113. Boland MP, Stoski DS, MacDonald NE, et al: Chronic jejunostomy feeding with a non-elemental formula in undernourished patients with cystic fibrosis. Lancet 1986; 1:232–234.
114. Drury D, Pianosi P, Kopelman H, et al: The effect of nutritional status on respiratory muscle strength and work capacity in cystic fibrosis. Pediatr Res 1990; 27(4):104A.
115. Vaisman N, Pencharz P, Corey M, et al: Energy expenditure of patients with cystic fibrosis. J Pediatr 1987; 111:496–500.
116. Buchdahl RM, Cox M, Fulleylove C, et al: Increased energy expenditure in cystic fibrosis. J Appl Physiol 1988; 64:1810–1816.
117. Shepherd RW, Holt TL, Vasques-Velasquez L, et al: Increased energy expenditure in young children with cystic fibrosis. Lancet 1988; 1:1300–1303.
118. Shepherd R, Cooksley WGE, Domville-Cooke WD: Improved growth and clinical, nutritional and respiratory changes in response to nutritional therapy in cystic fibrosis. J Pediatr 1980; 97:351–357.
119. Vaisman N, Levy L, Pencharz P, et al: Effect of salbutamol on resting energy expenditure in patients with cystic fibrosis. J Pediatr 1987; 111:137–139.
120. Bell L, Linton WL, Corey ML, et al: Nutrient intakes of adolescents with cystic fibrosis. J Can Diet Assoc 1981; 42:1–10.
121. Norman D, Elborn JS, Cordon SM, et al: Plasma tumour necrosis factor alpha in cystic fibrosis. Thorax 1991;46(2):91–95.
122. Sproul A, Huang N: Growth patterns in children with cystic fibrosis. J Pediatr 1964; 65:664–676.
123. Mitchell-Heggs P, Mearns M, Batten JC: Cystic fibrosis in adolescents and adults. Q J Med 1976; 45:479–504.
124. Peterson R, Peterson V, Robb R: Vitamin A deficiency with xerophthalmia and night blindness in cystic fibrosis. Am J Dis Child 1968; 116:662–665.
125. Keating J, Feigin R: Increased intracranial pressure associated with probable vitamin A deficiency in cystic fibrosis. Pediatrics 1970; 46:41–46.
126. Underwood B, Denning C: Blood and liver concentrations of vitamins A and E in children with cystic fibrosis of the pancreas. Pediatr Res 1972; 6:26–31.
127. Farrell P, Bieri J, Fratantoni J, et al: The occurrence and effects of human vitamin E deficiency. J Clin Invest 1977; 60:233–241.
128. Weinberg T, Gordon H, Oppenheimer E, et al: Myopathy in association with tocopherol deficiency in cases of congenital biliary atresia and cystic fibrosis of the pancreas. Am J Pathol 1958; 34:565–566.
129. Willison HJ, Muller DPR, Matthews S, et al: A study of the relationship between neurological function and serum vitamin E concentrations in patients with cystic fibrosis. J Neurol Neurosurg Psychol 1985; 48:1097–1102.
130. Hubbard V, Farrell P, di Sant'Agnese P: 25-hydroxycholecalciferol levels in patients with cystic fibrosis. J Pediatr 1979; 94:84–86.
131. Weisman Y, Reiter E, Stern R, et al: Serum concentrations of 25-hydroxyvitamin D in patients with cystic fibrosis. J Pediatr 1979; 95:416–418.
132. Hahn T, Squires A, Halstead L, et al: Reduced serum 25-hydroxyvitamin D concentration and disordered mineral metabolism in patients with cystic fibrosis. J Pediatr 1979; 94:38–42.
133. Tortenson O, Humphrey G, Edson J, et al: Cystic fibrosis presenting with severe hemorrhage due to vitamin K malabsorption: A report of three cases. Pediatrics 1970; 45:857–861.
134. Walters T, Koch F: Hemorrhagic diathesis and cystic fibrosis in infancy. Am J Dis Child 1972; 24:641–642.
135. Ater JL, Herbst JJ, Landaw SA, et al: Relative anemia and iron deficiency in cystic fibrosis. Pediatrics 1983; 71:810–814.
136. Solomons NW, Wagonfield JB, Rieger C, et al: Some biochemical indices of nutrition in treated cystic fibrosis patients. Am J Clin Nutr 1981; 34:462–474.
137. Green CG, Doershuk CF, Stern RC: Symptomatic hypomagnesemia in cystic fibrosis. J Pediatr 1985; 107:425–428.
138. Chase HP, Long MA, Lavin MH: Cystic fibrosis and malnutrition. J Pediatr 1979; 95:337–347.
139. Hubbard VS, Dunn GD, di Sant'Agnese P: Abnormal fatty acid composition of plasma lipids in cystic fibrosis. Lancet 1977; 2:1302–1304.
140. Lloyd Still JD, Johnson SB, Holman RT: Essential fatty acid status in cystic fibrosis and the effects of safflower oil supplementation. Am J Clin Nutr 1981; 34:1–7.
141. Parsons HG, O'Loughlin EV, Forbes D, et al: Supplemental calories improve essential fatty acid deficiency in cystic fibrosis patients. Pediatr Res 1988; 24:353–356.
142. Mansell AL, Andersen JC, Muttart CR, et al: Short term pulmonary effects of total parenteral nutrition in children with cystic fibrosis. J Pediatr 1984; 104:700–705.

Chapter 67

Congenital Diseases of the Exocrine Pancreas

RICHARD A. SCHREIBER

There are several congenital diseases of the exocrine pancreas (Table 67–1). Cystic fibrosis is by far the commonest hereditary disorder of the pancreas (see Chapter 66). Shwachman's syndrome is an infrequently occurring, multisystem disease initially defined by Bodian and associates[1] in 1964 and then by Shwachman and colleagues[2] also in 1964 to include patients who have exocrine pancreatic insufficiency, a normal sweat test, and bone marrow dysfunction. More recently, an entire constellation of signs and symptoms, including growth retardation, skeletal abnormalities, and hematologic, renal, hepatic, neurologic, and developmental disorders, has been associated with the syndrome (Table 67–2). This chapter discusses the clinical features, diagnosis, and treatment of Shwachman's syndrome. Other rare causes of congenital pancreatic exocrine insufficiency also are briefly reviewed.

SHWACHMAN'S SYNDROME

Although Shwachman's syndrome is the second most common hereditary abnormality of the exocrine pancreas after cystic fibrosis, its etiology and pathogenesis remain unknown. Several studies of affected families have pointed to an autosomal recessive mode of inheritance.[3] An autosomal dominant form with variable expression may exist in some cases.[4] No single gene defect has been described; however, a high frequency of spontaneous chromosomal breakage has been observed in a few patients.[5,6] As an ancillary hypothesis, one group has suggested that Shwachman's syndrome may be secondary to copper deficiency in the neonatal period.[7] Pancreatic atrophy has been observed in experimental copper deficiency, and some of the other manifestations of the syndrome, such as neutropenia and rib abnormalities, have been reported in children who were known to be copper deficient. Other authors have proposed that a cytoskeletal defect may account for some of the features of this disease.[8]

Table 67–1. CONGENITAL DISEASES OF THE EXOCRINE PANCREAS

Cystic fibrosis
Shwachman's syndrome
Johanson-Blizzard syndrome
Exocrine pancreatic dysfunction with refractory sideroblastic anemia
Isolated enzyme defects
Pancreatic agenesis
Congenital rubella

Clinical Features

Growth Retardation

Growth retardation, one of the cardinal manifestations of Shwachman's syndrome, is a primary feature that is present independently of the nutritional status or the severity of skeletal abnormalities described in these patients.[3] Most patients will eventually be below the third percentile for height, yet a normal growth velocity is usually maintained. Intrauterine growth retardation may occur, but in most patients growth parameters are normal at birth, and growth delay becomes clinically evident during the first year of life. Although two thirds of the 21 patients reviewed in one series had normal birth weights, all except one patient were below the third percentile for weight, height, and head circumference by toddler age.[3] Puberty is delayed in many of the older patients.

Table 67–2. FEATURES OF SHWACHMAN'S SYNDROME

Exocrine pancreatic hypoplasia
Short stature
Bone marrow dysfunction
Skeletal abnormalities
Recurrent infection
Impaired neutrophil chemotaxis
Renal tubular disorders
Chronic liver disease
Endocardial fibrosis
Dental abnormalities
Ichthyosis
Diabetes mellitus
Hirschsprung's disease

Pancreatic Hypoplasia

The hallmark of Shwachman's syndrome is pancreatic hypoplasia. Histologically, pancreatic acinar tissue is replaced by fat, but the pancreatic islets and ductular structures remain intact.[1, 2] As a consequence, quantitative pancreatic stimulation tests demonstrate diminished pancreatic enzyme secretion. The degree of pancreatic secretory impairment is quite variable, and not all patients have pancreatic insufficiency—defined as the presence of steatorrhea.[3, 9] Normal fat absorption appears to be the rule rather than the exception in patients older than 6 years of age. This finding is believed to be related to a marginal improvement in lipase secretion at an older age, yet all of these patients still demonstrate pancreatic dysfunction when formally tested by standard pancreatic stimulation techniques.[9] Symptoms of fat malabsorption usually are clinically evident in the first 6 months of life. Steatorrhea and associated fat-soluble vitamin deficiency or failure to thrive may be presenting features of Shwachman's syndrome in infancy. On the other hand, the absence of steatorrhea does not exclude a diagnosis of Shwachman's syndrome.

Skeletal Abnormalities

Metaphyseal dyschondroplasia, present in about 60% of patients, is usually detected after the first year of life and tends to resolve after puberty.[3] The hip is the most frequently affected site, but there may be involvement of the knees, humeral head, wrists, and ankles. Rib abnormalities are particularly common in infants. As a result, a narrow thoracic cage may be clinically evident, and some neonates may develop respiratory distress or asphyxiating thoracic dystrophy.[10, 11] Older children and adults may demonstrate restrictive or obstructive lung disease on pulmonary function testing.[12] Other skeletal changes include long bone tubulation and spinal abnormalities. Clinodactyly is a frequent finding.[3]

Bone Marrow Dysfunction

Hematologic abnormalities commonly manifesting as neutropenia but also as thrombocytopenia, hypoplastic anemia, or pancytopenia are classic features of Shwachman's syndrome.[3] Patients are also predisposed to lymphoproliferative malignancies.[13, 14] Because the neutropenia is most often cyclical, neutrophil counts should be obtained twice weekly for 3 consecutive weeks to detect this abnormality.[4] The etiology of the intermittent neutropenia is uncertain. Assays of bone marrow granulocyte colony-forming cells have yielded inconsistent results.[15] Whether there is a defect at the level of the stem cell has not been established. The neutropenia does not appear to be caused by circulating granulopoietic inhibitors.[15] A number of studies have confirmed that patients with Shwachman's syndrome have impaired mobility of polymorphonuclear leukocytes.[16–18] In addition to depressed chemotaxis, the neutrophils demonstrate increased chemiluminescence. It has been proposed that the aberrant chemotaxis may be secondary to autoxidation of the neutrophil.[19]

Patients with Shwachman's syndrome are prone to infection. Otitis media, sinusitis, pneumonia, osteomyelitis, and recurrent skin infections are often experienced.[3] Overwhelming sepsis is the leading cause of death in these patients. Shmerling and coworkers[20] have estimated a 25% mortality rate due to infection. The frequency and severity of infection, however, have not correlated with the degree of neutropenia. It is likely that susceptibility is related to the altered neutrophil function. Immunoglobulin deficiency has been reported in isolated cases.[3] The number of infectious episodes tends to diminish with age.

Other Manifestations

Renal abnormalities such as aminoaciduria, glycosuria, renal tubular acidosis, and nephrocalcinosis have been associated with Shwachman's syndrome.[21, 22] Chronic liver disease,[23] diabetes mellitus,[3] myocardial fibrosis,[24] central pontine myelinolysis,[25] and psychomotor retardation[3, 26] are other rare features reported with this condition.

Diagnosis

Pancreatic exocrine insufficiency should be considered in all children with failure to thrive. Fat malabsorption in an infant with bone marrow dysfunction and a negative sweat test suggests a diagnosis of Shwachman's syndrome. On the other hand, the older child who presents with short stature, normal fat absorption, skeletal abnormalities, and a history of repeated infections or isolated neutropenia should also be evaluated for Shwachman's syndrome. In the absence of pancreatic insufficiency, quantitative pancreatic stimulation tests to demonstrate pancreatic dysfunction are necessary to confirm the diagnosis. These studies are cumbersome and are not readily available in most centers. Alternatively, in the infant younger than 1 year of age with steatorrhea and a negative sweat test, the finding of a low serum immunoreactive trypsin concentration, coupled with a computed tomography scan demonstrating fatty infiltration of the pancreas, would secure the diagnosis and obviate the need for formal pancreatic function testing.[27, 28] Pancreatic needle biopsy guided by modern radiologic techniques, although now possible, is not warranted as a diagnostic maneuver.

Treatment

Once the diagnosis is established, the treatment of Shwachman's syndrome is generally supportive. Pancreatic enzyme replacement therapy for patients with fat malabsorption is required. Nutritional management with medium-chain triglycerides and the introduction of fat-soluble vitamin supplementation may also be necessary. With treatment, the degree of steatorrhea improves and weight gain may be evident, but height acceleration does not usually occur.[3] Most of these patients remain short in stature. Pancreatic enzyme therapy may eventually be discontinued, because most patients achieve normal fat absorption at a later age.[9] Infections usually respond to appropriate antimicrobial therapy. Because these patients are often neutropenic and have diminished neutrophil function, and because sepsis is a frequent cause of mortality, the onset of fever should demand a prompt and thorough investigation in search of a focus of infection. Prophylactic antibiotic therapy may be indicated, particularly in the young infant. Although no specific therapy for the neutrophil dysfunction can be recommended, in vitro and in vivo experiments have demonstrated that lithium may restore the defective chemotaxis seen in these patients' neutrophils.[29, 30] A recent report[31] has demonstrated successful treatment of aplastic anemia in Shwachman's syndrome with cyclosporin A.

JOHANSON-BLIZZARD SYNDROME

The Johanson-Blizzard syndrome is a rare disorder of exocrine pancreatic insufficiency and growth retardation. Only 28 cases have been reported to date.[32] The syndrome, first described by Johanson and Blizzard in 1971,[33] has striking clinical features and is quite easily recognized. Along with steatorrhea and failure to thrive, the classic features of this syndrome include microcephaly, midline scalp defects, an abnormal hair pattern, a small beaked nose with aplasia or hypoplasia of the nasal cartilage, small deciduous and absent permanent teeth, sensorineural hearing loss, mental retardation, an imperforate or anteriorly placed anus, and thyroid dysfunction. Other associated findings are cutaneous lacrimal fistulas, café au lait spots, accessory or absent nipples, congenital heart defects, and genitourinary anomalies. The condition is inherited in an autosomal recessive fashion.

EXOCRINE PANCREATIC DYSFUNCTION WITH REFRACTORY SIDEROBLASTIC ANEMIA

Four unrelated children have been characterized to have a unique syndrome affecting the bone marrow and the exocrine pancreas.[34] All these patients had a macrocytic anemia in early infancy associated with a low reticulocyte count and varying degrees of neutropenia and thrombocytopenia. In contrast with the bone marrow findings in patients with Shwachman's syndrome, bone marrow aspirates from these patients demonstrated a striking vacuolization of both erythroid and myeloid precursors, increased marrow hemosiderin, and the presence of ringed sideroblasts. Only one patient had steatorrhea, whereas two others had normal fat absorption. Pancreatic exocrine dysfunction was demonstrated in all three patients who underwent pancreatic stimulation tests. Two of the infants died, whereas the others had spontaneous improvement in their hematologic status. Postmortem examination of the pancreata showed acinar atrophy with fibrosis as opposed to the fatty infiltration described with Shwachman's syndrome. None of these children had skeletal abnormalities.

OTHER DISORDERS

The few remaining congenital diseases of the exocrine pancreas are exceedingly rare and are mentioned only for the sake of completeness. The few patients reported with selective lipase deficiency thrived despite having steatorrhea.[35] The cases of selective trypsin[36] or enterokinase deficiency[37] had severe growth retardation, hypoproteinemia, edema, and steatorrhea. Only one case of selective amylase deficiency has been described.[38] Pancreatic insufficiency has been associated with congenital rubella syndrome[39] and with pancreatic agenesis.[40]

REFERENCES

1. Bodian M, Sheldon W, Lightwood R: Congenital hypoplasia of the exocrine pancreas. Acta Pediatr Scand 1964; 53:282–293.
2. Shwachman H, Diamond LK, Oski FA, et al: The syndrome of pancreatic insufficiency and bone marrow dysfunction. J Pediatr 1964; 65:645–663.
3. Aggett PJ, Cavanagh NPC, Matthew DJ, et al: Shwachman's syndrome: A review of 21 cases. Arch Dis Child 1980; 55:331–347.
4. Burke V, Colebatch JH, Anderson CM, et al: Association of pancreatic insufficiency and chronic neutropenia in childhood. Arch Dis Child 1967; 42:147–157.
5. Fraccaro M, Scappaticci S, Arico M: Shwachman syndrome and chromosome breakage. Hum Genet 1988; 79:194.
6. Tada H, Ri T, Yoshida H, et al: A case of Shwachman syndrome with increased spontaneous chromosome breakage. Hum Genet 1987; 77:289–291.
7. Paterson CR, Wormsley KG: Hypothesis: Shwachman's syndrome of exocrine pancreatic insufficiency may be caused by neonatal copper deficiency. Ann Nutr Metab 1988; 32:127–132.
8. Rothbaum RJ, Williams DA, Daughtery CC: Unusual surface distribution of concanavalin A reflects a cytoskeletal defect in neutrophils in Shwachman syndrome. Lancet 1982; 2:800–801.
9. Hill RE, Durie PR, Gaskin KJ, et al: Steatorrhea and pancreatic insufficiency in Shwachman syndrome. Gastroenterology 1982; 83:22–27.
10. Michels VV, Donovan GK: Shwachman syndrome: Unusual presentation as asphyxiating thoracic dystrophy. Birth Defects 1982; 18:129–134.
11. Labrune M, Dommergues JP, Chaboche C, et al: Syndrome de Shwachman a manifestations thoraciques neonatales. Arch Fr Pediatr 1984; 41:561–563.
12. Wiggins J, Geddes DM: Respiratory aspects of Shwachman's syndrome in adults. Eur Respir J 1989; 2:285–288.
13. Caselitz J, Kloppel G, Delling G, et al: Shwachman's syndrome and leukaemia. Virchows Arch 1979; 385:109–116.
14. Woods WG, Roloff JS, Lukens JN, et al: The occurrence of leukemia in patients with the Shwachman syndrome. J Pediatr 1981; 99:425–428.
15. Saunders EF, Gall G, Freedman MH: Granulopoiesis in Shwachman's syndrome (pancreatic insufficiency and bone marrow dysfunction). Pediatrics 1979; 64:515–519.
16. Aggett PJ, Harries JT, Harvey BAM, et al: An inherited defect of neutrophil mobility in Shwachman syndrome. J Pediatr 1979; 94:391–394.
17. Thong YH: Impaired neutrophil kinesis in a patient with the Shwachman-Diamond syndrome. Aust Pediatr J 1978; 14:34–37.
18. Ruutu P, Savilahti E, Repo H, et al: Constant defect in neutrophil

locomotion but with age decreasing susceptibility to infection in Shwachman syndrome. Clin Exp Immunol 1984; 57:249–255.
19. Repo H, Savilahti E, Leirisalo-Repo M: Aberrant phagocyte function in Shwachman syndrome. Clin Exp Immunol 1987; 69:204–212.
20. Shmerling DH, Prader A, Hitzig WH, et al: The syndrome of exocrine pancreatic insufficiency, neutropenia, metaphyseal dysostosis, and dwarfism. Helv Paediatr Acta 1969; 24:547–575.
21. Marra G, Appiani AC, Romeo L, et al: Renal tubular acidosis in a case of Shwachman's syndrome. Acta Paediatr Scand 1986; 75:682–684.
22. D'Angio CT, Lloyd JK: Nephrocalcinosis in Shwachman's syndrome. Arch Dis Child 1989; 64:614–615.
23. Liebman WM, Rosental E, Hirshberger M, et al: Shwachman-Diamond syndrome and chronic liver disease. Clin Pediatr 1979; 18:695–696, 698.
24. Nivelton JL, Michiels R, Martres-Lassauniere MN, et al: Fibrose myocardique compliquant un syndrome de Shwachman: Discussion pathogenique de la complication cardiaque. Pediatrie 1978; 33:461–469.
25. Steinsapir KD, Vinters HV: Central pontine myelinolysis in a child with the Shwachman-Diamond syndrome. Hum Pathol 1985; 16:741–743.
26. Kent A, Murphy GH, Milla P: Psychological characteristics of children with Shwachman syndrome. Arch Dis Child 1990; 65:1349–1352.
27. Dossetor JF, Spratt HC, Rolles CJ, et al: Immunoreactive trypsin in Shwachman's syndrome. Arch Dis Child 1989; 64:395–396.
28. Kurdziel JC, Dondelinger R: Fatty infiltration of the pancreas in Shwachman's syndrome: Computed tomography demonstration. Eur J Radiol 1984; 4:202–204.
29. Azzara A, Carulli G, Ceccarelli M, et al: In vivo effectiveness of lithium on impaired neutrophil chemotaxis in Shwachman-Diamond syndrome. Acta Haematol 1991; 85:100–102.
30. Azzara A, Carulli G, Polidori R, et al: In vitro restoration by lithium of defective chemotaxis in Shwachman-Diamond syndrome. Br J Haematol 1988 70:502.
31. Barrios NJ, Kirkpatrick DV: Successful cyclosporin A treatment of aplastic anemia in Shwachman-Diamond syndrome. Br J Haematol 1990; 74:540–541.
32. Gershoni-Baruch R, Lerner A, Braun J, et al: Johanson-Blizzard syndrome: Clinical spectrum and further delineation of the syndrome. Am J Med Genet 1990; 35: 546–551.
33. Johanson A, Blizzard R: A syndrome of congenital aplasia of the nasal alae, deafness, hypothyroidism, dwarfism, absent permanent teeth, and malabsorption. J Pediatr 1971; 79:982–987.
34. Pearson HA, Lobel JS, Kocoshis SA, et al: A new syndrome of refractory sideroblastic anemia with vacuolization of marrow precursors and exocrine pancreatic dysfunction. J Pediatr 1979; 95:976–984.
35. Sheldon W: Congenital pancreatic lipase deficiency. Arch Dis Child 1964; 39:268–271.
36. Townes PL, Bryson MF, Miller G: Further observations on trypsinogen deficiency disease: Report of a second case. J Pediatr 1967; 71:220–224.
37. Hadorn B, Tarlow MJ, Lloyd JK, et al: Intestinal enterokinase deficiency. Lancet 1969; 1:812–813.
38. Lowe CU, May CD: Selective pancreatic deficiency. Am J Dis Child 1951; 82:459–464.
39. Donowitz M, Gryboski JD: Pancreatic insufficiency and the congenital rubella syndrome. J Pediatr 1975; 87:241–243.
40. Howard CP, Go VLW, Infante AJ, et al: Long-term survival in a case of functional pancreatic agenesis. J Pediatr 1980; 97:786–789.

Chapter 68

Acute Pancreatitis

ZVI WEIZMAN

Although acute pancreatitis occurs less frequently in children than in adults, it is probably more common in childhood than has previously been appreciated and may have significant morbidity and mortality. A survey of the English medical literature until 1967 presented data on 128 previously reported cases of childhood pancreatitis.[1] Most of the referenced publications consisted of limited case studies. Only recently have there been reports of larger patient groups.[2–6] Most prospective clinical studies in the literature are based on adult populations.

CLASSIFICATION

The term *pancreatitis* covers a wide spectrum of inflammatory conditions of the pancreas, ranging from severe to mild or even subclinical disease. In most patients, inflammation does not progress beyond the stage of edema and fatty necrosis. When the patient survives, these lesions are generally considered to be reversible. The terms *necrotizing* or *hemorrhagic pancreatitis* refer to severe disease with diffuse pancreatic necrosis and life-threatening systemic manifestations.

The most widely used clinical classification of pancreatitis distinguishes between acute and chronic pancreatitis. The phrase *acute, relapsing* is no longer used.[7] This chapter discusses the acute forms of the disease, including relapsing pancreatitis. In the acute types, pancreatic function and morphology are restored between acute attacks, whereas in the chronic forms there is nonreversible damage.

There have been several additional proposals in the literature for modified classifications of pancreatitis.[8] However, many of the criteria used are not applicable in childhood.

PATHOGENESIS

Pancreatitis is a disease of variable etiology. The exact mechanism by which each cause triggers acute inflammation is not always clear. It has been proposed that the initiating event either activates exocrine pancreatic enzymes or causes damage to the acinar cell. Pancreatic proteases are activated within the pancreas, probably owing to various factors such as trauma, ischemia, toxins, infections, and others. Activated zymogens, mainly trypsin, are able to activate other enzymes, and the result is autodigestion of the pancreas and surrounding tissues. There is digestion of cell membranes, vascular damage, edema, coagulation necrosis, and interstitial necrosis. Fat necrosis produces saponification of calcium.

Trypsin-activated phospholipase A_2 and elastase are believed to be responsible for some of these pathologic processes. Several observations have indicated that phospholipase A_2 might be the primary enzyme responsible for tissue necrosis in acute pancreatitis.[9] This enzyme is activated within the pancreas in experimental acute pancreatitis in animals, and its elevated catalytic activity in serum is associated with severe disease. However, the evidence is less clear in humans, and the causal relationship between phospholipase A_2 and the pathologic changes of human acute pancreatitis has not been established unequivocally. Vasoactive substances such as histamine, kinins, and kallikrein play a major role in increasing capillary permeability, resulting in transudation of fluids.

It remains unclear what constitutes the primary event leading to intrapancreatic proteolytic enzyme activation. Most speculation has centered around two hypotheses: (1) reflux of duodenal contents into the pancreatic duct, where enterokinase may activate trypsinogen or (2) pancreatic ductal hypertension, resulting from continued secretion into an obstructed duct leading to rupture of small ducts, extravasation of juices into the gland, and subsequent intraparenchymal activation of enzymes. Both hypotheses presume that enzyme activation occurs outside the acinar cell, but unequivocal evidence for either of these models is not available. Recent findings cast doubt on this concept and propose that enzymes become activated by lysosomal hydrolases within the pancreatic acinar cell itself.[10] Animal studies have evaluated two types of models, including mice fed choline-deficient diets supplemented with methionine and rats treated with excessive doses of cholecystokinin analogue. Both models demonstrated early intracellular admixture of digestive enzymes with lysosomal hydrolases (e.g., cathepsin B), which are able to activate trypsinogen.[11, 12]

Several studies have shown that oxygen free radicals play an important role in the development of inflammation in acute pancreatitis.[13, 14] Several researchers have found increased amounts of lipid peroxidation products, possibly derived from free radical oxidation, in the bile and pancreatic tissue of patients suffering from acute or recurrent disease. In addition, acetylcysteine, a well-known radical scavenger, caused significant improvement when administered to a patient with multiple organ failure due to severe acute pancreatitis. Thus, it seems reasonable to assume that oxygen free radicals are generated in acute pancreatitis in humans and that they add to the damage observed. Moreover, treatment with free radical scavengers could possibly interrupt these damaging mechanisms and improve outcome.

Two additional factors suggested as potentially contributing to the pathogenesis of pancreatitis include abnormalities in pancreatic microcirculation with resultant ischemia[15, 16] and emotional stress.[17]

ETIOLOGIES

There is a wide variety of causes of acute pancreatitis in the pediatric age group. In adults, biliary tract disease and alcoholism are the two commonest causes, and in many published series these represent the etiology in 70 to 80% of patients with acute pancreatitis.[18] In contrast, the causes of acute pancreatitis in childhood are quite different, and the commonest etiologic factors are trauma, multisystem disease, and drugs.[3, 4, 6] A detailed list of causes is given in Table 68–1. Viral infections, congenital structural anomalies, and metabolic diseases are also considered as common causes of acute pancreatitis in childhood. In as many as 25% of cases, no particular cause is identified. Only drugs reported to have well-documented association with acute pancreatitis are included in the table.[19] In recent years, more patients with acute pancreatitis associated with multisystem diseases have been reported, especially with Reye's syndrome[20, 21] and Kawasaki disease.[22]

Table 68–1. CAUSES OF ACUTE PANCREATITIS IN CHILDHOOD

Trauma
- Abdominal trauma
- Child abuse

Multisystem Disease
- Reye's syndrome
- Shock
- Hemolytic-uremic syndrome
- Crohn's disease
- Sarcoidosis
- Kawasaki disease

Drugs
- Chlorthalidone
- L-Asparaginase
- Azathioprine
- Sulfonamides
- Sulfasalazine
- Thiazides
- Furosemide
- Estrogens
- Tetracycline
- Valproic acid
- Phenformin
- Procainamide
- Corticosteroids
- Ethacrynic acid

Infections
- Sepsis
- Viruses (measles, mumps, Epstein-Barr virus, coxsackie B, rubella, hepatitis A and B, influenza, echovirus)
- *Mycoplasma pneumoniae*

Metabolic Disorders
- Hypercalcemia
- Hyperlipidemia
- Uremia
- $Alpha_1$-antitrypsin deficiency

Vasculitis
- Systemic lupus erythematosus
- Henoch-Schönlein purpura
- Kawasaki disease

Pancreatic Disorders
- Cystic fibrosis
- Diabetes
- Pancreas divisum
- Duplications
- Anomalies of ducts

Biliary Disorders
- Gallstones
- Choledochal cyst
- Biliary tree anomalies
- Duodenal obstruction
- Parasites
- After endoscopic retrograde cholangiopancreatography

Gastrointestinal Disorders
- Duodenal ulcer, penetrating
- Duplications

Nutritional Problems
- Malnutrition
- Rapid refeeding
- Bulimia

Toxic Conditions
- Alcohol
- Organophosphates
- Carbamates
- Borates
- Yellow scorpion bite

Transplantations
- Renal transplantation
- Graft-versus-host disease

Miscellaneous
- Hereditary
- Idiopathic
- Postoperative

As for congenital pancreatic anomalies, the commonest and most controversial entity has been pancreas divisum (dominant dorsal duct syndrome). Pancreas divisum occurs when the dorsal and ventral pancreatic ducts fail to fuse during embryogenesis. As a result, most of the pancreatic parenchyma is drained by the dorsal duct, with a relative obstruction to flow. Most experts consider this anatomic variant to be a significant cause of relapsing pancreatitis that should be treated by papillotomy.[23] However, other authors consider pancreas divisum a normal anatomic variant that is, at most, an infrequent cause of pancreatic pain. The indication for papillotomy according to these studies should be better defined.[24]

Among the toxic causative factors in childhood pancreatitis, two unrecognized entities have been described recently: organophosphate intoxication[25] and yellow scorpion bite.[26]

CLINICAL SPECTRUM

The cardinal symptom of pancreatitis is abdominal pain, which is most often epigastric in location. Other pain sites include the right upper or lower quadrant or the periumbilical area. The pain is usually sudden in onset; is usually sharp, constant and prolonged; and may last several days. Radiation of the pain is less often observed in childhood and may appear in the back, mid-lower or upper abdomen, and even at the lower anterior chest. Eating is a common aggravating factor. The pain is associated in most patients with nausea and vomiting, which is reported as bilious in about 10% of patients. Fever, when present, is usually mild (<38.5°C).

On physical examination the child appears anxious and quiet and often obtains relief when the trunk is flexed with the knees drawn up. Tachycardia is common, and hypotension and shock may be present in fulminating cases. Mild jaundice may be noted.

The abdomen is often slightly distended, with diffuse, mild tenderness noted. Guarding or localized rebound tenderness, or both, may sometimes appear in the upper abdomen. Bowel sounds are often decreased or absent. An epigastric mass is occasionally palpated in cases of pseudocyst formation. Ascites may be noted, associated with a bluish discoloration at the flanks (Grey Turner's sign) or around the umbilicus (Cullen's sign), indicating the presence of severe necrotizing pancreatitis. Some patients may develop pulmonary findings, including pleural effusion or adult-type respiratory distress syndrome.

DIAGNOSTIC MODALITIES

General Laboratory Tests

An elevated total white blood cell count is a frequent finding in acute pancreatitis, often with increased band forms. The erythrocyte sedimentation rate is often mildly elevated. Severe cases may show hemoconcentration. Damage to the endocrine islets during acute pancreatitis is reflected by transient hyperglycemia in 15 to 25% of patients. This is associated with an excess of glucagon rather than a deficit of insulin.[27] Hypocalcemia occurs in about 15% of patients. Serum alkaline phosphatase and aminotransferase levels may be transiently elevated with mild hyperbilirubinemia. Laboratory findings such as hyperglycemia, hypocalcemia, increased serum lactose dehydrogenase levels, azotemia, hypoalbuminemia, and hypoxemia may reflect more severe disease.

Plasma Levels of Pancreatic Enzymes

Measurement of serum amylase levels is still the most common test used to confirm a diagnosis of acute pancreatitis. Unfortunately, elevated serum total amylase is often associated with various nonpancreatic disorders. Hyperamylasemia often results from amylase of nonpancreatic origin, mainly salivary, or decreased metabolic clearance of this enzyme. Table 68–2 summarizes various conditions that are associated with hyperamylasemia.[28]

Because measuring serum total amylase activity presents a relatively low sensitivity and specificity in the diagnosis of acute pancreatitis, it has been suggested that measurement of urine total amylase levels and calculation of the amylase-creatinine clearance ratio might be a more specific test. However, according to several studies, this ratio offers little advantage over the serum total amylase level and correlates poorly with ultrasonic and clinical evidence of pancreatitis.[29] There appears to be no definite correlation between severity of pancreatitis and the degree of serum amylase level increase.

The measurement of serum pancreatic isoamylase level appears to offer a better clinical test. Multiple approaches have been developed for the discrimination of pancreatic and salivary isoamylases. The most widely used methods are electrophoretic separation and selective inhibition by plant proteins, mainly wheat germ lectins. Determination of pancreatic isoamylase levels is much more specific and sensitive than is total amylase measurement. However, only the production of monoclonal antibodies against pancreatic amylase allowed an approximately 100% separation of this isoenzyme.[30] Recently, monoclonal antibodies against pancreatic amylase have been developed.[31] An international multicenter evaluation of a double monoclonal antibody assay of pancreatic amylase, reported in 1988, revealed excellent selectivity.[32] Recently developed monoclonal antibody test strips may be used as a useful clinical screening tool.[33]

Serum lipase assay has been introduced in many clinical laboratories, because of its greater pancreas

Table 68–2. CONDITIONS ASSOCIATED WITH HYPERAMYLASEMIA

Disease	Likely Predominant Type of Serum Amylase
Pancreatic Diseases	
Pancreatitis—acute or chronic	P
Pseudocyst	P
Pancreatic ascites	P
Pancreatic trauma	
Blunt trauma	P
Abdominal or retroperitoneal surgery	P
Endoscopic retrograde pancreatography	P
Choledocholithiasis	P
Pancreatic cancer	P
Early cystic fibrosis	P
Salivary Diseases	
Parotitis	S
Trauma/surgery	S
Radiation	S
Calculi	S
Gut Diseases	
Perforated bowel	P
Mesenteric infarction	P
Intestinal obstruction	P
Appendicitis	P
Peritonitis	P
Liver Diseases	
Hepatitis	S and P
Cirrhosis	S and P
Alcoholism	S or P
Ectopic Amylase Production by Malignancies	S
Acidosis	
Ketoacidosis	S or P
Nonketotic	S
Renal Failure	S and P
Macroamylasemia	M
Female Genital Tract	
Ruptured ectopic pregnancy	S
Fallopian or ovarian cysts	S
Salpingitis	S
Postoperative	
Extracorporeal circulation	S or P
Nonabdominal surgery	S or P
Miscellaneous	
Pneumonia	S
Cerebral trauma	
Burns	
Abdominal aortic aneurysm	P
Drugs	S or P
Anorexia nervosa and/or bulimia	S

Abbreviations: P = pancreatic isoamylase; S = salivary-type isoamylase; M = macroamylase.

From Pieper-Bigelow C, Strocchi A, Levitt MD: Where does serum amylase come from and where does it go? Gastroenterol Clin North Am 1990; 19:793–810; with permission.

specificity, higher sensitivity, and prolonged elevation in plasma. A recent study shows that serum lipase determination combined with alkaline phosphatase measurement provides better diagnostic performance.[34] However, the degree of lipase increase in plasma also does not reflect the severity of acute pancreatitis.

Plasma immunoreactive cationic trypsin is another useful diagnostic method in pediatric acute pancreatitis. A recent study has clearly demonstrated the advantage of this test compared with serum total amylase determination. Cationic trypsin appeared to rise earlier in the disease process than did amylase and was consistently elevated during the first 5 days[6] (Figs. 68–1 and 68–2). The trypsin assay has the additional advantage of being able to detect active trypsin bound to the plasma inhibitors alpha$_1$-antitrypsin and alpha$_2$-macroglobulin by means of gel filtration techniques. In selected cases, this novel approach has been helpful in defining disease severity in children with acute pancreatitis.[35]

Pancreatic elastase I, measured by radioimmunoassay, showed a higher sensitivity in acute pancreatitis than did lipase, total amylase, or trypsin, mainly during the latter stages of the disease.[36] Phospholipase A_2 is another promising predictive enzyme. Its key role in the pathogenesis of acute pancreatitis has been mentioned earlier. Several studies show a significant correlation between plasma phospholipase A_2 level and severity of disease.[37]

Radiologic Studies

Plain abdominal roentgenograms may reveal changes such as colonic dilatation, obscured psoas margins, ileus, sentinel loop, or a radiolucent halo about the left kidney.

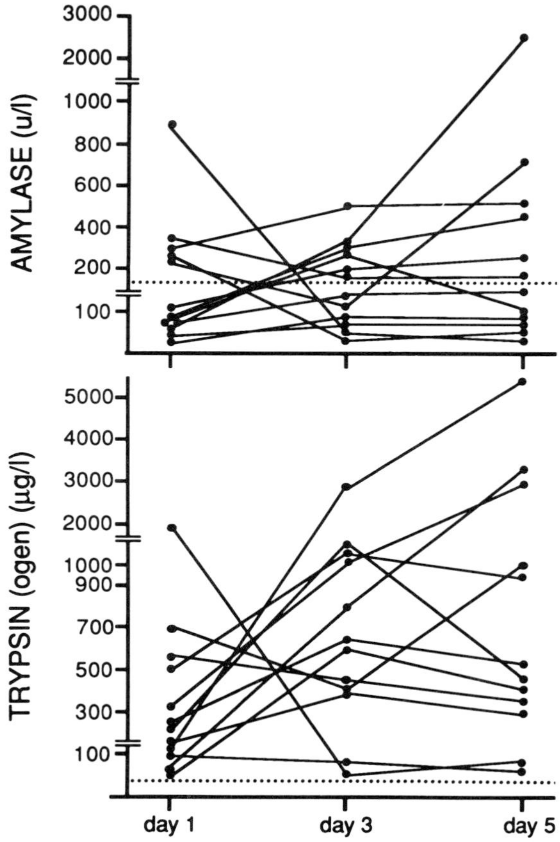

Figure 68–2. Serial determination of serum trypsin(ogen) and amylase levels in 12 patients with acute pancreatitis on days 1, 3, and 5 of hospital admission. In 7 of 12 patients, amylase values were normal on day 1, but became elevated in four patients by day 3. In three patients, serum amylase levels remained within normal range during the entire monitoring period. Serum trypsin(ogen) levels were elevated in all cases on Days 1, 3 and 5. (From Weizman Z, Durie PR: Acute pancreatitis in childhood. J Pediatr 1988; 113:24–29; with permission.)

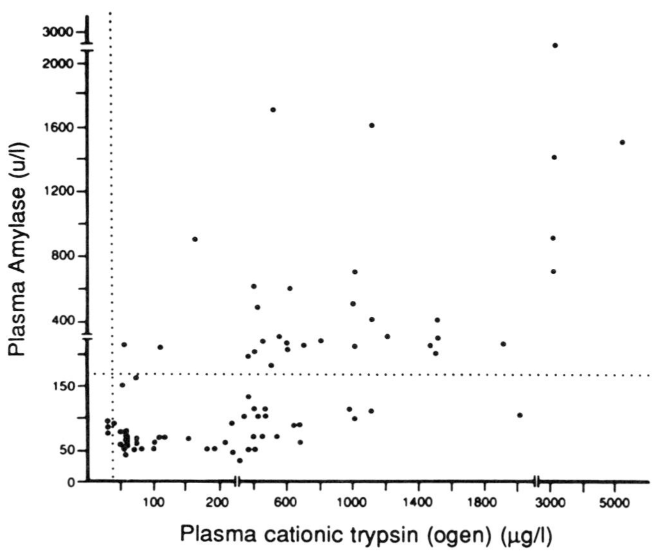

Figure 68–1. Comparison between levels of plasma cationic trypsin(ogen) and amylase (78 points in 32 patients) obtained within 48 hours of presentation. Upper limits of normal (+2 SD) for cationic trypsin(ogen) and amylase are shown. Forty-three data points (representing 11 patients) show elevated trypsin(ogen), but normal amylase values. (From Weizman Z, Durie PR: Acute pancreatitis in childhood. J Pediatr 1988; 113:24–29; with permission.)

Ultrasonography has been used as the radiologic procedure of choice in acute pancreatitis. The most widely used criteria for determining the presence of pancreatitis are based on alteration of pancreatic size, contour, and echotexture.[29] In a series of 36 pediatric cases of acute pancreatitis, this modality revealed abnormalities in 75%, the commonest finding being pancreatic edema or reduced echodensity.[6] However, a recent study has demonstrated that ultrasonographic pancreatic measurements in healthy children vary widely with each age group and also overlap with those of pancreatitis.[38] Evaluation of pancreatic size, configuration, and echogenicity was not reliable in the differentiation of the normal from the acutely inflamed pancreas. It was demonstrated that the presence of a dilated main pancreatic duct is the most useful sonographic feature suggesting acute pancreatitis.[38]

Computed tomography is considered to be the imaging procedure of choice to assess complications of acute pancreatitis, to guide aspiration and drainage procedures, and to provide detailed anatomic information before surgical intervention.[39]

Leukocyte scintigraphy with technetium-99m–hexamethyl propylene amine oxine as leukocyte label has been used recently in the assessment of acute pancreatitis. A correlation between severity of disease and leukocyte infiltration has been demonstrated.[40]

COMPLICATIONS

A detailed list of local and systemic complications of acute pancreatitis is given in Table 68–3.

Cardiovascular complications include hypovolemia and hypotension, sudden death, electrocardiographic changes, and pericardial effusion. Pulmonary complications develop in 10 to 15% of patients and include hypoxemia, atelectasis, pleural effusion, respiratory distress syndrome, and others. Renal failure due to acute tubular necrosis is another significant complication adversely affecting survival.

An inflammatory mass, such as pancreatic phlegmon, abscess, or pseudocyst may develop in the first 2 or 3 weeks following the acute stage. Serial ultrasonographic examinations allow early recognition of these complications. Pseudocyst formation is reported in 5 to 10% of cases. This complication occurs in cases with a wide variety of causes, but most commonly following trauma. Most pseudocysts resolve spontaneously, but some require a surgical drainage procedure. A pancreatic abscess or phlegmon is more likely to develop in severe cases of acute pancreatitis and is less often seen in the pediatric age group (see Chapter 69).

A wide range of mortality data is reported in different series. Mortality rates for acute mild (interstitial) pancreatitis were 5 to 17.5% and for acute fulminating (hemorrhagic) pancreatitis, 86 to 100%. High mortality rates were reported particularly in severe multisystem disorders, such as Reye's syndrome, shock, and sepsis, and in drug-induced pancreatitis.[4, 6]

PROGNOSIS

Most predictors for the severity of acute pancreatitis have been studied in adults, but may be applicable for severe cases in childhood as well. Ranson's multiple criteria[41] is a list of 11 risk factors to help predict severity of disease. Five factors are assessed on admission (increasing age, leukocytosis, hyperglycemia, and elevated serum lactic dehydrogenase and aspartate aminotransferase levels). Six other factors are evaluated within the first 48 hours (hematocrit decrease, azotemia, hypocalcemia, hypoxemia, acidosis, and fluid loss).[41] These criteria have been modified over the years and are also referred to as the *modified Glasgow* or the *Imrie criteria*. Recently, a more complex prognostic index called the *Acute Physiology and Chronic Health Evaluation Score (APACHE-II)* has been introduced.[42] This index is based on 12 physiologic variables, patient age, and history of major organ disease. The APACHE-II has been found to be more sensitive and more specific than previous criteria. Peritoneal tap may provide extra diagnostic information, but its ability to predict severity is similar. Computed tomography is being used with increasing frequency to determine severity of acute pancreatitis, but more studies are required to establish reliable criteria.[43]

Table 68–3. COMPLICATIONS OF ACUTE PANCREATITIS

I Local
- *A* Pancreatic phlegmon
- *B* Pancreatic abscess
- *C* Pancreatic pseudocyst
  - *1* Pain
  - *2* Rupture
  - *3* Hemorrhage
  - *4* Infection
- *D* Pancreatic ascites
  - *1* Disruption of main pancreatic duct
  - *2* Leaking pseudocyst
- *E* Involvement of contiguous organs by necrotizing pancreatitis
  - *1* Massive intraperitoneal hemorrhage
  - *2* Thrombosis of blood vessels
  - *3* Bowel infarction
- *F* Obstructive jaundice

II Systemic
- *A* Pulmonary
  - *1* Pleural effusion
  - *2* Atelectasis
  - *3* Mediastinal abscess
  - *4* Pneumonitis
  - *5* Adult respiratory distress syndrome
- *B* Cardiovascular
  - *1* Hypotension
    - *a* Hypovolemia
    - *b* Hypoalbuminemia
  - *2* Sudden death
  - *3* Nonspecific ST-T changes in electrocardiogram simulating myocardial infarction
  - *4* Pericardial effusion
- *C* Hematologic
  - *1* Disseminated intravascular coagulation (DIC)
- *D* Gastrointestinal hemorrhage*
  - *1* Peptic ulcer disease
  - *2* Erosive gastritis
  - *3* Hemorrhagic pancreatic necrosis with erosion into major blood vessels
  - *4* Portal vein thrombosis, variceal hemorrhage
- *E* Renal
  - *1* Oliguria
  - *2* Azotemia
  - *3* Renal artery and/or renal vein thrombosis
- *F* Metabolic
  - *1* Hyperglycemia
  - *2* Hypertriglyceridemia
  - *3* Hypocalcemia
  - *4* Encephalopathy
  - *5* Sudden blindness (Purtscher's retinopathy)
- *G* Central nervous system
  - *1* Psychosis
  - *2* Fat emboli
- *H* Fat necrosis
  - *1* Subcutaneous tissues (erythematous nodules)
  - *2* Bone
  - *3* Miscellaneous (mediastinum, pleura, nervous system)

*Aggravated by coagulation abnormalities (DIC).

From Greenberg NJ, Toskes PP, Isselbacher KJ: Diseases of the pancreas. *In* Braunwald E, Isselbacher KJ, Petersdorf RG, et al, eds: Harrison's Principles of Internal Medicine. 11th ed. New York, McGraw-Hill, 1987, p. 1375; with permission of McGraw-Hill, Inc.

Several other plasma parameters such as methemalbumin, ribonuclease, antiproteases, complement, and C-reactive protein have been used as predictors of severity in acute pancreatitis.

Some recent studies suggest two more markers with promising results.[43] One marker is urinary trypsinogen activated peptide, a five-amino-acid moiety that is liberated from trypsinogen on activation to trypsin. The other marker is granulocytic elastase. Preliminary data suggest that these two markers may be able to predict severity at the time of diagnosis.

TREATMENT

Treatment of acute pancreatitis consists of aggressive measures to counteract shock, respiratory failure, and protein catabolism and to relieve pain. In most patients, the disease is self-limited and subsides within a few days.

Intravenous fluids and colloids are administered to maintain normal intravascular volume. In addition, complete bowel rest is initiated and nasogastric suction performed in patients with persistent vomiting or ileus. Cimetidine has been proposed as a substitute for nasogastric suction, but its use offers no advantage. Total parenteral nutrition is used in severe cases for nutritional support. Although antibiotic therapy has been used in acute pancreatitis, it is probably of no benefit in most cases. Antibiotic therapy should be considered in patients with a strong clinical suspicion of secondary infection.

Administration of adequate pain relief is essential. In one series, 26% of pediatric patients required narcotic analgesia for control of severe pain.[6] Opiate analgesia may worsen the pain of acute pancreatitis by increasing spasm of the sphincter of Oddi. Because meperidine produces the least increase in intrabiliary pressure of all the pure opiate agonists, it has been recommended as the analgesic of choice for acute pancreatitis. An opiate analgesic with mixed antagonist-agonist actions, such as pentazocine, is another alternative.

Anticholinergic agents have been considered standard therapy in the past. The rationale has been to "put the pancreas at rest" and to decrease flow and enzyme secretion. However, there are no controlled studies demonstrating any advantage of these drugs over placebo.

Recently, a literature search was performed among English language publications to collect and analyze all controlled studies in which a therapeutic agent had been used to treat acute pancreatitis in both humans and laboratory animals.[44] Five therapeutic agents were included: aprotinin (Trasylol), glucagon, 5-fluorouracil, somatostatin, and peritoneal lavage. Whereas 81% of animal studies demonstrated improvement in survival, most well-designed human studies showed no positive effects of any agent on complications or survival. Because many of these studies did not have enough statistical power, the authors concluded that further multicenter studies with sufficient numbers of patients with severe pancreatitis are needed to evaluate these novel therapies in acute pancreatitis. In another study, somatostatin appeared to reduce the local complications of acute pancreatitis.[45]

Table 68–4. CAUSES OF ACUTE PANCREATITIS IN A SERIES OF 61 CHILDREN

Cause	No.	%	Recurrence No.	Recurrence %
Idiopathic	15	25	11	18
Multisystem disease	22	35	0	0
Reye's syndrome	10		0	
Sepsis/shock	6		0	
Hemolytic-uremic syndrome	3		0	
Viral infection	2		0	
SLE	1		0	
Traumatic	9	15	0	0
Structural	6	10	5	9
Biliary (cyst, stone, stricture)	5		4	
Pancreas divisum	1		1	
Metabolic	6	10	3	5
Hyperlipidemia (I, IIa, IV)	3		2	
Cystic fibrosis	2		1	
Hypercalcemia (TPN induced)	1		0	
Drugs (L-asparaginase, acetaminophen)	2	3	0	0
Familial	1	2	1	2
Total	61		20	

SLE, Systemic lupus erythematosus; TPN, total parenteral nutrition.
From Weizman Z, Durie PR: Acute pancreatitis in children. J Pediatr 1988; 113:24–29, with permission.

RELAPSING PANCREATITIS

In relapsing pancreatitis, there are acute bouts of pancreatic inflammation, but pancreatic function and morphology are usually restored between acute attacks. Recurrences are often noted in certain diagnostic categories, such as idiopathic pancreatitis, congenital anomalies of the pancreatobiliary tree, metabolic disorders (hyperlipidemia, hypercalcemia, and others), familial (hereditary) pancreatitis, and cystic fibrosis when pancreatic insufficiency is not fully developed (Table 68–4). Drug-induced disease should be considered as well in recurrent illness.

Endoscopic retrograde cholangiopancreatography is a useful technique in the investigation of relapsing disease. Delineation of pancreatic ductal anatomy may reveal surgically correctable abnormalities.

REFERENCES

1. Hartley RC: Pancreatitis under the age of five years: A report of three cases. J Pediatr Surg 1967; 2:419–423.
2. Sibert JR: Pancreatitis in children: A study in the north of England. Arch Dis Child 1975; 50:443–448.
3. Jordan SC, Ament ME: Pancreatitis in children and adolescents. J Pediatr 1977; 91:211–216.
4. Buntain WL, Wood JB, Wooley MM: Pancreatitis in childhood. J Pediatr Surg 1978; 13:143–149.
5. Tam PKH, Saing H, Irving IM, et al: Acute pancreatitis in children. J Pediatr Surg 1985; 20:58–60.
6. Weizman Z, Durie PR: Acute pancreatitis in childhood. J Pediatr 1988; 113:24–29.

7. Sarles H: Revised classification of pancreatitis—Marseille 1984. Dig Dis Sci 1985; 30:573–574.
8. Seligson U, Cho JW, Ihre T, et al: Evaluation of the diagnosis of pancreatitis. Scand J Gastroenterol 1982; 17:905–911.
9. Nevalainen TJ: Phospholipase A_2 in acute pancreatitis. Scand J Gastroenterol 1988; 23:897–904.
10. Steer ML, Meldolesi J, Figarella C: Pancreatitis: The role of lysosomes. Dig Dis Sci 1984; 29:934–938.
11. Lombardi B, Estes LW, Longnecker DS: Acute hemorrhagic pancreatitis (massive necrosis) with fat necrosis induced in mice by DL-methionine fed with a choline-deficient diet. Am J Pathol 1975; 79:465–476.
12. Lampel M, Kern H: Acute interstitial pancreatitis in the rat induced by excessive doses of a pancreatic secretagogue. Virchows Arch Pathol Anat Histol 1977; 373:97–117.
13. Schoenberg MH, Buchler M, Gaspar M, et al: Oxygen free radicals in acute pancreatitis of the rat. Gut 1990; 31:1138–1143.
14. Nonaka A, Manabe T, Kyogoku T, et al: Changes in lipid peroxide and oxygen radical scavengers in caerulein-induced acute pancreatitis: Imbalance between the offense and defense systems. Digestion 1990; 47:130–137.
15. Cobo JC, Abraham E, Bland RD, et al: Sequential hemodynamic and oxygen transport abnormalities in patients with acute pancreatitis. Surgery 1984; 95:324–330.
16. Kusterer K, Enghofer M, Zendler S, et al: Microcirculatory changes in sodium taurocholate-induced pancreatitis in rats. Am J Physiol 1991; 260:G346–G355.
17. Kaplan MH: Pathogenesis of pancreatitis: A unified concept. Int J Pancreatol 1986; 1:5–8.
18. Toskes PP, Greenberger NJ: Acute and chronic pancreatitis. *In* Cotsonas NJ, ed: Disease a Month. Chicago, Year Book Medical Publishers, 1983, pp 5–48.
19. Mallory A, Kern F: Drug-induced pancreatitis: A critical review. Gastroenterology 1980; 78:813–820.
20. Reye RDK, Morgan G, Baral J: Encephalopathy and fatty degeneration of the viscera: A disease entity in childhood. Lancet 1963; 2:749–752.
21. Ellis GH, Mirkin LD, Mills MC: Pancreatitis and Reye's syndrome. Am J Dis Child 1979; 133:1014–1016.
22. Stoler J, Biller JA, Grand RJ: Pancreatitis in Kawasaki disease. Am J Dis Child 1987; 141:306–308.
23. Warshaw AL: Dominant dorsal duct syndrome—pancreas divisum redefined. J Pediatr Gastroenterol Nutr 1990; 10:281–289.
24. Sugawa C, Walt AJ, Nunez DC, et al: Pancreas divisum: Is it a normal anatomic variant? Am J Surg 1987; 153:62–67.
25. Weizman Z, Sofer S: Acute pancreatitis in children with anticholinesterase insecticide intoxication. Pediatrics 1992; 90:204–206.
26. Sofer S, Shalev S, Weizman Z, et al: Acute pancreatitis in children following envenomation by the yellow scorpion *Leiurus quinquestriatus*. Toxicon 1991; 29:125–129.
27. Donowitz M, Hendler R, Spiro H, et al: Glucagon secretion in acute and chronic pancreatitis. Ann Intern Med 1975; 83:778–783.
28. Pieper-Bigelow C, Strocchi A, Levitt MD: Where does serum amylase come from and where does it go? Gastroenterol Clin North Am 1990; 19:793–810.
29. Cox KL, Ament ME, Sample WF, et al: The ultrasonic and biochemical diagnosis of pancreatitis in children. J Pediatr 1980; 96:407–411.
30. Schmidt E, Schmidt FW: Advances in the enzyme diagnosis of pancreatic diseases. Clin Biochem 1990; 23:383–394.
31. Rosenblum JL: Direct rapid assay of pancreatic isoamylase activity by use of monoclonal antibodies with low affinity for macroamylasemic complexes. Clin Chem 1988; 34:2463–2468.
32. Tietz NW, Burlina A, Gerhardt W, et al: Multicenter evaluation of specific pancreatic isoamylase assay based on double monoclonal antibody technique. Clin Chem 1988; 34:2069–2103.
33. Lorentz K: Isoamylase measurement with monoclonal antibody test strips. J Clin Chem Clin Biochem 1987; 25:309–311.
34. Viel JF, Foucault P, Bureau F, et al: Combined diagnostic value of biochemical markers in acute pancreatitis. Clin Chim Acta 1990; 189:191–198.
35. Durie PR, Gaskin KJ, Ogilvie JE, et al: Serial alterations in the forms of immunoreactive pancreatic cationic trypsin in plasma from patients with acute pancreatitis. J Pediatr Gastroenterol Nutr 1985; 4:199–207.
36. Ventrucci M, Pezzilli R, Naldoni P, et al: Serum pancreatic enzyme behavior during the course of acute pancreatitis. Pancreas 1987; 5:506–509.
37. Buchler M, Malfertheiner P, Schadlich H, et al: Role of phospholipase A_2 in human acute pancreatitis. Gastroenterology 1989; 97:1521–1526.
38. Siegel MJ, Martin KW, Worthington JL: Normal and abnormal pancreas in children: Ultrasound studies. Radiology 1987; 165:15–18.
39. Hill MC, Huntington DK: Computed tomography and acute pancreatitis. Gastroenterol Clin North Am 1990; 19:811–842.
40. Scholmerich J, Schumichen C, Lausen M, et al: Scintigraphic assessment of leukocyte infiltration in acute pancreatitis using technetium-99m–hexamethyl propylene amine oxine as leukocyte label. Dig Dis Sci 1991; 36:65–70.
41. Ranson JHC: Risk factors in acute pancreatitis. Hosp Pract 1985; 20:69–73.
42. Wilson C, Heath DI, Imrie CW: Prediction of outcome in acute pancreatitis: A comparative study of APACHE II, clinical assessment and multiple factor scoring systems. Br J Surg 1990; 77:1260–1264.
43. Steinberg WM: Predictors of severity of acute pancreatitis. Gastroenterol Clin North Am 1990; 19:849–861.
44. Steinberg WM, Schlesselman SE: Treatment of acute pancreatitis: Comparison of animal and human studies. Gastroenterology 1987; 93:1420–1427.
45. Choi RK, Mok F, Zhan WH, et al: Somatostatin in the treatment of acute pancreatitis: A prospective randomized controlled trial. Gut 1989; 30:223–227.

Chapter 69

Chronic Pancreatitis

DAVID PICCOLI

DEFINITION

Chronic pancreatitis is characterized by the progressive, insidious destruction of the pancreas due to repeated bouts of inflammation and necrosis. Repeated episodes of severe, mild, or subclinical pancreatitis cause a progressive loss of pancreatic function, which may result in pancreatic exocrine or endocrine insufficiency. There is some degree of recurrent or persistent abdominal pain, which may not be suggestive of pancreatic origin. The diagnostic categories of acute and chronic pancreatitis have been defined by the Marseille classification,[1, 2] but clinical differentiation can be difficult in the early course of recurrent disease. Many etiologies of chronic pancreatitis are similar to those of acute pancreatitis. There are a significant number of idiopathic cases in both groups. The more common etiologies of chronic pancreatitis are well documented and characterized. The causal role of numerous other diseases rarely reported with chronic pancreatitis is less well documented, and in many cases this may be a coincidental association.

PATHOLOGY

Chronic pancreatitis is characterized histologically by irregular sclerosis of the pancreas, with inflammation and destruction in a focal, segmental, or diffuse pattern. There may be damage to the ducts, with strictures and dilatation, protein deposition, and intraductal calcifications.[3] Proliferating fibroblasts, collagen, and lymphocytes surround pancreatic acini. Exocrine tissue is commonly lost before the islets of Langerhans are destroyed.

There are two morphologic patterns of chronic pancreatitis: chronic calcifying pancreatitis and chronic obstructive pancreatitis. Chronic calcifying pancreatitis results in atrophy of the acini, a marked increase in the interlobular fibrous tissue, and a chronic inflammatory infiltrate around the ducts and lobules (Fig. 69–1). The pancreas is grossly hard, with palpable areas of calcification and calculi. It has been suggested that calcifications are found in more significant cases of pancreatitis.[4] Pseudocyst formation is more common in chronic calcifying pancreatitis. This is the pattern commonly seen in adult alcohol-induced pancreatitis. Chronic calcifying pancreatitis in pediatric patients is most often due to juvenile tropical pancreatitis or hereditary pancreatitis.

In chronic obstructive pancreatitis the ductal epithelium is generally less severely damaged, and pancreatic calculi are uncommon. This type of chronic pancreatitis is more common with congenital or acquired obstructing lesions of the pancreatic duct (Fig. 69–2). It may improve after correction of the obstruction by surgery or sphincterotomy. Chronic obstructive pancreatitis is less common in children than chronic calcifying pancreatitis.

Chronic pancreatitis may occur with mechanical obstruction, with systemic disease, or as an isolated process. A careful history and physical examination can suggest some etiologies, but commonly the diagnosis requires extensive biochemical and radiologic evaluation. Although the range of etiologies parallels that of acute pancreatitis, a distinction should be made between recurrent acute pancreatitis and chronic pancreatitis.[5] This may not be possible early in the course of the disease, when recurrent acute episodes without pancreatic destruction cannot be differentiated from recurrent episodes with progressive damage. Usually, the initial episode of chronic pancreatitis is interpreted and treated as acute pancreatitis, unless there are specific findings to suggest a single chronic disorder (such as diabetes or a family history of pancreatitis).

The differential diagnosis of chronic pancreatitis is shown in Table 69–1. In pediatric patients, the most common etiologies are hereditary pancreatitis, obstructive pancreatitis due to congenital or acquired anomalies, and juvenile tropical pancreatitis. Other systemic diseases have very rarely been associated with chronic pancreatitis, but it is not known if the association is causal or chance. In a number of these associations, the difference between recurrent acute pancreatitis and chronic pancreatitis has not been well documented.

CLINICAL FEATURES

The most common initial clinical events in chronic pancreatitis are repeated episodes of acute pancreatitis. These bouts of acute pancreatitis are superimposed on a damaged pancreas, with progressively diminishing functional capacity. In some patients the exacerbations are not clinically evident. The pain may be absent, or not characteristic of pancreatitis. In these cases there is

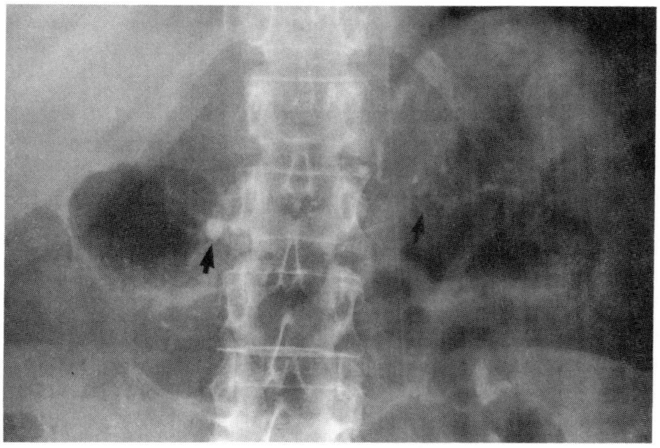

Figure 69–1. Plain film of the upper abdomen revealing multiple calcific densities lying within the pancreas *(arrows)*, due to chronic calcific pancreatitis.

an insidious progression of damage, and the disease becomes evident when the patient develops steatorrhea or diabetes mellitus.

Pain

The majority of children with chronic pancreatitis have either intermittent or chronic abdominal pain. The source of this pain is not well understood. The pain may be felt in the epigastrium, the upper quadrants, the back, or occasionally the periumbilical area. The pain may last, at varying intensities, for up to several weeks. As the disease progresses, the pain gradually lessens, and in many patients it resolves over time. This variable course of chronic pain should be considered when palliative surgery is considered, and when operative results are evaluated.

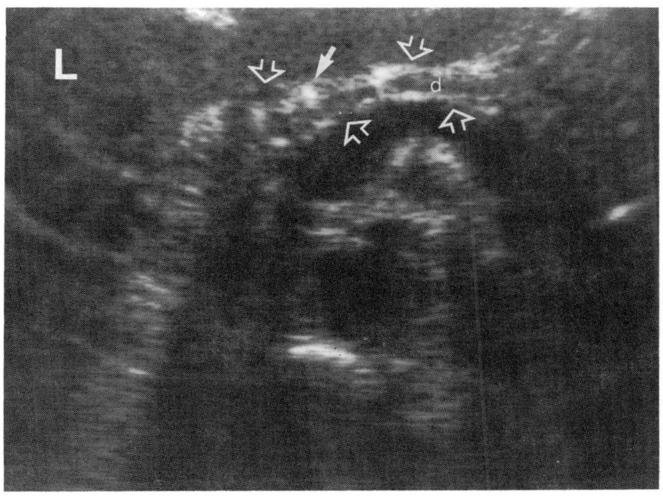

Figure 69–2. Abdominal ultrasound. Transverse sonographic image reveals an echogenic atrophic pancreas *(open arrows)* with a dilated, debris-filled pancreatic duct (*d*) and parenchymal calcifications *(closed arrows)*. *L*, liver.

Table 69–1. DIFFERENTIAL DIAGNOSIS OF CHRONIC PANCREATITIS

Congenital Lesions with Obstruction
Pancreas divisum
Annular pancreas
Choledochal cyst
Choledochocele
Intestinal duplication
Absence of the pancreatic duct
Absence or anomalous insertion of the common bile duct
Stenosis of the ampulla of Vater
Periampullary diverticulum
Anomalous choledochopancreaticoductal junction
Acquired Lesions with Obstruction
Pseudocyst
Gallstone pancreatitis
Benign and malignant tumors
Posttraumatic pancreatitis
Hereditary Disorders
Hereditary pancreatitis, with or without aminoaciduria
Cystic fibrosis
Hyperparathyroidism
Hyperlipoproteinemia types I and V
Mitochondropathy
Alpha$_1$-antitrypsin deficiency
Hemochromatosis
Systemic Diseases
Inflammatory bowel disease (Crohn's disease, ulcerative colitis)
Henoch-Schönlein purpura
Systemic lupus erythematosus
Malnutrition or refeeding
Sarcoidosis
Drug- or Toxin-Associated Pancreatitis
Alcohol
Hyperalimentation
Metabolic Disease
Hypercalcemia
Uremia
Hypertriglyceridemia
Miscellaneous
Juvenile tropical pancreatitis
Fibrosing pancreatitis
Postoperative pancreatitis
Posttransplantation
Idiopathic recurrent pancreatitis

Malabsorption and Failure to Grow

Weight loss and failure to grow are due to a combination of intake limited by postprandial pain and malabsorption. Glycosuria from diabetes mellitus may have a role in some patients. Although the secretion of pancreatic enzymes is diminished early in the course of chronic pancreatitis, clinically evident fat and protein malabsorption occurs only after more than 90% of pancreatic function is lost.[6] The steatorrhea is generally more pronounced than azotorrhea, due to a greater reduction of lipase than proteases early in the disease.[7] Carbohydrate malabsorption is less common, because salivary amylase is present, and pancreatic amylase secretion has a significant functional reserve. Fat-soluble vitamin malabsorption is not common, but nearly half of patients with pancreatic insufficiency have vitamin B_{12} (cobalamin) malabsorption. This is due to decreased degradation of the cobalamin-R protein complexes by pancreatic proteases, resulting in decreased cobalamin binding to intrinsic factor.[8, 9]

Diabetes Mellitus

Abnormalities of glucose metabolism due to the impaired release of both insulin and glucagon may be seen early in the course of the disease. Subsequently, the glucose tolerance test may be abnormal, and eventually overt diabetes may ensue. Diabetes mellitus is commonly the presenting abnormality in juvenile tropical pancreatitis. It is also seen in other forms of calcific pancreatitis, including alcohol-induced disease.

Pancreatic Malignancy

There is an increased incidence of pancreatic malignancy in patients with some types of chronic pancreatitis. This risk varies with different etiologies, which may be due in part to the nature of the chronic inflammation. There is also a reported increase in nonpancreatic malignancies in hereditary pancreatitis.

CHRONIC CALCIFYING PANCREATITIS

Hereditary Pancreatitis

Hereditary pancreatitis was first identified by Comfort and Steinberg in 1952.[10] It is inherited in autosomal dominant fashion, with incomplete penetrance, and is seen in various ethnic groups.[11–15] Hereditary pancreatitis is the second most common inherited disorder of the pancreas, and the second most common cause worldwide of recurrent pancreatitis in childhood.[16]

Pathology

Pathology specimens reflect the typical changes of long-standing chronic calcific pancreatitis, without any specific characteristic abnormalities. There is extensive acinar atrophy and interstitial fibrosis, with relatively normal appearing islet cells. There may be palpable calcifications along the ducts, intraductal stones, and obstruction.

Clinical Manifestations

The onset of pancreatitis occurs predominantly in the first two decades of life. The mean age of onset is 11 years, with a range from 11 months to late in adulthood.[16] Eighty percent of patients will have an initial episode of pancreatitis by 20 years of age.[12, 16, 17] By definition, this diagnosis is confirmed only when another member of the family has idiopathic recurrent pancreatitis. There is no specific characteristic of the clinical course early in this disease. Hereditary pancreatitis is characterized by recurrent attacks of severe upper abdominal pain, usually lasting several days.[18] Typical episodes of pancreatitis recur at intervals ranging from months to years. In general, the pancreatitis is of mild to moderate severity, but symptoms range from mild abdominal pain to severe hemorrhagic pancreatitis. Usually, there is spontaneous resolution of the symptoms after 3 to 8 days. The episodes of pain become less severe with age in many patients.[12] In others, however, the course of the disease is more severe, and surgery is required for palliation of pain and ductal obstruction.

Hereditary pancreatitis is an autosomal dominant disorder, with males and females equally affected. Estimates of penetrance are highly variable, ranging from 50 to 80% in different series.[16, 17] In families in which the prevalence of the disorder is less evident, other etiologies of pancreatitis should be considered. Manifestations are highly variable in different kindreds, and it is not clear that all groups will have a common metabolic or anatomic etiology. Three patterns of autosomal dominant–inherited pancreatitis have been reported: (1) with aminoaciduria of some variable type,[17, 19] (2) without aminoaciduria,[16] and (3) a rare entity with elevated sweat chloride unassociated with clinical cystic fibrosis.[20] These may be entirely different disorders, which will be further delineated only when their biochemical and genetic identities are determined.

Laboratory Evaluation

The diagnosis of hereditary pancreatitis is obvious if multiple family members have developed idiopathic recurrent pancreatitis at an early age. Ultrasound may demonstrate ductular dilatation before calculi are evident.[21] Radiographic examination of the pancreas may demonstrate large round calcifications in the pancreas, even in early childhood. Although calculi with varying distribution may be present in any form of chronic pancreatitis, the identification of large, discrete, rounded calcifications near the larger pancreatic ducts supports the diagnosis. Dilatation of the main duct may occur. Overall, approximately half of all patients demonstrate calcification of the pancreas. The occurrence of biliary calculi is unusual.[22] Endoscopic retrograde cholangiopancreatography (ERCP) may provide useful information by demonstrating large intraductal stones or dilatation.[23] Ultrasound and computerized tomography (CT) may demonstrate a shrunken and fibrotic pancreas.

The presence of increased urinary excretion of certain amino acids such as cysteine, lysine, arginine, glycine, or ornithine has been reported in some kindreds,[17, 19, 24, 25] but is absent in others.[16, 26] The presence of aminoaciduria does not appear to have an effect on the course of the disease, but may be useful diagnostically.

Complications

Hemorrhagic pancreatitis is a rare but severe complication of the recurrent episodes of pancreatitis.[17] Pancreatic pseudocysts are reported to occur in 5 to 50% of patients,[12, 23, 27] but appear to be nearly uniform in some kindreds.[28] Portal vein and splenic vein thrombosis have also been reported.[29] A rare patient has presented with pancreatic ascites.[30]

Pancreatic insufficiency may occur in up to half of patients, as demonstrated by a fecal fat collection, oral bentiromide absorption test, or pancreozymin-secretin stimulation test.[12, 16] Diabetes mellitus has been reported in up to 10 to 25% of patients with hereditary pancreatitis.[12, 16] Another 25% have abnormalities of the oral glucose tolerance test.[12, 16] In general, pancreatic diabetes is not clinically significant in the first two decades.

There is a significantly increased rate of malignancy in patients with hereditary pancreatitis.[16] Pancreatic adenocarcinoma has been reported at increased frequency in patients with hereditary pancreatitis, and also in family members without pancreatitis. Furthermore, there appears to be an increased incidence of other abdominal tumors in these kindreds.[16, 17]

Treatment

Treatment of the acute pancreatitis is similar to the supportive care administered for other etiologies of nonobstructive pancreatitis. Empiric therapy with low-fat diets and pancreatic supplementation has been recommended without controlled evaluations. Patients should avoid alcohol and other pancreatic toxins. In addition, medications with pancreatitis as a recognized side effect should be administered only when alternative therapies are unavailable. In cases with intractable pain or severe recurrent episodes of pancreatitis, an ERCP may delineate a clear obstructing ductular lesion that may respond to surgical intervention.

Approximately 20% of patients with significant hereditary pancreatitis have required surgery for attempted palliation of pain. Numerous procedures have been employed, including cholecystectomy with sphincterotomy, sphincteroplasty, caudal pancreatectomy, Puestow pancreaticojejunostomy,[31] and total pancreatectomy. Commonly patients require more than one procedure for palliation of pain, and overall results have been disappointing in many instances (see later).

Juvenile Tropical Pancreatitis

Juvenile tropical pancreatitis is the most common form of chronic pancreatitis in children, although it is rarely, if ever, seen far from the equator. It has been variously termed *fibrocalculous pancreatic diabetes, nutritional pancreatitis,* and *Afro-Asian pancreatitis.* Over 2,000 cases have been reported, which represent only a fraction of the incidence of this disease.[32–35] Juvenile tropical pancreatitis was first reported by Zuidema in 1955.[36] It has subsequently been identified in Asia, Africa, and South America, and the largest series has been reported by GeeVarghese and Pitchumoni from Kerala, India.[32, 35] The disease is characterized by chronic abdominal pain, diabetes mellitus, and pancreatic calculi. Although the pathophysiology of this disorder is not well characterized, malnutrition and diet in developing nations are clearly involved.[37]

Pathology

In juvenile tropical pancreatitis the pancreas is nodular, shrunken, and fibrotic, with multiple palpable calculi. There is ductular dilatation and stenosis, with variably sized intraductal stones composed chiefly of calcite.[38] Periductular fibrosis is common. The islets of Langerhans are initially well preserved, but later become atrophic. As is true of other etiologies of chronic calcifying pancreatitis, pseudocyst formation is common,[39] and pancreatic carcinoma occurs at increased frequency.[40]

Clinical Features

Juvenile tropical pancreatitis usually begins with nonspecific chronic abdominal pain late in the first decade of life. Three fourths of patients will have pain by age 25, although rare patients will remain pain free.[32] This pain usually precedes the onset of pancreatic diabetes, which typically occurs in the second decade or later. Initially the pain may be characteristic of pancreatitis, with associated vomiting. Later, the pain decreases or resolves, sometimes before the onset of diabetes mellitus. This pancreatic diabetes is secondary to generalized pancreatic destruction and is therefore distinct from insulin-dependent type I juvenile diabetes. It is brittle, with episodes of hypo- and hyperglycemia. Although some patients are highly responsive to insulin, insulin resistance has been identified. Microvascular complications do occur in pancreatic diabetes,[41] but other complications, such as ketosis and neuropathy, occur less commonly than in type I diabetes.

The clinical symptoms of exocrine pancreatic insufficiency are not striking, predominantly because of the low intake of fat and protein in the population afflicted with juvenile tropical pancreatitis.[32] If a high-fat diet is administered, the majority will demonstrate steatorrhea.

Etiology and Pathogenesis

Juvenile tropical pancreatitis is clearly associated with protein malnutrition, but the disease incidence does not coincide with the syndrome of kwashiorkor. In addition to protein deficiency, other nutritional deficiencies or toxins may play a role in the pathogenesis of this disorder. Cassava root is a carbohydrate source consumed in areas where tropical pancreatitis is endemic. The disease is uncommon in underdeveloped areas where rice is the staple carbohydrate. Cassava contains toxic cyanogenic glycosides that release hydrocyanic acid in the stomach, and animal models support the role of cassava in pancreatic damage.[42] Other studies have implicated sorghum or a low-fat diet itself.[43] Differences in food preparation and local dietary customs, as well as mineral, fat, and protein intake, may account for the variable incidence of this disease.

Diagnosis

The findings in juvenile pancreatitis are typical of other forms of chronic calcifying pancreatitis. The serum amylase results are variable and are commonly normal in advanced disease. The diagnosis in children from endemic areas is suggested by the association of diabetes mellitus and recurrent abdominal pain. Chronic calcifying pancreatitis can be identified on abdominal radiographs when the disease is advanced. Abdominal ultrasound and CT demonstrate smaller calcifications not evident on radiographs. Experience with ERCP is limited, but abnormalities of the ductular system are present. Steatorrhea may not be evident unless the diet includes sufficient fat. The pancreozymin-secretin stimulation test demonstrates a decrease in both volume and enzyme output. In younger patients, a high index of suspicion is necessary, as the symptoms and physical examination are nonspecific.

Treatment

Therapy is directed toward the repletion of nutritional deficits and the management of chronic pain. Diabetes may be treated with insulin or at times with oral hypoglycemic agents. Pancreatic enzyme supplementation will improve symptomatic steatorrhea, if present. Surgical therapy of tropical pancreatitis is complicated by the nutritional status of the patient, concomitant diabetes, and the incidence of pancreatic malignancy.[39, 44, 45]

CHRONIC OBSTRUCTIVE PANCREATITIS

Pancreas Divisum

Pancreas divisum results from the failure of the dorsal and ventral pancreas to fuse during the first trimester of gestation (see Chapter 64). As a result, the majority of the exocrine pancreatic flow enters the duodenum through the relatively smaller duct of Santorini and the accessory papilla. This anatomic variation is present in 5 to 14% of autopsy cases[46–49] and is found in 2 to 6% of patients undergoing endoscopic retrograde pancreatography.[50–55] The association of this relatively common lesion with chronic abdominal pain and chronic pancreatitis is still quite controversial. The association with pancreatitis has been reported in several series[50–53] but not in others.[56–59] In one ERCP series, the association of idiopathic pancreatitis with pancreas divisum was 25.6%, compared to a 5.8% overall incidence, suggesting a role for this lesion in pancreatic damage.[50] Other large series have demonstrated no difference in the incidence of pancreatitis.[60] Pancreatography does not demonstrate evidence of ductular dilatation or obstruction in most patients with pancreas divisum. It has been suggested that therapy in adults be attempted only when obvious duct dilatation is present.[60] Alternatively, opposing recommendations have been offered for symptomatic children[61] and adults without dilatation.[62] In an attempt to refine the indication for surgery, pancreatic stimulation tests have been used during imaging to demonstrate functional dilatation and to evoke a clinical response.[63] Ampullary manometry may give information about functional abnormalities of the sphincter.[64] Preliminary evidence suggests that the intraductal pressure at the minor sphincter is higher than that recorded in the major papilla in pancreas divisum.[65]

Histologic evidence for a focal pancreatitis has been provided from surgical specimens. In some cases, the area of the dorsal pancreas, drained through the accessory papilla, has demonstrated pancreatitis, while the ventral pancreas was spared.[50, 58]

The incidental finding of pancreas divisum without pancreatitis warrants conservative treatment. In the setting of recurrent pancreatitis, surgical and endoscopic approaches have been taken, including sphincteroplasty, sphincterotomy, stent placement, and pancreaticoduodenectomy.[52, 62, 66–71] The result of these interventions is variable. Surgery is most likely to provide clinical benefit if the pancreas divisum is associated with severe bouts of recurrent pancreatitis, or ductular dilatation, without any other etiology. Preoperative ERCP or intraoperative pancreatography[72] is essential to identify the lesion. If pancreas divisum is not correctly identified preoperatively, a sphincterotomy of only the major papilla may be erroneously performed.[50]

OTHER ETIOLOGIES OF CHRONIC PANCREATITIS

Hyperlipidemia

Familial hypertriglyceridemia is a well-established cause of recurrent acute pancreatitis that may also rarely result in chronic pancreatitis.[73] Approximately 30% of patients with type I disease, 15% with type IV disease, and 30 to 40% with type V disease have an associated acute pancreatitis, which may be recurrent. Pancreatic insufficiency has been reported only in type I and type V disease.[74, 75] Although the mechanism for injury is not established, it has been hypothesized that the lipolysis of excessive triglycerides in the pancreas results in the release of toxic triglycerides, with subsequent destruction.[76]

Diagnosis should be considered when there is a family history of hyperlipidemia and in patients with elevated triglyceride levels during acute pancreatitis. Although clinical and experimental data suggest that pancreatic damage can result from hyperlipidemia, it has been reported that pancreatitis itself may elevate plasma lipid levels.[77] Therefore, confirmation of the diagnosis should be attempted after the episode of pancreatitis has resolved.

Hyperparathyroidism and Hypercalcemia

The association of severe hypercalcemia and acute pancreatitis has been recognized in hyperparathyroidism, vitamin D intoxication, renal failure, total parenteral nutrition, and familial hypercalcemia.[78–80] The effect of moderate chronic hypercalcemia on the pancreas is not understood as well. In animal models, there is decreased volume and bicarbonate secretion in response to hormonal stimulation.[81] Patients with hyperparathyroidism may have limited or no hypocalcemia when evaluated during an acute attack of pancreatitis. Hypercalcemia is again evident after recovery. Pancreatic calculi and pancreatic insufficiency rarely result from repeated episodes of acute pancreatitis.

Alpha$_1$-Antitrypsin Deficiency

The rare association of chronic pancreatitis and alpha$_1$-antitrypsin deficiency has been reported.[82] The importance of this association in the pathogenesis of chronic pancreatitis is unclear.

Fibrosing Pancreatitis

Fibrosing pancreatitis is a rare idiopathic condition that may present with recurrent abdominal pain and biliary tract obstruction due to extrinsic compression by the head of the pancreas.[83–85] It should be considered during the evaluation for jaundice. Ultrasound demonstrates a dilated extrahepatic biliary tree with compression and tapering at the level of the pancreatic head.[85] The diagnosis can be confirmed by ERCP.[86] A choledochojejunostomy will relieve the obstruction.

Cystic Fibrosis

Recurrent acute pancreatitis may occur in a small number of patients with cystic fibrosis who do not have complete pancreatic insufficiency (see Chapter 66). With time, however, exocrine function may be lost, with subsequent pancreatic insufficiency.[87, 88]

Sclerosing Cholangitis

Sclerosing cholangitis has been associated with chronic pancreatitis.[89–91] The pancreatic damage is presumably due to chronic obstruction of the pancreatic duct at the level of the ampulla or via an abnormal choledochopancreaticoductal junction.

Congenital Obstructing Lesions

A number of congenital lesions of the pancreas, pancreatic ducts, bile duct, ampulla,[92] or the choledochopancreaticoductal junction[93, 94] have been reported to cause chronic obstructing pancreatitis. In each of these some combination of chronic obstruction and possible bile reflux has been postulated to cause chronic pancreatic damage.[11] Annular pancreas has been associated with chronic pancreatitis.[95, 96] Choledochal cyst, with or without an anomalous choledochopancreaticoductal junction, may result in recurrent acute pancreatitis or chronic pancreatitis.[94] Cysts in the duodenum or the head of the pancreas can result in chronic pancreatitis.[97] Benign and malignant tumors can present similarly. The role of chronic obstruction is supported by the finding that pancreatic stent placement may result in chronic pancreatitis.[98]

Posttraumatic Pancreatitis

Trauma to the pancreas usually results in acute pancreatitis. In severe cases, or those complicated by ductal rupture or pseudocyst, there may be localized fibrosis or chronic pancreatitis.[99] Although surgery is occasionally necessary to remove the damage, the majority of the gland is normal, and there is usually spontaneous resolution without chronic symptoms.

Mitochondrial Disorders

Chronic calcifying pancreatitis and pseudocyst formation have been reported in a child with cytochrome c oxidase deficiency and a mitochondrial myopathy.[100]

Inflammatory Bowel Disease

Chronic pancreatitis has been associated with both Crohn's disease and ulcerative colitis in rare instances.[101, 102]

Hyperalimentation

Chronic pancreatitis has been reported in patients on chronic hyperalimentation.[103] This may be due in part to nutritional deficiencies associated with intravenous feeding, underlying disease, or concomitant medical therapy.

DIAGNOSIS OF CHRONIC PANCREATITIS

Establishing the diagnosis of chronic pancreatitis can be difficult. In cases that present with apparent recurrent acute pancreatitis, noninvasive structural studies may lead to the diagnosis. In other cases with a presentation of chronic pain or pancreatic insufficiency, a clinical suspicion coupled with multiple studies may be required, and chronic disease may be evident only late in the natural history of the disease.

Serologic Tests

Because there is less inflammation than is usually found in acute pancreatitis, serum amylase and lipase measurements are not generally useful for the evaluation of chronic pancreatitis.[104] Tests of pancreatic function, rather than inflammation, are required for diagnosis.

Studies of Pancreatic Morphology

Abdominal Radiograph. A plain abdominal radiograph is useful if pancreatic calculi are present or if the mass effect of a large pseudocyst is evident.[105] These studies are relatively insensitive, but may be specific if positive (see Fig. 69–1).

Abdominal Ultrasound. Ultrasound should be the first imaging modality employed for the evaluation of chronic pancreatitis. Real time ultrasound provides excellent visualization of the pancreas in most patients and can provide information about other associated organs, including the hepatobiliary system. Pancreatic size can be accurately assessed by ultrasound.[106] The pancreas may become enlarged in an acute inflammatory process and may remain so for some time after symptoms have resolved.[107, 108] With time, the pancreas atrophies and eventually is smaller than normal[109, 110] (see Fig. 69–2). There is a heterogeneous pattern with areas of increased echogenicity and irregular contour. In some patients the atrophic gland is difficult to distinguish from surrounding retroperitoneal tissue.[111, 112] Calcifications may be evident on ultrasound, and newer technology has provided visualization of the pancreatic duct dilatation[113–115] (Fig. 69–3). Pancreatic cysts, pseudocysts, and abscesses are

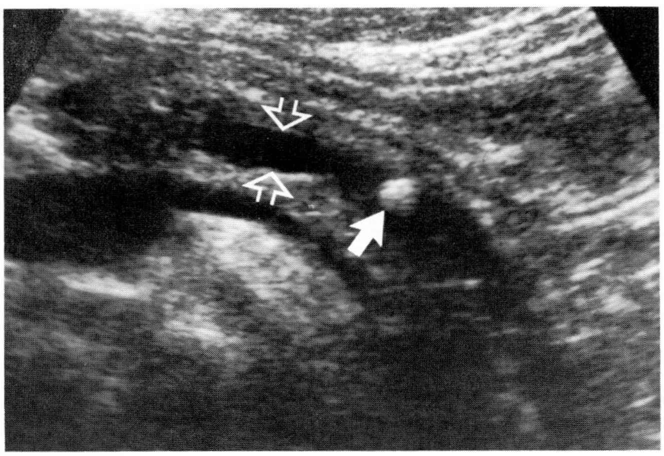

Figure 69–3. Abdominal ultrasound. Transverse sonographic image reveals a stone *(closed arrow)* lying within a dilated pancreatic duct *(open arrows)* in the body of the pancreas.

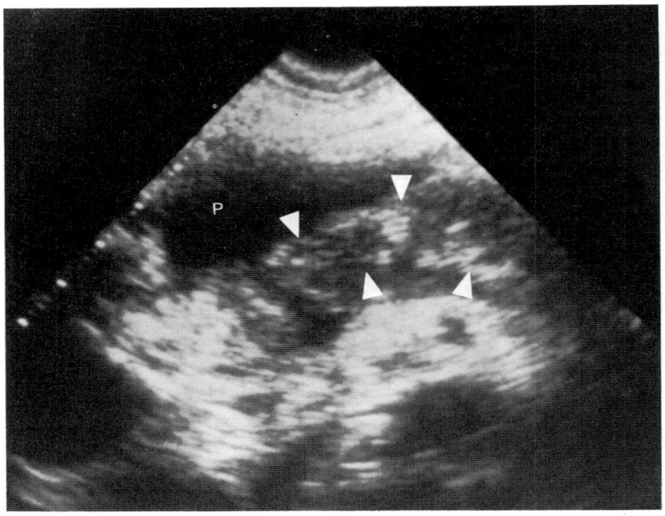

Figure 69–4. Abdominal ultrasound. Transverse image through the pancreatic head and body reveals multiple echogenic foci within the pancreas *(arrows)* and a fluid collection within the lesser sac, representing a pancreatic pseudocyst (*P*).

usually detected by ultrasound[116] (Fig. 69–4). Furthermore, retroperitoneal and hepatobiliary disease may provide information on the etiology of the pancreatitis. Finally, ultrasound guidance is frequently employed for pseudocyst and abscess drainage.[117–120] Although comparative studies have suggested that CT has better sensitivity and specificity in chronic pancreatic disease, the smaller size and lower incidence of significant obesity in pediatric populations allow high-quality sonographic imaging.

Abdominal Computerized Tomography. CT can detect calculi and calcifications that are not evident by other imaging studies[121] (Fig. 69–5). Additionally, CT may discriminate between a pancreatic pseudocyst and

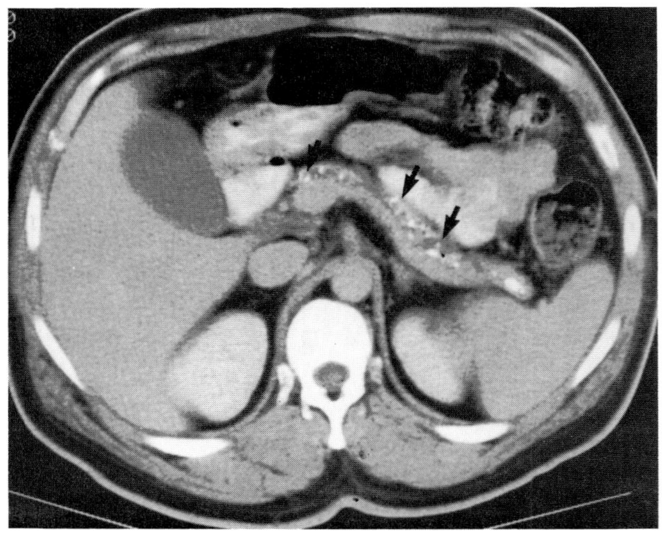

Figure 69–5. Abdominal CT scan. Transverse image through the pancreas reveals multiple discrete calcifications *(arrows)* throughout the entire pancreas.

an inflammatory phlegmon. Like ultrasound, it may be used to guide needle aspirations. Because of the exposure to radiation and the increased cost of CT, ultrasound should be the screening method of choice, followed by CT when the sonographic imaging is unsatisfactory.

Magnetic Resonance Imaging. Magnetic resonance imaging (MRI) is increasingly available for pancreatic imaging. Recent advances in imaging speed and newer imaging protocols have resulted in images of comparable quality to conventional CT without radiation exposure.[122] Techniques for fat suppression appear to allow further definition of pancreatic disease.[123] The importance of this modality will certainly increase in the near future.

Endoscopic Retrograde Cholangiopancreatography. The sensitivity and specificity of ERCP in adults with chronic pancreatitis have been reported to range from 71 to 93% and 89 to 100%, respectively.[124–126] Newer technology and pediatric endoscopes have allowed increased availability of this technique for pediatric populations.[127] The ERCP provides the most definitive information about the pancreatic ductular anatomy. Identification of dilatation and strictures, intraductular calcifications, and anomalies of insertion into the duodenum can best be identified by ERCP. Pancreas divisum can be detected primarily by ERCP (although dilated ducts have been identified by CT and ultrasound). Finally, therapeutic interventions such as dilation and sphincteroplasty can be performed at the time of the diagnostic study. Generally, ERCP is the last nonsurgical diagnostic test employed due to the expense, radiation, and technical difficulties involved. Nonetheless, it may be the only diagnostic test to demonstrate disease in noncalcified chronic pancreatitis.

Studies of Pancreatic Function. Pancreatic exocrine function can be quantitatively assessed via direct intubation and drainage of the duodenum during hormonal stimulation (Table 69–2). The data on the specificity of the less invasive indirect function tests are conflicting and inconclusive, given the variety of patients, control groups, and dosage schedules. In general, these noninvasive tests have been compared to the standard CCK-secretin test. Overall, the noninvasive tests have a sensitivity of 80 to 90% in patients with severe chronic pancreatitis and steatorrhea, but only 50% in patients with mild or early disease, despite a significant reduction in pancreatic secretory capacity. Details of pancreatic function tests are available in Chapter 65.

Table 69–2. DIAGNOSTIC TESTS FOR PANCREATIC FUNCTION IN CHRONIC PANCREATITIS

Direct stimulation tests
CCK-secretin test
Indirect tests via intubation
Lundh test
Duodenal aspiration
Indirect tests without intubation
72-hour fecal fat determination
NBT-PABA (bentiromide) test
Fluorescein dilaurate test
Fecal chymotrypsin determination
Labeled triglyceride breath tests
Dual-labeled Schilling's test
Serum evocative tests

The CCK-secretin test and its numerous modifications have been used to estimate pancreatic function for decades.[128–130] To calculate and correct for loss of duodenal contents, nonabsorbable markers have been employed with good success. However, the technical difficulties involved with performing this study in infants and children have led to the increased use of less invasive testing.

Other intubation tests have no significant advantage over the CCK-secretin stimulation test. The modified Lundh test has been used to assess physiologic pancreatic function in response to a standardized meal.[131, 132] Timed postprandial duodenal aspirates are assayed for proteolytic activity. The test cannot assess the volume of secretion or bicarbonate release and is less sensitive than the CCK-secretin test. Direct intubation of the duodenum and aspiration of stimulated secretions may be a useful screen in some patients in whom endoscopy or intubation is used for other indications.

Noninvasive testing has clear advantages in younger patients. A quantitative fecal fat determination is technically simple and readily available as a screening test. It is important that the fat intake be standardized and quantified during the evaluation. Unfortunately, the collection can be difficult in some instances, and the assay has limited sensitivity. The determination of fecal chymotrypsin in random or timed specimens has also been used to estimate pancreatic function.[133, 134]

The n-benzoyl-L-tyrosol-*p*-aminobenzoic acid test (NBT-PABA, or bentiromide test) uses a synthetic dipeptide linked to PABA for a simple estimation of chymotrypsin activity, which specifically cleaves the PABA moiety. The PABA is absorbed and excreted in the urine, where it is readily assayed.[135] Recently, modifications of this test using serum levels and different dosage schedules in infants have improved the reliability of the evaluation.[136]

In adults with severe pancreatic insufficiency, the sensitivity of the NBT-PABA test compared to the CCK-secretin test is 71%; in mild to moderate disease the sensitivity is only 46%.[137] Several foods, medications, and topical sunscreens can interfere with the reliability of this examination. A similar noninvasive test is the pancreolauryl test, or fluorescein dilaurate test (FDL). Fluorescein dilaurate is a synthetic ester that is hydrolyzed by pancreatic arylesterases, and the free fluorescein is absorbed and excreted in the urine. In both the FDL and the NBT-PABA a control meal using the free tracer (fluorescein or PABA) can estimate the kinetics of absorption, hepatic conjugation, and excretion, which may improve the sensitivity of these tests.

The dual-labeled Schilling test is abnormal in half of patients with exocrine pancreatic insufficiency.[8, 9] Cobalamin (vitamin B_{12}) is bound to R protein until it is partially degraded by pancreatic proteases. In pancreatic insufficiency it is not released from R protein, and thus cannot bind to intrinsic factor. Separately labeled [^{57}Co]-cobalamin-intrinsic factor and [^{58}Co]-cobalamin-R pro-

Table 69–3. THERAPY FOR CHRONIC PANCREATITIS

Pain control—narcotics
Diet
Pancreatic enzyme replacement
Insulin
Surgery
Sphincterotomy/sphincteroplasty
Drainage procedures (e.g., Puestow, Whipple)
Pseudocyst management
Limited or extensive resection
Transplantation

tein are administered orally with unlabeled cobinamide (which is given to bind any endogenous R protein) and intrinsic factor. Normally both labeled forms are absorbed in equal amounts. If the urinary assay of radiolabeled cobalamin-R protein is significantly lower than that of cobalamin-intrinsic factor (low $^{58}Co/^{57}Co$), there is evidence for pancreatic insufficiency.

THERAPY FOR CHRONIC PANCREATITIS

Therapy should be directed toward the alleviation of the symptoms and complications of chronic pancreatitis (Table 69–3).

Pain Control

During painful attacks, treatment should be similar to that for acute pancreatitis (see Chapter 68). In late chronic pancreatitis the recurrent episodes are less severe, unless complicated by pseudocyst or obstruction.

Chronic recurrent pain of significant degree is sometimes seen in chronic pancreatitis.[138] This may result in decreased intake and failure to grow. If routine analgesics are not effective, narcotics may be required for pain control. Attempts to destroy the pain pathway through the celiac plexus have produced variable results.[139] In some patients pain is decreased by the administration of pancreatic enzymes.[140, 141] This may be due to a feedback inhibition of pancreatic enzyme secretion.[142] For patients with intractable pain, surgery may be required (see later).

Malabsorption

The goal of dietary therapy should be to decrease symptoms and improve the overall nutritional status of the patient.[143] Some patients with pain will respond to a limited fat intake with a reduction in steatorrhea, bloating, and diarrhea. The diet should have sufficient calories and protein to provide for growth and maintenance. Smaller frequent meals and snacks may be required in some patients. Pancreatic enzyme supplementation (see Chapter 66) will result in a reduction in steatorrhea and azotorrhea.[144] In patients who do not improve on therapy, increased doses may be required. Since lipase is inactivated at pH less than 4, and since bicarbonate secretion is decreased in chronic pancreatitis, there may be limited active enzyme in the small intestine in some patients. Acid blockade with cimetidine can cause increased bioavailability of the pancreatic supplementation.[145] Enteric microencapsulation with a pH-dependent polymer is also used to improve delivery of active enzyme to the duodenum.[146, 147] If these measures do not improve steatorrhea, consideration should be given to the possibility of concomitant intestinal mucosal disease.

In patients with significant nutritional deficits or malnutrition, parenteral nutrition may be required to supplement enteral intake.[148, 149] In malnourished patients with limited tolerance for dietary fat, medium-chain triglycerides should be considered. Continuous nasogastric alimentation with elemental formulas may be required in some patients.

Pseudocysts

Space-occupying lesions of the pancreas occur in both acute and chronic pancreatitis. A pseudocyst is a cystic structure, commonly located in the lesser sac, that usually communicates with the pancreatic duct. The fluid contains high concentrations of pancreatic enzymes. Pseudocysts may occur insidiously and be found throughout the upper abdomen. A pseudocyst may be greater than a liter in volume, producing pain and palpable abdominal fullness. More commonly, the diagnosis is made by ultrasound or CT (Fig. 69–6). The abdominal CT is useful to distinguish a pseudocyst from an inflammatory pancreatic phlegmon. A pancreatic phlegmon is a mass of inflamed pancreas often containing patchy areas of necrosis. Bacterial infection of the devitalized tissue within and adjacent to the pancreas may be life threatening. A pancreatic abscess may have

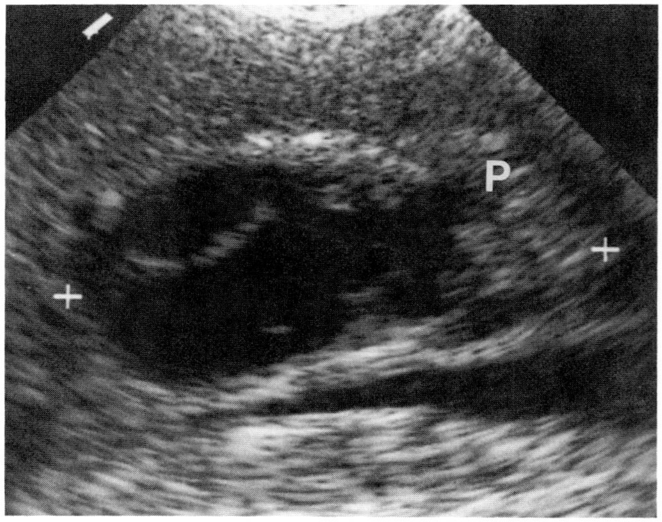

Figure 69–6. Abdominal ultrasound. Sagittal image through the pancreatic head and body reveals a large complex fluid collection posterior to the pancreas (*P*).

a similar appearance to a pseudocyst or phlegmon, but a patient with an abscess will have more signs of toxicity and sepsis.[150, 151] A pseudocyst can obstruct the pancreatic or common duct. Rupture of the cyst into the peritoneal cavity or an adjacent viscus can occur, with subsequent hemorrhage or peritonitis. Although the majority of pancreatic pseudocysts will resolve, those that persist longer than 6 weeks may require drainage.[152] This can be performed under ultrasound or CT guidance, or at laparotomy. Pseudocysts occurring in chronic pancreatitis may not carry the same risk as those in acute pancreatitis. Internal drainage, external drainage, and excision are the operative options for pseudocysts. Excision is commonly not technically possible. Internal drainage is the treatment of choice. An anastomosis is commonly made from the cyst to the jejunum, duodenum, or stomach, and the drained cyst cavity progressively obliterates. Recurrence can occur, but is not common.

Diabetes

The diabetes associated with chronic pancreatitis should be treated if there is significant glycosuria. In some patients, oral hypoglycemic agents may provide satisfactory control. In many others, however, insulin is required. Patients with pancreatic diabetes may be fairly brittle, with severe hypoglycemic episodes, even on small doses of insulin.[153] This may be due in part to a decreased glucagon secretion from the pancreas.[154] Because patients with diabetes secondary to chronic pancreatitis appear to have fewer vascular complications than those with idiopathic diabetes, therapy should be directed toward moderate control of blood glucose rather than normal blood sugar levels.

Renal Stones

Hyperoxaluria is a well-recognized complication of fat malabsorption. This can be treated by restriction of oxalate in the diet, calcium supplementation, pancreatic enzyme replacement, or aluminum supplementation. Actual renal stone formation in these patients is rare.

Obstruction of the Hepatobiliary Tree

Obstruction of the distal common duct may result in cholestasis, jaundice, biliary cirrhosis, or cholangitis.[155, 156] At times, these may be the presenting signs that alert the clinician to the possibility of chronic pancreatitis.[86]

Surgical Therapy

Surgical therapy is indicated for patients with chronic intractable pain, for obstruction of the common duct, and for complications of pseudocysts.[157, 158] In many patients, pain will improve with time; therefore, surgery should be used conservatively. Drainage procedures are employed if the preoperative studies demonstrate dilated pancreatic ducts. In selected cases, therapeutic ERCP can remove intraductal stones, place endoprostheses and nasobiliary drains, and perform sphincterotomies.[159, 160] A reduction in pain following an ERCP procedure may predict which patients will have favorable outcomes from definitive surgical drainage procedures.[161] A sphincterotomy can be performed endoscopically or surgically, if local distal obstruction is identified. For definitive drainage, the Puestow pancreaticojejunostomy uses an opened Roux-en-Y segment of jejunum sewn over the longitudinally opened main pancreatic duct.[31, 162] In cases of obstruction in the head of the pancreas that cannot be relieved by sphincteroplasty or stent placement, a Whipple pancreatoduodenectomy is required. A limited resection can be employed for local damage, especially if it is confined to the tail of the pancreas. In patients with severe unremitting pain, subtotal pancreatectomy may be required, although both exocrine and endocrine insufficiency may result. For patients with end organ failure (endocrine more than exocrine), pancreatic transplantation has recently become available.[163, 164] Overall, many patients will experience some significant relief of pain via operative or endoscopic therapy, but the wide variety of operative approaches and the reoperation rate signify that results are commonly suboptimal.[165] Efforts continue to identify which populations of patients are likely to benefit from surgery.

REFERENCES

1. Sarles H: Pancreatic symposium Marseilles. *In* Sarles H, ed: Biblotheca Gastroenterologica. fsc 7. Basel, New York, Karger, 1967.
2. Sarles H: Revised classification of pancreatitis—Marseille 1984. Dig Dis Sci 1985; 39:573–574.
3. Gyr KE, Singer MV, Sarles H: Pancreatitis: Concepts and Classification. Elsevier, Amsterdam, Excerpta Medica, 1984, pp xxi–xxv.
4. Scuro LA, Cavallini G, Benini L, et al: Pancreatic calcifications in patients with chronic pancreatitis. A sign of long-lasting or severe disease? Int J Pancreatol 1990; 6:139–150.
5. Sarles H, Bernard JP, Johnson C: Pathogenesis and epidemiology of chronic pancreatitis. Annu Rev Med 1989; 40:453–468.
6. DiMagno EP, Malagelada JR, Go VLW: Relationship between alcoholism and pancreatic insufficiency. NY Acad Sci 1975; 252:200–207.
7. DiMagno EP, Go VLW, Summerskill WHJ: Relations between pancreatic enzyme outputs and malabsorption in severe pancreatic insufficiency. N Engl J Med 1973; 288:813–815.
8. Allen RH, Seetharam B, Allen NC, et al: Correction of cobalamin malabsorption in pancreatic insufficiency with a cobalamin analogue that binds with high affinity to R protein but not to intrinsic factor: In vivo evidence that a failure to partially degrade R protein is responsible for cobalamin malabsorption in pancreatic insufficiency. J Clin Invest 1978; 61:1628–1634.
9. Allen RH, Seetharam B, Pedell E, et al: Effect of proteolytic enzymes on the binding of cobalamin to R protein and intrinsic factor: In vitro evidence that a failure to partially degrade R protein is responsible for cobalamin malabsorption in pancreatic insufficiency. J Clin Invest 1978; 61:47–54.
10. Comfort MW, Steinberg AG: Pedigree of a family with hereditary chronic relapsing pancreatitis. Gastroenterology 1952; 21:54–63.

11. Ghishan FK, Greene HL, Avant G, et al: Chronic relapsing pancreatitis in childhood. J Pediatr Surg 1983; 102:514–518.
12. Lilja P, Evander A, Ihse I: Hereditary pancreatitis—a report on two kindreds. Acta Chir Scand 1978; 144:35–37.
13. Rothstein FC, Wylie R, Gauderer MEL: Hereditary pancreatitis and recurrent abdominal pain of childhood. J Pediatr Surg 1985; 20:535–537.
14. Cucchiara S, Staiano A, Minella R, et al: Hereditary pancreatitis: Report of the second kindred in Italy. J Pediatr Gastroenterol Nutr 1990; 11:422–424.
15. Lin JT, Wang TH, Chen DS: Hereditary pancreatitis in a Chinese family. J Clin Gastroenterol 1990; 12:81–84.
16. Kattwinkel J, Lapey A, di Sant'Agnese PA, et al: Hereditary pancreatitis: Three new kindreds and a critical review of the literature. Pediatrics 1973; 51:55–69.
17. Riccardi VM, Shih VE, Holmes LB, Nardi GL: Hereditary pancreatitis. Arch Intern Med 1975; 135:822–825.
18. Gross JB: Hereditary pancreatitis. *In* Gambill EE, ed: Pancreatitis. St. Louis, CV Mosby, 1973, pp 109–114.
19. Gross JB, Ulrich JA, Jones JD: Urinary excretion of amino acids in a kindred with hereditary pancreatitis and aminoaciduria. Gastroenterology 1964; 47:41–48.
20. Hardy M, Cornet E, Dupon H, Gordeef A: Chronic pancreatitis associated with familial dilation of the pancreatic ducts: 6 operated cases. Bibl Gastroenterol 1965; 7:189–216.
21. Spencer JA, Lindsell DRM, Isaacs D: Hereditary pancreatitis: Early ultrasound appearances. Pediatr Radiol 1990; 20:293–295.
22. Appel MF: Hereditary pancreatitis. Arch Surg 1974; 108:63–65.
23. Perrault J, Gross JB, King JE: Endoscopic retrograde cholangiopancreatography in familial pancreatitis. Gastroenterology 1976; 71:138–144.
24. Logan A, Schlicke CP, Manning GB: Familial pancreatitis. Am J Surg 1968; 115:112–117.
25. Bergstrom K, Hellstrom K, Kallmer M, et al: Familial pancreatitis associated with hyperglycinuria. Scand J Gastroenterol 1973; 8:217–223.
26. Davidson P, Costanza P, Swieconek JA, et al: Hereditary pancreatitis: A kindred without gross aminoaciduria. Ann Intern Med 1968; 68:188–196.
27. Sato T, Saitoh Y: Familial chronic pancreatitis associated with pancreatic lithiasis. Am J Surg 1974; 127:511–517.
28. Fried AM, Selke AC: Pseudocyst formation in hereditary pancreatitis. J Pediatr 1978; 93:950–953.
29. McElroy R, Christiansen PA: Hereditary pancreatitis in a kinship associated with portal vein thrombosis. Am J Med 1972; 52:228–241.
30. Rao SS, Riley SA, Foster PN, et al: Hereditary pancreatitis presenting with ascites. Postgrad Med J 1986; 62:873–875.
31. Puestow CB, Gillespie WJ: Retrograde drainage of pancreas for chronic relapsing pancreatitis. Am Surg 1958; 76:898.
32. Pitchumoni CS: Special problems of tropical pancreatitis. Clin Gastroenterol 1984; 13:941–959.
33. GeeVarghese PJ, Pillai VK, Joseph MP, et al: The diagnosis of pancreatogenous diabetes mellitus. J Assoc Phys India 1962; 10:173–178.
34. GeeVarghese PJ: Pancreatic Diabetes. Bombay, Popular Prakashan, 1968.
35. GeeVarghese PJ: Calcific Pancreatitis. Trivandrum, St. Joseph's Press, 1986.
36. Zuidema PJ: Calcification and cirrhosis of the pancreas in patients with deficient nutrition. Doc Med Geogr Trop 1955; 7:229–251.
37. Pitchumoni CS: "Tropical" or "nutritional" pancreatitis. *In* Gyr KE, Singer MV, Sarles H, eds: Pancreatitis: Concepts and Classification. Elsevier, Amsterdam, Excerpta Medica, 1984, pp 359–363.
38. Schultz AC, Moore PB, GeeVarghese PJ, et al: X-ray diffraction studies of pancreatic calculi associated with nutritional pancreatitis. Dig Dis Sci 1986; 31(5):476–480.
39. Thomas PG, Augustine P, Ramesh H, et al: Observations and surgical management of tropical pancreatitis in Kerala and southern India. World J Surg 1990; 14(1):32–42.
40. Thomas PG, Augustine P: Pancreatic cancer in siblings with tropical pancreatitis. Indian J Gastroenterol 1987; 6:185–186.
41. Mohan V, Mohan R, Susheela L, et al: Tropical pancreatic diabetes in South India: Heterogeneity in clinical and biochemical profile. Diabetologia 1985; 28:229–232.
42. Pitchumoni CS, Jain NK, Lowenfels AB, et al: Chronic cyanide poisoning: Unifying concept for alcoholic and tropical pancreatitis. Pancreas 1988; 3:220–222.
43. Balakrishnan V, Sauniere JF, Hariharan M, Sarles H: Diet, pancreatic function, and chronic pancreatitis in south India and France. Pancreas 1988; 3:30–35.
44. Mabogunje OA, Lawrie JH: Surgery for chronic pancreatitis in Zaria, Nigeria. World J Surg 1990; 14:45–47.
45. Thomas PG, Augustine P: Surgery in tropical pancreatitis. Br J Surg 1988; 75:161–164.
46. Kleitsch WP: Anatomy of the pancreas: A study with special reference to the duct system. Arch Surg 1955; 71:795–802.
47. Dawson W, Langman J: An anatomical-radiological study on the pancreatic duct pattern in man. Anat Rec 1961; 139:59–68.
48. Berman LG, Prior JT, Abramow SM, Ziegler DD: A study of the pancreatic duct system in man by the use of vinyl acetate casts of postmortem preparations. Surg Gynecol Obstet 1960; 110:391–403.
49. Hand BH: An anatomical study of the choledochoduodenal area. Br J Surg 1963; 50:486–494.
50. Cotton PB: Congenital anomaly of pancreas divisum as cause of obstructive pain and pancreatitis. Gut 1980; 21:105–114.
51. Tulassy Z, Papp J: New clinical aspects of pancreas divisum. Gastrointest Endosc 1980; 26:143–146.
52. Richter JM, Schapiro RH, Mulley AG, et al: Association of pancreas divisum and pancreatitis and its treatment of sphincteroplasty of the accessory ampulla. Gastroenterology 1981; 81:1104–1110.
53. Sahel J, Cros R, Bourry J, et al: Clinicopathological conditions associated with pancreas divisum. Digestion 1982; 23:1–8.
54. Philip J, Koch H, Classen M: Variations and anomalies of the papilla of Vater, the pancreas and the biliary duct system. Endoscopy 1974; 6:70–77.
55. Kruse A: Pancreas divisum: A significantly high incidence in chronic pancreatitis? Scand J Gastroenterol 1977; 12(Suppl):45–52.
56. Delhaye M, Engelholm L, Cremer M: Pancreas divisum: Congenital anatomic variant or anomaly? Contribution of endoscopic retrograde dorsal pancreatography. Gastroenterology 1985; 89:951–958.
57. Rosch W, Koch H, Schaffner O, et al: The clinical significance of pancreas divisum. Gastrointest Endosc 1976; 22:206–207.
58. Mitchell J, Lintott DJ, Ruddell WSJ, et al: Clinical relevance of an unfused pancreatic duct system. Gut 1979; 20:1066–1071.
59. Hayakawa T, Kondo T, Shibata T, et al: Pancreas divisum. A predisposing factor to pancreatitis? Int J Pancreatol 1989; 5:317–326.
60. Burtin P, Person B, Charneau J, et al: Pancreas divisum and pancreatitis: A coincidental association? Endoscopy 1991; 23:55–58.
61. Wagner CW, Golladay ES: Pancreas divisum and pancreatitis in children. Am Surg 1988; 54:22–26.
62. Warshaw AL: Pancreas divisum: A case for surgical treatment. Adv Surg 1988; 21:93–109.
63. Madura JA: Pancreas divisum: Stenosis of the dorsally dominant pancreatic duct. A surgically correctable lesion. Am J Surg 1986; 151:742–745.
64. Satterfield ST, McCarthy JH, Geenen JE, et al: Clinical experience in 82 patients with pancreas divisum: Preliminary results of manometry and endoscopic therapy. Pancreas 1988; 3:248–253.
65. Staritz M, Meyer zum Buschenfelde KH: Elevated pressure in the dorsal part of pancreas divisum: The cause of chronic pancreatitis? Pancreas 1988; 3:108–110.
66. Cooperman M, Ferrera JJ, Fromkes JJ, et al: The surgical management of pancreas divisum. Am J Surg 1982; 143:107–112.
67. Warshaw AL, Richter JM, Schapiro RH: The cause and treatment of pancreatitis associated with pancreas divisum. Ann Surg 1983; 198:443–452.
68. Russell RCG, Wong NW, Cotton PB: Accessory sphincterotomy (endoscopic and surgical) in patients with pancreas divisum. Br J Surg 1984; 71:954–957.
69. Gregg JA, Monaco AP, McDermott WV: Pancreas divisum: Results of surgical intervention. Am J Surg 1983; 145:488–492.
70. Madura J, Fiore AC, O'Connor KW, et al: Pancreas divisum: Detection and management. Am Surg 1985; 51:353–357.
71. Blair AJ, Russell RCG, Cotton PB: Resection for pancreatitis in patients with pancreas divisum. Ann Surg 1984; 200:590–594.

72. Desa LA, Williamson RC: On-table pancreatography: Importance in planning operative strategy. Br J Surg 1990; 77:1145–1150.
73. Toskes PP: Hyperlipidemic pancreatitis. Gastroenterol Clin North Am 1990; 19:783–791.
74. Krauss RM, Levy AG: Subclinical chronic pancreatitis in type I hyperlipoproteinemia. Am J Med 1977; 62:144–149.
75. Salen S, Kessler JI, Janowitz HD: The development of pancreatic secretory insufficiency in a patient with recurrent pancreatitis and type V hyperlipoproteinemia. Mt Sinai J Med 1970; 37:103–107.
76. Saharia P, Margolis S, Zuidema GD, et al: Acute pancreatitis with hyperlipemia: Studies with an isolated canine pancreas. Surgery 1977; 82:60–67.
77. Pitchumoni CS, Agarwal N, Jain NK: Systemic complications of acute pancreatitis. Am J Gastroenterol 1988; 83(6):597–606.
78. Bess MA, Edis AJ, van Heerden JA: Hyperparathyroidism and pancreatitis. JAMA 1980; 243:246–247.
79. Mixter CG Jr, Keynes WM, Cope O: Further experience with pancreatitis as a diagnostic clue to hyperparathyroidism. N Engl J Med 1962; 266:265.
80. Werner S, Hjern B, Sjoberg HE: Primary hyperparathyroidism: Analysis of findings in a series of 129 patients. Acta Chir Scand 1974; 140:618–625.
81. Layer P, Hotz J, Schmitz-Moorman HP, Goebell H: Effects of experimental chronic hypercalcemia on feline exocrine pancreatic secretion. Gastroenterology 1982; 82:309–316.
82. Mihas AA, Hirschowitz BI: α1-Antitrypsin and chronic pancreatitis. Lancet 1976; 2:1032–1033.
83. McNeely RL, O'Neill JA, Ghishan F: Fibrosing pancreatitis—an obscure cause of painless obstructive jaundice: A case report and review of the literature. Pediatrics 1981; 67:136–139.
84. Elitsur Y, Siddiqui SY, Sloven D, et al: Chronic pancreatitis with diffuse fibrosis in early childhood. Pancreas 1989; 4:504–510.
85. Atkinson GO, Wyly JB, Gay BB, et al: Idiopathic fibrosing pancreatitis: A cause of obstructive jaundice in childhood Pediatr Radiol 1988; 18:28–31.
86. Wheatley MJ, Coran AG: Obstructive jaundice secondary to chronic pancreatitis in children: Report of two cases and review of the literature. Surgery 1988; 104:863–869.
87. Liu P, Daneman A, Stringer DA, et al: Large pancreatic cysts and pancreatic calcification in cystic fibrosis. J Can Assoc Radiol 1986; 37:279–282.
88. Gross V, Schoelmerich J, Denzel K, Gerok W: Relapsing pancreatitis as initial manifestation of cystic fibrosis in a young man without pulmonary disease. Int J Pancreatol 1989; 4:221–228.
89. Lillemoe KD, Pitt HA, Cameron JL: Primary sclerosing cholangitis. Surg Clin North Am 1990; 70:1381–1402.
90. Borkje B, Vetrik K, Odegaard S, et al: Chronic pancreatitis in patients with sclerosing cholangitis and ulcerative colitis. Scand J Gastroenterol 1985; 20:539–542.
91. Sood GK, Vij JC, Mohapatra JR, et al: Primary sclerosing cholangitis with chronic pancreatitis. Indian J Gastroenterol 1990; 9:309–310.
92. Moody FG, Vecchio R, Calabuig R, et al: Transduodenal sphincteroplasty with transampullary septectomy for stenosing papillitis. Am J Surg 1991; 161:213–218.
93. Misra SP, Dwivedi M: Pancreaticobiliary ductal union. Gut 1990; 31:1144–1149.
94. Perisic VN, Mihailovic T, Tomomasa T, et al: The role of the accessory pancreatic duct of Santorini in pancreatic drainage in children (with emphasis on choledochal cyst patients). Pediatr Radiol 1991; 21:258–261.
95. Dowsett JF, Rode J, Russell RC: Annular pancreas: A clinical, endoscopic, and immunohistochemical study. Gut 1989; 30:130–135.
96. Gilinsky NH, Lewis JW, Flueck JA, et al: Annular pancreas associated with diffuse chronic pancreatitis. Am J Gastroenterol 1987; 82:681–684.
97. Lowes JR, Rode J, Lees WR, et al: Obstructive pancreatitis: Unusual causes of chronic pancreatitis. Br J Surg 1988; 75:1129–1133.
98. Kozarek RA: Pancreatic stents can induce ductal changes consistent with chronic pancreatitis. Gastrointest Endosc 1990; 36:93–95.
99. Leppaniemi A, Haapiainen R, Kiviluoto T, et al: Pancreatic trauma: Acute and late manifestations. Br J Surg 1988; 75:165–167.
100. Kato S, Miyabayashi S, Ohi R, et al: Chronic pancreatitis in muscular cytochrome c oxidase deficiency. J Pediatr Gastroenterol Nutr 1990; 11:549–552.
101. Forbes D, Scott RB, Trevenen C, et al: Chronic pancreatitis associated with ulcerative colitis. Clin Invest Med 1987; 4:321–324.
102. Piontek M, Hengels KJ, Strohmeyer G: Crohn's disease: What about the pancreas? (editorial). J Clin Gastroenterol 1990; 12:491–493.
103. Izsak EM, Shike M, Roulet M, et al: Pancreatitis in association with hypercalcemia in patients receiving total parenteral nutrition. Gastroenterology 1980; 79:555–558.
104. Jordan SC, Ament ME: Pancreatitis in children and adolescents. J Pediatr 1977; 91:211–216.
105. Safrit HD, Rice R: Gastrointestinal complications of pancreatitis. Radiol Clin North Am 1989; 27:73–79.
106. Niederau C, Sonnenberg A, Mueller JE, et al: Sonographic measurements of the normal liver, spleen, pancreas and portal vein. Radiology 1983; 149:537–540.
107. Silverstein W, Isikoff MB, Hill MC, et al: Diagnostic imaging of acute pancreatitis: Prospective study using CT and sonography. Am J Roentgenol 1981; 137:457–502.
108. Hill MC, Barkin J, Isikoff MB, et al: Acute pancreatitis: Clinical vs CT findings. Am J Roentgenol 1982; 135:263–269.
109. Ferruci JT Jr, Wittenberg J, Black B, et al: Computed body tomography in chronic pancreatitis. Radiology 1979; 13:175–182.
110. Husband JE, Meire HB, Kreel L: Comparison of ultrasound and computer-assisted tomography in pancreatic diagnosis. Br J Radiol 1977; 50:855–863.
111. Cotton PB, Lees WR, Vallon AG, et al: Gray-scale ultrasonography and endoscopic pancreatography in pancreatic diagnosis. Radiology 1980; 134:453–459.
112. Freeny PC, Lawson TL: Radiology of the Pancreas. 1st ed. New York, Heidelberg, Berlin, Springer-Verlag, 1982.
113. Parulekar SG: Ultrasonic evaluation of the pancreatic duct. J Clin Ultrasound 1980; 8:457–463.
114. Gosink BB, Leopold GR: The dilated pancreatic duct: Ultrasonic evaluation. Radiology 1978; 125:475–478.
115. Weinstein DP, Weinstein BJ: Ultrasonic demonstration of the pancreatic duct: An analysis of 41 cases. Radiology 1979; 120:729–734.
116. Bolondi L, Li Bassi S, Gaiani S, et al: Sonography of chronic pancreatitis. Radiol Clin North Am 1989; 27:815–833.
117. Anderson B, Hancke S, Nielsen AD, et al: The diagnosis of pancreatic cyst by endoscopic retrograde pancreatography and ultrasonic scanning. Ann Surg 1988; 185:286–289.
118. Bradley EL III, Clements LJ Jr, Gonzalez AC: The natural history of pancreatic pseudocysts: A unified concept of management. Am J Surg 1979; 137:135–141.
119. Kressel HJ, Margulis AR, Gooding GW, et al: CT scanning and ultrasound in the evaluation of pancreatic pseudocysts: A preliminary comparison. Radiology 1979; 126:153–157.
120. Sarti DA, King W: The ultrasonic findings in inflammatory pancreatic disease. Semin Ultrasound 1980; 1:178–191.
121. Braganza JM, Fawcitt RA, Forbes WSC, et al: A clinical evaluation of isotope scanning, ultrasonography and computed tomography in pancreatic disease. Clin Radiol 1978, 29:639–646.
122. Smith FW, Reid A, Hutchinson JMS, et al: Nuclear magnetic resonance imaging of the pancreas. Radiology 1982; 142:677–680.
123. Mitchell DG, Vinirski S, Sapanaro S, et al: Liver and pancreas: Improved spin-echo T_1 contrast by shorter echo time and fat suppression at 1.5 T. Radiology 1991; 178:67–70.
124. Foley WD, Stewart ET, Lawson I, et al: Computed tomography, ultrasonography, and endoscopic retrograde cholangiopancreatography in the diagnosis of pancreatic disease: A comparative study. Gastrointest Radiol 1980; 5:29–35.
125. Braganza JM, Hunt LP, Warwick F: Relationship between pancreatic exocrine function and ductal morphology in chronic pancreatitis. Gastroenterology 1982; 82:1341–1347.
126. Caletti G, Brocchi E, Agostini D, et al: Sensitivity of endoscopic retrograde pancreatography in chronic pancreatitis. Br J Surg 1982; 69:507–509.

127. Allendorph M, Werlin SL, Geenen JE, et al: Endoscopic retrograde cholangiopancreatography in children. J Pediatr 1987; 110:206–211.
128. Lankisch PG: Exocrine pancreatic function tests. Gut 1982; 23:777–798.
129. Arvanitakis C, Cooke R: Diagnostic tests of exocrine pancreatic function and disease. Gastroenterology 1978; 74:932–948.
130. Wormsely KG: Tests of pancreatic secretion. Clin Gastroenterol 1978; 7:529–544.
131. Mottaleb A, Kapp F, Noguera ECA, et al: The Lundh test in the diagnosis of pancreatic disease: A review of five years' experience. Gut 1973; 14:835–841.
132. Braganza JM, Herman K, Hine P, et al: Pancreatic enzymes in human duodenal juice—a comparison of responses in secretin-pancreozymin and Lundh Borgstroem tests. Gut 1978; 19:358–366.
133. Ammann RW, Akovbiantz A, Haecki W, et al: Diagnostic value of the fecal chymotrypsin test in pancreatic insufficiency, particularly chronic pancreatitis: Correlation with the pancreozymin-secretin test, fecal fat excretion and final clinical diagnosis. Digestion 1981; 21:281–289.
134. Haverback BJ, Dyce BJ, Gutentag PJ, Montgomery DW: Measurement of trypsin and chymotrypsin in stool: A diagnostic test for pancreatic exocrine function. Gastroenterology 1963; 44:588–597.
135. Aravantis C, Greenberger NJ: Diagnosis of pancreatic disease by a synthetic peptide: A new test of exocrine pancreatic function. Lancet 1976; 1:663–666.
136. Laufer D, Cleghorn G, Forstner G, et al: The bentiromide test using plasma *p*-aminobenzoic acid for diagnosing pancreatic insufficiency in young children: The effect of two different doses and a liquid meal. Gastroenterology 1991; 101:207–213.
137. Niederau C, Grendell JH: Diagnosis of chronic pancreatitis. Gastroenterology 1985; 88:1973–1975.
138. Karanjia ND, Reber HA: The cause and management of the pain of chronic pancreatitis. Gastroenterol Clin North Am 1990; 19:895–904.
139. Bell S, Cole R, Robert-Thomson IC: Coeliac plexus block for control of pain in chronic pancreatitis. Br Med J 1980; 281:1604.
140. Isaksson G, Ihse I: Pain reduction by an oral pancreatic enzyme preparation in chronic pancreatitis. Dig Dis Sci 1983; 28:97–102.
141. Slaff J, Jacobson D, Tillman CR, et al: Protease-specific suppression of pancreatic exocrine secretion. Gastroenterology 1984; 87:44–52.
142. Brugge WR, Goff JS, Allen NC, et al: Development of a dual label Schilling test for pancreatic exocrine function based on the differential absorption of cobalamin bound to intrinsic factor and R protein. Gastroenterology 1980; 78:937–949.
143. Latifi R, McIntosh JK, Dudrick SJ: Nutritional management of acute and chronic pancreatitis. Surg Clin North Am 1991; 71:579–595.
144. Dobrilla G: Management of chronic pancreatitis. Focus on enzyme replacement therapy. Int J Pancreatol 1989; 5(Suppl):17–29.
145. Durie P, Bell L, Linton W, et al: Effect of cimetidine and sodium bicarbonate on pancreatic replacement theory in cystic fibrosis. Gut 1980; 21:778–786.
146. Gow R, Francis P, Bradbear R, et al: Comparative studies of varying regimens to improve steatorrhea and creatorrhea in cystic fibrosis: Effectiveness of an enteric coated preparation with and without antacids and cimetidine. Lancet 1981; 2:1071–1074.
147. DeYoung JL: Development of pancreatic enzyme microsphere technology and US findings with pancrease in the treatment of chronic pancreatitis. Int J Pancreatol 1989; 5:31–36.
148. Havala T, Shronts E, Cerra F: Nutritional support in acute pancreatitis. Gastroenterol Clin North Am 1989; 18:525–542.
149. Twersky Y, Bank S: Nutritional deficiencies in chronic pancreatitis. Gastroenterol Clin North Am 1989; 18:543–565.
150. Bassi C, Vesentini S, Nifosi F, et al: Pancreatic abscess and other pus-harboring collections related to pancreatitis: A review of 108 cases. World J Surg 1990; 14:505–511.
151. Lumsden A, Bradley EL: Secondary pancreatic infections. Surg Gynecol Obstet 1990; 170:459–467.
152. Warshaw AL, Rattner DW: Timing of surgical drainage for pancreatic pseudocyst. Clinical and chemical criteria. Ann Surg 1985; 202:720–724.
153. Sjoberg RJ, Kidd GS: Pancreatic diabetes mellitus. Diabetes Care 1989; 12:715–724.
154. Donowitz M, Hendler R, Spiro HM, et al: Glucagon secretion in acute and chronic pancreatitis. Ann Intern Med 1975; 83:778–781.
155. Rohrmann CA Jr, Baron RL: Biliary complications of pancreatitis. Radiol Clin North Am 1989; 27:93–104.
156. Wilson C, Auld CD, Schlinkert R, et al: Hepatobiliary complications in chronic pancreatitis. Gut 1989; 30:520–527.
157. Mannell A, Adson MA, McIlrath DC, et al: Surgical management of chronic pancreatitis: Long-term results in 141 patients. Br J Surg 1988; 75:467–472.
158. Synn AY, Mulvihill SJ, Fonkalsrud EW: Surgical management of pancreatitis in childhood. J Pediatr Surg 1987; 22:628–632.
159. Huibregtse K, Schneider B, Vrij AA, Tytgat GN: Endoscopic pancreatic drainage in chronic pancreatitis. Gastrointest Endosc 1988; 34:9–15.
160. Irani SK: Endoscopic management of pancreatic disorders. Gastroenterol Clin North Am 1990; 19:975–997.
161. Siegel JH, Ben-Zvi JS, Pullano W, Cooperman A: Effectiveness of endoscopic drainage for pancreas divisum: Endoscopic and surgical results in 31 patients. Endoscopy 1990; 22:129–133.
162. Crombleholme TM, deLorimier AA, Way LW, et al: The modified Puestow procedure for chronic relapsing pancreatitis in children. J Pediatr Surg 1990; 25:749–754.
163. Gruessner RW, Manivel C, Dunn DL, et al: Pancreaticoduodenal transplantation with enteric drainage following native total pancreatectomy for chronic pancreatitis: A case report. Pancreas 1991; 6:479–488.
164. Farney AC, Najarian JS, Nakhleh RE, et al: Autotransplantation of dispersed pancreatic islet tissue combined with total or near-total pancreatectomy for treatment of chronic pancreatitis. Surgery 1991; 110:427–437.
165. Ihse I, Borch K, Larsson J: Chronic pancreatitis: Results of operations for relief of pain. World J Surg 1990; 14:53–58.

Chapter 70

Secretory Neoplasms of the Pancreas

HILLEL NAON and DANIEL W. THOMAS

INTRODUCTION

Pancreatic neoplasms are exceedingly rare in children. The majority of childhood pancreatic tumors are benign endocrine neoplasms that secrete hormonally active peptides.[1, 2] A case of insulinoma was first described in 1927 by Wilder[3] in an adult with a metastatic islet cell carcinoma and profound hypoglycemia. Islet cell adenoma in a neonate was described by Sherman[4] in 1947 and was the first reported case of a secretory type of pancreatic neoplasm in pediatrics. This chapter focuses on functioning neoplasms of the pancreas occurring in childhood.

Functioning pancreatic neoplasms are composed primarily of islet cells that elaborate various endocrine secretory products. More than 50% of pancreatic endocrine neoplasms are multihormonal. However, clinical manifestations are nearly always derived primarily from hypersecretion of only one of the hormones that is produced.[5–7] The diagnosis of pancreatic islet cell neoplasms with excessive hormone production depends on the recognition of clinical syndromes associated with autonomous endocrine product secretion. The pancreatic islet A cells secrete glucagon; the B cells secrete insulin; the D cells secrete somatostatin; the F cells secrete vasoactive intestinal polypeptide (VIP), substance P, and possibly secretin; and the G cells secrete gastrin.[7, 8] There is much evidence to suggest that pluripotent stem cells in the pancreatic duct epithelium called *nesidioblasts* give rise under normal conditions to the aforementioned differentiated islet cell types. Nesidioblasts may differentiate into neoplasms, producing ectopic hormones under aberrant conditions.[7, 9, 10]

The development of highly specific and sensitive radioimmunoassays (RIAs) for detection of circulating peptides in the blood has facilitated the recognition and diagnosis of hormone-secreting neuroendocrine tumors. In children, the most common secretory pancreatic neoplasm is insulinoma associated with B cell adenoma or hyperplasia. Zollinger-Ellison syndrome associated with gastrinoma, VIPoma, and multiple endocrine neoplasia type 1 (MEN 1) have been described in children.[11] Glucagonoma and somatostatinoma have not been reported in children.[11] Table 70–1 lists such tumors and their characteristics.

MULTIPLE ENDOCRINE NEOPLASIA TYPE 1

Patients with MEN 1, also termed *Wermer's syndrome*, experience manifestations mainly originating from secretory neoplasms located in the parathyroid glands, pancreatic islets, or anterior pituitary. Disorders of the adrenal cortex and thyroid gland, bronchial and intestinal carcinoid tumors, and VIPomas have been included in this syndrome. Patients with MEN 1 may develop symptoms at any age, but the condition rarely presents in childhood or after the age of 60 years. Both sexes are affected with equal frequency.[12, 13] The disorder

Table 70–1. SECRETORY NEOPLASMS OF THE PANCREAS

Neoplasm	Hormone Secreted	Islet Cell Type	Major Clinical Features	% Malignant	Treatment
Insulinoma (adenoma, hyperplasia, nesidioblastosis)	Insulin	B	Hypoglycemia	10	Diazoxide, frequent feedings, octreotide acetate, surgery
Gastrinoma	Gastrin	G	Peptic ulcers, diarrhea	65	Gastric acid secretion, antagonists/blockers, surgery
VIPoma	VIP	F	Secretory diarrhea, hypokalemia, hypochlorhydria	50	Fluid and electrolyte replacement, octreotide acetate, steroids, surgery
Glucagonoma	Glucagon	A	Skin rash, stomatitis, diabetes	>75	Octreotide acetate, surgery

is inherited in an autosomal dominant mode with a high degree of penetrance.[14, 15] The MEN 1 gene has recently been mapped to chromosome 11.[16] There is evidence to suggest that tumor formation is associated with loss of a specific gene, which possibly unmasks a recessive mutation at this locus. Genetic markers for MEN 1 will undoubtedly soon become available.[16]

The clinical manifestations of MEN 1 are heterogeneous and depend on the endocrine organ involved and the functional nature of the secretory neoplasm. An extensive review of 88 patients, seven of whom were pediatric patients, by Ballard and coworkers[12] provided much of the early knowledge concerning the various features of MEN 1, which include (1) parathyroid gland hyperfunction (84%), (2) pituitary neoplasms (65%), (3) adenomas and hyperplasia of the adrenal cortex (38%), (4) thyroid disease (19%) (thyrotoxicosis, thyroid carcinoma, and nonfunctioning adenomas), and (5) peptic ulcers (58%). Ulcers were multifocal in more than half of the patients. Some patients had watery diarrhea or bronchial carcinoids. Pancreatic neoplasms were found in more than 75% of all the patients with MEN 1. These neoplasms were almost always multiple and consisted of both B cells, giving rise to insulinoma, and non-B cells, resulting in Zollinger-Ellison syndrome, or other neoplasms associated with glucagonoma, VIPoma, or somatostatinoma.

Genetic counseling and screening of family members with careful follow-up are important aspects in the management of patients with MEN 1. Treatment of pancreatic neoplasms associated with MEN 1 is discussed later in this chapter in sections dealing with the specific types of secretory tumors.

INSULINOMA

Insulinomas, though rare, are the most common form of hormone-secreting tumors of the pancreas in children and adults.[17] These are discrete pancreatic endocrine neoplasms composed mainly or exclusively of B cells. Insulinomas have been recognized as a cause of inappropriate insulin secretion for more than half a century. Whipple[18] described the typical triad of symptoms associated with this syndrome: insulin shock with fasting, a fasting blood sugar of less than half normal, and relief of symptoms with the administration of glucose. Over 100 cases of insulinoma, including islet B cell adenoma and hyperplasia, were compiled by Tudor in the *Childhood Disease Registry*.[19] The number of reports has increased considerably since the RIA for insulin became available for clinical use. Published cases of insulinoma indicate that an islet cell adenoma or hyperplasia may become manifest at any age during childhood, but there are two periods of peak incidence: the neonatal period through the first year of life; and after age 4 years, with a peak from 8 to 13 years of age. Insulinomas are more frequent in females.[19, 20] Eighty percent are solitary neoplasms, and over 90% are benign.[19, 21] Malignant insulinomas are exceedingly rare in children but have been reported.[2] Patients with insulinomas and the MEN 1 syndrome often have multiple insulinomas and are usually diagnosed at 15 to 25 years of age.[13] They account for about 10% of adult patients with insulinoma. In infants, diffuse adenomatosis or nesidioblastosis is frequently the cause of hyperinsulinemia.[22]

Insulinomas vary in size from lesions that are difficult to find even under dissection to huge tumors that are over 1,500 gm.[20] Ninety percent of insulinomas are less than 20 mm in diameter. Solitary tumors that are smaller than 5 mm in diameter are seldom associated with hypoglycemia.[20] They are usually encapsulated, firm, yellow-brown nodules that are histologically composed of cords and nests of well-differentiated B islet cells. Regardless of their size, insulinomas can be located anywhere in the pancreas and are rarely found outside the pancreas. Distinction between a benign or malignant insulinoma is difficult on the basis of histologic appearance alone.

The alpha chain of human chorionic gonadotropin (HCG-alpha) was recently reported[23] as a marker for malignancy in functioning endocrine neoplasms, including insulinomas. Since MEN 1 is the most common condition associated with multiple benign insulinomas, the presence of genetic markers for MEN 1[16] may alert the physician to the possibility of multiple insulinomas.

Symptoms of hypoglycemia such as headaches, visual disturbances, confusion, weakness, sweating, and palpitations are characteristic; convulsions or coma is a feature of significant prolonged hypoglycemia. Most symptoms occur after fasting and are often confused with neurologic or psychiatric disease. The finding of hypoglycemia that can be provoked with fasting remains the keystone in the recognition of the possibility of an insulinoma. Significant hypoglycemia can be demonstrated after a 12-hour overnight fast in over 90% of cases of proven insulinoma.[20] Plasma insulin levels are inappropriately elevated during hypoglycemia. Patients with insulinoma have insulin-connecting peptide (C-peptide) concentrations that parallel the elevated plasma insulin levels. Normally, when insulin is cleared from its precursor proinsulin, the C-peptide is released into the portal vein at a 1:1 ratio with insulin. Because insulinoma cells often process proinsulin incompletely, the serum often has a high ratio of proinsulin to insulin.[20] In normal subjects, serum insulin concentrations decrease to less than 5 microunits per ml when the blood sugar falls to 40 mg per dl or lower, and the ratio of plasma insulin (in microunits per ml) to serum glucose (in mg per dl) remains less than 0.3. In patients with insulinomas, the ratio is usually greater than 0.4 and increases with fasting.[24] Hypoglycemia in the absence of urinary ketones and the presence of low plasma beta-hydroxybutyrate are consistent with the diagnosis of insulinoma.

It is often difficult to localize insulinomas once the diagnosis has been made on clinical and laboratory grounds. Noninvasive studies, such as computed axial tomography (CT), ultrasound, and magnetic resonance imaging (MRI), are usually helpful when the insulinoma is greater than 2 cm. Experience with MRI of insulinomas has not been widely reported. Selective arteriography is usually performed if the noninvasive studies are negative. A hypervascular insulinoma can be detected by selective arteriography in 50 to 80% of cases.[24] In patients with negative noninvasive studies and nondiagnostic arteriography, portal venous sampling of blood for insulin is performed prior to surgery. Tumors that cannot be identified preoperatively can be either palpated during surgery or detected by intraoperative ultrasonography.[25, 26]

The treatment of choice for insulinoma is surgical ablation, which carries an excellent prognosis in most infants and children. At surgery, the islet cell tumor is often pink in color and firmer in consistency than the surrounding gland. The tumor is usually discrete and well encapsulated. The majority of these neoplasms can be simply enucleated. If the neoplasm cannot be localized, distal pancreatectomy with careful examination of sequential frozen sections of the gland is advisable. Resection of more than 80% of the gland is rarely required.[11]

In patients with MEN 1 syndrome who have extensive microadenomatosis, a 95% subtotal pancreatectomy is needed to achieve a cure.[1] The residual pancreatic tissue mass is usually sufficient to maintain normal function. Transient hyperglycemia is frequent in the immediate postoperative period.[27, 28] Diabetes mellitus with refractory hyperglycemia and ketonemia may occur soon after massive subtotal pancreatectomy.[28, 29] A recent report[30] suggests that diabetes mellitus can occur years after subtotal pancreatectomy. Improved medical treatment has recently facilitated postponement of blind pancreatectomy until the tumor can be identified. Regularly scheduled feedings combined with diazoxide therapy can be used to manage some patients for a prolonged period of time. Octreotide acetate (Sandostatin, Sandoz Ltd., Basel, Switzerland) is an eight-amino-acid synthetic peptide that possesses pharmacologic effects similar to those of the native hormone somatostatin, but has much longer duration of action. This drug effectively suppresses insulin release in approximately half the patients with insulinoma.[31] The agent most frequently used in the chemotherapy of malignant insulinoma is streptozotocin.[20]

NESIDIOBLASTOSIS

Nesidioblastosis or diffuse proliferation of nesidioblasts was first described and named by Laidlaw in 1938.[32] Nesidioblasts, meaning islet builders, are cells that differentiate from the pancreatic duct epithelium to form pancreatic islets.

About 100 cases of nesidioblastosis have been reported to date.[19] Since 1970, nesidioblastosis, sometimes also termed *neonatal hyperinsulinemic hypoglycemia,* has been diagnosed frequently in association with neonatal hypoglycemia. This resulted from advances in the understanding of pancreatic histology by special staining, electron microscopy, and specific hormonal immunofluorescent techniques.

The etiology of nesidioblastosis is unknown. Kloppel and Heitz[23] suggested that the histologic resemblance of pancreata with nesidioblastosis to those from immature fetuses occurred as a result of inappropriate control during the earliest phase of endocrine pancreatic development. A genetic component with an autosomal recessive inheritance pattern is suggested by the familial occurrence of neonatal nesidioblastosis and nesidioblastosis in familial endocrine adenomatosis.[22] Marks[20] suggested that in addition to the natural immaturity of the endocrine pancreas shown by all infants, those with hyperinsulinemic hypoglycemia may have subtle differences in their intraislet cellular relationships. Not only is the normal intraislet relationship between the insulin-secreting B cells and the somatostatin-secreting D cells disturbed, but there is also a reduction in the total number of intraislet D cells, which are thought to provide an inhibitory effect on insulin secretion. Unlike insulinomas, in which B cells appear to be unable to store and convert proinsulin to insulin efficiently, it seems that there is normal conversion of proinsulin into insulin in the B cells in cases of nesidioblastosis.

Clinically, hyperinsulinemic hypoglycemia is usually evident shortly after birth. Very rarely it presents after 3 months of age. Affected infants have the same broad spectrum of clinical manifestations as described for insulinoma and are equally refractory to medical therapy. They have a relatively high plasma insulin to glucose ratio.

The treatment of choice for neonatal hyperinsulinemic hypoglycemia is 95% pancreatectomy, which is successful in approximately 80 to 90% of infants with nesidioblastosis.[33] Somatostatin analogue is used for preoperative management as well as in infants who fail surgery.[31, 33] Providing permanent brain damage from hypoglycemia has not occurred, the prognosis of nesidioblastosis is good. This condition may be familial, especially when associated with leucine-reactive hypoglycemia. Therefore, it is important to monitor newborn siblings of affected children.

GASTRINOMA: ZOLLINGER-ELLISON SYNDROME

In 1955, Zollinger and Ellison[34] described one adult patient and a 16-year-old female who presented with the triad of gastric hypersecretion, fulminant and intractable peptic ulcer disease, and a non-B cell neoplasm of the pancreas. The hormone produced by the pancreatic tumor in this syndrome was recognized as gastrin more than 10 years later.[35, 36]

Tumors producing gastrin may be associated with symptoms other than those of Zollinger-Ellison syndrome, such as diarrhea, steatorrhea, and malabsorption.[37] Gastrinomas can originate in organs other than the pancreas, but they occur in the pancreas more often than any other site. The duodenum is the second most common site of origin.[38, 39]

There are at least four major peptide forms of gastrin that differ in the length of their polypeptide chains but have identical C-terminal peptide amides. The C-terminal tetrapeptide amide has been shown to constitute the physiologically active site of the gastrin molecule.[40] Each of the peptide forms of the gastrin molecule exists in sulfated and nonsulfated forms, which appears to confer no differences in physiologic activity or potency of the molecule. The principal form of gastrin in gastrinoma is a heptadecapeptide (G-17), which contains 17-amino-acid residues.[41, 42]

Zollinger-Ellison syndrome can develop at any age. It occurs most frequently, however, between ages 35 and 65 years and is more common in men than in women. Forty-six cases of childhood gastrinomas are reported in the *Childhood Disease Registry*.[19] Forty-one cases occurred in boys. The youngest patient reported was a 5-year-old girl who also had Marden-Walker syndrome.[43] The age range of Zollinger-Ellison syndrome reported in children is 5 to 16 years. Thirty-seven children had documented neoplasms, and hyperplasia was observed in six. Sixty-five percent of the tumors were malignant. This is similar to the findings in adults, in whom 60% of the cases are malignant, most of them having liver metastases at the time of diagnosis.[44] Twelve cases of gastrinoma in childhood were associated with islet cell carcinoma.[19] Although many adult patients with Zollinger-Ellison syndrome have accompanying diseases, such as MEN 1 syndrome, similar cases have not been reported in the pediatric age group.[11]

Symptoms in Zollinger-Ellison syndrome are due to the high circulating serum gastrin levels, which cause proliferation of the gastric parietal cell mass and stimulation of excessive gastric acid secretion. Children with Zollinger-Ellison syndrome invariably have volumes of gastric secretions ranging from 600 to 2,000 ml per day or more, with total acid production of 23 to 164 mEq per L.[45] Abdominal pain due to peptic ulcer disease is the most common clinical finding. Ulcers usually occur in the first portion of the duodenum or in the stomach. The ulcers are usually single but can be multiple. When multiple ulcers occur, they are frequently located not only in the first portion of the duodenum but also in the remainder of the duodenum or even the jejunum. Diarrhea is a frequent problem; it may precede ulceration in some patients or occur without ulcers in others. The diarrhea is due to the excessive amount of hydrochloric acid released into the duodenum. In addition to an osmotic diarrhea, the increased amounts of acid and pepsin entering the small bowel produce inflammatory changes of the intestinal mucosa. Steatorrhea is less common than diarrhea. Acidity of the duodenum and small intestine causes inactivation of pancreatic lipase, reduction of conjugated bile acids, and the above-mentioned mucosal damage.

The diagnosis of Zollinger-Ellison syndrome is based on the presence of gastric acid hypersecretion and hypergastrinemia.[46] Elevated fasting serum gastrin levels can also occur with massive small intestinal resection, pernicious anemia with gastric achlorhydria, renal failure, chronic gastritis, peptic ulcer disease, and antral G cell hyperplasia. Basal acid output (BAO) of greater than 15 mEq per hour in the unoperated patient should prompt suspicion of gastrinoma. There is a smaller increase between BAO and pentagastrin-stimulated gastric acid secretion in patients with gastrinoma. This test by itself cannot establish or exclude the diagnosis of Zollinger-Ellison syndrome because of the overlap in values with normal and peptic ulcer patients. Acid output is difficult to measure after ulcer surgery because it is difficult to recover all the acid and because bile and pancreatic juice often reflux into the stomach. Therefore, decreased acid secretion after partial gastric resection does not exclude the diagnosis of Zollinger-Ellison syndrome.

Utilizing RIA for gastrin, the upper limit of normal is 100 to 150 pg per ml. Gastrin levels greater than 500 pg per ml in a patient with acid hypersecretion are diagnostic of gastrinoma.[46] Several provocative tests have been used to evaluate patients with possible gastrinoma, especially those who do not exhibit serum gastrin levels higher than 500 pg per ml. These tests utilize measurements of serum gastrin levels in response to intravenous secretin, calcium infusion, or ingestion of a standard meal. The secretin stimulation test is by far the most valuable provocative test in identifying patients with Zollinger-Ellison syndrome.[46] Secretin, at a dose of 1 to 2 units per kilogram of body weight, is given intravenously over 30 to 60 seconds. Gastrin is measured in serum samples obtained before the injection of secretin and at 5-minute intervals thereafter for 30 minutes. In normal individuals and in patients with peptic ulcer disease, achlorhydria, or antral G cell hyperplasia, the infused secretin has little effect. In patients with Zollinger-Ellison syndrome, intravenous secretin induces a substantial and prompt increase of serum gastrin by at least 200 pg per ml, usually at 5 minutes, gradually returning to basal levels by 30 minutes. In patients with gastrinoma, intravenous calcium infusion causes an increase in serum gastrin of more than 400 pg per ml above the basal serum concentration. However, since this test does not add to the sensitivity or specificity of the secretin stimulation test and calcium infusion is potentially more hazardous, this test is not recommended. The third provocative test involves the feeding of a meal. In gastrinoma patients, serum gastrin levels increase little or not at all after a meal, but an increase in serum gastrin levels of more than 200% is observed in individuals with antral G cell hyperplasia.

Gastrinomas are difficult to find. In almost half the patients with clinical and laboratory evidence, the tumor cannot be identified at surgery.[39] Upper gastrointestinal series, CT scanning, hypotonic duodenography, selective angiography, and transhepatic portal venous sampling have been employed to locate gastrinomas preoperatively. Unfortunately, none of these procedures predict whether a tumor is resectable.

Treatment of Zollinger-Ellison syndrome involves control of the effects of hypergastrinemia, in particular peptic ulcer disease, as well as surgical treatment of the tumor, which is often malignant. Treatment should be individualized. In selecting the best therapy, the biologic behavior of these neoplasms and the clinical manifestations in each patient must be taken into consideration. Histamine$_2$ (H_2)-receptor antagonists are effective in reducing gastric acid secretion, producing relief from symptoms, and inducing ulcer healing in patients with Zollinger-Ellison syndrome. They are indicated as initial treatment of patients with gastrinoma, for prolonged treatment of those patients who are not candidates for tumor resection, and in those in whom total gastrectomy is not anticipated. High-dosage cimetidine, usually four to eight times the dose used in the treatment of common duodenal ulcer, is often required.[11, 46] Ranitidine and famotidine are more potent H_2-receptor blockers than cimetidine. These drugs require a comparable increase in dosage from that used in treatment of common duodenal ulcer. The dose of H_2-receptor antagonist required to maintain a satisfactory reduction in gastric acid secretion can be assessed by measuring the basal gastric acid output during the hour immediately prior to the next scheduled dose. The goal is to reduce gastric acid output to less than 10 mEq per hour during this interval.[46] This approach is based on endoscopic evidence that duodenitis and ulceration are absent when acid secretion is kept below 10 mEq per hour.[47]

The most effective drug in reducing gastric acid secretion and in inducing ulcer healing in patients with Zollinger-Ellison syndrome is omeprazole.[48, 49] Omeprazole's mechanism of action is to inhibit the potassium-hydrogen pump located in the apical membrane of the gastric parietal cell. Risks associated with the long-term use of such medications in children are unknown.

Complete surgical resection of the tumor should be performed when possible. Complete surgical removal of gastrinoma with cure has been achieved in approximately 30% of all patients with Zollinger-Ellison syndrome.[50, 51] Forty percent of patients with sporadic gastrinoma who have no evidence of metastatic disease have occult neoplasms that are most often found in the duodenal wall and are frequently not greater than 2 mm in diameter.[30] These microgastrinomas can be detected only after duodenotomy and intraluminal exploration.[39] Pancreatic gastrinomas are not completely resectable in most cases. When a metastatic or nonresectable gastrinoma is present, control of the ulcer disease may be accomplished in most cases by treatment with acid-production antagonists, perhaps with parietal cell vagotomy,[52] and in some patients by total gastrectomy.[44, 53, 54] Total gastrectomy is not a preferred option in the management of gastric hypersecretion in patients with Zollinger-Ellison syndrome, except in the minority of patients who are noncompliant or who are unable to take medications.[55] There is no convincing evidence that tumor progression is influenced by gastrectomy.[56] Success with chemotherapy using streptozotocin, 5-fluorouracil, and doxorubicin is limited.

VIPoma

Pancreatic cholera[57]—also called watery diarrhea, hypokalemia, and achlorhydria (WDHA) syndrome[58]—is a secretory diarrheal disorder associated with pancreatic neoplasms. Secretory diarrhea in conjunction with a non-B islet cell tumor in adults was first described by Verner and Morrison in 1958.[59] One of the patients they reported was a 19-year-old female. It is now widely accepted that VIP is the principal mediator involved in the pathogenesis of the diarrhea.[60] In adults, about 50% of VIP-producing tumors are malignant, and the remainder are due to pancreatic adenomas, hyperplasia, or nonpancreatic ganglioneuromas.[61] Most VIP-producing neoplasms in children are of neurogenic origin and include ganglioneuroblastomas, ganglioneuromas, and neuroblastomas.[19, 62, 63] Rare occurrences have been reported in association with neurofibromatosis and pheochromocytomas.[19] Sixty-four cases of childhood VIPoma have been reported.[19] Primary pancreatic islet cell lesions were evident in only two of these children. In 1979, Ghishan and coworkers[64] were the first to report on the association between sustained watery diarrhea and elevated levels of plasma VIP and pancreatic islet non-B cell hyperplasia. Their patient was a 3-month-old infant presenting with secretory diarrhea beginning at two weeks of age. After a 95% pancreatectomy, plasma VIP levels returned to normal. Brenner and associates[65] described a 15-year-old girl with massive watery and protein-losing diarrhea who was found to have an islet cell tumor secreting high levels of VIP. A subtotal pancreatectomy was needed to remove the tumor. There was no recurrence for up to 6 years later.

VIP is composed of 28 amino acids. Since the amino acid sequence of VIP is similar to those of secretin and glucagon,[66] it has endocrine functions similar to secretin, such as increased pancreatic bicarbonate excretion and inhibition of gastric acid secretion stimulated by pentagastrin and histamine. Vasoactive intestinal polypeptide also has a glucagon-like action of abnormal glucose tolerance. Additionally, the vasomotor action of VIP causes vasodilation in the systemic and splanchnic vascular beds. There is evidence to suggest that VIP stimulates cyclic adenosine monophosphate (cAMP) in intestinal epithelial cells, resulting in increased secretion of water and electrolytes into the small bowel that exceeds the normal absorptive capacity of the colon.[67] Localization of VIP is widespread throughout the body, being found normally in the ganglion cells of the autonomic nervous system, adrenal medulla, brain, bladder, and predominantly in the gastrointestinal tract.[68]

Clinically, the most prominent features of VIPoma are profuse diarrhea, hypochlorhydria, hypokalemia, and metabolic acidosis. Other described features include spontaneous cutaneous flushing, hypokalemic renal failure, reduced or absent gastric acid secretion, diabetes mellitus, hypomagnesemia, hypercalcemia, and excessive tearing.[68]

Diagnosis of VIPoma is made based on the clinical picture associated with increased plasma concentrations of VIP by RIA. Confirmatory laboratory findings include hypokalemic acidosis, prerenal azotemia, and decreased gastric secretion. When the diagnosis of VIPoma has been confirmed, it is then necessary to determine whether the tumor is situated in the pancreas or in another location such as a paraspinal ganglioneuroma. A CT scan and other specific radiologic examinations are indicated in the evaluation. If the pancreas remains the suspect organ, selective arteriography may localize the tumor. Transhepatic portal venous sampling for VIP may help localize the tumor preoperatively.[69] Surgical exploration is often necessary for diagnostic purposes.

Confirmation of the diagnosis is made by the immunocytochemical detection of neuron-specific enolase, VIP in the neoplasm, and electron microscopy for secretory granules.[1, 61]

It is important that dehydration and electrolyte imbalance be corrected preoperatively. Many palliative agents for symptomatic relief have been used with some success and may allow time for further diagnostic studies to localize the tumor (Table 70–2). The most potent pharmacologic antagonist of VIPomas is octreotide acetate. This drug has been given successfully to patients with VIPoma in order to suppress peptide secretion and watery diarrhea.[31, 60] The mechanism of action of this somatostatin analogue is to inhibit the release of VIP from the tumor and to inhibit intestinal secretion at the level of the enterocyte. The plasma concentrations of VIP in patients treated with octreotide acetate usually decline but normalize in only 30% of treated patients.[70] Although all patients treated with octreotide acetate responded initially with an improvement in their diarrhea and lower VIP plasma levels, some patients had a short-term effect. In other cases, a rebound situation was observed for the diarrhea as well as VIP levels.[70] In such cases, increased dosage of octreotide acetate in combination with steroids has proved to be helpful.[70] Indomethacin may be useful in cases of VIPoma associated with elevated prostaglandin E_2 levels.[71] Other pharmacologic agents, including clonidine, phenothiazine, lithium carbonate, propranolol, and interferon, may be helpful in selected cases in which other therapies have failed.

The most definitive treatment of VIPoma is surgery. Since most VIPomas in children are of neurogenic origin, they are usually found in the adrenals or retroperitoneal area. Removal of the tumor with or without adjunctive chemotherapy is indicated. The infant with VIPoma reported by Ghishan and coworkers[64] died from sepsis after a 95% pancreatectomy. The histopathology consisted of non-B islet cell hyperplasia. The 15-year-old girl with VIPoma described by Brenner and associates[65] was found to have a large tumor of the body and tail of the pancreas. Microscopic examination revealed a tumor of islet cells. Because the tumor was found in one of 25 perisplenic lymph nodes and also in a small pancreatic vein, the diagnosis was islet cell carcinoma. Eighty-five percent distal pancreatectomy achieved complete cure in this case. Since the experience with primary pancreatic VIPoma is extremely limited in children, information concerning this type of pancreatic neoplasm is derived from the adult literature. This type of secretory neoplasm is usually found in the distal two thirds of the pancreas. Isolated, single tumors have been reported in 80% of the patients. About half of all VIPomas are benign. Twenty-five percent of the tumors consist of islet cell hyperplasia.[68] A complete cure can be expected with subtotal (85%) pancreatectomy for biopsy-proven islet cell hyperplasia.[1, 68] Excision of the primary malignancy, even in the presence of liver metastases, is indicated to reduce the bulk of the tumor for subsequent chemotherapy. The combination of 5-fluorouracil and streptozotocin is reported to have a response rate of 65%.[72]

OTHER TUMORS

Glucagonoma and somatostatinoma have been reported only in adults to date. Glucagonoma is associated

Table 70–2. TREATMENT REGIMENS FOR VIPoma SYNDROMES

Modality	Comment
Acute-Supportive	
Intravenous fluids	May require >6 L per day
Correct hypokalemia, metabolic acidosis	>350 mEq per day often required
Peptide/Peptidomimetic	
Somatostatin/Sandostatin	First-line symptomatic therapy. Octreotide acetate is effective in the symptomatic improvement of the watery diarrhea syndrome in >90% of VIPoma patients.
Pharmacotherapy	
Corticosteroids	All enhance absorption; corticosteroids most effective. All inhibit secretion; lithium carbonate and phenothiazines may be slightly more effective. All are only transiently effective.
Alpha$_2$ agonists	
Angiotensin II	
Indomethacin	
Lithium carbonate	
Phenothiazines	
Opiates	
Propranolol	
Calcium channel blockers	
Adenylate cyclase inhibitors	
Surgery	Considered as both definitive therapy and, when possible, debulking therapy.
Chemotherapy	
Streptozotocin	Combination therapy is useful but does not produce permanent remission. Renal impairment can be very serious and is usually drug limiting.
5-Fluorouracil	
Chlorozotocin	
DTIC	

From O'Dorisio TM, Mekhjian HS, Gaginella TS: Medical therapy of VIPomas. Endocrinol Metab Clin North Am 1989; 18:549; with permission.

with increased levels of glucagon due to islet A cell tumors of the pancreas. Mallinson and colleagues[73] reported nine patients with pancreatic tumors who had a clinical complex consisting of diabetes mellitus, stomatitis, anemia, weight loss, diarrhea, and skin rash. Although the skin rash is not always present, it is the most characteristic feature of a glucagonoma. The rash is described as necrolytic with migratory erythema that most commonly involves the trunk, perineum, and thighs, but can also involve the face and legs. As the erythematous rash spreads, central necrosis and scales appear. The etiology of the skin rash is uncertain but is directly related to the hyperglucagonemia. It is possible that the panhypoaminoacidemia induced by chronic hyperglucagonemia may be the cause of the dermatologic findings. The youngest patient reported with glucagonoma was a 19-year-old female[74]; the average age of patients with glucagonoma is 56 years.[75, 76] Localization of the tumor is attempted by CT scan, ultrasonography, liver scan, transhepatic portal venous sampling for glucagon, and arteriography if knowledge of the tumor vascular supply is desired prior to surgery. The majority of the tumors are found in the body and tail of the pancreas, are at least 3 cm in diameter, and have distinctive characteristics.[76] Surgery is the treatment of choice. Chemotherapy for metastatic glucagonomas includes streptozotocin, with or without 5-fluorouracil. Occasionally DTIC (diaminotriazenoimidazole carboxamide) is used.[77]

Somatostatinoma has been designated the *inhibitory syndrome* because of its physiologic and pharmacologic effects of suppression on insulin, glucagon, gastrin, and cholecystokinin release.[1] Clinical findings include diabetes, cholelithiasis, steatorrhea, indigestion, hypochlorhydria, and occasional anemia.[78] The majority of tumors are found coincidentally at the time of cholecystectomy for cholelithiasis. However, the appearance of gallstones and steatorrhea in a diabetic patient should alert the physician to the remote possibility of somatostatinoma, necessitating exploration of the foregut organs for a tumor during the time of cholecystectomy. When found, the tumor is usually single, although it may metastasize to the liver. The diagnosis can be confirmed by RIA for an increased plasma concentration of somatostatin. Treatment is surgical removal of the tumor. Chemotherapy consists of streptozotocin and 5-fluorouracil.[1]

SUMMARY

Secretory pancreatic tumors are rare in children. Most are benign, tend to grow slowly, and are difficult to localize. More advanced diagnostic techniques will make the diagnosis of such tumors much easier once the condition is suspected. One such technique was recently reported by Lamberts and coworkers,[79] who described a receptor-scanning technique using a labeled analogue of octreotide as a radionuclide for the imaging of somatostatin receptor-positive tumors and their metastases. This technique is based on evidence that the majority of endocrine neoplasms that respond to octreotide therapy do so because they have abundant somatostatin receptors. The ability to target receptors on tumor cells raises the possibility of selectively directed chemotherapy or radiotherapy for inoperable or advanced tumors.

REFERENCES

1. Friesen SR: Update on the diagnosis and treatment of rare neuroendocrine tumors. Surg Clin North Am 1987; 67:379–393.
2. Grosfeld JL, Clatworthy HW, Hamoudi AB: Pancreatic malignancy in children. Arch Surg 1970; 101:370–375.
3. Wilder RM, Allan FN, Powell MH, et al: Carcinoma of islands of pancreas with hyperinsulinism and hypoglycemia. JAMA 1927; 89:348–355.
4. Sherman H: Islet cell tumor of pancreas in a newborn infant. Am J Dis Child 1947; 74:58–79.
5. Baylin SB, Mendelson G: Ectopic (inappropriate) hormone production by tumors: Mechanisms involved and the biological and clinical implications. Endocr Rev 1980; 1:45–77.
6. Polak JM, Bloom SR, Adrian TE, et al: Pancreatic polypeptide in insulinomas, gastrinomas, VIPomas and glucagonomas. Lancet 1976; 1:328–330.
7. Larsson LI, Schwartz T, Lundgrist G: Occurrence of human pancreatic polypeptide in pancreatic endocrine tumors. Am J Pathol 1976; 85:675–684.
8. Unger RH, Orci L: Glucagon and the cell: Physiology and pathophysiology. N Engl J Med 1981; 304:1518–1524.
9. Larson LI: Endocrine pancreatic tumors. Hum Pathol 1978; 9:401–416.
10. Heitz PU, Kasper M, Polak JM, et al: Pancreatic endocrine tumors: Immunocytochemical analysis of 125 tumors. Hum Pathol 1982; 13:263–271.
11. Grosfeld JL, Vane DW, Rescorla FJ, et al: Pancreatic tumors in childhood. J Pediatr Surg 1990; 25:1057–1062.
12. Ballard HS, Frame B, Hartsock RJ: Familial multiple endocrine adenoma-peptic ulcer complex. Medicine 1964; 43:481–516.
13. Rasbach DA, Van Harden JA, Telander RL, et al: Surgical management of hyperinsulinism in the multiple endocrine neoplasia type 1 syndrome. Arch Surg 1985; 120:584–589.
14. Wermer P: Genetic aspects of adenomatosis of the endocrine glands. Am J Med 1954; 16:363–371.
15. Schimke RN: Genetic aspects of multiple endocrine neoplasia. Annu Rev Med 1984; 35:25–31.
16. Larson C, Skogseid B, Oberg K, et al: Multiple endocrine neoplasia type 1 gene maps to chromosome 11 and is lost in insulinoma. Nature 1988; 332:85–87.
17. Buchanan KD, Johnston CF, O'Hare MT, et al: Neuroendocrine tumors: A European review. Am J Med 1986; 81(Suppl 6B):14.
18. Whipple AO: Adenoma of islet cells with hyperinsulinism. Ann Surg 1935; 101:1299–1355.
19. Tudor RB: Childhood Disease Registry. Q & R Clinic, Bismarck, ND, 1991.
20. Marks V: Hypoglycemia due to pancreatic causes. *In* Samols E, ed: The Endocrine Pancreas. New York, Raven Press, 1991, pp 207–227.
21. Liu TH, Tseng HC, Zhu Y, et al: Insulinoma: An immunocytochemical and morphologic analysis of 95 cases. Cancer 1985; 56:1420–1429.
22. Aynsley-Green A, Polak JM, Bloom SR, et al: Nesidioblastosis of the pancreas: Definition of the syndrome and management of the severe neonatal hyperinsulinemic hypoglycemia. Arch Dis Child 1981; 56:496–508.
23. Kloppel G, Heitz PU: Pancreatic endocrine tumors. Pathol Res Pract 1988; 183:155–168.
24. Boden G: Glucagonomas and insulinomas. Gastroenterol Clin North Am 1989; 18:831–845.
25. Grant CS, Van Heerden J, Charboneau JW, et al: Insulinoma: The value of intraoperative ultrasonography. Arch Surg 1988; 123:843–848.

26. Norton JA, Cromack DT, Shawker TH, et al: Intraoperative ultrasonographic localization of islet cell tumors: A prospective comparison to palpation. Ann Surg 1988; 207:160–168.
27. Thomas CG, Underwood LE, Carney CN, et al: Neonatal and infantile hypoglycemia due to insulin excess: New aspects of diagnosis and surgical management. Ann Surg 1977; 185:505–517.
28. Dunger DB, Burns C, Ghale GK, et al: Pancreatic exocrine and endocrine function after subtotal pancreatectomy for nesidioblastosis. J Pediatr Surg 1988; 23:112–115.
29. Greene SA, Aynsley-Green A, Soltesz G, et al: Management of secondary diabetes mellitus after total pancreatectomy in infancy. Arch Dis Child 1984; 59:356–359.
30. Labrune P, Lechevallier S, Rault M, et al: Diabetes mellitus 14 years after a subtotal pancreatectomy for neonatal hyperinsulinism. J Pediatr Surg 1990; 25(12):1246–1247.
31. Maton PN: The use of the long-acting somatostatin analogue, octreotide acetate, in patients with islet cell tumors. Gastroenterol Clin North Am 1989; 18:897–922.
32. Laidlaw GF: Nesidioblastoma, the islet cell tumor of the pancreas. Am J Pathol 1938; 14:125–134.
33. Frake DL, Norton JA: The role of surgery in the management of islet cells tumors. Gastroenterol Clin North Am 1989; 18:805–830.
34. Zollinger RM, Ellison EH: Primary peptic ulcerations of the jejunum associated with islet cell tumors of the pancreas. Ann Surg 1955; 142:709–728.
35. Gregory RA, Grossman MI, Tracy HJ, et al: Nature of the gastric secretagogue in Zollinger-Ellison syndrome tumors. Lancet 1967; 2:543–544.
36. Gregory RA, Tracy HJ, Agarwal KL, et al: Amino acid constitution of two gastrins isolated from Zollinger-Ellison tumor tissue. Gut 1969; 10:603–608.
37. Ellison EH, Wilson SD: The Zollinger-Ellison syndrome: Reappraisal and evaluation of 260 registered cases. Ann Surg 1964; 160:512–530.
38. Creutzfeldt W, Arnold R, Creutzfeldt C, et al: Pathomorphologic, biochemical and diagnostic aspects of gastrinomas (Zollinger-Ellison syndrome). Hum Pathol 1975; 6:47–76.
39. Thompson NW, Vinik AI, Eckhauser FE: Microgastrinomas of the duodenum: A cause for failed operations for the Zollinger-Ellison syndrome. Ann Surg 1989; 209:396–404.
40. Tracy HJ, Gregory RA: Physiological properties of a series of synthetic peptides structurally related to gastrin I. Nature 1964; 204:935–977.
41. Dockray GJ, Taylor IL: Heptadecapeptide gastrin: Measurement in blood by specific radioimmunoassay. Gastroenterology 1976; 71:971–977.
42. Power DM, Bunnett N, Turner AJ, et al: Degradation of endogenous heptadecapeptide gastrin by endopeptidase 24.11 in the pig. Am J Physiol 1987; 253:G33–G39.
43. Abe K, Niikawa N, Sasaki H: Zollinger-Ellison syndrome with Marden-Walker syndrome. Am J Dis Child 1979; 133:735–738.
44. Thompson JC, Lewis BG, Wiener I, et al: The role of surgery in Zollinger-Ellison syndrome. Ann Surg 1983; 197:594–605.
45. Schwartz DL, White JJ, Saulsbury F, et al: Gastrin response to calcium infusion: An aid to the improved diagnosis of Zollinger-Ellison syndrome in children. Pediatrics 1974; 54:599–602.
46. Deveney CW, Deveney KE: Zollinger-Ellison syndrome (gastrinoma): Current diagnosis and treatment. Surg Clin North Am 1987; 67:411–423.
47. Raufman JP, Collins SM, Pandol SJ, et al: Reliability of symptoms in assessing control of gastric acid secretion in patients with Zollinger-Ellison syndrome. Gastroenterology 1983; 84:108–113.
48. McArthur KE, Collen MJ, Maton PN, et al: Omeprazole: Effective, convenient therapy for Zollinger-Ellison syndrome. Gastroenterology 1985; 88:939–944.
49. Maton P, McArthur K, Wank S, et al: Long-term efficacy and safety of omeprazole in patients with Zollinger-Ellison syndrome. Gastroenterology 1986; 90:1537.
50. Wolfe MM, Jensen RT: Zollinger-Ellison syndrome: Current concepts in diagnosis and management. N Engl J Med 1987; 317:1200–1209.
51. Vogel SB, Wolfe MM, McGuigan JE, et al: Localization and resection of gastrinomas in Zollinger-Ellison syndrome. Ann Surg 1987; 200:550–555.
52. Richardson CT, Peters MN, Feldman M, et al: Treatment of Zollinger-Ellison syndrome with exploratory laparotomy, proximal gastric vagotomy and H_2-receptor antagonists. Gastroenterology 1985; 89:357–367.
53. Rothenberg RE, Radulescu OV, LaRaja RD, et al: The surgical treatment of the Zollinger-Ellison syndrome: An update. Am Surg 1987; 53:573–574.
54. Vinik AI, Thompson N: Controversies in the management of Zollinger-Ellison syndrome. Ann Intern Med 1986; 105:956–959.
55. Maton PN, Gardner JD, Jensen RT: Recent advances in the management of gastric acid hypersecretion in patients with Zollinger-Ellison syndrome. Gastroenterol Clin North Am 1989; 18:847–863.
56. Morowitz DA, Levine AE: Malignant Zollinger-Ellison syndrome: Remission of primary metastatic pancreatic tumor after gastrectomy: Report of a case and review of the literature. Am J Gastroenterol 1986; 81:471–473.
57. Matsumoto KK, Peter JB, Schultze RG, et al: Watery diarrhea and hypokalemia associated with pancreatic islet cell adenoma. Gastroenterology 1966; 50:231–242.
58. Marks IH, Banks S, Louw JH: Islet cell tumor of the pancreas with reversible watery diarrhea and achlorhydria. Gastroenterology 1967; 52:695–708.
59. Verner JV, Morrison AB: Islet cell tumor and a syndrome of refractory watery diarrhea and hypokalemia. Am J Med 1958; 25:374–380.
60. O'Dorisio TM, Mekhjian HS, Gaginella TS: Medical therapy of VIPomas. Endocrinol Metab Clin North Am 1989; 18:545–556.
61. Capella C, Polak JM, Buffa R, et al: Morphologic patterns and diagnostic criteria of VIP-producing endocrine tumors. Cancer 1983; 52:1860–1874.
62. Jansen-Goemans A, Engelhardt J: Intractable diarrhea in a boy with vasoactive intestinal peptide–producing ganglioneuroblastoma. Pediatrics 1977; 59:710–716.
63. Mitchell CH, Sinatra FR, Crast FW, et al: Intractable watery diarrhea, ganglioneuroblastoma and vasoactive intestinal peptide. J Pediatr 1976; 89:593–595.
64. Ghishan FK, Soper RT, Nassif EG, et al: Chronic diarrhea of infancy: Non-beta islet cell hyperplasia. Pediatrics 1979; 64:46–49.
65. Brenner RW, Sank LI, Kerner MB, et al: Resection of a VIPoma of the pancreas in a 15-year-old girl. J Pediatr Surg 1986; 21:983–985.
66. Mutt V: Isolation and structure of vasoactive intestinal polypeptide from various species. *In* Said SI, ed: Vasoactive Intestinal Peptide. New York, Raven Press, 1982, pp 1–10.
67. Racusen LC, Binder HJ: Alteration of large intestinal electrolyte transport by vasoactive intestinal polypeptide in the rat. Gastroenterology 1977; 73:790–796.
68. Krejs GJ: VIPoma syndrome. Am J Med 1987; 82(Suppl 5B):37–48.
69. Parkman HP, Malet PF, Ogorek CP, et al: Preoperative localization of a vasoactive intestinal peptide-secreting tumor by transhepatic portal venous sampling. Am J Gastroenterol 1988; 83:559–563.
70. Koelz A, Kraenzlin M, Gyr K, et al: Escape of the response to a long-acting somatostatin analogue (SMS 201–995) in patients with VIPoma. Gastroenterology 1987; 92:527–531.
71. Jaffe BM, Kopen DF, DeSchryver-Kecskemeti K, et al: Indomethacin-responsive pancreatic cholera. N Engl J Med 1977; 297:817–821.
72. Moertel CG, Hanley JA, Johnson LA: Streptozotocin alone compared with streptozotocin plus fluorouracil in the treatment of advanced islet cell carcinoma. N Engl J Med 1980; 303:1189–1194.
73. Mallinson CN, Bloom SR, Warin AP, et al: A glucagonoma syndrome. Lancet 1974; 2:1–5.
74. Riddle MC, Golper TA, Fletcher WS, et al: Glucagonoma syndrome in a 19-year-old woman. West J Med 1978; 129:68–72.
75. Stacpoole PW: The glucagonoma syndrome: Clinical features, diagnosis and treatment. Endocrinol Rev 1981; 2:347.
76. Higgins GA, Recant L, Fischman AB: The glucagonoma syndrome: Surgically curable diabetes. Am J Surg 1979; 137:142–148.
77. Prinz RA, Badrinath K, Banerji M, et al: Operative and chemotherapeutic management of malignant glucagon-producing tumors. Surgery 1981; 90:713–719.
78. Konomi K, Chijiiwa K, Katsuta T, et al: Pancreatic somatostatinoma: A case report and review of the literature. J Surg Oncol 1990; 43:259–265.
79. Lamberts SWJ, Bakker WH, Reubi JC, Krennig EP: Somatostatin-receptor imaging in the localization of endocrine tumors. N Engl J Med 1990; 323:1246–1249.

Chapter 71

Abnormalities of the Bile Ducts

JONATHAN S. EVANS

CLASSIFICATION

Pediatric bile tract disorders are a heterogeneous group that do not lend well to classification along conventional guidelines such as etiology or anatomy. A descriptive classification is given in Table 71–1 and will be followed in this chapter. Most disorders are rare, with few comprehensive pediatric reports described in the literature. When appropriate, information is provided from the adult literature.

ETIOLOGY

Two theories have been formulated to provide a unifying pathogenesis for the infantile cholangiopathies: the ductal plate malformation theory and the infantile obstructive cholangiopathy theory. Both theories attempt to explain via a common pathogenetic mechanism the overlapping clinical and pathologic pictures of diseases such as biliary atresia, neonatal hepatitis, choledochal cyst, and others.

Table 71–1. DESCRIPTIVE CLASSIFICATION OF PEDIATRIC BILIARY TRACT ABNORMALITIES

- Disorders of Fibrosis
  - Extrahepatic biliary atresia
  - Sclerosing cholangitis: primary or secondary
  - Pericholangitis
  - Congenital hepatic fibrosis*
  - Cystic fibrosis–associated hepatobiliary disease
- Disorders of Cyst Formation
  - Choledochal cysts
  - Caroli's disease
  - Infantile polycystic disease*
- Disorders of Paucity
  - Syndromatic paucity of interlobular bile ducts
  - Nonsyndromatic paucity of interlobular bile ducts: idiopathic or secondary
- Miscellaneous Disorders
  - Gallbladder perforation: idiopathic or secondary
  - Biliary tree stricture: idiopathic or secondary (extrinsic compression, cholelithiasis)
  - Congenital malformations
    - Agenesis
    - Septation
    - Duplication
    - Ectopic gallbladder
    - Accessory bile duct
    - Cholecystohepatic duct
    - Bronchobiliary fistula
    - Bile duct stricture

*Congenital hepatic fibrosis and infantile polycystic disease may be a single disease entity.

The ductal plate malformation theory first advanced by Jorgensen[1] has been recently reviewed by Desmet.[2] In this theory, the earliest form of the embryonic bile duct, the ductal plate, undergoes altered remodeling with persistence of excess structure and cannot achieve a normal final form. According to the time and the level at which the malformation occurs, the dysgenesis may be expressed as atresia (e.g., extrahepatic biliary atresia), paucity (e.g., Alagille syndrome), proliferation and fibrosis (e.g., congenital hepatic fibrosis, infantile polycystic disease), or cystic dilatation (e.g., choledochal cyst).

The concept of neonatal obstructive cholangiopathy was first proposed by Landing in 1974.[3] This theory postulates a common mechanism for biliary atresia, neonatal giant cell hepatitis, and choledochal cyst consisting of "a cholangiopathic process [that] is inflammatory with varying degrees of liver cell and bile duct epithelial injury, obliteration of biliary tree lumina, and later sclerosis determining the various possible outcomes."[3]

CLINICAL FEATURES

Most pediatric bile tract disorders present in a chronic fashion with mild symptomatology and physical signs. This often results in delayed diagnosis. Some children may present initially with a complication (e.g., cholangitis, variceal hemorrhage) that is the result of chronic progressive hepatobiliary disease. It is not unusual for suspicion to be raised on routine laboratory tests drawn for another reason.

EVALUATION AND DIAGNOSIS

Each child should be evaluated in a conventional manner beginning with a comprehensive history and physical examination. Biochemical testing is especially important to exclude nonbiliary tract causes of jaundice (e.g., viral hepatitis, $alpha_1$-antitrypsin deficiency, hemolysis). Pediatric gastroenterologists, radiologists, pathologists, and surgeons are often needed to pursue the evaluation and discriminate among the different causes of cholestasis. This may be best performed in a pediatric tertiary care center, where these specialists can collaborate and arrive at the correct diagnosis in an efficient and expeditious manner.

Visualization of the bile ducts is the key to diagnosis of pediatric biliary tract disorders. Historically this visualization was provided by the surgeon; however, new less invasive technologies are facilitating the evaluation and diagnosis. A list of these techniques is provided in Table 71–2, but the choice of a particular technique is dependent on the problem at hand, the availability of each technique, and the expertise of the people using them.

Histologic examination of liver tissue is usually abnormal but most often nondiagnostic due to the lack of disease-specific lesions. A notable exception is congenital hepatic fibrosis. The liver biopsy is nonetheless essential for prognostic reasons.

THERAPY

The goal of medical therapy in the treatment of pediatric biliary tract disorders is to prevent and treat the complications of each particular disease (e.g., vitamin E deficiency, bacterial cholangitis, malnutrition). Surgical therapy is the only modality to provide definitive treatment. Since the early 1980s, orthotopic liver transplantation has become a viable option for children with end-stage liver disease either as a result of failed primary repair or when primary repair was not possible.[4]

EXTRAHEPATIC BILIARY ATRESIA

Extrahepatic biliary atresia (EHBA) is an important clinical condition because early diagnosis and appropriate management affect overall prognosis. EHBA is defined as the absence of all or a portion of the extrahepatic biliary system. It results in complete obstruction of bile flow and, if untreated, leads to cirrhosis, liver failure, and death. There are a variety of anatomic forms that are best described in the classification adopted by the Japanese Society of Pediatric Surgery.[5] In this classification there are three principal types: atresia of the common bile duct, atresia of the common hepatic duct, and atresia of bile ducts at the porta hepatis. This last type corresponds to the "noncorrectable" form in previous classifications and represents greater than 80% of cases.[6] Nine subtypes further delineate the different anatomic variants.

Table 71–2. RECOMMENDED TECHNIQUES FOR THE EVALUATION OF PEDIATRIC BILIARY TRACT DISORDERS

Technique	References
Noninvasive	
Ultrasonography	27, 28, 30, 227, 265
Hepatobiliary scintigraphy	34–36, 265
Magnetic resonance imaging	
Computerized axial tomography	134
Nonoperative	
Duodenal intubation	32, 33
Endoscopic retrograde cholangiography	38–41, 125, 253, 254, 267
Percutaneous transhepatic cholangiography	37
Percutaneous cholecystic cholangiography	130, 131
Operative	
Operative cholangiogram	42
Laparotomy	42

Epidemiology

Biliary atresia is the second most frequent cause of neonatal cholestasis after idiopathic neonatal hepatitis.[7] Its overall incidence is estimated at 0.7 to 1.0 cases per 10,000 live births.[7, 8] The common belief that the disease is more prevalent among Japanese as compared to white populations was not supported when the incidence was studied in these populations on the island of Hawaii.[8] Furthermore, there does not appear to be an increased incidence of EHBA when Japanese populations in Hawaii and Sendai Japan were compared.[8]

Etiology

The cause of EHBA is still unknown. It was originally thought to be a congenital malformation, and this was supported by its known association with other congenital anomalies (e.g., polysplenia, preduodenal portal vein, intestinal atresia, and Turner's syndrome).[3] However, current theories support a progressive perinatal sclerotic process. Evidence for this is provided by the examination of surgical specimens removed during hepatic portoenterostomy, the operation that has been used since the 1960s for treatment of this disease.[9] This pathologic process is compatible with the infantile obstructive cholangiopathy theory described earlier.

Attempts to develop experimental models of biliary atresia have met with variable success. They have included perinatal injection of sclerosants and ligation of the bile duct,[10, 11] interruption of blood flow to the common bile duct,[12] and the use of infectious agents. In this last category, infection of mice with Reovirus type 3 has suggested a very convincing etiology for EHBA.[13] In this model, weanling mice infected with Reovirus type 3 showed ductular lesions at 2 weeks postinfection almost identical to those found in human bile duct remnants resected at portoenterostomy, but at a time when the virus could no longer be recovered from the mice. Furthermore, serologic evidence of Reovirus type 3 infection has been found in children with EHBA.[14] These last results have not, however, been supported by others,[15], and final acceptance or rejection of this theory is still awaited.[16] Well-documented time-space clustering of this disease also supports either an infectious or an environmental etiologic process.[17, 18]

Pathogenesis

EHBA is regarded as a progressive inflammatory cholangitis with sclerosis and obstruction.[9, 19, 20] It can involve the entire biliary system or it can be segmental with varying degrees of severity. Most frequently, the major bile ducts at the level of the porta hepatis are involved, and at diagnosis only fibrous tissue can be found as remnants of these structures (Fig. 71–1). Based upon the work of Kasai and his associates, microscopic biliary channels communicating with the intrahepatic bile ducts were found to exist within these fibrous remnants.[18, 21] This is the precept upon which surgical correction of this disease is based. It has been postulated that the diameter of these channels must exceed 150 μm in order for bile flow to be surgically re-established.[20, 22, 23] It is unclear whether the changes found on biopsy of the intrahepatic bile ducts and hepatic parenchyma are secondary to chronic distal obstruction or due to the primary pathologic process itself. These intrahepatic findings have been well described,[15, 24, 25] and a typical case at 9 weeks and 9 months of age is shown in Figures 71–2 and 71–3. The histologic findings on liver biopsy are variable and nonspecific. These include widening of portal tracts from edema and inflammatory cell infiltrate, destruction and degeneration of portal bile ducts with plugging, secondary bile ductular proliferation, and intraparenchymal inflammatory infiltrate with giant cell transformation found in 15%. Periportal fibrosis is progressive; in advanced cases, typical biliary cirrhosis is found, with bile lakes and increased intrahepatic copper stores. An experienced pathologist is critical to aid in the correct interpretation of these biopsies and to differentiate EHBA from other causes of cholestasis.

Clinical Features

The most typical presentation of EHBA is the child seen by the primary care physician during the first or second month of life with asymptomatic jaundice. The child has had an unremarkable perinatal course, appears well, and is thriving. Jaundice may have been present since birth, but in many cases it may reappear at two to three weeks of age after resolution of normal physiologic jaundice.

The stools are acholic (i.e., gray and unpigmented) with intermittent coloration, thought to be due to bilirubin-laden intestinal cells and secretions. The urine is yellow and dark, staining the diaper. The liver is enlarged, smooth, and firm. It is usually not as enlarged as in metabolic storage diseases. Splenomegaly may not develop until later.

In later stages of the disease, the jaundice deepens and develops a greenish hue; all secretions including tears and saliva become colored. Other stigmata of progressive cirrhosis are seen, including decreasing liver size, splenomegaly, abdominal distention with ascites, pruritus, peripheral edema, digital clubbing, bruising, rachitic rosary, dental dysplasia,[26] heart murmur secondary to pulmonary arteriovenous shunting, and malnutrition. Untreated, death is inevitable between 18 and 36 months of age.

Evaluation and Diagnostic Features

The diagnostic approach to a child with cholestasis has been discussed in the introduction. It should be

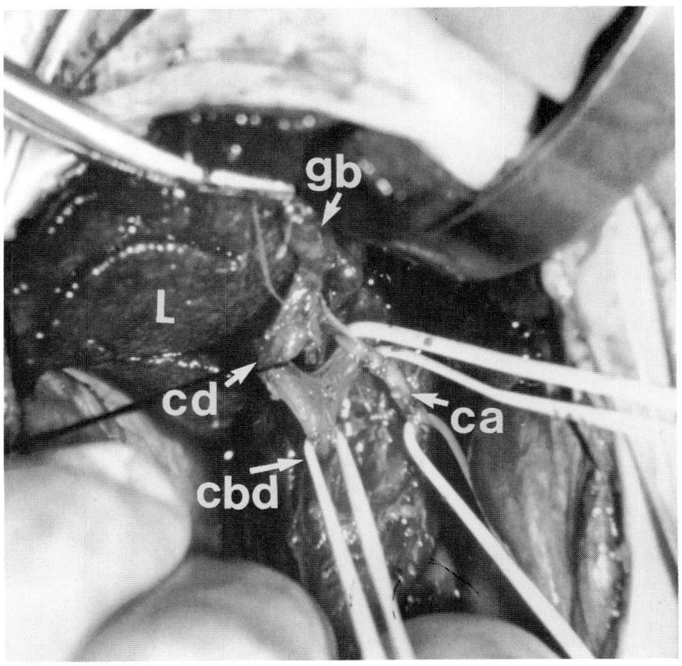

Figure 71–1. Exploratory laparotomy of an infant with extrahepatic biliary atresia. Operative view of the porta hepatis shows a green nodular liver (*L*) and an atretic gallbladder (*gb*). The common bile duct (*cbd*) and cystic duct (*cd*) were present but fibrotic and nonpatent. The cystic artery (*ca*) is also shown. (Courtesy of Dr. D. Mollit.)

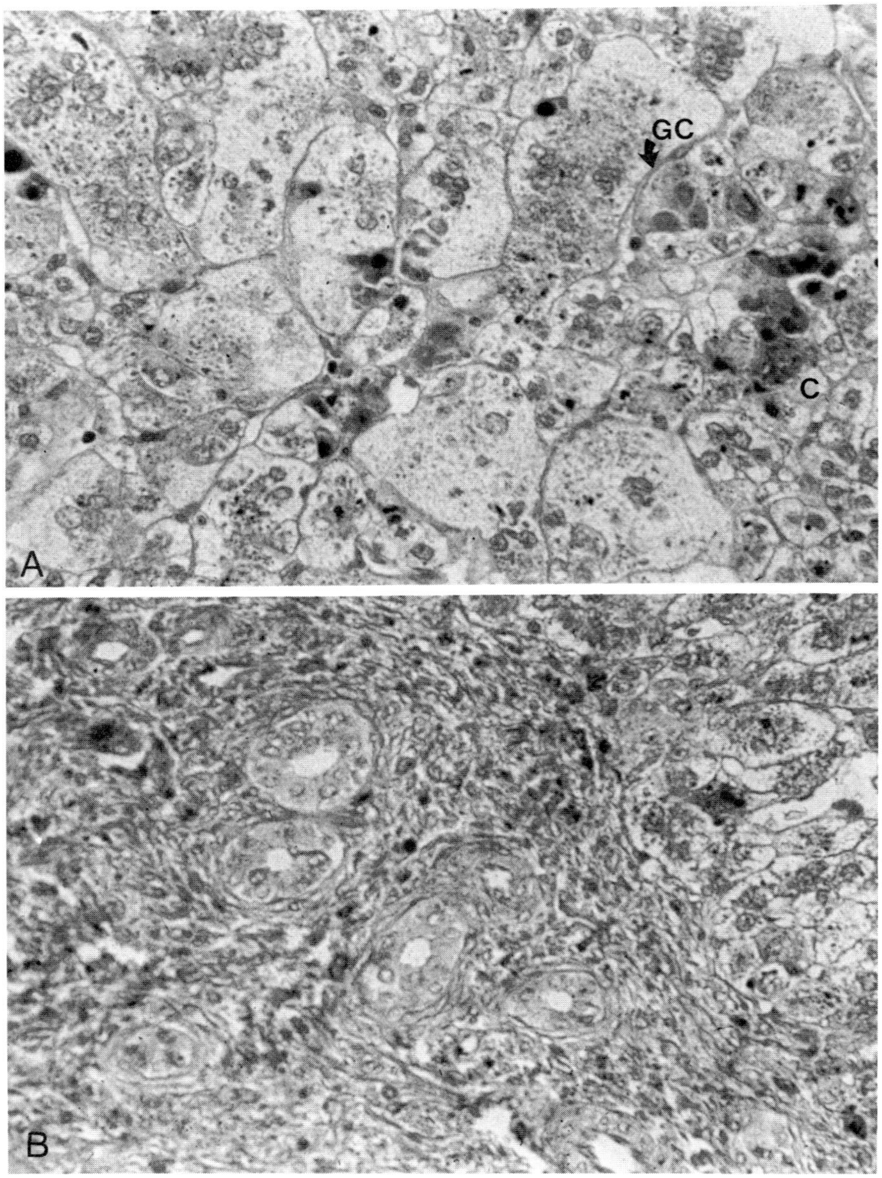

Figure 71–2. Liver histology in 9-week-old male with biliary atresia. *A,* Giant cell transformation of hepatocytes (*GC*) and intracytoplasmic cholestasis (*C*). Hematoxylin-eosin stain, × 250. *B,* A portal triad with bile ductular proliferation and fibrosis. Trichrome-Masson stain, × 100.

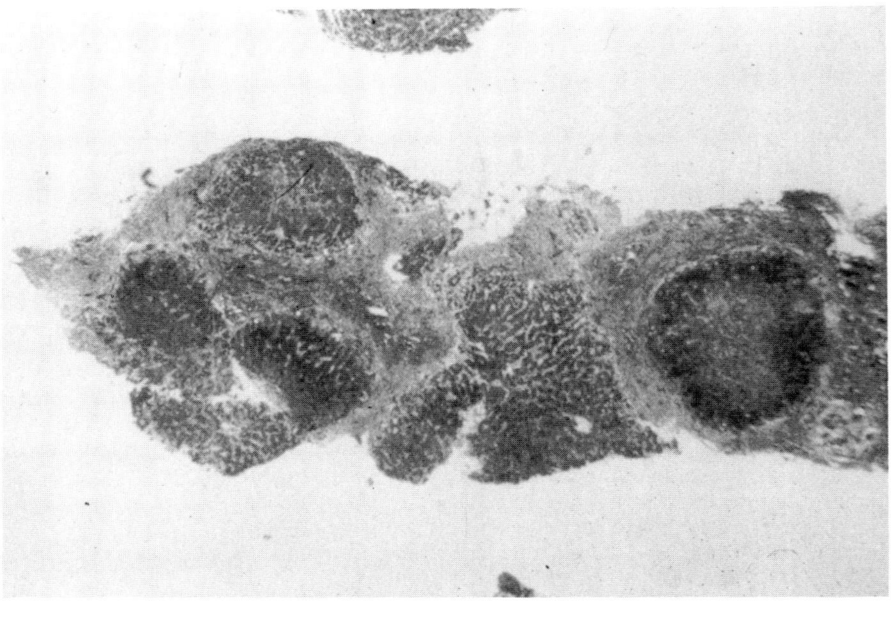

Figure 71–3. Same child as in Figure 71–2, biopsied at 9 months of age. Trichrome-Masson stain of liver tissue (× 25) shows well-established biliary cirrhosis.

emphasized, however, that early diagnosis in this disease improves surgical outcome (see later); a suggested evaluation protocol and schedule are provided in Table 71–3. Clinical features at presentation may be a helpful guide in directing the diagnosis (Table 71–4).

The absence of a gallbladder on abdominal ultrasound is helpful in guiding the diagnosis, but in 30% of cases, a normal gallbladder is visualized.[27, 28] In 22% of cases, the gallbladder remains in communication with the duodenum via patent cystic and common bile ducts.[28, 29] In these instances an oral feeding under ultrasonographic visualization of the gallbladder may not be as helpful as previously suggested.[30] Dilated bile ducts are not an ultrasonographic feature of EHBA.

Although the histologic features of EHBA are not necessarily diagnostic, a properly performed percutaneous needle liver biopsy is nonetheless helpful, adding important diagnostic data and excluding other diseases with characteristic findings (e.g, nonsyndromatic paucity of bile ducts).[31]

Duodenal intubation and collection of intestinal fluid have been reported by Greene and coworkers[32, 33] to be simple and direct. The presence of bile in the duodenal aspirate either by assay or by visual inspection confirms the patency of the extrahepatic bile ducts. An abdominal computerized tomography (CT) scan may be helpful to define abnormal anatomy (polysplenia, cysts, and so on).

Radionuclide hepatobiliary imaging using technetium-99M–labeled derivatives of iminodiacetic acid is now considered by many the "gold standard" to confirm patency of the extrahepatic bile ducts.[34–36] In the normal patient, this labeled molecule with a short half-life (6 hours) is taken up rapidly after intravenous injection by the liver (5 minutes) and then the gallbladder (15 minutes), and activity can be detected in the small bowel by 30 minutes and in the colon by 6 hours. Nonexcretion into the small bowel is found in patients with biliary obstruction, but also in severe intrahepatic cholestasis (e.g., $alpha_1$-antitrypsin deficiency, neonatal hepatitis). "Priming" of the liver with phenobarbital (5–10 mg per kg per day) for 5 days prior to testing increases the overall specificity from 63 to 94%, reducing the number of false positives (i.e., lack of excretion due to severe parenchymal disease despite a patent biliary tract).[35]

Based on the results of an evaluation suggesting extrahepatic obstruction to bile flow, direct visualization of the main bile ducts becomes essential. Percutaneous transhepatic cholangiography (PTC)[37] or endoscopic retrograde cholangiopancreatography (ERCP)[38–41] may in some centers provide this visualization. However, in most cases the child undergoes an exploratory laparotomy. This procedure often includes an open liver biopsy and involves a small right subcostal incision. If the gallbladder is fibrotic or contains white bile, then the incision is enlarged and full surgical exploration of the extrahepatic biliary tree is performed[42] (see Fig. 71–1). If the findings are consistent with EHBA, then a hepatic portoenterostomy is performed. In 30% of cases the gallbladder is patent and an operative cholangiogram is performed. Dilute contrast is injected under sufficient pressure to fill both the extrahepatic tree and the main intrahepatic branches of the common hepatic duct. In cases in which the common hepatic duct is not visualized, the distal common bile duct may be manually occluded and the injection repeated. In biliary hypoplasia secondary to prolonged severe intrahepatic cholestasis, the entire extrahepatic biliary tree is patent but the ducts are of small diameter. In these cases a cholecystostomy tube may be left in place for repeated imaging injections at a later date. If some or all of the extrahepatic bile ducts are nonpatent the surgeon proceeds with a hepatic portoenterostomy.

Table 71–3. SUGGESTED DIAGNOSTIC EVALUATION PROTOCOL FOR THE PATIENT WITH CONJUGATED HYPERBILIRUBINEMIA AND SUSPECTED EHBA

Day	Protocol
1	Laboratory evaluation
	Transaminases
	Alkaline phosphatase, gamma glutamyltranspeptidase, bilirubin (total/direct)
	Hepatitis A, B, C serology
	"TORCH" titers
	HIV screen
	$Alpha_1$-antitrypsin
	Urine metabolic screen
	Serum, urine amino acids
	Urine culture
	Thyroid profile
	Start phenobarbital (5–10 mg/kg/day)
2	Sweat chloride test
	Ultrasound of liver, gallbladder
3*	Percutaneous needle liver biopsy
	Duodenal intubation (optional)
	Abdominal CT scan (optional)
5	Hepatobiliary scintigraphy
6	Laparatomy ± operative cholangiogram

*Dependent on availability and indication. Percutaneous transhepatic cholangiography or endoscopic retrograde cholangiography may be performed on day 3 or 4.

Table 71–4. COMPARISON OF CLINICAL FEATURES AT PRESENTATION BETWEEN CHILDREN WITH INTRAHEPATIC AND EXTRAHEPATIC CAUSES OF CHOLESTASIS

Variable	Biliary Atresia	Neonatal Hepatitis
Birth	Term	Premature
Birth weight	Average for gestational age	Small for gestational age
Growth	Thriving	Failure
Appearance	Well	Ill
Stools	Acholic	Pigmented

Treatment

Treatment for EHBA is twofold: medical and surgical. Medical therapy involves the prevention and treatment of the complications of chronic cholestatic liver disease, portal hypertension, and malnutrition. Guidelines for medical therapy are given in Table 71–5.[43–57]

Surgical therapy for EHBA is essential, and techniques continue to evolve. Hepatic portoenterostomy is indicated for infants diagnosed before 8 to 10 weeks of age. Orthotopic liver transplantation is reserved for those children who fail primary repair or who are diagnosed after 12 to 14 weeks of age. Liver transplantation as first-line therapy for EHBA in all infants has been proposed, but remains controversial.[58]

Ladd is credited with the first successful repair of EHBA in 1928.[59] However, Morio Kasai in the 1950s was the first to understand the underlying pathogenesis of this disease (see earlier) and consistently provide bile drainage in these children. His disease concepts and surgical repair, the hepatic portoenterostomy, were not adopted in Japan until the 1960s and were not used in North America and Europe until the 1970s. The historical background and reasons for this slow acceptance are well described.[9] The hepatic portoenterostomy involves dissection of the fibrous porta hepatis at the level of the liver and portal vein bifurcation, identifying and preserving microscopic (>150 μm diameter) biliary ductules that will allow hepatic bile drainage. A Roux-en-Y intestinal conduit is constructed and anastomosed to the cut surface; a permanent biliary fistula evolves over time[9, 60–62] (Fig. 71–4). In 22% of cases,[29, 30] a patent gallbladder, cystic duct, and common bile duct may be used as a drainage conduit (hepatic portocholecystostomy).

Ascending bacterial cholangitis is the most frequent postoperative complication. Its occurrence implies patency between the intestinal conduit and hepatic parenchyma; it is thought to arise from intrahepatic bile stasis and an inevitable bacterial contamination of the intestinal conduit. Clinical features consist of unexplained fever, increased jaundice, decreased ostomy output in patients with an externalized conduit, decreased bile bilirubin content, and leukocytosis. Serum transaminases, bilirubin, and gamma glutamyltranspeptidase become further elevated, and the cholangitis may progress to overwhelming sepsis. Diagnosis is confirmed by liver biopsy. The infectious agent, in most cases a gram-negative enteric bacterium, can be identified by culture of blood and liver tissue in 75% of affected patients.[63, 64] Early broad-spectrum antibiotics (e.g., third-generation cephalosporin or combined ampicillin and gentamycin) are essential for good short- and long-term outcomes.

More than 15 modifications of the original Kasai operation have been developed to prevent ascending cholangitis. Most have involved temporary exteriorization of bile drainage through an intestinal conduit (see Fig. 71–4). Theoretically, this improved hepatofugal bile

Table 71–5. EXTRAHEPATIC BILIARY ATRESIA—GUIDELINES FOR MEDICAL THERAPY

Problem	Therapy	References	Comments
Chronic Cholestasis			
Cholestasis	Phenobarbital	43	
	Ursodeoxycholic acid	44, 45	Investigational
Pruritus	Bile acid binding agents	46	Efficacy of these agents is controversial or still under investigation
	Ultraviolet B light	47	
	Carbamazepine	43, 46	
	Rifampin	48	
	Antihistamines	43, 46	
Portal Hypertension			
Variceal hemorrhage	Transfusion		
	Vasopressin	49	
	Balloon tamponade	49, 50	
	Sclerotherapy	51, 52	
	Propranolol	53, 54	
Ascites ± peritonitis	Fluid restriction	46, 55	
	Furosemide, spironolactone		
	Albumin, paracentesis		
	Antibiotics		
Hypersplenism	Transfusion as needed		
	Erythropoietin (?)		
Malnutrition			
Intake	Oral, enteral, parenteral supplementation	56	Nutritionist's aid is invaluable
Carbohydrate	125–150% of needs	46, 57	
Protein	2–3 gm/kg/day if compensated 0.5–1 gm/kg/day if decompensated	46, 57	The value of branched-chain amino acids remains controversial
Fat	40–60% as medium-chain triglycerides	56, 57	Avoid essential fatty acid deficiency
Fat-soluble vitamins	A, D, E, K supplements	46	
Water-soluble vitamins	Multivitamin daily	57	No clinical deficiency described
Minerals	Supplements as needed	46, 57	Monitor as needed; no supplemental calcium
Trace elements	Supplements as needed		Monitor as needed

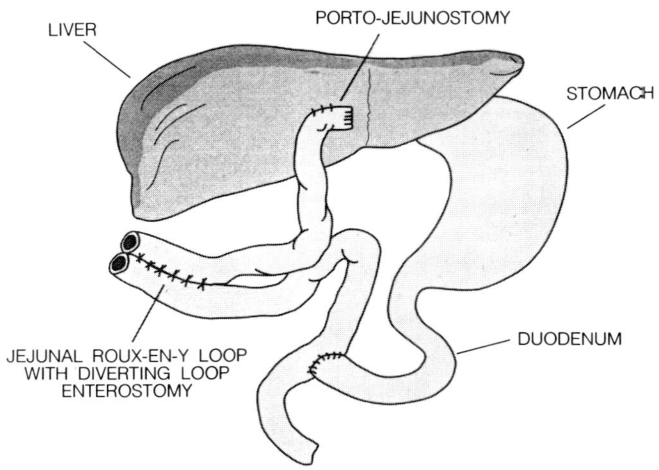

Figure 71–4. Schematic representation of a hepatic portoenterostomy (Kasai procedure) providing bile drainage in a case of extrahepatic biliary atresia. An externalized intestinal conduit is shown as one of the many modifications tried to prevent bacterial cholangitis.

flow, but in several studies it was not shown to be clinically effective and has now been abandoned in many centers.[62–64] More recent modifications to prevent bile reflux and cholangitis include the construction of a valved conduit[65–67] or an appendicoduodenostomy.[68]

Despite these surgical modifications, repeated episodes of cholangitis may occur, and the ensuing anastomotic and hepatic sclerosis with decreased bile flow adversely affects long-term outcome. Prophylactic antibiotics (e.g., trimethoprim-sulfamethoxazole, ampicillin) are widely used, but the controlled studies to determine their efficacy have not been performed; their usefulness is disputed by some.[9, 60] Corticosteroids and portoenterostomy revision have been used to re-establish bile flow after severe repeated episodes of bacterial cholangitis.

Portal hypertension is the other major complication following successful hepatic portoenterostomy. It may occur in 20% of patients with bile flow whether they have achieved an anicteric state or not. Signs and symptoms may first occur between the second and eighth year postoperatively and include splenomegaly and hypersplenism, ascites, and variceal hemorrhage.[60, 69, 70] Patients with externalized intestinal conduits may hemorrhage from peristomal varices.

Since 1980 and the advent of improved immunosuppressive therapy, orthotopic liver transplantation has become an important therapeutic modality in the treatment of children with EHBA. EHBA is the most frequent indication for pediatric liver transplantation, representing 40 to 55% of all pediatric liver transplants.[4, 71] Indications for referral to a pediatric transplant center include diagnosis after age 12 to 14 weeks, failure to excrete bile after hepatic portoenterostomy, and progressive severe liver disease despite a "successful" portoenterostomy. This last indication may be met years after the initial surgery and may be due to portal hypertension with unrelenting variceal hemorrhage or cirrhosis with hepatic synthetic failure. Recognition of poor prognostic factors may allow early referral prior to the onset of liver failure and malnutrition.

Results of Therapy and Prognosis

Hepatic portoenterostomy outcomes are variable among institutions but generally show improvement with increasing experience. Bile flow can be re-established in 50 to 85% of all patients, averaging 150 to 800 ml per day.[60, 72–74] Serum bilirubin levels return to normal in 45 to 80%.[70, 74–76] Four- and five-year survival rates post-hepatic portoenterostomy average 50%.[60, 72, 74, 77] Long-term survival rates are expected to improve with the advent of liver transplantation as a second line of therapy, but most major centers have recorded several 20-year survivors following hepatic portoenterostomy. Long-term morbidity, defined in one study as morbidity 5 to 15 years postportoenterostomy, includes ascending cholangitis (51%), variceal hemorrhage (20%), hepatomegaly (40%), hyperbilirubinemia (42%), and splenomegaly (52%).[70]

Age at operation and ascending cholangitis are the most significant prognostic factors affecting portoenterostomy results.[60, 66, 72, 78] Bile flow can be obtained in 80 to 86% of patients referred for portoenterostomy before 8 weeks of age; this falls to 45% beyond 10 weeks, and, although several "late" successful Kasai procedures have been reported,[78a] some believe that portoenterostomy is contraindicated beyond 12 weeks of age.[61, 79] Five-year survival increases from 50 to 91% in those children who do not develop ascending cholangitis postoperatively.[72] Additional favorable prognostic factors that have been reported include a postoperative bile bilirubin concentration greater than 8.8 mg per 100 ml[72] or 6 mg per day[66] and bile channels within the porta hepatis of a diameter greater than 150 μm.[20, 22]

Long-term survival (5 years) for all children undergoing liver transplantation approaches 70%,[4, 71] but may be less in children under 1 year of age (54 to 65%).[80, 81] One-year survival rates of children transplanted for EHBA vary between 55 and 88%.[58, 82, 83] Because of its overall good results, the question has been raised and is still debated whether liver transplantation should become the primary therapy for all children with EHBA.[58] Improving overall survival and the pool of organ donors through new surgical techniques, organ preservation fluids, and immunosuppressive therapy may in the future place liver transplantation at the forefront of therapy for children with EHBA.

SCLEROSING CHOLANGITIS

Sclerosing cholangitis is an inflammatory, obliterative fibrosis of the intra- and extrahepatic biliary tree.[84–88] Secondary sclerosing cholangitis is defined as those conditions in which a causal agent has been well established such as a postoperative stricture, choledocholithiasis, or caustic injury.[89, 90] Primary sclerosing cholangitis is a term reserved for those conditions in which a well-defined etiology cannot be discovered.[86] For example, although there is a complex relationship between chronic ulcerative colitis and sclerosing cholangitis (see later), a true causal relationship has not been proved, and the cholangitis remains primary. The remainder of this section is devoted to primary sclerosing cholangitis.

Epidemiology

Primary sclerosing cholangitis (PSC) is an uncommon disease described primarily in adults. Seventy percent of adult patients are men, and 66% are diagnosed under 45 years of age.[86] The incidence of pediatric PSC is unknown. Since 1980, only 96 children have been reported in the literature. The incidence of adult PSC is now 14 times greater than in the period 1956–1975. This is due in part to improved awareness and diagnostic techniques but also to a probable absolute increased incidence in the population.[87] An epidemiologic profile of pediatric PSC is given in Table 71–6.[84–87, 91–102] It is apparent that there is a lesser preponderance of males with PSC in the pediatric population as compared to adults. Also, children with inflammatory bowel disease (IBD) and PSC constitute 45% of the total as compared to 70% in adults ($P < 0.05$, chi square).

Etiology

The etiology of PSC is unknown but is thought to be multifactorial.[84, 86, 91] Insight into the pathogenesis of PSC is offered by the many clinical conditions associated with it (Table 71–7).[84, 95, 97, 99, 103–106] The relationships between PSC and these associated diseases are complex and still poorly understood. It is important to note that 10% of pediatric cases have no known associated condition.

Certainly the most frequent association is that of PSC with inflammatory bowel disease and specifically chronic ulcerative colitis. Inflammatory bowel disease is present in 70% of adult patients with PSC[87, 92, 107] but in only 45% of pediatric PSC patients. The prevalence of PSC within a population of adult IBD patients is only 4.5%.[106, 108] Chronic ulcerative colitis is the most prevalent form of inflammatory bowel disease in pediatric PSC, representing 74% of cases.

Table 71–6. EPIDEMIOLOGIC PROFILE OF 62 PUBLISHED PEDIATRIC PRIMARY SCLEROSING CHOLANGITIS CASES COMPARED WITH 293 PUBLISHED ADULT CASES

Variable	Pediatric	Adult
Number of patients	62	293
Average age at diagnosis (yr)	7	41
Males (%)	54	62
Females (%)	46	38
PSC + inflammatory bowel disease (%)*	45	70
References	84–86, 91, 93–102	87, 92, 99

*$P < 0.05$; chi square analysis.

Table 71–7. PRIMARY SCLEROSING CHOLANGITIS AND ASSOCIATED CLINICAL CONDITIONS COMPILED FROM 96 PUBLISHED PEDIATRIC CASES*

Variable	*n*	References
Inflammatory bowel disease		
Total	41	84, 102
Ulcerative colitis	31	
Crohn's disease	2	
Indeterminate colitis	8	
Histiocytosis X	15	84, 95
Congenital immunodeficiencies	11	84, 95, 97, 103
Neonatal cholestasis	10	84, 95
Cystic fibrosis	4	99, 104
Sickle-cell anemia	1	84
Autoimmune hemolytic anemia	1	105
Reticular sarcoma	1	84
No associated condition	12	84, 106
Total	96	

*Celiac disease has been associated with three adult cases of PSC[160] and acquired immunodeficiency syndrome (AIDS) with 26 adult cases.[123, 161] Both diseases are prevalent in the pediatric population but as yet are not reported to be associated with pediatric PSC.

The question has been raised whether PSC occurring in IBD patients maintains the same characteristics as in non-IBD patients. LaRusso[86] reported, based on clinical, pathologic, and cholangiographic data, that the characteristics were identical regardless of any association with IBD. Rabinowitz and associates,[107] however, studying 66 adults, found that PSC may be different when it occurs in association with inflammatory bowel disease. When it occurs in association with inflammatory bowel disease, PSC has a higher male to female ratio (2.9:1 versus 0.72:1) and more extensive biliary tree involvement.

As a consequence of the strong association between PSC and ulcerative colitis, investigators have postulated a cause-effect relationship between the two. In particular, they have suggested that low-grade portal bacteremia[109, 110] or medications used for therapy[111] may be important causal agents in the pathogenesis of PSC in IBD populations. However, the knowledge that PSC may develop long before chronic ulcerative colitis or years after proctocolectomy while on no medical agents disputes this.[86, 107, 108]

Immunodeficiency states also demonstrate a significant association with PSC, leading to several theories of causality; none have been confirmed. It is known, however, that immunoregulation in PSC is disturbed. Patients with PSC have higher levels of circulating immune complexes[112]; they may also have organ-specific and nonorgan-specific autoantibodies[113, 114] and disturbances of cellular immunity[115] and complement metabolism.[116]

A genetic component is thought to be involved in the pathogenesis as evidenced by well-documented familial recurrence of PSC.[117] PSC also has known associations with specific human leukocytye antigens (HLAs) (e.g., HLA-B8, HLA-DR3, and HLA-DR2, also implicated in several autoimmune diseases).[118–120]

Infection has been postulated to play a role in the pathogenesis of PSC. Specifically, Reovirus 3, hepatitis

B virus, cytomegalovirus, and cryptosporidium have been implicated, but either their causality has never been proved or these infections occurred in already immunocompromised patients.[86, 90, 103, 121–123]

The hepatic copper content in PSC is elevated and has been suggested to play a role in the pathogenesis. However, copper is also elevated in other cholestatic syndromes, and attempts to treat PSC with copper chelating agents have failed. Excess hepatic copper may be important, however, in perpetuating the hepatic lesion.[86]

Pathology

The majority of macroscopic hepatobiliary lesions are described using imaging techniques (see later). Isolated lobar atrophy may be noted at laparotomy.[103] Histologic lesions are found in almost all patients with PSC,[86, 106, 108, 124, 125] but they are nonspecific and in most cases nondiagnostic. They are important, however, for purposes of disease staging.[86, 90, 106, 108] The most important histologic feature is fibrous obliterative cholangitis, which can be seen in the early stages. This inflammatory cholangitis leads to replacement of duct segments by solid cords of connective tissue and eventually to complete loss of interlobular and adjacent septal bile ducts.[86] This periductal fibrosis may assume an "onion skin" appearance.

Progression of the disease has been described by Ludwig and colleagues,[124] who propose four stages. Stage 1, or portal stage, is described as a fibrous obliterative cholangitis with lymphocytic infiltration of the bile ducts. The bile ducts show narrowing, obliteration, and proliferation. The portal tracts become enlarged from edema and excess connective tissue. Stage 2, or periportal stage, shows extension of inflammation beyond the limiting plate into the hepatic parenchyma ("biliary piecemeal necrosis"). Stage 3, or septal fibrosis stage, involves extension of fibrous septa from the enlarged portal tracts. Bridging fibrosis may be seen. There are more marked ductal changes, especially obliteration and a decrease in ductal numbers. Some portal tracts may be found without any bile ducts. The fourth stage is reached when biliary cirrhosis with abnormal hepatic architecture and regenerative nodules is seen. The histology at this point may be indistinguishable from primary biliary cirrhosis. Sixty-four percent of adult PSC patients have histologic lesions consistent with stage 3 or 4.[92] This system of staging has not yet been accepted by all, due mainly to the wide spectrum of histologic changes that can be found in any individual patient.[108]

Selective copper stains (e.g., rhodamine, orcein) show increased copper stores in the periductular areas and are important in helping to differentiate PSC from chronic active hepatitis, especially when piecemeal necrosis is present.[88, 106]

The histologic lesions described mainly in adults can also be found in children, but the findings may be even less specific, making a histologic diagnosis even more difficult.[84, 88]

Clinical Features

Signs and symptoms reported in the pediatric and adult PSC populations are shown in Table 71–8.[84, 87, 92, 95, 97, 99, 102, 103, 119] The most frequent symptoms in children are chronic abdominal pain (38%) usually localized to the right upper quadrant, jaundice (35%) that is most often intermittent in nature, and chronic diarrhea (27%). The diarrhea is reported almost always in cases with associated inflammatory bowel disease. By comparison, fatigue, pruritus, and jaundice are the most frequent symptoms found in adults and are more prevalent than in children. Symptoms of PSC have an insidious onset and 80% of adult patients have had symptoms for an average of 2 years before diagnosis.[86] It is important to note that even though PSC is associated with inflammatory bowel disease, it may develop prior to the diagnosis of inflammatory bowel disease or years after a colectomy.[107]

Hepatomegaly and hepatosplenomegaly occur in 38% and 23% of children, respectively, and are the most frequent physical signs found. The examination is usually otherwise unremarkable except for signs of associated disease if present (e.g., hematochezia in ulcerative colitis). Seventeen percent of adults may present with cirrhosis and portal hypertension and 7% may be asymptomatic at presentation.[125]

The clinical complications most frequently reported in adults have been rarely described in children. Awareness of these complications, however, is important, as they should influence long-term therapeutic decisions.

Table 71–8. CLINICAL FEATURES OF 81 PUBLISHED PEDIATRIC CASES OF PRIMARY SCLEROSING CHOLANGITIS COMPARED WITH 227 ADULT CASES

Variable	Pediatric† (%)	Adult‡ (%)
Symptoms		
Abdominal pain	38	43
Jaundice	35	57
Chronic diarrhea*	27	—
Weight loss	22	36
Fever	17	41
Prolonged cholestasis	12	—
Pruritus	11	55
Fatigue	7	66
Nausea/vomiting	4	23
Hematochezia*	4	—
Skin rash	2	—
Delayed puberty	2	—
Arthralgia	1	—
Headache	1	—
Signs		
Hepatomegaly	38	51
Hepatosplenomegaly	23	—
Splenomegaly	1	31
Ascites	1	8
Anemia	2	—
Xanthomata	1	4
Acholic stools	1	—

*These symptoms may be more consistent with associated inflammatory bowel disease.
†Compiled from references 84, 87, 95, 97, 99, 102, 103, and 119.
‡Compiled from references 87 and 92.

Bile duct carcinoma has long been known to be associated with chronic ulcerative colitis but is also responsible for 19% of deaths in PSC.[92] It has been reported in 10 to 15% of adults with PSC.[126] Bacterial cholangitis occurring in the context of PSC can be the result of cholelithiasis or internal drainage procedures. It should be suspected in a known patient who develops unexplained fever, abdominal pain, and jaundice. Peristomal varices with bleeding may develop after proctocolectomy in patients with PSC and ulcerative colitis.[127]

Biochemical Features

Biochemical parameters most often present a cholestatic profile with increased alkaline phosphatase, gamma glutamyltranspeptidase, and direct bilirubin.[84, 86, 88, 90, 93] It is important to note that these values may fluctuate widely to the point of being normal in some patients despite strong cholangiographic findings.[86, 90, 128] The serum transaminases are only mildly elevated in the majority of patients.[86] Tests of copper metabolism including serum copper and ceruloplasmin, 24-hour urinary copper excretion, and quantitative hepatic copper are abnormal. The quantitative hepatic copper may reach levels found in primary biliary cirrhosis and Wilson's disease.[86]

Imaging Features

The most important diagnostic criterion of PSC is its cholangiographic appearance.[84, 86, 90, 129] Cholangiography in children may be obtained by a variety of techniques including endoscopic retrograde cholangiopancreatography, percutaneous transhepatic cholangiography, percutaneous cholecystography, and operative cholangiogram.[37, 39, 130, 131] The cholangiographic findings consist of diffusely distributed multifocal strictures alternating with normal or dilated segments (Fig. 71–5). The abnormalities may be multiple, involving all portions of the biliary tree, or may be localized to a unifocal stricture.[132] Highly specific biliary diverticulum and short bandlike strictures may be seen.[86] Cirrhosis may be suspected when thinning, tortuosity, and decreased arborization of the intrahepatic bile ducts are found.[125] Although not reported in children, cholangiocarcinoma may be detected by cholangiography in adults.[133] Other imaging modalities may be helpful but are not as specific as cholangiography.[134]

Diagnostic Features

PSC should be strongly suspected in any child presenting with clinical or laboratory parameters of liver disease and a known associated illness (see Table 71–7). Histologically it may be difficult to differentiate PSC from primary biliary cirrhosis, chronic active hepatitis, or Wilson's disease. Primary biliary cirrhosis may be a concern in the older adolescent female, but the presence of inflammatory bowel disease and the absence of anti-

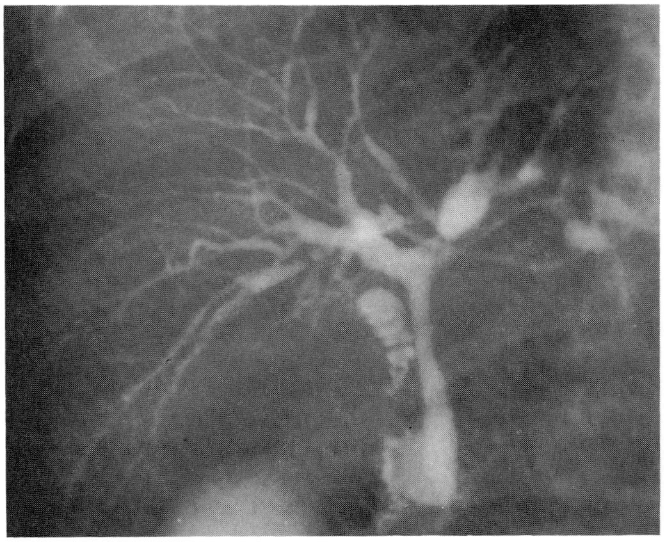

Figure 71–5. Fifteen-year-old female with sclerosing cholangitis. Cholangiographic views of the biliary tree show typical findings consisting of segmental strictures and dilatations of the bile ducts. (Courtesy of Drs. S. Markowitz and J. Hyams.)

mitochondrial antibodies will help eliminate this diagnosis.[90, 105] Copper stains of the liver may demonstrate a periportal distribution of copper rather than the diffuse distribution found in Wilson's disease. Cholangiography is the main diagnostic tool, and chronic active hepatitis, Wilson's disease, and primary biliary cirrhosis have normal cholangiographic findings. It is important to note that some patients with inflammatory bowel disease and histologic and clinical evidence of PSC demonstrate normal cholangiographic studies. These patients are classified as having "small-duct PSC."[86, 90, 126, 135]

Therapy

Therapy for PSC can be divided into medical, nonsurgical procedure, and surgical procedure categories (Table 71–9).[4, 90, 136–156] There have been no controlled trials to date that have shown effectiveness of any medical therapy to alter the course of disease.[86, 90, 126] Medical therapies that have been shown to be either ineffective or effective in only small uncontrolled studies are outlined in Table 71–9. Ursodeoxycholic acid is presently the most promising medical agent. Early reports show that it induces clinical, biochemical, and possibly cholangiographic improvement. The effects may be prolonged.[143, 146] Ursodeoxycholic acid is thought to act via displacement of potentially toxic bile acids from the bile acid pool. These toxic bile acids have been postulated to cause a self-perpetuating bile tract injury.[126] Long-term controlled studies are currently ongoing.[90] Because of the lack of any proven agent to impair disease progression, therapy in mild disease should aim at relieving symptoms and preventing the complications of chronic cholestatic disease. Ursodeoxycholic acid and rifampin have shown promise in relieving pruritus.[48] Fat-soluble vitamin deficiencies have been

Table 71–9. MEDICAL AND SURGICAL THERAPIES THAT HAVE BEEN USED IN THE TREATMENT OF PRIMARY SCLEROSING CHOLANGITIS

Therapy	References
Medical	
Immunosuppressants	
Corticosteroids (systemic)	136, 137
Azathioprine	138
Cyclosporine A	90, 139
Methotrexate	140
Colchicine	141
Bile acids	
Cholestyramine	142
Ursodeoxycholic acid	90, 126, 143–145
Antibiotics	146
Cupruretics	
Penicillamine	147
Nonsurgical Procedures	
Intraductal steroid lavage	148, 149
Percutaneous cholangioplasty	126, 150, 151
Endoscopic cholangioplasty	126, 152
Sphincteroplasty	126, 152
Surgical Procedures	
Proctocolectomy	153
Choledochoenterostomy	126, 154, 155
Biliary reconstruction	126, 154, 155
Liver transplantation	4, 90, 126, 155, 156

described in adults, and it is reasonable to provide oral supplements in all patients.[126]

Nonoperative procedures have become an important therapeutic modality when a dominant biliary stricture (i.e., a high-grade localized stricture) or an impacted stone is discovered. Both findings may lead to deterioration from obstruction or cholangitis. In these cases the stricture may be relieved using endoscopic or percutaneous balloon dilators. Biliary endoprostheses may be placed at the same time to prevent recurrence.[126, 150–152] Choledochal stones may be removed using the same nonoperative techniques.[126–151] Striking improvement in liver function tests and symptomatology following these procedures is reported.[126, 150–152]

Orthotopic liver transplantation is now a recommended therapeutic option for end-stage PSC as defined by portal hypertension with recalcitrant bleeding, refractory cholangitis, cirrhosis, and progressive liver failure.[90, 154, 156] End-stage PSC in children has been treated with transplantation, and the results are no different than for other conditions requiring transplantation.[4] Recurrence of sclerosing cholangitis in the allograft of an adult patient has been described.[156] Other nontransplant surgical procedures (e.g., colectomy, internal drainage) should be restricted, as they do not influence disease progression and may increase the disease complication rate.[90, 126, 153–155]

Prognosis

The natural history of PSC is not described in children, but studies in the adult population support the hypothesis that PSC in the overwhelming majority is a progressive disease even in patients who are asymptomatic at diagnosis.[92, 157] In adults, median survival from diagnosis is 6 to 12 years.[92, 125, 157] Wiesner and colleagues,[92] using multivariate analysis, showed that age, serum bilirubin, hemoglobin levels, the presence or absence of inflammatory bowel disease, and histologic liver biopsy stage were all independent predictors of disease outcome. If these variables are confirmed in adults and children, then patients can be stratified to low-, moderate-, or high-risk groups. This will have obvious benefits in planning individual therapies.

PERICHOLANGITIS

The term *pericholangitis* was first used by Mistilis in 1965 to describe the hepatic lesions found in adult patients with inflammatory bowel disease.[158, 159] It is a histologic diagnosis that has been reported as the most frequent hepatobiliary lesion in patients with chronic ulcerative colitis.[106, 108] Pericholangitis is a fibrosing inflammation of the portal tracts and is synonymous with other terms such as *portal triaditis, cholangiolitic hepatitis, interlobular hepatitis,* and *intrahepatic cholangitis.*[106, 108] Specifically, the portal tracts are expanded by edema and inflammatory infiltrate. The bile ducts may be increased in number and surrounded by concentric fibrosis in some areas or decreased in number in others. The morphologic features of pericholangitis may also resemble those of chronic active hepatitis, chronic persistent hepatitis, and nonspecific reactive hepatitis.[106]

Since the advent of the new nonoperative cholangiographic techniques, the boundaries between pericholangitis and primary sclerosing cholangitis have become unclear. For some, pericholangitis is the intrahepatic manifestation of PSC, and the term *small-duct PSC* should be used if cholangiographic evidence of large-duct PSC is lacking.[86, 90, 126, 135] In a study of 107 patients with chronic ulcerative colitis, the investigators found that 35% had pericholangitis and 17% had PSC; the spectrum of hepatic lesions between the two groups was indistinguishable.[135] These findings are supported by others.[90, 94]

CONGENITAL HEPATIC FIBROSIS

Congenital hepatic fibrosis (CHF) is an autosomal recessive disorder first described by Kerr and coworkers in 1961.[162] It is still unclear whether CHF and infantile polycystic disease (IPD) can be considered a single disease. For some they represent different clinical presentations of the same disease process, and this is supported by similar genetic inheritance patterns and lesions of the liver and kidneys.[163, 164] For others, and based on morphometric analysis of involved liver, CHF and IPD are two distinct diseases.[165] Recognizing that this controversy remains unsettled, each entity, for purposes of clarity, is described separately.

Etiology

CHF is an autosomal recessive disorder for which the underlying pathogenic mechanism remains unknown. CHF may result from a ductal plate malformation (see earlier).[166] Insight into its pathogenesis is provided by its association with other visceral lesions such as nephronophthisis,[167] congenital heart disease,[168] emphysema,[169] cerebral aneurysm,[170] mental retardation and dysmorphism,[171] protein-losing enteropathy,[172, 173] and choledochal cyst.[174] Recently, lesions similar to congenital hepatic fibrosis have also been described in adult autosomal dominant polycystic kidney disease.[175, 176]

Pathology

The characteristic histologic lesion of CHF is that of bile ductular proliferation within the context of a noninflammatory fibrosis.[162, 164, 166] The liver is divided by bands of mature fibrous tissue that surround groups of liver cells. The hepatocytes and lobular architecture appear normal. Inflammatory infiltrate throughout the liver is virtually absent. The portal tracts and fibrous bands contain increased numbers of bile ducts, which are characterized by their dysmorphic shapes and the absence of mitoses. The bile ducts may contain mucinous material or inspissated bile (Fig. 71–6). Duplication of the intrahepatic portal vein branches has been described and may be important in the development of portal hypertension.[177] In some cases, the disease may be localized to a single hepatic lobe.[178, 179] The renal lesions may be minimal and consist initially of dilatation of the medullary distal and collecting tubules. Cortical cysts develop later.[166]

Clinical Features

The clinical course of CHF is best characterized by the development of portal hypertension with preservation of normal hepatic synthetic and metabolic function. At the time of presentation, the signs and symptoms may vary from a virtually asymptomatic child to a dramatic inaugural variceal hemorrhage. In the majority of recorded cases, patients presented in the first decade of life with hepatosplenomegaly and/or signs of gastrointestinal bleeding (hematemesis, melena, anemia).[162, 164, 180] The children may also present with cholangitis.[180–182] A rare but significant complication of CHF is the development of malignancy in later life.[183–184] Cholangiocarcinoma is the type most frequently reported.[183] Clinical features due to renal involvement (palpable kidneys, arterial hypertension, etc.) may also present initially but usually develop later in life.[164, 167]

Biochemical Features

Biochemical parameters of liver function including serum bilirubin, alkaline phosphatase, albumin, and transaminases remain typically within the normal range. Excretion of Bromsulphalein may be delayed.[163, 164] Hematologic indices may be decreased secondary to hypersplenism. Renal function tests may also be abnormal.

Imaging Features

Imaging abnormalities are nonspecific except if angiography is performed, which may show duplication of the intrahepatic branches of the portal vein.[177] Ultrasonography and angiography are helpful in the evaluation of portal hypertension. Kidney ultrasound and intravenous pyelography demonstrate minor abnormalities in up to 90% of patients.[164]

Diagnosis

The diagnosis is confirmed by histologic examination of liver tissue showing the lesions described above (see

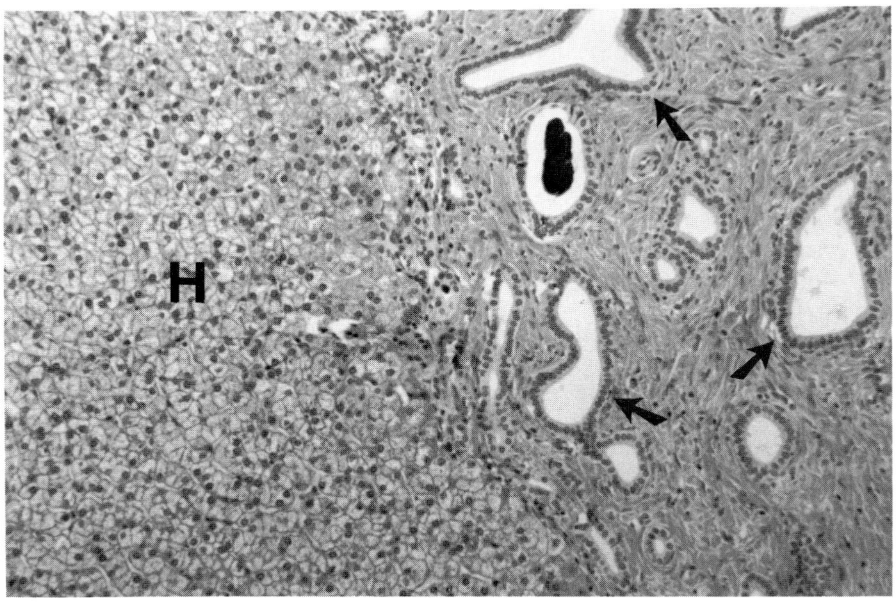

Figure 71–6. Congenital hepatic fibrosis. Liver biopsy (hematoxylin-eosin stain, × 100) shows a normal hepatic lobule (*H*) bordered by a wide band of mature, fibrous tissue. There is no inflammatory infiltrate; however, an increased number of abnormally shaped bile ducts are seen (*arrows*). (Courtesy of Dr. K. Barwick.)

Fig. 71–6). In rare cases, the diagnosis may be missed if the disease is isolated to the nonbiopsied lobe.[178, 179] A vitamin A level helps to discriminate between CHF and cases of hepatic fibrosis secondary to hypervitaminosis A.[185] All patients with CHF should be evaluated for renal disease and portal hypertension.

Treatment

Therapy is aimed at treating the complications of CHF. Cholangitis should be treated promptly with parenteral antibiotics, keeping in mind that a biliary tract stone may be initiating the infectious process. In these cases, an invasive procedure to remove the obstructing stone may be necessary.[186] The use of daily antibiotics and oral bile acid supplementation in the prophylaxis of recurring cholangitis has been described, but therapeutic efficacy awaits confirmation.[166, 187, 188]

Several comments regarding the treatment of portal hypertension in CHF are necessary. First, endoscopic sclerotherapy provides good short-term relief from esophageal variceal bleeding, but its long-term results in CHF have not been evaluated. Second, since its early description by Kerr in 1961, portosystemic shunt has been advocated for the treatment of portal hypertension in CHF.[162–164, 180, 189] Because hepatic metabolic function is maintained, the risk of encephalopathy after portosystemic shunting is less than for cirrhosis. Mortality from portosystemic shunting is estimated at 5% and recurrence of hemorrhage at 16%.[189] Finally, orthotopic liver transplantation is indicated in those patients who have failed the above options and continue to bleed.[4]

Prognosis

Long-term prognosis in CHF is unclear; however, it can be assumed that if the major complications (i.e., portal hypertension, cholangitis) are controlled, then long-term survival and quality of life should be good. In one study of 30 patients followed for 5 to 20 years after diagnosis, the overall mortality was 23%.[189] In another study, 27 patients were assessed as leading normal lives unless kidney failure was present.[164] It is clear that long-term survivors carry an undefined but increased risk of developing kidney disease or biliary tract malignancy and merit long-term surveillance.

INFANTILE POLYCYSTIC DISEASE

Infantile polycystic disease (IPD) is primarily a renal disorder with hepatic lesions identical to congenital hepatic fibrosis (CHF). Whether IPD and CHF are the same or different diseases remains an unresolved issue (see earlier).

IPD is an autosomal recessive disorder that occurs in 1 out of 4,000 to 1 out of 8,000 live births.[190, 191] Most patients present at birth with bilateral flank masses as a result of enlarged cystic kidneys. Due to inadequate intrauterine urine formation, there is often maternal oligohydramnios with associated respiratory insufficiency and Potter-type facies. In the typical case, the kidneys are grossly enlarged by a multitude of cysts originating in the collecting ducts. Renal failure usually occurs at an early age but in some cases may be delayed; these patients are then defined as having juvenile polycystic disease. The hepatic lesions of IPD are the same as those found in CHF (see earlier). Clinically they appear to cause fewer complications (e.g., portal hypertension) and occur at a later age than in CHF.[166] However, with improved care of end-stage renal disease, the increased long-term survival of these patients may lead to an increased incidence of clinically evident liver disease.

Portosystemic shunting has been recommended for those patients with significant portal hypertension.[192] Prognosis appears to be related to early pulmonary disease and later renal hypertension.[192]

CYSTIC FIBROSIS–ASSOCIATED HEPATOBILIARY DISEASE

Hepatobiliary abnormalities are described in up to 50% of patients with cystic fibrosis (CF); however, only 2% develop clinically apparent disease.[193–197] Cystic fibrosis–associated hepatobiliary disease (CFAHD) is a group of interrelated disorders resulting from the genetic defect causing cystic fibrosis. These disorders are outlined in Table 71–10; only those specifically relating to the biliary system are discussed here (see Chapter 66).

Etiology and Pathogenesis

Cystic fibrosis is inherited as an autosomal recessive disorder. A single disease locus has been identified on the long arm of chromosome 7 (region q31) where a 3 base pair deletion (F_{508}) has been identified as the mutation responsible for 70% of cases. At least 20 other mutations have also been described.[198] The variable clinical course between patients with CF may be attrib-

Table 71–10. SPECTRUM OF DISORDERS IN CYSTIC FIBROSIS–ASSOCIATED HEPATOBILIARY DISEASE

Parenchymal and Small Bile Duct Disorders
Hepatic steatosis
Neonatal cholestasis
Focal biliary cirrhosis
Multilobular biliary cirrhosis
Cardiovascular hepatopathy
Large Bile Duct Disorders
Inspissated bile syndrome
Cholelithiasis
Sclerosing cholangitis
Intrapancreatic common bile duct compression
Cholangiocarcinoma
Gallbladder Disorders
Cholelithiasis
Microgallbladder
Mucous hyperplasia (mucocele)

utable in part to the different expression for each mutation at the CF locus.[199] A recent study, however, has not found an association between a specific mutation and the development of hepatobiliary disease.[199a]

The protein synthesized by the CF gene has yet to be isolated but it appears to be involved in the regulation of apical epithelial cell chloride channels.[200] The resulting disorder in chloride secretion leads to underhydration of macromolecules produced by exocrine glands, including biliary mucus. This produces viscid, inspissated bile plugs, which have been hypothesized to play a central role in the pathogenesis of many of the hepatobiliary lesions described in CF.[193, 201]

Nonexocrine factors also appear to play a role in the pathogenesis of hepatobiliary disease as evidenced by histologic studies of involved liver.[202] These factors may be hepatocellular such as abnormal biliary lipid composition[203] or increased proportions of glycine conjugated, hydrophobic bile acids.[203–205] These abnormalities may lead to inflammation, sclerosis, and stone formation. Extrahepatic factors include compression of the common bile duct by a fibrotic pancreas[206] and an overall deficient nutritional, cardiac, and pulmonary status.[194–207] The hypothesized pathogenetic pathways for the development of hepatobiliary disease in cystic fibrosis are summarized in Figure 71–7.

Neonatal Cholestasis

The incidence of prolonged neonatal cholestasis has been reported to range from 2 to 20% of infants born with meconium ileus.[194, 208, 209] As outlined earlier, inspissated bile plugs may play a dominant role in the pathogenesis of prolonged neonatal cholestasis; however, it has also been associated with cytomegalovirus infection,[210] giant cell hepatitis,[211, 212] extrinsic biliary obstruction,[213, 214] and biliary atresia.[215] Meconium ileus is associated with up to 50% of cases.[210, 214]

Clinically the child may present with an early course consistent with cystic fibrosis (e.g., meconium ileus, meconium peritonitis, respiratory distress). In these infants the onset of jaundice may occur at birth or up to 3 weeks postnatally.[210] Signs and symptoms are consistent with a neonatal cholestatic syndrome (jaundice, hepatomegaly, acholic stools, etc.). In other infants the initial presentation may be neonatal cholestasis alone, and the evaluation is oriented toward the differentiation between intrahepatic and extrahepatic causes of cholestasis. A sweat chloride test is essential to establish the correct diagnosis.

Histologic features on biopsy are consistent with an extrahepatic biliary obstruction and include portal triads with inflammatory infiltrate, fibrosis, ductular proliferation, and eosinophilic bile plugs. The eosinophilic bile plugs represent inspissated biliary mucus. Intracytoplasmic cholestasis and giant cells may be seen. The findings may be suggestive of extrahepatic biliary atresia, and direct visualization of the extrahepatic biliary tree then becomes necessary to differentiate the two.[216] If the child undergoes exploratory laparotomy, the biliary tree is found to be normal but obstructed by thick tenacious inspissated bile. Radiographic visualization of the biliary tree may be helpful to eliminate extrinsic compression of the common bile duct.[213] Intraoperative biliary lavage may be attempted.

In most children recovery is spontaneous but may be prolonged and last up to 6 months.[194, 210] A small proportion of cases with periportal inflammation, fibrosis, and meconium ileus, however, will rapidly progress and die.[194, 201] For these children, there is no widely accepted therapy. Phenobarbital, cholecystokinin-octapeptide, and biliary lavage with normal saline, pancreatin, and *N*-acetylcysteine have been used with reasonable success in isolated cases.[210, 216–218]

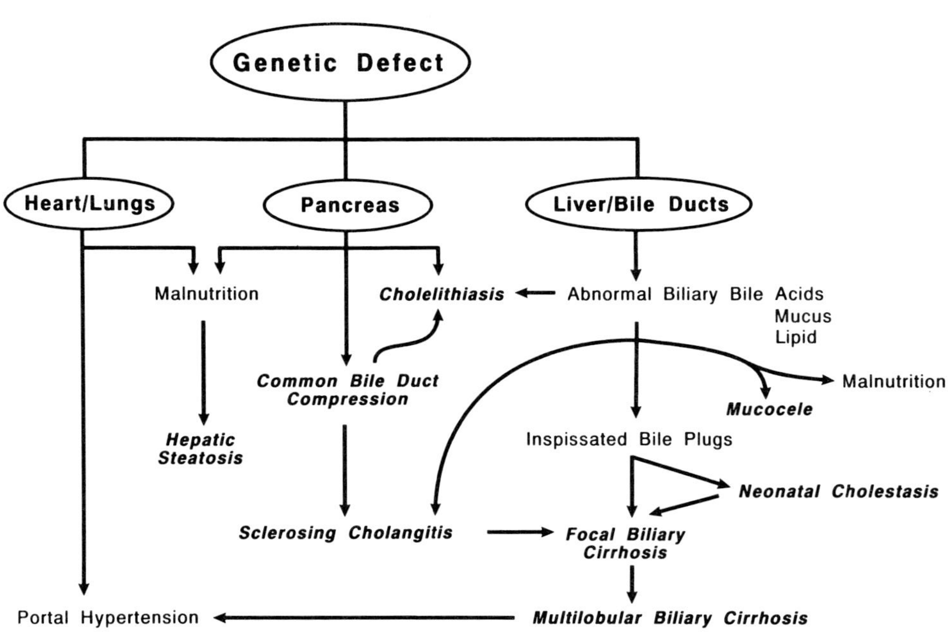

Figure 71–7. Pathogenetic mechanisms of cystic fibrosis–associated hepatobiliary disease.

Focal Biliary Cirrhosis and Multilobular Biliary Cirrhosis

Anderson in 1938 first reported hepatic disease in cystic fibrosis.[219] In 1944, Farber, using the term *mucoviscidosis,* described lesions secondary to mucus plugging in multiple organs, including the liver.[220] Bodian was the first to define "focal biliary fibrosis" as localized areas of eosinophilic mucus concretions and portal fibrosis interspersed among normal hepatic parenchyma.[221] di Sant'Agnese and Blanc then defined multilobular biliary cirrhosis in 1956 as the evolution of hepatic lesions in CF to a nodular, cirrhotic stage.[197]

The incidence of focal biliary cirrhosis, based on postmortem examinations, increases with age from 10% under 3 months to 27% beyond 1 year of age.[201] Histologically it is characterized by portal triads containing inspissated, granular eosinophilic material (biliary mucus), bile ductular proliferation, chronic inflammatory infiltrate, and variable fibrosis. A focal distribution is essential. The overall hepatic architecture is preserved (Figs. 71–8 and 71–9).[195–197, 201]

The early histologic stage of focal biliary cirrhosis, described by Oppenheimer and Esterly as excessive biliary mucus with mild portal changes (edema, chronic inflammatory infiltrate, and fibrosis), is reversible.[201] With time, however, focal biliary cirrhosis evolves to multilobular biliary cirrhosis characterized by the coalescence of involved foci to irregular, large, palpable nodules. The histology of this end stage to CF liver disease shows massive areas of fibrosis, regenerative nodules, and bile ductular proliferation adjacent to normal hepatic lobules. The normal architecture is disturbed. Centrilobular atrophy with or without hepatocellular necrosis may be seen and is a reflection of cor pulmonale.[195, 197]

Typically children with focal biliary cirrhosis are asymptomatic and have little if any clinical signs. Hepatomegaly may be present but is usually a feature of hepatic steatosis, which may be found in one third of patients.[194, 222]

Multilobular biliary cirrhosis is reported to occur in 4 to 6% of patients[207, 223] and becomes clinically relevant in 2 to 3%.[218, 224] Rarely, clinical hepatic disease may be the initial presentation of CF,[218, 224] but in most cases the diagnosis of CF is known, and clinical manifestations of liver disease present in the second decade of life.[193, 222] It can be speculated based on the studies of Oppenheimer and Esterly[201] and the increasing median age of survival in CF that the incidence of multilobular biliary cirrhosis will increase.

The clinical manifestations include firm, nodular hepatomegaly, splenomegaly, and other clinical signs of portal hypertension. In one study, 13 out of 15 cirrhotic patients presented with symptoms relating to portal hypertension, mainly variceal bleeding.[222] The clinical course may be complicated by ascites, jaundice, hypersplenism, coagulopathy, and encephalopathy.[194, 207, 222] As the disease progresses, the liver span decreases to become undetectable on clinical examination. Recurrent left upper quadrant pain may be due to repeated splenic infarction in the face of hypersplenism.[218] Adenocarcinoma of the extrahepatic biliary tree has been reported in a 27-year-old cirrhotic female.[225]

Biochemical parameters may be normal even when clinical evidence of cirrhosis is detected.[194, 207] Serum alkaline phosphatase (hepatic isoenzyme) may be elevated in up to 20% of patients with cystic fibrosis.[226]

Gamma glutamyltranspeptidase and serum transaminases may become elevated and fluctuate widely. Coagulation studies, complete blood counts, and vitamin levels need to be monitored for signs of coagulopathy, hypersplenism, and fat-soluble vitamin deficiency. Children with marginal vitamin K status require supplementation when placed on antibiotics due to suppression of colonic flora.

Multilobular biliary cirrhosis is demonstrated on ultrasound as a heterogeneous, echodense hepatic pattern

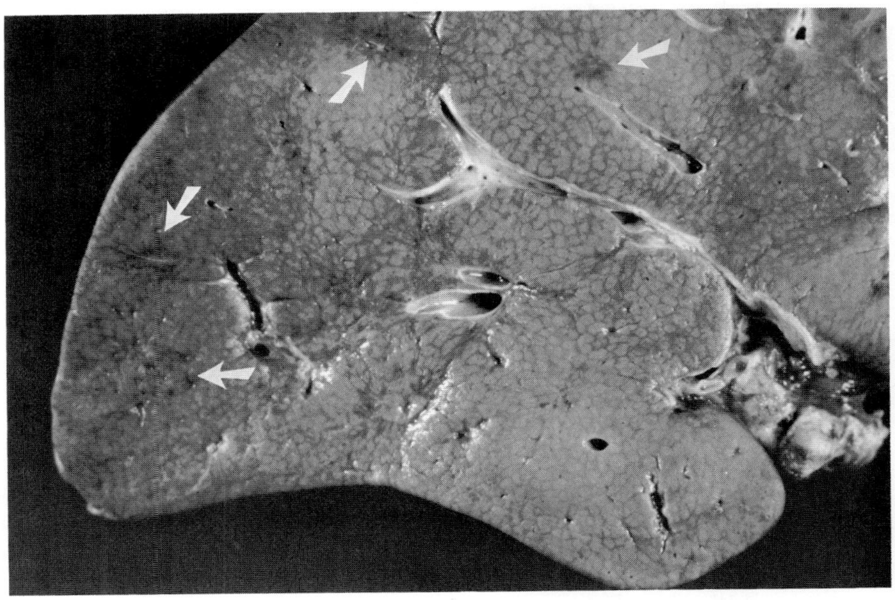

Figure 71–8. Eleven-year-old male with cystic fibrosis who died of pulmonary complications. Postmortem examination of the liver shows a diffusely congested liver with focal areas of biliary cirrhosis (*arrows*). (Courtesy of Dr. K. Barwick.)

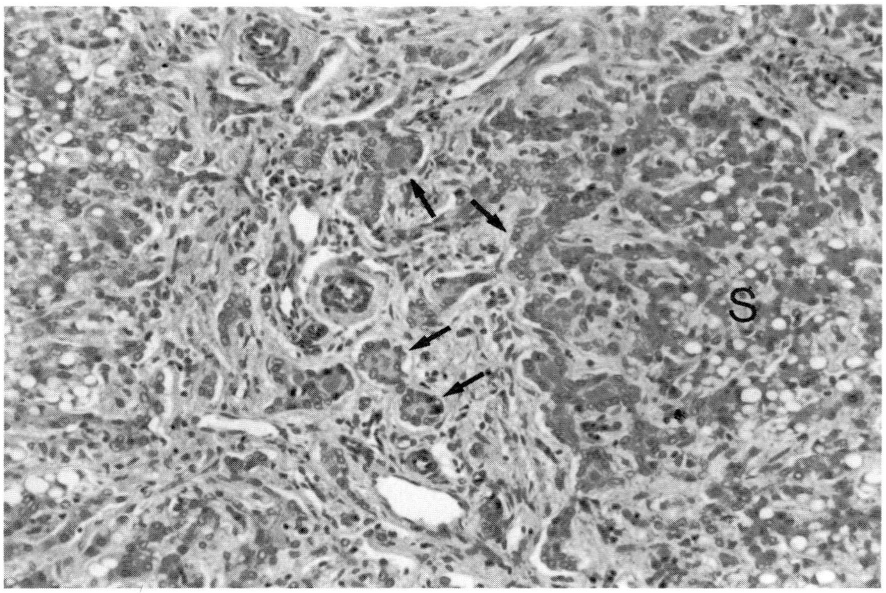

Figure 71–9. Liver biopsy demonstrating the lesions of biliary cirrhosis (hematoxylin-eosin stain, × 100). The portal triads are expanded by fibrosis and inflammatory infiltrate; there is also bile ductular proliferation (*arrows*) and eosinophilic material plugging several bile ducts. Hepatic steatosis (*S*) is also seen.

that reflects the regenerative nodules and fibrosis. The liver contour is irregular. Duplex sonography is helpful in evaluating established portal hypertension (e.g., reversal of flow, varices) and may become useful in detecting early liver disease.[227] A percutaneous liver biopsy may be misleading in early disease because of its focal nature. The sensitivity of the biopsy may be increased if "open" or laparoscopic biopsies are obtained.

Treatment goals for the symptomatic patient are aimed mainly at the complications of portal hypertension. Upper gastrointestinal bleeding should be treated aggressively and promptly. Endoscopic sclerotherapy, vasopressin, and balloon tamponade are well-accepted modalities in the pediatric population.[194, 207, 218, 223]

Portosystemic shunts have been performed in patients with CF for portal hypertension and hypersplenism.[194, 197, 218, 222, 223] Prior to the rebirth of liver transplantation in the early 1980s, portosystemic shunting was the only long-term option available but was contraindicated in the presence of severe hepatocellular and pulmonary disease. A distal splenorenal shunt (Warren shunt) is not a contraindication for future liver transplantation; however, prior consultation with a liver transplant center is helpful. The placement of a radiologically guided transjugular intrahepatic portosystemic shunt (TIPS) has recently been described as an alternative to traditional surgically created portosystemic shunts.[227a]

Children with cirrhosis secondary to CFAHD have been transplanted,[4, 228–230] and early reports indicate 70% survival rates—similar to non-CF transplanted patients.[228] In one study of 10 patients, mild to moderate lung disease was not associated with unusual complications; however, post-transplant pulmonary colonization with *Pseudomonas* was associated with two deaths.[228]

In rare cases, treatment for massive splenomegaly with resulting respiratory embarrassment or left upper quadrant pain may be indicated. An alternative to portosystemic shunting, splenic embolization, has been described.[218]

Investigations are ongoing to examine the effects of taurine and ursodeoxycholic acid supplementation on the progression of liver disease in CF. Both have been added to the diet, separately or together, to decrease the proportion of hydrophobic bile acids that are damaging to cell membranes. Early results show improvement in biochemical indices and hepatobiliary excretory function.[205, 231, 231a]

Intrapancreatic Compression of the Common Bile Duct

Pancreatic fibrosis causing compression of the common bile duct has been described since 1978.[206, 213, 232, 233] The most comprehensive study examined 50 patients with clinical and biochemical liver disease and, using hepatobiliary scintigraphy, found distal common bile duct obstruction in 96%.[206] Subsequent cholangiographies in 29 patients supported a similar high proportion of distal common bile duct compression. The authors concluded that distal common bile duct strictures in cystic fibrosis were common and possibly responsible for the development of biliary cirrhosis. It is important to note, however, that subsequent studies by different authors did not support the importance of common bile duct strictures.[234, 234a] In these studies, 17 of 23 patients with liver disease were found to have ultrasound and/or scintigraphy abnormalities; however, only 2 of the 15 who subsequently underwent cholangiography were found to have common bile duct strictures. From these studies, it appears that distal common bile duct compression plays a role in the pathogenesis of CFAHD, but its incidence and importance need further definition.

Up to 55% of patients with already established clinical or biochemical evidence of liver disease may experience recurrent right upper quadrant pain.[206] Biochemical parameters for liver disease may be normal despite significant cholangiographic findings. The diagnosis is established cholangiographically, but it should be noted from the above comments that the indications to pursue the evaluation with cholangiography may be subtle. Choledocholithiasis may be found on cholangiography.[234] Although not reported, endoscopic sphincterotomy would appear to be a reasonable first alternative to surgery, especially if pulmonary status is precarious. Cholecystojejunostomy has been reported, with good results, for relief of severe abdominal pain, cholangitis, or cholestasis.[206, 231]

Sclerosing Cholangitis

Sclerosing cholangitis is an additional expression of CFAHD but has been only rarely described.[99, 104] In the five reported cases presentation was no different from that in other forms of CFAHD, but sclerosing cholangitis was diagnosed in all five by cholangiography and supported by liver histology in four.

Gallbladder Disease

The frequency of gallbladder abnormalities in CF is high and increases with age, from 20% in children less than five to 60% in young adults.[194] Twelve to 20% of gallbladders cannot be visualized by intravenous cholecystography.[235, 236] Microgallbladders measuring less than 0.5 by 1.5 cm can be found radiologically in 14 to 20%[235, 236] and in 30% at postmortem.[194] Microgallbladders at postmortem may contain a thick white-colored bile. Mucous hyperplasia, or mucocele, is defined by mucus-filled cysts arising in the biliary epithelium. They may be large enough to be seen by cholecystography and are seen in up to 43% of gallbladders available for histology.[193] These gallbladder abnormalities are asymptomatic.

Cholelithiasis

Cholesterol stones of the gallbladder and intra- and extrahepatic biliary tree are well-documented complications of cystic fibrosis.[193, 194, 207, 224, 237] The incidence increases with age and overall is reported to be between 6 and 30%.[193, 194] The pathogenesis of gallstones in CF is complex and still poorly understood. Abnormal enterohepatic circulation of bile salts,[193, 194, 207] abnormal biliary lipid,[203] pancreatic insufficiency,[194] low taurine/glycine conjugation ratios of bile acids,[193, 203] and chronic cholestasis have all been implicated as factors in the pathogenesis. Gallstone formation does not appear to correlate with the severity of hepatic parenchymal disease.[235]

Cholelithiasis may remain asymptomatic in many patients with CF or present symptomatically as calculous cholecystitis.[224, 235] The symptomatology is most often chronic in nature, with a mean delay in diagnosis of 7 months.[224] The majority of symptoms—abdominal pain, food intolerance, or gastrointestinal upset—are nonspecific.[224] Ultrasonography is helpful in diagnosing gallbladder stones, but cholangiography may be needed if choledocholithiasis is suspected. The findings on ERCP have been well described.[237] Operative therapy should be reserved for those patients in whom there is good correlation between clinical and imaging findings. Nonvisualization of the gallbladder is not a sufficient imaging finding to recommend cholecystectomy.[193] Patients with precarious pulmonary status may benefit from the newer laparoscopic surgical techniques.[238] Choledocholithiasis may be amenable to endoscopic removal. Preventative measures include the avoidance of oral contraceptives in adolescent and adult females, because of the increase in cholesterol saturation of bile, and optimization of pancreatic enzyme supplements (see Chapters 66 and 72).

CHOLEDOCHAL CYSTS

Choledochal cysts are defined as a cystic dilatation of all or a portion of the intrahepatic and extrahepatic biliary tree. The first description of a choledochal cyst was recorded by A. Vater in 1723.[239]

Pathology

Choledochal cysts may vary in size measuring up to 10 liters in adults. Since the first classification by Alonso-Lej and associates in 1959[240] several modifications have been made,[241, 242] and currently five types of choledochal cysts are recognized (Fig. 71–10). Type I, representing 77% of cases, is a dilatation of the common bile duct. It may be diffusely fusiform (Fig. 71–11), large saccular, or small and localized.[243] Type II is a diverticulum of either the common bile duct or gallbladder and constitutes 2% of cases. Type III is a choledochocele, that is, a cystic dilatation of the intraduodenal portion of the

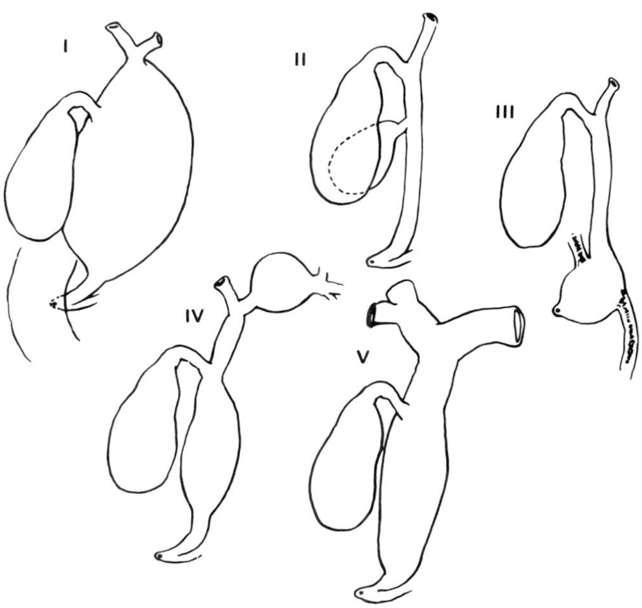

Figure 71–10. Classification of choledochal cysts. Type I: dilatation of the common bile duct. Type II: common bile duct diverticulum. Type III: choledochocele. Type IV: intrahepatic and extrahepatic bile duct cysts. Type V: diffuse dilatation of intrahepatic and extrahepatic bile ducts.

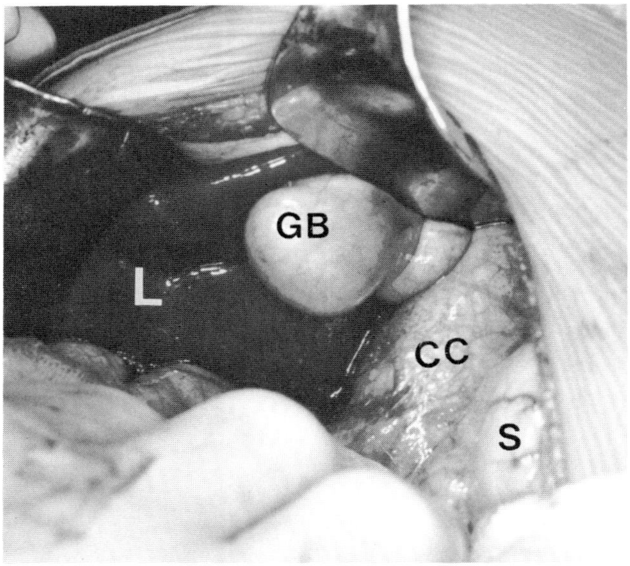

Figure 71–11. Operative view of a Type I choledochal cyst. *L,* liver; *GB,* cystic gallbladder; *CC,* fusiform choledochal cyst involving common bile duct; *S,* stomach. (Courtesy of Dr. D. Mollit.)

common bile duct (Fig. 71–12). It represents 1% of the total. Type IV represents 18% and is defined by multiple intrahepatic and extrahepatic cystic dilatations. Caroli's disease is included in Type IV and consists of multiple intrahepatic bile duct cysts that may or may not be confined to a single lobe. Type V is a fusiform dilatation of the entire intra- and extrahepatic biliary tree (Fig. 71–13) . Histologically the cyst wall is formed primarily of fibrous tissue, with variable amounts of smooth muscle and inflammatory cells. Most frequently an epithelial lining is absent, but when present, it appears as typical or flattened biliary epithelium.[240, 244] There are no pathognomonic findings on liver biopsy; it shows features also found in other biliary obstructive diseases (i.e., portal inflammation, fibrosis, bile ductular proliferation).

Epidemiology

Choledochal cysts are still considered rare, with an estimated incidence of 1 in 13,000 to 1 in 2,000,000.[245] The disease is more frequent in the Orient, with one third of cases reported in the Japanese literature.[245, 246] Seventy-five to 80% of patients are female.[243, 246] Although choledochal cysts have been diagnosed at all ages, including in fetuses and in octogenarians at autopsy,[245] 70% of patients are diagnosed under the age of 20, and 30% are diagnosed under the age of 1 year.[245–247]

Etiology

Choledochal cysts have long been considered a congenital malformation; however, acquired cases are well documented.[248–249] Common etiologies have been postulated to explain both choledochal cysts and other abnormalities of the biliary tree (see earlier). Yotsuyanagi in 1936[250] and other investigators since[244–247] have postulated an excess proliferation of biliary epithelial cells at an embryologic stage when the bile cords are solid. The subsequent canalization process of the bile cords is disturbed, and the ducts become abnormally dilated. If the excess proliferation is localized, the cyst is localized. This theory awaits confirmation, but is similar to the ductal plate malformation theory described above.

The common channel syndrome theory first advanced by Babbitt in 1973 and since supported by many others[248, 251–254] postulates that both congenital and acquired factors are necessary for the development of a biliary duct cyst. These investigators describe anomalous junctions between the pancreatic and biliary trees. In the normal individual the common bile duct and the canal of Wirsung join at their intraduodenal portions (Fig. 71–14). In patients with cystic bile ducts the formation of the common channel can occur 2 to 3 cm proximal to the ampulla of Vater. This anomalous junction facilitates the intermittent reflux of pancreatic secretions into the common bile duct, leading to stasis, inflammation, ulcerations, weakness, and dilatation of the biliary duct. This theory is supported by radiologic findings,[252–254] measurement of a high amylase content in bile aspirated from the cysts,[251–253] abnormal sphincter of Oddi function,[255] and a positive pressure gradient be-

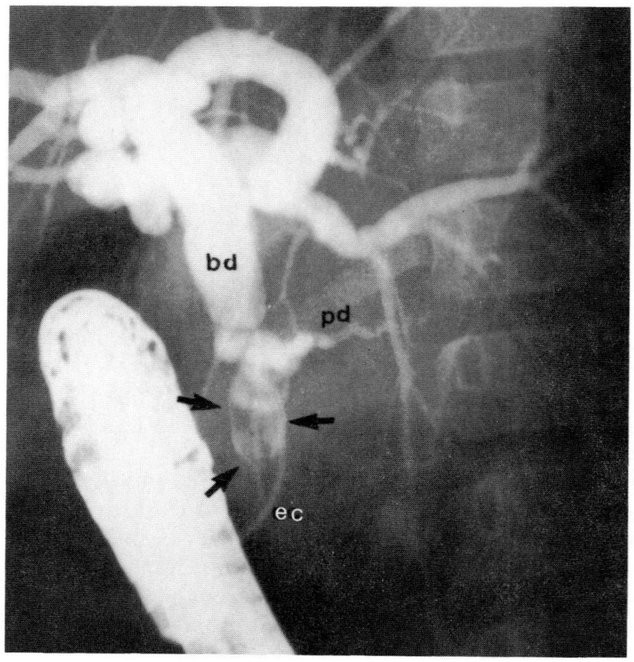

Figure 71–12. A symptomatic choledochocele in a 26-month-old child demonstrated by endoscopic retrograde cholangiopancreatography. This patient presented with acute pancreatitis and jaundice. Endoscopically, the ampulla appeared very enlarged and prominent. The choledochocele is outlined by arrows. The common bile duct (*bd*), pancreatic duct, partially filled (*pd*), and endoscopic cannula (*ec*) are also clearly visible. (Courtesy of Dr. J. Barnett.)

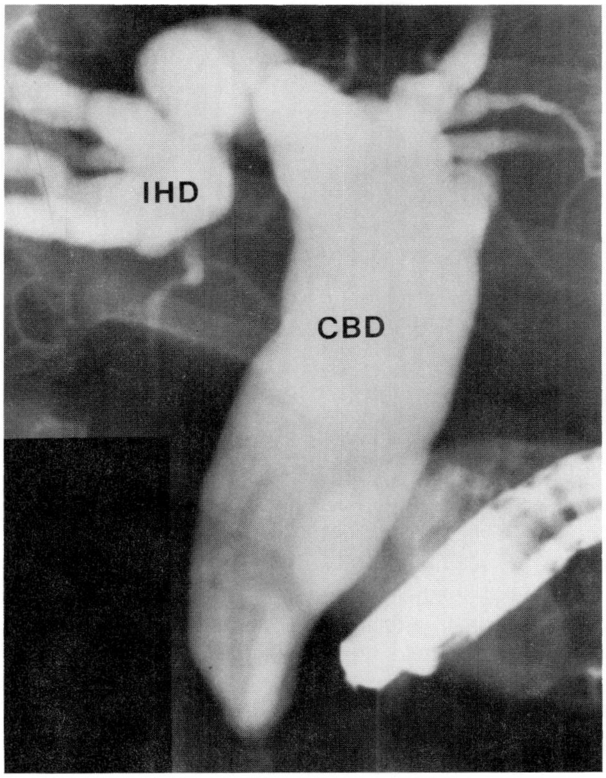

Figure 71–13. Seventeen-year-old black male evaluated for abnormal liver function tests and intermittent abdominal pain. Endoscopic retrograde cholangiopancreatography shows a Type V choledochal cyst. *CBD*, cystic common bile duct; *IHD*, cystic intrahepatic bile ducts.

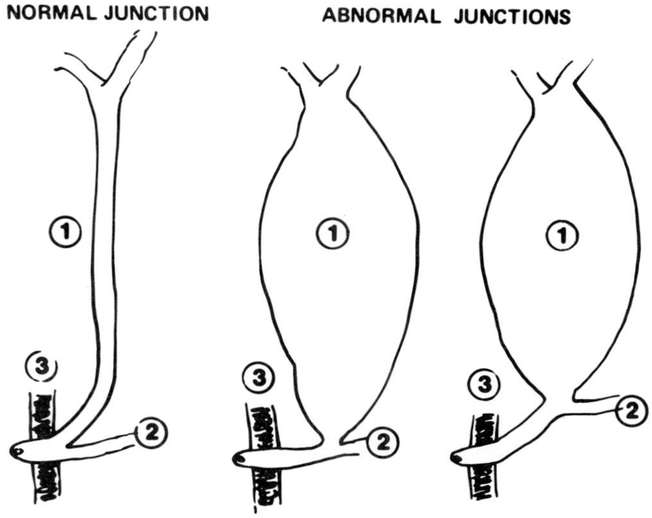

Figure 71–14. The common channel syndrome has been proposed as a potential etiology for the development of choledochal cysts. In this syndrome an anomalous pancreaticoduodenal junction exists. 1, common bile duct; 2, pancreatic duct; 3, duodenal wall.

tween the pancreatic duct and the biliary cyst.[256] However, it should be noted that an anomalous junction cannot be found in all cases.

Recently, oligoganglionosis with postganglionic neural dysfunction in the narrow portion distal to the cyst has been implicated in the genesis of choledochal cysts.[257, 258] Further investigations in this area are needed.

Clinical Features

Jaundice, abdominal pain, and abdominal mass form the classical clinical triad from which the diagnosis is suspected. However, reviews of large series of patients demonstrate that the triad may be present in only 12 to 30% of patients.[243, 244] This may be due to improved diagnostic techniques allowing earlier diagnosis. Table 71–11[243, 244, 247] lists the presenting signs and symptoms compiled from three large series of patients. The clinical features are nonspecific and may be intermittent. In adults they more frequently represent diseases such as acute cholecystitis, cholangitis, and pancreatic carcinoma. In the child, choledochal cyst may present as recurrent acute pancreatitis.[259] Mean duration of symptoms until diagnosis in one study was as long as 20 months (range 2 weeks to 12 years).[260]

Clinical complications due to chronic obstruction may involve ascending cholangitis with abscess formation and cholelithiasis. At presentation, periportal fibrosis may be found in 50% and cirrhosis in 25%.[260] Spontaneous perforation of the cyst with bile peritonitis may be an initial finding in 2%.[260a]

Carcinoma arising from the cyst or its remnants after partial excision is a significant risk estimated at 2 to 3% overall.[243, 246] An age-related incidence has been reported, with a child less than 10 years of age presenting a 0.7% risk and an adult beyond the second decade a 14% risk.[261] Tumor may also arise in the gallbladder, pancreas, or duodenum in 1%.[243] The most frequent histologic variety is adenocarcinoma.[243] It has been proposed that bile stagnation with increased secondary bile

Table 71–11. CLINICAL FEATURES AT PRESENTATION OF CHOLEDOCHAL CYSTS: 1,392 PATIENTS

Feature	Percentage
Abdominal pain	62
Jaundice	58
Abdominal mass	46
Dark urine	50
Fever	23
Nausea and vomiting	17
Anemia	17
Acholic stools	15
Hepatomegaly	8
Abdominal distention	4
Pruritus	3
Gastrointestinal hemorrhage	3
Peritonitis	2
Anorexia	2
Back pain	1
Fatigue	1
Weight loss	<1

Compiled from references 243, 244, and 247.

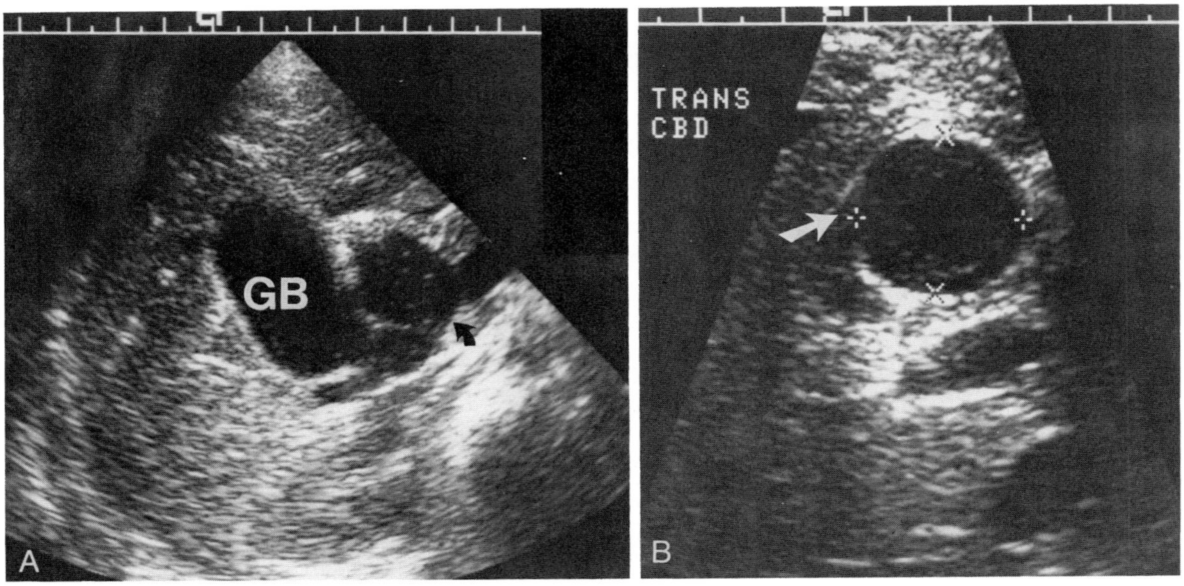

Figure 71–15. Seven-year-old white female presenting with abdominal pain, hyperamylasemia, and hyperbilirubinemia. Ultrasonography shows a normal gallbladder (*GB*) and a Type I choledochal cyst (*arrow*). Diameter of the cyst was 20 mm. *A,* longitudinal view; *B,* transverse view.

acid concentrations or chronic reflux of pancreatic secretions with inflammation may be responsible for biliary metaplasia and development of carcinoma.[262–264]

Biochemical Features

The diagnosis may be suggested from the biochemical evaluation of patients who present with obstructive jaundice (direct hyperbilirubinemia, increased alkaline phosphatase, and gamma glutamyltranspeptidase) and an elevated amylase.[247, 260]

Imaging Features

Imaging of the intrahepatic and extrahepatic biliary tree is necessary to confirm the diagnosis and may include ultrasonography[245, 247, 265, 266] (Fig. 71–15), abdominal CT scan (Fig. 71–16), hepatobiliary radionuclide scans,[260, 265, 266] endoscopic retrograde cholangiopancreatography[27, 253, 254, 267] (see Fig. 71–13), percutaneous transhepatic cholangiography, and operative cholangiography.[243, 247, 260] Alternative approaches, such as percutaneous injection, have been used to visualize the choledochal cyst (Fig. 71–17). The technique of choice is dependent on availability and expertise. It is helpful, when possible, to also delineate the main pancreatic ducts. Contrast studies of the upper intestine may demonstrate a choledochocele and, along with angiography, may be helpful in defining the anatomy preoperatively.[245, 260]

Diagnosis

The importance of establishing the correct preoperative diagnosis should be emphasized, as it allows a significant decrease in perioperative mortality.[268] The ability to accurately define the preoperative diagnosis has increased from 16% in 1956[268] to 75% today.[242]

Therapy

Definitive therapy is surgical. Past procedures for a Type I cyst have provided internal drainage, leaving the cyst in place (e.g. choledochocystduodenostomy, Roux-en-Y choledochocystojejunostomy; Fig. 71–18). However, with the present knowledge of pancreatic reflux

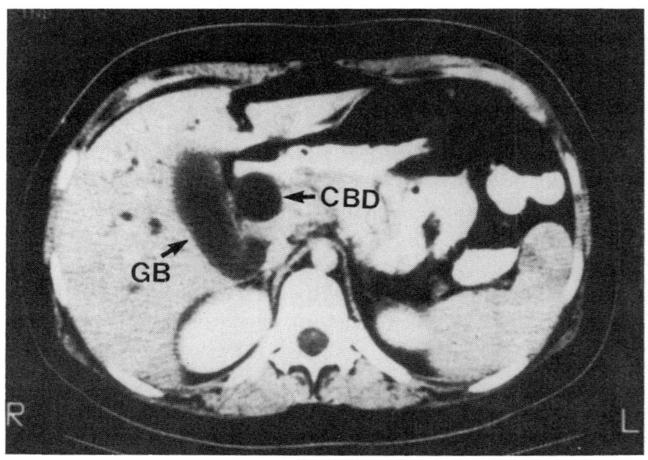

Figure 71–16. Fifteen-year-old white female presenting with chronic abdominal pain, hyperbilirubinemia, and hepatomegaly. CT scan shows a cystic common bile duct (*CBD*) and a dilated gallbladder (*GB*). ERCP confirmed a Type I choledochal cyst.

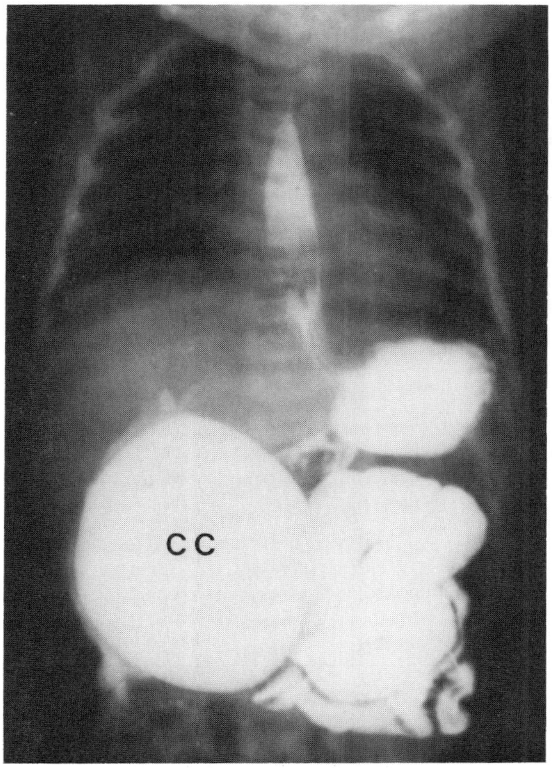

Figure 71–17. Sixteen-day-old male with jaundice and an abdominal mass. Percutaneous injection of the choledochal cyst (*CC*) was performed after upper gastrointestinal series. A Type I cyst was confirmed at laparotomy.

from anomalous pancreatobiliary junctions and an age-related incidence of carcinoma, total excision of the cyst is currently preferred. When possible, a choledochocystectomy with Roux-en-Y choledochojejunostomy or a Roux-en-Y hepaticojejunostomy is performed[244, 246, 247, 252, 253, 269–273] (see Fig. 71–18). The indication to perform a choledochojejunostomy as opposed to a hepaticojejunostomy depends on the degree of extension of the Type I cyst (e.g., saccular versus fusiform) and the ability to provide epithelial continuity between the two anastomotic segments. Variants of this procedure have been described including the use of a valved intestinal conduit to prevent recurrent cholangitis.[253, 269, 274] Because of the increased risk of cholangiocarcinoma, it has been recommended that reoperation with cystectomy be performed in those patients with retained cyst after an initial internal drainage procedure.[264] Postoperative morbidity is minimal (<10%),[275] and mortality now approaches 4%.[246]

Surgical therapy for Type II cysts involves excision of the diverticulum with ligation at the base of the stalk.[246, 270] Therapy for choledochocele may include transduodenal resection with choledochoduodenostomy or endoscopic sphincterotomy with extension of the incision over the cyst.[270, 272, 276–278] Due to its rarity, the incidence of carcinoma in choledochoceles is unknown; consequently, radical excision cannot be preferred over sphincterotomy.

The intrahepatic lesions of Type IV cyst, including Caroli's disease, may involve only one hepatic lobe which can be treated with lobectomy. Diffuse intrahepatic lesions may require liver transplantation.[271–276] There is insufficient reported experience to recommend a specific therapy for Type V choledochal cysts. However, due to their extensive nature, liver transplantation may be needed.

CAROLI'S DISEASE

Caroli's disease describes any condition with intrahepatic dilatation of the biliary tree, including some forms of choledochal cysts. It is important to note, however, that in Caroli's original description, he defined only two forms of intrahepatic biliary dilatation.[279, 280] Both types were associated with renal disease and familial inheritance. The first consisted of simple ductular ectasia. The second type also showed ductular ectasia but, in addition, periportal fibrosis, ductular proliferation, and portal hypertension. This second type is consistent with congenital hepatic fibrosis and/or infantile polycystic disease.

Few pediatric reports of Caroli's disease have been published. The disease may be lobar or panhepatic. The cystic dilatations are described as segmental, round, or lanceolate, measuring 1 to 4 cm in diameter.[280] Histologically the cyst walls show fibrosis with variable degrees of chronic and acute inflammation. The biliary epithelium may be normal, hyperplastic, ulcerated, or absent. Rarely carcinoma in situ may be found.[281] The liver may show features of congenital hepatic fibrosis.[282] The etiology of Caroli's disease is unknown. The ductal plate malformation theory and the infantile obstructive cholangiopathy theory have incorporated this disease into their respective pathogenetic mechanisms (see earlier).

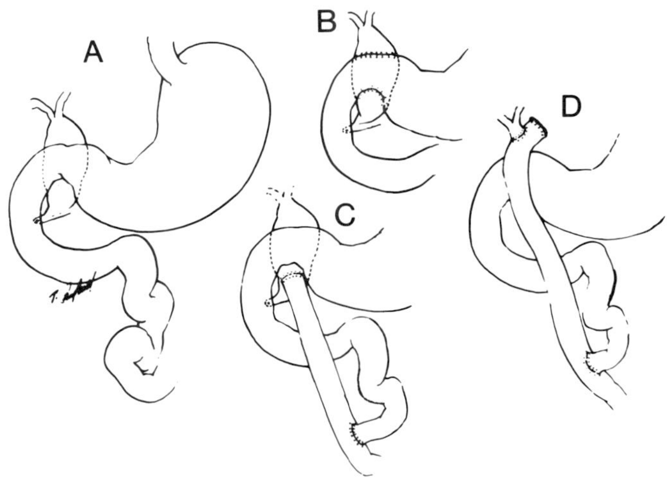

Figure 71–18. Surgical therapy for choledochal cyst, Type I. *A,* Preoperative anatomy; *B,* Choledochocystduodenostomy; *C,* Roux-en-Y choledochocystjejunostomy; and *D,* Cholecystectomy with Roux-en-Y choledochojejunostomy. The last operation is currently the procedure of choice.

Clinically, patients may present similarly to patients with choledochal cysts but without a palpable abdominal mass. Complications are also similar including cholelithiasis, cholangitis, cirrhosis, and carcinoma.[283–285]

The diagnosis is confirmed by biliary imaging techniques, including ultrasonography, endoscopic retrograde cholangiopancreatography, and percutaneous cholangiography. Liver biopsy and renal evaluation may be helpful in distinguishing this from congenital hepatic fibrosis. Definite therapy for panhepatic disease is limited and may involve liver transplantation, if and when cirrhosis becomes well established. Large cysts may benefit from internal or external drainage procedures. Hepatic lobectomy has been performed for isolated lobar disease.[270–277]

PAUCITY OF INTRAHEPATIC BILE DUCTS

Paucity of the interlobular bile ducts is defined as less than 0.5 bile ducts per portal triad on liver biopsy.[7] At least 10 portal triads are examined to ensure proper diagnosis.[286] Paucity of the interlobular bile ducts can be divided into syndromatic and nonsyndromatic varieties (Table 71–12).

Syndromatic Paucity of Interlobular Bile Ducts

Syndromatic paucity (SP) was first described by Watson and Miller in 1973 and in detail by Alagille in 1975.[287, 288] It may also be referred to in the literature as intrahepatic biliary atresia, arteriohepatic dysplasia, Alagille syndrome, or Alagille-Watson syndrome. The basic defect is obscure, but its inheritance is autosomal dominant with variable penetrance.[286] Recent studies suggest that the genetic defect can be assigned in some patients to a deletion of the short arm of chromosome 20.[289, 289a]

Table 71–12. DISORDERS WITH PAUCITY OF THE INTRAHEPATIC BILE DUCTS

I. Syndromatic paucity of intrahepatic bile ducts*
II. Nonsyndromatic paucity of intrahepatic bile ducts
  A. Idiopathic
  B. Nonidiopathic
    1. Infectious
      a. cytomegalovirus
      b. rubella
      c. reovirus type 3 (?)
      d. *Escherichia coli* (with mechanical obstruction)
    2. Genetic
      a. trisomy 21
      b. Zellweger's syndrome
      c. Ivemark's syndrome
    3. Metabolic
      a. $alpha_1$-antitrypsin deficiency
      b. cystic fibrosis (advanced stages)
      c. trihydroxycoprostanic acid excess
    4. Immunologic
      a. graft-versus-host disease
      b. hepatic allograft rejection
    5. Endocrine
      a. panhypopituitarism
    6. Other
      a. sclerosing cholangitis (stages 3 and 4)
      b. advanced biliary cirrhosis

*Synonyms are Alagille syndrome, Alagille-Watson syndrome, arteriohepatic dysplasia, and intrahepatic biliary atresia.

Table 71–13. SYNDROMATIC PAUCITY OF INTRAHEPATIC BILE DUCTS: CLINICAL AND DIAGNOSTIC FEATURES

Features	Frequency	Reference
Major		
Chronic cholestasis	91%	286
Characteristic facies	95%	286
Cardiac murmur: total	85%	286
Central and peripheral pulmonary stenosis	70%	286
Tetralogy of Fallot	9%	286
Vertebral anomalies	87%	286
Posterior embryotoxon	89%	286
Associated		
Growth retardation	50%	286
Mental retardation	20%	286
High-pitched voice		286
Renal mesangiolipidosis	74%	286
Hypogonadism (males)	86%	288
Cutaneous photosensitivity	Case report	290
Inner ear anomalies	Case report	291
Axenfeld (ocular) anomaly	Case report	292
Pigmentary retinopathy	Case report	292
Tubulointerstitial nephropathy	Case report	293
Nesidioblastosis	Personal observation	

Alagille, in a 1987 review of 80 cases, bases the diagnosis on five major clinical features (Table 71–13).[286, 288, 290–293] Thirty-five percent of patients present with the complete syndrome having all five features. Incomplete syndromic paucity is defined as chronic cholestasis with three major features and represents 48% of patients. All others, including 9% who do not present with cholestasis, require careful observation as some major features may become apparent with time.[286]

Chronic cholestasis may not appear until after the fourth month of life in 56%,[286] and paucity of interlobular bile ducts on biopsy may be a late finding apparent only after 6 months of life. Prior to 3 to 6 months of age, portal inflammation and intrahepatic cholestasis are the predominant histologic lesions.[294–296] When clear-cut clinical features are absent, it may be difficult on an early biopsy to differentiate this disease from extrahepatic biliary atresia. Some patients with arteriohepatic dysplasia and severely hypoplastic extrahepatic bile ducts have undergone hepatic portoenterostomies. As a result of the chronic cholestasis, gamma glutamyltranspeptidase, total bile acids, alkaline phosphatase, and cholesterol are elevated. The liver is enlarged and the children suffer from pruritus. Xanthomas usually develop by 4 years of age. The liver disease may progress to cirrhosis and portal hypertension.[286]

The facial abnormalities become more characteristic with advancing age and consist of a broad forehead, deeply set and widely spaced eyes, a nose that is either saddle shaped or long and straight, and an underdeveloped mandible resulting in a pointed chin (Fig. 71–19).

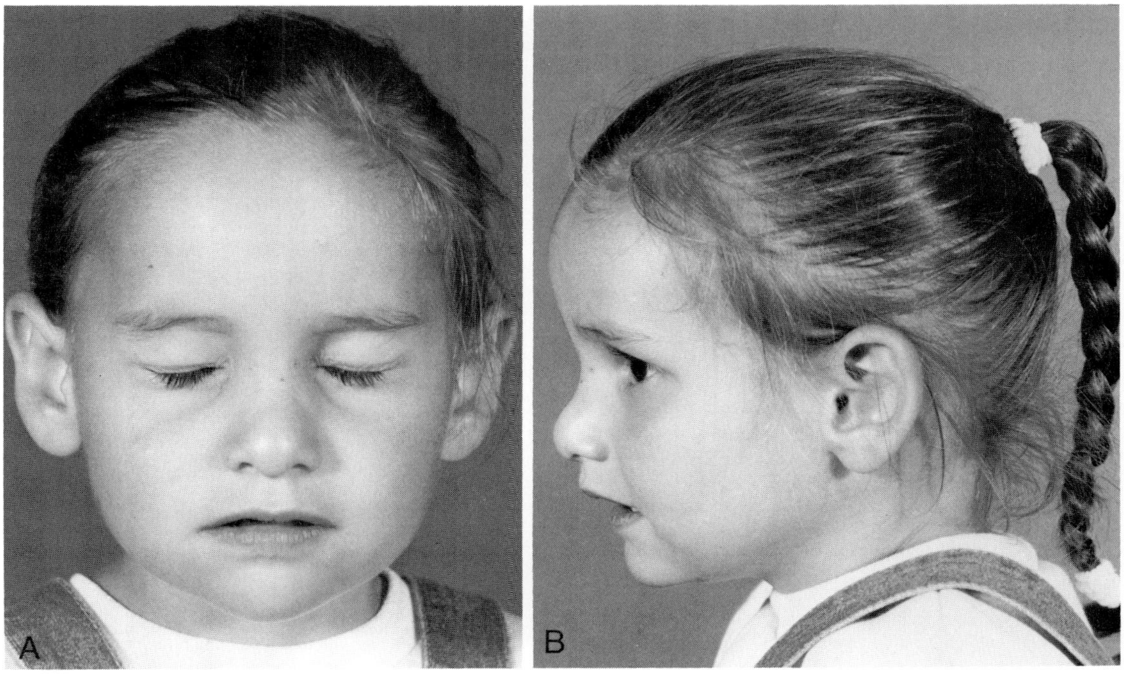

Figure 71–19. Three-year-old white female who presented at birth with cholestasis, tetralogy of Fallot, and nesidioblastosis. Evaluation, including serial liver biopsies, confirmed Alagille syndrome. Typical facial characteristics include deep-set eyes; small, pointed chin; and high, broad forehead (*A* and *B*).

Similar facial characteristics have been noted in children with other types of cholestatic syndromes.

The majority of cardiovascular anomalies are due to benign peripheral pulmonic stenosis, but lesions may be severe and involve the main pulmonary arteries or constitute a tetralogy of Fallot.

Vertebral anomalies are due to nonfusion of the anterior arches, giving a "butterfly" appearance on x-ray. Hemivertebra may also be seen. A posterior embryotoxon due to incomplete iridocorneal separation is frequently found on slit-lamp examination of the eye. Less common associations are described in Table 71–13.

The clinical course of patients with Alagille syndrome is variable. The cholestasis may progress in some to cirrhosis and portal hypertension. In others, the cholestasis may regress over time to become evident only by biochemical testing. In Alagille's initial experience of 80 patients, the overall mortality rate was 26%, with 30% of these due to cardiovascular complications and 20% due to hepatic complications.[286] This mortality is currently suspected to be much lower due to new cardiovascular surgical techniques and overall improving results in the management of children with severe liver disease.

The management of liver disease for these patients is entirely medical except in those who evolve to cirrhosis and become candidates for liver transplantation.[4]

Nonsyndromatic Paucity of Interlobular Bile Ducts

The term nonsyndromatic paucity of the interlobular bile ducts (NSP) is reserved for those conditions of bile duct paucity that do not fulfill the criteria for Alagille syndrome. NSP may be idiopathic in nature or associated with other disease states (see Table 71–12). Underlying etiologies such as alpha$_1$-antitrypsin deficiency,[286, 297] congenital rubella or cytomegalovirus infection,[286, 298] and Down's syndrome[299] have been described. Vanishing bile duct syndrome, the nonsyndromatic paucity seen in hepatic allograft rejection, may be related to donor-recipient HLA class mismatch. A disorder of HLA class 2 antigen expression can also be found in these patients as in graft-versus-host disease.[300] In both instances a nonsuppurative cholangitis leads to disappearance of interlobular bile ducts.

In one study, NSP represented 40% of all paucity cases.[286] Histologically, the findings are similar to Alagille syndrome, with bile duct paucity, fibrosis, giant cell transformation, and extramedullary erythropoiesis.[295] These features can be found, however, at a much earlier age than in syndromatic paucity (<90 days) and may facilitate differentiation between the two.[295] NSP may have a poorer prognosis than syndromatic paucity with a higher mortality rate from cirrhosis.[7]

BILE DUCT PERFORATION

Perforation of the extrahepatic biliary tree may be the result of trauma[301] or an acute intra-abdominal event such as necrotizing enterocolitis.[302] Spontaneous perforation of the common bile duct is, however, the most frequently encountered type and is the second most frequent cause of surgically correctable jaundice after biliary atresia.[303]

Spontaneous perforation of the common bile duct is found most frequently at the junction of the cystic duct and common hepatic duct.[303–307] Distal obstruction from stones, sludge, or stenosis and a mural defect due to an error of embryogenesis have been postulated to be important factors in the pathogenesis.[304, 306, 307] The perforation leads to bile ascites or the formation of a localized pseudocholedochal cyst. The disease most often presents between 1 week and 4.5 years of age[306] and is subacute in nature. Signs and symptoms consist of failure to thrive, abdominal distention, hernia formation, intermittent jaundice, and acholic stools. Rarely the child may present with signs of intestinal obstruction,[306] peritonitis,[303] or an abdominal mass.[304]

Biochemical parameters may be normal or mildly elevated. Ultrasonography confirms the presence of ascites, and hepatobiliary scintigraphy demonstrates leakage from the bile ducts into the peritoneum. Cholangiography localizes the point of rupture and outlines any possible distal obstruction. Therapy is surgical and, in most cases, simple drainage results in spontaneous closure.[304–307]

CONGENITAL MALFORMATIONS OF THE BILIARY TREE

Agenesis of the gallbladder is estimated to occur in one of every 2,500 to 6,000 live births.[308, 309] It may be associated with other congenital anomalies, especially cardiovascular, in which case it carries an early poor prognosis.[308] In most pediatric cases it is asymptomatic but may be responsible for biliary-type symptoms in adulthood.[308] The diagnosis can be suggested by ultrasonography or hepatobiliary scanning, but false-positive results may be encountered.[309, 310] Agenesis of the gallbladder has been reported as a non-sex-linked trait with variable penetrance.[311–313] Agenesis of the common bile duct and right and left hepatic ducts has been reported in very rare cases.[314]

The gallbladder may have an aberrant anatomic location. It has been described in various ectopic situations including intrahepatic, left sided, retroperitoneal, retrohepatic, and within the falciform ligament, among others.[308] Duplication of the gallbladder has also been described.[315]

Accessory bile ducts may be found connecting the right hepatic lobe to the cystic, left hepatic, right hepatic, or common bile ducts. Cholecystohepatic ducts, or sinuses of Luschka, are due to persistence of fetal connections between the gallbladder and hepatic parenchyma. They usually do not communicate with the gallbladder lumen. Rarely they may provide the main source of hepatic bile drainage.[315–317]

Other congenital anomalies include septation of the biliary tree,[316] bile duct stricture,[316,318] bronchobiliary fistulas,[319, 320] gastric heterotopia,[321] and abnormal insertion of the common bile duct into the duodenum.[322] Most congenital anomalies are asymptomatic in the pediatric age group, but knowledge of these anomalies is helpful for those children undergoing laparotomy for other reasons.

REFERENCES

1. Jorgensen M: The ductal plate malformation. Acta Pathol Microbiol Scand 1977; 257(Suppl): 1–88.
2. Desmet V: Cholangiopathies: Past, present and future. Semin Liver Dis 1987; 7:67–76.
3. Landing BH: Considerations of the pathogenesis of neonatal hepatitis, biliary atresia and choledochal cyst: The concept of infantile obstructive cholangiopathy. Prog Pediatr Surg 1974; 6:113–139.
4. Whittington P, Balistreri WF: Liver transplantation in pediatrics: Indications, contraindications and pretransplant management. J Pediatr 1991; 118:169–177.
5. Hays DM, Kimura K: Current classifications and forms of biliary atresia. *In* Hays DM, ed: Biliary Atresia: The Japanese Experience. Cambridge, Harvard University Press, 1980, pp 52–58.
6. Lilly JR, Pau CM, Ohi R: Historical background of the biliary atresia registry. *In* Daum F, ed: Extrahepatic Biliary Atresia. New York, Marcel Dekker, 1983, pp 73–77.
7. Balistreri, WF: Interrelationship between the infantile cholangiopathies and paucity of the intrahepatic bile ducts. *In* Balistreri WF, Stocker JT, eds: Pediatric Hepatology. New York, Hemisphere Publishing, 1990, pp 1–18.
8. Walton KT, Kasai M, Spence MA: Racial influence on the incidence of biliary atresia. Prog Pediatr Surg 1974; 6:53–62.
9. Hays DM, Kimura K: Biliary atresia: New concepts of management. *In* Ravitch M, ed: Current Problems in Surgery. Chicago, Year Book Medical Publishers, 1981, pp 546–608.
10. Holder TM, Ashcraft KW: The effects of bile duct ligation and inflammation in the fetus. J Pediatr Surg 1967; 2:35–39.
11. Ogawa T, Suruga K, Kajina Y, et al: Experimental study of the pathogenesis of infantile obstructive cholangiopathy and its clinical evaluation. J Pediatr Surg 1983; 18:131–135.
12. Pickett LK, Briggs HC: Biliary obstruction secondary to hepatic vascular ligation in the fetal sheep. J Pediatr Surg 1969; 4:95–101.
13. Morecki R, Glaser J, Horwitz M: Etiology of biliary atresia: The role of reo 3 virus. *In* Daum F, ed: Extrahepatic Biliary Atresia. New York, Marcel Dekker, 1983, pp 1–9.
14. Morecki R, Glaser J, Cho S, et al: Biliary atresia and reovirus type 3 infection. N Engl J Med 1982; 307:481–484.
15. Brown W, Sokol R, Levin M, et al: Lack of correlation between infection with Reovirus 3 and extrahepatic biliary atresia or neonatal hepatitis. J Pediatr 1988; 113:670–676.
16. Morecki R, Glaser J: Reovirus 3 and neonatal biliary disease: Discussion of divergent results. Hepatology 1989; 10:515–516.
17. Strickland A, Shannon K: Studies in the etiology of extrahepatic biliary atresia: Time space clustering. J Pediatr 1982; 100:749–753.
18. Danks D, Campbell P, Roger J, et al: Studies of the aetiology of neonatal hepatitis and biliary atresia. Arch Dis Child 1977; 52:360–367.
19. Altman PR: Biliary atresia. Pediatrics 1981; 68:896–898.
20. Chandra RS: Bile duct and hepatic morphology in biliary atresia: Correlation with bile flow following portoenterostomy. *In* Daum F, ed: Extrahepatic Biliary Atresia. New York, Marcel Dekker, 1983, pp 43–63.
21. Kasai M, Kimura S, Asakura Y, et al: Surgical treatment of biliary atresia. J Pediatr Surg 1968; 6:665–675.
22. Chandra RS, Altman RP: Ductal remnants in extrahepatic biliary atresia: A histopathologic study with clinical correlation. J Pediatr 1978; 93:196–200.
23. Kasai M, Watanabe I, Ohi R: Follow up studies of long term survivors after hepatic portoenterostomy for "non-correctable" biliary atresia. J Pediatr Surg 1975;10:173–182.
24. Haas JE: Bile duct and liver pathology in biliary atresia. World J Surg 1978; 2:561–569.
25. Ishak KG, Sharp HL: Developmental abnormality and liver disease in childhood. *In* MacSween R, Anthony P, Scheuer P, eds. Pathology of the Liver. New York, Churchill Livingstone, 1987, pp 66–98.
26. Rosenthal P, Ramos A, Mungo R: Management of children with hyperbilirubinemia and green teeth. J Pediatr 1986; 108:103–105.
27. Kasai M: Treatment of biliary atresia with special reference to

hepatic portoenterostomy and its modifications. Prog Pediatr Surg 1974; 6:5–52.
28. Grosfeld J, Fitzgerald J, Predaina R, et al: The efficacy of hepatoportoenterostomy in biliary atresia. Surgery 1989; 106:692–701.
29. Brunelle F: Biliary atresia and gallbladder contraction. AJR 1988; 150:694–695.
30. Weinberger E, Blumhagen J, Odell M: Gallbladder contraction in biliary atresia. AJR 1987; 149:401–402.
31. Brough AJ, Bernstein J: Liver biopsy in the diagnosis of infantile obstructive jaundice. Pediatrics 1969; 43:519–526.
32. Greene HL, Helinek GL, Moran R, et al: A diagnostic approach to prolonged obstructive jaundice by 24 hour collection of duodenal fluid. J Pediatr 1979; 95:412–414.
33. Greene HL, Helinek GL: Biliary atresia vs. neonatal hepatitis. J Pediatr 1980; 97:510–512.
34. Dick MD, Mowat AP: Biliary scintigraphy with DISIDA. A simpler way of showing bile duct patency in suspected biliary atresia. Arch Dis Child 1986; 61:191–192.
35. Majd M: Radionuclide studies in the evaluation of neonatal jaundice. *In* Daum F, ed: Extrahepatic Biliary Atresia. New York, Marcel Dekker, 1983, pp 23–32.
36. Wanke E, Karrer F, Brandt C, et al: Biliary atresia. Pediatr Rev 1989; 11:57–62.
37. Franken E, Smith W, Smith J, et al: Percutaneous cholangiography in infants. Am J Roentgenol 1978; 130:1057–1058.
38. Lebwohl O, Waye J: Endoscopic retrograde cholangiopancreatography in the diagnosis of extrahepatic biliary atresia. Am J Dis Child 1979; 133:647–649.
39. Allendorph M, Werlin SL, Geenen J: Endoscopic retrograde cholangiopancreatography in children. J Pediatr 1987; 110:206–211.
40. Heyman MB, Shapiro HA, Thaler MM: Endoscopic retrograde cholangiography in the diagnosis of biliary malformations in infants. Gastrointest Endosc 1988; 34:449–453.
41. Guelrud M, Jaen D, Torres P, et al: Endoscopic cholangiopancreatography in the infant: Evaluation of a new prototype pediatric duodenoscope. Gastrointest Endosc 1987; 33:4–8.
42. Lilly J, Karrer F: Contemporary surgery of biliary atresia. Pediatr Clin North Am 1985; 32:1233–1246.
43. Mowat AP: Liver disorders in childhood. Boston, Butterworths, 1987, p 44.
44. Nittono H, Tokita A, Hayashi M, et al: Ursodeoxycholic acid in biliary atresia. Lancet 1988; 1:528.
45. Ulrich D, Rating D, Schroter W, et al: Treatment with ursodeoxycholic acid renders children with biliary atresia suitable for liver transplantation. Lancet 1987; 2:1324.
46. Sokol R: Medical management of neonatal cholestasis. *In* Balistreri WF, Stocker J, eds: Pediatric Hepatology. New York, Hemisphere Publishing, 1990, pp 41–76.
47. Hanid M, Levi A: Phototherapy for pruritis in primary biliary cirrhosis. Lancet 1980; 2:530.
48. Cynamon H, Andres J, Iafrate R: Rifampin relieves pruritus in children with cholestatic liver disease. Gastroenterology 1990; 98:1013–1016.
49. Mowat AP: Liver disorders in childhood. Boston, Butterworths, 1987, p 316.
50. Chojkier M, Conn H: Esophageal tamponade in the treatment of bleeding varices: A decadal progress report. Dig Dis Sci 1980; 25:267–272.
51. Caulfield M, Wyllie R, Sivak M, et al: Upper gastrointestinal endoscopy in infants and children. J Pediatr 1989; 115:339–345.
52. Ament M, Berquist W, Vargas J, et al: Fiberoptic upper intestinal endoscopy in infants and children. Pediatr Clin North Am 1988; 35:141–155.
53. Sheen I, Chen T, Liaw Y: Randomized controlled study of propranolol for prevention of recurrent esophageal varices bleeding in patients with cirrhosis. Liver 1989; 9:1–5.
54. Ozsoylu S, Kocak N, Yuce N: Propranolol therapy for portal hypertension in children. J Pediatr 1985; 106:317–321.
55. Hesham A, Kadler H, Balistreri W: Cirrhosis. *In* Gellis S, Kagan B, eds: Current Pediatic Therapy. Philadelphia, WB Saunders, 1990, pp 206–207.
56. Kaufman S, Murray N, Wood P, et al: Nutritional support for the infant with extrahepatic biliary atresia. J Pediatr 1987; 110:679–686.
57. Greene HL: Nutritional aspects of biliary atresia. *In* Daum F, ed: Extrahepatic Biliary Atresia. New York, Marcel Dekker, 1983, pp 133–143.
58. Lilly JR, Hall R, Altman PR: Liver transplantation and Kasai operation in the first year of life: Therapeutic dilemma in biliary atresia. J Pediatr 1987; 110:561–562.
59. Ladd W: Congenital atresia and stenosis of the bile ducts. JAMA 1928; 91:1082–1085.
60. Lilly JR, Hernandez-Cano A, Hall R, et al: Surgery of biliary atresia. *In* Balistreri W, Stocker J, eds: Pediatric Hepatology. New York, Hemisphere Publishing, 1990, pp 19–27.
61. Kasai M: Hepatic portoenterostomy for the so-called "non-correctable" type of biliary atresia. *In* Daum F, ed: Extrahepatic Biliary Atresia. New York, Marcel Dekker, 1983, pp 79–90.
62. Lilly JR, Karrer FM, Hall RJ, et al: The surgery of biliary atresia. Ann Surg 1989; 210:289–296.
63. Ecoffey C, Rothman E, Bernard O, et al: Bacterial cholangitis after surgery for biliary atresia. J Pediatr 1987; 111:824–829.
64. Burnweit CA, Coln D: Influence of diversion on the development of cholangitis after hepatoportoenterostomy for biliary atresia. J Pediatr Surg 1986; 21:1143–1146.
65. Reynolds M, Luck S, Raffensberger J: The valved conduit prevents cholangitis: A follow-up. J Pediatr Surg 1985; 20:696–701.
66. Stewart BA, Hall RJ, Karrer FM, et al: Long term survival after Kasai's operation for biliary atresia. Pediatr Surg Int 1990; 5:87–90.
67. Yeh TJ, Chin TW, Tsai WC, et al: Mucosal intussusception to avoid ascending cholangitis. Br J Surg 1990; 77:989–991.
68. Crambleholme T, Harrison M, Langer J, et al: Biliary appendicoduodenostomy: A non-refluxing conduit for biliary reconstruction. J Pediatr Surg 1989; 24:665–667.
69. Hays D, Kimura K: Biliary atresia: The Japanese Experience. Cambridge, Harvard University Press, 1980, pp 122–132.
70. Koboyashi A, Itabashi F, Ohbe Y: Long term prognosis in biliary atresia after hepatic portoenterostomy: Analysis of 35 patients who survived beyond 5 years of age. J Pediatr 1984; 105:243–246.
71. Zitelli B, Gartner J, Malatuck J, et al: Liver transplantation. *In* Balistreri W, Stocker J, eds: Pediatric Hepatology. New York, Hemisphere Publishing, 1990, pp 363–376.
72. Houwen R, Zwierstra R, Soverijner R, et al: Prognosis of extrahepatic biliary atresia. Arch Dis Child 1989; 64:214–218.
73. Andrews H, Zwiren G, Caplon D, et al: Biliary atresia: An evolving perspective. S Med J 1986; 79:581–584.
74. Long term survival in biliary atresia (editorial). Lancet 1989; 2:597–598.
75. Kobayashi A, Utsonumiya T, Ohbe Y: Congenital biliary atresia: Analysis of 97 cases with reference to prognosis after hepatic portoenterostomy. Am J Dis Child 1976; 130:830–833.
76. Howard E, Driver M, McClement J, et al: Biliary atresia: The results of surgery in 88 consecutive cases. *In* Daum F, ed: Extrahepatic Biliary Atresia. New York, Marcel Dekker, 1983, pp 99–103.
77. Hitch D, Shikes R, Lilly JR: Determinants of survival after Kasai's operations for biliary atresia using actuarial analysis. J Pediatr Surg 1979; 14:310–314.
78. Lally K, Kanegaye J, Matsunura M, et al: Perioperative factors affecting the outcome following repair of biliary atresia. Pediatrics 1989; 83:723–726.
78a. Bielamowicz A, Weitzman JJ, Alshak NS, et al: Successful late Kasai portoenterostomy. J Pediatr Gastroenterol Nutr 1992; 14:232–236.
79. Mieli-Vergagni G, Howard E, Pastman B, et al: Late referral for biliary atresia—missed opportunity for effective surgery. Lancet 1989; 1:421–423.
80. Esquivel C, Koneru B, Karrer F, et al: Liver transplantation before one year of age. J Pediatr 1982; 110:545–548.
81. Sokal E, Veyckmans F, deVille de Goyet J, et al: Liver transplantation in children less than 1 year of age. J Pediatr 1990; 117:205–210.
82. Millis J, Broms J, Hiatt J, et al: Orthotopic liver transplantation for biliary atresia. Arch Surg 1988; 123:1237–1239.
83. Hall RJ, Karrer FM: Biliary atresia: Perspective on transplantation. Pediatr Surg Int 1990; 5:94–99.
84. Sisto A, Feldman P, Garel L: Primary sclerosing cholangitis in

children: Study of five cases and review of the literature. Pediatrics 1987; 80:918–923.
85. Werlin SL, Glicklich M, Jona J, et al: Sclerosing cholangitis in childhood. J Pediatr 1980; 96:433–435.
86. LaRusso NF, Wiesner RH, Ludwig J, et al: Primary sclerosing cholangitis. N Engl J Med 1984; 310:899–903.
87. Helzberg JH, Petersen JM, Boyer JL: Improved survival with primary sclerosing cholangitis: A review of clinicopathologic features and comparison of symptomatic and asymptomatic patients. Gastroenterology 1987; 92:1869–1875.
88. El-Shabrawi M, Wilkinson ML, Portmann B, et al: Primary sclerosing cholangitis in childhood. Gastroenterology 1987; 92:1226–1235.
89. Belghiti J, Benhamou JP, Houry S, et al: Caustic sclerosing cholangitis: A complication of the surgical treatment of hydatid disease of the liver. Arch Surg 1986; 121:1162–1165.
90. Ludwig J, LaRusso N, Wiesner RH: The syndrome of primary sclerosing cholangitis. Prog Liver Dis 1990; 9:555–566.
91. Mieli-Vergagni G, Lobo-Yeo A, McFarlane B, et al: Different immune mechanisms leading to autoimmunity in primary sclerosing cholangitis and autoimmune chronic active hepatitis of childhood. Hepatology 1989; 9:198–203.
92. Wiesner RH, Grambsch PM, Dickson ER, et al: Primary sclerosing cholangitis: Natural history, prognostic factors and survival analysis. Hepatology 1989; 10:430–436.
93. Classen M, Gotze H, Richter HJ, et al: Primary sclerosing cholangitis in children. J Pediatr Gastroenterol Nutr 1987;6:197–202.
94. Blackstone MO, Nemchansky BA: Cholangiographic abnormalities in ulcerative colitis–associated pericholangitis which resemble sclerosing cholangitis. Am J Dig Dis 1978; 23:579–585.
95. Maggiore G, DeGiacomo C, Ugazio A: Sclerosing cholangitis in childhood. Gastroenterology 1988; 94:551–552.
96. Johnson DA, Cattan EL, Hancock JE: Pediatric primary sclerosing cholangitis. Dig Dis Sci 1986; 31:773–777.
97. Gremse DA, Bucuvalas JC, Bongiovanni GL: Papillary stenosis and sclerosing cholangitis in an immunodeficient child. Gastroenterology 1989; 96:1600–1603.
98. Naveh Y, Mendelsohn H, Spira G, et al: Primary sclerosing cholangitis associated with immunodeficiency. Am J Dis Child 1983; 137:117–119.
99. Strandvik B, Hjelte L, Gabrielsson N, et al: Sclerosing cholangitis in cystic fibrosis. Scand J Gastroenterol 1985; 23:121–124.
100. Amedee-Manesme O, Bernard O, Brunelle F, et al: Sclerosing cholangitis with neonatal onset. J Pediatr 1987; 111:225–229.
101. DiPalma JA, Strobel CT, Farrow JG: Primary sclerosing cholangitis associated with hyperimmunoglobulin M immunodeficiency (dysgammaglobulinemia). Gastroenterology 1986; 19:464–468.
102. Kane W, Miller K, Sharp HL: Inflammatory bowel disease presenting as liver disease during childhood. J Pediatr 1980; 97:775–778.
103. Davis JJ, Heyman MB, Ferrell L, et al: Sclerosing cholangitis associated with chronic cryptosporidiosis in a child with a congenital immunodeficiency disorder. Am J Gastroenterol 1987; 82:1196–1202.
104. Benett I, Salh B, Haboubi NY, et al: Sclerosing cholangitis with hepatic microvesicular steatosis in cystic fibrosis and chronic pancreatitis. J Clin Pathol 1989; 42:466–469.
105. Baker SS, Compton CC: Case records of the Massachusetts General Hospital, case 3–1991. N Engl J Med 1991; 324:180–188.
106. Desmet VJ, Geboes K: Liver lesions in inflammatory bowel disorders. J Pathol 1987; 151:247–255.
107. Rabinowitz M, Gavaler JS, Schade RR, et al: Does primary sclerosing cholangitis occurring in association with inflammatory bowel disease differ from that occurring in the absence of inflammatory bowel disease? A study of sixty-six subjects. Hepatology 1990; 11:7–11.
108. Schrumpf E, Fausa O, Elgjo K, et al: Hepatobiliary complications of inflammatory bowel disease. Semin Liver Dis 1988; 8:201–209.
109. Brooke BN, Slaney G: Portal bacteremia in ulcerative colitis. Lancet 1958; 1:1206–1207.
110. Warren KW, Athanassiades S, Monge JI: Primary sclerosing cholangitis: A study of 42 cases. Am J Surg 1966; 111:23–28.
111. Eade MN: Liver disease in ulcerative colitis. Ann Intern Med 1970; 72:475–487.
112. Bodenheimer HC, LaRusso N, Thayer WR, et al: Elevated circulating immune complexes in primary sclerosing cholangitis. Hepatology 1984; 3:150–154.
113. Zauli D, Schrumpf E, Crespi L: An auto-antibody profile in primary sclerosing cholangitis. J Hepatology 1987; 5:14–18.
114. Chapman RW, Cottone M, Selby WS, et al: Serum autoantibodies, ulcerative colitis and primary sclerosing cholangitis. Gut 1986; 37:86–91.
115. MacFarlane IG, Wojicka BM, Tsantoulas DC, et al: Leukocyte migration inhibition in response to biliary antigens in primary biliary cirrhosis, sclerosing cholangitis and other chronic liver diseases. Gastroenterology 1979; 76:1333–1400.
116. Brinch L, Toisberg P, Schrumpf P, et al: The in vivo metabolism of C3 in hepatobiliary disease associated with ulcerative colitis. Scand J Gastroenterol 1982; 17:523–527.
117. Quigley EM, LaRusso N, Ludwig J, et al: Familial occurrence of primary sclerosing cholangitis and ulcerative colitis. Gastroenterology 1983; 85:1160–1165.
118. Schrumpf E, Fausa O, Forre O, et al: HLA antigens and immunoregulatory T cells in ulcerative colitis associated with hepatobiliary disease. Scand J Gastroenterol 1982; 17:187–191.
119. Chapman RW, Varghese Z, Gaul R, et al: Association of primary sclerosing cholangitis with HLA-B8. Gut 1983; 28:38–41.
120. Donaldson PT, Farrant JM, Wilkinson ML, et al: Dual association of HLA-DR2 and HLA-DR3 with primary sclerosing cholangitis. Hepatology 1991; 13:129–133.
121. Minuk GY, Paul RW, Lee PW: The prevalence of antibodies to Reovirus type 3 in adults with idiopathic cholestatic liver disease. J Med Virol 1985; 16:55–60.
122. Minuk GY, Rascanin N, Paul RW, et al: Reovirus type 3 infection in patients with primary biliary cirrhosis and primary sclerosing cholangitis. J Hepatology 1987; 5:8–13.
123. Celo JP: Acquired immunodeficiency syndrome cholangiopathy: Spectrum of disease. Am J Med 1989; 86:539–546.
124. Ludwig J, Barham SS, LaRusso N, et al: Morphologic features of chronic hepatitis associated with primary sclerosing cholangitis or chronic ulcerative colitis. Hepatology 1981; 1:632–640.
125. Chapman RW, Arborgh BA, Rhodes JM, et al: Primary sclerosing cholangitis: A review of its clinical features, cholangiography and hepatic histology. Gut 1980; 21:870–877.
126. Lindor KD, Wiesner RH, MacCarty RL, et al: Advances in primary sclerosing cholangitis. Am J Med 1990; 89:73–80.
127. Wiesner RH, LaRusso N, Dozois RR, et al: Peristomal varices after proctocolectomy in patients with primary sclerosing cholangitis. Gastroenterology 1986; 90:316–322.
128. Clements D, Rhodes JM, Elias E: Severe bile duct lesions without biochemical evidence of cholestasis in a case of sclerosing cholangitis. J Hepatol 1986; 3:72–74.
129. Krieger J, Seaman WB, Porter MR: The roentgenologic appearance of primary sclerosing cholangitis. Radiology 1970; 95:369–375.
130. Tepleck SK, Haskin PH, Sammon JK, et al: Common bile duct obstruction: Assessment by transcholecystic cholangiography. Radiology 1986; 161:138–139.
131. Brunelle F, Chaumont P: Cholecystographie percutanee chez l'enfant. Ann Radiol 1984; 27:111–116.
132. Sokal E, deVille J, Buts JP, et al: Unifocal stricture of the common bile duct in two children: A localized form of primary sclerosing cholangitis. J Pediatr Gastroenterol Nutr 1990; 11:268–274.
133. MacCarty RL, LaRusso N, May GR, et al: Cholangiocarcinoma complicating primary sclerosing cholangitis: Cholangiographic appearance. Radiology 1985; 156:43–46.
134. Teefey SA, Baron RL, Rohrmann CA, et al: Sclerosing cholangitis: CT findings. Radiology 1988; 169:635–639.
135. Wee A, Ludwig J: Pericholangitis in chronic ulcerative colitis: Primary sclerosing cholangitis of the small ducts? Ann Intern Med 1985; 102:581–587.
136. Burgert SL, Brown BP, Kirckpatrick RB, et al: Positive corticosteroid response in early primary sclerosing cholangitis (abstract). Gastroenterology 1984; 86:1037.
137. Myers RN, Cooper JG, Padis N: Primary sclerosing cholangitis: Complete gross and histologic reversal after long term steroid therapy. Am J Gastroenterol 1970; 53:527–538.

138. Wagner A: Azathioprine treatment in primary sclerosing cholangitis. Lancet 1971; 2:663–664.
139. Shelley D, Shelley WB: Cyclosporine therapy for pyoderma gangrenosum associated with sclerosing cholangitis and ulcerative colitis. J Am Acad Dermatol 1988; 18:1084–1088.
140. Knox TA, Kaplan MM: Methotrexate treatment of primary sclerosing cholangitis (abstract). Gastroenterology 1989; 96:614.
141. Leiser A, Kadish U: Beneficial effect of colchicine in a case of sclerosing cholangitis. Am J Med Sci 1986; 291:416–418.
142. Polter DE, Gruhl V, Eigenbrodt EH, et al: Beneficial effect of cholestyramine in sclerosing cholangitis. Gastroenterology 1980; 79:326–333.
143. Hayashi H, Higuchi T, Ichimiya H, et al: Asymptomatic primary sclerosing cholangitis treated with ursodeoxycholic acid. Gastroenterology 1990; 99:533–535.
144. O'Brien CB, Senior JR: Prolonged ursodiol effects in primary sclerosing cholangitis: A pilot study with two year follow-up (abstract). Gastroenterology 1991; 100:A782.
145. Kurosawa S, Kuwata H, Kushibiki K, et al: Ursodeoxycholic acid improved symptom and biochemical data as well as biliary tract sclerosis in primary sclerosing cholangitis (abstract). Gastroenterology 1991; 100:A764.
146. Chazouilleres O, Poupon R, Capron JP, et al: Is ursodeoxycholic acid an effective treatment of primary sclerosing cholangitis? (abstract). Gastroenterology 1989; 96:A583.
147. LaRusso N, Wiesner RH, Ludwig J, et al: Prospective trial of penicillamine in primary sclerosing cholangitis. Gastroenterology 1988; 95:1036–1042.
148. Grijm R, Hurbregtse K, Bartsolman J, et al: Therapeutic investigations in primary sclerosing cholangitis. Dig Dis Sci 1986; 31:792–798.
149. Allison MC, Burroughs AK, Noone P, et al: Biliary lavage with corticosteroids in primary sclerosing cholangitis: A clinical, cholangiographic and bacteriological study. Hepatology 1986; 3:118–122.
150. May GR, Bender CE, LaRusso N, et al: Non-operative dilation of dominant strictures in primary sclerosing cholangitis. AJR 1985; 145:1061–1064.
151. Skolkin MD, Alspaugh JP, Casarella WJ, et al: Sclerosing cholangitis: Palliation with percutaneous cholangioplasty. Radiology 1989; 170:199–206.
152. Johnson GK, Geenen JE, Venu RP, et al: Endoscopic treatment of biliary duct strictures in sclerosing cholangitis: Follow-up assessment of a new therapeutic approach. Gastrointest Endosc 1987; 33:9–12.
153. Cangemi JR, Wiesner RH, Beaver SJ, et al: Effect of proctocolectomy for chronic ulcerative colitis on the natural history of primary sclerosing cholangitis. Gastroenterology 1989; 96:790–794.
154. Martin FM, Rossi RL, Nugent FW, et al: Surgical aspects of sclerosing cholangitis. Results in 178 patients. Ann Surg 1990; 212:551–558.
155. Thompson JS, Wood P, Burnett DA, et al: The role of nontransplant procedures for sclerosing cholangitis. Am J Surg 1988; 156:506–508.
156. Marsh JW, Shunzaburo I, Makowka L, et al: Orthotopic liver transplantation for primary sclerosing cholangitis. Ann Surg 1988; 207:21–25.
157. Porayko MK, Wiesner RH, LaRusso N, et al: Patients with asymptomatic primary sclerosing cholangitis frequently have progressive disease. Gastroenterology 1990; 98:1594–1602.
158. Mistilis SP: Pericholangitis and ulcerative colitis. Pathology, etiology and pathogenesis. Ann Int Med 1965; 63:1–16.
159. Mistilis SP: Pericholangitis and ulcerative colitis. Clinical aspects. Ann Int Med 1965; 63:17–26.
160. Hay JE, Wiesner RH, Shorter RH, et al: Primary sclerosing cholangitis and celiac disease. Ann Int Med 1988; 109:713–717.
161. Schneiderman DJ, Cello JP, Laing FC: Papillary stenosis and sclerosing cholangitis in the acquired immunodeficiency syndrome. Ann Int Med 1987; 106:546–549.
162. Kerr DN, Harrison CV, Sherlock S, et al: Congenital hepatic fibrosis. J Med New Ser 1961; 30:91–117.
163. Sherlock S, ed: Diseases of the Liver and Biliary System. Boston, Blackwell Scientific Publications, 1981, p 406.
164. Alvarez F, Bernard O, Brunelle F, et al: Congenital hepatic fibrosis in children. J Pediatr 1981; 99:370–375.
165. Landing BH, Wells TR, Claireaux AE: Morphometric analysis of liver lesions in cystic diseases of childhood. Hum Pathol 1980; 11(suppl):549–560.
166. Witzleben C: Cystic diseases of the liver. *In* Zakim D, Boyer TD, eds: Hepatology. A Textbook of Liver Disease. Philadelphia, WB Saunders, 1990, pp 1395–1411.
167. Witzleben C, Sharp A: Nephronophthisis—congenital hepatic fibrosis: An additional hepatorenal disorder. Hum Pathol 1982; 13:728–733.
168. Naveh Y, Roguin N, Ludatscher R, et al: Congenital hepatic fibrosis with congenital heart disease. A family study with ultrastructural features of the liver. Gut 1980; 21:799–807.
169. Williams R, Scheuer PJ, Heard BE: Congenital hepatic fibrosis with an unusual pulmonary lesion. J Clin Pathol 1964; 17:135–142.
170. King K, Genta RM, Gianella RA, et al: Congenital hepatic fibrosis and cerebral aneurysm in a 32 year old woman. J Pediatr Gastroenterol Nutr 1986; 5:481–484.
171. Labrune P, Lange JC, Bodossum P, et al: Congenital hepatic fibrosis, cystic kidneys, mental retardation and facial dysmorphy: A new report of an autosomal recessive syndrome. J Pediatr Gastroenterol Nutr 1990; 10:540–545.
172. Pelletier VA, Galeano N, Brocha P, et al: Secretory diarrhea, protein-losing enteropathy, enterocolitis cystica superficialis, intestinal lymphangiectasia and congenital hepatic fibrosis: A new syndrome. J Pediatr 1985; 108:61–65.
173. Pederson PS, Tygstrap I: Congenital hepatic fibrosis combined with protein-losing enteropathy and recurrent thrombosis. Acta Pediatr Scand 1980; 69:571–574.
174. Evans-Jones G, Cudmore R: Choledochal cyst and congenital hepatic fibrosis. J Pediatr Surg 1990; 25:1259–1260.
175. Cobben JM, Breuning MH, Schoots C, et al: Congenital hepatic fibrosis in autosomal dominant polycystic kidney disease. Kidney Internat 1990; 38:880–885.
176. Matsuda O, Ideura T, Shinoda T, et al: Polycystic kidney of autosomal dominant inheritance, polycystic liver and congenital hepatic fibrosis in a single kindred. Am J Nephrol 1990; 10:237–241.
177. Odievre M, Chaumont P, Montagne PJ: Anomalies of the intrahepatic portal venous system in congenital hepatic fibrosis. Radiology 1977; 122:427–430.
178. Hausner RJ, Alexander RW: Localized congenital hepatic fibrosis presenting as an abdominal mass. Hum Pathol 1978; 5:473–476.
179. Farmer RG, Hermann RE, Sullivan BH: Congenital hepatic fibrosis of Riedel's lobe causing portal hypertension: Report of a case. Cleveland Clin Quart 1969; 36:143–148.
180. Fiorillo A, Migliorati R, Vajro P, et al: Congenital hepatic fibrosis with gastrointestinal bleeding in early infancy. Clin Pediatr 1982; 21:183–185.
181. Hewlett SA, Shulman ST, Ayoub EM: Cholangitis complicating congenital hepatic fibrosis. Am J Dig Dis 1975; 20:790–795.
182. Murray-Lyon IM, Shilkin KB, Laws JW: Cholangitis complicating congenital hepatic fibrosis. Gut 1972; 13:319.
183. Daroca PJ, Tuthill R, Reed RJ: Cholangiocarcinoma arising in congenital hepatic fibrosis. Arch Pathol 1975; 99:592–595.
184. Chen KT: Adenocarcinoma of the liver: Association with congenital hepatic fibrosis and Caroli's disease. Arch Pathol Lab Med 1981; 105:294–295.
185. Sorles J, Scheiner C, Sarran M, et al: Hepatic hypervitaminosis A: A familial observation. J Pediatr Gastroenterol Nutr 1990; 10:71–76.
186. Dusol M, Levi JU, Glasses K, et al: Congenital hepatic fibrosis with dilation of intrahepatic bile ducts. Gastroenterology 1976; 71:839–843.
187. Sanchez C, Gonzales E, Garau J: Trimethoprim-sulfamethoxazole treatment of cholangitis complicating congenital hepatic fibrosis. Pediatr Infect Dis 1986; 5:360–363.
188. Stillman AE, Earnest DC, Woolfenden JM: Hepatobiliary scintigraphy for cholestasis in congenital hepatic fibrosis. Am J Dis Child 1985; 139:41–45.
189. Kerr DN, Okonkwo S, Choa RG: Congenital hepatic fibrosis: The long term prognosis. Gut 1978; 19:514–520.
190. Kaplan BS, Kaplan P, Kotlus Rosenberg H, et al: Polycystic kidney disease in childhood. J Pediatr 1989; 115:867–880.

191. Avery ME, First LR: Pediatric Medicine. Baltimore, Williams and Wilkins, 1989, pp 616–621.
192. Lieberman E, Madrigal-Salina L, Gwinn JL, et al: Infantile polycystic disease of the kidneys and liver: Clinical, pathological, and radiological correlations and comparisons with congenital hepatic fibrosis. Medicine 1971; 50:277–318.
193. Isenberg JN: Cystic fibrosis: Its influence on the liver, biliary tree and bile salt metabolism. Semin Liv Dis 1982; 2:302–313.
194. Roy CC, Weber AM, Morin CL, et al: Hepatobiliary disease in cystic fibrosis: A survey of current issues and concepts. J Pediatr Gastroenterol Nutr 1982; 1:469–478.
195. Oppenheimer EH, Esterly JR: Pathology of cystic fibrosis: Review of the literature and comparison with 146 autopsied cases. Perspect Pediatr Pathol 1975; 2:241–275.
196. Craig JM, Haddad H, Shwachman H: The pathological changes in the liver in cystic fibrosis of the pancreas. Am J Dis Child 1957; 93:357–369.
197. di Sant'Agnese PA, Blanc WA: A distinctive type of biliary cirrhosis of the liver associated with cystic fibrosis of the pancreas: Recognition through signs of portal hypertension. Pediatrics 1956; 18:387–409.
198. Kerem BS, Rommens JM, Buchanan JA, et al: Identification of the cystic fibrosis gene: Genetic analysis. Science 1989; 245:1073–1080.
199. Kerem E, Casey M, Kerem BS, et al: The relation between genotype and phenotype in cystic fibrosis—analysis of the most frequent mutation. N Engl J Med 1990; 323:1517–1522.
199a. Duthie A, Doherty DG, Williams C, et al: Genotype analysis for DF508, G551D, and R553X mutations in children and young adults with cystic fibrosis with and without chronic liver disease. Hepatology 1992; 15:660–664.
200. Kopelman H, Corey M, Gaskin K: Impaired chloride secretion as well as bicarbonate secretion underlies the fluid secretory defect in the cystic fibrosis pancreas. Gastroenterology 1988; 95:349–355.
201. Oppenheimer EH, Esterly JR: Hepatic changes in young infants with cystic fibrosis: Possible relation to focal biliary cirrhosis. J Pediatr 1975; 86:683–689.
202. Hultcrantz R, Mongarelli S, Strandvik B: Morphological findings in the liver of children with cystic fibrosis: A light and electron microscopical study. Hepatology 1986; 6:881–889.
203. Roy CC, Weber AM, Morin CL, et al: Abnormal biliary lipid composition in cystic fibrosis: Effect of pancreatic enzymes. N Engl J Med 1977; 297:1301–1305.
204. Setchell KD, Smethurst P, Giunta A, et al: Serum bile acid composition in patients with cystic fibrosis. Clin Chim Acta 1985; 151:101–110.
205. Nakagawa M, Colombo C, Setchell KD: Comprehensive study of the biliary bile acid composition of patients with cystic fibrosis and associated liver disease before and after UDCA administration. Hepatology 1990; 12:322–334.
206. Gaskin KJ, Waters DC, Howman-Giles R, et al: Liver disease and common bile duct stenosis in cystic fibrosis. N Engl J Med 1988; 318:340–346.
207. Park RW, Grand RJ: Gastrointestinal manifestations of cystic fibrosis: A review. Gastroenterology 1981; 81:143–161.
208. Donnisson AB, Shwachman H, Gross RE: A review of 164 children with meconium ileus seen at the Children's Hospital Medical Center of Boston. Pediatrics 1966; 37:833–850.
209. Holsclaw DS, Eckstein HB, Nixon HH: Meconium ileus. Am J Dis Child 1965; 109:101–113.
210. Valman HB, France NE, Wallis PG: Prolonged neonatal jaundice in cystic fibrosis. Arch Dis Child 1971; 46:805–809.
211. Rosenstein BJ, Oppenheimer EH: Prolonged obstructive jaundice and giant cell hepatitis in an infant with cystic fibrosis. J Pediatr 1977; 91:1022–1023.
212. Psacharopoulos HT, Howard ER, Portman B, et al: Hepatic complications of cystic fibrosis. Lancet 1981; 2:78–80.
213. Vitullo BB, Rochon L, Seemayer TA: Intrapancreatic compression of the common bile duct in cystic fibrosis. J Pediatr 1978; 93:1060–1061.
214. Gatzimos CD, Jowitt RH: Jaundice in mucoviscidosis. Am J Dis Child 1955; 89:182–186.
215. Schwarz HP, Kramer R, Thurnheer U, et al: Liver involvement in cystic fibrosis. Helv Paediatr Acta 1978; 33:351–364.
216. Evans JS, George DE, Mollit D: Biliary infusion therapy in the inspissated bile syndrome of cystic fibrosis. J Pediatr Gastroenterol Nutr 1991; 12:131–135.
217. Davies C, Daneman A, Stringer DA: Inspissated bile in a neonate with cystic fibrosis. J Ultrasound Med 1986; 5:335–337.
218. Tanner MS: Current clinical management of hepatic problems in cystic fibrosis. J Soc Med 1986; 79(Suppl 12):30–43.
219. Anderson DH: Cystic fibrosis of the pancreas and its relation to celiac disease: A clinical and pathological study. Am J Dis Child 1938; 56:344–399.
220. Farber S: Pancreatic function and disease in early life: Pathologic changes associated with pancreatic insufficiency in early life. Arch Pathol 1944; 37:238–250.
221. Bodian M: Fibrocystic Disease of the Pancreas: A Congenital Disorder of Mucus Production—Mucosis. London, William Heineman Medical Books, 1952.
222. Stern RC, Stevens DP, Boat TF: Symptomatic hepatic disease in cystic fibrosis: Incidence, course, and outcome of portal systemic shunting. Gastroenterology 1976; 70:645–649.
223. Psacharopoulos HT, Portman B, Howard ER, et al: Hepatic complications of cystic fibrosis. Lancet 1981; 2:78–80.
224. Scott WJ, Block GE: Biliary stone disease in adults with cystic fibrosis. Surgery 1989; 105:671–673.
225. Abdul-Karim FW, King TA, Dahms BB, et al: Carcinoma of extrahepatic biliary system in an adult with cystic fibrosis. Gastroenterology 1982; 82:758–762.
226. Boat TF, Doershuk CF, Stern RC, et al: Serum alkaline phosphatase in cystic fibrosis. Clin Pediatr 1974; 13:505–512.
227. Haseman R, Grunert D, Reuter N, et al: Duplex sonography of the portal system and hepatic artery reveals early hepatic involvement in children with cystic fibrosis (abstract). Pediatr Pulmonol 1990; 5(Suppl):270.
227a. Zemel G, Katzen BT, Becker GJ, et al: Percutaneous transjugular portosystemic shunt. JAMA 1991; 266:390–393.
228. Cox KL: The role of liver transplantation in cystic fibrosis patients. Pediatr Pulmonol 1990; 5(Suppl):78–79.
229. Cox KL, Ward RE, Furgiuele TL, et al: Orthotopic liver transplantation in patients with cystic fibrosis. Pediatrics 1987; 80:571–574.
230. Mieles LA, Orenstein D, Tepermon L, et al: Liver transplantation in cystic fibrosis. Lancet 1989; 1:1073.
231. Colombo C, Setchell KD, Pedda M, et al: Effects of ursodeoxycholic acid therapy for liver disease associated with cystic fibrosis. J Pediatr 1990; 117:482–489.
231a. Colombo C, Castellani MR, Balistreri WF, et al: Scintigraphic documentation of an improvement in hepatobiliary excretory function after treatment with ursodeoxycholic acid in patients with cystic fibrosis and associated liver disease. Hepatology 1992; 15:677–684.
232. Lambert JR, Cole M, Crozier DN, et al: Intrapancreatic common bile duct compression causing jaundice in an adult with cystic fibrosis. Gastroenterology 1981; 80:169–172.
233. Patrick MK, Howman-Giles R, deSilva M, et al: Common bile duct obstruction causing right upper abdominal pain in cystic fibrosis. J Pediatr 1986; 108:101–102.
234. Nagel RA, Javaid A, Meire HB, et al: Liver disease and bile duct abnormalities in adults with cystic fibrosis. Lancet 1989; 2:1422–1425.
234a. O'Brien S, Keoga N, Casey M, et al: Biliary complications of cystic fibrosis. Gut 1992; 33:387–391.
235. Isenberg JN, L'Heureux PR, Warwick WJ, et al: Clinical observations on the biliary system in cystic fibrosis. Am J Gastroenterol 1976; 65:134–141.
236. Feigelson J, Mareschal JL, Sauvegrain J: Les anomalies de la vesicule biliaire dans la mucoviscidose. Med Chir Dig 1975; 4:121–124.
237. Bass S, Connon JJ, Ho CS: Biliary tree in cystic fibrosis. Biliary tract abnormalities in cystic fibrosis demonstrated by endoscopic retrograde pancreatography. Gastroenterology 1983; 84:1592–1596.
238. Edelman DS: Laparoscopic cholecystectomy under continuous epidural anesthesia in patients with cystic fibrosis. Am J Dis Child 1991; 145:723–724.
239. Vater A: Dissertatio inauguralis medica; Proes diss qua scirrhis viscerum disseret. University Library Edinburgh H22 1723; 70:1–24.
240. Alonso-Lej F, Rever W, Pessagno D: Congenital choledochal

cysts with a report of 2 and an analysis of 941 cases. Int Abst Surg 1959; 108:1–30.
241. Longmire W, Mandiola S, Gordon H: Congenital cystic disease of the liver and biliary system. Ann Surg 1971; 174:711–724.
242. Hadad A, Westbrook C, Campbell G, et al: Congenital dilatation of the bile ducts. Am J Surg 1976; 132:799–804.
243. Yamaguchi M: Congenital choledochal cyst: Analysis of 1433 patients in the Japanese literature. Am J Surg 1980; 140:653–657.
244. Saito S: Congenital choledochal cyst. Prog Pediatr Surg 1974; 6:63–90.
245. VanderPool D, Lane W, Winter J, et al: Choledochal cysts. Surg Gynecol Obstet 1988; 167:447–451.
246. Flanigan D: Biliary cysts. Ann Surg 1975; 182:635–643.
247. Kim S: Choledochal cyst: Survey of the surgical section of the American Academy of Pediatrics. J Pediatr Surg 1981; 16:402–407.
248. Cuschiere A, Davies R: Acute pancreatitis complicating a choledochal cyst. Br Med J 1969; 3:698.
249. Kozloff L, Joseph W: Cystic dilatation of the common bile duct in adults. Med Ann DC 1973; 42:595–598.
250. Yotsuyanagi S: Contribution to the etiology and pathology of idiopathic cystic dilatation of the common bile duct, with report of 3 cases. Gann 1936; 30:601–650.
251. Babbitt D, Starshak R, Clemmett A: Choledochal cyst: A concept of etiology. AJR 1973; 119:57–62.
252. Rattner D, Schapiro R, Warshaw A: Abnormalities of the pancreatic and biliary ducts in adult patients with choledochal cysts. Arch Surg 1983; 118:1068–1073.
253. Okada A, Oguchi Y, Kanata S, et al: Common channel syndrome—diagnosis with endoscopic retrograde cholangiopancreatography and surgical management. Surgery 1983; 93:634–642.
254. Wiedemeyer D, Stewart E, Dodds W, et al: Choledochal cyst: Findings on cholangiopancreatography with emphasis on ectasia of the common channel. AJR 1989; 153:969–972.
255. Iwai N, Tokiwa K, Tsuto T, et al: Biliary manometry in choledochal cyst with abnormal choledochopancreatic junction. J Pediatr Surg 1986; 21:873–876.
256. Tanaka M, Ikeda S, Kawakani K, et al: The presence of a positive pressure gradient from pancreatic duct to choledochal cyst: Clue to pancreatobiliary reflux. Endoscopy 1982; 14:45–47.
257. Kusanoki M, Saitoh N, Yamamusa T, et al: Choledochal cysts and oligoganglionosis in the narrow portion of the choledochus. Arch Surg 1988; 123:984–986.
258. Kusunoki M, Yanamura T, Takahashi T, et al: Choledochal cyst: Its possible autonomic involvement in the bile duct. Arch Surg 1987; 122:997–1000.
259. Stringel G, Filler R: Fictitious pancreatitis in choledochal cyst. J Pediatr Surg 1982; 17:359–361.
260. Sherman P, Kolster E, Davies C, et al: Choledochal cysts: Heterogeneity of clinical presentation. J Pediatr Gastroenterol Nutr 1986; 5:867–872.
260a. Treem WR, Hyams JS, McGowan GS, et al: Spontaneous rupture of a choledochal cyst: Clues to diagnosis and etiology. J Pediatr Gastroenterol Nutr 1991; 13:301–306.
261. Voyles C, Smadge C, Shands C, et al: Carcinoma in choledochal cysts: Age related incidence. Arch Surg 1983; 118:986–988.
262. Todani T, Watanabe Y, Toki A, et al: Reoperation for congenital choledochal cyst. Ann Surg 1988; 207:142–147.
263. Reveille R, Van Stiegmann G, Everson GT: Increased secondary bile acids in a choledochal cyst: Possible role in biliary metaplasia and carcinoma. Gastroenterology 1990; 99:525–527.
264. Todani T, Watanabe Y, Toki A, et al: Carcinoma related to choledochal cysts with internal drainage procedures. Surg Gynecol Obstet 1987; 164:61–64.
265. Parvey H, Eisenberg R, Wolfson J, et al: Complementary use of Doppler sonography and delayed right lateral scintigraphy for the diagnosis of choledochal cysts. S Med J 1990; 83:970–972.
266. Hurst R, MacGregor R, Brookemon V, et al: Choledochal cyst: Diagnosis in neonates. S Med J 1988; 81:1566–1568.
267. Thatcher B, Sivak M, Hermann R, et al: ERCP in evaluation and diagnosis of choledochal cyst: Report of 5 cases. Gastrointest Endosc 1986; 32:27–31.
268. Tsadardkas E, Robnett A: Congenital cystic dilatation of the common bile duct: Report of 3 cases, analysis of 57 cases and review of the literature. Arch Surg 1956; 72:311–327.
269. Stephenson B, Rees B: Choledochal cysts: Their management revisited. Br J Clin Pract 1990; 44:477–481.
270. Joseph V: Surgical techniques and long term results in the treatment of choledochal cyst. J Pediatr Surg 1990; 25:782–787.
271. Takiff H, Stone M, Fonkalsrud E: Choledochal cysts: Results of primary surgery and need for reoperation in young patients. Am J Surg 1985; 150:141–146.
272. Caudle S, Dimler M: The current management of choledochal cyst. Am J Surg 1986; 52:76–80.
273. Hershlag A, Lernan O, Bar Maor J, et al: Choledochal cyst: Review and report of four patients. Curr Surg 1984; 41:168–175.
274. Oweida S, Ricketts R: Hepatico-jejunoduodenostomy reconstruction following excision of choledochal cysts in children. Am Surg 1989; 55:2–6.
275. Karrer F, Hall R, Stewart B, et al: Congenital biliary tract disease. Surg Clin N Am 1990; 70:1403–1418.
276. Ghazi A, Slone E: Endoscopic management of choledochocele: A case report and review of the English literature. Surg Endosc 1987; 1:151–154.
277. O'Neill J, Templeton J, Schaufer L, et al: Recent experience with choledochal cyst. Ann Surg 1987; 205:533–540.
278. Sarris G, Tsang D: Choledochocele: Case report, literature review and proposed classification. Surgery 1989; 105:408–414.
279. Caroli J, Couinaud C: Une affection nouvelle, sans doubt congenitale, des voies biliaires. La dilatation kystique unilobaire des canaux hepatiques. Sem Hop Paris 1958; 14:496–502.
280. Caroli J: Diseases of the intrahepatic biliary tree. Clin Gastroenterol 1973; 2:147–161.
281. McSween RN, Anthony PP, Scheuer PJ, eds: Pathology of the Liver. New York, Churchill-Livingstone, 1987, p 179.
282. Mall J, Ghahremani G, Boyer J: Caroli's disease associated with congenital hepatic fibrosis and renal tubular ectasia. Gastroenterology 1974; 46:1029–1035.
283. Mercadier M, Chigot J, Clot J: Caroli's disease. WJ Surg 1984; 8:22–29.
284. Chen K: Adenocarcinoma of the liver: Association with congenital hepatic fibrosis and Caroli's disease. Arch Path Lab Med 1981; 105:294–295.
285. Bloutstein P: Association of carcinoma with congenital cystic diseases of the liver and bile ducts. Am J Gastroenterol 1977; 67:40–46.
286. Alagille D, Estrada M, Hadchouel M, et al: Syndromatic paucity of interlobular bile ducts (Alagille syndrome or arteriohepatic dysplasia): Review of 80 cases. J Pediatr 1987; 110:195–200.
287. Watson GH, Miller V: Arteriohepatic dysplasia: Familial pulmonary arterial stenosis with neonatal liver disease. Arch Dis Child 1973; 48:459–466.
288. Alagille D, Odievre M, Gautier M, et al: Hepatic ductular hypoplasia associated with characteristic facies, vertebral malformations, retarded physical, mental and sexual development and cardiac murmur. J Pediatr 1975; 86:63–71.
289. Zhang F, Deleuze J, Aurias A, et al: Interstitial deletion of the short arm of chromosome 20 in arteriohepatic dysplasia. J Pediatr 1990; 116:73–77.
289a. Desmaze C, Deleuze JF, Dutrillaux AM, et al: Screening of microdeletions of chromosome 20 in patients with Alagille syndrome. J Med Genet 1992; 29:233–235.
290. Poh-Fitzpatrick M, Zaider E, Sciales C, et al: Cutaneous photosensitivity and coproporphyrin abnormalities in the Alagille syndrome. Gastroenterology 1990; 99:831–835.
291. Okuno T, Takahashi H, Shibahara Y, et al: Temporal bone histopathologic findings in Alagille syndrome. Arch Otolaryngol Head Neck Surg 1990; 116:217–220.
292. Luxenberg M: Ocular findings in arteriohepatic dysplasia (Alagille's syndrome). Arch Ophthalmol 1989; 107:1077.
293. Hyams JS, Berman MM, Davis BH: Tubulointerstitial nephropathy associated with arteriohepatic dysplasia. Gastroenterology 1983; 85:430–434.
294. Dahms B, Petrelli M, Wyllie R: Arteriohepatic dysplasia in infancy and childhood: A longitudinal study of six patients. Hepatology 1982; 2:350–358.
295. Kahn E, Daum F, Markowitz J, et al: Non-syndromatic paucity of interlobular bile ducts: Light and electron microscopic evaluation of sequential liver biopsies in early childhood. Hepatology 1986; 6:890–901.

296. Kahn E, Daum F, Markowitz J, et al: Arteriohepatic dysplasia: Hepatobiliary morphology. Hepatology 1983; 3:77–83.
297. Hadchouel M, Gautier M: Histopathologic study of the liver in the early cholestatic phase of alpha–1-antitrypsin deficiency. J Pediatr 1976; 89:211–215.
298. Stern H, Tucker S: Cytomegalovirus infection in the newborn and early childhood: Three atypical cases. Lancet 1965; 2:1268–1271.
299. Puri P, Guiney E: Intrahepatic biliary atresia in Down's syndrome. J Pediatr Surg 1975; 10:423–424.
300. Sherlock S: The syndrome of disappearing intrahepatic bile ducts. Lancet 1987; 2:493–496.
301. Lee JG, Wherry DC: Traumatic rupture of the extrahepatic biliary ducts from external trauma. J Trauma 1961; 71:105–114.
302. Dolgin SE, Levine RL, Norton KI: Complete spontaneous disruption of the common bile duct: A late complication of necrotizing enterocolitis? J Pediatr Gastroenterol Nutr 1991; 12:379–382.
303. Lilly JR, Weintraub WH, Altman RP: Spontaneous perforation of the extrahepatic bile ducts and bile peritonitis in infancy. Surgery 1974; 75:664–671.
304. Haller JO, Condon VR, Berdan WE, et al: Spontaneous perforation of the common bile duct in children. Radiology 1989; 172:621–624.
305. Saltzman DA, Snyder CL, Leonard A: Spontaneous perforation of the extrahepatic biliary tree in infancy. Clin Pediatr 1990; 29:322–324.
306. Hammoudi SM, Alauddin A: Idiopathic perforation of the biliary tract in infancy and childhood. J Pediatr Surg 1988; 23:185–187.
307. Johnston JH: Spontaneous perforation of the common bile duct in infancy. Br J Surg 1961; 48:532–533.
308. Bennion RS, Thompson JE, Tompkins RK: Agenesis of the gallbladder without extrahepatic biliary atresia. Arch Surg 1988; 123:1257–1260.
309. Jackson RJ, McClellan D: Agenesis of the gallbladder: A cause of false positive ultrasonography. Am Surg 1989; 55:36–40.
310. O'Sullivan J, O'Brien PA, McFeely L, et al: Congenital absence of the gallbladder and cystic duct: Nonoperative diagnosis. Am J Gastroenterol 1987; 82:1190–1192.
311. Nadeau LA, Cloutier WA, Konecki JT, et al: Hereditary gallbladder agenesis: Twelve cases in the same family. J Maine Med Assoc 1972; 63:1–4.
312. Wilson JE, Dietrick JE: Agenesis of the gallbladder: Case report and familial investigation. Surgery 1986; 99:106–109.
313. Herrera-Ornelas L, Petrelli N, Mittelman A: Agenesis of the gallbladder. Surgery 1987; 101:770.
314. Markle GB: Agenesis of the common bile duct. Arch Surg 1981; 116:350–352.
315. Goor DA, Ebert PA: Anomalies of the biliary tree. Arch Surg 1972; 104:302–309.
316. Stokes TL, Old L: Cholecystohepatic duct. Am J Surg 1978; 135:703–705.
317. Kihne MJ, Schenken JR, Moor BJ, et al: Persistent cholecystohepatic ducts. Arch Surg 1980; 115:972–974.
318. Chapoy PR, Kendall RS, Fonkalsrud E, et al: Congenital stricture of the common hepatic duct: An unusual case without jaundice. Gastroenterology 1981; 80:380–383.
319. Neuhauser EB, Elkin M, Landing BH: Congenital direct communication between biliary system and respiratory tract. Am J Dis Child 1959; 83:654.
320. Weitzmann JJ, Cohen SR, Woods LO, et al: Congenital bronchobiliary fistula. J Pediatr 1968; 73:329–334.
321. Adam R, Fabiani B, Bismuth H: Hematobilia resulting from heterotopic stomach in the gallbladder neck. Surgery 1989; 105:564–569.
322. Lindner HH, Pena VA, Ruggeri VA: A clinical and anatomical study of anomalous terminations of the common bile duct into the duodenum. Ann Surg 1976; 184:626–632.

Chapter 72

Cholelithiasis and Cholecystitis

MARK A. GILGER

It is commonly perceived that gallbladder disease in children occurs infrequently and invariably is associated with underlying hemolytic disease, but neither of these perceptions is true. Although hemolytic disease predisposes children to gallstones, there is an increasing likelihood of finding other associated conditions such as total parenteral nutrition (TPN), prematurity, necrotizing enterocolitis, and cystic fibrosis. The advent of ultrasonography in the late 1970s has made the diagnosis of gallbladder disease simple and noninvasive, but perhaps more important, ultrasonography is a sensitive method for the diagnosis of stones. As a result, "incidental" or "silent" gallstones are now being detected more often in children. It is imperative to understand the pathogenesis and natural history of stones in infants and children to approach the treatment of pediatric gallbladder disease in a rational manner.

EPIDEMIOLOGY OF GALLSTONE DISEASE

Approximately 20 million adults in the United States have gallstones, and approximately 300,000 cholecystectomies are performed yearly.[1] Predominantly a disease of adulthood, gallstone disease ranges in prevalence from 4 to 11% in Western societies, with wide variations along racial and ethnic lines.[2–8] Incidence in adults is approximately 1 to 3%.[9] The incidence of gallstone disease is influenced by age, sex, culture, ethnicity, and a variety of medical factors,[6, 10–14] and it varies geographically. For instance, members of the Masai tribe of East Africa, whose bile is only half saturated with cholesterol, do not develop gallstones, whereas the Pima Indians of Arizona have an 80% prevalence.[5, 15]

The earliest reported case of cholelithiasis in a child was by Gibson in 1737.[16] On autopsy, multiple spongy, yellow gallstones were found in a 12-year-old boy, approximately 8 months after abdominal trauma. In a 1924 review of 888 cases of gallbladder disease, only 11 cases of biliary tract disease in patients younger than 20 years of age were reported.[17] Attempts to estimate the frequency of childhood gallstones included an extensive review of 5,037 cases in 1959, in which a prevalence of 0.15% in children younger than 16 years of age was noted.[18] During the early 1960s, fewer than 500 cases of gallbladder disease in children had been reported, giving rise to the concept that this is a rare disease in children.[19–24] The prevalence of gallbladder disease in children since the 1960s appears to be increasing.[25–30] In a study of 1,803 cholecystectomies performed from 1970 to 1974, an incidence of 4.3% in patients younger than 20 years of age, and 0.72% in children younger than 15 years of age was reported.[25] In a review of 708 infants referred for cholestasis between 1970 and 1981, an incidence of 1.4% was found.[30] Other reports have noted that 4% of all cholecystectomies are performed in patients younger than 20 years of age.[31, 32] Unfortunately, no detailed estimates of the incidence and prevalence of gallstone disease exist for children.

In a review of 693 cases of childhood gallstones reported since 1968, early infancy and adolescence were the commonest ages for diagnosis.[33] Infants younger than 6 months of age represented 10% of all cases in which the age was known. Children from 6 months to 10 years of age accounted for 21%, and adolescents (mostly female) 11 to 21 years of age represented 69% of all cases.[33] Most gallstones in children have an underlying predisposing condition, such as hemolytic disease, pregnancy, and TPN. Gallstones of infancy are typically found in "ill" infants receiving TPN. Stones found in children from the ages of 1 to 5 years are usually secondary to hemolysis, and stones found in adolescents are most likely associated with menarche, pregnancy, and the use of oral contraceptives.[33]

PATHOPHYSIOLOGY OF GALLSTONE DISEASE

Bile is composed of five major components: water, bilirubin, cholesterol, bile pigments, and phospholipids. Lecithin is the primary phospholipid. Calcium salts and some proteins are minor components of bile. Stone formation occurs owing to the precipitation of the insoluble constituents of bile, which are cholesterol, bile pigments, and calcium salts. Gallstones are classically divided into either cholesterol stones or pigment stones

Table 72–1. CHARACTERISTICS OF GALLSTONES IN CHILDREN

Characteristics	Cholesterol Stones	Pigment Stones: *Black*	Pigment Stones: *Brown*
Color	Yellow-white (often with dark core)	Black to brown	Brown to orange
Consistency	Hard Crystalline Layered	Hard, shiny Crystalline	Soft, greasy 50% amorphous; rest crystalline, inorganic salts Layered
Number and morphology	Multiple: 2—25 mm faceted, smooth Solitary: 2–4 cm (~10%) round, smooth	Multiple: <5 mm Irregular or smooth	Multiple: 10–30 mm Round, smooth
Composition	Cholesterol monohydrate >50% Glycoprotein Calcium salts	Bile pigment polymer ~40% Calcium carbonate or phosphate salts ~15% Cholesterol ~5% Mucin glycoprotein ~20%	Calcium bilirubinate ~60% Calcium palmitate and stearate soaps ~15% Cholesterol ~15% Mucin glycoprotein ~10%
Radiopaque	No	Yes ~50%	No
Location	Gallbladder ± common bile duct	Gallbladder	Common bile duct, intrahepatic ducts
Clinical associations	Hyperlipidemia Obesity Clofibrate Pregnancy Birth control pills Cystic fibrosis	Hemolytic anemia Cirrhosis TPN Ileal disease Ceftriaxone	Bacterial infection *(Escherichia coli)* Parasitic infection Bile duct anomaly
Recurrent	Yes	No	Yes
Sex	Female > Male	No difference	No difference
Age	Pubertal; increases with age	Any; increases with age	Any; increases with age
Bacteria	No	No	Yes (consistently found at core)
Soluble	Yes	No	No (minimally)

Data from references 30, 62, and 78–80.

(Table 72–1). Chemically pure gallstones are rare, and in any single stone the composition varies from the core to the crust. Most cholesterol stones contain calcium salts at their centers and often in some of the lamellae, as seen on cross-section (Fig. 72–1). The central nidus of calcium salts may imply a role in facilitating stone formation.[34] Most stones are "mixed" in composition, and the formation patterns of both cholesterol and pigment stones share many characteristics.

Cholesterol, the major sterol in bile, is nearly insoluble in water. It is made soluble in aqueous bile by aggregation with bile salts or lecithin. Bile salt monomers form first, until the critical micellar concentration is reached, and micelles begin to form.[35–38] Simple micelles (bile salts plus cholesterol) and mixed micelles (bile salt–lecithin-cholesterol aggregates) are thermodynamically stable. Vesicles or spherical unilamellar particles composed of a bilayer of lecithin and cholesterol with minimal bile salts form next. These vesicles are only partially stable or metastable and can fuse, forming biliary liquid crystals or liposomes (Figs. 72–2 and 72–3). As seen in Figure 72–3, micelles and vesicles coexist and undergo spontaneous interconversion.[39–41] This constant interplay of biliary aggregates maintains cholesterol solubility. When cholesterol is no longer soluble in any form, cholesterol monohydrate crystals precipitate from solution, a process known as *nucleation*.[42]

The interplay among the major bile components cholesterol, lecithin, and bile salts is depicted in an updated version of the classic triangular phase diagram shown in Figure 72–4. Each axis shows the molar percentages of cholesterol, lecithin, and bile salts. When the composition of bile lies in the micellar zone, the bile can solubilize additional cholesterol. As the cholesterol concentration continues to increase, the likelihood of cholesterol crystallization, and hence gallstone formation, increases. Clearly, a decrease in bile salt concentration or lecithin also predisposes to gallstones.

There appear to be three primary conditions that must be met to permit the formation of cholesterol gall-

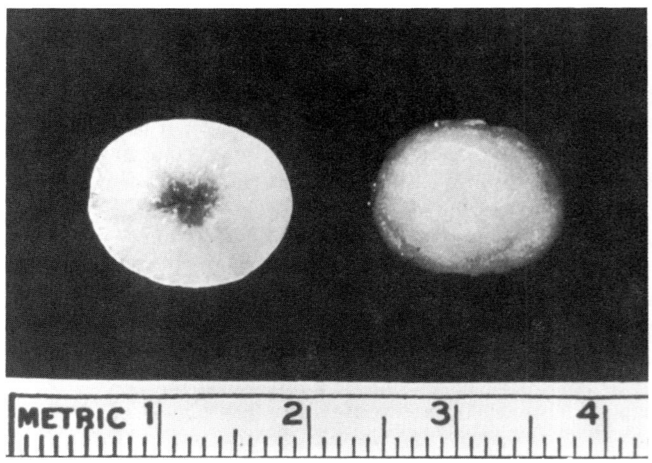

Figure 72–1. Typical cholesterol gallstone with pigmented core. (Courtesy of Dr. Milton J. Finegold.)

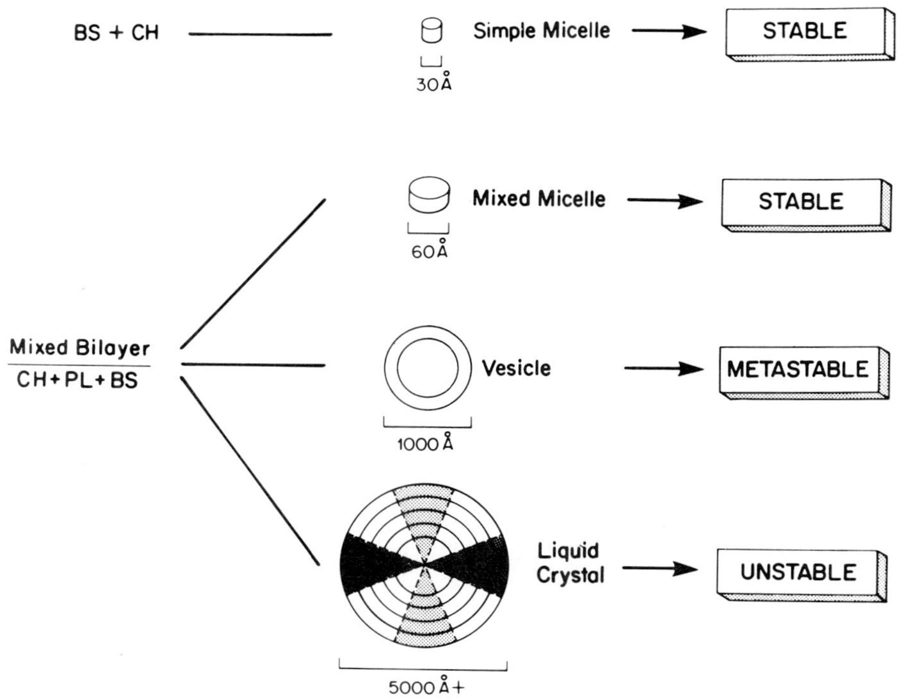

Figure 72–2. Schematic representation of the lipid aggregates in human bile. Bile salt monomers (not illustrated) solubilize a minute fraction of the cholesterol in bile. Simple micelles are small aggregates of bile salts and cholesterol whose structure has not been precisely defined. The other lipid aggregates probably have a cholesterol-bile salt-lecithin bilayer as their fundamental unit. In mixed micelles the bulky hydrophobic part of cholesterol is solubilized in the hydrocarbon matrix of the particles, whereas bile salt molecules are on the perimeter maintaining water solubility. Mixed micelles are thermodynamically stable. Vesicles are metastable spherical particles with a single lipid bilayer composed largely of cholesterol and lecithin molecules with only traces of bile salts. Liquid crystals are unstable particles composed of multiple concentric lipid bilayers that are believed to arise from the fusion of vesicles. These aggregates are birefringent and visible by polarized light microscopy and are therefore depicted schematically as Maltese crosses. CH, cholesterol; BS, bile salt; PL, phospholipid. (Modified from Carey MC, Cohen DE: Biliary transport of cholesterol in micelles and liquid crystals. *In* Paumgartner G, Stiehl A, Gerak W, eds: Bile Acids and the Liver. Lancaster, MTP Press, 1987, pp 287–300; with permission.)

stones.[43] First, the bile must be supersaturated with cholesterol, which then acts as the driving force behind crystal precipitation. Second, bile kinetics must be such as to allow nucleation, the transition to solid cholesterol crystals. Finally, gallbladder stasis must exist to allow agglomeration of cholesterol crystals into stones.[44] Two secondary conditions also appear to be critical in lithogenesis: gallbladder hypersecretion of mucus and excess arachidonyl lecithin (Fig. 72–5).[45–47]

Cholesterol supersaturation can result from the following conditions:

1. An increased delivery of cholesterol to the liver via increased lipoprotein (low-density lipoprotein and chylomicrons). This occurs in women secondary to estrogen or oral contraceptive use or to increased dietary cholesterol intake.[45, 48, 49]

2. An increased endogenous cholesterol synthesis secondary to 3-hydroxy-3-methylglutaryl coenzyme A (HMG-CoA) reductase activity. Obesity and hypertriglyceridemia are causes of increased HMG-CoA reductase activity.[50, 51]

3. A decrease in 7-alpha-hydroxylase activity, thus decreasing the conversion of cholesterol to bile acids.[52] This defect occurs most commonly with increasing age.

4. A decrease in the conversion of cholesterol to cholesterol esters from inhibited acyl-CoA cholesterol acyltransferase activity (ACAT).[45] Progesterone, either pregnancy induced or exogenous, and clofibrate are examples of ACAT inhibitors.

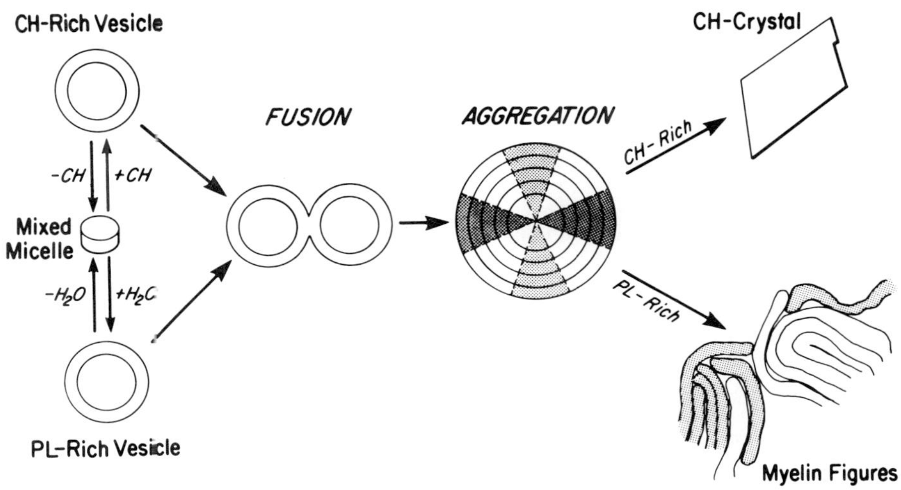

Figure 72–3. Interconversions and fate of biliary micelles and vesicles. Vesicles are formed when excess cholesterol or water is added to micellar solutions. The fusion of cholesterol-rich vesicles to form unstable liquid crystals ultimately leads to the formation of cholesterol monohydrate crystals. Liquid crystals rich in lecithin form tubelike lecithin bilayers called myelin figures. (Modified from Carey MC, Cohen DE: Biliary transport of cholesterol in micelles and liquid crystals. *In* Paumgartner G, Stiehl A, Gerak W, eds: Bile Acids and the Liver. Lancaster, MTP Press, 1987, pp 287–300; with permission.)

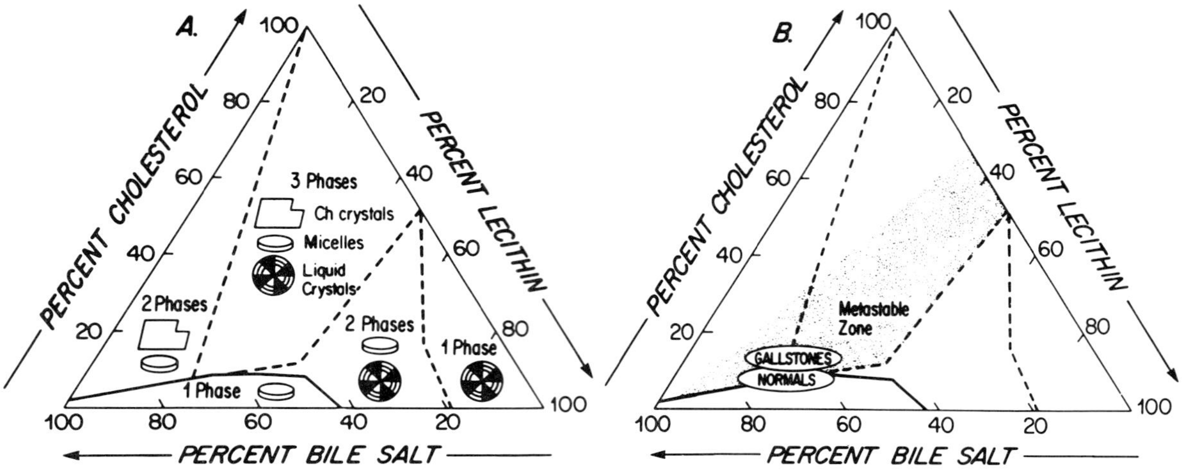

Figure 72–4. *A,* Triangular phase diagram showing phases present at equilibrium in biles of differing compositions. In the micellar zone (the area in the lower left of the triangle), all the cholesterol is held in solution as micelles. Biles with a composition outside the micellar zone, if allowed to come to equilibrium, would form liquid and/or solid cholesterol crystals (as depicted schematically in each of the zones). The micellar zone is larger for gallbladder bile (a 10% lipid solution shown here) than for hepatic bile (a 3% lipid solution not shown). *B,* Triangular phase diagram with schematic representations of ranges of lipid compositions found in gallbladder biles of normals and gallstone patients. Bile with a composition that falls in the metastable zone takes a prolonged time to come to equilibrium and thus appears to be stable. Excess cholesterol is "carried" in the metastable zone by cholesterol-rich unilamellar vesicles. The boundaries of the physiologically relevant metastable zone are approximate.[42a] (From Carey MC, Cohen DE: Biliary transport of cholesterol in micelles and liquid crystals. *In* Paumgartner G, Stiehl A, Gerak W, eds: Bile Acids and the Liver. Lancaster, MTP Press, 1987, pp 287–300; with permission.)

The potential defects leading to cholesterol supersaturation are thus numerous and overlapping.

Nucleation is not as well understood as cholesterol supersaturation. Nucleation times are strikingly different between gallstone patients and control subjects. In the bile of gallstone patients, nucleation occurs within 2 to 3 days, whereas bile from normal control subjects takes 1 to 2 weeks to nucleate or, often, it does not nucleate at all.[42] Gallbladder hypomotility seems to be involved in the crystallization process, since agitation prevents aggregation. Gallbladder stasis was proposed as the cause of gallstones as early as 1856.[53] Animal studies support hypomotility as an important causative factor.[54–57] Technetium-99m-dimethyl iminodiacetic acid gallbladder emptying studies in adult gallstone patients have documented diminished gallbladder emptying after meals.[58, 59]

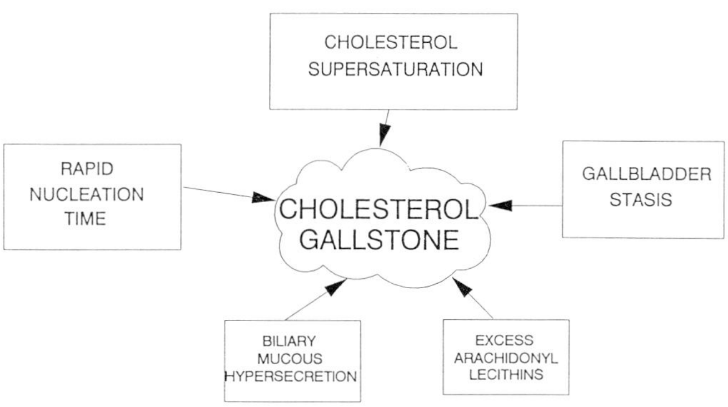

Figure 72–5. Current understanding of cholesterol gallstone formation. Cholesterol supersaturation is an essential prerequisite, which combined with a more rapid nucleation time and gallbladder stasis allows crystal formation. Excess biliary mucous provides a structural nidus for crystal growth, driven by increased dietary arachidonyl lecithins. (Adapted from Hay DW, Carey MC: Pathophysiology and pathogenesis of cholesterol gallstone formation. Semin Liver Dis 1990; 10:159–170; with permission.)

Biliary sludge, a collection of mucus, calcium bilirubinate, and cholesterol crystals, appears to precede the formation of gallstones in animal models.[42, 60] Mucin hypersecretion appears to be a primary event in sludge formation, and evidence suggests that prostanoids, such as arachidonyl lecithin, mediate the hypersecretion.[45–47] Mucin may serve as the nidus for nucleation and subsequent sludge formation owing to its hydrophobic domain, which binds phospholipid and cholesterol.[61]

Figure 72–5 summarizes the current understanding of the formation of cholesterol gallstones and, perhaps, of any gallstone. The process must have a supersaturated solution (either cholesterol or bilirubin pigment); a "still" environment, or gallbladder stasis; and crystal agglomeration or nucleation. The initial nucleating event creates the core of the stone, from which a self-perpetuating process ensues.

CHOLESTEROL STONES

Cholesterol gallstones are yellowish white in appearance, hard, crystalline, and layered (Fig. 72–6; see also Fig. 72–1).[62] They frequently have a brownish core, with a variety of substances found there, including calcium salts. "Rings" of protein (glycoproteins) and calcium salts (calcium bilirubinate, calcium hydroxyapatite, and calcium carbonate) form around the core, resulting in the layered appearance.[62] The cholesterol content is higher than 50%, with minimal calcium salt content. This composition is not radiopaque; thus, the stones are rarely seen on plain film radiographs. Cholesterol stones form within the gallbladder and are frequently multiple, ranging in size from approximately 2 to 25 mm in diameter.[62] The presence of cholesterol stones in the biliary tree is the result of migration. Cholesterol gallstones account for approximately 70% of all stones found in Western populations. The prevalence of cholesterol gallstones in children is unknown, but increases slowly with age in both sexes.[63] Pubertal changes, in particular early menarche, cause a dramatic increase in the incidence of cholesterol gallstones.[63, 64] This phenomenon has been attributed to the effect of estrogen and progesterone surges that occur during puberty; it has also been seen in pregnancy and with the use of oral contraceptives. Sex hormones appear to induce biliary stasis and cause cholesterol hypersecretion by the liver.[65–67] It remains unclear whether estrogen, the progestins, or a combination of both, are responsible, although estriol has been shown to produce lithogenic bile in rhesus monkeys.[68] There clearly is a genetic influence, with extraordinarily high prevalence rates seen in both children and adult Native Americans. Studies of the Pimas of Arizona have demonstrated the development of lithogenic bile containing excess cholesterol during adolescence.[64] Obesity has been shown to increase the likelihood of cholesterol gallstone formation, apparently from excessive hepatic cholesterol secretion secondary to increased cholesterol synthesis.[69]

Gallstones and gallbladder and biliary tract abnormalities are frequently found in patients with cystic fibrosis, and they increase with age.[70] "Microgallbladders" have been identified in as many as 16% of adult cystic fibrosis patients radiologically and in 30% of patients at autopsy.[71] Common bile duct stenosis has been identified in 96% of cystic fibrosis patients with liver disease, resulting in enlarged gallbladders and elevated serum bile acid levels, which may predispose to gallstone formation.[72] In cystic fibrosis patients, gallstones are found more frequently with increasing age, with an incidence of 6 to 12% in patients 12 years and older and 24% in adult autopsy studies.[70, 73] The abdominal pain associated with gallstones is frequently attributed to other causes, such as the distal ileal obstruction syndrome, thus illustrating the need for close inspection of the biliary tree in cystic fibrosis patients with abdominal pain. Gallstones in cystic fibrosis patients appear secondary to excessive bile acid loss resulting in a reduced bile acid pool. The bile composition becomes abnormal, with a relative excess of cholesterol associated with the decrease in bile salts, thus making the bile lithogenic.[74] The bile acid malabsorption and reduced bile salt pool respond to pancreatic enzyme therapy. Gallstones have not been found without pancreatic insufficiency.[75, 76] Recent attempts to identify gallbladder hypomotility in patients with cystic fibrosis have proven unsuccessful (see Chapter 66).[77]

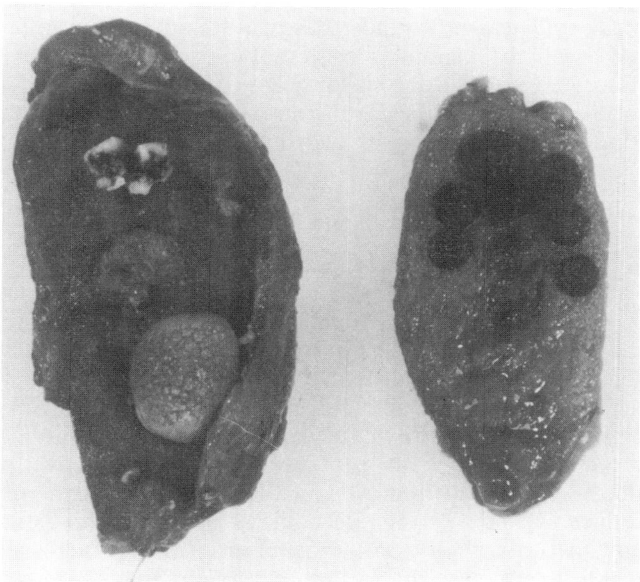

Figure 72–6. Two resected gallbladders contrasting multiple, large, pale cholesterol gallstones *(left)* and smaller black pigment gallstones *(right)*. (Courtesy of Dr. Milton J. Finegold.)

PIGMENT STONES

Pigment stones account for a much higher percentage of stones in prepubertal children, whereas cholesterol stones are predominant in adolescence and adulthood. Two types of pigment gallstones are found in children and are referred to as *black* and *brown*. In both black and brown stones, the pigment present is calcium bilirubinate, which interacts with mucin glycoproteins to form stones (see Table 72–1).[78, 79]

Black pigment stones are black to dark brown in color, small (usually <5 mm), occur multiply, and are typically hard, shiny, and crystalline (see Fig. 72–6).[80] They are composed primarily of highly cross-linked polymers of bilirubin with mucin glycoproteins and calcium salts of phosphate and carbonate.[81, 82] The high concentration of calcium salts (as compared with brown and cholesterol stones) accounts for the 50 to 75% radiopacity seen on plain radiographs. Black stones typically form within the gallbladder and do not recur after resection. They are usually associated with hemolytic diseases, of which sickle cell disease and hereditary spherocytosis are the most common. The duration of the hemolytic disease appears to be a significant risk factor for stone formation. Children younger than 10 years of age with sickle cell disease have a 14% prevalence of stones, whereas children 11 to 20 years of age have a 36% prevalence. Older adults with sickle cell disease have more than a 50% prevalence.[83, 84] Other disease states, such as thalassemia, Wilson's disease, and mechanical shearing of erythrocytes associated with artificial heart valves, have all been associated with black pigment stones.[85] Black pigment stones form within the gallbladder, and their presence in the common bile duct is the result of migration. Black stones are found in sterile bile and are not associated with infection.[86]

The formation of black stones results from altered gallbladder bile homeostasis and supersaturation of the bile. This process could occur by at least three mechanisms: an increase in bilirubin anions, an increase in unbound Ca^2, and a decrease in factors that solubilize bilirubin and calcium.[80] An increase in bilirubin anions has been shown to occur secondary to hemolysis.[80, 87] Increased unbound calcium could occur secondary to increased plasma ionized calcium or to a decrease in calcium-binding agents, such as micellar bile salts and lecithin-cholesterol vesicles.[87] The decrease in the bile salt pool secondary to an interruption of the enterohepatic circulation as seen in ileal resection or the NPO status accompanying TPN could result in this phenomenon.

Brown pigment stones are brown to orange in color, soft, soaplike or greasy in texture, and commonly assume the shape of their origin, the common bile duct.[80] The stone color is derived from calcium bilirubinate, and their greasy texture belies a significant component of fat (calcium palmitate or stearate derived from lecithin).[88, 89] The scarcity of calcium carbonate and phosphate accounts for their lack of opacity on radiography.[78] The cholesterol content ranges from 2 to 28%, which is higher than in black stones and allows in part for their increased solubility. The most distinct clinical feature of brown gallstones in both adults and children is the association with infection.[30, 90] These stones are a major public health problem in rural areas of Asian countries, where they are found secondary to parasitic infestation with such organisms as *Opisthorchis sinensis* and *Ascaris lumbricoides*.[91] They are an uncommon type of stone in Western society and are typically found in the common bile duct after cholecystectomy when the bile is infected. In some 85% of cases, the bile grows *Escherichia coli*.[92] In children, especially infants, these stones can be seen in association with other organisms such as *Staphylococcus, Enterobacter,* and *Citrobacter*.[90] Infection with stasis results in excessive secretion of mucin, which may serve as the glycoprotein nidus for stone formation.[87] Bacteria also release beta-glucuronidase, phospholipase A_1, and conjugated bile salt hydrolase, which hydrolyze bilirubin glucuronides, lecithin, and conjugated bile salts, producing unconjugated bilirubin, free saturated fatty acids, lysolecithin, and free bile acids.[93] With the exception of lysolecithin, these products precipitate with calcium to form stones.[87] Biliary tree abnormalities, such as stenosis, also may predispose to brown stone formation.

TOTAL PARENTERAL NUTRITION–ASSOCIATED STONES

The association between TPN and cholelithiasis is clearly established.[94–97] Gallstone formation in premature infants and neonates receiving TPN appears to have four stages: decreased hepatobiliary flow due to immaturity, stasis within the biliary tree, sludge formation, and finally, stone formation. Cholestasis, which increases with decreasing gestational age, is found in at least 50% of infants with a birth weight less than 1,000 gm.[98] After 2 months on TPN, 80% of infants have cholestasis.[98] This predisposition to cholestasis in infancy is multifactorial. Bile acid transport, bile secretion, and basal and stimulated bile salt flow rates are all immature.[99, 100] Bile salt–dependent and –independent flow are decreased, approximating only 50% of that in adults.[99, 101] The absence of oral feeding reduces the enterohepatic circulation of bile acids.[101] Fasting also inhibits the release of gut and biliary tree hormones, such as cholecystokinin, gastrin, secretin, motilin, and glucagon. In a study of 6-day-old premature infants receiving only TPN, no postnatal increase of these hormones was detected; however, after minimal feedings of human milk, elevations became clearly evident.[102] The formation of echogenic, thick, "molasses-like" biliary sludge within the gallbladder has been documented in both adults and children receiving TPN.[94–96, 103, 104] Serial ultrasound examinations of adults receiving continuous TPN infusion show sludge formation increasing from 6% of patients in the first week to 50% in the fourth week and 100% after 6 weeks.[94] Gallbladder enlargement may be the first physical sign of sludge formation in the infant.[95, 105, 106] Stagnant bile in a dilated gallbladder provides an ideal milieu for the development of both acalculous cholecystitis and cholelithiasis.[106] TPN-induced gallstones are pigment stones, typically black and usually found in the gallbladder. They often have a high calcium phosphate or carbonate content; however, stone analysis indicates that they are of a mixed bilirubin-cholesterol composition and perhaps belong to a special group of TPN-induced pigment stones.[97]

ILEAL DISEASE AND ILEAL RESECTION–ASSOCIATED STONES

The enterohepatic circulation constantly replenishes the bile acid pool, which in turn governs the rate of bile salt secretion. The terminal ileum serves as the site of nearly 98% of bile acid resorption. Terminal ileal disease, typically Crohn's disease, or congenital or surgical resection of the ileum can result in an interruption of this bile acid recycling. The bile salt pool is subsequently reduced, thus altering the balance of bile components and favoring cholesterol supersaturation and increased bile lithogenicity. The formation of gallstones secondary to ileal disease has been reported in both adults and children; although it is difficult to classify these stones as the pigment type, their composition favors this designation.[95, 107, 108]

FUROSEMIDE-ASSOCIATED STONES

The use of furosemide has been associated with an increased tendency to form gallstones. However, in all reported cases, numerous other contributing factors, such as prematurity, sepsis, and small bowel disease, were also noted. Thus, whether furosemide alone contributes to gallstone formation remains unclear.[109, 110]

SYMPTOMS OF GALLSTONE DISEASE

The classic symptom complex of right upper quadrant pain and vomiting is usually associated with stones only in older children and adolescents. Younger children tend to present with nonspecific symptoms. Jaundice is frequently encountered in "symptomatic" infants.[33] The most likely age for silent stones is infancy through the preschool years. Intolerance to fatty food is rarely reported in children. Fever is an unusual finding at any age, and, if present, indicates associated cholecystitis. Complications of gallstone disease include cholecystitis, choledocholithiasis, cholangitis, and gallbladder perforation, but these occur rarely in children.[111] Pancreatitis has been identified in 8% of children with gallstone disease and may represent the most common complication in children.[112]

Laboratory evaluation is usually unrewarding. Occasional patients will have a leukocytosis as well as mildly elevated hepatic transaminase levels. Plain film radiography is more useful in children than in adults, since about 50% of stones in children are radiopaque. Ultrasonography is the diagnostic procedure of choice, because it is noninvasive, sensitive, and quite specific. The ultrasonography also allows examination of the surrounding abdominal viscera, such as the pancreas and the biliary tree. Oral cholecystography has been largely replaced by ultrasound, but can occasionally be useful in the evaluation of gallbladder function. Endoscopic retrograde cholangiopancreatography (ERCP) is particularly useful in the evaluation of ductal stones. Percutaneous cholangiograms offer another approach but are seldom used in children.

TREATMENT OF GALLSTONE DISEASE

Observation may be the most prudent treatment in infants with asymptomatic gallstone disease. As the infant ages, the hepatobiliary enzyme systems mature and the potential for spontaneous stone dissolution exists.[113, 114] Spontaneous stone resolution also has been observed in TPN-induced gallstones. In children for whom the duration of TPN is expected to be limited and the stones are asymptomatic, observation is indicated. However, in children who are chronically dependent on TPN, such as in Crohn's disease, pseudo-obstruction syndrome, and the short bowel syndrome, stones should be removed.

Gallstones in older children should be removed, since spontaneous resolution does not occur. Cholecystectomy remains the procedure of choice in most children with symptomatic gallstone disease. Options to this traditional therapy include cholecystostomy and laparoscopic cholecystectomy. Cholecystostomy is indicated for acute drainage of the gallbladder and perhaps in seriously ill patients for whom only simple stone extraction is needed. Laparoscopic cholecystectomy results in a much smaller abdominal incision(s) and shorter hospitalization and may be performed under epidural anesthesia, thus offering a surgical approach to patients who are at high risk for general anesthesia, such as those with cystic fibrosis.[115]

Options for nonsurgical treatment of gallstone disease continue to proliferate and represent the driving force behind gallstone research. Despite the growing popularity of medical therapy for adults, there is no such approved medical treatment for gallstones in children (Table 72–2). Two bile acids currently exist for oral gallstone dissolution: chenodeoxycholic acid (chenodiol) and ursodeoxycholic acid (ursodiol). Both agents occur naturally and are present in bile. Chenodiol was first reported as effective in stone dissolution more than 20 years ago.[116, 117] The mechanism of action is through the inhibition HMG-CoA reductase, suppressing hepatic cholesterol synthesis.[116, 117] Side effects such as diarrhea and hepatotoxicity have limited its widespread use. Ursodiol has been used in Asian countries for centuries as an aphrodisiac and a digestive aid and is the major bile acid in bears, hence the prefix "urso." The mechanism of action is similar to chenodiol, inhibiting HMG-CoA reductase, and additionally, blocking intestinal absorption of cholesterol.[118] It has no hepatotoxicity and is currently under experimental use in chronic cholestatic diseases for treatment of pruritus and fatigue in both adults and children.[119–121] Diarrhea is rarely encountered. Combination use of both chenodiol and ursodiol appears more effective and allows a 50% reduction in dosage with fewer side effects.[122] Drawbacks to the use of such therapy include the long duration of therapy, recurrence after stopping, low success rate, and high cost. Only cholesterol stones are amenable to this therapy, thereby limiting its use in children.

Extracorporeal shock-wave lithotripsy (ESWL) was first used successfully in humans in 1980 to fragment renal calculi.[123] Application to gallstones followed in 1984, and since then thousands of patients have had successful gallstone fragmentation.[124] ESWL generates high-amplitude pressure waves that are focused on the stone by computerized ultrasonography. Because the stones are fragmented and must be expelled, a functioning gallbladder is essential. New-generation lithotriptors do not usually require the use of anesthesia or analgesia. Only symptomatic stones that are radiolucent can be treated with this method, again limiting its use in children. Best results are obtained with solitary stones, with success rates of 95 to 100% reported.[125] Oral dissolution therapy appears to be a rational addition to lithotripsy to achieve complete stone dissolution.[126] The two major complications of lithotripsy are cholecystitis and pancreatitis, reported in 1 to 2% of patients.[125, 126] Successful treatment of gallstones in children has been accomplished, although documentation is available only in anecdotal reports.

Table 72–2. TREATMENT ALTERNATIVES FOR GALLSTONES IN CHILDREN

Type	Comments	Approved in Children
Cholecystectomy	Method of choice in most cases	Yes
Cholecystostomy	Effective for acute gallbladder drainage (i.e., acalculous cholecystitis)	Yes
Laparoscopic cholecystectomy	Effective with severely ill patients, shortens hospitalization (i.e., cystic fibrosis)	Yes
ERCP		
Basket removal	Bile duct stone removal	Yes
Mechanical basket lithotripsy	Stone crushing within bile ducts (experimental)	No
Laser lithotripsy	Stone destruction within bile ducts (experimental)	No
ESWL	Limited experience (unpublished) only for cholesterol stones currently	No
Dissolution		
Oral	Ursodeoxycholic acid and chenodeoxycholic acid	No
	Block HMG-CoA, decreases cholesterol synthesis	
Contact	Methyl *tert*-butyl-ether (for cholesterol stones only)	No
	Bile acid EDTA (for pigment stones; experimental)	No
Preventive		
Enteral feeds	Even small amounts during TPN decrease stone risk	Yes
Weight loss	For obesity	Yes
Lovastatin and simvastatin	Block HMG-CoA reductase, decrease cholesterol synthesis (experimental)	No
Cholecystokinin	Stimulates gallbladder contraction while NPO (experimental)	No

EDTA, ethylene diaminetetraacetic acid.

Cholesterol gallstones can be dissolved in vitro within minutes to hours using methyl *tert*-butyl ether (MTBE).[127] MTBE is typically used as an octane enhancer in gasoline and a chromatography solvent in the laboratory; initial experimental results indicate that it can be used safely in humans.[128] The procedure first requires placement of a percutaneous transhepatic catheter into a contrast-enhanced gallbladder. MTBE is infused and aspirated over a 4- to 6-hour period, or until the stone is no longer visible fluoroscopically. A greater than 95% success rate in stone dissolution has been reported.[129] Complications include leakage of the MTBE, causing nausea, vomiting, and duodenitis, and intravascular hemolysis if the MTBE enters the vascular system.[129] Chemical dissolution of calcified cholesterol stones and brown pigment stones has been tried experimentally with bile acid ethylenediaminetetraacetic acid, but has shown only limited success.

The prevention of gallstones in children entails recognition of risk factors and an understanding of the pathophysiology of stone disease. The use of limited enteral feedings during TPN therapy, for example, stimulates gallbladder contraction, thus decreasing gallbladder stasis. Early use of pancreatic enzyme supplements in patients with cystic fibrosis decreases the propensity to stone formation. Informed use of contraceptives other than birth control pills, particularly in women with known gallstone risk factors, would seem advisable. Weight control in obese patients is advisable to decrease the risk of gallstone disease. Medical therapy with cholesterol-lowering agents, such as lovastatin and simvastatin, may be considered in high-risk patients, although no data exist for the use of this therapy in children (see Table 72–2).

CHOLECYSTITIS

Cholecystitis is a disease that results from inflammation of the gallbladder, typically secondary to gallstone obstruction of the cystic duct. Cholecystitis may be acute or chronic. Most cholecystitis in children is chronic and is associated with gallstones in 66% of cases.[130] The presentation of "acute" cholecystitis in children most likely represents a significant episode of an ongoing process of gallbladder distention and mucosal damage that culminated in cholecystitis.

The pathophysiology of cholecystitis parallels that of gallstone formation, with gallbladder stasis as the initiating event. The stasis is usually secondary to obstruction of the cystic duct by a gallstone or to local edema secondary to a stone. Other causes include external compression of the cystic duct by swollen lymph nodes, torsion of the gallbladder, congenital ductal abnormalities, and trauma. The basis for the inflammation is unclear, although mechanical distention, ischemia, bacteria, and lysolecithins have been implicated.[130] Experimental evidence suggests that phospholipase A, a gallbladder mucosal enzyme, hydrolyses lecithin into lysolecithin.[131] Lysolecithin stimulates local prostaglandin synthesis (prostaglandin E_2), disrupting the gallbladder mucosa and stimulating mucous production.[132, 133] Increased mucus causes gallbladder distention and cystic duct obstruction, triggering a cycle of mechanical and chemical events terminating in inflammation.

The typical presenting symptom is right upper quadrant abdominal pain, occasionally radiating to the back and associated with vomiting. When distended and inflamed, the gallbladder lies on the anterior abdominal wall between the ninth and tenth costal cartilages, causing localized tenderness on palpation and giving rise to the diagnostic Murphy's sign.[1] Jaundice and fever are seen in 25 to 30% of children and are more common in young infants. The onset of symptoms is usually over a period of 1 week, but lesser symptoms of biliary colic may occur over several years. The differential diagnosis should include hepatitis, hepatic abscess, tumor, gonococcal perihepatitis (Fitz-Hugh–Curtis syndrome), pancreatitis, appendicitis, peptic ulcer disease, pneumonia, pyelonephritis, and kidney stones.

Laboratory evaluation should include a complete blood count and differential; serum bilirubin, alkaline phosphatase or gamma-glutamyltransferase, serum aminotransferases, amylase levels; and urinalysis. Leukocytosis is frequently found. Elevated aminotransferase levels and mild hyperbilirubinemia are seen in 20% of patients. Elevated amylase levels are common even without pancreatitis. Marked elevation of the bilirubin, alkaline phosphatase, or gamma-glutamyltransferase levels may indicate stones in the biliary tree. The characteristic ultrasound finding is a discrete echo density indicating a stone, usually occupying a dependent position in the gallbladder, which changes or moves when the patient is moved and is associated with acoustic shadowing (Fig. 72–7). Gallbladder dilation, a thickened gallbladder wall, the presence of sludge, and biliary tree anomalies also may be seen (Fig. 72–8). Cholescintigraphy can be helpful to evaluate gallbladder function, revealing normal hepatic uptake but nonvisualization of the gallbladder at 1 hour.[134] False-positive results may occur with prolonged fasting, TPN, and hepatocellular disease. Oral cholecystography is used less frequently owing to several inherent drawbacks, such as failure to concentrate the dye (particularly if hyperbilirubinemia exists), a 6 to 8% false-negative rate, hypersensitivity to the dye, and radiation exposure.

Hospitalization with institution of intravenous fluids, cessation of oral feeding, gastric decompression, and analgesics is appropriate. Antibiotics are not needed in simple cases, but if fever persists or the condition worsens, their use is indicated. Ampicillin, gentamicin, and clindamycin are a common combination used to cover enteric organisms and provide good biliary excretion. Cefoperazone also is a logical choice owing to its excellent biliary excretion and broad spectrum of bacterial sensitivity.

Cholecystectomy is the procedure of choice in calculous cholecystitis. In children with sickle cell disease, hypertransfusion should be performed prior to surgery. Cholecystostomy with stone removal can be done in those patients for whom a functioning gallbladder is important, such as in patients with Crohn's disease or

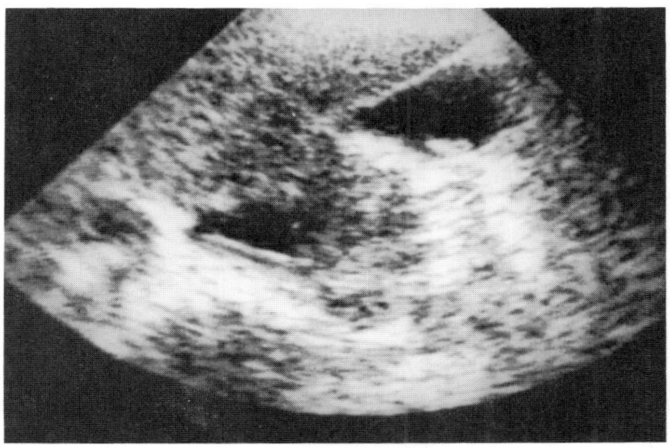

Figure 72–7. Ultrasound of gallstone within the gallbladder showing acoustic shadowing. (Courtesy of Dr. Robert V. Dutton.)

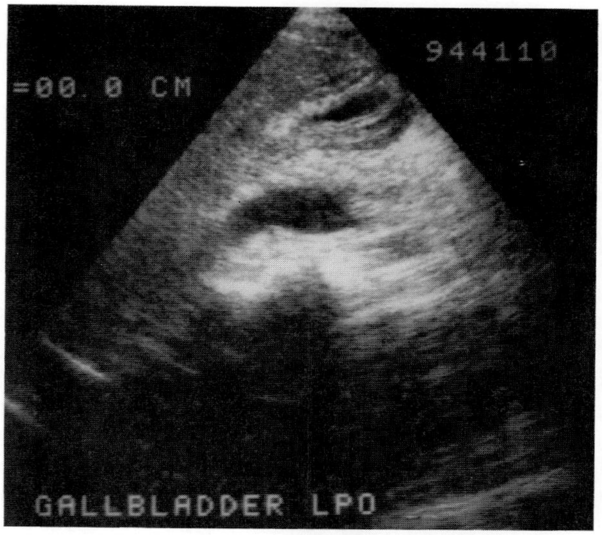

Figure 72–8. Ultrasound of dilated gallbladder with a thickened wall. (Courtesy of Dr. Robert V. Dutton.)

short gut syndrome. Table 72–2 lists the possible treatment options in children.

Most cases of cholecystitis usually resolve over several days. Complications occur in 30% of cases and include gallbladder perforation, abscess, or empyema formation. When fever persists or exceeds 102°F and pain or tenderness worsens, perforation is likely. Such perforations typically occur in the fundus of the gallbladder. A local perforation may wall off as an abscess, extend into the peritoneum as peritonitis, or lead to a cholecystoenteric fistula. Surgical intervention with vigorous antibiotic support is essential.

Chronic obstruction of the cystic duct may lead to the interesting finding of the "milk of calcium" gallbladder or "limy bile" syndrome (Fig. 72–9). In this situation, complete obstruction of the cystic duct leads to a hydropic gallbladder. Bile pigments are deconjugated to colorless compounds, and excess calcium is secreted, opacifying the bile to a white appearance both visually and radiographically.[62] Calcium accumulating in the wall of the gallbladder secondary to chronic cystic duct

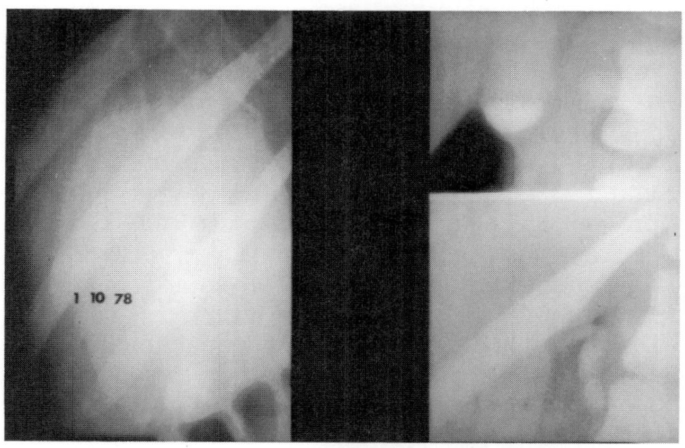

Figure 72–9. Milk of calcium or "limy bile," in a 9-year-old girl. (Courtesy of Dr. Robert V. Dutton.)

obstruction may produce the "porcelain gallbladder." This condition appears secondary to chronic cholecystitis and in adults leads to carcinoma in as many as 50% of cases.

CHOLEDOCHOLITHIASIS (COMMON BILE DUCT STONES)

Common bile duct stones are an unusual occurrence in children. Most ductal stones in children are black pigment stones, although cholesterol stones have been found. Both of these types of stones originate from the gallbladder. Less common are brown pigment stones, which form within the common bile duct secondary to infection.[90] Most ductal stones in children are believed to lodge within the common bile duct because of congenital narrowing or stenosis.[135] The usual clinical presentation of common bile duct stones in children is jaundice, progressing to symptoms similar to those of cholecystitis. Right upper quadrant pain with fever is common.

Laboratory evaluation may reveal leukocytosis, elevated aminotransferase levels, and specific elevations of biliary tract enzymes such as alkaline phosphatase and gamma-glutamyltransferase. If fever is present, blood cultures may be positive. Abdominal ultrasound is indicated to detect the presence of stones or ductal dilation.

The presence of fever requires broad-spectrum antibiotic coverage, as with cholecystitis. A dilated biliary tree with accompanying fever necessitates prompt surgical intervention, with drainage and stone removal. Although its use is still limited in children, ERCP offers an excellent tool for both diagnosis and therapy, including stone removal, dilation of a stenosis, or placement of a stent.[136]

ACALCULOUS CHOLECYSTITIS

Cholecystitis can occur without the presence of gallstones. This condition is rare in adults, but occurs with surprising frequency in pediatrics, usually in extremely ill children in intensive care units. The cause is not known, but is associated with the immediate postoperative state, trauma, or burns.[137–140] Sepsis from a variety of organisms, including *Leptospira*, group B streptococci, *Shigella*, *Salmonella*, and *E. coli,* has been associated with this condition, although no organism has emerged as definitive.[141] Because no obstructing stone is present, gallbladder stasis must play an important role. The stasis may be due to fever, dehydration, prolonged fasting, ileus, or TPN, which are common in the severely ill child.[141]

The clinical findings are usually fever, abdominal pain, and jaundice. Physical examination reveals a palpable abdominal mass, quite tender to touch. Laboratory studies are usually not helpful, but may reveal leukocytosis and elevated bilirubin levels. Diagnosis is aided by ultrasound identification of a large, distended gallbladder with a thickened wall and tenderness during the procedure (the ultrasonographic Murphy's sign). Biliary scintigraphy also is accurate, revealing normal liver uptake, but no visualization of the gallbladder. Unfortunately, false-negative results of both ultrasound and scintigraphy occur in as many as 20% of cases when no stone is seen.[142]

In most instances, the treatment of choice is emergency laparotomy, with either cholecystostomy or cholecystectomy. Since the incidence of gallbladder gangrene is rare in children as compared with adults, simple drainage may be the method of choice. If gangrene is suspected on inspection of the gallbladder at laparotomy, resection is necessary.

ACUTE HYDROPS OF THE GALLBLADDER

Hydrops of the gallbladder is characterized by distention but no inflammation. The distinction between acalculous cholecystitis and hydrops is therefore one of histology. Clinically, the differentiation of these two entities may be difficult. Most cases of acalculous cholecystitis are in severely ill patients, whereas hydrops tends to occur in a more benign setting, frequently involving a systemic vasculitis. The mucocutaneous lymph node syndrome (Kawasaki syndrome) is the commonest cause of gallbladder hydrops.[143, 144] Hydrops also has been associated with other vascular disorders, such as Sjögren's disease and systemic sclerosis, as well as nephrotic syndrome, familial Mediterranean fever, mesenteric adenitis, leptospirosis, and bacterial infection with *Staphylococcus* and *Streptococcus*.[62, 141, 145] The cause is unknown, although local lymph node enlargement around the cystic duct and local vasculitis causing gallbladder ischemia are possibilities.

The clinical presentation is acute right upper quadrant abdominal pain, nausea, and vomiting. Examination reveals upper abdominal tenderness, often with a palpable mass. Diagnosis is aided by ultrasound findings of a distended gallbladder with normal wall thickness and no echo densities. Biochemical studies are usually of little help. Surgical consultation should be obtained in all cases of suspected hydrops, although surgical intervention is *rarely* indicated. Medical management is supportive, with vigilant surgical observation. The development of fever or an increasingly tender abdomen suggests perforation and requires surgery. Most cases show steady resolution over about 2 weeks, with no known long-term sequelae.

UNUSUAL DISEASES OF THE GALLBLADDER

Carcinoma of the gallbladder has been reported in children, but is rare.[146] In adults, gallbladder carcinoma is usually associated with gallstones. Although commoner than carcinoma in children, benign gallbladder tumors also are rare. Adenomatous polyps have been described associated with Peutz-Jeghers syndrome.[147]

Adenomyomatosis, or hyperplastic gallbladder, denotes hyperplasia of the mucous membrane, thickening of the muscularis, and deep diverticular formations known as *Rokitansky-Aschoff sinuses*.[69] Odd deformities of the gallbladder, such as the phrygian cap, fish-hook anomaly, and Hartmann's pouch, are associated with adenomyomatosis of the gallbladder.[1] The cause of the hyperplasia is unknown, although increased intraluminal gallbladder pressure has been implicated. No specific symptoms have ever been attributed to this condition; therefore, no specific therapy is advised.

Cholesterolosis is characterized by accumulation of cholesterol esters in the mucosa and submucosa of the gallbladder. After resection, these areas are visible as yellow spots on a red mucosal background, giving the appearance of a strawberry, thus the term *strawberry gallbladder*. Occasionally, these areas enlarge and become polypoid, leading to cystic duct obstruction. Typically though, no symptoms are directly attributed to this condition, and thus no therapy is indicated. If symptoms do occur, cholecystectomy is indicated.

Metachromatic leukodystrophy or sulfatide lipidosis is an autosomal recessive disorder of sphingolipid metabolism. The biochemical defect in this disorder is the inability to degrade sphingolipid sulfatide or galactose-3 sulfate ceramide. The absence or deficiency of the lysosomal enzyme arylsulfatase A results in the accumulation of sulfatide in both neural and non-neural tissues, in particular the gallbladder. Gallstones have been reported in association with this disorder. The cause may involve gallbladder hypomotility secondary to sulfatide accumulation in the wall of the gallbladder or sulfatide granules serving as "seeds" for gallstone formation.[148]

Ceftriaxone can induce gallbladder concretions. Ceftriaxone is excreted in bile and has the ability to displace bilirubin from albumin-binding sites. Reports in both adults and children have noted biliary echo densities or sludge often causing symptoms of cholecystitis with right upper quadrant pain, nausea, and vomiting.[149, 150] Analysis of the sludge reveals high concentrations of a calcium salt of ceftriaxone, with traces of bilirubinate and cholesterol, thus resembling pigment stone composition.[151] The process of biliary concretion and the related symptoms are totally reversible when the drug is discontinued.

REFERENCES

1. Way LW, Sleisenger MH: Cholelithiasis: Chronic and acute cholecystitis. *In* Sleisenger MH, Fordtran JS, eds: Gastrointestinal Disease: Pathophysiology, Diagnosis, Management. Philadelphia, WB Saunders, 1989, p 1691.
2. Holland C, Heaton KH: Increasing frequency of gallbladder operations in the Bristol area. Br Med J 1972; 3:672.
3. Friedman GD, Kamel WB, Dawber TR: The epidemiology of gallbladder disease: Observations in the Framingham Study. J Chron Dis 1966; 19:273.
4. The Coronary Drug Project Research Group: The Coronary Drug project: Design, methods and baseline results. Circulation 1973: 47(Suppl 1):1.
5. Sampliner RE, Bennet PH, Comess LJ, et al: Gallbladder disease in the Pima Indians: Demonstration of high prevalence and early onset by cholecystography. N Engl J Med 1970; 283:1358.
6. Bainton D, Davies GT, Evans KT, et al: Gallbladder disease: Prevalence in a South Wales industrial town. N Engl J Med 1976; 294:1147.
7. Maurer KR, Everhart JE, Exxati TM, et al: Prevalence of gallstone disease in Hispanic populations in the United States. Gastroenterology 1989; 96:487.
8. Bates GC, Brown CH: Incidence of gallbladder disease in chronic hemolytic anemia (spherocytosis). Gastroenterology 1952; 21:104.
9. Barbara L, Festi D, Frabboni R, et al: Incidence and risk factors for gallstone disease: The Sirmione study (abstract). Hepatology 1988; 8:1256.
10. Barker DJP, Gardner MJ, Power C, et al: Prevalence of gallstones at necropsy in nine British towns: A collaborative study. Br Med J 1979; 2:1389.
11. Bateson MC, Bouchier IAD: Prevalence of gallstones in Dundee: Necropsy study. Br Med J 1975; 4:4271.
12. Layde PM, Vessey MP, Yeatles D: Risk factors for gallbladder disease: A cohort study of young women attending family planning clinics. J Epidemiol Commun Health 1982; 36:274.
13. Lindstrom CG: Frequency of gallstone disease in a well-defined Swedish population: A prospective necropsy study in Malmo. Scand J Gastroenterol 1977; 12:341.
14. Rome Group for the Epidemiology and Prevention of Cholelithiasis (GREPCO): Prevalence of gallstone disease in an Italian adult female population. Am J Epidemiol 1984; 119:796.
15. Biss K, Ho KJ, Mikkelson B, et al: Some unique biologic characteristics of the Masai of East Africa. N Engl J Med 1971; 284:694.
16. Gibson J: An extraordinary large gallbladder and hydropic cystis: Medical essays and observations. Philos Soc Edin 1737; 2:352.
17. Blalock A: A statistical study of 888 cases of biliary tract disease. Bull Johns Hopkins Hosp 1924; 35:391.
18. Glenn F: 25-year experience in the surgical treatment of 5037 patients with non-malignant biliary tract disease. Surg Gynecol Obstet 1959; 109:591–606.
19. Potter AH: Biliary disease in young subjects. Surg Gynecol Obstet 1938; 66:604.
20. Ulin AW, Nosal JL, Martin WC: Cholecystitis in childhood. Surgery 1952; 31:312.
21. Potter A: Gallbladder disease in young subjects. Surg Gynecol Obstet 1928; 46:795.
22. Gross RE: The Surgery of Infancy and Childhood. Philadelphia, WB Saunders, 1953, p 531.
23. Seiler I: Gallbladder disease in children. Am J Dis Child 1960; 99:662.
24. Swenson O: Pediatric Surgery. New York, Appleton-Century-Crofts, 1958, p 280.
25. Andrassy RJ, Treadwell TA, Ratner, IA, et al: Gallbladder disease in children and adolescents. Am J Surg 1976; 132:10.
26. Shafer AD, Ashley JV, Goodwin CD, et al: A new look at the multifactorial etiology of gallbladder disease in children. Am Surg 1983; 49:314.
27. Lau GE, Andrassy RJ, Mahour GH: A 30-year review of the management of gallbladder disease at a children's hospital. Am Surg 1983; 49:411.
28. Henschue CI, Littlewood-Teele R: Cholelithiasis in children: Recent observations. J Ultrasound Med 1983; 2:481.
29. Holcomb GW: Gallbladder disease. *In* Welch KJ, Randolph JA Jr, Rowe MI, eds: Pediatric Surgery. Vol 2. Chicago, Year Book Publications, 1986, p 1060.
30. Descos B, Bernard O, Brunelle F, et al: Pigment gallstones of the common bile duct in infancy. Hepatology 1984; 4:678.
31. Calabrese C, Pearlman DM: Gallbladder disease below the age of 21 years. Surgery 1971; 70:413.
32. Honore LH: Cholesterol cholelithiasis in adolescent females. Arch Surg 1980; 114:62.
33. Friesen CA, Roberts CC: Cholelithiasis: Clinical characteristics in children, case analysis and literature review. Clin Pediatr 1989; 28:294.
34. Salvioli G, Lugli R, Pellati M: Nucleation and aggregation of cholesterol crystals in the early phases of gallstone genesis. *In* Swobodnink W, Ditschuneit H, Soloway RD, eds: Gallstone Disease: Pathophysiology and Therapeutic Approaches. Berlin, Springer-Verlag, 1990, pp 11–25.

35. Renshaw PE, Janoff AS, Miller KW: On the nature of dilute aqueous cholesterol suspensions. J Lipid Res 1983; 24:47–51.
36. Carey MC, Cohen DE: Biliary transport of cholesterol in micelles and liquid crystals. *In* Paumgartner G, Stiehl A, Gerok W, eds: Bile Acids and the Liver. Lancaster, MTP Press, 1987, pp 287–300.
37. Chijiiwa K, Nagai M: Interaction of bile salt monomer and cholesterol in the aqueous phase. Biochim Biophys Acta 1989; 1001:111–114.
38. Hay DW, Carey MC: Pathophysiology and pathogenesis of cholesterol gallstone formation. Semin Liver Dis 1990; 10:159–170.
39. Sömjen GJ, Marikovsky Y, Lelkes P, et al: Cholesterol phospholipid vesicles in human bile: An ultrastructural study. Biochim Biophys Acta 1986; 879:14–21.
40. Halpern Z, Dudley MA, Kibe A, et al: Rapid vesicle formation and aggregation in abnormal human biles: A time-lapse video-enhanced contrast microscopy study. Gastroenterology 1986; 90:875–885.
41. Pattinson NR, Chapman BA: Distribution of biliary cholesterol between mixed micelles and nonmicelles in relation to fasting and feeding in humans. Gastroenterology 1986; 91:697–702.
42. Holan KR, Holzbach RT, Hermann RE, et al: Nucleation time: A key factor in the pathogenesis of cholesterol gallstone disease. Gastroenterology 1979; 77:611–617.
42a. Donovan JM, Carey MC: Separation and quantitation of cholesterol "carriers" in bile. Hepatology 1990; 12:945–1045.
43. Carey MC: Formation of cholesterol gallstones: The new paradigms. *In* Paumgartner G, Stiehl A, Gerok W, eds: Trends in Bile Acid Research. Dordrecht, Kluwer Academic Publishers, 1989, pp 259–281.
44. Forgacs IC: Pathogenesis of cholesterol gallstone disease: The motility defect. *In* Northfield T, Jazrawi R, Zentler-Munro P, eds: Bile Acids in Health and Disease. Dordrecht, Kluwer Academic Publishers, 1988, pp 135–153.
45. Carey MC, Cahalane MC: Whither biliary sludge? Gastroenterology 1988; 95:508–523.
46. Booker ML, Scott TE, LaMorte WW: Effect of dietary cholesterol on phosphatidylcholines and phosphatidylethanolamines in bile and gallbladder mucosa in the prairie dog. Gastroenterology 1989; 97:1261–1267.
47. Kajiyama G, Kubota S, Sasaki H, et al: Lipid metabolism in the development of cholesterol gallstones in hamsters: I. Study on the relationship between serum and biliary lipids. Hiroshima J Med Sci 1980; 29:133–141.
48. DenBesten L, Connor WE, Bell S: The effect of dietary cholesterol on the composition of human bile. Surgery 1973; 73:266–273.
49. Lee DWT, Gilmore CJ, Bonorris G, et al: Effect of dietary cholesterol on biliary lipids in patients with gallstones and normal subjects. Am J Clin Nutr 1985; 42:414–420.
50. Angelin B, Backman L, Einarsson K, et al: Hepatic cholesterol metabolism in obesity: Activity of microsomal 3-hydroxy-3-methylglutaryl coenzyme A reductase. J Lipid Res 1981; 23:770–773.
51. Ahlberg J, Angelin B, Bjorkhem I, et al: Hepatic cholesterol metabolism of normal and hyperlipidemic patients with cholesterol gallstones. J Lipid Res 1979; 20:107–115.
52. Einarsson K, Nilsel K, Leijd B, et al: Influence of age on secretion of cholesterol and synthesis of bile acids by the liver. N Engl J Med 1985; 313:277–282.
53. Meckel von Hemsback JH: Mikrogeologie: Ueber die Concremente im thierischen Organismus: Nach des Verfassers Tode herausgegeben und bevorwortet von Dr. Theodor Billroth. Berlin, Reimer, 1856.
54. Fridhandler TM, Davison JS, Shaffer EA: Defective gallbladder contractility in the ground squirrel and prairie dog during the early stages of cholesterol gallstone formation. Gastroenterology 1983; 85:830–836.
55. Doty JE, Pitt HA, Kuchenbecker SL, et al: Impaired gallbladder emptying before gallstone formation in the prairie dog. Gastroenterology 1983; 85:168–174.
56. Pellegrini CA, Ryan T, Broderick W, et al: Gallbladder filling and emptying during cholesterol gallstone formation in the prairie dog. Gastroenterology 1986; 90:143–149.
57. Li YF, Weisbrodt NW, Moody FG, et al: Calcium-induced contraction and contractile protein content of gallbladder smooth muscle after high-cholesterol feeding of prairie dogs. Gastroenterology 1987; 92:746–750.
58. Fisher RS, Stelzer F, Rock E, et al: Abdominal gallbladder emptying in patients with gallstones. Dig Dis Sci 1982; 27:1019–1024.
59. Behar J, Lee KY, Thompson WE, et al: Gallbladder contraction in patients with pigment and cholesterol stones. Gastroenterology 1989; 97:1479–1484.
60. Lee SP, Maher K, Nicholls JF: Origin and fate of biliary sludge. Gastroenterology 1988; 94:170.
61. Smith BF: Human gallbladder mucin binds biliary lipids and promotes cholesterol crystal nucleation in model bile. J Lipid Res 1987; 28:1088.
62. Shaffer EA: Gallbladder disease. *In* Walker WA, Durie PR, Hamilton JR, et al: Pediatric Gastrointestinal Disease: Pathophysiology, Diagnosis, Management. Philadelphia, BC Decker, 1991, pp 1152–1170.
63. Nilsson S: Gallbladder disease and sex hormones. Acta Chir Scand 1966; 132:275.
64. Bennion LJ, Knowler WC, Mott DM, et al: Development of lithogenic bile during puberty in Pima Indians. N Engl J Med 1979; 300:873.
65. Bennion LJ, Mot DM, Howard BV: Oral contraceptives raise the cholesterol saturation of bile by increasing biliary cholesterol secretion. Metabolism 1980; 29:18.
66. Berr F, Eckel RH, Kern F: Contraceptive steroids increase hepatic uptake of chylomicron remnants in healthy young women. J Lipid Res 1986; 27:645.
67. Kern F, Everson GT: Contraceptive steroids in cholesterol in bile: Mechanisms of actions. J Lipid Res 1987; 28:828.
68. Lynn J: Effects of estrogen upon bile: Implications with respect to gallstone formation. Ann Surg 1973; 178:514.
69. Warren KW, Williams CI, Tan EGC: Diseases of the Gallbladder and bile ducts. *In* Schiff L, Schiff ER, eds: Diseases of the Liver. Philadelphia, JB Lippincott, 1987, pp 1289–1335.
70. Warwick WJ, L'Heureux PR, Sharp HL, et al: Gallstones and cystic fibrosis. *In* Proceedings of the Seventh International Cystic Fibrosis Congress. Paris, 1976, pp 484–491.
71. Isenberg J, L'Heureux PR, Warwick W, et al: Clinical observations on the biliary system in cystic fibrosis. Am J Gastroenterol 1976; 65:134.
72. Gaskin KJ, Waters DLM, Howman-Giles R, et al: Liver disease and common-bile-duct stenosis in cystic fibrosis. N Engl J Med 1988; 318:340.
73. Vawter GF, Swachman H: Cystic fibrosis in adults: An autopsy study. Pathol Annu 1979; 14:357.
74. Roy CC, Weber AM, Morin CL, et al: Abnormal biliary lipid composition in cystic fibrosis: Effects of pancreatic enzymes. N Engl J Med 1977; 297:1301.
75. Weber AM, Roy CC, Morin CL, et al: Malabsorption of bile acids in children with cystic fibrosis. N Engl J Med 1973; 289:1001.
76. Watkins JB, Tercyak AM, Szczepanik P, et al: Bile salt kinetics in cystic fibrosis. Gastroenterology 1974; 67:385.
77. Santamaria F, Vajro P, Oggero V, et al: Volume and emptying of the gallbladder in patients with cystic fibrosis. J Pediatr Gastroenterol Nutr 1990; 10:303.
78. Crowther RS, Soloway RD: Pigment gallstone pathogenesis: From man to molecules. Semin Liver Dis 1990; 10:171.
79. Soloway RD, Trotman BW, Ostrow JD: Pigment gallstones. Gastroenterology 1977; 72:167.
80. Ostrow JD: The etiology of pigment gallstones. Hepatology 1984; 4:215S.
81. Black BE, Carr SH, Ostrow JD, et al: Equilibrium swelling of pigment gallstones: Evidence for network polymer structure. Biopolymers 1882; 21:601.
82. Burnett W, Dwyer KR, Kennard CHL: Black pigment in polybilirubinate gallstones. Ann Surg 1981; 193:331.
83. Sarnaik S, Slovis TI, Corbett DP, et al: Incidence of cholelithiasis in sickle cell anemia using the ultrasonic gray-scale technique. J Pediatr 1980; 96:1005.
84. Lackman BS, Lazerson J, Stashak RJ, et al: The prevalence of cholelithiasis in sickle cell disease as diagnosed by ultrasound and cholecystography. Pediatrics 1979; 64:501.

85. Merindino KA, Manhas DR: Man-made gallstones: A new entity following cardiac heart valve replacement. Ann Surg 1973; 177:694.
86. Tabata M, Nakayama F: Bacteria and gallstones: Etiological significance. Dig Dis Sci 1981; 26:218.
87. Cahalane MJ, Neubrand MW, Carey MC: Physical-chemical pathogenesis of pigment gallstones. Semin Liver Dis 1988; 8:317.
88. Robins SJ, Fasulo JM, Patton GM: Lipids of pigment gallstones. Biochem Biophys Acta 1982; 712:21.
89. Wosiewitz U, Schenk J, Sabinski F, et al: Investigations on common bile duct stones. Digestion 1983; 26:43.
90. Treem WR, Malet PF, Gourley GR, et al: Bile and stone analysis in two infants with brown pigment gallstones and infected bile. Gastroenterology 1989; 96:519.
91. Hikasa Y, Nagase M, Tanimura H, et al: Epidemiology and etiology of gallstones. Arch Jpn Chir 1980; 49:555.
92. Tabata M, Nakayama F: Bacteria and gallstones: Etiological significance. Dig Dis Sci 1981; 26:218.
93. Akiyoshi T, Nakayama F: Bile acid composition in brown pigment stones. Dig Dis Sci 1990; 35:27–32.
94. Benjamin DR: Hepatobiliary dysfunction in infants and children associated with long-term total parenteral nutrition: A clinicopathologic study. Am J Clin Pathol 1980; 81:276.
95. Roslyn JJ, Berquist WE, Pitt HA, et al: Increased risk of gallstones in children receiving total parenteral nutrition. Pediatrics 1983; 71:784.
96. Messing B, Bories C, Kunstlinger F, et al: Does total parenteral nutrition induce gallbladder sludge formation and lithiasis? Gastroenterology 1983; 84:1012.
97. Matos C, Avni EF, Van Gansbeke D, et al: Total parenteral nutrition (TPN) and gallbladder diseases in neonates: Sonographic assessment. J Ultrasound Med 1987; 6:243.
98. Beale EF, Nelson RM, Buccarelli RL, et al: Intrahepatic cholestasis associated with parenteral nutrition in premature infants. Pediatrics 1979; 64:347.
99. Suchy FJ, Bucavalas JC, Novak DA: Determinants of bile formation during development: Ontogeny of hepatic bile acid metabolism and transport. Semin Liver Dis 1987; 7:77.
100. Suita S, Ikeda K, Naito K, et al: Cholelithiasis in infants: Association with parenteral nutrition. J Parenter Enteral Nutr 1984; 8:569.
101. Suchy FJ, Mullick FG: Total parenteral nutrition–associated cholestasis. *In* Balistreri WF, Stocker JT, eds: Pediatric Hepatology. New York, Hemisphere Publishing, 1990, pp 29–40.
102. Lucas A, Bloom SR, Ayrisley-Green A: Gut hormones and minimal enteral feeding. Acta Paediatr Scand 1986; 75:719.
103. Enzenauer RW, Montrey JS, Barcia PJ, et al: Total parenteral nutrition cholestasis: A cause of mechanical biliary obstruction. Pediatrics 1985; 76:905.
104. Lilly JR, Sokol RJ: On the bile sludge syndrome or is total parenteral nutrition cholestasis a surgical disease? Pediatrics 1985; 76:992.
105. Bowen A: Ultrasound of the normal neonatal gallbladder. Diagn Imag Clin Med 1984; 53:231.
106. Doty JE, Pitt HA, Porter-Fink, et al: The pathophysiology of gallbladder disease induced by total parenteral nutrition (abstract). Gastroenterology 1982; 82:1046.
107. Heaton KW, Read AE: Gallstone in patients with disorders of the terminal ileum and disturbed bile salt metabolism. Br Med J 1969; 3:494.
108. Pellerin D, Bertin P, Nihoul-Fekete Cl, et al: Cholelithiasis and ileal pathology in childhood. J Pediatr Surg 1975; 10:35.
109. Whittington PF, Black DD: Cholelithiasis in premature infants treated with parenteral nutrition and furosemide. J Pediatr 1980; 97:647.
110. Callahan J, Haller JO, Cacciarelli AA, et al: Cholelithiasis in infants: Association with total parenteral nutrition and furosemide. Pediatr Radiol 1982; 143:437.
111. MacMillan RW, Schullinger JN, Santuli TV: Cholelithiasis in childhood. Am J Surg 1974; 127:689.
112. Reif S, Sloven DG, Lebenthal E: Gallstones in children: Characteristics by age, etiology and outcome. Am J Dis Child 1991; 146:105.
113. Keller MS, Markle BM, Laffey PA, et al: Spontaneous resolution of cholelithiasis in infants. Radiology 1985; 157:345.
114. Jacir NN, Anderson KD, Eichelberger M, et al: Cholelithiasis in infancy: Resolution of gallstones in three of four infants. J Pediatr Surg 1986; 21:567.
115. Edelman DS: Laparoscopic cholecystectomy under continuous epidural anesthesia in patients with cystic fibrosis. Am J Dis Child 1991; 145:723.
116. Danzinger RG, Hofmann AF, Schonfield, et al: Dissolution of cholesterol gallstones by chenodeoxycholic acid. N Engl J Med 1972; 286:1.
117. Salen G, Nicolau G, Shefer S: Chenodeoxycholic acid (CDCA) inhibits elevated hepatic HMG-CoA reductase activity in subjects with gallstones. Clin Res 1973; 21:523.
118. Salen G, Tint GS, Shefer S: Oral dissolution treatment of gallstones with bile acids. Semin Liver Dis 1990; 10:181.
119. Leuschner U, Leuschner M, Sieratzki J, et al: Gallstone dissolution with ursodeoxycholic acid in patients with chronic active hepatitis and two years follow-up: A pilot study. Dig Dis Sci 1985; 30:642.
120. Batta A, Salen G, Arora R, et al: Effect of ursodeoxycholic acid on bile acid metabolism in primary biliary cirrhosis. Hepatology 1989; 10:414.
121. Nittono H, Tokita A, Hayashi, et al: Ursodeoxycholic acid therapy in the treatment of biliary atresia. Biomed Pharmacother 1989; 43:37.
122. Podda M, Zuin M, Battezzati M, et al: Efficacy and safety of a combination of chenodeoxycholic and ursodeoxycholic acid for gallstone dissolution: A comparison with ursodeoxycholic acid alone. Gastroenterology 1989; 96:222.
123. Chaussy C, Schmiedt E, Joacham D, et al: First clinical experience with extracorporeally induced destruction of kidney stones by shock waves. J Urol 1980; 127:417.
124. Paumgartner G: Shock-wave lithotripsy of gallstones: Walter B. Cannon Lecture. AJR 1989; 153:235.
125. Sackman M, Delius M, Sauerbruch T, et al: Shock-wave lithotripsy of gallbladder stones—the first 175 patients. N Engl J Med 1988; 318:393.
126. Albert MB, Fromm H : Extracorporeal shock-wave lithotripsy of gallstones with the adjuvant use of cholelitholytic bile acids. Semin Liver Dis 1990; 10:197.
127. Allen MJ, Borody TJ, Thistle JL: In vitro dissolution of cholesterol gallstones: A study of factors influencing rate and a comparison of solvents. Gastroenterology 1985; 89:1097
128. Thistle JL: Topical dissolution treatment of cholesterol gallstones with methyl *tert*-butyl ether. Semin Liver Dis 1990; 10:187.
129. Thistle JL, Peterson BT, Bender CE, et al: Percutaneous dissolution of gallstones using methyl *tert*-butyl ether. Can J Gastroenterol 1990; 4:625.
130. Motil KJ: Cholecystitis. *In* Oski FA, DeAngelis CD, Feigin RD, et al, eds: Principles and Practices of Pediatrics. Philadelphia, JB Lippincott, 1990, pp 1779–1783.
131. Thronell E: Mechanisms in the development of acute cholecystitis and biliary pain: A study on the role of prostaglandins and effects of indomethacin. Scand J Gastroenterol 1982; 17(suppl 76):1.
132. Neiderhiser D, Thornell E, Bjorck S, et al: The effect of lysophosphatidylcholine on gallbladder function in the cat. J Lab Clin Med 1983; 101:699.
133. Thornell E, Jivegard L, Bukhave K, et al: Prostaglandin E_2 formation by the gallbladder in experimental cholecystitis. Gut 1986; 27:370.
134. Pare P, Shaffer EA, Rosenthall L: Nonvisualization of the gallbladder by 99mTc-HIDA cholescintigraphy as evidence of cholecystitis. Can Med Assoc J 1978; 118:384.
135. Lilly JR: Common bile duct calculi in infants and children. J Pediatr Surg 1980; 15:577.
136. Vennes JA: Management of calculi in the common duct. Semin Liver Dis 1983; 3:162.
137. Knudsen FJ, Fuber WF: Acute cholecystitis in the post-operative period. N Engl J Med 1963; 269:289.
138. Strode JE: Acute cholecystitis as a complication following surgery unrelated to the biliary tract. Surgery 1966; 59:195.
139. Munster AM, Goodwin MN, Pruitt BA Jr: Acalculous cholecystitis in burned patients. Am J Surg 1971; 122:591.
140. Weeder RS, Bashant GH, Muir RW: Acute noncalculous cholecystitis associated with severe injury. Am J Surg 1970; 119:729.

141. Ternberg JL, Keating JP: Acute acalculous cholecystitis: Complication of other illnesses in childhood. Arch Surg 1975; 110:543.
142. Shuman WP, Rogers JV, Rudd TG, et al: Low sensitivity of sonography and cholescintigraphy in acalculous cholecystitis. AJR 1984; 142:531.
143. Slovis TL, Hight DW, Philippart AI, et al: Sonography in the diagnosis and management of hydrops of the gallbladder in children with mucocutaneous lymph node syndrome. Pediatrics 1980; 65:789–794.
144. Grisoni E, Fisher R, Izant R: Kawasaki syndrome: Report of four cases with acute gallbladder hydrops. J Pediatr Surg 1984; 19:9–11.
145. Coperman PWM, Medd WE : Diffuse systemic sclerosis with abnormal liver and gallbladder. Br Med J 1967; 3:353.
146. Iwai N, Goto Y, Taniguchi H, et al: Cancer of the gallbladder in a 9-year-old girl. Kinderchir 1985; 40:106.
147. Foster DR, Foster DBE : Gallbladder polyps in Peutz-Jeghers syndrome. Postgrad Med J 1980; 56:373.
148. McKhann GM: Metachromatic leukodystrophy: Clinical and enzymatic parameters. Neuropediatrics 1984; 15(suppl):4.
149. Schaad UB, Tschaeppeler H, Lentze MJ, et al: Transient formations of precipitations in the gallbladder associated with ceftriaxone therapy. Pediatr Infect Dis 1988; 7:434.
150. Schaad UB, Wedgwood-Krucko J, Tschaeppler H: Reversible ceftriaxone-associated biliary pseudolithiasis in children. Lancet 1988; 2:1411.
151. Park HZ, Lee SP, Schy AL : Ceftriaxone-associated gallbladder sludge. Gastroenterology 1991; 100:1665.

Section Seven

GASTROINTESTINAL PROCEDURES

Chapter 73

Intestinal Biopsy

MARTIN MAKSIMAK and PETER J. CERA, JR.

The intestinal biopsy has become an invaluable tool in the practice of pediatric gastroenterology. Tissue samples from the gastrointestinal tract are often necessary to confirm or eliminate a clinical diagnosis. Even with the development and routine use of the fiber-optic endoscope in children and the improved mucosal detail seen with endoscopy and air-contrast radiographs, microscopic analysis is often critical. In this chapter, the various types of biopsy equipment, biopsy techniques, and possible complications are examined. Several topics of prime importance in pediatric gastroenterology are discussed along with the indications for tissue sampling, timing of such biopsies, and interpretation of these biopsies.

SMALL INTESTINE

Equipment

Since Wood and coworkers[1] designed their gastric biopsy tube in 1949, biopsies of the gastrointestinal tract have become routine. Similar but longer tubes were devised by Shiner[2] and Bramberg[3] that allowed access to the jejunum. Over the next several years many different intestinal biopsy tubes were invented, the most well-known being the Crosby-Kugler capsule[4] and the Carey capsule.[5] Even after the early 1960s improvements continued in small bowel biopsy equipment. Many instruments were adapted for use in children, such as decreasing the port size in the Crosby-Kugler capsule.[6] Also, a miniaturized version of the multipurpose biopsy tube was devised for infants by Ament and Rubin.[7] Both the Crosby capsule and the infant multipurpose biopsy tube were the standard instruments for pediatric intestinal biopsies for many years. In the mid-1970s a new steerable biopsy instrument was described for use in adults.[8] Subsequently, its successful use was reported in children by Ferry and Bending[9] and Vanderhoof and associates.[10] In the mid-1970s pediatric flexible endoscopy became a routine procedure to inspect the intestinal mucosa and to obtain tissue samples. Despite the ease of obtaining tissue samples with endoscopy, many continued to use other biopsy equipment because of concerns about tissue samples being crushed, too small, or obtained from the proximal duodenum, which was thought to affect interpretation.[10] Still others used a combination of a Crosby-Kugler capsule and a flexible endoscope to help position the capsule quickly in the small intestine while maximizing the "quality" of the tissue specimens.[11–14] Judging from the many recent studies on small bowel biopsy techniques, the flexible endoscope and the Crosby-Kugler capsule are the most commonly used equipment for small bowel biopsies. The Crosby-Kugler capsule placed via endoscopy has also proved to be very successful. Figure 73–1 shows several types of biopsy equipment. Table 73–1 elucidates the advantages and disadvantages of each biopsy system. Table 73–2 delineates the success rates and biopsy quality for each of the several types of small intestinal biopsy instruments. Table 73–3 lists clinical features associated with small bowel tissue abnormalities.

Biopsy Technique for Small Intestinal Biopsies

The techniques used during a small bowel biopsy are dependent on the equipment being used. With all types of equipment, sedation is helpful for the patient's comfort and cooperation. Many different sedatives have been used, including meperidine, diazepam, promethazine hydrochloride, and chlorpromazine; however, recent experience with midazolam has been favorable.[14] Midazolam is effectively administered intravenously and titrated for each individual patient. Children should be monitored before, during, and after the procedure while sedated.[23] Pulse oximetry is recommended as a simple means of assessing oxygenation during the procedure. Oxygen saturation most often decreases during initial intubation and with the passage of the instrument through the pylorus but can also occur prior to or even after the procedure if sedation is used.

A Crosby-Kugler capsule can be passed by itself; with the capsule tubing inside a shorter, larger-diameter, stiffer nasogastric "sleeve" to facilitate passage through the esophagus and stomach; with a Scott-Harden duodenal intubation tube[24]; or with a guide wire to assist with positioning in the small intestine.[25, 26] Prokinetic agents may be helpful to assist passage. Metoclopramide has been most commonly used for this purpose and can be given intravenously[27] or via the biopsy tube[28]; dom-

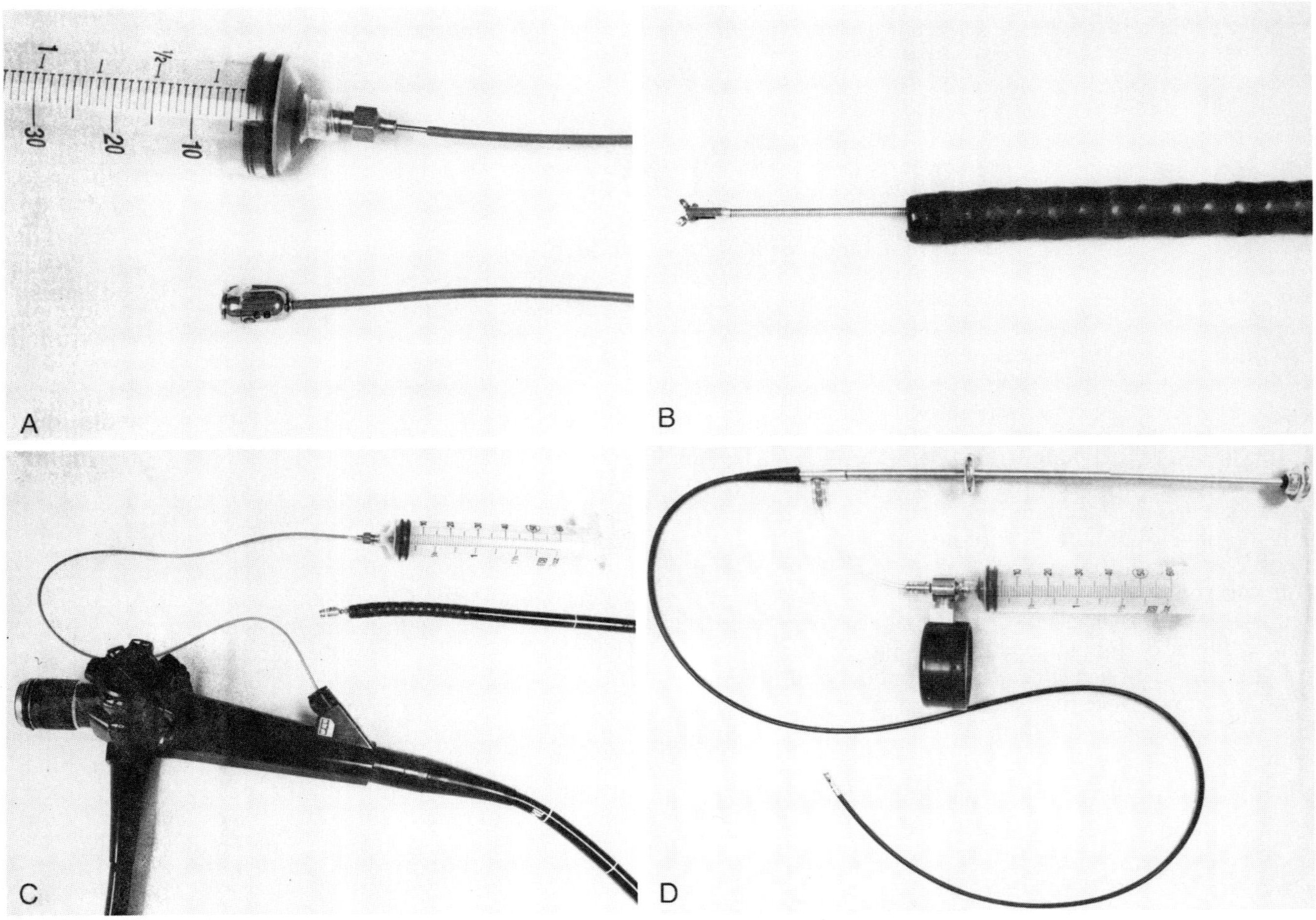

Figure 73–1. Biopsy instruments. *A,* Crosby-Kugler capsule. *B,* Endoscopic grasp forceps. *C,* Endoscopic placement of Crosby capsule. *D,* Pediatric multipurpose biopsy tube.

Table 73–1. ADVANTAGES AND DISADVANTAGES OF COMMONLY USED SMALL BOWEL BIOPSY SYSTEMS

Equipment	Advantages	Disadvantages
Crosby-Kugler capsule	1. Well-oriented tissue samples 2. Jejunal placement	1. Requires fluoroscopy 2. Success rate usually less than other methods listed 3. May require greater than 15 minutes to position the capsule 4. Sampling can be done only at a single site for each passage of the capsule 5. Malfunction of the capsule is not evident until the capsule is removed from the patient
Steerable small bowel biopsy instrument	1. Quick positioning 2. Well-oriented specimens 3. High success rate 4. Jejunal placement possible	1. Requires fluoroscopy 2. Very limited life span for the instrument 3. Sampling can be done only at a single site for each passage of the instrument
Endoscopic grasp biopsies	1. Quick placement 2. High sucess rate 3. No fluoroscopy needed 4. Biopsies from other parts of the upper gastrointestinal tract can be obtained	1. Most biopsies are duodenal not jejunal 2. At times, biopsies are poorly oriented 3. Multiple biopsies may be necessary to get an adequate sample, especially with small pediatric grasp biopsy forceps
Endoscopic placement of the Crosby-Kugler capsule	1. Quick placement 2. High success rate 3. No fluoroscopy needed 4. Jejunal biopsy possible 5. Well-oriented tissue samples	1. Sampling can be done only at a single site for each passage of the instrument 2. Malfunction of the capsule is not evident until the capsule is removed from the patient

Table 73–2. SUCCESS RATE WITH VARIOUS SMALL BOWEL BIOPSY INSTRUMENTS

Type of Instrument	Patient Type	Number of Procedures	Biopsy Success Rate (%)	Biopsies Obtained that Were Adequate (%)	Procedures with at Least One Adequate Biopsy (%)
Crosby-Kugler					
Greene et al[15]	Children	104	97	100	97
	Adults	3,765	94	100	94
Kauder and Bayless[16]	Children	60	80	—	—
Watson Capsule					
Odera and Ansaldi[17]	Children	137	88	90	81
Capsule via Endoscopy					
Maksimak[14]	Children	58	98	99	97
Sullivan et al[18]	Children	53	83	100	83
Mee et al[19]	Adults	80	90	83	75
Pediatric Grasp Forceps					
Odera[17]	Children	176	100	87.5	87.5
Mee et al[19]	Adults	40	100	43	90
Barakat et al[20]	Children	54	100	98	98
Standard Grasp Forceps					
Mee et al[19]	Adults	40	100	60	96
Korn and Foroozin[21]	Adults	22	100	76	100
Barkin et al[22]	Adults	38	100	—	100

peridone has also been used.[29] Intravenous erythromycin lactobionate[30] has been effectively utilized to pass small bowel motility catheters at a dose of 3 mg per kg over 1 hour and may prove helpful with biopsy tubes. Movement of the capsule past the pylorus can be enhanced by abdominal palpation, with the physician's hand protected from radiation with a radiopaque glove. As the tube is advanced toward the pylorus, palpation in a cephalad direction along the greater gastric curvature with the thumb or tip of several fingers directs the proximal tubing upward but the distal tubing and capsule downward. This downward deflection is often needed to pass the pylorus. Placing the patient in a right lateral decubitus position also is helpful. Once the tube is past the pylorus, its movement further into the duodenum is aided by changing the patient to a supine position with the head elevated. Finally, placing the patient in a left lateral decubitus position helps move the capsule to the jejunum, while more tubing is advanced. The capsule knife blade is triggered by applying suction to the capsule's tubing with a large syringe. Similar means are used to pass the multipurpose biopsy tube, Carey capsule, Watson capsule, and the steerable biopsy apparatus. However, with the steerable biopsy instrument, movement of the tip facilitates passage, with an average procedure time of approximately 6 minutes.[10] The technique of passage of an endoscope to obtain a grasp forceps biopsy needs no explanation; however, at times individual endoscopic biopsies may not be adequate for accurate analysis, especially with pediatric forceps. Biopsies can be improved by using the largest forceps possible,[19] taking multiple biopsies (at least four) from the small intestine,[19, 31] orienting the specimen on nylon mesh or filter paper,[19, 31–33] cutting numerous deeper tissue sections,[21, 33, 34] and obtaining tissue from a fold, which may increase the biopsy size.[20]

Table 73–3. SIGNS AND SYMPTOMS THAT MAY BE ASSOCIATED WITH SMALL INTESTINAL BIOPSY ABNORMALITIES

Chronic diarrhea
Decreased growth velocity
Foul-smelling stools (suspected steatorrhea)
Malnutrition
Ascites
Edema
Recurrent infection (suspected agammaglobulinemia, hypogammaglobulinemia)
Abdominal pain (suspected disaccharidase deficiency)

The Crosby-Kugler capsule placed via endoscopy essentially combines the ease of endoscope placement of the biopsy instrument with the excellent size and orientation of the Crosby capsule biopsy. An endoscope with at least a 2.8 mm channel is essential to insert the capsule tubing through the endoscope in a retrograde fashion. To properly ready the endoscope for capsule biopsies, a small pediatric forceps (e.g., Olympus XP forceps) is inserted in a normal fashion into the endoscope. The capsule tubing is then inserted onto the forceps, and the forceps is withdrawn in a normal fashion out of the handle of the endoscope. When the capsule tubing is pulled out of the biopsy port on the endoscope handle, a syringe is attached using a syringe adapter. The endoscope is then inserted in the usual fashion, with the biopsy capsule extending approximately 1 cm from the endoscope tip. When the mid esophagus has been reached, the capsule can be advanced further ahead of the endoscope to allow visualization of the gastrointestinal lumen. The endoscope and biopsy apparatus are then advanced into the duodenum. In a patient larger than 5 to 10 kg, the capsule is advanced further into the small intestine without moving the endoscope, allowing samples to be taken distal to the endoscope. In a small infant it may be difficult to pass an endoscope with an adequate size biopsy channel into the duodenum. In this situation the endoscope can be positioned just proximal to the pylorus, and the capsule can be pushed past the pylorus and into the duodenum or jejunum by advancing the capsule tubing. Once the capsule is correctly positioned, the capsule knife blade is fired in the normal fashion using a large syringe.

Complications

In general the various methods described are safe, but complications have been reported. Complications include respiratory compromise, bleeding,[35–37] small bowel hematomas,[38–40] prolonged retention of the biopsy capsule,[41] and perforation.[6, 37, 42, 43] Fortunately, these problems are rare and most of the literature comprises case reports. One of the most important studies of complications secondary to small bowel biopsies was reported by Partin and Schubert.[6] They showed that the major risk factor for perforation using the capsule suction biopsy was a biopsy port size of 3.0 mm. Port sizes of 1.5 or 2.0 mm were not associated with perforation.

Processing of the Intestinal Biopsy Samples

To determine the etiology of a patient's symptoms, several different criteria[28, 44] need to be evaluated to assure an accurate diagnosis. Table 73–4 illustrates what particular aspects of the biopsy need to be examined. Figure 73–2 shows a representative normal small bowel biopsy. Many specific lesions can be determined, as seen in Table 73–5.

Table 73–4. IMPORTANT FEATURES OF A SMALL INTESTINAL BIOPSY

Villous height
Crypt depth
Small bowel mucosal enzymes
Lamina propria cellular infiltrate
Epithelial abnormalities
Intraepithelial infiltrate
Periodic acid–Schiff stain of apical cytoplasm of the enterocyte

Intestinal samples are most commonly stained with hematoxylin and eosin; however, periodic acid–Schiff staining abnormalities of the apical cytoplasm may be indicative of microvillus atrophy.[28] In the normal small intestine, villus height is greater than crypt depth. If villus height equals crypt depth, then the damage is mild. If villus height is less than crypt death, then moderate damage exists. In severe injury the intestinal mucosa is flat.

In instances in which disaccharidase deficiency is suspected, biopsies can be taken for enzyme analysis. They should be placed in a small airtight container on ice until quick frozen with liquid nitrogen and kept at −22°C until analysis. Studies have shown that endoscopic biopsies are accurate for small intestinal disaccharidase assays.[45, 46] With three to six endoscopic biopsies, duplicate assays can be performed for lactase, sucrase, and maltase. Lee and coworkers found that the sucrose-lactose ratio may be the most helpful determination of primary lactose intolerance.[45] In a comparison study between endoscopic and capsule biopsies,[46] both were equally adequate for disaccharidase analysis. In patients less than 24 months of age, the degree of mucosal injury correlated inversely with lactase activity. In those greater than 24 months of age, the degree of

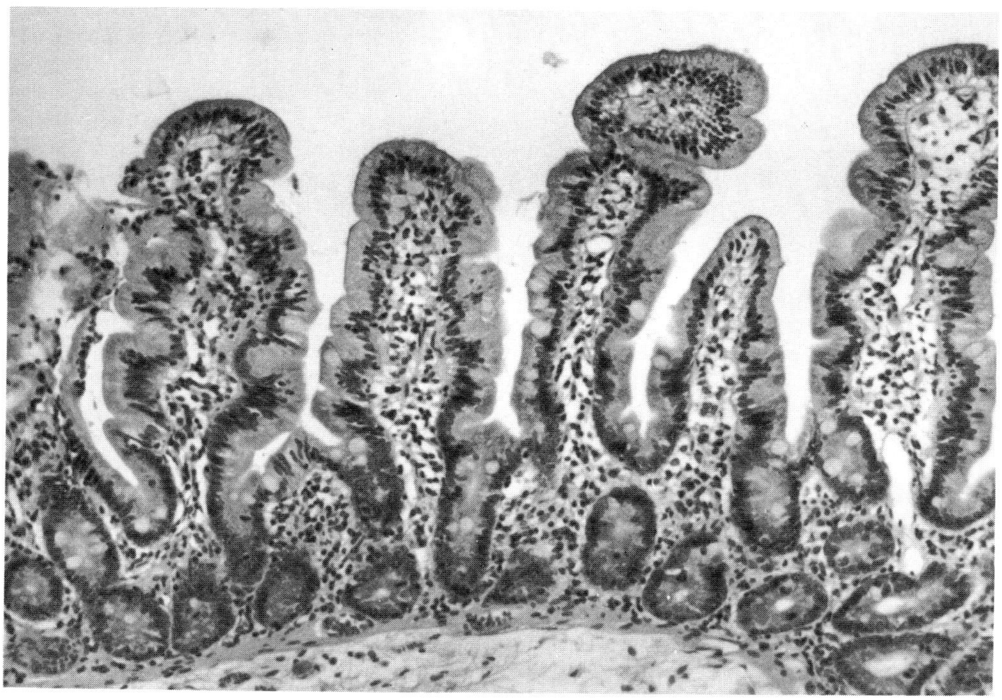

Figure 73–2. Normal jejunum. Cross section of the mucosa of normal jejunum. Hematoxylin-eosin stain, × 50.

Table 73–5. SMALL INTESTINAL ABNORMALITIES THAT MAY BE DELINEATED BY BIOPSY

Lesions Demonstrated Consistently on Biopsy (abnormalities may be nonspecific)	Lesions Inconsistently Demonstrated on Biopsy
Celiac disease	Hypogammaglobulinemia
Autoimmune enteropathy	*Giardia*
Abetalipoproteinemia	*Cryptosporidium*
Agammaglobulinemia	Postviral enteritis
Microvillus atrophy	Cow's milk/soy allergy
Disaccharidase deficiency	Eosinophilic gastroenteritis
	Lymphangiectasia
	CMV enteritis

mucosal injury inversely correlated best with maltase activity. The most common primary disaccharidase deficiencies are sucrase-isomaltase and lactase deficiency. In both instances intestinal morphology should be normal with decreased enzyme levels.[28]

In certain diseases the enterocyte is greatly affected. Normally this cell is columnar in morphology, but with celiac disease or postviral enteritis the enterocyte may become cuboidal.[34] In these two instances vacuolization can also be seen but is more prominent with a beta or hypobeta lipoproteinemia.[28, 44]

Normally a variety of cells exists in the lamina propria, including plasma cells, neutrophils, eosinophils, lymphocytes, and mast cells. Noting the degree of cellular infiltrate and the predominant cell type can be helpful in determining the etiology of mucosal injury. For example, normally there are less than 10 eosinophils per high-power field in the lamina propria.[47] An eosinophilic infiltrate greater than 20 per high-power field is suggestive of eosinophilic gastroenteritis or an allergic enteropathy. In agammaglobulinemia the villous architecture may vary, but the lamina propria lacks plasma cells.[28] The degree of cellular infiltrate in the intestinal epithelium may also be helpful. A value of 11.8 to 35 lymphocytes per 100 epithelial cells with a mean of 23.4 has been found to be normal for children.[48] A similar number has been found in adults. Increased numbers can be seen with celiac disease[49, 50] and occasionally giardiasis.[50]

Selected Small Bowel Abnormalities

Celiac Disease

Celiac disease is the classic illness that causes a flat proximal small bowel mucosal lesion. See Figure 73–3 for an example of celiac disease. Many other illnesses can give a flat intestinal lesion. Katz and Grand emphasized this point in their paper, "All That Flattens Is Not Sprue."[51] Table 73–6 lists disorders that may cause a flat mucosa.

Although most of the earlier investigators of celiac disease made a diagnosis via suction capsule biopsy or the multipurpose biopsy tube, the diagnosis can be made accurately via an endoscopic biopsy.[53] The histologic changes under light microscopy are characterized in Table 73–7.

With the presumptive diagnosis of celiac disease made on the basis of the biopsy and clinical features, the patient is placed on the gluten-free diet. In order to avoid a misdiagnosis and years of unnecessary dietary restriction, a repeat biopsy after at least 6 months of

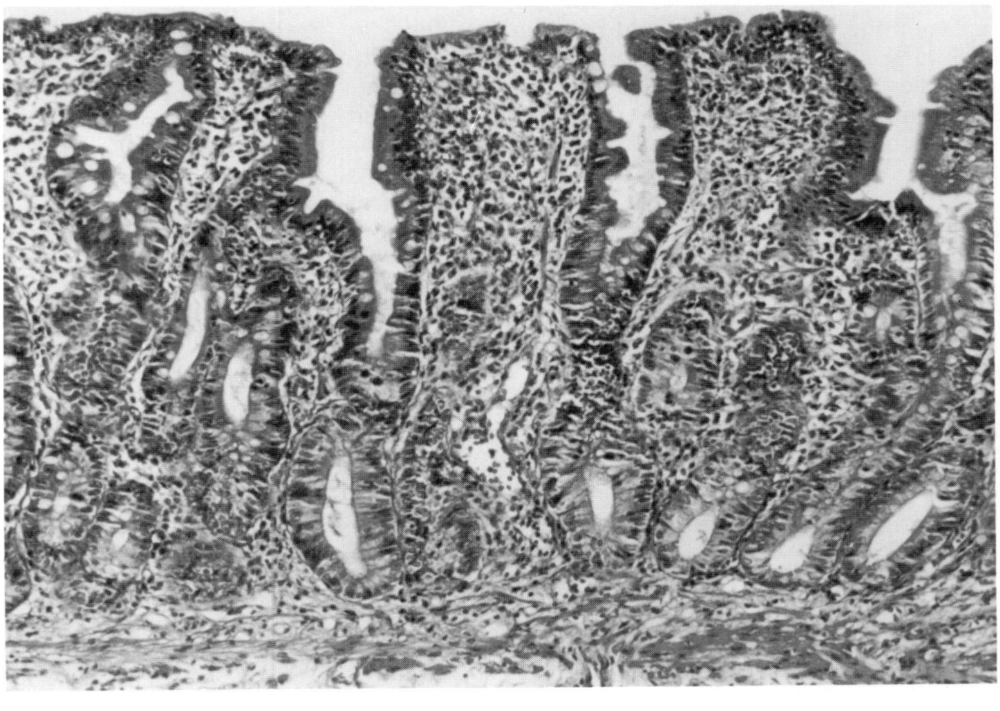

Figure 73–3. Celiac disease. Cross section of jejunal mucosa showing loss of villous pattern, inflammation in the upper lamina propria, and crypt hyperplasia. Hematoxylin-eosin stain, × 50.

Table 73–6. DISORDERS THAT MAY HAVE A FLAT MUCOSA[34, 52, 53]

Celiac disease
Tropical sprue
Viral or postviral enteritis
Allergic enteropathy
Malnutrition
Chemotherapy
Radiation therapy
Graft-versus-host disease
Folate/vitamin B_{12} deficiency
Immunodeficiency
Dermatitis herpatiformis
Bacterial overgrowth

gluten avoidance is recommended, particularly in children during the first year of life. In older children with compatible symptoms, repeat biopsy may not be necessary. If improvement is seen, then rechallenge and a third biopsy are needed for a definitive diagnosis of celiac disease in young patients.[54] The biopsy in celiac patients on a gluten-free diet for a short time shows variable features.[55] After a period of at least 6 months, the mucosa should show definite improvement to a normal or near normal appearance. Biopsy relapse should recur on reintroduction of gluten in celiac disease, although this may take months to even 2 years.[44] On reintroduction of gluten, the villous abnormalities may be patchy.[56]

Cow's Milk Allergy

Cow's milk protein intolerance is a common transient disorder that affects children usually in early infancy. Although the variability of symptoms can lead to both under diagnosis and overdiagnosis, the true incidence is approximately 1%.[57] Common symptoms include diarrhea, poor weight gain, colic, gastrointestinal bleeding, and vomiting. Dermatologic and respiratory manifestations may also occur. Mechanisms for hypersensitivity are believed to be type 1 (immediate hypersensitivity), type 3 (immune complex reaction), type 4 (cell-mediated delayed hypersensitivity), or a combination of mechanisms.

The diagnosis is usually made on the basis of clinical features and response to elimination and reintroduction of cow's milk, with confirmation by histopathology. There are no consistent specific laboratory parameters to rely on apart from biopsy. When considering a diagnosis of cow's milk sensitivity, it is always important to eliminate an infectious etiology as the cause for symptoms, although both infection and cow's milk sensitivity may coexist.[58]

Because of the transient nature of the problem (usually resolving by 1–3 years of age), many have been reluctant to impose serial biopsies as in celiac disease.[58, 59] The most accepted timing of the biopsies is to obtain tissue samples at the initial presentation, after which the patient is placed on milk elimination.[58] If the biopsy and the response to milk protein avoidance is consistent with the diagnosis, then avoidance of cow's milk products is recommended until 1 year of age or earlier if a rechallenge is desired. Salazar de Sousa and colleagues[59] have recommended performing two biopsies to make the diagnosis. In their study, after a presumptive diagnosis was made on the initial clinical features, the patient required a milk withdrawal period of at least 3.5 to 4 months before the mucosa returned to a normal histologic pattern. A milk challenge was then performed followed by an intestinal biopsy 1 to 2 days later. If the biopsy after 4 months of milk withdrawal was normal and changes were consistent with milk allergy postchallenge, then the diagnosis of milk sensitivity was confirmed. Table 73–8 delineates the histologic findings in cow's milk protein sensitivity.

If symptoms are suggestive of colonic involvement, with bloody diarrhea or antral lesions with recurrent vomiting, then biopsies of these areas may be indicated.

Eosinophilic Gastroenteritis

Eosinophilic gastroenteritis (EG), although probably allergic in nature, differs in many respects from cow's milk allergy.[58] In EG, the onset of symptoms tends to be later and is often associated with peripheral eosinophilia. EG usually does not respond to dietary manipulations and often requires corticosteroids for remission and at times for long-term control of symptoms.

Often the diagnosis rests on the demonstration of intestinal tissue eosinophilia. Eosinophilic infiltrates are not necessarily specific for EG. They can be found in other disorders such as esophagitis, cow's milk allergy, and inflammatory bowel disease.[64] With EG, the degree of tissue eosinophilia is much more severe. The Whitingtons[47] described a series of pediatric patients with EG. All had greater than 20 eosinophils per high-powered field under light microscopy. Table 73–9 shows the common histologic changes associated with EG.

Giardiasis

Giardia lamblia is a common intestinal parasite in both children and adults. This parasite can be found on stool examination for cysts or trophozoites or with an

Table 73–7. HISTOLOGIC CHANGES OF CELIAC DISEASE[34]

Absence of villi
Columnar epithelial cells become cuboidal
Increased intraepithelial lymphocytes
Lamina propria cellular infiltrate (mainly plasma cells)
Thickened crypts
Increased mitoses in crypts

Table 73–8. MUCOSAL FEATURES OF COW'S MILK ALLERGY

Severity of enteropathy—flat[60] to mild[61] (more typical) villous lesion
Thin mucosa[58]
Villous lesion tends to be patchy[56]
Intraepithelial cell counts—normal to slightly increased[62]
Eosinophilic lamina propria infiltrate may be present[63]
Histologic involvement of the antrum and colon is possible[63]

Table 73–9. HISTOLOGIC CHANGES ASSOCIATED WITH EOSINOPHILIC GASTROENTERITIS

Antrum and small bowel involvement most common[65]
Esophageal and colonic involvement possible[65]
Eosinophilic infiltrates greater than 20 per high-power field[47]
Epithelial damage[66]
Epithelial regeneration in antral biopsies[67]
Occasional marked villous shortening even simulating celiac disease[66]

Table 73–10. FEATURES OF GIARDIASIS SEEN ON SMALL INTESTINAL BIOPSY

Visualization of the trophozoite, which appears basophilic and pear-shaped following hematoxylin-eosin staining
Organisms most frequently seen between villi, at times attached to the surface epithelium, and occasionally in the crypts[44]
Villous appearance may vary from normal to severe blunting[68]
Villous abnormalities may be patchy[69]
Leukocyte infiltration may be seen in the lamina propria or epithelium, with or without villous abnormalities[44]

enzyme-linked immunoabsorbent assay (ELISA) of the stool. However, because *Giardia* colonization is heavy in the proximal small bowel, examination of duodenal juice, "touch preparations" of the duodenal or jejunal biopsies, a string test, mucosal brushings, and histologic biopsies are often valuable. Table 73–10 shows the features of *Giardia* that are seen on small intestinal biopsy. The organisms can be seen in Figure 73–4.

ESOPHAGUS

Esophageal diseases are commonly encountered in children. An esophageal biopsy is an important component in the diagnosis and determination of therapy. The different illnesses for which biopsies are helpful include common problems such as esophagitis secondary to gastroesophageal reflux and less common entities such as Barrett's esophagus or opportunistic infections in the immunocompromised child.

Equipment and Techniques

Prior to the introduction of the fiber-optic endoscope, evaluation of the esophagus was possible only by radiopaque contrast studies, rigid endoscopy under general anesthesia, or blind esophageal suction biopsy. Upper flexible endoscopy has been shown to be safe in children of all ages in the hands of an experienced examiner.[70, 71] Although flexible endoscopy is usually performed under sedation, most procedures can be performed without sedation in children less than 3 months of age. In patients less than 25 months of age, approximately half of the procedures were well tolerated without sedation. Endoscopically directed biopsies have several advantages. The procedure is quick and safe, and specific mucosal lesions can be biopsied. The two main disadvantages are the small size and poor orientation of the biopsy. Suction biopsies obtained with the Quintron multipurpose biopsy instrument are large and well oriented. However, suction biopsy specimens require fluoroscopic guidance or an estimation of esophageal length from the central incisors to the lower esophageal sphincter by calculation or prior esophageal motility study.[72]

It is important to obtain biopsies from the esophagus in the distal one fifth of the esophagus to avoid a false-negative result.[73] It is also important to avoid the distal

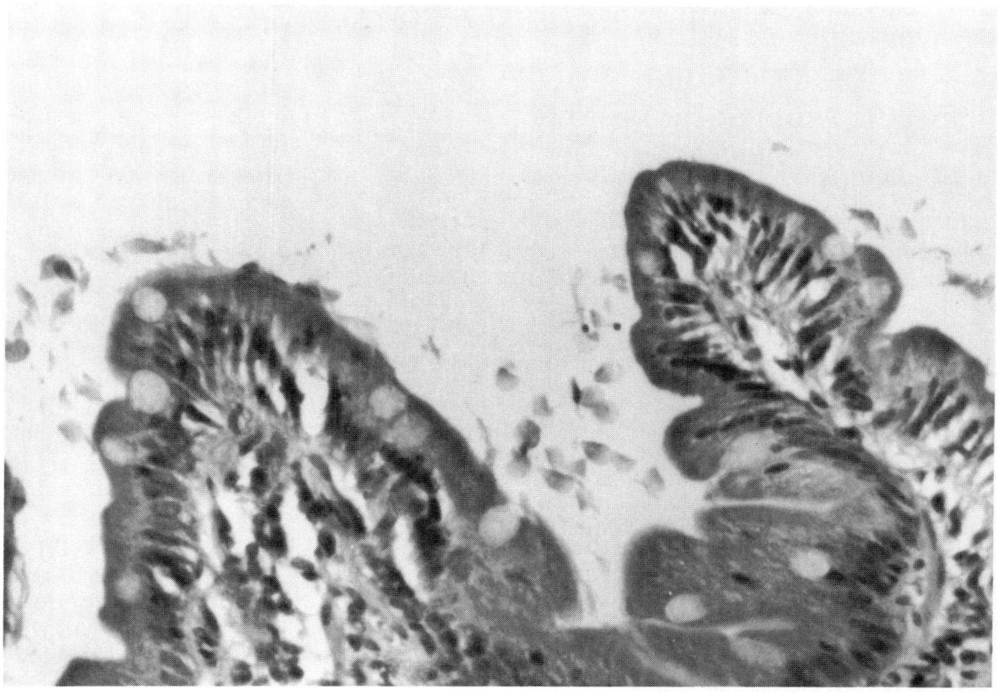

Figure 73–4. Giardiasis. Just above the brush border of the surface epithelial cells are many *Giardia lamblia* trophozoites of characteristic size and shape, including the typical side view. The nuclei are difficult to stain. There is very little inflammation in the mucosa. Hematoxylin-eosin stain, × 500.

2 cm to prevent obtaining a false-positive result,[74] since this area may contain inflammatory cells in patients without significant gastroesophageal reflux.

Indication for Esophageal Biopsy

Despite the widespread use of endoscopy, there is a definite need for esophageal tissue samples for an accurate diagnosis. In children with esophagitis, Biller and associates[75] showed that subtle endoscopic findings were not indicative of histologic esophagitis. Although the diagnosis of Barrett's esophagus is suggested by the sharp demarcation between the normal pale squamous mucosa and the red-brown columnar mucosa of Barrett's epithelium above the lower esophageal sphincter,[76] biopsy is necessary to confirm the suspected diagnosis. In infectious esophagitis, there may be a concomitant infection with more than one organism.[77] Biopsies may also identify a specific pathogen, such as cytomegalovirus (CMV) or herpes. Finally, in *Candida* esophagitis, only biopsies can reveal tissue invasion.[78]

Complications

Complications secondary to obtaining esophageal biopsies are uncommon with flexible endoscopy or hydraulic suction biopsy. In a study by Hargrove and coworkers,[70] only one episode of transient bradycardia during flexible endoscopy was seen in infants evaluated for suspected esophagitis. With hydraulic suction biopsies, Winchenbach and colleagues[79] reported a 0.1% incidence of significant hemorrhage in their extensive experience. However, one adult study revealed a 15% incidence of substernal chest discomfort within 24 hours after suction biopsy.[80] Other possible complications include aspiration, perforation, and infection, although they are rare.

Specific Esophageal Lesions

Esophagitis

Esophagitis secondary to gastroesophageal reflux is commonly encountered in pediatrics. Histopathologic lesions in children and adults have been well described in several reports. The various parameters for esophagitis are listed in Table 73–11.

Basal zone hyperplasia has been found to be one of the most sensitive parameters of esophagitis.[81, 82] However, increases in the basal zone and papillary height can be assessed accurately only with suction biopsy.[80] Black and associates[81] found that the sensitivity of predicting esophagitis when an increased basal zone layer was seen was 89%, with a specificity of 73%. These results were better than any other histologic marker. Dahms and Rothstein[86] have also included three other findings for esophagitis in addition to those mentioned in Table 73–11: (1) intraepithelial lymphocytes or squiggle cells, (2) basal cell nuclear changes—spongiosis, and (3) telangiectasia. However, they required at least two abnormalities in each biopsy to interpret the biopsy as esophagitis. Figure 73–5 reveals a high-power grasp biopsy in a patient with reflux esophagitis.

Table 73–11. HISTOLOGIC PARAMETERS OF PEPTIC ESOPHAGITIS

Basal zone hyperplasia greater than 25% (infants)[81] or 15% (adults)[80, 82] of the total epithelial thickness
Increased papillary height greater than 53% (infants)[12] or 66% (adults)[80, 82] of the total epithelial thickness
Intraepithelial eosinophilia[81, 83–85] and/or lamina propria eosinophilia[81]
Intraepithelial neutrophils[81, 84, 85]

Barrett's Esophagus

Barrett's esophagus occurs secondary to long-standing gastroesophageal reflux. Although the mean age of diagnosis is usually after the fourth decade,[87] it has been reported in children with severe gastroesophageal reflux.[88] The reason Barrett's esophagus generates such concern is the high incidence of adenocarcinoma (approximately 10%) associated with this lesion.[89] The red, brown, or salmon-pink color of Barrett's esophagus may be circumferential[90] or in patches.[78] The patchy lesions may represent an early finding, which may progress to a circumferential lesion.[78]

Histologic features have been categorized into three epithelial types:[76, 78] (1) atrophic gastric fundus-like mucosa with parietal and chief cells, often in the proximal portion of the Barrett's lesion; (2) specialized columnar epithelium that has a villus-like appearance with mucous glands and goblet cells; and (3) junctional-type epithelium that resembles the gastric cardia without parietal and chief cells. Most of the epithelium contains a mixture of these cell types.[91]

Despite the aggressive medical or surgical treatment of gastroesophageal reflux, the high incidence of adenocarcinoma in patients with Barrett's esophagus dictates the need for brush cytology and biopsy in all patients.[76] The proper frequency of endoscopic surveillance is unknown, but over a 19-year period, 2.5% of patients followed with Barrett's esophagus at the Mayo Clinic developed primary adenocarcinoma of the esophagus.[92] One patient with Barrett's esophagus reportedly developed an esophageal carcinoma over an 18-month period of follow-up.[93] Recommendations on endoscopic surveillance with brush cytology and biopsy range from every 6 to 12 months.[76, 94]

Infectious Esophagitis

The most common infectious causes of esophagitis are herpes, CMV, and *Candida.* These infections tend to occur in immunocompromised or debilitated patients.[78]

Herpes Esophagitis. The esophagus is the commonest part of the gastrointestinal tract infected with herpes. The classic early vesicular herpes lesions are very rarely seen, with the typical appearance being discrete,

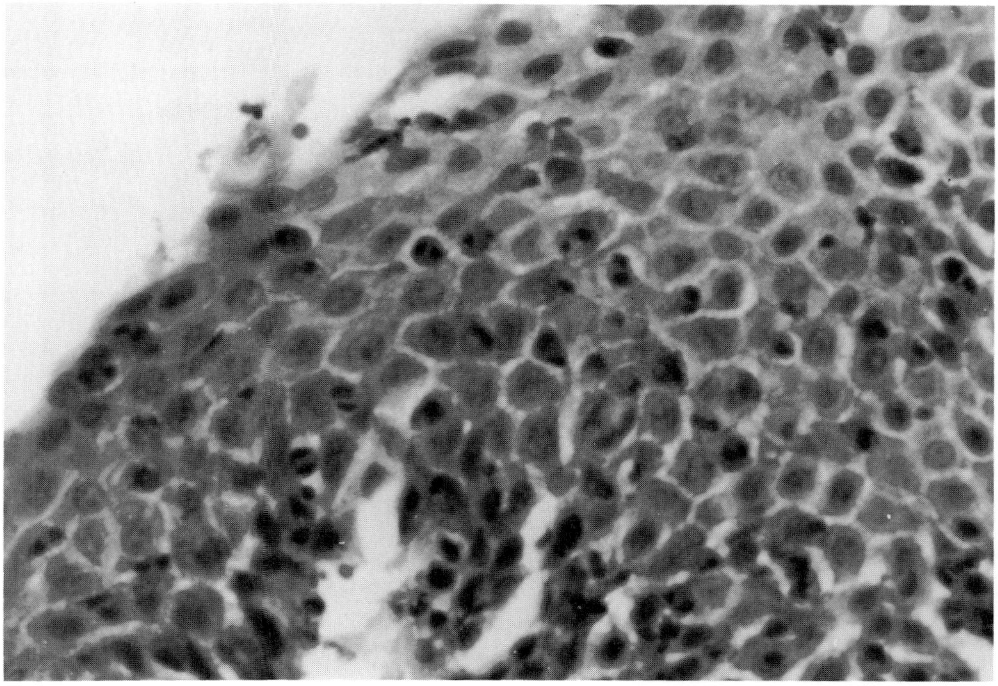

Figure 73–5. Reflux esophagitis. This high-power view reveals many binucleated cells (eosinophils) scattered among the esophageal squamous cells, indicating esophagitis. Hematoxylin-eosin stain, × 500.

punched-out ulcers covered by a white exudate and with raised erythematous margins. Lesions may be very similar to those caused by CMV. Excess exudate in the ulcer and extending into the esophageal lumen may resemble candida esophagitis.[78] With large areas of involvement, the esophagus may appear denuded. Typically, the lesion stops at the gastroesophageal junction.[78] Biopsies, cytologic brushings, and often viral and fungal cultures are needed for an accurate diagnosis.

For herpes, biopsies should be taken from the ulcer edge. The ulcer base reveals nonspecific inflammation and granulation tissue. The typical findings of esophageal herpes are[76, 86, 95] multinuclear giant cells, ground glass nuclei, and occasionally Cowdry type A inclusions, which are large acidophilic intranuclear inclusions surrounded by a halo. Figure 73–6 shows an example of herpes esophagitis.

CMV Esophagitis. Unlike herpes, the ulcer base is

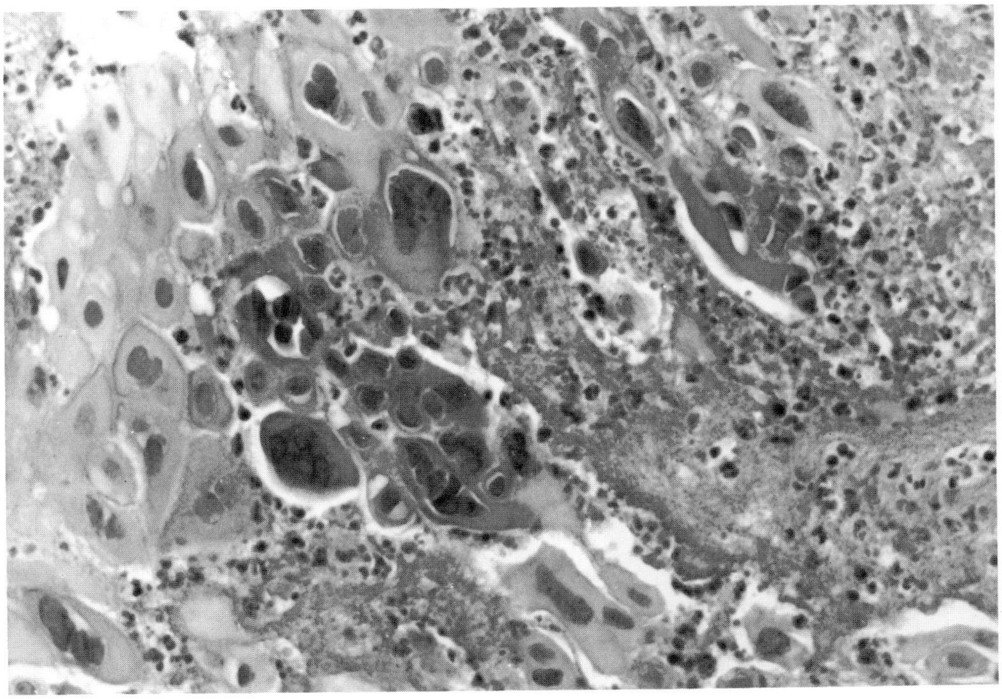

Figure 73–6. Herpes esophagitis. Multinucleated cells and single nucleated esophageal squamous cells contain enlarged homogenous (ground glass) nuclei presumed to occur because of proliferating herpes virus. Hematoxylin-eosin stain, × 313.

the best biopsy location to document CMV infection.[78] This is because the changes with CMV occur in the glandular epithelium, which is present in the endothelial cells and fibroblasts of the granulation tissue in this area. The endoscopic appearance of the ulcers is nonspecific; thus, biopsies are required of both the base and the margin to differentiate between herpes and CMV. The histologic characteristics of CMV are as follows:[78] (1) prominent acidophilic intranuclear inclusions, (2) increased cell size, and (3) occasional granular basophilic intracytoplasmic inclusions.

***Candida* Esophagitis.** *Candida* infections are common in the esophagus. Endoscopically, the fungal lesions appear as hyperemic or whitish plaques. In advanced cases, the esophagus may appear shaggy or cobblestoned.[78] Esophageal brushings of the lesions can reveal the presence of candida, but biopsies are required to show invasion. Histologically, the biopsies reveal acute and chronic inflammation with granulation tissue and ulceration. Both hyphae and budding yeast forms are commonly seen as in Figure 73–7.

STOMACH

Helicobacter Gastritis

Over the past several years, no other topic involving the stomach has generated as much interest as *Helicobacter pylori.* Although initially described in symptomatic adults,[96–98] there have been many subsequent studies showing the presence of this organism in children evaluated for gastrointestinal symptoms such as abdominal pain[99–105] and in asymptomatic adults.[106] The presence of *Helicobacter* in children with gastritis has ranged from 55 to 100%.[99, 102, 103] Kilbridge and coworkers[102] found a correlation between the severity of gastritis and the presence of the organism. None of the studies revealed a presence of the organism without gastritis.[99, 102, 103] The type of gastritis appears to be very important, since most studies show a strong association between the presence of primary gastritis and *Helicobacter.*[99–105] However, in patients with an identifiable cause for gastritis (secondary gastritis), it is uncommon to test positive for *Helicobacter.*[99]

Treatment with bismuth subsalicylate and amoxicillin has been associated with the clearance of the organism in 75%[101] to 100%.[100, 103] In those children in which *Helicobacter* was eradicated, the gastritis resolved in all patients.[100, 101, 103] Symptomatic improvement occurred in 75%[101] to 100%[100, 103] after the clearance of *Helicobacter.*

There are many methods to look for the presence of *Helicobacter* and its associated gastritis and duodenitis. Several noninvasive methods exist, such as an enzyme-linked immunoabsorbent assay (ELISA)[104, 107] and urease breath tests.[107] The ELISA for immunoglobulin (IgG) has a sensitivity in children from 75%[104] to 96%,[107] with a specificity of approximately 96%.[104, 107] The urease breath test using ^{13}C in children is extremely sensitive, but the label is expensive and the test requires the use of mass spectrometry.[107] A major disadvantage of a noninvasive test is that only one etiology is evaluated as the cause of the gastrointestinal symptoms. Endoscopy and appropriate biopsies are able to evaluate esophagitis, gastritis, and duodenitis with or without *Helicobacter*; ulcer disease; disaccharidase deficiency; and giardiasis.

In the diagnosis of *Helicobacter*, the endoscopist should not rely solely on the visual appearance of the antral and duodenal mucosa. Although a nodular antritis

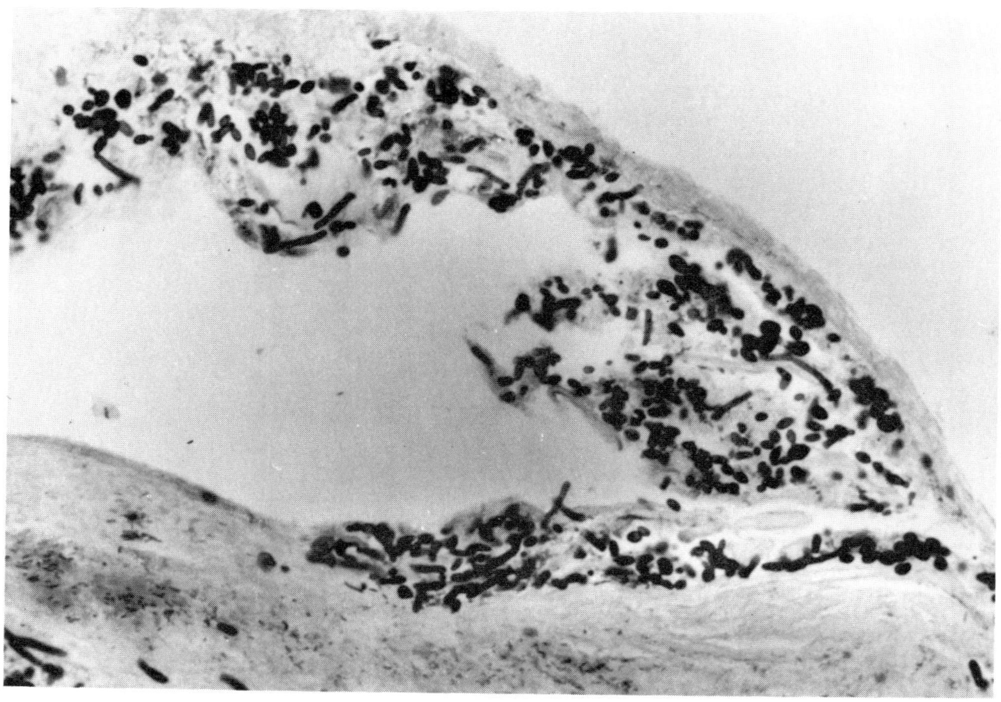

Figure 73–7. *Candida* esophagitis. Both yeast forms and hyphae are seen in the upper layers of the esophageal mucosa, indicating that the fungal organism is probably *Candida.* Grocott stain, × 313.

appears to be the classic macroscopic lesion of *Helicobacter,*[105, 108] the endoscopic appearance may vary and is often normal.[99, 102, 106, 108] Thus, biopsies are crucial to the diagnosis. Biopsies can be processed by several methods to reveal *Helicobacter*. The biopsy can be ground; then inoculated on blood agar, chocolate agar, or Shurow's median; and finally incubated under microaerophilic conditions for up to 7 days at 37°C.[99, 106, 107] However, only a few colonies may be present on a primary culture from children.[107]

An antral biopsy can also be placed into a urease test that is available commercially and has a sensitivity of approximately 90% in children.[109] However, the most widely used method involves actually staining the gastric biopsy. Montgomery and associates[110] reported that gram-stained touch preps of both the fundus and antrum correlated well with other diagnostic methods, with a sensitivity of 92% and specificity of 100%. Most studies have stained the actual biopsy sample with a silver stain,[103, 104, 109, 110] since the darkly stained organism is easy to see against a bright background (Fig. 73–8). Also, hematoxylin and eosin[103, 104, 109, 110] and Giemsa stains[102–109] are very accurate and widely used.

Histology

Most studies have shown a definite correlation between the presence of *Helicobacter* and gastritis. However, the histologic appearance of gastritis may vary considerably. Often the gastritis has been described to be superficial,[97, 98, 111, 112] with approximately 70 to 80% of antral biopsies with superficial gastritis yielding *Helicobacter* (Fig. 73–9). In some studies, the "activity" of the gastritis was irrelevant,[98] with 62% of the quiescent biopsies positive for *Helicobacter* and 68% of the actively inflamed biopsies being positive. Active inflammation means polymorphonuclear infiltrates; in quiescent biopsies, neutrophils were absent. Other studies have shown that there was an 84% incidence of *Helicobacter* with active gastritis and as low as a 33% incidence with chronic changes.[112] However, most studies have revealed a picture of a mixed acute and chronic gastritis predominating, which is often called active chronic gastritis.[102, 112–114] In most children, the chronic infiltration was predominant, with lymphocytic and plasma cell infiltrates in the lamina propria.[102] The acute changes are often focal and superficial.[112] The organisms are usually identified on the surface of the mucosa in the layer of mucus and/or in the gastric pits.[97]

COLON

Equipment

Several instruments are available for colonic biopsies in children. The choice of the instrument is usually dictated by the clinical problem, type of biopsy needed, and location of the biopsy. The most commonly used biopsy equipment includes the flexible sigmoidoscope, colonoscope, and the Rubin suction rectal biopsy tube. If biopsies are required of the entire colon and possibly the terminal ileum, a colonoscope is necessary. If only sigmoid and rectal specimens are needed, a flexible sigmoidoscope will suffice. But if a well-oriented specimen to rule out Hirschsprung's disease is necessary, a grasp biopsy obtained via an endoscope is usually insufficient. Suction biopsies would routinely yield a specimen of adequate depth and orientation to assess the presence of ganglion cells.

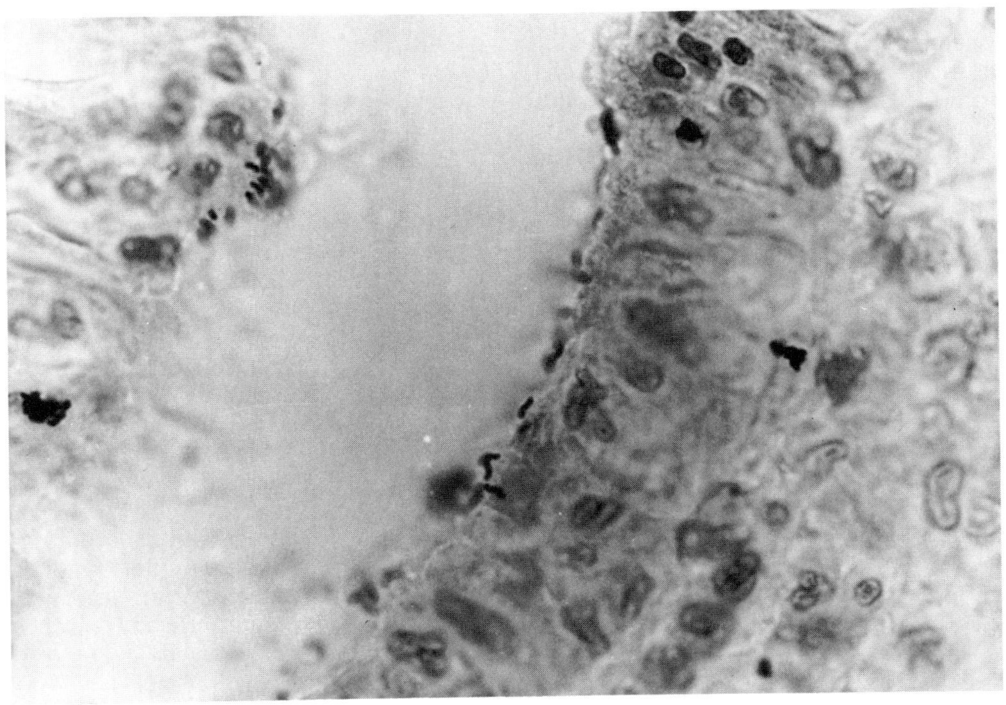

Figure 73–8. Acute gastritis with *Helicobacter.* The loose corkscrew configurations and the size distinguish the *Helicobacter* organisms seen commonly on the surface of the epithelium. Steiner silver stain, × 1008.

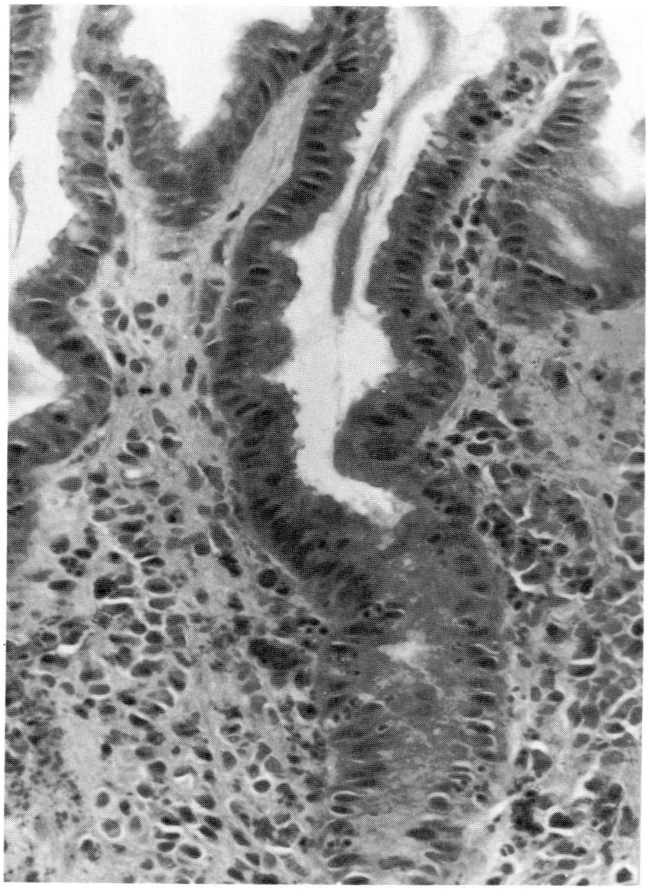

Figure 73–9. Superficial gastritis with *Helicobacter.* A mild superficial neutrophilic infiltrate is present in the antrum in a patient with *Helicobacter.* Hematoxylin-eosin stain, × 313.

There are many clinical situations in which colonic visualization along with biopsy would be helpful diagnostically and possibly therapeutically. Table 73–12 lists some of the common reasons for endoscopic evaluation of the colon along with biopsies.

In most children, colonoscopy can be performed with just sedation using a combination of meperidine and either diazepam or midazolam. Complications of colonoscopy and even polypectomy in children have been uncommon.[115, 116]

Table 73–12. INDICATIONS FOR COLONIC VISUALIZATION AND BIOPSY[28]

Symptoms of possible inflammatory bowel disease (chronic diarrhea with a negative infectious workup, bloody diarrhea, abdominal pain, weight loss)
Evaluation of the activity of inflammatory bowel disease (strictures, response to medical therapy, recurrences)
Cancer or dysplasia surveillance
Unexplained rectal bleeding
Polypectomy

Table 73–13. IMPORTANT COLONIC MUCOSAL BIOPSY FEATURES[117]

Degree of active disease from surface epithelial to crypt damage
Distribution of the inflammation
Nature of the inflammatory response
Signs of regeneration or repair
Signs of chronicity such as Paneth's cell or pyloric glandular metaplasia, crypt branching, or atrophy
Presence of microorganisms

Histology

When evaluating colonic biopsies, several mucosal features should be examined as shown in Table 73–13. However, even with the comprehensive analysis of the biopsy it may be difficult to make a definitive diagnosis. The results of the biopsy need to be correlated with the clinical picture and laboratory results.

Selected Childhood Colonic Diseases

Acute Self-Limited Colitis

Infectious colitis occurs frequently during childhood. Common bacterial organisms responsible include *Salmonella, Shigella, Campylobacter,* and *Escherichia coli. Yersinia* can mimic the clinical and pathologic findings of these organisms, but in children over five years of age the features are often more consistent with mesenteric lymphadenitis or terminal ileitis. In areas in which the bowel is infected with *Yersinia*, lymphoid follicles are massively enlarged and granulomas may be found. However, for most organisms that cause bacterial colitis, there are several typical features that are highly suggestive of self-limited disease and discriminate infectious colitis from idiopathic inflammatory bowel disease. The hallmarks of an acute bacterial colitis are neutrophilic infiltrates and edema.[78] The neutrophils are concentrated in the lamina propria, without the extensive involvement of the crypt epithelium or the numerous crypt abscesses seen in inflammatory bowel disease. Mononuclear cells may be present. Edema is most marked in the upper two thirds of the mucosa. Crypt distortion (branched glands), crypt atrophy, loss of crypt parallelism, and basal plasmacytosis commonly seen in inflammatory bowel disease are absent.[78] Figure 73–10 reveals early acute colitis. Inflammatory features become much less prominent within approximately 6 to 9 days after the onset of symptoms, and signs of repair become more obvious.[118] For example, mucosal edema, crypt inflammation, and neutrophilic lamina propria infiltration peak at zero to 4 days. At 6 to 9 days post onset, the crypt inflammation becomes less prominent and focal, along with only mild to moderate mucosal edema and neutrophilic infiltration. A lymphocytic predominance in lamina propria may be seen at this time. Other features may now be more obvious, such as mucin depletion,

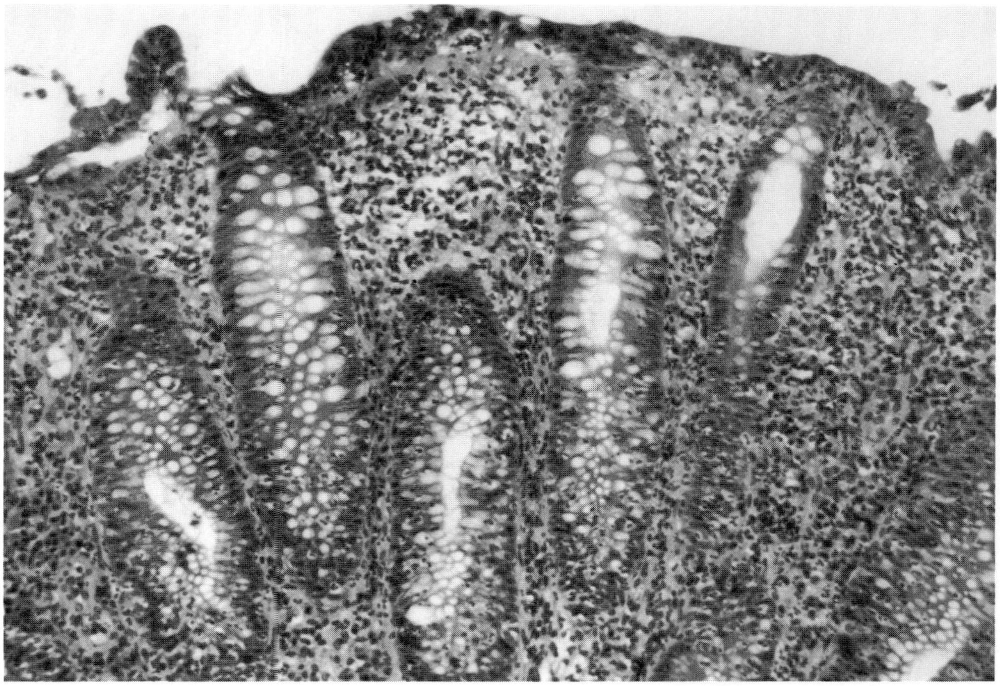

Figure 73–10. Acute (self-limited) colitis. A neutrophilic infiltrate is present in the lamina propria. The crypts are not distorted and remain parallel. Hematoxylin-eosin stain, × 125.

epithelial regeneration, and mitoses. After 9 days most of the described changes are absent to minimal. In no stage of acute self-limited colitis should crypt distortion or basal plasmacytosis be present.[78]

C. difficile *Colitis*

Clostridium difficile commonly inhabits the gastrointestinal tract of young infants but rarely causes symptoms in those less than a year of age. After one year of age this organism becomes less frequently found in the gastrointestinal tract of asymptomatic individuals. Although *C. difficile* can cause disease in a variety of settings, the strongest association has been with the use of antibiotics. The antibiotics allow overgrowth of the organism within the gastrointestinal tract with the production of three separate toxins—toxin A (enterotoxin), toxin B (cytotoxin), and toxin C (motility-altering factor)—along with a factor that inhibits neutrophil migration and phagocytosis.[64] These toxins cause the colonic abnormalities.

There are a variety of ways to diagnose *C. difficile* colitis. A *C. difficile* toxin titer correlates very well with culture of the organism and with the presence of pseudomembranes. However, this organism may be found in up to 40% of infants between 2 to 5 months of age without symptoms. Thus in a young infant an endoscopic exam of the colon with biopsies is often needed for definitive diagnosis. In instances of severe symptoms associated with antibiotic use, flexible sigmoidoscopy or colonoscopy may reveal the presence of a pseudomembrane, which can be confirmed histologically. These findings can result in a quicker diagnosis and institution of therapy. In many children pseudomembranes may not be present,[119] but the presence of symptoms, a positive *C. difficile* toxin titer, and the findings of acute colitis on a biopsy, along with the absence of any other infectious etiology, suggest that *C. difficile* is the likely diagnosis.

Three stages of colonic lesions are described for pseudomembranous colitis.[120] In type I (earliest lesion), inflammatory changes are restricted to the intraglandular surface epithelium and immediate adjacent lamina propria. There is often focal epithelial necrosis or irregularity with the presence of neutrophils, nuclear dust, and an eosinophilic exudate in the lamina propria. Type II lesions show the classic pseudomembrane. There is a well-defined group of distorted glands often distended by mucin and neutrophils. These glands are covered at the surface by a cloud of epithelial debris, fibrin, mucus, and neutrophils, which is the pseudomembrane. A type II lesion can be seen in Figure 73–11. In type III lesions there is complete structural necrosis of the mucosa with a thick covering of fibrin, mucus, and inflammatory debris. This stage is difficult to distinguish from other causes of colitis that cause extensive necrosis.

Ulcerative Colitis

The colonic biopsy is often critical to the diagnosis and long-term management of patients with ulcerative colitis. At initial presentation or with recurrence of symptoms in a patient with inflammatory bowel disease, the biopsy may help a clinician distinguish between a chronic and acute infectious colitis. If the clinical and laboratory parameters are unclear, sequential biopsies are also valuable. Many times clinical symptoms do not necessarily correlate with disease activity, and biopsies may aid in judging the patient's response to therapy.

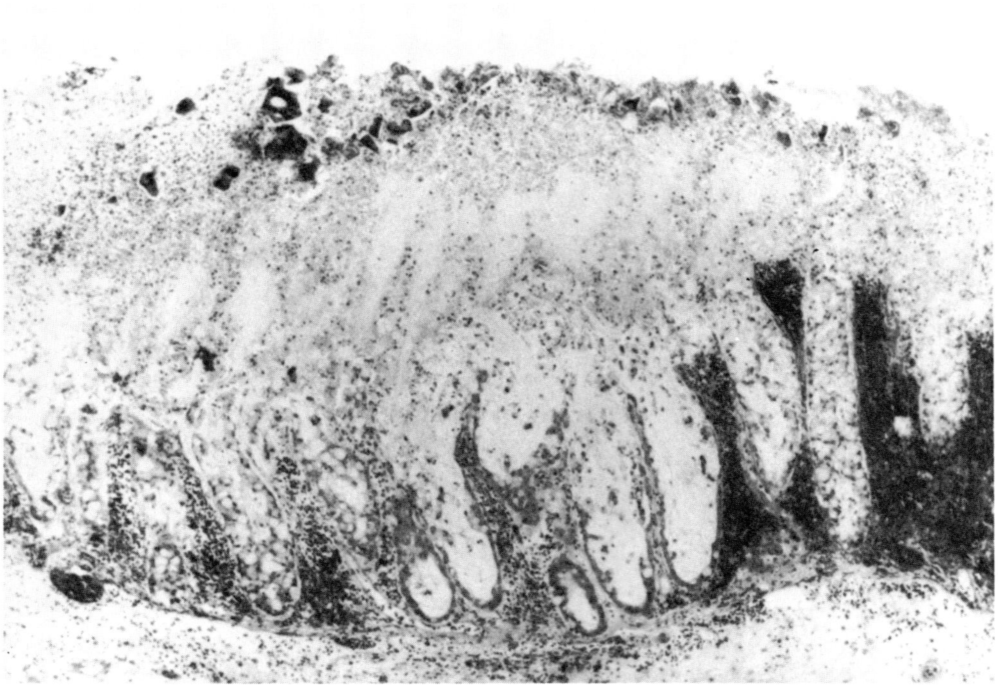

Figure 73–11. Pseudomembranous colitis. A layer of debris, bacterial colonies, mucous, and acute inflammatory cells is present above glands that are disintegrating with only a few intact epithelial cells in the crypts. Hematoxylin-eosin stain, × 50.

Often the histologic findings are divided into three different stages.[28, 78]

1. Active colitis. During this stage prominent vascular congestion and dilation with intramucosal hemorrhage are present. There is often epithelial necrosis and regeneration. Mucin is depleted and goblet cells are reduced or even absent. The lamina propria is infiltrated by heavy mixed inflammatory cells including lymphocytes, plasma cells, and foci of neutrophils. The neutrophils may collect within the crypt epithelium and result in cryptitis, crypt abscesses, and crypt rupture. Active ulcerative colitis is seen in Figure 73–12.

2. Resolving colitis. Even during the resolution of active colitis or in the remission stages of inflammatory bowel disease, the colonic biopsy should show features suggestive of ulcerative colitis. Acute inflammation and crypt abscesses resolve and the vascularity is reduced. There still may be acute and chronic inflammatory cells in the lamina propria, but less than during the acute

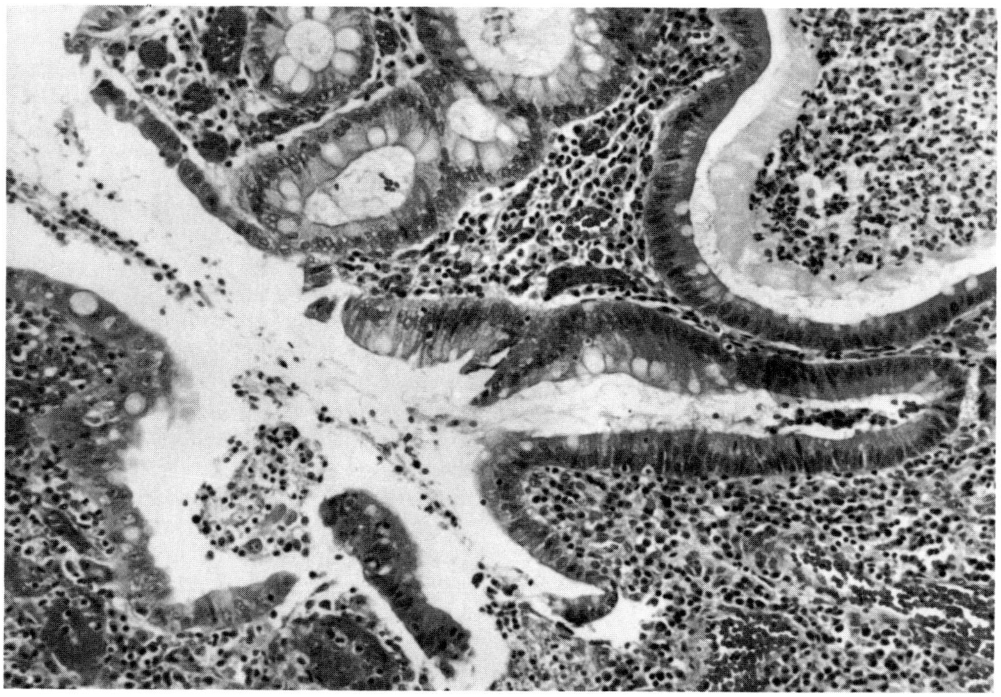

Figure 73–12. Active chronic ulcerative colitis. Crypt distortion, irregular regeneration, epithelial fragility, and chronic inflammation with a crypt abscess *(upper right)*. Hematoxylin-eosin stain, × 125.

phase. Crypt abnormalities are prominent with branching, an occasional villous pattern, and continued presence of mucus depletion. Reactive hyperplasia is visible at the base of the crypts.

3. Remission. Mucosal atrophy is present to a variable degree with continued crypt abnormalities. There is often crypt branching or loss of crypt parallelism. Goblet cells are easily seen, and Paneth cell metaplasia may be present. No active inflammation is visible.

Crohn's Disease

Crohn's disease has many clinical features that distinguish it from ulcerative colitis: extracolonic involvement, possible segmental distribution, presence of strictures or fistula, or both, presence of perianal disease, and differences in the endoscopic appearance. However, despite these differences, biopsies are often crucial to distinguish between Crohn's disease and ulcerative colitis. However, even with biopsies there are patients that are difficult to classify as having ulcerative colitis or Crohn's disease.

Granulomas are the hallmark of Crohn's disease in geographical areas where other causes of a granulomatous reaction in the gastrointestinal tract are rare. Granulomas are collections of epithelial cells that form loose or compact aggregates and contain multinucleated giant cells. These may be present in both the inflamed and normal mucosa. They are most often visualized in the submucosa.[78] The presence of granulomas in adults with Crohn's disease varies considerably among studies, from 0 to 30%,[28] with an incidence in children of 36% in one large study.[121] Some of the variability in the incidence of granulomas and Crohn's disease may be due to the different interpretation of what constitutes a granuloma.

Since Crohn's disease is a transmural disease, deep mucosal biopsies may reveal a mixed inflammatory infiltrate more prominent in the submucosa than the lamina propria.[64] Another important feature of Crohn's disease is the focal nature of the disease as compared to the diffuse pattern with ulcerative colitis. A colon biopsy in a patient with Crohn's disease is seen in Figure 73–13. The pathologist should receive multiple separately labeled tissue samples from both areas that appear both normal and those that appear abnormal.[64]

Unlike in ulcerative colitis, the goblet cell population in Crohn's disease is relatively maintained, with little crypt distortion except near areas of ulceration.[78] At an ulcer margin, crypt distortion, crypt abscesses, and epithelial cell degeneration and regeneration are often seen. Aphthoid ulcers and fissuring ulcers,[28, 64, 78] although rare, may be indicative of Crohn's disease. Aphthoid lesions are small areas of ulceration over lymphoid follicles; fissuring ulcers are ulcers that penetrate down into the submucosa.[78]

Hirschsprung's Disease

Hirschsprung's disease is a common disorder that occurs in approximately 1 out of 5,000 newborns.[122] Symptoms result from a lack of normal ganglion cells in the submucosa and myenteric plexuses, which causes poor relaxation in the affected bowel. In Hirschsprung's disease the ganglion cells are missing from the anus to a variable extent proximally. Most symptoms are present from early infancy and include delayed passage of meconium, abdominal distention, vomiting (often bilious), diarrhea, and poor weight gain. A variety of studies are available for diagnosis such as barium enema or anal manometry, but the rectal biopsy is the definitive means

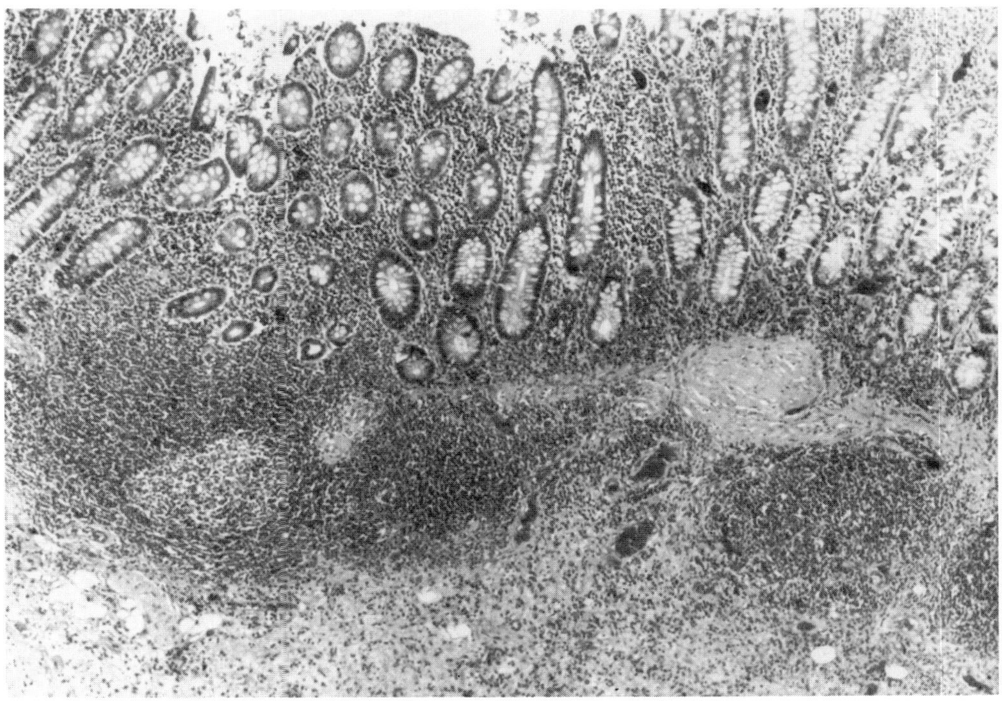

Figure 73–13. Crohn's disease of the colon. Chronic inflammation of the mucosa and deep submucosa with probable granulomas. The globlet cell population is relatively preserved. Hematoxylin-eosin stain, × 50.

of securing a diagnosis. Full-thickness surgical biopsies are most accurate, but screening for Hirschsprung's disease with a (Rubin) rectal suction biopsy is indicated in many cases (Fig. 73–14).

Normally there is a hypoganglionic zone extending up to 8 mm above the pectinate line in young children.[123] However, Campbell and Noblett[124] found that biopsies taken at 2 to 3 cm were less satisfactory than those taken at 3 to 4 cm above the pectinate line. They also recommended against the use of cleansing enemas prior to the biopsy, since these preparations can cause mucosal edema and result in less submucosa obtained at biopsy. Andrassy and associates[125] have accumulated a lot of experience using a rectal suction biopsy and have had only one misdiagnosis in 444 patients. They performed one biopsy at 2.5 cm and another at 3.5 cm in from the anal verge. The location of the two biopsies was high enough to avoid the normally hypoganglionic zone but low enough to avoid missing short segment involvement. In their study, the suction biopsy instrument knife blade was closed on insertion of the biopsy tube, then opened when the correct position was reached. Twenty centimeters of suction was applied for 20 seconds using the attached syringe before the knife blade was closed. Placing a finger gently in the anal canal sometimes helped the biopsy port contact the mucosa. The patients experienced no significant complications other than a mild transient bleeding.[125] However, there have been reports of serious complications such as perforations, bleeding requiring transfusion, peripheral limb gangrene, and even death.[126, 127]

The biopsies are examined normally under hematoxylin and eosin for the absence of submucosal ganglion cells and the presence of abnormally large nerve trunks in the aganglionic segment. Up to 50 to 100 sections may be needed to ensure accuracy of the diagnosis.[122] Mucosal biopsy staining for acetylcholinesterase may help confirm the diagnosis of Hirschsprung's disease.[128]

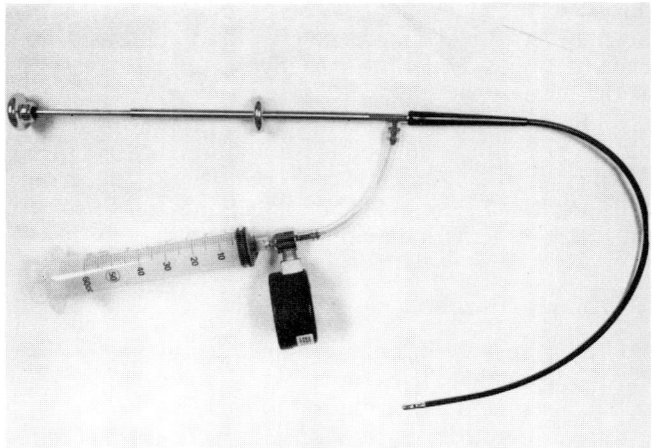

Figure 73–14. Rectal suction biopsy tube.

Colonic Polyps

Colonic polyps are a common cause of gastrointestinal bleeding in children.[129–131] It is estimated that as many as 1% of children have juvenile polyps. Besides bleeding, other presenting symptoms can include abdominal pain, rectal prolapse of the polyp, or occasionally intestinal obstruction. One study showed that 33% of patients had an iron-deficiency anemia.[131] Most children present with symptoms between 2 and 9 years of age, but the polyps have been found as early as 3 months of age.[131] Most juvenile polyps, 74 to 85%, are distal to the splenic flexure.[129–131] Up to 53% of the children may have multiple polyps.[130]

Until recently, all juvenile polyps were considered benign except for the local gastrointestinal symptoms. However, over the past several years there have been numerous reports of individuals with familial or nonfamilial generalized juvenile polyposis,[132–135] juvenile polyposis coli,[136] and even single juvenile polyps[137] with simultaneous or subsequent development of adenomas or adenocarcinoma. With generalized juvenile polyps there may also be a risk of gastrointestinal carcinoma of the stomach, duodenum, or pancreas.[133] Figures 73–15 and 73–16 show the microscopic features of a juvenile and adenomatous polyp, respectively.

A large study of 87 patients with juvenile polyposis was conducted by Jass and coworkers.[135] They found that 18 of 87 patients (20%) developed colorectal cancer at a mean age of 34 years, with the youngest only 15 years. The outcome was generally poor. Apparently 16% of the polyps removed had a multilobulated or villous configuration. Of these, 47% had dysplastic features, and only 9% of the typical juvenile polyps showed mild to moderate dysplasia. In addition, of the 1,032 polyps removed, 21 were adenomas. From their data, Jass and associates formulated a working definition to classify patients at risk. It was recommended that those with (1) greater than five juvenile polyps in the colon, (2) generalized gastrointestinal juvenile polyps, or (3) any number of juvenile polyps with a family history of juvenile polyposis undergo regular colonic surveillance to remove polyps and screen for early carcinoma.

Recommendations for juvenile polyposis coli are not as clear. From the study by Jass and colleagues,[135] it was not possible to separate patients with just colonic involvement from those with generalized polyposis. However, reports exist for the development of adenomatous changes and even adenocarcinoma with juvenile polyposis coli, although the risk is not clearly defined.[136, 138, 139]

The presence of five or fewer juvenile polyps in children cannot be assumed to be always associated with benign disease. Mazier and associates found that solitary adenomas were found in 5.2% of their patients less than 20 years of age with polyps, and solitary adenomas counted for 3.4% of all the polyps found in children less than 10 years of age.[140] In their study, all patients with any type of polyposis syndrome were eliminated from the study to eliminate any bias. Seven percent of the patients with polyps reported by Cynamon and coworkers had adenomatous features when patients with familial polyposis coli were excluded.[131] These risks support

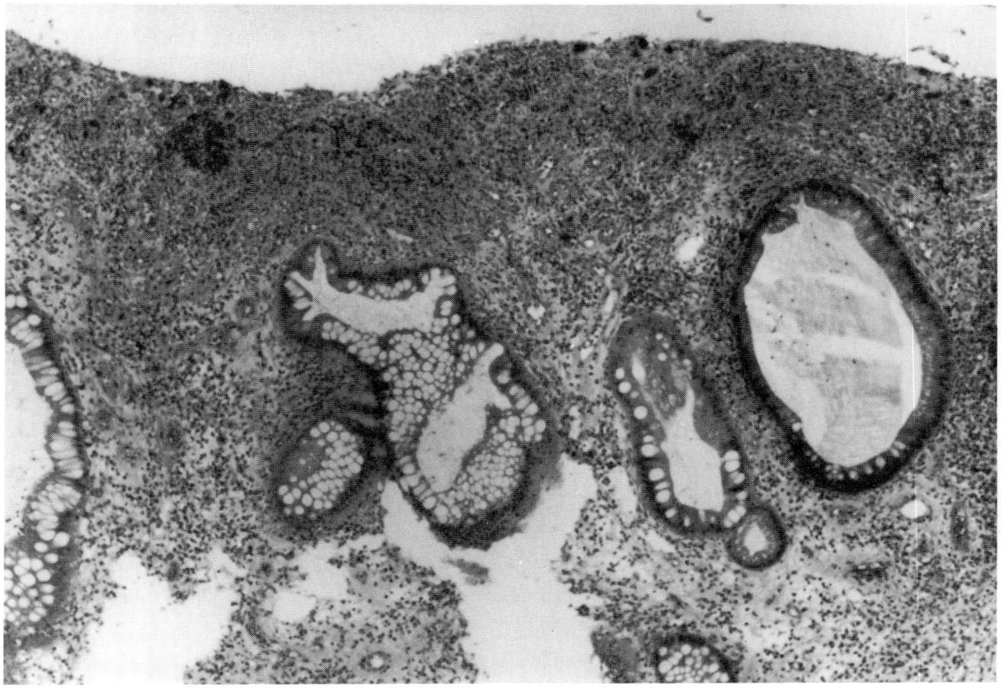

Figure 73–15. Juvenile polyp. The polyp is composed of numerous glands of varying size in a prominent stroma composed of numerous blood vessels and different cell types. There is no atypia seen in the epithelial cells. The surface is ulcerated. Hematoxylin-eosin stain, × 50.

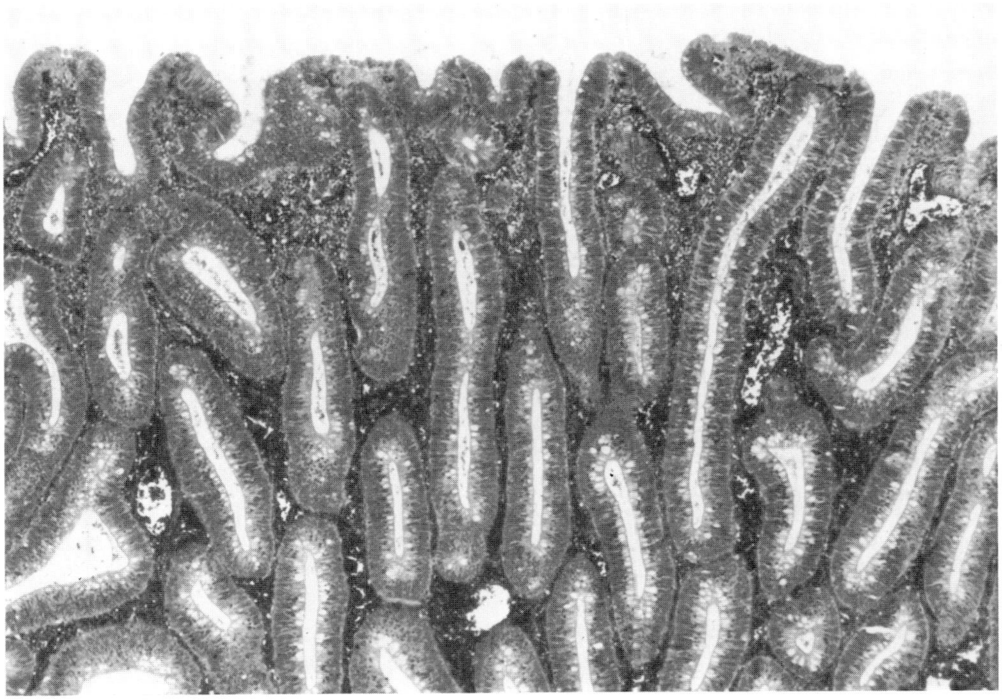

Figure 73–16. Adenomatous polyp. There is an increase in glands with crowding of the epithelial cells, significant loss of goblet cell mucosa, and nuclear atypia. The uniformity of gland size and gland lining thickness is characteristic. Hematoxylin-eosin stain, × 50.

the careful and aggressive evaluation of patients with suspected polyps. Because of the frequent proximal presence of polyps, a full colonoscopy is needed for adequate screening and removal. If more than five polyps are found or if adenomatous changes are present, frequent follow-up exams are needed. If five or fewer juvenile polyps are found and removed, the literature does not support aggressive follow-up at this time. However, if symptoms of rectal bleeding recur or there is evidence of iron deficiency with its potential risks, reevaluation should be undertaken.

ACKNOWLEDGMENT

The authors thank their secretary, Phyllis Scoz, and the typists in the word-processing department for their dedication and their patience with the many revisions.

REFERENCES

1. Wood IJ, Doig RK, Motteram R, et al: Gastric biopsy: Report on first five biopsies using a new flexible gastric biopsy. Lancet 1949; 270:1–18.
2. Shiner M: Jejunal-biopsy tube. Lancet 1956; 1:85.
3. Branborg LL, Rubin CE, Quinton WC: A multi-purpose instrument for suction biopsy of the esophagus, stomach, small bowel, and colon. Gastroenterology 1959; 37:1–16.
4. Crosby WH, Kugler HW: Intraluminal biopsy of the small intestine: The intestinal biopsy capsule. Am J Dig Dis 1959; 2:236–241.
5. Carey JB: A simplified gastrointestinal biopsy capsule. Gastroenterology 1964; 46:550–557.
6. Partin JC, Schubert WK: Precautionary note on the use of the intestinal biopsy capsule in infants and emaciated children. N Engl J Med 1966; 274:94–95.
7. Ament MZ, Rubin CE: An infant multipurpose biopsy tube. Gastroenterology 1973; 65:205–209.
8. Lindscheer WG, Abele JE: A new directable small bowel biopsy device. Gastroenterology 1976; 71:575–576.
9. Ferry GD, Bending DW: Peroral small bowel biopsies in infants and children using a directable biopsy instrument. Dig Dis Sci 1981; 80:938–941.
10. Vanderhoof JA, Hunt LI, Antonson DL: Rapid biopsy procedures for small intestinal biopsy in infants and children. Gastroenterology 1981; 80:938–941.
11. Sullivan PB, Phillips MB, Neale G: Endoscopic capsule biopsy of the small intestine. J Pediatr Gastroenterol Nutr 1988; 7:544–547.
12. Levy N, Sterner E: Endoscopic jejunal biopsy with the Crosby capsule. Br Med J 1984; 288:1914–1915.
13. Quak SH: Endoscopic capsule biopsy of the small intestine. J Pediatr Gastroenterol Nutr 1989; 8:276–277.
14. Maksimak M: A rapid safe small bowel biopsy technique in children. Gastrointest Endosc 1991; 37:358–361.
15. Greene HL, Rosenwing NS, Lufkin EG, et al: Biopsy of the small intestine with a Crosby-Kugler capsule. Dig Dis 1974; 19:189–198.
16. Kauder E, Bayless T: Peroral intestinal biopsy in children: A technique. Am J Dis Child 1964; 107:582–585.
17. Oderda G, Ansaldi N: Comparison of suction capsule and endoscopic biopsy of the small bowel mucosa. Gastrointest Endosc 1983; 33:265–266.
18. Sullivan PB, Phillips MB, Neale G: Endoscopic capsule biopsy of the small intestine. J Pediatr Gastroenterol Nutr 1988; 7:544–547.
19. Mee AS, Burke M, Vallon AG, et al: Small bowel biopsy for malabsorption: Comparison of the diagnostic adequacy of endoscopic forceps and capsule biopsy specimens. Br Med J 1985; 29:769–772.
20. Barakat MH, Ali SM, Badawi AR, et al: Peroral endoscopic duodenal biopsy in infants and children. Acta Pediatr Scand 1983; 72:563–569.
21. Korn ER, Foroozin P: Endoscopic biopsies of normal duodenum mucosa. Gastrointest Endosc 1974; 21:51–54.
22. Barkin JS, Schonfeld W, Thomsen S, et al: Enteroscopy and small bowel biopsy—an improved technique for the diagnosis of small bowel disease. Gastrointest Endosc 1985; 31:215–217.
23. Steffes CP, Sugawa C, Wilson RF, et al: Oxygen saturation monitoring during endoscopy. Surg Endosc 1990; 4:175–178.
24. Salter RH, Girdwood TG: Peroral jejunal biopsy with Watson capsule and Scott-Harden duodenal intubation tube. Lancet 1983; 2:1460.
25. Law RL: Guide wire manipulation of Crosby jejunal biopsy capsule under fluoroscopic control. Br Med J 1984; 288:286–287.
26. Make M: Guide wire manipulation of Crosby jejunal biopsy capsule. Br Med J 1984; 288:862–863.
27. Christir DL, Ament ME: A double-blind cross-over study of metoclopramide versus placebo for facilitating passage of multipurpose biopsy tube. Gastroenterology 1976; 70:726–728.
28. Walker-Smith JA, Phillips AD, Richman PI: Intestinal biopsy. *In* Walker WA, Durie PR, Hamilton JR, et al, eds: Pediatric Gastrointestinal Disease: Pathophysiology, Diagnosis, Management. Philadelphia, BC Decker, 1991, pp 1307–1323.
29. Barbezat GO, Wright JP: The use of domperidone to speed up the time taken for jejunal biopsy. SA Med J 1983; 64:626–627.
30. DiLorenzo C, Lachman R, Hyman PE: Intravenous erythromycin for post pyloric intubation. J Pediatr Gastroenterol Nutr 1990; 11:45–47.
31. Scott BB, Jenkins D: Endoscopic small intestinal biopsy. Gastrointest Endosc 1981; 27:162–167.
32. Kirberg A, Latorre JJ, Hartard ME: Endoscopic small intestinal biopsy in infants and children: Its usefulness in the diagnosis of celiac disease and other enteropathies. J Pediatr Gastroenterol Nutr 1989; 9:178–181.
33. Dandalides SM, Carey LUD, Petras R, et al: Endoscopic small bowel mucosal biopsy: A controlled trial evaluating forceps size and biopsy location in the diagnosis of normal and abnormal mucosal architecture. Gastrointest Endosc 1989; 35:197–200.
34. Cooper HS, Yogeshwar D, Gourley WK, et al: Proceedings of the 1988 subspecialty conference on gastrointestinal pathology at the USCAP: Diagnostic nonproblems in gastrointestinal biopsy pathology. Mod Pathol 1989; 2:244–259.
35. Lembcke B, Schneider, Lankish PG: How safe is small bowel biopsy? Endoscopy 1986; 18:80–83.
36. Schwachman H, Khaw TT, Antonowicz I: Diagnosis and treatment: Peroral intestinal biopsy. Pediatrics 1969; 43:460–462.
37. McDonald WG: Perforation and hemorrhage after gastrointestinal mucosal biopsy in a child. Gastroenterology 1966; 151:390–392.
38. Mullinger M, Wood BJ, Kliman MR, et al: Intramural hematoma of the duodenum: An unusual complication of small bowel biopsy. J Pediatr 1971; 78:323–326.
39. Tobin JJ, Schlang HA, James DR: Intramural hematoma of the duodenum associated with peroral small bowel biopsy. JAMA 1966; 198:787–789.
40. Ghishan FK, Werner M, Vieira P, et al: Intramural duodenal hematoma: An unusual complication of endoscopic small bowel biopsy. Am J Gastroenterol 1987; 82:368–370.
41. Bonamico M, Roggini M, Pierro A, et al: Superior mesenteric artery syndrome: An unusual cause of Watson biopsy capsule retention. J Pediatr Gastroenterol 1985; 4:146–147.
42. Gibbs DD, Keynes WM, Chir M: Perforation of a duodenal diverticulum by peroral suction. Gastroenterology 1963; 44:685–688.
43. Clarke SW: Jejunal perforation with the Crosby capsule. Lancet 1964; 2:727–728.
44. Variend S, Phillips AD, Walker-Smith JA: The small intestinal mucosal biopsy in childhood. Perspec Pediatr Pathol 1984; 1:57–78.
45. Lee JH, Griffiths WJ, Zantout I, et al: Adequacy of endoscopic biopsy specimens for disaccharidase assays. Dig Dis 1978; 23:1129–1131.
46. Heitlinger LA, Rossi TM, Lee P, et al: Human intestinal disaccharidase activities: Correlation with age, biopsy technique and degree of villous atrophy. J Pediatr Gastroenterol Nutr 1991; 12:204–208.

47. Whitington PF, Whitington GL: Eosinophilic gastroenteropathy in childhood. J Pediatr Gastroenterol Nutr 1988; 7:379–385.
48. Phillips AD, Rice SJ, France NE, et al: Small intestinal intraepithelial lymphocyte levels in cow's milk protein intolerance. Gut 1979; 20:509–512.
49. Ferguson A, Murray D: Quantitation of intraepithelial lymphocytes in human jejunum. Gut 1971; 12:988–994.
50. Mavromichalis J, Bruetin MJ, McNeish AJ, et al: Evaluation of intraepithelial lymphocyte count in the jejunum in childhood enteropathies. Gut 1976; 17:600–603.
51. Katz AJ, Grand RJ: All that flattens is not "sprue." Gastroenterology 1970; 76:375–377.
52. Gillberg R, Ahren C: Coeliac disease diagnosed by means of duodenoscopy and endoscopic duodenal biopsy. Scand J Gastroenterol 1977; 12:911–916.
53. Perera DR, Weinstein MW, Rubin CE: Small intestinal biopsy. Hum Pathol 1975; 6:157–217.
54. Meeuwisse GA: Diagnostic criteria in coeliac disease. Acta Paediatr Scand 1970; 59:461–463.
55. Yardley JH, Bayless TM, Norton JH, et al: Celiac disease. A study of jejunal epithelium before and after a gluten challenge. N Engl J Med 1962; 267:1173–1179.
56. Manuel PD, Walker-Smith JA, France NE: Patchy enteropathy in childhood. Gut 1979; 20:211–215.
57. Bahna SL, Heiner DC: Allergies to Milk. New York, Grune and Stratton, 1980.
58. Walker-Smith JA: Milk intolerance in children. Clin Allergy 1986; 16:183–190.
59. Salazar de Sousa J, da Silva A, Pereira MV, et al: Cow's milk protein-sensitive enteropathy: Number and timing of biopsies for diagnosis. J Pediatr Gastroenterol Nutr 1986; 5:207–209.
60. Kuitunen P, Visakorpi JK, Savilahti E, et al: Malabsorption syndrome with cow's milk intolerance: Clinical findings and course in 54 cases. Arch Dis Child 1975; 50:351–356.
61. Verkasalo M, Kuitunen P, Savilahti E, et al: Changing pattern of cow's milk intolerance. Acta Paediatr Scand 1981; 70:289–295.
62. Phillips AD, Rice SJ, Frances NE, et al: Changing pattern of cow's milk intolerance. Acta Paediatr Scand 1981; 70:289–295.
63. Katz AJ, Twarog FJ, Zeiger RS, et al: Milk-sensitive and eosinophilic gastroenteropathy: Similar clinical features with contrasting mechanisms and clinical course. J Allergy Clin Immunol 1984; 74:72–78.
64. Whitehead R, Livolsi V: Mucosal biopsy of the gastrointestinal Tract. 4th ed. Philadelphia, WB Saunders, 1990.
65. Goldman H, Provjansky R: Allergic proctitis and gastroenteritis in children. Am J Surg Pathol 1986; 10:75–86.
66. Walker WA, Winter H, Goldman H: Food sensitivity: Pathophysiology and practical approaches to diagnosis and treatment. Pediatric GI Nutr News 1987; 1:1–5.
67. Katz AJ, Goldman H, Grand RJ: Gastric mucosal biopsy in eosinophilic (allergic) gastroenteritis. Gastroenterology 1977; 73:705–709.
68. Ament ME, Rubin CE: Relation of giardiasis to abnormal intestinal structure and junction in gastrointestinal immunodeficiency syndrome. Gastroenterology 1972; 62:216–226.
69. Ament ME, Ochs HD, Davis SD: Structional junction of the gastrointestinal tract in primary immunodeficiency syndromes—A study of 39 patients. Medicine 1973; 52:227–248.
70. Hargrove CB, Ulshen MH, Shub MD: Upper gastrointestinal endoscopy in infants. Diagnostic usefulness and safety. Pediatrics 1984; 74:828–831.
71. Ament ME, Christie DL: Upper gastrointestinal fiberoptic endoscopy in pediatric patients. Gastroenterology 1977; 72:1244–1248.
72. Whitington PF, Orenstein SR: Manometric guidance in suction biopsy of the esophagus in children. J Pediatr Gastroenterol Nutr 1984; 3:535–538.
73. Ismail-Beigi F, Pope CE: Distribution of the histological changes of gastroesophageal reflux in the distal esophagus of man. Gastroenterology 1974; 66:1109–1113.
74. Weinstein WM, Bogoch ER, Bowes KL: The normal human esophageal mucosa: A histological reappraisal. Gastroenterology 1975; 68:40–44.
75. Biller JA, Winter HS, Gland RJ, et al: Are endoscopic changes predictive of histologic esophagitis in children? J Pediatr 1983; 103:215–218.
76. Sjogren RW Jr, Johnson LF: Barrett's esophagus: A review. Am J Med 1983; 74:313–321.
77. Hemstreet MPB, Reynolds DW, Meadows J: Oesophagitis—a complication of inhaled steroid therapy. Clin Allergy 1980; 10:733–738.
78. Fenoglio-Preiser CM, Lantz PE, Listrom MB, et al: Gastrointestinal Pathology—An Atlas and Text. New York, Raven Press, 1989.
79. Winchenbach CL, Fink SM, Berwick UW, et al: Significant hemorrhage as a complication of hydraulic suction biopsy of the esophagus. Am J Gastroenterol 1982; 77:897–898.
80. Knuff TE, Benjamin SB, Worsham GF, et al: Histologic evaluation of chronic gastroesophageal reflux. Dig Dis Sci 1984; 29:194–201.
81. Black DD, Haggitt RC, Orenstein SR, et al: Esophagitis in infants. Gastroenterology 1990; 98:1408–1414.
82. Collins BJ, Elliott H, Sloan JM, et al: Oesophageal histology in reflux oesophagitis. J Clin Pathol 1985; 38:1265–1272.
83. Shub MD, Ulshen MH, Hargrove CB, et al: Esophagitis: A frequent consequence of gastroesophageal reflux in infancy. J Pediatr 1985; 107:881–884.
84. Brown LF, Goldman H, Antonioli DA: Intraepithelial eosinophils in endoscopic biopsies of adults with reflux esophagitis. Am J Surg Pathol 1984; 8:899–905.
85. Winter HS, Madara JL, Stafford RJ, et al: Intraepithelial eosinophils: A new diagnostic criterion for reflux esophagitis. Gastroenterology 1982; 83:818–823.
86. Dahms BB, Rothstein FC: Mucosal biopsy of the esophagus in children. Perspect Pediatr Pathol 1987; 11:97–123.
87. Burgess JN, Payne WS, Anderson HA, et al: Barrett's esophagus. Mayo Clin Proc 1971; 46:728–734.
88. Hassall E, Weinstein WM, Ament ME: Barrett's esophagus in children. Gastroenterology 1985; 89:1331–1337.
89. Naef AP, Savary M, Ozzello L: Columnar lined lower esophagus in acquired lesion with malignant predisposition. J Thorac Cardiovasc Surg 1975; 20:826–835.
90. Meyer W, Vollman F, Bar W: Barrett's esophagus following total gastrectomy: A contribution to its pathogenesis. Endoscopy 1979; 2:121–126.
91. Thompson JJ, Zinsser KR, Enterline HT: Esophageal cancer and the premalignant changes of esophageal disease. *In* Cohen S, Soloway RD, eds: Diseases of the Esophagus. New York, Churchill Livingstone, 1982, p 293.
92. Hawe A, Payne WS, Weiland LH, et al: Adenocarcinoma in the columnar epithelial lined lower (Barrett) esophagus. Thorax 1973; 28:511–514.
93. Adler RH: The lower esophagus lined by columnar epithelian: Its association with hiatal hernia, ulcer structure and tumor. J Thorac Cardiovasc Surg 1963; 45:13–34.
94. Mangla JC: Barrett's esophagus. An old entity rediscovered. J Clin Gastroenterol 1981; 3:347–356.
95. Feiden W, Borchard F, Bürrig KF, et al: Herpes oesophagitis. Virchows Arch 1984; 404:167–176.
96. Warren JR, Marshall BJ: Unidentified curved bacilli in gastric epithelium with active chronic gastritis. Lancet 1983; 1:1273–1275.
97. Jones DM, Lessells AM, Eldridge J: *Campylobacter*-like organisms in the gastric mucosa: Culture, histological and serological studies. J Clin Pathol 1984; 37:1002–1006.
98. Price AB, Levi J, Dolby JM, et al: *Campylobacter pyloridis* in peptic ulcer disease: Microbiology, pathology and scanning electron microscopy. Gut 1985; 26:1183–1188.
99. Drumm B, Sherman P, Cutz E, et al: Association of *Campylobacter pylori* on the gastric mucosa with antral gastritis in children. N Engl J Med 1987; 316:1557–1561.
100. Eastham EJ, Elliott TSJ, Berkeley D, et al: *Campylobacter pylori* infection in children. J Infection 1988; 16:77–79.
101. Drumm B, Sherman P, Chiasson D, et al: Treatment of *Campylobacter pylori*-associated antral gastritis in children with bismuth subsalicylate and ampicillin. J Pediatr 1988; 113:908–912.
102. Kilbridge P, Dahms BB, Czinn SJ: *Campylobacter pylori*-associated gastritis and peptic ulcer disease in children. Am J Dis Child 1988; 142:1149–1152.

103. Glassman MS, Schwarz SM, Medow MS, et al: *Campylobacter pylori*-related gastrointestinal disease in children: Incidence and clinical findings. Dig Dis Sci 1989; 34:1501–1504.
104. Glassman MS, Dallal S, Berezin SH, et al: *Helicobacter pylori*-related gastroduodenal disease in children: Diagnostic utility of enzyme-linked immunoabsorbent assay. Dig Dis Sci 1990; 35:993–997.
105. Bujanover Y, Konickoff F, Baratz M: Nodular gastritis and *Helicobacter pylori*. J Pediatr Gastroenterol Nutr 1990; 11:41–44.
106. Dooley CP, Cohen H, Fitzgibbons PL: Prevalence of *Helicobacter pylori* infection and histologic gastritis in asymptomatic persons. N Engl J Med 1989; 321:1562–1566.
107. Drumm B: *Helicobacter pylori*. Arch Dis Child 1990; 65:1278–1282.
108. Queiroz DMM, Rocha GA, Mendes EN, et al: Differences in distribution and severity of *Helicobacter pylori* gastritis in children and adults with duodenal ulcer disease. J Pediatr Gastroenterol Nutr 1991; 12:178–181.
109. Odera G, Dell-olio D, Morra I, et al: *Campylobacter pyloric* gastritis: Long-term results of treatment with amoxicillin. Arch Dis Child 1989; 64:326–329.
110. Montgomery EA, Martin DF, Peura DA: Rapid diagnosis of *Campylobacter pylori* by Gram's stain. Am J Clin Pathol 1988; 90:606–609.
111. Börsch G, Schmidt G, Wegener M, et al: *Campylobacter pylori*: Prospective analysis of clinical and histological factors associated with colonization of the upper gastrointestinal tract. Eur J Clin Invest 1988; 18:133–138.
112. Nedenskov-Sorengen P, Bjorneklett A, Fausa O, et al: *Campylobacter pylori* infection and its relation to chronic gastritis. Scand J Gastroenterol 1988; 23:867–874.
113. Veereman-Wauters G, Ferrell L, Heyman M: Trends in *Campylobacter pylori* in pediatric and adult antral biopsies. West J Med 1984; 151:406–409.
114. Drumm B, O'Brien A, Cutz E, et al: *Campylobacter pyloridis*–associated primary gastritis in children. Pediatrics 1987; 80:192–195.
115. Gleason WA, Goldstein PD, Shatz BA, et al: Colonoscopic removal of juvenile colonic polyps. J Pediatr Surg 1975; 12:519–521.
116. Cadranel S, Rodesch P, Peeters JP, et al: Fiberendoscopy of the gastrointestinal tract in children. Am J Dis Child 1977; 131:41–45.
117. Goldman H, Antonioli DA: Mucosal biopsy of the rectum, colon and distal ileum. Hum Pathol 1982; 13:981–1012.
118. Surawicz CM, Belic L: Rectal biopsy helps to distinguish acute self limited colitis from idiopathic inflammatory bowel disease. Gastroenterology 1984; 86:104–113.
119. Sutphin JL, Grand RJ, Flores A, et al: *C. difficile*–associated chronic diarrhea in pediatrics. Am J Dis Child 1983; 137:275–278.
120. Price AB, Davies DR: Pseudomembraneous colitis. J Clin Pathol 1977; 30:112.
121. Chang SKF, Blackshaw AJ, Boyle J, et al: Histological diagnosis of chronic inflammatory bowel disease in childhood. Gut 1985; 26:55–59.
122. Boley SJ, Dinari G, Cohen MI: Hirschsprung's disease in the newborn. Clin Perinatol 1978; 5:45–60.
123. Aldridge RT, Campbell PE: Ganglion cell distribution in the normal rectum and anal canal: A basis for the diagnosis of Hirschsprung's disease by anorectal biopsy. J Pediatr Surg 1968; 3:475–489.
124. Campbell PE, Noblett HR: Experience with rectal suction biopsy in the diagnosis of Hirschsprung's disease. J Pediatr Surg 1969; 4:410–415.
125. Andrassy RJ, Isaacs H, Weitzman JJ, et al: Rectal suction biopsy for the diagnosis of Hirschsprung's disease. Ann Surg 1981; 193:419–424.
126. Rees BI, Azmy A, Nigam M, et al: Complications of rectal suction biopsy. J Pediatr Surg 1983; 18:273–275.
127. Jani BR, Brereton RJ, Dillon MJ: Peripheral limb gangrene following rectal biopsy. Clin Pediatr 1989; 28:585–588.
128. Huntley CC, Shaffner L, Challa VR, et al: Histochemical diagnosis of Hirschsprung's disease. Pediatrics 1982; 69:755–761.
129. Maksimak M: Childhood colonic polyps—diagnostic methods (abstract). Annual meeting, North American Society for Pediatric Gastroenterology and Nutrition, 1989.
130. Mestre JR: The changing pattern of juvenile polyps. Am J Gastroenterol 1986; 81:312–314.
131. Cynamon HA, Milor DE, Andres JM: Diagnosis and management of colonic polyps in children. J Pediatr 1989; 114:593–596.
132. Goodman ZD, Yardley JH, Milligan FD: Pathogenesis of colonic polyps—multiple juvenile polyps. Cancer 1979; 43:1906–1913.
133. Stemper TJ, Kent TH, Summers RW: Juvenile polyps and gastrointestinal carcinoma. Ann Int Med 1975; 83:639–646.
134. Longo WR, Touloukian JR, West B, et al: Malignant potential of juvenile polyposis coli. Dis Colon Rectum 1990; 33:980–984.
135. Jass JR, Williams CB, Bussey HJR, et al: Juvenile polyposis—a precancerous condition. Histopathology 1988; 13:619–630.
136. Tolia V, Chang CH: Adenomatous polyp in a four-year-old child. J Pediatr Gastroenterol Nutr 1990; 10:262–264.
137. Liu TH, Chen MC, Tseng HC, et al: Malignant change of juvenile polyp of colon. Clin Med J 1978; 4:434–439.
138. Mills SE, Fechner RE: Unusual adenomatous polyps in juvenile polyposis coli. Am J Surg Pathol 1982; 6:177–183.
139. Rosen P, Baratz M: Familial juvenile colonic polyposis with associated colon cancer. Cancer 1982; 49:1500–1503.
140. Mazier WP, Mackeigan JM, Billingham RP, et al: Juvenile polyps of the colon and rectum. Surg Gynecol Obstet 1982; 154:829–832.

Chapter 74

Esophagogastro-duodenoscopy, Colonoscopy, and Related Techniques

ROBERT WYLLIE and MARSHA KAY

The earliest gastrointestinal endoscopies were performed in the late 1880s using rigid instruments, looking initially at the esophagus and rectum. The semiflexible gastroscope was developed in the early 1930s by Schindler and Wolf utilizing a series of short focal-length lenses and a semiflexible tube.[1] Fiberoptic endoscopes, which were popularized in the late 1960s and early 1970s, are based on the principle of total internal reflection of light along cylindrical glass rods coated with a material of low refractive index. As light enters one end and strikes the interface between the highly refractive glass and the low refractive index of the glass coating, it is advanced by a series of internal reflections and emitted at the opposite end of the rod. Its position is maintained by maintaining the same relative position of each rod at both ends of the endoscope.[2] With the advent of fiberoptic endoscopes came the availability of both tip control and biopsy capability.[3] The first small-diameter instrument used for esophagogastroduodenoscopy (EGD) in a child was a fiberoptic bronchoscope.[4]

The development of the colonoscope followed that of upper panendoscopes. Rigid proctoscopes were developed in the late 1800s, and fiberoptic techniques were adapted to visualize the sigmoid and descending colon in the 1960s. In the 1970s the colonoscope was lengthened with four-way tip deflection, allowing for modern-day colonoscopic techniques.[3]

Gastrocameras were used for still photographs in the late 1940s, but video endoscopy has only been developed over the last two decades, with the first mass-produced video instruments introduced in the 1980s.[5] Currently, video endoscopes are used for EGD, endoscopic retrograde cholangiopancreatography (ERCP), and colonoscopy. Because of the requirement for narrower instrument diameter with preserved optic clarity, dedicated pediatric video endoscopes have only recently become available.

Pediatric gastrointestinal endoscopists are able to perform most of the endoscopic techniques of their adult counterparts. At the same time, they are developing unique applications of these techniques for pediatric patients. The advantage of pediatric gastrointestinal endoscopists is familiarity not only with age-related physiology but also with the spectrum of disease in pediatric patients. The referring physician and endoscopist should be familiar with the risks and benefits of endoscopy and those clinical situations in infants and children in which it is most likely to be useful.

PERSONNEL

Specially trained pediatric endoscopy assistants are an important component of the endoscopy team. Procedure anxiety can be diminished by an assistant who has previously met the child and parent(s), explained the procedure, and greeted them in the endoscopy suite. The same person can then hold and reassure the child throughout the procedure.[6] A second assistant is often needed to help obtain and process tissue during the procedure and assist with other equipment.

Physicians performing endoscopy on infants and children should have completed a pediatric gastroenterology fellowship or have experience with pediatric gastrointestinal diseases and adequate training in pediatric endoscopy. Intravenous sedation should be used only by physicians competent in administration of drugs and resuscitation in children.

FACILITIES

Routine endoscopy in infants and children is typically performed in an outpatient setting using parenteral sedation. Occasionally it is necessary to perform endoscopy at the hospital bedside or in an operating room. The endoscopy room should be equipped with instruments to monitor blood pressure, pulse, and oxygen

Table 74–1. UPPER GASTROINTESTINAL ENDOSCOPES AND SMALL BOWEL ENTEROSCOPES

Scope Name	Field of View	Depth of Field (mm)	Outer Diameter (mm)	Range of Tip Bending (in degrees)	Working Length (mm)	Channel Diameter (mm)
Nonvideo						
GIF × Q20	100°	3–100	9.8	210°/90° (up/down) 100°/100° (right/left)	1,025	2.8
GIF × P20	100°	3–100	7.9	210°/90° (up/down)	1,025	2
× P10			7.8	100°/100° (right/left)	1,025	
GIF × 5.2	90°	3–50	5.2	180°/90° (up/down) 100°/100° (right/left)	580	2
GIF 1T 20	100°	3–100	11.3	210°/90° (up/down) 100°/100° (right/left)	1,000	3.7
Video						
GIF 100	120°		9.5	210°/90° (up/down) 100°/100° (right/left)	1,040	2.8
GIF 1T 100	120°		11.0	210°/190° (up/down) 100°/100° (right/left)	1,040	3.7
SB Enteroscope						
Push-type SIF 10	120°	5–100	11.3	180°/180° (up/down)	1,675	2.8
Push-type SIF 20L	120°	5–100	10.5		2,175	2.8
Sonde-type SIF SW	120°	5–50	5.4	160°/160° (right/left)	2,790	1

Table 74–2. COLONOSCOPES AND SIGMOIDOSCOPES

Scope Name	Field of View	Depth of Field (mm)	Outer Diameter (mm)	Range of Tip Bending Maximum Tip Bending*	Working Length (mm)	Channel Diameter (mm)
Nonvideo						
CF20L	120°	5–100	13 (15 w/hood)	180°/180° (up/down) 160°/160° (right/left)	1,680	3.2
CF2OI	120°	5–100	13 (15 w/hood)	180°/180° (up/down) 160°/160° (right/left)	1,330	3.2
CFP20L	120°	5–100	12.2 (13.5 w/hood)	180°/180° (up/down) 160°/160° (right/left)	1,680	3.2
CFP20I	120°	5–100	12.2 (13.5 w/hood)	180°/180° (up/down) 160°/160° (right/left)	1,330	3.2
PCF10/20	120°	3–100	11.3	180°/180° (up/down) 160°/160° (right/left)	1,330	2.8
CF1T20L	120°	5–100	14.3 (l6 w/hood)	180°/180° (up/down) 160°/160° (right/left)	1,680	4.2
CF1T20I	120°	5–100	14.3 (16 w/hood)	180°/180° (up/down) 160°/160° (right/left)	1,330	4.2
Video						
PCF100	140°	3–100	11.3	180°/180° (up/down) 160°/160° (right/left)	1,330	2.8
CF100L	140°	5–100	15.4	180°/180° (up/down) 160°/160° (right/left)	1,670	3.2
CF100I	140°	5–100	15.4	180°/180° (up/down) 160°/160° (right/left)	1,320	3.2
CF-1T100L	140°	5–100	15.4	180°/180° (up/down) 160°/160° (right/left)	1,670	4.2
CF-1T100I	140°	5–100	15.4	180°/180° (up/down) 160°/160° (right/left)	1,235	4.2
Sigmoidoscopes						
Nonvideo						
P20S	120°	5–100	12.2 (13.5 w/hood)	180°/180° (up/down) 160°/160° (right/left)	630	3.2
OSF35-2	100°	3–100	12.2	180°/180° (up/down) 160°/160° (right/left)	350	3.2
Video						
CF-100S	140°	5–100	15.4	180°/180° (up/down) 160°/160° (right/left)	620	3.2

*Maximum tip bending is 230° unless otherwise indicated.

saturation. Pediatric resuscitation equipment including emergency medications, intravenous fluids, appropriately sized endotracheal tubes and laryngoscopes, oxygen, and resuscitation bags should be available.

EQUIPMENT

There are three main types of upper endoscopes: fiberoptic endoscopes, video endoscopes, and passive enteroscopes (Tables 74–1 and 74–2). Upper gastrointestinal endoscopes may also be divided on the basis of their angle of viewing—either forward or side viewing. Currently, side-viewing endoscopes are used only for ERCP and will be discussed in that context.

The endoscope is composed of an eyepiece mounted on a control handle that is attached to an insertion tube containing several thousand fiberoptic light bundles (Fig. 74–1). The control section is attached via a universal cord to a light, water, suction, and electrical source. The eyepiece may be focused by turning it to the left or the right according to the observer's diopter. An ancillary eyepiece may be mounted on the focusing ring, but it reduces the brightness of the image seen by the endoscopist. On the control handle there are two large dials mounted on the right-hand side of the instrument (Fig. 74–2). The larger, more medial dial controls the up-down angulation of the instrument tip. Turning the wheel toward the endoscopist flexes the tip upward. The smaller, lateral dial controls the left or right angulation of the tip. Turning the wheel toward the endoscopist flexes the tip to the left. Lateral to each dial is a locking mechanism that increases the resistance to turning the dial. On the proximal shaft of the endoscope there are two valves. The more proximal one is for suction, and the distal one controls air and water. The endoscopist activates the suction through the endoscope by depressing the more proximal button. The length of suctioning is determined by the amount of time the button is depressed. Air is insufflated through the endoscope by lightly occluding the distal button. Firmly pushing down on the button provides a stream of water for irrigation through the endoscope. Further down on the endoscope is a channel with a biopsy valve, through which can be passed various instruments including biopsy forceps, cytology brushes, needles for sclerotherapy or injection, guide wires, coagulation probes, heater probes, polypectomy snares, or other instruments. The field can be manually irrigated by using a blunt-ended needle attached to a syringe and manually flushing the channel. The rate of irrigation that can be achieved by this method is greater than the rate achieved by occluding the button on the endoscope. If the air button does not function properly during endoscopy, air can also be injected with a syringe via this channel to avoid switching endoscopes in mid-procedure. At the tip of the endoscope are five openings: an air-water outlet (for lens cleaning), the objective lens, two light guides, and an instrument channel for suction and biopsy forceps (Fig. 74–3). Large-diameter therapeutic instruments may contain an auxiliary water channel or a second suction/forceps channel, or both. The tip of the endoscope has a certain degree of angulation possible in an up or down, right or left direction. The flexible portion of the endoscope is the "working length" of the instrument.

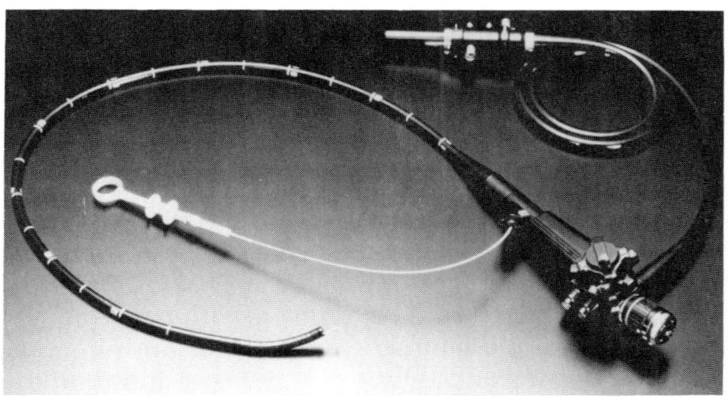

Figure 74–1. GIF × Q20 upper gastrointestinal fiberscope with biopsy forceps in biopsy channel. (Courtesy of Olympus Corporation.)

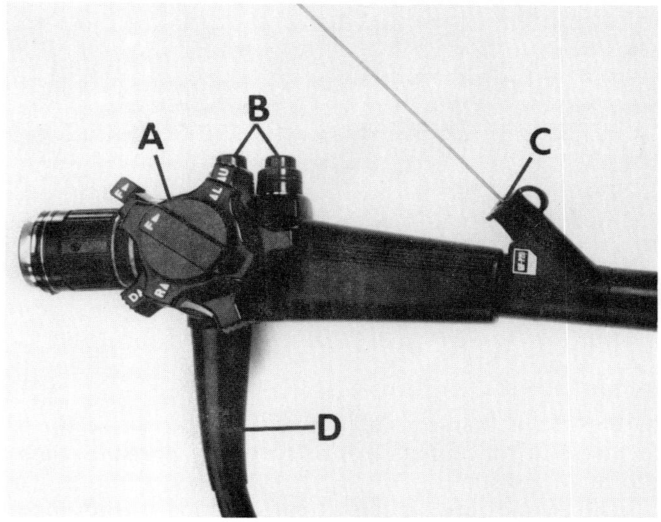

Figure 74–2. Control handle GIFP20 endoscope. *A,* Dials for directional control. *B,* Valves for suction and air/water. *C,* Biopsy channel. *D,* universal cord. (Courtesy of Olympus Corporation.)

The video endoscope represents an adaption of the fiberoptic instrument. Instead of an eyepiece, a sensing device in the instrument's distal tip transmits an image to a video processor for display on a television monitor[5] (Fig. 74–4). The control handle contains additional buttons to freeze or alter the image on the video screen. Parts or all of the procedure can be recorded for later review.

There are two main types of small bowel enteroscopes. The first is the push-type enteroscope, which represents a modification of the pediatric colonoscope with an increased working length (see Table 74–1). The second type of small bowel endoscope is the passive enteroscope, also known as the Sonde-type small intestinal fiberscope. It is of much smaller diameter than the push-type enteroscope and is a forward-viewing instru-

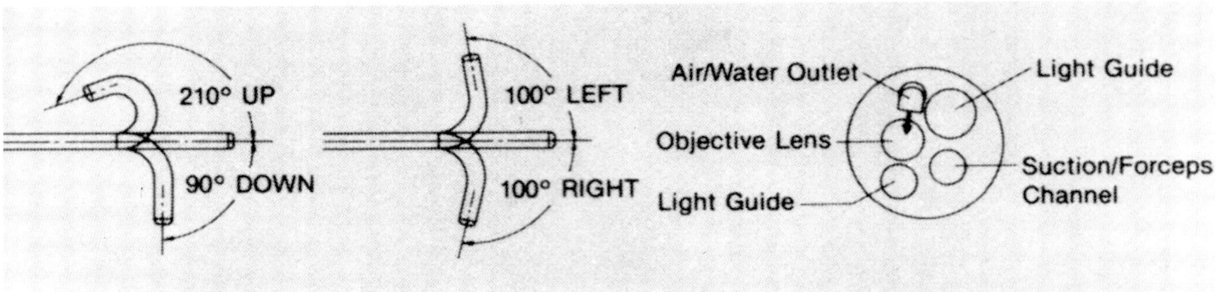

Figure 74–3. GIF × Q20 endoscope; degree of tip angulation and schematic of endoscope tip. (Courtesy of Olympus Corporation.)

ment with a balloon cuff located at the scope tip to facilitate advancement of the scope by peristalsis into the small intestine.

Colonscopes are similar in construction to the upper endoscopes with different diameters, instrument lengths, range of tip bending, and fields of view. Larger diameter instruments also have a hood at the distal end that aids in keeping the objective lens away from the mucosa.[7]

The most important issues related to pediatric endoscopy equipment are the diameter and length of the insertion tube, the degree of tip angulation, and the depth of field (see Tables 74–1 and 74–2). In term infants, the esophagus measures only 4 to 6 mm in diameter and 9 to 10 cm in length.[4] Some of the earliest EGDs were performed using small-diameter bronchoscopes with an insertion tube diameter of 5 mm. However, the tubes were too short to allow adequate visualization of the small bowel. Despite theoretical concerns of trauma, perforation, or airway compression, early pediatric endoscopists found that they could safely and effectively examine a neonate's digestive tract with an instrument of 7 mm in diameter without complication, due to distensibility of the esophagus. Newer gastrointestinal endoscopes, including forward- and side-viewing models, have a 5- to 6-mm outer diameter.

Colonoscopy in infants is usually performed with instruments designed for upper endoscopy because of their smaller diameter. Colonoscopy in normally developed children over 2 years of age can usually be performed with a colonoscope specifically designed for pediatric patients.

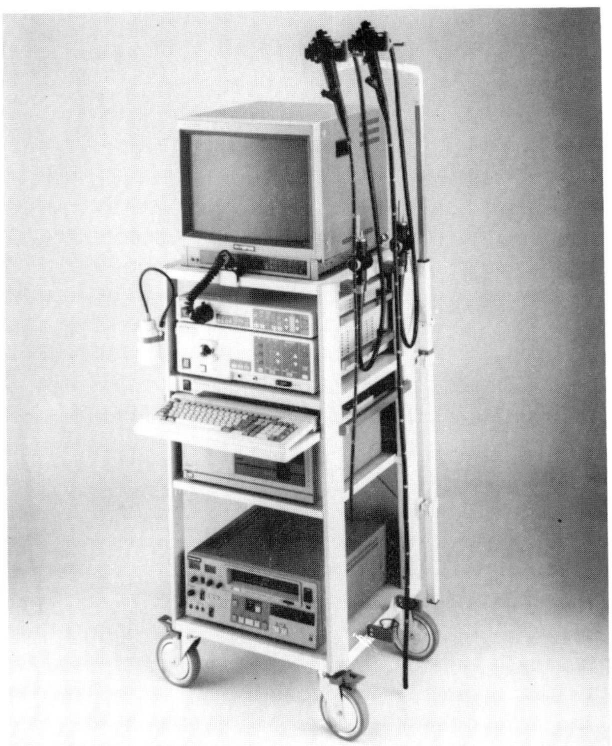

Figure 74–4. Video processor and power source for video endoscope. (Courtesy of Olympus Corporation.)

INDICATIONS

The indications for gastrointestinal endoscopy vary with the age of the patient. The need for endoscopy in neonates and infants is usually suggested by physical signs reported by parents or other observers and include vomiting, hematemesis, hematochezia, melena, hypotension, respiratory distress, abnormal posturing, or anemia. With toddlers and older children the history is of greater importance in identifying gastrointestinal disorders. The sensitivity of gastrointestinal endoscopy in establishing a diagnosis varies with the indication for the procedure (Table 74–3).

Esophagogastroduodenoscopy

The yield of upper endoscopic examination in pediatric patients differs with the age of the child and indication for the procedure. Chang and coworkers performed endoscopic examination in 38 infants less than 1 year of age. In 23 of the 27 infants (85%) with hematemesis, endoscopy demonstrated the source of bleeding. Endoscopy established the diagnosis in 27 of 38 infants overall, including 6 infants with normal upper gastrointestinal barium studies.[8] Similar results have been noted in other published series in infancy.[9, 10]

Ament and Christie reviewed their experience with 142 consecutive upper gastrointestinal endoscopies in children over a 33-month period.[11] Of the 36 patients

Table 74–3. INDICATIONS FOR ESOPHAGOGASTRODUODENOSCOPY AND COLONOSCOPY

Esophagogastroduodenoscopy
Acid peptic disease
Suspicion of mucosal inflammation (including infection); biopsy, brushing, and cytology examination
Acute epigastric or right upper quadrant pain
Hematemesis or melena
Dysphagia or odynophagia
Caustic ingestion or foreign body ingestion
Recurrent vomiting
Therapeutic intervention
- Cautery of bleeding lesion
- Stricture dilation
- Foreign body removal

Colonoscopy
Gastrointestinal hemorrhage
Chronic diarrhea
Suspected inflammatory bowel disease
Cancer surveillance
- Inflammatory bowel disease
- Polyposis syndromes

Therapeutic intervention
- Polyp removal
- Foreign body removal
- Decompression of toxic megacolon
- Dilation of stricture
- Cautery of bleeding lesion

who were endoscoped for hematemesis or melena, endoscopy identified the source in 28 of 36 (78%). Only one of three duodenal and one of five gastric ulcers identified by endoscopy were found by upper gastrointestinal x-ray. No source was identified in four patients (11.7%). Twelve of 31 (39%) patients with complaints of nausea, vomiting, dysphagia, odynophagia, or retrosternal pain who underwent endoscopy had esophagitis. Only one of 12 was diagnosed by simultaneous barium swallow.

Of the 66 patients who were studied for recurrent abdominal pain, a source was identified in 21 (32%). Four patients had gastric ulcers, eight had duodenal ulcers, four had gastritis, two had pancreatic rest, two had duodenitis, and one had Crohn's disease. Barium studies performed in all the patients identifed one of the four gastric ulcers, half of the duodenal ulcers, and none of the patients with gastritis. Forty-five patients had negative endoscopies. Seven patients in this group had upper gastrointestinal x-ray falsely suggestive of duodenal ulcer disease or pyloric channel inflammation.

Quak and colleagues recently reviewed their experience with 200 consecutive upper endoscopic examinations in children.[10] In patients presenting with hematemesis (mean age of 6.6 years), 21 of 29 (72%) had abnormal findings, and endoscopy was diagnostic in 45% of the patients with persistent vomiting. Ten of 26 (38%) patients endoscoped for acute abdominal pain had an abnormal endoscopy, and 82% of the patients who underwent endoscopy for chronic abdominal pain had a normal endoscopy. Younger patients with specific complaints appear to have an increased incidence of pathology on endoscopic examination.

Colonoscopy

The major indications for colonoscopy in infants and children include rectal bleeding, unexplained diarrhea, and abdominal pain with abnormal growth or weight loss. Prospective studies evaluating the efficacy of colonoscopy in children with rectal bleeding are not available, but retrospective series have been reported.[12–15] Quak and Prabhakaran evaluated 26 children passing blood from the rectum.[13] A source of bleeding was identified in 17, including 10 with colitis, five with polyps, and one each with lymphoid hyperplasia and a solitary sigmoid ulcer.

Colonoscopy is also performed to investigate abnormalities suspected on barium enema or small bowel follow-through. If inflammatory bowel disease is suspected, endoscopy can provide visual evidence of the nature and extent of disease, and biopsies obtained at the time of the procedure may define the nature of the underlying inflammation.[16, 17] In children with suspected polyps, colonoscopy provides a method of diagnosis and therapy with endoscopic removal of the lesions. In diseases associated with an increased rate of malignancy, such as ulcerative colitis or familial polyposis, colonoscopic surveillance for dysplastic changes is usually performed at regular intervals.[18, 19] Visualization and biopsy of the terminal ileum during colonoscopy is useful in the diagnosis of Crohn's disease, infectious ileitis, and lymphonodular hyperplasia.[20, 21] In some infections such as ileocecal tuberculosis, colonic schistosomiasis, and amebiasis, stool cultures are usually negative but the organisms can be identified on biopsy specimens or cytologic brushing.[22–25] Colonoscopy is usually not indicated in children complaining of chronic abdominal pain with unremarkable physical examinations and laboratory studies.

Indications for therapeutic colonoscopy include polypectomy, vascular ablation, and colonic decompression in toxic megacolon.[26–28] Colonic strictures can also be dilated through the endoscope using balloon dilators. Intussusception has been identified and reduced during colonoscopy, but barium enema or air-contrast reduction remains the procedure of choice.[29–32] Technically advanced therapeutic endoscopic procedures should be undertaken only by those with adequate experience.

CONTRAINDICATIONS

Absolute contraindications to gastrointestinal endoscopy include suspected perforation of the intestine and peritonitis in a toxic patient. There are several relative contraindications, including patients who are neutropenic or have bleeding disorders and chidren with a recent history of bowel surgery. In addition, patients with connective tissue disease, especially Ehlers-Danlos and Marfan's syndromes, are at increased risk of perforation during endoscopy.[33] Toxic dilation of the bowel carries an increased risk of perforation during colonoscopy, although the procedure may relieve the distention.[34, 35] Other relative contraindications include partial or complete bowel obstruction and aneurysm of the abdominal and iliac aorta. In all endoscopic procedures the clinician and the endoscopist must determine whether the potential information or therapeutic intervention outweighs the risk of the procedure (Table 74–4).

ANTIBIOTIC PROPHYLAXIS

The incidence of bacteremia after gastrointestinal endoscopy varies according to the procedure performed (EGD 2.2 to 12.5%, colonoscopy 0 to 15%, sclerotherapy and esophageal dilation up to 50%) and the patient's medical problem.[36, 37] Certain bacteria are more likely to be the cause of bacteremia after a procedure. These include *Escherichia coli, Bacteroides, Pseudomonas, Veillonella,* and *Peptostreptococcus,* especially after a lower gastrointestinal procedure.[38] However, other bacteria may be more virulent and more likely to cause endocarditis, especially *Streptococcus viridans* and enterococcus.[36] Prophylaxis is directed by the frequency and virulence of the anticipated organisms that may be encountered during the procedure.

The actual incidence of bacterial endocarditis following gastrointestinal procedures is quite low, with fewer than 20 cases reported.[36] There has been one prospective study in pediatric patients assessing the risk of bacteremia during endoscopy. Byrne and associates studied 50 patients who underwent esophagogastroduodenoscopy (including 36 who had biopsies) and 25 patients who had colonoscopy (including 7 who underwent biopsies and 15 who underwent snare polypectomies).[37] Blood cultures were obtained 5 minutes after intestinal intubation and then at 5 and 30 minutes after the procedure. One of the 50 patients who underwent EGD had a positive blood culture for group D streptococci. The patient, who had a duodenal ulcer that was biopsied, remained afebrile and had no sequelae. None of the patients who underwent colonoscopy with or without polypectomy had a positive blood culture.[37] Similar results have been reported in adult patients.[38]

Antibiotics are recommended for patients with prosthetic heart valves, a previous history of endocarditis, hypertrophic cardiomyopathy, mitral valve prolapse with valvular regurgitation, a surgically constructed systemic pulmonary shunt, and most congenital cardiac malformations. Prophylaxis is usually given prior to the procedure and repeated 6 to 8 hours after the procedure (Table 74–5).

Prophylaxis is not required in patients with physiologic or "innocent" murmurs; patients with a history of Kawasaki disease, mitral valve prolapse, or rheumatic heart disease without valvular dysfunction do not routinely require prophylaxis. Patients who are undergoing endoscopy at least 6 months after the repair of secundum atrial septal defects, ventricular septal defects, or patent ductus arteriosus without residual dysfunction also are not routinely given antibiotics prior to endoscopic procedures. The current antibiotic recommendations for prophylaxis are outlined in Table 74–5.

Table 74–4. CONTRAINDICATIONS TO ENDOSCOPY IN INFANTS AND CHILDREN

Absolute Contraindications
Suspected bowel perforation
Acute peritonitis

Relative Contraindications
Bleeding disorders and/or impaired platelet function
Neutropenia
Patients with increased risk of bowel perforation, including:
- Connective tissue disorders (Ehlers-Danlos and Marfan's syndromes)
- Caustic ingestion with a known tight stricture
- Toxic dilation of the bowel
- Partial or complete intestinal obstruction
- Recent bowel surgery

Table 74–5. REGIMEN FOR ENDOCARDITIS PROPHYLAXIS

1. Ampicillin 50 mg per kg intravenously or intramuscularly up to 2 gm plus gentamicin 2 mg per kg intravenously or intramuscularly up to 80 mg 30 minutes preprocedure, followed by amoxicillin 50 mg per kg by mouth up to 1.5 gm 6 hours after the procedure, or repeating the parenteral regimen 8 hours after the procedure.
2. *For those patients who are penicillin allergic:* Vancomycin 20 mg per kg intravenously 1 hour before the procedure (in addition to gentamicin) and 8 hours after the procedure to be administered over at least 60 minutes.
3. *Alternate low-risk patient regimen:* Amoxicillin 50 mg per kg up to 3 gm by mouth 1 hour before the procedure and 25 mg per kg up to 1.5 gm by mouth 6 hours after the initial dose.

From Dajani AS, Bisno AL, Chung KJ, et al: Prevention of bacterial endocarditis: Recommendations by the American Heart Association. JAMA 1990; 264:2919–2922; with permission. Copyright 1990, American Medical Association.

PREPARATION

Esophagogastroduodenoscopy

Preparation for upper gastrointestinal endoscopic procedures involves a period of fasting except in emergency situations. Infants less than 6 months of age are not fed for 2 to 4 hours prior to endoscopy, and children over 2 years of age fast for 6 to 8 hours.[39] Recently, Crawford and colleagues suggested that a shorter period of pre-endoscopy fasting may be possible. They found no difference in aspirated gastric volume (mean of 0.56 ml per kg) between those children fasted for 2 hours and those fasted for 6 hours.[40] With further corroboration, these data may be applied in the future to decrease the pre-endoscopy fasting interval, at least for clear liquids.

Colonoscopy

In addition to a period of fasting, lower panendoscopy can be successfully accomplished only if the colon is free of fecal debris. Large amounts of stool compromise the ability to negotiate the curves of the large bowel and prohibit complete visualization of the mucosa. Stool adherent to the lens often requires additional maneuvering and added air-water insufflation to clear the field of vision. Liquid stool can be aspirated through the suction channel but increases the examination time.

Many bowel preparations have been utilized to successfully cleanse the colon. The method depends on the age and cooperation of the child and the individual experience of the examiner. In infants who are totally breast or bottle fed, adequate preparation can usually be obtained with the use of small-volume enemas and substituting clear liquids for breast or bottle feeding for 12 to 24 hours. In older children and adolescents, the best preparation is usually obtained with the use of colonic lavage solutions that contain a nonabsorbable solution of polyethylene glycol, which causes an osmotic diarrhea[41–45] (Table 74–6). The risk of dehydration is minimal because of the limited transmural flux of sodium and water. To be effective, a large volume of solution must be ingested over a relatively short period of time. In adolescents of adult size, the usual regimen is 240 ml every 10 minutes until the fecal effluent is clear. This often requires 3 or 4 L of solution. Smaller volumes are recommended for younger children (Table 74–7). Occasionally, nasogastric administration may be necessary. The rate of nasogastric administration is 20 to 30 ml per minute or 1.2 to 1.8 L per hour in an older child or adolescent. Appropriate reductions of fluid can be made for infants and smaller children.

Oral cleansing solutions are effective in over 95% of the patients who drink adequate amounts of the fluid.[43, 45] An occasional patient may experience presumed allergic reactions manifested as dermatitis, urticaria, and rhinorrhea.[45]

If the child cannot comply with a large-volume lavage preparation, most endoscopists will use an alternative regimen of clear liquids for 48 to 72 hours accompanied by magnesium citrate the night before the procedure (Table 74–8). Saline enemas are usually administered the night before and the morning of the procedure to clear any residual stool.

SEDATION AND MONITORING

Sedation is used in most pediatric patients not only to minimize discomfort but also to provide amnesia for the procedure. This helps prevent the child from becoming fearful of contact with the physician, which is especially important in pediatric patients with chronic conditions that may require repeated procedures. In the last decade, most pediatric endoscopists have replaced general anesthesia with intravenous sedation for upper and lower endoscopy. Few studies are available comparing sedative medications in children[39, 46]; nevertheless, a combination of midazolam and meperidine is popular with pediatric gastroenterologists.

Meperidine, 1 to 2 mg per kg of body weight to a maximum of 100 mg, is administered by slow infusion followed by 0.1 to 0.2 mg per kg of body weight of midazolam. The dose of midazolam is titrated according to the patient's level of consciousness but rarely exceeds 5 mg as a total dose. Meperidine is usually given first to decrease the discomfort at the site of injection associated with intravenous midazolam. Younger children may require more midazolam per kilogram of body weight. Occasionally, it may be necessary to administer additional amounts of these medications during the procedure.

Transient reactions at the site of medication administration are not unusual and include cutaneous erythema distal to the site of injection not associated with clinically significant thrombophlebitis. Other reactions include coughing and a characteristic taste with meperidine infusion. In a prospective evaluation of this method of sedation in 100 pediatric endoscopic procedures at the Cleveland Clinic, approximately 50% of the patients had generalized cutaneous flushing, and urticaria without audible wheezing developed in 12 children. Rechallenge with the same sedative in two patients did not result in a more severe reaction.[39] Endoscopy in neo-

Table 74–6. COMPOSITION OF ORAL BOWEL CLEANSING SOLUTIONS

	Golytely	Nulytely	Colyte
Sodium (mmol/L)	125	65	125
Potassium (mmol/L)	10	5	10
Chloride (mmol/L)	35	53	35
Sulfate (mmol/L)	90	—	80
Bicarbonate (mmol/L)	20	17	20
Polyethylene glycol (mmol/L)	17.6	31.3	18
Osmolality (mOsm/L) (approximate)	280	280	280

Table 74–7. BOWEL PREPARATION USING ORAL SOLUTIONS

Weight of Child (kg)	Milliliter Each 10 Minutes Until Passage of Clear Fecal Effluent	Maximum Dose (ml)
<10	80	1,100
10–20	100	1,600
20–30	140	2,200
30–40	180	2,900
40–50	200	3,200
>50	240	4,000

Adapted from Bines JE, Winter HS: Lower endosocopy: *In* Walker WA, Durie PR, Hamilton JR, et al, eds: Pediatric Gastrointestinal Disease: Pathophysiology, Diagnosis, and Management. Philadelphia, BC Decker, 1990, p 1260; with permission.

Table 74–8. BOWEL PREPARATION

Children
Clear liquids for 48 to 72 hours
Magnesium citrate 1 oz per age in years to a maximum of 10 oz the night before the procedure
Saline enema the evening before and/or the morning of the procedure

Infants
Clear liquids for 12 to 24 hours
Nothing by mouth for 3 to 4 hours

nates may be performed with or without sedation, depending on the indication for the procedure. Sedation is helpful if the procedure will last more than a few minutes or interventional endoscopy is anticipated.

General anesthesia is necessary when a patient is uncooperative, will require a lengthy or complicated procedure, or has extenuating medical problems.

During the endoscopic procedure, arterial oxygen saturation and electrocardiographic tracings are routinely monitored. In a study by Castelle and coworkers, oxygen saturation was measured via pulse oximetry in 32 children undergoing upper gastrointestinal endoscopy.[47] Thirty of the patients were sedated utilizing a combination of intravenous meperidine and titrating doses of intravenous midazolam. The lowest oxygen saturations occurred during the endoscopic procedure. Twelve of the 32 (38%) developed oxygen saturations less than 90%. It was not necessary to terminate the procedure because of desaturation in any patient, and all the patients responded promptly to oxygen administration. There were no correlations found between the dose of meperidine or midazolam and the patient's age, weight, or mean and lowest saturation points during the monitoring period. Patients less than age one, when compared to those greater than age one, had a greater tendency to decrease their mean oxygen saturation. Patients with underlying cardiopulmonary disease also had lower mean saturation prior to and during the endoscopy.

Oxygen desaturation during sedation may occur without clinically apparent signs and symptoms.[48, 49] For this reason, pulse oximetry should be monitored during endoscopy. In some states, monitoring oxygen saturation is a requirement during general anesthetic procedures, and such statutes may soon be applied to endoscopy with intravenous sedation.[48] Neurologically impaired patients often have gastrointestinal problems that require endoscopy. Sedation in these patients can be unpredictable, and respiratory depression is more common. The dosage of meperidine is therefore reduced to 0.5 to 1.0 mg per kg, and the dosage of midazolam, if this drug is used, is titrated very slowly. Careful and attentive monitoring of the cardiopulmonary status is essential.[39] Medication dosages are also reduced in patients who have undergone a recent weight loss where the volume of distribution may be altered. These include patients with inflammatory bowel diseae, malignancy, or anorexia nervosa.

Naloxone is indicated only for narcotic-induced respiratory depression, because its use is usually associated with marked irritability in infants and young children. Flumazenil (Mazicon) is a newly available intravenous benzodiazepine antagonist that competitively blocks the effects of benzodiazepines on gamma-aminobutyric acid pathway–mediated inhibition in the central nervous system.[49a] Experience is limited with this agent; side effects with administration include facial erythema, dizziness, hyperexcitability, seizures, and serious cardiac arrhythmias. Because its half-life is shorter than the half-life of benzodiazepines, resedation after reversal of benzodiazepine sedation may occur, and patients should be monitored accordingly.

ANATOMY

Esophagogastroduodenoscopy

The esophagus is located posteriorly to the trachea in the neck. It ranges in size from 4 to 6 mm in diameter and 9 to 10 cm in length in the term infant, to a length of approximately 25 cm in the adult.[4, 50] It begins distal to the cricoid cartilage and ends at the cardiac orifice of the stomach.

The esophagus opens with swallowing, unlike the trachea, which is always open except with vocal cord movement. The esophageal opening appears lateral and posterior to each side of the trachea with swallowing. The trachea is easily distinguished from the esophagus by the presence of bilateral vocal cords on its anterolateral aspects and, if intubated, by the circular tracheal rings along its length.

The esophagus is narrowed at four locations: at the level of the cricopharyngeus, where the esophagus is crossed by the aortic arch, where it is crossed by the left mainstem bronchus, and at the lower esophageal sphincter. Of these, the regions just below the cricopharyngeus and just above the lower esophageal sphincter are often the sites where foreign bodies lodge after ingestion. The lower esophageal sphincter plays an important role in certain diseases such as achalasia and gastroesophageal reflux.

The stomach is usually located beneath the diaphragm and, in an adult, is approximately 40 cm distal to the incisors. The right aspect of the esophagus is in continuity with the lesser curvature of the stomach, while the left margin of the esophagus joins the greater curvature[50] (Fig. 74–5). The gastric rugae are most prominent along the greater curvature. The area of the stomach where the esophagus enters is known as the gastric cardia. That portion of the stomach above the junction of the esophagus and stomach is known as the fundus; it is also the most posterior aspect of the stomach. The majority of the stomach is known as the body of the stomach. On occasion, the esophagogastric junction is located above the diaphragm, which represents a hiatal hernia. Along the lesser curvature of the stomach is the

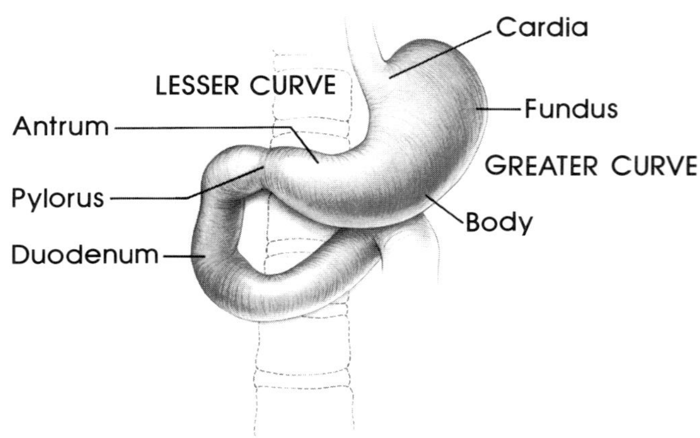

Figure 74–5. Endoscopic anatomy of the stomach and duodenum.

incisura. This notch divides the body of the stomach from the gastric antrum. The pylorus is the muscular junction between the stomach and the small intestine. The pyloric canal is 2 to 3 cm in length in the adult.[50] The diameter of the pyloric opening may vary according to patient age and size and may be affected or altered in certain disease states.

The most proximal portion of the small intestine is the duodenum. The average duodenal length in a full-term infant is 5 cm.[51] The duodenal bulb is an expanded region immediately distal to the pylorus. The duodenum then forms a C-shaped loop and, from the endoscopist's point of view, turns posteriorly and to the right for 2.5 cm in the older child and adult, then inferiorly for 7.5 to 10 cm (descending portion), then anteriorly and to the left for approximately 2.5 cm, finally connecting to the jejunum at the level of the ligament of Treitz. When it joins the jejunum, it turns abruptly forward.

The common bile duct and pancreatic duct obliquely enter the duodenal wall and join together in the ampulla of Vater, which opens into the descending portion of the duodenum via the duodenal papilla. The papilla is usually located approximately 8 to 10 cm distal to the pylorus in adults. The pancreatic duct may also empty via an accessory pancreatic duct, which is usually located proximal to the major duodenal papilla.[50] The duodenum, unlike the jejunum or ileum, does not have a mesentery.

The jejunum and ileum form a series of loops attached to the posterior abdominal wall via a mesentery. In a newborn, the average small intestinal length is 266 ± 56 cm.[52] In adults, the jejunum represents the proximal 2 meters and the ileum represents the distal 3 meters of the small bowel. Although the point of transition is often unclear, the jejunum is initially located in the left upper and left lower quadrants. Intraluminally, the jejunum is characterized by large thick folds, large villi, and a luminal diameter of approximately 4 cm. The ileum is thinner walled than the jejunum, with an inner diameter of 3.5 cm, smaller villi, and an increased amount of lymphoid tissue as compared to the jejunum.

Colonoscopy

The small intestine and transverse and sigmoid colons are attached to mesentery and shift positions freely[53] (Fig. 74–6). Their excursion during a procedure is limited by the length of bowel and length of their attachment. Disease processes, masses, or adhesions may influence their configuration or limit their mobility. The ascending colon and descending colon are relatively fixed in the retroperitoneum. The rectum is also relatively fixed as it passes through the pelvic connective tissue, with only a short segment free within the peritoneal cavity.

From the endoscopist's point of view, the anus is first intubated, then the rectum courses posteriorly to the coccyx and follows the gentle angle of the sacrum to the peritoneal reflection. Three "valves of Houston," two on the right and a middle one on the left, are encountered. These are crescentic, or semilunar, folds and are due to tension by the longitudinal muscle fibers of the teniae coli. These folds assume a more circular pattern in the sigmoid and descending colon and a characteristic triangular pattern in the transverse colon.

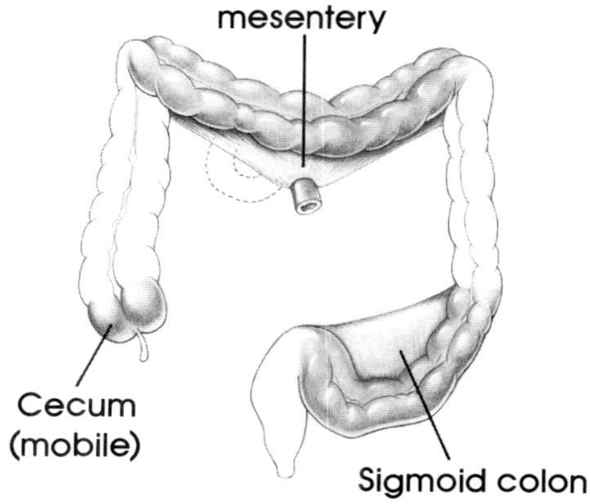

Figure 74–6. Mesenteric attachments of the colon. Mobile areas are darkened.

The sigmoid colon is attached to a mesentery and is relatively mobile. The descending colon is usually straight and ends at the splenic flexure, which forms an acute angulation with the transverse colon, turning abruptly to the right and anteriorly. The hepatic flexure forms the distal margin of the transverse colon and forms another abrupt, but inferior and posterior, angle with the descending colon. The transverse colon has a variable configuration and is suspended on a mesentery between the two fixed flexures. The ascending colon is fixed in the retroperitoneum and is relatively straight, ending in the mobile cecum. At the pole of the cecum the tenia fuse to cause a marked cecal haustration, often forming a "crow's foot" or "Mercedes Benz" sign. The appendiceal orifice is usually a crescentic opening slightly to the left of the midline. Occasionally it may appear as a tubular diverticulum. The postappendectomy opening appears identical unless the appendiceal stump has been inverted.

The ileocecal valve lies proximal to the cecal pole on the prominent ileocecal fold. It usually cannot be directly visualized but is recognizable by a slight irregularity of the fold, with the ileum passing obliquely downward from its cecal opening. The ileum is characterized by the circumferential valvular conniventes and a predominance of lymphoid tissue, especially in younger children.

TECHNIQUE

The endoscope is held in the left hand, with the thumb being used to turn the large dial; the index finger and sometimes the middle finger used to control the suction, air, and water valves; and the remaining fingers to hold the control handle. The insertion tube is held in the right hand. The lateral wheel, which controls right and left tip deflection, is usually manipulated with the right hand. The instruments used via the biopsy channel include sclerotherapy needles, biopsy forceps, cytology brushes, and syringes for irrigation and are usually inserted with the right hand. Prior to initiating a procedure the suction and air channels should be checked to ensure proper functioning.

Upper Endoscopy

The endoscopist usually stands on the patient's left during performance of esophagogastroduodenoscopy. After sedation in the supine position, the patient is turned to the left lateral decubitus position with the neck flexed downward in preparation for the procedure. Prior to insertion of the endoscope into the oral cavity, a bite block is placed in the patient's mouth. The endoscope dials are placed in a neutral position. Some individuals prefer to lock the right/left dial during esophageal intubation. The endoscope is guided through the bite block over the tongue to the back of the oropharynx by directing the endoscope tip posteriorly and somewhat laterally to the trachea; lateral motion is obtained by right and left torque on the shaft rather than by turning the dial. Some individuals use their forefinger to direct the tip and blindly advance the instrument. As the patient swallows, the cricopharyngeus relaxes and the esophagus, located posteriorly to the trachea and between the pyriform sinuses, can be intubated under direct vision. If the patient is unwilling or unable to swallow after the tip of the instrument is positioned at the esophageal inlet, gentle pressure will usually ease the tip through the cricopharyngeus into the proximal esophagus. The position of the endoscope during this procedure usually makes the patient gag, and if the instrument cannot be expeditiously passed it should be withdrawn.

After intubating the esophagus, the instrument is advanced down the esophageal lumen while simultaneously examining the mucosa for any lesions. The mucosa is examined as the instrument is inserted to avoid misinterpreting mucosal changes caused by passage of the endoscope. The esophagus is examined for evidence of inflammation, ulcerations, varices, hernias, and strictures. The location of the lower esophageal sphincter should be noted. The transition between squamous esophageal and gastric columnar mucosa is called the "Z line." At this point, the mucosa changes from a pale pink to a deep red. The diaphragmatic constriction of the gut lumen should be noted within 2 cm of the squamocolumnar junction unless a hiatal hernia or Barrett's esophagus is present.[54]

When the stomach is entered, suction is utilized to remove any residual gastric secretions. After the gastric secretions are removed, air is insufflated to separate the gastric rugae. The endoscope is then advanced while torquing to the right. This can be accomplished by applying pressure to the shaft or by the endoscopist twisting to the right; in the case of video instruments, torque can also be achieved by dropping the handle to the right or left, depending on the desired direction of torque. The endoscope is advanced along the lesser curve toward the pylorus, but it is usually necessary to fill the greater curvature with the endoscope prior to cannulating the pyloric canal (Fig. 74–7).

The pylorus appears as a small opening with radiating folds around it. Periodic antral waves may pass to the pylorus, changing its location and the size of the canal opening. The pylorus is entered by nudging the tip of the endoscope up to the opening and then directly cannulating the pyloric canal.

The duodenal bulb should be examined upon endoscope insertion rather than during withdrawal because of possible mucosal changes caused by passage of the instrument. After examination of all four quadrants, the scope is advanced to the posterior aspect of the bulb where the duodenum takes a sharp right and downward turn. The instrument is advanced using the dials and shaft torque, usually down and to the right followed by an upward spin of the dial, bringing the tip into the descending duodenum. Once the lumen of the descending duodenum is seen, a straightening maneuver is performed. This consists of pulling the endoscope slowly backward while maintaining the lumen in view. This reduces the loop along the greater curvature of the stomach and usually paradoxically advances the endoscope into the distal duodenum (Fig. 74–8). The duodenal mucosa, including ampulla of Vater, is examined while withdrawing the endoscope.

After adequate examination of the antrum, pylorus, and duodenum, the endoscope is retroflexed to look for lesions in the gastric cardia and fundus (Fig. 74–9). With the instrument looking toward the pylorus and located proximal to the incisura, the tip is deflected until the proximal stomach comes into view. The endoscope is then progressively withdrawn, bringing the cardia closer to the instrument tip while distending the cardia and fundus with air (Fig. 74–10). Patients will often burp during this maneuver, and cooperative children may be instructed to try to hold the air in the stomach. The endoscope is then rotated 180 degrees in each direction by torquing the insertion tube in a clockwise or counterclockwise manner.

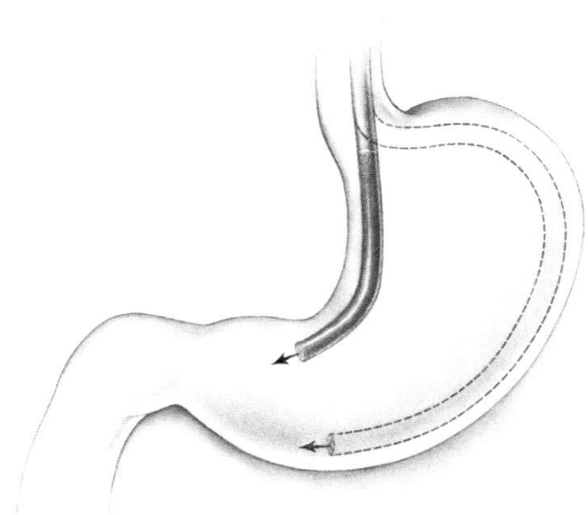

Figure 74–7. Advancement of the endoscope to the duodenum by filling the loop of the greater curvature.

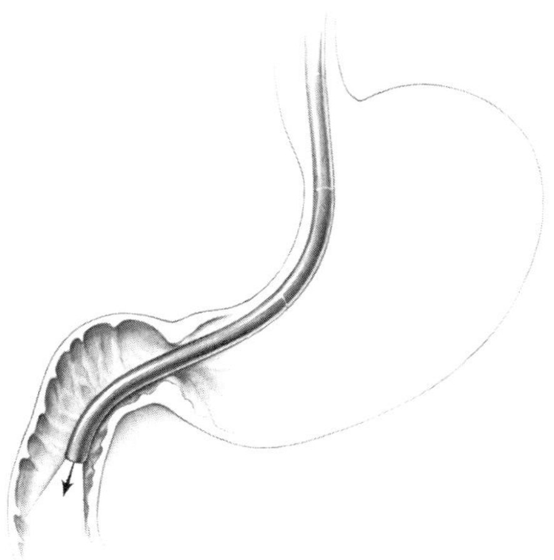

Figure 74–8. Duodenal straightening maneuver that paradoxically advances the endoscope into the distal duodenum by scope withdrawal.

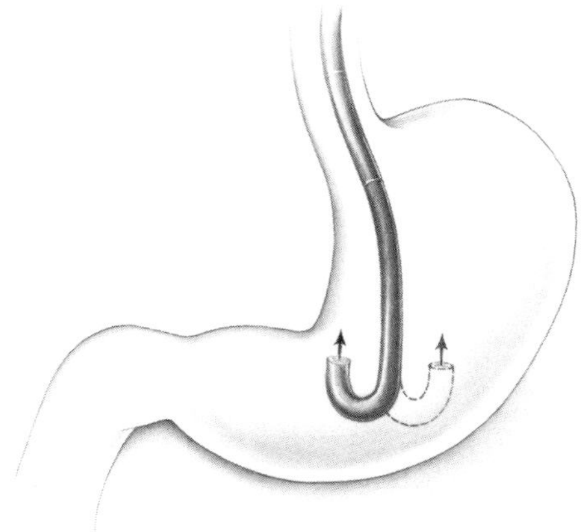

Figure 74–10. Examination of the gastric cardia and fundus by retroflexion, scope withdrawal, and rotation.

The instrument is then straightened, the remainder of the gastric mucosa is examined, and biopsies, if necessary, are performed. The endoscope is then withdrawn. Immediately prior to its leaving the stomach, air is aspirated from the stomach. The esophageal mucosa is once again examined. The endoscope is usually withdrawn rapidly in children when the level of the larynx is reached in order to increase patient comfort and diminish gagging.

Colonoscopy

Colonoscopy is traditionally performed in the left lateral decubitus position with knees bent. A lubricant is usually applied to the tip of the instrument prior to insertion into the anus. In patients with active perianal disease, lubrication with viscous lidocaine may relieve some discomfort. It is usually necessary to reapply lubricant during the procedure, as the lubricant tends to dry as the endoscope is serially advanced and withdrawn. The endoscopist may mistake the increased resistance secondary to poor lubrication as coming from the more proximal colon.

The anus is visually inspected, examining for fissures, fistulae, or skin tags, and the instrument is inserted into the anus and advanced into the rectum. The anal canal is 2 to 3 cm long (in the older child and adolescent) and is angled toward the umbilicus. The instrument is inserted until there is an abrupt decrease in resistance, indicating that the tip has passed from the anal canal into the rectal ampulla. Following insertion, the scope tip usually comes to rest near the anterior wall of the rectum, since the junction of the rectum and anal canal forms an angle of approximately 90 degrees. If the lumen is not in view, a small puff of air or withdrawing the endoscope a few centimeters will usually locate the lumen. Negotiating the colon is similar to the examination of the duodenum. The instrument should be subtly advanced using the dials for tip deflection, and the techniques of air insufflation and suction, rotation or torquing of the insertion tube, external pressure applied to the abdomen, and changing the position of the patient rather than simply "pushing." The elastic nature of the colon allows it to become long and tortuous when it is stretched by the colonoscope. Alternatively, it can be telescoped onto the instrument with little stretching by experienced endoscopists. The fundamentals of colonoscopy are (1) advance the endoscope under direct observation; (2) use as little air as possible while maintaining adequate visualization; (3) avoid forming loops, but when loops are formed, reduce them as quickly as possible; and (4) pull back and telescope the bowel onto the colonoscope whenever possible.[55]

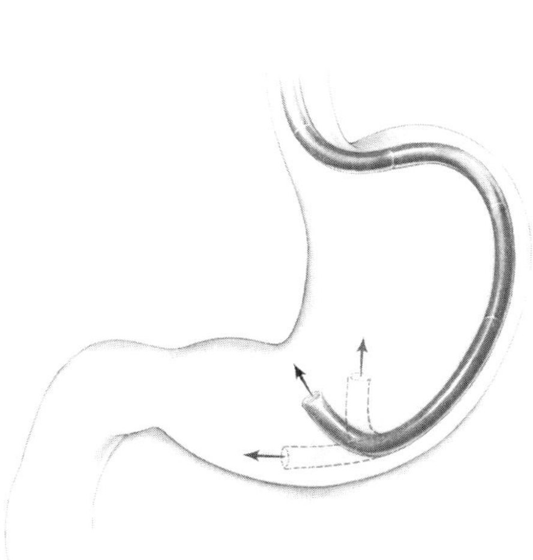

Figure 74–9. Examination of the antrum and incisura by upward deflection of the endoscope tip.

The most prominent landmarks in the rectum are the fixed "valves of Houston." These folds are accentuated haustral markings, and the lumen will veer toward the side of the fold. The endoscope is advanced with a series of short movements, jiggling motions, or torquing technique, depending on the skill and preference of the examiner. The junction of the rectum and sigmoid

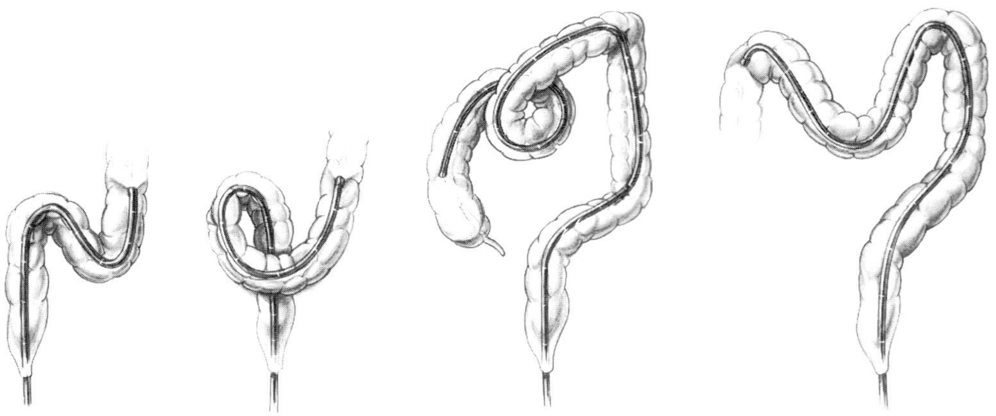

Figure 74–11. Common loops: "N" loop, alpha loop, gamma loop, and "U" loop.

usually presents the first major problem and opportunity to form a loop. If the endoscopist simply advances the instrument, the force of the colonoscope is transmitted to the wall of the colon, with progressive distention of the bowel and its mesentery; the patient usually experiences pain, and the examiner feels increasing resistance to forward motion. This is often accompanied by the failure of the tip to advance despite insertion of the colonoscope. Paradoxical movement may occur when the tip recedes as the instrument is advanced and a larger loop is formed.

Early colonoscopes with limited tip deflection and fields of view required a "slide by" technique, since the lumen could not always be kept in view. The instrument was advanced while the endoscopist had only a red field of view as the mucosa moved past the tip of the instrument. Advancement was halted when the mucosa was no longer slipping past the instrument tip or the mucosa took on a whitish hue, suggesting that compression of the bowel wall by the colonoscope was decreasing perfusion to the mucosa.

The instruments currently available reduce some of the technical difficulties, and the instrument should be advanced under direct visualization and not by the "slide by" technique. The skillful negotiation of the rectosigmoid junction is the key to successful colonoscopy. The experienced endoscopist will anticipate many of the potential problems. Several loops may be formed in the sigmoid colon. Names have been given to various configurations as they were seen under the fluoroscope with the patient positioned in the anterior posterior position (Fig. 74–11). The alpha loop resembles the Greek letter alpha and may occur in either a normal or reversed configuration. The most common loop is the "N" loop, which is shaped like the letter *N*. Each of these loops has a similar appearance when viewed from the lateral position. The sigmoid colon is usually directed upward and then forms a caudad-directed convex loop in the anterior posterior plane and a second cephalad convex loop with an oblique orientation to the anterior posterior plane (Fig. 74–12). Less common loops such as the double alpha loop can occur in a forward or backward orientation (Fig. 74–13). Regardless of the anatomy in the individual patient, the endoscopist is unaware of the anatomy unless fluoroscopy is used during the procedure. Since it is rarely needed to complete the procedure and exposes the patient, physician, and equipment to radiation, the experienced endoscopist will anticipate the potential problems rather than utilizing fluoroscopy.

Advancing the endoscope through the sigmoid colon should be a smooth and coordinated procedure. This often involves torquing the instrument along its shaft with the right hand and using the left hand to control the tip deflection. Repeated backward and forward motions are usually needed to telescope the colon onto the instrument. As the tip of the instrument reaches a bend, the dials or a combination of dials and torque is used to rotate the tip around the bend into the lumen. Withdrawing the instrument will often straighten the loop and allow advancement to the next bend. To reduce an alpha loop, the scope is withdrawn so the tip lies just distal to the rectosigmoid junction and then rotated 180 degrees (Fig. 74–14). Failure of "one to one" movement, increasing patient discomfort, and increased re-

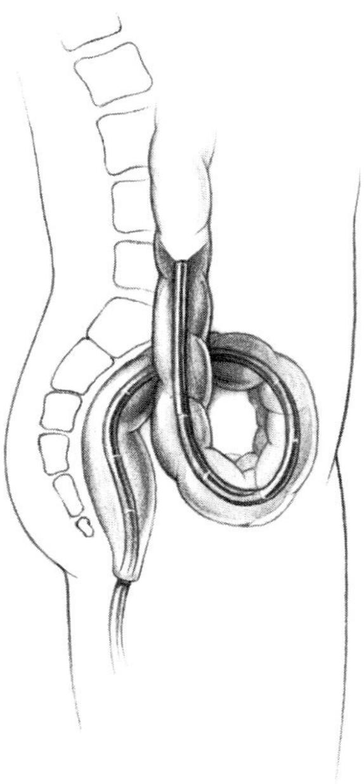

Figure 74–12. Lateral view of common loops.

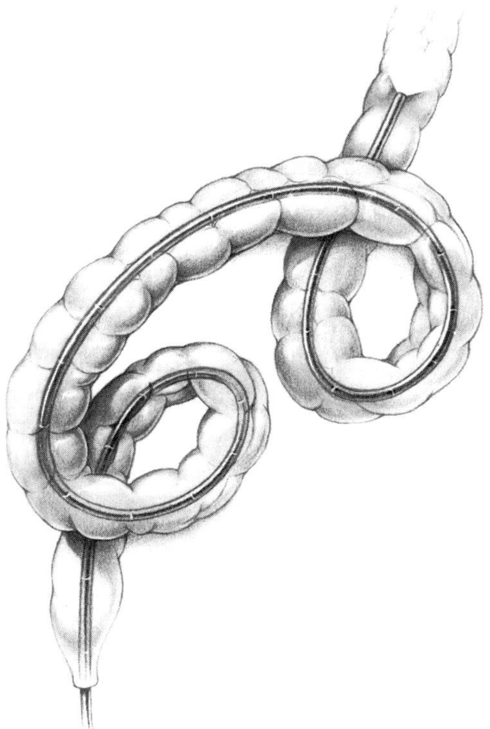

Figure 74–13. Double-alpha loop of the sigmoid colon.

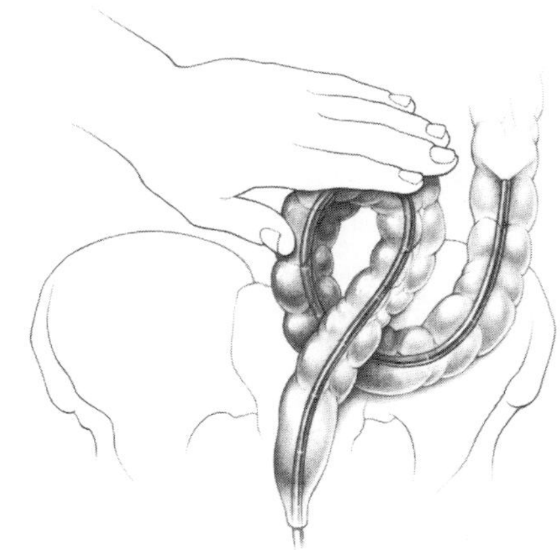

Figure 74–15. Anterior abdominal pressure may facilitate scope advancement by increasing resistance to loop formation.

sistance to insertion of the endoscope are usually signs of loop formation. Repeated attempts at loop removal are often necessary to traverse the sigmoid colon. In an occasional patient it may be necessary to push through the loop and then reduce it after the instrument reaches the more proximal colon. Hand pressure by an assistant on the anterior abdominal wall may be beneficial during this maneuver (Fig. 74–15). This should be done with caution only by an experienced endoscopist.

Alpha sigmoid loops, with the endoscope advanced into the distal descending colon, can be reduced by rotation (usually clockwise) and withdrawal. "N" loops can usually be removed with simple withdrawal. Occasionally an "N" loop will have to be converted to an alpha loop for reduction to be successful. This can be done by withdrawal and counterclockwise rotation. The conversion usually allows the endoscope to be advanced to the level of the descending colon, since most of the forward force on the "N" loop is directed at the apex of the loop and the forces in the alpha loop are more radially distributed. This permits advancement of the instrument despite the presence of the alpha loop. When the instrument reaches the descending colon the loop can be reduced. Attempted examination of the proximal colon is usually limited if there is a residual sigmoid loop.

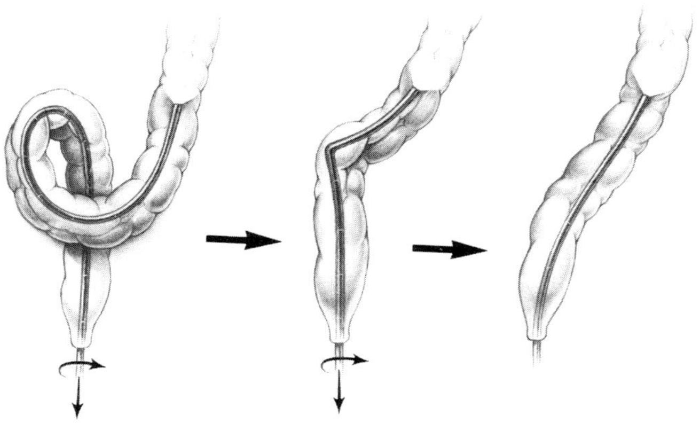

Figure 74–14. Alpha loop. Note initial posterior, then anterior configuration of the sigmoid colon. Clockwise torque and scope withdrawal allows reduction of the loop and straightening of the sigmoid colon.

There is no anatomical demarcation between the sigmoid and descending colon, but there is a tendency for the descending colon to be slightly smaller in diameter and to contain residual fecal debris because of its dependent position with the patient in the left lateral position. Often a long tunnel view may be obtained, and if the sigmoid loops have been reduced, the endoscope can usually be advanced to the level of the splenic flexure without difficulty. A straight sigmoid colon is essential for successful maneuvering around the splenic flexure. Paradoxical motion is often noted as the endoscope is advanced into the transverse colon. The configuration and forces resemble those of the "N" loop in the sigmoid colon. To reduce this tendency the patient is often rotated from the left lateral to the supine position. Clockwise rotation of the endoscope may also be helpful. The relationship of the transverse colon and splenic flexure also varies with respiration. Deep sustained inspiration in the cooperative child may decrease the acute angle of the splenic flexure and allow easier passage of the endoscope. If the endoscopist is unsuccessful, the instrument should be withdrawn to ensure reduction of a sigmoid loop that may not have been reduced or one that may have reformed during maneuvers to negotiate the flexure (Fig. 74–16). Multiple attempts by trial and error may be necessary to advance the instrument into the transverse colon.

The transverse colon is characterized by triangular-shaped haustral folds. The endoscope can usually be

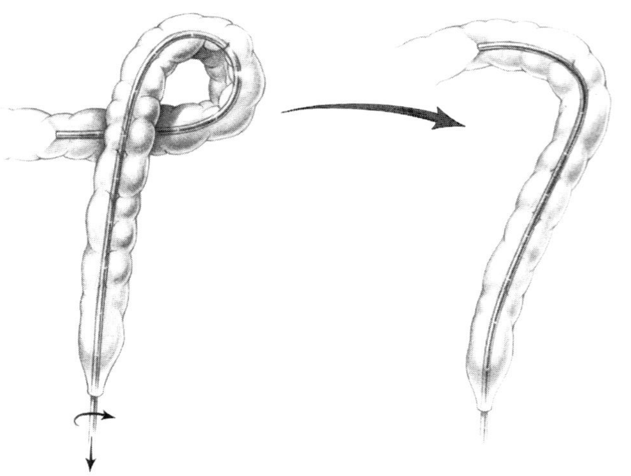

Figure 74–16. Reduction of the splenic flexure loop after intubation of the transverse colon. Without straightening, further advancement of the endoscope will be difficult and uncomfortable.

advanced to the hepatic flexure without difficulty, which is easily identified by the bluish discoloration of the outer wall caused by its close approximation to the liver. Occasionally a U-shaped loop is formed, which requires reduction prior to attempted negotiation of the hepatic flexure (see Fig. 74–11). If the transverse colon is redundant, a gamma loop may form. Reduction of this loop is difficult because rotational forces are poorly transmitted and the loop is usually large. Reduction is less difficult if the instrument can be advanced into the ascending colon and then withdrawn to reduce the loop.

The fixed position of the splenic flexure acts as a fulcrum while trying to negotiate the hepatic flexure. Suctioning in the region of the hepatic flexure usually draws the mucosa to the tip of the endoscope, and subsequently the tip can be maneuvered around the flexure into the ascending colon. If the flexure cannot be negotiated, withdrawal, manual rotation of the insertion tube, suctioning, manual compression of the abdominal wall, and/or sustained deep inspiration may be attempted to facilitate passage. If these measures fail it may still be possible to advance the endoscope, but the patient will usually experience some discomfort.

To advance the endoscope into the ascending colon, the tip of the instrument is usually turned into the lumen with the dials. Additional procedures such as withdrawal and rotation may be necessary if paradoxical movement is encountered. Deep inspiration may be effective in "pushing" the instrument into the ascending colon. After the tip is aligned with the lumen, suctioning will also collapse the cecum toward the tip of the instrument. If there have been any difficulties with the cleansing of the colon, they are most likely to become apparent in the ascending colon. Multiple washings of the mucosa and lens may be necessary to allow full examination of the mucosa. The cecum can be recognized by the typical anatomical landmarks of the triangular-shaped folds and the appendiceal orifice. With a standard endoscope or newer video endoscopes, the tip of the instrument can often be identified in the right lower quadrant as it transilluminates the anterior abdominal wall. Transillumination may not be successful with some video endoscopes. The ileocecal valve can be identified on the lateral surface of the prominent ileal fold as a slight irregularity of the valve contour. Occasionally the valve can be directly intubated, but usually it must be approached indirectly. The tip of the endoscope is brought to a position parallel to the valve, and the dials are used to deflect the tip 90 degrees toward the valve (Fig. 74–17). The maneuver is designed to catch the proximal lip of the valve with the tip of the endoscope. If the maneuver is successful, the lumen of the ileum will open, and adjustment of the tip will advance the instrument several centimeters. Several attempts may be needed to achieve success. Rotating the patient and suctioning the air from the cecum to draw the valve opening closer to the endoscope may be helpful. The mucosa of the ileum is easily identified by the presence of valvula conniventes and the presence of lymphoid aggregates, which appear as submucosal 2- to 4-mm mounds of tissue with normal overlying mucosa. The presence of lymphoid aggregates in adults has been associated with immunoglobulin A (IgA) deficiency but is normal in children; the amount tends to decrease with advancing age. If the valve cannot be cannulated and pathologic evaluation is needed, the forceps can sometimes be gently advanced through the valve and biopsy material obtained.

Examination of the mucosa is conducted principally as the instrument is withdrawn. All areas must be routinely examined, which means special attention must be given to the areas behind folds. Observation of areas around flexures may not be adequate if the scope slips back rapidly, and the instrument may have to be advanced back through areas not well visualized. Observation of the distal rectum requires a retroflexed maneuver for complete examination. This is done by turning the dials to their maximum deflection in the midrectum. The endoscope is then slowly rotated to obtain an unobstructed view. The scope must be straightened prior to removal from the anus.

Colostomies and ileostomies can usually be examined

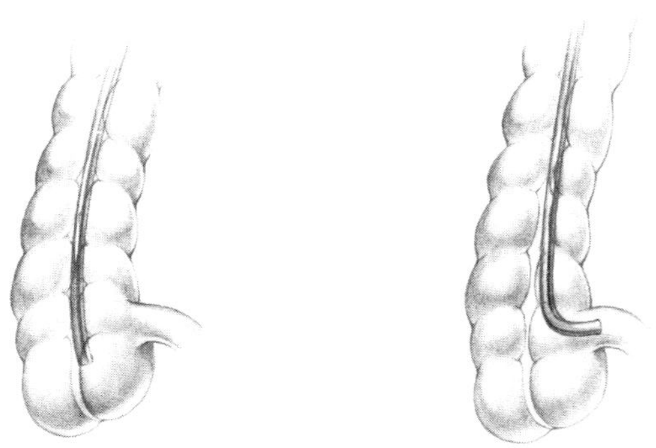

Figure 74–17. The ileocecal valve is intubated by tip deflection rather than en face.

as long as the openings are large enough to admit the tip of the instrument. Depending on the size, an appropriate scope should be chosen after a finger has been inserted into the opening. The length of bowel that can be examined is usually dependent on whether adhesions have formed. Advancement of the instrument around flexures in the bowel again involves repeated advancement, withdrawal, and torque of the insertion tube.

Flexible Proctosigmoidoscopy

Routine flexible proctosigmoidoscopy is useful in some pediatric patients. In compliant, usually older children with chronic illness such as ulcerative colitis, routine office examination to assess the extent and severity of disease when the history is in doubt or prior to initiating topical therapy for localized disease is useful. Examinations can be routinely performed with the same instruments that are used for full colonoscopy. Examination using either short (35 cm) or long (60 cm) flexible instruments in adults has produced similar pathologic yields.[56–61] No comparable information is available in the pediatric population, but if it is necessary to sedate pediatric patients for their comfort, it is usually appropriate to be prepared to perform a full colonoscopic examination. If pathology is encountered that is compatible with the patient's symptoms and therapeutic options do not rest on establishing the extent of the disease, the procedure can be terminated without attempting to examine the entire colon.

Anoscopy and Rigid Proctosigmoidoscopy

Anoscopy and rigid proctosigmoidoscopy are infrequently used procedures in the pediatric patient. Most pediatric gastroenterologists prefer flexible instruments when examination is required. The anoscope, however, remains a useful office instrument to better visualize the anal canal and identify sources of bleeding.[2]

BIOPSY TECHNIQUE

Histopathologic evaluation of the gastrointestinal tract is helpful in differentiating infectious, inflammatory, and malignant processes. Tissue biopsy is routinely obtained from suspicious lesions during endoscopic examination, but when the gross endoscopic appearance reveals a specific diagnosis, tissue analysis is unnecessary if the result will not alter therapy. Numerous techniques and devices have been designed to obtain tissue samples. There are a variety of pinch biopsy forceps available that are coordinated in size with endoscopic channel diameter. Some biopsy forceps are fenestrated with a needle so that two sequential biopsies may be performed without removing the forceps from the endoscope (Fig. 74–18). Fine needle biopsy may have an advantage when biopsy material from submucosal lesions is sought.[62] Suction biopsy, which has been adapted to the endo-

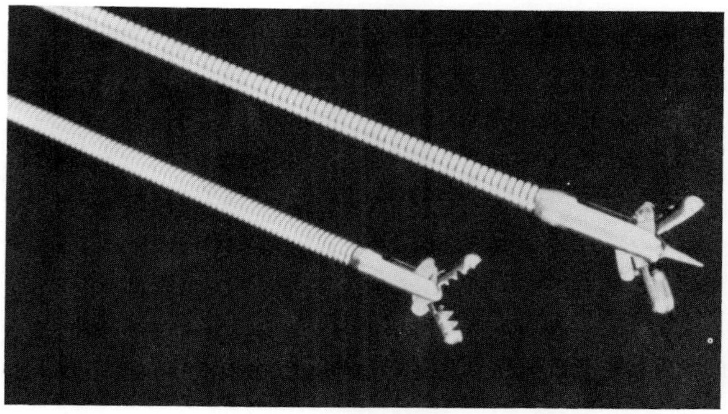

Figure 74–18. Biopsy forceps: alligator jaw forceps *(left)* for holding and removing objects and fenestrated forceps *(right)* for sequential biopsies. (Courtesy of Olympus Corporation.)

scope, is designed to obtain deeper samples. Larger sized biopsy specimens may also be obtained with a turn and suction technique.[63] Multiple biopsy specimens improve the diagnostic yield, but the size and location of the biopsies are probably more important.[64–66] Brush cytology or other combinations of techniques can increase diagnostic yield.[67] Snare excision is usually reserved for large polyps. For a more detailed discussion, see Chapter 73.

The technique of biopsy varies according to the lesion to be biopsied. To perform a routine biopsy, the closed pinch biopsy forceps are advanced through the biopsy channel to a point just past the tip of the endoscope, then they are opened immediately adjacent and perpendicular to the lesion if possible. This angulation may be difficult to achieve in the esophagus, small bowel, and terminal ileum. The open forceps are then closed and the tissue removed through the endoscope. The depth of biopsy is determined by the lesion being sought.

Esophagus

Reflux esophagitis is traditionally diagnosed by clinical criteria. Endoscopic biopsy is indicated in patients refractory to therapy or if the diagnosis remains unclear following visual examination of the mucosa.[68] The finding of Barrett's esophagus necessitates multiple biopsies to screen for dysplasia or adenocarcinoma.[69] Fungal and viral (cytomegalovirus, herpes simplex virus) esophagitis occurs in both immunocompromised and immunocompetent hosts.[70] Biopsy, cytology, and cultures aid in the diagnosis.[71] Malignant tumors of the esophagus are diagnosed by biopsy in the majority of cases. The addition of brush cytology increases the diagnostic yield in cancerous lesions.[72, 73]

Stomach

Gastric ulcers are not routinely biopsied because ulcerating gastric malignancies are rare in pediatric patients. If biopsies are performed, they should be obtained from the edge rather than the base of the lesion and are contraindicated if a visible vessel is present. Complications include perforation and bleeding.[74]

Gastritis secondary to drug administration does not usually require biopsy. Generalized gastritis may suggest the diagnosis of *Helicobacter pylori*, confirmed by Giemsa staining or urease testing of antral biopsies.[75–77]

Gastric biopsy may also aid in the diagnosis of idiopathic granulomatous gastritis, eosinophilic gastroenteritis, sarcoidosis, or Menetrier's disease.

Gastric neoplasia, although uncommon in pediatrics, may appear as an ulcerative, polypoid, or submucosal deformity or as thickened gastric folds. Pinch biopsy is the preferred technique for ulcerative or small polypoid lesions. Adenomas or hyperplastic polyps greater than 2.0 cm should be removed if feasible. Submucosal deformities may be evaluated by deep biopsies from a single site, with or without fine needle aspiration.

Small Intestine

Endoscopic pinch biopsy of the small bowel is helpful in the diagnosis of celiac disease, intestinal lymphangiectasia, and Crohn's disease.[78] Multiple directed specimens obtained from the descending duodenum or the more distal bowel have replaced capsule biopsy with comparable accuracy, increased patient comfort, and decreased risk of complications.[79–82] Jumbo forceps (open diameter 9 mm) or the turn and suction technique allows for larger sized specimens.[63] Distal biopsies can be obtained using small-caliber colonoscopes, enteroscopes, or endoscopically directed capsule biopsy, especially in lesions that characteristically have a patchy distribution.[83] Biopsy of macroscopically normal tissue may occasionally establish the diagnosis and allows for determination of disaccharidase levels if appropriate.[84, 85]

Small bowel parasitic infection may be identified by direct observation or pathologic identification of removed worms. Aspiration of duodenal contents and histologic examination can identify parasites such as *Giardia lamblia* or Strongyloides, which may not produce visual mucosal changes.[86] Duodenal tumors are rare and can be biopsied utilizing either the forward- or side-viewing endoscopes.

Ileum and Colon

The colonoscope can be used to obtain biopsy material and collect specimens for culture from the distal small bowel and colon. Histopathologic examination is useful in the differentiation of infectious, inflammatory, and malignant processes. Guidelines have outlined the general indications for colonoscopy and biopsy in patients with colonic polyps and inflammatory bowel disease.[66, 87, 88] Visual evidence of a suspicious lesion warrants histopathologic evaluation. Methods for obtaining tissue include snare excision, forceps biopsy, hot biopsy forceps, needle biopsy, and brush and salvage cytology. Needle biopsy, brush cytology, and salvage cytology are utilized mainly in the adult population to enhance the yield in patients with suspected colorectal malignancies.[67, 89] Needle biopsy has the theoretical advantage in ulcerated lesions of providing histologic material not only from the surface but also from areas deeper within the lesion. Needle biopsy may be useful in submucosal lesions that are difficult to access by biopsy forceps.[90–92] In most diseases involving pediatric patients, the forceps for pediatric size instruments or standard forceps provide adequate tissue for mucosal evaluation.

Endoscopy and biopsy can be useful in the diagnosis of infection and in the diagnosis and management of inflammatory bowel disease. Biopsy specimens (one or two using routine forceps) obtained during the acute phase of a bloody diarrheal illness may differentiate acute self-limited colitis from an initial or recurrent attack of chronic ulcerative colitis.[93–97] During the resolving phase of acute self-limited colitis, histologic changes may mimic those of Crohn's disease.[93] Bacterial cultures may be obtained during the procedure by the attachment of a "trap" to the suction equipment that gathers fecal effluent.

Terminal ileal examination may be useful in the diagnosis of Crohn's disease and the differentiation of Crohn's disease from lymphonodular hyperplasia.[21, 98, 99] Ileal visualization and biopsy may occasionally be useful in patients with infectious ileitis.[20, 100–102]

Ulcerative colitis is a predisposing risk factor for the development of colorectal cancer. Routine colonoscopy is usually initiated after 7 years in patents with pancolitis and after 15 years in those with left-sided disease. Biopsies should be taken from any suspicious areas, and serial biopsies should be taken from representative areas of the bowel for detection of dysplasia.[103–107]

Occasionally biopsies from macroscopically normal mucosa may be useful in the diagnosis of disease. Collagenous colitis with associated chronic diarrhea may present with macroscopically normal mucosa but characteristic histologic abnormalities.[108] Other diseases such as amyloidosis, inflammatory bowel disease, "microscopic colitis in children," and chronic schistosomiasis have been diagnosed by capsule or forceps biopsy of the colon when the mucosa has been macroscopically normal.[84, 108–117]

Complications after biopsy may include perforation and bleeding.[74] For a more detailed discussion see the section on complications.

THERAPEUTIC ENDOSCOPY

During the early years of gastrointestinal endoscopy, endoscopic examination was primarily a diagnostic tool. As technology advanced and procedural skills developed, the endoscope became a therapeutic instrument. Endoscopes have been used in children to remove foreign bodies and polyps, insert tubes into various organs, and stop bleeding lesions. For detailed discussions, the reader is referred to Chapters 13 (foreign bodies), 27 (esophageal varices), 33 (ulcers), and 73 (intestinal biopsy).

Acute gastrointestinal hemorrhage has become an indication for therapeutic endoscopic intervention, but emergent gastrointestinal endoscopy is associated with an increased risk of complications.[118] This includes a risk of aspiration of gastric contents and a higher risk associated with sedating an actively bleeding patient or a patient with decompensated cardiopulmonary or hepatic function.[118] Upper gastrointestinal lesions that may be amenable to endoscopic therapy include ulcers with evidence of active bleeding, oozing from beneath a clot overlying an ulcer (sentinel clot), or an ulcer with a visible vessel at its base that is not actively bleeding but appears as a red, blue, or white plug.

These same lesions have a high rate of rebleeding, approximately 50%, as compared to 10% or less incidence of rebleeding with other lesions, including those with an overlying clot without oozing or flat spots. Bleeding from esophageal varices can also be treated by endoscopic therapeutic intervention.[118, 119] Therefore, ongoing therapy to ablate distal esophageal varices is usually undertaken after the initial bleeding episode has resolved (see Chapter 27).[119, 120] Diffuse mucosal bleeding from duodenitis or gastritis is usually not responsive to endoscopic interventions. Colonic lesions treatable with endoscopic therapy include bleeding ulcers, angiomata, polyps and bleeding polyp stalks, an adherent clot in a single diverticulum, or an ulcerative lesion that is resistant to washing, with fresh blood nearby and no other visible lesion in the colon.[121, 122] As in upper gastrointestinal tract disease, diffusely bleeding colonic lesions cannot be successfully controlled by endoscopic intervention.

There are three well-established types of therapeutic intervention for acute gastrointestinal bleeding: injection, coagulation/heater probe, and laser therapy. The specific techniques employed depend on equipment availability and experience of the endoscopist. The techniques appear to have roughly equivalent efficacy.

Therapeutic endoscopy is most easily accomplished using a two-channeled therapeutic scope so that therapy (injection, coagulation, etc.) may be accomplished via one channel and simultaneous suction or irrigation may be performed using the second channel to keep the field in view. Unfortunately, therapeutic endoscopes are of a large diameter compared to standard pediatric endoscopes and often cannot be used in the pediatric patient. Therapeutic endoscopy may still be performed using a single-channel scope; however, it is technically more difficult.

INJECTION

Injection therapy is used for both variceal and nonvariceal bleeding. The technique of esophageal sclerotherapy for varices is discussed elsewhere (see Chapter 27). Nonvariceal injection therapy is usually performed by injecting a sclerosing agent at three to four sites around an exposed bleeding vessel (Fig. 74–19). Maximal volumes of sclerosant have been established in adults to minimize the risk of ulcer extension or perforation. Maximum volumes of sclerosants in pediatric patients have not been studied; however, maximal adult volumes should not be exceeded. Complications including perforation may occur with volumes of injection even less than the recommended maximum volumes. Table 74–9 lists the most commonly used solutions, their concentrations, and estimated maximal volumes. Several general principles should be noted. First, except under unusual circumstances, injection therapy should be confined to a single solution (single agent or a combination agent) during a given injection episode. Utilizing two sequential solutions may increase the risk of complication with smaller volumes of sclerosant than would be required by using a single agent alone. Second, the injection site (into vessel versus surrounding vessel versus submucosal) is specific for certain agents. Without appropriate clinical trials, changing the site of injection is probably hazardous. Third, the risks with injection therapy include increased bleeding, rebleeding, bowel ischemia, and perforation.[123] Fourth, precise volumes of injection are required. Those that involve smaller volumes may be more technically difficult. Fifth, injection therapy is not usually performed for colonic lesions, and volumes of injection have not been established for the large bowel.

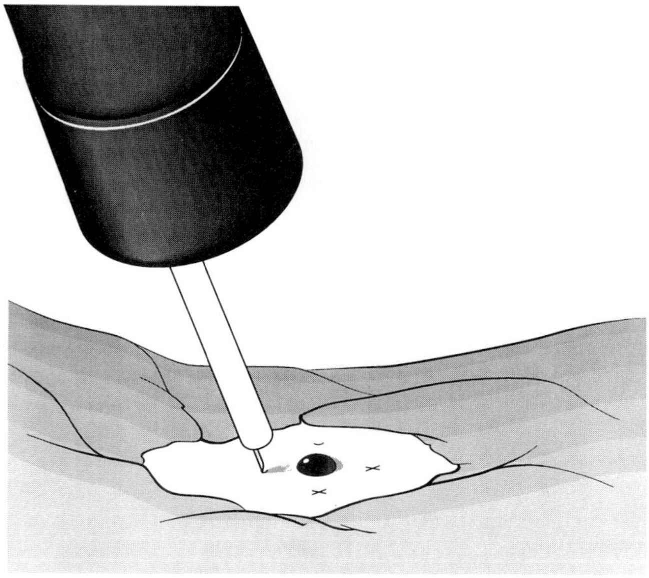

Figure 74–19. Injection circumferentially around a visible vessel in an ulcer base. Injection is performed at three to four sites around the exposed vessel.

THERMOCOAGULATION

A second method of establishing hemostasis is thermocoagulation, utilizing the heater probe or monopolar or bipolar (multipolar) coagulators (Table 74–10). The heater probe is composed of Teflon-coated hollow aluminum cylinders with an inner heater coil and a maximum internal temperature. The probe is water perfused to prevent tissue adherence, an advantage over monopolar coagulation, and heat is delivered via conduction to the tissue (Fig. 74–20). There are small (2.4 mm) and large (3.2 mm) diameter probes.[118] The patient should

Table 74–9. SCLEROSANTS FOR NONVARICEAL BLEEDING

Solution	Concentration	Volume/No. of Injections/Location	Maximum Total Volume	Comments
Hypertonic saline-epinephrine combination	3.6% saline + 1:20,000 epinephrine or 7.2% saline + 1:20,000 epinephrine*	3 ml/3–4 injections at base of bleeding vessel 1 ml/3–4 injections	9–12 ml	Repeat prophylactic injections if visible vessel present 24–48 hours after first hemostasis for lesions with extensive fibrosis*
Epinephrine with normal saline	1 ml of 1:10,000 epinephrine + 9 ml of normal saline	0.5–2.0 ml injected in multiple sites around bleeding vessel and into bleeding point itself	10 ml	Range 1.5–10 ml, mean = 4.1 ml; larger volumes in range for spurting vessels
Epinephrine followed by polidocanol	Epinephrine 1:10,000 5–10 ml Polidocanol 1% 5 ml	Inject epinephrine into the submucosa directly around blood vessel to achieve hemostasis by compression/vasoconstriction, then obliterate vessel with polidocanol	Epinephrine 5–10 ml Polidocanol 5 ml	May substitute bipolar coagulation or Nd:YAG laser for polidocanol
Thrombin in normal saline	100 IU thrombin/in 3 ml normal saline	Inject into bleeding vessel 10–15 ml total volume	10–15 ml	
Absolute ethanol	98% dehydrated ethanol	0.1–0.2 ml/injection at 3–4 sites surrounding bleeding vessel and 1–2 mm away from vessel	0.6–1.22 ml total	Inject via tuberculin syringe *slowly* (0.2 ml/3 seconds); extension/perforation significant risk if maximum volume exceeded; may be more technically difficult to control volume

*3.6%/.005% epinephrine prepared by combining 1 part Solution A (20 ml 15% NaCl solution and 1 ml of 0.1% epinephrine) to 3 parts of Solution B (20 ml distilled water, with 1 ml 0.1% epinephrine). 7.2%/.005% prepared by combining equal parts (1:1) of Solutions A and B.

Adapted from Sugawa C: Endoscopic diagnosis and treatment of upper gastrointestinal bleeding. Surg Clin North Am 1989; 69:1167–1183; with permission.

Table 74–10. THERMOCOAGULATION

Method	Site	Setting	Application Time	Number of Applications	Technique	Notes
Heater probe	Upper GI tract	30 joules		2–4	Firm tamponade, then coagulate around bleeding point, then on it	Decreased setting/time of application in colon or thinner gut wall
Monopolar	Upper GI tract	Midrange	1–2 sec/pulse		Directly on vessel <1 mm diameter; circumferentially around vessel >1 mm diameter	Perforation likely in colon
Bipolar/multipolar	Upper GI tract	15–25 watts	2 sec/pulse or up to 14 sec pulse	Multiple Single	Firm tamponade, then coagulate	Difficult angulation lesser curve or deformed duodenum
	Colon	5 watts	2 sec/pulse	Multiple		
Laser						
Nd:YAG	Upper GI tract	80 watts	0.5 sec/application		Distance: 1 cm from mucosa at least 2–3 mm away from arterial segments	
	Colon	40–80 watts	0.5–2.0 sec/application		Distance: 1.5–2.0 cm	Left-sided lesions only
Argon	Colon	2–8 watts	0.5 sec/application			May be used for right-sided lesions with caution
Hot biopsy forceps	Cecum and ascending colon	10–15 watts	1–2 sec		Tent mucosa away from muscle layer	Polyps ≤ 5 mm size; contraindicated in upper GI tract
	Left colon	15–20 watts	2 sec			

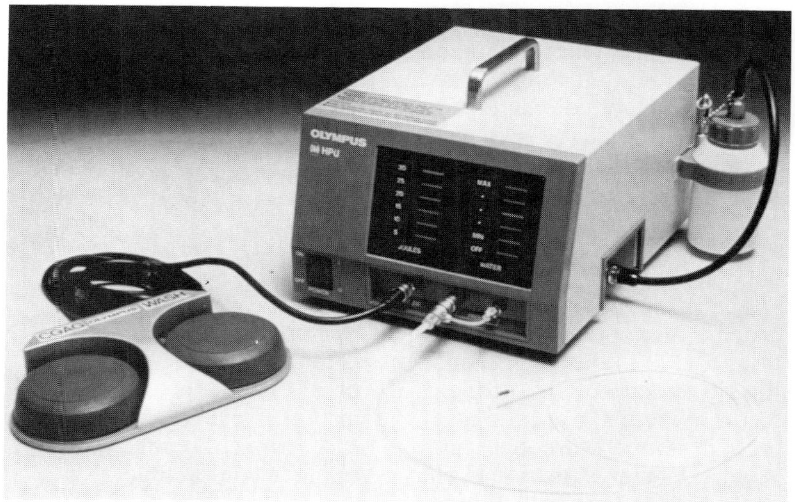

Figure 74–20. Heater probe unit with foot controls for coagulation and washing. Number of joules delivered is preset per application. (Courtesy of Olympus Corporation.)

be positioned so that the blood flows away from the ulcer base if possible. The probe is passed through the therapeutic channel, and coagulation is performed by tamponading the bleeding vessel by direct firm pressure using the heater probe and then coagulating the vessel (Fig. 74–21). Coagulation is usually performed in adults by two to four 30-joule pulses in succession.[120] Coagulation should be around the bleeding point first, and then directly on it. In studies of adult patients, the greatest success appears to be with firm tamponade on the ulcer bleeding point or nonbleeding visible vessel, and four pulses for a total of 120 joules in succession before the probe position is changed.[120, 124] This technique, however, may increase the risk of complications

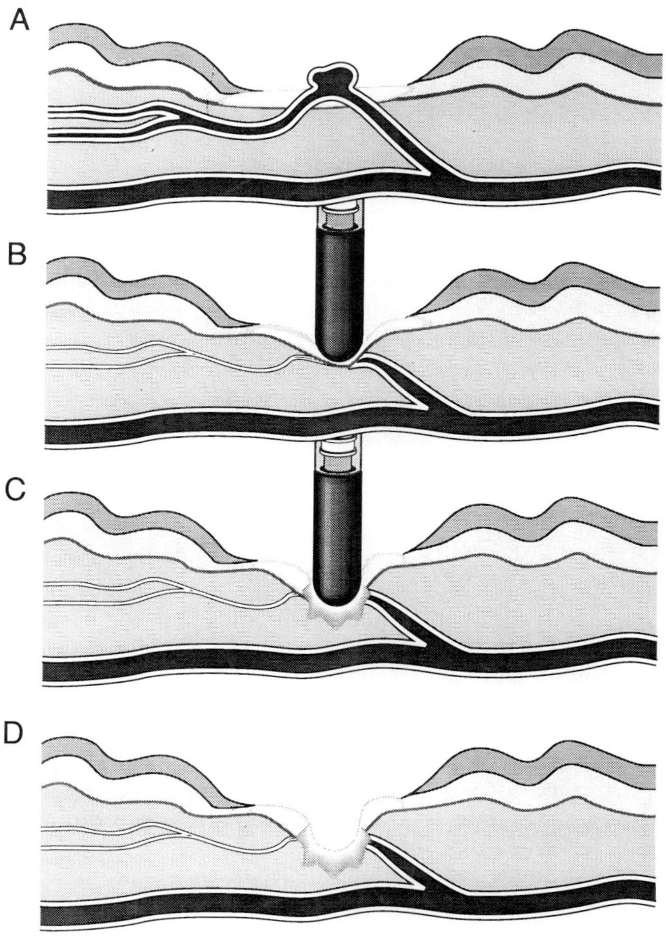

Figure 74–21. Coaptive coagulation utilizing the heater probe. *A,* Visible vessel in an ulcer base. Note vessel is not an end artery. *B,* Tamponade with probe initially. *C,* Coagulation after tamponade. *D,* "White footprint" at coagulation site.

when applied to other types of lesions, specifically Mallory-Weiss tears or angiomata, that occur in areas with a thinner gut wall.[120] The heater probe may also be used in cases of colonic bleeding. The number of joules per pulse should be reduced, especially in right-sided colonic lesions.[122, 125]

ELECTROCOAGULATION

There are two main types of electrocoagulation probes, monopolar and bipolar. In monopolar coagulation, a continuous or intermittent current is passed via the tip or side of the probe. The current is conducted to the patient's ground plate. The current is converted to high-temperature heat at the tissue contact point, which coagulates the tissue, causing collagen contraction and vessel shrinkage. For vessels less than 1 mm in diameter, the electrode is placed directly on the vessel and pressure is applied directly on the vessel to coapt it. With larger vessels, the coagulating current is placed circumferentially around the vessel until bleeding stops.[126] Usually a midrange setting is used for 1 to 2 seconds per pulse at a distance of 2 to 3 mm from the vessel. This is because an artery in an ulcer base may bleed from either side if it is not an end artery; therefore, a ring of tissue must be treated around the bleeding point to ensure adequate hemostasis. The aim is to achieve hemostasis of the underlying artery and not the overlying clot.[118] There are two main problems with monopolar coagulation. The first is that the depth of the burn is very difficult to regulate, and perforation is possible. This is especially true in the colon, where deep necrosis, perforation, and delayed massive bleeding have been reported with monopolar electrocoagulation.[122] The second problem is that there is a moderate amount of electrode adherence to the underlying tissue at the treated site and therefore poor visibility, especially in nonirrigated systems.[121] A third technical problem is the need to clean the tip of the probe as the coagulum accumulates during electrocoagulation.[126]

Currently bipolar or multipolar coagulation is the most popular method with endoscopists. Unlike monopolar coagulation, a grounding plate is not required. Current is transmitted from one electrode on the probe to another, and energy is delivered when any pair of electrodes is in contact with the bleeding target.[127] The BICAP (multipolar) probe has six points through which current can be passed; contact between any two is sufficient (Fig. 74–22). This has the advantage of allowing for tangential contact. The maximal temperature achieved with this method is significantly less than that of monopolar coagulation or the Nd:YAG laser, causing less tissue injury and having greater efficacy for vessels less than 2 mm in diameter.[128] There are two sizes of probes available, 2.3 mm and 3.2 mm. Like the heater probe, the correct technique is to compress the bleeding vessel first, then to coagulate. Forceful application of the larger-size probe appears to increase hemostatic bond strength and area and depth of coagulation.[128] The greatest depth of coagulation is usually achieved with a low to midrange setting (15 to 25 watts). Pulses should be applied as short, multiple pulses (2 seconds in duration) or a single long pulse up to 14 seconds in duration.[128] The longer, lower-voltage pulse is thought to work by increasing the depth of coagulation by decreasing tissue desiccation.[129] In adults, up to 40 seconds total of electrocoagulation are required.[128, 130, 131] Increased bleeding after bipolar coagulation has been reported in cases with a visible vessel; usually this bleeding is controllable with further bipolar coagulation, but on occasion surgery has been required.

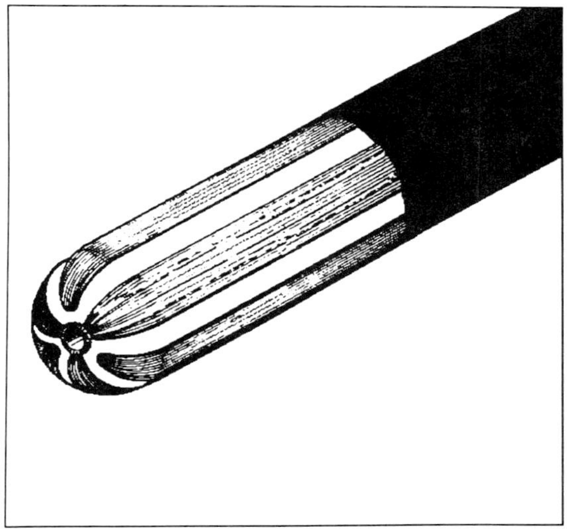

Figure 74–22. BICAP multipolar electrocoagulation probe. Note three pairs of alternating electrodes. (From Laine L: Bipolar-multipolar electrocoagulation of bleeding ulcers. Gastrointest Endosc Clin North Am 1991; 1:293; with permission.)

Bipolar electrocoagulation appears to be equally effective to the heater probe in terms of hemostasis, incidence of rebleeding, transfusion requirement, and need for emergency surgery. Several studies report a hemostasis rate in the 90% range for both modalities.[125, 128, 129, 132] It also appears to be as efficacious as the laser at a marked reduction in cost. The angulation of the probe, or use of a bipolar electrode compared to a laser, does not appear to affect the rebleeding rate. However, poor angulation along the lesser curvature of the stomach or in a deformed duodenum may make pressure application more difficult.[132]

Angiodysplasia, predominantly of the colon, has been treated successfully by endoscopic electrocoagulation. Hemorrhagic proctocolitis with recurrent bleeding after radiation therapy has also been successfully treated with a bipolar probe at a power setting of 5 with short 2-second pulses by coagulating at multiple bleeding sites.[133] Late rebleeding has been reported, which was treated successfully by repeat electrocoagulation. In some cases, surgery is still required.[134]

An additional coagulation technique used primarily in the colon is the hot biopsy forceps. This technique combines the principles of endoscopic biopsy and monopolar electrocoagulation. The lesion to be biopsied is grasped in the jaw of insulated biopsy forceps, including polyps up to 5 mm.[135] The forceps are used to tent the mucosa upward away from the colonic muscular layer (Fig. 74–23). A brief electrocoagulating current passes through the forceps to the mucosa and sometimes submucosa, causing coagulation at its base, while preserving the histologic integrity of the specimen. The unit is set on coagulation, at a setting of 10 to 15 W for 1 to 2 seconds in the cecum and ascending colon, up to 15 to 20 W for 2 seconds in the left colon. Higher settings or longer application times have been associated with an increased risk of perforation, especially in the right colon.[136, 137]

Perforation has been reported at an increased rate with application of the technique to the upper gastrointestinal tract, both in the stomach (secondary to increased gastric thickness, limiting tenting of the mucosa) and in the duodenum and ileum (secondary to thinness of the bowel wall and variable depth of penetration).[136] In the colon, the risk of perforation appears to be intermediate at .05%, less than that associated with snare polypectomy but greater than that of routine colonoscopy. However, for lesions greater than 5 mm, snare polypectomy is the preferred technique.[135]

Another complication of the hot biopsy forceps is major hemorrhage, which may occur in 0.41% of cases.[136] This is especially likely if the forceps are not held perpendicular to the mucosa. Short-circuiting of the current with massive hemorrhage, has been reported between the forceps tip and the noninsulated portion of the forceps, if the forceps are held at an angle of 15 degrees or less to the bowel wall.[137] Hemorrhage may be immediate or delayed up to 1 week after biopsy and may not respond to conservative therapy.[138]

Results of comparative trials of injection, coagulation, and heater probe therapy vary according to the method used. Utilizing the hypertonic saline/epinephrine solution in 158 ulcer patients, Hirao and associates achieved permanent hemostasis in 93.7% and temporary hemostasis in 4.4% of actively bleeding lesions or lesions with a visible vessel. The rate of emergency operation decreased from 21.7 to 0.8% when repeat prophylactic injection at 24 and 48 hours was performed.[123]

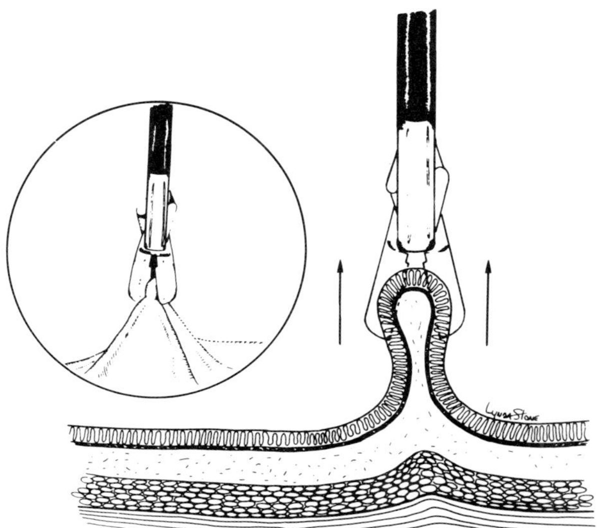

Figure 74–23. Insulated hot biopsy forceps. The mucosa is tented away from the colonic wall prior to electrocoagulation. (From Wadas D, Sanowski R: Complications of the hot biopsy forceps technique. Gastrointest Endosc 1988; 34(1):32–37; © by the American Society for Gastrointestinal Endoscopy; with permission.)

Multipolar electrocoagulation was used in 75 adult patients with evidence of an ulcer with a nonbleeding visible vessel.[128] The incidence of recurrent bleeding in the patients coagulated was 18% versus 41% in the nontreated controls, and the incidence of emergency surgery was 8% versus 30% in the untreated controls.

Waring and colleagues compared injection of absolute alcohol to the BICAP multipolar electrocoagulation unit in a randomized trial of actively bleeding ulcers or ulcers with stigmata of recent hemorrhage.[139] Initial success (93% BICAP, 97% injection), rebleeding rates (25% and 23%, respectively), need for emergency surgery (22% and 7%, respectively) mortality, and transfusion requirements were not statistically different. BICAP use and injection of absolute alcohol appear equally efficacious for use in therapeutic endoscopy. In some circumstances, one method may be technically easier. With BICAP probes, the depth of coagulation is limited to 2 mm, which limits its use with larger vessels. However, it has the advantage of a built-in wash system, aiding visibility with brisk bleeding as compared to injection therapy.[139]

Chung and coworkers randomized 132 patients with active ulcer bleeding to receive endoscopic epinephrine injection or heater probe treatment.[140] Endoscopy was repeated 24 hours later. The patients treated with epinephrine had initial success in 86% of spurting lesions and 100% of oozing lesions. Thirteen percent of the oozing lesions required retreatment at 24 hours. Seventeen percent of the patients in the injection group ultimately rebled and required surgery. There were no complications in this group. Of the patients treated with the heater probe, 75% of those with spurting lesions and 86% of those with oozing lesions had initial hemostatic success (83% initial success rate); 11% of the patients who stopped bleeding had a clinically significant rebleed, requiring surgery. There were two (3%) perforations noted in the heater probe group; both occurred in patients who required multiple heater probe applications within a 24-hour period. There was no difference in overall success rate utilizing a particular modality between gastric and duodenal ulcers; however, for both, the initial success rate was higher utilizing epinephrine.

The choice of therapeutic endoscopic technique depends to a significant extent on the training of the endoscopist and equipment availability. If the technique is properly performed, the results are similar using injection or thermal coagulation. Certain lesions, based on their anatomic location or briskness of bleeding, may be more amenable to one method than another.

LASER PHOTOCOAGULATION

Laser photocoagulation is another modality occasionally used to achieve endoscopic hemostasis. There are two main types of laser, the argon and the Nd:YAG laser. The argon laser's usefulness is limited because of light absorption by surrounding red blood. To use the argon laser, therefore, overlying blood must be eliminated with a coaxial air jet. Clinically, the argon laser is used primarily for right-sided colonic lesions. When compared with the Nd:YAG laser, it has a lower power and depth of tissue penetration.

The Nd:YAG laser is the most popular laser used in endoscopy. The laser admits a continuous wave of infrared light of a wave length of 1,064 with a power up to 100 W. This light is transmitted via a 600-micrometer glass fiber in a 2.5-mm Teflon catheter passed down the endoscope biopsy channel. Carbon dioxide is passed coaxially along the catheter to clear blood from the bleeding site and to keep the fiber tip cool and free from debris. A filter is attached to the eyepiece to prevent reflected laser light from entering the endoscopist's eye. The intense laser light is directed to coagulate tissue circumferentially around the bleeding site. The current recommendation for adults is to deliver 0.5-second pulses, at 80 W of energy, from a distance of 1 cm, and at least 2 to 3 mm away from visible arterial segments for upper gastrointestinal lesions.[141]

Lasers in colonoscopy and small bowel enteroscopy have been used for congenital vascular lesions (hereditary hemorrhagic telangiectasia, blue rubber bleb nevi syndrome) as well as superficial vascular lesions, including angiodysplasia, telangiectasia, and arteriovenous malformation.[121, 142–144] Asymptomatic, nonbleeding angiodysplasias are usually not treated.[122] One problem after laser photocoagulation of a lesion is that the histologic diagnosis is difficult to confirm.[118, 145]

Like the heater probe, laser therapy can also provoke bleeding, which can usually be stopped with further laser coagulation.[141] In addition, there is an increased chance of full-thickness perforation of the gut wall.[144] Application of the laser in the colon requires modification of both technique and power settings. The thermal effects of a laser beam on tissue vary according to the power density (the amount of energy converted to heat at the point where the laser beam strikes tissue) and the size of the contact area. Although the power setting and the exposure time can be preset, movement, especially in the right colon, and varying wall thickness, especially the thin ascending colon, can change the time of exposure required to produce perforation.[145] Instead of coagulating tissue, vaporization of tissue can occur.

There is a long learning curve associated with use of the laser, and this modality should be used only by experienced operators. Currently the laser seems to offer little advantage over the heater probe and BICAP, and because of its increased cost and decreased portability, the other two modalities are likely to predominate in the foreseeable future.

STRICTURE DILATION

Esophageal dilation can be performed with a variety of instruments, but only endoscopic dilation is discussed in this section. The advantage of endoscopic dilation is the ability to visualize the stenotic area, estimate its size, select an appropriately sized dilator, and, when necessary, pass a guide wire beyond the stenotic area. Savary Gillard dilators are among the most frequently used endoscopic dilating systems. The dilators themselves are hollow bougies of plastic-coated polyvinyl ranging in size from 5 to 15 mm (15 to 45 French). The tip is tapered and flexible, and the shaft is more rigid. Utilizing an endoscope with a therapeutic-sized channel (2.8 mm), the endoscopist inserts the endoscope to the level of the stenosis or beyond the stenosis if possible. A flexible-tipped guide wire is then advanced through the stricture under direct observation. When it passes the stricture, the endoscope is removed while the wire is kept in place by advancing the wire as the endoscope is withdrawn. The lubricated bougie is then threaded over the guide wire, which is held taut. Serial dilations are performed by progressively increasing the bougie size according to the amount of resistance encountered. The dilators should be checked for blood after each dilation. Strictures may need to be dilated over several sessions rather than on a single occasion. The guide wire must be held in place in between application of serial bougies in order to avoid slippage.[146]

In a large French-American series, larger-diameter dilations could be performed using the Savary system when compared with the Eder-Puestow dilating system. There was no statistically significant difference in the incidence of complications with each method.[146] The occurrence of esophageal perforation may relate more to the reason for dilation (e.g., caustic ingestion or malignancy as compared to peptic stenosis) than the dilating method used. Also, the success of dilation may relate to the indication. Dilating congenital stenosis is usually more effective than dilating achalasia or postsurgical stenosis.[147]

Endoscopic balloon dilation may also be performed utilizing the Gruntzig balloon catheter. This catheter was originally used for transluminal angioplasty. The catheter has a low-compliance inflatable polyvinyl balloon at its tip. The balloon is inflatable to a preset maximum diameter and pressure. If the pressure is exceeded, the balloon ruptures, reducing the risk of esophageal perforation. Inflation exerts only radially directed forces as opposed to the shearing longitudinal forces with conventional bougienage.[148] The catheter is positioned through the endoscope with or without the use of a guide wire. The balloon is inflated with either water or gastrograffin and held in inflation for 10 to 15 seconds, then deflated. Usually two or three inflations are performed per endoscopic session, and the sessions are repeated over several weeks or months with progressively larger-diameter catheters. This technique has been utilized for esophageal atresia with postoperative strictures and seems to be most helpful for strictures of recent onset.[149–152] Endoscopically directed hydrostatic balloon dilation has also been reported in obstructive gastroduodenal Crohn's disease.[153] Cicatrical anastomotic strictures of the colon have also been dilated with air- and water-filled balloons or with a mechanical dilator (e.g., Savary dilator) placed over an endoscopically directed guidewire.[154, 154a] These techniques may occasionally be accompanied by use of a sphincterotome.

Intralesional steroid injection of peptic esophageal strictures has been reported as an adjuvant to endoscopic dilation. Using small volumes of triamcinolone acetonide in four quadrants of the narrowest stricture segment, Kirsch and associates reported increased symptom-free intervals between endoscopic dilations.[155]

SMALL BOWEL ENTEROSCOPY

There are two major methods of small bowel enteroscopy currently applicable to pediatric patients. In children, this technique is used primarily for the evaluation of gastrointestinal bleeding of unknown origin. It may occasionally be indicated for small bowel biopsy, although this can usually be accomplished utilizing the standard upper endoscopes.

The most popular type of small bowel endoscopic examination is push enteroscopy. The limitation of this technique is that the angulation of the duodenum dissipates the propelling force transmitted to the shaft of the endoscope and subsequently creates a large loop in the stomach and duodenum. Gastroduodenal loops are occasionally able to be reduced by using a straightening tube.[156] Currently this type of enteroscopy is performed with either a sterilized pediatric colonoscope or a special push-type enteroscope—the SIF-10. Both of these endoscopes have a larger diameter than standard pediatric gastroscopes, limiting their usefulness in infants and small children. These endoscopes do, however, have a biopsy channel, and angulation of the tip is possible. Only the proximal jejunum in the adult, 90 cm from the ligament of Treitz, can be visualized with this endoscopic technique.[157, 158] After the scope is fully inserted, glucagon may be administered to decrease intestinal peristalsis.[158] The lumen is visualized primarily upon scope withdrawal, combining air insufflation and slow withdrawal of the scope. This technique is useful to detect a diffuse lesion and to detect causes of small bowel bleeding, especially arteriovenous malformations.[157, 158]

The second type of small bowel endoscopy is passive, using a Sonde-type enteroscope. The Sonde-type enteroscopes are passed intranasally. The instruments have a balloon at their tip and when it is inflated, bowel peristalsis acts to pull the endoscope through the small bowel (Fig. 74–24). This procedure may take 12 to 24 hours. As compared to the push-type enteroscopes, the Sonde scope has a much narrower diameter for greater patient comfort. It has no tip control for angulation, however, and has no biopsy channel.[156] The Lewis Way modification involves transnasal passage of the passive enteroscope with a suture at its tip. The pediatric colonoscope is then passed orally and the suture is grabbed using the biopsy forceps through the pediatric colonoscope channel. The pediatric colonoscope guides the passive enteroscope into the duodenum and is then carefully withdrawn. The balloon is inflated and its passage is monitored fluoroscopically. Metachlopromide and neostigmine may be given to facilitate scope movement.[159] As with the push-type enteroscope, the lumen is visualized using glucagon paralysis upon scope withdrawal.[156]

Tada and colleagues successfully visualized the distal small intestine up to 140 cm from the ligament of Treitz in three children by utilizing this technique. In only one, however, was pathology identified (Peutz-Jeghers polyps).[159] Current techniques have limited applicability to pediatric patients because children are unlikely to tolerate the long procedure time and the relatively large diameter of the instrument.

PERCUTANEOUS ENDOSCOPIC GASTROSTOMY AND PERCUTANEOUS ENDOSCOPIC JEJUNOSTOMY

The technique for percutaneous endoscopic gastrostomy (PEG) was originally described in 1980.[160] Though

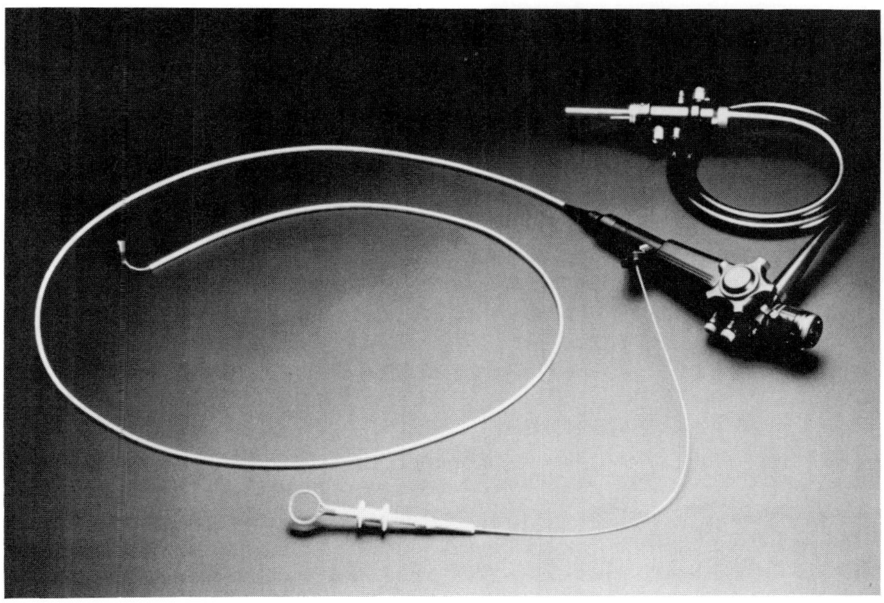

Figure 74–24. Sonde-type small bowel enteroscope. Note narrow diameter and decreased tip control. (Courtesy of Olympus Corporation.)

initially utilized in children, this technique has subsequently been applied to adults. The procedure is usually performed in those patients unable to swallow who require long-term enteral nutrition and who may be at high risk from either a prolonged anesthetic or an open surgical procedure. Placement of a PEG tube may have advantages compared to an open gastrostomy if general anesthesia is not required.[160]

The technique is performed as follows: A standard EGD is performed and the stomach is distended with air to oppose it to the anterior abdominal wall and to attempt to mobilize the liver, spleen, and colon away from the gastrostomy site.[160] Using the light from the endoscope tip, the stomach is transilluminated. After performing a sterile skin preparation and anesthetizing the skin using local anesthetic, a second physician introduces a 16-gauge medicut needle or stylet with needle percutaneously into the stomach. The usual site of entry is a point located at the junction of the middle two thirds and outer one third of a line drawn between the umbilicus and the midportion of the left inferior costal margin. Through the medicut or stylet a sturdy suture or guide wire is inserted into the stomach (Fig. 74–25A). This entire procedure is viewed simultaneously through the endoscope. The suture is grasped with a forceps or polypectomy snare, and the endoscope and snare are removed, with the suture pulled in a retrograde fashion out of the patient's mouth. The suture is held outside of the stomach at its entry point during this maneuver. The suture is then secured to the catheter and, with simultaneous application of traction on the abdominal portion of the suture, the catheter is pulled into the stomach and through the gastric and abdominal walls (Fig. 74–25B). Some individuals use both an internal and an external bumper to oppose the catheter to the abdominal wall, although modification of this technique has been reported[161] (Fig. 74–25C).

A modification of the percutaneous endoscopic gastrostomy technique was described by Russell and coworkers in 1984, utilizing a "peel-away" sheath to directly insert a Foley catheter into the stomach.[162, 163] A one-step button technique has recently been devised that threads a gastrostomy button over the suture in place of the catheter, avoiding the second procedure of converting the catheter to a button (Fig. 74–26).[163a]

Direct percutaneous endoscopic jejunostomy (PEJ) has also been reported.[164, 165] This technique is indicated in those patients prone to aspiration, with complete or partial gastric or duodenal obstruction or gastric motility disorders.[164] Because of the smaller jejunal size and its variable position, the technique is technically more difficult than the PEG technique. The procedure is performed utilizing a long push enteroscope, which is advanced into the jejunum up to 24 inches distal to the ligament of Treitz in adult-size patients. The endoscope tip is used to transilluminate the abdominal wall in a 2- to 3-cm area. The second physician uses direct fingertip pressure to identify a discrete intrajejunal indentation to the endoscopist. After sterile preparation and anesthesia of the skin, the stylet is introduced into the jejunum with a swift stab and the suture or guide wire is threaded through the stylet after removing the needle as with the PEG technique. The catheter is inserted in a similar fashion to the PEG catheter, except that an internal horizontal bar is not placed because it may cause obstruction of the narrower jejunal lumen or mucosal ulceration. A mushroom catheter is used to anchor its position to the abdominal wall.[164]

In some instances a PEJ tube may not be able to be placed because of inability to appose and transilluminate a jejunal segment adjacent to the abdominal wall. Theoretical problems with PEJ insertion include increased technical difficulty, including maintaining correct jejunal position and risk of needle entry into the abdomen either directly or through the posterior jejunal wall secondary to diminished luminal size. This technique

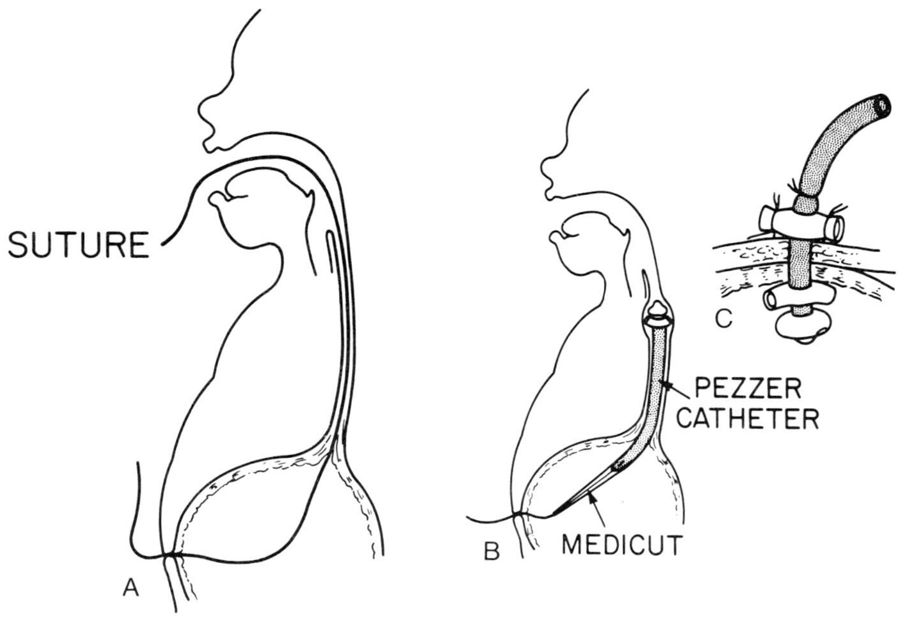

Figure 74–25. PEG placement. *A,* A suture or wire is brought out through the stomach and esophagus to the patient's mouth. *B,* While maintaining tension on the suture, the PEG catheter is passed over the suture into the stomach and through the anterior abdominal wall. *C,* The PEG catheter may be secured to the anterior abdominal wall with an external and internal bumper. (From Gauderer MW, Ponsky JL, Izant RJ Jr: Gastrostomy without laparotomy: A percutaneous endoscopic technique. J Pediatr Surg 1980; 15:874; with permission.)

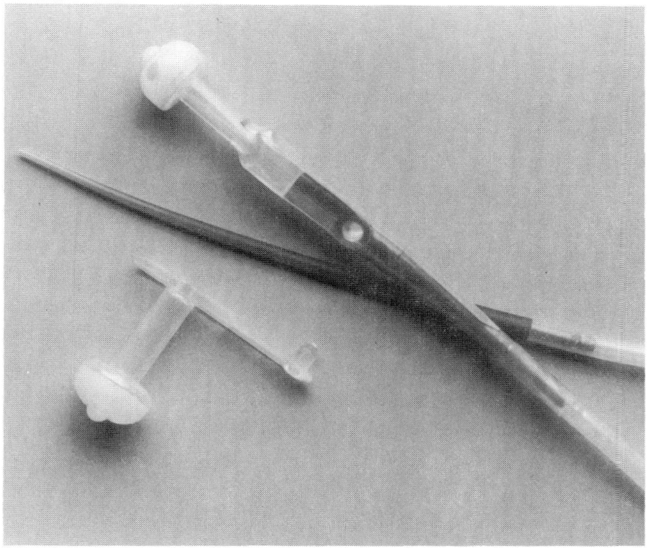

Figure 74–26. One-step percutaneous gastrostomy button. (Courtesy of Applied Medical Technology, Inc.)

may prove to be especially difficult in pediatric patients because of the reduced diameter of their intestinal lumen.[164] Before both the PEG and PEJ procedures, prophylactic antibiotics are routinely administered, directed against usual skin flora.[161, 164]

There have been a number of complications reported with insertion of PEG tubes. In addition, there are several relative contraindications to its use. Gauderer and associates reported their complications in 160 PEG procedures.[161] One patient with congenital heart disease died within 24 hours postoperatively, four patients (3%) developed minor catheter infections, and six patients (4%) required further surgery—two for catheter migration, one for peritoneal irritation, and three for gastrocolic fistulae. This type of fistula has been reported by other authors and may present up to several months after PEG placement.[166] With long-term follow-up, at least 50% of the patients in Gauderer's series with pre-PEG reflux ultimately required fundoplication. Fundoplication may also be required for reflux developing after or exacerbated by PEG placement. Grunow and colleagues studied 10 children with normal extended esophageal pH monitoring prior to PEG placement Six of the 10 developed gastroesophageal reflux after the PEG procedure.[167] Transgastric perforation of a PEG tube has also been reported, with leakage of gastric contents and feedings into the peritoneal cavity.[168]

Relative contraindications to a PEG tube include the following: (1) previous abdominal surgery in the region of the PEG tube, with a possibility of adhesions that alter the anatomy and relationship of the stomach and colon to the anterior abdominal wall or suspected intestinal malrotation (may also apply to a PEJ tube); (2) patients with documented gastroesophageal reflux in whom a simultaneous Nissen fundoplication would be indicated; and (3) patients who require retrograde dilation through a PEG tube for esophageal stenosis or stricture because of the possibility of separating the PEG from the anterior abdominal wall.[160]

POLYPECTOMY

The rationale for large bowel examination for suspected polyps in the adult patient is based on the assumption that cancers arise from preexisting adenomas or neoplastic polyps. Screening has been suggested for patients as they enter higher-risk age groups, for those who have a family or personal history of colon cancer, or for those who have an underlying disease process that would make them more susceptible to the development of carcinoma. Most polyps in the pediatric population are simple juvenile polyps and have no premalignant potential. Recently, however, a greater frequency of adenomas has been identified in pediatric patients.[169] In addition, up to one third of the patients with polyps develop an iron-deficiency anemia.[169] Identification of the source of bleeding in children also helps differentiate polyps from other sources of bleeding that require specific intervention to prevent sequelae.

Prior to polypectomy the patient must be cleansed of fecal debris. A poorly prepared colon results in poor visualization and increases the technical difficulty of the procedure. Excessive fecal debris or the use of certain gavage solutions such as mannitol places the patient at risk for explosion during attempted polypectomy.[169a] The risk of bleeding should be assessed by history. In certain situations it is prudent to perform a complete blood count and coagulation profile and have blood products available prior to polyp removal.

Diminutive polyps, or those less than 5 mm in diameter, are best removed with biopsy forceps. Hot biopsy monopolar forceps or routine forceps biopsy followed by coagulation, if necessary, allows histologic evaluation. Bipolar forceps and laser do not provide interpretable biopsy specimens.[170] If lesions are too numerous for removal, representative samples should be obtained for analysis.

Large polyps (greater than 5 mm) are usually removed with snare electrocautery.[171–174] The snare consists of a wire loop covered by a plastic tube. The snare is inserted into the endoscope with the plastic sheath completely covering the wire loop. The snare is then advanced down the operating channel of the endoscope until the sheath is seen protruding from the instrument. An assistant then opens the snare, and the wire loop can be visualized beyond the end of the sheath. The polyp is then lassoed and the sheath maneuvered to the stalk (Fig. 74–27). Most polyps in the pediatric population are pedunculated with a moderate to long stalk. To avoid a potential perforation and to be able to resnare the stalk in case of bleeding, the stalk should be snared 0.5 to 1 cm from the margin of the stalk and the bowel mucosa. The head of the polyp should be lifted off the mucosa prior to electrocautery, but contact between the head and the opposing mucosa should be avoided to prevent a collateral burn. After the polyp has been properly snared, a current is passed through the snare, which is slowly closed by the assistant. Rapid closure results in bleeding from vessels in the stalk that have been amputated but not coagulated. As the polyp coagulates there is a whitish discoloration of the polyp. In polyps with a short stalk the snare should be placed as

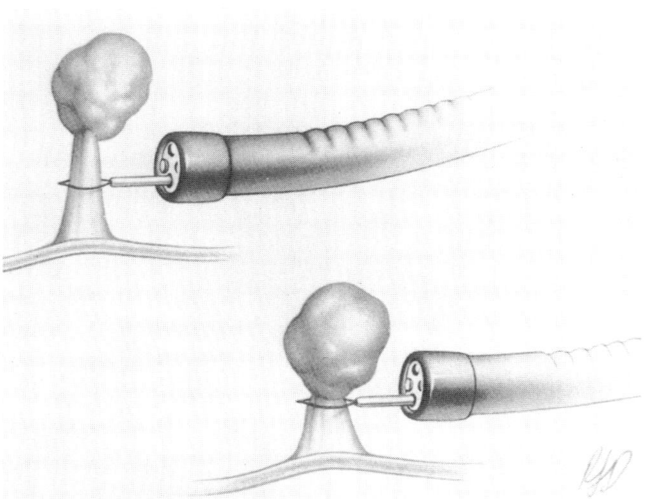

Figure 74–27. Snare polypectomy of a pedunculated polyp. After ensnarement, the loop is advanced to the polyp neck prior to closure, in order to allow sufficient length to resnare a bleeding polyp stalk and avoid thermal injury to the bowel wall. (From Shinya H: Colonoscopic polypectomy. *In* Shinya H, ed: Colonoscopy: Diagnosis and Treatment of Colonic Diseases. New York, Igaku-Shoin, 1982, p 182; with permission.)

close to the head of the polyp as possible. To remove polyps with large heads, it may occasionally be necessary to segmentally resect the polyp head (Fig. 74–28). After the head is reduced in size, it is usually possible to then snare the stalk and safely remove the remainder of the polyp. Broad-based polyps must be removed with care.

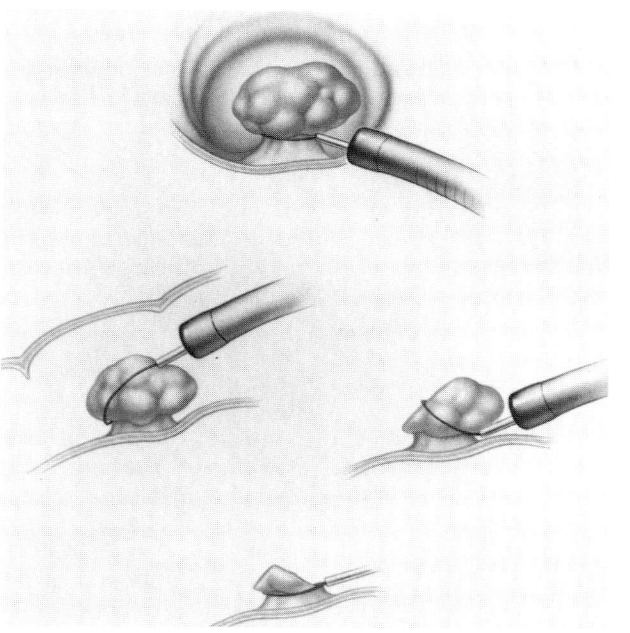

Figure 74–28. Snare polypectomy of the large sessile polyp by segmental excision of the head. (From Shinya H: Colonoscopic polypectomy. *In* Shinya H, ed: Colonoscopy: Diagnosis and Treatment of Colonic Diseases. New York, Igaku-Shoin, 1982, p 186; with permission.)

Transection of the polyp close to the bowel wall risks perforation. It is usually better to remove the polyp piecemeal. Piecemeal resection may also be necessary if the snare becomes lodged in the head of the polyp. Vigorous attempts at dislodging the wire may result in bleeding. In the case of large sessile polyps, the endoscopist must assess the risk of polypectomy and the nature of the information to be gained before deciding if the polyp should be removed endoscopically or transabdominally. Often segmental resection or multiple biopsies in sessile or broad-based polyps remove tissue adequate for pathologic differentiation. Occasionally large polyps may need to be reduced in multiple sessions for complete obliteration.

When multiple polyps are encountered, the most proximal should be removed first so that subsequent passage of the endoscope will not precipitate hemorrhage over the base of an already amputated polyp. In the patient with large numbers of polyps, representative polyps should be removed or biopsied for pathologic analysis.

After amputation polyps should be retrieved. Small polyps can be suctioned through the endoscope and the polyp retrieved in a trap. Large polyps may pose problems but can usually be retrieved with the snare, standard or foreign body forceps, or basket (Fig. 74–29). If the endoscopist is unable to retrieve the polyp, the patient can be given an enema or the parents can be asked to strain the stool and submit the tissue for later analysis.

Vascular lesions can be identified and cauterized during colonoscopy. Although these lesions are rare,[175–179] colonoscopy with therapeutic intervention can eliminate the need for surgery in many cases.[27, 28] There are two general varieties of lesions that have been identified: cavernous hemangiomas and small telangiectasias. The relatively small size of vascular lesions and their submucosal location limit the usefulness of barium studies in their identification, and radionuclide studies are helpful only if brisk bleeding is present. Many syndromes have been associated with vascular lesions in the gas-

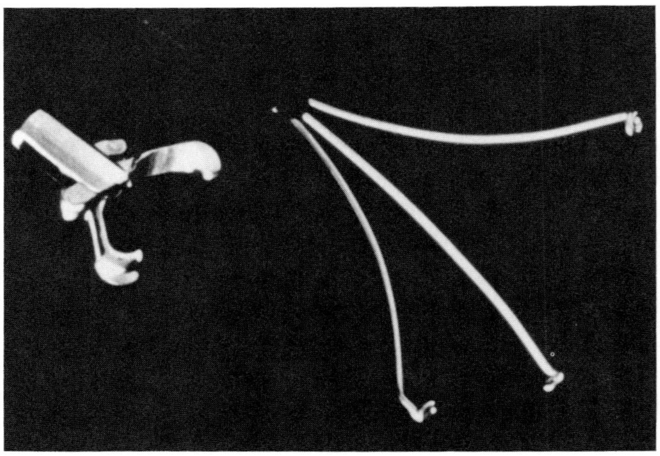

Figure 74–29. Foreign body forceps may be utilized for polyp retrieval. Rat/shark tooth forceps *(left)* and tripod polyp retriever *(right)*. (Courtesy of Olympus Corporation.)

trointestinal tract, among them Osler-Weber-Rendu, CREST syndrome (calcinosis cutis, Raynaud phenomenon, sclerodactyly, and telangiectasis), dyschondroplasia (Maffucci's syndrome), blue rubber bleb nevus syndrome, and diffuse neonatal hemangiomatosis.[180, 181] Telangiectasias may also occur in Turner's syndrome and pseudoxanthoma elasticum.[182, 183]

Lymphonodular hyperplasia of the colon may also be a cause of painless rectal bleeding.[184, 185] Thinning of the surface epithelium over the protruding lymphatic tissue with subsequent trauma from the passage of fecal material is thought to lead to ulceration and hematochezia. Prominent lymphatic nodules can be found throughout the large and small bowel. In children younger than 5 years of age, they may be found in up to 50% of large bowel examinations.[186] On colonoscopy they appear as smooth, round 2- to 4-mm nodules with normal overlying mucosa. Occasionally larger nodules may have central umbilication or an overlying erosion. This nodular lymph node tissue is thought to represent a self-limited response to antigenic stimulation and does not usually require any additional evaluation or therapy.

SPECIAL ENDOSCOPIC TECHNIQUES

Several new techniques performed through the endoscope have been reported. Okamatsu and colleagues performed a successful endoscopic membranectomy on a 60-day-old infant with trisomy 21 syndrome and a congenital duodenal membrane.[187]

The endoscope may also be used intraoperatively to guide surgical management. Humphrey and Dorazio reported a case of a 10-year-old male with intestinal malrotation in whom intraoperative endoscopy identified a web in the third portion of the duodenum.[188]

There has been a case report of endoscopic obliteration of a recurrent tracheoesophageal fistula in an infant by injection with Histoacryl into the fistula and 0.5% polidocanol around the fistula. The obliteration was endoscopically confirmed.[189] This technique requires further study prior to routine application.

COMPLICATIONS

Esophagogastroduodenoscopy

As with any procedure, the benefits of the endoscopic procedure and the diagnostic information obtained should outweigh the relative risk to the patient. Endoscopic complications can be classified into three types: those associated with sedation, those secondary to the procedure, and those associated with attempted therapeutic interventions. In some cases, the cause of the complication may remain indeterminate. Ament reported a prospective study of the complications associated with 2,046 upper intestinal endoscopies and 1,120 small intestinal biopsies in pediatric patients.[190] Complications occurred in 1.7% of upper intestinal endoscopies and in 0.5% of small intestinal biopsies. During endoscopy, bronchospasm, transient respiratory arrest, and phlebitis were the commonest complications. Fever and sedation complications (not specified) were commonest with small intestinal biopsy.[190] The American Society for Gastrointestinal Endoscopy (ASGE) has recently completed a review of 21,011 gastrointestinal endoscopies to determine the relative rate of drug-related complications. In a group consisting primarily of adult patients, the overall medication complication rate was 13.5 per 1,000 procedures; of these, 5.4 per 1,000 represented serious cardiac or respiratory complications, with a fatality rate of 0.3 per 1,000 procedures. Patients at highest risk for medication-related complications were those who received narcotics, were undergoing an emergent or urgent procedure, or were undergoing colonoscopy. The dosage of diazepam or midazolam did not appear to correlate with the complication rate.[191] Patients with cystic fibrosis may be particularly at risk for respiratory problems related to endoscopy or general anesthesia.[192]

There are a number of mechanical complications reported after upper gastrointestinal endoscopy. In a 1974 ASGE survey, there was a major complication rate of 1.32 per 1,000 upper endoscopies, including infection, perforation, bleeding, cardiopulmonary complications, and death.[74] In the same series, esophageal dilation was associated with a much higher complication rate, ranging from 4.25 per 1,000 cases using mercury bougies, to 6.1 per 1,000 using metal olives, and up to 18.1 per 1,000 when pneumatic or mechanical dilation was performed. Moghissi and Pender reviewed the results of 39 esophageal perforations occurring after diagnostic or therapeutic upper gastrointestinal endoscopy.[193] Twenty-three occurred during esophageal stricture dilation, ten during endoscopic removal of a foreign body, and six during diagnostic endoscopy. Perforations occurred with both rigid and flexible endoscopes, but were more likely if endoscopy was performed with a rigid instrument. Patients frequently presented with pain and dysphagia. All the patients had x-rays revealing subcutaneous emphysema, pneumomediastinum, or pneumothorax. The overall mortality rate was 33%. Mortality differed significantly between those presenting early (19% at less than 36 hours) and those presenting late (50% at greater than 36 hours).[193]

Intramural duodenal hematoma resulting in complete bowel obstruction and necessitating blood transfusions has been reported after duodenal biopsies.[194] Spontaneous bowel perforation has been reported in patients with Ehlers-Danlos syndrome type 4.[33] These patients may theoretically be at higher risk for perforation during or after gastrointestinal endoscopy.

Serious complications have also been reported after therapeutic injection. Full-thickness gastric necrosis has been reported after injection of 12 ml of 5% ethanolamine oleate (a sclerosant) into and around a benign actively bleeding ulcer,[195] and following injection of a combination of 4 ml of 1% polidocanol and 8 ml of a 1:10,000 epinephrine solution in a small posterior gastric ulcer.[196] Complications have also been reported after endoscopic laser therapy with an Nd:YAG laser with coaxial carbon dioxide, including free perforation, pneumoperitoneum (thought to occur because of dissection of high-pressure carbon dioxide gas through a laser-induced mucosal erosion and subsequent rupture of the gas-filled bleb), and delayed massive hemorrhage following laser coagulation of angiodysplasia.[197]

There have been two cases of fatal air embolism reported in pediatric patients who had undergone a Kasai procedure for biliary atresia and who were undergoing upper gastrointestinal endoscopy under general anesthesia. The first occurred in a 4-month-old undergoing endoscopy to determine the etiology of a diminished stomal bile output. Air apparently was infused into the bed of the porta hepatis, and the authors proposed that under pressure, this air dissected across diseased liver tissue into a large hepatic vein.[198]

A second similar case was reported in a 10-year-old female who, also after a Kasai procedure, developed a stricture at her anastomotic site with a stone above it. Under general anesthesia she underwent an endoscopic procedure to remove the stone and dilate the stricture through a percutaneous jejunal loop. The patient developed circulatory collapse and died of a massive air embolus.[199] Because the mechanism of death in these two cases is not entirely clear, extra caution is required in endoscopic procedures involving an exteriorized loop in a patient who has undergone a Kasai procedure.

Colonoscopy

Sedation complications during colonoscopy are similar to those reported during upper gastrointestinal tract examination. Several series have demonstrated a correlation between the frequency of technical complications during colonoscopy and the experience of the endoscopist.[200–202] Gastroenterologists treating adults have their highest complication rates during their first 50 to 100 colonoscopic procedures.[203]

Bleeding following colonoscopy is usually minimal but may follow mucosal biopsy or polypectomy. Bleeding following a diagnostic procedure has been reported in between 0.008 and 0.17% of procedures in adults[200, 201, 204] and is likely as rare in children.[12, 205–208] Bleeding following polypectomy is also uncommon. In a review of 1,000 colonoscopic polypectomies in patients ranging from 2 to 89 years, there was a 0.8% rate of minor bleeding, with no patient requiring a transfusion.[209]

Perforation is the most serious complication of colonoscopy in children; it has been reported at least four times and is usually related to polypectomy.[206, 210, 211] Of the cases reported, all were successfully managed with surgical intervention. The risk of perforation is increased in adult patients with severe active colitis, strictures, adhesions, or diverticula.[212] Recently, conservative management has been suggested in small lesions.[213] Clinically silent diastatic tears have been reported in children, but are thought to be unusual.[214]

REFERENCES

1. Gordon ME, Kirsner JB: Rudolf Schindler, pioneer endoscopist: Glimpses of the man and his work. Gastroenterology 1979; 77:354–361.
2. Rossi TR: Endoscopic examination of the colon in infancy and childhood. Pediatr Clin North Am 1988; 35:331–356.
3. Morrissey JF: Endoscopy—times past. *In* Proceedings of the 1991 National American Society for Gastrointestinal Endoscopy 50th Anniversary Postgraduate Course. New Orleans, American Society for Gastrointestinal Endoscopy; 1991, pp 7–18.
4. Freeman NV: Clinical evaluation of the fiberoptic bronchoscope (Olympus BF 5B) for pediatric endoscopy. J Pediatr Surg 1973; 8:213–220.
5. Sivak MV, Fleischer DE: Colonoscopy with a video endoscope: Preliminary experience. Gastrointest Endosc 1984; 30:1–5.
6. Caulfield M, Wyllie R, Sivak MV Jr, et al: Upper gastrointestinal tract endoscopy in the pediatric patient. J Pediatr 1989; 115:339–345.
7. Kawahara I, Ichikawa H: Fiberoptic instrument technology. *In* Sivak MV Jr, ed: Gastroenterologic Endoscopy. Philadelphia: WB Saunders, 1987, pp 20–41.
8. Chang MH, Wang TH, Hsu JY, et al: Endoscopic examination of the upper gastrointestinal tract in infancy. Gastrointest Endosc 1983; 29:15–17.
9. Hargrove CB, Ulshen MH, Shub MD: Upper gastrointestinal endoscopy in infants: Diagnostic usefulness and safety. Pediatrics 1984; 74:828–831.
10. Quak SH, Lam SK, Low PS: Upper gastrointestinal endoscopy in children. Singapore Med J 1990; 31:123–126.
11. Ament ME, Christie DL: Upper gastrointestinal fiberoptic endoscopy in pediatric patients. Gastroenterology 1977; 72:1244–1248.
12. Mougenot JF, Baldassarre ME, Mashako LM, et al: Polypes recto-coliques de l'enfant. Analyse de 183 cas. Arch Fr Pediatr 1989; 46:245–248.
13. Quak SH, Prabhakaran K: Colonoscopy in children with bleeding per rectum. Singapore Med J 1990; 31:454–456.
14. Tam PK: Pediatric colonoscopy—an experience of 102 cases. Z Kinderchir 1988; 43(Suppl)1:60–61.
15. Kawamitsu T, Nagashima K, Tsuchiya H, et al: Pediatric total colonoscopy. J Pediatr Surg 1989; 24:371–374.
16. Holmquist L, Ahren C, Fallstrom SP: Clinical disease activity and inflammatory activity in the rectum in relation to mucosal inflammation assessed by colonoscopy. A study of children and adolescents with chronic inflammatory bowel disease. Acta Paediatr Scand 1990: 79:527–534.
17. Alemayehu G, Jarnerot G: Colonoscopy during an attack of severe ulcerative colitis is a safe procedure and of great value in clinical decision making. Am J Gastroenterol 1991; 86:187–190.
18. Lashner BA, Kane SV, Hanauer SB: Colon cancer surveillance in chronic ulcerative colitis: historical cohort study. Am J Gastroenterol 1990; 85:1083–1087.
19. Lashner BA, Hanauer SB, Silverstein MD: Optimal timing of colonoscopy to screen for cancer in ulcerative colitis. Arch Intern Med 1988; 108:274–278.
20. Matsumoto T, Iida M, Matsui T, et al: Endoscopic findings in Yersinia enterocolitica enterocolitis. Gastrointest Endosc 1990; 36:583–587.
21. Coremans G, Rutgeerts P, Geboes K, et al: The value of ileoscopy with biopsy in the diagnosis of intestinal Crohn's disease. Gastrointest Endosc 1984; 30:167–172.
22. Tam PKH, Saing H, Lee JMH: Colonoscopy in the diagnosis of abdominal tuberculosis in children. Aust Paediatr J 1986; 22:143–144.
23. Bhargava DK, Shriniwas TC, Chawla TC, et al: Intestinal tuberculosis: Bacterial study of tissue obtained by colonoscopy and during surgery. J Trop Med Hyg 1985; 88:249–252.
24. Mohamed AR, al Karawi M, Yasawy MI: Schistosomal colonic disease. Gut 1990; 31:439–442.
25. Jammal MA, Cox K, Ruebner B: Amebiasis presenting as rectal bleeding without diarrhea in childhood. J Pediatr Gastroenterol Nutr 1985; 4:294–296.
26. Santos JC Jr, Aprilli F, Gulmaraes AS, et al: Angiodysplasia of the colon: Endoscopic diagnosis and treatment. Br J Surg 1988; 75:256–258.
27. Lanthier P, d'Harveng B, Vanheuverzwyn R, et al: Colonic angiodysplasia. Follow-up of patients after endoscopic treatment for bleeding lesions. Dis Colon Rectum 1989; 32:296–298.
28. Trudel JL, Fazio VW, Sivak MV: Colonoscopic diagnosis and treatment of arteriovenous malformations in chronic lower gas-

trointestinal bleeding. Clinical accuracy and efficacy. Dis Colon Rectum 1988; 31:107–110.
29. Roth SI, Helwig EB: Juvenile polyps of the colon and rectum. Cancer 1963; 16:468–479.
30. Shehitinin VE, Starygin OV, Stoliarov VIU, et al: Diagnostika i Khirurgicheskoe lechenie invaginatsii kishechnika u detei. Khirurgiia 1989; 11:65–68.
31. Maurer G, Kratochvil P, Brandstatter G: The value of colonoscopy and ultrasonography in the diagnosis of chronic intussusception in childhood. Endoscopy 1986; 18:29–30.
32. Shinya H, ed: Special applications of colonoscopy. *In* Colonoscopy, Diagnosis and Treatment of Colonic Diseases. New York, Igaku-Shoin, 1982.
33. Stillman AE, Painter R, Hollister DW: Ehlers-Danlos syndrome type IV: Diagnosis and therapy of associated bowel perforation. Am J Gastroenterol 1991; 86:360–362.
34. Overholt BF: Flexible fiberoptic sigmoidoscopy. CA 19:81, 1969.
35. Shinya H, ed: Indications and contraindications. *In* Colonoscopy, Diagnosis and Treatment of Colonic Diseases. New York, Igaku-Shoin, 1982.
36. Neu HC, Fleischer D: Recommendations for antibiotic prophylaxis before endoscopy. Am J Gastroenterol 1989; 84:1488–1491.
37. Byrne WJ, Euler AR, Campbell M, et al: Bacteremia in children following upper gastrointestinal endoscopy or colonoscopy. J Pediatr Gastroenterol Nutr 1982; 1:551–553.
38. Low DE, Shoenut JP, Kennedy JK, et al: Prospective assessment of risk of bacteremia with colonoscopy and polypectomy. Dig Dis Sci 1987; 32:1239–1243.
39. Wyllie R: Esophagogastroduodenoscopy in the pediatric patient. *In* Sivak MV Jr, ed: Gastroenterologic Endoscopy. Philadelphia, WB Saunders, 1987, pp 307–320.
40. Crawford M, Lerman J, Christensen S, et al: Effects of duration of fasting on gastric fluid pH and volume in healthy children. Anesth Analg 1990; 71:400–403.
41. Vila JJ, Gutierrez C, Garcia-Sala C, et al: Whole bowel irrigation: Experience in pediatric patients. J Pediatr Surg 1987; 5:447–450.
42. Lee JMH, Tam PKH, Saing H: Whole gut irrigation in infants and young children. Dis Colon Rectum 1987; 29:252–254.
43. Thomas G, Brozinski S, Isenberg JI: Patient acceptance and effectiveness of a balanced lavage solution (Golytely) versus the standard preparation for colonoscopy. Gastroenterology 1982; 82:435–437.
44. Caos A, Benner KG, Manier J, et al: Colonoscopy after Golytely preparation in acute rectal bleeding. J Clin Gastroenterol 1986; 8:46–49.
45. Michael KA, DiPiro JT, Bowden TA, et al: Whole bowel irrigation for mechanical colon cleansing. Clin Pharm 1985; 4:414–424.
46. Figueroa-Colon R, Grunow JE: Randomized study of premedication for esophagogastroduodenoscopy in children and adolescents. J Pediatr Gastroenterol Nutr 1988; 7:359–366.
47. Castelle HB, Fiedorek SC, Kiel EA: Arterial blood oxygen desaturation in infants and children during upper gastrointestinal endoscopy. Gastrointest Endosc 1990; 36:489–493.
48. Motoyama EK: Safety and outcome in pediatric anesthesia. *In* Motoyama EK, ed: Smith's Anesthesia for Infants and Children. Philadelphia, CV Mosby, 1990, pp 847–856.
49. Cote CJ, Goldstein EA, Cote MA, et al: A single blinded study of pulse oximetry in children. Anesthesiology 1988; 68:184–188.
49a. Votey SR, Bosse GM, Bayer MJ, et al: Flumazenil: A new benzodiazepine antagonist. Ann Emerg Med 1991; 20:181–188.
50. Warwick R, Williams PL, ed: Gray's Anatomy. Philadelphia, WB Saunders, 1973.
51. Benson CD: Resection and primary anastomosis of the jejunum and ileum in the newborn. Ann Surg 1955; 142:478–485.
52. Reiquam CW, Allen RP, Akers DR: Normal and abnormal small bowel lengths. Am J Dis Child 1965; 109:447–451.
53. Sakai Y: Technique of colonoscopy. *In* Sivak MV Jr, ed: Gastroenterologic Endoscopy. Philadelphia, WB Saunders, 1987, pp 840–867.
54. Sivak MV Jr: Technique of upper gastrointestinal endoscopy. *In* Sivak MV Jr, ed: Gastroenterologic Endoscopy. Philadelphia, WB Saunders, 1987, pp 272–295.
55. Cotton PB, Williams CB: Practical Gastrointestinal Endoscopy. Oxford, Blackwell, 1980, pp 99–141.
56. Dubow RA, Katon RM, Benner KG, et al: Short (35 cm) versus long (60 cm) flexible sigmoidoscopy: A comparison of findings and tolerance in asymptomatic patients screened for colorectal neoplasia. Gastrointest Endosc 1985; 31:305–308.
57. Sarles HE, Sanowski RA, Haynes WC, et al: The long and short of flexible sigmoidoscopy: Does it matter? Am J Gastroenterol 1986; 81:369–371.
58. Roosevelt J, Frankl H: Colorectal cancer screening by nurse practitioner using 60-cm flexible fiberoptic sigmoidoscopy. Dig Dis Sci 1984; 29:161–163.
59. Semerdjian G: Flexible sigmoidoscopy for screening in primary practice: A key to improved survival in colon cancer. Postgrad Med 1985; 78:47–50.
60. Yarborough GW, Waisbren BA: The benefits of systemic fiberoptic flexible sigmoidoscopy. Arch Intern Med 1985; 145: 95–96.
61. Rumans MC, Benner KG, Keffe EB, et al: Screening flexible sigmoidoscopy by primary care physicians: Effectiveness and costs in patients negative for fecal occult blood. West J Med 1986; 144:756–758.
62. Ingoldby CJH, Mason MK, Hall RI: Endoscopic needle aspiration cytology: A new method for the diagnosis of upper gastrointestinal cancer. Gut 1987; 28:1142–1144.
63. Levine DS, Reid BJ: Endoscopic biopsy technique for acquiring larger mucosal samples. Gastrointest Endosc 1991; 37:332–337.
64. Graham DY, Schwartz JT, Gain GD, et al: Prospective evaluation of biopsy number in the diagnosis of esophageal and gastric carcinoma. Gastroenterology 1982; 82:228–231.
65. Tissue sampling and analysis. Gastrointest Endosc 1991; 37: 663–665.
66. The role of colonoscopy in the management of patients with colonic polyps. Gastrointest Endosc 1988; 34:65–75.
67. Graham DY, Tabibian N, Michaletz PA, et al: Endoscopic needle biopsy: A comparative study of forceps biopsy, two different types of needles and salvage cytology in gastrointestinal cancer. Gastrointest Endosc 1989; 35:207–209.
68. Standards of Training and Practice Committee, American Society for Gastrointestinal Endoscopy: The role of endoscopy in the management of esophagitis. Gastrointest Endosc 1988; 34:9S.
69. Berenson MM, Riddell RH, Skinner DB, et al: Malignant transformation of esophageal columnar epithelium. Cancer 1978; 41:554–561.
70. Agha FP, Lee NH, Nostrant TT: Herpetic esophagitis: A diagnostic challenge in immunocompromised patients. Am J Gastroenterol 1986; 81:246–253.
71. Gazzard BG: HIV disease and the gastroenterologist. Gut 1988; 29:1497–1505.
72. Young JA, Hughes HE, Lee FD: Evaluation of endoscopic brush and biopsy touch smear cytology and biopsy histology in the diagnosis of carcinoma of the lower esophagus and cardia. J Clin Pathol 1980; 33:811–814.
73. Winawer SJ, Sherlock P, Belladonna JA, et al: Endoscopic brush cytology in esophageal cancer. JAMA 1975; 323: 1358–1364.
74. Mandelstam P, Sugawa C, Silvis SE, et al: Complications associated with esophagogastroduodenoscopy and with esophageal dilation. Gastrointest Endosc 1976; 23:16–19.
75. Dooley CP, Cohen H, Fitzgibbons PL, et al: Prevalence of *Helicobacter pylori* infection and histologic gastritis in asymptomatic persons. N Engl J Med 1989; 321:1562–1566.
76. Montgomery EA, Martin DF, Peura DA: Rapid diagnosis of *Campylobacter pylori* by Gram's stain. Am J Clin Path 1988; 90:606–609.
77. Marshall BJ, Warren JR, Francis GJ, et al: Rapid urease test in the management of *Campylobacter pylori*-associated gastritis. Am J Gastroenterol 1987; 82:200–210.
78. Holdstock G, Eade OE, Isaacson P, et al: Endoscopic duodenal biopsies in coeliac disease and duodenitis. Scand J Gastroenterol 1979; 14:717–720.
79. Achkar E, Carey WD, Petras R, et al: Comparison of suction capsule and endoscopic biopsy of small bowel mucosa. Gastrointest Endosc 1986; 32:278–281.
80. Scott BB, Jenkins D: Endoscopic small intestine biopsy. Gastrointest Endosc 1981; 27:162–167.
81. Sanfilippo G, Patane R, Fusto A, et al: Endoscopic approach to childhood coeliac disease. Acta Gastroenterol Belg 1986; 49:401–408.
82. Dandalides SM, Carey WD, Petras P, et al: Endoscopic small

bowel mucosal biopsy: A controlled trial evaluating forceps size and biopsy location in the diagnosis of normal and abnormal mucosal architecture. Gastrointest Endosc 1989; 35:197–200.
83. Parker HW, Agayoff JD: Enteroscopy and small bowel biopsy utilizing a peroral colonoscope. Gastrointest Endosc 1983; 29:139–140.
84. Mashako MN, Cezard JP, Navarro J, et al: Crohn's disease lesions in the upper gastrointestinal tract: Correlation between clinical, radiological, endoscopic and histologic features in adolescents and children. J Pediatr Gastroenterol Nutr 1984; 8:442–446.
85. Lee JH, Griffiths WJ, Zantout I, Welsh JD: Adequacy of endoscopic biopsy specimens for disaccharidase assays. Am J Dig Dis 1978; 23:1129–1131.
86. Monroe LS: The endoscopic encounter with parasites. Gastrointest Endosc 1984; 30:113–114.
87. The role of colonoscopy in the management of patients with inflammatory bowel disease. Gastrointest Endosc 1988; 34:10S–11S.
88. Fleischer DE, Goldberg SB, Browning TH, et al: Detection and surveillance of colorectal cancer. JAMA 1989; 261:580–585.
89. Jeevanandam V, Treat MR, Forde KA: A comparison of direct brush cytology and biopsy in the diagnosis of colorectal cancer. Gastrointest Endosc 1987; 33:370–371.
90. Lange P, Kock K, Lausten J, et al: Endoscopic fine needle aspiration cytology of the stomach. A new diagnostic procedure. Endoscopy 1987; 19:72–73.
91. Raskin JB, Welch P, Nadji M, et al: Transendoscopic needle aspiration cytology in the diagnosis of gastrointestinal malignancies. Gastrointest Endosc 1980; 26:75.
92. Raskin JB, Welch P, Zara J: Transendoscopic needle aspiration cytology. A comparison with standard biopsy techniques. Gastrointest Endosc 1981; 27:128.
93. Nostrant TT, Kumar NB, Appelman HD: Histopathology differentiates acute self-limited colitis from ulcerative colitis. Gastroenterology 1987; 92:318–328.
94. Kumar NB, Nostrant TT, Appelman HD: The histopathologic spectrum of acute self-limited colitis (acute infectious type colitis). Am J Surg Pathol 1982; 6:523–529.
95. Dickinson RJ, Gilmour HM, McClelland BL: Rectal biopsy in patients presenting to an infectious disease unit with diarrheal disease. Gut 1979; 20:141–148.
96. Surawicz CM, Belic L: Rectal biopsy helps to distinguish acute self limited colitis from idiopathic inflammatory bowel disease. Gastroenterology 1984; 86: 104–113.
97. Mee AS, Shild M, Burke M: *Campylobacter* colitis: Differentiation from acute inflammatory bowel disease. J Roy Soc Med 1985; 78: 217–223.
98. Gaisford WD: Fiberendoscopy of the cecum and terminal ileum. Gastrointest Endosc 1974; 21:13.
99. Nagasako K, Yazawa C, Takemoto T: Biopsy of the terminal ileum. Gastrointest Endosc 1972; 19:7.
100. Bradford WD, Noce PC, Gutman LT: Pathologic features of enteric infections with Yersinia enterocolitica. Arch Pathol 1974; 98:17.
101. Aoki G, Nagasako K, Nakae Y, et al: The fiberendoscopic diagnosis of intestinal tuberculosis. Endoscopy 1975; 7:113.
102. Bretholz A, Strasser H, Knoblauch M: Endoscopic diagnosis of ileocecal tuberculosis. Gastrointest Endosc 1978; 24:250.
103. Devroede G: Risk of cancer in inflammatory bowel disease *In* Winawere SJ, Schottenfeld D, Sherlock P, eds: Progress in Cancer Research and Therapy in Colorectal Cancer: Prevention, Epidemiology and Screening. New York, New York University Press, 1980, pp 325–334.
104. Greenstein AJ, Sachar DB, Smith H, et al: Cancer in universal and left-sided ulcerative colitis: Factors determining risk. Gastroenterology 1979; 77:290–294.
105. Collins R, Feldman M, Fordtran J: Colon cancer, dysplasia and surveillance in patients with ulcerative colitis. N Engl J Med 1987; 316:1654–1658.
106. Dobbins WO: Dysplasia and malignancy in inflammatory bowel disease. Ann Rev Med 1984; 35:33–48.
107. Fromm D: Endoscopic coagulation for gastrointestinal bleeding. N Engl J Med 1987; 316:1652–1653.
108. Salt WB, Llaneza PP: Collagenous colitis: A cause of chronic diarrhea diagnosed only by biopsy of normal appearing colonic mucosa. Gastrointest Endosc 1986; 32:421–423.
109. Read NW, Krejs GJ, Read MG, et al: Chronic diarrhea of unknown origin. Gastroenterology 1980; 78:264–271.
110. Surawicz CM, Meisel JL, Ylvisaker T, et al: Rectal biopsy in the diagnosis of Crohn's disease: Value of multiple biopsies and serial sectioning. Gastroenterology 1981; 81:66–71.
111. Krejs GJ, Fordtran JS: Diarrhea. *In* Sleisenger MH, Fordtran JS, eds: Gastrointestinal Disease. Philadelphia, WB Saunders, 1983, pp 257–280.
112. Heyman MB, Perman JA, Ferrell LD, et al: Chronic nonspecific inflammatory bowel disease of the cecum and proximal colon in children with grossly normal appearing colonic mucosal diagnosis by colonoscopic biopsies. Pediatrics 1987; 80:255–261.
113. Geboes K, Vantrappen G: The value of colonoscopy in the diagnosis of Crohn's disease. Gastrointest Endosc 1975; 22:18–23.
114. Kingham JGC, Levison DA, Ball JA, et al: Microscopic colitis—a cause of chronic watery diarrhea. Br Med J 1982; 285:1601–1604.
115. Elliott PR, Williams CB, Lennard-Jones JE, et al: Colonoscopic diagnosis of minimal change colitis in patients with a normal sigmoidoscopy and normal air-contrast barium enema. Lancet 1982; 1:650–651.
116. Sanderson IR, Boyle S, Williams CB, et al: Histologic abnormalities in biopsies from macroscopically normal colonoscopies. Arch Dis Child 1986; 61:274–277.
117. Mashako MN, Sonsino E, Navarro J, et al: Microscopic colitis: A new cause of chronic diarrhea in children? J Pediatr Gastroenterol Nutr 1990; 10:21–26.
118. Sugawa C: Endoscopic diagnosis and treatment of upper gastrointestinal bleeding. Surg Clin North Am 1989; 69:1167–1183.
119. Kovacs TO, Jensen DM: Endoscopic control of gastroduodenal hemorrhage. Annu Rev Med 1987; 38:267–277.
120. Jensen DM: Heat probe for hemostasis of bleeding peptic ulcers: Techniques and results of randomized controlled trials. Gastrointest Endosc 1990; 36:S42-S49.
121. Jensen DM, Machicado GA: Diagnosis and treatment of severe hematochezia. Gastroenterology 1988; 95:1569–1574.
122. Schrock TR: Colonoscopic diagnosis and treatment of lower gastrointestinal bleeding. Surg Clin North Am 1989; 69:1309–1325.
123. Hirao M, Kobayashi T, Masuda K, et al: Endoscopic local injection of hypertonic saline-epinephrine solution to arrest hemorrhage from the upper gastrointestinal tract. Gastrointest Endosc 1985; 31:313–317.
124. Lin HJ, Tsai YT, Lee SD, et al: A prospectively randomized trial of heat probe thermocoagulation versus pure alcohol injection in nonvariceal peptic ulcer hemorrhage. Am J Gastroenterol 1988; 83:283–286.
125. Jensen DM, Machicado GA, Kovacs TO, et al: Controlled, randomized study of heater probe and bicap for hemostasis of severe ulcer bleeding. Gastroenterology 1988; 94:A208.
126. Papp JP: Monopolar and electrohydrothermal treatment of upper gastrointestinal bleeding. Gastrointest Endosc 1990; 36:S34–S37.
127. Yamamoto H, Hajiro K, Matsui H, et al: Endoscopic bipolar electrocoagulation: Development of a new bipolar coagulator for stopping gastrointestinal bleeding. Gastroenterol Jpn 1982; 17:75–79.
128. Laine L: Bipolar/multipolar electrocoagulation. Gastrointest Endosc 1990; 36:S38-S41.
129. Jensen D, Hirabayashi K: A study of coagulation depths with bicap and heater probe to improve endoscopic hemostasis of bleeding peptic ulcers. Gastrointest Endosc 1989; 35:181.
130. Laine L: Multipolar electrocoagulation in the treatment of peptic ulcers with nonbleeding visible vessels. Ann Intern Med 1989; 110:510–514.
131. Laine L: Multipolar electrocoagulation in the treatment of active upper gastrointestinal tract hemorrhage. N Engl J Med 1987; 316:1613–1617.
132. Hui WM, Ng MM, Lok AS, et al: A randomized comparative study of laser photocoagulation, heater probe, and bipolar electrocoagulation in the treatment of actively bleeding ulcers. Gastrointest Endosc 1991; 37:299–304.
133. Mauhoury V, Brunetaud JM, Cortot A: Bipolar electrocoagula-

tion treatment for hemorrhagic radiation injury of the lower digestive tract. Gastrointest Endosc 1991; 37:492–493.
134. Rogers BH: Endoscopic electrocoagulation of vascular abnormalities of the gastrointestinal tract in 51 patients. Gastrointest Endosc 1982; 28:142–143.
135. Williams CB: Small polyps: The virtues and the dangers of hot biopsy. Gastrointest Endosc 1991; 37:394–395.
136. Wadas DD, Sanowski RA: Complication of the hot biopsy forceps technique. Gastrointest Endosc 1988; 34:32–37.
137. Quigley EM, Donovan JP, Linder J, et al: Delayed massive hemorrhage following electrocoagulating biopsy ("hot biopsy") of a diminutive colonic polyp. Gastrointest Endosc 1989; 35:S59-S63.
138. Nelson AM: Delayed hemorrhage following "hot biopsy" of a diminutive colonic polyp. Gastrointest Endosc 1990; 36:418.
139. Waring JP, Sanowski RA, Sawyer RL, et al: A randomized comparison of multipolar electrocoagulation and injection sclerosis for the treatment of bleeding peptic ulcer. Gastrointest Endosc 1991; 37:295–298.
140. Chung SC, Leung JW, Sung JY, et al: Injection or heat probe for bleeding ulcer. Gastroenterology 1991; 100:33–37.
141. Matthewson K, Swain CP, Bland M, et al: Randomized comparison of Nd:YAG laser, heater probe, and no endoscopic therapy for bleeding peptic ulcers. Gastroenterology 1990; 98:1239–1244.
142. Shahed M, Hagenmuller F, Rosch TH, et al: A 19-year-old female with blue rubber bleb nevus syndrome. Endoscopy 1990; 22:54–56.
143. Lanthier PH, D'Harveng B, Vanheuverzwyn R, et al: Colonic angiodysplasia. Dis Colon Rectum 1989; 32:296–298.
144. Noronha P, Leist M: Endoscopic laser therapy for gastrointestinal bleeding from congenital vascular lesions. J Pediatr Gastroenterol Nutr 1988; 7:375–378.
145. Buchi KN: Endoscopic laser surgery in the colon and rectum. Dis Colon Rectum 1988; 31:739–745.
146. Dumon JF, Meric B, Sivak MV Jr, et al: A new method of esophageal dilation using Savary-Gilliard bougies. Gastrointest Endosc 1985; 31:379–382.
147. Luzzani S, Valade A, Agliardi AC: Endoscopic treatment of oesophageal stenosis in children. Z Kinderchir 1988; 43(Suppl I):42–44.
148. London RL, Trotman BW, DiMarino AJ Jr, et al: Dilation of severe esophageal strictures by an inflatable balloon catheter. Gastroenterology 1981; 80:173–175.
149. Navarro FA Jr, Menasha M, Benjamin SB, et al: Transluminal dilation of esophageal strictures in infants following atresia repair. Gastrointest Endosc 1985; 31:200–201.
150. Goldthorn JF, Ball WS Jr, Wilkinson LG, et al: Esophageal strictures in children: Treatment by serial balloon catheter dilatation. Radiology 1984; 153:655–658.
151. Ball WS, Strife JL, Rosenkrantz J, et al: Esophageal strictures in children. Radiology 1984; 150:263–264.
152. Stringer PA, Pablot SM, Mancer K: Gruntzig angioplasty dilatation of an esophageal stricture in an infant. Pediatr Radiol 1985; 15:424–426.
153. Murthy VK: Repeated hydrostatic balloon dilation in obstructive gastroduodenal Crohn's disease. Gastrointest Endosc 1991; 37:484–485.
154. Begdoni G, Ricci E, Pedrazzoli C, et al: Endoscopic dilation of anastamotic colonic stenosis by different techniques: an alternative to surgery? Gastrointest Endosc 1987; 33:21–26.
154a. Nevfeld DM, Shemesh EI, Kodner IJ, et al: Endoscopic management of anastomotic colon strictures with electrocautery and balloon dilation. Gastrointest Endosc 1987: 33:24–26.
155. Kirsch M, Blue M, Desai RK, et al: Intralesional steroid injections for peptic esophageal strictures. Gastrointest Endosc 1991; 37:180–182.
156. Bowden TA Jr: Endoscopy of the small intestine. Surg Clin North Am 1989; 69:1237–1247.
157. Tada M, Kawai K: Small bowel endoscopy. Scand J Gastroenterol 1984; 19(Suppl 102):39–52.
158. Foutch PG, Sawyer R, Sanowski RA: Push-enteroscopy for diagnosis of patients with gastrointestinal bleeding of obscure origin. Gastrointest Endosc 1990; 36:337–341.
159. Tada M, Misaki F, Kawai K: Pediatric enteroscopy with a Sonde-type small intestinal fiberscope (SSIF-type VI). Gastrointest Endosc 1983; 29:44–47.
160. Gauderer MW, Ponsky JL, Izant RJ Jr: Gastrostomy without laparotomy: A percutaneous endoscopic technique. J Pediatr Surg 1980; 15:872–875.
161. Gauderer MW, Stellato TA, Olsen M, et al: Percutaneous endoscopic gastrostomy in 156 children: Indications, technique and complications. Z Kinderchir 1988; 43(Supp 1):38–40.
162. Russell TR, Brotman M, Norris F: Percutaneous gastrostomy. Am J Surg 1984; 148:132–137.
163. Miller RE, Winkler WP, Kotler DP: The Russell percutaneous endoscopic gastrostomy: Key technical steps. Gastrointest Endosc 1988; 34:339–342.
163a. Ferguson RD, Harig JM, Koznrek RA, et al: Placement of a feeding button (one-step button) as the initial procedure. Am J Gastroenterol (in press).
164. Shike M, Wallach C, Likier H: Direct percutaneous endoscopic jejunostomies. Gastrointest Endosc 1991; 37:62–65.
165. Lewis BS: Direct percutaneous endoscopic jejunostomy. Gastrointest Endosc 1991; 37:493.
166. Stefan MM, Holcomb GW, Ross AJ: Cologastric fistula as a complication of percutaneous endoscopic gastrostomy. JPEN 1989; 13:554–556.
167. Grunow JE, Al-Hafidh AS, Tunell WP: Gastroesophageal reflux following percutaneous endoscopic gastrostomy in children. J Pediatr Surg 1989; 24:42–45.
168. Willems MG: Transgastric perforation of a PEG and successful endoscopic management of the complication using the fibrin sealing technique. Endoscopy 1990; 22:288.
169. Cynamon HA, Milov DE, Andres JM: Diagnosis and management of colonic polyps in children. J Pediatr 1989; 114:593–596.
169a. Bigard MA, Gaucher P, Lassalle C: Fatal colonic explosion during colonoscopic polypectomy. Gastroenterology 1979; 177:1307–1310.
170. Kimmey MB, Silverstein FE, Saunders DR, et al: Endoscopic bipolar forceps: A potential treatment for the diminutive polyp. Gastrointest Endosc 1988; 34:38–41.
171. Gillespie PE, Chambers TJ, Chan KW, et al: Colonic adenomas: A colonoscopy survey. Gut 1979; 20:240.
172. Panish JF: Management of patients with polypoid lesions of the colon—current concepts and controversies. Am J Gastroenterol 1979; 71:315–324.
173. Shinya H, Wolff WI: Morphology, anatomic distribution and cancer potential of colonic polyps: An analysis of 7,000 polyps endoscopically removed. Ann Surg 1979; 109:679.
174. Knotson CO, Max MH: Diagnostic and therapeutic colonoscopy: A critical review of 663 examinations. Arch Surg 1979; 114:430.
175. Fischer SE, Harrison M, Adkins JC: Colonoscopic diagnosis of vascular anomalies in children. Clin Pediatr 1979; 18:299–303.
176. Abrahamson J, Shandling B: Intestinal hemangiomata in childhood and a syndrome for diagnosis: A collective review. J Pediatr Surg 1973; 8:487–495.
177. Rodesch P, Cadranel S, Peters JP, et al: Colonic endoscopy in children. Acta Pediatr Belg 1976; 29:181–184.
178. Skorgaard S, Sorensen FH: Bleeding hemangioma of the colon diagnosed by colonoscopy. J Pediatr Surg 1976; 11:83–84.
179. Soehendra N: Colonoscopy in children. Proctology 1979; 1:8–14.
180. Morris SJ, Kaplan SR, Ballan K, et al: Blue rubber bleb nevus syndrome. JAMA 1978; 239:1887.
181. Steffen RM, Wyllie R, Sivak MV Jr, et al: Colonoscopy in the pediatric patient. J Pediatr 1989; 115:507–514.
182. Goodman RM, Smith EW, Paton D, et al: Pseudoxanthoma elasticum: A clinical and histopathological study. Medicine 1963; 42:297–334.
183. Haddad HM, Wilkins L: Congenital anomalies associated with gonadal aplasia: A review of 55 cases. Pediatrics 1959; 23:885–902.
184. Capitanio MA, Kirkpatrick JA: Lymphoid hyperplasia of the colon in children. Radiology 1970; 94:323–327.
185. Kaplan B, Benson J, Rothstein F, et al: Lymphonodular hyperplasia of the colon as a pathologic finding in children with lower gastrointestinal bleeding. J Pediatr Gastroenterol Nutr 1984; 3:704–708.
186. Theander G, Tragardh B: Lymphoid hyperplasia of the colon in childhood. Acta Radiol (Diagn) 1976; 17:631–648.
187. Okamatsu T, Arai K, Yatsuzuka M, et al: Endoscopic membra-

nectomy for congenital duodenal stenosis. J Pediatr Surg 1989; 24:367–368.
188. Humphrey RW, Dorazio R: Correction of congenital duodenal obstruction assisted by intraoperative endoscopic guidance. Gastrointest Endosc 1984; 30:46–47.
189. Izzidien Al Samarrai AY, Jessen K, Haque K: Endoscopic obliteration of a recurrent tracheoesophageal fistula. J Pediatr Surg 1987; 22:993.
190. Ament ME: Prospective study of risks of complication in 6424 procedures in pediatric gastroenterology. Pediatr Res 1981; 15:524.
191. Arrowsmith JB, Gerstman B, Fleischer DE, et al: Results from the American Society for Gastrointestinal Endoscopy/U.S. Food and Drug Administration collaborative study on complication rates and drug use during gastrointestinal endoscopy. Gastrointest Endosc 1991; 37:421–427.
192. Richardson VF, Robertson CF, Mowat AP, et al: Deterioration in lung function after general anesthesia in patients with cystic fibrosis. Acta Paediatr Scand 1984; 73:75–79.
193. Moghissi K, Pender D: Instrumental perforations of the oesophagus and their management. Thorax 1988; 43:642–646.
194. Ghishan FK, Werner M, Vieira P, et al: Intramural duodenal hematoma: An unusual complication of endoscopic small bowel biopsy. Am J Gastroenterol 1987; 82:368–370.
195. Chester JF, Hurley PR: Gastric necrosis: A complication of endoscopic sclerosis for bleeding peptic ulcer. Endoscopy 1990; 22:287.
196. Loperfido S, Patelli G, La Torre L: Extensive necrosis of gastric mucosa following injection therapy of bleeding peptic ulcer. Endoscopy 1990; 22:285–286.
197. Johnston JH: Complications following endoscopic laser therapy. Gastrointest Endosc 1982; 28(2):135.
198. Lowdon JD, Tidmore TL Jr: Fatal air embolism after gastrointestinal endoscopy. Anesthesiology 1988; 69:622–623.
199. Desmond PV, MacMahon RA: Fatal air embolism following endoscopy of a hepatic portoenterostomy. Endoscopy 1990; 22:236.
200. Rogers BHG, Silvis SE, Nebel OT, et al: Complications of flexible fiberoptic colonoscopy and polypectomy: An analysis of the 1974 ASGE survey. Gastrointest Endosc 1975; 22:73–77.
201. Fruhmorgen P, Demling L: Complications of diagnostic and therapeutic colonoscopy in the Federal Republic of Germany: Results of an inquiry. Endoscopy 1979; 11:146–150.
202. Macrae FA, Tan KG, Williams CB: Towards safer colonoscopy: A report on the complications of 5000 diagnostic or therapeutic colonoscopies. Gut 1983; 24:376–383.
203. Rankin GB: Indications, contraindications, and complications of colonoscopy. *In* Sivak MV Jr, ed: Gastroenterologic Endoscopy. Philadelphia, WB Saunders, 1987, pp 868–880.
204. Gilbert DA, Hallstrom AP, Shaneyfelt SL, et al: The National ASGE Colonoscopy Survey: Complications of colonoscopy. Gastrointest Endosc 1984; 30:156.
205. Hassall B, Barclay GN, Ament ME: Colonoscopy in childhood. Pediatrics 1984; 73:594–549.
206. Habr-Gama A, Alves PRA, Gama-Rodriques JJ, et al: Pediatric colonoscopy. Dis Colon Rectum 1979; 22:530–535.
207. Williams CB, Laage NJ, Campbell CA, et al: Total colonoscopy in children. Arch Dis Child 1982; 57:49–53.
208. Kawamitsu T, Nagashima K, Tsuchiya H, et al: Pediatric total colonoscopy. J Pediatr Surg 1989; 24:371–374.
209. Demers RY, Stawick LE, Demers P: Relative sensitivity of the fecal occult blood test and flexible sigmoidoscopy in detecting polyps. Prev Med 1985; 14:55–62.
210. Gans SL, Ament M, Cristie DL: Pediatric endoscopy with flexible fiberscopes. J Pediatr Surg 1975; 10: 375–380.
211. Holgersen LO, Mossberg SM, Miller RE: Colonoscopy for rectal bleeding in childhood. J Pediatr Surg 1978; 13:83–85.
212. Hunt R: Towards safer colonoscopy. Gut 1983; 24:371–375.
213. Vincent M, Smith LE: Management of perforation due to colonoscopy. Dis Colon Rectum 1983; 26:61–63.
214. Livstone EM, Cohen GM, Troncale FJ, Touloukian RJ: Diastatic serosal lacerations: An unrecognized complication of colonoscopy. Gastroenterology 1974; 67:1245–1247.

Chapter 75

Endoscopic Retrograde Cholangiopancreatography

RITA STEFFEN, MOISES GUELRUD, and MICHAEL V. SIVAK, JR.

Endoscopic retrograde cholangiopancreatography (ERCP) is a technique used to acquire diagnostic information and to perform therapeutic maneuvers in the biliary tree and pancreas in patients of all ages. The procedure requires an endoscopist skilled in placement of a specialized side-viewing duodenoscope and provides direct radiographs of the biliary tree and pancreatic duct. Extensive experience with ERCP in the adult literature accrued in the 1970s, and the first reports of ERCP in infants and children were chiefly from adult gastroenterologists experienced with the technique. The development of prototype pediatric instruments, expansion of indications for the procedure in children, and the availability of skilled endoscopists have resulted in an increasing number of these procedures being performed in children.

Soon after the gastroscope was introduced and the papilla of Vater was visualized in the duodenum, placement of a catheter through the endoscope to cannulate the major papilla with subsequent injection of contrast material to fill the common bile duct and pancreatic ducts became possible. The first endoscopic cannulation of the ampulla of Vater was described by McCune and coworkers in 1968.[1] A lateral-viewing duodenoscope became available outside of Japan in 1970, and a burgeoning literature followed describing new aspects of diseases such as sclerosing cholangitis and sophisticated therapeutic applications. In 1976, Waye[2] reported the first ERCP in a pediatric patient by performing the procedure on a 6.0-kg, 14-week-old jaundiced infant with the standard adult cannulating instrument. Guelrud has performed the procedure successfully in infants weighing as little as 2.5 kg with a smaller instrument designed for pediatric patients.[3]

ERCP is safe in infants and children and can be performed with intravenous medication for conscious sedation or under general anesthesia for very young infants. Success rates of cannulating the relevant duct(s) in pediatric patients are as high as 95[4] to 96%.[5] Only 30 cases of ERCP examinations in children appeared in the English literature by 1980. Several authors have reported their series of ERCP examinations in infants and children,[3–13] for diagnostic yield, therapeutic uses, and safety in this young age group.

METHODS FOR IMAGING THE LIVER AND PANCREAS

There are several imaging modalities available for diagnosis of pancreaticobiliary diseases. Until the 1970s, oral cholecystography was the mainstay in the diagnosis of cholelithiasis; however, visualization of the common bile duct was not possible in the jaundiced patient or when the serum bilirubin level is greater than or equal to 3.0 mg per dl.[2] Ultrasonography is the screening method of choice for gallstones at any age and for pancreaticobiliary ductal dilatation and has a prominent role in pediatric gastroenterology because it is noninvasive, routinely available, and does not expose the patient to radiation. Computed tomography and magnetic resonance imaging are useful methods for hepatic parenchymal lesions, and these methods have application for defining liver and pancreatic abnormalities but are limited if information about ductal anatomy requires further delineation. Computed tomography and ultrasonography may not detect stones or lesions in the distal common bile duct.[14] Prospective comparisons of various liver imaging techniques are limited, and decisions for pediatric patients are guided by the suspected pathology, risks, benefits, and expense on an individual basis.

Appropriate selection of the imaging technique depends on the pathologic process.[15] Barium contrast examination may show displacement of the duodenal C-loop or stomach secondary to mass effect from pancreatic or biliary lesions but otherwise has a minor role in the diagnosis of pancreaticobiliary lesions. Radionuclide scanning with technetium 99m compounds is discussed in the section on biliary atresia.

Percutaneous transhepatic cholangiography (PTC) is another method used to image the biliary tree, but this invasive procedure requires adequate-sized or dilated bile ducts as the target for the needle to inject contrast material, may not image the distal common bile duct, cannot image the pancreatic duct (unless anomalous connection is present), and adds risk owing to liver puncture.[16] When the thinner Chiba needle was introduced, PTC gained wider acceptance because its use resulted in a decreased rate of complications. A randomized trial of 60 consecutive patients of ERCP versus

PTC found comparable success rates and complications, and both procedures need to be followed by surgical intervention if obstruction, which may lead to sepsis, is found.[17] PTC should be considered when prior surgical alterations and malrotations of the small bowel prevent duodenal intubation with the endoscope. Hemorrhage and bile peritonitis may complicate PTC, and a laparotomy may be needed for control and treatment.[18] Availability of these tests and local skills influence choices for initial evaluation.

Facilities

A well-equipped endoscopy suite, including equipment for monitoring vital signs, oxygen saturation, and resuscitation medications and equipment, is required for the procedure in patients of all ages. Occasionally ERCP is done in the operating theater, and fluoroscopic equipment must be present. Pediatric endoscopy assistants and specially trained nurses can help reduce preprocedure anxiety; monitor the clinical status of the patient; and assist in holding and reassuring the child,[19, 20] administering medications, handling biopsy forceps, and injecting contrast material.

Preparation and Sedation

The patient has the same preparation for ERCP as for upper gastrointestinal endoscopy[19] (see Chapter 74). A period of fasting precedes sedation and intubation with the endoscope, and this is age dependent. An intravenous line is placed in the right arm for sedation and administration of glucagon or other medications to prevent duodenal peristalsis.

Premedication is intended to sedate the child, minimize discomfort, and induce amnesia. General anesthesia may be necessary for very young infants or selected older patients. A combination of meperidine (1 to 2 mg per kg, to a maximum of 100 mg) and midazolam (0.1 mg per kg usually to a maximum of 5 mg) is slowly administered.[20] Occasionally atropine or glucagon is given when the duodenum is intubated to inhibit peristalsis for delicate cannulation of the ampulla. Somatostatin is being used in clinical trials during ERCP to assess its effect on decreasing gastrointestinal secretions[21] and producing transient small bowel atony.

Antibiotic prophylaxis for prevention of infective endocarditis is given according to the guidelines of the American Heart Association for children with congenital and rheumatic heart disease[22] (see Chapter 74). For adult patients with obstructive jaundice and pancreatic pseudocyst, antibiotics are also administered to prevent complications of sepsis from cholangitis and pancreatic abscess formation when injection of contrast material into an inadequately draining space is anticipated. Antibiotics have also been recommended when a stricture, stone, or space-occupying lesion is seen on ERCP.[23] There are no data to guide antibiotic prophylaxis for ERCP in children, and special situations in which a valvular prosthesis, vascular graft material, indwelling catheters, or transplanted organ in an immunosuppressed patient require individual consideration.

Equipment

The standard adult side-viewing duodenoscope and therapeutic adult-sized duodenoscopes have been used even in infants younger than 1 year of age.[2, 12] Specialized smaller caliber instruments have been developed and are now currently available (Olympus Corporation, Lake Success, NY). The initial pediatric side-viewing duodenoscope was manufactured without a cannula elevator mechanism and has been used successfully in very young infants.[3, 24] The commercial model includes an elevator and has an insertion tube 7.5 mm in diameter, an 80-degree field of view, and deflection capability of 120 degrees upward and 90 degrees to the right, left, and down. A 2-mm channel is designed to exit the side of the endoscope. Some authors believe the special pediatric endoscope is needed only for infants under 6 months of age.[4]

The endoscope is lateral-viewing so the ampulla and duct orifices may be cannulated from an en face position. The arrival of videoendoscopy using a charge-couple device with a television system has added several new dimensions of maneuverability and a lighter weight to the instrument as well as the ability to store and retrieve the endoscopic images.[25]

TECHNIQUE OF ERCP

Operator experience correlates with the degree of technical success in ERCP.[26] Care is taken to disinfect the equipment before each patient, but the procedure cannot be sterile because the insertion tube passes through the oropharynx. Routine use of pharyngeal sprays to anesthetize the pharynx is not necessary but used per the operator's discretion. After adequate intravenous sedation, a plastic bite-block is inserted between the teeth, and intubation of the esophagus is done "blindly." After the endoscope is guided into the descending duodenum, the papilla is brought into close position so the desired target duct may be cannulated from an en face position. The patient is lying in the left lateral decubitus position on a padded table and later adjusts to the prone position for more favorable angle of access to the papilla. A teflon catheter is skillfully manipulated into the papilla, and the gastrointestinal assistant injects contrast material through the primed tubing into the pancreatic and bile ducts. Care must be taken to remove any air in the syringe containing contrast material because introduction of air bubbles into the liver and pancreas will appear as rounded filling defects, simulating stones. Tilting the patient on the table will cause air to rise, and heavier filling defects to settle downward. Diluted contrast material is preferred for optimal visualization if filling defects are anticipated in the ducts. Special tapered tip cannulas should be available for pediatric patients and for negotiating the accessory papilla if necessary. Selected fluoroscopic images are recorded, and therapeutic maneuvers described earlier may then be performed.

After removal of the endoscope, placing the patient in the prone position and reverse Trendelenberg facilitates filling of the upper hepatic ducts by gravity.[2] Spot films may be taken fluoroscopically without the endoscope in the field. Photodocumentation of the ampullary region is possible by camera or videoendoscopy.

Small "daughter" or "baby" cholangioscopes have been designed to pass through the "mother" duodenoscope and into the biliary and pancreatic ducts for choledochoscopy, cholangioscopy, and pancreatoscopy. This technical advancement has limited application and has been described only in older patients.

Indications

In adults, gallstones and alcoholism are the two commonest causes of pancreatitis; however, in children the leading causes of pancreatitis are medications, trauma, infections, and ductal malformations.[22] The indications[8, 22, 27, 28] for ERCP in pediatric patients are (1) chronic pancreatitis or recurrent acute pancreatitis; (2) obstructive jaundice; and (3) preoperative ERCP, which is of value in defining ductal leaks from blunt abdominal trauma, localizing fistulous tracts from traumatic pseudocysts or pancreatic ascites, and outlining choledochal cysts.[29] Hepatitis and cirrhosis are diagnosed by other modalities and are not indications for ERCP; however, these conditions may be found on ERCP during investigation of other disorders by exclusion.

Diagnostic and Therapeutic Applications

ERCP is recognized as the best method of imaging the biliary tree and pancreatic ductal anatomy before operation. Alternative methods of imaging the liver and pancreas are available, and their choice depends on the suspected disease process as well as the therapeutic potential and the medical condition of the patient. Ultrasonography is the method of first choice for cholelithiasis and can help to estimate biliary and pancreatic ductal dilatation or pseudocysts but often fails to provide accurate information about the distal common bile duct and mid to distal pancreas owing to overlying bowel gas. A cholangiogram can identify areas of stricture, stones, sludge, polyps, and biliary-enteric fistulas and can demonstrate ascariasis, clonorchiasis, cholangiocarcinoma, and hepatocellular carcinoma. In patients whose liver is transplanted, the integrity of the anastomosis can be studied, and the area may be dilated if needed; in the same manner, bile leaks may be found.[30] Before ERCP, intraoperative pancreatography was the only method of opacifying the pancreatic duct.[31]

BILIARY DISORDERS

Biliary Atresia and Neonatal Hepatitis

The neonatal liver is susceptible to a wide variety of injuries, but the histologic reaction is often stereotypic: Liver biopsy will display cholestasis, giant cell transformation, inflammation, hepatocellular necrosis, extramedullary hematopoiesis, fibrosis, and bile duct proliferation, and findings of several cholestatic diseases of the liver may overlap in early infancy.[32] The differential diagnosis of idiopathic neonatal obstructive cholangiopathies is critical in the first weeks of life because early surgical management with the Kasai operation or hepatoportoenterostomy is known to improve morbidity and mortality.[33–38]

Exclusion of infectious, metabolic, and other causes of prolonged cholestasis in the newborn will leave 70 to 80% of patients for whom the key differentiation is extrahepatic biliary atresia (BA) versus neonatal hepatitis (NH).[39] Patients with BA will die without treatment, and rapid identification is necessary because the success rate of establishing bile flow declines after 2 months of age.[40] None of the available tests or combination of them has been 100% reliable in diagnosing BA; hence many of them have often been used, which can delay surgery.[41, 42] Even methods of collecting duodenal fluid for the presence of bile have been promising,[43] but false-negative diagnosis of BA has been described in an infant who produced green duodenal fluid at 2 weeks of age.[44]

Laparotomy with intraoperative cholangiography and wedge hepatic biopsy has been the best available method to establish the presence or absence of BA, and if the lesion was identified, the surgeon could proceed with a Kasai operation. The chief disadvantage of this approach is that many infants with NH will have undergone surgery to exclude BA, and some infants with other diseases causing cholestasis, such as arteriohepatic dysplasia (Alagille's syndrome),[45] will receive a hepatoportoenterostomy but remain cholestatic. A sweat chloride test is part of the evaluation of neonatal jaundice because some patients with cystic fibrosis have also undergone the Kasai procedure, emphasizing the difficulty and importance of accurate diagnosis.[46] Although failure of contrast material to flow retrograde into the liver despite clamping the distal common bile duct is accepted as diagnostic of BA, this cholangiographic appearance may also be seen with Alagille's syndrome. Proliferation of bile ducts is typical for BA, but percutaneous liver biopsy may result in insufficient tissue for diagnosis, and early biopsy may not be diagnostic. Another approach taken by some authors is laparoscopy by 4 weeks of age with liver biopsy and simultaneous cholangiography by transhepatic puncture of the gallbladder; Hirsig and Rickham[38] would then proceed to the Kasai operation under the same general anesthesia.

Cox and associates[40] in a prospective study of 33 neonates with conjugated hyperbilirubinemia compared the results of serum liver enzymes, ultrasonography, and liver biopsy with technetium 99m-disofenin scanning. When excretion of radioisotope was seen, BA was excluded, but scanning required a week and was less specific than ultrasonography and liver biopsy. Liver biopsy was 100% sensitive and 87% specific for BA, and technetium 99m-disofenin scanning was 100% sensitive and only 67% specific for BA. Ultrasonography was 78% sensitive and 75% specific. Liver enzymes in this study and their rate of rise in another[47] lacked sensitivity and specificity for BA. The authors concluded that radionuclide liver scanning was no more reliable than the other available tests and consumed valuable time in the preoperative period.

Administration of 5 mg per kg per day of phenobarbital for 5 days before scanning is known to enhance and accelerate biliary excretion of technetium tracer, thereby increasing the accuracy of the test. Phenobarbital pretreatment identified six infants with NH whose previous scans showed no liver excretion in one study.[48] When delayed or absent excretion of tracer is encountered, the scan has been carried out over 1 to 2 days, adding a week's time to the evaluation, when chances of a favorable response to a Kasai procedure may be decreasing.[49] Severe NH can also show lack of excretion of radionuclide label and cause a false-positive reading of BA. Absent gallbladder activity is characteristic of BA on the scan, but 20% of patients with BA will have a gallbladder demonstrated on ultrasonography.[48] Apparent gut excretion on technetium 99m-DISIDA has provided false-negative results for BA, which was later diagnosed on liver biopsy.[50]

In 1979, Lebwohl and Waye[51] published the first report of ERCP in a 4-month-old infant with biliary atresia, using the adult side-viewing instrument. There were no complications, and the authors believed the study would be of value in separating infants requiring surgery and could be done expediently in the first 1 to 2 months, when bile drainage has higher chances of being successful. Many examinations have been accomplished using standard lateral-viewing duodenoscopes in infants.[12] Problems described were duodenal erosions, abdominal distention, and retching from air insufflation, but these may be seen to accompany any upper endoscopic procedure and were not clinically significant.

In a series of 23 jaundiced infants ranging in age from 19 to 150 days, Guelrud and associates[3] used a miniaturized prototype pediatric duodenoscope to perform ERCP. The insertion tube is 8.5 mm in diameter and has a field view of 80 degrees. Four-way tip deflection to 120 degrees upward and 90 degrees in the other planes is possible. A forceps channel of 2 mm diameter is built into the instrument. Cannulation of the papilla was successful in 22 infants, and in 13 of 14 (93%) of patients with NH, the opacification of the common bile duct was thought to exclude BA. In six of seven (86%) infants with BA, only a pancreatogram was obtained, and BA was suspected; unnecessary surgery was avoided in most infants with neonatal jaundice. In very young infants, little or no sedation was needed. Size of these infants ranged from 2.4 to 7.3 kg. Examinations were performed quickly within a mean time of 8 minutes (range 2 to 18 minutes), and no complications were reported. Bile was seen in the duodenum in 12 patients, a finding believed to exclude BA; however, some infants with BA may have partial or segmental drainage.

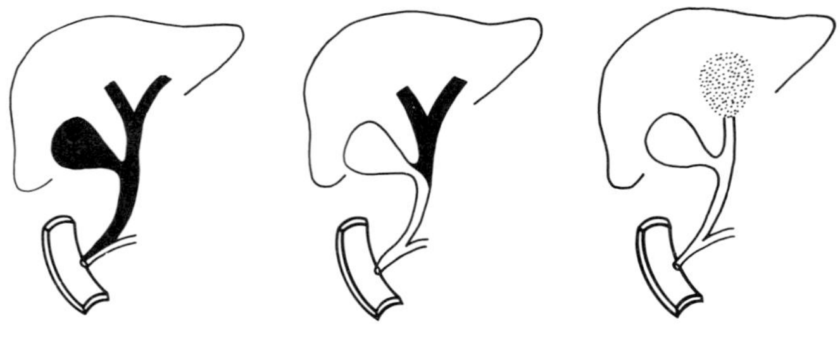

Figure 75–1. Schematic representation of the radiologic findings at ERCP in biliary atresia. Type 1, no visualization of biliary tree; type 2, opacification of the distal common duct and gallbladder without visualization of the main hepatic duct; and type 3, opacification of the distal common duct, the gallbladder, and a segment of the main hepatic duct with biliary lakes at the porta hepatis.

In their published larger series of 32 cholestatic infants in whom ERCP was performed with the Olympus PJF prototype duodenoscope, Guelrud and colleagues[6] distinguished three types of BA (Fig. 75–1): In type 1, there is no visualization of the biliary tree; type 2 BA describes visualization of the distal common bile duct and gallbladder, without the main hepatic or intrahepatic ducts; in type 3 BA, there is visualization of the distal common bile duct, gallbladder, and segment of the main hepatic duct with biliary lakes at the porta hepatis.[6] In some infants with biliary atresia with type 2 ERCP findings, there can be normal ultrasonographic emptying of the gallbladder in the absence of the main hepatic duct, which is a false-negative finding. Also in three of the six infants with type 3 ERCP findings, there was bile in the duodenum.[6] Neonatal hepatitis (Fig. 75–2) and biliary atresia (Figs. 75–3 to 75–5) are illustrated radiographically.

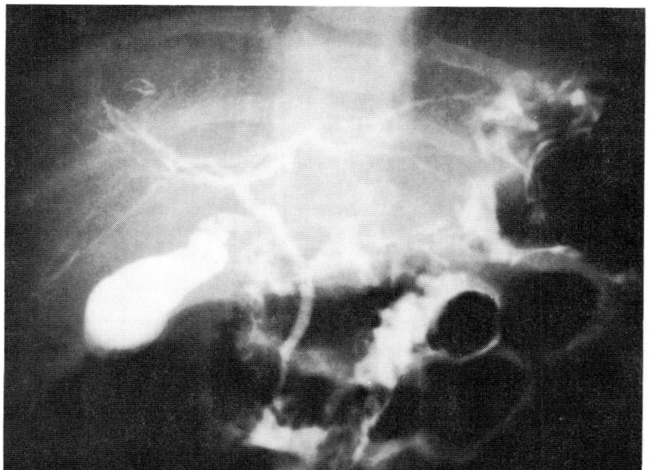

Figure 75–2. Neonatal hepatitis in a 41-day-old infant. A normal biliary tree is observed.

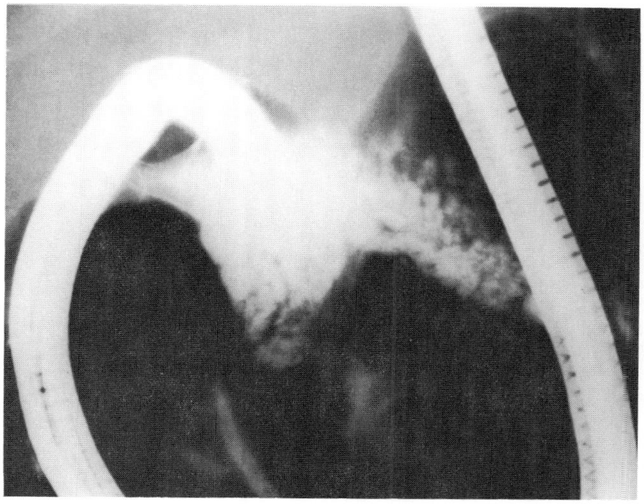

Figure 75–3. Biliary atresia in a 36-day-old infant with the type 1 ERCP finding. A pancreatogram with acinarization is observed. No opacification of the biliary tree is seen despite several maneuvers to opacify the common duct.

Matsuo and coworkers[52] used two modified fiberscopes with an outside diameter of 5 mm for assessment of the porta hepatis in a group of nine Japanese children with BA for postoperative evaluation of biliary drainage to determine success of the hepatic portoenterostomy. They described removal of bile clots from the tiny ducts and endoscopic washing or brushing to treat postoperative complications such as cholangitis.

ERCP is the most direct method of establishing a diagnosis of biliary atresia in the hands of these skilled endoscopists and may be appropriate as the first line test when such expertise and equipment are available.[53] Ultrasonography of jaundiced infants in the fasting and postprandial states demonstrating a decrease in gallbladder size after feeding virtually eliminates BA, whereas absence of a contracting gallbladder or common bile duct suggests the disease.[54] Presently, however, with the selection of tests available, 10 to 20% of infants require laparotomy, intraoperative cholangiogram, and wedge liver biopsy to make the diagnosis. In the future, ERCP may be used earlier in the diagnostic algorithm. Abnormal intrahepatic and extrahepatic ductal anatomy, site, and extent of disease in the liver and pancreas can be demonstrated by ERCP in a wide range of diseases.

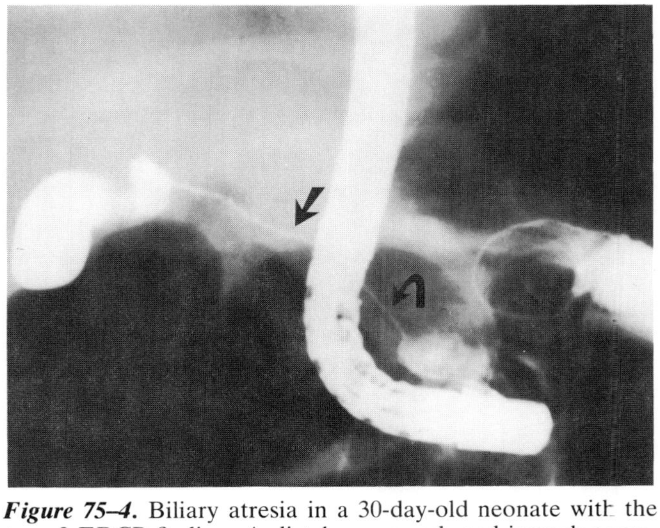

Figure 75–4. Biliary atresia in a 30-day-old neonate with the type 2 ERCP finding. A distal, narrowed, and irregular common duct is seen *(curved arrow)*. The cystic duct is wider than the common duct *(straight arrow)*. The gallbladder is normal. No opacification of the main hepatic duct or of the intrahepatic ducts is seen.

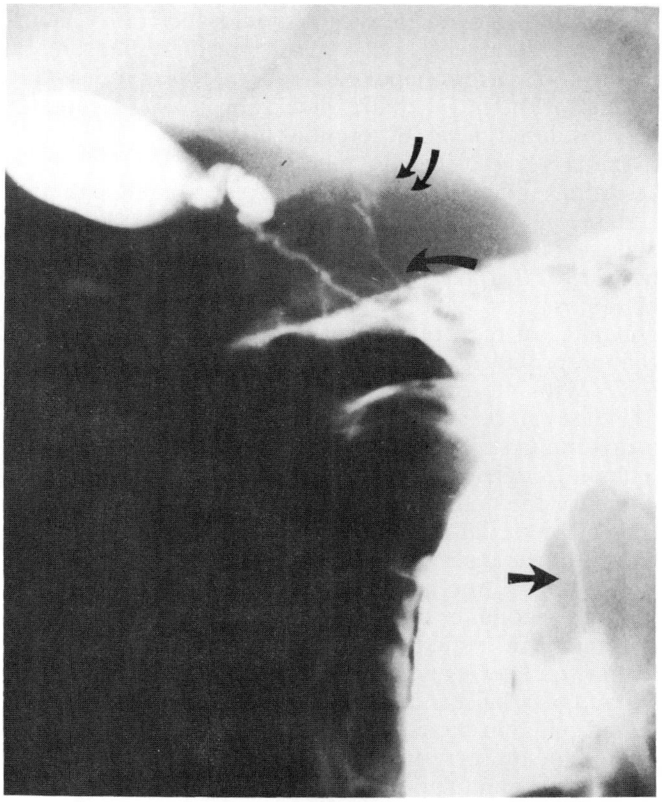

Figure 75–5. Biliary atresia in a 31-day-old infant with the type 3 ERCP finding. A distal narrowed common duct *(straight arrow)* and a main narrowed hepatic duct *(single curved arrow)* are visualized. Multiple biliary lakes are seen at the porta hepatis *(double curved arrows)*. The gallbladder is normal.

Other Biliary Disorders

Other biliary disorders have been studied with ERCP, and their characteristic anatomic forms give precise diagnosis. Caroli's disease, or congenital cystic dilatation of the intrahepatic bile ducts, with multiple segmental cylindrical or saccular dilatations of small biliary radicles can be demonstrated by ERCP.[55, 56] The extrahepatic biliary tree with possible coexistent strictures and calculi in Caroli's disease may also be seen.[57, 58]

The ERCP in Alagille's syndrome[59, 60] shows marked and diffuse narrowing of the extrahepatic biliary ducts with uniform narrowing of the intrahepatic ducts and reduced arborization. Hepatoportoenterostomy has been performed on patients with Alagille's syndrome and cystic fibrosis[46] for prolonged obstructive jaundice, and the diagnostic work-up should include a sweat chloride test and a search for the associated syndromatic findings of arteriohepatic dysplasia. Nonsyndromatic paucity of the intrahepatic ducts (Fig. 75–6) should also be considered in the differential diagnosis.

Primary sclerosing cholangitis (PSC)[61, 62] in children is accurately diagnosed with ERCP as in adult patients, and the majority of cases are associated with inflammatory bowel disease. The cholangiogram will show pruning of the peripheral biliary tree and irregular areas of stenosis and ectasia (Fig. 75–7). Liver histology can only suggest the presence of large duct obstruction but cannot provide a specific diagnosis, as can ERCP in PSC. With more advanced disease, palliative relief of jaundice can be accomplished by therapeutic dilation of a dominant stricture in a major duct with hydrostatic balloon bougienage.[63] ERCP is the most reliable technique for the diagnosis of PSC, and PTC may fail to get contrast material into the ducts owing to the sclerosing nature of the disease.

The biliary tree may have cystic dilatation and irregularities secondary to focal biliary cirrhosis or recurrent cholangitis in cystic fibrosis.[64] Stones may also be found within the liver as well as the extrahepatic bile ducts in CF and may be seen on ERCP. Collection of uncontaminated bile and pancreatic juice, with or without cholecystokinin or secretin stimulation, is possible with directed duct cannulation.[65]

Results of dilation of strictures of the biliary and pancreatic ducts or of the sphincter of Oddi with a hydrostatic balloon catheter passed through the endoscope have been described in a group of 24 patients, but more experience needs to be gathered to determine its efficacy and safety.[63] Congenital hepatic fibrosis in the infant will demonstrate a normal common bile duct and irregular intrahepatic ducts with multiple small cysts in the liver (Fig. 75–8).

Endoscopic biliary stenting was described by Soehen-

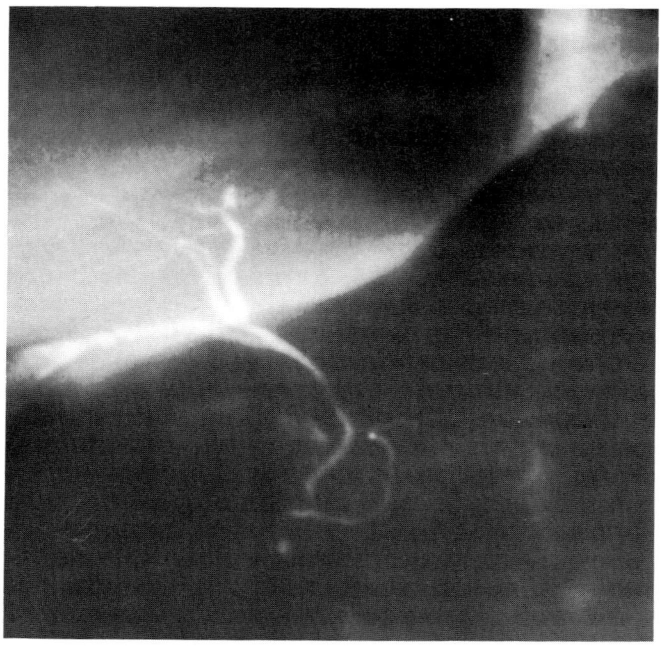

Figure 75–6. Nonsyndromatic paucity of bile ducts. A normal extrahepatic biliary duct is seen. Uniform narrowing of intrahepatic ducts and reduced arborization are visualized.

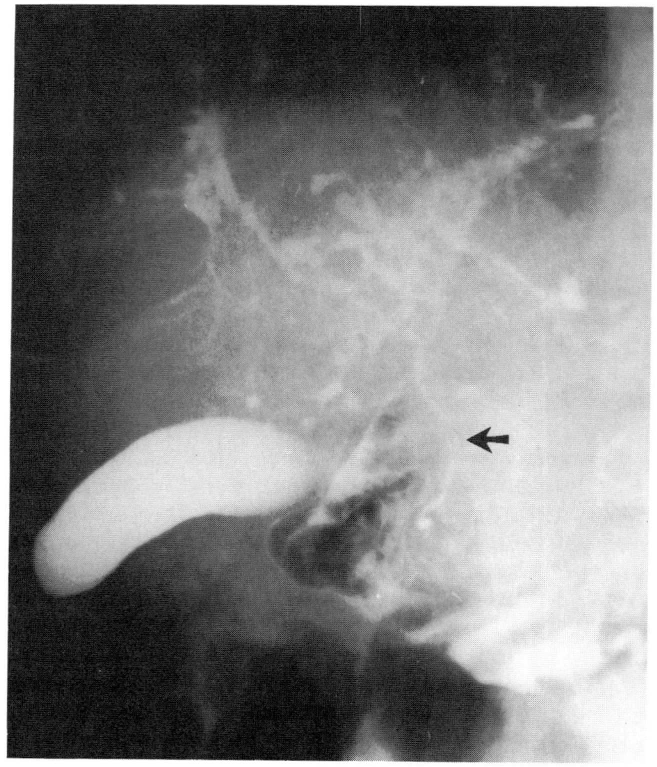

Figure 75–7. Primary sclerosing cholangitis in a 12-year-old female without an associated underlying condition. Note a narrow and irregular common duct *(arrow)* with pruning of the peripheral biliary tree and irregular areas of stenosis and ectasia.

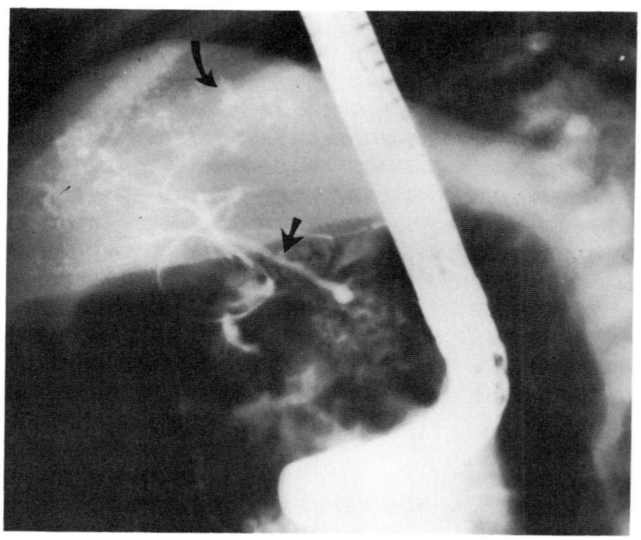

Figure 75–8. Congenital hepatic fibrosis in a 38-day-old infant. Note a normal common duct *(straight arrow)* and irregular intrahepatic ducts with multiple small cysts in the liver *(curved arrow)*.

dra and Reynders-Frederix in 1979,[66] for restoration of bile flow via placement of a plastic tube across a stricture. Endoscopic palliation of jaundice secondary to metastatic neuroblastoma by stent placement in a 2-year-old boy was successfully done by Bickerstaff and associates.[67] Guelrud and colleagues[68] reported the usefulness of ERCP for diagnosis and therapy in a 21-month-old child for stenting a malignant stricture in the common hepatic duct due to neuroblastoma. A papillotomy was done, and the stent was moved into position over a guide wire. Repeat ERCP with the prototype pediatric Olympus JFP duodenoscope 7 months later showed disappearance of the compression, and the biliary endoprosthesis was removed (Fig. 75–9). The diagnosis of cholangiocarcinoma in older patients may be obtained by biopsy forceps or brush cytology through the therapeutic channel on the duodenoscope.[69, 70] A "daughter" cholangioscope can be introduced through the "mother" duodenoscope for detailed cholangioscopy. ERCP can help differentiate extrinsic versus intrinsic compression by masses.

Rarely bleeding from the gastrointestinal tract is caused by hemobilia, or biliary tract hemorrhage, and localization of the site of bleeding to its exit from the papilla in the duodenum can be seen with the standard forward-viewing upper endoscope or the side-viewing duodenoscope.[71] Blood clots in the biliary tree may appear as irregularly shaped filling defects. Gallbladder papillomatosis is a rare condition that may cause bleeding from the biliary tract and can be diagnosed with ERCP.

Hydatid disease, a parasitic infection with *Echinococcus granulosus,* involves the liver and has been confirmed by cholangiogram and treated with endoscopic sphincterotomy in 10 patients with good decompression and no complications.[72] Before endoscopic sphincterotomy, stenosis of the papilla had to be treated surgically, but ERCP now has a place in the preoperative and

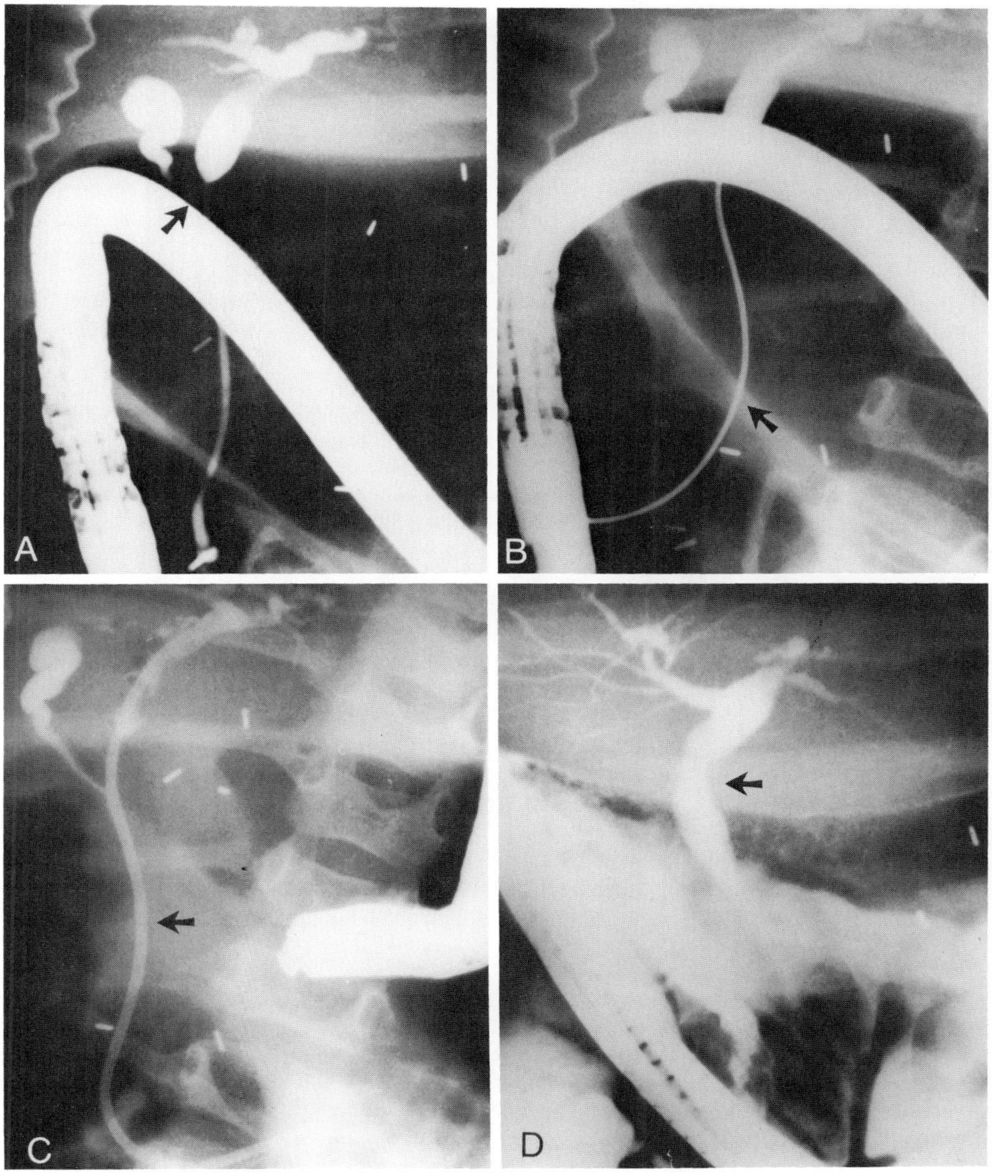

Figure 75–9. Malignant stricture at the common hepatic duct in a 21-month-old child with jaundice secondary to metastatic neuroblastoma. *A,* Note a stricture at the main hepatic duct *(arrow)* with dilation of intrahepatic ducts. The gallbladder and the common bile duct are normal. *B,* After sphincterotomy, a guide wire *(arrow)* is introduced into the left hepatic duct. *C,* A double pigtail biliary stent, 7 Fr in diameter, is placed *(arrow). D,* After 4 months of chemotherapy, the biliary stent was removed, and the common hepatic duct is free of stricture *(arrow).*

postoperative management in these patients. Therapeutic use of ERCP was reported from South Africa, where children averaging 12.4 kg with roundworm infestation had them removed from the duodenal papilla with the standard duodenoscope.[10] No complications were seen.

Choledocholithiasis

Common bile duct calculi occur rarely in both infants and children.[73] Conditions associated with the presence of stones include biliary tract malformations such as choledochal cyst, chronic liver disease,[74] hemolysis, and infection (Figs. 75–10 and 75–11). Rarely gallstones or calculi in the common bile duct occur without any known etiology, may be found incidentally during investigation of other organ systems, and may pass spontaneously. Larger stones, however, may have impact at the distal common bile duct and result in clinical and biochemical obstructive jaundice even in infants; endoscopic sphincterotomy with clearing of the duct by dragging out debris with a Fogarty catheter has been done successfully in a 3-year-old child.[75] Guelrud and colleagues[75a] have used endoscopic sphincterotomy to remove common bile duct stones in six jaundiced children (aged 6–12 years) who had previously undergone cholecystectomy. Endoscopic sphincterotomy is the procedure of choice in the management of retained and recurrent bile duct stones for adult patients in some centers.[76] Five pediatric patients have had endoscopic sphincterotomy in the series from Toronto for choledocholithiasis and for clearance of biliary debris in patients with cystic fibrosis.[4]

Manometric studies of sphincter of Oddi motor function have been combined with ERCP in the investigation of biliary dyskinesia, by sliding a water-perfused catheter

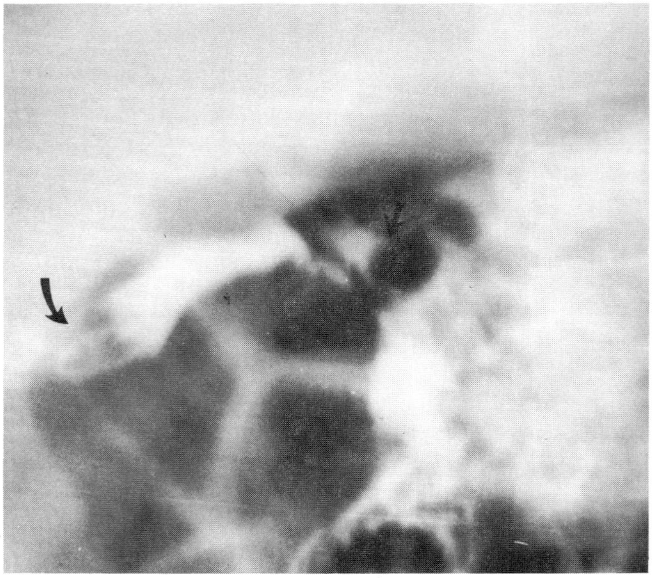

Figure 75–10. Cholelithiasis and common duct stone in a 29-day-old neonate with hemolytic anemia. Note a normal diameter common duct with a stone at the main hepatic duct *(straight arrow)* and dilated intraheptic ducts. The gallbladder is seen with stones *(curved arrow)*.

with a pressure transducer into the papilla and recording pressures during a pull-through maneuver. Normal values have been established,[77] and endoscopic sphincterotomy has been done during the procedure when elevated pressures have been documented, providing relief of symptoms in the majority of patients in this select subset.[78, 79] Allendorph and associates[13] report teenagers with right upper quadrant pain after cholecystectomy in

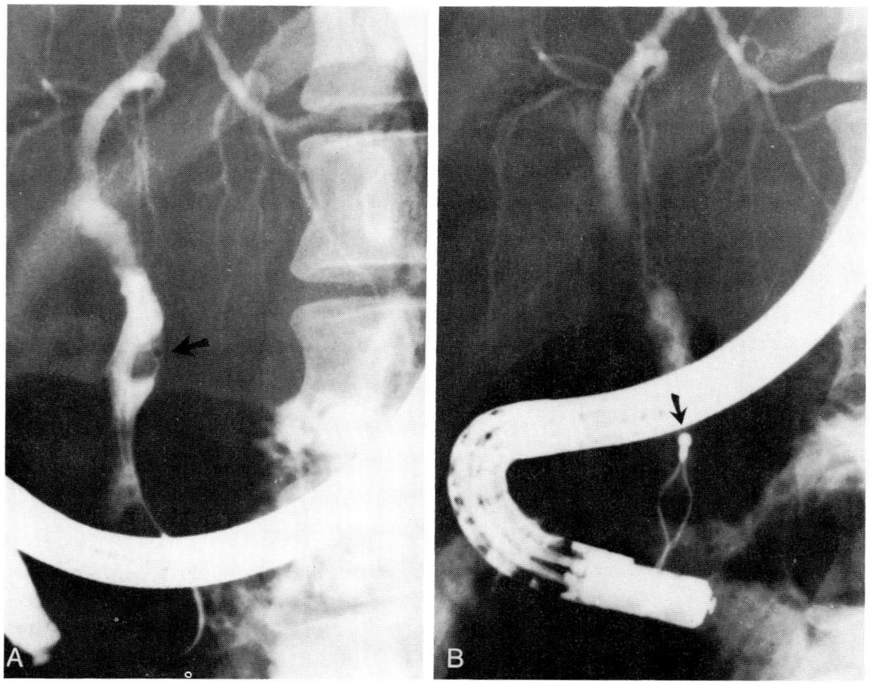

Figure 75–11. Choledocholithiasis in a 12-year-old patient with hemolytic anemia after cholecystectomy. *A,* Sludge and a common bile duct stone are visualized *(arrow)*. *B,* After endoscopic sphincterotomy, the common duct stone is retrieved with a basket *(arrow)*.

their series of 39 ERCP procedures in patients aged 6 months to 18 years and a mean age of 12.5 years. Opiates are not used for sedation because of their known effect on the smooth muscle of the sphincter, and higher doses of benzodiazepines are administered.

Vignote and colleagues[72] have recognized ERCP with endoscopic sphincterotomy (ES) to be the first choice treatment for surgical complications of hepatic hydatid disease as well as the drainage procedure of choice in patients with cholangitis owing to hydatid disease. The presence of *Ascaris* worms (Fig. 75–12) is also a cause of obstructive jaundice, and these worms may be pulled out of the biliary tree with a tripod snare and other special instruments.[10]

Choledochal Cyst

Considered to be a congenital malformation of the biliary tract, choledochal cysts were classified into three

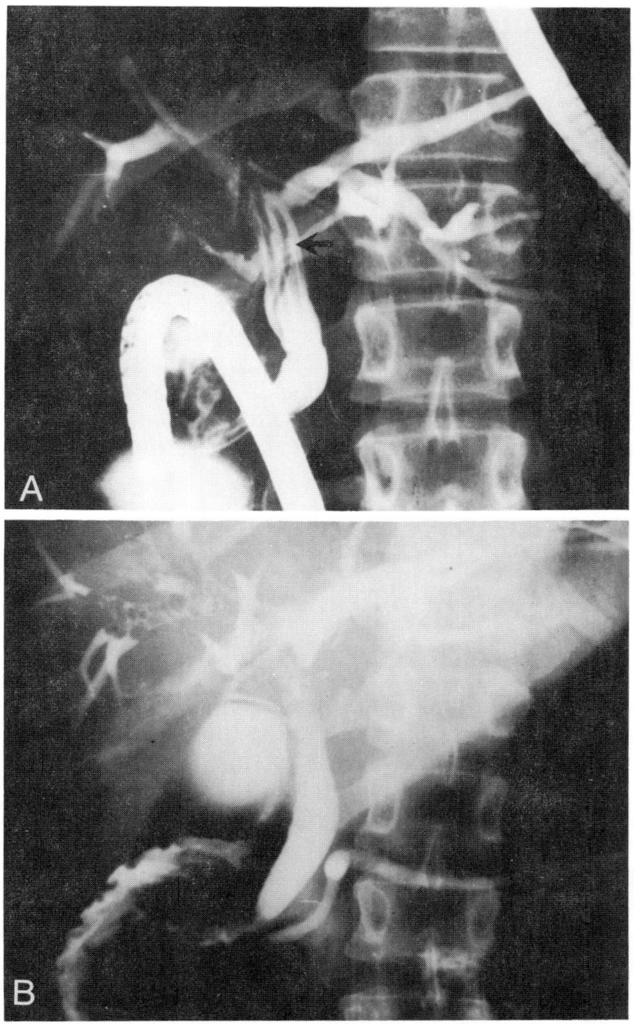

Figure 75–12. *Ascaris* in the common bile duct and right hepatic duct in a 17-year-old girl. *A,* Several tubular filling defects are visible *(arrow)*. *B,* After retrieving the worms with a tripod device, the common duct appears normal.

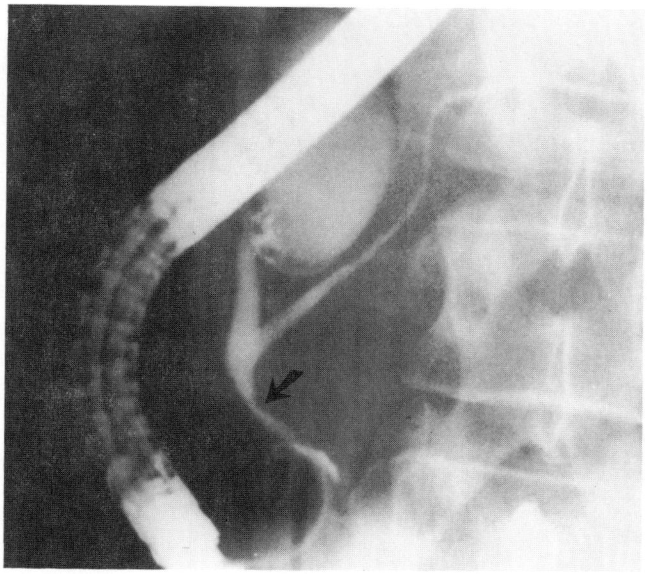

Figure 75–13. Choledochal cyst in an 11-year-old girl. Note an abnormal pancreaticobiliary duct junction with a long common channel *(arrow)* in a type A cyst.

types, which were classified by Alonso-Lej and colleagues in a review of the world's literature in 1959.[80] It is speculated that anomalous connection of the pancreatic and bile ducts is a factor in the development of a choledochal cyst, which is an abnormal localized dilatation of the biliary tract. A long common channel[81] distal to the anomalous junction of the pancreatic and biliary ducts is present, with or without stenosis at the papilla.[82] Okada and coworkers' series[83] of six patients were all very young children with common channel syndrome, each with jaundice, abdominal pain, vomiting, and fever and all cases diagnosed with ERCP. Only 20 to 40% of patients present with a triad of jaundice, right upper quadrant mass, and pain, and signs may be intermittent in appearance. Recurrent pancreatitis may also be secondary to a choledochal cyst or anomaly of the distal shared pancreaticobiliary duct.[84]

The first and most common type is congenital cystic dilatation of the common bile duct, in which the terminal common bile duct is frequently narrowed as it enters the duodenum (Figs. 75–13 to 75–15). The size of type I cysts is variable, their form is cylindrical or fusiform, and they account for 90% of all choledochal cysts.[85] Type II is a rare congenital diverticulum of the common bile duct; this lesion is not accompanied with jaundice. The term choledochocele is applied to a type III cyst that is limited to the small intraduodenal segment of the common bile duct, which herniates into the duodenal lumen. There is no mass, but nausea and vomiting are usually present. Todani and associates[86] expanded the classification in 1977 to include Caroli's disease as type IV-A biliary cystic dilation with multiple intrahepatic and extrahepatic cysts; type IV-B are cysts in the extrahepatic ductal system only. Solitary liver cysts are a type V lesion.

ERCP is of value in outlining these cysts and their

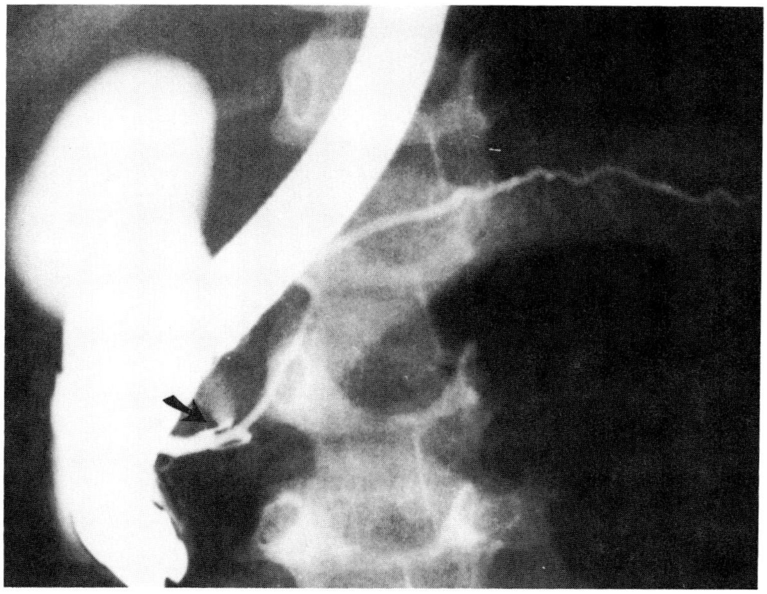

Figure 75–14. Choledochal cyst in a 3-year-old boy. Note the segmental choledochal dilatation with a stricture of the distal common duct *(arrow)*.

relationship to both ductal systems, providing a roadmap for the surgical approach.[87, 88] Ultrasonography,[89] computed tomography, and radionuclide scans cannot provide the same quality of anatomic detail as the ERCP, but these methods can provide data regarding size, contour, position, and presence of stones.[90] Cystolithiasis and cholangiocarcinoma[91] have been associated phenomena, presumably owing to biliary stasis, reflux of pancreatic secretions, and recurrent infections. Retrograde injection of contrast material into the ampulla of Vater or the minor (accessory) papilla in the anomalous pancreaticobiliary junction may simultaneously opacify both ductal systems. There are a few reported series describing therapeutic endoscopic sphincterotomy for type III cysts,[92] with a theoretical advantage of avoiding the postoperative complications of stagnation referred to as the sump syndrome.[93] Some authors consider anomalous drainage into a common channel a contraindication to endoscopic sphincterotomy.[63, 87]

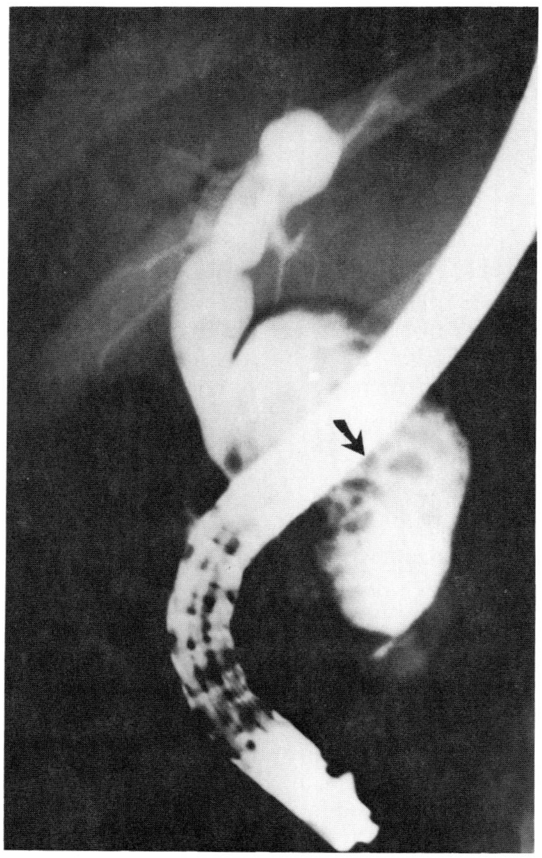

Figure 75–15. Choledochal cyst in a 12-year-old girl. Note multiple cystolithiasis *(arrow)* with a stricture of the distal common duct.

PANCREATIC DISORDERS

Congenital Malformations

Pancreas Divisum

Variants of the pancreatic duct system have been studied in autopsy series, and the most common variant is pancreas divisum (PD), occurring at a frequency of 3 to 10%.[94] The normal relationship of the main pancreatic duct is derived from union of the dorsal and ventral buds of pancreatic tissue in the embryo. When these buds do not fuse, a separate drainage system forms in which the accessory duct of Santorini becomes the main drainage for the gland, and the small ventral duct drains the head and uncinate process via the duct of Wirsung in the main papilla or through the ampulla of Vater. ERCP is the only way to diagnose PD, and cannulation of the minor papilla is necessary to demonstrate the complete pancreatic ductal system (Fig. 75–16). Some studies suggest that this anomaly occurs in equal frequency in patients with and without pancreatitis.[95] There

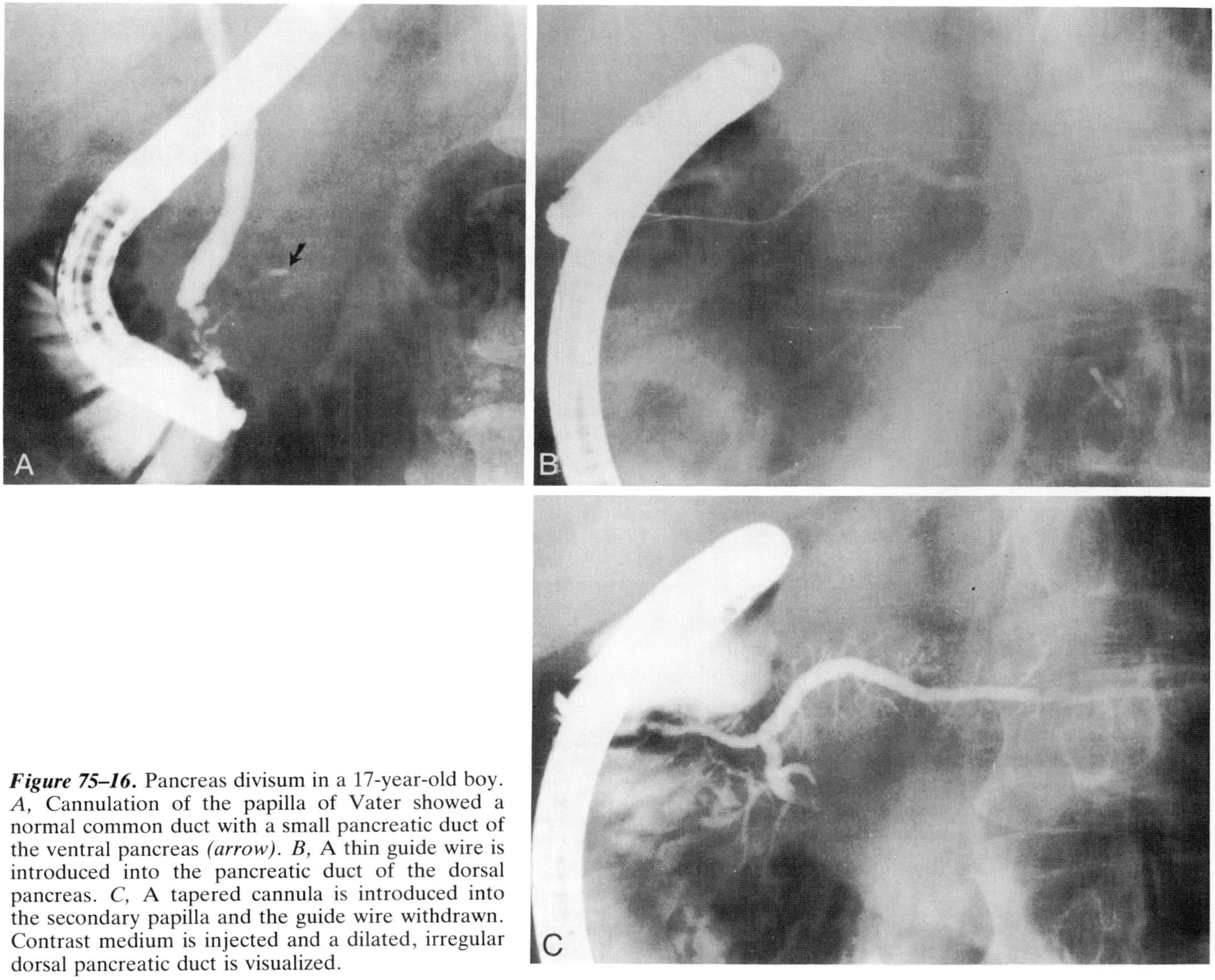

Figure 75–16. Pancreas divisum in a 17-year-old boy. *A,* Cannulation of the papilla of Vater showed a normal common duct with a small pancreatic duct of the ventral pancreas *(arrow). B,* A thin guide wire is introduced into the pancreatic duct of the dorsal pancreas. *C,* A tapered cannula is introduced into the secondary papilla and the guide wire withdrawn. Contrast medium is injected and a dilated, irregular dorsal pancreatic duct is visualized.

is controversy in the lilterature about PD as a cause of pancreatitis. Reports of divisum and pancreatitis in children[96–98] began to appear with the advent of ERCP. Cotton[99] found an incidence of PD of 3.6% of 169 patients with primary biliary tract disease, but of 78 patients with recurrent pancreatitis, the incidence was 25.6%. Considerable endoscopic talent is requisite to locating and cannulating the accessory papilla in PD when Santorini's duct is dominant and for patients who have juxta-ampullary diverticula. Recurrent pancreatitis has been reported in pediatric patients with PD,[98] and stones may be present in the pancreatic ducts.[100]

Secretions from a disrupted duct may irritate the peritoneal lining and result in pancreatic ascites, which is rare in children, but since ERCP has come into use to demonstrate ductal anatomy, reports of abnormalities, such as congenital intrapancreatic cyst and ascites in a 4-month-old, have recently appeared.[101] Levine and colleagues[102] reported usefulness of ERCP in preoperative evaluation of pancreatic ductal disruption causing pancreatic ascites. Large pediatric surgical series[103] corroborate the value of ductal definition in operative and nonoperative management of pancreatic disorders in this age group.

Annular pancreas is a term denoting a ring of pancreatic tissue surrounding the duodenum, which may cause symptoms to present from newborn to advanced age. The ERCP appearance of this congenital anomaly has been reported in a series of four patients from Japan.[104] A pancreatic rest is ectopic pancreatic tissue found in the gastrointestinal tract that is usually asymptomatic and often discovered incidentally in the stomach or duodenum by upper gastrointestinal endoscopy.[105]

Chronic Pancreatitis

Recurrent episodes of pancreatitis may be caused by anomalies and abnormalities of the pancreatic and biliary ducts,[84, 106, 107] which can now be defined precisely by ERCP, lessening the number of patients thought to have idiopathic pancreatitis.[108] Blustein and associates[109] recommend ERCP as the procedure of choice in children with relapsing pancreatitis because of the high yield of surgically correctable lesions. Another series of 10 children with chronic pancreatitis studied with ERCP emphasized that fibrosing pancreatitis needs to be considered in the differential diagnosis of obstructive jaundice.[110] A pancreatic or biliary ductal abnormality was found in 16 of 35 patients with recurrent pancreatitis in a series of children and adults who underwent ERCP.[111, 112] Surgical approach was based on the ERCP findings of potentially correctable lesions in these patients. A dilated, irregular main pancreatic duct with or without strictures and stones may be seen (Fig. 75–17 and 75–18). Therapeutic maneuvers such as placement of a nasobiliary drain[113] and nasopancreatic drain, placement of a pancreatic duct endoprosthesis, and pancreatic stone extraction done in 32 patients aged 12 to 68 years[114] are viable endoscopic alternatives to surgery.

Correlation between degree of structural changes seen on ERCP and functional impairment of the pancreas has been noted in pediatric and adult patients.[115] When pseudocysts complicate pancreatitis, the appropriate operation is determined by location and duration of the lesion,[116] and improvements in management of pediatric patients with acute and chronic pancreatitis have been attributed to ERCP.[117, 118] ERCP has been of value in demonstrating internal fistulization from a pancreatic pseudocyst to the pleural space in a child.[119]

Pancreatic Trauma

Injury by motor vehicle accidents and other causes of blunt or penetrating trauma may cause pancreatic ductal disruption in children and adults. Delayed recognition is not uncommon, especially since injuries to the body and tail of the pancreas may be indolent in their presentation.[120] The pancreas is positioned over the spine; hence its location makes the organ vulnerable to injury by blunt abdominal trauma, which may fracture or sever the ducts. The retroperitoneal location of the pancreas has made it relatively inaccessible to physical examination and difficult to image with older techniques before surgical exploration. ERCP is diagnostic for pancreatic duct laceration, showing extravasation of contrast material at the point of disruption.[121] Hall and colleagues[122] reported four cases of pancreatic trauma in children aged 2 to 13 years and recommended early cholangiogram to identify the presence and location of duct leakage for patients requiring urgent surgery. Traumatic pancreatitis and its sequelae have significant morbidity and mortality,[103, 120] and diagnosis with subsequent therapy should be accomplished as soon as possible to improve outcome.[123] Patients with normal ductograms are treated conservatively. ERCP in the diagnosis of an internal pancreatic fistula in a 5-year-old boy with pancreatic ascites greatly aided in the operative and medical management.[124] Again, there is potential for infection caused by injecting a fistula, which may communicate with a semiclosed pseudocyst, and prompt surgery is recommended by several authors. If a large pseudocyst is found, ERCP is probably unnecessary because this may be imaged by other means.[125] Spontaneous resolution of even very large pseudocysts is known to occur. Salinas and associates[126] suggest a role for ERCP in identifying pseudocysts likely to respond because they are connected to the main duct, and therapeutic dislodgment of proteinaceous plugs obstructing the duct may lead to resolution of the cyst.

Barkin and coworkers[127] did a prospective study to evaluate ERCP in both children and adults for suspected pancreatic ductal rupture after abdominal trauma. They found, as expected, both the sensitivity and the specific-

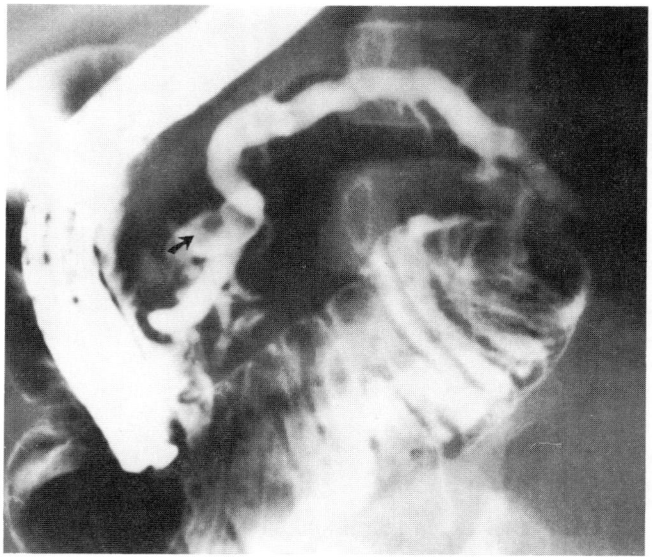

Figure 75–18. Chronic pancreatitis in a 9-year-old boy. Note severe dilation of the pancreatic duct with pancreatic stones *(arrow)*.

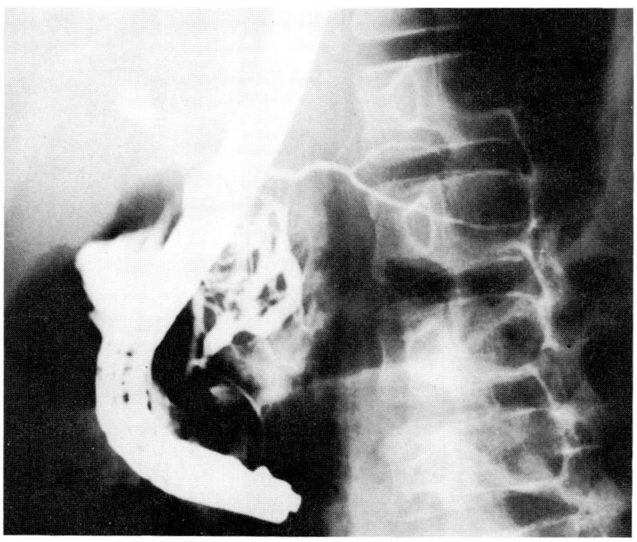

Figure 75–17. Chronic recurrent pancreatitis in a 14-year-old girl. An abnormal pancreaticobiliary junction is visualized. Note dilation of the pancreatic duct with dilated communicating branches at the head of the pancreas.

ity of ERCP to be 100% for pancreatic duct disruption, versus any combination of serum amylase, computed tomography scan, and peritoneal lavage for effective diagnosis. Neither the presence of hyperamylasemia nor the peak level separated patients with fractured pancreatic duct from those with intact ducts. Determination of location and extent of ductal tear directed surgical intervention in the pancreas, where contusion with edema, hematoma, surrounding injuries, and the retroperitoneal location of the organ may obscure injury.[128–130]

COMPLICATIONS

Reactions to medications used for sedation or general anesthesia may occur as with upper endoscopy; however, these are usually mild and infrequent (see Chapter 74). The most common complication following ERCP in adults is pancreatitis,[131] and reported incidence varies from 1 to 8%; however, clinical pancreatitis is rare. When measured, serum pancreatic enzymes are elevated, as expected following cannulation and injection of the pancreatic duct even in totally asymptomatic patients, and this is rarely of clinical significance.[132–134] Correlation has been noted between the force of injection of the pancreatic ducts with contrast material, degree of acinarization seen on fluoroscopy, urographic visualization,[135] and subsequent development of pancreatitis. Attempts to monitor the pressure of injection with manometers have been reported;[136] however, this has not proved to be practical or necessary. Care is taken to fill the ducts with minimal pressure, to stop the procedure if repeated injection of the pancreatic duct occurs when attempting to cannulate the bile duct,[137] and to establish the anatomy of the main pancreatic duct with as little filling of the secondary and tertiary pancreatic radicles as possible.

Bilbao and associates[138] retrospectively surveyed 10,435 ERCP examinations in a multicenter study and noted that experienced endoscopists had a 3% reported incidence of complications in adults, whereas inexperienced workers had four times the failure rate in cannulating the desired duct(s) and twice the complications (7%). Fluoroscopic time also decreases with growing experience of the endoscopist.[139] Data obtained on 2,884 examinations in Nebel's study[140] revealed a complication rate of 2.16%, with pancreatitis, cholangitis, cardiopulmonary problems, perforation, and bleeding being the chief complications in decreasing order of frequency. The incidence of complications in pediatric patients is unknown because there are only a few large series, in one of which oversedation and transient tracheal compression were reported in 10% of the infants. Mild pancreatitis occurred in two of 42 children undergoing ERCP, and endoscopic papillotomy was successful in five patients in this series.[4] In a series of 42 ERCP examinations in 37 children and one young adult, mild pancreatitis ensued in three patients (8%), all of whom had a history of pancreatitis.[12] Abnormalities were detected in 22 of 38 (58%) of patients in this series, 11 of whom required surgery.

In patients with pseudocyst formation, injection of the pancreatic duct with contrast material from an endoscope that has been passed through the unsterile oropharynx may potentially seed the cyst with bacteria and cause pancreatic abscess. There is controversy in the literature about ERCP in patients with pancreatic pseudocysts, but most authors favor waiting until the patient has recovered from the acute illness. When ERCP is done to plan operative approach, the interval to surgery should not exceed 24 hours.[125, 141] When ductal obstruction is found, prompt surgical intervention is recommended because of the risk of sepsis.[140]

Acute ascending cholangitis may complicate ERCP[142] and is potentially fatal; however, this risk was described in adults with malignant and other forms of stenotic obstruction to drainage of the biliary tree. Antibiotic prophylaxis is needed in this situation because 90% of cholangitis cases occur with biliary obstruction.[138] No deaths from ERCP have been reported in pediatric patients; in adults, septic complications and perforation have accounted for a mortality of 0.1 to 0.2%. Occasionally intramural injection of contrast material or extravasation of contrast material occurs, but in the pediatric ERCP literature this has not been noted as a complication.

An incision may be made in the sphincter of Oddi to provide improved drainage for biliary dyskinesia due to sphincter of Oddi dysfunction and to admit larger catheters with established therapeutic potential. Specialized instruments are available to pass through a channel in the endoscope, including balloons for removal of biliary stones and debris, Dormia wire baskets for closing around stones, stone-crushing devices, and standard and brush biopsy forceps for cytologic diagnosis of carcinomas in adult patients. Hydrostatic balloon catheters may be passed through a strictured area, then be inflated to dilate the stenotic area. Bleeding or hemorrhage may complicate endoscopic sphincterotomy in adults. In addition, perforation of the gastrointestinal tract or the common bile duct following instrumentation may complicate ERCP. Aspiration pneumonia may occur rarely.

Infections with *Pseudomonas aeruginosa* have been linked to contamination of endoscopes and closed water reservoirs,[143–145] and this has prompted changes and new guidelines for disinfection of the instruments and endoscopy suite. A randomized, controlled study of 61 patients found no statistical difference in the incidence of septic episodes (3% in each group) in controls versus patients who had gentamicin added to the contrast material.[146] Another prospective evaluation of 51 consecutive patients to determine the frequency of bacteremia with ERCP showed only one patient (2%) with multiple strictures of the main pancreatic duct who had transient bacteremia, but no septic illness ensued.[23] Any patient found to have a stricture was then given antibiotics after the procedure.

CONTRAINDICATIONS

Contraindications include inability of the patient to cooperate, perforation of a hollow viscus, shock, cervical spine injury, intestinal obstruction, and other cardiopulmonary conditions that would not permit safe use of intravenous sedation. Fever is a contraindication to ERCP in biliary obstruction unless followed by immediate ductal drainage.[142] Relative contraindications are coagulopathy, coma, and the presence of pancreatitis or cholangitis, unless therapeutic ERCP could treat the underlying cause of the infection. Certain structural abnormalities may preclude ERCP, such as esophageal stricture, postoperative changes in anatomy, and large paraesophageal hernia.[147]

SUMMARY

Approach to diagnostic studies of the pancreaticobiliary system depends on knowledge of available techniques and resources. ERCP has not been commonly used with pediatric patients, but advances in technology of prototype duodenoscopes and catheters used to cannulate the papilla in the past decade have established its role in obstructive jaundice and recurrent pancreatitis.[22] Because it is an invasive procedure, its place in the definition of pancreaticobiliary disease is reserved for cases that cannot be diagnosed with other methods such as ultrasonography. As yet the diagnostic yield for ERCP in otherwise unexplained abdominal pain is low, and it is not indicated for this, unless there is some evidence pointing to pathology in the area. Special advanced training and continuing experience in ERCP are needed beyond general endoscopic competence.[27] The procedure is of value in assessing surgically correctable lesions of the pancreas and biliary tree and has defined the cause of neonatal cholestasis in many infants, avoiding the need for surgery and intraoperative cholangiography. Careful patient selection and knowledge of available local skills and alternative methods will influence utilization and referral for ERCP in pediatric patients.

REFERENCES

1. McCune WS, Shorb PE, Moscovitz H: Endoscopic cannulation of the ampulla of Vater. Ann Surg 1968; 167:752–756.
2. Waye JD: Endoscopic retrograde cholangiopancreatography in the infant. Am J Gastroenterol 1976; 65:461–463.
3. Guelrud M, Jaen D, Torres P, et al: Endoscopic cholangiopancreatography in the infant: Evaluation of a new prototype pediatric duodenoscope. Gastrointest Endosc 1987; 33:4–8.
4. Buckley A, Connon JJ: The role of ERCP in children and adolescents. Gastrointest Endosc 1990; 36:360–372.
5. Cotton PB, Laage NJ: Endoscopic retrograde cholangiopancreatography in children. Arch Dis Child 1982; 57:131–136.
6. Guelrud M, Jaen D, Mendoza S, et al: ERCP in the diagnosis of extrahepatic biliary atresia. Gastrointest Endosc 1991; 37:522–526.
7. Wilkinson ML, Mieli-Vergani G, Ball C, et al: Endoscopic retrograde cholangiopancreatography in infantile cholestasis. Arch Dis Child 1991; 66:121–123.
8. Riemann JF, Koch H: Endoscopy of the biliary tract and pancreas in children. Endoscopy 1978; 10:166–172.
9. Heyman MB, Shapiro HA, Thaler MM: Endoscopic retrograde cholangiography in the diagnosis of biliary malformations in infants. Gastrointest Endosc 1988; 34:449–453.
10. van der Spuy S: Endoscopic retrograde cholangiopancreatography (ERCP) in children. Endoscopy 1978; 10:173–175.
11. Urakami Y, Seki H, Kishi S: Endoscopic retrograde cholangiopancreatography (ERCP) performed in children. Endoscopy 1977; 9:86–91.
12. Putnam PE, Kocoshis SA, Orenstein SR, Schade RR: Pediatric endoscopic retrograde cholangiopancreatography. Am J Gastroenterol 1991; 86:824–830.
13. Allendorph M, Werlin SL, Geenan JE, et al: Endoscopic retrograde cholangiopancreatography in children. J Pediatr 1986; 110:206–211.
14. Scharschmidt BF, Goldberg HI, Schmid R: Approach to the patient with cholestatic jaundice. N Engl J Med 1983; 308:1515–1519.
15. Riddlesberger MM: Diagnostic imaging of the hepatobiliary system in infants and children. J Pediatr Gastroenterol Nutr 1984; 3:653–664.
16. Schiff ER: Diagnostic percutaneous transhepatic cholangiography. Sem Liver Dis 1982; 2:49–56.
17. Elias E, Hamlyn AN, Jain S, et al: A randomized trial of percutaneous transhepatic cholangiography with the Chiba needle versus endoscopic retrograde cholangiography for bile duct visualization in jaundice. Gastroenterology 1976; 71:439–443.
18. Katon RM, Lee TG, Parent JA, et al: Endoscopic retrograde cholangiopancreatography (ERCP): Experience with 100 cases. Am J Dig Dis 1974; 19:295–306.
19. Caulfield M, Wyllie R, Sivak MV, et al: Upper gastrointestinal tract endoscopy in the pediatric patient. J Pediatr 1989; 115:339–345.
20. Steffen RM, Wyllie R, Sivak MV, et al: Colonoscopy in the pediatric patient. J Pediatr 1989; 115:507–514.
21. Guelrud M, Mendoza S, Viera L, Gelrud D: Somatostatin prevents acute pancreatitis after pancreatic duct sphincter hydrostatic balloon dilation in patients with idiopathic recurrent pancreatitis. Gastrointest Endosc 1991; 37:44–47.
22. Ament ME, Berquist WE, Vargas J, Perisic V: Fiberoptic upper intestinal endoscopy in infants and children. Pediatr Clin North Am 1988; 35:141–155.
23. Dutta SK, Cox M, Williams RB, et al: Prospective evaluation of the risk of bacteremia and the role of antibiotics in ERCP. J Clin Gastroenterol 1983; 5:325–329.
24. Mauer K, Waye JD: A new pediatric duodenoscope: Successful cannulation without a cannula elevator. Gastrointest Endosc 1989; 35:437–439.
25. Sivak MV: Video endoscopy. Clin Gastroenterol 1986; 15:205–234.
26. Classen M, Phillip J: Newer endoscopic techniques for image diagnosis and management of hepatobiliary disease. Sem Liver Dis 1982; 2:67–74.
27. Wigton RS, Vennes JA: Clinical competence in diagnostic endoscopic retrograde cholangiopancreatography. Ann Intern Med 1988; 108:142–144.
28. Guelrud M, Plaz-Abreu J: Endoscopic retrograde cholangiography. Lab Res Methods Biol Med 1983; 7:427–467.
29. Marshall JB, Halpin TC: Choledochocele as the cause of recurrent obstructive jaundice in childhood: Diagnosis by ERCP. Gastrointest Endosc 1982; 28:88–90.
30. Dominguez R, Young LW, Ledesma-Medina J, et al: Pediatric liver transplantation. Part II: Diagnostic imaging in postoperative management. Radiology 1985; 157:339–344.
31. Sivak MV: The normal retrograde pancreatogram and cholangiogram. *In* Sivak MV, ed: Gastroenterologic Endoscopy. Philadelphia, WB Saunders, 1987, pp 619–630.
32. Freese D: Intracellular cholestatic syndromes of infancy. Sem Liver Dis 1982; 2:255–270.
33. Alagille D: Cholestasis in the first three months of life. Prog Liver Dis 1979; 6:471–485.
34. Ferry GD, Selby MJ, Udall J, et al: Guide to early diagnosis of biliary obstruction in infancy. Clin Pediatr 1985; 24:305–311.
35. Mowat AP: Biliary disorders in childhood. Sem Liver Dis 1982; 2:271–281.
36. Odievre M, Hadchouel M, Landrieu P, et al: Long-term prognosis for infants with intrahepatic cholestasis and patent extrahepatic biliary tract. Arch Dis Child 1981; 56:373–376.
37. Mowat AP, Psacharopoulos HT, Williams R: Extrahepatic biliary

atresia versus neonatal hepatitis. Review of 137 prospectively investigated infants. Arch Dis Child 1976; 51:763–770.
38. Hirsig J, Rickham PP: Early differential diagnosis between neonatal hepatitis and biliary atresia. J Pediatr Surg 1980; 15:13–15.
39. Balistreri WF: Neonatal cholestasis. J Pediatr 1985; 106:171–184.
40. Cox KL, Stadalnik RC, McGahan JP, et al: Ruebner BH. Hepatobiliary scintigraphy with technetium–99m disofenin in the evaluation of neonatal cholestasis. J Ped Gast Nutr 1987; 6:885–891.
41. Manolaki AG, Larcher VF, Mowat AP, et al: The prelaparotomy diagnosis of extrahepatic biliary atresia. Arch Dis Child 1983; 58:591–594.
42. Kirks DR, Coleman RE, Filston HC, et al: An imaging approach to persistent neonatal jaundice. AJR 1984; 142:461–465.
43. Greene HL, Helinek GL, Moran R, O'Neill J: A diagnostic approach to prolonged obstructive jaundice by 24-hour collection of duodenal fluid. J Pediatr 1979; 95:412–414.
44. Dorney SFA, Kamath KR, Middleton AW, Kan A: Diagnosis of biliary atresia. N Engl J Med 1983; 308:968.
45. Markowitz J, Daum F, Kahn EI, et al: Arteriohepatic dysplasia I: Pitfalls in diagnosis and management. Hepatology 1983; 3:64–66.
46. Perkins WG, Klein GL, Beckerman RC: Cystic fibrosis mistaken for idiopathic biliary atresia. Clin Pediatr 1985; 24:107–109
47. Fung KP, Lau SP: Gamma-glutamyl transpeptidase activity and its serial measurement in differentiation between extrahepatic biliary atresia and neonatal hepatitis. J Pediatr Gastroenterol Nutr 1985; 4:208–213.
48. Majd M, Reba RC, Altman RP: Effect of phenobarbital on 99mTc-IDA scintigraphy in the evaluation of neonatal jaundice. Sem Nuc Med 1981; 11:194–204.
49. Kasai M, Suzuki H, Ohashi E: Technique and results of operative management of biliary atresia. World J Surg 1978; 2:571–580.
50. Williamson SL, Seibert JJ, Butler HL, Golladay ES: Apparent gut excretion of Tc–99m-DISIDA in a case of extrahepatic biliary atresia. Pediatr Radiol 1986; 16:245–247.
51. Lebwohl O, Waye JD: Endoscopic retrograde cholangiopancreatography in the diagnosis of extrahepatic biliary atresia. Am J Dis Child 1979; 133:647–649.
52. Matsuo S, Yoshiie K, Ikeda K: Endoscopic evaluation of the porta hepatis in patients with biliary atresia. Endoscopy 1985; 17:54–59.
53. Ament M: Is endoscopic cholangiopancreatography needed for the jaundiced infant? Gastrointest Endosc 1987; 33:49–52.
54. Green D, Carroll BA: Ultrasonography in the jaundiced infant: A new approach. J Ultrasound Med 1986; 5:323–329.
55. Perisic V: Role of PTC and ERCP in diagnostic imaging of the hepatobiliary tree: Caroli's disease in two siblings. J Pediatr Gastroenterol Nutr 1987; 6:647–648.
56. Perisic V: Role of percutaneous transhepatic cholangiography and endoscopic cholangiopancreatography in the diagnostic imaging of hepatobiliary system in infants and children. J Pediatr Gastroenterol Nutr 1985; 4:846–847.
57. Missavage AE, Sugawa C: Caroli's disease: Role of endoscopic retrograde cholangiopancreatography. Am J Gastroenterol 1983; 78:815–817.
58. Hermansen MC, Starshak RJ, Werlin SL: Caroli disease: The diagnostic approach. J Pediatr 1979; 94:879–882.
59. Morelli A, Pelli MA, Vedovelli A, et al: Endoscopic retrograde cholangiopancreatography study in Alagille's syndrome First report. Am J Gastroenterol 1983; 78:241–244.
60. Gorelick FS, Dobbins JW, Burrell M, Riely CA: Biliary tract abnormalities in patients with arteriohepatic dysplasia. Dig Dis Sci 1982; 25:815–820.
61. Classen M, Gotze H, Richter HJ, Bender S: Primary sclerosing cholangitis in children. J Pediatr Gastroenterol Nutr 1987; 6:197–202.
62. Johnson DA, Cattau EL, Hancock JE: Pediatric primary sclerosing cholangitis. Dig Dis Sci 1986; 31:773–777.
63. Siegel JH, Guelrud M: Endoscopic cholangiopancreatoplasty: Hydrostatic balloon dilation in the bile duct and pancreas. Gastrointest Endosc 1983; 29:99–103.
64. Bass S, Connon JJ, Ho CS: Biliary tree in cystic fibrosis: Biliary tract abnormalities in cystic fibrosis demonstrated by endoscopic retrograde cholangiography. Gastroenterology 1983; 84:1592–1596.
65. Cotton PB: Progress report: ERCP. Gut 1977; 18:316–341.
66. Soehendra N, Reynders-Frederix V: Palliative bile duct drainage. A new endoscopic method of introducing a transpapillary drain. Endoscopy 1980; 12:8–11.
67. Bickerstaff KI, Britton BJ, Gough MH: Endoscopic palliation of malignant biliary obstruction in a child. Br J Surg 1989; 76:1092–1093.
68. Guelrud M, Mendoza S, Zager A, Noguera C: Biliary stenting in an infant with malignant obstructive jaundice. Gastrointest Endosc 1989; 35:259–261.
69. Rustgi AK, Kelsey PB, Guelrud M, et al: Malignant tumors of the bile ducts: Diagnosis by biopsy during endoscopic cannulation. Gastrointest Endosc 1989; 35:248–251.
70. Soehendra N, Grimm H, Berger B, Nam VC: Malignant jaundice: Results of diagnostic and therapeutic endoscopy. World J Surg 1989; 13:171–177.
71. Howdle P, Miloszewski K, Glanville JN, Losowsky MS: Diagnosis of biliary tract hemorrhage (hemobilia) by endoscopy. Gastrointest Endosc 1976; 23:94–95.
72. Vignote ML, Mino G, de la Mata M, et al: Endoscopic sphincterotomy in hepatic hydatid disease open to the biliary tree. Br J Surg 1990; 77:30–31.
73. Shaw PJ, Spitz L, Watson JG: Extrahepatic biliary obstruction due to stone. Arch Dis Child 1984; 59:896–897.
74. Lilly JR: Common bile duct calculi in infants and children. J Pediatr Surg 1980; 15:577–580.
75. Man DWK, Spitz L: Choledocholithiasis in infancy. J Pediatr Surg 1985; 20:65–68.
75a. Guelrud M, Mendoza S, Jaen D, et al: ERCP and endoscopic sphincterotomy in infants and children with jaundice due to common bile duct stones. Gastrointest Endosc 1992; 38:450–453.
76. Broughan TA, Sivak MV, Hermann RE: The management of retained and recurrent bile duct stones. Surgery 1985; 98:746–751.
77. Guelrud M, Mendoza S, Rossiter G, Villegas MI: Sphincter of Oddi manometry in healthy volunteers. Dig Dis Sci 1990; 35:38–46.
78. Guelrud M: Papillary stenosis. Endoscopy 1988; 20:193–202.
79. Geenan JE, Hogan WJ, Dodds WJ, et al: The efficacy of endoscopic sphincterotomy after cholecystectomy in patients with sphincter-of-Oddi dysfunction. N Engl J Med 1989; 320:82–87.
80. Alonso-Lej F, Rever WB, Pessagno DJ: Congenital choledochal cyst, with a report of 2, and an analysis of 94 cases. Intern Abs Surg 1959; 108:1–30.
81. Wiedmeyer DA, Stewart ET, Dodds WJ, et al: Choledochal cyst: Findings on cholangiopancreatography with emphasis on ectasia of the common channel. AJR 1989; 153:969–972.
82. Wood WJ, Trump DS. Pancreaticobiliary common channel associated with common duct stricture. J Pediatr Surg 1986; 21:738–740.
83. Okada A, Oguchi Y, Kamata S, et al: Common channel syndrome—diagnosis with endoscopic retrograde cholangiopancreatography and surgical management. Surgery 1983; 93:634–642.
84. Karp MP, Jewett TC, Cooney DR: Chronic relapsing pancreatitis in childhood caused by pancreaticobiliary ductal anomaly. J Pediatr Gastroenterol Nutr 1983; 2:324–328.
85. Little KH, Loeb PM: Choledochal cyst. South Med J 1989; 82:255–258.
86. Todani T, Watanabe Y, Narusue MEA: Congenital bile duct cysts: Classification, operative procedures, and review of 37 cases including cancer arising from choledochal cyst. Am J Surg 1977; 134:263–269.
87. Thatcher BS, Sivak MV, Hermann RE, Esselstyn CB: ERCP in evaluation and diagnosis of choledochal cyst: Report of five cases. Gastrointest Endosc 1986; 32:27–31.
88. Guelrud M, Jaen D, Mendoza S, Torres P: Usefulness of endoscopic retrograde cholangiopancreatography in diagnosis of choledochal cysts in children. Gastroenter Endocrinol Nutric 1989; 43:9–12.
89. Chang M, Wang T, Chen C, Hung W: Congenital bile duct dilatation in children. J Pediatr Surg 1986; 21:112–117.
90. Sherman P, Kolster E, Davies C, et al: Choledochal cysts: Heterogeneity of clinical presentation. J Pediatr Gastroenterol Nutr 1986; 5:867–872.

91. Bloustein PA: Association of carcinoma with congenital cystic conditions of the liver and bile ducts. Am J Gastroenterol 1977; 67:40–46.
92. Venu RP, Geenan JE, Hogan WJ, et al: Role of endoscopic retrograde cholangiopancreatography in the diagnosis and treatment of choledochocele. Gastroenterology 1984; 87:1144–1149.
93. Siegel JH, Harding GT, Chateau F: Endoscopic incision of choledochal cysts (choledochocele). Endoscopy 1981; 13:200–202.
94. Sigfusson BF, Wehlin L, Lindstrom CG: Variants of pancreatic duct system of importance in endoscopic retrograde cholangiopancreatography. Observations on autopsy specimens. Acta Radiol Diagn Stockh 1983; 24:113–128.
95. Mitchell CJ, Lintott DJ, Ruddell WS, et al: Clinical relevance of an unfused pancreatic duct system. Gut 1979; 20:1066–1071.
96. Wagner CW, Golladay ES: Pancreas divisum and pancreatitis in children. Am Surg 1988; 54:22–26.
97. Yaffe MR, Gutenberger JE: Chronic pancreatitis and pancreas divisum in an infant: Diagnosed by endoscopic retrograde cholangiopancreatography and treated with somatostatin analog. J Pediatr Gastroenterol Nutr 1989; 9:108–111.
98. Yedlin ST, Dubois RS, Philippart AI: Pancreas divisum: A cause of pancreatitis in childhood. J Pediatr Surg 1984; 19:793–794.
99. Cotton PB: Congenital anomaly of pancreas divisum as cause of obstructive pain and pancreatitis. Gut 1980; 21:105–114.
100. Yvergneaux JP, Van den Boer H, De Keyser R, Brys R: Pancreas divisum: A teenager with calculi in the duct of Santorini. Report of a case treated by double drainage procedure. Acta Chir Belg 1985; 85:67–70.
101. Athow AC, Wilkinson ML, Saunders AJ, Drake DP: Pancreatic ascites presenting in infancy, with review of the literature. Dig Dis Sci 1991; 36:245–250.
102. Levine JB, Warshaw AL, Falchuk KR, Schapiro RH: The value of endoscopic retrograde pancreatography in the management of pancreatic ascites. Surgery 1977; 81:360–362.
103. Vane DW, Grosfeld JL, West KW, Rescorla FJ: Pancreatic disorders in infancy and childhood: Experience with 92 cases. J Pediatr Surg 1989; 24:771–776.
104. Yogi Y, Shibue T, Hashimoto S: Annular pancreas detected in adults, diagnosed by endoscopic retrograde cholangiopancreatography: Report of four cases. Gastroenterol Jpn 1987; 22:92–99.
105. Parker HW: Congenital anomalies of the pancreas. *In* Sivak MV, ed: Gastroenterologic Endoscopy. Philadelphia, WB Saunders, 1987, pp 770–779.
106. Perisic VN, Mihailovic T, Filipovic D: Congenital hepatic fibrosis, bile duct abnormality, long pancreaticobiliary common channel, and pancreatitis. J Pediatr Gastroenterol Nutr 1988; 7:790–791.
107. Crombleholme TM, deLorimier AA, Way LW, et al: The modified Puestow procedure for chronic relapsing pancreatitis in children. J Pediatr Surg 1990; 25:749–754.
108. Rosch W: ERCP in acute and chronic pancreatitis. *In* Sivak MV, ed: Gastroenterologic Endoscopy. Philadelphia, WB Saunders, 1987, pp 780–793.
109. Blustein PK, Gaskin K, Filler R, et al: Endoscopic retrograde cholangiopancreatography in pancreatitis in children and adolescents. Pediatrics 1981; 68:387–393.
110. Ghishan FK, Greene HL, Avant G, et al: Chronic relapsing pancreatitis in childhood. J Pediatr 1983; 102:514–518.
111. Cooperman M, Ferrara JJ, Carey LC, et al: Idiopathic acute pancreatitis: The value of endoscopic retrograde cholangiopancreatography. Surgery 1981; 90:666–670.
112. Cooperman AM, Sivak MV, Sullivan BH, Hermann RE: Endoscopic pancreatography: Its value in preoperative and postoperative assessment of pancreatic disease. Am J Surg 1975; 129:38–43.
113. Wurbs D, Phillip J, Classen M: Experiences with the long standing nasobiliary tube in biliary diseases. Endoscopy 1980; 12:219–223.
114. Huibregtse K, Schneider B, Vrij AA, Tytgat GNJ: Endoscopic pancreatic drainage in chronic pancreatitis. Gastrointest Endosc 1988; 34:9–15.
115. Girdwood AH, Hatfield ARW, Bornman PC, et al: Structure and function in noncalcific pancreatitis. Dig Dis Sci 1984; 29:721–726.
116. Cooney DR, Grosfeld JL: Operative management of pancreatic pseudocysts in infants and children: A review of 75 cases. Ann Surg 1975; 182:590–596.
117. Tam PKH, Saing H, Irving IM, Lister J: Acute pancreatitis in children. J Pediatr Surg 1985; 20:58–60.
118. O'Neill JA, Greene H, Grishan FK: Surgical implications of chronic pancreatitis. J Pediatr Surg 1982; 17:920–926.
119. Standaert L, Verstappen G, Malbrain H, et al: Hemorrhagic pleural effusion and mediastinal mass: Presenting symptoms in a child with pseudocyst of the pancreas. J Pediatr Gastroenterol Nutr 1983; 2:329–331.
120. Taxier M, Sivak MV, Cooperman AM, Sullivan BH: Endoscopic retrograde pancreatography in the evaluation of trauma to the pancreas. Surg Gynecol Obstet 1980; 150:65–68.
121. Rawlings W, Bynum TE, Pasternak G: Pancreatic ascites: Diagnosis of leakage site by endoscopic pancreatography. Surgery 1977; 81:363–365.
122. Hall RI, Lavelle MI, Venables CW: Use of ERCP to identify the site of traumatic injuries of the main pancreatic duct in children. Br J Surg 1986; 73:411–412.
123. Whittwell AE, Gomez GA, Byers P, et al: Blunt pancreatic trauma: Prospective evaluation of early endoscopic retrograde pancreatography. South Med J 1989; 82:586–591.
124. Filston HC, McLeod RM, Jones RS: Improved management of pancreatic lesions in children aided by ERCP. J Pediatr Surg 1980; 15:121–128.
125. Wind GG, Rubin P, Waye JD, Bauer JJ: Pancreatic pseudocyst: Is endoscopic retrograde cholangiopancreatography contraindicated? Mt Sinai J Med 1976; 43:558–564.
126. Salinas A, Rodriguez J, Guelrud M, et al: Resolution of pancreatic pseudocysts: When should we wait? Mt Sinai J Med 1986; 53:470–477.
127. Barkin JS, Ferstenberg RM, Panullo W, et al: Endoscopic retrograde cholangiopancreatography in pancreatic trauma. Gastrointest Endosc 1988; 34:102–165.
128. Belohlavek D, Merkle P, Probst M: Identification of traumatic rupture of the pancreatic duct by endoscopic retrograde pancreatography. Gastrointest Endosc 1978; 24:255–256.
129. Bozymski EM, Orlando RC, Holt JW: Traumatic disruption of the pancreatic duct demonstrated by endoscopic retrograde pancreatography. J Trauma 1981; 21:244–245.
130. Tim LO, Thompson PM, Segal I, Lawson HH: Endoscopic retrograde cholangiopancreatography in the management of traumatic pancreatic pseudocysts. South Am Med J 1979; 5:767–770.
131. LaFerla G, Gordon S, Archibald M, Murray WR: Hyperamylasaemia and acute pancreatitis following endoscopic retrograde cholangiopancreatography. Pancreas 1986; 1:160–163.
132. Okuno M, Himeno S, Kurokawa M, et al: Changes in serum levels of pancreatic isoamylase, lipase, trypsin, and elastase 1 after endoscopic retrograde pancreatography. Hepatogastroenterology 1985; 32:87–90.
133. Weaver HA, Sugawa C, Bouwman DL, Altshuler J: Isoamylase determinations in patients undergoing endoscopic retrograde cholangiopancreatography. Surg Gastroenterol 1984; 3:59–62.
134. Brandes JW, Scheffer B, Lorenz-Meyer H, et al: Complications and prophylaxis, a controlled study. Endoscopy 1981; 13:27–30.
135. Roszler MH, Campbell WL: Post-ERCP pancreatitis: Association with urographic visualization during ERCP. Radiology 1985; 157:595–598.
136. Kasugai T, Kuno N, Kizu M: Manometric endoscopic retrograde pancreatocholangiography. Am J Dig Dis 1974; 19:485–502.
137. Hamilton I, Lintott DJ, Rothwell J, Axon AT: Acute pancreatitis following endoscopic retrograde cholangiopancreatography. Clin Radiol 1983; 34:543–546.
138. Bilbao MK, Dotter CT, Lee TG, Katon RM: Complications of endoscopic retrograde cholangiopancreatography (ERCP). Gastroenterology 1976; 70:314–320.
139. van Husen N, Hogemann B, Egen V, Mehnert C: Radiation exposure in endoscopic retrograde cholangiopancreatography. Endoscopy 1984; 16:112–114.
140. Nebel OT, Silvis SE, Rogers G, et al: Complications associated with endoscopic retrograde cholangiopancreatography. Gastrointest Endosc 1975; 22:34–39.
141. O'Connor M, Kolars J, Ansel H, et al: Preoperative endoscopic retrograde cholangiopancreatography in the surgical management of pancreatic pseudocysts. Am J Surg 1986; 151:18–24.
142. Lai ECS, Lo C, Choi T, et al: Urgent biliary decompression

after endoscopic retrograde cholangiopancreatography. Am J Surg 1989; 157:121–125.

143. Classen DC, Jacobson JA, Burke JP, et al: Serious *Pseudomonas* infections associated with endoscopic retrograde cholangiopancreatography. Am J Med 1988; 84:590–596.

144. Doherty DE, Falko JM, Lefkovitz N, et al: *Pseudomonas aeruginosa* sepsis following retrograde cholangiopancreatography (ERCP). Dig Dis Sci 1982; 27:169–170.

145. Elson CO, Hattori K, Blackstone MO: Polymicrobial sepsis following endoscopic retrograde cholangiopancreatography. Gastroenterology 1975; 69:507–510.

146. Collen MJ, Hanan MR, Maher JA, Stubrin SE: Modification of endoscopic retrograde cholangiopancreatography (ERCP) septic complications by the addition of an antibiotic to the contrast media. Am J Gastroenterol 1980; 74:493–496.

147. Ferguson DR, Sivak MV: Indications, contraindications and complications of ERCP. *In* Sivak MV, ed: Gastroenterologic Endoscopy. Philadelphia, WB Saunders, 1987, pp 581–598.

Chapter 76

Gastrointestinal Motility

STEVEN L. WERLIN and CHRISTOPHER W. BROWN

MANOMETRIC TECHNIQUES

A variety of techniques have been developed for the study of gastrointestinal motility. This section reviews the key elements required for a successful clinical motility study. Techniques available only in specialized research laboratories, such as electrogastrography, the transcutaneous recording of gastric electrical activity, are not addressed in this chapter. The general overview of manometric techniques given in this section is followed by a detailed review of the individual tests.

The first element required for a successful study in a child is cooperation. Esophageal and gastroduodenal studies are uncomfortable because they require the passage of a rather large tube either through the mouth or nose. In children with a gastrostomy, gastroduodenal studies can be performed by passing a tube through the gastrostomy site. We prefer to sedate lightly the child who cannot be "talked through" a study with midazolam (0.1 to 0.2 mg per kg orally in cherry syrup or intravenously). Sedation is almost never needed for anorectal manometry.

The ideal upper gastrointestinal manometric tube has several characteristics. It must be soft, flexible, and small enough (<6 mm) for easy intubation and patient comfort. The infusion system must be of low compliance to record accurately the rapid changes in esophageal pressure without using a rapid infusion rate.[1–3] Because compliance is inversely related to lumen size, low compliance can be achieved only by limiting the internal diameter of the tube. Because a small catheter generates high-flow resistance, a compromise is necessary between the effects of flow rate and tube diameter.

We use a pneumohydraulic capillary infusion system that accurately records intraluminal pressures at infusion rates as low as 0.6 ml per minute.[3] The compliance of conventional syringe pump devices is so great that an infusion rate of 6 ml per minute is required to record accurately pressure transients in the esophagus. High infusion rates are undesirable for several reasons: they may increase the risk of aspiration in young patients, the large fluid volumes may induce secondary peristaltic waves, and absorption of the fluid will lead to bladder distention and patient discomfort.

The catheter is connected to pressure transducers and a polygraph.[2] The frequency response of commercial chart records and pressure transducers exceeds that necessary for accurate recording of the pressure transients generated during gastrointestinal manometry. Therefore selection may be made on the basis of price, reliability, or availability.

For esophageal manometry, we use a nine lumen polyvinyl manometric tube with an outer diameter of only 4.5 mm (Fig. 76–1). The tube has eight radial recording lumens, each 0.8 mm in diameter, surrounding a larger central lumen 1.6 mm in diameter. A distal sleeve sensor device is used to monitor lower esophageal sphincter (LES) pressure continuously.[4, 5] If a sleeve sensor is not available, instantaneous LES pressure can be determined using a "pull-through" technique.[6, 7] In the station pull-through technique, the manometry assembly is inserted until several of the side holes are in the stomach, as documented by recording gastric pressure that is higher than that of the esophagus. The assembly is then withdrawn in 1-cm increments. The location of the LES is determined by observing the appearance of a high-pressure zone. In the rapid pull-through technique, after insertion of the manometry tube into the stomach as explained previously, the assembly is withdrawn at a slow, steady continuous rate. The location of the LES is determined as explained previously. The advantage of the sleeve device is that it allows for the continuous monitoring of LES pressure during and between swallows.

Manometry can be performed using a tube with embedded microtransducers that directly sense pressure.[8] Because these tubes are generally thinner than water-perfused systems, they are well tolerated by patients. These probes have the additional advantage of not requiring perfusion, which as already mentioned can alter motility. This type of system has not gained widespread use because of its greater cost. Microtransducer-based tubes can be constructed for esophageal and gastroduodenal motility studies.

Although gastroduodenal manometry for the pediatric patient is not yet widely available, the limited studies published so far have generated new insights into the problems of gastroparesis and pseudo-obstruction.[9] Because gastroduodenal manometry requires the passage of a transpyloric tube, the manometry assembly must be long enough and flexible enough to reach the duodenum. When the child has a gastrostomy, the gastrostomy tube may be removed temporarily and the manometry assembly passed through the stoma. The manometry tube is placed so recording sites are located in the duodenum and antrum. The catheter is connected

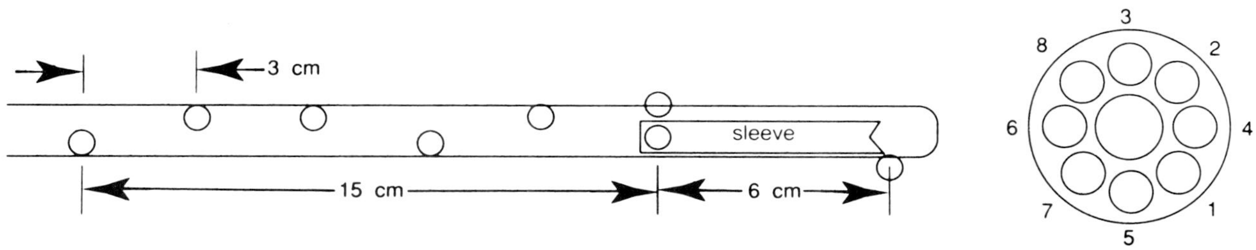

Figure 76–1. Esophageal manometry catheter with Dent sleeve. Eight radial lumens with inside diameter (ID) of 0.8 mm surround a center lumen of 1.8 mm ID. The manometry assembly has an outside diameter of 4.8 mm. Side hole openings, 0.8 mm in diameter, are located at 3-cm intervals. The Dent sleeve is located distally for continuous recording of lower esophageal sphincter pressure. (Courtesy of Arndorfer, Inc.)

to pressure transducers, a pneumohydraulic pump, and a polygraph.

For anorectal manometry, a variety of techniques are used, including pressure transducers, multiple balloons, and a single balloon attached to water-perfused catheters connected to pressure transducers and a pneumohydraulic pump.[10, 11] Sphincter electromyographic (EMG) activity can be monitored with skin electrodes. We use a single multilumen polyvinyl catheter with a distal balloon (Fig. 76–2). Three radially oriented side holes are located 0.5 cm apart distal to the balloon.

Manometry is safe and only rarely associated with significant complications (Table 76–1). Because esophageal and gastroduodenal manometry are uncomfortable procedures, sedation may be required. Aspiration or emesis may occur with insertion of the manometry catheter or may be a consequence of accumulation of perfused water, at the end of a long study and when the catheter is being withdrawn. A potential risk of perforation of the esophagus or stomach exists on introduction of the catheter assembly. The most significant risks are related to oversedation and allergic reactions to sedatives. A number of children, particularly those with spina bifida, have exhibited evidence of latex allergy.[12] Although symptoms are usually mild, anaphylaxis has occurred.

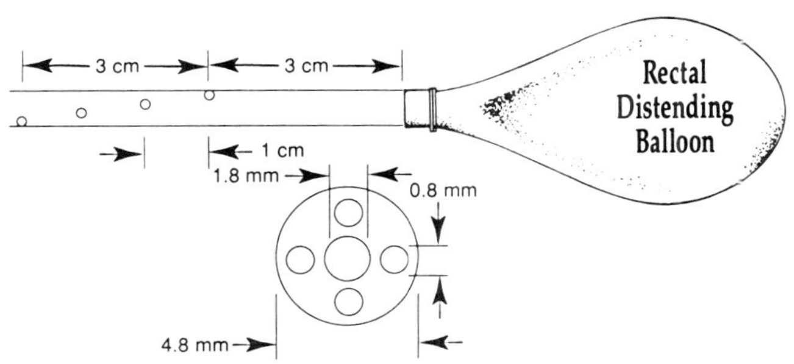

Figure 76–2. Anorectal manometry catheter. Four radial lumens with inside diameter (ID) of 0.8 mm surround a center lumen of 1.8 mm ID. The manometry assembly has an outside diameter of 4.8 mm. Attached to the distal end is a distending balloon with a maximal volume of 150 ml. Four radially oriented side hole openings of 0.8 mm are located 3 cm from the balloon at 1-cm intervals for recording pressure from the internal anal sphincter. (Courtesy of Arndorfer, Inc.)

ESOPHAGEAL MANOMETRY

The initiation of normal swallowing involves relaxation of the upper esophageal sphincter to allow passage of the food bolus into the body of the esophagus. Propulsion of the bolus to the stomach then requires coordinated, circumferential, peristaltic contractions along the body of the esophagus and anticipatory relaxation of the LES.[13, 14] The upper esophageal sphincter and LES are in a state of tonic contraction, and the body of the esophagus is usually relaxed.[14] Spontaneous (inappropriate) relaxations of the LES also occur episodically, unrelated to swallowing.[5, 14, 15] Consequently, evaluation of esophageal peristalsis and disorders of LES function require simultaneous measurement of pressure at three or more sites.

At our center, simultaneous pressure recordings are obtained from eight radially oriented and longitudinally distributed perfusion ports and a distal sleeve sensor device (see Fig. 76–1).[4] Smaller infants may not tolerate either the large external diameter or the relatively high total perfusion rate (0.5 ml per minute per port) associated with the nine lumen tube, so a smaller manometry catheter employing fewer ports may be required. To demonstrate peristalsis best, the perfusion ports are usually spaced from 2 to 5 cm apart. We use an interval of 3 cm, permitting most or all of the esophagus to be examined simultaneously, while allowing the sleeve device to remain in the LES.

A standard study employing a catheter with a sleeve device involves nasal or oral passage of the perfusion catheter until the distal perfusion port is present in the stomach.[16] The LES is located approximately 20 cm from the nares in infants and at about 40 cm from the nares in adults.[17, 18] The position may be verified by observance of respiratory pressure oscillations in oppos-

Table 76–1. COMPLICATIONS OF ESOPHAGEAL MANOMETRY

Aspiration
Discomfort
Emesis
Perforation
Side effects of sedation

ing direction to intrathoracic ports and by the higher pressure observed in the stomach. The catheter is then withdrawn until the sleeve device is positioned in the LES, which is identified as a high-pressure zone between the stomach and esophagus (Fig. 76–3). The catheter is then connected to the pneumohydraulic pump and strip chart recorder as described earlier. Continuous basal pressure recordings are obtained from the sleeve device and the multiple ports positioned in the esophageal body for 5 to 15 minutes. Esophageal body and LES responses to several wet and dry swallows are then recorded. If necessary, the catheter is partially withdrawn to permit evaluation of the proximal esophagus.

If a sleeve device is not available, the catheter is positioned with all ports in the stomach, and either a slow continuous (rapid pull-through) or incremental pull-through (station pull-through) technique is employed.[17] Because the LES is not radially symmetric, the LES pressure without a sleeve device is determined by averaging the pressures obtained from all ports as they pass through the sphincter. One disadvantage of the latter technique is the possible movement of the catheter in relation to the LES by axial displacement of the sphincter during swallowing and breathing, such that repeated measurements are required. The catheter may be repositioned with either the sleeve device or a distal perfusion port within the LES for evaluation of the effects of pharmacologic agents.

The normal upper esophageal sphincter is 3 to 4 cm long and forms a transverse slit. The zone of greatest pressure is directed along a posteroanterior axis. The

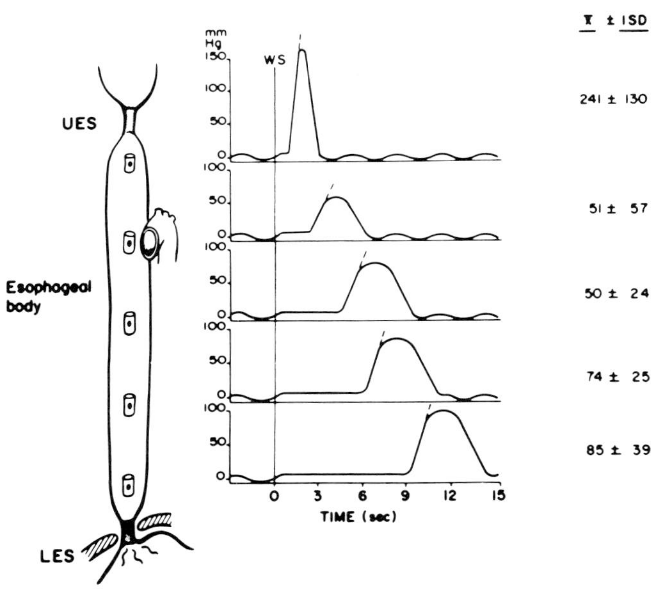

Figure 76–3. Normal esophageal manometry. Schematic representation of peristaltic pressure sequence associated with a wet swallow (WS). The dotted lines indicate the pressure rise rate slope. UES, upper esophageal sphincter; LES, lower esophageal sphincter. (From Dodds WJ, Stef JJ, Hogan WJ: Factors determining pressure measurement accuracy by intraluminal esophageal manometry. Gastroenterology 1976; 70:117–123; with permission.)

Table 76–2. INDICATIONS FOR ESOPHAGEAL MANOMETRY

Dysphagia
Intestinal pseudo-obstruction
Localization of the LES
Prior to antireflux surgery
Achalasia
Unexplained abnormal motility on radiologic studies

normal upper esophageal sphincter pressures range from 30 to 150 mm Hg. The contractions are generally of short duration. Primary peristalsis or swallow waves are initiated by the propulsion of a food or fluid bolus from the mouth toward the upper esophageal sphincter and are associated with relaxation of the upper sphincter.

Peristaltic waves are propagated along the esophagus at an average rate of 3 to 4 cm per second and last for less than 7 seconds (see Fig. 76–3).[14] The rate of propagation is fastest in the proximal esophagus, slows in the vicinity of the aortic arch, and increases again in the distal esophagus. The swallow wave also moves more slowly in response to a bolus than to a dry swallow.

Normal LES pressures are influenced by expiratory variation of intrathoracic pressures. It has been suggested that the end-expiratory LES pressure is most representative of the true value. The age of the subject also affects LES pressure. Normal values are 40 to 45 mm Hg for infants less than 1 year of age and 28 to 33 mm Hg after 1 year. The higher normal pressures noted in infants and neonates may be due, in part, to the relatively larger size of the catheter assembly, relative to the dimensions of the LES. Corresponding values in adults are 10 to 35 mm Hg. The LES demonstrates relaxation immediately after the onset of the swallow and remains relaxed until the contraction wave has passed, a duration of approximately 10 seconds. A postswallow augmentation of the LES pressure is then observed. If frequent repeated swallows occur, the LES may remain relaxed until several peristaltic waves have passed.

Two other forms of peristaltic swallow waves, termed secondary and tertiary peristalsis, may be seen in some circumstances and are defined according to their triggering stimuli. In contrast to primary peristalsis, which follows oropharyngeal initiation of a swallow, secondary peristalsis occurs in response to stimuli in the lumen of the esophagus, such as a persistent bolus or refluxed stomach acid.[15, 18] Although they may display lower amplitudes, these swallow waves are similar in appearance to those seen in primary peristalsis. Tertiary peristalsis is initiated by spontaneous depolarization of esophageal smooth muscle cells when communication with the swallowing center in the brain stem is disrupted.[18] Occasional simultaneous nonperistaltic contractions of the entire esophageal body, called tertiary contractions, may also occur.

The indications for esophageal manometry are listed in Table 76–2. Manometry is useful in the evaluation of known or suspected disorders of esophageal motility and in conditions that may be associated with disorders of esophageal function such as gastroesophageal reflux and pseudo-obstruction. It may also be useful in the evaluation of esophageal function before and after antireflux surgery and for the localization of the LES for positioning pH probes or obtaining biopsies.[17, 19]

Esophageal manometry has been extensively employed in the study of gastroesophageal reflux.[20, 21] Several factors have been found to be involved in this condition, and manometry in this setting may benefit from the simultaneous recording of gastroesophageal reflux. The major mechanisms for gastroesophageal reflux in the child are low basal LES pressure (<10 mm Hg) (Fig. 76–4), inappropriate relaxation of the LES (Fig. 76–5), and a rise of intra-abdominal pressure such as occurs with crying.[5] Of these three, inappropriate relaxation of the sphincter is probably the most common. Inappropriate relaxations are also observed in normal adult volunteers without clinically significant gastroesophageal reflux, so this finding in isolation is not diagnostic of pathological gastroesophageal reflux.[22] Inappropriate relaxations are often found in young infants and decrease in frequency with the growth and neurologic maturity of the child. In the clinical setting of significant gastroesophageal reflux associated with esophagitis, one may find evidence of a low LES pressure and occasional tertiary (simultaneous) contractions

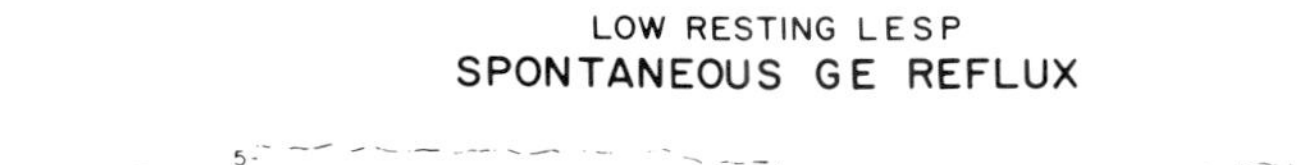

Figure 76–4. Spontaneous gastroesophageal reflux associated with low resting lower esophageal sphincter (LES) pressure. A micro pH probe exits the manometry assembly 3 cm above the LES. The LES pressure is continuously monitored with a Dent sleeve. Basal LES pressure varies within the low range of normal. Gastroesophageal reflux occurred during a 2-minute interval of very low LES pressure. (From Werlin SL, Dodds WJ, Hogan WJ, et al: Mechanisms of gastroesophageal reflux in children. J Pediatr 1980; 97:244–249; with permission.)

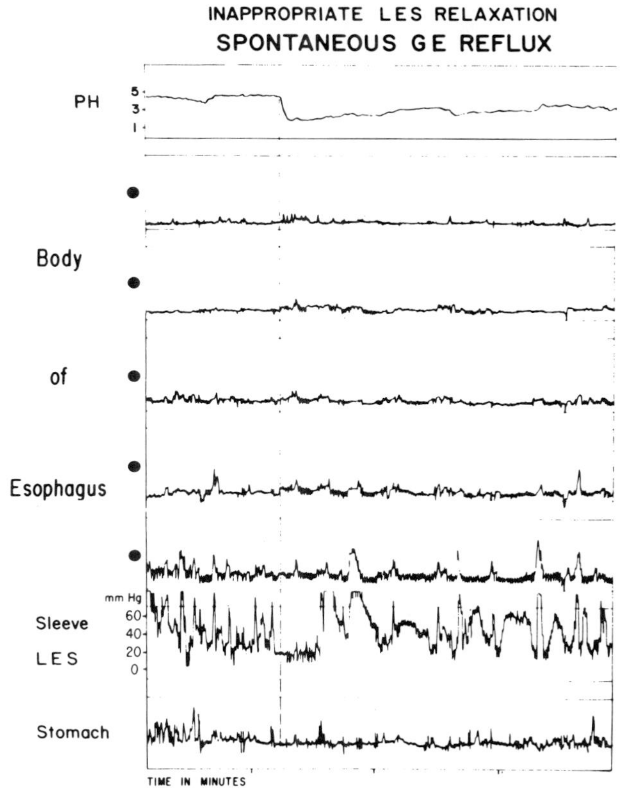

Figure 76–5. Spontaneous gastroesophageal reflux associated with inappropriate lower esophageal sphincter (LES) relaxation. A micro pH probe exits the manometry assembly 3 cm above the LES. The LES pressure is continuously monitored with a Dent sleeve. Basal LES pressure is in the normal range but undergoes a transient relaxation lasting 25 seconds. Acid reflux occurred during the interval of LES relaxation. (From Werlin SL, Dodds WJ, Hogan WJ, et al: Mechanisms of gastroesophageal reflux in children. J Pediatr 1980; 97:244–249; with permission.)

in the distal esophagus, which may improve after treatment of the esophageal inflammation.[23-25] Esophageal manometry may also be useful in preoperative evaluation if antireflux surgery is considered because decisions regarding the type or extent of surgery may be affected by findings of poor or absent peristalsis or of relatively high LES pressure.[19] Such information may be particularly important in patients who are at high risk of anesthetic complications. Although not yet extensively studied, manometry may be helpful in the evaluation of the effect of antireflux surgery on LES function.

Patients with repaired esophageal atresia often develop dysphagia, owing to aperistalsis of the perianastomotic esophagus (Fig. 76–6). The neural coordination of peristalsis is well demonstrated in these individuals because the swallow wave progresses normally down the entire body of the esophagus, despite the absence of contractions in the perianastomotic esophagus. Peristalsis may be absent from the proximal esophagus. Although normal LES function is preserved as determined by LES pressure, pathological gastroesophageal reflux is common in esophageal atresia. Poor clearance of

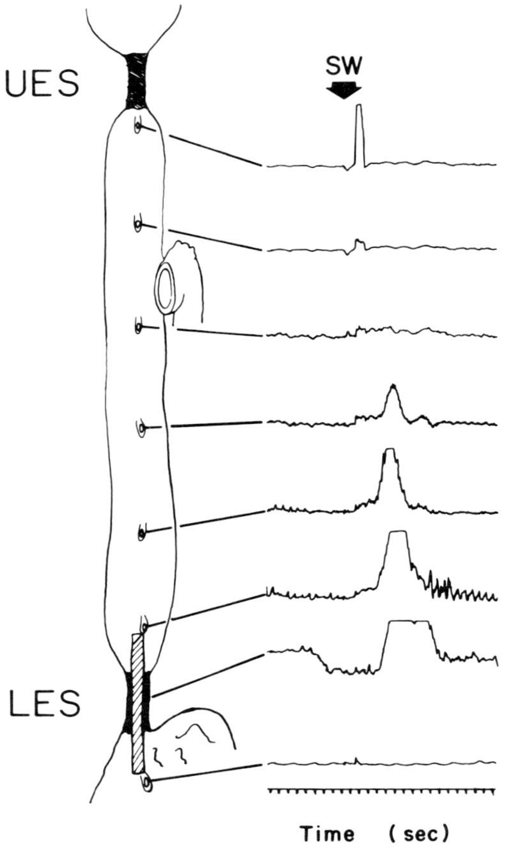

Figure 76–6. Esophageal atresia. Manometric recording of a peristaltic sequence. Six manometric recording sites spaced at 3 cm intervals span the entire esophagus. After swallowing (SW), a peristaltic pressure wave 80 mm Hg in amplitude is seen at the most proximal recording site, disappears at the aortic arch level, but reappears in the distal half of the esophagus. The LES functions normally. (From Werlin SJ, Dodds WJ, Hogan WJ, et al: Esophageal function in esophageal atresia. Dig Dis Sci 1981; 26:796–800; with permission).

refluxed gastric acid from the aperistaltic segment may contribute to esophagitis and stricture formation.

Esophageal manometry is necessary to confirm the radiologic diagnosis of achalasia. In achalasia, the LES fails to relax normally and exhibits a high resting pressure (Fig. 76–7).[18, 26] The body of the esophagus is often dilated, and low-amplitude simultaneous contractions, owing to a "common cavity" effect, are seen. Peristalsis is absent. There is often a high resting pressure in the body of the esophagus.

Several systemic neuromuscular disorders may have associated symptoms of dysphagia. The findings on esophageal manometry may reflect the type of muscle involvement. Because myotonic muscular dystrophy, congenital muscular dystrophy, myasthenia gravis, and infantile spinal muscular atrophy involve striated muscle, manometric abnormalities are found in the proximal esophagus and upper esophageal sphincter.[27, 28] Decreased upper esophageal sphincter pressure is found, along with decreased amplitude but normal duration of swallow waves in the proximal esophagus. Interestingly, no abnormal "myotonic" postswallow contractions are observed. Normal LES and distal esophageal function is preserved.[29, 30] In contrast, normal upper esophageal sphincter and upper esophageal function is seen with nonmyotonic muscular dystrophies.[30]

Abnormalities of esophageal motility may also be found in chronic idiopathic intestinal pseudo-obstruction. Decreased LES pressure, failure of LES relaxation with swallowing, low-amplitude pressure waves in the esophageal body with poor propagation, tertiary contractions, and retrograde contractions have all been reported, particularly in the distal two thirds of the esophagus.[31]

The distal esophagus may also be affected by progressive systemic sclerosis and mixed connective tissue disease.[18, 28, 32] Decreased LES pressure with normal relaxation may be found, along with tertiary contractions and diminished amplitude of swallow waves in the distal two thirds of the esophagus. The function of the proximal esophagus remains normal. No significant correlation has been demonstrated between the severity of the esophageal motor abnormalities and either the extent or duration of the systemic disease.

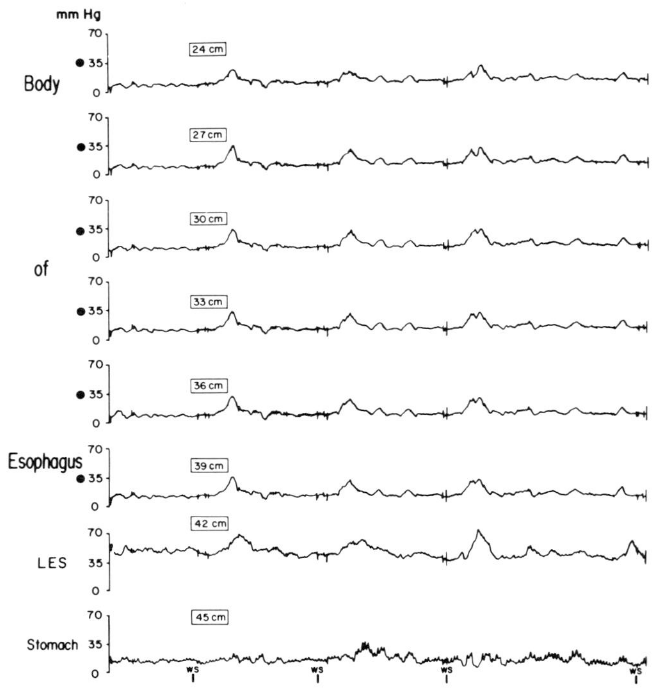

Figure 76–7. Achalasia. Manometric recording of a peristaltic sequence and lower esophageal sphincter (LES) pressure. Six manometric recording sites spaced 3 cm apart span the entire esophagus. A Dent sleeve spans the LES for continuous recording of LES pressure. A low pressure simultaneous contraction occurs after each wet swallow (WS). Normal peristalsis is not seen. The LES fails to relax with swallowing. Basal LES pressure is high. (Courtesy of Walter Hogan, MD.)

GASTRIC EMPTYING

Gastric emptying may be studied in several ways, none of which are ideal. The techniques used are based on a variety of principles including radiology, gastric aspiration, marker dilution, radionuclide imaging, and ultrasonography (Table 76–3).

Table 76–3. METHODS OF STUDY OF GASTRIC EMPTYING

Marker dilution
Radionuclide
Radiopaque meal
Ultrasonography

Gastric emptying of radiopaque meals, such as barium, can be used to estimate mechanical obstruction but give no useful physiologic information concerning the gastric emptying rate because it is impossible to estimate the amount of barium that has left the stomach at any given time. Despite this, the standard barium upper gastrointestinal series is the single most widely used and most useful study for the evaluation of gastric emptying. Mechanical obstruction, retained food, and excessively rapid or slow gastric emptying can be identified. For clinical purposes, more precise information is rarely needed.

Measurement of gastric emptying and volume by the sequential aspiration of gastric contents and measurement of either volume or the dilution of a nonabsorbable indicator dye or marker have been widely used in the past, primarily for research studies.[33] The underlying assumptions of dye dilution tests are that the marker is indeed not absorbed, mixing of the marker and meal is complete, and there is no gastric or salivary secretion. This technique is suitable only for the determination of gastric emptying of liquids. Information concerning the gastric emptying rates of various infant formulas and the effects of the various ingredients found in these formulas have been derived using these methods[34, 35] Unfortunately there has been no standardization of test meal volume or composition or frequency of sampling.

The most commonly used technique to measure gastric emptying in the pediatric patient is based on frequent imaging with a gamma camera for 60 to 120 minutes after the ingestion of a radiolabeled meal.[36] The emptying rate and half-emptying rates can be calculated. Most studies in children have reported emptying rates after 1 hour. It has been shown that the 1-hour emptying rate is not predictive of the 2-hour emptying rate.[37] Because infants are fed at intervals of greater than 1 hour, unless gastric emptying is rapid, the 1-hour emptying rate may not be of physiologic or clinical relevance. In many institutions, inadequate attention is paid to position and projection. In small infants, position is particularly important to prevent overlying of the stomach and small intestine. As already mentioned, there is great variability in published methods, making comparison of published studies difficult.

In our institution, we prefer to introduce the tracer into the stomach by nasogastric tube to avoid the possibility of aspiration. Technetium 99m sulfur colloid (200 to 500 μCi) is introduced into the stomach followed by a volume of formula (300 ml per 1.73 m^2).[36] The nasogastric tube is removed, and serial scans are obtained by a computer system for 2 hours. Gastric emptying is quantified by computer analysis. An area of interest is selected from the first and last 30-second frames. The small bowel is excluded. Count data are obtained, and the emptying rate is calculated (Figs. 76–8 and 76–9).

Although it is possible to study the emptying of liquids and solids, most pediatric studies are performed with labeled formula or juice and therefore estimate the gastric emptying only of liquids. This is unfortunate because patients with normal gastric emptying of liquids but significantly delayed emptying of a solid meal owing to abnormal antral contractility are not uncommon.[38]

Real-time ultrasonography has been used in adults as a noninvasive radioactive method for measuring antral contractions, antral duodenal coordination, and changes

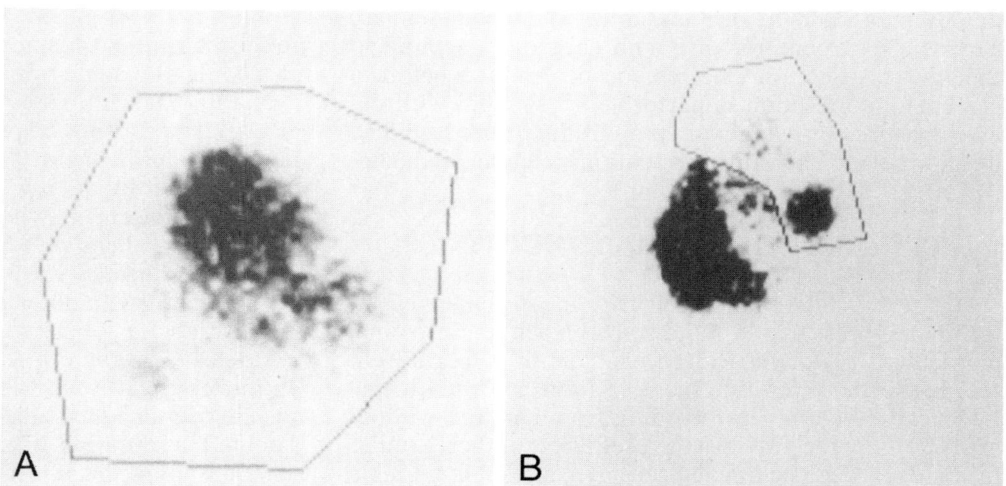

Figure 76–8. Gastric emptying evaluation, normal gastric emptying. *A*, Cursor over stomach at time 0. *B*, Cursor over stomach after 1 hour, only 23% of counts remain in stomach. (Courtesy of Robert Starshak, MD.)

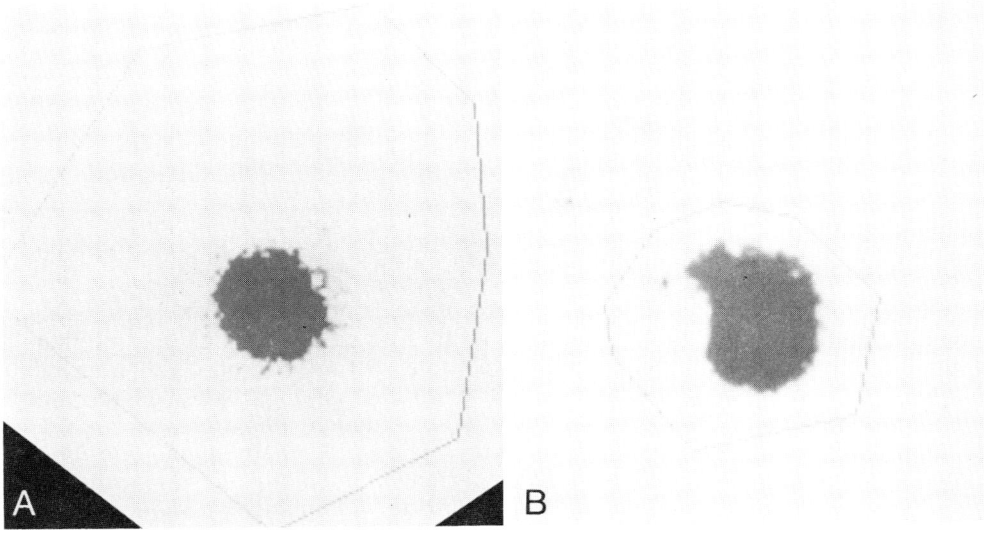

Figure 76–9. Gastric emptying evaluation, delayed gastric emptying. *A*, Cursor over the stomach at time 0. *B*, Cursor over the stomach after 1 hour, 87% of counts remain in stomach. (Courtesy of Robert Starshak, MD.)

in gastric volume after a meal.[39] The volume of the stomach at various times after a meal can be determined and the emptying rate calculated.

Because gastric emptying tests, particularly those based on radionuclide imaging, are more widely available than antroduodenal manometry, these tests are far more frequently used. Although many clinicians believe that manometry and tests of gastric emptying give equivalent information, in fact the information derived from each type of test is complementary, as manometry is used to define the disorder of gastric emptying. In healthy adults, there is reasonably good correlation between the results of gastric emptying tests and antroduodenal manometry. Poor postprandial gastric emptying of solids with normal emptying of liquids is usually associated with gastroduodenal hypomotility, whereas patients with primary intestinal pseudo-obstruction with normal gastroduodenal motility may have only subtle changes seen on a gastric emptying study. The lag phase before solid emptying is normal, but the rate of emptying may be delayed.

Gastric emptying should be determined in children with unexplained chronic nausea or gastric distention, with or without vomiting. Emptying of both solids and liquids may need to be measured. Many, but not all, pediatric gastroenterologists and surgeons recommend that the gastric emptying rate be determined before a Nissen fundoplication is performed.[40] A child with delayed gastric emptying and an antireflux procedure may develop severe abdominal distention, retching, and pain.

GASTRODUODENAL MANOMETRY

Gastroduodenal manometry, the measurement of intraluminal pressures in the distal stomach and proximal duodenum, is not yet widely available in pediatric centers in North America. This is in large part due to the technical difficulties in recording from children without artifact. Only recently has the usefulness of these studies in children become recognized. Because it is possible that many patients thought to have functional bowel disease may have disorders of gastrointestinal motility, it is anticipated that the use of this technique will gain widespread availability in the future. Studies have now been reported on infants and healthy children as well as those with pseudo-obstruction, recurrent abdominal pain, and chronic nonspecific diarrhea.[41–44] Although motility studies of the entire small intestine have been reported in adult subjects, such studies have not yet been performed in large numbers of children.

The patient is given a clear liquid meal the night before the study and receives no breakfast.[45] Intravenous fluids may need to be given to younger patients to prevent dehydration and hypoglycemia. Intravenous sedation may be given before insertion of the manometry assembly, particularly if it will be passed with endoscopic guidance. A multilumen motility catheter is passed transnasally or orally under fluoroscopic or endoscopic guidance so recording orifices are located in the distal, mid, and proximal duodenum and gastric antrum. If the child has a gastrostomy, the tube is removed, and the motility assembly can be passed through the gastrostomy site.

After the motility catheter is passed and its location verified fluoroscopically, the patient is taken to a quiet room. The patient remains supine with the head elevated at a 45 degree angle until the study is completed.

Normal fasting upper gastrointestinal motility is characterized by a triphasic pattern, known as the migrating motor complex (MMC) (Fig. 76–10).[46, 47] Phase I is characterized by quiescence or inactivity. Phase II contains intermittent activity consisting of contractions of random periodicity and amplitude. Phase III is defined as the presence of uninterrupted, regular contractions lasting about 5 minutes. The repeat rate of phase III contractions, 3 per minute in the stomach (antrum) and 11 to 13 per minute in the proximal small intestine, is an intrinsic feature of the enteric nervous system. Thus the gastric and intestinal pacemakers are driven separately. The duration of each phase varies according to location along the intestinal tract. A study should last at least as long as two to three complete cycles (100 minutes per cycle). Because abnormalities may be present in the fasting state, fed state or both, the fasting study period must be followed by the ingestion of a mixed solid-liquid meal. When the fasting MMC is interrupted by the ingestion of food, contractions develop that resemble phase II and last about 150 minutes. The disruption of fasting activity by a meal establishes the integrity of the enteroenteric reflexes.

About 50% of MMCs begin in the distal esophagus and 25% in the duodenum.[48] The rest of the MMCs begin more distally. The first postprandial MMC always begins in the stomach. There is also a diurnal variation. Approximately 40% of MMCs occur between 8 PM and 4 AM.[48] Considerable variability has been noted not only between patients, but even more importantly in individual patients when studied at different times.

When the primary symptoms relate to the stomach, e.g., nausea, vomiting, or distention, the condition is frequently called gastroparesis. When the symptoms are primarily intestinal, e.g., symptoms of bowel obstruction, the condition is called pseudo-obstruction. Despite these conventions, abnormalities of motility are frequently diffuse, even when symptoms appear to be localized.

Both quantitative and qualitative abnormalities have been reported in children with pathologic states suggestive of both myopathic and neuropathic abnormalities.[43–45] Qualitative abnormalities found have included retrograde contractions, low-amplitude contractions, absence of phase III, and nonpropagated bursts of duodenal contractions.

Quantitative abnormalities seen in children have included abnormalities in the frequency (tachygastria and bradygastria) and duration of phase III.[49] Low-amplitude contractions suggest a myopathic process (Fig. 76–11), whereas abnormalities of propagation and wave form suggest a neuropathic process. Abnormalities have been reported in intestinal pseudo-obstruction, recurrent abdominal pain, anorexia nervosa, diabetes mellitus, the dumping syndrome, following vagotomy, following Nissen fundoplication, possibly secondary to inadvertent damage to the vagus nerve, and associated with gastroesophageal reflux.[40, 43, 44, 50–52] Gastroparesis or delayed gastric emptying of solids has been described following viral infections.[42, 52]

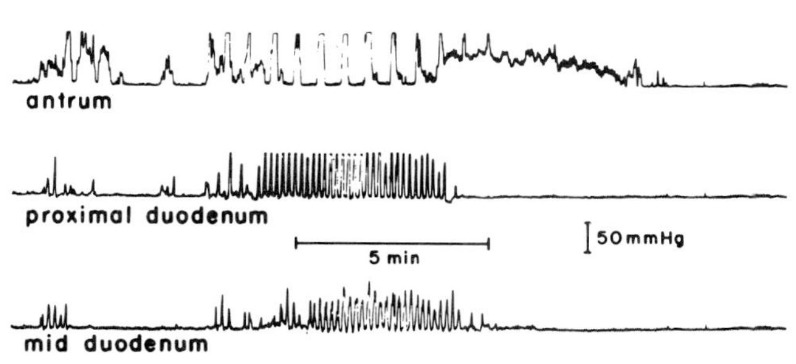

Figure 76–10. Normal fasting antroduodenal manometry. Phase III of the migrating myoelectric complex is present. Phase II is characterized by the irregular contractions preceding phase III and phase I by the absence of motility that follows phase III. (From Hyman PE: Absent postprandial duodenal motility in a child with cystic fibrosis: Correction of the symptoms and manometric abnormality with cisapride. Gastroenterology 1986; 90:1274–1279; with permission.)

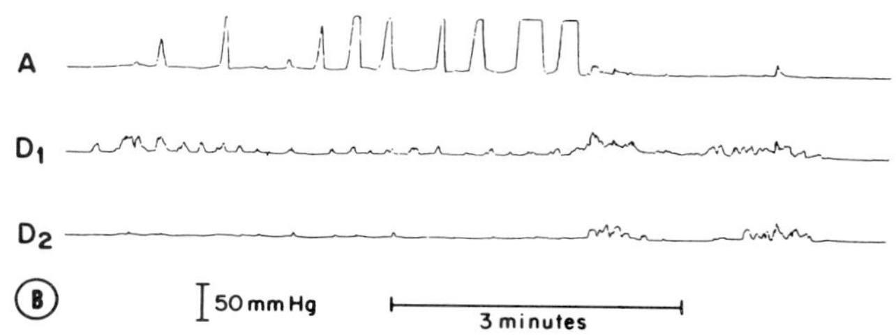

Figure 76–11. Fasting antroduodenal manometry, myopathic pseudo-obstruction. Duodenal contractions are too weak to establish presence of phase III activity . (From Hyman PE, McDiarmid SV, Napolitano J, et al: Antroduodenal motility in children with chronic intestinal pseudo-obstruction. J Pediatr 1988; 112:899–905; with permission.)

After a study, a patient will be assigned to one of three diagnostic categories: patients with normal motility; patients with abnormal gastric motor activity but normal intestinal motor activity; and patients with abnormal intestinal activity, which is usually associated with abnormal gastric activity.

Although the precise indications for performing gastroduodenal motility studies in children have yet to be defined, clear indications include intestinal pseudo-obstruction with abnormal or delayed gastric emptying and suspected gastroparesis (Table 76–4). Future indications may include the children with the following conditions when the standard evaluation is unrewarding: chronic nausea with or without associated vomiting, early satiety, postprandial epigastric fullness, recurrent abdominal pain, and anorexia. A suggested, although unproved, hypothesis states that many of the symptoms that are now attributed to functional gastrointestinal disease might ultimately be shown to be related to disorders of intestinal motility.

A variety of drugs may affect gastroduodenal motility so a careful history of drug use must be taken before a motility study is performed. These include anticholinergic agents such as tricyclic antidepressants and imipramine and opiates. These drugs should be stopped at least 48 hours before study.

INTESTINAL TRANSIT

A simple method of measuring intestinal transit is by following the passage of ingested radiopaque markers

Table 76–4. INDICATIONS FOR ANTRODUODENAL MANOMETRY

Abdominal distention
Abnormal gastric emptying
Chronic nausea (unexplained)
Chronic vomiting (unexplained)
Early satiety
Intestinal pseudo-obstruction
Postprandial epigastric fullness
Suspected gastroparesis

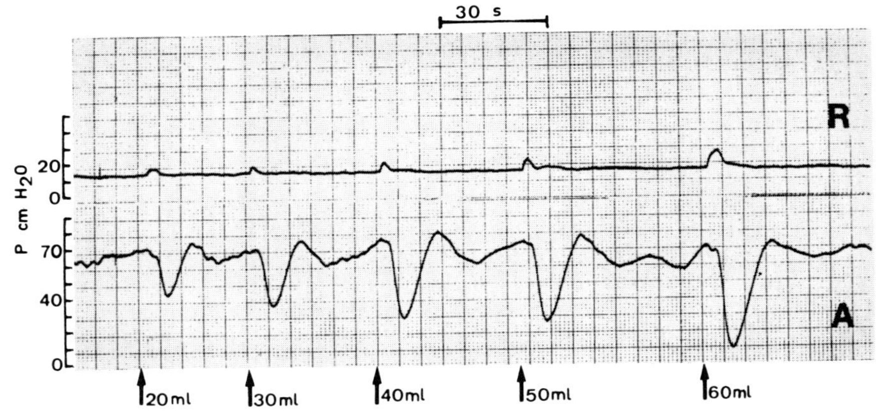

Figure 76–12. Normal anorectal manometry. Anorectal manometry tube with side hole in internal anal sphincter (*A*) and balloon in the rectum. Each rectal distention (*arrows*) induces relaxation of the internal anal sphincter and contraction of the rectum (*R*). The amplitude of the relaxation increases with increasing distention volumes. (From Meunier P, Mollard P: Control of the anal sphincter: Manometric study with human subjects. Pflugers Arch 1977; 370:233–239; with permission.)

by serial radiographs.[53–55] An abdominal radiograph is obtained immediately after the ingestion of a Sitzmark capsule and then on days 2 and 5. Transit through the small intestine is normal or only slightly prolonged, even in severe constipation, unless the patient has intestinal obstruction or pseudo-obstruction. Three patterns have been described: normal, delayed passage of the markers through the colon, and delayed passage of the markers from the rectum.[56] Delayed transit of markers through the ascending colon is rare. The most common finding in children is delay in the rectum. Occasionally a patient presents with constipation yet passes all markers normally. This type of patient (and family) needs psychiatric assistance.

ANORECTAL MANOMETRY

Normally the internal and external anal sphincters are in a state of tonic contraction.[56, 57] The internal anal sphincter (IAS) is 2 to 5.5 cm in length and located 3 to 7 cm proximal to the anus. The pressure of the IAS is 60 cm per H_2O (range 25 to 85), whereas that of the external anal sphincter (EAS) is lower, 30 cm per H_2O. During normal defecation, pressure rises in the rectum and simultaneously decreases in the anal canal (Fig. 76–12). Both the IAS and EAS relax. Following defecation, the closing reflex occurs, a slight rebound period of increased sphincter tone. The "anal wink" is a transient squeeze of the EAS in response to stimulation of the perianal skin.

Transient rectal distention induces relaxation of the IAS and contraction of the EAS, the "rectoanal reflex."[56, 57] In Hirschsprung's disease, the rectoanal reflex is absent.[10] The IAS fails to relax in response to rectal distention (Fig. 76–13). This lack of the rectoanal reflex has led to the widespread use of anorectal manometry for the diagnosis of Hirschsprung's disease. Because in Hirschsprung's disease the aganglionic segment always begins distally and extends a variable distance proximally, in theory anorectal manometry should be a perfect test. In practice, however, up to 20% of normal newborns, particularly low birth weight and premature infants, may have an abnormal rectoanal reflex.[58–60] In chronic (functional) constipation, the rectoanal inhibitory reflex is present.[61] The presence of the rectoanal inhibitory response makes Hirschsprung's disease unlikely.

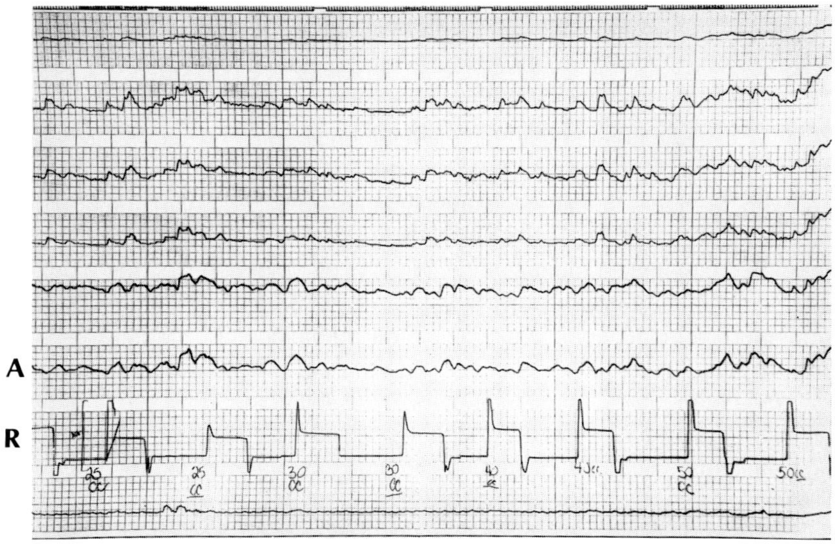

Figure 76–13. Anorectal manometry, Hirschsprung's disease. Anorectal manometry tube with side hole located in the internal anal sphincter (*A*) and balloon in the rectum (*R*). The internal anal sphincter fails to relax with distention of the rectum, demonstrating absence of the rectoanal reflex, characteristic of Hirschsprung's disease. (Courtesy of Walter Hogan, MD.)

As described earlier, a variety of techniques may be used in anorectal manometry. We use a single multilumen catheter with a distal balloon (see Fig. 76–2). Three side holes located 0.5 cm apart are distal to the balloon and are radially oriented. The size of the balloon may be varied, depending on the age and size of the patient. The catheter is connected to a pneumohydraulic pump and chart recorder. The balloon is connected to a 50-ml syringe. The patient is given a saline or phosphate enema before the examination.

The tube assembly is inserted through the anus until all the catheter orifices are located inside the anus. The locations of the IAS and the EAS are determined by the station pull-through technique. The catheters are perfused with water at a rate of 0.6 ml per minute. The pressure profile of the sphincters is determined by withdrawal of the catheter by increments of 0.5 to 1.0 cm at a steady, slow rate. Older, cooperative children are asked to squeeze the EAS at each station. The location of the IAS high-pressure zone is determined, and the catheter is reinserted with the balloon in the rectum and one or more side holes in the manometrically determined IAS. The balloon is then distended with increasing amounts of water or air, and the thresholds of sensitivity and relaxation of the IAS, the rectoanal inhibitory response, are determined.

A false abnormal result may be obtained in the newborn, especially the premature infant, if the balloon is not adequately inflated, if the patient is not adequately prepared, or if the patient is moving so that the balloon slips out of the proper location or artifact is produced.[58–60] Sedation may be helpful in the struggling younger child. All abnormal tests suggestive of Hirschsprung's disease should lead to histologic confirmation of the absence of ganglion cells with a rectal biopsy.

In chronic constipation, the basal anal pressure has been found to be normal, increased, and decreased.[61–68] The threshold for sensation is increased. In children with encopresis, relaxation of the IAS often occurs at volumes below the threshold of sensation. Because motility frequently returns to normal after treatment, the abnormalities of anorectal motility found in childhood constipation are probably the result, rather than the cause, of the constipation. Contraction, rather than relaxation, of the pelvic floor muscles may be seen in a subset of children with chronic constipation and encopresis.[64] These children may benefit from biofeedback therapy.

Abnormal anorectal manometry may also be found in children with megarectum caused by Hirschsprung's disease, anorectal malformations, spina bifida, other neurologic disorders, and intestinal pseudo-obstruction involving the colon (Table 76–5). Indications for anorectal manometry include suspicion of Hirschsprung's disease, as part of biofeedback training for the treatment of chronic constipation, atypical constipation, and the suspicion of intestinal pseudo-obstruction (Table 76–6).

Although anorectal manometry may be associated with mild discomfort, it is a simple and safe test to perform. The anxious child can easily be distracted by a television or by a story read by a parent.

Table 76–5. ABNORMAL ANORECTAL MANOMETRY

Anorectal malformations
Chronic constipation
Hirschsprung's disease
Megarectum
Neurologic disorders
Premature infant
Pseudo-obstruction
Spina bifida

Table 76–6. INDICATIONS FOR ANORECTAL MANOMETRY

Atypical constipation
Biofeedback
Suspected Hirschsprung's disease

REFERENCES

1. Stef JJ, Dodds WJ, Hogan WJ, et al: Intraluminal esophageal manometry: An analysis of variables affecting recording fidelity of peristaltic pressures. Gastroenterology 1974; 67:221–230.
2. Dodds WJ: Instrumentation and methods for intraluminal esophageal manometry. Arch Intern Med 1976; 136:515–523.
3. Arndorfer RC, Stef JJ, Dodds WJ, et al: Improved infusion systems for intraluminal esophageal manometry. Gastroenterology 1977; 73:23–27.
4. Dent J: A new technique for continuous sphincter pressure measurement. Gastroenterology 1976; 71:263–267.
5. Werlin SW, Dodds WJ, Hogan WJ, et al: Mechanisms of gastroesophageal reflux in children. J Pediatr 1980; 97:244–249.
6. Dodds WJ, Stewart ET, Hogan WJ, et al: Effect of esophageal movement on luminal esophageal pressure recording. Gastroenterology 1974; 67:592–600.
7. Dodds WJ, Hogan WJ, Stef JJ, et al: A rapid pull-through technique for measuring lower esophageal sphincter pressure. Gastroenterology 1975; 68:437–443.
8. Humphries TJ, Castell DO: Pressure profile of esophageal peristalsis in normal humans as measured by direct intraesophageal transducers. Dig Dis Sci 1977; 22:641–644.
9. Hyman PE, McDiarmid SV, Napolitano J, et al: Antroduodenal motility in children with chronic intestinal pseudo-obstruction. J Pediatr 1988; 112:899–905.
10. Tobon F, Reid NC, Talbert JL, et al: Nonsurgical test for the diagnosis of Hirschsprung's disease. N Engl J Med 1968; 278:188–193.
11. Rosenberg AJ, Vela AR: A new simplified technique for pediatric anorectal manometry. Pediatrics 1983; 71:240–245.
12. Nguyen DH, Burns MW, Shapiro GF, et al: Intraoperative cardiovascular collapse secondary to latex allergy. J Urol 1991; 146:571–574.
13. Weinstock LB, Clouse RE: Esophageal physiology: Normal and abnormal motor function. Am J Gastroenterol 1987; 82:399–405.
14. Diamant NE: Physiology of the esophagus. *In* Champion MC, McCallum RW, eds: Physiology, Diagnosis and Therapy in GI Motility Disorders. Philadelphia, The Medicine Publishing Foundation, 1987, pp 1–14.
15. Milla PJ: Gastrointestinal motility disorders in children. Pediatr Clin North Am 1988; 35:311–330.
16. Orlando RC: Esophageal manometry. *In* Drossman DA, ed: Manual of Gastroenterologic Procedures. New York, Raven Press, 1987, pp 30–44.
17. Scott B: Motility studies. *In* Walker WA, Durie PR, Hamilton JR, et al: Pediatric Gastrointestinal Disease. Philadelphia; BC Decker, 1991, pp 1324–1330.
18. Clouse RE: Motor disorders. *In* Sleisenger MH, Fordtran JS, eds: Gastrointestinal Disease. 4th ed. Philadelphia, WB Saunders, 1989, pp 561–562.

19. Vantrappen G: Diagnostic methodology of esophageal problems. *In* Champion MC, McCallum RW, eds: Physiology, Diagnosis and Therapy in GI Motility Disorders. Philadelphia, The Medicine Publishing Foundation, 1987, pp 51–60.
20. Grill BB, Hillemeier AC, Semeraro LA, et al: Effects of domperidone therapy on symptoms and upper gastrointestinal motility in infants with gastroesophageal reflux. J Pediatr 1985; 106:311–316.
21. Sondheimer JM, Arnold GL: Early effects of bethanechol on the esophageal motor function of infants with gastroesophageal reflux. J Pediatr Gastroenterol Nutr 1986; 5:47–51.
22. Armstrong D, Emde C, Bumm R: Twenty-four-hour pattern of esophageal motility in asymptomatic volunteers. Dig Dis Sci 1990; 35:1190–1197.
23. Cucchiara S, Staiano A, DiLorenzo C: Esophageal motor abnormalities in children with gastroesophageal reflux and peptic esophagitis. J Pediatr 1986; 108:907–910.
24. Herbst JJ: Gastroesophageal reflux. J Pediatr 1981; 98:859–870.
25. Jacob P, Kahrilas PJ, Vanagunas A: Peristaltic dysfunction associated with nonobstructive dysphasia in reflux disease. Dig Dis Sci 1990; 35:939–942.
26. Gelfand MD, Botoman VA: Esophageal motility disorders: A clinical overview. Am J Gastroenterol 1987; 82:181–186.
27. Christie DL: Pulmonary complications of esophageal disease. Pediatr Clin North Am 1984; 31:835–848.
28. Camilleri M: Disorders of gastrointestinal motility in neurologic diseases. Mayo Clin Proc 1990; 65:825–846.
29. Sack TL, Sleisenger MH: Myotonic dystrophy (myotonia dystrophica). *In* Sleisenger MH, Fordtran JS, eds: Gastrointestinal Disease. 4th ed. Philadelphia, WB Saunders, 1989, pp 516–517.
30. Eckardt VF, Nix W, Kraus W, et al: Esophageal motor function in patients with muscular dystrophy. Gastroenterology 1986; 90:628–635.
31. Vargas JH, Sachs P, Ament ME: Chronic intestinal pseudo-obstruction syndrome in pediatrics. J Pediatr Gastroenterol Nutr 1988; 7:323–332.
32. Flick JA, Boyke JT, Tuchman DN: Esophageal motor abnormalities in children and adolescents with scleroderma and mixed connective tissue disease. Pediatrics 1988; 82:107–111.
33. George JD: New clinical method for measuring the rate of gastric emptying: The double sampling test meal. Gut 1968; 9:237–242.
34. Siegal M, Lebenethal E, Topper W, et al: Gastric emptying in prematures of isocaloric feedings with differing osmolalities. Pediatr Res 1982; 16:141–147.
35. Sidebottom R, Curran JS, Williams PR, et al: Effects of long-chain vs medium-chain triglycerides on gastric emptying time in premature infants. J Pediatr 1983; 102:448–450.
36. Sty JR, Starshak RJ: The role of radionuclide studies in pediatric gastrointestinal disorders. Semin Nucl Med 1982; 12:156–172.
37. Gelfand MJ, Wagner GC. Gastric emptying in infants and children: Limited utility of 1-hour measurement. Pediatr Radiol 1991; 178:379–381.
38. Camilleri M, Brown ML, Malagelada JR: Relationship between impaired gastric emptying and abnormal gastrointestinal motility. Gastroenterology 1986; 91:94–99.
39. Hausken T, Odegaard S, Berstad A: Antroduodenal motility studied by real-time ultrasonography: Effect of Enprostil. Gastroenterology 1991; 100:59–63.
40. Maddern GJ, Jamieson GG, Chatterton BE, et al: Is there an association between failed antireflux procedures and delayed gastric emptying? Ann Surg 1985; 202:162–165.
41. Fenton TR, Harries JT, Milla PJ: Disordered small intestinal motility: A rational basis for toddler's diarrhea. Gut 1983; 24:897–903.
42. Tomomasa AT, Hyman PE, Itoh K, et al: Gastroduodenal motility in neonates: Response to human milk compared with cow's milk formula. Pediatrics 1987; 80:434–438.
43. Hyman PE, McDiarmid SV, Napolotano J, et al: Antroduodenal motility in children with chronic intestinal pseudo-obstruction. J Pediatr 1988; 112:899–905.
44. Pineiro-Carrero VM, Andres JM, Davis RH, et al: Abnormal gastroduodenal motility in children and adolescents with recurrent functional abdominal pain. J Pediatr 1988; 113:820–825.
45. Hyman PE, Napolitano JA, Diego A, et al: Antroduodenal manometry in the evaluation of chronic functional gastrointestinal symptoms. Pediatrics 1990; 86:39–44.
46. Szurszewski JH: A migrating electric complex of the canine small intestine. Am J Physiol 1969; 217:1757–1763.
47. Kelly KA: Motility of the stomach and gastroduodenal junction. *In* Johnson LR, ed: Physiology of the Gastrointestinal Tract. 2nd ed. New York, Raven Press, 1987, p 393.
48. Kellow JE, Borody TJ, Phillips SF, et al: Human interdigestive motility: Variations in patterns from esophagus to colon. Gastroenterology 1986; 191:386–395.
49. Milla PJ: Gastrointestinal motility disorders in children. Pediatr Clin North Am 1988; 2:311–329.
50. Malagelada JR, Rees WD, Mazzotta LJ, et al: Gastric motor abnormalities in diabetic and post-vagotomy gastroparesis: Effect of metoclopramide and bethanechol. Gastroenterology 1980;78:186.
51. McCallum RW, Grill BB, Lange R, et al: Definition of a gastric emptying abnormality in patients with anorexia nervosa. Dig Dis Sci 1985; 30:713–722.
52. Oh JH, Kim CH: Gastroparesis after a presumed viral illness: Clinical and laboratory features and natural history. Mayo Clin Proc 1990; 65:636–642.
53. Arhan P, Devroede G, Jehannin B, et al: Segmental colonic transit time. Dis Colon Rectum 1981; 24:625.
54. Arhan P, Devroede G, Bertrand J, et al. Idiopathic disorders of fecal continence in children. Pediatrics 1983; 71:774–779.
55. Hinton JM, Lennard-Jones JE, Young AC: A new method for studying gut transit times using radiopaque markers. Gut 1969; 10:842.
56. Schuster MM, Mendeloff AI: Motor action of rectum and anal sphincters in continence and defecation. *In* Code CF, Heidel W, eds: Handbook of Physiology. Sect 6, Vol IV. Washington, D.C., American Physiological Society, 1968, p 2121.
57. Deveroede G: Constipation. *In* Sleisenger MH, Fordtran JS, eds: Gastrointestinal Disease. 4th ed. Philadelphia, WB Saunders, 1989, pp 331–368.
58. Ito Y, Donahoe PK, Hendren WH: Maturation of the rectoanal response in premature and perianal infants. J Pediatr Surg 1977; 12:477–482.
59. Boston VE, Cywes S, Davies MRQ: Qualitative and quantitative evaluation of internal and sphincter function in the newborn. Gut 1977; 18:1036–1044.
60. Bowes KS, Kling S: Anorectal manometry in premature infants. J Pediatr Surg 1979; 14:533–535.
61. Loening-Baucke V, Younoszai MK: Abnormal anal sphincter response in chronically constipated children. J Pediatr 1982; 100:213–218.
62. Monar D, Taitz LS, Urwin OM, et al: Anorectal manometry results in defecation disorders. Arch Dis Child 1983; 58:257–261.
63. Loening-Baucke VA: Abnormal rectoanal function in children recovered from chronic constipation and encopresis. Gastroenterology 1984; 87:1299–1304.
64. Loening-Baucke VA, Cruikshank BM: Abnormal defecation dynamics in chronically constipated children with encopresis. J Pediatr 1986; 108:562–566.
65. Wald A, Chandra R, Chiponis D, et al: Anorectal function and continence mechanisms in childhood encopresis. J Pediatr Gastroenterol Nutr 1986; 5:346–351.
66. Meunier P, Mollard P, De Beaujeu MJ: Manometric studies of anorectal disorders in infancy and childhood: An investigation of the physiopathology of continence and defecation. Br J Surg 1976; 63:402–407.
67. Meunier P, Mollard P: Control of the internal anal sphincter (manometric study with human subjects). Pflugers Arch 1977; 370:233–239.
68. Hatch TF: Encopresis and constipation in children. Pediatr Clin North Am 1988; 35:257–280.

Chapter 77

Breath Testing

BENNY KERZNER

Breath testing has obvious advantages for a pediatric population in which painless, noninvasive investigations are especially appreciated. The challenge of introducing these tests into clinical practice has now been met by using sensitive technology to measure accurately minimal concentrations of gas and simple devices to gather samples from the full range of pediatric patients. Whether breath testing is used to evaluate intestinal, pancreatic, or hepatic function, the principles of the study are similar. The tests are dependent on the evolution of a gas from a substrate that is administered orally and selected because it challenges particular metabolic pathways often located in specific organs or organ components.

These tests may take advantage of the presence in breath of gases that are normally produced in the course of the body's metabolism; that are the products of the intestinal microflora; or that are unique and found only under test conditions. The most widely employed endogenously produced gas is carbon dioxide (CO_2). Carbon is ubiquitous in organic chemicals, and most aliphatic compounds that enter the body's metabolic pool have the potential to be oxidized to CO_2.[1] These breath tests have not gained wide application in pediatrics because to identify the critical carbon in breath one must choose ^{14}C, which is radioactive, or the heavy isotope ^{13}C, for which complex technology is necessary. Fortunately, the limitations of ^{14}C and ^{13}C technology do not apply to hydrogen breath tests, which have found remarkably wide application. Hydrogen is an exogenous gas, which originates from bacteria that inhabit the intestine.[2] The method has evolved from one too cumbersome for widespread application in children to a far more refined technique in which hydrogen concentration can be instantly measured in expired air.[3, 4] In this chapter, the physiology of hydrogen production, the application of hydrogen breath tests to clinical practice, and the bases for interpretation of results are discussed in some detail. The potential of CO_2 breath tests and those that depend on the evolution of a unique gas product, e.g., pentane, as an index of lipid peroxidation also hold promise and are mentioned.

HYDROGEN BREATH TEST

The hydrogen breath test (HBT) has become the method of choice for determining carbohydrate malabsorption.[5–7] It has been successfully used for population studies of congenital lactase deficiency,[5, 8–10] it provides a practical screening test for bacterial overgrowth,[11, 12] and the test is used to delineate small bowel transit time.[13, 14]

Physiology

The presence of hydrogen in flatus has been known for more than 100 years and in breath for the last 30, but its clinical application is a recent event.[3, 15, 16] In the early 1970s, Bond and Levitt[3] enunciated the principles that underlie the rationale for these studies: The HBT for carbohydrate malabsorption is analogous to a stool fat collection for steatorrhea in that the hydrogen evolved reflects the quantity of carbohydrate that is not absorbed. The colon produces virtually all of the body's hydrogen, and it has been determined that hydrogen in breath increases after the introduction of as little as 3 gm of carbohydrate into the organ.[17] The increase is directly related to the quantity of carbohydrate entering the colon because a constant proportion of the hydrogen enters the blood to be excreted in the breath.[3] The physiologic variables that affect hydrogen production in breath are those that influence the quantity, distribution, and quality of the bacterial flora; the substrates that are available for hydrogen production; the efficiency of the carbohydrate digestive absorptive mechanism; the rate and rhythm of intestinal peristalsis; and factors affecting the delivery of gas from the blood stream to the pulmonary alveoli for exhalation in breath.[18–20]

Bacterial Flora

For practical purposes, the intestinal microbial ecosystem that contributes hydrogen to breath is in the colon, although a limited amount of fermentation is reported from the oral cavity and the upper intestine when it is subject to bacterial overgrowth.[21] Important among these microbes are bacteroides, which produce succinate and propionate from carbohydrates; *Escherichia coli* are a lesser population.[22]

If HBTs are to be reliable, consistent, and comparable, the colonic flora should be relatively constant and available in unlimited supply to digest all of the malabsorbed carbohydrate. Indeed there are large numbers of bacteria in stool—approximately 1 x 10^{11} viable bacteria per gram of wet weight.[23] It has been shown, however, that differences in diet, therapy, and geographic location can radically affect the flora. Mechanical cleansing with enemas and laxatives will, as expected, quantitatively decrease the bacterial load and the production of hydrogen.[18] A wide variety of broad-spectrum antibiotics have an effect against the hydrogen-producing organisms.[24] The effect appears to be reversible within 2 weeks, but the impact may carry over for a month or more.[18] Failure of hydrogen production following oral lactulose or the addition of carbohydrate to stool in vitro indicates that hydrogen-producing organisms may be absent in 2 to 9% of the pediatric population at large and may be far more common in hospitalized patients.[25, 26]

Fermentation will proceed to yield hydrogen only under relatively alkaline conditions, making pH a major determinant of hydrogen production. Short-chain fatty acids result in product inhibition of the fermentation reactions by dropping the pH. Ironically, when carbohydrate malabsorption is severe and fatty acids are generated, the HBT is negative, although reducing substances are evident in the stool. Even when stools are alkaline, it is conceivable that acid in the cecum is inhibiting hydrogen evolution. The hydrogen-producing bacteria appear to persevere in the acid environment because hydrogen can be encouraged to reappear with an alkaline shift in the pH gradient.[27]

Diet

There is an orchestrated interaction between the dietary components, the products of fermentation, and intestinal function, which regulates hydrogen gas production. Most of the hydrogen evolved in the bowel lumen takes origin from unabsorbed carbohydrates, and the amount that reaches the bacteria is influenced by the frequency of meals and the quality and quantity of the ingested sugar.[28] Aside from lactose, which is often malabsorbed, relatively large amounts of poorly assimilated refined sugars such as fructose are being introduced into our diets.[29, 30] Carbohydrates not attacked by the mammalian enzyme system contribute substantially to gas production and include stachyose in beans, raffinose in cotton seed meal, and fibrous constituents of the diet: cellulose, hemicellulose, and pectins of vegetables and fruits.[31] We now appreciate that in a healthy person, the colonic flora are sustained by food that escapes digestion to reach the colon. Starch in particular reaches the terminal ileum, and estimates of the amount passing through as determined by hydrogen breath analysis or directly by measuring the sugar content of an ileostomy effluent are similar.[32, 33] Fermentation is encouraged by sugars reaching the colon. The bacterial enzymes necessary are induced, and the short-chain fatty acids produced exert a humoral effect, which hastens small bowel transit of carbohydrates to the colon. Short-chain fatty acids also exert humoral effects, which induce maturation and growth of the bowel.[34]

Increasing the fiber content of the meal decreases small bowel transit time and makes more starch available for hydrogen production.[35] Fat has an opposite effect. It slows gastric emptying and small bowel transit time, giving the normal digestive/absorptive processes a greater opportunity to assure assimilation.[36] Thus lactose in milk is far more readily tolerated than lactose in an aqueous solution.[37] Prolonged evolution of hydrogen from complex polysaccharides can contribute to high baseline breath test values.[22] Yet the prior diet could not be used to predict hydrogen production from starch, and it has little or no bearing on HBT values obtained after a period of starvation.[38]

Fasting Breath Hydrogen

Even after an appropriate meat and rice starch evening meal and an adequate fast, elevated hydrogen levels are frequently found and are difficult to explain. The resumption of peristalsis after sleep is thought to explain hydrogen evolution from unabsorbed dietary carbohydrates. These are propelled from the ileum to the cecum, or alternatively they are in the cecum and their fermentation is initiated when alkaline ileal contents enter the acid environment of the cecum.[39] The hydrogen may also be produced by anaerobic bacteria in the oropharynx.[40] An alternative explanation is the evolution of hydrogen from the carbohydrate moiety of intestinal glycoproteins. They are present in secretions, desquamated enterocytes, and also ingested meats. An influx of glycoproteins as a result of protein-losing enteropathy or accelerated turnover of enterocytes may explain the high baseline hydrogen breath values characteristic of bacterial overgrowth and conditions such as celiac disease.[41, 42]

Products of Fermentation

These are the short-chain organic acids acetate, propionate, and butyrate as well as hydrogen and CO_2. Most of the hydrogen produced in the large bowel is passed in flatus, is absorbed into the blood stream, or enters into a variety of metabolic pathways, i.e., methanogenesis, sulfate reduction, or acetogenesis.[43] Organisms capable of yielding methane are present in one third of the population. Methanogenesis is favored by a neutral pH and inhibited in an acid environment. Methane therefore is often produced from glycoproteins low in carbohydrate, which yield minimal quantities of hydrogen and allow the environment to be maintained at a neutral pH.[41] Possibly for the same reason, methane production is higher in slow transit situations. As both methane and hydrogen are produced from malabsorbed carbohydrate substrates, in ideal circumstances one would prefer to use the sum of their numbers to estimate the extent of carbohydrate malabsorption.[44, 45]

Development of Digestive Capacity

The pattern of development of carbohydrate digestive and absorptive pathways has special relevance for hydrogen production in the newborn period. Glucoamylase and sucrase activity are in place early in intrauterine life, whereas lactase activity reaches substantial levels only at or after birth. Some months pass before monosaccharide transport and endoamylase production reach adult levels.[46] Although these constraints on carbohydrate absorption rarely result in symptoms, evidence of carbohydrate malabsorption by way of hydrogen and stool analyses is frequently present. MacLean and Fink[47] have shown that by 3 weeks of life, all premature infants have hydrogen in their breath. A remarkable amount of the lactose they ingest enters the colon, and substantial quantities are lost in the stool.[47] In the full-term infant, hydrogen production peaks in the second month, and in the third, breath hydrogen increases late in the day in association with sleep. Evidence of malabsorption may disappear as early as 8 weeks in the breast-fed infant who enjoys the advantage of maturation factors in the milk, although in others it lasts for a number of months.[48, 49]

Motility

The more rapid the transit time in the small intestine and the longer the stasis in the colon, the greater the volume of hydrogen produced by the individual consuming fermentable carbohydrates. As a consequence, in patients with gastrectomies or those who are taking drugs such as metoclopramide, hydrogen evolution may be increased as a result of rapid gastric emptying.[3, 50] Conversely, when the carbohydrate is taken with a meal, particularly fat, which delays gastric emptying, hydrogen evolution is decreased.[37] As opposed to transit in the small intestine, delayed transit through the colon will accentuate hydrogen evolution, which may explain why hydrogen levels are much increased during sleep.[51]

Ventilation

Hypoventilation, as occurs in sleep, decreases hydrogen elimination from the body, and as blood levels increase, so do breath levels. Conversely, with exercise-induced hyperventilation, the hydrogen content of the body and breath fall.[51, 52]

The extent to which alveolar gas is diluted by inspired air can be calculated by considering the magnitude of the drop in the partial pressure of CO_2, which in the alveolus approaches 5%. A correction or "normalization" of breath hydrogen based on the breath CO_2 is therefore possible but only under steady-state conditions.[53] Hydrogen diffuses into the alveolus more rapidly than CO_2. Consequently, when minute ventilation suddenly changes, hydrogen levels cannot be predicted from CO_2 values.[20]

Methods

Sensors

The use of gas/solid phase chromatography made it practical to detect hydrogen in breath, and once the clinical applications were evident, rapid improvements in the technology followed. The original helium ionization sensors were replaced by the more sensitive thermal conductivity wires, and the use of molecular sieve columns with argon as the carrier gas became popular. Solid-state sensors were then introduced, and they are widely employed in portable, lightweight machines that use air as the carrier gas and eliminate the need to transport argon. Now electrochemical cells permit the use of hand-held instruments. The hydrogen is oxidized to water, and the electrochemical output is fed to a liquid crystal, which displays the hydrogen in parts per million. The sensitivity of this device ranges from 1 to 200 ppm.[3, 4, 54–56]

Collection Devices

When the HBT was introduced, the sensitivity of the technique depended on rebreathing air in a closed system over a given period in which the CO_2 was removed and the hydrogen concentrated. With improved sensitivity, "interval breath sampling" became possible. Here, at intervals, one or more exhalations are pooled to provide a representative sample of gas. This approach is less quantitatively accurate but simpler, more comfortable, and therefore practical.

A variety of masks and catheters have been employed to collect the gas, and probably because the HBT is sensitive, all have proved to be effective in the hands of their advocates. Face masks may cause discomfort and have not uniformly allowed for consistent results, particularly in small infants.[47] When attached to a polytef (teflon) bag by a low-resistance valve, however, they have been effective in eliminating the need for further manipulation of the sample.[57] Many believe that given the sensitivity of the technique, simply exhaling breath directly into a syringe or balloon, or in younger children drawing the breath into a syringe via nasopharyngeal catheters or nasal prongs, is adequate.[7] Others report, however, that the nasal prong technique yielded consistently lower hydrogen concentrations than oropharyngeal or nasopharyngeal catheters.[47]

Either all of the expired breath can be collected, or attempts can be made to obtain end-tidal air, given that this has the highest concentration of hydrogen and correlates best with the blood hydrogen levels. A variety of techniques have been proposed to achieve this end. Technicians can be trained to draw increments of the sample repetitively through a catheter toward the end of each inspiration. Using this technique, results with the nasal prong correlate closely with those using a Heldane-Priestly tube to draw end-expiratory volumes.[7] Alternatively, the subjects can exhale breath into a syringe with a distal hole through which the first portion of the exhalation escapes before the plunger is advanced to trap the end-tidal air.[58] More commonly, two balloons are fitted to a J-tube with a valve that ensures that once the first balloon is filled, the rest of the expired air enters the second for sampling. In the hand-held instrument, the end-expiratory air is trapped between two valves and diffuses directly to the detector.[4]

Infants offer a particularly challenging situation: cooperation is poor, respiration is rapid, tidal volumes are small, and contamination with dead-space and inspired air is likely. The use of end-tidal CO_2 is recommended, and an automatic sampling device that responds to the temperature changes in expired breath is now available. Expired air warms to temperatures approaching alveolar air, and at a critical point, the device triggers the plunger of a syringe to withdraw a fixed distance. In this way, 87% of the end-tidal volume is collected in the very small infant.[59]

Storage

The hand-held sensor used for hydrogen detection may eliminate the need for sample collection, but in most situations the gas must be stored for later analysis, and it is imperative that the gas does not escape in transit. A simple but practical solution for storage is the use of plastic or glass syringes; these vary in their retention efficiency and must be adequately sealed. Gas gradually diffuses through the body of plastic syringes, a tendency effectively diminished by keeping the syringes in a refrigerator at −20°C. Freezing the samples actually increases hydrogen loss between the barrel and the plunger. Gas does not diffuse through the wall of glass syringes; however, there is a rapid loss between the body and the plunger. This may be eliminated by applying a film of mineral oil or 0.1 N hydrochloric acid to the interface. Stoppers made of natural rubber are more effective than those made of silicone rubber.[60] A three-way stopcock fitted to the nozzle is effective only for up to 8 hours. Beyond that time, a tightly fitting seal such as a Critocap is needed.[61] When these precautions are taken, retention of gas in syringes is achieved for at least 48 hours, and can be extended up to a week. For more permanent storage, evacuated glass tubes are favored.[53] Although they involve more time, more manipulation, and greater expense, they are convenient when the samples are to be mailed from the home or a physician's office for analysis. Alternative collection devices include Mylar-coated foil bags and aerosol cans.[54, 55]

We have witnessed an evolution of technology from a relatively insensitive situation in which only 10 ppm of hydrogen could be detected to one in which 1 ppm can be found. More importantly, the technology is evolving to the point that lightweight field instruments are available, and storage of breath samples is not needed.

Tests

Tests for Carbohydrate Malabsorption

Lactose Breath Hydrogen Tests. Lactose is most commonly selected as a substrate for HBTs because lactase activity is rate-limiting for absorption and the enzyme is vulnerable. It is frequently lost as a genetically programmed phenomenon (congenital lactase deficiency) or in response to a wide variety of luminal toxins. The lactose tolerance test can therefore serve as an index of mucosal injury; it identifies malabsorbers, predicts those likely to respond to a lactose-free diet, correlates with abnormal mucosal lactase activity, and is more reliable than tests depending on serum measures of glucose.[62–64] Invasive techniques that depend on intestinal intubation and perfusion to measure absorption directly have been replaced by HBTs. Moreover, since its introduction, jejunal biopsy for morphology and measurement of disaccharidase activity is less essential.[65, 66]

Dose response curves for the various carbohydrate substrates used in HBTs have not been established. The doses used are an extrapolation from those traditionally employed in the standard glucose tolerance test: 2 gm per kg up to a maximum of 50 gm in a 10 or 20% aqueous solution. If the question under consideration is lactose tolerance rather than lactose malabsorption, a dose analogous to that of lactose in milk is preferred. Considering that 8 oz of milk contains 12 gm of lactose, there seems little point in going beyond twice that, i.e., 25 gm (one gm per kg of lactose to a maximum of 25 gm). A "physiologic" lactose tolerance test has been advocated using 0.5 gm of lactose per kilogram.[67] If the object of the test is to identify all patients with hypolactasia, however, the 2 gm per kg dose is preferable.[37, 64]

To assure low baseline values, the HBT must be conducted after an adequate fast. For older children, an overnight fast following a meat and rice dinner designed to avoid either excessive or complex carbohydrates is advised. A carbohydrate-free meal does cause a rise in hydrogen of approximately 2.5 ppm, but the baseline is re-established within 4 hours. In toddlers and infants, the fast may be reduced to 8 and 4 hours, respectively. If the zero value is higher than that obtained at 30 minutes, the latter is used to calculate the subsequent increment in hydrogen content.[64, 68]

In proved cases of hypolactasia, peak hydrogen values may be seen as early as 75 and as late as 210 minutes after the test dose. Nonetheless, it is generally agreed that the standard test should last only 2½ hours because although the early rise in hydrogen consistently identifies patients with hypolactasia, low late rises might signify incomplete assimilation by an intestine with normal lactase activity.[64] The greatest increase in breath hydrogen is most reliably observed between 120 and 180 minutes. This observation has prompted consideration of a simplified 2-hour breath test. Abramowitz and colleagues[69] found that levels at 0 and 120 minutes served to identify 95% of patients with lactose malabsorption. Others disagree and project more than a 20% reduction in positive results as well as an attendant loss of the ability to identify the biphasic pattern associated with bacterial overgrowth.[70, 71] A prolonged study is needed if physiologic conditions are simulated. Thus, Solomons and associates,[37] who incorporated a low test dose of lactose into milk, found the test to be sensitive for lactose intolerance provided that it was extended over 5 hours.

The criteria for identifying a positive HBT result have not been standardized or systematically changed in response to technologic advances. Increasingly, an increment of 20 ppm of hydrogen over the baseline, or the lowest recorded value, is accepted as a positive study.[72] Complete separation of patients with hypolactasia from controls, however, may be achieved only when an increase of greater than 10 ppm is observed.[64]

As stated previously, alveolar air is expired from the lung, and it is diluted by air in the dead-space or the environment. Thus to secure truly representative data on alveolar samples, end-expiratory air must be obtained, or, alternatively, the extent of dilution should be estimated by normalizing the hydrogen values with adjustments based on the concentration of CO_2, carbon monoxide, oxygen, or nitrogen in the sample.[73] Normalization is critical in young infants and in some children in whom timing of the collection is difficult, but it is usually not necessary in older patients. Because normalization against CO_2 is predicated on constant CO_2 evolution, it can be done only when ventilation is calm and constant, as dramatic shifts in minute ventilation will alter CO_2 concentration independent of hydrogen content.[20]

Sucrose Hydrogen Breath Test. A sucrose HBT offers a simple, reproducible, and accurate method to screen for primary sucrase isomaltase deficiency. The test does not replace jejunal biopsy for a definitive diagnosis, but a perseverent positive study is highly suggestive.[7, 74, 75] In contrast to secondary lactose intolerance, the role of hydrogen breath testing for delineation of secondary hyposucrasia is far more controversial. Secondary sucrase deficiency has not always been discernible, probably reflecting the high sucrase activity of the mucosa, which is approximately twice that of lactose, and the resilience of sucrase activity in the face of partial villous atrophy. A dose of 2 gm per kg up to 50 gm is recommended, but Davidson and Robb[77] suggested that a dose of at least 30 gm is necessary to identify secondary hyposucrasia. Additionally, they accept a sustained increase in hydrogen concentration as a positive result even if the elevation is considerably less than 20 ppm.[76, 77]

Monosaccharide Hydrogen Breath Test. With regard to monosaccharide malabsorption, parallel HBTs could theoretically be used. Limits in the assimilation of fructose and sorbitol have been delineated by these methods.[30, 78–81] Unfortunately, norms for the assimilation of these particular sugars have not as yet been defined, and as such, wide application of HBTs to define abnormalities in their absorption in the population at large cannot be made. HBTs have demonstrated that the assimilation of fructose is enhanced in the presence of glucose.[82]

Starch Hydrogen Breath Tests. Starch and glucose polymers have been effectively employed in HBTs but not to define the presence of specific illnesses. Rather, they are used to measure the body's efficiency in the assimilation of different varieties of starch and of different chain lengths of glucose polymers.[83, 84] A starch tolerance test has been proposed to determine pancreatic function. Its clinical application is limited because alternative digestive pathways, notably salivary and breast milk amylases, acting in concert with mucosal glucoamylase, detract from the exclusive measurement of pancreatic amylase activity. In starch tolerance tests, a considerable quantity of sugar is employed, i.e., 100 gm per test, and the test must be extended over 8 to 10 hours.[85]

Tests for Bacterial Overgrowth

Hydrogen breath testing for bacterial overgrowth has been effectively applied to pediatric populations with chronic diarrhea, immune deficiency, and lymphocytic leukemia.[86–88] HBTs yield positive results in bacterial overgrowth of the small intestine because although the bacterial colony is far smaller than in the colon, the gas evolved enters the blood stream rather than being passed in flatus. False-positive results are unusual, but there are reasons to anticipate false-negative studies. Certain strains of bacteria, such as anaerobic streptococci, do not produce hydrogen; others preferentially evolve methane, and occasionally the region of overgrowth is located so distal in the small bowel that the hydrogen peak produced cannot be distinguished from the normal "colonic peak."[89]

The routine lactose tolerance test may provide clues suggesting bacterial overgrowth: a high breath hydrogen value after an overnight fast or a rapid and sustained increase in hydrogen for several hours after the test dose.[86] Unfortunately, confirmatory tests are needed given that there are alternative reasons for an elevated baseline measurement, and both congenital and secondary lactase deficiency are common. Breath tests have proved valuable in this regard; lactulose is commonly used, and glucose is now receiving consideration as a substrate.

A High Baseline Value. The high baseline hydrogen concentration is presumably the consequence of bacterial action on intestinal glycoproteins; addition of carbohydrate to the diet does not elevate these values. A high baseline value is one greater than 2 standard deviations above the mean of a healthy population, and it usually approximates 15 ppm. It is an important screen for bacterial overgrowth, but there are frequent false-positive and false-negative results. High baseline values have also been identified in patients with cystic fibrosis, celiac disease, sickle cell anemia, pneumatosis intestinalis, and necrotizing enterocolitis. Conversely, as many as 40% of patients with bacterial overgrowth have normal values.[90, 91]

Lactulose Hydrogen Breath Test. The artificial sugar, lactulose, which escapes normal digestion and absorption, has proved to be a useful substrate, not only for identifying bacterial overgrowth but also as a probe to detect the absence of hydrogen-producing organisms and to measure small bowel transit time.

A dose of only 3 gm of lactulose results in hydrogen evolution, but for the test to be consistently positive a minimum of 6 and usually 10 gm is advocated. In the presence of bacterial overgrowth, lactulose yields "a double peak" hydrogen breath profile. The first increase is indicative of small bowel fermentation, and the second reflects further degradation of the substrate by the colonic bacteria. Separation of the two peaks is sometimes obscured, making differentiation of hydrogen evolution as a result of rapid small bowel transport to the colon difficult to distinguish from bacterial overgrowth.[12, 92] The lactulose breath test has been contrasted with ^{14}C choleglycine and found to be as effective. Both tests, however, have a low but definite false-negative test rate, so only taken together do they identify the majority of patients with bacterial overgrowth.[11]

Glucose Breath Test. Glucose or xylose can be employed as substrates in HBTs to detect bacterial overgrowth because they are efficiently absorbed and therefore not anticipated to reach the colon. The early appearance of hydrogen in breath after glucose administration suggests that bacteria have invaded the small intestine to make contact with the monosaccharide before its absorption. Moreover, this peak does not have to be distinguished from the colonic peak anticipated in a lactulose breath test.[93]

The glucose dose necessary to elicit responses in bacterial overgrowth has not been systematically determined, and a pediatric dose has not been firmly established. An early report using 10 gm of glucose in adult patients with bacterial overgrowth resulted in minimal quantities of hydrogen being produced. Increasing the dose to 50 gm provided positive results in approximately 50 to 70% of the patients, and going up to 80 gm increased sensitivity only to 75%.[94] Results with the glucose HBTs were equivalent to those obtained with $^{14}CO_2$ glucose and choleglycine breath tests. Only by applying two of the tests to patients were positive results obtained approaching those obtained by bacterial cultures. When an affirmative study is taken to be an increase of more than 12 ppm of hydrogen, rather than 20, positive results are detected 93% of the time and the specificity is 86%. In pediatrics, rather than the usual 2 gm per kg, up to 4 gm per kg of glucose have been advocated.[93]

Breath hydrogen studies have obvious advantages for identifying bacterial overgrowth, but they have limitations. By comparison to bacterial culture of the upper intestine, the specificity of the glucose and lactulose breath tests are only 83 and 44%.[92]

Transit Time

HBTs provide a simple method for measuring transit of a substrate or meal from the mouth to the cecum—a measure that has significant implications for absorption and can be associated with specific disease states.[95] Unabsorbed carbohydrates, including sorbitol, raffinose, and lactulose, are successfully used to measure orocecal transit time by timing the first appearance of gas, which denotes that the sugar has reached the colon to be fermented.[96] Lactulose is increasingly used to this end, but enthusiasm for its application has been tempered by the realization that the results vary greatly between individuals and on repetitive testing in any one patient. The explanation relates in part to the normal variations anticipated for gastric emptying and small bowel transit, but additional factors include the sugar's effect on transit time and the endogenous flora. Even very small concentrations of lactulose hasten transit time, and the practice of using a single dose for a wide age range ignores the impact of growth and maturation. A dose of 250 mg per kg of lactulose has been proposed, with a lower limit of 2 to 3 gm. The standard hydrogen breath test should be modified for measures of transit time. Breath should be sampled every 10 minutes; transit time is accepted as the time taken to record an increment of 10 or 15 ppm over baseline. The variability of the test is considerably improved by incorporating the lactulose into a standard meal containing protein and fat.[13, 14, 97]

Applications

Food Intolerance and Acceptance

The ability of the HBT to establish accurately the presence of carbohydrate malabsorption has clarified the role of malabsorption in the development of milk and food intolerance. Lactose malabsorption (LM) causes abdominal pain, gaseous distention, and diarrhea, and the symptoms improve when lactose is removed, hydrolyzed, or fermented.[98, 99] Yet patients with LM need not have a substantial amount of abdominal pain. Further, HBTs demonstrate that patients claiming to be intolerant of milk may have an incidence of LM no higher than that of controls.[100] LM is therefore only one cause of milk intolerance, and consequently discomfort is not always reversed with hydrolyzed formulas. Conversely, in patients with the irritable bowel syndrome and LM, the ingestion of milk may increase the incidence of symptoms only modestly.[101]

Consuming lactose as part of a balanced meal or in milk is important in modulating the symptoms of intolerance. The assimilation of the lactose in a meal is improved because delayed passage by the food allows for longer exposure to intestinal lactase and a more gradual presentation of the carbohydrate to the colonic flora. This effect is corroborated by finding diminished and late hydrogen production as well as fewer symptoms in patients receiving lactose in milk as opposed to water.[102] LM is not an absolute contraindication to the use of milk; patients with LM can tolerate at least 20 and up to 40 ml per kg of milk.[103] Even in protein-calorie malnutrition with severe hypolactasia, nitrogen retention and the clinical outcome are positively affected by milk consumption, although lactose may be less optimally used than a hydrolyzed lactose product. Tolerance is volume related: Although symptoms were induced only in 4.5% of lactose malabsorbers by 8 oz of milk, doubling the milk volume increased the incidence of symptoms fourfold.[104]

The HBT is also proving to be valuable in defining optimal diets for patients with LM. As one would predict, evaporated milks are better tolerated than skim milk products, which have a relatively higher lactose content and a more rapid transit time.[101, 105] Other findings, such as the ameliorating effect of cocoa on LM, are more difficult to explain.[106]

In tablet form, exogenous β-galactosidase dramatically decreases the hydrogen evolved following a standard lactose BHT. Twenty-four hours are required to hydrolyze more than 60% of the lactose in milk, but in both adults and children, β-galactosidase has been effective when added to milk just before consumption.[107] Hydrogen breath testing has demonstrated that acidophilic milk does not reduce hydrogen production; the lactase produced is trapped in the organism and unavailable to the substrate. Bile-vulnerable strains of acidophilic organisms that are lysed in the upper intestine may ultimately prove helpful in this regard.[108]

Yogurt, which is made by incubating milk with the β-galactosidase–producing organisms, is more effective than lactase tablets in reducing lactose content. The β-galactosidase activity depends on the viability of the organism at the time of consumption and gastric and intestinal pH; it is denatured below pH 3 and has a pH optimum between 6 and 7. The lactase activity in the bowel lumen is enhanced by the alkaline bile, although the β-galactosidase–producing organisms are not anticipated to grow in the lumen of the intestine. Despite these advantages of yogurt, HBT has made it possible to appreciate that yogurts are not equivalent in their ability to provide lactase activity, reduce hydrogen production, and relieve symptoms of intolerance. HBTs have demonstrated that the advantages of yogurt are limited by pasteurization and freezing; frozen yogurt is not much better than milk or ice cream. Moreover, flavored varieties are less efficacious. Adding yogurt to a lactose-containing diet does not improve carbohydrate absorption, indicating that the β-galactosidase enzyme is already saturated by the lactose in yogurt.[109]

Abdominal Pain

HBTs have a role in the management of patients with nonspecific recurrent abdominal pain because malabsorbed carbohydrates, be they lactose, sorbitol, stachyose, or other sugars, can cause pain even in the absence of diarrhea. Children with recurrent abdominal pain and LM by HBT improve on a milk-free diet.[110] The pain caused by LM, however, cannot be readily distinguished from that of irritable bowel syndrome.[111] Controlled studies suggest that LM is not a major cause of recurrent abdominal pain in our society. A similar incidence of LM is found among children with abdominal pain and control populations, and a similar proportion of children with and without LM improve with dietary therapy.[112, 113] There may, however, be an important interaction between organic pathology, LM, and abdominal pain. Patients with LM and irritable bowel syndrome or inflammatory bowel disease may develop symptomatic malabsorption on lower dietary levels of the offending carbohydrate. Although the identification of LM should not assure one that the explanation for abdominal pain has been defined, judicious withdrawal of lactose in these situations is indicated.[114]

Even less convincing is the association between LM and infantile colic. "Colic" is often ascribed to intestinal pathology, and a positive HBT has been described in some of these infants. A causal relationship is hard to prove because young infants are "physiologically" predisposed to carbohydrate malabsorption, the addition of soy polysaccharide to the formulas increases hydrogen production but not discomfort, and the increase in hydrogen could be due to accelerated small bowel transit in infants with colic.[115, 116]

Diarrhea

Hydrogen breath testing is used to elucidate the cause of diarrhea, which is the most evident symptom of carbohydrate malabsorption. Failure to assimilate lactose regularly causes diarrhea in such common childhood illnesses as enteric infection, protein allergy, gluten enteropathy, and malnutrition. Testing for LM is valid because continued administration of lactose in the face of chronic diarrhea increases losses of nitrogen and fat as well as carbohydrate calories; children with diarrhea persisting beyond 14 days grow poorly.[117, 118]

Children with acute infectious enteritis have a high incidence of false-negative HBT results, and the role of the test under these circumstances is therefore questionable.[37, 119] There are a number of possible explanations for the poor results: vomiting of the test dose, an inadequate fast with high baseline values, and the recent use of antibiotics. The most likely explanation, however, is the development of a low luminal pH and its effect on fermentation of unabsorbed carbohydrate. This effect is most evident when the diarrhea is at its worst; however, a window exists between normal and severe malabsorption in which the breath test is a sensitive index of the carbohydrate mass reaching the colon. Thus, in patients with acute enteritis, the HBT has been used to confirm the high incidence of secondary lactose and low incidence of secondary sucrose malabsorption, predict which infants will tolerate milk, predict which patients are likely to require a prolonged hospital stay, and demonstrate the advantage of continuous versus bolus feedings and the more efficient assimilation of glucose in contrast to glucose polymers.[120, 121]

CARBON DIOXIDE BREATH TESTS

CO_2 is an end product of substrate metabolism for energy production, and a relatively constant quantity of the gas is cleared in breath. An organic compound has the potential to be a substrate for these breath tests if its unique chemical structure permits it only to enter into metabolism by specific organs in relevant metabolic pathways that yield CO_2. The critical carbon must be labeled to allow its separation from the rest of expired CO_2. Labeling is accomplished by employing the radioactive beta-emitting ^{14}C isotope or the heavy ^{13}C isotope. For most tests, less than 10 μc of ^{14}C is necessary, a dose that offers less irradiation than a chest radiograph, but the ^{14}C can be incorporated in fat and cycled in the body for the duration of the patient's life. Therefore in pediatrics, ^{13}C substrates are preferred.[122] These heavy isotopes of carbon have an extra neutron in the nucleus, which increases their mass without affecting their chemical reactivity. A mass spectrometer is necessary to identify heavy carbon, and despite refinements in the technology, widespread application is limited by the expense of the substrates and the availability of the detector.[1, 123, 124]

An interval sampling procedure has considerably simplified the technique. The breath passes through a mixture of hyamine hydroxide and the indicator thaimolphthalein. The specific activity of ^{13}C in CO_2 is determined by mass spectrometry. CO_2 in millimeters per kilogram per hour is calculated, and the results are expressed as a percentage of the administered dose.[125] Considering the many factors that affect substrate assimilation, i.e., gastric emptying, intestinal transit time, digestion, and absorption; the variety of CO_2 pools in the body; and the variables that affect minute ventilation, the CO_2 breath tests are proving remarkably reliable. They have been applied to the evaluation of fat and carbohydrate absorption,[126, 127] bacterial overgrowth,[128] *Helicobacter* gastritis,[129] and assessment of liver function.[128]

Fat Absorption

A fat balance study, comparing oral intake and fecal losses, is presently considered the most accurate means of detecting steatorrhea, but breath testing would be a welcome replacement for these unpleasant, time-consuming investigations.[130] An ideal test would establish the presence of steatorrhea and whether the rate-limiting step in fat assimilation was lipolysis or mucosal absorption.[131] To accomplish this, triglycerides and cholesterol esters have been employed as substrates. The terminal carboxyl carbon of some or all of their fatty acids are labeled with either ^{14}C or ^{13}C carbon isotopes. Triolein, which incorporates medium-chain triglycerides, has gained acceptance as a sensitive screen for steatorrhea; it has been effectively applied to patients with pancreatic insufficiency, celiac, and Crohn's disease.[126, 132, 133] To distinguish defects in lipolysis from those resulting from mucosal disease, the test can be repeated with the triolein administered in conjunction with pancreatic lipase.[134] The specificity of this approach is, however, limited because the medium-chain fatty acids can be assimilated by the injured mucosa.[135] An alternative strategy is to do sequential breath tests with triolein; palmitic acid, a fatty acid that does not require lipolysis for absorption; and trioctanoin, a triglyceride whose short-chain fatty acids readily cross even an injured mucosa. All three substrates evolve CO_2 in normal individuals, only palmitic acid does so in patients with pancreatic insufficiency, and only trioctanoin and to a lesser extent triolein do so in patients with mucosal disease. A more recent innovation suggested to detect and follow the treatment of pancreatic disease is the use of ^{13}C octanoyl.[136] The labeled octanoic acid is attached to the second carbon of glycerol sandwiched between the two unlabeled long-chain fatty acids. The rate-limiting step is lipolysis, which must first release the outer fatty acids before having impact on ^{13}C octanoyl monoglyceride, whose absorption is not impeded by the mucosa. False-positive test results occur in celiac disease primarily because of failed pancreatic stimulation owing to inadequate release of cholecystokinin from the involved mucosa. Cholesteryl 1-^{14}C octanoate can also be used to assess pancreatic lipase activity, the advantage of the substrate being its resistance to hydrolysis by salivary and gastric lipase. It too has been effectively used to diagnose overt steatorrhea, but its efficiency for mild cases requires further study.[137]

Carbohydrate Absorption

The $^{13}CO_2$ breath tests have been applied to measure lactose, starch, glucose polymers, and glucose absorption. The tests have a role to play because many of the limitations of hydrogen breath testing, such as the high baseline values, lack of hydrogen-producing organisms in patients on antibiotics, and the need for unphysiologic carbohydrate doses, are overcome. Small doses of the carbohydrate substrate are used because only trace amounts of the label are necessary. An inexpensive, highly enriched source of ^{13}C lactose can be purchased. For starch, glucose polymers, and glucose, advantage is taken of corn's naturally enriched ^{13}C content. Discrimination is enhanced by ensuring that the test dose is given in a ^{13}C depleted formula or meal.[138] These tests are not a measure of carbohydrate malabsorption; rather, they are an index of carbohydrate assimilation and therefore the digestive absorptive efficiency of the small bowel. The cumulative percent of CO_2 recovered in 4 hours accurately discriminates normals from patients with impaired digestive absorptive pathways.[1, 139, 140] The sensitivity and specificity of these tests compare favorably with HBTs, and in the case of lactose malabsorption, the CO_2 breath test correlates closely with mucosal lactase activity.[141] A ^{13}C starch test has been successfully used to differentiate normal patients from those with pancreatic disease and to measure the relative absorption of different starches and glucose polymer substrates.[142] Lifschitz and colleagues[143] have applied $^{13}CO_2$ breath testing to glucose absorption by children. For glucose absorption, the HBT is limited because infants normally malabsorb dietary carbohydrate, they require to be fasted, and unphysiologic amounts of the carbohydrate need to be administered. The hydrogen produced reflects bacterial overgrowth or rapid transit of the glucose rather than limited absorptive capacity, and as mentioned, the test is frequently negative in the presence of severe diarrhea. The ^{13}C glucose breath test identifies patients with glucose-galactose malabsorption, and the pattern of glucose assimilation is similar to that for patients with severe diarrhea.[143]

Bacterial Overgrowth

The ability of bacteria to deconjugate bile salts can be used to identify bacterial overgrowth. A substrate of choline linked to labeled glycine is employed. Once the amino acid is separated from the bile salt, it is either fermented by luminal bacteria or absorbed and metabolized by the body to yield labeled CO_2. Therefore abnormally high concentrations of labeled breath CO_2 indicate deconjugation and implicate bacterial overgrowth. By comparison to luminal intubation, the ^{14}C choleglycine test has a specificity of 90% and a sensitivity of 70%. A ^{13}C choleglycine test has not been extensively used in children.[121] A potential source of error with the choleglycine test would be CO_2 evolution of the substrate by the colonic flora, as would be anticipated in patients with ileal resection or disease. An alternative to the choleglycine test is ^{14}C-labeled D-xylose, which is able to distinguish patients with overgrowth from controls. Xylose is a suitable substrate for luminal evolution of CO_2, but it does not enter the body's metabolic pool to yield endogenous carbon dioxide. A ^{13}C version of this promising substrate is yet to be tested in children.[128]

Urea Breath Tests

A CO_2 breath test has been developed as a simple noninvasive means for identifying *Helicobacter pylori*. This organism colonizes the stomach in association with gastric ulcers, duodenal ulcers, nonulcer dyspepsia, and gastritis. It has a remarkably high endogenous urease activity, which is exploited in the test by providing the patient ^{13}C or ^{14}C urea in a meal that has a considerable fat content to delay gastric emptying. The ^{13}C study is a highly sensitive and specific research tool for population surveys, and it effectively monitors *Helicobacter's* response to therapy. For the ^{14}C breath test, a rather small radioactive dose of 3 μc of ^{14}C is needed to obtain similar results.[129]

Aminopyrine and Erythromycin Breath Tests

Routine tests are inadequate measures of hepatic metabolic ability, and therefore a variety of drugs that depend on the integrity of the liver for metabolism have been proposed as sensitive probes of liver function. Aminopyrine and erythromycin are dependent on the hepatic microsomal P450 system for metabolism and can be used in breath tests because both yield CO_2 in proportion to their clearance from the blood stream. The clearance of aminopyrine from the blood stream is low, and CO_2 evolution is therefore dependent on its metabolism and not hepatic blood flow. The probe has proved to be a convincing measure of the severity of chronic hepatitis, cirrhosis, and acetaminophen poisoning and may provide the means to anticipate graft rejection after liver transplantation.[144-146] The erythromycin breath test has been ingeniously used to predict the dosing levels of cyclosporine necessary to maintain therapeutic blood levels. Because both erythromycin and cyclosporine depend on the liver P450IIIA system for metabolism, CO_2 production from erythromycin predicts cyclosporine blood levels and can be used to estimate initial dosing requirements.[147, 148]

UNIQUE BREATH GASES

There are a few breath tests characterized by the measurement of a gas not normally exhaled in breath. Examples include pentane, which is discussed, and others such as ammonia, which do not as yet have a significant role in clinical medicine.

Pentane Breath Test

Breath tests offer the potential to identify lipid peroxidation and to monitor the impact that free radical scavengers such as vitamin E have in restricting this injurious process. Peroxidation of omega-6 fatty acids produces pentane, and high levels of the gas can be dissipated on administration of vitamin E. Serum vitamin E levels relate directly to breath pentane levels.

Pentane can be reliably measured in breath after a 2-minute washout period during which hydrocarbon-free air is inhaled. A cumulative breath sample is obtained from which the hydrocarbon is concentrated by passage over cooling alumina. The sample is injected onto a stainless steel column containing Porasil-D, and the eluted pentane peak is detected by flame ionization.[149]

REFERENCES

1. Klein PD, Klein ER: Applications of stable isotopes to pediatric nutrition and gastroenterology: Measurement of nutrient absorption and digestion using ^{13}C. J Pediatr Gastroenterol Nutr 1985; 4:9–19.
2. Levitt MD: Production and excretion of hydrogen gas in man. N Engl J Med 1969; 281:122–127.
3. Bond JH, Levitt MD: Use of pulmonary hydrogen (H_2) measurements to quantitate carbohydrate absorption. Study of partially gastrectomized patients. J Clin Invest 1972; 51:1219–1225.
4. Fleming SC: Evaluation of a hand-held hydrogen monitor in the diagnosis of intestinal lactase deficiency. Ann Clin Biochem 1990; 27:499–500.
5. Nose O, Iada Y, Kai H, et al: Breath hydrogen test for detecting lactose malabsorption in infants and children. Prevalence of lactose malabsorption in Japanese children and adults. Arch Dis Child 1979; 54:436–440.
6. Hyams JS, Stafford RJ, Grand RJ, et al: Correlation of lactose breath hydrogen test, intestinal morphology, and lactase activity in young children. J Pediatr 1980; 97:609–612.
7. Perman JA, Barr RG, Watkins JB: Sucrose malabsorption in children: Noninvasive diagnosis by interval breath hydrogen determination. J Pediatr 1978; 93:17–22.
8. Flatz G, Henze HJ, Palabiyikoglu E, et al: Distribution of the adult lactase phenotypes in Turkey. Trop Geogr Med 1986; 38:255–258.
9. Brand JC, Darnton-Hill I, Gracey MS, et al: Lactose malabsorption in Australian Aboriginal children. Am J Clin Nutr 1985; 41:620–622.
10. Caskey DA, Payne-Bose D, Welsh JD, et al: Effects of age on lactose malabsorption in Oklahoma native Americans as determined by breath H_2 analysis. Am J Dig Dis 1977; 22:113–116.
11. Rhodes JM, Middelton P, Jewell DP: The lactulose hydrogen breath test as a diagnostic test for small-bowel overgrowth. Scand J Gastroenterol 1979; 14:333–336.
12. King CE, Toskes PP: Breath tests in the diagnosis of small intestine bacterial overgrowth. CRC Crit Rev Clin Lab Sci 1984; 21:269–281.

13. Bond JH, Levitt MD: Investigation of small bowel transit time in man utilizing pulmonary hydrogen meaurements. J Lab Clin Med 1975; 85:546–555.
14. Korth H, Muller I, Erckenbrecht WM: Breath hydrogen as a test for gastrointestinal transit. Hepatogastroenterology 1984; 31:282–284.
15. Ruge E: Bewitrage zur Kentniss der Darmgase. Chem-Zentrabl 1862; 7:347–351.
16. Nielsen JP: Trace constituents in breath as related to flatulence. Proceedings of the Fifth Annual Bean Research Conference. Denver, Western Regional Research Laboratory, U.S. Department of Agriculture, 1961, p 49.
17. Vreugdenhil G, Sinaasappel M, Bouquet J: A comparative study of the mouth to caecum transit time in children and adults using a weight adapted lactulose dose. Acta Paediatr Scand 1986; 75:483–488.
18. Gilat T, BenHur H, Gelmen-Malachi E, et al: Alterations of the colonic flora and their effect on the hydrogen breath test. Gut 1978; 19:602–605.
19. Solomons NW, Viteri F, Rosenberg IH: Development of an interval sampling hydrogen (H_2) breath test for carbohydrate malabsorption in children: Evidence for a circadian pattern of breath H_2 concentration. Pediatr Res 1978; 12:816–823.
20. Perman JA, Modler S, Engel RR: Effect of ventilation on breath hydrogen measurements. J Lab Clin Med 1985; 105:436–439.
21. Metz G, Gassuei MA, Doasar BS: Breath hydrogen-test for small intestinal bacterial colonization. Lancet 1976; 1:668–669.
22. Wollan MJ: Fermentation in the rumen and human large intestine. Science 1981; 213:1463–1468.
23. Glober GA, Kamiyama S, Nomura A, et al: Bowel transit-time and stool weight in populations with different colon-cancer risks. Lancet 1977; 2:110–111.
24. Murphy EL, Calloway DH: The effect of antibiotic drugs on the volume and composition of intestinal gas from beans. Am J Dig Dis 1972; 17:639–642.
25. Metz G, Jenkins DJA, Blendis LM: Lactose hydrogen (H_2) breath test in health and disease. Gut 1976; 17:397.
26. Joseph F, Rosenberg A: Breath hydrogen testing: Disease versus normal patients. J Pediatr Gastroenterol Nutr 1988; 7:787–788.
27. Perman JA, Modler S, Olson AC: Role of pH production of hydrogen from carbohydrates by colonic bacterial flora. J Clin Invest 1981; 67:643–650.
28. Stephen AM, Wiggins HS, Englyst HN, et al: The effect of age, sex, and level of intake of dietary fibre from wheat on large-bowel function in thirty healthy subjects. Br J Nutr 1986; 56:349–361.
29. Rumessen JJ, Gudmand-Hoyer E: Functional bowel disease: Malabsorption and abdominal distress after ingestion of fructose, sorbitol, and fructose-sorbitol mixtures. Gastroenterology 1988; 95:694–700.
30. Nelis GF, Vermeeren MA, Jasen W: Role of fructose-sorbitol malabsorption in the irritable bowel syndrome. Gastroenterology 1990; 99:1016–1020.
31. Englyst HW, Cummings JH: Digestion of the polysaccharides of some cereal foods in the human small intestine. Am J Clin Nutr 1985; 42:778–787.
32. Stephen AM, Haddad AC, Phillips SF: Passage of carbohydrate into the colon. Direct measurements in humans. Gastroenterology 1983; 85:589–595.
33. Flourie B, Leblond A, Florent CH, et al: Starch malabsorption and breath gas excretion in healthy humans consuming low- and high-starch diets. Gastroenterology 1988; 95:356–363.
34. Koruda MJ, Rolandelli RH, Zimmaro DM, et al: Parenteral nutrition supplemented with short-chain fatty acids: Effect on the small bowel mucosa in normal rats. Am J Clin Nutr 1990; 51:685–689.
35. Shinnick FL, Hess RL, Fischer MH, et al: Apparent nutrient absorption and upper gastrointestinal transit with fiber-containing enteral feedings. Am J Clin Nutr 1989; 49:471–475.
36. Welch IM, Cunningham KM, Read NW: Regulation of gastric emptying by ileal nutrients in humans. Gastroenterology 1988; 94:401–404.
37. Solomons NW, Garcia-Ibanez R, Viteri FE: Reduced rates of breath hydrogen (H_2) excretion with lactose tolerance tests in young children using whole milk. Am J Clin Nutr 1979; 32:783–786.
38. Perman JA, Modler S, Barr RG, et al: Fasting breath hydrogen concentration: Normal values and clinical application. Gastroenterology 1984; 87:1358–1363.
39. Read NW, Miles CA, Fisher D, et al: Transit of a meal through the stomach, small intestine, and colon in normal subjects and its role in the pathogenesis of diarrhea. Gastroenterology 1980; 79:1276–1282.
40. Mastropaola G, Rees WDW: Evaluation of the hydrogen breath test in man: Definition and elimination of the early hydrogen peak. Gut 1987; 28:721–725.
41. Perman JA, Modler S: Glycoproteins as substrates for production of hydrogen and methane by colonic bacterial flora. Gastroenterology 1982; 83:388–393.
42. Corazza GR, Strocchi A, Gasbarrini G: Fasting breath hydrogen in celiac disease. Gastroenterology 1987; 93:53–58.
43. Gibson GR, Cummings JG, MacFarlane GT, et al: Alternative pathways for hydrogen disposal during fermentation in the human colon. Gut 1990; 31:679–683.
44. Cloarec D, Bornet F, Gouilloud S: Breath hydrogen response to lactulose in healthy subjects: Relationship to methane producing status. Gut 1990; 31:300–304.
45. Flick JA, Perman JA: Nonabsorbed carbohydrate: Effect on fecal pH in methane-excreting and nonexcreting individuals. Am J Clin Nutr 1989; 49:1252–1257.
46. Mobassaleh M, Montgomery RK, Biller JA, et al: Development of carbohydrate absorption in the fetus and neonate. Pediatrics 1985; 75:160–166.
47. MacLean WC, Fink BB: Lactose malabsorption by premature infants: Magnitude and clinical significance. J Pediatr 1980; 97:383–388.
48. Barr RG, Hanley J, Patterson DK, et al: Breath hydrogen excretion in normal newborn infants in response to usual feeding patterns: Evidence for "functional lactase insufficiency" beyond the first month of life. J Pediatr 1984; 104:527–533.
49. Heine W, Zunft HJ, Muller-Bethow W, et al: Lactose and protein absorption from breast milk and cow's milk preparations and its influence on the intestinal flora. Acta Paediatr Scand 1977; 66:699–703.
50. Staniforth DH, Rose D: Statistical analysis of the lactulose/breath hydrogen test in the measurement of orocaecal transit: Its variability and predictive value in assessing drug action. Gut 1989; 30:171–175.
51. Solomons NW, Viteri FE: Breath hydrogen during sleep. Lancet 1976; 2:636.
52. Payne DL, Welsh JD, Claypool PL: Breath hydrogen (H_2) response to carbohydrate malabsorption after exercise. J Lab Clin Med 1983; 102:147–150.
53. Niu H, Schoeller DA, Klein PD: Improved gas chromatographic quantitation of breath hydrogen by normalization to respiratory carbon dioxide. J Lab Clin Med 1979; 94:755–763.
54. Solomons NW: Application of a simple gas chromatographic technique for measuring breath hydrogen. J Lab Clin Med 1977; 90:856–862.
55. Howall JN, van Der Fecht R, Flatz G: Hydrogen breath test for lactose tolerance adapted to population screening. Clin Chim Acta 1980; 103:229–231.
56. Stevenson DK, Cohen RS, Ostrander CR, et al: A sensitive analytical apparatus for measuring hydrogen production rates. II. Application to studies in human infants. J Pediatr Gastroenterol Nutr 1982; 1:233–237.
57. Kien CL, Liechty EA, Myerberg DZ, et al: Effects in premature infants of normalizing breath hydrogen concentrations with CO_2: Increased H_2 concentration and reduced interaliquot variation. J Pediatr Gastroenterol Nutr 1986; 6:286–289.
58. Kneepens CMF, Bijleveld MA, Vonk RJ, et al: The daytime breath hydrogen profile in children with abdominal symptoms and diarrhoea. Acta Paediatr Scand 1986; 75:632–638.
59. Young CY, Ma YP, Wong FHW, et al: Automatic end-expiratory air sampling device for breath hydrogen test in infants. Lancet 1991; 337:90–93.
60. Rumessen J, Gudmand-Hoyer E: Retention and variability of hydrogen (H_2) samples stored in plastic syringes. Scand J Lab Invest 1987; 47:627–630.
61. Murry RD, Kerzner B, MacLean WC, et al: Efficient storage system for breath hydrogen. J Pediatr Gastroenterol Nutr 1985; 4:711–713.

62. Newcomer AD, McGill DB, Thomas PI, et al: Prospective comparison of indirect methods for detecting lactase deficiency N Engl J Med 1975; 293:1232–1236.
63. Metz G, Blendis LM, Jenkins DJA: Hydrogen breath test for lactase deficiency. N Engl J Med 1976; 294:730.
64. Barr RG, Watkins JB, Perman JA: Mucosal function and breath hydrogen excretion: Comparative studies in the clinical evaluation of children with nonspecific abdominal complaints. Pediatrics 1981; 68:526–533.
65. Davidson GP, Robb TA: Value of breath hydrogen analysis in management of diarrheal illness in childhood: Comparison with duodenal biopsy. J Pediatr Gastroenterol Nutr 1985: 4:381–387.
66. Hyams JS, Stafford RJ, Grand RJ, et al: Correlation of lactose breath hydrogen test, intestinal morphology, and lactase activity in young children. J Pediatr 1980; 97:609–612.
67. Ting CW, Hwang B, Wu TC: Developmental changes of lactose malabsorption in normal Chinese children: A study using breath hydrogen test with a physiological dose of lactose. J Pediatr Gastroenterol Nutr 1988; 7:848–851.
68. Flatz G, Kuhnau W, Naftali D: Breath hydrogen test for lactose absorption capacity: Importance of timing of hydrogen excretion and of high fasting hydrogen concentration. Am J Clin Nutr 1984; 39:752–755.
69. Abramowitz A, Granot E, Tamir I, et al: Two-hour lactose breath hydrogen test. J Pediatr Gastroenterol Nutr 1986; 5:130–133.
70. Ceriani R, Zuin G, Paccagninis S: Two-hour lactose breath hydrogen tests. J Pediatr Gastroenterol Nutr 1986; 6:995–996.
71. Robb TA, Davidson GP: Two-hour lactose breath hydrogen test (letter). J Pediatr Gastroenterol Nutr 1987; 6:481–482.
72. Solomons NW, Barillas C: The cut-off criterion for a positive hydrogen breath test in childen: A reappraisal. J Pediatr Gastroenterol Nutr 1986; 5:920–925.
73. Robb TA, Davidson GP: Advances in breath hydrogen in quantitation in pediatric sample collection and normalization to constant oxygen and nitrogen levels. Clin Chim Acta 1981; 111:281–283.
74. Douwes AC, Fernandes J, Jongbloed AA: Diagnostic value of sucrose tolerance test in children evaluated by breath hydrogen measurement. Acta Paediatr Scand 1980; 69:79–82.
75. Ford RPK, Barnes GL: Breath hydrogen test and sucrase isomaltase deficiency. Arch Dis Child 1983; 58:595–597.
76. Metz G, Jenkins JA, Newman A, et al: Breath hydrogen in hyposucrasia. Lancet 1976; 1:119–120.
77. Davidson GP, Robb TA: Detection of primary and secondary sucrose malabsorption in children by means of breath hydrogen technique. Med J Aust 1983; 2:29–32.
78. Ravich WJ, Bayless TM, Thomas M: Fructose: Incomplete intestinal absorption in humans. Gastroenterology 1983; 84:26–29.
79. Barnes G, McKellar W, Lawrance S: Detection of fructose malabsorption by breath hydrogen test in a child with diarrhea. J Pediatr 1983; 103:575–577.
80. Kneepens CM, Vonk RJ, Fernandes J: Incomplete intestinal absorption of fructose. Arch Dis Child 1984; 59:735–738.
81. Hyams JS: Sorbitol intolerance: An unappreciated cause of functional gastrointestinal complaints. J Pediatr 1983; 84:30–33.
82. Truswell AS, Seach JM, Thorburn AW: Incomplete absorption of pure fructose in healthy subjects and the facilitating effect of glucose. Am J Clin Nutr 1988; 48:1424–1430.
83. Levine AS, Tallman JR, Grace MK: Effect of breakfast cereals on short term food intake. Am J Clin Nutr 1989; 50:1303–1307.
84. Shulman RJ, Kerzner B, Sloan HR, et al: Absorption and oxidation of glucose polymers of different lengths in young infants. Pediatr Res 1986; 20:740–743.
85. Kerlin P, Wong L, Harris B, et al: Rice flour, breath hydrogen, and malabsorption. Gastroenterology 1984; 87:578–585.
86. Davidson GP, Robb TA, Kirubakaran CP: Bacterial contamination of the small intestine as an important cause of chronic diarrhea and abdominal pain: Diagnosis by breath hydrogen test. Pediatrics 1984; 74:229–235.
87. Piquata C, Budillon G, Manaco G, et al: Jejunal bacterial overgrowth and intestinal permeability in children with immune deficiency syndrome. Gut 1990; 31:879–882.
88. Smith GM, Chester IM, Asquith P, et al: Small intestinal bacterial overgrowth in patients with chronic lymphocytic leukemia. J Clin Pathol 1990; 43:57–59.
89. Metz G, Gassull MA, Drasar BS, et al: Breath-hydrogen test for small-intestinal bacterial colonisation. Lancet 1976; 1:668–669.
90. Perman JA, Modler S: Glycoproteins as substrates for production of hydrogen and methane by colonic bacterial flora. Gastroenterology 1982; 83:388–393.
91. Perman JA, Modler S, Barr RG, et al: Fasting breath hydrogen concentration: Normal values and clinical application. Gastroenterology 1984; 87:1358–1363.
92. Corazza GR, Menozzi MG, Stocchi A, et al: Diagnosis of small bowel bacterial overgrowth. Reliability of jejunal culture and inadequacy of breath hydrogen testing. Gastroenterology 1990; 98:302–309.
93. Kerlin P, Wong L: Breath hydrogen testing in bacterial overgrowth of the small intestine. Gastroenterology 1988; 95:982–988.
94. King CE, Toskes PP: Comparison of the 1-gram [^{14}C] xylose, 10-gram lactulose-H_2 and 80-gram glucose H_2 breath tests in patients with small intestine bacterial overgrowth. Gastroenterology 1986; 91:1447–1451.
95. Read NW: Small bowel transit time of food in man: Measurement, regulation and possible importance. Scand J Gastroenterol 1984; 19(Suppl 96):77–85.
96. Saunders DR, Wiggins HS: Conservation of mannitol, lactulose and raffinose by the human colon. Am J Physiol 1981; 241:397–402.
97. Staniforth DH: Comparison of orocaecal transit times assessed by the lactulose/breath hydrogen and the sulphasalazine/sulphapyridine methods. Gut 1989; 30:978–982.
98. Davidson GP: Lactase deficiency: Diagnosis and management. Med J Aust 1984; 141:442–443.
99. Rosado JL, Solomons NW, Lisker R, et al: Enzyme replacement therapy for primary adult lactase deficiency. Gastroenterology 1984; 87:1072–1082.
100. Tor'un B, Solomons NW, Viteri FE: Lactose malabsorption and lactose intolerance: Implications for general milk consumption. Arch Latinoam Nutr 1979; 29:445–494.
101. Lisker R, Aguilar L, Lares I, et al: Double blind study of milk lactose intolerance in a group of rural and urban children. Am J Clin Nutr 1980; 33:1049–1053.
102. Martini MC, Kukielka D, Savaiano DA: Lactose digestion from yogurt: Influence of a meal and additional lactose. Am J Clin Nutr 1991; 53:1253–1258.
103. Brown KH: Nutritional consequences of low dose milk supplements consumed by lactose-malabsorbing children. Am J Clin Nutr 1980; 33:1054–1063.
104. Kwon PH Jr, Rorick MH, Scrimshaw NS: Comparative tolerance of adolescents of differing ethnic backgrounds to lactose-containing and lactose-free dairy drinks. II. Improvement of a double-blind test. Am J Clin Nutr 1980; 33:22–26.
105. Payne DL, Welsh JD, Manion CV, et al: Effectiveness of milk products in dietary management of lactose malabsorption. Am J Clin Nutr 1981; 34:2711–2715.
106. Lee CM, Hardy CM: Cocoa feeding and human lactose intolerance. Am J Clin Nutr 1989; 49:840–844.
107. Medow MS, Thek KD, Newman LJ, et al: β-Galactosidase tablets in the treatment of lactose intolerance in pediatrics. Am J Dis Child 1990; 144:1261–1264.
108. Savaiano DA, AbouElAnouar A, Smith DE, et al: Lactose malabsorption from yogurt, pasteurized yogurt, sweet acidophilus milk, and cultured milk in lactase-deficient individuals. Am J Clin Nutr 1984; 40:1219–1223.
109. Martini MC, Kukielka D, Savaiano DA: Lactose digestion from yogurt: Influence of a meal and additional lactose. Am J Clin Nutr 1991; 53:1253–1258.
110. Barr RG, Levine MD, Watkins JB: Recurrent abdominal pain of childhood due to lactose intolerance. N Engl J Med 1979; 300:1449–1452.
111. Newcomer AD, McGill DB: Irritable bowel syndrome. Role of lactase deficiency. Mayo Clin Proc 1983; 58:339–341.
112. Lebenthal E, Rossi TM, Nord KS, et al: Recurrent abdominal pain and lactose absorption in children. Pediatrics 1981; 67:828–832.

113. Wald A, Chandra R, Fisher SE, et al: Lactose malabsorption in recurrent abdominal pain of childhood. J Pediatr 1982; 100:65–68.
114. Kirschner BS, DeFavaro MV, Jensen W: Lactose malabsorption in children and adolescents with inflammatory bowel disease. Gastroenterology 1981; 81:829–832.
115. Liebman WM: Infantile colic. Association with lactose and milk intolerance. JAMA 1981; 245:732–733.
116. Treem WR, Hyams JS, Blankschen E, et al: Evaluation of the effect of a fiber-enriched formula on infant colic. J Pediatr 1991; 119:695–701.
117. Penny ME, Paredes P, Brown KH: Clinical and nutritional consequences of lactose feeding during persistent postenteritis diarrhea. Pediatrics 1989; 84:835–844.
118. Black RE, Brown KH, Becker S: Effects of diarrhea associated with specific enteropathogens on the growth of children in rural Bangladesh. Pediatrics 1984; 73:799–805.
119. Gardiner AJ, Tarlow MJ, Sutherland IT, et al: Lactose malabsorption during gastroenteritis, assessed by the hydrogen breath test. Arch Dis Child 1981; 56:364–367.
120. Davidson GP, Goodwin D, Robb TA: Incidence and duration of lactose malabsorption in children hospitalized with acute enteritis: Study in a well-nourished urban population. J Pediatr 1984; 105:587–590.
121. Lifschitz CH, Irving CS, Gopalakrishna GS: Carbohydrate malabsorption in infants with diarrhea studied with the breath hydrogen test. J Pediatr 1983; 102:371–375.
122. Phaysen EH: Diagnostic value of the ^{13}C-cholylglycine breath test. Clin Gastroenterol 1977; 6:277–245.
123. McGaw BA, Milne E, Duncan GJ: A rapid method for the preparation of combustion samples for stable carbon intake analysis by isotope ratio mass spectrometry. Biomed Environ Mass Spectrom 1988; 16:269–273.
124. Schoeller DA, Schneider JF, Solomons NW: Clinical diagnosis with the stable isotope ^{13}C in CO_2 breath tests: Methodology and fundamental considerations. J Lab Clin Med 1977; 90:412–421.
125. Schoeller DA, Klein PD: A simplified technique for collecting breath CO_2 for isotope ratio mass spectrometry. Biomed Mass Spectrom 1978; 5:29–31.
126. Butler RN, Lawson MI, Gohling NJ, et al: Clinical evaluation of the ^{14}C-triolein breath test: A critical analysis. Aust NZ Med 1984; 14:111–113.
127. Ghoos Y, Vantrappen G, Rutgeerts P: The ^{13}C lactose breath test using naturally labelled lactose for the diagnosis of lactose malabsorption. Gastroenterology 1986; 90:1426.
128. Hepner GW, Vessel ES: Quantitative assessment of hepatic function by breath analysis after oral administration of [^{14}C] aminopyrine. Ann Intern Med 1975; 83:632–638.
129. Marshall BJ, Plankey MW, Hoffman SR, et al: A 20 minute breath test for Helicobacter pylori. Am J Gastroenterol 1991; 86:438–445.
130. Levy-Gigi C, Madelowitz N, Peled Y, et al: Is the fat breath test effective in the diagnosis of fat malabsorption and pancreatic disease? Digestion 1978; 18:77–85.
131. Strange RC, Reid J, Holton D, et al: The glyceryl (^{14}C) ripalmitate breath test: A reassessment. Clin Chim Acta 1980; 103:317–323.
132. Newcomer AD, Hofmann AF, Dimagno EP, et al: Triolein breath test. A sensitive and specific test for fat malabsorption. Gastroenterology 1979; 76:6–13.
133. Einarsson K, Bjorkhem I, Eklof R, et al: ^{14}C-triolein breath test as a rapid and convenient screening test for fat malabsorption. Scand J Gastroenterol 1983; 18:9–12.
134. Goff JS: Two-stage triolein breath test differentiates pancreatic insufficiency from other causes of malabsorption. Gastroenterology 1982; 83:44–46.
135. Watkins JB, Klein PD, Schoeller DA, et al: Diagnosis and differentiation of fat malabsorption in children using ^{13}C-labeled lipids: Trictonoin, triolein, and palmitic acid breath tests. Gastroenterology 1982; 82:911–917.
136. Vantrappen GR, Rutgeerts PJ, Ghoos YF, et al: Mixed triglyceride breath test: A noninvasive test of pancreatic lipase activity in the duodenum. Gastroenterology 1989; 96:1126–1134.
137. Cole SG, Rossi S, Stern A, et al: Cholesteryl octanoate breath test. Preliminary studies on a new noninvasive test of human pancreatic exocrine function. Gastroenterology 1987; 93:1372–1380.
138. Boutton TW, Hopkinson JM, Benton DA, et al: Background levels of carbon–13 reduced in breath and stool by new infant formula. J Pediatr Gastroenterol Nutr 1988; 7:723–731.
139. Klein PD: Clinical applications of $^{13}CO_2$ measurements. Fed Proc 1982; 41:2698–2701.
140. Lacroix M, Masora F, Pontus M, et al: Glucose naturally labeled with carbon 13: Use for metabolic studies in man. Science 1973; 181:445–446.
141. Hiele M, Ghoos Y, Rutgeerts P, et al: $^{13}CO_2$ breath test using naturally enriched lactose for the detection of lactase deficiency in patients with gastrointestinal symptoms. J Lab Clin Med 1988; 112:193–200.
142. Liele M, Ghoos Y, Rutgeerts P, et al: $^{13}CO_2$ breath test to measure the hydrolysis of various starch formulations in healthy subjects. Gut 1990; 31:175–178.
143. Lifschitz CH, Boutton TW, Carrazza F, et al: A carbon-13 breath test to characterize glucose absorption and utilization in children. J Pediatr Gastroenterol Nutr 1988; 7:842–847.
144. Oakland CD, Hickman R, Terblanche J: The aminopyrine breath test predicts the outcome of hepatic transplantation in pigs. Hepatology 1989; 9:602–605.
145. Baker AL, Kotake AH, Schoeller DA: Clinical ability of breath tests for the assessment of hepatic function. Semin Liver Dis 1982; 3:318–329.
146. Bircher J, Kupfer A, Gikalov I, et al: Aminopyrine demethylation measured by breath analysis in cirrhosis. Clin Pharmacol Ther 1976; 20:484–492.
147. Watkins PB, Murray SA, Winkelman LG, et al: Erythromycin breath test as an assay of glucocorticoid-inducible liver cytochromes P-450. J Clin Invest 1989; 83:688–697.
148. Watkins PB, Hamilton TA, Annesley TM, et al: The erythromycin breath test as a predictor of cyclosporine blood levels. Clin Pharmacol Ther 119; 48:120–129.
149. Lemoyne M, Van Gossum A, Kurian R, et al: Breath pentane analysis as an index of lipid peroxidation: A functional test of vitamin E status. Am J Clin Nutr 1987; 46:267–272.

Chapter 78

Gastrointestinal Imaging

SIMON C. S. KAO and E. A. FRANKEN, JR.

INTRODUCTION

The explosion in new imaging technologies during the last several years has substantially improved clinicians' ability to characterize many gastrointestinal diseases of children. As with many other disciplines, pediatric gastrointestinal imaging has become subspecialized. Except at the most comprehensive pediatric care institutions, it becomes necessary to modify the approach of imaging of pediatric disease. For instance, endoscopy by a skilled pediatric gastroenterologist is clearly a superior method for evaluating mucosal disease of the esophagus. However, in an institution without such a specialist, barium examination of the esophagus by a pediatric radiologist may be preferred to endoscopy by a physician not skilled in pediatric diagnosis. In like fashion, various imaging modalities, such as nuclear medicine, ultrasound, or magnetic resonance (MR) imaging, may be chosen for use at a particular hospital for a specific patient based more on the skills of the consulting radiologist than on the theoretical value of the particular type of study.

It is important that the attending physician gives considerable thought to the need for imaging in individual patients. In general, imaging examinations are requested when clinical diagnosis is uncertain and the study offers the possibility of raising the likely clinical diagnosis beyond action threshold.[1] Examination is often unnecessary if the clinical diagnosis is already confirmed or highly suspected. For example, ultrasound evaluation of possible appendicitis has its greatest value in those patients not already scheduled for emergency laparotomy. Conversely, to perform an ultrasound examination on those patients for whom surgery is already planned is redundant. Similarly, once one imaging study has allowed a firm diagnosis, a second study is usually unnecessary. An example would be performing an MR imaging examination to delineate a liver abscess that has already been detected by computed tomographic (CT) examination. However, additional imaging studies are sometimes needed for disease staging in patients in whom the diagnosis is already evident. Examples include small bowel enema for the initial staging of Crohn's disease and work-up for metastases in a patient with a known primary neoplasm.

Unfortunately, many pediatric patients are unable or unwilling to cooperate for their imaging study. For plain films and most barium examinations, immobilization using a variety of homemade or commercial devices may be necessary.[2] For those examinations that require considerable periods of time and in which patient motion is a significant adverse factor, sedation may be required. CT and MR imaging are often in this category.

At the authors' own institution, they have initiated protocols, in conjunction with consultants from the clinical services and from anesthesiology, so that sedation may be customized according to the child's needs and response. One must avoid the temptation not to involve the anesthesiologist when that physician's skills are needed for optimal patient safety. The authors' system involves identifying high-risk patients prospectively who will be handled primarily by the anesthesiologist. Examples would include patients on high dosages of barbiturates, those with known prior contrast reactions, acute trauma patients, and children who have had prior failures with regular sedation regimens.

Monitoring is necessary for patients receiving sedation in the radiology department and is particularly critical in MR imaging because it is difficult to observe patients directly.[3] Ideally, blood pressure, temperature, heart rate, respiratory rate, oxygen saturation, and tidal carbon dioxide should be monitored. Elements of a sedation program that must be in place include appropriate resuscitation facilities, parental involvement, a system for monitoring during scanning, and a routine for care and observation after completion of the examination.

Most radiologists sedate children for imaging procedures with chloral hydrate at a dose of 75 to 100 mg per kg orally with a maximum dose of 1 gm per dose or 2 gm per 24 hours. Intravenous nembutal to a sedative dose of about 5 mg per kg is recommended by other investigators. A variety of "cocktails" using narcotics and sedatives have been used over the years. Intravenous drugs such as diazepam (Valium) and very-short-acting narcotics are useful but are generally in the province of the anesthesiologist.

Contrast agents used for imaging examinations of children are in essence the same as those used for adults, with some important modifications as indicated later.[4] The type of contrast agent needed for examination of the pediatric gastrointestinal tract varies as to the type of examination desired and information required. Room air is sufficient to confirm esophageal atresia and duodenal atresia and to delineate the proximal bowel. If one does not overdistend the part being examined, there is no hazard.

Barium preparations are generally the agents of choice for examination of the esophagus, stomach, small bowel, and colon, unless perforation is suspected. Complications may result if there is leakage outside the gut, and occasionally if there is significant absorption of water from low-osmolar barium suspension.[4] Mucosal surfaces in infants are not as well visualized with barium suspensions as in adults. Although this may be partly due to lack of skill of the pediatric radiologist, characteristic differences in the child's gastrointestinal tract, particularly the mucous coating of the stomach, probably play a more important role. For upper gastrointestinal examinations, barium preparations with a weight/volume (wt/vol) of 50 to 100% are usually employed. For single-contrast examinations of the colon, a 15 to 25% wt/vol barium suspension is adequate. Double-contrast examinations require using a 200 to 250% wt/vol barium preparation. For enteroclysis, a 30% wt/vol suspension of barium is recommended.

Water-soluble contrast material is sometimes used to evaluate the pediatric gastrointestinal tract. These agents are more damaging than barium if aspirated but cause fewer problems when leaked from the gastrointestinal tract. The low osmolar agents are recommended for infants because of less risk of water depletion and its attendant difficulties. Iohexol in a concentration of 180 to 300 mg of iodine per ml can be used in patients in whom barium is not advised.[5]

Intravenous contrast enhancement is used in most abdominal CT examinations. The authors' usual routine is to administer a bolus injection of 0.5 ml per kg up to a maximum of 50 ml in most pediatric patients.[4] The authors' current practice is to use low osmolar contrast material for neonates, sedated children, and those children with prior history of contrast reaction. About 50% of the authors' pediatric patients now receive low osmolar contrast agents.

Dilute barium mixtures used in CT examinations to opacify the stomach, small bowel, and colon are used in the same circumstances as those of adults.

Gadopentetate dimeglumine (Gd-DTPA) in an intravenous dose of 0.1 mmol per kg is useful in many MR imaging examinations of infants and children. Its full use in abdominal imaging has not yet been defined.

IMAGING TECHNIQUES

Plain Radiography

The abdominal plain film (KUB, flat plate) remains a valuable tool for the evaluation of abdominal disease. It is a necessary preliminary examination for many imaging studies of the abdomen, particularly to evaluate an abdominal mass. The plain film is the most useful examination to assess bowel gas as to its distribution and amount when intestinal obstruction is being considered. The plain film is the usual method of assessing calcification within the abdomen. Supine and horizontal beam films of the abdomen are the basis for evaluation of the acute abdomen, either traumatic or nontraumatic in nature. There are at least three areas in which the plain film has little use: evaluation of the patient with chronic vague abdominal pain, assessment of liver size, and quantitation of the amount of fecal material.

It is critical in performing the abdominal plain film that patient motion be kept to a minimum. This requires a screen film system and imaging unit so that the examination can be performed in 0.01 second or less. Appropriate collimation, with exclusion of the chest, is necessary for a quality examination. In the neonate, portable examination usually suffices and a grid is unnecessary. If bowel perforation is suspected, a horizontal beam film is essential in addition to the supine film. Either upright, left lateral decubitus (right side up) or cross-table lateral film will suffice.

It is axiomatic that the personnel must be skilled in performing radiography in children. Restraints may be needed for the uncooperative patient. Gonad shields are used for males but generally not recommended for females. Particular attention should be given to protecting the thermal environment of the premature neonate.[6]

The abdominal radiograph is not particularly accurate for recognizing specific abnormalities except for identification of free air, intestinal obstruction, and type of abdominal calcification. At the same time, it is most valuable to the radiologist for orientation prior to other imaging studies.[6]

The risk of plain radiography is essentially that of the radiation employed. This is minimized by using appropriate parameters for examination and incorporating gonad shields.

Fluoroscopy

Fluoroscopy is involved in most radiologic procedures accompanying conventional radiography. It is rarely used on an isolated basis. Fluoroscopy of infants and children should be performed with particular attention to minimizing the amount of radiation. This includes using variable field size image intensifiers, pulsed radiation, and modified lenses on the image tube. Videotape recording of fluoroscopic studies saves repetition. The radiation dose involved with fluoroscopy is substantial, with a few seconds' exposure resulting in a dose more than 100 times that of plain radiography. Thus, fluoroscopy should be used only when indicated.

Contrast Studies of the Gastrointestinal Tract

Pediatric diseases vary from those of adults, and the cooperation level of children is different. Therefore, examinations are performed in a considerably different fashion from those for adults. Double-contrast studies to evaluate mucosal details are less often needed in children. Indications and techniques for contrast studies vary according to the age of the patient, the suspected diagnosis, and, to some extent, the skills of the radiologist. For example, because stomach cancer is virtually unknown in children but malrotation is a common problem, a routine upper gastrointestinal series is modified substantially from the procedure performed in adults. Similarly, the suspected diagnosis (e.g., hypertrophic pyloric stenosis as opposed to possible peptic ulcer) results in a considerably different examination in the individual child.

Although examinations vary substantially according to age and indication, the following general comments are valid. For the esophagus, stomach, and duodenum, barium is the usual agent employed. Water-soluble agents are potentially dangerous if aspirated, are more costly, and do not have the mucosal coating capabilities of barium. Thus, barium is the preferred agent unless extravasation is suspected or colon obstruction is likely. Immobilization of even the most uncooperative child is usually possible, and sedation is rarely needed. If the child is unwilling or unable to swallow contrast, delivery via a nasogastric tube is the least traumatic method to complete the study. The amount of barium to be used varies according to age of the patient. In a neonate or infant, 30 to 100 ml may suffice. In an older child, 250 to 500 ml of barium might be used, especially if the small bowel is to be studied. Children have difficulty with swallowing the crystals, which induce gas formation within the stomach. Therefore, if double-contrast examination is indicated, the authors generally introduce air through a nasogastric tube.

Dietary restrictions for infants prior to an upper gastrointestinal series are few. In patients younger than 1 year of age, withholding feedings for 3 to 4 hours is usually sufficient. Beyond age 2, feedings should be withheld from midnight for a morning examination. For those children to be examined in the afternoon, a clear liquid breakfast is allowed. In most instances, these restrictions will result in an empty stomach at the time of examination.

Although each examination is customized according to the suspected clinical diagnosis and condition of the patient, the following guidelines can be used. For examination of the esophagus, the swallowing mechanism and esophageal peristalsis should be evaluated, as should the gastroesophageal junction with the patient supine. Fluoroscopic observation of the filled esophagus in anteroposterior (AP) and lateral positions or other positions at right angles to one another is usual. For the stomach, each portion is evaluated both filled with barium and with an air contrast view of the same area. In infants and younger children, the entire examination is performed with the table horizontal; in older children and adolescents, a portion of the examination may be performed with the patient upright. If additional air is needed for the air contrast views in infants, the authors customarily pass a nasogastric tube and inject air directly into the stomach. In a cooperative adolescent, gas-generating crystals may be used. The duodenal bulb is evaluated with filled views at right angles to one another, as well as with air contrast spot films. Note is made of the rest of the duodenum, particularly the position of the ligament of Treitz. At the completion of the examination, an AP and usually lateral overhead radiographs are exposed to record the position of the stomach, duodenum, and proximal small bowel.

In those occasional instances in which double-contrast evaluation of the esophagus, stomach, or duodenum is needed in children, the authors follow the recommendations of Stringer.[7] This evaluation requires administration of high-density barium followed by gas producing pills or granules. The esophagus is generally studied with the patient standing; the subsequent evaluation of the stomach and duodenum is performed with the table horizontal and the patient positioned for coating of the mucosal surface with barium and subsequent filling of the lumen with gas.

Barium is the agent of choice for examination of the small bowel unless there is suspicion of perforation. Most examinations are performed following standard study of the stomach and duodenum. When the small bowel is to be examined, a sufficient (large) amount of barium is necessary. Although the amount varies with age, up to 500 ml would be routine in an adolescent, with proportionately less in a younger person. With relatively large amounts of barium, transit through the small bowel is usually more rapid, distention is better, and fewer films are needed. It is important that the radiologist monitor the small bowel examination with review of each film after it is taken. Fluoroscopic evaluation of the terminal ileum and ileocecal valve is the final step in the small bowel examination.[2]

If there is suspicion of localized disease of the small bowel or if staging for known Crohn's disease is indicated, enteroclysis examination may be of value. This requires placement of a tube to the level of the duodenojejunal junction, with subsequent infusion of dilute barium. Although enteroclysis study is uncomfortable and does add radiation, it is of considerable value in delineating regional small bowel pathology.[8] The authors are hesitant to use this study in infants because of the possibility of water intoxication. Substantial water absorption in these examinations has been documented in adults.[9] Care must be taken during enteroclysis to avoid gross reflux into the stomach.

Colon examinations in children are substantially different from those of adults except for investigation of gastrointestinal bleeding. The extensive purging to cleanse the lower bowel is not necessary in most children. In general, the fecal content of the bowel should be somewhat reduced so that barium can flow freely through the colon and mucosal detail noted on the postevacuation study. Thus, the authors' own routine is to suggest no purging of the colon as preparation for barium enema for children younger than 3 years of age. For older children, a laxative, sometimes followed by a low enema, is generally performed.[10] Cleansing enemas should be given to children with some caution. Commercial enema preparations that are high in phosphate are not recommended for children younger than 2 years of age. As a general guide to the amount of fluid to be given for cleansing enemas, the publication of Hernandez and associates[10] may be consulted. In those patients studied for suspected Hirschsprung's disease, no prior preparation is given.

Thorough preparation is necessary only in children being evaluated for polyps (with lower gastrointestinal bleeding) or inflammatory bowel disease. In patients with acute ulcerative colitis, a low-residue diet 24 hours before examination may suffice. In other instances, considerable cleansing of the colon is necessary.[2]

The child undergoing a colon examination is immobilized in the same fashion as for other fluoroscopic studies. Balloon-type enema tips should not be used because they can perforate the pediatric colon. Concentric taping around the tube utilizing the adjacent buttocks usually suffices.

Addition of 1 tablespoon of salt (15 mg) to 1 L of barium suspension is routine for enema fluid. This gives an approximate sodium concentration of 70 mEq per L in the barium suspension, with less risk of water intoxication.

Double-contrast colon examination is useful to detect colon polyps and to evaluate mucosal detail in suspected inflammatory bowel disease. As mentioned, thorough cleansing of the colon is necessary both to show mucosal detail and to discover intraluminal masses. This usually requires a combination of low-residue diet, laxatives, and enemas according to the age and condition of the patient.[2, 7] A high-density barium with good mucosal coating abilities such as HD-85 or Polybar is ideal. The barium suspension is introduced into the colon as far as the splenic flexure. Subsequently, air is inflated into the system and the patient positioned to move barium and air throughout the colon. When filling is complete, anteroposterior, posteroanterior, and both lateral decubitus abdominal radiographs are performed. A lateral view of the rectum and special views of the sigmoid colon may be needed.

Diagnostic colon examination using water-soluble agents is occasionally performed in the neonate. Ideally, low-osmolar contrast material diluted to isotonicity should be used. Most radiologists administer water-soluble material in this situation via a syringe.

Computed Tomography

CT is central to diagnostic imaging of the pediatric abdomen. Its advantages[11] are several:

1. CT allows discrimination of tissue density of about 0.5%. This is 10 times the discrimination of plain films.
2. Images can be presented in various planes.
3. Correct measurement of tissue densities may be made related to the fat or water content of a suspected lesion. Although this is not 100% accurate, it represents a considerable improvement in tissue discrimination over plain film.

Using CT has some disadvantages in children. The relatively long time for collection of data when compared with that for plain radiography makes motion degradation a problem. The amount of radiation is substantially more than that of plain radiography. The relative paucity of fat in the pediatric abdomen makes discrimination of various organs more difficult.

There are a variety of indications for abdominal CT. In general, it should be considered for all those patients in whom simpler studies are not definitive (as discussed in subsequent sections). For certain lesions—abdominal mass, evaluation of liver and pancreas, abdominal trauma, and intra-abdominal abscess—CT may play a primary role. It is axiomatic that all prior imaging studies be reviewed by the radiologist prior to performance of CT, both to confirm the necessity for the study and to tailor the examination.

Although CT scanners are not designed specifically for children, the most effective are those with a short scan time. This allows less motion artifact, the possibility for dynamic scanning, and a more efficient and faster procedure. Immobilization, sedation, monitoring, and environmental protection for the child undergoing CT scan are as outlined previously.

In most circumstances, the gut lumen is opacified for abdominal CT. This allows identification of stomach, duodenum, and small bowel. It is particularly helpful in separating the pancreas, retroperitoneum, and mesentery. A variety of methods are used to produce contrast filling of bowel for CT; none are completely successful. Although several radiologists recommend water-soluble iodine-containing agents in low concentration (e.g., 3% meglumine diatrizoate [Gastrografin]), barium mixtures in a 1 to 1.5% wt/vol suspension are now available. These have higher acceptance rates among patients and comparable bowel opacification.[12] The oral contrast material is usually given in two sessions: one 45 to 60 minutes in advance of the study to opacify the distal small bowel and one 15 minutes before the scan for opacification of the stomach and duodenum.[13] The volume to be used depends on the size of the patient. In neonates, 50 to 100 ml suffices; in adolescents, 500 to 750 ml is necessary. If one desires to have the colon opacified, administration of contrast material the night before the examination does this but frequently causes streak artifacts. An enema utilizing dilute contrast material can be given on the examination table.[14] In many instances, there is sufficient fecal material in the colon to identify it as such, so that contrast material is not necessary.

Intravenous contrast agents are used almost universally to augment body CT examinations in children. Reasons for this include the ability to determine vascular anatomy and to accentuate differences between tumor and host tissues (Fig. 78–1). Administration of contrast material in a bolus gives the best opacification of vessels but has the disadvantage that the entire area of interest usually cannot be scanned before the bolus disappears. Most investigators compromise, commonly injecting one half to two thirds of the contrast material in bolus fashion with subsequent intravenous drip.

Agents used for intravenous contrast are those used elsewhere in the body. Usually, 2 ml per kg is sufficient intravenous contrast material. If the kidneys are the only area to be examined, 1 ml per kg may suffice. The low-osmolar agents are probably the drugs of choice for infants and should be considered in other special situations.

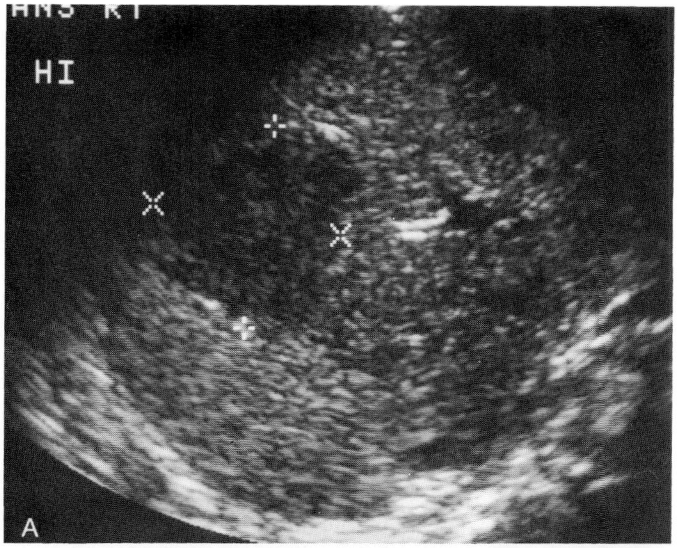

Figure 78–1. A 9-month-old boy with an incidental finding of a liver mass. *A,* Ultrasound of the liver shows a hypoechoic mass (marked by *cursors*) without distal acoustic enhancement. *B* and *C,* Enhanced axial CT scans of liver show characteristic progressive and complete peripheral-to-central enhancement *(arrows)* of an initially hypodense nodule, characteristic of a hepatic hemangioma.

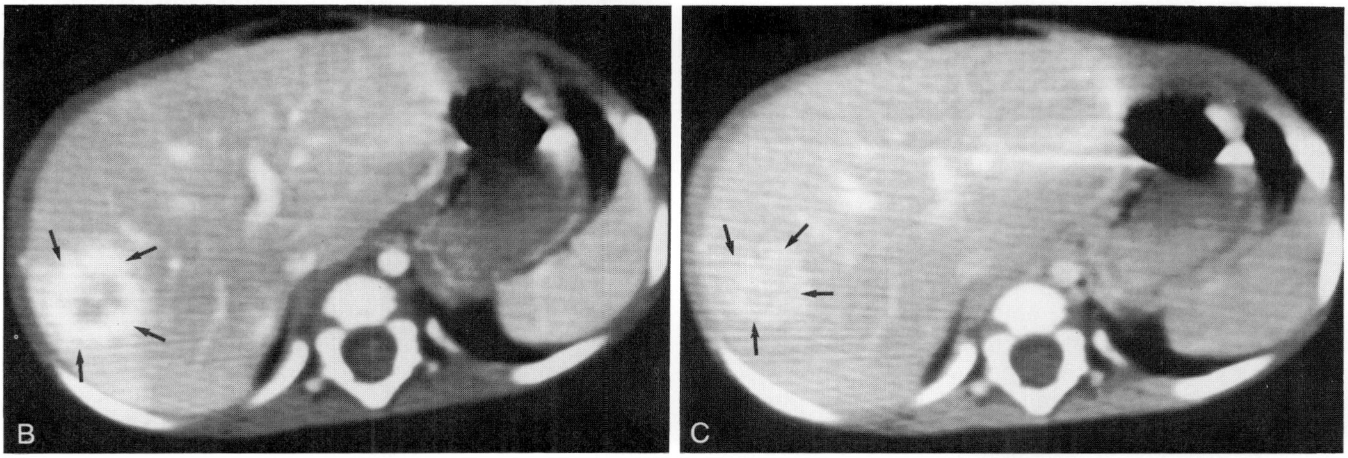

A preliminary digital radiograph of the abdomen is usually performed for orientation and to determine the limits of the axial scans. For infants and in those situations in which fine definition is needed, contiguous axial scans are generally 5 mm in thickness. In most children, contiguous axial scans of 1 cm thickness are performed.[13, 14] Specific guidelines have been developed for scan protocols in various clinical situations.[15]

Although coronal and sagittal images can be directly obtained in infants, in most circumstances reconstructions from axial scans are the more accepted procedure. Three-dimensional reconstructions can be of value.

A variety of window width and window level settings may be used according to suspected diagnosis. For instance, liver images are usually recorded with a more narrow width than the rest of the abdomen to detect the potential minimal differences between hepatic lesions and normal parenchyma. In addition, it is useful to measure densities of abnormalities discovered during the CT scan.

It is customary to obtain another digital radiograph of the abdomen or perhaps a plain radiograph after completion of the CT study, eliminating the need for an excretory urogram.

Ultrasound

Ultrasound is in many ways an ideal modality for examining the pediatric abdomen.[13] There is no radiation damage or known pathologic biologic effect. The paucity of fat planes in children is a potential advantage in ultrasound; also, because of the real-time nature of current ultrasound equipment, respiratory motion is less important. The ability to perform multiplanar imaging is particularly advantageous in infants and children. Finally, small patient size is an advantage. For a given unit, the higher the transducer frequency, the better the image resolution but with decreased penetration. Thus, in children one can routinely use a transducer with a higher frequency than for examination of the same anatomic area in adults.

Most ultrasound examinations are performed using a real-time transducer. In infants, the examination may be performed at the bedside. A 3.5 mHz transducer may be necessary for obese children, but in all others a 5 mHz transducer usually suffices. Newer types of transducers include intraluminal probes useful for endovaginal or transrectal examinations, as well as those probes associated with endoscopes.

Operator skills are critical to the performance of quality ultrasound imaging in infants and children. There is probably no other area of diagnostic imaging in which the special skills of the pediatric radiologist to evaluate and to demonstrate disease in this age group are more important.

Ultrasound is the modality of choice for examination of the pediatric liver and biliary tract. Similarly, the pancreas and spleen are probably evaluated in better fashion by the skilled sonographer than by utilizing CT. Vascular structures of the abdomen, including the portal vein and its tributaries, are best evaluated by ultrasound. Discovery and quantitation of ascitic fluid are most efficiently evaluated by sonographic methods. Ultrasound adds a considerable dimension to evaluation of the gut wall, so that in some circumstances (e.g., hypertrophic pyloric stenosis), it offers a diagnostic dimension beyond that of barium studies.

Doppler ultrasound makes use of the shift in frequency due to motion to determine the direction of a moving target. By varying the delay between transmission and reception of the echo, measurement of flow can be determined at defined points in the diagnostic image. Color Doppler expands this concept so that colors are based on the direction of a phase shift throughout the image. Stationary objects are assigned a "gray" scale, with movement toward or from the transducer assigned different colors.

Technique of ultrasound examination varies substantially from one patient to another, depending on suspected clinical diagnosis, ability to obtain windows of access to the organ of interest according to patient anatomy, and skills of the operator. In general, each area of interest is examined in at least two planes at right angles to one another, with a systematic approach to ensure that the entire region of interest is examined.

In many situations, ultrasound has a sensitivity or specificity greater than that of most other imaging modalities. Thus, examinations of the liver for mass lesions, evaluation of the biliary tract and gallbladder, and assessment of portal vein abnormalities, pancreatic size and lesions, pylorus, and small bowel wall are often best performed with ultrasound. Detection of ascites is an area in which ultrasound generally excels. It is the prime modality for separating cystic from solid lesions of all intra-abdominal organs.

Complications of ultrasonography are few and are generally related to operator skills in evaluating the pediatric patient for suspected disease.

Nuclear Medicine

Nuclear medicine studies are useful for certain gastrointestinal diseases of infants and children. In general, they are safe and minimally invasive. In addition to the morphologic information available from other imaging studies, nuclear medicine has the advantage of obtaining functional data that may be of quantifiable nature.[15]

Most nuclear medicine examinations are more organ specific than are other studies in diagnostic imaging. As the new modalities of diagnostic imaging have evolved, the morphologic information from nuclear medicine has become of less clinical value, but the need for functional information has increased in corresponding fashion. There are new radiopharmaceuticals now available with short half-lives that are more specific for target organs. Nuclear medicine is a diagnostic modality that has adapted well to the age of the computer, so that the vast majority of examinations are now computer assisted, offering more refined qualitative and quantitative analysis than was previously possible.

Ideally, a wide variety of equipment is needed for good pediatric nuclear medicine. A gamma camera with a large field of view allows imaging of neonates to adolescents. At the same time, small cameras that are mobile and can be used at the bedside are useful for neonates.

Magnification techniques are frequently needed for examination in small infants. Pinhole collimation provides the best spatial resolution and is useful for static imaging. The converging collimator provides magnification without loss of count sensitivity and is thus valuable for dynamic images with short collection times.

Liver-spleen scans are of limited value in today's imaging environment because a spatial resolution of 1.5 to 2 cm is required to detect mass lesions. However, these scans can be used to quantify liver size in patients with diffuse disease.

Hepatobiliary scintigraphy is widely used in both neonates and older children. Indeed, this modality has been a principal method by which knowledge of biliary disease in children has increased. The neonate with obstructive jaundice is a prime indication for hepatobiliary scintigraphy. In older children, cholestatic jaundice is the principal indication for the hepatobiliary scan, which can provide functional information regarding patency of the biliary tracts, filling of the gallbladder, and so forth (Fig. 78–2). There is also a role for such studies in hepatobiliary trauma and in the postoperative period.

Nuclear medicine is of considerable value in evaluating the child with gastroesophageal reflux (GER). Like all other modalities, it suffers from lack of a "gold standard" in the evaluation of this disease. Advantages of nuclear medicine include ability to quantify reflux, to study gastric emptying at the same time, and to allow prolonged observation, as well as the noninvasive nature of the modality.

Because Tc-99m-pertechnetate concentrates in the gastric mucosa, it can identify those Meckel's diverticula with such ectopic mucosa such as those that present with bleeding. Sensitivity of the study is approximately 85% with specificity of 95% in children with the appropriate clinical situation, that is, painless lower gastrointestinal bleeding.

Nuclear medicine techniques can be quite helpful in identifying the source of bleeding in children with occult blood loss from the gastrointestinal tract (see later discussion).

Magnetic Resonance Imaging

MR imaging has revolutionized diagnostic imaging in all areas and age groups. Positive attributes of MR

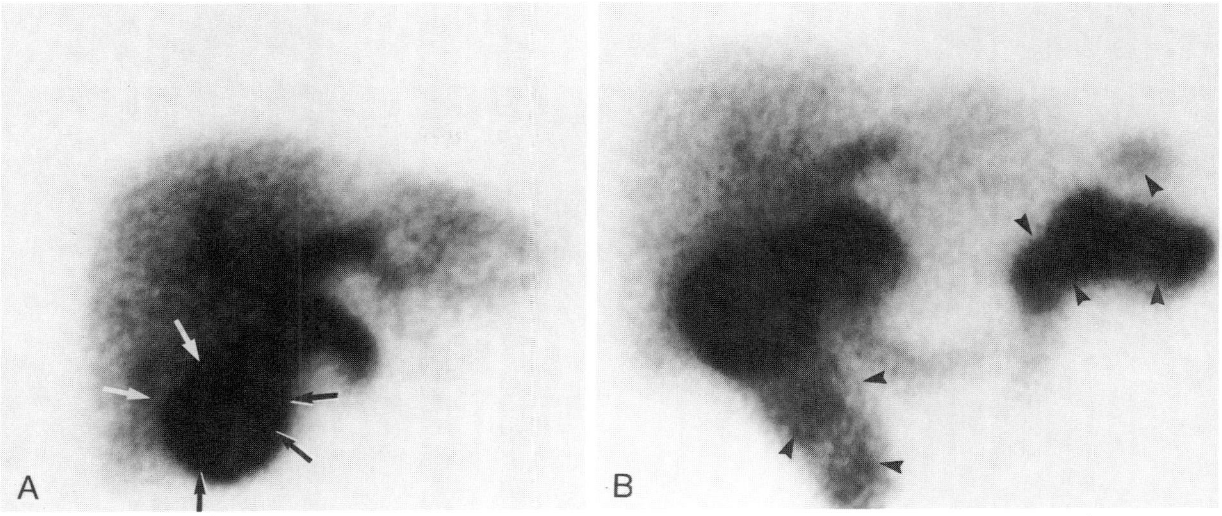

Figure 78–2. A 15-year-old boy with clinical suspicion of acute cholecystitis. Twenty-minute *(A)* and 30-minute *(B)* images of Tc 99m hepatobiliary scintigraphy show normal visualization of the gallbladder *(arrows)* and subsequent filling of the small bowel *(arrowheads)*, excluding an obstructive process in the biliary tree.

imaging that are now clinically useful and that will become more so include (1) tissue characterization beyond that of conventional imaging, (2) multiplanar imaging, (3) high soft tissue contrast resolution, and (4) visualization of vessels.[16] MR imaging of the abdomen has lagged behind that of head imaging because of motion degradation and poor visualization of the bowel. The appearance of various structures varies in MR imaging according to pulse sequences employed. In the gut, peristaltic activity and intraluminal contents may alter the image. The liver is well visualized, particularly if techniques minimizing respiratory motion artifacts are used. Pancreas, spleen, and kidney are reasonably well characterized using MR imaging. Although the gallbladder is identified on MR imaging examinations, the signal from bile varies considerably according to its length of time in the gallbladder. The gut is the least well visualized because of motion artifact and because of similarity of T_1 and T_2 signals to adjacent tissue.

Indications for MR imaging expand each year. In the liver, identification of mass lesions is now quite good, if motion suppression techniques are used (Fig. 78–3). For certain tumors, such as liver hemangioma, MR imaging offers definitive diagnosis.[17] Cystic lesions such as bowel duplication and choledochal cyst are well visualized on MR imaging. In anal atresia, MR imaging provides valuable information regarding the position of the rectum and adjacent pelvic musculature[18] (Fig. 78–4).

The use of contrast agents in MR imaging of the abdomen is preliminary. Intravenous gadolinium is of considerable assistance in localizing tumors and their recurrence. Development of intraluminal contrast agents is in an early phase.

Developments in MR imaging include new techniques to decrease motion artifacts, detection coils designed to improve signal-to-noise ratio, and fast-scan imaging techniques. MR angiography and spectroscopy are now available. All of these techniques will expand capability in the immediate future.

Angiography

Angiographic studies are infrequently needed for diagnostic imaging of abdominal disease in children. The newer modalities have generally replaced the need for angiography in liver tumors. Endoscopy and nuclear medicine techniques are the methods of choice for the evaluation of most cases of gastrointestinal bleeding. Computed tomography and ultrasound have replaced angiography in imaging the traumatized child. Portal hypertension can be evaluated in a satisfactory fashion by ultrasound, CT, and sometimes MR imaging.

There remains a role for therapeutic angiography in some cases, such as embolization of vascular tumors, ablation of esophageal varices, and transluminal angioplasty.

CLINICAL PROBLEMS REQUIRING IMAGING

Acute Abdomen

The first duty of diagnostic imaging in the acute abdomen is to determine whether the patient has medical or surgical disease. The second goal is to determine the type of medical or surgical disease present.

The imaging work-up of the patient with an acute abdomen varies according to likely diagnosis, which in turn differs by patient age. Necrotizing enterocolitis is the major cause in the premature neonate. In term

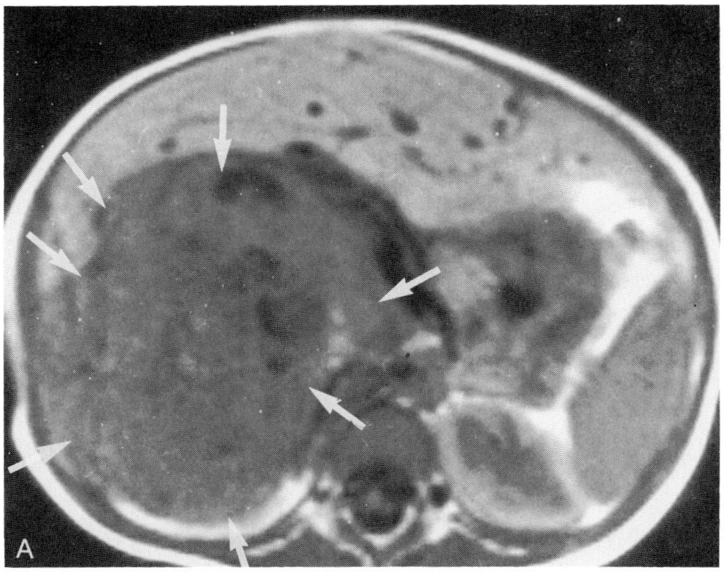

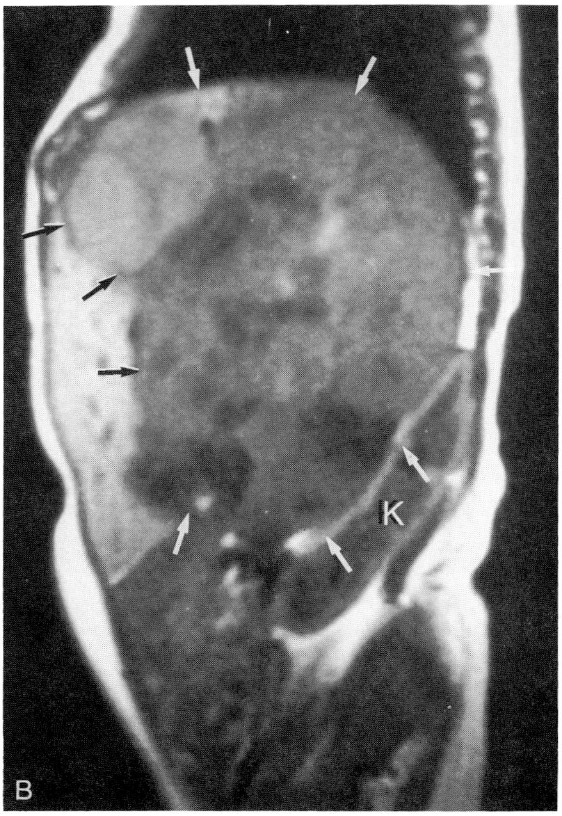

Figure 78–3. A 15-month-old girl with a large hepatoblastoma. Axial *(A)* and sagittal *(B)* T_1-weighted MR scans show a large hypointense mass *(arrows)* arising from the right lobe, with compression of the normal liver parenchyma and displacement of the kidney *(K)*.

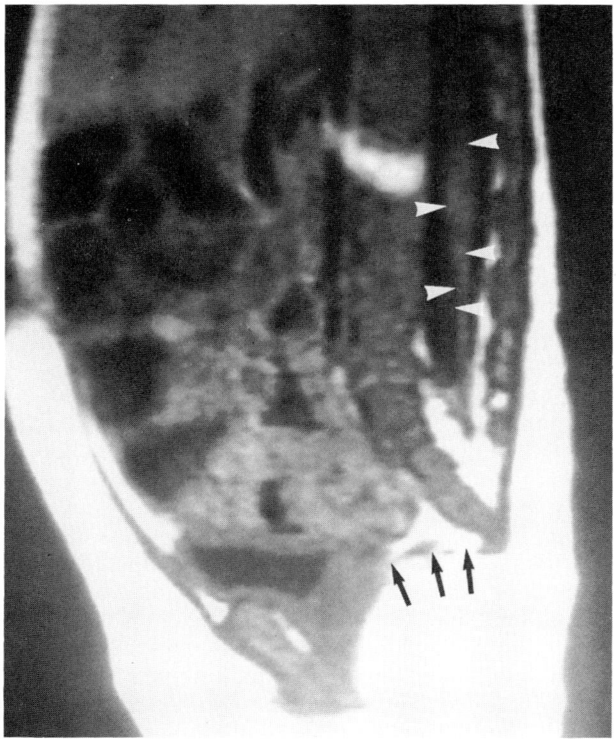

Figure 78–4. A 4-month-old girl with imperforate anus. Midsagittal T_1-weighted image shows termination of the rectum just above the pelvic floor musculature *(arrows)* and evidence of a tethered cord *(arrowheads)*, an anomaly not infrequently associated with anorectal anomalies.

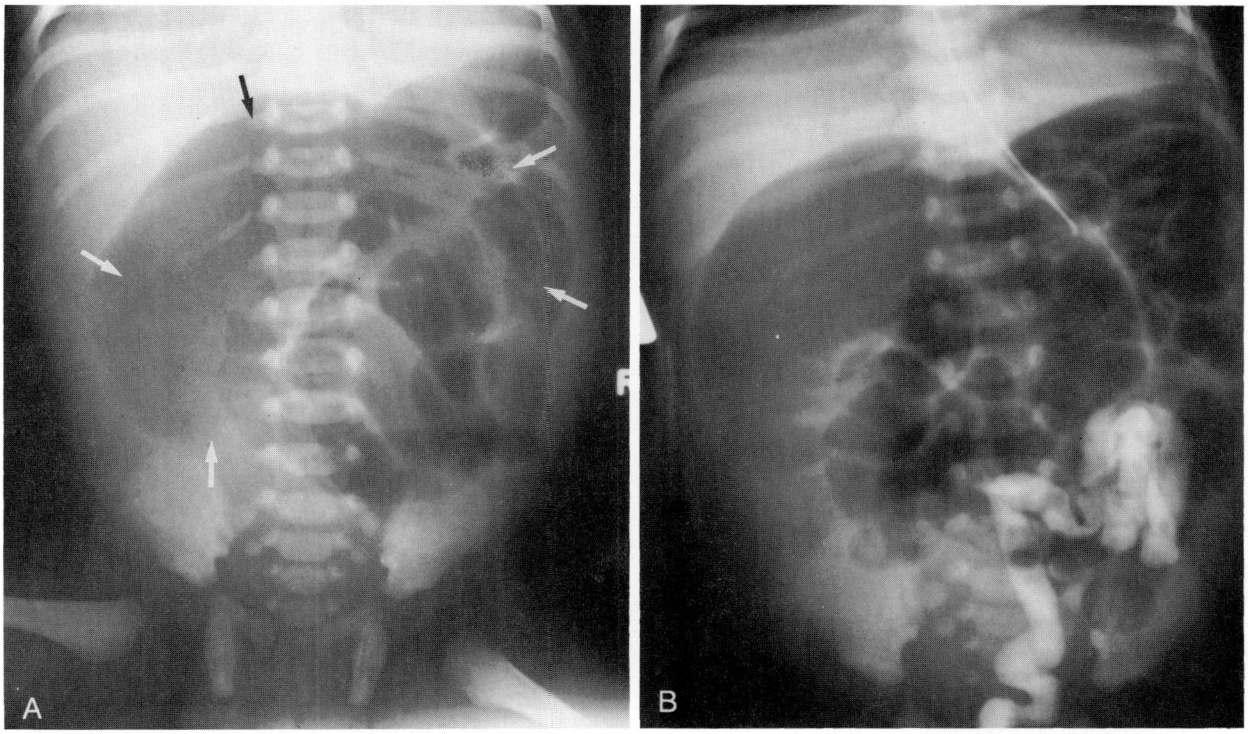

Figure 78–5. Colon atresia in a 2-day-old girl. *A,* The abdominal radiograph shows numerous distended loops of bowel, with one particularly large loop *(arrows)* in the mid-abdomen. *B,* Barium enema shows an unused "microcolon," with cessation of retrograde flow in the descending colon. This confirms colonic obstruction.

neonates, intestinal obstruction (Fig. 78–5) and paralytic ileus associated with sepsis are the most likely diagnoses. After the neonatal period, intussusception, strangulated hernia, inflamed Meckel's diverticulum, and malrotation with volvulus are the principal surgical causes.[19] Beyond the infant age group, appendicitis is the major cause of the acute abdomen requiring surgery.

Supine and horizontal beam radiographs of the abdomen as well as the chest film form the basis for imaging evaluation of the acute abdomen. Unless the clinical findings or the results from the plain film suggest otherwise, ultrasound evaluation is usually the next modality to be considered. CT is needed in some situations.

Appendicitis, although the commonest acute surgical ailment of infants and children, may have obscure clinical manifestations, particularly in infants. Appendiceal perforation is more likely in the pediatric age group. Plain abdominal radiographs are normal in about half of the cases of appendicitis. Contemporary sonography utilizing graded compression of the lower abdomen allows direct visualization of the inflamed appendix (Fig. 78–6). The authors' experience with this technique indicates that the examination is of particular value in the child in whom clinical suspicion is low: either to make a definitive diagnosis of appendicitis or to exclude it with confidence.[20] Barium enema can be used to aid in the diagnosis of appendicitis. CT is often the study of choice for discovery of appendiceal abscess.

Chronic Abdominal Pain

With recurrent abdominal pain a common complaint in children,[21] a critical problem is how to choose which patients need imaging evaluation. In most instances, the possibility of functional disease is reinforced by appropriate clinical history. Organic disease can be suspected if the pain had its onset before age 4 years or after age 13 years, if the pain is located away from the midline, or if there is a family history of gastrointestinal disease. The presence of genitourinary symptoms should prompt work-up of that system in a patient with chronic abdominal pain. Gastrointestinal diseases in which recurrent abdominal pain can be a predominant symptom include peptic ulcer and inflammatory bowel disease. Current experience indicates that endoscopy is the procedure of choice to detect peptic ulcer. Inflammatory bowel disease requires thorough contrast examination of the small bowel and colon.

Diarrhea

The child with acute diarrhea seldom needs radiographic examination. In those occasional instances in which radiographs are obtained, small bowel dilatation can somewhat resemble intestinal obstruction. The role of diagnostic imaging in the patient with chronic diarrhea is limited. Barium studies of the small bowel are needed

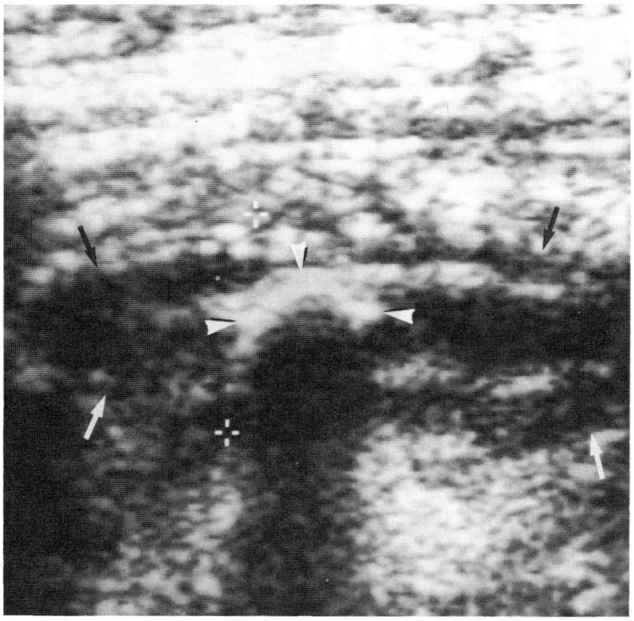

Figure 78–6. An 18-year-old girl with right lower quadrant pain. Graded compression of the right lower quadrant shows a distended appendix *(arrows)* with thickened wall and an appendicolith *(arrowheads)* producing acoustic shadowing.

to diagnose inflammatory bowel disease such as regional enteritis or anatomic abnormalities. Some anatomic causes of chronic diarrhea are blind loop syndrome, enteric fistula, malrotation, partial intestinal obstruction, and short gut syndrome.

Constipation and Reduced Stooling

Functional intestinal obstruction in neonates is a complex problem in which plain radiography and contrast examinations of the colon play a major role.[22] Paralytic ileus is diagnosed according to the clinical situation and plain radiography, with occasional resort to barium enema. Other functional disturbances such as meconium plug syndrome, small left colon syndrome, "inspissated milk" syndrome, and similar conditions usually require contrast examination of the colon for diagnosis. In many cases, the contrast examination will elicit stooling with subsequent patient recovery.

Hirschsprung's disease, an important cause of functional obstruction in the neonate, is well demonstrated on barium enema (Fig. 78–7).

In the older child with recurrent constipation, Hirschsprung's disease remains in the differential diagnosis. The barium enema is a major tool in allowing recognition of this disease.[23]

Abdominal Mass

In most infants and children with abdominal mass, imaging studies are not needed because surgical intervention is usually not indicated. For instance, hepatosplenomegaly with acute leukemia does not need further imaging investigation.

Most surgical masses of children involve retroperitoneal structures, particularly the kidney. In neonates, an even larger number of masses may be extraperitoneal,[24] with hydronephrosis and cystic kidney the most frequent diagnoses. In older children, Wilms' tumor and neuroblastoma are the usual tumors. Other masses include neoplasms of the lower urinary tract, liver, gut, and other soft tissue of the abdomen.[25]

Investigation of the surgical abdominal mass starts with the plain film. Most radiologists would subsequently proceed with ultrasound examination to confirm the presence of a mass and to show its origin. If the mass is found to be cystic on sonography (e.g., hydronephrosis), the diagnostic work-up is different than for solid lesions. Further studies would depend primarily on suspected diagnosis, expertise of the radiologist, and locally available facilities. CT is frequently needed, and nuclear medicine is occasionally of value (Fig. 78–8). MR imaging plays an increasing and important role in the evaluation of abdominal mass.[26]

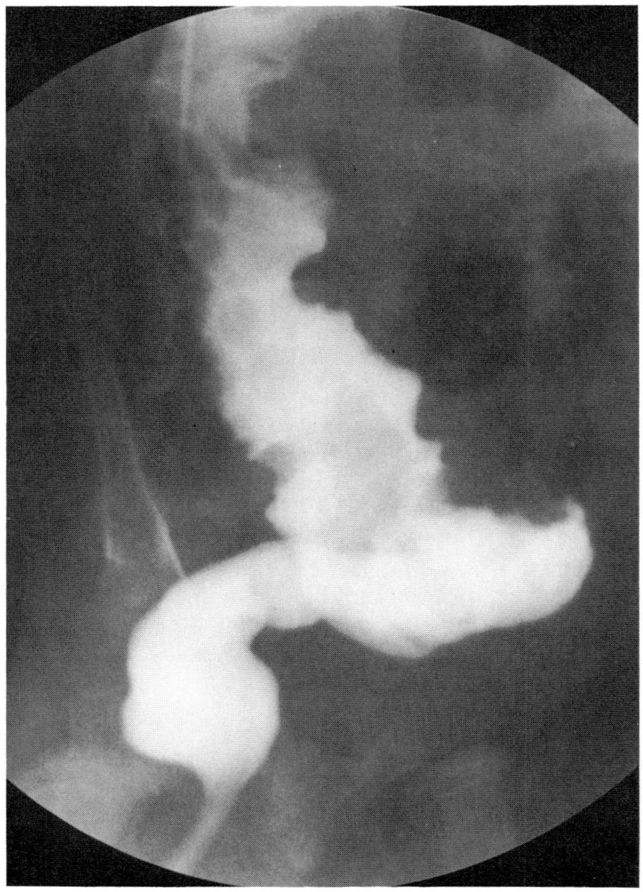

Figure 78–7. A 5-month-old boy with bloody diarrhea. Barium enema shows an irregular nodular mucosal surface in the dilated (relative to the rectum) descending colon, compatible with colitis complicating Hirschsprung's disease. Subsequent rectal biopsy confirmed this diagnosis.

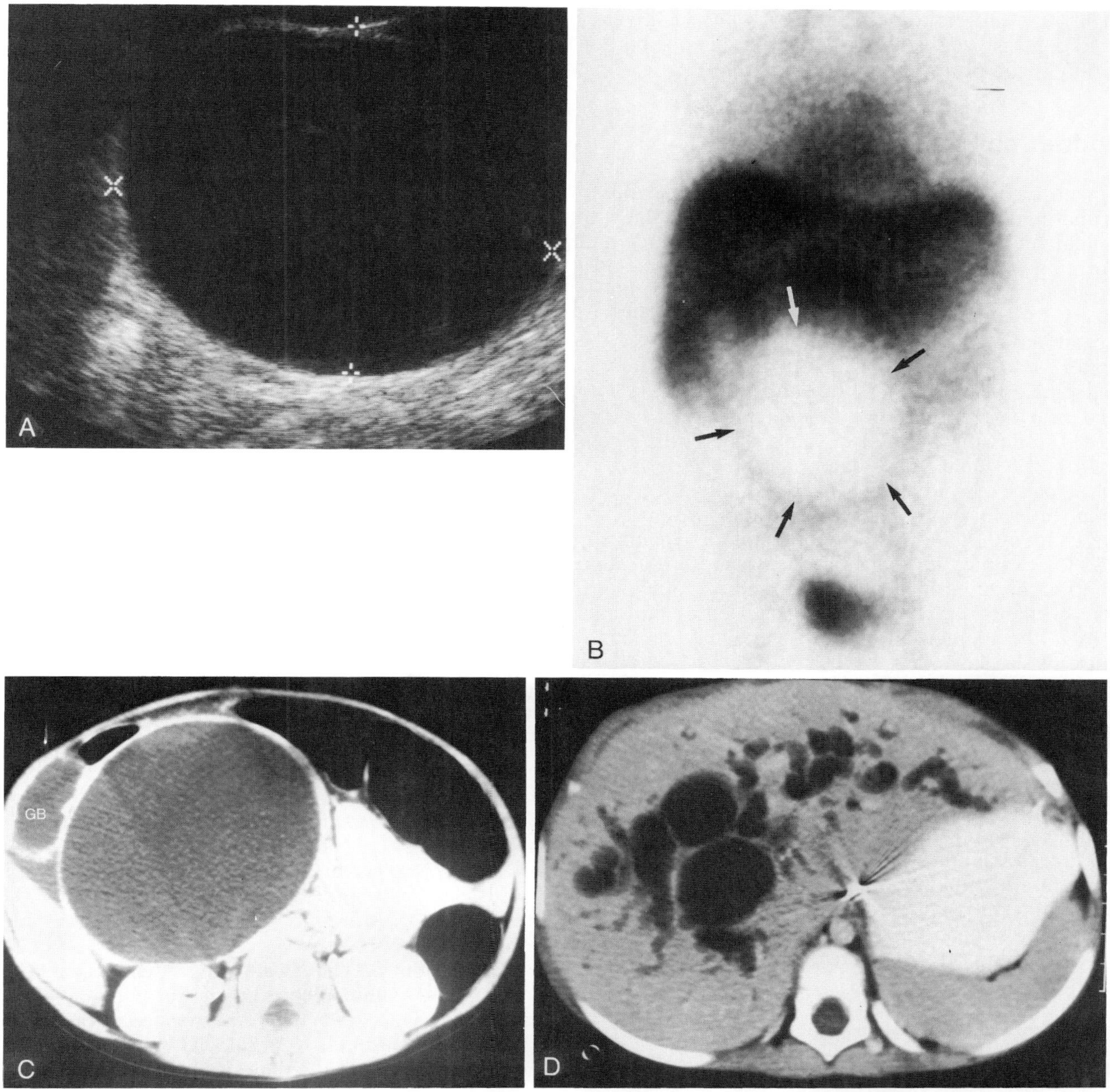

Figure 78–8. A 4-year-old girl with a large choledochal cyst and dilated intrahepatic bile ducts. *A,* Ultrasound scan of the right upper abdomen shows a large anechoic (cystic) mass (marked by *cursors*). *B,* Tc-99m-labeled hepatobiliary scintigraphy shows a large photopenic area inferior to the liver *(arrows)*. *C* and *D*, CT scans of the liver show a large mass with low attenuation medial to the gallbladder *(GB)* and diffuse dilatation of the intrahepatic biliary tree.

Vomiting and Abdominal Distention

Abdominal plain films are the foundation for evaluation of neonates with suspected intestinal obstruction. The plain film usually indicates if obstruction is present and the site of obstruction. In some cases (e.g., duodenal atresia), further imaging studies may not be required prior to surgery. In general, the more gas-filled bowel loops, the greater the difficulty in telling the site of obstruction and in distinguishing mechanical intestinal obstruction from paralytic ileus.

Total obstruction in the upper gastrointestinal tract can be confirmed with additional air if necessary. Oral contrast may be required to confirm partial obstruction. Suspected distal small bowel or colon obstruction is best evaluated by contrast enema and opacifying the colon (see Fig. 78–5). If obstruction is confirmed, the site is identified (small bowel or colon) and frequently a specific diagnosis obtained (e.g., meconium ileus). Although there are certain circumstances in which water-soluble contrast might be used for the enema, barium generally is the preferred agent.[12]

Abdominal Trauma

Diagnostic imaging is of considerable value in children with abdominal trauma. The supine abdominal film with complementary horizontal beam film to exclude gut perforation is the first examination of choice. In most institutions, CT is performed as the primary diagnostic modality for abdominal trauma because the quality of the examination is less dependent on the skills of the operator. If a specific abnormality is to be evaluated (e.g., splenic hematoma), ultrasound examination by a skilled practitioner may be the imaging procedure of choice. CT has the ability to evaluate the entire abdomen from the dome of the diaphragm to the perineum; this is a particular advantage in most traumatized children in whom location of suspected trauma is imprecise. If the child with abdominal trauma is hemodynamically stable, CT examination is generally safe. Administration of contrast material is not advised in an unstable child. In any event, contrast material will not enter the renal system if the glomerular filtration rate has decreased because of shock.

Clinical evaluation remains the primary means to determine whether children need a CT examination to detect intra-abdominal injury following blunt trauma.[27] In the past, there was a tendency to request abdominal CT in traumatized children with an "unevaluable abdomen," usually children with head injury. This is not an efficacious procedure unless there are clinical indications of abdominal trauma. In general, CT can detect free air, ascites, or hemoperitoneum and other generalized manifestations of trauma. It is usually diagnostic of a specific organ injury such as hepatic laceration, splenic hematoma, renal fracture, etc. (Fig. 78–9).

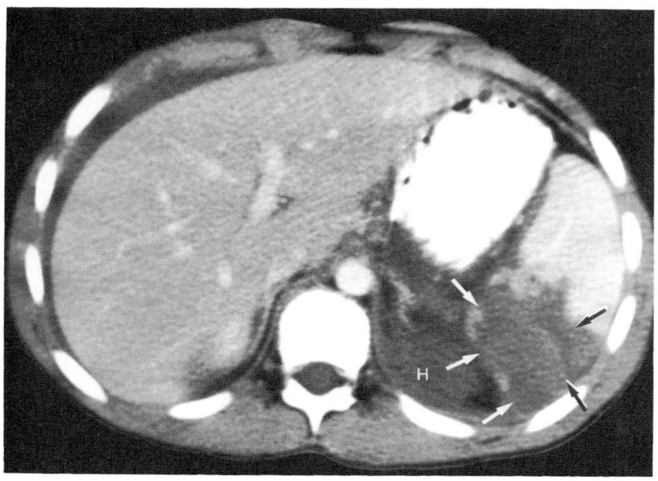

Figure 78–9. A 14-year-old boy with abdominal trauma. Enhanced axial CT scan of abdomen shows laceration and hematoma in the posterior portion of the spleen *(arrows)*. A hematoma *(H)* is also seen at the upper pole of left kidney.

Gastrointestinal Bleeding

The causes of gastrointestinal bleeding in children vary considerably from those in adults and differ within the pediatric age group according to the location of the bleeding.[28] In neonates, gastrointestinal bleeding is usually related to stress ulcer, and in most such cases bleeding ceases within 24 to 48 hours. Diagnostic imaging is seldom required. In the infant age group, substantial gastrointestinal bleeding from the lower gastrointestinal tract usually indicates Meckel's diverticulum or stress ulcer. In the child older than 1 year of age, causes of bleeding become more diverse. Portal hypertension and its associated complications occur, bleeding colon polyps may be identified, and Meckel's diverticulum is less frequent.

There is a major role for nuclear medicine studies in the imaging of gastrointestinal bleeding in children.[29] Such studies detect the presence of active bleeding and help to localize the site. A bleeding rate as low as 0.1 ml per minute can sometimes be detected. Meckel's diverticulum may be well shown on nuclear medicine studies (Fig. 78–10). The double-contrast enema is an excellent method for the detection of colon polyps. Endoscopy is useful for the evaluation of massive gastrointestinal bleeding. Angiography is reserved only for those children in whom endoscopy is not practical or in whom other methods have failed.

Swallowing Disorders

Dysphagia may arise from intrinsic or extrinsic anatomic causes, neuromuscular disease, or a combination of both. Esophageal disease producing feeding difficulties is classically studied with the barium swallow. Ultrafast CT is of substantial value to document vascular rings in these patients.

Evaluation of the swallowing mechanism requires real-time dynamic recording of the event and careful analysis.[30] This is classically performed with feeding of a bolus of barium (by nipple when appropriate) and with recording on videotape. It is important not to use water-soluble contrast material for such studies, because there is risk of aspiration. A new development in the evaluation of dysphagia is the use of real-time ultrasound. Experience to date indicates that specific ultrasound patterns may be associated with specific types of oral dysphagia.[31]

Gastroesophageal Reflux

The role of diagnostic imaging in GER is somewhat imprecise in that there is no universally accepted gold standard to separate the GER that occurs in the normal person from that of the pathologic situation. It seems clear that GER is related to subsequent peptic esophagitis and stricture and that at least one factor in producing GER is relaxation of the lower esophageal sphincter.[32] Other poorly defined factors may be of equal

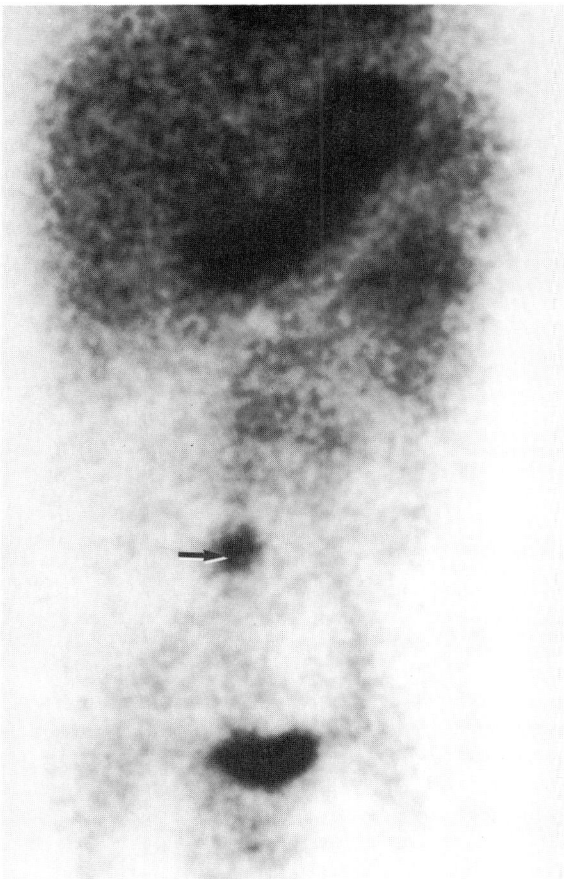

Figure 78–10. A 6-year-old girl with lower gastrointestinal bleeding. Tc-99m-pertechnetate scan shows a focal area of abnormal uptake *(arrow)* at the right lower quadrant of abdomen, characteristic of a Meckel's diverticulum.

importance in producing esophagitis. These include delay in gastric emptying, clearing of esophageal contents via peristalsis, spontaneous deglutition, salivary buffering, and mucosal resistance to acid.

Barium studies in GER are useful to detect structural anomalies such as hiatus hernia. They are less valuable to identify GER because of poor sensitivity and specificity and the short observation time inherent in fluoroscopy studies. Radionuclide scintigraphy has the advantages of having a long observation period and being reasonably noninvasive. Ultrasound evaluation of GER has several advantages. These include being totally noninvasive and having the ability to extend real-time observation for GER over a long period.

Gastric Outlet Obstruction in Infants

Hypertrophic pyloric stenosis (HPS) is the commonest cause of gastric outlet obstruction and the most frequent indication for laparotomy in infancy. Clinical manifestations and subsequent diagnosis are usually in the third to fifth week of life. As in many other situations, imaging evaluation of HPS depends greatly on the expertise of the physicians caring for the patient. Careful examination by an experienced pediatric surgeon will suffice in many cases. Most radiologists are well versed in the barium meal study of suspected pyloric stenosis and have an average accuracy of more than 90% in diagnosis.[33] The disadvantages of this method are the radiation involved and the slight risk of aspiration. Many radiologists with interest in pediatric ultrasound now rely on sonography to diagnose HPS.[34] Careful measurement of muscle thickness and attention to the real-time examination confirming gastric outlet obstruction allow confident diagnosis in most cases (Fig. 78–11).

Intussusception

Intussusception is the commonest abdominal emergency in the first 2 years of life beyond the neonatal period. Plain radiography is of value in the diagnosis of intussusception and is essential to discover complications such as intestinal obstruction or gut perforation. For many years, the contrast enema has been the standard method to confirm the clinical diagnosis of intussuscep-

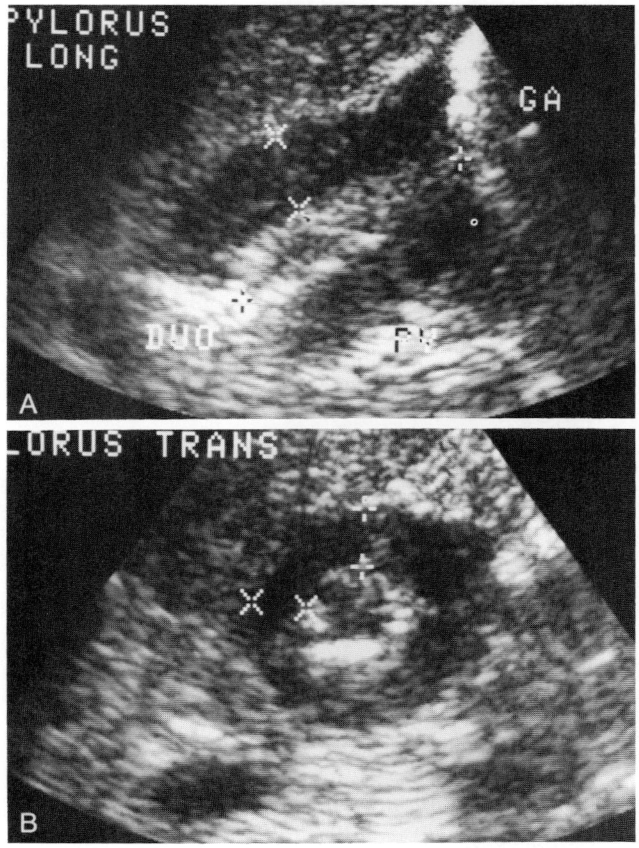

Figure 78–11. A 2-month-old girl with projectile vomiting. *A*, Longitudinal scan of the pylorus *(PY)* shows thickening of the muscle wall *(x–x)* to 6 mm with elongation *(+–+)* of the canal to 2.6 cm *(GA,* gastric antrum; *DUO,* duodenum). *B*, Transverse scan of the pylorus appears as a thickened donut, with the hypoechoic muscle marked by *cursors*.

tion. Techniques for diagnosis and reduction of intussusception are well established.[35] More recently, radiologists skilled in ultrasound have shown that sonography may be equal to the contrast enema in diagnostic accuracy.[36]

Classic treatment of uncomplicated ileocolic intussusception (without peritonitis, gangrene, or perforation) has been by barium enema under fluoroscopic control (Fig. 78–12). There is now substantial interest in the reduction of intussusception by insufflation of rectal gas. Preliminary results indicate a reduction rate comparable with that of the hydrostatic enema with perhaps even greater safety. To the authors' knowledge, controlled series to evaluate this problem are not yet reported.

Necrotizing Enterocolitis

Necrotizing enterocolitis (NEC) is the commonest cause of an acute abdomen in the premature neonate. Morbidity and mortality of the disease are related to birth weight and maturity. The abdominal plain film is the principal method of diagnosis of NEC. In most cases, pneumatosis of the bowel wall is visible, with perforation evident by intraperitoneal air[37] (Fig. 78–13). It is mandatory that there be a horizontal beam radiograph (decubitus, upright, or cross-table lateral) in addition to a supine film to detect intraperitoneal air.

Because of the variation in clinical manifestations and interobserver inconsistencies in the diagnosis of NEC, the authors frequently perform contrast enemas to establish the diagnosis.[38, 38a] The authors have now used contrast enemas in more than 100 cases and have found them to be a valuable method to confirm or exclude a diagnosis of NEC and without significant hazard of perforation (Fig. 78–14).

Ultrasound can sometimes aid in the diagnosis of NEC by detecting microbubbles of gas within the portal venous system or the liver parenchyma.

Anorectal Malformation

Classic clinical and surgical concepts of imperforate anus have included defining whether the gut terminates above or below the pelvic musculature and identifying associated fistulas. Surgical repair, whether a combined abdominoperineal approach or a simpler perineal surgical procedure, has been based on these determinations.

Further refinements in pathologic anatomy in imperforate anus have made note of the importance of the sphincteric musculature of the pelvic floor (striated muscle complex) for directing surgical placement of the neorectum and for relating this to prognosis for subsequent fecal continence.

MR imaging of the pelvis and perineum, particularly images in the transaxial plane, is invaluable to evaluate location of the striated muscle complex and the appropriate approach for surgical repair (see Fig. 78–4). The examination is especially valuable in the postoperative patient with incontinence being considered for surgical revision.[18]

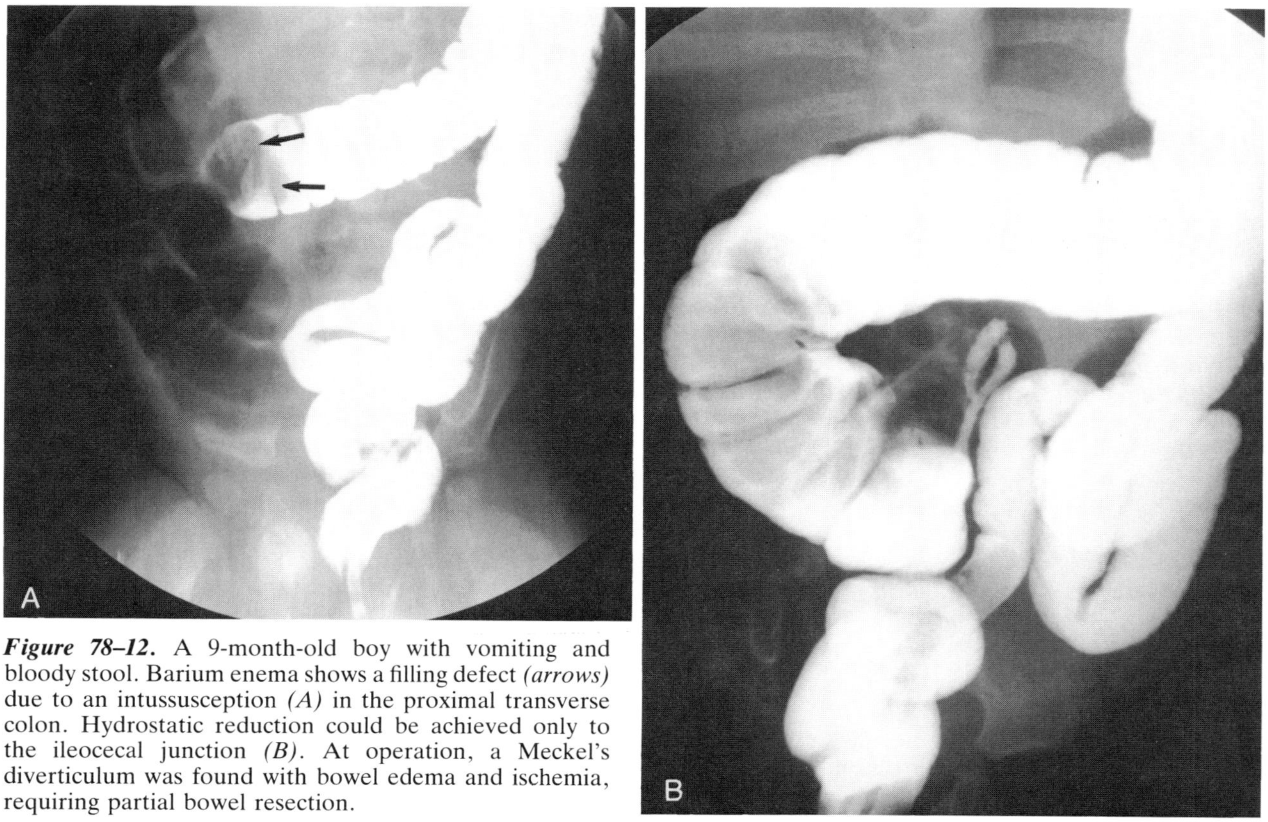

Figure 78–12. A 9-month-old boy with vomiting and bloody stool. Barium enema shows a filling defect *(arrows)* due to an intussusception *(A)* in the proximal transverse colon. Hydrostatic reduction could be achieved only to the ileocecal junction *(B)*. At operation, a Meckel's diverticulum was found with bowel edema and ischemia, requiring partial bowel resection.

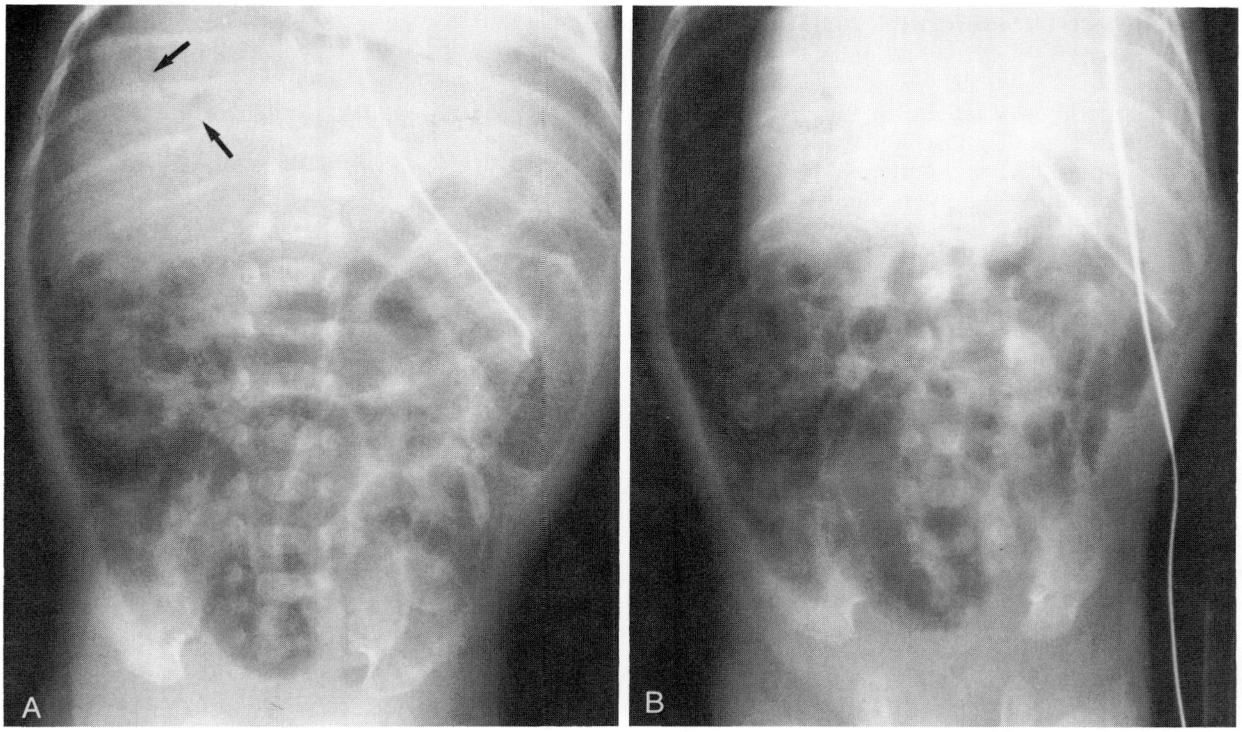

Figure 78–13. A 21-day-old premature boy with acute abdominal distention and bloody stool. Supine *(A)* and left lateral decubitus (displayed as upright) *(B)* views of abdomen show mottling in the right flank, portal venous air *(arrows),* and pneumoperitoneum. Operation showed necrotizing enterocolitis involving the right colon with a small perforation.

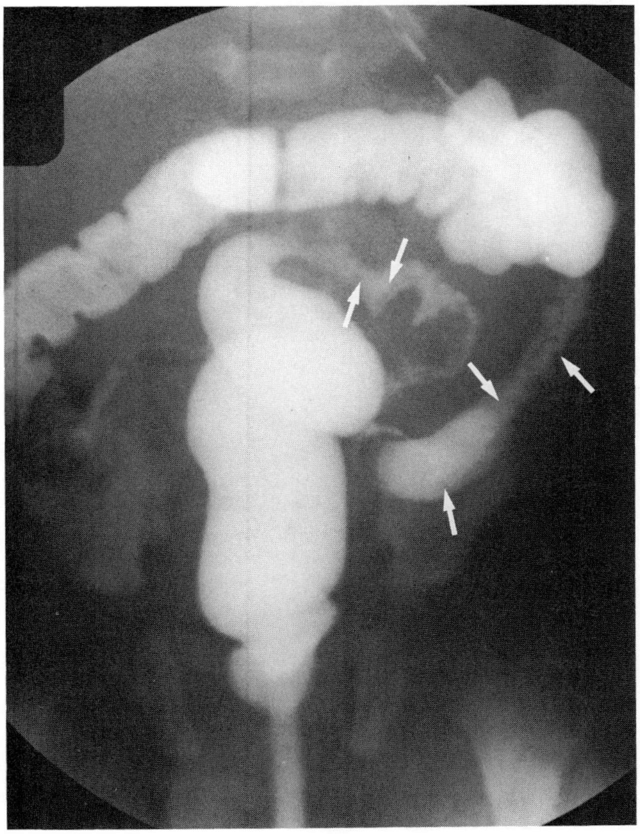

Figure 78–14. A 4-day-old neonate presenting with bloody stool. Plain abdominal radiograph shows no pneumatosis, portal venous gas, or pneumoperitoneum. Barium enema shows spasm and irregularities *(arrows)* in the descending and proximal sigmoid colon, a common finding in necrotizing enterocolitis.

Chronic Liver Disease and Portal Hypertension

Noninvasive methods of diagnostic imaging now offer reasonable precision in diagnosis and evaluation of liver disease. Sonography, CT, and perhaps MR imaging are all capable of evaluating the liver parenchyma for liver size and shape, segmental location of mass lesions, and status of the biliary tract and vascular structures of the liver.

Evaluation of the neonate with jaundice usually includes sonography to exclude choledochal cyst, followed by radionuclide studies to separate biliary atresia and neonatal hepatitis.[39] Mass lesions of the liver can be handled by a variety of imaging modalities, depending on the individual physician's skill. For diseases of the gallbladder and bile ducts, ultrasound is usually the first examination.

Most children with portal hypertension have extrahepatic occlusion of the portal vein. In those children with portal hypertension secondary to chronic liver disease, manifestations of the primary disease are usually present. Although barium studies can detect esophageal varices, sonography usually offers more definitive information, showing an occluded portal vein, collateral vessels within the porta hepatis, and venous varices elsewhere (Fig. 78–15). Doppler examination offers an even more sophisticated method of studying collateral vessels.[40] The portal vein occlusion and the associated collateral vessels can also be seen on CT and sometimes on MR imaging. Angiography rarely is called for in a child requiring surgery for portal hypertension.

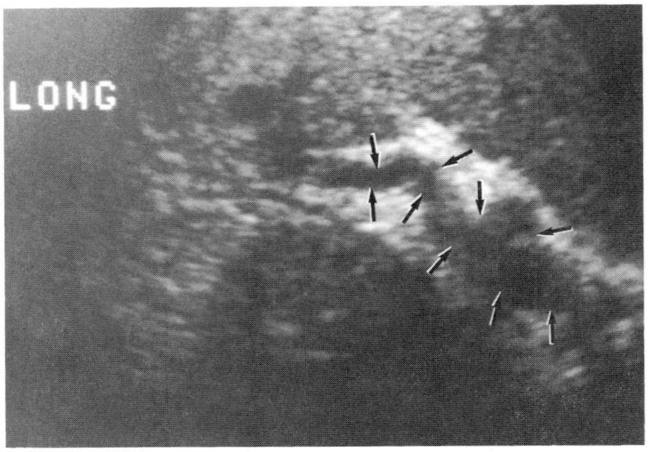

Figure 78–15. A 12-year-old boy with repeated hematemesis. Sonogram of the portal tract shows serpiginous vessels *(arrows)* replacing the normal portal vein. Splenoportovenogram (not shown) confirms the presence of portal vein thrombosis with cavernous transformation to maintain hepatopedal blood flow.

Liver Transplantation

The frequency of liver transplantation continues to increase in the pediatric age group. Recipients are those with end-stage liver disease from a variety of causes, particularly failed surgery for biliary atresia. Extensive preoperative evaluation in these patients is needed, the object being to show the anatomy of the liver and porta hepatis as well as to assess any findings of portal hypertension present. Much of this evaluation can be per-

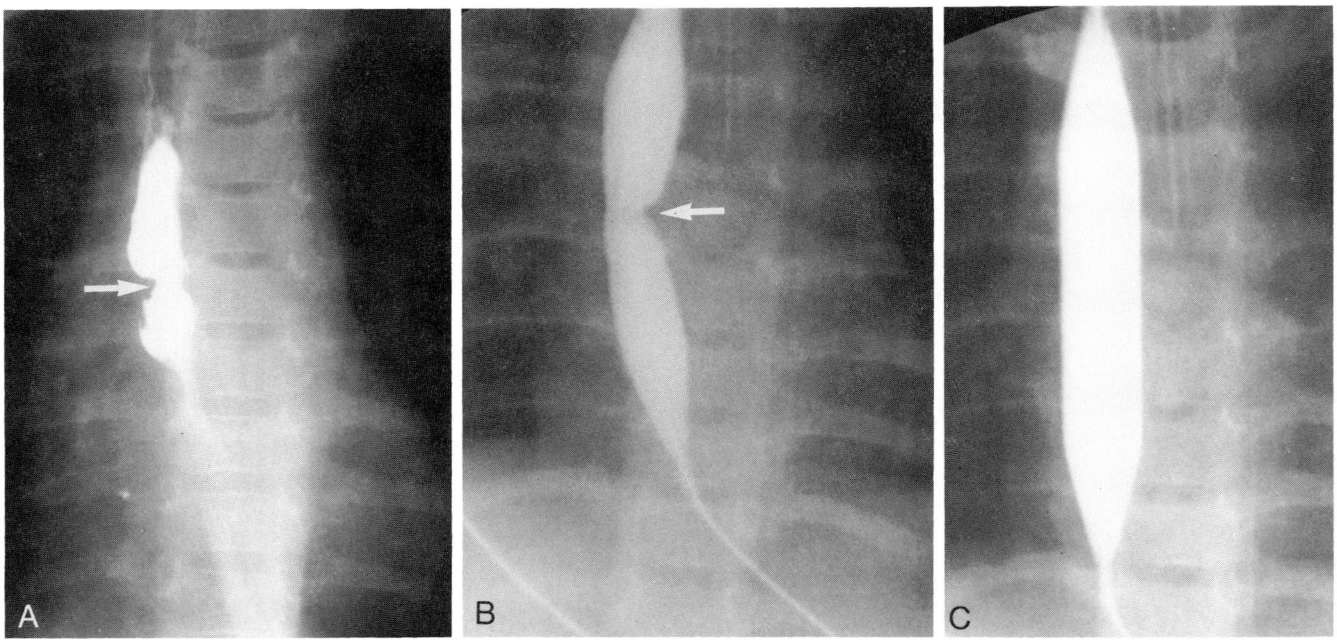

Figure 78–16. A 21-month-old girl with balloon dilatation of an esophageal stricture following repair of tracheoesophageal fistula. *A,* Initial barium swallow shows an irregular focal stricture *(arrow)* of the mid-esophagus. *B,* A partially distended balloon is seen crossing the stricture, with a waist indentation *(arrow)* at its middle. *C,* With full distention of the balloon, the waist is obliterated.

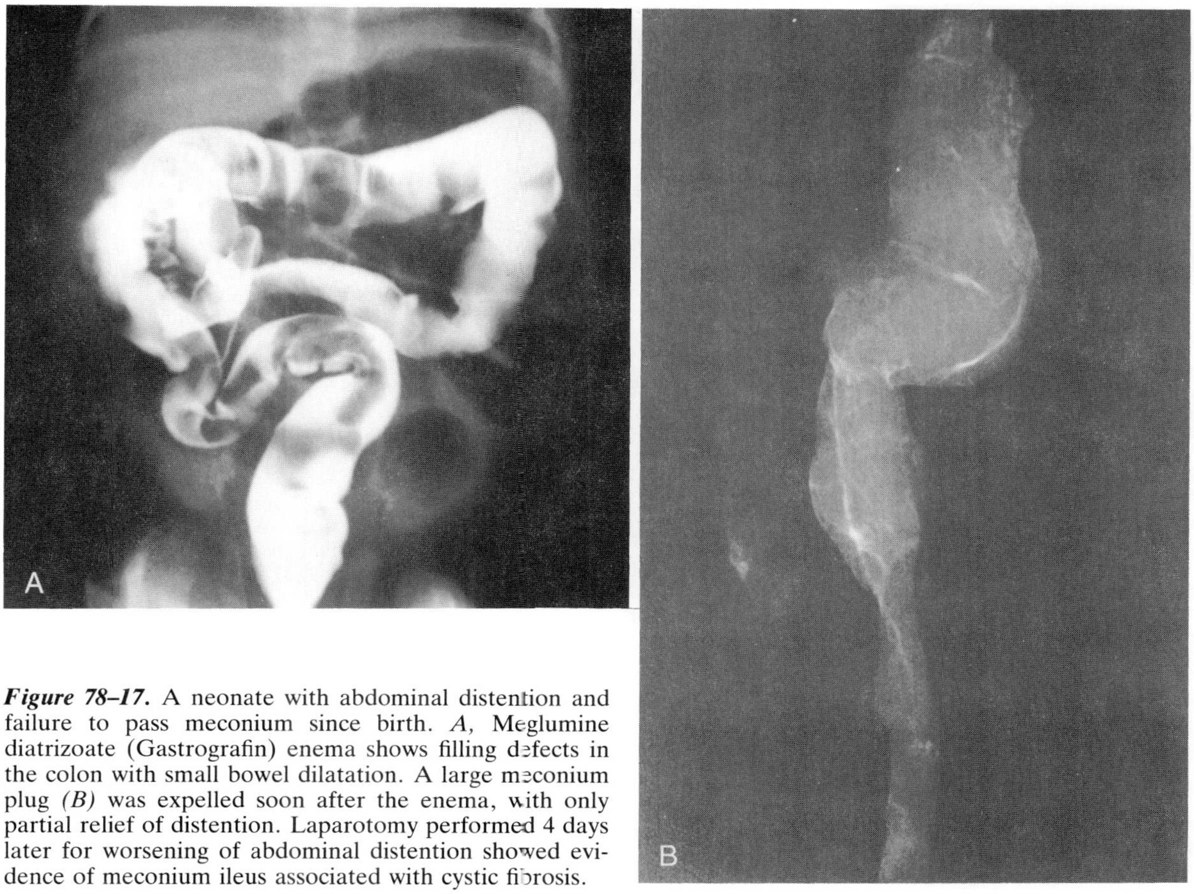

Figure 78–17. A neonate with abdominal distention and failure to pass meconium since birth. *A,* Meglumine diatrizoate (Gastrografin) enema shows filling defects in the colon with small bowel dilatation. A large meconium plug *(B)* was expelled soon after the enema, with only partial relief of distention. Laparotomy performed 4 days later for worsening of abdominal distention showed evidence of meconium ileus associated with cystic fibrosis.

formed with sonography, although CT and MR imaging are used in some patients.

Postoperative complications of liver transplantation include thrombosis of the hepatic artery or portal vein with or without infarction, obstruction or leak of the biliary anastomosis, rejection phenomena, and postoperative infection. Almost all the diagnostic imaging modalities useful to evaluate liver disease are needed for these patients.[41]

Esophageal Dilatation

Strictures in the esophagus may follow chemical, reflux, or infective esophagitis; repair of esophageal atresia; and trauma (Fig. 78–16). Such strictures can be dilated in the radiographic suite with the use of transluminal angioplasty balloons placed across the stricture.[42] Advantages of the procedure are several: radially directed forces are theoretically less dangerous than the longitudinal shearing forces used with bougienage; general anesthesia is not always necessary; and the stricture may respond after only one or two procedures.

Water-Soluble Enemas in the Treatment of Meconium Ileus

Almost all white infants with meconium ileus have associated cystic fibrosis. Laparotomy can often be avoided in infants with uncomplicated meconium ileus and associated gastrointestinal obstruction by the administration of contrast enema.[4] Consensus indicates a need to produce an osmotic diarrhea with the contrast enema pulling body water into the bowel to "flush" the inspissated material from the colon and distal small bowel (Fig. 78–17). A variety of contrast agents have been recommended. They include Gastrografin (meglumine diatrizoate), which also has a surface wetting agent, as well as diatrizoate and similar water-soluble agents. It is likely that the osmotic diarrhea produced by such hypertonic agents has a major role in eliminating the abnormal meconium from the gut. Using the procedure, considerable attention to the fluid and electrolyte balance is necessary because dehydration is a real possibility.

Other Therapeutic Procedures

Gastrostomy can be performed via a percutaneous approach in many children. Such a technique avoids prolonged anesthesia and surgery in a child who is chronically ill. The procedure appears to be safe and applicable to the pediatric age group.[43]

Drainage of abscess and biopsy of individual organs (Fig. 78–18) are feasible in all age groups. Most of the techniques useful in adults are applicable, with modification, to children.

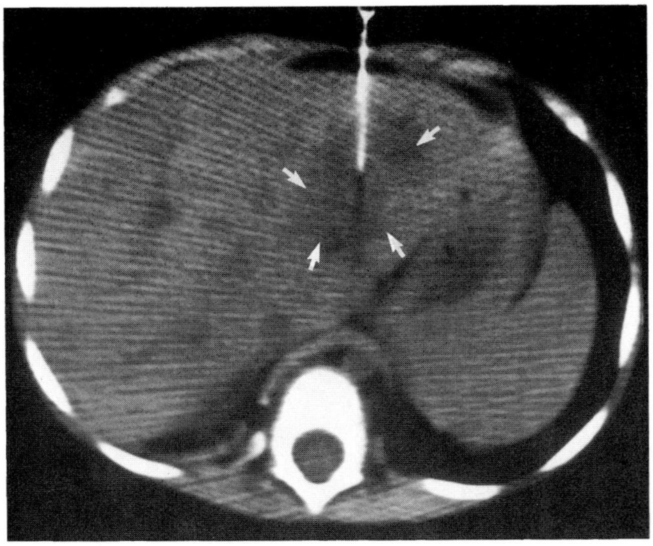

Figure 78–18. A 34-month-old girl with histiocytosis and sclerosing cholangitis. Unenhanced axial CT scan of liver shows a hypoechoic mass *(arrows)* in the left lobe. Fine-needle biopsy under CT guidance showed no evidence of recurrence of histiocytosis or neoplasm. Subsequent operation showed a large fibrotic mass secondary to sclerosing cholangitis.

REFERENCES

1. Weinstein MC, Fineberg HB: Clinical Decision Analysis. Philadelphia, WB Saunders, 1980.
2. Franken EA Jr, Smith WL: Gastrointestinal Imaging in Pediatrics, 2nd ed. Philadelphia, Harper & Row, 1982, pp 2–15.
3. Kuharik MA: Sedation, anesthesia, and patient monitoring. *In* Cohen MD, Edwards MK, eds: Magnetic Resonance Imaging of Children. Philadelphia, BC Decker, 1990, pp 75–84.
4. Smith WL, Sato Y, Franken EA Jr: Pediatric contrast agents. *In* Katzberg R, ed: The Contrast Media Manual. Baltimore, Williams & Wilkins, 1992, pp 219–220.
5. Cohen MD, Towbin R, Baker S, et al: Comparison of Iohexol with barium and gastrointestinal studies of infants and children. AJR 1991; 156:345–350.
6. Rational Use of Diagnostic Imaging in Paediatrics. Geneva, World Health Organization, 1987, pp 40–49.
7. Stringer DA: Pediatric gastrointestinal examinations. *In* Dobranowski J, Stringer DA, Somer SS, Stevenson GH, eds: Procedures in Gastrointestinal Radiology. New York, Springer-Verlag, 1990, pp 107–166.
8. Stringer DA, Cloutier S, Daneman A, et al: The value of the small bowel enema in children. Can Assoc Radiol J 1986; 37:13–16.
9. Barloon TJ, Franken EA Jr: Plasma electrolyte status after small bowel enteroclysis. AJR 1986; 146:323–325.
10. Hernandez R, Gutowski D, Guire KE: Capacity of the colon in children. AJR 1979; 133:683–685.
11. Berger PE: Computerized tomography. *In* Franken EA Jr, Smith WL, eds: Gastrointestinal Imaging in Pediatrics, 2nd ed. Philadelphia, Harper & Row, 1982, pp 490–529.
12. Franken EA Jr, Sato Y, Smith WL: Pediatric use of contrast agents. *In* Skucas J, ed: Radiographic Contrast Agents. 2nd ed. Rockville, MD, Aspen, 1989, pp 462–485.
13. Middleton WD: Physical principle and instrumentation. *In* Siegel MJ, ed: Pediatric Sonography. New York, Raven Press, 1991, pp 1–7.
14. Daneman A: Pediatric Body CT. New York, Springer-Verlag, 1987.
15. Treves ST: Pediatric Nuclear Medicine. New York, Springer-Verlag, 1985, pp 129–190.
16. Cohen MD: Gastrointestinal system. *In* Cohen MD, Edwards MK, eds: Magnetic Resonance Imaging of Children. Philadelphia, BC Decker, 1990, pp 611–678.
17. Boechat MI, Kangarloo H, Ortega J, et al: Primary liver tumors in children: Comparison of CT and MR imaging. Radiology 1988; 169:727–732.
18. Sato Y, Pringle KC, Bergman RA, et al: Congenital anorectal anomalies: MR imaging. Radiology 1988; 168:157–162.
19. Franken EA Jr, Kao SCS, Smith WL, et al: Imaging of the acute abdomen in infants and children. AJR 1989; 153:921–928.
20. Kao SCS, Smith WL, Abu-Yousef MM, et al: Acute appendicitis in children: Sonographic findings. AJR 1989; 153:375–379.
21. Kao SCS, Franken EA Jr: The child with abdominal pain. *In* Hilton SV, Edwards DA, eds: Practical Pediatric Radiology, 2nd ed. Philadelphia, WB Saunders (in press).
22. Franken EA Jr, Smith WL, Frey EE, et al: Intestinal motility disorders of infants and children: Classification, clinical manifestations and roentgenology. Crit Rev Diagn Imaging 1987; 27:203–236.
23. Rosenfield NS, Ablow RC, Markowitz RI, et al: Hirschsprung disease: Accuracy of the barium enema examination. Radiology 1984; 150:393–400.
24. Teele RL, Share JC: The abdominal mass in the neonate. Semin Roentgenol 1988; 23:175–184.
25. Sty JR, Wells RG: Other abdominal and pelvic masses in children. Semin Roentgenol 1988; 23:216–231.
26. Fletcher BD, Kopiwoda SY, Strandjord SE, et al: Abdominal neuroblastoma: Magnetic resonance imaging and tissue characterization. Radiology 1985; 155:699–703.
27. Taylor GA, Eichelberger MR, O'Donnell R, et al: High and low yield indications for abdominal CT in children following blunt trauma. Ann Surg 1991; 213:212–218.
28. Oldham KT, Lobe TE: Gastrointestinal hemorrhage in children: A pragmatic update. Pediatr Clin North Am 1985; 32:1247–1263.
29. Hyams JS, Leichtner AM, Schwartz AN: Recent advances in diagnosis and treatment of gastrointestinal hemorrhage in infants and children. J Pediatr 1985; 106:1–8.
30. Ardran GM, Kemp FH: Normal and disturbed swallowing. Prog Pediatr Radiol 1969; 2:151–169.
31. Smith WL, Erenberg A, Nowak A, et al: Physiology of sucking in the normal term infant using real-time ultrasound. Radiology 1985; 156:379–381.
32. Sondheimer JM: Gastroesophageal reflux: Update on pathogenesis and diagnosis. Pediatr Clin North Am 1988; 35:103–116.
33. Breaux CW, Georgeson KE, Royal SA, et al: Changing patterns in the diagnosis of hypertrophic pyloric stenosis. Pediatrics 1988; 81:213–217.
34. Blumhagen JD, Maclin L, Krauter D, et al: Sonographic diagnosis of hypertrophic pyloric stenosis. AJR 1988; 150:1367–1370.
35. Bisset GS III, Kirks DR: Intussusception in infants and children: Diagnosis and therapy. Radiology 1988; 168:141–146.
36. Pracros JP, Tran-Minh VA, Morin de Finfe CH, et al: Acute intestinal intussusception in children: Contribution of ultrasonography (145 cases). Ann Radiol 1987; 30:525–530.
37. Frey EE, Smith WL, Franken EA Jr, et al: Analysis of bowel perforation in necrotizing enterocolitis. Pediatr Radiol 1987; 17:380–382.
38. Uken P, Smith W, Franken EA Jr, et al: Use of the barium enema in the diagnosis of necrotizing enterocolitis. Pediatr Radiol 1988; 18:24–27.

38a. Kao SCS, Smith WL, Franken EA Jr, et al: Contrast enema diagnosis of necrotizing enterocolitis. Pediatr Radiol 1992; 22:115–117.

39. Kirks DR, Coleman RE, Filston HC, et al: An imaging approach to persistent neonatal jaundice. AJR 1984; 142:461–465.
40. Patriquin H, Lafortune M, Burns P, et al: Duplex Doppler examination in portal hypertension: Technique and anatomy. AJR 1987; 149:71–76.
41. Herbener T, Zajko AB, Campbell WL, et al: Diagnostic imaging in the evaluation of postoperative complications in liver allograft recipients: Experience with over 1,200 transplantations. Scientific exhibit, RSNA, Chicago, 1988.
42. Sato Y, Frey EE, Smith WL, et al: Balloon dilatation of esophageal stenosis in children. AJR 1988; 150:639–642.
43. Towbin RB, Ball WS Jr, Bisset GS III: Percutaneous gastrostomy and percutaneous gastrojejunostomy in children: Antegrade approach. Radiology 1988; 168:473–476.

Chapter 79

Gastrointestinal Mucosal Biopsy

BEVERLY BARRETT DAHMS

INTRODUCTION

Successful histopathologic interpretations of mucosal biopsy material require cooperation and communication between gastroenterologist and pathologist. Biopsy interpretation is both an art and a science, involving a synthesis of the clinical history, endoscopic findings, and histologic observations. Pathologists do more than "read" the findings on the slide; therefore, a diagnosis based solely on histologic observations is often incomplete. If this interpretive process is to take place, the gastroenterologist must provide clinical information in addition to the biopsy specimen, including history, radiologic abnormalities, physical findings, endoscopic observations, and differential diagnosis. This process is best accomplished by use of a special submission form for endoscopic biopsies sent to the surgical pathology department that is completed by the physician rather than by a technical assistant unfamiliar with these details.

In nearly every instance, an indication for endoscopy in a child is an indication for biopsy. Even when no endoscopic abnormalities are apparent, the biopsy often reveals important findings. If the biopsy specimen is normal, that can serve to comfort the parents or the child. The endoscopist should aim to maximize the information provided by the biopsy by procuring the largest piece of tissue possible. Optimally, each organ examined should be biopsied at several levels, and multiple pieces of tissue obtained at each level. It is important that specimens from different levels be placed in separate containers and that the level be indicated for the pathologist. In most situations, standard fixation, paraffin embedding, and hematoxylin-eosin staining are all that are necessary. Biopsy studies on samples requiring fresh or frozen tissue are, of course, not placed in fixative. Possible special procedures include (1) cultures for *Helicobacter pylori*, cytomegalovirus (CMV), herpesvirus, or other infectious agents; (2) glutaraldehyde fixation for electron microscopy; (3) snap-frozen tissue for acetylcholinesterase staining in evaluation of Hirschsprung's disease; and (4) frozen tissue for enzyme or biochemical analysis.

Standard fixation varies from laboratory to laboratory. Ten percent buffered formalin is the standard fixative used by surgical pathologists and is acceptable for endoscopic biopsies. Some pathologists prefer alternate fixatives, such as Bouin's, Zenker's, and Hollande solutions, because these render the tissue firmer and less susceptible to damage during processing and also result in sharper contrast after staining. However, duration of fixation is limited with special fixatives, and specimens cannot be left in them for several days as they can be in formalin. The choice of fixative is best left to the discretion of the pathologist. When tissue is removed from the forceps or suction tube and placed directly into fixative, it contracts and curls permanently and cannot be well oriented later by the histotechnologist. Random embedding and tangential sectioning result in numerous artifacts that often make histologic interpretation difficult. Optimally, gastrointestinal biopsy specimens are sectioned (cut) perpendicular to the surface and muscularis mucosae. Proper orientation prior to fixation is particularly important in the small intestine, otherwise villous and crypt architecture cannot be evaluated well. It is best for the endoscopist to orient the biopsy, surface up, on a piece of Millipore filter, Gelfoam, or nylon mesh prior to placing it in the container of fixative. With practice, this is easily accomplished with the naked eye. In some hospitals, the endoscopy nurse or assistant assumes this function and becomes rapidly proficient.

Sectioning of tissue at 5 μm or less is mandatory for evaluation of endoscopic biopsy specimens. If the section is too thick, small structures such as infectious organisms and submucosal ganglion cells may be missed. Ideally, the histotechnologist working with endoscopic biopsy specimens should use fresh disposable knife blades and limit a cutting session to small biopsy specimens, or at least cut the small specimens before the larger ones. It is impossible to achieve good sections if small biopsy specimens are alternated with large specimens. The technologist must get into the center of the biopsy; the first sections cut from the block usually contain only fragments of mucosa. Three to five glass slides, each containing a serial ribbon of at least 10 tissue sections, should be generated from each paraffin block (Fig. 79–1). In addition to providing abundant tissue to examine, serial sectioning may overcome the drawback of random orientation, since a few optimally oriented sections usually appear somewhere on the glass slides if many sections are cut.

Standard hematoxylin-eosin staining is often the only stain required. Special stains are best left to the discretion of the pathologist, who is guided in the selection by the differential diagnosis provided. Different brands and dye lots of stain, and slight differences in fixatives, section thickness, and staining procedures result in some variations in the slides produced from one laboratory to another. Clinicians quickly become adept at recognizing eosinophils, infectious organisms, and other sought-after features in their own laboratory's slides.

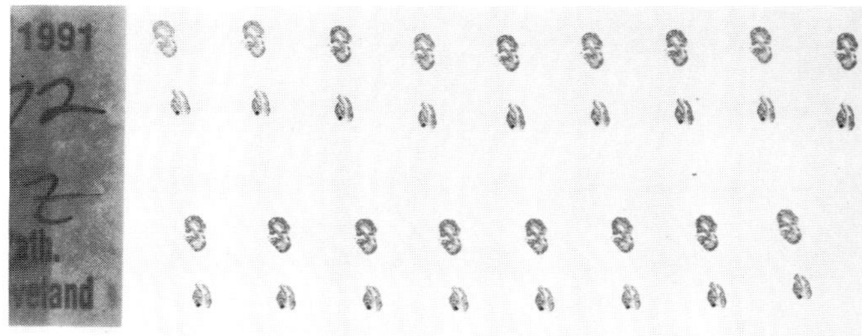

Figure 79–1. Photograph of a glass microscopic slide containing a "ribbon" of serial tissue sections cut from a paraffin block. Optimally, at least three such glass slides are examined from each paraffin block to ensure that the histotechnologist has reached the center of the tissue, the pathologist has sufficient tissue to examine, and focal lesions such as granulomas or crypt abscesses are not missed. × 1.8.

ESOPHAGUS

Technical Considerations and Normal Esophageal Mucosa

Infants and children undergoing upper endoscopy usually have biopsy specimens taken from two levels of the distal esophagus, the first approximately 2 to 3 cm proximal to the visualized lower esophageal sphincter (LES) and the second level approximately 4 to 5 cm above the LES. It is mandatory that for each level, the endoscopist uses a different container, with the location relative to the LES clearly labeled. This precaution is necessary so that the pathologist does not overread normal background inflammatory cells near the LES or an irregular but normal squamocolumnar junction as Barrett's esophagus.

In most cases of suspected infectious esophagitis, it is advisable that additional tissue samples be submitted for fungal and viral cultures. If esophageal involvement is focal, it is possible that cultures will be positive without diagnostic features appearing in histologic sections. If ulcerations are apparent through the endoscope, it is best to sample the margins of an ulcer as well as intervening nonulcerated mucosa.

Normal esophageal mucosa (Fig. 79–2) is covered by nonkeratinizing stratified squamous epithelium; beneath this is a lamina propria of loose connective tissue containing capillaries and, still deeper, a thin muscularis mucosae. The basal layer of epithelium, where mitosis and cell replication occur, constitutes no more than 15 to 20% of total epithelial thickness. Basal cells are recognizable by their large, round nuclei and relatively sparse basophilic cytoplasm compared with the more superficial epithelial cells. As epithelial cells mature, they move closer to the lumen and develop a flattened contour, compressed nucleus, and abundant, pale cytoplasm. Papillae of lamina propria project into the base of the epithelium, but normally do not extend upward more than 50% of total epithelial thickness. Occasional intraepithelial lymphocytes are normally found, but eosinophils and neurophils are not normally present.

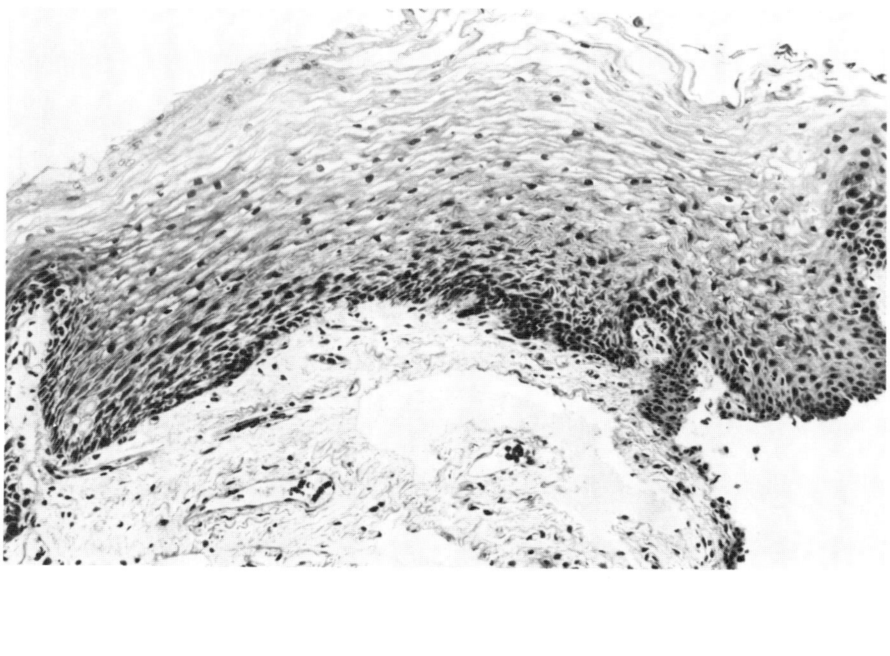

Figure 79–2. This normal esophageal biopsy shows a thin epithelial basal layer with dark, rounded nuclei. Most of the epithelium shows maturation, as indicated by abundant cytoplasm and flattened nuclei. Lamina propria papillae are sparse, and inflammation is absent. Compare with Fig. 79–3. Hematoxylin-eosin stain, × 140.

Reflux Esophagitis

Confirmation of reflux esophagitis is the commonest indication for endoscopy of the upper gastrointestinal tract in infants and children. Endoscopy and biopsy are the most sensitive diagnostic procedures available for documenting this condition. Approximately 30% of pediatric patients with symptomatic and histologic evidence of reflux esophagitis fail to demonstrate gross endoscopic evidence of esophagitis, such as erythema, granularity, and ulceration.[1] Therefore, biopsy is recommended in a child with symptoms severe enough to warrant endoscopy, even when endoscopy appears "negative."

The histologic features of reflux esophagitis[2-6] form a spectrum in severity that may vary from level to level in given patients, or even within one level at different points on the mucosal circumference (Table 79–1 and Fig. 79–3). Multiple biopsy specimens ensure a greater chance of documenting the presence and range of histologic abnormalities. Intraepithelial inflammation with lymphocytes, neutrophils, and "squiggle cells" is found in nearly every case of reflux esophagitis in infants and children. Squiggle cells are distorted, elongated inflammatory cells of indeterminate type, probably lymphocytes or degranulated neutrophils or eosinophils, and are numerous in most biopsies of reflux esophagitis.[2] Sparse intraepithelial lymphocytes alone do not constitute inflammation; they may be found normally near the LES. However, obviously increased numbers of lymphocytes or squiggle cells (i.e., more than two or three per high-power field in multiple adjacent fields) support the diagnosis of esophagitis. Intact neutrophils within the epithelium are not often found, except in severe inflammation or when ulceration is present. Inflammation in the lamina propria is often present in association with intraepithelial inflammation but is not diagnostically significant, since it can be observed in normal children.

Table 79–1. HISTOLOGIC FINDINGS IN REFLUX ESOPHAGITIS

Intraepithelial inflammation
Eosinophils, squiggle cells, neutrophils, lymphocytes
Basal cell hyperplasia >30% of epithelial thickness
Papillary elongation >50% of epithelial thickness
Basal layer spongiosis, mitoses
Telangiectasia
Balloon cells

Intraepithelial eosinophils are highly correlated specifically with prolonged acid bathing of the esophageal mucosa and are the single most helpful histologic feature of reflux esophagitis. Because their bilobate nucleus and bright pink granular cytoplasm are so highly visible on routine hematoxylin-eosin staining, eosinophils can be readily identified on extremely small, poorly oriented, and even fragmented biopsies. However, only 30 to 50% of children with reflux esophagitis demonstrate intraepithelial eosinophils[2, 7]; the absence of this finding does not rule out the diagnosis. Eosinophils may be sparse and focal or so numerous that they constitute the dominant intraepithelial inflammatory cell. The reason for such variable populations of eosinophils in reflux esophagitis is unknown. Even though intraepithelial eosinophils are characteristic of reflux esophagitis, they are

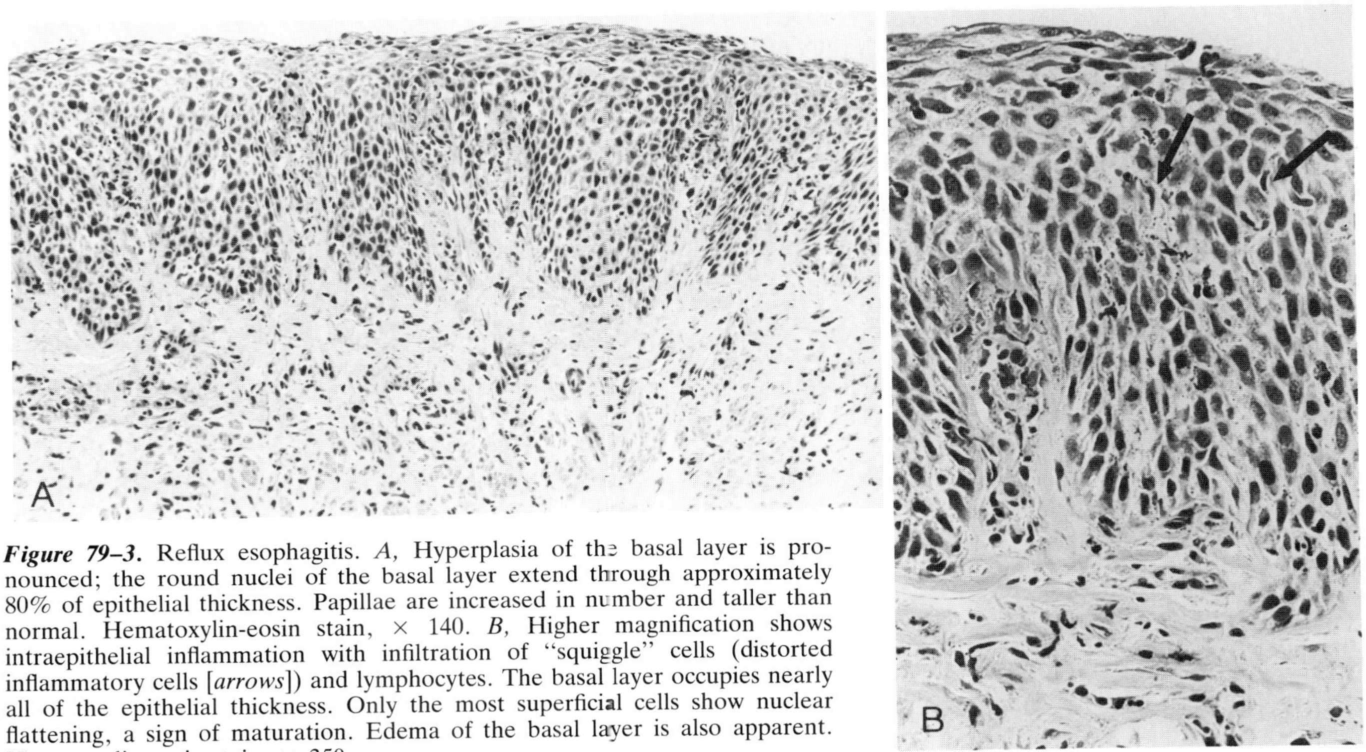

Figure 79–3. Reflux esophagitis. *A,* Hyperplasia of the basal layer is pronounced; the round nuclei of the basal layer extend through approximately 80% of epithelial thickness. Papillae are increased in number and taller than normal. Hematoxylin-eosin stain, × 140. *B,* Higher magnification shows intraepithelial inflammation with infiltration of "squiggle" cells (distorted inflammatory cells [*arrows*]) and lymphocytes. The basal layer occupies nearly all of the epithelial thickness. Only the most superficial cells show nuclear flattening, a sign of maturation. Edema of the basal layer is also apparent. Hematoxylin-eosin stain, × 350.

not pathognomonic for this condition. Esophageal eosinophilic infiltration may also be found in infectious esophagitis and eosinophilic gastroenteritis.

With persistent acid bathing of the esophageal mucosa, rapid epithelial turnover results in a series of squamous epithelial changes helpful in the diagnosis of reflux esophagitis (see Fig. 79–3). The basal layer, normally occupying only 15 to 20% of epithelial thickness, undergoes hyperplasia to constitute more than 30% and, in severe reflux esophagitis, as much as 100% of total epithelial thickness. Lamina propria papillae, normally projecting less than 50% through the width of the epithelium, elongate and extend closer to the surface. Papillae also appear more numerous than normal in reflux esophagitis. Accurate evaluation of basal layer hyperplasia and papillary elongation requires optimal orientation of biopsy specimens during embedding, because orientation can result in an artifactually thickened basal layer or elongated papillae. Many pediatric esophageal biopsy specimens are too small for proper orientation, limiting the application of these criteria. Basal layer spongiosis (edema), nuclear enlargement, and an increased mitotic rate are often found in severe cases of esophagitis.

Dilated capillaries within papillae are another sign of esophagitis. Tangential sections of papillae, which are frequent on randomly oriented biopsy material, often make telangiectatic capillaries appear to be isolated blood lakes within the squamous epithelium. This artifact, although helpful in diagnosing reflux esophagitis, is not specific and may be found in numerous other causes of esophageal irritation. Balloon cells are pale, distended squamous cells containing intracytoplasmic plasma proteins that have presumably leaked from capillaries rendered more permeable than usual by inflammation. They have been described in reflux esophagitis.[8]

The histologic differential diagnosis of reflux esophagitis is limited. In otherwise healthy children, an occasional case of herpes esophagitis will present with symptoms similar to those of gastroesophageal reflux. In oncology patients and immunosuppressed persons, infection is more likely to cause esophagitis than is reflux. Other diagnostic possibilities include eosinophilic (allergic) gastroenteritis, caustic ingestion (usually lye-containing cleaning agents), Crohn's disease, and dermatologic conditions (toxic epidermal necrolysis, epidermolysis bullosa, erythema multiforme, and pemphigus). In general, in such patients, the clinical setting is different, other problems are usually obvious, and the differential diagnosis is not difficult.

Barrett's Esophagus

Barrett's esophagus is acquired columnar metaplasia of the distal esophagus resulting from chronic gastroesophageal reflux. The association between gastroesophageal reflux and Barrett's esophagus has been recognized for decades in adults, but only recently has it become widely accepted that, in children, the pathogenesis is the same and is not the result of a congenital abnormality. The incidence of Barrett's esophagus is reported to be approximately 10% of pediatric patients with gastroesophageal reflux.[6, 9–11]

In Barrett's esophagus, the entire thickness of mucosa is transformed. Surface epithelial cells resemble gastric epithelial cells, uniform tall columnar cells with basal nuclei, and an abundant mucus-containing apical cytoplasm. A prominent glandular layer is present, with glands resembling mucous glands of gastric cardia or, alternatively, gastric fundic glands with parietal and chief cells. Three histologic types of Barrett's esophagus have been described, although mixed types are also common[12, 13]: (1) gastric fundic type, (2) junctional type resembling gastric cardia, and (3) specialized columnar type with a prominent villiform surface and goblet cells interspersed with columnar surface epithelial cells (Fig. 79–4). Special histologic stains, especially periodic acid–Schiff combined with Alcian blue at pH 2.5, enhance recognition of goblet cells and also show focal positivity of occasional surface epithelial cells containing intestinal-type mucins, as opposed to gastric-type mucins, which are found in most surface epithelial cells in Barrett's esophagus.[11, 14]

Of the three histologic types, gastric fundic and junctional types of Barrett's esophagus are the most commonly encountered in children. The specialized colum-

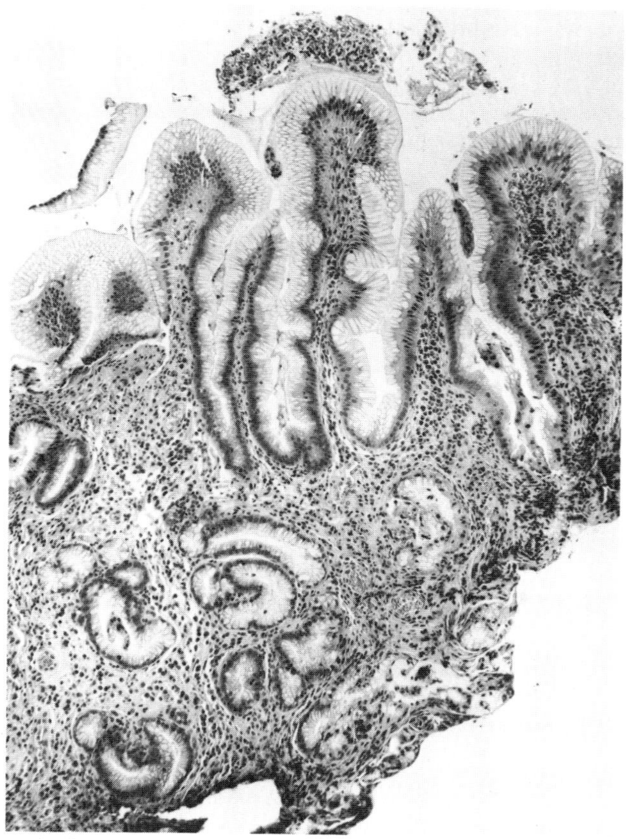

Figure 79–4. Barrett's esophagus from a biopsy of the mid-esophagus in an adolescent with a long history of reflux esophagitis. This example has villous projections, tall columnar epithelium, distorted mucous glands, and diffuse inflammatory infiltration of the lamina propria. Hematoxylin-eosin stain, × 120.

nar type is usually restricted to those in the adolescent age group or older. All three types of Barrett's mucosa often show inflammation and glandular distortion or shortening that prevent confusion with normal stomach, but this is not a reliable criteria. Of the three histologic types, only the specialized columnar type is sufficiently distinctive so as not to be confused with normal gastric mucosa at the squamocolumnar junction. Certainty in the diagnosis of Barrett's esophagus rests on the location of the biopsy in relation to the LES, as well as histologic findings. Because the normal squamocolumnar junction is variable and may show a zigzag configuration of gastric and squamous mucosa at the interface, the diagnosis of Barrett's esophagus is doubtful within 2 or 3 cm proximal to the LES when only gastric mucosa is present. In equivocal cases, multiple additional biopsies may be required from different levels and different points on the esophageal circumference to determine whether or not a Barrett's esophagus is present. Identification of specialized columnar epithelium at any level of the esophagus, or identification of gastric fundic or junctional types of mucosa 3 cm or more proximal to the LES, permits more certain diagnosis of Barrett's esophagus.

Once the diagnosis of Barrett's esophagus has been considered or made with certainty, it is important to monitor the patient regularly. In adults, a progression from dysplasia with Barrett's esophagus to adenocarcinoma is thought to occur.[13] Dysplasia and adenocarcinoma are rare in children, but they do occur.[15, 16]

Infectious Esophagitis

Fungi, chiefly *Candida* species and viruses, may cause esophagitis but rarely do so in normal immunocompetent children. Those groups at greatest risk are congenitally immunodeficient children, patients with acquired immunodeficiency syndrome (AIDS), organ transplantation patients, cancer patients, and long-term hospitalized patients treated with antibiotics or steroids. Esophageal biopsy material in immunocompromised children should be carefully examined for viral inclusions and fungi. Fungal identification is greatly enhanced by use of special stains, especially Gomori's methanamine silver and periodic acid–Schiff. Immunostaining (immunoperoxidase) may be helpful in instances in which viral inclusion bodies are not seen, but viral infection is suspected and morphology is equivocal. Viral culture of endoscopically obtained tissue may permit a diagnosis of herpes or CMV esophagitis in the absence of diagnostic tissue changes and is recommended in high-risk patients.

Candida *esophagitis*[17, 18] usually occurs in the distal one third of the esophagus and appears as white plaques, with or without surrounding hyperemia and ulcerations. Histologically, plaques and ulcer beds show a tangle of yeast forms and pseudohyphae amid acute inflammatory cells and necrotic cellular debris. The surrounding mucosa shows acute and chronic inflammation and epithelial changes that may resemble the changes of reflux esophagitis. *Aspergillus*, *Mucormycosis,* and *Cryptococcus* have also been reported as infectious agents in fungal esophagitis.

Herpes esophagitis is the most commonly encountered viral infection of the esophagus.[19] It may occur in otherwise normal children accompanying primary herpetic gingivostomatis,[20] but is commoner as a reactivation of previously encountered herpesvirus infection in immunosuppressed or debilitated persons. Multiple small, well-circumscribed ulcers covered by white exudate and surrounded by normal mucosa may be seen anywhere in the esophagus; in severe cases, ulceration is confluent. Ulcers consist chiefly of necrotic debris and usually do not contain diagnostic herpesvirus inclusions. Inclusions are found in intact squamous cells at ulcer margins and are of two types: Cowdry type A inclusions are large, single intranuclear inclusions surrounded by a clear halo and are usually less numerous than the Cowdry type B inclusions, which are homogeneous ground-glass intranuclear inclusions with a smudged appearance, often found within multinucleated giant cells. The small sample size of mucosal biopsies may not permit demonstration of characteristic inclusions. Herpes infection may be suspected by the findings of severe neutrophilic infiltration, discohesion of epithelial cells, and bland necrosis, all of which are usual in reflux esophagitis. If endoscopically normal-appearing mucosa is biopsied, histologic changes may be mild and nonspecific, or the biopsy may be normal.

CMV esophagitis is rare, even in immunosuppressed patients. When present, it is often part of a more generalized gastrointestinal or systemic CMV infection. Microscopically, the giant intranuclear inclusions are easily recognizable on routine hematoxylin-eosin stain. If inclusions are present, they are located in endothelial cells and fibroblasts of ulcer bed or lamina propria rather than in squamous cells.

STOMACH

Technical Considerations and Normal Gastric Mucosa

The chief use of gastric mucosal biopsy in children is to establish the presence of gastritis and to determine whether it is a nonspecific or a distinctive entity, such as *H. pylori* infection, eosinophilic gastroenteritis, or Crohn's disease. Children usually do not develop many of the entities diagnosed on adult gastric biopsies, including atrophic gastritis, intestinal metaplasia, and adenocarcinoma. Endoscopically abnormal areas of the stomach should be sampled or, if lesions are not grossly apparent, both the body of the stomach and the antrum should be biopsied. Often, gastritis is histologically apparent first in the antrum and, if generalized, is severer in the antrum than elsewhere. Multiple tissue samples of the antrum are better than a single sample for demonstration of *H. pylori*, which may be focally distributed.

All areas of the stomach are covered by uniform tall columnar surface epithelium which dips into pits, into which empty the secretions of a thick layer of complex glands. Glands in the fundus and the body are long and straight, but because of an oblique orientation and sectioning of mucosal biopsy specimens are often seen in cross-section. Glands are packed with large eosinophilic parietal cells and paler chief cells. Antral (pyloric) glands are much shorter, approximately the same length as the gastric pits. Uniform mucous cells line the straight or loosely coiled antral glands. The histologic transition from body to antrum may differ from the grossly apparent transition area, and there may be a zone of variable length where mixed antral and fundic glands are found. The glandular layer of the stomach increases in thickness throughout childhood. Grasp biopsies in infants may secure the entire mucosa and even some submucosa. In adolescents, it is more usual that only the surface epithelium and superficial portions of the glandular layer are obtained. Lamina propria is most apparent just beneath the surface epithelium and adjacent to gastric pits; there is normally little space between glands, especially in the body of the stomach. The lamina propria contains a small number of diffusely distributed plasma cells and lymphocytes. Lymphoid aggregates or follicles are distinctly rare in young children, but may be seen occasionally in adolescents. Neutrophils are not normally present at any age.

Chronic Nonspecific Gastritis

The term *chronic gastritis* has been used in many different ways to describe diverse conditions including dyspepsia, persistent gastritis of various causes, and histologic gastritis with a chronic cellular infiltrate composed of lymphocytes and plasma cells. For years, the classification scheme of Whitehead provided the histologic standard by which gastritis was classified and graded.[21] More recently, simpler pathogenetically based classifications have been used.[22] For practical purposes, gastritis is characterized as chronic according to duration of symptoms and type of inflammatory infiltrate. Gastritis is said to be "specific" when it can be identified as a known disease, such as Crohn's disease, or eosinophilic gastroenteritis. *Chronic nonspecific gastritis* refers to a clinical and histologic picture for which no cause is known, although it is suspected to be within the spectrum of acid peptic disease. Affected patients may have associated peptic ulcers, and the gastritis often responds to antacids or histamine H_2 antagonists. It is commonly diagnosed in school-aged children who present with persistent epigastric pain and sometimes vomiting. Typically, the antrum is involved earliest and usually remains more severely affected when the process spreads to the body of the stomach.

At endoscopy, the mucosa in chronic nonspecific gastritis is erythematous, edematous, and friable. Histologically, the lamina propria is diffusely infiltrated with lymphocytes and plasma cells, often causing separation of the normally tightly packed glands (Fig. 79–5). Lymphoid aggregates and follicles may be superimposed on diffuse background inflammation. In severe cases a focal neutrophilic infiltrate is present, usually surrounding acutely inflamed glands. Small glandular abscesses, glandular distortion, and even focal glandular destruction are seen in the severest cases. When polymorphonucelar leukocytes are present, the gastritis is said to be "active"; this finding is associated with clinical exacerbations. The surface epithelium is usually intact, although it may appear more cuboidal than usual. Erosions are present in extremely severe cases.

The differential diagnosis of chronic nonspecific gastritis includes all of the entities with more distinctive histologic findings, including *H. pylori* gastritis, eosinophilic gastroenteritis, and Crohn's disease.

Helicobacter Pylori Gastritis

H. pylori (formerly *Camplylobacter pylori* or *Campylobacter*-like organisms) may be responsible for most cases of chronic gastritis and duodenal ulcer disease in children and adolescents.[23–27] It is rarely found in children younger than 5 years of age, but has been demonstrated in the stomach of 50 to 70% of children with chronic gastritis and is also found in the stomach of 90% of children and adolescents with duodenal ulcers. *H.*

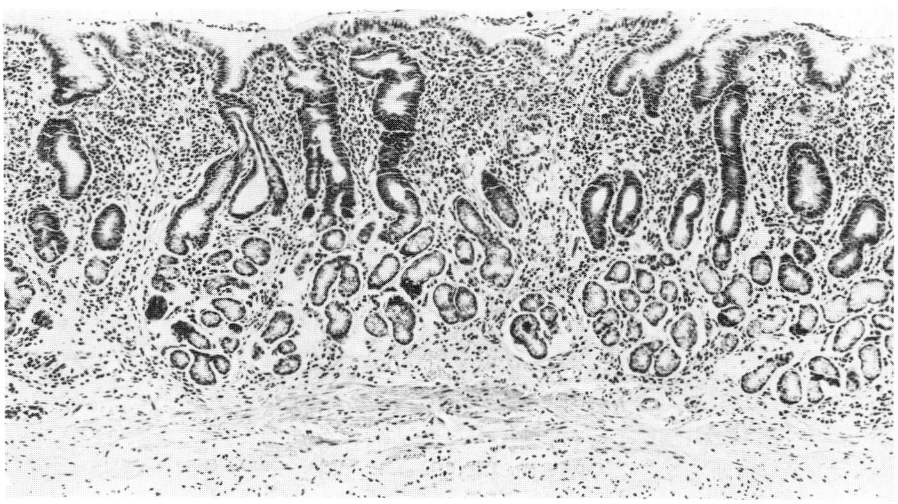

Figure 79–5. Chronic nonspecific gastritis. The lamina propria of the antrum is filled with chronic inflammatory cells, causing separation and distortion of the glands. Surface epithelium is flattened. Hematoxylin-eosin stain, × 88.

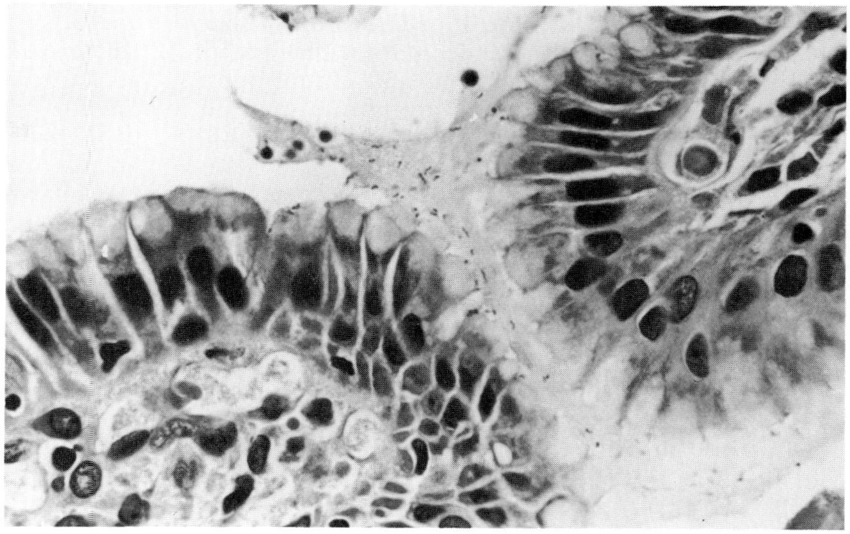

Figure 79–6. *Helicobacter pylori* gastritis. Numerous slender bacilli can be discerned within the mucous coat overlying gastric epithelial cells. This is the appearance of *H. pylori* on high magnification (× 1,200) with hematoxylin-eosin staining.

pylori is not found in the absence of histologic gastritis, although the gastritis may not always be symptomatic. The organism is present only in cases of primary gastritis; patients with gastritis secondary to Crohn's disease or eosinophilic gastroenteritis do not carry the organism.

Histologic demonstration of the organism is currently the easiest and most direct way to make the diagnosis.[28] At low magnification, the histology is identical to that of chronic nonspecific gastritis: diffuse chronic gastritis with plasma cells and lymphocytes uniformly filling the lamina propria, intact surface epithelium and rare foci of neutrophilic infiltration surrounding acutely inflamed glands. Foci of acute inflammation are seen much less frequently in children than in adults with *H. pylori* gastritis. The organisms are most reliably found in the antrum, although by the time a biopsy is performed, many patients have fundal gastritis as well.

Organisms are seen as rows and groups of slender bacilli, 3 to 5 μm long under high dry magnification (× 400) in the superficial mucous coat overlying surface epithelium and within the superficial portions of gastric pits (Fig. 79–6). Hematoxylin-eosin–stained slides are perfectly adequate to identify the bacteria, if tissue is well fixed and thinly sectioned to 5 μm or less. Under oil immersion the organisms can be seen better since their loose S-shape or curved structure is more apparent. The organisms can also be visualized with a number of special stains, including Giemsa, Warthin-Starry, Brown-Hopps, acridine orange, Steiner, Diff-Quick, and a number of modifications of the Gram stain. The organism cannot be seen on standard tissue Gram stains such as Brown-Brenn.

The appearance of the organisms in the mucous coat is distinctive and correlates exactly with a positive culture of the organism in medical centers where cultures are performed. Failure to see the organism when it is present (false negative) may be a problem if technical quality of the slides is poor, especially if the section is more than 5 μm thick. In some laboratories special stains may be necessary to visualize the bacilli with certainty. Giemsa stain is the simplest of those currently used for this purpose.

Eosinophilic Gastroenteritis

Eosinophilic gastroenteritis is a rare disease characterized by segmental eosinophilic infiltration of the gastrointestinal tract. It involves the gastric antrum and proximal small intestine in at least two thirds of patients. The diagnosis requires systemic findings, including peripheral blood eosinophilia, extraintestinal allergic manifestations such as eczema or asthma, and usually increased serum immunoglobulin E (IgE). A poorly understood allergic reaction is thought to cause the disease.[29–33] Gastrointestinal involvement may be transmural, mucosal, or, rarely, only serosal in location. In most cases the gastric antrum is the most severely affected site in the gastrointestinal tract and should be one of the sites biopsied when the diagnosis is considered. Mucosal biopsy specimens show patchy or diffuse inflammation of the lamina propria with a predominance of eosinophils. The number of eosinophils in the antrum is often striking, with 10 to 50 or more present in a single high-power microscopic field.[33] There is always an associated eosinophilic infiltration of surface epithelium and glands. Eosinophilic aggregates in lamina propria and glandular lumens are seen in severe cases.

The strict laboratory and histologic diagnostic criteria cited should be met before a diagnosis of eosinophilic gastroenteritis is made. Lesser numbers of eosinophils may be found in the stomach when subacute or chronic inflammation occurs, including instances of Crohn's disease, infections in immunosuppressed patients, cow's milk protein intolerance, and chronic nonspecific gastritis.

Gastric Crohn's Disease

Crohn's disease of the stomach usually occurs in association with disease in the more usual location, that is, the ileum and the colon. Crohn's disease occasionally may present in the stomach. In such cases, the antrum is usually involved, often in continuity with proximal duodenum. Gastric histology is similar to that of Crohn's disease in other sites.[34] Diffuse or patchy chronic inflammation with numerous plasma cells in the lamina propria infiltrate, small noncaseating granulomas, lymphoid aggregates, and ulcerations are all characteristic. In adults, isolated granulomatous gastritis not associated with Crohn's disease has been described rarely.[35] Additional but rare causes of gastric granulomatous inflammation include tuberculosis, fungal infections, sarcoidosis, and chronic granulomatous disease.

Ménétrier's Disease

Although often mentioned in the differential diagnosis of gastric outlet obstruction, Ménétrier's disease is extremely rare in children. It has been associated with CMV infection, and unlike Ménétrier's disease in adults,[36] is usually self-limited. Histologic features include mucous cell hyperplasia and elongation of gastric pits, mucous cell-lined cysts between the gastric pits and glandular layer, and glandular atrophy. In children, other causes of gastric outlet obstruction, such as peptic ulcer disease, *H. pylori* gastritis, Crohn's disease, eosinophilic gastroenteritis and chronic granulomatous disease,[37] are more likely to be encountered than is Ménétrier's disease.

SMALL INTESTINE

Technical Consideration and Normal Small Intestinal Mucosa

It is most important that of all gastrointestinal mucosal sites biopsied in children, those from the small intestine be properly handled in the endoscopy suite and histology laboratory. Accurate histologic diagnosis depends on evaluation of villus height and structure, which can only be achieved if the specimen is properly oriented and sectioned at right angles to the surface. The endoscopist or a designated assistant should carefully remove the specimen from the capsule and place it, submucosal side down, on filter paper or similar material prior to placing it in fixative. The histotechnologist is then able to orient the specimen accurately and section it properly. If this step is omitted, tangential sectioning results in artifactual shortening and widening of villi, leading to possible misinterpretation (Fig. 79–7*A*). Obliquely cut mucosa can be recognized by cross sectioning of the usually straight tubular glands and, in extremely tangential sections, artifactual multilayering of the normally basal single layer of nuclei in surface cells (Fig. 79–7*B*). A row of at least three contiguous villi is necessary for optimal evaluation. Some of the deficiencies of tangential sectioning can be recouped by examination of serial sections, but this process is tedious and never entirely satisfactory.

Optimally oriented sections of duodenum and jejunum show a ratio of villus height to crypt length of 3 to 1 in infants and 4 to 1 in older children. Villi are slightly more slender and uniform in the jejunum than in the duodenum, where villi over Brunner's glands may appear stretched or shortened. Villi are covered by tall columnar surface enterocytes for the most part, with goblet cells interspersed. With optimally thin sections, the brush border of surface enterocytes can be discerned under high dry magnification. Only rare lymphocytes and no neutrophils are normally present in surface glandular epithelium. The lamina propria contains a uniformly dispersed population of lymphocytes, plasma cells, and occasional eosinophils and histiocytes. Mitosis takes place in the crypts of Lieberkühn, where mitotic figures are seen occasionally in crypt epithelium. Migration and differentiation of immature crypt cells to villus tips take approximately 5 to 6 days.

In addition to villus architecture, a small intestinal biopsy is also evaluated for the presence, type, and distribution of inflammation, including the absence of plasma cells (a possible clue to immunodeficiency), the presence of infectious organisms, such as *Giardia lamblia*, and abnormal infiltrations, such as the storage cells of Wolman disease or the foamy histiocytes of *Mycobacterium avium-intracellulare* infection. Special stains are not routinely done, but may be necessary if examination of hematoxylin-eosin sections suggests the presence of certain infectious organisms or storage materials. Electron microscopy is rarely done on small intestinal biopsy sections; the chief indication for this in children is in the evaluation for intractable diarrhea of infancy, when congenital microvillus atrophy is being considered. In some patients with malabsorption, a frozen-tissue sample may be saved for analysis of enzyme activity, particularly when disaccharidase deficiency is being considered.

Small intestinal mucosal biopsies are performed when three main clinical diagnostic categories are suspected: peptic duodenitis, malabsorption, and unusual infections.

Peptic Duodenitis

Patients with acid-induced inflammation of the duodenum are usually older children who present with recurrent episodes of epigastric pain. In severe cases, duodenal ulcer is also present. The duodenal biopsy findings of this common condition are nonspecific and consist chiefly of chronic inflammation in the lamina propria and variable but mostly mild villous atrophy. During clinical exacerbations, neutrophils are often superimposed, mixed with the chronic inflammatory infiltrate in the lamina propria and infiltrating glandular or surface epithelium. The more specific findings of gastric metaplasia and Brunner's gland hyperplasia described in adults with this condition are almost never seen in children.[22] Biopsy findings of peptic duodenitis are not diagnostic by themselves but rather serve to support and quantify clinical and endoscopic impressions. In pediatric patients, biopsy results are likely to be reported as "nonspecific acute and chronic inflammation of duodenal mucosa" rather than as a more specific finding. Documentation of duodenal inflammation permits separation of patients with acid-peptic disease from those with functional epigastric complaints.

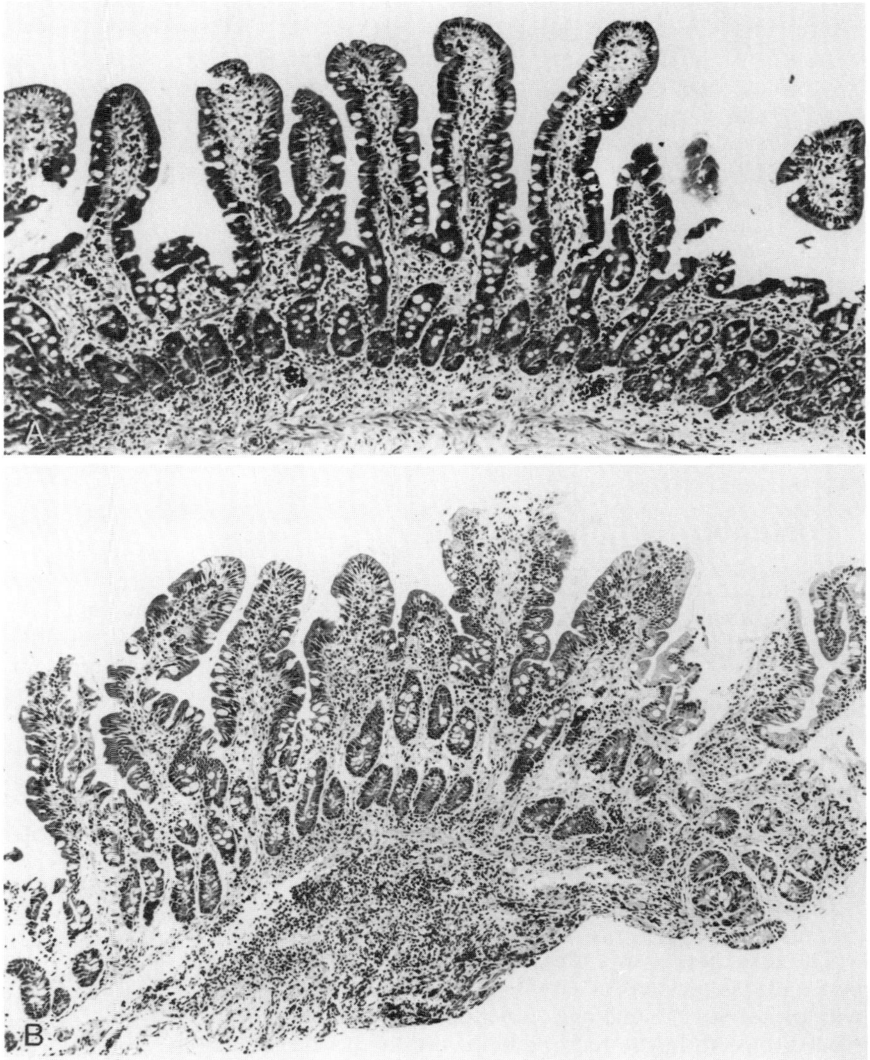

Figure 79–7. Normal small intestinal biopsy. *A,* Optimal orientation and sectioning perpendicular to the surface demonstrates normal villus-to-crypt ratio and tall slender villi. Note that the glands are longitudinally sectioned. Hematoxylin-eosin stain, × 88. *B,* Oblique sectioning of the same biopsy specimen as *A* at another location in the serial section. Note that the glands are cross-sectioned, an indication of oblique orientation. Villi are artifactually shortened relative to glandular depth, artifactually widened, and variable in height. Hematoxylin-eosin stain, × 88.

Celiac Disease

No laboratory test has replaced serial intestinal biopsies for diagnosing celiac disease. Celiac disease can be strongly suspected from a single small intestinal biopsy, but the most conservative approach to establishing the diagnosis is the three-biopsy, or "on-off-on" gluten, protocol: (1) clinical demonstration of malabsorption and an initial abnormal biopsy while the patient is on an unrestricted diet containing gluten, (2) resolution of symptoms and histologic findings on a gluten-free diet, and (3) recurrence of symptoms and biopsy abnormalities with dietary gluten challenge. Because celiac disease is a lifelong illness requiring an inconvenient diet, and because there is an increased risk of gastrointestinal lymphoma and carcinoma in affected adults, diagnosis should be established with certainty by following this protocol when the diagnosis is made during the first year of life. In older children with typical biopsy abnormalities and a characteristic response to gluten withdrawal, repeat biopsy may not be necessary.

In untreated celiac disease ("on gluten"), proximal small intestine (Fig. 79–8) shows (1) total or nearly total villous atrophy; (2) flattening of surface epithelial cells and a tendency toward pseudostratification of nuclei; (3) compensatory crypt hypertrophy, that is, elongation of glands and increased mitotic activity in crypt epithelial cells; (4) diffuse heavy infiltration of lamina propria by plasma cells and lesser numbers of lymphocytes and eosinophils; (5) intraepithelial infiltration by lymphocytes; and (6) uniformity of villous atrophy and diffuse inflammation throughout the biopsy.[38–41]

A second biopsy taken after clinical response to a gluten-free diet ("off gluten") shows marked improvement in the villus to crypt ratio and resolution of most of the inflammation, but almost never is there restoration of completely normal morphology. The third, or gluten challenge, biopsy shows relapse of findings.

At the author's center and in many others in the United States, celiac disease is not commonly seen. Most small intestinal biopsies performed for clinical evidence of malabsorption are diagnosed as another entity. See Table 79–2 for other causes of villous atrophy in infants and children.

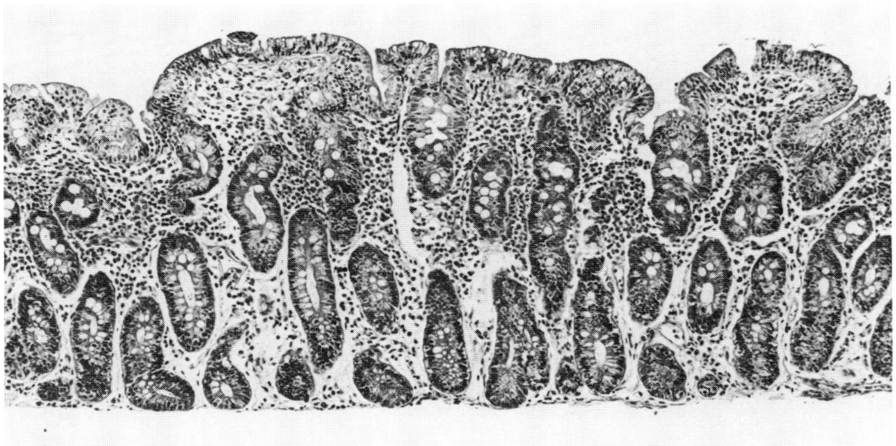

Figure 79–8. Celiac disease. This jejunal biopsy from an untreated patient shows nearly complete villous atrophy, elongation of the glandular layer, diffuse infiltration of the lamina propria by plasma cells and lymphocytes (which cannot be resolved at this magnification), and intraepithelial inflammatory cell infiltration. Compare with Fig. 79–7*A*. The uniformity and severity of villous atrophy and the diffuse nature of the inflammation are characteristic of celiac disease. Hematoxylin-eosin stain, × 88.

Postenteritis Enteropathy

An infant or child who recovers from an episode of apparent viral gastroenteritis will occasionally lapse into a malabsorptive state lasting weeks to months. Usually the clinical tests of malabsorption and biopsy findings are not as uniformly or severely abnormal as in celiac disease. Villous atrophy and inflammation are usually nonuniform in severity from one area to another, that is, the enteropathy is patchy (Fig. 79–9).[42, 43]

Cow's Milk and Soy Protein Intolerance

The history of cow's milk and soy protein intolerance is usually suggestive of cow's milk protein intolerance, with either very young age (<6 months) or recent switch from breast to bottle feeding being characteristic. Small intestinal biopsies often show varying severity of changes from area to area, or one tissue sample may demonstrate variable and usually subtotal villous atrophy and chronic inflammation of lamina propria, that is, patchy enteropathy (Figs. 79–9 and 79–10).[31, 44–49] Eosinophils may be increased in the lamina propria and present within surface and glandular epithelium, or they may be completely absent. If eosinophils are particularly numerous (>60 eosinophils per 10 high-power microscopic fields), the diagnosis of eosinophilic gastroenteritis should be considered. However, eosinophilic gastroenteritis occurs rarely in infants compared with cow's milk protein enteropathy, and its diagnosis requires systemic manifestations described later. The distinction between cow's milk protein enteropathy, which responds to dietary elimination of the offending protein, and eosinophilic gastroenteritis, which does not respond to dietary measures, may be difficult at times.[31]

Table 79–2. CAUSES OF VILLOUS ATROPHY IN INFANTS AND CHILDREN

Peptic duodenitis
Celiac disease
Infectious enteritis
Postenteritis enteropathy
Cow's milk and soy protein intolerance
Eosinophilic gastroenteritis
Immunodeficiency: congenital, acquired, AIDS
Crohn's disease
Protein-calorie malnutrition
Bacterial overgrowth or stasis
Microvillus inclusion disease
Intractable diarrhea of infancy

Eosinophilic Gastroenteritis

Children with the rare condition of eosinophilic gastroenteritis usually present after infancy and may manifest malabsorption or protein-losing enteropathy due to small intestinal involvement. Peripheral blood eosinophilia and other extraintestinal allergic manifestations may be present as well. Histologic diagnostic criteria are the same as discussed in the section on the stomach. Although intestinal changes are rarely as severe as those in the gastric antrum, patchy villous atrophy is present in cases with severe intestinal involvement. Small intestinal involvement, when present, is usually in the duodenum and proximal jejunum and may be focal. Multiple biopsies at different levels are suggested if the diagnosis is suspected.

Immunodeficiency

Either primary immunodeficiency or AIDS can present as malabsorption, diarrhea, and failure to thrive. Selective IgA deficiency and common variable hypogammaglobulinemia are the two commonest, superceded by AIDS in some hospitals. Variable degrees of villous atrophy and inflammation are seen on biopsy in many immunodeficient states.[50–52] In contrast with celiac disease, plasma cells are conspicuously absent, and enteropathy is patchy in some immunodeficiencies, such as common variable hypogammaglobulinemia, severe combined immunodeficiency, and X-linked agammaglobulinemia. Patients with immunodeficiency are particularly prone to giardiasis.

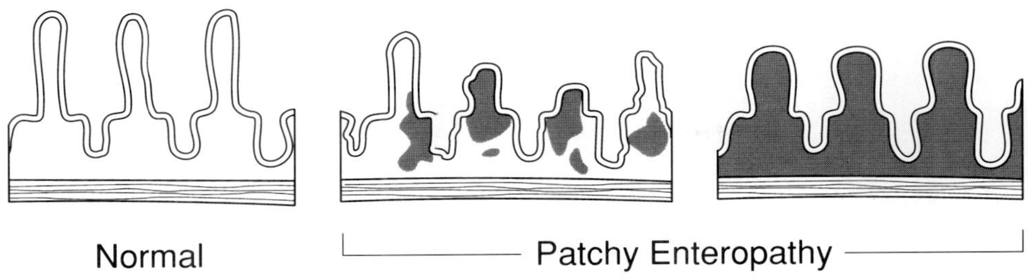

Figure 79–9. Patchy enteropathy refers to variable and usually subtotal villous atrophy and inflammation, which may vary in severity from area to area within the tissue section. Compare with Fig. 79–8, which shows uniform total villous atrophy and diffuse inflammation in celiac disease. Patchy enteropathy is nonspecific and may be found in postenteritis enteropathy, dietary protein intolerance, immunodeficiency states, Crohn's disease, some enteric infections, intractable diarrhea of infancy, and other conditions.

AIDS Enteropathy

Failure to thrive, diarrhea, and malabsorption often occur during the course of AIDS. In some patients with AIDS, intestinal infection with bacteria, *Giardia*, *Cryptosporidium*, *M. avium-intracellulare*, *Candida,* and CMV clearly exacerbate gastrointestinal symptoms. In other AIDS patients, diligent clinical and histologic search for these agents is negative, and bacterial pathogens are ruled out by culture, yet the patients have a histologic picture of subtotal villous atrophy and chronic inflammation of the lamina propria, so-called AIDS enteropathy (Fig. 79–11). Direct infection of the intestine by the HIV–1 virus is believed responsible, but this has not been validated.[53–56]

M. avium-intracellulare is an opportunistic systemic infection of AIDS patients with a distinctive filling of the lamina propria by foamy histiocytes packed with masses of bacilli. The histiocytes are able to ingest the organisms, but because of impaired cellular immunity, cannot kill them. Although the nearly pathognomonic histiocytes are easily identified on routine hematoxylin-eosin stain, a Ziehl-Neelsen stain is necessary to demonstrate the acid-fast bacilli.[57, 58] Infants with congenital AIDS usually do not become infected with *M. avium-intracellulare,* but infection with the organism occurs in older pediatric patients and adults with AIDS.

Other Infections

Some infectious agents causing diarrhea and malabsorption can be recognized on small intestinal biopsies, although most intestinal infections are better diagnosed by culture, serology, or stool examination. Trophozoites of *G. lamblia* are visible at the surface of small intestinal enterocytes or in the mucus coat, particularly between villi. The trophozoites have an arched or curved appearance at high magnification and are 10 to 18 μm long (Fig. 79–12). Immunocompetent children may show slight to moderate villous atrophy and chronic inflammation on biopsy; immunodeficient patients often show more severe changes.[59, 60] *Cryptosporidium* likewise may be found in normal persons, but is commoner in immunodeficient patients, particularly those with AIDS. The organisms are quite small (3–4 μm in diameter),

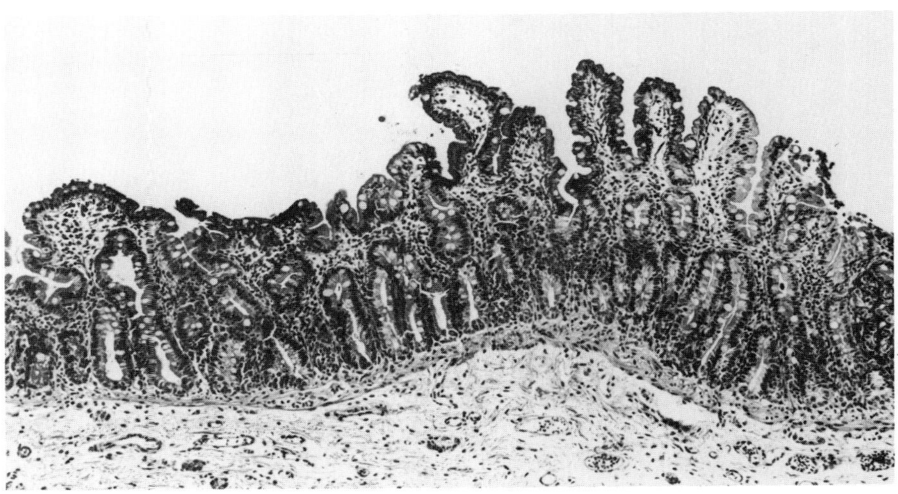

Figure 79–10. Cow's milk protein intolerance. This duodenal biopsy from an infant shows variable villous atrophy and nonuniform inflammation of the lamina propria. Hematoxylin-eosin stain, × 88.

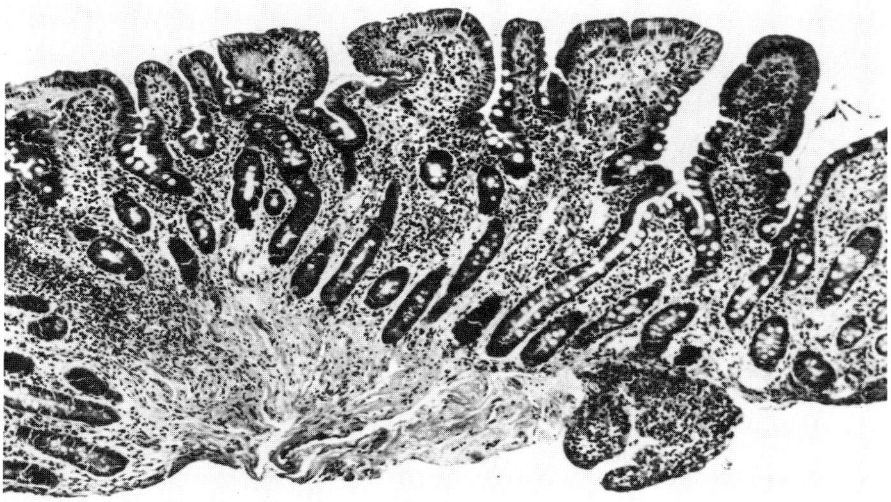

Figure 79–11. AIDS enteropathy. This duodenal biopsy from a 1-year old child with AIDS and chronic diarrhea shows nonspecific partial villous atrophy, villous blunting, and chronic inflammation. Bacterial and other pathogens were ruled out by negative bacterial and viral cultures and negative stool examination. Hematoxylin-eosin stain, × 88.

but can be seen on high dry magnification on hematoxylin-eosin–stained sections as a row of spherical basophilic structures.[61–63] Fungal diseases of the gastrointestinal tract are almost always limited to debilitated and immunosuppressed patients.

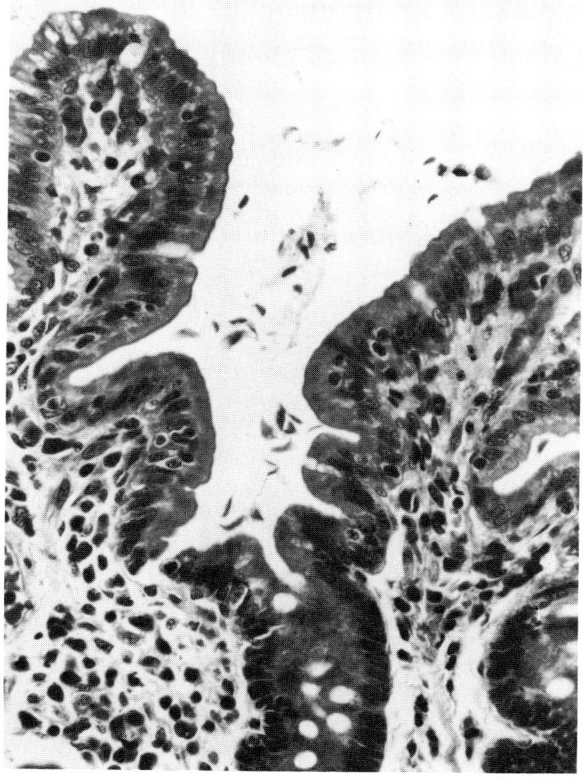

Figure 79–12. Giardiasis. The small, curved trophozoites of *Giardia lamblia* are present, overlying the surface epithelium between two villi in this duodenal biopsy. Hematoxylin-eosin stain, × 350.

Crohn's Disease

Small intestinal Crohn's disease may present with malabsorption, although other symptoms and signs usually are also apparent. The histology is described in the following section.

Intestinal Lymphangiectasia

Dilated lymphatic vessels in the lamina propria characterize the group of conditions known as *intestinal lymphangiectasia.* Primary intestinal lymphangiectasia is rare and often accompanied by extraintestinal lymphatic abnormalities. Secondary lymphangiectasia results from lymphatic obstruction due to cardiac conditions, tumors, and inflammatory bowel disease (IBD). The appearance of the biopsy specimen for both primary and secondary forms is similar, with dilated lymphatic vessels usually located near the tips of villi. Dilated lymphatic vessels must be distinguished from artifactual separation of surface epithelium from underlying lamina propria, which results from suction during the biopsy procedure. Lymphatic vessels are contained by endothelial cells, whereas artifactual tears are not.[64, 65]

Short Bowel Syndrome

Patients with marked dimunition of intestinal length following surgical resection often experience malabsorption from an inadequate absorptive surface area. In addition, administration of prolonged intravenous nutrition without peroral feedings contributes to villous atrophy and chronic inflammation. The mechanism of these changes is probably a combination of malnutrition and stasis.

Intractable Diarrhea of Infancy

Intractable diarrhea of infancy is a diagnostic category describing a young infant with diarrhea, malabsorption, and malnutrition lasting weeks to months and showing villous atrophy and chronic inflammation on small intestinal biopsy.[66, 67] The causes are unknown and include postinfectious diarrhea, dietary protein intolerance, familial disorders, and other now poorly understood disorders. The presence of serum autoantibodies to small intestinal epithelium in approximately half of affected patients[68, 69] and the clinical response to azathioprine and cyclosporine[70, 71] suggest that autoimmunity plays an etiologic role.

The role of biopsy in this condition is limited to documentation of clinically suspected small intestinal disease and elimination of known causes of diseases with similar symptoms, including giardiasis, eosinophilic gastroenteritis, microvillus inclusion disease, and immunodeficiency. The diagnosis is chiefly one of exclusion not only of the entities just mentioned but of a large number of others that can be eliminated as diagnostic possibilities only by exhaustive clinical laboratory testing.

The histologic findings seen in intractable diarrhea of infancy are variable from patient to patient and also differ from biopsy to biopsy in the same patient. By the time they are biopsied after several weeks of diarrhea, most infants show severe if not total villous atrophy, crypt hypertrophy, and patchy infiltration of the lamina propria by lymphocytes and plasma cells. In some instances, eosinophils are also noticeably increased, but they do not infiltrate epithelium. Neutrophils may also be mildly increased in the lamina propria. Cuboidal surface epithelial cells, edema, and mild secondary lymphangiectasia are often seen.[72–74] In many patients, pathologic changes are not limited to the small intestine. The colon and even the stomach may show chronic inflammation, epithelial flattening, and glandular distortion.

In infants with onset of secretory diarrhea within the first few weeks of life and severe abnormalities on small intestinal biopsy, it is necessary to rule out congenital microvillus atrophy (see later discussion).

Microvillus Inclusion Disease

Microvillus inclusion disease is a rare familial disease that presents at birth[75–77] with severe secretory diarrhea and must be distinguished from other causes of intractable diarrhea of infancy. The small intestinal mucosa is atrophic, with villous atrophy, crypt hypoplasia, and nonspecific chronic inflammation. It cannot be distinguished by light microscopy from many other conditions showing villous atrophy. The pathognomonic finding is seen only on electron microscopy of surface enterocytes, in which are found cytoplasmic inclusions surrounded by a distinctive brush border rim.

COLON

Technical Considerations and Normal Colonic Mucosa

Normal colonic mucosa has a flat surface without villi. It is dominated by closely aligned parallel crypts of Lieberkühn, which extend at right angles from the surface deep to the muscularis mucosae. The glandular appearance in histologic sections has been likened to the fingers of a glove, with little space, or lamina propria, between each finger. Most of the length of the crypts is lined by goblet cells, which are so numerous that at first glance they seem to constitute all the epithelial cells of the colon. However, the bases of the crypts contain immature columnar cells without mucin; tall columnar absorptive cells are distributed along the length of the crypts and, occasionally, on the luminal surface between crypts. Normally, mitosis is limited to the basal one half of the crypts, and no more than one or two mitotic figures per crypt are seen. The presence of more superficial or more numerous mitotic figures is a clue to increased cellular turnover. As cells mature, they are pushed up from the bases of the crypts and onto the surface. Abundant superficial goblet cells and tall columnar absorptive cells indicate normal maturation; goblet cell depletion and reduced height of absorptive cells indicate rapid turnover, which may be an acute or chronic process. Tangential sectioning of crypts, commonly seen in randomly oriented biopsy specimens, results in an appearance of numerous round glandular structures. In this instance, it is necessary to search serial sections for an area where the crypts are more optimally (longitudinally) sectioned, or else architectural changes such as crypt shortening, branching, or distortion may be missed.

The lamina propria in normal children contains diffusely distributed plasma cells, lymphocytes, histiocytes, and occasional eosinophils. Neutrophils are not normally present, nor are eosinophil clusters or intraepithelial eosinophils. The density of inflammatory cells depends on the age of the patient and the location within the lamina propria. The superficial zone just beneath the epithelium often contains more cells than do the deeper areas of lamina propria. Cellularity is less in neonates than in older infants and children. Lymphoid aggregates and follicles are seen occasionally in normal children. Muciphages are distinctive foamy histiocytes with abundant pale cytoplasm, filled with mucin released during goblet cell dissolution. The presence of these muciphages in large numbers may indicate a pathologic degree of epithelial cell destruction; however, they may also be found following laxative use or enemas.

Colitis

Evaluation of colonic mucosal biopsy specimens for the presence and type of colitis is often more difficult than evaluation of inflammation from other sites owing to the wide range of normal, the frequent appearance of artifacts mimicking inflammation, the nonspecificity of many of the histologic findings, and the numerous diagnostic possibilities.[78–80] Thickness of the tissue section, intensity of staining, age of the patient, and normal variation in the number of cells in the lamina propria influence the interpretation of cellularity. Familiarity with a given laboratory's range of normal appearance is crucial. A diagnosis of colitis requires more than a mild or moderate increase in the number of lymphocytes or plasma cells or the presence of an occasional lymphoid follicle in the lamina propria. Definite evidence of colitis includes (1) inflammatory cell infiltration of surface or crypt epithelium, (2) neutrophils in epithelium or lamina propria, (3) crypt damage, (4) degenerating or regenerating cuboidal epithelial cells, (5) epithelial nuclear enlargement and hyperchromatism with loss of apical mucin and goblet cells, (6) an unequivocal increase of inflammatory cells in the lamina propria, and (7) erosion or ulceration. An artifact encountered on colonic biopsies that mimics an erosion or ulcer is focal separation of surface epithelium. A true erosion has accentuated inflammatory cells and numerous netrophils in the subjacent lamina propria, whereas artifactual separation of epithelium does not. Epithelial cells overlying a lymphoid follicle often show flattening and intraepithelial lymphocytes, which is normal. Mild degrees of edema, congestion, and hemorrhage can be induced by the grasp or suction procedure of the biopsy; these must not be overinterpreted.

Once it is ascertained that colitis is present, an attempt is made to categorize it and, if possible, to make a precise diagnosis. Chronic changes that indicate likely ulcerative colitis or Crohn's disease are sought (see later). Histologic categorization beyond nonspecific inflammation often is not possible, and the gastroenterologist must interpret this in conjunction with history, cultures, endoscopic findings, and radiologic changes.

Infectious Colitis

When infectious colitis is being considered,[78–81] most infections are best diagnosed by stool culture and examination or an increase in a specific antibody titer, not by biopsy. Many infections produce a similar pattern of nonspecific acute inflammation in the mucosa. The biopsy helps with differential diagnosis in puzzling situations in which distinguishing the patterns of pure acute inflammation suggestive of infection helps to rule out a specific finding, such as allergic proctitis, underlying Crohn's disease, and ulcerative colitis. Only rarely is a specific infectious diagnosis such as amebiasis or pseudomembranous colitis possible. In the absence of specific histologic features or a positive microbiologic identification of the offending organism, the constellation of changes seen on biopsy in acute infections is known as *acute self-limited colitis*.[82, 83] These findings include neutrophilic infiltration of lamina propria and epithelium, crypt abscesses, edema, hyperemia and, in severe cases, erosions and ulcerations (Fig. 79–13). The background

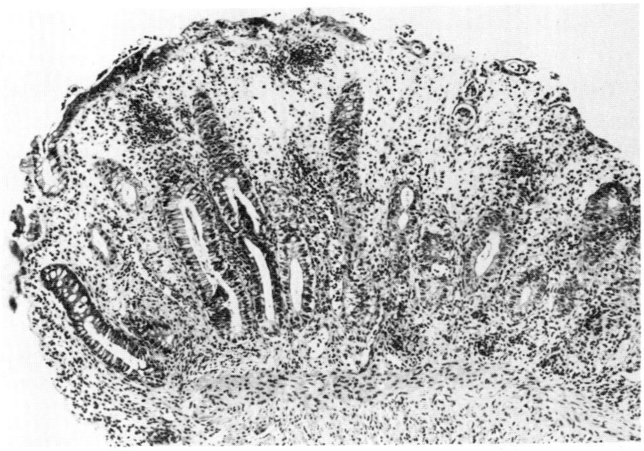

Figure 79–13. Infectious colitis. The colonic biopsy of this patient with *Salmonella typhimurium* shows focal superficial ulceration, edema, crypt abscesses, and inflammation of the lamina propria. The inflammatory infiltrate consists chiefly of neutrophils, which cannot be resolved at this magnification. Hematoxylin-eosin stain, × 88.

increase in chronic inflammatory cells characteristic of Crohn's disease and ulcerative colitis is absent (see later). Epithelial regenerative changes may be seen, but chronic crypt changes are not.

Pseudomembranous Colitis

Pseudomembranous colitis is a severe form of antibiotic-associated diarrhea resulting from overgrowth of *Clostridium difficile* in the colon, following alteration of normal intestinal flora.[84–86] In patients with Hirschsprung's disease, and rarely in others, pseudomembranous colitis can arise without antibiotic usage and may present as toxic megacolon.[87, 88] *C. difficile* can be cultured from stool with some difficulty using special microbiologic media; it is also diagnosed by documenting the presence of its fecal toxin (toxin B). Endoscopy often shows discrete 0.2- to 1-cm diameter yellow plaques on the colonic mucosal surface, with coalescence of the plaques into a shaggy membrane in the severest cases. Histologically, the plaques consist of neutrophils, necrotic debris, and mucus in continuity with similar exudate in dilated crypts. The superficial mucosa underlying the plaques is necrotic. At low magnification, the pseudomembrane forms a distinctive mushroom or cloud focally distributed over the surface, with intervening areas nearly normal in appearance (Fig. 79–14). However, this appearance is not always present with *C. difficile* infection; different phases of the disease may vary in appearance.

Chronic Inflammatory Bowel Disease (Ulcerative Colitis or Crohn's Disease)

In a patient with colonic symptoms of recent or uncertain onset, inconclusive radiographs, and nonspe-

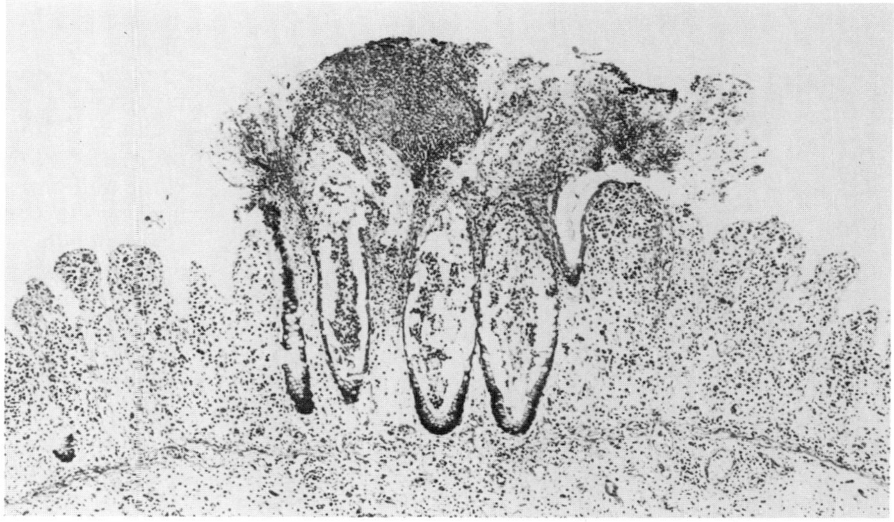

Figure 79–14. Pseudomembranous colitis. A plaque or membrane composed of neutrophils, necrotic epithelial cells, and inflammatory debris is present on the surface of the colon. The membrane may be focal, as in this example, or diffuse, and is often contiguous with subjacent crypt abscesses. Hematoxylin-eosin stain, × 56.

cific endoscopic findings, the pathologist is often asked to distinguish between chronic IBD[78, 89–93] (i.e., ulcerative colitis or Crohn's disease), and other conditions, including infectious colitis, acute self-limited colitis, irritable colon syndrome, and other causes of colonic symptoms. The distinction may be impossible on the first biopsy in many cases, although in some patients chronic changes permit assignment to the category of chronic IBD. These changes (Fig. 79–15) include the following:

1. Distortion of crypt architecture. This is one of the most reliable criteria for identification of IBD. Nonparallel crypts with vertical or horizontal branching, leaning crypts, missing crypts ("wide open spaces"), dilation, and short crypts (not extending deep to the muscularis mucosae) indicate chronic IBD.

2. Increase in chronic inflammatory cells (plasma cells and lymphocytes) in the lamina propria. Eosinophils may also be prominent. This change may be diffuse or focal; the distribution may help distinguish between ulcerative colitis and Crohn's disease. Acute inflammation may also be found in IBD and, in some patients, may be so severe that neutrophils dominate the inflammatory response. In such instances, the lamina propria still shows a net increase in chronic inflammatory cells. In most cases of infectious colitis, neutrophils more completely dominate the inflammatory response.

3. Noncaseating (sarcoid) granuloma (Fig. 79–16). This finding is nearly pathognomonic for Crohn's disease; however, fewer than 20% of patients with Crohn's disease present this finding on their first mucosal biopsy. Rarely, granulomas or giant cells are present without Crohn's disease; in such instances, the granulomas are usually single and specifically related to a ruptured crypt or surface ulceration.

4. A villous or undulating surface. This finding reflects present or previous crypt pathology with irregular shortening or other distortion.

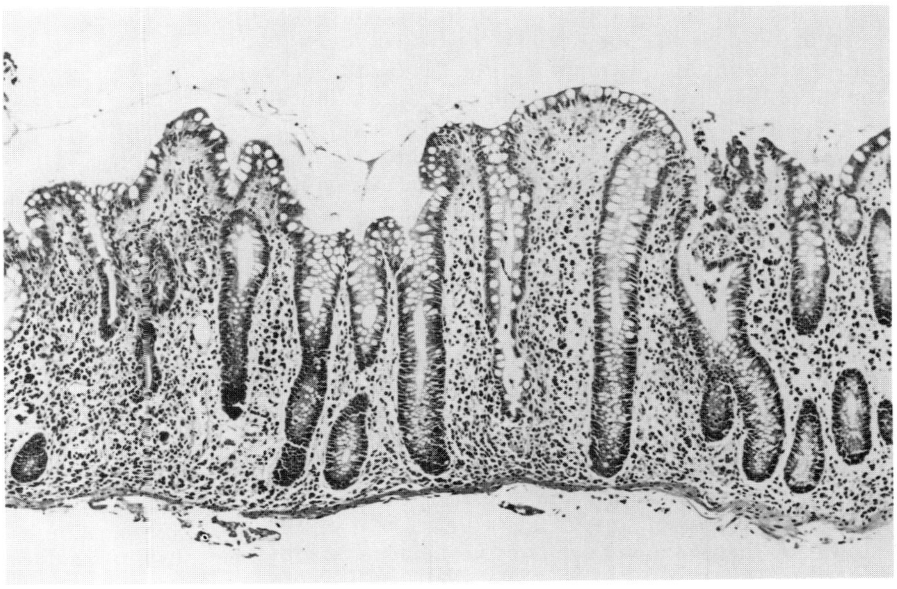

Figure 79–15. Chronic inflammatory bowel disease (ulcerative colitis). This was the first biopsy on an adolescent with recent onset of bloody diarrhea, yet chronic distortion of crypt architecture is apparent. On the left, several crypts extend only part way to the muscularis mucosae. A branching crypt is seen on the right. Crypt changes result in an undulating rather than a normally flat surface. The lamina propria shows a diffuse increase in plasma cells and lymphocytes (not identifiable at this magnification). These changes indicate disease chronicity and are characteristic of chronic inflammatory bowel disease. Hematoxylin-eosin stain, × 88.

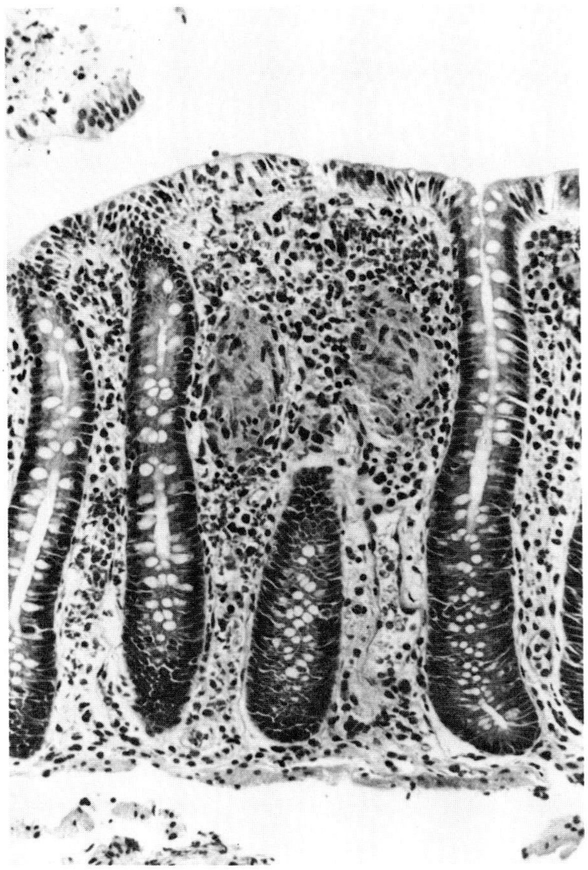

Figure 79–16. Crohn's disease. Two small granulomas are present in the lamina propria of this colonic biopsy. The noncaseating microgranulomas found in mucosal biopsies often consist of only a rounded, well-circumscribed collection of histiocytes. Granulomas indicate Crohn's disease, but are present less than 20% of the time in mucosal biopsies of patients with Crohn's disease. Hematoxylin-eosin stain, × 220.

5. Paneth cell metaplasia. Paneth cells are usually limited to small intestinal glands, with some spillover into the cecum and ascending colon. Their presence in the more distal parts of the colon is often an indication of chronic IBD.

6. A previous biopsy diagnosis of "moderate nonspecific colitis" with persistence or recurrence of symptoms over several months or longer, followed by a second biopsy with similar changes. In many patients with IBD, chronicity of symptoms and pathologic changes are the only way to make the diagnosis. Changes on any one biopsy may not be diagnostic of IBD, but persistence of low-grade chronic changes over months indicates IBD. There is a spectrum of severity in IBD—not all patients have progressive or fulminant disease. Of course, other histologic features are often found in chronic IBD, such as acute inflammation, cryptitis and crypt abscesses, erosions and ulcerations, and goblet cell depletion and increased mitoses of superficial and glandular epithelia. However, these changes are not too specific and may be found in infectious colitis and acute self-limited colitis.

Distinguishing between ulcerative colitis and Crohn's disease may be impossible by mucosal biopsy alone. Clinical observations, such as small intestinal or gastric involvement by symptoms, or radiologic studies and endoscopic findings, such as skip areas and pseudopolyps, are often instrumental in making the distinction. If the pathologist receives biopsy specimens from several levels of the colon, the distribution and the severity of pathology in each area are often a clue. Crohn's disease characteristically shows skip areas, a tendency to be worst in the right colon, rectal sparing, granulomas, and focal variations in the intensity of inflammation from one part of a given tissue section to another (microscopic skip areas; Fig. 79–17). Ulcerative colitis is almost always worst in the rectum and left colon and does not demonstrate skip areas. Microscopically, chronic inflammation in ulcerative colitis tends to be evenly distributed over the tissue section.

Allergic Proctitis and Allergic Colitis

Allergic proctitis and allergic colitis are common conditions that should be considered when infants, usually younger than 6 months of age, present with rectal bleeding, with or without diarrhea. Cow's milk or soy protein is the offending agent in most instances, although the condition is also recognized occasionally in breast-fed infants. Endoscopic abnormalities are usually limited to the rectum and left colon and include erythema, petechiae and, in severe cases, erosions. Biopsy material shows a diffuse and often striking increase in eosinophils in the lamina propria. Baseline criteria include a quantitative count of more than 60 eosinophils per 10 high power fields in addition to eosinophilic infiltration of surface and crypt epithelium. Intraepithelial eosinophils are usually focal, and examination of serial sections is often required to locate them. Eosinophilic aggregates in the lamina propria and eosinophilic crypt abscesses may be present. Hemosiderin-containing

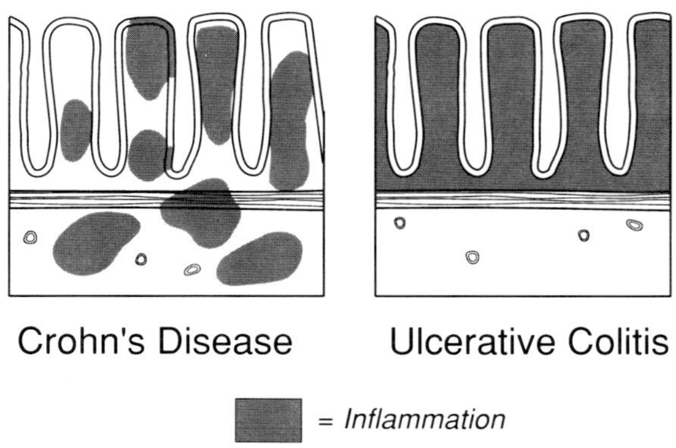

Figure 79–17. Patterns of inflammation in Crohn's disease *(left)* versus ulcerative colitis *(right)*. In ulcerative colitis, inflammation is diffuse, uniform, and limited to the mucosa. In Crohn's disease, the inflammation may be focal and variable, extending to the depths of the submucosa on the biopsy.

macrophages denote chronic bleeding into the lamina propria.[29, 45, 94, 95]

This condition must be distinguished from infectious colitis, which does not show the characteristic predominance of eosinophils in the inflammatory infiltrate. Occasional eosinophils may be found normally in lamina propria, and a mild increase in eosinophils may be found in any subacute or chronic inflammatory process of the colon.

Infants with allergic proctitis do not have the systemic manifestations or gastric antral and small intestinal involvement seen in eosinophilic gastroenteritis, although both conditions share the same striking degree of eosinophilic tissue infiltration, and both may have peripheral blood eosinophilia.[29]

Hemolytic-Uremic Syndrome

The gastrointestinal prodrome of hemolytic-uremic syndrome includes diarrhea and hematochezia. Infection with verotoxin-producing *Escherichia coli* and *Shigella* is associated with the development of hemolytic-uremic syndrome, and bacterial toxins are believed to be responsible for colonic mucosal inflammation and ulceration.[96, 97] Pseudomembranous colitis and toxic megacolon may occur in severe cases. Biopsy findings show nonspecific acute inflammation.

Hirschsprung's Disease

In Hirschsprung's disease, defective craniocaudad migration of neural crest cells during embryogenesis results in congenital absence of intramural parasympathetic ganglion cells, including those of the submucous (Meissner's) plexus, in the distal gastrointestinal tract.[98, 99] Histologic evaluation of rectal suction biopsy has become the standard diagnostic technique for evaluation of Hirschsprung's disease.[99, 100] If ganglion cells are seen in the submucous plexus, the diagnosis is ruled out, whereas absence of ganglion cells (aganglionosis) in the submucous plexus of a properly performed biopsy indicates Hirschsprung's disease. When rectal suction biopsy first became widely used for this purpose, it was regarded as a screening procedure, and it was thought necessary to confirm the diagnosis with demonstration of aganglionosis in the myenteric (Auerbach's) plexus of a transmural or muscularis propria biopsy. In many centers, the excellent correlation between mucosal and muscularis biopsy findings over years of experience has led to a change of opinion; diverting colostomies and "pull-through" procedures are now often done on the basis of aganglionosis in suction (mucosal) biopsies alone in patients with classic symptoms and an abnormal radiograph. This practice varies from hospital to hospital, however, depending on local practice, the experience and preference of the surgeon, the availability of suction biopsy, and the experience of the pathologist in interpreting the submucosal plexus in infants. Ganglion cells in the submucosal plexus are smaller and more difficult to identify than are those in the myenteric plexus; accurate and confident interpretation of the submucosal plexus requires experience on the part of the pathologist. Before placing a colostomy, some surgeons still rely on confirmation of aganglionosis in the myenteric plexus in a full-thickness or muscularis biopsy obtained under anesthesia.

It is imperative that a rectal biopsy for the evaluation of Hirschsprung's disease be taken at least 2 cm above the mucocutaneous junction. Nearer to the sphincter, normal persons demonstrate aganglionosis, which can easily be misinterpreted if the location is not recognized. Any squamous epithelium or striated muscle on the biopsy disqualifies it as too distal to interpret for Hirschsprung's disease. Multiple biopsies at a given level increase the probability of obtaining a good specimen. An adequate biopsy should contain at least as much tissue (submucosa) below the muscularis mucosae as above it. Ganglion cells should be carefully sought on four or five slides, each containing a ribbon of sections (at least 50 sections in all) before being interpreted as negative for ganglion cells. For certain identification, it is best to identify the "neural units" of Yunis and associates,[100] consisting of a nerve twig and several ganglion cells characteristically clustered around its perimeter. Ganglion cells are polygonal with abundant cytoplasm, an eccentric nucleus, and a prominent nucleolus. In neonates, the nucleolus is not present most of the time, and the amount of cytoplasm is less than in children and adults, making recognition more difficult. Endothelial cells, histiocytes and smooth muscle cells can all be mistaken for single ganglion cells. In Hirschsprung's disease the nerve fibers of the plexus are present, but ganglion cells are absent. Unusually large, prominent, and numerous nerve trunks are seen in approximately half of patients with Hirschsprung's disease. However, hypertrophic nerves are not a reliable indicator of Hirschsprung's disease, and when they are seen, the same methodic examination of serial sections should proceed as when large nerve trunks are absent. The submucosal plexus from a normal infant is compared with that of a patient with Hirschsprung's disease in Figure 79–18.

Mucosal biopsies require paraffin embedding and examination of serial sections for evaluation of ganglion cells. Frozen-section examination of mucosal biopsies is inadvisable, because only a limited amount of submucosa can be examined and resolution of ganglion cells is often inadequate. Frozen-section diagnosis of Hirschsprung's disease may be necessary in emergencies such as suspected Hirschsprung's enterocolitis or colonic perforation. Demonstration of aganglionosis by frozen section requires transmural biopsy or a biopsy of muscularis propria for visualization of the myenteric plexus, since in the myenteric plexus, ganglion cells are larger and are recognized with more certainty on frozen section than are submucosal ganglion cells.

Because the diagnosis of aganglionosis is a negative finding, and recognition of submucosal ganglion cells can be difficult, some laboratories perform acetylcholinesterase staining of frozen tissue sections in conjunction with examination of conventional hematoxylin-eosin–stained slides.[98, 101, 102] In Hirschsprung's disease, acetyl-

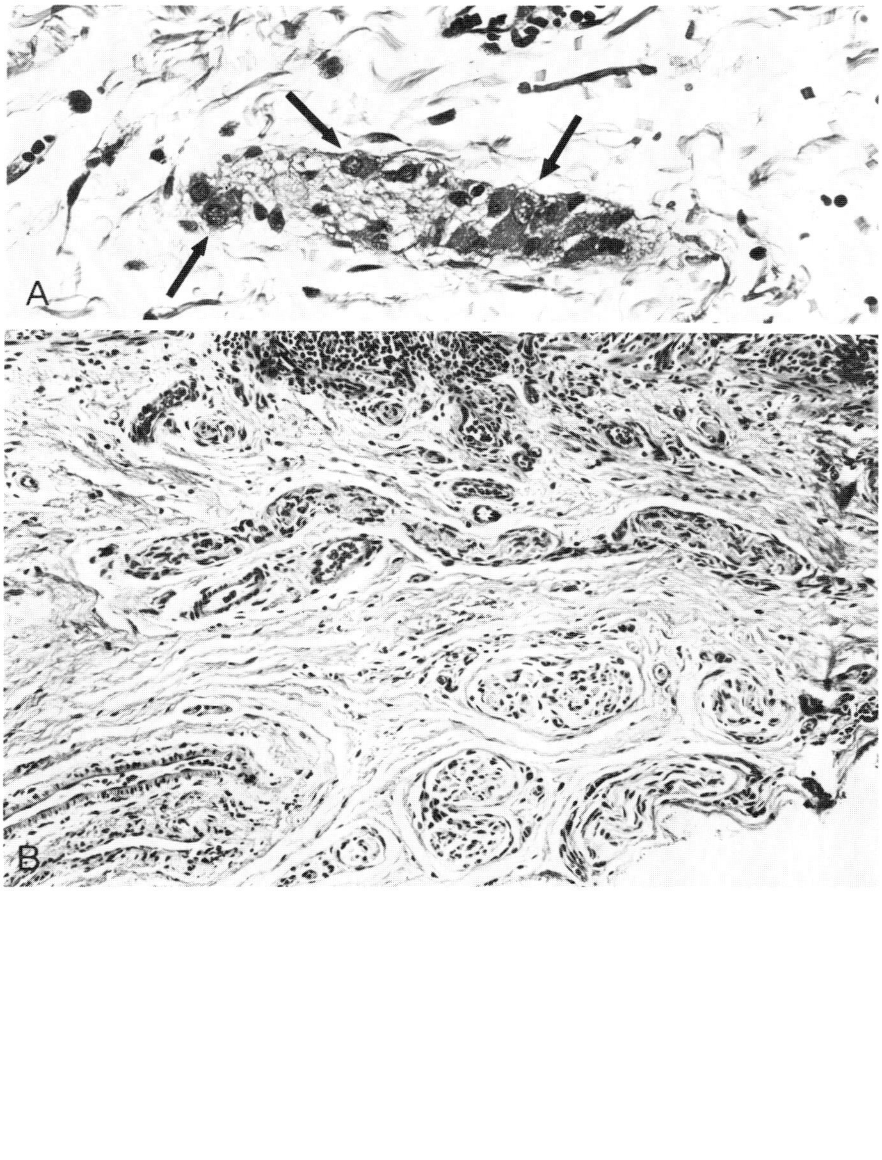

Figure 79–18. *A,* Normal submucosal (Meissner's) plexus from a rectal suction biopsy of an infant. The plexus consists of an elongate nerve fiber with several ganglion cells *(arrows)* clustered around its perimeter. Ganglion cell nuclei are eccentric and, in neonates, usually lack a nucleolus. Hematoxylin-eosin stain, × 350. *B,* Submucosal plexus in an infant with Hirschsprung's disease. The plexus consists of nerve fibers only, without ganglion cells. In this example, the nerve trunks are abnormally numerous, and those at the bottom of the photograph are larger than normal. Hematoxylin-eosin stain, × 140.

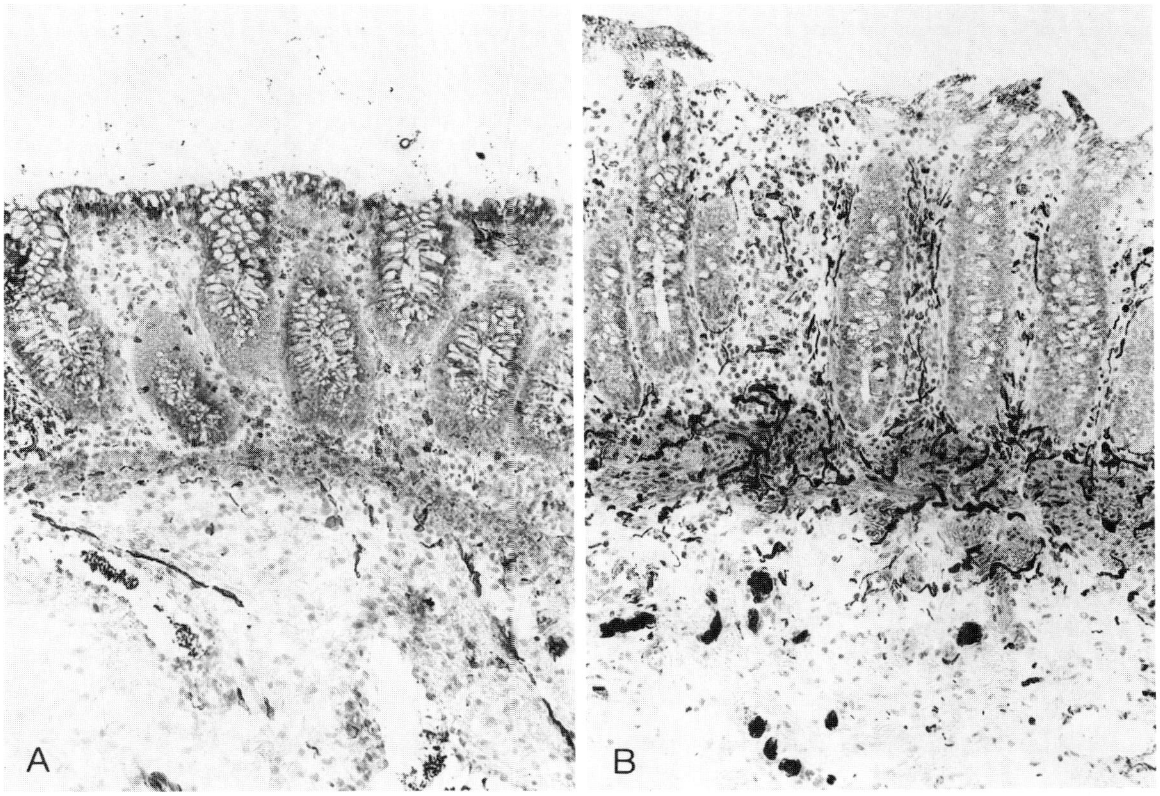

Figure 79–19. *A,* Acetylcholinesterase staining of a frozen section of rectal suction biopsy from a normal infant. Staining is negative, except for rare slender nerve fibers in the muscularis mucosae. Acetylcholinesterase stain, × 110. (Courtesy of A. James McAdams, MD.) *B,* Acetylcholinesterase staining of a rectal suction frozen section from a patient with Hirschsprung's disease. A network of black nerve fibers is present in muscularis mucosae and, to a lesser extent, in the lamina propria. Compare with *A.* Acetylcholinesterase stain, × 110. (Courtesy of A. James McAdams, MD.)

cholinesterase stain shows an increase in coarse cholinergic nerve fibers in the muscularis mucosae and sometimes extending into the lamina propria when compared with normal patients (Fig. 79–19). This provides a positive finding for the diagnosis of Hirschsprung's disease, which many pathologists and gastroenterologists find reassuring. Shortcomings of the technique are that it requires preparation of frozen sections, use of histochemical staining, and careful interpretation of the result. The pattern of acetylcholinesterase staining changes with age, and false-negative results may occur. Acetylcholinesterase staining cannot replace conventional hematoxylin-eosin staining of paraffin-embedded tissue, but may be helpful when done in conjunction with it.

Recently, immunoperoxidase staining for neuron-specific enolase and S100 protein has been advocated to facilitate the recognition of the immature submucosal plexus in paraffin-embedded sections.[103, 104] Most pathologists who frequently interpret mucosal biopsies for Hirschsprung's disease do not find this offers any advantage over examination of serial sections conventionally stained with hematoxylin-eosin.

Identification of even sparse numbers of ganglion cells in a mucosal suction biopsy taken 2 cm or more proximal to the mucocutaneous junction is evidence enough to eliminate Hirschsprung's disease as a diagnostic possibility. Rare cases of hypoganglionosis have been reported in patients presenting with symptoms similar to those of Hirschsprung's disease.[99] Hypoganglionosis is defined as a 10-fold decrease in normal numbers of ganglion cells in the myenteric plexus. In these patients, the entire plexus, nerve fibers as well as ganglion cells, is hypoplastic. Diagnosis of hypoganglionosis requires examination of the myenteric plexus[98]; mucosal biopsies cannot be used to quantitate ganglion cells.

REFERENCES

1. Biller JA, Winer HS, Grand RJ, et al: Are endoscopic changes predictive of histologic esophagitis in children? J Pediatr 1983; 103:215–218.
2. Dahms BB, Rothstein FC: Mucosal biopsy of the esophagus in children. Perspect Pediatr Pathol 1987; 11:97–123.
3. Dayal Y: Reflux esophagitis. *In* Cooper HS, Dayal Y, Gourley WK, eds: Proceedings of the 1988 Subspecialty Conference on Gastrointestinal Pathology at the USCAP. Mod Pathol 1989; 2:244–259.
4. Groben PA, Siegal GP, Shub MD, et al: Gastroesophageal reflux and esophagitis in infants and children. Perspect Pediatr Pathol 1987; 11:124–151.
5. Herbst JJ: Gastroesophageal reflux. J Pediatr 1981; 98:859–870.

6. Shub MD, Ulshen MH, Hargrove CB, et al: Esophagitis: A frequent consequence of gastroesophageal reflux in infancy. J Pediatr 1985; 107:881–884.
7. Winter HS, Madara JL, Stafford RJ, et al: Intraepithelial eosinophils: A new diagnostic criterion for reflux esophagitis. Gastroenterology 1982; 83:818–823.
8. Jessurun J, Yardley JH, Giardiello FM, et al: Intracytoplasmic plasma proteins in distended esophageal squamous cells (balloon cells). Mod Pathol 1988; 1:175–181.
9. Curtis DJ, Hassall E, Weinstein WM, et al: Barrett's esophagus in childhood. Gastroenterology 1985; 89:1331–1337.
10. Dahms BB, Rothstein FC: Barrett's esophagus in children: A consequence of chronic gastroesophageal reflux. Gastroenterology 1984; 86:318–323.
11. Qualman SJ, Murray RD, McClung J, et al: Intestinal metaplasia is age related in Barrett's esophagus. Arch Pathol Lab Med 1990; 114:1236–1240.
12. Paull A, Trier JS, Dalton MD, et al: The histologic spectrum of Barrett's esophagus. N Engl J Med 1976; 295:476–480.
13. Hamilton SR: Reflux esophagitis and Barrett's esophagus. *In* Goldman H, Apelman HD, Kaufman N, eds: Gastrointestinal Pathology. Baltimore, Williams & Wilkins, 1990, pp 11–68.
14. Lee RG: Mucins in Barrett's esophagus: A histochemical study. Am J Clin Pathol 1984; 81:500–503.
15. Cooper JE, Spitz L, Wilkins BM: Barrett's esophagus in children: A histologic and histochemical study of 11 cases. J Pediatr Surg 1987; 22:191–196.
16. Hoeffel JC, Nihoul-Fekete C, Schmitt M: Esophageal adenocarcinoma after gastroesophageal reflux in children. J Pediatr 1989; 115:259–261.
17. Mathieson R, Dutta SK. *Candida* esophagitis. Dig Dis Sci 1983; 28:365–370.
18. Scott BB, Jenkins D: Gastro-oesophageal candidiasis. Gut 1982; 23:137–139.
19. Nash G, Ross JS: Herpetic esophagitis, a common cause of esophageal ulceration. Hum Pathol 1974; 5:339–345.
20. Ashenburg C, Rothstein FC, Dahms BB: Herpes esophagitis in the immunocompetent child. J Pediatr 1986; 108:584–587.
21. Whitehead R, Trulove SC, Gear MWL: The histologic diagnosis of chronic gastritis in fiberoptic gastroscope biopsy specimens. J Clin Pathol 1972; 25:1–11.
22. Yardley JH: Pathology of chronic gastritis and duodenitis. *In* Goldman H, Appelman HD, Kaufman N, eds: Gastrointestinal Pathology. Baltimore, Williams & Wilkins, 1990, pp 69–143.
23. DeGiacomo C, Fiocca R, Villani L: *Helicobacter pylori* infection and chronic gastritis. J Pediatr Gastroenterol Nutr 1990; 11:310–316.
24. Drumm B, O'Brien A, Cutz E, et al: *Campylobacter pyloridis*-associated gastritis in children. Pediatr 1987; 80:192–195.
25. Drumm B, Sherman P, Cutz E, et al: Association of *Campylobacter pylori* on the gastric mucosa with antral gastritis in children. N Engl J Med 1987; 316:1557–1561.
26. Kilbridge PM, Dahms BB, Czinn SJ: *Campylobacter pylori*-associated gastritis and peptic ulcer disease in children. Am J Dis Child 1988; 142:1149–1152.
27. Mahony MJ, Wyatt JI, Littlewood JM: *Campylobacter pylori* gastritis. Arch Dis Child 1988; 63:654–655.
28. Yardley JH, Paull G: *Campylobacter pylori*: A newly recognized infectious agent in the gastrointestinal tract. Am J Surg Pathol 1988; 12(Suppl 1):89–99.
29. Goldman H, Proujansky R: Allergic proctitis and gastroenteritis in children. Am J Surg Pathol 1986; 10:75–86.
30. Katz AJ, Goldman H, Grand RJ: Gastric mucosal biopsy in eosinophilic (allergic) gastroenteritis. Gastroenterology 1977; 73:705–709.
31. Katz AJ, Twarog FJ, Zeiger RS, et al: Milk sensitive and eosinophilic gastroenteropathy: Similar clinical features with contrasting mechanisms and clinical course. J Allergy Clin Immunol 1984; 74:72–78.
32. Trounce JQ, Tanner MS: Eosinophilic gastroenteritis. Arch Dis Child 1985; 60:1186–1188.
33. Whitington PF, Whitington GL: Eosinophilic gastroenteropathy in children. J Pediatr Gastroenterol Nutr 1988; 7:379–385.
34. Haggitt RC, Meissner WA: Crohn's disease of the upper gastrointestinal tract. Am J Clin Pathol 1973; 59:613–622.
35. Fahimi HD, Deren JJ, Gottlieb LS, et al: Isolated granulomatous gastritis: Its relationship to disseminated sarcoidosis and regional enteritis. Gastroenterology 1963; 45:161.
36. Coad NAG, Shah AJ: Ménétrier's disease in childhood associated with cytomegalovirus infection: A case report and review of the literature. Br J Radiol 1986; 59:615–620.
37. Dickerman JD, Colletti RB, Tampas JP: Gastric outlet obstruction in chronic granulomatous disease of childhood. Am J Dis Child 1986; 140:567–570.
38. Lebenthal E, Branski O: Childhood celiac disease—a reappraisal. J Pediatr 1981; 98:681–690.
39. Perera DR, Weinstein WM, Rubin CE: Small intestinal biopsy. Hum Pathol 1975; 6:157–217.
40. Variend S, Phillips AD, Walker-Smith JA: The small intestinal mucosal biopsy in childhood. Perspect Pediatr Pathol 1984; 8:57–78.
41. Walker-Smith J: Coeliac disease. *In* Diseases of the Small Intestine in Childhood. 2nd ed. Kent, England, Pitman Medical Publishing, 1979, pp 91–138.
42. Barnes GL, Townley RRW: Duodenal mucosal damage in 31 infants with gastroenteritis. Arch Dis Child 1973; 48:343–349.
43. Manuel PD, Walker-Smith JA, France NE: Patchy enteropathy in childhood. Gut 1979; 20:211–215.
44. Fontaine JL, Navarro J: Small intestinal biopsy in cow's milk protein allergy in infancy. Arch Dis Child 1975; 50:357–362.
45. Grybowski JD: Gastrointestinal milk allergy in infants. Pediatrics 1967; 40:354–362.
46. Kuitunen P, Rapola J, Savilahti E, et al: Response of the jejunal mucosa to cow's milk in the malabsorption syndrome with cow's milk intolerance. Acta Paediatr Scand 1973; 62:586–595.
47. Kuitunen P, Visakorpi JK, Savilahti E, et al: Malabsorption syndrome with cow's milk intolerance: Clinical findings and course in 54 cases. Arch Dis Child 1975; 50:351–356.
48. Maluenda C, Phillips AD, Briddon A, et al: Quantitative analysis of small intestinal mucosa in cow's milk-sensitive enteropathy. J Pediatr Gastroenterol Nutr 1984; 3:349–356.
49. Walker-Smith J, Harrison M, Kilby A, et al: Cow's milk-sensitive enteropathy. Arch Dis Child 1978; 53:375–380.
50. Ament ME, Ochs HD, Davis SD: Structure and function of the gastrointestinal tract in primary immunodeficiency syndromes: A study of 39 patients. Medicine (Baltimore) 1973; 52:227–248.
51. Ament ME: Immunodeficiency syndrome and gastrointestinal diseases. Pediatr Clin North Am 1975; 22:807–825.
52. Doe WF: Immunodeficiency and the gastrointestinal tract. Clin Gastroenterol 1983; 12:839–853.
53. Dworkin B, Wormer GP, Rosenthal WS, et al: Gastrointestinal manifestations of the acquired immunodeficiency syndrome: A review of 22 cases. Am J Gastroenterol 1985; 80:774–778.
54. Kotler DP, Gaetz HP, Lange M, et al: Enteropathy associated with the acquired immunodeficiency syndrome. Ann Intern Med 1984; 101:421–428.
55. McLoughlin LC, Nord KS, Joshi VV, et al: Severe gastrointestinal involvement in children with the acquired immunodeficiency syndrome. J Pediatr Gastroenterol Nutr 1987; 6:517–524.
56. Powell KR: Approach to gastrointestinal manifestations in infants and children with HIV infection. J Pediatr 1991; 119(Suppl):534–540.
57. Horsburgh CR: *Mycobacterium avium* complex infection in the acquired immunodeficiency syndrome. N Engl J Med 1991; 324:1332–1338.
58. Klatt EC, Jensen DF, Meyer PR: Pathology of *Mycobacterium avium-intracellulare* infection in acquired immunodeficiency syndrome. Hum Pathol 1987; 18:709–714.
59. Hartong WA, Gourley WK, Arvanitakis C: Giardiasis: Clinical spectrum and functional-structural abnormalities of the small intestinal mucosa. Gastroenterology 1979; 77:62–68.
60. Rosekrans PCM, Lindeman J, Meijer CJLM: Quantitative histological and immunohistochemical findings in jejunal biopsy specimens in giardiasis. Virchows Arch (Pathol Anat) 1981; 393:145–151.
61. Alpert G, Bell LM, Kirkpatrick CE, et al: Cryptosporidiosis in a day care center. N Engl J Med 1984; 311:860.
62. Lefkowitch JH, Krumholz S, Feng-Chen KC, et al: Cryptosporidiosis of the human small intestine: A light and electron microscopic study. Hum Pathol 1984; 15:746–752.

63. Navin TR, Juranek DD: Cryptosporidiosis: Clinical, epidemiologic and parasitologic review. Rev Infect Dis 1984; 6:313–327.
64. Abramowsky C, Hupertz V, Kilbridge P, et al: Intestinal lymphangiectasia in children: A study of upper gastrointestinal endoscopic biopsies. Pediatr Pathol 1989; 9:289–297.
65. Vardy PA, Lebenthal E, Schwachman H: Intestinal lymphangiectasis: A reappraisal. Pediatrics 1975; 55:842–851.
66. Rossi TM, Lebenthal E, Nord KS, et al: Extent and duration of small intestinal mucosal injury in intractable diarrhea of infancy. Pediatrics 1980; 66:730–735.
67. Vanderhoof JA: The protracted diarrhea syndrome. *In* Balistreri WF, Vanderhoof JA, eds: Pediatric Gastroenterology and Nutrition. London, Chapman and Hill Medical, 1990, pp 123–131.
68. Mirakian R, Richardson A, Milla PJ, et al: Protracted diarrhea of infancy: Evidence in support of an autoimmune variant. Br Med J 1986; 293:1132–1136.
69. Colletti RB, Guillot AP, Rosen S, et al: Autoimmune enteropathy and nephropathy with circulating anti-epithelial cell antibodies. J Pediatr 1991; 118:858–864.
70. Coulthard M, Searle J, Patrick M: Cyclosporin-responsive enteropathy and protracted diarrhea. J Pediatr Gastroenterol Nutr 1990; 10:257–261.
71. Seidman EG, Lacaille F, Russo P, et al: Successful treatment of autoimmune enteropathy with cyclosporine. J Pediatr 1990; 117:929–932.
72. Schwachman H, Lloyd-Still JD, Khaw K, et al: Protracted diarrhea of infancy by intravenous alimentation: II. Studies of small intestinal biopsy results. Am J Dis Child 1973; 125:365–368.
73. Goldgar CM, Vanderhoof JA: Lack of correlation of small bowel biopsy and clinical course of patients with intractable diarrhea of infancy. Gastroenterology 1986; 90:527–531.
74. Shiner M, Putman M, Nichols VN, et al: Pathogenesis of small-intestinal mucosal lesions in chronic diarrhea of infancy: I. A light microscopic study. J Pediatr Gastroenterol Nutr 1990; 11:455–463.
75. Davidson GP, Cutz E, Hamilton JR, et al: Familial enteropathy: A syndrome of protracted diarrhea from birth, failure to thrive and hypoplastic villus atrophy. Gastroenterology 1978; 75:783–790.
76. Cutz E, Rhoads JM, Drumm B, et al: Microvillus inclusion disease: An inherited defect of brush-border assembly and differentiation. N Engl J Med 1989; 320:646–651.
77. Phillips AD, Jenkins P, Raafat F, et al: Congenital microvillous atrophy: Specific diagnostic features. Arch Dis Child 1985; 60:135–140.
78. Goldman H, Antonioli A: Mucosal biopsy of the rectum, colon and distal ileum. Hum Pathol 1982; 13:981–1012.
79. Haggitt RC: Differential diagnosis of colitis. *In* Goldman H, Appleman HD (eds): Gastrointestinal Pathology (International Academy of Pathology Monograph). Baltimore, Williams & Wilkins, 1990, pp 325–355.
80. Fenoglio-Preiser CM, Lantz PE, Listrom MB, et al: The non-neoplastic large intestine. *In* Gastrointestinal Pathology: An Atlas and Text. New York, Raven Press, 1989, pp 619–725.
81. Buchino JJ, Suchy FJ, Snyder JW: Bacterial diarrhea in infants and children. Perspect Pediatr Pathol 1984; 8:163–180.
82. Surawicz CM, Belic L: Rectal biopsy helps to distinguish acute self-limited colitis from idiopathic inflammatory bowel disease. Gastroenterology 1984; 86:104–113.
83. Nostrant TT, Kumar NB, Appelman HD: Histopathology differentiates acute self-limited colitis from ulcerative colitis. Gastroenterology 1987; 92:318–328.
84. Price AB, Davies DR: Pseudomembranous colitis. J Clin Pathol 1977; 30:1–12.
85. Buts P, Weber AM, Roy CC, et al: Pseudomembranous enterocolitis in childhood. Gastroenterology 1977; 73:823–827.
86. Viscidi RP, Bartlett JG: Antibiotic-associated pseudomembranous colitis in children. Pediatrics 1981; 67:381–386.
87. Thomas DFM, Fernie DS, Bayston R, et al: Enterocolitis in Hirschsprung's disease: A controlled study of the etiologic role of *Clostridium difficile*. J Pediatr Surg 1986; 21:22–25.
88. Brearly S, Armstrong GR, Nairn R, et al: Pseudomembranous colitis: A lethal complication of Hirschsprung's disease unrelated to antibiotic usage. J Pediatr Surg 1987; 22:257–259.
89. Ament ME: Inflammatory disease of the colon: Ulcerative colitis and Crohn's disease. J Pediatr 1975; 86:322–334.
90. Chong SK, Blackshaw AJ, Boyle S, et al: Histological diagnosis of chronic inflammatory bowel disease in childhood. Gut 1985; 26:55–59.
91. Price AB, Morson BC: Inflammatory bowel disease: The surgical pathology of Crohn's disease and ulcerative colitis. Hum Pathol 1975; 6:7–29.
92. Whitehead R: Ulcerative colitis, Crohn's colitis, ischaemic colitis, pseudomembranous and antibiotic-associated colitis. *In* Mucosal Biopsy of the Gastrointestinal Tract. Philadelphia, WB Saunders, 1990, pp 290–341.
93. Yardley JH, Donowitz M: Colo-rectal biopsy in inflammatory bowel disease. *In* Yardley JH, Morson BC, Abell MR, eds: The Gastrointestinal Tract. Vol 18, Monographs in Pathology. Baltimore, Williams & Wilkins, 1977, pp 50–94.
94. Jenkins HR, Pinicott JR, Soothill JF, et al: Food allergy: The major cause of infantile colitis. Arch Dis Child 1984; 59:326–329.
95. Winter HS, Antonioli DA, Fukagawa N, et al: Allergy-related proctocolitis in infants: Diagnostic usefulness of rectal biopsy. Mod Pathol 1990; 3:5–10.
96. Berman W: The hemolytic-uremic syndrome: Initial clinical presentation mimicking ulcerative colitis. J Pediatr 1972; 81:275–278.
97. Whitington PF, Friedman AL, Chesney RW: Gastrointestinal disease in the hemolytic-uremic syndrome. Gastroenterology 1979; 76:728–733.
98. Meier-Ruge W: Hirschsprung's disease: Its aetiology, pathogenesis and differential diagnosis. Curr Top Pathol 1974; 59:131–179.
99. Weinberg AC: Hirschsprung's disease—a pathologist's view. Perspect Pediatr Pathol 1975; 2:207–239.
100. Yunis EJ, Dibbins EW, Sherman FE: Rectal suction biopsy in the diagnosis of Hirschsprung's disease in infants. Arch Pathol Lab Med 1976; 100:329–333.
101. Lake BD, Puri P, Nixon HH, et al: Hirschsprung's disease: An appraisal of histochemically demonstrated acetylcholinesterase activity in suction rectal biopsy specimens as an aid to diagnosis. Arch Pathol Lab Med 1978; 102:244–247.
102. Wakely PE, McAdams AJ: Acetylcholinesterase histochemistry and the diagnosis of Hirschsprung's disease: A 3½-year experience. Pediatr Pathol 1984; 2:35–46.
103. Hall CL, Lampert PW: Immunocytochemistry as an aid in the diagnosis of Hirschsprung's disease. Am J Clin Pathol 1985; 83:177–181.
104. Vinores SA, May E: Neuron-specific enolase as an immunocytochemical tool for the diagnosis of Hirschsprung's disease. Am J Surg Pathol 1985; 9:281–285.

Section Eight

NUTRITIONAL MANAGEMENT

Chapter 80

The Practical Use of Infant Formulas

ANA ABAD-SINDEN and JAMES L. SUTPHEN

HISTORY

Human breast milk has always been considered to be the ideal food for neonates. When our ancestors were unable to breast feed their own infants, they employed wet nurses. In fact, the wet nurse was an integral member of ancient societies, including those of Mesopotamia, Egypt, Greece, and the Roman empire. During the Industrial Revolution in the mid-eighteenth century, women were employed for the first time in factories, and the time available for nursing their infants diminished. Moreover, the salary for a factory worker was greater than that of a wet nurse.[1] This disparity led to a decline in the number of available wet nurses. When a wet nurse was not available, and artificial formula was used, there was an appalling infant mortality, which was variously quoted in foundling hospitals in the eighteenth and nineteenth centuries at rates from 80 to 99.6% during the first year of life. Fresh animal milk was generally not available owing to the lack of refrigeration. Therefore, liquid substitutes, including beer and "slops," were fed to infants. These malted carbohydrate foods were available as byproducts of the beer brewing industry. The popularity of malted products extended into the later use of malted milk in early infant feeding practices.[2] "Pap," a thick suspension of bread in milk or water, was also used.

The preservation of milk by canning preceded the development of refrigeration techniques. In 1835, William Newton developed a method of evaporating milk to yield a condensed milk product. This was adapted by Gale Borden in 1853, when he patented evaporated milk with supplemental sugar as Eagle Brand Condensed Milk. In 1883, Myenberg further modified condensed milk by sterilizing the milk at high temperatures.[3] The heat process modified the casein to produce a finer and, it was thought, more digestible curd. Evaporated milk became a popular component of home-made infant formula during the early twentieth century. In 1915, the first modified cow's milk formula was developed and subsequently marketed 4 years later as SMA (synthetic milk adapted).[4] This initial mixture was modified to contain 0.9% protein, 4.6% fat, and 6.5% carbohydrate, a basic formula that is still present although extensively modified by many products currently available.[5]

As the dairy industry expanded and refrigeration became available, modifications of standard cow's milk were made by diluting whole cow's milk by one half or two thirds and adding additional carbohydrate in the form of simple sugars or starches. This had the effect of decreasing the high protein load. However, these initial formulations still contained quite high phosphorus loads and an elevated renal solute load. Moreover, the amounts of vitamins were variable in the initial products, and deficiencies of vitamins D and C were a problem. This led to the use of cod liver oil and fresh fruits in the diets of infants. Gradually, infant formulas become more "complete," and the need for supplemental vitamins and other infant feedings diminished. However, the experiences of the last century and the early part of this century have left a heavy mark on infant feeding practices, and the persistent use of cereal products, vitamin supplements, and fruit juices as supplements to infant formula during the first 6 months of life continue to be a common practice.

There are five cow's milk–based infant formulas currently on the market in the United States: SMA (Wyeth), Similac (Ross), Enfamil (Mead Johnson), Gerber Baby Formula (Gerber), and Good Start (Carnation). Infant formulas are available as powders, concentrates, or ready-to-feed formulas. Powder is the most convenient product in terms of cost and storage. However, it requires some care to ensure that the appropriate concentration is achieved. After reconstitution, powdered formula may be stored in the refrigerator for 24 hours. Similarly, formula concentrate, once reconstituted, must be stored in the refrigerator for no longer than 24 hours. Although occasionally infants seem to have preferences for particular infant formulas, more often the infant is easily persuaded to switch from one to another, assuming parental and physician bias can be overcome. Therefore, it is prudent to instruct parents to look for sales and special offers when shopping for infant formula. The common practice of offering starter packages of infant formula on discharge from newborn nurseries often has the effect of unintentional endorsement of a particular product by the medical establishment. New parents should be cautioned against assuming that sample discharge packs of formula must be continued throughout the first year of life.

If parents select formula feeding, it is prudent during the initial stages of feeding to stress involvement by both parents. Although is has long been appreciated that breast-feeding improves maternal-infant bonding, the effects of bottle-feeding by fathers has not been similarly investigated. Fathers should be encouraged to participate in feeding during prenatal visits and later at discharge from the newborn nursery. If both parents work, shared feeding responsibility is quite equitable and probably beneficial.

Prior to initiating the feeding, the parent should be certain to have all necessary equipment assembled. This generally will include a towel or blanket to shield the parent from, and wipe up, the inevitable spills associated with feedings. The bottle should be held in a position that allows formula to fill the nipple. Prior to initiating the feeding, the flow of formula from the nipple should be ascertained by holding the bottle upside down. A proper-sized nipple should allow occasional drips from the nipple. If the hole is too small, the infant will become frustrated during the feeding. If the hole is too large, too much formula may enter the infant's mouth and lead to choking. During initial feedings, the size of the feeding will probably not exceed 1 or 2 ounces. Consequently, feedings will have to be administered at relatively frequent intervals, for example, every 2 to 3 hours. Gradually, the size of the feedings may be adjusted upward and the interval between feedings gradually increased to allow the infant and parents to sleep through the night without a feeding.

During the feeding, the infant inevitably swallows some air. This may be exacerbated if the bottle is held incorrectly, frequently removed from the mouth, or offered at such infrequent intervals that the infant eats voraciously and swallows air during the feedings. Alternatively, prolonged forced feeding may lead to swallowed air at the end of the feeding. Excessive air swallowing during feedings may be a component of colic. Proper burping technique is essential to alleviate unwanted swallowed air. After every 1 or 2 ounces, depending on the severity of the problem, the feeding should be interrupted and the infant gently supported in a semi-sitting position while a hand is gently rubbed or tapped on the back. If this does not produce a burp within a relatively short period, the infant should be gently extended out of the sitting position so that the esophagogastric angle and gastric bubble position will change slightly. These efforts should continue until a burp is obtained. Inexperienced parents may often be frustrated and give up too easily. Other factors that may help alleviate air swallowing include changing the nipple or switching to collapsible plastic bag–type feeders that do not require the passage of air through the nipple to relieve an accumulated vacuum in the bottle.

The issue of sterilizing feeding equipment has been of considerable concern for parents. It is seldom necessary to sterilize equipment completely, assuming that the usual standards of hygiene are employed and that the water supply is not contaminated. Given the strong bias for sterilization, often it is easier to allow sterilization than to counsel against it. Similarly, standard wisdom dictates that infant formula must be warmed before it can be fed. Although some infants do seem to prefer formula at room temperature, many infants do not seem to appreciate the difference. For these lucky parents, it is needless to insist that the formula be warmed to room temperature. If a microwave oven is used to facilitate the warming, it is important to remember that different microwave ovens heat formula at different rates and that bottles placed at different positions within a given microwave may also heat at different rates. The parent should be advised to test the temperature of the formula prior to feeding the infant if a microwave has been used.

At approximately 4 to 6 weeks of age, infants will begin to appreciate environmental stimuli other than bottle feeding. Parents must be encouraged to have age-appropriate stimuli for infants at this time (for example, dangle toys, mobiles, and music boxes). Otherwise, infant boredom may be confused with hunger. This confusion is commonest at 4 to 6 weeks of age. If an infant is crying and the usual entertainment measures have not helped, feedings should then be offered.

Failure to consider alternatives to hunger as causes of infant distress may lead to overfeeding and obesity. This can be a particular problem if the parents are obese. Other factors that may potentiate obesity include overly aggressive feeding of solids and the use of infant feeders to administer extremely high-caloric density feedings to infants. It is important to remember that actual weight gain, not calorie intake, is the final diagnostic criteria for obesity. Some infants who are crossing linear growth curves in an upward fashion may have transient growth rates that are two to three times more than normal for short periods. This can translate into as much as 200 to 300 extra calories per day for a 4- to 6-month-old child who is rapidly crossing growth curves. As long as this is in the context of good linear growth, concern regarding obesity is not warranted.

Although the infant is capable of swallowing liquids in utero, the extrusion reflex prevents coordination of swallowing of solid foods until 4 to 6 months of age. This primitive reflex was probably designed to keep foreign objects out of the baby's mouth prior to the time when they might be introduced as dietary constituents. However, it is improper to abstract from this a teleologic argument for a requirement for solids when the extrusion reflex disappears. Currently, the American Academy of Pediatrics advises that there is no advantage to solid food supplements for human milk or formula feeding before 4 to 6 months of age.[6] Probably it is the introduction of supplemental foods that induces weaning in human infants. After introduction of solids, the intake of formula or human milk decreases while the total caloric intake remains roughly constant.[7]

The nutrient contents of term cow's milk infant formulas available in the United States are remarkably similar (Table 80–1). The protein content of all formulas is primarily derived from nonfat milk. Enfamil and SMA are enriched by the addition of demineralized whey to alter the final whey to casein ratio. The carbohydrate component of all standard infant formulas is lactose, the normal sugar in breast milk. The argument for adopting lactose as the primary carbohydrate in infant formulas is derived from comparison to breast and animal milk.

Table 80–1. NUTRIENT LEVELS PER 100 KCAL FOR INFANT FORMULAS

Nutrient	Minimum	Maximum
Protein (g)	1.8	4.5
Fat (g)	3.3	6.0
Linoleic acid	0.3*	—
Vitamin A (IU)	250	750
Vitamin D (IU)	40	100
Vitamin E (IU)	0.7†	—
Vitamin K (μg)	4	—
Vitamin C (mg)	8	—
Thiamin (μg)	40	—
Riboflavin (μg)	60	—
Vitamin B_6 (μg)	35‡	—
Vitamin B_{12} (μg)	0.15	—
Niacin (μg)	250	—
Folic acid (μg)	4	—
Pantothenic acid (μg)	300	—
Biotin (μg)	1.5	—
Choline (mg)	7	—
Inositol (mg)	4	—
Calcium (mg)	60	—
Phosphorus (mg)	30	—
Magnesium (mg)	6	—
Sodium (mg)	20	60
Potassium (mg)	80	200
Chloride (mg)	55	150
Iron (mg)	0.15	3
Zinc (mg)	0.5	—
Manganese (μg)	5	—
Copper (μg)	60	—
Iodine (g)	5	75

*2.7% of calories.
†0.7 IU/gm linoleic acid.
‡15 μg/gm protein.
Data from Food and Drug Administration: Rules and regulations: Nutrient requirements for infant formulas. Fed Register 1985; 50:45106–45108 (21 CFR Part 107).

Although there are some data to suggest improved calcium absorption with lactose, there are no feeding data to support lactose as a clearly superior carbohydrate source in standard infant formula.

The fat content of infant formula is composed of blends of soy and coconut oil. SMA also uses safflower oil and oleo. Some adjustment in these fat blends may be expected as knowledge of the influence of infantile dietary fat on eventual development of atherosclerotic heart disease expands. All term infant formulas have identical caloric densities and nearly identical osmolalities (Table 80–2).

Although whole cow's milk is available in plentiful supply in the United States, its use is currently reserved for children older than 12 months of age. Early feeding of whole cow's milk is associated with the development of milk protein sensitization, gastrointestinal blood loss, hypoproteinemia, poor iron absorption, and, if fed exclusively, scurvy and other vitamin deficiencies. In addition to intestinal blood loss associated with whole cow's milk, the iron content of the milk is low, and what iron is available from other dietary sources is absorbed poorly because of the high phosphorus content of the milk. Finally, the high protein and mineral content of the milk leads to an unacceptable potential renal solute load that may present significant problems in summer months when hydration may be an issue.[8]

When whole cow's milk is fed to infants older than 1 year of age, it is currently recommended that the regular butterfat concentration be used. Feeding milk of lower butterfat concentration to infants younger than 2 years of age may be associated with inadequate calorie intake. The compensatory ingestion of large volumes of low-fat milk to adjust for caloric density may lead to much higher protein intakes with its attendant high potential renal solute load. These factors are most important for infants who consume milk as a major component of the diet. As the infant ages into the second year of life, assuming an adequate distribution of nonmilk calories, the relative disadvantage of lower fat milks becomes less certain and is currently a matter of considerable debate.[8]

PRACTICAL USE OF INFANT FORMULAS

Specialized Infant Formulas

A number of specialized formulas are commercially available for infants who have malabsorption or formula intolerance to the carbohydrate, fat, or protein components of standard infant formulas. In addition, specialized formulas have been developed to meet the unique physiologic requirements of the preterm infant. The following discussion reviews the rationale for the selection and indications for the various specialized formulas currently available.

Soy Infant Formulas

Soy infant formulas are considered to be the formula of choice for the treatment of uncomplicated lactose intolerance and, providing that an allergy to intact soy protein does not exist, cow's milk protein allergy as well. Except for carbohydrate and protein, soy protein formulas are nutritionally similar to standard infant formulas and provide adequate growth, minerals, and nitrogen balance. The fat is composed of vegetable oils blended to simulate the ratio of polyunsaturated to saturated fats of breast milk. Vitamins and minerals are added to soy formulas in accordance with the recommendations set by the American Academy of Pediatrics (AAP),[8] the Infant Formulas Act of 1980,[9] and subsequent modifications.[10] Soy formulas are fortified with iron at a level that provides 2 mg per kg for the infant consuming approximately 120 kcal per kg. These formulas contain a refined soy protein isolate that has been heat treated for the enhancement of protein digestibility and mineral bioavailability.[11] However, zinc may be less biologically available in soy formula, possibly owing to the presence of phytate.[11] Because soy protein also has a lower bioavailability than do casein and whey, its concentration in infant formulas has been increased to 1.8 to 2.1 gm per dl and fortified with methionine to improve the protein quality.[11, 12] Carnitine, which plays a role in the transport and oxidation of long-chain fatty acids, has also been added to all soy formulas owing to

Table 80–2. INFANT FORMULAS (UNITED STATES)

	kcal/oz	mOsm/kg	Carbohydrate (gm/100 ml)	Fat (gm/100 ml)	Protein (gm/100 ml)	Components
Term Cow's Milk Protein Formulas						
Similac	20	290	7.2	3.6	1.5	Lactose; soy, coconut oil; nonfat milk
Enfamil	20	278	6.9	3.8	1.5	Lactose; coconut oil, soy; nonfat milk, demineralized whey
SMA	20	300	7.2	3.6	1.5	Oleo, lactose; coconut, safflower, soy oil; nonfat milk, demineralized whey
Gerber	20	320	7.3	3.7	1.5	Lactose, soy, coconut oil, nonfat milk
Soy-Based Formulas						
Isomil	20	250	6.8	3.6	2.0	Corn syrup solids, sucrose; soy and coconut oil; soy protein isolate, L-methionine
Prosobee	20	200	6.9	3.6	2.0	Corn syrup solids, soy and coconut oil; soy protein isolate, L-methionine
Nursoy	20	296	6.9	3.6	2.1	Sucrose; oleo, coconut, safflower, soy oils; soy protein isolate, L-methionine
Preterm Infant Formulas						
Similac Special Care	24	300	8.6	4.4	2.2	Corn syrup solids, lactose; MCT oil, corn and coconut oil; nonfat milk, demineralized whey
Enfamil Premature	24	300	8.9	4.1	2.4	Same as above
"Preemie" SMA	24	268	8.6	4.4	2.0	Lactose, maltodextrins; MCT oil, coconut, oleo, soy oil; nonfat milk, demineralized whey
Specialized Formulas						
Nutramigen	20	480	8.8	2.6	2.2	Sucrose, modified tapioca starch; corn oil; casein hydrolysate
Portagen	20	220	7.8	3.2	2.4	Corn syrup solids, lactose; MCT oil and corn oil; sodium caseinate
Pregestimil	20	350	9.1	2.7	1.9	Corn syrup solids, modified tapioca starch; corn oil and MCT oil; casein hydrolysate with amino acids
Good Start H.A.	20	265	7.4	3.4	1.6	Lactose maltodextrins; palm oil, safflower oil, coconut oil; hydrolyzed whey
Alimentum	20	370	6.8	3.7	1.8	Tapioca starch, sucrose; MCT oil, safflower oil, soy oil, casein hydrolysate with amino acids

its negligible amounts in the unsupplemented product.[12] Soy formulas contain either corn syrup solids (glucose polymers and hydrolyzed corn starch), sucrose, or a combination of both as the carbohydrate source. Because of a higher molecular weight, the corn syrup solids act to reduce the osmolality of the formulas.[12, 13] The sweetness of sucrose may make the formula more palatable to some infants.

There are a number of indications for the use of soy formulas in infant feeding. The rare infant with primary lactase deficiency or galactosemia should be started on soy formulas. More commonly, however, soy formulas are used for the nutritional management of infants with secondary lactose intolerance following gastroenteritis, protein-calorie malnutrition, or other causes of mucosal injury.[11, 12] In chronic nonspecific or postinfectious diarrhea that does not result in lactose intolerance, the use of lactose containing formula may be preferable or at least acceptable.[14] For infants who also develop a relative sucrase deficiency following a bout of severe gastroenteritis, Isomil SF (Ross) or Prosobee (Mead Johnson), which are both sucrose free, would be the formulas of choice. Soy formulas can also be used for the nutritional management of cow's milk protein sensitivity; however, from 8 to about 50% of children with cow's milk protein allergy experience a sensitivity to intact soy protein as well.[15, 16] These children would best be managed with a hydrolysate formula instead. Children with cow's milk allergy may demonstrate anemia or gastrointestinal, dermatologic, respiratory, neurologic, or vascular symptoms, or all of these. These children should be taken off milk and then rechallenged for establishment of a diagnosis. Milk can generally be reintroduced into the diet within 6 months to 2 years, depending on the severity of the cow's milk protein sensitivity.[15, 16]

Soy formulas, like standard formulas, are available in ready-to-feed, concentrated, or powered forms. The ready-to-feed form is generally the most expensive, whereas the powdered form is the least expensive. An additional advantage of the concentrate and powdered forms is that they can be readily mixed to the 24-kcal per ounce concentration for the nutritional management of infants who take inadequate volumes or are fluid restricted.

Hydrolysate Formulas

Nutramigen (Mead Johnson) is indicated for the nutritional management of infants who have allergies to intact protein from either cow's milk or soy. The protein in Nutramigen consists of casein hydrolyzed to free amino acids and polypeptides that has been charcoal treated for the reduction of its allergenicity.[12] Nutramigen is also essentially lactose free, with approximately 2% sucrose and 28% tapioca starch as the carbohydrate sources. Corn oil is the source of fat, and the formula is also iron fortified. Nutramigen has been reformulated to reduce its osmolality to approximately 320 mOsm per kg and is usually well tolerated by the term infant at a concentration of 20 kcal per ounce. Nutramigen, which is available as a powder concentrate or ready-to-feed liquid form, costs approximately twice as much as standard infant formula.

Pregestimil (Mead Johnson) is one of the formulas of choice for infants with generalized malabsorption of both protein and fat, for example, short gut syndrome of severe villous injury. This formula, which is considered elemental in both its protein and fat components, is commonly used for the nutritional management of infants with newly diagnosed cystic fibrosis. Pregestimil is composed of casein hydrolysates with added L-cystine, L-tyrosine, and L-tryptophan as its protein source.[12] The fat is a blend of 60% corn oil and 40% medium-chain triglycerides (MCT). The carbohydrate component is provided by 85% corn syrup solids and 15% modified tapioca starch. This carbohydrate blend helps to maintain the osmolality at 350 mOsm per kg when mixed to a concentration of 20 kcal per ounce. Pregestimil, which is only available in the powdered form, has a cost twice that of standard formula.

Alimentum (Ross) is a recent addition to the line of hypoallergenic formulas. It is similar to Pregestimil (Mead Johnson). This product is also indicated for the nutritional management of the infant with generalized malabsorption. The protein consists of enzymatically hydrolyzed charcoal-treated casein containing approximately 60% free amino acids. The formula's hypoallergenicity has been tested through both animal challenge tests and immunosorbent inhibition assays. The fat blend consists of 50% MCT, 40% safflower oil and 10% soy oil. Unlike Pregestimil, this formula contains a carbohydrate blend consisting of both tapioca starch and sucrose. Alimentum is also supplemented with taurine and carnitine at the levels found in human milk. Alimentum is currently available in the ready-to-feed form at a concentration of 20 kcal per ounce. With an osmolality of 370 mOsm per kg and a renal solute load of 124 mOsm per L, this formula is well tolerated by the term infant.

Good Start (Carnation) has recently been introduced as a hypoallergenic formula. The protein component of Good Start is whey hydrolyzed by heat treatment and enzyme modification to an average peptide length of 5.6 amino acids. The product's hypoallergenicity has been tested in animal sensitization and challenge tests (Carnation product monograph). Clinical studies by Chandra and associates[17] and Vandenplas and colleagues[18] have demonstrated that the incidence of intolerance, including skin, respiratory, and gastrointestinal symptoms, was significantly reduced in infants with a family history of allergy when fed this whey hydrolysate formula. In a recent study by Merritt and coworkers[19] of infants with gastrointestinal symptoms of cow's milk- or soy protein–based formula intolerance, the whey hydrolysate formula was found to be an acceptable alternative to soy or casein hydrolysate formulas in most instances. Although Good Start is marketed as a hypoallergenic formula, a recent study documented that Good Start had 100 to 700 times the number of identifiable milk protein antigens as did Nutramigen and Alimentum.[20] Good Start is composed of a carbohydrate blend of lactose (70%) and maltodextrins (30%). Lactose has been demonstrated to inhibit chronic nonspecific or infectious diarrhea in infants previously managed with soy formula.[21] The fat component is a blend of palm oil (60%), high oleic safflower oil (22%), and coconut oil (18%), with a resulting polyunsaturated to saturated fat ratio similar to that found in human milk (Carnation, Product Monograph). The cost of Good Start is approximately the same as that of standard infant formula.

Fat-Modified Formula

Portagen (Mead Johnson) is indicated for the nutritional management of infants with steatorrhea due a limited bile salt pool, that is, biliary atresia, or with other forms of fat malabsorption or intolerance. This formula contains 88% MCT and 12% corn oil. MCT, which contain fatty acids 8 to 12 carbons in length, is to a small extent directly absorbed into the hepatic portal vein instead of exclusively through the lymphatic system.[10, 11] A substantial amount of MCT absorption occurs in the stomach after hydrolysis by gastric and lingual lipase. The intestinal absorption of MCT is therefore less dependent on pancreatic lipase and bile salts.[22] Portagen contains intact protein in the form of sodium caseinate and contains 73% corn syrup solids and 25% sucrose as the carbohydrate sources. At the concentration of 20 kcal per ounce, Portagen has an osmolality of 220 mOsm per kg. Also available in the powdered form, this formula is well tolerated by infants with fat malabsorption or intolerance primarily due to cholestatic liver disease.

Preterm Infant Formulas

Preterm formulas have been developed that are uniquely suited to meet the specialized physiologic and gastrointestinal needs of these infants. The three commercially available preterm formulas currently in use are Enfamil Premature Formula (Mead Johnson), Similac Special Care (Ross), and "Preemie" SMA (Wyeth). Numerous studies have demonstrated that these formulas are nutritionally adequate and safe and can support intrauterine growth rates in the preterm infant.[23, 24] In the very-low-birthweight infant weighing less than 1,000 gm, preterm formula should be introduced and advanced cautiously, paying close attention to signs of gastrointestinal intolerance. Aggressive advancement of enteral feedings in the very-low-birthweight infant is associated with feeding intolerance and necrotizing enterocolitis.[25]

The nutrient composition of preterm formulas has been modified to meet the specific needs of the preterm infant. Lactose, which is the predominant carbohydrate in human milk and standard infant formulas, is not well utilized by the preterm infant, because intestinal lactase is deficient.[24] Preterm formulas contain 40 to 50% lactose and the remaining 50 to 60% of the carbohydrate as glucose polymers, which are well digested and utilized in the preterm infant.[26] Preterm formulas contain more protein than do standard formulas at a level of 2.2 to 2.4 gm per dl to meet the elevated requirements of preterm infants.[24] In addition, the protein in preterm formulas consists of 60% whey and 40% casein. Whey protein, which contains more cystine and less methionine than casein, may be better suited for the needs of the preterm neonate. Because preterm infants have low levels of bile acids, they are less able to digest and absorb the long-chain triglycerides found in standard infant formulas. Preterm formulas contain 10 to 50% of fat as MCT. MCT has been demonstrated to improve fat digestion and absorption in low-birthweight infants, resulting in improved rates of weight gain[27] and enhanced calcium absorption,[28] although more recent studies have shown insignificant advantages in fat absorption.[22]

Because preterm infants consume such a small volume of milk, they would not receive their recommended dietary allowances for vitamins and minerals if consuming standard formula. Table 80–3 summarizes calorie, protein, and selected vitamin and mineral needs of preterm and term infants.[24, 29, 30] Enfamil Premature Formula and Similac Special Care are specially fortified, and additional vitamin supplementation is not required. An exception to this can be found with vitamin D, however. The AAP Committee on Nutrition recommends an intake of 500 UI per day of vitamin D in the preterm infant.[29] Because of individual variations in the sensitivity to vitamin D, two of the formula manufacturers (Wyeth and Ross) have chosen relatively conservative levels of vitamin D in their formulas. Preemie SMA, for example, contains 480 IU of vitamin D per liter, whereas Similac Special Care contains 1,220 IU per liter (product monographs). Achievement of the AAP recommendations of vitamin D for the preterm infant[24, 29] would require the use of a vitamin D supplement containing 400 IU when using these two formulas. A recent study by Ziegler and associates,[31] however, evaluated vitamin D status and calcium balance in preterm infants fed preterm formula containing either 552 IU or 2,360 IU of vitamin D per liter. Serum vitamin D levels were within normal ranges for both groups, and there were no significant differences in calcium absorption. More recent investigations have emphasized the greater importance of increasing calcium and phosphorus concentrations in infant formulas over increasing vitamin D levels for the enhancement of bone mineralization in the preterm infant.[29, 32] Vitamin E, a biologic antioxidant, has been considered to play an important role in neonatal nutrition because preterm infants are born with low body stores, have wide variability in absorption, and are thus prone to deficiency. Current preterm formulas contain approximately three times the level recommended by the AAP.[23] Because the human fetus deposits significant calcium and phosphorous in the form of new bone during the last trimester, the preterm infant has elevated requirements for both calcium and phosphorus that cannot be met by the levels in either human milk or standard infant formula. The preterm formulas Enfamil Premature Formula and Similac Special Care have elevated levels of both calcium and phosphorous. Balance studies using these formulas have demonstrated calcium retention rates comparable with fetal accretion rates.[23] Owing to immature kidneys and excessive urinary losses, preterm infants often develop hyponatremia during the first weeks of life. Preterm formulas have elevated levels of sodium over that of human milk or standard formulas to meet the elevated requirements of the preterm infant.[23] Preterm formulas contain between 32 and 41 mg of sodium per 100 ml compared with a range of 15 to 22 mg of sodium per 100 ml of standard infant formula (product monograph). Preterm infants receiving less than 2 kg may develop physiologic anemia due to their compromised iron

Table 80–3. RECOMMENDED DAILY NUTRIENT INTAKES OF TERM AND PRETERM INFANTS

Nutrient	Term Infant	Preterm Infant
Energy	98–108 kcal/kg	120–150 kcal/kg
Protein	1.5–2.2 gm/kg	3–4 gm/kg
Vitamin A	500 IU	1400 IU
Vitamin D	400 IU	500–600 IU
Vitamin E	5 IU	5–25 IU
Vitamin C	20 mg	50–60 mg
Vitamin K	15 μg	15 μg
Thiamine	0.2 mg	0.2 mg
Riboflavin	0.4 mg	0.4 mg
Pyridoxine	0.4 mg	0.4 mg
Niacin	5 mg	5 mg
Vitamin B_{12}	1.5 μg	1.5 μg
Folic acid	50 μg	50–100 μg
Iron	6–10 mg	2 mg/kg/day (after 6–8 weeks of age)

Data from references 24, 29, and 30.

stores. The lower an infant's birthweight and initial hemoglobin concentration, the greater the need for supplemented iron.[33] Although early iron supplementation for preterm infants predisposed them to hemolytic anemia, this is no longer a concern with adequate vitamin E levels found in current preterm formulas.[34] Preterm formulas with iron provide approximately 2 mg per kg of iron per day, when infants are fed 120 kcal per kg. The AAP recommends that preterm infants begin to receive iron-fortified formula no later than 6 to 8 weeks of age.[33]

Human Milk Fortifiers

Even though mature human milk provides a number of nutritional, physiologic, and immunologic advantages over infant formulas, it does not meet the elevated calorie, protein, vitamin, and mineral needs of the preterm infant. Preterm human milk, however, which is higher in protein, sodium, chloride, magnesium, and iron than is mature human milk, may be more suitable for the feeding of the preterm infant.[35–37] Despite these advantages, preterm milk is still relatively deficient in calcium and phosphorus for the needs of the growing very-low-birthweight infant.[23] Two fortifiers, Enfamil Human Milk Fortifier (Mead Johnson) and Similac Natural Care (Ross), are currently available to supplement human milk to the nutrient levels found in preterm formulas. Enfamil Human Milk Fortifier is a powder supplement that adds carbohydrate, whey protein, vitamins, and minerals to human milk. The addition of one packet of this fortifier to 25 ml of human milk adds 4 kcal per ounce while increasing the osmolality by 30 mOsm per kg. Studies using fortified human milk have shown significantly improved weight gain and lower alkaline phosphatase levels in preterm infants (Mead Johnson product literature). An additional advantage of this specific fortifier is that it does not dilute the immunologic properties of human milk.[38] Similac Natural Care is a liquid supplement that is mixed in a one to one ratio with expressed human milk. As with the powdered supplement, this fortifier increases the calorie, protein, calcium, and phosphorus, and vitamin concentration of human milk (Ross Laboratories product literature). Natural Care provides the additional advantage of lower osmolality but does dilute the anti-infective properties of human milk.

Formula Supplementation

Although standard and specialized infant formulas generally meet the nutritional requirements of full-term infants, there are a number of special circumstances that may warrant the additional supplementation of these formulas with caloric, vitamin and mineral, or enzymatic additives.

Vitamin Supplementation

Standard infant formulas have been designed to meet the recommended dietary allowance (RDA) for infants when consumed at a level of approximately 1 quart per day.[39] As such, healthy term infants consuming standard, soy, or specialized infant formulas do not need to receive vitamin supplementation. Infants older than 6 months of age receiving iron-fortified formula and cereal generally do not develop vitamin or mineral deficiencies. Because vitamin D is present in low quantities in human milk, breast-fed infants who do not receive adequate sunlight should receive an additional 400 IU of vitamin D per day. It should be noted, however, that the incidence of vitamin D deficiency in breast-fed term infants is extremely low. Infants with clinical bronchopulmonary dysplasia, congenital heart disease, cystic fibrosis, or chronic renal disease may require multivitamin supplementation owing to their limited formula intake, decreased absorption, increased vitamin requirements, or a combination of these. In addition, preterm infants who are switched to standard formulas on achieving a weight of 2 kg generally require multivitamin supplementation until they are able to take in 1 quart of formula per day. With the exception of the earlier mentioned conditions or disease states, healthy infants do not require vitamin supplements. Recent surveys such as the Gerber Nutrition Survey[40] and the Ross Laboratories Infant Nutrition Survey,[23] for example, suggest that most infants have more than adequate vitamin and mineral intakes. Despite these findings, approximately one third to one half of infants 6 months to 12 months old receive nutrient supplements in the form of vitamin A, C, and D or multivitamin preparations.[42]

Iron Supplementation

According to the Food and Nutrition Board of the National Academy of Sciences, the RDA for iron for term infants is 10 mg per day. This RDA is based on an estimate of 10% absorption of dietary iron. Iron-fortified standard infant formulas contain iron at a level that provides approximately 2 mg per kg for the infant consuming approximately 120 kcal per kg. This level of iron meets or exceeds most infants' RDAs. Despite the availability of iron-fortified formulas, in 1987 the U.S. Centers for Disease Control reported that 15.9% of low-income children 6 to 24 months of age were anemic as defined by a hemoglobin concentration less than 11 gm per dl.[43, 44] Infants in the first 2 years of life are susceptible to iron deficiency anemia if given formula or foods low in iron content or foods containing iron of low bioavailability.[43] The effect of iron deficiency during infancy on behavioral development has been shown in a number of studies from a variety of cultures.[43–48] These studies that used the Bayley Scales of Infant Development to measure mental and motor development demonstrated lower mental test scores in anemic infants.[43] In some of these studies,[45–47] the reversal of the anemic state had little discernible effect on the indices of mental and psychomotor development. The AAP Committee on Nutrition as well as other international organizations recommend that iron-fortified formula be used for all formula fed infants[49] to prevent iron deficiency anemia. Some physicians, however, are reluctant to recommend feeding of iron-fortified infants because of the concern over adverse reactions including increased fussiness, regurgitation, loose stools, and constipation. In this regard, a recent study failed to substantiate significant feeding-related behaviors with iron fortification.[50]

Caloric Additives

Infants with various chronic disease states, such as bronchopulmonary dysplasia, congenital heart disease, and cystic fibrosis, often are unable to meet their caloric and protein requirements owing to inadequate intake, fluid restriction, malabsorption, or a combination of these. In these clinical situations, standard or specialized infant formulas may be supplemented with caloric modular components, including protein, fat, and carbohydrate modules. Formula can be initially concentrated to 24 kcal per ounce using less free water when mixing the powder or concentrate form. Concentrating a formula to a caloric density greater than 24 kcal per ounce, however, should generally be avoided during the first year of life, because elevated renal solute load and osmolality may become a concern. Increased caloric densities can be achieved through formula supplementation with caloric modular components. Modular protein products such as ProMod (Ross) and Casec (Mead Johnson) may be used to increase formula protein density. Fat modulars such as vegetable oils for the orally fed infant or emulsified products such as Microlipid (Cheseborough-Ponds) for the pump- or tube-fed infant may be added to formulas to increase their caloric density. Fat should not exceed 60% of total calories to prevent ketosis. Excessive fat intake can also lead to formula intolerance by significantly decreasing gastric emptying. The addition of glucose polymers such as Polycose (Ross) or Moducal (Mead Johnson) as supplemental carbohydrates can also increase formula caloric density while promoting gastrointestinal tolerance. When adding more than one modular component for maintenance of caloric distribution, a gradual and stepwise addition of each of these components individually can help promote better tolerance. The selection of appropriate nutrient modules depends on the specific needs of the infant as well as the composition, digestibility, and availability of the product.[51]

Enzymatic Additives

Infants with either primary or secondary lactose intolerance may still be nutritionally managed with breast milk or standard infant formula providing that the lactose is appropriately hydrolyzed to galactose and glucose. Lactase, commercially available as Lactaid, is derived from the fungus *Kluyveromyces lactis*. The addition of 5 drops of Lactaid to 1 quart of milk or infant formula followed by an incubation time of 24 hours in the refrigerator results in 70% lactose hydrolysis. For severe lactose intolerance, 10 drops of Lactaid enzyme will essentially hydrolyze all the lactose. Lactaid can be used with whole, low-fat, skim, canned, and reconstituted nonfat dry milk and in infant formulas. Lactose-hydrolyzed milk is well tolerated by children with lactose intolerance and, in one study, improved calcium absorption over lactose-free alternative diets with extra calcium supplementation.[52] Lactase is also available as Lactrase, which is derived from the fungus *Aspergillus oryzae*. The advantage of this form over Lactaid is that it is stable over a wider range of pH (4–8), is heat stable, and thus may be considered to be more effective at lactose hydrolysis just prior to milk ingestion.

REFERENCES

1. Barness LA: History of infant feeding practices. Am J Clin Nutr 1987; 46:168–170.
2. Radbill SX: Infant feeding through the ages. Clin Pediatr 1981; 20:613–621.
3. Anderson SA, Chinn HI, Fisher KD: History and current status of infant formulas. Am J Clin Nutr 1982; 35:381–397.
4. Gertenberger HJ, Ruh HO: Studies in the adaptation of an artificial food to human milk: II. A report of three years' clinical experience with the feeding of S.M.A. (synthetic milk adapted). Am J Dis Child 1919; 171:1–37.
5. Gertenberg HJ, Haskins HD, McGregor HH, et al: Studies in the adaptation of an artificial food to human milk. Am J Dis Child 1915; 10:249–265.
6. Barnes LA: Bases of weaning recommendations. J Pediatr 1990; 117:S84–S85.
7. Garza C, Butte NF: Energy intakes of human milk-fed infants during the first year. J Pediatr 1990; 117:S124–S131.
8. Committee on Nutrition: Commentary on breast-feeding and infant formulas, including proposed standards of formulas. Pediatrics 1976; 57:278.
9. United States Congress: Infant Formulas Act of 1980. Public Law 96–359, September 26, 1980.
10. Food and Drug Administration: Rules and regulations: Nutrient requirements for infant formulas. Fed Register 1985; 50:45106–45108 (21 CFR part 107).
11. American Academy of Pediatrics, Committee on Nutrition: Soy-protein formulas: Recommendations for use in infant feeding. Pediatrics 1983; 72:359.
12. Brady MS, Rickard KA, Fitzgerald JF, et al: Specialized formulas and feedings for infants with malabsorption or formula intolerance. J Am Diet Assoc 1986; 85:191.
13. Lebenthal E, Heitlinger L, Lee PC, et al: Corn syrup sugars: In vitro and in vivo digestibility and clinical tolerance in acute diarrhea of infancy. J Pediatr 1983; 103:29.
14. Donovan GK, Torres-Pinedo R: Chronic diarrhea and soy formulas. Am J Dis Child 1987; 141:1069.
15. Bock SA, Atkins FM: Patterns of food hypersensitivity during sixteen years of double-blind, placebo-controlled food challenges. J Pediatr 1990; 117:561–567.
16. Bishop JM, Hill DJ, Hosking CS: Natural history of cow milk allergy: Clinical outcome. J Pediatr 1990; 116:862–867.
17. Chandra RK, Singh G, Shridhara B: Effect of feeding whey hydrolysate, soy and conventional cow milk formulas on incidence of atopic disease in high risk infants. Ann Allergy 1989; 63:102.
18. Vandenplas Y, Malfroot A, Dab I: Short-term prevention of cow's milk protein allergy in infants. Immunol Allergy Pract 1989; 430:17.
19. Merritt RJ, Carter M, Haight M, et al: Whey protein hydrolysate formula for infants with gastrointestinal intolerance to cow milk and soy protein in infant formulas. J Pediatr Gastroenterol Nutr 1990; 11:78.
20. Sampson HA, Bernhisel-Broadbent J, Yang E, et al: Safety of casein hydrolysate formula in children with cow milk allergy: I. J Pediatr 1991; 118:520–525.
21. Donovan GK, Torres-Pinedo R: Chronic diarrhea and soy formulas. Am J Dis Child 1987; 141:1069.
22. Hamosh M, Bitman J, Liao TH, et al: Gastric lipolysis and fat absorption in preterm infants: Effect of medium-chain triglyceride- or long-chain triglyceride–containing formulas. Pediatrics 1989; 83:86–92.

23. Brady MS, Rickard KA, Ernst JA, et al: Formulas and human milk for premature infants: A review and update. J Am Diet Assoc 1982; 81:547.
24. Committee on Nutrition, American Academy of Pediatrics: Nutritional needs of the low-birth-weight infant. Pediatrics 1985; 75:976.
25. Brown EG, Sweet AY: Preventing necrotizing enterocolitis in neonates. JAMA 1978; 240:2452.
26. Cicco R, Holzman IR, Brown DR, et al: Glucose polymers tolerance in premature infants. Pediatrics 1981; 67:498.
27. Roy CC, Ste-Marie M, Chartrand L, et al: Correction of malabsorption of the preterm infant with a medium-chain triglyceride formula. J Pediatr 1975; 86:446.
28. Andrews BF, Lorch V: Improved fat and calcium absorption in LBW infants fed a medium chain triglyceride–containing formula. Pediatr Res 2974; 8:104.
29. Greer FR, Tsang RC: Calcium, phosphorus, magnesium, and vitamin D requirements for the preterm infant. *In* Tsang RC, ed: Vitamin and Mineral Requirements in Preterm Infants. New York, Marcel Dekker, 1985, pp 99–136.
30. National Research Council, Food and Nutrition Board: Recommended Dietary Allowances. 8th ed. Washington, DC, National Academy of Sciences, 1980.
31. Ziegler EE, Johnson KJ, Nelson SE, et al: Formula vitamin D content and mineral balance in preterm infants. Am J Clin Nutr 1990; 51:528.
32. Greer FR, Tsang RC: Calcium and vitamin metabolism in term and low-birth-weight infants. Perinatol Neonatol 1986; 9:14.
33. Oski FA: Iron requirements of the premature infant. *In* Tsang RC, ed: Vitamin and mineral requirements in preterm infants. New York, Marcel Dekker, 1985, pp 9–22.
34. Williams MJ, Shott RJ, O'Neal PL, et al: Role of dietary iron and fat on vitamin E deficiency of infancy. N Engl J Med 1975; 292:887.
35. Lemon JA, Moye L, Hall D, et al: Differences in the composition of preterm and term human milk during early lactation. Pediatrics Res 1982; 16:113.
36. Gross SJ, David RJ, Bauman L, et al: Nutritional composition of milk produced by mothers delivering preterm. J Pediatr 1980; 96:641.
37. Anderson GH, Atkinson SA, Bryan MH: Energy and macronutrient content of human milk during early lactation from mothers giving birth prematurely and at term. Am J Clin Nutr 1981; 34:258.
38. Kerner JA, Yang CC, Stevenson DK: Effects of nutritional supplementation of anti-infective factors in human milk. Gastroenterology 1988; 223:94.
39. Benkov KJ, LeLeiko NS: A rational approach to infant formulas. Pediatr Ann 1987; 16:225.
40. Purvis GA, Bartholmey SJ: Infant feeding practices: Commercially prepared baby foods. *In* Tsang RC, Nichols BF, eds: Nutrition During Infancy. Philadelphia, Hanley & Belfus 1988, pp 399–417.
41. Martinez GA, Ryan AS, Malec DJ: Nutrient intakes of American infants and children fed cow's milk or infant formula. Am J Dis Child 1985; 139:1010.
42. Curtis DM: Infant nutrient supplementation. J Pediatr 1990; 117:S110.
43. Filler LJ: Iron needs during rapid growth and mental development. J Pediatr 1990; 117:S143.
44. Yip R: Iron nutritional status defined. *In* Filer LJ, ed: Dietary Iron: Birth to Two Years. New York, Raven Press, 1989, pp 19–36.
45. Walter T, Kovalskys J, Stekel A: Effect of milk iron deficiency on infant mental development scores. J Pediatr 1983; 102:519.
46. Lozoff B, Brittenham GW, Wolf AW, et al: Iron deficiency anemia and iron therapy effects on infant developmental test performance. Pediatrics 1987; 79:981.
47. Lozoff B, Brittenham GW, Viteri FE, et al: The effects of short-term oral iron therapy on developmental deficits in iron-deficient anemic infants. J Pediatr 1982; 100:351.
48. Oski FA, Honig AS, Helu B, et al: Effect of iron therapy on behavior in nonanemic, iron-deficient infants. Pediatrics 1983; 71:877.
49. Committe on Nutrition: Iron-fortified infant formulas. Pediatrics 1989; 84:1114.
50. Nelson SE, Ziegler EE, Copeland AM, et al: Lack of adverse reactions to iron-fortified formula. Pediatrics 1988; 83:360.
51. Smith JL, Heymsfield SB: Enteral nutrition support: Formula preparation from modular ingredients. J Parenter Enteral Nutr 1983; 7:280.
52. Nielson OH, Schiotz PO, Rasmussen SN, et al: Calcium absorption and acceptance of low-lactose milk among children with primary lactase deficiency. J Pediatr Gastroenterol Nutr 1984; 3:219.

Chapter 81

Nutritional Assessment

WILLIAM J. KLISH

The hospitalized child with a diagnosis of failure to thrive will normally have a thorough nutritional assessment to determine the etiology of the problem, but nutritional assessment should be an integral part of the evaluation of every hospitalized child, regardless of diagnosis.[1] During a prolonged hospital stay, nutritional disturbances can occur even in the previously well-nourished child. This is particularly true when oral intake is suspended or limited. Clinicians rely heavily on sophisticated and highly technical medical and surgical intervention, but adequate nutrition is sometimes forgotten even though it is critically important in promoting adequate wound healing, resistance to infection, and recovery from illness. Nutritional status should therefore be continually assessed in the hospitalized patient. This chapter discusses nutritional assessment methods and their practical application.

DIET HISTORY

A detailed diet history is of obvious importance, because it cannot be assumed that all children eat normally. Children on a strict vegetarian diet may develop protein deficiency if their meals are not properly planned, and their intake of vitamin B_{12}, iron, or pyridoxine may be only marginally adequate. Adolescents often skip meals or eat erratically. Children active in athletics may not get the extra energy required or may become involved in sport "fad" diets. Older children and adolescents may attempt weight loss through starvation or develop anorexia nervosa or bulimia. The most accurate way to assess dietary intake is with a diet diary kept for 3 to 5 days. This period will account for most of the daily variation in intake and also eliminate the subjectiveness present in diet recall records. Food preference evaluations are also sometimes helpful. Dietary analysis is effectively accomplished by a registered dietician.

A history of medication use is essential, since some medications can cause specific nutritional disturbances. Table 81–1 provides some examples of nutritional alterations related to specific drugs.

Table 81–1. NUTRITIONAL DISTURBANCES ASSOCIATED WITH CERTAIN MEDICATIONS*

Medication	Nutritional Disturbances
Antacids	Inhibit absorption of phosphate
Phenytoin	Folate deficiency
	Vitamin C deficiency
	Rickets (increased vitamin D turnover)
Barbiturates	Vitamin C deficiency
	Rickets (increased vitamin D turnover)
Aspirin	Increased excretion of vitamin C
Trimethoprim	Folate deficiency
Methotrexate	Folate deficiency
Isoniazid	Pyridoxine (B_6) deficiency
	Tryptophan and niacin deficiency
Oral contraceptives	Folate deficiency
Vitamin A	Excessive use may cause toxicity
Oral antibiotics	Interfere with intestinal vitamin K production

*Many other examples exist.

ANTHROPOMETRY

Anthropometric measurements can be used to assess growth, either cross-sectionally to measure distance or longitudinally to measure growth velocity. If children are measured once, their growth status can be assessed by comparing this measurement to distance reference values. However, if it is possible to measure the person more than once, growth velocity data can be obtained, which is more valuable because it reflects change. Table 81–2 provides guidelines for the time intervals between measurements that are necessary to develop meaningful incremental data.

Accurate measurements are particularly important when obtaining velocity data, because there is twice the chance of error in calculating the growth increment.

Table 81–2. RECOMMENDED TIME INTERVALS FOR VELOCITY MEASUREMENTS

Measurement	Interval
Weight	7 days
Length	4 weeks
Stature	8 weeks
Head circumference	7 days (infants)
	4 weeks (up to 4 years old)
Mid-arm circumference	4 weeks

Length and Stature

Length, or stature, is by far the most useful indication of growth status. It is a stable measure of linear body growth that results from the interaction of genetics and environment. In spite of the difficulty in obtaining an accurate measurement (particularly in infants), this measurement should be made. In infants and children younger than 2 years of age, recumbent length is measured. This should be accomplished using a measuring table or board that consists of a rigid headboard affixed at a right angle, a movable footboard, and a wooden rule attached at one side. Any apparatus that does not include each of these elements will sacrifice accuracy. To perform the measurement, the infant lies on the long axis of the measuring board. The measurer should be assisted by someone holding the crown of the infant's head against the headboard so that the external auditory meatus and the lower margin of the eye orbit are perpendicular. The measurer then grips both ankles with one hand and positions the heels firmly against the foot board, which is manipulated with the other hand. The knees, which are slightly flexed, are then firmly pressed down on the table with the lateral edge of the hand. If the head is no longer against the headboard at this point, it should be brought back gently but firmly. In this way the infant is gently stretched to overcome any voluntary contraction of the frame. The recumbent length should be recorded to the nearest 0.5 cm.

Stature is measured in children older than 2 years of age. Several apparatus are available to affix to a wall and vary from expensive commercial stadiometers to handmade models.* Measurements are made with the child's feet bare, and the child should stand erect with the heels, buttocks, and shoulders all touching the measuring board. The heels should be together with the feet at a 45-degree angle with each other. The axis of vision should be horizontal with the child looking straight ahead. The upper margin of the external auditory meatus and the lower margin of the orbit should be horizontal. From the side, the auditory meatus, acromion process, trochanter of the hip, and lateral malleolus should all be in the same perpendicular line. The child should be told to make him- or herself "as tall as possible, keeping the heels on the ground." The measurer should check to see if the heels are properly positioned and then slide the head projection firmly down onto the crown of the head. The stature is then recorded to the nearest 0.5 cm. When possible, the parents' stature should be obtained. If only one parent's stature is obtainable, maternal stature is more valuable. Reference values for length and stature should be placed in all pediatric units and clinics and are available for both distance (Figs. 81–1 to 81–4) and velocity (Figs. 81–5 and 81–6).[2–5]

*Examples include (1) the Harpender Infantometer, a portable instrument measuring with a range of 300 to 940 mm that has counter recording instrumentation (Holtain Ltd, Crosswell, Crymmych, Dyfed, Wales, UK [US agents: Pfister Imports, 450 Barell Avenue, Carlstadt, NJ 07072]) and (2) Accustat, which is produced by Genentech, Inc., 800 Forbes Boulevard, S., San Francisco, CA 94080.

Weight

There are various types of apparatus available to measure body weight, such as infant scales, beam-balance scales, and read-out scales. Whichever type is used, it needs to be regularly calibrated to maintain accuracy. Weight should always be recorded as nude weight. If the subject is not weighed nude, then the estimated weight of the clothing should be subtracted from the total weight. Reference values for body weight both as distance (see Figs. 81–1 to 81–4) and velocity curves (Figs. 81–7 and 81–8) and in relation to length and stature are available.[2, 3]

Weight for Height

The ratio of actual weight to the ideal weight for height (usually referred to as *weight for height*) can be used as an indicator to differentiate the stunted child from the wasted child and is independent of age. Stunting is caused by genetic or endocrine abnormalities and results in a child who is small for age but has a body weight that is proportional to the child's length. Wasting results from nutritional deprivation, and body weight is depleted out of proportion to length, making the weight-for-height ratio low. Undernutrition is defined as a weight-for-height ratio of less than 90%, and severe marasmus has a ratio of less than 65%. Obesity is defined by a weight for height greater than 120%. Reference values for prepubescent normal children are available in chart form (Figs. 81–9 to 81–12).[3]

The ratio of mid-arm circumference to head circumference was developed by Ranawati and McLaren[6] as a method to estimate weight for height when the proper apparatus for measuring weight or height is not available. Mid-arm circumference is significantly influenced by subcutaneous fat and therefore fluctuates with total body weight. The head circumference in an infant and young child parallels the child's linear growth. Therefore, the mid-arm to head circumference ratio varies directly with the weight-for-height ratio and can be used as a substitute until head growth slows at about 3 years of age. A ratio greater than 0.31 is considered normal, and one less than 0.25 is indicative of severe malnutrition (Fig. 81–13). Various degrees of undernutrition lie between.

Head Circumference

Head circumference can be a useful measurement until about 3 years of age, when head growth slows. It must be measured with a narrow and nonstretchable metal or plastic measuring tape. To obtain an accurate measurement, the tape must cross the frontal bone area just above the supraorbital ridges passing around the head at the same level on both sides to the occiput. It is then moved up or down slightly to obtain the maximum circumference. The tape should have sufficient tension to press the hair against the skull. Normal

Text continued on page 1104

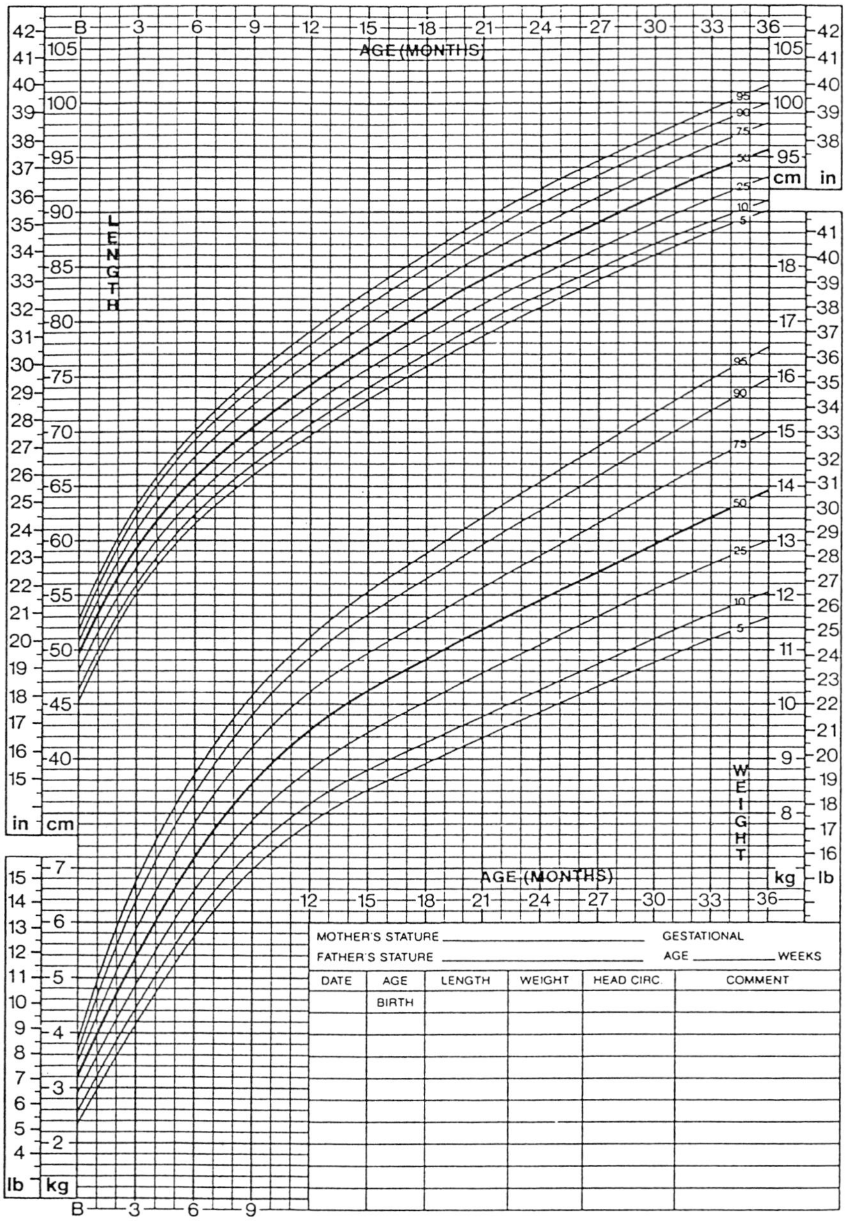

Figure 81–1. Girls: Birth to 36 months physical growth NCHS percentiles. (Adapted from Hamill PV, Drizd TA, Johnson CL, et al: Physical growth: National Center for Health Statistics percentiles. Am J Clin Nutr 1979; 32:607–629. © Am. J. Clin. Nutr. American Society for Clinical Nutrition.)

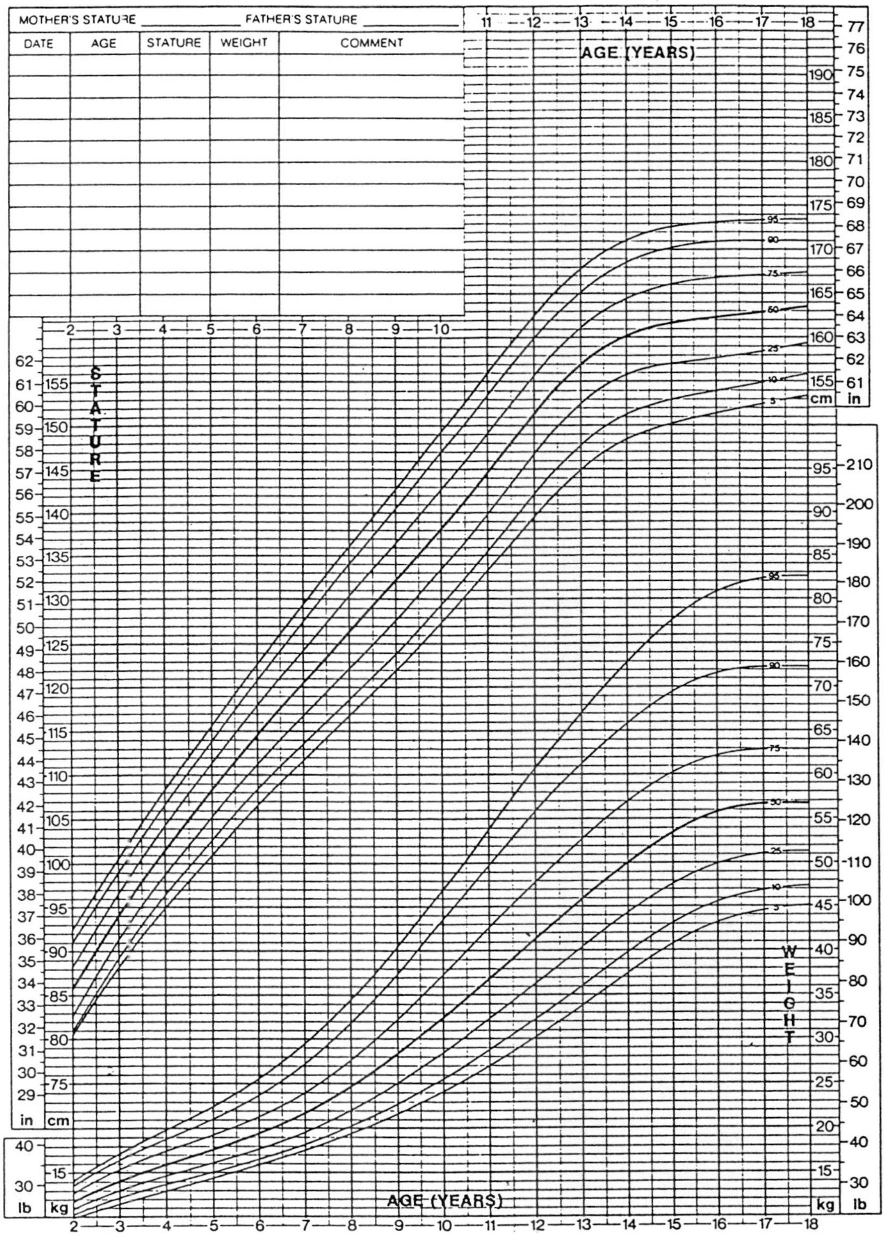

Figure 81–2. Girls: 2 to 18 years physical growth NCHS percentiles. (Adapted from Hamill PV, Drizd TA, Johnson CL, et al: Physical growth: National Center for Health Statistics percentiles. Am J Clin Nutr 1979; 32:607–629. © Am. J. Clin. Nutr. American Society for Clinical Nutrition.)

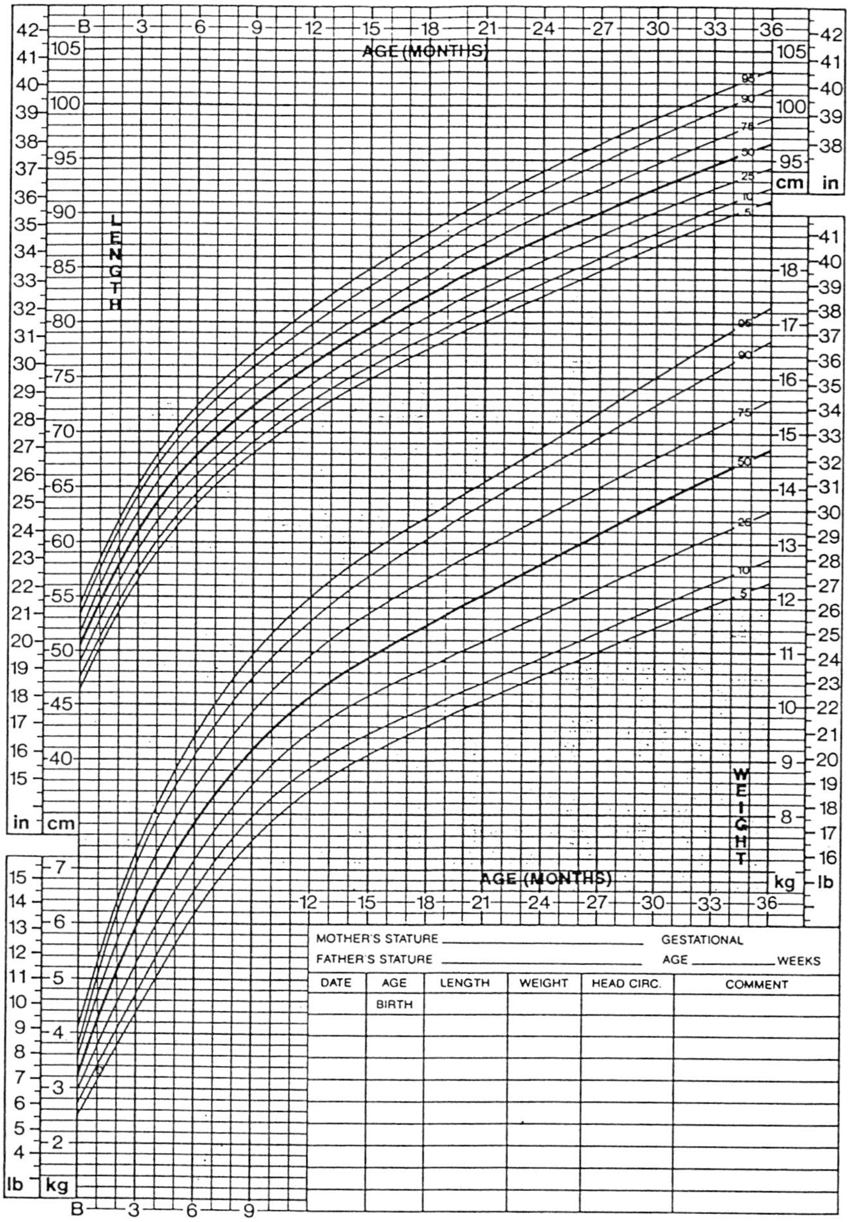

Figure 81–3. Boys: Birth to 36 months physical growth NCHS percentiles. (Adapted from Hamill PV, Drizd TA, Johnson CL, et al: Physical growth: National Center for Health Statistics percentiles. Am J Clin Nutr 1979; 32:607–629. © Am. J. Clin. Nutr. American Society for Clinical Nutrition.)

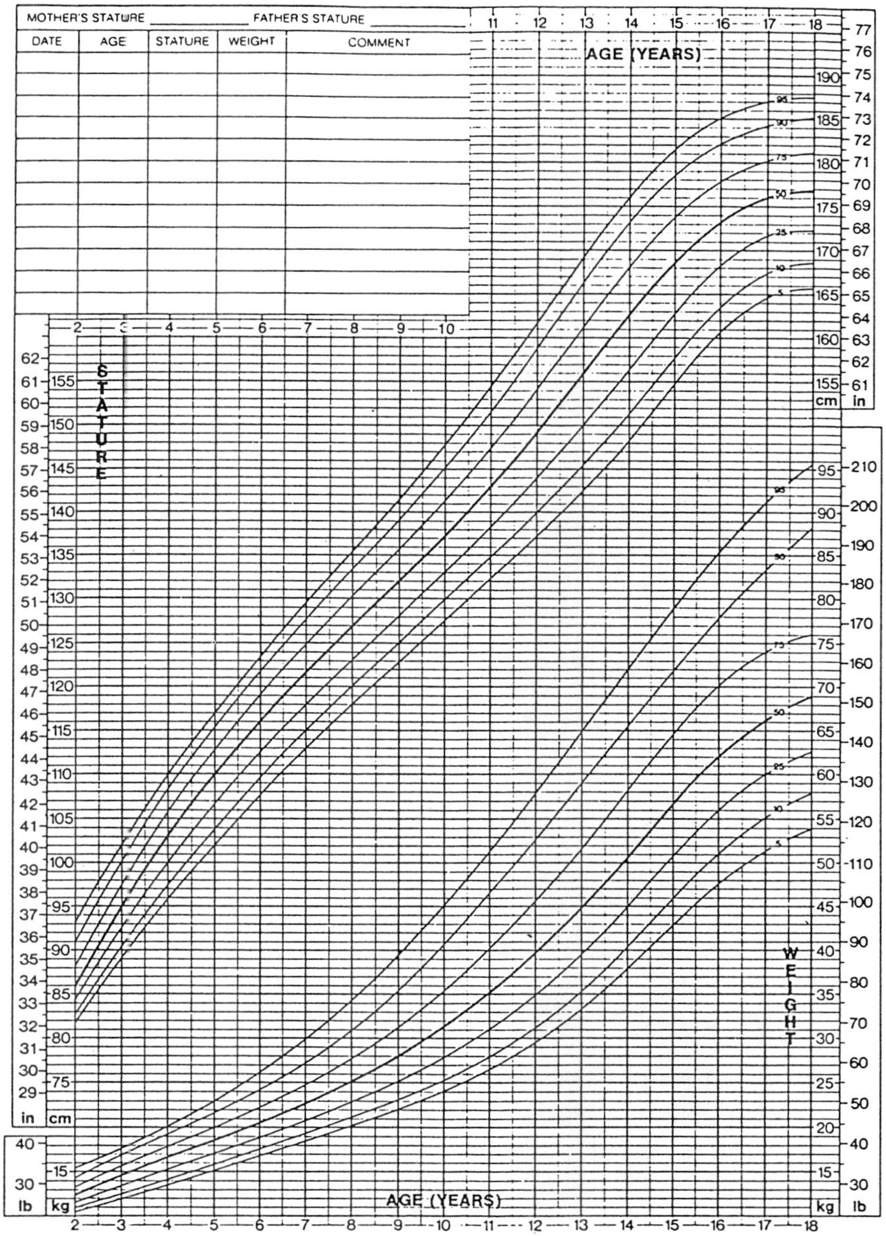

Figure 81–4. Boys: 2 to 18 years physical growth NCHS percentiles. (Adapted from Hamill PV, Drizd TA, Johnson CL, et al: Physical growth: National Center for Health Statistics percentiles. Am J Clin Nutr 1979; 32:607–629. © Am. J. Clin. Nutr. American Society for Clinical Nutrition.)

HEIGHT VELOCITY, GIRLS

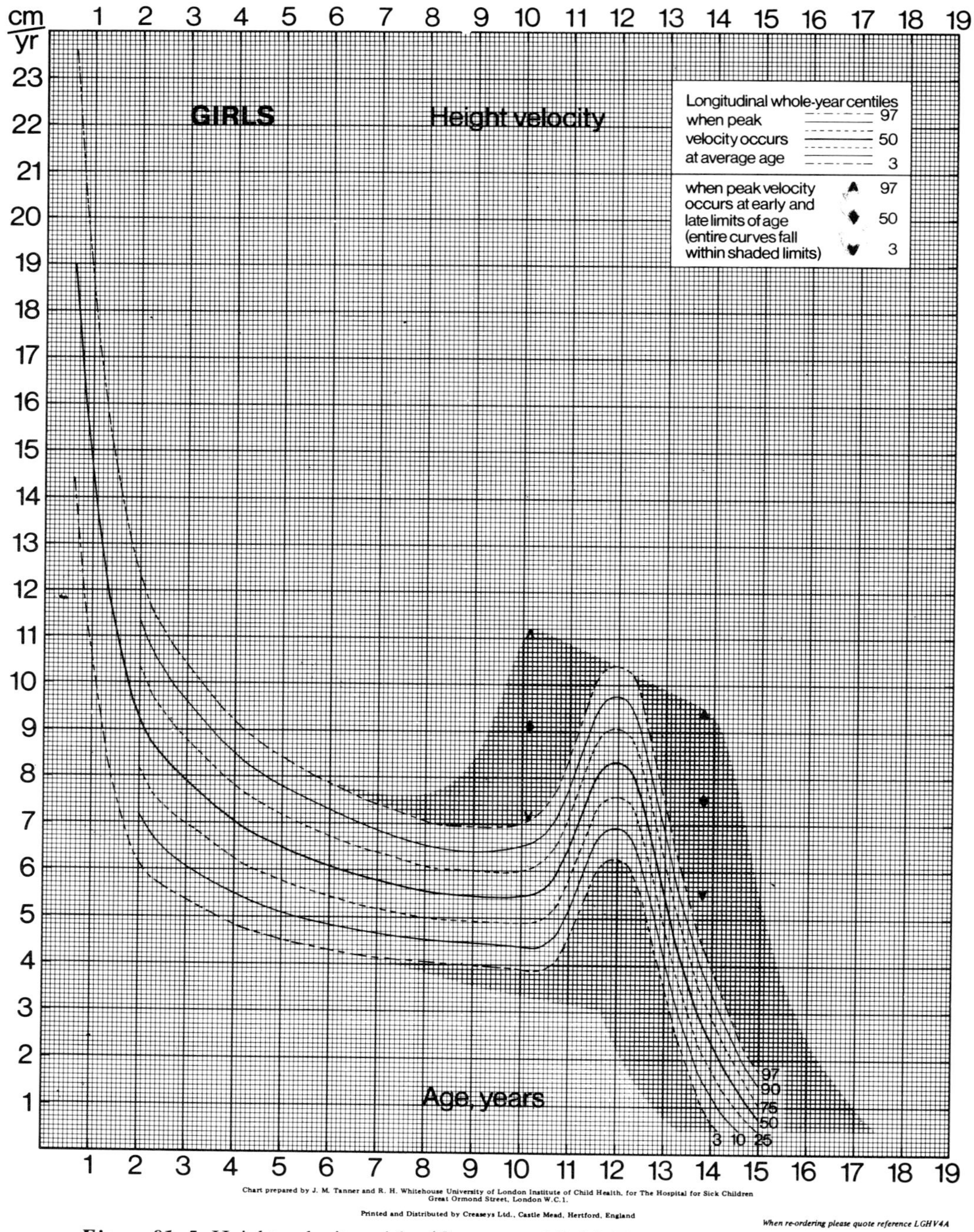

Figure 81–5. Height velocity, girls. (Courtesy of J. M. Tanner and R. H. Whitehouse.)

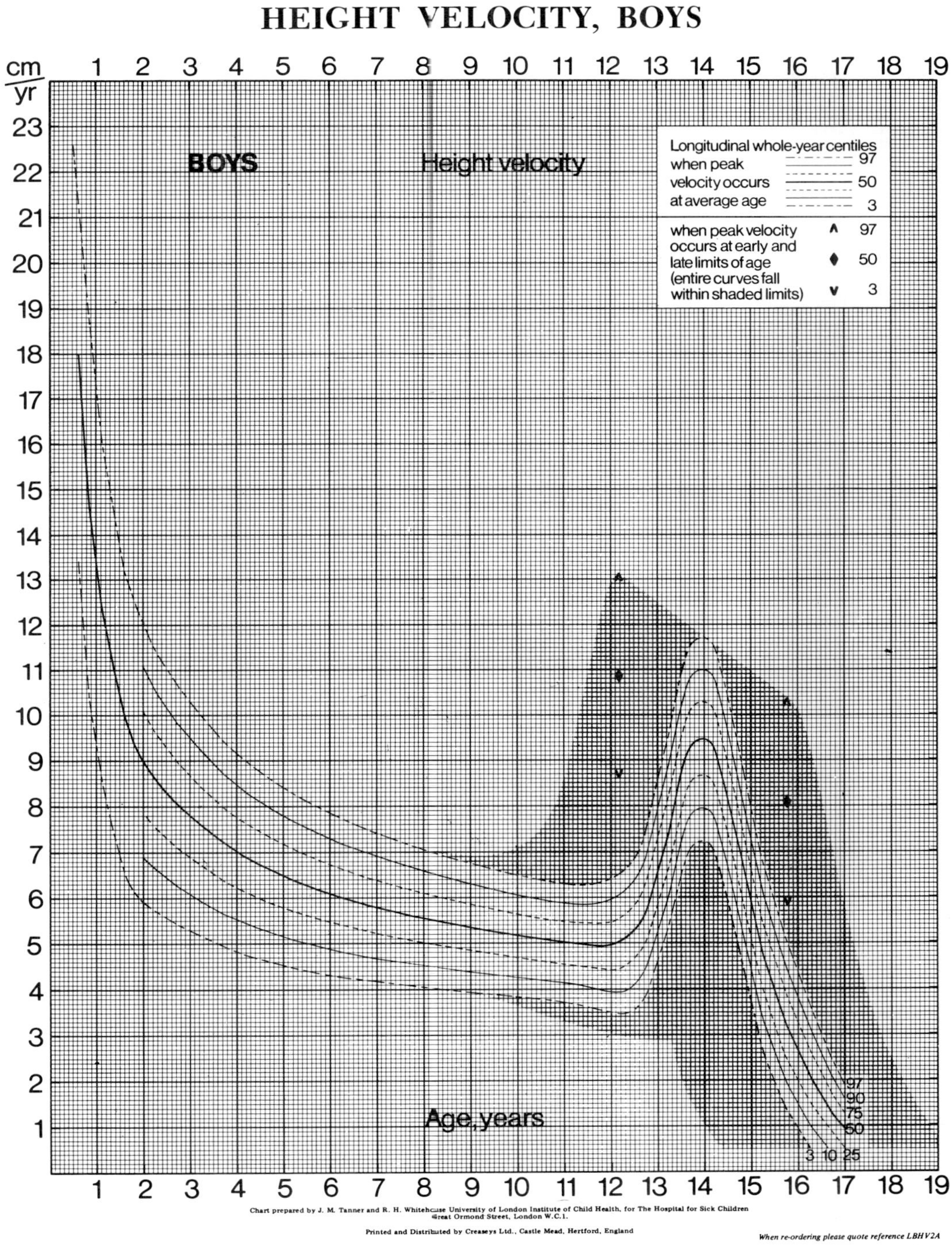

Figure 81–6. Height velocity, boys. (Courtesy of J. M. Tanner and R. H. Whitehouse.)

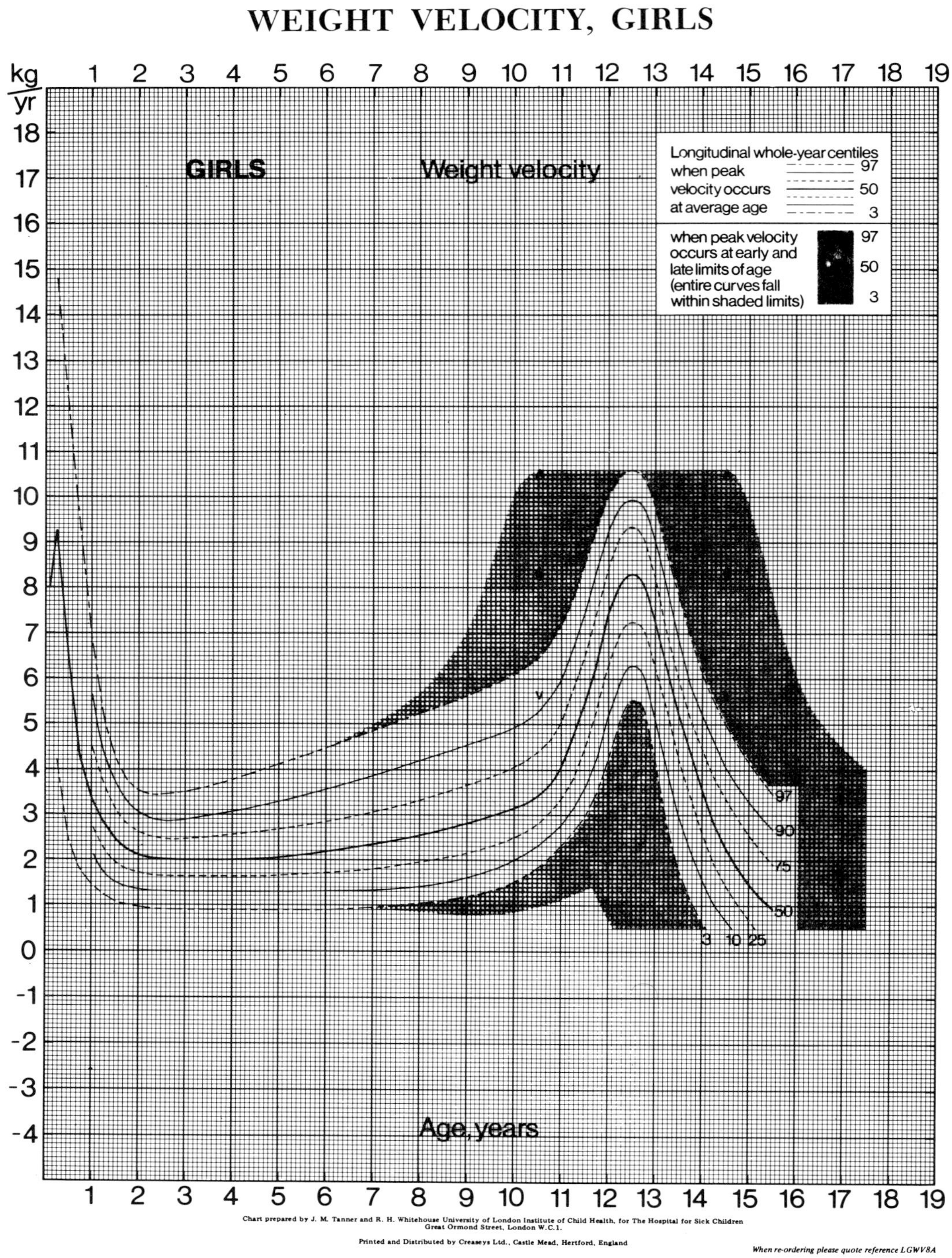

Figure 81–7. Weight velocity, girls. (Courtesy of J. M. Tanner and R. H. Whitehouse.)

WEIGHT VELOCITY, BOYS

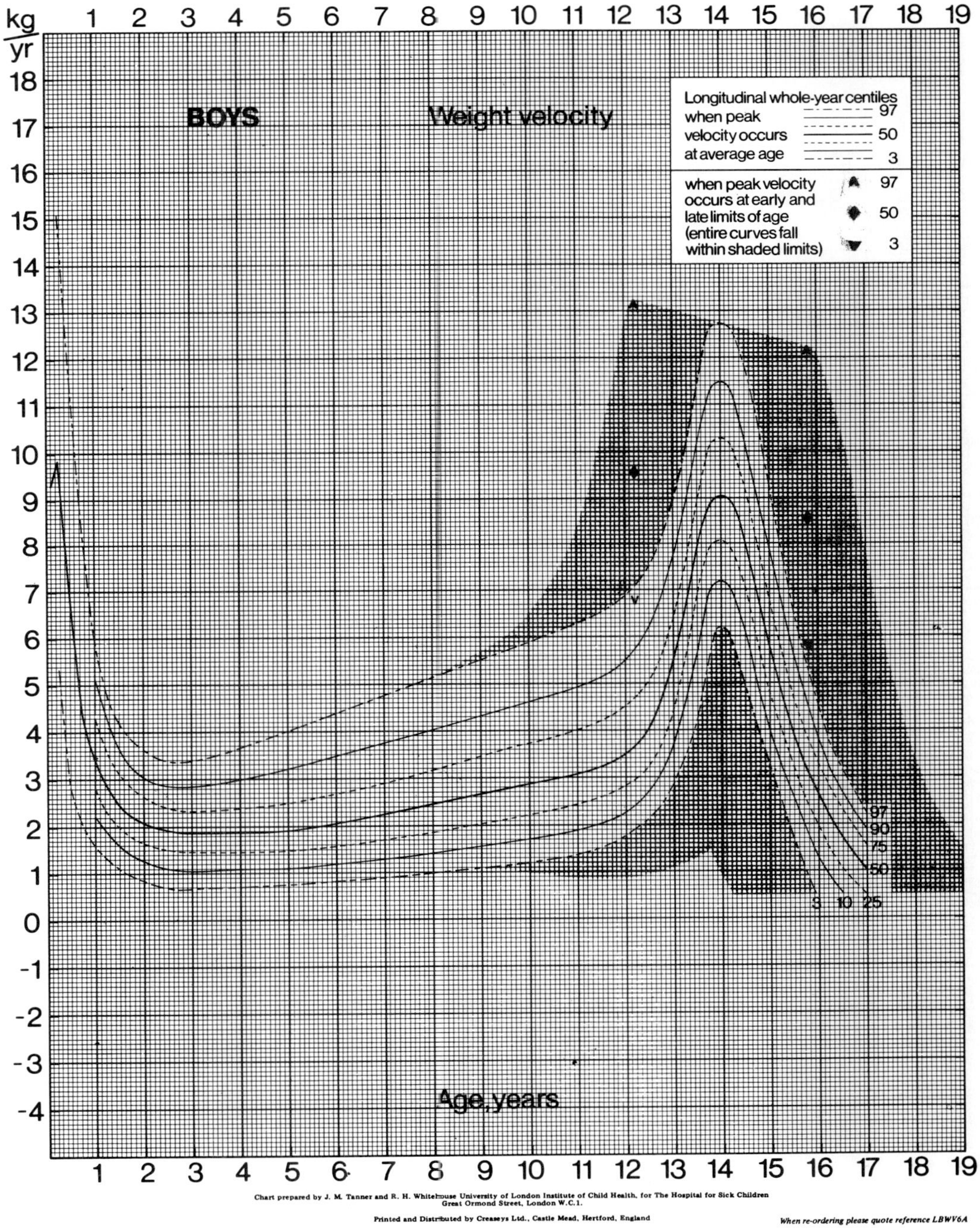

Figure 81–8. Weight velocity, boys. (Courtesy of J. M. Tanner and R. H. Whitehouse.)

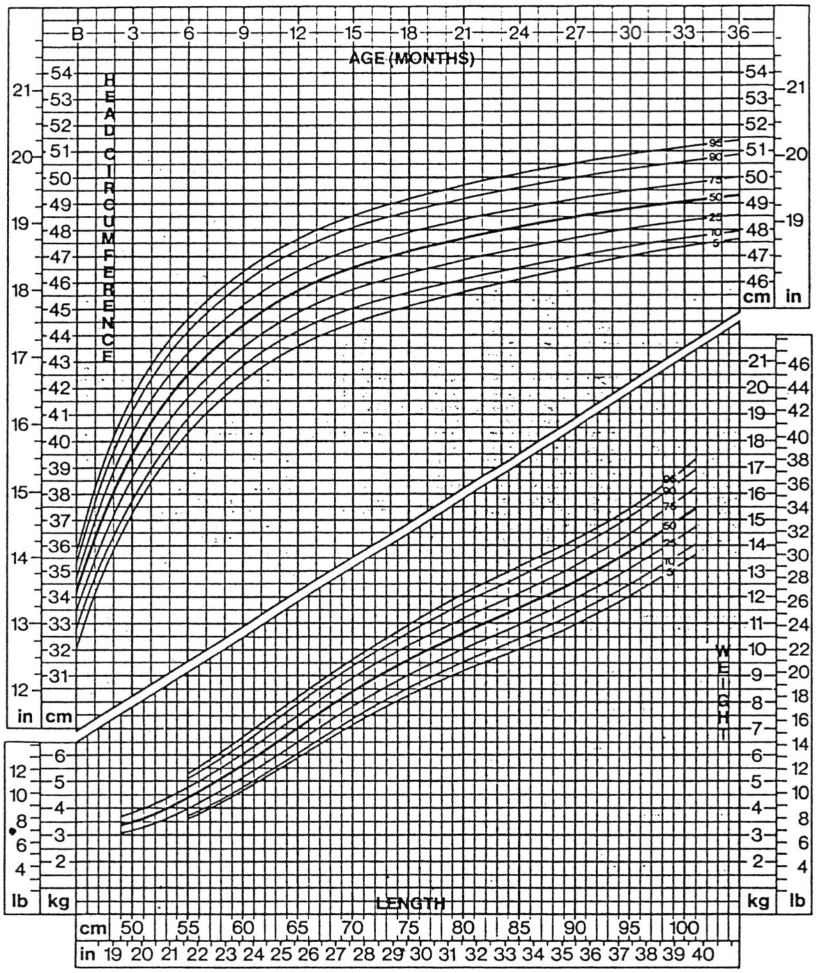

Figure 81–9. Girls: birth to 36 months physical growth NCHS percentiles. (Adapted from Hamill PV, Drizd TA, Johnson CL, et al: Physical growth: National Center for Health Statistics percentiles. Am J Clin Nutr 1979; 32:607–629. © Am. J. Clin. Nutr. American Society for Clinical Nutrition.)

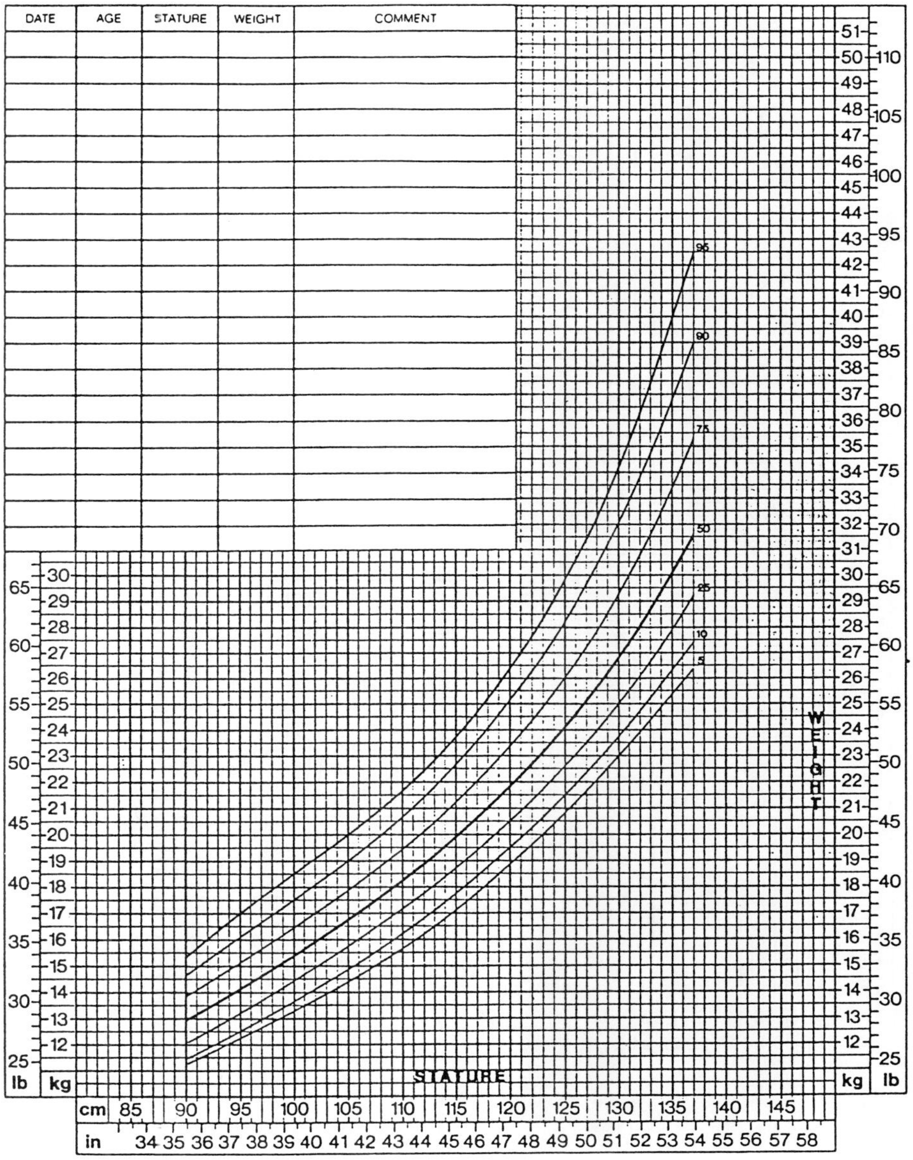

Figure 81–10. Girls: prepubescent physical growth NCHS percentiles. (Adapted from Hamill PV, Drizd TA, Johnson CL, et al: Physical growth: National Center for Health Statistics percentiles. Am J Clin Nutr 1979; 32:607–629. © Am. J. Clin. Nutr. American Society for Clinical Nutrition.)

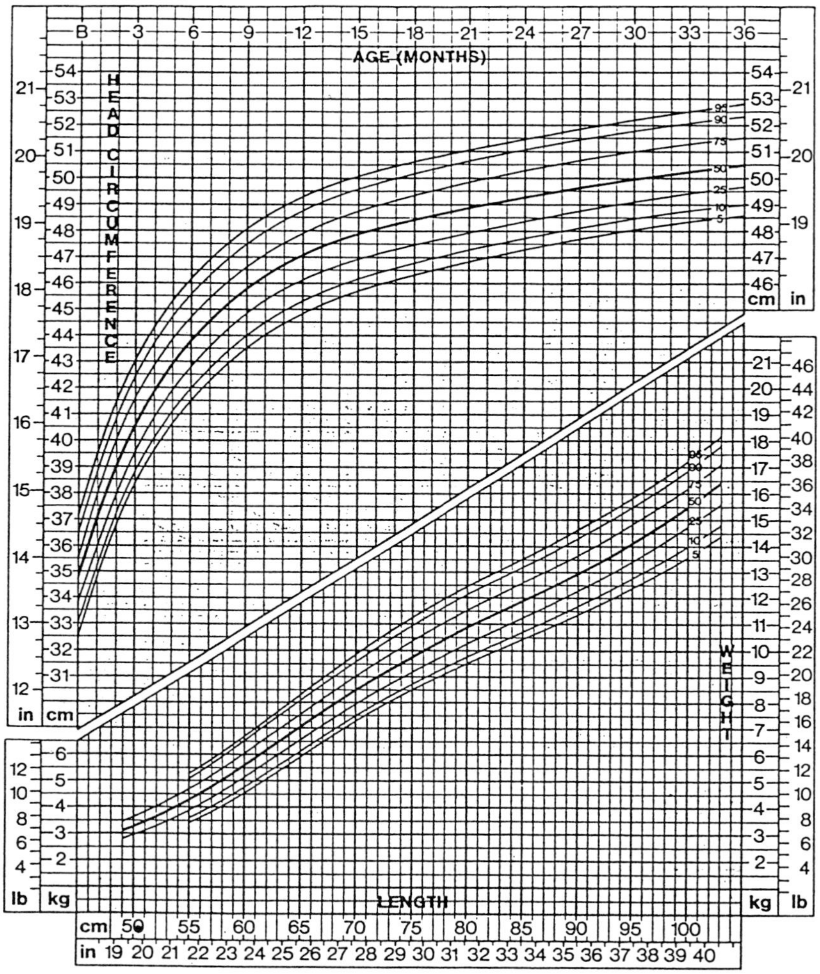

Figure 81–11. Boys: birth to 36 months physical growth NCHS percentiles. (Adapted from Hamill PV, Drizd TA, Johnson CL, et al: Physical growth: National Center for Health Statistics percentiles. Am J Clin Nutr 1979; 32:607–629. © Am. J. Clin. Nutr. American Society for Clinical Nutrition.)

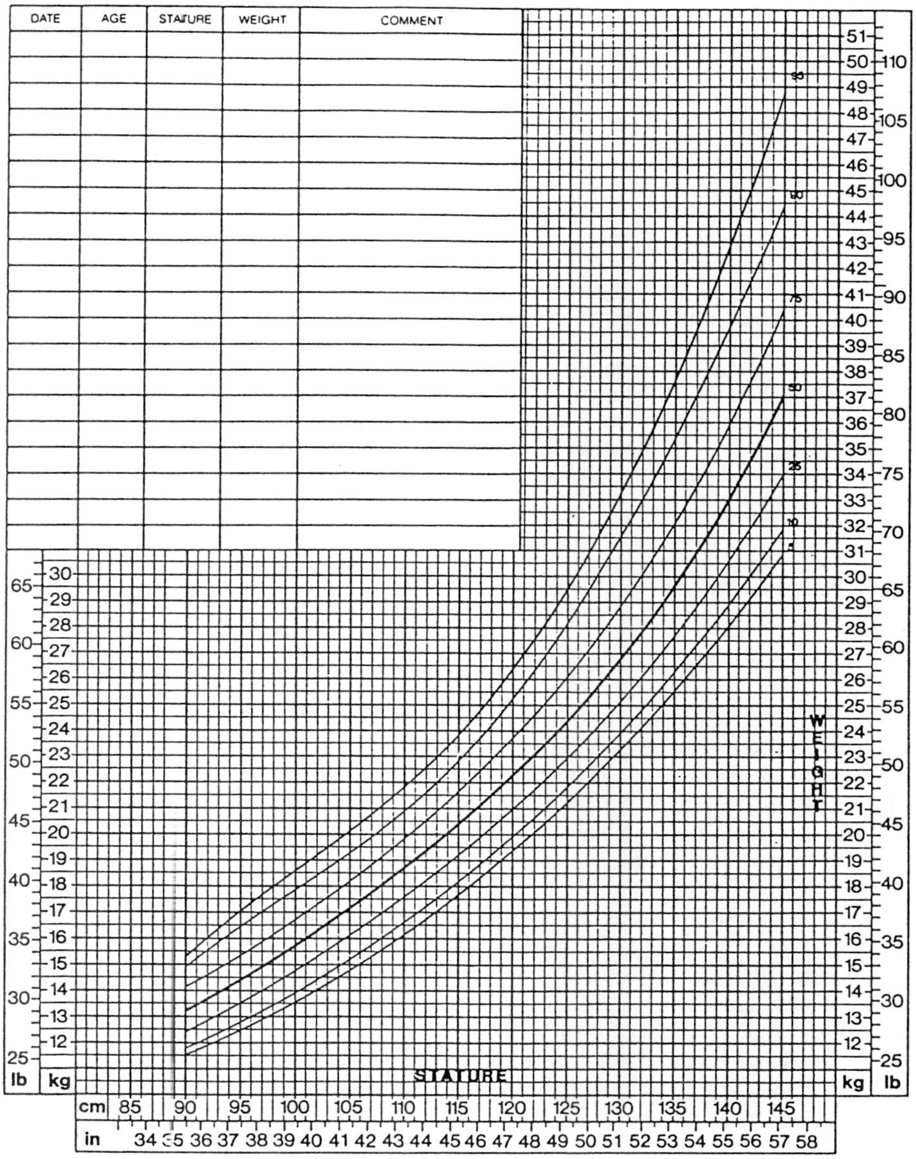

Figure 81–12. Boys: prepubescent physical growth NCHS percentiles. (Adapted from Hamill PV, Drizd TA, Johnson CL, et al: Physical growth: National Center for Health Statistics percentiles. Am J Clin Nutr 1979; 32:607–629. © Am. J. Clin. Nutr. American Society for Clinical Nutrition.)

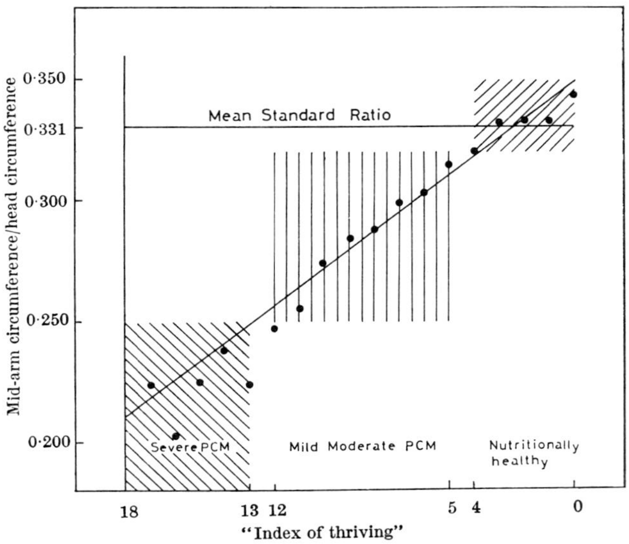

Figure 81–13. Mid-arm circumference to head circumference ratio compared with an "index of thriving" based on weight, height, head circumference, and mid-arm circumference in relation to international standards in 1,276 children. $r = 0.75$. PCM, protein-calorie malnutrition. (Reprinted with permission from *Nature* [Kanawate A, McLaren DS: Assessment of marginal malnutrition. Nature 1970; 228:573–574]. Copyright 1970 Macmillan Magazines Limited.)

reference values exist from birth to 3 years for both distance (see Figs. 81–9 and 81–11) and velocity.[2, 3]

Mid-Arm Circumference

The mid–upper arm circumference is an indicator of muscle growth in all ages. The left arm is usually measured by convention. The tape to be used should be the same as that used to measure the head circumference. A point is marked midway between the acromion and the olecranon on the vertical axis of the upper arm (with the arm bent at a right angle) and between the lateral and medial surface of the arm. The child should then stand or sit with the arm hanging loose at the side. The tape is passed around the arm at the level marked and is tightened so that it touches but does not compress the skin or alter the contour of the arm (Fig. 81–14). Because the arm on cross-section is not an exact circle, some difficulty is usually met in ensuring that the tape touches the arm on the medial surface. To accomplish this, the middle finger of the left hand can be used gently to press the tape to the skin. Normal reference values for distance are available for children aged 1 year and older.[7]

NUTRITIONAL ASSESSMENT THROUGH THE MEASUREMENT OF BODY COMPOSITION

The major form of stored energy in the body is fat. A small amount of carbohydrate in the form of glycogen is present, but this can be depleted after only 1 or 2 days of starvation. Protein can also be used for energy, but all protein in the body is present only as functional tissue, so its utilization results in a decrease in the functional body mass. Because fat is used preferentially by the body as an energy source during starvation or periods of metabolic stress, the accurate measurement of this body compartment would be the ideal method to assess a child's nutritional status. Longitudinal measurements would allow estimates of nutritional sufficiency during periods of recovery from disease. Many methods of measurement of the fat and fat-free compartments of the body exist; however, most of them are not applicable to the child, because they are either too inaccurate or too cumbersome to be used in this age group.[8] New methods that provide an easy way to measure fat and fat-free mass are being developed.[9, 10] If these methods prove practical, they will revolutionize the surveillance of the nutritional status of the hospitalized patient.

A

B

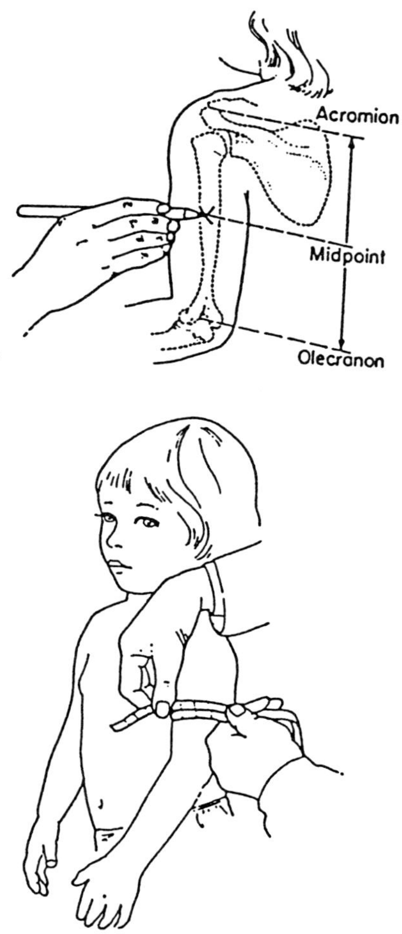

Figure 81–14. Technique for measuring mid–upper arm circumference. The midpoint between the acromium and the olecranon is determined *(A)*, and the circumference is measured at that point *(B)*. Measurements should be made to the nearest 0.1 cm. (From Jeliffee DB: The assessment of the nutritional status of the community. Geneva; World Health Organization, Monograph Series No. 53, 1966; with permission.)

Fatfold Measurements

Currently, the most frequently used method to estimate body fatness in the hospitalized patient is skin fatfold measurement. This method is limited because of two assumptions: (1) that the subcutaneous fat mantle reflects the total amount of fat in the body and (2) that the measurement sites selected represent the average thickness of the entire mantle. Neither of these assumptions is true. There are two studies of humans that address the first assumption. Forbes and associates[11] showed that only 42% of the total body fat of a full-term neonate resides in the subcutaneous compartment, and Moore and colleagues[12] found the value to be 32% in an adult woman. The second assumption can be discredited simply by observing the regional variation of subcutaneous fat among individual persons. Some people have truncal distribution of fat with thin arms and legs, whereas others have the reverse. The variation in body form is tremendous, resulting in endless permutations of fat distribution.

In the infant and young child, the use of skin fatfold measurements as an index of total body fat has not been fully validated by an alternate method.[13] Accurately and reproducibly measuring a skin fatfold is difficult in a normal person and perhaps impossible in an edematous or obese one. These problems make this measurement limited in its usefulness as a tool for nutritional assessment of an individual. It is sometimes useful, however, for the longitudinal assessment of a patient's response to nutritional therapy. The calipers recommended for fatfold measurements include the Holtain caliper* and the Lange caliper (Cambridge Instruments, Silver Spring, MD). All measurements are taken on the left side of the child. The fold of skin should be firmly grasped between the left thumb and forefinger (for right-handed persons) and then lifted up. A firm grip, not exceeding the pain threshold, eliminates or at least reduces the variations in the apparent thickness of skinfold that could result from differences in the pulling force of the fingers. The width of the skin that is enclosed between the fingers is an important factor. It cannot be standardized, in its absolute size, for all the sites of the body. With a thick subcutaneous layer, a wider segment of the skin must be "pinched" to form a fold than if the adipose tissue is poorly developed, as it is on the dorsum of the hand. For a given site, the width of the skin should be the smallest amount that will yield a well-defined fold. The fold is pinched and lifted several times to make certain that no musculature is grasped. The skinfold is held with the thumb and finger while the contact surface of the calipers is placed over the fold. The grip on the caliper should be released completely, allowing the spring to compress the fold (Fig. 81–15). When the movement of the needle on the caliper dial stops, a reading is taken to the nearest millimeter. Normative data are available for children in the first 3 years of life[13a] and for childhood through adulthood.[13b] The position on the skinfold where the calipers are placed requires comment. The two sides of the fold are not completely parallel. When the skin is lifted, the fold will be narrower near the crest and spread out near the base. If the calipers are placed at the base, the resulting measurement is too large. The correct distance from the crest to place the calipers is where the surfaces are approximately parallel to each other, usually just below the fingers. It is extremely important to measure skinfolds accurately. Even after extensive practice, it is possible to make errors owing to slight misplacement of the caliper or misreading of the dial. To avoid such errors, the following procedures are recommended. Skinfolds should be lifted two or three times to determine the fold to be measured before placing the calipers. It is natural to become anxious to put the calipers in place before determining what is to be measured. The jaws of the calipers must be on the same site if repeated measurements are done. The skin must be released between each of the measurements.

*The Holtain caliper is a newer version of the original Harpender caliper and is available from Holtain and Pfister (see earlier footnote).

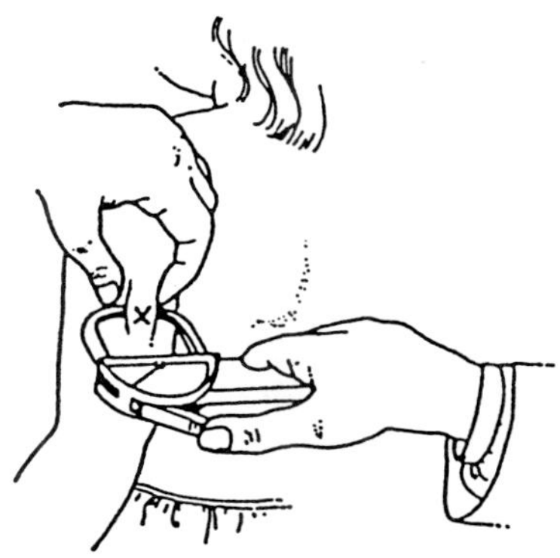

Figure 81–15. Technique for measuring triceps skinfold thickness. The midpoint of the upper arm is marked as described for Figure 81–14. (From Jeliffee DB: The assessment of the nutritional status of the community. Geneva; World Health Organization, Monograph Series No. 53, 1966; with permission.)

The two most frequent sites of skinfold measurements are the triceps and the suprailiac crest. The level for the triceps skinfold is the same level as where the upper arm was marked with the felt pen for a circumference measurement (midway between the acromion and the olecranon with the arm bent at a right angle). With the arm dropped and hanging loosely, the skinfold is then lifted away from the underlying muscle fascia with a sweeping motion of the fingers with the observer gripping the "neck" of the fold between middle finger and thumb. The skinfold caliper is then applied to the fold. The point of measurement for the suprailiac skinfold is 1 cm above and 2 cm medial to the anterior superior iliac spine. This postion is best palpated with the subject standing facing the observer and is marked with a pen. The skinfold is picked up as a vertical skinfold and the caliper applied below the fingers.

Hydrodensitometry

The oldest method of estimating the relative proportion of lean and fat in the human body is densitometry, which was introduced in 1942 by Albert Behnke.[14] This method uses the Archimedes principle to determine the density of a person by dividing the actual weight by the amount of weight lost when the person is completely submerged in water. Because the density of fat and the lean compartments of the body are assumed to be constants, it is possible to calculate mathematically the proportion of each when the density of the whole body is known. This method is widely used to measure body fat in adults. Its use in children, however, is limited by the fact that young children cannot be submerged under water. Even in older children, the method is limited by the fact that during maturation, the density of the lean body mass changes, thus invalidating one of the basic assumptions of the method.[15] In the hospitalized patient, this method becomes useless because one cannot expect sick children, or adults for that matter, to subject themselves to submersion in water even if the problems of intravenous lines, dressings, and so forth could be dealt with. Newer methods using this principle of air rather than water displacement are being developed; however, no data exist as yet to determine their practicality.

Total Body Potassium

Another method that has become a gold standard for the measurement of lean body mass and body fat in adults is the measurement of total body potassium.[16, 17] This method takes advantage of the fact that naturally occurring potassium (^{39}K) contains a fixed proportion (0.0118%) of the radioactive isotope ^{40}K. In determining lean body mass, the subject is placed in a specially designed scintillation chamber and the number of radioactive emissions from ^{40}K is recorded during a 30- to 60-minute period. Total body potassium is then calculated from the amount of ^{40}K present. Because potassium resides only in the lean body mass and not in fat, and its proportion in the lean mass is relatively fixed, an estimation of the total amount of lean body mass can be derived. Fat can then be calculated by the subtraction of lean body mass from total body weight. This technique has the advantage of being noninvasive; however, it presents several limitations, particularly for the hospitalized patient. The counting time is long and requires isolation in a special chamber, which may not be possible with a child or an ill subject. Few machines are available that have sufficient sensitivity to measure infants or small children. Since small children have little lean body mass, they have relatively fewer radioactive disintegrations per unit time than adults. If the counting instrument is not sufficiently shielded from background radiation (cosmic radiation, radon gas, and others), the small number of counts emanating from an infant or small child can be "lost" in the background. Finally, the assumption is made that the potassium content of all elements of lean body mass is constant. This is known not to be true, since the potassium content of the liver tends to be less than that of skeletal muscle. Also, since the relative weight of visceral organs to skeletal muscle varies with age, this method may be too imprecise for use in children.

Total Body Water

Because neutral fat does not bind water, the measurement of total body water offers a means for estimating the nonfat compartment of the body.[18] This can be accomplished in a fairly noninvasive manner by orally administering water labeled with a known amount of either radioactive tritium (^{3}H) or the stable isotopes deuterium (^{2}H) or oxygen 18. Total body water then can be estimated by determining the dilution of the isotope within a body fluid such as serum, urine, saliva, and others after a suitable period of equilibration. Because the water content of lean body mass is relatively constant, this compartment can be estimated. Even though this method is simple, its application to clinical problems is limited by the fact that the assays for deuterium and oxygen 18 are cumbersome and radioactive tritium is not suitable for use in children. A basic methodologic problem also exists, because the water content of lean body mass changes with age and may also vary slightly among people of the same age. Isotopes of hydrogen also appear to exchange with nonaqueous hydrogen, resulting in an overestimation of body water content. Oxygen 18 appears not to have the same problem but is an expensive substance.

Body Imaging

Body imaging techniques have been used to estimate fatness. Computed tomographic scanning can provide an accurate assessment of the thickness of the subcutaneous fat mantle at selected body sites but is subject to the same errors and assumptions inherent to skin- and fatfold measurements. Magnetic resonance imaging holds promise for the future, since it might be possible to program the imaging instrument to quantitate fat in any given cross-sectional image of the body. Total body scanning, though, would be time consuming and therefore expensive.

Neutron Activation

Many elements can be made radioactive by bombarding them with neutrons. The neutron activation method of total body analysis takes advantage of this principle by activating the body with a known amount of neutron energy and counting the induced radioactivity in a whole-body counting chamber. A given dose of neutrons will generate a known amount of activity within a defined mass of substance. The total activity will therefore reflect the total mass of the substance; therefore, a particular element can be identified by the characteristic energy of the electromagnetic radiation it emits. This method can be used to determine the amount of a number of elements in the body, including calcium, sodium, chlorine, phosphorus, magnesium, and nitrogen. Total body nitrogen can be used to estimate lean body mass. This method should allow a much better understanding of human body composition through its use as a research tool; however, its clinical use will be limited by the great expense of a neutron activation facility. Also, even though the radiation exposure by this method is small (approximately 30 mrad), the fact that there is radiation exposure will limit its use in children.

Bioelectrical Impedance Analysis

More recently, several electrical techniques have been developed to measure lean body mass.[19–22] Bioelectrical impedance analysis (BIA) has become somewhat popular both as a research tool as well as a health spa component. This method is based on the principle that a weak electrical current passes through the body by way of the lean compartment rather than fat. The relation of impedance to electrical flow is directly proportional to the amount of lean tissue present. This method has been validated with hydrodensitometry and total body water by isotope dilution in adults. It is noninvasive, portable, and relatively cheap; however, it appears to be imprecise. Small changes in body water, such as diurnal variation, appear to make significant differences in the estimate of lean body mass. Placement of the electrodes (wrist and ankle) that inject and record the electrical current is critical. As a result, the standard error of the estimate is rather high (2–2.5 kg in adults). BIA has not yet been accurately applied to infants. The changing water content and distribution of the lean body mass of growing children should cause the impedance to change progressively with age, making this method extremely difficult to use in these age groups.

Total Body Electrical Conductivity

A recently developed electrical method that shows great promise is total body electrical conductivity (TOBEC),[23, 24] which is based on the principle that organisms placed in an electromagnetic field perturb the field. The degree of perturbation depends on the amount and volume of distribution of electrolytes present within the body. Electrolytes reside exclusively in the lean body mass, thus allowing estimation of this body compartment. This method is safe—the total energy dissipated in a subject measured is at least 100 times less than what has been established as a safety standard for exposure to electromagnetic energy. The instrument consists of a hollow chamber, open at both ends, the walls of which contain transducer coils that generate the appropriate electromagnetic field. To obtain a reading, the subject is passed through the chamber and current is applied for less than 1 minute in the adult machine and approximately 1 second in the infant machine. The infant machine has been calibrated against the fat-free mass of infant miniature pigs as determined by chemical analysis. The older child and adult machine has been calibrated against hydrodensitometry, total body water by isotope dilution, and total body potassium. The standard error of the estimate of lean body mass for this method is 70 gm for infants and 930 gm for adults. TOBEC is proving to be a rapid, safe, and noninvasive method for accurately determining body composition. Its major limitation is its lack of portability. The TOBEC method shows the greatest promise for becoming a practical tool for nutritional assessment of the hospitalized child.

Photon and X-Ray Absorptiometry

Abnormalities in bone mineralization as a complication of prematurity or disease (such as renal or hepatic) are being recognized with increasing frequency. The traditional method to assess this parameter has been radiologic, but radiographs are not a sensitive indicator of bone density. The development of photon absorptiometry and, more recently, x-ray absorptiometry may provide a tool for the assessment of this parameter. In this technique, the bone is scanned transversely by a low-energy photon beam generated by ^{125}I or an x-ray beam, and the transmission is monitored by a scintillation detector. The change in transmission of the beam as it is moved across the bone is a function of the bone density in the region. There is evidence that the bone density of the distal radius can be related to the total skeletal mass, at least in adults. Dual photon or x-ray absorptiometry of the spine provides an index of the density of trabecular bone. Further study is needed, but these methods show promise as sensitive means to assess abnormalities in bone growth and development.

NUTRITIONAL ASSESSMENT THROUGH THE MEASUREMENT OF BIOCHEMICAL PARAMETERS

Serum and urine assays can be helpful in the assessment of the nutritional status of an individual person, but their usefulness is limited by their wide variation within normal groups and the lack of easy availability of many of the vitamin assays. Normal values for some of the biochemical measurements are shown in Table 81–3. Since many values either vary with age or might be perceived to, they are listed by age group in this table. Values for protein stature may or may not reflect the degree of nutritional deficiency. In simple starvation (marasmus), there is a tendency to maintain the circulatory pool of visceral proteins at the expense of somatic protein. The blood urea nitrogen level tends to decrease in starvation; however, in patients in whom water intake is restricted, such as those with anorexia nervosa, the serum value may actually be elevated.

Serum sodium is frequently decreased in malnutrition as a dilutional effect, since total body water is physiologically increased as a consequence of starvation. This value is seldom lower than 135 mEq/L, however. The

Table 81–3. NORMAL VALUES: BIOCHEMICAL MEASUREMENTS OF SPECIFIC NUTRITIONAL STATUS

Tests	Age and Sex Group						
	Low Birth Weight Infant	***Neonate*** *Birth–1 mo*	***Infant*** *1–12 mo*	***Child*** *1–4 yr*	***Child*** *4–9 yr*	***Male*** *9–18 yr*	***Female*** *9–18 yr*
Protein							
Blood							
Serum albumin (g/dl)	≥2.5	≥2.5	≥3	≥3.5	≥3.5	≥3.5	
Retinol-binding protein (mg/dl)	2–3	2–3	2–3	2–3	2–3	3–6	3–6
Blood urea nitrogen (mg/dl)	7–22	7–22	7–22	7–22	7–22	7–22	
Thyroxine-binding protein (mg/dl)	20–50	20–50	20–50	20–50	20–50	20–50	20–50
Transferrin (mg/dl)	170–250	170–250	170–250	170–250	170–250	170–250	
Fibronectin (mg/dl)	30–40	30–40	30–40	30–40	30–40	30–40	
Urine							
Creatinine/height index	—	>0.9	>0.9	>0.9	>0.9	>0.9	—
3-Methyl histidine (μmol/kg)	—	4.2 ± 1.3	—	—	—	3.2 ± 0.6	2.1
3-Methyl histidine (μmol/g creatinine)	—	253 ± 78	—	—	—	126 ± 32	92
Hydroxyproline index	—	>2	>2	>2	>2	>2	—
Vitamin A							
Plasma retinol (μg/dl)	≥30	≥30	≥30	≥30	≥30	≥30	—
Plasma retinol-binding protein (mg/dl)	2–3	2–3	2–3	2–3	2–3	2–3	2–3
Vitamin D							
25-OH-D_3 (ng/ml)	≥20	≥20	≥20	≥20	≥20	≥20	—
Riboflavin							
Red cell glutathione reductase stimulation effect (%)	<20	<20	<20	<20	<20	<20	—
Vitamin B_6							
Red cell transaminases Plasma pyridoxal phosphate Xanthurenic acid excretion	Feasible for use in all age groups. Although a useful measurement, it is not readily available and not practical in children younger than 9 years of age.						
Folacin							
Serum folate (ng/ml)	>6	>6	>6	>6	>6	>6	—
Red blood cell folate (ng/ml)	>160	>160	>160	>160	>160	>160	—
Vitamin K							
Prothrombin time (seconds)	11–15	11–15	11–15	11–15	11–15	11–15	—
Vitamin E							
Plasma alpha-tocopherol (mg/dl)	≥0.7	≥0.7	≥0.7	≥0.7	≥0.7	≥0.7	≥0.7
Red blood cell hemolysis test (%)	≤10	≤10	≤10	≤10	≤10	≤10	—
Vitamin C							
Plasma (mg/dl)	>0.2	>0.2	>0.2	>0.2	>0.2	>0.2	>0.2
Leukocyte (μg/108 cells)	Difficult to perform on infants and children owing to sample requirements.						
Thiamine							
Red blood cell transketolase stimulation effect (%)	<15	<15	<15	<15	<15	<15	<15
Vitamin B_{12}							
Serum vitamin B_{12} (pg/ml)	≥200	≥200	≥200	≥200	≥200	≥200	—
Absorption test	Excretion of more than 7.5% of the orally ingested labeled vitamin B_{12}.						
Iron							
Hematocrit (%)	31	31	33	36	39	36	
Hemoglobin (g/dl)	11	12	12	13	14	13	
Serum ferritin (ng/ml)	>10	>10	>10	>10	>10	>10	
Serum iron (μg/dl)	>30	>30	>40	>50	>60	>60	
Serum total iron-binding capacity (μg/dl)	350–400	350–400	350–400	350–400	350–400	350–400	350–400
Serum transferrin saturation (%)	>12	>12	>12	>14	>15	>16	>16
Serum transferrin (mg/dl)	170–250	170–250	170–250	170–250	170–250	170–250	
Erythrocyte protoporphyrin (μg/dl red blood cells)	<80	<80	<75	<70	<70	<70	<70
Zinc							
Serum zinc (μg/dl)	80–120	80–120	80–120	80–120	80–120	80–120	
Erythrocyte zinc	Erythrocytes contain approximately 10 times more zinc than does plasma.						

dilution effect can also be seen with the hematologic parameters such as hematocrit and hemoglobin.

Table 81–3 is by no means all inclusive. Other vitamins, such as biotin and niacin, as well as essential fatty acids can be measured. These measurements are seldom clinically indicated, though. Assessment of the levels of minerals such as calcium, magnesium, phosphorus, iodine, copper, and selenium are readily available in most laboratories and sometimes are important to measure as part of the nutritional assessment.

REFERENCES

1. Fomon SM: Nutritional disorders of children: Prevention, screening, and followup. DHEW Publication No (HSA) 77–5104. Bethesda, MD, Department of Health and Human Services, 1977.
2. Hamill PV, Drizd TA, Johnson CL, et al: Physical growth: National Center for Health Statistics percentiles. Am J Clin Nutr 1979; 32:607–629.
3. Roche AF, Himes JH: Incremental growth charts. Am J Clin Nutr 1980; 33:2041–2052.
4. Tanner JM, Davies PSW: Clinical longitudinal standards for height and height velocity for North American children. J Pediatr 1985; 107:317–328.
5. Himes JA, Roche AF, Thissen D, et al: Parent-specific adjustments for evaluation of recumbent length and stature of children. Pediatrics 1985; 75:304–313.
6. Ranawati AA, McLaren DS: Assessment of marginal malnutrition. Nature 1970; 228:573–574.
7. Frisancho AR: New norms for upper limit fat and muscle areas for assessment of nutritional status. Am J Clin Nutr 1981; 34:2540–2545.
8. Kagan, BM, Stanincova V, Felix NS, et al: Body composition of premature infants: Relation to nutrition. Am J Clin Nutr 1972; 25:1153–1164.
9. Lohman TG: Research progress in validation of laboratory methods of assessing body composition. Med Sci Sports Exerc 1984; 16:596–605.
10. Lohman TG: Applicability of body composition techniques and constants for children and youths. Exerc Sport Sci Rev 1986; 14:325–357.
11. Forbes RM, Cooper AR, Mitchell HH: The composition of the human body as determined by chemical analysis. J Biol Chem 1953; 203:359–366.
12. Moore FD, Lister J, Boyden CM, et al: The skeleton as a feature of body composition: Values predicted by isotope dilution and observed by cadaver dissection in an adult female. Hum Biol 1968; 40:135–188.
13. Infant body composition by skinfold measurements. Nutr Rev 1975; 33:7–9.

13a. Karlberg P, Engstrom I, Lichtenstein H, et al: The development of children in a Swedish urban community: A prospective longitudinal study. III. Physical growth during the first three years of life. Acta Paediatr Scand (Suppl) 1968; 187:48.

13b. Frisancho AR: New norms of upper limb fat and muscle areas for assessment of nutritional status. Am J Clin Nutr 1981; 34:2540.

14. Lohman TG: Skinfolds and body density and their relation to body fatness: A review. Hum Biol 1981; 53:181–225.
15. Forbes GB: Body composition in adolescence. Prog Clin Biol Res 1981; 61:55–72.
16. Forbes GB, Schultz F, Cafarelli C, et al: Effects of body size on potassium-40 measurement in the whole body counter (tilt-chair technique). Health Phys 1968; 15:435–442.
17. Remenchik AP, Miller CE, Kessler WV: Body composition estimates derived from potassium measurements. Publication No. ANL-7461. US Atomic Energy Commission Argonne Natl Lab, 1968, pp 73–90.
18. Lukaski HC, Johnson PE: A simple inexpensive method of determining total body water using a tracer dose of D_2O and infrared absorption of biological fluids. Am J Clin Nutr 1985; 41:363–370.
19. Katch FI, Solomon RT, Sayevitz M, et al: Validity of bioelectrical impedance to estimate body composition in cardiac and pulmonary patients (letter). Am J Clin Nutr 1986; 43:972–973.
20. Lukaski HC, Bolonchuk WW, Hall CB, et al: Validation of tetrapolar bioelectrical impedance method to assess human body composition. J Appl Physiol 1986; 60:1327–1332.
21. Lukaski HC, Johnson PE, Bolonchuk WW, et al: GI assessment of fat-free mass using bioelectrical impedance measurements of the human body. Am J Clin Nutr 1985; 41:810–817.
22. Rinke WJ: Electrical impedance: A new technique to assess human body composition. Milit Med 1986; 151:338–341.
23. Cochran WJ, Klish WJ, Wong WW, et al: Total body electrical conductivity used to determine body composition in infants. Pediatr Res 1986; 20:561–564.
24. Fiorotto ML, Cochran WJ, Funk RC, et al: Total body electrical conductivity measurements: Effects of body composition and geometry. Am J Physiol 1987; 252:R794–R800.

Chapter 82

Vitamins and Trace Elements

J. ROBERTO MORAN

The term *vitamin* describes a group of organic compounds, essential for life, which are required in small amounts for normal metabolic function. Vitamins were identified by alphabetical letters following their discovery and are generally subdivided into fat-soluble and water-soluble groups. The fat-soluble vitamins include vitamins A (retinol), D (ergocalciferol and cholecalciferol), E (tocopherol), and K (phylloquinone). The water-soluble vitamins include vitamins B_1 (thiamine), B_2 (riboflavin), B_6 (pyridoxine), B_{12} (cyanocobalamin) and C (ascorbic acid). Selective nutritional requirements are listed in Tables 82–1 to 82–4.

FAT-SOLUBLE VITAMINS

Vitamins A, D, E, and K differ from the water-soluble vitamins in several respects. Absorption of the fat-soluble vitamins is subject to the mechanisms of fat absorption. Thus, people with pancreatic insufficiency or cholestasis are prone to deficiency. Fat-soluble vitamins also require a carrier system, usually lipoproteins, for solubility in blood. The depletion times of these vitamins are longer than those of the water-soluble vitamins, with the possible exception of vitamin B_{12}. Additionally, there is a potential for toxicity with excessive intake over a prolonged period.

Vitamin A

Metabolism

The parent compound in the vitamin A group is called all-*trans*-retinal. In a nutritional sense the vitamin A family includes all naturally occurring compounds with the biologic activity of retinol. Carotenoids are retinol precursors and are nutritionally active; however, only 50 of approximately 600 carotenoids found in nature are converted into vitamin A. Common dietary sources of preformed vitamin A are dairy products, liver, and fish. Sources of provitamin A carotenoids are carrots, yellow squash, dark-green leafy vegetables, corn, and oranges.

Preformed vitamin A in foods is present largely as retinyl ester. During proteolytic digestion in the stomach, retinyl ester and carotenoids are released from foods and aggregate with other lipids. In the small intestine, because of the combined action of bile and pancreatic esterases, the retinol esters are hydrolyzed. Retinol and hydrocarbon carotenoids form micelles and are then transported (probably by a passive process) across the absorptive epithelial cells.[1] The rate of absorption of dietary vitamin A in healthy persons who ingest significant amounts of fat is higher than 80%. Dietary carotenoids are absorbed approximately half as well as vitamin A. As the amount of carotenoids in the diet increases, the absorption efficiency decreases.[2] The absorption of carotenoids is more critically dependent on the presence of bile salts than is that of vitamin A.[1] Most of the beta-carotene and other carotenoids are eventually converted to retinol within the intestinal epithelia. Retinol is re-esterified and, together with a small amount of carotenoids, is incorporated into chylomicrons that are released into the lymph. The formed esters are taken up predominantly by the liver for storage, mostly as retinyl palmitate.

Vitamin A is well stored in the body, with more than 90% of the total being found in the liver. Retinol is subsequently liberated for its delivery to target tissues

Table 82–1. RECOMMENDED DIETARY ALLOWANCES FOR FAT-SOLUBLE VITAMINS

	Age (yr)	Vitamin A (μg)	Vitamin D (μg)	Vitamin E (mg)	Vitamin K (μg)
Infants	0.0–0.5	375	7.5	3	5
	0.5–1.0	375	10	4	10
Children	1–3	400	10	6	15
	4–6	500	10	7	20
	7–10	700	10	7	30
Males	11–14	1000	10	10	45
	15–18	1000	10	10	65
	19–24	1000	10	10	70
Females	11–14	800	10	8	45
	15–18	800	10	8	55
	19–24	800	10	8	60

Adapted with permission from RECOMMENDED DIETARY ALLOWANCES: 10TH EDITION. Copyright 1989 by the National Academy of Sciences. Published by the National Academy Press, Washington, D.C.

Table 82–2. RECOMMENDED DIETARY ALLOWANCES FOR WATER-SOLUBLE VITAMINS

	Age (yr)	Vitamin C (mg)	Thiamine (mg)	Riboflavin (mg)	Niacin (mg NE)	Vitamin B_6 (mg)	Folate (μg)	Vitamin B_{12} (μg)	Biotin (μg)	Pantothenic Acid (mg)
Infants	0.0–0.5	30	0.3	0.4	5	0.3	25	0.3	10	2
	0.5–1.0	35	0.4	0.5	6	0.6	35	0.5	15	3
Children	1–3	40	0.7	0.8	9	1.0	50	0.1	20	3
	4–6	45	0.9	1.1	12	1.1	75	1.0	25	3–4
	7–10	45	1.2	1.3	13	1.4	100	1.4	30	4–5
Males	11–14	50	1.3	1.5	17	1.7	150	2.0	30–100	4–7
	15–18	60	1.5	1.8	20	2.0	200	2.0	30–100	4–7
	19–24	60	1.5	1.7	19	2.0	200	2.0	30–100	4–7
Females	11–14	50	1.1	1.3	15	1.4	150	2.0	30–100	4–7
	15–18	60	1.1	1.3	15	1.5	180	2.0	30–100	4–7
	19–24	60	1.1	1.3	15	1.6	180	2.0	30–100	4–7

Adapted with permission from RECOMMENDED DIETARY ALLOWANCES: 10TH EDITION. Copyright 1989 by the National Academy of Sciences. Published by the National Academy Press, Washington, D.C.

through a highly regulated process. The parenchymal cells synthesize retinol binding protein (RBP), and the major form of circulating vitamin A is a 1:1 complex of all-*trans*-retinal with retinol binding protein (holo-RBP). Liver parenchymal disease lowers plasma RBP levels, but only when liver reserves of vitamin A are nearly depleted do plasma concentrations of retinol decrease significantly. Deficiency is commonly associated with protein-calorie malnutrition, a low intake of fat, and malabsorption syndromes. Low concentrations (<0.035 mmol/L) of plasma retinol are closely associated with clinical signs of deficiency. Levels greater than 3.5 mmol/L are indicators of a toxic state.[3]

Functions

Vitamin A is necessary for preservation of vision, and clinical signs of deficiency include night blindness and various stages of xerophthalmia. Vitamin A has been implicated in other physiological processes, including spermatogenesis, fetal development, immune response, growth, and others. Most of these processes depend directly or indirectly on the second major function of vitamin A: cellular differentiation. The actions of vitamin A, including its deficiency, on these specific processes have been reviewed elsewhere.[4, 5]

Table 82–3. RECOMMENDED DIETARY ALLOWANCES FOR MINERALS

	Age (yr)	Calcium (mg)	Phosphorus (mg)	Magnesium (mg)
Infants	0.0–0.5	400	300	40
	0.5–1.0	600	500	60
Children	1–3	800	800	80
	4–6	800	800	120
	7–10	800	800	170
Males	11–14	1,200	1,200	270
	15–18	1,200	1,200	400
	19–24	1,200	1,200	350
Females	11–14	1,200	1,200	280
	15–18	1,200	1,200	300
	19–24	1,200	1,200	280

Adapted with permission from RECOMMENDED DIETARY ALLOWANCES: 10TH EDITION. Copyright 1989 by the National Academy of Sciences. Published by the National Academy Press, Washington, D.C.

Vitamin D

Metabolism

Vitamin D_3 is produced photochemically by the action of sunlight from a precursor sterol present in the skin, 7-dehydrocholesterol. Vitamin D_3 is also present in the diet, and the major source is fortified milk. Intraluminal bile salts are required for adequate absorption. Transport in the small intestine is believed to involve a passive mechanism.[6]

In terms of its structure and mode of action, vitamin D is similar to the classic steroid hormones, for example, aldosterone and cortisone. Vitamin D_3 is, in reality, a prohormone. In the liver, vitamin D_3 undergoes its initial transformation under the action of D-25-hydroxylase, a cytochrome P-450–like enzyme present in the microsomes and mitochondria. The metabolite formed is $25(OH)D_3$, which is the major circulating form of vitamin D. Whether severe hepatic disease interferes with 25-hydroxylation extensively enough to be clinically significant is uncertain. However, rickets may develop in severe childhood cholestasis, and subnormal concentrations of $25(OH)D_3$ are found.

From the liver, $25(OH)D_3$ is returned to the circulatory system where it is transported to the kidney by a specific transport protein, the vitamin D–binding protein.[7] In the kidney a second hydroxyl group is added, yielding the product $1,25(OH)_2D_3$. The most important point of regulation of the vitamin D endocrine system occurs through the control of the activity of the enzyme responsible for this transformation, the renal 1-hydroxylase. In this way the production of the hormone $1,25(OH)_2D_3$ can be modulated according to the calcium needs. The main factors stimulating synthesis are parathyroid hormone and low circulating concentrations of $1,25(OH)_2D_3$, calcium, and phosphate.[8] Renal failure impairs the synthesis of $1,25(OH)_2D_3$ (Fig. 82–1).

Functions

The primary role of vitamin D is to stimulate absorption of calcium and phosphorus from the small intestine. The direct regulator of active calcium transport is $1,25(OH)_2D_3$, and its action involves the four aspects of

Table 82–4. ESTIMATED SAFE AND ADEQUATE DAILY DIETARY INTAKE OF SELECTED TRACE ELEMENTS

	Age (yr)	Iron (mg)	Zinc (mg)	Copper (mg)	Manganese (mg)	Fluoride (mg)	Chromium (μg)	Molybdenum (μg)	Iodine (μg)	Selenium (μg)
Infants	0–0.5	6	5	0.4–0.6	0.3–0.6	0.1–0.5	10–40	15–30	40	10
	0.5–1.0	10	5	0.6–0.7	0.6–1.0	0.2–1.0	20–60	20–40	50	15
Children and	1–3	10	10	0.7–1.0	1.0–1.5	0.5–1.5	20–80	25–50	70	20
adolescents	4–6	10	10	1.0–1.5	1.5–2.0	1.0–2.5	30–120	30–75	90	20
	7–10	10	10	1.0–2.0	2.0–3.0	1.5–2.5	50–200	50–150	120	30
	11–14	12–15	12–15	1.5–2.5	2.0–5.0	1.5–2.5	50–200	75–250	150	40–45
Adults		10–15	12–15	1.5–3.0	2.0–5.0	1.5–4.0	50–200	75–250	150	50–70

Adapted with permission from RECOMMENDED DIETARY ALLOWANCES: 10TH EDITION. Copyright 1989 by the National Academy of Sciences. Published by the National Academy Press, Washington, D.C.

calcium movement across the cell: (1) entry across the brush border, (2) binding at immobile sites, (3) intracellular movement, and (4) extrusion across the basolateral membrane. Intracellular calcium movement is the rate-limiting step in calcium transport and is facilitated by a vitamin D–dependent calcium-binding protein named *calbindin-D*. The effects of vitamin D on the other three aspects of transport are less dramatic.[9] Vitamin D also promotes the mobilization and accretion of calcium and phosphorus from bone and the reabsorption of calcium and phosphorus in the kidney.

Vitamin D intoxication can be a concern in patients being treated with vitamin D or vitamin D analogues. Patients suffering from hypervitaminosis D have been shown to exhibit a 15-fold increase in plasma 25(OH)D_3

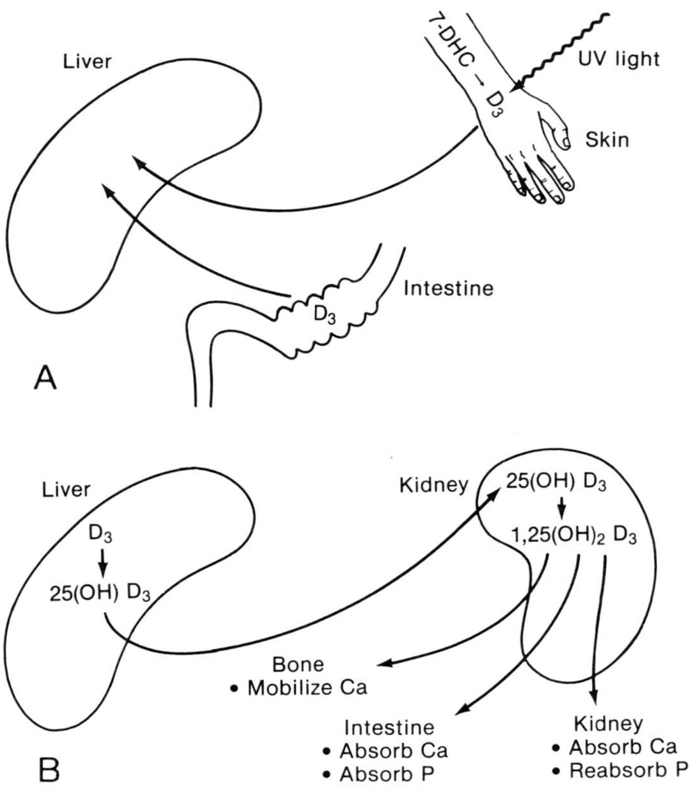

Figure 82–1. Metabolism of Vitamin D. *A,* Vitamin D_3 synthesis. 7-DHC, 7-dehydrocholesterol. *B,* Vitamin D_3 activation and functions.

levels; however, 1,25(OH)$_2$$D_3$ concentrations are not substantially altered.[10] Symptoms include hypercalcemia, hypercalciuria, anorexia, nausea, vomiting, muscular weakness, diffuse demineralization of bones, and general disorientation. If intoxication is allowed to go unchecked, death will eventually occur.

Vitamin E

Metabolism

In the early isolation of vitamin E from plant oils, four similar compounds were found. The name *tocopherol* was proposed, and the four components were designated by the letters alpha, beta, gamma, and delta. Their structures have two primary parts, a complex ring and a long, saturated side chain. The four tocopherols differ only in the number and position of the methyl groups on the ring. Alpha-tocopherol is the most commonly occurring and also the most active form. Tocopherols are readily oxidized by air, especially in the presence of iron. When oxidized, a quinone without biologic activity is formed. To prevent this oxidation, most nutritional supplements of alpha-tocopherol are esterified to yield alpha-tocopherol acetate. This form is resistant to oxidation but has no biologic activity until hydrolyzed by gastrointestinal esterases. The freed tocopherol is then absorbed.

The absorption of vitamin E is associated with fat absorption. Efficiency, however, is relatively low compared with triglyceride absorption. Studies in humans show a wide range, from 20 to 80%, with an average of approximately 50% absorption at normal intakes of 5 to 15 mg/dl.[11] Further, the percentage of absorption decreases as the amount ingested increases.[12] The absorption of commonly available preparations of vitamin E (alpha-tocopherol, tocopheryl acetate, and tocopheryl succinate) is hampered by insufficient concentrations of intraluminal bile acids. Additionally, if pancreatic function is not normal, fat digestion and tocopherol absorption will be impaired. A different formulation of vitamin E, D-alpha-tocopheryl polyethylene glycol succinate (TPGS) has been investigated. In this preparation, the vitamin E is linked to polyethylene glycol, which readily passes through the intestinal epithelium. TPGS has been found to be efficacious for treatment of vitamin E deficiency in children with chronic cholestatic liver disease.[13]

Free tocopherol appears in chylomicrons and rapidly equilibrates with other lipoproteins as the chylomicrons are cleared. There is a high correlation between plasma tocopherol concentration and plasma total lipid levels. A normal vitamin E to total lipid ratio is greater than 0.6.[14] For practical purposes, the ratio of tocopherol to cholesterol plus triglycerides is as useful as the ratio to total lipids for evaluating vitamin E status.[15] Liver, adipose tissue, and muscle slowly accumulate tocopherol by transfer from plasma lipoproteins. These stores, however, are not readily mobilized during times of deficiency.[16]

Functions

Vitamin E functions primarily as an antioxidant by inhibiting the peroxidation of polyunsaturated fatty acids (PUFAs) present in the lipid layers of cell membranes. Diets with high concentrations of PUFAs result in corresponding changes in the PUFA content of cell membranes and thus exhibit a greater susceptibility to fatty acid peroxidation. This, in turn, increases the requirements for vitamin E. The peroxidation of cell membranes may be catalyzed by iron, which is the primary reason why the addition of iron to the diet increases the vitamin E requirements. During the 1960s, hemolytic anemia developed in preterm infants fed formulas that were high in PUFAs and low in vitamin E. This nutrient imbalance was corrected, and the syndrome soon disappeared.[17] The mechanism by which vitamin E deficiency produces neuromuscular degeneration is largely unknown.

Vitamin K

Metabolism

There are several compounds with vitamin K activity. Phylloquinone, vitamin K_1, is the major dietary form of the vitamin. Menaquinones are synthesized by bacteria. Menadione, a synthetic compound, is not important in human nutrition, but a water-soluble derivative (Synkayvite) is available commercially. Absorption of phylloquinone is influenced by lipid absorption. The vitamin is rapidly concentrated in liver, but in contrast with the other fat-soluble vitamins, it has a rapid turnover in this organ. The human gut contains large quantities of bacterially produced menaquinones. However, the extent of absorption of these menaquinones from the large intestine and their role in human nutrition are not clearly established, particularly in neonates who are breastfed.[18] The principal homologue in plasma is phylloquinone.

Vitamin K stores are low at birth because of poor placental transfer. The low vitamin K content of breast milk and low milk intake are contributing factors to vitamin K deficiency in the neonate.[19] Formulas are now routinely supplemented with vitamin K, and the American Academy of Pediatrics recommends intramuscular administration of phylloquinone at birth.[20]

Functions

In the liver, the vitamin functions as a cofactor for the conversion of intracellular precursor proteins to the active forms of the clotting factors II, VII, IX, and X.

Vitamin K deficiency was reported in patients on long-term total parenteral nutrition, and supplementation of the vitamin is advised under these circumstances. Depression of the vitamin K–dependent coagulation factors has also been found in malabsorption syndromes, short bowel syndrome, and biliary obstruction. There is no known toxicity associated with the administration of high doses of phylloquinone.[21] Administration of menadione to infants was shown to be associated with hemolytic anemia and liver toxicity, and phylloquinone is now prescribed to prevent hemorrhagic disease of the neonate.

WATER-SOLUBLE VITAMINS

The water-soluble vitamins function as cofactors for enzyme reactions. Their needs are dependent on the energy and content of the diet, as well as the rate of energy utilization. These vitamins are not stored to any great extent, and toxicity is rare.

Ascorbic Acid

Metabolism

Ascorbic acid (vitamin C) is a six-carbon compound resembling a monosaccharide. The vitamin is synthesized by many plants from carbohydrate precursors, including glucose. During evolution, some vertebrates lost the enzyme responsible for the terminal step in the conversion of glucose to ascorbic acid. Thus, humans and other primates are among the few species unable to synthesize the vitamin and require it in the diet. Human milk supplies sufficient ascorbic acid to full-term infants. Cows synthesize ascorbic acid, but their milk contains a low concentration of the vitamin. Thus, commercially available infant formulas are fortified to levels similar to those in human milk.

Being a derivative of glucose, most ascorbic acid is transported by a sodium-dependent active transport system (K_m of approximately 1 mmol/L). After accumulating inside the cell, ascorbic acid moves by an undetermined mechanism across the basolateral cell membrane toward the blood. Dosages of as much as 100 mg of ascorbic acid per day are 80 to 90% absorbed. However, when high luminal concentrations of vitamin prevail, the carrier mechanism becomes saturated, and additional ascorbic acid is absorbed only by simple diffusion, which proceeds at a low rate. Therefore, high doses of ascorbic acid are likely to be incompletely absorbed by the intestine.[22]

Vitamin C is labile to oxidation, which may be enhanced by the presence of iron, zinc, and copper. Dehydroascorbic acid, the oxidative product of ascorbic acid, appears to be transported by diffusion. High intakes of iron, copper, zinc, and pectin were observed to have an adverse effect on vitamin C metabolism.[23] It is uncertain whether these effects reflect a direct influence on the absorption of ascorbic acid or represent changes in the amount of the vitamin oxidized before absorption.

For most people ascorbic acid has a low toxicity. With excessive intake the absorbed ascorbic acid is largely excreted into the urine. Only a small amount is metabolized to oxalate. However, people who form kidney stones should avoid the intake of high doses of vitamin C.[24] This also is true for patients with renal impairment or those who are on chronic hemodialysis.[25]

Functions

Ascorbic acid serves as a reducing agent in a number of important hydroxylation reactions. Deficiency in ascorbic acid results in an impairment of collagen synthesis, because the vitamin participates in the hydroxylation of proline to hydroxyproline and of lysine to hydroxylysine. The defect in collagen synthesis is reflected in the failure of wounds to heal, defects in tooth formation, and rupture of capillaries. Scurvy was described by ancient civilizations and was historically a scourge of explorers and warriors. In developed countries, the rare occurrence of scurvy is associated with alcoholism, nutritional ignorance, and poverty.

Other functions of ascorbic acid are to participate in the synthesis of carnitine, adrenal hormones, and vasoactive amines; microsomal drug metabolism; leukocyte functions; and tyrosine and folate metabolism. Vitamin C has also been considered a nutrient with gastric and esophageal cancer prevention properties.[26]

Thiamine

Metabolism

Thiamine is widely distributed in foods. However, milk of mothers with poor diets or alcoholism is deficient in the vitamin.

Thiamine absorption occurs by at least two mechanisms[27]: At low concentrations, the vitamin is absorbed by an active, carrier-mediated, sodium-dependent transport system; and at high concentrations, absorption is primarily by passive diffusion. The vitamin is phosphorylated in the jejunal mucosa. Phosphorylation helps maintain a favorable gradient for subsequent substrate entry, and it is the rate-limiting step in thiamine absorption.[28] Thiamine in excess of tissue needs is excreted in the urine.

Functions

In its phosphorylated form, thiamine pyrophosphate, the vitamin serves as a coenzyme for the decarboxylation reactions involving carbohydrates in the Krebs' cycle and in the formation of ketoses of the pentose phosphate pathway. Therefore, the needs for thiamine increase as carbohydrate intake increases.

Thiamine is also involved in the decarboxylation of branched-chain amino acids and may have a specific function in nerve conduction and synaptic transmission.[29]

Severe deficiency results in the disease beriberi, which is characterized by extensive damage to the nervous and cardiovascular systems. In infants, symptoms include cyanosis, tachycardia, and aphonia (soundless crying). Death often occurs from cardiac failure.

Riboflavin

Metabolism

Riboflavin is a yellow compound that is widely distributed throughout the plant and animal kingdoms. The two major coenzyme forms of the vitamin, riboflavin-5-phosphate (flavin mononucleotide; FMN) and riboflavin-5′-adenosine diphosphate (flavin adenine dinucleotide; FAD) constitute the bulk of dietary riboflavin.

After ingestion of these coenzymes, riboflavin is released by nonspecific hydrolytic activities in the gastrointestinal tract. Enterocytes in the upper small bowel absorb riboflavin by initial rapid uptake that is sodium dependent and inhibited by ouabain, reflecting an adenosine triphosphate–involved active cotransport system.[30] The presence of a carrier was suggested.[31] Some consideration has been given to developmental aspects of riboflavin transport associated with maturation and aging.[32, 33] Conversion to FMN and FAD within the mucosa occurs before release in the circulation.

Circulatory transport is by tight complexing with immunoglobulins as well as some loose association with albumin.[34] Metabolism of riboflavin depends on dietary intake and saturation of tissue stores. Absorption of large doses of the vitamin is limited by the small intestine, and excesses are rapidly excreted in the urine. Low tissue levels of the vitamin are extensively protein bound. Because of this affinity and extensive renal tubular reabsorption, tissue flavin levels do not decrease to less than acceptable limits except in severe deficiency states.

Functions

The riboflavin coenzymes are essential components of several enzymes involved in electron transport. Some of the reactions in which these enzymes are present include energy metabolism, glycogen synthesis, production of erythrocytes by the bone marrow, and transformation of folic acid to its coenzyme.

Deficiency is encountered almost invariably in combination with deficits of other water-soluble vitamins. In fact, classically described deficiency syndromes such as glossitis and dermatitis may have resulted from other complicating deficiencies. Biochemical deficiency has been reported in neonates during phototherapy.[35, 36] Further studies are needed, however, before routine supplementation is recommended.

Vitamin B_6

Metabolism

The vitamin B_6 group is composed of three natural compounds: pyridoxine, pyridoxamine and pyridoxal. The three forms are absorbed in the jejunum by a nonsaturable process. After absorption, most of the vitamin B_6 is transported to the liver, where it is converted to the principal active form of the vitamin, pyridoxal-5′-phosphate (PLP). Pyridoxal and PLP are released into circulation for use by other tissues (Fig. 82–2).

Isoniazid and penicillamine form inactive compounds with PLP. Long-term treatment with these drugs can result in a deficiency of the vitamin[37]; hence, the recommended therapy is concurrently to administer vitamin B_6 supplements. Plasma PLP is significantly lower in cirrhosis and other hepatic and biliary diseases, apparently because of increased turnover of circulating PLP.[38, 39] It is not clear, however, whether this apparent vitamin B_6 deficiency contributes to the abnormal metabolism of amino acids and other compounds.

Functions

PLP is utilized by more than 60 enzymes.[40] The interconversions of amino acids and their respective alpha-ketoacids by aminotransferases (e.g., alanine aminotransferase, aspartate aminotransferase, and so forth) are central to the biosynthesis and catabolism of amino acids. These enzymes provide a simple link between the amino acid and intermediates of glycolysis (e.g., alanine and pyruvate) and the tricarboxylic acid cycle (e.g., aspartate and oxaloacetate). Synthesis of nicotinamide from tryptophan requires a PLP-dependent enzyme. Other examples of vitamin B_6 functions include the decarboxylation of precursor amino acids for the synthesis of polyamines, histamine, and neurotransmitters.

Isolated dietary deficiency is uncommon. Most of the vitamin in milk is in the form of pyridoxal or pyridoxamine, both of which are quite sensitive to heat. Such destruction was probably responsible for vitamin B_6 deficiency and seizures observed in infants fed a liquid infant formula in the 1950s.[41] For this reason, the relatively heat-stable pyridoxine is used for the fortification of formulas. Consumption of amounts exceeding several hundred milligrams per day may induce side effects such as neurotoxicity manifested by peripheral neuropathy, ataxia, and, in neonates, hypotonia requiring assisted ventilation.[42, 43]

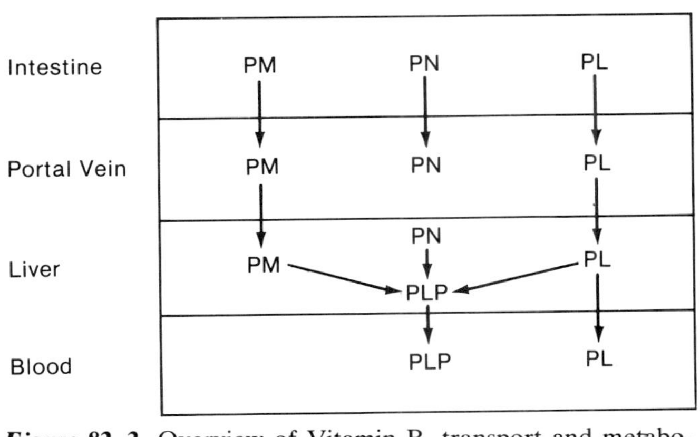

Figure 82–2. Overview of Vitamin B_6 transport and metabolism. PM, pyridoxamine; PN, pyridoxine; PL, pyridoxal; PLP, pyridoxal-5′-phosphate.

Niacin

Metabolism

Niacin is the generic term that describes nicotinic acid and nicotinamide, which are biologically equivalent as vitamins. These compounds are rapidly absorbed in the proximal intestine. At low concentrations, absorption occurs as a sodium-dependent, facilitated diffusion, but at higher concentrations passive diffusion predominates.[44] Niacin is also biosynthesized from dietary tryptophan, and this pathway is an important route for meeting the body's niacin requirement. Deficiencies of vitamin B_6 or riboflavin slow the conversion, because these enzymes are essential cofactors in the synthetic pathway.[45]

Niacin is distributed widely in plant and animal foods. In plants, niacin may be bound to macromolecules and be unavailable. New varieties of corn, however, contain more tryptophan and niacin than do conventional sources. Further, the bioavailability of bound niacin is increased by pretreatment with lime water, a procedure used in Central America and Mexico for preparation of tortillas.[37]

The active coenzyme forms of niacin are the pyridine nucleotides nicotinamide-adenine dinucleotide (NAD) and nicotinamide-adenine dinucleotide phosphate (NADP), and they are synthesized in all tissues from nicotinic acid or nicotinamide, or both. Although these cofactors are widely distributed, no true storage occurs.

Functions

NAD functions as an electron carrier for intracellular respiration. NADP functions as a hydrogen donor in reductive biosyntheses, such as in fatty acid and steroid synthesis. The coenzymes participate as codehydrogenases with enzymes involved in the oxidation of fuel molecules such as lactate, pyruvate, alcohol, and glucose-6-phosphate. Thus, the features of the deficiency state (pellagra) are complex and involve the skin, digestive tract, and nervous system, causing dermatitis, diarrhea, and dementia, respectively. Pellagra is rarely seen in the modern world but is still present in corn-eating regions. Death occurs if the deficiency is not treated.

Pharmacologic doses of nicotinic acid decrease low-density lipoprotein cholesterol and increase high-density lipoprotein cholesterol concentrations. The lipid-lowering effect of nicotinic acid is not known, but it does not appear to be related to any vitamin coenzyme function, because nicotinamide does not have a similar effect.[46]

Biotin and Pantothenic Acid

The requirements of biotin and pantothenic acid are not well defined, and deficiency states have been described only under special circumstances, such as prolonged total parenteral nutrition without supplementation and generalized malnutrition.

The functions of biotin have been reviewed recently.[47] Most of the biotin in foods appears to be protein bound. Biotinidase, an enzyme present in pancreatic juice and in intestinal mucosa, releases biotin during digestion.[48] Absorption of the vitamin occurs primarily in the upper small intestine via a carrier-mediated process that is sodium dependent and electroneutral and that is capable of accumulating biotin against a concentration gradient.[49] Biotin has coenzyme functions in the metabolism of fat, carbohydrate, and some amino acids. Deficiency induces alopecia, periorificial dermatitis, conjunctivitis, and developmental delay.

Pantothenic acid is a widely distributed vitamin whose biochemical function is expressed in coenzyme A. Deficiency can be produced in experimental animals, but only with difficulty in humans. No recommended daily allowance for pantothenic acid has yet been set.

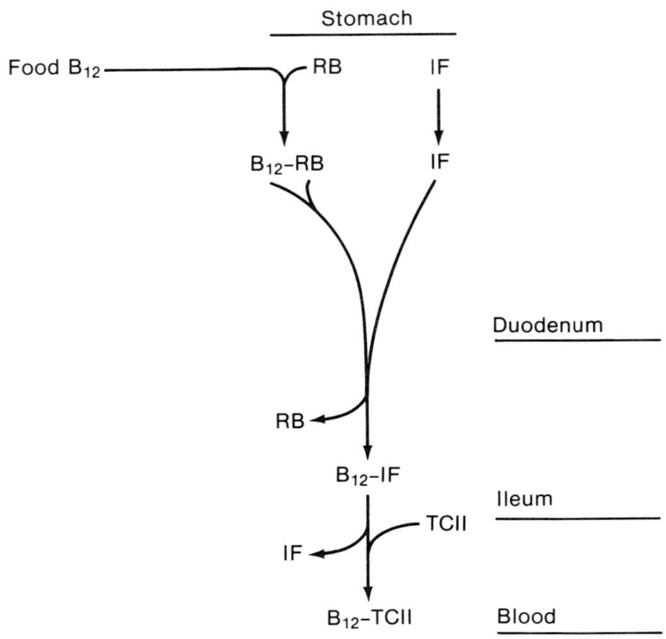

Figure 82–3. Overview of vitamin B_{12} metabolism. RB, R-binders; IF, intrinsic factor. TC II, transcobalamin II.

Vitamin B_{12}

Metabolism

Dietary vitamin B_{12} is present in amounts considerably in excess of requirements. However, the vitamin is lacking in plants, and strict vegetarians generally develop vitamin B_{12} deficiency slowly over a period of many years. These persons may have a markedly subnormal concentration of vitamin B_{12} in milk and eventually induce deficiency in the nursing infant[50] (Fig. 82–3).

Vitamin B_{12} is released from its protein bond by gastric juice, and absorption takes place in the ileum after the vitamin forms a complex with a glycoprotein produced by the parietal cells of the stomach (intrinsic factor [IF]). In the low pH of the stomach, however, vitamin B_{12} possesses a higher affinity for proteins called *R-binders* than for IF. R-binders are present in saliva, gastric juice, and milk. In the higher pH of the duodenum, pancreatic proteases degrade R-binders, releasing the bound vitamin, at which point it combines with IF.[51, 52] Therefore, malabsorption of vitamin B_{12} may result when there is impairment of gastric secretory function, pancreatic insufficiency, an acidic intestinal pH, or an abnormal ileum (Table 82–5).

The IF–vitamin B_{12} complex probably enters the ileal absorptive cell in intact form. The vitamin is then freed from IF, and it binds to transcobalamin II (TC II) either within or at the serosal surface of the enterocyte. TC II turns over rapidly in plasma and appears to modulate the delivery of vitamin B_{12} to cells that require it.[53]

Vitamin B_{12} is the only water-soluble vitamin that is stored. The total body content is 2 to 5 mg in an adult man; of this amount, approximately 1 mg is in the liver. Bile is a primary route of excretion, and enterohepatic circulation is of great importance.[54] Feces contain a large amount of vitamin B_{12}, because microorganisms in the colon synthesize large amounts of the vitamin. The vitamin, however, is not absorbed from the colon.

Functions

Vitamin B_{12} is required for normal hematopoiesis by facilitating the cyclic metabolism of folic acid, which is essential for thymidine and thus deoxyribonucleic acid (DNA) synthesis (see later). The vitamin's activity in reactions requiring transfer of methyl groups, such as synthesis of methionine, is essential for a normally functioning nervous system.[55]

Table 82–5. SOME PHYSIOLOGIC CAUSES OF VITAMIN B_{12} DEFICIENCY

Physiologic Process	Associated Disorder
Diet intake	Reduced in vegetarians
Gastric phase	
Release from food	Gastrectomy, achlorhydria
IF secretion	Pernicious anemia, gastrectomy, congenital absence
Intestinal phase	
Release by pancreatic proteases	Pancreatic insufficiency
Intestinal transit	IF–vitamin B_{12} taken by fish, tapeworm, or bacterial overgrowth
Attachment to ileal receptors	Ileal disease (Crohn's disease) Resection
Passage through ileal wall	Familial vitamin B_{12} malabsorption
Plasma transport by TC II	TC II deficiency

Folic Acid

Metabolism

Folic acid (pteroylglutamic acid) has a double-ringed structure (pteroic acid) and glutamic acid. When pteroic acid is linked to two or more glutamic acid residues, polyglutamates are formed. Most of the folates in nature occur in this form, for example, pentaglutamates and hexaglutamates predominate in animal tissues.

Intraluminal polyglutamates are hydrolyzed to monoglutamates by an intestinal enzyme found in the brush border. This pteroylpolyglutamate hydrolase is an exopeptidase that cleaves the polyglutamyl chain one residue at a time. It has a pH optimum near neutrality and is activated by zinc.[56] A dual system of folate uptake (saturable and nonsaturable) by the intestine has been postulated; however, there is no conclusive proof that folic acid accumulates in free form against an electrochemical gradient.[57] Methylfolate is the predominant form in the liver, and stores are depleted relatively rapidly.

Availability from foods varies greatly, with levels of 25 to 96% reported. Human and cow's milk (unlike goat's milk, which is folate free) are good sources of the vitamin.

Functions

Tetrahydrofolic acid (THF), the coenzyme form of the vitamin, participates in one-carbon transfers needed for the biosynthesis of nucleotide metabolism, essential for ribonucleic acid (RNA) and DNA synthesis and, hence, for cell replication. Thus, the main metabolic consequence of folate deficiency results in arrest or prolongation of cell division in a variety of tissues, particularly those with the highest rates of cell multiplication (bone marrow and intestine).

THF is regenerated from methylfolate by the action of a vitamin B_{12}–containing enzyme. Thus, vitamin B_{12} deficiency results in folate being trapped as methylfolate, becoming metabolically useless. The folate-trap hypothesis explains the fact that the hematologic damage of vitamin B_{12} deficiency is indistinguishable from that of folate deficiency. In both instances, the defective synthesis of DNA results from the same final common pathway defect, namely, an inadequate quantity of THF to participate in DNA synthesis.[58]

Nutritional folate deficiency is one of the commonest hypovitaminosis conditions in humans, and it is commonest under circumstances that increase folate requirements, such as rapid growth in the preterm infant.[59, 60] Megaloblastic changes and hypersegmentation of neutrophils on blood smears are generally noted. Toxicity of folic acid in moderate doses is virtually nonexistent.

MAJOR MINERALS

Calcium, Phosphorus, and Magnesium

Calcium, phosphorus and magnesium are essential for tissue structure and function. They are found in largest quantities in bone, as part of the minerals that provide bone structure and density. Bone also serves as a storage pool from which the rest of the body can draw. The physiology and metabolism of these three elements are interrelated, and their role outside of the bone is just as important.

Metabolism

The amount of calcium absorbed is dependent on the proportions of chelating and precipitating agents in the diet, which determine the amount of calcium available for absorption, and the degree of vitamin D stimulation of the intestinal mucosa, which determines the rate of calcium uptake. Calcium content is high in dairy products, nuts, and whole grains. Plant foods may have high calcium content, but the calcium may be unavailable because of high concentrations of oxalate (spinach and tea) or phytates (cereals) that form water-insoluble salts with calcium and magnesium. Chelating agents that retain calcium in water-soluble form increase its availability. Glucose, lactose, certain amino acids, citrate, and hydrogen ion have been reported to serve this function.[61] The effect of lactose on calcium absorption is still controversial, but there seems to be evidence that lactose malabsorption does not impair intestinal calcium absorption and retention.[62, 63]

Phosphate is abundant in cow's milk, meats, processed foods, and soft drinks. Phosphorus is readily absorbed in the form of free inorganic phosphate, after digestive hydrolysis and release from foodstuffs. Only the phosphorus that is part of dietary phytate is not well hydrolyzed and therefore unavailable. Absorption occurs throughout the small intestine by simple diffusion and by an active transport process.

The calcium to phosphorus ratio varies widely in foods. The approximate ratio for human milk is 2 to 1, for commercial infant formula is 1.3–1.8 to 1 and for cow's milk is 1.2 to 1. The high phosphorus content of cow's milk with its lower calcium to phosphorus ratio is one factor in the pathogenesis of neonatal tetany. Studies in adult humans fed large amounts of phosphorus have failed to show clear-cut adverse effects.[64]

Magnesium is widely distributed in foods. It is absorbed primarily in the small intestine by two separate transport systems. One system is carrier mediated that becomes saturated at low intraluminal concentrations. The other mechanism is simple diffusion and occurs at higher concentrations of the mineral. Absorption with usual diets is reported to be in the range of 46 to 73% in infants and 25 to 60% in adults.[65] Intestinal absorption is reduced in malabsorption syndromes, particularly those associated with steatorrhea, such as celiac disease and short bowel syndrome. Increased amounts of fatty acids in the intestinal lumen form insoluble soaps with magnesium, leading to loss from dietary and endogenous sources. Thus, malnourished adolescents with Crohn's disease given nutritional supplements have further increased fecal magnesium but not fecal nitrogen or calcium levels.[66]

Absorbed magnesium is retained either for tissue growth or as turnover replacement; the remainder is excreted in the urine. When magnesium intake is restricted, magnesium output becomes extremely low within 5 to 7 days.[67] Increased excretion is influenced by hypercalciuria, renal tubular dysfunction, and diuresis either induced by diuretics such as furosemide, or osmotic as seen in diabetes. Therefore, the intestinal and renal excretory mechanisms in normal people permit homeostasis over a wide intake of dietary magnesium.

Functions

Calcium has a structural function because it is the major component of bone and tooth structure. It also plays an important role in transmission of nervous, mechanical, and hormonal impulses, enzyme regulation, and blood clotting.

Phosphorus is also important in bone and tooth structure. It is part of adenosine triphosphate, RNA, and DNA and it is intimately involved in energy metabolism, storage, and regulation. It functions as an intracellular buffer, and it is part of the cell membrane phospholipid.

Magnesium plays an essential role in a wide range of cellular reactions, including those involving the phosphorylation of glucose, the citric acid cycle, and the synthesis of DNA. It is also involved in neuromuscular transmission.

Nutrition-specific deficiency of calcium alone is rarely diagnosed. Deficiencies of calcium and phosphorus presumably are the major contributors to rickets and fractures in very-low-birthweight infants.[68] Nutritional deficiency of phosphorus specifically contributes to bone demineralization and rickets in small preterm infants, especially those who receive human milk feedings.[69] Conditions that impair intestinal absorption and renal tubular reabsorption of magnesium are associated with symptomatic deficiency. Decreased magnesium intake or inadequate amounts of magnesium in parenteral or enteral preparations may be a complicating factor. Symptoms of deficiency include tetany, anorexia, nausea, vomiting, and personality changes. Convulsions and coma occur more frequently in infants.

TRACE ELEMENTS

Trace elements and *micronutrients* are terms describing elements that have in common the characteristic of being present in low tissue concentration. Trace elements function primarily in enzyme systems, where their role ranges from weak, ionic effects to specific associations with protein. Iron is the most abundant of these elements. With the exception of iron, trace element deficiency has been reported primarily in association with unsupplemented total parenteral nutrition, in malnutrition in general, and in persons with unusual dietary practices (Table 82–6).

Definition of specific biochemical functions in higher animals for the ultratrace elements (boron, silicon, vanadium, nickel, and arsenic) still has not been achieved, although these elements have been described as being essential nutrients. A recent review[70] describes potential sites of essential action for these elements. If any of these functions are widely proved, the element involved will be firmly established as having a nutritional requirement. Based on animal findings, the dietary requirement is likely to be small, on the order of micrograms per day.

Of the trace elements, iron, zinc, and copper are discussed in some detail. Comprehensive reviews have been published recently.[71–73]

Iron

Metabolism

Iron metabolism is unusual in the degree to which dietary iron absorption differs and in the efficiency with which iron is retained once it has been absorbed. The bioavailability of iron, that is, the amount absorbed from food, can vary from less than 1% to more than 50%.[74] The percentage that is absorbed depends on both the nature of the diet and the regulatory mechanisms in the intestinal mucosa that reflect the body's physiologic need for iron.

Most of the iron in the diet is present as nonheme, inorganic (mainly ferric [Fe^{+3}]) complexes. Ferric iron is insoluble in aqueous solutions more alkaline than pH 3, unless it is chelated or reduced to the ferrous (Fe^{+2}) form. Gastric acid solubilizes ferric iron and makes it available for chelation with substances such as peptides that keep iron dissolved and allow its absorption in the alkaline environment of the small intestine. Other agents present in the diet, such as carbonates, oxalates, phosphates, and phytates, combine with iron to form insoluble precipitates and macromolecules that are poorly absorbed. Therefore, the absorption of nonheme iron is strongly influenced by its solubility in the upper part of the small intestine, which, in turn, depends on how the composition of the meal as a whole affects iron solubility. For example, nonheme iron absorption from a meal containing enhancers of absorption, such as meat, fish, or chicken, is good.[75] However, absorption tends to be poor from meals in which whole grain cereals and legumes predominate. Vitamin C reduces Fe^{+3} to Fe^{+2}, and the addition of relatively small amounts of meat or a source of vitamin C substantially increases nonheme iron absorption from the entire meal.[76] Human milk is low in iron, but its iron is relatively well absorbed in comparison with that in unfortified cow's milk formula.[77] The presence of lactoferrin, an iron-binding protein in human milk, and the presence of lactoferrin receptors on the intestinal mucosa may explain why iron is so well absorbed from human milk.[78]

Heme iron is derived primarily from the hemoglobin and myoglobin in meat, poultry, and fish. Heme iron plays a quantitatively important role; a much greater percentage of heme iron is absorbed, and its absorption is less affected by other dietary constituents.[79] The heme is taken up as such by the intestinal cells; subsequently, the iron is released from the porphyrin in the intestinal mucosa and enters the circulation as iron. Unlike inorganic iron, heme iron is soluble in alkaline solutions and

Table 82–6. SELECTED TRACE ELEMENTS

Element	Usual Sources	Function	Excess Syndromes	Deficiency Syndromes	Comments
Chromium	Spices, meats, vegetables, fruit, cheese, whole grains, brewers' yeast	Potentiates insulin action	Lung cancer	Malnourishment, insulin resistance, elevated serum cholesterol, atheromata, peripheral neuropathy	Abnormal glucose tolerance responsive to chromium supplement; depletion of chromium stores with increased age Unsupplemented TPN is risk factor for malnutrition
Cobalt	Leafy green vegetables	Component of vitamin B_{12}	In animals: anemia, growth retardation	Animals: growth retardation, hepatic and renal disease	
Copper	Oysters, nuts, liver, kidney, dried legumes, water	Component of copper metalloenzymes: cytochrome *c* oxidase, lysyl oxidase, tyrosinase, ascorbic acid oxidase	Wilson's disease/ cirrhosis, neurologic abnormalities, glycosuria, aminoaciduria, cataracts, osteomalacia, rickets, coagulation defects, hypophosphatemia, pancytopenia	Congenital: Menkes' kinky hair syndrome, hypothermia, blood vessel rupture/tortuosity, decreased myelination, seizures, mental retardation Acquired: nutritional anemia, neutropenia, osteopenia, hypercholesterolemia	Concentration in water is variable Decreased absorption with: ascorbic acid, sulfides, undenatured protein, large doses of zinc, phytate, calcium, cadmium, iron, and molybdenum Serum level may not correlate with tissue level
Fluoride	Fluoridated water Food content-variable	Incorporated into crystalline hydroxyapatite Increased resistance to caries	Acquired: nausea, vomiting, epigastric pain, ptyalism, headache, dizziness, weakness, metallic taste, severe coma, hemolytic anemia, mottling and brown staining of teeth	Poor dentition, caries, osteoporosis	Inhibition by milk, aluminum antacids
Iodine	Iodized table salt, salt water, shellfish, fish, breast milk, infant formulas	Component of triiodothyronine and thyroxine Cellular growth and oxidation	Thyrotoxicosis	Cretinism, goiter	
Manganese	Plant foods, cereal, nuts, leafy vegetables, whole grains, tea Low content: meat + milk	Component of metalloenzymes: pyruvate carboxylases, mitochondrial superoxide dismutase Cofactor of cellular enzymes (e.g., glycosyltransferase)	Psychiatric and neurologic disorders	Impaired growth, neonatal ataxia Structural abnormalities: liver, kidney, heart Mitochondrial abnormalities	Calcium, phosphorus, soy protein may interfere with absorption and utilization
Molybdenum	Meats, grains, legumes	Constituent of flavin-dependent enzymes: xanthine oxidase, aldehyde oxidases, sulfite oxidase	Goutlike syndrome	Growth retardation (animals), amino acid intolerance, tachycardia, tachypnea, central scotomas, irritability, decreased uric acid	
Selenium	Fish, barley, whole wheat, meat; soil Low content: fruits and vegetables	Antioxidant as a component of glutathione peroxidase	Loss of hair, brittle nails, garlic breath, fatigue, irritability, irritation of mucous membranes	Impaired neutrophil function, cardiomyopathy Animals: liver necrosis, muscular dystrophy	Keshan's disease, includes cardiomyopathy
Zinc	Shellfish, dried beans, peas, nuts, cereal, pasta, liver, meat, colostrum Human milk, infant formula	Component of metalloenzymes: alkaline phosphatase, carboxypeptidases, carbonic anhydrase, superoxide dismutase, RNA/ DNA polymerase, elongation factor 1, thymidine kinase	Abdominal pain, diarrhea, fever	Congenital: acrodermatitis enteropathica, dermatitis, alopecia, diarrhea, infection, cachexia, death Acquired: nutritional dwarfism, anorexia, anemia, hypogonadism, dermatitis, lethargy, geophagia, impaired wound healing, hypogeusia, impaired chemotaxis, decreased retinol binding protein levels	Symptoms of acrodermatitis appear after weaning from breast-feeding Sickle cell disease/TPN risk factor; Regular exogenous supply required (stores not readily mobilized) Absorption decreased by phytic acid, calcium, fiber, ferrous iron

is not affected by many substances that enhance (vitamin C) or diminish the absorption of inorganic iron.

When both forms of iron in the diet are considered, an average of approximately 6% of total dietary iron is absorbed by men and approximately 13% by women in their childbearing years. The higher absorption by women is related to their lower body iron stores.[78] Thus, iron repletion is regulated mainly by keeping absorptive processes attuned to body needs. However, the mechanism by which iron absorption is regulated remains in dispute.[79, 80]

The delivery of iron to the tissues involves transferrin in the plasma and a system of cell membrane receptors that are specific for transferrin.[81] The receptors bind the transferrin-iron complex at the cell membrane and carry it into the cell, where iron is released. Tissues that have a high uptake of iron, such as erythroid precursors and liver, contain large numbers of transferrin receptors. Although the affinity of the receptors appears to be constant in various tissues, the number of receptors is highly regulated.[82] When cells are in an iron-poor surrounding, the number of receptors increases, and vice versa.

The major storage compounds are ferritin and hemosiderin, which are present primarily in the liver, reticuloendothelial cells, and bone marrow. Storage iron may be almost entirely depleted before iron-deficiency anemia develops. Conversely, a more than 20-fold increase over normal average stores may occur before there is evidence of tissue damage. As liver iron stores become abnormally large, hemosiderin makes up an increasingly greater proportion of total iron.

Functions

The essential iron compounds consist primarily of heme proteins. Those proteins have an iron-porphyrin prosthetic group, and their function is related to oxidative energy metabolism. Hemoglobin is the most abundant, and its function is to transport oxygen to the tissues. Myoglobin, the red pigment of muscle, transports and stores oxygen for use during muscle contraction. Cytochromes are enzymes involved in electron transport and are located in the mitochondria and in other organelles.

Another group of iron enzymes involved in oxidative metabolism in which iron is not in the form of heme are NAD dehydrogenase and succinic dehydrogenase. Iron is also required by some enzymes in other metabolic process such as the tricarboxylic acid cycle and gluconeogenesis pathways.

Iron deficiency is the commonest nutritional deficiency worldwide,[83] and it can be successfully prevented on a large scale. The major causes of iron deficiency are insufficient assimilation of iron from the diet, dilution of body iron by rapid growth, and loss of blood. At approximately 4 months of age, iron stores are first likely to become depleted. During infancy, total iron in the body should more than double to accommodate the rapid rate of growth and an increase in red blood cell mass.[84] Excessive cow's milk consumption is associated with iron deficiency in infants. Milk is a poor source of iron and is frequently associated with occult intestinal blood loss in early infancy.[85]

Severe iron poisoning is characterized by damage to the intestinal mucosa, which can cause bloody diarrhea. Acidosis, liver failure, and shock may follow. Chronic iron overload results primarily from a genetic disorder, hemochromatosis, characterized by increased iron absorption and manifested by diabetes and liver and heart failure in men older than 60 years. Frequent transfusions for thalassemia and aplastic anemia also induce chronic iron overload.

Zinc

Metabolism

Despite considerable research, the mechanism of zinc absorption has not been fully delineated.[86] There has been speculation regarding the roles of intraluminal zinc-binding ligands in the absorption process. Agents that may have functional significance include fatty acids, prostaglandins, citric acid, and picolinic acid. There is little doubt that exogenous (dietary) or endogenous (pancreatic, biliary, or mucosal) ligands affect zinc absorption from a meal. It is unlikely, however, that the presence of ligands is required for zinc to be absorbed.

Absorption takes place primarily in the small intestine, and all segments may have functional importance. Absorption involves two kinetic processes: a carrier-mediated component (saturable at higher luminal zinc concentrations) and a nonsaturable diffusion component. Maximal transport rate by the carrier-mediated process is enhanced during periods of low zinc intake. In contrast, the diffusion component is unaffected by zinc deficiency, and absorption is proportional to luminal zinc concentration.[87]

Regulation of zinc absorption appears to be related to the synthesis of intestinal metallothionein, a small protein that binds zinc, copper, and other divalent cations. Expression of the metallothionein gene is induced by high dietary levels of zinc, particularly when copper intake is low.[88] Metallothionein seems to act as an inducible ligand that buffers zinc absorption. For example, zinc absorption decreases and intestinal metallothionein increases during periods of high zinc intake. Conversely, during zinc deficiency, metallothionein concentrations are low, and release of zinc from the intestine to the portal circulation increases.[89]

A link between the pancreas and zinc absorption may exist during bowel or pancreatic disease. Zinc secretion from enterocytes to the lumen has been shown experimentally,[90] and osmotic changes in the gastrointestinal tract may alter the absorption-secretion balance for zinc. Pancreatic insufficiency will reduce the enzymatic hydrolysis of food components, which then limits zinc release and availability for cellular uptake. Further, pancreatic secretions may contain constituents that increase zinc uptake by the intestine.[91]

Zinc is rapidly transported via the plasma, which constitutes 10 to 20% of the zinc in whole blood. The major portion of zinc in blood is contained in erythrocytes. Albumin appears to be the principal metabolically active, exchangeable zinc pool in blood and constitutes approximately 80% of the zinc in plasma. Plasma zinc concentrations tend to reflect intake when dietary zinc amounts are low. However, the plasma level exhibits circadian variations, decreases during stress, and is subject to transitory postprandial depression.

Although extracellular fluids represent a metabolically important body zinc compartment, only less than 0.5% of total body zinc is found in blood.[92] Therefore, zinc is primarily an intracellular ion. Zinc concentrations in bone, testes, hair, and blood tend to reflect dietary zinc intake. Other tissues, such as muscle, brain, and heart, have relatively stable concentrations of zinc, unresponsive to amounts of dietary intake over most ranges of intake.

Functions

The number of zinc-requiring enzymes is at least 60. Structural and functional roles for many metalloenzymes, encompassing each enzyme class, as well as a role in stabilization of macromolecules (including receptor molecules) have been described.[93] Further, the interaction of zinc with nuclear proteins that bind to promoter sequences of specific genes and thus regulate transcription suggests another spectrum of biologic effects for zinc.

Lesions resulting from severe zinc deficiency are manifestations of altered physiologic processes. Many of these lesions occur in tissues that contain some of the highest levels of zinc, such as skin (dermatitis), bone (skeletal anomalies), and reproductive organs (altered reproductive performance). Other signs include retarded growth, depressed immune function, anorexia, diarrhea, and alopecia.[93] Mild chronic zinc deficiency may be indicated by impaired immune function and reduced rate of growth in children. The low plasma levels of zinc in conjunction with some of the symptoms mentioned earlier and amelioration in response to increased zinc intake confirm the deficiency state. Because there is no major body store of zinc, response to repletion can be rapid.[94]

Copper

Metabolism

Copper is absorbed from all segments of the gastrointestinal tract, including the stomach and large intestine.[95] Although the sites of absorption are species dependent, the duodenum appears to be the major site for all species. The mechanism of copper absorption is not clear, but it is regulated at the intestinal mucosa. As in zinc, metallothionein appears to serve primarily as a negative regulator of copper absorption.

Zinc exerts an antagonistic effect on copper bioavailability. This effect appears to be mediated primarily at the intestinal mucosa via metallothionein, which binds copper more strongly than it does zinc. Thus, intestinal metallothionein, induced in response to high zinc intake, may preferentially bind dietary copper in a nonabsorbable form. Copper deficiency in adult humans has been induced by ingestion of at least 150 mg of zinc or more per day.[96]

Copper is taken up by the liver and converted to ceruloplasmin, which is the major transport protein for copper. Ceruloplasmin donates copper to nonhepatic tissues for synthesis of cuproenzymes, and there is evidence that peripheral cells possess specific binding sites for this protein.[97] Copper is excreted primarily via the gastrointestinal tract, and bile contributes the major portion of endogenous fecal copper. Bile from normal humans contains a high-molecular-weight substance that is absent in Wilson's disease.[98] The role of this protein may be to decrease copper reabsorption normally.

Functions

Several cuproenzymes play critical metabolic roles. Although specific pathologic states have not been identified for all cuproenzymes, their activities are generally depressed by copper deprivation. Acquired copper deficiency was first described by Cordano and coworkers in 1964.[99] The cases had prolonged periods of malnutrition and repeated episodes of diarrhea. All had been nutritionally rehabilitated using cow's milk, which is low in copper. The same syndrome occurs in persons maintained on long-term parenteral nutrition using copper-deficient solutions, in premature infants, and in neonates.[100]

Anemia was the first-described sign of copper deficiency. It results, at least in part, from faulty iron metabolism; however, the exact biochemical mechanism by which copper prevents anemia is still unclear. Copper deficiency results in low lysyl oxidase activity and consequent failure of elastin and collage crosslinking, resulting in vascular rupture and osteoporosis. Hypercholesterolemia, ataxia, and impaired immune competence have been described with copper deficiency, but the biochemical defects are unknown.

REFERENCES

1. Olson JA: Vitamin A, retinoids and carotenoids. *In* Shils ME, Young VR, eds: Modern Nutrition in Health and Disease. 7th ed. Philadelphia, Lea & Febiger, 1988, pp 293–312.
2. Brubacher G, Weiser H: The vitamin A activity of beta-carotene. Int J Vitam Nutr Res 1985; 55:5.
3. Olson JA: Vitamin A. *In* Brown ML, ed: Present knowledge in nutrition. Washington, DC, International Life Sciences Institute, Nutrition Foundation, 1990, pp 96–107.
4. Underwood BA: Vitamin A in animal and human nutrition. *In* Roberts AB, Sporn MB, eds: The Retinoids. Orlando, Academic Press, 1984, pp 281–392.
5. Bauernfeind JC: Vitamin A Deficiency and Its Control. Orlando, Academic Press, 1987.
6. Hollander D: Intestinal absorption of vitamin A, E, D, and K. J Lab Clin Invest 1981; 97:449.
7. van Baelen H, Bouillon R: Purification of the serum vitamin D-binding protein (9DBP) from different species. *In* Forest MG, Pugeat M, eds: Binding Proteins of Steroid Hormones. London, John Libbey, 1986, pp 69–83.
8. Henry HL, Norman AW: Vitamin D: Metabolism and biological actions. Annu Rev Nutr 1984; 4:493.

9. Broner F: Calcium absorption. *In* Johnson LR, ed: Physiology of the Gastrointestinal Tract. New York, Raven Press, 1987, pp 1419–1435.
10. Hughes MR, Baylink DJ, Jones PG, et al: Radioligand receptor assay for 25-hydroxyvitamin D_2/D_3. J Clin Invest 1976; 58:61.
11. MacMahan MT, Neale G: The absorption of alphatocopherol in control subjects and in patients with intestinal malabsorption. Clin Sci 1970; 38:197.
12. Lambert GH, Papp LA, Paton JB: Megadoses of vitamin E in oxygen-dependent premature newborn infants. J Perinatol 1985; 5:44.
13. Sokol RJ, Heubi JE, Butlersimon N, et al: Treatment of vitamin E deficiency during chronic childhood cholestasis with oral D-alpha-tocopheryl polyethylene glycol–1000 succinate. Gastroenterology 1987; 93:975.
14. Sokol RJ, Butlersimon NA, Bettis D, et al: Tocopheryl polyethylene glycol 1000 succinate therapy for vitamin E deficiency during chronic childhood cholestasis: Neurologic outcome. J Pediatr 1987; 111:830.
15. Thurnham DI: The use of different lipids to express serum tocopherol: Lipid ratios for the measurement of vitamin E status. Ann Clin Biochem 1986; 23:514.
16. Machlin L, ed: Handbook of Vitamins: Nutritional, Biochemical, and Clinical Aspects. New York, Marcel Dekker, 1984, pp 99–145.
17. Bier JG, Carash L, Hubbard VS: Medical uses of vitamin E. N Engl J Med 1983; 308:1063.
18. Greer FR, Mummahschendel LL, Marshall S, et al: Vitamin K_1 (phylloquinone) and vitamin K_2 (menaquinone) status in newborns during the first week of life. Pediatrics 1988; 81:137.
19. Motohara K, Matsukura M, Matsuda I, et al: Severe vitamin K deficiency in breast-fed infants. J Pediatr 1984; 105:943.
20. American Academy of Pediatrics, Committee on Nutrition: Vitamin K supplementation for infants receiving milk substitute infant formulas and for those with fat malabsorption. Pediatrics 1971; 48:483.
21. National Research Council: Vitamin tolerance of animals. Washington, DC, National Academy Press, 1987.
22. Rose RC: Transport of ascorbic acid and other water-soluble vitamins. Biochim Biophys Acta 1988; 979:335.
23. Sauberlich HE: Ascorbic acid. *In* Brown ML, ed: Present Knowledge in Nutrition. Washington, DC, International Life Sciences Institute, Nutrition Foundation, 1990, pp 96–107.
24. Chalmers AH, Cowley DM, Brown JM: A possible etiological role for ascorbate in calculi formation. Clin Chem 1986; 32:333.
25. Balchke P, Schmidt P, Zazgornik J, et al: Ascorbic acid aggravates secondary hyperoxalemia in patients on chronic hemodialysis. Ann Intern Med 1984; 101:344.
26. Glatthaar B, Hornig DH, Moser U: The role of ascorbic acid in carcinogenesis. Adv Exp Med Biol 1986; 206:357.
27. Bowman BB, McCormick DB, Rosenberg IH: Epithelial transport of water-soluble vitamins. Annu Rev Nutr 1989; 9:187.
28. Rindi G: Thiamin absorption by small intestine. Acta Vitaminol Enzymol 1984; 6:47.
29. Haas RH: Thiamin and the brain. Annu Rev Nutr 1988; 8:483.
30. Akiyama T, Selhub J, Rosenberg IH: FMN phosphatase and FAD pyrophosphatase in rat intestinal brush borders: Role in intestinal absorption of dietary riboflavin. J Nutr 1982; 112:263.
31. Said HM, Arianas P: Characteristics of riboflavin transport in human intestinal brush border membrane residues. Gastroenterology 1990; 98:A554.
32. Said HM, Hollander D: Does aging affect the intestinal transport of riboflavin? Life Sci 1985; 36:69.
33. Said HM: Development maturation of riboflavin intestinal transport in rat. Pediatr Res 1985; 19:1175.
34. Innis WSA: Variations in riboflavin binding by human plasma: Identification of immunoglobulins as the major proteins responsible. Biochem Med 1985; 34:151.
35. Lucas A, Bates C: Transient riboflavin depletion in preterm infants. Arch Dis Child 1984; 59:837.
36. Sisson TR: Photodegradation of riboflavin in neonates. Fed Proc 1987; 46:1883.
37. Moran JR, Greene H: Nutritional biochemistry of water-soluble vitamins. *In* Grand RJ, Sutphen JL, Dietz WH Jr, eds: Pediatric Nutrition: Theory and Practice. Boston, Butterworths, 1987, pp 51–68.
38. McCormick DB: Vitamin B_6. *In* Shils ME, Young VN, eds: Modern Nutrition in Health and Disease. Philadelphia, Lea & Febiger, 1988, pp 376–382.
39. Merrill AH, Henderson JM: Diseases associated with defects in vitamin B_6 metabolism or utilization. Annu Rev Nutr 1987; 7:137.
40. Dolphin D, Poulson R, Avramovic O, eds: Pyridoxal Phosphate: Chemical, Biochemical and Medical Aspects. Parts A and B, Vol 1A and 1B. New York, John Wiley & Sons, 1986.
41. Molony CJ, Parmelee AH: Convulsions in young infants as a result of pyridoxine (vitamin B_6) deficiency. JAMA 1954; 154:405.
42. Schaumberg H, Kaplan J, Windebank A, et al: Sensory neuropathy from pyridoxine abuse: A new megavitamin syndrome. N Engl J Med 1983; 309:445.
43. Kroll JS: Pyridoxine for neonatal seizures: An unexpected danger. Dev Med Child Neurol 1985; 27:377.
44. Bechgaard H, Jespersen S: GI absorption of niacin in humans. J Pharm Sci 1977; 66:871.
45. Satyanarayana U, Narasinga Rao BS: Dietary tryptophan level and the enzymes of tryptophan-NAD pathway. Br J Nutr 1980; 43:107.
46. Canner PL, Berge KG, Wenger NK, et al: Fifteen-year mortality in Coronary Drug Project patients: Long-term benefit with niacin. J Am Coll Cardiol 1986; 8:1245.
47. Mock DM: Biotin. *In* Brown ML, ed: Present Knowledge in Nutrition. Washington, DC, International Life Sciences Institute, Nutrition Foundation, 1990, pp 96–107.
48. Wolf B, Heard GS, McVoy JRS, et al: Biotinidase deficiency: The possible role of biotinidase in the processing of dietary protein-bound biotin. J Inherited Metab Dis 1984; 7(suppl 2):121.
49. Said HM, Redha R, Nylander W: Biotin transport in the human intestine: Site of maximum transport and effect of pH. Gastroenterology 1988; 95:1312.
50. Higginbottom MC, Sweetman L, Nyan WL: A syndrome of methylmalonic aciduria, homocystinuria, megaloblastic anemia and neurologic abnormalities in vitamin B_{12}–deficient breast-fed infant of a strict vegetarian. N Engl J Med 1978; 299:317–323.
51. Donaldson RM: Intrinsic factor and the transport of cobalamin. *In* Johnson LR, ed: Physiology of the Gastrointestinal Tract. New York, Raven Press, 1987, pp 959–973.
52. Kapadia CR, Donaldson RM: Disorders of cobalamin (vitamin B_{12}) absorption and transport. Annu Rev Med 1985; 36:93.
53. Hall C: The proteins of transport of the cobalamins. *In* Zittoun JA, Cooper BA, eds: Folates and Cobalamins. New York, Springer-Verlag, 1989, pp 53–70.
54. Kanazawa S, Herbert V, Herzlich B, et al: Removal of cobalamin analogue in bile by enterohepatic circulation. Lancet 1983; 1:707.
55. Scott JM, Dinn JJ, Wilson P, et al: Pathogenesis of subacute combined degeneration: A result of methyl group deficiency. Lancet 1981; 2:334.
56. Chandler CJ, Wang TTY, Halsted CH: Pteroylpolyglutamate hydrolase from human jejunal brush borders: Purification and characterization. J Biol Chem 1986; 261:928.
57. Rose RC: Intestinal absorption of water-soluble vitamin. *In* Johnson LR, ed: Physiology of the Gastrointestinal Tract. New York, Raven Press, 1987, pp 1581–1596.
58. Eto I, Krumdieck CL: Determination of three different pools of reduced one-carbon substituted folates: II. Quantitation and chain-length determination of the pteroylpolyglutamates of rat liver. Anal Biochem 1981; 115:138.
59. Matoh Y, Zehavi I, Topper E, et al: Folate nutrition and growth in infancy. Arch Dis Child 1979; 54:699–702.
60. Ek J, Behnke L, Halvorsen KS, et al: Plasma and red cell folate values and folate requirements in formula-fed premature infants. Eur J Pediatr 1984; 142:78–82.
61. Knowles JB, Wood RJ, Rosenberg IH: Response of fractional calcium absorption in women to various coadministered oral glucose doses. Am J Clin Nutr 1988; 48:1471–1474.
62. Nielsen OH, Schiotz PO, Rasmussen SN, et al: Calcium absorption and acceptance of low-lactose milk among children with primary lactase deficiency. J Pediatr Gastroenterol Nutr 1984; 3:219–223.
63. Tremaine WJ, Newcomer AD, Riggs BL, et al: Calcium absorption from milk in lactase-deficient and lactase-sufficient adults. Dig Dis Sci 1986; 4:376–378.

64. Committee on Nutrition, American Academy of Pediatrics: Calcium phosphorus, and magnesium. *In* Forbes GB, Woodruff CW, eds: Pediatric Nutrition Handbook. 2nd ed. Chicago, American Academy of Pediatrics, 1985, pp 111–122.
65. Greer FR, Tsang RC: Calcium, phosphorus, magnesium, and vitamin D requirements for the preterm infant. *In* Tsang RC, ed: Vitamin and Mineral Requirements in Preterm Infants. New York, Marcel Dekker, 1985, pp 99–136.
66. Motil KJ, Altschuler SI, Grand RJ: Mineral balance during nutritional supplementation in adolescents with Crohn's disease and growth failure. J Pediatr 1985; 107:473–479.
67. Shils ME: Experimental human magnesium depletion. Medicine 1969; 48:61–85.
68. Koo WWK, Tsang RC: Bone mineralization in infants. Prog Food Nutr Sci 1984; 8:229–302.
69. Koo WWK, Antony G, Stevens LHS: Continuous nasogastric phosphorus infusion in hypophosphatemic rickets of prematurity. Am J Dis Child 1984; 138:172–175.
70. Nielsen FH: Nutritional requirements for boron, silicon, vanadium, nickel, and arsenic: Current knowledge and speculation. FASEB J 1991; 5:2661–2667.
71. Hurley LS, Keen CL: Manganese. *In* Underwood E, Mertz W, eds: Trace Elements in Human Health and Animal Nutrition. New York, Academic Press, 1987, pp 185–223.
72. Offenbacher EG, Pi-Sunyer FX: Chromium in human nutrition. *In* Olson RE, ed: Annual Reviews of Nutrition. Palo Alto, CA, Annual Reviews Inc, 1988, pp 543–563.
73. Litov RE, Combs GF: Selenium in pediatric nutrition. Pediatrics 1991; 87:339–351.
74. Charlton RW, Bothwell TH: Iron absorption. Annu Rev Med 1983; 34:55.
75. Cook JD, Monsen ER: Food iron absorption in human subjects: III. Comparison of the effect of animal proteins on non-heme iron absorption. Am J Clin Nutr 1979; 29:859.
76. Siegenberg D, Baynes RD, Bothwell TH, et al: Ascorbic acid prevents the dose-dependent inhibitory effects of polyphenols and phytates on nonheme-iron absorption. Am J Clin Nutr 1991; 53:537.
77. Saarinen UM, Simes MA, Dallman PR: Iron absorption in infants: High bioavailability of breast milk iron as indicated by the extrinsic tag method of iron absorption and by the concentration of serum ferritin. J Pediatr 1977; 91:36.
78. Davidson LA, Lonnerdal B: Specific binding of lactoferrin to brush-border membrane: Ontogeny and effect of glycon chain. Am J Physiol 1988; 254:G580.
79. Hallberg L: Bioavailability of iron in man. Annu Rev Nutr 1981; 1:123.
80. Peters TJ, Raja KB, Simpson RJ, et al: Mechanisms and regulation of iron absorption. Ann NY Acad Sci 1988; 526:141.
81. Huebers HA, Finch CA: The physiology of transferrin and transferrin receptors. Physiol Rev 1987; 67:520.
82. Casey JL, Hentze MW, Koeller DM, et al: Iron-responsive elements: Regulatory RNA sequences that control in RNA levels and translation. Science 1988; 240:924.
83. DeMaeyer E, Adiels-Tegman M, Rayston E: The prevalence of anemia in the world. World Health Stat Q 1985; 38:302.
84. Dallman, PR, Simes MA, Stekel A: Iron deficiency in infancy and childhood. Am J Clin Nutr 1980; 33:86–118.
85. Fomon SJ: Cow milk feeding in infancy: Gastrointestinal blood loss and iron nutritional status. J Pediatr 1981; 98:540.
86. Lonnerdal B: Intestinal absorption of zinc. *In* Mills CF, ed: Zinc in Human Biology. New York, Springer-Verlag, 1989, pp 33–55.
87. Hoadley JE, Leinart AS, Cousins RJ: Kinetic analysis of zinc uptake and serosal transfer by vascularly perfused rat intestine. Am J Physiol 1987; 252:G825.
88. Blalock TL, Dunn MA, Cousins RJ: Metallothionein gene expression in rats: Tissue-specific regulation by dietary copper and zinc. J Nutr 1988; 118:222.
89. Hoadley JE, Leinart AS, Cousins RJ: Relationship of ^{65}Zn absorption kinetics to intestinal metallothionein in rats: Effects of zinc depletion and fasting. J Nutr 1988; 118:497.
90. Oestreicher P, Cousins RJ: Copper and zinc absorption in the rat: Mechanism of mutual antagonism. J Nutr 1985; 115:159.
91. Solomons NW, Cousins RJ: Zinc. *In* Solomons NW, Rosenberg IH, eds: Absorption and Malabsorption of Mineral Nutrients. New York, Alan R. Liss, 1984, pp 125–197.
92. Cousins RJ: Systemic transport of zinc. *In* Mills CF, ed: Zinc in Human Biology. New York, Springer-Verlag, 1989, pp 79–93.
93. Hambidge KM, Casey CE, Krebs NF: Zinc. *In* Mertz W, ed: Trace Elements in Human and Animal Nutrition. Vol 2, 5th ed. Orlando, Academic Press, 1986, pp 1–137.
94. Hambidge KM: Mild zinc deficiency in human subjects. *In* Mills CF, ed: Zinc in Human Biology. New York, Springer-Verlag, 1989, pp 281–296.
95. Davis GK, Mertz W: Copper. *In* Mertz W, ed: Trace Elements in Human and Animal Nutrition. 5th ed. New York, Academic Press, 1986, pp 301–364.
96. Hoffman HN, Phyliky RL, Fleming CR: Zinc-induced copper deficiency. Gastroenterology 1988; 94:508.
97. Stevens MD, Di Silvestro RA, Harris ED: Specific receptor for ceruloplasmin in membrane fragments from aortic and heart tissues. Biochemistry 1984; 23:261–266.
98. Iyengar V, Brewer GJ, Dick RD, et al: Studies of cholecystokinin-stimulated biliary secretions reveals a high molecular weight substance in normal subjects that is absent in patients with Wilson's disease. J Lab Clin Med 111:267, 1988.
99. Cordano A, Baertl JM, Graham GG: Copper deficiency in infancy. Pediatrics 1964; 34:324.
100. Baker SS: Nutritional biochemistry of minerals-micronutrient. *In* Grand RJ, Sutphen JL, Dietz WH Jr, eds: Pediatric Nutrition Theory and Practice. Boston, Butterworths, 1987, pp 51–68.

Chapter 83

Enteral Nutrition

NEAL S. LeLEIKO, PATRICE BURKE, and CEWIN CHAO

The first route for the nutritional support of a sick child is via the alimentary canal. Enteral alimentation provides the most acceptable and effective method for maintaining and repleting the nutritional state of pediatric patients who have functioning gastrointestinal tracts. In this chapter, we discuss the background necessary for implementating successful enteral nutrition therapy as well as the indications, methods, and expected results of therapy.

The development of the subspecialty of pediatric gastroenterology has been accompanied by a renewed appreciation of the importance of proper nutrition for sick infants and children. Specialists in pediatric gastroenterology by definition must be well schooled in the basic principles of clinical nutrition. Much of their work will be concerned with the assessment of the nutritional status of the pediatric patient and with the prevention of nutritional depletion in these patients. When malnutrition already exists, whether primarily involving disease of the gastrointestinal tract or secondary to nongastrointestinal causes, pediatric gastroenterologists work with the rest of the medical team to prescribe special nutritional regimens to replete the patient.

There are two ways that special nutritional regimens may be administered: via the enteral pathway, i.e., through the gastrointestinal (alimentary) tract, or via the parenteral route, i.e., intravenously. The enteral pathway is the preferred route.[1–5] It maintains and when necessary helps to return the integrity of the gastrointestinal mucosa (which parenteral nutrition does not do), and it is safer than parenteral nutrition.

Successful alimentation may be achieved using the oral route or a nasogastric, nasojejunal, gastrostomy, or jejunostomy feeding tube. The choice of the route depends on the primary medical problem and the clinical status of the child who is being supported. Defined formula diets (which are often and inappropriately referred to as "elemental" diets) provide flexibility in nutrient composition, caloric density, and osmolarity as well as taste. The biochemical assessment and monitoring of the child receiving enteral alimentation should be approached in the same manner as the assessment of the child receiving total parenteral nutrition.

Patients who require nutritional support are suffering from either primary gastrointestinal disease or from the secondary gastrointestinal side effects of their primary disease (Table 83–1). There is evidence that both types of patients may derive specific advantages if their nutrition is delivered through the gastrointestinal tract as opposed to the parenteral route. Specifically studies after experimental intestinal resection[6–10] have shown that the return of normal gastrointestinal function is related to intraluminal (i.e., alimentary tract) nutrition. Studies[11] of laboratory animals who were given identical nutritionally complete formulas either orally or through the parenteral route have shown that the mucosal weight of the gastrointestinal tract as well as the total protein and DNA content were all greater in the animals receiving enteral nutrition. The brush border enzymes, which are important in digestion, were also higher in those animals that were fed. It has been shown[8, 9, 12] that exclusive parenteral nutrition results in decreased intestinal mucosal cell turnover and thereby a decreased height of the mucosal villi. The intestinal atrophy or hypotrophy produced by total parenteral nutrition appears to be preventable by the infusion of cholecystokinin and secretin.[13] The infusion of small amounts of nutrients intraluminally similarly seems to have a protective effect on the intestinal mucosa.

From the metabolic view, there are several consequences that clearly relate to the pathway (enteral versus parenteral) of nutrition. After ingestion of a protein-

Table 83–1. CLINICAL USES OF DEFINED FORMULA DIETS

	References
Chronic illness with failure to thrive	3, 4
Home nutritional support	71–74
Malabsorption syndromes	3, 73
Short bowel syndrome	3
Cancer patients with malnutrition	75, 76
Gastrointestinal fistula	3, 28
Intractable diarrhea	77
Congenital heart disease with failure to thrive	78
Early postoperative feeding	79
Inflammatory bowel disease	3, 4, 23, 80, 81
Chronic liver disease	82, 83
Renal failure	84, 92
Low birth weight and premature infants	85, 86
Glycogen storage disease	87–90
Burns	91
Diagnostic studies	3
Metabolic test meals	3
Pancreatitis	27

containing meal, the cells of the intestinal mucosa absorb the protein as oligopeptides and free amino acids. The oligopeptides are hydrolyzed to amino acids within the epithelial cells, and then the amino acids are transported to the liver via the portal vein. Within the epithelial cells, glutamine and glutamic acid are metabolized, yielding alanine for transport into the portal system. The liver metabolizes most amino acids during first pass, with the exception of the branched-chain amino acids, which are catabolized primarily in the muscle, kidneys, adipose, and brain. Studies of parenterally administered amino acids, especially branched chains,[11, 14] suggest that careful attention needs to be paid to implications of parenteral versus enteral feeding. The studies in aggregate suggest that for the short term, aberrations in protein metabolism are less related to route of administration than to amounts administered; for long-term therapy, however, the enteral route is preferable. This is especially important when the effects of route of feeding are assessed in terms of effect on insulin and glucagon secretion. The use of unbalanced mixtures of nutrients is greater in the parenterally fed patient. Currently little is known about the effects of route of administration on vitamin requirements, but there is evidence that the net availability of trace elements administered parenterally is unpredictable.[15] It seems evident that the intestine has a regulatory function for the absorption and elimination of many minerals.

Laboratory work on the availability of purines for nucleic acid synthesis in the gastrointestinal tract[16–20] suggests that the lack of preformed dietary purines may limit the ability of the sick intestinal mucosa to recover and regenerate normal function. Purines are not currently available in parenteral formulas.

Thus, there is a metabolic price to be paid for receiving nutrition via the parenteral route. Many aberrant findings are caused by nonphysiologic patterns and amounts of nutrients[21] rather than the actual route of delivery. It is clear, however, that we currently lack sufficient understanding to provide for the optimal nutritional needs of our patients via the parenteral route when compared with the enteral route. Further, these problems are most likely to be of consequence for the patient who will receive long-term nutritional therapy. Therefore it is important to try to understand how such a patient may be managed via the enteral route.

DEFINED FORMULA DIETS

The large number of defined formula diets commercially available provides the clinical nutritionist with a diverse number of alternative regimens from which to choose. Numerous manufacturers actively compete in what has become an extremely lucrative business.

Although the use of prepared formulas has many advantages, the practitioner must guard against new, inadequately announced changes in "known" formulations. In this regard, it is inappropriate to select a formula by "name"; instead it is preferable to consider the pertinent components of the diet first. Then those components should be sought in a particular formula. As a general rule, the least synthetic and least "predigested" or "elemental" formula that meets the patient's expected needs will be the safest and best formula. This generic approach is much more rational and much more appropriate than considering brand name. With regard to selecting the generic formula, an assessment of the integrity of the patient's gastrointestinal tract, which is part of a thorough nutritional assessment, should reveal the known or suspected absorptive defects or other problems that might impede normal nutrition. For general reference, a partial list of enteral nutrition products that are commonly used is given in Table 83–2. It is evident from the listing that we rely on specialized infant formulas for much of our special enteral needs. Beyond those formulas, only a few special enteral products are used.

Each advantage cited for any particular defined formula diet implies potential problems. For example, one

Table 83–2. ENTERAL FEEDING PRODUCTS*

Special Infant Formula by Type of Formula	
Protein Hydrolysates	
Nutramigen	100% LCT—Lactose-free
Pregestimil	60% MCT—Lactose-free
Alimentum	50% MCT—Lactose-free
Good Start	100% LCT—70% lactose
MCT Predominant	
Portagen	85% MCT—Corn syrup solids
Lactose-free	All current soy formulas
Low Sodium	
SMA	Regular infant formula
Premature Formula (24 cal/oz)	
Enfamil Premature	Ca/P 2:1 Lactose-free
Similac Special Care	Ca/P 2:1 50% MCT
SMA Premature	CA/P 2:1 13% MCT, 50% Lactose
Special Enteral Products by Manufacturer	
Ross	
Enrich	Standard tube feeding with fiber
Ensure	Flavored for oral use
Osmolite	Low sodium
Ross SLD	High protein, clear liquid
TwoCal	2 cal/oz
Jevity	High protein and fiber
Vital HN	Partially hydrolyzed protein with low fat
Pediasure	Designed for 1–6 year age group
Mead Johnson	
Isocal	Standard tube feeding (1 cal/ml)
Isocal HCN	High protein and high calorie (2 cal/ml)
Sustacal	High protein—standard tube feeding (1 cal/ml)
Criticare HN	Protein hydrolysate (1 cal/ml)
Clintec	
Peptamen	High protein hydrolysate with 70% MCT
O'Brien/KMI	
Reabilan	Protein hydrolysate with 40% MCT
Norwich Eaton	
Vivonex Ten	Free amino acids and 2.8 gm of LCT/L
Sandoz	
Compleat	Meat-based blenderized tube feeding
Impact	Possible immune system modulators
Sherwood Medical	
Magnacal	High calorie tube feeding (2 cal/ml)

*Formulas are listed with general characteristics; for precise constituents, check with manufacturer, since these are all subject to change with minimal or no notice.

MCT, medium-chain triglyceride; LCT, light-chain triglyceride.

problem that tends to limit nutrient density is the problem of osmolality. Our experience suggests that even the child without intrinsic gastrointestinal disease may begin to complain of gastrointestinal symptoms when the osmolality of the formula approaches 600 mOsm per L. This experience is consistent with that of investigators[22] who have reported delayed gastric emptying when the osmolality of the duodenal contents is 560 mOsm per L.

The specific therapeutic benefits of defined formula diets are those that accrue from good nutrition. Special claims regarding the therapeutic benefits of any of these diets have not been adequately distinguished from the nutritional effects. It is therefore prudent to regard any specific claim with some degree of skepticism. To clarify the issue, expert groups have tried to meet to discuss available data. Potential therapeutic applications of enteral nutritional treatment for patients with inflammatory bowel disease have been extensively reviewed and reported in a state-of-the-art review.[23] Whether further work will better define a primary therapeutic role for any particular enteral formula remains to be seen.

Nonetheless, formulas can be tailored to take advantage of the physiologic properties of the constituents. For example, the protein content of the formula has been demonstrated to be directly proportional to its acid-secreting potential.[24] Gastrin release itself is related to the presence of specific amino acids and small peptides.[25] The administration of intragastric amino acids results in significant pancreatic stimulation, which can be minimized if the infusion is intrajejunal and at neutral pH.[26] The decreased pancreatic output that results suggests a possible explanation for the apparent efficacy of defined formula diets in the treatment of pancreatitis[27] and high-output intestinal fistulas.[28–30]

Other considerations regarding the fat and carbohydrate contents of the diets and routes of delivery may also be pertinent. Overall it must be emphasized that the comparison of studies using different formulas under nonstandard conditions is usually not valid. It is evident that careful and critical evaluation of each apparently relevant report is absolutely essential to place it in its proper therapeutic role.

The use of commercial preparations of a known composition facilitates the accurate measurement of nutrient intake. They are therefore of great value in metabolic studies and in critical care situations, in which accurate intake measurements are necessary.

Because of the flexibility of these formulas, it is common to have constituents vary in relation to one another. This occasionally leads to inappropriate amounts of energy and protein intake. With insufficient protein intake, positive nitrogen balance is impossible, and similarly adequate energy must be supplied to allow for protein synthesis. The term nitrogen/calorie ratio is frequently used in this regard, but it should be remembered that this is only a simplistic attempt to convey the importance of meeting both the patient's energy and protein needs. Munro[21] has pointed out in a review of oral versus parenteral nutrient metabolism that major deviations that occur in parenterally nourished patients are often the result not of the route of delivery of the nutrient but rather of the unusual pattern of nutrients administered. The clear implication is that similar aberrations are to be expected through the injudicious use of the enteral pathway.

CONSTITUENTS OF DEFINED FORMULA DIETS

Fat

Fat has the highest caloric density of any nutrient. The intake of fat is important because our experience suggests that for most pediatric patients the limiting nutrient is energy (or caloric) intake. Patients who suffer unusual losses of protein-rich fluid will require increased amounts of protein, but even in those patients energy intake will ultimately be limiting. Triglycerides composed of glycerol esterified to long-chain fatty acids yield approximately 9 calories per gm when they are oxidized. They are therefore highly desirable nutrients for any nutritionally depleted patient. The major considerations with regard to choosing the amount or type of dietary fat include (1) the use and absorption of long-chain triglycerides; (2) the use and absorption of synthetic medium-chain triglycerides; and (3) the requirements for essential fatty acids.

Dietary fat consists of predominantly long-chain triglycerides. The process of digestion and absorption of long-chain triglycerides is divided into several stages (Fig. 83–1). Within the lumen of the gastrointestinal tract, the long-chain fat must be emulsified and acted on by gastrointestinal (predominantly pancreatic) lipases. The lipases break down the triglyceride to free fatty acids and glycerol. Bile salts from the liver are necessary to form micelles to solubilize the free fatty acids for transport in the intestinal lumen to the brush border membrane. At the brush border membrane, the fatty acids are absorbed into the enterocyte. Within the enterocyte, fatty acids are re-esterified with glycerol to form a triglyceride again. With the addition of apolipoproteins, phospholipid, cholesterol ester, and cholesterol, chylomicrons are formed, which are then released into the lymphatics.

The assimilation of long-chain fat is disrupted in several clinical situations: pancreatic insufficiency resulting in decreased lipases; bile duct obstruction or hepatitis resulting in decreased bile flow to the intestine and thereby decreased micelle formation; gastrointestinal mucosal damage resulting in decreased surface area for the absorption of fatty acids; metabolic derangements inhibiting the formation of chylomicrons; and diseases or obstruction of the lymphatics inhibiting the transport of lymph back into the circulation. In some circumstances, it is acceptable to allow the increased fat malabsorption that results from increased fat intake to take advantage of the increased caloric density of the fat that does get absorbed. In other circumstances, long-chain fat must be largely excluded from the diet.

Medium-chain triglycerides are synthetic fats that contain a glycerol backbone esterified to fatty acids that are

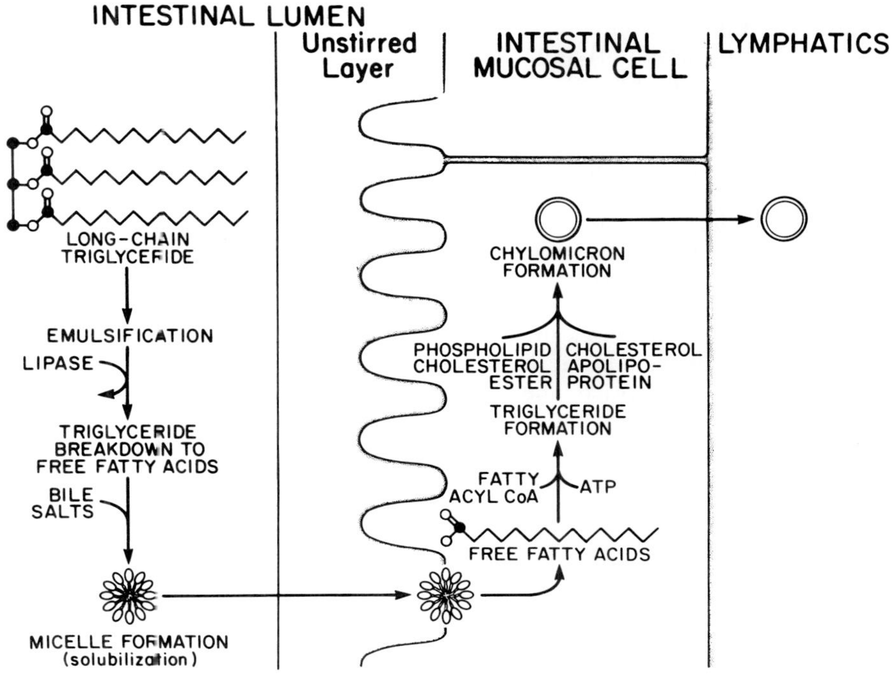

Figure 83–1. Digestion and absorption of long-chain triglyceride. Within the lumen of the small intestine, the long-chain triglyceride is emulsified and acted on by lipases. The resulting free fatty acids (FFAs) are formed into micelles along with the bile salts. As micelles, the FFA (and glycerol) diffuse through the intestinal unstirred layer and are absorbed into the enterocytes. Within the enterocytes, the FFAs are re-esterified and then combined with phospholipid, cholesterol ester, cholesterol, and apolipoprotein B to form a chylomicron. The chylomicra pass out of the enterocyte and via the lymphatic circulation into the blood stream.

8 to 10 carbons in length. Medium-chain triglycerides yield 8.3 calories per gm on oxidation and are therefore essentially as useful as long-chain fat from an energy point of view. Medium-chain triglycerides (Fig. 83–2) are hydrolyzed more rapidly than long-chain fats in the small intestine when pancreatic lipases are present and are converted almost exclusively into free fatty acids and glycerol. If no pancreatic lipase is present, the medium-chain triglyceride can be found in the intestinal mucosa mainly as unhydrolyzed triglyceride.[31, 32] Thus, even in the absence of pancreatic lipase and bile salts, medium-chain triglycerides are transported through the intestinal lumen and through the brush border into the enterocyte intact. The unusual behavior of medium-chain triglyceride in the intestinal lumen and its absorption characteristics are due to the greater water solubility of medium-chain triglyceride and its products. The lower interfacial tension of the smaller triglyceride molecules with water facilitates its emulsification, so the formation of micelles is not necessary.

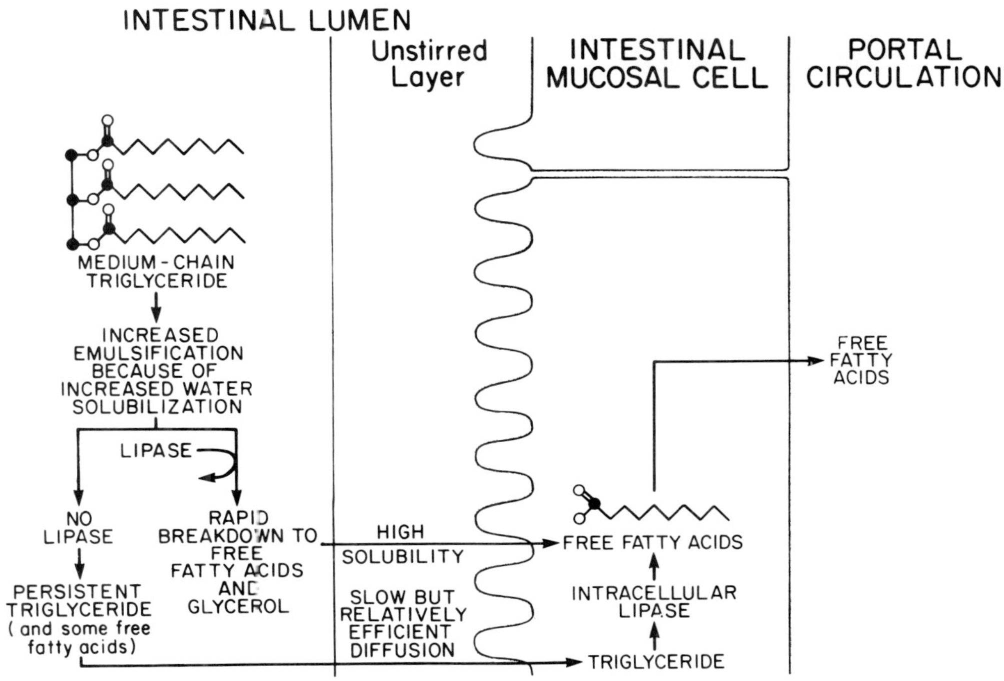

Figure 83–2. Digestion and absorption of medium-chain triglyceride. Within the lumen of the small intestine, the medium-chain triglyceride is rapidly and efficiently emulsified. If lipases are present, there is the risk of rapid breakdown to free fatty acids (FFAs) and glycerol with a resulting high local osmotic pressure. Without lipase or bile salts, the medium-chain triglyceride (and some FFAs) slowly but efficiently diffuse through the unstirred layer and are taken up intact by the enterocytes. Within the lumen of the mucosal cell, the triglyceride is broken down to FFAs, and these FFAs are transported via the portal circulation to the liver.

The exact mechanism and the rate-limiting step in the absorption of these different fats are unknown. The relatively high solubility of intact medium-chain triglycerides enhances their diffusion to the brush border of the enterocyte. The triglyceride and the medium-chain free fatty acids are readily taken up into the enterocyte. Within the enterocyte, the triglyceride is acted on by intracellular lipases, and the resulting free fatty acids are released directly into the portal circulation.[33] The clinical indications for the use of medium-chain triglycerides are based on these characteristics (Table 83–3).

There are circumstances under which one, the other, or both types of fat become highly desirable as constituents of the prescribed diet. It has been demonstrated[31, 34] that the maximum absorption of long-chain fat is decreased when medium-chain triglycerides are added. The total triglyceride absorbed when both are present, however, is greater than the maximum absorption of either alone. Absorption of medium-chain triglycerides from the rat cecum[35] and the dog colon[36] has been reported. The importance of this phenomenon and whether it has any implications for the human are unclear.

The true capacity of the gastrointestinal tract to absorb fat has not been precisely measured. It is generally accepted that the rate of fat absorption is proportional to the amount of fat ingested, and the more fat ingested the more absorbed.

If there are no specific defects in fat absorption demonstrated or anticipated, the fat of choice for a defined formula diet is regular, long-chain (dietary) fat. The use of medium-chain triglycerides in patients who have intact mechanisms for the normal digestion of fat can lead to osmotic diarrhea resulting from the rapid lipolysis of the medium-chain triglycerides to glycerol (and medium-chain free fatty acids). This diarrhea may potentiate the symptoms for which the formula was prescribed and result in unfortunate consequences. Additionally, there are a few patients who seem to have an unexplained or idiosyncratic reaction resulting in severe diarrhea when they ingest even small amounts of medium-chain triglycerides. Patients who require increased calories may conceivably be helped by a mixture of both medium-chain triglycerides and long-chain triglycerides. Ideally fecal fat determinations can be used as a guide to determine the optimal combination of medium-chain triglyceride, long-chain triglyceride, or both to be given to the patient.

Essential fatty acids are all long-chain fatty acids and therefore absent in medium-chain triglycerides. Because the administration of medium-chain triglycerides may decrease the absorption of long-chain triglyceride, the addition of small amounts of linoleic acid to a medium-chain triglyceride formula may be insufficient to prevent essential fatty acid insufficiency. The exact requirements for essential fats are disputed, but it is clear that the clinician must guard against the development of essential fatty acid deficiency. If long-chain fat absorption is severely compromised, the parenteral administration of lipid emulsions containing essential fats must be considered.

Table 83–3. POTENTIAL INDICATIONS FOR REPLACEMENT OF SOME OR ALL OF DIETARY LONG-CHAIN FATS WITH MEDIUM-CHAIN TRIGLYCERIDE*

Cholestasis including
Cholestatic jaundice secondary to total parenteral nutrition or medications
Hepatitis (any type)
Bile duct obstruction
Biliary atresia
Bile salt depletion
Terminal ileal dysfunction or disease
Prematurity
Congenital deficiency of bile salts
Pancreatic insufficiency including
Cystic fibrosis
Interruption of lymph drainage including
Congenital lymphangiectasia
Chylothorax
Chylous ascites
Decreased villous surface area including
Severe enteritis
Short gut syndrome
Metabolic derangements of long-chain fat assimilation including
Abetalipoproteinemia

*Note: Replacement of long-chain triglyceride with medium-chain triglyceride may lead to or even contribute to essential fatty acid deficiency.

Carbohydrates

Complex carbohydrates are broken down to individual monosaccharides by the brush border oligosaccharidases. The individual monosaccharides are then absorbed into the enterocytes via specific transport systems. There are four distinct brush border oligosaccharidases.[37] Three are clinically significant enzymes (Fig. 83–3): (1) maltase (glucoamylase); (2) sucrase-isomaltase (sucrase α-dextrinase); and (3) lactase. The fourth, trehalase (acts on the sugar trehalose, which is found only in young mushrooms and insects), is of little clinical significance.

Maltase (glucoamylase) is the most abundant oligosaccharidase in the gastrointestinal tract. Sucrase is present in intermediate amounts, and lactase, which splits lactose into glucose and galactose, is present in the least quantities.

All of the disaccharidases may be expected to be depressed when there is mucosal disease of the small intestine. Lactase appears to be the most sensitive to injury and the last of the disaccharidases to recover full activity after mucosal damage.[7, 38, 39]

Because the disaccharidases are present in older enterocytes, any process that causes rapid intestinal regeneration and therefore repopulation of the intestinal villi with young cells (i.e., recovery from acute gastroenteritis) will represent a period of relative disaccharidase deficiency for the patient. Additionally, starvation alone may be sufficient to lower disaccharidase activity because it results in decreased cell turnover, mucosal hypotrophy, and therefore decreased surface area. It may therefore be important to limit dietary sources of lactose in the malnourished child or in the child recuperating from gastrointestinal insult for a short period of time. Restriction beyond a brief period necessary to demonstrate mucosal recovery is, however, not warranted. Breath hydrogen testing (when clinically indicated) is a noninvasive method to determine the status of carbohydrate absorption (e.g., lactose, sucrose) so resumption of acceptable amounts of dietary carbohydrates is not delayed.

In selecting a carbohydrate for a defined formula diet, it is important to note that the use of glucose significantly increases the osmotic concentration of a formula. A disaccharide will provide, on a gram for gram basis, one half the osmotic load of a monosaccharide. The use of synthetic glucose polymers may contribute as little as one fifth to the total osmotic load of a similar amount of glucose. Many defined formula diets therefore use glucose polymers and long-chain starches as their carbohydrate source. The assimilation of these long-chain carbohydrates appears to proceed so the osmolarity of the intestinal contents is not adversely affected. Although it has been shown[40, 41] that sucrose or fructose feedings may cause increases in the intestinal level of sucrase and maltase, no such dietary effect on lactase activity has ever been demonstrated.

It is important to document the existence of carbohydrate malabsorption when it is suspected and a formula change is contemplated. This may be done by testing for the presence of hydrogen in breath samples or by searching for reducing substances in fresh (preferably less than 5 minutes old) stool. Reducing substances may be checked[42] by placing five drops of liquid stool in a test tube along with 10 drops of water, then by adding one Clinitest (Ames) tablet. The color that is evolved is compared with the package insert. Normally there are no reducing substances present. A reading of 1/2% is abnormal; a reading of 1/4% is considered potentially not significant. If the patient's formula contains a nonreducing sugar (i.e., sucrose), it must first be hydrolyzed. This is accomplished by using 0.1 N hydrochloric acid instead of water and by briefly heating the test tube over a flame until the solution boils (for 30 seconds). The solution is then tested by adding the Clinitest tablet. Generally, if carbohydrate fermentation products are present in the stool of an infant with diarrhea, the stool has an acid pH, and it seems to "burn" the infant's diaper area regardless of how meticulous the caretaker is. This finding is not invariably present, and it would not be expected when lactose-containing milk is reintroduced after a prolonged milk-free period. Under such circumstances, it may take a few days for the colonic bacterial population to change to an acid-forming flora.

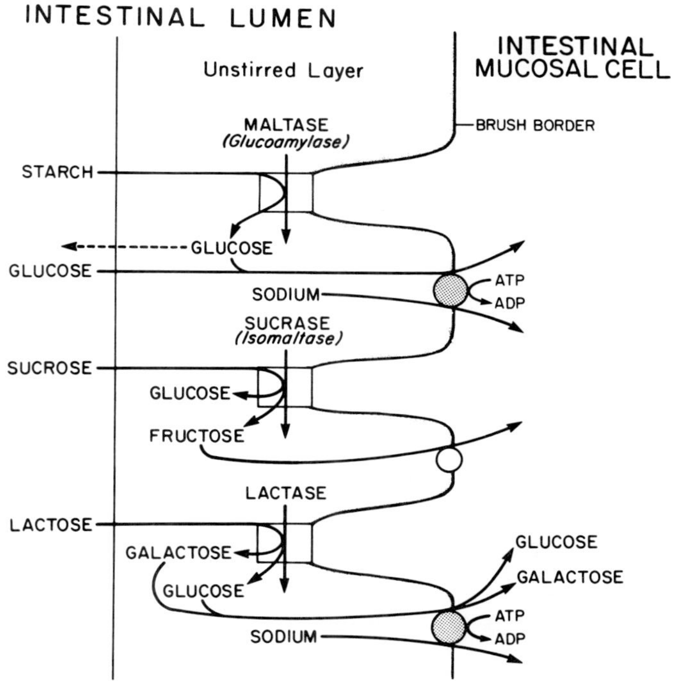

Figure 83–3. Digestion and absorption of carbohydrate. Within the intestinal lumen the carbohydrates diffuse through the unstirred layer to the intestinal brush border. There they are acted on by their respective carbohydrases and broken down to component monosaccharides. The monosaccharides are absorbed via active and passive routes.

Protein

A child's protein requirements may be met by using intact proteins, protein hydrolysates, individual amino acids, or a combination of these. Patients who have no known deficiency of the exocrine pancreatic function and no suspected major absorptive defect or protein allergy should receive high-quality intact protein. Intact protein is considerably less expensive than other dietary forms, is much more palatable, and does not contribute significantly to a formula's osmolarity. Within a given volume and osmolarity, the formula containing intact protein will allow for significantly greater nutrient density. Patients who are unable to tolerate intact protein because of protein allergy, exocrine pancreatic deficiency, or severe intestinal mucosal disease should receive a protein hydrolysate, a more readily absorbed form of protein.

For many years, nutritionists believed that amino acids represented the optimal form of predigested protein and that a protein source containing only amino acids would be "most" easily absorbed. This was an oversimplified and incorrect view of the mechanism of protein absorption. The absorption of small peptides, especially dipeptides, has been shown to play a significant role in the digestion of protein.[43] Perhaps one quarter of absorbed protein in health is absorbed in the form of oligopeptides.[44] The oligopeptides, especially dipeptides, are absorbed and then hydrolyzed by brush border and cytoplasmic hydrolases to free amino acids.[45] The mechanism of transport of the individual amino acids has been shown to be energy dependent and active and in many cases dependent on true carrier proteins with some degree of specificity for neutral, basic, and acidic amino acids. A lack of competition between

Table 83–4. MEDIAN HEIGHTS AND WEIGHTS AND RECOMMENDED ENERGY INTAKE

Category	Age (years) or Condition	Weight (kg)	Weight (lb)	Height (cm)	Height (in)	REE[a] (kcal/day)	Average Energy Allowance (kcal)[b] Multiples of REE	Per kg	Per day[c]
Infants	0.0–0.5	6	13	60	24	320		108	650
	0.5–1.0	9	20	71	28	500		98	850
Children	1–3	13	29	90	35	740		102	1,300
	4–6	20	44	112	44	950		90	1,800
	7–10	28	62	132	52	1,130		70	2,000
Males	11–14	45	99	157	62	1,440	1.70	55	2,500
	15–18	66	145	176	69	1,760	1.67	45	3,000
	19–24	72	160	177	70	1,780	1.67	40	2,900
	25–50	79	174	176	70	1,800	1.60	37	2,900
	51+	77	170	173	68	1,530	1.50	30	2,300
Females	11–14	46	101	157	62	1,310	1.67	47	2,200
	15–18	55	120	163	64	1,370	1.60	40	2,200
	19–24	58	128	164	65	1,350	1.60	38	2,200
	25–50	63	138	163	64	1,380	1.55	36	2,200
	51+	65	143	160	63	1,280	1.50	30	1,900
Pregnant	1st trimester								+0
	2nd trimester								+300
	3rd trimester								+300
Lactating	1st 6 months								+500
	2nd 6 months								+500

[a]Calculation based on FAO equations (Table 3–1 [in original source]), then rounded.
[b]In the range of light to moderate activity, the coefficient of variation is ± 20%.
[c]Figure is rounded.
Reprinted with permission from RECOMMENDED DIETARY ALLOWANCES: 10TH EDITION. Copyright 1989 by the National Academy of Sciences. Published by the National Academy Press, Washington, D.C.

amino acid uptake and the uptake of peptides suggests that separate carriers for absorption are present. It has thus become clear that in the severely damaged mucosa, the ideal form of protein for absorption will be found in a mixture of oligopeptides and individual free amino acids.

The clinical importance of peptide transport has been demonstrated in certain diseases; for example, in patients with Hartnup's disease (in which there is a specific inability to transport some neutral amino acids such as tryptophan), normal development can occur,[46] and this has been similarly demonstrated in cystinuria (another disorder involving amino acid transport).[47, 48] It is conceivable that in the damaged mucosa, similar transport mechanisms are important. Some investigators[49, 50] have shown that in surgically shortened intestines there are marked decreases in capacity to absorb free amino acids. Further, there appears to be significantly less impairment in the absorption of dipeptides. Rats with exocrine pancreatic deficiency have been shown[51] to use a diet containing 85% of the protein as oligopeptides significantly better than when fed a similar diet as either intact protein or as free amino acids.

From a practical point of view, it is necessary first to estimate the protein needs of the sick child. Then an appropriate form of protein must be selected. When possible, this should be a high-quality intact protein. There is no evidence that the use of formulas containing only amino acids offers any advantage to patients with decreased protein absorption. On the contrary, evidence suggests that such formulas may represent a significant problem for the patient. They may be poorly tolerated either because of bad taste or high osmolar load. The use of oligopeptides (protein hydrolysates) and formulas that are mixtures of oligopeptides and free amino acids is usually adequate for the enteral support of most patients in need of the specialized defined formula diets who cannot tolerate intact proteins.

Energy and Protein Requirements

In most clinical situations, energy requirements for children are estimated from age. The pediatric population is divided into five groups: the preterm infant (less than 40 weeks' gestational age, infants (0 to 12 months), preschoolers (1 to 5 years old), school-aged children (5 to 11 years old), and adolescents (11 to 18 years old). These five groups are identified to categorize functional and developmental change and to estimate nutritional requirements. Each general grouping implies size, activity, and rate of growth.

Actual energy requirements vary widely among healthy individuals and as one might imagine are even more variable in disease. For the healthy individual, energy requirements may be estimated from the guidelines provided by the National Academy of Sciences, National Research Council (also known as the Recommended Dietary Allowances [RDAs])[52] (Table 83–4). From birth through age 10 years, the RDA for energy is estimated from intakes associated with normal growth in children of the developed world (data compiled by World Health Organization [WHO] on energy intakes of healthy children in the United States, Canada, the United Kingdom, and Sweden).[53] Above age 10, separate allowances are identified for boys and girls because of the onset of puberty.

The 10th edition RDA[52] recommends a mean of 108 kcal per kg per day for infants up to 6 months of age and 98 kcal per kg per day for infants 6 to 12 months of age. Although these numbers are based on studies of "normal intake," actual energy intakes vary widely in this range. Dewey and Lonnerdal[54] report that intakes averaged 107 kcal per kg per day at 1 month of age and declined to 85 kcal per kg per day over the next 6 months.

Stewart and associates[55] report a range of 52 to 152 kcal per kg per day consumed by a group of infants studied at 3-month intervals, with total average intakes declining with age. These reports clearly emphasize that the RDA values provide only an estimate of caloric needs. When determinations of energy requirements are crucial to the management of a particular patient, they must never be determined by charts or "rule-of-thumb" calculations. Instead, the clinical response to feeding (appropriate weight gain or loss or change over time in objective measurements of body composition such as skin-fold thickness) is the most valuable indicator of caloric adequacy. If techniques for assessing resting energy expenditure are available, they must be interpreted with caution but may provide valuable assistance in determining energy requirements.

In many clinical settings, the simple application of the RDAs as a screening evaluation of caloric requirements may be sufficient for the well-nourished child. The RDAs are not an adequate tool, however, for the determination of energy needs for sick or malnourished children, such as patients with the conditions listed in Table 83–1.

Activity and injury "factors" have been suggested for calculating the increase in energy expenditure with various types of injury in the patient population. Although these values have not been validated in the pediatric population, they have been used in the pediatric clinical setting to account for observed differences in energy needs during illness and stress.[56]

Occasionally estimation of energy requirements is complicated by the presence of multiple processes occurring simultaneously, for example, when increased needs caused by infection complicate postoperative wound healing, or decreased needs result from inactivity or increased body fat. Special circumstances such as these may warrant special assessment techniques such as indirect calorimetry.

Any discussion of energy requirements requires consideration of protein requirements as well, and vice versa. The present RDAs (10th edition) for protein requirements are in part influenced by recent data on observed intakes of healthy children but are also affected by estimates derived from data on nitrogen-balance studies in the age group 6 months to 9 years.[52] Because there are large gaps in the experimental data, a modified factorial approach was used by the WHO group to estimate a "safe level of intake." This safe level is defined as the average requirement plus 2 standard deviations. This is in contrast to estimates of energy requirements, which are based on the average requirement of a group of normal, healthy individuals. It is important to understand this fundamental difference in recommendations of the RDA. The different approaches were deemed appropriate because if all individuals consumed protein at levels equal to or moderately greater than the "safe level of intake," there would be little chance that any would have inadequate intake or be subject to harmful effects. On the other hand, a level of energy intake that ensures a low probability of inadequate intake (median plus 2 standard deviations) is also a level that would ensure that some individuals would overconsume, become obese, and become predisposed to disease states of the obese. Again, one must keep in mind that RDAs for protein intake are intended to apply only to healthy individuals whose energy intake is adequate. In considering the ideal protein needs in diseased and stressed states, it should be recognized that protein and energy metabolism are interrelated.

Vitamins and Minerals

Vitamin and mineral requirements for the pediatric population are listed in the RDA[52] (Table 83–5). In general, individuals who consume a varied diet that is adequate for the macronutrients (total energy, protein, and fat) are at a low risk for vitamin and mineral deficiencies.

Potential vitamin and mineral deficiencies in the pediatric population may occur even with adequate caloric intake, in the presence of fat malabsorption, drug/nutrient interactions, and with prolonged tube feeding with highly specialized diets.

PRETERM INFANTS

Optimizing the delivery of protein and energy is of paramount importance for the management of the preterm, small-for-gestational age and low-birth-weight infant. The nutritional requirements of these infants are higher per kilogram body weight than those of normal weight full-term infants, as is their surface area, relative to weight. In addition, they have an accelerated rate of growth. Premature birth, in particular, increases energy, protein, and mineral needs for growth. During the last 10 weeks of gestation, normal fetal weight doubles, length increases by 25%, and two thirds of mineral deposition in the fetal skeleton occurs.[57]

Because exact energy requirements for the preterm infant are unknown, the goal of nutrition in this high-risk group has been to approximate the growth in utero of a normal fetus at the postconception age.[57a] Numerous studies of energy expenditure and protein-energy balance have been conducted to determine the dietary requirements of the preterm infant because utilization of observed mean intakes is an inappropriate method in this population. In addition to a more rapid rate of growth and limited energy stores, there is no reason to believe that preterm infants possess an adequately developed appetite mechanism to modulate intake as does the healthy full-term infant.[58]

Although different expert committees estimate the mean energy requirements with generally good agreement, it is worth noting the large range in energy expenditure cited by the European Society of Paediatric Gastroenterology and Nutrition Committee (ESPGNC)

TABLE 83–5. FOOD AND NUTRITION BOARD, NATIONAL ACADEMY OF SCIENCES—NATIONAL RESEARCH COUNCIL RECOMMENDED DIETARY ALLOWANCES (Revised 1989)[a]
Designed for the maintenance of good nutrition of practically all healthy people in the United States

Category	Age (yr) or Condition	Weight[b] (kg)	Weight[b] (lb)	Height[b] (cm)	Height[b] (in)	Protein (g)	Fat-Soluble Vitamins: Vitamin A (μg RE)[c]	Vitamin D (μg)[d]	Vitamin E (mg α-TE)[e]	Vitamin K (μg)
Infants	0.0–0.5	6	13	60	24	13	375	7.5	3	5
	0.5–1.0	9	20	71	28	14	375	10	4	10
Children	1–3	13	29	90	35	16	400	10	6	15
	4–6	20	44	112	44	24	500	10	7	20
	7–10	28	62	132	52	28	700	10	7	30
Males	11–14	45	99	157	62	45	1,000	10	10	45
	15–18	66	145	176	69	59	1,000	10	10	65
	19–24	72	160	177	70	58	1,000	10	10	70
	25–50	79	174	176	70	63	1,000	5	10	80
	51+	77	170	173	68	63	1,000	5	10	45
Females	11–14	46	101	157	62	46	800	10	8	55
	15–18	55	120	163	64	44	800	10	8	60
	19–24	58	128	164	65	46	800	10	8	65
	25–50	63	138	163	64	50	800	5	8	65
	51+	65	143	160	63	50	800	5	8	65
Pregnant						60	800	10	10	65
Lactating	1st 6 months					65	1,300	10	12	65
	2nd 6 months					62	1,200	10	11	65

[a]The allowances, expressed as average daily intakes over time, are intended to provide for individual variations among most normal persons as they live in the United States under usual environmental stresses. Diets should be based on a variety of common foods in order to provide other nutrients for which human requirements have been less well defined. See text [in original source] for detailed discussion of allowances and of nutrients not tabulated.

[b]Weights and heights of Reference Adults are actual medians for the U. S. population of the designated age, as reported by NHANES II. The median weights and heights of those under 19 years of age were taken from Hamill et al: (1979) (see pages 16–17 [in original source]).The use of these figures does not imply that the height-to-weight ratios are ideal.

[c]Retinol equivalents. 1 retinol equivalent (RE) = 1 μg retinol or 6 μg β-carotene. See text [in original source] for calculation of vitamin A activity of diets as retinol equivalents.

as compared with the recommendations provided by the American Academy of Pediatrics Committee on Nutrition (Table 83–6). The large variability cited stresses the importance of carefully considering the "individual" when estimating energy expenditure in the clinical setting. For example, for an infant who is unusually active, who is handled frequently, and who may be malabsorbing, intake should be appropriately adjusted upward.[59]

The estimated requirements of protein are based on the net fetal accretion rate of protein, 3.5 to 4.0 gm per kg per day (Table 83–7). Care must be taken to avoid increasing the protein content of the preterm diet because excessive protein can potentially be harmful. This is because of the immaturity of the preterm infant's metabolic and excretory functions.[60] Gaull and associates[61] report that infants fed whey-predominant (60:40) formulas, with whey-casein protein ratios similar to those of human milk, had metabolic indices and plasma amino acid levels closer to those of infants fed pooled, mature human milk.[61]

Selected vitamin and mineral requirements for the preterm infant are outlined in Table 83–7. Requirements are based on body weight/gestational age (800 to 1,200 gm versus 1,200 to 1,800 gm) and are based on rates of retention of individual nutrients and minerals.

ADMINISTRATION OF SPECIAL DIETS

The first principle of nutrition support is to use the enteral rather than the parenteral route. Some patients' nutritional requirements may be met by manipulating their regular diet. Others may require supplements to provide the needed nutrition. If the patient is either unable or unwilling to take adequate nutrition through the normal oral route, one of the alternatives (nasogastric feeding, gastrostomy, nasojejunal feeding, jejunostomy) must be used.

Nasogastric feeding is the procedure of choice for most infants and children who have functioning gastrointestinal tracts but are either unable or unwilling to take food orally. We use a 6 or an 8 Fr soft polyurethane feeding tube, weighted at the tip, for tube feeding. This tube may be left in place for many days without irritation or other adverse affects. This soft, flexible tube has made long-term nasogastric feeding a viable modality of nutritional treatment. (If such a soft tube is not available and harder clear plastic tubes must be employed, prolonged nasogastric feeding is contraindicated.)

Many people report difficulty in passing the newer polyurethane nasogastric tube because it is so soft. Some manufacturers now provide an indwelling stylet that gives the tube more rigidity and therefore makes it easier to pass. It is our experience that the use of this stylet is unnecessary but likely to be preferred by the patient and staff. The proper way to pass the soft nasogastric tube involves the slow and often meticulous process of passing the tube to the nasopharynx via the nares and then having the patient swallow the tube. For a few children, this seems very difficult. For most, it is easily accomplished the first time. We suggest the use of viscous (2%) lidocaine (Xylocaine) jelly on the tip of

TABLE 83–5. FOOD AND NUTRITION BOARD, NATIONAL ACADEMY OF SCIENCES—NATIONAL RESEARCH COUNCIL RECOMMENDED DIETARY ALLOWANCES (Revised 1989)[a] *Continued*

Designed for the maintenance of good nutrition of practically all healthy people in the United States

Water-Soluble Vitamins							Minerals						
Vitamin C (mg)	*Thiamin (mg)*	*Riboflavin (mg)*	*Niacin (mg NE)*[f]	*Vitamin B_6 (mg)*	*Folate (μg)*	*Vitamin B_{12} (μg)*	*Calcium (mg)*	*Phosphorus (mg)*	*Magnesium (mg)*	*Iron (mg)*	*Zinc (mg)*	*Iodine (μg)*	*Selenium (μg)*
30	0.3	0.4	5	0.3	25	0.3	400	300	40	6	5	40	10
35	0.4	0.5	6	0.6	35	0.5	600	500	60	10	5	50	15
40	0.7	0.8	9	1.0	50	0.7	800	800	80	10	10	70	20
45	0.9	1.1	12	1.1	75	1.0	800	800	120	10	10	90	20
45	1.0	1.2	13	1.4	100	1.4	800	800	170	10	10	120	30
50	1.3	1.5	17	1.7	150	2.0	1,200	1,200	270	12	15	150	40
60	1.5	1.8	20	2.0	200	2.0	1,200	1,200	400	12	15	150	50
60	1.5	1.7	19	2.0	200	2.0	1,200	1,200	350	10	15	150	70
60	1.5	1.7	19	2.0	200	2.0	800	800	350	10	15	150	70
60	1.2	1.4	15	2.0	200	2.0	800	800	350	10	15	150	70
50	1.1	1.3	15	1.4	150	2.0	1,200	1,200	280	15	12	150	45
60	1.1	1.3	15	1.5	180	2.0	1,200	1,200	300	15	12	150	50
60	1.1	1.3	15	1.6	180	2.0	1,200	1,200	280	15	12	150	55
60	1.1	1.3	15	1.6	180	2.0	800	800	280	15	12	150	55
60	1.0	1.2	13	1.6	180	2.0	800	800	280	10	12	150	55
70	1.5	1.6	17	2.2	400	2.2	1,200	1,200	300	30	15	175	65
95	1.6	1.8	20	2.1	280	2.6	1,200	1,200	355	15	19	200	75
90	1.6	1.7	20	2.1	260	2.6	1,200	1,200	340	15	16	200	75

[d]As cholecalciferol. 10 μg cholecalciferol = 400 IU of vitamin D.
[e]α-Tocopherol equivalents. 1 mg *d*-α tocopherol = 1 mg α-TE. See text for variation in allowances and calculation of vitamin E activity of the diet as α-tocopherol equivalent.
[f]1 NE (niacin equivalent) is equal to 1 mg of niacin or 60 mg of dietary tryptophan.
Reprinted with permission from RECOMMENDED DIETARY ALLOWANCES. 10TH EDITION. Copyright 1989 by the National Academy of Sciences. Published by the National Academy Press, Washington, D.C.

the tube. In addition, before insertion, a little jelly may be applied via a cotton-tip applicator to the nares. The applicator may be advanced a short way so the patient's anterior nares are completely anesthetized. This will enhance the initial insertion of the tube. The older child is given some ice chips to hold in a cup. The younger child is suitably restrained. The nasogastric tube coated with the anesthetic ointment is slowly inserted to the back of the nasopharynx and gradually, over 1 to 2 minutes, advanced through the nasopharynx and into the esophagus. If the youngster seems unduly distressed, further advancement is delayed until the area is anesthetized from the anesthetic jelly. If a stylet is employed, the increased rigidity speeds the passage and allows the exertion of more forward force to expedite passage through the nasopharynx and into the esophagus.

The proper position of the tube in the stomach is checked by injecting air while listening over the abdomen. If there is any question about the position of the tube, a radiograph is taken. Nasobronchial insertion without significant respiratory distress has been described[62] with the use of a small-diameter feeding tube (inserted with the "help" of a stylet). After the first one or two insertions, the anesthetic jelly is unnecessary. Properly done, the procedure is not traumatic and is generally readily accomplished. The entire process is analogous to the placement of an intravenous needle, only less traumatic. For most children, starting an intravenous line is not difficult; for some, it is more of a problem; and for a few, it requires a great deal of patience and expertise. Overall most children greatly prefer the tube to intravenous therapy, as do most hospital staff, once they have gained some experience with the technique. Occasionally the nasogastric tube will be vomited and will come out through the mouth. The observation of the tube going into the nose and coming out of the mouth may be distressing to the patient or the patient's family. The situation should be handled in a calm, firm way, with the tube retrieved an appropriate length and the child made to swallow the tube again.

A few children will vomit several times in the first 12 to 24 hours. For these children, the tube should be immediately and matter-of-factly replaced. Virtually all children tolerate the tube after the first 24 to 36 hours.

Table 83–6. ESTIMATIONS OF ENERGY REQUIREMENT (kcal/kg/day) FOR THE PREMATURE INFANT

Factor	American Academy of Pediatrics*	European Society of Paediatric Gastroenterology and Nutrition†	
		Average	*Range*
Energy expenditure			
Resting metabolic rate	50	52.5	45–60
Activity	15	7.5	5–10
Cold stress	10	7.5	5–10
Synthesis/thermic effect of food	8	17.5	10–25
Energy stored	25	25.0	20–30
Energy excreted	12	20.0	10–30
Estimated energy requirement	120	130	95–165

*Data adapted from Forbes GB, Woodruff CW: Pediatric Nutrition Handbook. 2nd ed. Elk Grove, IL, American Academy of Pediatrics, 1985; with permission.
†Data from Committee on Nutrition of Preterm Infant, European Society of Paediatric Gastroenterology and Nutrition and Feeding of Preterm Infants. Oxford, Blackwell Scientific, 1987.

Table 83–7. ESTIMATED REQUIREMENTS AND ADVISABLE INTAKES FOR PRETERM INFANTS FOR PROTEIN AND MAJOR MINERALS

Requirement	Tissue Increment (per day)	Estimated Requirement (per day)	Advisable Intake *per day*	Advisable Intake *per kg**	Advisable Intake *per 100 kcal†*
Body weight 800 to 1,200 gm (26–28 weeks' gestational age)					
Protein (gm)	2.32	3.64	4.0	4.0	3.1
Sodium (mEq)	1.63	3.22	3.5	3.5	2.7
Chloride (mEq)	1.23	2.79	3.1	3.1	2.4
Potassium (mEq)	0.87	2.52	2.5	2.5	1.9
Calcium (mg)	116.0	188.0	210.0	210.0	160.0
Phosphorus (mg)	75.0	126.0	140.0	140.0	108.0
Magnesium (mg)	3.2	8.7	10.0	10.0	7.5
Body weight 1,200 to 1,800 gm (29–31 weeks' gestational age)					
Protein (gm)	3.01	4.78	5.2	3.5	2.7
Sodium (mEq)	1.77	4.08	4.5	3.0	2.3
Chloride (mEq)	1.30	3.47	3.8	2.5	2.0
Potassium (mEq)	1.03	3.45	3.4	2.3	1.8
Calcium (mg)	154.0	251.0	280.0	185.0	140.0
Phosphorus (mg)	98.0	171.0	185.0	123.0	95.0
Magnesium (mg)	4.0	11.7	13.0	8.5	6.5

*Assuming body weight of 1,000 and 1,500 gm for the 800 to 1,200 and 1,200 to 1,800 gm infants.
†Assuming calorie intake of 130 kcal/kg per day.
Adapted from Ziegler EE, Biga RL, Fomon SJ: Nutritional requirements of the preterm infant. *In* Suskind RM, ed: Textbook of Pediatric Nutrition. New York, Raven Press, 1981, p 32; with permission.

The vast majority tolerate it immediately. The cooperation and determination of the nursing and medical staff are of paramount importance. The family's role is also important. Generally speaking, when the importance of the tube to the child's nutrition is explained, the family is supportive. The tube must not be presented as a punishment. Frequently children are informed that if they do not eat the appropriate amount of calories, they "will need the tube." This approach is unwarranted and leads to poor results. A matter-of-fact, direct approach when tube feeding becomes necessary is much more appropriate.

If it is desirable to pass the tube through the pylorus, the patient should be placed in the right lateral position. The tube is passed, the position is checked on a radiograph to make sure there is adequate tubing in the stomach, and the patient is allowed to pass the tube spontaneously or with the aid of an appropriate dose of metoclopramide. The tube is generally expected to pass within the first 24 to 36 hours, if not much sooner.

Once a tube is in place, the patient may, if the physicians are agreeable, eat around the tube. In other words, the child may eat or drink via the mouth and may be supplemented by the nasogastric tube. Some children, particularly adolescents, have such strong feelings against the tube that they choose to remove the tube and to drink the formula without the tube. Although this is unusual, it is definitely not rare. Such children should be afforded the opportunity to do this.

The use of nasojejunal feedings has been described[63–67] as a successful and safe method for the nutritional support of sick, low-birth-weight infants as well as older children. Simply, the principle is to deposit the formula beyond the pylorus so the pyloric sphincter prevents regurgitation. Theoretically the relatively large surface area of the intestinal villi should allow for the rapid absorption of iso-osmolar solutions. A small weighted silicone rubber tube can easily pass into the jejunum of a newborn. Placement of the tube in the jejunum, however, does result in some reflux of formula back into the stomach. The use of a needle-catheter jejunostomy has been described for adults,[68] and we have begun to employ this technique in children, although our experience is still limited.

The nasojejunal or jejunostomy infusion should be managed in the same manner as the nasogastric tube feeding, with a gradual increase in rate and formula concentration until a child's nutritional requirements are met. Constant infusion over a 24-hour period results in greater tolerance than bolus feedings. In general, because the formula is passing directly into the jejunum and bypassing the important control mechanisms in the stomach and proximal duodenum, the formula should be designed to be readily assimilated. Pain, nausea, distention, flatulence, hypermotility, and diarrhea may result from challenging the small intestine with feedings of intact protein, complex carbohydrates, long-chain triglyceride, or even an appropriate formula with too high an osmolarity or volume. Nonetheless, we have generally been surprised at how well jejeunostomy feedings are tolerated without the need to resort to specialized formulas. Before beginning any feeding in the premature or newborn infant, the risks of necrotizing enterocolitis must be assessed.

Patients with severe neurologic impairment, severe gastroesophageal disease, in a postoperative period after gastroesophageal surgery, or with severe cardiorespiratory disease may have functioning gastrointestinal tracts but require placement of either a temporary or permanent feeding gastrostomy. The considerations of using this route are similar to those using the nasogastric tube. Additionally, the patient is evaluated for gastroesophageal reflux with a pH probe. According to the results, a percutaneous endoscopic gastrostomy or a surgical gastrostomy is considered. The presence of gastroesophageal reflux does not contraindicate the placement of a gastrostomy. If the reflux is severe, however, a surgical gastrostomy with fundoplication is considered. Once established, care must be taken to prevent accidental dislodgment of the gastrostomy feeding tube. Bleeding, significant discomfort, and generalized peritonitis secondary to leakage of formula from the gastrostomy site may result from the purposeful or accidental dislodgment of the gastrostomy by the patient. We have employed the technique of percutaneous endoscopic gastrostomy successfully in a large number of children and infants and find this a highly acceptable method for patients who will require long-term tube feeding.

Starting the Feeding

Formula infusion by any of the above-mentioned routes may be either intermittent or continuous. Our experience strongly indicates that continuously infused feedings are better tolerated than bolus feedings. Further, we as well as others[69] have found that the amount of calories that can be administered to a sick patient is greater when the formula is infused continuously rather than intermittently. The attempted use of bolus feedings in the sick child represents an unwarranted delay for the sick child in need of nutrition. With bolus feedings, there is more nausea and vomiting and more cramping and diarrhea. More importantly, when patients who are not tolerating bolus feedings are switched to continuous feedings, there is frequently a marked improvement in, if not complete cessation of, their symptoms.

Continuous feedings should be instituted by beginning the infusion with a dilute formula, at a rate of just a few milliliters per hour. If this rate is tolerated, it may be advanced rapidly over the next several hours, perhaps doubling the rate every 2 or 3 hours until a maintenance fluid level is achieved. Once a satisfactory volume is being infused, the concentration of the solution may be increased until adequate nutrition is achieved. This process may take hours or months depending on the integrity of the gastrointestinal tract mucosa. In cases in which it is impossible to deliver an adequate volume of formula or an adequate amount of nutrition via the gastrointestinal tract, supplemental parenteral fluid or nutrition may have to be provided.

When vomiting is a problem, the cause of the vomiting should be determined as soon as possible. In determining cause, it is important that an observer be present when vomiting occurs. Consideration must first be given to medications, overfeeding, intrinsic disease, psychogenic factors, patient position, and improper formula. Only after these factors have been ruled out should "tube intolerance" be considered. At that point, the history must be rechecked with regard to the frequency of vomiting before the tube feeding and the relationship of vomiting to the administration of any particular medication. Vomiting in itself is not an absolute contraindication to tube feeding.

Once a special enteral feeding is begun, we recommend that the patient be monitored as if he or she were receiving total parenteral nutrition. The frequency of laboratory work must be individualized, but the safest course is to observe the patient extremely closely during the first days of any special enteral nutritional regimen. Table 83–8 lists complications of special enteral feeding.

A deep commitment from all involved in the care of the child is essential for successful tube feeding. Occasionally there is a period early in the therapy when frequent tube insertion seems necessary. If this occurs, the patient and more frequently the staff become frustrated. Tube feeding must be viewed as an important or even life-saving therapy. The use of the nasogastric tube is the least invasive of a variety of alimentation techniques, including gastrostomy and parenteral alimentation. As pediatric centers become more experienced with the use of central hyperalimentation, the use of a parenteral route becomes simple, nonmessy, and even easy. The use of parenteral alimentation in a child whose gastrointestinal tract is functioning or can be made to provide adequate nutrition is clearly inappropriate.

Home Tube Feeding

Before a patient becomes a candidate for home tube feedings, there are many factors to consider. The nutrition support nurse who will follow the patient and act as a coordinator of the patient's care must develop a rapport with the patient and caregiver to provide a comfortable environment. The nutrition support team, consisting of the attending physician(s) (pediatrician, pediatric gastroenterologist, pediatric surgeon, other pediatric subspecialists), fellows, nurses, nutritionists, and social workers, generally discuss the feasibility of home enteral feedings on rounds or during discharge planning. Many aspects of the patient's care must be considered, including the effects of the therapy on medications, chemotherapy, travel to office visits, planned vacations, camp, and so forth. One member of the team, usually the nutrition support nurse, is responsible for taking the initiative for providing support to the patient or caregiver in the decision to learn home enteral feedings. The team addresses the physical and emotional needs of the patient, the availability and competency of the caregiver, the family and home

Table 83–8. COMPLICATIONS OF SPECIAL ENTERAL FEEDING

Overhydration (especially with concurrent parenteral fluid administation)
Hyperglycemia
Azotemia (with excessively increased protein intakes)
Hypovitaminosis K
Dehydration secondary to diarrhea
Mineral and electrolyte disorders (especially secondary to vomiting and diarrhea)
Failure to gain weight secondary to inadequate energy intake
Aspiration
Nutrient deficiency (secondary to formula error)

environment, the community, and the financial resources of the patient.

Patients are referred for home tube feedings because they no longer need inpatient care beyond that required for special nutritional support. In the hospital setting, as already described, the patient is placed on tube feedings at a slow rate via an enteral pump until able to tolerate an adequate amount of formula for nutritional needs. This affords the opportunity to see how the patient and family are likely to respond to problems they may encounter at home. Changes in weight and caloric intake are carefully followed so changes that occur at home can be better anticipated.

The nutrition support nurse instructs the caregiver or patient to use safely and independently a nasogastric tube (or nasojejunal tube, gastrostomy, or jejeunostomy) for home tube feedings. Although this generally requires several days, we usually plan on 5 days for training. The first lesson is a demonstration. The caregiver or patient is provided with a diagram of the basic anatomy of the head, neck, stomach, and lungs. The patient or caregiver is encouraged to discuss fears and understanding of the nasogastric feedings. Individuals often have misconceptions, which are clarified. Written educational materials are also provided.

First, the importance of handwashing is stressed as the most effective means of decreasing contamination. Next, the nasogastric tube is taken from its package and inspected. As in the hospital tube feeding, a no. 6 or a no. 8 Fr polyurethane tube is used, and a stylet is advised. The caregiver is instructed to inspect the tube for any defects, to check the feeding hole and weighted end, and to pull on the wire stylet to see if it can be freely removed. The tube is then measured and marked from the feeding hole. The actual length is assessed as the distance from the nostril to the tip of the ear and then to the midpoint between the xiphoid process and the umbilicus. The tube is marked at this point with a piece of contrasting colored tape. The process is repeated during the training period to ensure accuracy. Caregivers are encouraged to participate in these activities and are continuously given positive reinforcement.

When ready, the patient is positioned for insertion of the nasogastric tube. (Patients and their parents have usually, although not always, had extended experience with tube feeding in the hospital.) An infant would be swaddled and placed on a 45 degree angle or in an infant's seat. A toddler could be swaddled in the same matter. A school-aged child and adolescent would be encouraged to place the tube themselves with supervision. Often this is not practical for the first one or two passages. The tube is lubricated with a water-soluble lubricant and held in the hand by the thumb and index finger. It is placed in the nostril and advanced through the nasal opening and threaded down until the mark is reached. Patients gag, tear, and cry during insertion. If their reaction is excessive, the tube may be removed and insertion attempted at another time. Once the tube is passed to the prescribed length, the wire stylet is removed, and the tube is taped laterally to the nares with a piece of hypoallergenic tape. The tube is not taped to the nostril or pulled tightly against it because even with a soft tube this could lead to pressure sores. It is necessary to tape the tube as close to the nostril as possible. This is important because the area often becomes moist from mucus, tears, and saliva, and the ease with which a young child may remove the tube is increased when the tape is distant from the insertion site.

During and even after insertion, the patient is continuously monitored for signs and symptoms of incorrect tube placement. The caregiver is instructed to assess the patient for excessive coughing, breathing difficulty, and color changes. If there is any concern, the tube is removed immediately. After placement, the patient is comforted and held by the caregiver to provide security and to be quieted. This is the perfect time to check placement. A 60-ml syringe is used to instill 4 ml of air, which exerts a gentle pressure on the tube. It is not recommended to use smaller syringes because of the increased force they exert on the tube. A teaching stethoscope with two sets of ear pieces may be used during the lessons in the hospital, so the caregiver can recognize the sound of air instillation into the tube when listening left of the umbilicus. If the sound is not heard, the air is instilled again. If it is still not heard, the tube is removed.

The nasogastric tube is then used for feeding, using a regimen that has been well tolerated in the past. The first days of patient instruction are not the best time for initiation of changes in the tube feeding, especially if those changes are likely to be difficult to tolerate. This is most often true for changes from continuous to bolus feeds. The physical therapy, speech pathology, and occupational therapy departments may have to be consulted to evaluate the patient and provide oral stimulation. The caregivers are taught exercises that are repeated at home, so sucking and swallowing skills are not forgotten.

During the following lessons, the caregiver is encouraged to place the nasogastric tube with the assistance of the instructor. The lessons are individualized to each patient. Caregivers are encouraged "to room in" if possible, so they can feel comfortable giving the feedings and learn the normal patterns of the patient, i.e., bowel, bladder, sleep, spit up, in a controlled hospital environment.

Caregivers are instructed on the use of an enteral pump. The pump should be the same pump that will be used at home. This usually requires two to three lessons for the caregiver to prepare independently enteral feeding bags, program pump, and troubleshoot alarms.

Supplies and formula are usually provided by an infusion company. If the patient has multiple needs such as medications, monitoring, oxygen, suctioning, occupational therapy, or physical therapy, he or she may be referred to a certified home health agency, which delivers the supplies and services to the home. These should be the identical supplies used by the instructor, so the caregiver has mastered their use. A nursing visit is generally provided within the first 24 hours of discharge, and the caregiver is given all important phone numbers: the physician, the nutrition support nurse, the nutritionist, and a 24-hour hotline number that is available from the infusion company for any technical crisis that may occur with equipment. Discharge is planned for early in the day, so if a problem arises at home there are many resources available. The nutrition support nurse telephones the patient or caregiver the day of discharge to offer reassurance.

Follow-up care of the patient is provided by the members of the nutrition support team. The patient is seen as an outpatient for continuing assessment of nutritional status, compliance, and emotional status. The nutrition support nurse maintains regular contact with patients to monitor their progress.

If the patient requires long-term tube feeding (in excess of 3 months) or the patient or caregiver cannot tolerate insertion of the tube, a gastrostomy is considered. When a patient has a gastrostomy, the patient or caregiver is instructed how to care for the gastrostomy in the hospital. This requires 2 to 3 days. The patient or caregiver changes the dressing, gives the feedings, learns the operation of the enteral pump if indicated, and troubleshoots possible complications. On our service, patients are not discharged until the nutrition support team feels comfortable that the patient and caregiver are capable of independent care of the gastrostomy.

A low-profile gastrostomy connecting device is considered for patients who are active. These small devices, although expensive, are highly regarded by parents and patients alike. The low-profile device is individually measured and ordered from the manufacturer. The gastrostomy track must traditionally be healed before any attempt at insertion of the low-profile device (generally 4 to 6 weeks after placement). The gastrostomy tube is removed, and the device is placed by the physician. The patients and caregivers often prefer this small device as compared with the long gastrostomy tube. The low-profile device typically is supplied as a set, which contains special adapters that fit into the device and allow the gastrostomy feedings to be given.[70] Recently, placement of a low-profile gastrostomy tube as the initial procedure has been described.[93]

Using the approach discussed, we have discharged hundreds of children for long-term home enteral "tube" therapy with outstanding tolerance and excellent results of treatment.

SUMMARY

The first route for the nutritional support of a sick child is via the alimentary canal. Enteral alimentation provides an acceptable and effective method for maintaining and repleting the nutritional state of pediatric patients who have functioning gastrointestinal tracts.

Successful alimentation may be achieved using the oral route or a nasogastric, nasojejunal, gastrostomy, or jejunostomy feeding tube. The choice of the route depends on the primary medical problem and the clinical status of the child who is being supported. Defined formula diets provide flexibility in nutrient composition, caloric density, and osmolarity as well as taste. The biochemical assessment and monitoring of the child receiving enteral alimentation should be approached in the same manner as the assessment of the child receiving total parenteral nutrition. Once successful special alimentation has been established for an inpatient, the patient may be a candidate for continued care at home.

REFERENCES

1. Heimburger DC: Enteral feeding. If the gut works, use it. Ala J Med Sci 1982; 19:387.
2. Lake AM, Kleinman RE, Walker WA: Enteric alimentation in specialized gastrointestinal problems: An alternative to total parenteral nutrition. Adv Pediatr 1981; 28:319.
3. LeLeiko NS, Murray CA, Munro HN: Enteral support of the hospitalized child. *In* Suskind R, ed: Textbook of Pediatric Nutrition. New York, Raven Press, 1981, pp 357–374.
4. Merritt RJ, Sinatra FR, Smith GA: Nutritional support of the hospitalized child. Adv Nutr Res 1983; 5:77.
5. Kennedy-Caldwell C: Pediatric nutritional support. *In* Kennedy-Caldwell C, Grant J, eds: Nutritional Support in Nursing. Philadelphia, WB Saunders, 1988, pp 233–262.
6. Altmann GG: Demonstration of a morphological control mechanism in the small intestine. Role of pancreatic secretions and bile. *In* Dowling RH, Riecken EO, eds: Intestinal Adaptation. New York, Schauttauer Verlag, 1974, pp 33–46.
7. Dworkin LD, Levine GM: Oral intake maintains small intestinal mass, in part, by factors other than direct contact with the small bowel. Clin Res 1975; 23:576A.
8. Feldman EJ, Dowling RH, McNaughton J, Peters TJ: Effects of oral versus intravenous nutrition on intestinal adaptation after small bowel resection in the dog. Gastroenterology 1976; 70:712.
9. Johnson LR, Copeland EM, Dudrick SJ, et al: Structural and hormonal alterations in the gastrointestinal tract of parenterally fed rats. Gastroenterology 1975; 68:1177.
10. Johnson LR: The trophic action of gastrointestinal hormones. Gastroenterology 1976; 70:278.
11. Dworkin LD, Levine GM, Farber NJ, Spector MH: Small intestinal mass of the rat is partially determined by indirect effects of intra-luminal nutrition. Gastroenterology 1976; 71:626.
12. Eastwood GL: Small bowel morphology and epithelial proliferation in intravenously alimented rabbits. Surgery 1977; 82:613.
13. Hughes CA, Bates T, Dowling H: Cholecystokinin and secretin prevent intestinal mucosal hypoplasia of total parenteral nutrition in the dog. Gastroenterology 1978; 75:34.
14. Wahren J, Felig P, Hagenfeldt L: Effect of protein ingestion on splanchnic and leg metabolism in normal man and in patients with diabetes mellitus. J Clin Invest 1976; 57:978–999.
15. Jacobson S, Wester PO: Balance study of twenty trace elements during total patenteral nutrition in man. J Nutr 1977; 37:107–126.
16. LeLeiko NS, Bronstein A, Baliga BS, Munro HN: De novo purine nucleotide synthesis in the rat small and large intestine: Effect of dietary protein and purines. J Pediatr Gastroenterol Nutr 1983; 2:313–319.
17. LeLeiko NS, Martin BA, Walsh MJ, et al: Tissue specific gene expression results from a purine and pyrimidine-free diet and 6-mercaptopurine in the rat small intestine and colon. Gastroenterology 1987; 93:1014–1020.
18. LeLeiko NS, Baliga BS, Wilkins D, et al: Comparison of purine biosynthetic pathways in the small and large bowel (abstract). Gastroenterology 1978; 74:1054.
19. LeLeiko NS, Bronstein A, Munro HN: Effect of dietary purines on de novo synthesis of purine nucleotides in the small intestinal mucosa (abstract). Pediatr Res 1979; 13:403.
20. Walsh MJ, Sanchez-Pozo A, LeLeiko NS: A regulatory element is characterized by purine-mediated and cell-type specific gene transcription. Molec Cell Biol 1990; 10:4356–4364.
21. Munro HN: Differences in metabolic handling of orally versus parenterally administered nutrients. *In* Green M, Greene HL, eds: The Role of the Gastrointestinal Tract in Nutrient Delivery. New York, Academic Press, 1984, pp 183–198.
22. Meeroff JC, Phillips SF: Control of gastric emptying by osmolality of duodenal contents. Gastroenterology 1975; 68:1144.
23. Seidman E, LeLeiko NS, Ament M, et al: Nutritional issues in pediatric inflammatory bowel disease. J Pediatr Gastroenterol Nutr 1991; 12:424–438.
24. Saint Hilaire S, Lavers M, Kennedy J, Code C: Gastric acid secretory value of different foods. Gastroenterology 1960; 39:1.
25. Elwin CE: Gastric acid responses to antral application of some amino acids, peptides, and isolated fractions of a protein hydrolysate. Scand J Gastroenterol 1974; 9:239.

26. Ragins H, Levenson SM, Signer R, et al: Intrajejunal administration of an elemental diet at neutral pH avoids pancreatic stimulation: Studies in dog and man. Am J Surg 1973; 126:606.
27. Voitk AJ, Brown RA, McArdle AH, et al: Use of an elemental diet in the treatment of complicated pancreatitis. Am J Surg 1973; 125:223.
28. Bury KD, Stevens RV, Randall HT: Use of a chemically defined, liquid elemental diet in nutritional management of fistulas of the alimentary tract. Am J Surg 1971; 121:174.
29. Porter JM, Snowe RJ, Silver D: Tuberculous enteritis with perforation and abscess formation in childhood. Surgery 1972; 71:254.
30. Voitk AJ, Brown RA, McArdle AH, et al: Clinical uses of an elemental diet—preliminary studies. Can Med Assoc J 1972; 107:123.
31. Clark SB, Holt PR: Inhibition of steady-state absorption of long chain triglyceride by medium-chain triglyceride on the unanesthesized rat. Gastroenterology 1969; 56:214.
32. Greenberger NJ, Rodgers JB, Isselbacher KJ: Absorption of medium and long chain triglycerides: Factors influencing their hydrolysis and transport. J Clin Invest 1966; 45:217.
33. Playoust MC, Isselbacher KJ: Studies on the intestinal absorption and intramucosal lipolysis of a medium chain triglyceride. J Clin Invest 1964; 43:878.
34. Clark SB, Holt PR: Rate-limiting steps in steady-state intestinal absorption of trioctanoin-1-14C. J Clin Invest 1968; 47:612.
35. Valdivieso VD, Schwabe AD: Absorption of medium-chain lipids from the rat cecum. Am J Dig Dis 1966; 11:474.
36. Pihl BG, Glotzor DJ, Patterson JF: Absorption of medium-chain fatty acids by the dog colon. J Appl Physiol 1966; 21:1059.
37. Van Dyke RW: Mechanisms of digestion and absorption of food. *In* Sleisenger MH, Fordtran JS, eds: Gastrointestinal Disease. Vol 2. 4th ed. Philadelphia, WB Saunders, 1989, pp 1062–1088.
38. Plotkin GR, Isselbacher KJ: Secondary disaccharidase deficiency in adult celiac disease (nontropical sprue) and other malabsorption states. N Engl J Med 1964; 271:1033.
39. Welsh JD, Zschiesche OM, Anderson J, Walker A: Intestinal disaccharidase activity in celiac sprue. (Gluten-sensitive enteropathy.) Arch Intern Med 1969; 123:33.
40. Rosensweig NS, Herman RH: Time response of jejunal sucrase and maltase activity to a high sucrase diet in normal man. Gastroenterology 1969; 56:500.
41. Rosensweig NS, Herman RH: Control of jejunal sucrase and maltase activity by dietary sucrose and fructose in man. J Clin Invest 1968; 47:2253.
42. Kerry KR, Anderson CM: A ward test for sugar in feces. Lancet 1964; 1:981.
43. Adibi SA, Soleimanpour M: Functional characterization of dipeptide transport system in human jejunum. J Clin Invest 1974; 53:1368.
44. Alpers D: Digestion and absorption of carbohydrates and proteins. *In* Johnson L, ed: Physiology of the Gastrointestinal Tract. 2nd ed. New York, Raven Press, 1987, pp 1469–1487.
45. Kim YS, Birtwhistle W, Kim YW: Peptide hydrolases in the brush border and soluble fractions of small intestinal mucosa of rat and man. J Clin Invest 1972; 51:1419.
46. Navab F, Asatoor AM: Studies on intestinal absorption of amino acids and a dipeptide in a case of Hartnup disease. Gut 1970; 11:373.
47. Asatoor AM, Harrison BDW, Milne MD, Prosser DI: Intestinal absorption of an arginine-containing peptide in cystinuria. Gut 1972; 13:95.
48. Hellier MD, Holdsworth CD, Perrett D, Thirumalai C: Intestinal dipeptide transport in normal and cystinuric subjects. Clin Sci 1972; 43:659.
49. Adibi SA, Fogel MR: Comparison of free amino acid and dipeptide absorption in the jejunum of sprue patients. Gastroenterology 1974; 67:586.
50. Fogel MR, Ravitch MM, Adibi SA: Free amino acid and dipeptide absorption in the jejunum of patients with jejunoileal bypass for obesity. Gastroenterology 1975; 68:894.
51. Imondi AR, Stradley RP: Utilization of enzymatically hydrolyzed soybean protein and crystalline amino acid diets by rats with exocrine pancreatic insufficiency. J Nutr 1974; 104:793.
52. National Research Council: Recommended Dietary Allowances. 10th ed. Washington DC, National Academy Press, 1989.
53. Energy and Protein Requirements. FAO/WHO/UNU Expert Consultation. Geneva, World Health Organization, 1985.
54. Dewey KG, Lonnerdal B: Nutrition. Growth and fatness of breast-fed infants from one to six months. Fed Proc 1982; 41:352.
55. Stewart RA, Bond J, et al, eds: Infant and Child Feeding. New York, Academic Press, 1981, pp 123–133.
56. Long CL, Shaffel N, Geiger JN, et al: Metabolic response to injury and illness: Estimation of energy and protein needs from indirect calorimetry and nitrogen balance. J Paren Ent Nutr 1979; 3:452–456.
57. Ziegler EE, Bigra RL, Fomon SJ: Nutritional requirements of the premature infant. *In* Suskind RM, ed: Textbook of Pediatric Nutrition. New York, Raven Press, 1981, pp 29–39.
57a. Forbes GB, Woodruff CW: Pediatric Nutrition Handbook. 2nd ed. Elk Grove Village, IL, American Academy of Pediatrics, 1985.
58. Hay W Jr: Neonatal Nutrition and Metabolism. St Louis, Mosby-Year Book, 1991.
59. Committee on Nutrition of Preterm Infant, European Society of Paediatric Gastroenterology and Nutrition and Feeding of Preterm Infants. Oxford, Blackwell Scientific Publications, 1987.
60. Raiha NCR, Heinonen K, Rassin DK, et al: Milk protein quantity and quality in low-birth weight infants: I. Metabolic responses and effects on growth. Pediatrics 1976; 57:659–674.
61. Gaull GE, Rassin PK, Raiha NCR, et al: Milk protein quantity and quality in LBW infants: IV. Effects on sulfur amino acids in plasma and urine. J Pediatr 1977; 90:348.
62. Schorlemmer GR, Battaglini JW: An unusual complication of naso-enteral feeding with small diameter feeding tubes. Ann Surg 1984; 199:104.
63. Beddis I, McKenzie S: Transpyloric feeding in the very low birthweight (1500 G and below) infant. One year's experience in an intensive care neonatal unit. Arch Dis Child 1979; 54:213.
64. Cheek JA, Staub GF: Nasojejunal alimentation for premature and full-term newborn infants. J Pediatr 1973; 82:955.
65. McLean GK, Rombeau JL, Caldwell MD, et al: Transgastrostomy jejunal intubation for enteric alimentation. AJR 1982; 139(6):1129.
66. Rhea JW, Ghazzawi O, Weidman O: Nasojejunal binding: An improved device and intubation technique. J Pediatr 1973; 82:951.
67. Wells DH, Zachman RD: Nasojejunal feedings in low-birth-weight infants. Pediatrics 1975; 87:276.
68. Page CP, Carlton PK, Andrassy RJ, et al: Safe, cost-effective postoperative nutrition. Defined formula diet via needle-catheter jejunostomy. Am J Surg 1979; 138:939.
69. Parker P, Stroop S, Greene H: A controlled comparison of continuous versus intermittent feeding in the treatment of infants with intestinal disease. J Pediatr 1981; 99:360.
70. Huth MM, O'Brien ME: The gastrostomy feeding button. Pediatr Nurs 1987; 13:241–245.
71. Chrysomilides SA, Kaminski MV Jr: Home enteral and parenteral nutritional support: A comparison. Am J Clin Nutr. 1981; 34:2271.
72. Greene HL, Helinek GL, Folk CC, et al: Nasogastric tube feeding at home: A method for adjunctive nutritional support of malnourished patients. Am J Clin Nutr 1981; 34:1131.
73. Heymsfield SB, Smith-Andrews JL, Hersch I: Home nasoenteric feeding for malabsorption and weight loss refractory to conventional thrapy. Ann Intern Med 1983; 98:168.
74. Navarro J, Cezard JP, Vargas J: Nasogastric tube feeding at home in gastroenterological pediatric practice (letter). Am J Clin Nutr 1982; 35:408.
75. Rickard KA, Baehner RL, Contes TD, et al: Supportive nutritional intervention in pediatric cancer. Can Res 42 (Suppl):766s.
76. Rickard KA, Kirksey A, Baehner RL, et al: Effectiveness of enteral and parenteral nutrition in the nutritional mangement of children with Wilms' tumors. Am J Clin Nutr 1980; 33:2622.
77. Weizman Z, Schmueli A, Deckelbaum RJ: Continuous nasogastric drip elemental feeding: Alternative for prolonged parenteral nutrition in severe prolonged diarrhea. Am J Dis Child 1983; 137:253.
78. Vanderhoof JA, Hofschire PJ, Baluff MA: Continuous enteral feedings. An important adjunct to the management of complex congenital heart disease. Am J Dis Child 1982; 136:825.
79. Ryan JA Jr, Page CP, Babcock L: Early postoperative jejunal feeding of elemental diet in gastrointestinal surgery. Am Surg 1981; 47:393.
80. Morin CL, Roulet M, Roy CC, Weber A: Continuous elemental enteral alimentation in children with Crohn's disease and growth failure. Gastroenterology 1980; 79:1205.

81. Morin CL, Roulet M, Roy CC, et al: Continuous elemental enteral alimentation in the treatment of children and adolescents with Crohn's disease. J Paren Ent Nutr 1982; 6:194.
82. Morgan MY: Enteral nutrition in chronic liver disease. Acta Chir Scand 1981; 507 (Suppl):81.
83. Smith J, Horowitz J, Henderson JM, Heymsfield S: Enteral hyperalimentation in undernourished patients with cirrhosis and ascites. Am J Clin Nutr 1982; 35:56–72.
84. Takala J: Growth failure due to uremia and congenital nephrosis: Growth enhancement by aggressive nutritional therapy. J Paren Ent Nutr 1982; 6:388.
85. Drew JH, Johnston R, Finocchiaro C, et al: A comparison of nasojejunal with nasogastric feedings in low-birth-weight infants. Aust Paediatr J 1979; 15:98.
86. Milner RD, Minoli I, Moro G, et al: Growth and metabolic and hormonal profiles during transpyloric and nasogastric feeding in preterm infants. Acta Paediatr Scand 1981; 70:9.
87. Greene HL, Parker PH, Slonim AE, Burr IM: Resolution of the need for continuous nocturnal feeding in a patient with severe type I glycogen storage disease. J Pediatr 1981; 99:602.
88. Greene HL, Slonim AE, Burr IM, Moran JR: Type I glycogen storage disease: Five years of management with nocturnal intragastric feeding. J Pediatr 1980; 96:590.
89. Michels VV, Beaudet AL, Potts VE, Montandon CM: Glycogen storage disease: Long-term follow-up of nocturnal intragastric feeding. Clin Genet 1982; 21:136–140.
90. Perlman M, Aker M, Slonim AE: Successful treatment of severe type I glycogen storage disease with neonatal presentation by nocturnal intragastric feeding. J Pediatr 1979; 94:772.
91. Kauste A: Parenteral and enteral nutrition of the thermally injured patient. Ann Chir Gynaecol 1980; 69(5):197.
92. Abras E, Walser M: Nitrogen utilization in uremic patients fed by continuous nasogastric infusion. Kidney Int 1982; 22(4):392.
93. Ferguson RD, Harig JM, Koznrek RA, et al: Placement of a feeding button (one-step button) as the initial procedure. Am J Gastroenterol (in press)

Chapter 84

Parenteral Nutrition in Infants and Children

MARVIN E. AMENT, LAURIE REYEN, and WILLIAM J. GUSS

INTRODUCTION

Parenteral nutrition is a technique for providing the body's nutritional needs through the intravenous route. The nutrients that are typically administered consist of water, dextrose, amino acids, lipid emulsion, minerals, vitamins, and trace metals. Intravenous nutrition has been available for the past 25 years and has become a well-accepted medical practice. Metabolic, mechanical, and infectious complications can occur with its usage. When done in a careful manner, however, these potential complications can be reduced to a minimum.

Parenteral nutrition should not be used in patients who have adequate intestinal function who may be fed orally, enterally, or by gastrostomy feedings. Many patients who traditionally might have been candidates for total parenteral nutrition (TPN) can now be managed as effectively using specialized elemental enteral formulas.[1]

In most instances, parenteral nutrition should not be used for a duration of less than 5 days. It is also usually not considered in patients who are near death and have little or no chance of recovery[2] (Table 84–1). Parenteral nutrition is supportive therapy for burn patients and those with chronic diarrhea, malabsorption, and malnutrition. Infants with congenital gastrointestinal anomalies such as gastroschisis, omphalocele, tracheoesophageal fistula, multiple intestinal atresias, meconium ileus and peritonitis, malrotation and volvulus, or diaphragmatic hernia usually require prolonged intravenous support. TPN may be considered as primary therapy for patients with short bowel syndrome secondary to intestinal resection, for patients with Crohn's disease refractory to medical management, and for patients who have gastrointestinal fistulas.

Newer uses for parenteral nutrition include patients with hepatic failure awaiting liver transplantation and in the posttransplantation period, malnourished oncology patients and patients undergoing bone marrow transplantation, and cardiac patients who are malnourished before surgery and require nutritional support before and after surgery. The use of intravenous nutrition in these complex patients has been associated with a reduced incidence of sepsis and an acceleration of wound healing, and in patients not anergic because of chemotherapy there is evidence of a more rapid return of immune function.[3] Parenteral nutrition is supportive therapy and in itself is not sufficient to reverse the underlying disease process.

Parenteral nutrition has been increasingly used for patients who have acquired immunodeficiency syndrome (AIDS). Parenteral support may be beneficial provided the patient has not had serious or irreversible central nervous system damage.[4] Although it is beneficial in slowing or reversing the malnutrition associated with this condition, it does not measurably improve the immune function of affected patients.

Patients unable to tolerate continuous enteral elemental feeding should be considered for parenteral nutrition. Term infants and children who do not receive oral nutrition for 5 days should have parenteral nutrition started. Very low birth weight (VLBW) infants may become rapidly nutritionally depleted when not fed because of limited endogenous fat stores. Parenteral

Table 84–1. INDICATIONS FOR PARENTERAL NUTRITION*

Intestine Dysfunction	Examples Where Expected to Last >7 Days
Intractable vomiting	Severe acute pancreatitis
Diarrhea	Severe acute flare of inflammatory bowel disease, enteral feeding intolerance
Mucositis	Chemotherapy
Ileus	Severe trauma/major abdominal surgery when adequate enteral diet is not expected to resume within 10 days, sepsis
Small bowel obstruction	Owing to cancer, adhesions, intestinal pseudo-obstruction
Malabsorption	Severe mucosal injury, short bowel syndrome, radiation enteritis, protein losing enteropathy
NPO for 7 or more days	Enterocutaneous fistula, anastomotic leak, ileus, transplantation

*Total parenteral nutrition may be indicated if the intestine is dysfunctional or inaccessible, and this condition is expected to continue beyond 7 to 10 days (3 days in severe malnutrition). Specific indications are listed.
NPO, nothing by mouth.

feedings in these infants, however, may need to be reduced because of limited tolerance to both glucose and lipids. Growth and weight gain in infants and children receiving central venous TPN is equivalent to those fed human milk or standard formulas.[5] This technique has been responsible for improving survival of distressed infants, especially those with gastroschisis and intractable diarrhea of infancy. The development of parenteral nutrition has decreased mortality in these patients from 75 to 90% to less than 10%.[6]

PARENTERAL NUTRITION REQUIREMENTS

Calories (Energy)

Infants generally require more enteral than parenteral calories because a portion of the enterally supplied calories is lost in the stool and expended in the process of digestion and absorption. This is especially true in the immature infant.[7] The typical intravenous caloric requirements based on weight are shown in Table 84–2. For children over 10 years of age, the Harris-Benedict equation may be used to determine basal energy expenditure if the patient's height, weight, and age are known. An equation has been developed that uses the same principles for infants.[8, 9]

Boys: $\text{kcal per 24 hr} = 66 + (13.7 \times W) + (5 \times H) + (6.8 \times A)$

Girls: $\text{kcal per 24 hr} = 655 + (9.6 \times W) + (1.8 \times H) - (4.7 \times A)$

Infants: $\text{kcal per 24 hr} = 22 + (31 \times W) + (1.2 \times H)$

where W = weight in kg; H = height in cm; and A = age in years.

Total energy expenditure in the healthy child can be determined by multiplying the value obtained for basal energy expenditure by a factor of 1.6 to 1.75 for males and 1.5 to 1.65 for females.

Table 84–2. CALORIC REQUIREMENT BY WEIGHT

Patient Age Group	Estimated Daily Calorie Requirement*
Neonatal	
Low birth weight	150 kcal/kg
Normal birth weight	100–120 kcal/kg
Pediatric	
0–10 kg	100 kcal/kg
11–20 kg	1000 kcal + 50 kcal/kg for every kg >10 kg
>20 kg	1500 kcal + 20 kcal/kg for every kg >20 kg
or	
1–7 years old	75–90 kcal/kg
7–12 years old	60–75 kcal/kg
12–18 years old	30–60 kcal/kg
Adult	
Maintain lean body mass	30–35 kcal/kg (33 kcal/kg)
Rebuild lean body mass	35–40 kcal/kg (40 kcal/kg)

*Kilocalories per kilogram ideal body weight. In patients who are severely underweight, actual body weight should be used in place of ideal body weight in the initial days of parenteral nutrition.

Certain conditions are known to increase caloric requirements: fever (12% for each degree above 37° C), cardiac failure (15 to 25%), major surgery (20 to 30%), burns (up to 100%), severe sepsis (25%), and long-term growth failure (50 to 100%). After one determines the basal energy expenditure, caloric needs can be adjusted depending on the degree of stress, nutritional depletion, and activity level found in such patients (mild stress, 1.25; moderate stress, 1.50; and severe stress, 2.0).[10] In the premature infant, the overall requirements for energy may be reduced, and therefore the correction factor due to stress may not be as great.[11]

To establish positive nitrogen balance, both dextrose and amino acids must be provided. Studies in premature infants with weights appropriate for gestational age demonstrate that two isocaloric intravenous feeding regimens will result in substantially different nitrogen balance depending upon whether or not crystalline amino acids are provided.[11] Premature infants gained weight at intravenous intakes of 70 to 90 kcal per kg per day if amino acids were provided at a rate of 2.7 to 3.5 gm per day with growth rates similar to those in utero.[12]

Indirect calorimetry has become increasingly available as a tool to measure resting energy expenditure in adults and children. There are technical problems, however, with measuring oxygen consumption and carbon dioxide production of infants on respirators. Measurements become increasingly inaccurate in patients who require high oxygen concentration, e.g., FIO_2 greater than 40%. Indirect calorimetry can easily be used in infants who are not on respirators, provided the equipment can measure small changes in air flow. It remains unclear whether indirect calorimetry materially alters the amount of nutrients provided to the patient or affects outcome. Our clinical experience suggests that approximately 10% of patients may benefit from its determination.

Central venous parenteral nutrition allows for greater caloric delivery than the peripheral route because more concentrated solutions of dextrose can be used. In patients with respiratory, cardiac, and renal disease who are fluid restricted, central intravenous nutrition may be the only way to provide adequate calories. Concentrations of dextrose up to 30 to 35% may be necessary to provide sufficient carbohydrate calories. Peripheral parenteral nutrition can maximally deliver 80 kcal per kg per day to the patient. In infants, this provides maintenance calories but cannot supply adequate calories for catch-up growth. Because of the lower concentration of dextrose used in peripheral parenteral nutrition, increased amounts of fat are used to provide calories. The ideal mixture, whether central or peripheral, is one in which fat and carbohydrate are both used as energy sources. Intravenous fats are especially useful in patients who have lung disease, such as hyaline membrane disease and cystic fibrosis. Higher fat infusions allowing lower carbohydrate administration decrease carbon dioxide production and the respiratory quotient, decrease fluid administration, and may prevent fatty infiltration of the liver.

Fluids

Multiple factors determine the fluid requirements of infants and children. These include hydration status, size, age, environmental factors, and underlying disease.[13] The typical daily fluid maintenance requirements for pediatric patients are 100 ml per kg for the first 10 kg of body weight, 1,000 ml plus 50 ml per kg for every kilogram above 10 kg, and 1,500 ml plus 20 ml per kg for every kilogram above 20 kg. The fluid requirements of premature infants are unique.[8, 14] Infants of 1,000 gm or less should receive 140 ml per kg per day by the third day of life and 150 ml per kg per day by the beginning of the third week. Fluid requirements are increased in infants and children with elevated body temperature, diarrhea, glycosuria, use of radiant warmers and conventional single-walled incubators, diuretic treatment, phototherapy, respiratory distress, infection, and an ambient temperature above the neutral thermal range.

Conditions that reduce fluid requirements include bubble-walled incubators, heat shields, thermal blankets, relatively high humidity, oliguria, and the use of humidified air via an endotracheal tube. Patent ductus arteriosus,[15] bronchopulmonary dysplasia,[16] necrotizing enterocolitis,[17] and intraventricular hemorrhage[18] have been associated with excessive fluid intake greater than 150 ml per kg per day. In newborns free of renal disease, urine volumes of less than 2 ml per kg per hour and a urine specific gravity of greater than 1.010 suggest an inadequate state of hydration.

Carbohydrates

Dextrose is the major source of nonprotein calories in parenteral nutrition. It provides 3.4 kcal per gm in the monohydrate form. This differs from enteral glucose, which provides 4 kcal per gm. The osmolality of parenteral nutrition solutions depends primarily on the dextrose concentration. The limitation of peripheral parenteral nutrition is phlebitis associated with the use of dextrose concentrations greater than 10 to 12.5%. Even with low concentration dextrose solutions, peripheral intravenous catheters have a relatively short life span. Successfully maintaining intravenous access often becomes a problem in patients who require prolonged nutritional support.

Carbohydrate administration is initiated in a stepwise fashion to allow the body to respond with endogenous insulin production and to prevent glycosuria with a secondary osmotic diuresis. In central venous parenteral nutrition, concentrations of 10 to 15% are initially started and then increased until the final concentration is achieved.[19, 20] When glucose is the sole caloric source, it leads to a greater degree of water retention and is more likely to lead to hepatic steatosis than if it is combined with intravenous lipids.[21] Carbon dioxide production is also significantly higher when glucose is the sole source of nonprotein calories.[22] Optimally parenteral nutrition should be balanced, with 20 to 30% of the calories administered as a fat emulsion.

In the neonate, the initial rate of administration of dextrose should not exceed 6 to 8 mg per kg per minute to avoid hyperglycemia. Premature infants develop hyperglycemia at lower rates of dextrose infusion than do term infants.[23] We do not recommend the administration of insulin to premature infants receiving parenteral nutrition because they are often profoundly sensitive to small amounts of insulin, leading to hypoglycemia with associated complications.[24] In a recent retrospective study of VLBW infants, however, insulin infusion did improve glucose tolerance and energy intake.[25]

Amino Acids

Amino acid requirements vary with age. Representative parenteral amino acid solutions are listed in Table 84–3. In premature infants, excessive amino acid administration may result in azotemia, especially in low birth weight infants. Premature neonates require 2.5 to 3 gm per kg per day of protein. Infants from birth to 1 year of age require 2.5 gm per kg per day of protein; children 2 to 13 years of age, 1.5 to 2 gm per kg per day; adolescents and adults, 1 to 1.5 gm per kg per day. Heird and coworkers have developed an amino acid solution for neonates and infants (TrophAmine) that results in amino acid levels in the blood similar to those in healthy, breast-fed, 1-month-old infants.[26, 27] TrophAmine provides adequate amounts of the essential amino acids, including taurine, tyrosine, and histidine, as judged by a normalized plasma amino acid profile, as well as providing aspartic acid, glutamic acid, and dicarboxylic acids. Helms and colleagues[28] compared TrophAmine with the standard amino acid formula FreAmine III in 25 neonates who required parenteral nutrition. The mean birth weight was 1.37 ± 0.23 kg in the TrophAmine group and 1.69 ± 0.72 kg in the FreAmine III group. Infants were studied for no less than 5 days and for a maximum of 21 days with either central or peripheral catheters. Those who received TrophAmine had significantly greater weight gain and nitrogen retention than the FreAmine III group. Further, the neonates who received TrophAmine demonstrated normal plasma amino acid profiles. Typically 30 to 50% of those infants who receive parenteral nutrition for more than 2 weeks are expected to develop some degree of cholestasis. TrophAmine has had a dramatic effect in reducing the frequency of cholestasis, perhaps because of the addition of taurine.[28] Studies comparing Aminosyn PF and TrophAmine in preterm infants suggest TrophAmine is superior in that age group.[28] Currently we recommend TrophAmine during the first year of life and standard amino acid solutions in older children and adolescents.

One-half gram per kilogram per day of protein should be used to initiate parenteral nutrition in neonates and then increased by 0.5 gm per kg per day until the desired goal is reached. Older infants and children can start

Table 84–3. REPRESENTATIVE PARENTERAL AMINO ACID SOLUTIONS

Preparation	Concentrations Available (gm Nitrogen/100 ml)	% Essential Amino Acids*	Special Characteristics	Manufacturer
Aminosyn	3.5% (0.55); 5% (0.79); 7% (1.1); 8.5% (1.34); 10% (1.57)	46	Premature formulas available that contain taurine	Abbott
Aminess	5.2% (0.66)	100	Only essential amino acids; used predominantly for renal failure	Clintec
BranchAmin	4% (0.44)	100	Only components isoleucine, leucine, valine	Clintec
FreAmine	3% (0.46); 6.9% (0.97); 8.5% (1.3); 10% (1.53)	49.1	High branch chain formulations available	McGaw
HepatAmine	8% (1.2)	55	Increased amount branch chain amino acids	McGaw
Nephramine	5.4% (0.64)	99.6	Almost exclusively essential amino acids	McGaw
Novamine	11.4% (1.8); 15% (2.37)	50.7	Highest protein concentration available	Clintec
Renamin	6.5% (1.0)	66.5		Clintec
Travasol	2.75% (0.46); 3.5% (0.59); 4.25% (0.71); 5.5% (0.93); 8.5% (1.43); 10% (1.65)	45.3	Alanine and glycine predominant nonessential amino acids	Clintec
TrophAmine	6% (0.93); 10% (1.55)	57.3	Contains taurine, increased amount in 10% form	McGaw

*Essential amino acids: histidine, leucine, isoleucine, lysine, methionine, phenylalanine, threonine, tryptophan, valine.
Note: Solutions contain varying electrolytes. Percentages and values given are approximate; manufacturer's labeling should be consulted for exact values.

with 1.0 gm per kg per day and increase by 0.5 gm per kg per day until the desired level is attained. Improved weight gain and normal plasma amino acid patterns have been demonstrated using amino acid preparations specifically designed for neonates as compared with standard formulations.[27, 28]

From 150 to 200 nonprotein calories are required per gram of nitrogen to promote efficient net protein utilization. Otherwise, amino acids will be used as an energy source. One gram of nitrogen is equal to approximately 6.25 gm of protein. The ratio is calculated by the following equation:

$$\frac{\text{nonprotein calories}}{\text{gm nitrogen}}$$

and is optimally greater than or equal to 150:1.

Lipids

Intravenous fat provides essential fatty acids necessary for the growth of the infant or child and to promote normal development of the nervous system.[29] Fats also provide calories in a concentrated form. Intravenous fat preparations are available as 10% solutions, which supply 1.1 kcal per ml, and 20% solutions, which supply 2 kcal per ml. It is possible to provide sufficient calories for growth in preterm neonates and infants with peripheral nutrition if maximal volumes of fats are used, i.e., 60% of total calories. Close monitoring of triglyceride levels must be done to ensure that fats are effectively cleared. In addition, the infant must be able to tolerate fluid volumes of 140 ml per kg per day. The advantage of using intravenous fat preparations in peripheral parenteral nutrition regimens is that it may prolong the life span of small veins by allowing a reduction in the dextrose concentration. Fat-free TPN without enteral feedings leads to essential fatty acid deficiency.[30] The earliest biochemical changes of fatty acid deficiency may appear in the neonate within 2 days.[31] Clinical signs of deficiency include reduced growth rate, flaky dry skin, poor hair growth, thrombocytopenia, increased susceptibility to infections, and impaired wound healing and are always preceded by biochemical evidence of deficiency.[32] Essential fatty acid deficiency can be determined by calculating the ratio of 5,8,11-icosatrianoic to arachidonic acid (triene-to-tetraene ratio). A ratio greater than 0.4 is indicative of essential fatty acid deficiency.[32] At least 2 to 4% of total calories must be administered as intravenous fat to prevent essential fatty acid deficiency. This dose can be achieved by using 0.5 to 1.0 gm per kg per day of a lipid emulsion. Intravenous fat emulsions may be administered separately from the parenteral nutrition or may be mixed with protein and carbohydrates to provide a "three-in-one" emulsion. Solutions that contain three in one mixtures *cannot* be filtered.

Because the intravenous fat particles act like chylomicrons, their rate of elimination and metabolic fate are similar. The clearance from plasma of infused fats is dependent on the activity of lipoprotein lipase in the capillary endothelial cells of muscle and adipose tissue. Intravenous fat is optimally provided over several hours.[33, 34] Infusion rates of 0.7 gm per kg per hour or more result in greater fluctuation of plasma lipid levels than rates of 0.12 gm per kg per hour or less. Rapid infusion rates have also been associated with decreased oxygen saturation and pulmonary embolization.

Until recently linoleic acid was thought to be the only essential fatty acid. Currently linolenic acid is also thought to be an essential fatty acid, especially in the developing neonate, as demonstrated by its presence in the developing brain. The intravenous fat preparations currently available for use are shown in Table 84–4. Studies comparing pure soybean oil preparations with those containing a mixture of safflower and soybean oil show no difference in the incidence of hypertriglycerid-

Table 84–4. FAT EMULSIONS FOR PARENTERAL NUTRITION

	Base	% Linoleic Acid	% Linolenic Acid	Cholesterol mg/L	Concentration	gm/L	cal/ml
Intralipid	Soybean oil	54	8	400–600	10%	100	1.1
					20%	200	2.0
Liposyn	Safflower oil	77	<0.5	trace	10%	100	1.1
					20%	200	2.0
Travemulsion	Soybean oil	56	6	trace	10%	100	1.1
					20%	200	2.0

emia between the two products, and resultant fatty acid profiles are similar.[35, 36] Carnitine is necessary for optimum oxidation of fatty acids, and infants maintained on parenteral nutrition solutions may have decreased total plasma carnitine levels. A study in neonates demonstrated that intravenous administration of L-carnitine resulted in normal plasma carnitine and lower peak triglyceride levels after delivery of a fat bolus.[37] Other studies using supplemental carnitine have not shown significant improvement in the metabolism of fat emulsions.[38] Preparations using medium-chain triglycerides (MCT) have been developed but currently are not recommended because MCT preparations do not provide the essential fatty acids.

Twenty percent intravenous fat is indicated when there is a need to restrict fluid volume. The dose of these preparations should not exceed 0.15 gm per kg per hour. We believe that the 20% intravenous fat emulsion is advantageous because it provides twice the amount of triglyceride as compared with a 10% solution with no increase in the amount of phospholipid. Phospholipid is believed to inhibit lipoprotein lipase, the main enzyme responsible for intravenous fat clearance.

Electrolytes

Table 84–5 shows the range of recommended daily intakes of electrolytes and minerals for parenteral nutrition solutions in infants and children. Preterm infants have much greater calcium and phosphorus requirements as compared with term infants, older children, and adults.[39] Because calcium and phosphorus are incorporated into the bone matrix during the last 6 to 8 weeks of gestation, premature infants without adequate supplementation are at a greater risk for developing rickets and fractures. Serum calcium and phosphorus levels should therefore be obtained weekly in these high-risk infants. Because serum calcium is maintained at the expense of bone mineralization, a normal serum calcium does not necessarily mean that adequate amounts of calcium are being delivered. The serum phosphorus level fluctuates less rapidly and is a better indicator of total body stores of phosphorus. Levels of alkaline phosphatase up to five times the normal adult reference are acceptable in preterm infants; a value greater than this suggests rickets.

Calcium and phosphorus requirements in some preterm infants may exceed the solubility of these two elements in the parenteral nutrition solutions. This typically occurs during fluid restriction. The amount of calcium and phosphorus that can be added to a parenteral nutrition solution is determined primarily by the pH of the solution, which is also affected by the amino acid product and concentration. The two pediatric mixtures, TrophAmine and Aminosyn PF, have an acidic pH to allow for adequate amounts of calcium and phosphorus to be added to the solutions.[40] Continuous infusion of calcium in TPN solutions is preferable to bolus administration. Infusion of both calcium and phosphorus should occur simultaneously and results in stable calcium and phosphorus concentrations.[41]

Vitamins

In 1989, the Food and Nutrition Board of the National Academy for Sciences, National Research Council re-

Table 84–5. DAILY INTRAVENOUS ELECTROLYTE REQUIREMENTS IN PATIENTS WITH ADEQUATE RENAL FUNCTION

	Usual Adult Dose per 24 hr	Pediatric Dose per kg/24 hr	Infant Dose per kg/24 hr
Sodium	100–150 mEq	3–4 mEq	2–8 mEq
Potassium	60–120 mEq	2–3 mEq	2–6 mEq
Chloride	100–150 mEq	2–4 mEq	0–6 mEq
Calcium*	9–22 mEq	0.5–1.0 mEq	0.9–2.3 mEq 200–500 mg†
Phosphate*	15–30 mM	2 mM	1–1.5 mM
Magnesium	8–24 mEq	0.25–0.5 mEq	0.25–0.5 mEq‡

*The product obtained by multiplying the total number of mEq of calcium per liter by the total number of mEq of phosphate per liter must not exceed *200* to prevent precipitation of the calcium phosphate complex. Must include calcium and phosphate content of base solutions. Increased concentration of administration on the basis of fluid restriction may result in precipitation.

†Given as calcium gluconate salt, 215.25 mg/mEq: maximum for infants 2 g/24 hr.

‡Given as magnesium sulfate salt; 60.15 mg/mEq.

Table 84–6. SUGGESTED INTAKES OF PARENTERAL VITAMINS IN INFANTS AND CHILDREN, AMERICAN SOCIETY FOR CLINICAL NUTRITION, 1988

Vitamin	Term Infants and Children Dose per day*	Preterm Infants Dose/kg Body Weight (maximum not to exceed term infant dose)	
		Current Suggestions†	*Best Estimate for New Formulation*‡
Lipid-soluble			
A (μg)§	700	280	500
E (mg)§	7	2.8	2.8
K (μg)	200	80	80
D (μg)§	10	4	4
(IU)	400	160	160
Water-soluble			
Ascorbic acid (mg)	80	32.0	25
Thiamin (mg)	1.2	0.48	0.35
Riboflavin (mg)	1.4	0.56	0.15
Pyridoxine (mg)	1.0	0.4	0.18
Niacin (mg)	17	6.8	6.8
Pantothenate (mg)	5	2.0	2.0
Biotin (μg)	20	8.0	6.0
Folate (μg)	140	56.0	56.0
Vitamin B_{12} (μg)	1.0	0.4	0.3

*Identical to those of the AMA (NAG). MVI-Pediatric (Armour) meets these guidelines. Recent data indicate that 40 IU/kg/day of vitamin D (maximum of 400 IU/day) is adequate for term and preterm infants. The higher dose of 160 IU/kg/day has not been associated with complications and maintains blood levels within the reference range for term infants fed orally. This dosage therefore appears acceptable until further studies using the lower dose formulation indicate its superiority.

†A practical guide (2 ml of MVI-Pediatric per kg body weight) providing adequate levels of vitamins E, D, and K; low levels of retinol; and excess levels of most B vitamins. The maximum daily dose is 5 ml for any infant.

‡Because of elevated water-soluble vitamin levels, the current proposal is to reduce water-soluble vitamins and increase retinol (see text in reference).

§700 μg RE = 2300 international units (IU); 7 mg a-tocopherol = 7 IU; 10 μg vitamin D = 400 IU.

Modified from Greene HL, Hambridge KM, Schanler R, et al: Guidelines for the use of vitamins, trace elements, calcium, magnesium, and phosphorus in infants and children receiving total parenteral nutrition. Am J Clin Nutr 1988; 48:1324–1342; with permission. © Am. J. Clin. Nutr. American Society for Clinical Nutrition.

viewed and recommended daily allowances for the fat-soluble vitamins for infants, children, and adults. They also made similar recommendations for the water-soluble vitamins. These recommendations are shown in Table 84–6. Currently there are two formulations of intravenous vitamins available for use: MVI 12 and MVI Pediatric, manufactured by Armour Pharmaceutical (Kankakee, IL) (Table 84–7).

MVI Pediatric should be used in children up to 10 years of age. Above that age, the adult formulation meets the needs of the older child more adequately. The adult formulation lacks vitamin K, however, and in patients who require prolonged parenteral nutrition, it may have to be supplemented.

Currently there is no clinically available formulation for high-risk premature infants. Our current practice is to give one vial of MVI Pediatric per day for term infants and children up to 10 years of age and 40% of a vial per kg body weight for preterm infants.[42]

Lipid-Soluble Vitamins

Synthetic detergents, such as polysorbate, are used to solubilize the lipid-soluble vitamins in an aqueous mixture and are available outside of the United States. VitaLipid made by Kabi Vitrum (Stockholm, Sweden) contains vitamins A, D, E, and K dissolved in fractionated soybean oil and emulsified with fractionated egg phospholipid. Infants can receive water-soluble vitamins in the glucose–amino acid solution and the lipid-soluble vitamins with intravenous fat. This preparation is currently not available in the United States.

Several of the vitamins used in parenteral nutrition are lost either through adsorption to the plastic TPN bags or tubing or by light exposure. Up to 40% of

Table 84–7. COMPOSITION OF INTRAVENOUS MULTIVITAMIN PREPARATIONS

		MVI-12*	MVI-Pediatric†
Lipid-soluble‡			
A (mg)		1	0.7
E (mg)		10	7
K (μg)		—	200
D (μg)		5	10
Water-soluble			
Ascorbic acid	(mg)	100	80
Thiamin	(mg)	3	1.2
Riboflavin	(mg)	3.6	1.4
Pyridoxine	(mg)	4	1
Niacin§	(mg)	40	17
Pantothenate¶	(mg)	15	5
Biotin	(μg)	60	20
Folate	(μg)	400	140
Vitamin B_{12}	(μg)	5	1

*Amounts given are per 10 ml.

†Amounts given are per 5 ml.

‡1 mg vitamin A = 3,300 USP units; 5 μg vitamin D (ergocalciferol) = 200 USP units; 10 mg vitamin E = 10 USP units.

§As niacinamide.

¶As dexpanthenol (*d*-pantothenyl alcohol).

Values given are approximate. Manufacturer's labeling should be consulted for exact values and formulation changes.

vitamin A may be lost because of its adherence to the intravenous tubing and because of degradation owing to light.[43] Pyridoxine is decomposed by exposure to ordinary light conditions.[44] Substantial amounts of vitamins A, D, and E may also be lost over a period of 24 hours.[45, 46] The problem of vitamin loss from parenteral nutrition solutions may be the most severe in VLBW infants because of the light intensity used in nurseries and the smaller volume of TPN solution exposed to the administration tubing for longer periods of time. Infants weighing less than 1 kg should receive 1.5 ml per day of MVI Pediatrics.

Forty percent of a vial of MVI Pediatric will provide 2.8 mg of alpha-tocopherol per kg per day. Physicians must monitor the vitamin E levels in patients, particularly small infants. Inadequate dosing of vitamin A may lead to a lack of retinol in VLBW infants. Studies have demonstrated both a higher incidence of bronchopulmonary dysplasia with low plasma retinol levels, and a significant reduction in the incidence of bronchopulmonary dysplasia in patients treated with vitamin A intramuscularly in the neonatal period.[46, 47]

MVI Pediatric contains 200 μg per vial of phylloquinone, a lipid-soluble vitamin K preparation. If MVI 12 is used in older children, the patient will need supplemental vitamin K, which can be given by intravenous supplementation (1 mg IV) or a weekly intramuscular injection (5 to 10 mg IM).[45] Vitamin K does not necessarily have to be given on a daily basis if the patient is not receiving antibiotics. In patients who have intact gastrointestinal tracts, the natural production of vitamin K by the bacteria in the colon and distal small intestine may obviate the need for routine vitamin K supplementation.

Water-Soluble Vitamins

The use of MVI Pediatric for the younger infant and MVI 12 for the older child should prevent water-soluble vitamin deficiency.[11, 12] Even though riboflavin may be inactivated by light, there have been no cases reported of riboflavin deficiency in patients receiving parenteral nutrition. Although the recommended parenteral dose of pyridoxine in full-term infants, 1 mg per day, may be more than is necessary, it has not resulted in any identifiable toxicity. In preterm infants who receive 40% of MVI Pediatric, the levels of water-soluble vitamins appear to be more than adequate, and no recognized toxicity has been demonstrated. Biotin deficiency secondary to TPN use is no longer reported since biotin has been added to the MVI Pediatric preparation.[48] Biotin deficiency was characterized by the presence of scaly dermatitis, thinning of hair, pallor, irritability, and lethargy, many features similar to those seen in zinc deficiency.[48]

Trace Elements

Recommendations for trace elements have been published[49] (Table 84–8). Persistent diarrhea or excessive gastrointestinal losses from ostomy sites greatly increase the loss of zinc.[50, 51] From adult studies, we know that approximately 17 mg of zinc are lost per kilogram of stool or ileostomy output and 12 mg per L of small bowel fluid lost via fistulas or stomas. No similar studies have been done in pediatric patients.

Table 84–8. SUGGESTED DAILY INTRAVENOUS INTAKE OF TRACE ELEMENTS IN INFANTS AND CHILDREN*

Element	Infants μg/kg/day		Children μg/kg/day (maximum μg/day)
	Preterm†	*Term*	
Zinc	400	250 <3 mo 100 >3 mo	50 (5000)
Copper‡	20	20	20 (300)
Selenium§	2.0	2.0	2.0 (30)
Chromium§	0.20	0.20	0.20 (5.0)
Manganese‡	1.0	1.0	1.0 (50)
Molybdenum§	0.25	0.25	0.25 (5.0)
Iodide	1.0	1.0	1.0 (1.0)

*When TPN is only supplemental or limited to <4 wk, only Zn need be added. Thereafter, addition of the remaining elements is advisable.

†Available concentrations of Mo and Mn are such that dilution of the manufacturer's product may be necessary. Neotrace (Lyphomed Co, Rosemont, IL) contains a higher ratio of Mn to Zn than suggested in this table (i.e., Zn = 1.5 mg, and Mn = 25 μg in each milliliter).

‡Omit in patients with obstructive jaundice.

§Omit in patients with renal dysfunction.

Modified from Greene HL, Hambridge KM, Schanler R, et al: Guidelines for the use of vitamins, trace elements, calcium, magnesium, and phosphorus in infants and children receiving total parenteral nutrition. Am J Clin Nutr 1988; 48:1324–1342; with permission. © Am. J. Clin. Nutr. American Society for Clinical Nutrition.

Selenium deficiency in pediatric patients may be recognized both clinically and by certain laboratory tests. Erythrocyte macrocytosis, loss of pigmentation in the hair and skin, and muscle weakness are characteristic of deficiency. Elevated serum transaminase and creatinine levels may also be found.[52] Cardiomyopathy has been described. Intravenous supplementation with 2 μg per kg per day of selenium can reverse the signs and symptoms of selenium deficiency. Myopathy secondary to selenium deficiency may be reversed with therapy within a period of 6 weeks.[53] Selenium should always be included as a required trace metal in patients with chronic diarrhea and large ostomy outputs.

The recommendations for chromium in parenteral nutrition may be excessive, and the use of 0.20 μg per kg per day given intravenously may lead to elevated chromium levels.[54] Some centers no longer recommend supplemental chromium or iodide in parenteral nutrition solutions.[55, 56] Typically iodide is a component of the water used to mix parenteral solutions and is a natural contaminant of the salts added to the solutions. Iodide from antiseptic solutions used to clean the catheter entrance site may be absorbed through the skin and contribute to the normal iodide levels. In more than two decades, we have never seen a patient with iodide deficiency who was on parenteral nutrition.

Iron

Intravenous iron needs to be provided to patients unable to absorb it through the enteral route. Because iron is absorbed proximally in the duodenum and jejunum, a trial of an oral iron preparation should always be given first. Dilute forms of iron dextran have been added to TPN solutions without serious consequences. We have seen no adverse consequences as a result of providing 0.5 to 1 mg of an iron dextran preparation daily.[57] To document that sufficient iron is being provided, serum iron, total iron binding capacity, and percent saturation should be monitored. Overdoses of intravenous iron dextran have resulted in the development of secondary hemochromatosis with resultant cirrhosis of the liver (personal observation).

Aluminum

Although TPN solutions may be contaminated with small amounts of aluminum, the levels are less than they were a decade ago.[58] Experience has shown that infants and children receiving long-term parenteral nutrition have serum aluminum levels similar to age-matched and sex-matched controls eating diets appropriate for age [59] In the past, the major source of aluminum contamination was casein hydrolysate. With the use of crystalline amino acids, sterile water, and dextrose, the contamination of the solutions is relatively low. Calcium salts contribute up to 80% of the total aluminum load in current TPN solutions. Similar contamination can occur from the ingestion of food. In the past when aluminum contamination was excessive, concerns were raised in children regarding impaired bone matrix formation and mineralization.[60]

ROUTE OF ADMINISTRATION—CENTRAL VERSUS PERIPHERAL VEIN

Complication rates of children receiving parenteral nutrition in peripheral veins differ from those who receive it through central veins. Approximately 10% of those who receive central venous TPN incur a septic complication, whereas it is uncommon in the peripheral vein group. Morbidity may occur, however, when peripheral parenteral nutrition solutions are infused into the soft tissues with resultant tissue sloughing.

The complication rate and duration of therapy are higher for central venous TPN than for peripheral venous administration. If the number of days of therapy per patient is compared, however, the complication rate between the two groups is similar.[61] Caloric need is the primary determinant of the route of nutritional support. Centrally alimented patients may receive more calories and gain more weight on a daily basis. The use of peripheral TPN may result in fewer calories being provided than ordered, secondary to infiltration and loss of venous access. It is difficult to maintain peripheral parenteral nutrition for more than 2 weeks. It is better to choose central TPN from the onset of nutritional therapy if it is anticipated that the enteral route will be unavailable for 2 or more weeks. Central venous TPN must usually be used to achieve normal growth and weight gain in older infants and children.[62]

Central Venous Parenteral Nutrition

To minimize the risk of venous thrombosis and phlebitis, large caliber veins with a high volume of blood flow must be used. Silastic catheters have been available for more than two decades. We do not recommend other catheters because polyvinyl or polyurethane tubing tends to become more rigid after intravenous placement, leading to more frequent complications.

For long-term parenteral nutrition, either Hickman or Broviac catheters are frequently used. They may be placed by either a cutdown or a percutaneous method.[63] These catheters provide better stability and decrease the risk of infection because the end of the catheter is subcutaneously tunneled to exit at a distant site. The catheter is trimmed to an appropriate length so it terminates in the superior vena cava. These catheters differ from traditional ones by having a reinforced polytef (Teflon) neck to reduce the risk of cracking, a distal Luer-Lok connector, which allows them to be screw capped when not in use, and a Dacron cuff attached to the midportion of the catheter. This material stimulates the formation of dense fibrous adhesions that anchor the catheter securely subcutaneously and create a barrier for ascending bacteria. It takes approximately 2 weeks after catheter placement for this type of adhesion to develop; sutures are left in place until that time.

Parenteral nutrition catheters can also be placed percutaneously using the internal jugular vein, brachial vein, cephalic vein, or inferior epigastric veins. Once inserted, the catheter is advanced into the superior vena cava to its junction with the right atrium. Cardiac arrhythmias can be precipitated if the catheter is in the atrium, so it is preferable for the catheter to float in the superior vena cava. Other complications occurring with right atrial catheter placement include incorporation into the endocardium and perforation of the atrium with secondary cardiac tamponade.[64] Tamponade can occur even with Silastic catheters. Catheter placement should be confirmed by radiographic studies before infusion of solution. Central venous catheters should be placed in the operating room or in special patient care areas using sterile technique. To prevent infections of both the catheter and the catheter exit site, dressings should be changed at least three times per week, and nursing guidelines for catheter care and its cleaning should be established.[65, 66] Catheters are used primarily for the delivery of parenteral nutrition. They may also be used, however, for blood transfusions and for medication administration.

It is possible with proper aseptic technique to minimize infection of these catheters. Long-term venous access has been successful in infants with birth weights of less than 1,000 gm.[67] If a central venous catheter becomes infected, in most instances the infection can be successfully treated with antibiotics without catheter removal. Staphylococcal infections are the most common infections and are readily susceptible to treatment. Fungal infections in the catheter are usually an indication for catheter removal. Double and triple lumen catheters may be particularly useful in pediatric oncologic and transplantation patients and require considerably more care than single lumen catheters. If cracks or breaks occur in Hickman or Broviac double or triple lumen catheters, repair kits are available that allow a new end piece to be spliced to the old catheter. Catheters in long-term parenteral nutrition patients have been in place for more than a decade without serious complications.[68]

We do not recommend that umbilical artery catheters be used for the administration of parenteral nutrients. Parenteral nutrition solutions may thrombose veins and cause phlebitis, leading to portal venous thrombosis and extrahepatic portal hypertension. In addition, arterial damage can occur. If parenteral nutrition is required in infants and peripheral veins are either not usable or inadequate, subcutaneous subclavian catheterization or cutdown should be used. We believe that the risk of complications associated with the use of umbilical arteries and veins does not justify their use.

INITIATION OF PARENTERAL NUTRITION THERAPY

Ideally before starting parenteral nutrition, a complete nutritional assessment is performed. In routine practice, most individuals do not perform anthropometric measurements other than height and weight. Nutritional assessment techniques have been extensively reviewed[69–72] (see Chapter 81). For preterm infants, skinfold thickness reference data are available as are midarm circumference data.[73] The use of the midarm circumference to head circumference ratio provides a method for evaluation of intrauterine growth and a noninvasive technique for monitoring somatic protein stores in the growing preterm infant.[74]

TYPE OF THERAPY

Maintenance

Maintenance nutrition is appropriate in the patient without an underlying chronic illness or nutritional deficit, who will not experience stressful metabolic conditions in the hospital.

Maintenance and Partial Repletion

Maintenance and partial repletion nutritional therapy is indicated if the patient has a serum albumin level of less than 3 gm per dl, the transferrin level is less than 150 μg per dl, or the lymphocyte count is less than 1.5 $\times$ 10^9 per L. Body measurements suggesting the need for repletion therapy include a weight to height ratio greater than 2 standard deviations below normal or less than 80% of standard, arm muscle area below the fifth percentile, or a creatinine height index less than 80% of standard. This group requires close monitoring for evidence of further nutritional depletion and at least maintenance nutritional support if full repletion is not possible. If these patients have associated sepsis secondary to surgery or major injury, they should be treated as if they require full repletion therapy.

Maintenance and Full Repletion

Maintenance and full repletion nutritional support is appropriate if the serum albumin level is less than 2.5 gm per dl, the transferrin level is less than 100 μg per dl after 6 months of age, the lymphocyte count is less than 1.0 $\times$ 10^9 per L except in patients on chemotherapy or radiation therapy, or if anergy persists beyond infancy in patients not on corticosteroids. Body measurements suggesting the need for full nutritional repletion include the presence of a weight to height ratio greater than 2 standard deviations below normal or less than 80% of standard, an arm muscle area below the fifth percentile, or a creatinine height index less than 60% of standard. Full repletion plus maintenance therapy is also indicated in any patient markedly stressed with marginal skeletal or visceral protein stores.

Standard amino acids and electrolyte concentrations for parenteral nutrition solutions have been developed to meet most patients' needs. These solutions generally provide 1.0 to 1.5 gm per kg per day of amino acids as well as maintenance quantities of electrolytes and vitamins administered in sufficient volumes to meet the patient's fluid requirements, roughly 1,500 ml per m^2 per day. Calories may be adjusted to meet the individual patient's needs by varying the rate of delivery of the parenteral nutrition solutions, the dextrose concentration, and the fat emulsion dosage. The electrolyte and mineral contents of these standard formulations are listed in Table 84–9. The advantages of standard solutions include lower cost, less wastage, and improved quality control. Custom solutions tailored to the individual needs of a patient are available in most institutions.

Table 84–9. COMPOSITION OF STANDARD HOME PARENTERAL NUTRITION SOLUTIONS

Ingredients	Units	Concentrations		
Amino acids	%	2.0	3.5	4.25
Formula code		Pediatric	Adult	Adult
Sodium	mEq/L	30	35	35
Potassium	mEq/L	25	30	30
Calcium	mEq/L	10	5	5
Magnesium	mEq/L	10	10	10
Chloride	mEq/L	30	35	35
Phosphate	mmol/L	7.5	10	10
Acetate	mEq/L	35	55	64
Copper	mg/L	1	1	1
Zinc	mg/L	2	2	2
Selenium	μg/day	20	40	40

Chromium has been deleted as a standard additive to home TPN solutions.

A custom solution is prepared when an electrolyte is ordered at an increased or decreased concentration, when the amino acid concentration differs from available standards, or when special amino acid preparations are needed. Preprinted parenteral nutrition order forms are available at most major centers that care for children. These order forms usually require the patient's weight, total intake of fluids for the day, the amount of fat emulsion to be used as well as the concentration, the desired protein intake, and the concentration of dextrose. Trace elements, vitamins, and electrolytes are ordered in amounts per day or amounts per kilogram per day. For adolescents and teenagers, adult standard solutions may be used. An example of an order form is shown in Figure 84–1. Most hospitalized patients receive parenteral nutrition 24 hours per day. Cyclical TPN is used if the patient is stable and is going to remain hospitalized for a prolonged interval of time or when home TPN is anticipated. The patient should have stable metabolic status, normal electrolytes, and a steady weight gain for at least 2 to 4 days on continuous TPN before this is instituted.

TRANSITION FROM PARENTERAL TO ENTERAL NUTRITION

Animal studies have demonstrated the importance of providing enteral nutrients to maintain the structural and functional integrity of the gastrointestinal tract.[75] The trophic effects on the mucosa may be directly mediated by gastrointestinal hormones. Even in patients with a very short small intestine, it is desirable to provide at least a small amount of enteral nutrition to help maintain the intestinal mass and normal enzyme levels.

The change from parenteral nutrition to enteral feeding must be gradual and may take days, weeks, or months. The transition time in part depends on the length of the intestine as well as the degree of mucosal damage in those with intractable diarrhea. Continuous enteral feedings may be required to change from parenteral to enteral nutrition. The conversion from parenteral to enteral and oral therapy will depend on the volume of diarrhea passed as well as the degree of absorption that takes place.[76] Some patients will fail to make the transition simply because they do not have sufficient mucosal mass. Small volumes of oral feedings are given to stimulate the infant to develop the skills of sucking and swallowing. In infants with a compromised mucosa or in whom there is deficient bowel, however, continuous perfusion of the gastrointestinal tract is usually the initial means by which the feeding is delivered.

COMPLICATIONS OF PARENTERAL NUTRITION

There are three general types of complications that can occur from the use of parenteral nutrition: technical, infectious, and metabolic. Complications can often be avoided by careful monitoring and fastidious aseptic technique. Complications are reduced when parenteral nutrition protocols are administered by those familiar with the technique. Technical catheter complications usually occur at the time of insertion and include pneumothorax, hemothorax, subclavian artery injury, subclavian hematoma, innominate or subclavian vein lacerations, catheter embolization, cardiac perforation and tamponade, and nerve injuries.[65, 66, 77–79]

Catheter Occlusion

There are no controlled studies that demonstrate the benefit of heparin in parenteral nutrition. It is used to prevent thrombosis and usually is given at a dosage of 1 unit per ml of TPN solution. Some practitioners also believe heparin may reduce the incidence of catheter-related sepsis. Heparin does stimulate the release of the enzyme lipoprotein lipase, which may enhance the clearance of intravenous fat.

Other agents are used to restore patency to thrombosed or occluded catheters. Urokinase may be administered either as a bolus or a prolonged low-dose intravenous infusion.[80, 81] It works by activating plasminogen that is converted to plasmin, which can lyse the fibrin clot. Boluses typically are in the range of 5,000 to 10,000 units for adult patients. Continuous low-dose infusion has been studied at a dosage of 200 U per kg per lumen per hour up to 24 hours in pediatric patients without adverse sequelae. Streptokinase works by the same mechanism as urokinase, but it is a bacterially derived product and therefore may be antigenic.[81] Other bolus catheter clearing agents include 0.1 N hydrochloric acid (0.2 to 1.0 ml in adults) and tissue plasminogen activator (tPA) (2 mg per 2 ml in adult patients as a bolus administration).[82, 83]

Central Venous Catheter Infections

The most frequent catheter-related complication after successful insertion is infection. An indwelling catheter serves as a portal of entry, and a malnourished or debilitated infant or child is a good host for infection. Stringent aseptic technique is of utmost importance in minimizing the risk of infection.

If a fever greater than 38.5° C develops during the administration of parenteral nutrition, a close examination for a focal source must be undertaken. In particular, phlebitis, pulmonary infection, urinary tract infection, and abdominal sepsis should be considered. Fevers may also be associated with reactions to the nutrients such as fat emulsions, other drugs, or possible contamination of the solutions.

If no focal infection is identified, blood cultures, both bacterial and fungal, should be drawn both from the catheter and peripherally, and antibiotics should be started. Sterile technique is particularly important. A complete blood count with differential, urine culture,

UCLA Medical Center
PEDIATRIC PARENTERAL NUTRITION ORDER

Write firmly—you are making 2 copies.
(See information on reverse side.)

Room: ☐ Check here if existing TPN may not be used.

****INDICATION** ______

ASSESSMENT

**Height ______ inches **Current Weight ______ kg Usual Weight ______ kg

Percentiles: Height ______ %ile Weight for Height ______ %ile Weight for Age ______ %ile

Albumin ______ gm% Prealbumin ______ mg%

ESTIMATED NEEDS

AGE (yr)	CALORIES/KG/DAY	PROTEIN(g)/KG/DAY
0-1	90-120	2.0 - 2.5
1-7	75-90	1.5 - 2.0
7-12	60-75	1.5 - 2.0
12-18	30-60	1.0 - 1.5

DAILY CALORIES = ______

DAILY PROTEIN = ______

****FIRST-TIME ORDERS WITHOUT INDICATION, HEIGHT, AND WEIGHT WILL NOT BE HONORED.**

TPN SOLUTION

DEXTROSE (circle one)

%	10	15	20	25	30	35
(kcal/L)	(340)	(510)	(680)	(850)	(1020)	(1190)

☐ PERIPHERAL
☐ CENTRAL

RATE (choose one)

☐ Infuse at ____ ml/hr. Check chemstick glucose every ____ hr. Call M.D. if > ____ mg%.

☐ Start central TPN at _____ml/hr x _____hr, increase to _____ml/hr x _____hr, then increase to _____ml/hr thereafter. Check chemstick glucose before each rate increase and every ____ hr thereafter. Call M.D. if > ____ mg%.

☐ Start central TPN at _____ ml/hr D10%. Increase by 5% dextrose every _____ liter(s) up to _____% dextrose. Check chemstick glucose every ___ hr until at final dextrose concentration, then every _____. Call M.D. if > ____ mg%.

AMINO ACIDS, ELECTROLYTES AND TRACE ELEMENTS

☐ 2.0% Amino Acids
Standard Pediatric Electrolytes
Contents per liter:

Na	30	mEq	Cl	30	mEq
K	25	mEq	Ac	35	mEq
Ca	10	mEq	Zn	2	mg
Mg	10	mEq	Cu	1	mg
PO4	7.5	mMol			

☐ 3.5% Amino Acids
Standard Adult Electrolytes
Contents per liter:

Na	35	mEq	Cl	35	mEq
K	30	mEq	Ac	55	mEq
Ca	5	mEq	Zn	2	mg
Mg	10	mEq	Cu	1	mg
PO4	10	mMol			

☐ ______% Amino Acids (complete below)
Write complete contents PER LITER below:

Na	mEq	PO4	mMol	Cl & Ac Std; OR
K	mEq	Zn	mg	☐ max Ac, std Cl ☐ max Ac, min Cl
Ca	mEq	Cu	mg	☐ max Cl, std Ac
Mg	mEq			☐ max Cl, min Ac

VITAMINS ☐ Pediatric MVI 5 ml/day OR ☐ Adult MVI 10 ml/day (pharmacist rounds dose to nearest 1.0 ml/L).

ADDITIVES

Regular Human Insulin ______ units/L. Other:

FATS

20% (2.0 kcal/ml) (0.2g/ml) Infuse _______ ml over _______ hrs every _______.

Give test dose of 3 ml/hr for first 10 mins.
Do not exceed 1.25 ml/kg/hr = 0.25 g/kg/hr.

NURSING CARE

☐ Flush central venous catheter daily with heparin ______ units per lumen diluted to 3ml with 0.9% NaCl (see back for dosing).
☐ Daily weights, strict inputs and outputs.
☐ Temperature every 8 hours.
☐ Urine glucose (contact M.D. if 2 consecutive urines are ≥ 2+) q ______.

LAB TESTS

☐ Prealbumin -- day 1 & 4, then q Mon.
☐ Na, K, Cl, CO2 content, Glucose, Ca, Mg, P -- day 1 & 2, then q Mon, Thur.
☐ Triglyceride -- day 1 & 4, then q Mon (draw > 6 hours post infusion).
☐ BUN, Creatinine -- day 1 & 2, then q Mon.
☐ CBC with differential -- day 1, then q Mon, Thurs.
☐ Total Protein, Albumin, PT, PTT -- day 1, then q Mon.
☐ AST, ALT, Alk Phos, Total & Direct Bilirubin -- day 1, then q Mon.

Physician Signature ____________ Pager # ____________ Date & Time ____________

3310 PHA (1/91) J3-3310
MR C/003 (I)

MEDICAL RECORD

PEDIATRIC PARENTERAL NUTRITION ORDER

Figure 84–1. Pediatric parenteral nutrition order form used by the UCLA Medical Center.

and chest radiograph should also be performed. If the fever stops within hours or a focus is found, the parenteral nutrition solution can be restarted. If fever continues without an identifiable cause or the patient becomes toxic, repeat central and peripheral blood cultures for bacteria and fungi should be obtained, and the physician should consider removing the catheter.

Catheter infection in home TPN patients is usually treated by administering parenteral antibiotics for at least 4 weeks. Many patients are dependent on the catheters and TPN for survival, and potential problems arise secondary to limited central venous access with repeated catheter replacement. In general, therapy is most effective in cases of gram-positive bacteremia, but success in treating gram-negative organisms is not uncommon.[84, 85] The most common cause of infection is gram-positive bacteria (including oxacillin-resistant, coagulase-negative staphylococci), followed by gram-negative bacteria, fungi, and less frequently mycobacteria. Empiric antibiotic therapy is initiated after blood cultures are drawn. Catheter removal is required in the presence of fungal infection, septic shock, endocarditis, embolism, persistent fever, or disseminated intravascular coagulation. In addition, infections of the tunnel tract usually require catheter removal. If a catheter is removed, antimicrobial therapy is continued for 5 to 7 days, and a new catheter is placed when the patient has been afebrile with negative blood cultures for at least 72 hours. The TPN solution itself is an uncommon source of infection because the hypertonicity and acidity of the solutions limit the short-term growth and survival of bacteria. Bacteria that grow poorly in TPN solutions, however, can proliferate when the same reservoir is used to infuse solution for more than 24 hours. Therefore care should be taken in handling TPN solutions to minimize the risk of solution contamination. Vancomycin is often a component of the initial therapy in suspected catheter infection. Typically gentamicin or other gram-negative coverage is added to the initial regimen pending final culture and sensitivity reports.[84]

Metabolic Complications

Hyperglycemia

If a patient receiving parenteral nutrition spills 2,000 mg per dl (2 plus) or greater glucose on urine testing on two or more consecutive occasions, the physician should rule out drug interactions causing a false-positive test, verify the infusion rate, ensure that no "catching up" has been attempted, and check the urine and serum potassium because glucosuria may be secondary to hypokalemia. Hyperglycemia may also herald the onset of sepsis and precede temperature elevation by several hours. If there is no evidence of a false-positive test, altered infusion rate, or sepsis, the rate of dextrose administration must be decreased or insulin added.

If insulin is used to control hyperglycemia, initially 1 U of regular insulin is added per 10 gm of dextrose, e.g., 10 U for 1 L of 10% dextrose. The insulin dose should be adjusted with a sliding scale based on blood glucose determinations if 1 U of insulin per 10 gm of dextrose is insufficient. It is usually inappropriate to attempt to regulate the patient's serum glucose if it is less than 150 mg per dl. Finer control is rarely possible and places the patient at risk for developing hypoglycemia.

Hypoglycemia

Hypoglycemia may occur with abrupt cessation of parenteral nutrition infusions. Infusions of greater than 10% dextrose should be tapered before cessation to prevent hypoglycemia. The infusion can be tapered by decreasing the rate by 50% every 15 minutes for the last 30 minutes of fluid administration. In the unusual child who becomes hypoglycemic while tapering over 30 minutes, a longer taper over 1 or 2 hours may be necessary.

Electrolyte Imbalances

The most common electrolyte disturbances are related to potassium, phosphorus, and magnesium, which often decline during periods of active protein synthesis. If acidosis or alkalosis develops, an attempt should be made to identify the underlying cause before manipulating the parenteral nutrition solution. Hyperchloremic metabolic acidosis may be remedied by the substitution of acetate for the chloride salts of sodium and potassium. Bicarbonate is not added to parenteral nutrition solutions owing to its incompatibility with calcium. *In general, a tendency to "chase" slight variations in laboratory tests with frequent changes in the electrolyte content of parenteral nutrition solutions should be avoided.* This is a common cause of wastage to the pharmacy. Wherever possible, acute deficiencies should be corrected with separately "piggy-backed" bolus infusions. Increased electrolyte requirements may be met by addition to the parenteral nutrition solution. Sources of electrolytes other than parenteral nutrition solutions should be identified as well. Extraneous fluid losses (e.g., nasogastric suction, fistula drainage) should be replaced with the appropriate intravenous solution. Most importantly, iatrogenic electrolyte problems can be minimized by close monitoring whenever an electrolyte is removed, reduced, or increased in the parenteral nutrition formulation.[62, 65, 71]

Hepatic Dysfunction

During the past decade, there has been a dramatic reduction in the incidence of TPN-induced liver disease, which coincides with the formulation of balanced amino acid solutions specifically designed for infants.[86–88] Patients and particularly infants who are placed on TPN should be monitored for evidence of liver dysfunction. This can be done by measuring the gamma-glutamyl transpeptidase (GGTP), 5′-nucleotidase, or serum bile acid levels. If these are not available, direct bilirubin measurement can be done on a weekly basis.

Abnormal Liver Function Tests

Elevation of alanine aminotransferase (ALT), aspartate aminotransferase (AST), and alkaline phosphatase to five times the upper limit of normal without jaundice may occur within 2 to 14 days after initiating parenteral nutrition therapy. These test results generally return to near normal without discontinuing parenteral nutrition. Providing too many calories, insufficient fat emulsion to meet essential fatty acid requirements, and pre-existing liver disease can contribute to persistently elevated liver function tests. Rarely liver function test abnormalities associated with acute right upper quadrant pain and hepatomegaly may occur. This may be due to excessive calories or acute fatty infiltration of the liver associated with the conversion of glucose to fat. Decreasing the total or carbohydrate calories generally leads to prompt resolution.

Cholelithiasis

The risk of development of gallstones in patients of all ages on parenteral nutrition is substantially increased. This risk increases further with ileal disease or resection. The risk of developing gallbladder sludge as a consequence of TPN is almost 100% after patients have been on TPN for 6 full weeks. In a study of 246 infants and children receiving parenteral nutrition for more than 4 weeks, nearly 15% of those who underwent ultrasound examination of the gallbladder had cholelithiasis. Six of these required cholecystectomy for relief of chronic abdominal pain, pancreatitis, or empyema of the gallbladder; one had a cholecystostomy, one had abdominal colic, one died of hepatic insufficiency, and two of the remaining patients were asymptomatic.[89] Long-term studies of patients receiving parenteral nutrition have revealed cholelithiasis in as many as 40%. If parenteral nutrition is contemplated for longer than 90 days, baseline and repeat ultrasound examinations of gallbladder for sludge may be appropriate.[90, 91] Any infant or child who is on parenteral nutrition for more than 30 days and has abdominal pain should be assessed for evidence of biliary sludge or stones. Stimulation of the gallbladder with enteral feeding may substantially reduce the risk of sludge or stone formation.

Bone Disease

Osteopenia without associated symptoms is characteristic of patients who receive long-term parenteral nutrition. In the past, a clinical syndrome seen in patients on long-term TPN consisting of bone pain, hypercalcemia with normal serum phosphate, 1,25-dihydroxy-vitamin D levels, and 25-dihydroxy-vitamin D levels was associated with aluminum toxicity. We have not seen any cases of this symptomatic bone disease because all our patients have been placed on crystalline amino acid solutions. These solutions are contaminated with small amounts of aluminum.

Premature infants are subject to a condition called osteopenia of prematurity, characterized by decreased bone mineralization. In most instances, it is subclinical and is often diagnosed only after the development of bone fractures or overt rickets. It is currently believed that deficiencies of calcium and phosphorus are responsible for the osteopenia rather than a defect in vitamin D metabolism.[92] Fluoride deficiency has also been implicated in the pathogenesis.[93] Rickets in the premature infant can be assessed by measuring the serum alkaline phosphatase level. If it exceeds six times the adult normal value, further evaluation is indicated.

Refeeding Syndrome

Severely malnourished patients are at risk for mineral and electrolyte abnormalities when nutritional repletion in initiated.[94] A decrease in the serum phosphate level owing to the intracellular movement of phosphate can lead to acute respiratory failure. Serum potassium and magnesium can also drop acutely secondary to intracellular shifts. Phosphate, potassium and magnesium levels should be monitored at least daily for the first week of nutritional therapy in severely depleted patients. Initiating therapy too quickly may lead to fluid overload, increased metabolic rate, and increased cardiac workload, resulting in congestive heart failure and respiratory compromise, especially in severely malnourished patients in whom somatic protein catabolism can further compromise respiratory function.

A marked increase in carbon dioxide production occurs with glucose administration. If the amount of carbon dioxide produced exceeds the ventilatory capacity, the arterial PCO_2 will increase. This is especially important in patients with chronic pulmonary disease on ventilators. Alternate sources of calories, i.e., fat, are associated with less carbon dioxide production and should be considered. Excess calories in patients with respiratory compromise should be avoided.

Hyperlipidemia

It is important to provide intravenous fat as a component of the parenteral nutrition solutions. At a minimum, it should be provided to avoid essential fatty acid deficiency, and optimally in peripheral parenteral nutrition it should be used to provide adequate calories for maintenance. The only effective way to monitor the use of intravenous lipids is by measuring serum triglycerides, cholesterol, and fatty acids.[95] Initially patients should have triglyceride and cholesterol determinations weekly. The level of serum triglyceride should be kept under 200 mg per dl and the cholesterol below 250 mg per dl. If either value is elevated, the intravenous fat dosage should be adjusted. Serum triglyceride values should be obtained 24 hours after a dosage increase to ensure patient tolerance of the new dosage. A sudden increase in the triglyceride level at a dose that was previously tolerated should raise the suspicion of sepsis.

In infants with respiratory or cardiac disease, a decrease in the intravenous fat dose should be considered with worsening oxygen saturation. Intravenous fat should be used cautiously in all low birth weight infants with respiratory or cardiovascular disease. Some investigators claim chronic lung disease is more likely to develop and be more severe after lipid administration.[95] It may be prudent to avoid its use during the first week of life. Neonates receiving bolus doses of heparin (10 U per kg) in addition to heparin (1 U per ml) mixed with parenteral nutrition have a significantly lower triglyceride concentration than patients receiving the bolus dosage alone.[97] In premature infants, there are no guidelines with regard to the use of heparin in the parenteral nutrition solutions. One potential problem is that more free fatty acids will be released than can be metabolized, resulting in elevated serum lipids.

Although there has been concern in jaundiced infants of potentiating the development of kernicterus, intravenous fat emulsions do not appear to displace bilirubin from albumin circulating in the plasma. The American Academy of Pediatrics currently recommends that infants with bilirubin levels of 8 to 10 mg per dl, assuming an albumin concentration of 2.5 to 3.0 gm per dl, should receive the amount of intravenous fat required to prevent essential fatty acid deficiency.[98]

Sepsis and Lipids

In a year long prospective study of 50 children on home TPN, Dahlstrom and colleagues[99] noted significantly increased serum triglyceride levels, and elevated prothrombin and partial thromboplastin times in six children who were acutely ill. In patients who are acutely ill, we therefore recommend lowering the dosage of intravenous fat.

Thrombocytopenia

Although it has been reported, in our experience over 18 years we have not seen any patients on long-term parenteral nutrition receiving daily fat who developed significant thrombocytopenia.[100]

Monitoring of Carbohydrate and Protein Infusions

While on parenteral nutrition patients should have their urine checked for glucose. If the urine glucose concentration is 2% or greater, the blood glucose should be determined. The dextrose content of the TPN solution may need to be decreased or the rate of infusion reduced to prevent an osmotic diuresis. There is infrequently an indication to use more than 2.5 gm per kg per day of amino acids in patients on parenteral nutrition. The use of excessive amino acids results in metabolic acidosis and excess ammonia production. Patients with kidney or liver disease are at an increased risk for development of these problems. Blood ammonia and blood urea nitrogen (BUN) determinations should be performed if there is a suspicion of protein intolerance to ensure that the administered protein does not overwhelm the synthetic capacity of the liver. In clinical practice, we do not routinely do urine urea nitrogen for nitrogen balance because it is difficult to obtain accurate 24-hour urine collections. If desired, nitrogen balance can be determined by collecting a 24-hour urine sample for urea nitrogen and by knowing the amount of parenteral protein administration. The formula for nitrogen balance is:

$$N_2 \text{ balance} = \text{grams of protein (intake)} \div 6.25 - (\text{urinary urea nitrogen} + 3)$$

MONITORING

Proper monitoring of patients receiving parenteral nutrition is necessary to detect and prevent complications, determine if adequate nutritional ingredients are being infused, and document positive clinical benefits. Most metabolic complications can be prevented or detected before they cause serious consequences if an adequate biochemical monitoring regimen is rigidly followed. During hospitalization, the patient should have an initial height and weight measurement and then daily weights and accurate measurements of intake and output. Temperature should be taken three times daily and all urine tested for glucose and acetone. Baseline blood studies including electrolytes, magnesium, calcium, phosphorus, glucose, complete blood count with differential and quantitative platelets, iron and total iron binding capacity, prothrombin time, activated partial thromboplastin time, total protein, albumin, prealbumin, BUN, creatinine, AST, ALT, bilirubin, alkaline phosphate, and triglycerides should be monitored frequently. Electrolytes, BUN, creatinine, magnesium, calcium, and phosphorus should be measured daily during the first several days of therapy. Glucose should be measured when initiating central venous TPN, and glucose levels should be monitored before and after every rate or concentration increase. Once the patient is stable, tests need not be repeated more than twice weekly. Trace elements should be obtained at the beginning of therapy if a patient is malnourished or has excessive ostomy output to determine if supplemental zinc, selenium, or other trace elements should be provided. They should also be periodically monitored during therapy. If the patient does not have liver disease or renal disease, the prealbumin typically demonstrates an increase by the fourth day of TPN if adequate protein and calories are being provided.

USE OF LONG-TERM PARENTERAL NUTRITION

It is important for children placed on parenteral nutrition who do not have an ileus or fistula that prevents the usage of the gastrointestinal tract to receive some oral or enteral nutrition on a regular basis. This is done to promote the infant's skill at sucking and swallowing as well as to stimulate mucosal development. Patients who require parenteral nutrition on a long-term basis can be discharged from the hospital after the family is educated in the techniques for the care of the central line and infusion pumps. Home TPN is indicated in a variety of patients with short bowel syndromes, serious mucosal injury, or pseudo-obstruction syndromes.[68]

Children on home TPN can lead productive lives and do most things that other children do.

As small intestinal transplantation becomes more successful, it may become possible that patients who formerly anticipated living their life on parenteral nutrition will be able to return to enteral feedings and a more normal existence.

REFERENCES

1. Booth IW, Shaw V: Parenteral nutrition. *In* Milla PJ, Muller DRR, eds: Harries' Pediatric Gastroenterology. Edinburgh, Churchill Livingstone, 1988, p 588.
2. Weinsier RL, Heimburger DC, Butterworth CE: Handbook of Clinical Nutrition. St. Louis, CV Mosby, 1989, p 99.
3. Reimer SL, Michener WM, Steiger E: Nutritional support of the critically ill child. Pediatr Clin North Am 1980; 27:647–660.
4. Singer P, Katz DP, Dillon L, et al: Nutritional aspects of the acquired immunodeficiency syndrome. Am J Gastroenterol 1992; 87: 265–273.
5. Candy DCA: Parenteral nutrition in paediatric practice: A review. J Hum Nutr 1980; 34:287–296.
6. Levy JS, Winters RW, Heird WC: Total parenteral nutrition in pediatric patients. Pediatr Rev 1980; 4:99–106.
7. Reichman B, Chessex P, Putet G, et al: Diet, fat accretion, and growth in premature infants. N Engl J Med 1981; 305:1495–1500.
8. Wheeler N. Parenteral nutrition: *In* Kelts DG, Jones RD, eds: Manual of Pediatric Nutrition. Boston, Little, Brown, 1984, p 151.
9. Caldwell MO, Kennedy CC: Normal nutritional requirements. Surg Clin North Am 1981; 61:491–498.
10. Zlotkin SH, Stallings VA, Pencharz PB: Total parenteral nutrition in children. Pediatr Clin North Am 1985; 32:381–400.
11. Baker JP, Detsky AS, Stewart S, et al: Randomized trial of total parenteral nutrition in critically ill patients: Metabolic effects of varying glucose-lipid ratios as the energy source. Gastroenterology 1984; 87:53–59.
12. Zlotkin SH, Bryan MH, Anderson CH: Intravenous nitrogen and energy intakes required to duplicate in utero nitrogen accretion in prematurely born human infants. J Pediatr 1981; 99:115–120.
13. Cochran EB, Phelps SJ, Helms RA: Parenteral nutrition in pediatric patients. Clin Pharmacol 1988; 7:351–366.
14. Adamkin DH: Total parenteral nutrition in hyaline membrane disease. *In* Lebenthal E, ed: Total parenteral nutrition: Indications, utilization, complications, pathophysiologic considerations. New York, Raven Press, 1986, p 305.
15. Bell EF, Warburton D, Stonestreet BS, et al: Effect of fluid administration on the development of symptomatic patent ductus arteriosus and congestive heart failure in premature infants. N Engl J Med 1980; 302:598–604.
16. Brown ER, Start A, Sosenko I, et al: Bronchopulmonary dysplasia: Possible relationship to pulmonary edema. J Pediatr 1978; 92:982–984.
17. Goldman HI: Feeding and necrotizing enterocolitis. Am J Dis Child 1980; 134:553–555.
18. Goldbert RN, Chung D, Goldman SL, et al: The association of rapid volume expansion and intraventricular hemorrhage in the preterm infant. J Pediatr 1980; 96:1060–1063.
19. Kerner JA: Carbohydrate requirements. *In* Kerner JA Jr, ed: Manual of Pediatric Parenteral Nutrition. New York, John Wiley & Sons, 1983, p 79.
20. Committee on Nutrition, American Academy of Pediatrics: Parenteral nutrition. *In* Forbes GB, Woodruff CW, eds: Pediatric Nutrition Handbook. Chicago, American Academy of Pediatrics, 1985, p 154.
21. Committee on Nutrition, American Academy of Pediatrics: Commentary on parenteral nutrition. Pediatrics 1983; 71:547–552.
22. Bursztein S, Elwyn DH, Askanazi J, Kinney JM, eds: The theoretical framework of indirect calorimetry and energy balance. *In* Energy, Metabolism, Indirect Calorimetry and Nutrition. Baltimore, Williams & Wilkins, 1989, pp 27–83.
23. Pereira GR, Glassman M: Parenteral nutrition in the neonate. *In* Rombeau JL, Caldwell MD, eds: Parenteral Nutrition. Philadelphia, WB Saunders, 1986, p 702.
24. Schwartz R: Should exogenous insulin be given to very low birth weight infants? J Pediatr Gastroenterol Nutr 1982; 1:287–288.
25. Vaucher YE, Walson PD, Morrow G: Continuous insulin infusion in hyperglycemic, very low birth weight infants. J Pediatr Gastroenterol Nutr 1982; 1:211–217.
26. Wu PYK, Edwards NB, Storm MC: Characterization of the plasma amino acid pattern of normal term breast-fed infants. J Pediatr 1986; 109:347–349.
27. Heird WC, Dell RB, Helms RA, et al: Amino acid mixture designed to maintain normal plasma amino acid patterns in infants and children requiring parenteral nutrition. Pediatrics 1987; 80:401–408.
28. Helms RA, Christensen ML, Mauer EC: Comparison of pediatric versus standard amino acid formulation in preterm neonates requiring parenteral nutrition. J Pediatr 1987; 110:466–470.
29. Cashore WJ, Sedaghatian MR, Usher RH: Nutritional supplements with intravenously administered lipid, protein hydrolysate, and glucose in small premature infants. Pediatrics 1975; 56:8–16.
30. O'Neill JA, Caldwell MD, Meng HC: Essential fatty acid deficiency in surgical patients. Ann Surg 1977; 185:536–543.
31. Friedman Z, Danon A, Stahlman MT, et al: Rapid onset of essential fatty acid deficiency in the newborn. Pediatrics 1976; 58:640–649.
32. Friedman Z, Schochat SJ, Maisels JM, et al: Correction of essential fatty acid deficiency in newborn infants by cutaneous application of sunflower seed oil. Pediatrics 1976; 58:650–654.
33. Brans YW, Andrews DS, Carrillo DW, et al: Tolerance of fat emulsions in very-low-birth-weight infants. Am J Dis Child 1988; 142:145–152.
34. Cooke RJ, Burckhart GJ: Hypertriglyceridemia during the intravenous infusion of a safflower-oil based fat emulsion. J Pediatr 1983; 103:959–961.
35. Nizar L, Vyhmeister N, Fisher L, Grill B: The risk of hypertriglyceridemia increases with the duration of intravenous fat administration (abstract). Clin Res 1990; 38:191A.
36. Grill B, Yoon S, Fisher L, et al: Prospective comparison of two intravenous lipid emulsions in premature infants: Effects on plasma fatty acids (abstract). JPEN 1990; 14:115.
37. Helms RA, Borum PR, Hay WW, et al: Intravenous (IV) carnitine during parenteral nutrition (PN) in neonates. JPEN 1987; 11(Suppl):9.
38. Helms RA, Whitington PF, Mauer EC, et al: Enhanced lipid utilization in infants receiving oral L-carnitine during long-term parenteral nutrition. J Pediatr 1986; 109:984–988.
39. Poole RL: Electrolyte and mineral requirements. *In* Kerner JA Jr, ed: Manual of Pediatric Parenteral Nutrition. New York, John Wiley & Sons, 1983, p 129.
40. Lenz GT, Mikrut BA: Calcium and phosphate solubility in neonatal parenteral nutrient solutions containing Aminosyn-PF or Trophamine. Am J Hosp Pharm 1988; 45:2367–2371.
41. Kimura S, Nose O, Seino Y: Effects of alternate and simultaneous administration of calcium and phosphorus on calcium metabolism in children receiving total nutrition. JPEN 1986; 10:513–516.
42. Moore MC, Green HL, Phillips B, et al: Evaluation of a pediatric multiple vitamin preparation for total parenteral nutrition in infants and children: I. Blood levels of water-soluble vitamins. Pediatrics 1986; 77:530–538.
43. Greene HL, Phillips BL, Franck L, et al: Persistently low blood retinol levels during and after parenteral feeding of very low birth weight infants—examination of losses into IV administration sets and a method of prevention by addition to a lipid emulsion. Pediatrics 1987; 79:894–900.
44. Chen MF, Boyce HW Jr, Triplett L: Stability of the B vitamins in mixed parenteral nutrition solutions. JPEN 1983; 7:462–464.
45. Gillis J, Jones G, Pencharz P. Delivery of vitamins A, D and E in parenteral nutrition solutions. JPEN 1983; 7:11–14.
46. Shenai JP, Kennedy KA, Chytil F, Stahlman MT: Clinical trial of vitamin A supplementation in infants susceptible to bronchopulmonary dysplasia. J Pediatr 1987; 111:269–277.

47. Shenai JP, Chytil F, Stahlman MT: Vitamin A status of neonates with bronchopulmonary dysplasia. Pediatr Res 1985; 19:185–188.
48. Mock DM, DeLorimer AA, Liebman WM, et al: Biotin deficiency: An unusual complication of parenteral alimentation. N Engl J Med 1981; 304:810–812.
49. Greene HL, Hambridge KM, Schanler R, Tsang RT: Guidelines for the use of vitamins, trace elements, calcium, magnesium, and phosphorus in infants and children receiving total parenteral nutrition: Report of the Subcommittee on Pediatric Parenteral Nutrition Requirements from the Committee on Clinical Practice Issues of the American Society for Clinical Nutrition. Am J Clin Nutr 1988; 48:1324–1342.
50. Wolman SL, Anderson GH, Marliss EB, Jeejeebhoy KN: Zinc in total parenteral nutrition: Requirements and metabolic effects. Gastroenterology 1979; 76:458–467.
51. Ruz M, Solomons N: Fecal zinc excretion during oral rehydration therapy for acute infectious diarrhea (abstract). Fed Proc 1987; 46:748.
52. Vinton NE, Dahlstrom KA, Strobel CT, Ament ME: Macrocytosis and pseudoalbinism: Manifestations of selenium deficiency. J Pediatr 1987; 111:711–717.
53. Kelly DA, Coe AW, Shenkin A, et al: Symptomatic selenium deficiency in a child on home parenteral nutrition. J Pediatr Gastroenterol Nutr 1988; 7:783–785.
54. Moukarzel A, Vargas J, Buchman AL, Ament ME: Chromium requirements of patients on long term parenteral nutrition are not the recommended chromium intake (abstract). Clin Res 1991; 39:652A.
55. Moukarzel AA, Song MK, Buchman AL, et al: Excessive chromium intake in children receiving total parenteral nutrition. Lancet 1992; 339:385–388.
56. Moukarzel AA, Buchman AL, Salas JS, et al: Iodine supplementation in children receiving long-term parenteral nutrition. J Pediatr 1992; 121:252–254.
57. Wan KK, Tsallas G: Dilute iron dextran formulation for addition to parenteral nutrient solutions. Am J Hosp Pharm 1980; 37:206–210.
58. Vargas J, Klein G, Ament ME, et al: Metabolic bone disease of total parenteral nutrition: Course after changing from casein to amino acids in parenteral solutions with reduced aluminum content. Am J Clin Nutr 1988; 48:1070–1078.
59. Moukarzel A, Ament ME, Vargas J, et al: Non aluminum dependent osteopathy in children on long-term parenteral nutrition (abstract). Am J Clin Nutr 1990; 51:520.
60. Koo WW, Kaplan LA: Aluminum and bone disorders: With specific reference to contamination of infant nutrients. J Am Coll Nutr 1988; 7:199–214.
61. Ziegler M, Jakobowski D, Hoelzer D, et al: Route of pediatric parenteral nutrition: Proposed criteria revision. J Pediatr Surg 1980; 15:472–476.
62. Heird WC: Parenteral nutrition. *In* Grand RJ, Sutphen JL, Dietz WH, eds: Pediatric Nutrition. Boston, Butterworths, 1987, p 747.
63. Rubenstein R, Michalak J, Stegman R, et al: Hickman catheter insertion via the percutaneous subclavian route. Nutr Support Serv 1982; 2(6):9–10.
64. Leibovitz E, Ashkenazi A, Levin S, Nissim F: Fatal cardiac tamponade complicating total parenteral nutrition via a Silastic central vein catheter (letter). J Pediatr Gastroenterol Nutr 1988; 7:306–307.
65. Morrow AL, Poirier-Kerner L, Andolina AS, Walsh ME: Nursing care of the pediatric patient on parenteral nutrition. *In* Kerner JA Jr, ed: Manual of Pediatric Parenteral Nutrition. New York, John Wiley & Sons, 1983, p 329.
66. Forlaw L, Torosian MH: Central venous catheter care. *In* Rombeau JL, Caldwell MD, eds: Parenteral Nutrition. Philadelphia, WB Saunders, 1986, p 306.
67. Warner BW, Gorgone P, Schilling S, et al: Multiple purpose central venous access in infants less than 1,000 grams. J Pediatr Surg 1987; 22:820–822.
68. Vargas J, Ament ME, Berquist WE: Long term home parenteral nutrition in pediatrics: Ten years' experience in 102 patients. J Pediatr Gastroenterol Nutr 1987; 6:24–32.
69. Hattner JAT, Kerner JA Jr: Nutritional assessment of the pediatric patients. *In* Kerner JA Jr, ed: Manual of Pediatric Parenteral Nutrition. New York, John Wiley & Sons, 1983, p 19.
70. Ney D: Nutritional assessment. *In* Kelts DG, Jones RD, eds: Manual of Pediatric Nutrition. Boston, Little, Brown, 1984, p 99.
71. Walker WA, Hendricks K: Manual of Pediatric Nutrition. Philadelphia, WB Saunders, 1985.
72. Merritt RJ, Blackburn GL: Nutritional Assessment and Metabolic Book of Pediatric Nutrition. New York, Raven Press, 1981, p 285.
73. Vaucher YE, Harrison GG, Udal JN, et al: Skinfold thickness in North American infants 24–41 weeks gestation. Hum Biol 1984; 5:713–731.
74. Sasanow SR, Georgieff MK, Pereira GR: Mid-arm circumference and mid-arm/head circumference ratios: Standard curves for anthropometric assessment of neonatal status. J Pediatr 1987; 109:316–321.
75. Heird WC: Effects of total parenteral alimentation on intestinal function. *In* Sunshine P, ed: Gastrointestinal Development and Neonatal Nutrition: Report of the 72nd Ross Conference on Pediatric Research. Columbus, OH, Ross Laboratories, 1977, pp 68–72.
76. Ament ME, Barclay GN: Chronic diarrhea. Pediatr Ann 1982; 11(1):124–131.
77. Jewett TC Jr: Techniques with catheters and complications of total parenteral nutrition. *In* Lebenthal E, ed: Total Parenteral Nutrition: Indications, Utilization, Complications, and Pathophysiological Considerations. New York, Raven Press, 1986, p 185.
78. Grant JP: Catheter access. *In* Rombeau JL, Caldwell MD, eds: Parenteral Nutrition. Philadelphia, WB Saunders, 1986, p 306.
79. Kerner JA Jr: Technical complications. *In* Kerner JA Jr, ed: Manual of Pediatric Parenteral Nutrition. New York, John Wiley & Sons, 1983, p 193.
80. Haire WD, Lieberman RP: Thrombosed central venous catheters: Restoring function with 6-hour urokinase infusion after failure of bolus urokinase. JPEN 1992; 16:129–132.
81. Bagnall HA, Gomperts E, Atkinson JB: Continuous infusion of low-dose urokinase in the treatment of central venous catheter thrombosis in infants and children. Pediatrics 1989; 83:963–966.
82. Shulman RJ, Reed T, Pitre D, Laine L: Use of hydrochloric acid to clear obstructed central venous catheters. JPEN 1988; 12:509–512.
83. Atkinson JB, Bagnall HA, Gomperts E: Investigational use of tissue plasminogen activator (t-PA) for occluded central venous catheters. JPEN 1990; 14:310–311.
84. Nahata MC, King DR, Powell DA, et al: Management of catheter related infections in pediatric patients. JPEN 1988; 12:58–59.
85. Wang EEL, Prober CG, Ford-Jones L, Gold R: The management of central intravenous catheter infections. Pediatr Infect Dis 1984; 3:110–113.
86. Marino L, Hack M, Dahms B: Two year follow-up: Growth and neonatal PN-associated liver disease (abstract). JPEN 1981; 5:569.
87. Kibort PM, Ulich TR, Berquist WE, et al: Hepatic fibrosis and cirrhosis in children on long term parenteral nutrition (abstract). Clin Res 1982; 30:115.
88. Hodes JE, Grosfeld JL, Weber TR, et al: Hepatic failure in infants on total parenteral nutrition (TPN): Clinical and histopathologic observations. J Pediatr Surg 1982; 17:463–468.
89. King DR, Ginn-Pease ME, Lloyd TV, et al: Parenteral nutrition with associated cholelithiasis: Another iatrogenic disease of infants and children. J Pediatr Surg 1987; 22:593–596.
90. Roslyn JJ, Pitt HA, Mann LL, et al: Gallbladder disease in patients on long-term parenteral nutrition. Gastroenterology 1983; 84:148–154.
91. Whitington PF, Black DD: Cholelithiasis in premature infants treated with parenteral nutrition and furosemide. J Pediatr 1980; 97:647–649.
92. Tsang RC: The quandary of vitamin D in the newborn infant. Lancet 1983; 1:1370–1372.
93. Moukarzel AA, Buchman AL, Vargas J, et al: Is fluoride deficiency related to the bone disease of parenteral nutrition (PN)? Gastroenterology (in press).
94. Nichols BL, Alvarado J, Rodriguez J, et al: Therapeutic implications of electrolyte, water and nitrogen losses during recovery from protein-calorie malnutrition. J Pediatr 1974; 84:759–768.

95. Schreiner RL, Glick MR, Nordschow CD, Gresham EL: An evaluation of methods to monitor infants receiving intravenous lipids. J Pediatr 1979; 94:197–200.
96. Hammerman C, Aramburo MJ: Decreased lipid intake reduces morbidity in sick premature neonates. J Pediatr 1988; 113:1083–1088.
97. Zaiden H, Dhanireddy R, Hamosh M, et al: Effect of continuous heparin administration of Intralipid® clearing in very-low-birth-weight infants. J Pediatr 1982; 101:599–602.
98. Committee on Nutrition, American Academy of Pediatrics: Use of intravenous fat emulsions in pediatric patients. Pediatrics 1981; 68:738–743.
99. Dahlstrom KA, McIntosh N, Ament ME: A comparison of two 20% lipid emulsions. JPEN 1987; 11(2):149–151.
100. Cohen IT, Dahms B, Hays DM: Peripheral total parenteral nutrition employing a lipid emulsion (Intralipid®): Complications encountered in pediatric patients. J Pediatr Surg 1977; 12:837–845.

Chapter 85

Management of Acute Diarrhea

MATHURAM SANTOSHAM, CHRISTOPHER DUGGAN, KENNETH H. BROWN, and WILLIAM B. GREENOUGH III

INTRODUCTION

Diarrheal diseases are a major cause of pediatric mortality and morbidity worldwide, with 1.5 billion episodes and 4 million deaths estimated to occur yearly in developing countries.[1] Even in an industrialized country such as the United States, more than 200,000 children are hospitalized annually because of diarrhea, and more than 500 childhood deaths occur.[2]

During the past two decades, a number of infectious agents that cause acute diarrhea have been identified.[3] The mechanisms by which these organisms cause disease and the ensuing pathophysiologic disturbances that occur in the host have also been carefully delineated.[4] Probably the single most important recent achievement related to control of diarrhea-induced mortality has been the demonstration of the safety and efficacy of oral rehydration solutions (ORS). Another major advance has been our increased knowledge about the appropriate dietary management of diarrhea. The term oral rehydration therapy (ORT) is used to mean both the appropriate fluid and electrolyte management and dietary therapy. In this chapter, the major historical events that have led up to our understanding of ORT and its current status as the mainstay of diarrheal therapy are described.

Dehydration, the most serious acute complication of diarrhea, refers literally to a water deficit only (Gr., *hydor* = water) but is taken to mean a deficiency of both water and solutes when used to describe patients with diarrhea. This distinction is important historically because the design of fluids to treat dehydration successfully was possible only after the volume and solute composition of diarrheal stools were known.

Vibrio cholerae infections, the most extreme type of dehydrating diarrhea, struck England and Russia in the early 19th century, thus providing the incentive for the first attempts at the intravenous fluid therapy.[5,6] O'Shaughnessy (as quoted[7]) was the first to describe the physiologic disturbances in diarrhea and to outline the rationale for intravenous therapy as an attempt "first to restore the blood to its natural specific gravity; second to restore its deficient saline matters." Latta,[8] who is credited with the first use of such treatment, employed a solution with approximately 58 mmol per L of sodium, 49 mmol per L of chloride, and 9 mmol per L of bicarbonate. He had some initial success with injections of this fluid; because of lack of sterile technique, however, chills and sepsis frequently resulted after intravenous fluid therapy. In addition, patients selected for intravenous treatment were usually near death from hypovolemia and often succumbed despite treatment. Not surprisingly, widespread acceptance of intravenous therapy for cholera was delayed until the 20th century.[7]

Mortality from cholera was eventually reduced from 60 to 30% with the use of intravenous solutions, and a further reduction occurred following the addition of sodium bicarbonate to the fluid.[9] This success was possible despite errors in measuring the solute concentration in choleric stools, a mistake that led to the use of a hypertonic solution for many years.[10] Accurate stool analysis eventually permitted the formulation of a more appropriate intravenous solution, so that all cases of cholera in Thailand in 1958 were treated successfully.[11] Between 1962 and 1967 in Dhaka, Bangladesh, a standard intravenous solution was given to cholera patients with excellent results, even under adverse field conditions. Simultaneously, a team in Calcutta from The Johns Hopkins University and the All India Institute of Tropical Medicine and Hygiene developed effective intravenous replacement therapy and further described the pathophysiological derangements produced by cholera.[12]

Because many of the studies documenting the effectiveness of intravenous therapy for diarrheal dehydration were conducted in economically disadvantaged populations, there was a strong impetus to develop less expensive but equally effective oral solutions, which would be more accessible to the poor. Oral solutions would also have the advantage of being less invasive and of reducing the need for admission to the hospital. The first sophisticated ORS were developed by Harrison in Baltimore and Darrow at Yale in the 1940s. Harrison's solution contained (in mmol per L): sodium 62, potassium 20, chloride 52, lactate 30, and glucose 183 (3.3%).[13] A commercial preparation (Lytren, Mead Johnson Company) was soon available in the United

States, but its widespread use in the 1950s coincided with an apparent increased incidence of hypernatremia.[14] Whether the product's relatively high carbohydrate concentration (8%), incorrect mixing, or suboptimal dietary practices (e.g., ingestion of boiled skim milk) were to blame, ORS soon fell out of favor in the North American pediatric community.

Meanwhile, basic studies on intestinal solute transport mechanisms were pointing the way to a more physiologic solution. At Oxford University, it was shown that the addition of glucose to solutions of sodium chloride resulted in an accelerated movement of fluid across the rabbit intestinal mucosa.[15] Further studies from Harvard University[16] and the U.S. Air Force[17] indicated that the absorption of 1 molecule of glucose was linked with that of 1 ion of sodium and that this process took place at the brush border of the intestinal epithelium. It was later shown that the other organic molecules, such as amino acids, dipeptides, and tripeptides, could also participate in this "cotransport" phenomenon,[18] and that this process remained intact during acute diarrhea.[19]

Clinical data supporting these results were soon obtained. Investigators at the Cholera Research Laboratory in Dhaka, at the Johns Hopkins Research Unit in Calcutta, and in Thailand were all making clinical observations of cholera patients.[12] In 1965 in Dhaka, it was demonstrated that intestinal perfusion of cholera patients with glucose altered the transepithelial membrane potential in a way consistent with an active cotransport process.[20] Subsequently, studies both in Dhaka and Calcutta confirmed that the addition of glucose to sodium-containing solutions resulted in net movement of salt and water from the intestinal lumen to the blood stream of patients with severe cholera.[21, 22] Safe, practical, and physiologically appropriate solutions were then formulated,[23] with the first field testing of ORS occurring in the rural Bangladesh area of Matlab Bazaar.[24] This trial established oral rehydration as an effective method of treating diarrhea patients, even those with severe cholera. Further evidence for the efficacy of ORS was obtained under adverse field conditions during the War of Liberation of Bangladesh in 1971. Millions of refugees fled to camps near Calcutta, where an epidemic of cholera occurred. Use of ORS reduced mortality rates from more than 50% to less than 5% and eventually, when combined with initial intravenous therapy, to less than 1%.[25]

PHYSIOLOGIC BASIS FOR THE COMPOSITION OF ORAL REHYDRATION SOLUTIONS

A discussion of the physiologic basis of ORS composition requires some understanding of the pathophysiology of diarrheal disease (see Chapter 15). Briefly, because diarrhea may be defined as a state of increased fecal water excretion, and because net solute movement largely determines water movement, the secretion and absorption of electrolytes are crucial in the pathogenesis of diarrhea.[26] Cholera, whose toxin stimulates cyclic adenosine monophosphate (cAMP)-mediated chloride secretion into the gut lumen, is a prime example of a secretory diarrhea. As already noted, the determination of the solute concentration of diarrheal stools was crucial in the design of appropriate replacement fluids. In severe cholera, the composition of stools can approach that of an ultrafiltrate of plasma, with further potassium and bicarbonate added by colonic secretion. Thus, the original ORS compositions, based as they were on data in cholera patients, contained 100 to 120 mmol per L of sodium.

Because many of the landmark studies of ORS were done on patients suffering from cholera, concern was raised whether a solution designed for the treatment of a severe, secretory diarrhea would be appropriate for the treatment of the more common, but less severe, viral infections. In these patients, diarrhea occurs not as a result of active secretion of electrolytes and fluids as much as the reduced absorptive capabilities of damaged intestinal villi.[27] Sodium and water losses are less than those of cholera patients (Table 85–1). Of note in such conditions when absorptive capacity is reduced is the ability of osmotic forces in the gastrointestinal lumen to exacerbate fluid afflux from the blood stream into the intestine. Clinical implications of these pathophysiologic factors are as follows:

1. Children with high purging rates have an increased requirement for sodium in the replacement fluid; if given only water, they are at risk for hyponatremia and resultant central nervous system dysfunction.
2. If hyperosmotic oral solutions (such as those high in either salts or sugar) are offered instead, the increased osmotic load may worsen the diarrhea. Hypernatremia may ensue, which can lead to central nervous system thromboses and permanent neurologic sequelae.[29] Thus, an osmotically balanced solution is necessary for optimal results.

Considerations such as these led some to argue for the development and production of two types of ORS: one of higher sodium content for cholera and other conditions with high stool outputs and another lower in salts for viral gastrointestinal infections.[30] In 1975, a

Table 85–1. MEAN STOOL OUTPUT AND STOOL SODIUM CONCENTRATION IN CHILDREN WITH CHOLERA, ENTEROTOXIGENIC *ESCHERICHIA COLI*, AND ROTAVIRUS DIARRHEA

Organism	Stool Output (ml/kg/8 hours)	Stool Sodium on Admission† (mEq/L)
Cholera (n = 37)	60.1 ± 40.1	88.9 ± 27.9
ETEC (n = 38)	39.2 ± 22.2	53.7 ± 28.0
Rotavirus (n = 45)	33.1 ± 19.0	37.2 ± 22.0

*Cholera versus ETEC and rotavirus, $P < 0.01$.
†Cholera versus ETEC and rotavirus, $P < 0.001$.
ETEC, enterotoxigenic *Escherichia coli*.
From Molla AM, Rahaman M, Sarker SA, et al: Stool electrolyte content and purging rates in diarrhea caused by rotavirus, enterotoxigenic *E. coli* and *V. cholerae* in children. J Pediatr 1981; 98:835–838; with permission.

Table 85–2. COMPOSITION OF COMMERCIAL ORAL REHYDRATION SOLUTIONS AS WELL AS FREQUENTLY USED ORAL SOLUTIONS

Liquid	Carbohydrate (gm/100 ml)	Sodium in (mEq/L)	Potassium in (mEq/L)	Chloride in (mEq/L)	Bicarbonate* in (mEq/L)
WHO-ORS	2.0	90	20	80	30
Hydra-Lyte	1.2	84	10	59	10
Rehydralyte	2.5	75	20	65	30
Pedialyte	2.5	45	20	35	30
Lytren	2.0	50	25	45	30
Resol	2.0	50	20	50	34
Infalyte	2.0	50	20	40	30
Apple juice	11.9	0.43	25	—	—
Coca-Cola	10.0	3.6	—	—	13.4
Gatorade	4	23.5	2.5	17	—
7-UP	10.0	0.5	—	—	—
Water (Baltimore city)	—	3	0.5	4	—

*Actual or potential bicarbonate, such as lactate, citrate, or acetate.
Adapted from Santosham M, et al. Pediatr Rev. Reproduced by permission of Pediatrics, vol. 8, p. 276, 1987.

group of investigators who were interested in reducing diarrheal mortality by promoting ORS met to resolve this controversy. At this meeting, it was agreed that both the World Health Organization (WHO) and UNICEF would promote a single solution (WHO-ORS) containing (in mmol per L): sodium 90, potassium 20, chloride 80, bicarbonate 30, and glucose 111 (2%). The dry ingredients of the WHO-ORS were distributed in convenient packages containing (in gm) sodium chloride 3.5, sodium bicarbonate 2.5, potassium chloride 1.5, and glucose 20, with instructions to mix each packet with 1 L of water. A single solution was promoted because of the realization that it would be simpler and ultimately safer to train health workers at all levels of education in different countries to use just one solution appropriately. The WHO-ORS, which represents a compromise between the optimal sodium concentration desired for the rapidly purging cholera patients and the lower sodium concentration needed by those with viral gastroenteritis, has in fact been found to be safe and efficacious for both cholera and noncholera diarrhea, and in all age ranges of patients.[23]

CLINICAL STUDIES

During the late 1960s and 1970s a number of studies were conducted in developing countries using the WHO-ORS. These studies clearly established the safety and efficacy of WHO-ORS in treating diarrhea of all causes in adults and children.[19] It was also shown that proper use of the WHO-ORS can safely correct hypernatremia and hyponatremia,[31] thus helping to allay concerns about possible induction of hypernatremia by oral rehydration. Based on these studies, WHO recommended the use of WHO-ORS for the treatment of diarrhea in children and adults, regardless of the cause of the diarrhea or initial serum sodium value. This form of therapy has been widely used and well accepted in developing countries.

The first clinical studies to evaluate the use of ORT in more affluent countries were conducted on the Apache Indian Reservation in Arizona in the early 1970s.[32, 33] These studies confirmed the previous findings in developing countries, but reluctance to use ORS in the U.S. pediatric community continued, primarily because of the unsubstantiated fear that WHO-ORS might induce hypernatremia. Consequently, pediatricians in the United States continued to use intravenous therapy for treatment of hospitalized patients with diarrhea. They also recommended a variety of "clear liquids," which contained an inappropriately low concentration of sodium and high concentration of carbohydrate (Table 85–2). The ORS commercially available at that time also had relatively low sodium concentration (25 to 30 mmol per L) and high carbohydrate concentration (5 to 8%). To assess these concerns, Santosham and coworkers[35] conducted a randomized, controlled clinical trial of well-nourished Panamanian and U.S. children hospitalized with acute diarrhea. Fifty children received the WHO-ORS, 48 received a similar solution with 50 mmol per L of sodium instead of 90, and 48 received standard intravenous therapy. There were no differences in stool output or duration of diarrhea among the three groups, and all patients with hypernatremia or hyponatremia had safe resolution of these electrolyte imbalances with ORS alone. Other investigators likewise confirmed the safety and efficacy of ORS for infants hospitalized in the United States.[36]

Studies evaluating ORS for the outpatient management of mild diarrhea in children from the United States have also been done. In one,[37] four different oral solutions (whose sodium concentrations ranged from 90 to 30 mmol per L) were given to outpatients with less than 5% dehydration. Ninety-eight percent (137 of 140) of the subjects were successfully treated as outpatients, and no differences in duration of diarrhea or amount of fluid ingested were found among the groups. Other investigators have shown that the use of oral rather than intravenous fluid therapy for infantile diarrhea in a U.S. hospital emergency room can lead to substantial cost savings with equal efficacy.[38]

Based on these studies conducted in the United States, the American Academy of Pediatrics (AAP) made the following recommendations for the treatment of diarrhea in developed countries.[39] For rehydration therapy, oral solutions should contain 2 to 2.5% (110 to 140 mmol per L) of glucose, 75 to 90 mmol per L of sodium, 20 mmol per L potassium, 20 to 30% of anions as base, and the remainder as chloride. For maintenance therapy, the sodium content should be reduced to 40 to 60 mmol per L. Alternatively, a solution such as the WHO-ORS could be used for both hydration and maintenance if during the latter period low sodium fluids, such as water, low osmolar juices, or breast milk, are taken in equal amounts as the rehydration solution.

LIMITATIONS OF ORAL REHYDRATION THERAPY

Although oral rehydration therapy is recommended for all age groups and for diarrhea of any cause, some restrictions to its use do exist, as described in the following:

Severe Dehydration. Patients in shock or near shock should be treated with intravenous solutions. When pulse, blood pressure, state of consciousness, and ability to drink return to normal, rehydration therapy can be continued orally. Likewise, patients with abdominal ileus should not be given oral fluids until bowel sounds are audible.

Intractable Vomiting. Almost all patients with acute diarrhea present with vomiting as well. The vast majority, however, can be successfully rehydrated with oral fluids if small volumes of ORS (5 to 10 ml) are given every 5 minutes, with a gradual increase in the amount consumed. A common mistake is to allow a thirsty infant to drink large volumes ad libitum from a cup or a feeding bottle; the caretaker should be instructed to give ORS in small amounts via a spoon or syringe. Continuous nasogastric drip infusion of ORS is also sometimes helpful in the vomiting child. Often, correction of acidosis during the first few hours of rehydration therapy will reduce the rate of vomiting, although occasionally intractable vomiting will prevent successful oral rehydration and necessitate recourse to intravenous therapy.

High Stool Output. The chances of a patient being able to maintain positive fluid balance decline with increasing stool output; one study in patients with cholera[40] found that the success rate of oral therapy decreased from greater than 90% to about 67% when stool outputs exceeded 10 ml per kg per hour. No patient should be denied ORT therapy simply because of a high purging rate, as most patients will respond to oral treatment.

Carbohydrate Malabsorption. The presence of glucose or reducing substances in the stools accompanied by a dramatic increase in stool output with the administration of ORS is an indication of carbohydrate malabsorption. The presence of stool-reducing substances alone is not sufficient to make the diagnosis because many such infants can be successfully managed by oral therapy. Patients with true glucose malabsorption will also show an immediate reduction in stool output when ORS is replaced with intravenous therapy. The incidence of clinically significant glucose malabsorption during acute diarrhea is approximately 1% in most populations, although rates as high as 8% have been reported in selected studies.[41]

PREPARATION AND PACKAGING OF ORAL REHYDRATION SOLUTIONS

ORS may be distributed premixed with water or as dry ingredients in packets. The latter type of preparation is more common in developing countries, where low cost, long shelf life, and ease of transport make it more suitable. The disadvantage of packets is the potential for mixing with inappropriate volumes of water. The resulting ORS may then be too dilute or too concentrated.[42] For the reconstitution of ORS in packets, the cleanest available source of water should be used. In areas with contaminated water, cooled, boiled water is recommended. Oral rehydration should never be withheld from a dehydrated child solely because of concerns over water purity.

The bicarbonate component of the WHO-ORS has been replaced with the bicarbonate precursor, citrate, owing to its longer shelf life. Citrate-containing solutions are as efficacious as ones containing bicarbonate,[41] and both bases aid in the intestinal absorption of sodium and water.[43] In the past 5 years, manufacturers of ORS in the United States have altered their formulations to contain appropriate concentrations of carbohydrate (see Table 85–2). The sodium concentrations of the fluids have also been increased compared with previously available ORS.

DIETARY THERAPY

The nutritional management of the child with acute diarrhea has been the subject of renewed debate during the past several years. A patient with diarrhea is at nutritional risk for several reasons: anorexia and food withdrawal may prevent adequate energy and nutrient intakes; gastrointestinal absorption of carbohydrates, fats, proteins, and micronutrients may be decreased; excess urinary and stool nitrogen losses are likely, even in subclinical infections; and metabolic demands may be higher with fever and systemic illness.[44] Community-based studies in Latin America, Africa, and Asia[45, 46, 47] have documented adverse nutritional consequences and eventual growth retardation secondary to repeated gastrointestinal infections. Subsequently, researchers have sought the best way of preventing these nutritional complications.

Two alternative dietary approaches have been considered: reduction of feeding during illness (to avoid osmotic diarrhea secondary to intestinal malabsorption) versus continued enteral feeding (to avoid the adverse nutritional consequences of fasting).[48] The advantage of the traditional advice of "resting the gut" is the reduced stool output commonly seen in fasting infants. Fasting also leads directly to reduced enterocyte renewal,[49] however, an effect that is not reversed with parenteral (versus enteral) nutrition.[50] Enteral nutrition stimulates intestinal cell renewal in several ways. In the short bowel syndrome, for example, villous hypertrophy and increased absorptive capability are stimulated by the direct effects of nutrients on the mucosa and by the nutrient-induced secretion of trophic hormones in the gastrointestinal tract.[51] Further, intestinal permeability is increased in fasted (as opposed to fed) children with acute diarrhea.[52] Thus, there are several theoretical reasons to avoid fasting.

Two clinical trials, using lactose-free formulas, have compared these two approaches to dietary therapy in well-nourished infants with diarrhea. In Arizona,[53] Apache infants less than 12 months old received initial rehydration therapy before being randomized to one of two maintenance diets. One group received a full-strength, soy-protein isolate, lactose-free formula at 150 ml per kg per 24 hours throughout the maintenance phase. The control group received WHO-ORS and water (each at 75 ml per kg per 24 hours) for the first 48 hours of maintenance therapy; half-strength, soy formula for the next 24 hours; and finally full-strength formula for the remainder of the study. Both the stool output and the duration of diarrhea were reduced by approximately 50% in the infants who were given full-strength formula immediately after rehydration when compared with the control group. The authors concluded that soy-based, lactose-free formulas can be safely used during acute diarrhea and that their use actually improves outcome in comparison with maintenance therapy using just rehydration solutions.

In Peru,[54] four different feeding regimens were compared in a group of 128 children aged 3 to 36 months with acute diarrhea. After oral rehydration, group one received a full-strength formula (casein, sucrose, corn syrup solids, and vegetable oil) at 110 kcal per kg per 24 hours; group two received a similar formula at half-strength (55 kcal per kg per 24 hours) for 48 hours before being advanced to full-strength formula; and group three received glucose ORS alone for 48 hours, half-strength formula for 48 hours, then full-strength formula. Although stool output in the last group was significantly lower than that in the other groups for the first 48 hours, the difference disappeared when these patients were fed. Moreover, the duration of diarrhea and failure rates among all four groups were similar. Interestingly, nitrogen balance, energy absorption, weight gain, and change in arm circumference and skinfold thickness were all positively related to the level of dietary energy intake (i.e., groups one and two had the best outcome in these categories). This study was taken as further evidence for the recommendation of continued enteral feeding during an episode of diarrhea.

Young infants who receive most of their nutrients from cow's milk or milk-derived formulas (but are not yet consuming solid foods) require special consideration. Lactose in these products must be digested by mucosal lactase before being absorbed by the small intestine. Lactase is the disaccharidase most easily injured during enteric infections, being the first to decrease and the last to reappear.[55] Incompletely absorbed lactose can exacerbate diarrhea and contribute to systemic acidosis.[56]

Conway and Ireson[57] compared four different patterns of feeding in 200 well-nourished infants: One group received ORS for 24 hours before being gradually advanced to a full-strength, lactose-containing formula over 72 hours, whereas patients in the other three groups received full-strength formulas immediately on rehydration, the formulas differing only in their lactose content (regular, low-lactose, or lactose-free). Better weight gain was seen at 2 and 5 days in the latter three groups when compared with the first group, although lower stool output was seen in the low-lactose group. Most studies generally support the conclusion that lactose-free diets are better tolerated by children hospitalized for diarrhea than are lactose-containing ones,[58] although some investigators have found no difference in the clinical outcome among children fed lactose-containing diets.[59] Moreover, mixed diets containing some milk are generally well tolerated even by known lactose malabsorbers.[60]

Considering this set of results, we recommend that full-strength, lactose-free or lactose-reduced diets be given to well-nourished, bottle-fed infants immediately on rehydration in amounts sufficient to satisfy energy and nutrient requirements. If such formulas are unavailable, full-strength, lactose-containing formulas should be used under supervision to ensure that carbohydrate malabsorption does not complicate the clinical course. Suspected lactose malabsorption can be assessed by stool pH and reducing substances; stool pH less than 6.0 and reducing substances greater than 0.5% are suggestive of carbohydrate malabsorption. Appropriate therapy includes temporary reduction or removal of lactose from the diet.

Despite concerns about lactose malabsorption in breast-fed children with diarrhea, continued breast-feeding during illness appears to be clinically advantageous. A study of breast fed patients randomized to either ORS alone or ORS plus continued breast-feeding during the first 24 hours of hospital treatment found that the breast-fed group had reduced stool output.[61] Continued breast-feeding during diarrhea is advantageous for several possible reasons. First, breast fed infants generally consume smaller amounts of milk more frequently than bottle-fed infants. Thus, the reduced amount of milk presented to the intestine per unit time may be less likely to exceed the gut's absorptive capacity. Second, the many anti-infective properties of human milk may mitigate the course of the disease as well as prevent secondary infections. In addition to these beneficial effects of breast-feeding on the outcome of diarrhea, suckling is needed to release prolactin and oxytocin, without which continued milk production is not possible. Thus, continued breast-feeding should be advocated to protect subsequent lactation, if for no other reason.*

*Of possible significance to the issue of breast-feeding during diarrhea are studies of casein-derived opioid peptides (beta-casomorphins), in which decreased peristalsis and increased ion transport across the intestinal epithelium have been seen in animal models.[62]

Older children receiving semi-solid or solid foods should continue to receive their usual diet during diarrhea. Cereal-milk and cereal-legume diets have been used successfully for the dietary management of these patients.[63, 64] Little information is available on the absorption and retention of micronutrients during childhood diarrhea, although two studies suggest that the net balance of trace elements may be decreased.[65, 66] The therapeutic implications of these observations have not yet been critically examined.

When anorexia or severe malabsorption interferes with nutritional management, dietary therapy must continue through the phase of convalescence. Energy-rich and nutrient-rich diets must be provided in amounts ranging from about 10 to 100% greater than usual requirements to ensure rapid compensatory growth.[67] The actual amount of additional food required depends on the individual's pre-existing nutritional status, amount of weight lost during the illness, and the desired rapidity of nutritional recovery.

HOME FLUID THERAPY FOR DIARRHEA

Appropriate home treatment of a child with diarrhea can obviate the need for further medical intervention by preventing dehydration and by reducing nutritional complications. The cornerstone of such management, as noted earlier, includes adequate replacement of fluid losses plus continued enteral feeding.

Two schools of thought concerning the formulation of home replacement fluids emerged at a recent symposium on ORT.[68] One group stressed the need to encourage an adequate volume of fluid intake early in the course of illness so as to prevent dehydration, with less attention given to the specific formulation of the fluid. Others emphasized the importance of using a physiologically correct solution (i.e., one with adequate sodium content), despite the recognized difficulties with standardization of fluids mixed at home.[42, 69] In line with the physiologic principles noted earlier, however, it would seem that as long as hydration and renal perfusion are maintained, reasonable variations in the sodium content of home hydration fluids may be acceptable.

A conference was held to discuss the appropriate household management of diarrhea.[70] The following recommendations were issued for selection of appropriate home fluids:

1. The most important aspect of home management to prevent dehydration is the administration of increased volumes of fluids. The choice of recommended fluids should be guided by this objective.
2. Specific home fluids recommended for the prevention of dehydration may include food-based fluids (e.g., gruels, soups) and plain fluids (e.g., water) and must be given with an appropriate diet. Although ORS solution is designed for treatment of dehydration, it may also be used as a home fluid to prevent dehydration.
3. If food-based fluids are recommended, the ones selected should be readily available (the ingredients are easy to obtain and inexpensive; preparation is easy); readily given in large volumes (considered a "drink"); acceptable for use during diarrhea (no cultural prohibitions, acceptable taste); familiar (the basic recipe is widely known); and safe (the recipe provides an appreciable margin of safety to accommodate possible errors in preparation, so fluids are unlikely to be excessively concentrated or to have too much sodium).
4. If possible, home fluids (or the foods given during diarrhea) should contain salt, to improve their effectiveness, especially in areas where access to ORS is poor. Recipes are preferred that *normally* contain a safe amount of salt. If the food-based fluid and the diet do not contain sufficient salt, it may be added to the fluid (3.0 gm per L), provided that this is considered feasible under program conditions.
5. If provision of salt in a home fluid is not feasible, unsalted foodbased fluids or a plain fluid such as water should be given along with food.
6. Sugar-salt solutions may be recommended if they are already being used and have been demonstrated to be safely prepared and effectively used in a particular setting.
7. If sugar-salt solutions are used, it is recommended that they contain 3.0 gm per L of salt and 18 gm per L of sugar. This formula provides a substantial margin of error before solutions would become potentially dangerous owing to overconcentration.
8. When food-based fluids are used for home treatment, special efforts must be made to ensure that use of the fluids does not lead to reduced intake of nutrients. This requires added emphasis on the importance of feeding during and after diarrhea.
9. Recommended home fluids should not be prepared by diluting conventional weaning foods, e.g., cereals, or soups. If for any reason weaning foods are diluted during diarrhea, vigorous efforts may be necessary to ensure that this practice ends when diarrhea stops.

An ideal strategy would be one in which mothers could be taught to use appropriate home fluids as soon as diarrhea begins and to continue feeding infants with appropriate diets. In addition, the strategy should include messages to stop administering additional fluids when diarrhea stops and to encourage infants to increase their dietary intake. Successful transfer of this information requires well-planned health education efforts.

DEVELOPMENT OF IMPROVED ORAL REHYDRATION SOLUTIONS

If the 1970s saw the widespread use of ORS, which *The Lancet* termed one of the most important medical advances of the 20th century,[71] the 1980s have witnessed further efforts to develop more efficacious solutions, especially for use in the developing world, where the problem of diarrhea is particularly severe. Among the recognized problems of the current WHO-ORS are the following:

1. Glucose-based ORS has been widely demonstrated

to be effective in treating and preventing dehydration, but it has no effect on the duration of diarrhea or stool output. Thus, many caretakers and practitioners still make recourse to multiple, costly, and often ill-advised therapeutics in an effort to reduce diarrhea.

2. Although from 1983 to 1987 the worldwide production of ORS packets has more than tripled (from 100 million to 350 million),[68] the sheer scale of the incidence of diarrhea makes even this large number insufficient to meet the world's needs. Each of the developing world's 240 million children less than 3 years old is expected to have six to 10 episodes of enteric infections annually.[72] It would be impossible to produce and distribute adequate numbers of packets for each episode.

3. The distribution by health centers and practitioners of special packets for diarrhea is thought by some to create further dependency on the health care system for an illness that can, with sufficient education, be treated successfully at home.

Cereal-based ORS, in which complex carbohydrate sources, such as rice, wheat, maize, or potato, are used in place of the simple carbohydrate glucose, have the potential to remedy all three of these drawbacks. Reasoning along the physiologic principles of cotransport (see earlier), researchers in Dhaka and Calcutta hoped to improve intestinal absorption of fluid and electrolytes by presenting more carrier molecules to the gastrointestinal mucosa. Simply adding more glucose or peptide carriers to the solution was one approach, and a glycine-based ORS has been subjected to clinical trials[73, 74] with mixed results. A study in which the WHO-ORS was compared with a solution containing alanine showed a 40% reduction in stool output among those who received alanine.[75]

Alternatively, glucose polymers, starch, and proteins could be added, which in turn would be hydrolyzed into carrier units of glucose and peptides by the action of digestive enzymes such as amylase and peptidase.[76] Use of these polymers would not increase luminal osmotic forces (which would be counterproductive to the absorption of water and electrolytes), as would happen if the individual carrier molecules were added from the start. Studies have demonstrated that glucose polymer–based ORS are at least as efficacious as glucose-based ORS.[77]

Successful use of cereal-based ORS (in which 50 gm per L of cooked rice powder was substituted for 20 gm per L of glucose in the formulation of ORS) was first reported by Patra and associates[78] and Molla and colleagues,[79] both in 1982. In the first study, 26 children aged 3 months to 5 years with acute, dehydrating diarrhea were given a rice-based solution. Compared with matched controls, study children had lower purging rates during the first 24 hours and a shorter duration of diarrhea. Confirmatory results have been forthcoming.[80, 81] Thus, cereal-based ORS, with its potential for reducing stool output and its ability to be made at home with common sources of starch,[82] seems to be an excellent alternative to glucose-based ORS.

Cereal-based ORT, however, is not without its own problems: (1) Preparation of the solution takes time and, if not made from pre-cooked ingredients, cooking fuel; (2) without refrigeration, bacterial contamination is likely within several hours; (3) caretakers may wrongly perceive that cereal-based solutions contain adequate energy and nutrients, with underfeeding a result; and (4) standardization of cereal-based solutions may prove difficult (chemical analyses of several food-based solutions made by mothers in India, for example, showed a wide range of sodium content and generally inadequate amounts of base and glucose).[83]

Moreover, critical analysis of studies supporting the use of cereal-based ORS reveals that the quantity and quality of the maintenance diet was often not standardized or measured adequately, leaving open the possibility that variations in diet accounted for the results. As noted previously, it has also been shown that early feeding reduces the severity, duration, and nutritional consequences of diarrhea. It has been suggested by some that the relative advantages of cereal-based ORS over glucose-based ORS will not be seen if food is provided immediately after rehydration to both groups of individuals.[68, 81] Large-scale studies comparing cereal-based ORS with glucose-based ORS, in which all subjects receive standardized, early feedings, are currently ongoing in Egypt and Pakistan. It seems likely that instead of entirely replacing glucose-based ORS as treatment for acute diarrhea, cereal-based solutions will prove to be an effective therapeutic alternative, especially in those areas where distribution of packets is limited or where cultural acceptance of cereal-based solutions is higher.

RECOMMENDATIONS FOR THE TREATMENT OF ACUTE DIARRHEA

Fluid therapy in acute diarrhea is given in two phases: rehydration and maintenance (Table 85–3). During rehydration, the estimated fluid deficit based on clinical assessment is replaced. Although many symptoms and signs have been used for this purpose, evidence[84] indicates that some signs (e.g., deep breathing, decreased peripheral perfusion, and decreased skin elasticity) may be more accurate than others (e.g., sunken eyes, sunken fontanelle, absent tears). Laboratory values (high blood urea nitrogen, low venous pH) may also be helpful. Patients with mild to moderate dehydration should be given 50 to 100 ml per kg of ORS over a 4-hour period. A solution similar to the WHO-ORS is recommended for rehydration. For severe dehydration, intravenous fluids (e.g., lactated Ringer's solution) 40 ml per kg per hour should be given until pulse, blood pressure, and state of consciousness return to normal, at which point oral rehydration may be started. In addition to replacing the estimated deficit, replacement of ongoing losses on a 1:1 basis with ORS should occur during rehydration. If stool and losses owing to vomiting cannot be measured accurately, approximately 10 ml per kg of ORS should be given for each stool passed and 2 ml per kg for each episode of vomiting. Clinical reassessment should be

Table 85–3. DIARRHEA TREATMENT CHART

Degree of Dehydration	Signs*	Rehydration Therapy (within 4 hours)	Replacement of Stool Losses	Maintenance Therapy†
Mild	Slightly dry buccal mucous membranes, increased thirst	ORS 50 ml/kg	10 ml/kg or ½ to 1 cup of ORS for each diarrheal stool	Breast feeding, ½ strength lactose-containing milk or formula, undiluted lactose-free formula, juices
Moderate	Sunken eyes, sunken fontanelle, loss of skin turgor, dry buccal mucous membranes	ORS 100 ml/kg	Same as above	Same as above
Severe	Signs of moderate dehydration plus one of the following: rapid thready pulse, cyanosis, rapid breathing, lethargy, coma	IV fluids (Ringer's lactate), 40 ml/kg/hr until pulse and state of consciousness return to normal and then give 50–100 ml/kg of ORS	Same as above	Same as above

*If no signs of dehydration are present, rehydration therapy is not required; proceed with maintenance therapy and replacement of stool losses.
†Infants and children who receive solid food may continue their usual diet.

done at least every 4 hours. If dehydration persists, or recurs, another phase of rehydration therapy is indicated.

Once hydration is achieved, the maintenance phase begins, in which maintenance fluid and energy and nutrient requirements are met. During maintenance, replacement of ongoing losses owing to stool and vomiting must continue. These excess fluid losses can be replaced with either low-solute ORS (containing 30 to 60 mEq sodium) or by standard WHO-ORS. If the WHO-ORS or similar fluid is used for replacement therapy during maintenance, an additional source of a low-sodium fluid is recommended. Breast-fed infants should receive breast milk ad libitum, and formula-fed infants should receive approximately 150 ml per kg per day of their maintenance diet. Infants receiving lactose-containing formulas before their illness should be switched to lactose-free formulas for several days or monitored closely for signs of intolerance. If lactose-free formulas are not available, lactose-containing ones can be diluted approximately 1:1 with another source of energy and nutrients, such as cereal flour, to maintain the same energy density of the formula while reducing its lactose content. If the milk formulas are diluted only with water, the full-strength diet should be resumed as soon as possible, preferably within 1 or 2 days.

Older children should receive their usual mixed diets and fluids, as desired. Ongoing fluid losses (stool and vomiting) should be replaced until diarrhea resolves (Table 85–3).

TOWARD THE FUTURE

Successful and routine implementation of ORT is only now becoming widespread. WHO estimates that less than 10% of the developing world's children had access to ORS in 1982, whereas by 1988, 61% had access, with an estimated 32% of diarrheal illnesses being treated with ORS or a home solution. It has been estimated that this 32% use rate may have averted 1 million childhood deaths in 1988 alone.[1] Data from Egypt[85] indicate a substantial drop in diarrhea-related mortality since the institution of that country's National Control of Diarrheal Diseases Project.

Despite this tremendous success, millions of children remain susceptible to diarrheal disease and its consequences of dehydration, malnutrition, and death. If the wealth of knowledge acquired in the past three decades can be successfully used to implement ORT (fluid and electrolyte therapy plus appropriate feeding) programs, these devastating consequences of diarrhea can be avoided.

REFERENCES

1. Claeson M, Merson MH: Global progress in the control of diarrheal disease. Pediatr Infect Dis J 1990; 9:345–355.
2. Ho MS, Glass RI, Pinsky PF, Anderson LJ: Rotavirus as a cause of diarrheal morbidity and mortality in the United States. J Infect Dis 1988; 158:1112–1116.
3. Moellering RC Jr, Gorbach SL: Infectious diarrhea. Infect Dis Clinics North Am, 1988, 2(3).
4. DuPont HL, Pickering LK: Infections of the gastrointestinal tract; microbiology, pathophysiology, and clinical features. *In* Greenough WB III, Merigan TC, series eds. Current Topics in Infectious Disease. New York: Plenum, 1980, 21–226.
5. Jaenichen: Memoire sur le choler-morbus qui regne en Russie. Gazette Med Paris 1830–1831; 85: 1–2.
6. O'Shaughnessy WB: Proposal for a new method of treating the blue epidemic cholera. Lancet 1831; 1:366.
7. Cosnett JE: The origins of intravenous fluid therapy. Lancet 1989; 1:768–771.
8. Latta T: Malignant cholera: Documents communicated by the Central Board of Health London, relative to the treatment of cholera by the copious injection of aqueous and saline fluids into the veins. Lancet 1832; 2:274.
9. Sellards AW: Tolerance for alkalies in Asiatic cholera. Philippine J Sci 1910; 5:363.
10. Rogers LE: Bowel disease in the Tropics. London, Froude, Hadden & Stoughton, 1921.
11. Watten RH, Morgan FM, Songkhla VN, et al: Water and electrolyte studies in cholera. J Clin Invest 1959; 38:1879–1889.
12. Van Heyningen WE, Seal JR: Cholera: The American scientific experience 1947–1980. Boulder, CO, Westview Press, 1983.
13. Finberg L: The role of oral electrolyte-glucose solutions in hydration for children: international and domestic aspects. J Pediatr 1980; 96:51–54.
14. Paneth N: Hypernatremic dehydration of infancy: An epidemiologic review. Am J Dis Child 1980; 134:785–791.

15. Fisher RB, Parsons DS: Glucose movements across the wall of the rat small intestine. J Physiol 1953; 119:210–223.
16. Curran PF: Na, Cl and water transport by rat ileum in vitro. J Gen Physiol 1960; 43:1137–1148.
17. Schultz SG, Zalusky R: Ion transport in isolated rabbit ileum. II. The interaction between active sodium and active sugar transport. J Gen Physiol 1964; 47:1043–1059.
18. Schultz SG: Sodium-coupled solute transport by small intestine: A status report. Am J Physiol 1977; 233:249.
19. Hirschhorn N: The treatment of acute diarrhea in children: An historical and physiological perspective. Am J Clin Nutr 1980; 33:637–663.
20. Sachar DB, Taylor JO, Saha JR, Phillips RA: Intestinal transmucosal electric potential and its response to glucose in acute and convalescent cholera. Gastroenterology 1969; 56:512–531.
21. Hirschhorn N, Kinzie JL, Sachar DB, et al: Decrease in net stool output in cholera during intestinal perfusion with glucose-containing solutions. N Engl J Med 1968; 279:176–181.
22. Pierce NF, Banwell JG, Mitra RC, et al: Effect of glucose electrolyte infusion upon water and electrolyte balance in Asiatic cholera. Gastroenterology 1968; 55:333–343.
23. Pierce NF, Hirschhorn N: Oral fluid is a simple weapon against dehydration: How it works and how to use it. WHO Chronicle 1977; 31:87–93.
24. Cash RA, Nalin DR, Rochat R, et al: A clinical trial of oral therapy in a rural cholera treatment center. Am J Trop Med Hyg 1970; 19:653–656.
25. Mahalanabis D, Choudri AB, Bagchi NG, et al: Oral fluid therapy of cholera among Bangladesh refugees. Johns Hopkins Med J 1973; 132:197–205.
26. Casteel HB, Fiedorek SC: Oral rehydration therapy. Pediatr Clin North Am 1990; 37:295–311.
27. Butler DG, Gall DG, Kelly MH, Hamilton JR: Mechanisms responsible for diarrhea in an acute viral enteritis in piglets. J Clin Invest 1974; 53:1335–1342.
28. Molla AM, Rahaman M, Sarker SA, et al: Stool electrolyte content and purging rates in diarrhea caused by rotavirus, enterotoxigenic *E. Coli* and *V. cholerae* in children. J Pediatr 1981; 98:835–838.
29. Finberg L, Luttreil C, Redd H: Pathogenesis of lesions in the central nervous system in hypernatremic states. II. Experimental studies of gross anatomical changes and alterations in the chemical composition of the tissues. Pediatrics 1959; 23:46–53.
30. Nichols BL, Soriano HA: A critique of oral therapy of dehydration due to diarrheal syndromes. Am J Clin Nutr 1977; 30:1457.
31. Pizarro D, Posada G, Villavicencio N, et al: Oral rehydration in hypernatremic and hyponatremic diarrheal dehydration: treatment with oral glucose/electrolyte solution. Am J Dis Child 1983; 137:730.
32. Hirschhorn N, Cash RA, Woodward WE, Spivey GH: Oral fluid therapy of Apache children with acute infectious diarrhoea. Lancet 1972; 2:15–18.
33. Hirschhorn N, McCarthy BJ, Ranney B, et al: Ad libitum oral glucose-electrolyte therapy for acute diarrhea in Apache children. J Pediatr 1973; 83:562–571.
34. Greene MG, ed: The Harriet Lane Handbook. 12th ed. St. Louis, Mosby-Year Book, 1991, pp 274, 375.
35. Santosham M, Daum RS, Dillman L, et al: Oral rehydration therapy of infantile diarrhea: A controlled study of well-nourished children hospitalized in the United States and Panama. N Engl J Med 1982; 306:1070–1076.
36. Tamer AM, Friedman LB, Maxwell SRW, et al: Oral rehydration of infants in a large urban U.S. medical center. J Pediatr 1985; 107:14–19.
37. Santosham M, Burns B, Nadkarni V, et al: Oral rehydration therapy for acute diarrhea in ambulatory children in the United States: A double-blind comparison of four different solutions. Pediatrics 1985; 76:159–166.
38. Listernick R, Zieserl E, Davis AT: Outpatient oral rehydration in the United States. Am J Dis Child 1986; 140:211–215.
39. American Academy of Pediatrics Committee on Nutrition: Use of oral fluid therapy and post-treatment feeding following enteritis in children in a developed country. Pediatrics 1985; 75:358–361.
40. Sack DA, Islam S, Brown KH, et al: Oral therapy in children with cholera: A comparison of sucrose and glucose electrolyte solutions. J Pediatr 1980; 96:20–26.
41. Salazar-Lindo E, Sack RB, Chea-Woo E, et al: Bicarbonate versus citrate in oral rehydration therapy in infants with watery diarrhea: A controlled clinical trial. J Pediatr 1986; 108:55–60.
42. Santosham M, Foster S, Rousey DB, et al: Outpatient use of oral rehydration solutions in an Apache population: Effect of instructions on preparation and contamination. J Pediatr Gastroenterol Nutr 1984; 3:687–691.
43. Turnberg LA, Fordtran JS, Carter NW, et al: Mechanisms of bicarbonate absorption and its relationship to sodium transport in the human jejunum. J Clin Invest 1970; 49:548.
44. Lifshitz F: Interrelationship of diarrhea and infant nutrition. *In* Lebenthal E, ed: Textbook of Gastroenterology and Nutrition in Infancy. 2nd ed. New York, Raven Press, 1989, p 659.
45. Martorell R, Habicht J-P, Yarbrough C, et al: Acute morbidity and physical growth in rural Guatemalan children. Am J Dis Child 1975; 129:1296–1301.
46. Rowland MGM, Cole TJ, Whitehead RG: A quantitative study into the role of infection in determining nutritional status in Gambian village children. Br J Nutr 1977; 37:441–450.
47. Black RE, Brown KH, Becker S: Effects of diarrhea associated with specific enteropathogens on the growth of children in rural Bangladesh. Pediatrics 1984; 173:799–805.
48. Brown KH, MacLean WC Jr: Nutritional management of acute diarrhea: An appraisal of the alternatives. Pediatrics 1984; 73:119–125.
49. Brown HO, Levine ML, Lipkin M: Inhibition of intestinal cell renewal and migration induced by starvation. Am J Physiol 1963; 205:868–872.
50. Johnson LR, Copeland EM, Dudrick SJ, et al: Structural and hormonal alterations in the gastrointestinal tract of parenterally fed rats. Gastroenterology 1975; 68:1177–1183.
51. Vanderhoof JA: Short bowel syndrome. *In* Lebenthal E, ed: Textbook of Gastroenterology and Nutrition in Infancy. 2nd ed. New York, Raven Press, 1989, p 794.
52. Isolauri E, Juntunen M, Wiren S, et al: Intestinal permeability changes in acute gastroenteritis: Effects of clinical factors and nutritional management. J Pediatr Gastroenterol Nutr 1989; 8:466–473.
53. Santosham M, Foster S, Reid R, et al: Role of soy-based, lactose-free formula during treatment of acute diarrhea. Pediatrics 1985; 76:292–298.
54. Brown KH, Gastanaduy AS, Saavedra JM, et al: Effect of continued oral feeding on clinical and nutritional outcomes of acute diarrhea in children. J Pediatr 1988; 112:191–200.
55. Sunshine P, Kretchmer N: Studies of small intestine during development. III. Infantile diarrhea associated with intolerance to disaccharides. Pediatrics 1964; 34:38–50.
56. Torres-Pinedo R, Lavastida M, Rivera CL, et al: Studies on infant diarrhea. I. A comparison of the effects of milk feeding and intravenous therapy upon the composition and volume of the stool and urine. J Clin Invest 1966; 45:469–480.
57. Conway SP, Ireson A: Acute gastroenteritis in well-nourished infants: Comparison of four feeding regimens. Arch Dis Child 1989; 64:87–91.
58. Brown KH, Lake A: Appropriate use of human and non-human milks for the dietary management of children with diarrhea. J Diarrh Dis Res 1991; 9:168–185.
59. Isolauri E, Vesikari T, Saha P, Viander M: Milk versus no milk in rapid refeeding after acute gastroenteritis. J Pediatr Gastroenterol Nutr 1986; 5:254.
60. Brown KH, Khatun M, Parry L, Ahmed MG: Nutritional consequences of low dose milk supplements consumed by lactose-malabsorbing children. Am J Clin Nutr 1980; 33:1054–1063.
61. Khin-Maung-U, Wai-N, Myo-Khin, et al: Effect on clinical outcome of breast feeding during acute diarrhea. Br Med J 1985; 290:587–589.
62. Hautefeuille M, Brantl V, Dumontier AM, Desjeux JF: In vitro effects of beta-casomorphins on ion transport in rabbit ileum. Am J Physiol 1986; 250:G92–G97.
63. Brown KH, Perez F, Gastanaduy AS: Clinical trial of modified whole milk, lactose-hydrolyzed whole milk, or cereal-milk mixtures for the dietary management of acute childhood diarrhea. J Pediatr Gastroenterol 1991; 12:340–350.
64. Alacon P, Montoya R, Perez F, et al: Clinical trial of home available, mixed diets versus a lactose-free, soy-protein formula for the dietary management of acute childhood diarrhea. J Pediatr Gastroenterol Nutr 1991; 12:224–232.

65. Castillo-Duran C, Vial P, Uauy R: Trace mineral balance during acute diarrhea in infants. J Pediatr 1988; 113:452–457.
66. Ruz M, Solomons NW: Mineral excretion during acute, dehydrating diarrhea treated with oral rehydration therapy. Pediatr Res 1990; 27:170–175.
67. Committee on International Nutrition Programs, Food and Nutrition Board, National Research Council: Nutritional Management of Acute Diarrhea in Infants and Children. Washington, DC: National Academy Press, 1985.
68. Elliott K, Attawell K, Wilson R, et al, eds: Cereal-based Oral Rehydration Therapy for Diarrhoea. London, Pegasus Press, Aga Khan Foundation and International Child Health Foundation, 1990.
69. Harland P: Composition of oral solutions prepared by Jamaican mothers for treatment of diarrhoea. Lancet 1981; 1:600–601.
70. Household Management of Diarrhea and Acute Respiratory Infections. Report of a Scientific Meeting at The Johns Hopkins School of Hygiene and Public Health in collaboration with the United Nations Children's Fund and the Diarrhoeal Diseases and Acute Respiratory Infections Control Programs of the World Health Organization. Occasional Paper No. 12, November, 1990.
71. Water with sugar and salt. Lancet 1978; 2:300–301.
72. Black RE, Brown KH, Becker S, Yunus M: Longitudinal studies of infectious disease and physical growth of children in rural Bangladesh. I. Patterns of morbidity. Am J Epidemiol 1982; 115:305–314.
73. Patra FC, Mahalanabis D, Jalan KN, et al: In search of a super solution: Controlled trial of glycine-glucose oral rehydration solution in infantile diarrhea. Acta Pediatr Scand 1984; 73:18.
74. Santosham M, Burns B, Reid R, et al: Glycine-based oral rehydration solution: Reassessment of safety and efficacy. J Pediatr 1986; 109:795–801.
75. Patra FC, Sack DA, Islam A, et al: Oral rehydration formula containing alanine and glucose for treatment of diarrhoea: A controlled trial. Br Med J 1989; 198:1353–1356.
76. Greenough WB III: Pancreatic and hepatic hypersecretion in cholera. Lancet 1965; 2:991–994.
77. Pizarro D, Posada G, Sandi L, Moran JB: Rice-based oral electrolyte solutions for the management of infantile diarrhea. N Engl J Med 1991; 324:517–521.
78. Patra FC, Mahalanabis D, Jalan KN, et al: Is oral rice electrolyte solution superior to glucose electrolyte solution in infantile diarrhea? Arch Dis Child 1982; 57:910–912.
79. Molla AM, Sarker SA, Hussain M, et al: Rice-powder electrolyte solution as oral therapy in diarrhoea due to *Vibrio cholerae* and *Escherichia coli*. Lancet 1982; 1:1317–1319.
80. Molla AM, Ahmad SM, Greenough WB III: Rice-based oral rehydration solution decreases stool volume in acute diarrhea. Bull WHO 1985; 63:751–756.
81. Santosham M, Fayad IM, Hashem M, et al: A comparison of rice-based oral rehydration solution and "early feeding" for the treatment of acute diarrhea in infants. J Pediatr 1990; 116:868–875.
82. Rahman ASM, Bari A, Molla AM, Greenough WB III: Mothers can prepare and use rice salt oral rehydration solution in rural Bangladesh. Lancet 1985; 2:539–540.
83. Rolston DDK, Mathew P, Mathan VI: Food-based solutions are a viable alternative to glucose-electrolyte solutions for oral hydration in acute diarrhoea—studies in a rat model of secretory diarrhoea. Trans Roy Soc Trop Med Hyg 1990; 84:156–159.
84. Mackenzie A, Barnes G, Shann F: Clinical signs of dehydration in children. Lancet 1989; 2:605–607.
85. El-Rafie M, Hassouna WA, Hirschhorn N, et al: Effect of diarrhoeal disease control on infant and childhood mortality in Egypt. Lancet 1990; 335:334–338.

Index

Note: Page numbers in *italics* refer to illustrations; page numbers followed by (t) refer to tables.